BLOOD AND ITS DISORDERS

BLOOD AND ITS DISORDERS

EDITED BY

R. M. HARDISTY

MD, FRCP, FRCPath
Professor of Haematology
Institute of Child Health
University of London;
Honorary Consultant Haematologist
The Hospital for Sick Children
Great Ormond Street, London

AND

D. J. WEATHERALL

MA, MD, FRCP, FRCPath, FRS
Nuffield Professor of
Clinical Medicine
University of Oxford;
Honorary Director
Medical Research Council
Molecular Haematology Unit
University of Oxford

SECOND EDITION

BLACKWELL SCIENTIFIC PUBLICATIONS
OXFORD LONDON EDINBURGH
BOSTON MELBOURNE

© 1974, 1982 by Blackwell Scientific Publications
Editorial offices:
Osney Mead, Oxford OX2 0EL
8 John Street, London WC1N 2ES
9 Forrest Road, Edinburgh EH1 2QH
52 Beacon Street, Boston, Massachusetts 02108, USA
99 Barry Street, Carlton, Victoria 3053, Australia

First published 1974
Second edition 1982

Printed in Great Britain at
The Alden Press, Oxford and
bound by Butler & Tanner Ltd, Frome, Somerset

DISTRIBUTORS

USA
  Blackwell Mosby Book Distributors
  11830 Westline Industrial Drive
  St Louis, Missouri 63141

Canada
  Blackwell Mosby Book Distributors
  120 Melford Drive, Scarborough
  Ontario, M1B 2X4

Australia
  Blackwell Scientific Book Distributors
  214 Berkeley Street, Carlton
  Victoria 3053

British Library
  Cataloguing in Publication Data

Blood and its disorders.—2nd ed.
  1. Blood—Diseases
  I. Hardisty, R.M.   II. Weatherall, D.J.
  616.1′5   RC636

  ISBN 0-632-00833-4

Contents

v

Contents

Contributors

BARBARA BAIN MD, FRACP, MRCPath, *Senior Lecturer in Haematology, St Mary's Hospital Medical School, London*

G.W.G. BIRD DSc, PhD, MB, BS, FRCPath, *Director and Consultant Pathologist of the Regional Blood Transfusion Service, Birmingham; Consultant Associate in Clinical Haematology, United Birmingham Hospitals; Honorary Lecturer in Experimental Pathology, University of Birmingham*

A.L. BLOOM MD, MRCP, FRCPath, *Professor of Haematology, Welsh National School of Medicine; Consultant Haematologist, University Hospital of Wales, Cardiff; Director, Cardiff Haemophilia Centre*

A.J. BOWDLER MD, PhD, BSc, MRCP, *Professor of Medicine, Marshall University, Huntington, West Virginia, USA*

M.C. BRAIN DM, FRCP, FRCP(C), *Professor of Medicine, McMaster University, Hamilton, Ontario, Canada*

C. BUNCH MB, ChB, MRCP, *Clinical Reader in Medicine, University of Oxford; Nuffield Department of Clinical Medicine, John Radcliffe Hospital, Headington, Oxford*

S.T.E. CALLENDER DSc, MD, FRCP, *formerly Clinical Reader and Consultant Physician, University of Oxford; Nuffield Department of Clinical Medicine, John Radcliffe Hospital, Headington, Oxford*

J.M. CHESSELLS MD, FRCP, *Consultant Clinical Haematologist, The Hospital for Sick Children, Great Ormond Street, London*

C.M. CHESTERMAN MB, BS, DPhil, FRACP, *Reader in Medicine, St Vincent's Hospital, Fitzroy 3065, Australia*

J.B. CLEGG PhD, *Member of MRC External Staff, MRC Molecular Haematology Unit, University of Oxford*

J.A. DAVIES MD, MRCP, *Senior Lecturer, University Department of Medicine, The Martin Wing, The General Infirmary, Leeds*

P.M. EMERSON MD, MRCS, MRCPath, *Consultant Haematologist, United Oxford Hospitals; Gibson Laboratories, The Radcliffe Infirmary, Oxford*

P.T. FLUTE MD, FRCP, FRCPath, *Professor of Haematology, St George's Hospital Medical School, London*

C.D. FORBES MD, FRCP, *Senior Lecturer and Honorary Consultant Physician, Department of Medicine, Royal Infirmary, Glasgow*

D.A.G. GALTON MD, FRCP, *Honorary Director, MRC Leukaemia Unit, Royal Postgraduate Medical School, Hammersmith Hospital, London*

A. GOLDBERG DSc, MD, FRCP, FRFPS, *Professor of Materia Medica, University of Glasgow*

J.M. GOLDMAN BM, BCh, FRCP, *Consultant Physician, MRC Leukaemia Unit, Royal Postgraduate Medical School, Hammersmith Hospital, London*

E.C. GORDON-SMITH MA, MSc, MRCP, *Senior Lecturer and Honorary Consultant Physician, Department of Haematology, Royal Postgraduate Medical School, Hammersmith Hospital, London*

A.J. GRIMES PhD, *Professor of Experimental Haematology, St Thomas' Hospital and Medical School, London*

R.M. HARDISTY MD, FRCP, FRCPath, *Professor of Haematology, Institute of Child Health, The Hospital for Sick Children, Great Ormond Street, London*

A.R. HAYWARD PhD, MB, MRCP, *Associate Professor of Pediatrics, University of Colorado Medical Center, Denver, Colorado 80220, USA*

A.V. HOFFBRAND DM, MRCP, MRCPath, *Professor of Haematology, Royal Free Hospital School of Medicine, London*

E.R. HUEHNS MD, PhD, *Professor of Haematology, University College Hospital Medical School, London*

NEVIN C. HUGHES JONES MA, DM, PhD, MRCP, *Member of Scientific Staff, MRC Unit for Mechanisms in Tumour Immunity, MRC Research Centre, Hills Road, Cambridge*

A. JACOBS MD, FRCPath, *Professor of Haematology, Welsh National School of Medicine, University Hospital of Wales, Cardiff*

H.E.M. KAY MD, FRCP, FRCPath, *Consultant Haematologist, Department of Clinical Pathology, Royal Marsden Hospital, London*

L.G. LAJTHA MD, DPhil, FRCPath, *Professor, Paterson Laboratories, Christie Hospital and Holt Radium Institute, Manchester*

S.M. LEWIS MD, BSc, FRCPath, DCP, *Reader in Haematology, Royal Postgraduate Medical School, Hammersmith Hospital, London*

K.E.L. McCOLL MD, MRCP, *Lecturer in Medicine, Western Infirmary, Glasgow*

T.J. McELWAIN MB, BS, FRCP, *Consultant Physician and Head, Division of Medicine, Institute of Cancer Research, Royal Marsden Hospital, Sutton, Surrey*

I.C.M. MacLENNAN PhD, MRCPath, *Professor of Immunology, University of Birmingham Medical School, Birmingham*

G.P. McNICOL PhD, MD, FRCP, FRCPath, *Principal and Vice-Chancellor, University of Aberdeen; late Professor of Medicine, The General Infirmary, Leeds*

D.Y. MASON DM, FRCPath, *Lecturer in Haematology, University of Oxford; Consultant Haematologist, Nuffield Department of Clinical Medicine, John Radcliffe Hospital, Headington, Oxford*

M.R. MOORE BSc, PhD, *Senior Lecturer in Medicine, Western Infirmary, Glasgow*

D.C. NICHOLSON PhD, FRIC, FRCPath, *Reader in Chemical Pathology, King's College Hospital Medical School, London*

T.C. PEARSON MD, MRCPath, *Senior Lecturer in Haematology, St Thomas' Hospital and Medical School, London*

D.G. PENINGTON MA, DM, FRCP, FRACP, FRCPA, *Professor of Medicine, University of Melbourne; St Vincent's Hospital, Fitzroy, Australia*

M.J. PIPPARD MB, ChB, MRCP, *Wellcome Research Fellow, Nuffield Department of Clinical Medicine, John Radcliffe Hospital, Headington, Oxford*

C.R.M. PRENTICE MD, FRCP, *Reader in Medicine and Honorary Consultant Physician, Department of Medicine, Royal Infirmary, Glasgow*

A.W. SEGAL PhD, MD, MRCP, *Senior Lecturer in Haematology, University College Hospital, London*

J.P. SLOANE MB, BS, MRCPath, *Consultant Histopathologist, Royal Marsden Hospital, Sutton, Surrey*

J.F. SOOTHILL MA, FRCP, FRCPath, *Hugh Greenwood Professor of Immunology, Institute of Child Health, London*

G.H. TOVEY CBE, MD, FRCP, FRCPath, *formerly Director of the South West Regional Blood Transfusion Centre, Bristol and the National Tissue Typing Reference Laboratory; formerly Clinical Lecturer in Haematology, University of Bristol*

D.J. WEATHERALL MA, MD, FRCP, FRCPath, FRS, *Nuffield Professor of Clinical Medicine, University of Oxford; Honorary Director, MRC Molecular Haematology Unit, University of Oxford*

G. WETHERLEY-MEIN MD, BA, FRCP, FRCPath, *Professor of Haematology, St Thomas' Hospital and Medical School, London*

J.M. WHITE MD, MB, ChB, MRCPath, *Professor of Haematology, King's College Hospital Medical School, London*

S.N. WICKRAMASINGHE PhD, MB, BS, MRCPath, *Professor of Haematology, St Mary's Hospital Medical School, London*

W.G. WOOD PhD, *MRC Staff Member, MRC Molecular Haematology Unit, University of Oxford*

The late SHEILA WORLLEDGE MB, BS, FRCPath, *Department of Haematology, Royal Postgraduate Medical School, Hammersmith Hospital, London*

M. WORWOOD BSc, PhD, *Senior Lecturer in Haematology, Welsh National School of Medicine, University Hospital of Wales, Cardiff*

Preface to second edition

Important advances have been made in many areas of haematology during the eight years since the first edition of this book, and this alone has necessitated the complete re-writing of most of the chapters. We have also heeded the advice of many friends and reviewers, and have done our best to fill the gaps and correct the unevenness of many parts of the first edition. New chapters have been added on developmental haematology, thrombosis and anti-thrombotic therapy, and on the practical clinical approach to patients with blood disorders. The sections on leucocytes and haemostasis have been expanded and reorganized so as to relate descriptions of normal structure and function more closely to the corresponding disorders, a pattern which was largely confined to the red cell section in the first edition. To counteract the increase in size resulting from these changes—already at the limit of tolerance for a single volume—our publishers have agreed to a radical change of format, whereby the expanded whole has been encompassed within slightly reduced physical dimensions. In this way we hope that we have reassured those of our colleagues who suggested to us that if future editions of this book weighed as much as the first edition, haematology in the United Kingdom might become restricted only to those who had achieved some previous proficiency in weight-lifting!

Two-thirds of our original contributors remain with us, and to them we have added twenty-four new collaborators. Of those we have lost, it is extremely sad to recall the untimely deaths of Carl de Gruchy and Gordon Hamilton Fairley, and, more recently, of Sheila Worlledge who had already agreed to contribute again to this edition. We are particularly grateful to Drs Hughes Jones and Barbara Bain for revising Sheila Worlledge's chapter at such short notice.

We would both like to express our extreme gratitude to our secretaries, Lata Popat, Janet Watt and Liz Gunson, for all their hard work and help in preparing this edition. As before, the venture has been encouraged at every step by our publishers and we would like to thank Per Saugman, John Robson, Erica Ison and Simon Rallison for allowing this edition to see the light of day.

Roger Hardisty
David Weatherall

Preface to first edition

The last few years have seen an extraordinarily rapid accumulation of knowledge about the disorders which affect mainly the blood and blood-forming organs. Indeed it is now extremely difficult to define the boundaries of haematology since the subject encompasses disciplines which range from molecular biology to the clinical management of the acute complications of malignant disease; an understanding of the former subject requires a working knowledge of most of the basic sciences while the latter encompasses the whole of internal medicine! It is not surprising therefore that both in the United Kingdom and the U.S.A. haematology is going through a difficult phase of redefinition, particularly with respect to the relative roles to be played by the clinician and laboratory worker in its future development. It is against this difficult and rather ill-defined background that undergraduate and postgraduate teaching programmes in haematology must be developed.

These considerations make it clear that no single textbook can hope to act as a complete work of reference for diseases of the blood. For this reason a large number of excellent monographs have been published during recent years which deal in great depth with specific classes of blood disorders, but while these are excellent sources of reference for the specialist and research worker, it is difficult for the postgraduate or practising clinician to abstract the real essentials of the subject from such sources. In the present book we have attempted to bridge the gap between these works and the shorter textbooks of haematology. Thus we have tried to present a relatively complete summary of the disorders of the blood and of the physiological and biochemical concepts which are required for their full understanding. In the production of this book we have had in mind particularly postgraduates training in clinical or laboratory haematology or in internal medicine and related fields, and because of the physiological approach throughout the book we hope that it may also interest undergraduates and graduates in the basic sciences whose work touches upon various aspects of haematology.

No pair of authors can now hope to cover unaided the whole field of haematology in any depth. For a book of this sort multiple authorship is now inevitable, whatever the theoretical disadvantages of different styles and approaches. We pride ourselves on having amassed a very strong team, mostly of practising haematologists, on which we could depend for an account both of the physiology and biochemistry of the blood and blood-forming organs and of the clinical effects and management of disorders affecting them. Although some of the physiological aspects—haemopoiesis, leucocyte function, haemostasis and the blood groups—have been gathered into an introductory section, we have felt it appropriate to relate many other aspects of normal function more closely to the accounts of their defects. Many of the chapters on blood disorders, therefore, are introduced by a section dealing specifically with the normal function of the organ or cell type under discussion.

The multi-author approach has meant a certain amount of repetition but in such a rapidly growing field we did not think that the presentation of more than one approach, particularly in controversial areas, would do any harm. Because of the recent production of several superb atlases of haematology we did not feel that there was any need for extensive illustration of the peripheral-blood or bone-marrow appearances described in this book. Similarly, we have decided against the inclusion of a section on laboratory techniques, believing that these are more readily available in smaller volumes convenient for reference at the bench.

In a rapidly moving field such as haematology it is an unfortunate fact that textbooks are out of date before they are published. For this reason we are particularly grateful to the publishers for allowing so many alterations and additions at the proof stage in an attempt to avoid this. We are also grateful to the many authors, editors and publishers who have have allowed us to reproduce previously published figures; these are acknowledged individually in the relevant figure legends. Finally we wish to thank our secretaries, particularly Mrs Anne Attwater and Mrs Elizabeth Hole, for their invaluable help. Mr Per Saugman and Mr J. L. Robson of Blackwell Scientific Publications Ltd have encouraged the venture at every stage.

April 1974   R.M.H., D.J.W

x

SECTION 1
INTRODUCTION

Chapter 1
The constituents of normal blood and bone marrow

S. M. LEWIS

Blood is a fluid containing various chemicals in solution and a variety of cells in suspension. It circulates throughout all the blood vessels of the body and participates in all organ activities. It provides the means for respiration and nutrition and for the control of infection and of haemorrhage. Clearly, it is the essence of life and it is not surprising that blood has been regarded with awe since human life itself began.

HAEMOPOIESIS*

Blood comprises about eight per cent of the total body weight. In health the cellular component is approximately 45% and the fluid component 55%. The cells are derived from 'haemopoietic' organs, namely bone marrow, spleen, liver and lymph nodes; the process by which cells proliferate, mature and ultimately reach the circulating blood is termed 'haemopoiesis'. More specifically, red cells develop by erythropoiesis and white cells by leucopoiesis, this latter process being further separated into lymphopoiesis and granulopoiesis. Yet another cell line is that of megakaryocytes, which produce platelets. The interrelationship of the cell lines has been a subject of much debate, and several schools have favoured different views which can be summarized as follows:

1 all cells, including lymphocytes, stem from a single totipotential primitive blood cell which may give rise to any type of blood cell (monophyletic theory of Maximow [1], Bloom & Bartelmez [2] and others);

2 different blood cells are derived from completely differentiated blast cells (polyphyletic theory of Ferrata and others, subsequently reviewed by Knoll & Pingel [3]);

3 modified polyphyletic theory propounded by Naegeli, who suggested that granulocytes, monocytes and megakaryocytes are derived from the myeloblast;

4 a further modification by Schilling, who excluded monocytes which he considered as developing independently from reticulo-endothelial cells;

* Etymologically 'haematopoiesis' is the exact form, but in current practice either word is acceptable.

5 Doan [4] and Sabin et al. [5] considered that a different stem cell was responsible for each cell line but they conceived a primitive multipotential reticulum cell as a precursor to the stem cells of myeloblast, lymphoblast and monoblast, and another primitive cell, derived from endothelial cells lining the intersinusoidal capillaries of the bone marrow, as the precursor to erythroid series and histiocytes.

In the past decade analysis of haemopoietic cells by culture, cytochemistry, immunology and more refined techniques of electron microscopy has thrown much light on the origins, development and interrelationship of the various haemopoietic cells. It is now clear that there are multipotential haemopoietic stem cells (CFU-S), present in marrow and spleen (see Chapter 2). As a result of response to a specific stimulus these stem cells give rise to the earliest precursor cells of one of the haemopoietic cell lines. The committed cells are known as colony-forming cells (CFC); it is possible that they are the cells which have previously been classified as haemocytoblasts. Sometimes two lines, e.g. erythroid and myeloid, may be stimulated at the same time, and recent experimental evidence indicates that there is a close relationship between the granulocytes and monocytes [6, 7]. It is not clear whether the stem cells in the spleen and the marrow are identical; normally it seems likely that development along haemopoietic lines will occur only in the environment of the marrow where the haemopoietic stem cell becomes essentially a fixed tissue cell with extensive reproductive capacity [8]. These topics are dealt with in greater detail in Chapter 2.

An acceptable concept of the origin and relationships of the blood cells is illustrated in Table 1.1.

Haemopoiesis during fetal development (Fig. 1.1) (see also Chapter 3)

Mesenchymal cells first appear in the yolk sac in two-week-old embryos. They are found in the blood islets in the area vasculosa; this is a tubular structure composed of two layers—an outer layer which forms a primitive vascular structure and an inner layer which forms the primitive endothelial cells and gives rise to

Table 1.1. The morphological classification of blood cell development

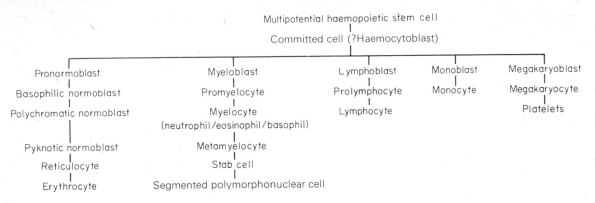

the haemopoietic stem cells. In this phase only mega-loblast-like erythroid cells develop. Although these cells have some morphological features of erythro-blasts, including haemoglobinization, they are gigantic cells with a volume of 1800–2400 fl [3]. As development continues these cells are replaced by smaller normoblasts. As the latter in turn develop and mature, their nuclei disappear and erythrocytes are formed. This process takes place in the fetal vascular system, and continues for about six to nine weeks.

The liver becomes the main site of haemopoiesis by the 12th–16th week and remains active until a few weeks before birth. At first haemopoiesis is confined to erythropoiesis, but soon granulopoiesis can also be seen and by the 16th week granulocytes are quite numerous. The spleen is a relatively minor organ of erythropoiesis and granulopoiesis, starting at about the same time as the liver, continuing to the 20th week and then often, albeit to a small extent, until birth. The spleen is rather more active in lymphopoiesis. During this period the thymus is also a transient site for haemopoiesis, primarily of lymphocytes, but also of some myelocytes and erythroblasts.

The bone marrow becomes a site of haemopoiesis from about the 20th week. At first it is concerned chiefly with granulocyte formation, but shortly thereafter rapid proliferation of erythropoietic tissue occurs, and by the 30th week the marrow is fully cellular with all lines represented. At this stage the marrow becomes the predominant source of blood cells.

Postnatal haemopoiesis (see also Chapter 3)
At birth actively haemopoietic (red) marrow occupies the entire capacity of the bones, and this remains so for two to three years. During this time the spleen, liver

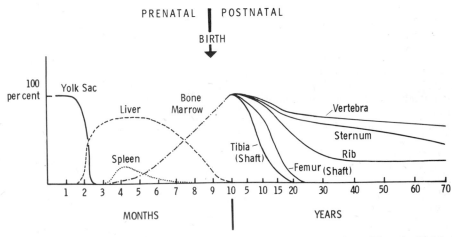

Fig. 1.1. Sites of haemopoiesis during fetal development and after birth (adapted from Wintrobe M.M. (1967) *Clinical Haematology*, 6th edn., pp. 2, 17. Henry Kimpton, London).

and other extramedullary sites of haemopoiesis are inert, but because the marrow capacity is fully extended, any excessive demand for blood production, e.g. by haemorrhage or haemolysis, will result in the reactivation of these extramedullary sites. From childhood there is a gradual replacement of the red marrow by fatty (yellow) marrow. The long bones begin to develop fatty marrow in their diaphyseal portions. This process increases from the distal to the proximal ends of bones until, at the age of about 20–22 years, red marrow is confined to the upper ends of femur and humerus and to the flat bones of the sternum, ribs, vertebrae, cranium and pelvis (Fig. 1.2); the total amount of active red marrow in the body remains almost identical in the child and the adult. In the adult, even in those areas where there is red marrow, there are likely to be specks of fatty marrow, especially in the anterio-superior part of the manubrium, sacrum, iliac crest, and acetabular side of the ilium [9]. In the elderly the sites of adult red marrow become increasingly replaced by fatty marrow. Experimental studies suggest that the type of marrow which is normally present in different areas is determined genetically, although an increased requirement for blood production can override this mechanism [10, 11]. When extramedullary haemopoiesis occurs it is most likely to be in the spleen but ectopic haemopoiesis will also be seen in the liver and in many other sites, including lymph nodes, kidney, adrenal glands, lungs and pleura, pancreas and even in skin, subcutaneous tissue and muscle. It is important, but often difficult, to distinguish between extramedullary haemopoiesis which occurs as a compensatory mechanism when increased demands cannot be met by marrow hyperplasia alone, and that which occurs when there is a haemoproliferative disease affecting different organs.

The extent and site(s) of erythropoietic activity are demonstrable by radioactive screening after administration of ^{52}Fe (Fig. 1.3) [12]. In general, granulopoiesis parallels erythropoiesis in the marrow. The

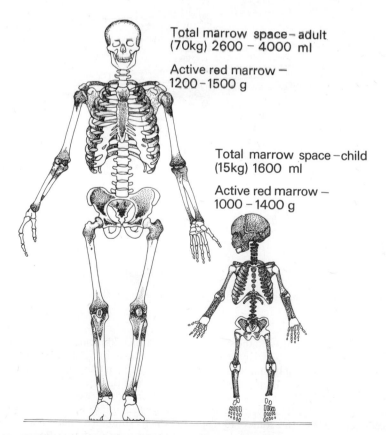

Total marrow space – adult
(70kg) 2600 – 4000 ml

Active red marrow –
1200 – 1500 g

Total marrow space – child
(15kg) 1600 ml

Active red marrow –
1000 – 1400 g

Fig. 1.2. Comparison of red marrow areas in the child and adult. There is an almost identical amount of red marrow in each, despite a fivefold difference in body weight. (From Bierman H.R. (1961) Homeostasis of the blood cell elements. In: *Functions of the Blood* (ed. MacFarlane R.G. & Robb-Smith A.H.T.), p. 357. Blackwell Scientific Publications, Oxford.)

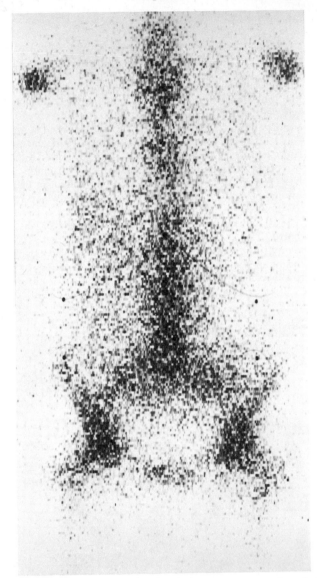

Fig. 1.3. Bone scan showing areas of erythropoietic activity in an adult, after administration of ^{52}Fe.

origins and distribution of lymphocytes and the significance of the marrow population is discussed in detail in Chapter 17. It is now believed that all lymphocytes are ultimately derived from the stem cells of the bone marrow and that the other lymphoid tissues, e.g. thymus, spleen, lymph nodes and gastrointestinal tract, are populated by cells derived from this source [13–16]. Nodules of lymphatic tissue are normal components of human bone marrow and lymphopoiesis in the bone marrow has been demonstrated by a variety of experimental techniques. The amount of nodular and diffuse lymphatic tissue is relatively large in infants, disappears partly in adolescence, and tends to reappear at the age of 40–50 years [17, 18].

Monocytes are not normally present in bone marrow in large numbers but may be seen in certain conditions which stimulate their response, e.g. tuberculosis, leprosy, lipoid storage diseases and subacute bacterial endocarditis. The developmental relationship of monocytes to granulocytes is discussed in Chapter 15.

HAEMOPOIETIC-CELL MORPHOLOGY

In this section a brief account will be given of the morphological features of the normal cells of the haemopoietic system. Further details and a description of cells altered by disease or genetic abnormalities will be described in later chapters. When individual cells are described it must be remembered that a gradation exists between the immature cell and its mature descendants so that in practice it may be difficult to give any particular cell a precise name. Nevertheless, as cells mature, specific features develop so that their appearance will indicate that the cell has reached a certain stage of development. Transformation from an immature cell to a mature one involves changes in both cytoplasm and nucleus which, in health, occur synchronously.

Cytoplasmic differentiation is associated with changes in nucleic acid content. When stained by a Romanowsky stain the cytoplasm of an immature cell is deeply basophilic because of a high content of ribonucleic acid. As the cell matures loss of cytoplasmic RNA leads to reduction in its basophilia. In the erythroid cells there is an additional unique change in that haemoglobin is synthesized so that the cell becomes polychromatic and then pink. In the granulocytes cytoplasmic differentiation is influenced by the appearance of enzyme-related granules which give the cells their unique eosinophilic, basophilic or neutrophilic character.

Nuclear maturation results in reduction in nuclear size with condensation of chromatin and loss of RNA-positive nucleoli. There may be associated shape changes, for example lobulation of granulocyte nuclei, while the cell as a whole undergoes a reduction in size. In general, nucleus to cytoplasm (N/C) ratio is found to be higher in younger cells than in more mature ones.

Marrow cells whose relationship to stem cells and the committed compartments is uncertain

Reticulum cell (Fig. 1.4)
Syn. Haemohistioblast, Ferrata cell

The relationship of this cell to blood-cell development and to the multipotential stem cell is uncertain. It is 15–25 μm in diameter, occasionally bigger, with an irregular outline and with blunt protoplasmic projections. The nucleus is oval with finely reticulated chromatin which stains purple-red, and there are nodular thickenings where the chromatin strands cross. There are three to six nucleoli with irregular hazy outline. The cytoplasm is blue and not generally granular although it may contain a few large azurophil granules. A large number of red granules or strands are characteristic of the fixed histiocyte cells, and in these cells the irregularity of the cell margin is especially marked because the cells are torn away from their nest when the marrow is collected. The N/C ratio is 1:1 or less.

By electron microscopy, Golgi apparatus, vacuoles of endoplasmic reticulum and cytosomes are well shown and there are prominent microtubules and fibrillary structures. Mitochondria are few and of small size and ribosomes are rarely found.

Haemocytoblast (Fig. 1.4)
As is the case for the marrow reticulum cell, the relationship of this cell to those of the committed compartments, i.e. red- and white-cell precursors, is uncertain. It is 20–30 μm in diameter and has the same type of reticulated nucleus and nucleoli as the reticulum cell. The cytoplasm is less deeply stained, however, especially near the nucleus; it is non-granular and the cell outline is more rounded. The N/C ratio is about 1–1·5:1. By contrast to the reticulum cell, this cell has a

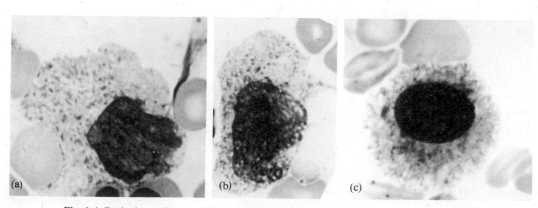

Fig. 1.4. Reticulum cells (a and b) and haemocytoblast (c), by light microscopy (× 1170).

greater number of mitochondria, although ribosomes and polyribosomes are still relatively sparse.

The red-cell series (see also Chapter 4)

Pronormoblast (Fig. 1.5)
Syn. Pro-erythroblast; rubriblast

This is the youngest cell identifiable with the red-cell series. It is 14–19 μm in diameter. The nucleus is light purple, vesicular and granular with evenly distributed chromatin. There are one to three prominent nucleoli. The cytoplasm is granular and light blue, although as the cell matures it stains more darkly and tends to condense at the periphery. The cell is ovoid, often with a slightly irregular outline.

Electron microscopy shows numerous large mitochondria and there are abundant ribosomes, mainly in the form of polyribosomes. There is a prominent centrosome composed of centrioles and Golgi bodies and there are a few microtubules and fibrils. There may be ferritin molecules scattered throughout the cytoplasm, with some present in the mitochondria (Fig. 1.6).

Basophilic normoblast (Fig. 1.5)
Syn. Early erythroblast

The nucleoli disappear and the nuclear chromatin condenses to form coalescent clumps.

Polychromatic normoblast (Fig. 1.5)
Syn. Intermediate erythroblast

It is in this cell that haemoglobin first appears, and the cytoplasm takes on a lighter bluish-red colour. The nucleus has blue-black coarsely clumped chromatin. The cell is 12–15 μm in diameter and the N/C ratio has decreased.

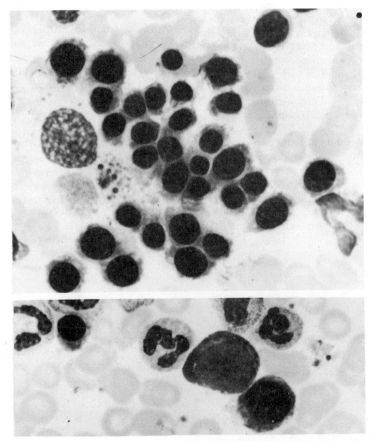

Fig. 1.5. Above: Nest of erythroblasts adjacent to a reticulum cell. Ferritin is present in the vicinity of the cells. The normoblasts are at all stages of development from basophilic to pyknotic. Below: Pronormoblast, basophilic normoblast and polychromatic normoblast (× 1100).

Electron microscopy shows the presence of abundant mitochondria and ribosomes mainly as polyribosomes, whilst residual ferritin becomes grouped into small (siderotic) clusters. Microtubules are no longer a feature (Fig. 1.6).

Pyknotic normoblast (Fig. 1.5)
Syn. Orthochromic normoblast; acidophilic normoblast; oxyphilic normoblast

By now the cell has become rounded and small, 8–12 μm in diameter. The nucleus is dark and homogeneous with condensed chromatin in a structureless mass. The cytoplasm is increasingly haemoglobinized. The N/C ratio is further decreased and the nucleus becomes eccentric, moving to the periphery of the cell prior to expulsion.

At this stage the cell has reached the end of its active DNA synthesis and is incapable of further division.

Reticulocyte (Fig, 1,7)
This non-nucleated cell, 7–10 μm in diameter, still contains some RNA and ribosomes which account for its polychromatic staining character (diffuse basophilia) when stained by a Romanowsky method, and its reticular appearance when stained by new methylene blue or other 'reticulocyte' stains (Fig. 1.7a). The ribosomes are present mostly as polyribosomes; there are small mitochondria and, at least in the earlier stages, occasional vesicles, remnants of cellular organelles and ferritin (Fig. 1.7b and c). As the reticulocyte matures the reticulum becomes scanty and in the most mature cells it may appear as only a few scattered granules. The cell has an irregular margin, reflecting active cellular movement.

Erythrocyte (Figs 1.8–1.10)
In two to three days the reticulocyte matures into the erythrocyte. This is normally a biconcave-shaped cell, 7–8 μm in diameter (Fig 1.8). At first sight it seems to be a structureless bag containing haemoglobin. By electron microscopy of a cut section, the cytoplasm of the erythrocyte is electron dense and homogeneous (Fig. 1.9a); a small proportion of normal erythrocytes contains autophagic vacuoles and degenerate particles of cell organelles (Fig. 1.9b) [19]. In haemoglobin-free sections it is sometimes possible to see an intracellular network (stroma?) continuous with the membrane (Fig. 1.10) [20].

The membrane is a three-layered structure consisting of an electron-translucent layer bounded on either side by an electron-dense border (for review, see Ref. 267). This appearance is consistent with the lipid–protein mosaic model developed by Singer [22] on the basis of earlier concepts by Davson & Danielli [21, 265]

and Robertson [266]. In this there are presumed to be two layers of lipid molecules arranged so that their non-polar (hydrophobic) hydrocarbon chains, which face either the outer or inner surface of the cell, are polar, charged and hydrophilic (see also Chapter 10).

These outer layers are protein bound, and there is some penetration of the entire membrane from plasma to cytoplasm by the protein; some of the protein is mobile within the lipid matrix [22]. Glycophorin, actin, and spectrin are three proteins of particular importance as they provide the framework for maintaining red-cell shape and normal deformability. Actin makes up about five per cent of the protein composition of the red-cell membrane; it has characteristics of smooth muscle [23]. Spectrin constitutes 25% of the membrane protein; it is a filamentous protein of high molecular weight [24], and it combines with actin to provide the contractile lattice work at the inner aspect of the red-cell membrane. Glycophorin is a glycoprotein which spans the membrane, attaching to spectrin on its cytoplasmic surface; it contains neuraminic (sialic) acid and thus provides the negative surface charge. Calcium also plays an important role in maintaining functional integrity of the cell membrane and it is present at specific sites within the protein structure of the membrane [259].

Between the cytoplasm of the cell on the one side and the intercellular space on the other, the cell membrane is involved in various events which depend on dynamic contact between cells; these include the flow of nutrients and nucleotides into the cell, communication between cells and control of the movement of cells in relation to their environment [260]. Unlike the majority of tissues in the body where cells remain in close apposition, haemopoietic cells separate from each other at an early stage of maturation. Failure of erythroid cells to separate and the persistence of intercellular junctions characterizes dyserythropoiesis (see Chapter 4, pages 124 and 125).

The nuclear membrane also has a dynamic function and is not merely a static partition between nucleus and cytoplasm. It controls the ordered arrangement of chromatin in the nucleus during interphase, and an intact nuclear membrane appears to be a prerequisite for normal mitosis. The nuclear membrane has a controlling influence on synthesis of DNA, and competent nuclear-pore function is necessary for assembly of polyribosomes, transport of RNA and protein synthesis [261–263]. The nuclear membrane and cell membrane are functionally interrelated. Thus, when the nuclear membrane is damaged, for example by toxic agents, there are extensive ultrastructural abnormalities and functional defects including disruption of the cell membrane; conversely, there is evidence that a normally functioning cell membrane is a necessary

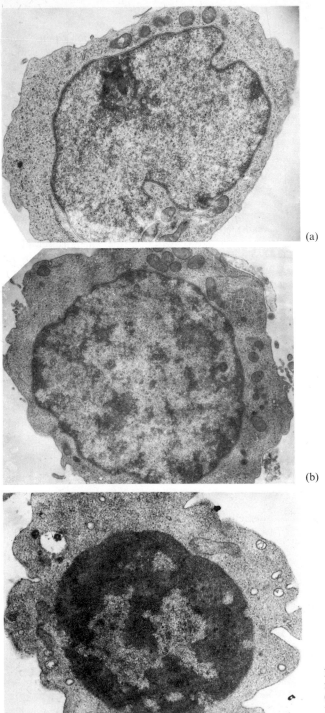

(a)

(b)

(c)

Fig. 1.6. Erythroid cells as seen by transmission electron microscopy (× 14 000), showing stages of development. (a) Pronormoblast; (b) and (c) early normoblasts; (d) pyknotic normoblast; (e) extrusion of nucleus from late normoblast.

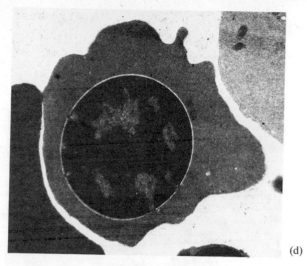

(d)

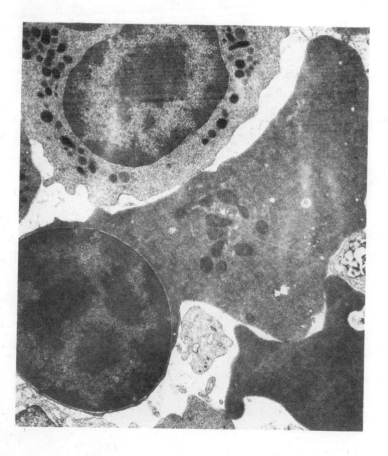

(a)

(c)

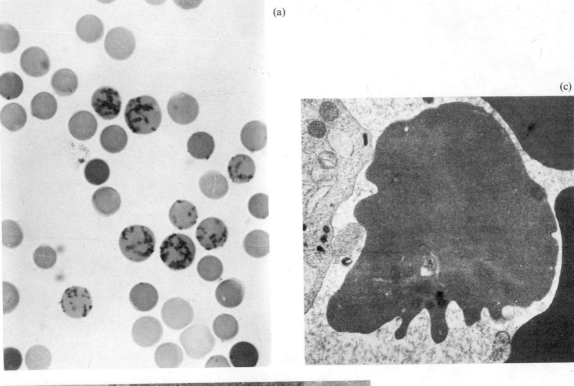

(b)

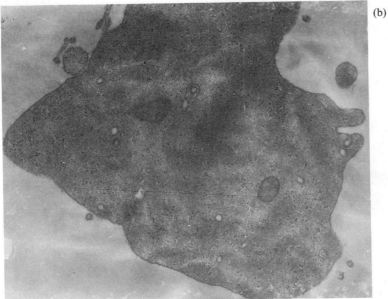

Fig. 1.7. Reticulocytes: (a) stained with new methylene blue (×1200); (b) and (c) sections as seen by electron microscopy (×13 500). The reticulocyte shown in (b) is younger, and contains mitochondria and abundant ribosomes, whereas (c) contains only a few organelles.

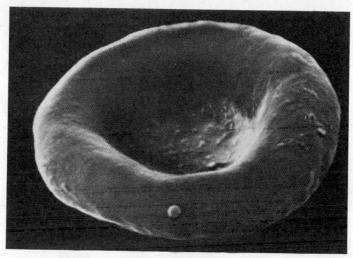

Fig. 1.8. Erythrocyte as seen by scanning electron microscope (×15 000).

(a)

(b)

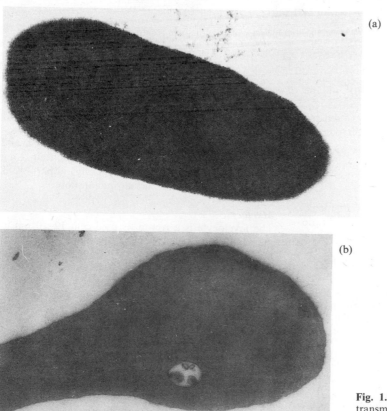

Fig. 1.9. Sections of erythrocytes as seen by transmission electron microscopy (×36 000): (a) is homogeneously electron-dense; (b) contains an autophagic vacuole with inclusions.

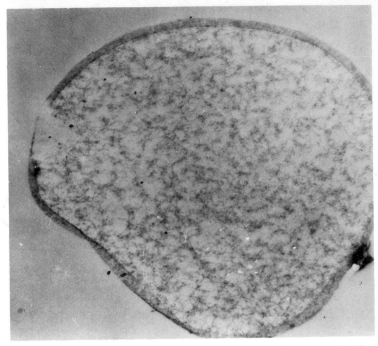

Fig. 1.10. Section of 'ghost' of erythrocyte after lysis. The cell membrane (? with some residual haemoglobin) has become apparent (× 23 000).

prerequisite for maintaining the integrity of the nuclear membrane [264].

The structure/function relationships of the red-cell membrane are discussed in more detail in Chapter 10.

Granulocyte series (Figs 1.11 and 1.12)

Myeloblast
The myeloblast is a round cell, 12–20 μm in diameter. The nucleus occupies most of the cell with a N/C ratio of 6:1. The nucleus has a fine reticular, evenly distributed chromatin and contains two or more distinct pale blue nucleoli. The cytoplasm is light blue with a thin, deeply basophilic rim. It contains no specific granules, but may occasionally contain one or more red-staining rods (Auer bodies). By electron microscopy one can see numerous large mitochondria and ribosomes, mainly in the form of rosettes. The Golgi area is not very prominent.

Promyelocyte
Syn. Progranulocyte

This cell is slightly larger than the myeloblast, with a large ovoid, perhaps slightly indented nucleus, the chromatin of which stains light purple. The N/C ratio

is 4:1. The cytoplasm is lightly basophilic with a few relatively large dark-blue granules. There are two or more nucleoli, which are pale blue and less distinct than in the myeloblast.

There are still numerous large mitochondria and abundant free ribosomes. The cytoplasm contains long cisternae or ergastoplasm. The Golgi apparatus is situated in the area of nuclear indentation.

Myelocyte
The myelocyte is a round or oval cell, 12–20 μm in diameter. The nucleus is similarly shaped with slight indentation; its chromatin is light purple and moderately clumped; there are no nucleoli. The N/C ratio is 2:1. The cytoplasm is bluish-pink with numerous small granules which may be undifferentiated azurophilic or differentiated into eosinophilic, basophilic or neutrophilic. By electron microscopy the specific granules are less dense than the azurophilic granules.

Metamyelocyte
This cell is slightly smaller than the myelocyte and with a more pronounced nuclear indentation. The N/C ratio is 1·5:1 and the nuclear chromatin is becoming increasingly condensed. As these changes continue there arises the *band form* (stab cell) which is

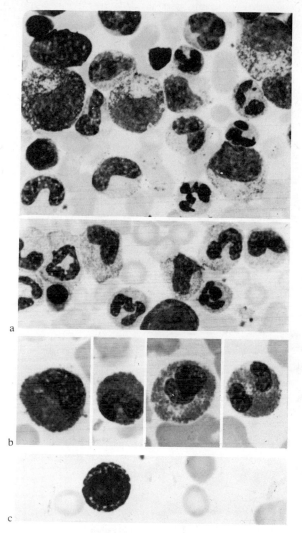

Fig. 1.11. Granulopoiesis, by light microscopy (×1040): (a) cells at various stages of maturation, including promyelocytes, myelocytes, metamyelocytes, stab cells and mature polymorph neutrophils; (b) eosinophil series; (c) a mature basophil.

horseshoe-shaped, and then the segmented *poly-morphonuclear granulocyte* which is the last cell of the series. It may be difficult to distinguish between the stab cell and the early segmented cell; in the former the sides of the nucleus should have parallel edges with no widening anywhere along the length to suggest a beginning of the lobulation which characterizes the polymorph. Eventually the nucleus will consist of two or more lobes separated by thin filamentous chromatin strands. The eosinophil and basophil usually have bilobed nuclei: the neutrophil has three to five lobes. The neutrophil granules are small, violet-pink, whereas the eosinophil has large yellow-red granules and the basophil coarse blue-black granules that almost fill the cytoplasm and frequently obscure the nucleus. The specific granules have a characteristic electron-microscope appearance [25–27]. By scanning electron microscopy, the granulocyte surface shows prominent ridge-like profiles and small ruffles, frequently polarized to one edge of the cell (Fig. 1.13). Eosinophils and basophils also have a varying number of microvilli: these may be particularly prominent in the basophil leading to misidentification as lymphocytes [28].

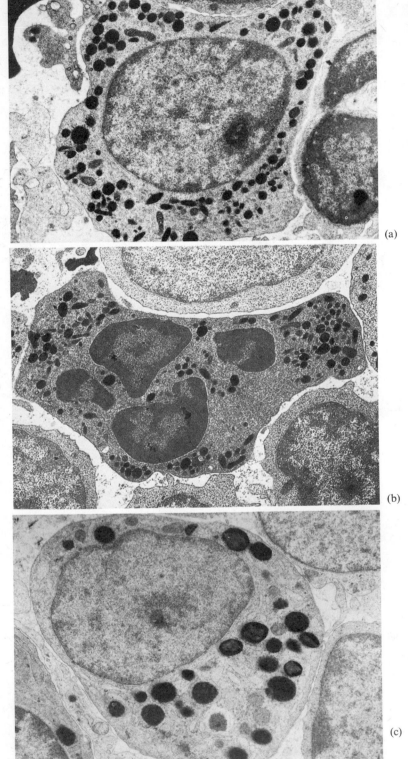

(a)

(b)

(c)

Fig. 1.12. Granulocytes as seen by transmission electron microscopy (a) neutrophil myelocyte ($\times 11\,250$); (b) neutrophil polymorph ($\times 9750$); (c) eosinophil ($\times 11\,250$); (d) basophil ($\times 15\,000$). Note the characteristic appearances of the specific granules.

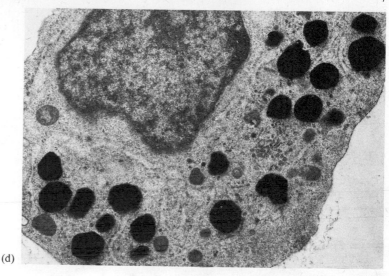

(d)

Lymphocyte series (Figs 1.14–1.16)

Lymphoblast

This cell is 10–18 μm in diameter. The nucleus occupies most of the cell and the N/C ratio is 6:1. The nuclear chromatin is dark purple and aggregated along the nuclear membrane; there are one or two indistinct nucleoli. The cytoplasm is deep blue, often with a paler perinuclear area; there are occasional azurophil granules.

Prolymphocyte

This cell is slightly smaller (9–17 μm) than the lymphoblast with a N/C ratio of 4–5:1. There is

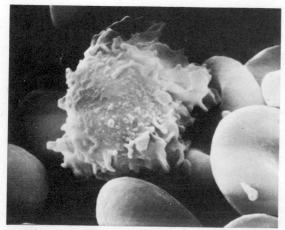

Fig. 1.13. Granulocytes as seen by scanning electron microscopy (×8500). (By courtesy of Professor A. Polliack.)

usually one nucleolus. The cytoplasm is light to dark blue.

Lymphocyte

By light microscopy, on the basis of size, two forms of lymphocyte may be seen. The large lymphocyte has a diameter of 8–16 μm; the small one 7–9 μm. They are round cells with a round nucleus which is central or slightly eccentric. The chromatin is dark purple-blue, coarse and clumped. The nuclear membrane is sharply defined. There are no nucleoli. The cytoplasm is light blue; it may be relatively abundant, possibly with a nuclear-clear zone and with a N/C ratio of 1·2:1 to 1·5:1. In small lymphocytes, however, the cytoplasm may be present in only a rim round the nucleus. Occasional azurophil granules are present in the large lymphocyte which has prominent ergastoplasm, a few small mitochondria and infrequent ribosomes. The small lymphocyte has large mitochondria and cytosomal electron-dense granules, which correspond to the azurophil granules seen by light miscoscopy, as well as other larger but less dense bodies. Ribosomes are abundant in the small lymphocyte with high-density cytoplasm: they are few in number in the cells which have light cytoplasm.

Atypical or reactive lymphocytes are pleomorphic cells which occur in infectious mononucleosis and a number of other conditions. They are described in Chapters 17, 18 and 33 and are mentioned here because large lymphocytes may, at times, be confused with them, although it is possible that when lymphocytes showing atypical features are present in apparently healthy individuals they represent a mildly reactive state. Moreover, distinguishing reactive lymphocytes

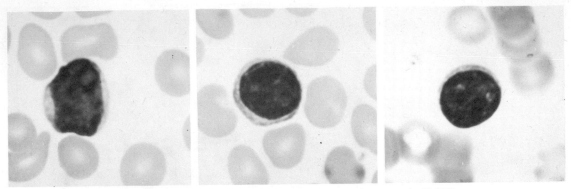

Fig. 1.14. Lymphoblast and lymphocytes by light microscopy (× 13 000).

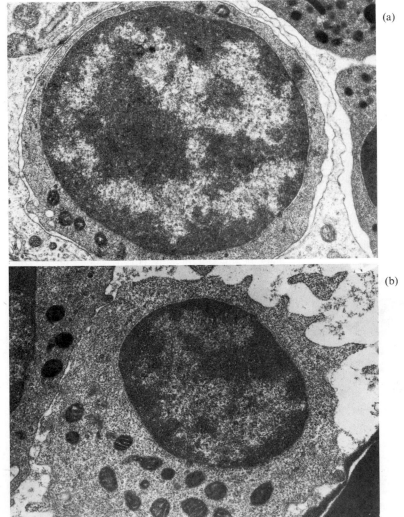

(a)

(b)

Fig. 1.15. Lymphocytes as seen by transmission electron microscopy (× 22 500): (a) large lymphocytes with few mitochondria; (b) small lymphocytes with abundant mitochondria and other electron-dense bodies.

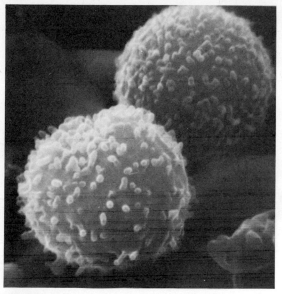
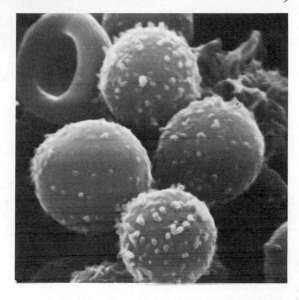

Fig. 1.16. Lymphocytes as seen by scanning electron microscopy. The microvilli vary between cells, as illustrated on the right (×8500). (By courtesy of Professor A. Polliack.)

from normal large lymphocytes is to some extent subjective and influenced by the method of preparation and staining of the blood film.

The majority of lymphocytes in a normal blood film are T lymphocytes. They can be readily distinguished from B lymphocytes by surface markers and *in-vitro* function tests (see Chapter 17) but it is debatable whether they can be defined by morphological features in a routine Romanowsky-stained film. By scanning electron microscopy (SEM) the lymphocyte shows multiple microvilli, usually present in profusion over the entire surface, although some lymphocytes have a smoother appearance with few microvilli (Fig. 1.16). It has been suggested that it is the T cell which has the abundance of microvilli and hence that B and T cells

can thus be distinguished by SEM [28]; this view is not shared by all and, at least to some extent, differences in surface structure may be induced artefactually by the method of preparation of the materials prior to examination.

Plasma cells (Figs 1.17 and 1.18)

Plasmablasts are not a feature of normal blood or bone marrow. The mature plasma cell (plasmacyte) is elliptical, with an eccentric nucleus which is ovoid and usually sited in the smaller end of the cell. Its chromatin is purplish, very coarse and clumped in a characteristic way, resembling a cartwheel. The N/C ratio is 1:2 and there are no obvious nucleoli. The cytoplasm is deep blue with a pale perinuclear halo

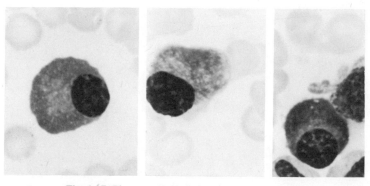

Fig. 1.17. Plasma cells by light microscopy (×1300).

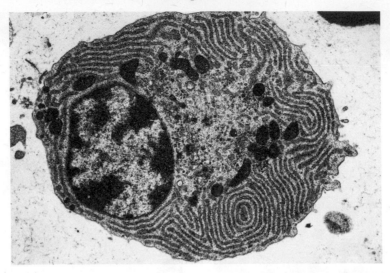

Fig. 1.18. Plasma cells as seen by transmission electron microscopy (× 13 500).

especially near one side of the nucleus. Vacuoles are present near the periphery of the cell. The electron-microscopic appearance is characterized by a pattern of parallel concentric sacs of ribosome-lined ergastoplasm [25–27]. The Golgi apparatus is well developed and is located at the cytoplasmic side of the nucleus. Mitochondria are large, with strikingly dense matrix. Small nucleoli may be seen in an appropriate plane of section.

Monocytes (Figs 1.19 and 1.20)

The monoblast is 12–20 μm in diameter with a large round or ovoid nucleus with light purple-pink staining fine and delicate chromatin. It contains one to two nucleoli. There is a distinct nuclear membrane. The N/C ratio is 1·5:1 to 2:1. The cytoplasm is deep blue and agranular.

The monocyte

This is the largest of the normal cells in the peripheral blood. It is 10–12 μm in diameter. The nucleus is oval, notched or horseshoe-shaped, with a light purple-pink staining delicate chromatin which tends to condense along the nuclear membrane. There are no nucleoli. The N/C ratio is 2·5:1. The cytoplasm is slate-coloured with some lilac-coloured granules. The most characteristic electron-microscope features [27] are irregular finger-like processes which enable phagocytosis to take place, with the production, at the cell periphery, of phagocytic vacuoles. Other small vacuoles occur near the nucleus and the Golgi apparatus. There are short profiles of ergastoplasm, small electron-dense round or rod-shaped granules enclosed by a double membrane, and small mitochondria. Bundles of fibrils may also be seen in the cytoplasm. As seen by SEM, the

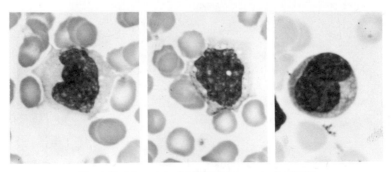

Fig. 1.19. Monocytes by light microscopy (× 1300).

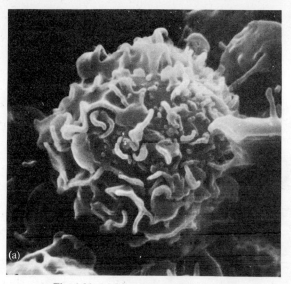
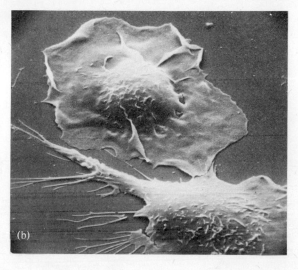

Fig. 1.20. (a) Monocyte and (b) spreading macrophage (× 8500). (By courtesy of Professor A. Polliack.)

monocyte is a large irregular cell, the membrane of which has prominent coarse ruffles and few (or no) microvilli (Fig. 1.20).

Platelets

Megakaryocyte (Figs 1.21 and 1.22)
This is the largest cell of the haemopoietic system. Immature forms are 10–24 μm and mature forms up to 50 μm in size with a mean diameter of 24 μm [29]. It varies enormously in appearance, so as to defy description of a single typical form. As a rule it has a

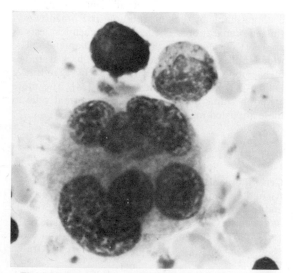

Fig. 1.21. Megakaryocyte by light microscopy (× 1300).

multiplicity of nuclei with coarse, irregularly clumped chromatin. At first the cytoplasm is abundant and pale blue with fine azurophil granules. As the cell matures, the cytoplasm becomes eosinophilic and the granules become more abundant. There may be pseudopod-like projections with granules extending into their periphery and sometimes platelets may be seen to be derived therefrom. Electron microscopy (Fig. 1.22) shows many α granules scattered throughout the cytoplasm, some with dense cores (nucleoids), the so-called bull's-eye granules; there are also electron-dense glycogen granules, and small round mitochondria. In the early stages the cell has tubular endoplasmic reticulum, which is replaced in the later stages by platelet demarcation vesicles which delineate the granule-containing cytoplasmic fragments which enter the circulation as platelets.

Platelet (see also Chapter 26)
Syn. thrombocyte

The platelet is a disc-shaped object, 2–3 μm in diameter. Conventional light microscopy yields little useful information on its structure but extensive electron-microscopic studies have revealed the complexities of structure within this apparently simple cell [30]. These include a triple-layered membrane, mitochondria, lysosomes, electron-dense bodies and α granules, glycogen granules, microtubules and microfibrils, filamentary bundles and a system of vacuoles and vesicles which seem to make up a canalicular system connecting with the exterior (Fig. 1.23).

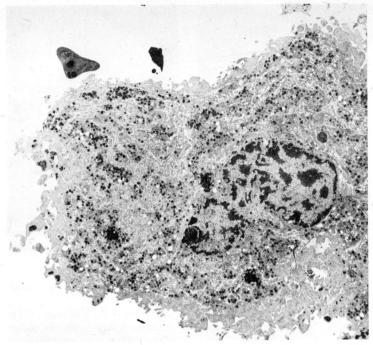

Fig. 1.22. Mature megakaryocyte as seen by transmission electron microscopy. (By courtesy of Mme. J. Breton-Gorius.)

This section has been intended to outline the essential morphological features of haemopoietic cells. Of necessity it is not possible to describe all the variations in cell morphology which occur, nor to include descriptions of non-haemopoietic cells which may be seen in a bone-marrow preparation, such as osteoblasts and tissue mast cells. For further reference the reader is referred to atlases of haematology (e.g. Refs 31, 32). Similarly, only cursory descriptions of electron-microscopic features have been given and reference should be made to more extensive reviews [25–27]. In modern haematological practice light microscopy and electron microscopy are linked with cytochemical studies in order to relate function to morphology and to identify blood cells which have been altered by disease, or to distinguish cell lines when the cells under scrutiny are not sufficiently mature to be distinguishable by their morphology in Romanowsky-stained preparations. The use of cytochemical tests as applied to leucocytes is described in Chapter 15. The wider applications of cytochemical methods in studies of haemopoiesis have been reviewed by Flandrin & Daniel [33] and by Dacie & Lewis [34]. The more common stains and the reaction of normal cells to these are listed in Table 1.2.

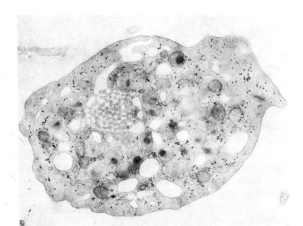

Fig. 1.23. Platelet as seen by transmission electron microscopy. (By courtesy of Mme. J. Breton-Gorius.)

THE BONE MARROW

General organization

An understanding of the structure of the bone marrow and the spatial relationship of its cellular components has been advanced by ulstrastructural studies, SEM and three-dimensional reconstruction based on serial sections [35–37]. The essential features are illustrated in Figures 1.24 and 1.25.

The human bone marrow contains a matrix which

Table 1.2. Cytochemical reactions of normal human blood cells

Cell	Alkaline phosphatase	Peroxidase	Lipid	PAS (glycogen)	Esterase NAS-DC	Esterase NAS-DA	NAS-DAF
Blasts	0	0	0–1	1	0	0	0
Myelocytes	1	4	2–4	1	2–4	2–4	2–4
Metamyelocytes	1–2	4	2–4	2	2–4	2–4	2–4
Neutrophils	1–4	4	2–4	4	2–4	2–4	2–4
Eosinophils	0	4	2–4	0	0	0	0
Basophils	0	0	2–4	0	0	0	0
Lymphocytes	0	0	0	1	0	0	0
Monocytes	0	1–3	2–3	2	2–4	1–3	0–1
Pronormoblasts	0	0	0	0	0	0	0
Normoblasts	0	0	0	0	0	0	0
Megakaryocytes	1	0	1	2	0	2–3	1–2

0 = negative, 1 = trace, 2 = slight, 3 = moderate, 4 = intense.
NAS-DC: Napthol AS D chloracetate.
NAS-DA: Napthol AS D acetate.
NAS-DAF: NAS-DA inhibited by fluoride.

consists of fat cells, vascular structures and their lining endothelial cells, reticulum cells, mast cells, plasma cells and fibrils [35]. The fat cells are abundant large cells about 80 μm in diameter, and they form a major component comprising, in health, one-third to two-thirds of the marrow volume. They are arranged in spheres in a three-dimensional pack. The spaces between the fat cells are filled by sheets of developing haemopoietic cells and by vessels and sinusoids. The sinusoids are arranged in interconnecting polygonal networks which in turn are connected with small venules which unite to form larger collecting venules. Arterioles provide the afferent blood supply to these networks either directly or through capillaries. These vessels frequently pass through bone before entering the marrow spaces to connect the sinusoids. The sinusoids are lined by a thin continuous layer of endothelial cells and a discontinuous adventitial layer.

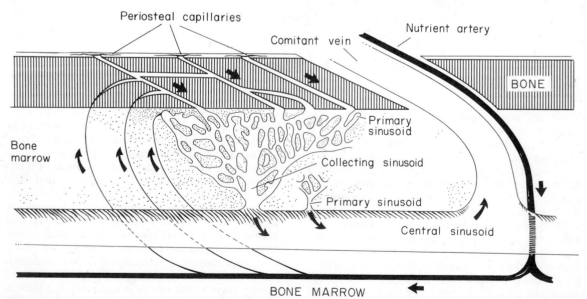

Fig. 1.24. Diagram of circulation in the bone marrow. The arterial supply is primarily through osteal vessels and venous drainage is through the large central sinusoid via primary and collecting sinusoids. (From de Bruyn P.P.H., Breen P.C. & Thomas T.B. (1970) The microcirculation of the bone marrow. *The Anatomical Record*, **168**, 55.)

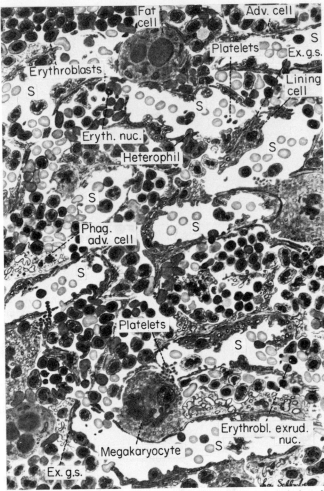

Fig. 1.25. Structural organization of bone marrow, showing distribution of haemopoietic cells in relation to sinuses (S). Ex.g.s. = extracellular ground substance. (From L. Weiss [36] with permission.)

There are also abundant fixed macrophages. The reticular cells are flattened, irregularly-shaped cells which extend from the surface of the fat cells to the sinusoids and serve as centres for clusters of haemopoietic cells, although erythropoiesis is not restricted to the sinuses but occurs over the entire marrow space. Plasma cells are in close contact with the sinusoidal wall, where they tend to proliferate and become stretched out along the sinusoidal membrane (Fig. 1.26). The mast cell is a constant feature of bone-marrow architecture. These cells are not numerous but because of their characteristic abundant metachromatic granules they are readily recognized. They are usually situated in the vicinity of the vascular structures.

There is evidence that the microvascular system is in a state of dynamic change [42]. During increased haemopoietic activity resulting, for example, from haemorrhage, an increased number of arterioles and capillaries originating from vessels within bone spicules enter the marrow space, the sinusoids become dilated and there is increased resorption of bone spicules surrounding the marrow spaces, so that there is an increase in the size of the spaces. The increased area becomes filled with haemopoietic cells as well as with fat. At the end of a period of stimulus, fat and haemopoietic elements regress and increased growth of bone decreases the size of the marrow spaces. Bone formation appears to be necessary for the functional integrity of bone-marrow tissue [43]. Whether erythropoietin plays a part in this is uncertain, but there is evidence that it has an effect on the micro-environment, making it conducive for erythropoiesis. There is an indirect vasodilator effect, with increased per-

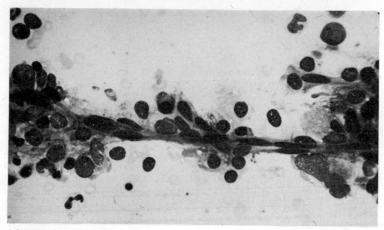

Fig. 1.26. Bone-marrow sinusoid lined by endothelial cells and with plasma cells in contact.

meability of the microvasculature, resulting in increased blood flow and erythropoietic cell release [44]. Also developing erythroblasts must have adequate oxygenation to respond maximally [45] and this oxygen supply might be provided by the increased numbers of arterioles that result from the erythropoietin-induced stimulus. The chemical composition of the stroma influences haemopoiesis, and this may be affected directly as a response of stromal cells to changes in tissue oxygenation and pH [44].

The reticulum cell has been described above in relation to haemopoiesis. As an element of the reticulo-histiocytic or reticulo-endothelial (RE) system it has, in addition, a particular role in phagocytosis and iron metabolism. When colloid particles are introduced into the bloodstream they are taken up largely by the RE cells of the liver, and to a lesser degree by spleen and lungs. A very small percentage is taken up by the bone marrow. The marrow is an active site of phagocytosis of normal red cells at the end of their lifespan [46] and it may become a major site of erythro-phagocytosis when there is extramedullary cell destruction or when the liver and spleen are inadequate to cope with severe haemolysis. Marrow reticulum cells contain iron, set free from phagocytosed erythrocytes, which in turn passes, apparently by rhopheocytosis, into the erythroblasts which are in contact with the reticulum cell or its projections. The reticulum cell has one further function; its projections embrace the sinusoids of the marrow, sometimes forming a second layer of sinus wall. These structures resemble fibroblasts and may participate in procollagen synthesis and the formation of reticulin fibres. In this way they play a part in mechanical stabilization of the marrow.

Release of blood cells into circulation

Each day some 2×10^{11} erythrocytes, 1×10^{11} granulocytes and 4×10^{11} platelets enter the circulation. The mechanism whereby this occurs is still a subject for speculation. It has been postulated that the endothelial lining of the sinus wall is capable of translating a humoral signal which indicates the requirements of the body for the type of cell to be delivered [47]. When a cell begins to migrate it exerts pressure on the endothelial membrane of the luminal side. The two membranes fuse and then separate in a different plane to open a pore for the cell. Dilatation of the lumen to meet an outpouring of cells is achieved by the layers of overlapping endothelial cells overriding each other [47] (Fig. 1.27). This is possible because, unlike other endothelial cells, these do not have tight junctions [48]. As a nucleated erythrocyte migrates through this barrier its nucleus is removed and the cytoplasm can then squeeze through the pore [49]. Reticulocytes, too, will be released into circulation when they have lost enough of their inclusions (mitochondria, etc.) to become sufficiently plastic. As far as leucocytes are concerned, motility of the mature cells may play an important role in this process helped, in the case of granulocytes with segmented nuclei, by their ability to align their nuclear segments. Megakaryocytes throw out pseudopodia which become nipped off to form platelets in the circulation. An alternative view is that the sinusoidal capillaries open intermittently to release mature cells and then close again while new cells develop. It has been suggested that immature cells are retained within the marrow during this process as they are embedded in a thick jelly-like substance which liquefies as the cells mature. These explanations of the release into the circulation of mature cells do not offer a reason for the presence of nucleated red cells and immature myeloid cells in the peripheral blood in certain diseases. In most cases this leuco-erythroblastic reaction is thought to be due to extramedullary

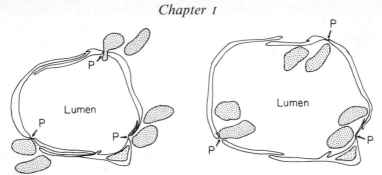

Fig. 1.27. Concept of mechanism whereby endothelial cells slide over each other to increase size of lumen of sinus and facilitate cell migration through the pores (P). (From M. Tavassoli & M. Shaklai [48] with permission.)

haemopoiesis with a less well-controlled release of cells from the spleen and other extramedullary sites than from the marrow. However, a similar loss of control might perhaps occur in the marrow, too, when an architectural alteration of the microvascular system results from proliferation. Control of the mechanism of cell release appears to be mediated by erythropoietin and other hormonal and humoral factors, with the spleen playing a significant part in the process.

Bone-marrow biopsy

Bone-marrow biopsy is an indispensable part of haematology, both for diagnostic purposes and for studying the progression of disease and the effects of therapy. It requires material which can be spread into a smear for studying cell morphology, as well as sections for assessing the extent of cellularity and for making a histological diagnosis. The need for repeated sampling makes it especially important that a technique be used which gives the patient the least possible discomfort and is free of hazard. To obtain material for smears, needle aspirations are simple, safe (even in thrombocytopenia), relatively painless, can be repeated many times, and can even be performed on outpatients. There are a number of needles, each marginally different, designed for marrow puncture. They include the well-known Salah and Klima needles [34]. Particles of marrow which are obtained by aspiration can be concentrated and sectioned. For a more definitive section of marrow tissue, however, it is necessary to use a trephine. Microtrephines such as the Turkel [50] can be used at any site almost as easily as an aspiration needle but they suffer the disadvantage that the specimen thus obtained is minute. Slightly larger needles such as the Gardner [39] and Vim–Silverman [51, 52] are suitable for use in posterior iliac-crest punctures. To some extent these needles tend to compress the material, resulting in an alteration of architecture. This artefact can be avoided by using a needle with a tapering end such as the Jamshidi–Swaim [53, 54]. Larger trephines of the iliac crest, such as the

Sacker–Nordin type of trephine [55, 56] are of particular value when there is some doubt whether a sample obtained by aspiration or by microtrephine is truly representative. In aplastic anaemia or myelosclerosis, for example, or when a marrow-infiltrating neoplasm is suspected, a larger trephine is frequently necessary (Fig. 1.28).

SITES OF MARROW BIOPSY
Bone-marrow aspiration can be carried out from the sternum, iliac crest, anterior or posterior iliac spines or the spinous process of the lumbar vertebrae. In children under the age of two years the upper end of the tibia is a convenient site. The usual site for sternal puncture is the manubrium or the first or second portions of the body of the sternum. If several punctures are being performed a different site should, if possible, be selected for each in order to avoid marrow which might be disorganized by haemorrhage resulting from the previous puncture. Similarly, sites of accidental trauma and of X-ray therapy must be avoided. It should be remembered that marrow cellularity varies at different sites in relation to age, so that an assessment of cellularity requires experience of what might be expected at that site in that particular age group. Of all the sites the sternum probably provides the best representative material. The fact that one aspiration may not provide a representative sample must always be borne in mind. Obviously, a large-section biopsy is less likely to be unrepresentative than an aspirated sample (Fig. 1.29). Marrow smears should be stained by a Romanowsky stain, and also for iron and for appropriate cytochemical reactions. Sections should be stained by haematoxylin and eosin, by silver impregnation for reticulin and Perls' reaction for iron. Methods of biopsy and handling the specimens are described by Dacie & Lewis [34].

QUANTITATIVE ANALYSIS OF BONE-MARROW SPECIMENS
A wide range of figures has been given in the literature

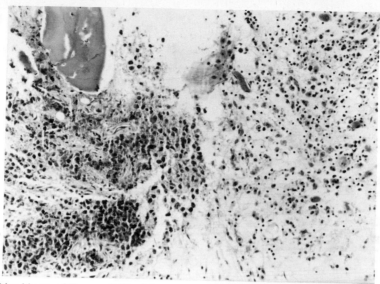

Fig. 1.28. Trephine biopsy of iliac crest, showing presence of infiltrating neoplasm (on left) (H & E stain, ×150).

for the total cell content of aspirated normal bone marrow [34]. This is not surprising in view of the fact that marrow is usually aspirated in the form of particles of varying size together with free cells and is diluted with a relatively uncontrolled amount of peripheral blood. For these reasons there is little point in carrying out a quantitative cell count. The degree of cellularity can be assessed within broad limits by inspection of marrow particles in the stained film. If less than one-quarter of the particle is occupied by haemopoietic cells it is probably hypocellular. It is

difficult to assess the significance of a single particle as adjacent particles may vary enormously in their cellularity. Of course, when no fragments have been obtained it is not possible to evaluate the degree of cellularity with even this degree of certainty, nor to know whether a 'dry tap' has been due to bone-marrow abnormality (myelosclerosis, aplastic anaemia, infiltrative tumour) or to technical failure. In these cases especially, the degree of cellularity can only be judged with any certainty in sections.

Physiological variation must be taken into account.

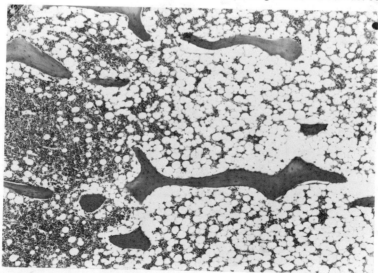

Fig. 1.29. Trephine biopsy of bone marrow from patient with aplastic anaemia, showing variable marrow cellularity (H & E stain, ×150).

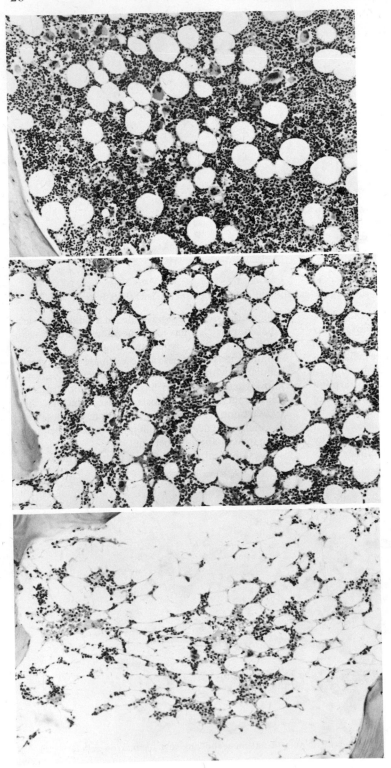

Fig. 1.30. Range of cellularity found in iliac-crest bone biopsies in normal adults (H & E stain, ×135).

Marrow cellularity is affected by age. The greater extent of haemopoietic (red) marrow in children has already been discussed; the proportion of fat cell to active cellular components in the red marrow is also less in children than in adults. In subjects of 70 years of age or more the marrow tends to become still more fatty both at the iliac crest [57] and, especially, at the manubrium sterni [34]. In pregnancy there is slight to moderate hyperplasia [58]. The range of cellularity at the iliac crest in normal adults is illustrated in Figure 1.30. Generally, in normal subjects haemopoietic cells occupy between one-third and two-thirds of the section, the rest of the area consisting of fat tissue; cellularity greater than 75% of the area indicates hyperplasia, and if less than 25%, hypoplasia. It is, of course, essential to remember that 'cellularity' as such is of little diagnostic significance without knowing the proportion due to erythropoiesis, myelopoiesis or some other cellular components.

Reticulin

A small amount of reticulin is to be seen in all bone-marrow sections. An increased amount may be seen in a variety of disorders. In some it is associated with fibroblast proliferation as the primary disorder whilst reticulin deposition also occurs as a secondary reactive phenomenon, in association with neoplasms, infections (notably tuberculosis), irradiation and toxic exposure to chemicals such as benzol. A gross increase in reticulin occurs characteristically in myelosclerosis (agnogenic myeloid metaplasia) but a variably in-creased amount occurs in cases of acute and chronic leukaemias, polycythaemia vera and other myeloproliferative conditions [59–61]. The pattern of the reticulin is characteristically thick and wavy in myelosclerosis and related conditions (Fig. 1.31).

Iron

A marrow smear or section stained for iron provides important information, and a Prussian-blue stain (Perls' reaction) should be carried out routinely on marrow films. Normally erythroblasts contain only a few small scattered iron-containing (siderotic) granules, and some of this 'storage' iron may be seen to be in RE cells. The extent of marrow iron is an indicator of body iron stores [62]; when reduced or absent it is a sensitive indication of iron-deficiency even when there is no overt anaemia. The number of nucleated red cells containing obvious siderotic granules is related to the iron stores of the body and the serum iron level [63]. When there is disturbance in haemoglobin synthesis the granules become larger and more numerous; these cells are then referred to as sideroblasts. Any discrepancy in the balance between the iron contained in erythroblasts and that in RE cells or present as free iron stores points to some disturbance in iron metabolism and/or haemoglobin synthesis. In infections, for example, iron stores may be increased and there will be abundant siderotic material in the RE cells but few or no siderotic granules in erythroblasts.

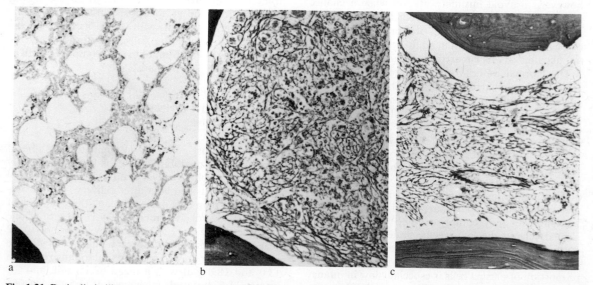

Fig. 1.31. Reticulin in iliac-crest trephine biopsies, as demonstrated by silver-impregnation staining method (× 120): (a) normal; (b and c) increased; (c) was from a patient with definite myelosclerosis; (b) was from a patient with a less clearly defined myeloproliferative disorder.

The myelogram

It is a matter of opinion whether any useful purpose is served by carrying out a differential cell count on bone-marrow smears. First of all there is the problem of sampling error, leading to serious inaccuracy. Thus there may be a different cell distribution in different parts of the smear (e.g. in the trail compared to the central part); then, again, the fixed reticulum cells and the largest cells, such as megakaryocytes, tend to resist aspiration and remain in the marrow or embedded in marrow fragments; moreover, dilution of the aspirated marrow with peripheral blood leads to an unavoidable, variable error. A second problem is the fact that it may be impossible to know at what precise state of development a cell is, or even to be sure to which system it belongs. It would seem more realistic to examine a film systematically and to interpret the marrow from its general appearance, backed by a knowledge of the patient's peripheral-blood count and clinical features. For diagnostic purposes it will, as a rule, suffice to have a description of general cellularity, type of erythropoiesis (i.e. whether normoblastic or megaloblastic), and whether maturation of erythropoietic and leucopoietic cells is proceeding normally, together with an estimate of the relative numbers of each series (myeloid/erythroid ratio). It may be of some value to have an approximate count of the proportion of cells of one or other type in special circumstances, e.g. the proportion of primitive cells when early leukaemia is suspected or of plasma cells in the diagnosis of myelomatosis. Care must be taken, however, to avoid misinterpretation when a chance aspiration at the site of a lymph follicle might result in a film with an unusually high proportion of lymphocytes; although infrequent in adults lymph follicles are not uncommon in the marrow of infants and children.

The normal values for a differential count on aspirated bone marrow given in Table 1.3 are those given for adults by Dacie & Lewis [34]. Marked variations occur in children [64]. During the first month after birth the erythroid cells decrease so that only about 10% of the nucleated cells are erythroblasts at two to three weeks, whilst myeloid cells increase during the first two weeks of life, following which a sharp drop occurs at about the third week. At the end of the first month about 60% of the cells are myeloid; this value remains stationary until the age of 20. Lymphocytes may comprise up to 40% of the nucleated cells in the first weeks, gradually decreasing during the first and second year, thereafter comprising about 15% of the cells during the rest of childhood. The proportion of plasma cells is especially low in infancy and up to the age of five years [65]. The myeloid/erythroid ratio is low at birth, but increases rapidly during the first two weeks to values as high as 11:1 and then

Table 1.3. Normal range for differential count on aspirated bone marrow (%)

Reticulum cells	0·1–2
Haemocytoblasts	0·1–1
Myeloblasts	0·1–3·5
Promyelocytes	0·5–5
Myelocytes	
Neutrophil	5–20
Eosinophil	0·1–3
Basophil	0–0·5
Metamyelocytes	10–30
Polymorphonuclears	
Neutrophil	7–25
Eosinophil	0·2–3
Basophil	0–0·5
Lymphocytes	5–20
Monocytes	0–0·2
Megakaryocytes	0·1–0·5
Plasma cells	0·1–3·5
Pronormoblasts	0·5–5
Basophilic and polychromatic normoblasts	2–20
Pyknotic normoblasts	2–10

gradually, during the first year, decreases to 3:1, and this ratio is retained during childhood. In adults the ratio is usually 3:1 or 4:1, although it varies widely and a range of 2·5–15:1 represents the full scale of normality [34]. These changes are discussed further in Chapter 3.

During normal pregnancy quantitative changes in the bone-marrow cellularity occur, mainly in the third trimester [58]. There is hyperplasia, which affects both erythropoiesis and granulopoiesis, the latter proportionately less, though with some increase in the percentage of immature cells. A return to normal begins in the puerperium but is not completed until at least six weeks post partum.

THE BLOOD COUNT

Haemoglobin

This is the most common determination in clinical medicine. Haemoglobin content is high immediately after birth, reaching a level of up to 20 g/dl, especially when the cord is tied later after delivery. The haemoglobin level then falls during the first three months of life to 10–11 g/dl. It is reported as 11–13 g/dl at one year, increasing to 11·5–14·8 g/dl by the age of 10–12 years, and reaching adult levels by the age of 15. The usual values for normal men are said to range between 13·0 and 18·0 g/dl with a mean of 15 g/dl, and for women 11·5–16·5 g/dl with a mean of 13·5 g/dl [34, 66]. In old age the haemoglobin is reported to fall, in men, to a mean level of 13·4 g (±1·6) at 65, 12·9 g (±1·6) at

75 and 12·2 g ($\pm$1·4) of the age of 85 [67]. By contrast, in elderly women the level tends to rise, so that a sex difference of 2 g/dl in younger age groups is reduced to 1 g/dl in old age [68]. These differences have, however, not been shown in one study on a large number of subjects over the age of 65 [69].

The range of so-called normal haemoglobin levels has been a matter of controversy for a long time, and the range given here is so wide as to be of relatively little value in assessing the signficance of a measurement at the limits of the range. There are several reasons for the difficulty in establishing normal levels. In the past, variation in technique, use of unreliable methods with artificial standards often based on misconception, and lack of an international haemoglobin reference preparation have been blamed for discrepancies in data from different laboratories. These problems have been largely overcome by the use of the reference preparation introduced by the International Committee for Standardization in Haematology [70] and a standardized method of haemoglobinometry [34, 71]. A second reason is the difficulty in establishing criteria for perfect health to ensure that a normal reference population means precisely that. The presence of chronic ill health in an entire community may result in the acceptance of that state of health as normal until it is shown in its true perspective by comparison with a higher standard of health [72–76]. Indeed, this raises the fundamental question of the difference between 'normal' and 'usual' in establishing clinical significance (see p. 132). The next factor to consider is that of physiological variations, including the influence of age and sex, physical exercise and posture and environment.

Age differences have been described in the previous paragraph. Sex differences become apparent after puberty. Their cause is not completely understood. The lower level in women is partly due to hormonal differences, whilst continuing blood loss at menstruation might lead to a degree of iron deficiency [77], although loss of as much as 100 ml of blood with each period does not appear to cause a significant decrease in haemoglobin concentration even though it results in a low serum iron with a high iron-binding capacity [78]. Oral contraceptives given to healthy women result in an increase in serum iron and iron-binding capacity, but do not affect the haemoglobin level [68, 79], so it is possible that the lower serum iron of women is due to oestrogen and/or progestogen influences and does not necessarily betoken iron deficiency. In normal pregnancy the haemoglobin is on average 1 g/dl lower than in the same age non-pregnant woman, but this is due to an increase in plasma volume and not to a reduction in the circulating red cells, unless there is an associated true anaemia from iron or folate deficiency. The

red-cell indices (see p. 33) show no significant differences between the sexes.

Muscular exercise, if at all strenuous, raises the haemoglobin level transiently, either because of re-entry of red cells into the capillaries or through loss of circulating plasma. Athletes tend to have slightly lower haemoglobin levels than non-athletes, but this is probably not significant [85]. Athletes do, however, have significantly higher red cell and plasma volumes, with total blood volumes on average 20% higher than in non-athletes [85]. Posture, too, causes transient alterations in red-cell concentration; there is an increase of about five to ten per cent in haemoglobin (and PCV) within 20 minutes after changing from a recumbent to a standing position [81, 82], while it has been shown [83] that alteration in the position of the arm alone during sample collection, i.e. whether dependent or at the atrial level, affects cell concentration. As far as sampling is concerned it should be remembered that capillary blood has approximately five per cent higher concentration of red cells than does venous blood [34], and stasis by a tourniquet before venepuncture will also cause haemoconcentration. Stasis also causes discrepancies between ear-lobe and finger-tip samples of 'capillary' blood [84].

Diurnal variation is usually slight [80] but fluctuations of as much as 15% have been reported [86], with highest levels in the morning. It has been suggested that seasonal variations also occur although evidence for this has been conflicting [87, 88]. Altitude results in an increased haemoglobin level, the magnitude of which depends on the duration and extent of the anoxic stimulus [89]. In general, at an altitude of 2 km (6500 feet) the figure is said to be about 1 g/dl higher than at sea level, and at 3 km (10 000 feet) it is 2 g/dl higher. In one study the increase was found to be in the order of 1 g/dl for each kilometre, with slightly higher increase in men than in women [257]. This appears in part to be a true increase because of increased erythropoiesis, but a secondary factor is a decrease in plasma volume which occurs at high altitudes [90]. Erythropoiesis appears to be affected by cigarette smoking, and this results in a slightly higher haemoglobin concentration amongst smokers, apparently especially women, and a slightly higher packed cell volume in both men and women [91]. It may even result in frank polycythaemia [92]. There is a direct association between smoking and carboxyhaemoglobin concentration in the blood; smokers are liable to have up to 10% by contrast to one to two per cent in non-smokers [93, 94].

Haemoglobinometry
The oxygen-combining capacity of blood is 1·34 ml O_2/g haemoglobin. As a functional estimation of

haemoglobin, measurement of oxygen capacity provides the most meaningful information, but it is hardly practicable in clinical practice. Iron content of haemoglobin can be estimated accurately by spectrophotometry, titrimetric methods and X-ray emission spectrography [95, 96]. Iron content is converted into haemoglobin content by the relationship 100 g haemoglobin $\equiv 0.347$ g iron [70]. Although these methods are impracticable for routine clinical purposes they have provided absolute chemical values from which it has been possible to derive an accurate relationship of millimolar extinction coefficient to haemoglobin content. The International Committee for Standardization in Haematology established specifications for a cyanmethaemoglobin (hemiglobincyanide) standard on a basis of a molecular weight of 64 458 and a millimolar extinction coefficient of 44·0 [70]. This has a stability of at least six years and it has been adopted by the World Health Organization as an International Reference Preparation. Because of the availability of this reliable and stable standard the cyanmethaemoglobin method had been widely adopted in routine practice. A further advantage is that all forms of haemoglobin except sulphaemoglobin are readily converted to cyanmethaemoglobin. A disadvantage of the method is the need for a reaction time of up to several minutes to ensure complete conversion of the pigment. By contrast, the oxyhaemoglobin method is the simplest and quickest method for general use with a photo-electric colorimeter, as total conversion occurs in a matter of seconds. Its disadvantage, however, is that it is not possible to prepare a stable oxyhaemoglobin standard and it is not a satisfactory method in the presence of carboxyhaemoglobin, methaemoglobin or sulphaemoglobin [34]. An alkaline-haematin method, although somewhat more elaborate, is a useful ancillary method as it gives a true estimate of total haemoglobin. Other methods, e.g. Sahli's acid haematin and Haldane's carboxyhaemoglobin, are now obsolete.

Haemoglobin concentration is usually expressed as mass concentration in g/dl or g/l; it has been proposed that expression might alternatively be as substance concentration using the unit mole [97]. Thus, as an example of this latter system, 15 g/dl = 9·3 mmol/l, assuming that the elementary entity of the haemoglobin molecule is a monomer.

Red-cell count

At birth the red-cell count is $4.0–6.0 \times 10^{12}/l$ or even higher. The count falls in childhood parallel with haemoglobin (see above). At one year of age it is $3.6–5.0 \times 10^{12}/l$, and at 10–12 years it is $4.2–5.2 \times 10^{12}/l$. In adults the normal range is generally accepted to be $4.5–6.5 \times 10^{12}/l$ in men and $3.9–5.6 \times 10^{12}/l$ in women. This wide range was established mainly from manual haemocytometer counts and although these figures have been sanctified by long usage they must be questioned when account is taken of the error of the method and the unavoidable cell-distribution errors which occur when relatively few cells are counted. The advent of automatic cell counters increased enormously the practicability of red-cell counting which now has a precision of one to two per cent, and an accuracy of two to three per cent, provided that adequate attention is paid to instrument calibration and quality control procedures [98–100]. The result of this refinement is that the cell count rather than haemoglobin is now frequently used as the primary measurement of the blood count. The various counting systems are based on different principles, but, in general, they incorporate a procedure by which a suspension of blood flows in a stream and the cells are counted as light impulses as they pass a condenser, or as scattered light when they interrupt a beam, or as electric pulses when they change the conductivity by passing between electrodes and suspending medium. The count may vary slightly on the same sample by different counting systems, unless they have been calibrated appropriately.

Reticulocyte counts

The normal reticulocyte count is 0·5–1·5% in adults and children, and two to six per cent in full-term infants at birth [34, 66]. In absolute numbers the count has been reported as varying between 25×10^9 and $85 \times 10^9/l$ [34, 66, 101]. The reticulocyte count is usually taken as a fairly accurate reflection of erythropoietic activity, and it has been suggested that a count below $40 \times 10^9/l$ should be taken as an indication of depressed erythropoiesis [102]. However, any deduction of marrow activity from reticulocyte turnover assumes that reticulocytes remain in circulation for a constant period of time. This is not, in fact, necessarily true. Normally reticulocytes mature in two to three days, 24 hours of which are spent in the circulation. However, if the reticulocytes are released into circulation prematurely, as might be expected in conditions of increased demand, the maturation time in circulation of these so-called 'shift' or stimulated reticulocytes will be prolonged for up to three days. In such cases it is more informative to relate the reticulocyte count to the stage of development as indicated by RNA content, or by calculating a true reticulocyte count from an estimated maturation time, i.e.

True reticulocyte count =

$$\frac{\text{Absolute reticulocyte count/l}}{\text{Maturation time (days)}} \quad [103]$$

By comparing the corrected reticulocyte count with the normal count, a reticulocyte-production index is obtained; from this it is possible to assess if marrow response is appropriate to the degree of anaemic stimulus. The normal marrow response is as follows [104]:

PCV	Production index	Maturation time in circulation (days)
0·45	1	1·0
0·35	2–3	1·5
0·25	3–5	2·0
0·15	3–5	2·5

When the reticulocyte count is reported as a percentage and the total RBC is not known it is necessary to apply a further correction factor to compensate for the fact that the observed count depends on both the rate of production and the total number of red cells diluting the reticulocytes in circulation. It is calculated by multiplying the observed count by the PCV (or Hb) as a fraction of normal, i.e.

$$\left(\frac{PCV}{0·45} \text{ or } \frac{Hb(g/dl)}{15}\right).$$

Packed cell volume (PCV)

Four methods are in use for determining the PCV. These include two methods in which blood is centrifuged, a conductivity method and a method in which PCV is derived from measurement of erythrocyte cell volume and numbers of red cells by an electronic counting system (e.g. Coulter S). For the centrifugation methods blood is centrifuged either in a Wintrobe tube (bore 2·55 mm) at 2000–2300 g for 30 minutes [34, 105] or in a capillary tube at 10 000 g for five minutes [34, 105]. The errors of these methods and their limitations have been discussed in a series of papers by the International Committee for Standardization in Haematology [106–108]. With the microhaematocrit method, technical errors can be reduced to ±1% [105]. It is essential to avoid excess anticoagulation, as more than 2 mg/ml of EDTA is liable to cause cell shrinkage with a lowering of PCV [109–111]. Other factors to be taken into account are the trapping of plasma and the effect of centrifugal force on cell shape. With normal blood, trapped plasma appears to be in region of two to three per cent with microhaematocrit [112–113] and somewhat higher with lower-speed centrifugation [114]. Trapping is greater with polycythaemic blood [34, 114] and also in spherocytosis [115], thalassaemia [116], hypochromic anaemias and sickled blood [117]. In all these conditions, haematocrit measurement of PCV might be expected to give erroneously high results unless corrected for trapped plasma. Whether centrifu-

gation results in alteration in cell shape and/or loss of intracellular fluid to any significant extent is not clear [118]. If it does, this may also affect the measurement of PCV. A reference method has been established which is based on centrifugation in a Wintrobe tube, and correction for trapped plasma by an isotope method [119]. This provides a high degree of accuracy and precision, but it is impractical for routine use.

When the PCV is computed by an electronic counter the results are not influenced by the concentration of anticoagulant in the blood specimen [120], by oxygenation, nor by the excessive trapped plasma which occurs with centrifugation of some abnormal bloods. Thus, PCV estimation by this means should be potentially more accurate, but this is dependent on reliable instrument calibration. Conductivity methods are based on measurement of electrical conductivity of whole blood. These are, however, liable to serious error when there are pathological alterations of proteins [106] and when there is slight variation in the relative concentration of anticoagulant in the blood specimen. The PCV is expressed as a fractional volume. It implies the measured volume of the red cells per litres of whole blood (in l/l).

Absolute values

So-called absolute values (or indices) are mean cell volume (MCV), mean cell haemoglobin (MCH), and mean cell haemoglobin concentration (MCHC). Their derivation from cell-count parameters is as follows:

$$MCV = PCV \div RBC/l \times 10^{15}$$
expressed as femtolitres (fl)
$$MCH = Hb(g/l) \div RBC(/l) \times 10^{12} \text{ or } Hb(g/dl)$$
$$\div RBC/l \times 10^{13}$$
expressed as picograms (pg)
$$MCHC = Hb(g/l) \div PCV$$
expressed as g/l
or $Hb(g/dl) \div PCV$
expressed as g/dl

The normal ranges are as follows [34]:

	3 months	1 year	10–12 years	Adults (men and women)
MCV (fl)	83–110	77–101	77–95	76–96
MCH (pg)	24–34	23–31	24–30	27–32
MCHC (g/dl)	27–34	28–33	30–33	30–35

Obviously, the accuracy and significance of these data depend on the accuracy of the measurement from which they have been derived. Thus, the reliability of MCV and MCH must be as much in question as that of the RBC. In the past this has led to a tendency to discard both the RBC and the indices derived from the RBC from routine blood counts, whereas MCHC derived from the reputedly more accurate measurements of Hb and PCV has been considered a more reliable index. The advent of automatic cell counters has, however, now provided a means for greater accuracy and critical evaluation of normal ranges, and a discriminant function which can be used for screening for various conditions, e.g. β thalassaemia [121–124] and also for α thalassaemia [125]. Identification of minor degrees of macrocytosis by MCV has become an important means for detecting the earliest stages of megaloblastosis associated with vitamin-B_{12} or folate deficiency [126, 127] and a range of diseases associated with dyserythropoiesis [128]. The MCV is also reliable for recognizing iron deficiency at an early stage [126, 127, 129] and for distinguishing between iron deficiency and the anaemia of chronic disorder [130]. The MCV has also been found to be useful as an indicator of chronic alcoholism in apparently normal non-anaemic subjects with an unexplained increased MCV in a health screening programme [131].

Measurements by Coulter S indicate that MCH and MCHC are remarkably constant in health, MCH being about 30 pg and MCHC 33 g/dl with a coefficient of variation of two per cent of these figures. MCV is found to be somewhat higher by Coulter S than by traditional methods. There is need for assessment of the differences between methods [132] and the reasons for these differences, before establishing reference values. It is desirable to have reference standards to ensure instrument calibration and to establish a correlation between methods.

Red-cell size distribution

The size of individual red cells, expressed as their diameter (RCD), and the degree of variation in size may be estimated by diffraction methods [133] or measured directly with the aid of an eye-piece micrometer [34] or particle-size analyser [134]. The Price-Jones curve is a size-distribution analysis. It had a period of great popularity in the 1930s when it was considered to be an essential part of the investigation of anaemia, although the labour expended contributed nothing to the understanding of the case and merely provided a graphic record of what was to be seen by inspection of a stained film. The normal red-cell diameter is given as 6·7–7·7 μm (mean 7·2 μm) in dry films and somewhat larger (mean 8·3–8·7 μm) for cells examined in rouleaux or as single cells in wet preparations [34]. Other parameters derived from cell size are cell thickness and surface area. Cell thickness has been reported to be 1·5–1·9 μm (mean 1·7 μm) [135] or 1·5–1·7 μm (mean 1·6 μm) [136] in wet preparations, and 1·7–2·5 μm in dry films [34]. Surface area has been said to be 128–144 μm² (mean 134 μm²) [135] or 132–160 μm² (mean 145 μm²) [136] by different

workers. There is a close correlation between the ratio of diameter/thickness and MCH, and also MCHC [137]. With the advent of electronic counters which include facilities for particle-size analysis, e.g. Coulter Channelyzer and the S Plus Counting System it is now possible to obtain erythrocyte size-distribution curves rapidly and with a precision enabling even minor deviations from the normal graph to be identified [138, 139]. This is a potentially important tool for studying the pathophysiology of the red cell [140]; it has diagnostic value, for example as a rapid screening test for thalassaemia trait [141] or in a multiple haematinic factor deficiency [142] where MCV may be misleadingly normal. The use of an analysing computer allows an even greater range of measurement including quantification of red-cell morphological characteristics of size, shape, and staining intensity as a reflection of haemoglobin concentration [143, 144].

WHOLE BLOOD AND PLASMA

Plasma is the fluid component of blood and comprises approximately 55% of the whole-blood volume in health. It is complex liquid consisting of proteins in a dilute aqueous solution of salts. Its composition is shown in Table 1.4. The plasma proteins are important in regulating blood volume and the body's fluid balance, and they contribute to blood viscosity. An interrelationship of red cells and the plasma proteins determines the sedimentation rate of blood. Fibrinogen is the precursor of fibrin and it functions in blood clotting. When blood is allowed to clot the plasma, now devoid of fibrinogen, becomes serum. Plasma and serum are, in health, light straw-coloured. A deeper yellow colour is a sign of jaundice. Iron deficiency results in a very pale appearance. When blood is centrifuged other characteristic appearances which may help diagnostically include the occurrence of opacity in lipaemia, and a cloudiness occurring at low temperatures in cases where there is a cold-precipitable protein (cryoglobulin): this has been encountered in multiple myeloma and also in cases of chronic lymphocytic leukaemia and other disorders. In haemolytic anaemias in which intravascular haemolysis occurs (e.g. paroxysmal nocturnal haemoglobinuria, paroxysmal cold haemoglobinuria) there may be a pink tinge to the plasma, and similarly lysis may occur *in vitro* to the specimen or may be seen in the plasma as a result of its occurrence *in vivo* in cases where the red cells are susceptible to mechanical trauma, such as in sickle-cell anaemia and spherocytosis. In a centrifuged sample of blood, the plasma is separated from the red cells by a thin reddish-grey layer of packed leucocytes and platelets, the buffy coat. This is increased in size as

Table 1.4. Composition of plasma

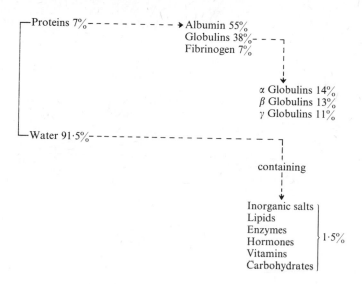

a result of leucocytosis, and becomes a notable feature in leukaemias. Platelets give rise to a cream-coloured layer on top of the buffy layer, and this becomes a distinct feature when the platelet count is unduly high, as in thrombocythaemia.

Specific gravity

The normal specific gravity of whole blood as determined by weight is given as 1·048–1·066 (mean 1·057) for men and slightly lower (mean 1·053) for women, and there is a normal diurnal variation of 0·003 [145]. The specific gravity of serum is 1·026–1·031 and of red cells 1·092–1·095 [146]. The specific gravity of blood depends on a number of factors, particularly haemoglobin concentration in the red cells and protein concentration in the plasma. By centrifuging blood with inert liquids, e.g. benzyl benzoate [147] or mixtures of phthalate esters [148] of known density, it is possible to measure the density of a blood cell population. When this procedure is carried out with a range of oils a density distribution of cells can be obtained [148]. In normal subjects the red cells vary considerably in their density. The lightest cells are 1·100, the heaviest 1·222 whilst a median population has a range between 1·106 and 1·112 [148, 149]. The distribution of density is sigmoidal when plotted on arithmetic graph paper, with a pattern similar and parallel to that produced by osmotic haemolysis (Fig. 1.32). In general, reticulocytes are the lightest cells and are most resistant to osmotic lysis whereas the most fragile cells, which tend to be spherical, are the

heaviest. There are rare discrepancies in this relationship, notably in paroxysmal nocturnal haemoglobinuria [149] and in familial Mediterranean fever [148].

The relationship of haemoglobin concentration to specific gravity has been used as the basis for a haemoglobin screening test [150]; for this the specific gravity of blood is assessed by introducing a drop of the blood into a copper sulphate solution of known specific gravity. By using a range of specific gravities it is possible to estimate haemoglobin with some degree of accuracy. Although this is, today, an obsolete procedure, the use of a single solution (e.g. sp. gr. 1·046) to separate 'anaemic' from 'normal' bloods (at a level of approximately 10 g/dl) is still used to some extent, especially in blood transfusion services. However, this method does not stand up well to critical evaluation [151]. In one study it was found that whereas 10% of prospective blood donors were rejected as 'anaemic' by the copper-sulphate method, at least half of them were subsequently shown to be normal by haemoglobin and PCV measurements [152].

Erythrocyte sedimentation rate

Erythrocyte sedimentation rate (ESR) or blood sedimentation rate (BSR) is a measure of the suspension stability of red cells in blood. Various methods have been devised for its measurement, but nowadays that of Westergren [153] is almost universally used [156]. In this method a tube 30 cm in length and 2·5 mm in diameter is filled with blood diluted with 32·8 g/l trisodium citrate (109 mmol/l) in the proportion of one

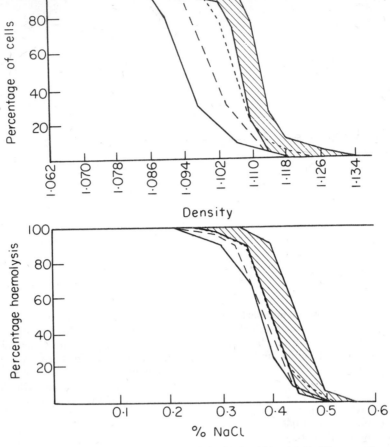

Fig. 1.32. Density distribution (above) and osmotic fragility (below) of red blood cells. The normal ranges are indicated by hatched-line areas; the other curves are from patients with hypochromic anaemias: (- - - - -) MCHC 29 g/dl; (– – – –) MCHC 27 g/dl; (———) MCHC 25 g/dl.

part citrate to four parts of blood, and then set upright. The numerical value in mm is obtained by measuring the distance from the surface meniscus to the upper limit of the red-cell layer in the column of blood after 60 minutes. The rate of sedimentation is influenced by a number of interrelated factors. Basically it depends upon the difference in specific gravity between red cells and plasma, but it is also influenced very greatly by the extent to which the red cells form rouleaux, as large clumps of cells sediment more rapidly than single cells. Other factors which might affect sedimentation include the degree of anaemia, any tilt of the tube, the dimensions of the tube (bore and length) and possibly the composition of the tube (glass or plastic) and the nature of the anticoagulant used. These factors influence the relationship of the downward force of the falling erythrocytes to the opposing retarding force which comes from displacement of the plasma by the erythrocytes (Fig. 1.33).

The all-important rouleaux formation is increased by high concentrations of fibrinogen and other acute phase proteins and immunoglobulins; it is retarded by albumin. The acute-phase proteins are a heterogeneous group which include fibrinogen, haptoglobin, ceruloplasmin, α_1 acid glycoprotein, α_1 antitrypsin and C-reactive protein. They are synthesized in increased amounts as a response or reaction to (a) acute tissue damage cause by physical or chemical toxins, trauma, infection, infarction and immunological injury, (b) chronic inflammation of chronic infection and collagen diseases, (c) malignant disease and (d) pregnancy and the puerperium.

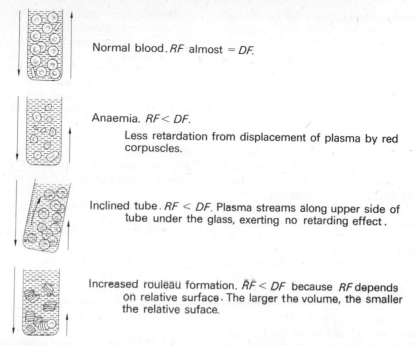

Normal blood. *RF* almost = *DF*.

Anaemia. *RF* < *DF*.
Less retardation from displacement of plasma by red corpuscles.

Inclined tube. *RF* < *DF*. Plasma streams along upper side of tube under the glass, exerting no retarding effect.

Increased rouleau formation. *RF* < *DF* because *RF* depends on relative surface. The larger the volume, the smaller the relative suface.

Fig. 1.33. Factors which influence the erythrocyte sedimentation rate. RF = retarding force, DF = downward force of red cells. (From Wintrobe M.M. (1967) *Clinical Hematology*, 6th edn, p. 356. Henry Kimpton, London.)

Although the ESR is an empirical test, it is easy to perform with relatively simple equipment and facilities; thus, it is widely used in clinical medicine as a non-specific reaction giving information of a general character with the same usefulness as, for example, body temperature, pulse rate and leucocyte count. It is a measure of the presence and severity of inflammatory and other morbid processes: there is a fairly close correlation between the ESR and disease activity and it provides a means for monitoring progress and response to therapy in chronic diseases. At times, it may be much more sensitive than other means in detecting an abnormal state and may draw attention to an otherwise occult disease.

The normal ESR is stated by Dacie & Lewis [34] to be up to 5 mm for men and up to 7 mm for women. Different normal ranges have been reported in other studies [157]. Taking all these figures into account, most normal men would be expected to have an ESR less than 12 mm and normal women an ESR less than 19 mm and in both men and women over the age of 60 an ESR less than 19 mm. In both men and women over the age of 60 an ESR over 20 mm may be found without any obvious cause [154, 155] and levels as high as 40 mm have been reported in normal subjects over the age of 65. In newborn infants ESR has been found

to be less than 2 mm but this was based on a micromethod [166]. By the standard Westergren method the ESR in childhood appears to be the same as for normal men with no difference between boys and girls [158]. Ten per cent of apparently normal children have an increased rate [159]. Physiological increases in ESR occur in pregnancy; the increase begins at about the 10th–12th week and does not return to normal until the third to fourth week post partum [160]. These wide ranges emphasize the fact that the test may be influenced by environmental and technical factors as well as by a number of inherent variables. Ambient temperature is an important factor, whilst even a small deviation of the tube from the vertical may lead to major discrepancies; for reproducible results it is thus essential to pay meticulous attention to a standard technique [34], and to use Westergren tubes of specified dimensions [156, 161].

While a normal ESR cannot be taken to exclude organic disease, the vast majority of acute or chronic infections, neoplastic diseases, collagen diseases, renal insufficiency and other diseases associated with changes in the plasma proteins will lead to an acceleration of sedimentation. Anaemia may of itself increase sedimentation, and attempts have been made to apply formulae in order to correct for the anaemia, but as the effect of the anaemia on the ESR is irregular these are not generally considered worthwhile and, moreover, the anaemia represents part of the overall clinical picture.

Plasma viscosity

Globulins, especially fibrinogen, are large non-spherical molecules which, in solution, are more viscous than the smaller spherical albumin molecules, so that a higher relative concentration of the former components will result in an increased plasma viscosity. The measurement of plasma viscosity is thus a nonspecific test of organic disease which largely parallels the ESR [162, 163]. It has some advantages over the ESR in that it is not affected by anaemia, and the degree of viscosity is claimed to reflect severity of disease more closely than ESR, with fewer discrepancies [162]. Moreover, specimens of blood can be examined for several days after collection and the test can be standardized with EDTA as the anticoagulant. It does, however, require a more complex and expensive piece of apparatus [164, 165] than that required for ESR. A comprehensive review by Harkness [162] describes various types of viscometers and the results of an extensive series of tests on normal subjects and patients with various diseases.

Normal plasma from EDTA blood has a viscosity (at 25°C) of 1·50–1·72 cP (mean 1·64, s.d. 0·052) with no significant differences between men and women. It is affected by age, being low in infants and possibly slightly higher in old age; it is also affected by exercise and is increased in pregnancy but it is remarkably constant in health with little or no diurnal variation, so that a change of only 0·03–0·05 cP in an individual subject probably has clinical significance. As with ESR, plasma viscosity is influenced predominantly by plasma fibrinogen and it is increased under the same conditions as is the ESR, although it has been suggested that changes in ESR lag behind those of plasma viscosity by 24–48 hours in the acute-phase reaction. Reduced plasma viscosity occurs when there are low levels of immunoglobulins but unlike ESR it is not affected by red-cell abnormalities and it is not reduced in polycythaemia. Major discrepancies between the two tests occur when raised plasma globulin levels are associated with falling albumin; this pattern would tend to increase the ESR but to reduce the plasma viscosity.

Whole-blood viscosity is a function of the amount and quality of blood cells as well as the various plasma proteins; it is controlled by the interaction between these components and so provides information of a different order. It is influenced especially by PCV and MCHC. Whole-blood viscosity provides interesting data on the rheological behaviour of blood in polycythaemia, when there is alteration in red-cell flexibility or deformability and in hyperviscosity syndromes. Studies of factors which influence whole-blood viscosity may provide useful information with therapeutic implications but it must be appreciated that flow of the blood sample in a rigid capillary is far removed from flow through blood vessels *in vivo*, and whole-blood viscosity has, as yet, little place in routine investigations [157, 167].

Blood volume

Measurement of haemoglobin, PCV and red-cell count provides information on the relative red-cell concentration in the blood but does not necessarily reflect the absolute red-cell volume, and it does not take into account fluctuations in the total volume of circulating blood or situations where there is a disproportionate increase or reduction in the plasma volume. There are a number of diseases in which this may occur and will result in an erroneous clinical assessment on the basis of the blood count (Table 1.5). The correlation between the peripheral-blood PCV and circulating red-cell volume is curvilinear with a single exponential function providing a good approximation (Fig. 1.34) [168]. However, individual observations are scattered fairly widely; it is thus apparent that in order to obtain a correct haematological picture it is often necessary to determine the blood volume. In practice this has its greatest use:

1 in polycythaemia, when the demonstration of an absolute increase in red-cell volume is necessary for diagnosis and for assessment of severity;
2 in the investigation of the effects of blood loss on the circulation in the management of surgical patients, especially when the prevention of post-operative cardiac failure and shock requires restoration of blood-volume equilibrium, and in the management of patients suffering from burns;
3 in the elucidation of obscure anaemias when the possibility of a pseudo-anaemia, because of an increase in plasma volume, must be considered.

The subject of blood volume and its measurement has a large literature and there have been several extensive reviews [169–171].

Red-cell volume (RCV) and plasma volume (PV) can be measured by dilution techniques. For RCV isotope-labelled red cells are used; a number of different isotopes have been tried, but ^{51}Cr in the form of sodium chromate and sodium pertechnate ($^{99}Tc^m$) obtained from a ^{99}Mo generator are the most widely used labels [172]. There are a few circumstances in which a second label is required; ^{51}Cr and $^{99}Tc^m$ can be used for this as the radioactivity due to each can be separated when they are present in combination [172]. Moreover, as $^{99}Tc^m$ has a half-life of six hours, it can be used at short intervals for consecutive studies. For plasma volume a number of dyes have been used, for example T1824 (Evans' Blue), but these have been superseded by the use of isotope-labelled albumin and other plasma proteins such as transferrin [173]. As a protein label ^{125}I is the most suitable [172]; plasma labelled with ^{125}I and red cells labelled with [99]Tc[m] or ^{51}Cr can be used in combination in order to measure plasma and red-cell volumes concurrently.

failure [175] or in shock [176]. In such cases sampling should be delayed for 60 minutes.

Plasma volume

This is calculated in a similar way, by comparing the radioactivity in 1 ml of the labelled protein with 1 ml of post-injection sample. By contrast to red-cell labels there is a continual loss of label from protein, so that early loss may occur before mixing in the plasma has

Table 1.5. Clinical effect of variable relationship between red-cell and plasma volumes

Red-cell volume	Plasma volume	Cause	Effect
Normal	High	Pregnancy (2nd–3rd trimesters) Cirrhosis Nephritis	Pseudo-anaemia
Normal	Low	Congestive cardiac failure Stress Essential hypertension Peripheral circulatory failure Dehydration Oedema High altitude (first 2 weeks) Prolonged bed rest	Pseudo-polycythaemia
Low	Normal	Anaemia	Accurate reflection of degree of anaemia
Low	High	Anaemia	Clinical anaemia less severe than indicated by blood count
Low	Low	Haemorrhage Severe anaemia (when PCV below 0·2)	Clinical anaemia more severe than indicated by blood count
High	Normal to low	Polycythaemia vera Secondary polycythaemia ('erythrocytosis')	Accurate reflection of clinical state or polycythaemia less severe than apparent
High	High	Polycythaemia (when PCV more than 0·5)	Polycythaemia more severe than apparent
Normal or even high	High	Marked splenomegaly	Pseudo-anaemia

Red-cell volume

Red-cell volume is calculated by comparing the radioactivity of 1 ml of the labelled red cells (as a standard) with the radioactivity of 1 ml of a post-injection sample of (packed) red cells. In practice, measurement is usually made on whole blood and the result is converted to activity per millilitre of red cells by multiplying by the PCV as measured by a standard procedure and corrected, if necessary, for trapped plasma (see p. 33). The post-injection sample is usually obtained after 10 or 20 minutes. This time is chosen to ensure equilibration throughout the vascular space. A delayed mixing time occurs in patients with gross splenomegaly [174] or when the patient is in cardiac

been completed. Assuming a constant rate of loss, a number of samples can be taken at intervals over the first 30 minutes after injection and by extrapolation a zero-time estimation can be deduced. However, this assumption is not necessarily valid, and some workers utilize a single sample collected at 10 minutes with the (equally questionable) assumption that there is little loss of the label at this time. Another problem concerns the fact that, unlike the red-cell volume, the plasma volume is difficult to define anatomically. It is labile and since it contains approximately 90% water, the large exchange of water across the capillary bed which normally takes place will influence the plasma volume continuously. Furthermore, there is a possibility that a

Chapter I

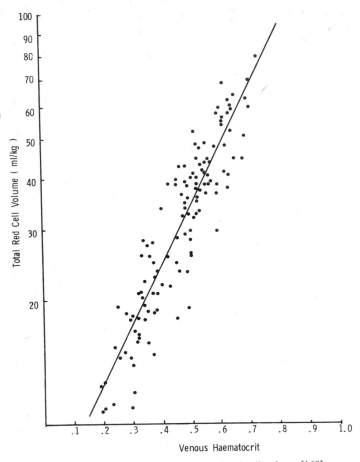

Fig. 1.34. Correlation between PCV and red-cell volume [168].

small fraction of the injected albumin exchanges with a small rapidly exchanging pool and as this occurs during the mixing period it cannot be corrected for. Clearly, then, plasma volume as measured is less reliable than red-cell volume.

Total blood volume (BV)
From the direct measurement of RCV and venous PCV it should in theory be possible to calculate the total blood volume. Unfortunately this is not the case as the whole-body PCV (H_B) is not identical with the venous PCV (H_V); this is mainly because of a lower haematocrit of blood in capillaries as compared with that in the larger vessels. In normal subjects the ratio H_B/H_V is approximately 0·9 [172] but the ratio does not apply in splenomegaly, when it is raised. It is lower than normal in cases of cirrhosis, nephritis and cardiac failure and it is increased in pregnancy [34]. Even in some normal subjects it varies [177], and it is especially increased in normal subjects at high altitudes [172].

Expression of results of blood-volume estimation
The blood volume of normal subjects varies considerably in relation to height and weight. Thus, for the clinical interpretation of blood-volume data only relatively large increases or decreases can be diagnosed with any certainty unless the subject's blood volume has been estimated on a previous occasion. Results can be expressed in ml/kg of total body weight, in ml/kg lean body weight, in relation to height and weight, or as a total volume together with the predicted volume for a normal subject of the same height, weight and age.

The commonest method for expressing blood-volume estimation is in terms of body weight. An objection is that the fat is relatively, but not entirely, avascular so that low values are obtained in obese subjects. To overcome this problem some workers relate blood volume to fat-free lean body weight as determined experimentally [179]. Alternatively, excess fat can be discounted by using an estimate of so-called 'idea! weight' as obtained by reference to standard tables based on height, age, build and sex, or from a calculation: weight (kg) = height (in cm) − 100. These methods are somewhat arbitrary and tend to over-correct for the avascularity of fat.

There have been several methods proposed for estimating normal blood volume on the basis of height–weight relationship or body surface area, but none gives a result with a 95% confidence better than ±10%, so that only fairly large deviations from normal values can be established. Moreover, by these methods an obese subject's observed total blood volume may be as much as one litre less than the predicted value, and in a muscular subject the observed total blood volume may be one litre greater than that predicted. However, in most cases formulae using surface area [180–182] appear to be fairly reliable [172].

Normal values

Based on weight alone, normal values with 95% confidence limits are as follows [34, 172]:

Red-cell volume, men	30 ± 5 ml/kg
women	25 ± 5 ml/kg
Plasma volume, men and women	45 ± 5 ml/kg
Total blood volume (BV)	70 ± 10 ml/kg

Obviously, the absolute volume varies enormously and no 'normal range' can be given. At birth, total blood volume is about 300 ml [183]. During the first year the value is said to fluctuate [184], but it is not clear whether this is a true observation or due to technical problems of measurement. After infancy, blood volume increases until puberty, when the volume increases more rapidly in males than in females (Fig. 1.35). In pregnancy both plasma and total blood volumes increase; the plasma volume increases especially in the first trimester, although the greatest increase of total volume occurs during the second half of pregnancy. By term, plasma volume may have increased by 40% and the total blood volume by 32% or more. Post partum the blood volume returns to normal within a week [185–187].

As a rule the blood volume remains remarkably constant and quick adjustments take place even after blood transfusion or intravenous administration of other fluids. Thus, the total blood volume usually returns to its pretransfusion level within 24 hours of the end of a transfusion. Bed rest is associated with a reduction in blood volume, due almost entirely to a contraction of the plasma volume [188].

Spleen red-cell mass

Estimation of the size of the red-cell pool in the spleen can be made from the difference in blood-volume measurements before and after splenectomy, from simultaneous RCV and PV estimation using ^{51}Cr and ^{125}I labels respectively [179], from blood-flow measurements following injection of isotope-labelled red cells [189], and by quantitative scanning of the spleen after administration of isotope-labelled red cells [190, 191]. The normal spleen has a red-cell mass of approximately 30–70 ml representing two to five per cent of the total red cells in circulation. Increased volumes occur consistently in polycythaemia vera [192], and in various myeloproliferative and lymphoproliferative disorders [193, 194].

LEUCOCYTES AND THE LEUCOCYTE COUNT

The total number of leucocytes in the circulating blood as measured by the white-blood-cell count (WBC) varies widely in health. The wide normal range is to a large extent real but in interpreting the WBC it must be recognized that the method on which most normal

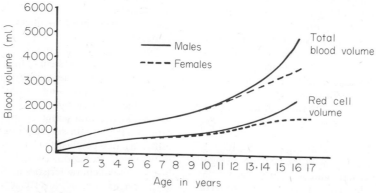

Fig. 1.35. Age and sex variations in total blood volume and red-cell volume. Only mean values are given, derived from various published data.

ranges have been based is haemocytometer counts, with which a variation of 12–20% is not unusual. But by electronic counter and the use of reference preparations it is possible to reduce the analytic coefficient of variation to 2·5% [98, 195, 196]; this means that there is an increasing awareness of possible clinical significance in relatively small fluctuations and deviation of the count from the normal (reference) values.

Normal range [34, 197]
The normal range for the leucocyte count (mean and 2 s.d.) is as follows:

Infant at birth	$15 \pm 5 \times 10^9/l$
Infant, 1 year	$12 \pm 6 \times 10^9/l$
Children, 4–7 years	$11 \pm 5 \times 10^9/l$
Children, 8–12 years	$9 \pm 4 \times 10^9/l$
Adults	$7 \pm 3 \times 10^9/l$

The range shown above includes 95% of healthy persons, but a count as low as $1·5 \times 10^9/l$ may occasionally be found in an apparently normal subject. Normal and abnormal overlap so that a value well within the normal range may be pathological in a particular subject, and vice versa. It is, thus, important to try to establish an individual's own baseline of normality in order to assess the signficance of a count.

Physiological variations
The effect of age is indicated above. There appear to be some sex differences with higher counts in women under the age of 50 years, while after this age the total leucocyte count becomes lower in women than in men [198–200]. There are, possibly, rhythmic variations related to the menstrual cycle although the extent of this is uncertain [201, 202]. Diurnal variations of up to 10–15% also occur, with the minimum counts in the morning with the subject at rest [196]. Light activity may raise the count slightly whilst strenuous exercise causes increases of up to $30 \times 10^9/l$. Other causes of a variable increase include emotional stress and the taking of food. It is essential to establish standardized conditions for blood collection to avoid these biological variations, but even so, minor infections and allergies also effect the leucocyte count so that it may be difficult to establish the 'normal' range in a group of people with certainty. There are racial differences due to variations in one or other of the cell types (see below).

A moderate leucocytosis of up to $15 \times 10^9/l$ is common during pregnancy, with the peak about eight weeks before parturition, and returning to normal levels a week or so after delivery [203]. Some forms of oral contraception have been reported to raise the WBC [198]. Cigarette smoking increases the count by up to 30% with a clear relationship between the amount of smoke inhaled and the leucocyte count [204, 205].

Differential leucocyte count
The differential leucocyte count is usually expressed in percentages of the various types of cells in a blood film. Relative counts do not, however, indicate whether there is a true increase or decrease of cell population, and data should be expressed in absolute figures per microlitre or litre of blood. The differential count depends to some extent on artificial differences in distribution due to the process of preparation. In a wedge smear, polymorphs tend to concentrate in the tail of the film, lymphocytes in the centre. Even in well-made films a variance of $\pm 10\%$ is to be expected [34] while it is a waste of time attempting to do a differential count on a badly made smear. An instrument is now available which produces uniform smears by a centrifugation procedure [206].

A second problem with the differential count is the random error in estimating the proportion of the various cell types: in a 100-cell count the 95% confidence limits are so wide that the result is only meaningful when there is gross elevation in the numbers of cells, and it is of little value for estimating cells seen in low proportions. Even 500-cell counts are of limited value for estimating the low-proportion cells with any degree of reliability. Automation is the only possible method for counting the large number of cells necessary to obtain an accurate differential leucocyte count. Recent developments in instruments have produced a variety of automated differential cell counters. One type is a pattern-recognition computer which identifies cells in a stained-blood film and classifies them in accordance with a program to which the computer has been trained. The early models have been limited in that they were unable to classify immature cells and their performance was slow, requiring at least a minute to find and classify 100 cells. There have, however, been significant advances in performance in later models.

Another approach is that of the Technicon Haemalog D, which uses a system of differential cytochemical staining with subsequent electronic counting of cells in suspension. An advantage of this system is the speed with which a large number of cells can be identified, thus making a differential count on 10^4 cells a simple procedure. Its main shortcoming is that a number of cells may not be classified by the cytochemical reactions which are used, and as leucocytes vary in their histochemical characteristics in disease, errors in classification may occur. Nevertheless, this instrument and other processes for differential cell counting are likely to become established as practical methods for routine use. There have been several recent reviews [198, 207–210].

Normal differential count

Most reports are based on the traditional procedure, but despite the limitations in accuracy mentioned above, physiological variations can be appreciated in the data of these various studies which have, in general, been based on 200-cell counts. The normal range is wide, and the count varies at different ages. In adults it is as follows:

Neutrophils	40–75%; 2500–7500 × 10^6/l
Lymphocytes	20–45%; 1500–3500 × 10^6/l
Monocytes	2–10%; 200–800 × 10^6/l
Eosinophils	1–6%; 40–440 × 10^6/l
Basophils	0–1%; 0–100 × 10^6/l

Average counts in infants and children based on various reported series [34, 211, 212] are shown in Figure 1.36.

Physiological and diurnal variations may be expected, as the variation of total leucocyte count referred to above will, as a rule, be due to an effect of one or other cell type selectively. An appreciation of the function of the different cells will indicate which cell is likely to be affected by a physiological or pathological process. The functions of the various types of leucocytes are described in Chapters 16 and 17. It is not clear whether there are any environmental influences, other than the secondary effects of endemic disease, or hereditary influences. In some areas of Africa, for example, there is a tendency for a reversal of neutrophil/lymphocyte ratios, with the total count at the lower levels of normal [213, 214]. Obviously, in areas where there are endemic, parasitic or protozoal diseases, reactive eosinophilia or monocytosis may be sufficiently common to be regarded as a 'normal' state (Chapter 33). However, a similar racial difference has been noted in the USA, with a lower neutrophil and higher lymphocyte mean count in black Americans by comparison with Caucasians [258]. A sex difference has been reported with a cyclical variation in women with a consistent fall in the neutrophil count at menstruation. The monocyte shows a similar variation. After the menopause the total leucocyte count and the neutrophil count are lower than in men of a similar age [198–200, 259].

In pregnancy, the neutrophil count rises in parallel with total leucocyte count, with a peak at about eight weeks before parturition, whereas the lymphocyte count remains fairly steady throughout pregnancy, apart from a slightly lower mean count in the first trimester [203].

There is a diurnal variation in all cell types [196]. The eosinophils are said to be especially subject to diurnal variation, with differences as much as 100% between the lowest counts, which occur in the day, and the highest counts which occur at night [34]. The height of the eosinophil count is controlled, at least to some extent, by the adrenal cortex; the diurnal fluctuations parallel diurnal glucocorticoid fluctuation.

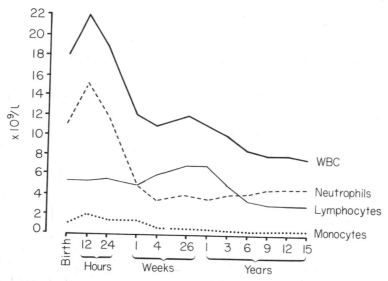

Fig. 1.36. Variations in total leucocyte count and differential count in infants and children; based on data from various sources [34, 211, 212].

PLATELET COUNT

Methods

There are many methods for platelet counts in use [216], and their number is doubtless due to the difficulty of counting small bodies which aggregate and break up easily and which may be difficult to distinguish from extraneous debris. The methods in common use today include visual methods especially with phase contrast microscopy [34, 217] and electronic counting methods [34, 218, 219]. For counting platelets by electronic methods it is important to use particle-free filtered diluents and careful selection of appropriate calibration settings to ensure that only the platelet-sized particles are counted. It is necessary in some electronic methods to separate the platelets from other blood corpuscles. Several methods have been described; that of Bull *et al.* [218, 220], in which separation is carried out in small-bore plastic tubing, is used extensively. An alternate method of augmented sedimentation with Boyum's methyl cellulose-Isopaque mixture at sp.gr. 1·08 has been reported to give consistently satisfactory results [217].

Normal values

The normal value of platelets varies with the method used. In the literature it has been given as $150–600 \times 10^9/l$ or even more [221]. With standardized methods [34] the normal range in health is approximately $150–400 \times 10^9/l$. There is a sex difference; in women the count is higher by about $40–70 \times 10^9/l$ [222]; a fall in platelets is said to occur about the time of menstruation, with highest levels at mid-cycle and there is some evidence of a cycle with a 21–35-day rhythm [223]. There is no evidence that oral contraceptives affect the platelet count. In individual subjects the count is relatively constant [221], without any obvious diurnal variation in men, although there is a suggestion of slight diurnal variation in women, with a lower level in the morning than in the evening [222]. Within the wide normal range there are no obvious age differences; however, at birth and in infancy the platelet count tends to be at the lower levels.

A reduced platelet count, of less than $100 \times 10^9/l$, is invariably an indication of a definite abnormality affecting haemopoiesis or platelet survival. Increased platelet counts may occur in myeloproliferative disorders, especially the condition referred to as essential thrombocythaemia (see Chapter 32) and it may also occur transiently after haemorrhage, trauma, surgical operations, infections and in malignant diseases. Following splenectomy the platelet count rises sharply, often within a matter of hours, reaching a peak in one to two weeks, and then returns to normal values over a period of weeks or months. In some cases, especially in patients with anaemia, e.g. in haemolysis which has failed to respond to splenectomy, the platelet count may remain high indefinitely [224]. In thrombocythaemia the platelet count is greater than $1000 \times 10^9/l$, sometimes $2000–3000 \times 10^9/l$; in the other conditions in which the platelet count is increased, it is usually of the order of $500–800 \times 10^9/l$.

Methods are now available for measuring the relative volume of platelets per unit volume of blood as a plateletcrit, and also the platelet size distribution [225, 226]. As they age, platelets become smaller, and have lower functional capability. There is evidence that platelet function in circulation correlates with their total volume rather than with their numbers [227], and that measurement of their volume may provide a sensitive index of the platelet abnormality which leads to bleeding manifestations [227, 228, 255, 256].

EVALUATION OF THE BLOOD COUNT

What is meant by the 'blood count', and the approach to its interpretation, depends on the facilities available for carrying out the analysis, and the workload within the laboratory. There are, today, three levels of activity depending on the availability of:
1 only manual–visual techniques;
2 electronic cell counter; and
3 full automation.

When an electronic cell counter is not available, counting of leucocytes (WBC) and red cells (RBC) is laborious. The 'routine blood count' in such circumstances consists, at least, of haemoglobin and/or PCV, WBC and examination of a blood film. As far as possible, both haemoglobin and PCV should be measured, partly to provide a check one against the other and also to allow deduction of MCHC. The most important part of the examination is inspection of the blood film. The diagnosis of a blood disease may often be made from the film, as it is the appreciation of the various forms of abnormality and combinations of abnormalities in the morphology of blood cells which leads to the correct diagnosis. To exclude a leucocyte abnormality, a total white count is essential, as inspection of the film can give only a very crude, and often misleading, estimate of a quantitative normality, or otherwise, of the leucocytes. On the other hand, a rapid survey of a well-made film will indicate to the trained observer the pattern of the differential distribution of leucocytes without need for an actual differential count, and will enable him to identify abnormalities of cells, or to recognize cells which are not usual inhabitants of the peripheral blood.

As far as platelets are concerned, here too a

quantitative count is necessary to exclude an abnormality as a report that the platelets are present in normal numbers on a film is crude and may be inaccurate and misleading. Because platelet counting by a visual method is time-consuming it should not be undertaken unless there is clinical evidence of a haemorrhagic disorder or other reason to suspect that the count might be abnormal. Hence, the platelets are not included in the 'routine blood count'.

The red-cell count alone rarely gives information of decisive importance. The errors of the estimation by visual methods are unavoidably large and thus the absolute values of MCH and MCV derived therefrom cannot be relied upon to pick out the minor abnormalities of mild iron deficiency or megaloblastic anaemias. When hypochromasia or macrocytosis becomes sufficiently marked to be defined beyond doubt by quantitative measurement it is, as a rule, readily identified in the blood film. The reticulocyte count is more useful than the red-cell count in providing information about the state of erythropoiesis [102, 103], although the total red-cell count is useful in converting the percentage of reticulocytes into an absolute count.

The advent of the electronic cell counter has changed the pattern of the blood count, in that a red-cell count can now be carried out easily and with a much greater accuracy than hitherto. Thus, absolute values can attain an importance in diagnosis. In mild megaloblastic anaemias the haemoglobin and PCV may be normal or only just subnormal and the degree of macrocytosis slight. This may be missed on inspection of the stained film but might be picked up if the MCV is estimated accurately.

A revolutionary advance in the laboratory has been the automated counting system [99, 123, 229]. While the electronic counter made significant impact in terms of increased precision, accuracy and workload capacity, the level of automatic action was limited as long as human intervention was required for sample preparation, recording of results and computing of interrelated indices. There are now several instruments available for carrying out blood counts including platelet counts by automation and there have been an increasing number of reviews and evaluation reports (e.g. Refs 98, 123, 132, 225, 230, 231).

Further refinements include data-processing computer programs linked to the counting systems to enable data to be transmitted rapidly to the clinician and also to be retained on record for future extraction and for subsequent review and analysis. Another function of the computer is to provide a facility for the statistical aspects of the laboratory's quality control programme, with continuous monitoring so that there can be early warning that the laboratory and/or instrument performance has gone out of control (see p.

47). The use of computers for these purposes in haematology has been the subject of much thought, and extensive feasibility studies in several institutions. The need for correct programming and the selection of an appropriate computer for the specific requirements of the haematologist are important considerations [232–237].

In an automated laboratory, a factor to be considered is the inclusion of a blood film as part of the blood count. Clearly, when an entire blood count can be carried out in 30 seconds, supervised by a single technician, the limiting factor is the need to make, stain and examine a blood film. However, there can be no question that inspection of a blood film, followed if necessary by bone-marrow examination, remains the basis of diagnostic haematology; thus a blood count should include a film, and it is in the analysis of the film that the practice of laboratory haematology at a routine level retains its need for human expertise and experience, notwithstanding the advances in instrument technology. Indeed, the value of automation is the fact that it relieves the skilled workers from tedious, time-consuming chores, and thus provides better opportunity for attending to those tasks such as film examination which do require their skill.

EXAMINATION OF THE BLOOD FILM

In attempting to arrive at a diagnosis from inspection of a blood film the presence or absence of abnormalities affecting red cells, leucocytes and platelets must all be taken into account. The film must be well spread and stained and it must be looked at methodically. In later chapters the morphological features of various diseases will be described. In this section only brief mention will be made of the abnormalities which should be looked for.

Red cells

Anisocytosis. Variation in size: a small degree of anisocytosis is present normally; this is a reflection of the variable age of the red cells in circulation, as the youngest cells are larger than older ones and the peripheral-blood film will normally include occasional reticulocytes which are the largest non-nucleated red cells. In almost any blood disorder there is an increased amount of anisocytosis as a non-specific feature.

Macrocytosis. Cells that are larger than normal: found in megaloblastic anaemia due to vitamin-B_{12} or folate deficiency; also in aplastic anaemia and dysplastic anaemia and in liver disease. If due to an increased proportion of reticulocytes (as in haemolytic anaemias) their distinctive colour (see below) should distinguish them.

Microcytosis. Cells that are smaller than normal: they occur in iron deficiency, thalassaemia and other defects of iron metabolism as hypochromic cells. In haemolytic anaemias, orthochromic or hyperchromic microcytes are found.

Poikilocytosis. Variation in cell shape: occurs in any dyserythropoiesis including dysplastic anaemias and megaloblastic anaemias and also as the result of damage to circulating red cells in drug-induced haemolysis, microangiopathic haemolytic anaemias, etc. It is a prominent feature in myelofibrosis.

Hypochromasia. Palely staining cells: these result from haemoglobin deficiency; iron deficiency is the most common cause but haemoglobin and iron utilization disorders, for example thalassaemia or sideroblastic anaemia, also produce pale erythrocytes.

Polychromasia. Some cells staining a different colour: caused by the presence of reticulocytes which are usually bluish-grey by the time they appear in circulation, even in states of intense erythropoiesis. Deep blue polychromasia is found when there is gross disturbance in erythropoiesis, especially when there is extramedullary haemopoiesis.

Leptocytes and target cells. Unusually thin cells, with unstained centres or a centrally stained area which gives it the name of target cell: indicative of a haemoglobin defect (i.e. failure to form haemoglobin or a haemoglobinopathy) and occurs especially in Hbs C, S and E, thalassaemia and iron deficiency. It is also seen in liver disease or in the absence of a functioning spleen.

Sickle cells. Occur in varying proportions in homozygous sickle-cell disease and in sickle-cell combination with other abnormal haemoglobins. They are increased in blood from such conditions if subjected to anoxia before the film is made.

Spherocytes. Spheroidal cells: they occur in many types of haemolytic anaemia including hereditary spherocytosis, immune haemolytic anaemia, Hb C disease and in burns. Spherical forms may occur as an artefact of crenation, even in normal blood, especially when stored.

Elliptocytes. Normally 10–15% of the red cells are elliptical. A greater number, 90% or more, occur in hereditary elliptocytosis. However, elliptocytes (really poikilocytes) are also found in myelosclerosis, megaloblastic anaemias, iron deficiency and thalassaemia.

Stomatocytosis. A slit instead of central concavity in the red cell: occurs in a rare form of congenital haemolytic anaemia and rarely as an acquired defect in liver disease and in lead poisoning.

Irregularly contracted cells. Triangular-shaped cell fragments (schistocytes), helmet-shaped cells and spiculated cells with conspicuous spines (burr cells) are characteristic of microangiopathic haemolytic anaemias and haemolytic uraemic syndrome. Other forms occur in drug- or chemical-induced haemolytic anaemias. In newborn infants a small number, referred to as pyknocytes, are seen. Schistocytes are also found in various congenital haemolytic anaemias, severe megaloblastic anaemias, in thalassaemia, in association with burns, and in mechanical haemolytic anaemia.

Acanthocytes. Crenated cells with surface projections: an inherited defect associated with abnormal phospholipid metabolism. Similar cells, occurring in cirrhosis and in anorexia nervosa, are called 'spur' cells.

Other abnormalities to be noted in the red cells include the presence of inclusions (Howell–Jolly bodies, punctate basophilia, Pappenheimer bodies, Cabot's rings), normoblasts, rouleaux and agglutination. These various phenomena are extensively illustrated by Dacie & Lewis [34].

Leucocytes

The main points to look for in relation to leucocytes are their numbers—leucocytosis or leucopenia—the differential count and the presence of immature or abnormal forms. These are described in Chapters 15–18.

Platelets

Although it is not possible to assess platelet numbers with any degree of confidence from a film, one can, nevertheless, get a rough assessment of markedly decreased or increased numbers of platelets in a well-made film. Morphological appearances to be noted are abnormal variation in size which is often a conspicuous feature in thrombocythaemia, myelosclerosis and megakaryocytic myelosis (see Chapter 32). In these conditions megakaryocytic nuclei or fragments thereof may be seen in the peripheral-blood film. In thrombocytopenic purpura the quantitative increase is usually obvious; the platelets which are seen are frequently larger than normal.

Platelet satellism is a phenomenon in which platelets adhere to neutrophils [238, 239]. It occurs *in vitro* with EDTA blood and is usually considered to have no clinical significance, but it has also been reported in association with platelet antibodies in lymphoma [240] and in thrombocytopenia [241]. It may give rise to spurious platelet counts with an electronic counter.

STANDARDIZATION AND QUALITY ASSURANCE

Standardization and quality assurance are interrelated processes which ensure good laboratory practice. The aim is to recognize errors and to minimize them, so that laboratory tests will be reliable, their results valid, and comparable with results obtained for the same tests in other laboratories. Reliability of a test is defined by its accuracy and precision.

Accuracy is a measure of the closeness of an estimated value to the true values, whereas *precision* is the closeness with which repeat measurements on one sample agree with each other, irrespective of the true value. Precision can be checked by repeated tests on selected routine specimens. Accuracy can be checked only by use of reference materials with known contents.

Reference material is sometimes known as a 'standard'. There are international reference preparations which have been developed by international agencies such as the World Health Organization (WHO), and national reference preparations are also produced in many countries. The WHO international reference preparations relevant to haematology include haemoglobincyanide, erythropoietin, blood-typing antisera, immunoglobulins, blood coagulation factors (VIII and IX), urokinase, thrombin and human thromboplastin [242]. Their clinical and physical characteristics are defined and the concentration or units of activity ('assigned value') is obtained from measurements performed by a number of expert laboratories using a reference technique.

A calibrator is a material based on a reference preparation; by comparing results obtained with the calibrator and the reference preparation in an appropriate test, a value is assigned to the calibrator so that it can then be used to calibrate an instrument, graduate an item of equipment or adjust a measurement [243]. Calibrators would be of particular value with blood-counting systems, but unfortunately materials are not yet available which are entirely satisfactory, except for measurement of haemoglobin [244, 245]. A calibrator can consist of an artificial substance or natural blood with some form of preservative or stabilizer.

A control is a material which is used for checking precision of a method in routine practice. It is not intended to check accuracy, and its actual value is irrelevant, although its concentration must be within a practical range. It must be stable during the period of use, and it should behave like natural blood in the test system.

Internal quality control
The procedure which should be included in a comprehensive system will vary with the test undertaken, the instruments used, the extent of automation. Apart from carrying out tests on patients' specimens in duplicate and regular checks of precision and instrument calibration as described above, there are three procedures to be considered.

Use of control material
The mean value and standard deviation of a control material is established by 20 replicate measurements. Thereafter the material is tested daily or several times per day if appropriate. Results should fluctuate around the mean, remaining within 2 s.d. of the mean. Values outside 2 s.d. will indicate performance error; if several values occur consecutively on one side of the mean, even if within 2 s.d., this indicates a deterioration in performance. Plotting the results on a graph provides a visual display which makes it easy to detect loss of control. The test can be made more sensitive for detecting the day-to-day variation by applying the Cusum procedure [246]; this is a statistical manoeuvre in which the running total of the differences between each measurement and the mean is recorded, taking the plus and minus signs into account. As random changes tend to cancel each other out, in a stable situation the Cusum oscillates around zero; a small but consistent trend of error will become progressively magnified.

Statistical quality control
This is based on the principle that for certain tests the normal range remains constant. Thus, for example, MCV, MCH and MCHC should not vary significantly in healthy individuals; also, there is a constancy of distribution of their value in a patient population in any medium- to large-sized hospital, handling a sufficiently large number of tests. Thus, once the means for these tests have been established in a clinical laboratory an altered figure on any occasion will point to error.

Plotting graphs of the behaviour of all the indices in combination will show characteristic patterns which can be used not only to determine that a defect has occurred but also to identify the cause of error and even to pinpoint the precise location of the machine malfunction [247, 248]. By appropriate computer facilities interphased with the counting system this monitoring can be carried out continuously in order to provide early warning that the laboratory and/or instrument performance has gone out of control [232, 233, 247].

Correlation assessment

An essential component of haematological practice is to ensure that the laboratory test makes sense in terms of clinical correlation. By the use of a cumulative report form it is possible to see at a glance if there has been any change in a patient's blood values. The trend of the blood count is even better appreciated when the data are plotted on time-related logarithmic charts [34]. In patients receiving cytotoxic therapy, for example, it is possible to predict the expected blood-count changes from the linear trend; any plot showing gross divergence from the result expected should arouse suspicion of a laboratory error, requiring checking. Finally, correlation of the blood film with the blood-count measurement provides control of these two tests reciprocally.

External quality assessment

In interlaboratory trials, control samples are received periodically from an outside source in order to compare accuracy levels of different laboratories. It complements internal quality control, and is especially necessary for preventing the situation in which an individual laboratory might have an excellent precision but still be inaccurate. Interlaboratory trials also provide a means for assessing the 'state of the art' at a national (or regional) level by identifying inferior methods, poor reagents and faulty instruments. National schemes have already been established in a number of countries [249–251].

Reference values

Interpretation of an isolated value of a laboratory test is not possible without comparing it with a reference value and the reference distribution. The concept of a range to include all apparently normal subjects and the use of an arithmetical mean is of limited value, as this fails to take account of physiological variations, environmental effects and variations due to different diets. Establishing reference values in a population requires a well-defined protocol to take account of (a) age, sex, race and genetic factors of the reference population, (b) physiological conditions and environmental states—time of day, season, altitude, contraceptives, stage of menstrual cycle, how soon

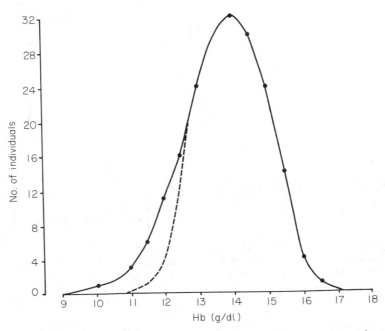

Fig. 1.37. Reference values: A frequency curve has been drawn for haemoglobin measurement in an apparently normal population of women in a community at sea level (solid line). The interrupted line represents a normalized Gaussian distribution after excluding outliers. Derived from this, the reference value (mean) is 14·0 g/dl, s.d. 1·1 g/dl. Thus 95% (2 s.d.) limits are 11·8–16·2 g/dl and 99% (3 s.d.) limits 10·7–17·3 g/dl. The skewness of the original distribution curve indicates that this community was not entirely 'healthy'.

after a meal, alcohol, smoking, etc., and (c) analytic conditions—venous or capillary blood, anticoagulant and treatment of the specimen [252, 253].

In the process of obtaining the reference data it is, of course, necessary to exclude subjects suffering from pathological conditions; it is, however, not always easy to be certain that the subjects in *apparently* good health are really normal. The bias of selection can, to an extent, be discounted by applying statistical principles and using a small random sample to represent the parent population, provided that the population is at least free from overt ill health [72, 75, 254]. By plotting a frequency curve, taking the modal value as the point of reference, and superimposing a Gaussian curve on the mode, a normal range can be defined without being influenced by outlying data which should not belong to a truly normal population (Fig. 1.37). From the Gaussian curve a mean can be estimated with reasonable accuracy even when there is a skew distribution curve. The mean ± 2 s.d. gives the reference value and the reference limits between which 95% of normal subjects should belong.

REFERENCES

1 MAXIMOW A.A. (1924) Relation of blood cells to connective tissue and endothelium. *Physiological Reviews*, **4**, 533.

2 BLOOM W. & BARTELMEZ G.W. (1940) Hematopoiesis in young human embryos. *American Journal of Anatomy*, **67**, 21.

3 KNOLL W. & PINGEL E. (1949) Der Gang der Erythropoiese beim menschlichen Embryo. *Acta Haematologica*, **2**, 369.

4 DOAN C.A. (1932) Current views on the origin and maturation of cells of the blood. *Journal of Laboratory and Clinical Medicine*, **17**, 887.

5 SABIN F.R., MILLER F.R., SMITHBURN K.C., THOMAS R.M. & HUMMEL I.E. (1936) Changes in the bone marrow and blood cells of developing rabbits. *Journal of Experimental Medicine*, **64**, 97.

6 METCALF D. (1978) The control of neutrophil and macrophage production at the progenitor cell level. In: *Experimental Hematology Today* (ed. Baum S.J. & Ledney G.D.), p. 35. Springer-Verlag, New York.

7 METCALF D. (1979) Detection and analysis of human granulocyte-monocyte precursors using semi-solid cultures. *Clinics in Haematology*, **8**, 263.

8 SCHOFIELD R. (1978) The relationship between the spleen colony-forming cells and the haemopoietic stem cell. *Blood Cells*, **4**, 7.

9 HASHIMOTO M. (1960) The distribution of active marrow in the bones of a normal adult. *Kyushu Journal of Medical Science*, **11**, 103.

10 TAVASSOLI M. & CROSBY W.H. (1970) Bone marrow histogenesis: a comparison of fatty and red marrow. *Science*, **169**, 291.

11 MANIATIS A., TAVASSOLI M. & CROSBY W.H. (1971) Factors affecting the conversion of yellow to red marrow. *Blood*, **37**, 581.

12 ANGER H.O. & VAN DYKE D. (1964) Human bone marrow distribution shown *in vivo* by iron-52 and the positron scintillation camera. *Science*, **144**, 1587.

13 FORD C.E. (1966) Traffic of lymphoid cells in the body. In: *The Thymus: Experimental and Clinical Studies, Ciba Foundation Symposium* (ed. Wolstenholme G.E.W. & Porter R.), p. 131. Churchill, London.

14 MICKLEM H.S., FORD C.E., EVANS E.P. & GRAY J. (1966) Interrelationships of myeloid and lymphoid cells: studies with chromosome-marked cells transfused into lethally irradiated mice. *Proceedings of the Royal Society, Series B*, **165**, 78.

15 McGREGOR D.D. (1968) Bone marrow origin of immunologically competent lymphocytes in the rat. *Journal of Experimental Medicine*, **127**, 78.

16 AUERBACH R. (1964) In: *The Thymus in Immunobiology* (ed. Good R.A. & Gabrielsen A.E.), p. 95. Hoeber, New York.

17 BLOOM W. & FAWCETT D.W. (1962) *A Textbook of Histology*, W.B. Saunders Co., Philadelphia and London.

18 MAEDA K., HYUN B.H. & REBUCK J.W. (1977) Lymphoid follicles in bone marrow aspirates. *American Journal of Clinical Pathology*, **67**, 41.

19 KENT G., MINICK O.T., VOLINI F.I. & ORFEI E. (1966) Autophagic vacuoles in human red cells. *American Journal of Pathology*, **48**, 831.

20 LEWIS S.M. & STUART P.R. (1970) Ultrastructure of the red blood cell. *Proceedings of the Royal Society of Medicine*, **63**, 465.

21 DAVSON H. & DANIELLI J.F. (1952) *The Permeability of Natural Membranes*, 2nd edn. Cambridge University Press, Cambridge.

22 SINGER S.J. (1974) The molecular organisation of membranes. *Annual Review of Biochemistry*, **43**, 805.

23 TILNEY L.G. & DETMERS P. (1975) Actin in erythrocyte ghosts and its association with spectrin. *Journal of Cell Biology*, **66**, 508.

24 MARCHESI V.T. & STEERS E. (1968) Selective solubilization of a protein component of the red cell membrane. *Science*, **159**, 203.

25 HUHN D. & STICH W. (1969) *Fine Structure of Blood and Bone Marrow*, p. 33. Lehmanns Verlag, Munich.

26 BESSIS M. (1973) *Living Blood Cells and their Ultrastructure*, p. 298. Springer-Verlag, Berlin.

27 TANAKA Y. & GOODMAN J.R. (1972) *Electron Microscopy of Human Blood Cells*, p. 89. Harper & Row, New York.

28 POLLIACK A. (1977) *Normal Transformed and Leukaemic Leukocytes*. Springer-Verlag, Berlin.

29 LEVINE R.F. (1980) Isolation and characterization of normal human megakaryocytes. *British Journal of Haematology*, **45**, 487.

30 TURPIE A.G.G., McNICHOL G.P. & DOUGLAS A.S. (1971) Platelets: haemostasis and thrombosis. In: *Recent Advances in Haematology* (ed. Goldberg A. & Brain M.C.), p. 249. Churchill Livingstone, Edinburgh and London.

31 UNDRITZ E. (1973) *Atlas of Haematology*, 2nd edn. Sandoz Ltd., Basel.

32 McDONALD G.A., DODDS T.C. & CRUICKSHANK B.

(1978) *Atlas of Haematology*, 4th edn. Churchill Livingstone, Edinburgh.

33 FLANDRIN G. & DANIEL M-T. (1981) Cytochemistry in the classification of leukaemias. In: *Methods in Haematology, Vol. 1: the Leukaemic Cell* (ed. Catovsky D.), p. 29. Churchill Livingstone, Edinburgh.

34 DACIE J.V. & LEWIS S.M. (1975) *Practical Haematology*, 5th edn., p. 120. Churchill Livingstone, Edinburgh.

35 TRUBOWITZ S. & MASEK B. (1970) The structural organization of the human marrow matrix in thin sections. *American Journal of Pathology*, **53**, 908.

36 WEISS L. (1965) The structure of bone marrow. Functional interrelationships of vascular and hematopoietic compartments in experimental hemolytic anemia. An electron microscope study. *Journal of Morphology*, **117**, 467.

37 MOHANDAS N. & PRENANT M. (1978) Three dimensional model of bone marrow. *Blood*, **51**, 633.

38 McCUSKEY R.S., McCLUGAGE S.G. & YOUNKER W.J. (1971) Microscopy of living bone marrow in situ. *Blood*, **38**, 87.

39 DE BRUYN P.P.H., BREEN P.C. & THOMAS T.B. (1970) The microcirculation of the bone marrow. *Anatomical Record*, **168**, 55.

40 BRÅNEMARK P.I. (1959) Vital microscopy of bone marrow in rabbits. *Scandinavian Journal of Clinical and Laboratory Investigation*, **11** (Suppl. 38), 1.

41 KINOSITA R., OHNO S. & BIERMAN H.R. (1961) Studies on bone marrow dynamics: observations on microcirculation in rabbit bone marrow in situ. *Bibliotheca Anatoma*, **1**, 106.

42 McCLUGAGE S.G., McCUSKEY R.S. & MEINEKE H.A. (1971) Microscopy of living bone marrow *in situ*. II. Influence of microenvironment on hemopoiesis. *Blood*, **38**, 96.

43 AMSEL A., MANIATIS A. & CROSBY W.H. (1969) The significance of intramedullary cancellous bone formation in the repair of bone marrow tissue. *Anatomical Record*, **164**, 101.

44 McCUSKEY R.S. & MEINEKE H.A. (1977) Erythropoietin and the hemopoietic microenvironment. In: *Kidney Hormones, Vol. II, Erythropoietin* (ed. Fisher J.W.), p. 311. Academic Press, London and New York.

45 STOHLMAN F. & BRECHER G. (1957) Humoral regulation of erythropoiesis. III. Effect of exposure to simulated altitude. *Journal of Laboratory and Clinical Medicine*, **49**, 890.

46 MARTON P.F. (1970) Erythrophagocytosis in the human bone marrow. *Scandinavian Journal of Haematology*, **7**, 177.

47 TAVASSOLI M. (1979) The marrow–blood barrier. *British Journal of Haematology*, **41**, 297.

48 TAVASSOLI M. & SHAKLAI M. (1979) Absence of tight junctions in endothelium of marrow sinuses: possible significance for marrow cell egress. *British Journal of Haematology*, **41**, 303.

49 TAVASSOLI M. & CROSBY W.H. (1973) Fate of the nucleus of marrow erythroblast. *Science*, **173**, 912.

50 TÜRKEL H. & BETHELL F.H. (1953) Biopsy of bone marrow performed by a new and simple instrument. *Journal of Laboratory and Clinical Medicine*, **28**, 1246.

51 CONRAD M.E. & CROSBY W.H. (1961) Bone marrow biopsy: modification of the Vim–Silverman needle. *Journal of Laboratory and Clinical Medicine*, **57**, 642.

52 MILLER G.C. & DENNIS D.T. (1968) Bone and marrow biopsy with saw-toothed modification of Vim–Silverman needle. *Lancet*, **ii**, 1278.

53 JAMSHIDI K. & SWAIM W.R. (1971) Bone marrow biopsy with unaltered architecture. *Journal of Laboratory and Clinical Medicine*, **77**, 335.

54 INWOOD M.J. (1975) Jamshidi bone marrow needle modification. *Journal of Laboratory and Clinical Medicine*, **86**, 535.

55 SACKER L.S. & NORDIN B.E.C. (1963) A simple bone-biopsy needle. *Lancet*, **i**, 347.

56 WILLIAMS J.A. & NICHOLSON G.I. (1963) A modified bone-biopsy drill for outpatient use. *Lancet*, **i**, 1408.

57 HARTSOCK R.J., SMITH, E.B. & PETTY C.S. (1965) Normal variation with aging of the amount of haemopoietic tissue in bone marrow from the anterior iliac crest. *American Journal of Clinical Pathology*, **42**, 436.

58 LOWENSTEIN L. & BRAMLAGE C.A. (1957) The bone marrow in pregnancy and the puerperium. *Blood*, **12**, 261.

59 BURSTON J. & PINNIGER J.L. (1963) The reticulin content of bone marrow in haematological disorders. *British Journal of Haematology*, **9**, 1972.

60 SANERKIN N.G. (1964) Stromal changes in leukaemia and related bone marrow proliferations. *Journal of Clinical Pathology*, **17**, 541.

61 ROBERTS B.E., MILES D.W. & WOODS C.G. (1969) Polycythaemia vera and myelosclerosis: a bone marrow study. *British Journal of Haematology*, **16**, 75.

62 RATH C.E. & FINCH C.A. (1948) Sternal marrow hemosiderin: a method for the determination of available iron stores in man. *Journal of Clinical Medicine*, **33**, 81.

63 HANSEN H.A. & WEINFIELD A. (1959) Haemosiderin estimations and sideroblast counts in the differential diagnosis of iron deficiency and other anaemias. *Acta Medica Scandinavica*, **165**, 333.

64 GLASER K., LIMARZI L.R. & PONCHER H.G. (1950) Cellular composition of the bone marrow in normal infants and children. *Pediatrics*, **6**, 789.

65 STEINER M.L. & PEARSON H.A. (1966) Bone marrow plasmacyte values in childhood. *Journal of Pediatrics*, **68**, 562.

66 O'SULLIVAN M.B. (1979) Laboratory Hematology Procedures. *CRC Handbook Series in Clinical Laboratory Science*, **1**, 5.

67 SMITH, J.S. & WHITELAW D.M. (1971) Hemoglobin values in aged men. *Canadian Medical Association Journal*, **105**, 816.

68 CRUICKSHANK J.M. (1970) Some variations in the normal haemoglobin concentration. *British Journal of Haematology*, **18**, 523.

69 ELWOOD P.C., SHINTON N.K., WILSON C.I.D., SWEETNAM P. & FRAZER A.C. (1971) Haemoglobin, vitamin B_{12} and folate levels in the elderly. *British Journal of Haematology*, **21**, 557.

70 INTERNATIONAL COMMITTEE FOR STANDARDIZATION IN HAEMATOLOGY (1978) Recommendations for reference method for haemoglobinometry in human blood (ICSH Standard EP 6/2: 1977) and specifications for international haemiglobincyanide reference preparation

(ICSH Standard EP 6/3:1977). *Journal of Clinical Pathology*, **31**, 139.

71 VAN ASSENDELFT O.W., HOLTZ A.H. & LEWIS S.M. (1971) Determination of the hemoglobin content of blood. *World Health Organization Document*, WHO/BS/71.1026.

72 LEWIS S.M. (1970) Problems of establishing the normal haemoglobin values in a community. In: *Standardization in Hematology* (ed. Astaldi G., Sirtori C. & Vanzetti G.). Franco Angeli Editore, Milan.

73 LAYRISSE M. (1970) Normal haemoglobin values versus observed values: selecting the population sample. In: *Standardization in Hematology* (ed. Astaldi G., Sirtori C. & Vanzetti G.), p. 101. Franco Angeli Editore, Milan.

74 LEWIS S.M. (1970) Problems of establishing the normal haemoglobin values in a community. In: *Standardization in Hematology* (ed. Astaldi G., Sirtori C. & Vanzetti G.), p. 92. Franco Angeli Editore, Milan.

75 VITERI F.E., DE TUNA V. & GUZMÁN M.A. (1972) Normal haematological values in the Central American population. *British Journal of Haematology*, **23**, 189.

76 VITERI F.E. & GUZMÁN M.A. (1972) Haematology status of the Central American population: prevalence of individuals with haemoglobin levels below 'normal'. *British Journal of Haematology*, **23**, 725.

77 FIELDING J., KARABUS C. & BRUNSTRÖM G.M. (1968) Storage iron depletion in male blood donors: its significance for iron status in women. *Journal of Clinical Pathology*, **21**, 402.

78 HALBERG L., HÖGDAHL A.M., NILSSON L. & RYBO G. (1961) Menstrual blood loss and iron deficiency. *Acta Medica Scandinavica*, **180**, 369.

79 BURTON J.L. (1967) Effect of oral contraceptives on haemoglobin, packed cell volume, serum iron and total iron-binding capacity in healthy women. *Lancet*, **i**, 978.

80 ELWOOD P.C. (1962) Diurnal haemoglobin variation in normal male subjects. *Clinical Science*, **23**, 379.

81 MOLLISON P.L. (1979) *Blood Transfusion in Clinical Medicine*, 6th edn., p. 128. Blackwell Scientific Publications, Oxford.

82 EKELUND L.-G, EKLUND B. & KAIJSER L. (1971) Time course for the change in hemoglobin concentration with change in posture. *Acta Medica Scandinavica*, **190**, 335.

83 EISENBERG S. (1963) The effect of posture and position of the venous sampling site on the hematocrit and serum protein concentration. *Journal of Laboratory Medicine*, **61**, 755.

84 CHATTERJEE G. & MAASER R. (1971) Ein vergleich von Hämoglobin — und Hämatocrit — Bestimmugen im Blut aus dem Ohrlappchen und aus der Fingerbeere von Kindern. *Deutsche Medizinische Wochenschrift*, **96**, 789.

85 BROTHERHOOD J., BROZOVIC B. & PUGH L.G.C. (1975) Haematological status of middle and long distance runners. *Clinical Science and Molecular Medicine*, **48**, 139.

86 STENGLE J.M. & SCHADE A.L. (1957) Diurnal nocturnal variations of certain blood constituents in normal human subjects: plasma iron, siderophilin, bilirubin, copper, total serum protein and albumin, haemoglobin and haematocrit. *British Journal of Haematology*, **3**, 117.

87 NATVIG H., BJERKEDAL T. & JONASSEN Ø. (1963) Studies on hemoglobin values in Norway. III. Seasonal variations. *Acta Medica Scandinavica*, **174**, 351.

88 SAUNDERS C. (1965) Some erythrocyte parameters on a cross section of UKAEA employees. *Laboratory Practice*, **14**, 1390.

89 HURTADO A., MERINO C. & DELGADO E. (1964) Influence of anoxemia on the hemopoietic activity. *Archives of Internal Medicine*, **75**, 284.

90 LEVIN N.W., METZ J., HART D., VAN HEERDEN P.D.R., BROADMAN R.G. & FARBER S.A. (1960) The blood volume of healthy adult males resident in Johannesburg (altitude 5740 feet). *South African Journal of Medical Science*, **28**, 132.

91 ISAGER H. & HAGERUP L. (1971) Relationship between cigarette smoking and high packed cell volume and haemoglobin levels. *Scadinavian Journal of Haematology*, **8**, 241.

92 SMITH J.R. & LANDOW S.A. (1978) Smokers' polycythemia. *New England Journal of Medicine*, **298**, 6.

93 SHIELDS C.E. (1971) Elevated carbon monoxide level from smoking in blood donors. *Transfusion* (Philadelphia), **11**, 89.

94 RUSSELL M.A.H., WILSON C., COLE P.V. & IDLE M. (1973) Comparison of increases in carboxyhaemoglobin after smoking 'extra mild' and 'non mild' cigarettes. *Lancet*, **ii**, 687.

95 ZIJLSTRA W.G. & VAN KAMPEN E.J. (1960) Standardization of haemoglobinometry. *Clinica Chimica Acta*, **5**, 719.

96 MORNINGSTAR D.A., WILLIAMS G.Z. & SUUTARINEN P. (1966) The millimolar extinction coefficient of cyammethaemoglobin from direct measurements of hemoglobin iron by X-ray emission spectrography. *American Journal of Clinical Pathology*, **46**, 403.

97 WORLD HEALTH ORGANIZATION (1977) *The SI for the Health Professions*. WHO, Geneva.

98 LEWIS S.M. (1972) Enumeration of blood cells and bacteria. In: *Biomedical Technology in Hospital Diagnosis* (ed. Elder A.T. & Neill D.W.), p. 211. Pergamon Press, Oxford.

99 KAPLOW L.S., SCHAUBLE M.K. & BECKTEL J.M. (1979) Validity of hematologic data in VA hospital laboratories. A veterans administration cooperative study. *American Journal of Clinical Pathology*, **71**, 291.

100 KOEPKE J.A. (1975) Interlaboratory trials: the quality control survey programme of the College of American Pathologists. In: *Quality Control in Haematology* (ed. Lewis S.M. & Coster J.F.), p. 53. Academic Press, London.

101 MYHRE E. (1961) Reticulocyte count. *Nordisk Medicin*, **65**, 37.

102 CLINE M.J. & BERLIN N.I. (1963) The reticulocyte count as an indicator of the rate of erythropoiesis. *American Journal of Clinical Pathology*, **39**, 121.

103 HILLMAN R.S. (1969) Characteristics of marrow production and reticulocyte maturation in normal man in response to anemia. *Journal of Clinical Investigation*, **48**, 443.

104 HILLMAN R.S. (1969) The control of marrow production by the level of iron supply. *Journal of Clinical Investigation*, **48**, 454.

105 BRITISH STANDARDS INSTITUTION (1968) Specification

for apparatus for measurement of packed cell volume. BS 4316, 1968.

106 DE BOROVICZENY D.G. (1966) Standardization of packed cell volume determination. In: *Standardization in Haematology. II. Bibliotheca Haematologica*, **24**, 83.

107 CROSLAND TAYLOR P. (1975) Problems of the red cell volume. In: *Quality Control in Haematology* (ed. Lewis S.M. & Coster J.F.), p. 97. Academic Press, London.

108 CHANARIN I. (1975) Critical appraisal of the PCV. In: *Quality Control in Haematology* (ed. Lewis S.M. & Coster J.F.), p. 103. Academic Press, London.

109 LAMPASSO J.A. (1965) Error in hematocrit value produced by excessive ethylenediaminetetraacetate. *American Journal of Clinical Pathology*, **44**, 109.

110 PENNOCK C.A. & JONES K.W. (1966) Effect of ethylenediaminetetraacetic acid (dipotassium salt) and heparin on the estimation of packed cell volume. *Journal of Clinical Pathology*, **19**, 196.

111 LEWIS S.M. & STODDART C.T.H. (1971) Effects of anticoagulants and containers (glass and plastic) on the blood count. *Laboratory Practice* **10**, 787.

112 RUSTAD H. (1964) Correction for trapped plasma in micro-haematocrit determinations. *Scandinavian Journal of Clinical and Laboratory Investigation*, **16**, 677.

113 SWAN H. & NELSON A.W. (1968) Canine trapped plasma factors at different microhaematocrit levels. *Journal of Surgical Research*, **8**, 551.

114 CHAPLIN H. & MOLLISON P.L. (1952) Correction for trapped plasma in the red cell column of the hematocrit. *Blood*, **7**, 1227.

115 FURTH F.W. (1956) Effect of spherocytosis on value of trapped plasma in red cell column of capillary and Wintrobe hematocrits. *Laboratory Clinical Medicine*, **48**, 421.

116 ECONOMOU-MAVROU C. & TSENGHI C. (1965) Plasma trapped in the centrifuged red cells of children with severe thalassaemia. *Journal of Clinical Pathology*, **18**, 203.

117 ENGLAND J.M., WALFORD D.N. & WATERS D.A.W. (1972) Re-assessment of the reliability of the haematocrit. *British Journal of Haematology*, **23**, 247.

118 RAMPLING M. & SIRS J.A. (1970) The effect of hematocrit and anticoagulants on the rate of packing of erythrocytes by a centrifuge. *Physics in Medicine and Biology*, **15**, 15.

119 INTERNATIONAL COMMITTEE FOR STANDARDIZATION IN HAEMATOLOGY (1980) Recommendations for reference method for determination by centrifugation of packed cell volume of blood. *Journal of Clinical Pathology*, **33**, 1.

120 BRITTIN G.M., BRECHER G. & JOHNSON C.A. (1969) Elimination of error in hematocrit produced by excessive EDTA. *American Journal of Clinical Pathology*, **52**, 780.

121 MAZZA U., SAGLIO G., CALIGARIS CAPPIO F., CAMASCHELLA C., NERETTO G. & GALLO E. (1976) Clinical and haematological data in 254 cases of beta-thalassaemia trait in Italy. *British Journal of Haematology*, **33**, 91.

122 PEARSON H.A., O'BRIEN R.T. & MCINTOSH S. (1973) Screening for thalassaemia trait by electronic measurement of MCV. *New England Journal of Medicine*, **288**, 351.

123 LEWIS S.M. (1979) Clinical implications of automation in cell counting systems. *Clinical and Laboratory Haematology*, **1**, 1.

124 KLEE G.G., FAIRBANKS V.F., PIERRE R.V. & O'SULLIVAN M.B. (1976) Routine erythrocyte measurements in diagnosis of iron-deficiency anemia and thalassemia minor. *American Journal of Clinical Pathology*, **66**, 870.

125 HEGDE U.M., WHITE J.M., HART G.H. & MARSH G.W. (1977) Diagnosis of α-thalassaemia trait from Coulter counter 'S' indices. *Journal of Clinical Pathology*, **30**, 884.

126 CROFT R.F., STREETER A.M. & O'NEILL B.J. (1974) Red cell indices in megaloblastosis and iron deficiency. *Pathology*, **6**, 107.

127 GRINER P.F. & ORANBURG P.R. (1978) Predictive values of erythrocyte indices for tests of iron, folic acid and vitamin B_{12} deficiency. *American Journal of Clinical Pathology*, **70**, 748.

128 DAVIDSON R.J.L. & HAMILTON P.J. (1978) High mean red cell volume: its incidence and significance in routine haematology. *Journal of Clinical Pathology*, **31**, 493.

129 ENGLAND J.M., WARD S.M. & DOWN M.C. (1976) Microcytosis, anisocytosis and the red cell indices in iron deficiency. *British Journal of Haematology*, **34**, 589.

130 RAPER C.G.L., ROSEN C. & CHOUDHURY M. (1977) Automated red cell indices and marrow iron reserves in geriatric patients. *Journal of Clinical Pathology*, **30**, 353.

131 UNGER K.W. & JOHNSON D. (1974) Red blood cell mean corpuscular volume: a potential indicator of alcohol usage in a working population. *American Journal of Medical Science*, **267**, 281.

132 LEWIS S.M. & BENTLEY S.A. (1977) Haemocytometry by laser-beam optics: evaluation of the Hemac 630L. *Journal of Clinical Pathology*, **30**, 54.

133 CHILD J.A., KING J., NEWMAN T.H. & WATERFIELD R.L. (1967) A diffraction method for measuring the average volumes and shapes of red blood cells. *British Journal of Haematology*, **13**, 364.

134 BEHLEN L. & BOROVICZENY K.G. (1963) Eine halbautomatische Methode zur Bestimmung der Price–Jones — Kurven. *Schweizerische Medizinische Wochenschrift*, **42**, 1509.

135 HOUCHIN D.N., MUNN J.L. & PARNELL B.L. (1958) A method for the measurement of red cell dimensions and calculation of mean corpuscular volume and surface area. *Blood*, **13**, 1185.

136 WESTERMAN M.P., PIERCE L.E. & JENSEN W.N. (1961) A direct method for the quantitative measurement of red cell dimensions. *Journal of Laboratory and Clinical Medicine*, **57**, 819.

137 CHILD J.A., BOWRY W.M.P. & KNOWLES J.P. (1970) Abnormality of red-cell diameter/thickness ratio: findings in iron-deficiency anaemia. *British Journal of Haematology*, **19**, 251.

138 ENGLAND J.M. & DOWN M.C. (1974) Red cell volume distribution curves and the measurement of anisocytosis. *Lancet*, **i**, 701.

139 BESSMAN J.D. & JOHNSON R.K. (1975) Erythrocyte volume distribution in normal and abnormal subjects. *Blood*, **46**, 369.

140 BESSMAN D. (1977) Erythropoiesis during recovery from macrocytic anemia: macrocytes, normocytes and microcytes. *Blood*, **50**, 995.

141 TORLONTANO G., TATA A. & CAMPAGNA A. (1972) A

rapid screening test for thalassaemia trait. *Acta Haematologica* (Basel), **48**, 234.

142 PROCTOR S.J., COX J.R. & SHERIDAN T.J. (1976) Anisocytosis and the C-1000 Channelyzer in macrocytic anaemia. *Journal of Clinical Pathology* **29**, 719.

143 BENTLEY S.A. & LEWIS S.M. (1975) The use of an image analysing computer for the quantitation of red cell morphological characteristics. *British Journal of Haematology*, **29**, 81.

144 JAMES V. & GOLDSTEIN D.J. (1974) Haemoglobin content of individual erythrocytes in normal and abnormal blood. *British Journal of Haematology*, **28**, 89.

145 POLOWE D. (1929) The specific gravity of the blood: its clinical significance. *Journal of Laboratory and Clinical Medicine*, **14**, 811.

146 LEAKE C.D., KOHL M. & STEBBINS G. (1927) Diurnal variations in the blood specific gravity and erythrocyte count in healthy human adults. *American Journal of Physiology*, **81**, 493.

147 REZNIKOFF P. (1923) A method for the determination of the specific gravity of red blood cells. *Journal of Experimental Medicine*, **38**, 441.

148 DANON D. & MARIKOWSKY Y. (1964) Determination of density distribution of red cell population. *Journal of Laboratory and Clinical Medicine*, **64**, 668.

149 LEWIS S.M. & VINCENT P.C. (1968) Red cell density in paroxysmal nocturnal haemoglobinuria. *British Journal of Haematology*, **14**, 513.

150 PHILLIPS R.A., VAN SLYKE D.D., HAMILTON P.B., DOLE V.P., EMERSON K. & ARCHIBALD R.M. (1943) Copper sulphate method for measuring specific gravities of whole blood and plasma. *Bulletin of the US Army Medical Department*, **71**, 66.

151 PIROFSKY B. & NELSON H.M. (1964) The determination of hemoglobin in blood banks. *Transfusion* (Philadelphia), **4**, 45.

152 KEATING L.J., GORMAN R. & MOORE R. (1967) Hemoglobin and hematocrit values of blood donors. *Transfusion* (Philadelphia), **7**, 420.

153 WESTERGREN A. (1921) Studies of the suspension stability of the blood in pulmonary tuberculosis. *Acta Medica Scandinavica*, **54**, 247.

154 BOTTIGER L.E. & SVEDVERG C.A. (1967) Normal erythrocyte sedimentation rate and age. *British Medical Journal*, **ii**, 85.

155 BOYD R.V. & HOFFBRAND B.I. (1966) Erythrocyte sedimentation rate in elderly hospital in-patients. *British Medical Journal*, **i**, 901.

156 INTERNATIONAL COMMITTEE FOR STANDARDIZATION IN HAEMATOLOGY (1977) Recommendation for measurement of erythrocyte sedimentation rate of human blood. *American Journal of Clinical Pathology*, **68**, 505.

157 LEWIS S.M. (1980) The erythrocyte sedimentation rate and plasma viscosity. *ACP Broadsheet* No. 94.

158 LASCARI A.D. (1972) The erythrocyte sedimentation rate. *Pediatric Clinics of North America*, **19**, 1113.

159 HOLLINGER N.F. & ROBSON S.J. (1953) A study of the erythrocyte sedimentation rate for well children. *Journal of Pediatrics*, **42**, 304.

160 WINTROBE M.M. (1967) *Clinical Hematology*, 6th edn., p. 360. Henry Kimpton, London.

161 BRITISH STANDARDS INSTITUTION (1968) Specification for Westergren tube for measurement of erythrocyte sedimentation rate, BS 2554, 1968.

162 HARKNESS J. (1972) The viscosity of human blood plasma; its measurement in health and disease. *Biorheology*, **8**, 171.

163 HUTCHISON R.M. & EASTHAM R.D. (1977) A comparison of the erythrocyte sedimentation rate and plasma viscosity in detecting changes in plasma proteins. *Journal of Clinical Pathology*, **30**, 345.

164 HARKNESS J. (1963) A new instrument for the measurement of plasma-viscosity. *Lancet*, **ii**, 280.

165 JACOBS H.R. (1969) A low shear tube viscometer for blood. *Biorheology*, **6**, 121.

166 ADLER S.M. & DENTON R.L. (1975) The erythrocyte sedimentation rate in the newborn period. *Journal of Pediatrics*, **86**, 942.

167 DINTENFASS L. (1976) *Rheology of Blood in Diagnostic and Preventive Medicine*. Butterworth, London.

168 BENTLEY S.A. & LEWIS S.M. (1976) The relationship between total red cell volume, plasma volume and venous haematocrit. *British Journal of Haematology*, **33**, 301.

169 MOLLISON P.L. (1979) *Blood Transfusion in Clinical Medicine*, 6th edn., p. 114. Blackwell Scientific Publications, Oxford.

170 GREGERSEN M.I. & RAWSON T.A. (1959) Blood volume. *Physiological Review*, **39**, 307.

171 NAJEAN Y. & CACCHIONE R. (1977). Blood volume in health and disease. *Clinics in Haematology*, **6**, 543.

172 INTERNATIONAL COMMITTEE FOR STANDARDIZATION IN HAEMATOLOGY (1980) Recommended methods for measurement of red-cell and plasma volume. *Journal of Nuclear Medicine*, **21**, 793.

173 RICKETTS C. & CAVILL I. (1978) Measurement of plasma volume using ^{59}Fe-labelled transferrin. *Journal of Clinical Pathology*, **31**, 196.

174 TIZIANELLO A. & PANNACCIULLI I. (1959) The effect of splenomegaly on dilution curves of tagged erythrocytes and red blood cell volume. *Acta Haematologica* (Basel), **21**, 346.

175 REILLY W.A., FRENCH R.M., LAW F.Y.K., SCOTT K.G. & WHITE W.E. (1954) Whole blood volume determined by radio-chromium-tagged red cells: comparative studies on normal and congestive heart failure patients. *Circulation*, **9**, 571.

176 NOBLE R.P. & GREGERSEN M.I. (1946) Blood volume in clinical shock. *Journal of Clinical Investigation*, **25**, 158.

177 BROZOVIC B., KORUBIN V., LEWIS S.M. & SZUR L. (1966) Simultaneous red cell and plasma volume determinations by a differential absorption method. *Journal of Laboratory and Clinical Medicine*, **68**, 142.

178 METZ J., LEVIN N.W. & HART D. (1962) Effect of altitude on the body/venous hematocrit ratio. *Nature (London)*, **194**, 483.

179 MULDOWNEY F.P. (1957) The relationship of total red cell mass to lean body mass in man. *Clinical Science*, **16**, 163.

180 RETZLAFF J.A., TAUSCE W.N., KIELY J.M. & STROEBEL C.F. (1969) Erythrocyte volume, plasma volume, and lean body mass in adult men and women. *Blood*, **33**, 649.

181 HURLEY P.J. (1975) Red cell and plasma volumes in normal adults. *Journal of Nuclear Medicine*, **16**, 46.

182 WENNESLAND R., BROWN E., HOPPER J. JR., HODGES

J.L. JR, GUTTENTAG O.E., SCOTT K.G., TUCKER I.N. & BRADLEY B. (1959) Red cell, plasma and blood volume in healthy men measured by radiochromium (Cr^{51}) cell tagging and hematocrit: influence of age, somatotype and habits of physical activity on the variance after regression of volumes to height and weight combined. *Journal of Clinical Investigation*, **38**, 1065.

183 MOLLISON P.L., VEALL N. & CURBUSH M. (1950) Red cell and plasma volumes in newborn infants. *Archives of Diseases in Childhood*, **25**, 242.

184 SISSON T.R.C., LUND C.J., WHALEN L.E. & TELEK A. (1960) The blood volume in infants. *Journal of Pediatrics*, **56**, 43.

185 LUND C.J. & SISSON T.R.C. (1958) Blood volume and anemia of mother and baby. *American Journal of Obstetrics and Gynecology*, **76**, 1013.

186 CHESLEY L.C. (1972) Plasma and red cell volumes during pregnancy. *American Journal of Obstetrics and Gynecology*, **112**, 440.

187 LANGE R.D. & DYNESIUS R. (1973) Blood volume changes during normal pregnancy. *Clinics in Haematology*, **2**, 433.

188 TAYLOR H.L., ERICKSON L., HENSCHEL A. & KEYS A. (1945) The effect of bed rest on the blood volume of normal young men. *American Journal of Physiology*, **144**, 227.

189 TOGHILL P.J. (1964) Red-cell pooling in enlarged spleens. *British Journal of Haematology*, **10**, 347.

190 GLASS H.I., DE GARRETA A.C., LEWIS S.M., GRAMMATICOS P. & SZUR L. (1968) Measurement of splenic red-blood-cell mass with radioactive carbon monoxide. *Lancet*, **i**, 669.

191 HEGDE U.M., WILLIAMS E.D., LEWIS S.M., SZUR L., GLASS H.I. & PETTIT J.E. (1973) Measurement of splenic red cell volume and visualisation of the spleen with Technetium-99. *Journal of Nuclear Medicine*, **14**, 769.

192 BATEMAN S., LEWIS S.M., NICHOLAS A. & ZAAFRAN A. (1978) Splenic red cell pooling: a diagnostic feature in polycythaemia. *British Journal of Haematology*, **40**, 389.

193 PETTIT J.E., WILLIAMS E.D., GLASS H.I., LEWIS S.M., SZUR L. & WICKS C.J. (1971) Studies of splenic function in the myeloproliferative disorders and generalised malignant lymphomas. *British Journal of Haematology*, **20**, 575.

194 LEWIS S.M., CATOVSKY D., HOWS J.M. & ARDALAN B. (1977) Spenic red cell pooling in hairy cell leukaemia. *British Journal of Haematology*, **35**, 351.

195 LEWIS S.M. (1972) Developing a blood cell standard. In: *Modern Concepts in Haematology* (ed. Izak G. & Lewis S.M.), p. 217. Academic Press, New York.

196 STATLAND B.E., WINKEL P., HARRIS S.C., BURDSALL M.J. & SAUNDERS A.M. (1978) Evaluation of biologic souces of variation of leukocyte counts and other hematologic quantities using very precise automated analyzers. *American Journal of Clinical Pathology*, **69**, 48.

197 BAIN B.J. & ENGLAND J.M. (1975) Normal haematological values: sex difference in neutrophil count. *British Medical Journal*, **i**, 306.

198 ENGLAND J.M. & BAIN B.J. (1976) Total and differential leucocyte count. *British Journal of Haematology*, **33**, 1.

199 ALLAN R.N. & ALEXANDER M.K. (1968) A sex difference in the leucocyte count. *Journal of Clinical Pathology*, **21**, 691.

200 CRUICKSHANK J.M. & ALEXANDER M.K. (1970) The effect of age, sex, parity, haemoglobin level and oral contraceptive preparations on the normal leucocyte count. *British Journal of Haematology*, **18**, 541.

201 MORLEY A.A. (1966) A neutrophil cycle in healthy individuals. *Lancet*, **ii**, 1220.

202 MORLEY A. (1973) Correspondence. *Blood*, **41**, 329.

203 CRUICKSHANK J.M. (1970) The effects of parity on the leucocyte count in pregnant and nonpregnant women. *British Journal of Haematology*, **18**, 531.

204 TIBBLIN E., BENGTSSON C., HALLBERG L. & LENNARTSSON J. (1979) Haemoglobin concentration and peripheral blood cell counts in women. The population study of women in Göteburg, 1968–1969. *Scandinavian Journal of Haematology*, **22**, 5.

205 CORRE F., LELLOUCH J. & SCHWARTZ D. (1971) Smoking and leucocyte counts: results of an epidemiological survey. *Lancet*, **ii**, 632.

206 NOURBAKHSH M., ATWOOD J.G., RACCIO J. & SELIGSON D. (1978) An evaluation of blood smears made by a new method using a spinner and diluted blood. *American Journal of Clinical Pathology*, **70**, 885.

207 BENTLEY S.A. & LEWIS S.M. (1980) Aspects of automated differential leucocyte counting. In: *Topical Reviews in Haematology, Vol. 1* (ed. Roath S.), p. 50. Wight, Bristol.

208 BENTLEY S.A. & LEWIS S.M. (1977) Automated differential leucocyte counting: the present state of the art. *British Journal of Haematology*, **35**, 481.

209 KOEPKE J.A. (ed.) (1979) Differential leukocyte counting: *CAP Conference Aspen 1977*. College of American Pathologists, Skokie Ill.

210 MELAMED M.R., MULLANEY P.F. & MENDELSOHN M.L. (eds) (1979) *Flow Cytometry and Sorting*, J. Wiley & Sons, New York.

211 KATO K. (1935) Leucocytes in infancy and childhood: a statistical analysis of 1081 total and differential counts from birth to 15 years. *Journal of Pediatrics*, **7**, 7.

212 ALTMAN P.L. & DITTMER D.S. (eds) (1964) *Biology Data Book*, p. 272. Federation of American Societies for Experimental Biology, Washington.

213 SHAPER A.G. & LEWIS P. (1971) Genetic neutropenia in people of African origin. *Lancet*, **ii**, 1021.

214 WOODLIFF H.J., KATASHA P.K., TIBALEKA A.K. & NZARO E. (1972) Total leucocyte count in Africans. *Lancet*, **ii**, 875.

215 MUCHMORE H.G., BLACKBURN A.B., SHURLEY J.T., PIERCE C.M. & McKOWN B.A. (1970) Neutropenia in healthy men at the South Polar Plateau. *Archives of Internal Medicine*, **125**, 646.

216 WERTZ R.W. & KOEPKE J.A. (1977) A critical analysis of platelet counting methods. *American Journal of Clinical Pathology*, **68**, 195.

217 LEWIS S.M., WARDLE J., COUSINS S. & SKELLY J.W. (1979) Platelet counting—development of a reference method and a reference preparation. *Clinical and Laboratory Haematology*, **1**, 227.

218 BULL B.S., SCHNEIDERMAN M.A. & BRECHER B. (1965) Platelet counts with the Coulter Counter. *American Journal of Clinical Pathology*, **44**, 678.

219 GLASS U.H., WETHERLEY-MEIN G., MILLS R.T. & PRIEST C.J. (1971) Automated platelet counting. *British Journal of Haematology*, **21**, 529.

220 BULL B.S. (1970) Aids to electronic platelet counting. *American Journal of Clinical Pathology*, **4**, 37.

221 SLOAN A.W. (1951) The normal platelet count in man. *Journal of Clinical Pathology*, **4**, 37.

222 STEVENS R.F. & ALEXANDER M.K. (1977) A sex difference in the platelet count. *British Journal of Haematology*, **37**, 295.

223 MORLEY A. (1969) A platelet cycle in normal individuals. *Australasian Annals of Medicine*, **18**, 127.

224 HIRSH J. & DACIE J.V. (1966) Persistent post-splenectomy thrombocytosis and thrombo-embolism. *British Journal of Haematology*, **12**, 44.

225 ROWAN R.M., FRASER C., GRAY J.H. & McDONALD G.A. (1979) The Coulter Counter Model S Plus: the shape of things to come. *Clinical and Laboratory Haematology*, **1**, 29.

226 MUNDSCHENK D.D., CONNELLY D.P., WHITE J.G. & BRUNNING R.D. (1976) An improved technique for the electronic measurement of platelet size and shape. *Journal of Laboratory and Clinical Medicine*, **88**, 301.

227 KARPATKIN S. (1978) Heterogeneity of human platelets. VI. Correlation of platelet function with platelet volume. *Blood*, **51**, 307.

228 ROPER P.R., JOHNSTON D., AUSTIN J., AGARWAL S.S. & DREWINKO B. (1977) Profiles of platelet volume distribution in normal individuals and in patients with acute leukemia. *American Journal of Clinical Pathology*, **68**, 449.

229 WHITEHEAD T.P. (Ed.) (1969) *Automation and Data Processing in Pathology* (Symposium organized by College of Pathologists). Published by *Journal of Clinical Pathology*, London.

230 BINET J.L. (1978) L'Automatique en hématologie. *Nouvelle Revue française d'Hématologie*, **20**, 145.

231 BRITTIN G.M., BRECHER G. & JOHNSON C.A. (1969) Evaluation of the Coulter Counter Model 'S'. *American Journal of Pathology*, **52**, 679.

232 BRECHER G. & WATTENBURG W.H. (1972) Evaluation of laboratory computers—what can they do for us? In: *Modern Concepts in Hematology* (ed. Izak G. & Lewis S.M.), p. 244. Academic Press, New York.

233 PAGE C.F. & ENGLAND J.M. (1979) A minicomputer laboratory data-management system: the St. Mary's system and its haematology applications. *Clinical and Laboratory Haematology*, **1**, 165.

234 CAVILL I., RICKETTS C. & JACOBS A. (1975) *Computer in Haematology*. Butterworth, London.

235 YOUNESS E. & DREWINKO B. (1978) A computer-based reporting system for bone marrow evaluation. *American Journal of Clinical Pathology*, **69**, 333.

236 DREWINKO B., WALLACE B., FLORES C., CRAWFORD R.W. & TRUJILLO J.M. (1977) Computerised hematology. Operation of a high-volume hematology laboratory. *American Journal of Clinical Pathology*, **67**, 64.

237 BURMESTER H.B.C. & CROW G.S. (1979) 'On line' data handling in a routine haematology department. *Journal of Clinical Pathology*, **32**, 254.

238 FIELD E.J. & MACLEOD I. (1963) Platelet adherence to polymorphs. *British Medical Journal*, **ii**, 388.

239 SKINNIDER L.F., MUSCLOW C.E. & KAHN W. (1978) Platelet satellitism—an ultrastructural study. *American Journal of Hematology*, **4**, 179.

240 WHITE L.A., BRUBAKER L.H., ASHER R.H., HENRY P.H. & ADELSTEIN E.H. (1978) Platelet satellitism and phagocytosis by neutrophils: association with antiplatelet antibodies and lymphoma. *American Journal of Hematology*, **4**, 313.

241 GREIPP P.R. & GRALNICK H.R. (1976) Platelet to leukocyte adherence phenomena associated with thrombocytopenia. *Blood*, **47**, 513.

242 WORLD HEALTH ORGANIZATION (1977) Biological substances: international standards, reference preparations, and reference reagents. WHO, Geneva.

243 CROSLAND TAYLOR P.J., ALLEN R.W.B., ENGLAND J.M., FIELDING J.F., LEWIS S.M., SHINTON N.K. & WHITE J.M. (1979) Draft protocol for testing calibration and quality control material used with automatic blood-counting apparatus. *Clinical and Laboratory Haematology*, **1**, 61.

244 GILMER P.R., WILLIAMS L.J., KOEPKE J.A. & BULL B.S. (1977) Calibration methods for automated hematology instruments. *American Journal of Clinical Pathology*, **68** (S), 185.

245 LEWIS S.M. (1975) Standards and reference preparations. In: *Quality Control in Haematology* (ed. Lewis S.M. & Coster J.F.), p. 79. Academic Press, London.

246 CAVILL I. & JACOBS A. (1973) Quality Control in Haematology. *ACP Broadsheet No. 75*. Association of Clinical Pathologists, London.

247 BULL B.S., ELASHOFF R.M., HEILBRON D.C. & COUPERUS J. (1974) A study of various estimates for the derivation of quality control procedures from patient erythrocyte indices. *American Journal of Clinical Pathology*, **61**, 473.

248 BULL B.S. (1975) A statistical approach to quality control. In: *Quality Control in Haematology* (ed. Lewis S.M. & Coster J.F.), p. 111. Academic Press, London.

249 LEWIS S.M. & COSTER J.F. (1975) (eds) *Quality Control in Haematology*, p. 13. Academic Press, London.

250 MAJEWSKI E. & SÖKER M. (1977) Über Ringversuche. *Zeitschrift des Deutscher Verband Technischer Assistenten in der Medizin*, **11**, 435.

251 LAWSON N.S. & HAVEN G.T. (1976) The role of regional quality control programmes in the practice of laboratory medicine in the United States. *American Journal of Clinical Pathology*, **66**, 268.

252 INTERNATIONAL FEDERATION OF CLINICAL CHEMISTRY (1978) Provisional recommendations on the theory of reference values. *Clinica Chimica Acta*, **87**, 459F.

253 SUNDERMAN F.W. (1975) Current concepts of 'normal values', 'reference values' and 'discrimination values' in clinical chemistry. *Clinical Chemistry*, **21**, 1873.

254 GARBY L. (1970) Annotation: The normal haemoglobin level. *British Journal of Haematology*, **19**, 429.

255 LE TOHIC F., PROST-DVOJAKOVIC R.J., LE MENN R. & SAMAMA M. (1978) Problèmes posés par la mesure des volumes plaquettaires dans les grandes thrombopénies. *Nouvelle Revue française d'Hématologie*, **20**, 155.

256 KHAN I., ZUCKER-FRANKLIN D. & KARPATKIN S. (1975) Microthrombocytosis and platelet fragmentation associated with idiopathic/autoimmune thrombocytopenic purpura. *British Journal of Haematology*, **31**, 449.

257 WALKER A.R.P. (1956) Correction of haematological

data for altitude. *Transactions of Royal Society of Tropical Medicine and Hygiene*, **50,** 510.

258 VAN ASSENDELFT O.W., McGRATH C., MURPHY R.S. & SCHMIDT R.M. (1977). The differential distribution of leukocytes. In: *Differential Leukocyte Counting* (ed. Koepke J.A.), p. 11. *CAP Conference Aspen 1977*, College of American Pathologists, Skokie, Ill.

259 FRISCH B. & LEWIS S.M. (1978) Localization and role of calcium in the erythrocyte coat: effects of enzymes and storage. *British Journal of Haematology*, **40,** 541.

260 STAEHLIN L.A. (1974) Structure and function of intercellular junctions. *International Review of Cytology*, **39,** 191.

261 WISCHNITZER S. (1973). The submicroscopic morphology of the interphase nucleus. *International Review of Cytology*, **34,** 1.

262 FELDHERR C.M. (1972) Structure and function of the nuclear envelope. *Advances in Cellular and Molecular Biology*, **2,** 273.

263 FRANKE W.W. (1974) Nuclear envelopes. Structure and biochemistry of the nuclear envelope. The electron microscopy and composition of biological membranes and their ultrastructure. *Philosophical Transactions of the Royal Society, London Branch*, **268,** 67.

264 LEWIS S.M. & FRISCH B. (1976) Congenital dyserythropoietic anemias: electron microscopy. In: *Congenital Disorders of Erythropoiesis*, p. 171. Ciba Foundation Symposium No. 37 (New Series). Elsevier-Excerpta Medica/North Holland, Amsterdam and Oxford.

265 DANIELLI J.F. & DAVSON H. (1935) A contribution to the theory of permeability of thin films. *Journal of Cellular Comparative Physiology*, **5,** 495.

266 ROBERTSON J.D. (1959) The ultrastructure of cell membranes and their derivation. *Biochemical Society Symposium*, **16,** 3.

267 WEINSTEIN R.S. & McNUTT N.S. (1970) Ultrastructure of red cell membranes. *Seminars in Hematology*, **7,** 259.

Chapter 2
Cellular kinetics of haemopoiesis

L. G. LAJTHA

The study of cellular kinetics is the study of cell populations; the sequence of changes, in time and space, in the composition or size of the population, due to processes of proliferation, differentiation or other physiological or non-physiological causes. The aim of such studies is first to develop assay methods with which such changes can be quantitatively measured, then to describe the normal state (i.e. in dynamic equilibrium) and the way perturbations influence, and are corrected by, the steady state, and finally to identify those factors and mechanisms which control the steady state maintenance.

There are few cell populations in the adult organism more appropriate for cell kinetic studies than the haemopoietic tissue. It consists of a complex of interlinked cell populations, most of which (though not all) are in a state of fast proliferation. Cell differentiation (and maturation) act as physiological 'removal' of cells from and into subpopulations. Demands for proliferation and differentiation can vary greatly under conditions of haemopoietic stress (haemorrhage, infection or cytotoxic therapy), or pathological conditions (anaemias, leukaemias, etc.). It is necessary to understand the cellular kinetic mechanisms and their controlling factors in order to be able to manipulate them for therapeutic purposes.

According to present concepts, the haemopoietic tissue can be divided into three cell population groups: stem cells, morphologically unrecognized precursor cells, and morphologically recognizable precursor cells. The descendants of the latter are the haemic cells, which will be dealt with in later Chapters.

STEM CELLS

For the purposes of definition, 'stem' cells represent a cell type which, in the adult organism, can maintain its own numbers in spite of physiological or artificial removal of cells from the population. The operative definition is 'maintain its own numbers', implying that this is achieved by proliferation within the population and not by the entry of cells from another population.

This definition is not only applicable to haemopoietic stem cells, but to all cell populations which are capable of turnover and/or regeneration through their own proliferative capacity, to maintain their numbers throughout healthy adult life [1, 2].

The physiological 'removal' in the case of haemopoietic stem cells is a differentiation step—the first step in the chain of events during the process of blood cell formation. The initial differentiation step may still leave opportunities for more than one subsequent differentiation step, and increasing maturation may restrict these [3].

The history of the haemopoietic stem cell is almost as old as cellular haematology itself. In the early decades of this century, a truly 'battle royal' was raged between the great haematological schools of Maximow, Doan, Sabin, Downey, Naegeli, Ferrata and others, concerning the morphological identity of the haemopoietic stem cells, and concerning the question of whether they are totipotential, pluripotential or monopotential, i.e. provide all, some, or only one line of the differentiating marrow cells. Tenuous morphological arguments and the equally tenuous *post hoc ergo propter hoc* principle could not settle a problem which required direct experimental proof. It was the transplantation technique which has provided this experimental evidence—at least in the small rodent, and new cytogenetic and isoenzyme methodologies in man.

Evidence for a pluripotent stem cell in the mouse
The first evidence for a pluripotent haemopoietic stem cell came from the work of Ford, Loutit and their colleagues [4, 5] which showed that a single chromosomally marked cell clone can repopulate the entire haemopoietic system of lethally irradiated and subsequently marrow-grafted mice. This evidence was followed by a quantification of stem cells in haemopoietic cell suspension by Till and McCulloch and their colleagues [6–9] who have shown that graded injections of bone-marrow cells form macroscopically visible nodules in the spleens of lethally irradiated recipient mice, and that each of these nodules consti-

tutes a clone (colony) originating from a single cell which is capable of giving rise to erythroid, myeloid or megakaryocytic lines of cells.

The term 'colony-forming unit' (CFU-S) is used to describe those cells in the original marrow suspension which 'arrive' to the spleen and are successful in forming haemopoietic colonies. These CFU-S represent therefore a certain fraction of the total potentially colony-forming cells (CFC-S). The overall plating efficiency of these cells can be determined with two procedures, one is the f number determination, the other the ω factor determination.

The f factor [7], i.e. the fraction of CFC-S which arrives to the spleens, is determined by a retransplantation method. The number of colonies which are produced in the spleen of irradiated recipients of haemopoietic cell suspension (bone marrow, embryonic liver) are linearly dependent on the number of cells injected. If one takes an animal which has been irradiated and given enough bone-marrow cells to produce 50–100 colonies in its spleen, the latter can be taken out of the animal (instead of allowing eight to nine days for visible development of colonies) within two to three hours of injection of the cells. A suspension of this spleen can then be injected into a second, irradiated recipient animal. Since it is known that the donor spleen contains a certain number of colony-forming cells, the fraction which arrives into the spleen of the secondary recipient and forms visible colonies nine days later gives the f number. The shrinkage of the spleen shortly after irradiation will influence the number of CFU-S it can contain, or which can be recovered from it [10], hence the interpretation of the f number determinations will be different in recipients which had been irradiated two or 24 hours before.

The determination of the ω factor (describing the fraction of stem cells which, though 'arriving', are unsuccessful in forming a colony) is based on the knowledge that the CFC-S is giving rise to differentiating descendants while forming the colonies. Indeed, cytological inspection of excised colonies indicates that about 90% of the cells are recognizable normoblasts or granulocytes (or megakaryocytes). When a CFC-S 'settles' in the spleen, the subsequent fate of its descendants will be determined by two processes: proliferation and differentiation. At any cell division there will be a finite chance that one or both daughter cells of the dividing CFC-S may differentiate—and thus cease to be a CFC-S. This represents a balance between 'birth' and 'death' of CFC-S [7]. Since the number of CFC-S increases in the recipient spleen with time after grafting, the 'birth' probability is higher than the 'death' (differentiation) probability. There is a finite chance, however, that at an early stage, say in the first or second divisions, all daughter cells differentiate.

The differentiating cells having a limited proliferation potential (see below), this would result in the 'extinction' of a potential colony. The extinction probability, ω, can be deduced from the coefficient of variation of the CFU-S number in the colonies [11].

It should be recalled here that in early concepts about the stem cells it was proposed that they possess a capacity for an asymmetric cell division which would result in one daughter cell remaining a stem cell, the other becoming a differentiated cell. This rigid asymmetric division concept is untenable since it would never allow recovery of stem-cell numbers after a depletion with, for example, radiation or other cytotoxic agents, or during colony growth, all of which are, however, properties well attested in experimental systems. Osgood has invoked [12, 13] a switch between the asymmetric α–α, η and the symmetric α–2α division to allow for this. However, since the rate of differentiation of the CFU-S is primarily from noncycling (G_o) cells in the steady state and continuously variable, the concept of 'tying' differentiation to an asymmetric cell division is untenable.

Other stem-cell tests

While the colony-forming assay is an absolute measure of the pluripotential CFU-S (or CFC-S) in a cell population, other methods have been used for the detection of 'repopulating' cells. These are also based on grafting, and subsequent determination of either:
1 the spleen weight [14];
2 erythroid cellularity or erythrocyte production [15, 16];
3 granulocyte production [17];
4 total DNA synthesis exhibited by the graft in, for example, the spleen or marrow of the recipient [18]; or
5 the protective value of the graft in lethally irradiated animals.

A common disadvantage of all these tests is that they do not give a measure of the absolute number of stem cells, and that the end points they measure are not entirely dependent on the number of stem cells injected: they are affected by states and demands for differentiation. Also, their performance is not simpler or cheaper than that of the colony-forming assay. However, since good splenic colonies can be detected only in the mouse, and only questionably good ones in the rat, their value lies in assays of repopulating capacity of grafted haemopoietic tissues in other animals. For obvious ethical reasons none of these tests are applicable to man.

Recently, Metcalf *et al.* [20], described the occurrence of two to 10% mixed colonies (containing erythroid, neutrophilic, eosinophilic, megakaryocytic and macrophage cells) in agar cultures of mouse haemopoietic tissue, and attributed their presence to the seeding and differentiation of pluripotent stem cells. The exact frequency of cells forming such mixed colonies in culture is, however, difficult to assess, and the phenomenon has not as yet been demonstrated with human marrow. The long-term bone-marrow culture, in which mouse stem cells can be maintained proliferating and differentiating for several months [21], is in the process of being adapted for human haemopoietic tissues. If successful, the method could be used for studies on human haemopoietic stem cells.

PROPERTIES OF THE CFU-S

Cycle kinetics

In the mouse, the f number of CFU-S is about 0·1 (ranging from 0·05 to 0·2 depending on transplantation conditions) and the ω factor about 0·6, therefore the 'plating efficiency' of the CFU-S is around six per cent. Since the CFU-S concentration in the marrow is between 200 and 400 CFU-S/10^6 cells (dependent on the strain and sex of the mice used*), this means some 3500–6500 CFC-S/10^6 bone-marrow cells. In normal steady state the great majority of these cells are not in a state of proliferation, i.e. their population turnover is very slow. In experiments with high doses of ^{3}H-thymidine given *in vitro* or *in vivo*, it was found that only about 10% (or less) of the CFU-S are killed (i.e. were in the DNA synthetic stage of the cell cycle), but this figure increases to over 50% during induced states of CFU-S proliferation, such as after sublethal irradiation of the mouse, or after lethal irradiation followed by marrow grafting [22, 23]. This finding confirms the view that the pluripotent haemopoietic stem-cell population is primarily a non-cycling or G_0 population that can, however, be triggered into cell cycle on demand for proliferation [24].

This low cycling of the population is understandable in view of the two amplifying transit populations (the committed precursors and the recognizable erythroid cells) which represent some 10 cell cycles' worth of proliferation, i.e. an amplification of approximately × 1000. Thus, for each stem cell differentiating into the erythroid line the eventual ouput can be 1000 reticulocytes. The stem population can, of course, cycle fast too; under maximal conditions of demand for growth, i.e. in the lethally irradiated and marrow-grafted mice, the population doubling time for CFU-S is about 20–24 hours [25]. It must be remembered, however, that population doubling time and cell cycle time are not the same concepts. Even under maximal demand for CFU-S growth there is a 'loss' of CFU-S for

differentiation (see the above-mentioned 'birth' and 'death' process) and therefore the cell cycle of the maximally proliferating CFU-S is still significantly shorter than the observed population doubling time [26]. As will be illustrated later (Fig. 2.4) the rate of 'loss' for differentiation is apparently limited—under conditions of maximum demand for proliferation *and* differentiation—to about 40% per cell cycle.

The G_0 state (state of no cycling) in the majority of CFU-S in normal steady state has also been demonstrated with drugs that act specifically in some phases of the cell generation cycle in contrast to the fast-cycling mouse leukaemia cells [27, 28]. The therapeutic gain, however, useful as it is, is insufficient for curative effect in even moderately advanced leukaemia.

From the cell kinetic point of view the pluripotent CFU-S population is illustrated in Figure 2.1.

The study of the control of stem-cell proliferation (i.e. the triggering from G_0 into cycle) has yielded some interesting results recently. Control appears to be 'local' in nature, with an active radius of about six to seven cell diameters [29–32]. Thus, in a shielded part of the bone marrow, the stem cells retain their normal numbers and low cycling rate at a time when in the unshielded rest of the marrow of, for example, an irradiated animal, the stem cells are proliferating intensively. Both inhibitory and stimulatory factors have been isolated from haemopoietic tissues [33–36]; these factors are produced by cells other than the stem cells [37], and their effect appears to be a stem-cell specific, reversible, switching on/off mechanism [38]. Purification and characterization of these stem-cell proliferation controlling factors, and studies of their mechanisms of action are in progress. However, extremely low concentrations of non-specific pharmacological agents (e.g. β-adrenergic and cholinergic compounds) can also induce stem-cell cycling [39–41] and their physiological and potential therapeutic role deserves further studies.

Genetic control

Recent information has thrown interesting light on the role of genetic influences on CFU-S growth control. In the genetically anaemic WW^v mice, the number of CFU-S is almost undetectably low, i.e. when WW^v bone marrow is grafted into recipient animals (irradiated normal littermates of genotype WW, or unirradiated WW^v) no colony formation is detected apart from a very low number (less than 1/1000 of normal) of very small colonies. The fault lies in the WW^v cells and not in the WW^v internal environment, since if the normal WW marrow is grafted into even unirradiated WW^v recipients, it takes and corrects the anaemia, and repopulates the WW^v host with WW CFU-S in near-normal numbers. This indicates that the fault is a

---

* In female mice significant oscillations of CFU-S numbers occur, depending on the stage of oestrus.

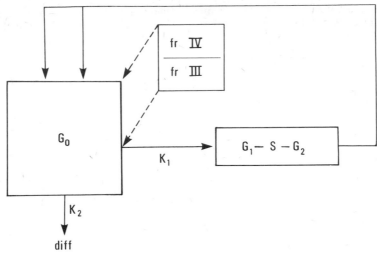

Fig. 2.1. Kinetic model of the pluripotential stem-cell population. The majority of cells in steady state are in a non-cycling (G_0) state. Differentiation stimuli remove cells from the population at rate K_2 and, in response, the population-size control mechanism (e.g. the balance between the stimulatory factor III and the inhibitory factor IV [33, 36] triggers cells into cycle at rate K_1. Once in cycle the cells pass through the pre-DNA-synthetic G_1 phase (i.e. the commencement of a net synthesis of structural proteins), then enter into DNA synthesis (S phase), then into the pre-mitotic G_2 phase before commencing the prophase stage of mitosis. In the 'average' human haemopoietic cells the duration of the G_1 phase ranges between eight and 15 hours, that of the DNA synthetic phase about eight to 12 hours, and that of the G_2 phase about three to five hours. On completion of the mitotic processes the triggered cells enter the G_0 population at rate $2K_1$.

lack of normal proliferative capacity of the WW^v CFU-S [42].

An opposite situation exists in another strain of anaemic mice, of the genotype Sl/Sl^d. When the marrow of such mice is grafted into irradiated normal littermates, it can form colonies at normal frequency, i.e. it contains a normal number of CFU-S. The Sl/Sl^d cells, when grafted into unirradiated WW^v recipients, will cure the anaemia by colonizing the WW^v host with essentially normal CFU-S. However, when normal marrow is grafted into Sl/Sl^d or Sl^d/Sl^d recipients, its colony yield will be low. The fault in this case lies in the Sl/Sl^d 'environment' in which, apparently, normal CFU-S growth is markedly retarded. This fault lies truly in the microenvironment of the Sl/Sl^d host, since parabiosis with the normal genetic counterpart fails to affect both the inability of Sl/Sl^d parabiont, and the ability of the normal parabiont, to support CFU proliferation [43].

These conclusions have been reinforced by *in-vitro* studies in the long-term bone-marrow cultures, in which WW^v haemopoietic tissue can form effective milieu for WW or Sl/Sl^d stem-cell proliferation, while Sl/Sl^d micromilieu (the adherent supporting layer in the cultures) causes a run-down of normal stem cells seeded on it [44].

A third genetic abnormality occurs in the flexed-tailed mice of genotype *f/f* in which CFU-S growth

(and numbers) are normal, but the capacity of the *f/f* CFU-S to give rise to erythroid cells appears to be impaired [45].

These studies, which hopefully will be extended with time to other conditions, begin to illustrate the independent multigenic control of the various aspects of stem-cell function.

Spatial organization of CFU-S

The distribution of CFU-S in the femoral marrow of the mouse is not entirely homogeneous. It has been shown that the concentration (CFU-S/10^5 bone-marrow cells) increases, from the central axis of the femoral marrow to the endosteal surface, by at least a factor of 2. This concentration gradient appears to obey a square-law relationship, and the 'endosteal' CFU-S appear to proliferate faster—in normal steady state—than the 'central' ones [46, 47]. It is particularly noteworthy that the spatial distribution of the pluripotent stem cells is different from that of their immediate descendants. A special 'stem-cell environment' may also be indicated by the long-term bone-marrow cultures [21, 48], in which the adherent layer has to develop 'pockets' of giant fat cells before the culture is ready to receive pluripotent stem cells and support their proliferation. These giant cells appear to act as foci, in the close vicinity of which active stem-cell proliferation and differentiation takes place (Fig. 2.2).

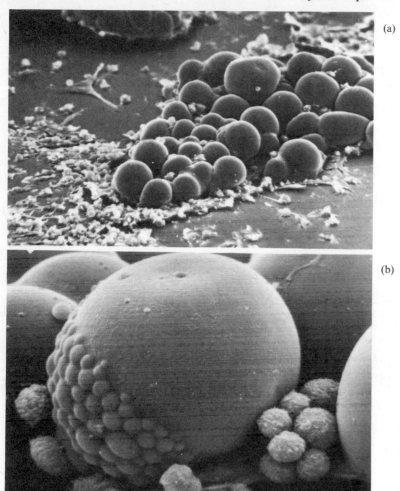

(a)

(b)

Fig. 2.2. Relationship of the giant fat cells and haemopoietic cells in the 'adherent layer' of the long-term marrow cultures [21, 48]. (a) 'Nest' of fat cells and flattened 'epitheloid' cells on which the haemopoietic cells settle, and (b) close spatial relationship between giant fat cells and clusters of haemopoietic cells.

Mobility of CFU-S

While the bone marrow is the main source of CFU-S, the spleen (a haemopoietic organ in the adult mouse) also contains CFU-S, although the concentration is only about one-tenth of that of the bone marrow. Hence the total number of CFU-S in a normal mouse spleen is not more than in one femur. Some migration is indicated by the fact that the peripheral blood also contains some CFU-S, about $1/10^6$ nucleated blood cells.

During embryogenesis, considerable migration of the CFU-S population takes place. They first appear in the yolk sac [49] which is the only site of genuine *de-novo* formation of haemopoiesis (i.e. the site of the embryonic differentiation or 'true' birth of stem cells.) From the yolk sac they migrate into the embryonic liver, which at certain stages of embryogenesis behaves like the adult bone marrow. Indeed, the same CFU-S which in the yolk sac produces erythroid progeny carrying embryonic haemoglobin, will produce adult haemoglobin when growing in the liver or spleen [50–52]. The migrating capacity of CFU-S persists in the adult mouse as well, and the rate of migration from the marrow to the spleen can be quantitatively measured [53, 54]. The rate of this migration is increased under stress conditions such as administration of bacterial endotoxin [55] or sometimes following acute or chronic irradiation [23].

Radiation and drug sensitivity

The pluripotent haemopoietic stem cells are among the most radiosensitive cells in the body [56] and their sensitivity is influenced by their turnover state [57, 58]. They exhibit similarly high sensitivity to cytotoxic

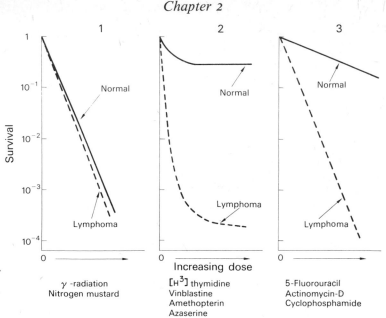

Fig. 2.3. The form of dose–survival curves for normal haemopoietic and lymphoma-colony forming cells exposed to nine different anticancer agents for 24 hours *in vivo* [59].

drugs, and although this is also influenced by their turnover state, important differences have been found between the sensitivity of normal CFU-S and leukaemic cells with certain drugs [59]. This is illustrated in Figure 2.3. Although the sensitivity difference with the drugs so far tested is not enough to be curative for advanced leukaemia, it is the first quantitative demonstration of a genuine drug sensitivity difference between normal and malignant cells of similar origin.

Proliferative potential

The pluripotent stem cell has very considerable proliferative potential. Some of this can be illustrated by the following calculation: assuming that when the first CFC-S is formed in the yolk sac, it is not a single phenomenon but simultaneously, say, 100 CFC-S are differentiating from some embryonic mesenchymal cell population. During embryonic and neonatal growth their number increases to reach some $2–4 \times 10^6$ CFC-S in a 10–12-week-old mouse (see above, re CFC-S concentration in the marrow). This would mean approximately 15 population doublings. In terms of cell cycles this amounts to much more, since this population growth is achieved against a continuous loss ('death') of CFC-S for differentiation to establish and to maintain haemopoiesis in the developing foetus and growing young animal. A conservative estimate would be some 35–40 cell cycles. During adult life the CFC-S population has a steady-state turnover to provide the differentiating cells, and with a five-day

turnover (as seems to be the case with most strains of mice) and a two-year average life span, some 140 more cell cycles will be performed by the population, i.e. a total of over 180 cycles from the original 'stock' CFC-S [60].

With repeated cytotoxic damage (e.g. whole-body irradiation) or, even better, by grafting marrow into lethally irradiated mice, a significant number of additional cycles can be 'forced' in the CFC-S population. Serial grafting at suitable intervals can add at least another 100 cycles or so to the total which the population can perform [61–63]. This is a significant excess over the rather limited figure which has been postulated as the maximum number of cell cycles possible for somatic mammalian cells [64].

It should be appreciated that this figure of 180 (plus potentially another 100 or more) refers to the mouse. In man, with a life span some 35 times longer, even assuming a cell cycle time 3·5 times longer, the total number of cycles per *average* stem cell during a lifetime could be 10 times higher. Since there is no evidence for stem-cell depopulation with ageing, the proliferative capacity of the haemopoietic stem cells is clearly very high.

In view of these figures, it is perhaps a surprising fact that on serial grafting, the protective capacity of the marrow graft can be exhausted [65–67]. In most of these serial grafting experiments, however, the number of transferred stem cells was not kept constant. With decreasing effective stem-cell graft size the proliferation of these cells will be chronically increased, and it is known that the self-replicating capacity of the stem cells can be impaired by over-forcing proliferation [68]. It has been proposed that for the maintenance of full reproductive capacity, suitable periods of non-cycling states (G_o state) may be required [1]. Furthermore, an interrelationship between the proliferative activity of stem cells and their micromilieu ('stem-cell niches') has also been postulated [2, 68] and it appears that if this is not interfered with and consequently the appropriate periods of the non-cycling G_o states can be maintained, extensive and prolonged stimulation of the stem cells can be maintained without loss of proliferative capacity [69].

Conclusions from animal studies

From the evidence described above it is clear that, in the mouse at least, there is a pluripotent stem cell for haemopoiesis. This cell, the 'colony-forming cell' (CFC-S) fulfils the criteria in the sense that it is capable of maintaining its own numbers during adult life, in spite of continued requirement for cell loss; i.e. differentiation into various 'transit' cell lines. That in the mouse this cell can provide erythrocytic, granulocytic, thrombocytic and lymphoid descendants is amply proved by chromosome-marker evidence [4, 5, 9].

How much of the data can be extrapolated for man is not known; clearly the CFU-S methodology is not applicable. Quantitative differences are certain to be expected; cell cycle and population doubling times are usually longer in man than in the small rodent by about a factor of two to three. In spite of the possible (but cautious) extrapolation from mouse to man, it is essential that more quantitative information should be obtained about the human haemopoietic stem cell. While this will depend on new methodological advances, one of the great haematological debates is certainly over: the haemopoietic stem cell *is* a pluripotential cell.

'COMMITTED' PRECURSOR CELLS

The old stem-cell concepts envisaged a relatively simple situation: a (pluripotential) stem cell which, on appropriate demand, can differentiate into a recognizable (e.g. erythroid or granulocytic, etc.) cell. There is a steadily mounting body of experimental data, however, which suggests that this is not so, and that between the pluripotent stem cell and the recognizable differentiating precursor cells there may be intermediate, less pluripotential (i.e. more committed) but morphologically still unrecognized cell populations. The evidence for these is discussed below.

Erythropoietic precursor cells

When the humoral factor erythropoietin was first used for the assay of the haemopoietic stem-cell population [70, 71] it was thought to be a measure of *the* stem cells. With the introduction of the spleen colony method as an absolute measure of the pluripotent stem cells [6–9], certain differences between the two assay methods have been noticed. First, the recovery pattern of the 'stem cells' after a small dose of radiation (e.g. 150 rad whole-body dose) was different: a fast recovery, within six days, to normal level with the erythropoietin test, but a delayed recovery, following a four- to five-day postradiation 'dip' with the colony-forming test [72–74]. This, and the observation that, following erythropoietic demand, the reticulocyte peak occurs much earlier than changes in the number of CFU-S, led to the proposal that the CFU-S and the 'erythropoietin-responsive cell' (ERC) may not be identical [75]. This was confirmed by the '[³H] thymidine-suicide' experiments which showed that in steady state the CFU-S is a slowly turning-over cell population [22, 23], while the ERC is a very fast cycling population, even in the absence of erythropoietic demand [23, 76].

Further evidence for the non-identity of CFU-S and ERC is obtained from simple calculation of daily demands for cell production. In the mouse, taking a 50-day RBC life span, some $1–2 \times 10^8$ RBC are formed daily. The number of cell cycles in the nucleated red-cell series can be taken as six to seven (i.e. an amplification of approximately $\times 100$) which means a demand for $1–2 \times 10^6$ cells entering the erythron per day. The total number of CFC-S ($=$CFU-S corrected for f number and ω factor) is about $1–2 \times 10^6$, of which not much more than 10%, i.e. $1–2 \times 10^5$, appear to turn over (i.e. leave the population) per day. This turnover amounts only to about one-tenth of the daily requirement for entry into the erythron, therefore the CFC-S cannot be the cell which enters the erythron and it has to be amplified; this is achieved by entry into, and dividing during transit in, another cell population, the ERC population.

Investigation of the kinetics of the splenic colonies in grafted mice gives further information. By the sixth day after grafting, individual colonies may contain in excess of 10^5 nucleated cells. This implies a population doubling time of less than eight hours. However, from the sixth day onwards the population doubling time of the colonies is about 20–24 hours (Fig. 2.4) and, in fact, it may proceed at this slower rate *before* the sixth day (but the colonies are too small to allow accurate cell counting). The CFU-S population doubling time, however, remains at 20–24 hours from the first day onwards. This slow population doubling is the result of two processes: a cell-cycle time shorter than 20–24 hours, and a loss of cells from the CFU-S population

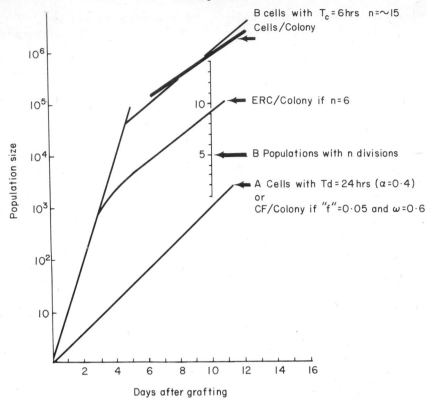

Fig. 2.4. Model of the spleen colony growth. The growth of the pluripotent stem cells corrected for the *f* factor and ω factor gives the growth curve designated 'A-cells'. This implies a cell-cycle time (T_c) of about six to seven hours, with a loss for differentiation at the rate of about 40% per cell cycle. The differentiating 'B' cells, with a similar cell-cycle time, undergo some 15 cycles—nine as ERC and a further six as nucleated red cells—before reaching a non-dividing stage. The size of the B population depends on the number of cell cycles it undergoes during its amplifying transit to the final non-dividing stage [26].

for differentiation into ERC. The latter must have a cell-cycle time shorter than eight hours and must undergo an amplification under these conditions of some 1000-fold (nine to 10 cell cycles).

This fast ERC growth suggested that the ERC population may not be homogeneous, it may have an 'age structure', i.e. that the 'early' ERC may not respond to erythropoietin like the 'late' ERC (last few cycles). This is clear from the consideration that if all ERC, 'early' and 'late' were available for differentiation into the erythron, then the observed ERC growth—like CFU-S growth—would be due to a combination of (a) proliferation and (b) loss of cells from the population (for differentiation). But this would only be possible if the cell cycle of the ERC would be considerably less than three to four hours which is an unlikely figure even in the small rodent [26]. This being so, the ERC population may be considered as a dividing transit population [77] which 'matures' from a 'potential' or 'pre'-ERC stage, as it proceeds

through its amplifying cell cycles, and only the late stages of this maturation process may be able to respond to erythropoietin, i.e. become 'real' ERC.

This concept has been further strengthened with the development of methods for erythroid colony growth *in vitro* [78–80]. A cardinal feature of these methods is that the erythroid colonies which develop *in vitro* have a transient existence; after the initial growth of two to three days they disappear within the next three to four days (in the case of mouse haemopoietic tissue—the time scale is longer in man). This feature allows the detection of relatively late cells (e.g. early pronormoblasts) which can form small erythroid colonies within two to three days in the case of mouse cells, or six to seven days in the case of human cells (soon after which time they disappear)—or progressively larger colonies, and/or 'bursts' of colonies developing from days five to 10 or 10 to 20 (with mouse or human cells respectively), developing from earlier precursor cells.

The nomenclature used in the literature is somewhat

confusing, since the cell which forms colonies early in the culture (two to three days), termed CFU-E (colony-forming unit erythroid), is in fact a cell late in the development of the erythroid 'lineage'. That it is probably not earlier than an early pronormoblast, and it is not an ERC, is indicated by the fact that CFU-E numbers are sharply affected by bleeding or hypertransfusion, unlike ERC [81]. The cells which form the larger and later-occurring colonies (or bursts of colonies) are earlier cells in the lineage, denoted BFU-E (burst-forming cells erythroid); their number is largely unaffected by quick changes in demand for erythropoiesis—they correspond to the pre-ERC–ERC population described earlier. Evidence for the 'age structure' can be demonstrated in the BFU-E population by comparing, for example, the cycling rates of early BFU-E (which take nine to 10 days to form haemoglobinized bursts of colonies) with that of late BFU-E (five to seven days erythroid bursts). In a normal steady state the cycling rate of early BFU-E is low (approximately 20%) while that of the late BFU-E is high (approximately 50%). During regeneration from cytotoxic damage the cycling rates of early BFU-E, like that of the low cycling stem cells, can increase [82], thus explaining the growth curve illustrated in Figure 2.4.

The detailed experimental evidence concerning the properties of this *in-vitro* detectable 'committed' erythroid precursor population has been reviewed recently [83, 84]. Nothing is known as yet about the stimulus for the differentiation of early BFU-E from the pluripotent stem cells (CFU-S) but it is known that early BFU-E require a factor (or factors) termed burst-promoting activity (BPA) or burst-feeding activity (BFA) for their *in-vitro* growth [85, 86], and under certain conditions they require 'cooperation' from T cells [87, 88]. The requirement for BPA appears to decrease with the maturation from early to late BFU-E, in contrast to erythropoietin requirement which appears to be virtually nil in early BFU-E, but increases with maturation to late BFU-E [85], probably explaining the previous *in-vivo* findings of erythropoietin stimulation of ERC [89].

In normal steady state, unlike during colony growth, the degree of amplification, that is the number of cell cycles from the earliest to the 'real' ERC (i.e. through the early to late BFU-E transit), may be smaller, and the cell-cycle times in the population may be longer than during regeneration. Removal of cells from the ERC population (e.g. by erythropoietin) appears to result, in time, in an increased 'feed' of CFU-S into the committed precursor line, with a concomitant increased CFU-S turnover [90]. The cell population system operates by a 'two-step' differentiation: (a) from the self-maintaining CFU-S into the first ampli-

fying and 'maturing' transit population, the ERC, mediated by some feedback information from the ERC to the CFU-S, and (b) from the 'late' ERC into the second amplifying and maturing transit population, the erythron, mediated by erythropietin; this latter step appears to be very highly sensitive to actinomycin D [91]. The scheme is illustrated in Figure 2.5, and the details of the last stage, the erythron itself, in Figure 2.6.

In-vitro granulocytic colony-forming cell

In 1966, Bradley and Metcalf described a method (similar to that which had been used for the culture of mast cells *in vitro* [92]), which produced maintenance of growth for 1–2 weeks yielding granulocytic colonies from explanted bone-marrow cells [93]. These 'colony-forming units of cells in culture' (CFU-C or CFC-C) have been found to occur in human marrow and peripheral blood also [94–97]. The essence of the culture method is that the cells are suspended in a semi-solid medium (agar, methylcellulose or fibrin) in which microscopically (and even macroscopically) visible colonies develop. For such colony growth, a colony-stimulating activity or factor (CSA or CSF) must be incorporated into the culture medium. The CSA has been demonstrated by using a 'feeder' layer of embryonic cells or media in which embryonic cells have been grown. Similarly, sera from leukaemic endotoxin-treated or irradiated neutropenic animals contains CSA [98]. The factor also appears in urine, including human urine [99] and in media 'conditioned' by human leukocytes [100], and is elevated in some pathological human sera [101]. Some sera appear to contain a specific inhibitory factor of CSA, the concentrations of which appear to vary in the various pathological states [102, 103].

As to the identity of the CFU-C as opposed to the pluripotential spleen colony-forming CFU-S, there is a considerable body of evidence strongly indicating that they represent different cell populations. Thus the radiosensitivity of CFU-S is different from that of CFU-C (D_o = 90 *vs* 160 rad γ rays), CFU-C turnover state is higher, a suitable dose of [^{3}H] thymidine or hydroxyurea kills 40% of CFU-C while only about 10% of CFU-S [23, 104], neutropenic states can cause a significant increase in the number of CFU-C without much effect on CFU-S [105], in the genetically anaemic WW^v mice CFU-S numbers are almost undetectably low, but the CFU-C numbers are within normal limits [106], and under conditions in which the CFU-C can exhibit moderate proliferative capacity *in vitro*, the CFU-S cannot [107].

In spite of these differences, there is good evidence from transplantation and cytogenetic studies that the CFU-C is derived from the pluripotent CFU-S [108].

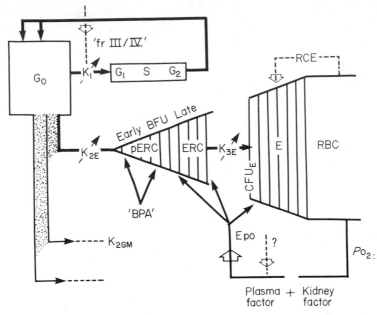

Fig. 2.5. Scheme of the erythropoietic system. The pluripotent stem cells (see also Fig. 2.1) give rise to the earliest 'committed' erythroid precursor (pre-ERC, or early BFU-E) which undergoes amplifying divisions during its 'maturation', for example from BPA dependence to Epo responsiveness (see text). Epo also induces the second differentiation step from the late ERC to the early pronormoblast (CFU-E). Cell-cycle time in the erythron is modulated by cell-line-specific material obtained from red cells (RCE). The degree of amplification (i.e. the number of cell cycles during transit) can be varied on demand, thus increasing or decreasing output without necessarily changing input from the stem cells. BPA = burst-promoting activity; Epo = erythropoietin; other abbreviations as defined in the text.

Since its presence can be demonstrated in the earliest site of haemopoiesis (the yolk sac) at a time when there is no detectable granulopoiesis [49], the CFU-C cannot be equated with any of the morphologically identifiable granulocyte precursors. The most likely explanation is that the CFU-C, like the ERC mentioned earlier, constitutes an intermediate 'committed' precursor-cell population between the multipotential stem cells and the morphologically and functionally recognizable granulocyte series. Unlike the ERC, there is no good *in-vitro* method to assess how many cell cycles (i.e. how much amplification) exist in the CFU-C population, but preliminary data indicate that it is less than in the case of ERC. Nevertheless, some control of CFU-C proliferation exists as evidenced from the apparently increased turnover rate of the population in regenerating marrow [109].

The original description of CFU-C (and CSF) referred to cells which yielded granulocyte/macrophage colonies. The proportion of these cells depended to a great extent on the type and quantity of CSF used. However, with refinements of the techniques, better defined media and better characterized colony-stimulating preparations, evidence is accumulating that a spectrum of *in-vitro* colony-forming cells and colony-stimulating factors (activities) may exist [110, 111]. Thus an eosinophilic CFU-C population (EO-CFU-C) has been reported, which requires specific EO-CSF for its colony forming [112, 113], and similarly, megakaryocyte colony formation may require a specific factor or factors [114, 115].

A note of caution is needed, however, in the interpretation of these reports. The fact that granulocytic, erythroid, etc. colonies can be observed *in vitro* does not necessarily mean that the particular colony (or colonies) originate from 'committed precursor' cells! This is illustrated in the description of erythroid colony formation discussed earlier, in which it has been demonstrated that while the BFU-E clearly fulfils the criteria for committed precursor cells, the CFU-E is more likely to be an early pronormoblast (or a very late ERC at the most).

Thus, the granulocyte/monocyte colony former (GM-CFU-C) is likely to be a committed precursor, but whether the 'purified' G-CFU-C or M-CFU-C, or the Eo-CFU-C (and particularly the Mega-CFU-C) are also such committed precursors, or already differentiated early members of the morphologically

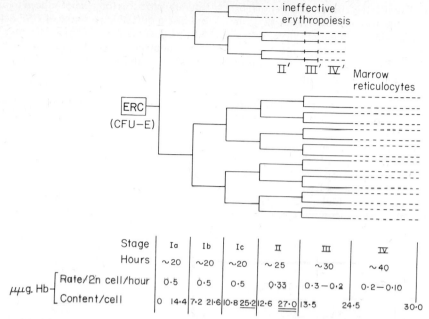

Fig. 2.6. Kinetic model of the human erythron. The erythropoietin-responsive cell gives rise to the first cell in the erythron, which undergoes a number of cell cycles while it accumulates haemoglobin. With increasing concentration of haemoglobin the lengths of cell cycles increase and, at a critical concentration, the cell loses its proliferative potential. Since halving of the haemoglobin content (not concentration!) occurs after each cell division, if an early division is prevented by premature increase in haemoglobinization the cell will proceed on the 'skipped division' pathway, arriving at the reticulocyte stage earlier, i.e. saving time but at the expense of numbers. The term 'ineffective erythropoiesis' denotes the occasional cell death during this amplifying transit process. (After Lajtha L.G. & Oliver R. (1960) Studies on the kinetics of erythropoiesis: A model of the erythron. Ciba Foundation Symposium, *Haemopoiesis*, p. 289. Churchill, London.)

recognizable series of cells, is open to question. Colony size, while not definitive, can be an indicator. Small colonies (or clusters) of less than 20–50 cells, which may be the result of pronormoblasts, early promyelocytes, or megakaryoblasts, the earlier committed precursor cells, could be expected to yield larger colonies by the greater proliferative capacities of such cells (earlier in the developmental lineage).

Humoral regulation of CFU-C

In view of the above-mentioned uncertainties on the identities of the specific target cells, it is not surprising that the mechanisms of action of the various 'colony-stimulating activities' are not clear. With *in-vitro* cell systems, in artificial media, a conscious differentiation has to be made between cell-line-specific regulating factors, and mere *in-vitro* permissive factors (which enable the particular cell type to survive the particular culture conditions imposed on it).

Even with the reasonably well-defined and committed precursor of granulocytic/monocytic colonies (the GM-CFU-C), it is not clear in what way its colony-stimulating factor (the GM-CSF) operates on the population—whether by increasing the numbers and/or speed of cell cycles in the population, or by increasing the rate of differentiation of the pluripotent CFU-S into CFU-C, or that of CFU-C into recognizable granulocyte precursors. The concentration of this factor certainly increases sharply in the serum during infections [116], in response to antigenic stimulation [117, 118] and at certain times, after whole-body irradiation [119]. When injected *in vivo*, it causes not only an increase of CFU-C numbers, but also monocytosis and increased granulopoiesis [120]. It must be remembered, however, that, at the time of writing, many of the references to 'CSF' in the literature are operational terms, denoting only partially purified preparations. Furthermore, the marrow contains a significant granulocytic reserve which, on demand, can be released into the circulation [121, 122] and a 'neutrophil-releasing' or 'leukocytosis-inducing' factor has been demonstrated to operate in perfused femora [123, 124].

Lately some considerably purified preparations of 'CSF-s' have been reported (see review by Moore[111]) but their roles and cell-line (and species) specificities

Chapter 2

are not yet fully elucidated. It is also noteworthy that in the long-term bone-marrow culture system [21], in which continuous production and proliferation of CFU-C and active granulopoiesis exists for months, there is no detectable CSF activity in the culture medium. However, since in these cultures there is a close spatial relationship between the proliferation cells and the 'adherent layer' of cells (containing macrophage elements) the inter-cell transfer of such factors cannot be excluded.

While, therefore, the question of what exactly is regulated by the various levels of circulating CSF (or CSF-s) remains unanswered, there is evidence accumulating for the existence of complex feedback loops in the humoral regulation of granulopoiesis [111]. It appears that the monocyte/macrophage population

not only produces (or can be induced to produce) CSF, but also a diffusible inhibitor of CSF action (likely to be prostaglandin E (PGE)). The monocyte/macrophage population may be functionally heterogeneous in respect of obligatory CSF producers, inducible CSF producers and PGE producers. The 'loops' may be further complicated by factors contained and potentially released by mature granulocytes. While the specific granylocyte proliferation modulator does not affect CFU-C proliferation [125], a glycoprotein, possibly lactoferrin, effectively (and reversibly) inhibits CSF production by macrophages [111].

The fine structure and the regulating mechanisms of granulocyte/monocyte production are only beginning to be understood; thus the scheme illustrated in Figure 2.7, while attempting to bring the available informa-

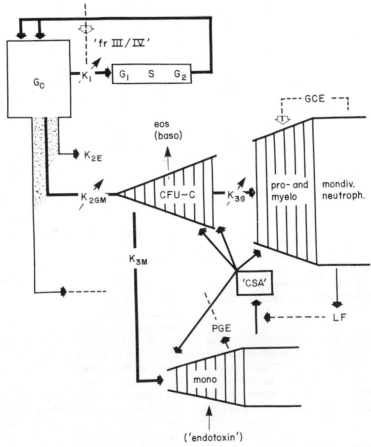

Fig. 2.7. Scheme of the granulopoietic system. The pluripotent stem cells give rise to an early 'committed' precursor of the granulocyte–monocyte system. CSA, produced by activated monocytes/macrophages stimulates proliferation (? and induces differentiation into the promyelocytic stage). Feedback loops are constituted by PGE balancing CSA effect in monocytes, and by LF released from granulocytes regulating CSA production. Modulation of granulocyte proliferation is effected by cell-line-specific material obtained from mature granulocytes (GCE).

tion together, should be considered an oversimplification.

Due to the lack of a comparable marker of maturation to haemoglobin, no granulocytopoietic scheme of similar accuracy to Figure 2.6 can be constructed as yet. Two recent reviews, however, present the evidence available today on the quantitative aspects of flow kinetics within the recognizable granulocytic cells [126, 127].

CONCLUSIONS

The type of study of the cell populations discussed above has been called by McCulloch 'a chapter of haematology without the microscope'. This is not surprising since definitions like CFU, ERC, BFU, etc. are all operationally determined, and the number of these cells—due to the amplification in the last, i.e. the morphologically recognizable cell populations—is obviously a small fraction of the total cells in the marrow (certainly under 10%). The majority of the 'recognizable' bone-marrow cells belong to the last amplifying series of cells, the nucleated red-cell series or the granulocytic series (see Table 2.1). Even if the 'typical' bone-marrow lymphocytes are included in the 'recognizable' cells, there are sufficient numbers of cells without enough morphologically distinctive features (i.e. no reliable morphological criteria for assignment of function) to hide the required number of pluripotent stem cells and committed precursor cells among them.

It is not the subject of this chapter to discuss the recognizable precursor cells—these will be dealt with in detail by subsequent chapters on erythropoiesis, granulopoiesis and thrombopoiesis, respectively. Nor is the subject of lymphopoiesis discussed here, since the question of origin of B and T cells respectively is still being actively debated. There seems to be a consensus of opinion that B cells are ultimately derived from pluripotential stem cells [5, 128], but the techniques for the study of their developmental pathways are just becoming available [129]. The ontogeny of the T lymphocytes is more uncertain—partly because of

chromosomal evidence in chronic myeloid leukaemia [130] indicating either different stem cells, or a very long-lived precursor population. Recent evidence from the long-term bone-marrow cultures, in which pre-T cells appear to be generated [131] does, however, favour the concept of their origin from the pluripotent stem cells—as does isoenzyme marker indicating monoclonal origin of myeloid and lymphoid cells [132].

In spite of notable recent progress in the field, our knowledge of the early cellular kinetics of haemopoiesis has some equally notable gaps. No information is available on the pre-megakaryocytic stages of thrombopoiesis and very little, as mentioned above, on lymphopoiesis. The nature of controlling factors is just beginning to be understood. Some of the molecular events involved in the mechanism of action of erythropoietin are just beginning to be elucidated, as is the dissociation between the phenomena of differentiation and proliferation.

Nevertheless, the recent advances in methodology have brought not only a better insight into the cellular dynamics of haemopoiesis, but also some clinically relevant developments. The *in-vitro* systems for the detection of the granulopoietic committed precursor cells (GM-CFU-C) can be used to extend data obtained from the conventional morphological studies. The matter has been reviewed in detail [110, 133, 134]. There are situations in which the methodology is particularly applicable. First there is the assessment of 'marrow reserves' by determining the number/concentration of *in-vitro* colony-forming cells. This may give useful information, either on a patient's reserve status during a course of intensive cytotoxic therapy, or on the potential usefulness of a sample of haemopoietic tissue intended for grafting (e.g. assessment of functional viability of stored cells for autografting). Secondly, determination of the growth potential of explanted cells, particularly of the ratio of clusters (< 30 cells) and colonies (> 50 cells) may be used as an early indication of blast-cell crisis in chronic myelocytic leukaemia, or of relapse in acute leukaemia. Finally, other applications, still awaiting further improvements in the standardization of granulocytic and erythroid

Table 2.1. Illustration of the effect of amplification during steady-state transit in a line of two hypothetical successive transit (e.g. ERC-erythron) cell populations originating from the stem cells

Stem cells →	'committed' precursors	1st	2nd	3rd	4th	5th	cycle →	'recognizable' precursors	1st	2nd	3rd	4th	5th	cycle
? 10–20 × input in 'store'	1	2	4	8	16	32			64	128	256	512	1024	cells
? 1–2%		0.097%				1.56%			3.12%				50%	of total

precursor-cell cultures, include a more meaningful analysis of underlying defects in neutropoiesis and anaemias (congenital or acquired).

Some of the recent developments which could, potentially, both sharpen up and speed up investigations on haemopoietic precursor cells involve the combination of flow cytometry with the use of suitably labelled monoclonal antibodies. The use of cell sorters is already becoming standard methodology [135], and antisera against various leukaemic cells [136] and even stem cells [137, 138] have been isolated. With the new and powerful analytical tool of making of monoclonal antibodies [139] and their use in cell-sorting systems, there is, in principle, every possibility of dissecting the various subpopulations of cells in very precise, and eventually, functional terms.

The haemopoietic cell population, representing a two-step differentiation system, from the pluripotent stem cells to the 'committed' precursors, and from the 'committed' to the 'recognizable' precursors, each step followed by maturation as well as proliferation, presents a complex cell regulatory system, both of practical and fundamental interest. The practical interest is in the control of the haemopoietic functions and their correction in disease; the fundamental interest is in the eventual understanding and control of differentiation and proliferation in general terms.

REFERENCES

1 LAJTHA L.G. (1979) Stem cell concepts. *Differentiation*, **14**, 23.

2 POTTEN C.S., SCHOFIELD R. & LAJTHA L.G. (1979) A comparison of cell replacement in bone marrow, testis and three regions of surface epithelium. *Biochimica et Biophysica Acta*, **56**, 281.

3 LAJTHA L.G. & SCHOFIELD R. (1974) On the problem of differentiation in haemopoiesis. *Differentiation*, **2**, 313.

4 FORD C.E., HAMERTON J.L., BARNES D.W.H. & LOUTIT J.F. (1956) Cytological identification of radiation-chimaeras. *Nature (London)*, **177**, 452.

5 BARNES D.W.H., FORD C.E., GRAY S.M. & LOUTIT J.F. (1959) Spontaneous and induced changes in cell populations in heavily irradiated mice. *Progress in Nuclear Energy, Series VI*, **2**, p. 1. Pergamon Press, London.

6 TILL J.E. & McCULLOCH E.A. (1961) A direct measurement of the radiation sensitivity of normal mouse bone-marrow cells. *Radiation Research*, **14**, 213.

7 TILL J.E., McCULLOCH E.A. & SIMINOVITCH L. (1964) A stochastic model of stem-cell proliferation, based on the growth of spleen colony-forming cells. *Proceedings of the National Academy of Sciences*, **51**, 29.

8 BECKER A.J., McCULLOCH E.A. & TILL J.E. (1963) Cytological demonstration of the clonal nature of spleen colonies derived from transplanted mouse marrow cells. *Nature (London)*, **197**, 452.

9 WU A.M., TILL J.E., SIMINOVITCH L. & McCULLOCH E.A. (1967) A cytological study of the capacity for differentiation of normal haemopoietic colony-forming cells. *Journal of Cellular Physiology*, **69**, 177.

10 LORD B.I. (1971) The relationship between spleen colony production and spleen cellularity. *Journal of Cell and Tissue Kinetics*, **4**, 211.

11 VOGEL H., NIEWISCH H. & MATIOLI G. (1968) The self renewal probability of hemopoietic stem cells. *Journal of Cellular Physiology*, **72**, 221.

12 OSGOOD E.E. (1957) A unifying concept of the etiology of the leukemias, lymphomas and cancer. *Journal of the National Cancer Institute*, **18**, 155.

13 OSGOOD E.E. (1959) Blood cell survival in tissue cultures. *Annals of the New York Academy of Sciences*, **77**, 777.

14 POPP R.A., CONGDEN C.C. & GOODMAN J.W. (1965) Spleen weight as a measure of marrow-cell growth in irradiated mice. *Proceedings of the Society of Experimental Biology and Medicine*, **120**, 395.

15 SMITH L.H. (1964) Marrow transplantation measured by uptake of Fe^{59} by spleen. *American Journal of Physiology*, **206**, 1244.

16 HODGSON G.S. (1962) Erythrocyte Fe^{59} uptake as a function of bone marrow dose injected in lethally irradiated mice. *Blood*, **19**, 460.

17 HELLMAN S. & GRATE H.E. (1967) Production of granylocytic progeny by transplanted bone marrow in irradiated mice. *Blood*, **30**, 103.

18 CUDKOWICZ G., UPTON A.C., SMITH L.H., GOSSLEE D.G. & HUGHES W.L. (1964) An approach to the characterization of stem cells in bone marrow. *Annals of the New York Academy of Sciences*, **114**, 571.

19 McCULLOCH E.A. & TILL J.E. (1960) The radiation sensitivity of normal mouse bone-marrow cells determined by quantitative marrow transplantation into irradiated mice. *Radiation Research*, **13**, 115.

20 METCALF D., JOHNSON G.R. & MANDEL T.E. (1979) Colony formation in agar by multipotential haemopoietic cells. *Journal of Cellular Physiology*, **98**, 401.

21 DEXTER T.M., ALLEN T.D. & LAJTHA L.G. (1977) Conditions controlling the proliferation of haemopoietic stem cells *in vitro*. *Journal of Cellular Physiology*, **91**, 335.

22 BECKER A.J., McCULLOCH E.A., SIMINOVITCH L. & TILL J.E. (1965) The effect of differing demands for blood cell production on DNA synthesis by hemopoietic colony-forming cells of mice. *Blood*, **26**, 296.

23 LAJTHA L.G., POZZI L.V., SCHOFIELD R. & FOX M. (1969) Kinetic properties of haemopoietic stem cells. *Journal of Cell and Tissue Kinetics*, **2**, 39.

24 LAJTHA L.G. (1963) On the concept of the cell cycle. *Journal of Cellular and Comparative Physiology*, **67** (Suppl. 1), 143.

25 McCULLOCH E.A. & TILL J.E. (1964) Proliferation of hemopoietic colony-forming cells transplanted into irradiated mice. *Radiation Research*, **22**, 383.

26 LAJTHA L.G., GILBERT C.W. & GUZMAN E. (1971) Kinetics of haemopoietic colony growth. *British Journal of Haematology*, **20**, 343.

27 VALERIOTE F.A., BRUCE W.E. & MEEKER B.E. (1966) Comparison of the sensitivity of normal hematopoietic and transplanted lymphoma colony-forming cells of mice to vinblastine administered *in vivo*. *Journal of the National Cancer Institute*, **36**, 21.

28 BRUCE W.R., MEEKER B.E., POWERS W.E. & VALERIOTE F.A. (1969) Comparison of the dose- and time-survival curves for normal hematopoietic and lymphoma colony-forming cells exposed to vinblastine, vincristine, arabinosylcytosine, and amethopterin. *Journal of the National Cancer Institute*, **42**, 1015.

29 CROIZAT H., FRINDEL E. & TUBIANA M. (1970) Proliferative activity of the stem cells in the bone marrow of mice after single and multiple irradiations. *International Journal of Radiation Biology and Related Studies in Physics, Chemistry and Medicine*, **18**, 347.

30 RENCRICCA N.G., RIZZOLI V., HOWARD D., DUFFY P. & STOHLMAN F., JR (1970) Stem cell migration and proliferation during severe anaemia. *Blood*, **36**, 764.

31 PATT H.M. & MALONEY M.A. (1972) Relationship of bone-marrow cellularity and proliferative activity: a local regulatory mechanism. *Cell and Tissue Kinetics*, **5**, 303.

32 GIDALI J. & LAJTHA L.G. (1972) Regulation of haemopoietic stem cell turnover in partially irradiated mice. *Cell and Tissue Kinetics*, **5**, 147.

33 LORD B.I., MORI K.J., WRIGHT E.G. & LAJTHA L.G. (1976) An inhibitor of stem-cell proliferation in normal bone marrow. *British Journal of Haematology*, **34**, 441.

34 FRINDEL E., CROIZAT H. & VASSORT F. (1976) Stimulating factors liberated by treated bone marrow. *Experimental Hematology*, **4**, 56.

35 FINDEL E. & GUIGON M. (1977) Inhibition of CFU entry into cycle by a bone marrow extract. *Experimental Hematology*, **5**, 74.

36 LORD B.I., MORI K.J. & WRIGHT E.G. (1977) A stimulator of stem-cell proliferation in regenerating bone marrow. *Biomedicine*, **27**, 223.

37 WRIGHT E.G. & LORD B.I. (1978) Production of stem-cell proliferation stimulators and inhibitors by haemopoietic cell suspensions. *Biomedicine*, **28**, 156.

38 WRIGHT E.G., LORD B.I., DEXTER T.M. & LAJTHA L.G. (1969) Mechanisms of haemopoietic stem-cell proliferation control. *Blood Cells*, **5**, 247.

39 BYRON J.W. (1975) Manipulation of the cell cycle of the hemopoietic stem cell. *Experimental Hematology*, **3**, 44.

40 BYRON J.W. (1977) Analysis of receptor mechanisms involved in the hemopoietic effects of androgens: use of the Tfm mutant. *Experimental Hematology*, **5**, 429.

41 BYRON J.W. (1977) Mechanism for histamine H$_2$-receptor induced cell-cycle changes in the bone-marrow stem cell. *Agents Actions*, **7**, 209.

42 McCULLOCH E.A., SIMINOVITCH L. & TILL J.E. (1964) Spleen-colony formation in anemic mice of genotype WW. *Science*, **144**, 844.

43 McCULLOCH E.A., SIMINOVITCH L., TILL J.E., RUSSELL E.S. & BERNSTEIN S.E. (1965) The cellular basis of the genetically determined hemopoietic defect in anemic mice of genotype S1/S1^d. *Blood*, **26**, 399.

44 DEXTER T.M. & MOORE M.A.S. (1977) *In vitro* duplication and 'cure' of haemopoietic defects in genetically anaemic mice. *Nature (London)*, **269**, 412.

45 FOWLER J.H., TILL J.E., McCULLOCH E.A. & SIMINOVITCH L. (1967) The cellular basis for the defect in haemopoiesis in flexed-tailed mice. II. The specificity of the defect for erythropoiesis. *British Journal of Haematology*, **13**, 256.

46 LORD B.I. & HENDRY J.H. (1972) The distribution of haemopoietic colony forming units in the mouse femur and its modification by X-rays. *British Journal of Radiology*, **45**, 110.

47 LORD B.E., TESTA N.D. & HENDRY J.H. (1975) The relative spatial distribution of CFU-S and CFU-C in the normal mouse femur. *Blood*, **46**, 65.

48 DEXTER T.M. (1979) Cell interactions *in vitro*. In: *Clinics in Haematology, Vol. 8*, No. 2, p. 453. W. B. Saunders, London.

49 MOORE M.A.S. & METCALF D. (1970) Ontogeny of the haemopoietic system: Yolk sac origin of *in vivo* and *in vitro* colony forming cells in the developing mouse embryo. *British Journal of Haematology*, **18**, 279.

50 RUSSELL E.S. & BERNSTEIN S.E. (1966) Blood and blood formation. In: *Biology of the Laboratory Mouse*, 2nd edn. (ed. Green E.L.), p. 351. McGraw-Hill, New York.

51 KOVACH J.S., MARKS P.A., RUSSELL E.S. & EPLER H. (1967) Erythroid cell development in foetal mice: ultrastructural characteristics and hemoglobin synthesis. *Journal of Molecular Biology*, **25**, 131.

52 BARKER J.E. (1968) Development of the mouse hematopoietic system. I. Types of hemoglobin produced in embryonic yolk sac and liver. *Development Biology*, **18**, 14.

53 HANKS G.E. (1964) *In vivo* migration of colony-forming units from shielded bone marrow in the irradiated mouse. *Nature (London)*, **203**, 1393.

54 ROBINSON C.V., CUMMERFORD S.L. & BATEMAN J.L. (1965) Evidence for the presence of stem cells in the tail of the mouse. *Proceedings of the Society for Experimental Biology and Medicine*, **119**, 222.

55 HANKS G.E. & AINSWORTH E.J. (1967) Endotoxin protection and colony-forming units. *Radiation Research*, **32**, 367.

56 McCULLOCH E.A. & TILL J.E. (1962) The sensitivity of cells from normal mouse bone marrow to gamma radiation *in vitro* and *in vivo*. *Radiation Research*, **16**, 822.

57 DUPLAN J.F. & FEINENDEGEN L.E. (1970) Radiosensitivity of the colony-forming cells. *Proceedings of the Society for Experimental Biology and Medicine*, **134**, 319.

58 HENDRY J.H. & HOWARD A. (1971) The response of haemopoietic colony-forming units to single and split doses of γ-rays or D-T neutrons. *International Journal of Radiation Biology*, **19**, 51.

59 BRUCE W.R. (1967) The action of chemotherapeutic agents at the cellular level and the effects of these agents on hematopoietic and lymphomatous tissue. *Proceedings of VII Canadian Cancer Research Conference, 1966*, **7**, p. 53. Pergamon Press, London.

60 SCHOFIELD R. & LAJTHA L.G. (1976) Cellular kinetics of erythropoiesis. In: *Congenital Disorders of Erythropoiesis*. Ciba Foundation Symposium 37, p. 3. Elsevier, Excerpta Medica, North Holland, Amsterdam.

61 LAJTHA L.G. & SCHOFIELD R. (1971) Regulation of stem cell renewal and differentiation: possible significance in aging. In: *Advances in Gerontological Research*, Vol. 3, p. 131. Academic Press, New York.

62 HARRISON D.E. (1973) Normal production of erythrocytes by mouse bone marrow continues for 73 months. *Proceedings of the National Academy of Sciences, USA*, **70**, 3184.

63 Pozzi L.V., Andreozzi U. & Silini G. (1973) Serial transplantation of bone-marrow cells in irradiated isogenic mice. *Current Topics in Radiation Research*, **8**, 259.

64 Hayflick L. (1965) The limited *in vitro* lifetime of human diploid cell strains. *Experimental Cell Research*, **37**, 611.

65 Barnes D.W.H., Forc C.E. & Loutit J.F. (1959) Greffes en série de moelle osseuse homologue chez des souris irradiés. *Le Sang*, **30**, 762.

66 van Bekkum D.W. & Weyzen W.W.H. (1961) Serial transfer of isologous and homologous hematopoietic cells in irradiated hosts. *Pathologie-Biologie, Semaine Hôpital*, **9**, 888.

67 Siminovitch L., Till J.E. & McCulloch E.A. (1964) Decline in colony-forming ability of marrow cells subjected to serial transplantation into irradiated mice. *Journal of Cellular and Comparative Physiology*, **64**, 22.

68 Schofield R. (1978) The relationship between the spleen colony forming cell and the haemopoietic stem cell. *Blood Cells*, **4**, 7.

69 Ross & Micklem (to be published).

70 Gurney C.W., Lajtha L.G. & Oliver R. (1962) A method for investigation of stem-cell kinetics. *British Journal of Haematology*, **8**, 461.

71 Lajtha L.G., Oliver P. & Gurney C.W. (1962) Kinetic model of a bone marrow stem-cell population. *British Journal of Haematology*, **8**, 442.

72 Alexanian R., Porteous D.D. & Lajtha L.G. (1963) Stem-cell kinetics after irradiation. *International Journal of Radiation Biology*, **7**, 87.

73 Till J.E. (1963) Quantitative aspects of radiation lethality at the cellular level. *American Journal of Roentgenology*, **90**, 917.

74 Blackett N.M., Roylance P.J. & Adams K. (1964) Studies of the capacity of bone-marrow cells to restore erythropoiesis in heavily irradiated rats. *British Journal of Haematology*, **10**, 453.

75 Bruce W.R. & McCulloch E.A. (1964) The effect of erythropoietic stimulation on the hemopoietic colony-forming cells of mice. *Blood*, **23**, 216.

76 Porteous D.D. & Lajtha L.G. (1968) Restoration of stem-cell function after irradiation. *Annals of the New York Academy of Sciences*, **149**, 151.

77 Gilbert C.W. & Lajtha L.G. (1965) The importance of cell population kinetics in determining response to irradiation of normal and malignant tissue. In: *Cellular Radiation Biology*, p. 474. Williams and Wilkins, Baltimore.

78 Stephenson J.R., Axelrad A.A., McLeod D.L. & Shreeve M.M. (1971) Introduction of colonies of hemoglobin-synthesizing cells by erythropoietin *in vitro*. *Proceedings of the National Academy of Sciences, USA*, **68**, 1542.

79 Axelrad A.A., McLeod D.L., Shreeve H.M. & Heath D.A. (1974) Properties of cells that produce erythrocytic colonies *in vitro*. In: *Hemopoiesis in Culture* (ed. Robinson W.), p. 226. U.S. Government Printing Office, Washington.

80 Iscove N.N. & Sieber, F. (1975) Erythroid progenitors in mouse bone marrow detected by macroscopic colony formation in culture. *Experimental Hematology*, **3**, 32.

81 Gregory C.J., McCulloch E.A. & Till J.E. (1973) Erythropoietic progenitors capable of colony formation in culture: state of differentiation. *Journal of Cellular Physiology*, **81**, 411.

82 Gregory C.J. & Eaves A.C. (1978) Three stages of erythropoietic progenitor cell differentiation distinguished by a number of physical and biologic properties. *Blood*, **51**, 527.

83 Iscove N.N. (1978) Regulation of proliferation and maturation of early and late stages of erythroid differentiation. In: *Cell Differentiation and Neoplasia* (ed. Sanders G.F.), p. 195. Raven Press, New York.

84 Testa N.G. (1979) Erythroid progenitor cells: their relevance for the study of haematological disease. *Clinics in Haematology*, **8** (Suppl. 2), 311.

85 Iscove N.N. & Guilbert L.J. (1978) Erythropoietin independence of early erythropoiesis and a two-regulator model of proliferative control in the hemopoietic system. In: *In Vitro Aspects of Erythropoiesis* (ed. Murphy M.L.), p. 3. Springer-Verlag, New York.

86 Wagemaker G. (1978) Cellular and soluble factors influencing the differentiation of primitive erythroid progenitor cells (BFU-E) *in vitro*. In: *In Vitro Aspects of Erythropoeisis* (ed. Murphy M.L.), p. 44. Springer-Verlag, New York.

87 Nathan D.G., Chess L., Hillman D.G., Clarke B., Breard J., Merler E. & Houseman D.E. (1978) Human erythroid burst-forming unit: T cell requirement for proliferation *in vitro*. *Journal of Experimental Medicine*, **147**, 324.

88 Nathan D.G., Hillman D.G., Chess L., Alter B.P., Clarke B.J., Breard J. & Houseman D.E. (1978) Normal erythropoietic helper T cells in congenital hypoplastic (Diamond–Blackfan) anemia. *New England Journal of Medicine*, **298**, 1049.

89 Reissman K.R. & Udupa K.B. (1972) Effect of erythropoietin on erythropoietin-responsive cells. *Journal of Cell and Tissue Kinetics*, **5**, 481.

90 Guzman E. & Lajtha L.G. (1970) Some comparisons of the kinetic properties of femoral and splenic haemopoietic stem cells. *Journal of Cell and Tissue Kinetics*, **3**, 91.

91 Reissman K.R. & Ito K. (1966) Selective eradication of erythropoiesis by actinomycin D as the result of interference with hormonally controlled effector pathway of cell differentiation. *Blood*, **28**, 201.

92 Pluznik D.H. & Sachs L. (1965) The cloning of normal 'mast' cells in tissue culture. *Journal of Cellular and Comparative Physiology*, **66**, 319.

93 Bradley T.R. & Metcalf D. (1966) The growth of mouse bone marrow cells *in vitro*. *Australian Journal of Experimental Biology and Medical Science*, **44**, 287.

94 Senn J.S., McCulloch E.A. & Till J.E. (1967) Comparison of colony-forming ability of normal and leukaemic human marrow in cell culture. *Lancet*, **ii**, 597.

95 McCredie K.B., Hersh E.M. & Freireich E.J. (1971) Cells capable of colony formation in the peripheral blood of man. *Science*, **171**, 293.

96 Kurnick J.E. & Robinson W.A. (1971) Colony growth of human peripheral white blood cells *in vitro*. *Blood*, **37**, 136.

97 Chervenick P.A. & Boggs D.R. (1971) *In vitro* growth of granulocytic and mononuclear cell colonies from blood of normal individuals. *Blood*, **37**, 131.

98 ROBINSON W.A., METCALF D. & BRADLEY T.R. (1967) Stimulation by normal and leukemic mouse sera of colony formation *in vitro* by mouse bone-marrow cells. *Journal of Cellular and Comparative Physiology*, **69**, 83.

99 STANLEY E.R. & METCALF D. (1969) Partial purification and some properties of the factor in normal and leukaemic human urine stimulating mouse bone-marrow colony growth *in vitro*. *Australian Journal of Experimental Biology and Medical Sciences*, **47**, 467.

100 ISCOVE N.N., SENN J.S., TILL J.E. & McCULLOCH E.A. (1971) Colony formation by normal and leukemic human marrow cells in culture: effect of conditional medium from human leukocytes. *Blood*, **37**, 1.

101 FOSTER R., METCALF D., ROBINSON W.A. & BRADLEY T.R. (1968) Bone marrow colony-stimulating activity in human sera. Results of two independent surveys in Buffalo and Melbourne. *British Journal of Haematology*, **15**, 147.

102 CHAN S.H. & METCALF D. (1970) Inhibition of bone marrow colony formation by normal and leukaemic human serum. *Nature (London)*, **227**, 845.

103 METCALF D., CHAN S.H., GUNZ F.W., VINCENT P. & RAVICH R.B.M. (1971) Colony-stimulating factor and inhibitor levels in acute granulocytic leukemia. *Blood*, **38**, 143.

104 RICKARD K.A., SHADDUCK R., HOWARD D.E. & STOHLMAN F., JR (1970) A differential effect of hydroxyurea on hemopoietic stem cell colonies *in vitro* and *in vivo*. *Proceedings of the Society of Experimental Biology and Medicine*, **134**, 152.

105 RICKARD K.A., MORLEY A., HOWARD D. & STOHLMAN F., JR (1971) The *in vitro* colony-forming cell and the response to neutropenia. *Blood*, **37**, 6.

106 BENNETT M., CUDKOWICZ G., FOSTER R.S., JR & METCALF D. (1968) Hemopoietic progenitor cells of W anemic mice studied *in vivo* and *in vitro*. *Journal of Cellular Physiology*, **71**, 211.

107 TESTA N.E.G. & LAJTHA L.G. (1973) Comparison of the kinetics (CFUₛ) and culture (CFU꜀). *British Journal of Haematology*, **24**, 367.

108 WU A.M., SIMINOVITCH L., TILL J.E. & McCULLOCH E.A. (1968) Evidence for a relationship between mouse hemopoietic stem cells and cells forming colonies in culture. *Proceedings of the National Academy of Sciences*, **59**, 1209.

109 ISCOVE N.N., TILL J.E. & McCULLOCH E.A. (1970) The proliferative states of mouse granulopoietic progenitor cells. *Proceedings of the Society of Experimental Biology and Medicine*, **134**, 33.

110 METCALF D. (1979) Detection and analysis of human granulocyte-monocyte precursors using semi-solid cultures. In: *Clinics in Haematology, Vol. 8*, No. 2. p. 263. W. B. Saunders, London.

111 MOORE M.A.S. (1979) Humoral regulation of granulopoiesis. In: *Clinics in Haematology, Vol. 8*, No. 2. p. 287. W. B. Saunders, London.

112 METCALF D., PARKER J., CHESTER M.M. & KINCADE P.W. (1974) Formation of eosinophilic-like granulocytic colonies by mouse bone-marrow cells *in vitro*. *Journal of Cell Physiology*, **84**, 275.

113 JOHNSON G.R., DRESCH C. & METCALF D. (1977) Heterogeneity in human neutrophil, macrophage and eosinophil progenitor cells demonstrated by velocity sedimentation separation. *Blood*, **50**, 823.

114 METCALF D., MACDONALD N.R., ODARTCHENKI N. & SORCHAT B. (1975) Growth of mouse megakaryocyte *in vitro*. *Proceedings of the National Academy of Sciences, USA*, **72**, 1744.

115 McLEOD D.L., SHREEVE M.M. & AXELRAD A.A. (1976) Induction of megakaryocyte colonies with platelet formation *in vitro*. *Nature (London)*, **261**, 492.

116 METCALF D. & WAHREN B. (1968) Bone marrow colony-stimulating activity of sera in infectious mononucleosis. *British Medical Journal*, iii, 99.

117 McNEILL T.A. (1970) Antigenic stimulation of bone marrow colony-forming cell. III. Effect *in vivo*. *Immunology*, **18**, 61.

118 METCALF D. (1971) Acute antigen-induced elevation of serum colony stimulation factor (CSS) levels. *Immunology*, **21**, 427.

119 MORLEY A., RICKARD K.A., HOWARD D. & STOHLMAN F., JR (1971) Studies on the regulation of granulopoiesis. Possible humoral regulation. *Blood*, **37**, 14.

120 METCALF D. & STANLEY E.R. (1971) Haematological effects of mice of partially purified colony-stimulating factor (CSF) prepared from human urine. *British Journal of Haematology*, **21**, 481.

121 CRADDOCK C.G., JR, ADAMS W.S., PERRY S., SKOOG W.A. & LAWRENCE J.S. (1955) Studies of leukopoiesis. The technique of leukopheresis and the response of myeloid tissue in normal and irradiated dogs. *Journal of Laboratory and Clinical Medicine*, **45**, 881.

122 BIERMAN H.R., KELLY K.H., BYRON R.L. & MARSHALL G.J. (1961) Leucapheresis in man. I. Haematological observations following leucocyte withdrawal in patients with non-haematological disorders. *British Journal of Haematology*, **7**, 51.

123 GORDON A.S., NERI R.O., SIEGEL C.D., DORNFEST B.S., HANDLER E.S., LoBUE J. & EISLER M. (1960) Evidence for a circulating leucocytosis inducing factor (LIF). *Acta Haematologica*, **23**, 323.

124 KATZ R., GORDON A.S. & LAPIN D.M. (1966) Mechanisms of leukocyte production and release. VI. Studies on the purification of the leucocytosis-inducing factor. *Journal of the Reticulo-endothelial Society*, **3**, 103.

125 LORD B.I., TESTA N.G., WRIGHT E.G. & BANERJEE R.K. (1977) Lack of effect of a granulocyte proliferation inhibitor on their committed precursor cells. *Biomedicine*, **26**, 163.

126 VINCENT P.C. (1977) Granulocyte kinetics in health and disease. *Clinics in Haematology, Vol. 6*, No. 3. p. 695. W. B. Saunders, London.

127 CRONKITE E.P. (1979) Kinetics of granulocytopoiesis. In: *Clinics in Haematology, Vol. 8*, No. 2. p. 351. W. B. Saunders, London.

128 MILLER R.G. & PHILLIPS R.A. (1975) Development of B lymphocytes. *Federation Proceedings*, **34**, 145.

129 MICKLEM H.S. (1979) B lymphocytes, T lymphocytes and lymphopoiesis. *Clinics in Haematology, Vol. 8*, No. 2. p. 395. W. B. Saunders, London.

130 TRUJILLO J.M. & OHNO S. (1963) Chromosomal alteration of erythropoietic cells in chronic myeloid leukaemia. *Acta Haematologica*, **29**, 311.

131 PHILLIPS R.B. & JONES E. (personal communication).

132 PRCHAL J.T., THROCKMORTON D.W., CAROL A.J. III., FUSON E.W., GAMS R.A. & PRCHAL J.F. (1978). A common progenitor for human myeloid and lymphoid cells. *Nature (London)*, **274**, 590.

133 METCALF D. & MOORE M.A.S. (1971) Haemopoietic cells. *Frontiers of Biology, 24*. North Holland, Amsterdam.

134 METCALF D. (1977) *Hemopoietic Colonies.* p. 277. Springer-Verlag, Berlin, Heidelberg, New York.

135 MILLER R.G. & PRICE G.B. (1979) Cell separation and surface markers. In: *Clinics in Haematology, Vol. 8, No. 2.* p. 421. W. B. Saunders, London.

136 GREAVES M.F. (1975) Clinical application of cell surface markers. In: *Progress in Hematology, Vol. 9* (ed. Brown G.B.), p. 255. Grune and Stratton, New York.

137 VAN DEN ENGH G.J. & GOLUB E.S. (1974) Antigenic differences between hemopoietic stem cells and myeloid precursors. *Journal of Experimental Medicine*, **139**, 1621.

138 VAN DEN ENGH G.J., RUSSELL J. & DECICCO D. (1978) Surface antigens of hemopoietic stem cells: the expression of BAS, Thy-1, and H-2 antigens on CFU-S. In: *Experimental Hematology Today 1978* (ed. Baum S.J. & Ledney G.D.), p. 9. Springer-Verlag, New York.

139 KÖHLER G. & MILSTEIN C. (1975) Continuous cultures of fused cells secreting antibody of predefined specificity. *Nature (London)*, **256**, 495.

Chapter 3
Developmental haemopoiesis

W. G. WOOD

Haemopoiesis in the developing fetus follows the same general pattern as that in the adult (described in the previous chapter), in which the erythrocytic, granulocytic and megakaryocytic cell lineages are all derived from a common pluripotential stem cell. Nevertheless, differences are imposed upon this scheme by the fact that the intrauterine stages of development are marked by rapid growth, and in order to maintain sufficient numbers of both stem cells and their differentiated progeny during this period, haemopoiesis must be considerably accelerated relative to the steady-state condition of normal adult life.

Developmental changes in haemopoiesis are particularly marked in the erythroid cells. In view of the changes in the availability of oxygen in embryonic, fetal and postnatal life it is not surprising that the characteristics of fetal erythrocytes show marked differences from their adult counterparts and that changes in the pattern of production should accompany birth.

In this chapter the features of normal haemopoiesis which are characteristic of the fetal and neonatal periods are presented and contrasted with the situation in normal adults. Haematological problems particularly associated with the perinatal period are discussed elsewhere in their appropriate chapters.

DEVELOPMENTAL CHANGES IN ERYTHROPOIESIS

Sites of erythropoiesis
The pre-implantation embryo obtains oxygen by diffusion and it has been calculated that once the thickness of the embryo exceeds 0·3 mm, this process is inadequate and that a circulatory system is essential to maintain respiration *in utero* [1]. Erythropoiesis in the human fetus begins in the second to third week after conception by the formation of blood islands, mainly in the area vasculosa of the yolk sac [2]. By analogy with blood island formation in the chick and mouse, it is likely that this process of differentiation requires the

intimate association of mesodermal and endodermal tissues [3, 4], and results in the production of tight clusters of basophilic cells which continue to divide and mature until they resemble early erythroblasts. As haemoglobin synthesis begins, the cells become polychromatic and enter the newly formed circulatory system during the third week of gestation, when the heart starts pumping. Proliferation and maturation of these cells continues in the circulation until they are fully haemoglobinized macrocytes with a highly condensed nucleus, which is retained within the cell. In the chick and mouse these primitive red cells develop as a fairly well synchronized cohort of cells with a limited lifespan and no self-renewal capability. In all species which have been examined, the primitive red cells produced during yolk-sac erythropoiesis contain haemoglobins which are largely or totally restricted to this period of development, the embryonic haemoglobins.

These differences in the morphological features, self-renewal capability and haemoglobin content separate the primitive red cells of yolk-sac origin from the definitive red cells which replace them when erythropoiesis shifts to intraembryonic sites. As pointed out by Ingram [5], the crucial question in terms of understanding the determination event in this process is the relationship of the precursor cells of these two lines. Both primitive and definitive line cells may have diverged from a common pluripotent stem cell, with the primitive cell line developing as a single cohort while the definitive cell line retains its self-renewal capabilities. Alternatively the stem cells which produce the primitive line cells may themselves be precursors of the definitive line stem cells. Numerous experiments have been carried out in chicks and in mice in attempts to answer this question and at the present time the results are equivocal [6–10]. It appears that pluripotent haemopoietic cells are present within chick embryos (but perhaps not in mouse embryos) prior to the development of the circulation but that once a circulatory system is established there is migration of stem cells between the embryo proper and the yolk sac in both directions. The intraembryonic stem cells may not, however, reside in the future haemopoietic sites but migrate there from other sites in the embryo, although migration from the yolk sac by an interstitial route has not been excluded.

The liver is the major site of erythropoiesis during most of fetal life in man, taking over from the yolk sac during the fifth week of gestation [2, 11, 12]. The earliest recognizable erythroid cells develop extravascularly among the mesenchyme cells but in intimate contact with the endodermal epithelium. By the eighth week of gestation, cells at all stages of erythroid maturation are present and at the height of hepatic erythropoiesis erythroid cells may comprise up to 50% of the cells in the fetal liver [15]. Although pluripotent stem cells and granulocyte precursor cells (CFU-C) are present in the liver during this erythroid phase (at least in the mouse [6]), there is no evidence of granulopoiesis. Occasional foci of megakaryopoiesis have been observed in human fetal liver [2, 11]. This restriction to largely erythropoiesis is presumably under localized control since differentiation along all three haemopoietic cell lines occurs contemporaneously in the bone marrow.

In addition to hepatic erythropoiesis, secondary sites of red-cell production are found in the thymus, kidney, various connective tissues and the spleen [2]. Splenic erythropoiesis occurs extravascularly and begins at about the same time as hepatic red-cell production [13]. The relative contribution of the spleen and other secondary sites of erythropoiesis to the total red-cell production is unknown but is probably quite small. Towards term, erythropoiesis declines in the liver but persists until shortly after birth [14]. During the last trimester, the fetal bone marrow begins to assume the major role. Haemopoiesis begins in the bone marrow as early as nine to 11 weeks' gestation [2, 16], and erythroid, myeloid and lymphoid cells are fairly equally represented [16]. Later in gestation the proportion of lymphocytes present is much lower and between 30 weeks' gestation and term, erythroid cells account for about 40% and myeloid cells for 40–50% of the total [17].

Control of erythropoiesis in fetal life
Little is known about the control of haemopoiesis and erythropoiesis in fetal life. During the rapid growth of the fetus, there is a demand to increase the size of the stem-cell compartment, while at the same time increasing numbers of terminally differentiated cells must be produced. The kinetics of this process are not understood since we know very little about the rates of production and destruction of red cells during this period. It is clear, however, from animal studies that a much higher proportion of pluripotent stem cells are in

cycle in the fetus than in the adult [18–20]. A shorter cell-cycle time of the committed erythroid precursor cells (BFU-E and CFU-E) is implied by the production of haemoglobinized colonies in culture earlier than their adult counterparts, at similar or lower erythropoietin concentrations, a phenomenon which has been observed in several animal species [21–23] as well as in man [24, 25].

It is not known at present whether the increased rate of erythropoiesis in the fetus is accompanied by increased levels of erythropoietin or whether the erythroid precursor cells show increased sensitivity to the hormone. The sensitivity of current assays of erythropoietin in serum may not be sufficient to detect an increased level in the fetus compared to normal adult values. Nevertheless, it seems clear that the erythroid cells of the human fetus are responsive to erythropoietin. The hormone has been detected in the cord blood of full-term and premature newborns [26, 27], although these may be elevated by hypoxia during delivery [22]. Increased levels are found in hypoxic human newborns whether the hypoxia is due to fetal anaemia, placental dysfunction or maternal hypoxaemia [28].

Studies in animals have shown that fetal erythropoiesis is independently regulated. Hypertransfusion of pregnant mice failed to decrease fetal erythropoiesis [29], while administration of large doses of erythropoietin to pregnant rats failed to stimulate fetal erythropoiesis [30]. Similar results have been obtained in sheep and goats [22], in which it has also been shown that bleeding of catheterized fetuses results in increased fetal erythropoietin levels but no demonstrable transfer across the placenta [31]. Although fetal erythropoiesis is independently controlled, it is sensitive to changes in the maternal circulation which affect its oxygen supply. Indeed, goat fetuses appear to be more sensitive, or respond more rapidly, to maternal phlebotomy; erythropoietin becoming detectable in the fetal circulation after 15 minutes but not until 15 hours in the maternal serum [22, 32].

It also appears that in the fetus, the site of erythropoietin production may differ from the adult. Bilateral nephrectomy of fetal goats [32] or newborn rats [33, 34] failed to reduce erythropoietin production in response to bleeding. This could be achieved though by subtotal hepatectomy [22, 34], implicating the liver as the major site of erythropoietin production in the fetus. As in the adult, erythropoietin production in the sheep fetus is enhanced by testosterone and thyroxin [35]. The change over to the kidney as the major site of erythropoietin production occurs after birth. It is not known whether a similar change of site also occurs in man, but infants with renal agenesis are not anaemic.

NORMAL ERYTHROID PARAMETERS DURING DEVELOPMENT

Intrauterine life

The changes in haemoglobin level, haematocrit and red-cell count during human fetal development have been reported by several authors [36–40] although naturally there is a shortage of data between 22 and 34 weeks' gestation. The results are summarized in Table 3.1.

At 10 weeks' gestation the haemoglobin level is around 10 g/dl and over the next 12 weeks this rises steadily to about 14 g/dl. This level appears to remain relatively constant since at 34 weeks the level is around 15 g/dl after which it increases again to reach the normal cord blood level of about 17 g/dl (Fig. 3.1). The red-cell count follows the haemoglobin level, increasing from around $1 \cdot 0 – 1 \cdot 5 \times 10^{12}/l$ at 10 weeks' gestation to around $4 \cdot 5 \times 10^{12}/l$ at term. The red-cell count shows a greater increase between 22 and 34 weeks than the haemoglobin level due to the decrease in the MCH during this period (see below). The haematocrit shows a similar pattern but with a wider scatter of values reported.

During intrauterine development the size of the red cells produced decreases, with a sharp drop from about

Table 3.1. Mean red-cell values during gestation (from Ref. 40, with permission)

Age (in weeks)	Hb (gm/100 ml)	Haematocrit (%)	RBC (10^6/cu.mm)	Mean corpusc. vol. (fl)	Mean corpusc. Hb (pg)	Mean corpusc. Hb conc. (%)	Nuc. RBC (% of RBCs)	Retic. (%)	Diam. (μm)
12	8·0–10·0	33	1·5	180	60	34	5·0–8·0	40	10·5
16	10·0	35	2·0	140	45	33	2·0–4·0	10–25	9·5
20	11·0	37	2·5	135	44	33	1·0	10–20	9·0
24	14·0	40	3·5	123	38	31	1·0	5–10	8·8
28	14·5	45	4·0	120	40	31	0·5	5–10	8·7
34	15·0	47	4·4	118	38	32	0·2	3–10	8·5

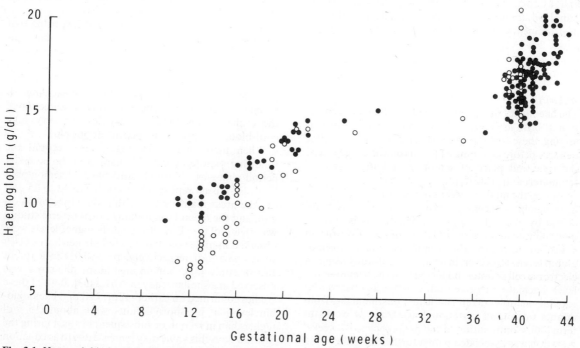

Fig. 3.1. Haemoglobin levels in the human fetus during gestation. The data are combined from Refs 38 (●) and 39 (○).

200 fl to 130 fl between 10 and 24 weeks' gestation (although the earliest samples probably include the macrocytic, primitive erythroid cells) and then declines more gradually to reach normal cord blood levels of 110–120 fl. There is concomitant drop in the mean cell haemoglobin from about 60 pg to 35–40 pg, such that the MCHC remains relatively constant throughout this period (Table 3.1).

Nucleated RBC may constitute up to 10% of erythroid cells in the peripheral blood at 10 weeks' gestation, decreasing to around one per cent at 20 weeks. The number of nucleated cells continues to drop reaching about 0·01% at term. The reticulocyte count shows a similar decrease, from about 40% at 10 weeks reaching five to 10% by 20 weeks and three to seven per cent at term. It is not possible from the above information to gain an accurate picture of the rate of red-cell production during gestation since we have no information about the blood volume, red-cell mass or red-cell lifespan during this period. Approximate estimates based on the limited information available, however, suggest that the absolute number of new red cells produced per day rises throughout gestation but when expressed as the rate of red-cell production/kg body weight or /red-cell mass, such calculations give highest values early in gestation and decline with development [41]. When the rate of red-cell production has been measured at term, based either on the number and lifespan of reticulocytes [42], the kinetics of radioiron uptake into red cells and plasma [43] or by measurements of the red-cell mass [44], a figure of about 2·5–3·5% of the red-cell mass/day is obtained, about three to five times the rate of an adult in the steady state.

At birth
The haemoglobin, haematocrit and red-cell concentration at birth are affected by various factors. Principal among these are the gestational age, the time after delivery before clamping of the umbilical-cord vessels, the time and place of sampling and the degree of fetomaternal transfusions.

During the final two weeks of development the mean haemoglobin concentration has been reported to increase by about 1–3 g/dl [37, 45]. If this is correct, uncertainties in the gestational age of the newborn will contribute to the variability in the cord blood haemoglobin levels. However, in a more recent study using an electronic cell counter, no increase in the haemoglobin level, haematocrit or red-cell count was observed in capillary samples taken on the first postnatal day from infants ranging in gestational age from 24 weeks to term [46]. Continuation of the pregnancy to 42 weeks' gestation was associated with a further increase of 1–5 g/dl in the study of Walker & Turnbull [37], but was not observed by Marks *et al.* [47], or Rooth & Sjöstedt [45].

At birth, one-quarter to one-third of the fetal blood volume is contained in the placental and cord vessels, but at the end of the first minute about one-half of this is transfused to the newborn [48, 49]. Delayed clamping of the cord therefore results in a higher red-cell mass and haemoglobin concentration. At 72 hours of age, infants with immediate cord clamping had a red-cell mass of 31 ml/kg compared to 49 ml/kg in infants with delayed clamping [48, 49].

The site of blood sampling at birth also affects the results since capillary samples give a consistently higher haemoglobin concentration than cord blood or venous samples. The difference is generally of the order of five to 10% but may be occasionally much higher (see Ref. 40). The difference between venous blood and capillary samples is greater in infants with delayed cord clamping [50] suggesting that transudation of the plasma from a sluggish circulation may be responsible for the difference. Venous blood sampling in the first few hours after birth shows a rise in haemoglobin concentration compared with cord blood levels. In part this also depends upon the size of the placental transfusion since the total blood volume of the infant adjusts rapidly by decreasing the plasma volume and hence increasing the red-cell and haemoglobin concentration [48, 50, 51]. However, even with immediate cord clamping some increase in haemoglobin can be observed over the first eight hours [51].

As a result of these factors, it is not surprising that the normal values for cord-blood haemoglobin concentration show wide variability. While most values fall within the range of 14–20 g/dl, more extreme values are occasionally observed. It has been suggested that in these cases there is an abnormally large exchange of blood between the fetus and its mother, the direction of the exchange resulting in very low or very high cord-blood haemoglobin concentrations [40].

When these factors are taken into account the following picture of red-cell changes in the neonatal period emerges. Normal cord-blood haemoglobin levels have been reported to range from 12 to 25 g/dl but the great majority fall within the range of 14–20 g/dl, and the mean level obtained over several studies was 16·8 g/dl (see Ref. 40). Slightly higher levels were observed in male compared to female newborns (16·9 versus 16·5 g/dl respectively, $p = <0·01$) in a recent British study [52], but no significant difference was observed in a similar study in Africa [53]. Both of these studies confirmed an earlier report [54] that haemoglobin levels in first-born infants were about 0·5 g/dl higher than in second or subsequent births. During the first few days this value may increase due to a reduction in the plasma volume, particularly in infants with delayed clamping of the cord, but thereafter remains relatively constant during the first week of life. The haematocrit and red-cell count show similar changes, increasing during the first few hours and declining to the cord blood level by the end of the first week (Table 3.2).

At birth the reticulocyte count is generally within the range of two to seven per cent with a mean of about five per cent [40, 42, 46, 55]. This level is maintained over the first three days but then decreases abruptly and the proportion is normally less than one per cent at the end of the first week. Nucleated red blood cells (largely late normoblasts) are also normally present in cord blood at a level of about $5 \times 10^8/l$, or about one per 10 000 erythrocytes. Values expressed as a percentage of the white cells are of little value because of the great variability in the white-cell count. Nucleated red cells disappear by the fourth day of life in normal infants.

The red cells at birth are considerably larger than those of normal adults and display a much greater variability in their size distribution. The average mean cell volume is about 118 fl [37, 56], but the normal range may be as great as 105–130 fl. The average MCH is about 37 pg, also higher than in adult cells so that the MCHC is similar in the newborn and adult. The red-cell indices measured with electronic cell counters tend to be rather higher than those obtained by manual methods.

Along with most of the other haematological parameters at birth, the blood volume also shows great variability. In normal full-term infants during the first day of life, values ranging from 50 to 100 ml/kg have been obtained [48, 57] with a mean of about 85 ml/kg, slightly higher than the mean adult values of 77 ml/kg. Again, delayed clamping of the cord results in higher values [48], and the blood volume is positively correlated with the haematocrit [57]. The red-cell volume shows similar variability with values ranging from 23 to 58 ml/kg with a mean of 42 ml/kg [57]. Its relationship to the haematocrit can be simply expressed as: red-cell mass (ml/kg) = venous haematocrit − 12, with a standard error of about 10% [58].

In premature infants the blood volume/kg body weight tends to be somewhat higher than in full-term newborns, largely due to an increased plasma volume, since the red-cell volume remains largely unchanged [59, 60].

The red-cell lifespan of premature and full-term neonates has been measured by a variety of techniques including the differential agglutination technique of Ashby, the disappearance of red cells labelled with ^{51}Cr, [^{32}P]DFP or ^{59}Fe and by the disappearance of fetal haemoglobin containing erythrocytes transfused into adults. Each of these techniques has its inherent problems and limitations of sensitivity. In addition there are problems of interpreting the results since the increased rate of red-cell production prior to birth

Table 3.2. Red-cell indices in the first 12 weeks of life (from Ref. 56, with permission)

Age	No. of cases	Hb gm/dl ±S.D.	RBC × 10¹²/l ±S.D.	HCT (%) ±S.D.	MCV fl ±S.D.	MCHC (%) ±S.D.	Retic. (%) ±S.D.
Days							
1	19	19·3±2·2	5·14±0·7	61±7·4	119±9·4	31·6±1·9	3·2±1·4
2	19	19·0±1·9	5·15±0·8	60±6·4	115±7·0	31·6±1·4	3·2±1·3
3	19	18·8±2·0	5·11±0·7	62±9·3	116±5·3	31·1±2·8	2·8±1·7
4	10	18·6±2·1	5·00±0·6	57±8·1	114±7·5	32·6±1·5	1·8±1·1
5	12	17·6±1·1	4·97±0·4	57±7·3	114±8·9	30·9±2·2	1·2±0·2
6	15	17·4±2·2	5·00±0·7	54±7·2	113±10·0	32·2±1·6	0·6±0·2
7	12	17·9±2·5	4·86±0·6	56±9·4	118±11·2	32·0±1·6	0·5±0·4
Weeks							
1–2	32	17·3±2·3	4·80±0·8	54±8·3	112±19·0	32·1±2·9	0·5±0·3
2–3	11	15·6±2·6	4·20±0·6	46±7·3	111±8·2	33·9±1·9	0·8±0·6
3–4	17	14·2±2·1	4·00±0·6	43±5·7	105±7·5	33·5±1·6	0·6±0·3
4–5	15	12·7±1·6	3·60±0·4	36±4·8	101±8·1	34·9±1·6	0·9±0·8
5–6	10	11·9±1·5	3·55±0·2	36±6·2	102±10·2	34·1±2·9	1·0±0·7
6–7	10	12·0±1·5	3·40±0·4	36±4·8	105±12·0	33·8±2·3	1·2±0·7
7–8	17	11·1±1·1	3·40±0·4	33±3·7	100±2·6	33·7±2·6	1·5±0·7
8–9	13	10·7±0·9	3·40±0·5	31±2·5	93±12·0	34·1±2·2	1·8±1·0
9–10	12	11·2±0·9	3·60±0·3	32±2·7	91±9·3	34·3±2·9	1·2±0·6
10–11	11	11·4±0·9	3·70±0·4	34±2·1	91±7·7	33·2±2·4	1·2±0·7
11–12	13	11·3±0·9	3·70±0·3	33±3·3	88±7·9	34·8±2·2	0·7±0·3

leads to a higher proportion of young cells in the cord blood. Unless this factor is taken into account, values for the red-cell lifespan in this period will tend to be overestimated. Partly because of these problems, the results of the various studies on red-cell lifespan in neonates have shown wide variability and sometimes conflicting results. Nevertheless, the overall picture which has emerged from these studies (reviewed in Refs 40, 61, 62) appears to have produced a consensus agreement that the red cells of the newborn have a considerably shortened survival, perhaps as low as 45–70 days.

Similar studies on premature newborns are less numerous, but in four studies involving a total of 26 infants, the half life of ^{51}Cr-tagged cells range from 10 to 20 days (mean 16 d) compared to a normal adult range of about 25–33 days as measured by these techniques [63–66]. In a further study of 33 premature infants a mean ^{51}Cr half-life of 22 days was obtained [67]. There seems little doubt therefore that the red cells produced at earlier stages in gestation have clearly shortened survival times.

The red cells formed after birth appear to have a lifespan similar to that of adult red cells [68, 69].

The red-cell picture during the first few weeks after birth
Following the transient changes in haemoglobin, haematocrit and red-cell levels immediately after birth, there is a steady decline in these parameters during the first two months of life in healthy full-term newborns (Table 3.2). The nadir is reached at about seven to nine weeks, at which stage the haemoglobin level has fallen to 9·5–11 g/dl, the haematocrit to 30–33%, and the red-cell count to about $3·4 \times 10^{12}$/l [56, 70, 72]. This decline is matched by the reticulocyte count which remains at less than one per cent from the end of the first week until about six weeks postnatally [42, 56]. Examination of the bone marrow shows that erythroid-cell precursors decline sharply during the first week [71, 72] matched by a decrease in the uptake of radioactive iron into haemoglobin [73]. Erythropoietin levels become undetectable during this period [26, 74]

and it has also been suggested that inhibitors of erythropoiesis might be produced [75].

The sharp decline in erythropoietic activity following birth is accepted as a physiological adaptation to the greater availability of oxygen following birth. Together with the shortened red-cell survival at this time and the increasing haemodilution due to growth, the reduced rate of red-cell production accounts for the decrease in haemoglobin concentration and the decline in the red-cell mass. As discussed later, however, oxygen delivery to the tissues actually increases during this period due to a shift in the oxygen dissociation curve. The newborn is capable of responding to increased demand during the first few weeks, and anaemic or hypoxic infants do not show the decrease in marrow erythroid activity seen in normal newborns [72] and continue to produce detectable levels of erythropoietin [26, 76]. Furthermore, the level to which the haemoglobin falls does not depend on the initial cord blood level. Both high and low normal haemoglobin concentrations decline to about 10–11 g/dl before recovery begins [47].

In premature infants the decline in haemoglobin level and red-cell count during the first few weeks of life tends to occur earlier and more rapidly, decreasing to levels of about 6·5–9·0 g/dl (Table 3.3) [70, 77, 78]. Plasma erythropoietin levels in normal premature infants measured by the *in-vivo* polycythaemic-mouse assay were undetectable at the time when the haemoglobin levels were at their nadir [76, 79]. However, by radioimmunoassay (a technique which is more sensitive but which measures both biologically active and inactive forms of the hormone) a significant inverse correlation was found between plasma erythropoietin levels and either haemoglobin concentration or oxygen-unloading capacity of the blood in 45 premature infants, although the hormone levels were considerably less than would be expected for similar degrees of anaemia in older individuals [80]. These data suggest that the premature newborn responds appropriately to the decreased level of haemoglobin and that, as in the full-term neonate, the early anaemia of prematurity is

Table 3.3. Serial haemoglobin values in low-birth-weight infants (from Ref. 78, with permission)

Birth Weight (g)	Age (weeks)				
	2	4	6	8	10
800–1000	16·0 (14·8–17·2)	10·0 (6·8–13·2)	8·7 (7·0–10·2)	8·0 (7·1–9·8)	8·0 (6·9–10·2)
1001–1200	16·4 (14·1–18·7)	12·8 (7·8–15·3)	10·5 (7·2–12·3)	9·1 (7·8–10·4)	8·5 (7·0–10·0)
1201–1400	16·2 (13·6–18·8)	13·4 (8·8–13·3)	10·9 (8·5–13·3)	9·9 (8·0–11·8)	9·8 (8·4–11·3)
1401–1500	15·6 (13·4–17·8)	11·7 (9·7–13·7)	10·5 (9·1–11·9)	9·8 (8·4–12·0)	9·9 (8·4–11·4)
1501–2000	15·6 (13·5–17·7)	11·0 (9·6–14·0)	9·6 (8·8–11·5)	9·8 (8·4–12·1)	10·1 (8·6–11·8)

physiological. However, among the most premature infants, particularly these born before 32 weeks' gestation, clinical consequences of this anaemia may develop [81].

Although deficiencies of iron, folic acid, vitamin B_{12} and vitamin E can aggravate the degree of anaemia in premature infants, the lack of these nutritional factors does not normally play a major role in the decline in haemoglobin levels [78, 82, 83]. In the majority of cases, premature infants do not have low serum iron or decreased transferrin saturation and do not respond to the early administration of oral iron [84]. Preterm babies are, however, at risk of developing iron deficiency anaemia after five to six months (the so-called late anaemia of prematurity) since the major iron source of the newborn resides in haemoglobin [82]. The red-cell mass of premature infants may not be sufficient to provide an adequate iron supply after erythropoiesis resumes and although iron is absorbed from breast milk more readily than from artificial formulas [85, 86], supplemental iron may be necessary [87].

The reasons for the greater drop in haemoglobin in premature compared with full-term infants are still not clear. It has been ascribed [78, 82] to lower oxygen consumption by the preterm babies, in turn related to a reduced respiratory quotient and metabolic rate. However, measurements of oxygen consumption have produced contradictory results with some studies supporting this hypothesis [88–91], while others have observed higher levels of oxygen consumption in preterm infants [92, 93].

The erythroid precursor content of the bone marrow remains low for about three to four weeks [71, 72] but there is a further delay in the recovery of the peripheral red-cell count and haemoglobin level, as the rate of red-cell destruction continues to exceed production and continued growth results in expansion of the blood volume. By eight to 12 weeks after birth, however, erythropoietin is once more detectable in the serum [27, 74], the marrow erythroid content has increased to adult proportions [72] and the haemoglobin level begins to rise.

Haemoglobin and red-cell indices in infancy and childhood

The postnatal decline in haemoglobin concentration levels off at about two to three months and then increases slightly by six months of age to a mean level

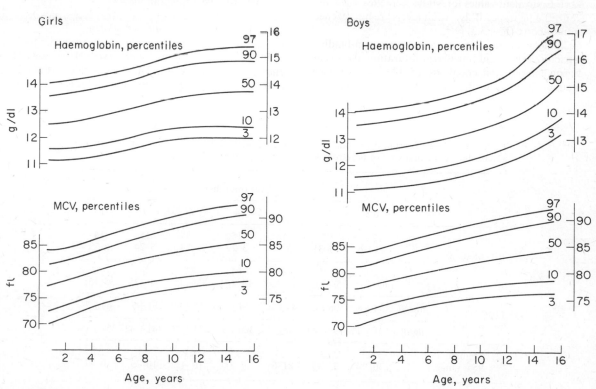

Fig. 3.2. Haemoglobin and MCV percentile curves for girls and boys during childhood (from Ref. 95, with permission).

of about 12·5 g/dl in normal infants in whom iron deficiency has been excluded [94]. This level is maintained until about two years of age and then shows a gradual increase up to puberty (Fig. 3.2) [95]. At the onset of puberty the haemoglobin level reaches a plateau in girls but continues to rise in boys, the haematocrit being related to the degree of sexual maturity [95, 96]. In determining normal haemoglobin values during childhood, racial differences must also be borne in mind, since it has been shown that Negro children consistently show mean haemoglobin levels which are about 0·5–1·0 g/dl lower than Caucasian or Oriental children [97, 98], a difference which is maintained into adult life and which does not appear to depend on social or nutritional status [99].

In addition to the changes in haemoglobin and red-cell levels during childhood, changes in the MCV and MCH have also been demonstrated in children in whom iron deficiency and thalassaemia had been excluded [100]. The MCV and MCH continue to fall during the first year of life with a mean level (± 2 SD) of 77 ± 7 fl in infants aged 10–17 months rising slightly to 81 ± 5 fl in children between 1·5 and seven years of age. Approximately half of the children in this later age group fall below the lower limit of normal for adults of 80 fl. Equivalent values for MCH were $26 \cdot 1 \pm 2 \cdot 8$ and $27 \cdot 6 \pm 3 \cdot 4$ pg respectively. Adult levels are not reached until puberty (Fig. 3.2) [95].

Changes in the serum iron, total iron-binding capacity (TIBC) and transferrin saturation also occur during infancy and childhood (Table 3.4) (see also Chapter 5). At birth the serum iron level shows wide variability and is correlated with the maternal level [53]. During the first six months the mean level drops from 22 μmol/l to 14 μmol/l (range 5–24 μmol/l), during which time there is a rise in the TIBC from 34 to 60 μmol/l. Thus the transferrin saturation decreases from about 70% at birth to about 25% by six months of age [101]. During childhood the serum iron and transferrin saturation level gradually rise, reaching adult levels at puberty [102].

DEVELOPMENTAL CHANGES IN ERYTHROCYTE CHARACTERISTICS

The differences in the sites and kinetics of erythropoiesis during normal development are accompanied by marked differences in the mature erythrocytes which are produced. These include the changes in the red-cell size and lifespan discussed in the previous section, as well as differences in membrane function, antigenic properties and metabolism between fetal and adult red cells. The major difference between the cell types, of course, lies in the types of haemoglobin produced. These changes are discussed in detail in Chapter 8 and only the major points need be summarized here to give an overall view.

Developmental changes in haemoglobins

In the earliest human embryos examined, three embryonic haemoglobins are observed—Hbs Gower 1 and 2 and Hb Portland. These haemoglobins disappear by about 12 weeks' gestation and it is likely that

Table 3.4. Values of serum iron, total iron-binding capacity and transferrin saturation in 47 infants during the first year of life (from Ref. 101, with permission)

		Age (months)						
		0·5	1	2	4	6	9	12
SI Median 95% range	μmol/l	22 11–36	22 10–31	16 3–29	15 3–29	14 5–24	15 6–24	14 6–28
	μg/dl	120 63–201	125 58–172	87 15–159	84 18–164	77 28–135	84 34–135	78 35–155
TIBC (mean$\pm$SD)	μmol/l	34 ± 8	36 ± 8	44 ± 10	54 ± 7	58 ± 9	61 ± 7	64 ± 7
	μg/dl	191 ± 43	199 ± 43	246 ± 55	300 ± 39	321 ± 51	341 ± 42	358 ± 38
S% Median 95% range		68 30–99	63 35–94	34 21–63	27 7–53	23 10–43	25 10–39	23 10–47

SI = Serum iron; TIBC = total iron-binding capacity; S% = transferrin saturation.

they are largely, if not totally, restricted to the erythrocyte population of yolk-sac origin. The Hb F is also present in blood from embryos of six to 12 weeks' gestation but since both primitive and definitive line cells are present at this stage it is not clear whether Hb F (or even Hb A) is present in the yolk-sac cells.

From the inception of hepatic erythropoiesis, Hb F ($\alpha_2\gamma_2$) forms the major haemoglobin throughout intra-uterine life. However, there is about five to 10% of the major adult haemoglobin Hb A ($\alpha_2\beta_2$) produced during this period also. The intercellular distribution of these haemoglobins has not been studied in detail during this period although it appears that Hb A is present in most, if not all, of the red cells but that the amount may vary from cell to cell [103, 104]. At about 32–36 weeks' gestation, the proportion of Hb A increases, matched by a concomitant decline in Hb F production. The decrease in Hb F occurs fairly sharply at first and by three months after birth accounts for less than 10% of the newly synthesized haemoglobin. Thereafter, the decline continues more slowly and adult levels of Hb F (less than one per cent) may not be reached until the end of the first year of life or even later. The minor adult haemoglobin, Hb A_2, is detectable at birth and reaches its adult level of about 2·5% by about six months of age [105, 106].

The cellular and molecular basis of this change-over is the subject of much current interest [107, 108]. However, studies on haemoglobin synthesis and the intracellular distribution of Hbs F and A during the neonatal period have not produced a clear picture of events at the cellular level during this period. Interpretation of the results are complicated by the very low level of erythropoiesis immediately after birth, with few red cells being produced during a critical part of the switching period. This may explain why the decline in Hb F after birth has been attributed to an abrupt transition to Hb A production [109], and why the intercellular distribution of the two haemoglobins in infants over two months of age appears to demonstrate their presence in distinct populations of red cells [110]. In contrast, measurements of haemoglobin synthesis during the switchover period have suggested a gradual replacement of Hb F by Hb A [111, 112], and this is supported by the demonstration that up to 50% of the cells in young infants appear to contain appreciable amounts of both haemoglobins [110, 113–115].

Changes in red-cell metabolism during development
The metabolism of human embryonic red cells or red cells from the early stages of fetal development have not been studied but cord-blood erythrocytes from full-term and premature infants have been extensively examined and show many differences from adult red cells. Studies of this nature require careful interpretation, however, since apparent differences in enzyme activities may simply reflect the younger mean red-cell age of cord blood. The activities of many enzymes decline with red-cell age, and comparisons can only be made with adult cells of comparable age. Electrophoresis of red-cell enzymes from fetal material has failed to identify any specific isozymes associated with this stage of development, and although the intensities of various isozymes of enolase, guanylate kinase, hexokinase, lactate dehydrogenase, nucleoside phosphorylase and phosphofructokinase differ between fetal and adult red cells; this has been attributed to the differences in the age structure of the red cells [116].

Glycolysis
Taking into account the higher proportion of young red cells in cord blood, their rate of glucose consumption is decreased relative to adult cells [117]. Despite this, the activities of four of the glycolytic enzymes, glucose phosphate isomerase, glyceraldehyde-3-phosphate dehydrogenase, phosphoglycerate kinase and enolase, are increased. These enzymes are not believed to be rate-limiting steps in glycolysis, and of the two critical enzymes, the activity of hexokinase is similar to that of adult cells, while that of phosphofructokinase is decreased to about 70% of comparable adult levels [118–120]. That the reduced activity of phosphofructokinase may be responsible for the decreased glycolysis of red cells from newborns is supported by the observation that manipulation of the cells to maximize the activity of this enzyme has a much greater effect on cord-blood cells than on adult cells [121].

Changes in the levels of glycolytic enzymes and intermediates during the first year of life have recently been documented [235, 236] and correlated with the decline in Hb F levels and the plasma inorganic phosphorus content [237].

Newborn and adult red cells also differ in the metabolism of 2,3-diphosphoglycerate (2,3-DPG). This compound plays an important role in modulating the oxygen affinity of Hb A but shows little interaction with Hb F (see following section). In adult cells much of the 2,3-DPG is bound by deoxyhaemoglobin whereas in fetal cells with high levels of Hb F (which has a markedly lowered affinity for 2,3-DPG) relatively little 2,3-DPG is bound to haemoglobin. Nevertheless, the levels of 2,3-DPG are similar in cord blood and adult cells (about 5 μmol/l). This is surprising since 2,3-DPG is a potent inhibitor of its own formation, acting at the level of the DPG-mutase enzyme. Furthermore, incubation of cord cells in air leads to a much more rapid rundown in 2,3-DPG levels than occurs in adult cells, although the mechanism of this is not clear. It has been suggested that it may be due to the relative block in glycolysis resulting from reduced phosphofructokinase activity [122]. Alternatively it has been ascribed to increased flow from 1,3-DPG to 3 phosphoglycerate as a result of the increased activity of phosphoglycerate kinase [123], or to increased breakdown of 2,3-DPG [121, 124]. In the face of this accelerated run-down of 2,3-DPG and the decreased binding to haemoglobin F to reduce feedback inhibition, the high levels in cord-blood cells remain to be explained.

In contrast to glucose metabolism, galactose utilization is higher in the red cells of the newborn than in adult cells, with a considerable increase in galactokinase activity [125].

Pentose-phosphate pathway

The red cells of the newborn are particularly susceptible to oxidant-induced injury, as for instance after the application of oxidant drugs or other compounds liable to increase endogenous peroxide formation [126]. This susceptibility results in glutathione instability, the development of methaemoglobinaemia and Heinz-body formation.

The detoxification of peroxide in adult red cells is accomplished by a series of reactions involving glutathione, whose reduction is dependent on the enzymes glutathione perioxidase and glutathione reductase. These reactions require the presence of NADPH which is generated by the pentose-phosphate pathway (hexose monophosphate shunt) and hence are dependent upon G6PD activity.

The activity of the hexose monophosphate shunt in cord-blood cells appears to be normal and is capable of stimulation by oxidants [127, 128]. The levels of glutathione peroxidase are inappropriately low for the metabolic age of the red cells [128, 131], but no direct relationship between this deficiency and the peroxide sensitivity of newborn red cells has been established. These cells also have reduced levels of methaemoglobin reductase (diaphorase) and catalase, two other enzymes associated with detoxification of oxidized compounds.

It has also been suggested that the reduced level of membrane —SH groups may be a factor in the vulnerability of the red cells at this age [132], possibly accentuated by decreased levels of membrane antioxidants such as vitamin E. It may be the cumulative effect of several deficiencies, rather than one major factor which is responsible for the cells' sensitivity to oxidant damage.

Energy metabolism in newborn red cells

The ATP levels are elevated in cord-blood cells [118, 133, 134], but only to a level consistent with their younger mean cell age. During *in-vitro* incubation of the cells, the levels of ATP decrease, unlike normal adult cells [134], and uptake of orthophosphate into ATP and 2,3-DPG is reduced compared to adult cells [122, 135]. It is not clear whether these changes in metabolism are related to some of the membrane changes described below, such as decreased potassium influx and decreased membrane flexibility, factors which in adult cells are associated with older cells containing lower levels of ATP.

Developmental changes in other red-cell enzymes

Lower levels of catalase [136], acetyl cholinesterase [120, 136, 137] and adenylate kinase [120] have also been reported for cord-blood red cells. In addition, there is a very marked reduction in the two red-cell carbonic anhydrases [138, 139]. Next to haemoglobin, carbonic anhydrase is the most abundant protein found in adult erythrocytes but its levels are very low in fetal life and only begin to increase after 32 weeks' gestation. At birth the activity of the more abundant, but less active, CA I is only five to 15% that of adult levels while CA II activity is about 20–30% that of adult red-cell values. However, these levels seem quite adequate to maintain the normal physiological function.

Membrane structure and function in red cells of the neonate

Structural examination of the red-cell membranes by polyacrylamide gel electrophoresis has shown no gross difference in the major protein and glycoprotein components of newborn and adult red cells [140, 141]. Nevertheless, functional differences in membrane properties have been demonstrated. These include decreased levels of ouabain-sensitive ATPase [142], decreased permeability to non-electrolytes such as glycerol and thiourea [143], decreased content of linoleic acid [144], decreased active influx of potassium leading to increased leakage of potassium on storage [145], and increased affinity for glucose [146]. In addition the red cells of the newborn are less deformable [147, 148] and morphological abnormalities are common during short periods of incubation *in vitro* [134, 149]. The majority of cord-blood red cells are slightly more resistant to osmotic lysis than adult cells, but a small population of abnormally fragile cells also appears to be present [149–152]. The biochemical basis of these differences remains to be explained and it is also unclear whether any of the membrane differences (or metabolic alterations) play any role in the reduced lifespan of the red cells of the newborn.

Developmental changes in membrane antigens have been described for the closely related substances of the ABO, Ii Lewis and P blood groups [153]. The A and B antigens are detectable on red cells in early fetal life but are not fully developed at birth and reach adult levels by the age of two to four years.

The antigens of the Lewis group are expressed very weakly at birth, developing after a few weeks and with Le[a] appearing earlier than Le[b]. Lewis substances are absorbed onto the red cells from the serum, and the red cells of neonates are rapidly transformed by plasma from adults, so these changes probably reflect low concentrations of Lewis substances in the serum of neonates and are not a characteristic of the red cells.

The most marked antigenic changes between neonatal and adult red cells occurs in the Ii-antigen system. Cord-blood cells react strongly with anti-i and weakly with anti-I whereas adult cells show the opposite pattern of reactivity [154]. The change-over occurs largely during the first 18 months of life. It has been suggested that these differences may be due to conformational changes in the red-cell membrane, but the biochemical basis of these antigens has recently been determined and the change in the developmental pattern has been ascribed to the increased activity of an enzyme which allows branching of the carbohydrate chains [155].

OXYGEN DELIVERY IN THE FETUS AND NEONATE

The oxygen dissociation curve of fetal blood is shifted to the left of the adult curve indicating that fetal red cells have a higher oxygen affinity than their adult counterparts. The P_{50} (the partial pressure of oxygen at which 50% of the haemoglobin is saturated) of fetal cells is 6–8 mmHg lower than adult cells [156]. However, when purified solutions of Hb A and Hb F are studied under the same conditions, the oxygen affinity of Hb F is slightly lower than that of Hb A [157–159]. This discrepancy was explained when it was discovered that the oxygen affinity of haemoglobin was considerably reduced on interaction with a variety of organic phosphates, particularly 2,3-DPG [160, 161] and that the reduction in the oxygen affinity of Hb F was only 20–40% of that produced by the same concentration of 2,3-DPG binding to Hb A [157, 162, 165]. This also explains the poor correlation between the oxygen dissociation curve of fetal blood with the proportion of fetal haemoglobin. When the effect of 2,3-DPG is taken into account, together with the relative proportions of Hbs A and F, a good correlation with the P_{50} of the whole blood is obtained [166, 167].

The effect on the fetus of this decreased interaction of 2,3-DPG with Hb F lies in preventing a rightward shift in the oxygen dissociation curve to compensate for the relative hypoxia *in utero*, ensuring that the oxygen affinity of the fetus does not drop below that of its mother. The higher oxygen affinity of fetal blood allows it to bind oxygen from the maternal circulation as it passes through the placental villi. Assuming a placental P_{O_2} of about 40 mmHg, fetal red cells are able to become about 80% saturated with oxygen. Since the tissue oxygen levels in the fetus are lower than those of the adult—maybe as low as 15 mmHg—more than half of this oxygen can be released. However, infants who have been transfused *in utero* with adult red cells suffer no obvious deleterious effects [170]. Similarly the offspring of mothers with high-oxygen-affinity haemoglobin variants appear to be normal [171, 172].

The oxygen affinity of fetal blood does not stay constant during intrauterine development. Measurement of the P_{50} of cord blood of premature infants from 24 weeks' gestation onwards showed a significant rise with gestational age [166–168]. The proportion of Hb A increases during this period, and a rise in the level of 2,3-DPG has also been reported [166, 167]. It has been suggested [167] that the binding of 2,3-DPG to the increasing amounts of Hb A may be responsible for the increase in 2,3-DPG levels during this period, by the removal of feedback inhibition of its own synthesis, an effect which has been demonstrated *in vitro* [169]. However, in a further study [168], no such increase in 2,3-DPG was observed when non-stressed normal fetuses of 24–42 weeks' gestational age were examined. This study also showed no change with gestational age in the pH difference between plasma and red cells although there was a significant inverse correlation between the red-cell hydrogen ion concentration and 2,3-DPG levels. This negative correlation could explain the discrepancy with the previous studies [166, 167] if in those cases the more premature infants had a greater tendency to acidosis.

Following birth the oxygen dissociation curve shifts progressively to the right, brought about by changes in 2,3-DPG levels and by the replacement of Hb F by Hb A. During the first week of life there is a transient increase in 2,3-DPG levels following which the levels remain relatively constant during the first six months at about 5·0–5·5 mmol/l packed red cells, similar to adult values [166, 173]. In the second half of the first year, however, these increase to about 7·4 mmol/l. During the first few months of life the amount of haemoglobin drops from about 17 to 11 g/dl, yet because of the increased availability of oxygen after birth and the progressive shift to the right in the oxygen dissociation curve, the three-month-old infant can deliver more oxygen to the tissue than at birth (Fig. 3.3).

In premature infants with higher Hb F levels and possibly lower levels of 2,3-DPG at birth, a greater

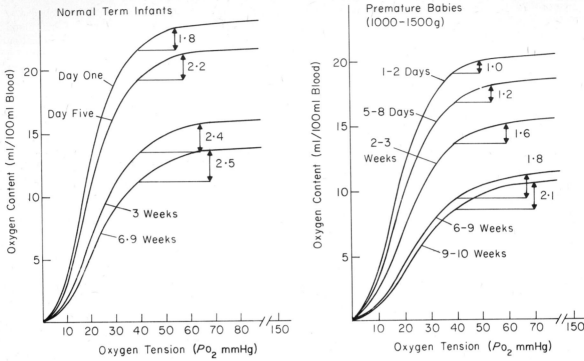

Fig. 3.3. The blood oxygen-releasing capacity at various ages from the time of birth in term and premature infants (from Ref. 166, with permission).

increase in 2,3-DPG levels occurs during the first few weeks of life. This may tend to decrease the oxygen affinity of the red cells by decreasing the intracellular pH. However, in those with severe respiratory distress, particularly the most acidotic, the 2,3-DPG levels are considerably reduced [166, 174] since low pH inhibits 2,3-DPG production. These infants therefore are incapable of compensating for their hypoxic state by increasing 2,3-DPG levels and may benefit from exchange transfusions with fresh adult red cells [166, 175].

DEVELOPMENTAL CHANGES IN WHITE-CELL PRODUCTION AND FUNCTION

Compared with erythropoiesis, very little is known about myelopoiesis during different stages of development and even less about associated changes in the funtion of the different white cells.

Myelopoiesis can be seen in some areas of fetal connective tissue as early as the seventh week of gestation and begins in the bone marrow at about the 10–11th week of gestation [2]. Circulating neutrophils can be observed in small numbers by the 11th week

[176]. Lymphopoiesis has not been observed in the yolk sac but occurs in the lymph plexuses at nine weeks and in the lymph glands by 11 weeks. Circulating lymphocytes are present by nine weeks. The proportion of T lymphocytes in cord blood, as judged by indirect immunofluorescence, is similar to adult controls, but if estimated by rosette formation it is smaller. B cells are present in similar proportions to adults. However, because the total lymphocyte count is higher than adult blood the total numbers of B, T and null cells is higher than in adults [177].

Changes in the total white-cell count and differential count during development
The changes in the total white-cell count and differential count at different stages of postnatal development are summarized in Table 3.5. The absolute numbers of polymorphonuclear neutrophils rises in both term and premature infants in the first 24 hours of life. The count remains relatively level during the first few days and then starts to fall by the end of the first week. It is not uncommon to see immature white cells in the blood of normal newborns; these may include promyelocytes and even blast cells, and they are more frequent in premature than in term infants. After the first week the

Table 3.5. Ranges and means (in parentheses) for differential white-cell counts at different stages of development. The values are expressed as white blood cells $\times 10^9$/l. (Adapted with permission from Altman P.L. & Dittmer D.S. (eds) *Blood and Other Body Fluids*. Federation of American Societies for Experimental Biology, Washington, 1961)

Age	Total WCC	Neutrophils	Eosinophils	Basophils	Lymphocytes	Monocytes
Birth	9·0–30·0 (18·1)	6·0–26·0 (11·0)	0·20–0·85 (0·40)	0·0–0·64 (0·1)	2·0–11·0 (5·5)	0·4–3·1 (1·05)
7 days	5·0–21·0 (12·0)	1·5–10·0 (5·5)	0·70–1·1 (0·5)	0·0–0·25 (0·05)	2·0–17·0 (5·0)	0·3–2·7 (1·1)
14 days	5·0–20·0 (11·4)	1·0–9·5 (4·5)	0·7–1·0 (0·35)	0·0–0·23 (0·05)	2·0–17·0 (5·5)	0·2–2·4 (1·0)
1 year	6·0–17·5 (11·4)	1·5–8·5 (3·5)	0·05–0·71 (0·30)	0·0–0·20 (0·05)	4·0–10·5 (7·0)	0·05–1·1 (0·55)
4 years	5·5–15·5 (9·1)	1·5–8·5 (3·8)	0·02–0·65 (0·25)	0·0–0·20 (0·05)	2·0–8·0 (4·5)	0·0–0·80 (0·45)
6 years	5·0–14·5 (8·5)	1·5–8·1 (4·3)	0·0–0·65 (0·23)	0·0–0·20 (0·05)	1·5–7·0 (3·5)	0·0–0·8 (0·40)
10 years	4·5–13·5 (8·1)	1·8–8·0 (4·4)	0·0–0·60 (0·20)	0·0–0·20 (0·04)	1·5–6·5 (3·1)	0·0–0·8 (0·35)
21 years	4·5–11·0 (7·4)	1·8–7·7 (4·4)	0·0–0·45 (0·20)	0·0–0·20 (0·04)	1·0–4·8 (2·5)	0·0–0·8 (0·30)

white-cell count falls progressively and over the next few years the lymphocytes predominate (Table 3.5).

Because of these normal alterations in the neutrophil count, immediately after birth the total and differential white-cell count is of limited clinical value for the diagnosis of neonatal infection. This problem has recently been reviewed in detail [178]. Perinatal factors other than bacterial infection which significantly alter neutrophil response during the early days of life include maternal hypertension, maternal fever prior to delivery, haemolytic disease, and periventricular haemorrhage. Neutropenia in the presence of respiratory distress in the first 72 hours has a high likelihood of signifying bacterial disease, whereas neutropenia in the presence of asphyxia is significantly less likely to reflect an infective cause. Clearly the interpretation of apparent abnormal neutrophil counts during the first few days of life must include consideration of both infectious and non-infectious perinatal disorders and must take into account the broad range in the total and differential white-cell count immediately after birth even in normal neonates. An attempt to discriminate between different neonatal pathology based on the white-cell count has been reported by Manroe *et al.* [178]; these studies have emphasized the remarkable variability in the white-cell changes in normal neonates, and just how much overlap there is between normality and the various perinatal disorders which may alter the total or differential white-cell counts.

Neutrophil function at birth and in infancy

White-cell function is considered in detail in Chapter 15. Although the absolute neutrophil count of premature and term infants is usually higher than that found in older children and in adults, there is no doubt that there is an increased susceptibility to bacterial and other infections at this stage of development. As described in detail in Chapter 15, destruction of bacteria by neutrophils requires that the organisms are taken up and destroyed, a process which depends on opsonin activity of the plasma, chemotaxis, phagocytosis and the killing capacity of the cells.

There is effective opsonin activity for certain organisms in full-term infants, and in some cases this is related to decreased amounts of specific antibodies and complement factors. Neutrophil function in neonates is reviewed in detail by Boxer [177]. Random neutrophil mobility and chemotaxis in response to chemotactic factors generated from pooled sera is reduced. Locomotive capacity and response to lymphokines is similar for cord-blood and adult monocytes. Cord-blood neutrophils have a normal recognition system and ingest latex and immune-coated particles as efficiently as adult cells. They have similar densities of Fc and complement receptors to adult cells. Neonatal neutrophils ingest bacteria as well as their adult counterparts; there is still considerable controversy as to whether their killing capacity is equal to that of adult neutrophils, however.

Cellular immunity

The different components of the cellular immune system are described in detail in Chapter 17. Here we will summarize briefly the early development of this system.

The cellular immune system is derived from haematopoietic stem cells in the fetal liver and spleen; these enter the thymus at about the eighth week of gestation where they acquire surface alloantigens [179]. It appears that during the migration from the cortex to the medulla of the thymus some cells undergo maturation whereas others die. The thymus-derived cells (T cells) are then distributed throughout the body where they concentrate in areas such as the lymph nodes and spleen (see Ref. 177). Fetal thymocytes acquire phytohaemagglutin (PHA) responsiveness at about 12 weeks' gestation and blood lymphocytes about two weeks later.

Neonatal lymphocytes undergo a greater degree of spontaneous transformation into blasts and, up to three months of age, incorporate greater amounts of thymidine than adult lymphocytes. Although they are responsive to PHA stimulation, the lymphocytes of newborn infants may be less active than those of adults in other effector functions such as lymphokine release and direct lymphocyte-killing ability. A variety of other differences betwen neonatal and adult lymphocytes as regards their effector function are reviewed by Boxer [177].

Humoral immune system

As mentioned earlier, circulating immunoglobulin-bearing lymphocytes have been observed in the human fetus as early as nine weeks' gestation. IgM production from fetal lymphoid tissue has been observed by 10 weeks [180] and IgG and IgA synthesis by 12 and 13 weeks respectively [177]. IgG transferred passively from the maternal circulation has been found as early as the 38th day of gestation. the IgG level remains at about 100 mg/dl until 17 weeks at which time it increases proportionately to gestational age. At 40 weeks the cord-blood IgG concentration is usually greater than the maternal IgG level although nearly all cord-blood IgG is of maternal origin. After birth the maternal IgG disappears from the circulation with a half-life of about 25 days. By four to six months, neonatal IgG reaches its lowest level but steadily rises thereafter as the infant's capacity to synthesize antibody increases, so that by the age of one year the IgG level is about 60% of the normal adult level (reviewed in Ref. 177).

Although synthesis of IgA is initiated at 30 weeks' gestation it proceeds at a very low level so that it is not usually detectable until several days after birth. By the end of the first year, serum IgA levels have only reached about 10% of the normal adult level.

Although normally the fetus synthesizes small amounts of immunoglobulins, it is able to produce IgM and IgA given an appropriate stimulus; these antibodies are present in many newborn infants who have had severe perinatal infection. The degree of IgM response is related to the type of infection, its severity and the maturity of the infant. Since IgM does not cross the placenta, the presence of specific IgM antibodies indicates that the infant is synthesizing the antibody and is, or has been, infected. These responses are extremely variable, and intrauterine infections such as rubella do not always activate the fetal immune system [177].

Other factors involved in the susceptibility of neonates to infection

Relative splenic hypofunction may be another factor which makes newborn infants prone to infection. Although their red cells contain relatively few Howell–Jolly bodies, the number of cells with surface pits, which are indicative of splenic hypofunction, is significantly increased in full-term newborns and in premature infants [181].

DEVELOPMENTAL CHANGES IN THE HAEMOSTATIC MECHANISM

PLATELETS IN THE FETUS AND NEONATE

Platelet production and numbers

Little is known of platelet production during early fetal life: megakaryocytes have not been found in the human yolk sac [182]. They are seen in the haemopoietic tissue of the liver and spleen by about 12 weeks' gestation, and are prominent in the bone marrow during the last trimester [17]. Platelets have been seen in the fetal circulation from 11 weeks' gestation onwards [183]: the mean platelet count appears to be slightly above $100 \times 10^9/l$ at around 20 weeks' gestation [184, 185], rising to about $200–250 \times 10^9/l$ at term [186, 187]; pre-term infants have similar [188, 189] or slightly lower counts [190], depending largely on their birth weight. The platelet count has been found to be higher in the umbilical vein than the umbilical artery [191], and tends to rise to $300–400 \times 10^9/l$ during the first three to four weeks of postnatal life in both full-term and premature infants [187, 188]. Neonatal platelet counts of less than $100 \times 10^9/l$ should be regarded as subnormal, and demand explanation whatever the degree of prematurity.

Platelet function

Very few attempts have been made to study the functional capacity of fetal platelets: prolonged bleeding from puncture wounds has been noted at around 20 weeks' gestation [183], and studies on the platelets of a small group of fetuses at this stage of development showed a profound defect of aggregation in response to adrenaline and collagen, and a lesser defect of ADP aggregation, relative to adult platelets [184]. The platelets of normal newborn infants are defective compared with adult platelets in a number of respects: they have a reduced glycogen content and platelet factor-3 availability [192], respond less well to ADP, adrenaline and collagen [192–194], and have a defect of release of their dense-body contents [194–196], most marked in response to adrenaline [197]. The underlying mechanism of these defects has not been fully explained: it is evidently not due to storage-pool deficiency [194] or to cyclo-oxygenase deficiency [198], but may be attributable to a lack of metabolic ATP [194, 197]. Whatever the cause, the defects are of little clinical significance, since they evidently do not produce a bleeding tendency on their own. They may result, however, in an unusual susceptibility of neonatal platelets to the additional defect imposed by the maternal ingestion of aspirin, which may lead to neonatal bleeding [199].

FETAL AND PERINATAL BLOOD COAGULATION

Fibrinogen

Clotting of fetal blood has been observed from about 11 to 12 weeks' gestation [200]. The difficulty of obtaining clean samples of blood from earlier fetuses makes results of clotting tests very unreliable, but fibrinogen synthesis has been demonstrated in cultures of fetal liver as early as five and a half weeks [201]. Holmberg *et al.* [185] found very low levels of fibrinogen in the blood of two fetuses at around 12–14 weeks, and a mean value of just under 1 g/l for fetuses between this age and 24 weeks. Premature infants from this stage of gestation onwards have been found to have mean fibrinogen levels well within the adult range (Fig. 3.4), though the scatter is understandably wider in the smaller infants. The lower limit of normal may reasonably be taken as 1·5 g/l at birth, whatever the degree of prematurity.

Clotting methods for the determination of fibrinogen often give somewhat lower results in fetuses and neonates than those based on protein determination or heat precipitation. These observations, and the prolonged thrombin clotting time of cord blood [202, 203], have led to a prolonged argument as to whether fetal fibrinogen is structurally distinct from its adult counterpart [204], or whether the findings on fetal

samples are attributable to partial degradation of fibrinogen resulting from incipient clotting and/or fibrinolysis [203]. The discussion continues, but the evidence for the existence of fetal fibrinogen is accumulating: Witt and her colleagues [205, 206] found that it chromatographed differently from adult fibrinogen on DEAE-cellulose, and that fingerprints of its tryptic digest showed three different peptide spots; it was found to contain twice as much phosphorus as adult fibrinogen and to be less susceptible to the action of thrombin, particularly at alkaline pH. Although some of these findings have been disputed [207], Witt & Tesch [208] now claim to have localized the difference between adult and fetal fibrinogen to the Aα chain. They believe that it is synthesized until about one week after birth.

The vitamin-K-dependent clotting factors [209]

In fetuses removed by hysterotomy at around 20 weeks' gestation, factor IX levels of 14–40% (mean 23%) and factors II, VII and X (assayed together as 'prothrombin and proconvertin') of 12–35% (mean 25%) have been found [185]. In pure fetal blood samples obained by fetoscopy at 15–22 weeks, the mean factor IX was 12·5% (range 8–18%) [210]. All these factors remain well below normal adult levels at term, and unless vitamin K is given to the mother during labour, or to the neonate, all of them fall further during the first few days of life; they then gradually rise to reach adult levels by about one to three months (Fig. 3.4). Levels of 25–60% are usual at term, factor IX being more often towards the lower end of this range. The numerous published reports have been summarized [183, 209]. While the delay in achieving adult plasma concentrations is presumably attributable to immaturity of biosynthetic enzyme systems in the liver, the immediate post-natal fall is due to a superimposed vitamin-K deficiency. Contributory factors to this include insufficient intake of the vitamin (particularly in breast-fed infants) and poor alimentary absorption before the establishment of the normal post-natal bacterial flora. Haemorrhagic disease of the newborn (see Chapter 29) simply represents an exaggeration of this transient deficiency.

Factor V

Plasma factor V concentrations in the fetus are only slightly below the normal adult range, even as early as 12–24 weeks' gestation [185, 189]. In neonates, whether full-term or premature, factor-V levels do not differ signficantly from those of older children or adults [209].

Factor VIII

The best estimates of factor-VIII activity in early fetal

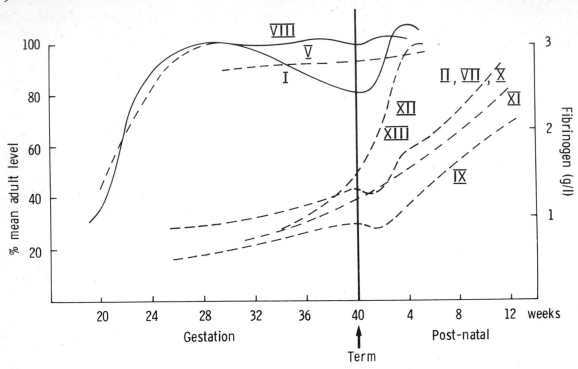

Fig. 3.4. Approximate mean levels of clotting factors in pre-term and full-term infants, and during the first weeks of postnatal life.

life are those obtained by fetoscopic sampling of pure fetal blood [210, 211]: at about 20 weeks' gestation, mean values in 20 normal fetal samples were VIIIC, 43·5 u/dl; VIIICAg, 22·3 u/dl; and VIIIRAg, 60·1 u/dl. Similar concentrations were found in non-haemophilic fetuses whose mothers were obligate or putative carriers of the haemophilia gene. Factor-VIIIC levels correlated with VIIIRAg, but not with VIIICAg. Similar VIIIC concentrations have been found in abortuses at the same period of gestation [185].

In the newborn, VIIIC values are within the normal adult range [189, 191, 212], and are not related to the maternal VIIIC concentration, which is usually raised at the time of delivery, since factor VIII does not cross the placenta. There is some evidence for a gestational-age dependency: Sell & Corrigan [189] found that mean VIIIC values increased from 90 u/dl at 27–30 weeks' gestation to 168 u/dl at full-term. Factor VIIIRAg has also been found to be normal or raised in newborn infants, both full-term and premature [185, 209], and the ristocetin cofactor (von Willebrand factor) is also raised [196]. Factor VIII with both these activities, though not VIIIC, has been shown to be synthesized *in vitro* by vascular endothelial cells from the umbilical cord (see Chapters 27 and 28).

Contact factors

All the factors involved in the initial, contact-activated phase of the intrinsic coagulation system—factors XII and XI, prekallikrein (Fletcher factor) and HMW kininogen (Fitzgerald factor)—are present at lower concentrations in cord than in adult blood [209]; mean values for factors XII and XI are shown in Fig. 3.4. It has been suggested that factor-XII concentrations in premature infants are dependent on gestational age [213]. Few data are available concerning the rate at which adult levels are achieved after birth; Hilgartner & Smith [214] found that mean factor-XI concentrations approximately doubled, from 36% in cord blood to 73%, within two to five months; their assay method was probably also sensitive to Fletcher factor [209].

Factor XIII

Although a few investigators have reported normal adult concentrations of factor XIII in cord blood, the weight of evidence now suggests that mean concentrations in the newborn are about half those found in adults [215, 216]. Values in fetuses at 17–24 weeks' gestation were found to be about half those of full-term neonates, and adult levels were reached about three weeks after birth [215].

Antithrombin III
Details of antithrombin activity in the blood of newborns and during infancy are given in Refs 217 and 218.

Screening tests of coagulation in the neonate
The combined effect of these changes in individual clotting factors on the results of the usual screening tests of the coagulation mechanism in neonates may be summarized as follows: the kaolin-activated partial thromboplastin time (KPTT) is prolonged, owing to the deficiency of factors IX and X, and perhaps also of the contact factors; the prothrombin time is prolonged, as a result of the deficiency of factors II, VII and X; and the thrombin time may also be slightly prolonged, owing to the delayed conversion of fibrinogen, and perhaps the presence of fibrinogen/fibrin degradation products, if steps are not taken to inhibit *in-vitro* fibrinolysis in the sample (see below). The thrombotest provides the most sensitive overall measurement of the vitamin-K-dependent factors, and is convenient for use on capillary blood samples: results in newborn infants are usually between about 15 and 40% of a normal adult conrol.

FIBRINOLYSIS IN THE FETUS AND NEONATE
Ekelund and his colleagues have reported a series of investigations on the fibrinolytic mechanism in fetuses, pre-term and full-term neonates and infants during the first year of life [219–222]. They found marked fibrinolytic activity, as reflected in a short euglobulin lysis time, from as early as 16 weeks' gestation. Plasminogen activator activity was high from this time until birth, when it fell rapidly to reach adult levels within about four hours; this postnatal fall was accompanied by a progressive lengthening of euglobulin lysis time. Mean plasminogen concentrations rose progressively from 20% between 12 and 24 weeks' gestation to 43% at term, and reached adult levels by about six months of age. Inhibitors of plasminogen activation were above adult levels throughout the second half of fetal life, and gradually declined to the adult range during about the first six months after birth. Mean α_2-macroglobulin concentrations rose progressively from 36% in the earliest fetuses studied to 170% at term, and remained high throughout infancy, while normal adult levels of progressive antiplasmin were observed at all stages of fetal and postnatal life. The fibrinolytic mechanism is thus very active in the newborn infant for a few hours after birth, but provided that samples are taken into proteolytic inhibitors to prevent *in-vitro* fibrinolysis, levels of fibrinogen/fibrin degradation products in neonatal blood are comparable to those found in healthy adults [221, 223].

CHANGES IN HAEMOPOIESIS DURING ADULT LIFE AND IN THE AGED

Although the most striking changes in the patterns of haemopoiesis are seen during fetal development and in the first few years of life, there is increasing evidence that the normal haemopoietic system is never absolutely static and that subtle changes continue to occur throughout adult life and into old age. Although many of these physiological alterations are still ill-defined, some patterns are emerging. It is important for the haematologist to appreciate these changes as they have considerable relevance in attempting to define what is 'normal' for any particular group [224].

The bone marrow
The cellularity of the bone marrow decreases with increasing age, at least as estimated from studies of trephine biopsies. For example, sections of the anterior iliac-crest marrow have demonstrated a progressive decrease in cellularity; if this is classified as 100% during the first year of life, it drops to about 50% over the first 30 years [225]. In the posterior iliac-crest marrow there is a plateau at about 50% up to the age of 65 years with a decrease in cellularity to about 30% over the next decade [226]. All these changes are due to an increase in fat together with a reduction in the volume of cancellous bone.

Haemoglobin level
The changes in the haemoglobin level during childhood and adolescence were considered earlier in this chapter. It seems to remain at a plateau until middle age after which there is a significant fall which is more marked in males than females. Pooling data from several large series it appears that the mean haemoglobin level in men over 60 years of age has ranged between 12·4 and 14·9 g/dl, and in females of a similar age from 11·7 to 13·8 g/dl [224]. However, there is still little reliable data about what is a 'normal' haemoglobin level for a particular age group. Hence in any individual case, anaemia in an elderly patient should be assumed to be due to some definable pathological cause rather than to age itself, until proved otherwise.

Other red-cell changes
As mentioned earlier in this chapter, the fetal haemoglobin level probably goes on falling throughout adolescence. There have been no really good studies of haemoglobin F levels in the aged. Red-cell 2,3-diphosphoglycerate also falls significantly although the associated change in oxygen affinity is probably too small to be of physiological importance [227]. There tends to be a slight increase in the mean cell volume (MCV) with increasing age and there is some evidence that this is more marked in smokers than non-smokers [224].

White cells

The white-cell count seems to remain relatively constant from adolescence through middle life but there is a small but significant fall in the total leucocyte count after the age of 65 years [228]. There is some evidence for changes in the relative proportion of T and B cells in the blood of elderly patients as compared with those of young populations although many of the studies show rather conflicting data [229, 230]. Similarly there is data which suggests that such lymphocyte functions as response to various mitogens, cutaneous hypersensitivity reactions and levels of transfer factor, are reduced in the elderly [229]. Immunoglobulin levels show so much variation even within healthy populations that it is difficult to be sure whether there is a genuine change with age. It appears that IgG and IgM levels reach a peak in early adult life and then fall slowly so that by the sixth to seventh decade they are significantly lower than those in young adults [231, 232]. Most studies have shown an increase in γ-globulin levels after this time. Monoclonal plasma immunoglobulins are found with increasing frequency with age, reaching an incidence of six per cent in individuals over the age of 80 years (see Chapter 19) [233].

Erythrocyte sedimentation rate (ESR)

The ESR is significantly increased in a number of healthy men and women over the age of 60 years. Values ranging from 2 to 42 mm/hour have been found in hospitalized patients above the age of 65 years in whom no cause could be found; in 30% of these patients sedimentation rates exceeded 20 mm/hour [234].

Coagulation factors

Factor VIII and fibrinogen levels have been reported to increase with age [224].

REFERENCES

1 BARTELS H. (1970) Prenatal respiration. *North-Holland Research Monographs—Frontiers in Biology, Vol. 17.* North-Holland, Amsterdam.

2 GILMOUR J.R. (1941) Normal haemopoiesis in intrauterine and neonatal life. *Journal of Pathology,* **52,** 25.

3 WILT F.H. (1974) The beginnings of erythropoiesis in the yolk sac of the chick embryo. *Annals of the New York Academy of Sciences,* **241,** 99.

4 RIFKIND R.A., CHUI D. & EPLER H. (1969) An ultrastructural study of early morphogenetic events during the establishment of fetal hepatic erythropoiesis. *Journal of Cell Biology,* **40,** 343.

5 INGRAM V.M. (1972) Embryonic red blood cell formation. *Nature (London),* **235,** 338.

6 MOORE M.A.S. & METCALF D. (1970) Ontogeny of the haemopoietic system: yolk sac origin of *in vivo* and *in vitro* colony forming cells in the developing mouse embryo. *British Journal of Haematology,* **18,** 279.

7 JOHNSON G.R. & MOORE M.A.S. (1975) Role of stem cell migration on initiation of mouse foetal liver haemopoiesis. *Nature (London),* **258,** 726.

8 LE DOUARIN N.M. (1978) Ontogeny of hematopoietic organs studied in avian embryo interspecific chimeras. In: *Differentiation of Normal and Neoplastic Hemopoietic Cells* (ed. Clarkson B., Marks P.A. & Till J.E.). Cold Spring Harbor Conferences on Cell Proliferation, Vol. 5, p. 6. Cold Spring Harbor Laboratories.

9 MARTIN C., BEAUPAIN D. & DIETERLEN-LIEVRE F. (1978) Development relationship between vitelline and intra-embryonic haemopoiesis studied in avian 'yolk sac chimeras'. *Cell Differentiation,* **7,** 115.

10 BEAUPAIN D., MARTIN D. & DIETERLEN-LIEVRE F. (1979) Are developmental hemoglobin changes related to the origin of stem cells and site of erythropoiesis? *Blood,* **53,** 212.

11 ZAMBONI L. (1965) Electron microscopic studies of blood embryogenesis in humans. II. The hemopoietic activity in the fetal liver. *Journal of Ultrastructural Research,* **12,** 525.

12 DJALDETTI M., OVADIA J., BESSLER H., FISHMAN P. & HALBRECHT I. (1975) Ultrastructural study of the erythropoietic events in human embryonic livers. *Biology of the Neonate,* **26,** 367.

13 DJALDETTI M. (1979) Hemopoietic events in human embryonic spleens at early gestational stages. *Biology of the Neonate,* **36,** 133.

14 LANGLEY F.A. (1951) Haemopoiesis and siderosis in the foetus and newborn. *Archives of Disease in Childhood,* **26,** 64.

15 THOMAS D.B., RUSSELL P.M. & YOFFEY J.M. (1960) Pattern of haemopoiesis in the foetal liver. *Nature (London),* **187,** 876.

16 YOFFEY J.M. & THOMAS D.B. (1964) The development of bone marrow in the human fetus. *Journal of Anatomy,* **96,** 425.

17 KALPAKTSOGLOU P.K. & EMERY J.L. (1965) Human bone marrow during the last three months of intrauterine life. *Acta Haematologica,* **34,** 228.

18 BECKER A.J., McCULLOCH E.A., SIMINOVITCH L. & TILL J.E. (1965) The effect of differing demands for blood cell production on DNA synthesis by hemopoietic colony forming cells of mice. *Blood,* **26,** 296.

19 KUBANEK B., RENRICCA N., PORCELLINI A., HOWARD D. & STOHLMAN F. (1970) The pattern of stem cell repopulation in heavily irradiated mice receiving transplants of fetal liver. *Blood,* **35,** 64.

20 SCHOFIELD R. (1970) A comparative study of the repopulating potential of grafts from various haemopoietic sources: CFU repopulation. *Cell Tissue Kinetics,* **3,** 119.

21 RICH I.N. & KUBANEK B. (1979) The ontogeny of erythropoiesis in the mouse detected by the erythroid colony-forming technique. *Journal of Embryology and Experimental Morphology,* **50,** 57.

22 ZANJANI E.D., POSTER J., MANN L.I. & WASSERMAN L.R. (1977) Regulation of erythropoiesis in the fetus. In: *Kidney Hormones. II. Erythropoietin* (ed. Fisher J.W.), p. 463. Academic Press, London and New York.

23 DARBRE P.D., ADAMSON J.W., WOOD W.G., WEATHER-ALL D.J. & ROBINSON J.S. (1979) Patterns of globin chain synthesis in erythroid colonies grown from sheep marrow of different developmental stages. *British Journal of Haematology*, **41**, 459.

24 HASSAN M.W., LUTTON J.D., LEVERE R.D., RIEDER R.F. & CEDERQVIST L.L. (1979) *In vitro* culture of erythroid colonies from human fetal liver and umbilical cord blood. *British Journal of Haematology*, **41**, 477.

25 STAMATOYANNOPOULOS G., ROSENBLUM B.B., PAPAYANNOPOULOU T, BRICE M., NAKAMOTO B. & SHEPARD T.H. (1979) Hb F and Hb A production in erythroid cultures from human fetuses and neonates. *Blood*, **54**, 440.

26 HALVORSEN S. (1963) Plasma erythropoietin levels in cord blood and in blood during the first weeks of life. *Acta Paediatrica*, **52**, 425.

27 HALVORSEN S. & FINNE P.H. (1968) Erythropoietin production in the human fetus and newborn. *Annals of the New York Academy of Sciences*, **149**, 576.

28 FINNE P.H. (1966) Erythropoietin levels in cord blood as an indicator of intrauterine hypoxia. *Acta Paediatrica*, **55**, 478.

29 JACOBSON L.O., GOLDWASSER E., GURNEY C.W., FRIED W. & PLZAK L. (1959) Studies of erythropoietin: the hormone regulating red cell production. *Annals of the New York Academy of Sciences*, **77**, 551.

30 MATOTH Y. & ZAIZOV R. (1971) Regulation of erythropoiesis in the fetal rat. *Israel Journal of Medical Science*, **7**, 839.

31 GORDON A.S., ZANJANI E.D., PETERSON E.N., GIDARI A.S., LOBUE J. & CAMISCOLI J.F. (1971) Studies on fetal erythropoiesis. In: *Regulation of Eyrthropoiesis* (ed. Gordon A.S., Condorelli M. & Peschle C.), p. 188. Ponte, Milan.

32 ZANJANI E.D., PETERSON E.N., GORDON A.S. & WASSERMAN L.R. (1974) Erythropoietin production in the fetus: role of kidney and maternal anaemia. *Journal of Laboratory and Clinical Medicine*, **83**, 281.

33 LUCARELLI G., PORCELLINI A., CARNEVALI C., CARMENA A. & STOHLMAN F. (1968) Fetal and neonatal erythropoiesis. *Annals of the New York Academy of Sciences*, **149**, 544.

34 PESCHLE C. & CONDORELLI M. (1976) Regulation of fetal and adult erythropoiesis. In: *Congenital Disorders of Erythropoiesis. CIBA Foundation Symposium 37*, p. 25. Elsevier, Excerpta Medica, North-Holland, Amsterdam.

35 ZANJANI E.D. & BANISADRE M. (1979) Hormonal stimulation of erythropoietin production and erythropoiesis in anephric sheep fetuses. *Journal of Clinical Investigation*, **64**, 1181.

36 WINTROBE M.M. & SCHUMACKER H.B. (1935) Comparison of hematopoiesis in the fetus and during recovery from pernicious anemia together with a consideration of the relationship of fetal hematopoiesis to macrocytic anemia of pregnancy and anemia in infants. *Journal of Clinical Investigation*, **14**, 837.

37 WALKER J. & TURNBULL E.P.N. (1953) Haemoglobin and red cells in the human foetus and their relation to the oxygen content of the blood in the vessels of the umbilical cord. *Lancet*, **ii**, 312.

38 TURNBULL E.P.N. & WALKER J. (1955) Haemoglobin and red cells in the human foetus. *Archives of Diseases in Childhood*, **30**, 102.

39 THOMAS D.B. & YOFFEY J.M. (1962) Human foetal haemopoiesis. I. The cellular composition of foetal blood. *British Journal of Haematology*, **8**, 290.

40 OSKI F.A. & NAIMAN J.L. (1972) *Haematologic Problems in the Newborn* (2nd edn). W. B. Saunders, Philadelphia.

41 WOOD W.G. (1982) Erythropoiesis and haemoglobin production during development. In: *Biochemical Development of the Fetus and Neonate. I. The Fetus* (ed. Jones C.T.). Elsevier-North Holland, Biomedical Press. In press.

42 SEIP M. (1955) The reticulocyte level, and the erythrocyte production judged from reticulocyte studies, in newborn infants during the first week of life. *Acta Paediatrica*, **44**, 355.

43 GARBY L., SJOLIN A. & VUILLE J.C. (1963) Studies on erythrokinetics in infancy. III. Plasma disappearance and red cell uptake of intravenously injected radioiron. *Acta Paediatrica*, **52**, 537.

44 BRATTEBY L.E. (1968) Studies on erythrokinetics in infancy. X. Red cell volume of newborn infants in relation to gestational age. *Acta Paediatrica*, **57**, 132.

45 ROOTH G. & SJÖSTEDT S. (1957) Haemoglobin in cord blood in normal and prolonged pregnancy. *Archives of Diseases in Childhood*, **32**, 91.

46 ZAIZOV R. & MATOTH Y. (1976) Red cell values on the first postnatal day during the last 16 weeks of gestation. *American Journal of Hematology*, **1**, 275.

47 MARKS J., GAIRDNER D. & ROSCOE J.D. (1955) Blood formation in infancy. III. Cord blood. *Archives of Diseases in Childhood*, **30**, 117.

48 USHER R., SHEPHARD M. & LIND J. (1963) The blood volume of the newborn infant and placental transfusion. *Acta Paediatrica*, **52**, 497.

49 YAO A.C., LIND J., TIISALA R. & MICHELSSON K. (1969) Placental transfusion in the premature infant with observations on clinical course and outcome. *Acta Paediatrica*, **58**, 561.

50 OH W. & LIND J. (1966) Venous and capillary haematocrit in newborn infants and placental transfusion. *Acta Paediatrica*, **55**, 38.

51 GAIRDNER D., MARKS J., ROSCOE J.D. & BRETTELL R.O. (1958) The fluid shift from the vascular compartment imediately after birth. *Archives of Diseases in Childhood*, **33**, 489.

52 LIND T., GERRARD J., SHERIDAN T.S. & WALKER W. (1977) Effect of maternal parity and infant sex upon the haematological values of cord blood. *Acta Paediatrica*, **66**, 33.

53 REINHARDT M.C. & MARTI H.R. (1978) Haematological data of African newborns and their mothers in Abidjan. *Helvetica Paediatrica Acta*, **33** (Suppl. 41), 85.

54 GUEST G.M. & BROWN E.W. (1957) Erythrocytes and hemoglobin of the blood infancy and childhood. *American Journal of Diseases in Childhood*, **93**, 486.

55 ZINKHAM W.J. (1963) Peripheral blood and bilirubin values in normal full-term primaquine sensitive Negro infants: effects of vitamin K. *Pediatrics*, **31**, 983.

56 MATOTH Y., ZAIZOV R. & VARSANO I. (1971) Postnatal changes in some red cell parameters. *Acta Paediatrica Scandinavica*, **60**, 317.

57 MOLLISON P.L., VEALL N. & CUTBUSH M. (1950) Red cell and plasma volume in newborn infants. *Archives of Diseases in Childhood*, **25**, 242.

58 BRATTEBY L.E. (1968) Studies on erythrokinetics in infancy. IX. Prediction of red cell volume from venous hematocrit in early infancy. *Acta Paediatrica Scandinavica*, **57**, 125.

59 SCHULMAN I., SMITH C.H. & STERN G.S. (1954) Studies on the anemia of prematurity. *American Journal of Diseases in Childhood*, **88**, 567.

60 USHER R. & LIND J. (1965) Blood volume of the newborn premature infant. *Acta Paediatrica Scandinavica*, **54**, 419.

61 BRATTEBY L.-E., GARBY L., GROTH T., SCHNEIDER W. & WADMAN B. (1968) Studies on erythro-kinetics in infancy. XIII. The mean life span and the life span frequency function of red blood cells formed during feotal life. *Acta Paediatrica Scandinavica*, **57**, 311.

62 PEARSON H.A. (1967) Life-span of the fetal red blood cell. *Journal of Pediatrics*, **70**, 166.

63 GILARDI A. & MIESCHER P. (1957) Die Lebensdauer von autolagen und homologen Erythrocyten bei früngeboremen und älteren Kindern. *Schweizerische Medizinische Wochenschrift*, **87**, 1456.

64 FOCONI S. & SJOLIN S. (1959) Survival of Cr^{51}-labelled red cells from newborn infants. *Acta Paediatrica*, **48**, 18.

65 VEST M.F. (1959) Cited by Kaplan & Hsu (1961) *Pediatrics*, **27**, 354.

66 KAPLAN E. & HSU K.S. (1961) Determination of erythrocyte survival in newborn infants by means of Cr^{51}-labelled erythrocytes. *Pediatrics*, **27**, 354.

67 VEST M.F. & GRIEDER H.R. (1961) Erythrocyte survival in the newborn infant, as measured by chromium^{51} and its relationship to the postnatal serum bilirubin levels. *Journal of Pediatrics*, **59**, 794.

68 GARBY L., SJOLIN S. & VUILLE J.C. (1964) Studies on erythrokinetics in infancy. V. Estimation of the life span of red cells in the newborn. *Acta Paediatrica*, **53**, 165.

69 VEST M., STREBEL L. & HAUENSTEIN L. (1965) The extent of 'shunt' bilirubin and erythrocyte survival in the newborn infant measured by the administration of ^{15}N glycine. *Biochemical Journal*, **95**, 11C.

70 O'BRIEN R.T. & PEARSON H.A. (1971) Physiologic anemia of the newborn infant. *Journal of Paediatrics*, **79**, 132.

71 GAIRDNER D., MARKS J. & ROSCOE J.D. (1952) Blood formation in infancy. I. The normal bone marrow. *Archives of Diseases in Childhood*, **27**, 128.

72 GAIRDNER G., MARKS J. & ROSCOE J.D. (1952) Blood formation in infancy. II. Normal erythropoiesis. *Archives of Diseases in Childhood*, **27**, 214.

73 GARBY L., SJOLIN S. & VUILLE J.C. (1963) Studies on erythrokinetics in infancy. III. Plasma disappearance and red cell uptake of intravenously injected radioiron. *Acta Paediatrica*, **52**, 537.

74 MANN D.L., SITES M.L., DONATI R.M. & GALLAGHER N.I. (1965) Erythropoietic stimulating activity during the first ninety days. *Proceedings of the Society of Experimental Biology and Medicine*, **118**, 212.

75 SKJAELAAEN P., HALVORSEN S. & SEIP M. (1970) Inhibition of erythropoiesis by plasma from newborn infants. *Israel Journal of Medical Science*, **7**, 857.

76 MCINTOSH S. (1975) Erythropoietin excretion in the premature infant. *Journal of Pediatrics*, **86**, 202.

77 GAIRDNER D., MARKS J. & ROSCOE J.D. (1955) Blood formation in infancy. IV. The early anaemia of prematurity. *Archives of Diseases in Childhood*, **30**, 203.

78 STOCKMAN J.A. (1975) Anemia of prematurity. *Seminars in Hematology*, **12**, 163.

79 BUCHANAN G.R. & SCHWARTZ A.D. (1974) Impaired erythropoietin response in anemic premature infants. *Blood*, **44**, 347.

80 STOCKMAN J.A., GARCIA J.F. & OSKI F.A. (1977) The anemia of prematurity. *New England Journal of Medicine*, **296**, 647.

81 WARDROP C.A.J., HOLLAND B.M., VEALE K.E.A., JONES J.G. & GRAY O.P. (1978) Nonphysiological anaemia of prematurity. *Archives of Diseases in Childhood*, **53**, 855.

82 STOCKMAN J.A. & OSKI F.A. (1978) Physiological anaemia of infancy and the anaemia of prematurity. *Clinics in Haematology*, **7**, 3.

83 CHESSELLS J.M. (1979) Blood formation in infancy. *Archives of Diseases in Childhood*, **54**, 831.

84 BROZOVIC B., BURLAND W.L., SIMPSON K. & LORD J. (1974) Iron status of preterm low birthweight infants and their response to oral iron. *Archives of Diseases in Childhood*, **49**, 386.

85 MCMILLAN J.A., LANDAW S.A. & OSKI F.A. (1976) Iron sufficiency in breast fed infants and the availability of iron from human milk. *Pediatrics*, **58**, 686.

86 SAARINEN U.M., SIIMES M.A. & DALLMAN P.R. (1977) Iron absorption in infants: high bioavailability of breast milk iron as indicated by the extrinsic method of iron absorption and by the concentration of serum ferritin. *Journal of Pediatrics*, **91**, 36.

87 LUNDSTRÖM V., SIIMES M.A. & DALLMAN P.R. (1977) At what age does iron supplementation become necessary in low birthweight infants? *Journal of Pediatrics*, **91**, 878.

88 ADAMS F.J., FUJIWARA T., SPEARS R. & HODGMAN J. (1964) Temperature regulation in premature infants. *Pediatrics*, **33**, 487.

89 MESTYAN J., FEKETE M., BATA G. & JARAI I. (1964) The basal metabolic rate of premature infants. *Biology of the Neonate*, **7**, 11.

90 SINCLAIR J.C. & SILVERMAN W.A. (1966) Intrauterine growth in active tissue mass of the human fetus with particular reference to the undergrown baby. *Pediatrics*, **38**, 48.

91 SINCLAIR J.C., SCOPER J.W. & SILVERMAN W.A. (1967) Metabolic reference standards for the neonate. *Pediatrics*, **39**, 724.

92 HILL J.F. & ROBINSON D.C. (1968) Oxygen consumption in normally grown, small for dates and large for dates newborn infants. *Journal of Physiology*, **199**, 685.

93 HEY E.N. (1969) The relation between environmental temperature and oxygen consumption in the newborn baby. *Journal of Physiology*, **200**, 589.

94 SAARINEN U.A. & SIIMES M.A. (1978) Developmental changes in red blood cell counts and indices of infants after exclusion of iron deficiency by laboratory criteria and continuous iron supplementation. *Journal of Pediatrics*, **92**, 412.

95 DALLMAN P.R. & SIIMES M.A. (1979) Percentile curves for hemoglobin and red cell volume in infancy and childhood. *Journal of Pediatrics*, **94**, 26.

96 DANIEL W.A. (1973) Hematocrit: maturity relationship in adolescence. *Pediatrics*, **52**, 388.

97 OWEN G.M., LUBIN A.H. & GARRY P.J. (1973) Hemoglobin levels according to age, race and transferrin saturation in preschool children of comparable socioeconomic status. *Journal of Pediatrics*, **82**, 850.

98 DALLMAN P.R., BARR G.D., ALLEN C.M. & SHINEFIELD H.R. (1978) Hemoglobin concentration in white, black and oriental children: is there a need for separate criteria in screening for anemia? *American Journal of Clinical Nutrition*, **31**, 377.

99 GARN S.M., SMITH N.J. & CLARK D.C. (1975) Lifelong differences in hemoglobin levels between blacks and whites. *Journal of the National Medical Association*, **67**, 91.

100 KOERPER M.A., MENTZER W.C., BRECHER G. & DALLMAN P.R. (1976) Developmental change in red blood cell volume: implication in screening infants and children for iron deficiency and thalassemia trait. *Journal of Pediatrics*, **89**, 580.

101 SAARINEN U.M. & SIIMES M.A. (1977) Developmental changes in serum iron, total iron binding capacity, and transferrin saturation in infancy. *Journal of Pediatrics*, **91**, 875.

102 KOERPER M.A. & DALLMAN P.R. (1977) Serum iron concentration and transferrin saturation in the diagnosis of iron deficiency in children: normal development changes. *Journal of Pediatrics*, **91**, 870.

103 STAMATOYANNOPOULOUS G. (1978) Discussion of paper by Stamatoyannopoulous G. & Papayannopoulou T. In: *Cellular and Molecular Regulation of Hemoglobin Switching* (ed. Stamatoyannopoulous G. & Nienhuis A.W.), p. 342. Grune & Stratton, New York.

104 BOYER S.H. & DOVER G.J. (1978) The in vivo biology of F cells in man. In: *Cellular and Molecular Regulation of Hemoglobin Switching* (ed. Stamatoyannopoulous G. & Nienhuis A.W.), p. 47. Grune & Stratton, New York.

105 MASERA G. (1968) Diagnosi de eterozigotismo per la β talassemia nel primo anno di vita. *Minerva Pediatrica*, **20**, 686.

106 SERJEANT B.E., MASON K.P. & SERJEANT G.R. (1978) The development of haemoglobin A₂ in normal Negro infants and in sickle cell disease. *British Journal of Haematology*, **39**, 259.

107 WOOD W.G., CLEGG J.B. & WEATHERALL D.J. (1977) Developmental biology of human hemoglobins. In: *Progress in Haematology, Vol. X* (ed. Brown E.B.), p. 43. Grune & Stratton, New York.

108 STAMATOYANNOPOULOUS G. & NIENHUIS A.W. (eds) (1978) *Cellular and Molecular Regulation of Hemoglobin Switching*. Grune & Stratton, New York.

109 COLOMBO B., KIM B., ATENCIO R.P., MOLINA C. & TERRENATO L. (1976) The pattern of foetal haemoglobin disappearance after birth. *British Journal of Haematology*, **32**, 79.

110 SHEPARD M.K., WEATHERALL D.J. & CONLEY C.L. (1962) Semi-quantitative estimation of the distribution of fetal hemoglobin in red cell populations. *Bulletin of the Johns Hopkins Hospital*, **110**, 293.

111 BARD H., MAKOWSKI E.L., MESCHIA G. & BATTAGLIA F.C. (1970) The relative rates of synthesis of hemoglobins A and F in immature red cells of newborn infants. *Pediatrics*, **45**, 766.

112 BARD H. (1975) The postnatal decline of hemoglobin F synthesis in normal full-term infants. *Journal of Clinical Investigation*, **55**, 395.

113 BETKE K. & KLEIHAUER E. (1958) Fetaler und bleibender blutfarbstoff in erythrozyten und erythroblasten von menschliden feten und neugeborenen. *Blut*, **4**, 241.

114 FRASER I.D. & RAPER A.B. (1962) Observations on the change from foetal to adult erythropoiesis. *Archives of Diseases in Childhood*, **37**, 289.

115 ZIPURSKY A., NEELANDS P.J. CHOWN B. & ISRAELS L.G. (1962) The distribution of fetal hemoglobin in the blood of normal children and adults. *Pediatrics*, **30**, 262.

116 CHEN S.-H., ANDERSON J.E., GIBLETT E.R. & STAMATOYANNOPOULOUS G. (1977) Isozyme patterns in erythrocytes from human fetuses. *American Journal of Hematology*, **3**, 23.

117 OSKI F.A. & SMITH C.A. (1968) Red cell metabolism in the premature infant. III. Apparent inappropriate glucose consumption for cell age. *Pediatrics*, **41**, 473.

118 GROSS R.T., SCHROEDER E.A.R. & BROUNSTEIN S.A. (1963) Energy metabolism in the erythrocytes of premature infants compared to full term newborn infants and adults. *Blood*, **21**, 755.

119 OSKI F.A. (1969) Red cell metabolism in the newborn infant. V. Glycolitic intermediates and glycolytic enzymes. *Pediatrics*, **44**, 84.

120 KONRAD P.N., VALENTINE W.N. & PAGLIA D.E. (1972) Enzymatic activities and glutathione content of erythrocytes in the newborn: comparison with red cells of older normal subjects and those with comparable reticulocytosis. *Acta Haematologica*, **48**, 193.

121 OSKI F.A. & KOMAZAWA M. (1975) Metabolism of the erythrocytes of newborn infants. *Seminars in Hematology*, **12**, 209.

122 ZIPURSKY A., LA RUE T. & ISRAELS L.G. (1960) The in vitro metabolism of erythrocytes from newborn infants. *Canadian Journal of Biochemical Physiology*, **38**, 727.

123 SCHRÖTER W. & WINTER P. (1967) Der 2,3-Diphosphoglyceratsloffwichsel in den Erythrozyten neugeborenen und erwachsener. *Klinische Wochenschrift*, **45**, 255.

124 TRUEWORTHY R.C. & LOWMAN J.T. (1971) Intracellular control of 2,3-diphosphoglycerate concentration in fetal red cells. *Proceedings of the Society of Pediatric Research*, p. 86.

125 NG W.G., DONNEL G.N. & BERGEN W.R. (1965) Galactokinase activity in human erythrocytes of individuals at different ages. *Journal of Laboratory and Clinical Medicine*, **66**, 115.

126 STOCKS J., OFFERMAN E.L., MODELL C.B. & DORMANDY T.L. (1972) The susceptibility to autoxidation of human red cell lipids in health and disease. *British Journal of Haematology*, **23**, 713.

127 OSKI F.A. (1967) Red cell metabolism in the premature infant. II. The pentose phosphate pathway. *Pediatrics*, **39**, 689.

128 GLADER B.E. & CONRAD M.E. (1972) Decreased glutathione peroxidase in neonatal erythrocytes: lack of relation to hydrogen peroxide metabolism. *Pediatric Research*, **6**, 900.

129 GROSS R.T., BRACCI R., RUDOLPH N., SCHRODER E. & KOCHEN J.A. (1967) Hydrogen peroxide toxicity and detoxification in the erythrocytes of newborn infants. *Blood*, **29**, 481.

130 BRACCI R., BENEDETTI P.A. & CIAMBELLOTTI V. (1970) Hydrogen peroxide generation in the erythrocytes of newborn infants. *Biology of the Neonate*, **15**, 135.

131 WHAUN J.M. & OSKI F.A. (1970) Relation of red blood cell glutathione peroxidase to neonatal jaundice. *Journal of Pediatrics*, **76**, 555.

132 SCHRÖTER W. (1971) Drug susceptibility and the development of erythrocyte enzyme systems. In: *Nutricia Symposium: Metabolic Processes in the Fetus and Newborn Infant* (ed. Jonxis J.H.P. & Visser H.K.A.), p. 73. Stenfert-Kroese NV, Leiden.

133 DeLUCA C., STEVENSON J.H. & KAPLAN E. (1962) Simultaneous multiple-column chromatography: its application to the separation of the adenine nucleotides of human erythrocytes. *Annals of Biochemistry*, **4**, 39.

134 OSKI F.A. & NAIMAN J.L. (1965) Red cell metabolism in the newborn infant. I. Adenosine triphosphate levels, adenosine triphosphate stability and glucose consumption. *Pediatrics*, **36**, 104.

135 GREENWALT J.T., AYERS V.E. & MORELL S.A. (1962) Phosphate partition in the erythrocytes of normal newborn infants and infants with erythroblastosis fetalis. III. P^{32} uptake and incorporation. *Blood*, **19**, 468.

136 JONES P.E.H. & McCANCE R.A. (1949) Enzyme activities in the blood of infants and adults. *Biochemical Journal*, **45**, 464.

137 BURMAN D. (1961) Red cell cholinesterase activity in infancy and childhood. *Archives of Diseases in Childhood*, **32**, 362.

138 WEHINGER H. (1973) Zur Natur und ontogenetischem Entwicklung von Carboanhydrase-Isoenzymen in menschlichen Erythrozyten. *Blut*, **27**, 172.

139 SELL J.E. & PETERING H.G. (1974) Carbonic anhydrases from human neonatal erythrocytes. *Journal of Laboratory and Clinical Medicine*, **84**, 369.

140 SCHEKMAN R. & SINGER S.J. (1976) Clustering and endocytosis of membrane receptors can be induced in mature erythrocytes of neonatal but not adult humans. *Proceedings of the National Academy of Sciences, USA*, **73**, 4075.

141 SHAPIRO D.L. & PASQUALINI P. (1978) Erythrocyte membrane proteins of premature and full-term newborn infants. *Pediatric Research*, **12**, 176.

142 WHAUN J. & OSKI F.A. (1969) Red cell stromal adenosine triphosphatase (ATPase) of newborn infants. *Pediatric Research*, **3**, 105.

143 HOLLAN S.R., SZELENYI J.G., BREUER J.G., MEDGYESI G. & SOTER V.N. (1968) Structural and functional differences between human foetal and adult erythrocytes. *Haematologica*, **1**, 409.

144 CROWLEY J., WAYS P. & JONES J.W. (1965) Human fetal erythrocyte and plasma lipids. *Journal of Clinical Investigation*, **44**, 989.

145 BLUM S.F. & OSKI F.A. (1969) Red cell metabolism in the newborn infant. IV. Transmembrane potassium flux. *Pediatrics*, **43**, 396.

146 MOORE T.J. & HALL N. (1971) Kinetics of glucose transport in adult and fetal human erythrocytes. *Pediatric Research*, **5**, 356.

147 LaCELLE P.L. & WEED R.I. (1970) Low oxygen pressure: a cause of erythrocyte membrane rigidity. *Journal of Clinical Investigation*, **49**, 54a.

148 GROSS G.P. & HATHAWAY W.E. (1972) Fetal erythrocyte deformability. *Pediatric Research*, **6**, 593.

149 SJOLIN S. (1954) The resistance of red cells *in vitro*. A study of the osmotic properties, the mechanical resistance and the storage behaviour of red cells of fetuses, children and adults. *Acta Paediatrica*, **43**, 1.

150 CRAWFORD M., CUTBUSH M. & MOLLISON P.L. (1953) Hemolytic disease of newborn due to anti A. *Blood*, **8**, 620.

151 DANON Y., KLEINMAN A. & DANON D. (1970) The osmotic fragility and density distribution of erythrocytes in the newborn. *Acta Haematologica*, **43**, 242.

152 LUZATTO L., ESAN G.J.F. & OGIEMUDIA S.E. (1970) The osmotic fragility of red cells in newborns and infants. *Acta Haematologica*, **43**, 248.

153 MOLLISON P.L. (1972) *Blood Transfusion in Clinical Medicine* 5th edn. Blackwell Scientific Publications, Oxford.

154 MARSH W.L. (1961) Anti-i: a cold antibody defining the Ii relationship in human red cells. *British Journal of Haematology*, **7**, 200.

155 FUKUDA M., FUKUDA M.N. & HAKOMORI S. (1979) Developmental change and genetic defect in the carbohydrate structure of band 3 glycoprotein of human erythrocyte membrane. *Journal of Biological Chemistry*, **254**, 3700.

156 ANSELMINO K.T. & HOFFMAN F. (1930) Die Ursachen des Icterus Neonatorum. *Archiv für Gynäkologie*, **143**, 477.

157 ALLEN D.W., WYMAN T. & SMITH C.A. (1953) The oxygen equilibrium of fetal and adult hemoglobin. *Journal of Biological Chemistry*, **203**, 84.

158 TYUMA I. & SHIMIZU K. (1969) Different response to organic phosphates of human fetal and adult hemoglobins. *Archives of Biochemistry and Biophysics*, **129**, 404.

159 TYUMA I. & SHIMIZU K. (1970) Effect of organic phosphates on the difference in oxygen affinity between fetal and adult human haemoglobin. *Federation Proceedings (Federation of American Societies for Experimental Biology)*, **29**, 1112.

160 BENESCH R. & BENESCH R.E. (1967) The effect of organic phosphates from the human erythrocyte on the allosteric properties of hemoglobin. *Biochemical and Biophysical Research Communications*, **26**, 162.

161 CHANUTIN A. & CURNISH R.R. (1967) Effect of organic and inorganic phosphates on the oxygen equilibrium of human erythrocytes. *Archives of Biochemistry*, **121**, 96.

162 BAUER C., LUDWIG I. & LUDWIG M. (1968) Different effects of 2,3-diphosphoglycerate and adenosine triphosphate on the oxygen affinity of adult and foetal human hemoglobin. *Life Sciences*, **7**, 1339.

163 DeVERDIER C-H. & GARBY L. (1969) Low binding of 2,3-dipohosphoglycerate to haemoglobin F. Contribution to the knowledge of the binding site and explanation for the high oxygen affinity of fetal blood. *Scandinavian Journal of Clinical Investigation*, **23**, 149.

164 MAURER H.S., BEHRMAN R.C. & HONIG G.R. (1970) Dependance of the oxygen affinity of blood on the presence of foetal or adult haemoglobin. *Nature (London)*, **227**, 388.

165 BUNN H.F. & BRIEHL R.W. (1970) The interaction of 2,3-diphosphoglycerate with various human haemoglobins. *Journal of Clinical Investigation*, **49**, 1088.

166 DELIVORIA-PAPADOPOULOS M., RONCEVIC N.P. & OSKI

F.A. (1971) Postnatal changes in oxygen transport of term, premature, and sick infants: the role of red cell 2,3-diphosphoglycerate and adult hemoglobin. *Pediatric Research*, **5**, 235.

167 ORZALESI M.M. & HAY W.W. (1971) The regulation of oxygen affinity of fetal blood. I. In vitro experiments and results in normal infants. *Pediatrics*, **48**, 857.

168 BARD H. & TEASDALE F. (1979) Red cell oxygen affinity, hemoglobin type, 2,3-diphosphoglycerate and pH as a function of fetal development. *Pediatrics*, **64**, 483.

169 OSKI F.A., GOTTLEIB A.J., MILLER W.W. & DELIVORIA-PAPADOPOULOS M. (1970) The effects of deoxygenation of adult and fetal hemoglobin on the synthesis of red cell 2,3-diphosphoglycerate and its in vivo consequences. *Journal of Clinical Investigation*, **49**, 400.

170 NOVY M.J., FRIGOLETTO F.D., EASTERDAY C.L., UMANSKY I. & NELSON N.M. (1971) Changes in cord blood oxygen affinity after intrauterine transfusions for erythroblastosis. *New England Journal of Medicine*, **285**, 589.

171 PARER J.T. (1970) Reversed relationship of oxygen affinity in maternal and fetal blood. *American Journal of Obstetrics and Gynecology*, **108**, 323.

172 CHARACHE S., JACOBSON R., BRIMHALL B., MURPHY E.A., HATHAWAY P., WINSLOW R., JONES R., RATH C. & SIMKOVICH J. (1978) Hb Potomac (101 Glu replaced by Asp): speculation on placental oxygen transport in carriers of high affinity hemoglobins. *Blood*, **51**, 331.

173 HJELM M. (1969) The content of 2,3-diphosphoglycerate and some other phosphocompounds in human erythrocytes during the neonatal period. *Försvarsmedicin*, **5**, 195.

174 WIMBERLEY P.D., WHITEHEAD M.D. & HEUHNS E.R. (1977) The effect of acidosis on red cell 2,3-DPG and oxygen affinity of whole foetal blood. *Les colloques de l'INSERM: interactions moleculaires de l'hémoglobine*, **70**, 295.

175 OSKI E.A. (1973) The unique red cell and its function. *Pediatrics*, **51**, 494.

176 PLAYFAIR J.H.L., WOLFENDALE M.R. & KAY H.E.M. (1963) The leucocytes of peripheral blood in the human foetus. *British Journal of Haematology*, **9**, 336.

177 BOXER L.A. (1978) Immunological function and leucocyte disorders in newborn infants. *Clinical Haemtology*, **7**, 123.

178 MANROE B.L., WEINBERG A.G., ROSENFELD C.R. & BROWNE R. (1979) The neonatal blood count in health and disease. I. Reference values for neutrophilic cells. *Journal of Pediatrics*, **99**, 89.

179 OWEN J.T. & RAFF M.C. (1970) Studies on the differentiation of thymus-derived lymphocytes. *Journal of Experimental Medicine*, **132**, 1216.

180 GITLIN D. & BLASUCCI A. (1969) Development of gamma G, gamma N, gamma M, beta 1Cl, beta 1A, Ci esterase inhibition, ceruloplasmin, transferrin, hemopexin, haptoglobin, fibrinogen, plasminogen, alpha-1-antitrypsin, orosmucoid, beta-lipoprotein, alpha-2-macroglobin, and pre-albumin in the human conceptus. *Journal of Clinical Investigation*, **48**, 1433.

181 SCHWARTZ E. & GILL F.M. (1977) Hematology of the newborn. In: *Hematology* (ed. Williams W.J., Beutler E., Erslev A.J. & Rundles R.W.) 2nd edn, p. 37. McGraw-Hill, New York.

182 HESSELDAHL H. & LARSEN F.J. (1971) Hemopoiesis and blood vessels in human yolk sac. An electron microscopic study. *Acta Anatomica*, **78**, 274.

183 BLEYER W.A., HAKAMI N. & SHEPARD T.H. (1971) The development of hemostasis in the human fetus and newborn infant. *Journal of Pediatrics*, **79**, 838.

184 PANDOLFI M., ÅSTEDT B., CRONBERG L. & NILSSON I.M. (1972) Failure of fetal platelets to aggregate in response to adrenaline and collagen. *Proceedings of the Society for Experimental Biology & Medicine*, **141**, 1081.

185 HOLMBERG L., HENRIKSSON P., EKELUND H. & ÅSTEDT B. (1974) Coagulation in the human fetus. Comparison with term newborn infants. *Journal of Pediatrics*, **85**, 860.

186 ABLIN A.R., KUSHNER J.H., MURPHY A. & ZIPPIN C. (1961) Platelet enumeration in the neonatal period. *Pediatrics*, **28**, 822.

187 ALEXANDRE P., ANDRE E. & STREIFF F. (1974) Etude sur sang capillaire de la coagulation du nouveau-né à terme et du nourrison. *Archives françaises de Pédiatrie*, **31**, 739.

188 ABALLI A.J., PUAPONDH Y. & DESPOSITO F. (1968) Platelet counts in thriving premature infants. *Pediatrics*, **42**, 685.

189 SELL E.J. & CORRIGAN J.J. JR (1973) Platelet counts, fibrinogen concentrations, and factor V and factor VIII levels in healthy infants according to gestational age. *Journal of Pediatrics*, **82**, 1028.

190 MEDOFF H.S. (1964) Platelet counts in premature infants. *Journal of Pediatrics*, **64**, 287.

191 FOLEY M.E., CLAYTON J.K. & McNICOL G.P. (1977) Haemostatic mechanisms in maternal, umbilical vein and umbilical artery blood at the time of delivery. *British Journal of Obstetrics & Gynaecology*, **84**, 81.

192 HRODEK O. (1969) L'agrégration des plaquettes chez le nouveau-né. *Nouvelle Revue française d'Hématologie*, **9**, 569.

193 MULL M.M. & HATHAWAY W.E. (1970) Altered platelet function in newborns. *Pediatric Research*, **4**, 229.

194 CORBY D.G. & ZUCK T.F. (1976) Newborn platelet dysfunction: a storage pool and release defect. *Thrombosis and Haemostasis*, **36**, 200.

195 WHAUN J.M. (1973) The platelet of the normal infant: 5-hydroxtryptamine uptake and release. *Thrombosis et Diathesis Haemorrhagica*, **30**, 327.

196 TS'AO C., GREEN D. & SCHULTZ K. (1976) Function and ultrastructure of platelets of neonates: enhanced ristocetin aggregation of neonatal platelets. *British Journal of Haematology*, **32**, 225.

197 WHAUN J.M. & LIEVAART P. (1980) The platelet of the newborn infant—adenine nucleotide metabolism and release. *Thrombosis and Haemostasis*, **43**, 99.

198 STUART M.J. (1978) The neonatal platelet: evaluation of platelet malonyl dialdehyde formation as an indicator of prostaglandin synthesis. *British Journal of Haematology*, **39**, 83.

199 BLEYER W.A. & BRECKENRIDGE R.T. (1970) Studies on the detection of adverse drug reactions in the newborn. II. The effects of prenatal aspirin on newborn hemostasis. *Journal of the American Medical Association*, **213**, 2049.

200 ZILLIACUS H., OTTELIN A-M. & MATSSON T. (1966) Blood clotting and fibrinolysis in human fetuses. *Biologica Neonatorum*, **10**, 108.

201 GITLIN D. & BIASUCCI A. (1969) Development of $_\gamma$G, $_\gamma$A, $_\gamma$M, β_{1c}/β_{1a}, C'1 esterase inhibitor, ceruloplasmin, transferrin, hemopexin, haptoglobin, fibrinogen, plasminogen, α_1-antitrypsin, orosomucoid, β-lipoprotein, α_2-macroglobulin and prealbumin in the human conceptus. *Journal of Clinical Investigation*, **48**, 1433.

202 LARRIEU M.J., SOULIER J.P. & MINKOWSKI A. (1952) Le sang du cordon ombilical: étude complète de sa coagulabilité, comparaison avec le sang maternel. *Etudes Neonatales*, **1**, 39.

203 VON FELTEN A. & STRAUB P.W. (1969) Coagulation studies of cord blood, with special reference to 'fetal fibrinogen'. *Thrombosis et Diathesis Haemorrhagica*, **22**, 273.

204 KUNZER W. (1961) Fetales fibrinogen. *Klinische Wochenschrift*, **39**, 536.

205 WITT I., MÜLLER H. & KÜNZER W. (1969) Evidence for the existence of foetal fibrinogen. *Thrombosis et Diathesis Haemorrhagica*, **22**, 101.

206 WITT I. & MÜLLER H. (1970) Phosphorus and hexose content of human fetal fibrinogen. *Biochimica et Biophysica Acta*, **221**, 402.

207 TEGER-NILSSON A-C. & EKELUND H. (1974) Fibrinogen to fibrin transformation in umbilical cord blood and purified neonatal fibrinogen. *Thrombosis Research*, **5**, 601.

208 WITT I. & TESCH R. (1979) Molecular characterization of human foetal fibrinogen. *Thrombosis and Haemostasis* (Abstract), **42**, 79.

209 HATHAWAY W.E. & BONNAR J. (1978) *Perinatal Coagulation*, p. 53. Grune & Stratton, New York.

210 MIBASHAN R.S., RODECK C.H., THUMPSTON J.K., EDWARDS R.J., SINGER J.D., WHITE J.M. & CAMPBELL S. (1979) Plasma assay for fetal factors VIIIC and IX for prenatal diagnosis of haemophilia. *Lancet*, **ii**, 1309.

211 MIBASHAN R.S., PEAKE I.R., RODECK C.H., THUMPSTON J.K., FURLONG R.A., GORER R., BAINS L., & BLOOM A.L. (1980) Dual diagnosis of prenatal haemophilia A by measurement of fetal factor VIIIC and VIIIC antigen (VIIICAg). *Lancet*, **ii**, 994.

212 PRESTON A.E. (1964) The plasma concentration of factor VIII in the normal population. I. Mothers and babies at birth. *British Journal of Haematology*, **10**, 110.

213 CORRIGAN J.J. JR, SELL E.J. & PAGEL C. (1977) Hageman factor and disseminated intravascular coagulation (DIC) in newborns and rabbits. *Pediatric Research*, **11**, 916.

214 HILGARTNER M.W. & SMITH C.H. (1965) Plasma thromboplastin antecedent (factor XI) in the neonate. *Journal of Pediatrics*, **66**, 747.

215 HENRIKSSON P., HEDNER U., NILSSON I.M., BOEHM J., ROBERTSON B. & LORAND L. (1974) Fibrin-stabilizing factor (factor XIII) in the fetus and the newborn infant. *Pediatric Research*, **8**, 789.

216 YAMADA K., SHIRAHATA A. & MEGURO T. (1976) The comparative studies of factor XIII of newborn infants obtained by three methods: clot solubility, immunological and fluorescent assays. *Acta Haematologica Japonica*, **39**, 79.

217 HATHAWAY W.E., NEUMANN L.L., BORDEN C.A. & JACOBSON L.J. (1978) Immunologic studies of antithrombin III heparin cofactor in the newborn. *Thrombosis and Haemostasis*, **39**, 624.

218 TEGER-NILSSON A.C. (1975) Antithrombin in infancy and childhood. *Acta Paediatrica Scandinavica*, **64**, 624.

219 EKELUND H., HEDNER U. & ASTEDT B. (1970) Fibrinolysis in human foetuses. *Acta Paediatrica Scandinavica*, **59**, 369.

220 EKELUND H. & FINNSTROM O. (1972) Fibrinolysis in pre-term infants and in infants small for gestational age. *Acta Paediatrica Scandinavica*, **61**, 369.

221 EKELUND H., HEDNER U. & NILSSON I.M. (1970) Fibrinolysis in newborns. *Acta Paediatrica Scandinavica*, **59**, 33.

222 EKELUND H. (1972) Fibrinolysis in the first year of life. *Acta Paediatrica Scandinavica*, **61**, 5.

223 CHESSELLS J.M. (1971) This significance of fibrin degradation products in the blood of normal infants. *Biology of the Neonate*, **17**, 219.

224 WILLIAMS W.J. (1977) Hematology in the aged. In: *Hematology* (ed. Williams W.J., Beutler E., Erslev A.J. & Rundles R.W.) 2nd edn, p. 49. McGraw-Hill, New York.

225 HARTSTOCK R.J., SMITH E.B. & PETTY C.S. (1965) Normal variations with aging on the amount of hematopoietic tissue in bone marrow from the anterior iliac crest. *American Journal of Clinical Pathology*, **43**, 326.

226 CALLENDER S.T. & SPRAY G.H. (1962) Latent pernicious anaemia. *British Journal of Haematology*, **8**, 230.

227 PURCELL Y. & BROZOVIC B. (1974) Red cell 2,3-diphosphoglycerate concentration in man decreases with age. *Nature (London)*, **251**, 511.

228 CAIRD F.I., ANDREWS G.R. & GALLIE T.B. (1972) The leucocyte count in old age. *Age and Ageing*, **1**, 239.

229 WEKSLER M.E. & HUTTEROTH T.H. (1972) Impaired lymphocyte function in aged humans. *Journal of Clinical Investigation*, **53**, 99.

230 AUGENER W., COHNEN E., REUTER A. & BRITTINGER E. (1974) Decrease of T lymphocytes during aging. *Lancet*, **i**, 1164.

231 BUCKLEY C.E. III & DORSEY F.C. (1979) The effect of aging on human serum immunoglobin concentrations. *Journal of Immunology*, **105**, 964.

232 BUCKLEY C.E. III & DORSEY F.C. (1971) Serum immunoglobulin levels throughout the life-span of healthy man. *Annals of Internal Medicine*, **75**, 673.

233 AXELSSON U., BACHMANN R. & HALLEN J. (1966) Frequency of pathological proteins (M-components) in 6995 sera from an adult population. *Acta Medica Scandinavica*, **179**, 235.

234 BOTTIGER L.E. & SVEDBERG C.A. (1967) Normal erythrocyte sedimentation rate and age. *British Medical Journal*, **ii**, 85.

235 TRAVIS S.F., KUMAR S.P., PAEZ P.C. & DELIVORIA-PAPADOPOULOS M. (1980) Red cell metabolic alterations in postnatal life in term infants: glycolytic enzymes and glucose-6-phosphate dehydrogenase *Pediatric Research*, **14**, 1349.

236 TRAVIS S.F., KUMAR S.P. & DELIVORIA-PAPADOPOULOS M. (1981) Red cell metabolic alterations in postnatal life in term infants: glycolytic intermediates and adenosine triphosphate. *Pediatric Research*, **15**, 34.

237 TRAVIS S.F., KUMAR S.P. & DELIVORIA-PAPADOPOULOS M. (1981) Red cell metabolic alterations in post-natal life in term infants: possible control mechanisms. *Pediatric Research*, **15**, 133.

SECTION 2
THE RED CELL
AND ITS DISORDERS

Chapter 4
The pathophysiology of erythropoiesis

S. N. WICKRAMASINGHE AND D. J. WEATHERALL

The term erythron is used to describe the circulating red blood cells and their precursors. The erythron of the normal adult is an example of a steady-state cell-renewal system in which a continuous loss of circulating red cells by senescence is precisely balanced by new red-cell production within the bone marrow. This chapter deals with some aspects of the anatomy, physiology, biochemistry and cell kinetics of erythropoiesis. It also reviews the methods available for the investigation and quantification of erythropoiesis in humans and provides an overall view of anaemia and the mechanisms underlying the perturbation of erythropoiesis in various diseases.

MODEL OF THE ERYTHRON

There are two categories of red-cell precursors; the early precursor cells which have not yet been recognized morphologically with certainty but which can be investigated by functional tests and which are described as the 'unrecognized' precursors, and the morphologically recognizable precursors. The morphologically unrecognized precursors which include the multipotent haemopoietic stem cells (CFU-S), erythroid burst-forming units (BFU-E) and erythroid colony-forming units (CFU-E) are discussed in detail in Chapter 2. The morphologically recognizable red-cell precursors include the proerythroblasts, basophilic erythroblasts, early and late polychromatic erythroblasts and reticulocytes. The members of the latter group of cells have been unequivocally identified as belonging to the erythron by virtue of the fact that they take up significant quantities of radioactive iron when incubated with ^{55}Fe- or ^{59}Fe-labelled transferrin and the fact that they contain cytochemically detectable quantities of haemoglobin.

The basic features of the red-cell renewal system are illustrated in Figure 4.1. Red cells are ultimately derived from multipotent haemopoietic stem cells. The latter develop into erythropoietin-responsive cells (ERC) via several intervening cell generations. The ERC become proerythroblasts under the influence of the hormone erythropoietin. The proerythroblasts, which are the most immature of the morphologically recognizable red-cell precursors, then progress through several cytological classes and mature into reticulocytes. The cytological classes in between pro-erythroblasts and reticulocytes are, in order of increasing maturity, the basophilic erythroblasts, the early polychromatic erythroblasts and the late polychromatic erythroblasts. After a period in the marrow, the reticulocytes enter the circulation within which they mature into fully formed erythrocytes.

Cell proliferation occurs in the various types of morphologically unrecognized red-cell precursors and in proerythroblasts, basophilic erythroblasts and early polychromatic erythroblasts but not in more mature cells. By contrast, the results of progressive cytodifferentiation are manifest in all classes of red-cell precursors, both proliferating and non-proliferating.

Erythrocytes have a lifespan of about 120 days; the majority of the senescent red cells are removed from the circulation by the cells of the mononuclear phagocyte system.

The rate of red-cell production is regulated mainly via alterations in the level of erythropoietin in the plasma. Except in certain pathological situations, the level of this hormone bears an inverse relationship to the oxygen-carrying capacity of the circulating red-cell mass. The main effect of erythropoietin is to stimulate erythropoiesis by increasing the rate of maturation of ERC into proerythroblasts.

ANATOMY OF THE ERYTHRON

In normal adults, erythropoiesis occurs extravascularly in the haemopoietic bone marrow. The distribution of haemopoietic bone marrow within the normal adult human skeleton is given on page 5.

PROBABLE MORPHOLOGY OF THE UNRECOGNIZED CELLS
Although a definite morphological identification of the multipotent haemopoietic stem cell has not yet been

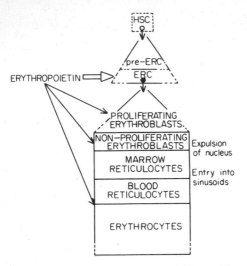

Fig. 4.1. A model of the erythron. HSC: multipotent haemopoietic stem cells; pre-ERC: pre-erythropoietin-sensitive cells; ERC: erythropoietin-responsive cells.

made, a variety of investigators have provided strong circumstantial evidence that in the mouse, this cell resembles a medium-sized or large lymphocyte. For example, using density gradients, van Bekkum *et al.* and Dicke *et al.* [1–3] prepared fractions of marrow cells in which over 20% of the cells were multipotent haemopoietic stem cells as defined by the spleen colony assay described in Chapter 2. From ultrastructural studies of such preparations, these authors concluded that the candidate stem cell was 7–10 μm in diameter, had rounded outlines, contained relatively little cytoplasm, and possessed a large nucleus with one or two large nucleoli and a few masses of nuclear membrane-associated heterochromatin. The possibility that murine multipotent stem cells have the morphological features of large lymphocytes has also been supported by studies of subpopulations of bone-marrow cells which have been separated on the basis of light scatter measurements on a light-activated cell sorter [4].

The morphology of the multipotent haemopoietic stem cells of humans may be similar to that of mice. Barr and his colleagues [5] have shown that a subpopulation of mononuclear cells obtained from human peripheral blood is multipotent. More than 95% of this subpopulation consisted of large lymphocytes without T-cell markers. When cultured within Millipore diffusion chambers which were implanted intraperitoneally in lethally irradiated mice, this subpopulation of cells proliferated and matured into megakaryocytes, granulocyte precursors and erythroblasts.

Recent electron-microscope autoradiographic studies of human bone-marrow cells which had been

incubated with serum-bound ^{55}Fe have revealed an occasional ^{55}Fe-labelled cell profile which displayed the labelling characteristics of early erythroblasts but which failed to show some of the ultrastructural characteristics usually attributed to proerythroblasts [6]. Such cells had large, very irregular or deeply indented nuclei with small to moderate quantities of heterochromatin and prominent nucleoli (Fig. 4.2). They sometimes failed to show rhopheocytotic activity at their cell surface. It has been suggested that these cells, which would not have been recognized as members of the erythroid series in the absence of the overlying autoradiograph, may represent erythropoietin-responsive cells which are on the way to developing into proerythroblasts.

MORPHOLOGY OF RECOGNIZABLE ERYTHROPOIETIC CELLS

Light-microscope appearances

The morphological appearances of the various red-cell precursors were outlined in Chapter 1. Different authors still tend to use somewhat different criteria for subdividing the morphologically recognizable red-cell precursors in Romanowsky-stained marrow smears into different cytological classes. One set of criteria which has been used for this purpose is given in Table 4.1. An important area of variability in the classifications used by different workers is the method of distinguishing between the proliferating, early polychromatic erythroblasts and the non-proliferating late polychromatic erythroblasts. This variability stems from the absence of a reliable way of distinguishing between the proliferating and non-proliferating polychromatic erythroblasts in stained marrow smears. The use of a nuclear diameter of 6·5 μm as the point of demarcation between early and late polychromatic cells (Table 4.1) is based on the observation that the majority of the polychromatic cells with a nuclear diameter of less than 6·5 μm have diploid DNA contents and do not incorporate [^{3}H]thymidine [7, 8].

The term orthochromatic erythroblast is sometimes used more or less synonymously with the term late polychromatic erythroblast. This usage is misleading as totally orthochromatic erythroblasts are rarely seen in well-stained smears of normal marrow. In normal individuals, virtually all of the most mature nucleated erythroblasts have a slightly polychromatic cytoplasm and these cells mature into polychromatic red cells. The latter appear as reticulocytes when stained supravitally with brilliant cresyl blue.

The cell and nuclear sizes in each of the various classes of proliferating erythroblast vary considerably and this variation is partly due to the fact that there is a significant increase in both cell and nuclear size as a

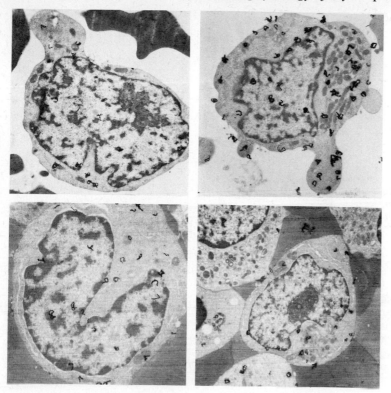

Fig. 4.2. Electron microscope autoradiographs of four immature-looking human bone-marrow cells which have incorporated ^{55}Fe after incubation with serum-bound $^{55}FeCl_3$ at 37°C for three hours. These cells do not show the ultrastructural characteristics usually attributed to proerythroblasts and may represent precursors of the proerythroblasts.

Table 4.1. Classification of morphologically recognizable human red-cell precursors in Romanowsky-stained marrow smears

Cell type	Identifying features	Quantity of condensed chromatin	Proliferation status
Basophilic erythropoietic cells*	Basophilic cytoplasm	Small	In cell cycle
Early polychromatic erythroblasts	Slightly or moderately polychromatic cytoplasm and nuclear diameter $\geqslant 6\cdot5$ μm	Moderate	In cell cycle
Late polychromatic erythroblasts	Polychromatic cytoplasm and nuclear diameter $<6\cdot5$ μm	Moderate or large	Non-dividing
Reticulocytes	Polychromatic cytoplasm and absence of nucleus	—	Non-dividing

* Includes proerythroblasts and basophilic erythroblasts.

haemopoietic cell progresses through interphase. However, this increase is always less than twofold so that there is a progressive reduction in mean cell and nuclear size in successive generations of erythroblasts of increasing maturity (Fig. 4.3). The reduction in cell and nuclear size continues during the maturation of the non-dividing, late polychromatic erythroblasts. It is probable that a reduction in cell volume also occurs during the maturation of reticulocytes within the marrow. There is a 17% reduction in mean cell volume during the maturation into red cells of blood reticulocytes produced during normal steady-state erythropoiesis [9].

Electron-microscopic appearances
The ultrastructural features of human proerythro-

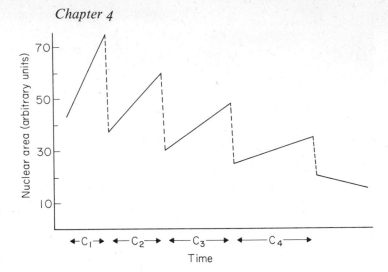

Fig. 4.3. Schematic representation of the changes in nuclear area which occur in an erythropoietic cell as it progresses through four successive cell cycles (C_1–C_4). The interrupted lines indicate the positions of mitoses.

blasts and their progeny have been described by several authors [10–12]. The proerythroblast possesses a large rounded nucleus with little or no peripheral chromatin condensation and one or more very large irregularly shaped nucleoli which are frequently associated with the nuclear margin. The nuclear outline is usually somewhat irregular and may show a moderately deep indentation adjacent to a relatively small centrosome.

The centrosome is made up of two centrioles surrounded by the sacs of a fairly well-developed Golgi apparatus (Fig. 4.4). The cytoplasm contains numerous ribosomes, several mitochondria, a large number of scattered ferritin molecules, a few pleomorphic acid-phosphatase-positive cytoplasmic granules, a few strands of rough endoplasmic reticulum, some microtubules and occasionally, a fen-

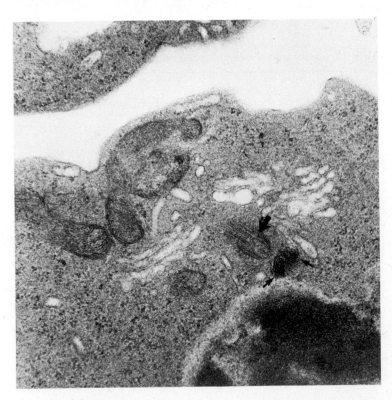

Fig. 4.4. Centrosome in a polychromatic erythroblast. The centriole (large arrow) is surrounded by the flattened saccules of the Golgi apparatus. The two membrane-bound electron-dense granules (small arrows) probably represent lysosomes ($\times 72\,400$).

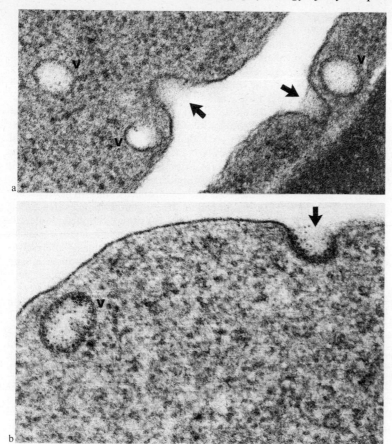

Fig. 4.5. Rhopheocytotic surface depressions (arrows) and vesicles (marked v) in erythroblasts (×142 000). (a) Two adjacent cells from a normal bone marrow. (b) Erythroblast from the hypersiderotic marrow of a patient with hereditary spherocytosis. Note that there are ferritin molecules associated with the rhopheocytotic surface depressions and vesicles in (b) but not in (a).

estrated lamellar complex. The ribosomes, which are frequently arranged as polysomes and sometimes in short spirals are easily seen against the relatively electron-lucent cytoplasm. The lysosomal granules, which are found near the Golgi saccules, are 0·3–0·5 μm in diameter, consist of moderately electron-dense amorphous material bounded by a single membrane and may occasionally contain ferritin molecules. As in the case of all the other morphologically recognizable red-cell precursors, the proerythroblasts show characteristic surface invaginations which develop into small intracytoplasmic vesicles (rhopheocytotic vesicles). The walls of the latter (Fig. 4.5) consist of a single membrane whose inner surface is coated with some material which may be mucopolysaccharide or glycoprotein. In the marrow, the process of rhopheocytosis is considered to be virtually unique to erythroblasts; however, it is also rarely seen in myelocytes and plasma cells. Ferritin molecules are infrequently found within the rhopheocytotic vesicles of normal erythroblasts but are frequently found in this situation in the eryth-

roblasts of patients whose plasma total iron-binding capacity is nearly saturated.

The maturation of a proerythroblast into a late polychromatic erythroblast is accompanied by a variety of ultrastructural changes. These include a progressive increase in the amount of nuclear membrane-associated condensed chromatin, the appearance of increasingly large foci of condensed chromatin in the nucleoplasm, a gradual diminution in the number and size of the nucleoli and an alteration in their fine structure, a reduction in the number of nuclear pores, a progressive decrease in the number of ribosomes, a decrease in the number and size of the mitochondria after the early polychromatic erythroblast stage, a tendency for the intracytoplasmic ferritin molecules to aggregate into siderosomes, some of which are membrane-bound, and a progressive increase in the electron density of both the cytoplasm and the nucleoplasm due to the accumulation of haemoglobin. The most mature erythroblasts possess micronucleoli which usually show a segregation of the fibrillar and granular nucleolar components [13]. According to Yataganas *et al.* [14], 33–40% of the total haemoglobin content of a normal mature human erythroblast is located within the nucleus.

In normal human bone marrow, the late polychromatic erythroblasts develop into reticulocytes by extruding their nuclei. Electron-microscope studies have shown that the nuclear membrane of an extruded nucleus is always surrounded by a very thin rim of haemoglobin-containing cytoplasm enclosed within a cytoplasmic membrane. According to Bessis *et al.* [15], the amount of haemoglobin-containing cytoplasm expelled with each nucleus is about five to 10% of that contained in a newly formed reticulocyte. In ultrathin sections, reticulocytes have irregular outlines and contain some ribosomes, a few mitochondria and occasionally, vestiges of the centrosome. The profiles of reticulocytes (and red cells) may also show membrane-bound acid-phosphatase-positive autophagic vacuoles containing mitochondria, ribosomes and membranes at varying stages of degradation [16]. The circulating erythrocytes have a biconcave shape and do not contain any intracellular organelles apart from the occasional autophagic vacuole (see Chapter 1, p. 13).

Erythroblastic islands
In the bone marrow, the erythroblasts are organized into discrete erythroblastic islands composed of one or two central macrophages surrounded by one or two layers of erythroblasts [17]. Ultrastructural studies have shown that thin cytoplasmic processes arise from the periphery of the central macrophage and extend between individual erythroblasts. In a recent study, Mohandas & Prenant [18] report a three-dimensional reconstruction of erythroblastic islands in rat bone marrow based on a study of 0·5-μm-thick serial sections of Epon-embedded blocks of marrow tissue. These authors find that the number of erythroblasts in each individual erythroblastic island is either two, four, eight, 16 or 32 and that although a macrophage is invariably present in close association with each island, it is not located centrally as has been previously reported. Mohandas & Prenant also make the interesting observation that in the marrow of hypertransfused rats, all of the erythroblasts within a single erythroblastic island are at the same stage of maturation and suggest that the finding of erythroblasts at different stages of maturity in the erythroblastic islands of normal marrow results from the mixing of cells from neighbouring erythroblastic islands in a tissue with a much higher erythropoietic activity than in the polycythaemic marrow. These authors also show that the erythroblastic islands are not spatially restricted to the immediate vicinity of the marrow sinuses and that

although immature erythroblasts are tightly grouped, the more mature erythroblasts appear to move apart so that by the time the late polychromatic erythroblast stage is reached they are found dispersed amongst other cells.

The functional significance of the close association between a macrophage and the cells of an erythroblastic island is still not clear. There is little doubt that the macrophage is involved in the phagocytosis and degradation of extruded erythroblast nuclei, abnormal erythroblasts (p. 124) and aged or pathological erythrocytes (p. 116). Although it has been suggested that ferritin may be transferred between the macrophage and the adjacent erythroblasts, this hypothesis has been questioned and there is now some evidence that ferritin molecules found at sites of rhopheocytotic surface depressions and within rhopheocytotic vesicles may be produced by the erythroblasts themselves [19–21]. The speculations that the macrophage may in some way influence the nature of erythropoietic activity within an erythroblastic island and that this effect may be mediated via the production of erythropoietin remain to be substantiated. Recent studies have demonstrated that mouse peritoneal macrophages exert a stimulating effect on the formation of erythroid colonies when the macrophages are co-cultured with mouse bone-marrow cells in a semi-solid medium containing erythropoietin [22].

Both the frequency distribution of erythroblasts in rat erythroblastic islands and the observation that all the cells within an erythroblastic island are at the same stage of maturity suggest that, at least in the rat, the erythroblastic islands are derived from a single erythropoietic cell which undergoes four or five divisions. In view of the limited number of divisions which appear to occur within an erythroblastic island, it seems likely that the erythropoietic cell which becomes associated with a macrophage and subsequently proliferates to form an erythroblastic island is the erythropoietin-responsive cell.

Number of erythroblasts
The best available estimates for the total numbers of erythroblasts, marrow reticulocytes, blood reticulocytes and circulating red cells in normal individuals are given in Table 4.2 [23] and figures for the relative frequencies of the various types of erythroblasts in normal marrow are given on page 23. Messner *et al.* [24] subdivide the erythroblasts from normal human marrow into five groups (E_1–E_5), on the basis of the observation that the frequency distribution of the nuclear diameters of erythroblasts shows five peaks, and find that the number of erythroblasts nearly doubles from one cytological class to the next. Categories E_1,

Table 4.2. Average values for some parameters of the recognizable red-cell precursors in normal individuals

Cell type	Total number/ kg body weight	Maturation time or lifespan (days)
Erythroblasts	$\simeq 3 \times 10^9$	4·5
Marrow reticulocytes	$3–5 \times 10^9$	2·5
Blood reticulocytes	$\simeq 3 \times 10^9$	1–2
Erythrocytes	300×10^9	120

E_2 and E_3 correspond to basophilic erythropoietic cells, and categories E_4 and E_5 roughly correspond to early and late polychromatic erythroblasts, respectively. The data of Messner *et al.* are consistent with the idea that, on average, there are three cell divisions in the basophilic erythropoietic cells and one division in the early polychromatic erythroblasts. If the classification given in Table 4.1 is used, the numbers of basophilic erythropoietic cells, early polychromatic erythroblasts and late polychromatic erythroblasts in normal marrow are in the ratio $1:1\cdot3:2\cdot7$.

CELL PROLIFERATION DURING ERYTHROPOIESIS

The proliferative activity of the morphologically unrecognized and recognized erythroid precursors serves to markedly increase the number of red cells produced from each multipotent haemopoietic stem cell. It is currently thought that in normal humans there are, on average, four cell divisions in the proliferating erythroblast compartment. Each proerythroblast would, therefore, develop into 2^4 or 16 red cells, provided that there is no cell death between these two stages. The number of additional cell divisions which occur within the morphologically unrecognized precursor pool is not known but if this number is given the value n the total amplification within the erythron would be $2^{(4+n)}$. If $n = 4$, each multipotent stem cell would develop into as many as 256 red cells.

The cell-cycle time (generation time) is the interval of time between the formation of a daughter cell following the completion of mitosis in a parent cell and the completion of mitosis in the newly formed daughter cell. In continuously proliferating diploid mammalian cells, the cell generative cycle can be divided into four phases:

1 a post-mitotic, pre-DNA synthetic period (G_1, the first gap) during which the nucleus has a diploid (2c) DNA content;

2 the DNA synthesis (S) period during which the nucleus doubles its DNA content;

3 a post-DNA-synthetic, premitotic period (G_2, the second gap) during which the nucleus has a tetraploid (4c) DNA content; and

4 mitosis (M).

Several biochemical processes other than the replication of nuclear DNA are more or less confined to various parts of the cell cycle and some of these are essential for the normal movement of a cell through its cell cycle and hence for cell proliferation [25]. For example, the synthesis of a species of RNA and of specific 'G_1 proteins' must take place during the G_1 phase before a G_1 cell enters the S phase. It is also known that the synthesis of histones occurs concurrently with the synthesis of DNA and that inhibition of protein synthesis early in S is rapidly followed by a cessation of DNA synthesis. An impairment of the synthesis of RNA or protein during G_2 prevents the entry of G_2 cells into mitosis.

Only 10% or less of the multipotent haemopoietic stem cells present in the bone marrow of normal adult mice are in the S phase. This finding indicates that the majority of the stem cells are either temporarily out of cell cycle (i.e. in G_0) or are slowly proliferating with a long cell-cycle time (presumably due to the presence of a long G_1 phase). The normally quiescent multipotent haemopoietic stem cells are triggered into active proliferation ($> 50\%$ of cells in S) in certain experimentally induced perturbations of haemopoiesis [26]. Although similar data are not available for human multipotent haemopoietic stem cells, there are no reasons to believe that the stem cells of humans are behaviourally very different from those of mice.

Whereas the majority of the multipotent stem cells of adult rodents are normally in a quiescent state, the pre-ERC and ERC are more actively engaged in proliferation. The percentage of S-phase cells amongst the pre-ERC is 30 in normal, bled or hypertransfused mice and this value increases to 63 during marrow regeneration in irradiated host mice [27]. There are 60–80% of S-phase cells amongst the ERC [26, 27], proerythroblasts, basophilic erythroblasts and early polychromatic erythroblasts in normal bone marrow. This high percentage probably indicates that all the members of these four cytological classes are in active cell cycle.

Quantitative cytochemical studies of Feulgen-stained cells have shown that the majority of the proliferating erythroblasts in normal human bone marrow have DNA contents of 2–4c and are, therefore, diploid cells. As the percentage of cells of a given type in any particular phase of the cell cycle is a function of the average duration of that phase relative to the average duration of the total inter-mitotic time, it can be concluded from the data shown in Table 4.3 that proliferating erythroblasts have a relatively short G_1 period

Table 4.3. Distribution of proliferating erythroblasts in the various stages of interphase in five haematologically normal patients [23]

Cell type	Percentages*				S/G_2*	No. of nuclei assessed*
	G_1	S	G_2	U†		
Basophilic erythropoietic cells‡	32 (24–36)	62 (58–70)	6 (3–7)	0·4 (0–0·9)	10·7 (9·2–25·5)	166 (78–334)
Early polychromatic erythroblasts	11 (4–14)	81 (77–85)	8 (4–10)	0·2 (0–0·7)	10·9 (8·3–21·2)	174 (145–206)

* Average values with ranges given in parentheses.
† Cells which appear to have been arrested after progressing through part of the S phase.
‡ Proerythroblasts plus basophilic erythroblasts.

and a very short G_2 period when compared with the duration of the S phase. The duration of S in the erythroblasts of haematologically normal patients has been studied after a single intravenous injection of [³H]thymidine, using the *in-vivo* labelled mitoses technique, and appears to be 12–14 hours [28]. The upper limit for the duration of mitosis *in vivo* has been calculated to be one hour [29].

The biochemical mechanisms underlying the cessation of proliferation after the early polychromatic erythroblast stage are unknown. The association between a rising level of intracellular haemoglobin and the cessation of cell division during erythropoiesis has led to the still-unproven hypothesis that cell division is inhibited when a critical intracellular haemoglobin content or concentration is achieved [30, 31], perhaps by some direct effect of intranuclear haemoglobin. Yataganas *et al.* [32] have shown that erythroblasts with an intracellular haemoglobin concentration greater than 22% do not synthesize DNA.

RESULTS OF DIFFERENTIATION: BIOCHEMISTRY OF THE ERYTHRON

Differentiation
It is likely that the biochemical process of differentiation primarily involves a differential release and repression of the activity of DNA so that a selected set of genes is either activated or is made capable of being activated at the appropriate time and in the appropriate microenvironment. The biochemical basis underlying such a regulation of gene activity is uncertain but acidic nuclear proteins have been implicated in this process [33] (see Chapter 9). The process of differentiation must operate at the level of the multipotent haemopoietic stem cell when such a cell becomes committed to the red-cell renewal system. Some investigators have postulated that there is a second erythropoietin-mediated differentiation step which operates at the level of the ERC. Although it is generally considered that the *process* of differentiation occurs in one or more steps within the morphologically unrecognized precursor pool, the *results* of differentiation are manifest in both the morphologically unrecognizable and the recognizable precursor pools. The results of differentiation include various biochemical and functional changes which occur throughout erythropoiesis, as well as all the morphological (including ultrastructural) changes described earlier in this chapter which follow from some of the biochemical changes. The biochemical changes include both the synthesis of some species of molecules and the regulated degradation of others.

The most striking consequence of differentiation in the recognizable erythropoietic cells is a progressive increase in the mean intracellular haemoglobin concentration in successive cytological classes. This is associated with a progressive decrease in mean dry mass, total RNA content and total RNA concentration per cell (Fig. 4.6). The changes in total RNA are largely due to changes in ribosomal RNA as the latter accounts for most of the RNA in a cell. Other results of differentiation include the gradual reduction in mean cell and nuclear size in successive cytological classes [23], a progressive increase in the amount of heterochromatin in successive cytological classes (p. 103), the loss of proliferative activity after the early polychromatic erythroblast stage (p. 103), the extrusion of the nucleus of the late polychromatic erythroblast (p. 104), alterations in intracellular enzymes (p. 111), changes in cell deformability [34] and in the fluorescence anisotropy (fluidity) of the cell membrane [35], and changes in the composition of the cell membrane such as the appearance of the D antigen (p. 111).

The definitive description of the biochemistry of

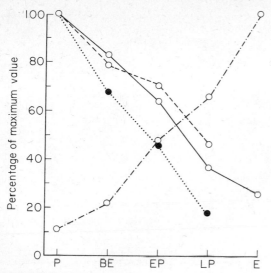

Fig. 4.6. Changes in mean dry mass (——), RNA content (····), RNA concentration (– – –), and haemoglobin concentration (–·–·–) per cell during normal human erythropoiesis. P = proerythroblasts, BE = basophilic erythroblasts, EP = early polychromatic erythroblasts, LP = late polychromatic erythroblasts, E = erythrocytes. (From Ref. 32.)

erythropoiesis will have to include an explanation for the orderly expression of the various results of differentiation at specific times during erythropoiesis. It is not yet certain whether the various structural genes involved in various facets of cytodifferentiation are activated in one or more blocks in the morphologically unrecognized precursor pool or whether these structural genes are activated throughout erythropoiesis in the sequence in which their gene products are required. It is possible that several aspects of cytodifferentiation are not regulated by the timing of gene activation but by other mechanisms such as alterations of the rates at which a precursor of mRNA is processed into functional mRNA or by feedback systems affecting pre-existing intracytoplasmic metabolic pathways (without alterations in the rates of synthesis of mRNA for particular enzymes). Further information on the regulation of the biochemistry of erythropoiesis may well be obtained from current studies of Friend cells. The latter are obtained by culturing splenic tissue from mice infected with the Friend virus complex and seem to be ERCs which have been transformed by the virus so that they are no longer responsive to erythropoietin. They may, however, be induced to differentiate down the erythropoietic pathway by treatment with dimethylsulphoxide (DMSO) or several other agents [36].

DNA/RNA metabolism

DNA replication. The entry of mammalian cells from G_1 into S is at least partly controlled by events occurring in the G_1 phase [25]. As in other cell types, the replication of DNA during the S phase of erythroblasts occurs near the junction between condensed chromatin (heterochromatin) and expanded chromatin (euchromatin) (Fig. 4.7). Because none of the early polychromatic erythroblasts have a totally euchromatic nucleus, it is likely that, at least in the nuclei of these cells, areas of heterochromatin decondense, replicate and then recondense during the S phase [37]. During DNA replication, the two strands of the DNA double helix unwind and a new daughter strand is synthesized on each of the two separated parental strands using the parental strands as templates. The synthesis of new DNA involves the polymerization of the four deoxyribonucleoside triphosphates (deoxyadenosine, deoxyguanosine, deoxythymidine and deoxycytidine triphosphates) in the appropriate sequence under the influence of DNA polymerases. The replication of DNA commences at several sites and occurs in many short stretches along the length of each very long DNA molecule; each replicating unit or replicon is between 10 and 250 μm long. Further details of the biochemistry of DNA replication are given in Chapter 6.

The susceptibility of the ERCs to undergo further cytodifferentiation may be cell-cycle-dependent as there is some evidence that the maturation of Friend cells into haemoglobin-containing erythroblasts requires at least one period of DNA synthesis in the presence of the inducing agent, DMSO [36, 38]. In most cell-renewal systems there is an inverse relationship between proliferative activity and the extent of cytodifferentiation and this is also true of the erythropoietic system. The mechanisms leading to the cessation of cell proliferation after the early polychromatic erythroblast stage are still uncertain.

RNA metabolism. The synthesis of RNA occurs at the junction between heterochromatin and euchromatin (Fig. 4.7). Light- and electron-microscope autoradiographic studies have revealed that during normal human erythropoiesis, the rate of synthesis of total cellular RNA declines markedly with increasing maturation until it is very low in the late polychromatic erythroblasts [39–42]. Reticulocytes have no nucleus and consequently are incapable of RNA synthesis. There is evidence that 30–70% of the RNA molecules which are synthesized within human erythroblasts are short-lived and rapidly degraded within the nucleus [39]. This intranuclear RNA degradation is a general feature of eukaryotic cells and is not confined to erythroblasts. It has been shown that several eukaryotic

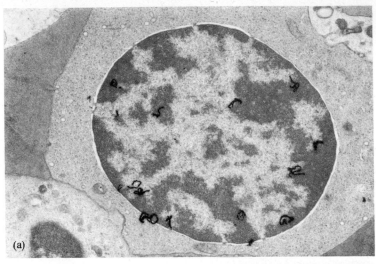

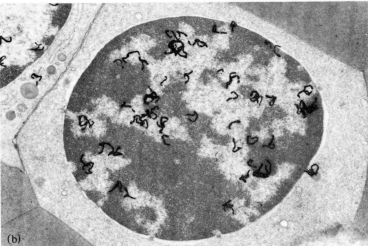

Fig. 4.7. Electron-microscope auto-radiographs of two early polychromatic erythroblasts illustrating that DNA synthesis (a), and RNA synthesis (b), occur predominantly near the junction between condensed chromatin (heterochromatin) and expanded chromatin (euchromatin). The cell in (a) had been incubated with [6-³H] thymidine (20 μCi per ml; specific activity 26 Ci/mmol) for 15 minutes and that in (b) with [5-³H] uridine (150 μCi per ml; specific activity 24 Ci/mmol) for 15 minutes.

mRNAs, including avian and mouse globin mRNA, are initially synthesized as very large molecules which are called heterogeneous nuclear RNA (HnRNA) and which are 10–20 times larger than the functional messenger RNA (mRNA) molecules (see Chapter 9). The non-mRNA material in these HnRNA molecules is degraded intranuclearly [43–46]. Despite the continuous intranuclear degradation of newly synthesized RNA, the proliferating erythroblasts show an increase in total RNA content as they progress through interphase [32].

Investigations employing anaemic rabbits and mice have suggested that although all species of RNA (i.e. ribosomal RNA, mRNA and transfer RNA) are synthesized in all types of erythroblast, ribosomal RNA is synthesized predominantly in the proerythroblasts and basophilic erythroblasts and mRNA in the more mature cells [47, 48]. More recently, two groups of workers have studied the appearance of globin mRNA during erythropoiesis in the fetal mouse liver [49–51]. These workers detected mRNA both by using the technique of hybridization with globin cDNA (a radioactive transcript of globin mRNA prepared using reverse transcriptase) and by translation of the mRNA in the Krebs ascites system and concluded that proerythroblasts contain negligible quantities of globin mRNA and that the synthesis of globin mRNA normally commences in the basophilic erythroblasts. Further investigations have shown that high levels of erythropoietin stimulate the appearance of globin mRNA in the proerythroblasts of fetal livers both *in vivo* and *in vitro* [52].

Protein synthesis

The biochemistry of protein synthesis and a detailed account of haemoglobin synthesis are given in Chapter 9. Autoradiographic studies of normal human bone marrow have shown that protein synthesis occurs in all types of recognizable red-cell precursors, including reticulocytes [53]. As the reticulocytes do not contain a nucleus, they must depend on pre-formed RNA for protein synthesis. The rate of synthesis of protein decreases progressively in successive cytological classes of increasing maturity and this decrease is particularly marked in the proliferating erythroblast pool [39–41]. Mature red cells do not contain ribosomes and are therefore incapable of protein synthesis.

The haemoglobin content of basophilic erythropoietic cells and early polychromatic erythroblasts increases during interphase to reach a maximum during the early part of the S phase and changes little thereafter. By contrast the dry mass of these cells increases throughout interphase. It appears that haemoglobin is synthesized mainly during G_1 and early S and that the increase in dry mass after the early part of the S phase is due to an increase in non-haemoglobin proteins and nucleic acids [32].

Studies in anaemic rabbits have shown that the activities of a number of enzymes show considerable variations as erythroid cells progress down the erythropoietic pathway and that the pattern of changing activity differs for different enzymes [54]. For example there is little carbonic anhydrase activity in the basophilic cells but this activity increases progressively with increasing maturity to reach maximum values in the reticulocytes. By contrast, the catalase activity of an erythroid cell remains more or less constant during erythropoiesis except for an increase at the reticulocyte stage. The activities of glucose-6-phosphate dehydrogenase, 6-phosphogluconate dehydrogenase, adenosine deaminase and nucleoside phosphorylase are relatively high in the proliferating erythroblasts but show a steep decline between the proliferating early polychromatic erythroblast stage and the non-dividing late polychromatic erythroblast stage. Other enzyme changes which have been described during erythropoiesis in anaemic rabbits are a small decline in lactate dehydrogenase activity and a 60% increase in adenylate kinase activity as a cell passed from the dividing compartments into the non-dividing compartments.

There are some data which suggest that in mice, the different proteins found in the cell membranes of mature erythrocytes are synthesized by precursor cells at different stages of maturity. It appears that the bulk of the spectrin and actin polypeptides are synthesized before the major transmembrane glycoprotein and that the synthesis of glycoprotein ceases before that of several minor proteins found on the inner surface of the red-cell membrane [55].

Development of red-cell antigens

The A, B and H antigens as well as antigens belonging to the Rh, MNSs, P, Lutheran, Kell, Duffy, Kidd and Ii systems have been demonstrated on human erythroblasts at all stages of maturity, including proerythroblasts [56–58]. The quantity of D antigen as judged by binding to ^{125}I-labelled anti-D in proerythroblasts, basophilic erythroblasts, early polychromatic erythroblasts, late polychromatic erythroblasts and mature red cells is in the ratio $1/4 : 1/2 : 2/3 : 3/4 : 1$, respectively [59]. This progressive increase in antibody binding could be due either to a progressive increase in the number of D-antigen sites with increasing maturity or to alterations which affect antibody binding such as changes in the composition of the membrane or in the orientation of the D antigen.

Nutritional requirements for erythropoiesis

Anaemia usually develops late during the course of the development of dietary deficiencies. Iron, folic acid and vitamin B_{12} are the three nutrients which are most frequently involved in nutritional anaemias in man.

Iron. This is an essential constituent of the haemoglobin molecule and is consequently an important nutritional requirement for erythropoiesis. A discussion of iron metabolism and the haematological effects of iron deficiency may be found in Chapter 5.

Vitamin B_{12} and folic acid. The active forms of these two vitamins are required for DNA synthesis and cell proliferation. A deficiency of either vitamin B_{12} or folate induces megaloblastic haemopoiesis in humans. This type of haemopoiesis is characterized by a gross perturbation of erythroblast proliferation and a marked increase in ineffective erythropoiesis. The metabolic functions of the vitamin-B_{12} and folate coenzymes and the biochemical and haematological consequences of vitamin-B_{12} or folate deficiency are discussed elsewhere (Chapter 6).

Vitamin B_6 or pyridoxine. Pyridoxine is converted in the liver to the active coenzyme pyridoxal phosphate which has several functions in amino-acid metabolism. The coenzyme also participates in haem synthesis by promoting the formation of δ-aminolaevulinic acid from glycine and succinyl-coenzyme A. A deficiency of pyridoxine in animals causes a hypochromic anaemia. Although a nutritional pyridoxine deficiency is very rare in humans, abnormalities in pyridoxine metabolism are present in some patients with sideroblastic anaemia. Various aspects of pyridoxine metabolism

Chapter 4

and an account of the sideroblastic anaemias are given in Chapter 13.

Riboflavin. A normochromic normocytic anaemia has been induced in humans by a combination of riboflavin deprivation and the administration of the riboflavin antagonist, galactoflavin [60]. In this situation the bone marrow shows erythroid hypoplasia and vacuolation of erythroblasts. Naturally occurring riboflavin deficiency in humans is usually found as part of a complex nutritional deficiency state. However, occasional patients have been described in whom the anaemia and erythroid hypoplasia have responded to riboflavin and not to other nutrients [61].

Vitamin C (ascorbic acid). Patients with scurvy have a normocytic, macrocytic or microcytic anaemia with erythroid hyperplasia in the marrow [62, 63]. However, as such patients suffer from deficiencies of several essential nutrients other than vitamin C, it is difficult to attribute the anaemia to a deficiency of vitamin C. Humans deliberately fed on a vitamin-C-deficient diet for up to 39 months do not develop anaemia [64]. However, there are reports of cases of scurvy in which the anaemia has failed to respond to iron, vitamin B_{12} and folate but has subsequently responded to ascorbic acid [65] (see Chapter 6).

Vitamin E (α tocopherol). A deficiency of this vitamin in premature infants [66] and in occasional patients with malabsorption [67] is associated with low serum tocopherol levels, a haemolytic state and an abnormal sensitivity of erythrocytes to peroxide-induced haemolysis (see Chapter 7). Vitamin-E deficiency causes a marked perturbation of erythropoiesis in monkeys and swine but not in humans.

Copper. Anaemia and neutropenia due to copper deficiency have been reported in malnourished children [69], a patient with coeliac disease [70] and in patients receiving long-term parenteral nutrition after extensive bowel resections [71]. The haematological features found in these patients have varied from case to case and have included a high MCV, normoblastic or megaloblastic erythropoiesis, the formation of ring sideroblasts and the vacuolation of erythroblasts. Studies in experimental animals have indicated that copper deficiency causes an increase in ineffective erythropoiesis.

Other minerals and vitamins. Although an anaemia occurs in certain experimental animals made deficient in cobalt, pantothenic acid and nicotinic acid, there is no clear evidence that the deficiency of these substances plays an important role in the pathogenesis of the anaemia in nutritional deficiency states in man. A deficiency of selenium causes a reduction in the activity of the selenium-containing enzyme glutathione peroxidase but this does not seem to cause a haemolytic anaemia [72].

Amino acids. An anaemia associated with either erythroid hypoplasia or a pure red-cell aplasia develops in protein-deficient humans and animals. Detailed studies in experimental animals indicate that this anaemia is largely caused by an impairment of the production of erythropoietin rather than an impairment of the synthesis of globin or other red-cell proteins [73, 74]. However, there is some shortening of red-cell lifespan in protein-deficient rats and this appears to be at least partly due to an abnormality in the structure of the red cells [75]. Patients with kwashiorkor (severe protein deficiency) and marasmus usually suffer from a variety of nutritional deficiencies in addition to a protein deficiency and are also prone to suffer from infections. Therefore, the pathogenesis of the anaemia in such patients is often quite complex.

Carbohydrates. Patients with severe anorexia nervosa suffer from a marked deficiency of carbohydrates and calories but, usually, little protein deficiency. Such patients frequently have an anaemia which may be associated with a neutropenia and a thrombocytopenia. The bone marrow is hypocellular and the fat cells are completely replaced by a gelatinous extracellular material consisting of acidic mucopolysaccharide [76]. The mechanisms by which a severe deficiency of carbohydrates and calories induce these disturbances in haemopoiesis are not known.

ENTRY OF RETICULOCYTES INTO THE CIRCULATION

As the denucleation of late polychromatic erythroblasts usually occurs within the marrow parenchyma, the majority of the reticulocytes must travel across the wall of the marrow sinusoids to enter the circulation. The luminal surface of a marrow sinusoid is virtually completely covered by a single layer of a 'primitive' type of endothelial cell. Tight junctions are absent at sites of overlap between adjacent endothelial cells and it is possible that this feature permits large changes in the volumes of the marrow sinusoids [77]. Even in electron micrographs of well-fixed marrow tissue, several small gaps are seen in the layer of endothelial cells but these gaps are now considered to be artefacts. The abluminal surfaces of the endothelial cells of marrow sinusoids are partially covered by an incomplete layer of adventitial cells.

The migration of reticulocytes from the marrow

parenchyma into the lumina of the marrow sinusoids has been studied in experimental animals both by transmission and scanning electron microscopy [78–82]. It is now considered that this migration occurs not through pre-existing channels, as had been previously thought, but through channels which develop across the endothelial cells at the time of reticulocyte transit. These transendothelial channels, which are frequently found near the junction between two endothelial cells, are quite narrow. Consequently, reticulocytes have to undergo a marked deformation during their passage through such channels. The greater deformability of the reticulocyte as compared with its nucleated precursor [34] and the motility of the reticulocyte [83] must both be of considerable importance for the egress of this cell through the sinusoidal wall. There is no adventitial cell cover at sites of egress of reticulocytes through the endothelium.

The mechanisms which regulate the release of reticulocytes into the circulation are not yet fully understood. At least in theory, alterations in the rates of entry of new blood cells into the sinusoids may be determined by some effect either on the cells of the marrow parenchyma or on the sinusoidal walls. Erythropoietin stimulates the discharge of reticulocytes from the isolated perfused limbs of animals [84, 85], but the way in which this is brought about is still not clear. The administration of erythropoietin leads to a reduction in the adventitial cell cover of the marrow sinusoids thereby facilitating the access of all types of maturing cells including reticulocytes to the abluminal surfaces of the endothelial cells. As the reduction in adventitial cell cover cannot account for the *selective* increase in the rate of release of reticulocytes from the marrow, it is probable that erythropoietin also has some other effect on the release mechanisms.

Marrow sinusoids show peculiar slow rhythmic volume changes *in vivo* [86]. The possibility that these rhythmic movements play a role in the egress of reticulocytes into the circulation is suggested by studies of animals made polycythaemic by the transfusion of red cells. Such animals show a marked distension of the sinusoids due to packing with red cells and this sinusoidal packing is associated with a reduction in the number of reticulocytes in transit through the sinusoidal wall [80].

RATES OF FLOW OF ERYTHROPOIETIC CELLS

For the investigation of the rates of flow of cells during erythropoiesis, the erythron must be considered to consist of a number of serially connected cytological compartments in which cell division occurs at the boundaries between adjacent compartments [87, 88]. The principles underlying this type of analysis have been outlined in relation to the investigation of granulocyte kinetics in Chapter 15. In studies of the kinetics of erythropoiesis, the morphologically recognizable cells have been divided into five cytological compartments, E_1–E_5 (p. 106) into any one of these compartments (K_{IN}) is equal to the rate of efflux of cells (K_{OUT}) out of the preceding compartment. The birth rate (K_B) in any particular compartment is equal to N_S/t_S where N_S is the number of cells in the S phase and t_S the average duration of the S phase in that compartment. Provided that the rate of cell death within a cytological compartment is negligible, K_{OUT} will be equal to K_{IN} plus K_B for that compartment. The relative rates of flow of cells into and out of various compartments calculated by the above approach (and assuming that K_{IN} into E_1 is virtually zero) are given in Table 4.4. The calculated rate of efflux of cells from the E_4 compartment (i.e. early polychromatic erythroblast compartment) agreed closely with the observed rate of influx of radioactive cells into the non-dividing E_5 compartment after a single intravenous injection of [³H]thymidine [89]. This agreement provides good evidence that the amount of cell death during normal erythropoiesis is quite small.

INEFFECTIVE ERYTHROPOIESIS

The loss of potential erythrocytes as a consequence of the death of some red-cell precursors is referred to as ineffective erythropoiesis. Although it is indisputable that some cells die in any actively proliferating cell

Table 4.4. Calculated relative rates of flow of erythroblasts (per hour) into and out of various cytological compartments, assuming that $t_s = 12$ hours (from Ref. 89)

	E_1	E_2	E_3	E_4	E_5
PD*	100	218	610	810	1910
LI%*	100	77	82	50	0
N_s*	100	168	500	405	—
K_{IN}*	†	8·2	22·2	64·0	101‡
K_B*	8·2	14·0	41·8	33·8	
K_{OUT}*	8·2	22·2	64·0	97·8	

* PD = proportional distribution of erythroblasts in the different cytological compartments. LI, N_s, K_{IN}, K_B and K_{OUT} are defined in the text.
† Assumed to be zero.
‡ Calculated using PD = 1910 and an observed rate of influx of [³H]TdR-labelled cells of 5·3% per hour.

system, the studies of the kinetics of red-cell production referred to in the previous section have suggested that the extent of ineffective erythropoiesis in haematologically normal individuals is very small [89]. By contrast, data from studies of bilirubin production and from ferrokinetic studies indicate that four to 12% [90] and 14–34% [91–93] respectively, of the total erythropoietic activity is ineffective in normal individuals. The explanation of this discrepancy lies in the fact that, unlike cell kinetic studies, neither bilirubin production studies nor ferrokinetic studies actually measure cell death. The latter two techniques give information on the effectiveness with which haemoglobin synthesized by red-cell precursors or iron taken up by these cells, respectively, are utilized for incorporation into mature red cells and therefore only provide a very indirect measure of ineffective erythropoiesis. The high estimates for the extent of ineffective erythropoiesis in normal individuals given by bilirubin production and ferrokinetic studies are at least partly due to the fact that these two techniques detect as ineffective erythropoiesis, the degradation of the narrow rim of haemoglobin-containing cytoplasm which surrounds each extruded erythroblast nucleus. The loss of some-haemoglobin-containing cytoplasm at the time of nuclear extrusion does not lead to a reduction of the *number* of potential erythrocytes and should, therefore, not be included as a component of ineffective erythropoiesis.

Whereas ineffective erythropoiesis appears to account for a very small fraction of total erythropoietic activity in normal individuals, it accounts for a substantial fraction in several diseases such as homozygous β thalassaemia, the congenital dyserythropoietic anaemias and the megaloblastic and sideroblastic anaemias (see p. 135).

TIME PARAMETERS OF ERYTHROPOIESIS

The time parameters during the morphologically recognizable phase of human erythropoiesis in the normal steady state have been determined mainly by cell kinetic studies in individuals who have been given a single intravenous injection of [^{3}H]thymidine [23]. The time taken for a proerythroblast to develop into reticulocytes and for the resultant reticulocytes to enter the bloodstream is about seven days [94]. Approximately half of this time is spent in the pool of proliferating erythroblasts; the remainder is spent in the non-dividing precursor pool. Within the non-dividing pool, about 20 hours is spent in the late polychromatic erythroblast pool [24, 95] and about 2·5 days in the marrow

reticulocyte pool. The blood reticulocytes develop into erythrocytes over a period of one to two days.

LIFESPAN AND FATE OF RED BLOOD CELLS

Assessment of red-cell lifespan
A variety of methods have been used to determine the lifespan of the circulating red cell. These methods fall into two categories, indirect and direct. Two of the three indirect methods depend on complex calculations based on ferrokinetic measurements made during the first two weeks after an injection of ^{59}Fe-labelled transferrin [93, 96]. The third indirect method is based on measurements of bilirubin turnover [97]. One of the disadvantages of these indirect methods is that they can only be applied to the study of the lifespan of a subject's cells in his own circulation. There are three types of direct methods; the cross-transfusion technique of Ashby, and the cohort-labelling and random-labelling techniques. Although the various methods available for the determination of red-cell lifespan give slightly different results, the data suggest that the average red-cell lifespan in a normal adult is 110–120 days.

Cross-transfusion technique of Ashby
In the Ashby technique [98–101], a large volume of compatible red cells is transfused into a recipient. The transfused red cells must be antigenically distinguishable from the red cells of the recipient, usually on the basis of differences in the ABO, MN or Rh antigens. The subsequent survival of the cells is studied by the technique of differential agglutination or haemolysis using appropriate antibodies. Two of the major disadvantages of this technique are that it is time-consuming and that it cannot be used to determine the survival of patients' red cells in their own circulation.

Cohort-labelling methods
In the cohort-labelling methods [102–106] a group of newly produced erythrocytes is labelled with a radioactive precursor of haem (e.g. [^{15}N]glycine, [^{14}C]glycine, ^{59}Fe) or globin (^{75}Selenomethionine). The radioactive compound is only available for incorporation into newly formed red cells over a relatively short period so that the radioactive red cells can be considered to be of almost the same age. The labelling is usually performed *in vivo* and the subsequent fate of the labelled cohort of red cells is followed by serial sampling of the blood. In normal individuals, the radioactivity in the red cells shows an initial rapid increase and then remains more or less constant until the cohort approaches the end of its lifespan after which the radioactivity falls very rapidly (Fig. 4.8). The time interval between the mid-points of the ascending and

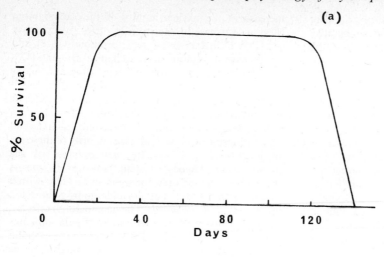

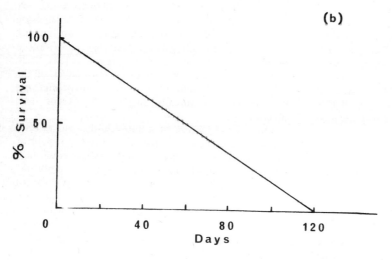

Fig. 4.8. Red-cell-survival curves which would be expected with the ideal cohort-labelling technique (a) and the ideal random-labelling technique (b).

descending portions of the graph is usually taken as the average lifespan of the red cells. When the red cell survival is normal, the blood has to be sampled for as long as 130–150 days to demonstrate the destruction of the radioactive cohort. The interpretation of data obtained from the cohort-labelling methods depends on the assumptions that the label remains within the red cells throughout their lifespan and that there is no reutilization of the label for the formation of new red cells following the degradation of cells belonging to the original radioactive cohort. ^{59}Fe is a much less satisfactory cohort label than labelled glycine as a high proportion of the iron released during the catabolism of haemoglobin is reutilized for haemoglobin synthesis.

Random-labelling methods
Red cells with a random age-distribution are labelled using a suitable radioactive compound and the survival of the radioactive red cells is then followed by serial sampling of the blood. If there is no elution of the label from the red cells and provided that the degree of random destruction of red cells is insignificant, the red-cell radioactivity curve would be linear and the time at which the radioactivity falls to zero would be the mean cell lifespan (Fig. 4.8).

Labelling of red cells with ^{51}Cr. This is the most commonly used method for the determination of red-cell lifespan [107–109]. Unlike the Ashby technique, it can be used to study the survival of very small volumes of red cells and the patient's red cells in his own circulation. The radioactive chromate anion (^{51}CrO$_4^{2-}$) enters the red cell and is converted into the trivalent cation (^{51}Cr^{3+}) which binds predominantly to β and γ

chains of haemoglobin molecules. As cationic Cr does not penetrate into red cells, any ^{51}Cr which is liberated from the degradation of labelled red cells does not reattach itself to other red cells. A serious disadvantage of the Cr method is that the label does not bind sufficiently firmly to the haemoglobin; the ^{51}Cr elutes at the rate of about one per cent per day. During the first two to three days there is also an additional loss, so that in normal individuals the survival at 24 hours is only about 96% of the survival at 10 minutes. As a result of the roughly exponential elution of Cr from red cells, the normal red-cell ^{51}Cr survival curve, plotted on arithmetical graph paper, is not linear but curvilinear. In view of the difficulties caused by Cr elution, many workers express their results in terms of the time in days at which the red-cell ^{51}Cr count-rate falls to 50% of its initial value ($T_{\frac{1}{2}}$Cr or T_{50}Cr) rather than as a true red-cell lifespan. The normal range for T_{50}Cr depends on the details of the red-cell labelling technique used and should be determined for each laboratory; it is around 27–36 days. A true red-cell lifespan could be obtained from ^{51}Cr data if the method of red-cell labelling is carefully standardized and appropriate correction factors are applied to the observed ^{51}Cr survival data to correct for Cr elution [110]. However, even after the data are corrected in this way, a slightly curvilinear survival curve may be found in some normal individuals.

Labelling of red cells with DF^{32}P. Di-isopropyl fluorophosphonate, which binds to the cholinesterase within red cells, has been used to label red cells both *in vitro* [111–112] and *in vivo* [113]. Unlike Cr, DFP binds very firmly to red cells and does not elute from them after the first 24–48 hours. In normal individuals, the loss of red-cell radioactivity is, therefore, linear from about 24–48 hours after the injection of either *in-vitro* labelled cells or DF^{32}P into the circulation. [^{3}H]DFP may be used instead of DF^{32}P [114].

Fate of red blood cells

Red cells undergo a number of biochemical and biophysical changes as they age within the circulation. The activity of several intracytoplasmic enzymes decreases with increasing red-cell age but these changes are not necessarily rate-limiting with respect to the various reactions in which the enzymes participate. There is a reduction in the activity of the enzymes involved in the anaerobic glycolytic pathway (Embden–Meyerhof pathway) and the pentose phosphate pathway and a reduction in the overall rate of glycolysis [115–117]. Other changes which occur with ageing include a decrease in surface area, lipid content and negative charge of the cell membrane [118–122], a decreased ability to reduce methaemoglobin [123], an increase in the oxygen affinity of the haemoglobin [124], an increase in density [125, 126], a decrease in size [119, 127], a reduction in deformability [128], and an increase in osmotic and mechanical fragility [127, 129]. The changes in the cell membrane and in the density and size of ageing red cells appear to be caused by the shedding of haemoglobin-containing exocytic microvesicles at the cell surface [130].

In normal adults about 3×10^6 red cells reach the end of their lifespan each second. The majority of these are phagocytosed intact by the macrophages of the mononuclear phagocyte system. However, it appears that some effete red cells undergo osmotic lysis within the circulation and that others undergo fragmentation prior to their phagocytosis. The haemoglobin released from red cells which lyse within the circulation combines with a specific haemoglobin-binding α_2 globulin present in the plasma, which is called haptoglobin (see p. 138). The haemoglobin–haptoglobin complexes are subsequently ingested by macrophages. Studies using ^{59}Fe- and ^{51}Cr-labelled red cells have shown that the majority of aged red cells are destroyed in the spleen in the rat and in the marrow in the rabbit [131, 132]. The relative importance of the macrophages of the spleen, marrow and liver in the destruction of effete red cells in normal humans has not at present been determined.

The unique feature of a 110–120-day-old normal erythrocyte which is recognized by a macrophage prior to erythrophagocytosis is still unknown. It could be a physical or chemical change in the red-cell membrane. Marton [133] has shown that the macrophages present in the parenchyma of rat bone marrow protrude cytoplasmic processes through the sinusoidal walls into the intravascular spaces and that these intrasinusoidal protrusions engulf circulating aged or heat-damaged red cells.

The haemoglobin molecules in the red cells, red-cell fragments and haptoglobin–haemoglobin complexes which are phagocytosed by macrophages are degraded into bilirubin (Fig. 4.9). This process involves the removal of the globin chains, the release of iron from the haem and the opening of the porphyrin ring with the formation of biliverdin. The porphyrin ring is opened by oxidation of the α-methene bridge. The conversion of the porphyrin ring to biliverdin is mediated by the microsomal enzyme *haem oxygenase* [134], requires both oxygen and NADH, and represents a rate-limiting step in the degradation of haem. One molecule of carbon monoxide is formed with the opening of each porphyrin ring and this forms the basis of the use of carbon-monoxide production as an index of haemoglobin catabolism (p. 124). The biliverdin is converted to bilirubin in the presence of NADPH and the cytoplasmic enzyme *biliverdin reductase* [134, 135].

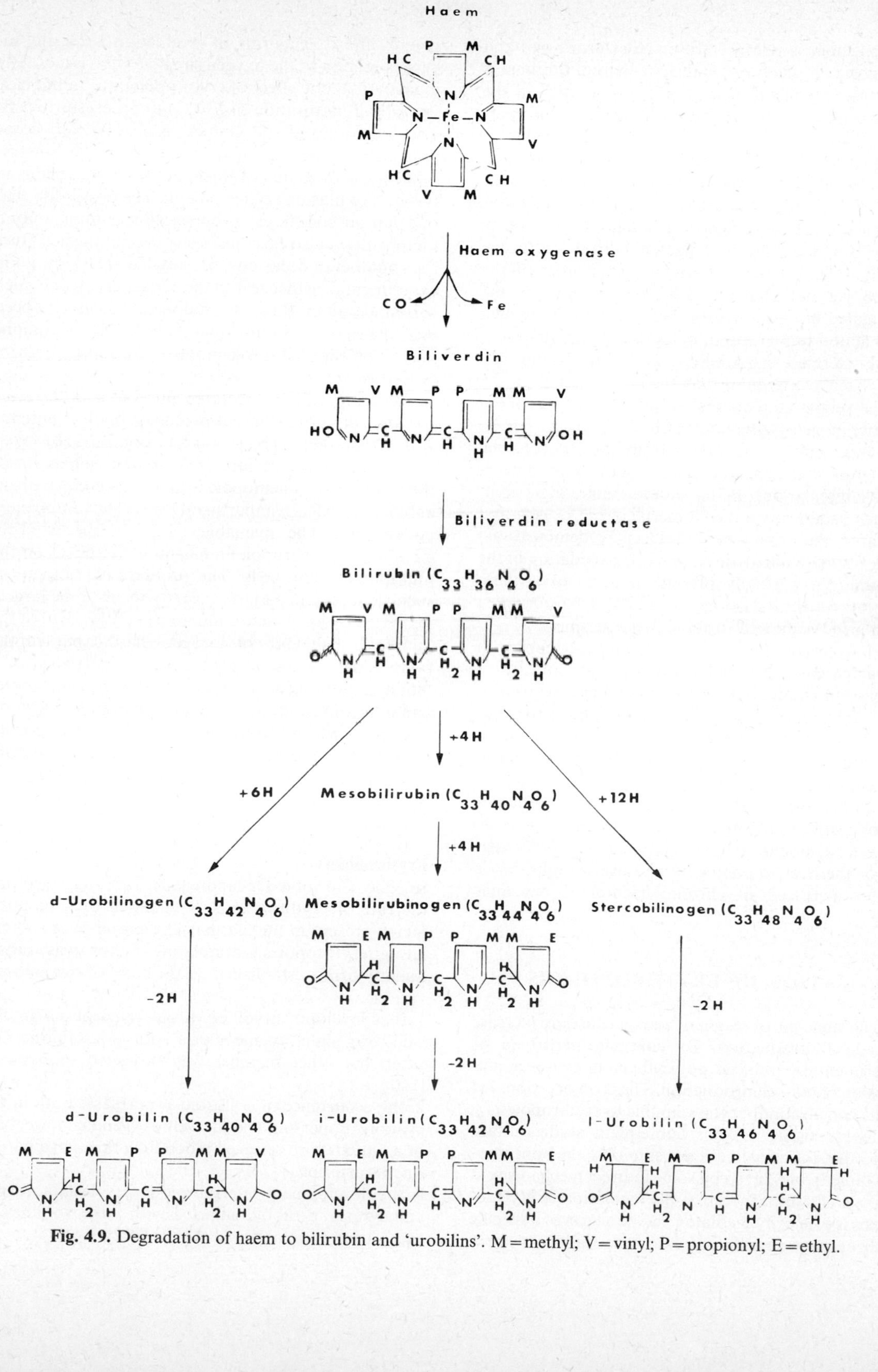

Haem

Haem oxygenase

CO ← → Fe

Biliverdin

Biliverdin reductase

Bilirubin $(C_{33}H_{36}N_4O_6)$

+4H

+6H   Mesobilirubin $(C_{33}H_{40}N_4O_6)$ +12H

+4H

d-Urobilinogen $(C_{33}H_{42}N_4O_6)$ Mesobilirubinogen $(C_{33}H_{44}N_4O_6)$ Stercobilinogen $(C_{33}H_{48}N_4O_6)$

−2H   −2H   −2H

d-Urobilin $(C_{33}H_{40}N_4O_6)$ i-Urobilin $(C_{33}H_{42}N_4O_6)$ l-Urobilin $(C_{33}H_{46}N_4O_6)$

Fig. 4.9. Degradation of haem to bilirubin and 'urobilins'. M = methyl; V = vinyl; P = propionyl; E = ethyl.

The bilirubin is released from the macrophages and transported to the liver via the circulation. Bilirubin is insoluble in aqueous solutions and is carried in the plasma bound to the albumin. Within the hepatic parenchymal cells, the bilirubin is made water-soluble by conjugation with acidic radicles. Most of the bilirubin is converted to bilirubin diglucuronide under the influence of the microsomal enzyme *glucuronyl transferase* but some is converted to the monoglucuronide or to the sulphate. The conjugated bilirubin is transported to and across the canalicular border of the hepatocyte and excreted in the bile. In the gut, the conjugated bilirubin is progressively reduced by bacterial action to a group of colourless compounds collectively termed 'stercobilinogens' or 'urobilinogens'. The '-ogen' compounds may then be converted to the orange-yellow 'stercobilins' or 'urobilins'. Most of the stercobilinogen passes out of the body in the faeces. However, some is absorbed from the gut into the circulation and then re-excreted by the liver (enterohepatic circulation). Being water-soluble, these compounds pass through the glomeruli of the kidneys and appear in the urine where they can be demonstrated using Ehrlich's aldehyde reagent. The oxidation of the urobilinogen normally present in urine to urobilin accounts for the darkening of urine which is observed when urine is allowed to stand in a container.

In haemolytic states the body attempts to cope with the increased rate of red-cell destruction both by an increase in the number of macrophages involved in erythrophagocytosis and by increasing the intracellular activity of the enzymes involved in the catabolism of haemoglobin. The activity of the enzyme haem oxygenase in rat hepatic microsomes is increased by a factor of two to seven after the injection of haemoglobin or methaemalbumin and after an experimentally induced haemolytic anaemia [136]. Similarly, the capacity of the liver to conjugate and excrete bilirubin is greatly increased in chronic haemolytic anaemias [137].

REGULATION OF ERYTHROPOIESIS

Anoxic, anaemic or stagnant anoxia causes an increase in red-cell production. By contrast, hyperoxia or experimentally induced polycythaemia causes a suppression of red-cell production. These observations led to the conclusion that the stimulus to erythropoiesis is related to tissue anoxia. Subsequent studies established that the anoxia did not stimulate the bone marrow directly but did so by some indirect mechanism. It is now well established that the regulation of erythropoiesis is primarily mediated via the action of a specific erythropoiesis-stimulating hormone called erythropoietin and that its rate of production is usually inversely related to the oxygen supply to the tissues. The main cytokinetic effect of erythropoietin is to increase the rate of maturation of ERC into proerythroblasts. The secretions of the endocrine glands exert some influence on the rate of red-cell production but this influence is mediated at least partly via alterations in the level of plasma erythropoietin. The possibility that one or more specific erythropoiesis-inhibiting humoral factors might also exist has been raised in the literature on a number of occasions. Although there is now good experimental evidence for the existence of one such substance, an erythrocytic chalone, it has not yet been established with certainty that the erythrocytic chalone plays a physiological role in the regulation of erythropoiesis *in vivo*.

There must be considerable alterations in the morphologically unrecognized precursor pool of patients with a sustained increase in erythropoiesis. However, the mechanisms regulating the size and behaviour of the multipotent haemopoietic stem-cell compartment and the pre-ERC compartment are still not completely understood. The available data are discussed in Chapter 2. Erythropoietin has no direct effect on the multipotent stem cells. The proliferative activity of such stem cells in a marrow cavity seems to be largely regulated by local factors and to be independent of the number or behaviour of stem cells in other parts of the body. There is also evidence for the existence of a 'burst-promoting activity' in horse or fetal calf serum and in media conditioned by human peripheral-blood leucocytes which is quite distinct from erythropoietin and which influences the proliferative activity of both the pre-ERC and the multipotent haemopoietic stem cell.

Erythropoietin

In 1906, Carnot & Deflandre [138, 139] suggested that the rate of erythropoiesis is regulated by a humoral factor present in the plasma. The existence of a circulating erythropoiesis-stimulating factor was subsequently firmly established on the basis of three observations:

1 the development of erythroid hyperplasia in the well-oxygenated member of a pair of parabiotic rats when the other member was subjected to hypoxia [140];

2 the occurrence of erythroid hyperplasia both in the cyanotic upper half and the well-oxygenated lower half of a patient with reversed blood flow through a patent ductus arteriosus [141];

3 the development of erythroid hyperplasia and reticulocytosis in rabbits injected with large volumes of the plasma from anaemic rabbits [142].

Chemistry and purification of erythropoietin

Erythropoietin is a non-dialysable, relatively heat-stable sialic-acid-containing glycoprotein which has the electrophoretic mobility of an α globulin. Its biological activity *in vivo* is dependent on the presence of sialic acid [143]. The native form of human erythropoietin has an apparent molecular weight of 39 000 and the asialo form of 34 000 when studied by sodium dodecyl sulphate (SDS) polyacrylamide gel electrophoresis [144].

Human erythropoietin derived from the urine of patients with aplastic anaemia has now been purified to apparent homogeneity employing a seven-step procedure which incorporates ion exchange chromatography, ethanol precipitation, gel filtration and adsorption chromatography [144]. This purified hormone runs as a single electrophoretic component in polyacrylamide gels at pH 9, in the presence of SDS at pH 7 and in the presence of Triton X-100 at pH 6. It has a potency of 70 400 iu of erythropoietin per milligram of protein.

Two relatively impure WHO International Reference Preparations of erythropoietin prepared from the pooled urine of anaemic patients are now available for the purpose of standardization of erythropoietin assays. One iu of erythropoietin is defined as the activity in 1·48 mg of the first international reference preparation [145] or in 0·5 mg of the second preparation [146]. The international unit roughly corresponds to the earlier cobalt unit which was based on the erythropoietin activity induced by a standard dose of cobalt chloride.

Measurement of erythropoietin

Bioassays. The original methods used for the assay of erythropoietin were bioassays [147]. In these assays the ability of a biological preparation to increase red-cell production in a suitable animal is compared with the effect of a known volume of a standard preparation of erythropoietin. The various assays which have been used differ in the method employed to measure the increase in erythropoietic activity, in the species and strain of experimental animal used, in the methods used to prepare such animals prior to the assay and in the way in which the test substance is administered. The most sensitive method of measuring the increase in erythropoietic activity is to study the incorporation of parenterally administered ^{59}Fe into the haemoglobin of circulating red cells. Several methods have been used to depress the production of endogenous erythropoietin in the test animals and thereby increase the sensitivity of the bioassay. These include starvation [148], the establishment of transfusion-induced polycythaemia [148, 149], exposure to hypoxia [150], or some combination of these procedures. The minimum detectable dose of erythropoietin by the most sensitive bioassay which is currently available (in which polycythaemic mice are used and the increase in erythropoietic activity is assessed by measuring ^{59}Fe utilization) is 0·05–0·1 iu. This degree of sensitivity only permits the measurement of erythropoietin in the plasma of severely anaemic patients (PCV $\leqslant$ 0·3); it does not allow the measurement of moderately elevated, normal or subnormal erythropoietin levels in untreated plasma. Other disadvantages of bioassays are that they are both time-consuming and costly and require considerable technical expertise. Erythropoietin can be detected in normal plasma using bioassays provided that the hormone in about 200 ml of plasma is first concentrated by a procedure which includes boiling for five minutes.

Cell-culture techniques. Krantz and his colleagues [151] developed an *in-vitro* assay which was based on the principle that the incorporation of ^{59}Fe into haem is stimulated by the addition of as little as about 0·05 iu of human or sheep erythropoietin per millilitre of marrow culture prepared either from rat or human bone marrow. An even more sensitive *in-vitro* assay based on the same principle has been described more recently in which mouse fetal liver cells are used instead of adult bone-marrow cells [152, 153]. The latter assay is capable of detecting 0·001 iu (1 milliunit) of erythropoietin and gives levels of 0·15 ± 0·1 iu per millilitre of serum (mean ± 2 s.d.) in normal subjects. One theoretical difficulty of these tissue culture assays lies in the fact that the effect of erythropoietin which is measured, namely the stimulation of haem synthesis, is quite different from that measured in the bioassays. It is therefore difficult to be certain that these two types of assay measure the same chemical substance. This difficulty is underlined by the observation that the removal of sialic acid from erythropoietin results in a loss of activity when measured by a bioassay but not by a tissue culture assay [151]. Nevertheless, from a study in a variety of clinical situations, Napier *et al.* [153] have shown that the erythropoiesis-stimulating factor which is measured by the fetal liver cell assay varies in a manner which is consistent with its having a function as an *in-vivo* regulator of erythropoiesis.

Immunological methods. Attempts have been made to develop erythropoietin assays based on double diffusion [154], haemagglutination inhibition [155, 156] and radioimmunoassay [157–159] techniques. In the past, such attempts have been hampered by the lack of a sufficiently pure antigen. However, with the development of methods for the production of pure preparations of erythropoietin, a specific and sensitive radioimmunoassay which can detect both normal and subnormal levels of serum erythropoietin has now been developed [160, 161]. This radioimmunoassay resembles the tissue culture assay in that it does not distinguish between native erythropoietin which is biologically active and desialated erythropoietin which is biologically inactive *in vivo*. The radioimmunoassay of Garcia *et al.* [161] can detect as little as 0·4 milliunits of erythropoietin and gives a mean value of 0·022 units per millilitre of serum in normal individuals.

Production of erythropoietin

The kidney is the major source of erythropoietin production in adult animals and humans. It is still not clear whether it produces the hormone directly, a pro-erythropoietin or a renal erythropoietic factor (REF) which interacts with a serum factor to form erythropoietin. The liver appears to be the primary organ concerned with erythropoietin production in the fetus. There is some extrarenal erythropoietin production in anephric adult animals and humans and the available data implicate the liver and spleen in this process.

Renal erythropoietin. Jacobson and his colleagues [162] showed that the appearance of erythropoietin in the plasma of adult rodents subjected to hypoxia was inhibited by previous bilateral nephrectomy and concluded that the organ concerned with erythropoietin production was the kidney. This conclusion was subsequently supported by the demonstration that the production of erythropoietin is stimulated when isolated kidneys are perfused with poorly oxygenated blood [163–166].

There is some evidence that a particulate subcellular fraction of the kidneys of hypoxic animals contains REF which generates erythropoietin when incubated with normal plasma or serum [167–170]. This reaction shows no species-specificity [171]. The REF does not usually have any erythropoietin-like biological activity *in vivo* but some REF preparations may contain erythropoietin [172]. Furthermore, REF and erythropoietin are immunochemically dissimilar. Thus anti-erythropoietin antibodies do not cross-react with REF and anti-REF antibodies do not cross-react with erythropoietin [173]. Gordon and his colleagues have proposed that REF is an enzyme (erythrogenin) and that the serum substrate is a precursor of erythropoietin (a pro-erythropoietin). However, it has been pointed out that the available data are also consistent with two other possibilities, i.e. that REF is a pro-erythropoietin which is activated on incubation with normal serum [168, 174] or that preparations of REF contain both the active erythropoietin molecule and an inhibitor of erythropoietin and that the latter is inactivated after incubation with normal serum. The possibility that

REF is a pro-erythropoietin has recently been supported by the data of Peschle *et al.* [172] who have shown that REF may be converted to erythropoietin in the absence of serum by a variety of physical procedures such as prolonged storage at $-20°C$, freeze-drying and repeated freeze-thawing.

There is still some uncertainty regarding the localization of REF production within the kidney. Investigations employing the immunofluorescence technique have demonstrated the presence of erythropoietin in the glomerular tufts or the glomerular epithelial cells [175–179] thereby suggesting that the glomerulus is probably the site of erythropoietin production or storage. However, the relevance of these data is limited by the fact that the anti-erythropoietin antibodies used in such studies would have been impure.

The serum factor involved in the generation of erythropoietin from REF remains to be characterized. The liver appears to be the source of the serum factor as partially hepatectomized animals have a subnormal capacity to produce erythropoietin when exposed to hypoxia [180]. There is some indirect evidence that hypoxia might act as a stimulus for the production of the serum factor [180].

Extrarenal erythropoietin in the adult. Several studies have demonstrated that bilaterally nephrectomized rodents [181], baboons [182] and humans [183–185] are capable of producing some erythropoietin in response to hypoxia. The quantity of erythropoietin which can be produced in anephric adult animals is small: for example, nephrectomized rats exposed to hypoxia produce only 10–15% of the amount of erythropoietin produced by non-nephrectomized control animals [186–188]. However, both extrarenal and renal erythropoietin are immunochemically similar in that an antibody raised against renal erythropoietin was effective in neutralizing the biological activity of extrarenal erythropoietin [187, 188]. The major source of extrarenal erythropoietin in adult anephric animals appears to be the liver as the extrarenal erythropoietin response is almost completely abolished if nephrectomy is combined with subtotal hepatectomy prior to exposure to hypoxia [189]. The importance of the liver in extrarenal erythropoietin production has been supported by the demonstration of an REF-like substance in hepatic and splenic homogenates from nephrectomized animals subjected to hypoxia [190, 191]. Peschle *et al.* [192] have demonstrated an enhanced production of extrarenal erythropoietin in anephric rats with experimentally induced hyperplasia of the Kupffer cells and have implicated these cells as the source of extrarenal erythropoietin.

The possibility that the liver is involved in extrarenal erythropoietin production in man is supported by the finding of high erythropoietin levels in the plasma, urine and tumour extracts of patients with hepatocellular carcinoma [193].

Erythropoietin production in the fetus (see Chapter 3). Fetal goats [194] and neonatal rats [195] who have been subjected to bilateral nephrectomy do not suffer from an impairment in their capacity to produce erythropoietin in response to various types of hypoxia. By contrast, neonatal and weanling rats subjected to partial hepatectomy show a significant reduction in the production of erythropoietin in response to hypoxia [196]. These data indicate that the major source of erythropoietin in fetal life is the liver and not the kidney. Detailed studies of erythropoietin production in neonatal and weanling rats have revealed that the liver is the primary site of erythropoietin production in the first two weeks of life and that the kidneys start producing erythropoietin in the third week and become the major site of erythropoietin production in the eighth week [179]. A substance with the biological activity of erythropoietin is synthesized in cultures of fetal mouse liver cells [197, 198] and human fetal liver cells [199]. Immunofluorescence studies have suggested that the erythropoietin-containing cells in fetal mouse liver cultures are the Kupffer cells [179].

Some aspects of the erythropoietin response. The rate of synthesis of erythropoietin is thought to be regulated by the amount of oxygen delivered to those cells involved in the synthesis of REF. After acute hypoxia in man [200], cobalt administration in rats [201] and a few hours after acute blood loss in the rat [202], there is a respiratory alkalosis with an increase in blood pH, a decrease in Pa,co_2 and an increase in the affinity of the intracellular haemoglobin for oxygen. These changes precede the production of erythropoietin. Furthermore, the prevention of the respiratory alkalosis which occurs after hypoxia or blood loss by the inhalation of five per cent CO_2 causes a hypercarbia and a marked reduction in the levels of plasma erythropoietin [203]. Miller and her colleagues have interpreted these data as indicating either that the cells producing REF are sensitive to changes in pH or Pa,co_2 or both (rather than to the Pa,o_2) or that the fall in Pa,co_2 in anaemic or hypoxic hypoxia leads to vasoconstriction with a decrease in blood flow to, and consequently the Pa,o_2 at, the sites of production of REF.

In rats whose PCVs are acutely reduced from 0·44 to 0·25 by bleeding, an increase in plasma erythropoietin is detected six hours after the bleeding. The erythropoietin levels are maximal at 12 hours and return to control values by 48 hours, despite the persistence of anaemia [202]. This fall in erythropoietin levels is associated with, but not necessarily caused by, an increase

in red-cell 2,3 DPG and a decrease in the affinity of the intracellular haemoglobin for oxygen. Whatever its cause might be, the transient nature of the erythropoietin response to acute hypoxia poses the question as to how an increased output of red cells from the marrow is maintained after the erythropoietin levels return to normal. A possible explanation is that only slight increases in erythropoietin levels (which cannot be detected by bioassays) are required to maintain an increased rate of red-cell production. Alternatively, the initial high erythropoietin level may increase the numbers and alter the properties of the morphologically unrecognized cells which are committed to erythropoiesis in such a way that an increased red-cell production persists in the presence of a very small increase in erythropoietin level. A third possibility is that erythropoietin levels do not necessarily reflect rates of production (and 'utilization') of erythropoietin, and that the latter remain high after the levels have returned to normal.

The increased generation of erythropoietin after the exposure of rats to a brief period of hypoxia is inhibited by the injection of actinomycin D before but not after the exposure to hypoxia indicating that the stimulation of erythropoietin synthesis by hypoxia requires DNA-dependent RNA synthesis [187].

Biochemical changes induced by erythropoietin
It seems likely that erythropoietin stimulates the conversion of ERCs to proerythroblasts and subsequently into mature red cells by inducing or stimulating the synthesis of specific mRNA molecules required for the synthesis of a variety of proteins. This view is supported by the observation that erythropoietin increases RNA synthesis in the erythropoietin-responsive cells of polycythaemic mice *in vivo* [204, 205]. It also stimulates the synthesis of mRNA, rRNA and tRNA in bone-marrow cells both *in vitro* [206, 207] and *in vivo* [208]. Recent studies have shown that erythropoietin stimulates the appearance of globin mRNA in proerythroblasts.

In addition to its effects on RNA synthesis, erythropoietin has been shown to stimulate the synthesis of ALA synthetase [209] and haem [151] in suspension cultures of bone-marrow cells, enhance the rate of DNA synthesis in ERC [205] and the recognizable red-cell precursors [210], increase the rate of iron uptake from transferrin [211], increase the rate of glycolysis via the hexose monophosphate shunt [212] and increase the incorporation of ^{14}C-glucosamine into the acid-soluble fraction of marrow cells [213]. The stimulation of the synthesis of ALA synthetase and haem and of the uptake of iron are inhibited by actinomycin D, indicating that these effects are based on DNA-dependent RNA synthesis.

Cytokinetic changes induced by erythropoietin

From a cell kinetics point of view the most important effect of erythropoietin is to increase the rate of conversion of ERC into proerythroblasts [214–217]. In other words, this hormone increases the number of red-cell production lines operating within the marrow and thereby increases the output of red cells. Studies in bled mice and in polycythaemic mice given a single injection of BCNU or busulphan have also revealed that high concentrations of erythropoietin have another important effect within the marrow, namely to increase the size of the ERC compartment apparently by an effect on erythropoietin-sensitive precursors of the ERC [27, 218]. Thus, it appears that when there is a need for a substantial increase in the rate of red-cell production, the increased levels of erythropoietin which are generated not only stimulate the formation of proerythroblasts from ERCs but also the production of ERCs from their immediate precursors (see Chapter 2).

Erythropoietin also has several effects on the cell kinetics in the morphologically recognizable red-cell-precursor pool. These include a reduction in the mean and median cell-cycle times of proliferating erythroblasts [23, 219, 220], a reduction in the spread in the cell-cycle times of proliferating erythroblasts [220], a shortening of the total maturation time in the recognizable red-cell-precursor pool [221, 222], a reduction in the adventitial cell cover of marrow sinusoids and an accelerated release of reticulocytes from the marrow (p. 112). Whether or not a specific level of erythropoietin causes an alteration in the number of cell divisions within the proliferating erythroblast pool depends on the relationship between the degree of shortening of the mean cell-cycle time and the degree of shortening of the average maturation time in this cell pool. An increase in the average number of cell divisions would result in the production of an increased number of red cells from each ERC. Conversely, a reduction in the average number of cell divisions would result in a decrease in the number of red cells produced from each ERC. However, the disadvantage of this loss of amplification would be partly offset by a considerable shortening of the time taken for the maturation of a proerythroblast into red cells.

The erythron has a considerable physiological reserve. In patients with congenital or acquired haemolytic anaemia, the various cytokinetic alterations mentioned above could result in a six- to ninefold increase in the rate of red-cell production [223].

Macrocytes are produced when rats are subjected to acute haemorrhage, hypoxia or phenylhydrazine-induced haemolysis [224] and when large doses of erythropoietin are injected into normal or hypertransfused rats [225, 226]. An erythropoietin-induced macrocytosis which is unrelated to a secondary folate deficiency is also seen in patients with severe haemolytic anaemias. The mechanisms underlying the macrocytosis which occurs in the presence of high levels of erythropoietin are uncertain. However, Stohlman and his colleagues have postulated that this macrocytosis results from a reduction in the average number of cell divisions within the proliferating erythroblast pool as a consequence of an acceleration of haemoglobin synthesis and the premature acquisition of a critical intracellular haemoglobin concentration at which cell division ceases. The macrocytes produced in animals and patients with a marked increase in erythropoiesis are short-lived [227]. Such cells are derived from the maturation of macroreticulocytes which are much larger than reticulocytes produced during normal steady-state erythropoiesis. Macroreticulocytes are two to three times larger in volume than normal red cells.

Role of endocrine glands

The importance of the endocrine glands in the maintenance of normal erythropoiesis is suggested by the clinical observations that patients with hypofunction of the anterior lobe of the pituitary gland, thyroid, testes or adrenal glands may suffer from an anaemia which responds only to therapy with the deficient hormone or hormones. Rats subjected to hypophysectomy also develop an anaemia which disappears after treatment with a combination of growth hormone, ACTH, corticosteroids, thyroid hormones and testosterone [228]. Extensive studies in animals subjected to hypophysectomy, orchidectomy, thyroidectomy or adrenalectomy have revealed that such animals are capable of making an erythropoietic response to severe hypoxia [229–231] and that the endocrine glands modify rather than initiate the regulation of erythropoiesis [157, 232]. However, the influence of the secretions of the endocrine glands on the regulation of erythropoiesis is emphasized by the observation that rats which have been hypophysectomized three to seven months previously show a subnormal erythropoietin response to hypoxia when compared with sham-operated controls [172].

Studies in experimental animals have shown that androgens, growth hormone and thyroxine stimulate erythropoiesis by an effect on the kidneys which leads to an increased production of REF and, consequently, of erythropoietin [233–237]. However, androgens have additional erythropoietin-independent effects on erythropoiesis in that they have been shown to stimulate resting multipotent haemopoietic stem cells into cell cycle directly and to expand the size of the pre-ERC pool [238–241]. Furthermore, the *in-vitro* studies of Singer & Adamson [242] have shown that fluoxymesterone, a synthetic androgen, enhances the number of erythroid colonies formed in the presence of suboptimal concentrations of erythropoietin by an effect on rapidly cycling ERC. By contrast, etiocholanolone, a naturally occurring non-androgenic metabolite of testosterone, enhances the number of erythroid colonies formed in the presence of all (including optimal) concentrations of erythropoietin by an effect on non-S-phase cells.

Low concentrations of ACTH and glucocorticoids augment erythropoiesis and high concentrations depress it [243, 244]. The stimulation of erythropoiesis by corticosteroids appears to be partly mediated via the elevation of erythropoietin levels [245] and partly via a direct stimulatory effect on erythropoiesis [246].

Prolactin stimulates erythropoiesis in polycythaemic mice, normal mice and post-partum, non-lactating mice [247, 248] but the mechanisms underlying these effects remain to be clarified.

Whereas all the above-mentioned hormones stimulate the production of red cells, low doses of oestrogens inhibit erythropoiesis at least in certain species. Oestrogens appear to act on the erythron by more than one mechanism. It has been shown that low doses of oestrogens inhibit erythropoietin production in response to hypoxia in female rats and in mice [249, 250]. Oestrogens also antagonize the effect of erythropoietin on the ERCs [251, 252]. Furthermore, oestrogen-treated mice show a reduction of the number of multipotent haemopoietic stem cells (spleen colony-forming cells) in the marrow and spleen presumably due to some damaging influence on these cells [253], and a reduction in the number of *in-vitro* erythroid colony-forming cells in the marrow [250]. The second of these effects could be caused by a diminished response of ERCs to erythropoietin *in vitro*. In mice, high doses of oestrogens do not impair the erythropoietin response induced by hypoxia to any appreciable extent [250]. Pharmacological doses of oestrogens have been reported to cause osteosclerosis in rodents [254].

Erythrocytic chalone

The proliferation of the cells of certain tissues is under the regulation of substances called chalones. A chalone is a tissue-specific inhibitor of proliferation which is produced by the mature cells of the cell system upon which it acts. Chalones are not species-specific and the effects of a chalone on its target cells are short-lived so that the inhibition of cell proliferation is reversible. There is now some evidence for the existence of an erythrocytic chalone which is produced by mature erythrocytes and which inhibits erythroblast proliferation. Thus, several workers have shown that when extracts of fresh normal rat serum, serum from polycythaemic rats or supernatants of suspension cultures of rat erythrocytes (erythrocyte supernatants) are incubated with normal rat bone-marrow cells for three to

18 hours, there is a significant suppression of the [3H]thymidine-labelling index of erythroblasts; the suppression is greater with polycythaemic serum than with normal serum [255–257]. The presence in rat erythrocyte supernatants of a substance which affects proliferating erythroblasts but not proliferating lymphoid or granulocytopoietic cells has also been shown by the technique of fluorescence polarization which gives a measure of the structure of the cytoplasmic matrix [258].

The possibility that the *in-vitro* effects mentioned above may be relevant in the regulation of erythropoiesis *in vivo* has been recently supported by the studies of Lord *et al.* [259]. These workers have demonstrated that the injection of as little as 10–300 μg of material from an erythrocyte supernatant into a mouse influences the *in-vivo* proliferation of the morphologically recognizable red-cell precursors but not of the erythropoietin-responsive cells. The main cytokinetic effect of the red-cell supernatant appeared to be a reversible prolongation of the cell-cycle time, largely due to a prolongation of G_1. It is possible that the inhibitor of erythropoiesis which has been reported to be present in extracts of the plasma of humans who have returned to sea level after living at high altitudes [260, 261] will eventually be shown to be erythrocytic chalone.

THE ASSESSMENT OF ERYTHROPOIESIS

Morphological studies of bone-marrow cells

Evidence of dyserythropoiesis

In normal bone marrow, the vast majority of the erythroblasts are uninucleate, display a considerable degree of synchrony between nuclear and cytoplasmic maturity, and show no peculiar cytological features. However, even in normal marrow, $1 \cdot 36 \pm 0 \cdot 40$ (1 s.d.) per 1000 erythroblasts are binucleate [262] and a very occasional erythroblast shows an irregularly shaped nucleus, karyorrhexis, Howell–Jolly bodies or an unusual degree of dissociation between nuclear and cytoplasmic maturity. The electron microscope reveals two additional features in a very few erythroblasts from normal marrow, namely intercellular spindle bridges and small intranuclear clefts. The presence of more than one nucleus per erythroblast and of the other unusual cytological features mentioned above presumably results from abnormalities both of proliferation and of cytodifferentiation and are consequently described as dyserythropoietic changes. In several diseases these abnormalities are encountered in an unusually high proportion of the erythroblasts, thus providing evidence of a perturbation of erythropoiesis. In addition, some of the erythroblasts of patients with these diseases display a variety of other dyserythropoietic changes such as internuclear chromatin bridges or perinuclear rings of coarse siderotic granules, which are either not encountered at all or are seen only extremely rarely in normal marrow.

It is evident from the preceding discussion that the assessment of erythropoiesis should include a careful examination of Romanowsky-stained marrow smears for the presence of dyserythropoietic changes in an abnormally high proportion of the erythroblasts. Useful data on the prevalence of dyserythropoietic changes may also be obtained from ultrastructural studies of the erythroblasts. The various dyserythropoietic changes which can be detected under the light and electron microscopes are summarized in Tables 4.5 and 4.6 respectively, and some of the ultrastructural features indicative of dyserythropoiesis are illustrated in Figures 4.10–4.12. It is emphasized that these changes are seen in a variety of aetiologically unrelated disorders and are, therefore, best considered as non-specific stigmata of perturbations of proliferation and cytodifferentiation. However, some of these dyserythropoietic changes are found in an unusually high proportion of the erythroblasts in certain specific clinically defined conditions or groups of disorders. For example, although a short stretch of double membrane may be found parallel to the cell membrane in an occasional erythroblast in several diseases, the presence of a more or less complete double membrane 40–60 nm away from, and parallel to, the cell membrane in a high proportion of the erythroblasts, is a characteristic feature of some patients with congenital dyserythropoietic anaemia.

Evidence of ineffective erythropoiesis
The most direct way of establishing that there is an increase in ineffective erythropoiesis is to demonstrate the presence of phagocytosed erythroblasts at various stages of degradation within the cytoplasm of the bone-marrow macrophages. This can be done by electron-microscope studies of freshly aspirated marrow fragments (Fig. 4.13).

Investigation of proliferative activity
The majority of the methods available for obtaining information regarding the duration of the phases of the cell cycle depend on the use of radioactive thymidine as an autoradiographic marker for cells in the S phase. The radioactive thymidine can be used either *in vitro* or *in vivo*. When injected intravenously, the thymidine is only available for incorporation into cells over a period of 10–40 minutes. Two *in-vitro* methods which have been used to study human erythroblasts are:
1 a double-labelling technique in which cells are exposed first to [^{3}H]thymidine and then to [^{14}C]thymidine with a known interval of time between the two exposures [263–265];
2 a technique in which cells are pre-incubated with fluorodeoxyuridine to block the *de-novo* synthesis of thymidylate prior to a quantitative autoradiographic study of the rate of incorporation of [^{14}C]thymidine [266]. The second of these methods permits the duration of the S phase to be determined in single cells. The most useful *in-vivo* method is the labelled mitoses technique. In this method, several marrow aspirations are performed at intervals of time after a single intravenous injection of [^{3}H]thymidine and the percentage of labelled (radioactive) mitotic figures in each of these aspirates is determined. The theoretical considerations behind all of the above-mentioned techniques as well as the method of calculating the various time parameters of the cell cycle for each technique may be found in the monograph by Wickramasinghe [23].

Table 4.5. Dyserythropoietic changes which may be detected under the light microscope

1	Irregularly shaped nuclei
2	Karyorrhexis
3	Howell–Jolly bodies
4	Bi- or multinuclearity
5	Intercellular cytoplasmic bridges
6	Megaloblasts
7	Macronormoblasts
8	Poor haemoglobinization of cytoplasm
9	Basophilic stippling of cytoplasm
10	Increased proportion of orthochromatic erythroblasts
11	Vacuolation of cytoplasm
12	Excess of coarse acid ferrocyanide-positive siderotic granules (abnormal sideroblasts)
13	Ring sideroblasts
14	Gigantoblasts (mononucleate or multinucleate)
15	Internuclear chromatin bridges

Table 4.6. Dyserythropoietic changes other than those listed in Table 4.5 which may be detected under the electron microscope. Some of the features listed below are very occasionally seen in normal marrow but are found with an abnormally high frequency in pathological states

1   Membrane-bound intranuclear clefts
2   Absence, myelinization or reduplication of parts of the nuclear membrane
3   Separation of the nuclear membrane from the nucleus
4   Widening of the space between the two layers of the nuclear membrane
5   Intranuclear inclusions (mitochondria, myelin figures)
6   Deposition of electron-dense material, sometimes resembling ribosomes, on the cytoplasmic surface of the nuclear membrane
7   Different ultrastructural appearance of different nuclei within the same multinucleate cell
8   Fusion of two or more nuclei in a multinucleate cell
9   Swiss-cheese appearance of heterochromatin
10   Mitochondrial degeneration (iron-loading, swelling, loss of cristae)
11   Giant siderosomes
12   Intracytoplasmic autophagic vacuoles, sometimes containing degenerating mitochondria or myelin figures
13   Intercellular spindle bridges
14   Lipid-laden intracytoplasmic vacuoles
15   Free intracytoplasmic myelin figures
16   Annulate lamellae
17   Abnormalities in some regions of contact between erythroblasts
18   Presence of a double membrane 40–60 nm away from and parallel to the cell membrane
19   Reduction in electron density of cytoplasmic matrix
20   Scarcity of ribosomes
21   Clustering of degenerating cytoplasmic organelles near the nucleus

Technique of combined Feulgen microspectrophotometry and [³H]thymidine autoradiography

Most of the available information regarding abnormalities in the proliferation of the morphologically recognizable haemopoietic cells has resulted from the application of the technique of combined Feulgen microspectrophotometry and [³H]thymidine autoradiography [7, 23]. This technique enables one to use an aliquot of marrow obtained during a diagnostic marrow aspiration to determine the percentage distribution of any particular cell type in the different stages of interphase G_1, S and G_2. The marrow cells are incubated with [³H]thymidine for 30 minutes prior to the preparation of smears which are then stained by a Romanowsky method. A photographic map is prepared of a selected area of a slide and the position and type of every cell in the area is recorded on the map. The Romanowsky stain is then leached out, the slide restained by the Feulgen method and the absorbances of individual Feulgen-stained nuclei are measured using a microspectrophotometer. Finally, an autoradiograph is prepared and the S-phase cells are identified by virtue of their incorporation of [³H]thymidine. As the Feulgen reaction is both a specific and stoichiometric staining reaction for nuclear DNA, the Feulgen absorbance of a nucleus is proportional to its DNA content. Cells which fail to incorporate [³H]thymidine

(i.e. non-S cells) can therefore be separated into G_1 or G_2 cells by virtue of the fact that G_2 cells have double the DNA content of G_1 cells. As mentioned earlier, the interpretation of data on the percentage distribution of erythroblasts in different phases of the cell cycle is based on the fact that the percentage of cells in any particular phase is a function of the average duration of that phase relative to the average duration of the total intermitotic period. The demonstration of an abnormality in the cell-cycle distribution implies a disturbance in the normal progression of cells through the cell cycle.

Table 4.7 summarizes the data obtained with the technique of combined Feulgen microspectrophotometry and [³H]thymidine autoradiography in four diseases associated with a marked increase in ineffective erythropoiesis. The major limitation of this technique is that it only gives information about the cell-cycle distribution at one point in time and does not give definite information as to how an abnormal distribution has developed. For example, the increased proportion of cells in G_2 found in vitamin-B_{12} deficiency (Table 4.7) may in theory be due to a prolongation of the G_2 phase, an arrest (temporary or permanent) after a period in G_2 or a shortening of G_1 plus S (with a normal G_2 phase). The conclusions on the most probable kinetic aberrations given in Table 4.7 are based both on the abnormalities in the cell-cycle distribution as well as on evidence from other investigations

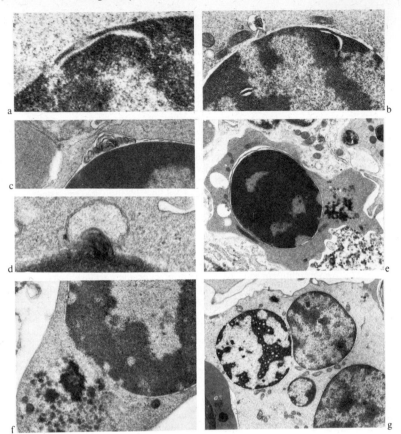

Fig. 4.10. Some ultrastructural abnormalities affecting erythroblast nuclei. (a) and (b) Intranuclear clefts in hereditary spherocytosis (a) and azathioprine-induced megaloblastic erythropoiesis (b). (c) and (d) Myelinization of the nuclear membrane in β-thalassaemia trait and primary acquired sideroblastic anaemia, respectively. (e) Duplication of the nuclear membrane in β-thalassaemia trait. (f) Loss of nuclear membrane adjacent to a mass of precipitated α chains in homozygous β thalassaemia. (g) Swiss-cheese appearance of one of four nuclei in a multinucleate erythroblast in CDA, type III.

into bone-marrow function in the diseases under study. Such investigations include:

1 ferrokinetic and erythrokinetic studies;

2 light-microscope autoradiographic studies of the rates of protein synthesis in individual cells;

3 studies on the relationship between morphological or biosynthetic abnormalities and the position of the abnormal cell in the cell cycle;

4 ultrastructural studies;

5 electron-microscope autoradiographic studies of the relationship between ultrastructural abnormalities and biosynthetic activities.

Quantification of erythropoiesis

A detailed quantitative analysis of erythropoiesis of the type shown in Table 4.4 involves the intravenous injection of [³H]thymidine and the performance of serial marrow aspirations. Although this type of direct analysis of the kinetics of erythropoiesis provides invaluable information, its application to clinical problems is severely limited because of the possible radio-

biological hazards from injecting [³H]thymidine. Cell kinetic studies are also technically complex and time-consuming. A number of alternative and less direct methods are available for the quantification of the overall activity of cell production and destruction within the erythron of patients (Table 4.8). These methods vary in their complexity and have their own shortcomings which frequently stem from the indirectness of the approach (e.g. the lack of correlation between ferrokinetic indices and erythropoietic activity). Some of the methods measure total (effective plus ineffective) erythropoietic activity and others assess effective erythropoietic activity. The amount of ineffective erythropoiesis is usually assessed by the degree of discrepancy between indices of total and effective erythropoiesis.

Measurement of effective erythropoiesis

Reticulocyte count. The reticulocyte percentage can be used as a clinically useful index of effective erythropoiesis provided that corrections are applied to take

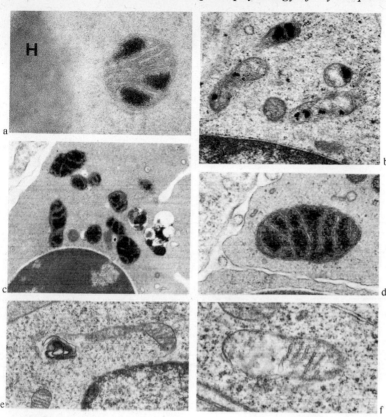

Fig. 4.11. Some ultrastructural abnormalities affecting the mitochondria of erythroblasts and reticulocytes. (a)–(d) Iron-laden mitochondria in Hb H disease (a), primary acquired sideroblastic anaemia (b), and hereditary sideroblastic anaemia (c and d). The electron-dense iron-containing material is present in between the mitochondrial cristae. (e) and (f) Myelin figure (e) and electron-lucent areas showing a loss of cristae (f) in mitochondria from a severely iron-deficient patient. H = mass of precipitated β chains.

account of variations in the number of circulating red cells and in the reticulocyte maturation times in different patients. The reticulocyte count is initially determined and expressed as the number of reticulocytes per 100 mature red cells plus reticulocytes in a supravitally stained blood film. The reticulocyte percentage can then be manipulated to take account of variations in the red-cell count or PCV by using it to calculate either the absolute reticulocyte count or the absolute reticulocyte percentage (see Chapter 1, p. 32). The absolute reticulocyte count is determined from the reticulocyte percentage and total red-cell count and is expressed as the number of reticulocytes per μl of blood. The absolute reticulocyte percentage is the patient's reticulocyte percentage related to a PCV of 0·45 and is determined by multiplying the crude reticulocyte percentage by (Patient's PCV/0·45). The number of red cells turned over per day per μl of blood (i.e. the rate of effective erythropoiesis) is equal to the number of reticulocytes per μl of blood divided by the average maturation time of blood reticulocytes in days. It is evident from this relationship that if the maturation time of blood reticulocytes is assumed to be constant, the rate of effec-

tive erythropoiesis is proportional to the absolute reticulocyte count (and also to the absolute reticulocyte percentage). Although in clinical practice a constant reticulocyte maturation time is frequently assumed, it is known that the maturation time is inversely proportional to the degree of anaemia. Hillman & Finch [268, 269] have suggested that in order to obtain the most reliable information on the rate of effective erythropoiesis from reticulocyte values, the latter should also be corrected for alterations in blood reticulocyte maturation time, and have proposed that 1·0, 1·5, 2·0 and 2·5 days should be used as the average maturation times corresponding to PCVs of 0·45, 0·35, 0·25 and 0·15, respectively. The maturation correction is made by dividing the absolute reticulocyte count or percentage by the estimated maturation time. The resulting figure is called the reticulocyte-production index.

Red-cell turnover based on the mean cell lifespan. Provided that the erythron is in a steady-state, the rate of entry of reticulocytes into the circulation (i.e. the rate of effective erythropoiesis) is equal to the rate of loss of red cells from the erythron. The rate of effective

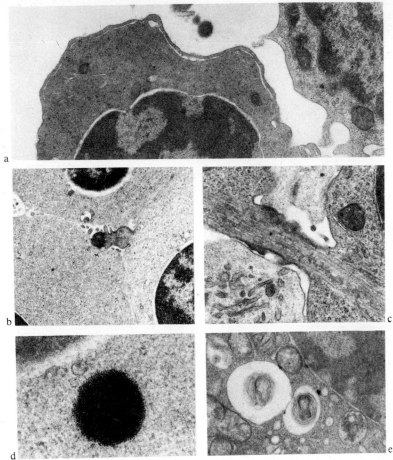

Fig. 4.12. Some ultrastructural abnormalities affecting the cytoplasm of erythropoietic cells. (a) Double membrane aligned parallel to the cell membrane in CDA, type II. (b) and (c) Inter-erythroblastic cytoplasmic bridges containing microtubules in a patient with azathioprine-induced megaloblastic erythropoiesis (b), and in a case of CDA, type II (c). (d) and (e) A siderosome (d) and intracytoplasmic autophagic vacuoles containing myelin figures (e) in erythroblasts from a patient with Hb H disease.

erythropoiesis can therefore be estimated indirectly from the total number of red cells in the circulation and the mean red-cell lifespan.

Red-cell ^{59}Fe utilization and red-cell iron turnover. Another method of assessing effective erythropoietic activity is to measure the amount of radioactive iron which appears within the circulating red-cell mass 10–14 days after a single intravenous injection of ^{59}Fe-labelled transferrin. However, the red-cell ^{59}Fe utilization is influenced by the diversion of part of the injected radioactive iron to non-erythropoietic tissues and the reutilization of iron refluxed from the marrow. For these reasons this parameter may give misleading information on the rate of effective erythropoiesis, particularly in certain diseases. The red-cell iron turnover is derived from the red-cell ^{59}Fe utilization so as to take account of the complexities of the flow of iron to and from the plasma and is considered to be a more reliable index of effective erythropoietic activity than the red-cell ^{59}Fe utilization (see section on ferrokinetic studies on p. 163).

Measurement of total erythropoiesis

Total number of erythroblasts. A technique based on the radioisotope dilution principle is available for the determination of the total number of erythroblasts in the body. However, this technique is not suitable for routine clinical use as it requires the intravenous administration of a fairly high dose of radioactive iron [270–272].

Plasma iron turnover (PIT) and total marrow iron turnover (MIT). Of the various indices of total erythropoiesis listed in Table 4.8, the PIT and MIT are the most useful and reliable. The PIT is calculated from the initial disappearance rate of intravenously injected ^{59}Fe-labelled transferrin and the concentration of transferrin iron in the plasma. As the turnover of non-erythroid iron usually accounts for only a small

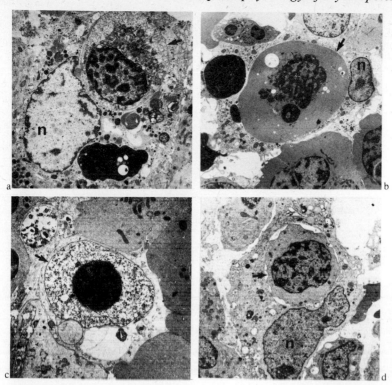

Fig. 4.13. Electron micrographs showing the phagocytosis of erythroblasts by bone-marrow macrophages in untreated vitamin-B_{12} deficiency (a); congenital dyserythropoietic anaemia-type III (b); pyoderma gangrenosum with ineffective erythropoiesis preceding the development of pure red-cell aplasia (c) and *Plasmodium falciparum* malaria (d). The nuclei of the macrophages are marked and the phagocytosed erythroblasts, which show various ultrastructural abnormalities, are arrowed.

fraction of the PIT, the PIT may be used as an index of total erythropoiesis in many clinical situations. However, the PIT gives an overestimate of total erythropoiesis in some diseases (e.g. aplastic anaemia) with an increase in non-erythroid iron turnover. The MIT which is calculated from the PIT is derived in such a way that it takes account of variations in non-erythroid iron turnover and is therefore considered to be a more reliable index of total erythropoiesis than the PIT (see section on ferrokinetic studies on p. 163).

Faecal urobilinogen excretion. Most of the urobilinogen excreted in the faeces is ultimately derived from the catabolism of the haemoglobin within circulating red cells when these are broken down at the end of their lifespan (p. 115). The remainder of the faecal urobilinogen is derived from the degradation of the narrow rim of haemoglobin-containing cytoplasm surrounding extruded erythroblast nuclei, from the intramedullary degradation of abnormal erythroblasts and from the turnover of porphyrins in non-erythroid tissues. Because the contribution from non-erythroid tissues is small, the rate of excretion of urobilinogen in the faeces may be used as an index of total erythropoietic activity. However, the use of this index has been limited because of the difficulties of obtaining complete faecal collections over several days and the unpleasantness of working with such collections. As faecal urobilinogen results from the effects of gut bacteria on conjugated bilirubin, the rate of excretion of faecal urobilinogen may give misleading information on total erythropoietic activity in patients with antibiotic-induced alterations in the bacterial flora within the bowel and in patients with marked abnormalities in the gastro-intestinal transit time. The normal range reported by Giblett *et al.* [223] for the total daily excretion of faecal urobilinogen is 157 ± 54.4 mg (1 s.d.).

Carbon-monoxide production. The catabolism of 1 mol of haem results not only in the formation of 1 mol of bilirubin which is degraded and excreted as urobilinogen in the faeces but also of 1 mol of carbon monoxide (p. 116) which is lost through the lungs. As the catabolism of haem is the sole endogenous source of carbon monoxide, total erythropoietic activity can be assessed by estimating the rate of loss of carbon monoxide from the lungs. This may be done by measuring the rate of increase of carbon monoxide in the blood when the patient is breathing in a closed system. As in the case of faecal urobilinogen excretion, carbon-monoxide production is a measure of total

Table 4.7. Data from the technique of combined Feulgen microspectrophotometry and ^{3}H-thymidine autoradiography and the conclusions derived from them in some clinical situations [23, 267]

Diagnosis	Abnormalities in cell-cycle distribution of erythroblasts	Probable cytokinetic aberrations
Vitamin-B_{12}-deficiency or primary acquired sideroblastic anaemia	1 Increase in percentage of U cells* and G_2 cells 2 Decrease in S/G_2 ratio 3 Decrease in percentage of S cells and slight increase in percentage of G_1 cells 4 Cell-cycle abnormalities most marked in early polychromatic cells	Arrest of early polychromatic cells at all stages of interphase, particularly in S and G_2
Homozygous β thalassaemia	1 Marked increase in percentage of G_1 cells with corresponding decrease in percentage of S cells 2 Increase in U cells 3 Decrease in S/G_2 ratio 4 Cell-cycle abnormalities confined to early polychromatic cells	Substantial prolongation of G_1 with arrest in entry of G_1 cells into S Some cells which enter S become arrested in S or G_2
Congenital dyserythropoietic anaemia, type III	1 Increase in percentage of U cells amongst mononucleate early polychromatic erythroblasts 2 Presence of some mononucleate cells with DNA contents of 4–20c 3 Presence of multinucleate cells with total DNA contents of 2–40c	Arrest of polychromatic cells after a period in S Development of markedly polyploid mononucleate and multinucleate cells due to an arrest in the progress of cells through various points in mitosis

* Cells which appear to have been arrested after progressing through part of the S phase.

Table 4.8. Indices employed for the quantification of erythropoietic activity (other than cell kinetic indices)

Erythropoietic activity assessed	Index
Effective erythropoiesis	Reticulocyte counts Red-cell turnover based on the mean cell lifespan Red-cell ^{59}Fe utilization Red-cell iron turnover
Total erythropoiesis	Total number of erythroblasts Plasma iron turnover Total marrow iron turnover Faecal urobilinogen excretion Carbon-monoxide production M/E ratio
Ineffective erythropoiesis	Discrepancy between indices of total and effective erythropoiesis Early-labelled bilirubin production

erythropoiesis plus the turnover of non-erythroid (mainly hepatic) haem [273, 274].

Myeloid/erythroid ratio (M/E ratio). In clinical practice the M/E ratio is the most commonly used index of total erythropoietic activity. This is the ratio between the number of granulocytes and their precursors and the number of erythroblasts in a marrow smear. The M/E ratio gives a rough idea of the number of nucleated red cells in the bone marrow provided that the number of marrow granulocytes and their precursors is normal and the total volume of haemopoietic marrow is unaltered. Two further difficulties with the use of this index are the wide range of values for the M/E ratio in normal individuals and the inaccuracy introduced by the presence of contaminating blood granulocytes in the marrow aspirate. Glaser *et al.* [275] found an average M/E ratio of 2·94 (range, 1·22–11·78) in 92 normal individuals with an age range of one to 20 years.

Index of ineffective erythropoiesis

Early labelled bilirubin production. When [^{15}N]glycine is given to humans it becomes incorporated into the haem which is synthesized within the erythropoietic cells and appears in the haemoglobin of a cohort of newly formed circulating red cells. At the end of the life span of this labelled cohort, the ^{15}N can be recovered in faecal urobilinogen. There is, however, an early peak of labelled bilirubin and faecal urobilinogen during the first few days after the administration of labelled glycine [276, 277]. This early labelled fraction is comprised of two components:

1 a non-erythropoietic component which peaks between 12 and 14 hours and seems to be derived from the turnover of hepatic haem; and

2 an erythropoietic component which peaks within three to five days [278, 279].

The erythropoietic component is probably derived from ineffective erythropoiesis, the degradation of the haemoglobin within and around extruded erythroblast nuclei and the degradation of some haemoglobin within the autophagic vacuoles of viable erythropoietic cells. The magnitude of the non-erythropoietic component may be determined by studying the incorporation of [^{15}N]δ-aminolaevulinic acid (ALA) into early labelled bilirubin, as ALA is incorporated into hepatic haem but not into erythroid haem. Thus from a study of the incorporation of [^{15}N]glycine and [^{15}N]ALA into early labelled bilirubin it is possible to assess the magnitude of the erythropoietic component of the early labelled bilirubin peak and use this as an index of ineffective erythropoiesis [280]. This method is technically very complex and is unsuitable for routine clinical use.

Localization of erythropoiesis

Radioactive iron may be used to localize sites of erythropoiesis within the body. Non-quantitative information regarding the distribution of erythropoietic tissue can be obtained by surface-counting during the first few hours after the intravenous administration of 5 μCi of ^{59}Fe attached to transferrin [281, 282]. Quantitative information may be obtained after the administration of about 200 μCi of the much shorter-lived isotope ^{52}Fe by using a rectilinear scanner or γ-camera [283–286]. Because of its short lifespan, ^{52}Fe has to be generated in a cyclotron unit immediately before its use.

PATHOPHYSIOLOGY OF THE ERYTHRON

We have seen in previous sections how the erythron is regulated so that the circulating red-cell mass is able to meet the oxygen requirements of the tissues. By far the commonest disorder of this finely tuned system is a reduction in the number of circulating red cells or anaemia. The opposite occurrence, i.e. an increased red-cell mass or polycythaemia, is much less common. In the sections which follow we shall deal with some general aspects of the pathophysiology of anaemia so as to form a basis for a detailed description of each of the common forms of anaemia which follow in subsequent chapters. The pathophysiology of the polycythaemias is considered in detail in Chapter 32.

Anaemia

In functional terms anaemia can be defined as a state in which the number of circulating red cells is insufficient to supply the oxygen requirements of the tissues. However, as we shall see later there are numerous compensatory mechanisms which can be brought into play to restore the oxygen supply to the vital centres and therefore in clinical practice this functional definition is of limited value. For this reason anaemia is usually defined as a reduction of the haemoglobin concentration, red-cell count or haematocrit to below normal levels.

The definition of anaemia

It has been extremely difficult to establish a normal range of haematological values (see Chapter 1, p. 31) and the definition of anaemia usually involves the adoption of rather arbitrary criteria. For example, the World Health Organization recommends that anaemia should be considered to exist in those adults whose haemoglobin levels are lower than 13 g/dl (males) or 12 g/dl (females). Children aged six months to six years are considered anaemic at haemoglobin levels below 11 g/dl and those aged six to 14 years below 12 g/dl. [287]. The disadvantage of such arbitrary criteria for defining anaemia is that there may be many apparently normal individuals whose haemoglobin concentration is below their optimal level. Furthermore, a glance at the 'normal values' for adults shown in Chapter 1, page 30 indicates that there is such a large standard deviation that many adult females must be considered normal even though they have haemoglobin levels below 12 g/dl. For this reason Natvig and his colleagues [288, 289] have defined the normal limits of haemoglobin values at different ages and in both sexes as the mean haemoglobin concentration following iron supplementation ± twice the standard deviation. They consider anaemia to be present when the haemoglobin concentration is below this range but as far as any individual is concerned this still remains an arbitrary criterion. Indeed statistical considerations indicate that 2·5% of normal individuals will have haemoglobin values less than the mean minus two standard deviations.

It must not be assumed that haemoglobin values within the normal range denote normality for the individual and they certainly do not exclude occult deficiencies such as latent iron deficiency or latent pernicious anaemia which are revealed only by specific tests. For example, in a random sample of the adult population in Wales investigated during 1967 (see Chapter 5) there was clear evidence of iron deficiency in subjects with haemoglobin concentrations well within the conventional normal range.

Prevalence of anaemia

The prevalence of anaemia has been studied in many population groups but it is difficult to compare data from different sources because of variations in methodology, standardization and the criteria adopted. Certain patterns emerge, however. An early survey carried out in Great Britain during 1943 [290] established that haemoglobin levels were low in a significant proportion of the population, particularly susceptible groups being children under the age of five years, pregnant women and those in social classes IV and V. Another random population study in the UK was reported for a South Wales mining community in the Rhondda Fach [291]. The prevalence of anaemia was found to be 14% for women aged 55–64 years and three per cent for men aged 35–64 years. These and similar studies have shown that anaemia is commonest in women between the ages of 15 and 44 years and then becomes relatively less frequent, although the prevalence increases again in the 75-years-and-over age group. Interestingly it is only in the latter group that

the prevalence in males and females is almost the same. Where the cause of the anaemia has been analysed in these surveys the majority of cases have been due to iron deficiency. No doubt these prevalence-of-anaemia data vary considerably between the developed countries but, as will be discussed in greater detail in Chapter 5, nutritional anaemia is relatively common in most populations at specific periods during development, and late in life.

Analysis of the prevalence of anaemia in tropical populations is extremely complex because, although there is no doubt that it is widespread, in many cases it simply reflects the high incidence of other diseases rather than climatic and social factors [292]. This is shown very clearly by the studies of Bray in West Africa who found that there was a marked seasonal variation in haemoglobin values in young children and that this was related to the seasonal variability in the activity of *P. falciparum* malaria [293]. The problem of the prevalence of anaemia in the tropics has been analysed in detail in several extensive reviews [292].

Adaptation to anaemia

The function of the red cell is to carry oxygen between the lungs and the tissues. However, tissue oxygenation is the result of an extremely complicated series of interactions of different organ systems of which the erythron is only one [294]. Obviously the cardiac output, ventilatory function and state of the capillaries are of critical importance as well. Each of these supply systems is regulated differently. Ventilation responds to changes in pH, CO_2 and hypoxia. Cardiac output responds to the amount of blood entering the heart and this is regulated mainly by the effects of the metabolism of peripheral tissues on the resistance to blood flow in the microvasculature. The erythron itself responds to changes in haemoglobin concentration, arterial oxygen saturation and to the oxygen affinity of the circulating haemoglobin. Thus, in terms of tissue oxygenation a decreased capacity of any of these components may be compensated for by increased activity of the others [294].

A decrease of arterial oxygen loading due to a lowered oxygen tension in the environment or to lung disease results in increased ventilation, an increased haemoglobin concentration and a right shift in the oxygen dissociation curve. When increased ventilation occurs, a respiratory alkalosis is produced which in time is corrected by an increased loss of base through the kidneys. On the other hand, a decreased cardiac output is not usually associated with an increased haemoglobin concentration but rather by shunting of blood from areas of high flow to more critical tissues together with a shift in the oxygen dissociation curve to the right. In cases of mild to moderate anaemia the oxygen dissociation curve shifts to the right and there is redistribution of blood to the vital centres; at more extreme levels of anaemia there is an increase in cardiac output and some degree of hyperventilation. Thus, when considering the adaptive changes to anaemia and its likely effects in an individual patient all the factors involved in tissue oxygenation have to be considered.

Compensation by the red cell. Since each gram of haemoglobin carries 1·34 ml of oxygen the circulating blood in anaemic patients with haemoglobin levels higher than 5 g/dl will contain more oxygen than is consumed by the tissues, i.e. about 6 ml of oxygen per 100 ml of blood [295]. However, an increased oxygen extraction would aggravate rather than ameliorate tissue hypoxia because it would further reduce the oxygen tension at the venous end of the capillary and hence increase the relative degree of tissue hypoxia. As pointed out by Erslev [295], as is the case for other kinetic systems such as water, steam or electricity, the total amount of potential energy is of little importance unless combined with pressure or voltage as a driving force.

It appears that in many types of anaemia the oxygen dissociation curve is shifted to the right. The reduction in oxygen affinity allows more oxygen to be released at relatively higher pressures. This change is not pH-dependent but appears to result from increased production of 2,3 diphosphoglycerate (2,3 DPG). The way in which elevated levels of the latter cause a decreased oxygen affinity of haemoglobin is considered in detail in Chapter 8. The mechanism of increased 2,3 DPG synthesis in response to anaemia is not absolutely certain but it has been suggested that because deoxygenated haemoglobin is present at higher than normal concentrations it binds more 2,3 DPG and therefore removes product inhibition from the rate-limiting enzyme required for 2,3 DPG synthesis, i.e. 2,3 diphosphoglycerate mutase [296]. The degree to which this mechanism can help compensate for any particular level of anaemia depends to some extent on the type of haemoglobin and metabolic activity of the red cell. For example, it must be relatively unimportant in the fetus because haemoglobin F interacts to only a very limited degree with 2,3 DPG (see Chapter 3, p. 85). On the other hand, in certain inherited haemolytic anaemias where there is a block in the glycolytic pathway associated with an accumulation of 2,3 DPG, compensation may be extremely efficient (see Chapter 7, p. 270).

Local changes in tissue perfusion. The blood volume does not change grossly in anaemia and therefore increased tissue perfusion has to be achieved by shunting of blood from less to more vital organs. There is vasoconstriction of the vessels of the skin and kidney; this

mechanism has little effect on renal function. The organs which gain from the redistribution seem to be mainly the myocardium, brain and muscle [297].

Cardiovascular changes. It seems likely that mild degrees of anaemia are compensated for by shifts in the oxygen dissociation curve and some degree of redistribution of blood flow. However, when the haemoglobin level falls below 7–8 g/dl there is a measurable increase in cardiac output both at rest and after exercise [297, 298]. There may be an increase in the stroke rate and a hyperkinetic circulation develops characterized by tachycardia, arterial and capillary pulsation, a wide pulse pressure, and haemic murmurs. The circulation time is shortened, left ventricular stroke work is increased and coronary flow increases in proportion to the increased cardiac output [297]. The haemodynamic responses in chronic anaemia have been investigated by studying the effects of orthostatic stress or pressor amines [299]. It has been found that there is an acute reversal of the high output state in chronic anaemia by both these approaches. These observations suggest that redistribution of blood volume and vasodilation with reduced afterload play a dominant role in hyperkinetic circulatory responses to chronic anaemia and indicate that this state is labile rather than fixed. The mechanism of the vasodilation is not known. An additional factor which may be of some importance in increasing cardiac output is the reduction in blood viscosity produced by a relatively low red-cell mass.

While the normal myocardium may tolerate sustained hyperactivity of this type indefinitely, patients with associated coronary artery disease or those with extreme anaemia may have impaired oxygenation of the myocardium. In such cases cardiomegaly, pulmonary oedema, ascites and peripheral oedema may occur and a state of high output cardiac failure is established. At this stage the plasma volume is almost always increased.

Pulmonary function. Since blood, regardless of its oxygen-carrying capacity, is almost completely oxygenated in the lungs, the oxygen pressure of arterial blood in an anaemic patient should be the same as that in a normal individual and hence an increase in respiratory rate would not be expected to improve the oxygenation of the tissues. Curiously, however, severe anaemia is associated with exertional dyspnoea. Although in some patients this may be related to incipient cardiac failure in most cases it appears to be an inappropriate response to hypoxia which is centrally mediated [300].

Compensation by the erythron. As mentioned earlier in the chapter, the kidney responds to hypoxia by increasing the output of erythropoietin. Assuming that the bone marrow is capable of responding, this results in increased erythroid activity which is manifested by erythroid hyperplasia and a reticulocytosis. We will consider this response further when we deal with the pathophysiology of haemolytic anaemia.

Clinical effects of anaemia

Since anaemia reduces tissue oxygenation it is not surprising that it is associated with widespread organ dysfunction and hence an extremely varied clinical picture. The latter depends, of course, on whether the anaemia is of rapid or more insidious onset.

After acute blood loss the haemoglobin and plasma are reduced proportionately and the symptoms are mainly of volume depletion. Depending on the fluid intake, there may be a minor drop in the packed cell volume during the first 10 hours; volume replacement is not accomplished until between 60 and 90 hours by the influx of albumin from the extravascular compartment. Thus the picture of rapid blood loss is characterized by the typical syndrome of shock with collapse, dyspnoea, tachycardia, a poor volume pulse, reduced blood pressure and marked peripheral vasoconstriction.

With anaemia of more insidious onset, the compensatory mechanisms outlined in the previous sections have time to develop. In mild anaemia there may be no symptoms or simply increased fatigue and slight pallor. In more severe degrees of anaemia the symptoms and signs are more marked. Pallor is best discerned in the mucous membranes; the nail beds and palmar creases, although often said to be useful sites for detecting anaemia, are relatively insensitive for this purpose. Cardiorespiratory symptoms and signs include exertional dyspnoea, tachycardia, palpitations, angina or claudication, night cramps, increased arterial pulsation, capillary pulsation, a variety of cardiac bruits [297], reversible cardiac enlargement [297] and, if cardiac failure occurs, basal crepitations, peripheral oedema and ascites. Neuromuscular involvement is reflected by headache, vertigo, lightheadedness, faintness, tinnitus, roaring in the ears, cramps, increased cold sensitivity and haemorrhages in the retina. Gastrointestinal symptoms include loss of appetite, nausea, constipation and diarrhoea. Genito-urinary involvement causes menstrual irregularities, urinary frequency and loss of libido.

It is often said that a low-grade fever may be caused by anaemia *per se*. Certainly dramatic alterations in the body temperature may follow the administration of folic acid or vitamin B_{12} to patients with megaloblastic anaemia but it is extremely difficult to dissociate the effects of the cause of any particular anaemia from the effects of the anaemia itself on temperature regulation.

Curiously, good experimental data are lacking on this long-standing clinical problem.

It is clear from these considerations that transfusion of patients with long-standing anaemia, particularly if they are in early high-output cardiac failure, can be extremely hazardous. At this stage the total blood volume is normal or increased and transfusion may result in the rapid onset of pulmonary oedema. The administration of powerful diuretics at the same time as the blood can effect a reduction in plasma volume and help prevent this complication; in extreme cases an exchange transfusion may be required.

The causes of anaemia

Since more than one underlying defect of the erythron is involved in almost all cases of anaemia, it is extremely difficult to provide a really adequate classification of the causes. For example, some of the congenital haemolytic anaemias result from genetically determined intrinsic defects of red-cell metabolism yet they need an external agent such as a drug to provoke haemolysis. Similarly, although the megaloblastic anaemias of vitamin-B_{12} or folate deficiency result largely from a major degree of ineffective erythropoiesis there is also a significant amount of peripheral haemolysis. Thus, any classification of the anaemias based on the pathophysiology of the erythron must be designed in the knowledge that it will only present a very incomplete picture of the different mechanisms involved.

Clearly, a reduction in the red-cell mass can result from either an abnormality in the production of red cells or an increased rate of loss of cells either by destruction or bleeding. An impaired production of red cells may result from

1 an absolute decrease in total erythropoietic activity or an increase inappropriate to the degree of anaemia or

2 a marked increase in the intramedullary destruction of red-cell precursors (i.e. in ineffective erythropoiesis).

Based on this approach we can derive a simple classification of anaemia as shown in Table 4.9 in which the causes are divided into decreased or inappropriately increased total erythropoiesis, greatly increased ineffective erythropoiesis, haemolysis and blood loss. The methods available for the quantitation of total and ineffective erythropoiesis are discussed on page 126.

Table 4.9. The main groups of anaemias

Impaired red-cell production
   Decreased or inappropriately increased total erythropoiesis
   Greatly increased ineffective erythropoiesis
Increased rate of red-cell destruction (haemolysis)
Loss of red cells from the circulation (bleeding)

Table 4.10. Main groups of anaemias due to a decrease or inappropriate increase of total erythropoietic activity

Iron-deficiency anaemia
Anaemia of chronic disorders
Reduced erythropoietin production
   Renal disease
   Hypofunction of endocrine glands
   Reduced O_2 affinity of haemoglobin
Aplastic anaemia
Pure red-cell hypoplasia
Infiltrative disorders
   Leukaemia
   Lymphoma
   Secondary carcinoma
   Myeloma

Various disorders in each of these groups of anaemias will be discussed in detail in later chapters. Here we will consider the general classification and pathophysiology of each major type.

Decreased or inappropriately increased total erythropoiesis
The anaemias which fall into this category are summarized in Table 4.10. The most common of these result from an inadequate supply of iron to the erythron. In several of the conditions listed in Table 4.10 there is some increase in ineffective erythropoiesis but this is not the major abnormality in the pathophysiology of the erythron.

Iron deficiency results in abnormal maturation of the red-cell precursors due to defective haemoglobin synthesis. There is only a slight increase in total erythropoiesis even in patients with a moderate or marked anaemia. The abnormal maturation is associated with dyserythropoietic changes which are largely confined to the late erythroblasts and with a relatively minor degree of ineffective erythropoiesis [294, 301]. Chronic inflammatory disorders and related conditions also interfere with the iron supply to red-cell precursors, probably by blocking the release of catabolized red-cell iron from reticulo-endothelial cells. In these conditions, known collectively as the anaemias of chronic disorders, there is a slightly shortened red-cell survival and therefore increased erythron iron requirements. The basic defect in iron deficiency anaemia and that due to inflammation is similar therefore, in that the plasma iron level is inadequate to support the requirements for erythropoiesis.

Impairment of total erythropoietic activity can also result from infiltration of the marrow with leukaemic or other neoplastic cells and from various lesions of the haemopoietic stem cells or red-cell precursors. An ab-

normality in the haemopoietic stem-cell compartment appears to be the usual cause of the reduced total erythropoiesis in cases of congenital and acquired hypoplastic anaemia and the presence of an anti-erythropoietin antibody or a cytotoxic antibody against erythroblasts in cases of pure red-cell hypoplasia.

Finally, an absolute or relative decrease in total erythropoiesis may occur in any disorder associated with erythropoietin deficiency. By far the commonest group are the anaemias of renal failure. A deficiency of erythropoietin appears to be partly responsible for the anaemia seen in various endocrine deficiencies such as hypothyroidism and hypopituitarism (see Chapter 33). It may also explain the mild anaemia associated with haemoglobin variants with decreased oxygen affinity.

As a group the anaemias characterized by a decrease or inadequate increase in total erythropoietic activity are associated with a low reticulocyte count. The red cells are usually normochromic and normocytic although there may be a mild macrocytosis with some deeply staining macroreticulocytes (shift cells) in those cases where erythropoietin production is increased. If granulopoiesis is normal the defect in red-cell production may be reflected by an increase in the M/E ratio.

Greatly increased ineffective erythropoiesis
The anaemias which result primarily from a major degree of ineffective erythropoiesis are summarized in Table 4.11.

The causes of ineffective erythropoiesis are numerous. They include abnormalities of DNA synthesis and defective cytoplasmic maturation. Abnormal DNA synthesis usually results from vitamin-B_{12} or folic-acid deficiency or the administration of drugs such as the antipurines and antipyrimidines. The

Table 4.11. Main groups of anaemias resulting primarily from greatly increased ineffective erythropoiesis

Abnormality of DNA synthesis
   Vitamin-B_{12} deficiency
   Folate deficiency
   Drugs (antipurines, antipyrimidines)
Defective cytoplasmic maturation
   Disorders of globin synthesis
      Thalassaemia
   Disorders of haem and/or iron metabolism
      Sideroblastic anaemia
Unknown mechanism
   Erythroleukaemia
   Congenital dyserythropoietic anaemias
   'Refractory anaemia with hyperplastic marrow'
   Certain infections (*P. falciparum* malaria)
   Some chemicals

important causes of defective cytoplasmic maturation include the inherited disorders of globin synthesis, the thalassaemia syndromes, and the genetic and acquired defects of iron metabolism which make up the sidero-blastic anaemias. A major degree of ineffective erythropoiesis is also present in a group of disorders of unknown aetiology known collectively as the congenital dyserythropoietic anaemias and in erythroleukaemia. Furthermore, there is increasing evidence that some drugs and certain infections may cause a marked increase in ineffective erythropoiesis.

The characteristic finding in the disorders listed in Table 4.11 is marked erythroid hyperplasia with a striking reduction in the M/E ratio associated with a low peripheral reticulocyte count and reticulocyte index. Mainly because of the significant intramedullary destruction of precursors there is usually an elevated bilirubin and LDH level. Furthermore, there are nearly always morphological abnormalities of the red-cell precursors (see p. 124 and Chapter 31). Megaloblastic erythropoiesis and a macrocytic red-cell population are encountered in patients with abnormal DNA synthesis, in erythroleukaemia and in some cases of congenital dyserythropoietic anaemia. By contrast, the conditions caused by abnormal cytoplasmic maturation are characterized by normoblastic hyperplasia and microcytic red cells. However, even in the latter cases there is marked anisocytosis and there may be a proportion of abnormal macrocytes in the peripheral circulation. Furthermore, megaloblastic changes may develop as a result of a secondary folate deficiency.

In summary, this group of anaemias is characterized by a marked increase in total erythropoiesis mediated through increased erythropoietin production, and a significant intramedullary destruction of red-cell precursors. This destruction is frequently associated with a severe disorder of erythroblast proliferation (see p. 124). There is usually a mild haemolytic component due to abnormalities in those cells which do reach the peripheral blood. These changes are reflected by marked ferrokinetic abnormalities including an elevated plasma iron level, increased plasma iron turnover, decreased incorporation into circulating haemoglobin and accumulation of iron in bone-marrow macrophages together with increased iron stores in the liver and other tissues. A fascinating and unexplained enigma is why these anaemias are often associated with a marked increase in iron absorption in the presence of normal or elevated body iron stores.

The abnormalities in bilirubin metabolism associated with ineffective erythropoiesis are mainly the result of intramedullary destruction of large numbers of red-cell precursors and hence the breakdown of haemoglobin with increased bilirubin production. If a radioactively labelled amino acid which is incorpor-

ated into haem such as [^{14}C]-glycine is injected into normal individuals some bilirubin is labelled within five days (early-labelled bilirubin) while the majority is labelled late from 80 to 120 days [302] (see p. 131). The origin of the early labelled fraction is uncertain although it probably originates partly in the liver and partly in the marrow. This fraction is markedly increased in the presence of ineffective erythropoiesis; presumably this reflects intramedullary breakdown of haemoglobin. In some varieties of dyserythropoietic anaemia increased amounts of abnormal pyrroles are excreted in the urine; these are also thought to be products of haem metabolism.

The haemolytic anaemias
The major groups of haemolytic anaemias are summarized in Table 4.12 and the pathophysiology of haemolysis is summarized in Figure 4.14.

Haemolytic mechanisms. Premature destruction of red cells may occur either because the membrane is abnormal in structure and function, the cells are exposed to excessive physical trauma in the circulation, or because they are unusually rigid due to the

Table 4.12. Main groups of haemolytic anaemias

Genetic disorders of the red cell
    Membrane
        Hereditary spherocytosis
        Hereditary ovalocytosis
        Stomatocytosis
        Other 'leaky' membrane disorders
        Acanthocytosis
    Haemoglobin
        Sickling disorders
        Haemoglobins C, D and E
        Unstable haemoglobins
        Thalassaemia syndromes
    Energy pathways
        Hexose monophosphate shunt
        Embden–Meyerhof pathway
Acquired disorders of the red cell
    Immune
        Isoimmune—Rh or ABO
        Autoimmune—warm or cold antibody
    Non-immune
        Trauma: Microangiopathy
                Valve prosthesis
                Body surface contact
        Membrane defects: PNH, liver disease
        Parasitic disorders
        Bacterial infection
        Physical agents, drugs and chemicals
        Hypersplenism
        Due to defective red-cell maturation

---

precipitation or abnormal molecular configuration of haemoglobin.

For a red cell to survive it must be able to maintain a normal shape and permeability and to undergo plastic deformation in the microcirculation [302]. The latter characteristic depends mainly on the cell surface/volume ratio which in turn is dependent on the integrity of its membrane. Normal membrane function relies on the production of energy for active transport of sodium and potassium in and out of the cells and for the maintenance of the protein sulphydryl groups in their reduced state. It also depends on the existence of a system for the renewal of membrane lipids to preserve a normal lipid composition. If any of these functions fail the red cell tends to assume a spherical shape, i.e. to develop a small surface area for a given volume, and hence is not easily deformed. The resulting loss of plasticity leads to selective sequestration in the spleen and other parts of the reticulo-endothelial system. This type of pathological process occurs in genetic disorders of the red-cell membrane such as hereditary spherocytosis and in conditions in which there is a reduced amount of energy production or abnormal lipid metabolism. The membrane may also be damaged by the interaction of antibodies on the cell surface with macrophages of the reticulo-endothelial system and by the direct action of complement, trauma, chemicals, bacterial products or parasites.

The red cells may be damaged by excessive trauma. This may occur in several ways including excessive turbulence created by cardiac-valve prostheses, rigid fibrin strands in the microvasculature (microangiopathy) or due to excessive pressure on body surfaces.

Finally, red cells which contain abnormally aggregated or precipitated haemoglobin molecules become less deformable and may be damaged or destroyed in the marrow, spleen or microcirculation. This type of process occurs in the sickling and thalassaemia disorders and in conditions associated with a genetic instability of the haemoglobin molecule. Precipitation of haemoglobin with the production of Heinz bodies may follow the action of a variety of oxidant agents. Oxidative haemolysis is potentiated by deficiencies of enzymes such as glucose-6-phosphate dehydrogenase which make the cell more prone to oxidant damage. The ways in which oxidative damage is mediated are complicated and only partly understood. They include reduction in red-cell glutathione levels, haemoglobin instability, generation of superoxides and other intermediates, deficiency of antioxidants such as vitamin E, and accumulation of iron (see Chapter 7, p. 276).

Sites of red-cell destruction. The red cells may be destroyed either intravascularly or extravascularly or in both sites. The particular site of destruction depends on the type and degree of damage to the cells. For example, complement-damaged cells have large holes in the membrane and are destroyed intravascularly whereas IgG-coated cells are removed by interaction with macrophages in the reticulo-endothelial elements of the spleen and liver.

The constant bombardment of the reticulo-endothelial elements of the spleen by abnormal red cells causes splenomegaly, a phenomenon which has been called 'work hypertrophy'. This subject is considered in greater detail in Chapter 20.

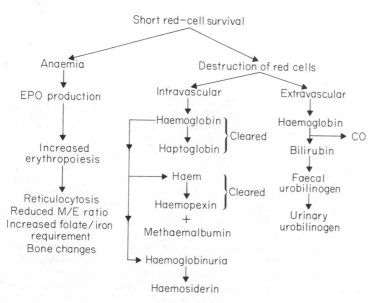

Fig. 4.14. Summary of the pathophysiology of haemolysis. EPO = erythropoietin.

Breakdown of haemoglobin. About 80% of the haem liberated by the breakdown of haemoglobin is converted to bilirubin. The fate of bilirubin was considered earlier in the chapter (p. 116). In haemolytic states there is an increased production of bilirubin and also of urinary and faecal urobilinogen. However, measurements of the latter as an indication of the rate of haemolysis are unreliable because bilirubin may be derived from ineffective erythropoiesis and also because the level of faecal urobilinogen is dependent on the activity of micro-organisms in the gut (see p. 117).

The bilirubin level in the peripheral blood of patients with haemolysis depends on the rate of haemolysis and on the ability of the liver to conjugate and excrete bilirubin. Thus, in the neonatal period, immaturity of the fetal liver may lead to very high levels of bilirubin in association with relatively low-grade haemolysis. Unconjugated bilirubin does not appear in the urine and therefore the hyperbilirubinaemia of haemolysis is sometimes described as an 'acholuric' jaundice.

Haemoglobin metabolism in the circulation and the kidneys. When haemoglobin is liberated into the circulation it is bound to haptoglobin and the haemoglobin–haptoglobin complex is rapidly removed. Thus, the most sensitive guide to intravascular haemolysis is a reduction in serum haptoglobin level. This occurs even when the haemolysis is primarily extravascular, possibly because there is some leak of free haemoglobin into the circulation. If the binding capacity of haptoglobin is exceeded haemoglobin appears in the plasma where it is degraded and the liberated haem binds to haemopexin.

There are still many deficiencies in our knowledge about the haemoglobin and haem-binding proteins of the blood. Haptoglobin is a collective term applied to a group of α globulins which are synthesized in the liver [303]. Several molecular varieties have been identified by their electrophoretic migration and it is known that their structure is genetically determined by two allelic systems. Three phenotypes are recognized, i.e. 1–1, 2–2 and 2–1; they are made up of similar subunits but differ with respect to molecular weight, haemoglobin-binding capacity and clearance rates. Normally sufficient haptoglobin is present to bind 100–140 mg of haemoglobin/100 ml of plasma. Haemoglobin–haptoglobin complex has a molecular weight such that it is not excreted by the kidney, but is cleared from the plasma at a rate of approximately 15 mg haemoglobin/100 ml/hour by the reticulo-endothelial system. It should be remembered that haptoglobin levels are modified by other factors than haemolysis including infection, liver disease and malignancy. Furthermore, their level is under genetic control and congenital ahaptoglobinaemia occurs in some populations.

Haemopexin [304] is a β glycoprotein which consists of two components, I and II; I is a monomer and II, which contains four electrophoretic bands, is a polymeric form. Its normal concentration is approximately 80 mg/100 ml of plasma. The haemopexin–haem complexes are removed from the circulation by the liver.

When the haemoglobin-binding capacity of haptoglobin and haem-binding capacity of haemopexin is saturated, free haemoglobin appears in the plasma where it is rapidly oxidized to methaemoglobin and the haematin is bound to albumin to form methaemalbumin. The latter is responsible for the dirty brown colour of the plasma associated with severe intravascular haemolysis. Albumin selectively binds up to two haem groups per molecule.

In cases of marked intravascular haemolysis, haemoglobin may be present in the plasma in sufficient quantities to saturate its haptoglobin, haemopexin and albumin-binding capacities and hence may appear in the urine. This occurs because tetrameric haemoglobin freely dissociates into αβ dimers with a molecular weight of about 32 000 which is small enough to permit glomerular filtration [306]. At plasma haemoglobin levels of 30 mg/ml or less, no haemoglobin appears in the urine because it is reabsorbed in the proximal renal tubules. At levels in excess of this free haemoglobin is found in the urine. Porphyrin and globin are rapidly catabolized in the renal tubule cells and some iron is transferred into capillary blood. However, much of it is converted into haemosiderin. Cells containing the latter are cast off and appear in the urine; the presence of haemosiderin in spun-down urinary sediment is by far the most reliable indication of a state of chronic intravascular haemolysis. Haemosiderinuria may be demonstrated in the urinary sediment by the Prussian-blue reaction.

Compensatory mechanisms. The normal red-cell life-span is approximately 120 days. If this is shortened the circulating haemoglobin level falls, relatively less oxygen is transported to the kidney, there is an increased output of erythropoietin and the rate of erythropoiesis increases. Assuming that the marrow is healthy the circulating red-cell mass is restored to normal. This condition is called a compensated haemolytic state. Indeed, with a healthy bone marrow, the red-cell survival can be reduced by as much as eight times without a drop in the haemoglobin level. However, if the red-cell survival time is less than 15 days even a healthy marrow cannot compensate and a haemolytic anaemia results. If the bone marrow is abnormal or if there is an inadequate supply of iron or other substances required for red-cell production, anaemia may result when the red-cell survival is considerably greater than 15 days.

Within a few days of the onset of haemolysis, reticulocyte count increases and erythroid hyperplasia becomes measurable by a decrease in the M/E ratio. With sustained haemolysis there is an expansion of the erythroid marrow and within two to three months the rate of erythropoiesis may rise to 10–15 times normal [306]. This process is mirrored by a marked reticulocytosis and the spilling over of normoblasts into the peripheral blood. The stained peripheral-blood film characteristically shows variation in colour of the cells and the presence of variable numbers of grey-staining macrocytes.

This increase in erythroid proliferation has important consequences. In particular there is an increased demand for iron and maximum proliferation cannot occur in the presence of a limited iron supply [301]. Similarly there is a marked increase in folate requirements. There is spread of erythroid marrow down the long bones and, especially if haemolysis occurs from early life, some degree of extramedullary haemopoiesis in the spleen, liver and lymph nodes. Expansion of the marrow in this way can lead to bone deformity similar to that observed in the severe dyserythropoietic anaemias.

The degree of compensation may be modified by the oxygen affinity of the red cells. For example, some haemoglobin variants which produce haemolytic anaemia such as sickle haemoglobin have a low oxygen affinity and therefore the anaemia is well compensated. Similarly, in association with genetic defects of the glycolytic pathway the level of 2,3 diphosphoglycerate may be elevated and this also causes a right shift in the oxygen dissociation curve with increased delivery of oxygen.

REFERENCES

1 VAN BEKKUM B.W., VAN NOORD M.J., MAAT B. & DICKE K.A. (1971) Attempts at identification of hemopoietic stem cells in mouse. *Blood*, **38**, 547.

2 DICKE K.A., VAN NOORD M.J., MAAT B. SCHAEFER U.W. & VAN BEKKUM D.W. (1973) Attempts at morphological identification of the haemopoietic stem cell in primates and rodents. In: *Haemopoietic Stem Cells* (ed. Wolstenholme G.E.W. & O'Connor M.). Associated Scientific Publishers, Amsterdam.

3 DICKE K.A., VAN NOORD M.J. & VAN BEKKUM D.W. (1973) Attempts at morphological identification of the hemopoietic stem cell in rodents and primates. *Experimental Hematology*, **1**, 36.

4 VAN DEN ENGH G., VISSER J. & TRASK B. (1979) Identification of CFU-s by scatter measurements on a light-activated cell sorter. In: *Experimental Hematology*

Today 1979 (ed. Baum S.J. & Ledney G.D.), p. 19. Springer-Verlag, New York.

5 BARR R.D., WHANG-PENG J. & PERRY S. (1975) Hemopoietic stem cells in human peripheral blood. *Science*, **190**, 284.

6 WICKRAMASINGHE S.N. & HUGHES M. (1979) Intracellular localization of ^{55}Fe after serum-mediated uptake by human erythropoietic cells. *Scandinavian Journal of Haematology*, **22**, 67.

7 WICKRAMASINGHE S.N., CHALMERS D.G. & COOPER E.H. (1967) Disturbed proliferation of erythropoietic cells in pernicious anaemia. *Nature (London)*, **215**, 189.

8 WICKRAMASINGHE S.N., COOPER E.H. & CHALMERS D.G. (1968) A study of erythropoiesis by combined morphologic, quantitative cytochemical and autoradiographic methods. Normal human bone marrow, vitamin B_{12} deficiency and iron deficiency anemia. *Blood*, **31**, 304.

9 KILLMANN S.A. (1964) On the size of normal human reticulocytes. *Acta Medica Scandinavica*, **176**, 529.

10 BESSIS M. (1964) Hemopoietic tissue and blood. In: *Electron Microscopic Anatomy* (ed. Kurtz S.M.). Academic Press, New York.

11 TANAKA Y. & GOODMAN J.R. (1972) *Electron Microscopy of Human Blood Cells.* Harper & Row, New York.

12 CAWLEY J.C. & HAYHOE F.G.J. (1973) *Ultrastructure of Haemic Cells. A Cytological Atlas of Normal and Leukaemic Blood and Bone Marrow.* W. B. Saunders, London, Philadelphia and Toronto.

13 SMETANA K., GYORKEY F., GYORKEY P. & BUSCH H. (1975) Studies on nucleoli of maturing human erythroblasts. *Experimental Cell Research*, **91**, 143.

14 YATAGANAS X., GAHRTON G. & THORELL B. (1974) Intranuclear hemoglobin in erythroblasts of β-thalassemia. *Blood*, **43**, 243.

15 BESSIS M., BRETON-GORIUS J. & THIERY J.P. (1961) Rôle possible de l'hémoglobine accompagnant le noyau des erythroblasts dans l'origine de la stercobiline éliminée précocement. *Compte Rendu de l'Académie des Sciences, Paris*, **252**, 2300.

16 KENT G., MINICK O.T., VOLINI F.I. & ORFEI E. (1966) Autophagic vacuoles in human red cells. *American Journal of Pathology*, **48**, 831.

17 BESSIS M. (1958) L'ilôt erythroblastique, unité fonctionnelle de la moelle osseuse. *Revue d'Hématologie*, **13**, 8.

18 MOHANDAS N. & PRENANT M. (1978) Three-dimensional model of bone marrow. *Blood*, **51**, 633.

19 TANAKA Y., BRECHER G. & BULL B. (1966) Ferritin localization on the erythroblast cell membrane and ropheocytosis in hypersiderotic human bone marrow. *Blood*, **28**, 758.

20 TANAKA Y. & BRECHER G. (1971a) Effect of surface digestion and metabolic inhibitors on appearance of ferritin in guinea pig erythroblasts *in vitro*. Evidence for the production of apoferritin on the erythroblast cell membrane. *Blood*, **37**, 211.

21 TANAKA Y. & BRECHER G. (1971b) Micropinocytotic ferritin in erythroid cells: species dependency and relation to serum iron levels. *Blood*, **38**, 431.

22 MURPHY M.J. & URABE A. (1978) Modulatory effect of macrophages on erythropoiesis. In: *In Vitro Aspects of Erythropoiesis* (ed. Murphy M.J. Jr), p. 189. Springer-Verlag, New York.

23 WICKRAMASINGHE S.N. (1975) *Human Bone Marrow.* Blackwell Scientific Publications, Oxford.

24 MESSNER H., FLIEDNER T.M. & CRONKITE E.P. (1969) Kinetics of erythropoietic cell proliferation in pernicious anaemia. *Series Haematologica*, **II/4**, 44.

25 WICKRAMASINGHE S.N. (1979) Studies on the cell cycle in human bone marrow. In: *Quantitative Cytochemistry and its Applications* (ed. Pattison J.R., Bitensky L. & Chayen J.), p. 9. Academic Press, London.

26 LAJTHA L.G., POZZI L.V., SCHOFIELD R. & FOX M. (1969) Kinetic properties of haemopoietic stem cells. *Journal of Cell and Tissue Kinetics*, **2**, 39.

27 ISCOVE N.N. (1977) The role of the erythropoietin in regulation of population size and cell cycling of early and late erythroid precursors in mouse bone marrow. *Journal of Cell and Tissue Kinetics*, **10**, 323.

28 STRYCKMANS P., CRONKITE E.P. FACHE J., FLIEDNER T.M. & RAMOS J. (1966) Deoxyribonucleic acid synthesis time of erythropoietic and granulopoietic cells in human beings. *Nature (London)*, **211**, 717.

29 KILLMANN S.A., CRONKITE E.P., FLIEDNER T.M. & BOND V.P. (1964) Mitotic indices of human bone-marrow cells. III. Duration of some phases of erythrocytic and granulocyte proliferation computed from mitotic indices. *Blood*, **24**, 267.

30 LAJTHA L.G. & OLIVER R. (1960) Studies on the kinetics of erythropoiesis: a model of the erythron. In: *Ciba Foundation Symposium on Haemopoiesis* (ed. Wolstenholme G.E.W. & O'Connor M.), p. 289. Churchill, London.

31 STOHLMAN F. (1964) Humoral regulation of erythropoiesis. XIV. A model for abnormal erythropoiesis in thalassaemia. *Annals of the New York Academy of Sciences*, **119**, 578.

32 YATAGANAS X., GAHRTON G. & THORELL B. (1970) DNA, RNA and hemoglobin during erythroblast maturation. A cytophotometric study. *Experimental Cell Research*, **62**, 254.

33 GILMOUR S. (1973) New look at chromatin. *Nature (London)*, **246**, 8.

34 LEBLOND P.F., LA CELLE P.L. & WEED R.I. (1971) Cellular deformability: a possible determinant of the normal release of maturing erythrocytes from the bone marrow. *Blood*, **37**, 40.

35 ARNDT-JOVIN D.J. & JOVIN T.M. (1976) Cell separation using fluorescence emission anisotrophy. *Journal of Supramolecular Structure*, **5** (Suppl. 1), 123.

36 HARRISON P.R. (1976) Analysis of erythropoiesis at the molecular level. *Nature (London)*, **262**, 353.

37 MILNER G.R. (1969) Nuclear morphology and the ultrastructural localization of deoxyribonucleic acid synthesis during interphase. *Journal of Cell Science*, **4**, 569.

38 LEVY J., TERADA M., RIFKIND R.A. & MARKS P.A. (1975) Induction of erythroid differentiation in cells infected with Friend Virus: relationship to the cell cycle. *Proceedings of the National Academy of Sciences, USA*, **72**, 28.

39 TORELLI U., GROSSI G., ARTUSI T., EMILIA G., ATTIYA I.R. & MAURI C. (1964) RNA and protein metabolism in normal human erythroblasts and granuloblasts. *Acta Haematologica*, **32**, 271.

40 SCHMID J.R., KIELY J.M., TAUXE W.N. & OWEN C.A., JR (1966) *In vitro* DNA and RNA synthesis in human bone-marrow cells: a study of 12 normal subjects and 12 patients with lymphoplasmocytic disorders. *Blood*, **27**, 310.

41 YOSHIDA Y., TODO A., SHIRAKAWA S., WAKISAKA G. & UCHINO H. (1968) Proliferation of megaloblasts in pernicious anemia as observed from nucleic acid metabolism. *Blood*, **31**, 292.

42 WICKRAMASINGHE S.N. (1977) Normal erythropoiesis: mechanisms of disturbance in disease. In: *Dyserythropoiesis* (ed. Lewis S.M. & Verwilghen R.L.), p. 21. Academic Press, New York.

43 DARNELL J.E., JELINEK W.R. & MOLLOY G.R. (1973) Biogenesis of mRNA: genetic regulation in mammalian cells. *Science*, **181**, 1215.

44 IMAIZUMI T., DIGGELMANN H. & SCHERRER K. (1973) Demonstration of globin messenger sequences in giant nuclear precursors of messenger RNA of avian erythroblasts. *Proceedings of the National Academy of Sciences, USA*, **70**, 1122.

45 RUIZ-CARRILO A., BEATO M., SCHUTZ B., FEIGELSON P. & ALLFREY V.G. (1973) Cell free translation of the globin message within polydisperse high-molecular-weight ribonucleic acid of avian erythrocytes. *Proceedings of the National Academy of Sciences, USA*, **70**, 3641.

46 WILLIAMSON R., DREWIENKIEWICZ C.E. & PAUL J. (1973) Globin messenger sequences in high molecular weight RNA from embryonic mouse liver. *Nature (New Biology)*, **241**, 66.

47 EVANS M.J. & LINGREL J.B. (1969) Hemoglobin messenger ribonucleic acid. Synthesis of 9S and ribosomal ribonucleic acid during erythroid cell development. *Biochemistry*, **8**, 3000.

48 GASKILL P. & KABAT D. (1971) Unexpectedly large size of globin messenger ribonucleic acid. *Proceedings of the National Academy of Sciences, USA*, **68**, 72.

49 RAMIREZ F., GAMBINO R., MANIATIS G.M., RIFKIND R.A., MARKS P. & BANK A. (1975) Changes in globin mRNA content during erythroid cell differentiation. *Journal of Biological Chemistry*, **250**, 6054.

50 TERADA M., CANTOR L., METAFORA S., RIFKIND R.A., BANK A. & MARKS P.A. (1972) Globin messenger RNA activity in erythroid precursor cells and the effect of erythropoietin. *Proceedings of the National Academy of Sciences, USA*, **69**, 3575.

51 HARRISON P.R., CONKIE D., AFFARA N. & PAUL J. (1974) *In situ* localisation of globin messenger RNA formation. I. During mouse foetal liver development. *Journal of Cell Biology*, **63**, 402.

52 CONKIE D., KLEIMAN L., HARRISON P.R. & PAUL J. (1975) Increase in the accumulation of globin mRNA in immature erythroblasts in response to erythropoietin *in vivo* or *in vitro*. *Experimental Cell Research*, **93**, 315.

53 WICKRAMASINGHE S.N. & CHALMERS D.G. (1968) Protein synthesis in megaloblastic erythropoiesis caused by vitamin B$_{12}$ deficiency. *Nature (London)*, **218**, 463.

54 DENTON M.J., SPENCER N. & ARNSTEIN H.R.V. (1975) Biochemical and enzymic changes during erythrocyte differentiation. The significance of the final cell division. *Biochemical Journal*, **146**, 205.

55 CHANG H., LANGER P.J. & LODISH H.F. (1976) Asynchronous synthesis of erythrocyte membrane proteins.

Proceedings of the National Academy of Sciences, USA, **73,** 3206.

56 YUNIS J.J. & YUNIS E. (1963) Cell antigens and cell specialization. I. A study of blood group antigens on normoblasts. *Blood,* **22,** 53.

57 YUNIS J.J. & YUNIS E. (1964) Cell antigens and cell specialization. II. Demonstration of some red-cell antigens of human normoblasts. *Blood,* **24,** 522.

58 YUNIS J.J. & YUNIS E. (1964) Cell antigens and cell specialization. IV. On the H substance of normoblasts, megakaryocytes and platelets. *Blood,* **24,** 531.

59 REARDEN A. & MASOUREDIS S.P. (1977) Blood group D antigen content of nucleated red-cell precursors. *Blood,* **50,** 981.

60 LANE M. & ALFREY C.P. JR (1965) The anemia of human riboflavin deficiency. *Blood,* **25,** 432.

61 FOY H., KONDI A. & MACDOUGALL L. (1961) Pure red-cell aplasia in marasmus and Kwashiorkor treated with riboflavin. *British Medical Journal,* **i,** 937.

62 GOLDBERG A. (1963) The anaemia of scurvy. *Quarterly Journal of Medicine,* **32,** 51.

63 COX E.V., MEYNELL M.J., NORTHAM B.E. & COOKE W.T. (1967) The anaemia of scurvy. *American Journal of Medicine,* **42,** 220.

64 CRANDON J.H., LUND C.C. & DILL D.B. (1940) Experimental human scurvy. *New England Journal of Medicine,* **223,** 353.

65 BRONTE-STEWART B. (1953) The anaemia of adult scurvy. *Quarterly Journal of Medicine,* **22,** 309.

66 GROSS S. & MELHORN D.K. (1972) Vitamin E, red-cell lipids and red-cell stability in prematurity. *Annals of the New York Academy of Sciences,* **203,** 141.

67 BINDER H.J., HERTING D.C., HURST V., FINCH S.C. & SPIRO H.M. (1965) Tocopherol deficiency in man. *New England Journal of Medicine,* **273,** 1289.

68 POWELL L.W. (1973) Vitamin E deficiency in human liver disease and its relation to haemolysis. *Australian and New Zealand Journal of Medicine,* **3,** 355.

69 CORDANO A., BAERTL J.M. & GRAHAM G.G. (1964) Copper defiency in infancy. *Pediatrics,* **34,** 324.

70 PORTER K.G., MCMASTER D., ELMES M.E. & LOVE A.H.G. (1977) Anaemia and low serum copper during zinc therapy. *Lancet,* **ii,** 774.

71 DUNLAP W.M., JAMES G.W. & HUME D.M. (1974) Anemia and neutropenia caused by copper deficiency. *Annals of Internal Medicine,* **80,** 470.

72 PERONA G., GUIDI G.C., PIGA A., CELLERINO R., MILANI G., COLAUTTI P., MOSCHINI G. & STIEVANO B.M. (1979) Neonatal erythrocyte glutathione peroxidase deficiency as a consequence of selenium imbalance during pregnancy. *British Journal of Haematology,* **42,** 567.

73 REISSMAN K.R. (1964) Protein metabolism and erythropoiesis. I. The anaemia of protein deprivation. II. Erythropoietin formation and erythroid responsiveness in protein deprived rats. *Blood,* **23,** 137 and 146.

74 ADAMS E.B. (1970) Anaemia associated with protein deficiency. *Seminars in Haematology,* **7,** 55.

75 DELMONTE L., ASCHKENASY A. & EYQUEM A. (1964) Studies on the hemolytic nature of protein-deficiency anemia in the rat. *Blood,* **24,** 49.

76 MANT M.J. & FARAGHER B.S. (1972) The haematology of anorexia nervosa. *British Journal of Haematology,* **23,** 737.

77 TAVASSOLI M. & SHAKLAI M. (1979) Absence of tight junctions in endothelium of marrow sinuses: possible significance for marrow-cell egress. *British Journal of Haematology,* **41,** 303.

78 CAMPBELL F.R. (1972) Ultrastructural studies of transmural migration of blood cells in the bone marrow of rats, mice and guinea pigs. *American Journal of Anatomy,* **135,** 521.

79 CHAMBERLAIN J.K., LEBLOND P.F. & WEED R.I. (1975) Reduction of adventitial cell cover: an early direct effect of erythropoietin on bone-marrow ultrastructure. *Blood Cells,* **1,** 655.

80 CHAMBERLAIN J.K., WEISS L. & WEED R.I. (1975) Bone-marrow sinus cell packing: a determinant of cell release. *Blood,* **46,** 91.

81 DE BRUYN P.P.H., MICHELSON S. & THOMAS T.B. (1971) The migration of blood cells of the bone marrow through the sinusoidal wall. *Journal of Morphology,* **133,** 417.

82 WEISS L. (1970) Transmural cellular passage in the vascular sinuses of rat bone marrow. *Blood,* **36,** 189.

83 BESSIS M. & BRICKA M. (1952) Aspect dynamique des cellules du sang. Son étude par la microcinématographie en contraste de phase. *Revue d'Hématologie,* **7,** 407.

84 GORDON A.S., LOBUE J., DORNFEST B.S. & COOPER G.W. (1962) Reticulocyte and leucocyte release from isolated perfused rat legs and femurs. In: *Erythropoiesis* (ed. Jacobson L.O. & Doyle M.), p. 321. Grune & Stratton, New York and London.

85 FISHER J.W., LAJTHA G., BUTTOO A.S. & PORTEOUS D.D. (1965) Direct effects of erythropoietin on the bone marrow of the isolated perfused hind limbs of rabbits. *British Journal of Haematology,* **11,** 342.

86 BRANEMARK P.I. (1959) Vital microscopy of bone marrow in rabbit. *Scandinavian Journal of Clinical and Laboratory Investigation,* **11** (Suppl.), 38.

87 KILLMAN S-A., CRONKITE E.P., FLIEDNER T.M. & BOND V.P. (1962) Mitotic indices of bone-marrow cells. I. Number and cytologic distribution of mitoses. *Blood,* **19,** 743.

88 PATT H.M. & MALONEY M.A. (1963) An evaluation of granulocytopoiesis. In: *Cell Proliferation* (ed. Lamerton L.F. & Fry R.J.M.), p. 157. Blackwell Scientific Publications, Oxford.

89 CRONKITE E.P., FLIEDNER T.M., STRYCKMANS P., CHANANA A.D., CUTTNER J. & RAMOS J. (1965) Flow patterns and rates of human erythropoiesis and granulocytopoiesis. *Series Haematologica,* **5,** 51.

90 SAMSON D., HALLIDAY D., NICHOLSON D.C. & CHANARIN I. (1976) Quantitation of ineffective erythropoiesis from the incorporation of ^{15}N delta-aminolaevulini acid and ^{15}N-glycine into early labelled bilirubin. I. Normal subjects. *British Journal of Haematology,* **34,** 33.

91 POLLYCOVE M. & MORTIMER R. (1961) The quantitative determination of iron kinetics and hemoglobin synthesis in human subjects. *Journal of Clinical Investigation,* **40,** 753.

92 COOK J.D., MARSAGLIA G., ESCHBACH J.W., FUNK D.D. & FINCH C.A. (1970) Ferrokinetics: a biological model for iron exchange in man. *Journal of Clinical Investigation,* **49,** 197.

93 RICKETTS C., JACOBS A. & CAVILL I. (1975) Ferrokine-

tics and erythropoiesis in man: the measurement of effective erythropoiesis, ineffective erythropoiesis and red-cell life-span using ^{59}Fe. *British Journal of Haematology*, **31**, 65.

94 LOCKNER D. (1966) Quantitation of erythropoiesis by a new method. I. Studies on healthy subjects. *Scandinavian Journal of Clinical and Laboratory Investigation*, **18**, 493.

95 BOND V.P., FLIEDNER T.M., CRONKITE E.P., RUBINI J.R. & ROBERTSON J.S. (1959) Cell turnover in blood and blood-forming tissues studied with tritiated thymidine. In: *The Kinetics of Cellular Proliferation* (ed. Stohlman F., Jr), p. 188. Grune & Stratton, New York and London.

96 DAGG J.H., HORTON P.W., ORR J.S. & SHIMMINS J. (1972) A direct method of determining red-cell life-span using radioiron: an application of the occupancy principle. *British Journal of Haematology*, **22**, 9.

97 BERK P.D., BLOOMER J.R., HOWE R.B. & BERLIN N.I. (1970) The life-span of the cell as determined with labeled bilirubin. In: *Formation and Destruction of Blood Cells*, p. 91. J. B. Lippincott, Philadelphia.

98 ASHBY W. (1919) Determination of length of life of transfused blood corpuscles in man. *Journal of Experimental Medicine*, **29**, 267.

99 WIENER A.S. (1934) Longevity of the erythrocyte. *Journal of the American Medical Association*, **102**, 1779.

100 MOLLISON P.L. & YOUNG I.M. (1942) The *in vitro* survival in the human subject of transfused erythrocytes after storage in various preservative solutions. *Quarterly Journal of Experimental Physiology*, **31**, 359.

101 HURLEY T.H. & WEISSMAN R., JR (1954) Determination of the survival of transfused red cells by the method of differential haemolysis. *Journal of Clinical Investigation*, **33**, 835.

102 SHEMIN D. & RITTENBERG D. (1946) The life-span of the human red blood cell. *Journal of Biological Chemistry*, **166**, 627.

103 BERLIN N.I., LAWRENCE J.H. & LEE H.C. (1954) The pathogenesis of the anaemia of chronic leukaemia: measurement of the life-span of the red blood cell with glycine-2-C^{14}. *Journal of Laboratory and Clinical Medicine*, **44**, 860.

104 BERLIN N.I., BEEKMANS M., ELMLINGER P.J. & LAWRENCE J.H. (1957) Comparative study of the Ashby differential agglutination, carbon^{14} and iron^{59} methods for determination of red-cell life-span. *Journal of Laboratory and Clinical Medicine*, **50**, 558.

105 FINCH C.A., WOLFF J.A., RATH C.E. & FLUHARTY R.G. (1949) Iron metabolism: erythrocyte iron turnover. *Journal of Laboratory and Clinical Medicine*, **34**, 1480.

106 PENNER J.A. (1966) Investigation of erythrocyte turnover with selenium-75-labelled methionine. *Journal of Laboratory and Clinical Medicine*, **67**, 427.

107 EBAUGH F.G., JR, EMERSON C.P. & ROSS J.F. (1953) The use of radioactive chromium 51 as an erythrocyte tagging agent for the determination of red cell survival *in vivo*. *Journal of Clinical Investigation*, **32**, 1260.

108 MOLLISON P.L. & VEALL N. (1955) The use of the isotope ^{51}Cr as a label for red cells. *British Journal of Haematology*, **1**, 62.

109 DONOHUE D.M., MOTULSKY A.G., GIBLETT E.R., PIRZIO-BIROLI G., VIRANUVATTI V. & FINCH C.A. (1955)

The use of chromium as a red-cell tag. *British Journal of Haematology*, **1**, 249.

110 MOLLISON P.L. (1979) *Blood Transfusion in Clinical Medicine*, 6th edn. Blackwell Scientific Publications, Oxford.

111 COHEN J.A. & WARRINGA M.G.P.J. (1954) The fate of P^{32}-labelled di-isopropyl-fluorophosphonate in the human body and its use as a labelling agent in the study of the turnover of blood plasma and red cells. *Journal of Clinical Investigation*, **33**, 459.

112 BRATTEBY L-E. & WADMAN B. (1968) Labelling of red blood cells *in vitro* with small amounts of di-iso-propyl-fluorphosphonate (DF ^{32}P). *Scandinavian Journal of Clinical and Laboratory Investigation*, **21**, 197.

113 HEIMPEL H., ERDMANN H., HOFFMAN G. & KEIDERLING W. (1964) Tierexperimentelle Untersuchungen zur Markierung von Erythrozyten mit radioaktiven Diisopropylfluorophosphat (DFP^{32}). *Nuclear Medicine* (Amsterdam), **4**, 32.

114 CLINE M.J. & BERLIN N.I. (1962) Measurement of red cell survival with tritiated di-isopropyl fluorophosphate. *Journal of Laboratory and Clinical Medicine*, **60**, 826.

115 BERNSTEIN R.E. (1959) Alterations in metabolic energetics and cation transport during aging of red cells. *Journal of Clinical Investigation*, **38**, 1572.

116 BISHOP C. & VAN GASTEL C. (1969) Changes in enzyme activity during reticulocyte maturation and red-cell aging. *Haematologica*, **3**, 29.

117 CHAPMAN R.G. & SCHAUMBURG L. (1967) Glycolysis and glycolytic enzyme activity of aging red cells in man. *British Journal of Haematology*, **13**, 665.

118 WESTERMAN M.P., PIERCE L.E. & JENSEN W.N. (1963) Erythrocyte lipids: a comparison of normal young and old populations. *Journal of Laboratory and Clinical Medicine*, **62**, 394.

119 VAN GASTEL C., VAN DEN BERG D., DE GIER J. & VAN DEENEN L.L.M. (1965) Some lipid characteristics of normal red blood cells of different age. *British Journal of Haematology*, **11**, 193.

120 WALTER H. & SELBY F.W. (1966) Counter-current distribution of red blood cells of slightly different ages. *Biochimica et Biophysica Acta*, **112**, 146.

121 WEED R.I., LA CELLE P.L. & MERRIL E.W. (1969) Metabolic dependence of red-cell deformability. *Journal of Clinical Investigation*, **48**, 795.

122 WINTERBOURN C.C. & BATT R.D. (1970) Lipid composition of human red cells of different ages. *Biochimica et Biophysica Acta*, **202**, 1.

123 KEITT A.S., SMITH T.W. & JANDL J.H. (1966) Red cell 'pseudo-mosaicism' in congenital methemoglobinaemia. *New England Journal of Medicine*, **275**, 397.

124 HAIDAS S., LABIE D. & KAPLAN J.C. (1971) 2,3 Diphosphoglycerate content and oxygen affinity as a function of red-cell age in normal individuals. *Blood*, **38**, 463.

125 DANON D. & MARIKOVSKY Y. (1964) Determination of density distribution of red-cell population. *Journal of Laboratory and Clinical Medicine*, **64**, 668.

126 PIOMELLI S., LURINSKY G. & WASSERMAN L.R. (1967) Relationship between cell age and specific gravity evaluated by ultracentrifugation in a discontinuous density gradient. *Journal of Laboratory and Clinical Medicine*, **69**, 659.

127 HOFFMAN J.F. (1958) On the relationship of certain erythrocyte characteristics to their physiological age. *Journal of Cellular Physiology*, **51**, 415.

128 LA CELLE P.L. & ARKIN B. (1970) Acquired rigidity: a possible determinant of normal RBC life-span. *Blood*, **36**, 837.

129 MARKS P.A., JOHNSON A.B., HIRSHBERG E. & BANKS J. (1958) Studies on the mechanism of aging human red blood cells. *Annals of the New York Academy of Sciences*, **75**, 95.

130 GREENWALT T.J., LAU F.O., SWEENEY-HAMMOND K., MITTEN J. & CHO M.S. (1979) The role of microvesiculation in erythrocyte aging. *Proceedings of 32nd Annual Meeting of the American Association of Blood Banks*, p. 3.

131 HUGHES-JONES N.C. & CHENEY B. (1961) The use of ^{51}Cr and ^{59}Fe as red-cell labels to determine the fate of normal erythrocytes in the rat. *Clinical Science*, **20**, 323.

132 HUGHES-JONES N.C. (1961) The use of ^{51}Cr and ^{59}Fe as red-cell labels to determine the fate of normal erythrocytes in the rabbit. *Clinical Science*, **20**, 315.

133 MARTON P.F. (1975) Ultrastructural study of erythrophagocytosis in the rat bone marrow. *Scandinavian Journal of Haematology*, **23** (Suppl.).

134 TENHUNEN R., MARVER H.S. & SCHMID R. (1968) The enzymatic conversion of heme to bilirubin by microsomal heme oxygenase. *Proceedings of the National Academy of Sciences, USA*, **61**, 748.

135 LANDAW S.A., CALLAHAN E.W., JR & SCHMID R, (1970) Catabolism of heme *in vivo*: comparison of the simultaneous production of bilirubin and carbon monoxide. *Journal of Clinical Investigation*, **49**, 914.

136 TENHUNEN R., MARVER H.S. & SCHMID R. (1970) The enzymatic catabolism of hemoglobin stimulation of microsomal heme oxygenase by hemin. *Journal of Laboratory and Clinical Medicine*, **75**, 410.

137 LESTER R. & TROXLER R.F. (1969) Recent advances in bile pigment metabolism. *Gastroenterology*, **56**, 143.

138 CARNOT P. & DEFLANDRE G. (1906) Sur l'activité hémopoïétique du sérum au cours de la régénération du sang. *Compte Rendu de l'Académie des Sciences, Paris*, **143**, 384.

139 CARNOT P. & DEFLANDRE C. (1906) Sur l'activité hemopoïétique des différents organes au cours de la régénération du sang. *Compte Rendu de l'Académie des Sciences, Paris*, **143**, 432.

140 REISSMANN K.R. (1950) Studies on the mechanisms of erythropoietic stimulation in parabiotic rats during hypoxia. *Blood*, **5**, 372.

141 STOHLMAN F., JR, RATH C.E. & ROSE J.C. (1954) Evidence for a humoral regulation of erythropoiesis. Studies on a patient with polycythemia secondary to regional hypoxia. *Blood*, **9**, 721.

142 ERSLEV A.J. (1953) Humoral regulation of red-cell production. *Blood*, **8**, 349.

143 SCHOOLEY J.C. & MAHLMANN L.J. (1971) Inhibition of the biologic activity of erythropoietin by neuraminidase *in vivo*. *Journal of Laboratory and Clinical Medicine*, **78**, 765.

144 MIYAKE T., KUNG C.K.H. & GOLDWASSER E. (1977) Purification of human erythropoietin. *Journal of Biological Chemistry*, **252**, 5558.

145 COTES P.M. & BANGHAM D.R. (1966) An international reference preparation for bioassay of erythropoietin. *Bulletin of the World Health Organization*, **35**, 751.

146 ANNABLE L., COTES P.M. & MUSSETT M.V. (1972) The second international reference preparation of erythropoietin, human, urinary, for bioassay. *Bulletin of the World Health Organization*, **47**, 99.

147 COTES P.M. (1971) Measurement of erythropoietin. In: *Kidney Hormones* (ed. Fisher J.W.), p. 243. Academic Press, London and New York.

148 FRIED W., PLZAK L.F., JACOBSON L.O. & GOLDWASSER E. (1957) Studies on erythropoietin. III. Factors controlling erythropoietin production. *Proceedings of the Society of Experimental Biology and Medicine*, **94**, 237.

149 JACOBSON L.O., GOLDWASSER E. & GURNEY C.W. (1960) Transfusion-induced polycythaemia as a model for studying factors influencing erythropoiesis. In: *Ciba Foundation Symposium on Haemopoiesis* (ed. Wolstenholme G.E.W. & O'Connor M.), p. 423. Churchill, London.

150 COTES P.M. & BANGHAM D.R. (1961) Bio-assay of erythropoietin in mice made polycythaemic by exposure to air at a reduced pressure. *Nature (London)*, **191**, 1065.

151 KRANTZ S.B., GALLIEN-LARTIGUE O. & GOLDWASSER E. (1963) The effect of erythropoietin on heme synthesis by marrow cells *in vitro*. *Journal of Biological Chemistry*, **238**, 4085.

152 DUNN C.D.R., JARVIS J.H. & GREENMAN J.M. (1975) A quantitative bioassay for erythropoietin using mouse fetal liver cells. *Experimental Hematology*, **3**, 65.

153 NAPIER J.A.F., DUNN C.D.R., FORD T.W. & PRICE V. (1977) Pathophysiological change in serum erythropoiesis stimulating activity. *British Journal of Haematology*, **35**, 403.

154 GOUDSMIT R., KRUGERS DAGNEAUX P.G.L.C. & KRIJNEN H.W. (1967) Een immunochemische bepaling van erythropoietine. *Folia Medica Neerlandica*, **10**, 39.

155 LANGE R.D., MCDONALD T.P., JORDAN T.A., MITCHELL T.J. & KETCHMAR A.L. (1971) The haemagglutination inhibition assay for erythropoietin. *Israel Journal of Medical Science*, **7**, 861.

156 JORDAN T.A., POTTER T.P. & ESSARY B.H. (1975) Erythropoietin assay by haemagglutination inhibition. *American Journal of Medical Technology*, **41**, 146.

157 FISHER J.W., ROH B.L., MALGOR L.A., SAMUELS A.I., THOMPSON J., NOVECK R. & ESPADA J. (1971) Chemical agents which stimulate erythropoietin production. In: *Kidney Hormones* (ed. Fisher J.W.), p. 343. Academic Press, London and New York.

158 COTES P.M. (1973) Erythropoietin. In: *Peptide Hormones* (ed. Berson S.A. & Yalow R.S.), p. 1110. North-Holland Publishing Company, Amsterdam.

159 LERTORA J.J., DARGON P.A., REGE A.B. & FISHER J.W. (1975) Studies on a radioimmunoassay for human erythropoietin. *Journal of Laboratory and Clinical Medicine*, **86**, 140.

160 SHERWOOD J.B. & GOLDWASSER E. (1979) A radioimmunoassay for erythropoietin. *Blood*, **54**, 885.

161 GARCIA J.F., SHERWOOD J. & GOLDWASSER E. (1979) Radioimmunoassay of erythropoietin. *Blood Cells*, **5**, 405.

162 JACOBSON L.O., GOLDWASSER E., FRIED W. & PLZAK L.

(1957) Role of kidneys in erythropoiesis. *Nature (London)*, **179**, 633.

163 KURATOWSKA Z., LEWARTOWSKI B. & MICHALAK E. (1961) Studies on the production of erythropoietin by isolated perfused organs. *Blood*, **18**, 527.

164 REISSMANN K.R. & NOMURA T. (1962) Erythropoietin formation in isolated kidneys and liver. In: *Erythropoiesis* (ed. Jacobson L.O. & Doyle M.), p. 71. Grune & Stratton, New York and London.

165 ZANGHERI E.O., CAMPANA H., PONCE F., SILVA J.C. FERNANDEZ F.O. & SUAREZ F.R. (1963) Production of erythropoietin by anoxic perfusion of the isolated kidney of a dog. *Nature (London)*, **199**, 572.

166 FISHER J.W. & LANGSTON J.W. (1968) Effects of testosterone, cobalt and hypoxia on erythropoietin production in the isolated perfused dog kidney. *Annals of the New York Academy of Sciences*, **149**, 75.

167 KURATOWSKA Z. & LEWARTOWSKI B. (1962) Studies on the active principle released by the hypoxic kidney into Tyrode's solution. In: *Erythropoiesis* (ed. Jacobson L.O. & Doyle M.), p. 101. Grune & Stratton, New York and London.

168 KURATOWSKA Z., LEWARTWOSKI B. & LIPIŃSKI B. (1964) Chemical and biologic properties of an erythropoietin-generating substance obtained from perfusates of isolated anoxic kidneys. *Journal of Laboratory and Clinical Medicine*, **64**, 226.

169 CONTRERA J.F. & GORDON A.S. (1966) Erythropoietin: production by a particulate fraction of rat kidney. *Science*, **152**, 653.

170 CONTRERA J.F., GORDON A.S. & WIENTRAUB A.H. (1966) Extraction of an erythropoietin-producing factor from a particulate fraction of rat kidney. *Blood*, **28**, 330.

171 GORDON A.S. & ZANJANI E.D. (1971) Studies on the renal erythropoietic factor (REF). In: *Kidney Hormones* (ed. Fisher J.W.), p. 295. Academic Press, London and New York.

172 PESCHLE C., MAGLI M.C., CILLO F., LETTIERI F., PIZZELLA F., MIGLIACCIO G., SORICELLI A., SCALA G., MASTROBERARDINO G. & SASSO G.F. (1978) Recent advances in erythropoiesis physiology. In: In Vitro *Aspects of Erythropoiesis* (ed. Murphy M.J., Jr), p. 227. Springer-Verlag, New York.

173 MCDONALD T.P., ZANJANI E.D., LANGE R.D. & GORDON A.S. (1971) Immunological studies of the renal erythropoietic factor (erythrogenin). *British Journal of Haematology*, **20**, 113.

174 PESCHLE C. & CONDORELLI M. (1975) Biogenesis of erythropoietin: evidence for proerythropoietin in a subcellular fraction of kidney. *Science*, **190**, 910.

175 FISHER J.W., TAYLOR G. & PORTEOUS D.D. (1965) Localization of erythropoietin in glomeruli of sheep kidney by the fluorescent antibody technique. *Nature (London)*, **205**, 611.

176 FRENKEL E.P., SUKI W. & BAUM J. (1968) Some observations on the localization of erythropoietin. *Annals of the New York Academy of Sciences*, **149**, 292.

177 BUSUTTIL R.W., ROH B.L. & FISHER J.W. (1971) The cytological localization of erythropoietin in the human kidney using the fluorescent antibody technique. *Proceedings of the Society for Experimental Biology and Medicine*, **137**, 327.

178 BUSUTTIL R.W., ROH B.L. & FISHER J.W. (1972) Localization of erythropoietin in the glomerulus of the hypoxic dog kidney using a fluorescent antibody technique. *Acta Haematologica*, **47**, 238.

179 GRUBER D.F., ZUCALI J.R., WLEKLINSKI J., LA RUSSA V. & MIRAND E.A. (1977) Temporal transition in the site of rat erythropoietin production. *Experimental Hematology*, **5**, 399.

180 KATZ R., COOPER G.W., GORDON A.S. & ZANJANI E.D. (1968) Studies on the site of production of erythropoietin. *Annals of the New York Academy of Sciences*, **149**, 120.

181 MIRAND E.A. & PRENTICE T.C. (1957) Presence of plasma erythropoietin in hypoxic rats with or without kidney(s) and/or spleen. *Proceedings of the Society for Experimental Biology and Medicine*, **96**, 49.

182 MIRAND E.A., STEVENS R.A., GROENEWALD J.H., VAN ZYL J.J.W. & MURPHY G.P. (1969) Extra-renal erythropoietin production in the baboon. *Proceedings of the Society for Experimental Biology and Medicine*, **130**, 685.

183 NATHAN D.G., SCHUPACK E., STOHLMAN F., JR & MERRILL J.P. (1964) Erythropoiesis in anephric man. *Journal of Clinical Investigation*, **43**, 2158.

184 ERSLEV A.J., MCKENNA P.J., CAPELLI J.P., HAMBURGER R.J., COHN H.E. & CLARKE J.E. (1968) Rate of red-cell production in two nephrectomized patients. *Archives of Internal Medicine*, **22**, 230.

185 NAETS J.P. & WITTEK M. (1968) Presence of erythropoietin in the plasma of one anephric patient. *Blood*, **31**, 249.

186 FRIED W., KILBRIDGE T., KRANTZ S., MCDONALD T.P. & LANGE R.D. (1969) Studies on extra-renal erythropoietin. *Journal of Laboratory and Clinical Medicine*, **73**, 244.

187 SCHOOLEY J.C. & MAHLMANN L.J. (1972) Evidence for the *de novo* synthesis of erythropoietin in hypoxic rats. *Blood*, **40**, 662.

188 SCHOOLEY J.C. & MAHLMANN L.J. (1972) Erythropoietin production in the anephric rat. I. Relationship between nephrectomy, time of hypoxic exposure, and erythropoietin production. *Blood*, **39**, 31.

189 FRIED W. (1972) The liver as a source of extra-renal erythropoietin production. *Blood*, **40**, 671.

190 PESCHLE C., D'AVANZO A., RAPPAPORT I.A., RUSSO-LILLO S., MARONE G. & CONDORELLI M. (1973) Role of erythrogenin from liver and spleen in erythropoietin production in the anephric rat. *Nature (London)*, **243**, 539.

191 KAPLAN S.M., ROTHMANN S.A., GORDON A.S., RAPPAPORT I.A., CAMIOCOLI J.F. & PESCHLE C. (1973) Extra-renal sites of erythrogenin production. *Proceedings of the Society for Experimental Biology and Medicine*, **143**, 310.

192 PESCHLE C., MARONE G., GENOVESE A., MAGLI C. & CONDORELLI M. (1976) Hepatic erythropoietin: Enhanced production in anephric rats with hyperplasia of Kupffer cells. *British Journal of Haematology*, **32**, 105.

193 MIRAND E.A. & MURPHY G.P. (1971) Erythropoietin alterations in human liver disease. *New York State Journal of Medicine*, **71**, 860.

194 ZANJANI E.D., PETERSON E.N., GORDON A.S. & WASSERMAN L.R. (1974) Erythropoietin production in the

fetus: role of the kidney and maternal anemia. *Journal of Laboratory and Clinical Medicine*, **83**, 281.

195 CARMENA A.O., HOWARD D. & STOHLMAN F., JR (1968) Regulation of erythropoiesis. XXII. Erythropoietin production in the newborn animal. *Blood*, **32**, 376.

196 SCHOOLEY J.C. & MAHLMANN L.J. (1974) Extrarenal erythropoietin production by the liver in the weanling rat. *Proceedings of the Society for Experimental Biology and Medicine*, **145**, 1081.

197 ZUCALI J.R., STEVENS V. & MIRAND E.A. (1975) *In vitro* production of erythropoietin by mouse fetal liver. *Blood*, **46**, 85.

198 ZUCALI J.R., McGARRY M.P. & MIRAND E.A. (1977) Stimulation of erythropoiesis in a grafted animal by mouse fetal liver culture media. *Experimental Haematology*, **5**, 103.

199 CONGOTE L.F. (1977) Regulation of fetal liver erythropoiesis. *Journal of Steroid Biochemistry*, **8**, 423.

200 MILLER M., RORTH M., PARVING H.H., HOWARD D., REDDINGTON I., VALERI C.R. & STOHLMAN F., JR (1973) pH effect on erythropoietin response to hypoxia. *New England Journal of Medicine*, **288**, 706.

201 MILLER M.E., HOWARD D., STOHLMAN F., JR & FLANAGAN P. (1974) Mechanism of erythropoietin production by cobaltous chloride. *Blood*, **44**, 339.

202 MILLER M.E., RORTH M., STOHLMAN F., JR, VALERI C.R., LOWRIE G. & HOWARD D. (1976) Mechanism of erythropoietin production after acute haemorrhage in the rat. *British Journal of Haematology*, **33**, 379.

203 MILLER M.E. & HOWARD D. (1979) Modulation of erythropoietin concentrations by manipulation of hypercarbia. *Blood Cells*, **5**, 389.

204 PERRETTA M. & TIRAPEUGI C. (1968) Effect of erythropoietin on nucleic acid metabolism from polycythaemic rat bone marrow. *Experientia*, **24**, 680.

205 ORLIC D., GORDON A.S. & RHODIN J.A.G. (1968) Ultrastructural and autoradiographic studies of erythropoietin-induced red-cell production. *Annals of the New York Academy of Sciences*, **149**, 198.

206 KRANTZ S.B. & GOLDWASSER E. (1965) On the mechanism of erythropoietin-induced differentiation. II. The effect on RNA synthesis. *Biochimica et Biophysica Acta*, **103**, 325.

207 GROSS M. & GOLDWASSER E. (1969) On the mechanism of erythropoietin-induced differentiation. V. Characterization of the ribonucleic acid formed as a result of erythropoietin action. *Biochemistry*, **8**, 1795.

208 PAVLOV A.D. (1969) Molecular aspects of action of endogenous erythropoietin. The effects of erythropoietic stimuli on synthesis of ribonucleic acids in rabbit bone marrow. *Biochimica et Biophysica Acta*, **195**, 156.

209 BOTTOMLY S.S. & SMITHEE G.A. (1969) Effect of erythropoietin on bone-marrow δ-amino-levulinic acid synthetase and heme synthetase. *Journal of Laboratory and Clinical Medicine*, **74**, 445.

210 DUKES P.P. (1968) *In vitro* studies on DNA synthesis of bone-marrow cells stimulated by erythropoietin. *Annals of the New York Academy of Sciences*, **149**, 437.

211 HRINDA M.E. & GOLDWASSER E. (1969) On the mechanism of erythropoietin-induced differentiation. VI. Induced accumulation of iron by marrow cells. *Biochimica et Biophysica Acta*, **195**, 165.

212 PEETS E.A. & GORDON A.S. (1968) Effects of erythropoietin on glucose utilization by bone-marrow cells. *Life Sciences*, **7**, 561.

213 DUKES P.P., TAKAKU F. & GOLDWASSER E. (1963) *In vitro* studies on the effect of erythropoietin on glucosamine-1-^{14}C incorporation into rat bone-marrow cells. *Endocrinology*, **74**, 960.

214 JACOBSON L.O., GOLDWASSER E., PLZAK L.F. & FRIED W. (1957) Studies on erythropoiesis. IV. Reticulocyte response of hypophysectomized and polycythaemic rodents to erythropoietin. *Proceedings of the Society for Experimental Biology and Medicine*, **94**, 243.

215 ALPEN E.L. & CRANMORE D. (1959) Observations on the regulation of erythropoiesis and on cellular dynamics by Fe^{59} autoradiography. In: *The Kinetics of Cellular Proliferation* (ed. Stohlman F., Jr), p. 290. Grune & Stratton, New York.

216 FILMANOWICZ E. & GURNEY C.W. (1961) Studies on erythropoiesis. XVI. Response to a single dose of erythropoietin in polycythaemic mouse. *Journal of Laboratory and Clinical Medicine*, **57**, 65.

217 ERSLEV A.J. (1964) Erythropoietin *in vitro*. II. Effect on 'stem cells'. *Blood*, **24**, 331.

218 UDUPA K.B. & REISSMANN K.R. (1979) *In vivo* erythropoietin requirements of regenerating erythroid progenitors (BFU-e, CFU-e) in bone marrow of mice. *Blood*, **53**, 1164.

219 HANNA I.R.A. (1968) An early response of the morphologically recognisable erythroid precursors to bleeding. *Journal of Cell and Tissue Kinetics*, **1**, 91.

220 HANNA I.R.A., TARBUTT R.G. & LAMERTON L.F. (1969) Shortening of the cell-cycle time of erythroid precursors in response to anaemia. *British Journal of Haematology*, **16**, 381.

221 TARBUTT R.G. (1969) Cell population kinetics of the erythroid system in the rat: the response to protracted anaemia and to continuous γ-irradiation. *British Journal of Haematology*, **16**, 9.

222 HILLMAN R.S. (1969) Characteristics of marrow production and reticulocyte maturation in normal man in response to anemia. *Journal of Clinical Investigation*, **48**, 443.

223 GIBLETT E.R., COLEMAN D.H., PIRZIO-BIROLI G., DONOHUE D.M., MOTULSKY A.G. & FINCH C.A. (1956) Erythrokinetics: quantitative measurements of red-cell production and destruction in normal subjects and patients with anemia. *Blood*, **11**, 291.

224 BRECHER G. & STOHLMAN F., JR (1962) The macrocytic response to erythropoietic stimulation. In: *Erythropoiesis* (ed. Jacobson L.O. & Doyle M.), p. 216. Grune & Stratton, New York and London.

225 BRECHER G. & STOHLMAN F., JR (1961) Reticulocyte size and erythropoietic stimulation. *Proceedings of the Society for Experimental Biology and Medicine*, **107**, 887.

226 STOHLMAN F., JR, BRECHER G. & MOORES R.R. (1962) Humoral regulation of erythropoiesis. VIII. The kinetics of red-cell production and the effect of erythropoietin. In: *Erythropoiesis* (ed. Jacobson L.O. & Doyle M.), p. 162. Grune & Stratton, New York and London.

227 STRYCKMANS P.A., CRONKITE E.P., GIACOMELL G., SCHIFFER L. & SCHNAPAUFF H. (1968) The maturation and fate of reticulocytes after *in vitro* labelling with tritiated amino acids. *Blood*, **31**, 33.

228 CRAFTS R.C. & MEINEKE H.A. (1959) The anemia of hypophysectomized animals. *Annals of the New York Academy of Sciences*, **77**, 501.

229 FEIGIN W.M. & GORDON A.S. (1950) Influence of hypophysectomy on the hemopoietic response of rats to lowered barometric pressures. *Endocrinology*, **47**, 364.

230 VAN DYKE D.C., CONTOPULOS A.N., WILLIAMS B.S., SIMPSON M.E., LAWRENCE J.H. & EVANS H.M. (1954) Hormonal factors influencing erythropoiesis. *Acta Haematologica*, **11**, 203.

231 PILIERO S.J. (1959) Influence of hypoxic stimuli upon blood formation in endocrine-deficient animals. *Annals of the New York Academy of Sciences*, **77**, 518.

232 GORDON A.S. (1957) Influence of humoral factors on erythropoiesis. *American Journal of Clinical Nutrition*, **5**, 461.

233 FRIED W. & GURNEY C.W. (1968) The erythropoietic-stimulating effects of androgens. *Annals of the New York Academy of Sciences*, **149**, 356.

234 MEINEKE H.A. & CRAFTS R.C. 1968) Further observations on the mechanism by which androgens and growth hormone influence erythropoiesis. *Annals of the New York Academy of Sciences*, **149**, 298.

235 GORDON A.S., MIRAND E.A., WENIG J., KATZ R. & ZANJANI E.D. (1968) Androgen actions on erythropoiesis. *Annals of the New York Academy of Sciences*, **149**, 318.

236 PESCHLE C., ZANJANI E.D., GIDARI A.S., McLAURIN W.D. & GORDON A.S. (1971) Mechanism of thyroxine action on erythropoiesis. *Endocrinology*, **89**, 609.

237 PESCHLE C., RAPPAPORT I.A., SASSO G.F., GORDON A.S. & CONDORELLI M. (1972) Mechanism of growth hormone (GH) action of erythropoiesis. *Endocrinology*, **91**, 511.

238 BYRON J.W. (1970) Effect of steroids on the cycling of haemopoietic stem cells. *Nature (London)*, **228**, 1204.

239 BYRON J.W. (1972) Comparison of the action of ^{3}H-thymidine and hydroxyurea on testosterone-treated hemopoietic stem cells. *Blood*, **40**, 198.

240 GORSHEIN D., HAIT W.N., BESSA E.C., JEPSON J.H. & GARDNER F.H. (1974) Rapid stem-cell differentiation induced by 19-nortestosterone decanoate. *British Journal of Haematology*, **26**, 215.

241 PESCHLE C., MAGLI M.C. CILLO C., LETTIERI F., PIZZELLA F., GENOVESE A. & SORICELLI A. (1977) Enhanced erythroid burst formation in mice after testosterone treatment. *Life Sciences*, **21**, 773.

242 SINGER J.W. & ADAMSON J.W. (1976) Steroids and hematopoiesis. III. The response of granulocytic and erythroid colony-forming cells to steroids of different classes. *Blood*, **48**, 855.

243 COHEN P. & GARDNER F.H. (1965) Effect of massive triamcinolone administration in blunting the erythropoietic response to phenylhydrazine hemolysis. *Journal of Laboratory and Clinical Medicine*, **65**, 88.

244 GLADER B.E., RAMBACH W.A. & ALT H.L. (1968) Observations on the effect of testosterone and hydrocortisone on erythropoiesis. *Annals of the New York Academy of Sciences*, **149**, 383.

245 MALGOR L.A., TORELES P.R., KLAINER E., BARRIOS L. & BLANC. C.C. (1974) Effects of dexamethasone on bonemarrow erythropoiesis. *Hormone Research* (Basel), **5**, 269.

246 GOLDE D.W., BERSCH N. & CLINE M.J. (1976) Potentiation of erythropoiesis *in vitro* by dexamethasone. *Journal of Clinical Investigation*, **57**, 57.

247 JEPSON J.H. & LOWENSTEIN L. (1965) Erythropoiesis during pregnancy and lactation. I. Effect of various hormones on erythropoiesis during lactation. *Proceedings of the Society for Experimental Biology and Medicine*, **120**, 500.

248 JEPSON J. & LOWENSTEIN L. (1966) Erythropoiesis during pregnancy and lactation in the mouse. II. Role of erythropoietin. *Proceedings of the Society for Experimental Biology and Medicine*, **121**, 1077.

249 PESCHLE C., RAPPAPORT I.A., SASSO G.F., CONDORELLI M. & GORDON A.S. (1973) The role of estrogen in the regulation of erythropoietin production. *Endocrinology*, **92**, 358.

250 PESCHLE C., MAGLI M.C., CILLO C., LETTIERI F., CACCIAPUOTI A., PIZZELLA F. & MARONE G. (1977) Erythroid colony formation and erythropoietin activity in mice treated with estradiol benzoate. *Life Sciences*, **21**, 1303.

251 JEPSON J. & LOWNSTEIN L. (1966) Inhibition of the stem-cell action of erythropoietin by estradiol. *Proceedings of the Society for Experimental Biology and Medicine*, **123**, 457.

252 JEPSON J. & LOWENSTEIN L. (1967) Inhibition of the stem-cell action of erythropoietin by estradiol valerate and the protective effect of 17α-hydroxy-progesterone caproate and testosterone propionate. *Endocrinology*, **80**, 430.

253 FRIED W., TICHLER T., DENNENBERG I., BARONE J. & WANG F. (1974) Effects of estrogens on hematopoietic stem cells and on hematopoiesis of mice. *Journal of Laboratory and Clinical Medicine*, **83**, 807.

254 GARDNER W.U. & PFEIFFER L.A. (1943) Influence of estrogens and androgens on the skeletal system. *Physiological Reviews*, **23**, 139.

255 KIVILAAKSO E. & RYTÖMAA T. (1970) The effect of polycythaemic serum on the proliferation of rat bonemarrow cells *in vitro*. *Journal of Cell and Tissue Kinetics*, **3**, 385.

256 KIVILAAKSO E. & RYTÖMAA T. (1971) Erythrocyte chalone, a tissue-specific inhibitor of cell proliferation in the erythron. *Journal of Cell and Tissue Kinetics*, **4**, 1.

257 BATEMAN A.E. (1974) Cell specificity of chalone-type inhibitors of DNA synthesis released by blood leucocytes and erythrocytes. *Journal of Cell and Tissue Kinetics*, **7**, 451.

258 LORD B.I., CERCEK L., CERCEK B., SHAH G.P., DEXTER T.M. & LAJTHA L.G. (1974) Inhibitors of haemopoietic cell proliferation?: specificity of action within the haemopoietic system. *British Journal of Cancer*, **29**, 168.

259 LORD B.I., SHAH G.P. & LAJTHA L.G. (1977) The effects of red blood cell extracts on the proliferation of erythrocyte precursor cells, *in vivo*. *Journal of Cell and Tissue Kinetics*, **10**, 215.

260 REYNAFARJE C., RAMOS J., FAURA J. & VILLAVICENCIO D. (1964) Humoral control of erythropoietic activity in man during and after altitude exposure. *Proceedings of the Society for Experimental Biology and Medicine*, **116**, 649.

261 REYNAFARJE C. (1968) Humoral regulation of the erythropoietic depression of high altitude polycythemic

subjects after return to sea level. *Annals of the New York Academy of Sciences*, **149**, 472.

262 NEMEC J. & POLAK H. (1964) Erythropoietic polyploidy. I. The morphology of polyploid erythroid elements and their incidence in healthy subjects. *Folia Haematologica, Internationales Magazin für Klinische und Morphologische Blutforschung* (Leipzig), **84**, 24.

263 WIMBER D.E. & QUASTLER H. (1963) A ^{14}C- and ^{3}H-thymidine double labelling technique in the study of cell proliferation in tradescantia root tips. *Experimental Cell Research*, **30**, 8.

264 KESSE-ELIAS M., HARRISS E.B. & GYFTAKI E. (1967) *In vitro* study of DNA-synthesis time and cell cycle-time in erythrocyte precursors of normal and thalassaemic subjects, using a ^{3}H- and ^{14}C-thymidine double labelling technique. *Acta Haematologica*, **38**, 170.

265 KLEIN H.O., LENNARTZ K.J., EDER M. & GROSS R. (1970) *In vitro* verfahren zur autoradiographischen Bestimmung der Zellkinetik der Erythroblasten bei Tier und Mensch. *Histochemie*, **21**, 369.

266 DÖRMER P. (1973) Kinetics of erythropoietic cell proliferation in normal and anemic man. A new approach using quantitative ^{14}C-autoradiography. *Progress in Histochemistry and Cytochemistry* (Stuttgart), **6**, 1.

267 WICKRAMASINGHE S.N. & GOUDSMIT R. (1979) Some aspects of the biology of multinucleate and giant mononucleate erythroblasts in a patient with CDA, type III. *British Journal of Haematology*, **41**, 485.

268 HILLMAN R.S. & FINCH C.A. (1967) Erythropoiesis: normal and abnormal. *Seminars in Hematology*, **4**, 327.

269 HILLMAN R.S. & FINCH C.A. (1969) The misused reticulocyte. *British Journal of Haematology*, **17**, 313.

270 SUIT H.D. (1957) A technique for estimating the bone-marrow cellularity *in vivo* using ^{59}Fe. *Journal of Clinical Pathology*, **10**, 267.

271 DONOHUE D.M., GABRIO B.W. & FINCH C.A. (1958) Quantitative measurement of hematopoietic cells of the marrow. *Journal of Clinical Investigation*, **37**, 1564.

272 SKÅRBERG K.O. (1974) Cellularity and cell proliferation rates in human bone marrow. I. An *in vivo* method to estimate the total marrow cellularity in man. *Acta Medica Scandinavica*, **195**, 291.

273 WHITE P., COBURN R.F., WILLIAMS W.J., GOLDWEIN M.I., ROTHER M.L. & SHAFER B.C. (1967) Carbon monoxide production associated with ineffective erythropoiesis. *Journal of Clinical Investigation*, **46**, 1986.

274 BERK P.D., RODKEY F.L., BLASHCKE T.F., COLLISON H.A. & WAGGONER J.G. (1974) Comparison of plasma bilirubin turnover and carbon monoxide production in man. *Journal of Laboratory and Clinical Medicine*, **83**, 29.

275 GLASER K., LIMARZI L.R. & PONCHER H.G. (1950) Cellular composition of the bone marrow in normal infants and children. *Paediatrics*, **6**, 789.

276 LONDON I.M., WEST R., SHEMIN D. & RITTENBERG D. (1950) On the origin of bile pigment in normal man. *Journal of Biological Chemistry*, **184**, 351.

277 GRAY C.H., NEUBERGER A. & SNEATH P.H.A. (1950) Studies in congenital porphyria. II. Incorporation of ^{15}N in the stercobilin in the normal and in the porphyric. *Biochemical Journal*, **47**, 87.

278 ISRAELS L.G., YAMAMOTO T., SKANDERBEG J. & ZIPURSKY A. (1963) Shunt bilirubin: evidence for two components. *Science*, **139**, 1054.

279 YAMAMOTO T., SKANDERBEG J., ZIPURSKY A. & ISRAELS L.G. (1965) The early appearing bilirubin: evidence for two components. *Journal of Clinical Investigation*, **44**, 31.

280 SAMSON D., HALLIDAY D., NICHOLSON D.C. & CHANARIN I. (1976) Quantitation of ineffective erythropoiesis from the incorporation of [^{15}N]δ-aminolaevulinic acid and [^{15}N]glycine into early-labelled bilirubin. II. Anaemic patients. *British Journal of Haematology*, **34**, 45.

281 SZUR L. & LEWIS S.M. (1975) Iron kinetics in polycythaemia vera and myelofibrosis. *Clinics in Haematology*, **4**, 407.

282 CHADHURI T.K., EHRHART J.C., DEGOWIN R.L. & CHRISTIE J.H. (1974) ^{59}Fe whole body scanning. *Journal of Nuclear Medicine*, **15**, 667.

283 ANGER H.O. & VAN DYKE D. (1964) Human bone-marrow distribution shown *in vivo* by iron-52 and the positron scintillation camera. *Science*, **144**, 1587.

284 MCINTYRE P.A., LARSON S.M., EIKMAN E.A., COLEMAN M., SHEFFER U. & HODKINSON B. (1974) Comparison of the metabolism of iron-labelled transferrin and indium-labelled transferrin by the erythropoietic marrow. *Journal of Nuclear Medicine*, **15**, 856.

285 MERRICK M.V., GORDON-SMITH E.C., LAVENDER J.P. & SZUR L. (1975) A comparison of ^{111}In with ^{52}Fe and ^{99}Tc^{m} sulphur colloid for bone-marrow scanning. *Journal of Nuclear Medicine*, **16**, 66.

286 PETTIT J.E., LEWIS S.M., WILLIAMS E.D., GRAFTON C.A., BOWRING C.S. & GLASS H.I. (1976) Quantitative studies of splenic erythropoiesis in polycythaemia vera and myelofibrosis. *British Journal of Haematology*, **34**, 465.

287 WORLD HEALTH ORGANIZATION (1968) *Nutritional Anaemias*. Technical Report Series No. 405, Geneva.

288 NATVIG H., VELLAR O.D. & ANDERSON J. (1967) Studies on haemoglobin values in Norway. VII. Haemoglobin, haematocrit and MCHC values among boys and girls aged 7–20 years in elementary and grammar schools. *Acta Medica Scandinavica*, **182**, 183.

289 NATVIG H. & VELLAR O.D. (1967) Studies on haemoglobin values in Norway. VIII. Haemoglobin, haemotocrit and MCHC values in adult men and women. *Acta Medica Scandinavica*, **182**, 193.

290 MEDICAL RESEARCH COUNCIL (1945) *Haemoglobin levels in Great Britain in 1943*. Special Report Series No. 252. H.M.S.O., London.

291 KILPATRICK G.S. & HARDISTY R.M. (1961) The prevalence of anaemia in the community. A survey of a random sample of the population. *British Medical Journal*, **i**, 778.

292 PITNEY W.R. (1971) Anaemia in the tropics. In: *Recent Advances in Haematology* (ed. Goldberg A. & Brain M.C.), p. 337. Churchill Livingstone, London.

293 MCGREGOR I.A., GILLES H.M., WALKERS J.H., DAVIES A.H. & PEARSON F.A. (1956) Effects of heavy and repeated malarial infections on Gambian infants and children. *British Medical Journal*, **ii**, 686.

294 HILLMAN R.S. & FINCH C.A. (1974) *Red Cell Manual*, 4th edn. F. A. Davies Company, Philadelphia.

295 Erslev A.J. (1972) General effects of anemia. In: *Hematology* (ed. Williams W.J., Beutler E., Erslev A.J. & Rundles R.W.) 2nd edn, p. 251. McGraw-Hill, New York.

296 Oski F.A., Gottlieb A.J., Miller W.W. & Delivoria-Papadopoulos M. (1970) The effects of deoxygenation of adult and fetal hemoglobin on the synthesis of red cell 2,3 diphosphoglycerates and its *in vivo* consequences. *Journal of Clinical Investigation*, **49**, 400.

297 Varat M.A., Adolph R.J. & Fowler N.O. (1972) Cardiovascular effects of anemia. *American Heart Journal*, **83**, 415.

298 Sharpey-Schafer E.P. (1944) Cardiac output in severe anaemia. *Clinical Science*, **5**, 125.

299 Duke M. & Abelmann W.H. (1969) The hemodynamic response to chronic anemia. *Circulation*, **39**, 503.

300 Sproule B.J., Mitchell J.H. & Miller W.F. (1960) Cardiopulmonary physiologic responses to heavy exercise in patients with anemia. *Journal of Clinical Investigation*, **39**, 378.

301 Hillman R.S. (1969) Characteristics of marrow production and reticulocyte maturation in normal man in response to anemia. *Journal of Clinical Investigation*, **48**, 443.

302 Cooper R.A. & Shattil S.J. (1971) Mechanisms of hemolysis—the minimal red-cell defect. *New England Journal of Medicine*, **285**, 1514.

303 Javid J. (1967) Human serum haptoglobins. *Seminars in Hematology*, **4**, 35.

304 Müller-Eberhard U. & English E.C. (1967) Purification and partial characterization of human hemopexin. *Journal of Laboratory and Clinical Medicine*, **70**, 619.

305 Bunn H.F. & Jandl J. (1969) Renal excretion of hemoglobin. *Journal of Experimental Medicine*, **129**, 925.

306 Harris J.W. & Kellermeyer R.W. (1978) Red cell destruction and the hemolytic disorders. In: *The Red Cell—Production, Metabolism, Destruction: Normal and Abnormal*. Revised edn. Harvard University Press, Cambridge.

Chapter 5
Iron metabolism, iron deficiency and overload

A. JACOBS AND M. WORWOOD

The importance of iron in human metabolism is its central role in erythropoiesis and in many intracellular redox reactions. Its study has been stimulated by the common occurrence of iron deficiency and, more recently, by increasing interest in iron overload.

CHEMISTRY

Iron is one of the group of transition metals which share two important properties—the ability both to exist in several oxidation states and to form stable complexes. It is these properties which have made the transition elements important components of electron- and oxygen-carrying proteins. The most common valency states for iron are Fe^{2+} and Fe^{3+}. In acid solution these ions can exist as the free ion surrounded by six molecules of water, but neutralization of such solutions results in progressive hydrolysis with eventual precipitation of ferric hydroxide. If the water molecules are replaced by appropriate ligands a stable complex can be formed which is soluble at neutral pH. Both Fe^{2+} and Fe^{3+} generally form octahedral complexes in which the central metal ion is surrounded by six ligands. The biological chemistry of iron is the chemistry of these complexes. Although many sugars, amino-acids and nucleotides will form complexes with iron almost all the iron in the body is found in very specific protein complexes.

Oxygen- and electron-transport proteins
Table 5.1 lists the more important known iron compounds in the body, many of which are associated with oxygen transport both in the blood and in the tissues. In the haemoproteins, of which haemoglobin is the most abundant, iron is present in haem with two additional ligands, one above and one below the flat tetrapyrrole ring. In haemoglobin one of these ligands is histidine in the protein chain and in oxyhaemoglobin oxygen acts as the other. Haemoglobin iron is in the ferrous state and oxidation to the ferric state to form methaemoglobin prevents oxygen binding. The oxygen-carrying property of haem is found only in haemoglobin and myoglobin and is absent when it is complexed with other proteins. The haemoglobin molecule consists of four haem groups linked to four polypeptide chains and it can bind four molecules of oxygen (see also Chapter 8). It has MW 64 500. Myoglobin has MW 17 000 and consists of a single polypeptide chain with one haem group. It has a higher affinity for oxygen than haemoglobin and behaves as an oxygen store in muscle cells. When oxygen supply is limited it is released to cytochrome oxidase which has a higher affinity for oxygen than myoglobin.

Mitochondria contain a system for the transport of electrons from intracellular substrates to molecular oxygen with the simultaneous generation of ATP. This pathway contains a number of iron compounds, including the cytochromes, which transmit electrons by means of reversible valency changes of their iron atoms. Failure of this system due to lack of oxygen supply to the tissues, enzyme depletion or blocking with metabolic inhibitors such as cyanide, leads to defective energy production and an accumulation of intermediate metabolites with eventual cell death. One of the most closely studied cytochromes, cytochrome c, has MW 12 500 and contains a single haem group together with an associated polypeptide chain. The free binding sites of its haem iron are linked to histidine and methionine and the haem complex is placed deeply within the molecule. These characteristics prevent cytochrome c from binding free oxygen while allowing the iron atom to alternate between the ferric and ferrous states. Cytochrome P_{450} occurs in endoplasmic reticulum and in adrenal mitochondria. It takes part in hydroxylation reactions associated with drug detoxication and sterol synthesis. Iron sulphur proteins also take part in electron transport (Table 5.1). They contain 'non-haem' iron which is covalently bound to acid-labile sulphide or cysteinyl sulphur [2].

The iron content of the body
Table 5.2 shows the approximate amount of iron present in different forms in the body. It is difficult to obtain accurate estimates, particularly of tissue enzymes, and few direct measurements of total body

Table 5.1. Some mammalian iron-containing proteins (taken from Ref. 1, with permission)

Protein	Mol. wt	No. of Fe atoms per molecule	Distribution	Function
Haem containing				
Haemoglobin	65 000	4 protohaem	Red blood cells	O_2 carrier
Myoglobin	17 000	1 protohaem	Muscle	O_2 carrier
Cytochrome aa_3	180 000*	2 haem a	Mitochondria	Terminal oxidase
b	18 000–30 000*	1 protohaem	Mitochondria	Electron transport
c_1	37 000*	1 haem c	Mitochondria	Electron transport
c	12 000	1 haem c	Mitochondria	Electron transport
b_5	12 000	1 protohaem	Endoplasmic reticulum	Electron transport
P_{450}		protohaem	Endoplasmic reticulum	Steroid, drug, hydroxylation
Catalase	240 000	4 protohaem	Red blood cells, peroxisomes	Peroxide breakdown
Lactoperoxidase	93 000	1 protohaem	Milk	Peroxide breakdown
Tryptophan pyrrolase	—	haem dependent	Liver cytosol	L-tryptophan→formylkynurenine
Non-haem				
Aconitase	66 000	2 Fe 3 S	Pig heart†	Citric acid cycle
(Phenylalanine hydroxylase)	100 000	2 Fe	Rat liver†	Phenylalanine→tryosine
Adrenodoxin	12 500	2 Fe 2 S	Adrenal mitochondria	Steroid hydroxylation
(Complex III Fe-S protein)	30 000	2 Fe 2 S	Mitochondria	Electron transport
(Succinate dehydrogenase Fe-S protein)	27 000	2 Fe 2 S	Mitochondria	Electron transport
(Succinate dehydrogenase flavoprotein)	70 000	4 Fe 4 S 1 FAD	Mitochondria	Electron transport
NADH dehydrogenase		23–28 (Fe + S) FMN	Mitochondria	Electron transport
Xanthine oxidase	275 000	8 Fe 8 S 2 FAD 2 Mo	Milk†, tissue	Hypoxanthine→uric acid
Transferrin	77 000	2	Plasma	Iron transport
Lactoferrin	77 000	2	Milk, secretions	Iron transport
Ferritin	450 000–900 000 000	0–4000	All tissues	Iron storage
Haemosiderin		Up to 37% Fe (dry wt.)	Liver, spleen, bone marrow	Iron storage

A number of iron-dependent enzymes or processes have not been included.
* Soluble preparations of membrane-bound cytochromes.
† Enzyme isolated from this source. Found in other tissues.

Table 5.2. Distribution of iron in the body of a 70 kg man* (taken from Ref. 3, with permission)

Protein	Tissue	Fe concentration (µg/g wet tissue unless stated otherwise)	Total iron (mg)	Basis of calculation of total iron	Ref.
Haemoglobin	Red blood cells	0·52 µg/ml blood	2600	15 g haemoglobin/dl blood. Blood volume = 5000 ml	456
Myoglobin	Muscle	See ref.	400	Myoglobin content of various muscles	
Mitochondrial cytochromes	All tissues	See ref.	17	Calculated from the cytochrome c content of the human body [457] and ratios of cytochrome aa_3, b and c_1 to cytochrome c in rat tissues [458]	459
'Microsomal' cytochromes (b_5 and P_{450})	Liver	1·2–2·4	2–4	Assuming equal concentration of cytochromes b_5 and P_{450}	457
Catalase	Liver and red blood cells		5		457
Transferrin	Plasma and extravascular fluid	1 µg/ml plasma	8	231 mg transferrin/kg body weight. 30% saturated with iron	16
Non-haem iron (including ferritin haemosiderin)	Liver	230	410	Liver weight 1800 g	460
	Spleen	240	48	Spleen weight 200 g	460
	Kidney	35	11	Kidney weight 310 g	460
	Skeletal muscle	26	730	Muscle weight 28 000 g	461
	Bone marrow	2·7 µg/mg marrow protein	300	Marrow weight 1200 g	243
	Brain	10–210	60		462

* Obviously this table is incomplete (particularly for tissues such as the intestines). In muscle the low iron content and high weight may result in an inaccurate total iron content. The amounts of storage iron in the tissues measured chemically are considerably higher than the total amount of 'mobilizable iron' [260]. This suggests that not all tissue storage iron is readily available for haemoglobin synthesis.

iron have been published [4]. Many subjects have much less storage iron than is indicated by these calculations.

Storage iron

All the cells of the body require iron for the synthesis of metabolically active compounds. Cells also have the ability to store excess iron. There are two forms of storage iron: the soluble form known as ferritin, and insoluble haemosiderin. Ferritin is a well-defined molecule consisting of a protein shell which encloses an iron core. Haemosiderin appears to be a degraded form of ferritin in which the protein shells have partly disintegrated allowing the iron cores to aggregate [5]. Haemosiderin deposits are readily seen with the aid of the light microscope as areas of Prussian-blue staining when tissue sections are stained with potassium ferrocyanide in the presence of acid. Normally, much of the body's store of iron is present as ferritin but with increasing iron deposition in the tissues the proportion present as haemosiderin increases [5].

Ferritin is found in all cells and in particularly high concentrations in liver, spleen and bone marrow. The protein was first crystallized from horse spleen by Laufberger in 1937. The apoprotein has MW 450 000 and is composed of 24 identical subunits each with MW 18 500. The latter form a nearly spherical shell which encloses a central core containing up to 4500 atoms of iron in the form of ferric hydroxyphosphate (for a review of the structure of ferritin see Harrison *et al.* [6]). Much of the amino-acid sequence is known [7] and X-ray crystallographic analysis at 2·8 Å resolution has demonstrated the arrangement of the subunits within the molecule, channels between the subunits and their quaternary structures [8] (Fig. 5.1).

Ferritin, like many other proteins, shows considerable heterogeneity of size and charge. Purified preparations may contain about 10% of the protein in the form of dimers, trimers, etc. Polymerization seems to be at least partly dependent on concentration [9] but its biological significance is unknown. Apoferritins from horse, rat, man and various plants differ in amino-acid composition [7]. There are also differences in isoelectric point: ferritins from horse heart, liver and spleen having lower isoelectric points than the corresponding rat or human ferritins. On isoelectric focusing ferritin from any tissue shows heterogeneity. Thus, human liver and spleen ferritins have a range of 'isoferritins' with isoelectric points between 5·3 and 5·8; heart contains isoferritins in the range 4·8–5·2 and kidney has isoferritins with intermediate pI [10]. Drysdale and colleagues [11, 12] have proposed that this heterogeneity is seen because ferritin molecules are made up of varying proportions of two types of subunit: an H subunit which predominates in the acidic isoferritins and has MW 21 000 and an L

subunit which predominates in liver ferritin and has MW 19 000. This explanation is not yet universally accepted [13]. Changes in the isoelectric focusing pattern of human ferritins have been described in tissues from patients with iron overload and cancer [11] with preferential accumulation of more basic isoferritins in response to excess iron and accumulation of more acidic isoferritins in tumours.

In vitro, ferritin shows all the properties required of an iron storage protein (for a review see [14]). Apoferritin takes up Fe^{2+}, oxidizes it and deposits Fe^{3+} within the iron core. Initially, oxidation takes place at catalytic sites on the inner surface of the protein but the surface area of the iron core is also an important factor controlling rates of iron uptake and release. Release of iron is effected by reducing agents including sodium dithionite and thioglycollic acid; $FMNH_2$* and $FADH_2$† are particularly effective and may have physiological significance. Studies in animals and cultured cells show that apoferritin is synthesized in response to iron administration [15]. The process may involve an increase in the proportion of the total mRNA available for protein synthesis or an increase in the proportion of subunits converted to apoferritin.

Transferrin

Iron in the plasma is almost entirely bound to transferrin (Fig. 5.2) which is a β globulin of MW 80 000 containing six per cent carbohydrate [16]. Transferrin has two binding sites each able to bind one atom of FeIII. The iron-transferrin complex has a characteristic salmon-pink colour with an absorption maximum at 470 nm. At pH 7·0 the affinity of transferrin for iron is very high but there is 50% dissociation at pH 4·8 which is complete at about pH 4·5. The plasma concentration of transferrin is normally about 2·4 g/l and each mg of transferrin can bind 1·45 μg iron. As the iron-binding sites are usually about 30% saturated a total of 3 mg iron is found in the plasma.

Serum transferrins have been purified from many species and each consists of a single polypeptide chain. Much of the amino-acid sequence of human transferrin has been determined [17]. There are 676 residues and comparison of the C- and N-terminal halves of the molecule has revealed strong internal homology with approximately 40% of the amino acids in corresponding positions being identical. MacGillivray *et al.* [17] suggest that transferrin may have evolved from a precursor with a single metal binding site. The carbohydrate is present in the form of two identical and nearly symmetrical branched heterosaccharide chains

---

* Reduced form of flavin mononucleotide.
† Reduced form of flavin adenine dinucleotide.

(a)

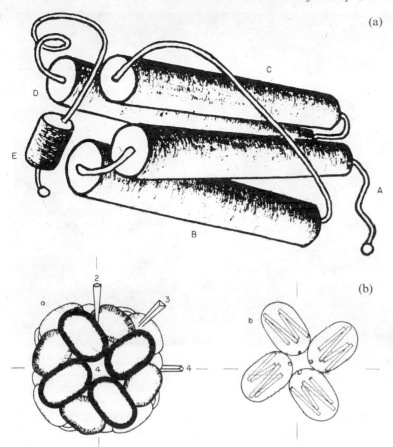

(b)

Fig. 5.1. (a) Schematic drawing of an apoferritin subunit. The subunit contains four nearly parallel helices 34–42 Å long and a short helix, E, at right angles to these. Non-helical segments connecting the helices are indicated. (b) Schematic drawings of the subunit arrangement in an apoferritin molecule viewed down a fourfold axis. a, Complete molecule showing some of its symmetry axes. b, Subunits related by a fourfold axis. (From Ref. 8 with permission.)

each ending with N-acetyl-neuraminic acid [18]. Both chains are present in the C-terminal region of the protein linked to asparagine residues 415 and 608 [17].

One iron-binding site is on the C-terminal protein of the molecule and one on the N-terminal protein. Tyrosyl-hydroxyl, imidazole nitrogen and water provide the six iron-chelating ligands at the binding sites. In addition an anion, usually HCO_3^-, is bound along with iron [19]. In the absence of the anion, strong binding of iron does not take place. Other metals also bind specifically (i.e. in the same way as iron): Cu(II), Cr(III), Co(III), Ga(III) and Mn(III). Many other metals also bind to transferrin but may not satisfy the conditions for specific binding [19].

There has been much experimentation and speculation about differences between the iron-binding sites of transferrin particularly since the hypothesis put forward by Fletcher & Huehns in 1968 [20] about differences between the two sites in delivering iron to cells. The earliest studies of iron-binding by transferrins suggested that the apparent formation constant

for the binding of the first Fe(III) ion was much smaller than that for the binding of the second Fe(III) ion [21]. This implies that two iron atoms would bind to the protein so that solutions of transferrin would contain only apotransferrin and diferric transferrin. However, the existence of monoferric transferrins rules out this model [22]. Later studies suggested that the formation constants are similar [23] and until recently it was accepted that the iron-binding sites are equivalent and independent and that there is random binding of iron to each site [19]. However, in the last five years much evidence has accumulated which indicates that there are differences in the binding of iron at the two sites [19]. It has also become possible to study the occupancy of the two sites directly by using the urea electrophoresis technique of Makey & Seal [24] which separates the four species of transferrin: apotransferrin, Fe_C transferrin, Fe_N transferrin and diferric transferrin (C and N refer to the C- and N-terminal halves of the protein). Formation constants for the various Fe-transferrin species have been calculated by Aisen *et*

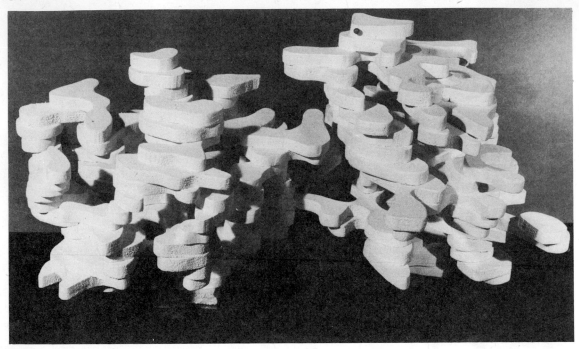

Fig. 5.2. A view of a balsa wood model demonstrating bilobal structure of human transferrin at 6 Å. (From Ref. 472 with permission.)

al. [25]. They are of the order of 10^{20} mol^{-1} under physiological conditions of pH and PCO$_2$. The distribution of iron between the two sites is dependent on the form of iron presented to the protein [25, 26]. In serum there appears to be preferential binding to the N-terminal site [27].

Although chemical and physical differences between the binding sites have been clearly demonstrated, functional differences in the delivery of iron to red cells have not been confirmed, Harris & Aisen [28] found that the iron-binding sites of human transferrin were equivalent in their ability to donate iron to human reticulocytes, that rabbit transferrin sites were equivalent with rabbit cells but that differences were seen when human transferrin was incubated with rabbit reticulocytes. Awai *et al.* [29] found differences in the uptake of radioiron from the two sites of transferrin after injection of labelled transferrin into the intact rat but later studies from the same group indicated that these results were caused by differences between the two isotransferrins of rat plasma [30]. The story is further complicated by the large number of genetically controlled variants of transferrin in human and animal populations [31]. All the variants appeared to function in an equivalent way [32] but now that differences between the binding sites are more clearly appreciated

it is necessary to re-examine functional differences between the iron-binding sites and differences between transferrin variants.

Transferrin synthesis occurs mainly in the liver in adult animals although synthesis has been demonstrated in many tissues [16]. The protein is synthesized on ribosomes of the rough endoplasmic reticulum with attachment of carbohydrate during passage through the smooth endoplasmic reticulum and Golgi vesicles before secretion into the plasma. Distribution and turnover studies have been reviewed by Morgan [16]. In normal subjects the fractional catabolic rate for transferrin is about 0·16 plasma pools/day. No single tissue appears to predominate in the degradation of transferrin.

The transferrin family of single-chain, two-sited metal-binding glycoproteins also includes the iron-binding protein of egg-white, *conalbumin* or *ovotransferrin* and the iron-binding protein of milk which is known as *lactoferrin* or *lactotransferrin* (for a discussion of nomenclature and relationships between these proteins see Ref. 19).

Lactoferrin is found in neutrophils and in other secretions [33, 34] as well as in milk. It has similar iron-binding properties to transferrin but the formation constant for the monoferric–lactoferrin complex is greater than that for monoferric–transferrin [35]. There is little immunological cross-reaction between the two proteins [36]. The function of lactoferrin is uncertain but it may have a bacteriostatic activity because of its affinity for iron [33] and its activity as a regulator of myelopoiesis is under investigation [465]. Plasma levels may be assayed by radioimmunoassay [37, 38].

IRON BALANCE

The iron content of the body is normally kept constant by a delicate balance between the amount absorbed and the amount lost. Iron losses from the body are limited and there is no physiological mechanism for regulating the excretion of excess amounts [39]. This is a reflection of the ease with which iron forms intracellular complexes and the absence of free or loosely bound iron in the body. The factors determining balance are complex and relate to the subject, the diet and the environment [40].

Attempts have been made to measure total iron losses by administering a radioactive tracer and observing its rate of disappearance. Finch [41] injected ^{55}Fe intravenously and followed blood levels for several years. After the first year, when the isotope became gradually distributed throughout slowly exchangeable pools, the blood level showed an exponential decrease which was assumed to reflect total body iron loss. These data suggested a daily iron loss of 0·6 mg in men and non-menstruating women and 1·2 mg in menstruating women, and concord with other estimates [42] using ^{59}Fe and measuring total losses by whole body counting. A further application of the ^{55}Fe method to four groups of males living in different parts of the world showed a remarkable consistency of results in those with a normal body load despite differences of race and climatic conditions [43]. In South African Bantu the mean iron loss was 2·2 mg daily compared with 0·9–1·0 mg daily in the other three groups. This is probably related to the increased iron load in these subjects, with a consequent increase in iron content of exfoliating cells and macrophages, particularly from the gut. Iron loss from the skin was probably over-estimated in this study [44] and the gastro-intestinal tract appears to be the major site of iron loss in normal males, about 0·3–0·4 mg being derived from blood loss, 0·25 mg from biliary excretion and 0·1 mg from exfoliated epithelial cells [43]. Urinary iron losses are less than 0·1 mg daily [45].

In menstruating women there is a variable blood loss. Hallberg *et al.* [46] found a mean menstrual loss of 43·4 ml, equivalent to about 0·7 mg iron daily, but more than 10% of women had losses in excess of 80 ml, equivalent to over 1·4 mg daily, and therefore a mean daily total iron loss in excess of 2·3 mg. Menstrual loss in excess of 80 ml is commonly associated with iron deficiency. The factors influencing menstrual loss are not fully understood but the concordance of measurements in monozygotic compared to dizygotic twins suggests some genetic control. There is a relationship between endometrial plasminogen activator and menstrual loss and it has been suggested that fibrinolytic activity may be the basis for genetic regulation of menstrual loss [47]. Women suffering from iron-deficiency anaemia are usually found to have a loss greater than normal and iron deficiency itself has been implicated as a cause of menorrhagia [48]. A more probable explanation of the association is that increased losses lead to iron deficiency. The production of iron-deficiency anaemia by repeated phlebotomy does not cause menorrhagia and treatment of anaemic subjects with iron results in an increase of blood loss rather than a decrease [49, 50].

Iron requirements are determined by the total losses from the body and if these can be assessed then nutritional needs should be a simple matter of replacement. However, while it is possible to calculate the amount of iron that needs to be absorbed, the availability of iron in different foods varies and this together with differences in intraluminal reactions and the absorptive capacity of the intestinal mucosa makes it difficult to determine the amount of food iron required. It is generally assumed that under normal conditions about five to 10% of the dietary iron is absorbed [51] and if the average iron content of the British diet is 13·5 mg daily [52] then it should not be difficult for a man with normal iron losses to maintain himself in positive balance. When iron losses are minimal then a dietary iron absorption of less than 10% may be adequate. The iron requirements of normal menstruating women may be in excess of 2 mg daily and in this case the amount and availability of food iron must be such that a compensatory increase on the level of intestinal absorption will allow iron balance to be maintained. The average dietary intake in the UK is lower in those families with children and decreases as the number of children increases, suggesting a more remote effect of pregnancy on iron balance. The iron absorption mechanism is extremely sensitive to changes in iron status, even in healthy non-anaemic subjects, and it seems likely that the majority of people in the population can adapt to different iron intakes by regulation of absorption. A study of normal women revealed no difference in haemoglobin or serum iron concentrations in subjects with dietary iron intakes varying from 6 to 28 mg daily [53]. Anaemia was found only in menstruating women and was not related to dietary intake. Beaton *et al.* [54] suggest that it is possible to compensate for normal menstrual iron losses when dietary intake is about 11 mg daily and in normal women haemoglobin levels are only significantly reduced in those with a menstrual loss in excess of 80 ml [46].

Direct measurements of iron absorption in normal adults, using foods labelled biologically with radio-active iron, have shown considerable differences in availability [51] with a mean absorption of about 10%, and measurements in children using milk, eggs and liver as the sources of iron also showed a mean value of about 10% [55]. The mean absorption from bread milled from wheat grown with radioactive iron has been estimated at about 4·5% in normal subjects and 7·8% in those with iron deficiency [56]. Layrisse *et al.* [57] carried out studies on a number of foods and found a low absorption of 1·7–7·9% from wheat, corn, black beans, lettuce and spinach. Higher absorptions of 15·6–20·3% were found from soya beans, fish, veal and haemoglobin. Not only does the absorption of iron from different foods vary but there is a variable increase in absorption occurring as a response to anaemia [51, 56].

Interaction between foods is an important source of variation in iron absorption. Absorption is impaired by egg [58] and potentiated by orange juice [59] or alcohol [60]. This interaction is well demonstrated by the inhibition of iron absorption from veal in the presence of corn or beans, while iron in corn or beans is better absorbed when given together with either veal or fish [61]. The stimulating effect of fish on iron absorption from black beans appears to be due to the presence of cysteine in the digestive products of fish [62].

If the mean absorption of food iron is taken to have an upper value of 20% in normal subjects [63], then an adequate iron supply in the diet can be calculated from data on iron losses. This ignores wide variations in the iron content of the same food obtained from different sources and calculations are made even more difficult by the disparity between values given in published tables and those found by analysis [64–66]. However, various recommendations on dietary iron requirements have been made. The FAO/WHO group recommend different iron intakes depending on the proportion of the diet consisting of animal food (Table 5.3), but it should be remembered that a diet with enough iron to prevent iron deficiency entirely would contain excess iron for many and it could be argued that supplementation for vulnerable groups is more logical than food fortification [40]. Many countries have adopted enrichment of flour as a national policy in an attempt to maintain the level of intake. Criticisms of these policies have been based on the apparent ineffectiveness of present methods for the fortification of foods [66] and the possible dangers of iron overload [67, 68].

Pregnancy

There are a number of physiological situations in which iron requirements are in excess of those indicated and a negative iron balance can give rise to latent or clinical iron deficiency. The demands of pregnancy and lactation are particularly great. When adequate iron is available the red-cell mass may increase by about 30% [69, 70] taking up an additional 500 mg of iron as haemoglobin. In addition about 250–300 mg of iron is transferred across the placenta to the fetus.

Table 5.3. Recommended daily intake of iron [63]

	Daily iron absorption required	Daily dietary intake required according to diet		
		Calories derived from animal food (% of total calorie intake)		
		<10%	10–25%	>25%
	mg	mg	mg	mg
Infants 0–4 months	0·5	*	*	*
Infants 5–12 months	1·0	10	7	5
Children 1–12 years	1·0	10	7	5
Boys 13–16 years	1·8	18	12	9
Girls 13–16 years	2·4	24	18	12
Menstruating women	2·8	28	19	14
Men and non-menstruating women	0·9	9	6	5

*Breast milk assumed adequate.

During delivery and the puerperium blood loss of 500 ml or more [71], together with placental iron, may account for an additional drain of about 300 mg iron. The net iron requirements are somewhat reduced as the expanded red-cell mass returns to normal after delivery but the total cost is about 500 mg. Iron requirements during pregnancy cannot be easily calculated as many non-pregnant women have little or no reserve iron and may already be overtly iron deficient. Supplementation with medicinal iron is necessary to ensure adequate iron status and 30 mg of elemental iron given daily in the form of ferrous fumarate is effective in maintaining haemoglobin levels throughout pregnancy [72].

The transfer of iron from the mother to the fetus takes place almost entirely during the last trimester of pregnancy, and prematurity results in a shortening of this transfer period. The total amount of iron in the newborn infant is closely related to birth weight [73]. Most of this iron is in the form of circulating haemoglobin, and late clamping of the cord after delivery can result in an increase of over 50% in this fraction [74]. A detailed study of the effects of iron supplementation during pregnancy on the haematological status of the infant in the first 18 months of life showed that in a well-nourished population there was little effect from either oral or parenteral iron [75]. The haemoglobin levels achieved in infancy were, however, higher than those in an under-privileged group, but in all cases the levels fell short of what appeared to be a physiological maximum. The administration of 250 mg parenteral iron to the infant at the age of nine months achieved complete elimination of anaemia by the age of 12 months and this effect persisted for at least six months longer. It was concluded from these results that the most important factor in the infant's iron economy that can be influenced by medical treatment is its post-natal iron intake. The administration of iron to the pregnant woman has relatively little influence on the infant's iron stores.

Infancy and childhood

Iron balance during growth is reviewed by Burman [76]. During the transition from infancy to adult life the total body iron content increases approximately from 300 to 4000 mg and if there was a uniform rate of growth this would mean a daily iron increment of 0·5 mg in addition to the normal replacement of physiological losses. In fact, there are considerable differences in iron metabolism and growth rate during this period which affect requirements. Sjölin & Wranne [77] have calculated the total body iron and the amount in the major body compartments during the first 12 years of life assuming no limitation of supply (Fig. 5.3). During the first six weeks of life there is a marked decrease in haemoglobin mass. Some of the iron from this source is probably utilized for myoglobin synthesis but most enters the storage pool and is reflected by the increase in liver iron content found at this time [78]. Injected iron is poorly utilized for haemoglobin synthesis during the first eight weeks of life but after this time erythropoiesis becomes more active [79].

When ^{55}Fe was administered to fetuses *in utero* there was no dilution of the labelled haemoglobin in the peripheral blood until after this time signifying that no absorption and utilization of exogenous iron had occurred [80]. Endogenous iron still accounted for 70% of body iron at the end of the first year and 40% at the end of the second year. While some authors have found only three per cent absorption of radioative ferrous iron in premature and full-term infants in the first three months of life [81], others have shown a higher level of iron absorption in infants below the age of three months than at any other age and there is some evidence that the level of absorption is related to growth rate and thus to iron requirements [82, 83]. The investigation of ferrous iron absorption in infancy by whole body counting shows that when normal amounts of stainable iron are present in the bone marrow the percentage absorption is comparable to normal replete adults in both premature and full-term infants [84]. In premature infants iron absorption increases at the age of about three months as iron deficiency develops, and later in the first year a similar phenomenon is seen in full-term infants. Iron requirements appear to be minute during the first four months of life but increase rapidly after that time, and a daily dietary intake of about 10 mg between eight and 12 months will produce an optimal haemoglobin concentration in most normal infants [85]. The mean absorption of food iron in infants appears to be similar to that in adults [56]. The American Academy of Pediatrics [86] has recommended a daily dietary intake of 1 mg/kg body weight for full-term infants and 2 mg/kg body weight for premature infants, with a maximum intake of 15 mg/day. Dietary requirements in the second year of life are probably about 5–7 mg daily provided that there is a good state of nutrition at the end of the first year [87].

Iron requirements are related to growth rate throughout childhood and adolescence and after the high incremental growth rate in the first year there is a subsequent decrease. A second growth spurt occurs in adolescence, particularly in males, when iron requirements rise above normal adult levels for a short period and iron deficiency is sometimes seen at this time [88, 89]. In the adolescent female iron requirements are increased by the menarche.

The foregoing considerations of iron balance apply largely to western populations, in which prevailing

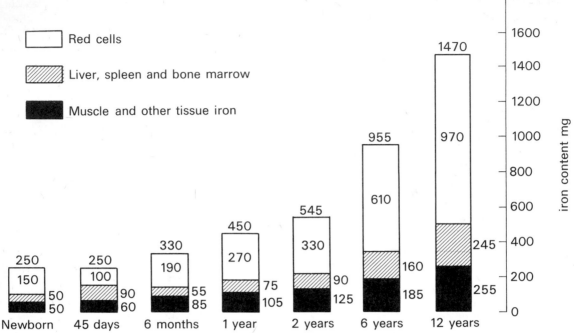

Fig. 5.3. Iron content of different body compartments during childhood (after Sjölin and Wranne [77]).

socio-economic conditions result in a moderately satisfactory nutritional status. In many tropical areas there is a greater probability of iron depletion. Though the quantity of meat eaten is often low, the prime cause of iron deficiency is excess iron loss due to hookworm infestation [90]. Many other factors, such as protein and riboflavin deficiency and infection, are important in the aetiology of tropical anaemia, but these are not considered here.

IRON ABSORPTION

There is insufficient space in this chapter to provide a review of the many experimental studies of iron absorption in the last 30 years. The various experimental animals and techniques employed have contributed to the many conflicting opinions about the nature and control of iron absorption. The reader is referred to a recent and detailed review of the topic [91] for further information. Physiological control over iron balance is normally maintained by the regulation of iron absorption. The intestinal epithelium is extremely sensitive to the iron requirements of the body and can reject unwanted dietary iron or absorb increased amounts when stores are low. Much of the intensive work carried out on the absorption mechanism is related to

the behaviour of simple iron salts. When absorption from increasing doses of inorganic iron is measured in man, the amount of iron absorbed increases although the percentage of the dose absorbed decreases [92]. The absorption of inorganic iron is highest when given alone in the fasting state and is reduced by food in proportion to the size of the meal [93].

Although data obtained with simple iron salts are relevant to normal physiological processes, dietary iron does not always behave in the same way. Food iron is released into the gastric juice either as the Fe^{2+} and Fe^{3+} ions or as a haem complex and the intra-luminal behaviour of these is different. The amount of food iron available for absorption depends on its release during the digestive process and its interactions in the gastro-intestinal lumen. Less than half the total amount of iron in food is released by peptic digestion and, except in the case of meat, this is largely in the form of ionizable iron. The amount released is considerably reduced in subjects with gastric atrophy [94].

The fate of released iron depends largely on its chemical reactions within the gut lumen. Ferric ions undergo increasing polymerization as the pH rises towards neutrality, eventually forming a ferric hydroxide precipitate. Ferrous ions do not undergo such marked polymerization and their solubility is greater than ferric ions at any given pH, which accounts at least partly for their greater availability. The unpolymerized ions of both types found at pH 1–2 are chemically reactive and when the gastric contents pass into the jejunum and neutralization occurs, they combine with ligands present in solution to form complexes which may or may not be available for absorption. Both phytate and phosphate limit iron absorption through the formation of insoluble complexes, but this can be overcome by an increased level of either iron or calcium [95, 96]. The inhibitory effect of natural phytate is less than that of pure sodium phytate. The stimulating effect of ascorbic acid on iron absorption is partly related to the fact that it reduces iron to the more soluble ferrous form and partly to the formation of soluble iron-ascorbate chelates [94]. Fructose also forms iron chelates which remain soluble at an alkaline pH and may pass across the epithelial cell membrane. Food iron absorption may be reduced by orally administered desferrioxamine [97]; the extent of the reduction probably depends on the amount released in the ferric form.

Abnormal components of the diet may sometimes remove iron from solution and thus make it unavailable. In patients with pica, clay eating may result in the formation of insoluble complexes in the gut and animal experiments suggest that aluminium hydroxide, calcium carbonate and magnesium trisilicate have a similar effect [98, 99]. The simultaneous administration of iron salts and tetracycline results in a gross impairment of absorption of both substances, probably due to the formation of unavailable iron chelates in the gut lumen [100, 101]. Tea is a potent inhibitor of iron absorption [102] but has not been implicated as a cause of iron deficiency.

Effect of gastric juice

There has been much conflicting evidence regarding the effect of gastric juice on iron absorption but there seems little doubt that hydrochloric acid itself plays an important part. Patients with iron-deficiency anaemia and normal acid secretion absorb more ferric iron from a test dose than those with a histamine-fast achlorhydria [103]. Iron absorption in subjects with complete achlorhydria is greater when the dose is administered with 0·05M hydrochloric acid than with water [104]. This effect is greater for ferric than for ferrous iron but haemoglobin iron is not affected. A low gastric pH ensures that inorganic iron remains available for binding with potential receptors in the stomach to produce complexes that can remain soluble at the neutral pH in the gut lumen.

A number of workers in the past have suggested that gastric secretions contain specific factors responsible for promoting or inhibiting absorption by the small intestine but these hypotheses have not received general support [105]. More recently it has been suggested that both transferrin [106] and lactoferrin [107] are involved in the uptake of iron by gut mucosal cells. Under normal circumstances most of ionizable iron released from the food in the stomach probably either binds to the mucoprotein in the gastric secretions or becomes unavailable on neutralization. Only in exceptional circumstances, when large amounts of a potential chelating agent such as ascorbic acid or citric acid are ingested, do other low-molecular-weight complexes form [105]. The iron–mucoprotein complex behaves as an intraluminal carrier system enabling non-haem iron to reach the absorbing epithelium in a soluble state, though it is not absorbed in this form.

In the presence of chelating agents such as cysteine or ascorbic acid, iron is detached from its mucoprotein carrier to form a low-molecular-weight iron complex and similar complex-formation also occurs with other amino acids [94]. Examination of the jejunal contents during the two hours following ingestion of a normal meal shows that iron first appearing in the lumen is in the form of a higher-molecular-weight complex, but the amount of iron complexed to small molecules gradually increases until, two hours after the meal, this comprises 30–40% of the total ionizable iron present [108]. Sugars and amino acids which could act as iron chelators are also formed in the brush border of the absorbing intestinal cells and the high local concentrations between the microvilli give optimal conditions for chelation and absorption. Carrier proteins secreted by the epithelial cells would also be available for iron binding at this site.

There is no clear evidence that pancreatic secretions have any direct effect on iron absorption [109]. Their importance is indirect. The digestion of polypeptides by pancreatic enzymes results in the appearance of amino acids and dipeptides in the upper jejunum. The absorption of pure haemin iron is relatively poor unless protein-degradation products are also present to prevent polymerization of the haem complex [110], possibly by complex formation.

Uptake and transport of iron by the intestinal epithelial cells

Iron is absorbed primarily in the duodenum and upper jejunum. It is generally accepted that transfer of iron across the intestinal mucosal cell is a two-stage process involving rapid uptake of iron by the cell and subsequent transfer of some of this iron to the plasma. Early studies indicated that both steps were dependent on oxidative metabolism [111–113] but that the second stage was rate-limiting [113]. Small doses of iron seemed to be absorbed by a carrier-mediated process but, for larger doses, the mechanism appeared to be simple diffusion [114]. More recently, the availability of isolated epithelial cells, brush-border membrane preparations and the measurement of initial uptake rates has made it possible to examine the first stage uptake of iron by the cell. Some studies have shown that uptake of iron is by passive diffusion and that changes in the iron status of the animal have no effect on the rate of iron uptake [115, 116]. Other investigators have found the opposite. Acheson & Schultz [117] found that iron deficiency caused increased uptake by small-intestinal segments. Greenberger *et al.* [118] and Kimber *et al.* [119] found that alteration in the iron stores of rats changed the amount of iron taken up by isolated brush borders.

The stages between iron uptake at the brush border and transfer across the serosal membrane are difficult to define. Before considering the behaviour of absorbed radioactive iron in the cell it is necessary to examine the subcellular distribution of iron within the epithelial cell. In iron-replete and iron-loaded animals Richmond *et al.* [120] found that the highest concentration of iron was in the mitochondrial fraction but there was a substantial proportion of the cellular iron in the so-called soluble fraction (i.e. iron not associated with membranes). In homogenates of epithelial cells prepared from iron-deficient rats the iron content was much lower and iron was concentrated in the membrane fractions, particularly the mitochondrial fraction. The process of iron transport across the epithelial cell is very rapid and it is likely that little of the radioactive iron seen in a cell homogenate after administering radioiron to the gut lumen will be iron in transit across the cell. Much of the radioiron will have interacted with the mucosal cell and been taken up by organelles such as the mitchondria or incorporated into ferritin.

Subcellular fractionation of rat small-intestinal mucosa within one hour of giving small doses of iron labelled with ^{59}Fe showed that the mucosal radioactivity was largely present in the soluble fraction [121, 122]. In iron-replete rats it was mostly bound to ferritin but, in rats kept on an iron-deficient diet, there was less 'soluble' iron and most of this was associated with a transferrin-like protein [123–125]. This differs from plasma transferrin immunologically, in isoelectric point and in amino-acid composition [126]. Huebers *et al.* [123] have proposed that this protein is an intracellular iron carrier on the absorption pathway. Electron-microscopic autoradiography in mouse and rat tissues has demonstrated the uptake of labelled iron at the brush border with concentration of label in cytoplasm rich in rough endoplasmic reticulum and free ribosomes during the early, rapid phase of iron absorption [127–129]. This is compatible with the incorporation of absorbed iron into soluble protein. Neither subcellular fractionation nor electron-microscope studies have suggested that mitchondria play a role in transfer of iron across the epithelial cell, but recently Hopkins & Peters [130] have described significant and rapid uptake of absorbed iron by mitchondria in guinea-pig intestinal cells. These authors did not comment on iron content of the cell or the subcellular distribution of endogenous iron.

Iron transfer across the serosal surface of the intestinal epithelial cell is also extremely difficult to study in isolation. Nevertheless, a number of authors have suggested that this is a carrier-mediated active transport process, inhibited by other metals such as cobalt and manganese [131] and is the site in the epithelial cell at which iron absorption is controlled. Serosal transfer includes delivery of iron to transferrin in the plasma. Iron release from isolated epithelial cells is enhanced by addition of apotransferrin to the medium [132] but transferrin is not essential. Even in the absence of transferrin rapid transfer of iron from a duodenal loop to the perfusion medium is obtained [133].

An alternative mechanism has been proposed for iron transfer from intestinal lumen to the plasma which depends on the formation of low-molecular-weight iron chelates [134]. Their progress across the cell depends on their interaction with intracellular ligands or macromolecules. Most iron chelates appearing at the serosal surface of the epithelium are likely to react rapidly with transferrin because of its high binding constant, but in some cases, such as iron-EDTA, the reaction with transferrin is slow and some of the chelate is lost in the urine.

Uptake and transfer of haem iron

Most of the haem iron liberated from food enters the absorbing cells as the intact haem complex [135]. It takes rather longer to appear in the plasma than iron derived from non-haem sources and this lag is probably due to the release of iron within the cell by the enzyme haem oxygenase [136] (see also p. 168). Iron released from haem within the epithelial cells probably follows the same metabolic pathway as other forms of absorbed iron. Haem iron behaves as a stable chelate until it has entered the mucosa and its absorption is unaffected by many of the intraluminal factors which influence ionizable iron.

Control mechanisms

Some of the factors which influence iron absorption, such as the availability of dietary iron, have already been discussed. The amount of iron absorbed increases with the amount presented to the intestinal mucosa, but the percentage absorbed decreases with increasing quantities of haem and non-haem iron [135, 137].

The amount of iron absorbed is also closely related

to the iron requirements of the body (i.e. to body iron stores), but the regulatory mechanism between the iron stores and the intestinal epithelial cell remains hypothetical. It is possible that the major control mechanism lies in the intestinal mucosa itself. Crosby [138] has suggested that the iron status of the body primes the cell to allow passage of more or less iron according to the body's need. The mechanisms within the cell could be related to the rate of ferritin synthesis [138], the degree of saturation of a carrier [139], or the iron requirement of the cell for haem synthesis [140]. Measurements of the iron content of the whole gut wall confirmed the relationship between iron content of the gut and iron status [141, 142], but more recent studies have shown that there is no direct relationship between the iron content of the epithelial cell and iron absorption [120, 143, 144]. It is possible that changes in plasma iron turnover [142] as well as in plasma iron concentration control mucosal iron concentration and iron uptake.

Other possible control mechanisms involve the two different binding sites of transferrin [20] and unidentified humoral factors. Little evidence has been found for either of these. Cavill *et al.* [145] have suggested that the search for particular 'signals' or control mechanisms to explain the regulation of iron absorption is unnecessary and that serosal transfer of iron may be regarded simply as part of the equilibrium between plasma iron and 'exchangeable iron' in all tissues ('exchangeable iron' meaning iron available for binding by circulating transferrin). The total exchangeable iron in the body is related to the amount of storage iron; if the plasma iron turnover remains constant, any decrease in total exchangeable iron in the major storage organs will be compensated by increased transfer from the small intestine in order to maintain equilibrium. Increased plasma iron turnover leads to increased iron removal from all tissues, including the intestinal epithelium, and so causes increased iron absorption. In some haemolytic anaemias there may be iron accumulation in the reticulo-endothelial system, thus providing a counterbalance to the increased plasma iron turnover. The balance between these two factors will decide whether iron absorption is increased or not.

Anaemia or anoxia can stimulate a rise in iron absorption by at least two separate mechanisms. The first follows an increase in erythropoietin levels, which, experimentally, is followed by an increase in erythropoiesis accompanied by an increased iron turnover and a rise in iron absorption. When the marrow is destroyed before erythropoietin administration no increase in absorption occurs, suggesting that increased iron turnover rather than erythropoietin itself is the real stimulus to absorption [146]. The second

mechanism is not dependent on erythropoietin, as mice with marrow aplasia still respond to anoxia by increasing iron absorption, even though no erythropoietin response in the marrow can be elicited. In patients with aplastic anaemia iron absorption is higher when haemoglobin concentrations are low than when the haemoglobin concentrations are raised by transfusion [147, 148]. This is probably related to the suppression of erythropoesis (and therefore the reduction in plasma iron turnover) caused by transfusion [149].

IRON TRANSPORT

Iron is transported round the body by the plasma and extravascular fluids. Plasma iron has been studied rather more thoroughly than that of extravascular fluids. Although only about 4 mg of iron is present in the plasma at any one time the daily turnover is about 30 mg [150]. Most of the iron entering plasma is released from reticulo-endothelial cells following the breakdown of time-expired red cells. Smaller amounts enter the plasma pool from intestinal absorption, from the mobilization of storage compounds and from parenchymal iron pools.

The exchange of radioactive iodinated transferrin between plasma and the extravascular fluid has been demonstrated in man. When equilibrium has been established after four to six days, approximately equal amounts of transferrin are present in each compartment [151]. About 85% of ^{59}Fe tracer carried by transferrin is taken up by developing red-cell precursors and less than 15% by other tissues of the body [152], of which liver, muscle and skin are the most notable [153]. This process can be followed by a combination of plasma, whole-blood and surface counting after the intravenous injection of ^{59}Fe-labelled transferrin (Fig. 5.4). In normal subjects about 34% of the iron leaving the plasma pool refluxes from a non-fixed extravascular compartment [154] and is only incorporated in mature red cells after recycling. Transferrin is the major carrier of non-haem iron in plasma and most investigators have not found any evidence for the participation of other proteins, either in iron binding or transport [155]. It has been suggested, however, that citrate may bind small amounts of iron in plasma and that some binding to other protein fractions also occurs [156]. There may also be small amounts of circulating ferritin iron (see p. 169). There has recently been some interest in the presence of non-transferrin iron in the serum of patients with transfusional iron overload [151].

The range of iron concentration in plasma is normally quite wide with an average of about 125 μg/dl in men and 100 μg/dl in women [158]. A random

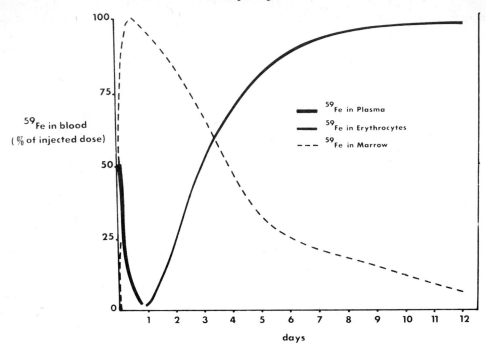

Fig. 5.4. Plasma, red-cell and marrow radioactivity following the intravenous injection of ^{59}Fe bound to transferrin.

sample of the Welsh population showed a mean value of 101 μg/dl in men and 90 μg/dl in women [159]. The sex difference in plasma iron concentration does not appear to be related to iron deficiency. It first makes its appearance at puberty when the plasma iron level rises in males but remains constant in females. The menstrual cycle has no effect on plasma iron levels in females and the sex difference is not decreased by six weeks of iron therapy [160]. The average plasma iron level at birth in infants studied by Sturgeon [161] was 193 μg/dl and this fell rapidly during the first few hours of life to about 50 μg/dl. It had risen to about 100 μg/dl by the end of the first week of life but had fallen to about 50 μg/dl at three to six months. By two years the mean value had risen to about 100 μg/dl, approaching adult values [161]. The plasma iron level tends to decrease with age in women but this may be related to iron deficiency [159]. There is normally a marked diurnal variation in plasma iron levels, the highest values being found in the morning and the lowest values in the latter half of the day [162, 163]. The diurnal variation in plasma iron appears to be due to variations in the release of iron from the reticulo-endothelial system [164].

The values for total iron-binding capacity found in normal adults vary between 300 and 400 μg/dl and this is usually about one-third saturated with iron. Levels were found to be slightly higher in women than in men in a randomly selected population [159], but this is probably related to the higher incidence of iron deficiency in women. The iron-binding capacity in infants at birth is within the normal adult range but it falls rapidly during the first day of life to about 50 μg/dl. It rises to about 200 μg/dl by the end of the first week of life [161]. At this time the transferrin saturation may be 100% but this gradually falls to the median level of about 25% found in childhood [466, 467].

Variations in the serum iron and total iron-binding capacity (TIBC)

Changes in serum iron and iron-binding capacity are found in a wide variety of disease states but its measurement for diagnostic purposes is of limited value because of unpredictable fluctuations *in vivo*. The serum iron concentration may be decreased, either because of iron deficiency or possibly because of impaired release of iron from the reticulo-endothelial system. This latter state is found in chronic inflammatory conditions and malignancy or, more transiently, following acute infections or surgery [165, 166]. Serum iron levels may be increased in a number of conditions. These may be associated with decreased erythropoiesis, as in aplastic anaemias or acute leukaemias;

haemolytic anaemia; ineffective erythropoiesis, as in pernicious anaemia; or a gross increase in the amount of iron in the body, as in haemochromatosis or transfusional overload.

The serum TIBC is usually low in acute and chronic infections and this may be due either to an increase in catabolism or a decrease in transferrin synthesis, but the rapid fall in transferrin level following the injection of endotoxin indicates that some other mechanism may also be involved [166]. Other general conditions associated with impaired protein synthesis or increased loss, such as kwashiorkor or the nephrotic syndrome, are also associated with low transferrin levels. The serum iron-binding capacity is frequently reduced in patients with iron overload, giving percentage saturations of 60–100%. An abnormally high TIBC is seen as a characteristic feature of iron deficiency, in many cases in the absence of anaemia. An increased level may also be found in pregnancy and in patients taking oral contraceptives [167]. The mechanism controlling the amount of iron-binding protein is not clear. In rats and rabbits increased plasma transferrin levels can be produced by hypoxia [168] but no such changes can be produced in human subjects [169]. In man there is an inverse relationship between storage iron and plasma TIBC and it has been suggested that the storage iron level may be the main factor controlling plasma TIBC [170]. Recent studies with rats have confirmed this [171]. In cases of congenital atransferrinaemia there is increased deposition of iron at extra-medullary sites but impaired uptake by developing erythroid cells. This results in a hypochromic microcytic anaemia with marked iron deposition and cirrhosis of the liver [172, 173].

Iron transport across the placenta is rapid and unidirectional [174]. During pregnancy the maternal serum iron level either remains constant or falls, but the transferrin concentration usually rises. Serum iron concentrations in the fetus are usually high and the transferrin level is low compared with those of the mother [175], but this does not appear to be due to differences in the binding capacity of fetal and maternal transferrin [176]. Transferrin does not cross the placenta in significant amounts and the placental transfer of iron is associated with the formation of haemosiderin and ferritin [177]. Maximum transfer occurs in late pregnancy and is probably related to the growth of the fetus [177].

FERROKINETICS

Much of the existing information about the movement of iron in the body has been obtained by the use of radioactive tracers. The major pathways of iron metabolism are shown in Figure 5.5. ^{59}Fe, an easily counted γ-emitting nuclide with a half-life of 45 days, is the most commonly used isotope. Particularly detailed studies have been made of the redistribution of radioactive transferrin-bound iron injected into the peripheral circulation. Information obtained in this way is useful in studying the plasma iron pool, marrow utilization of iron for erythropoiesis and the distribution of iron in the tissues.

Most of the iron leaving the plasma is utilized for erythropoiesis in the bone marrow. In normal subjects there is initially a rapid exponential decrease in plasma radioactivity with removal of half the ^{59}Fe in about 60–90 minutes. After a short period a slower rate of clearance is found and the clearance curve can be broken down into two or more additional exponential components. These components usually become obvious when over 90% of the plasma ^{59}Fe has already disappeared and indicate a return of labelled iron from the tissues and extravascular fluid. Although it is agreed that the multi-exponential pattern of plasma ^{59}Fe clearance is due to the exchange of ^{59}Fe between plasma and extravascular iron pools there are many opinions on the nature and size of these pools [178]. In the original observations of Huff *et al.* [179], measurements of plasma radioactivity were limited to the first few hours after the administration of the tracer and no feedback was observed. The resulting clearance pat-

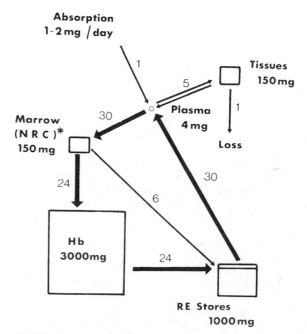

Fig. 5.5. Major pathways of iron metabolism. * NRC = nucleated red cells.

tern was seen as a single exponential function and was interpreted as being entirely due to bone-marrow uptake. Pollycove & Mortimer [180] used data from the multi-exponential ^{59}Fe-clearance curve and a mathematical model of body kinetics to calculate the rate of exchange between plasma and extravascular iron. Their results were consistent with the existence of a labile erythropoietic pool fed from the plasma and from which iron could transfer either into the developing red cells or back into the plasma. This labile pool was thought to be situated on the membrane of immature normoblasts [181]. The model also included an exchange with a labile storage pool, although this appeared to be negligible except in cases of iron overload. Other authors have suggested ferrokinetic models which include iron exchange between plasma, interstitial fluid and a number of intracellular pools of which the marrow iron pool is quantitatively the most important. The validity of these models can only be checked by measuring the sizes of the pools and comparing the values with the predicted pool sizes. Because these pools are often difficult to define chemically or anatomically this has so far not been possible.

More recently, new approaches have been developed which do not require the definition of unknown and inaccessible compartments [154, 182]. These are based on the calculation of ^{59}Fe reflux into the plasma following its initial clearance. The ^{59}Fe which does not return to the plasma is retained either in circulating red cells, or in non-erythroid tissues. Many older concepts have proved to be no longer acceptable. The half-time ($T_{\frac{1}{2}}$) of plasma iron clearance, which has been widely used as measure of erythroid activity can give an erroneous estimate [183]. Plasma iron turnover (PIT) has also been used for the same purpose though it does not differentiate between an erythroid or a non-erythroid destination for iron leaving the plasma. It also takes no account of iron reflux, which amounts to about 35% of the iron leaving the plasma pool in normal subjects and may be very much greater where there is ineffective erythropoiesis or hypoplasia [183]. Similarly the percentage ^{59}Fe utilization by red cells has been widely used as a measure of effective erythropoiesis though the re-utilization of refluxed ^{59}Fe from both erythroid and non-erythroid sources, the patient's iron status and the red-cell lifespan can all influence the results. It is not possible to equate the red-cell utilization with effective erythropoiesis [183] and the erythrocyte iron turnover (EIT) derived from the percentage utilization and the PIT is equally fallacious. However, when the red-cell utilization is corrected for reflux and related to the PIT it can provide a valid measure of effective red-cell iron turnover [183], provided that there has been no

significant loss of ^{59}Fe from the mature red cells during the study.

Analysis of an accurately determined plasma iron clearance curve and incorporation of ^{59}Fe in red cells allows the calculation of total marrow iron turnover (MIT), red-cell iron turnover (RCIT) which reflects effective erythropoiesis, ineffective iron turnover (IIT) in which ineffective erythropoiesis contributes the major component, and mean red-cell lifespan (MRCLS).

Methods for obtaining these measurements and their interpretation have been reviewed [184] and normal values are given in Table 5.4. It is also possible to calculate extravascular iron turnover and non-erythroid tissue iron turnover, though these are not of such frequent clinical value.

Ferrokinetic measurements

The main use of ferrokinetics has been as an index of erythropoietic activity. Clinical studies should be based on an accurate definition of the behaviour of iron specifically bound to transferrin in the plasma and reliable results can only be obtained when specific precautions are taken to ensure that all the radioactive tracer is initially bound to the protein carrier and that only ^{59}Fe transferrin, and not traces of labelled haem, are measured subsequently [184]. After the first day of such studies plasma radioactivity has usually fallen to less than one per cent of the initial value and correction for fluctuations in plasma iron concentration is essential. The major sources of reflux are recirculation from extravascular fluid, which accounts for about eight per cent of iron leaving the plasma and has a $T_{\frac{1}{2}}$ of about 10 hours, and a second slower process involving iron temporarily incorporated into tissues (mainly erythroid cells) before return to the plasma with a $T_{\frac{1}{2}}$ of about eight days. This second component accounts for about 25% of the PIT and largely represents ineffective erythropoiesis. Variations in the clearance and refluxes result in differences in the plasma radioactivity curve (Fig. 5.6). Methods for analysing these curves have been described by a number of authors and are reviewed by Cavill & Ricketts [184].

The meticulous technique and somewhat specialized analysis required to obtain useful results restricts the use of ferrokinetic techniques to those patients posing major clinical problems. In haemolytic anaemias it is possible to quantitate both red-cell lifespan and erythroid output and in dyserythropoietic disorders it is useful to obtain an index of ineffective erythropoiesis. In patients with refractory or aplastic anaemia it is particularly useful to have a quantitative measure of erythroid turnover, ineffective erythropoiesis and red-cell lifespan.

Table 5.4. Erythroid iron turnover in normal subjects (taken from Ref. 184, with permission)

Authors		Number of subjects	Plasma iron turnover (µmol/l blood/d)	Marrow iron turnover (µmol/l blood/d)	Red-cell iron turnover (µmol/l blood/d)	Ineffective iron turnover (µmol/l blood/d)	(%)	Mean red-cell lifespan (days)
Barosi *et al.* [468]	Mean	8	119	90	84	6	6	109
	Range		99–143	78–105	73–100	1–12	1–14	88–124
Cavill *et al.* [469]	Mean	10	129	107	82	25	22	103
	Range		89–183	73–159	54–105	14–54	13–34	74–153
Dinant & de Maat [470]	Mean	17	118	95	76	20	20	118
	Range		66–203	59–155	55–118	5–35	8–29	82–149

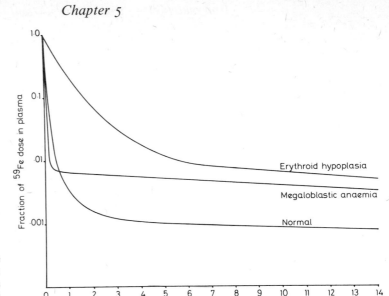

Fig. 5.6. ^{59}Fe-clearance curves from the plasma of a normal subject, a patient with megaloblastic anaemia and a patient with refractory hyperplastic anaemia. (From Ricketts *et al.* [182] with permission.)

Surface counting techniques

Following the injection of ^{59}Fe-labelled transferrin, measurements of the amount of radioactivity in various organs can be made by placing a collimated scintillation counter over the appropriate sites. Measurements are usually made over the heart, liver, spleen and sacrum. This technique is particularly useful in determining the sites of iron sequestration in patients with refractory anaemia or in determining the site of extramedullary erythropoeisis in patients with myelosclerosis. The distribution of erythropoietic marrow has also been studied by using the short-lived isotope ^{52}Fe (half-life 8·3 hours) and obtaining pictures with a positron camera [185]; quantification is possible using rectilinear scanning [186]. An alternative, but less satisfactory method of studying the distribution of iron uptake following the intravenous administration of ^{59}Fe is by the use of a linear scanner to measure radioactivity in the narrow segments of the whole body [187].

Reticulo-endothelial function

Impairment of red-cell production is known to occur in chronic inflammatory conditions and in malignancy despite a normal or even an accelerated utilization of transferrin-bound iron. This may be due partly to a failure of iron re-utilization after senescent red cells have been taken up by the recticulo-endothelial system [165, 166]. The block in iron release from reticulo-endothelial cells has been demonstrated following the administration of radioiron-labelled red cells [188], but this procedure presents practical difficulties. An alternative method in which reticulo-endothelial iron

release has been measured following the simultaneous administration of ^{55}Fe-labelled Imferon and ^{55}Fe-labelled transferrin [189], still requires the injection of amounts of iron greater than tracer quantities. Attempts to formulate a mathematical model for the determination of a rate of iron release from reticulo-endothelial cells have not been entirely successful and it is likely that highly specific activity probes will be necessary to provide data suitable for analysis [190].

INTRACELLULAR MECHANISMS

Cellular uptake of transferrin-bound iron

This has been most thoroughly studied with human reticulocytes and the findings have been summarized by Morgan [16]. The cell membrane has 'receptors' which bind transferrin molecules and release them after removal of iron. Iron uptake requires an intact cell, is temperature dependent, and is inhibited by certain metabolic inhibitors and by treatment of the cells with trypsin or chymotrypsin. The receptors are not present on erythrocytes. The greatest rates of transferrin and iron uptake are shown by early and intermediate normoblasts, and as the cell matures iron uptake and the number of receptors decline in parallel [191, 192]. The number of receptors has been estimated as about 100 000 for the reticulocyte [193]. There is evidence that some of the transferrin associated with the cell membrane is taken within the cell by a process of endocytosis [194, 195] although whether this step is essential for iron delivery to the cell is not certain. A number of attempts to isolate the transferrin receptor from the red-cell membrane have been made by solubilizing membrane proteins in detergent. The conflicting results obtained have been reviewed [19].

Although red cells can take iron from iron chelates for haem synthesis [196] an interaction with transferrin may still occur as cells depleted of membrane-bound transferrin by repeated incubation in transferrin-free medium at 37°C were unable to incorporate iron from low-molecular-weight chelates [197]. The way in which iron is released from the transferrin-receptor complex is not known but removal of bicarbonate anion, reduction of Fe^{3+} to Fe^{2+} or a reduction of pH are possible mechanisms [198].

Uptake of transferrin iron by guinea-pig, rabbit, rat and human placenta also shows similarities to red-cell iron uptake [16] but in species with non-haemochorial placentas, such as the cat, iron is obtained from red cells trapped within the placenta [199]. It is not certain how widespread the transferrin receptor is in cells with lower iron requirements, but iron delivery with reversible binding of transferrin has been described for rat liver [200] and for cultured rat liver cells [201, 202].

The reticulo-endothelial system is largely responsible for the breakdown of haemoglobin and cellular requirements for iron are probably satisfied from this source. It is usually assumed that transferrin removes iron from these cells, and there is some uncertainty about the ability of phagocytic cells to obtain iron from transferrin. Uptake of transferrin iron by rat liver is thought to be confined to the hepatocytes [203]. Uptake of transferrin iron has been described for rabbit pulmonary macrophages [204] and human monocytes [205]. However, the amount of iron taken up per cell is not comparable with that achieved by immature red cells, and transferrin uptake might be by endocytosis and catabolism. This has been described in the case of the L132 cell derived from human fetal lung [206] and for human macrophages [207]. The isolated epithelial cells from rat small intestine appear to have a greater affinity for apotransferrin than transferrin and this suggests that transferrin may act as a direct acceptor for absorbed iron [132] although, as mentioned earlier (p. 160), it does not seem to be essential.

Intracellular iron exchange
The way in which iron is exchanged between membranes and proteins is not known but three types of intermediate have attracted interest:
1 *Low-molecular-weight iron chelators.* It has been postulated that there is a 'labile' or 'chelatable' pool of iron which mediates exchange [208–210]. Such iron may be in the form of complexes with sugars, nucleotides [211], amino acids, etc., or may be loosely associated with protein. Concentrations of iron are likely to be very low [212]. The existence of a labile pool

of iron may be inferred from knowledge of the chemistry of iron and from *in-vivo* and *in-vitro* experiments [210] but attempts to extract and purify components of the pool will almost certainly disturb the equilibrium between various forms of iron chelates. Studies of the exchange of iron between transferrin molecules and between transferrin and ferritin provide some insight into the role of low-molecular-weight chelators. It is known that citrate enables a rapid exchange of iron to take place between transferrin molecules, possibly through the formation of an intermediate ternary complex of Fe^{3+}, transferrin and citrate [213]. The fraction of total iron bound to citrate at any instant in time is negligible. *In-vitro* studies of iron exchange between transferrin and ferritin have shown that a reducing agent is necessary to assist in the removal of iron from transferrin and to ensure that iron is in the ferrous state for uptake by ferritin [214]. A number of chelating agents enhances the transfer and it is possible that a ferrous chelate is formed as an intermediate between transferrin and ferritin. The requirement of ATP for iron transfer from transferrin to ferritin in liver slices and homogenates may be a result of its acton as a chelating agent rather than as a source of energy [214].

2 *Transferrin.* There has been particular interest in the function of transferrin as an intracellular iron transport protein in two cell types—the intestinal epithelial cell and the immature red cell. In the intestinal cell there seems to be a specific transferrin, differing in amino-acid composition from plasma transferrin, which carries iron across the cell during its absorption (see p. 160). Although several authors have reported that after incubation of red cells with ^{59}Fe much of the soluble non-haem radioiron is associated with transferrin, others have not confirmed this finding and Romslo [215] has pointed out that the percentage of non-haem iron bound to transferrin decreases with increasing centrifugal force applied to sediment membranes, suggesting that the transferrin in cell supernatants is actually membrane-bound.

3 *Ferritin.* Ferritin has been demonstrated within nucleated red cells and reticulocytes and haemosiderin can also be found in small amounts [216, 217]. As the cell reaches its full haemoglobin content the ferritin disappears. When [^{14}C]-leucine is used as a radioactive tracer apoferritin synthesis can be demonstrated within normoblasts and reticulocytes [218]. Curiously, the rate of apoferritin synthesis is maximal before the rate of iron uptake reaches a maximum [219]. It has been suggested, as a result of electron-microscope examination of bone marrow, that immature red cells cluster around macrophages and obtain iron from them by a process analagous to pinocytosis which has been called rhopheocytosis [217]. However, it seems

unlikely that this represents an important source of iron for the cell in view of the ability of immature red cells to acquire sufficient iron from transferrin. It is even less likely that the cell would acquire intact ferritin molecules in this way.

Immature red cells contain an 'acidic' ferritin (of similar pI to heart ferritin) [220]. Gabuzda & Pearson [221] labelled rabbit reticulo-endothelial cells with ^{55}Fe and heat-damaged red cells and marrow erythroblasts with $^{59}FeCl_3$ injected into the plasma. On anion exchange chromatography they found that the two isotopes of iron were readily separated with the ^{59}Fe being associated with the more acidic ferritin. Thus, although the red cell contains more acidic isoferritin than reticulo-endothelial cell ferritin, its function is still unclear.

Mazur & Carleton [222] incubated rat marrow cells with ^{59}Fe-labelled transferrin *in vitro* and found that the maximum incorporation of ^{59}Fe into ferritin took place before the maximum incorporation into haem. Nunez *et al.* [223] and Speyer & Fielding [224] have also found evidence that ferritin acts as an inter- mediate in the transfer of iron to the mitochondrion for haem synthesis. However, Zail *et al.* [225], Primosigh & Thomas [226] and Borova *et al.* [227] were not able to show that ferritin acted as an intermediate. In these and other studies [228, 229] iron-binding fractions other than ferritin, transferrin or haem were described as intermediates on the pathway to haem synthesis. These 'intermediates' were usually of rela- tively low molecular weight.

Iron uptake by mitochrondria and haem synthesis
Most of the iron entering the red cell is eventually incorporated into haem. The last stage in this process is catalyzed by the enzyme ferrochelatase which is found on the inner mitochondrial membrane with its active site on the inner surface [230]. This means that the substrate, Fe^{2+} and porphyrin, and the product, haem, have to cross the mitochondrial membranes. Under suitable conditions intact, isolated mitochondria take up iron from Fe(III) sugar complexes, from transferrin and from ferritin. This topic has been critically reviewed by Romslo [215].

Haem breakdown (see also Chapter 4)
Haemoglobin in old or damaged red cells is catabo- lized in the recticulo-endothelial cells of the spleen, liver, bone marrow and other tissues, but haptoglobin- bound and 'free' haemoglobin in plasma is removed from the circulation by the hepatic parenchymal cells [231]. Similarly, haem in plasma is taken up by hepatocytes after dissociation from haemopexin at specific receptors on the cell surface [232]. Normally, however, most of the haem degraded by hepatocytes comes from the breakdown of intracellular haemo- proteins such as cytochrome P_{450}. Haemoglobin enters the hepatic lysosomal system where breakdown of the protein takes place with the release of haem [233]. Haem is degraded to biliverdin and CO by the enzyme haem oxygenase which is found in the endoplasmic reticulum [234]. Biliverdin IX formed by haem oxy- genase is reduced to bilirubin IX by biliverdin reductase [235]. The iron released by the action of haem oxy- genase presumably enters the intracellular labile pool. Haem oxygenase is dependent on NADPH and mole- cular oxygen and requires oxidation of ferrous iron and separation of haem from its protein for maximum activity. The enzyme was originally thought to require cytochrome P_{450} as a terminal oxidase but several studies have demonstrated that this is not so [236, 237].

Primstone *et al.* [238] demonstrated the importance of the reticulo-endothelial system in this process by showing that administration of methaemalbumin, haemoglobin or haem *in vivo* induced very high levels of enzyme activity in pure populations of macrophages from peritoneal cavity of rats and lungs of rabbits. In pure macrophage populations the specific activity of the enzyme, after induction with haem, was higher than that in whole liver or spleen from the same animals. (For a discussion of non-enzymic oxidation of haem see Jackson [239].)

IRON STATUS

Variations in iron balance may sometimes lead to considerable changes in the total amount of iron in the body, with consequent iron deficiency or overload. The optimal amount of iron is usually thought to be present when the synthesis of physiologically active compounds is not limited. Ferritin and haemosiderin are usually considered to be reserve compounds which are synthesized when the amount of iron present in the body is in excess of active metabolic requirements. In iron overload it is these compounds which are present in increased amounts. The claim that iron stimulates haemoglobin formation in normal subjects has not been borne out by critical examination [240]. In iron depletion all the iron-containing compounds of the body may be reduced in amount, though they do not all become affected at the same time. The parameter of iron status chosen for study in any given clinical situation will depend on the precise objective and whether iron overload or deficiency is suspected.

Measurement of storage iron

Quantitative phlebotomy
Iron stores represent the amount of iron in the body

available for mobilization when requirements are increased. The most direct method for measuring this is to determine the amount available for haemoglobin formation following rigorous phlebotomy. This procedure was first described by Haskins *et al.* [241] and bleeding was carried out at such a rate that the greater part of the iron utilized for haemoglobin formation was obtained from stores rather than by absorption. After repeated venesections the subjects were unable to maintain their haemoglobin levels and at this point it was assumed that available iron stores had been depleted. The amount of iron removed in the form of blood was then calculated. This method for measuring iron stores is only suitable in exceptional circumstances. It has two minor theoretical drawbacks: one is the observation that in patients with greatly increased iron stores there may be difficulty in mobilizing all the haemosiderin from the reticulo-endothelial cells, so that iron-deficiency anaemia may occur while haemosiderin aggregates are still visible in the bone marrow; in addition Torrance *et al.* [242] have suggested that storage iron in muscle is not as readily available for mobilization as that at other sites.

Estimation of tissue iron concentrations

The liver and bone marrow are the most important storage sites and the amount of iron present in these organs can be estimated chemically, visually, using the Prussian-blue reaction on tissue sections, by indirect tests with chelating agents or by isotope dilution techniques. The chemical estimation of non-haem iron in human bone-marrow aspirates has been described by Trubowitz *et al.* [243] and the use of needle biopsy samples of liver for iron estimation has been found useful in the diagnosis of overload [244]. In a study of adult Bantu and white subjects dying in hospital, the concentration of non-haem iron in the bone marrow showed a close correlation with the concentration in the liver over a wide range [245], suggesting that the liver and marrow have an equal capacity to store iron under normal circumstances. Other studies have shown a greater scatter of results although the overall relationship still holds [170]. In the South African study, histological assessment of haemosiderin in bone-marrow particles was found to show good agreement with chemical estimations over a wide range of values [245], but greater variation has been found by other workers [170, 243].

The most convenient method of estimating reticulo-endothelial iron stores in bone marrow is by examining histological sections of aspirated particles [246]. A semi-quantitative assessment may be made by grading the visible Perls-positive granules [247]. A similar semi-quantitative assessment of stainable iron may be made in liver sections, though in this case parenchymal

as well as reticulo-endothelial iron has to be taken into account [248].

Normal red-cell precursors contain some Prussian-blue staining granules in their cytoplasm and these are diminished in iron deficiency [216]. In practice accurate sideroblast counts are tedious and laborious and for this reason are rarely carried out. The absence of sideroblasts is not diagnostic of iron deficiency but rather of an impairment of iron delivery to developing red-cell precursors [249]. An increase in the sideroblasts indicates an abnormality of haem synthesis rather than an increase in storage iron.

Chelatable iron

A number of workers have attempted to assess iron stores indirectly by measuring urinary iron excretion following an injection of the iron-chelating agent desferrioxamine. The intramuscular injection of 500 mg of desferrioxamine is followed by an increase in the urinary iron excretion during the following six hours [250]. The amount is significantly increased in patients with iron overload. Fielding [251] suggested that the amount of iron excreted in the urine does not always bear a constant relationship to the amount chelated *in vivo* and recommended a differential ferrioxamine test which enables the amount of iron chelated *in vivo* to be calculated. Other workers [252], however, found that the desferrioxamine-induced urinary iron excretion correlated well with the amount of iron chelated in the body in both normal and iron-deficient subjects. Balcerzak *et al.* [253] found a close linear correlation between desferrioxamine-induced iron excretion and iron stores measured by the phlebotomy technique. Harker *et al.* [248] also found a correlation between total iron stores and iron-chelate excretion but felt that this relationship applied more specifically to liver parenchymal iron than to reticulo-endothelial stores. They suggest that chelate-induced iron excretion is a useful test of liver parenchymal overload. Barry & Sherlock [244], using diethylenetriamine penta-acetic acid (DTPA) as a chelating agent, found a good correlation between urinary iron excretion and liver iron concentration in normal subjects and in those with iron overload. The correlation between chelate-induced iron excretion in the urine and body iron stores is most useful when stores are increased. Haemolysis and ineffective erythropoiesis may be associated with some increase in chelatable iron, possibly through an increase in a non-ferritin chelatable pool in reticulo-endothelial cells [208].

Serum ferritin

Measurement of serum ferritin concentration also provides information about storage-iron levels. Addison *et al.* [254] were the first to describe an assay sensitive enough to measure ferritin concentrations in normal serum although ferritinaemia in patients with liver disease had previously been described [255]. The immunoradiometric (or labelled-antibody) assay of Addison *et al.* [254], and (especially) the two-site immunoradiometric assay described by Miles *et al.* [256] have been widely used. More recently radioimmunoassays and enzyme-linked methods have been introduced. Immunoassay techniques for ferritin have been recently reviewed [257].

Normal subjects. In normal adults serum-ferritin concentrations are in the range 15–300 $\mu g/l$ but concentrations are both age- and sex-dependent. Some examples of normal ranges are given in Table 5.5. Although ranges reported by two groups of workers have been selected the normal ranges reported by other authors are very similar. Further information is given in recent reviews [258, 259].

At birth, serum ferritin concentrations are relatively high (as are non-haem iron concentrations in the liver). During the first weeks of life the haemoglobin concentration in the blood falls to 10–11 g/dl due to the removal of fetal red cells from the circulation at the time when the rate of erythropoiesis is relatively low [76]. The iron released by the destruction of red cells is stored in the tissues and causes an increased concentration of serum ferritin. In the next two months synthesis of adult haemoglobin causes a rapid fall in the concentration of non-haem iron in the tissues and in serum ferritin concentration. Both remain low throughout childhood and adolescence. Serum ferritin concentrations tend to be higher in men than in women of child-bearing age and reflect known differences in storage-iron levels, but ferritin concentrations are higher in older women than in younger women because of the increase in storage-iron levels which follows cessation of menstruation and child-bearing. Walters *et al.* [260] reported a good correlation between 'mobilizable storage iron' (measured by phlebotomy) and serum ferritin concentrations in 22 normal subjects.

Iron-deficiency anaemia. Patients with simple iron-deficiency anaemia have a microcytic anaemia, a low serum iron concentration, a high total iron-binding capacity, an absence of stainable iron in the bone marrow and a subsequent response to therapeutic iron. In such patients serum ferritin concentrations are almost invariably less than 15 $\mu g/l$ [258].

Iron overload. Serum ferritin concentrations are high in patients with idiopathic haemochromatosis. Concentrations are usually in the range 1000–10 000 $\mu g/l$ but may be lower in patients presenting early in the course of the disease [258]. The value of the assay in detecting minor degrees of iron overload in relatives of patients is discussed later. Serum ferritin appears to be useful in screening relatives of patients and in particular in detecting more advanced iron overload. However, careful comparison with ferritin levels in age- and sex-matched controls is essential.

In patients with secondary iron overload, serum ferritin concentrations are usually high. Concentra-

Table 5.5. Serum ferritin concentration in normal subjects (taken from Ref. 257, with permission)

Age and sex	No. of subjects	City or state	Median ferritin conc. ($\mu g/l$)	Range
Newborn babies	21	San Francisco [463]	101	12–200*
Infants (1 month)	11	San Francisco	356	60–800*
Infants (1–2 months)	9	San Francisco	160	5–220*
Infants (3–5 months)	18	San Francisco	80	6–230*
Children (6 months–15 years)	514	San Francisco	30	7–142†
Adolescent (12–18 years)	251	Washington State [289]	22‡	10–63§
Women (18–45 years)	370	Washington State	25	7–140§
Women (over 45 years)	215	Washington State	89	12–170§
Men (18–45 years)	240	Washington State	94	34–196§
Men (over 45 years)	165	Washington State	124	29–455§

Babies, infants and children from San Francisco were healthy and not anaemic.
Subjects from Washington State were from lower-income families.
* Approximate value estimated from a figure.
† 95% confidence range.
‡ Approximate value, data from male and female children given separately, but no significant differences were found between the two groups.
§ 10–90 percentile.

tions of up to 20 000 μg/l may be found in children with homozygous β thalassaemia who have received 400–500 units of blood. However, concentrations in excess of about 4000 μg/l probably reflect the presence of liver damage as well as iron deposition [261].

Another group of patients who may develop iron overload, although to a much lesser extent, are those on maintenance haemodialysis for treatment of renal disease. Regular intravenous infusion of iron is frequently used to prevent blood losses during the dialysis procedure causing iron deficiency. Serum ferritin concentrations have been shown to correlate with the grade of stainable iron in the bone marrow and the assay is of value in monitoring iron therapy, and so preventing iron overload [262–265].

High serum ferritin levels due to causes other than iron overload

Liver disease. The liver contains about one-third of the storage iron in the body and much ferritin so it is not surprising that high levels of serum ferritin are often found in patients with liver disease. The highest levels (concentrations up to 27 600 μg/l have been reported) are found in patients with massive hepatic necrosis. Prieto *et al.* [266] found that there were parallel reductions in serum ferritin concentration and aspartate transaminase activity in patients recovering from drug or viral-induced hepatitis. They also found a linear relationship between the ratio of serum ferritin concentration : aspartate transaminase activity and liver iron concentration in 37 patients with a wide range of liver iron concentrations. Although the value of the serum ferritin : aspartate transaminase ratio has not been confirmed [267] the finding of a normal serum ferritin concentration in a patient with raised aspartate transaminase activity is good evidence against iron overload in that patient.

Infection, inflammation and chronic disease. Acute infection or inflammation causes a rapid drop in the serum iron concentration and a rise in serum ferritin levels [268]. As a low serum iron concentration is found in most patients with chronic inflammation, infection or malignant disease measurement of serum iron concentrations gives little information about storage-iron levels. A correlation between grade of stainable iron in the marrow and serum ferritin concentrations has been demonstrated in patients with inflammation [269] and rheumatoid arthritis [270] and the assay is thus of value in assessing levels of storage iron in such patients. However, Lipschitz *et al.* [269] found that serum ferritin concentrations were higher for each grade of stainable iron than in patients without

inflammation or infection, and in patients with an absence of stainable iron in the bone marrow, serum ferritin may be higher than the values of 15 μg/l found in patients with simple iron-deficiency anaemia. Bentley & Williams [270] suggested that this was because the serum-ferritin assay was a more sensitive indicator of storage iron in the bone marrow than the histochemical method but deposition of iron at other sites [271] and changes in the rate of synthesis, release or clearance of ferritin must also be considered.

Malignant disease. Serum ferritin concentrations are often elevated in patients with malignant disease, particularly acute myeloid leukaemia [272], hepatoma [273] or carcinoma of the pancreas [274]. Although there may be both quantitative and qualitative changes in ferritin synthesis in a tumour, serum ferritin levels generally appear to provide merely an indicator of disease activity. The use of antibodies to acidic ferritins to detect 'tumour ferritins' has not been of value [275] and attempts to use serum ferritin levels in order to predict relapse in children with acute lymphoblastic leukaemia [276] or in women with breast cancer have failed [277]. In most cases raised levels of serum ferritin in cancer appear to be due to increased levels of storage iron in anaemic patients and (in later stages) to cellular damage.

The origin of serum ferritin and its removal from the plasma. Both clinical and experimental evidence indicate that much of the plasma ferritin originates from reticulo-endothelial cells [258]. Serum ferritin has a relatively low iron content [278] and much of the circulating protein is glycosylated [279], suggesting that secretion rather than leakage through cell membranes takes place. Massive hepatic necrosis provides an example of a situation where liver parenchymal cells provide most of the circulating ferritin. Ferritin is rapidly removed from the plasma by hepatic parenchymal cells [258].

Clinical use of the serum-ferritin assay. The assay of serum ferritin provides a useful and convenient way of assessing the level of storage iron in normal subjects. In simple iron-deficiency anaemia, ferritin concentrations are less than 15 μg/l.

Unfortunately, many patients do not present with simple clinical syndromes. In the presence of infection, inflammatory disease, tissue damage or malignancy there is still a relationship between the serum-ferritin concentration and the level of iron stores. However, in such patients ferritin concentrations are higher than those in 'control' subjects with similar levels of storage iron. Thus ferritin concentrations of up to 50 μg/l may be found in patients with no stainable iron in the bone marrow. Liver damage is especially associated with high serum ferritin levels which obscure the diagnostic value of the assay in iron deficiency but in patients with liver damage a normal serum ferritin concentration is good evidence against iron overload.

Serum iron and total iron-binding capacity (TIBC)
Traditionally measurements of serum iron concentration and TIBC have been made in order to assess levels of storage iron. From the discussion on page 171 it is obvious that the serum iron concentration is not directly related to the level of storage iron. However, in some circumstances characteristic changes in serum iron concentration may be found. In patients with iron-deficiency anaemia the serum iron concentration is low, the TIBC is raised and the transferrin saturation is less than 16%. The increased TIBC is characteristic of a deficiency of storage iron. However, in most hospital patients anaemia is secondary to another disease process and such patients will have a low serum iron concentration and percentage saturation even in the presence of adequate amounts of storage iron. For this reason measurement of serum iron and transferrin saturation is of limited value. In patients with iron overload, serum iron concentrations are raised and the TIBC may be reduced, giving a percentage saturation greater than 60%. A high percentage saturation is found in the earliest stages of idiopathic haemochromatosis and the assay of serum iron and TIBC is of particular use in making this diagnosis. There are also many other conditions such as marrow aplasia, haemolytic anaemia or hepatic necrosis in which a high percentage saturation is found but is not of specific diagnostic importance.

Numerous methods have been evolved for the estimation of serum iron. Those which are generally used are based on the separation of iron from its carrier protein, followed by its colorimetric measurement. Methods based on atomic absorption spectroscopy have not been widely accepted as they have the defect of including any haem iron which may be present. The principles involved have been reviewed by Bothwell *et al.* [91]; the common colour-developing agents used have been 2, 2′-dipyridyl, tripyridyl triazine and bathophenanthroline. The International Committee for Standardization in Haematology has recently published a standard method for the estimation of serum iron [280].

The total iron-binding capacity (TIBC) is usually measured by determining the amount of iron required to saturate the iron-binding protein present in the serum sample. A number of methods have been used for absorbing the excess iron, absorbing with magnesium carbonate being the most satisfactory [91, 281]. Immunological methods for determining transferrin

are available but are not commonly used in the assessment of iron status.

Normal iron stores
Most normal subjects have some storage iron and under these conditions it is assumed that iron lack is not a limiting factor in the synthesis of biologically active compounds. There is no evidence to indicate that a large amount of storage iron is preferable to a small amount and indeed there is considerable evidence regarding the harmful effects of excess iron. The optimum store is presumably that which will act as a buffer against normal physiological variations in iron requirements in the rest of the body.

Mean values for total mobilizable iron measured by venesection [260] are 767 mg in normal men and 232 mg in normal women. It is unusual to find more than 1500 mg of storage iron. Gale *et al.* [245] measured total bone-marrow iron stores in a large number of human subjects by the use of radioisotope dilution technique and found the mean value in 24 white males to be about 300 mg. Finch [41] allowed radioiron to mix with body pools for a period of three to five years and calculated a mean value of about 600 mg for total storage iron in men. This was less than the value found by the venesection technique and it was concluded that the radioactive tracer had not mixed completely with the storage-iron pool. Weinfeld [282] has calculated the average non-haem iron content of liver to be 400 mg for men, 235 mg for post-menopausal women and 130 mg for menstruating women. Scott & Pritchard [283] estimated the iron stores in 114 healthy white college women by evaluating stainable iron in the bone marrow and equating the results with available stores following phlebotomy. They found that in 24% of subjects there was stainable iron present in the bone marrow and that in a further 42% there was only a minimal amount. Those with no stainable iron were able to convert less than 150 mg of iron to haemoglobin following phlebotomy and those with minimal stainable iron less than 350 mg. These results suggest that two-thirds of normal, healthy women are able to mobilize less than 350 mg of iron and frequently appreciably less.

Charlton *et al.* [284] have attempted to assess the iron nutritional state of different population groups by determining the storage-iron concentration in nearly 4000 specimens of liver obtained at necropsy in 18 different countries. There was a positive correlation between liver iron concentration and age in South African Bantu males but no such correlation was found in other groups. Iron concentrations in females under the age of 40 years were lower than in males in all countries, but over the age of 50 years storage-iron levels in women were similar to those found in men.

The effect of age on storage-iron concentrations was thought to depend on the amount of available iron in the diet and on sex; the lowest storage concentrations were found in subjects from India and New Guinea and significant differences between the storage-iron status of different groups in western countries were also found. In the USA, there is a significant increase in mean liver iron concentration with age in women but not in men [285]. Non-haem iron levels below 50 μg/g liver indicate depletion of the storage pool to the extent that iron-deficiency anaemia is either present or to be anticipated; 4·3% of males and 10% of females between the ages of 10 and 20 years fall in this range. Up to nine per cent of males and 26% of females above the age of 20 are in this depleted state. In menstruating women the incidence of iron concentrations in this range reaches 40%, though it falls to 13% in those of 50 years of age [285].

IRON DEFICIENCY

The diagnosis of severe iron-deficiency anaemia presents no difficulty. There is, however, a need to define and diagnose iron deficiency before it reaches this extreme state. Depletion of body iron reserves makes the subject more likely to become depleted of active iron compounds if iron loss continues. Erythropoiesis and synthesis of tissue enzymes may be impaired from lack of iron for some time before the characteristic picture of a hypochromic microcytic anaemia results. Unfortunately this diagnostic no-man's-land has been littered with a number of descriptive terms that have not always been clearly defined and whose physiological significance is not always clear.

The evolution of iron deficiency
Iron deficiency should be defined in relation to the major iron-containing compartments of the body. These are
1 storage iron;
2 transport iron;
3 erythrocyte iron; and
4 tissue iron-containing proteins.

When iron losses exceed iron absorption there is gradual mobilization of iron stores and the sequence of events in other compartments depends to some extent on the rapidity of iron loss. Hagberg *et al.* [286] examined 136 apparently healthly male blood donors. Those who have given between one and four donations during the previous year showed a significance rise in serum iron level compared to unbled donors, and it was not until five or more donations were given in a year that serum iron levels became significantly reduced and accompanied by a simultaneous rise in TIBC. The increase in serum iron following venesec-

tion was interpreted as an increase in iron transport, presumably due to mobilization of stores. Conrad & Crosby [287] carried out a more intensive venesection regime on a small number of subjects and removed 500 ml of blood one to three times weekly until a total of 2–7·5 litre had been removed. The initial change was a fall in haemoglobin concentration which then remained steady at a reduced level as the frequency of venesection was reduced. When haemoglobin production kept pace with blood loss an average haemoglobin production of three to four times normal was maintained and the reticulocyte count in the peripheral blood increased for a short time. Serum iron concentration gradually fell but did not reach subnormal level until at least 500 mg of iron had been removed. Increased production of haemoglobin persisted until the subject had lost approximately 1·5 g of iron, when the haemoglobin concentration in the peripheral blood again fell if phlebotomy was continued. At this point storage iron was presumably depleted. When venesections were stopped the characteristic changes of iron deficiency gradually disappeared. Haemoglobin concentration returned to normal first, followed by the MCV, serum iron and iron-binding capacity, bone-marrow iron and iron absorption in that order. Jacobs *et al.* [288] showed that serum ferritin concentration was a good index of iron stores and that the level fell rapidly after the start of a venesection regime, followed later by a fall in the transferrin saturation. This is a particularly useful measure of storage iron in population surveys [289–291], in blood donors [292], and following iron therapy [293].

A number of phases in the development of iron deficiency can be defined. The first is sometimes referred to as prelatent iron deficiency [84] indicating absence of iron stores but with a normal plasma iron concentration. There is no evidence regarding the state of tissue iron enzymes at this stage but iron absorption is increased [84]. Further iron depletion is characterized by the development of latent iron deficiency in which the plasma iron concentration and transferrin saturation fall but the haemoglobin concentration remains normal. Although transferrin saturation is invariably less than 16% in iron-deficient patients, this is not diagnostic of iron depletion and may be found in chronic infections when there is sequestration of iron in the reticulo-endothelial cells. The delivery of iron to the red-cell precursors of the marrow is impaired at a transferrin saturation below 16% and this has been described by Bainton & Finch [249] as iron-deficient erythropoiesis. It eventually results in impaired haem synthesis and the development of hypochromic anaemia. There is an increase in erythrocyte protoporphyrin resulting from a lack of iron for haem synthesis. Protoporphyrin is lost from circulating red cells only as they are replaced by new cells and the persistence of raised levels after the treatment of iron deficiency may even allow a retrospective diagnosis to be made [294]. The importance of latent iron deficiency is that it may be a stage in the development of a more severe depletion. A group of 26 women in whom latent iron deficiency had been diagnosed were re-examined two years later by Dagg *et al.* [295] who then found that 10 had become anaemic.

Classical iron-deficiency anaemia occurs when the depletion of storage iron and the continuation of iron-deficient erythropoiesis has resulted in the formation of microcytic red cells which become increasingly poorly haemoglobinized in the course of time. Eventually, grossly abnormal red cells are produced and ineffective erythropoiesis together with a reduced red-cell lifespan result in a fall in total red-cell count.

The depletion of tissue iron enzymes in the iron-deficient state has been recognized both in animals and in human subjects [296]. These changes are relatively common in the presence of severe iron-deficiency anaemia but may also occur before the onset of anaemia. The pathological importance of these phenomena has yet to be fully appreciated but it seems probable that they result in widespread, though undramatic morbidity [296].

Prevalence of iron deficiency

Prevalence studies of iron deficiency in the past have usually used haemoglobin concentration as an index. Iron-deficiency anaemia indicates the most severe cases of depletion and is therefore some guide to the overall prevalence. The use of this index is justified in those populations where iron deficiency is the main cause of anaemia and this appears to be true in the countries of north-western Europe and in the USA [298–302]. Anaemia can be defined in a number of ways for the purpose of estimating prevalence. In a random sample of the industrial population of South Wales arbitrary levels of haemoglobin were chosen below which 'anaemia' was diagnosed—12·5 g/dl or less in man and 12 g/dl in women. Three per cent of adult men and 14% of post-menopausal women were found to be anaemic by this criterion. The prevalence of iron deficiency in a Norwegian population has been obtained by studying the haemoglobin distribution in different population groups before and after the administration of iron supplements [300]. A normal range was based on mean values after iron supplementation ± twice the standard deviation and on this basis anaemia was considered to exist when the haemoglobin concentration was less than 14 g/dl in men and 12·5 g/dl in women with slightly lower limits for children. The prevalence of iron-deficiency anaemia was 3·1% in adult men and 5·3% in adult women and between 2·0

and 3·4% in children between the ages of 11 and 16 [303]. Garby *et al.* [304] point out the disadvantages of using arbitrary criteria for the definition of iron-deficiency anaemia which include the difficulty of comparing different estimates. A study in Uppsala showed that 30% of women of fertile age give a significant haemopoietic response to iron supplementation. Although these women have not necessarily benefited from the procedure it is suggested that the criterion of response to iron supplementation is less arbitrary than one based on a fixed haemoglobin concentration [297]. In tropical countries iron-deficiency anaemia is a major problem. In India, Ceylon and East Africa haemoglobin levels were so low that Foy & Kondi [305] expressed the incidence of anaemia as the percentage of the population with haemoglobin concentrations below 8 g/dl. In Assam 16·5% of the population had a haemoglobin concentration below this level and in Portuguese East Africa 32·3% of the population were affected. A comparable survey in the Seychelles showed that anaemia was not so prevalent here and this was attributed partly to the lower hookworm rates and loads following control programmes. Information on the prevalence of iron-deficiency anaemia is to be found in a number of reviews [40, 306–308].

More recently, serum-ferritin estimations have been used to evaluate iron status in population studies involving both adults and children [289–291]. In one of these [289] a comparison betwen serum ferritin, transferrin saturation and erythrocyte protoporphyrin showed clearly the difficulty of defining iron deficiency as a specific condition which is either present or absent. It is only possible to evaluate specific aspects of iron status which may reflect different stages in the development of iron deficiency.

Iron-deficiency anaemia

Although the ordered sequence of iron depletion which follows a steady iron loss [287] may sometimes be seen, many cases do not fit this picture. If iron loss is rapid then depletion of the plasma and red-cell compartments may be evident while storage iron is still present. Tissue iron depletion is not necessarily the final stage of iron deficiency and may be found even in the absence of anaemia. The picture is also often confused by the results of previous iron therapy.

Symptoms and signs

Many of the signs and symptoms of iron-deficiency anaemia are non-specific. Beveridge *et al.* [309] studied 371 patients and found an abnormality of the tongue in 39%. Glossitis was found more commonly in patients over the age of 40 years and those considered to have a poor diet. In many cases there was complete or almost complete absence of filiform papillae. Angular stomatitis was present in 14% of patients, but absence of teeth and badly fitting dentures was probably a cause in many cases. Koilonychia was found in 18% of patients. Other associated disturbances are those commonly found in all patients with anaemia such as pallor, breathlessness and tachycardia. In severe cases, angina and myocardial failure with oedema may occur. Pica has been described as an important feature of iron deficiency in both children [310] and adults who may ingest clay, soap, paper or ice. The last condition is referred to as pagophagia [311]. The term 'sideropenia' was coined by Waldenstrom [312] to describe iron deficiency affecting the tissues but not producing anaemia, and a therapeutic trial on non-anaemic subjects complaining of chronic fatigue indicated a symptomatic improvement on the administration of iron but not by a placebo [313]. This improvement appeared to be related to the presence of sideropenia. The association of symptoms such as fatigue, headache, irritability and palpitations with minor degrees of iron deficiency has not been confirmed but more elaborate functional tests have revealed impairment of exercise efficiency, intellectual capacity and work performance in iron-deficient subjects. These changes are reviewed by Beutler & Fairbanks [314] and are discussed on page 177.

Haematological changes

Severe iron-deficiency anaemia is characterized haematologically by a reduced haemoglobin concentration and red-cell count in the peripheral blood. The erythrocytes are microcytic (MCV less than 80 fl) and the red cells are often distorted. In addition to poorly haemoglobinized red cells containing only a rim of pigment around their perimeter, target cells, cigar-shaped cells and other bizarre shapes are often found. A reticulocytosis is not usually found unless there is active bleeding and iron stores have not yet been completely depleted. The platelet count may be increased and occasionally nucleated red cells are seen in the peripheral blood [315]. Thrombocytopenia which responds to iron therapy has also been reported [316].

While absolute indices are useful in the diagnosis of severe iron-deficiency anaemia the diagnosis cannot be excluded on the basis of normal values, especially in early cases. Patients with iron deficiency show an overlap in values for MCV, MCH and MCHC with those of normal subjects. Fairbanks [259] has studied observer error in examining peripheral-blood films and concludes that the diagnosis of iron-deficiency anaemia from examination of the peripheral blood is difficult and not very reliable. The introduction of automatic cell counting equipment has also necessitated a re-evaluation of the significance of absolute indices. The Coulter S automatic cell counter is extremely sensitive to hypochromia as expressed by the MCH and microcytosis as measured by the MCV, mild degrees of abnormality being detected when no abnormality can be seen on the blood film.

Bone-marrow examination usually shows a moderate degree of normoblastic hyperplasia. The developing red-cell precursors show poor haemoglobinization and the later forms often have a ragged vacuolated cytoplasm. Sideroblastic granules are found in less than 10% of red-cell precursors and often not at all [249]. The absence of stainable iron from reticulo-endothelial cells in the bone marrow is diagnostic of iron-deficiency anaemia. Occasionally, however, if blood loss has been particularly rapid, haemosiderin may not be mobilized rapidly enough for red-cell formation and a hypochromic picture may result even though stainable iron remains in the marrow. Large doses of iron dextran may also result in the formation of unavailable iron stores in reticulo-endothelial cells and if patients who have been treated in this way subsequently develop iron deficiency, stainable iron deposits will still be visible in the bone marrow. Serum ferritin concentration is invariably low (p. 169).

The serum iron concentration is usually low and values below 5 μmol/l are not uncommon. The TIBC is usually increased and the transferrin saturation is usually less than 16% [249]. The utilization of transferrin-bound iron for erythropoiesis is rapid and increased compared to normal subjects. The turnover time for labelled plasma iron is reduced and this appears to be related to the severity of the anaemia. The marrow iron turnover is not normally reduced despite the reduction in circulating red-cell mass but much of the iron taken up by erythroid tissue returns to the plasma for reutilization as a result of ineffective erythropoiesis [318].

Catabolized iron is released rapidly from reticulo-endothelial cells into the plasma and re-utilized for erythropoiesis [188, 189].

The malformed red cells of iron-deficiency anaemia may have a reduced lifespan [319], and in rats experimental iron-deficiency anaemia appears to be associated with ineffective erythropoiesis [320] and early rapid destruction of newly formed cells in the peripheral blood [321]. Similar changes are found in iron-deficient patients. Iron-deficient erythrocytes have an impaired ability to pass through millipore filters *in vitro* and this may be associated with *in-vivo* changes leading to splenic sequestration and trapping by reticulo-endothelial cells [322].

Tissue changes

Widespread tissue changes occur outside the haemopoietic system in patients with iron-deficiency anaemia. The oral mucosa of iron-deficient patients may be atrophic and sometimes shows evidence of abnormal keratinization. There may be associated nuclear abnormalities [323]. Cytochrome-oxidase depletion in the epithelial cells occurs both in patients with severe iron-deficiency anaemia and those in whom anaemia has not yet developed [324]. While treatment with iron results in a rapid reappearance of enzyme activity in the buccal mucosa, atrophic changes do not heal rapidly and there is no clear association between enzyme and morphological abnormalities. Koilonychia is characteristic of iron deficiency though its incidence varies in different series of patients. The nails in this condition are deficient in cysteine [325], an abnormality in sulphur-containing amino acids similar to that seen in the oral mucosa [326]. The Paterson–Kelly syndrome of post-cricoid obstruction and dysphagia is a premalignant condition which has long been accepted as a consequence of iron deficiency [327]. The condition is found mainly in middle-aged women though some cases have been reported in adolescence [328]. Its precise pathogenesis is obscure. Gastric atrophy, defective vitamin-B_{12} absorption and pyridoxine deficiency have also been found [329, 330] and the condition has been recorded in patients with pernicious anaemia. The increased prevalence of post-cricoid lesions in patients after gastrectomy suggests that a nutritional deficiency is a factor in the causation of this condition though it is difficult to specify a particular nutrient [331].

Changes in the stomach, varying in degree from superficial gastritis to gastric atrophy, are found in the majority of patients with iron-deficiency anaemia. This appears to be reversible below the age of 30 but progressive in older patients [332, 333]. Gastric atrophy, when it occurs, is often associated with the presence of circulating parietal-cell antibody [334] and in this group of patients the risk of developing pernicious anaemia is high [335]. The relative rarity of achlohydia and gastric atrophy in Indians compared with Caucasians with iron-deficiency anaemia suggests a racial difference in susceptibility of the gastric mucosa to iron deficiency [336].

Children with iron-deficiency anaemia may show stunting of the duodenal villi which may revert to normal after treatment [337, 338]. This is not found in adults [339]. Intestinal absorption of ^{59}Fe haemoglobin in children with severe dietary iron deficiency is said to be lower than in control subjects [340].

Iron deficiency gives rise to defective synthesis of haem enzymes in many tissues and may result in impaired activity of other iron-dependent systems. There is no consistent pattern of depletion for specific enzymes or for particular tissues of the body [295, 341].

When iron deficiency is produced in rats by a combination of repeated bleeding and a deficient diet, cytochrome-c concentration in the liver and kidneys is reduced before there is any significant fall in haemoglobin concentration in the peripheral blood. Succinate dehydrogenase activity is impaired in the myocardium but not in other organs. Rats weaned on an iron-deficient diet have a retarded growth rate and rapidly become anaemic. A parallel reduction of myoglobin and cytochrome-c concentration occurs in the muscles and in the small-intestinal epithelium there is a reduction in cytochrome-oxidase activity [342, 343]. There is no reduction in the cytochrome-c content of the brain. When anaemic rats are treated with iron, the skeletal muscle concentration of myoglobin does not reach normal levels until 40 days after the start of treatment, though normal haemoglobin concentrations are attained after four days. Cytochrome-c concentration returns to normal within two days in the intestinal mucosa but takes 40 days to reach normal level in muscle. Cytochrome-oxidase activity in iron-deficient jejunal epithelium returns within two days of iron treatment but only newly formed cells contain normal amounts of the enzyme and the older cells remain depleted. There is some evidence of a similar phenomenon in human subjects. The slow repair of tissue cytochrome deficiencies in long-lived cells such as skeletal muscle may have a greater potential for resulting in permanent damage. In addition to haem enzyme depletion, structural changes in mitochondria may occur in iron-deficient myocardium, liver, and red-cell precursors [344]. Other enzyme defects found in iron deficiency involve catalase, glutamate formimino-transferase, xanthine oxidase, peroxidases, aconitase, oxidative phosphorylation, catecholamine metabolism, and α-glycerophosphate dehydrogenase [314]. In addition G6PD glutamic-oxaloacetic transaminase, phosphoglucomutase [314] and small-intestinal disaccharidase activity [345] also appear to be depleted in iron deficiency. None of the last group of enzymes is thought to be directly iron-dependent.

It has been suggested that iron deficiency results in a secondary defect of folate metabolism [346]. This would account for the increased urinary excretion of formiminoglutamic acid following a histidine load [347] and the neutrophil hypersegmentation that is sometimes found in the blood of iron-deficient patients. Use of the deoxyuridine suppression test on bone marrow and transformed lymphocytes from iron-deficient subjects revealed a functional folate deficiency in eight out of 15 cases even in the presence of a normal serum folate concentration [348]. The results did not, however, reveal clearly whether there was a concurrent dietary deficiency of folic acid, a secondary malabsorption or an intrinsic effect of iron deficiency on folate metabolism.

Considerable evidence has now accumulated that iron deficiency, even of a relatively minor degree, affects activity, exercise tolerance and work capacity. Edgerton *et al.* [349] found diminished ability of anaemic rats in exercising on a motor treadmill. Diminution in exercise tolerance was proportional to the degree of anaemia. Finch *et al.* [350] also used a motor-driven treadmill to show that iron deficiency, even in the absence of anaemia, significantly reduced muscular performance in rats and the performance was rapidly improved by the administration of iron, even though during a four-day period there was no increase in haemoglobin concentration. The return of exercise ability appeared to correlate with changes in α-glycerophosphate dehydrogenase activity in skeletal muscle rather than changes in the cytochrome pigments or myoglobin. Even in unstressed rats left to move spontaneously within their cages there is a considerable reduction in activity in iron-deficient animals compared with controls and recovery occurs within two days even in those animals which are not anaemic [351].

In man the deleterious effects of even mild anaemia on physical work capacity have been demonstrated both clinically and experimentally [352]. Studies in rubber plantation workers in West Java showed a correlation between results of the Harvard step test and haemoglobin concentrations. It was also found that the earnings of rubber tappers, who were paid according to work output, correlated with the haemoglobin concentration. Treatment with 100 mg of elemental iron daily for 60 days resulted in a significant improvement in haematological status, Harvard-step-test performance and work output.

Dallman *et al.* [353] found that iron deficiency in weanling rats was followed by a reduction of iron concentration in the brain and that this persisted even if repletion of iron stores in the body was carried out at a later date. Iron-deficient rats select drinking water fortified with iron in preference to distilled water [354]. In man the suggestion that iron deficiency may result in neurological or cerebral deficits has been difficult to substantiate [355]. Studies in children have, however, revealed some suggestive evidence [356]. Lower scholastic achievement in iron-deficient children of families of low socio-economic class, lower mean IQ scores in iron-deficient, socially deprived children and an increased incidence of behavioural disturbances have all been recorded. In all cases, however, the inter-relationship of poverty, malnutrition, retarded intellectual development and anaemia have been difficult to unravel.

The association between iron-deficiency anaemia and an enhanced susceptibility to infection was first observed by McKay in 1928 [357]. The importance of this phenomenon has been disputed ever since. While the antibacterial effect of unsaturated transferrin has been clearly demonstrated, severe iron deficiency is associated with defects in both polymorph and lymphocyte function [314]. On balance, the evidence seems to indicate that iron deficiency has a greater effect in promoting infection than does iron supplementation, but the issue cannot be considered settled [314].

Aetiology

Adults. The aetiology of iron-deficiency anaemia in 371 patients has been analysed by Beveridge *et al.* [309]. The age and sex distribution of patients coming into hospital is shown in Figure 5.7. Blood loss from the gastro-intestinal tract was found in 149 patients. It was significantly more common in patients over 50 years of age and the most common causes were haemorrhoids, salicylate ingestion, peptic ulceration, hiatus hernia and diverticulosis. A gastro-intestinal neoplasm was found in two per cent of patients. In 16% of patients the occult blood test was positive but no cause could be found; 38 patients in the series had had a previous gastric operation and idiopathic steatorrhea was present in 21 patients. Menorrhagia was considered an aetiological factor in the anaemia of 37% of female patients and three patients had post-menopausal bleeding. In 17% of patients no cause for the iron

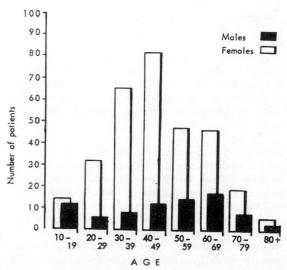

Fig. 5.7. Age and sex of 371 patients with hypochromic iron-deficiency anaemia attending hospital [309]. Courtesy of Professor L. J. Witts.

deficiency could be found. The age and sex distribution of these patients did not differ from the group as a whole.

Infancy and childhood. Iron status is determined by the combined effect of neonatal stores, growth, dietary intake and losses. Dietary insufficiency is commonest in countries with low nutritional standards but occurs in most populations. There is usually a fall of haemoglobin in the second six months of life associated with a low MCHC [358]. Moe [85] found that 12% of infants aged 12 months have a haemoglobin concentration less than 10 g/dl. In Mauritius, Stott [359] found a haemoglobin concentration below 10·8 g/dl in 60% of children between the ages of one and two years and 33% of children between the ages of four and five years. Of children between the ages of five and 15 years, 21% had a haemoglobin concentration less than 11·5 g/dl. Davis *et al.* [360] observed the incidence of iron-deficiency anaemia in European and West Indian infants living in a similar environment in London. While the incidence of iron-deficiency anaemia was 53·3% in West Indian immigrants, in their white neighbours it was only 22·4%. There is some suggestion that improving nutritional standards of some European countries may be reducing the prevalence of iron deficiency. Valhquist [361] reported haemoglobin concentrations in pre-school-age children in Sweden, Ethiopia and Ceylon which showed striking differences. The mean haemoglobin concentration in Swedish children was 12·4 g/dl, in Ethiopia 11·9 g/dl and in Ceylon 7·4 g/dl. Similar differences were shown in children between the ages of six and 10 years. Sturgeon [161] suggested that the rapid growth of well-nourished children might be a factor promoting iron deficiency in those with an optimal economic background. Other factors of importance in the aetiology of childhood anaemia are gastro-intestinal haemorrhage (e.g. from Meckel's diverticulum), intestinal parasites and possibly blood loss after tonsillectomy. Malabsorption syndromes may also be important.

Adolescence. Adolescence is a time of increased growth rate in both sexes and the onset of menstruation in women. Severe iron-deficiency anaemia in young women at this age appears to have been extremely common in the nineteenth century, when the syndrome of chlorosis was in its heyday [362]. The disappearance of this condition is presumably the result of improved nutritional standards. There is still, however, a somewhat increased incidence of iron-deficiency anaemia in this age group. In a survey of 14-year-old schoolchildren a haemoglobin concentration of less than 12·5 g/dl was found in three per cent of boys; in those girls who had not reached the menarche the incidence was 2·1% but in those who had already started menstruation the incidence was 9·2% [363]. Measurement of haemoglobin concentrations in 4221 recruits entering the Royal Air Force between the ages of 18 and 20 years showed 50 to have a concentration of less than 12 g/dl and 49 of these had iron-deficiency anaemia [88]. In two of these men the anaemia was presumed to be due to bleeding from the gastro-intestinal tract but in the remaining 47 no obvious cause was discovered. Examination of 2000 recruits to the Royal Army Medical Corps aged between 17 and 21 years showed 1·1% to have a haemoglobin concentration of less than 12 g/dl. In a similar examination of 1000 trained men of an airborne division only 0·1% had this degree of anaemia [89].

Pregnancy. The inevitable depletion of body iron commonly results in the transformation of a state of adequacy to one of deficiency. The incidence of iron-deficiency anaemia in pregnancy is high but not always significantly higher than in the non-pregnant female population, many of whom have already been depleted by previous pregnancies. Stott [359] found 60% of pregnant women in Mauritius to be anaemic compared with 57% of non-pregnant women. In India, Sood & Ramalingaswami [364] found a haemoglobin concentration of less than 12 g/dl in 88·3% of pregnant women compared to 75·3% of non-pregnant women. In populations with a lower incidence of iron deficiency the incidence of anaemia in pregnancy is also lower. Pritchard & Hunt [365] showed that 47% of pregnant women who had received no iron supplement had haemoglobin concentrations below 11 g/dl at term and Chisholm [366] found 37% of a similar group to have haemoglobin concentrations below this level. The incidence of haemoglobin concentrations below 11 g/dl was reduced to less than six per cent by the administration of iron during the last trimester. Serum ferritin concentration usually falls to iron-deficient levels by 30 weeks of pregnancy unless supplemental iron has been given [367]. Fetal requirements for iron are maximal during the last three months of pregnancy and iron deficiency in the mother may result in lower neonatal iron stores [367]. When adequate iron supplementation is given during pregnancy, haemoglobin concentrations at term are the same as those at the beginning of pregnancy [368], though there may be a fall between 21 and 36 weeks due to plasma-volume changes [369].

Gastro-intestinal bleeding. Less than 1 ml of blood is normally lost each day from the gastro-intestinal tract [43]. Increased losses can be compensated by an increase in iron absorption but this will be limited by the amount and availability of iron in the diet. The detection of blood loss from the gastro-intestinal tract may present difficulties and chemical tests for occult blood are often unsatisfactory [370]. Elwood *et al.* [371] found nine per cent of postive results in non-anaemic women and there was often disagreement regarding the interpretation of the test by two independent observers. False negative results may be due to intermittent blood loss. Chemical tests vary in their sensitivity but 60% positive results may be expected when the stools contain over 20 ml blood [370]. Blood loss can be measured by whole-body counting following the administration of ^{59}Fe, and a study of patients with hiatus hernia [372] showed some correlation between the haemoglobin level and the daily amount of blood loss. The stools of seven anaemic patients shown by this method to be losing blood were found to give consistently negative results by the usual occult blood tests.

In the UK the commonest lesions giving rise to gastro-intestinal loss are haemorrhoids and peptic ulceration [309], but malignancy and colonic ulceration are not uncommon. Normal therapeutic doses of salicylates give rise to a mean daily blood loss of about 2–3 ml. In patients taking higher doses the loss may be increased and a haemorrhagic gastritis may result. Holt *et al.* [372] found that nearly half their patients with hiatus hernia were losing blood at the rate of more than 16 ml daily and they suggest that this explains the occasional resistance to treatment of this type of anaemic patient and the frequency of relapse.

The major cause of alimentary blood loss outside Europe and North America is hookworm infestation. The amount of blood lost is proportional to the worm load but is not related to the haemoglobin level [90, 373]. Expulsion of the worms always results in cessation or diminution of blood loss but there is not usually any improvement in the haemoglobin level unless iron is also administered. The daily faecal blood loss per worm has been estimated as 0·03 ml. It has been suggested that in atrophic gastritis and the coeliac syndrome, blood loss from the gastro-intestinal tract may be due to an increased turnover of epithelial cells and by exudation rather than simple blood loss [374].

Post-gastrectomy anaemia. It has been estimated that in England and Wales in 1967 there were at least 150 000 patients who had had a partial gastrectomy [375], and for them iron deficiency remains an important nutritional problem. The incidence of anaemia increases with time after the operation and the fall in haemoglobin is faster in women than in men, particularly in those below the age of 50 years [376]. The two main factors in pathogenesis are blood loss and malabsorption of iron. Kimber *et al.* [377] examined

eight patients with post-gastrectomy iron-deficiency anaemia and found significant intermittent blood loss in seven of them while decreased iron absorption was found in only five. Holt *et al.* [378] investigated 11 post-gastrectomy patients and five were shown to be losing blood at a rate of over 150 ml/month. A blood loss of more than 60 ml/month was confined to those patients with a history of anaemia. Baird *et al.* [379], however, found no excessive blood loss in 18 patients with post-gastrectomy anaemia and concluded that occult bleeding was not an important factor in pathogenesis.

There is considerable evidence that malabsorption of iron occurs in post-gastrectomy patients [380–382]. Chronic gastritis and reduction in hydrochloric acid secretion by the gastric remnant probably results in an impaired release of iron from food with a subsequent reduction in availability [94]. A study of 51 patients before and after gastric surgery has failed to produce any evidence that an autoimmune gastritis occurs [383]. In no case was circulating parietal-cell antibody detected after operation which had not been found in the pre-operative serum. Impaired iron absorption due to disease of the gastro-intestinal tract is uncommon except after gastrectomy. Even in patients with idiopathic steatorrhoea, iron deficiency may be associated with apparently unimpaired absorption but an increased loss of iron from the mucosal surface [384].

Treatment
The management of iron-deficiency anaemia has two aims:
1 to discover and treat the cause of the underlying negative iron balance which has produced anaemia; and
2 to provide an adequate supply of iron for the restoration of normal values of circulating haemoglobin and tissue iron, and to supply the body with a small reserve of storage iron.

The most common cause of iron deficiency is blood loss from the body; identification of the site of bleeding may allow specific treatment and thus modify the long-term therapeutic approach. Reconstitution of the normal body iron content can be carried out in most patients using an oral iron preparation. There are numerous preparations available and the choice should be governed by effectiveness, lack of side-effects and expense [385]. A meticulous study by Brise & Hallberg [386] has shown that ferrous sulphate, ferrous succinate, ferrous fumarate and ferrous gluconate, amongst others, are all absorbed to a comparable extent. The side-effects of ferrous salts are related to the dose administered [387] and when the daily dose of iron is reduced to 100 mg, side-effects are rare. One way of reducing side-effects is by giving the iron in a poorly released form. This has the disadvantage that it is also poorly absorbed; this occurs in the cases of ferrous carbonate and some of the sustained-release preparations [388, 389].

A number of substances have been recommended for their action in increasing iron absorption. When 500 mg of ascorbic acid is given with a standard dose of 30 mg ferrous sulphate there is a 50% increase in absorption [390]. It is probably due to formation of an iron–ascorbate chelate in the lumen of the gut. Succinic acid has a similar effect on iron absorption but the mechanism here is not clear [391]. Maximum supply of iron to the bone marrow for erythropoiesis is obtained by giving frequent doses to maintain a high serum–iron level [392]. The treatment of iron-deficiency anaemia is, however, rarely a matter of extreme urgency and the risk of increased side-effects discourages the use of high oral doses. Three tablets daily of ferrous gluconate produce a haematological response equal to that obtained by the intramuscular injection of 1 g of iron dextran [365]. Anaemic women taking ferrous sulphate, ferrous gluconate or ferrous fumarate in amounts containing 180–220 mg iron daily increase their haemoglobin concentrations by 0·25 g/dl/day compared with 0·28 g/dl/day in women receiving intramuscular iron dextran [393]. The major difficulty in treating iron deficiency with oral preparations is the uncertainty of knowing whether the patient is actually taking the treatment. There is some evidence that as many as one-third of patients may not take the iron tablets prescribed for them [394] and this may be a major factor in deciding on parenteral therapy. Other indications are failure of iron absorption, gastro-intestinal intolerance or continued uncontrollable bleeding at a rate which makes oral therapy inadequate.

Iron dextran is an extensively used preparation and it may be administered as a series of intramuscular injections or by total-dose infusion [395, 396]. Iron-sorbitol-citrate can also be administered parenterally but has the disadvantage that 18–53% of the iron may be excreted in the urine [397] and there is a possible risk of provoking urinary-tract infection [398]. One of the disadvantages of iron-dextran therapy is that it is often not completely utilized and some may remain either at the site of the injection or sequestered in reticulo-endothelial cells in the bone marrow.

There is no general agreement on when to stop treatment with iron. While building up of iron stores is often recommended, they have no value other than to act as a buffer against future iron depletion. While the buffer should be adequate to deal with physiological fluctuations in requirements, an excessive store may allow prolonged bleeding to go unrecognized for a considerable time before anaemia develops. A normal haemoglobin concentration is usually attained after eight weeks' iron therapy, whatever the initial level, and the continuation of oral iron for a further two months gives a twofold increase in iron stores as indicated by serum ferritin concentration [293]. Failure of the patient to respond adequately to iron therapy should lead to a re-evaluation. Providing that the correct diagnosis has been made and the treatment has been taken there may be continued bleeding or an associated condition such as infection, renal failure or rheumatism.

Anaphylactic reactions to parenteral iron may rarely occur and in the case of intravenous infusions this usually happens after only a small amount of the preparation has been given [399]. For this reason infusions should always be started very slowly and the patient watched carefully for the first few minutes. Reactions have been noted specifically in patients with malabsorption [400] and rheumatoid arthritis [401]. In some cases a syndrome of arthralgia and a lympha-denopathy develops [402].

IRON OVERLOAD

In the normal adult the amount of iron in the body remains fixed, iron losses being balanced by a delicate adjustment of iron absorption. Iron overload may result from an abnormal increase in the amount of iron absorbed, from the parenteral administration of iron or from blood transfusion. Rarely there may be focal accumulations of iron due to a pathological process in a single organ. Iron may be deposited either primarily in parenchymal cells, particularly in the liver, or in reticulo-endothelial cells, though there is often deposition in both. The classification of iron overload is necessarily somewhat arbitrary though convenient for descriptive purposes (Table 5.6).

Primary idiopathic haemochromatosis

Definition
A precise definition has eluded all observers and in the absence of any direct knowledge of the biochemical

Table 5.6. The main causes of iron overload

Primary overload
  Idiopathic haemochromatosis
Secondary overload
  Transfusion siderosis
  Refractory anaemia
  Increased iron ingestion from diet
  Alcoholic cirrhosis
  Therapeutic overload

---

disorder in this condition the diagnosis rests on clinical and laboratory studies showing increased iron-loading and inappropriately high iron absorption in the absence of any other pathological process. It is characterized by parenchymal rather than reticulo-endothelial iron deposits and, usually, a high serum iron and serum ferritin concentration. Eventually organ damage occurs. Usually the term 'haemo-chromatosis' is restricted to the primary (idiopathic) form of iron overload but other authors have extended its use to include any form of *parenchymal* cell iron overload [403].

Aetiology

Sheldon's monumental work on this condition [404] concluded that it was the result of an inborn error of metabolism and this view has been held by most workers since that time. Williams *et al.* [405] examined 46 close relatives of 16 patients with idiopathic haemo-chromatosis and found excess iron in liver biopsy sections in 28, though clinical signs of the disease were minimal and only one relative had definite cirrhosis. They suggested that the disorder might be inherited, those with the disease being the homozygotes and the mildly affected relatives the heterozygous carriers. It is possible that the very long time required for iron accumulation to produce clinical signs of disease is the reason why cases are infrequently described in different generations of the same family. MacDonald and his colleagues [406] suggested that idiopathic haemo-chromatosis is simply a variant of nutritional or alcoholic cirrhosis. They have pointed out the frequent findings of haemosiderin deposits in cases of portal cirrhosis and the frequent association of alcoholism with haemochromatosis which was originally noted by Sheldon [404]. Many alcoholic drinks, particularly red wine, have a high iron content and alcohol may also act as a stimulus to iron absorption [60]. However, Celada *et al.* [407] were not able to confirm this effect of alcohol. These factors may play a part in accelerating the disease process even if they do not initiate it. The recent documentation of a strong association between idiopathic haemochromatosis and HLA antigens [408], specifically HLA-A3, has enabled the prediction of both homozygous and heterozygous cases within a family before there were any manifestations of the disease [409–411]. The reason for the association remains unclear. The present consensus seems to be that primary haemochromatosis represents the end-point of a process in which a genetic defect results in excessive iron absorption over many years, with the gradual accumulation of parenchymal iron and subsequent tissue damage [403]. In fully developed cases, iron absorption is normal or only marginally increased [412], but as the iron load is removed by venesection

iron absorption gradually increases until it is well above the normal range. As the total body load increases after the completion of venesection, iron absorption falls, with the eventual result that the patient with a severe load remains in equilibrium. Some of the excess iron is excreted into the gut by the migration of iron-laden macrophages from the mucosa into the lumen. Iron absorption is increased in about half the relatives of patients with idiopathic haemo-chromatosis [413].

Clinical and pathological features

The disease is more common in males than in females and whereas in males it may be detected at any time in adult life, in females it is usually first seen after the menopause probably owing to the increased physio-logical iron losses before that time. At the time of Sheldon's work in 1935 no case had been reported under the age of 20 years. In his series of collected cases, diabetes was the first symptom in 25·7% of cases, abdominal symptoms related to an enlarged liver in 25·7% of cases and pigmentation of the skin in 25·7% of cases; impotence was noticed as a relatively rare mode of presentation. The pathological features of the organs [158, 404] are striking in fully developed cases. Widespread haemosiderin deposits are found in the parenchymal cells of many organs. The concentrations of iron in liver and pancreas may be 50–100 times normal, with the liver alone containing 10–20 g of iron. The concentration in the thyroid is usually 25 times normal and that in the heart and adrenals 10–15 times normal. Iron concentrations are somewhat lower in the spleen, kidneys, skin and stomach and much of the pigmentation present here is haemofuscin. In the skin, iron deposits are associated with increased deposits of melanin which account for much of the visible pigmentation. The liver is usually enlarged and has a rusty red colour. Portal cirrhosis is often found but may be in a relatively early stage of development. The first changes to be seen are probably the presence of finely dispersed iron-staining deposits in the parenchymal cells throughout the liver lobules. Fatty changes may occur and there may also be some iron deposition in Kupffer cells. When cirrhosis is marked, less pigment is found in the regenerating liver lobules and primary car-cinoma of the liver is found in some cases.

The pancreas has haemosiderin deposits in acinar cells and to a lesser extent in the islets of Langerhans. There is usually marked fibrosis and degeneration of acinar epithelium. The islets are reduced in number and may show scarring. The myocardium contains haemosiderin deposits in about 90% of cases and the heart is usually enlarged. Myocardial fibrosis has been reported. Haemosiderin deposits are present in the epithelial cells of the thyroid, parathyroid, anterior pituitary and adrenal cortex, though fibrosis does not usually occur. The testes contain only small amounts of haemosiderin, but testicular atrophy is common and may be present in about 70% of cases at the time of diagnosis [414]. Other sites of iron deposition are in the mucosal cells of the stomach and macrophages in the lamina propria of the small intestinal mucosa. The F bodies described by Hartman *et al.* [415] in the epithelium of the small intestine of normal subjects are absent in haemochromatosis [138] and this has been held to imply a failure of ferritin formation at this site of subsequent excess iron absorption.

Diabetes mellitus eventually develops in 80% of all patients with idiopathic haemochromatosis but it seems that factors other than the severity and duration of iron overload are involved in its development. There is an increased incidence of diabetes in the families of haemochromatotic patients with diabetes compared with those patients without diabetes. Insulin resistance is common, unlike primary pancreatic diabetes. Cardiac failure develops in about 15% of patients and in the younger age group is a common cause of death. Arthropathy is common [414].

Diagnosis
The classic view is that the diagnosis of idiopathic haemochromatosis must be established by demonstrating excessive iron stores together with parenchymal cell damage [403]. However, in the early stages of the disease a number of screening tests may be helpful. Serum-iron concentration is usually high and the circulating transferrin is usually completely or almost completely saturated. The TIBC of serum is usually somewhat reduced. Serum ferritin may be increased though this is not invariably the case early in the iron-loading process. A combination of all these investigations is necessary in screening for the disease. Stainable iron in the bone marrow is not usually increased until very late in the development of iron loading [416, 417] and at this stage iron may also be seen as small stainable aggregates in circulating macrophages [418]. Increased iron stores may be demonstrated by measuring the post-desferrioxamine urinary excretion. In screening relatives of patients known to have the disease, the greatest predisposition is found in those with the same HLA haplotype as the propositus [410].

Treatment
The beneficial effects of removing excess iron by venesection [420] suggest that iron plays a prime role in the pathogenesis of tissue damage. While the treatment of idiopathic haemochromatosis is directed towards reducing the body iron stores, control of secondary features such as diabetes is important. Regular, fre-

quent, phlebotomies should be carried out and, after an initial fall in haemoglobin level, increased erythroid activity in the bone marrow will result in the gradual mobilization of storage iron. An index of the amount of abnormal iron stores can be gained by measuring the total amount of blood removed by venesection before there are signs of depletion. The progress of treatment can be gauged by periodic measurement of serum ferritin concentration. Both serum iron and ferritin concentrations return to normal if treatment is adequate. In addition to subjective improvement of many patients on this regime there is usually an objective improvement of skin pigmentation, hepatomegaly and liver function tests. In a few cases improvement in the histological pattern of liver biopsies has been described [421]. Some patients show improvement in diabetes mellitus and a reduction in hepatic fibrosis, but other manifestations such as hypogonadism and arthropathy are only rarely improved [414, 420]. The mean survival of untreated patients is 18% after five years and six per cent after 10 years. With treatment the survival is 66% at five years and 32% at 10 years [420].

Transfusion siderosis
Patients with chronic refractory anaemia often receive repeated blood transfusions and the iron released from these red cells results in gradually increasing deposits of iron in reticulo-endothelial cells. This type of iron overload is often seen in idiopathic hypoplastic anaemia, in sideroblastic anaemia and in thalassaemia. In many cases where the total iron load has been measured directly, this has been found to be in excess of the amount of iron administered by transfusion [422] and it must be assumed that there has been excessive absorption in response to the anaemia. When patients are transfused to high haemoglobin levels, absorption of iron from food is not increased until the haemoglobin falls below 9–10 g/dl [423].

While the reticulo-endothelial deposits of iron in this condition are relatively harmless, parenchymal deposition may eventually result in a clinical picture of diabetes, cardiac and liver damage and pigmentation almost indistinguishable from primary haemochromatosis. Buja & Roberts [424] found myocardial siderosis in all patients who had received more than 100 units of blood. Five out of 19 patients had had chronic congestive cardiac failure and those with atrial iron deposits had suffered from supraventricular arrhythmias. Modell [425] found the first signs of iron toxicity in patients with thalassaemia major on a high transfusion regime to be the failure of normal growth and development at puberty. At the age of 14 years, boys were at the third percentile for height and had a retarded bone age. In eight deaths due primarily to iron overload, two were due to acute cardiac failure in patients who were not heavily loaded and six followed a long period of chronic cardiac failure. The chronic overload state was usually associated with hepatomegaly and ascites, retarded sexual development and multiple endocrine abnormalities including hypoparathyroidism and adrenal failure. In a few cases of chronic refractory anaemia, iron absorption may be increased to such an extent that overload occurs even in the absence of transfusion [426].

Attempts to decrease the iron load in these patients may include the adoption of a vegetarian diet, the taking of food known to inhibit iron absorption such as tea [423] and splenectomy, where transfusion requirements are in excess of theoretical needs [425].

Iron chelation therapy was introduced as a method of removing iron from patients suffering with iron overload nearly 20 years ago, but it was not until the study of homozygous β-thalassaemia patients by Barry *et al.* [427] that clear evidence was obtained that iron load could be reduced. It has become apparent in recent years that desferrioxamine given by slow infusion, either intravenously or subcutaneously, results in far more effective chelation and iron excretion than when the same dose is given as a single injection [428–430]. When the scorbutic state which commonly develops in iron-loaded patients is corrected by ascorbic-acid supplements, this may result in up to a threefold increase in iron excretion following desferrioxamine [431–433]. Significant amounts of iron excretion can only be obtained with intramuscular injections after a critical iron load has already accumulated [434] but use of the infusion technique has resulted in negative balance being achieved at any level of iron loading and it should be technically possible to prevent iron overload by an early introduction of regular chelation therapy [430]. The inconvenience and expense of permanent infusions of iron chelator has resulted in the investigation of many alternatives to desferrioxamine but none of these has yet proved completely successful therapeutically [435].

Dietary iron overload

This condition has been studied in the greatest detail in the case of Bantu siderosis. Bothwell & Isaacson [436] found that only 30% of adult males examined at autopsy in the Johannesburg area had hepatic iron concentrations in the normal range and 37% had severe siderosis with concentrations of iron comparable to those found in idiopathic haemochromatosis. In women only 12% had severe siderosis. This iron loading is due to a high intake of iron in food and beer prepared in iron pots. The high fructose content of the diet may also contribute to the load through the formation of easily absorbable iron–fructose chelates

[437]. The average adult male Bantu has an intake of about 50–100 mg iron daily from beer and the low pH of this beverage ensures that the iron is in an ionized and absorbable form. The amount absorbed is more than enough to account for the degree of iron load found in these subjects [438]. However, changes in social conditions, and in particular the drinking of beer brewed commercially, are ensuring that 'Bantu siderosis' is becoming less common [439]. In the earliest phase of this condition haemosiderin granules are found in the parenchymal cells particularly in the periportal areas [158]. As the condition progresses, iron is found throughout the lobules and also in the Kupffer cells. Iron in the spleen is found in the macrophages in the pulp. The differentiation from idiopathic haemochromatosis is that in the latter condition reticulo-endothelial deposits are not prominent even in advanced stages. Epithelial deposits are not a significant finding. In a small proportion of advanced cases hepatic siderosis is severe and associated with cirrhotic changes and these patients may have widespread parenchymal deposits. Other rare sources of dietary iron overload are prolonged oral iron therapy [440, 441] and the generalized siderosis occurring in Manchuria due to the high iron content of water and food (Kashin–Beck disease).

Chronic iron toxicity

The precise relationship between iron overload and parenchymal damage remains a mystery [464]. Iron does not exist in tissues in the free state and its acccumulation in cells stimulates ferritin and haemosiderin formation. Such deposits are usually present for a very long time before secondary pathological changes develop. Iron given parenterally in the form of repeated transfusions usually remains localized in reticulo-endothelial cells with little toxic effect. It has been suggested that parenchymal deposits of iron arise from iron absorbed through the gut but this alone does not necessarily give rise to toxicity: adult Bantu accumulate large amounts of parenchymal iron in this way without usually developing cirrhosis. It is possible that other factors are necesssary for parenchymal damage to occur. Cirrhosis is rapidly induced in iron-overloaded animals given ethionine or a low-protein diet [442, 443]. In human subjects alcohol and malnutrition may well be precipitating factors and iron overload is thought to increase susceptibility to vitamin-E deficiency [444, 445] and increase the likelihood of a scorbutic state. Iron overload increases ascorbic-acid catabolism and, in the Bantu, can induce scurvy with secondary osteoporosis [446, 447]. The possible mechanisms of iron toxicity have been fully reviewed [464].

Acute iron toxicity

The essential ingredients leading to acute iron toxicity are a curious child who is able to walk and a bottle or box of iron tablets [448]. The likelihood of a toddler eating tablets is increased if they are attractively coloured and sugar-coated. The ideal preparation is probably an unattractive grey-coloured, unsweetened tablet individually wrapped in a foil pack so that the number removed is easily seen. Acute poisoning can be divided into four stages [448]:

Phase 1. The first symptoms appear about 30 minutes after eating the tablets—the child complains of abdominal pain and may vomit, the stomach contents are brown and may be blood-stained. This is followed by the signs and symptoms of cardiovascular collapse and there may be diarrhoea characterized by green or black stools with a watery consistency. Collapse may become profound, with 'air hunger' and coma leading to death in a few hours; 20% of children die in this phase.

Phase 2. If the patient survives the first phase, clinical improvement usually occurs as the iron is taken up by the reticulo-endothelial system. This phase lasts 10–14 hours.

Phase 3. At about eight to 24 hours after the ingestion of iron there is often a sudden severe clinical relapse with profound shock followed by coma. This is due to release of iron from the reticulo-endothelial system. The majority of deaths occur in this phase.

Phase 4. If the patient recovers from the acute toxic effects there may be late manifestations due to scarring; of the 24 survivors reported by Aldridge [448] six later developed signs of stenosis of the stomach or duodenum.

Riessmann *et al.* [449] simulated fatal iron poisoning in children by the administration of iron salts by stomach tube to rabbits and dogs. Toxic doses were rapidly absorbed and histological changes were seen even when there was a fatal outcome. Some intestinal bleeding occurred in a few instances by diapedesis from congested capillaries. Serum iron levels of several mg/dl developed within an hour and most of this was in the ferric state and not bound to transferrin. The rise in serum iron was proportional to the dose ingested and the survival time varied with the dose. Riessmann & Coleman [450] showed that a metabolic acidosis was produced and this was thought to reflect an interference with the Krebs-cycle mechanism.

A severe necrotizing gastritis occurs in virtually every case [448]. The mucosal surfaces are haemorrhagic with extensive sloughing. There is an infiltration with polymorphonuclear leucocytes and mononuclear cells, platelet thrombi are numerous in sub-mucosal capillaries and veins and both ferrous and ferric iron have been detected histochemically in the tissues. Similar changes occur in the small intestinal mucosa.

In the liver there may be cloudy swelling and haemorrhagical periportal necrosis. The presence of a coagulation defect with thrombocytopenia and hypoprothrombinemia together with the histological appearances of disseminated platelet thrombi suggest that intravascular coagulation may occur [451].

A mortality rate of 45–50% was found in the group reviewed by Aldridge [448]. Severe cases characterized by coma and shock who receive no treatment appear to have a 100% mortality [452]. The use of desferrioxamine in the treatment of acute iron poisoning has led to a considerable improvement in prognosis. Only one fatality occurred in 16 cases of accidental poisoning in children treated by Barr & Frazer [453] and this was associated with delay in the onset of specific chelation therapy. Diagnosis is based on clinical history, high serum iron, or the appearance of 'vin rosé' urine after an injection of desferrioxamine. A rapid test for excess iron in gastric fluid has been devised [454]. Gastric lavage should be carried out using one per cent sodium bicarbonate solution to neutralize gastric contents and reduce the solubility of any iron present. This should be followed by the instillation of 5 g desferrioxamine into the stomach to chelate any remaining iron and prevent further absorption. An initial intramuscular dose of desferrioxamine (1 g in children, 2 g in adults) should be given. If it is known that only two or three tablets have been taken and there are no symptoms, then further treatment may not be necessary. Whitten *et al.* [452] found that 26 patients who never manifested shock or coma survived despite the fact that chelating agents were used in four cases only. In the absence of any symptoms the severity of the iron load can be gauged by observing urine after the intramuscular dose of desferrioxamine has been given and the estimation of serum iron concentration. Red urine or a serum iron concentration in excess of 500 μg/100 ml indicates serious poisoning. If these signs are present or there are clinical symptoms an intravenous drip should be set up and desferrioxamine administered by continuous infusion at a rate not exceeding 15 mg/kg/h with a maximum dose of 80 mg/kg in 24 h. Treatment should be continued for as long as the urine remains discoloured by ferrioxamine excretion or the serum iron concentration remains greater than 200 μg/100 ml. Current estimates of mortality when treatment is instituted early are in the range of one per cent or less [455].

REFERENCES

1 WORWOOD M. (1977) The clinical biochemistry of iron. *Seminars in Hematology*, **14**, 3.

2 HALL D.O., CAMMACK R. & ROA K.K. (1974) Non-

haem iron proteins. In: *Iron in Biochemistry and Medicine* (ed. Jacobs A. & Worwood M.), p. 279. Academic Press, London.

3 JACOBS A. & WORWOOD M. (1979) Normal iron metabolism. In: *Metals and the Liver* (ed. Powell L.W.). Marcel Dekker Inc., New York.

4 MOORE C.V. & DUBACH R. (1962) Iron. In: *Mineral Metabolism*, Vol. 2B (ed. Comar C.L. & Bonner F.), p. 287. Academic Press, London.

5 JACOBS A. (1977) Iron overload—clinical and pathologic aspects. *Seminars in Hematology*, **14**, 89.

6 HARRISON P.M., CLEGG G.A. & MAY K. (1980) Ferritin: structure and function. In: *Iron in Biochemistry and Medicine II* (ed. Jacobs A. & Worwood M.), p. 131. Academic Press, London.

7 CRICHTON R.R., COLLET-CASSART D., PONCE-ORTIZ Y., WAUTERS M., ROMAN F. & PAQUES E. (1977) Ferritin: comparative structural studies, iron deposition and mobilisation. In: *Proteins of Iron Metabolism* (ed. Brown E.B., Aisen P. Fielding J. & Crichton R.R.), p. 13. Grune & Stratton, New York.

8 BANYARD S., STAMMERS D.K. & HARRISON P.M. (1978) Electron density map of apoferritin at 2·8Å resolution. *Nature (London)*, **271**, 282.

9 LEE S.S.C. & RICHTER G.W. (1976) The monomers and oligomers of ferritin and apoferritin: association and dissociation. *Biochemistry*, **15**, 65.

10 POWELL L.W., ALPERT E., ISSELBACHER K.J. & DRYSDALE J.W. (1975) Human isoferritins: organ specific iron and apoferritin distribution. *British Journal of Haematology*, **30**, 47.

11 DRYSDALE J.W. (1977) Ferritin phenotypes: structure and metabolism. In: *Iron Metabolism*, Ciba Foundation Symposium 51 (New Series). Elsevier/Excerpta Medica/North Holland, Amsterdam.

12 AROSIO P., ADELMAN T.G. & DRYSDALE J.W. (1978) On ferritin heterogeneity. Further evidence for heteropolymers. *Journal of Biological Chemistry*, **253**, 4451.

13 RUSSELL S.M., HARRISON P.M. & SHINJO S. (1978) Discrete bands in ferritin electrofocusing patterns. *British Journal of Haematology*, **38**, 296.

14 HARRISON P.M. (1977) Ferritin: an iron storage molecule. *Seminars in Hematology*, **14**, 55.

15 BOMFORD A.B. & MUNRO H.N. (1980) Biosynthesis of ferritin and isoferritins. In: *Iron in Biochemistry and Medicine II* (ed. Jacobs A. & Worwood M.), p. 173. Academic Press, London and New York.

16 MORGAN E.H. (1974) Transferrin and transferrin iron. In: *Iron in Biochemistry and Medicine* (ed. Jacobs A. & Worwood M.), p. 29. Academic Press, London.

17 MACGILLIVRAY R.T.A., MENDEZ E. & BREW K. (1977) Structure and evolution of serum transferrin. In: *Proteins of Iron Metabolism* (ed. Brown E.B., Aisen P., Fielding J. & Crichton R.R.), p. 133. Grune & Stratton, New York.

18 SPIK G. & MAZURIER J. (1977) Comparative structural and conformational studies of polypeptide chain, carbohydrate moiety and binding sites of human serotransferrin and lactoferrin. In: *Proteins of Iron Metabolism* (ed Brown E.B., Aisen P., Fielding J. & Crichton R.R.), p. 143. Grune & Stratton, New York.

19 AISEN P. (1980) The transferrins. In: *Iron in Biochemistry and Medicine II* (ed. Jacobs A. & Worwood M.), p. 87. Academic Press, London.

20 FLETCHER J. & HUEHNS E.R. (1968) Function of transferrin. *Nature (London)*, **218**, 1211.

21 WARNER R.C. & WEBER I. (1953) The metal combining properties of conalbumin. *Journal of American Chemical Society*, **75**, 5094.

22 WENN R.V. & WILLIAMS J. (1968) The isoelectric fractionation of hen's-egg ovotransferrin. *Biochemical Journal*, **198**, 69.

23 AASA R., MALMSTRÖM B.G., SALTMAN P. & VÄNNGARD T. (1963) The specific binding of iron(III) and copper(II) to transferrin and conalbumin. *Biochimica et Biophysica Acta*, **75**, 203.

24 MAKEY D.G. & SEAL U.S. (1976) The detection of four molecular forms of human transferrin during the iron-binding process. *Biochimica et Biophysica Acta*, **453**, 250.

25 AISEN P., LEIBMAN A. & ZWEIER J. (1978) Stoichiometric and site characteristics of the binding of iron to human transferrin. *Journal of Biological Chemistry*, **253**, 1930.

26 EVANS R.W. & WILLIAMS J. (1978) Studies of the binding of different iron donors to human serum transferrin and isolation of iron-binding fragments from the N- and C-terminal regions of the protein. *Biochemical Journal*, **173**, 543.

27 WILLIAMS J. & MORETON K. (1980) The distribution of iron between the metal-binding sites of transferrin in human serum. *Biochemical Journal*, **185**, 483.

28 HARRIS D.C. & AISEN P. (1975) Functional equivalence of the two iron-binding sites of human transferrin. *Nature (London)*, **257**, 821.

29 AWAI M., CHIPMAN B. & BROWN E.B. (1975) *In-vivo* evidence for the functional heterogeneity of transferrin-bound iron. I. Studies in normal rats. *Journal of Laboratory and Clinical Medicine*, **85**, 769.

30 OKADA S., JARVIS B. & BROWN E.B. (1979) *In-vivo* evidence for the functional heterogeneity of transferrin-bound iron. V. Isotransferrins: an explanation of the Fletcher-Huehns phenomenon in the rat. *Journal of Laboratory and Clinical Medicine*, **93**, 189.

31 WANG A., SUTTON H.E. & SCOTT I.D. (1967) Transferrin D$_1$: identity in Australian aborigines and American negroes. *Science*, **156**, 936.

32 TURNBULL A. & GIBLETT E.R. (1961) The binding and transport of iron by transferrin variants. *Journal of Laboratory and Clinical Medicine*, **57**, 450.

33 MASSON P.L., HEREMANS J.F. & DIVE C.H. (1966) An iron-binding protein common to many external secretions. *Clinica Chimica Acta*, **14**, 735.

34 MASSON P.L., HEREMANS J.F. & SCHONNE E. (1969) Lactoferrin, an iron binding protein in neutrophilic leucocytes. *Journal of Experimental Medicine*, **130**, 643.

35 AISEN P. & LEIBMAN A. (1972) Lactoferrin and transferrin: a comparative study. *Biochimica et Biophysica Acta*, **257**, 314.

36 KINKADE J.M. JR, KENDALL MILLER W.W. III & SEGARS G.M. (1976) Isolation and characterization of murine lactoferrin. *Biochimica et Biophysica Acta*, **446**, 407.

37 HANSEN N.E., MALMQUIST J. & THORELL J. (1975) Plasma myeloperoxidase and lactoferrin measured by radioimmunoassay: relation to neutrophil kinetics. *Acta Medica Scandinavica*, **198**, 437.

38 BENNETT R.M. & CHITRA M. (1976) A solid-phase radioimmunoassay for the measurement of lactoferrin in human plasma: variations with age, sex and disease. *Journal of Laboratory and Clinical Medicine*, **88**, 156.

39 McCANCE R.A. & WIDDOWSON E.M. (1937) Absorption and excretion of iron. *Lancet*, **i**, 680.

40 BEATON G.H. (1974) Epidemiology of iron deficiency. In: *Iron in Biochemistry and Medicine* (ed. Jacobs A. & Worwood M.), p. 477. Academic Press, London and New York.

41 FINCH C.A. (1959) Body iron exchange in man. *Journal of Clinical Investigation*, **38**, 392.

42 SAITO H., SARGENT T., PARKER H.G. & LAWRENCE J.H. (1964) Whole body iron loss in normal man measured with a Gamma spectrometer. *Journal of Nuclear Medicine*, **5**, 571.

43 GREEN R., CHARLTON R., SEFTEL H., BOTHWELL T., MAYET F., ADAMS B., FINCH C. & LAYRISSE M. (1968) Body iron excretion in man. A collaborative study. *American Journal of Medicine*, **45**, 336.

44 CAVILL I., JACOBS A., BEAMISH M. & OWEN G.M. (1969) Iron turnover in skin. *Nature (London)*, **222**, 167.

45 DAGG J.H., SMITH J.A. & GOLDBERG A. (1966) Urinary excretion of iron. *Clinical Science*, **30**, 495.

46 HALLBERG L., HÖGDAHL A.M., NILSSON L. & RYBO G. (1966) Menstrual blood loss—a population study. *Acta Obstetrica and Gynaecologica Scandinavica*, **45**, 25.

47 RYBO G. (1970) Menstrual loss of iron. In: *Iron Deficiency* (ed. Hallberg L., Harwerth H.-G. & Vannotti A.), p. 163. Academic Press, London.

48 TAYMOR M.L., STURGIS S.H. & YAHAI C. (1964) The etiological role of chronic iron deficiency in production of menorrhagia. *Journal of the American Medical Association*, **187**, 323.

49 PRITCHARD J.A. (1966) Absence of menorrhagia in induced iron deficiency anaemia. *Obstetrics and Gynaecology*, **27**, 541.

50 JACOBS A. & BUTLER E.B. (1965) Menstrual blood loss in iron deficiency anaemia. *Lancet*, **ii**, 407.

51 MOORE C.V. (1964) Iron nutrition. In: *Iron Metabolism* (ed. Gross F.). Springer-Verlag, Berlin.

52 NATIONAL FOOD SURVEY COMMITTEE (1970) *Household food consumption and expenditure: 1980.* HMSO, London.

53 DAVIES R.H., JACOBS A. & RIVLIN R. (1967) Dietary iron and haematological status in normal subjects. *British Medical Journal*, **iii**, 711.

54 BEATON G.H., THEIN M., MILNE H. & VEEN M.J. (1970) Iron requirements of menstruating women. *American Journal of Clinical Nutrition*, **23**, 275.

55 SCHULZ J. & SMITH N.J. (1968) A quantitative study of the absorption of food iron in infants and children. *Journal of Diseases of Children*, **95**, 109.

56 HUSSAIN R., WALKER R.B., LAYRISSE M., CLARK P. & FINCH C.A. (1965) Nutritive value of food iron. *American Journal of Clinical Nutrition*, **16**, 464.

57 LAYRISSE M., COOK J.D., MARTINEZ C., ROCHE M., KUHN I.N., WALKER R.B. & FINCH C.A. (1969) Food iron absorption: a comparison of vegetable and animal foods. *Blood*, **33**, 430.

58 ELWOOD P.C., NEWTON D., EAKINS H.D. & BROWN D.A. (1968) Absorption of iron from bread. *American Journal of Clinical Nutrition*, **21**, 1162.

59 CALLENDER S.T.E. (1970) Food iron utilisation. In: *Iron Deficiency* (ed. Hallberg L., Harwerth H.-G. & Vannotti A.), p. 75. Academic Press, London.

60 CHARLTON R.W., JACOBS P., SEFTEL H. & BOTHWELL T.H. (1964) Effect of alcohol on iron absorption. *British Medical Journal*, **ii**, 1427.

61 LAYRISSE M., MARTINEZ-TORRES C. & ROCHE M. (1968) Effect of interaction of various foods on iron absorption. *American Journal of Clinical Nutrition*, **21**, 1175.

62 MARTINEZ-TORRES C. & LAYRISSE M. (1970) Effect of amino acids on iron absorption from a staple vegetable food. *Blood*, **35**, 669.

63 WORLD HEALTH ORGANISATION (1970) *Requirements of ascorbic acid, vitamin D, vitamin B_{12}, folate, and iron.* Technical Reports Series No. 452, Geneva.

64 JACOBS A. & GREENMAN D.A. (1969) Availability of food iron. *British Medical Journal*, **i**, 673.

65 WRETLIND A. (1970) Food iron supply. In: *Iron Deficiency* (ed. Hallberg L., Harwerth H.-G. & Vannotti A.), p. 39. Academic Press, London.

66 ELWOOD P.C. (1963) A clinical trial of iron fortified bread. *British Medical Journal*, **i**, 224.

67 NORMAL C. (1974) FDA halts scheme to combat anaemia. *Nature (London)*, **247**, 498.

68 CROSBY W.H. (1978) The safety of iron fortified food. *Journal of the American Medical Association*, **239**, 2026.

69 PRITCHARD J.A. & SCOTT D.E. (1970) Iron demands during pregnancy. In: *Iron Deficiency* (ed. Hallberg L., Harwerth H.-G. & Vannotti A.), p. 173. Academic Press, London.

70 DE LEEUW N.K.W., LOWENSTEIN L. & HSIEH Y. (1966) Iron deficiency and hydremia in normal pregnancy. *Medicine (Baltimore)*, **45**, 291.

71 NEWTON M. (1966) Post partum hemorrhage. *American Journal of Obstetrics and Gynecology*, **94**, 711.

72 CHANARIN I. & ROTHMAN D. (1971) Further observations on the relation between iron and folate status in pregnancy. *British Medical Journal*, **ii**, 81.

73 WIDDOWSON E.M. & SPRAY C.M. (1951) Chemical development *in utero*. *Archives of Diseases of Childhood*, **26**, 205.

74 YAO A.C., MOINIAN M. & LIND J. (1969) Distribution of blood between infant and placenta after birth. *Lancet*, **ii**, 871.

75 STURGEON P. (1959) Studies of iron requirements in infants. III. Influence of supplemental iron during normal pregnancy on mother and infant. (b) The infant. *British Journal of Haematology*, **5**, 45.

76 BURMAN D. (1974) Iron metabolism in infancy and childhood. In: *Iron in Biochemistry and Medicine* (ed. Jacobs A. & Worwood M.), p. 543. Academic Press, London.

77 SJÖLIN S. & WRANNE L. (1968) Iron requirements during infancy and childhood. In: *Occurrence, Causes and Prevention of Nutritional Anaemias* (ed. Blix G.), p. 148. Swedish Nutrition Foundation.

78 LINTZEL W., RECHENBERGER J. & SCHAIRER E. (1944) Uber den Eizenstofweksel des Neugeborenen und des Säuglings. *Zeitschrift Gesamte Experimentalle Medizin*, **113**, 591.

79 GARBY L., SJÖLIN S. & VUILLE J.-C. (1963) Studies on erythrokinetics in infancy. III. Disappearance from

plasma and red cell uptake of radioactive iron injected intravenously. *Acta Paediatrica*, **52**, 537.

80 SMITH C.A., CHERRY R.B., MALETSKOS C.J., GIBSON J.G. II, ROBY C.C., CATON W.L. & REID D.E. (1955) Persistence and utilisation of maternal iron for blood formation during infancy. *Journal of Clinical Investigation*, **34**, 1391.

81 OETTINGER L., MILLS W.B. & HAHN P.F. (1954) Iron absorption in premature and full term infants. *Journal of Paediatrics*, **45**, 302.

82 GARBY L. & SJÖLIN S. (1959) Absorption of labelled iron in infants less than three months old. *Acta Paediatrica*, **48** (Suppl. 117), 24.

83 GORTEN M.K., HEPNER R. & WORKMAN J.B. (1963) Iron metabolism in premature infants. I. Absorption and utilisation of iron as measured by isotope studies. *Journal of Paediatrics*, **63**, 1063.

84 HEINRICH H.C. (1970) Intestinal iron absorption in man. In: *Iron Deficiency* (ed. Hallberg L., Harwerth H.-G. & Vannotti A.), p. 213. Academic Press, London.

85 MOE P.J. (1963) Iron requirements in infancy. *Acta Paediatrica* (Suppl.), **150**.

86 AMERICAN ACADEMY OF PEDIATRICS (1969) Committee on nutrition. Iron balance and requirements in infancy. *Pediatrics*, **43**, 134.

87 MOE P.J. (1964) Iron requirements in infancy. II. The influence of iron fortified cereals given during the first year of life, on the red blood picture of children at $1\frac{1}{2}$–3 years of age. *Acta Paediatrica*, **53**, 423.

88 LEONARD P.J. (1954) Hypochromic anaemia in RAF recruits. *Lancet*, **i**, 899.

89 BRUMFITT W. (1960) Primary iron deficiency anaemia in young men. *Quarterly Journal of Medicine*, **29**, 1.

90 TASKER P.W.G. (1961) Blood loss from hookworm infection. *Transactions of the Royal Society of Tropical Medicine and Hygiene*, **5**, 36.

91 BOTHWELL T.H., CHARLTON R.W., COOK J.D. & FINCH C.A. (1979) *Iron Metabolism in Man*. Blackwell Scientific Publications, Oxford.

92 SMITH M.D. & PANNACCUILLI I.M. (1958) Absorption of inorganic iron from graded doses: its significance in relation to iron absorption tests and the mucosal block theory. *British Journal of Haematology*, **4**, 428.

93 BRISE H. (1962) Influence of meals on iron absorption in oral iron therapy. *Acta Medica Scandinavica*, **171** (Suppl.), 376.

94 JACOBS A. & MILES P.M. (1969) Intraluminal transport of iron from stomach to small intestinal mucosa. *British Medical Journal*, **iv**, 778.

95 APTE S.V. & VENKATACHALAM P.S. (1964) The influence of dietary calcium on absorption of iron. *Indian Journal of Medical Research*, **52**, 213.

96 HUSSAIN R. & PATWARDHAN V.N. (1959) The influence of phytate on the absorption of iron. *Indian Journal of Medical Research*, **47**, 676.

97 KUHN I.N., LAYRISSE M., ROCHE M., MARTINEZ C. & WALKER R.B. (1968) Observations on the mechanism of iron absorption. *American Journal of Clinical Nutrition*, **21**, 1184.

98 MINNICH V., OKCUOĞLU A., TARCON Y., ARCASOY A., CIN S., YÖRÜKOĞLU O., RENDA F. & DEMIRAĞ B. (1968) Pica in Turkey. II. Effect of clay upon iron absorption. *American Journal of Clinical Nutrition*, **21**, 78.

99 FREEMAN S. & IVY A.C. (1942) The influence of antacids upon iron retention by the anaemic rat. *American Journal of Physiology*, **137**, 706.

100 GREENBERGER N.J., RUPPERT R.D. & CUPPAGE F.E. (1967) Inhibition of intestinal iron transport induced by tetracycline. *Gastroenterology*, **53**, 590.

101 NEUVONEN P.J., GOTHONI G., HACKMAN R. & BJÖRKSTEN K. (1970) Interference of iron with the absorption of tetracyclines in man. *British Medical Journal*, **iv**, 532.

102 DISLER P.B., LYNCH S.R., CHARLTON R.W., TORRANCE J.D., BOTHWELL T.H., WALKER R.B. & MAYET F. (1975) The effect of tea on iron absorption. *Gut*, **16**, 193.

103 GOLDBERG A., LOCHHEAD A.C. & DAGG J.H. (1963) Histamine-fast achlorhydria and iron absorption. *Lancet*, **i**, 848.

104 JACOBS P., BOTHWELL T. & CHARLTON R.W. (1964) Role of hydrochloric acid on iron absorption. *Journal of Applied Physiology*, **19**, 187.

105 JACOBS A. (1970) Digestive factors in iron absorption. In: *Progress in Gastroenterology*, Vol. II (ed. Glass G.B.J.), p. 221. Grune & Stratton, New York.

106 HUEBERS H. (1979) Die enterale Resorption von Transferrin-Eisen: Bedeutung für die Eisenresorption. Inauguraldissertation zur Erlangung der Doktorwürde. Universität des Saarlandes.

107 COX T.M., MAZURIER J., SPIK G., MONTREUIL J. & PETERS T.J. (1979) Iron binding proteins and influx of iron across the duodenal brush border. Evidence for specific lactotransferrin receptors in the human intestine. *Biochima et Biophysica Acta*, **588**, 120.

108 GLOVER J. & JACOBS A. (1971) Observations on the jejunal lumen after a standard meal. *Gut*, **12**, 369.

109 MURRAY M.J. & STEIN N. (1966) Does the pancreas influence iron absorption? *Gastroenterology*, **51**, 694.

110 CONRAD M.E., BENJAMIN B.I., WILLIAMS H.L. & FOY A.L. (1967) Human absorption of haemoglobin iron. *Gastroenterology*, **53**, 5.

111 DOWDLE E.B., SCHACHTER D. & SCHENKER H. (1960) Active tranport of ^{59}Fe by everted segments of rat duodenum. *American Journal of Physiology*, **198**, 609.

112 JACOBS P., BOTHWELL T.H. & CHARLTON R.W. (1966) Intestinal iron transport: studies using a loop of gut with an artificial circulation. *American Journal of Physiology*, **210**, 694.

113 MANIS J.G. & SCHACHTER D. (1962) Active transport of iron by intestine: features of the two-step mechanism. *American Journal of Physiology*, **203**, 73.

114 GITLIN D. & CRUCHARD A. (1962) On the kinetics of iron absorption in mice. *Journal of Clinical Investigation*, **41**, 344.

115 SHEEHAN R.G. (1976) Unidirectional uptake of iron across intestinal brush border. *American Journal of Physiology*, **231**, 1438.

116 SAVIN M.A. & COOK J.D. (1978) Iron transport by isolated rat intestinal mucosal cells. *Gastroenterology*, **75**, 688.

117 ACHESON A. & SCHULTZ S.G. (1972) Iron influx across the brush border of rabbit duodenum: effects of anaemia and iron loading. *Biochima et Biophysica Acta*, **255**, 479.

118 GREENBERGER N.J., BALCERZAK S.P. & ACKERMAN G.A. (1969) Iron uptake by isolated brush borders: changes

induced by alterations in iron stores. *Journal of Laboratory and Clinical Medicine*, **73**, 711.

119 KIMBER C.L., MUKHERJEE T. & DELLER D.J. (1973) *In-vitro* iron attachment to the intestinal brush border: effect of iron stores and other environmental factors. *American Journal of Digestive Diseases*, **18**, 781.

120 RICHMOND V.S., WORWOOD M. & JACOBS A. (1972) The iron content of intestinal epithelial cells and its subcellular distribution: studies on normal, iron-loaded and iron-deficient rats. *British Journal of Haematology*, **23**, 605.

121 HUEBERS H., HUEBERS E., SIMON J. & FORTH W. (1971) A method for preparing stable density gradients and their application for fractionation of intestinal mucosal cells. *Life Sciences*, **10** (Part II), 377.

122 WORWOOD M. & JACOBS A. (1971) The subcellular distribution of orally administered ^{59}Fe in rat small intestinal mucosa. *British Journal of Haematology*, **20**, 587.

123 HUEBERS H., HUEBERS E., FORTH W. & RUMMEL W. (1971) Binding of iron to a non-ferritin protein in the mucosal cells of normal and iron-deficient rats during absorption. *Life Sciences*, **10** (Part I), 1141.

124 WORWOOD M. & JACOBS A. (1971) Absorption of ^{59}Fe in the rat: iron binding substances in the soluble fraction of intestinal mucosa. *Life Sciences*, **10** (Part I), 1363.

125 HALLIDAY J.W., POWELL L.W. & MACK U. (1976) Iron absorption in the rat: the search for possible intestinal mucosal carriers. *British Journal of Haematology*, **34**, 237.

126 HEUBERS H., HEUBERS E., RUMMEL W. & CRICHTON R.R. (1976) Isolation and characterization of iron-binding proteins from rat intestinal mucosa. *European Journal of Biochemistry*, **66**, 447.

127 BÉDARD Y.C., PINKERTON P.H. & SIMON G.T. (1971) Radio autographic observations on iron absorption by the normal mouse duodenum. *Blood*, **38**, 232.

128 BÉDARD Y.C., PINKERTON P.H. & SIMON G.T. (1973) Radioautographic observations on iron absorption by the duodenum of mice with iron overload, iron deficiency and X-linked anemia. *Blood*, **42**, 131.

129 HUMPHRYS J., WALPOLE B. & WORWOOD M. (1977) Intracellular iron transport in rat intestinal epithelium: biochemical and ultrastructural observations. *British Journal of Haematology*, **36**, 209.

130 HOPKINS J.M.P. & PETERS T.J. (1979) Subcellular distribution of radio-labelled iron during intestinal absorption of guinea-pig enterocytes with special reference to the mitochondrial localization of the iron. *Clinical Science*, **56**, 179.

131 THOMSON A.B.R. & VALBERG L.S. (1972) Intestinal uptake of iron cobalt and manganese in the iron-deficient rat. *American Journal of Physiology*, **223**, 1327.

132 LEVINE P.H., LEVINE A.J. & WEINTRAUB L. (1972) The role of transferrin in the control of iron absorption: studies on a cellular level. *Journal of Laboratory and Clinical Medicine*, **80**, 333.

133 JACOBS P., BOTHWELL T.W. & CHARLTON R.W. (1966) Internal iron transport: studies using a loop of gut with an artificial circulation. *American Journal of Physiology*, **210**, 697.

134 HELBOCK H.J. & SALTMAN P. (1967) The transport of iron by rat intestine. *Biochima et Biophysica Acta*, **135**, 979.

135 CONRAD M.E., WEINTRAUB L.R., SEARS D.A. & CROSBY W.H. (1966) Absorption of hemoglobin iron. *American Journal of Physiology*, **211**, 1123.

136 RAFFIN S.B., WOO C.H., ROOST K.T., PRICE D.C. & SCHMID R. (1974) Intestinal absorption of hemoglobin iron-heme cleavage by mucosal heme oxygenase. *Journal of Clinical Investigation*, **54**, 1344.

137 BANNERMAN R.M. (1965) Quantitative aspects of hemoglobin-iron absorption. *Journal of Laboratory and Clinical Medicine*, **65**, 944.

138 CROSBY W.H. (1963) The control of iron balance by the intestinal mucosa. *Blood*, **22**, 441.

139 PINKERTON P.H. (1969) Control of iron absorption by the intestinal epithelial cell: review and hypothesis. *Annals of Internal Medicine*, **70**, 401.

140 JACOBS A. (1973) The mechanisms of iron absorption. In: *Clinics in Haematology*, Vol. 2 (ed. Callender S.T.), p. 323. W.B. Saunders, London.

141 CONRAD M.W., WEINTRAUB L.R. & CROSBY W.H. (1964) The role of the intestine in iron kinetics. *Journal of Clinical Investigation*, **43**, 963.

142 WEINTRAUB L.R., CONRAD M.E. & CROSBY W.H. (1964) The significance of iron turnover in the control of iron absorption. *Blood*, **24**, 19.

143 BALCERZAK S.P. & GREENBERGER M.J. (1968) Iron content of isolated intestinal epithelial cells to iron absorption. *Nature (London)*, **220**, 270.

144 MATTII R., MIELKE C.H. JR, LEVINE P.H. & CROSBY W.B. (1973) Iron in the duodenal mucosa of normal, iron-loaded and iron-deficient rats. *Blood*, **42**, 959.

145 CAVILL I., WORWOOD M. & JACOBS A. (1975) Internal regulation of iron absorption. *Nature (London)*, **256**, 328.

146 MENDEL G.A. (1961) Studies on iron absorption. I. The relationships between the rate of erythropoiesis, hypoxia and iron absorption. *Blood*, **18**, 727.

147 SCHIFFER L.M., PRICE D.C. & CRONKITE E.P. (1965) Iron absorption and anemia. *Journal of Laboratory and Clinical Medicine*, **65**, 316.

148 HEINRICH H.C., GABBE E.E., OPPITZ K.H., WHANG D.H., BENDER-GÖTZE C., SCHÄFER K.H., SCHRÖTER W. & PFAU A.A. (1973) Absorption of inorganic and food iron in children with heterozygous and homozygous β-thalassaemia. *Zeitschrift Kinderheit*, **115**, 1.

149 CAVILL I., RICKETTS C., JACOBS A. & LETSKY E. (1978) Erythropoiesis and the effect of transfusion in homozygous β-thalassemia. *New England Journal of Medicine*, **298**, 776.

150 BOTHWELL T.H., HURTADO A.V., DONOHUE D.M. & FINCH C.A. (1957) Erythrokinetics. IV. The plasma iron turnover as a measure of erythropoiesis. *Blood*, **12**, 409.

151 AWAI M. & BROWN E.G. (1963) Studies of metabolism of I^{131}-labelled human transferrin. *Journal of Laboratory and Clinical Medicine*, **61**, 363.

152 CAVILL I., RICKETTS C. & JACOBS A. (1979) Erythropoiesis, iron stores and tissue iron exchange in man. *Clinical Science*, **56**, 223.

153 CHENEY B.A., LOTHE K., MORGAN E.H., FOOD S.K. & FINCH C.A. (1967) Internal iron exchange in the rat. *American Journal of Physiology*, **212**, 376.

154 COOKE J.D., MARSAGLIA G., ESCHBACH J.W., FUNK

D.D. & FINCH C.A. (1970) Ferrokinetics: a biologic model for plasma iron exchange in man. *Journal of Clinical Investigation*, **49**, 197.

155 HOSAIN F. & FINCH C.A. (1964) Ferrokinetics: a study of transport iron in plasma. *Journal of Laboratory and Clinical Medicine*, **64**, 905.

156 SARKAR B. (1970) State of iron(III) in normal serum: low molecular weight and protein ligands besides transferrin. *Canadian Journal of Biochemistry*, **48**, 1339.

157 HERSHKO C., GRAHAM G., BATES G.W. & RACHMILE-WITZ E.A. (1978) Non-specific serum iron in thalassaemia: an abnormal serum iron fraction of potential toxicity. *British Journal of Haematology*, **40**, 255.

158 BOTHWELL T.H. & FINCH C.A. (1962) *Iron Metabolism*. Churchill, London.

159 JACOBS A., WATERS W.E., CAMPBELL H. & BARROW A. (1969) A random sample from Wales. III. Serum iron, iron binding capacity and transferrin saturation. *British Journal of Haematology*, **17**, 581.

160 VERLOOP M.C., BLOKHUIS E.W.M. & BOS C.C. (1959) Causes of the differences in haemoglobin and serum iron between men and women. *Acta Haematologica*, **21**, 199.

161 STURGEON P. (1954) Studies of iron requirements in infants and children. I. Normal values for serum iron, copper and free erythrocyte protoporphyrin. *Paediatrics*, **13**, 107.

162 BOWIE E.J.W., TAUXE W.N., SJOBERG W.E. & YAMAGUCHI M.Y. (1963) Daily variation in the concentration of iron in serum. *American Journal of Clinical Pathology*, **40**, 491.

163 BOTHWELL T.H. & MALLETT B. (1955) Diurnal variation in the turnover of iron through the plasma. *Clinical Science*, **14**, 235.

164 FUNK O.D. (1970) Plasma iron turnover in normal subjects. *Journal of Nuclear Medicine*, **11**, 107.

165 CARTWRIGHT G.E. (1966) The anaemia of chronic disorders. *Seminars in Haematology*, **3**, 351.

166 CARTWRIGHT G.E. & LEE G.R. (1971) The anaemia of chronic disorders. *British Journal of Haematology*, **21**, 147.

167 BURTON J.L. (1967) Effect of oral contraceptives on haemoglobin, packed cell volume, serum iron, and total iron binding capacity in healthy women. *Lancet*, **i**, 978.

168 MORGAN E.H. (1962) Factors regulating plasma total iron binding capacity in rat and rabbit. *Quarterly Journal of Experimental Physiology*, **47**, 57.

169 MORGAN E.H. (1970) Effect of hypoxia on serum concentration of transferrin and other serum proteins in human subjects. *Journal of Laboratory and Clinical Medicine*, **75**, 1006.

170 WEINFELD A. (1964) Storage iron in man. *Acta Medica Scandinavica* (Suppl.), 427.

171 MORTON A.G. & TAVILL A.S. (1977) The role of iron in the regulation of hepatic transferrin synthesis. *British Journal of Haematology*, **36**, 383.

172 HEILMEYER L., KELER W., VIVELL W., KEIDERLING W., BETKE K., WOHTER F. & SCHULZE A.G. (1961) Congenital transferrin deficiency in a seven year old girl. *German Medical Monthly*, **6**, 385.

173 GOYA N., MIYAZAKI S., KODATE S. & USHIO B. (1972) A family of congenital atransferrinemia. *Blood*, **40**, 239.

174 BOTHWELL T.H., PRIBILLA W.F., MEBUST W. & FINCH C.A. (1958) Iron metabolism in the pregnant rabbit. Iron transport across the placenta. *American Journal of Physiology*, **193**, 615.

175 LAURELL C.-B. (1947) Studies of transportation and metabolism of iron in the body. *Acta Physiological Scandinavica*, **14** (Suppl.), 46.

176 FLETCHER J. & SUTER P.E.N. (1969) The transport of iron by the human placenta. *Clinical Science*, **36**, 209.

177 KAUFMAN N. & WYLLIE J.C. (1970) Materno-foetal iron transfer in the rat. *British Journal of Haematology*, **19**, 515.

178 CAVILL I. & RICKETTS C. (1974) The kinetics of iron metabolism. In: *Iron in Biochemistry and Medicine* (ed. Jacobs A. & Worwood M.), p. 613. Academic Press, London.

179 HUFF R.L., HENNESSEY T.G., AUSTIN R.E., GARCIA J.F., ROBERTS B.M. & LAWRENCE J.H. (1950) Plasma and red cell iron turnover in normal subjects and in patients having various hematopoietic disorders. *Journal of Clinical Investigation*, **29**, 1041.

180 POLLYCOVE M. & MORTIMER R. (1961) The quantitative determination of iron kinetics and haemoglobin synthesis in human subjects. *Journal of Clinical Investigation*, **40**, 753.

181 POLYCOVE M. & MAQSOOD M. (1962) Existence of an erythropoietic labile iron pool in animals. *Nature (London)*, **194**, 152.

182 RICKETTS C., JACOBS A. & CAVILL I. (1975) Ferrokinetics and erythropoiesis in man: the measurement of effective erythropoiesis, ineffective erythropoiesis and red cell lifespan using ^{59}Fe. *British Journal of Haematology*, **31**, 65.

183 RICKETTS C., CAVILL I., NAPIER J.A.F. & JACOBS A. (1977) Ferrokinetics and erythropoiesis in man: an evaluation of ferrokinetic measurements. *British Journal of Haematology*, **35**, 41.

184 CAVILL I. & RICKETTS C. (1980) Human iron kinetics. In: *Iron in Biochemistry and Medicine II* (ed. Jacobs A. & Worwood M.), p. 573. Academic Press, London.

185 VAN DYKE T. & ANGER H.O. (1965) Patterns of marrow hypertrophy and atrophy in man. *Journal of Nuclear Medicine*, **6**, 109.

186 BRUCE-TAGOE A.A., HOFFBRAND A.V., SHORT M.D. & SZUR L. (1973) 52 studies of the effects of treatment on erythropoiesis in megaloblastic anaemia. *British Journal of Haematology*, **25**, 341.

187 ALFREY C.P., LYNCH E.C. & HETTIG R.A. (1969) Studies of iron kinetics using a linear scanner. I. Distribution of sites of uptake of plasma iron in haematological disorders. *Journal of Laboratory and Clinical Medicine*, **73**, 405.

188 NOYES W.D., BOTHWELL T.H. & FINCH C.A. (1960) The role of the reticulo-endothelial cell in iron metabolism. *British Journal of Haematology*, **6**, 43.

189 BEAMISH M.R., DAVIES A.G., EAKINS J.D., JACOBS A. & TREVETT D. (1971) The measurement of reticulo-endothelial iron release using iron dextran. *British Journal of Haematology*, **21**, 617.

190 BENTLEY D.P., CAVILL I., RICKETTS C. & PEAKE S. (1979) A method for the investigation of reticulo-endothelial iron kinetics in man. *British Journal of Haematology*, **43**, 619.

191 NUNEZ M.T., GLASS J., FISCHER S., LAVIDOR L.M.,

LENK E.M. & ROBINSON S.H. (1977) Transferrin receptors in developing murine erythroid cells. *British Journal of Haematology*, **36**, 519.

192 VAN BOCKXMEER F. & MORGAN E.H. (1979) Transferrin receptors during rabbit reticulocyte maturation. *Biochimica et Biophysica Acta*, **584**, 76.

193 VAN BOCKXMEER F. & MORGAN E.H. (1977) Indentification of transferrin receptors in reticulocytes. *Biochimica et Biophysica Acta*, **468**, 437.

194 MORGAN E.H. & APPLETON T.C. (1969) Autoradiographic localization of ^{125}I-labelled transferrin in rabbit reticulocytes. *Nature (London)*, **223**, 1371.

195 SULLIVAN A.L., GRASSO J.A. & WEINTRAUB L.R. (1976) Micropinocytosis of transferrin by developing red cells: an electron microscopic study utilizing ferritin conjugated transferrin and ferritin conjugated antibodies to transferrin. *Blood*, **47**, 133.

196 MORGAN E.H. (1971) A study of iron transfer from rabbit transferrin to reticulocytes using synthetic chelating agents. *Biochimica et Biophysica Acta*, **244**, 103.

197 HEMMAPLARDH D. & MORGAN E.H. (1974) The mechanism of iron exchange between synthetic iron chelators and rabbit reticulocytes. *Biochimica et Biophysica Acta*, **373**, 84.

198 AISEN P. & BROWN E.B. (1975) Structure and function of transferrin. *Progress in Hematology*, **9**, 25.

199 WONG C.T. & MORGAN E.H. (1974) Source of foetal iron in the cat. *Australian Journal of Experimental Biology and Medical Science*, **52**, 413.

200 GARDINER M.E. & MORGAN E.H. (1974) Transferrin and iron uptake by the liver in the rat. *Australian Journal of Experimental Biology and Medical Science*, **52**, 723.

201 BEAMISH M.R., KEAY L., OKIGAKI T. & BROWN E.B. (1975) Uptake of transferrin-bound iron by rat cells in tissue culture. *British Journal of Haematology*, **31**, 479.

202 GROHLICH D., MORLEY C.G.D., MILLER R.J. & BEZKOROVAINY A. (1977) Iron incorporation into isolated rat hepatocytes. *Biochemical and Biophysical Research Communications*, **76**, 682.

203 HERSHKO C., COOK J.D. & FINCH C.A. (1973) Storage iron kinetics. III. Study of desferrioxamine action by selective radioiron labels of RE and parenchymal cells. *Journal of Laboratory and Clinical Medicine*, **81**, 876.

204 MACDONALD R.A., MACSWEEN R.M.N. & PECHET G.S. (1969) Iron metabolism by reticuloendothelial cells *in vitro*. Physical and chemical conditions. Lipotrope deficiency and acute inflammation. *Laboratory Investigation*, **21**, 236.

205 SUMMERS M.R. & JACOBS A. (1976) Iron uptake and ferritin synthesis by peripheral blood leucocytes from normal subjects and patients with iron deficiency and the anaemia of chronic disease. *British Journal of Haematology*, **34**, 221.

206 HEMMAPLARDH D. & MORGAN E.H. (1974) Transferrin and iron uptake by human cells in culture. *Experimental Cell Research*, **87**, 207.

207 O'SHEA M.J., KERSHENOBICH D. & TAVILL A.S. (1973) Effects of inflammation on iron and transferrin metabolism. *British Journal of Haematology*, **25**, 707.

208 KARABUS C.D. & FIELDING J. (1967) Desferrioxamine chelatable iron in haemolytic, megaloblastic and sideroblastic anaemias. *British Journal of Haematology*, **13**, 924.

209 LIPSCHITZ D.A., DUGARD J., SIMON M.O., BOTHWELL T.H. & CHARLTON R.W. (1971) The site of action of desferrioxamine. *British Journal of Haematology*, **20**, 395.

210 JACOBS A. (1977) An intracellular transit iron pool. In: *Iron Metabolism* (ed. Fitzsimmons D.W.), p. 91. Ciba Foundation Symposium No. 51.

211 BARTLETT G.R. (1976) Iron nucleotides in human and rat red cells. *Biochemical and Biophysical Research Communications*, **70**, 1063.

212 MAY P.M. & WILLIAMS D.R. (1980) The inorganic chemistry of iron metabolism. In: *Iron in Biochemistry and Medicine II* (ed. Jacobs A. & Worwood M.). Academic Press, London.

213 BATES G.W., BILLUPS C. & SALTMAN P. (1967) The kinetics and mechanism of iron(III) exchange between chelates and transferrin. *Journal of Biological Chemistry*, **242**, 2810.

214 MILLER J.P.G. & PERKINS D.J. (1969) Model experiments for the study of iron transfer from transferrin to ferritin. *European Journal of Biochemistry*, **10**, 146.

215 ROMSLO I. (1980) Intracellular iron transport. In: *Iron in Biochemistry and Medicine II* (ed. Jacobs A. & Worwood M.), p. 325. Academic Press, London.

216 DOUGLAS A.S. & DACIE J.V. (1953) The incidence and significance of iron containing granules in human erythrocytes and their precursors. *Journal of Clinical Pathology*, **6**, 307.

217 BESSIS M.C. & BRETON-GORIUS J. (1962) Iron metabolism in the bone marrow as seen by electron microscopy. A critical review. *Blood*, **19**, 635.

218 MATIOLI G.T. & EYLAR E.H. (1964) The biosynthesis of apoferritin by reticulocytes. *Proceedings of the National Academy of Sciences, USA*, **52**, 508.

219 KONIJN A.M., HERSHKO C. & IZAK G. (1979) Ferritin synthesis and iron uptake in developing erythroid cells. *American Journal of Hematology*, **6**, 373.

220 WORWOOD M., AHERNE W., DAWKINS S. & JACOBS A. (1975) The characteristics of ferritin from human tissues, serum and blood cells. *Clinical Science and Molecule Medicine*, **48**, 441.

221 GABUZDA T.G. & PEARSON J. (1969) Metabolic and molecular heterogeneity of marrow ferritin. *Biochimica et Biophysica Acta*, **194**, 50.

222 MAZUR A. & CARLETON A. (1963) Relation of ferritin iron to heme synthesis in marrow and reticulocytes. *Journal of Biological Chemistry*, **238**, 1817.

223 NUNEZ M.T., GLASS J. & ROBINSON S.H. (1978) Mobilization of iron from the plasma membrane of the murine reticulocyte. The role of ferritin. *Biochimica et Biophysica Acta*, **509**, 170.

224 SPEYER B.E. & FIELDING J. (1979) Ferritin as a cytosol iron transport intermediate in human reticulocytes. *British Journal of Haematology*, **42**, 255.

225 ZAIL S.S., CHARLTON R.W., TORRANCE J.D. & BOTHWELL T.H. (1964) Studies on the formation of ferritin in red cell precursors. *Journal of Clinical Investigation*, **43**, 670.

226 PRIMOSIGH J.V. & THOMAS E.D. (1968) Studies on the partition of iron in bone marrow cells. *Journal of Clinical Investigation*, **47**, 1473.

227 BOROVA J., PONKA P. & NEUWIRT J. (1973) Study of intracellular iron distribution in rabbit reticulocytes with normal and inhibited heme synthesis. *Biochimica et Biophysica Acta*, **320**, 143.

228 ALLEN D.W. & JANOL J.H. (1960) Kinetics of intracellular iron in rabbit recticulocytes. *Blood*, **15**, 71.

229 GREENOUGH W.B., PETERS T. & THOMAS E.D. (1962) An intracellular protein intermediate for hemoglobin formation. *Journal of Clinical Investigation*, **41**, 1116.

230 JONES M.S. & JONES O.T.G. (1969) The structural organization of haem synthesis in rat liver mitochondria. *Biochemical Journal*, **113**, 507.

231 BISSELL D.M. (1975) Formation and elimination of bilirubin. *Gastroenterology*, **69**, 519.

232 SMITH A. & MORGAN W.T. (1979) Haem transport to the liver by haemopexin. Receptor-mediated uptake with recycling of the protein. *Biochemical Journal*, **182**, 47.

233 KORNFELD S., CHIPMAN B. & BROWN E.B. (1969) Intracellular catabolism of hemoglobin and iron dextran by rat liver. *Journal of Laboratory and Clinical Medicine*, **73**, 181.

234 TENHUNEN R., MARVER H.S. & SCHMID R. (1969) Microsomal heme oxygenase. Characterization of the enzyme. *Journal of Biological Chemistry*, **244**, 6388.

235 TENHUNEN R., ROSS M.E., MARVER H.S. & SCHMID R. (1970) Reduced nicotinamide-adenine dinucleotide phosphate dependent biliverdin reductase: partial purification and characterization. *Biochemistry*, **9**, 298.

236 MAINES M.D. & KAPPAS A. (1974) Cobalt induction of hepatic heme oxygenase; with evidence that cytochrome P-450 is not essential for this enzyme activity. *Proceedings of the National Academy of Sciences, USA*, **71**, 4293.

237 YOSHIDA T., TAKAHASHI S. & KIKUCHI G. (1974) Partial purification and reconstitution of the heme oxygenase system from pig spleen microsomes. *Journal of Biochemistry*, **75**, 1187.

238 PIMSTONE N.R., TENHUNEN R., SERTZ P.T., MARVER H.S. & SCHMID R. (1971) The enzymatic degradation of hemoglobin to bile pigments by macrophages. *Journal of Experimental Medicine*, **13**, 1264.

239 JACKSON A.H. (1974) Haem catabolism. In: *Iron in Biochemistry and Medicine* (ed. Jacobs A. & Worwood M.), p. 145. Academic Press, London.

240 DELEEUW N.K.M. & LOWENSTEIN L. (1966) The effect of intramuscular iron therapy on haematological values in normal men and women. *Canadian Medical Association Journal*, **95**, 554.

241 HASKINS D., STEVENS A.R., FINCH S. & FINCH C.A. (1952) Iron metabolism. Iron stores in man as measured by plebotomy. *Journal of Clinical Investigation*, **31**, 543.

242 TORRANCE J.D., CHARLTON R.W., SCHAMAN A., LYNCH S.R. & BOTHWELL T.H. (1968) Storage iron in muscle. *Journal of Clinical Pathology*, **21**, 495.

243 TRUBOWITZ S., MILLER W.L. & SAMORA J.C. (1970) The quantitative estimation of non-heme iron in human marrow aspirates. *American Journal of Clinical Pathology*, **54**, 71.

244 BARRY M. & SHERLOCK S. (1971) Measurement of liver-iron concentration in needle biopsy specimens. *Lancet*, **i**, 100.

245 GALE E., TORRANCE J. & BOTHWELL T. (1963) The quantitative estimation of total iron stores in human bone marrow. *Journal of Clinical Investigation*, **42**, 1076.

246 DACIE J.V. & LEWIS S.M. (1975) *Practical Haematology*, 5th edn. Churchill, London.

247 CONRAD M.E. & CROSBY W.H. (1962) The natural history of iron deficiency induced by phlebotomy. *Blood*, **20**, 173.

248 HARKER L.A., FUNK D.D. & FINCH C.A. (1961) Evaluation of storage iron by chelates. *American Journal of Medicine*, **45**, 105.

249 BAINTON D.F. & FINCH C.A. (1964) The diagnosis of iron deficiency anemia. *American Journal of Medicine*, **37**, 62.

250 WOHLER F. (1964) Diagnosis of iron storage diseases with desferrioxamine (Desferal test). *Acta Haematologica*, **32**, 321.

251 FIELDING J. (1965) Differential ferrioxamine test for measuring chelatable body iron. *Journal of Clinical Pathology*, **18**, 88.

252 HALLBERG L. & HEDENBURG L. (1967) Desferrioxamine-induced urinary iron excretion in normal and iron deficient subjects. *Scandinavian Journal of Haematology*, **4**, 11.

253 BALCERZAK S.P., WESTERMAN M.P., HEINLE E.W. & TAYLOR F.H. (1968) Measurement of iron stores using deferoxamine. *Annals of Internal Medicine*, **68**, 518.

254 ADDISON G.M., BEAMISH M.R., HALES C.N., HODGKINS M., JACOBS A. & LLEWELLIN P. (1972) An immunoradiometric assay for ferritin in the serum of normal subjects and patients with iron deficiency and iron overload. *Journal of Clinical Pathology*, **25**, 326.

255 REISSMANN K.R. & DIETRICH M.R. (1956) On the presence of ferritin in the peripheral blood of patients with hepatocellular disease. *Journal of Clinical Investigation*, **35**, 588.

256 MILES L.E.M., LIPSCHITZ D.A., BIEBER C.P. & COOK J.D. (1974) Measurement of serum ferritin by a 2-site immunoradiometric assay. *Analytical Biochemistry*, **61**, 209.

257 WORWOOD M. (1980) Serum ferritin. In: *Methods in Hematology* (ed. Cook J.), p. 59. Churchill Livingstone, New York.

258 WORWOOD M. (1979) Serum ferritin. *Critical Reviews in Clinical and Laboratory Sciences*, **10**, 171.

259 WORWOOD M. (1980) Serum ferritin. In: *Iron in Biochemistry and Medicine II* (ed. Jacobs A. & Worwood M.), p. 203. Academic Press, London.

260 WALTERS G.O., MILLER F.M. & WORWOOD M. (1973) Serum ferritin concentration and iron stores in normal subjects. *Journal of Clinical Pathology*, **26**, 770.

261 WORWOOD M., CRAGG S.J., JACOBS A., McLAREN C., RICKETTS C. & ECONOMIDOU J. (1980) Binding of serum ferritin to concanavalin A: patients with homyzgous β thalasaemia and transfusional iron overload. *British Journal of Haematology*, **46**, 409.

262 ALJAMA P., WARD M.K., PIERIDES A.M., EASTHAM E.J., ELLIS H.A., FEEST T.G., CONCEICAO S. & KERR D.N.S. (1978) Serum ferritin concentration: a reliable guide to iron overload in uremic and hemodialyzed patients. *Clinical Nephrology*, **10**, 101.

263 HOFMAN V., DESCOEUDRES C., MONTANDON A., GALEAZZI R.L. & STRAUB P.W. (1978) Serumferritin bei Neireninsuffizienz Hämodialyse und nach Neiretransplantation. *Schweizerische Medizinische Wochenschrift*, **108**, 1835.

264 HUSSEIN S., PRIETO J., O'SHEA M., HOFFBRAND A.V., BAILLOD R.A. & MOORHEAD J.F. (1975) Serum ferritin assay and iron status in chronic renal failure and haemodialysis. *British Medical Journal*, i, 546.

265 MIRAHMADI K.S., PAUL W.L., WINER R.L., DABIR-VAZIRI N., BYER B., GORMAN J.T. & ROSEN S.M. (1977) Determinant of iron requirement in hemodialysis patients. *Journal of the American Medical Association*, **238**, 601.

266 PRIETO J., BARRY M. & SHERLOCK S. (1975) Serum ferritin in patients with iron overload and with acute and chronic liver diseases. *Gastroenterology*, **68**, 525.

267 VALBERG L.S., GHENT C.N., LLOYD D.A., FREI J.V. & CHAMBERLAIN M.J. (1978) Diagnostic efficacy of tests for the detection of iron overload in chronic liver disease. *Canadian Medical Association Journal*, **119**, 229.

268 ELIN R.J., WOLF S.M. & FINCH C.A. (1977) Effect of induced fever on serum iron and ferritin concentrations in man. *Blood*, **49**, 147.

269 LIPSCHITZ D.A., COOK J.D. & FINCH C.A. (1974) A clinical evaluation of serum ferritin as an index of iron stores. *New England Journal of Medicine*, **290**, 1213.

270 BENTLEY D.P. & WILLIAMS P. (1974) Serum ferritin concentrations as an index of storage iron in rheumatoid arthritis. *Journal of Clinical Pathology*, **27**, 786.

271 ANON (1968) Iron in rheumatoid synovium. *Lancet*, ii, 340.

272 WORWOOD M., SUMMERS M., MILLER F., JACOBS A. & WHITTAKER J.A. (1974) Ferritin in blood cells from normal subjects and patients with leukaemia. *British Journal of Haematology*, **28**, 27.

273 KEW M.C., TORRANCE J.D., DERMAN D., SIMON M., MACNAB G.M., CHARLTON R.W. & BOTHWELL T.H. (1978) Serum and tumour ferritins in primary liver cancer. *Gut*, **19**, 294.

274 KOHGO Y., NIITSU Y., WATANABE N., OHTSUKA S., KOSETI H., SHIBATA K. & URUSHIZAKI I. (1976) Studies on radioimmunoassay of serum ferritin and its clinical implication in diseases of the digestive organs. *Japanese Journal of Gastroenterology*, **73**, 1553.

275 JONES B.M., WORWOOD M. & JACOBS A. (1980) Serum ferritin in patients with cancer: determination with antibodies to HeLa cell and spleen ferritin. *Clinica Chimica Acta*, **106**, 203.

276 PARRY D.H., RICKETTS C. & JACOBS A. (1978) Serum ferritin during unmaintained remission in acute lymphoblastic leukaemia. *British Medical Journal*, ii, 1341.

277 COOMBS R.C., POWLES T.J., GAZET J.-C., FORD H.T., MCKINNA A., ABBOTT M., GEHRKE C.W., KEYSER J.W., MITCHELL P.E.G., PATEL S., STIMSON W.H., WORWOOD M., JONES M. & NEVILLE A.M. Screening for metastases in breast cancer: an assessment of biochemical and physical methods. *Cancer*, (In press).

278 WORWOOD M., DAWKINS S., WAGSTAFF M. & JACOBS A. (1976) The purification and properties of ferritin from human serum. *Biochemical Journal*, **157**, 97.

279 CRAGG S.J., WAGSTAFF M. & WORWOOD M. (1980) Sialic acid and the microheterogeneity of human serum ferritin. *Clinical Science*, **58**, 259.

280 INTERNATIONAL COMMITTEE FOR STANDARDIZATION IN HAEMATOLOGY (Iron Panel) (1978) Recommendations for the measurement of serum iron in human blood. *British Journal of Haematology*, **38**, 291.

281 INTERNATIONAL COMMITTEE FOR STANDARDIZATION IN HAEMATOLOGY (Iron Panel) (1978) The measurement of total and unsaturated iron-binding capacity in serum. *British Journal of Haematology*, **38**, 281.

282 WEINFELD A. (1970) Iron stores. In: *Iron Deficiency: Pathogenesis, Clinical Aspects, Therapy* (ed. Hallberg L., Harwerth H.-G. & Vannotti A.), p. 329. Academic Press, London.

283 SCOTT D.E. & PRITCHARD J.A. (1967) Iron deficiency in healthy young college women. *Journal of the American Medical Association*, **199**, 897.

284 CHARLTON R.W., HAWKINS D.M., MAVOR W.O. & BOTHWELL T.H. (1970) Hepatic iron storage concentrations in different population groups. *American Journal of Clinical Nutrition*, **23**, 358.

285 STURGEON P. & SHODEN A. (1971) Total liver storage iron in normal populations of the USA. *American Journal of Clinical Nutrition*, **24**, 469.

286 HAGBERG B., WALLENIUS G. & WRANNE L. (1958) Latent iron deficiency after repeated removal of blood in blood donors. *Scandinavian Journal of Clinical and Laboratory Investigation*, **10**, 63.

287 CONRAD M.E. & CROSBY W.H. (1962) The natural history of iron deficiency induced by phlebotomy. *Blood*, **20**, 173.

288 JACOBS A., MILLER F., WORWOOD M., BEAMISH M.R. & WARDROP C.A. (1972) Ferritin in the serum of normal subjects and patients with iron deficiency and iron overload. *British Medical Journal*, iv, 206.

289 COOK J.D., FINCH C.A. & SMITH N.J. (1976) Evaluation of the iron status of a population. *Blood*, **48**, 449.

290 VALBERG L.S., SORBIE J., LUDWIG T. & PELLETIER D. (1976) Serum ferritin and the iron status of Canadians. *Canadian Medical Association Journal*, **114**, 417.

291 DERMAN D.P., LYNCH S.R., BOTHWELL T.H., CHARLTON R.W., TORRANCE J.D., BRINK B.A., MARGO G.M. & METZ J. (1978) Serum ferritin as an index of iron nutrition in rural and urban South African children. *British Journal of Nutrition*, **39**, 383.

292 FINCH C.A., COOK J.D., LABBE R.F. & CULALA M. (1977) Effect of blood donation on iron stores as evaluated by serum ferritin. *Blood*, **50**, 441.

293 BENTLEY D.P. & JACOBS A. (1975) Accumulation of storage iron in patients treated for iron-deficiency anaemia. *British Medical Journal*, i, 64.

294 DAGG J.H., GOLDBERG A. & LOCHHEAD A. (1966) Value of erythrocyte protoporphyrin in the diagnosis of latent iron deficiency (sideropenia). *British Journal of Haematology*, **12**, 326.

295 DAGG J.H., MARROW J.J., MACFARLANE B. & GOLDBERG A. (1967) Sideropenia (latent iron deficiency). *Quarterly Journal of Medicine*, **36**, 600.

296 JACOBS A. (1969) Tissue changes in iron deficiency. *British Journal of Haematology*, **16**, 1.

297 GARBY L., IRNELL L. & WERNER I. (1969) Iron deficiency in women of fertile age in a Swedish community. III. Estimation of prevalence based on response to iron supplementation. *Acta Medica Scandinavica*, **185**, 113.

298 KILPATRICK G.S. & HARDISTY R.M. (1961) The prevalence of anaemia in the community. *British Medical Journal*, i, 778.

299 JACOBS A., KILPATRICK G.S. & WITHEY J.L. (1965) Iron deficiency anaemia in adults: prevalence and prevention. *Postgraduate Medical Journal*, **41**, 418.

300 NATVIG H. & VELLAR O.D. (1967) Studies on hemoglobin values in Norway. VIII. Hemoglobin, hematocrit and MCHC values in adult men and women. *Acta Medica Scandinavica*, **182**, 193.

301 COMMITTEE ON IRON DEFICIENCY (1968) Iron deficiency in the United States. *Journal of the American Medical Association*, **203**, 407.

302 HALLBERG L., HALLGREN J., HOLLENDER A., HOGDAHL A.M. & TIBBLIN G. (1968) Occurrence of iron deficiency anaemia in Sweden. In: *Occurrence, Causes, and Prevention of Nutritional Anaemias* (ed. Lix G.), p. 19. Swedish Nutrition Foundation.

303 NATVIG H., VELLAR O.D. & ANDERSON J. (1967) Studies on hemoglobin values in Norway. VII. Hemoglobin, hematocrit and MCHC values among boys and girls aged 7–20 years in elementary and grammar schools. *Acta Medica Scandinavica*, **182**, 183.

304 GARBY L., IRNELL L. & WERNER I. (1969) Iron deficiency in women of fertile age in a Swedish community. *Acta Medica Scandinavica*, **185**, 107.

305 FOY H. & KONDI A. (1957) Anaemia of the tropics. Relation to iron intake, absorption and losses during growth, pregnancy and lactation. *Journal of Tropical Medicine and Hygiene*, **60**, 105.

306 BLIX G. (ed.) (1958) *Occurrence, Causes and Prevention of Nutritional Anaemias*. Swedish Nutrition Foundation.

307 HALLBERG L., HARWERTH H.-G. & VANNOTTI A. (1970) *Iron deficiency: Pathogenesis, Clinical Aspects, Therapy*, Academic Press, London.

308 COWAN B. & BHARUCHA C. (1973) Iron deficiency in the tropics. In: *Clinics in Haematology*, Vol. 2: *Iron Deficiency and Iron Overload* (ed. Callender S.T.). W. B. Saunders, London.

309 BEVERIDGE B.R., BANNERMAN R.M., EVANSON J.M. & WITTS L.J. (1965) Hypochromic anaemia. A retrospective study and follow-up of 378 in-patients. *Quarterly Journal of Medicine*, **34**, 145.

310 LANZKOWSKY P. (1959) Investigation into the etiology and treatment of pica. *Archives of Diseases in Childhood*, **34**, 140.

311 REYNOLDS R.D., BINDER H.J., MILLER M.B., CHANG W.W.Y. & HORAN S. (1968) Pagophagia and iron deficiency anemia. *Annals of Internal Medicine*, **69**, 435.

312 WALDENSTRÖM J. (1938) Iron and epithelium. Some clinical observations. I. Regeneration of the epithelium. *Acta Medica Scandinavica* (Suppl. 90), p. 380.

313 BEUTLER E., LARSH S.E. & GURNEY C.W. (1960) Iron therapy in chronically fatigued nonanemic women: a double blind study. *Annals of Internal Medicine*, **52**, 378.

314 BEUTLER E. & FAIRBANKS V.F. (1980) The effects of iron deficiency. In: *Iron in Biochemistry and Medicine II* (ed. Jacobs A. & Worwood M.), p. 393. Academic Press, London.

315 KASPER C.K., WHISSELL D.Y.E. & WALLERSTEIN R.O. (1965) Clinical aspects of iron deficiency. *Journal of the American Medical Association*, **191**, 359.

316 LOPAS H. & RABINER S.F. (1966) Thrombocytopenia association with iron deficiency anemia. *Clinical Pediatrics*, **5**, 609.

317 BEUTLER E. (1959) The red cell indices in the diagnosis of iron-deficiency anemia. *Annals of Internal Medicine*, **50**, 313.

318 CAVILL I., RICKETTS C., NAPIER J.A.F. & JACOBS A. (1977) Ferrokinetics and erythropoiesis in man: red cell production and destruction in normal and anaemic subjects. *British Journal of Haematology*, **35**, 33.

319 LAYRISSE M., LINARES J. & ROCHE M. (1965) Excess hemolysis in subjects with severe iron deficiency anemia associated and non-associated with hookworm infection. *Blood*, **25**, 73.

320 ROBINSON S.H. (1969) Increased formation of early-labelled bilirubin in rats with iron deficiency: evidence for the ineffective erythropoiesis. *Blood*, **33**, 909.

321 McKEE L.C. JR, WASSON M. & HEYSSEL R.M. (1968) Experimental iron deficiency in the rat. The use of ^{51}Cr, DF^{32}P and ^{59}Fe to detect haemolysis of iron deficient cells. *British Journal of Haematology*, **14**, 87.

322 CARD R.T. & WEINTRAUB L.R. (1971) Metabolic abnormalities of erythrocytes in severe iron deficiency. *Blood*, **37**, 725.

323 BODDINGTON M.M. (1959) Changes in buccal cells in anaemias. *Journal of Clinical Pathology*, **12**, 222.

324 DAGG J.H., JACKSON J.M., CURRY B. & GOLDBERG A. (1966) Cytochrome oxidase in latent iron deficiency (sideropenia). *British Journal of Haematology*, **12**, 331.

325 JALILI M.A. & AL-KASSAB S. (1959) Koilonychia and the cysteine content of nails. *Lancet*, **ii**, 108.

326 JACOBS A. (1961) Carbohydrates and sulphur-containing compounds in the anaemic buccal epithelium. *Journal of Clinical Pathology*, **14**, 610.

327 AHLBOM H.E. (1936) Simple achlorhydric anaemia, Plummer–Vinson syndrome and carcinoma of the mouth, pharynx and oesophagus in women. *British Medical Journal*, **ii**, 331.

328 CRAWFURD M.D'A., JACOBS A., MURPHY B. & PETERS D.K. (1965) Paterson–Kelly syndrome in adolescence: a report of five cases. *British Medical Journal*, **i**, 693.

329 JACOBS A. & KILPATRICK G.S. (1964) The Paterson–Kelly syndrome. *British Medical Journal*, **ii**, 79.

330 JACOBS A. & CAVILL I.A.J. (1968) Pyridoxin and riboflavin status in the Paterson–Kelly syndrome. *British Journal of Haematology*, **14**, 153.

331 JACOBS A., VATERLAWS L., LAWRIE B. & CAMPBELL H. (1960) Post-gastrectomy anaemia and the Paterson–Kelly syndrome. *British Journal of Haematology*, **17**, 615.

332 JACOBS A., LAWRIE J.H., ENTWISTLE C.C. & CAMPBELL H. (1966) Gastric acid secretion in chronic iron-deficiency anaemia. *Lancet*, **ii**, 190.

333 LEES F. & ROSENTHAL S.D. (1958) Gastric mucosal lesions before and after treatment in iron-deficiency anaemia. *Quarterly Journal of Medicine*, **27**, 19.

334 DAGG J.H., GOLDBERG A., ANDERSON J.R., BECK J.S. & GRAY K.G. (1964) Autoimmunity in iron-deficient anaemia. *British Medical Journal*, **i**, 1349.

335 DAGG J.H., GOLDBERG A., GIBBS W.N. & ANDERSON J.R. (1966) Detection of latent pernicious anaemia in iron-deficiency anaemia. *British Medical Journal*, **ii**, 619.

336 DESAI H.G., MEHTA B.C., BARKAR A.C. & JEEJEEBHOY K.N. (1967) Measurement of gastric acid secretion with

histamine infusion tests in iron-deficiency anaemia. *Indian Journal of Medical Research*, **5**, 1051.

337 NAIMAN J.L., OSKI F.A., DIAMOND L.K., VAWTER G.F. & SCHWACHMAN H. (1964) The gastrointestinal effect of iron-deficiency anemia. *Pediatrics*, **33**, 83.

338 GUHA D.K., WALIA B.N.S., TANDON B.N., DEO M.G. & GHAI O.P. (1968) Small bowel changes in iron-deficiency anaemia of childhood. *Archives of Diseases in Childhood*, **43**, 239.

339 RAWSON A. & ROSENTHAL F.D. (1960) The mucosal of the stomach and small intestine in iron-deficiency. *Lancet*, **i**, 730.

340 KIMBER C. & WEINTRAUB L.R. (1968) Malabsorption of iron secondary to iron-deficiency. *New England Journal of Medicine*, **279**, 453.

341 BEUTLER E. (1964) Tissue effects of iron-deficiency. In: *Iron Metabolism* (ed. Gross F.), p. 256. Springer-Verlag, Berlin.

342 DALLMAN P.R. & SCHWARTZ H.C. (1965) Distribution of cytochrome C and myoglobin in rats with dietary iron-deficiency. *Pediatrics*, **35**, 677.

343 DALLMAN P.R. & SCHWARTZ H.C. (1965) Myoglobin and cytochrome response during repair of iron-deficiency in the rat. *Journal of Clinical Investigation*, **44**, 1631.

344 DALLMAN P.R. & GOODMAN J.R. (1970) Enlargement of mitochondrial compartment in iron and copper deficiency. *Blood*, **35**, 496.

345 HOFFBRAND A.V. & BROITMAN S.A. (1969) Effect of chronic nutritional iron-deficiency on the small intestinal disaccharidase activities of growing dogs. *Proceedings of the Society of Experimental Biology and Medicine*, **130**, 595.

346 VITALE J.J., RESTREPO A., VELEZ H., RIKER J.B. & HELLERSTEIN E.E. (1966) Secondary folate deficiency induced in the rat by dietary iron-deficiency. *Journal of Nutrition*, **88**, 315.

347 CHANARIN I., BENNETT M.C. & BERRY V. (1962) Urinary excretion of histidine derivatives in megaloblastic anaemia and other conditions and a comparison with the folic acid clearance test. *Journal of Clinical Pathology*, **15**, 269.

348 DAS K.C., HERBERT V., COLMAN N. & LONGO D.L. (1978) Unmasking covert folate deficiency in iron-deficient subjects with neutrophilhypersegmentation: dU suppression tests on lymphocytes and bone marrow. *British Journal of Haematology*, **39**, 357.

349 EDGERTON V.R., BRYANT S.L., GILLESPIE C.A. & GARDNER G.W. (1972) Iron deficiency anemia and physical performance and activity of rats. *Journal of Nutrition*, **102**, 381.

350 FINCH C.A., MILLER L.R., INAMDAR A.R., PERSON R., SEILER K. & MACKLER B. (1976) Iron deficiency in the rat. Physiological and biochemical studies of muscle dysfunction. *Journal of Clinical Investigation*, **58**, 447.

351 JACOBS A. & GLOVER J. (1972) The activity pattern of iron deficient rats. *British Medical Journal*, **ii**, 627.

352 VITERI F.E. & TORUN B. (1974) Anaemia and physical work capacity. In: *Clinics in Haematology*, Vol. 3 (ed. Garby L.), p. 609. W. B. Saunders, London.

353 DALLMAN P.R., SIIMES M.A. & MANIES E.C. (1975) Brain iron: persistent deficiency following short-term

354 WOODS S.C., VASSELLI J.R. & MILAM K.M. (1977) Iron appetite and latent learning in rats. *Physiology and Behaviour*, **19**, 623.

355 FAIRBANKS V.F., FAHEY J.L. & BEUTLER E. (1971) *Clinical Disorders of Iron Metabolism*, 2nd edn. Grune & Stratton, New York.

356 POLLITT E. & LEIBEL R.L. (1976) Iron deficiency and behaviour. *Journal of Pediatrics*, **88**, 372.

357 MACKAY H.M.M. (1928) Anaemia in infancy: prevalence and prevention. *Archives of Diseases in Childhood*, **3**, 117.

358 BURMAN D. (1971) Iron requirements in infancy. *British Journal of Haematology*, **20**, 243.

359 STOTT G. (1960) Anaemia in Mauritius. *Bulletin of the World Health Organization*, **23**, 781.

360 DAVIES L.R., MARTEN R.H. & SARKANY I. (1960) Iron-deficiency anaemia in European and West Indian infants in London. *British Medical Journal*, **ii**, 1426.

361 VAHLQUIST B. (1968) Occurrence of nutritional anaemias in children. In: *Occurrence, Causes and Prevention of Nutritional Anaemias* (ed. Blix G.). Swedish Nutrition Foundation.

362 SCHWARTZ D. (1951) Chlorosis: a retrospective investigation. *Acta Medica Belgica* (Suppl.).

363 ELWOOD P.C., WITHEY J.L. & KILPATRICK G.S. (1964) Distribution of haemoglobin level in a group of school children and its relation to height, weight and other variables. *British Journal of Preventive and Social Medicine*, **18**, 125.

364 SOOD S.K. & RAMALINGASWAMI V. (1968) The interaction of multiple dietary deficiencies in the pathogenesis of anaemia of pregnancy. In: *Occurrence, Causes and Prevention of Nutritional Anaemias* (ed. Blix G.), p. 135. Swedish Nutrition Foundation.

365 PRITCHARD J.A. & HUNT C.S. (1958) A comparison of the hematologic responses following the routine prenatal administration of intramuscular iron and oral iron. *Surgery, Gynaecology and Obstetrics*, **106**, 516.

366 CHISHOLM M. (1966) A controlled clinical trial of prophylactic folic acid and iron in pregnancy. *Journal of Obstetrics and Gynaecology of the British Commonwealth*, **73**, 191.

367 FENTON V., CAVILL I. & FISHER J. (1977) Iron stores in pregnancy. *British Journal of Haematology*, **37**, 145.

368 MORGAN E.H. (1961) Plasma iron and haemoglobin levels in pregnancy. The effect of oral iron. *Lancet*, **i**, 9.

369 CHANARIN I., ROTHMAN D. & BERRY V. (1965) Iron-deficiency and its relation to folic-acid status in pregnancy. *British Medical Journal*, **i**, 480.

370 ROSS G. & GRAY C.H. (1964) Assessment of routine tests for occult blood in faeces. *British Medical Journal*, **i**, 1351.

371 ELWOOD P.C., WATERS W.E., GREEN W.J. & WOOD M.M. (1967) Evaluation of a screening survey for anaemia in adult non-pregnant women. *British Medical Journal*, **iv**, 714.

372 HOLT J.M., MAYET F.G.H., WARNER G.T., CALLENDER S.T. & GUNNING A.J. (1968) Iron absorption and blood loss in patients with hiatus hernia. *British Medical Journal*, **ii**, 22.

373 FOY H. & KONDI A. (1960) Hookworms in the aetiology

iron deprivation in the rat. *British Journal of Haematology*, **31**, 209.

of tropical iron deficiency anaemia. Radio-isotope studies. *Transactions of the Royal Society of Tropical Medicine and Hygiene*, **54**, 419.

374 CROFT D.N. (1970) Body iron loss and cell loss from epithelia. *Proceedings of the Royal Society of Medicine*, **63**, 1221.

375 JONES F.A. (ed.) (1967) *Post-gastrectomy Nutrition*. A Glaxo Symposium. Lloyd-Luke, London.

376 BAIRD I.M., BLACKBURN E.K. & WILSON G.M. (1959) The pathogenesis of anaemia after partial gastrectomy. I. Development of anaemia in relation to time after operation, blood loss and diet. *Quarterly Journal of Medicine*, **28**, 21.

377 KIMBER C., PATTERSON J.F. & WEINTRAUB L.R. (1967) The pathogenesis of iron deficiency anemia following partial gastrectomy. A study of iron balance. *Journal of the American Medical Association*, **202**, 935.

378 HOLT J.M., GEAR M.W.L. & WARNER G.T. (1970) The role of chronic blood loss in the pathogenesis of post-gastrectomy iron deficiency anaemia. *Gut*, **11**, 847.

379 BAIRD I.M., ST JOHN D.J.B. & NASSER S.S. (1970) Role of occult blood loss in anaemia after partial gastrectomy. *Gut*, **11**, 55.

380 STEPHENS A.R., PIRZIO-BIROLI G., HARKINS H.N., NYHUS L.M. & FINCH C.A. (1959) Iron metabolism in patients after partial gastrectomy. *Annals of Surgery*, **149**, 534.

381 BAIRD I.M. & WILSON G.M. (1959) The pathogenesis of anaemia after partial gastrectomy. II. Iron absorption after partial gastrectomy. *Quarterly Journal of Medicine*, **28**, 35.

382 CHOUDHURY M.R. & WILLIAMS J. (1959) Iron absorption and gastric operation. *Clinical Science*, **18**, 527.

383 ASHURST P.M. (1968) Parietal cell antibodies in patients undergoing gastric surgery. *British Medical Journal*, **ii**, 647.

384 WEBB M.G.T., TAYLOR M.R.H. & GATENBY P.B.B. (1967) Iron absorption in coeliac disease of childhood and adolescence. *British Medical Journal*, **ii**, 151.

385 CALLENDER S.T. (1974) Treatment of iron deficiency. In: *Iron in Biochemistry and Medicine* (ed. Jacobs A. & Worwood M.), p. 529. Academic Press, London.

386 BRISE H. & HALLBERG L. (1962) Absorbability of different iron compounds. *Acta Medica Scandinavica*, **376**, (Suppl.), 23.

387 HALLBERG L., RYTTINGER L. & SÖLVELL L. (1966) Side effects of oral iron therapy. A double blind study of different iron compounds in tablet form. *Acta Medica Scandinavica*, **459** (Suppl.), 3.

388 MIDDLETON E.J., NAGY E. & MORRISON A.B. (1966) Studies on the absorption of orally administered iron from sustained-release preparations. *New England Journal of Medicine*, **274**, 136.

389 CALLENDER S.T. (1970) Oral iron therapy. *British Journal of Haematology*, **18**, 123.

390 BRISE H. & HALLBERG L. (1962) Effect of ascorbic acid on iron absorption. *Acta Medica Scandinavica*, **376** (Suppl.), 51.

391 BRISE H. & HALLBERG L. (1962) Effect of succinic acid on iron absorption. *Acta Medica Scandinavica*, **376** (Suppl.), 59.

392 HILLMAN R.S. & HENDERSON P.A. (1969) Control of marrow production by the level of iron supply. *Journal of Clinical Investigation*, **48**, 454.

393 PRITCHARD J.A. (1966) Hemoglobin regeneration in severe iron-deficiency anemia. *Journal of the American Medical Association*, **195**, 717.

394 BONNAR J., GOLDBERG A. & SMITH J.A. (1969) Do pregnant women take their iron? *Lancet*, **i**, 457.

395 VARDE K.N. (1964) Treatment of 300 cases of iron deficiency of pregnancy by total dose infusion of iron dextran complex. *Journal of Obstetrics and Gynaecology of the British Commonwealth*, **71**, 919.

396 BONNAR J. (1965) Anaemia in obstetrics: an evaluation of treatment by iron-dextran infusion. *British Medical Journal*, **ii**, 1030.

397 WETHERLEY-MEIN G., BUCHANAN J.G., GLASS U.H. & PEARCE L.C. (1962) Metabolism of ^{59}Fe sorbitol complex in man. *British Medical Journal*, **i**, 1796.

398 BRIGGS J.G., KENNEDY A.C. & GOLDBERG A. (1963) Urinary white cell excretion after iron-sorbitol-citric acid. *British Medical Journal*, **ii**, 352.

399 CLAY B., ROSENBERG B., SAMPSON N. & SAMUELS S.I. (1965) Reactions to total dose intravenous infusion of iron dextran (Imferon). *British Medical Journal*, **i**, 29.

400 KARHUNEN P., HARTEL G., KIVIKANGAS V. & REINIK-AINEN M. (1970) Reaction to iron sorbitol injection in 3 cases of malabsorption. *British Medical Journal*, **ii**, 521.

401 LLOYD K.N. & WILLIAMS P. (1970) Reactions to total dose infusion of iron dextran in rheumatoid arthritis. *British Medical Journal*, **ii**, 323.

402 THEODOROPOULOS G., MAKKOUS A. & CONSTANTOU-LAKIS M. (1968) Lymph node enlargement after a single massive infusion of iron dextran. *Journal of Clinical Pathology*, **21**, 492.

403 POWELL L.W. & HALLIDAY J.W. (1980) Idiopathic haemochromatosis. In: *Iron in Biochemistry and Medicine II* (ed. Jacobs A. & Worwood M.), p. 461. Academic Press, London.

404 SHELDON J.H. (1935) *Haemochromatosis*. Oxford University Press, Oxford.

405 WILLIAMS R., SCHEUER P.J. & SHERLOCK S. (1962) The inheritance of idiopathic haemochromatosis. *Quarterly Journal of Medicine*, **321**, 249.

406 MACDONALD R.A. (1964) *Hemochromatosis and Hemosiderosis*. C. C. Thomas, Springfield, Illinois.

407 CELADA A., RUDOLF H. & DONATH A. (1978) Effect of a single ingestion of alcohol on iron absorption. *American Journal of Hematology*, **5**, 225.

408 SIMON M., BOUREL M., FAUCHET R. & GENETET B. (1976) Association of HLA-A3 and HLA B14 antigens with idiopathic haemochromatosis. *Gut*, **17**, 332.

409 SIMON M., BOUREL M., GENETET B. & FAUCHET R. (1977) Idiopathic hemochromatosis. Demonstration of recession transmission and early detection by family HLA typing. *New England Journal of Medicine*, **297**, 1017.

410 BEAUMONT C., SIMON M., FAUCHET R., HESPEL J.-P., BRISSOT P., GENETET B. & BOUREL M. (1979) Serum ferritin as a possible marker of the hemochromatosis allele. *New England Journal of Medicine*, **301**, 169.

411 CARTWRIGHT G.E., EDWARDS C.Q., KRAVITZ K., SKOL-NICK M., AMOS D.B., JOHNSON A. & BUSKJAER L. (1979) Hereditary hemochromatosis: phenotypic expression of the disease. *New England Journal of Medicine*, **301**, 175.

412 WILLIAMS R., MANENTI S., WILLIAMS H.S. & PITCHER C.S. (1966) Iron absorption in idiopathic haemochromatosis before, during and after venesection therapy. *British Medical Journal*, **ii**, 78.

413 WILLIAMS R., PITCHER C.S., PARSONSON A. & WILLIAMS H.S. (1965) Iron absorption in the relatives of patients with idiopathic haemochromatosis. *Lancet*, **i**, 1243.

414 WILLIAMS R. (1971) Haemochromatosis. In: *Seventh Symposium on Advanced Medicine* (ed. Bouchier I.A.D.), p. 199. Pitman Medical, London.

415 HARTMAN R.S., CONRAD M.E., HARTMAN R.E., JOY R.J.T. & CROSBY W.H. (1963) Ferritin-containing bodies in human small intestinal epithelium. *Blood*, **22**, 397.

416 BRINK B., DISLER P., LYNCH S., JACOBS P., CHARLTON R. & BOTHWELL T. (1976) Patterns of iron storage in dietary iron overload and idiopathic hemochromatosis. *Journal of Laboratory and Clinical Medicine*, **88**, 725.

417 VALBERG L.S., SIMON B., MANLEY P.N., CORBETT W.E. & LUDWIG J. (1975) Distribution of storage iron as body iron stores expand in patients with hemochromatosis. *Journal of Laboratory and Clinical Medicine*, **86**, 479.

418 YAM L.T., FINKEL H.E., WEINTRAUB L.R. & CROSBY W.H. (1968) Circulating iron containing macrophages in hemochromatosis. *New England Journal of Medicine*, **279**, 512.

419 BOMFORD A. & WILLIAMS R. (1976) Long term results of venesection therapy in idiopathic haemochromatosis. *Quarterly Journal of Medicine*, **45**, 611.

420 WILLIAMS R., SMITH P.M., SPICER E.J.F., BARRY K. & SHERLOCK S. (1969) Venesection therapy in idiopathic haemochromatosis. *Quarterly Journal of Medicine*, **38**, 1.

421 BOMFORD A. & WILLIAMS R. (1976) Long term results of venesection therapy in idiopathic haemochromatosis. *Quarterly Journal of Medicine*, **45**, 611.

422 OLIVER R.A.M. (1959) Siderosis following transfusions of blood. *Journal of Pathology and Bacteriology*, **77**, 171.

423 DE ALARCON P.A., DONOVAN M.A., FORBES G.B., LANDAW S.E. & STOCKMAN J.A. III (1979) Iron absorption in the thalassaemia syndromes and its inhibition by tea. *New England Journal of Medicine*, **300**, 5.

424 BUJA L.M. & ROBERTS W.C. (1971) Iron in the heart. Etiology and clinical significance. *American Journal of Medicine*, **51**, 209.

425 MODELL B. (1977) Total management of thalassaemia major. *Archives of Diseases of Childhood*, **52**, 489.

426 PIPPARD M.J., CALLENDER S.T., WARNER G.T. & WEATHERALL D. (1979) Iron absorption and loading in β-thalassaemia intermedia. *Lancet*, **ii**, 819.

427 BARRY M., FLYNN D.M., LETSKY E.A. & RISDON R.A. (1974) Long-term chelation therapy in thalassaemia major: effect on liver iron concentration, liver histology and clinical progress. *British Medical Journal*, **ii**, 16.

428 PROPPER R.D., SHURIN S.B. & NATHAN D.G. (1976) Reassessment of the use of desferrioxamine B in iron overload. *New England Journal of Medicine*, **294**, 1421.

429 HUSSAIN M.A.M., FLYNN D.M., GREEN N., HUSSEIN S. & HOFFBRAND A.V. (1976) Subcutaneous infusion and intramuscular injection of desferrioxamine in patients with transfusional iron overload. *Lancet*, **ii**, 1278.

430 PIPPARD M.J., CALLENDER S.T., LETSKY E.A. & WEATHERALL D.J. (1978) Prevention of iron loading in transfusion dependent thalassaemia. *Lancet*, **i**, 1178.

431 NIENHUIS A.W., DE LEA C., AAMODT R., BARTTER F. & ANDERSON W.F. (1976) Evaluation of desferrioxamine and ascorbic acid for the treatment of chronic iron overload. In: *Iron Metabolism and Thalassemia* (ed. Bergsman D., Cerami A., Peterson C.M. & Graziano J.H.). Alan R. Liss Inc., New York.

432 HUSSAIN M.A.M., GREEN N., FLYNN D.M. & HOFFBRAND A.V. (1977) Effect of dose, time and ascorbate on iron excretion after subcutaneous desferrioxamine. *Lancet*, **i**, 977.

433 PROPPER R.D. & NATHAN D.G. (1977) Use of desferrioxamine and "the pump". In: *Chelation Therapy in Chronic Iron Overload* (ed. Zaino E.C. & Roberts R.H.). Symposia Specialists Inc., Miami.

434 MODELL C.B. & BECK J. (1974) Long-term desferrioxamine therapy in thalassemia. *Annals of the New York Academy of Sciences*, **232**, 201.

435 HOFFBRAND A.V. (1980) Transfusion siderosis and chelation therapy. In: *Iron in Biochemistry and Medicine II* (ed. Jacobs A. & Worwood M.), p. 499. Academic Press, London.

436 BOTHWELL T.H. & ISAACSON C. (1962) Siderosis in the Bantu. A comparison of incidence in males and females. *British Medical Journal*, **i**, 522.

437 CHARLEY P.J., SARKAR B., STITT C.F., SALTMAN P. (1963) Chelation of iron by sugars. *Biochimica et Biophysica Acta*, **69**, 313.

438 BOTHWELL T.H., SEFTELL H., JACOBS P., TORRANCE J.D. & BAUMSLAG N. (1964) Iron overload in Bantu subjects. Studies on the availablilty of iron in Bantu beer. *American Journal of Clinical Nutrition*, **14**, 47.

439 MACPHAIL A.P., SIMON M.D., TORRANCE J.D., CHARLTON R.W., BOTHWELL T.H. & ISAACSON C. (1979) Changing patterns of dietary iron overload in black South Africans. *American Journal of Clinical Nutrition*, **32**, 1272.

440 JOHNSON B.F. (1968) Hemochromatosis resulting from prolonged oral iron therapy. *New England Journal of Medicine*, **278**, 1100.

441 TURNBERG L.A. (1965) Excessive oral iron therapy causing haemochromatosis. *British Medical Journal*, **i**, 1360.

442 GOLBERG L. & SMITH J.P. (1960) Iron overloading and hepatic vulnerability. *American Journal of Pathology*, **36**, 125.

443 ORFEI E., VOLINI F.I., MADERA-ORSINI F., MINICK O.T. & DENT G. (1968) Effect of iron loading on the hepatic injury induced by ethionine. *American Journal of Pathology*, **52**, 547.

444 TOLLERZ G. & LANNEK N. (1964) Protection against iron toxicity in vitamin E deficient piglets and mice by vitamin E and synthetic anti-oxidants. *Nature (London)*, **201**, 846.

445 MELHORN D.K. & GROSS S. (1969) Relationships between iron dextran and vitamin E in iron deficiency anemia in children. *Journal of Laboratory and Clinical Medicine*, **74**, 789.

446 LYNCH S.R., SEFTELL H.C., TORRANCE J.D., CHARLTON R.W. & BOTHWELL T.H. (1967) Accelerated oxidative catabolism of ascorbic in siderotic Bantu. *American Journal of Clinical Nutrition*, **20**, 641.

447 LYNCH S.R., BERELOWITZ I., SEFTELL H.C., MILLER

G.B., KRAWITZ P., CHARLTON R.W. & BOTHWELL T.H. (1967) Osteoporosis in Johannesburg Bantu males. Its relationship to siderosis and ascorbic acid deficiency. *American Journal of Clinical Nutrition*, **20**, 799.

448 ALDRIDGE R.A. (1958) Acute iron toxicity. In: *Iron in Clinical Medicine* (ed. Wallerstein R. & Mettier S. R.). University of California, Berkeley.

449 REISSMANN K.R., COLEMAN T.J., BUDAI B.S. & MOR-IARTY L.R. (1955) Acute intestinal iron intoxication. I. Iron absorption, serum iron and autopsy findings. *Blood*, **10**, 35.

450 REISSMANN K.R. & COLEMAN T.J. (1955) Acute intestinal iron intoxication. II. Metabolic, respiratory and circulatory effects of absorbed iron salts. *Blood*, **10**, 46.

451 WILSON S.J., HEATH H.E., NELSON P.L. & ENS G.G. (1958) Blood coagulation in acute iron intoxication. *Blood*, **13**, 483.

452 WHITTEN C.F., GIBSON G.W., GOOD M.H., GOODWYN J.F. & BROUGH A.J. (1965) Studies in acute iron poisoning. I. Desferrioxamine in the treatment of acute iron poisoning. Clinical observations, experimental studies, and theoretical considerations. *Pediatrics*, **36**, 322.

453 BARR D.G.D. & FRAZER D.K.B. (1968) Acute iron poisoning in children: Role of chelating agents. *British Medical Journal*, **1**, 737.

454 McGUIGAN M.A., LOVEJOY F.H. JR, MARINO S.K., PROPPER R.D. & GOLDMAN P. (1979) Qualitative deferoxamine color test for iron ingestion. *Journal of Pediatrics*, **94**, 940.

455 WAXMAN H.S. & BROWN E.B. (1969) Clinical usefulness of iron chelating agents. In: *Progress in Haematology*, Vol. 6 (ed. Brown E.B. & Moore C.V.). Heinemann, London.

456 ÅKESON A., BIÖRCH G. & SIMON R. (1968) On the content of myoglobin in human muscles. *Acta Medica Scandinavica*, **183**, 307.

457 DRABKIN D.L. (1951) Metabolism of the hemin chromoproteins. *Physiological Reviews*, **31**, 345.

458 WILIAMS J.N. JR (1968) A comparative study of cytochrome ratios in mitochondria from organs of the rat, chicken and guinea pig. *Biochimica et Biophysica Acta*, **162**, 175.

459 SCHOENE B., FLEISCHMANN R.A., REMINER H. & OLDERSHAUSEN H.F. (1972) Determination of drug metabolizing enzymes in needle biopsies of human liver. *European Journal of Clinical Pharmacology*, **4**, 65.

460 CHANG L.L. (1973) Tissue storage iron in Singapore. *American Journal of Clinical Nutrition*, **26**, 952.

461 TORRANCE J.D., CHARLTON R.W., SCHMAN A., LYNCH S.R. & BOTHWELL T.H. (1968) Storage iron in muscle. *Journal of Clinical Pathology*, **21**, 495.

462 HALLGREN B. & SOURANDER P. (1958) The effect of age on the non-haemin iron in the human brain. *Journal of Neurochemistry*, **3**, 41.

463 SIIMES M.A., ADDIEGO J.E. & DALLMAN P.R. (1974) Ferritin in serum: diagnosis of iron deficiency and iron overload in infants and children. *Blood*, **43**, 581.

464 JACOBS A. (1980) The pathology of iron overload. In: *Iron in Biochemistry and Medicine II* (ed. Jacobs A. & Worwood M.), p. 427. Academic Press, London.

465 BOXMEYER H.E., DeSOUSA M., SMITHYMAN A., RALPH P., HAMILTON J., KURLAND J.I. & BOGNACKI J. (1980) Specificity and modulation of the action of lactoferrin, a negative feedback regulator of myelopoiesis. *Blood*, **55**, 324.

466 KOERPER M.A. & DALLMAN P.R. (1977) Serum iron concentration and transferrin saturation in the diagnosis of iron deficiency in children: normal development change. *Journal of Pediatrics*, **91**, 870.

467 SAARINEN U.M. & SIIMES M.A. (1977) Development changes in serum iron, total iron-binding capacity and transferrin saturation in infancy. *Journal of Pediatrics*, **91**, 875.

468 BAROSI G., CAZZOLA M., MARCHI A., MORANDI S., PERANI V., STEFANELLI M. & PERUGINI S. (1978) Iron kinetics and erythropoiesis in Fanconi's anaemia. *Scandinavian Journal of Haematology*, **21**, 29.

469 CAVILL I., RICKETTS C., NAPIER J.A.F. & JACOBS A. (1977) Ferrokinetics and erythropoiesis in man: red cell production and destruction in normal and anaemic subjects. *British Journal of Haematology*, **35**, 33.

470 DINANT H.J. & DE MAAT C.E.M. (1978) Erythropoiesis and mean red cell lifespan in normal subjects and in patients with the anaemia of active rheumatoid arthritis. *British Journal of Haematology*, **39**, 437.

471 FAIRBANKS V.F. (1971) Is the peripheral blood film reliable for the diagnosis of iron-deficiency anemia? *American Journal of Clinical Pathology*, **55**, 447.

472 GORNSKY B., HORSBURGH C., LINDLEY P.F., MOSS D.S., PARKER M. & WATSON J.L. (1979) Evidence for the bilobal nature of diferric rabbit plasma transferrin. *Nature (London)*, **281**, 157.

Chapter 6
Vitamin B$_{12}$ and folate metabolism: the megaloblastic anaemias and other nutritional anaemias

A. V. HOFFBRAND

The megaloblastic anaemias are a group of disorders in which the bone-marrow morphology assumes a distinctive appearance. The anaemia is usually caused by deficiency of vitamin B$_{12}$ (referred to as B$_{12}$) or of folate, and the major part of this chapter concerns the physiological and biochemical processes in which these two vitamins are involved and the diseases which cause their deficiency. The metabolism of B$_{12}$, the syndromes causing B$_{12}$ deficiency and its diagnosis are considered first. The general clinical, morphological and biochemical features of megaloblastic anaemia and of B$_{12}$ neuropathy are described under the heading of pernicious anaemia. Nutritional and biochemical aspects of folate and the causes and diagnosis of folate deficiency are dealt with next. The management of patients suffering from megaloblastic anaemia due either to abnormalities of B$_{12}$ or folate metabolism or to faults in DNA synthesis not caused by B$_{12}$ or folate deficiency or abnormality are then dealt with. The final section discusses the possible biochemical basis of megaloblastic anaemia and B$_{12}$ neuropathy.

General aspects of megaloblastic anaemias are dealt with by Chanarin [1] and Hoffbrand [2] and a number of monographs or large reviews have covered particular aspects of the subject [3–19].

VITAMIN B$_{12}$

STRUCTURE AND CHEMICAL FORMS
The existence of an anti-pernicious anaemia factor in liver was suspected from earlier experiments on feeding large amounts of liver to patients with pernicious anaemia [20], but B$_{12}$ itself was only crystallized as cyanocobalamin in 1948 [21, 22]. Cyanocobalamin forms dark red prisms, has a molecular weight of 1355 (C$_{63}$H$_{88}$O$_{14}$N$_{14}$PCo) and a molecular radius of 8 nm. It is water soluble (about 1·2% at room temperature), forms a weakly basic solution and is relatively stable. Aqueous solutions show absorption maxima at 278, 361 and 550 nm. The structure of all the cobalamins consists of a planar, corrin ring with a nucleotide portion, 5,6-dimethylbenzimidazole attached to ribose phosphate set nearly at right angles to it (Fig. 6.1). The term 'corrinoid' is used to described all compounds containing the corrin ring, which consists of four reduced pyrrole rings with a central cobalt atom. Three of the rings are linked by bridged carbon atoms (as in the porphyrin nucleus) but a direct bond exists between the α portion of rings A and D (Fig. 6.1). All but six of 19 carbon atoms constituting the corrin ring are fully substituted with methyl, acetamide or propionamide side chains. The phosphate of the nucleotide portion is esterified with 1-amino-2-propanol, which also joins in amide linkage to the propionic-acid side chain on ring D of the planar group. The cobalt atom is coordinated to one of the nitrogen atoms of the benzimidazole and, in cyanocobalamin, to a cyanide (—CN) group.

The term 'vitamin B$_{12}$' may be used to describe *cyanocobalamin* alone but is often used (as here) to include other forms of the vitamin in which the —CN is replaced by another side group (Table 6.1). In nature, B$_{12}$ exists largely as the two forms, *methylcobalamin* (methyl-B$_{12}$) and *5'-deoxyadenosylcobalamin* (ado-B$_{12}$). These are extremely labile since they are converted to a fourth form of B$_{12}$, *hydroxocobalamin* (hydroxo-B$_{12}$), after exposure to light for a few seconds. These forms are separated by paper chromatography and identified by bioautography, protection from light being essential [23–25]. Forms of B$_{12}$ which have also been identified in natural materials include *sulphitocobalamin* and *phosphorocobalamin* and other related compounds with variations in the ligand attached to the cobalt atom have been produced chemically. Biosynthesis of natural coenzymes from hydroxocobalamin requires enzymes reducing the cobalt atom from the tri- to di- and mono-valent states, and then enzymatic addition of the 5'-deoxyadenosyl group or methyl group which is donated in the homocysteine-methionine reaction via S-adenosylmethionine from methyltetrahydrofolate [7]. The different oxidation states of the cobalt atom in cobalamin are designated: vitamin B$_{12}$ or Cob(III)alamin (oxidized), vitamin B$_{12r}$ or Cob(II)alamin and vitamin B$_{12s}$

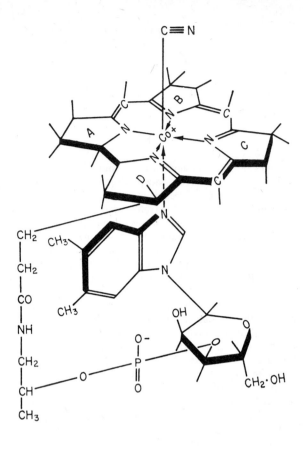

Fig. 6.1. The structure of cyanocobalamin. In methyl-, hydroxo- and deoxyadenosyl-cobalamin, the —CN group is replaced by —CH₃, —OH, and 5′-deoxyadenosyl groups respectively.

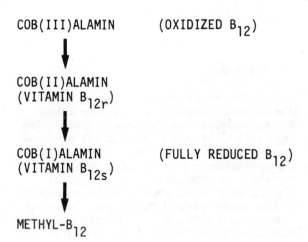

Fig. 6.2. Reduction of oxidized cobalamin (Cob(III)alamin) and formation of fully reduced methyl-cobalamin (methyl-B₁₂).

Table 6.1. Some characteristics of vitamin B_{12} and folate

	Vitamin B_{12}	Folate
Parent form	Cyanocobalamin	Pteroylglutamic acid (folic acid)
Molecular weight	1355	441
Natural forms	Methycobalamin, deoxy-adenoxylcobalamin, hydroxocobalamin	Reduced, methylated or formylated pteroylpolyglutamates
Foods	Animal origin only (liver, meat, fish, dairy produce)	Yeast, liver, green vegetables, nuts, cereals, fruit, etc.
Effect of cooking	Little or no effect	May destroy completely
Adult daily requirements	1–2 μg	100–200 μg
Normal daily intake	3–30 μg	400–500 μg
Body stores	3–5 mg (2–4 years' supply)	6–20 mg (4 months' supply)
Site of absorption	Ileum	Duodenum and jejunum
Mechanism	Gastric intrinsic factor	Deconjugation, reduction and methylation
Enterohepatic circulation	Yes	Yes

or Cob(I)alamin (fully reduced) (Fig. 6.2). A number of analogues ('pseudo-vitamin B_{12}'s') which lack one or other on the planar or nucleotide portions of vitamin B_{12} exist in nature. Cobamides contain substitutions in place of ribose (e.g. adenosine, guanine or hypoxanthine) while in anilides propionamide side chains are replaced by substituted amides. Cobinamides are corrinoids with no nucleotide portion at all. The demonstration of B_{12} analogues in human serum causing high B_{12} levels measured by radioassay has led to recent increased interest in the analogues.

B_{12} is produced commercially as a by-product in the manufacture of streptomycin, since *Streptomyces griseus* is one of the many micro-organisms which synthesize the vitamin; radioactive B_{12} is obtained if the organism is grown in the presence of radioactive cobalt.

BIOCHEMICAL REACTIONS IN MAN

Only three reactions have been shown to require B_{12} in humans:

1 methionine synthesis;
2 isomerization of methylmalonyl CoA to succinyl CoA; and
3 interconversion of β leucine and α leucine.

Homocysteine-methionine methyl transferase (methionine synthetase)

The enzyme concerned is homocysteine-methionine methyltransferase and the reaction requires 5 methyl-tetrahydrofolate (methyl-THF) as methyl donor, S-adenosyl methionine (SAM) and a reducing agent ($FADH_2$) as well as methyl-B_{12} as coenzyme (Fig. 6.3). Methyl-THF probably donates the methyl group to methyl-B_{12} bound to the protein apoenzyme, which then passes the methyl group to homocysteine. The

apoenzyme may normally be undersaturated with B_{12}. Weissbach & Taylor [26] suggest that SAM has a 'priming' action when, in the presence of the reducing agent, it methylates molecules of the reduced B_{12}–enzyme complex.

B_{12}-dependent methionine synthesis is important in the regeneration of THF from methyl-THF. Methionine is an essential amino acid but the generation of methionine and SAM by this reaction may also be relevant to the clinical effects of B_{12} deficiency or inactivation (see p. 245). A second B_{12}-independent mechanism of synthesis of methionine from homocysteine has been shown to occur in certain micro-organisms which utilize the triglutamate form of methyl-THF [27] but this mechanism is not present in the one mammalian system, rat liver, so far tested.

Isomerization of methylmalonyl CoA to succinyl CoA

The conversion of propionate to succinate involves three enzymes (Fig. 6.4). Carboxylation of propionyl CoA to D-methylmalonyl CoA by propionyl carboxylase requires biotin. The enzyme methylmalonyl CoA racemase then converts the inactive D isomer to the active L enantiomorph. The third reaction, which uses two molecules of deoxyadenosylcobalamin (ado-B_{12}) per molecule of apoenzyme as prosthetic group, consists of the isomerization of L-methylmalonyl CoA to succinyl CoA. The amount of B_{12} normally present is probably sufficient for this reaction and is not rate limiting. This reaction is part of a route by which cholesterol and odd-chain fatty acids, as well as a number of amino acids and thymine, may be used for energy requirements via the Krebs cycle, for gluconeogenesis or to form δ-aminolaevulinic acid (Fig. 6.4). The pathway is of particular importance in ruminants which obtain much of their energy from

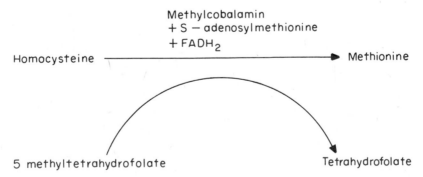

Fig. 6.3. The conversion of homocysteine to methionine. This is the only known biochemical reaction which requires both vitamin C and folate.

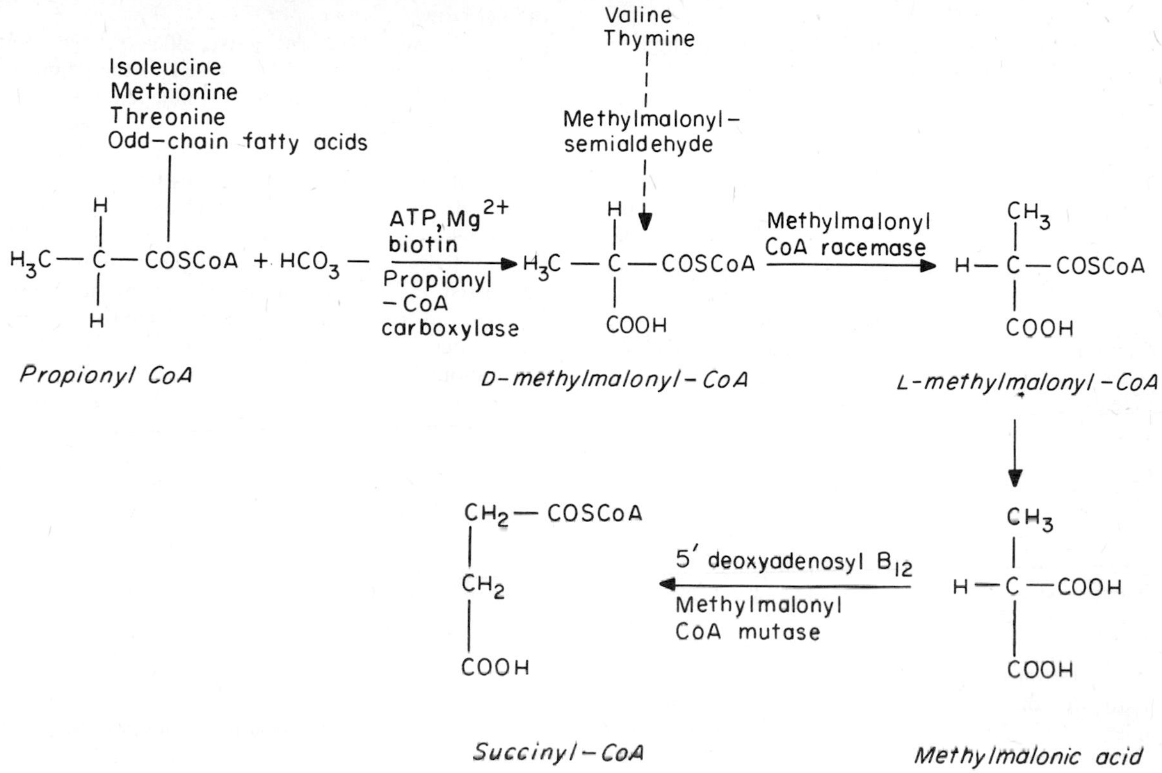

Fig. 6.4. The metabolism of propionate to succinate. The exact site at which valine and thymine feed into the pathway is unknown.

propionic acid produced by micro-organisms in their rumen. The importance of these reactions in humans is best illustrated by the syndromes that have recently been described in infants suffering from inborn errors of metabolism involving them (see p. 238) [28, 29].

Isomerization of β leucine to α leucine
The enzyme catalysing the reversible migration of an amino group from a terminal carbon atom in α leucine to an adjacent one in β leucine has been identified in human tissues [30]. In B$_{12}$ deficiency, β leucine accumulates while α leucine is decreased, implying that the normal reaction is in the β→α leucine direction [31].

BIOCHEMICAL REACTIONS IN BACTERIA
In addition to the three reactions already described, B$_{12}$ takes part in a number of other reactions in various micro-organisms. *Methylcobalamin* is required for transmethylation or other reactions involving methyl or carboxyl groups (e.g. synthesis of methane and the formation of acetate from carbon dioxide). *Deoxyadenosylcobalamin* is required for reactions involving transfer of hydrogen atoms and their replacement by an adjacent group as in the isomerization of L-glutamic acid to threo-β-methyl-L-aspartic acid, oxidation of 1,2-diols (1,2-propanediol, and 1,2-ethanediol) by the enzyme diol-dehydrase to the corresponding aldehydes, the conversion of ethanolamine to acetaldehyde and ammonia, reduction of ribonucleoside triphosphates to deoxyribonucleoside triphosphates and conversion of lysine to butyrate, acetate and ammonia. None of these reactions has been found to require B$_{12}$ in mammalian systems. In humans, ribonucleotide reduction occurs at the diphosphate level and activation of the enzyme requires iron rather than B$_{12}$. Single reports have suggested that cobalamins are involved in methylation of RNA in the rat and in protein synthesis but both await confirmation. B$_{12}$-deficient chicks have been found to have elevated hepatic levels of pantothenate. If true, this could be due to a disturbance of coenzyme-A metabolism due to reduced isomerization of methylmalonyl CoA.

DIETARY SOURCES

A normal Western diet contains between three and 30 μg B_{12} daily, usually 5–10 μg; the amount increases by-and-large with the cost and quality of the diet, since the vitamin is found solely in foods of animal origin (Table 6.1). All natural B_{12} arises from synthesis by micro-organisms, and animals derive it either by direct absorption from the intestine (as in ruminants), by coprophagy (as in herbivores such as the rabbit and fowl) or in food (as in humans). The highest concentrations are found in liver (which contains about 1 μg/g), kidney, shellfish, muscle meats, fowl and dairy produce including milk, which in humans has 0·1 μg/100 g. There is probably no B_{12} in fruit, vegetables, nuts and cereals, unless these have been contaminated by bacteria. Soil and natural waters also contain B_{12} due to bacterial contamination. In general, B_{12} is not destroyed by cooking but, under alkaline conditions and in the presence of vitamin C, some may be lost at high temperatures (e.g. on boiling fresh milk), while severe heating of meat and meat products may also partly degrade B_{12}. Large doses of vitamin C may also degrade B_{12} *in vivo* [32].

HUMAN STORES AND REQUIREMENTS

Estimates of total human adult body B_{12} stores by microbiological and isotope-dilution techniques have shown levels ranging from two to 11 mg with a mean usually in the range of 3–5 mg. The highest concentration is in liver, with about 20% of this concentration in kidney, adrenal, pancreas and lower levels in other organs. The cerebro-spinal fluid contains only 30 ng/l. Most liver B_{12} and B_{12} in other cells is in mitochondria, as ado-B_{12}. Small amounts of methyl-B_{12} are present in cell cytoplasm and this is the main form in plasma. Small amounts of hydroxo- and cyano-B_{12} also occur in plasma. In the fetus, the highest concentrations are in liver, adrenal, kidney and lung; plasma, spleen, lung and colon have higher levels than in the adult [33].

Daily requirements are thought to be about 2–3 μg, though a smaller dose, between 0·1 and 1 μg will produce an haematological response in a patient with megaloblastic anaemia due to B_{12} deficiency. Losses occur mainly in the urine and in faeces but the human body does not seem able to degrade B_{12}. Heysell *et al.* [33a] have suggested that body B_{12} is lost at a constant rate in proportion to body B_{12} stores of the order of 0·1%/day. If this is so, absolute losses would be less as the body becomes depleted and this would help to protect patients from severe deficiency. In practice, it takes from two to four years for megaloblastic anaemia to develop following total gastrectomy—which causes sudden cessation of B_{12} absorption. Stores are lower in subjects existing on a vegan diet (e.g. in India) and less B_{12} is then needed to maintain the status quo.

ABSORPTION

Two mechanisms exist, one active, efficient, mediated by intrinsic factor (IF) and localized to the ileum in man, the other passive, inefficient, independent of IF and non-specific to site. Virtually all dietary B_{12} appears to be available for absorption. It is released from protein and peptide complexes in the stomach and duodenum and mainly attaches to IF. A portion also attaches to non-IF 'R' binder (see below). This has less selectivity than IF for true B_{12} compounds and may assist in the prevention of absorption of B_{12} analogues in food or synthesized in some subjects by upper intestinal organisms [34–36]. The R binder forms about 20% of the B_{12} binding capacity of normal gastric juice, IF forming about 60% partly degraded IF the remainder. Intrinsic factor is a glycoprotein of MW 44 000–48 000 with about 15% carbohydrate, which is actively secreted by the parietal cells of the body and fundus of the stomach in humans, the cells which also secrete hydrochloric acid. Cyclic nucleotides in gastric mucosa regulate the secretion [37]. The existence of this protein was first demonstrated by the important studies of Castle published in 1929 and 1930 in patients with pernicious anaemia [38]. Most animals (but not the dog) secrete an IF but this shows some species specificity [39]. One molecule of IF binds one molecule of B_{12} but the complex readily dimerizes. Intrinsic factor binds equally well all the neutral cobalamins, and Gräsbeck [40] considers that the nucleotide portion of B_{12} fits into a pit on the surface of IF, the —CN, —OH, or other group attached to the cobalt being outermost. Hippe *et al.* [41] have shown that IF (and the transcobalamins) bind to cyanocobalamin in the region of the edge of the corrin ring, probably with overlap to the adjoining part of the dimethylbenzimidazole. B_{12} analogues such as cobamides and cobinamides are not bound by IF.

The complex B_{12}–IF has a smaller molecular radius (32 nm) than free IF (36 nm) and it is likely that surface peptide bonds of IF, easily attacked by proteolytic enzymes (e.g. pepsin) in the digestive tract, are protected in the complex by infolding of the molecule. Nevertheless, some free IF is present in the upper small intestinal lumen and may bind biliary B_{12} and, it has been postulated, B_{12} produced by some small intestinal bacteria [42]. Binding of B_{12} by IF is rapid, the equilibrium constant for the reaction at 26°C is estimated at 6×10^9 M, the same from pH 2 to 10 and more recently as $1·5 \times 10^9$ M [43]. At pH values above 10–12, IF is destroyed.

One unit of IF is defined as that which binds 1 ng of B_{12}. Basal secretion by young adult males is about 3000 units/hour, or about 36 units/ml; females secrete a similar concentration but about half the total amount, while in older subjects, the average secretion falls to about 50% over the age of 50. Following histamine, gastrin, pentagastrin or insulin stimulation, secretion increases to 16 000 units/hour, or to 100 units/ml in concentration in young adult males. There is a relation between amount of acid and IF secreted, except in the first 15 minutes after stimulation, when IF secretion rises disproportionately, due to release of preformed IF.

Maximum absorption from a $1 \cdot 0$ μg dose of B_{12} requires 500–1000 units of IF. Thus the body secretes a vast excess and the normal limiting factor on absorption appears to be in the ileum [44, 45], which in humans is capable of absorbing only $1 \cdot 5$ μg B_{12} from a single oral dose of IF–B_{12} complex. Following this, the ileum is refractory to further B_{12} absorption for about three to four hours. At neutral pH and in the presence of calcium ions, IF–B_{12} complex passively attaches to receptor sites on the brush border membrane of the ileal mucosal cells. The ileal receptor is a macromolecule, $MW > 1 \times 10^6$, a lipoprotein consisting of two subunits [46–50]. Approximately $0 \cdot 3$–$4 \cdot 9 \times 10^{12}$ molecules are present per gram of mucosa [51]. The steps that occur in the transfer of B_{12} across the ileal cell are still not completely understood. It is likely that an energy-requiring step is involved and B_{12} enters either the mitochondria or lysosomes of the cell and remains there during a period of mucosal delay, in man about six hours, the peak blood level being reached only eight to 12 hours after an oral dose [52–54]. Thereafter B_{12} is transferred to the portal blood, where it is found attached mainly to transcobalamin (TC)II [55]. The TCII involved may be produced locally by the ileum [56, 57]; in congenital TCII deficiency there is malabsorption of B_{12} [58]. Intrinsic factor does not enter portal blood but whether it is digested off at the brush border, or also enters the cell [59] is uncertain although recent work suggests that lysosomal digestion is a probable mechanism [60]. Cyano-B_{12} enters plasma largely or completely unchanged [61]. Without IF only $0 \cdot 5$–$1 \cdot 5\%$ of a single oral dose of the order of 30–300 μg of B_{12} is absorbed in man by the second mechanism—i.e passively. This occurs through the duodenum and jejunum (or nasal, buccal or respiratory-tract mucosae) and is rapid, with a rise in serum level in one hour.

Role of pancreatic secretion

Trypsin digests R protein (see below) secreted in gastric juice which competes with IF for food B_{12}. The R binder is capable of binding B_{12} as tightly as IF and competes with IF particularly effectively at low pH. Thus the alkali pH of the pancreatic secretion as well as proteolytic enzymes aids B_{12} transfer from R binders to IF [35].

Entero-hepatic circulation

Variable estimates have been given of the amount of B_{12} in bile, ranging from less than 1 μg to as high as 43 μg/day. Further B_{12} enters the gut lumen from gastric, pancreatic and intestinal secretions and from sloughed intestinal cells. In all patients with malabsorption of B_{12}, it is all lost in faeces; in normal subjects and vegans a large proportion of this B_{12} is presumably reabsorbed and this may explain the less rapid clearance of B_{12} from the body in normals and vegans compared to pernicious anaemia noted in some studies [62].

PLASMA TRANSPORT OF VITAMIN B_{12}

Two proteins which carry B_{12} in plasma are reasonably well characterized, TCI and TCII, and each binds B_{12}, one molecule for one molecule, probably attaching to the B group in the corrin nucleus [63] (Fig 6.5).

Transcobalamin I (TCI)

Transcobalamin I is one of a number of closely related proteins (R binders, also termed 'cobalothins') [64] present in many cells of the body as well as in plasma, bile, saliva, CSF and gastric juice. The R-B_{12} binding proteins, present in saliva, milk, pleural and amniotic fluids, appear to have identical polypeptide portions defined by amino-acid composition and immune reactivity. The terminal amino acids have been sequenced in two R binders and found to be identical [65, 66]. The carbohydrate consists of sialic acid, fucose, galactose, mannose, galactosamine and glucosamine in differing proportions. The serum protein is thought to be largely secreted by granulocytes and their precursors and is released when these cells die [67]. Its concentration in plasma appears to be related to the size of the total blood (and possibly marrow and splenic) granulocyte pool [68, 69]. It has a molecular weight (MW), as estimated by gel filtration, of about 121 000 [70]. More recent studies after purification by affinity chromatography show the MW to be 56 000–58 000 with a Stokes' radius of $51 \cdot 3$ nm [71, 72]. It migrates on electrophoresis as an α_1 globulin, and in normal serum is thought to be capable of carrying about 700–800 ng B_{12}/l. It carries nearly all the B_{12} normally present in serum [73] and is capable, on average, of binding another 200–300 ng/l, being 50–70% saturated. The TCI gains B_{12} which is released from tissues, especially the liver. The amount attached to TCI (which largely accounts for the serum B_{12} level) therefore relates to body stores of B_{12}. The TCI gives up B_{12} only slowly to tissues. It has been considered to be a storage form of B_{12} and absence of this binder from plasma has been reported to cause a low level of B_{12} in serum but no clinical abnormality [74]. The TCI-B_{12} has a half-life in plasma of nine to ten days.

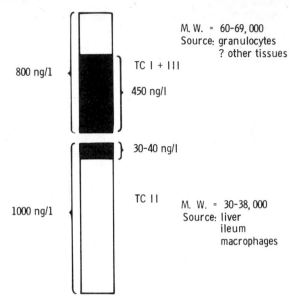

M. W. = 60–69,000
Source: granulocytes
? other tissues

TC I + III

800 ng/l

450 ng/l

30–40 ng/l

TC II

1000 ng/l

M. W. = 30–38,000
Source: liver
ileum
macrophages

Fig. 6.5. The transcobalamins (serum-B_{12}-binding proteins) indicating the amount of endogenous B_{12} normally attached to them (solid rectangles) and their unsaturated binding capacity (open rectangles).

The half-life of TCI apo-protein is similar to that of TCI-B_{12}.

Transcobalamin III (TCIII)

This is the name given to a glycoprotein identical to TCI except for minor variations in the sugar composition [75–77]. It separates from TCI on ion exchange chromatography but not on Sephadex-gel filtration. There is evidence that it arises mainly from mature neutrophils whereas TCI is derived mainly from neutrophil precursors [78]. In contrast to TCI, the half-life is only three minutes (human TCIII in rabbit), it is not catabolized in the liver and a proportion is excreted intact in bile. Recent work suggests that one role of TCI and TCIII is to bind B_{12} analogues (which may be absorbed from the diet) and to transport these to the liver for excretion in the bile [34]. TCII, like IF, is a more selective binder for 'true' B_{12} and does not bind or enhance marrow uptake of B_{12} analogues. Gullberg [79] suggests that the R binders in plasma secretions and milk may also have a bacteriostatic action by depriving micro-organisms of B_{12}.

Transcobalamin II (TCII)

The second B_{12}-binding protein in plasma has an estimated MW of 38 000 by centrifugation after purification by affinity chromatography [80], a Stokes' radius of 25·5 nm and a similar electrophoretic mobility to β globulin. It is synthesized in the liver [81], macrophages [81] and probably in the ileum [56, 57]. Studies following bone-marrow transplantation suggest that macrophages are the major source since the

TCII iso-protein pattern (see below) of the recipient largely assumes that of the donor [82]. The protein normally carries about 50 ng/l of B_{12} (5–10% of plasma B_{12}) but is capable of binding about 1000 ng/l and, being unsaturated, binds most of the B_{12} leaving cells [83, 84]. Uptake of B_{12} from TCII by haemopoietic cells requires calcium or magnesium ions and active cellular protein synthesis, and is reduced if cells are B_{12} deficient, but normal or increased when cells are folate deficient [85, 86].

After entering liver cells from TCII, B_{12} accumulates mainly in mitochondria but a transient lysosomal phase has also been demonstrated [87]. Specific receptors on the cell surface for TCII-B_{12} have been isolated from plasma membranes of rat liver, human placenta and fibroblasts [88, 89]. It is likely that TCII-B_{12} complex enters cells by pinocytosis, with release of B_{12}, mainly to enter mitochondria, after digestion of TCII by proteolysis. Congenital deficiency of TCII causes the development of megaloblastic anaemia at a few weeks of age because of inability to transfer B_{12} from plasma to the marrow. Semi-purified TCII has been reported to have a half-life of as little as five to 90 minutes and not to be re-utilized, but whether this half-life applies to undenatured TCII is uncertain [6, 71]. An antibody to TCII has been described in patients receiving long-term therapy with depot B_{12} preparations of hydroxocobalamin and such patients show extremely high (> 10 μg/l) serum B_{12} levels [90]. Five iso-proteins of TCII (TCII, 1–5) have been identified which are inherited in a Mendelian recessive pattern [91, 92]. There is no evidence for a functional difference in these TCII iso-proteins in the transport of B$_{12}$.

Other vitamin-B$_{12}$-binding proteins

A number of other binding proteins have been described. An α-globulin binder occurs in fetal serum and in the sera of patients with polycythaemia vera, which differs qualitatively from normal TCI but it is not clear whether or not this is identical to TCIII. 'R' binders (which have a sugar composition different from TCI or TCIII) have also been described in the sera of patients with tumours [93–95]. An abnormal TCII has also been described in one patient [96].

DISTURBANCES OF VITAMIN-B$_{12}$-BINDING PROTEINS IN DISEASE

Transcobalamin I and III

Changes in the concentration of the serum-B$_{12}$-binding proteins may occur in a variety of diseases and may or may not be associated with changes in the serum B$_{12}$ level. The most important abnormality is a rise in TCI which occurs in chronic granulocytic leukaemia (CGL) and also in other myeloproliferative diseases such as myelosclerosis, polycythaemia vera and acute myeloid leukaemia (AML). The serum B$_{12}$ level in CGL is usually in the range of 1000–10 000 ng/l [97]. There is some evidence that the binder in these conditions may be qualitatively abnormal since it may bind B$_{12}$ so firmly that the serum B$_{12}$ level may remain normal even if the patient also develops pernicious anaemia with megaloblastic anaemia [98]. In polycythaemia vera, where the increase is largely of mature cells, TCIII rather than TCI is usually raised [99, 100]. Benign diseases associated with a chronic leucocytosis may also be accompanied by a rise in serum unsaturated-B$_{12}$-binding capacity (UB$_{12}$BC) due mainly to a rise in TCIII, as in chronic inflammatory bowel diseases [101]. The TCIII is released from granulocytes *in vitro* after blood has been taken, however, and care must be taken to avoid this *in-vitro* artefact which is particularly marked with lithium heparin anti-coagulant [102, 103].

High serum B$_{12}$ levels occur in patients with carcinoma of various types [104, 105] when the liver cells are breaking down in association with acute hepatitis, active cirrhosis, liver abscess, hepatoma and other forms of acute liver damage [106] and can be used to follow response to therapy of these diseases [107]. Part of the B$_{12}$ may be free, but rises in both β(TCII) and α-globulin (TCI and III) binders have also been described, as well as a variant of TCI in children with hepatoma. A hepatoma binder with similar polypeptide but different sugar composition to normal TCI has been identified [66, 93]. Raised TCI with a raised serum B$_{12}$ level may also occur in renal failure [108].

Transcobalamin II

There is an increase in serum UB$_{12}$BC in untreated pernicious anaemia but a decrease in total B$_{12}$BC due to a fall in the level of TCII. In pregnancy, on the other hand, there is an increase in TCII. Increase in TCII has also been described in autoimmune diseases [109], Gaucher's disease [110], myeloma [111] and in acute myeloblastic leukaemia with monocytic differentiation [99]. In autoimmune diseases, it is suggested that TCII levels may be used to monitor the response to therapy [112]. The serum B$_{12}$ level is often normal in these conditions despite the raised TCII levels. Both congenital absence of TCII [58] and familial raised TCII levels have been described [113].

VITAMIN B$_{12}$ DEFICIENCY

The deficiency arises either because of inadequate ingestion or because of malabsorption of the vitamin (Table 6.2).

INADEQUATE INTAKE

Adults

Inadequate intake is a rare cause of deficiency in Western communities, since it only occurs in strict vegans or in subjects taking a wholly inadequate diet for economic or psychiatric reasons. It is, however, common in Hindu individuals in India, East Africa, Britain and elsewhere who, for religious and often economic reasons, avoid all animal foods such as meat, fish and dairy produce. Such a diet contains virtually

Table 6.2. Causes of vitamin-B$_{12}$ deficiency

Veganism

Gastric lesions: (Adult) pernicious anaemia; congenital intrinsic factor deficiency or abnormality; total or partial gastrectomy

Intestinal lesions: Stagnant-loop syndrome (blind-loop, fistula, jejunal diverticulosis, stricture, etc.); ileal resection and Crohn's disease; selective malabsorption with proteinuria; chronic tropical sprue; fish tapeworm, transcobalamin-II deficiency

---

no B_{12} and in one subject, who developed megaloblastic anaemia, the measured B_{12} in her diet was only 0·5 μg daily [114]. Milk or eggs help to protect against nutritional B_{12} deficiency, but boiling milk, as is usually practised by Hindus, reduces its B_{12} content. The incidence of mild B_{12} deficiency (or low B_{12} stores) in Indian vegans (assessed by Western normal standards) is extemely high (e.g. 50% of normal young adult Hindu medical students were found to have serum B_{12} levels less than 100 ng/l, but only a small proportion developed clinical symptoms of megaloblastic anaemia [115, 116]. The main fall in the serum B_{12} level occurs within the first two years on a vegan diet (as B_{12} levels fall geometrically) and subsequent falls may not occur even after many further years, and the subject may remain in perfect health. Red-cell B_{12} levels have been found normal in most subjects despite reduced serum B_{12} levels [117]. Possibly, the intact entero-hepatic circulation reduces losses of B_{12} [62]. Moreover, absolute losses are reduced in relation to stores and thus minute quantities of B_{12} eaten may maintain haemopoiesis at an adequate level despite stores being low.

In Hindu vegans, folate deficiency is also frequent, apparently due to the low folate content of the diet, which consists largely of polished rice and well-cooked vegetables. Iron deficiency is also frequent, particularly in females. On the other hand, westerners who take a strict vegetarian diet tend to have high blood folate levels, probably because of a high folate diet. Such subjects may present with B_{12} neuropathy which is extremely rare in Hindu vegans [118].

Infants

Infants born and breast-fed by B_{12}-deficient mothers due to veganism, sprue or, more rarely, unrecognized pernicious anaemia, may develop megaloblastic anaemia as early as four months of age [119, 120]. This responds to oral B_{12} in doses as little as 0·1 μg daily [119]. Lack of B_{12} transfer *in utero* as well as in milk appears to be the cause.

MALABSORPTION OF VITAMIN B_{12}

The conditions which cause B_{12} deficiency sufficient to cause megaloblastic anaemia are described first. These are relatively few and by far the most important of these in Western countries is Addisonian pernicious anaemia (Table 6.2). Conditions which usually only cause mild degrees of B_{12} deficiency or transient malabsorption of B_{12} are dealt with subsequently.

ADULT PERNICIOUS ANAEMIA (PA)

This is defined as severe malabsorption of B_{12} due to lack of IF following atrophic gastritis.

Incidence

The peak age at diagnosis is 60 years, and only about 10% of patients present before 40 years. In most series, there has been a preponderance of women to men of about 10:7. The highest incidence occurs in northern Europeans, and in Scandinavia the incidence is 100–130 per 100 000 population. In Britain there are quite marked regional differences with over 200 cases per 100 000 in parts of Scotland, less than 100 per 100 000 in south-east England. Probably no race is immune to the disease which has been reported in Chinese, Indians, Indonesians, American Indians and Negroes, as well as in all countries and races of Europe.

There is an increased incidence of PA in persons of blood group A—in one series 44·9% of patients were blood group A compared to 40·3% of controls. It is also more common in those with light-coloured eyes, early greying of the hair and vitiligo. There is also a marked familial tendency with an incidence in close relatives about 20 times that in controls, a positive family history in 20–30% of patients, and an increased incidence in the monozygotic twin of a patient. First- and second-degree relatives of patients show an increased incidence either of overt PA or of one or more abnormality found in PA such as gastric achlorhydria, atrophic gastritis, malabsorption of B_{12}, or parietal-cell antibody in serum.

Overall, no association between PA and any particular HLA-histocompatibility group has been observed in several studies, although when a subgroup of PA associated with endocrine diseases was considered alone, an association with HLA-B8, B12 and BW15 was found.

Latent pernicious anaemia. This term was used to describe patients with no anaemia but atrophic gastritis, malabsorption of B_{12} and mild B_{12} deficiency [121]. Parietal-cell antibodies are usually present, IF antibodies present in about 50% of patients. There seems little need to distinguish this group from early PA and they should be treated similarly.

Associated diseases

Endocrine disease. There is a marked clinical and immunological overlap between PA and thyrotoxicosis, primary myxoedema and Hashimoto's disease. Not only is the incidence of these three diseases increased in PA patients, but also thyroid antibodies occur in 55% of PA patients and are common in their relatives, while PA occurs in about 10%, and gastric-parietal-cell antibody in about 33% of patients with primary myxoedema including Hashimoto's disease [122]. There are also definite associations between PA and Addison's disease and hypoparathyroidism in which PA has been reported in between five and 10% of cases [123, 124] (see also Chapter 33). Vitiligo occurs in 90% of PA patients while there is an increased incidence of PA and parietal-cell antibody in vitiligo.

Other diseases. Macrocytic anaemia was found in 27 of 2544 patients (1·05%) with rheumatoid arthritis [125]. Not all these patients were studied in detail and a proportion were probably not cases of PA. This study does not suggest a significant association of rheumatoid arthritis and PA, nor is PA particularly common in patients with myasthenia gravis. The association of PA with diabetes mellitus is also not well-established statistically, since the two diseases are common in older age groups. Nevertheless, serum-parietal-cell antibody definitely occurs with an increased incidence, and serum IF antibody has also been described in the absence of PA in patients with diabetes mellitus [126].

There is a definite association between PA and hypo-γ-globulinaemia, however [127]. This may be of the primary acquired or congenital types and affect all three immunoglobulins or IgA selectively. Pernicious anaemia is similar to that in other patients but manifests relatively early, at less than 40 years in half the patients and may, in some cases, be preceded by a history of recurring infections. The patients usually lack serum antibodies to gastric antigens, but these may be present in those with selective IgA deficiency, and plasma cells are absent from the inflammatory infiltrate in the gastric mucosa. There is an increased incidence of intestinal malabsorption in these patients, in some due to giardiasis, and there may be little or no correction of malabsorption with B$_{12}$ therapy. The incidence in PA in hypo-γ-globulinaemia is three per cent or less but the incidence of atrophic gastritis in hypo-γ-globulinaemia is probably much higher [127].

In children, PA (and other organ-specific auto-immune diseases) may be associated with chronic monilial infection of skin, mucous membranes and nails. This appears to be due to defective T-cell function. Other probable associations with PA are pure red-cell aplasia and dermatitis herpetiformis; associations which have been suggested and not proven include myeloma, polycythaemia vera and myelofibrosis. The association of PA with iron-deficiency anaemia is complex. There is no doubt an increased incidence of PA, atrophic gastritis and parietal-cell antibody in iron-deficiency-anaemia patients. Iron therapy may increase acid secretion without any improvement in the histology of the stomach. How far the changes are due to defective cell-mediated immunity in iron deficiency, a direct effect of iron lack on the stomach, or early PA leading to iron deficiency due to atrophic gastritis is difficult to analyse.

Carcinoma of the stomach. The incidence of gastric cancer, estimated from post-mortem studies, is about four to six per cent with a two to three per cent incidence in clinical studies of patients followed for varying periods of time, about three times that in the normal population [128]. It is more common in men than women and significantly reduces the life-expectancy of males with PA. The tumour is found more commonly in the body and fundus of the stomach as compared with pylorus and antrum, and gastric polypi at these sites are also frequent.

Clinical features

The onset is usually insidious, often with definite symptoms for only a few weeks, preceded by years of ill-health only recognized after successful therapy. The symptoms vary greatly according to the degree of anaemia and the age of the patient. When anaemia is severe, the patient usually shows general weakness, pallor, tiredness, shortness of breath, anorexia and weight-loss. In older subjects, features of congestive heart failure, angina of effort or intermittent claudication may be present. Younger subjects often have surprisingly few symptoms despite severe anaemia. A sore tongue is common even without anaemia; the tongue is either bald or red, raw and painful. An association with aphthous ulceration inside the mouth has been suggested but not proven [129]. Paraesthesiae are also frequent even in patients without objective evidence of a neuropathy. Diarrhoea, episodic or continuous, may occur. An infection, particularly of the chest or urinary tract, may precipitate symptoms. Infertility is usual in both sexes and may be the presenting feature. Melanin pigmentation around the nail beds, over the face and trunk, particularly in skin creases, may occur and reverses rapidly with B$_{12}$ therapy. Mild jaundice, which together with pallor gives the patient a 'lemon-yellow' tint and a mild fever are common findings. The spleen is palpable in about half the severely anaemic patients. When anaemia is mild or absent there may be no clinical features and the diagnosis may only be made when a blood count and film are examined for other reasons.

Vitamin-B$_{12}$ neuropathy

Patients with B$_{12}$ deficiency or inactivation of B$_{12}$ (e.g. by nitrous oxide) may present with neurological disease as well as, or instead of, anaemia. The usual symptoms are paraesthesiae in the feet, or feet and hands, difficulty in walking ('walking on cotton wool') and, more rarely, difficulty with use of the hands. Sensations of numbness, cold or of lightning pains in the limbs and loss of bladder and rectal control are less common and late features. The symptoms arise because of a peripheral neuropathy, associated in some cases with degeneration of the posterior and lateral tracts of the spinal cord. The basic pathology is demyelination which in more severe cases is accompanied by degeneration of axis cylinders. The posterior columns are affected before the lateral tracts. The legs are always more severely affected than arms. Loss of vibration and position sense with an ataxic gait and positive Romberg sign are features of posterior column and peripheral nerve loss. Superficial pain and touch sensation are lost. Loss of vibration sense is marked but deep-pain sensation preserved. Spastic paresis may occur with knee and ankle reflexes increased due to lateral-tract loss, but flaccid weakness may also occur with these reflexes lost but the Babinski response extensor. Visual disturbances with retrobulbar neuritis or optic neuropathy may be present. Mental symptoms are usually mild, consisting of forgetfulness, irritability and inertia. Rarely an organic dementia with delirium is present but psychotic features usually only occur in those with an underlying predisposition. Electro-encephalogram changes have been described which improve with therapy [130].

The neuropathy is more common in men than women and always signifies a severe degree of B_{12} deficiency, assessed biochemically, even when anaemia is mild or absent. The usual cause is PA, but it may arise in patients suffering from severe B_{12} deficiency from other causes such as gastrectomy, the intestinal stagnant-loop syndrome, chronic tropical sprue and veganism. The biochemical basis for B_{12} neuropathy remains obscure, though recently attempts have been made to relate this to a disturbance in the homocysteine–methionine reaction (see p. 202).

Haematological findings

Like the clinical features, the peripheral blood and bone-marrow appearances vary markedly according to the severity of anaemia. When the haemoglobin is extremely low (4–6 g/dl) the peripheral blood shows marked variation in size and shape of red cells with many oval macrocytes, cell fragments and distorted cells (Fig. 6.6). The number of red cells is reduced to a greater extent than the haemoglobin and the MCV is usually raised to levels between 110 and 140 fl, although in some severely anaemic cases, the MCV may be normal, probably due to presence of many small fragmented cells. The proportion of cells containing Howell–Jolly bodies is slightly raised but only markedly so if the spleen is atrophied or has been removed. Punctate basophilia is present and reticulocytes stain deeply and the MCHC is normal, but a proportion of the distorted cells may appear hypochromic. The leucocyte count is reduced to $1\cdot5$–$4\cdot0 \times 10^9$/l due to a fall in both neutrophils and

lymphocytes and a proportion of the neutrophils show hypersegmented nuclei (i.e. more than five lobes) and eosinophils show more than two lobes. Very large neutrophils with eight or more lobes (macropolycytes) may be present. The platelet count is moderately reduced, usually to levels of 50–150×10^9/l. Patients with leucocyte counts less than 1×10^9/l and platelet counts of $15\cdot0 \times 10^9$/l or less are recorded and may be misdiagnosed as having aplastic anaemia or acute leukaemia. Megaloblasts and myelocytes (due to extra-medullary haemopoiesis) may be found in the peripheral blood, particularly if buffy-coat films are examined.

When anaemia is less severe, macrocytosis is still the main feature but the distortion of red cells and the fall in leucocytes and platelets is less marked. In mildly anaemic or non-anaemic cases, only a few macrocytes and hypersegmented neutrophils and a raised MCV may suggest the diagnosis.

Macrocytosis may also occur due to alcohol ingestion, liver disease, myxoedema, aplastic anaemia, acquired sideroblastic anaemia, myeloma, etc., and in any patient with a raised reticulocyte count (e.g. due to haemolytic anaemia or acute haemorrhage) (Table 6.3). Hypersegmented neutrophils are also seen in renal failure and as a familial disorder. They may occur

Table 6.3. Macrocytosis usually without megaloblastic anaemia

1 Alcohol
2 Liver disease
3 Myxoedema
4 Cytotoxic drugs
5 Reticulocytosis (e.g. after haemorrhage, haemolysis)
6 Aplastic anaemia and pure red-cell aplasia
7 Primary acquired sideroblastic anaemia
8 Myeloma and other maligant diseases
9 Pregnancy
10 New born
11 Chronic airways disease
12 Pre-leukaemia ('myelodysplastic syndromes')

in iron deficiency, but then there is usually associated B_{12} or folate deficiency.

The blood appearances are identical in megaloblastic anaemia due to B_{12} or folate deficiencies whatever the causes, but the picture may be modified by associated conditions (see Fig. 6.6). When iron deficiency is also present, the MCV may be normal and the peripheral blood assumes a dimorphic appearance with small hypochromic cells and well-filled macrocytes. Infections, particularly in patients with conditions of increased folate requirement such as pregnancy, chronic haemolysis and myelosclerosis, may precipitate an 'aplastic arrest' of haemopoiesis with possibly rapidly developing pancytopenia. In such cases there may be little evidence of megaloblastic haemopoiesis in the peripheral blood and although the marrow is usually megaloblastic, it may occasionally show an erythroblastopenia. Megaloblastic anaemia may also be superimposed on diseases such as myelosclerosis, haemolytic anaemia, carcinoma or myeloma, which modify the blood film and cause the anaemia to be out of proportion to the degree of megaloblastic change.

The bone marrow in the severely anaemic case is hypercellular, usually with a lowered or reversed myeloid/erythroid ratio, though occasionally erythroid hypoplasia may occur [131]. The extent of haemopoietic marrow is increased, particularly in younger subjects, and red marrow may be found in the tibiae and bones of the forearm. There is an increased proportion of early cells, erythroblasts and myeloblasts. The erythroid cells at all stages have a megaloblastic appearance. The cells are large, the nucleus has an open, stippled or lacy appearance (Fig. 6.6). The cytoplasm is relatively more mature than the nucleus and this dissociation is best seen in the later cells, since fully orthochromatic cells may be present with nuclei that are still not fully condensed. Mitoses are frequent and sometimes abnormal, and nuclear remnants, Howell–Jolly bodies, bi- and tri-nucleated cells and dying cells all indicate gross dyserythropoiesis.

There is an increased number and size of siderotic granules in the developing erythroblasts, and marrow iron stores usually appear normal or increased. Ring sideroblasts are unusual except in alcoholic megaloblastic anaemia. The abnormalities of granulocyte precursors are best seen in the metamyelocytes, which are abnormally large (giant), and may assume peculiar shapes since their nuclei are twisted and bent. Hypersegmented polymorphs may be seen and the megakaryocytes show an increase in nuclear lobes. Iron deficiency may partly mask the changes in the red cells but not in the white cells.

The severity of megaloblastic change is related to the degree of anaemia. In less anaemic cases, hypercellularity of the marrow with an increased proportion of early erythroid cells is less marked or absent. The main features are the abnormal nuclear pattern and asynchrony between nuclear and cytoplasmic development of red-cell precursors and the giant metamyelocytes. The megaloblastic changes in less anaemic cases may be described as 'intermediate', 'early', 'mild' or 'transitional' [132]. The term 'megaloblastoid' is best avoided altogether as it has been used in several ways—to denote mild changes, or changes not responsive to B$_{12}$ or folate, or changes the nature of which the observer is unsure.

GENERAL LABORATORY FINDINGS IN MEGALOBLASTIC ANAEMIA

The specific changes in B$_{12}$ or folate deficiency are discussed elsewhere. The general abnormalities are mainly due to a shortened red-cell survival and increased death of cells in the marrow (ineffective haemopoiesis). Red-cell survival is reduced due to both intra- and extracorpuscular defects. Serum bilirubin is usually in the range 17–50 μmol/l with an increase mainly in the prehepatic (unconjugated) component. There is an increased stercobilinogen excretion compared to the circulating haemoglobin mass and there is elevated early excretion of labelled bilirubin after an injection of [^{15}N]-glycine [133] due to an increase in the later (marrow) rather than early (hepatic) component of the early excretion peak [134]. The direct Coombs test is positive in about 10% of cases due to complement only [135] and the cells show other membrane abnormalities such as an increase in the I and i antigens and of sensitivity to cold lysis and a disturbance of red-cell membrane proteins [135a]. There is a raised plasma methaemalbumin level with a positive Schumm's test in over 50% of severe cases. Haemosiderinuria is uncommon but absence of haptoglobins usual. The serum lactic-dehydrogenase level is raised to between 1000 and 10 000 iu [136] due to an increase mainly in the first and second (heat-stable) isoenzymes [137]. The rise has been attributed to an increase in enzyme level in individual megaloblasts as well as to increased cell destruction, but this is not established. Serum γ-hydroxybutyrate dehydrogenase, SGOT, phosphohexose isomerase, aldolase, isocitric dehydrogenase and malic dehydrogenase among other enzymes may also be raised and there is a moderate rise in serum lysosome (muramidase) [138]. The activities of many enzymes in red cells are increased in megaloblastic anaemia and fall with specific therapy. There is a generally increased level of amino acids in blood and urine and increased urea excretion though serum levels of methionine are low and those of valine are normal [139]. Serum cholesterol is reduced.

Iron metabolism

The serum iron is raised in the more anaemic patients, and with transferrin levels somewhat reduced, about 50% of the total iron-binding capacity (TIBC) is saturated. Plasma iron clearance is rapid, iron turnover raised but incorporation into red cells reduced [140]. The maturation time of red cells, studied by ^{59}Fe incorporation is prolonged [141]. Serum ferritin levels are raised in the more anaemic cases and fall with therapy within the first 24–48 hours [142].

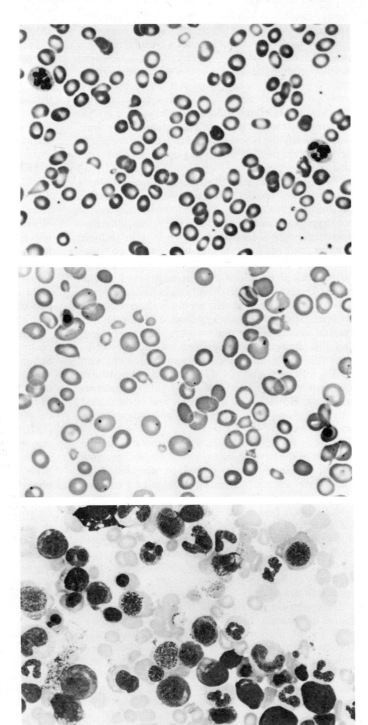

Fig. 6.6a. Peripheral-blood film of a 32-year-old female with nutritional megaloblastic anaemia; haemoglobin 6·1 g/dl, serum vitamin B_{12} 120 pg/ml. The film shows gross anisocytosis and poikilocytosis, oval macrocytes and three hyper-segmented polymorphs (May–Grünwald–Giemsa, × 492).

Fig. 6.6b. Peripheral-blood film of a 58-year-old female with adult coeliac disease, splenic atrophy and megaloblastic anaemia; serum vitamin B_{12} 144 pg/ml; serum folate 1·4 ng/ml. The film shows gross anisocytosis, poikilocytosis and Howell–Jolly bodies, target cells, crenated cells and two circulating megaloblasts (May–Grünwald–Giemsa, × 492).

Fig. 6.6c. Bone marrow of same patient as Fig. 6.6a. This field shows developing megaloblasts at all stages, giant metamyelocytes and a hyperseg-mented polymorph (May–Grünwald–Giemsa, × 492).

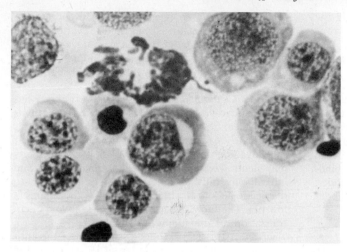

Fig. 6.6d. Bone marrow of same patient as Fig. 6.6a. at higher power (× 1066) to show a clump of developing megaloblasts.

GENERAL TISSUE EFFECTS OF VITAMIN-B₁₂·
AND FOLATE DEFICIENCIES

Either deficiency may affect all rapidly proliferating cells causing macrocytosis and nuclear abnormalities (e.g. clumped or finely dispersed chromatin and multiple cell nuclei). These changes occur in epithelial-cell surfaces (e.g. of the tongue, mouth, gastric, intestinal, respiratory, urinary and genital tracts [143]). Macrocytosis of the jejunal mucosal cells with shortening of the villi occur in untreated PA [144] but there are conflicting reports of the effect of nutritional folate deficiency [145, 146]. Both deficiencies may cause malabsorption of B₁₂ given with IF [147, 148]. A low serum alkaline phosphatase has been described in untreated PA and ascribed to decreased production from osteoblasts [149], while reduced liver regeneration in active liver disease has been reported in severe folate deficiency [150]. Chronic methotrexate toxicity may predispose to hepatic fibrosis or cirrhosis [151]. The remarkable observation that large oral (but not parental) doses of folic acid cause an increased level of jejunal glycolytic enzymes in normal subjects [152] awaits confirmation.

Vitamin-B₁₂ deficiency may cause organic nervous damage (see above) but this has not been established for severe folate deficiency, although a number of reports, usually on a few patients, have suggested improvement of a neuropathy with folic-acid therapy [153, 154] and an 18% incidence of peripheral neuropathy has been found in folate-deficient megaloblastic anaemia [155]. Folate deficiency is frequently associated with irritability, forgetfulness, slowing of mental processes and possibly organic dementia [156]. A role for folate in synthesis of brain 5-hydroxy-tryptamine has been proposed [157]. Mixed folate deficiency is common, however, in patients with psychiatric disorders, and nutritional folate deficiency is not uncommon in patients with chronic neurological disorders. Thus it remains uncertain whether folate deficiency actually causes an organic neuropathy. Melanin skin pigmentation may occur in patients with deficiency of either B₁₂ or folate and is reversed with appropriate therapy but its cause is still obscure.

PATHOGENESIS OF PERNICIOUS ANAEMIA

The stomach lesion

A severe degree of gastric atrophy, usually or always of immune origin, almost certainly underlies the disease. The gastric lesion is called gastric atrophy if glandular elements are completely lost, atrophic gastritis when severe but some glandular elements remain and superficial gastritis when the lesion is mild. The stomach is infiltrated with lymphocytes and plasma cells and the mucosa may show intestinal metaplasia. All coats of the wall are atrophic. Small numbers of parietal cells may remain in about 20–33% of PA patients. The number of endocrine-secreting cells and in particular G cells (gastrin-secreting cells) in both antrum and fundus is increased [158]. Radiological evidence of gastric atrophy is present in about 70% of all cases. The changes seen are absence or reduction of folds in the greater curve and fundus, and the stomach may assume a long, tubular shape.

Achlorhydria is present in all cases. The resting juice usually has a pH of seven or greater and there is little or no change after maximal stimulation. The volume of gastric juice secreted is also low and peptic activity subnormal.

About 80% of patients with PA have raised serum gastrin, often to levels found in the Zollinger–Ellison syndrome [159]. The source of the high gastrin levels is thought to be an increased number of G cells in the stomach which are hypersecreting because of failure of the normal inhibitory action of gastric acid.

Intrinsic factor (IF) is usually absent but can be detected in low concentration in about one-third of patients. Secretion is always less than 250 units/hour after stimulation and the concentration less than 10 units/ml. It is possible that some patients secrete larger amounts, but this is neutralized by IF antibody in the juice [160].

Non-intrinsic-factor B_{12} binders are also present in gastric juice, normally about 10% of the total B_{12}-binding capacity. In PA, the concentration of this binder, which is closely related to TCI, may be increased about three times.

Antibodies in pernicious anaemia

Three antibodies have been detected to gastric components:

Parietal-cell antibody. This reacts with the microsomal or endoplasmic-reticulum component of parietal cells of human, rat or other species [161]. It can be detected by a complement-fixation technique, or by the more sensitive immunofluorescent technique and is present in the sera of about 90% of patients. In serum it is an IgG but it has been detected in gastric juice as IgA [162].

The antibody is not rare in the general population since it occurs in two per cent of unselected persons aged less than 30 years, in eight per cent of those aged 30–60, and in as many as 16% of females aged over 60. In general, subjects with the antibody show some degree of gastritis, the incidence increasing with the severity of the lesion. The antibody has been detected in occasional subjects without gastritis however.

Parietal-cell antibody is common in close relatives of patients with PA and in many conditions other than PA—for example thyroid disorders, Addison's disease, chronic active hepatitis and chronic iron deficiency [163].

Intrinsic factor (IF) antibodies. Two apparently distinct antibodies have been described: blocking (type I) antibody which prevents the attachment of B_{12} to IF but has no effect on the complex, and binding (type II, precipitating, co-precipitating) antibody which combines with IF whether or not it is attached to B_{12} and blocks the attachment of IF to ileal receptor sites. The blocking antibody occurs in the sera of about 55% of patients and the binding antibody in about 37%, but rarely alone, so that some 45% of patients show neither antibody [164]. The patients showing both antibodies tend to have the highest titres of blocking antibody, suggesting that they are either the 'best' autoantibody producers or have had most antigenic stimulation with

IF, and that of the two antigenic sites of IF, the B_{12}-binding site is the stronger. The antibodies in serum are IgG and may cross the placenta, and infants have been described with transplacentally acquired antibody and delayed production of free IF [165].

Gastric juice antibodies. Intrinsic factor antibody has been found in the gastric juice in PA in 16 of 28 patients [160]. The antibody may be secretory IgA [160] and is thought to be produced locally by the mononuclear cells invading the gastric mucosa [166]. The antibody may neutralize small amounts of remaining IF and indeed may only be detected if steps are taken to dissociate it from IF [106]. The complex dissociates at low pH. Therefore, gastric achlorhydria favours neutralization of remaining IF by antibody *in vivo*, whereas gastric acid favours dissociation of the antibody and, therefore, association of IF with B_{12}, and thus B_{12} absorption. The presence of IF antibodies in gastric and possibly intestinal juices explains why PA patients do not absorb B_{12} from B_{12}–IF complex as well as controls.

There is no relation between the presence of IF antibody in gastric juice and in serum, but there is evidence that the presence of antibody in the gastric juice, and less certainly in serum, diminishes the absorption of administered IF–B_{12} complex [167].

Intrinsic factor antibodies occur very rarely in patients without PA. Ten of eleven such subjects in one study had thyrotoxicosis and nine had a family history of other autoimmune disease; all had atrophic gastritis, even though they secreted IF and showed normal absorption of B_{12}. Follow-up of the patients for three to seven years has not shown progression to PA [168].

Cell-mediated immunity to intrinsic factor

Positive results against IF using the leucocyte migration inhibition test have been found in 30 of 35 PA cases [169].

Response to steroids

Steroid therapy may cause an improvement in the gastric mucosal lesion. There may be reduction in inflammatory-cell infiltrate, regeneration of glands, a fall in titre of serum IF antibody, secretion of small amounts of acid and IF, and haematological remission [170].

Development of pernicious anaemia

The disease is thought to arise on the basis of atrophic gastritis which may be due to a local, genetically determined, cell-mediated 'autoimmune' reaction, but it may also be that the gastritis can occur in some subjects entirely because of acquired factors (e.g. chronic iron deficiency). Most, but not all, patients with PA differ mainly from other patients with severe atrophic gastritis by developing IF antibodies which may be active, not only in the stomach, but also in the small intestine since small amounts of IF do not seem as active in promoting B$_{12}$ absorption in PA as in gastrectomy patients. Why some subjects with atrophic gastritis develop antibodies to IF but others do not, remains obscure.

CHILDHOOD PERNICIOUS ANAEMIA

Congenital intrinsic-factor deficiency
About 44 children have now been described who were born without functioning IF, but with a normal gastric biopsy and acid and pepsin secretion. Antibodies to parietal cell or IF are absent [171]. The child usually presents with megaloblastic anaemia or neuropathy between the fourth and 28th months of life, but may present in teenage. The disease is transmitted as an autosomal recessive. Five pairs of siblings and four other possible pairs have been recorded; in several, the parents were related.

An interesting variant has been reported [172]. This boy, a child of consanguineous marriage, presented at the age of 13 years with megaloblastic anaemia and was found to have all the characteristics of congenital IF deficiency, except IF was detectable (60 units/ml) in the gastric juice by radioimmunoassay. The IF was found to behave chromatographically, by precipitation techniques and by isoelectric focusing electrophoresis exactly like normal human IF. The patient had an abnormal IF, and this was possibly due to an amino-acid substitution at the ileal rather than B$_{12}$-binding site [173]. In the light of these findings, it is possible that previously reported patients with congenital IF deficiency may have had structurally abnormal IF which could render the protein undetectable by both radioimmunoassay and by functional tests, i.e. if the defect were at the B$_{12}$-binding site.

Childhood occurrence of 'autoimmune' pernicious anaemia
A form of PA, resembling that in adults, may occur in children. They show gastric atrophy with achlorydria, but differ from adult cases by having a higher incidence of IF antibody (90%) but lower incidence of parietal-cell antibody (10%) in serum and by often having an associated endocrinopathy such as hypoparathyroidism, myxoedema or Addison's disease which may present before or after the anaemia [171]. Mucocutaneous candidiasis, vitiligo, alopecia areata and diabetes mellitus may also be present. Siblings may show an endocrinopathy such as myxoedema, hypoparathyroidism or adrenal atrophy and some patients and siblings have suffered from steatorrhoea [174].

These children thus have a genetically determined tendency to develop organ-specific antibodies which is similar, but more marked, than that in adults with PA.

TOTAL GASTRECTOMY
Severe B$_{12}$ deficiency due to lack of IF is the inevitable result of this operation, the peak incidence of megaloblastic anaemia or neuropathy being from two to eight years after the operation but, rarely, it can develop after 10 years. Serum B$_{12}$ levels have been found to fall steeply a few months after the operation, but definitely subnormal levels are usually reached later. This correlates with the known logarithmic loss of body B$_{12}$ stores.

PARTIAL GASTRECTOMY
Anaemia has been found in as many as 53% of 292 patients [175]. Almost all patients, and particularly pre-menopausal women, show iron deficiency which is the principal cause of their anaemia. This deficiency is probably due to poor diet, malabsorption and blood loss, before, at the time of, or following the operation.

The exact incidence of megaloblastic anaemia is difficult to estimate because B$_{12}$ or folate deficiency are usually complicated by iron deficiency and the anaemia is dimorphic, but in one large study it occurred in six per cent of 265 patients [176]. In Britain, B$_{12}$ deficiency accounts for about 80% and folate deficiency, 20% or less of these megaloblastic anaemias. Subnormal serum B$_{12}$ levels occur in up to 18% of the patients and so many patients show subnormal serum B$_{12}$ levels without overt megaloblastic anaemia and may remain with 'subclinical deficiency' for many years. The response to B$_{12}$ is variable and can only be properly assessed after iron deficiency has been corrected. In some patients, subnormal levels of serum B$_{12}$ are found (even below 100 ng/l) by microbiological assay, despite normal levels by isotope dilution assay. The explanation for this discrepancy and which result is correct in the individual cases is still uncertain, although the presence of B$_{12}$ analogues in serum, possibly produced by small intestinal bacteria which compete with B$_{12}$ for binding protein used in the radioassay, appears to be the most likely explanation [177]. In a few other post-gastrectomy patients, serum B$_{12}$ levels have been reported to rise spontaneously with iron therapy [178].

The cause of the B$_{12}$ deficiency is usually lack of IF and the onset is usually from two to four years after the operation, but many present at 10–15 years. Inhibition of IF by duoedenal juice may play a part [179] and the most important factor determining the incidence of B$_{12}$ deficiency is size of the resection [180]. In some, but not all, series the deficiency was more common after an operation for a gastric rather than a duodenal ulcer.

Vitamin-B_{12} absorption is usually corrected by giving IF but may also improve in some patients if food or histamine is given simultaneously [181]. On the other hand, there is evidence that some patients who may be able to absorb crystalline B_{12} normally are unable to absorb B_{12} bound to protein in food [182]. In a few patients, the main cause is an intestinal stagnant-loop syndrome due to a blind loop created at the time of operation. In others, minor degrees of malabsorption of B_{12} given with IF may be caused by an abnormal jejunal bacterial flora [183].

SMALL-INTESTINAL DISEASE

Intestinal stagnant-loop syndrome

The normal upper small intestine in the fasting state usually contains small numbers of bacteria, particularly *Aerobacter*, *Streptococci* and *Lactobacilli* at concentrations of 10^3 organisms or less per ml of intestinal juice. In a number of disorders of the small intestine, the number and type of organism is altered and the abnormal flora causes malabsorption of B_{12}, fat and possibly of other nutrients [184]. The anatomical lesion may be small-intestinal diverticulosis or a stricture, fistula, anastomosis, surgically produced blind loop or resection. In addition, an abnormal upper-gut flora may be present in scleroderma, Whipple's disease, PA and simple atrophic gastritis, after vagotomy or gastro-enterostomy and during administration of ganglion-blocking drugs. In all these conditions, the number of faecal organisms in the jejunal juice may rise to 10^6–10^9. The most common cause of B_{12} deficiency among these conditions is multiple jejunal diverticulosis which usually presents in later life with a long-standing history of gastro-intestinal upset rather than with anaemia [185].

The cause of malabsorption of B_{12} is thought to be utilization of dietary B_{12} by the organisms which probably compete with IF for the vitamin [186]. Both *E. coli* and *E. bacteroides* have been implicated, even though these organisms, *in vitro*, ingest B_{12} bound to IF far less readily than free B_{12}. Vitamin B_{12} is malabsorbed in the stagnant-loop syndrome even when it is given with IF, but the absorption can be corrected by a short course of a broad-spectrum antibiotic (e.g. tetracycline or lincomycin), and this may cause a temporary improvement in anaemia. Conversion of dietary B_{12} to inactive analogues may be another effect of the bacteria [36]. Steatorrhoea is largely due to deconjugation of bile salts by colonic bacteria, particularly the anaerobic flora.

Ileal resection

Removal of as little as four to six feet of terminal ileum in an adult may cause malabsorption of B_{12}. In some cases, the resection is for Crohn's disease and remaining ileal disease or fistula or blind loops may aggravate the malabsorption. In children, it is uncertain how much ileum is needed to maintain normal B_{12} absorption, but it is possible that they fare relatively better than adults. With larger ileal resections, patients not only malabsorb B_{12}, but also fat and protein which may also cause secondary deficiencies of calcium, magnesium and potassium [187]. Jejuno-ileal by pass and ileostomy also may lead to malabsorption of B_{12}, usually without anaemia. Interestingly, resection of the upper small intestine leads to an increased absorptive capacity for B_{12} by the distal gut [188].

Crohn's disease

The incidence of severe B_{12} deficiency in patients without resections or fistulae is unknown but is probably extremely low, even though some degree of malabsorption of B_{12} is frequent in such patients. Low serum B_{12} levels, or megaloblastic anaemia requiring B_{12} therapy, mainly due to ileal resection or a stagnant-loop syndrome, have been described in 23 of 43 patients [189] and in 13 of 54 patients [190]. Folate deficiency is at least as common as B_{12} deficiency as a cause of megaloblastic anaemia in active Crohn's disease [190].

Specific malabsorption with proteinuria (Imerslund's disease; Imerslund–Gräsbeck's disease)

This autosomal recessive congenital disease has a widespread occurrence especially in inbred communities in Scandinavia and Israel and, like congenital IF deficiency, usually presents in the first few years of life with anaemia, failure to thrive and gastro-intestinal symptoms [191–193]. The gastric biopsy, gastric-acid and IF secretion are normal, but B_{12} from IF–B_{12} complex is not absorbed and thus an ileal defect is thought to be present. The ileum appears normal, however, by both light and electron microscopy and, in one case, took up IF–B_{12} complex normally *in vitro* [194]. Absorption of other substances and small-bowel X-ray are normal. Suggestions that malabsorption of B_{12} is due to an inhibitor in intestinal juice, to bacteria or to an immune mechanism have not been substantiated. A failure of pinocytotic or lysosomal mechanisms in both ileum and kidney seems most likely.

Proteinuria, which is mild, non-specific, benign and mainly albumin, is present in nearly all cases, though three have not shown this feature. The renal tract and renal biopsy are usually normal [193]. However Imerslund [191] found congenital abnormalities of the kidneys and ureters and a mild amino-aciduria in some of her cases, albeit from a highly inbred community.

The patients remain well on maintenance B$_{12}$ therapy and failure to provide this has allowed relapse.

Tropical sprue

This disease is endemic in parts of the West Indies, Sri Lanka, Africa and southern Asia, and may occur in Europeans who live in or visit these countries for as little as a few weeks [195, 196]. It presents as a generalized malabsorption syndrome in which, in contrast to coeliac disease, the upper (jejunal) and lower (ileal) portions of the small intestine are virtually equally affected, histologically showing partial villous atrophy. In the most acute form, the disease presents largely as a gastro-intestinal upset with diarrhoea, but deficiencies occur rapidly and megaloblastic anaemia is common and some degree of folate and/or B$_{12}$ deficiency, universal [197]. In the earlier stages, anaemia is due to folate deficiency. Malabsorption of B$_{12}$ occurs from the start of the illness, and the longer the duration of the illness, the more severe the B$_{12}$ deficiency. Indeed, in some cases, the upper small-intestinal function returns to normal with incomplete therapy, but the ileal defect persists. Thus patients with chronic tropical sprue may show megaloblastic anaemia or, rarely, neuropathy due to B$_{12}$ deficiency [198]. Malabsorption of B$_{12}$ may be corrected like the rest of the disease in early cases by folic acid and/or broad-spectrum antibiotic therapy, while B$_{12}$ itself may have a beneficial effect on gut function.

Fish tapeworm (Diphyllobothrum latum) infestation [199]

D. latum is a common infestation in humans in Finland and also around the Great Lakes of the USA, and around the lakes in Switzerland, Germany, Italy, Russia, and other European countries and Japan, but it is only in Finland that the infestation causes severe B$_{12}$ deficiency. Man is infested by eating inadequately cooked fish, which contain larvae in their muscles. The worms attach to the mid-ileum, measure 3–10 m with 3000 or more segments, and excrete as many as a million or more eggs in 24 hours. The eggs infect minute crustacea in water, develop into larvae which enter the fish if it should eat the crustacea. In Finland, malabsorption of B$_{12}$ has been found in up to 92% of carriers, subnormal serum B$_{12}$ levels in 38%, megaloblastic changes in about nine per cent, and overt megaloblastic anaemia in two per cent [200]. Neuropathy has also occurred. Expulsion of the worm (e.g. by oral administration of 3–4 g of *Extractum filicis*) causes a spontaneous improvement in both the serum B$_{12}$ level and B$_{12}$ absorption; absorption may take several weeks to become normal, while serum B$_{12}$ levels may not become normal for many months or even years. The deficiency is ascribed to uptake of the vitamin by the worm which itself has a high B$_{12}$ content (2·3 μg/g dry weight) and appears to be able to take up B$_{12}$ from IF almost as easily as from the free vitamin.

CAUSES OF MALABSORPTION OF VITAMIN B$_{12}$ (USUALLY) WITHOUT SEVERE VITAMIN B$_{12}$ DEFICIENCY (Table 6.4)

Gastritis without pernicious anaemia

The incidence of severity of gastritis increases with age and is often accompanied by achlorhydria, which may be histamine fast, by decreased pepsin secretion and by the presence of parietal-cell antibody and increased gastrin concentration in serum [201, 202]. Intrinsic-factor secretion is reduced in a rough correlation with the severity of the gastritis, but quite severe reduction can occur without impaired B$_{12}$ absorption. Carbachol (carbamylcholine chloride) was thought to stimulate secretion of IF in gastritis but direct assays have given conflicting results. About half the patients with severe atrophic gastritis show impaired B$_{12}$ absorption, though this is usually in a borderline range and occasional patients have subnormal serum B$_{12}$ levels, again usually in the borderline zone. A proportion of patients progress to overt PA after 10–15 years of follow-up [203]. The distinction of severe forms of simple gastritis from early or latent PA is difficult in some cases. The presence of haematological or neurological changes due to B$_{12}$ deficiency, a serum B$_{12}$ level less than 100 ng/l, raised methylmalonic-acid excretion, IF antibodies or a severely impaired B$_{12}$ absorption, however, all suggest that genuine PA is present.

Other gastric lesions

Malabsorption of B$_{12}$, with or without B$_{12}$ deficiency, has been described in patients with corrosive gastritis

Table 6.4. Causes of malabsorption of B$_{12}$ not usually leading to severe B$_{12}$ deficiency

Simple atrophic gastritis, other gastric lesions, adult coeliac disease, severe chronic pancreatitis and cystic fibrosis, Zollinger–Ellison syndrome, drugs (neomycin, colchicine, slow-release potassium chloride, metformin, phenformin, anticonvulsants, ? para-amino salicylate), deficiencies of folate, B$_{12}$ or protein, giardiasis, reduced gut mobility (e.g. scleroderma, Whipple's disease, radiation damage) and operations in which the stomach has been bypassed. On the other hand, vagotomy with pyloroplasty does not seem to cause impaired B_{12} absorption.

Adult coeliac disease (gluten-induced enteropathy)
B_{12} absorption is impaired in between 40 and 50% of patients with untreated adult coeliac disease, particularly in those with marked steatorrhoea [204, 205], and subnormal serum B_{12} levels occur in about one-third, but in fewer children with coeliac disease. The B_{12} deficiency is probably never the main cause of megaloblastic anaemia in this disease, however, since accompanying folate deficiency due to the upper-intestinal lesion is always more severe. In contrast to tropical sprue, a response of the anaemia in coeliac disease uncomplicated by other gastro-intestinal disease, even partial, to physiological doses of B_{12} has never been shown.

Pancreatic disease
Malabsorption of B_{12} has been described in about half the patients with severe chronic pancreatitis [206, 207] and more frequently in cystic fibrosis [208]. It was initially ascribed to lowered pH in the ileum or to lowered calcium-ion concentration due to the formation of insoluble calcium soaps. It is more likely that trypsin in pancreatic secretion has a more specific role in B_{12} absorption, removing B_{12} from attachment to non-IF-binding protein found in gastic juice. Alkali may help, favouring B_{12} binding to IF in preference to binding to the R-type protein [35].

Zollinger–Ellison syndrome
Vitamin-B_{12} malabsorption in this syndrome is likely to be due to lowered pH in the ileum.

Drugs [209, 210]
Neomycin causes malasorption of B_{12} probably by a direct toxic action on the ileal mucosa, though the drug also interferes with absorption of lipids by an intra-luminal action of precipitating micelles. Colchicine also acts by damaging ileal function. Slow-release potassium-chloride tablets have been shown to cause transient malabsorption, and this has been ascribed to acidification of the ileum lumen to a suboptimal pH for B_{12} absorption. Subnormal serum B_{12} levels were reported in patients taking oral contraceptives [211], and in four of 71 diabetic patients taking metformin; malabsorption of B_{12} occurred in 21 (30%) of these patients [212] and in 46% of patients taking phenformin. One patient with megaloblastic anaemia due to B_{12} deficiency ascribed to phenformin has now been described [213] Anticonvulsant drugs cause malabsorption of B_{12}, reversible by folate therapy even if the drugs are continued [214]. Alcohol has also been reported to cause transient B_{12} malabsorption [215]. Other drugs reported to reduce B_{12} absorption include para-amino salicylate [216], cholestyramine, large doses of vitamin C [217, 218] and cimetidine [219].

Nutritional deficiencies
It is likely that both B_{12} and folate deficiencies may, in certain patients, cause a reversible malabsorption of B_{12} due to an ileal defect which may, surprisingly, take several weeks or months to recover. Protein deficiency may have a similar effect.

Giardiasis
About half the patients with *Giardia lamblia* infection show malabsorption of B_{12} which improves when the infection is treated [220]. The mechanism is probably an effect on the ileal enterocyte.

DIAGNOSIS OF VITAMIN-B_{12} DEFICIENCY
When a patient is suspected of B_{12} deficiency because of megaloblastic anaemia, glossitis, neuropathy or other clinical or laboratory findings, its presence may be confirmed by one of four methods (Table 6.8, page 234). The deoxyuridine suppression test is described on page 242.

Therapeutic trial
This is valuable in a patient with uncomplicated megaloblastic anaemia in determining whether B_{12} or

Table 6.5. Interconversion of folates

Enzyme	Conversion
Dihydrofolate reductase	$DHF \rightarrow THF$
5,10-methylene-THF reductase	$5,10—CH_2—THF \rightarrow 5—CH_3—THF$
5,10-methylene-THF dehydrogenase	$5,10—CH_2—THF \rightarrow 5,10=CH—THF$
5,10-methenyl-THF cyclohydrase	$5,10=CH_2—THF \rightarrow 10—CHO—THF$
5-formimino-THF cyclodeaminase	$5—CH=NH—THF \rightarrow 5,10=CH—THF$
10-formyl-THF synthetase	$THF \rightarrow 10—CHO—THF$

folate deficiency is the cause [221]. Physiological doses of B$_{12}$ (1 or 2 μg intramuscularly) or of folic acid (100 or 200 μg orally or intramuscularly) are given for 10 days. The patient should be maintained during this time and, if possible, for a week before commencing therapy, on a diet of low folate or B$_{12}$ content. This largely means omitting liver and kidney from the hospital diet. In patients with megaloblastic anaemia associated with alcohol, spontaneous remission may occur on a hospital diet when alcohol is stopped, unless a diet containing virtually no B$_{12}$ or folate is given.

Optimal response. The reticulocytes begin to rise on the second or third day and reach a peak on the sixth or seventh day of therapy (Fig. 6.7). The height of the peak is related to the initial severity of anaemia, being about 40% when the initial red-cell count is 1×10^{12}/l, about 30% when $1 \cdot 5 - 2 \times 10^{12}$/l, about 20% when $2 \cdot 5 - 3 \cdot 0 \times 10^{12}$/l, and up to 10% when this is $3 - 4 \times 10^{12}$/l. The reticulocytosis may last for about three weeks with successive but lower reticulocyte peaks, presumably due to later release from the marrow of cells derived from stem cells rendered effective by therapy.

The red-cell count rises to over $3 \cdot 0 \times 10^{12}$/l by the third week and to over 4×10^{12}/l by the fifth week. The white-cell count becomes normal by the fifth to seventh day and platelets rise, often to levels of $400 - 800 \times 10^9$/l simultaneously with the reticulocytosis. Hypersegmented neutrophils disappear from the peripheral blood on the 10–14th day, marrow erythropoiesis is largely normoblastic within 48 hours of starting therapy, and leucopoiesis normal after 10–14 days.

Biochemical changes. The serum iron falls within 24 hours and may remain subnormal for several weeks even in the absence of iron deficiency. The serum ferritin also falls within 48 hours. The serum folate falls rapidly in B$_{12}$-deficient patients given B$_{12}$. In folate deficiency, the serum B$_{12}$ may rise spontaneously with the reticulocyte response. The serum LDH is also useful for following the response since this falls steadily to reach normal levels within about two weeks of starting specific therapy.

Poor response. This will occur if the incorrect vitamin is given in a physiological dose. The patient is then given

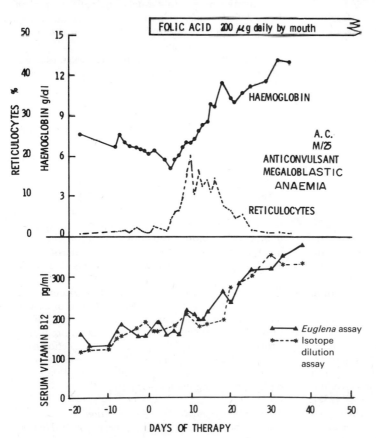

Fig. 6.7. The haematological response of a patient with anticonvulsant megaloblastic anaemia to a physiological dose of folic acid. The serum B$_{12}$ level rose simultaneously with the reticulocytosis. In this case, both assays of vitamin B$_{12}$ gave consistently similar results (by courtesy of the *British Journal of Haematology*).

a physiological dose of the other vitamin for a further period of 10 days. The response will be suboptimal even if the correct vitamin is given if there is double deficiency of both vitamins, associated iron deficiency, or if an infection or another disease (e.g. carcinoma) is present which may inhibit the marrow response.

The therapeutic trial is not often performed nowadays since it is time-consuming, particularly if the inappropriate vitamin happens to be given first. It is of most value in patients with subnormal levels of both B_{12} and folate in order to analyse how far each deficiency contributes to anaemia.

Serum vitamin B_{12}

Measurement. Microbiological techniques employ the organisms *Lactobacillus leichmannii*, *Euglena gracilis* ('z' strain), *Escherichiae coli* and *Ochromonas malhamensis*, and the normal range is approximately from 160 to 925 ng/l [222]. Isotope dilution methods are now more widely used. These use normal serum, pure or crude IF, chick serum, or chronic granulocytic leukaemia serum to bind B_{12}, and albumin-coated or haemoglobin-coated charcoal [223, 224], DEAE cellulose, Sephadex filtration or dialysis to separate free and bound B_{12}. In general, the results with the isotope dilution and microbiological assays give a fair agreement [225]. However, the radioassays have been found to give somewhat higher results in normal subjects (e.g. a normal range from 200 to 1000 ng/l) [224] and overlap between results in normals and untreated pernicious anaemia [226]. Even larger discrepancies have been found with the sera of some patients following partial gastrectomy, with folate deficiency, pregnancy and other conditions [224]. One explanation for the higher serum B_{12} levels with radioassays than microbiological assays is that B_{12} analogues are present in serum that compete with true B_{12} for the binding protein used in the radioassay, but are not active for the microbiological assay organisms [227]. Pure IF, it is thought, will give results more comparable with the microbiological assays since it is more selective than other B_{12} binders in its binding for true B_{12}. Alternatively, radioassays have been modified by adding a B_{12} analogue (e.g. cobinamide) to the binding protein to block binding sites for B_{12} analogues and this has led to results more close to those of the microbiological assays [228].

Results in megaloblastic anaemia. Patients with megaloblastic anaemia due to B_{12} deficiency show subnormal serum vitamin levels, usually below 100 ng/l, with the *E. gracilis* assay [229, 230]. There is a selective fall in the methyl-B_{12} component of serum B_{12} [231]. Extremely low levels (less than 50 ng/l) are the rule in patients with severe B_{12} neuropathy, even if little or no anaemia is present, and in patients with severe anaemia [230], but may occur in the absence of anaemia or neuropathy.

Patients with megaloblastic anaemia due to folate deficiency may also show subnormal serum B_{12} levels, usually in the borderline (100–160 ng/l) range [232]. These occur in about one-third of patients with anaemia due to nutritional folate deficiency, particularly in the most anaemic patients. The B_{12} level may rise spontaneously to normal with folic-acid therapy [230] (Fig. 6.7). A similar low serum B_{12} level may also occur in severe folate deficiency from other causes (e.g. malabsorption, pregnancy, anticonvulsant drugs or pyrimethamine therapy). Explanations which have been proposed include poor dietary intake of B_{12}, malabsorption of B_{12}, redistribution of B_{12} or its individual coenzyme forms between plasma and cells, but none have been established. Liver B_{12} is normal in most, but may be slightly reduced in some [233], and red-cell B_{12} was reduced from a normal mean of 155 ng/l to a mean of 80 ng/l in one series [244]. *In-vitro* tests suggest that the low serum B_{12} in folate deficiency may well further impair marrow DNA synthesis [232].

In many severely folate-deficient patients, genuine B_{12} deficiency may also be present (e.g. in tropical sprue, partial gastrectomy or adult coeliac disease). In such patients, the serum B_{12} may be extremely low and rise slightly but remain subnormal with folic-acid therapy alone and only become normal when B_{12} is also given.

Subnormal serum vitamin B_{12} levels without megaloblastic anaemia. These are frequent in patients with a number of conditions (e.g. veganism, atrophic gastritis, partial gastrectomy and pregnancy). In some, these probably indicate a minor degree of B_{12} deficiency shown by haematological abnormalities, but in other subjects their exact significance is uncertain, particularly when isotope-dilution assay reveals a normal result and the blood appears normal. A number of antibiotics and antimetabolites, when given in large doses, inhibit the microbiological assay of B_{12} and cause artificially low serum B_{12} levels [235–237].

Raised serum vitamin-B_{12} levels. These occur principally when the serum concentration of one or other of the B_{12}-binding proteins is raised, and the clinical causes have been discussed above (p. 207). Frequently, a raised serum B_{12} level is caused by an injection of B_{12} (e.g. for a Schilling test) given days or weeks before the blood is taken, or due to contamination of the serum by B_{12}-producing bacteria *in vitro*.

Methylmalonic-acid (MMA) excretion
The biochemical pathways have been decribed on page

202 (Fig. 6.4). Methylmalonic acid (MMA) may be measured by gas, paper or thin-layer chromatography or by spectrophotometric assay, and the usual normal range is 0–4 mg/24 hours. The excretion of MMA is raised in patients with B_{12} deficiency but is normal in folate deficiency, liver disease and all other conditions so far tested, with the sole exception of certain inborn errors of metabolism involving B_{12} or methylmalonyl CoA isomerase [238].

In B_{12} deficiency, but not in normals, the excretion of MMA can be increased by loading the patient with L-valine (10 g) or isoleucine [239]. Virtually all patients with megaloblastic anaemia or neuropathy due to B_{12} deficiency have raised excretion levels, as do a proportion of patients with subnormal serum B_{12} levels with only minor haematological changes. The MMA excretion is not so sensitive to B_{12} deficiency as the serum B_{12} level since a large number of patients with subnormal serum B_{12} levels and mild megaloblastic changes may have normal MMA excretion. It has been suggested that MMA may be toxic to the nervous system and cause the neuropathy or spinal-cord damage, or that a disturbance of fatty-acid metabolism due to defective MMCoA metabolism may lead to the neuropathy [240]. There is no direct evidence for these theories and, indeed, children with congenital methylmalonic aciduria show no evidence of neurological damage similar to that due to B_{12} deficiency, whereas monkeys exposed to nitrous oxide develop a neuropathy without raised MMA excretion.

Other organic acids. Excretion of propionic and acetic acids may be raised in B_{12} deficiency and blood levels of pyruvate and α-oxoglutarate may be increased, but their measurement is not a reliable test for the deficiency [241, 242].

Congenital methylmalonic aciduria. A number of infants with this disorder have been described since the first case was reported in 1968. They present in the first few months of life with vomiting, metabolic acidosis and ketotic hyperglycinaemia and may excrete up to 6 g of MMA in 24 hours. Two sub-groups have been delineated by clinical and biochemical studies [238, 243]: one, which does not respond to B_{12} and is either due to deficiency of the apoenzyme methylmalonyl-CoA mutase or to deficiency of methylmalonyl-CoA racemase; a second responds to massive doses of B_{12}. The latter infants are thought to fail to synthesize ado-B_{12} [244].

Four infants, two of whom were brothers, who showed homocystinuria in addition to methylmalonic aciduria have been described [245, 246]. In each case, the primary defects appeared to be in methylation of homocysteine and in isomerization of methylmalonyl

CoA, due to a defect in the uptake or early metabolism of B_{12} to either of its coenzyme forms. Of great interest, only one of these children showed megaloblastic anaemia [246].

TESTS FOR THE CAUSE OF VITAMIN B_{12} DEFICIENCY (Table 6.8, page 234)
Some of these have already been discussed and others are mentioned in a final section on the management of megaloblastic anaemia (p. 235).

Vitamin-B_{12} absorption studies deserve special mention here. Radioactive B_{12} is used, employing either the ^{58}Co or ^{57}Co label. Five techniques are available, whole-body absorption, hepatic uptake, faecal excretion, urinary excretion, and plasma levels. Each test may be carried out giving the dose to fasting subjects alone and then together with an IF preparation [247, 248]. The size of the oral dose will determine the normal range; 1·0 μg is widely employed, from which normal subjects absorb 30–80%, and usually more than 50%. The urinary-excretion (Schilling) test requires a flushing dose of 1000 μg non-radioactive B_{12} and this involves treatment of a patient, but this is not needed in the other techniques. Reduced excretion occurs if there is impaired renal function. A recently introduced time-saving technique (Dicopac) involves the simultaneous administration of B_{12} labelled with two isotopes, one of which is attached to IF. Differential counting is then carried out [249]. Due to exchange of isotopes, this gives less clear discrimination, in PA, between the results with the dose alone and with IF, than the tests performed separately [250, 251]. It is most useful in elderly subjects when urine collection may be incomplete.

Doscherholmen *et al.* [252] recommended a B_{12}-labelled absorption test in which the labelled dose is given with a standard food (ovalbumin) rather than as a crystalline dose since some patients following gastrectomy, or with atrophic gastritis, can then be shown to malabsorb B_{12}, even though they absorb crystalline B_{12} normally [253].

Vitamin-B_{12} absorption tests are used not only to elucidate the cause of B_{12} deficiency (gastric or intestinal, and if intestinal, bacterial or non-bacterial by re-testing after antibiotic therapy), but also as a test of small-intestinal function.

FOLATE

HISTORY [254]
The existence of an anti-anaemia factor in 'Marmite' was first proposed by Lucy Wills and she further established that this factor could correct nutritional anaemia in monkeys, so it was later called 'vitamin M'

[185, 186]. Other lines of research also pointed to the existence of folates. A factor needed for growth of chicks was termed vitamin Bc and 'factor U', while the 'Norit eulate factor' was a term used for growth factor for *L. casei*, which could be adsorbed onto and eluted from charcoal. Mitchell *et al*. [257] used 'folic acid' to describe the pure compound they isolated from spinach, which was a growth factor for *Streptococcus latis R (S. faecalis)*, and folic acid was first synthesized chemically in 1945.

NATURAL FORMS

Folic acid (pteroylglutamic acid) is the parent compound of a large group of naturally occurring, structurally related compounds, collectively called 'folates'. In theory, well over 100 compounds may exist and it is likely that the number present in any cell is large. Folic acid itself has a molecular weight of 441·4, forms yellow, spear-shaped crystals and is sparingly soluble in water but dissolves readily in dilute alkali, the solution showing absorption maxima at 256, 282 and 36 nm. The molecule consists of three portions: pteridine, para-aminobenzoic acid and L-glutamic acid (Fig. 6.8). Pteroylglutamic acid probably does not exist in nature; bacteria which synthesize folates use dihydropteroic acid as substrate. The natural folate compounds differ from folic acid in three respects:

1 three states of reduction of the pteridine ring can occur;
2 six different one-carbon units may be present at positions N_5 or N_{10} or both; and
3 a chain of variable length which consists of addi-

tional L-glutamic acid residues may be linked in a series by γ-peptide bonds to the glutamic acid.

The polyglutamyl side chain is usually three, five or seven residues in length, but the exact number varies from one tissue to the next and, within a given tissue, many different chain lengths may be present. Folate is transported in body fluids as a monoglutamate. The main form in human plasma and cerebrospinal fluid is 5-methyltetrahydrofolate [258] although traces of 10-formyl folate have also been identified [259], but in liver 75–80% of the folates are pteroylpolyglutamates [260, 261], in the rat most containing five glutamates per molecules, about 20% pteroyltriglutamates and only traces of mono- and di-glutamates are present [260]. Mature leucocytes contain from 40 to 120 ng folate/ml packed cells [262] and whether mature or immature, contain about 85% pteroylpolyglutamates. Red cells contain at least 90% pteroylpolyglutamates with 4, 5, 6 glutamates [263, 264] while yeast folates are about 97% pteroylpolyglutamates [265].

Microbiological activity

At the low concentration of folates present in most natural tissues, chemical methods of analysis are inadequate. The growth responses of the different folates for the three micro-organisms usually used to measure and identify them, *Lactobacillus casei (L. casei)*, *Streptococcus faecalis (S. faecalis)* and *Pediococcus cervisiae (P. cervisiae)* are listed by Chanarin [1]. Pteroylpolyglutamates with more than three glutamate residues are not microbiologically active but deconjugation to mono-, di- or tri-glutamates renders them active. The enzymes that bring about deconjuga-

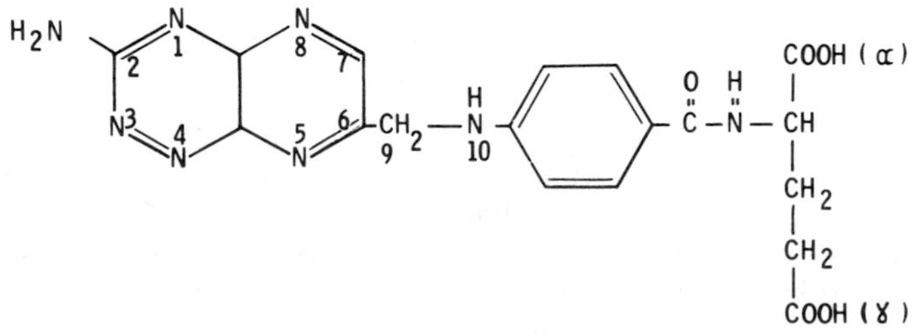

Folic acid (pteroylglutamic acid)

Dietary folates may contain :-

1) Additional hydrogen atoms at positions 7 & 8 (dihydrofolate) or 5, 6, 7 & 8 (tetrahydrofolate)

2) A formyl group at N_5 or N_{10} or a methyl group at N_5 or other single carbon unit

3) Additional glutamate moieties attached to the γ carboxyl group of the glutamate moiety

Fig. 6.8. The structural formula of folic acid (pteroylglutamic acid).

tion are present in all tissues and are called (inappropriately) 'conjugases' and are discussed next.

FOLATE DECONJUGATION AND CONJUGATION

Folate conjugase (also termed γ-glutamyl-γ-carboxy-peptidase or pteroylpolyglutamate hydrolase [266]) hydrolyses glutamate residues off pteroylpolyglutamates. The enzyme present in human and most other animal tissues has a pH optimum of 4·5–4·6, shows preference to pteroylpolyglutamates of longer chain length, removes the glutamate residues singly, and deconjugates folates to the monoglutamate form. The enzyme is localized principally in lysosomes [266]. It shows specificity to the γ-peptide bond, but the terminal glutamate can be exchanged for another amino acid, such as leucine or aspartate, without complete loss of enzyme activity providing the linkage is the γ bond [267]. The enzyme present in most bird tissues (e.g chick pancreas) has a pH optimum around seven to eight and deconjugates folates only as far as the diglutamate derivatives.

Pteroylpolyglutamates are built up by addition of single glutamate moieties in mammalian liver after folic acid has first been reduced and methylated or formylated [261]. Reduction, however, is not essential for polyglutamate formation to occur [268]. Conjugation occurs in the cytoplasm or mitochondria of the cells and its takes several days for injected labelled folic acid to equilibrate with endogenous folate [268, 269]. Folinic acid, however, is rapidly converted to polyglutamate forms [270]. The optimal substrate for polyglutamate formation in mammalian cells is unknown although recent studies suggest dihydrofolate (DHF), tetrahydrofolate (THF) and formyl tetrahydrofolate (formyl THF) are all active whereas methyl THF is a poor substrate [271, 272]. This is relevant to the action of B$_{12}$ deficiency on folate metabolism (see p. 243).

BIOCHEMICAL REACTIONS OF FOLATES

Folates are concerned with transfer of single carbon unit moieties in reactions in amino-acid metabolism and synthesis of purines and pyrimidines (Fig. 6.9). The attached unit may be methyl (—CH$_3$), methylene (—CH$_2$—), methenyl (=CH—), formyl (—CHO) or formimino (—CH=NH—) at the N$_5$, N$_{10}$, or N$_{5-10}$ positions. The folate is in the active tetrahydro- (THF) form in which it is maintained by the enzyme DHF reductase. In all reactions tested, the polyglutamate forms of the folate coenzyme are more active than the corresponding monoglutamate [273, 274].

Reduction: dihydrofolate reductase

This enzyme reduces dihydrofolic acid (DHF) and, much less effectively, folic acid to the functionally active THF state. A principal function is to reduce DHF, produced during synthesis of thymidylate (Fig. 6.10) and also reduce ingested folic acid or DHF. The enzyme has a molecular weight of between 21 000 and 24 000, and is present in all animal, bacterial and viral tissues examined, localized to the cytoplasmic-microsomal fraction. The enzyme has two pH optima, 4·5 and 7·5, with DHF as substrate but an optimum only at the lower pH with folic acid as substrate [275].

A number of pharmacologically important compounds (e.g. methotrexate, pyrimethamine and trimethoprim) inhibit the enzyme and are discussed later (see p. 240).

Interconversion of folates

The enzymes involved in interconversion of folates in mammalian tissues and the reactions they carry out are

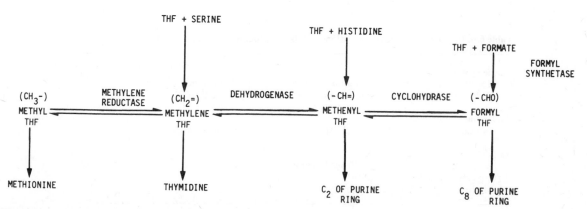

Fig. 6.9. Interconversion of the different folate coenzymes. In natural materials, these coenzyme forms largely exist as their polyglutamate derivatives. THF = tetrahydrofolate.

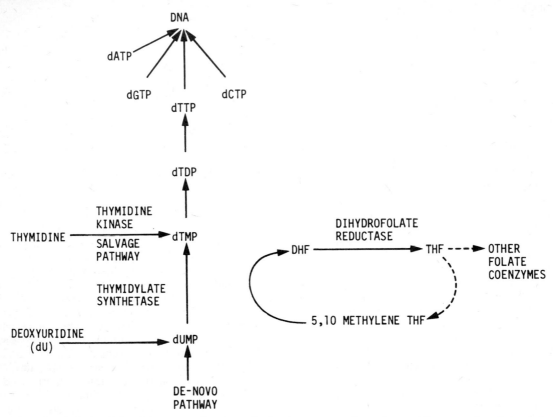

Fig. 6.10. The synthesis of thymidine monophosphate via the *de-novo* route from deoxyuridine monophosphate or from preformed thymidine (salvage pathway). Dihydrofolate reductase reduces dihydrofolate (DHF) produced during thymidylate synthesis to tetrahydrofolate (THF); d = deoxyribose; A = adenine; G = guanine; T = thymidine; C = cytosine; MP = monophosphate; DP = diphosphate; TP = triphosphate.

Table 6.6. Biochemical synthetic reactions of folates in mammalian cells

Purine synthesis
(a) Formylation of glycinamide ribotide for formyl glycinamide ribotide
(b) Formylation of aminoimidazole carboxamide ribotide (AICAR) to FICAR

Pyrimidine synthesis
Methylation of deoxyuridine monophosphate to thymidylate monophosphate

Amino-acid interconversion
(a) Removal of formimino group from formimonoglutamic acid (Figlu) to form glutamic acid
(b) Glycine–serine interconversion
(c) Methylation of homocysteine to methionine

shown in Figure 6.9 and Table 6.5 (p. 218). The reactions concerned with transfer of single carbon units are shown in Table 6.6 and are discussed below.

Utilization of formate
The enzyme formyl-THF synthetase or the formate-activating enzyme, which is present in mammalian cells, brings about synthesis of 10-formyl THF from formate, ATP and THF. The main formate donors in mammalian cells are methionine, sarcosine and S-methyl-cysteine [276].

Purine and pyrimidine synthesis
Folates are concerned in two reactions in purine synthesis which involve insertion of carbon atoms 8 and 2 respectively in the purine ring. They are also involved in one reaction in pyrimidine synthesis, the methylation of deoxyuridylate monophosphate (dUMP) to thymidylate monophosphate (dTMP), mediated by the enzyme thymidylate synthetase. The folate coenzyme is oxidized to DHF and this enzyme system is coupled with DHF reductase (Fig. 6.10). Thymidylate synthetase is rate-limiting for DNA synthesis in mammalian tissues. The level of the enzyme increases in rapidly proliferating tissues and the reaction is sensitive to folate antagonists and to folate deficiency (see below). The cell may also acquire thymidylate by uptake and phosphorylation of pre-formed thymidine under the action of the enzyme, thymidine kinase (the so-called 'salvage' pathway (Fig. 6.9)).

Amino-acid interconversions

Histidine breakdown. One of the pathways of histidine metabolism involves its degradation to glutamic acid. The first step in the reaction sequence involves conversion of histidine to urocanic acid. Urocanic acid is then converted to formiminoglutamic acid (Figlu) via the intermediate 4-imidizolone-5-propionic acid by the enzyme urocanase. Folate is required for removal of the formimino group which is transferred to THF. Urocanase is sensitive to protein lack, Figlu transferase to folate deficiency and both enzymes are disturbed by diseases of the liver.

Serine–glycine conversion. This reversible reaction involves both THF and pyridoxal 5-phosphate as co-enzymes. The reaction in mammalian tissues seems to be in the direction of serine synthesis. 5,10-methylene-THF donates an additional hydroxymethyl group and pyridoxal 5-phosphate acts as intermediate coenzyme. This reaction has formed the basis of a biochemical test for folate deficiency [277, 278].

Methionine synthesis. Methionine may be synthesized by methylation of homocysteine; 5-methyl-THF acts as methyl donor and methyl-B$_{12}$ as intermediate coenzyme (Fig. 6.3). This reaction is also discussed on pages 244 and 246.

Other reactions. A folate coenzyme has been shown to formylate methionyl-sRNA in *E. coli* and phage particles to N-formylmethionyl-sRNA, a compound thought to initiate protein synthesis in these organisms. As yet there is no evidence that folate is needed for these reactions in mammalian cells. Folate is also needed to formylate glycine in certain organisms but probably not in man.

Function of naturally occurring folate polyglutamates
It is likely that folate–polyglutamate derivatives play a major role in biochemical reactions in mammalian and other cells and the monoglutamates are transport forms but may also serve as models for the natural coenzymes [14]. Serine hydroxymethylase from a number of sources appears to react better in the presence of reduced folate polyglutamate than with corresponding reduced monoglutamate derivative [279]. Other folate–polyglutamate coenzymes which have been found to be more active than the corresponding monoglutamate in mammalian systems include methionine synthetase and thymidylate synthetase [274]. Polyglutamate addition to folates may also help to retain them in cells, the monoglutamate forms being more easily transported out of cells. The T-even bacteriophage of *E. coli* has been found to have an absolute requirement for the penta-γ-glutamyl derivative of dihydrofolic acid for phage assembly and infectivity and the corresponding tetra- or hexa-derivatives inhibit *in-vitro* phage assembly [280]. Thus, the exact proportion of the different polyglutamate forms may be important for determining the speed and direction of folate-requiring reactions.

DIETARY INTAKE AND REQUIREMENTS
Adults require about 100–200 µg folate daily [181]. Fifty µg will produce a haematological response in some folate-deficient patients but as much as 200 µg may be needed to maintain a normal status quo. Total body stores are from 6 to 20 mg, situated mainly in the liver, which contains on average about 10 µg/g [282]. Thus, stores are sufficient only for a few months and, indeed, a human developed early megaloblastic anaemia in four months when maintained experimentally on a diet lacking folate [281]. Losses of folate occur in the urine (up to 15 µg daily) [283, 284], in saliva and sweat and probably in cells desquamating from skin, gut and other epithelial tissues. Most of the folate in faeces is synthesized by bacteria and this is not

available for absorption. The body can degrade folate by cleavage at the C_9—N_{10} bond to give rise to aminobenzoylglutamate and pteridines. In rats p-acetamidobenzoylglutamate appears in urine [285]. Pterin-6-aldehyde has been identified in human urine, the excretion being raised in neoplasia [286] and losses of folate breakdown compounds occur in urine, bile and probably from other sites. In conditions with increased cell synthesis and breakdown, folate consumption, and therefore requirements, are increased.

A normal Western diet probably provides around 400 μg folate daily (although estimates have varied widely from 200 to over 1000 μg), mostly in the polyglutamate form [287–290]. Folate is present in virtually all foods, the highest concentrations occurring in liver, yeast, green vegetables, chocolate and nuts, which all usually contain more than 30 μg/100 g wet weight. Folates may be easily destroyed by cooking, particularly at high temperatures, in large volumes of water and, if reheating is practised (when the protective effect of ascorbate in food is lost), up to 90–100% folate may be lost.

ABSORPTION AND TRANSPORT

Absorption

Folate absorption occurs mainly through the duodenum and jejunum. Little is absorbed from the ileum and none from the large gut [291]. Folates ingested in the amounts normally present in the diet all enter the portal blood as a single compound, 5-methyl-THF [292]. At least three biochemical reactions are needed to convert the natural forms to this compound (Fig. 6.11):

1 deconjugation;
2 reduction; and
3 methylation.

Deconjugation is brought about by folate conjugase which is present in small amounts in saliva, succus entericus and, in much higher concentrations, in the small-intestinal mucosa. The amounts in the lumen of the small intestine are low and it seems possible that deconjugation of dietary folate occurs partly in the mucosal cell [293–295]. The presence of a folate conjugase with a neutral pH optimum at the brush border of the intestinal cell has been suggested but not certainly identified [296]. Perfusion studies have suggested folate deconjugation occurs at, or close to, the surface of the mucosa [297]. The brush border of the small intestine does contain a specific folate-binding protein which may indeed act as a receptor for dietary folate [298, 299].

The greater the number of glutamate residues in the chain, the less well the compound is absorbed [300, 301]. Reduced monoglutamate derivatives are virtually 100% absorbed at normal doses [302]. At higher doses, the proportion absorbed falls. The rate-limiting step is probably transfer of the compounds across the luminal surface membrane of the cell, rather than deconjugation. Natural materials may contain inhibitors of folate absorption, either by binding folates in insoluble form or by inhibition of deconjugation [303].

Dietary, partly reduced (dihydro-) or non-reduced compounds are converted to the THF derivative by the enzyme dihydrofolate reductase. Formylated and other non-methylated compounds are all converted to the 5-methyl derivative [292]. Folic acid itself is a poor substrate for dihydrofolate reductase and except in small physiological doses, is largely transferred across the intestinal mucosa unchanged and subsequently reduced in the liver [304]. There is still disagreement about whether folic acid and reduced folate monoglutamates presented to the small intestine are actively or passively reabsorbed. The balance of animal experi-

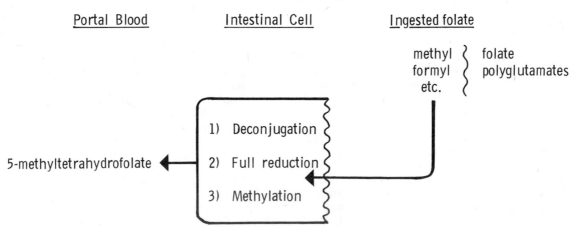

Fig. 6.11. Three biochemical steps involved in absorption of dietary folates.

mental evidence now favours a passive process, possibly with facilitated diffusion or solvent drag [294] but support for the existence of a specific 'permease' for folate in man comes from studies showing greater absorption of L- than D-5-methyl-tetrahydrofolate [305] and from the existence of the condition, specific malabsorption of folate [306].

There is no completely satisfactory test of folate absorption. Microbiological assay of serum or urine with *L. casei* or *S. faecalis* after an oral dose of non-radioactive folic acid, reduced pteroylmonoglutamates or natural or synthetic pteroylpolyglutamates have been used. On the other hand, tritiated folic acid, reduced monoglutamates or polyglutamates may be used with measurement of faecal or urinary excretion or plasma levels of radioactivity [293, 294].

Plasma transport
About two-thirds of 5-methyl-THF in plasma is loosely attached to α_2 macroglobulin, albumin and transferrin and may be easily dialysed away. A small proportion is highly bound to a specific folate-binding protein. A similar binding protein occurs in milk, bile and saliva [307]. It binds preferentially oxidized folates and pteridines and does not facilitate folate entry to cells other than the liver and possibly intestine [306a]. Its role appears to be transport of unwanted folates to the liver for breakdown and excretion, or for conversion into fully active, reduced forms [308]. The role of intracellular folate binders which have been identified in liver [309, 310], in intestinal mucosa, brush-border membranes, and in normal and leukaemic leucocytes remains uncertain.

Serum folate arises partly by displacement of endogenous folate from liver by newly absorbed folate. Folates enter marrow cells by an active carrier-mediated uptake process, mainly into the more primitive, rapidly proliferating cells [311, 312]. Separate mechanisms exist for transport of reduced folates (and methotrexate) and folic acid. Reduced forms enter cells by an active, energy-dependent, carrier-mediated mechanism, inhibited by a rise in cell cyclic AMP [313–316]. The transport is several times greater than for folic acid. A specific binding protein for folates is present on membranes of cells which transport folates [316]. The concentration of methyl folate in CSF is about three times that of plasma due to active secretion in the choroid plexus [317, 318].

Entero-hepatic circulation
The daily excretion of folate in bile has been estimated as 60–90 μg and this is largely in the form of reduced methyl and formyl folates which are largely reabsorbed and maintain serum folate [319].

Renal excretion
This has only been studied in detail in the dog [320]. There is tubular reabsorption of folate with some storage in the kidney at low plasma levels but at higher levels there is complete glomerular filtration of unbound folate with little reabsorption. Urinary losses of folate in man are normally less than 13 μg daily but may be increased considerably in liver diseases or heart failure. Urine also contains breakdown products of folates (see p. 226).

CLINICAL AND HAEMATOLOGICAL FEATURES OF
FOLATE DEFICIENCY
The symptoms of anaemia due to folate deficiency are similar to those of megaloblastic anaemia due to B$_{12}$ deficiency. Glossitis and pigmentation of the skin are features of either deficiency. Apart from possible minor mental changes, however, folate deficiency has not been proved to cause a neuropathy (see p. 246). Often the symptoms of folate deficiency progress rapidly once they have appeared, and this is particularly so in conditions of increased folate consumption such as pregnancy and is aggravated if an infection supervenes. Indeed folate deficiency in pregnancy or the early puerperium may result in an acute illness characterized by fever, and rapidly falling haemoglobin with severe malaise, a clinical picture which can present considerable diagnostic problems. In some patients an underlying condition such as coeliac disease or epilepsy with anticonvulsant therapy is known to be present, but in others an underlying disease is first diagnosed clinically or by laboratory tests only when megaloblastic anaemia occurs.

The peripheral blood and bone marrow changes are identical to those found in B$_{12}$ deficiency and, in general, give a good indication of the severity of folate deficiency since the more severe the anaemia, the greater the morphological change in the blood and marrow, and the greater the degree of folate deficiency measured biochemically (Fig. 6.6). In patients who develop the anaemia extremely rapidly, however, the peripheral blood film may show surprisingly little change, apart from pancytopenia, even though anaemia is marked and the marrow shows florid megaloblastosis. Rarely, patients show selective aplasia of the red-cell series; the marrow may then appear entirely leucopoietic and can be mistaken for acute myeloblastic leukaemia. The fall in white cells and platelets is usually in keeping with the degree of anaemia but occasional patients may show relatively severe degrees of leucopenia or thrombocytopenia. This may occur when there is arrest of haemopoiesis due to methotrexate, alcohol or other antifolate drugs, where an infection produces an 'arrest' of haemopoiesis, or where folate deficiency supervenes on myelosclerosis.

CAUSES OF FOLATE DEFICIENCY
(Table 6.7)

Poor nutrition

Inadequate dietary intake is the commonest cause of folate deficiency, particularly if a poor diet is taken in the face of increased demands for folate (e.g. in pregnancy, chronic inflammatory or malignant disorders). It is more common in races who cook food at high temperatures, especially if this is done repeatedly. It is probably on this basis that the deficiency is more common, for instance, in India than China, or in England than the USA. It is also common in Burma, Malaya, Africa and South America. Very few direct analyses of the folate content of the diets have been made and estimates from tables are unreliable. Nevertheless, it seems likely that subjects with nutritional megaloblastic anaemia due to folate deficiency take less than 50 μg, and often less than 20 μg, total folate daily. This is particularly likely in the poor, aged,

lonely, edentulous, dietary faddists, alcoholics, patients with chronic diseases which reduce appetite and following partial gastrectomy and with other oesophageal or gastro-intestinal disorders. It has also been decribed in the emotionally or psychiatrically disturbed and other subjects living in institutions, particularly when they are also taking barbiturates [321, 322].

The diet of patients with severe nutritional folate deficiency in Western countries consists largely of tea, bread and butter, with small amounts of meat, fish or fowl. Liver, green vegetables, nuts, fruit and cheese are notably lacking. Vitamin-C deficiency is often also present and there may be clinical scurvy [323].

The diagnosis is made from the history and by excluding other causes of folate deficiency, particularly coeliac disease in Western communities and tropical sprue where this is frequent, by tests for intestinal malabsorption and by jejunal biopsy. Differential

Table 6.7. Causes of folate deficiency*

Poor diet
  e.g. poverty, mentally ill, chronic illness, special diets, alcoholics, goat's milk, scurvy, kwashiorkor, etc.

Malabsorption
  Gluten-induced enteropathy (adult or child)
  Dermatitis herpetiformis
  Tropical sprue
  Specific malabsorption
  Systemic infections
  Minor factor in jejunal resection, partial gastrectomy, Crohn's disease, congestive heart failure, drugs (e.g. cholestyramine,
    salazopyrine)
  Also described in alcoholism, lymphoma

Increased utilization
  Pregnancy and lactation
  Prematurity and infancy
  Haemolytic anaemia (e.g. sickle-cell anaemia, thalassaemia major)
  Myelosclerosis
  Malignancy (e.g. carcinoma, myeloma, leukaemia)
  Inflammatory diseases (e.g. Crohn's, rheumatoid arthritis, tuberculosis, malaria, widespread eczema)

Increased losses
  e.g. congestive heart failure, liver necrosis, haemodialysis, peritoneal dialysis

Drugs
  Anticonvulsants, barbiturates, ? oral contraceptives

Metabolic
  Homocystinuria

Mixed causes
  e.g. liver disease, alcoholism

---

* Poor diet is a factor in most cases of severe folate deficiency.

diagnosis from tropical sprue may, however, be particularly difficult. Indeed, cases of megaloblastic anaemia due to folate deficiency with no, or minimal evidence of, malabsorption and normal jejunal-mucosa appearance, in whom there is failure to elicit a definite history of poor diet, have been labelled 'temperate sprue' [324], but it is likely that most of these patients are suffering from nutritional megaloblastic anaemia.

Infancy. Folate deficiency in infancy, as in many other conditions, is due to dietary intake being insufficient to meet demands, particularly if intake is reduced or demands are increased for any reason. Newborn infants show serum and red-cell folate levels two to three times those of adults [325]. These fall exponentially to normal levels over the first few weeks of life. The folate content of breast milk is approximately 50 μg/l but powdered milks, particularly if these are boiled, may contain much less than this [1, 326] and so provide insufficient folate for the newborn infant which has demands which have been estimated as 10 times those of an adult on a body weight basis.

Premature babies. These show particularly steep falls in folate levels in the first few weeks of life, due probably to consumption of folate during growth and also, perhaps, due to excess urinary-folate excretion [327, 328]. A proportion—in one series seven of 54 babies studied—particularly those of lowest birth weight, develop megaloblastic anaemia at about six to 10 weeks [329]. The smallest babies (weighing less than 1200 g at birth) and those who have infections, feeding difficulties or exchange transfusions are particularly prone to this complication and prophylactic folic acid is probably worthwhile in all such infants.

Nutritional megaloblastic anaemia in full-term infants usually occurs later (six months to three years), typically in generally malnourished children who develop infections of the respiratory or urinary tracts and childhood viral infections. In some cases this anaemia may be associated with scurvy or kwashiorkor.

Goat's milk anaemia. This is a type of nutritional folate deficiency which has been described in Germany, Italy, New Zealand, the USA and other countries. It occurs in infants fed goat's milk, which has a much lower folate content than that of cow's or artificial milk (approximately 50 μg/l) since it contains only 6 μg folate/l [1, 326]. As in other megaloblastic anaemias of infancy, an infection often precipitates the onset of clinical symptoms.

Malabsorption

Relatively few diseases cause a severe degree of malabsorption of folate (Table 6.7), but minor degrees of malabsorption may contribute to the deficiency in other conditions.

Adult coeliac disease. Virtually all patients with this disease show folate deficiency [330]. It occurs most commonly between the ages of 30 and 50 and many of the patients give a definite or suggestive history of coeliac disease in childhood. Most of the patients give a history of persistent or episodic diarrhoea but this is absent in about 20% of otherwise typical cases. The stools are typically pale, offensive and tend to float. Osteomalacia, pigmentation, clubbing of the fingers, haemorrage due to prothrombin deficiency and weakness due to hypokalaemia are common features. The diagnosis is established by jejunal biopsy, which is always abnormal and usually shows sub-total villous atrophy but, in less than 10% of patients, partial villous atrophy. Tests of fat excretion, absorption of xylose, glucose and B$_{12}$, and intestinal X-ray are also useful but less diagnostic. The lesion is always most marked in the upper small intestine and the ileal mucosa may appear normal. The gut lesion responds to a gluten-free diet and relapses on reintroduction of gluten. In some otherwise typical cases, the response to gluten withdrawal is poor and these patients may have a severe illness with protein deficiency and a poor prognosis. The blood picture on presentation varies. Some 10–20% of patients present with megaloblastic anaemia. More frequently anaemia is due to combined iron and folate deficiency [330]. Some 10–15% of all cases show changes of splenic atrophy in the blood but sensitive isotope studies reveal that some degree of splenic atrophy is present in nearly all cases [331].

Serum and red-cell folate levels are almost always low, and these tests may be used for following the response to treatment since they improve spontaneously if a gluten-free diet is given.

The cause of the deficiency is thought to be mainly malabsorption of dietary folate. This is not due to a lack of folate conjugase in the mucosa but more probably to damage to, and reduction of, the absorptive surface of the duodenal and jejunal mucosa [332, 333]. It is also likely that in this condition, and in other conditions of folate malabsorption, biliary folate and folate present in sloughing intestinal cells is also lost excessively. Surprisingly, megaloblastic anaemia in these patients, in some cases responds to folic acid given orally in as low a dose as 50–200 μg. Presumably, dietary folate is much less well absorbed than folic acid. As mentioned earlier, mild B$_{12}$ deficiency is present in some of the patients, but this is probably never the main cause of megaloblastic anaemia [330].

Most cases will require iron as well as folic acid to correct the anaemia, but it is unusual for additional B_{12}, vitamin B_6 or other haematinic therapy to be necessary.

Childhood coeliac disease. The incidence of folate deficiency in these children assessed by serum and red-cell folate is probably equal to that in adults. However, the children are almost all iron deficient and it is unusual for them to develop uncomplicated megaloblastic anaemia. Serum B_{12} levels are usually normal and splenic atrophy rare [330, 334].

Tropical sprue. In the early months of this disease megaloblastic anaemia due to folate deficiency is present in almost all the patients. The cause of the deficiency is a combination of malabsorption and poor diet. As in coeliac disease, malabsorption of dietary folate is more marked than malabsorption of folic acid but jejunal folate-conjugase concentration is normal [335]. There is some evidence that folate deficiency may predispose visitors to the tropics to develop the disease, and better evidence that folic acid therapy corrects not only the megaloblastic anaemia but also the glossitis, anorexia, diarrhoea and malabsorption of xylose, fat, B_{12} and folate [336]. Most of the patients, particularly those with more chronic disease, also require antibiotic and B_{12} therapy for a complete cure. Iron deficiency is unusual while splenic atrophy has occurred but is much less common than in adult coeliac disease. Tropical sprue may also occur in children when the incidence of folate deficiency and response to folic acid seem to be similar to that in adults.

Dermatitis herpetiformis. It is now clear from intestinal structural and functional tests, haematological and immunological studies and the effects of gluten withdrawal that almost all patients with this skin disease also have an upper intestinal lesion indistinguishable from that seen in adult coeliac disease [337]. This, and the skin condition, may respond to gluten withdrawal [338]. Splenic atrophy is also common [339]. Most patients show subnormal serum folate levels but only 50% have subnormal red-cell folate and overt megaloblastic anaemia is the exception. The severity of folate deficiency has been found to correlate with the severity of the jejunal lesion and both are usually less than in coeliac disease. The deficiency is probably due to malabsorption of dietary folate [332]. Patients receiving dapsone may show a haemolytic anaemia due to the oxidizing effect of this drug on red cells but this drug probably has no direct effect on folate status or the gut lesion.

Specific malabsorption of folate. Only five patients with this interesting congenital defect have been described, and two of these were siblings. Megaloblastic anaemia developed in early infancy or childhood. The best-documented cases showed malabsorption of all forms of folate tested, including folic acid, folinic acid or pteroyltriglutamic acid, failure to transport folate into the cerebrospinal fluid, with megalobastic anaemia, mental retardation and cerebral calcification [305, 340].

Other conditions. When megaloblastic anaemia due to folate deficiency occurs in the following conditions it is likely that the major cause is poor diet. Mild degrees of malabsorption of folate may occur after jejunal resection and in Crohn's disease. Folate deficiency occurs in most patients with active Crohn's disease on the basis of poor diet and increased requirements for folate as well as possible mild malabsorption. Change in pH in the small intestine has been suggested but not proven to contribute to the malabsorption [341, 342]. Salicylazosulphapyridine may also cause malabsorption of folate [343] but megaloblastic anaemia due to folate deficiency is rare in ulcerative colitis treated with this drug. The deficiency is unusual when Crohn's disease is quiescent [190]. In extreme cases, megaloblastic anaemia may occur but in these cases the anaemia, which is partly due to inflammatory disease itself and sometimes to iron deficiency, is not completely corrected by folic-acid therapy alone [190].

Mild folate deficiency is common following partial gastrectomy but severe folate deficiency is unusual and mainly of dietary origin [344]. Only five per cent of 292 cases in London had serum folate levels less than 3·0 μg/l and only six of the 292 had anaemia partly or completely due to folate deficiency [175]. In this series, patients with iron-deficiency anaemia showed lower serum folate levels than iron-replete patients but iron therapy did not improve the folate status suggesting poor diet might contribute to both deficiencies. Mild degrees of malabsorption of natural folate has been found in some of the patients.

Mild malabsorption of folate has been described in patients with chronic lymphocytic leukaemia, lymphomas, congestive heart failure and alcoholism [1, 293]. It has also been suggested that folate deficiency due to malabsorption may occur in the intestinal stagnant-loop syndrome, but it is likely that the deficiency in these cases is of dietary origin. Folate excess due to bacterial contamination of the upper small intestine is better established in the stagnant-loop syndrome [345]. High serum, red-cell and urinary folate have been described and there is a rough correlation between the concentration of bacteria in jejunal juice and the height of the serum folate (which may reach levels of 40–50 μg/l). Moreover, the folate levels fall when antibiotic therapy is given [345]. On the other hand, systemic bacterial infections cause impaired absorption of folate [346].

Excess folate consumption

A large number of conditions may predispose to folate deficiency. It is presumed that degradation of the vitamin is increased. Of these, the most important is pregnancy.

Pregnancy. This has been the subject of several major studies [347–349]. Until the advent of prophylactic folic acid, the incidence of megaloblastic anaemia in pregnancy varied from about 0·5% in Western countries to 50% in southern India. Requirements for folate are thought to increase by about 100–300 μg daily, due to folate transfer to the fetus, which causes a fall in serum and red-cell folate, most marked in the last trimester, when low serum folate levels may occur in 50% of patients, low red-cell folate in about 30%. In normal pregnancy, it is unlikely that malabsorption of folate or increased urinary folate losses are important causes of the deficiency and, indeed, red-cell folate in late pregnancy has been found to correlate with dietary folate intake and poor diet may account, in some cases, for the tendency of the deficiency to recur. In other cases, however, this is due to another underlying cause of the deficiency (e.g. coliac disease), anticonvulsant therapy or a chronic haemolytic anaemia.

Severe folate deficiency in pregnancy is more common in patients who are also iron deficient, in twin pregnancies, if serum and red-cell folate levels are low in early pregnancy, in multiparae compared to primiparae and possibly, in Britain, in late winter and early spring. Megaloblastic anaemia may also be precipitated by infection, usually of the urinary tract, in which case megaloblastic 'arrest' of haemopoiesis has been described. Some patients present with megaloblastic anaemia in the post-partum period. Folate is lost during lactation, and this may be an additional drain on already depleted stores.

A number of complications of pregnancy—stillbirths, prematurity, recurrent abortion, ante-partum and post-partum haemorrhage and congenital malformation of the fetus, have been suggested to occur in association with severe folate deficiency. None are completely established, though prophylactic folic-acid therapy does appear to reduce the incidence of prematurity in a malnourished population [350].

A fall in serum B$_{12}$ level occurs in normal pregnancy (in the absence of folate deficiency) with the lowest level at term and a spontaneous rise three to five weeks after delivery; approximately 20% of women may have subnormal levels in the last trimester.

The case for the prophylactic administration of folic acid in pregnancy is strong and this is now practised routinely in Great Britain. The dose of folic acid usually given is 300–400 μg daily. Larger doses carry the risk, albeit rare, of masking megaloblastic anaemia due to B$_{12}$ deficiency and possibly precipitating B$_{12}$ neuropathy. Folate alone does not improve the mean haemoglobin level in pregnancy; iron is required in addition and it is convenient to give a combined iron and folate tablet, provided this is not expensive.

Haemolytic anaemia. Folate deficiency is likely to occur in most types of haemolytic anaemia but particularly in those with ineffective erythropoiesis, since primitive cells contain and utilize more folate than mature cells. The deficiency may produce an apparent arrest of haemopoiesis, the nature of which is revealed by bone-marrow examination. In a few cases with megaloblastic anaemia, daily doses of folic acid larger than the usual adult requirements have been required to produce a response [351]. Very low serum folate levels have been found in 25% and positive Figlu tests were present in 16 of 22 patients with sickle-cell anaemia [352] and the deficiency is common in other major haemoglobinopathies such as haemoglobin H disease, haemoglobin SC and in thalassaemia major. The deficiency is also frequent in warm-type autoimmune haemolytic anaemia and also in mechanical, drug-induced and micro-angiopathic haemolytic anaemia. Megaloblastic anaemia due to folate deficiency has been recorded in hereditary spherocytosis on a number of occasions but is probably less common in this disease. The deficiency is even less frequent in patients with pyruvate-kinase deficiency and in paroxysmal nocturnal haemoglobinuria, in which, indeed, folate clearance is usually slower than normal.

Chronic myelosclerosis. This is an important cause of megaloblastic anaemia in Britain. Among a series of 49 patients, most of whom had been studied over many years, nearly one-third at some stage developed marked megaloblastic changes, and another third showed mild changes [353]. The deficiency is particularly common where myelosclerosis follows polycythaemia vera and in some patients occurred during the transition phase between the two diseases. The complication may be missed because pancytopenia may be due to the disease itself and because of the difficulty in obtaining marrow. The deficiency may present primarily with thrombocytopenia, increased transfusion requirements or rapidly developing pancytopenia following an intercurrent infection (Fig. 6.12). The cause is thought to be inadequate diet in the face of ineffective erythropoiesis, leucopoiesis and thrombopoiesis, causing increased utilization. In the United States, folate deficiency appears to be much less

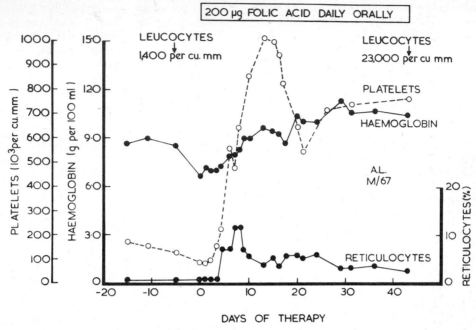

Fig. 6.12. The haematological response of a patient with thrombocythaemia and myelosclerosis who developed pancytopenia following an intercurrent infection and was treated with folic acid 200 μg daily by mouth (by courtesy of the *Quarterly Journal of Medicine*).

common in this disease and this may be related to the generally better dietary folate intake. In contrast, polycythaemia vera is not a significant cause of folate deficiency and the patients who have developed megaloblastic anaemia have been incidental cases of PA or nutritional megaloblastic anaemia or had undergone partial gastrectomy.

Sideroblastic anaemia. Mild folate deficiency is common in the acquired forms of this disease, particularly when there is an associated disease which may also cause the deficiency (e.g. myelosclerosis), alcoholism or rheumatoid arthritis [354]. The cause is probably increased folate utilization due to ineffective haemopoiesis and about one-third of patients show some response, albeit small, to folic-acid therapy. In some patients, however, megaloblastic changes are refractory to both folate and B_{12} therapy.

Leukaemia. Mild folate deficiency is common in acute leukaemia and less common in the chronic forms, but it is unusual for the deficiency to aggravate anaemia, and folic acid which might 'feed the tumour' should not be given unless there is a good chance of real benefit. Megaloblastic changes in myeloid leukaemia and erythroleukaemia may also occur which are refractory to folic acid and B_{12} therapy.

Myeloma. Low serum levels are common in this condition and a small proportion of the patients develop marked megaloblastic anaemia. Such patients usually are in the late stage of the disease and the response to folic acid is disappointing [355]. Low serum B_{12} levels also occur even in patients with normal B_{12} absorption and there is probably no significant association between myeloma and PA [356].

Carcinoma, lymphoma. Despite the high incidence of low serum folate levels and positive Figlu tests in these diseases, the incidence of severe folate deficiency is quite low. Indeed, the mean red-cell folate level in unselected carcinoma patients is normal, although occasional patients with widespread disease or with tumours of the oesophagus or stomach may develop severe deficiency, largely of dietary origin.

Inflammatory diseases. Patients with active tuberculosis may develop the deficiency which improves spontaneously with successful chemotherapy. None of the anti-tuberculous drugs has been shown to cause the deficiency. Though mild megaloblastic changes are common, anaemia, if present, is usually due to impaired iron utilization and possibly iron deficiency as well as folate deficiency [357]. Gough *et al.* [358] found a high incidence of mild folate deficiency in rheumatoid arthritis and a few patients had megaloblastic anaemia due to the deficiency. Psoriasis, exfoliative dermatitis, erythrodermia and widespread eczema may be associated with mild folate deficiency but alone do not cause megaloblastic anaemia. Megaloblastic anaemia due to folate deficiency appears to be more frequent in malaria [359].

Mixed causes

Congestive heart failure. Urinary loss of folate may reach 100 μg in 24 hours or more in congestive heart failure (or active liver disease) and is presumably due to release of folate from liver to plasma [360]. Mild malabsorption of folate has also been described and megaloblastic haemopoiesis is common [361], though it is unusual for this to cause megaloblastic anaemia.

Renal failure. Mild folate deficiency is common and due to a combination of anorexia, vomiting and removal of folate from plasma by peritoneal or haemodialysis [362]. Hypersegmented polymorphs, not due to folate or B$_{12}$ deficiency may also occur in uraemic patients. Folate therapy is usually given to all patients receiving regular haemodialysis, estimated to remove approximately 52 μg on each dialysis [363].

Liver disease and alcoholism. Folate deficiency has been described in all forms of liver disease, but is particularly common in alcoholics and in haemochromatosis [364]. Of 40 patients with liver disease in one study, the four who had megaloblastic anaemia were all alcoholics [365]. Low liver folate levels (less than 5 μg/g) occurred in 14 of 20 patients with alcoholic cirrhosis in another study while the serum folate was low in at least half these patients [366]. The cause of the deficiency is probably multiple. Excess urinary folate loss occurs in active liver disease such as active cirrhosis or infective hepatitis. Poor storage of folate and inadequate dietary intake may also be important. Alcohol also seems to have a toxic effect on haemopoiesis, causing impaired iron utilization, vacuolization of the cytoplasm and nuclei of precursor cells generally. Ingestion of spirits may cause megaloblastic changes within 4–10 days if pre-existing folate deficiency is present, and arrest of haemopoiesis in patients with megaloblastic anaemia, responding to physiological doses of folic or folinic acid [367] (see Chapter 33). Sideroblastic changes may also appear [368] and thombocytopenia may appear without megaloblastic anaemia. Alcohol appears to interfere with delivery of folate to plasma from storage areas but it may have other effects on folate utilization [369].

Intensive-care units. Pancytopenia due to megaloblastic anaemia has been described in patients undergoing intensive care (e.g. following cardiac surgery). A number of mechanisms have been implicated: folate deficiency due to increased consumption, alcohol in intravenous nutrition, nitrous-oxide anaesthesia (see below) and an effect on the marrow of the amino-acid mixture infused [370, 371]. In some units, folic acid is given routinely and prolonged N$_2$O anaesthesia is avoided.

Metabolic causes

Homocystinuria. Children with homocystinuria due to cystathionase deficiency show a high incidence of folate deficiency which is most severe in those with the severest forms of the disease [372]. The cause of the deficiency is probably increased folate utilization due to increased conversion of homocysteine to methionine, folate absorption and excretion being normal [372]. Folic-acid therapy causes increased excretion of methionine and decreased excretion of homocysteine [372]. Pyridoxine therapy causes a reduction in folate levels, possibly by increasing homocysteine conversion to methionine. Homocystinuria may also occur in association with methylmalonic aciduria due to a derangement in B$_{12}$ metabolism (see p. 238).

Iron deficiency. There are several conditions which are associated with a deficiency of both iron and folate. For instance, in pregnancy, and following partial gastrectomy, iron-deficient patients show a higher incidence of folate deficiency than iron-replete subjects [373, 374]. In neither situation does iron therapy correct folate deficiency and it is likely that the two deficiencies occur together in the subjects with the poorest nutrition or absorption. It has been suggested that iron deficiency *per se* can cause increased Figlu excretion, hypersegmented polymorphonuclear leukocytes and giant metamyelocytes, a raised red-cell folate and increased folate utilization, but none of these effects is established [375]. On the other hand, iron deficiency may mask the morphological changes of megaloblastosis in the bone marrow and, *in vitro*, both iron deficiency and desferrioxamine reduce the abnormality of thymidylate synthesis in megaloblastic cells [376] probably due to inhibition of ribonucleotide reductase [377].

Miscellaneous. Increased clearance of folate has been described in thyrotoxicosis but a true deficiency is unusual. Folate deficiency, the cause of which is obscure but probably mainly dietary, has also been recorded in patients with myxoedema, Paget's disease of bone, and chronic neurological and psychiatric diseases [378].

Anticonvulsant and other antifolate drugs

Anticonvulsants. Megaloblastic anaemia occurs in patients receiving diphenylhydantoin, primidone and barbiturates. The incidence of folate deficiency in patients receiving these drugs depends on the dose, type of drug and probably on the diet of the patient [379]. Subnormal red-cell folate levels occur in about one-third of patients and this is the incidence of megaloblastic changes in the marrows of unselected patients [380]. Subnormal serum B_{12} levels occur in a few non-anaemic patients but are usual in those with megaloblastic anaemia.

Poor diet is always a factor in those with megaloblastic anaemia but the role of the drugs in producing the deficiency is uncertain. Explanations proposed include inhibition of folate coenzyme synthesis or function, inhibition of absorption of folic acid or specifically of pteroylpolyglutamates by inhibition of intestinal conjugase, induction of ribosomal enzymes with excessive folate utilization or displacement of folate from its transport protein in plasma. None of these theories has, however, been confirmed although recent studies in mice show that diphenylhydantoin does increase folate catabolism [381]. The drugs do not affect transport of folate in the cerebrospinal fluid or bone marrow [382]. There is also some evidence that they may interfere with pyrimidine synthesis in bacteria. Reynolds [383] has suggested that treatment with folic acid improves certain mental symptoms with an increase in alertness and drive, but increases the number of fits and, indeed, a case of status epilepticus, apparently precipitated by folic acid, has been de-scribed. However, there is no evidence on the basis of a double blind trial for these theories [384].

Other possible folate antagonists. Oral contraceptives have been suggested to cause folate deficiency [385] but there is no evidence to support this [386, 387]. Nitro-furantoin has not been confirmed as a folate anta-gonist but a few reports suggest triamterene as a weak antagonist [1, 388]. Sulphonamides inhibit bacterial synthesis of folate but do not affect folate metabolism in humans who rely on the preformed vitamin. The effect of alcohol on folate metabolism is discussed on page 233.

DIAGNOSIS OF FOLATE DEFICIENCY
(Table 6.8)

It is always likely that folate deficiency is present in a patient with megaloblastic haemopoiesis and a normal serum B_{12} level. Folate deficiency may be confirmed by a therapeutic trial or by direct laboratory tests for folate deficiency, and the best and most widely used tests are measurement of serum and red-cell folate.

Serum folate

This may be measured microbiologically using *L. casei* or by radioassay [389–391]. Most laboratories would agree that levels below $3 \cdot 0 \ \mu g/l$ are low, $3 \cdot 0–5 \cdot 0 \ \mu g/l$ borderline, and levels about $5 \cdot 0$ or $6 \cdot 0 \ \mu g/l$ definitely normal [392]. The upper limit of normal is poorly defined and values between $7 \cdot 0$ and $31 \cdot 0 \ \mu g/l$ have been quoted. Certain sera, particularly from coeliac disease patients, contain an antibody which agglutinates *L. casei* and this may reduce growth of the organism in whole-serum assays. Care must also be taken to avoid excess exposure of the assay medium to light, other-wise growth of the organism will be poor because of

Table 6.8. Steps in the diagnosis of megaloblastic anaemia

Suspicion: Raised MCV, anaemia, glossitis, paraesthesiae, neuropathy, psychiatric disturbance, poor diet, malabsorption, abdominal disease or operation, residence in tropics, anticonvulsant drugs, alcohol, family history of anaemia, etc.

Diagnosis of megaloblastic haemopoiesis: Examination of peripheral blood and bone marrow. Measurement of serum bilirubin, LDH

Differentiation of B_{12} or folate deficiency:* Measurement of serum B_{12}, serum and red-cell folate, therapeutic trial, deoxyuridine-suppression test

Tests for cause of deficiency:
(a) *General*: Diet history, barium meal and follow-through X-ray
(b) *Vitamin B_{12}*: Gastric secretion of acid and intrinsic factor, endoscopy and gastric biopsy, B_{12}-absorption studies, tests for parietal-cell and intrinsic-factor antibodies, jejunal bacteriology, proteinuria, etc.
(c) *Folate*: Jejunal biopsy, small-intestinal absorption, tests for underlying disease

---

* Methylmalonic-acid and Figlu-excretion tests now obsolete.

lack of riboflavin. Radioassays for serum folate use labelled (^{3}H or ^{14}C) folic acid or 5-methyl THF or labelled seleno-methionine folate, with β lactoglobulin or crude milk protein as binder. The results correlate reasonably well with those obtained by microbiologic assay [393, 393a].

The serum folate assay is a sensitive, reliable guide to the presence of folate deficiency. It is subnormal in all patients with the deficiency and is normal or raised in B$_{12}$-deficient patients who are not also folate deficient. The serum folate gives little guide to the severity of folate deficiency since it may be equally low in gross megaloblastic anaemia and in patients with normoblastic haemopoiesis. The level falls when a normal subject takes a folate-free diet for a few days and is extremely low after a few weeks on such a diet. The rapid fall has been attributed to lack of displacement of liver folate, the normal source of serum folate, by recently ingested folate. Raised serum folate levels are found, not only in some patients by B$_{12}$ deficiency, but may also be found in the intestinal stagnant-loop syndrome, in patients with liver damage and renal failure, as well as in patients receiving folate or in bacterially contaminated sera.

Red-cell folate

This is measured as a serum folate with *L. casei* or by radioassay. The normal range is from 160 to 640 μg/l and the result is subnormal in patients with megaloblastic anaemia due to folate deficiency (particularly in the most anaemic patients) and in patients with significant tissue depletion of folate without megaloblastic anaemia, but is normal in patients with normoblastic haemopoiesis, even if the serum folate is low [394]. The red-cell folate is subnormal in about 60% of patients with megaloblastic anaemia due to B$_{12}$ deficiency, and this is particularly so in the most anaemic patients [394]. Reticulocytes contain more folate than mature cells and raised red-cell folate may occur in patients with a reticulocytosis from any cause such as haemolysis and haemorrhage, and the overall red-cell folate may be normal in these conditions, despite the presence of megaloblastic anaemia [394]. Normal red-cell folate levels may also occur in patients with severe folate deficiency who have been transfused in the weeks before blood was taken for assay, since the folate in mature red cells is not released until the cells die.

Figlu (formiminoglutamic acid) excretion

The biochemical pathway involved was described on page 225. Normal subjects excrete from 0 to 16 mg of Figlu in eight hours after an oral load of 15 g of histidine and the excretion is raised in patients with severe folate deficiency. The test is no longer used since positive results are also obtained in 50–60% of patients with severe B$_{12}$ deficiency [395] as well as in many patients with liver disease, carcinoma, tuberculosis, sarcoidosis, polyarteritis nodosa, scleroderma, myelosclerosis and thyrotoxicosis in the absence of folate deficiency. Moreover, the Figlu test may be negative despite severe folate deficiency in pregnancy and in patients with severe protein deficiency (kwashiorkor) in which lack of urocanase causes a block in Figlu production from urocanic acid [396]. Increased excretion of urocanic acid also occurs in other diseases—e.g. carcinoma and tuberculosis with liver damage when it bears no relation to folate deficiency.

MANAGEMENT OF MEGALOBLASTIC ANAEMIA

INVESTIGATION
(Table 6.8)
The first step is suspicion that megaloblastic anaemia or B$_{12}$ or folate deficiency is present, even in the absence of megaloblastic anaemia. Suspicion may arise because of symptoms of anaemia, neuropathy or of gastro-intestinal disease or other conditions which may predispose to one or other deficiency (Tables 2.2, 2.3 and 2.4). Suspicion is often aroused by the finding of a raised MCV in the peripheral blood. Causes of raised MCV other than megaloblastic anaemia are listed in Table 6.3. These may be distinguished from true megaloblastic anaemia by the absence of oval cells and hypersegmented neutrophils and by the presence of associated blood abnormalities (e.g. target cells and acanthocytes in liver disease). The higher the MCV, the more likely it is that true megaloblastic anaemia is present. A raised MCV, in the absence of anaemia and of other changes of B$_{12}$ or folate deficiency suggests excess alcohol ingestion. Examination of the patient may reveal not only pallor or jaundice or the features of B$_{12}$ neuropathy but may also show evidence of a condition such as myxoedema which is particularly associated with PA or an underlying disease which is the cause of folate deficiency (e.g. coeliac disease or a chronic inflammatory or malignant disease). The next step is a close examination of the peripheral-blood film, a blood count including haemoglobin estimation, red-cell, white-cell and platelet counts and, if necessary, examination of the bone marrow, which will not only establish whether or not megaloblastosis is present but will also reveal the iron status of the patient. If the clinical and haematological features are suggestive, assays of serum B$_{12}$ and folate, and red-cell folate will establish whether B$_{12}$ or folate deficiency, or both deficiencies, are present. Further tests are then necessary to determine the cause of the deficiency. In either

case, a diet history and barium meal and follow-through X-ray examination (or endoscopy) will be needed. Gastric function and B_{12} absorption studies, tests for parietal cell and IF antibody in serum, gastric biopsy or jejunal biopsy if sprue is suspected, are valuable for elucidating the cause of B_{12} deficiency, Tests for the cause of folate deficiency include jejunal biopsy, xylose, folate and fat absorption tests, and tests for underlying haematological, inflammatory or malignant disease, though these are usually obvious when severe folate deficiency occurs.

Mild folate deficiency is far more common than megaloblastic anaemia due to the deficiency. The decision whether a patient with, for instance, a subnormal serum folate level has deficiency of a severity to warrant full investigation and treatment is determined largely by the blood and bone-marrow findings and, if this can be measured, on the red-cell folate level. On the other hand, a subnormal serum B_{12} level is a highly significant finding and always requires full investigation in Western countries.

GENERAL TREATMENT (Table 6.9)

If possible, treatment should be delayed until the cause of the anaemia or vitamin deficiency is known. In the severely anaemic or thombocytopenic patient, therapy may be required as soon as samples of blood and marrow necessary for diagnosis have been obtained. If so, both B_{12} (hydroxocobalamin) and folic acid should be given. If *cardiac failure* is present this should be treated in the usual way with diuretics. Blood transfusion should be avoided but if it is essential because of tissue anoxia, not more than 250 ml of packed cells

may be given slowly, possibly with drawing 100 ml or so of blood from the other arm.

A mild *fever* is present in most anaemic cases and falls to normal with therapy. Temperatures greater than 39·5°C or fever persisting despite correct therapy suggest that infection, often of the respiratory or urinary tract, is present. *Hypokalaemia* during the response to therapy has recently been described [397]. Serum potassium levels should be monitored during the first 10 days of treatment and, if necessary, potassium therapy given promptly, particularly if heart failure is already present. Gout may present on or about the sixth day of therapy due to increased purine breakdown. This requires the usual immediate treatment; long-term treatment may be necessary as these subjects usually have a gouty predisposition.

TREATMENT OF VITAMIN-B_{12} DEFICIENCY

Most patients who develop B_{12} deficiency require life-long B_{12} therapy. The underlying cause can be corrected in only a few circumstances such as expulsion of the fish-tapeworm, surgical removal of an intestinal blind-loop, or antibiotic, folate and B_{12} therapy in tropical sprue. In all patients, initial saturation of body stores with B_{12} is required and this is best carried out with at least six intramuscular injections of 1000 μg hydroxocobalamin, spaced at two or three day intervals. Hydroxocobalamin binds tightly to body proteins and is retained in the body three times as well as cyanocobalamin. Because it is better retained, hydroxocobalamin is also preferable to cyanocobalamin for maintenance therapy and a number of different regimes are used, varying from 500 μg once every three months to 1000 μg once every two months, or four injections of 1000 μg over a period of

Table 6.9. Treatment of megaloblastic anaemia

	Vitamin-B_{12} deficiency	Folate deficiency
Initial*	100 μg hydroxocobalamin intramuscularly × 6 over 2–3 weeks	5 mg folic acid daily for 4 months
Maintenance	100 μg hydroxocobalamin intramuscularly once every 3 months	Correct underlying cause (e.g. gluten-free diet). Folic acid 5 mg daily or weekly
Prophylaxis	Total gastrectomy, ileal resection	Pregnancy, prematurity, severe haemolytic anaemia, myelosclerosis, haemo- and peritoneal dialysis, parenteral feeding (e.g. intensive care)

* N.B. Other therapy which may be needed initially includes diuretics, potassium supplements, platelet concentrates. Blood transfusion is best avoided.

two weeks once each year. It is the author's practice to give 1000 µg once every three months. Larger and more frequent doses have been used for patients with B$_{12}$ neuropathy but there is no evidence that this is of greater benefit.

The haematological response to treatment has been described (p. 218). The patient feels better in 48–72 hours with a return of appetite and relief of pain from the tongue. The temperature falls in a few days, and gastro-intestinal symptoms disappear within a week or two. The nervous system improves more slowly and may not be maximum until six months [398]. Improvement is not complete if there is spinal-cord damage, particularly if symptoms were present for more than a few months before treatment started.

Prophylactic B$_{12}$ therapy. This is given from the time of operation in patients undergoing total gastrectomy or ileal resection.

Sensitivity to B$_{12}$ injections. This is rare and may present as anaphylactoid reactions or urticaria and may be confirmed by intradermal testing. It usually involves all forms of the vitamin. Such patients must be given oral B$_{12}$ therapy. Antibody to transcobalamin (TC)II has been detected in the sera of patients given depot preparations of cyano- or hydroxocobalamin and these preparations should be avoided.

There is no evidence that B$_{12}$ therapy is of any value in any non-B$_{12}$-deficient state except in some cases of congenital methylmalonic aciduria (p. 221), and in TCII deficiency and nitrous oxide inactivation of B$_{12}$. It is widely used, however, as a tonic. A number of workers have claimed that frequent large doses of hydroxocobalamin improve patients with tobacco amblyopia and with Leber's optic atrophy on the basis that B$_{12}$ becomes inactivated in the cyanocobalamin form in these conditions. There is no evidence, on the basis of a double-blind trial, for the value of hydroxocobalamin therapy in the absence of true B$_{12}$ deficiency in these conditions.

Oral B$_{12}$ therapy. This is, in general, less satisfactory than parenteral therapy since, even in normal subjects, daily absorption is limited to a few micrograms and thus stores cannot be saturated for years, while therapy is required daily for maintenance. In patients with malabsorption of B$_{12}$, 2–3 µg can be absorbed passively through the upper small intestine each day, provided 500–1000 µg oral doses are given; this regime is used for patients sensitive to B$_{12}$ injections, who refuse injections or have a bleeding disorder in which injections would cause haemorrhage. Smaller daily oral doses (e.g. 30–50 µg) may be given to vegans instead of

injections. Oral preparations with attached IF are not used at all since resistance to the IF soon develops.

TREATMENT OF FOLATE DEFICIENCY

Initial treatment and replenishment of stores
Though it is possible to obtain an optimal response in most patients with 100–200 µg folic acid daily, it is usual to treat deficient patients with larger doses: 5–15 mg daily. This may be given orally in all patients who can swallow tablets, since even in those with severe malabsorption, sufficient folate is absorbed from this dose to replenish stores. Before folic acid is given in these large doses it is always necessary to ensure that B$_{12}$ deficiency is not present. It is uncertain how long initial folic-acid therapy should be continued, though it is usual to give the vitamin for several months until a new population of red cells has been formed. Folinic acid is reserved for combating the toxic effects of dihydrofolate-reductase inhibitors, methotrexate, pyrimethamine or trimethoprim.

Long-term management
It is often possible to correct the cause of folate deficiency and thus to prevent the deficiency recurring (e.g. by an improved diet, a gluten-free diet in coeliac disease, or by treatment of an inflammatory disease such as tuberculosis or Crohn's disease) (Table 6.7). In these cases, there is no need to continue folic acid for life. In other situations, however, it is advisable to give folic acid continually to prevent the deficiency recurring (e.g. in chronic myelosclerosis, chronic haemolytic anaemia such as thalassaemia major, or in patients with adult coeliac disease who do not respond to a gluten-free diet). Moreover, dietary folate deficiency itself tends to recur and it is advisable to follow patients who have developed nutritional megaloblastic anaemia at yearly intervals to make sure the deficiency has not recurred.

Prophylactic folic-acid therapy. This is given in pregnancy, to premature infants, to patients undergoing regular dialysis, and to patients in intensive care. It is also usually given to patients with severe chronic haemolytic anaemias (e.g. thalassaemia major or sickle-cell anaemia).

Side-effects and contra-indications
Folic acid is remarkably non-toxic and reports of effects on the mental state of normal subjects and epileptics have not been confirmed. In all patients who take folic acid for many years, it is advisable to measure the serum B$_{12}$ or B$_{12}$ absorption in order to ensure that B$_{12}$ deficiency is not masked. It is inadvisable to give folic acid to patients with malignant

diseases unless severe folate deficiency is present and there is some definite short-term benefit to be gained since it is possible that folic acid will accelerate growth of the tumour.

MEGALOBLASTIC ANAEMIA DUE TO ABNORMALITIES OF VITAMIN B_{12} OR FOLATE METABOLISM

VITAMIN B_{12}
(Table 6.10)

Congenital

Transcobalamin II (TCII) deficiency. This was first recognized in 1971 by Hakami *et al.* [1958] in two sibs and a number of subsequent cases have been described [399–402]. The syndrome may occur in either sex, being inherited as an autosomal recessive. Megaloblastic anaemia typically occurs within a few weeks of birth. Serum B_{12} and folate levels are normal and thus cases may be misdiagnosed. The deoxyuridine suppression test is, however, abnormal and corrected by high concentrations of B_{12} *in vitro*, provided autologous plasma is added but is not corrected by methyl THF. Chromatography reveals no B_{12} binding in the TCII region while the sera of both parents show approximately 50% of normal TCII binding. The infant's serum is unable to promote uptake of B_{12} into normal cells but the infant's cells are able to take up normal amounts of B_{12} from normal serum. Vitamin-B_{12} absorption is reduced. In one case, immunoglobulins were absent until B_{12} therapy was given suggesting the intracellular deficiency affected lymphocyte development and function [400].

The anaemia responds to massive parenteral doses of B_{12} (e.g. 1000 μg hydroxocobalamin one to three times weekly, which presumably enables sufficient B_{12} to enter marrow cells from plasma by passive diffusion [403]. If patients are not treated sufficiently early and with adequate doses of B_{12}, a severe neuropathy may develop [401, 402].

An interesting variant of this syndrome has been described in a Negress aged 31 who had megaloblastic anaemia since infancy responding to large doses of B_{12} and to folate. This was shown to be due to an abnormal TCII (TCII Cardeza) that would bind B_{12} but was incapable of enhancing its entry to cells [96]. The serum B_{12} was extremely high even in the absence of B_{12} therapy. Apoprotein studies in congenital TCII deficiency have shown the protein is usually absent or substantially reduced in concentration but in one case, TCII was present but unable to bind B_{12} [404].

Methylmalonic (MM) aciduria (MMA). This is a group of inborn errors of metabolism, in some but not all, associated with megaloblastic anaemia. The syndrome may be due to a fault of the enzyme MM racemase which converts D-MMCoA to L-MMCoA, MM mutase which converts MMCoA to succinyl CoA or to a selective failure of synthesis of ado-B_{12}. In these conditions the infants show a metabolic ketoacidosis and protein intolerance but no anaemia. High doses of B_{12} are beneficial only if selective lack of ado-B_{12} is the fault (p. 202).

Another rare group of infants with MMA show homocystinuria in addition and are thought to lack both ado-B_{12} and methyl-B_{12}. These may have normoblastic or megaloblastic haemopoiesis. The explanation for normoblastic haemopoiesis is not known; whether it is due to selective retention of B_{12}-coenzyme activity in the marrow compared to the liver, to the length of time the condition has been present before diagnosis or to other factors remains to be determined.

Acquired

Nitrous oxide (N_2O) inhalation. Although pancytopenia with megaloblastic erythropoiesis due to N_2O anaesthesiae was first recognized in 1956 [405], it was

Table 6.10. Megaloblastic anaemia due to abnormalities of vitamin-B_{12} or folate metabolism

	Vitamin B_{12}	Folate
Inherited	1 Transcobalamin-II deficiency 2 Methylmalonic aciduria with homocystinuria (some cases)	1 5-methyl-THF transferase deficiency 2 Dihydrofolate-reductase deficiency 3 Folate-transport defect 4 Specific folate malabsorption
Acquired	Nitrous oxide	Dihydrofolate reductase inhibitors: Methotrexate, pyrimethamine, DDMP, DDEP, triamterene, (trimethoprim)

only in 1978 when Amess *et al.* [406] clearly showed that this was due to inactivation of B$_{12}$ that considerable interest in this action arose. Nitrous oxide oxidizes transition-metal complexes, converting B$_{12}$ from the active reduced cob(I)alamin form to cob(III)alamin, which condenses to the inactive cob(II)alamin (Fig. 6.13). Methyl-B$_{12}$ is rapidly inactivated with a block in methionine synthase in bone marrow, brain and other tissues, both in experimental animals and human cells [407–409]. It takes several hours for the enzyme activity to recover once exposure to N$_2$O is discontinued [407]. On the other hand, ado-B$_{12}$ is not inactivated [410] and MMA excretion does not occur in experimental animals even after many months of exposure [407, 411].

Nitrous oxide causes an abnormal dU-suppression test indicating reduced thymidylate synthetase activity in experimental animals (mice, rats and monkeys) as well as in humans [406, 412]. Humans not only develop megaloblastic anaemia but may also show a peripheral neuropathy resembling that of B$_{12}$ deficiency. This has been described in dentists and others chronically exposed to N$_2$O [414–416]. Experimental animals show an abnormal dU-suppression test corrected by B$_{12}$ but do not develop megaloblastic anaemia. Monkeys, however, have been found to develop a neuropathy with spinal-cord damage closely resembling human subacute combined degeneration of the cord [411]. Thus, an animal model of B$_{12}$ deficiency is available for studying the biochemical basis of B$_{12}$ neuropathy as well as of B$_{12}$-folate interrelations (see below).

Cyanate inactivation of B$_{12}$. The theory that clinical syndromes may arise because of inactivation of body B$_{12}$ as cyano-B$_{12}$ (due to excessive ingestion of cyanate or cyanide in the diet, e.g. in cassava, inhalation in tobacco smoke or due to inborn errors in cyanate metabolism) has not been substantiated either in humans or experimental animals. The theory attempted to explain the widely differing syndromes of tobacco amblyopia, Leber's optic atrophy, and certain congenital or acquired peripheral neuropathies on this basis, but the massive accumulation of cyanocobalamin expected has not been demonstrated using sensitive chromatographic techniques [417]. Nor have patients with these conditions been shown by double-blind trials to respond better to hydroxocobalamin than to cyanocobalamin or indeed to a placebo.

FOLATE METABOLISM

Congenital

A number of congenital disorders of folate metabolism have been described but their extreme rarity and difficulty in documentation has not established their existence beyond doubt [13].

5-methyltetrahydrofolate transferase deficiency. The one Japanese infant described had dilated cerebral ventricles, brain atrophy and megaloblastic anaemia associated with a high serum folate and responded to therapy with folic acid and pyridoxine. Japanese infants with cerebral atrophy and mental retardation have also been described who were thought to have cyclohydrase and formino-transferase deficiencies but these did not show megaloblastic anaemia.

Dihydrofolate-reductase deficiency. Only two cases have been described in detail [418] and subsequent follow-up of the second case of that report has shown the correct diagnosis to be TCII deficiency [402]. The existence of this syndrome in which, as in methotrexate toxicity, there is a response to folinic acid but not to folic acid depends, therefore, on a single case.

Congenital specific malabsorption of folate (see p. 229)

Acquired

Inhibitors of dihydrofolate reductase. An excellent symposium dealing with these compounds has been published [419] and only a brief synopsis is given here.

Methotrexate, the best known, differs structurally from folic acid by having an amino group at position 4 of the pteridine ring and a methyl group attached at N$_{10}$ (Fig. 6.14). It is easily absorbed from the gut, binds firmly to dihydrofolate reductase (from which it can displace other folates) and is then retained in the body for several months, though some is excreted in the urine in the first 24 hours after administration. The drug preferentially enters and kills proliferating haemopoietic cells, probably by a carrier-mediated mechanism partly related to that for transport of reduced folates [315]. It causes the haematological, chromosomal and biochemical features of megaloblastic anaemia, though leucopenia and thrombocyto-

$$COB(I) \xrightarrow{\ \ N_2O\ \ } COB(III) \ + \ N_2$$

$$COB(III) \ + \ COB\ I \longrightarrow 2COB(II)$$

Fig. 6.13. Oxidation of vitamin B$_{12}$ by nitrous oxide.

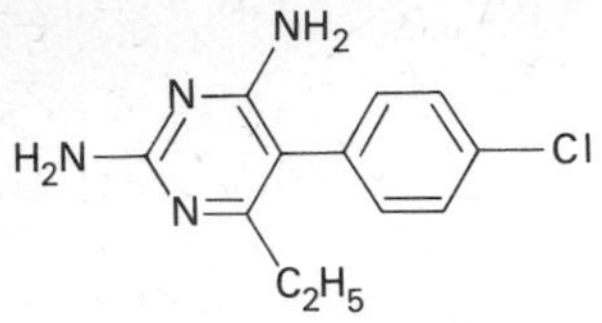

PYRIMETHAMINE

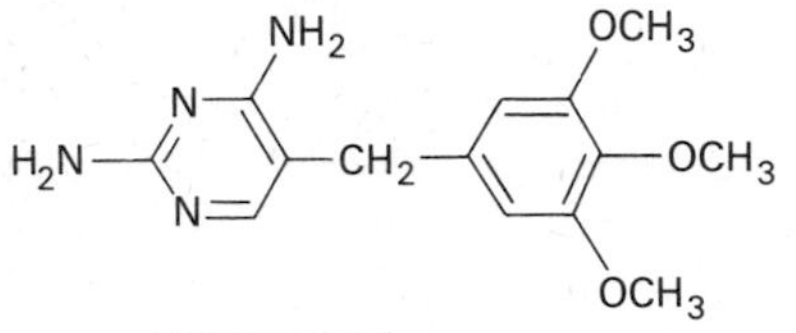

TRIMETHOPRIM

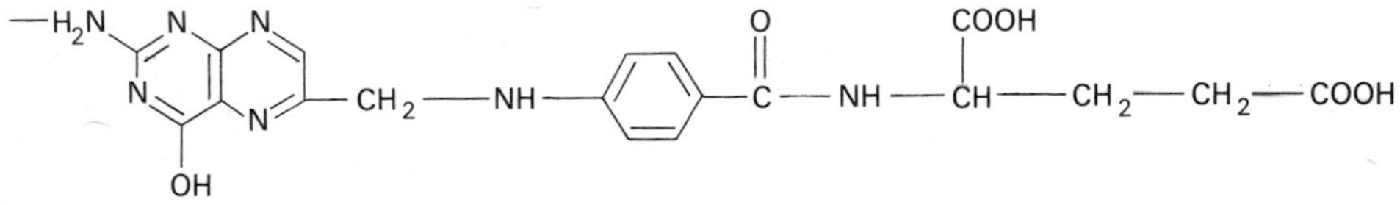

FOLIC ACID

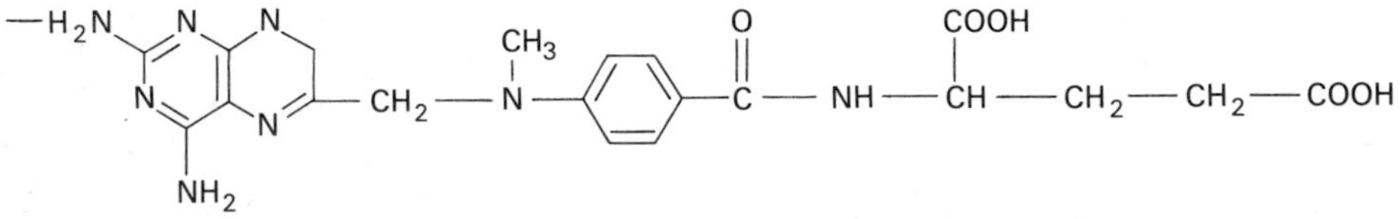

METHOTREXATE

Fig. 6.14. The structural formulae of folic acid, methotrexate, pyrimethamine and trimethoprim.

penia tend to be particularly marked. It is used for treatment of acute leukaemia, meningeal leukaemia, lymphomas and other solid tumours, including chorionic carcinoma, and for psoriasis. Toxicity usually presents as a gastro-intestinal disturbance with ulceration of the mouth and pharynx and can be overcome by administering the reduced folate, folinic acid, which is sometimes given to improve the therapeutic index of methotrexate [420], or to protect the bone marrow when methotrexate is given intrathecally for meningeal leukaemia. Long-term methotrexate therapy, as practised for psoriasis, may cause hepatic fibrosis or cirrhosis.

The drug reduces thymidylate synthesis and lowers cell concentration of thymidine triphosphate (dTTP) and so may increase uptake of preformed thymidine due to reduced inhibition of thymidine kinase [421]. Inhibition of purine, lipid and protein synthesis may also occur and may be important. Resistance is associated with an increased dihydrofolate-reductase level in the malignant cells which does not occur in normal cells [419]. Decreased transport of methotrexate into cells and intracellular alteration of the drug or of the target enzyme have also been shown in some cell systems [419].

Aminopterin closely resembles methotrexate structurally and functionally but it is not used therapeutically because it appears to be more toxic. Pyrimethamine is one of a group of 2,4-diaminopyrimidines which is used as a malarial prophylactic at a dose of 25 mg weekly, but at more frequent doses it has been used for treating polycythaemia vera and toxoplasmosis. It causes features of folate deficiency in man and has proved fatal when used in large doses or when given to subjects already folate deficient. Trimethoprim acts as a bacteriostatic by competitively inhibiting bacterial dihydrofolate reductase at different site from methotrexate. Equivalent inhibition of the human enzyme requires a concentration about 50 000 times greater. The recommended daily dose is 320 mg but the drug is usually given with a sulphonamide, usually sulpha-methoxazole, which acts synergistically by inhibiting synthesis of folate by bacterial but not by human cells. *In-vitro* studies have shown that the drug, like metho-trexate, interferes with thymidylate synthesis by human bone-marrow cells, but the inhibition is slight unless a concentration 10 times that found in plasma with normal therapeutic doses is used [422, 423]. Despite its low affinity for the human enzyme, there is evidence that trimethoprim may produce haematolo-gical side-effects and these can be severe in patients with pre-existing folate or B$_{12}$ deficiency. Slight changes in haemoglobin concentration, neutrophil and platelet counts with raised Figlu excretion have been noted with doses of 500–1000 mg daily. More dramatic changes, apparently due to the drug, have been seen in patients with untreated megaloblastic anaemia who have shown rapidly increasing pancyto-penia, or a poor response to specific therapy [424, 425].

Triemterene and pentamidine also probably act as dihydrofolate-reductase inhibitors in man but the evidence for this is scant [423]. DDMP and DDEP are two more recently developed drugs which inhibit dihydrofolate reductase and have potential use as anti-human agents.

Defect of folate transport. A patient with aplastic anaemia, megaloblastosis and a defect of cell uptake of methyl-THF has been described. Five other relatives showed a similar defect of cell uptake of folate without pancytopenia; abnormal membrane folate transport has also been described in hereditary dyserythropoiesis [420, 427] and also in the condition of specific malabsorption of folate (p. 230).

MEGALOBLASTIC ANAEMIA NOT DUE TO FOLATE OR VITAMIN-B$_{12}$ DEFICIENCY OR ALTERED METABOLISM

Orotic aciduria

This is a rare but well-characterized syndrome in which there is usually an inherited deficiency of two consecu-tive enzymes (concerned in pyrimidine synthesis), orotidylic pyrophosphosylase and orotidylic decar-boxylase. The disease is transmitted as an autosomal recessive and presents in the first year or two of life with failure to thrive, mental retardation and megalo-blastic anaemia unresponsive to B$_{12}$ or folate. The diagnosis is made by finding crystals of orotic acid in the urine; excretion of orotic acid reaches 6 g/24 hours due to failure of orotic-acid utilization and to excessive orotic-acid synthesis consequent on failure of end-product inhibition by uridine.

The first child diagnosed died [428] but subsequent cases have been treated successfully with uridine in large oral doses (e.g. 300 mg five times daily) [429]. The relatively high frequency of heterozygotes (with slightly raised orotic-acid excretion) suggests that some affected fetuses die *in utero* [430]. A biochemical variant of the condition, with identical clinical findings is now recognized with deficiency of only one enzyme [431].

Thiamine-responsive megaloblastic anaemia

Three children with this disorder have been described. The first presented at 11 years. The megaloblastic anaemia appeared to be due to excess thiamine utilization [432]. The child showed no clinical evidence of thiamine deficiency and the cellular levels of three enzymes known to require thiamine were normal. The biochemical basis for the anaemia is unknown.

Congenital familial megaloblastic anaemia

Two sisters with megaloblastic anaemia, presenting at three and seven weeks, have been described by Lamp-kin *et al.* [433]. The anaemia responded well to B$_{12}$ and folic acid given together in large doses, even though neither deficiency had been demonstrated, but the anaemia relapsed if either vitamin was discontinued. The elder sister showed severe mental retardation. The site of the biochemical defect is unknown but thymidy-

---

Table 6.11. Megaloblastic anaemia not due to folate or vitamin-B$_{12}$ deficiency

Congenital
(a) Orotic aciduria (uridine-responsive)
(b) Thiamine-responsive
(c) Requiring massive doses of vitamin B$_{12}$ and folate
(d) Congenital dyserythropoietic anaemia (some types)
(e) ? Lesch–Nyhan syndrome (adenine-responsive)

Acquired
(a) Erythroleukaemia, other myeloid leukaemias, primary acquired sideroblastic anaemia
(b) Drugs—cytosine arabinoside, 5-fluorouracil, hydroxyurea, 6-mercaptopurine, etc.

late synthesis and orotic-acid excretion were both normal.

Lesch–Nyhan syndrome

This consists of mental retardation, self-mutilation and gout and is due to congenital defect of the enzyme hypoxanthine-guanine phosphoribosyltransferase, which is concerned with purine synthesis. There is no adequately documented case of megaloblastic anaemia in this syndrome but a case with megaloblastic anaemia which apparently responded to adenine was briefly reported and another case with megaloblastosis with normal serum B_{12} and folate levels has been mentioned [434].

Erythroleukaemia, myeloid leukaemias, acquired sideroblastic anaemia

Megaloblastic anaemia, unresponsive to B_{12} and folate therapy may occur in these conditions and has also been described in congenital dyserythropoietic anaemia (see Chapter 31). The marrow appearances may be indistinguishable but usually white-cell changes are less marked, and the picture is modified by the underlying haemopoietic disorder (e.g. an increase in myeloblasts, distorted forms, ring sideroblasts). Biochemical studies have shown that the defect is not at thymidylate synthesis and the exact defect responsible for megaloblastosis is unknown. Folate deficiency may also occur in all these diseases.

Drugs

A number of anti-pyrimidine drugs (as well as dihydrofolate-reductase inhibitors), notably cytosine arabinoside, which inhibits DNA polymerase, 5-fluorouracil, which inhibits thymidylate synthetase and hyroxyurea which inhibits ribonucleotide reductase, cause megaloblastosis without interfering directly with folate or B_{12} metabolism. Anti-purine drugs (e.g. 6-mercaptopurine and azathioprine) cause megaloblastosis less frequently. Drugs which interfere with DNA metabolism other than synthesis (e.g. alkylating agents) do not cause megaloblastosis.

Vitamin E

Megaloblastic anaemia responding to vitamin E was described in malnourished children in Jordan [435], but coincidental folate deficiency with a response to dietary folate was not completely excluded.

BIOCHEMICAL BASIS OF MEGALOBLASTIC ANAEMIA

The exact explanation for the peculiar morphology of the megaloblast is still uncertain. A number of cytogenetic and biochemical studies suggest that the primary fault concerns DNA replication and this is usually due to starvation of one or other precursor, most commonly thymidine triphosphate (dTTP). A primary defect in DNA replication is consistent with the morphological observation of delay in, and abnormality of, nuclear maturation with normal cytoplasmic development. Moreover, similar morphological features with an increase in nuclear and cell volume and dispersal of condensed chromatin can be induced in a temperature-sensitive mutant mouse-cell line when DNA replication is inhibited.

CHROMOSOME FINDINGS

Dividing bone marrow cells and lymphocytes from patients with megaloblastic anaemia show the following abnormalities [436, 437]:
1 the chromosomes are elongated, despirallated, more delicate and slender than normal;
2 there is an increase in the number of random breaks;
3 the centromere is spread; and
4 there are increased numbers of cells in prophase in colchicine-treated marrows. Earlier reports of increased aneuploidy are confirmed by recent studies.

The changes are corrected within a few days with appropriate therapy and are associated with a prolongation of S and G2 phases of the cell cycle [438] (see Chapter 2). An increased number of cells with an intermediate amount of DNA between 2C and 4C are in a resting phase [438]. Giant metamyelocytes often have intermediate DNA content and are unable, therefore, to give rise to hypersegmented neutrophils which have a 2C DNA content [439].

BIOCHEMICAL FINDINGS

Thymidylate synthesis: the deoxyuridine (dU)-suppression test

The base composition of normal and megaloblastic marrow DNA is similar [440]. The ratio of RNA to DNA in megaloblastic cells is, however, increased [441]. Cells from patients with severe B_{12} or folate deficiency show an abnormality of thymidylate synthesis suggesting that reduced supply of dTTP, an immediate DNA precursor, leads to the fault in DNA replication. The fault in thymidylate synthesis has been demonstrated indirectly by the dU-suppression test. This consists of incubating cells with non-radioactive dU *in vitro*. This can be shown to have a different effect on the uptake of [³H]thymidine into DNA by normal and megaloblastic cells [442–444] in that dU has considerably less blocking effect on [³H]thymidine incorporation into megaloblasts than into normoblasts. The difference is thought to be due to failure of methylation of deoxyuridine monophosphate (dUMP) to thymidylate monosphosphate (dTMP) in megaloblastic cells, due to reduced thymidylate-synthetase activity (Fig. 6.10). dUMP is derived by phosphorylation of the added dU. The level of thymidine triphosphate (dTTP) (derived by phosphorylation of dTMP) in the cells is thought to control, by feedback inhibition, the action of thymidine kinase and thus uptake of [³H]thymidine added *in vitro*. Also dTMP derived from non-radioactive dU will dilute [³H]TMP derived from labelled thymidine and thus reduce label entering DNA. The dU-suppression test is normal in megaloblastic anaemia where the fault is not at thymidylate synthesis (e.g. with 6-mercaptopurine therapy) [445]. Methotrexate added *in vitro* to normal cells produces an effect like B_{12} or folate deficiency on deoxyuridine suppression of [³H]thymidine uptake [443] and has indeed been shown to lower cell dTTP levels rapidly [446]. The effect of dU on [³H]thymidine uptake is obviously complex since even when thymidylate synthesis is totally inhibited by 5-fluorouracil, dU still blocks [³H]thymidine uptake, suggesting a direct effect of dU or dUMP on thymidine kinase [447]. Thymidine-kinase activity is substantially increased in megaloblasts, compared to normoblasts, and megaloblasts take up more labelled thymidine than normoblasts, even in the absence of dU [445, 448]. The thymidine kinase is of the fetal type [447a]. More recently, a pile up of dUMP in megaloblasts which can be rapidly relieved *in vitro* with the appropriate folate or B_{12} compound has been shown directly [449].

Recent studies have also shown in some detail the nature of the defective DNA replication which results from starvation of a DNA precursor and this is considered next.

Normal DNA replication
DNA replication in mammalian cells begins at many points or origins along the chromosome. These are points at which the two parent strands separate to form a replication fork from which new DNA is synthesized in both directions using both parent strands as templates with base pairing (A—T, T—A, G—C, C—G). The distance between two adjacent origins is called a replicon. Initiation requires prior insertion of a short RNA 'primer' and DNA is synthesized on the free OH′ end of the primer by the main replicative enzyme, the α DNA polymerase. This only synthesizes in the 5′–3′ direction according to the sugar–phosphate linkages. The two opposing strands run in opposite directions. One new strand of DNA is therefore synthesized 'back' to the replication fork in the 5′–3′ direction in short (Okazaki) pieces, approximately 120–200 bases long. The RNA primer is ultimately digested by the RNAase and the gap left filled with new DNA. A DNA ligase links up the new

segments of DNA, whether Okazaki piece or replicon-sized.

DNA replication in megaloblastic anaemia
Slowing of all these processes of DNA replication has been shown in megaloblastic cells, including rate of Okazaki-piece formation, average rate of replication-fork movement and rate of linking up small DNA pieces to form chromosomal-sized DNA [450–452]. These defects can also be produced in normal cells by exposing them to drugs (e.g. methotrexate or hydroxyurea), which reduce supply of dTTP or one of the other three deoxynucleoside-triphosphate DNA precursors. The DNA polymerase itself is present in normal or increased concentration in megaloblastic anaemia due to B_{12} or folate deficiencies and DNA ligation and repair is normal [453, 454]. Megaloblastic changes can also be produced in mammalian cells in which DNA synthesis is slowed by temperature alterations [454a].

The observation of a normal overall dTTP concentration in B_{12} or folate deficient megaloblasts [455] was a surprising finding in view of the solid evidence for reduced thymidylate synthesis. More recently this observation has been explained as due to functional compartmentalization of dTTP and the other DNA precursors in human cells. It is suggested that small pools of dTTP and the other three DNA precursors are present at high concentration at the DNA replication fork. These are produced locally by a multi-enzyme complex including a number of key enzymes concerned in supply of the deoxynucleoside triphosphates (dNTP) whereas much larger pools at lower concentrations are present in the rest of the nucleus or even cytoplasm of the cells [456–458]. These large pools are probably destined mainly for degradation or DNA repair. In megaloblasts the overall cell dTTP is thought to be normal because the large low-concentration pool is normal, even though there is reduced supply of dTTP at the point where it is needed in high concentration for DNA synthesis (i.e. at the DNA replication fork).

Role of vitamin B₁₂: methyl-folate-trap hypothesis
The reduced blocking action of dU on [³H]thymidine uptake in megaloblasts *in vitro* can be corrected by adding large doses of folic or folinic acid *in vitro*, whether the anaemia is due to folate or B_{12} deficiency. The concentration of the apoenzyme, thymidylate synthetase, is normal or increased in megaloblasts [459]. The role of folate as its 5,10-methylene-THF coenzyme form for thymidylate synthesis is well established (Fig. 6.10). The role of B_{12} is less clear. It is not needed directly for thymidylate synthetase.

Vitamin-B_{12}-deficient cells are known to have a reduced folate content and to show reduced activity of all reactions requiring folate coenzymes. In particular, B_{12} deficiency appears to secondarily affect thymidylate synthesis by reducing the intracellular level of 5,10-methylene-THF. The most widely accepted view is that this is due to 'trapping' of folate in the form 'methyl-folate' [460, 461] (Fig. 6.15). This theory suggests that lack of B_{12} causes folate to accumulate as 5-methyl-THF due to failure of the reaction in which homocysteine is methylated by methyl-THF to methionine. This deprives the cells of THF and all other forms of folate. Methyl-THF is the form in which folate enters all body cells; dietary folates are all converted to this form by the intestinal cells (see p. 226). It is supposed that unless methyl-THF is demethylated, it largely accumulates in plasma and is excreted (e.g. in urine). In the monoglutamate form it probably cannot accumulate in cells from which it readily diffuses.

This theory presupposes that methyl-THF can only be 'demethylated' by the homocysteine–methionine reaction in which B_{12} is involved. Methyl-THF can also be converted directly to methylene-THF. However, at neutral pH, the reaction lies sufficiently in the methyl-THF rather than methylene-THF direction so that escape of methyl-THF directly to methylene-THF in B_{12} deficiency is probably slight [462]. Methyl-THF can also be oxidized to give formaldehyde and THF, with conversion of the biogenic amines dopamine and tryptamine to give an isoquinolone and carboline respectively [463, 464]. In favour of the 'methyl-folate-trap' theory, it has been shown that methionine aggravates the defect of dU blocking of [³H]thymidine uptake by B_{12}-deficient megaloblasts *in vitro*, whereas homocysteine, presumably by acting as a receptor of the methyl group from the trapped methyl-THF, reduces the defect [465]. Moreover, methyl-THF, unlike other forms of folate, will not correct the defect of thymidylate synthesis in B_{12}-deficient cells [443, 446, 467]. Entry of plasma methyl-THF to cells is reduced in B_{12} deficiency [468]. Whether this reduced entry is secondary to failure of subsequent methyl-THF metabolism inside the cell or is due to a more specific

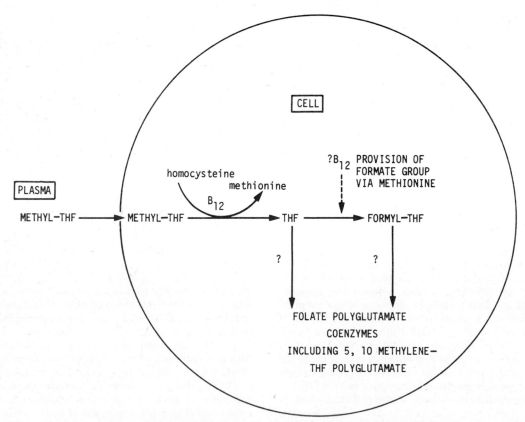

Fig. 6.15. Suggested role of vitamin B_{12} in synthesis of folate polyglutamate coenzymes. Methyl-tetrahydrofolate (methyl-THF) enters cells from plasma in the monoglutamate form and the methyl group is donated to homocysteine to form methionine. Folate polyglutamates are then synthesized either from THF or from formyl-THF (see text).

effect of B$_{12}$ deficiency on methyl-folate transport into cells is unknown.

All intracellular folate coenzymes, including THF, 5,10-methylene-THF, 5,10-methenyl-THF and 10-formyl-THF become depleted in B$_{12}$ deficiency and the reactions in which these folate compounds take part are all disturbed. The most widely accepted explanation is that these coenzyme forms exist in cells and function largely as their polyglutamate derivatives, that methyl-THF entering cells in the monoglutamate form is not a direct substrate for polyglutamate synthetase [270, 469–471], hence that B$_{12}$ is needed in the pathway of conversion of folate from methyl-THF in the monoglutamate form to all the folate coenzymes in the polyglutamate form. Reduced concentrations of folate polyglutamates in relation to monoglutamate forms occur in all cells tested in humans or rats with B$_{12}$ deficiency or in rats with B$_{12}$ inactivated by N$_2$O [472–474]. Thus, failure of demethylation of methyl-THF due to B$_{12}$ deficiency is thought to deprive cells of the correct folate substrate for folate-polyglutamate synthesis. Hoffbrand [14] proposed this to be THF in human cells and *in-vitro* studies confirm that methyl-THF is a poor substrate in mammalian cells whereas DHF, THF and formyl-THF are good substrates [272, 475].

On the other hand, studies in rats exposed to N$_2$O have suggested that formyl-THF rather than THF is the preferred substrate [470, 471]. THF itself could not be converted to polyglutamate forms in the livers of rats with B$_{12}$ inactivation due to N$_2$O exposure. Together with the excellent correction by formyl-THF of the dU-suppression test in B$_{12}$ deficiency or B$_{12}$ inactivation, this observation has led Chanarin *et al.* [476] to suggest that B$_{12}$ is necessary for provision of the formate group of formyl-THF rather than for provision of THF itself (Fig. 6.15). In their studies THF corrected the dU-suppression test less well in B$_{12}$ deficiency than in folate deficiency, and less well than formyl-THF in B$_{12}$-deficient or N$_2$O-treated cells. Formyl-THF (folinic acid) corrects equally well in B$_{12}$- or folate-deficient cells [477, 478]. Whether or not this is due to increased stability or increased transport across the cell membranes of formyl-THF compared to THF in the *in-vitro* systems used remains uncertain. All studies show that THF corrects substantially better than methyl-THF in B$_{12}$-deficient cells suggesting that failure of demethylation of methyl-THF is at least partly responsible for the defect in folate metabolism produced by B$_{12}$ deficiency.

If B$_{12}$ is indeed necessary in the provision of formate to convert THF to formyl-THF this could be by its role in synthesis of methionine, a known formate donor. Methionine has indeed been shown to increase folate-polyglutamate synthesis in B$_{12}$-deficient animals [479].

However, this is an alternative explanation for this observation. Methionine may be converted to S-adenosylmethionine (SAM) and this is known to inhibit reduction of 5,10-methylene-THF to methyl-THF. Thus, increased cell SAM concentration due to methionine administration could shift the equilibrium of folates in the direction of formyl-THF and away from methyl-THF. This has been suggested by Krebs *et al.* [480]. It thus remains to be elucidated whether the methionine effect on folate-polyglutamate synthesis in B$_{12}$ deficiency is by provision of formate or by increasing cell SAM levels. The failure of methionine to improve the dU suppression in B$_{12}$ deficiency is difficult to explain on the 'provision of formate' hypothesis alone. It may be that there are three effects on folate-polyglutamate coenzyme synthesis caused by a block in homocysteine conversion to methionine due to B$_{12}$ deficiency:

1 diminished supply of THF from methyl-THF (a functionally 'dead' compound);

2 diminished conversion of THF to formyl-THF due to lack of methionine donation of formate; and

3 a shift in equilibrium between methenyl-THF and methyl-THF in favour of methyl-THF due to a lowering in cell SAM concentration.

Reduced folate-polyglutamate coenzyme synthesis from methyl-THF is proposed as the explanation not only of reduced thymidylate synthesis in B$_{12}$ deficiency but also of the increased excretion of Figlu [481] and aminoimidazole-carboxamide-ribotide (AICAR) [482], and of reduced serine formation from formate [483].

CLINICAL OBSERVATIONS

The degree of anaemia in B$_{12}$ deficiency seems to be determined by the folate status of patients, since for comparable degrees of B$_{12}$ deficiency assessed by serum B$_{12}$ level or methylmalonic-acid excretion, the most anaemic patients show the lowest serum and red-cell folate levels, the fastest clearance of folic acid and the highest incidence of positive Figlu tests [484]. The explanation for the variation in folate levels between one patient with pernicious anaemia (PA) and the next is uncertain. It may be partly related to dietary intake of folate, partly due to folate losses in urine and bile, and partly related to the degree of ineffective erythropoiesis which develops, since increased cell turnover could consume folate excessively. Treatment of B$_{12}$-deficient patients with folic acid is well known to partly or completely correct anaemia due to B$_{12}$ deficiency. This is thought to be due to raising intracellular folate content by mass action. Neuropathy is not corrected and may even be precipitated, but whether this is due to alteration in B$_{12}$ distribution between different tissues or between its various biochemical forms, or some other effect, is unknown. Large doses of B_{12}, however, produce little or no response in folate-deficient patients unless there is coincidental B_{12} deficiency.

RNA AND PROTEIN SYNTHESIS

Though folates are required for two steps in purine synthesis, and AICAR excretion is raised in folate and B_{12} deficiency, the balance of evidence suggests that neither folate nor B_{12} deficiency cause an overall defect of RNA synthesis in humans and, indeed, the RNA:DNA content ratio of megaloblasts is greater than normal [485], though a reduced mean RNA synthesis has been noted in B_{12}-deficient phytohaemagglutin-transformed lymphocytes as compared to normal [86]. The high RNA content and large size of the megaloblasts has been ascribed to prolongation of the intermitotic interval, but whether this is the whole story is uncertain. Protein synthesis by reticulocytes in megaloblastic anaemia appears to be normal [486]. Altered histone composition in megaloblastic bone marrow has been described but is likely to be due to relative immaturity of the cells, rather than to a primary defect [8].

Vitamin-B₁₂ neuropathy

The biochemical basis for this remains to be determined but now that an experimental animal model, the nitrous-oxide treated Rhesus monkey, is available [411], it is possible that this puzzle may be resolved. Earlier work had attempted to relate the neuropathy to methylmalonic-acid accumulation in the nervous system which in some way might interrupt fatty-acid synthesis in nervous tissue [487, 488]. However, the observation of B_{12} neuropathy in patients with TCII deficiency [401, 402] and in monkeys exposed to N_2O [411] without MMA excretion makes this unlikely to be the mechanism. Similar neurological lesions can be produced in rats exposed to cycloleucine [489] which blocks conversion of methionine to S-adenosylmethionine (SAM). Since N_2O exposure or B_{12} deficiency may interfere with methionine, and hence SAM synthesis, by producing a block in homocysteine–methionine conversion, it has been postulated that B_{12} neuropathy is due to lack of SAM in nervous tissue leading to defective methylation reactions in lipid (e.g phosphatidylcholine) synthesis [490]. This theory fails to explain why a similar nerve lesion does not occur in severe folate deficiency, or indeed why folic-acid therapy appears to aggravate rather than improve the lesion. It seems unlikely that the neuropathy can be related to the alteration in leucine metabolism which occurs in B_{12} deficiency since this reaction requires ado-B_{12} which does not seem to be affected by N_2O exposure.

OTHER DEFICIENCY ANAEMIAS

ANAEMIA OF SCURVY

Patients with scurvy are often anaemic and this anaemia responds to small doses of vitamin C (ascorbic acid) alone or, in a minority of cases, in combination with other haematinics. Nevertheless, the exact role of ascorbic acid in haemopoiesis remains uncertain.

Biochemical aspects

It is apparent that ascorbic acid is necessary for the maintenance of intercellular material of skin, cartilage, periosteum and bone. It may also have a role in the hydroxylation of proline to hydroxyproline, needed for collagen synthesis [491]. The adrenals have a high ascorbate content and ACTH causes this to fall, but the biochemical significance of this, as well as the reason for the high ascorbate content of leucocytes, which falls with infection, is unknown, though it has been postulated that the vitamin is concerned in the body's reaction to stress. Vitamin C is also thought to have direct roles in folate metabolism and more generally in redox systems in the body (e.g. coupled with glutathione, cytochromes, pyridine or flavin nucleotides). Iron-deficient patients tend to have raised ascorbate levels and iron-overloaded subjects have low levels. Excess iron probably causes oxidative degradation of ascorbate [492]. Changes in iron metabolism may occur because ascorbic acid is needed, together with ATP, for incorporation of transferrin-bound iron into ferritin and for release of iron from ferritin [493] (see Chapter 5). Serum ferritin is lower than expected for the estimated iron stores in vitamin-C deficiency while vitamin-C therapy raises the serum ferritin in experimental animals [494] and man [495] and increases the amount of iron available for chelation [496]. It also increases parenchymal iron at the expense of RE iron [492].

Nutritional aspects

Vitamin C is found in nature as the reduced form, L-ascorbic acid, and at much lower concentrations as the oxidized form, dehydroascorbic acid (Fig. 6.16). Both are biologically active, and are easily destroyed by oxidizing agents and alkalis. Man, primates and guinea-pigs are the only animals to require the preformed vitamin. Ten milligrams or less of vitamin C daily will prevent clinical scurvy in adults, but a larger daily amount (20–70 mg) has been recommended and even more in pregnancy and lactation, and on a body-weight basis in infants, children and adolescents. Nevertheless, in some experiments, it has taken almost six months for clinical changes to occur in adults

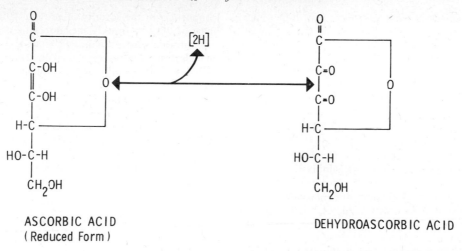

Fig. 6.16. Structure of ascorbic acid and its oxidation.

receiving only 1 mg vitamin C daily [497]. Losses of ascorbate, as such, occur in urine and faeces and the vitamin is also lost in urine after degradation to oxalate.

The highest concentrations of the vitamin—in some cases 200 mg or more per 100 g, but usually in the range 30–100 mg/100 g—are found in green plants, citrus fruits, berries, tomatoes and in liver and kidney, with lesser amounts in potatoes, but there is little in cereals, dairy produce, meat and most fish. Like folate, the vitamin is easily destroyed by cooking, particularly in alkaline conditions, and is also lost on storage of food, particularly if it is exposed to air.

Absorption occurs throughout the length of the small-intestinal tract but mainly from the duodenum and jejunum. The body has a great capacity to absorb the vitamin, and deficiency has not been observed to arise through malabsorption. The normal level in plasma ranges from 0·1 to 1·5 mg/100 ml, and in whole blood from 0·2 to 0·7 mg/100 ml, the exact levels depending on dietary intake.

Vitamin-C deficiency sufficiently severe to cause clinical scurvy arises because of insufficient dietary intake. In Western countries, this is most common among the aged, particularly those living alone in impoverished circumstances on diets lacking fresh vegetables, fruit and liver. It also occurs rarely in infants on totally inadequate diets, particularly those with infections, or who take foods in which the vitamin has been completely destroyed by heat in preparation. Low vitamin-C levels are common in patients with thryrotoxicosis, malignant diseases, peptic ulceration, during pregnancy and in patients with iron overload, but rarely progress to overt clinical scurvy.

Blood picture

Anaemia is present in about 80% of patients and in virtually all with clinically severe disease [495, 498]. The anaemia is usually normochromic, but may be hypochromic if there is associated iron deficiency, or macrocytic because of a reticulocytosis (which usually varies between two and 11%) or because of megalo-blastosis. The white cells and platelets are usually normal, unless they are affected by associated severe megaloblastosis, infection or haemorrhage. No consistent coagulation defect has been found and the most likely explanation for the bleeding diathesis is a capillary defect which has been attributed to both defective synthesis of cement substance and to depolymerization of collagen. The bone marrow is usually normocellular or hypercellular, rarely hypocellular. It is usually normoblastic but frank megaloblastosis occurs in about 10% of cases and megaloblastic changes in an additional proportion are mild.

The anaemia seems to be mainly due to a direct effect of ascorbic-acid deficiency on erythropoiesis. Three factors (haemolysis, iron and folate deficiencies) may also contribute in some cases but even together they cannot completely account for the anaemia. Extravascular haemolysis results from widespread haemorrhage into the skin, subcutaneous tissues, joints and periosteum. This probably accounts for the reticulocytosis, raised bilirubin and increased excretion of urobilinogen in the faeces and urine found in many cases. Intravascular haemolysis has also been suggested [498] but the normal haptoglobin levels found in a large proportion of cases do not support this [500]. Many cases with little or no evidence of haemolysis show anaemia while in others, rest in bed may reduce extravascular haemolysis considerably without affecting the anaemia.

Iron is usually present in the marrow and the total iron-binding capacity is normal, though the serum iron is often low. External haemorrhage rarely occurs and occult blood tests are negative. The serum B_{12} level and B_{12} absorption are normal. All cases show some degree of folate deficiency and low serum folate levels are usual, though the red-cell folate may be 'falsely normal' due to the reticulocytosis. The deficiency may be sufficiently severe to cause megaloblastic anaemia which responds to folic acid. However, in most patients to whom physiological doses of folic acid have been given and the diet controlled, vitamin C has also been necessary to correct the megaloblastic anaemia. One patient apparently showed a complete response to folic acid, 50 μg, alone [501], while vitamin C alone has also been found to correct megaloblastic anaemia in other patients, apparently taking a diet of low folate content [502]. Certainly in the experimental animal fed a diet deficient in both folate and vitamin C, megaloblastosis reverted to normal when either vitamin was given [503].

Whether there is an biochemical interrelation between folate and vitamin C is still undecided. Vitamin C has been suggested to be necessary to maintain folate in the fully reduced, active state, but there is no biochemical evidence for this. Patients with scurvy have been found to excrete slightly raised amounts of folate in the urine and this excretion was found to fall dramatically with ascorbic-acid therapy; however, the explanation for this finding remains obscure [499, 500].

ANAEMIA OF PROTEIN DEFICIENCY

Anaemia occurs in the stage of severe protein malnutrition known as 'kwashiorkor' and in protein-calorie malnutrition or 'marasmus'. These conditions are most common in the tropics, particularly in young infants and pregnant women, but may also occur in older children and adults of either sex. Adult 'kwashiorkor' also occurs in Western countries (e.g. in patients with gastro-intestinal disorders) [504]. The severity of the anaemia varies widely, but the mean haemoglobin levels in series reported from India, South Africa, Kenya and Uganda have ranged from 8·0 to 9·1 g/dl. The anaemia is usually normochromic and normocytic. The reticulocyte percentage is normal or low and the marrow is of normal or reduced cellularity with erythropoiesis selectively reduced in some cases. In many patients, an anaemia undoubtedly partly due to protein deficiency is complicated by infection and other deficiencies (e.g. folate and iron). In these cases, the severity of anaemia is out of proportion to the severity of protein deficiency. The marrow may be frankly megaloblastic or may show obvious changes only in the leucocytes (e.g. giant metamyelocytes and hypersegmented neutrophils), with the changes in the red cells mild and difficult to recognize. Vitamin-E deficiency has also been described in some patients, and is said to cause macrocytic anaemia, while riboflavin deficiency has been said to cause aplastic arrest in a few patients during the haematological response to protein [505]. Complete correction of the anaemia often requires antibiotics, iron and folic acid as well as a high-protein diet.

Pathogenesis

The exact way in which protein deficiency causes anaemia is still uncertain. A deficiency of amino acids for globin formation is probably not the mechanism. More probably the anaemia is due to lack of erythropoietin drive on the marrow consequent on lack of stimulus to erythropoietin release. It is not due to lack of protein for erythropoietin synthesis [506]. When the patient with kwashiorkor is fed a high-protein diet, there is a rapid rise in plasma erythropoietin levels [507]. Experimental protein deficiency in animals causes a similar anaemia to that seen in man and it responds to exogenous erythropoietin or to androgens (which augment the action of endogenous erythropoietin).

MISCELLANEOUS DEFICIENCY ANAEMIAS

Experimental riboflavin deficiency in humans causes an anaemia resembling that of protein deficiency (i.e. normochromic, normocytic, with a low reticulocyte count and marrow erythroid hypoplasia) [508, 509]. Vacuolation of the pronormoblasts may also occur [509]. It is unlikely that cases of pure riboflavin-deficiency anaemia occur clinically, but the deficiency has been suggested to contribute to anaemia in subjects with multiple deficiencies, particularly those with kwashiorkor [505]. A disturbance of riboflavin metabolism has been suggested to occur in congenital hypoplastic anaemia but these patients do not respond to riboflavin therapy [510]. Vitamin-E deficiency has been suggested to cause a haemolytic anaemia in the premature infant and a macrocytic, megaloblastic anaemia in patients with protein-calorie malnutrition. Pyridoxine deficiency is discussed in Chapter 13. Deficiencies of nicotinic and pantothenic acids have been found to cause anaemia in experimental animals, but not in humans.

REFERENCES

1 CHANARIN I. (1979) *The Megaloblastic Anaemias.* 2nd edn. Blackwell Scientific Publications, Oxford.

2 HOFFBRAND A.V. (1976) Megaloblastic anaemia. *Clinics in Haematology*, **5**, 471.

3 SMITH E.L. (1965) *Vitamin B₁₂.* 3rd edn. Methuen, London.

4 ARNSTEIN H.R.V. & WRIGHTON R.J. (1971) *The Cobalamins.* A Glaxo Symposium. Churchill-Livingstone, London.

5 PRATT J.M. (1972) *Inorganic Chemistry of Vitamin B₁₂.* Academic Press, London.

6 ALLEN R.H. (1975) Human vitamin B₁₂ transport proteins. In: *Progress in Hematology*, Vol. IX (ed. Brown E.B.), p. 57. Grune & Stratton, New York.

7 BABIOR B.M. (ed.) (1975) *Cobalamin: Biochemistry and Pathophysiology.* John Wiley & Sons, New York.

8 KASS L. (1976) Pernicious anemia. *Major Problems in Internal Medicine*, Vol. VII. Saunders, Philadelphia.

9 ZAGALAK B. & FRIEDRICH W. (eds.) (1979) *Vitamin B₁₂.* Walter de Gruyter, Berlin.

10 CASTLE W.B. (1980) The conquest of pernicious anemia. In: *Blood, Pure and Eloquent* (ed. Wintrobe M.M.), p. 283. McGraw-Hill, New York.

11 CHANARIN I. (1980) Cobalamins and nitrous oxide: a review. *Journal of Clinical Pathology*, **33**, 909.

12 BLAKLEY R.L. (1969) *The Biochemistry of Folic Acid and Related Pteridines*, p. 139. North-Holland/Amsterdam.

13 ERBE R.W.(1975) Inborn errors of folate metabolism. *New England Journal of Medicine*, **293**, 753 and 807.

14 HOFFBRAND A.V. (1975) Synthesis and breakdown of natural folates (folate polyglutamates). In: *Progress in Haematology*, Vol. IX (ed. Brown E.B.), p. 85. Grune & Stratton, New York.

15 (1977) *Biochemistry and Physiology in Relation to the Human Nutrition Requirement.* National Academy of Sciences, Washington.

16 PFLEIDERER W. (ed.) (1975) *Chemistry and Biology of Pteridines.* Walter de Gruyter, Berlin.

17 KISLIUK R.L. & BROWN G.M. (ed.) (1978) Chemistry and Biology of Pteridines. In: *Developments in Biochemistry*, Vol. IV. Elsevier/North-Holland, New York.

18 BOTEZ M.I. & REYNOLDS E.H. (eds.) (1979) *Folic Acid in Neurology, Psychiatry and Internal Medicine.* Raven Press, New York.

19 HERBERT V. (ed.) (1980) Hematologic complications of alcoholism. *Seminars in Hematology*, **17.**

20 MINOT G.R. & MURPHY W.P. (1927) A diet rich in liver in the treatment of pernicious anaemia: study of 105 cases. *Journal of the American Medical Association*, **89**, 759.

21 SMITH E.L. & PARKER L.F.J. (1948) Purification of antipernicious anaemia factor. *Biochemical Journal*, **43**, viii.

22 RICKES E.L., BRINK N.G., KONIUSZY F.R., WOOD T.R. & FOLKERS K. (1948) Crystalline vitamin B₁₂. *Science*, **107**, 396.

23 LINDSTRAND K. (1964) Isolation of methylcobalamin from natural source material. *Nature (London)*, **204**, 188.

24 LINNELL J.C., HOFFBRAND A.V., PETERS T.J. & MATHEWS D.M. (1969) Estimation of individual plasma B₁₂ compounds in normal subjects and states of deranged B₁₂ metabolism. *Journal of Clinical Pathology*, **22**, 742.

25 LINNELL J.C. (1975) The fate of cobalamin *in vivo.* In: *Cobalamin: Biochemistry and Pathophysiology* (ed. Babior B.M.), p. 287. John Wiley & Sons, New York.

26 WEISSBACH H. & TAYLOR R.T. (1968) Metabolic role of vitamin B₁₂. *Vitamins and Hormones*, **26**, 395.

27 WOODS D.D., FOSTER M.A. & GUEST J.R. (1965) Cobalamin-dependent and independent methyl-transfer in methionine biosynthesis. In: *Transmethylation and Methionine Biosynthesis* (ed. Shapiro S.K. & Schienk F.), p. 138. University of Chicago Press, Chicago.

28 WILLARD H.F. & ROSENBERG L.E. (1979) Inborn errors of cobalamin metabolism—effect of cobalamin supplementation in culture on methylmalonyl CoA mutase activity in normal and mutant human fibroblasts. *Biochemical Genetics*, **17**, 57.

29 MAHONEY M.J., HART A.C., STEEN V.D. & ROSENBERG L.E. (1975) Methylmalonicacidemia: biochemical heterogeneity in defects of 5'-deoxyadensoylcobalamin synthesis. *Proceedings of the National Academy of Sciences, USA*, **72**, 2799.

30 POSTON J.M. (1976) Leucine 2,3-aminomutase, an enzyme of leucine catabolism. *Journal of Biological Chemistry*, **251**, 1859.

31 POSTON J.M. (1980) Cobalamin-dependent formation of leucine and β-leucine by rat and human tissue: changes in pernicious anemia. *Journal of Biological Chemistry*, **255**, 10067.

32 HERBERT V., JACOB E. & WONG K.-T.J. (1977) Destruction of vitamin B₁₂ by vitamin C. *American Journal of Clinical Nutrition*, **30**, 297.

33 RAPPAZZO M.E., SALMI H.A. & HALL C.A. (1970) The content of vitamin B₁₂ in adult and foetal tissue: a comparative study. *British Journal of Haematology*, **18**, 425.

33a HEYSSEL R.M., BOZIAN R.C., DARBY W.J. & BELL M.C. (1966) Vitamin B₁₂ turnover in man. *American Journal of Clinical Nutrition*, **18**, 176.

34 KOLHOUSE J.T. & ALLEN R.H. (1977) Absorption, plasma transport and cellular retention of cobalamin analogues in the rabbit. *Journal of Clinical Investigation*, **60**, 1381.

35 ALLEN R.H., SEETHARAM B., PODELL E. & ALPERS D.H. (1978) Effect of proteolytic enzymes on the binding of cobalamin to R protein and intrinsic factor. *Journal of Clinical Investigation*, **61**, 47.

36 BRANDT L.J., GOLDBERG L., BERNSTEIN L.H. & GREENBERG G. (1979) The effect of bacterially produced vitamin B₁₂ analogues (cobamides) on the in vivo absorption of cyanocobalamin. *American Journal of Clinical Nutrition*, **18**, 1832.

37 KAPADIA C.F., SCHAFER D.E., DONALDSON R.M. & EBERSOLE E.R. (1979) Evidence for involvement of cyclic nucleotides in intrinsic factor secretion by isolated rabbit gastric mucosa. *Journal of Clinical Investigation*, **64**, 1044.

38 CASTLE W.B., TOWNSEND W.C. & HEATH C.W. (1930) Observations in the etiologic relationship of achylia gastrica to pernicious anaemia. III. The nature of the reaction between normal human gastric juice and beef

muscle, leading to clinical improvement and increased blood formation similar to the effect of liver feeding. *American Journal of Medical Science*, **180**, 305.

39 GLASS G.B.J. (1963) Gastric intrinsic factor and its function in the metabolism of vitamin B_{12}. *Physiological Reviews*, **43**, 529.

40 GRÄSBECK R. (1969) Intrinsic factor and the other vitamin B_{12} transport proteins. In: *Progress in Hematology*, Vol. 6 (ed. Brown E.B. & Moore C.V.), p. 233. Grune & Stratton, New York.

41 HIPPE E., HABER E. & OLESEN H. (1971) Nature of vitamin B_{12} binding. II. Steric orientation of vitamin B_{12} on binding and number of combining sites of human intrinsic factor and the transcobalamins. *Biochimica et Biophysica Acta*, **243**, 75.

42 KAPADIA C.R., MATHAN V.I. & BAKER S.J. (1976) Free intrinsic factor in the small intestine in man. *Gastroenterology*, **70**, 704.

43 STENMAN U.-H. (1976) Intrinsic factor and the vitamin B_{12} binding proteins. *Clinics in Haematology*, **5**, 473.

44 BOOTH C.C. & MOLLIN D.L. (1959) The site of absorption of vitamin B_{12} in man. *Lancet*, **i**, 18.

45 DONALDSON R.M. (1975) Mechanisms of malabsorption of cobalamin. In: *Cobalamin: Biochemistry and Pathophysiology* (ed. Babior B.M.), p. 335. John Wiley & Sons, New York.

46 HOOPER D.C., ALPERS D.H., BURGER R.L., MEHLMAN C.S. & ALLEN R.H. (1973) Characterization of ileal vitamin B_{12} binding using homogeneous human and hog intrinsic factors. *Journal of Clinical Investigation*, **52**, 3074.

47 KATZ M. & COOPER B.A. (1974) Solubilized receptor for vitamin B_{12}-intrinsic factor complex from human intestine. *British Journal of Haematology*, **26**, 569.

48 OKUDA K. & FUJII T. (1977) Solubilization of the ileal receptor for intrinsic factor-vitamin B_{12} complex in the rat. *Journal of Laboratory and Clinical Medicine*, **89**, 172.

49 COTTER R. & ROTHENBERG S.P. (1976) Solubilization, partial purification and radioassay for the intrinsic factor receptor from the ileal mucosa. *British Journal of Haematology*, **34**, 477.

50 KOUVONEN I. & GRÄSBECK R. (1981) Topology of the hog intrinsic factor receptor in the intestine. *Journal of Biological Chemistry*, **256**, 154.

51 HAGEDORN C.H. & ALPERS D.H. (1977) Distribution of intrinsic factor-vitamin B_{12} receptors in human intestine. *Gastroenterology*, **73**, 1019.

52 BOOTH C.C. & MOLLIN D.L. (1956) Plasma, tissue and urinary radioactivity after oral administration of ^{56}Co-labelled vitamin B_{12}. *British Journal of Haematology*, **2**, 223.

53 DOSCHERHOLMEN A. & HAGEN P.S. (1956) Radioactive vitamin B_{12} absorption studies: results of direct measurement of radioactivity in the blood. *Journal of Clinical Investigation*, **35**, 699.

54 PETERS T.J. & HOFFBRAND A.V. (1970) Absorption of vitamin B_{12} by the guinea-pig. I. Subcellular localization of vitamin B_{12} in the ileal cell during absorption. *British Journal of Haematology*, **19**, 369.

55 HALL C.A. & FINKLER A.E. (1965) The dynamics of transcobalamin II. A vitamin B_{12} binding substance in plasma. *Journal of Laboratory and Clinical Medicine*, **65**, 459.

56 CHANARIN I., MUIR M., HUGHES A. & HOFFBRAND A.V. (1978) Evidence for intestinal origin of transcobalamin II during vitamin B_{12} absorption. *British Medical Journal*, **i**, 1453.

57 ROTHENBERG S.P., WEISS J.P. & COTTER R. (1978) Formation of transcobalamin II-vitamin B_{12} complex by guinea-pig ileal mucosa in organ culture after in vivo incubation with intrinsic factor-vitamin B_{12}. *British Journal of Haematology*, **40**, 401.

58 HAKAMI N., NEIMAN P.E., CANELLOS G.P. & LAZERSON K. (1971) Neonatal megaloblastic anemia due to inherited transcobalamin II deficiency in two siblings. *New England Journal of Medicine*, **285**, 1163.

59 ROTHENBERG S.P., WEISBERG H. & FICARRA A. (1972) Evidence for the absorption of immunoreactive intrinsic factor into the intestinal epithelial cell during vitamin B_{12} absorption. *Journal of Laboratory and Clinical Medicine*, **79**, 587.

60 JENKINS W.J., EMPSON R., JEWELL D.P. & TAYLOR K.B. (1981) The subcellular localization of vitamin B_{12} during absorption in guinea pig ileum. *Gut* (in press).

61 LINNELL J.C., HOFFBRAND A.V., PETERS T.J. & MATTHEWS D.M. (1971) Chromatographic and bioautographic estimation of plasma cobalamins in various disturbances of vitamin B_{12} metabolism. *Clinical Science*, **40**, 1.

62 AMIN S., SPINKS T., RANICAR A., SHORT M.D. & HOFFBRAND A.V. (1980) Long-term clearance of ^{57}Co-cyanocobalamin in vegans and pernicious anaemia. *Clinical Science*, **58**, 101.

63 HIPPE E. & OLESEN H. (1971) Nature of vitamin B_{12} binding. III. Thermodynamics of binding to human intrinsic factor and transcobalamins. *Biochimica et Biophysica Acta*, **243**, 83.

64 STENMAN U.H. (1975) Vitamin B_{12} binding proteins of R-type cobalamins. *Scandinavian Journal of Haematology*, **14**, 91.

65 BURGER R.L. & ALLEN R.H. (1974) Characterization of vitamin B_{12}-binding proteins isolated from human milk and saliva by affinity chromatogrpahy. *Journal of Biological Chemistry*, **250**, 7700.

66 BURGER R.L., WAXMAN S., GILBERT H.S., MEHLMAN C.S. & ALLEN R.H. (1975) Isolation and characterization of a novel vitamin B_{12}-binding protein associated with hepatocellular carcinoma. *Journal of Clinical Investigation*, **56**, 1262.

67 SIMONS K. & WEBER T. (1966) The vitamin B_{12}-binding protein in human leucocytes. *Biochimica et Biophysica Acta*, **117**, 201.

68 CHIKKAPA G., CORCINO J., GREENBERG M.L. & HERBERT V. (1971) Correlation between various blood white cell pools and the serum B_{12}-binding proteins. *Blood*, **37**, 142.

69 CATOVSKY D., GALTON D.A.G., GRIFFIN C., HOFFBRAND A.V. & SCUR L. (1971) Serum lysozyme and vitamin B_{12} binding capacity in myeloproliferative disorders. *British Journal of Haematology*, **21**, 661.

70 HOM B.L. & AHLUWALIA B.K. (1968) The vitamin B_{12} binding capacity of transcobalamin I and II of normal human serum. *Scandinavian Journal of Haematology*, **5**, 64.

71 ALLEN R.H. & MAJERUS P.W. (1972) Isolation of vitamin B_{12}-binding proteins using affinity chromatography. II. Purification and properties of a human granulocyte vitamin B_{12}-binding protein. *Journal of Biological Chemistry*, **247**, 7702.

72 NEXØ E. (1978) Transcobalamin I and other human R-binders: purification, structural, spectral and physiological studies. *Scandinavian Journal of Haematology*, **20**, 221.

73 ENGLAND J.M., DOWN M.C., WISE I.L. & LINNELL J.C. (1976) The transport of endogenous vitamin B_{12} in normal human serum. *Clinical Science and Molecular Medicine*, **51**, 47.

74 CARMEL R. & HERBERT V. (1969) Deficiency of vitamin B_{12}-binding alpha globulin in two brothers. *Blood*, **33**, 1.

75 CARMEL R. (1972) The presence of a third vitamin B_{12}-binding protein in serum. *British Journal of Haematology*, **22**, 53.

76 BLOOMFIELD F.J. & SCOTT J.M. (1972) Identification of a new vitamin B_{12} binder (transcobalamin III) in normal human serum. *British Journal of Haematology*, **22**, 33.

77 ALLEN R.H. (1976) The plasma transport of vitamin B_{12}. *British Journal of Haematology*, **33**, 161.

78 ZITTOUN J., MARQUET J. & ZITTOUN R. (1975) The intracellular content of the three transcobalamins at various stages of normal and leukaemic myeloid cell development. *British Journal of Haematology*, **31**, 299.

79 GULLBERG R. (1976) Review: biological functions of the vitamin B_{12}-binding protein characterized by large molecular size. *Scandinavian Journal of Gastroenterology*, **11**, 225.

80 ALLEN R.H. & MAJERUS P.W. (1972) Isolation of vitamin B_{12}-binding proteins using affinity chromatography. III. Purification and properties of human plasma transcobalamin II. *Journal of Biological Chemistry*, **247**, 7709.

81 RACHMILEWITZ B., RACHMILEWITZ M., CHAOUAT M. & SCHLESINGER M. (1978) Production of TCII (Vitamin B_{12} transport protein) by mouse mononuclear phagocytes. *Blood*, **52**, 1089.

82 FRATER-SCHRODER M., NISSEN C., GMUR J. & HITZIG W.H. (1980) Bone marrow participates in the biosynthesis of human transcobalamin II. *Blood*, **56**, 560.

83 HALL C.A. (1975) Transcobalamins I and II as natural transport proteins of vitamin B_{12}. *Journal of Clinical Investigation*, **56**, 1125.

84 SCHNEIDER R.J., BURGER R.L., MEHLMAN C.S. & ALLEN R.H. (1976) Role and fate of rabbit and human transcobalamin II in plasma transport of vitamin B_{12} in rabbit. *Journal of Clinical Investigation*, **57**, 27.

85 RETIEF F.P., GOTTLIEB C.W. & HERBERT V. (1966) Mechanism of vitamin B_{12} uptake by erythrocytes. *Journal of Clinical Investigation*, **45**, 1907.

86 HOFFBRAND A.V., TRIPP E. & DAS K.C. (1973) Uptake of vitamin B_{12} by phytohaemagglutinin-transformed lymphocytes. *British Journal of Haematology*, **24**, 147.

87 PLETSCH Q.A. & COFFEY J.W. (1971) Intracellular distribution of radioactive vitamin B_{12} in rat liver. *Journal of Biological Chemistry*, **246**, 4619.

88 SELIGMAN P.A. & ALLEN R.H. (1978) Characterization of the receptor for transcobalamin II isolated from human placenta. *Journal of Biological Chemistry*, **253**, 1766.

89 YOUNDAHL-TURNER P., ROSENBERG L.E. & ALLEN R.H. (1978) Binding and uptake of transcobalamin II by human fibroblasts. *Journal of Clinical Investigation*, **61**, 133.

90 SKOUBY A.P., HIPPE E. & OLESEN H. (1971) Antibody to transcobalamin II and B_{12} binding capacity in patients treated with hydroxocobalamin. *Blood*, **38**, 769.

91 DAIGER S.P., LABOWE M.L., PARSONS M., WANG L. & CAVALLI-SFORZA L.L. (1978) Detection of genetic variation with radioactive ligands. III. Genetic polymorphism of transcobalamin II in human plasma. *American Journal of Human Genetics*, **30**, 202.

92 FRADER-SCHRODER M., HITZIG W.H. & BUTLER R. (1979) Studies on transcobalamin (TC)I. Detection of TCII isoproteins in human serum. *Blood*, **53**, 193.

93 WAXMAN W. & GILBERT H.S. (1974) Characteristics of a novel serum vitamin B_{12} binding protein associated with hepatocellular carcinoma. *British Journal of Haematology*, **27**, 229.

94 NEXØ E., OLESEN H., CHRISTENSEN J.M., THOMSEN J. & KRISTIANSEN K. (1975) Characterization of a cobalamin-binding plasma protein from a patient with hepatoma. *Scandinavian Journal of Clinical and Laboratory Investigation*, **35**, 683.

95 NEXØ E., OLESEN H., NØRREDAM K. & SCHWARTZ M. (1975) A rare case of megaloblastic anaemia caused by disturbances in the plasma cobalamin binding proteins in a patient with hepatocellular carcinoma. *Scandinavian Journal of Haematology*, **14**, 320.

96 HAURANI F.I., HALL C.A. & RUBIN R. (1979) Megaloblastic anemia as a result of an abnormal transcobalamin II (Cardeza). *Journal of Clinical Investigation*, **64**, 1253.

97 HERBERT V. (1968) Diagnostic and prognostic values of measurement of serum vitamin B_{12}-binding proteins. *Blood*, **32**, 305.

98 BRITT R.P. & ROSE D.P. (1966) Pernicious anemia with a normal serum vitamin B_{12} level in a case of chronic granulocytic leukemia. *Archives of Internal Medicine*, **117**, 32.

99 BLOOMFIELD F.J., SCOTT J.M., SOMERVILLE J.J.F. & WEIR D.G. (1973) Levels in normal, pathological, and foetal sera of the three transcobalamins. *Irish Journal of Medical Science*, **142**, 51.

100 ZITTOUN J., ZITTOUN R., MARQUET J. & SULTAN C. (1975) The three transcobalamins in myeloproliferative disorders and acute leukaemia. *British Journal of Haematology*, **31**, 287.

101 CARMEL R. (1972) Vitamin B_{12}-binding protein abnormality in subjects without myeloproliferative disease. I. Elevated serum vitamin B_{12}-binding capacity levels in patients with leucocytosis. *British Journal of Haematology*, **22**, 43.

102 SCOTT J.M., BLOOMFIELD J.F., STEBBINS R. & HERBERT V. (1974) Studies on derivation of transcobalamin III from granulocytes. Enhancement by lithium and elimination by fluorides of in vitro increments in vitamin B_{12}-binding capacity. *Journal of Clinical Investigation*, **53**, 228.

103 CARMEL R. (1978) Vitamin B_{12}-binding proteins in serum and plasma in various disorders. Effect of anticoagulants. *American Journal of Clinical Pathology*, **69**, 319.

104 GIMSING P. & HIPPE E. (1978) Increased concentration of transcobalamin I in a patient with metastatic carcinoma of the breast. *Scandinavian Journal of Haematology*, **21**, 243.

105 CARMEL R. (1975) Extreme elevation of serum transcobalamin I in patients with metastatic cancer. *New England Journal of Medicine*, **292**, 282.

106 WAXMAN S., LIU C.-K., SCHREIBER C. & HELSON L. (1977) The clinical and physiological implications of hepatoma B_{12} binding proteins. *Cancer Research*, **37**, 1908.

107 KANE S.P., MURRAY-LYON I.M., PARADINAS F.J., JOHNSON P.K., WILLIAMS R., ORR A.H. & KOHN J. (1978) Vitamin B_{12} binding protein as a tumour marker for hepatocellular carcinoma. *Gut*, **19**, 1105.

108 HALL C.A. (1975) Measurement of vitamin B_{12} binding protein of plasma. II. Interpretation of patterns in disease. *Blood*, **45**, 287.

109 FRATER-SCHRODER M., GROB P.J., HITZIG W.H. & KENNY A.B. (1978) Increased unsaturated transcobalamin II in active autoimmune disease. *Lancet*, **ii**, 238.

110 GILBERT H.S. & WEINRED N. (1976) Increased circulating levels of transcobalamin II in Gaucher's Disease. *New England Journal of Medicine*, **295**, 1096.

111 CARMEL R. & HOLLANDER D. (1978) Extreme elevation of transcobalamin II levels in multiple myeloma and other disorders. *Blood*, **51**, 1057.

112 FRATER-SCHRODER M., HITZIG W.H., GROSS P.K. & KENNY A.B. (1978) Elevated transcobalamin II in autoimmune diseases: influence of immunosuppressive therapy. *Schweizerische Medizinische Wochenschrift*, **108**, 1604.

113 KANE S.P., HOFFBRAND A.V., ALLEN R.H. & NEALE G. (1976) A familial abnormality of circulating vitamin B_{12} binding proteins: occurrence in a family of high serum concentrations of transcobalamin II. *British Journal of Haematology*, **33**, 249.

114 STEWART J.S., ROBERTS P.D. & HOFFBRAND A.V. (1970) Response of dietary vitamin-B_{12} deficiency to physiological oral doses of cyanocobalamin. *Lancet*, **ii**, 542.

115 BANERJEE D.K. & CHATTERJEA J.B. (1960) Serum vitamin B_{12} in vegetarians. *British Medical Journal*, **ii**, 992.

116 MEHTA B.M., REGE D.V. & SATOSKAR R.S. (1964) Serum vitamin B_{12} and folic acid activity in lactovegetarian and non-vegetarian healthy adult Indians. *American Journal of Clinical Nutrition*, **15**, 77.

117 INAMDAR-DESHMUKH A.B., JATHAR V.S., JOSEPH D.A. & SATOSKAR R.S. (1976) Erythrocyte vitamin B_{12} activity in healthy Indian lactovegetarians. *British Journal of Haematology*, **32**, 395.

118 WOKES F., BADENOCH J. & SINCLAIR H.M. (1955) Human dietary deficiency of vitamin B_{12}. *American Journal of Clinical Nutrition*, **3**, 375.

119 JADHAV M., WEBB J.K.G., VAISHNAVA S. & BAKER S.J. (1962) Vitamin B_{12} deficiency in Indian infants. A clinical syndrome. *Lancet*, **ii**, 903.

120 LAMPKIN B.C., SHORE N.A. & CHADWICK D. (1966) Megaloblastic anemia of infancy secondary to maternal pernicious anemia. *New England Journal of Medicine*, **274**, 1168.

121 CALLENDER S.T. & SPRAY G.H. (1962) Latent pernicious anaemia. *British Journal of Haematology*, **8**, 230.

122 DONIACH D., ROITT I.M. & TAYLOR K.B. (1965) Autoimmunity in pernicious anemia and thyroiditis: a family study. *Annals of the New York Academy of Sciences*, **124**, 605.

123 BLIZZARD R.M., CHEE D. & DAVIS W. (1967) The incidence of adrenal and other antibodies in the sera of patients with idiopathic adrenal insufficiency (Addison's disease). *Clinical and Experimental Immunology*, **2**, 19.

124 BLIZZARD R.M., CHEE D. & DAVIS W. (1966) The incidence of parathyroid and other antibodies in the sera of patients with idiopathic hypoparathyroidism. *Clinical and Experimental Immunology*, **1**, 119.

125 PARTRIDGE R.E.H. & DUTHIE J.J.F. (1963) Incidence of macrocytic anaemia in rheumatoid arthritis. *British Medical Journal*, **i**, 89.

126 UNGAR B., STOCKS A.E., MARTIN F.I.R., WHITTINGHAM S. & MACKAY I.R. (1968) Intrinsic factor antibody, parietal cell antibody and latent pernicious anaemia in diabetes mellitus. *Lancet*, **ii**, 415.

127 TWOMEY J.J., JORDAN P.H., JARROLD T., TRUBOWITZ S., RITZ N.D. & CONN H.O. (1969) The syndrome of immunoglobulin deficiency and pernicious anemia. A study of ten cases. *American Journal of Medicine*, **47**, 340.

128 ZAMCHECK N., GRADLE E., LEY A. & NORMAL L. (1955) Occurrence of gastric cancer among patients with pernicious anemia at the Boston City Hospital. *New England Journal of Medicine*, **252**, 1103.

129 WRAY D., FERGUSON M.M., MASON D.K., HUTCHEON A.W. & DAGG J.H. (1975) Recurrent apthae: treatment with vitamin B_{12}, folic acid, and iron. *British Medical Journal*, **ii**, 490.

130 WALLACE P.W. & WESTMORELAND B.F. (1976) The electroencephalogram in pernicious anemia. *Mayo Clinic Proceedings*, **51**, 281.

131 WALTON J.N., KILOH L.G., OSSELTON J.W. & FARRALL J. (1954) The electroencephalogram in pernicious anaemia and subacute combined degeneration of the cord. *Electroencephalography and Clinical Neurophysiology*, **6**, 45.

132 DACIE J.V. & WHITE J.C. (1949) Erythropoiesis with particular reference to its study by biopsy of human bone marrow: a review. *Journal of Clinical Pathology*, **2**, 1.

133 LONDON I.M. & WEST R. (1950) The formation of bile pigment in pernicious anemia. *Journal of Biological Chemistry*, **184**, 359.

134 YAMAMOTO T., SKANDERBERG J., ZIPURSKY A. & ISRAELS L.G. (1965) The early appearing bilirubin: evidence for two components. *Journal of Clinical Investigation*, **44**, 31.

135 FORSHAW J. & HARWOOD D.L. (1965) The direct antiglobulin (Coombs) test in megaloblastic anaemia. *Journal of Clinical Pathology*, **18**, 119.

135a BALLAS S.K. (1978) Abnormal erythrocyte membrane protein pattern in severe megaloblastic anemia. *Journal of Clinical Investigation*, **61**, 1097.

136 HOFFBRAND A.V., KREMENCHUZKY S., BUTTERWORTH P.J. & MOLLIN D.L. (1966) Serum lactic dehydrogenase activity and folate deficiency in myelosclerosis and other haematological diseases. *British Medical Journal*, **i**, 577.

137 EMERSON P.M., WITHYCOME W.A. & WILKINSON J.H. (1967) The origin of the elevated serum lactate dehydro-

genase in megaloblastic anaemia. *British Journal of Haematology*, **13**, 656.

138 PERILLIE P.E., KAPLAN S.S. & FINCH S.C. (1967) Significance of changes in serum muramidase activity in megaloblastic anemia. *New England Journal of Medicine*, **277**, 10.

139 PARRY T.E. (1969) Serum valine and methionine levels in pernicious anaemia under treatment. *British Journal of Haematology*, **16**, 221.

140 FINCH C.A., COLEMAN D.H., MOTULSKY A.G., DONOHUE D.M. & REIFF R.H. (1956) Erythrokinetics in pernicious anemia. *Blood*, **11**, 807.

141 NATHAN D.G. & GARDNER F.H. (1962) Erythroid cell maturation and hemoglobin synthesis in megaloblastic anemia. *Journal of Clinical Investigation*, **41**, 1086.

142 HUSSEIN S., LAULICHT M. & HOFFBRAND A.V. (1978) Serum ferritin in megaloblastic anaemia. *Scandinavian Journal of Haematology*, **20**, 241.

143 BODDINGTON M.M. & SPRIGGS A.I. (1959) The epithelial cells in megaloblastic anaemia. *Journal of Clinical Pathology*, **12**, 228.

144 FOROOZAN P. & TRIER J.S. (1967) Mucosa of the small intestine in pernicious anemia. *New England Journal of Medicine*, **277**, 553.

145 WINAWER S.J., SULLIVAN L.W., HERBERT V. & ZAMCHECK N. (1965) The jejunal mucosa in patients with nutritional folate deficiency and megaloblastic anemia. *New England Journal of Medicine*, **272**, 892.

146 BIANCHI A., CHIPMAN D.W., DRESKIN A. & ROSENWEIG N.S. (1970) Nutritional folic acid deficiency with megaloblastic changes in the small bowel epithelium. *New England Journal of Medicine*, **282**, 859.

147 MOLLIN D.L., BOOTH C.C. & BAKER S.J. (1957) The absorption of vitamin B₁₂ in control subjects, in Addisonian pernicious anaemia and in the malabsorption syndrome. *British Journal of Haematology*, **3**, 412.

148 SCOTT R.B., KAMMER R.B., BURGHER W.F. & MIDDLETON F.G. (1968) Reduced absorption of vitamin B₁₂ in two patients with folic acid deficiency. *Annals of Internal Medicine*, **69**, 111.

149 VAN DOMMELEN C.K.V. & KLASSEN C.H.L. (1964) Cyanocobalamin-dependent depression of the serum alkaline phosphatase level in patients with pernicious anemia. *New England Journal of Medicine*, **271**, 541.

150 LEEVY C.M., BAKER H., TENHOVE W., FRANK O. & CHERRICK C.R. (1965) B complex vitamins in liver disease of the alcoholic. *American Journal of Clinical Nutrition*, **16**, 339.

151 ROENIGK H.R. JR, BERGFELD W.F., ST. JACQUES R., OWENS F.J. & HAWK W.A. (1971) Hepatotoxicity of methotrexate in the treatment of psoriasis. *Archives of Dermatology*, **103**, 250.

152 ROSENWEIG N.S., HERMAN R.H., STIFEL F.B. & HERMAN Y.F. (1969) Regulation of human jejunal glycolytic enzymes by oral folic acid. *Journal of Clinical Investigation*, **48**, 2038.

153 MANZOOR M. & RUNCIE J. (1976) Folate-responsive neuropathy: report of 10 cases. *British Medical Journal*, **i**, 1176.

154 BOTEZ M.I., CADOTTE M., BEAULIEU R., PICHETTE L.P. & PISON C. (1976) Neurologic disorders responsive to folic acid therapy. *Journal of the Canadian Medical Association*, **115**, 217.

155 SHOVRON S.D., CARNEY M.W.P., CHANARIN I. & REYNOLDS E.H. (1980) The neuropsychiatry of megaloblastic anaemia. *British Medical Journal*, **281**, 1036.

156 HERBERT V. (1962) Experimental nutritional folate deficiency in man. *Transactions of the Association of American Physicians*, **75**, 307.

157 BOTEZ M.I., YOUNG S.N., BACHEUAER J. & GAUTHIER S. (1979) Folate deficiency and decreased brain-5-hydroxytryptamine synthesis in man and rat. *Nature (London)*, **278**, 182.

158 CREUTZFELDT W., ARNOLD R., CREUZFELDT C., FEURLE G. & KETTERER H. (1971) Gastrin and G-cells in the antral mucosa of patients with pernicious anaemia, acromegaly and hyperparathyroidism and in a Zollinger–Ellison tumour of the pancreas. *European Journal of Clinical Investigation*, **1**, 461.

159 MCGUIGAN J.E. & TRUDEAU W.L. (1970) Serum gastrin concentrations in pernicious anemia. *New England Journal of Medicine*, **282**, 358.

160 ROSE M. & CHANARIN I. (1969) Dissociation of intrinsic factor from its antibody: application to study of pernicious anaemia gastric juice specimens. *British Medical Journal*, **i**, 468.

161 WARD H.A. & NAIRN R.C. (1972) Gastric parietal cell autoantigen: physical, chemical and biological properties. *Clinical and Experimental Immunology*, **10**, 435.

162 FISHER J.M., REES C. & TAYLOR K.B. (1965) Antibodies in gastric juice. *Science*, **150**, 1467.

163 IRVINE W.J., DAVIES S.H., TEITELBAUM S., DELAMORE I.W. & WYNN WILLIAMS A. (1964) The clinical and pathological significance of gastric parietal cell antibody. *Annals of New York Academy of Sciences*, **124**, 657.

164 SAMLOFF I.M., KLEIMAN M.S., TURNOER M.D., SOBEL M.V. & JEFFRIES G.H. (1968) Blocking and binding antibodies to intrinsic factor and parietal cell antibody in pernicious anemia. *Gastroenterology*, **55**, 575.

165 BAR-SHANY S. & HERBERT V. (1967) Transplacentally acquired antibody to intrinsic factor with vitamin B₁₂ deficiency. *Blood*, **30**, 777.

166 BAUR S., FISHER J.M., STRICKLAND D.G. & TAYLOR K.B. (1968) Autoantibody-containing cells in the gastric mucosa in pernicious anaemia. *Lancet*, **ii**, 887.

167 SCHADE S.G., FEICK P., MUCKERHEIDE M. & SCHILLING R.F. (1966) Antibody to B₁₂-IF complex which inhibits B₁₂ absorption. *New England Journal of Medicine*, **275**, 528.

168 ROSE M.S., CHANARIN I., DONIACH D., BROSTOFF J. & ARDEMAN S. (1971) Intrinsic-factor antibodies in absence of pernicious anaemia. 3–7 year follow up. *Lancet*, **ii**, 9.

169 CHANARIN I. & JAMES D. (1974) Humoral and cell-mediated intrinsic-factor antibody in pernicious anaemia. *Lancet*, **i**, 1078.

170 ARDEMAN S. & CHANARIN I. (1965) Steroids and Addisonian pernicious anaemia. *New England Journal of Medicine*, **273**, 1352.

171 MCINTYRE O.R., SULLIVAN L.W., JEFFRIES G.H. & SILVER R.H. (1965) Pernicious anemia in childhood. *New England Journal of Medicine*, **272**, 981.

172 KATZ M., LEE S.K. & COOPER B.A. (1972) Vitamin B₁₂ malabsorption due to a biologically inert intrinsic factor. *New England Journal of Medicine*, **287**, 425.

173 KATZ M., MEHLMAN C.S. & ALLEN R.H. (1974) Isolation and characterization of an abnormal intrinsic factor. *Journal of Clinical Investigation*, **53**, 1274.

174 WUEPPER K.D. & FUDENBERG H.H. (1967) Moniliasis, autoimmune polyendocrinopathy and immunologic family study. *Clinical and Experimental Immunology*, **2**, 71.

175 HINES J.D., HOFFBRAND A.V. & MOLLIN D.L. (1967) The hematologic complications following partial gastrectomy. A study of 292 patients. *American Journal of Medicine*, **43**, 555.

176 DELLER D.J. & WITTS L.J. (1962) Changes in the blood after partial gastrectomy with special reference to vitamin B_{12}. I. Serum vitamin B_{12} haemoglobin serum, iron and bone marrow. *Quarterly Journal of Medicine*, **31**, 71.

177 KOLHOUSE J.F., KONDO H., ALLEN N.C., PODELL E. & ALLEN R.H. (1978) Cobalamin analogues are present in human plasma and can mask cobalamin deficiency because current radioisotope dilution assays are not specific for the cobalamin. *New England Journal of Medicine*, **299**, 785.

178 COX E.V., MEYNELL M.J., GADDIE R. & COOKE W.T. (1959) Interrelation of vitamin B_{12} and iron. *Lancet*, **ii**, 998.

179 COTTER R., ROTHENBERG S.P. & WEISS J.P. (1979) Dissociation of the intrinsic factor vitamin B_{12} complex by bile—contributing factor to B_{12} malabsorption in pancreatic insufficiency. *Scandinavian Journal of Gastroenterology*, **14**, 545.

180 JOHNSON H.D. & HOFFBRAND A.V. (1970) The influence of extent of resection, type of anastomosis, and of ulcer site on the haematological side effects of gastectomy. *British Journal of Surgery*, **57**, 33.

181 DELLER D.J., GERMAR H. & WITTS L.J. (1961) Effect of food on absorption of radioactive vitamin B_{12}. *Lancet*, **i**, 574.

182 DOSCHERHOLMAN A., McMAHON J. & RIPLEY D. (1976) Inhibitory effect of eggs on vitamin B_{12} absorption: description of a simple ovalbumin ^{57}Co-vitamin B_{12} absorption test. *British Journal of Haematology*, **33**, 261.

183 TABAQCHALI S., OKUBADEJO O.A., NEALE G. & BOOTH C.C. (1966) Influence of abnormal bacterial flora on small intestinal function. *Proceedings of the Royal Society of Medicine*, **59**, 1244.

184 TABAQCHALI S. (1970) The pathophysiological role of small intestinal bacterial flora. *Scandinavian Journal of Gastroenterology*, **5** (Suppl.), 6.

185 COOKE W.T., COX E.V., FONE D.J., MEYNELL M.J. & GADDIE R. (1963) The clinical and metabolic significance of jejunal diverticulae. *Gut*, **4**, 115.

186 GIANNELLA R.A., BROITMAN S.A. & ZAMCHECK N. (1972) Competition between bacteria and intrinsic factor for vitamin B_{12}: implications for vitamin B_{12} malabsorption in intestinal bacterial overgrowth. *Advances in Internal Medicine*, **16**, 191.

187 BOOTH C.C. MACINTYRE I. & MOLLIN D.L. (1964) Nutritional problems associated with extensive lesions of the distal small intestine in man. *Quarterly Journal of Medicine*, **33**, 401.

188 DOWLING R.H. (1967) Compensatory changes in intestinal absorption. *British Medical Bulletin*, **23**, 275.

189 MEYNELL M.J., COOKE W.T., COX E.V. & GADDIE R. (1957) Serum-cyanocobalamin level in chronic intestinal disorders. *Lancet*, **i**, 901.

190 HOFFBRAND A.V., STEWART J.S., BOOTH C.C. & MOLLIN D.L. (1968) Folate deficiency in Crohn's disease; Incidence, pathogenesis and treatment. *British Medical Journal*, **ii**, 71.

191 IMERSLUND O. (1960) Idiopathic chronic megaloblastic anaemia in children. *Acta Paediatrica*, **49** (Suppl. 119), 1.

192 GRÄSBECK R., GORDIN R., KANTERO I. & KUHLBÄCK B. (1960) Selective vitamin B_{12} malabsorption and proteinuria in young people. A syndrome. *Acta Medica Scandinavia*, **167**, 289.

193 BEN-BASSAT I., FEINSTEIN A. & RAMOT B. (1969) Selective vitamin B_{12} malabsorption with proteinuria in Israel. *Israel Journal of Medical Science*, **5**, 62.

194 MacKENZIE I.L., DONALDSON R.M., TRIER J.S. & MATHAN V.I. (1972) Ileal mucosa in familial selective vitamin B_{12} malabsorption. *New England Journal of Medicine*, **286**, 1021.

195 KLIPSTEIN F.A. (1968) Tropical sprue. *Gastroenterology*, **54**, 275.

196 WELLCOME TRUST COLLABORATIVE STUDY (1971) *Tropical Sprue and Megaloblastic Anaemia*. Churchill-Livingstone, London.

197 KLIPSTEIN F.A. (1970) Recent advances in tropical malabsorption. *Scandinavian Journal of Gastroenterology*, **5** (Suppl. 6), 93.

198 MOLLIN D.L. & BOOTH C.C. (1971) Chronic tropical sprue in London. In: *Tropical Sprue and Megaloblastic Anaemia*. Wellcome Trust Collaborative Study, p. 61. Churchill-Livingstone, London.

199 VON BONDSDORFF B. (1977) *Diphyllobothriasis in Man*. Academic Press, London.

200 PALVA I.P. (1962) Vitamin B_{12} deficiency in fish tapeworm carriers. A clinical and laboratory study. *Acta Medica Scandinavica*, **171** (Suppl. 374), 1.

201 JOSKE R.A., FINCKH E.S. & WOOD I.K. (1955) Gastric biopsy: a study of 1000 consecutive successful gastric biopsies. *Quarterly Journal of Medicine*, **24**, 269.

202 COGHILL N.F., DONIACH D., ROITT I.M., MOLLIN D.L. & WILLIAMS A.W. (1965) Auto-antibodies in simple atrophic gastritis. *Gut*, **6**, 48.

203 SIURALA M., VARIS K. & WILJASALO M. (1966) Studies of patients with atrophic gastritis: a 10–15 year follow-up. *Scandinavian Journal of Gastroenterology*, **1**, 40.

204 MOLLIN D.L. (1959) The megaloblastic anaemias. *Lectures on the Scientific Basis of Medicine*, **7**, 94.

205 STEWART J.S., POLLOCK D.J., HOFFBRAND A.V., MOLLIN D.L. & BOOTH C.C. (1967) A study of proximal and distal intestinal structure and absorption function in idiopathic steatorrhoea. *Quarterly Journal of Medicine*, **36**, 425.

206 MATUCHANSKY C., RAMBAUD J.C., MODIGLIANI R. & BERNIER J.J. (1974). Vitamin B_{12} malabsorption in chronic pancreatitis. *Gastroenterology*, **67**, 406.

207 VON DER LIPPE G., ANDERSEN K.-J. & SCHJÖNSBY H. (1976) Intestinal absorption of vitamin B_{12} in patients with chronic pancreatic insufficiency and the effect of human duodenal juice on the intestinal uptake of vitamin B_{12}. *Scandinavian Journal of Gastroenterology*, **11**, 689.

208 DEREN J.J., ARORA B., TOSKES P.P., HANSELL J. &

SIBINGA M.S. (1973) Malabsorption of crystalline vitamin B₁₂ in cystic fibrosis. *New England Journal of Medicine*, **288**, 949.

209 WAXMAN S., CORCINO J. & HERBERT V. (1970) Drugs, toxins and dietary amino-acids affecting vitamin B₁₂ or folic acid absorption or utilization. *American Journal of Medicine*, **48**, 599.

210 SCOTT J.M. & WEIR D.G. (1980) Drug-induced megaloblastic change. *Clinics in Haematology*, **9**, 587.

211 WERTALIK L.F., METZ E.N., LOBULIO A.F. & BALCERZAK S.P. (1972) Decreased serum B₁₂ levels with oral contraceptive use. *Journal of the American Medical Association*, **221**, 1371.

212 TOMKIN G.H., HADDEN D.R., WEAVER J.A. & MONTGOMERY D.A.D. (1971) Vitamin-B₁₂ status of patients on long-term metformin therapy. *British Medical Journal*, **ii**, 685.

213 CALLAGHAN T.S., HADDEN D.R. & TOMKIN G.H. (1980) Megaloblastic anaemia due to vitamin B₁₂ malabsorption associated with long-term metformin treatment. *British Medical Journal*, **280**, 1214.

214 REYNOLDS E.H., HALLPIKE J.F., PHILLIPS B.M. & MATTHEWS D.M. (1965) Reversible absorptive defects in anticonvulsant megaloblastic anaemia. *Journal of Clinical Pathology*, **18**, 593.

215 LINDENBAUM J. & LIEBER C.S. (1969) Alcohol-induced malabsorption of vitamin B₁₂ in man. *Nature (London)*, **224**, 806.

216 LINE D.H., SEITANIDES B., MORGAN J.O. & HOFFBRAND A.V. (1971) The effect of chemotherapy on iron, folate and vitamin B₁₂ metabolism in tuberculosis. *Quarterly Journal of Medicine*, **40**, 331.

217 HERBERT V., LANDAU L., BASH R., GROSBERG S. & COLMAN N. (1979) Ability of megadoses of vitamin C to destroy vitamin B₁₂ and cobinamide and to reduce absorption of vitamin B₁₂ (with a note on B₁₂ radioassays). In: *Vitamin B₁₂* (ed. Zagalak B. & Friedrich W.), p. 1059. De Gruyter, Berlin.

218 HINES J.D. (1975) Ascorbic acid and vitamin B₁₂ deficiency. *Journal of the American Medical Association*, **234**, 24.

219 STEINBERG W., KING C. & TOSKES P. (1978) Cimetidine inhibits absorption of food bound B₁₂. *Gastroenterology*, **74**, 1099.

220 WRIGHT S.G., TOMKINS A.M. & RIDLEY D.S. (1977) Giardiasis: clinical and therapeutic aspects. *Gut*, **18**, 343.

221 MARSHALL R.A. & JANDL J.H. (1960) Responses to 'physiologic' doses of folic acid in the megaloblastic anemias. *Archives of Internal Medicine*, **105**, 352.

222 ANDERSON B.B. (1964) Investigations into the Euglena method for the assay of vitamin B₁₂ in serum. *Journal of Clinical Pathology*, **17**, 14.

223 LAU K.-S., GOTTLIEB C., WASSERMAN C.R. & HERBERT V. (1965) Measurement of serum vitamin B₁₂ level using radioisotope dilution and coated charcoal. *Blood*, **26**, 202.

224 RAVEN J.L., ROBSON M.B., MORGAN J.O. & HOFFBRAND A.V. (1972) Comparison of three methods for measuring vitamin B₁₂ in serum: radioisotopic, *Euglena gracilis* and *Lactobacillus leichmannii*. *British Journal of Haematology*, **22**, 21.

225 MOLLIN D.L., HOFFBRAND A.V., WARD P.G. & LEWIS S.M. (1980) Interlaboratory comparison of serum vitamin B₁₂ assay. *Journal of Clinical Pathology*, **33**, 243.

226 COOPER B.A. & WHITEHEAD V.M. (1978) Evidence that some patients with pernicious anemia are not recognized by radiodilution assay for cobalamin in serum. *New England Journal of Medicine*, **299**, 816.

227 KOLHOUSE J.F., KONDO H., ALLEN N.C., PODELL E. & ALLEN R.H. (1978) Cobalamin analogues are present in human plasma and can mask cobalamin deficiency because current radioisotope dilution assays are not specific for true cobalamin. *New England Journal of Medicine*, **299**, 785.

228 KUBASIK N.P., RICOTTA M. & SINE H.E. (1980) Commercially-supplied binders for plasma cobalamin (vitamin B₁₂) analysis—'purified' intrinsic factor, 'cobinamide'-blocked R-protein binder, and non-purified intrinsic factor-R protein binder—compared to microbiological assay. *Clinical Chemistry*, **26**, 598.

229 MOLLIN D.L., WATERS A.H. & HARRISS E.B. (1962) Clinical aspects of the metabolic inter-relationships between folic acid and vitamin B₁₂. In: *Vitamin B₁₂ and Intrinsic Factor*. 2nd European Symposium (ed. Heinrich H.C.), p. 737. Enke Verlag, Stuttgart.

230 MOLLIN D.L., ANDERSON B.B. & BURMAN J.F. (1976) The serum vitamin B₁₂ level: its assay and significance. *Clinics in Haematology*, **5**, 521.

231 LINNELL J.C., HOFFBRAND A.V., HUSSEIN H.A.-A., WISE I.J. & MATTHEWS D.M. (1974) Tissue distribution of coenzyme and other forms of vitamin B₁₂ in control subjects and patients with pernicious anaemia. *Clinical Science and Molecular Medicine*, **46**, 163.

232 VAN DER WEYDEN M.B., ROTHER M. & FIRKIN B.G. (1972) The metabolic significance of reduced serum B₁₂ in folate deficiency. *Blood*, **40**, 23.

233 ANDERSON B.B. (1965) Investigations into the Euglena method of assay of vitamin B₁₂: the results obtained in human serum and liver using an improved method of assay. Ph.D. thesis, University of London.

234 HARRISON R.J. (1971) Vitamin B₁₂ levels in erythrocytes in anaemia due to folate deficiency. *British Journal of Haematology*, **20**, 623.

235 LIE J.T., UNGAR B. & COWLING D.C. (1969) Effect of anti-microbial agents on the Euglena method of serum vitamin B₁₂ assay. *Journal of Clinical Pathology*, **22**, 554.

236 POWELL D.E.B., THOMAS J.H., MANDELL A.R. & DIGNAM C.T. (1969) Effect of drugs on vitamin B₁₂ levels obtained using the Lactobacillus leichmannii method. *Journal of Clinical Pathology*, **22**, 672.

237 STREETER A.M., SHUM H.Y. & O'NEILL B.J. (1970) The effect of drugs on the microbiological assay of serum folic acid and vitamin B₁₂ levels. *Medical Journal of Australia*, **1**, 900.

238 MAHONEY M.J. & ROSENBERG L.E. (1975) Inborn error of cobalamin metabolism. In: *Cobalamin: Biochemistry and Pathophysiology* (ed. Babior B.M.), p. 369. John Wiley & Sons, New York.

239 GOMPERTZ D., HYWELL-JONES J. & KNOWLES J.P. (1967) Metabolic precursors of methylmalonic acid in vitamin B₁₂ deficiency. *Lancet*, **i**, 424.

240 GREENFIELD J.G. & MEYER A. (1963) Vitamin B₁₂ neuropathy (subacute combined degeneration of the spinal cord). In: *Greenfield's Neuropathology* (ed. Blackwood W. *et al.*). Edward Arnold, London.

241 BUCKLE R.M. (1966) Blood pyruvic and α-oxoglutaric acids in vitamin B_{12} deficiency. *Clinical Science*, **31**, 181.

242 COX E.V., ROBERTSON-SMITH D., SMALL M. & WHITE A.M. (1968) The excretion of propionate and acetate in vitamin B_{12} deficiency. *Clinical Science*, **35**, 123.

243 MORROW G., BARNESS L.A., CARDINALE G.J., ABELES R.H. & FLAKS S.G. (1969) Congenital methylmalonic acidemia: enzymatic evidence for two forms of the disease. *Proceedings of the National Academy of Sciences, USA*, **63**, 191.

244 ROSENBERG L.E., LILLJEQVIST A.-C., HSIA Y.E. & ROSENBLOOM F.M. (1969) Vitamin B_{12} dependent methylmalonicaciduria: defective B_{12} metabolism in cultured fibroblasts. *Biochemical and Biophysical Research Communications*, **37**, 607.

245 GOODMAN S.I., MOE P.G., HAMMOND K.B., MUDD S.H. & UHLENDORF B.W. (1970) Homocystinuria with methylmalonic aciduria: two cases in a sibship. *Biochemical Medicine*, **4**, 500.

246 DILLON M.J., ENGLAND J.M., GOMPERTZ D., GOODEY P.A., GRANT D.B., HUSSEIN H.A.-A., LINNELL J.C., MATTHEWS D.M., MUDD S.H., NEWNS G.H., SEAKINS J.W.T., UHLENDORF B.W. & WISE I.J. (1974) Mental retardation, megaloblastic anaemia, methylmalonic aciduria and abnormal homocysteine metabolism due to an error in vitamin B_{12} metabolism. *Clinical Science and Molecular Medicine*, **47**, 43.

247 MOLLIN D.L. & WATERS A.H. (1968) The study of vitamin B_{12} absorption using labelled cobalamins. *Medical Monographs*, **6**. The Radiochemical Centre, Amersham, England.

248 GLASS G.B.J. (1974) *Gastric Intrinsic Factor and Other Vitamin B_{12} Binders*. Thieme, Stuttgart.

249 KATZ J.H., DIMASE J. & DONALDSON R.M. JR (1963) Simultaneous administration of gastric juice-bound and free radioactive cyanocobalamin: rapid procedure for differentiating between intrinsic factor deficiency and other causes of vitamin B_{12} malabsorption. *Journal of Laboratory and Clinical Medicine*, **61**, 266.

250 BREWSTER A., MARCON N., LOUX H., FLETCHER J. & ZAMCHECK N. (1970) Hemoglobin iron (HbFe^{59}) absorption in pernicious anemia (PA) and total gastrectomized patients unimproved by crude intrinsic factor (IF) or normal gastric juice (GJ). *Clinical Research*, **18**, 377.

251 KNUDSEN L. & HIPPE E. (1974) Vitamin B_{12} absorption evaluated by a dual isotope test (Dicopac). *Scandinavian Journal of Haematology*, **13**, 287.

252 DOSCHERHOLMAN A., McMAHON J. & RIPLEY D. (1976) Inhibitory effect of eggs on vitamin B_{12} absorption: description of a simple ovalbumin ^{57}Co-vitamin B_{12} absorption test. *British Journal of Haematology*, **33**, 261.

253 STREETER A.M., SHUM H.-Y., DUNCOMBE V.M., HEWSON J.W. & THORPE M.E.C. (1976) Vitamin B_{12} malabsorption associated with a normal Schilling test result. *Medical Journal of Australia*, **1**, 54.

254 JUKES T.H. & STOKSTAD E.L.R. (1948) Pteroylglutamic acid and related compounds. *Physiological Reviews*, **28**, 51.

255 WILLS L. (1931) Treatment of 'pernicious anaemia of pregnancy' and 'tropical anaemia'. *British Medical Journal*, **i**, 1059.

256 WILLS L. & EVANS B.D.F. (1938) Tropical macrocytic anaemia: its relation to pernicious anaemia. *Lancet*, **ii**, 416.

257 MITCHELL H.K., SNELL E.E. & WILLIAMS R.J. (1941) The concentration of 'folic acid'. *Journal of American Chemical Society*, **63**, 2284.

258 HERBERT V., LARRABEE A.R. & BUCHANAN J.M. (1962) Studies on the identification of a folate compound of human serum. *Journal of Clinical Investigation*, **41**, 1134.

259 RATANASTHIEN K., BLAIR J.A., LEEMING R.J., COOKE V.T. & MELIKIAN V. (1974) Folates in human serum. *Journal of Clinical Pathology*, **27**, 875.

260 SHIN Y.S., WILLIAMS M.A. & STOKSTAD E.L.R. (1972) Identification of folic acid compounds in rat liver. *Biochemical and Biophysical Research Communications*, **47**, 35.

261 CORROCHER R., BHUYAN B.K. & HOFFBRAND A.V. (1972) Composition of pteroylpolyglutamates (conjugated folates) in liver and their formation from folic acid. *Clinical Science*, **43**, 799.

262 HOFFBRAND A.V. & NEWCOMBE B.E.A. (1967) Leucocyte folate content in vitamin B_{12} and folate deficiency in leukaemia. *British Journal of Haematology*, **13**, 954.

263 NORONHA J.M. & ABOOBAKER V.S. (1963) Studies on the folate compounds of human blood. *Archives of Biochemistry and Biophysics*, **101**, 445.

264 SCHERTEL M.E., BOEHNE J.W. & LIBBY D.A. (1965) Folic acid derivatives in yeast. *Journal of Biological Chemistry*, **240**, 3154.

265 PERRY J. & CHANARIN I. (1977) Abnormal folate polyglutamate ratios in untreated pernicious anaemia corrected by therapy. *British Journal of Haematology*, **35**, 397.

266 HOFFBRAND A.V. & PETERS T.J. (1969) The subcellular localization of pteroylpolyglutamate hydrolase and folate in guinea-pig intestinal mucosa. *Biochimica et Biophysica Acta*, **192**, 479.

267 BAUGH C.M. & KRUMDIECK C.L. (1971) Naturally occurring folates. *Annals of the New York Academy of Sciences*, **186**, 7.

268 CORROCHER R. & HOFFBRAND A.V. (1972) Subcellular localization and effect of methotrexate on the incorporation of radioactive folic acid into liver folate. *Clinical Science*, **43**, 815.

269 LESLIE G.I. & BAUGH C.M. (1974) The uptake of pteroyl (^{14}C) glutamic acid into rat liver and its incorporation into the natural pteroylpoly-γ-glutamates of that organ. *Biochemistry*, **13**, 4957.

270 HOFFBRAND A.V., TRIPP E. & LAVOIE A. (1976) Synthesis of folate polyglutamates in human cells. *Clinical Science and Molecular Medicine*, **50**, 61.

271 TAYLOR R.T. & HANNA M.L. (1977) Folate-dependent enzymes in cultured Chinese hamster cells: folylpolyglutamate synthetase and its absence in mutants auxotrophic for glycine + adenosine + thymidine. *Archives of Biochemistry and Biophysics*, **181**, 331.

272 MORAN R.G. & COLMAN P.D. (1980) Studies on mammalian folate poly-γ-glutamate synthetase. *Proceedings of the American Association for Cancer Research*, **21**, 25 (Abstract).

273 COWARD J.K., CHELLO P.L., CASHMORE A.R., PARAMESWARAN K.N., DEANGELIS L.M. & BERTINO J.R. (1975) 5-methyl-5,6,7,8-tetrahydropteroyl oligo-γ-L-glutamates:

synthesis and kinetic studies with methionine synthetase from bovine brain. *Biochemistry*, **14**, 1548.

274 KISLIUK R.L. GAUMONT Y. & BAUGH C.M. (1974) Polyglutamyl derivatives of folate as substrates and inhibitors of thymidylate synthetase. *Journal of Biological Chemistry*, **249**, 4100.

275 BERTINO J.R., SILBER R., FREEMAN M., ALENTY A., ALBRECHT M., GABRIO B.W. & HUENNEKENS F.M. (1963) Studies on normal and leukemic leucocytes. IV. Tetrahydrofolate dependent enzyme systems and dihydrofolic reductase. *Journal of Clinical Investigation*, **42**, 1899.

276 WEINHOUSE S. & FRIEDMANN B. (1952) Study of precursors of formate in the intact rat. *Journal of Biological Chemistry*, **197**, 733.

277 ELLEGAARD J. & ESMANN V. (1972) Folate deficiency in malnutrition, malabsorption, and during phenytoin treatment diagnosed by determination of serine synthesis in lymphocytes. *European Journal of Clinical Investigation*, **2**, 315.

278 TIKERKAE J. & CHANARIN I. (1978) Folate-dependent serine synthesis in lymphocytes from controls and patients with megaloblastic anaemia: the effect of therapy. *British Journal of Haematology*, **38**, 353.

279 BLAKELEY R.L. (1957) Interconversion and glycine: some further properties of the enzyme system. *Biochemical Journal*, **65**, 342.

280 KOZLOFF L.M., LUTE M. & CROSBY L.K. (1970) Bacteriophage tail components. III. The use of synthetic pteroylhexaglutamate for T4D tail plate assembly. *Journal of Virology*, **6**, 754.

281 HERBERT V. (1962) Minimal daily adult folate requirement. *Archives of Internal Medicine*, **110**, 649.

282 CHANARIN I., HUTCHINSON M., McLEAN A. & MOULE M. (1966) Hepatic folate in man. *British Medical Journal*, **i**, 396.

283 RETIEF F.P. & HUSKISSON Y.J. (1969) Serum and urinary folate in liver disease. *British Medical Journal*, **ii**, 150.

284 HOFFBRAND A.V., TABAQCHALI S., BOOTH C.C. & MOLLIN D.L. (1971) Small intestine bacterial flora and folate status in gastrointestinal disease. *Gut*, **12**, 27.

285 MURPHY M., KEATING M., BOYLE P., WEIR D.G. & SCOTT J.M. (1976) The elucidation of the mechanism of folate catabolism in the rat. *Biochemical and Biophysical Research Communication*, **71**, 1017.

286 HALPERN R., HALPERN B.C., STEA B., DUNLOP A., CONKLIN K., CLARK B., ASHE M., SPERLING L., HALPERN J.A., HARDY D. & SMITH R.A. (1977) Pterin-6-aldehyde. A cancer cell catabolite: identification and application in diagnosis and treatment of human cancer. *Proceedings of the National Academy of Sciences, USA*, **74**, 587.

287 BUTTERWORTH C.E. JR, SANTINI R. JR & FROMMEYER W.B. JR (1963) The pteroylglutamate components of American diets as determined by chromatographic fractionation. *Journal of Clinical Investigation*, **42**, 1929.

288 CHANARIN I., ROTHMAN D., PERRY J. & STRATFULL D. (1968) Normal dietary folate, iron, and protein intake, with particular reference to pregnancy. *British Medical Journal*, **ii**, 394.

289 PERRY J. (1971) Folate analogues in normal mixed diets. *British Journal of Haematology*, **21**, 435.

290 HOPPNER K., LAMPI B. & PERRIN D.E. (1973) Folacin activity of frozen convenience foods. *Journal of the American Dietetic Association*, **63**, 536.

291 HEPNER G.W., BOOTH C.C., COWAN J., HOFFBRAND A.V. & MOLLIN D.L. (1968) Absorption of crystalline folic acid in man. *Lancet*, **ii**, 302.

292 PERRY J. & CHANARIN I. (1970) Intestinal absorption of reduced folate compounds in man. *British Journal of Haematology*, **18**, 329.

293 HOFFBRAND A.V. (1971) Folate absorption. *Journal of Clinical Pathology*, **24** (Suppl. 5), 66.

294 ROSENBERG I.H. (1976) Absorption and malabsorption of folates. *Clinics in Haematology*, **5**, 589.

295 HALSTED C.H. (1979) The intestinal absorption of folates. *American Journal of Clinical Nutrition*, **32**, 846.

296 REISENAUER A.M., KRUMDIECK C.L. & HALSTED C.H. (1977) Folate conjugase: Two separate activities in human jejunum. *Science*, **198**, 196.

297 HALSTED C.H., REISENAUER A.M., ROMERO J.J., CANTOR D.S. & RUEBNER B. (1977) Jejunal perfusion of simple and conjugated folates in coeliac sprue. *Journal of Clinical Investigation*, **59**, 933.

298 LESLIE G.I. & BAUGH C.M. (1974) The uptake of pteroyl (^{14}C) glutamic acid into rat liver and its incorporation into the natural pteroylpoly-γ-glutamates of that organ. *Biochemistry*, **13**, 4957.

299 COLMAN N., HETTIARACHCHY N. & HERBERT V. (1981) Detection of a milk factor that facilitates folate uptake by intestinal cells. *Science*, **211**, 1427.

300 BUTTERWORTH C.E. JR, BAUCH C.M. & KRUMDIECK C. (1969) A study of folate absorption and metabolism in man utilizing carbon-14-labelled polyglutamates synthesised by the solid phase method. *Journal of Clinical Investigation*, **48**, 1131.

301 BAUGH C.M., KRUMDIECK C.L., BAKER H.J. & BUTTERWORTH C.R. JR (1971) Studies on the absorption and metabolism of folic acid. I. Folate absorption in the dog after exposure of isolated intestinal segments to synthetic pteroylpolyglutamates of various chain lengths. *Journal of Clinical Investigation*, **50**, 2009.

302 NIXON P.F. & BERTINO J.R. (1972) Effective absorption and utilization of oral formyltetrahydrofolate in man. *New England Journal of Medicine*, **286**, 175.

303 TAMURA T., SHIN Y.S., BUEHRING K.U. & STOKSTAD E.L.R. (1976) The availability of folates in man: effect of orange juice supplement on intestinal conjugase. *British Journal of Haematology*, **32**, 123.

304 WHITEHEAD V.M. & COOPER B.A. (1967) Absorption of unaltered folic acid from the gastro-intestinal tract in man. *British Journal of Haematology*, **13**, 679.

305 WEIR D.G., BROWN J.P., FREEDMAN D.S. & SCOTT J.M. (1973) The absorption of the diastereoisomers of 5-methyltetrahydropteroylglutamate in man: a carrier-mediated process. *Clinical Science and Molecular Medicine*, **45**, 625.

306 LANZKOWSKY P. (1970) Congenital malabsorption of folate. *American Journal of Medicine*, **48**, 580.

307 ROTHENBERG S.P. & da COSTA M. (1976) Folate binding proteins and radioassay for folate. *Clinics in Haematology*, **5**, 569.

308 FERNANDES-COSTA F. & METZ J. (1979) Role of serum folate binders in the delivery of folate to tissues and to the fetus. *British Journal of Haematology*, **41**, 335.

309 CORROCHER R., DE SANDRE G., PACOR M.L. & HOFF-

BRAND A.V. (1974) Hepatic protein binding of folate. *Clinical Science and Molecular Medicine*, **46**, 551.

310 ZAMIEROWSKI M.M. & WAGNER C. (1977) Identification of folate binding proteins in rat liver. *Journal of Biological Chemistry*, **252**, 933.

311 DAS K.C. & HOFFBRAND A.V. (1970) Studies of folate uptake by phytohaemagglutinin-stimulated lymphocytes. *British Journal of Haematology*, **19**, 203.

312 CORCINO J.J., WAXMAN S. & HERBERT V. (1971) Uptake of tritiated folates by human bone marrow cells *in vitro*. *British Journal of Haematology*, **20**, 503.

313 GOLDMAN I.D. (1971) The characteristics of the membrane transport of amethopterin and the naturally occurring folates. *Annals of the New York Academy of Sciences*, **186**, 400.

314 HOFFBRAND A.V., TRIPP E., CATOVSKY D. & DAS K.C. (1973) Transport of methotrexate into normal haemopoietic cells and into leukaemic cells and its effects on DNA synthesis. *British Journal of Haematology*, **25**, 497.

315 HUENNEKENS F.M., VITOLS K.S. & HENDERSON G.B. (1978) Transport of folate-compounds in bacterial and mammalian cells. *Advances in Enzymology and Related Areas of Molecular Biology*, **47**, 313.

316 McHUGH M. & CHENG Y.-C. (1979) Demonstration of a high affinity folate binder in human cell membranes and its characterization in cultured human KB cells. *Journal of Biological Chemistry*, **254**, 1312.

317 CHEN C.-P. & WAGNER C. (1975) Folate transport in the choroid plexus. *Life Sciences*, **16**, 1571.

318 SPECTOR R. (1979) Affinity of folic acid for the folate-binding proteins of choroid plexus. *Archives of Biochemistry and Biophysics*, **194**, 632.

319 STEINBERG S., CAMPBELL C. & HILLMAN R.S. (1979) Kinetics of the normal enterohepatic cycle. *Journal of Clinical Investigation* **50**, 910.

320 GORESKY C.A., WATANABE H. & JOHNS D.G. (1963) The renal excretion of folic acid. *Journal of Clinical Investigation*, **42**, 1841.

321 MONTO R.W., KAVANAGH D. & REBUCK J.W. (1958) Severe nutritional macrocytic anemia in emotionally disturbed patients. *American Journal of Clinical Nutrition*, **6**, 105.

322 GOUGH K.R., READ A.E., McCARTHY C.F. & WATERS A.H. (1963) Megaloblastic anaemia due to nutritional deficiency of folic acid. *Quarterly Journal of Medicine*, **32**, 243.

323 ZALUSKY R. & HERBERT V. (1961) Megaloblastic anemia in scurvy with response to 50 micrograms of folic acid daily. *New England Journal of Medicine*, **265**, 1033.

324 COOKE W.T., FONE D.J., COX E.V., MEYNELL M.J. & GADDIE R. (1963) Acute folic acid deficiency of unknown aetiology: temperate sprue. *Gut*, **4**, 292.

325 VANIER T.M. & TYAS J.F. (1966) Folic acid status in normal infants during the first year of life. *Archives of Disease in Childhood*, **41**, 658.

326 HOPPNER K., LAMPI B. & PERRIN D.E. (1972) The free and total folate activity in foods available on the Canadian market. *Canadian Institute of Food Technology Journal*, **5**, 60.

327 SHOJANIA A.M. & GROSS S. (1964) Folic acid deficiency and prematurity. *Journal of Pediatrics*, **64**, 323.

328 VANIER T.M. & TYAS J.F. (1967) Folic acid status in premature infants. *Archives of Disease in Childhood*, **42**, 57.

329 STRELLING M.K., BLACKLEDGE G.D., GOODALL H.H. & WALKER C.H.M. (1966) Megaloblastic anaemia and whole blood folate levels in premature infants. *Lancet*, **i**, 898.

330 HOFFBRAND A.V. (1974) Anaemia in adult coeliac disease. *Clinics in Gastroenterology*, **3**, 71.

331 MARSH G.W. & STEWART J.S. (1970) Splenic function in adult coeliac disease. *British Journal of Haematology*, **19**, 445.

332 HOFFBRAND A.V., DOUGLAS A.P., FRY L. & STEWART J.S. (1970) Malabsorption of dietary folate (pteroylpolyglutamates) in adult coeliac disease and dermatitis herpetiformis. *British Medical Journal*, **iv**, 85.

333 HALSTED C.H., REISENAUER A.M., SHANE B. & TAMURA T. (1978) Availability of monoglutamyl and polyglutamyl folates in normal subjects and in patients with coeliac sprue. *Gut*, **19**, 886.

334 DORMANDY K.M., WATERS A.H. & MOLLIN D.L. (1963) Folic-acid deficiency in coeliac disease. *Lancet*, **i**, 632.

335 HOFFBRAND A.V., NECHELES T.F., MALDONADO N., HORTAS E. & SANTINI R. (1969) Malabsorption of folate polyglutamates in tropical sprue. *British Medical Journal*, **ii**, 543.

336 O'BRIEN W. & ENGLAND N.W.J. (1964) Folate deficiency in acute tropical sprue. *British Medical Journal*, **ii**, 1573.

337 FRY L., KEIR P., McMINN R.M.H., COWAN J.D. & HOFFBRAND A.V. (1967) Small intestinal structure and function and haematological changes in dermatitis herpetiformis. *Lancet*, **ii**, 729.

338 FRY L., McMINN R.M.H., COWAN J.D. & HOFFBRAND A.V. (1969) Gluten-free diet and reintroduction of gluten in dermatitis herpetiformis. *Archives of Dermatology*, **60**, 129.

339 PETTIT J.E., HOFFBRAND A.V., SEAH P.P. & FRY L. (1972) Splenic atrophy in dermatitis herpetiformis. *British Medical Journal*, **ii**, 438.

340 SAUBERLICH H.E. (1949) The effect of folic acid upon the urinary excretion of the growth factor required by *Leuconostoc citrovorum*. *Journal of Biological Chemistry*, **181**, 467.

341 LUCAS M.L., COOPER B.T., LEI F.H., JOHNSON I.T., HOLMES G.K.T., BLAIR J.A. & COOKE W.T. (1978) Acid microclimate in coeliac and Crohn's disease: a model for folate malabsorption. *Gut*, **19**, 735.

342 RUSSELL R.M., DHAR G.J., DUTTA S.K. & ROSENBERG I.H. (1979) Influence of intraluminal pH on folate absorption: studies in control subjects and in patients with pancreatic insufficiency. *Journal of Laboratory and Clinical Medicine*, **93**, 428.

343 FRANKLIN J.L. & ROSENBERG I.H. (1973) Impaired folic acid absorption in inflammatory bowel disease: effects of salicylazosulfapyridine (azulfidine). *Gastroenterology*, **64**, 517.

344 DELLER D.J., IBBOTSON R.N. & CROMPTON B. (1964) Metabolic effect of partial gastrectomy with special reference to calcium and folic acid. II. The contribution of folic acid deficiency to the anaemia. *Gut*, **5**, 225.

345 HOFFBRAND A.V., TABAQCHALI S. & MOLLIN D.L. (1966) High serum folate levels in intestinal blind-loop syndrome. *Lancet*, **i**, 1339.

346 COOK G.C., MORGAN J.O. & HOFFBRAND A.V. (1974) Impairment of folate absorption by systemic bacterial infections. *Lancet*, **ii**, 1416.

347 HANSEN H.A. (1964) *On the Diagnosis of Folic Acid Deficiency*, p. 90. Almqvist & Wiskell, Stockholm.

348 GILES C. (1966) An account of 335 cases of megaloblastic anaemia of pregnancy and the puerperium. *Journal of Clinical Pathology*, **19**, 1.

349 CHANARIN I., ROTHMAN D., WARD A. & PERRY J. (1968) Folate status and requirement in pregnancy. *British Medical Journal*, **ii**, 390.

350 BAUMSLAG N., EDELSTEIN T. & METZ J. (1970) Reduction of incidence of prematurity by folic acid supplementation in pregnancy. *British Medical Journal*, **i**, 16.

351 LINDENBAUM J. & KLIPSTEIN F.A. (1963) Folic-acid deficiency in sickle-cell anemia. *New England Journal of Medicine*, **269**, 875.

352 PEARSON H.A. & COBB W.T. (1964) Folic acid studies in sickle-cell anemia. *Journal of Laboratory and Clinical Medicine*, **64**, 913.

353 HOFFBRAND A.V., CHANARIN I., KREMENCHUZKY S., SZUR L., WATERS A.H. & MOLLIN D.L. (1968) Megaloblastic anaemia in myelosclerosis. *Quarterly Journal of Medicine*, **37**, 493.

354 MOLLIN D.L. & HOFFBRAND A.V. (1968) Sideroblastic anaemia. In: *Recent Advances in Clinical Pathology*, *Series V* (ed. Dyke S.C.), p. 273. Churchill, London.

355 HOFFBRAND A.V., HOBBS J.R., KREMENCHUZKY S. & MOLLIN D.L. (1967) Incidence and pathogenesis of megaloblastic erythropoiesis in multiple myeloma. *Journal of Clinical Pathology*, **20**, 699.

356 HANSEN O.P., DRIVSHOLM A. & HIPPE E. (1977) Vitamin B₁₂ metabolism in myelomatosis. *Scandinavian Journal of Haematology*, **18**, 395.

357 ROBERTS P.D., HOFFBRAND A.V. & MOLLIN D.L. (1966) Iron and folate metabolism in tuberculosis. *British Medical Journal*, **ii**, 198.

358 GOUGH K.R., MCCARTHY C., READ A.E., MOLLIN D.L. & WATERS A.H. (1964) Folic-acid deficiency in rheumatoid arthritis. *British Medical Journal*, **i**, 212.

359 STRICKLAND G.T. & KOSTINAS J.E. (1970) Folic acid deficiency complicating malaria. *American Journal of Tropical Medicine and Hygiene*, **19**, 910.

360 BRODY J.I., SOLTYS H.D. & ZINSSER H.F. (1969) Folic acid deficiency in congestive heart failure. *British Heart Journal*, **31**, 741.

361 HYDE R.D. & LOEHRY C.A.E.H. (1968) Folic acid malabsorption in cardiac failure. *Gut*, **9**, 717.

362 HAMPERS C.L., STREIFF R., NATHAN D.G., SYNDER D. & MERRILL J.P. (1967) Megaloblastic hemopoiesis in uremia and in patients on long-term hemodialysis. *New England Journal of Medicine*, **276**, 551.

363 SIDDIQUI J., FREEBURGER R. & FREEMAN R.M. (1970) Folic acid, hypersegmented polymorphonuclear leukocytes and the uremic syndrome. *American Journal of Clinical Nutrition*, **23**, 11.

364 HERBERT V., ZALUSKY R. & DAVISON C.S. (1963) Correlation of folate deficiency with alcoholism and associated macrocytosis, anemia and liver disease. *Annals of Internal Medicine*, **58**, 977.

365 KLIPSTEIN F.A. & LIMDENBAUM J. (1965) Folate deficiency in chronic liver disease. *Blood*, **25**, 445.

366 LINDENBAUM J. & LIEBER C.S. (1969) Hematologic effect of alcohol in man in the absence of nutritional deficiency. *New England Journal of Medicine*, **281**, 333.

367 SULLIVAN L.W. & HERBERT V. (1964) Suppression of hematopoiesis by ethanol. *Journal of Clinical Investigation*, **43**, 2048.

368 HINES J.D. (1969) Reversible megaloblastic and sideroblastic marrow abnormalities in alcoholic patients. *British Journal of Haematology*, **16**, 87.

369 LINDENBAUM J. (1980) Folate and vitamin B₁₂ deficiencies in alcoholism. *Seminars in Hematology*, **17**, 119.

370 WARDROP C.A.J., HEATLEY R.V., TENNANT G.B. & HUGHES L.E. (1975) Acute folate deficiency in surgical patients on aminoacid-ethanol intravenous nutrition. *Lancet*, **ii**, 640.

371 WARDROP C.A.J., LEWIS M.H., TENNANT G.B., WILLIAMS R.H.P. & HUGHES L.E. (1977) Acute folate deficiency associated with intravenous nutrition with aminoacid-sorbitol-ethanol: prophylaxis with intravenous folic acid. *British Journal of Haematology*, **37**, 521.

372 CAREY M.C., FENNELLY J.J. & FITZGERALD O. (1968) Homocystinuria. II. Subnormal serum folate levels, increased folate clearance and effects of folic acid therapy. *American Journal of Medicine*, **45**, 26.

373 CHANARIN I., ROTHMAN D. & BERRY V. (1965) Iron deficiency and its relation to folic acid status in pregnancy: results of a clinical trial. *British Medical Journal*, **i**, 480.

374 HOFFBRAND A.V., HINES J.D., HARRISON R. & MOLLIN D.L. (1967) B₁₂ and folate deficiency following partial gastrectomy. In: *Post-Gastrectomy Nutrition* (ed. Krikler D.M.), p. 1. Lloyd-Luke, London.

375 OMER A., FINLAYSON N.D.C., SHEARMAN D.J.C., SAMSON R.R. & GIRDWOOD R.H. (1970) Plasma and erythrocyte folate in iron deficiency and folate deficiency. *Blood*, **35**, 821.

376 VAN DER WEYDEN M., ROTHER M. & FIRKIN B. (1972) Megaloblastic maturation masked by iron deficiency: a biochemical basis. *British Journal of Haematology*, **22**, 299.

377 HOFFBRAND A.V., GANESHAGURU K., HOOTON J.W.L. & TATTERSALL M.H.N. (1976) Effect of iron deficiency and desferrioxamine on DNA synthesis in human cells. *British Journal of Haematology*, **33**, 517.

378 CARNEY M.W.P. (1967) Serum folate values in 423 psychiatric patients. *British Medical Journal*, **iv**, 512.

379 KLIPSTEIN F.A. (1964) Subnormal serum folate and macrocytosis associated with anticonvulsant drug therapy. *Blood*, **23**, 68.

380 BECROFT D.M.O. & HOLLAND J.T. (1966) Goat's milk and megaloblastic anaemia of infancy. *New Zealand Medical Journal*, **65**, 303.

381 KELLY D., WEIR D., REED B. & SCOTT J. (1979) Effect of anticonvulsant drugs on the rate of folate catabolism in mice. *Journal of Clinical Investigation*, **64**, 1089.

382 CHANARIN I., PERRY J. & REYNOLDS E.H. (1974) Transport of 5-methyltetrahydrofolic acid into the cerebrospinal fluid in man. *Clinical Science and Molecular Medicine*, **46**, 369.

383 TAGUCHI H., ABDUL-CADER Z., PERRY J., REYNOLDS E.H. & CHANARIN I. (1977) Effect of anticonvulsants on the uptake of 5-methyltetrahydrofolic acid by the

choroid plexus in rabbits. *Clinical Science and Molecular Medicine*, **53**, 75.

384 BOWE J.C., CORNISH E.J. & DAWSON M. (1971) Evaluation of folic acid supplements in children taking phenytoin. *Developmental Medicine and Child Neurology*, **13**, 343.

385 SHOJANIA A.M., HORNADY G.J. & BARNES P.H. (1971) The effect of oral contraceptives on folate metabolism. *American Journal of Obstetrics and Gynecology*, **111**, 782.

386 PAINE C.J., GRAFTON W.D., DICKSON G.L. & EICHNER E.R. (1975) Oral contraceptives, serum folate, and hematologic status. *Journal of the American Medical Association*, **231**, 731.

387 STEPHENS M.E.M., CRAFT I., PETERS T.J. & HOFFBRAND A.V. (1972) Oral contraception and folate metabolism. *Clinical Science*, **42**, 405.

388 CORCINO J., WAXMAN S. & HERBERT V. (1970) Mechanism of triamterene-induced megaloblastosis. *Annals of Internal Medicine*, **73**, 419.

389 BAKER H., HERBERT V., FRANK O., PASHER I., HUTNER S.H., WASSERMAN L.R. & SOBOTKA H. (1959) A microbiological method for detecting folic acid deficiency in man. *Clinical Chemistry*, **5**, 275.

390 WATERS A.H. & MOLLIN D.L. (1961) Studies on the folic acid activity of human serum. *Journal of Clinical Pathology*, **14**, 335.

391 JALALUDDIN M., CAMPBELL J.B., SANHUEZA J. & SESLER A. (1977) Observations on the determination of serum and red-cell folate levels by a radiometric assay method. *Clinical Biochemistry*, **10**, 38.

392 HERBERT V. (1966) The aseptic addition method for *L. casei* assay of folate activity in human serum. *Journal of Clinical Pathology*, **19**, 12.

393 DAWSON D.W., DELAMORE I.W., FISH D., FLAHERTY T.A., GOWENLOCK A.H., HUNT L.P., HYDE K., MacIVER J.E., THORNTON J.A. & WATERS H.M. (1980) An evaluation of commercial radioisotope methods for the determination of folate and vitamin B_{12}. *Journal of Clinical Pathology*, **33**, 234.

393a JONES P., GRACE C.S. & ROZENBERG M.C. (1979) Interprepation of serum and red cell folate results. A comparison of microbiological and radioisotopic methods. *Pathology*, **11**, 45.

394 HOFFBRAND A.V., NEWCOMBE B.F.A. & MOLLIN D.L. (1966) Method of assay of red cell folate activity and the value of the assay as a test for folate deficiency. *Journal of Clinical Pathology*, **19**, 17.

395 ZALUSKY R. & HERBERT V. (1961) Failure of forminoglutamic acid (FIGLU) excretion to distinguish vitamin B_{12} deficiency from nutritional folic acid deficiency. *Journal of Clinical Investigation*, **40**, 1091.

396 ALLEN D.M. & WHITEHEAD R.G. (1965) The excretion of urocanic acid and formiminoglutamic acid in megaloblastosis accompanying kwashiorkor. *Blood*, **25**, 283.

397 LAWSON D.H., MURRAY R.M. & PARKER J.L.W. (1972) Early mortality in the megaloblastic anaemias. *Quarterly Journal of Medicine*, **41**, 1.

398 UNGLEY C.C. (1949) Subacute combined degeneration of the cord. I. Response to liver extracts. II. Trials with vitamin B_{12}. *Brain*, **78**, 382.

399 HITZIG W.H., DOHMANN U., PLUSS H.J. & VISCHER D. (1974) Hereditary transcobalamin II deficiency: clinical findings in a new family. *Journal of Pediatrics*, **85**, 622.

400 HITZIG W.H. & KENNY A.B. (1975) The role of vitamin B_{12} and its transport globulins in the production of antibodies. *Clinical and Experimental Immunology*, **20**, 105.

401 BURMAN J.F., MOLLIN D.L., SOURIAL N.A. & SLADDEN R.A. (1979) Inherited lack of transcobalamin II in serum and megaloblastic anaemia: a further patient. *British Journal of Haematology*, **43**, 27.

402 HOFFBRAND A.V., TRIPP E., JACKSON B.F.A. & LUCK W.E. (1981) Hereditary transcobalamin II deficiency previously diagnosed as congenital dihydrofolate reductase deficiency. *New England Journal of Medicine* (in press).

403 HALL C.A., HITZIG W.H., GREEN P.D. & BEGLEY J.A. (1979) Transport of therapeutic cyanocobalamin in the congenital deficiency of transcobalamin II (TCII). *Blood*, **53**, 251.

404 SELIGMAN P.A., STEINER L.L. & ALLEN R.H. (1980) Studies of a patient with megaloblastic anemia and an abnormal transcobalamin II. *New England Journal of Medicine*, **303**, 1209.

405 LASSEN H.C.A., HENRIKSEN E., NEUKIRCH F. & KRISTENSEN H.S. (1956) Treatment of tetanus. Severe bone-marrow depression after prolonged nitrous-oxide anaesthesia. *Lancet*, **i**, 527.

406 AMESS J.A.L., BURMAN J.F., REES G.M., NANCEKIEVILL D.G. & MOLLIN D.L. (1978) Megaloblastic haemopoiesis in patients receiving nitrous oxide. *Lancet*, **ii**, 339.

407 DEACON R., LUMB M., PERRY J., CHANARIN I., MINTY B., HALSEY M.J. & NUNN J.F. Selective inactivation of vitamin B_{12} in rats by nitrous oxide. *Lancet*, **ii**, 1023.

408 LINNELL J.C., QUADROS E.V., MATTHEWS D.M., JACKSON B. & HOFFBRAND A.V. (1978) Nitrous oxide and megaloblastosis: biochemical mechanism. *Lancet*, **ii**, 1372.

409 DEACON R., LUMB M., PERRY J., CHANARIN I., MINTY B., HALSEY M.J. & NUNN J.F. (1980) Inactivation of methionine synthase by nitrous oxide. *European Journal of Biochemistry*, **104**, 419.

410 QUADROS E.V., JACKSON B., HOFFBRAND A.V. & LINNELL J.C. (1979) Interconversion of cobalamins in human lymphocytes *in vitro* and the influence of nitrous oxide on synthesis of cobalamin coenzymes. In: *Vitamin B_{12}* (ed. Zagalak B. & Friedrich W.), p. 1045. De Gruyter, Berlin.

411 DINN J.J., McCANN S., WILSON P., REED B., WEIR D. & SCOTT J. (1978) Animal model for subacute combined degeneration. *Lancet*, **ii**, 1154.

412 DEACON R., CHANARIN I., PERRY J. & LUMB M. (1980a) Impaired deoxyuridine utilization in the B_{12}-inactivated rat and its correction by folate analogues. *Biochemical and Biophysical Research Communications*, **93**, 516.

413 SAHENK Z., MENDELL J.R., COURI D. & NACHTMAN J. (1978) Polyneuropathy from inhalation of N_2O cartridges through a whipped-cream dispenser. *Neurology*, **28**, 485.

414 KRIPKE B.J., TALARICO L., SHAH N.K. & KELMAN A.D. (1977) Hematologic reaction to prolonged exposure to nitrous oxide. *Anesthesiology*, **47**, 342.

415 LAYZER R.B. (1978) Myeloneuropathy after prolonged exposure to nitrous oxide. *Lancet*, **ii**, 1227.

415a LAYZER R.B., FISHMAN R.A. & SCHAFTER J.A. (1978) Neuropathy following abuse of nitrous oxide. *Neurology*, **28**, 504.

416 GUTMAN L., FARRELL B., CROSBY T.W. & JOHNSON D. (1979) Nitrous oxide-induced myelopathy-neuropathy: potential for chronic misuse by dentists. *Journal of the American Dental Association*, **98**, 58.

417 LINNELL J.C., SMITH A.D.M., SMITH C.L., WILSON J. & MATTHEWS D.M. (1968) Effects of smoking on metabolism and excretion of vitamin B$_{12}$. *British Medical Journal*, **ii**, 215.

418 TAURO G.P., DANKS D.M., ROSE P.B., VAN DER WEYDEN M.B., SCHWARZ M.A., COLLINS V.L. & NEAL B.W. (1976) Dihydrofolate reductase deficiency causing megaloblastic anemia in two families. *New England Journal of Medicine*, **294**, 466.

419 BERTINO J.R. (ed.) (1971) Folate antagonists as chemotherapeutic agents. *Annals of New York Academy of Sciences*, **186.**

420 BERTINO J.R., LEVITT M., McCULLOUGH J.L. & CHABNER B. (1971) New approaches to chemotherapy with folate antagonists. Use of leucovorin 'rescue' and enzymic folate depletion. *Annals of New York Academy of Sciences*, **186**, 486.

421 HOFFBRAND A.V. & TRIPP E. (1972) Unbalanced deoxyribonucleotide synthesis caused by methotrexate. *British Medical Journal*, **ii**, 140.

422 SIVE J., GREEN R. & METZ J. (1972) Effect of trimethoprim on folate-dependent DNA synthesis in human bone marrow. *Journal of Clinical Pathology*, **25**, 194.

423 STEBBINS R. & BERTINO J.R. (1976) Megaloblastic anaemia produced by drugs. *Clinics in Haematology*, **5**, 619.

424 CHANARIN I. & ENGLAND J.M. (1972) Toxicity of trimethoprim-sulphamethoxazole in patients with megaloblastic haemopoiesis. *British Medical Journal*, **i**, 651.

425 SALTER A.J. (1973) The toxicity profile of trimethoprim/sulphamethoxazole after four years of widespread use. *Medical Journal of Australia*, **1** (Suppl. 2), 70.

426 BRANDA R.F., MOLDOW C.F., MACARTHUR J.R., WINTROBE M.M., ANTHONY B.K. & JACOBS H.S. (1978) Folate induced remission in aplastic anemia with familial defect of cellular folate uptake. *New England Journal of Medicine*, **298**, 469.

427 HOWE R.B., BRANDA R.F., DOUGLAS S.D. & BRUNNING R.D. (1979) Hereditary dyserythropoiesis with abnormal membrane folate transport. *Blood*, **54**, 1080.

428 HUGULEY C.M. JR, BAIN J.A., RIVERS S.L. & SCOGGINS R.B. (1959) Refractory megaloblastic anemia associated with excretion of orotic acid. *Blood*, **14**, 615.

429 BECROFT D.M.O., PHILLIPS L.I. & SIMMONDS A. (1969) Hereditary orotic aciduria: long-term therapy with uridine and a trial of uracil. *Journal of Pediatrics*, **75**, 885.

430 ROGERS L.E., NICOLAISEN A.K. & HOLT J.G. (1975) Hereditary orotic aciduria: results of a screening survey. *Journal of Laboratory and Clinical Medicine*, **85**, 287.

431 JADHAV M., WEBB J.K.G., VAISHNAVA S. & BAKER S.J. (1962) Vitamin B$_{12}$ deficiency in Indian infants. A clinical syndrome. *Lancet*, **ii**, 903.

432 ROGERS L.E., PORTER F.S. & SIDBURY J.B. JR (1969) Thiamine-responsive megaloblastic anemia. *Journal of Pediatrics*, **74**, 494.

433 LAMPKIN B.C., PYESMANY A., HYMAN C.B. & HAMMOND D. (1971) Congenital familial megaloblastic anemia. *Blood*, **37**, 615.

434 VAN DER ZEE S.P.M., LOMMEN E.J.P., TRIJBELS J.M.F. & SCHRETLEN E.D.A.M. (1970) The influence of adenine on the clinical features and purine metabolism in the Lesch–Nyhan syndrome. *Acta Paediatrica Scandinavica*, **59**, 259.

435 MAJAJ A.S., DINNING J.S., AZZAM S.A. & DARBY W.J. (1963) Vitamin E responsive megaloblastic anemia in infants with protein-calorie malnutrition. *American Journal of Clinical Nutrition*, **12**, 374.

436 HEATH C.W. (1966) Cytogenetic observations in vitamin B$_{12}$ and folate deficiency. *Blood*, **27**, 800.

437 MENZIES R.C., CROSSEN P.E., FITZGERALD P.H. & GUNZ F.W. (1966) Cytogenetic and cytochemical studies on marrow cells in B$_{12}$ and folate deficiency. *Blood*, **28**, 581.

438 WICKRAMASINGHE S.N., CHALMERS D.G. & COOPER E.H. (1968) Disturbed proliferation of erythropoietic cells in pernicious anaemia. *Nature (London)*, **215**, 189.

439 WICKRAMASINGHE S.N. (1972) Kinetics and morphology of haemopoiesis in pernicious anaemia. *British Journal of Haematology*, **22**, 111.

440 HOFFBRAND A.V. & PEGG A.E. (1972) DNA base composition in normoblastic and megaloblastic marrow. *Nature (New Biology)*, **235**, 187.

441 THORELL B. (1947) Studies on the formation of cellular substances during blood cell production. *Acta Medica Scandinavica*, **128** (Suppl. 200), 1.

442 KILLMANN S.A. (1964) Effect of deoxyuridine on incorporation of tritiated thymidine: Difference between normoblasts and megaloblasts. *Acta Medica Scandinavica*, **175**, 483.

443 METZ J., KELLY A., CHAPPINSWETT V., WAXMAN S. & HERBERT V. (1968) Deranged DNA synthesis by bone marrow from vitamin B$_{12}$-deficient humans. *British Journal of Haematology*, **14**, 575.

444 DAS K.C. & HOFFBRAND A.V. (1970) Lymphocyte transformation in megaloblastic anaemia: morphology and DNA synthesis. *British Journal of Haematology*, **19**, 459.

445 WICKRAMASINGHE S.N., DODSWORTH H., RAULT R.M.J. & HULME B. (1974) Observations on the incidence and cause of macrocytosis in patients on azathioprine therapy following renal transplanation. *Transplantation*, **18**, 443.

446 TATTERSALL M.H.N., LAVOIE A., GANESHAGURU K., TRIPP E. & HOFFBRAND A.V. (1975) Deoxyribonucleoside triphosphates in human cells: changes in disease and following exposure to drugs. *European Journal of Clinical Investigation*, **2**, 191.

447 PELLINIEMI T.-T. & BECK W.S. (1980) Biochemical mechanisms in the Killmann experiment in human lymphocyte cultures: a critique of the 'Deoxyuridine suppression test'. *Journal of Clinical Investigation*, **65**, 449.

447a ELLIMS P.H., HAYMAN R.J. & VAN DER WEYDEN M.B. (1979) Expression of fetal thymidine kinase in human cobalamin or folate deficient lymphocytes. *Biochemical and Biophysical Research Communications*, **89**, 103.

448 HOOTON J.W.L. & HOFFBRAND A.V. (1976) Thymidine kinase in megaloblastic anaemia. *British Journal of Haematology*, **33**, 527.

449 TAHERI R., WICKREMASINGHE R.G. & HOFFBRAND A.V. (1981) Metabolism of thymine nucleotides synthesised via the *de novo* mechanism in normal and megaloblastic human cells. *Biochemical Journal*, **196**, 225.

450 WICKREMASINGHE R.G. & HOFFBRAND A.V. (1979) Defective DNA synthesis in megaloblastic anaemia: studies employing velocity sedimentation in alkaline sucrose density gradients. *Biochimica et Biophysica Acta*, **563**, 46.

451 WICKREMASINGHE R.G. & HOFFBRAND A.V. (1980) Reduced rate of DNA replication fork movement in megaloblastic anemia. *Journal of Clinical Investigation*, **65**, 26.

452 WICKREMASINGHE R.G. & HOFFBRAND A.V. (1980) Conversion of partially single stranded replicating DNA to double-stranded DNA in delayed in megaloblastic anaemia. *Biochemica et Biophysica Acta*, **607**, 411.

453 HOFFBRAND A.V., GANESHAGURU K., HOOTON J.W.L. & TRIPP E. (1976) Megaloblastic anaemia: initiation of DNA synthesis in excess of DNA chain elongation as the underlying mechanism. *Clinical Haematology*, **5**, 727.

454 HOOTON J.W.L. & HOFFBRAND A.V. (1977) DNA synthesis in isolated lymphocyte nuclei. Effects of megaloblastic anaemia due to folate or vitamin B_{12} deficiency or antimetabolite drugs. *Biochimica et Biophysica Acta*, **477**, 250.

454a DARDICK I., SHEININ R. & SETTERFIELD G. (1978) Mutant mouse L-cells: a model for megaloblastic anaemia. *British Journal of Haematology*, **39**, 483.

455 HOFFBRAND A.V., GANESHAGURU K., LAVOIE A., TATTERSALL M.H.N. & TRIPP E. (1974) Thymidylate concentration in megaloblastic anaemia. *Nature (London)*, **248**, 602.

456 REDDY G.P.V. & MATTHEWS C.K. (1978) Functional compartmentation of DNA precursors in T_4 phage-infected bacteria. *Journal of Biochemical Chemistry*, **253**, 3461.

457 REDDY C.P.V. & PARDEE A.B. (1980) Multienzyme complex for metabolic channeling in mammalian DNA replication. *Proceedings of the National Academy of Sciences, USA*, **77**, 3312.

458 TAHERI R., WICKREMASINGHE R.G. & HOFFBRAND A.V. (1981) Alternative metabolic fates of thymine nucleotides in human cells. *Biochemical Journal*, **194**, 451.

459 SAKAMOTO S., NIINA M. & TAKAKU F. (1975) Thymidine synthetase activity in bone marrow cells in pernicious anemia. *Blood*, **46**, 699.

460 HERBERT V. & ZALUSKY R. (1962) Interrelation of vitamin B_{12} and folic acid metabolism: folic acid clearance studies. *Journal of Clinical Investigation*, **41**, 1263.

461 NORONHA J.M. & SILVERMAN M. (1962) On folic acid, vitamin B_{12}, methionine and formiminoglutamic acid metabolism. In: *Vitamin B_{12} and Intrinsic Factor II*. Europäisches Symposium (ed. Heinrich H.C.), p. 728. Enke, Stuttgart.

462 DAS K.C. & HERBERT V. (1976) Vitamin B_{12}-folate interrelations. *Clinics in Haematology*, **5**, 697.

463 STEBBINS R.D., MELLER F., ROSENGARTEN H., FRIEDHOFF A. & SILBER R. (1976) Identification of N^5N^{10} methylene tetrahydrofolate reductase as the enzyme involved in the 5-methyltetrahydrofolate-dependent formation of a β-carboline derivative of 5-hydroxytryptamine in human platelets. *Archives of Biochemistry and Biophysics*, **173**, 673.

464 PEARSON A.G.M. & TURNER A.J. (1975) Folate dependent I-carbon transfer to biogenic amines mediated by methylenetetrahydrofolate reductase. *Nature (London)*, **258**, 173.

465 WAXMAN S., METZ J. & HERBERT V. (1969) Defective DNA synthesis in human megaloblastic bone marrow: effects of homocysteine and methionine. *Journal of Clinical Investigation*, **48**, 284.

466 GANESHAGURU K. & HOFFBRAND A.V. (1978) The effect of deoxyuridine, vitamin B_{12}, folate and alcohol on the uptake of thymidine and on the deoxynucleoside triphosphate concentrations in normal and megaloblastic cells. *British Journal of Haematology*, **40**, 29.

467 ZITTOUN J., MARQUET J. & ZITTOUN R. (1978) Effect of folate and cobalamin compounds on the deoxyuridine suppression test in vitamin B_{12} and folate deficiency. *Blood*, **51**, 119.

468 TISMAN G. & HERBERT V. (1973) B_{12} dependence of cell uptake of serum folate: an explanation for high serum folate and cell folate depletion in B_{12} deficiency. *Blood*, **41**, 465.

469 McGING P., REED B., WEIR D.G. & SCOTT J.M. (1978) The effect of vitamin B_{12} inhibition *in vivo*. Impaired folate polyglutamate biosynthesis indicating that 5-methyltetrahydropteroylglutamate is not its usual substrate. *Biochemical and Biophysical Research Communication*, **82**, 540.

470 PERRY J., CHANARIN I., DEACON R. & LUMB M. (1979) The substrate for folate polyglutamate biosynthesis in the vitamin B_{12}-inactivated rat. *Biochemical and Biophysical Research Communication*, **91**, 678.

471 LUMB M., DEACON R., PERRY J., CHANARIN I., MINTY B., HALSEY M.J. & NUNN J.F. (1980) The effect of nitrous oxide inactivation of vitamin B_{12} on rat hepatic folate. Implications for the methylfolate-trap hypothesis. *Biochemical Journal*, **186**, 933.

472 THENEN S.W. & STOKSTAD E.L.R. (1973) Effect of methionine on specific folate coenzyme pools in vitamin B_{12} deficient and supplemented rats. *Journal of Nutrition*, **103**, 363.

473 JEEJEEBHOY K.N., PATHARE S.M. & NORONHA J.M. (1965) Observations on conjugated and unconjugated blood folate levels in megaloblastic anemia and the effects of vitamin B_{12}. *Blood*, **26**, 354.

474 PERRY J. & CHANARIN I. (1977) Abnormal folate polyglutamate ratios in untreated pernicious anaemia corrected by therapy. *British Journal of Haematology*, **35**, 397.

475 SPRONK A.M. (1974) Tetrahydrofolate polyglutamate synthesis in rat liver. *Federation Proceedings*, **32**, 471.

476 CHANARIN I., DEACON R., LUMB M. & PERRY J. (1980) Vitamin B_{12} regulates folate metabolism by the supply of formate. *Lancet*, **ii**, 505.

477 DEACON R., CHANARIN I., PERRY J. & LUMB M. (1981) Marrow cells from untreated pernicious anaemia can-

not use tetrahydrofolate normally. *British Journal of Haematology*, **46**, 523.

478 TAHERI R., WICKREMASINGHE R.G. & HOFFBRAND A.V. (1981) Metabolism of deoxyuridine-derived nucleotides by megaloblastic marrow cells. *British Journal of Haematology* (in press).

479 KUTZBACH C., GALLOWAY E. & STOKSTAD E.L.R. (1967) Influence of vitamin B$_{12}$ and methionine on levels of folic acid compounds and folate enzymes in rat liver. *Proceedings of the Society of Experimental Biology and Medicine*, **124**, 801.

480 KREBS H.A., HEMS R. & TYLER B. (1976) The regulation of folate and methionine metabolism. *Biochemical Journal*, **158**, 341.

481 HERBERT V. & SULLIVAN L.W. (1963) Formiminoglutamic aciduria in humans with megaloblastic anemia: diminution by methionine or glycine. *Proceedings of the Society of Experimental Biology and Medicine*, **112**, 304.

482 HERBERT V., STREIFF R., SULLIVAN L. & McGEER P. (1964) Accumulation of a purine intermediate (aminoimidazole-carboxamide) (AIC) in megaloblastic anemias associated with vitamin B$_{12}$ deficiency, folate deficiency with alcoholism and liver disease. *Federation Proceedings*, **23**, 188.

483 ELLEGAARD J. & ESMANN V. (1973) Folate deficiency in pernicious anaemia measured by determination of decreased serine synthesis in lymphocytes. *British Journal of Haematology*, **24**, 571.

484 HOFFBRAND A.V. (1971) The megaloblastic anaemias. In: *Recent Advances in Haematology* (ed. Goldberg A. & Brain M.C.), p. 1. Churchill, London.

485 LAJTHA L.G. & KUMATORI T. (1957) Nucleic acid metabolism in megaloblastic marrows *in vitro*. *Nature (London)*, **180**, 991.

486 BURKA E.R. & MARKS P.A. (1967) Protein synthesis in human reticulocytes induced by therapy of megaloblastic anemia. *Blood*, **30**, 405.

487 FRENKEL E.P. (1973) Abnormal fatty acid metabolism in peripheral nerves of patients with pernicious anemia. *Journal of Clinical Investigation*, **52**, 1237.

488 FRENKEL E.P., KITCHENS R.L. & JOHNSTON J.M. (1973) The effect of vitamin B$_{12}$ deprivation on the enzymes of fatty acid synthesis. *Journal of Biological Chemistry*, **248**, 7540.

489 JACOBSON W., GANDY G. & SIDMAN R.L. (1973) Experimental subacute combined degeneration of the cord in mice. *Journal of Pathology*, **109**, xiii.

490 DINN J.J., WEIR D.G., McCANN S., REED B., WILSON P. & SCOTT J.M. (1980) Methyl group deficiency in nerve tissue: a hypothesis to explain the lesion of subacute combined degeneration. *Irish Journal of Medical Science*, **149**, 1.

491 UDENFRIEND S. (1966) Formation of hydroxyproline in collagen. *Science*, **152**, 1335.

492 LIPSCHITZ D.A., BOTHWELL T.H., SEFTEL H.C., WAPNICK A.A. & CHARLTON R.W. (1971) The role of ascorbic acid in the metabolism of storage iron. *British Journal of Haematology*, **20**, 155.

493 MAZUR A., GREEN S.Z. & CARLETON A. (1960) Mechanism of plasma iron incorporation into hepatic ferritin. *Journal of Biological Chemistry*, **235**, 595.

494 ROESER H.P., HALLIDAY J.W., SIZEMORE D.J., NIKLES A. & WILLGOSS D. (1980) Serum ferritin in ascorbic acid deficiency. *British Journal of Haematology*, **45**, 459.

495 CHAPMAN R.W., HUSSAIN M.A.M., GORMAN A.G., POLITIS D., FLYNN D.M., SHERLOCK S. & HOFFBRAND A.V. *Journal of Clinical Pathology* (submitted).

496 HUSSAIN M.A.M., FLYNN D.M., GREEN N. & HOFFBRAND A.V. (1977) Effect of dose, time, and ascorbate on iron excretion after subcutaneous desferrioxamine. *Lancet*, **i**, 977.

497 MEDICAL RESEARCH COUNCIL (1948) Vitamin-C requirements of human adults. Experimental study of vitamin-C deprivation in man. *Lancet*, **i**, 853.

498 GOLDBERG A. (1963) The anaemia of scurvy. *Quarterly Journal of Medicine*, **32**, 51.

499 COX E.V. (1968) The anaemia of scurvy. *Vitamins and Hormones*, **26**, 635.

500 COX E.V., MEYNELL M.J., NORTHAM S.E. & COOKE W.T. (1967) The anemia of scurvy. *American Journal of Medicine*, **42**, 220.

501 ZALUSKY R. & HERBERT V. (1961) Megaloblastic anemia in scurvy with response to 50 microgram of folic acid daily. *New England Journal of Medicine*, **265**, 1033.

502 ASQUITH P., OELBAUM M.H. & DAWSON D.W. (1967) Scorbutic megaloblastic anaemia responding to ascorbic acid alone. *British Medical Journal*, **iv**, 402.

503 MAY C.D., HAMILTON A. & STEWART C.T. (1953) Experimental megaloblastic anaemia and scurvy in the monkey. *Journal of Nutrition*, **49**, 121.

504 NEALE G., ANTCLIFFE A.C., WELBOURN R.B., MOLLIN D.L. & BOOTH C.C. (1967) Protein malnutrition after partial gastrectomy. *Quarterly Journal of Medicine*, **36**, 369.

505 FOY H. & KONDI A. (1968) Comparison between erythroid aplasia in marasmus and kwashiorkor and the experimentally induced erythroid aplasia in baboons by riboflavin deficiency. *Vitamin and Hormones*, **26**, 653.

506 ADAMS E.B. (1970) Anemia associated with protein deficiency. *Seminars in Hematology*, **7**, 55.

507 McKENZIE D., FRIEDMAN R., KATZ S. & LANZKOWSKY P. (1967) Erythropoietin levels in anemia and kwashiorkor. *South African Medical Journal*, **41**, 1044.

508 LANE M. & ALFREY C.P. JR (1965) The anemia of human riboflavin deficiency. *Blood*, **25**, 432.

509 ALFREY C.P. JR & LANE M. (1970) The effect of riboflavin deficiency on erythropoiesis. *Seminars in Hematology*, **7**, 49.

510 ALTMAN K.I. & MILLER G. (1953) A disturbance of tryptophane metabolism in congenital hypoplastic anaemia. *Nature (London)*, **172**, 868.

Chapter 7
Red-cell metabolism: hereditary enzymopathies

PAULINE M. EMERSON AND A. J. GRIMES

NORMAL RED-CELL METABOLISM

Normal, human and mature red cells survive in the circulation for 110–120 days [1] and are maintained in a physiological state simply by the flux of glucose through the Embden–Meyerhof (EMP) and pentose-phosphate (PPP) pathways. In this respect the metabolism of adult red cells is much less complex than that of their nucleated precursors which are capable of division, DNA, RNA, haem, protein and lipid synthesis, and contain glycogen, a respiratory chain and Krebs cycle. Red-cell precursors contain all the components and subcellular organelles present in any nucleated cell, but almost all of them atrophy with the loss of the nucleus. Remnants of the cells' former metabolic capacity are detectable during the reticulocyte phase but on maturation to adult cells only the EMP and PPP are retained. This decline of the cells' metabolic capacity is shown in Table 7.1.

Collated data on the contents of mature red cells [2] show the presence of nearly 100 enzymes but only some 25 are known to be required in the two glycolytic pathways and their associated reactions. It seems likely that those enzymes for which no function has been designated in mature red cells are locked in and remain detectable only so long as their activity persists. Whether relevant or not to metabolism there is no mechanism for enzyme synthesis in mature red cells and so each enzyme decays at its characteristic rate throughout the lifespan of the cell. This decline in enzyme activity is certainly one of the mechanisms of red-cell ageing because eventually the glycolytic rate becomes inadequate to maintain the concentrations of glycolytic intermediates several of which are indispensable to the function of the cell.

Some 25 phosphate esters are present in the cell and their concentration is maintained by glucose flux through the EMP and PPP. Two of them, ATP and 2,3-DPG, are concerned with special functions in the cell (Table 7.2). Three others, namely NADH, NADPH and GSH have specific roles in maintaining the *status quo* of mature cells (Table 7.2).

Utilization of glucose
D-Glucose is the normal substrate required by the cell although it can utilize galactose, fructose or mannose. Pentoses and disaccharides are not metabolized. Red cells can also use the nucleosides inosine, adenosine and guanosine because a nucleoside phosphorylase present in the cells will cleave the nucleoside to give ribose 1-phosphate and this is converted by phosphoribosylmutase to ribose 5-phosphate, an intermediate of the PPP (see Fig 7.3).

D-glucose passes into the cell by facilitated diffusion,

Table 7.1. Metabolic characteristics of red cells during maturation [610]

	Nucleated cell	Reticulocyte	Mature cell
Division	+	0	0
DNA synthesis	+	0	0
RNA synthesis	+	0	0
RNA present	+	+	0
Lipid synthesis	+	+	0
Haem synthesis	+	+	0
Protein synthesis	+	+	0
Cytochrome and electron transfer	+	+	0
Krebs cycle	+	+	0
EMP	+	+	+
PPP	+	+	+

Table 7.2. Role of key glycolytic intermediates in red-cell function

	EMP	PPP
Cell shape and flexibility Membrane function	ATP	GSH
Regulation of oxygen transport	2,3-DPG ATP	
Reducing potential	NADH	NADPH GSH

a mechanism which requires no energy, is unaffected by insulin, and occurs independently of cellular metabolism. Pentoses and hexoses can also enter the cell but disaccharides like sucrose, lactose and maltose are essentially impermeant.

Glycogen

Normal red cells have no glycogen deposits and depend upon the plasma glucose to maintain glycolysis. The enzymes necessary for the synthesis and breakdown of glycogen are present in the cell and indeed glycogen turnover normally takes place; it does not accumulate because glycogen synthetase activity is too low [3, 4]. Only in some of the glycogen storage diseases where the degradative enzymes are present in low-activity mutant forms does glycogen appear in the cells [5–8]. Its presence appears to have little consequence, for although glucose consumption is increased, the reticulocyte count and cell survival are normal [9, 10].

Embden–Meyerhof pathway

The pathway is shown in Figure 7.1. The normal substrate, D-glucose, passes through the pathway at a rate of 1–2 mmols/litre of red cells/hour at 37°C and maintains the phosphorylated intermediates at the concentrations shown in Table 7.3. This rate is well

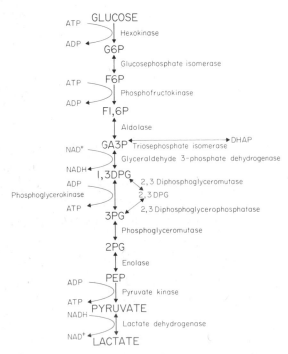

Fig. 7.1. The Embden–Meyerhof pathway (EMP).

below the maximum indicated by the maximum velocities of the individual enzymes assayed in dilute haemolysates (Table 7.4). Such values, although comparable with other published data, do not reflect the situation within the cell for they are maximum activities obtained in dilute solution in the presence of excess substrate and cofactors. Nevertheless, they demonstrate that the maximum activities differ by three orders of magnitude and that Hx displays the least activity which is only threefold greater than the glycolytic rate in intact cells. This fact, together with the close correspondence between the rate of decline of Hx activity and the fall in the rate of glycolysis as red cells mature [11] has suggested that Hx is a pacemaker of glycolysis. However, the situation is more complex than this because several of the glycolytic enzymes are acting under constraints imposed by the presence of inhibitors.

Regulation of the glycolytic rate

The rather complex multi-step control of glycolysis has been dealt with in detail [12] and is considered here only in outline. Most of the glycolytic enzymes operate in the cell near to equilibrium and are reversible. The three kinases Hx, PFK, and PK are not in this category, they work far removed from equilibrium and are essentially irreversible; they also have low activities (Table 7.4) and are under restraint from a number of effectors (Table 7.5). One of the aims of glycolysis is to produce ATP from ADP and to maintain the concentration of the former in the cell. ATP stimulates Hx activity but is an inhibitor both of PFK and PK activity. In stimulating Hx activity the product (G6P) exerts an inhibitory effect on the enzyme. The overall result of an increase in the ATP concentration is a reduction in the rate of glycolysis, whereas a fall in the ATP concentration stimulates the glycolytic rate.

Such a mechanism for the control of the glycolytic rate is likely to be an oversimplification because small changes in ATP concentration are probably too slight to provoke alterations in the glycolytic rate. However, the concentrations of the three nucleotides ATP, ADP and AMP are related via the adenylate kinase (AK) reaction:

$$2ADP \underset{AK}{\rightleftharpoons} AMP + ATP$$

ADP and AMP, but particularly the latter, are present in the cells at low concentration compared with ATP (Table 7.3). Thus, a small change in ATP concentration gives a large fractional change in AMP, and AK responds by acting so as to prevent leakage of adenine nucleotides down to irrecoverable products of nucleotide breakdown. In this way AK is a device for 'topping up' the ATP concentration. In addition AMP is one of

Table 7.3. Average concentration of EMP intermediates in fresh, human, mature red cells*

Intermediate	Abbreviation	Concentration (μmol/dl red cells)
Glucose 6-phosphate	G6P	3·4
Fructose 6-phosphate	F6P	1·3
Fructose 1,6-diphosphate	F1,6P	0·5
Glyceraldehyde 3-phosphate	GA3P	0·55
Dihydroxyacetone phosphate	DHAP	1·3
2,3-diphosphoglycerate	2,3-DPG	450
3-phosphoglycerate	3PG	4·7
2-phosphoglycerate	2PG	1·0
Phosphoenolpyruvate	PEP	1·4
Adenosine 5'-triphosphate	ATP	130
Adenosine 5'-diphosphate	ADP	13
Adenosine 5'-monophosphate	AMP	3·4

* Data compiled from Refs. 16, 28, 30 and 454.

the effectors of PFK and a small change in the ATP concentration produces a large fractional change in the AMP concentration by which PFK is affected. In this way AMP acts as an amplifier of small changes in ATP and thereby offers a more sensitive mechanism for the control of glycolysis. Such a role for AMP is not proven in red cells but has experimental support from experiments in other tissues [13]. This fine control could integrate with the multi-step regulation provided by Hx, PFK and PK.

Table 7.4. Maximum velocities of glycolytic enzymes assayed in haemolysates*

Enzyme	Abbreviation	Velocity
Hexokinase	HX	10
Glucosephosphate isomerase	GPI	151
Phosphofructokinase	PFK	82
Aldolase	Aldolase	31
Glyceraldehydephosphate dehydrogenase	GAPD	800
Triosephosphate isomerase	TPI	5100
Phosphoglycerate kinase	PGK	1910
2,3-diphosphoglycerate mutase	DPGM	
2,3-diphosphoglycerate phosphatase	DPGase	
Phosphoglycerate mutase	PGM	228
Enolase	Enolase	95
Pyruvate kinase	PK	158
Lactate dehydrogenase	LDH	1257

* Units of activity are mmols of substrate converted per litre of red cells per hour at 25°C. All enzymes were assayed at pH 8·1, the value of overall maximum glycolytic activity in intact red cells. Data compiled from Ref. 15.

Factors affecting the glycolytic rate

The velocity of glucose flux through the EMP is affected by several factors of physiological significance including pH, inorganic phosphate, oxygen tension and temperature. In pathological conditions which are not connected with any red cell defects any of these four factors may be outside the normal range and will change the glycolytic rate and may alter the concentrations of glycolytic intermediates. In general, such changes in glycolysis would not be expected to derange cell metabolism to the point of provoking haemolysis.

Influence of pH. The glycolytic rate has long been known to be sensitive to pH; a rise of blood pH increases the rate to a maximum at *c.* 8·1 while a fall of pH diminishes it [14–16].

Table 7.5. Effectors of EMP enzymes

Enzyme	Activators	Inhibitors
Hx		
GPI		
PFK	G1,6P, AMP, NH_4^+, P_i, ADP	ATP, H^+, t^0, 2,3-DPG
Aldolase		
GAPD		NADH, 2,3-DPG
TPI		
PGK		
DPGM		2,3-DPG
DPGase		3PG
PGM		
Enolase		
PK	F1,6P, H^+	ATP, 2,3-DPG
LDH		

A rise of pH has different effects at several points in the pathway. These include:

1 a fall in ATP concentration without an equivalent rise in ADP level so that there is a fall in the total nucleotide pool;

2 a marked rise in the F1,6P concentration due to a release of the pH-sensitive ATP inhibition of PFK;

3 a fall in inorganic phosphate concentration;

4 a decrease in the $NAD^+/NADH$ ratio—such changes once implicated GAPD in the regulation of glycolysis but the reaction is reversible and is not now thought to be involved; and

5 a decrease in the G6P concentration which releases Hx from product inhibition and increases its activity despite the lowered ATP level.

A decrease in the blood pH diminishes the glycolytic rate in two ways. First, the G6P concentration is increased which diminishes Hx activity. In addition, an accumulation of pyruvate causes increased PK activity due to the effector action of an increased H^+. This increase in activity does not overcome the inhibition of Hx and PFK activity.

Influence of inorganic phosphate. It is well known that the glycolytic rate is stimulated by the presence of inorganic phosphate [17–25]. The data of the last author suggests that a significant rise in the rate of glycolysis requires an increase of inorganic phosphate to several times the physiological level (1 mM). Hypophosphataemia, induced by dietary manipulation, depresses the glycolytic rate and decreases the concentrations of both ATP and 2,3-DPG [12, 26]. At physiological pH values an increased inorganic phosphate also raises the ATP concentration as well as those of all intermediates between F1,6P and PEP [20]. The G6P concentration is unaffected but ADP is somewhat decreased which serves to stimulate Hx activity. Despite the raised ATP concentration, PFK activity is increased because inorganic phosphate releases ATP inhibition of the enzyme.

Influence of oxygen tension. Under anaerobic conditions the glycolytic rate is significantly increased [16, 27, 28]. This occurs because deoxyhaemoglobin is a stronger base than oxyhaemoglobin and protons combine with the deoxy form, raising the intracellular pH and thus the glycolytic rate. Values for the concentrations of glycolytic intermediates also suggest that anaerobic conditions increase the intracellular pH because crossover points occur at both PFK and PK steps [12, 28, 29]. However, an explanation based on pH alone is not adequate because of the involvement of 2,3-DPG with haemoglobin. The total content of this ester is higher in red cells under anaerobic conditions but the amount of the free ester which is available in the EMP is less because of the binding to deoxyhaemoglobin. 2,3-DPG exerts an inhibitory effect at several points in the pathway—at the GAPD, 2,3-DPGM and PK steps—and this will modify the phosphate ester pattern.

Influence of temperature. The glycolytic rate rises with a rise of temperature to a maximum at 48°C independent of pH [14]. At 2–6°C, the usual temperature range for the storage of banked blood, the rate of glucose consumption of red cells stored in ACD is *c.* 0·05 mmols/litre of red cells/hour, or about 2·5% of the rate at 37°C [1]. The pattern of change of the phosphate ester concentration at low temperature has been studied in considerable detail with a view to preventing or reversing the storage lesion which appears when blood is stored for up to 21 days prior to transfusion. It is not intended to consider this topic here [1]. Over short periods of storage at low temperature, sufficient only to allow the EMP to achieve equilibrium, a crossover point occurs at PFK with accumulation of F1,6P and triose phosphates [30].

Role of ATP

The nucleotide pool in mature red cells consists mainly of ATP, ADP and AMP whose concentrations are in the ratio 40:4:1 (Table 7.3). Other nucleotides are also present at low concentration (e.g. GTP and ITP) and there is some interplay between the purine compounds in the cell, but ATP is the cells' major nucleotide in both quantitative and functional terms.

Two moles of ATP are generated per mole of glucose consumed to yield a steady-state concentration of 80–140 μmol/dl of packed cells, that is 0·8–1·4 mM with respect to packed cells, or 1·2–2·1 mM with respect to cell water. ATP is the prime energy source in the cell and is associated particularly with three cellular activities. These are:

1 the maintenance of the cation and water content of the cell, a process mediated by the sodium and calcium pumps;

2 as a substitute for 2,3-DPG in modulating the position of the oxygen dissociation curve (see Chapter 8); and

3 in the preservation of cell shape and flexibility (see Chapter 10).

The sodium pump

Red cells are similar to other cell types in containing a low sodium (Na^+) and high potassium (K^+) concentration (Table 7.6). Passage of both Na^+ and K^+ occurs down their concentration gradients and, in the absence of any device preventing it, Na^+ would accumulate while K^+ would be lost from the cell. The net entry rate of Na^+ exceeds the net rate of K^+ efflux

Table 7.6. Red-cell and plasma concentrations of important cations*

Ion	Plasma	Cell
Sodium (Na$^+$)	130–140 mM	6–20 mM
Potassium (K$^+$)	3–4·5 mM	90 mM
Calcium (Ca^{2+})	1–11 mM	16–41 μM

* Data on other cations are given in Ref. 455.

so that the cellular content of Na$^+$+K$^+$ would increase and net entry of water take place in order to reduce the cation concentration. This would result in cell swelling and eventual lysis. The purpose of the Na$^+$ pump is to prevent cell swelling by reversing the passive influx of Na$^+$ and efflux of K$^+$. Such a reversal requires that the cations shall be passed uphill against their concentration gradients, an active transport process that requires ATP as an energy source.

Red-cell membranes contain a Na$^+$- and K$^+$-dependent ATPase [31, 32] and this is the site for the outward transport of Na$^+$ and the inward transport of K$^+$ in a coupled and asymmetric reaction expressed as follows:

$$3Na + ATP + 2K \longrightarrow 2K + ADP + P_i + 3Na$$

$$\underbrace{\qquad}_{\text{Inside} \quad \text{Outside}} \qquad \underbrace{\qquad}_{\text{Inside} \quad \text{Outside}}$$

Magnesium (Mg^{2+}) is also required in the reaction because ATP functions as the Mg^{2+} salt. The rate of pumping is sensitive to external K$^+$ and to internal Na$^+$, these are the sides of the membrane from which the respective ions are pumped. The pump is inhibited by cardioactive steroids such as ouabain, strophanthin, digoxin and scillaren [33] which act upon the external side of the membrane at the site of entry of K$^+$. A phosphorylated intermediate is involved in the simultaneous transport of Na$^+$ and K$^+$ and the simplest reaction sequence to express this is given by [34]:

$$ATP + E \xrightarrow[\text{Mg}^{2+}, \text{Na}^+]{} E_1 - P + ADP$$

$$E_1 - P \xrightarrow[\text{Mg}^{2+}]{} E_2 - P$$

$$E_2 - P \xrightarrow[\text{K}^+]{} E + P_i$$

where $E_1 - P$ and $E_2 - P$ are two phosphorylated forms of an intermediate protein. Thus a Na$^+$-dependent phosphorylation of the protein and a K$^+$-dependent release of P$_i$ occurs, and it is the latter reaction which is inhibited by cardiac glycosides.

The ATP required in the initial Na$^+$-dependent phosphorylation step appears to be sited in a membrane compartment [35–37] and it may be relevant that the EMP enzymes are also located at the membrane rather than freely dispersed in the cytoplasm. The ATP generated in the PGK reaction is probably the source for Na$^+$ and K$^+$ transport and clearly the sodium pump depends to this extent upon glycolysis. In any situation in which glycolysis ceases, either through metabolic depletion or by the presence of inhibitors such as fluoride or iodoacetate, active transport also stops because of an interruption in the flow of ATP. The converse is also true because sodium-pump activity affects the rate of glycolysis. This has been demonstrated in three ways and the results have led to the notion that the pump is a pacemaker of glycolysis [35, 38, 39]. Under normal conditions some 15–20% of the ATP generated by glycolysis is needed for Na$^+$ pumping [38, 40]; this can be increased to *c.* 75% if the pump is stimulated as, for example, by a rise in internal Na$^+$.

The two types of cation movement so far described are unmediated passive leakage and the counteracting active transport process. These two mechanisms do not describe fully the observed kinetic behaviour, and other forms of Na$^+$ and K$^+$ movement have been proposed. These include:

1 exchange diffusion of Na$^+$ without a net change in the intracellular level, a process which is sensitive to both ouabain and extracellular K$^+$;

2 exchange diffusion of K$^+$, also ouabain-sensitive and giving no net change of K$^+$; and

3 exchange diffusion of Na$^+$, insensitive to ouabain and K$^+$ and giving no net change in the intracellular Na$^+$ concentration.

Evidence for these five modes of cation transport is given in detail by Whittam & Wheeler [34].

The calcium pump

The plasma concentration of calcium (Ca^{2+}) is between 10^3 and 10^4 times greater than that of red cells (Table 7.6). Despite this enormous concentration gradient the diffusion of Ca^{2+} into red cells is very slow [41] and the bulk of cellular Ca^{2+} is bound to the cell membrane which is not normally saturated [42–50]. The presence of Ca^{2+} in red cells appears to be necessary in order to maintain their low permeability towards Na$^+$ and K$^+$; on the other hand, an increase in the cellular content also increases the cells' permeability towards K$^+$. These two opposing effects may arise through the attachment of Ca^{2+} to different binding sites; it has been suggested that the site at which low permeability towards K$^+$ is maintained is within the membrane, while Ca^{2+} binding to the inner surface promotes increased K$^+$ leakage [51].

The low intracellular and high extracellular Ca^{2+}, together with the increased permeability of red cells to this cation in conditions of metabolic depletion, suggest that Ca^{2+} can be transported out of the red cells against a concentration gradient. Early evidence of a Ca^{2+}-activated ATPase [32, 52–54] was augmented by the findings of Schatzmann and his group [41, 55–57] and it is now established that red-cell membranes contain a Ca^{2+}, Mg^{2+}-ATPase which extrudes Ca^{2+} from the cell against a concentration gradient in an energy-requiring reaction which utilizes ATP; the extrusion is independent of K^+ or Na^+ and is unaffected by Na^+-pump inhibitors. The Ca^{2+} pump is asymmetric in that there is no coupled movement of other ions. The mechanism of the pump action has some similarities to the Na^+ pump in that the presence of Ca^{2+}, Mg^{2+} and ATP causes an enzyme phosphorylation to take place with a conformational change to a structure of low Ca^{2+} affinity which permits Ca^{2+} to be released to the cell exterior. It differs from the Na^+ pump in that the dephosphorylation occurs without the stimulus of a second cation and the enzyme reverts to its original state with high affinity Ca^{2+} sites facing the cell interior.

Failure of the Ca^{2+} pump to expel excess Ca^{2+} results in a net leakage of K^+ and shrunken, inflexible, sphered or echinocytic cells. These cell changes are also likely to occur under any conditions which permit net Ca^{2+} entry into cells and so the precise effects of excess Ca^{2+} alone are not easy to determine. Use of the Ca^{2+} ionophore A23187 [58] has helped to clarify the particular effects of Ca^{2+} because it allows this cation alone to enter the cell and so any consequences to the cell are due to the presence of this particular cation. Incubation of red cells with the Ca^{2+} ionophore produces echinocytes with an increased membrane content of 1,2-diacylglycerol and a loss of ATP [59–62]. The echinocyte spicules bud off into microvesicles of diameter *c*. 100 nm which contain 50% of

the 1,2-diacylglycerol [63] originating, it is thought, from phosphatidylcholine which is depleted. The loss of ATP is considered to be due to the increased Ca^{2+} pumping and it is intriguing that the number of spicules formed on echinocytes (30–50) is similar to the calculated number of Ca^{2+}-pumping sites [64].

Abnormal amounts of Ca^{2+} in red cells become bound to protein and in particular to spectrin, which lies as a network on the inner side of the membrane [65–68] (see Chapter 10). Recent evidence suggests that the stiffening effect of Ca^{2+} on the membrane may arise through stimulation of a transglutaminase [69]. This enzyme catalyses the formation of γ-glutamyl ε-lysine bridges between membrane proteins. Normally the enzyme is inactive but is stimulated by the presence of low levels of Ca^{2+} such as occur, for example, in senescent red cells, sickle cells or normal red cells which are metabolically depleted. As a consequence of the polymerization of protein brought about by transglutaminase the cell becomes more rigid. There is contrary evidence, however, that suggests the enzyme decays rapidly, at any rate in depleted cells [70].

Thus, the exclusion of Ca^{2+} from red cells is mediated via active Ca^{2+} transport and the preservation of a low internal Ca^{2+} is vital in order to preserve the monovalent cation status, cell deformability and shape. Both the content and flux of Ca^{2+} are disturbed in sickle cells (see Chapter 8).

Role of 2,3-DPG

2,3-DPG is the most abundant of the red-cell phosphate esters (see Table 7.3) and although characterized 55 years ago [71] its ability to modulate the position of the oxygen dissociation curve was discovered only in 1967 [72, 73]. It is produced from 1,3-diphosphoglycerate in that section of the EMP called the Rapoport–Luebering shuttle (Fig. 7.2); 1,3-DPG is also the

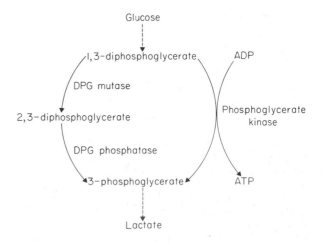

Fig. 7.2. The Rapoport–Luebering shuttle.

substrate for the PGK reaction and the common product is 3-phosphoglycerate (3PG) which passes through to lactate. The concentration of 2,3-DPG is about 100 times greater than that of 3PG but under normal conditions only about 20% of 1,3-DPG is converted to 2,3-DPG [74]. The ester inhibits several enzymes in the EMP (Table 7.5) but in particular 2,3-DPGM so that it inhibits its own synthesis; in addition, 3PG is a cofactor for the mutase reaction. The shuttle functions as a self-regulating system which maintains the concentration of 2,3-DPG and ATP, the one at the expense of the other.

The level of 2,3-DPG is sensitive to the factors which affect the glycolytic rate, particularly pH, and a fall or rise in intracellular pH, either *in vivo* or *in vitro*, results in a decrease and increase respectively in the concentration of this ester [75–79]. A fall in the pH specifically increases DPG-phosphatase activity which also results in a decrease in the 2,3-DPG concentration. Hypoxia increases the 2,3-DPG level in two ways; as mentioned earlier (p. 267) there is an increase in intracellular pH which is the major effect, but also increased binding of the ester to deoxyhaemoglobin occurs which diminishes the free pool of ester, decreases product inhibition of DPG-mutase activity and results in increased production.

The importance of 2,3-DPG in red cells is its ability to react, on a mole-for-mole basis, about 100 times more readily with the deoxy- form of haemoglobin than with the oxy- form. Other esters will do this, in particular ATP, and it is significant that the molar concentration of 2,3-DPG + ATP is about 4 mM, which is similar to the molar concentration of haemoglobin in the cells. The reaction of 2,3-DPG with deoxyhaemoglobin lowers its oxygen affinity, that is, shifts the dissociation curve to the right. The ester is bound by salt bridges within the central cavity of the haemoglobin molecule between the two β-chains and on oxygenation, when the cavity contracts, the ester is expelled.

The position of the dissociation curve is well known to be affected by changes of pH and CO_2, as well as by 2,3-DPG, and the simultaneous effects of these three variables have been investigated [80]. Abnormalities in the position of the curve arise in a number of clinical or environmental situations; these abnormalities are a consequence of changes of pH, CO_2, Po_2, 2,3-DPG or the presence of an abnormal haemoglobin, and are dealt with in Chapter 8.

Role of NADH
NADH is produced from NAD^+ at the GAPD step in the EMP (Fig. 7.1). It is converted to NAD^+ in the final step of the pathway, catalysed by LDH. The concentrations of the two forms of the coenzyme in the cell are low, NAD^+ is 0.03–0.07 mM [81–84] and NADH less than 0.002 mM [12] so that the ratio of NAD^+ to NADH is about 25:1.

Apart from its role in the EMP, NADH is a co-enzyme for NADH-linked methaemoglobin reductase (diaphorase) which is the major route for methaemoglobin (MetHb) reduction in red cells (see p. 275). Such reduction is accompanied by an accumulation of pyruvate because NADH is withdrawn from the LDH reaction but pyruvate, like lactate, can diffuse readily from the cell.

$$\text{Pyruvate} \xleftarrow{\quad} \begin{array}{c} \text{NADH} \\ \text{LDH} \end{array} \xrightarrow{\quad} \begin{array}{c} Fe^{3+}(\text{MetHb}) \\ \text{Diaphorase} \end{array}$$
$$\text{Lactate} \xrightarrow{\quad} \text{NAD}^+ \xleftarrow{\quad} Fe^{2+}(\text{Hb})$$

Pentose-phosphate pathway (PPP)
The pentose-phosphate pathway (PPP) in red cells serves two main functions: to maintain the level of NADP and to provide ribose 5-phosphate (R5P) which acts in the restricted pathway of purine metabolism present in the cell. Like NADH, NADP is present in both oxidized ($NADP^+$) and reduced (NADPH) forms but both are in low concentration; $NADP^+$ is about 1 μM while NADPH is about 45 μM [85].

The several steps in the pathway are shown in Figure 7.3. It is cyclic, leading off from the product of the Hx reaction (G6P) and producing eventually F6P and GA3P, both of which are intermediates in the main pathway of glycolysis, the EMP. The first step is catalysed by glucose-6-phosphate dehydrogenase (G6PD) and leads to 6-phosphogluconate (6PG) in a two-step reaction which is essentially irreversible [86]. The reaction requires $NADP^+$ which is reduced to NADPH and the activity of the whole pathway is controlled by the availability of $NADP^+$ [87]. The pathway can be stimulated by the presence of an electron acceptor such as methylene blue. The maximum rate of stimulation is in constant ratio to the activity measured in dilute haemolysates of a number of G6PD mutants with subnormal activity [88], which suggests that the enzyme also exerts an effect on the rate of the pathway.

The second step in the PPP is catalysed by 6-phosphogluconate dehydrogenase (6PGD) which also requires $NADP^+$ as coenzyme. The oxidation of 6PG to ribulose 5-phosphate (Ru5P) results in the liberation of CO_2 with the conversion of a six-carbon into a five-carbon sugar. This is the only metabolic reaction in mature red cells yielding CO_2 and the mole-for-mole liberation of CO_2 as $^{14}CO_2$ from ^{14}C-1-glucose is used to determine the activity of the pathway in intact red cells incubated *in vitro*.

The product of the 6PGD reaction is Ru5P which is

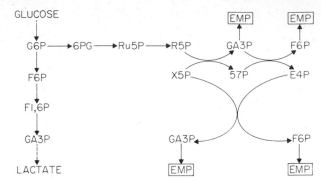

Fig. 7.3. The pentose-phosphate pathway (PPP).

the substrate for two reactions catalysed by an epimer-ase and an isomerase and leading to xylulose 5-phos-phate and ribose 5-phosphate (R5P) respectively (Fig. 7.3). Each of the products can react together to form sedoheptulose 7-phosphate and GA3P in a reaction catalysed by transketolase. Transketolase requires Mg^{2+} and thiamine pyrophosphate (vitamin B_1) for full activity. One of the products, GA3P, is an intermediate in the EMP and re-entry to the EMP along this route offers an ATP-sparing effect by bypassing PFK. The products of the transketolase reaction, sedoheptulose 7-phosphate and GA3P, can react under the influence of a transaldolase to yield F6P and erythrose 4-phosphate and the former pro-duct is also a constituent of the EMP which provides a second re-entry point to the pathway. The final reaction of the pathway is catalysed by transketolase and yields GA3P and F6P from xylulose 5-phosphate and erythrose 4-phosphate.

Factors influencing PPP activity
The activity of this pathway is expressed either as a percentage of the overall glucose consumption or as an amount of glucose passing through the pathway in unit time. Values obtained depend upon the *in-vitro* condi-tions but in the absence of stimulants of the pathway are usually less than 11% of the overall glucose consumption [4, 89–92].

Unlike the main glycolytic pathway (see p. 266) the PPP is not sensitive to pH [14, 28]. It is, however, stimulated by a wide range of oxidant compounds including those substances which are haemolytic in G6PD deficiency (Table 7.7). Thus, as well as meth-ylene blue, compounds such as cysteine, ascorbate, acetylphenylhydrazine, 1- and 2-naphthol and nitro-furantoin will increase PPP activity *in vitro* [93]. The mechanism of action of these and other substances depends upon their structure and the metabolites which they form but, either directly or indirectly, the availability of $NADP^+$, which is a major regulator of

PPP activity, is increased [87, 94]. Some stimulants act through their electron-acceptor properties and, by direct reaction with NADPH, convert it to $NADP^+$ so that the ratio $NADP^+:NADPH$ is increased which also increases PPP activity. Others act through a less specific oxidation of a number of red-cell sites, includ-ing GSH, and the PPP is stimulated in restoring this compound to its steady-state level.

An alternative view [86] on the regulation of PPP activity is that NADPH exerts an inhibitory effect on G6PD activity. The ratio $NADP^+:NADPH$ is nor-mally low and any inducement to increase PPP activity acts via an increase in the ratio so that the fall in NADPH de-inhibits G6PD rather than the rise in $NADP^+$ causing a stimulus to the pathway.

Glutathione (GSH) and associated reactions
Glutathione (GSH) is a tripeptide of glycine, cysteine and glutamate with the proper name γ-L-glutamyl-L-cysteinylglycine. Its biosynthesis, first shown in rat liver [95], has also been demonstrated in mature human red cells [96, 97]. It occurs in two stages, the first being the formation of glutamylcysteine followed by the attachment of glycine. The enzyme responsible for the first step is glutamylcysteine synthetase which requires ATP, Mg^{2+} and the presence of intact —SH groups; the second stage is catalysed by GSH synthe-tase which is rate-limiting for the overall reaction and also requires Mg^{2+} and ATP but not the presence of —SH groups [98].

The biosynthesis of GSH by mature red cells enables them to maintain a high intracellular concentration (approximately 70 mg/dl or 2·2 mM). The cell mem-brane is impermeable to GSH and the plasma concen-tration is negligible; also the oxidized form (GSSG) cannot enter red cells but at high concentration can leave them in an energy-dependent reaction [99–103]. The GSSG concentration is usually low, about 10% of the GSH + GSSG level, and it is not clear whether GSSG leakage is a normal occurrence. GSH has a

Table 7.7. Drugs associated with haemolysis in G6PD deficiency [252]

Established as haemolytic	Not established as haemolytic in therapeutic doses
Acetanilide	Acetaminophen (paracetamol)
Acetylphenylhydrazine	Acetophenetidine (phenacetin)
Methylene blue	Acetylsalicyclic acid (aspirin)
Naphthalene (moth balls)	Aminopyrine (pyramidon)
Nalidixic acid (Negram)	Antazoline (antistine)
Niridazole (Ambilhar, *Ciba*)	Antipyrine
Nitrofurantoin (Furadantin, *Eaton*)	Ascorbic acid (vitamin C)
Pamaquin (Plasmoquine)	Benzhexol (Artane, *Lederle*)
Pentaquine	Chloramphenicol
Primaquine	Chlorguanidine (Paludrine, *ICI*)
Sulphacetamide	Chloroquine
Sulphamethoxazole	Colchicine
Sulphanilamide	Diphenylhydramine (Benadryl, *Parke, Davis*)
Sulphapyridine	Isoniazide
Thiazosulphone (Promizole)	L-DOPA
Toluidine blue	Menadione
Trinintrotoluene (TNT)	Menaphthone
	p-Aminobenzoic acid
	Phenylbutazone
	Phenytoin
	Probenecid (Benemid, *Merck Sharp & Dohme*)
	Procainamide HCL (Pronestyl, *Squibb*)
	Pyrimethamine (Daraprim, *Wellcome*)
	Quinidine
	Quinine
	Streptomycin
	Sulfacytine
	Sulphadiazine
	Sulphaguanidine
	Sulphamethoxypyridazine (Lederkyn, Midicel, Kynex)
	Sulphisoxazole (Gantrisin, *Roche*)
	Trimethoprim
	Tripelennamine (Pyribenzamine, *Ciba*)
	Vitamin K

half-life of about three days [104] which indicates that it is turned over; this may be a consequence of degradation because red cells contain glutathionase [105] but it could also be because of a loss from the cells of the oxidized dimer. A high concentration of GSSG is undesirable in red cells because:

1 it has no function;
2 it may leak from the cells and be unavailable for reduction to GSH;
3 it may inhibit Hx [106]; and
4 it can bind to haemoglobin [107].

Purpose of GSH. The major role of GSH in red cells is to protect protein —SH groups against oxidation and to trap unwanted metallic ions by forming mercap-

tides. The protein moiety of red cells is distributed between the enzymes, membrane and haemoglobin, with more than 97% accountable to haemoglobin. A number of enzymes contain —SH groups at their active sites, and loss of these groups renders the enzyme inactive. Membrane proteins require that their —SH groups be intact in order to preserve cell flexibility, to permit the controlled diffusion of cations, and to allow the passage of glucose and other low-molecular-weight substances. Failure to maintain the six —SH groups of haemoglobin in the reduced state can lead to the formation of Heinz bodies (see p. 275).

Apart from this well-studied function of GSH in —SH protection and, less well understood, in scavenging free radicals [108], GSH participates in three other cellular activities. One is the glyoxalase reaction for the conversion of methylglyoxal to lactate in which GSH acts as a cofactor; the purpose of this reaction in red cells is unknown [109–113]. Another of its activities is as a prosthetic group bound to glyceraldehyde-3-phosphate dehydrogenase (GAPD) [114]. GSH is also involved in the detoxication of certain foreign compounds; this occurs by conjugation, acetylation and removal of the glycine and glutamate to yield mercapturic acids [115]. It is of interest that although this detoxicating mechanism has not been demonstrated in red cells, a number of haemolytic compounds such as the polycyclic hydrocarbons are known to form mercapturic acids.

Glutathione reductase (GR). This enzyme catalyses the reduction of GSSG to 2GSH using NADPH or NADH as hydrogen donor:

$$GSSG + NADPH + H^+ \rightarrow 2GSH + NADP^+$$
$$\text{or,} \quad GSSG + NADH + H^+ \rightarrow 2GSH + NAD^+$$

NADPH is the preferred cofactor and the relative activity compared with NADH is between five and eight to one; the K_m values for NADPH and NADH are 11 and 270 μM respectively [116, 117]. GR appears to be a single enzyme because extensive fractionation has failed to separate the activity with the two cofactors, and electrophoresis of either the normal or mutant enzyme shows only a single band [116, 118–120]. The enzyme is inhibited by chromate and by 2,5-dinitrobenzoic acid [121–124].

GR contains FAD as a prosthetic group [116, 119, 121, 125] and it is possible to increase red-cell GR activity *in vitro* by the addition of FAD to haemolysates, or *in vivo* by ingestion of 5 mg daily of riboflavin [126, 127]. GSSG is not a unique substrate of GR which will reduce dihydrolipoic acid [116] and also the mixed disulphides formed between GSH and protein —SH groups [128]; the latter reaction was demonstrated with mixed disulphides of haemoglobin and was thought to be of significance when red cells are assaulted by oxidative agents.

Glutathione peroxidase (GSH-Px). Decomposition of the highly toxic H_2O_2 is carried out in two reactions catalysed by catalase and by GSH-Px:

The relative contribution made by the two enzymes depends upon the generation of H_2O_2; at low rates GSH-Px is the major route while at higher rates catalase becomes more important [129]. GSH-Px is highly specific for GSH but less so for the acceptor and several other peroxides (e.g. steroid hydroperoxides, linoleic hydroperoxide and ethyl hydroperoxide) are also reduced [130, 131]. The enzyme has been crystallized from bovine blood and consists of four subunits each of approximate MW 21 000 with selenium attached to each subunit [132–134].

Catalase
The catalase molecule has an approximate MW of 250 000 with four Fe^{3+}-containing porphyrin groups. H_2O_2 is broken down in a rapid two-stage reaction [135]:

$$\text{Protein-}Fe^{3+}\text{-OH} + H_2O_2 \rightarrow$$
$$\text{Protein-}Fe^{3+}\text{-O—OH} + H_2O$$
$$\text{(Complex I)}$$

then,

$$\text{Protein-}Fe^{3+}\text{-O—OH} + H_2O_2 \rightarrow$$
$$\text{Protein-}Fe^{3+}\text{-OH} + H_2O + O_2$$
$$\text{(Complex II)}$$

The enzyme can, however, function as a peroxidase and catalyse reactions of the type:

$$AH_2 + H_2O_2 \rightarrow A + 2H_2O$$

in which A may be a phenol, an alcohol or ascorbate. The peroxidase reaction occurs in more than one stage [136, 137] starting with the attachment of H_2O_2 to the enzyme to form Complex I as before.

$$\text{Protein-}Fe^{3+}\text{-OH} + H_2O_2 \rightarrow$$
$$\text{Protein-}Fe^{3+}\text{-O—OH} + H_2O$$
$$\text{(Complex I)}$$

Complex I is green and before further reaction can take place is converted into a red Complex II which can then react with a suitable hydrogen donor:

$$\text{Protein-}Fe^{3+}\text{-O—OH} + AH_2 \rightarrow$$
$$\text{Protein-}Fe^{3+}\text{-OH} + H_2O + A$$
$$\text{(Complex II)}$$

Thus, the catalytic activity of catalase described previously is a special case in which H_2O_2 is both substrate and acceptor.

The formation of Complex I is sensitive to oxidants which may produce an inactive Complex II [138]. The inactive Complex II can be reactivated by several substances (e.g. ethanol, NADPH or NADH) [139, 140]. Small amounts of Complex II are present in red cells [139, 141] and its reactivation by NADPH links catalase activity with the PPP so that both routes for H_2O_2 breakdown can be linked to glycolysis. It is of interest in this respect that primaquine administered to G6PD-deficient subjects produces about a 35% fall in catalase activity within seven days, followed by a rise to normal values; a change that is too early to be due to red-cell destruction and reticulocytosis. It was thought [139] that the change in catalase activity was linked to the cells' metabolic activity in that the inhibition was relieved by NADPH associated with a stimulation of the PPP.

The peroxidatic activity of catalase is due to its prosthetic group, a porphyrin ring containing Fe^{3+} iron. Haemoglobin also displays peroxidatic activity when the iron is in the ferric state to give methaemoglobin, and this property is exploited in testing for faecal blood. Addition of peroxide to faeces in the presence of the chromogen benzidine will produce a strongly coloured product if blood is also present to decompose the peroxide.

Competition for H_2O_2

The three routes for H_2O_2 breakdown in red cells, namely catalase, GSH-Px and non-enzymically by methaemoglobin are all linked to glycolysis. The relative contributions made by these three options depends upon the rate of generation of H_2O_2; at low rates GSH-Px is the major route while at high rates, or with bursts of H_2O_2 at lower rates, catalase preponderates [129, 142].

It is clear from several pieces of evidence that whilst catalase can play a part in the breakdown of H_2O_2 it is not essential to the survival of red cells. It is absent from duck red cells and when inhibited in human red cells they remain viable. Also, in congenital acatalasaemia in humans there is no detectable haemolysis whereas in GSH-Px deficiency there can be an associated haemolytic anaemia [143, 144]. GSH-Px appears essential to cell survival, a view supported by the fact that in the Swiss type of acatalasaemia PPP activity is about three times normal and the red cells can withstand the oxidative stress of incubation with 5 mM ascorbate [145], a concentration which increases PPP activity some 12-fold in acatalasaemic red cells but does not stimulate in normal red cells. Thus, in the absence of catalase, GSH-Px activity is the primary route for the disposal of H_2O_2 and this is manifested by an increased turnover of GSH. It is of interest, therefore, that in the acatalasaemic duck, the GSH concentration in the red cells is around three times that in normal human red cells and GSH reductase activity is about five times greater [146].

Oxidation of haemoglobin

There are two sites in the haemoglobin molecule which are prone to oxidation, the Fe^{2+} atom in the haem ring which forms Fe^{3+} and the —SH groups of the globin moiety which can be converted to —S—S— bridges. Under physiological conditions human red cells are capable of reversing oxidation at either site and indeed can do so even when the cell is besieged by oxidative agents.

Methaemoglobin (MetHb)

Oxidation of the haem iron yields MetHb and the reaction is given by:

$$Fe^{2+} \rightarrow Fe^{3+} + 1e^-$$

that is, a loss to some acceptor of one electron from ferrous iron gives ferric iron. MetHb has no physiological function for it cannot combine with oxygen. It is a brown pigment which is distinguishable from oxy- or deoxyhaemoglobin by an absorption maximum at 630 nm, a property used for its assay. There are several synonyms for MetHb, namely, hemiglobin, ferrihaemoglobin or ferriprotoporphyrin IX-globin, but MetHb or methaemoglobin remain as the familiar names.

The iron lies in the central cavity (about 2 Å in radius) of the porphyrin ring to which it is bound by four covalent bonds via the four pyrrol nitrogen atoms. Haem is in the form of a planar disc with a slightly rumpled surface and is attached to the globin chain by a fifth covalent bond between iron and the proximal histidine residue of the globin chain. It lies in a pocket of the globin chain like a penny pushed into a ball of plasticine with only the rim showing. The pocket is composed of 20 hydrophobic amino acids and the polar propionate side chains of the haem are on the exposed portion of the rim. Thus, the Fe^{2+} lies within a hydrophobic environment which is a necessary condition to preserve the stability of the iron–haem–globin complex; reactions with invading polar compounds like water are made less probable.

The iron atom in the deoxy- form of haemoglobin lies about 0·5 Å outside the haem ring [147] but binding with oxygen results in a contraction of the iron which can then enter the plane of the haem ring [148, 149]. This switch of the iron atom initiates the series of conformational changes which occur throughout the haemoglobin molecule as it is oxygenated.

The formation of oxyhaemoglobin from deoxyhaemoglobin is an oxygenation rather than an oxidation, that is, an electron is shared reversibly between the oxygen and the iron atom and when oxygen is released from haemoglobin at low oxygen tension the electron is retained by the iron atom. Complete transfer of an electron from iron to oxygen can occasionally occur [150]:

$$Fe^{2+} + O_2 \rightleftharpoons Fe^{2+} \cdot O_2 \rightleftharpoons Fe^{3+} \cdot O_2^-$$

This produces MetHb with bound oxygen and their opposite charges will discourage dissociation. However, some dissociation will occur to give MetHb and the highly reactive superoxide iron O_2^- (see Ref. 151).

The slow formation of MetHb which occurs in haemolysates or intact cells when the usual means for its prevention are absent may arise from this autoxidative reaction [152]. This loss of an electron from the iron atom can be facilitated by a number of agents and the presence of abnormal amounts of MetHb, greater than one per cent, in blood containing normal haemoglobin is an indication of drug-induced oxidation in both congenitally defective and normal cells.

The superoxide anion can arise in red cells by the mechanism just described but also through free radicals formed from oxidative drugs. In either event the cells are protected from this reactive and potentially hazardous agent by the presence of a superoxide dismutase (SOD):

$$O_2^- + O_2^- + 2H^+ \xrightarrow{SOD} H_2O_2 + O_2$$

By this means O_2^- is reduced to H_2O_2 which can be degraded by catalase or GSH-Px (see p. 273).

Reduction of methaemoglobin

The normal MetHb concentration in whole blood (less than one per cent) is a balance between formation and reduction [153–155]. In the absence of NADH-linked MetHb-reductase activity, which is the principal means for its reduction, MetHb accumulates at the rate of about three per cent per day [156]. The reducing systems for MetHb decrease in activity with ageing of red cells but it is not clearly established that the small amount of MetHb normally present in red cells is located in the older cohort (for summary of earlier data see Ref. 157).

The reduction of MetHb can take place along four routes. The major route (NADH-linked MetHb reductase) reduces about 67% [158] while the second route of quantitative importance is via NADPH-linked MetHb reductase which is linked, via NADPH, with the PPP. The other two routes are minor, non-enzymic reactions in which direct reduction takes place with ascorbate or GSH. Reduction by GSH has been observed *in vitro* only [159, 160] and for several reasons is not considered to be of physiological significance. Thus, a low red-cell GSH is not a feature of congenital methaemoglobinaemia and MetHb is not notable when GSH is congenitally or artificially low in red cells. Similarly ascorbate reduction of MetHb is too slow under physiological conditions to be of importance [161–163]. A comparison of the four reductive routes [155, 158] gives values for NADH-, NADPH-linked reductase, ascorbate and GSH activity of 67, 5, 16 and 12%, respectively.

NADPH-linked methaemoglobin reductase. This minor route for MetHb reduction is linked to the PPP via NADPH. The enzyme system is distinct from that

catalysing the NADH-linked reduction [158, 164–171] and is stimulated by riboflavin, flavin mononucleotide or FAD; it is reported to be a flavin reductase [172].

A number of extrinsic agents will reduce MetHb in red cells but the two in clinical use are ascorbate and methylene blue. The former acts by a direct chemical reduction but the latter exerts its effect in conjunction with NADPH. It is known that oxidized methylene blue acts as an electron acceptor to convert NADPH to $NADP^+$ and thereby stimulate the PPP and increase the turnover of $NADP^+$ to NADPH. Reduction of the dye may be enzymically linked to the NADPH-linked MetHb reductase rather than to direct chemical oxidation of NADPH. The reduced dye then may directly reduce MetHb [173, 174].

Heinz bodies

Heinz bodies are seen in red cells as irregular, refractile inclusions which lie attached to the membrane and vary in size up to about 3 μm. Several small bodies may be seen in a single cell but larger bodies tend to occur singly. They are the last stage in the oxidative breakdown of haemoglobin and consist of insoluble aggregates of degraded haemoglobin containing occluded cellular fragments of lipid and some enzyme protein. First described by Heinz [175] who observed them following the action of phenylhydrazine on red cells, there exists an extensive early literature reviewed in 1949 [176]. Their chemical and physical nature has been examined by a number of workers since (e.g. Refs. 177, 178) and these studies have confirmed and extended the earlier views. Heinz bodies are attached to the membrane and may protrude through it; the bonding was thought to be through disulphide bridges [179, 180] but others [181] suggest that weaker binding forces are involved.

Heinz bodies may be produced in normal or in congenitally defective red cells by a variety of extrinsic agents; they appear spontaneously in small numbers in normal cells following splenectomy and in considerable numbers after splenectomy in cells containing a congenitally unstable haemoglobin.

Normal cells. The Heinz bodies found in the cells of normal but splenectomized subjects are probably in the older cohort of cells in which the reductive capacity is fading. Their presence demonstrates the ability of the spleen to remove inclusions, which it can do without sequestering the cells [182]. Heinz bodies may also occur as a transient incidence in the normal cells of unsplenectomized subjects who have ingested a sufficient amount of an oxidant drug such as phenacetin or codeine; in this situation the reducing capacity of the cells, particularly in the older ones, has been swamped by the drug and/or its metabolites.

Abnormal cells. There are several congenital defects of red cells which have in common an inability to maintain an adequate GSH concentration or to regenerate GSH at a sufficient rate during an oxidative onslaught. In such a situation there is a shortfall in —SH group protection and H_2O_2 detoxication by GSH-Px (see p. 273) and so such cells are abnormally sensitive to oxidant drugs. This group of sensitive cells comprises G6PD, 6PGD, GSH, GSH-Px and GSH-reductase deficiency. Heinz bodies are not normally present except after the ingestion of those drugs which are haemolytic in G6PD deficiency (Table 7.7).

Red cells which contain a congenitally unstable haemoglobin (e.g. Köln, Hammersmith, Zürich or H), form inclusion bodies by the continuous precipitation of the labile haemoglobin. They are observed in blood films only after splenectomy, a further demonstration of the spleen's ability to remove them. Although inclusions arising from unstable haemoglobins are not Heinz bodies in the purist sense, because they are not the product of an external attack by an oxidant upon Hb A, they are chemically and morphologically indistinguishable from Heinz bodies.

The imbalance of globin-chain synthesis in thalassaemia produces excess α or β chains in the maturing cells and these form inclusions [183] which consist of degraded, insoluble and coalesced α or β chains which stain, like Heinz bodies, with methyl violet.

Mechanism of Heinz-body formation. From a study of normal red cells treated *in vitro* with acetylphenylhydrazine a reaction scheme was proposed [184] for the production of Heinz bodies from Hb A. The initial step is the formation of MetHb followed by oxidation of the two accessible —SH groups of β_{93} cysteine, one in each β chain. Both these oxidations are reversible provided that the cells are glycolysing because MetHb reductase will reduce MetHb and GSH will reduce the oxidized —SH groups. Any further oxidation is considered to be irreversible because it affects the remaining four —SH groups submerged within the molecule; oxidation of these would disturb the tertiary and quaternary structure and lead to uncoiling of the molecule to render it increasingly insoluble and polymerized so that eventually it is precipitated as a Heinz body.

This scheme has been somewhat modified following later studies on the congenitally unstable haemoglobins which spontaneously degrade into Heinz bodies without the intervention of added oxidants. These studies have focused on two aspects, the part played by the haem moiety and the involvement of —SH groups [185].

Role of haem. Most of the unstable haemoglobins have a weakened haem–globin binding on the β chain, a defect which is secondary to a structural instability in or near to the haem pocket. The presence of haem on the globin confers stability and its removal increases the chance that globin will lose its helical component and become insoluble. Heating of haemolysates at 50°C accelerates this process [186] and provides the basis of a screening test for the detection of an unstable haemoglobin [187]. At 50°C or below HbA is stable but unstable haemoglobins like Zürich, Köln, Hammersmith, Sydney and Christchurch are precipitated from solution at rates which are some measure of their instability [185, 188]. The heat-precipitated material from different haemoglobins varies in colour from pale to dark red-brown, an indication of the haem content. A synthetic analogue of Hb A in which the β chains are free of haem ($\alpha_2^{haem} \beta_2^0$) is also heat-labile but acquires the heat-stable properties of Hb A if the haem groups are replaced [185, 189, 190]. Thus, in the formation of inclusions a weakened haem–globin binding puts the globin at risk by increasing its propensity to precipitate; haem depletion increases this tendency towards instability.

Role of —SH groups. The preservation of the —SH groups in globin is necessary for the stabilization of haemoglobin and GSH is an essential protective agent in this process. In an early study [184] GSH was shown to form mixed disulphides with haemoglobin during the treatment of Hb A with phenylhydrazine. Examination of one of the first known unstable haemoglobins (Ube-1) suggested [191] that the two reactive —SH groups of the β_{93} cysteine were blocked; this was later found to occur in haemoglobins Köln and Hammersmith [179, 180]. Evidence that these two —SH groups are important and may be blocked by GSH is as follows:

1 during treatment of Hb A with phenylhydrazine GSH disappears and forms mixed disulphides with two —SH groups on Hb A [184];

2 fresh red cells containing Hb Hammersmith or Köln have a somewhat low GSH concentration [179, 186, 190, 192];

3 incubation at 50°C of red cells containing Hb Köln or Hammersmith results in precipitation of the unstable haemoglobin together with a loss of GSH; in normal red cells both the haemoglobin and GSH are stable [180];

4 treatment of Hb A with *p*-CMB (p-chlormercuribenzoate) renders the haemoglobin thermally labile when more than two —SH groups are blocked [180]; and

5 heat treatment of Hb Köln, Sydney or Christchurch causes two of the —SH groups to become oxidized [188].

Role of MetHb and haemichromes. Despite considerable study, it remains uncertain whether MetHb formation is an obligatory first step for the production of Heinz bodies. According to some [184, 193], MetHb is the initial and required step. It is clear that the particular oxidant used as well as the experimental conditions affect the amount of MetHb formed [194, 195]. Some investigators, however, have queried the presence of MetHb as a necessary prerequisite for drug-induced Heinz-body formation [195–197]. Some of the divergent findings could be attributed to the variable, sometimes rapid disappearance of MetHb during haemoglobin oxidation [198]. In the case of the unstable haemoglobins, small amounts of MetHb are usually to be found in fresh red cells because the congenital abnormality in the vicinity of the haem pocket results in the readier access of water; this facilitates both MetHb and superoxide formation. The presence of superoxide (see p. 275), or of its product H_2O_2, is a hazard because haemoglobin can be auto-oxidized in addition to undergoing oxidation from H_2O_2 [199].

During slow or mild oxidation of normal or congenitally unstable haemoglobin, the absorption spectra of haemolysates reveal the presence of unstable intermediates called haemichromes. These are haem-containing molecules or subunits of haemoglobin in which the ferric iron has an additional bond to the distal histidine E7 [200]. During the degradation of haemoglobin a reversible haemichrome appears but later an irreversible one forms in which the additional ferric–iron bond is attached to an amino-acid residue other than histidine [200] (see Chapters 8 and 9).

All these data, which are derived from studies of the congenitally unstable haemoglobins, have been incorporated into a model (Fig. 7.4) to describe the spontaneous formation of Heinz bodies from unstable haemoglobins [188]. Whether or not haem-depleted globin is produced depends upon the particular haemoglobin.

Oxidation of red cells (Fig. 7.5)

From the preceding description it is clear that haemoglobin is a primary target for the oxidative hazard to which the whole cell is exposed. The amount of haemoglobin in the cell together with its auto-oxidative properties have caused it to be studied more than other cellular proteins but the latter are also susceptible to —SH oxidation. The cell lipids, all located on the membrane, are also oxidizable and the major sites of reaction are the —C=C— double bonds on the fatty-acid chains of the phospholipid component. Their oxidation yields lipid peroxides and these are normally maintained at low concentration by the presence in plasma of the anti-oxidant vitamin E. Oxidation of —SH groups is prevented or reversed by GSH (see p. 272) which is in turn maintained in the reduced state by GR (see p. 273) and MetHb is reduced as earlier described (see p. 275).

One potent oxidant to which red cells are exposed is H_2O_2 and the competition to detoxicate this substance has been described (p. 274). Part at least of the H_2O_2 in the cells arises from the superoxide ion, O_2^-, through the action of the dismutase SOD. The superoxide ion is a well-characterized radical whose danger to the cell is rapidly disarmed through conversion to H_2O_2. It is very probable that other reactive oxidant radicals are produced which are in equilibrium with O_2^- but these

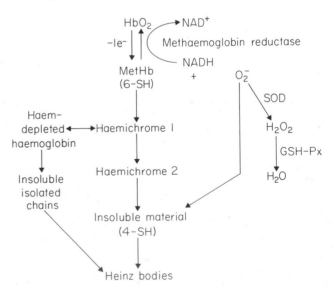

Fig. 7.4. Model for Heinz-body formation [188].

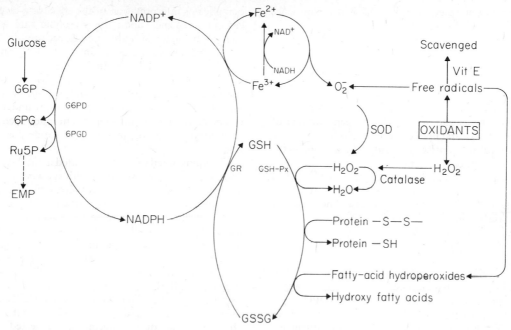

Fig. 7.5. The oxidation-reduction system in red cells.

are maintained at a low level by the continuous drain of O_2^- to H_2O_2.

This ability of the red cell to cope with oxidant stress is vital for its survival and when the oxidation–reduction status is impaired (e.g. in diaphorase or G6PD deficiency), the lifespan or function of the cell is restricted.

Purine metabolism in red cells

Interest in purine metabolism in red cells has been stimulated in recent years by three factors: the need to sustain or regenerate nucleotide concentrations in cold-stored blood used for transfusion, the existence of a rare congenital abnormality, the Lesch–Nyhan syndrome, for which red cells can be used as the diagnostic tissue and the disturbed purine and adenine metabolism in renal failure and in pyrimidine 5′-nucleotidase deficiency.

Mature red cells cannot synthesize nucleotides *de novo* although adenine nucleotides are turned over within the cell. They can, however, be built up from the adenine level and the idea is emerging that red cells are a transport system for some bases which originate in the liver.

The first step of nucleotide synthesis in human red cells is the conversion of a purine base to the corresponding nucleotide (AMP, IMP or GMP), a reaction catalysed by a phosphoribosyl transferase and requiring 5-phosphoribosyl-l-pyrophosphate (PRPP):

$$PRPP \begin{array}{l} + \text{adenine} \xrightarrow{\text{APRT}} AMP + \\ + \text{guanine} \\ + \text{hypoxanthine} \end{array} \Big\} \xrightarrow{\text{HGPRT}} \left\{ \begin{array}{l} GMP+ \\ IMP+ \end{array} \right\} P\text{-}P$$

APRT is adenine phosphoribosyl transferase and HGPRT, also called HPRT, is hypoxanthine guanosine or hypoxanthine phosphoribosyl transferase. In the Lesch–Nyhan syndrome there is a deficiency of HPGRT (or HPRT) activity with increased APRT activity and a red-cell PRPP concentration about 10 times normal.

PRPP is produced from ribose 5-phosphate (R5P), formed in the PPP, and ATP:

$$R5P + ATP \xrightarrow[\text{synthetase}]{PRPP} PRPP + ATP$$

The reaction is catalysed by PRPP synthetase (also called ribose phosphate pyrophosphokinase, RPK) which is markedly stimulated by the presence of phosphate and inhibited by ADP, GDP or 2,3-DPG. It has a low activity in pyrimidine 5′-nucleotidase deficiency (see p. 291).

Thus, given that adenine base is available to red cells the presence of RPK and APRT allows the elevation of one mole of base to AMP with the consumption of one mole of ATP:

$$R5P + ATP + \text{adenine} \rightarrow 2AMP$$

AMP can be elevated further to ADP by the presence of adenylate kinase (AK):

$$AMP + ATP \underset{AK}{\rightleftarrows} 2ADP$$

and the glycolytic pathway can raise ADP to ATP.

Ageing of red cells

Mature red cells lack the mechanism for synthesis of protein or lipid and so there is a steady decline of enzyme activity and lipid content of cells following the reticulocyte stage until their eventual destruction in the reticulo-endothelial system.

Almost all the enzymes which have been studied show a diminished activity in older cells. Exceptions are LDH, nucleoside phosphorylase and possibly glyoxalase. Some of the red-cell enzymes consist of a number of isozymes, more than in other cells and this may be due to the comparatively long life of the cells and also to chemical modifications such as de-amidation [201–205]. The concentrations of inter-mediates have been little studied with respect to age of cells; such data as are reported (e.g. 2,3-DPG [206]) suggest that there is a decline in ester level with cell ageing. The greatest difference in a cell constituent as a function of age is shown by creatine which offers the best criterion to date of a successful *in-vitro* separation of cells into young and old fractions [207].

The MetHb found in normal blood (about one per cent) represents the balance between production and reduction. As mentioned (see p. 275) it is not certain whether the older cells contain more MetHb although the reducing capacity of red cells certainly decreases with age. When the MetHb concentration is increased in cells by an oxidative assault the older cells contain more MetHb than the younger cells as, for example, in a drug-induced episode in G6PD deficiency when MetHb appears in the older cells although transiently and in small amount because the older cells are preferentially destroyed.

The Hb A_3 of blood is located in the older cells [208]. This is the derivative of Hb A which contains GSH as a mixed disulphide on one of the β-chain —SH groups.

The glycolytic rate diminishes with red-cell age whether assessed by glucose consumption or lactate production and the activity of the PPP also declines with age. There is a close correspondence between the falling rate of glucose consumption and hexokinase activity during cell ageing [26] and in view of the low activity of Hx (see p. 265) this decline has implicated Hx as a pacemaker of glycolysis. The activity of the other glycolytic enzymes also falls, at characteristic rates, during ageing of the cells but all are present in considerable excess by comparison with the glycolytic rate.

The increased glycolytic activity of younger red cells complicates interpretation of the effect of a glycolytic enzyme deficiency upon the glycolytic rate when a haemolytic anaemia is also present because the higher activity of the young cells can mask the subnormal activity in the old cells. In such cases the rate of glycolysis is compared with control samples which have high reticulocyte counts but are otherwise normal. The age of any red-cell population under study can be assessed by a time-dependent index such as the reticulocyte count or, better, the creatine concentration.

The lipids of red cells are all located in the membrane and the concentration declines with age whether values are expressed per cell, per unit volume or unit surface area of cells [209–211]. The principal loss of lipids occurs during the reticulocyte stage while the cells are undergoing remodelling; all classes of lipids are affected and the profile is similar in cells of all ages. The surface of red cells also decreases to give cells with a smaller volume and H_2O content, decreased K^+ (expressed a cell H_2O) and an increased Na^+ content, osmotic fragility and mechanical fragility [206], as well as an increased rigidity [212, 213]. That surface changes occur during ageing is suggested by an increasing susceptibility to haemolysis by immune antibodies and complement [214].

LABORATORY DETECTION OF RED-CELL ENZYME DEFECTS

An enzyme abnormality should be suspected in any patient with a non-spherocytic haemolytic anaemia for which there is no acquired basis. The clinical and haematological features of this type of anaemia are described in detail later. Enzyme abnormalities which are not associated with haemolysis are also considered because of the light they have shed into some of the mechanisms operating in normal red-cell metabolism.

The two commonest deficiencies are due to mutants of G6PD and pyruvate kinase (PK); all others are rare. There are several screening tests for G6PD deficiency (see p. 299) and an assay kit (Boehringer, Mannheim) and spot test for PK deficiency [215].

Preliminary screening tests (Table 7.8)
In a well-equipped laboratory, geared to metabolic studies and enzyme kinetics, the assay of all red-cell enzymes known to occur as mutants will usually provide a diagnosis. Most laboratories are not so directed but a number of simple screening tests can be carried out to restrict the possibilities.

Osmotic fragility. This test is carried out on both fresh

Table 7.8. A sequence for the laboratory diagnosis of congenital haemolytic anaemias

Blood film:	May be normal. Polychromasia usually present. Occasionally acanthocytes, stomatocytes, target cells or spherocytes* may be seen
Osmotic fragility:	Fresh and incubated blood but especially the latter. A left-shifted curve is given by hypochromic or young cells, right-shifted curve given by fragile cells
Autohaemolysis test:	Type I* or II. An abnormal result suggests further study
Heinz bodies:	Suggest defect in PPP or an unstable haemoglobin

↓

G6PD screen:	For a heterozygote having a haemolytic episode a cytochemical test is necessary if the screening test is normal
PK assay:	PK deficiency is the commonest of the EMP disorders
Heat stability:	Detection of an unstable haemoglobinopathy
GSH, GSH stability:	An abnormal result indicates a gross deficiency (including G6PD) of the PPP or its associated reactions

↓

Assay of glycolytic esters including ATP and 2,3-DPG. A build-up of sequential ester concentration suggests an enzyme block following the increased ester concentration. High ATP level suggests pyrimidine 5′-nucleotidase deficiency (an artefact due to high GTP level)

↓

Assay of deficient enzyme:	Characterization of variant

* Diagnosis of hereditary spherocytosis in mild form by laboratory testing may be inconclusive. HS is further suggested by an increased Na^+ and K^+ flux and a decreased acidified-glycerol lysis time.

and incubated blood and provides two pieces of information. An increased resistance indicates the presence of young cells or cells with a low MCHC. An increased fragility, often seen as a tail, indicates the presence of an abnormal cohort of cells or spherocytes. An increased fresh-blood osmotic fragility worsened by incubation is, of course, a diagnostic criterion of hereditary spherocytosis but acquired spherocytosis also gives this picture.

The increase osmotic fragility following 24 hours of incubation occurs also with normal cells and is a consequence of cell swelling. Following exhaustion of the endogenous glucose after a few hours, net Na^+ leakage occurs into cells at a greater rate than net K^+ leakage from cells. Water enters the cells and increases the volume to bring them closer to their critical haemolytic volume so that when placed in hypotonic solution they are less able than fresh cells to withstand the osmotic stress. Microspherocytes are particularly susceptible since they are closer than normal cells to the critical haemolytic volume. Hypochromic cells, on the other hand, actually shrink following 24 hours of incubation because of the abnormal cation leakage which occurs [216] and the incubated osmotic-fragility

curve indicates an osmotic resistance even greater than that shown by the fresh cells. An increased incubated osmotic fragility of red cells from patients with non-sperocytic haemolytic anaemia indicates either abnormal cation leakage by the cells or defective cell membranes.

Autohaemolysis. This test involves the incubation of sterile, defibrinated blood for 48 hours in the presence and absence of added glucose [217, 218]. Under these conditions normal red cells give little lysis (< 5%) and even less (< 0·5%) with added glucose present. Abnormal cells may undergo considerable lysis which is diminished by the presence of added glucose (Type I; as in hereditary spherocytosis) or is unaffected or even worsened by its presence (Type II; as in PK deficiency). One of the originators of the test suggested in 1964 [219] that it had outlived its usefulness, a view repeated 14 years later by Beutler [220]. Doubtless the test will become redundant eventually but it continues to retain the merit, not of offering a diagnosis, but of indicating defective red cells, which assists the decision to refer the blood for enzyme assay.

Methaemoglobin, GSH and Heinz bodies. The significance attaching to abnormal levels of any of these three substances is considered at relevant points in the text. In general, an increased MetHb concentration, a low GSH level or the presence of Heinz bodies suggest an oxidative assault on the red cells by drugs, a congenital defect in the mechanism for reducing MetHb or maintaining GSH, an unstable haemoglobin or the presence of free globin chains.

Examination of enzyme variants

Following the preliminary screening tests outlined above, further investigation requires assay of specific enzymes. For the two commonest deficiencies, G6PD and PK, spot tests are available [215] and for G6PD several screening tests and an assay kit are available.

The quantitative assay of an enzyme is normally determined in dilute buffered solution containing an excess of substrate(s) and cofactor(s) so that the enzyme is the rate-limiting factor. The reaction is led, if possible, through a further set of enzyme reactions which require NADH or NADPH as coenzyme because the conversion of the coenzyme from the oxidized to the reduced form (or vice versa) can be followed at 340 nm and monitored against time to give the velocity of the reaction. This value, equivalent to the maximum activity of the enzyme, is expressed in suitable units and related to unit number or volume of red cells or to unit weight of haemoglobin. A diminished reaction velocity indicates a deficiency of the enzyme; this means a mutant enzyme is present whose concentration may or may not be normal— many mutants are less stable than the normal enzyme—but whose activity is diminished because of molecular structural abnormalities. Further characterization of the mutant requires a study of its charge characteristics, stability and kinetic behaviour as described below.

Electrophoresis of haemolysates or partially purified extracts is carried out, usually on starch gel, with the intention of revealing abnormal bands. This indicates an abnormal net charge on the molecule and is evidence of an abnormal structure. The technique has been useful for the detection of a number of variants, especially G6PD.

An enzyme variant may be less stable than its normal counterpart and may decay more rapidly when stored *in vitro* at any temperature. The rate of decay is faster at higher temperatures (above 37°C) and thermal stability has been used to detect mutants by following the thermally induced decline in activity over a few hours.

Enzyme activity is pH-sensitive because of ionizable groups on both the substrate and enzyme molecule. As a consequence, an enzyme shows a characteristic pH-activity curve and deviations from it provide non-specific evidence of a mutant enzyme.

The Michaelis constant (K_m) of an enzyme is the dissociation constant of the enzyme–substrate complex; numerically it is that substrate concentration which yields the half-maximal reaction velocity. The graph of reaction velocity against substrate concentration is a hyperbola but linear relationships may be calculated (see Ref. 221) which permit the K_m value to be obtained. A low K_m value implies a high affinity of the substrate for the enzyme and vice versa and each enzyme has a characteristic value for its substrate(s) and another for its cofactor or coenzyme. An abnormal K_m value suggests a peculiarity around the active centre of the enzyme which affects its affinity. The K_m value has proved a useful index for the identification of mutants.

Some enzymes will react with analogues of their true substrate (e.g. 2-deoxyglucose 6-phosphate can replace G6P in the G6PD reaction) and this offers a further test because the K_m value can be determined for the abnormal substrate. The characterization of PK mutants has been assisted by the use of an activator, fructose 1,6-diphosphate, which stimulates mutant enzymes differently from normal [222, 223].

Because of the number of mutants of PK which have been reported a need has arisen for standardization of techniques. This has been attempted [224] and full details are available for the preparation of partially purified extracts, enzyme assay and techniques for characterization of the enzyme.

ENZYMOPATHIES OF THE EMBDEN–MEYERHOF PATHWAY (EMP)

In this section the biochemical changes and clinical features associated with enzyme deficiencies of the EMP are described. With the exception of pyruvate-kinase deficiency [225] they are all rare, the second most common being glucose phosphate isomerase deficiency. The conditions may arise as a result of gene deletions, structural mutations or post-translational modifications but as yet the mechanisms are not fully understood, most defects being so rare as to prohibit attempts at exact classification. In addition, there is marked heterogeneity within the same group. In the absence of consanguinity, homozygotes are usually compound heterozygotes for two separate mutant enzymes, making biochemical definition difficult. The majority of deficiencies show an autosomal recessive pattern of inheritance, homozygotes exhibiting full expression whereas heterozygotes have intermediate levels of enzyme activity but are clinically symptom-free. An exception is phosphoglycerate kinase deficiency which is sex-linked; in some other types the precise mode of inheritance is yet to be established.

These conditions are grouped together under the title of congenital non-spherocytic haemolytic anae-mias (CNSHA) after the description by Selwyn & Dacie in 1954 [217] of two congenitally anaemic patients whose red cells showed absence of appreciable spherocytosis, normal osmotic fragility and spon-taneous lysis upon incubation which was not corrected by the presence of added glucose (Type II). These patients were subsequently found to be suffering from pyruvate-kinase deficiency (see p. 288). Since then defects have been described in most of the EMP enzymes.

The haematological abnormality common to most is a shortened red-cell survival which may produce a variable degree of anaemia ranging from severe hae-molysis in infancy and childhood to full compensation in a symptom-free adult homozygote. In association with this haemolysis are the usual findings of erythroid hyperplasia, reticulocytosis, variable jaundice, early pigment gallstone formation, splenomegaly and ex-acerbation of the anaemia by infection or other intercurrent illness. Fortunately, aplastic crises are rare and haemosiderosis is not a problem in untrans-fused patients. When other tissues carry the enzyme defect there may be muscular or neurological abnor-malities. Generally, white-cell function appears to be normal in the few cases where it has been assessed. Drug sensitivity is not a problem as in defects of the PPP.

The red-cell morphological changes are non-specific and frequently not marked; nevertheless mild to moderate anisocytosis and poikilocytosis with macro-cytosis, polychromasia, basophilic stippling, target cells, fragmented cells and occasional spherocytes are often described from the stained peripheral blood smear [226]. A fairly characteristic feature has been the presence of crenated cells (burr cells) in small numbers. As splenectomy has often been performed, post-splenectomy changes are commonly seen. The Direct Coombs' Test is negative, haemoglobin electrophor-esis normal and the unincubated osmotic fragility normal or only slightly shifted.

The red-cell survival is shortened and an interesting finding in some patients is the paradoxical further reduction of the half-life following splenectomy. This is due to the survival of a severely compromised cohort of cells which would previously have been destroyed in the spleen. Similarly, the reticulocyte count often rises after splenectomy in the presence of clinical improve-ment.

There is as yet no specific treatment for these conditions and therapy consists of blood transfusion for symptomatic comfort, folate supplement and prompt treatment of infections. Splenectomy has been shown to be beneficial in some cases and should certainly be considered where transfusion require-ments are high. Ante-natal diagnosis is possible and adequate genetic counselling should be given when the carrier status of prospective parents is known.

Hexokinase (Hx) deficiency

Normal Hx. This enzyme catalyses the initial step in the EMP to yield glucose 6-phosphate (G6P) which is also the entry point to the PPP (Fig. 7.1). Hexokinase (Hx) operates far from equilibrium and is essentially irreversible. It is inhibited by its product (G6P) [227] but this is relieved by an increased ATP level. Activity is affected by small ATP changes [228]. The decay rate of Hx closely follows the decline in glycolytic activity as red cells age and the enzyme has the lowest capacity of all the glycolytic enzymes [12, 229]; this has suggested that the enzyme is a pacemaker of glycolysis [26].

Hexokinase (Hx) exists in isozymic form. Type I is the major isozyme which accounts for about 90% of the total activity; a Type III and a trace of Type II are also present [230, 231]. The three types conform electrophoretically to some of the several isozymes of other tissues. Type II isozyme is associated with Hb F; it is present in the red cells of neonates, was absent in a neonate's red cells which lacked Hb F, and present in a family with a hereditary persistence of Hb F.

Variant forms of Hx. A decreased Hx activity was first described in three patients from two unrelated families with a Fanconi-type aplastic anaemia without haemo-lysis [232, 233]. Red cells, platelets and white cells were affected and the red-cell enzyme had 24–60% of normal activity. Lactate production and ATP were also low. The decreased Hx activity in these patients is likely to have been a consequence of chromosomal breakages [234].

Hexokinase (Hx) deficiency presenting as a primary disorder and associated with a congenital haemolytic anaemia was first described by Valentine *et al.* [235] in an 11-year-old girl of English and Polish extraction. The measured activity of the enzyme was about 60% of normal but markedly lower when correction was made for the young red-cell population present (reticulocyte count 14·5%). Red-cell ATP concentration was normal as were the K_m values for either substrate. Glucose and fructose consumption were subnormal even without correction for the young cell population. The PPP activity was almost that expected for the age of the cells when expressed as the amount of glucose passing through but appeared to be increase when expressed as a percentage of the subnormal overall glucose consumption. Methylene blue (10^{-6} M) was less stimulatory to the PPP than in normal blood. Only the major Type I isozyme was demonstrable in the red cells of this patient [236]. The incubated osmotic fragility was increased but became normal following splenectomy. Autohaemolysis showed a Type I pattern and inheritance of the defect was autosomal recessive.

Following the description of this carefully studied case, several others were reported [237–242]. Despite the young red-cell population present, glucose consumption of the cells was decreased in several of the reports but also has been found slightly increased [242]. The ATP concentration has usually been low [232, 238, 240, 242] but also normal [235]. The 2,3-DPG concentration has been low [238] or normal [242]. The presence of a low 2,3-DPG results in a leftward shift of the oxygen-dissociation curve and this is disadvantageous because oxygen delivery to the tissue is diminished. This is reflected in the physical behaviour of the patients who are incapacitated more than the extent of their anaemia would indicate [243]. In the first described case of Hx deficiency the enzyme showed normal kinetic behaviour but subsequent reports indicate that the enzyme exists in mutant forms. This is apparent not only by a decreased affinity for glucose [237–239] and a diminished rate of glucose consumption, but also by a decreased affinity for ATP [238, 240]. In two cases [238] the storage characteristics of the enzyme suggested that it was a mutant and in one case [241] the enzyme was unstable at 4° and 46°C.

Diagnosis. The autohaemolysis pattern is Type I or normal and the osmotic fragility and red-cell morphology have been normal. Diagnosis of the deficiency requires care because Hx shows significant age dependency and mature red cells have an activity only two to three per cent that of reticulocytes [244]. As a consequence, examination of a young red-cell population can mask the presence of a mutant with low activity. It is important to determine in parallel the activity in a blood sample comprising cells of equivalent age. Also it is advisable to assay an age-dependent enzyme other than Hx; the ratio of the two activities will indicate whether Hx activity is subnormal. A further difficulty is that mutants show elevated K_m values for glucose and may yield normal values in the presence of excess substrate (e.g. Refs. 237, 239). The enzyme should therefore also be assayed at low glucose concentration.

Glucosephosphate-isomerase (GPI) deficiency

Normal GPI. The second step in the EMP is freely reversible and provides fructose 6-phosphate (F6P) which is also one of the end products of the PPP (Fig. 7.3). The G6P is the entry point to the PPP, and F6P is one of the exit points and so GPI can be bypassed through the pathway. The enzyme has been isolated from a variety of tissues and is dimeric with a MW of 94 000–132 000; the K_m value for G6P is in the range $1 \cdot 2 \times 10^{-3} - 10^{-4}$ M [245–247]. The GPI appears to occur without isozymic variation as several tissues give the same electrophoretic mobility for the enzyme [248–250] and for this reason GPI deficiency in red cells can be accompanied by diminished activity in plasma and white cells. However, electrophoresis at pH 8·6 of heterozygote blood can show three bands resulting from random selection of two subunits (i.e. two homodimers and one heterodimer) [248].

Variant forms of GPI. A considerable number of GPI mutants are known and many which show electrophoretic differences do not have low activities and are not associated with haematological abnormalities [248, 251]. Mutants which have low activities and are associated with haemolytic anaemia tend to have normal K_m values for G6P and F6P and a normal pH optimum but show decreased heat stability (see Ref. 252, p. 201).

The first reported case of GPI deficiency [253] in a male infant with haemolytic anaemia (reticulocytes approx. 28%) gave a red-cell activity for GPI of about 20% normal. Both plasma and white-cell activities were low and family studies suggested an autosomal-recessive inheritance. Glucose consumption and the ATP concentration were increased in accord with the young red-cell population present. Autohaemolysis was Type I and the incubated osmotic fragility was increased. A later report from the same group [254] described GPI deficiency with severe haemolysis in three siblings from a family unrelated to their first case. The GPI activity was 13–40% of normal and the reticulocyte count was in the range 40–70%. The K_m values for red- and white-cell enzymes were normal but electrophoresis of haemolysates showed an abnormal band without minor bands. Red cells were inefficient in recycling glucose through the PPP. Both parents and four clinically asymptomatic siblings gave low red- and white-cell activities but the parents showed normal electrophoretic bands.

Following these first reports many others have appeared and are reviewed [252, 255]. Glucose consumption is usually increased although some reports suggest that this is not in proportion to the young cell population [253, 256–259]. The ATP concentration is usually low to normal, G6P is increased and F6P near normal, while GA3P and DHAP are normal [256–266].

An unusual case of combined GPI and G6PD deficiency is reported [260]. Both parents showed partial GPI deficiency and the mother was a heterozygote for G6PD deficiency. Two brothers were hemizygous for G6PD deficiency and one was homozygous for GPI deficiency; a sister was heterozygous for both deficiencies. The propositus, a male with haemolytic anaemia (reticulocytes 7–20%), had 24% of normal GPI activity while the heterozygotes in the family had 42–65% of normal activity. Glycolysis in the affected male was about twice the normal value and the G6P concentration was nearly five time normal. Glycolytic esters distal to the block were low, except for 2,3-DPG which was increased. The ATP concentration was low after correction for the young cell population. The G6PD activity in the affected patients' red cells was reduced to only 80% of normal and GSH stability was normal; the Heinz-body test gave an abnormal result, however, and the patient was drug-sensitive. The GPI deficiency has also been reported in association with increased hepatic glycogen storage and mental retardation [267].

Diagnosis. There is a considerable variation in the severity of the haemolytic anaemia. Severe GPI deficiency has presented as hydrops fetalis and pre-natal diagnosis by examination of the amniotic cells is possible [268]. The stained peripheral blood film shows anisocytosis and poikilocytosis; spiculated cells and ovalocytes have also been observed [269] and both young and old cells have a markedly increased rigidity [270]. The osmotic fragility is usually normal and the autohaemolysis normal of Type I, but with less correction of lysis by glucose than in other disorders. Splenectomy has often been beneficial. Attempts at treatment with methylene blue, to bypass the EMP block and pass substrate through the PPP, have been unsuccessful.

Most variants appear to be due to a single amino-acid substitution resulting from a point mutation but a recent case has been described [271] where the enzyme had a significantly lowered MW, though to be due to a deletion mutation.

Phosphofructokinase (PFK) deficiency

Normal PFK. The phosphorylation of F6P in the presence of ATP and PFK yields fructose 1,6-diphosphate (F1,6P) (Fig. 7.1). The PFK is a major control step in glycolysis (see p. 265) and its activity is modified by a number of regulators (Table 7.5). The enzyme has allosteric properties and its kinetic behaviour varies in different tissues. Whilst ATP is one of the substrates it is also an inhibitor; its K_m value is 25 μM (red-cell ATP concentration is 0·8–1·5 mM) and the enzyme is not notably pH-sensitive. However, ATP inhibition of the enzyme is very sensitive to pH and is marked at low pH; this inhibition reduces the affinity of the enzyme

for its other substrate, F6P. It has been calculated [12] that under cellular conditions of substrate concentration the enzyme operates at 0·1% of its capacity. ATP inhibition occurs through the Mg^{2+}-ATP complex, the normal mode of action of ATP, which is less inhibitory than the free nucleotide.

The enzyme is tetrameric with MW 330 000. It exists in isozymic form and red cells contain two types of subunit known as muscle type and liver type [272].

Unlike most glycolytic enzymes, PFK activity in cord blood is appreciably lower than in adult blood and it is probable that a fetal PFK exists with different kinetic properties [283].

Variants of PFK. Diminished PFK activity with almost complete muscle enzyme deficiency (Type VII glycogen-storage disease) and evidence of haemolysis was described in three Japanese patients [273, 274]. The red cells showed 50% of normal activity and only one of the two components present in red cells, the missing component being that present in normal muscle. In a later report [275] red-cell esters following the block, including 2,3-DPG, were found to be low while F6P was near twice the normal value.

A patient with 60% of normal red-cell PFK activity and a haemolytic anaemia but with normal muscle activity and no apparent muscle disorder has been described [276, 277]. The osmotic fragility, autohaemolysis, lactate production, red-cell Na^+, K^+, and Na^+ flux were all normal. The mother and maternal grandmother of the propositus also showed a diminished red-cell PFK activity but no haemolytic anaemia. Other cases of the deficiency associated with haemolytic anaemia are reported [278–281] and the subject has been reviewed [282].

Generally, patients present with a lifelong history of fatigue and exercise intolerance which cannot be corrected by raising the blood glucose. Skeletal muscles contain excess glycogen and there is no rise in lactate after ischaemic exercise. Patients are not anaemic but there is evidence of a compensated haemolytic anaemia. Platelets and granulocytes are not affected.

Aldolase deficiency

Normal aldolase. This enzyme catalyses the reversible cleavage of F1,6P to give glyceraldehyde 3-phosphate (GA3P) and its isomer dihydroxyacetone (DHAP). The equilibrium favours the backward reaction, the formation of the diphosphate.

Variants of aldolase. A deficiency of this enzyme has been reported only once [284], in a mentally handicapped child, the offspring of first cousins, both of whom had normal activities of the red-cell enzyme. The patient had a mild haemolytic anaemia and increased liver glycogen deposits.

Triose-phosphate-isomerase (TPI) deficiency

Normal TPI. The two triose phosphates, DHAP and GA3P, which are produced in the aldolase reaction are interconvertible in the presence of TPI. The equilibrium lies towards the formation of DHAP and in normal red cells the ratio of DHAP to GA3P is about 3:1. The GA3P is the sole substrate for the next enzyme in metabolic sequence and so there is a flow of substrate as shown:

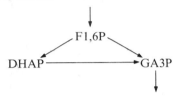

The capacity of TPI is the greatest of all the glycolytic enzymes in the red cell and is two orders of magnitude greater than that of Hx (Table 7.4). In red cells the enzyme is a dimer present as three isozymes [285]. It was thought originally that the three bands represented two homopolymers with an intermediate heteropolymer but it is now considered that the most cathodic band is the primary form of the enzyme and the other two are secondary isozymes due to post-translational changes [286], possibly the result of de-amidation [287]. The gene marker for TPI is located on chromosome 12 [288].

Variants of TPI. A red-cell deficiency of this enzyme (10% of normal activity) was first described in an infant of French and Negro ancestry [289]. The mutant enzyme was associated with a chronic haemolytic anaemia (Hb 10g/dl; reticulocytes 13%) and a progressive muscular disorder. Both parents showed intermediate TPI activity but were haematologically normal. A second case, strikingly similar to the first, and with both parents heterozygotes, was described shortly after [290, 291]. The two cases were thought to be related. A third case, of Anglo-Caucasian extraction, and unrelated to the other cases but with a similar condition, is also reported [291]. In all patients white cells were also affected and in one the serum, CSF and muscle showed low activity. Red-cell glucose was unexpectedly high even after correction for the young cell population present while the ATP concentration was normal or only slightly low. The DHAP was more than 20 times the level in normal cells and methylene blue had a smaller effect on overall glucose consumption than in normal or reticulocyte-rich blood. Four

further examples of this deficiency are reported by the original group [293, 294] and others [294, 295]. The last-named group described six members of one family, including both parents, who showed heterozygote values for TPI activity. The red cells of the propositus had increased concentrations of F1,6P, GA3P and DHAP and also, as in the earlier cases, a raised glucose consumption. The PPP activity was somewhat low but showed significant stimulation with methylene blue.

The notable abnormality in TPI deficiency is the very high concentration of DHAP and it has been suggested [226] that this intermediate is toxic to the cell. Unlike the cells of other tissues, red cells are unable to convert DHAP to glycerol phosphate. Otherwise the cause of the haemolytic anaemia is unknown. Most other tissues also carry the defect including leucocytes and thymus but neutrophil function appears to be normal when examined despite the frequency of infectious complications [292, 296]. The most common finding in kinetic studies has been thermal instability of the enzyme and the absence of immunologically cross-reacting material; it is suggested that the defect is due to enzyme instability rather than to reduced specific activity [297].

In some members of the family in the original report [292] double heterozygosity for TPI and G6PD deficiency and Hb S existed without ill effects; and in two females who had triple deficiencies with anaemia there was no good evidence that the low haemoglobin was due to the co-existing defects.

Diagnosis. Clinically patients present with a severe haemolytic anaemia from birth, and death in the neonatal period is common [292]. Neurological complications appear at six months or later and comprise progressive impairment of motor development with general spasticity or, more commonly, muscle weakness and flaccidity with absent tendon jerks. Speech becomes unintelligible and seizures may occur. The incidence of severe intercurrent infection is higher than in other congenital non-spherocytic haemolytic anaemias and death from repeated respiratory infections and respiratory insufficiency is the rule—most patients die in infancy although one has survived 21 years [293].

Peripheral blood appearances, osmotic fragility and autohaemolysis are not helpful in diagnosis which must be made on the results of enzyme assay.

Glyceraldehyde-3-phosphate-dehydrogenase (GAPD) deficiency

Normal GAPD. The conversion of GA3P to 1,3-diphosphoglycerate (1,3-DPG) is effected by GAPD in the presence of NAD^+ and inorganic phosphate (Fig. 7.1). This well-studied enzyme consists of four subunits and has MW 144 000. It contains —SH groups essential for activity and the inhibition of glycolysis by iodoacetate is due to reactivity of the inhibitor with these groups. The K_m value for GA3P is 7.8×10^{-5} M [298] and the enzyme is stabilized by NAD^+. The complex that NAD^+ normally forms with the enzyme can be dissociated with physiological concentrations of ATP [299]. The equilibrium of the reaction lies well over towards the formation of 1,3-DPG and the enzyme is one of the more active in the pathway (Table 7.4). It was formerly believed to be regulatory; this is not so, although changes brought about in the NAD^+:NADH ratio can change the phosphate ester profile. The activity of the enzyme is sensitive to pH as a consequence of changes in the coenzyme ratio; at alkaline pH values NADH increases and F1,6P accumulates, while at acid pH both F1,6P and DHAP fall with a rise in 3PG, 2,3-DPG and PEP [300].

There is good evidence that GAPD is bound within the red cell to the membrane (e.g. Refs 301, 302) and it seems probable that it is normally located on the cytoplasmic face with 3×10^5 molecules bound to high-affinity sites [303, 304]. The gene locus for GAPD is assigned to chromosome 12.

Variants of GAPD. A deficiency of this enzyme was first reported in the red cells of a father and son of English descent [305]. The GAPD activity was 20–30% of normal and there was an associated haemolytic anaemia (reticulocytes 10–15%) with a normal osmotic fragility and a Type-I autohaemolysis. The ATP and phosphoglyceric acids were decreased in concentration and the F1,6P was increased.

An unusual family has been reported with a partial GAPD deficiency (50%) and hereditary spherocytosis [306]. Four members had both low GAPD activity and hereditary spherocytosis, three had low GAPD activity alone, two had normal GAPD activity and hereditary spherocytosis, and the remainder were normal. Those members with a diminished GAPD activity alone were not anaemic and so a causal relationship between the enzyme deficiency and haemolysis remains to be established in this family.

Phosphoglycerate-kinase (PGK) deficiency

Normal PGK. The dephosphorylation of 1,3-DPG to 3-phosphoglycerate (3PG) is catalysed by PGK in the presence of ADP (Fig. 7.1). At this step ATP is formed from ADP and since 1,3-DPG is a three-carbon compound originating from six-carbon glucose, two moles of ATP are produced per mole of glucose consumed. Under intracellular conditions PGK operates near equilibrium which is towards the formation of 3PG. The enzyme requires Mg^{2+} (or Mn^{2+}) to form the metal salt but will act also with IDP (inosine diphosphate). It has a K_m value for ADP of 0·2–0·4 mM [26]; with Mg^{2+}-ATP the affinity is increased and the K_m value is 0·1 mM [12]. The K_m value for the other substrate, 1,3-DPG is 2 μM and so the enzyme is sensitive under intracellular conditions to variations in the concentration of this ester. The enzyme is inhibited by ATP at physiological concentrations. As with GAPD, PGK is thought to be membrane-bound, in close functional association with the sodium pump [301].

The PGK constitutes one branch of the Rapoport–Luebering shuttle (Fig. 7.2) and 1,3-DPG is the common substrate for the two branches, the other branch leading to the formation of 2,3-DPG.

Variants of PGK. A moderate deficiency of red-cell PGK in a Caucasian woman with a non-spherocytic haemolytic anaemia was first described in 1968 [307]. The white cells were not affected. A gross deficiency in the red cells of two male Chinese children with haemolytic anaemia and mental retardation was reported shortly after [308]. Splenectomy in the more affected of the two children was followed by a rise in the haemoglobin and freedom from transfusion requirements. The red-cell PGK activity was about five per cent of normal and white cells also showed subnormal activity in the more affected patient. Autohaemolysis was Type II as is often found in other patients. The ATP was somewhat low and the 2,3-DPG concentration was notably increased, while glucose consumption and lactate production were normal.

Following these two reports, further cases have been described [309–314]. Transmission of the defect is sex-linked and female heterozygotes have two red-cell populations, one normal and one enzyme-deficient. White cells are also affected and neurological abnormalities common. Red-cell ATP levels are normal or somewhat low and the 2,3-DPG concentration is normal or increased. The concentration of some phosphate esters preceding the block, namely, triose phosphates and F1,6P is increased.

The anaemia associated with the deficiency varies in severity from severe to mild and in one family seven affected males in two generations had no overt clinical symptoms or anaemia although their PGK activities were about 21% of normal [315]. Splenectomy gave no improvement in the first reported case [307] but other reports suggest some improvement [308, 310, 311]. The kinetic properties of the enzyme have been found to be normal [310, 314].

2,3-diphosphoglycerate mutase (2,3-DPGM) deficiency

Normal 2,3-DPGM. The conversion of 1,3-DPG to 2,3-DPG is catalysed by the presence of 2,3-DPGM and the reaction requires the presence of 3PG or 2PG as a phosphate acceptor [316, 317]. The K_m value for 1,3-DPG is 0·5 μM [318, 319] which is in the region of the intracellular concentration of the ester ($< 1 \mu$M) so that 2,3-DPG production is affected by small changes in the concentration of 1,3-DPG. It is calculated that the enzyme operates at less than one per cent of its maximal activity in the cell because 2,3-DPG is strongly inhibitory [318, 320]. Thyroxine and its analogues are also inhibitory, 95% inhibition is imposed by 50 μM triiodothyronine and 50% by 75 μM thyroxine [321].

Variants of 2,3-DPGM. The unequivocal diagnosis of this deficiency has been delayed by the lack of an enzyme assay. The first description relied upon the abnormal and irreversible loss of 2,3-DPG during the incubation of red cells from two patients with congenital non-spherocytic haemolytic anaemia. Further indirect evidence was obtained in three unrelated patients, also with non-spherocytic haemolytic anaemia, whose red cells showed a diminished ATP concentration and lactate production [322]. Direct assay of the enzyme was carried out on the red cells of a German family, the male propositus of which had a severe and eventually fatal congenital haemolytic anaemia [323]. Both parents, a sister and the father's mother were asymptomatic but had a 2,3-DPGM activity in their red cells which was only 55–66% of normal and a 2,3-DPG concentration of about 50% of normal.

A detailed study of a family, six members of whom were affected, with partial 2,3-DPGM deficiency associated with a compensated haemolytic anaemia has been described [324]. Only recently has a case of complete deficiency been recorded [325, 326] in a 42-year-old male of French origin who presented with polycythaemia (Hb 19·0 g/dl) and ruddy cyanosis but was otherwise asymptomatic. Red-cell morphology was normal and there was no evidence of haemolysis. No enzyme was detectable and the 2,3-DPG concentration was less than three per cent of normal, giving a marked increase in oxygen affinity of the haemoglobin. Disphosphoglycerate phosphatase activity was also extremely low and monophosphyglycerate mutase activity reduced by 50%. The GSH, ATP, F1,6P and triose phosphates were all elevated but G6P and F6P were low in concentration. Two offspring had intermediate levels of enzyme activity and haemoglobin and 2,3-DPG values at the upper and lower limits of

normal respectively. The patient was treated by phlebotomy and the condition was well tolerated. This case is of interest in that the findings are those predictable from a complete absence of the enzyme and it demonstrates the ability of a subject to compensate for a low 2,3-DPG concentration without gross debility. That the deficiency arose from the presence of a mutant enzyme is suggested by the abnormal stability and electrophoretic mobility of the enzyme [327].

2,3-Diphosphoglycerate phosphatase (2,3-DPGase) deficiency

Normal 2,3-DPGase. The dephosphorylation of 2,3-DPG to form 3-phosphoglycerate (3PG) is catalysed by 2,3-DPGase (Fig. 7.1). The activity of the enzyme is very low in intact red cells; only about 60 μmol of ester is converted by one litre of cells per hour at 37°C [319]. Both Cl$^-$ and inorganic phosphate activate the enzyme under physiological conditions, but pathological levels of phosphate are not thought to affect enzyme activity. Other halides, several S-containing compounds, HCO$_3^-$ and particularly glycolate 2-phosphate are also stimulatory [319, 328–332]. The K_m value at activating concentrations of Cl$^-$ and inorganic phosphate is 0·05 μM [319] and so the enzyme, unlike 2,3-DPGM, is insensitive to small changes in the cellular concentration of 2,3-DPG.

Variants of 2,3-DPGase. A deficiency of this enzyme has been reported in two unrelated infants with non-spherocytic haemolytic anaemia and a number of associated clinical disorders [333]. The 2,3-DPG concentration was normal but both ATP and ADP were increased to 50% above the normal value.

Phosphoglyceromutase and enolase deficiency

Neither of these enzymes has been convincingly shown to occur in mutant form.

Pyruvate-kinase (PK) deficiency

Normal PK. This enzyme is responsible for the effectively irreversible conversion of phosphoenolpyruvate (PEP) to pyruvate with the simultaneous transfer of a phosphate group on to ADP to give ATP (Fig. 7.1). The enzyme requires both Mg^{2+} and K^+ as cofactors, the affinity of the enzyme for ADP being increased by the presence of K^+ [334]. It has been suggested [335] that PK has two binding sites each of which can bind K^+, substrate or product and binding at one site promotes binding at the second.

There are some similarities between the red-cell (R) and liver (L) enzymes; both are the product of the same gene, have similar MWs of about 230 000 and exist as tetramers with four identical subunits [336, 337]. Electrophoresis of partially purified normal red-cell PK shows two bands [338] which have been designated L'_4 (PK R_1) and $L_2L'_2$ (PK R_2), the former preponderating in erythroblasts and young cells [339, 340]. It is suggested that as red cells age, partial proteolysis transforms the L' subunits to the L form so that the $L_2L'_2$ type becomes predominant in mature cells [338]. In hepatocytes a very active proteolytic system possibly produces early transformation of the L'_4 enzyme to the L_4 type [338]. Two other isozymic forms of PK are M_1 and M_2, the former preponderating in muscle and the latter in white cells; in addition liver cells have a minor M_2 component [341].

PK shows allosteric properties, and of several effectors F1,6P is the most potent. Under normal intracellular conditions the enzyme should be saturated with the effector because the concentration for half maximal stimulation is $0.05-0.2 \mu M$ [339, 342–344] while the intracellular concentration is considerably greater than this (Table 7.3). The L'_4 (PK R_1) and L_4 forms show different kinetic properties in their affinity for PEP, inhibition by ATP and regulation by F1,6P. The L'_2L_2 (PK R_2) form gives intermediate values supporting the suggestion that there are two kinetically different forms of PK in red cells [345]. Following the original proposition [346] that allosteric enzymes have two conformations which are in equilibrium, R and T forms, different properties are ascribed to the R and T forms of PK [342, 347, 348]. In the R form the enzyme shows increased affinity for PEP, a decreased K_m value for the positive effector F1,6P and weak inhibition by ATP, whereas in the T form there is a low affinity for PEP and F1,6P but strong inhibition by ATP. A left shift in the equilibrium towards the active R form is produced by low concentrations of F1,6P.

The capacity of PK in normal cells is greater than 50 times the requirement as judged by the rate of lactate production, and the enzyme is normally unsaturated with respect to its two substrates (Table 7.4) [349]. Both inorganic phosphate and 2,3-DPG inhibit the reaction [350–354] and it is of interest that in those species with low 2,3-DPG levels PK activity is high [12].

Pyruvate-kinase (PK) deficiency. The first cases of PK deficiency to be reported were those of Valentine *et al.* [355], in three males with congenital non-spherocytic haemolytic anaemia. Since that time more than 300 cases have been recorded and it is the commonest deficiency affecting the EMP.

Metabolic abnormalities. The three homozygotes for PK deficiency first reported by Valentine's group gave a Type II autohaemolysis pattern and in their original description of this test [217] the authors reported on two patients who were the prototypes of the Type II classification; these two patients were subsequently shown to be PK-deficient [356]. Many reports of PK deficiency with a Type II autohaemolysis pattern appeared in the early sixties which gave rise to the notion that the two findings were invariably linked. Given an allowance for bias, inexperience and local variations of technique this is not true, for Type I and even normal patterns can be found. An improvement in the technique [218] increased the number of Type II cases earlier described as Type I but which were known to be PK-deficient. The ready assay of the enzyme has relegated the autohaemolysis test to a secondary role for the diagnosis of this deficiency.

Glucose consumption of red cells in PK deficiency is impaired [217, 356–360]. Observed values are normal or slightly raised but are low after correction for the young red-cell population present. Both pyruvate levels and lactate production are low, the pyruvate:lactate ratio remaining normal [357–363] and phosphate esters preceding the block are raised [357, 359, 362, 363].

2,3-DPG was first reported as increased in concentration in three cases [364], a finding which suggested a glycolytic block following the production of this ester before PK deficiency had been described. It has since been amply confirmed that homozygous PK deficiency is accompanied by an increased 2,3-DPG concentration. This offers a degree of compensation for the anaemia (see Chapters 4 and 8) because the oxygen-dissociation curve is displaced to the right, indicating a lowered oxygen affinity of the haemoglobin.

The ATP concentration in red cells was originally reported as low [356, 361, 362, 364–369] although not notably so in the case of one group [364]. Subsequently, a number of cases were described with normal or even increased levels [358, 360, 370–375]. It is now considered that typically the ATP concentration is in the normal or low–normal range. The NAD^+ and NADH concentrations are low but the ratio is normal [356, 362, 376].

Under normal circumstances the ATP in red cells is produced exclusively by the EMP; in gross PK deficiency the cells have a severely restricted lifespan and the peripheral blood contains a high proportion of reticulocytes which retain a residual though fading Krebs cycle. This offers an alternative source for ATP generation upon which the red cells may well depend for their survival. This was established [358] first, by incubation of enzyme-deficient cells in the absence of glucose which gave no loss of ATP over a few hours; secondly, by the demonstration that the presence of 10 mM inorganic phosphate in the absence of glucose raised the ATP concentration; and thirdly, by showing that the presence of 5 mM cyanide in abnormal cells resulted in a loss of ATP but left normal cells unaffected in this respect. Thus, PK-deficient red cells were shown to depend upon oxidative phosphorylation for the maintenance of ATP. Other observers have also noted the cyanide sensitivity and mitochondrial dependence of PK-deficient cells [377–379].

PK-deficient red cells undergo marked lysis during *in-vitro* incubation in the absence of glucose, more than do normal cells. This suggests that in addition to the enzyme deficiency there is a secondary abnormality associated with the membrane. Circumstantial evidence that this is so is the increased K^+ leakage and flux in older PK-deficient cells [357, 380]; this is observed *in vitro* together with a loss of water and cell shrinkage, a process of desiccocytosis [381].

Heterozygotes. The PK deficiency associated with congenital non-spherocytic anaemia represents the gross or homozygous form of the disease. Intermediate levels of PK activity not generally associated with haemolysis are found in heterozygotes. The disease is inherited as an autosomal-recessive disorder with a calculated frequency greater than 0·005% [382].

Variants of PK. A considerable number of kinetically abnormal forms of PK have been characterized. The disease is likely to be heterogeneous because inheritance of abnormal genes appears to offer no environmental advantages, unlike G6PD deficiency. In addition the enzyme is expressed by two genes, and the presence of two abnormal gene products is likely to give rise to hybrid enzymes (see Ref. 252, p. 171). The first indication that in PK deficiency there was an abnormal enzyme present was the finding of an abnormal K_m value for PEP [368]. Later reports on four patients gave normal K_m values for both substrates [383, 384]. It is now clear that although the K_m value for ADP is usually normal [339, 385–389] that for PEP may be normal [339, 385, 386, 389–393], increased [339, 348, 373, 378, 385, 388, 390–392, 394] or even decreased [385, 390, 391, 395].

Studies of the other properties of enzymes with diminished activity have revealed mutants with slow, increased or normal electrophoretic mobility; normal or abnormal pH optima curves; increased thermal lability; decreased, normal or even increased urea stability, and normal or increased K_m values for the effector F1,6P.

True homozygotes arise only from consanguineous parents but most subjects are doubly heterozygous for two separate genes thus increasing the biochemical complexity of the condition. The simple assay of the enzyme under the usual conditions may be inadequate to establish a diagnosis. For example, four patients

from two unrelated families gave normal or only slightly low activities for the enzyme when assayed under routine conditions with excess substrate [396]. However, the K_m values for PEP were 10 times greater than normal and assay of the enzyme using intracellular concentrations of substrate revealed a low activity. Later studies on these patients [222, 223] revealed abnormal behaviour of the enzyme in the presence of F1,6P. In another case [397], assay revealed the PK activity to be supranormal and yet the concentrations of the glycolytic esters were raised, except for ATP, particularly near the PK step. This case was subsequently established as a PK mutant by finding that the partially purified enzyme gave an abnormal K_m value. Such observations mean that a normal assay result does not eliminate the possibility of a mutant enzyme. A further complication in the assay of suspect blood is the need to remove white cells which otherwise may give an erroneously high assay value.

Attempts have been made to classify variants according to whether they are stabilized in the T or R form [346]* and also according to their electrophoretic mobility and behaviour on *in-vitro* proteolysis in an attempt to correlate the findings with the clinical severity of the disease [398]. This work is in its early stages but generally, if the residual enzyme activity is below 15–20% of normal, there is marked haemolysis whatever kinetic abnormalities are displayed by the enzyme.

The exact mechanism by which haemolysis occurs is not known with any certainty but the common denominator is thought to be a failure of energy metabolism and this arises from structural gene mutations.

Because of all these factors, together with the need to standardize the data and rationalize the nomenclature, instructions have been made available for the full characterization of the enzyme [224].

Clinical features. The disorder shows considerable variation in severity, ranging from a severe haemolytic anaemia, presenting in early infancy, to a compensated haemolytic disorder of adults [225]; it has presented as a neonatal anaemia [399] severe enough to require exchange transfusion. Growth retardation may occur in severely affected children. Occasionally it presents in

---

* Allosteric proteins are composed of a number of separate protein subunits which are associated in such a way that they occupy equivalent positions in the oligomer and the protein possesses at least one axis of symmetry. The conformation of each subunit is constrained by its association with other subunits. At least two conformations of the oligomeric protein exist in the absence of substrate and these conformational states are in equilibrium with each other. The two conformations are called the R (relaxed) and T (tensed) states and possess different kinetic properties

late childhood or early adult life. The typical manifestations are those of a congenital haemolytic anaemia, namely jaundice and slight to moderate splenomegaly but in less severely affected patients presenting in their second and third decades, clinical jaundice may be absent. Hepatomegaly may be present, especially in patients who have received numerous transfusions; cholelithiasis is common. The clinical severity tends to remain constant in an individual patient in the absence of infection or surgery. Whilst death in the first few years of life has been reported, survival to adulthood is common. Affected women have undergone pregnancy without significant complications [360]. In spite of reduced liver-enzyme activity, hepatic dysfunction has not been recorded and so it is probable that the small amount of M enzyme present is adequate. Leucocyte function appears also to be unaffected.

Blood picture. Haemoglobin values show considerable variation, ranging from 5 to 12 g/dl. The reticulocyte count also varies between patients; before splenectomy it is usually slight to moderate, but post-splenectomy counts of more than 50% are common [358]. This increase in reticulocytosis after splenectomy is thought to be due to the survival of severely compromised cells which would previously have been sequestered in the spleen. PK-deficient reticulocytes are very sensitive to haemolysis and it has been suggested that the unfavourable kinetics of the L'_4 (PK R_1) type of PK present in young cells aggravates the deficiency [398]. In most cases the red cells show a fairly uniform macrocytosis of moderate to marked degree and little or no poikilocytosis. The cells are either normally haemoglobinized or very slightly hypochromic; polychromasia is usual and a variable number of nucleated red cells may be present. Bizarre echinocytes which may resemble acanthocytes are also seen, particularly after splenectomy [357, 358, 380, 400]. A greater degree of morphological change may occur in infants or young children [360]. Post-splenectomy, siderocytes and Pappenheimer bodies are commonly present.

The osmotic fragility of fresh blood is normal or slightly decreased; that of incubated blood is usually, but not invariably, increased. The autohaemolysis pattern has already been considered (see p. 280). The antiglobulin (Coombs) test and the Hams test are negative. Heinz bodies, abnormal haemoglobins, increased Hb A_2 or F are not present. The white cell and platelet counts are normal but may be increased, especially after splenectomy.

The half-time for ^{51}Cr-labelled red cells is usually markedly reduced, but moderate reduction has been reported [360]. The pattern of surface counting with ^{51}Cr-labelled cells has been reported in detail [401].

Diagnosis. Deficiency of PK is the commonest of the EMP defects and is the likeliest cause of a congenital non-spherocytic haemolytic anaemia with recessive inheritance. The diagnosis can usually be made by observing the decreased activity of the red-cell enzyme. In affected homozygotes, values are in the range 5–20% of the normal mean value but are sometimes higher. After correction for the young cell population present assay values are very low. Diagnosis can be difficult in some cases (see p. 289) and full kinetic studies may be necessary to make the diagnosis. Supportive evidence for PK deficiency is provided by an increased 2,3-DPG concentration and a Type-II autohaemolysis pattern.

Treatment. The main form of treatment is blood transfusion as required for symptomatic comfort. Requirements vary considerably and are increased during infective episodes and other intercurrent illness. However, some patients never require transfusion. Many patients tolerate moderately severe anaemia extremely well because of the associated decreased oxygen affinity of the haemoglobin.

Splenectomy should be considered in any patient requiring regular transfusion and in other patients with severe anaemia as it has now been shown to be beneficial although the haemoglobin rarely returns to normal. Surface counting has shown an improved survival of young cells [401]. Folic-acid supplement is advisable and patients should be alerted to the need for prompt treatment of infections.

Other treatments tried in this condition have been the administration of steroids, immunosuppressive agents, AMP and riboflavin, but without any real therapeutic benefit. Infusions of inosine and adenine have been reported as improving the anaemia in one patient (see Ref. 252, p. 187).

Acquired PK deficiency. In other haemolytic disorders PK activity is normal or increased but rare cases are described in which the activity is mildly decreased [402, 403]. Acquired PK deficiency is reported in a number of haematological disorders including acute leukaemia, cytopenia, refractory anaemia, aplasia, PNH and pernicious anaemia (see Ref. 252, p. 172). In general, the level of activity is that seen in heterozygotes for the congenital deficiency and is rarely less than 50% of normal.

Lactate-dehydrogenase (LDH) deficiency

Normal LDH. The two final products of the EMP, pyruvate and lactate, are both unphosphorylated and can diffuse freely across the red-cell membrane. Both are required in the cell for continuing glycolysis

because the conversion of pyruvate to lactate, catalysed by LDH, is associated with the oxidation of
NADH to NAD^+ and the latter form of the enzyme is
required by GAPD. Also, NADH is required for the
reduction of MetHb. The capacity of LDH is about
one mole of pyruvate reduced per litre of red cells
per hour at $37°C$ (Table 7.4) and it is one of the more
active enzymes. Its activity with NADPH is only
about six per cent of that with NADH [12]; this is
increased in the presence of excess pyruvate [404] but
the former coenzyme has no physiological role in the
LDH reaction. The reaction is reversible but the
intracellular equilibrium is not readily determinable
because of the technical difficulties in determining the
$NADH/NAD^+$ ratio.

LDH exists in a number of isozymic forms, all with
an approximate MW of 134 000, and comprising
tetramers of two types of subunits called M (muscle)
and H (heart). All possible forms exist, namely M_4,
M_3H_1, M_2H_2, M_1H_3 and H_4. Human red cells contain
all five isozymes in the proportion M_4 1, M_3H_1 2, M_2H_2
14, M_1H_3 39 and H_4 44% [12].

Variants of LDH. Deficiency of LDH as been described [405] in a 64-year-old diabetic Japanese male
without any haematological abnormalities. Red-cell
LDH activity was near five per cent of the normal
average and the residual activity was due to the M
subunit, H being absent, so that the only isozyme
present was M_4. A brother and five offspring of the
propositus had LDH activity which was half the
normal mean and showed a 5% deficit of H_4. The red
cells of the homozygote had increased levels of F1,6P,
DHAP and GA3P with a low blood lactate and normal
pyruvate. This increased ester level was suggested to be
a result of a decreased $NAD^+:NADH$ ratio which
caused a restriction at the GAPD step.

Congenital abnormalities associated with red-cell ATP

When a congenital non-spherocytic haemolytic anaemia is associated with a primary defect in the EMP a
low red-cell ATP concentration might be predicted as a
secondary effect. In fact, this occurs only in Hx, TPI,
GAPD, PGK and in some cases of PK deficiency. In
GPI, 2,3-DPGM and 2,3-DPGase deficiency the
values are in accord with the age of the red-cell
population; in other defects the values are not available. The presence of reticulocytes in a blood sample is
likely to obscure a low ATP level because the young
cells have some capacity for producing ATP from the
Krebs cycle, while the mature cells with low ATP
levels, as in PK deficiency, are unlikely to survive for
very long. Estimation of the ATP concentration is easy
and gives some measure of the metabolic state of the

red cells; its significance is more difficult to interpret
because it represents the steady-state result of a
number of variables.

An ethnic difference in the red-cell concentration of
ATP occurs in American male Negroes whose mean
level is significantly lower than that of male Caucasians
[406]. The same author earlier described [407, 408] an
American Negro family in which there was a congenital elevation of the red-cell ATP to twice the normal
value. Study of a large family with β thalassaemia
revealed that 18 non-thalassaemic and 13 thalassaemic
members had red-cell ATP levels that were almost
twice the normal value [409].

Pyrimidine 5′-nucleotidase (P5N) deficiency

Pyrimidine 5′-nucleotidase (P5N) catalyses the hydrolytic dephosphorylation of pyrimidine 5′-ribose monophosphate to freely diffusible pyrimidine nucleoside.

A deficiency of this enzyme has been reported in the
red cells of four members of three separate families
[410]. The red cells of affected individuals contained up
to six times the normal concentration of nucleotides of
which 80% were pyrimidines. Normally red cells
contain only trace amounts of pyrimidine nucleotides,
the major component being purine nucleotides. These
patients had earlier been described as having high
red-cell ATP levels because of the erroneous identification of pyrimidines as adenine.

Since then several other cases have been reported
(see Ref. 252, p. 229). The condition presents generally
as a congenital non-spherocytic haemolytic anaemia
of mild to moderate degree and the notable feature in the
blood film is the presence of basophilic stippling which
is thought to be due to impaired ribosome degeneration [410]. As with lead poisoning, this may be
missed unless fresh blood is examined; it disappears
from blood collected into EDTA after storage for three
hours [411]. The red cells contain uniquely high
concentrations of cytidine and uridine nucleotides and
there is an associated, but as yet unexplained, increased GSH concentration and a partial deficiency of
ribosephosphate pyrophosphokinase (PRPP synthe-
tase). In one case globin synthesis was abnormal (α/β
ratio 1:5) due possibly to excess α-chain production
[411]. Partial purification of a mutant enzyme showed
an increased K_m for cytidine 5′-monophosphate, a
marked shift in the pH optimum curve to the acid side
but normal electrophoretic mobility and heat stability,
suggesting a structural gene mutation [412].

Family studies show an autosomal-recessive mode
of inheritance and heterozygotes have intermediate
levels of activity. There is a rapid and simple screening
test but the diagnosis should be confirmed by enzyme
assay. Splenectomy has not resulted in marked clinical
improvement [413–415].

A secondary deficiency of P5N occurs in patients with lead poisoning whose cells also show basophilic stippling and an abnormal accumulation of pyrimidine nucleotides [416]. This accumulation can be such as to account for up to 80% of the total nucleotide pool and correlates directly with the blood lead concentration. Inhibition of P5N activity may be as high as 95% in severe cases and the reticulocyte response is dampened in anaemic patients possibly because of a direct effect on haemopoiesis.

Adenylate-kinase (AK) deficiency

Adenylate-kinase (AK) deficiency is described in an Arab family coexisting with G6PD deficiency [417]. Both parents of the propositus had a partial deficiency but were haematologically normal; two of the children had severe AK deficiency, six were partially deficient and one was deceased. The two children with severe deficiency also had a haemolytic anaemia. Total adenine nucleotides were increased but only in accord with the young cell population present. The ADP was somewhat higher than expected. A second example of this disorder, also associated with haemolysis, is reported from France [418].

Adenosine deaminase (ADA)

An increase in ADA activity is reported in two families with well-tolerated haemolysis [419–421]. The ATP and total adenine nucleotide concentration was decreased by 50% and the ADA activity was increased up to 75 times normal. The enzyme appeared kinetically to be normal and the hyperactivity was ascribed to over-production of the normal enzyme. The cause of this dominantly inherited defect remains unexplained but may be due to a failure of a feedback mechanism. There is no associated immunological deficiency as occurs with ADA deficiency of lymphocytes and red cells [422].

NADH-linked methaemoglobin reductase (diaphorase) deficiency

The major route for the reduction of MetHb in red cells is that catalysed by diaphorase, a cytochrome b_5 reductase, which uses NADH as a coenzyme. A number of mutants of the enzyme have been reported and whilst none is associated with haemolysis the condition is of haematological interest because of the accumulation of MetHb which occurs in patients with diminished diaphorase activity. The presenting feature is cyanosis due to MetHb in the red cells. This is apparent when the level reaches 1·5–2·0 g/dl of whole blood [423]. Blood samples appear dark when more than about 10% of MetHb is present and the colour does not change on shaking the blood vigorously in air. The tolerable level varies between patients but does not

usually exceed 45–50%. Compensatory erythrocytosis may also occur. Levels of MetHb below about 25% can be tolerated without ill effects, above 35–40% some exertional dyspnoea and occasional headaches may occur.

Cyanosis is also the predominating feature in Hb M disease, but the inheritance of Hb M follows a dominant pattern and this, together with the abnormal absorption spectra of Hb M and the failure of either ascorbate or methylene blue to reduce the level of the 630 nm absorbing material, serves to distinguish the two disorders.

Ascorbate (500 mg daily) or methylene blue (1–2 mg/kg body weight) corrects the methaemoglobinaemia due to diaphorase deficiency. Ascorbate is a direct reductant of MetHb while methylene blue, which has a faster action, stimulates the PPP and increases the action of NADPH-linked MetHb reductase whose contribution to MetHb reduction is otherwise minor (see p. 275).

Early descriptions of diaphorase deficiency are reviewed [424] and currently some 450 cases are on record [425]. The family histories indicate an autosomal-recessive mode of inheritance with both sexes affected. Homozygotes have 10–15% of normal activity and heterozygotes about 60%; the latter do not usually have methaemoglobinaemia but are prone to it from oxidant drug action. Europeans are affected and there is a high incidence among Alaskan Eskimos (15 cases in 20 000 subjects) and Indians [426].

In several reports of diaphorase deficiency there is a leftward shift of the oxygen dissociation curve indicating an increased oxygen affinity of the haemoglobin [427]. This is a consquence of MetHb in the blood and occurs because the ferric-iron component of the total haemoglobin iron is distributed throughout the haemoglobin of the blood; the presence of one ferric iron in a haem group increases the oxygen affinity of the remaining haem groups and this is manifested as a left-shifted dissociation curve. Such a shift does not always occur; in a patient with 20% MetHb most of it was localized in the older cells [428] and the dissociation curve was normal. The accumulation of MetHb in the older cells was a consequence of their diminished ability to reduce it.

The major abnormality in the red cells remains that shown originally [429] namely, that in diaphorase-deficient red cells MetHb accumulates because of the inability of diaphorase to reduce it.

Variants

The advent of a reliable starch-gel technique permitted extensive surveys to be conducted which revealed several variants (e.g. Refs 430, 431). According to one group [431] most normal subjects have a normal band, designated Dia 1, but a few have one of five different phenotypes. The commonest mutant is Boston Fast whose activity is only slightly decreased and whose mobility is similar to Dia 2 found in normal subjects. Mutants with low activity are also reported [432–435]. An association between diaphorase deficiency in children and mental retardation has been noted [436–438].

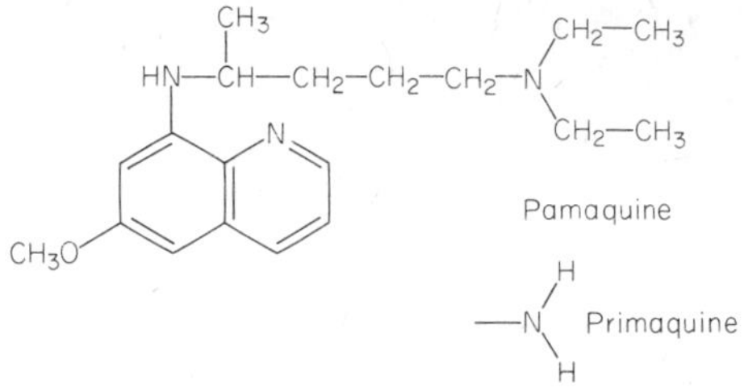

ENZYMOPATHIES OF THE PENTOSE-PHOSPHATE PATHWAY (PPP) AND ITS ASSOCIATED REACTIONS

In this section are described the haemolytic disorders associated with G6PD deficiency and deficiencies of GSH metabolism, namely, GSH synthetase, reductase and peroxidase. By far the most common and important is G6PD deficiency; it is often remarked that 100 million persons carry the trait.

Other defects are rarer than originally thought, for many of the reported cases of GSH reductase and peroxidase deficiency are now known to be due to lack of riboflavin and selenium respectively. However, genetically inherited defects do occur occasionally and are described in the appropriate sections.

The chronic haemolytic disorders due to these deficiencies differ broadly from those due to EMP defects in that:
1 they tend to be less severe;
2 the red-cell ATP concentration is usually normal;
3 the Heinz-body and GSH stability tests are usually positive;
4 haemolysis may be exacerbated by drugs and fava beans; and
5 red-cell morphological changes are slight or absent.

In only relatively few reported cases has splenectomy been performed; it has either been without effect or has caused slight improvement.

Glucose-6-phosphate dehydrogenase (G6PD) deficiency

Historical
Several accounts [252, 439, 440] have set out the sequential findings which led to the discovery of G6PD deficiency by Carson *et al.* [441] and the salient features are considered below.

An acute haemolytic episode following ingestion of the 8-aminoquinoline Pamaquine (Fig. 7.6) was noted first by Cordes [442–444] in six of 250 American male Negroes; one of the affected cases proved fatal. Others noted a haemolytic effect of the drug accompanied by cyanosis, methaemoglobinaemia and Heinz-body formation [445–448]. That pigmented rather than white-

Fig. 7.6. Structures of Pamaquine and Primaquine.

skinned ethnic groups were selectively affected by Pamaquine and other antimalarial drugs was also noted. Thus, male Indians were reported to be more susceptible than male Britons to Mepacrine, quinine and Pamaquine [449–452] and of 10 000 male Indians receiving these drugs, 0·13% developed haemoglobinuria. In America further reports appeared: it was noted [453] that of 3000 Caucasian and Negro subjects who received similar drugs, 10, all Negroes, developed haemoglobinuria, as did seven of 157 Negroes receiving Pamaquine during a two- to 14-day period [454]. Haemolysis can be provoked in drug-sensitive Negroes by the administration of 30 mg of Primaquine base daily whereas white adults can tolerate up to 240 mg without any haematological consequences. This predisposition of pigmented ethnic groups towards certain drugs has now been amply demonstrated.

Injection of ^{51}Cr-labelled cells from drug-sensitive individuals into normal recipients who then received Primaquine resulted in destruction of the transfused cells only and so it was established that the donor cells carried an intrinsic defect [455, 456]. Older cells are more susceptible to drugs than young ones [457].

The first chemical abnormality described was a slight depression in the GSH concentration of Primaquine-sensitive cells and these cells were also shown to be particularly sensitive to incubation *in vitro* with acetylphenylhydrazine which produced a marked fall in the GSH concentration whereas normal cells were little affected [458–460]. Other unrelated compounds such as ascorbate, hydroxylamine, Primaquine, furantion, naphthols and napthaquinone, also diminished the GSH level [460–465].

Further investigation into the biochemical pathway concerned with GSH metabolism led to the first precise description of G6PD deficiency by Carson *et al.* in 1956 [441]; this was soon confirmed by others. The antimalarial then in common use was Primaquine (Fig. 7.6) and so the deficiency was designated 'Primaquine sensitivity'. Most of the early studies were carried out on American Negroes but many other racial groups are known to be affected including Sephardic Jews, Chinese, Indians, Malays, Thais, Filipinos and

Melanesians [439]. In particular, Mediterranean subjects with favism (see p. 296) were shown to be G6PD-deficient. A full description of the ethnic distribution, mechanism of haemolysis, associated red-cell abnormalities and kinetic properties of G6PD variants is given by Beutler [252].

Genetics

G6PD deficiency is inherited in a sex-linked fashion, transmission occurring from mother to son but not from father to son. Full expression of the defect occurs in hemizygous males in whom the single X chromosome carries the mutant gene and in homozygous females who carry the defect on both chromosomes.

Values for G6PD activity in heterozygous females vary from very low, approaching those found in hemizygous males, to entirely normal. This variability in activity arises because their blood contains two populations of red cells, one normal and one G6PD-deficient; the proportion of each is characteristic for the subject and determines the activity in a sample of their blood [466]. It arises because one of the two X chromosomes in females is inactivated [467]. The Lyon hypothesis assumes that both female X chromosomes are initially active after fertilization but, early in embryonic development, one of them becomes inactive so that a condition of mosaicism arises with some cells having active genes from the father and others those from the mother. The ratio of normal to deficient cells depends upon such factors as the stage of development at which inactivation occurs, the relative proliferative capacity of the two types of cells and their respective ability to cope with survival.

Haemophilia A is closely linked on the X chromosome to the G6PD locus and this fact has been used for the prenatal diagnosis of haemophilia [468].

Variants of G6PD

At the time of writing some 180 different variants of G6PD have been described [469–471] and new ones continue to be reported. They are characterized by their *in-vitro* activity, electrophoretic mobility, heat stability, affinities for substrate and substrate analogues and inhibition by NADPH.

The commonest form of the enzyme is G6PD B and this is presumed to be the normal form. It probably exists as a dimer *in vitro* with a MW of approximately 105 000 daltons. Starch-gel electrophoresis yields a single band designated the B band, but in clinically normal subjects of African ancestry a second faster band, designated the A band, may also be present. The two variants have similar kinetic properties and differ by one amino-acid substitution. The red cells of African males contain either the A or B type of G6PD with a frequency of about 70% B and 18% A [472, 473].

Females may have either A, B or both bands and the presence of two bands in an individual has proved useful as a clonal marker. Of the many other variants now known the A − and Mediterranean type will be described in detail because these two account for over 95% of affected individuals.

African types, A − variant. In G6PD-deficient males no bands are seen using crude haemolysates, but with purified preparations the small amount of G6PD activity present runs in the position of the A band; for this reason it was designated A −. In American male Negroes the frequency of the deficiency is about 12% and about three per cent of females are homozygous. American Negroes derive from Africa but the African population is not homogeneous; surveys have shown considerable variation in the frequency of the A − variant and also the occurrence of rare other mutants. Even so, the A − variant is by far the commonest and is called the African type of G6PD deficiency.

The activity of G6PD in whole blood of affected individuals is 8–20% while in heterozygous females it varies between normal and values for the fully expressed males. The A − variant has the same catalytic activity as the A and B types but is more unstable. In young cells the activity and concentration are normal but the decay rate is greater than that of the A or B variants [474–478]. Their separation by chromatography suggests that the A and A − variants are different in structure [477, 479, 480]. White cells in G6PD A − have a near normal activity, explained by the fact that they have a shorter lifespan than red cells and therefore the activity decays to a lower level in the latter cells [481–484]. Platelets, the eye lens and liver show low activities of the enzyme [485–487].

This mutation was the one found in individuals originally described as having Primaquine sensitivity but this is a misleading term because it implies that G6PD-deficient subjects with other variants may not be sensitive to Primaquine.

Mediterranean type. This form of G6PD deficiency has been known for centuries as a familial condition affecting natives of the Mediterranean littoral because of its association with favism (see p. 296). The Mediterranean mutant has altered K_m values for G6P and $NADP^+$, diminished heat stability, faster decay rate and increased utilization of other substrates such as 2-deoxyglucose 6-phosphate and galactose 6-phosphate. Assayable activity is lower than in the A − type, usually less than five per cent of normal and decreased values are found in young as well as old cells. This low activity explains the particular sensitivity of affected individuals towards haemolytic agents.

The white cells also have decreased activity of the

enzyme but this is not as marked as in the red cells, homozygotes having about 50% and heterozygotes normal activity [488, 489].

Other variants. In an extensive review, Beutler lists the kinetic properties of 150 well-defined variants and has also a useful guide, produced by classifying variants into classes on the basis of their activity, drug sensitivity, susceptibility of subjects to favism and infections, the likelihood of neonatal jaundice and presentation as a chronic haemolytic disorder (see Ref. 252, p. 57).

Mechanism of drug-induced haemolysis
Drugs which are known to provoke a haemolytic crisis (Table 7.7) vary in their chemical structure and there is no obvious common route by which they or their metabolites might provoke haemolysis. However, many of them are responsible for an increased generation of H_2O_2 either directly, via their metabolites or through the generation of the superoxide ion (O_2^-). The amounts generated are sufficient to destroy G6PD-deficient cells because they are unable to maintain an adequate GSH concentration in the face of such oxidative stress.

The precise effects of an increased H_2O_2 concentration in red cells depend upon the concentration and exposure time. The prime targets for oxidation are GSH, protein —SH groups, haem ferrous iron and possibly lipids. Hydrogen peroxide is degraded by catalase but at low concentration the more important pathway is via GSH-Px which has an absolute requirement for GSH (see p. 273). It is probable [129] that GSH is oxidized to GSSG first followed by MetHb formation. The impotence of G6PD-deficient cells in the face of an oxidative assault becomes apparent when the endogeneous GSH is exhausted because GSH reductase, which requires a steady supply of NADPH, cannot reduce GSSG back to GSH at the required rate. The turnover of NADPH is limited by the ability of the PPP to be accelerated and in G6PD deficiency this ability is severely restricted. In normal red cells, the pathway can be stimulated by some 40 times, but in deficient cells only several times, insufficient for the necessary rapid reformation of GSH. In addition, catalase activity falls and weakens the defence against peroxide attack.

The exposure of G6PD-deficient cells to haemolytic agents *in vivo* results in less MetHb formation than occurs in normal cells, an unexpected result in view of the normal NADH-requiring MetHb reductase activity in both types of cells. However, greater amounts of MetHb are formed in the older cells and these are selectively damaged in G6PD deficiency and rapidly removed from the circulation.

The presence of Heinz-bodies in cells, arising from

an oxidative assault, is probably a key factor in rendering them effete but the exact mechanism of destruction is not known. Cellular inclusions certainly produce membrane rigidity and cation leakage, factors which promote sequestration in the spleen. In addition, other proteins may be oxidized and a recent report has demonstrated the presence of polypeptide aggregates containing spectrin but not globin attached to the cell membrane in patients with congenital non-spherocytic haemolytic anaemia due to G6PD deficiency [490]. Lipid peroxidation has also been implicated [491–493].

Clinical features
The vast majority of G6PD-deficient patients are symptomless, normal on physical examination and have a normal haemoglobin and blood picture. Their main problems arise from a susceptibility to various adverse factors which promote haemolysis; this can vary from mild to very severe, requiring urgent admission to hospital. The clinical manifestations of G6PD deficiency and their relationship to enzyme activity are summarized in Figure 7.7.

Drug-induced haemolysis. This is the commonest manifestation of the disorder. The extent to which individuals are affected shows considerable variation even within the groups carrying the same genetic defect. The patient usually gives a history of having ingested an offending drug one to three days before symptoms occur and these may vary from mild lethargy to severe weakness, with lumbar or abdominal pain and the passage of dark urine; very occasionally renal failure ensues. The only abnormal findings are pallor, jaundice and, rarely, a palpable spleen. In general, haemolysis tends to be more severe in Caucasians than Negro subjects.

After about a week, the patient begins to feel better and the haemolytic state ceases. In the first detailed study of the clinical course in which Negro volunteers (A— type) received 30 mg of Primaquine base daily for a prolonged period, the haemolytic state ceased spontaneously and the haemoglobin level rose to normal by 20–30 days despite continued administration of the drug [494]. The self-limiting nature of the haemolysis occurs because drug sensitivity is a function of cell age; older cells are destroyed while young cells and reticulocytes with their higher activity are more resistant. Haemolysis settles at a particular level for a given level of drug but the resistance of young cells is relative and haemolysis increases if the level of drug increases [495]. Similar studies on subjects with G6PD Mediterranean have demonstrated that the haemolysis tends to be more severe for a given dose of Primaquine and that it

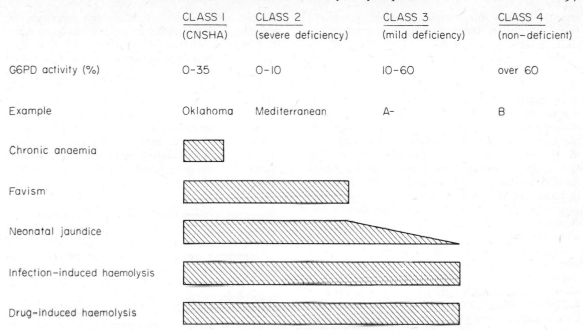

	CLASS I (CNSHA)	CLASS 2 (severe deficiency)	CLASS 3 (mild deficiency)	CLASS 4 (non–deficient)
G6PD activity (%)	0–35	0–10	10–60	over 60
Example	Oklahoma	Mediterranean	A–	B

Fig. 7.7. Likelihood of the major clinical consequences of G6PD deficiency (after Beutler [252]).

may not be self-limiting in the face of continued drug administration [496].

Red-cell morphological changes may be minimal but in very severe cases red-cell fragmentation and spherocytosis can be seen. The earliest abnormality is the presence of Heinz bodies followed by the rapid development of anaemia, and free haemoglobin appears in the urine. After about three to five days the number of Heinz bodies decreases sharply and a reticulocytosis occurs followed by a gradual rise in haemoglobin.

Favism. This is one of the most serious complications of G6PD deficiency and before the advent of blood transfusions was associated with an appreciable mortality. For centuries the disorder of favism has been recognized in inhabitants of territories bordering on the Mediterranean and is now known to be an acute haemolytic anaemia of sudden onset which occurs in some G6PD-deficient persons sensitive to the fava bean (*Vicia faba*) either on ingestion of the raw, cooked or dried bean or following inhalation of the pollen from the blossom of the plant. Attacks occur most commonly in the spring [497, 498].

When haemolysis is due to pollen inhalation, not as common as once thought [498], it may be fulminating and begin within a few minutes of exposure, but when due to bean ingestion there is a latent period of six to 30 hours before the onset of the haemolysis. The fava bean is the common European broad bean but haemolysis can be provoked by other plants [499, 500]. The active factor is secreted in the breast and favism has been seen in a nursing infant [498].

The condition does not occur in individuals carrying the A − variant but has been described in many other population groups [252] most commonly in Italy and Greece where G6PD Mediterranean is the commonest genotype [498, 501]. It usually affects children, maximum age incidence between one and six years and is relatively rare in adults [498]. Not all persons with a similar G6PD variant are affected and haemolysis may occur in individuals who have previously eaten the bean without ill effects [498].

The symptoms are of acute onset and include fever, headache, nausea, vomiting, lumbar pain and general malaise followed in a few hours by haemoglobinuria and jaundice. The fall in haemoglobin varies from slight to profound and life-threatening [497]. Renal failure, requiring dialysis, and vitreoretinal haemorrhages may occur [502, 503]. Distorted red cells and contraction of the haemoglobin from the cell membrane may be seen on the blood film. The attack ceases after two to six days and there are no long-term ill effects. If death occurs this is usually within the first 48 hours following exposure.

Heterozygotes may also suffer from favism [504]. In a recent survey of 51 girls requiring hospitalization, 61% were heterozygotes, the remainder being homozygotes [505]. Only three of the heterozygotes required blood transfusion. The proportion of deficient cells in their circulation ranged from 45 to 55% and was similar to the assay activity. It was estimated that 1·3% of heterozygotes in the general population were at risk from favism.

The mechanism by which favism occurs still awaits elucidation but three factors are necessary to produce haemolysis, namely G6PD deficiency, an as yet unidentified constituent of *Vicia faba* and a 'sensitivity' in the individual. In 1966 the results of a large survey of 500 families in Greece demonstrated an undoubted familial aggregation of cases and the data fitted the hypothesis of Mendelian segregation of an autosomal gene which when found together with G6PD deficiency predisposed to the development of haemoglobinuric favism [506].

G6PD deficiency is not the only enzyme defect to be associated with favism and it has been described with glutathione synthetase deficiency (see p. 300). In addition it has been suggested that a mild form of favism can occur without haemoglobinuria in individuals with normal G6PD activity [605]. Impaired D-glutaric acid production is another possibly associated factor [507].

Pyrimidine aglycones and L-dopa have been considered as toxic agents within the bean itself [606, 607] but conclusive evidence for either has yet to be produced. An immunological mechanism seems unlikely [508].

G6PD deficiency in the newborn. Normal neonates have a raised G6PD activity at birth. The precise extent to which G6PD deficiency compromises the newborn infant appears to differ in reports from various parts of the world. American infants carrying the A − variant appear to be generally unaffected although the risk of hyperbilirubinaemia increases with prematurity [509–512]. However, reports on deficient Africans suggest that the risk is high, and in one series 60% of Nigerian infants who developed a serum bilirubin above 170 μmol/l were G6PD-deficient [513].

In a series of large studies from Greece the following conclusions were reached [514–518]. First, by comparing haemoglobin, reticulocyte and bilirubin values with those of normal infants it was concluded that the lifespan of deficient erythrocytes is shortened in the neonatal period but that anaemia was not a problem. Secondly, it was confirmed that G6PD deficiency is associated with neonatal jaundice in the absence of other predisposing factors such as prematurity, bloodgroup incompatibility and exposure to potentially toxic agents such as vitamin-K analogues and naphthalene. However, the incidence of severe jaundice (serum bilirubin levels > 270 μmol/l) varied markedly

between regions and the data strongly supported the existence of an additional icterogenic, probably genetic factor transmitted independently of G6PD deficiency but which when present in the same individual was likely to cause severe hyperbilirubinaemia. This work confirmed the results of an early report of a familial incidence in isolated cases [519].

Similar studies on Chinese and Thai infants have shown that severe jaundice may occur with G6PD deficiency and it is recommended that any infant from any area with severe unexplained neonatal hyperbilirubinaemia should be screened for G6PD deficiency [520, 521].

Congential non-spherocytic haemolytic anaemia
As mentioned earlier, some variants (Beutler, Type I) may be associated with a chronic haemolytic state. These patients are rare compared with the vast majority of symptomless individuals and the history and presentation is similar to that found in other congenital non-spherocytic haemolytic anaemias; also it varies in severity.

Neonatal jaundice, sometimes requiring exchange transfusion, has been described [522–524] and the other clinical features include a variable degree of anaemia, mild jaundice, splenomegaly, pigment-stone formation and the occasional occurrence of cataracts [522, 523]. The haemoglobin level may be normal in fully compensated cases or as low as 6·0 g/dl, but most patients do not require regular transfusion except during haemolytic crises which may be precipitated by infections, drugs or fava beans. These crises may be very severe requiring urgent medical treatment and haemoglobin levels as low as 2·1 g/dl have been reported [525].

The blood film shows the criteria of a chronic haemolytic state with macrocytosis, polychromasia, anisocytosis and poikilocytosis. The reticulocyte count varies with the severity of the condition. In most patients ^{51}Cr-labelling of the red cells has shown equal uptake by the spleen and liver [523, 526]. Heterozygotes are usually unaffected.

Other predisposing factors
A wide varity of infections, both bacterial and viral, may cause haemolysis in deficient subjects without the administration of drugs or may accentuate the haemolysis provoked by drugs [527]. The degree of haemolysis is variable but rarely severe. Amongst the conditions in which haemolysis commonly occurs are bacterial pneumonia, typhoid fever and Gram-negative infections. Viral hepatitis is often associated with marked hyperbilirubinaemia due to impaired liver function but this does not necessarily augur badly for

the patient [528]. Acute renal failure may occur during the course of an infection.

Haemolysis also occurs in diabetic ketoacidosis but ceases when the patient has been controlled [529]. The anaemia is probably due to a combination of biochemical abnormalities and/or infections.

In all these conditions recovery of the haemoglobin level may be delayed due to associated bone-marrow suppression.

Association with other congenital red-cell defects
Patients with sickle-cell trait and G6PD deficiency are not compromised by the combined deficiency. In a large survey of 65 000 black male patients admitted to hospital, 0·9% suffered from both defects but this had no adverse effect on length of hospital stay or mortality when compared with normal patients and those carrying either one of the defects [530]. Similar findings are reported in patients with homozygous sickle-cell disease and G6PD deficiency [531].

G6PD deficiency has been reported in association with autoimmune haemolytic anaemia, hereditary spherocytosis and elliptocytosis, GPI deficiency, and adenylate kinase and heterozygous PK deficiency [417, 532–535]. In none of these patients did the presence of G6PD deficiency appear to increase the severity of the disorder and response to splenectomy in the patient with HS was complete.

Malaria
Since 1960, it has been suggested [536, 537] that G6PD-deficient red cells are protected against invasion by malarial parasites. Studies on heterozygous females have shown that at the cellular level the rate of parasitization of G6PD(+) cells was greater than in G6PD(−) cells [538]. Other evidence supports the idea of a selective advantage of enzyme-deficient cells with respect to *P. falciparum* [539, 540]. The mechanism remains obscure as parasitic development is normal *in vivo* in G6PD(−) males [541]. It is reported that the development of *P. falciparum* in G6PD(−) cells is inhibited under conditions of oxidative stress [542]. The development of a technique for the culture of malarial parasites *in vitro* [608] has made it possible to study the mechanisms of parasite invasion of, and intracellular growth in, red cells and their failure to survive in abnormal environments [609]. It seems probable that the inadequacy of G6PD-deficient red cells to detoxicate the oxidation products of parasite metabolism creates an unfavourable environment in which the parasites themselves cannot thrive.

The question often arises as to which drugs can safely be given to patients with G6PD deficiency. Of the drugs commonly used in prophylaxis and treatment, chloroquine, chlorguanidine, pyrimethamine, quinine, sulphathiazine and sulphadoxine can be given in full therapeutic doses. However, the possible use of primaquine for the eradication of hepatic schizonts in *P. vivax* and *P. ovale* malaria from African subjects carrying the A− variant poses a problem. This is certainly the most effective therapeutic agent and providing the recipients are closely monitored, it is probably safe to give at the recommended dosage in view of the self-limiting nature of the haemolysis. Dapsone is sometimes prescribed in combination with pyrimethamine or chlorguanidine for prophylaxis against *P. falciparum* where resistant strains are common. The haemolytic effect is mild in G6PD-deficient individuals but the drug is best avoided if other agents are available.

Tumour markers
Female G6PD-B/G6PD-A heterozygotes have proved useful for demonstrating the monoclonal origin of certain malignant conditions in that tumours arising from a single cell carry only one enzyme type, that is, A or B, but not both. Among haematological conditions shown to be monoclonal by this technique are chronic granulocytic leukaemia [543, 544], PNH [545], polycythaemia rubra vera [546] and recently a common progenitor for human myeloid and lymphoid cells has been shown in a patient with acquired sideroblastic anaemia [547].

Treatment
For the vast majority of patients with G6PD deficiency no treatment is required. Management consists of reassurance, genetic counselling and sensible advice regarding the avoidance of drugs, chemicals and, where relevant, fava beans. Most people with G6PD deficiency are unaware of the defect.

When haemolysis does occur following exposure to drugs or infections then hospitalization may be required but again, removal of the offending drug or treatment of the infection is often all that is required. In cases where there is a severe haemolysis and profound anaemia blood transfusion is essential or, as mentioned earlier, exchange transfusion may be necessary to prevent kernicterus.

Patients with congenital non-spherocytic haemolytic anaemia are a more difficult problem but rarely require regular transfusion. Supplementary dietary folate is advisable as in other chronic haemolytic anaemias. Splenectomy has been carried out in a number of cases but only in one-third has it proved beneficial [548].

Laboratory detection of G6PD deficiency
Osmotic fragility and autohaemolysis tests are not helpful in diagnosis, nor are there any specific features

of red-cell morphology. The direct antoglobulin test is negative.

Techniques available for the full investigation and characterization of a mutant are described [252, 549] but this is not necessary for clinical purposes where the prime need is an unequivocal diagnosis of G6PD deficiency. Diagnostic techniques are outlined below.

Heinz-body test. This was the first test to be devised for the diagnosis of drug-sensitive individuals; it is simple to perform but difficult to standardize and whilst reliable in hemizygotes and female homozygotes, false positives can be obtained (e.g. in thalassaemia, the unstable haemoglobinopathies and in GSH and GSH-reductase deficiency). The test consists of the aerobic incubation of red cells with acetylphenylhydrazine for two hours. Under these conditions normal red cells contain one or more Heinz bodies and less than about 30% of the cells contain more than five inclusions. With G6PD-deficient cells more than half contain many small inclusions.

The GSH stability test. The somewhat low GSH concentration found in drug-sensitive cells [458] is not sufficiently abnormal to be of diagnostic use. However, the incubation of drug-sensitive cells with acetyl-phenylhydrazine results in a marked fall of GSH whereas normal cells are little affected [459, 460]. This is the basis of the GSH stability test. False positives may be obtained if too little glucose is present or the samples are over-oxygenated. Haemoglobin E thalassaemia also gives positive results [550]. Hemizygous males show almost complete disappearance of GSH after two hours' incubation while heterozygous females give intermediate values.

Neither of the above tests is much used with the availability of the following more direct tests.

Screening tests. The brilliant-cresyl-blue test [551] continues to be much used and is entirely reliable provided the incubation is carried out under anaerobic conditions and the haematocrit is standardized to a fixed value. In 1977 the International Committee for Standardization in Haematology (ICSH) recommended the fluorescent-spot test as the most reliable [552]. A small amount of red cells are added to a mixture of G6P, NADP$^+$, GSSG and saponin in tris-HCl buffer. After 10 minutes the reaction mixture is spotted onto filter paper and examined under UV light. The NADPH formed produces a bright fluorescence in normal subjects while deficient subjects show little or no fluorescence. The test is particularly useful in population studies as dried blood spotted onto filter paper will give satisfactory results.

Quantitative assays. The recommended method is that agreed by ICSH in 1977 [552]. The G6PD activity is measured in buffered haemolysates prepared from washed cells and supplemented with G6P, Mg^{2+} and NADP$^+$. The reaction is followed by the rate of formation of NADPH at 340 nm. Hemizygotes, even during a haemolytic crisis, show reduced activity but heterozygotes, because of the double red-cell population, may give normal results. The histochemical test described below [553] permits more accurate diagnosis in females since the presence of G6PD in individual cells is detected.

Histochemical test. Intact red cells in which the haemoglobin has been converted to methaemoglobin by the addition of nitrite are incubated with tetrazolium MTT in phosphate-buffered glucose. The MTT is reduced by haemoglobin, but not methaemoglobin, to form insoluble purple granules of monoformazan. The rate of reduction of methaemoglobin back to haemoglobin via NADPH reductase depends upon the NADPH produced by the stimulated PPP. In G6PD-deficient individuals NADPH production is inadequate to reduce the methaemoglobin and so the cells contain fewer granules. In heterozygotes, two populations can be seen, one containing abundant, and one devoid of, granules. Cells are scored for the presence of granules and characteristic graphs are drawn. Because G6PD activity in individual cells is observed it becomes possible to diagnose a deficiency in heterozygote blood during a haemolytic episode when the blood contains young, normal cells with supranormal activity.

6-Phosphogluconate-dehydrogenase (6PGD) deficiency

This enzyme catalyses the second step of the PPP, the conversion of 6-phosphoglyconate (6PG) to ribulose 5-phosphate (Fig. 7.3).

An inherited variant of the enzyme, displaying normal activity was described in 1963 [554] and a year later several members of a Negro family were found to have only 50% of normal activity but no haematological abnormalities [555]. Affected members were all heterozygotes, the inheritance was autosomal and the family also had G6PD deficiency which segregated independently of 6PGD.

Since then two large surveys of over 5000 individuals have revealed several genetic variants with some individuals having about 50% of normal activity but none with haemolysis [556–558]. The administration of 60 mg of Primaquine daily to one subject did not provoke a haemolytic crisis [556]. Thus, it seems unlikely that this deficiency exists in association with a haemolytic anaemia either spontaneous or induced by drugs (but see Refs 559, 560). Other variants of the enzyme have also been reported [561–564].

GSH deficiency

The biosynthesis of GSH takes place in two stages:

1 γ-L-glutamate + L-cysteine → γ-L-glutamylcysteine; then

2 γ-L-glutamylcysteine + L-glycine → γ-L-glutamylcysteinylglycine (GSH)

The first stage is catalysed by γ-L-glutamylcysteine synthetase (GC-S) and the second by GSH synthetase (GSH-S); both steps require ATP.

Non-spherocytic haemolytic anaemia has been described in five members of a Dutch family, in whom the GSH concentration was less than 10% of normal [565, 566]. The haemolysis was fairly well compensated, red-cell morphological changes minimal, normal osmotic fragility and ATP concentration, but the Heinz-body test was positive. Several other reports followed and it is now known that GSH deficiency results from a failure of one of the two enzymes responsible for GSH synthesis [566, 567].

A defect in the first stage of synthesis, that is, in GC-S, is very rare and is associated with haemolytic anaemia and neurological complications [568]. The GSH is very low in the red cells and the condition is inherited as an autosomal-recessive disorder.

There are two different clinical syndromes associated with deficiencies in the second stage of GSH biosynthesis that are catalysed by GSH-S. In the first, a mild haemolytic anaemia is associated with a chronic metabolic acidosis, usually of neonatal onset and the passage of large amounts of 5-oxoproline (pyroglutamic acid) in the urine [569, 570]; some cases have associated neurological disturbances. The haemolysis is worsened by the ingestion of oxidant drugs and favism has been reported. The red cells show anisocytosis and polychromasia and form large numbers of small Heinz bodies during incubation with phenylhydrazine. The GSH concentration is very low in the red cells but the γ-glutamylcysteine level is not raised because of conversion to 5-oxoproline. The accumulation of 5-oxoproline is considered to be due to a failure in the normal feedback mechanism by which GSH formation prevents the build-up of γ-glutamylcysteine; as a consequence massive oxoprolinuria occurs. The red cells and serum also contain increased amounts of threonine, proline and tyrosine [571]. There is no specific treatment for the disorder but splenectomy may lessen the haemolysis [572] and the metabolic acidosis can be controlled by oral bicarbonate [571].

In the second type of GSH-S deficiency [566, 567] the only manifestation is mild haemolysis. The red cells have a decreased enzyme activity and GSH concentration but in contrast to the first type, leucocytes and skin fibroblasts show near normal activity [573]. The enzyme is unstable *in vivo* and has a shortened survival in intact red cells. Absence of oxoprolinuria is attributed to the fact that nucleated red cells are able to maintain sufficient enzyme activity and GSH to prevent the over-production of 5-oxoproline.

The GSH-S deficiency is very rare and consanguinity has been a feature of several of the reported families. It is inherited as an autosomal recessive disorder and heterozygotes, although exhibiting intermediate activity, can maintain normal amounts of GSH. The GSH-deficient red cells are easily damaged by chromium and for this reason the measurement of the red-cell lifespan by the chromium technique gives unreliable results.

Glutathione-reductase (GR) deficiency

Glutathione reductase (GR) is an unusually stable enzyme which catalyses the reduction of oxidized glutathione (GSSG) using either NADH or NADPH as hydrogen donors. The preferred cofactor is NADPH in red cells and the enzyme appears to be a single molecular species. The enzyme is a dimer of two identical subunits each of MW 50 000; it is inhibited by chromate and requires flavin adenine nucleotide (FAD) as a prosthetic group, each of the two subunits of the enzyme containing two FAD molecules. The activity of the enzyme can be increased *in vitro* by the addition to haemolysates of FAD and also *in vivo* by the administration of 5 mg daily of riboflavin [126, 127]. The baseline in normal subjects is said to correlate directly with the dietary intake of riboflavin.

Abnormal GR activity

It is clear that many of the early cases of low GR activity were due to riboflavin deficiency [574] and mutant forms of the enzyme are actually quite rare [575]. The first two cases reported were associated with a haemolytic anaemia following the administration of sulphoxone or 8-aminoquinolines, and the susceptibility of the deficient cells was proven in one case by cross-transfusion studies [576, 577]. In this case the activity of the enzyme was 57% of normal and the GSH concentration low although its stability was normal. Numerous reports followed and by 1968 61 patients were on record [578] of whom 14 had no haematological abnormalities and the remainder had a haemolytic anaemia that was either spontaneous or drug-induced. The GR deficiency has also been recorded in association with Hb C disease, α thalassaemia, haemophilia B and leukaemia [578–580].

It now seems probable that most of these early cases were associated with riboflavin deficiency. Surveys in north Thailand and Malaysia have shown deficiencies in GR activity which were corrected by riboflavin supplements [581, 582] and a number of reports have shown this dependence on riboflavin in both *in-vivo* and *in-vitro* studies.

Mutants of GR in which there are molecular abnormalities of the enzyme do, however, exist. A patient with panmyelopathy had a GR activity in the red cells of about 60% and while this was raised to normal by riboflavin *in vivo*, or FAD *in vitro*, this stimulation was less than is seen with normal cells and electrophoresis demonstrated the presence of a mutant enzyme [583]. In the best-documented case virtually complete absence of GR activity was noted in the red cells of three children of a consanguineous marriage [584]. Intermediate values were found in the parents' red cells and the activity of the enzyme could not be restored either by the addition of FAD *in vitro* or the administration of riboflavin *in vivo*. The GSH concentration of the cells was normal but its stability was decreased on incubation with phenylhydrazine. Clinically the condition presented as an attack of favism in a sister. The blood pictures of the affected members were entirely normal but the leucocyte and platelet activity of GR was markedly reduced and two of the three children had cataracts.

A genetic variant with increased activity and fast electrophoretic mobility has also been described [585] affecting Negroes and possibly associated with gout.

Glutathione-peroxidase (GSH-Px) deficiency

Gluthathione peroxidase (GSH-Px) is one of the two enzymes responsible in red cells for the decomposition of H_2O_2, catalase being the other. The relative contribution made by these two enzymes has already been considered. The GSH-Px is an atypical enzyme in that it lacks haem and flavin but contains selenium, one atom per four subunits.

Abnormal GSH-Px activity

The presence in red cells of a mutant enzyme with reduced activity which is causally related to haemolysis has not been satisfactorily established.

Both premature and full-term infants have reduced levels of GSH-Px activity but values as low as 30% of normal have been recorded without evidence of haemolysis [586, 587]. The activity approaches normal at about six months of age. That adult females have higher values of GSH-Px activity than males has been shown by several workers [588, 589].

A close correlation has been shown between blood selenium concentration and low GSH-Px activity in New Zealand where the soil content of this element is low [590], and two recent surveys have demonstrated reduced selenium levels in pregnant women and cord blood which correlated well with the enzyme activities

in mother and infant [589, 591]. The GSH-Px activity can also be increased *in vivo* and *in vitro* by the administration or addition of selenium [592].

The red cells of neonates are particularly sensitive to oxidative assault but the mechanisms are incompletely understood. However, in vitamin E-sufficient, premature infants diets rich in polyunsaturated fatty acids (PUFA) and iron but deficient in selenium, which may thus affect GSH-Px activity, may be contributory causes [611].

A genetic variant for low GSH-Px activity, designated GSH-Px^L, has been described and is particularly common in people of Mediterranean ancestry [593]. Homozygotes have about 50% of normal activity but no evidence of any haematological abnormality.

Because of the factors which can affect GSH-Px activity, the early cases of diminished enzyme activity associated with haemolysis, either spontaneous or drug-induced, need to be re-evaluated.

Raised activities of GSH-Px are reported in megaloblastic anaemia, α thalassaemia and G6PD deficiency [594, 595], and low activities in iron-deficiency anaemia [596].

Catalase deficiency

A diminished activity of red-cell catalase was first described in a young Japanese girl with oral gangrene but no evidence of any haematological abnormality [597]. By 1952 nine cases from three families were known, seven with oral gangrene, and an hereditary transmission of the defect seemed likely [598, 599]. The singular property of the red cells was their blackening on treatment with H_2O_2 solution, an effect later exploited in a simple screening test for the disorder [600]. Whilst the defect was first observed in red cells, other tissues are affected (e.g. liver, bone marrow and nasal tissue). Acatalassaemia in Japan was reviewed in 1968 when 77 cases from 39 Japanese families were recorded together with three from a Korean family; approximately half had oral gangrene [601]. Catalase activity in the red cells of affected subjects was low, from zero to about three per cent of normal; in addition several family members had intermediate (about 50%) values and these were presumed heterozygotes. Transmission of the defect appeared to follow an autosomal recessive pattern.

The existence of catalase deficiency in Switzerland emerged from the screening of 18 459 blood samples from Swiss males when two cases were found [600], and a further case after screening a total of 73 661 subjects. Family studies on the first two cases revealed eight more to make a total of eleven [602]. In addition, a number of presumed heterozygotes with intermediate values (60–85% of normal) were located. None of the homozygous Swiss subjects had oral gangrene nor any observable haematological disorder. Red-cell catalase activity in the homozygotes was zero to 1·3% of normal [603]. The different values among Swiss and Japanese heterozygotes, together with the absence of gangrene in the former, has suggested that the genetic defect is different in the two groups.

The significance of catalase is considered on page 273. The fact that acatalasic subjects show no haematological abnormalities shows that the enzyme is not essential to the red cell; this is because GSH-Px decomposes H_2O_2 under normal conditions and only when the peroxide level rises to high values is catalase necessary.

REFERENCES

1 MOLLISON P.L. (1979) *Blood Transfusion in Clinical Medicine*, 6th edn., p. 22. Blackwell Scientific Publications, Oxford.

2 PENNELL R.B. (1974) Composition of normal human red cells. In: *The Red Blood Cell* (ed. Surgenor D.M.), p. 93. Academic Press, London.

3 MOSES S.W., BASHAN N. & GUTMAN A. (1972) Glycogen metabolism in the normal red blood cell. *Blood*, **40**, 836.

4 MOSES S.W., BASHAN N. & GUTMAN A. (1972) Properties of glycogen synthetase in erythrocytes. *European Journal of Biochemistry*, **30**, 205.

5 SIDBURY J.B., CORNBLATH M., FISHER J. & HOUSE E. (1961) Glycogen in erythrocytes of patients with glycogen storage disease. *Pediatrics*, **27**, 103.

6 LEVIN S., MOSES S.W., CHAYOTH R., JAGODA N. & STEINITZ K. (1967) Glycogen storage disease in Israel. A clinical, biochemical and genetic study. *Israel Journal of Medical Sciences*, **3**, 397.

7 VAN HOOF F. (1967) Amylo-1, 6-glucosidase activity and glycogen content of the erythrocytes of normal subjects, patients with glycogen storage disease and heterozygotes. *European Journal of Biochemistry*, **2**, 271.

8 MOSES S.W. & GUTMAN A. (1972) Inborn errors of glycogen metabolism. *Advances in Pediatrics*, **19**, 95.

9 MOSES S.W., CHAYOTH R., LEVIN S., LAZAROVITZ E. & RUBINSTEIN D. (1968) Glucose and glycogen metabolism in erythrocytes from normal and glycogen storage disease Type III subjects. *Journal of Clinical Investigation*, **47**, 1343.

10 MOSES S.W., BASHAN N., GUTMAN A. & OCKERMAN P.A. (1974) Glycogen metabolism in glycogen-rich erythrocytes. *Blood*, **44**, 275.

11 HINTERBERGER U., OCKEL E., GERISCHER-MOTHES W. & RAPOPORT S. (1961) Grösse und pH-Abhängigkeit der anaeroben Glykolyse und der Hexokinase-Aktivität von Erythrocyten und Retikulocyten des Kaninchens. *Acta Biologica et Medica Germanica*, **7**, 50.

12 JACOBASCH G., MINAKAMI S. & RAPOPORT S.M. (1974) Glycolysis of the erythrocyte. In: *Cellular and Molecular Biology of Erythrocytes* (ed. Yoshikawa H. & Rapoport S.M.), p. 55. University Park Press, Baltimore.

13 SACKTOR B. & HURLBUT E.C. (1966) Regulation of metabolism in working muscle *in vivo*. II. Concentra-

tions of adenine nucleotides, arginine phosphate and inorganic phosphate in insect flight muscle during flight. *Journal of Biological Chemistry*, **241**, 263.

14 MURPHY J.R. (1960) Erythrocyte metabolism. II. Glucose metabolism and pathways. *Journal of Laboratory and Clinical Medicine*, **55**, 286.

15 CHAPMAN R.G., HENNESSY M.A., WALTERSDORPH A.M., HUENNEKENS F.M. & GABRIO B.W. (1962) Erythrocyte metabolism. V. Levels of glycolytic enzymes and regulation of glycolysis. *Journal of Clinical Investigation*, **41**, 1249.

16 YOSHIKAWA H. & MINAKAMI S. (1968) Regulation of glycolysis in human red cells. *Folia Haematologica*, **89**, 357.

17 ROSE I.A., WARMS J.V.B. & O'CONNELL E.L. (1964) Role of inorganic phosphate in stimulating the glucose utilisation of human red blood cells. *Biochemical and Biophysical Research Communications*, **15**, 33.

18 TSUBIO K.K. & FUKUNAGA K. (1965) Inorganic phosphate and enhanced glucose degradation by the intact erythrocyte. *Journal of Biological Chemistry*, **240**, 2806.

19 MINAKAMI S. & YOSHIKAWA H. (1965) Inorganic phosphate and erythrocyte glycolysis. *Biochimica et Biophysica Acta*, **99**, 175.

20 MINAKAMI S. & YOSHIKAWA H. (1966) Studies on erythrocyte glycolysis, III. The effects of active transport, pH and inorganic phosphate concentration on erythrocyte glycolysis. *Journal of Biochemistry*, **59**, 145.

21 RIZZO S.C. & ECKEL R.E. (1966) Control of glycolysis in human erythrocytes by inorganic phosphate and sulfate. *American Journal of Physiology*, **211**, 429.

22 JACOBASCH G. (1968) Elnfluss des Phosphates und des Magnesiums auf die Regulation der Glykolyse. *Folia Haematologica*, **89**, 376.

23 GERCKEN G. (1968) Der Einfluss der anorganischen Phosphatkonzentration auf den Adeninnukleotidgehalt und die Glykolysegeschwindigkeit von Kaninchenerythrozyten. *Folia Haematologica*, **89**, 400.

24 ROSE I.A. & WARMS J.V.B. (1970) Control of red cell glycolysis. The cause of triose phosphate accumulation. *Journal of Biological Chemistry*, **245**, 4009.

25 OSUOHA S.M. (1976) Red Cell Metabolism in Renal Disease. Ph.D. thesis, University of London.

26 RAPOPORT S. (1968) The regulation of glycolysis in mammalian erythrocytes. In: *Essays in Biochemistry* (ed. Campbell P.N. & Greville G.D.), p. 69. Academic Press, London.

27 ASAKUTA T., SATO Y., MINAKAMI S. & YOSHIKAWA H. (1966) Effect of deoxygenation of intracellular hemoglobin on red cell glycolysis. *Journal of Biochemistry*, **5**, 524.

28 RATTANAPANONE V. (1976) Human Red Cell Metabolism and Viability under Different Conditions of pH and of Oxygen Tension. Ph.D Thesis, University of London.

29 HAMASAKI N., ASAKURA T. & MINAKAMI S. (1970) Effect of oxygen tension on glycolysis in human erythrocytes. *Journal of Biochemistry*, **68**, 157.

30 MINAKAMI S., SUZUKI C., SAITO T. & YOSHIKAWA H. (1965) Studies on erythrocyte glycolysis. I. Determination of the glycolytic intermediates in human erythrocytes. *Journal of Biochemistry*, **58**, 543.

31 POST R.L., MERRITT C.R., KINSOLVING C.R. &

ALBRIGHT C.D. (1960) Membrane adenosine triphosphatase as a participant in the active transport of sodium and potassium in the human erythrocyte. *Journal of Biological Chemistry*, **235**, 1796.

32 DUNHAM E.T. & GLYNN I.M. (1961) Adenosine triphosphatase activity and the active movements of alkali metal ions. *Journal of Physiology*, **156**, 274.

33 SCHATZMANN H.J. (1953) Herzglykoside als Hemmstoffe für den aktiven Kalium-und Natrium-Transport durch die Erythrocyten-Membran. *Helvetica Physiologica et Pharmacologica Acta*, **11**, 346.

34 WHITTAM R. & WHEELER K.P. (1970) Transport across cell membranes. *Annual Reviews of Physiology*, **32**, 21.

35 PARKER J.C. & HOFFMAN J.F. (1967) The role of membrane phosphoglycerate kinase in the control of glycolytic rate by active cation transport in human red blool cells. *Journal of General Physiology*, **50**, 893.

36 PROVERBIO F. & HOFFMAN J.F. (1972) Differential behaviour of the Mg-ATPase and the Na, Mg-ATPase of human red cell ghosts. *Federation Proceedings*, **31**, 215.

37 HOFFMAN J.F. (1973) Molecular aspects of the Na^+, K^+-pump in red blood cells. In: *Organisation of Energy-Transducing Membranes* (ed. Nakao M. & Packe L.), p. 9. University of Tokyo Press, Tokyo.

38 WHITTAM R. & AGER M.E. (1965) The connexion between active cation transport and metabolism in erythrocytes. *Biochemical Journal*, **97**, 214.

39 POST R.L. & JOLLY P.C. (1957) The linkage of sodium, potassium and ammonium active transport across the human erythrocyte membrane. *Biochimica et Biophysica Acta*, **25**, 118.

40 MURPHY J.R. (1963) Erythrocyte metabolism. V. Active cation transport and glycolysis. *Journal of Laboratory and Clinical Medicine*, **61**, 567.

41 SCHATZMANN H.J. & VINCENZI E.F. (1969) Calcium movements across the membrane of human red cells. *Journal of Physiology*, **201**, 369.

42 GENT W.L.G., TROUNCE J.R. & WALSER M. (1964) The binding of calcium ion by the human erythrocyte membrane. *Archives of Biochemistry and Biophysics*, **105**, 582.

43 HARRISON D.G. & LONG C. (1968) The calcium content of human erythrocytes. *Journal of Physiology*, **199**, 367.

44 FORSTNER J.F. & MANERY J.F. (1970) Calcium binding sites in human erythrocyte ghosts. *Federation Proceedings*, **29**, 664.

45 FORSTNER J.F. & MANERY J.F. (1971) Calcium binding by human erythrocyte membranes. *Biochemical Journal*, **124**, 563.

46 FORSTNER J.F. & MANERY J.F. (1971) Calcium binding by human erythrocyte membranes, significance of carboxyl, amino and thiol groups. *Biochemical Journal*, **125**, 343.

47 LONG C. & MOUAT B. (1971) The binding of calcium ions by erythrocyte and 'ghost'-cell membranes. *Biochemical Journal*, **123**, 829.

48 TOLBERG A.B. & MACEY R.I. (1972) The release of membrane-bound calcium by radiation and sulfhydryl reagents. *Journal of Cellular Physiology*, **79**, 43.

49 BUCKLEY J.T. & HAWTHORNE J.N. (1972) Erythrocyte membrane polyphosphoinositide metabolism and the regulation of calcium binding. *Journal of Biological Chemistry*, **247**, 7218.

50 DUFFY M.J. & SCHWARZ V. (1973) Calcium binding by the erythrocyte membrane. *Biochimica et Biophysica Acta*, **330**, 294.

51 PORZIG H. (1977) Studies on the cation permeability of human red cell ghosts. *Journal of Membrane Biology*, **31**, 317.

52 CAFFREY R.W., TREMBLAY R., GABRIO B.W. & HUENNEKENS F.M. (1956) Erythrocyte metabolism. II. Adenosinetriphosphatase. *Journal of Biological Chemistry*, **223**, 1.

53 OHNISHI T. (1962) Extraction of actin and myosin-like proteins from erythrocyte membranes. *Journal of Biochemistry*, **52**, 307.

54 NAKAO T., NAGANO K., ADACHI K. & NAKAO M. (1963) Separation of two adenosine triphosphatases from erythrocyte membrane. *Biochemical and Biophysical Research Communications*, **13**, 444.

55 SCHATZMANN H.J. (1966) ATP-dependent Ca^{++}-extrusion from human red cells. *Experientia*, **22**, 364.

56 SCHATZMANN H.J. (1973) Dependence on calcium concentration and stiochiometry of the Ca pump in human red cells. *Journal of Physiology*, **235**, 551.

57 SCHATZMANN H.J. (1975) Active calcium transport and Ca^{2+}-activated ATPase in human red cells. *Current Topics in Membrane Transport*, **6**, 126.

58 REED P.W. & LARDY H.A. (1972) A23187: a divalent cation ionophore. *Journal of Biological Chemistry*, **247**, 6970.

59 ALLAN D. & MICHELL R.H. (1975) Accumulation of 1,2-diacylglycerol in the plasma membrane may lead to echinocyte transformation of erythrocytes. *Nature (London)*, **258**, 348.

60 KIRKPATRICK F.H., HILLMAN D.G. & LACELLE P.L. (1975) A23187 and red cells: changes in deformability, K^+, Mg^{2+}, Ca^{2+} and ATP. *Experientia*, **31**, 653.

61 TAYLOR D., BAKER R. & HOCHSTEIN P. (1977) The effect of calcium ionophore A23187 on the ATP level of human erythrocytes. *Biochemical and Biophysical Research Communications*, **76**, 205.

62 PLISHKER G. & GITELMAN H.J. (1976) Calcium transport in intact human erythrocytes. *Journal of General Physiology*, **68**, 29.

63 ALLAN D., BILLAH M.M., FINEAN J.B. & MICHELL R.H. (1976) Release of diacylglycerol-enriched vesicles from erythrocytes with increased intracellular $[Ca^{2+}]$. *Nature (London)*, **261**, 58.

64 LACELLE P.L., WEED R.I. & SANTILLO P.A. (1976) Pathophysiologic significance of abnormalities of red cell shape. In: *Membranes and Disease* (ed. Bolis L., Hoffman J.F. & Leaf A.), p. 1. Raven Press, New York.

65 NAKAO M., NAKAO T., TATIBANA C. & YOSHIKAWA H. (1960) Shape transformation of erythrocyte ghosts on addition of adenosine triphosphate to the medium. *Journal of Biochemistry*, **47**, 694.

66 WINS P. & SCHOFFENIELS E. (1966) $ATP + Ca^{++}$-linked contraction of red cell ghosts. *Archives Internationales de Physiologie et de Biochemie*, **74**, 812.

67 PALEK J., CURBY W.A. & LIONETTI F.J. (1971) Effects of calcium and adenosine triphosphate on volume of human red cell ghosts. *American Journal of Physiology*, **220**, 19.

68 PALEK J., CURBY W.A. & LIONETTI F.J. (1971) Relation of Ca^{++}-activated ATPase to Ca^{++}-linked shrinkage of human red cell ghosts. *American Journal of Physiology*, **220**, 1028.

69 LORAND L., SIEFRING G.E. & LOWE-KRENTZ L. (1979) Enzymatic basis of membrane stiffening in human erythrocytes. *Seminars in Hematology*, **16**, 65.

70 COETZER T.L. & ZAIL S.S. (1979) Cross-linking of membrane proteins of metabolically-depleted and calcium-loaded erythrocytes. *British Journal of Haematology*, **43**, 375.

71 GREENWALD I. (1925) A new type of phosphoric acid compound isolated from blood, with some remarks on the effect of substitution on the rotation of L-glyceric acid. *Journal of Biological Chemistry*, **63**, 339.

72 CHANUTIN A. & CURNISH R.R. (1967) Effect of organic and inorganic phosphates on the oxygen equilibrium of human erythrocytes. *Archives of Biochemistry and Biophysics*, **121**, 96.

73 BENESCH R. & BENESCH R.E. (1967) The effect of organic phosphates from the human erythrocyte on the allosteric properties of hemoglobin. *Biochemical and Biophysical Research Communications*, **26**, 162.

74 GERLACH E. & DUHM J. (1972) Regulation of the concentration of 2,3-diphosphoglycerate in the erythrocyte. *Scandinavian Journal of Clinical and Laboratory Investigation*, **29** (Suppl. 126), 5.

75 RAPOPORT S. (1936) Über Phosphorglycerinsäure als Transport Substanz des Blutphosphorus und ihr Verhalten bei experimenteller Ammonchloridazidose I. *Biochemische Zeitschrift*, **289**, 411.

76 RAPOPORT S. & GUEST G.M. (1939) The decomposition of diphosphoglycerate in acidified blood: its relationship to reactions of the glycolytic cycle. *Journal of Biological Chemistry*, **129**, 781.

77 ASAKUTA T., SATO Y., MINAKAMI S. & YOSHIKAWA H. (1966) pH dependency of 2,3-diphosphoglycerate content in red blood cells. *Clinica Chimica Acta*, **14**, 840.

78 RÖRTH M. (1970) Dependency on acid-base status of blood of oxyhemoglobin dissociation and 2,3-diphosphoglycerate level in human erythrocytes. I. *In-vitro* studies on reduced and oxygenated blood. *Scandinavian Journal of Clinical and Laboratory Investigation*, **26**, 43.

79 ASTRUP P., RÖRTH M. & THORSHAUGE C. (1970) Dependency on acid-base status of oxyhemoglobin dissociation and 2,3-diphosphoglycerate level in human erythrocytes. *Scandinavian Journal of Clinical and Laboratory Investigation*, **26**, 47.

80 KILMARTIN J.V. (1976) Interaction of haemoglobin with protons, CO_2 and 2,3-diphosphoglycerate. *British Medical Bulletin*, **32** (No. 3), 209.

81 BISHOP C., RANKINE D.M. & TALBOT J.H. (1959) The nucleotides in normal human blood. *Journal of Biological Chemistry*, **234**, 1233.

82 YOSHIKAWA H., NAKANO M., MIYAMOTO K. & TATIBANA M. (1960) Phosphorus metabolism in human erythrocyte. II. Separation of acid-soluble phosphorus compounds incorporating P^{32} by column chromatography with ion exchange resin. *Journal of Biochemistry*, **47**, 635.

83 OMACHI A., SCOTT C.B. & MILLMAN M.S. (1970) Influence of prior storage on pyridine nucleotide metabolism of human erythrocytes incubated in *vitro*. *Journal of Laboratory and Clinical Medicine*, **76**, 668.

84 OMACHI A., SCOTT C.B. & FORD D.L. (1972) Pyridine nucleotide metabolism in stored human erythrocytes. *Clinica Chimica Acta*, **37**, 351.

85 OMACHI A., SCOTT C.B. & HEGARTY H. (1969) Pyridine nucleotides in human erythrocytes in different metabolic states. *Biochimica et Biophysica Acta*, **184**, 139.

86 EGGLESTON L.V. & KREBS H.A. (1974) Regulation of the pentose phosphate cycle. *Biochemical Journal*, **138**, 425.

87 CAHILL G.F., HASTINGS A.B., ASHMORE J. & ZOTTU S. (1958) Studies on carbohydrate metabolism in rat liver slices. X. Factors in the regulation of pathways of glucose metabolism. *Journal of Biological Chemistry*, **230**, 125.

88 GAETANI G.D., PARKER J.C. & KIRKMAN H.N. (1974) Intracellular restraint: a new basis for the limitation in response to oxidative stress in human erythrocytes containing low-activity variants of glucose-6-phosphate dehydrogenase. *Proceedings of the National Academy of Sciences, USA*, **71**, 3584.

89 BARTLETT G.R. & MARLOW A.A. (1953) Erythrocyte carbohydrate metabolism. I. The flow of C^{14}- glucose carbon into lactic acid, carbon dioxide, cell polymers, and carbohydrate intermediate pool. *Journal of Laboratory and Clinical Medicine*, **42**, 178.

90 DE LOECKER W.C.J. & PRANKERD T.A.J. (1961) Factors influencing the hexose monophosphate shunt in red cells. *Clinica Chimica Acta*, **6**, 641.

91 GRIMES A.J. (1963) Glycolysis in young and mature normal human erythrocytes. *Nature (London)*, **198**, 1312.

92 WORATHUMRONG N. (1975) Some Effects of Salicylate on Human Red Cells. Ph.D. thesis. University of London.

93 SZEINBERG A. & MARKS P.A. (1961) Substances stimulating glucose catabolism by the oxidative reactions of the pentose phosphate pathway in human erythrocytes. *Journal of Clinical Investigation*, **40**, 914.

94 ROSE I.A. (1961) The use of kinetic isotope effects in the study of metabolic control. *Journal of Biological Chemistry*, **236**, 603.

95 BLOCH K. (1964) The synthesis of glutathione in isolated liver. *Journal of Biological Chemistry*, **179**, 1245.

96 HOCHBERG A., RIGBI M. & DIMANT E. (1961) The incorporation in *vitro* of glycine and L-glutamic acid into glutathione of human erythrocytes. *Biochimica et Biophysica Acta*, **90**, 464.

97 BOIVIN P. & GALAND C. (1965) La synthèse du glutathion au cours de l'anémie hémolytique congénitale avec déficit en glutathion réduit. Déficit congenital en glutathion-synthétase erythrocytaire. *Nouvelle Revue française d'Hématologie*, **5**, 707.

98 MINNICH V., SMITH M.B., BRAUNER M.J. & MAJERUS P.W. (1971) Glutathione biosynthesis in human erythrocytes. I. Identification of the enzymes of glutathione synthesis in hemolysates. *Journal of Clinical Investigation*, **50**, 507.

99 ELDJARN L., BREMER J. & BÖRRESEN H.C. (1962) The reduction of disulphides by human erythrocytes. *Biochemical Journal*, **82**, 192.

100 SRIVASTAVA S.K. & BEUTLER E. (1967) Permeability of normal and glucose-6-phosphate dehydrogenase defi-

cient erythrocytes to glutathione. *Biochemical and Biophysical Research Communications*, **28**, 659.

101 Srivastava S.K. & Beutler E. (1969) The transport of oxidized glutathione from human erythrocytes. *Journal of Biological Chemistry*, **244**, 9.

102 Srivastava S.K. & Beutler E. (1969) The transport of oxidized glutathione from the erythrocytes of various species in the presence of chromate. *Biochemical Journal*, **114**, 833.

103 Beutler E. & Srivastava S.K. (1968) The efflux of GSSG from human erythrocytes. In: *Metabolism and Membrane Permeability of Erythrocytes and Thrombocytes* (ed. Deutsch E., Gerlach E. & Moser K.), p. 91. Geo. Thieme, Stuttgart.

104 Dimant E., Landsberg E. & London I.M. (1955) The metabolic behaviour of reduced glutathione in human and avian erythrocytes. *Journal of Biological Chemistry*, **213**, 769.

105 Rouser G., Jelinek B. & Samuels A.J. (1956) Amino acid metabolism in human blood cells. *Federation Proceedings*, **15**, 342.

106 Eldjarn L. & Bremer J. (1962) The inhibitory effect at the hexokinase level of disulphides on glucose metabolism in human erythrocytes. *Biochemical Journal*, **84**, 286.

107 Huisman T.H.J. & Doxy A.M. (1962) Studies on the heterogeneity of hemoglobin. V. Binding of hemoglobin with oxidized glutathione. *Journal of Laboratory and Clinical Medicine*, **60**, 302.

108 Kosower N.S. & Kosower E.M. (1974) Protection of membranes by glutathione. In: *Glutathione* (ed. Flohé L., Benöhr H.C., Sies H., Waller H.D. & Wendel A.), p. 216. Geo. Thieme, Stuttgart.

109 Lohmann K. (1932) Beitrag zur enzymatischen Umwandlung von synthetischem Methylglyoxal in Milchsäure. *Biochemische Zeitschrift*, **254**, 332.

110 Jowett M. & Quastel J.H. (1933) LXX. The glyoxalase activity of the red blood cell. The function of glutathione. *Biochemical Journal*, **27**, 486.

111 Cohen P.P. & Sober E.K. (1945) Glyoxalase activity of erythrocytes from cancerous rats and human subjects. *Cancer Research*, **5**, 631.

112 Klebanoff S.J. (1956) Glutathione metabolism. I. The glyoxalase activity of mature mammalian erythrocytes. *Biochemical Journal*, **64**, 425.

113 Valentine W.N. & Tanaka K.R. (1961) The glyoxalase content of human erythrocytes and leucocytes. *Acta Haematologica*, **26**, 303.

114 Kirmsky I. & Racker E. (1952) Glutathione, a prosthetic group of glyceraldehyde-3-phosphate dehydrogenase. *Journal of Biological Chemistry*, **198**, 721.

115 Chasseaud L.F. (1974) Glutathione S-transferases. In: *Glutathione* (ed. Flohé L., Benöhr H.C., Sies H., Waller H.D. & Wendel A.), p. 90. Geo. Thieme, Stuttgart.

116 Scott E.M., Duncan I.W. & Ekstrand V. (1963) Purification and properties of glutathione reductase of human erythrocytes. *Journal of Biological Chemistry*, **238**, 3928.

117 Waller H.D. (1968) Glutathione reductase deficiency. In: *Hereditary Disorders of Erythrocyte Metabolism* (ed. Beutler E.), p. 185. Grune & Stratton, New York.

118 Beutler E. & Yeh M.K.Y. (1963) Erythrocyte glutathione reductase. *Blood*, **21**, 573.

119 Icén A. (1967) Glutathione reductase of human erythrocytes. Purification and properties. *Scandinavian Journal of Clinical and Laboratory Investigation*, **20** (Suppl. 96), 1.

120 Kaplan J.C. (1968) Electrophoretic study of glutathione reductase in human erythrocytes and leucocytes. *Nature (London)*, **217**, 256.

121 Buzard J.A. & Kopko F. (1963) The flavin requirement and some inhibition characteristics of rat tissue glutathione reductase. *Journal of Biological Chemistry*, **238**, 464.

122 Koutras G.A., Hattori M., Schneider A.S., Ebaugh F.G. & Valentine W.N. (1964) Studies on chromated erythrocytes. Effect of sodium chromate on erythrocyte glutathione reductase. *Journal of Clinical Investigation*, **43**, 323.

123 Koutras G.A., Schneider A.S., Hattori M. & Valentine W.N. (1965) Studies on chromated erythrocytes. Mechanisms of chromate inhibition of glutathione reductase. *British Journal of Haematology*, **11**, 360.

124 Chan P.S., Chandler M. & Beck L.V. (1969) Chromate inhibition, in erythrocytes, of chemically stimulated increases in glucose oxidation via the hexose monophosphate pathway (HMP). *Proceedings of the Society for Experimental Biology and Medicine*, **130**, 257.

125 Stall G.E.J., Helleman P.W., Dewael J. & Veeger C. (1969) Purification and properties of an abnormal glutathione reductase from human erythrocytes. *Biochimica et Biophysica Acta*, **185**, 63.

126 Beutler E. (1969) Effect of flavin compounds on glutathione reductase activity: *in-vivo* and *in-vitro* studies. *Journal of Clinical Investigation*, **48**, 1957.

127 Beutler E. (1969) Gluthathione reductase: stimulation in normal subjects by riboflavin supplementation. *Science*, **165**, 613.

128 Srivastava S.K. & Beutler E. (1970) Glutathione metabolism of the erythrocyte. The enzyme cleavage of glutathione-haemoglobin preparations by glutathione reductase. *Biochemical Journal*, **119**, 353.

129 Aebi H. & Suter H. (1974) Protective function of reduced glutathione (G-SH), against the effect of prooxidative substances and of irradiation in the red cell. In: *Glutathione* (ed. Flohé L., Benöhr H.C., Sies H., Waller H.D. & Wendel A.), p. 192, Geo. Thieme, Stuttgart.

130 Little C. & O'Brien P.J. (1968) An intracellular GSH-peroxidase with a lipid peroxode substrate. *Biochemical and Biophysical Research Communications*, **31**, 145.

131 Little C. (1972) Steroid hydroperoxides as substrates for glutathione peroxidase. *Biochimica et Biophysica Acta*, **284**, 375.

132 Mills G.C. (1959) The purification and properties of glutathione peroxidase of erythrocytes. *Journal of Biological Chemistry*, **234**, 502.

133 Rotruck J.T., Hoekstra W.G., Pope A.L., Ganther H., Swanson A. & Hafeman D. (1972) Relationship of selenium to GSH peroxidase. *Federation Proceedings*, **31**, 691.

134 Flohé L. & Gunzler W.A. (1974) Glutathione peroxidase. In: *Glutathione* (ed. Flohí L., Benöhr H.C., Sies H., Waller H.D. & Wendel A.), p. 132. Geo. Thieme, Stuttgart.

135 DEISSEROTH A. & DOUNCE A.L. (1970) Catalase: physical and chemical properties, mechanism of catalysis, and physiological role. *Physiological Reviews*, **50**, 319.

136 CHANCE B. (1949) The enzyme-substrate compounds of horse-radish peroxidase and peroxides. II. Kinetics of formation and decomposition of the primary and secondary complexes. *Archives of Biochemistry and Biophysics*, **22**, 224.

137 CHANCE B. (1949) The properties of the enzyme-substrate compounds of horse-radish and lacto-peroxidase. *Science*, **109**, 204.

138 CHANCE B. (1947) Intermediate compounds in the catalase-hydrogen peroxide reaction. *Acta Chemica Scandinavica*, **1**, 236.

139 EATON J.W., BORAAS M. & ETKIN N.L. (1972) Catalase activity and red cell metabolism. In: *Hemoglobin and Red Cell Structure and Function* (ed. Brewer G.J.), p. 21. Plenum Press, New York.

140 EATON J.W. & SHAFFER E. (1974) Quoted in Pentose Phosphate Metabolism, Eaton J.W. and Brewer G.J., p. 451. In: *The Red Cell*, **1** (ed. Surgenor D.M.). Academic Press, New York.

141 LIEBOWITZ J. & COHEN G. (1968) Increased hydrogen peroxide levels in glucose 6-phosphate dehydrogenase deficient erythrocytes exposed to acetylphenylhydrazine. *Biochemical Pharmacology*, **17**, 983.

142 NICHOLLS P. (1972) Contributions of catalase and glutathione peroxidase to red cell peroxide removal. *Biochimica et Biophysica Acta*, **279**, 306.

143 NECHELES T.F., BOLES T.A. & ALLEN D.M. (1968) Erythrocyte glutathione-peroxidase deficiency and hemolytic disease of the newborn infant. *Journal of Pediatrics*, **72**, 319.

144 NECHELES T.F., MALDONADO N., BARQUET-CHEDIAK A. & ALLEN D.M. (1969) Homozygous erythrocyte glutathione-peroxidase deficiency: clinical and biochemical studies. *Blood*, **33**, 164.

145 JACOB H.S., INGBAR S.H. & JANDL J.H. (1965) Oxidative hemolysis and erythrocyte metabolism in hereditary acatalasia. *Journal of Clinical Investigation*, **44**, 1187.

146 MARTI H.R. (1965) Quoted by Aebi *et al.* (1968) In: *Hereditary Disorders of Erythrocyte Metabolism* (ed. Beutler E.), p. 41. Grune & Stratton, New York.

147 HOARD J.L. (1968) Some aspects of heme stereochemistry. In: *Structural Chemistry and Molecular Biology* (ed. Rich A. & Davidson N.), p. 573, Freeman & Co., San Francisco.

148 HUBER R., EPP O. & FORMANEK H. (1969) The environment of the haem group in erythrocruorin (chironomus thummi). *Journal of Molecular Biology*, **42**, 591.

149 PERUTZ M.F. (1970) Stereochemistry of co-operative effects in haemoglobin. *Nature (London)*, **228**, 726.

150 WEISS J.J. (1964) Nature of the iron-oxygen bond in oxyhaemoglobin. *Nature (London)*, **202**, 83.

151 SALTZMAN H.A. & FRIDOVICH I. (1973) Oxygen toxicity. Introduction to a protective enzyme: superoxide dismutase. *Circulation*, **48**, 921.

152 MISRA H.P. & FRIDOVICH I. (1972) The generation of superoxide radical during the autoxidation of hemoglobin. *Journal of Biological Chemistry*, **247**, 6960.

153 PAUL W.D. & KEMP C.R. (1944) Methemoglobin: a normal constituent of blood. *Proceedings of the Society for Experimental Biology and Medicine*, **56**, 55.

154 PETERS J.P. & VAN SLYKE D.D. (1946) In: *Quantitative Clinical Chemistry*, 2nd edn. p. 373. Baillière, Tindall & Cox, London.

155 SCOTT E.M. (1968) Congenital methemoglobinemia due to DPNH-diaphorase deficiency. In: *Hereditary Disorders of Erythrocyte Metabolism* (ed. Beutler E.), p. 102. Grune & Stratton, New York.

156 EDER H.A., FINCH C. & MCKEE R.W. (1949) Congenital methemoglobinemia. A clinical and biochemical study of a case. *Journal of Clinical Investigation*, **28**, 265.

157 JAFFÉ E.R. (1964) Metabolic processes involved in the formation and reduction of methemoglobin in human erythrocytes. In: *The Red Blood Cell* (ed. Bishop C. & Surgenor D.M.), p. 347. Academic Press, New York.

158 SCOTT E.M., DUNCAN I.W. & EKSTRAND V. (1965) The reduced pyridine nucleotide dyhydrogenases of human erythrocytes. *Journal of Biological Chemistry*, **240**, 481.

159 MORRISON D.B. & WILLIAMS E.F. (1938) Methemoglobin reduction by glutathione or cysteine. *Science*, **87**, 15.

160 BARCROFT H., GIBSON Q.H., HARRISON D.C. & MCMURRAY J. (1945) Familial idiopathic methaemoglobinaemia and its treatment with ascorbic acid. *Clinical Science*, **5**, 145.

161 GIBSON Q.H. (1943) The reduction of methaemoglobin by ascorbic acid. *Biochemical Journal*, **37**, 615.

162 FINCH C.A. (1948) Methemoglobinaemia and sulfhemoglobinemia. *New England Journal of Medicine*, **239**, 470.

163 BARCROFT H., GIBSON Q.H. & HARRISON D.C. (1949) Methaemoglobinaemia. In: *Haemoglobin—Barcroft Memorial Conference*, p. 223. Butterworth Scientific Publications, London.

164 SASS M.D., CARUSO C.J. & FARHANGI M. (1967) TPNH—methemoglobin reductase deficiency: a new red-cell enzyme defect. *Journal of Laboratory and Clinical Medicine*, **70**, 760.

165 KAPLAN J.C. & BEUTLER E. (1967) Electrophoresis of NADH- and NADPH- diaphorases in normal subjects and patients with congenital methemoglobinemia. *Biochemical and Biophysical Research Communications*, **29**, 605.

166 BLOOM G.E. & ZARKOWSKY H.S. (1969) Heterogeneity of the enzymatic defect in congenital methemoglobinemia. *New England Journal of Medicine*, **281**, 919.

167 KAJITA A., KERWAR G.K. & HEUNNEKENS F.M. (1969) Multiple forms of methemoglobin reductase. *Archives of Biochemistry and Biophysics*, **130**, 662.

168 NIETHAMMER D. & HUENNEKENS F.M. (1971) Bound TPN as the determinant of polymorphism in methemoglobin reductase. *Biochemical and Biophysical Research Communications*, **45**, 345.

169 NIETHAMMER D. & HUENNEKENS F.M. (1971) Electrophoretic separation and characterization of the multiple forms of methemoglobin reductase. *Archives of Biochemistry and Biophysics*, **146**, 564.

170 HSIEH H.S. & JAFFÉ E.R. (1971) Electrophoretic and functional variants of NADH — methemoglobin reductase in hereditary methemoglobinemia. *Journal of Clinical Investigation*, **50**, 196.

171 MATSUKI T., YUBISUI T., TOMODA A., YONEYAMA Y., TAKESHITA M., HIRANO M., KOBAYASHI K. & TANI Y. (1978) Acceleration of methaemoglobin reduction by

riboflavin in human erythrocytes. *British Journal of Haematology*, **39**, 523.

172 YUBISHI T., MATSUKI T., TANISHIMA K., TAKESHITA M. & YONEYAMA Y. (1977) NADPH— flavin reductase in human erythrocytes and the reduction of methemoglobin through flavin by the enzyme. *Biochemical and Biophysical Research Communications*, **76**, 174.

173 BEUTLER E. & BALUDA M.C. (1962/3) The role of methemoglobin in oxidative degradation of hemoglobin. *Acta Haematologica*, **27**, 321.

174 SASS M., CARUSO C.J. & AXELROD D.R. (1969) Mechanism of the TPNH-linked reduction of methemoglobin by methylene blue. *Clinica Chimica Acta*, **24**, 77.

175 HEINZ R. (1890) Morphologische Veränderungen der rothen Blutkörperchen durch Gifte. *Virchows Archiv*, **122**, 112.

176 WEBSTER S.H. (1949) Heinz body phenomenon in erythrocytes. A review. *Blood*, **4**, 479.

177 BEAVEN G.H. & WHITE J.C. (1954) Oxidation of phenylhydrazine in the presence of oxyhaemoglobin and the origin of Heinz bodies in erythrocytes. *Nature (London)*, **173**, 389.

178 JENSEN W.N. & LESSIN L.S. (1970) Membrane alterations associated with hemoglobinopathies. *Seminars in Hematology*, **7**, 409.

179 JACOB H.S., BRAIN M.C. & DACIE J.V. (1968) Altered sulfhydryl reactivity of hemoglobins and red blood cell membranes in congenital Heinz body hemolytic anemia. *Journal of Clinical Investigation*, **47**, 2664.

180 JACOB H.S., BRAIN M.C. & DACIE J.V. (1968) Abnormal haem binding and globin SH group blockade in unstable haemoglobins. *Nature (London)*, **218**, 1214.

181 WINTERBOURN C.C. & CARRELL R.W. (1973) The attachment of Heinz bodies to the red cell membrane. *British Journal of Haematology*, **25**, 585.

182 WEED R.I. & REED C.F. (1966) Membrane alterations leading to red cell destruction. *American Journal of Medicine*, **41**, 681.

183 FESSAS PH. (1963) Inclusions of hemoglobin in erythroblasts and erythrocytes of thalassemia. *Blood*, **21**, 21.

184 ALLEN D.W. & JANDL J.H. (1961) Oxidative hemolysis and precipitation of hemoglobin. II. Role of thiols in oxidant drug action. *Journal of Clinical Investigation*, **40**, 454.

185 JACOB H.S. (1970) Mechanisms of Heinz body formation and attachment to red cell membrane. *Seminars in Hematology*, **7**, 341.

186 GRIMES A.J. & MEISLER A. (1962) Possible cause of Heinz bodies in congenital Heinz body anaemia. *Nature (London)*, **194**, 190.

187 GRIMES A.J., MEISLER A. & DACIE J.V. (1964) Congenital Heinz body anaemia: further evidence on the cause of Heinz body production in red cells. *British Journal of Haematology*, **10**, 281.

188 WINTERBOURN C.C. & CARRELL R.W. (1974) Studies of hemoglobin denaturation and Heinz body formation in the unstable hemoglobins. *Journal of Clinical Investigation*, **54**, 678.

189 WINTERHALTER K.H. (1966) Sequence of linkage between the prosthetic groups and the polypeptide chains of haemoglobin. *Nature (London)*, **211**, 932.

190 WINTERHALTER K.H. & DERANLEAU D.A. (1967) The structure of a hemoglobin carrying only two hemes. *Biochemistry*, **6**, 3136.

191 SHIBATA S., IUCHI I., MIYAJI T., UEDA S. & TAKEDA I. (1963) Hemolytic disease associated with the production of abnormal hemoglobin and intraerythrocytic Heinz bodies. *Acta Haematologica Japonica*, **26**, 164.

192 VAUGHAN JONES R., GRIMES A.J., CARRELL R.W. & LEHMANN H. (1967) Köln haemoglobinopathy. Further data and a comparison with other hereditary Heinz body anaemias. *British Journal of Haematology*, **13**, 394.

193 ITANO H.A., HOSOKAWA K. & HIROTA K. (1976) Induction of haemolytic anaemia by substituted phenylhydrazines. *British Journal of Haematology*, **32**, 99.

194 HARLEY J.D. & MAUER A.M. (1960) Studies on the formation of Heinz bodies. I. Methemoglobin production and oxyhemoglobin destruction. *Blood*, **16**, 1722.

195 MILLER A. & SMITH H.C. (1970) The intracellular and membrane effects of oxidant agents on normal red cells. *British Journal of Haematology*, **19**, 417.

196 RENTSCH G. (1968) Genesis of Heinz bodies and methemoglobin formation. *Biochemical Pharmacology*, **17**, 423.

197 BEUTLER E. (1969) Drug-induced hemolytic anemia. *Pharmacological Reviews*, **21**, 73.

198 NAGEL R.L. & RANNEY H.M. (1973) Drug-induced oxidative denaturation of hemoglobin. *Seminars in Hematology*, **10**, 269.

199 CARRELL R.W. (1967) The unstable haemoglobins. Ph.D. thesis, University of Cambridge.

200 RACHMILEWITZ E.A., PEISACH J. & BLUMBERG W.E. (1971) Studies on the stability of oxyhemoglobin A and its constituents chains and their derivatives. *Journal of Biological Chemistry*, **246**, 3356.

201 PIOMELLI S., CORASH L.M., DAVENPORT D.D., MIRAGLIA J. & AMOROSI E.L. (1968) In-vivo lability of glucose-6-phosphate dehydrogenase in Gd^{A-} and $Gd^{Mediterranean}$ deficiency. *Journal of Clinical Investigation*, **47**, 940.

202 FISHER R.A. & HARRIS H. (1969) Studies on the purification and properties of the genetic variants of red cell acid phosphohydrolase in man. *Annals of the New York Academy of Sciences*, **166**, 380.

203 FUNAKOSHI S. & DEUTSCH H.F. (1969) Human carbonic anhydrases. II. Some physicochemical properties of native isozymes and of similar isozymes. *Journal of Biological Chemistry*, **244**, 3438.

204 EDWARDS Y.H., HOPKINSON D.A. & HARRIS H. (1971) Inherited variants of human nucleoside phosphorylase. *Annals of Human Genetics*, **34**, 395.

205 TURNER B.M., FISHER R.A. & HARRIS H. (1974) The age related loss of activity of four enzymes in the human erythrocyte. *Clinica Chimica Acta*, **50**, 85.

206 BERNSTEIN R.E. (1959) Alterations in metabolic energetics and cation transport during aging of red cells. *Journal of Clinical Investigation*, **38**, 1572.

207 GRIFFITHS W.J. & FITZPATRICK M. (1967) The effect of age on the creatine in red cells. *British Journal of Haematology*, **13**, 175.

208 MEYERING C.A., ISRAELS A.L.M., SEBENS T. & HUISMAN T.H.J. (1960) Studies on the heterogeneity of hemoglobin. II. The heterogeneity of different human hemoglobin types in carboxymethyl cellulose and in Amberlite

IRC-50-chromatography; quantitative aspects. *Clinica Chimica Acta*, **5**, 208.

209 PRANKERD T.A.J. (1958) The ageing of red cells. *Journal of Physiology*, **143**, 325.

210 WESTERMAN M.P., PIERCE L.E. & JENSEN W.N. (1963) Erythrocyte lipids: a comparison of normal young and normal old populations. *Journal of Laboratory and Clinical Medicine*, **62**, 394.

211 VAN GASTEL C., VAN DEN BERG D., DEGIER J. & VAN DEENEN L.L.M. (1965) Some lipid characteristics of normal red blood cells of different age. *British Journal of Haematology*, **11**, 193.

212 LACELLE P.L., KIRKPATRICK F.H., UDKOW M.P. & ARKIN B. (1973) Membrane fragmentation and Ca^{++}-membrane interaction: potential mechanisms of shape change in the senescent red cell. In: *Red Cell Shape* (ed. Bessis M., Weed R.I. & Leblond P.E.,), p. 69. Springer-Verlag, New York, Heidelberg and Berlin.

213 LACELLE P.L., KIRKPATRICK F.H. & UDKOW M. (1973) Relation of altered deformability, ATP, DPG and Ca^{++} concentrations in senescent erythrocytes. In: *Erythrocytes, Thrombocytes, Leukocytes* (ed. Gerlach E., Moser K., Deutsch E. & Wilmanns W.), p. 49. Geo. Thieme, Stuttgart.

214 GRIGGS R.C. & HARRIS J.W. (1961) Susceptibility to immune hemolysis as related to age of human and dog red blood cells. *Blood*, **18**, 806.

215 BEUTLER E. (1966) A series of new screening procedures for pyruvate kinase, glucose-6-phosphate dehydrogenase deficiency and glutathione reductase deficiency. *Blood*, **28**, 553.

216 CHAPMAN S.J. & ALLISON J.V. & GRIMES A.J. (1974) Abnormal cation movements in human hypochromic red cells incubated *in vitro*. *Scandinavian Journal of Haematology*, **10**, 225.

217 SELWYN J.G. & DACIE J.V. (1954) Autohaemolysis and other changes resulting from the incubation *in vitro* of red cells from patients with congenital hemolytic anemia. *Blood*, **9**, 414.

218 GRIMES A.J., LEETS I. & DACIE J.V. (1968) The autohaemolysis test: appraisal of the method for the diagnosis of pyruvate kinase deficiency and the effect of pH and additives. *British Journal of Haematology*, **14**, 309.

219 DAVIE J.V. (1964) The hereditary non-spherocytic haemolytic anaemias. *Acta Haematologica*, **31**, 177.

220 BEUTLER E. (1978) Why has the autohemolysis test not gone the way of the cephalin flocculation test? *Blood*, **51**, 109.

221 THORN M.B. (1968) Enzyme kinetics. In: *Biochemists' Handbook* (ed. Long C.), p. 205. E. & F. N. Spon, London.

222 MUNRO G.F. & MILLER D.R. (1970) Mechanism of fructose diphosphate activation of a mutant pyruvate kinase from human red cells. *Biochimica et Biophysica Acta*, **206**, 87.

223 PAGLIA D.E. & VALENTINE W.N. (1971) Additional kinetic distinctions between normal pyruvate kinase and a mutant isozyme from human erythrocytes. Correction of the kinetic anomaly by fructose 1,6-diphosphate. *Blood*, **37**, 311.

224 MIWA S., BOIVIN P., BLUME K.G., ARNOLD H., BLACK J.A., KAHN A., STAAL G.E.J., NAKASHIMA K., TANAKA K.R., PAGLIA D.E., VALENTINE W.N., YOSHIDA A. &

225 BEUTLER E. (1979) International Committee for Standardisation in Haematology: recommended methods for the characterization of red cell pyruvate kinase variants. *British Journal of Haematology*, **43**, 275.

225 TANAKA K.R. & PAGLIA D.E. (1971) Pyruvate kinase deficiency. *Seminars in Hematology*, **8**, 367.

226 JAFFÉ E.R. (1970) Hereditary hemolytic disorders and enzymatic deficiencies of human erythrocytes. *Blood*, **35**, 116.

227 ROSE I.A. & O'CONNELL E.L. (1964) The role of glucose 6-phosphate in the regulation of glucose metabolism in human erythrocytes. *Journal of Biological Chemistry*, **239**, 12.

228 RAPOPORT S. (1974) Control mechanisms of red cell glycolysis. In: *The Human Red Cell in vitro* (ed. Greenwalt T.J. & Jamieson G.A.), p. 153. Grune & Stratton, New York.

229 BREWER G.J. (1974) General red cell metabolism. In: *The Red Blood Cell* (ed. Surgenor D.M.) **1**, p. 387.

230 HOLMES E.W., MALONE J.I., WINEGRAD A.I. & OSKI F.A. (1967) Hexokinase isoenzymes in human erythrocytes: association of Type II with fetal hemoglobin. *Science*, **156**, 646.

231 MALONE J.I., WINEGRAD A.I., OSKI F.A. & HOLMES E.W. (1968) Erythrocyte hexokinase isoenzyme patterns in hereditary haemoglobinopathies. *New England Journal of Medicine*, **279**, 1071.

232 LÖHR G.W., WALLER H.D., ANSCHÜTZ F, & KNOPP A. (1964–5) Blochemische Defekte in den Blutzellen bei familiärer Panmyelopathie (Typ Fanconi). *Humangenetik*, **1**, 383.

233 LÖHR G.W., WALLER H.D., ANSCHÜTZ F, & KNOPP A. (1965) Hexokinase-mangel in Blutzellen bie einer Sippe mit familiarer Panmyelopathie (Typ Fanconi). *Klinische Wochenschrift*, **43**, 870.

234 SCHRÖEDER T.M. (1966) Cytogenetische und cytologische Befunde bei enzymopenischen Panmyelopathien und Pancytopenien. *Humangenetik*, **2**, 287.

235 VALENTINE W.N., OSKI F.A., PAGLIA D.E., BAUGHAN M.A., SCHNEIDER A.S. & NAIMAN J.L. (1967) Hereditary hemolytic anemia with hexokinase deficiency. *New England Journal of Medicine*, **276**, 1.

236 ALTAY C., ALPER C.A. & NATHAN D.G. (1970) Normal and variant isoenzymes of human blood cell hexokinase and the isoenzyme patterns in hemolytic anemia. *Blood*, **36**, 219.

237 NECHELES T.F., RAI U.S. & ALLEN D.M. (1968) A hexokinase variant associated with congenital nonspherocytic hemolytic disease. *Clinical Research*, **16**, 540.

238 KEITT A.S. (1969) Hemolytic anemia with impaired hexokinase deficiency. *Journal of Clinical Investigation*, **48**, 1997.

239 NECHELES T.F., RAI U.S. & CAMERON D. (1970) Congenital nonspherocytic hemolytic anemia associated with an unusual erythrocyte hexokinase abnormality. *Journal of Laboratory and Clinical Medicine*, **76**, 593.

240 MOSER K., CIRESA M. & SCHWARZMEIER J. (1970) Hexokinasemangel bei hëmolytischer Anämie. *Medizinische Weir*, **21**, 1977.

241 BOARD P.G., TRUEWORTHY R. & SMITH J.E. & MOORE K. (1978) Congenital nonspherocytic hemolytic anemia with an unstable hexokinase variant. *Blood*, **51**, 111.

242 BEUTLER E., DYMENT P.G. & MATSUMOTO F. (1978) Hereditary nonspherocytic hemolytic anemia and hexokinase deficiency. *Blood*, **57**, 935.

243 OSKI F.A., MARSHALL B.E., COHEN P.J., SUGERMAN H.J. & MILLER L.D. (1971) Exercise with anaemia. The role of the left-shifted or right-shifted oxygen-hemoglobin equilibrium curve. *Annals of Internal Medicine*, **74**, 44.

244 ROGERS P.A., FISHER R.A. & HARRIS H. (1975) An examination of the age-related patterns of decay of the hexokinase of human red cells. *Clinica Chimica Acta*, **65**, 291.

245 SLEIN M.W. (1968) In: *Biochemists' Handbook* (ed. Long C.), p. 436. E. and F. N. Spon, London.

246 ARNOLD H., BLUME K.G. & LÖHR G.W. (1974) Glucose phosphate isomerase deficiency with congenital nonspherocytic hemolytic anemia: a new variant (Type Nordhorn). II. Purification and biochemical properties of the defective enzyme. *Pediatric Research*, **8**, 26.

247 TILLEY B.E., GRACY R.W. & WELCH S.G. (1974) A point mutation increasing the stability of human phosphoglucose isomerase. *Journal of Biological Chemistry*, **249**, 4571.

248 DETTER J.C., WAYS P.O., GIBLETT E.R., BAUGHAN M.A., HOPKINSON D.A., POVEY S. & HARRIS H. (1968) Inherited variations in human phosphohexose isomerase. *Annals of Human Genetics*, **31**, 329.

249 PAYNE D.M., PORTER D.W. & GRACY R.W. (1972) Evidence against the occurrence of tissue-specific variants and isoenzymes of phosphoglucose isomerase. *Archives of Biochemistry and Biophysics*, **151**, 122.

250 NAKASHIMA K., MIWA S., ODA S., ODA E., MATSUMOTO N., FUKOMOTO Y. & YAMADA T. (1973) Electrophoretic and kinetic studies of glucose-phosphate isomerase (GPI) in two different Japanese families with GPI deficiency. *American Journal of Human Genetics*, **25**, 294.

251 GIBLETT E.R. (1969) *Genetic Markers in Human Blood*, p. 527. Blackwell Scientific Publications, Oxford.

252 BEUTLER E. (1978) *Hemolytic Anemia in Disorders of Red Cell Metabolism*, p. 201. Plenum Medical Book Co., New York.

253 BAUGHAN M.A., VALENTINE W.N., PAGLIA D.E., WAYS P.O., SIMON E.R. & DEMARSH Q.B. (1968) Hereditary hemolytic anemia associated with glucose-phosphate isomerase (GPI) deficiency—a new enzyme defect of human erythrocytes. *Blood*, **32**, 236.

254 PAGLIA D.E., HOLLAND P., BAUGHAN M.A. & VALENTINE W.N. (1969) Occurrence of defective hexosemonophosphate isomerization in human erythrocytes and leukocytes. *New England Journal of Medicine*, **280**, 66.

255 PAGLIA D.E. & VALENTINE W.N. (1974) Hereditary glucosephosphate isomerase deficiency. A review. *American Journal of Clinical Pathology*, **62**, 740.

256 ARNOLD H., BLUME K.G., BUSCH D., LEUKEITT U., LÖHR G.W. & LUBS E. (1970) Klinische und biochemische Untersuchungen zur Glucose-phosphatisomerase normaler menschlicher Erythrocyten und bei Glucose-phosphatisomerasemangel. *Klinische Wochenschriften*, **48**, 1299.

257 ARNOLD H., ENGLEHARDT R. & LÖHR G.W. (1973) Glucosephosphat-isomerase Typ Reeklinghausen: Eine neue Defektvariante mit hämolytischer Anämie. *Klinische Wochenschriften*, **51**, 1198.

258 SCHRÖTER W., KOCH H.H., WONNEBERGER B., KALINOWSKY W., ARNOLD A., BLUME K.G. & HUTHER W. (1974) Glucose-phosphate isomerase deficiency with congenital non-spherocytic hemolytic anemia: a new variant (Type Nordhorn). I. Clinical and genetic studies. *Pediatric Research*, **8**, 18.

259 PAGLIA D.E., PAREDES R., VALENTINE W.N., DORANTES S. & KONRAD P.N. (1975) Unique phenotypic expression of glucosephosphate isomerase deficiency. *American Journal of Human Genetics*, **27**, 62.

260 SCHRÖTER W., BRITTINGER G., ZIMMERSCHMITT E., KÖNIG E. & SCHRADER D. (1971) Combined glucose phosphate isomerase and glucose-6-phosphate dehydrogenase deficiency of the erythrocyte: a new haemolytic syndrome. *British Journal of Haematology*, **20**, 249.

261 MIWA S., NAKASHIMA K., ODA S., ODA E., MATSUMOTO N., OGAWA H. & FUKOMOTO Y. (1973) Glucosephosphate isomerase (GPI) deficiency hereditary nonspherocytic hemolytic anemia. Report of the first case found in Japanese. *Acta Haematologica Japan*, **36**, 65.

262 MIWA S., NAKASHIMA K., ODA S., MATSUMOTO N., OGAWA H., KOBAYASHI R., KOTANI M., HARATA A., ONAYA T. & YAMADA T. (1973) Glucosephosphate isomerase (GPI) deficiency hereditary nonspherocytic hemolytic anemia. Report of the second case found in Japanese. *Acta Haematologica*, **36**, 70.

263 BEUTLER E., SIGALOVE W.H., MUIR W.A., MATSUMOTO F. & WEST C. (1974) Glucosephosphate-isomerase (GPI) deficiency: GPI Elyria. *Annals of Internal Medicine*, **80**, 730.

264 MIWA S., NAKASHIMA K., TAJIRI M., ONO J., ABE S., ODA E., NONAKA H., MATSUOKA I., SHIMOYAMA S., HIRATA Y., AMAKI I., HORIUCHI A., YAMAGUCHI H. & NISHINA T. (1975) Three cases in two families with congenital nonspherocytic hemolytic anemia due to defective glycosephosphate isomerase: GPI Matsumoto. *Acta Haematologica Japan*, **38**, 238.

265 VAN BIERVLIET J.P.G.M. (1975) Glucosephosphate isomerase deficiency in a Dutch family. *Acta Paediatrica Scandinavica*, **64**, 868.

266 VAN BIERVLIET J.P.G.M., VAN MILLIGEN-BOERSMA L. & STAAL G.E.J. (1975) A new variant of glucosephosphate isomerase deficiency (GPI-Utrecht). *Clinica Chimica Acta*, **65**, 157.

267 VAN BIERVLIET J.P.G.M. & STAAL G.E.J. (1977) Excessive hepatic glycogen storage in glucose phosphate isomerase deficiency. *Acta Paediatrica Scandinavica*, **66**, 311.

268 WHITELAW A.G.L., ROGERS P.A., HOPKINSON D.A., GORDON H., EMERSON P.M., DARLEY J.H., REID C. & CRAWFORD M.d'A. (1979) Congenital haemolytic anaemia resulting from glucose phosphate isomerase deficiency: genetics, clinical picture and pre-natal diagnosis. *Journal of Medical Genetics*, **16**, 189.

269 VIVES-CORRONS J.L., ROZMAN C., KAHN A., CARRERA A. & TRIGINER J. (1975) Glucose phosphate isomerase deficiency with hereditary hemolytic anemia in a Spanish family: clinical and familial studies. *Humangenetik*, **29**, 291.

270 SCHRÖTER W. & TILLMAN W. (1977) Decreased deformability of erythrocytes in haemolytic anaemia asso-

ciated with glucose-phosphate isomerase deficiency. *British Journal of Haematology*, **36**, 475.

271 YUAN P.M., ZAUN H.R., KESTER M.V., SNIDER C.E., JOHNSON M. & GRACY R.W. (1979)A deletion mutation in glucosephosphate isomerase (GPI Denton). *Clinica Chimica Acta*, **92**, 481.

272 MEIENHOFER M.C., LAGRANGE J.L., COTTREAU D., LENOIR G., DREYFUS J.C. & KAHN A. (1979) Phosphofructokinase in human blood cells. *Blood*, **54**, 389.

273 TARUI S., OKUNO G., IKURA Y., TANAKA T., SUDA M. & NISHIKAWA M. (1965) Phosphofructokinase deficiency in skeletal muscle. A new type of glycogenosis. *Biochemical and Biophysical Research Communications*, **19**, 517.

274 TARUI S., KONO N., NASU T. & NISHIKAWA M. (1969) Enzymatic basis of the co-existence of myopathy and haemolytic disease in inherited phosphofructokinase deficiency. *Biochemical and Biophysical Research Communications*, **34**, 77.

275 TARUI S., KONO N. & KUMAJIMA M. (1976) Interrelation between phosphofructokinase activity and 2,3-diphosphoglycerate level in erythrocytes: studies on hereditary phosphofructokinase deficiency and diabetic ketoacidosis. 16th Congress of the International Society of Haematology, Kyoto, p. 2.

276 WATERBURY L. & FRENKEL E.P. (1969) Phosphofructokinase deficiency in congenital nonspherocytic hemolytic anemia. *Clinical Research*, **17**, 347.

277 WATERBURY L. & FRENKEL E.P. (1972) Hereditary non-spherocytic hemolysis with erythrocyte phosphofructokinase deficiency. *Blood*, **39**, 415.

278 MIWA S., SATO T., MURAO H., KOZURU M. & IBAYASHI H. (1972) A new type of phosphofructokinase deficiency hereditary nonspherocytic hemolytic anemia. *Acta Haematologica Japan*, **35**, 113.

278 LUTCHER C.L. & BIGLEY R.L. (1974) Hemolytic anemia due to phosphofructokinase (PFK) deficiency. *Clinical Science*, **22**, 66a.

280 KAHN A., ETIEMBLE J., MIENHOFER M.C. & BOIVIN P. (1975) Erythrocyte phosphofructokinase deficiency associated with an unstable variant of muscle phosphofructokinase. *Clinica Chimica Acta*, **61**, 415.

281 ODA S., ODA E. & TANAKA K.R. (1977) Erythrocyte phosphofructokinase (PFK) deficiency: characterization and metabolic studies. *Clinical Research*, **25**, 344a.

282 TARUI S., KONO N., KUWAJIMA M. & IKURA Y. (1978) Type VII glycogenosis (muscle and erythrocyte phosphofructokinase deficiency). *Monographs in Human Genetics*, **9**, 42.

283 KAHN A., BOYER C., COTTREAU D., MARIE J. & BOIVIN P. (1977) Immunologic study of the age related loss of activity of six enzymes in the red cells from newborn infants and adults. Evidence for a fetal type of erythrocyte phosphofructokinase. *Pediatric Research*, **11**, 271.

284 BEUTLER E., SCOTT S., BISHOP A., MARGOLIS N., MATSUMOTO F. & KUHL W. (1973) Red cell aldolase deficiency and hemolytic anemia; a new syndrome. *Transactions of the Association of American Physicians*, **86**, 154.

285 KAPLAN J.C., TEEPLE L., SHORE N. & BEUTLER E. (1968) Electrophoretic abnormality in triose phosphate isomerase deficiency. *Biochemical and Biophysical Research Communications*, **31**, 768.

286 TURNER B.M., FISHER R.A. & HARRIS H. (1975) In: *Isozymes* (ed. Makert C.), p. 781. Academic Press, New York.

287 CORRAN P.H. & WALEY S.G. (1975) The amino acid sequence of rabbit muscle triose phosphate isomerase. *Biochemical Journal*, **145**, 335.

288 BALTIMORE CONFERENCE (1975) *Third International Workshop on Human Gene Mapping Birth Defects* XII, 7. New York, The National Foundation, 1976.

289 SCHNEIDER A.S., VALENTINE W.N., HATTORI M. & HEINS H.L. (1965) Hereditary hemolytic anemia with triose phosphate isomerase deficiency. *New England Journal of Medicine*, **272**, 229.

290 SHORE N.A., SCHNEIDER A.S. & VALENTINE W.N. (1965) Erythrocyte triosephosphate isomerase deficiency (abstract). *Journal of Pediatrics*, **67**, 939.

291 SCHNEIDER A.S., VALENTINE W.N., BAUGHAN M.A., PAGLIA D.E., SHORE N.A. & HEINS H.L. (1968) Triose phosphate isomerase deficiency. I. A multi-system inherited enzyme disorder. Clinical and genetic aspects. In: *Hereditary Disorders of Erythrocyte Metabolism* (ed. Beutler E.), p. 265. Grune & Stratton, New York.

292 VALENTINE W.N., SCHNEIDER A.S., BAUGHAN M.A., PAGLIA D.E. & HEINS H.L. (1966) Hereditary hemolytic anemia with triose phosphate isomerase deficiency. *American Journal of Medicine*, **41**, 27.

293 HARRIS S.R., PAGLIA D.E., JAFFÉ E.R., VALENTINE W.N. & KLEIN R.L. (1970) Triosephosphate isomerase deficiency in an adult. *Clinical Research*, **18**, 529.

294 FREYCON F., LAURAS B., BOVIER-LAPIERRE F., DORCHE C.L. & GODDON R. (1975) Congenital hemolytic anemia with triose phosphate isomerase deficiency. *Pediatria*, **30**, 55.

295 BELLINGHAM A.J., ROBINSON L.A. & MARTIN J. (1977) Triose phosphate isomerase deficiency. *Proceedings of British Society of Haematology*, 14 Jan.

296 VIVES-CORRONS J.-L., RUBINSON-SKALA H., MATEO M., ESTELLA J., FELIU E. & DREYFUS J.-C. (1978) Triose phosphate isomerase deficiency with hemolytic anemia and severe neuromuscular disease. Familial and biochemical studies of a case found in Spain. *Human Genetics*, **42**, 171.

297 SKALA H., DRYFUS J.C., VIVES-CORRONS J.-L., MATSUMOTO F. & BEUTLER E. (1977) Triose phosphate isomerase deficiency. *Biochemical Medicine*, **18**, 226.

298 WOLNY M., WOLNY E. & BARANOWSKI T. (1968) Preparation and some properties of crystalline D-glyceraldehyde-3-phosphate dehydrogenase from human erythrocytes. *Bulletin de l'Académie Polonaise des Sciences*, **16**, 13.

299 STANCEL G.M. & DEAL W.C. (1968) Metabolic control and structure of glycolytic enzymes. V. Dissociation of yeast glyceraldehyde-3-phosphate dehydrogenase into subunits. *Biochemical and Biophysical Research Communications*, **31**, 398.

300 ARESE P., PESCARMONA G.P., BOSIA A. & CAVALLERO M. (1972) Regolazione dell'attivita glyceraldeidefosfato deidrogena sica eritrocitaria de parte della concentrazione idrogenionica. *Bolletino della Societa Italiana di Biologia Sperimentale*, **48**, 4.

301 SCHRIER S.L. (1963) Studies of the metabolism of human erythrocyte membranes. *Journal of Clinical Investigation*, **42**, 756.

302 GREEN D.E., MURER E., HULTIN H.O., RICHARDSON S.H., SALMIN B., BRIERLEY G.P. & BAUM H. (1965) Association of integrated metabolic pathways with membranes. I. Glycolytic enzymes of the red blood corpuscle and yeast. *Archives of Biochemistry and Biophysics*, **112**, 635.

303 KANT J.A. & STECK T.L. (1973) Specificity in the association of glyceraldehyde 3-phosphate dehydrogenase with isolated human erythrocyte membranes. *Journal of Biological Chemistry*, **248**, 8457.

304 McDANIEL C.F., KIRTLEY M.E. & TANNER M.J.A. (1974) The interaction of glyceraldehyde-3-phosphate dehydrogenase with human erythrocyte membrane. *Journal of Biological Chemistry*, **249**, 6478.

305 HARKNESS D.R. (1966) A new erythrocytic enzyme defect with hemolytic anemia: glyceraldehyde-3-phosphate dehydrogenase deficiency. *Journal of Laboratory and Clinical Medicine*, **68**, 879.

306 McCANN S.R., FINKEL B., CADMAN S. & ALLEN D.W. (1976) Study of a kindred with hereditary spherocytosis and glyceraldehyde-3-phosphate dehydrogenase deficiency. *Blood*, **47**, 171.

307 KRAUS A.P., LANGSTON M.F. & LYNCH B.L. (1968) Red cell phosphoglycerate kinase deficiency. A new cause of non-spherocytic hemolytic anemia. *Biochemical and Biophysical Research Communications*, **30**, 173.

308 VALENTINE W.N., HSIEH H.S., PAGLIA D.E., ANDERSON H.M., BAUGHAN M.A., JAFFÉ E.R. & GARSON O.M. (1969) Hereditary hemolytic anemia associated with phosphoglycerate kinase deficiency in erythrocytes and leukocytes. *New England Journal of Medicine*, **28**, 528.

309 HJELM M. & WADMAN B. (1970) Non-spherocytic haemolytic anaemia with phosphoglycerate kinase deficiency. *XIIIth Congress of the International Society of Haematology*, p. 21. Munich.

310 CARTIER P., HABIBI B., LEROUX J.-P. & MARCHAND J.-C. (1971) Anémie hémolytique congénitale associée à un déficit en phosphoglycerate-kinase dans les globules rouge, les polynucléaires et les lymphocytes. *Nouvelle Revue française d'Hématologie*, **11**, 565.

311 MIWA S., NAKASHIMA K., ODA S., OGAWA H., NAGUFUJI H., ARIMA M., OKUNA T. & NAKASHIMA T. (1972) Phosphoglycerate kinase (PGK) deficiency hereditary non-spherocytic hemolytic anemia. Report of a case found in a Japanese family. *Acta Haematologica Japonica*, **35**, 571.

312 KONRAD P.N., McCARTHY D.J., MAUER A.M., VALENTINE W.N. & PAGLIA D.E. (1973) Erythrocyte and leukocyte phosphoglycerate kinase deficiency with neurologic disease. *Journal of Pediatrics*, **82**, 456.

313 ARESE P., BOSIA A., GALLO E., MAZZA U. & PESCARMONA G.P. (1973) Red cell glycolysis in a case of 3-phosphoglycerate kinase deficiency. *European Journal of Clinical Investigation*, **3**, 86.

314 BIOVIN P., HAKIM J., MANDEREAU J., GALAND C., DEGOS F. & SCHAISON G. (1974) Erythrocyte and leucocyte 3-phosphoglycerate kinase deficiency. Study of the properties of the enzyme, phagocytic activity of the polymorphonuclear leucocytes and a review of the literature. *Nouvelle Revue française d'Hématologie*, **14**, 495.

315 KRIETSCH W.K., KRIETSCH H., KAISER W., DÜNWALD M., KUNTZ G.W., DUHM J. & BÜCHER T. (1977) Hereditary deficiency of phosphoglycerate kinase: a new variant in erythrocytes and leucocytes, not associated with haemolytic anaemia. *European Journal of Clinical Investigation*, **7**, 427.

316 RAPOPORT S. & LUEBERING J. (1950) The formation of 2,3-diphosphoglycerate in rabbit erythrocytes: the existence of a diphosphoglycerate mutase. *Journal of Biological Chemistry*, **183**, 507.

317 RAPOPORT S. & LUEBERING J. (1952) An optical study of disphosphoglycerate mutase. *Journal of Biological Chemistry*, **196**, 583.

318 ROSE Z.B. (1968) The purification and properties of diphosphoglycerate mutase from human erythrocytes. *Journal of Biological Chemistry*, **243**, 4810.

319 ROSE Z.B. (1970) Enzyme controlling 2-3-diphosphoglycerate in human erythrocytes. *Federation Proceedings*, **29**, 1105.

320 GERLACH E. & DUHM J. (1972) Regulation of the concentration of 2,3-diphosphoglycerate in the erythrocyte. *Scandinavian Journal of Clinical and Laboratory Investigation*, **29** (Suppl. 126), 5.

321 LAPPIN T.R. (1976) Hormones and erythrocytic 2,3 DPG metabolism. *British Journal of Haematology*, **33**, 151.

322 LÖHR G.W. & WALLER H.D. (1963) Zur biochemie einiger Angeborener hämolytischen Anämien. *Folia Haematologica*, NF, **8**, 377.

323 SCHRÖTER W. (1965) Kongenitale nichtsphärocytäse hämolytische Anämie bei 2,3-diphosphoglyceratemutase-mangel der Erythrocyten im frühen Sänglingsalter. *Klinische Wochenschriften*, **43**, 1147.

324 TRAVIS S.F., MARTINEZ J., GARVIN J., ATWATER J. & GILLMER P. (1978) Study of a kindred with partial deficiency of red cell 2,3-diphosphoglycerate mutase (2,3-DPGM) and compensated hemolysis. *Blood*, **51**, 1107.

325 ROSA R., NAJEAN Y., PREHU M., BEUZARD Y. & ROSA J. (1977) Total deficiency of red cell disphosphoglycerate mutase (DPGM). *Blood*, **50** (Suppl. 1) 84. (Abstract).

326 ROSA R., PREHU M.O., BEUZARD Y. & ROSA J. (1978) The first case of a complete deficiency of diphosphoglycerate mutase in human erythrocytes. *Journal of Clinical Investigation*, **62**, 907.

327 PETERSON L.L. (1978) Red cell diphosphoglycerate mutase. Immunochemical studies in vertebrate red cells, including a human variant lacking 2,3-DPG. *Blood*, **52**, 953.

328 DUHM J., DEUTICKE B. & GERLACH E. (1968) Bildung und Abbau der 2,3-diphosphoglycerinesäure in Menschenerythrocyten unter verschiedenen experimentellen Bedingungen. In: *Metabolism and Membrane Permeability of Erythrocytes and Thrombocytes* (ed. Deutsch E., Gerlach E. & Moser K.), p. 69. Geo. Thieme, Stuttgart.

329 DUHM J., DEUTICKE B. & GERLACH E. (1968) Metabolism of 2,3-diphosphoglycerate and glycolysis in human red blood cells under the influence of dipyridamole and inorganic sulfur compounds. *Biochimica et Biophysica Acta*, **170**, 452.

330 PARKER J.C. (1969) Influence of 2,3-diphosphoglycerate metabolism on sodium-potassium permeability in human red blood cells: studies with bisulfite and other redox agents. *Journal of Clinical Investigation*, **48**, 117.

331 ROSE Z.B. & LIEBOWITZ J. (1970) 2,3-Diphosphoglycer-

Red-cell metabolism: hereditary enzymopathies 313

ate phosphatase from human erythrocytes. *Journal of Biological Chemistry*, **245**, 3232.

332 DUHM J. & GERLACH E. (1974) Metabolism and function of 2,3-diphosphoglycerate in red blood cells. In: *The Human Red Cell in vitro* (ed. Greenwalt T.J. & Jamieson G.A.), p. 111. Grune & Stratton, New York.

333 SYLLM-RAPOPORT I., JACOBASCH G., ROIGAS H. & RAPOPORT S. (1965) 2,3-PGasemangel als mögliche ursache erholten ATP-gehaltes. *Folia Haematologica*, **83**, 363.

334 BEUTLER E., MATSUMOTO F. & GUINTO E. (1974) The effect of 2,3-DPG on red cell enzymes. *Experientia*, **30**, 190.

335 KOLER R.D. & VAN BELLINGHEN P. (1968) The mechanism of precursor modulation of human pyruvate kinase. *Advances in Enzyme Regulation*, **6**, 127.

336 MARIE J., KAHN A. & BOIVIN P. (1976) L-type pyruvate kinase from human liver. Purification by double affinity elution, electrofocusing and immunological studies. *Biochimica et Biophysica Acta*, **438**, 393.

337 MARIE J., KAHN A. & BOIVIN P. (1977) Human erythrocyte pyruvate kinase. Total purification and evidence for its antigenic identity with L-type enzyme. *Biochimiea et Biophysica Acta*, **481**, 96.

338 KAHN A., MARIE J., GARREAU H. & SPRENGERS E.D. (1978) The genetic system of the L-type pyruvate kinase in man. Subunit structure, interrelation and kinetic characteristics of the pyruvate kinase enzymes from erythrocytes and liver. *Biochimica et Biophysica Acta*, **523**, 59.

339 BLUME K.G., HOFFBAUER R.W., BUSCH D., ARNOLD H. & LÖHR G.W. (1971) Purification and properties of pyruvate kinase in normal and in pyruvate kinase deficient human red blood cells. *Biochimica et Biophysica Acta*, **227**, 364.

340 IMAMURA K., TANAKA T., NISHINA T., NAKASHIMA K. & MIWA S. (1973) Studies on pyruvate kinase (PK) deficiency. II. Electrophoretic, kinetic and immunological studies on pyruvate kinase of erythrocytes and other tissues. *Journal of Biochemistry*, **74**, 1165.

341 MARIE J., KAHN A. & BOIVIN P. (1976) Pyruvate kinase isozymes in man. I. M-type isozymes in adult and foetal tissues, electrofocusing and immunological studies. *Human Genetics*, **31**, 35.

342 GARREAU H. & BUC-TEMKINE H. (1972) Allosteric activation of human erythrocyte pyruvate kinase by fructose-1,6-disphosphate. *Biochimie*, **54**, 1103.

343 BLUME K.G., ARNOLD H., LÖHR G.W. & BEUTLER E. (1973) Additional diagnostic procedures for the detection of abnormal red cell pyruvate kinase. *Clinica Chimica Acta*, **43**, 443.

344 BLUME K.G., ARNOLD H., LÖHR G.W. & SCHOLZ G. (1974) On the molecular basis of pyruvate kinase deficiency. *Biochimica et Biophysica Acta*, **370**, 601.

345 BOIVIN P., GALAND C. & DEMARTIAL M.C. (1972) Co-existence de deux types de pyruvate-kinase cinétiquement differents dans les globules rouges humains normaux. *Nouvelle Revue française d'Hématologie*, **11**, 565.

346 MONOD J., WYMAN J. & CHANGEUX J.-P. (1965) On the nature of allosteric transitions: a plausible model. *Journal of Molecular Biology*, **12**, 88.

347 STAAL G.E.J., KOSTER J.F., KAMP H., VAN MILLIGEN-

BOERSMA L. & VEEGER C. (1971) Human erythrocyte pyruvate kinase. Its purification and some properties. *Biochimica et Biophysica Acta*, **227**, 86.

348 STAAL G.E.J., CEERDINK R.P., VLUG A.M.C. & HAMELINK M.L. (1976) Defective erythrocyte pyruvate kinase. *Clinica Chimica Acta*, **68**, 11.

349 ROSE I.A. (1971) Regulation of human red cell glycolysis: a review. *Experimental Eye Research*, **11**, 264.

350 ROSE I.A. & WARMS J.V.B. (1966) Control of glycolysis in the human red cell. *Journal of Biological Chemistry*, **241**, 4848.

351 STAAL G.E.J., KOSTER J.F. & VAN MILLIGEN-BOERSMA L. (1970) Some properties of abnormal red blood cell pyruvate kinase. *Biochimica et Biophysica Acta*, **220**, 613.

352 BLACK J.A. & HENDERSON M.H. (1972) Activation and inhibition of human erythrocyte pyruvate kinase by organic phosphates, amino acids, dipeptides and anions. *Biochimica et Biophysica Acta*, **284**, 115.

353 JACOBASCH G. & RAPOPORT S. (1965) Phosphoglyzerinsäureveranderungen in Retikulozyten und Erythrozyten von Schafen. *Folia Haematologica*, **83**, 389.

354 PONCE J., ROTH S. & HARKNESS D.R. (1971) Kinetic studies on the inhibition of glycolytic kinases of human erythrocytes by 2,3-diphosphoglyceric acid. *Biochimica et Biophysica Acta*, **250**, 63.

355 VALENTINE W.N., TANAKA K.R. & MIWA S. (1961) A specific erythrocyte glycolytic enzyme defect (pyruvate kinase) in three subjects with congenital non-spherocytic hemolytic anemia. *Transactions of the Association of American Physicians*, **74**, 100.

356 GRIMES A.J., MEISLER A. & DACIE J.V. (1964) Hereditary non-spherocytic haemolytic anaemia. A study of red-cell carbohydrate metabolism in twelve cases of pyruvate kinase deficiency. *British Journal of Haematology*, **10**, 403.

357 NATHAN D.G., OSKI F.A., SIDEL V.W. & DIAMOND L.K. (1965) Extreme hemolysis and red-cell distortion in erythrocyte pyruvate kinase deficiency II. Measurements of erythrocyte glucose consumption, potassium flux and adenosine triphosphate stability. *New England Journal of Medicine*, **272**, 118.

358 KEITT A.S. (1966) Pyruvate kinase deficiency and related disorders of red cell gycolysis. *American Journal of Medicine*, **41**, 762.

359 OSKI F.A. & BOWMAN H. (1968) A low K_m phosphoenolypyruvate mutant in the Amish with red cell pyruvate kinase deficiency. *British Journal of Haematology*, **17**, 289.

360 TANAKA K.R. & VALENTINE W.N. (1968) Pyruvate kinase deficiency. In: *Hereditary Disorders of Erythrocyte Metabolism* (ed. Beutler E.), p. 229. Grune & Stratton, New York.

361 PRANKERD T.A.J. (1963) Inherited enzyme defects in congenital haemolytic anaemia. *Proceedings of the IXth Congress of the European Society of Haematology, Lisbon*, **2**, p. 735. Karger, Basel.

362 BUSCH D. (1963) Erythrocyte metabolism in three persons with hereditary non-spherocytic anemia, deficient in pyruvate kinase. *Proceedings of the IXth Congress of the European Society of Haematology, Lisbon*, **2**, p. 783. Karger, Basel.

363 BUSCH D. (1964) Congenitale nichtsphärozytase hamo-

lytische Anämie mit Mangel an erythrozytaren Pyruv-kinase. *Folia Haematologica*, NF, **9**, 89.

364 ROBINSON M.A., LODER P.B. & DEGRUCHY G.C. (1961) Red-cell metabolism in non-spherocytic congenital hae-molytic anaemia. *British Journal of Haematology*, **7**, 327.

365 LARIZZA P., BRUNETTI P. & GRIGNANI F. (1963) Bio-chemical and genetic aspects of erythrocyte pyruvate kinase deficiency. *Proceedings of the IXth Congress of the European Society of Haematology, Lisbon*, **2**, p. 745. Karger, Basel.

366 SHAFER A.W. (1963) Glycolytic intermediates in eryth-rocytes in non-spherocytic hemolytic anemia with defi-ciency of glucose 6-phosphate dehydrogenase (G6-PD) or pyruvate kinase (PK). *Clinical Research*, **11**, 103.

367 BRUNETTI P., PUXEDDU A., NENCI G. & MIGLIORNI E. (1963) Congenital non-spherocytic haemolytic anaemia due to pyruvate-kinase deficiency. *Acta Haematologica*, **30**, 88.

368 WALLER H.D. & LÖHR G.W. (1964) Hereditary non-spherocytic enzymopenic hemolytic anemia with pyru-vate kinase deficiency. *Proceedings of the IXth Congress of the International Society of Haematology, Mexico City*, **1**, p. 257. Grune & Stratton, New York.

369 BESTEATTI A., ROSSI U., LOOS J.A. & PRINS H.K. (1964) A case of congenital atypical haemolytic anaemia with pyruvate kinase deficiency. *Vox Sanguinis*, **9**, 492.

370 TWOMEY J., MOSER R., HUDSON W., O'NEAL F. & ALFREY C. (1966) ATP metabolism in pyruvate kinase (PK) deficient erythrocytes. *Clinical Research*, **14**, 437.

371 COLLIER H.B., ASHFORD D.R. & BELL R.E. (1966) Three cases of hemolytic anemia with erythrocyte pyruvate kinase deficiency in Alberta. *Canadian Medical Associ-ation Journal*, **95**, 1188.

372 BUSCH D. & HEIMPEL H. (1969) Hereditäre nichtsphäro-zytare hämolytische Anämie mit hohem Erythrozyten-ATP. *Blut*, **19**, 293.

373 GULBIS E., WEBER A., DECHAMPS L., DENYS P., SOKAL G., LÖHR G., RUDIGER H., BLUME K., PIRET L. & DUNJIC A. (1970) Contribution à l'étude de l'anémie hémolytique congenitale avec deficit en pyruvate-kinase. *Archives française Pediatrie*, **27**, 31.

374 MIWA S. & NISHINA T. (1974) Studies on pyruvate kinase (PK) deficiency. I. Clinical, haematological and erythrocyte enzyme studies. *Acta Haematologica Japonica*, **37**, 1.

375 PAGLIA D.E., KONRAD P.N., WOLFF J.A. & VALENTINE W.N. (1976) Biphasic reaction kinetics in an anomalous isozyme of erythrocyte pyruvate kinase. *Clinica Chimica Acta*, **73**, 395.

376 LODER P.B. & DE GRUCHY G.C. (1965) Red-cell enzymes and co-enzymes in non-spherocytic congenital haemo-lytic anaemias. *British Journal of Haematology*, **11**, 21.

377 MENTZER W.C., BAEHNER R.L., SCHMID-SCHÖNBEIM H., ROBINSON S.H. & NATHAN D.G. (1971) Selective reticu-locyte destruction in erythrocyte pyruvate kinase defi-ciency. *Journal of Clinical Investigation*, **50**, 688.

378 SCHRÖTER W. (1972) Clinical heterogeneity of erythro-cyte pyruvate kinase deficiency. *Helvetica Paediatrica Acta*, **27**, 471.

379 MIWA S. (1973) Hereditary hemolytic anemia due to erythrocyte enzyme deficiency. *Acta Haematologica Japonica*, **36**, 573.

380 OSKI F.A., NATHAN D.G., SIDEL V.W. & DIAMOND L.K. (1964) Extreme hemolysis and red-cell distortion in erythrocyte pyruvate kinase deficiency. I. Morphology, erythrokinetics and family studies. *New England Jour-nal of Medicine*, **270**, 1023.

381 NATHAN D.G. & SHOHET S.B. (1970) Erythrocyte ion transport defects and hemolytic anemia: 'hydrocytosis' and 'desiccytosis'. *Seminars in Hematology*, **7**, 381.

382 BLUME K.G., LÖHR G.W., PRAETSCH O., RÜDIGER H.W. & WENDT G.G. (1968) Beitrag zur Populations genetik der pyruvatkinase menschlicker Erythrocyten. *Human Genetics*, **6**, 261.

383 CAMPOS J.O., KOLER R.D. & BIGLEY R.H. (1965) Kinetic differences between human red cells and leuco-cyte pyruvate kinase. *Nature (London)*, **208**, 194.

384 WIESEMANN U. & TÖNZ O. (1966) Investigations of the kinetics of red cell pyruvate kinase in normal individuals and in a patient with pyruvate kinase deficiency. *Nature (London)*, **209**, 612.

385 STAAL G.E.J., KOSTER J.F. & NIJESSEN J.G. (1972) A new variant of red blood cell pyruvate kinase deficiency. *Biochimica et Biophysica Acta*, **258**, 685.

386 SCHRÖTER W. & TILLMANN W. (1975) Membrane-localized pyruvate kinase of red blood cells in hemolytic anemia associated with pyruvate kinase deficiency. *Klinische Wochenschrift*, **53**, 1106.

387 PAGLIA D.E., VALENTINE W.N. & RUCKNAGEL D.L. (1972) Defective erythrocyte pyruvate kinase with im-paired kinetics and reduced optimal activity. *British Journal of Haematology*, **22**, 651.

388 PAGLIA D.E., KONRAD P.N., WOLFF J.A. & VALENTINE W.N. (1976) Biphasic reaction kinetics in an anomalous isozyme of erythrocyte pyruvate kinase. *Clinica Chimica Acta*, **73**, 395.

389 KAHN A., MARIE J. & BOIVIN P. (1976) Pyruvate kinase isozymes in man. II. L type and erythrocyte-type isozymes. Electrofocusing and immunological studies. *Human Genetics*, **33**, 35.

390 MIWA S., NAKASHIMA K., ARIYOSHI K., SHINOHARA K., ODA E. & TANAKA T. (1975) Four new pyruvate kinase (PK) variants and a classical PK deficiency. *British Journal of Haematology*, **29**, 157.

391 BOIVIN P., GALAND C. & DEMARTIAL M.C. (1972) Etudes sur la pyruvate-kinase erythrocytaire. II. Hetero-geneite enzymologique des deficits etudes a propos de 28 cas avec anemie hemolytique congenitale. *Nouvelle Revue française d'Hématologie*, **12**, 569.

392 BUC H., NAJMAN A., COLUMELLI S. & CARTIER P. (1972) Deficit en congenital pyruvate kinase erythrocytaire: étude cinetique de l'enzyme et consequences meta-boliques. *Clinica Chimica Acta*, **38**, 131.

393 GHERARDI M., VERGNES H., CORBERAND J. & REGNIER C. (1974) Deficit en pyruvate kinase erythrocytaire accompagne d'une anemie hemolytique neonatale severe. Etude familiale et caracterisation biochimique de l'enzyme. *Acta Haematologica*, **52**, 248.

394 YAMADA K., ADACHIBARA A., NAKAZAWA S., SHINKAI A., NISHINA T. & MIWA S. (1974) Erythrocyte pyruvate kinase deficiency associated with kinetically aberrant isozyme. *Acta Haematologica Japonica*, **37**, 17.

395 BRANDT N.J. & HANEL H.K. (1971) Atypical pyruvate kinase in a patient with haemolytic anaemia. *Scandina-vian Journal of Haematology*, **8**, 126.

396 PAGLIA D.E., VALENTINE W.N., BAUGHAN M.A., MILLER D.R., REED C.F. & McINTYRE O.R. (1968) An inherited molecular lesion of a kinetically abberant isozyme associated with premature haemolysis. *Journal of Clinical Investigation*, **47**, 1929.

397 OHYAMA H., KUMATORI T., NISHINA T. & MIWA S. (1969) Functionally abnormal pyruvate kinase in congenital hemolytic anemia. *Acta Haematologica Japonica*, **32**, 330.

398 KAHN A., KAPLAN J.-C. & DREYFUS J.-C. (1979) Advances in hereditary red cell enzyme anomalies. *Human Genetics*, **50**, 1.

399 BOWMAN H.S. & PROCOPIO F. (1963) Hereditary non-spherocytic hemolytic anemia of the pyruvate-kinase deficient type. *Annals of Internal Medicine*, **58**, 567.

400 LEBLOND P.F., LYONNAIS J. & DELAGE J.-M. (1978) Erythrocyte populations in pyruvate kinase deficiency anaemia following splenectomy. I. Cell morphology. *British Journal of Haematology*, **39**, 55.

401 NATHAN D.G., OSKI F.A., MILLER D.R. & GARDNER F.H. (1968) Life-span and organ sequestration of the red cells in pyruvate kinase deficiency. *New England Journal of Medicine*, **278**, 73.

402 LODER P.B. & DE GRUCHY G.C. (1965) Red-cell and co-enzymes in non-spherocytic congenital haemolytic anaemias. *British Journal of Haematology*, **11**, 21.

403 TANAKA K.R. (1969) Pyruvate kinase. In: *Biochemical Methods in Red Cell Genetics* (ed. Yunis J.J.), p. 167. Academic Press, New York.

404 WARRENDORF E.M. & RUBINSTEIN D. (1973) The elevation of adenosine-triphosphate levels in human erythrocytes. *Blood*, **42**, 637.

405 MIWA S., NISHINA T., KAKEHASHI Y., KITAMURA M., HIRATSUKA A. & SHIZUME K. (1971) Studies on erythrocyte metabolism in a case with hereditary deficiency of H-subunit of lactate dehydrogenase. *Acta Haematologica Japonica*, **34**, 228.

406 BREWER G.J. (1967) Genetic and population studies of quantitative levels of adenosine triphosphate in human erythrocytes. *Biochemical Genetics*, **1**, 25.

407 BREWER G.J. (1964) A new inherited abnormality of human erythrocytes characterized by elevated levels of adenosine triphosphate (ATP). *Journal of Clinical Investigation*, **43**, 1287.

408 BREWER G.J. (1965) A new inherited abnormality of human erythrocytes—elevated erythrocytic adenosine triphosphate. *Biochemical and Biophysical Research Communciations*, **18**, 430.

409 ZÜRCHER C., LOOS J.A. & PRINS H.K. (1965) Hereditary high ATP content of human erythrocytes. Proceedings of the Xth Congress of International Society of Blood Transfusion, Stockholm. *Bibliotheca Haematologica*, **23**, 549.

410 VALENTINE W.N., FINK K., PAGLIA D.E., HARRIS S.R. & ADAMS W.S. (1974) Hereditary hemolytic anemia with human erythrocyte pryimidine-5'-nucleotidase deficiency. *Journal of Clinical Investigation*, **54**, 866.

411 BEN-BASSAT I., BROK-SINONI F., KENDE G., HOLTZMANN F. & RAMOT B. (1976) A family with red cell pyrimidine-5-nucleotidase deficiency. *Blood*, **47**, 919.

412 FUJII H., NAKASHIMA K., MIWA A. & NOMURA K. (1979) Electrophoretic and kinetic studies of a mutant red cell pyrimidine 5'-nucleotidase. *Clinica et Chimica Acta*, **95**, 89.

413 VALENTINE W.N., ANDERSON H.M., PAGLIA D.E., JAFFÉ E.R., KONRAD P.N. & HARRIS S.R. (1972) Studies on human erythrocyte nucleotide metabolism. II. Non-spherocytic haemolytic anaemia, high red cell ATP, and ribose phosphate pyrophosphokinase deficiency. *Blood*, **39**, 674.

414 VALENTINE W.N., BENNETT J.M., KRIVIT W., KONRAD P.N., LOWMAN J.T., PAGLIA D.E. & WAKEM C.J. (1973) Non-spherocytic haemolytic anaemia with increased red cell adenine nucleotides, glutathione and basophilic stippling and ribose-phosphate pyrophosphokinase (RPK) deficiency: studies on two new kindreds. *British Journal of Haematology*, **24**, 157.

415 ROCHANT H., DREYFUS B., ROSA R. & BOIVIN M. (1975) First case of pyrimidine 5' nucleotidase deficiency in a male. *International Society of Haematology, European and African Third Meeting, London* (Abstract **1**, 19).

416 PAGLIA D.E., VALENTINE W.N. & FINK K. (1977) Lead poisoning. Further observations of erythrocyte pyrimidine nucleotidase deficiency and intracellular accumulation of pyrimidine nucleotidase deficiency and intracellular accumulation of pyrimidine nucleotides. *Journal of Clinical Investigation*, **60**, 1362.

417 SZEINBERG A., KAHAN D., GAVENDO S., ZAIDMAN J. & BEN-EZZER J. (1969) Hereditary deficiency of adenylate kinase in red blood cells. *Acta Haematologica (Basel)*, **42**, 111.

418 BOIVIN P., GALAND C., HAKIM J., SIMONY D. & SELIGMAN M. (1971) Une nouvelle erythroenzymopathie. Anemie hémolytique congénitale non spherocytaire et deficit en adenylate-kinase erythrocytaire. *Presse Medicale*, **79**, 215.

419 PAGLIA D.E., VALENTINE W.N., TARTAGLIA A.P. & KONRAD P.N. (1970) Adenine nucleotide reactions associated with a dominantly transmitted form of non-spherocytic anaemia. *Blood*, **36**, 837.

420 VALENTINE W.N., PAGLIA D.E., TARTAGLIA A.P. & GILSAN F. (1977) Hereditary haemolytic anaemia with increased red cell adenosine deaminase (45- to 75-fold) and decreased adenosine triphosphate. *Science*, **195**, 783.

421 MIWA S., FUJII H., NAKATSUJI T., MIURA Y., ASANO H. & ASANO S. (1978) A case of red cell adenosine deaminase over-production associated with hereditary haemolytic anaemia. *17th Congress of the International Society for Haematology, Paris 1978* (Abstract **1**, 245).

422 GIBLETT E.L., ANDERSON J.E., COHEN F., POLLARA B. & MEUWISSEN H.J. (1972) Adenosine-deaminase deficiency in two patients with severely impaired cellular immunity. *Lancet*, **ii**, 1067.

423 FINCH C.A. (1948) Methemologlobinemia and sulfhemoglobinemia. *New England Journal of Medicine*, **239**, 470.

424 JAFFÉ E.R. (1966) Hereditary methemoglobinemias associated with abnormalities in the metabolism of erythrocytes. *American Journal of Medicine*, **41**, 786.

425 HSIEH H.-S. & JAFFÉ E.R. (1975) Metabolism of methemoglobin. In: *The Red Blood Cell* (ed. Surgenor D.M.) **2**, p. 802. Academic Press, New York.

426 SCOTT E.M. & HOSKINS D.D. (1958) Hereditary methe-

moglobinemia in Alaskan eskimos and Indians. *Blood*, **13**, 795.

427 GIBSON Q.H. & HARRISON D.C. (1947) Familial idiopathic methaemioglobinaemia. Five cases in one family. *Lancet*, **ii**, 941.

428 KEITT A.S., SMITH T.W. & JANDL J.H. (1966) Red-cell 'pseudomosaicism' in congenital methemoglobinemia. *New England Journal of Medicine*, **275**, 397.

429 GIBSON W.H. (1948) The reduction of methaemoglobin in red blood cells and studies on the cause of idiopathic methaemoglobinaemia. *Biochemical Journal*, **42**, 13.

430 DETTER J.C., ANDERSON J.E. & GIBLETT E.R. (1970) NADH diaphorase: an inherited variant associated with normal methemoglobin reduction. *American Journal of Human Genetics*, **22**, 100.

431 HOPKINSON D.A., CORNEY G., COOK P.J.L., ROBSON E.B. & HARRIS H. (1970) Genetically determined genetic variants of human red cell NADH diaphorase. *Annals of Human Genetics*, **34**, 1.

432 WEST C.A., GOMPERTS B.D., HUEHNS E.R., KESSEL I. & ASHBY J.R. (1967) Demonstration of an enzyme variant in a case of congenital methaemoglobinaemia. *British Medical Journal*, **ii**, 212.

433 KAPLAN J.C. & BEUTLER E. (1967) Electrophoresis of NADH- and NADPH-diaphorases in normal subjects and patients with congenital methemoglobinaemia. *Biochemical and Biophysical Research Communications*, **29**, 605.

434 SCHWARTZ J.M., PARESS P.S., ROSS J.M., DIPILLO F. & RIZEK R. (1972) Unstable variant of NADH methemoglobin reductase in Puerto Ricans with hereditary methemoglobinemia. *Journal of Clinical Investigation*, **51**, 1594.

435 GONZALEZ R., ESTRADA M., WADE M., DE LA TORRE E., SVARCH E., FERNANDEZ O., ORTIZ R., GUZMAN E. & COLOMBO B. (1978) Heterogeneity of hereditary methemoglobinaemia: a study of four Cuban families with NADH-methemoglobin reductase deficiency including a new variant (Santiago di Cuba variant). *Scandinavian Journal of Haematology*, **20**, 385.

436 FIALKOW P.J., BROWDER J.A., SPARKES R.S. & MOTULSKY A.G. (1965) Mental retardation in methemoglobinemia due to diaphorase deficiency. *New England Journal of Medicine*, **273**, 840.

437 JAFFÉ E.R., NEUMANN G., ROTHBERG H., WILSON F.T., WEBSTER R.M. & WOLF J.A. (1966) Hereditary methemoglobinemia with and without mental retardation. A study of three families. *American Journal of Medicine*, **41**, 42.

438 KAPLAN J.C., LEROUX A., BAKOURI S., GANGARD J.P. & BENABADJI M. (1974) La lésion enzymatique dans la méthémoglobinémie congenitale nécessive avec encéphalopathie. Description d'une nouvelle variante déficitaire de NADH-diaphorase (variante Beni-Massous). *Nouvelle Revue française d'Hématologie*, **14**, 755.

439 BEUTLER E. (1966) Glucose-6-phosphate dehydrogenase deficiency. In: *Metabolic Basis of Inherited Disease* (ed. Stanbury J.B., Wyngaarden J.B. & Fredrickson D.S.) 2nd edn, Chapter 47. McGraw-Hill, New York.

440 DACIE J.V. (1967) *The Haemolytic Anaemias, Part IV*, 2nd edn., p. 999. Churchill, London.

441 CARSON P.E., FLANAGAN C.L., ICKES C.E. & ALVING A.S. (1956) Enzymatic deficiency in primaquine-sensitive erythrocytes. *Science*, **124**, 484.

442 CORDES W. (1926) Experiences with plasmochin in malaria. *United Fruit Company 15th Annual Report*, p. 66.

443 CORDES W. (1927) Observations on the toxic effect of plasmochin. *United Fruit Company 16th Annual Report*, p. 62.

444 CORDES W. (1928) Zwischen Fälle bei der Plasmochin-behandlung. *Archive für Schiffs- und Tropen-Hygiene*, **32**, 143.

445 MANSON-BAHR P. (1926–7) In discussion on the haemoglobinurias. *Transactions of the Royal Society of Tropical Medicine and Hygiene*, **20**, 411.

446 MANSON-BAHR P. (1927) The action of plasmochin on malaria. *Proceedings of the Royal Society of Medicine*, **20**, 919.

447 EISELBERG K.P. (1927) Plasmochinvergiftung. *Wiener Klinische Wochenschrift*, **40**, 525.

448 PALMA M.D. (1928) Study of plasmochin therapy in malaria. *Riforma Medica*, **44**, 753.

449 MANIFOLD J.A. (1931) Report on a trial of plasmoquine and quinine in the treatment of benign tertian malaria. *Journal of the Royal Army Medical Corps*, **56**, 321.

450 AMY A.C. (1934) Haemoglobinuria: a new problem on the Indian frontier. *Journal of the Royal Army Medical Corps*, **62**, 178.

451 SMITH S. (1943) Haemoglobinuria following the administration of plasmoquine. *Transactions of the Royal Society of Tropical Medicine and Hygiene*, **37**, 155.

452 DIMSON S.M. & McMARTIN R.B. (1946) Pamaquine haemoglobinuria. *Quarterly Journal of Medicine*, **15**, 25.

453 SWANTZ H.E. & BAYLISS M. (1945) Haemoglobinuria: report of ten cases of its occurrence in Negroes during convalescence from malaria. *War Medicine*, **7**, 104.

454 EARLE D.P., BIGELOW F.S., ZUBROD C.G. & KANE C.A. (1948) Studies on the chemotherapy of the human malarias. IX. Effect of pamaquine on the blood cells of man. *Journal of Clinical Investigation*, **27** (suppl.), 121.

455 WEINSTEIN I.M., DERN R.J. & TALMAGE D.W. (1953) Studies on the mechanism of hemolysis in primaquine-sensitive negroes. *Journal of Clinical Investigation*, **32**, 609.

456 DERN R.J., BEUTLER E. & ALVING A.S. (1954) The hemolytic effect of primaquine. II. The natural course of the hemolytic anemia and the mechanism of its self-limited character. *Journal of Laboratory and Clinical Medicine*, **44**, 171.

457 BEUTLER E., DERN R.J. & ALVING A.S. (1954) The hemolytic effect of primaquine. IV. The relationship of cell age to hemolysis. *Journal of Laboratory and Clinical Medicine*, **44**, 439.

458 BEUTLER E., DERN R.J. & ALVING A.S. (1955) The hemolytic effect of primaquine. VI. An *in-vitro* test for sensitivity of erythrocytes to primaquine. *Journal of Laboratory and Clinical Medicine*, **45**, 40.

459 BEUTLER E. (1956) *In-vitro* studies of the stability of red cell glutathione: a new test for drug sensitivitiy. *Journal of Clinical Investigation*, **35**, 690.

460 BEUTLER E. (1957) The glutathione instability of drug-sensitive red cells. A new method for the *in-vitro*

detection of drug-sensitivity. *Journal of Laboratory and Clinical Medicine*, **49**, 84.

461 BEUTLER E. (1956) *In-vitro* studies of the stability of red cell glutathione: a new test for drug sensitivity. *Journal of Clinical Investigation*, **35**, 690.

462 KIMBRO E.L., SACHS M.V. & TORBERT J.V. (1957) Mechanism of hemolytic anemia induced by nitrofurantion (Furadantin). *Bulletin of the Johns Hopkins Hospital*, **101**, 245.

463 ZINKHAM W.H. & CHILDS B. (1957) Effect of vitamin K and naphthalene metabolites on glutathione metabolism of erythrocytes from normal newborns and patients with naphthalene hemolytic anaemia. *American Journal of Diseases of Children*, **94**, 420.

464 ZINKHAM W.H. & CHILDS B. (1957) Effect of naphthalene derivatives on glutathione metabolism of erythrocytes from patients with naphthalene hemolytic anemia. *Journal of Clinical Investigation*, **36**, 938.

465 ZINKHAM W.H. & CHILDS B. (1958) A defect of glutathione metabolism in erythrocytes from patients with a naphthalene-induced hemolytic anemia. *Pediatrics*, **22**, 461.

466 BEUTLER E. & BALUDA M.C. (1964) The separation of glucose-6-phosphate dehydrogenase-deficient erythrocytes from the blood of heterozygotes for glucose-6-phosphate dehydrogenase deficiency. *Lancet*, i, 189.

467 LYON M.F. (1962) Sex chromatin and gene action in the mammalian X-chromosome. *American Journal of Human Genetics*, **14**, 135.

468 EDGELL G.J.S., KIRKMAN H.N., CLEMONS E., BUCHANAN P.D. & MILLER C.H. (1978) Prenatal diagnosis by linkage: Haemophilia A and polymorphic glucose-6-phosphate dehydrogenase. *American Journal of Human Genetics*, **30**, 80.

469 YOSHIDA A., BEUTLER E. & MOTULSKY A.G. (1971) Human glucose-6-phosphate dehydrogenase variants. *Bulletin WHO*, **45**, 243.

470 BEUTLER E. & YOSHIDA A. (1973) Human glucose-6-phosphate dehydrogenase variants: a supplementary tabulation. *Annals of Human Genetics*, **37**, 151.

471 YOSHIDA A. & BEUTLER E. (1978) Human glucose 6-phosphate dehydrogenase variants: a supplementary tabulation. *Annals of Human Genetics*, **41**, 347.

472 BOYER S.H. & PORTER I.H. (1962) Electrophoretic heterogeneity of glucose-6-phosphate dehydrogenase and its relationship to enzyme deficiency. *Journal of Clinical Investigation*, **41**, 1347.

473 EATON J.W. & BREWER G.J. (1974) Pentose phosphate metabolism. In: *The Red Blood Cell* (ed. Surgenor D.M.) **1**, p. 456. Academic Press, New York.

474 MARKS P.A., SZEINBERG A. & BANKS J. (1961) Erythrocyte glucose 6-phosphate dehydrogenase of normal and mutant human subjects. Properties of the purified enzyme. *Journal of Biological Chemistry*, **236**, 10.

475 KIRKMAN H.N. & CROWELL B.B. (1963) Molecular deficiency of glucose-6-phosphate dehydrogenase in primaquine sensitivity. *Nature (London)*, **197**, 286.

476 KIRKMAN H.N. (1966) Deficiency of the mutant protein in persons with glucose-6-phosphate dehydrogenase defects. *Federation Proceedings*, **25**, 337.

477 YOSHIDA A., STAMATOYANNOPOULOS G. & MOTULSKY A.G. (1967) Negro variant of glucose-6-phosphate

dehydrogenase deficiency (A−) in man. *Science*, **155**, 97.

478 YOSHIDA A. (1968) The structure of normal and variant human glucose-6-phosphate dehydrogenase. In: *Hereditary Disorders of Erythrocyte Metabolism* (ed. Beutler E.), p. 146. Grune & Stratton, New York.

479 LUZZATO L. & ALLAN N.C. (1965) Different properties of glucose-6-phosphate dehydrogenase from human erythrocytes with normal and abnormal enzyme levels. *Biochemical and Biophysical Research Communications*, **21**, 547.

480 LUZZATTO L. & OKOYE V.C.N. (1967) Resolution of genetic variants of human erythrocyte glucose-6-phosphate dehydrogenase by thin-layer chromatography. *Biochemical and Biophysical Research Communications*, **29**, 705.

481 MARKS P.A., GROSS R.T. & HURWITZ R.E. (1959) Gene action in erythrocyte deficiency of glucose-6-phosphate dehydrogenase deficiency: tissue enzyme levels. *Nature (London)*, **183**, 1266.

482 MARKS P.A. & GROSS R.T. (1959) Erythrocyte glucose-6-phosphate dehydrogenase deficiency: evidence of differences between Negroes and Caucasians with respect to this genetically determined trait. *Journal of Clinical Investigation*, **38**, 2253.

483 SABINE J.C., JUNG E.D., FISH M.B., PESTANER L.C. & RANKIN R.E. (1963) Observations on the inheritance of glucose-6-phosphate dehydrogenase deficiency in erythrocytes and in leucocytes. *British Journal of Haematology*, **9**, 164.

484 KAHN A., HAKIM J., BOIVIN P., BOUCHEROT J., DURAND D. & TROUBE H. (1974) Leucocytes et déficits en G-6-PD érythrocytaire. *Nouvelle Revue française d'Hématologie*, **14**, 291.

485 WURZEL H., MCCREARY T., BAKER L. & GUMERMAN L. (1961) Glucose-6-phosphate dehydrogenase activity in platelets. *Blood*, **17**, 314.

486 ZINKHAM W.H. (1961) A deficiency of glucose-6-phosphate dehydrogenase activity in lens from individuals with primaquine-sensitive erythrocytes. *Bulletin of Johns Hopkins Hospital*, **109**, 206.

487 ORZALESI N., SORCINELLI R. & BINAGHI F. (1976) Glucose-6-phosphate dehydrogenase in cataracts of subjects suffering from favism. *Ophthalmic Research*, **8**, 192.

488 BONSIGNORE A., FORNAINI G., LEONCINI G. & FANTONI A. (1966) Electrophoretic heterogeneity of erythrocyte and leucocyte glucose-6-phosphate dehydrogenase in Italians from various ethnic groups. *Nature (London)*, **211**, 876.

489 BONSIGNORE A., FORNAINI G., LEONCINI G., FANTONI A. & SEGNI P. (1966) Characterization of leukocyte glucose-6-phosphate dehydrogenase in Sardinian mutants. *Journal of Clinical Investigation*, **45**, 1865.

490 JOHNSON G.J., ALLEN D.W., CADMAN S., FAIRBANKS V.F., WHITE J.G., LAMPKIN B.C. & KAPLIN M.E. (1979) Red cell membrane polypeptide aggregates in glucose-6-phosphate dehydrogenase mutants with chronic hemolytic anemia. *New England Journal of Medicine*, **301**, 522.

491 STOCKS J., KEMP M. & DORMANDY T.L. (1971) Increased susceptibility of red blood cell lipids to autoxidation in haemolytic states. *Lancet*, i, 266.

492 DIMOPOULOS C., MORAKIS A., DIMOPOULOS B., ZERVAS A., PANAYIOTIDES N. & DOUTSIAS A. (1973) Anémie hémolytique aiguë consécutive à l'administration de nitrofurane et de novalgine chex deux malades présentat un déficit en glucose-6-phosphate-dehydrogenase érythrocytaire. *Journal D'Urologie et de Nephrologie (Paris)*, **79**, 524.

493 GOLDSTEIN B.D. & DONAGH E.M. (1976) Spectrofluorescent detection of *in vivo* red cell lipid peroxidation in patients treated with diaminodiphenylsulfone. *Journal of Clinical Investigation*, **57**, 1302.

494 DERN R.J., WEINSTEIN I.M., LEROY G.V., TALMAGE D.W. & ALVING A.S. (1954) The hemolytic effect of primaquine. I. The localization of the drug-induced hemolytic defect in primaquine-sensitive individuals. *Journal of Laboratory and Clinical Medicine*, **43**, 303.

495 KELLERMEYER R.W., TARLOV A.R., BREWER G.J., CARSON P.E. & ALVING A.S. (1962) Hemolytic effect of therapeutic drugs: clinical considerations of the primaquine-type hemolysis. *Journal of the American Medical Association*, **180**, 388.

496 SALVIDIO E., PANNACCIULLI I., TIZIANELLO A. & AJMAR F. (1967) Nature of hemolytic crises and the fate of G6PD deficient, drug-damaged erythrocytes in Sardinians. *New England Journal of Medicine*, **276**, 1339.

497 LUISADA A. (1941) Favism: singular disease affecting chiefly red blood cells. *Medicine*, **20**, 229.

498 KATTAMIS C.A., KYRIAZAKOU M. & CHAIDAS S. (1969) Favism, clinical and biochemical data. *Journal of Medical Genetics*, **6**, 34.

499 LARIZZA P., BRUNETTI P. & GRIGNANI F. (1960) Anemie emolitiche enzimopeniche. *Haematologica*, **45**, 1.

500 MOTULSKY A.G. (1965) Theoretical and clinical problems of glucose-6-phosphate dehydrogenase deficiency. In: *Abnormal Haemoglobins in Africa* (ed. Jonxis J.H.P.), p. 143. Blackwell Scientific Publications, Oxford.

501 SANSONE G., PIGA A.M. & SEGNI G. (1958) Il favismo. *Minerva Medica*, Torino.

502 SYMVOULIDIS A., VOUDICLARIS S., MOUNTOKALAKIS T. & POUGOUNIAS H. (1972) Acute renal failure in G-6-PD deficiency. *Lancet*, **ii**, 819.

503 SORCINELLI R. & GUISO G. (1979) Vitreoretinal haemorrhages after ingestion of fava bean in G-6-PD deficient subject. *Ophthalmologica*, **178**, 259.

504 RUSSO G., MOLLICA F., PAVONE L. & SCHILIRO G. (1972) Hemolytic crises in Sicilian females heterozygous for G-6-PD deficiency. *Pediatrics*, **49**, 854.

505 SANNA G., DEVIRGILIIS S., PALMAS C., ARGIOLOU F., FRAU F. & CAO A. (1979) Favism in Gd Mediterranean heterozygous females. *Pediatric Research*, **13**, 812.

506 STAMATOYANNOPOULOS G., FRASER G.R., MOTULSKY A.G., FESSAS P., AKRIVAKIS A. & PAPAYANNOPOULO T.H. (1966) On the familial predisposition to favism. *American Journal of Human Genetics*, **18**, 253.

507 CASSIMOS C.H.R., ZAFIRU M.K. & TSIURES J. (1974) Urinary D-glutaric acid excretion in normal and G-6-PD deficient children with favism. *Journal of Paediatrics*, **84**, 871.

508 FIORELLI G., PODDA M., CORRIAS A. & FARGION S. (1974) The relevance of immune reactions in acute favism. *Acta Haematologica*, **51**, 211.

509 ZINKHAM W.H. (1963) Peripheral blood and bilirubin values in normal full-term primaquine-sensitive negro infants: effect of vitamin K. *Pediatrics*, **31**, 983.

510 O'FLYNN M.E.D. & HSIA D.Y. (1963) Serum bilirubin levels and glucose-6-phosphate dehydrogenase activity in newborn American negroes. *Journal of Pediatrics*, **63**, 160.

511 PERKINS R.P. (1976) The significance of glucose-6-phosphate dehydrogenase deficiency in pregnancy. *American Journal of Obstetrics and Gynecology*, **125**, 215.

512 ESHAGHPOUR E., OSKI F.A. & WILLIAMS M. (1967) The relationship of glucose-6-phosphate dehydrogenase activity to hyperbilirubinaemia in negro premature infants. *Journal of Pediatrics*, **70**, 595.

513 BIENZLE U., EFFIONG C. & LUZZATTO L. (1976) Erythrocyte glucose-6-phosphate dehydrogenase deficiency (G-6-PD type A−) and neonatal jaundice. *Acta Paediatrica Scandinavica*, **65**, 70.

514 DOXIADIS S.A., FESSAS PH. & VALAES T. (1960) Erythrocyte enzyme deficiency in unexplained Kernicterus. *Lancet*, **ii**, 44.

515 DOXIADIS S.A., FESSAS PH. & VALAES T. (1961) Glucose-6-phosphate dehydrogenase deficiency. A new aetiological factor of severe neonatal jaundice. *Lancet*, **i**, 297.

516 FESSAS PH., DOXIADIS S.A. & VALAES T. (1962) Neonatal jaundice in glucose-6-phosphate dehydrogenase deficient infants. *British Medical Journal*, **ii**, 1359.

517 DOXIADIS S.A. & VALAES T. (1964) The clinical picture of glucose-6-phosphate dehydrogenase deficiency in early infancy. *Archives of Diseases of Childhood*, **39**, 545.

518 VALAES T., KARAKLIS A., STRAVRAKAKIS D., BAVELA-STRAVRAKAKIS K., PERAKIS A. & DOXIADIS S.A. (1969) Incidence and mechanism of neonatal jaundice related to glucose-6-phosphate dehydrogenase deficiency. *Pediatric Research*, **3**, 448.

519 PANIZON F. (1960) Erythrocyte enzyme deficiency and unexplained icterus. *Lancet*, **ii**, 1093.

520 FLATZ G., SRINGAM S., PREMYOTHIN C., PENBHARKKUL S., KETUSINGH R. & CHULAJATA R. (1963) Glucose-6-phosphate dehydrogenase deficiency and neonatal jaundice. *Archives of Diseases of Childhood*, **38**, 566.

521 YUE P.C.K. & STRICKLAND M. (1965) Glucose-6-phosphate dehydrogenase deficiency and neonatal jaundice in Chinese male infants in Hong Kong. *Lancet*, **i**, 350.

522 WESTRING D.W. & PISCIOTTA A.V. (1966) Anaemia, cataracts and seizures in a patient with glucose-6-phosphate dehydrogenase activity. *Archives of Internal Medicine*, **118**, 385.

523 HELGE H. & BORNER K. (1966) Kongenitale nichtsphaerozytaere haemolytische Anamie, Katarakt und glucose-6-phosphate dehydrogenase-mangel. *Deutsche Medizinische Wochenschrift*, **91**, 1584.

524 BEUTLER E., GROOMS A.M., MORGAN S.K. & TRINIDAD F. (1972) Chronic severe hemolytic anemia due to G-6-PD Charleston: a new deficient variant. *Journal of Pediatrics*, **80**, 1005.

525 JOHNSON G.J., KAPLAN M.E. & BEUTLER E. (1977) G-6-PD Long Prairie: a new mutant exhibiting normal sensitivity to inhibition by NADPH and accompanied by non-spherocytic hemolytic anemia. *Blood*, **49**, 247.

526 MOHLER D.N. & WILLIAMS W.J. (1964) Hereditary hemolytic disease secondary to glucose-6-phosphate

dehydrogenase deficiency. Report of three cases with special emphasis on ATP metabolism. *Blood*, **23**, 427.

527 CARSON P.E. & FRISCHER H. (1966) Glucose-6-phosphate dehydrogenase deficiency and related disorders of the pentose phosphate pathway. *American Journal of Medicine*, **41**, 744.

528 KATTAMIS C.A. & TJORTJATON F. (1970) The hemolytic process of viral hepatitis in children with normal or deficient glucose-6-phosphate dehydronegase activity. *Journal of Pediatrics*, **77**, 422.

529 GELLADY A. & GREENWOOD R.D. (1972) G-6-PD hemolytic anemia complicating diabetic ketoacidosis. *Clinical Research*, **9**, 27.

530 HELLER P., BEST W.R., NELSON R.B. & BECKTEL J. (1979) Clinical implications of sickle-cell trait and glucose-6-phosphate dehydrogenase deficiency in hospitalized black patients. *New England Journal of Medicine*, **300**, 1001.

531 GIBBS W.N., WARDLE J. & SERJEANT G.R. (1980) Glucose-6-phosphate dehydrogenase deficiency in homozygous sickle cell disease in Jamaica. *British Journal of Haematology*, **45**, 73.

532 MOSKOWITCH R.M. (1970) Auto-immune haemolytic anaemia in a patient with a deficiency of red cell glucose-6-phosphate dehydrogenase. *Johns Hopkins Medical Journal*, **126**, 139.

533 STAAL G.E.J., PUNT K., GEERDINK R.A., BOS C.C. & BARTSTRA H. (1970) A possible new variant of G-6-PD with decreased activity (G-6-PD Utrecht) in a Dutch family with hereditary spherocytosis. *Scandinavian Journal of Haematology*, **7**, 401.

534 OEZER L. & MILLS G.C. (1964) Elliptocytosis with haemolytic anaemia. *British Journal of Haematology*, **10**, 468.

535 SHROETER W., BRITTINGER G., ZIMMERSCHMITT E., KOENIG E. & SCHRADER D. (1971) Combined glucose phosphate isomerase and glucose-6-phosphate dehydrogenase deficiency of the erythrocytes: a new haemolytic syndrome. *British Journal of Haematology*, **20**, 249.

536 ALLISON A.C. (1960) Glucose-6-phosphate dehydrogenase deficiency in red blood cells of East Africans. *Nature (London)*, **186**, 531.

537 MOTULSKY A.G. (1960) Metabolic polymorphisms and the role of infectious disease in human evolution. *Human Biology*, **32**, 28.

538 LUZZATTO L., USANGA E.A. & REDDY S. (1969) Glucose-6-phosphate dehydrogenase deficient red cells. Resistance to infection by malarial parasites. *Science*, **164**, 839.

539 LUZZATTO L. & TESTA U. (1978) Human erythrocyte glucose-6-phosphate dehydrogenase: structure and function in normal and mutant subjects. *Current Topics in Haematology*, **1**, 1.

540 BIENZLE U., OKOYE V.C.N. & GOEGLER H. (1972) Haemoglobin and glucose-6-phosphate dehydrogenase variants. Distribution and relation to malarial endemicity in a Togolese population. *Tropenmedizin und Parasitologie (Stuttgart)*, **23**, 56.

541 MARTIN S.K., MILLER L.K., ALLING D., OKOYE V.C., ESAN G.J.F., OSUNKOYA B.O. & DEANE M. (1979) Severe malaria and glucose-6-phosphate dehydrogenase deficiency: a re-appraisal of the malarial G-6-PD hypothesis. *Lancet*, **i**, 524.

542 FRIEDMAN M.J. (1979) Oxidant damage mediates variant red cell resistance to malaria. *Nature (London)*, **280**, 245.

543 FIALKOW P.J., GARTLER S.M. & YOSHIDA A. (1967) Clonal origin of chronic myelocytic leukaemia in man. *Proceedings of the National Academy of Sciences, USA*, **58**, 1468.

544 FIALKOW P.J. (1964) The origin and development of human tumors studied with cell markers. *New England Journal of Medicine*, **291**, 26.

545 ONI S.B., OSUNKOYA B.O. & LUZATTO L. (1970) Paroxysmal nocturnal haemoglobinuria. Evidence for monoclonal origin of abnormal red cells. *Blood*, **36**, 145.

546 ADAMSON J.W., FIALKOW P.J., SCOTT M., JAROSLOV F.P. & STEINMANN L. (1976) Polycythemia vera: stem-cell and probable clonal origin of disease. *New England Journal of Medicine*, **295**, 913.

547 PRCHAL J.T., THROCKMONTON D.W., CARROLL A.J., FUSON E.W. & GAMS R.A. (1978) A common progenitor for human myeloid and lymphoid cells. *Nature (London)*, **274**, 590.

548 BEN-BASSAT J. & BEN-ISHAY D. (1969) Hereditary hemolytic anemia associated with glucose-6-phosphate dehydrogenase deficiency (Mediterranean type). *Israel Journal of Medical Science*, **5**, 1053.

549 MOTULSKY A.G. & YOSHIDA A. (1969) Methods for the study of red cell glucose-6-phosphate dehydrogenase. In: *Biochemical Methods in Red Cell Genetics* (ed. Yunis J.J.), p. 51. Academic Press, New York.

550 SWARUP S., GHOSH S.K. & CHATTERJEA J.B. (1960) Glutathione stability test in haemoglobin E-thalassemia disease. *Nature (London)*, **188**, 153.

551 MOTULSKY A.G. & CAMPBELL-KRAUT J.M. (1961) Population genetics of glucose-6-phosphate dehydrogenase deficiency of the red cell. *Proceedings of the Conference on Genetic Polymorphisms and Geographic Variations in Disease* (ed. Blumberg B.S.), p. 159. Grune & Stratton, New York.

552 BEUTLER E., BLUME K.G., KAPLAN J.C., LÖHR G.W., RAMOT B. & VALENTINE W.N. (1977) International Committee for Standardization in Haematology: recommended methods for red-cell enzyme analysis. *British Journal of Haematology*, **35**, 331.

553 FAIRBANKS V.F. & LAMPE L.T. (1968) A tetrazolium-linked cytochemical method for estimation of glucose-6-phosphate dehydrogenase activity in individual erythrocytes: applications in the study of heterozygotes for glucose-6-phosphate dehydrogenase deficiency. *Blood*, **31**, 589.

554 FILDES R.A. & PARR C.W. (1963) Human red cell phosphogluconate dehydrogenase. *Nature (London)*, **200**, 890.

555 BREWER G.J. & DERN R.J. (1964) A new inherited enzymatic deficiency of human erythrocytes: 6-phosphogluconate dehydrogenase deficiency. *American Journal of Human Genetics*, **16**, 472.

556 DERN R.J., BREWER G.J., TASHIAN R.E. & SHOWS T.B. (1966) Hereditary variation of erythrocyte 6-phosphogluconate dehydrogenase. *Journal of Laboratory and Clinical Medicine*, **67**, 255.

557 PARR C.W. (1966) Erythrocyte phosphogluconate dehydrogenase polymorphism. *Nature (London)*, **210**, 487.

558 CARTER N.D., FILDES R.A., FITCH R.A. & PARR C.W. (1968) Genetically determined electrophoretic variations of human phosphogluconate dehydrogenase. *Acta Genetica et Statistica Medica*, **18**, 109.

559 LAUSECKER CH., HEIDT P., FISCHER D., HARTLEY B.H. & LÖHR G.W. (1965) Anémie hémolytique constitutionelle avec déficit en 6-phospho-gluconate deshydrogenase. *Archives française de Pediatrie*, **22**, 789.

560 SCIALOM C., NAJEAN Y. & BERNARD J. (1966) Congenital nonspherocytic haemolytic anaemia with incomplete deficit in 6PGD *Nouvelle Revue française d'Hématologie*, **6**, 452.

561 GORDON H., KERAAM M.M. & VOOIJS M. (1967) Variants of 6-phosphogluconate dehydrogenase within a community. *Nature (London)*, **214**, 466.

562 DAVIDSON R.G. (1967) Electrophoretic variants of human 6-phosphogluconate dehydrogenase: population and family studies and description of a new variant. *Annals of Human Genetics*, **30**, 335.

563 BLAKE N.M. & KIRK R.L. (1969) New genetic variant of 6-phosphogluconate dehydrogenase in Australian aborigines. *Nature (London)*, **221**, 278.

564 GORDON H., KERAAN M.M., WOODBURNE V. & SOPHANGISA E. (1969) Quantitative variation of 6-phosphogluconate dehydrogenase in an African population. *Nature (London)*, **221**, 96.

565 OORT M., LOOS J.A. & PRINS H.K. (1961) Hereditary absence of reduced glutathione in the erythrocytes—a new clinical and biochemical entity. *Vox Sanguinis*, **6**, 370.

566 PRINS H.K., OORT M., LOOS J.A., ZÜRCHER C. & BECKERS T. (1966) Congenital nonspherocytic hemolytic anemia associated with glutathione deficiency of the erythrocytes. Hematologic, biochemical and genetic studies. *Blood*, **27**, 145.

567 BOIVIN P., GALAND C., ANDRÉ R. & DEBRAY J. (1966) Anémies hémolytiques congenitales avec déficit isolé en glutathion réduit par déficit en glutathione synthetase. *Nouvelle Revue française d'Hématologie*, **6**, 859.

568 KONRAD P.N., RICHARDS F., VALENTINE W.N. & PAGLIA D.E. (1972) γ-Glutamylcysteine synthetase deficiency. A cause of hereditary hemolytic anemia. *New England Journal of Medicine*, **286**, 557.

569 JELLUM E., KLUGE T., BORRESEN H.C., STOKKE O. & ELDJARN L. (1970) Pyroglutamic aciduria—a new inborn error of metabolism. *Scandinavian Journal of Clinical and Laboratory Investigation*, **26**, 327.

570 LARSSON A. & ZETTERSTROEM R. (1974) Pyroglutamic aciduria (5-oxoprolinuria), an inborn error in glutathione metabolism. *Pediatric Research*, **8**, 852.

571 HANGENFELDT L., LARSSON A. & ANDERSSON R. (1978) The γ-glutamyl cycle and amino acid transport. Studies of free amino acids, γ-glutamyl-cystein and glutathione in erythrocytes from patients with 5-oxoprolinuria (glutathione synthetase deficiency). *New England Journal of Medicine*, **229**, 587.

572 MOHLER D.N., MAJERUS P.W., MINNICH V., HESS C.E. & GARRICK M.D. (1970) Glutathione synthetase deficiency as a cause of hereditary hemolytic disease. *New England Journal of Medicine*, **283**, 1253.

573 SPIELBERG S.P., GARRICK M.D., CORASH L.M., BUTLER J., TIETZE F., ROGERS L. & SCHULMAN J.D. (1978) Biochemical heterogeneity in glutathione synthetase

deficiency. *Journal of Clinical Investigation*, **61**, 1417.

574 BEUTLER E. (1974) Glutathione reductase. In: *Gluthathione* (ed. Flohé L., Benöhr H.Ch., Sies H., Waller H.D. & Wendel A.), p. 109. Geo. Thieme, Stuttgart.

575 LÖHR G.W., BLUME K.G., RÜDIGER H.W. & ARNOLD H. (1974) Genetic variability in the enzymatic reduction of oxidized glutathione. In: *Glutathione* (ed. Flohé L., Benöhr H.Ch., Sies H., Waller H.D. and Wendel A.), p. 165. Geo. Thieme, Stuttgart.

576 DESFORGES J.F., THAYER W.W. & DAWSON J.P. (1959) Hemolytic anemia induced by sulfoxone therapy, with investigations into the mechanisms of its production. *American Journal of Medicine*, **27**, 132.

577 CARSON P.E., BREWER G.J. & ICKES C. (1961) Decreased glutathione reductase with susceptibility to hemolysis. *Journal of Laboratory and Clinical Medicine*, **58**, 804.

578 WALLER H.D. (1968) Glutathione reductase deficiency. In: *Hereditary Disorders of Erythrocyte Metabolism* (ed. Beutler E.), p. 185. Grune & Stratton, New York.

579 STAAL G.E.J., HELLEMAN P.W., VAN MILLIGEN-BOERSMA L. & VERLOOP M.C. (1968) Properties of glutathione reductase purified from erythrocytes with normal and with diminished activity of the enzyme. *Nederlands Tijdschrift Geneeskunde*, **112**, 1008.

580 JAFFÉ E.R. (1968) In: *Hereditary Disorders of Eyrthrocyte Metabolism* (ed. Beutler E.), p. 206. Grune & Stratton, New York.

581 FLATZ G. (1971) Population study of erythrocyte glutathione reductase activity. *Human Genetics*, **11**, 269.

582 WALLER H.D. (1974) In: *Glutathione* (ed. Flohé L., Benöhr, H.Ch., Sies H., Waller H.D. & Wendel A.), p. 173. Geo. Thieme, Stuttgart.

583 BENÖHR H.C. & WALLER H.D. (1970) Activation of glutathione reductase with flavin adenine dinucleotide (FAD). *XIIIth Congress of the International Society of Haematology, Munich*, p. 120.

584 LOOS H., ROOS D., WEENING R. & HOUWERZIJL J. (1976) Familial deficiency of glutathione reductase in human blood cells. *Blood*, **48**, 53.

585 LONG W.K. (1967) Glutathione reductase deficiency in red blood cells: variant associated with gout. *Science*, **155**, 712.

586 GROSS R.T., BRACCI R., RUDOLPH N., SCHROEDER E. & KOCHEN J.A. (1967) Hydrogen peroxide toxicity and detoxification in the erythrocytes of newborn infants. *Blood*, **29**, 481.

587 EMERSON P.M., MASON D.Y. & CUTHBERT J.E. (1972) Erythrocyte glutathione peroxidase content and serum tocopherol levels in newborn infants. *British Journal of Haematology*, **22**, 667.

588 BOIVIN P., DEMARTIAL M.C., GALAND C. & FARADAYI M. (1971) Differences d'activité de la glutathione-peroxidase érythrocytaire selon le sexe chez la souris et chez l'homme. *Nouvelle Revue française d'Hématologie*, **11**, 167.

589 RUDOLPH N. & WONG S.L. (1978) Selenium and glutathione peroxidase activity in maternal and cord plasma and red cells. *Pediatric Research*, **12**, 789.

590 THOMPSON C.D., REA H.M. DOESBURG V.M. & ROBINSON M.F. (1977) Selenium concentration and glutathione peroxidase activity in whole blood of New Zealand residents. *British Journal of Nutrition*, **37**, 457.

591 PERONA G., GUIDI G.C., PIGA A., CELLERINO R.,

MILANI G., COLAUTTI P., MOSCHINI G. & STIEVANO B.M. (1979) Neonatal erythrocyte glutathione peroxidase deficiency as a consequence of selenium imbalance during pregnancy. *British Journal of Haematology*, **42**, 567.

592 PERONA G., GUIDI G.G., PIGA A., CELLERINO R., MENNA R. & ZATTI M. (1978) *In vivo* and *in vitro* variations of human erythrocyte glutathione peroxidase activity as a result of cells ageing, selenium availability and peroxide activation. *British Journal of Haematology*, **39**, 399.

593 BEUTLER E. & MATSUMOTO F. (1975) Ethnic variation in red cell glutathione peroxidase activity. *Blood*, **46**, 103.

594 CELLERINO R., GUIDI G. & PERONA G. (1976) Plasma iron and erythrocytic glutathione peroxidase activity. *Scandinavian Journal of Haematology*, **17**, 111.

595 BEUTLER E. (1977) Glucose-6-phosphate dehydrogenase deficiency and red cell glutathione peroxidase. *Blood*, **49**, 467.

596 HOPKINS J. & TUDHOPE G.R. (1973) Glutathione peroxidase in human red cells in health and disease. *British Journal of Haematology*, **25**, 563.

597 TAKAHARA S. & MIYAMOTO H. (1948) Three cases of progressive oral gangrene due to lack of catalase in the blood. *Journal of the Otorhinolaryngological Society of Japan*, **51**, 163.

598 TAKAHARA S. (1952) Progressive oral gangrene probably due to lack of catalase in the blood (acatalasemia). *Lancet*, **II**, 1101.

599 KAZIRO K., KIKUCH G., NAKAMURA H. & YOSHIWA M. (1952) Die Frage nach der physiologen Funktion der Katalase im menschlichen Organismus; Notiz 'ber die Entdeckung einer Konstitutionsanomalie 'anenzymia catalasea'. *Chemische Berichte*, **85**, 886.

600 AEBI H., HEINIGER J.P., BÜTLER R. & HÄSSIG A. (1961) Two cases of acatalasia in Switzerland. *Experientia*, **17**, 466.

601 TAKAHARA S. (1968) Acatalasemia in Japan. In: *Hereditary Disorders of Erythrocyte Metabolism* (ed. Beutler E.), p. 21. Grune & Stratton, New York.

602 AEBI H., BOSSI E., CANTZ M., MATSUBARA S. & SUTER H. (1968) Acatalas(em)ia in Switzerland. In: *Hereditary Disorders of Erythrocyte Metabolism* (ed. Beutler E.), p. 41. Grune & Stratton, New York.

603 AEBI H., BAGGIOLINI M., DEWALD B., LAUBER E., SUTER H., MICHELI A. & FREI J. (1964) Observations in two Swiss families with acatalasia. II. *Enzymologica Biologica et Clinica*, **4**, 121.

604 YOSHIDA A. (1967) A single amino-acid substitution (asparagine to aspartic acid) between normal (B+) and the common negro variant (A+) of human glucose-6-phosphate dehydrogenase. *Proceedings of the National Academy of Sciences, USA*, **57**, 835.

605 SARTORI E. (1971) On the pathogenesis of favism. *Journal of Medical Genetics*, **8**, 462.

606 MAGER J., GLASER G., RAZIN A., ISAK G., BIEN S. & NOAM M. (1965) Metabolic effects of pyrimides derived from Fava bean glycosides on human erythrocytes deficient in glucose-6-phosphate dehydrogenase. *Biochemical and Biophysical Research Communications*, **20**, 235.

607 KOSOWER N.S. & KOSOWER E.M. (1967) Does 3,4-dihydroxyphenylalaline play a part in favism? *Nature (London)*, **215**, 285.

608 PHILLIPS R.S., TRIGG P.I., SCOTT-FINNIGAN T.J. & BARTHOLOMEW R.K. (1972) Culture of *Plasmodium falciparum in vitro*: a subculture technique for demonstrating antiplasmodial activity in serum from some Gambians, resident in an endemic malarious area. *Parasitology*, **65**, 525.

609 PASVOL G. & WEATHERALL D.J. (1980) The red cell and the malarial parasite. *British Journal of Haematology*, **46**, 165.

610 HARRIS J.W. & KELLERMEYER R.W. (1972) In: *The Red Cell*, 2nd edn. Harvard University Press, Cambridge, Massachusetts.

611 GROSS S. (1976) Hemolytic anaemia in premature infants: Relationship to Vitamin E, selenium, glutathione peroxidase and erythrocyte lipids. *Seminars in Hematology*, **13**, 187.

Chapter 8
The structure and function of haemoglobin: clinical disorders due to abnormal haemoglobin structure

E. R. HUEHNS

The main functions of the red cell are the transport of oxygen to the tissues and carbon dioxide to the lungs, and its organization is geared almost exclusively to these ends. In order to carry out these activities the cell is filled with haemoglobin, the oxygen-carrying pigment of the blood, and its metabolic pathways are adapted to service the haemoglobin molecule so that its function is maintained satisfactorily.

There are three main types of pathological processes which can affect haemoglobin and thus cause disease:
1 reduction in or absence of synthesis of the molecule;
2 synthesis of an abnormal protein (the haemoglobinopathies); and
3 abnormalities of the enzyme systems of the red cell servicing the protein molecule.

Reduction in or absence of synthesis of the haemoglobin molecule is caused by deficient synthesis of either globin or haem. The former is almost exclusively inherited and comprises the thalassaemias described in Chapter 9. Deficient synthesis of globin has also been found in some patients with erythroleukaemia (Chapter 9).

Reduction of haem synthesis is, in most cases, due to iron deficiency (Chapter 5) or, much more rarely, to abnormalities of porphyrin synthesis (Chapter 14). In this chapter, diseases caused by inherited structural abnormalities of the protein part of the molecule, the haemoglobinopathies, will be described, as well as the acquired conditions, methaemoglobinaemia, sulphaemoglobinaemia and carbonmonoxyhaemoglobinaemia, as well as HbAIc.

NORMAL HAEMOGLOBIN

Structure of haemoglobin
Haemoglobins are large, complex protein molecules, the function of which is to transport oxygen from the lungs to the tissues and CO_2 from the tissues to the lungs. Recent work by Perutz and his collaborators [1–6] has shown not only the overall arrangement of the molecule, but also the details of the orientation of the amino-acid side chains in each subunit. Further-

more, they have been able to show that the two forms of haemoglobin, deoxy- and oxyhaemoglobin, differ considerably in their structure, and this has helped greatly in understanding the function of the molecule.

In shape, the molecule resembles a spheroid 64 Å × 55 Å × 50 Å, with a molecular weight of about 65 000. Each molecule consists of four polypeptide chains with a haem group (Fig. 8.1) attached to each chain. There are two pairs of identical chains, called α and β chains, so that its structure can be written $\alpha_2\beta_2$. The α chains consist of 141 amino acids and the β chains have 146. The amino-acid sequence of the two human chains is given in Table 8.1. The internal arrangement of both chains is very similar; each is wound up into eight spiral or helical segments connected by short, non-helical segments to give each subunit a roughly spherical shape (Fig. 8.2). For descriptive purposes the helices are labelled alphabetically by the letters A–H starting at the free amino end, called the N terminus; the non-helical segments are labelled by the letters of the helices they connect, i.e. the EF segment is the piece of chain connecting the E and F helices. There are also non-helical segments at the N-terminal end, called the NA segment, and at the

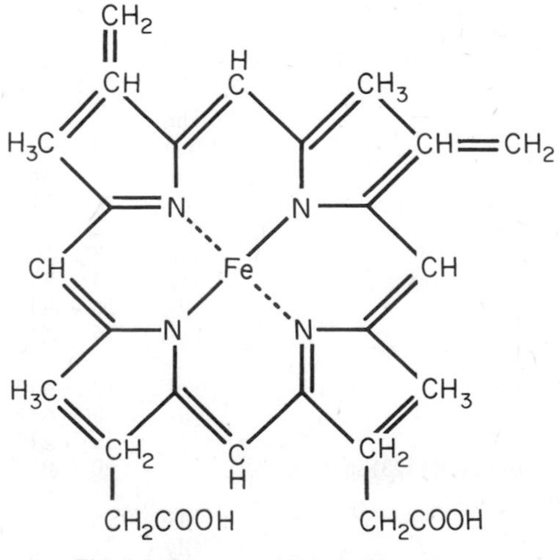

Fig. 8.1. Structure of the haem group.

Table 8.1. Amino-acid sequence of the human globin chains with notes on the position and function of the residues.
    The interactions between residues in the $\alpha_1\beta_1$ and $\alpha_1\beta_2$ contacts are discussed in Refs 1, 3 and 9.
Abbreviations:

E External	SB Salt Bridge	oxy: oxy form only
I Internal	HB Hydrogen Bond	deoxy: deoxy form only

This table has been compiled from the literature, the sequence data come from Refs 12–16 and the structural data come from various papers by Dr Perutz and his co-workers [1–9, 17–22]. I am also very grateful to Dr Perutz for invaluable help in compiling the table, and for some unpublished data.

α chain — position in molecule and notes	amino acid	residue number	Helical notation	residue number	amino acid	β chain — position in molecule and notes	γ chain of Hb F (differences from β chain)	δ chain of Hb A₂ (differences from β chain)
Central cavity, α—α contact deoxy: SB to α—COOH Arg HC3 (141) the other α chain Bohr & cooperativity	Val	1	NA1	1	Val	Internal cavity; DPG binding oxy: SB to His HC3 (146) other β chain, Bohr	Gly	
Central cavity, side chain internal	Leu	2	NA2	2	His	Internal cavity, DPG binding		
	—	—	NA3	3	Leu	Surface crevice	Phe	
E	Ser	3	A1	4	Thr	E		
E	Pro	4	A2	5	Pro	E	Glu	
E	Ala	5	A3	6	Glu	E		
E, SB to Lys H10 (127) same α chain, close to α—COOH Arg HC3 (141) other α chain	Asp	6	A4	7	Glu	E	Asp	
E	Lys	7	A5	8	Lys	E, deoxy SB to Asp EF3 (79) same β chain		
E	Thr	8	A6	9	Ser	E	Ala	Thr
E	Asn	9	A7	10	Ala	E	Thr	
I	Val	10	A8	11	Val	I	Ileu	
E	Lys	11	A9	12	Thr	Surface crevice		Asn
E	Ala	12	A10	13	Ala	E	Ser	
I	Ala	13	A11	14	Leu	Surface crevice		
I, between helices A & E	Try	14	A12	15	Try	I, between helices A & E		
E	Gly	15	A13	16	Gly	E		
E	Lys	16	A14	17	Lys	E, SB to Glu GH4 (121) same β chain		
I	Val	17	A15	18	Val	I		
E	Gly	18	A16	—	—			
E	Ala	19	AB1	—	—			
E, SB to Glu B4 (23) same α chain	His	20	B1	19	Asn	E		
E	Ala	21	B2	20	Val	E		
E	Gly	22	B3	21	Asp	E, SB to Lys E5 (61) same β chain	Glu	

TABLE 8.1—*(continued)*

α chain					β chain	γ chain of Hb F (differences from β chain)	δ chain of Hb A₂ (differences from β chain)
position in molecule and notes	amino acid	residue number	Helical notation	residue number	amino acid	position in molecule and notes	
E, SB to His B1 (20) same α chain	Glu	23	B4	22	Glu	E	Asp	Ala
OH external, ring internal	Tyr	24	B5	23	Val	I	Ala	
I	Gly	25	B6	24	Gly	I		
E	Ala	26	B7	25	Gly	E		
E	Glu	27	B8	26	Glu	E, SB to His G18 (116) same β chain		
I	Ala	28	B9	27	Ala	I	Thr	
I	Leu	29	B10	28	Leu	I		
$\alpha_1\beta_1$ contact, SB to His CD8 (50) same α chain	Glu	30	B11	29	Gly	I		
$\alpha_1\beta_1$ contact	Arg	31	B12	30	Arg	$\alpha_1\beta_1$ contact		
I, haem contact	Met	32	B13	31	Leu	I, haem contact		
I	Phe	33	B14	32	Leu	I		
E, $\alpha_1\beta_1$ contact	Leu	34	B15	33	Val	Surface pocket, $\alpha_1\beta_1$ contact		
I, $\alpha_1\beta_1$ contact	Ser	35	B16	34	Val	Surface pocket, $\alpha_1\beta_1$ contact		
I, $\alpha_1\beta_1$ contact	Phe	36	C1	35	Tyr	$\alpha_1\beta_1$ contact		
E, $\alpha_1\beta_2$ contact	Pro	37	C2	36	Pro	E, oxy: $\alpha_1\beta_2$ contact		
E, $\alpha_1\beta_2$ contact	Thr	38	C3	37	Try	I, $\alpha_1\beta_2$ contact		
haem contact	Thr	39	C4	38	Thr	I, haem contact		
E, deoxy: $\alpha_1\beta_2$ contact; cooperativity	Lys	40	C5	39	Gln	E, oxy: $\alpha_1\beta_2$ contact		
E, $\alpha_1\beta_2$ contact	Thr	41	C6	40	Arg	E, $\alpha_1\beta_2$ contact		
Main chain external, side chain internal; $\alpha_1\beta_2$ contact, haem contact. HB to Phe G5 (98) same α chain	Tyr	42	C7	41	Phe	Surface crevice, haem contact		
Main chain external, side chain internal, haem contact	Phe	43	CD1	42	Phe	Surface crevice, haem contact		
E, deoxy: $\alpha_1\beta_2$ contact	Pro	44	CD2	43	Glu	E	Asp	
E, haem contact to —COOH of propionic acid	His	45	CD3	44	Ser	E, haem contact to —COOH of propionic acid		
E, haem contact	Phe	46	CD4	45	Phe	Main chain external, side chain internal, haem contact		
E	Asp	47	CD5	46	Gly	E		
Surface crevice	Leu	48	CD6	47	Asp	E	Asn	
E	Ser	49	CD7	48	Leu	Surface crevice		
E, SB to Glu B11 (30) same α chain	His	50	CD8	49	Ser	E		
E	Gly	51	CD9	—	—			

T ABLE 8.1—*(continued)*

α chain position in molecule and notes	α chain amino acid	α chain residue number	Helical notation	β chain residue number	β chain amino acid	β chain position in molecule and notes	γ chain of Hb F (differences from β chain)	δ chain of Hb A₂ (differences from β chain)
	—	—	D1	50	Thr	E	Ser	Ser
	—	—	D2	51	Pro	E, $\alpha_1\beta_1$ contact	Ala	
	—	—	D3	52	Asp	E	Ser	
	—	—	D4	53	Ala	E		
	—	—	D5	54	Val	I	Ile	
	—	—	D6	55	Met	E, $\alpha_1\beta_1$ contact		
	—	—	D7	56	Gly	E		
E	Ser	52	E1	57	Asn	E		
E	Ala	53	E2	58	Pro	E		
E	Gln	54	E3	59	Lys	E		
I	Val	55	E4	60	Val	I		
E	Lys	56	E5	61	Lys	E, SB to Asp B3 (21) same β chain		
E	Gly	57	E6	62	Ala	E		
Haem contact ('Distal His')	His	58	E7	63	His	Surface crevice, haem contact ('Distal His')		
I	Gly	59	E8	64	Gly	I		
E	Lys	60	E9	65	Lys	E		
E	Lys	61	E10	66	Lys	E, ? haem contact with —COOH of propionic acid		
I, haem contact	Val	62	E11	67	Val	I, haem contact		
Surface crevice	Ala	63	E12	68	Leu	I		
E	Asp	64	E13	69	Gly	E		Thr
E	Ala	65	E14	70	Ala	E, haem contact		Ser
I	Leu	66	E15	71	Phe	I, haem contact		Leu
E	Thr	67	E16	72	Ser	E		Gly
E	Asn	68	E17	73	Asp	E		
I	Ala	69	E18	74	Gly	E		Ala
Surface crevice	Val	70	E19	75	Leu	I		Ile
E	Ala	71	E20	76	Ala	E		Lys
E	His	72	EF1	77	His	E		
Surface crevice	Val	73	EF2	78	Leu	I		
E	Asp	74	EF3	79	Asp	E, deoxy: SB to Lys A5 (8) same β chain		
E	Asp	75	EF4	80	Asn	E		Asp
I	Met	76	EF5	81	Leu	I		
E	Pro	77	EF6	82	Lys	Surface of central cavity, DPG binding		
E	Asn	78	EF7	83	Gly	E		
E	Ala	79	EF8	84	Thr	E		

T ABLE 8.1—(*continued*)

α chain — position in molecule and notes	amino acid	residue number	Helical notation	residue number	amino acid	β chain — position in molecule and notes	γ chain of Hb F (differences from β chain)	δ chain of Hb A₂ (differences from β chain)
Surface crevice	Leu	80	F1	85	Phe	I		
E	Ser	81	F2	86	Ala	E		Ser
E	Ala	82	F3	87	Thr	E	Gln	Gln
Surface crevice, haem contact	Leu	83	F4	88	Leu	Surface crevice, haem contact		
I	Ser	84	F5	89	Ser	I		
E	Asp	85	F6	90	Glu	E		
E, haem contact	Leu	86	F7	91	Leu	Surface crevice, haem contact		
I, haem contact ('Proximal His')	His	87	F8	92	His	Haem contact ('Proximal His')		
Surface crevice	Ala	88	F9	93	Cys	E, reactive sulphydryl		
E	His	89	FG1	94	Asp	E, deoxy: SB to His HC3 (146) same β chain, Bohr		
E	Lys	90	FG2	95	Lys	E		
E, oxy: $\alpha_1\beta_2$ contact	Leu	91	FG3	96	Leu	Surface crevice, haem contact		
E, $\alpha_1\beta_2$ contact	Arg	92	FG4	97	His	E, $\alpha_1\beta_2$ contact		
I, haem contact; oxy: $\alpha_1\beta_1$ contact, deoxy: HB to Tyr HC2 (140) same α chain	Val	93	FG5	98	Val	I, side chain haem contact, main chain $\alpha_1\beta_2$. deoxy: HB to HC2 (145) same β chain		
Central cavity, oxy: $\alpha_1\beta_2$ contact	Asp	94	G1	99	Asp	$\alpha_1\beta_2$ contact. HB to Glu G3 (101) same β chain		
Central cavity, $\alpha_1\beta_2$ contact	Pro	95	G2	100	Pro	Facing internal cavity, deoxy: $\alpha_1\beta_2$ contact		
Central cavity, $\alpha_1\beta_2$ contact	Val	96	G3	101	Glu	Facing internal cavity, $\alpha_1\beta_2$ contact. HB to Asp G1 (99) same β chain		
Haem contact	Asn	97	G4	102	Asn	Haem contact, oxy: $\alpha_1\beta_2$ contact		
Haem contact; HB to Tyr C7 (42) same α chain	Phe	98	G5	103	Phe	I, haem contact		
Central cavity	Lys	99	G6	104	Arg	Central cavity	Lys	
Surface crevice, central cavity	Leu	100	G7	105	Leu	Internal cavity, surface crevice		
I, haem contact	Leu	101	G8	106	Leu	I, haem contact		
Central cavity	Ser	102	G9	107	Gly	I		
Central cavity, $\alpha_1\beta_1$ contact	His	103	G10	108	Asn	Internal cavity, $\alpha_1\beta_1$ contact		
I, $\alpha_1\beta_1$ contact	Cys	104	G11	109	Val	I, close to $\alpha_1\beta_1$ contact		
I	Leu	105	G12	110	Leu	I		
I, $\alpha_1\beta_1$ contact	Leu	106	G13	111	Val	I		

TABLE 8.1—(*continued*)

α chain			Helical notation	β chain			γ chain of Hb F (differences from β chain)	δ chain of Hb A₂ (differences from β chain)
position in molecule and notes	amino acid	residue number		residue number	amino acid	position in molecule and notes		
I, $\alpha_1\beta_1$ contact	Val	107	G14	112	Cys	I, $\alpha_1\beta_1$ contact	Thr	
I	Thr	108	G15	113	Val	I		
I	Leu	109	G16	114	Leu	I		
I	Ala	110	G17	115	Ala	I, $\alpha_1\beta_1$ contact		
Surface crevice, $\alpha_1\beta_1$ contact	Ala	111	G18	116	His	Surface crevice, $\alpha_1\beta_1$ contact SB to Glu B8 (26) same β chain	Ile	Arg
E	His	112	G19	117	His	E		Asn
Surface crevice	Leu	113	GH1	118	Phe	Surface crevice		
E, $\alpha_1\beta_1$ contact	Pro	114	GH2	119	Gly	E, $\alpha_1\beta_1$ contact		
E	Ala	115	GH3	120	Lys	E		
E	Glu	116	GH4	121	Glu	E, SB to Lys A14 (17) same β chain		
I, $\alpha_1\beta_1$ contact	Phe	117	GH5	122	Phe	I, $\alpha_1\beta_1$ contact		
E	Thr	118	H1	123	Thr	E, $\alpha_1\beta_1$ contact		
E, $\alpha_1\beta_1$ contact	Pro	119	H2	124	Pro	E, $\alpha_1\beta_1$ contact		Gln
E	Ala	120	H3	125	Pro	E, $\alpha_1\beta_1$ contact	Glu	
Surface crevice	Val	121	H4	126	Val	Surface crevice		Met
I, $\alpha_1\beta_1$ contact Bohr	His	122	H5	127	Gln	I, $\alpha_1\beta_1$ contact		
E, $\alpha_1\beta_1$ contact	Ala	123	H6	128	Ala	I, $\alpha_1\beta_1$ contact		
Surface crevice	Ser	124	H7	129	Ala	Surface crevice	Ser	
I	Leu	125	H8	130	Tyr	I	Try	
Central cavity, $\alpha_1\beta_1$ contact cooperativity; Bohr deoxy: SB to Arg HC3 (141) other α chain	Asp	126	H9	131	Gln	I, $\alpha_1\beta_1$ contact		
Central cavity, SB to Asp A4 (6) same α chain, deoxy: SB to —COOH Arg HC3 (141) other α chain	Lys	127	H10	132	Lys	Surface crevice, between β chains		
I	Phe	128	H11	133	Val	I		Met
I, haem contact	Leu	129	H12	134	Val	I		
Central cavity	Ala	130	H13	135	Ala	Central cavity		Thr
Central cavity	Ser	131	H14	136	Gly	Central cavity		Gly/Ala
I, haem contact	Val	132	H15	137	Val	I, haem contact		
Central cavity	Ser	133	H16	138	Ala	Central cavity		
Central cavity	Thr	134	H17	139	Asn	Central cavity	Ser	
Surface crevice, central cavity	Val	135	H18	140	Ala	Central cavity		
I, haem contact	Leu	136	H19	141	Leu	I, haem contact		
Central cavity	Thr	137	H20	142	Ala	Central cavity	Ser	

TABLE 8.1—(*continued*)

α chain position in molecule and notes	amino acid	residue number	Helical notation	residue number	amino acid	β chain position in molecule and notes	γ chain of Hb F (differences from β chain)	δ chain of Hb A₂ (differences from β chain)
Central cavity	Ser	138	H21	143	His	Central cavity, DPG binding (N.B. Ser of γ chain does not bind DPG), Bohr	Ser	
E	Lys	139	HC1	144	Lys	E		Arg
Deoxy: HB to Val FG5 (93) same α chain; held between helices F & H Oxy: mobile; cooperativity	Tyr	140	HC2	145	Tyr	Deoxy: HB to Val FG5 (98) same β chain held between helices F & H Oxy: mobile; cooperativity		
E, deoxy: SBs to Asp H9 (126), Lys H10 (127) and αNH₂Val NA1 (1) other α chain Oxy: mobile; Bohr	Arg	141	HC3	146	His	α₁β₂ contact; deoxy SBs to Lys C5 (40) α chain and Asp FG1 (94) same β chain V. der W to Pro C2 (37) α oxy: mobile; SB to Val NA1 (1) other β chain Bohr & cooperativity		

C-terminal end, called the HC segment. Because of the folding of the polypeptide chain and the helical structure, amino acids far apart in the amino-acid sequence may be very close together in the three dimensional model of the molecule, and many different parts of the chain can come together in one region of the molecule. The haem group in each subunit lies in a deep pocket lined by 20 hydrophobic (non-polar) residues derived from the B, C, E, F, G and H helices as well as the CD and FG segments. The non-polar edge of the haem group with the vinyl side chains is internal, while the proprionic side chains make polar contacts with residues CD3 and E10. The iron of the haem group is covalently bonded to histidine F8 (eighth amino acid of the F helix, α87 or β92). These residues are often referred to as the proximal histidines, and although they do not occupy the same position along the α and the β chain, the homology of their position in the molecule is obvious when using the helical notation.

The oxygen molecule sits on the other side of the haem group opposite histidine E7 (α58, β63), the so-called distal histidines. Examination of the distribution of amino acids shows that only those with hydrophobic side chains point to the interior of a subunit, while all the charged amino acids are external. Thus the tertiary structure of the polypeptide chain is stabilized by hydrophobic interactions on the interior of each subunit as well as those around the haem group. There are also specific bonds holding the helices together. The interactions between the α and β subunits (at the α₁β₁ contact, see below) are also important in maintaining the stability of the subunit.

The four subunits lie on the four corners of a tetrahedron (triangular-based pyramid). There is little contact between the like chains (i.e. α—α or β—β), while there is close contact between unlike chains. From Figure 8.3 it can be seen that there are four contacts between α and β chains, the αβ contacts. These are of

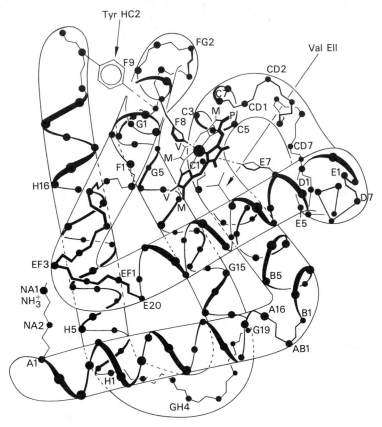

Fig. 8.2. Diagrammatic sketch showing the course of the polypeptide chain in the β subunit. (From Ref. 9.)

two types: $\alpha_1 \equiv \beta_1$ (or $\alpha_2 \equiv \beta_2$) and $\alpha_1 - \beta_2$ (or $\alpha_2 - \beta_1$). The $\alpha_1 \equiv \beta_1$ contact contains about 34 residues which partly interlock with each other, allowing very little movement between subunits. The $\alpha_1 - \beta_2$ contact contains about 20 residues, and the interaction between the two subunits is less firm. It is at this contact that haemoglobin dissociates ($\alpha_2\beta_2 \rightleftharpoons \alpha_1 \equiv \beta_1 + \alpha_2 \equiv \beta_2$) [10] and that an important part of the quaternary rearrangement of the molecule between the oxy- and deoxy- forms of haemoglobin described below occurs.

The oxy- and deoxy- forms of haemoglobin
During the uptake of oxygen by haemoglobin the affinity for oxygen increases and similarly as oxygen is released the affinity decreases. This effect is due to the haem–haem interactions, a measure of which is given by the 'n' value of the Hill equation. Interrelated to the haem–haem interactions is the environmental control of the oxygen affinity by such factors as pH (the Bohr shift), CO_2 and 2,3-diphosphoglycerate (2,3-DPG). The fundamental basis of these properties is the ability of haemoglobin to take up various conformations

which differ in their affinity for oxygen. Physiologically, these changes are important because the former, pH and CO_2, tend to decrease affinity in the tissues, thus facilitating oxygen release, while in the lungs oxygen affinity is increased, facilitating oxygen uptake. The interaction with 2,3-DPG adjusts the oxygen affinity to its optimum in certain physiological and pathological states.

Each individual subunit may take up a number of conformations, the most extreme having a very high or very low relative oxygen affinity. These two (extreme) conformations are in equilibrium with each other. However, when oxygen is bound the subunits are almost all in the high-affinity form, while without oxygen the low-affinity form is favoured.

Similarly the whole tetramer molecule exists in two main states: a low- and a high-affinity form. In the whole molecule the presence of subunits in the low-affinity form (without oxygen) would tend to push the tetramer conformation into its low-affinity form and this in turn tends to push the other subunits into their low-affinity form. The reverse happens as oxygen is

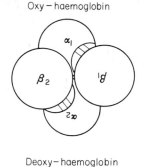

Oxy – haemoglobin

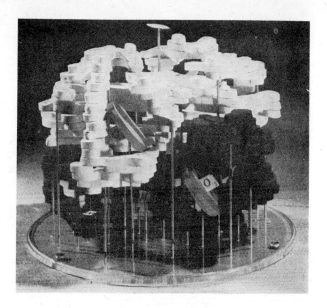

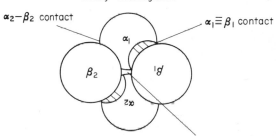

Deoxy – haemoglobin

$\alpha_2 - \beta_2$ contact

$\alpha_1 \equiv \beta_1$ contact

position of 2,3 DPG
between the β-chains

Fig. 8.3. Models of the haemoglobin molecule. (a) Model of haemoglobin at 5 Å resolution; α chains white, β chains black (photograph kindly supplied by Dr M. F. Perutz). (b) Diagrammatic representation of the conformational change of haemoglobin on oxygenation to show 2,3-DPG-binding site between the β chains. (From Ref. 11.)

bound. These equilibria are shown diagrammatically in Figure 8.4.

As the oxygen affinity of a haemoglobin solution depends on the proportion of low- and high-affinity molecules it can be seen that as oxygen is bound the oxygen affinity increases and *vice versa*, thus producing the sigmoid oxygen dissociation curve.

An increase in 2,3-DPG, CO_2 and H^+ (fall of pH) as well as a rise in temperature stabilize the low-affinity form of haemoglobin, reducing oxygen affinity. For changes in oxygen affinity in the physiological range brought about by these factors no change in the co-operativity in the binding of oxygen occurs.

From the above it can be deduced that deoxy-haemo-globin is almost completely in the low-affinity form, while oxy-haemoglobin is almost completely in the high-affinity form. Perutz [18, 191] has determined the structure of these and has been able to deduce the 'function' of various residues in the molecule.

The change from the deoxy- to the oxy- form (or *vice versa*) is initiated by a change of position of the iron relative to the plane of the porphyrin ring. In the deoxy- form the iron atom is slightly out of the plane of the porphyrin on the proximal histidine side. This is because the effective radius of the iron atom is larger in the deoxy- than the oxy- form and, in effect, is pushed

outside the plane of the porphyrin ring in the former. When oxygen is bound, the iron atom moves into the plane of the porphyrin ring. As the position of the iron is fixed by its bond to histidine F8 the porphyrin ring tilts in relation to the globin part of the molecule. This, in turn, produces a shift in helical regions of the chain of the order of 2–3 Å, breaking the hydrogen bond between valine FG5 and the penultimate tyrosine (HC2) which is now expelled from the pocket between the F and H helices occupied in the deoxy- form. This frees the C-terminal residues of the now oxygenated chain, tending to break certain salt linkages with the other chains in the molecule, and makes the deoxy-structure of the other subunits less stable, thus increasing their oxygen affinity. The quaternary deoxy- structure also becomes less stable and when approximately three subunits are in the oxy- form the quaternary oxy-conformation is preferred. This change consists of a rotation of the $\alpha^1 \equiv \beta^1$ dimers in the whole (tetramer) molecule over each other at the α_1/β_2 contact, there being considerable rearrangement of the bonds holding the molecule together in this contact. In addition, the space between the β chains present in the deoxy-form of haemoglobin becomes smaller.

These changes in structure explain the way both 2,3-DPG and pH affect the oxygen affinity. 2,3-DPG

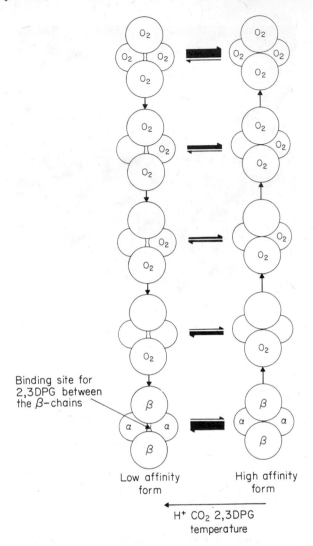

Binding site for
2,3DPG between
the β−chains

Low affinity   High affinity
form   form

H⁺ CO₂ 2,3DPG
temperature

Fig. 8.4. Diagrammatic representation of the equilibrium between the low- and high-affinity forms of haemoglobin. It can be seen that as oxygen is bound the equilibrium shifts to the right increasing the oxygen affinity. Interaction with H^+, CO_2 and 2,3-DPG or an increase in temperature stabilizes the low-affinity form reducing the oxygen affinity. (From Ref. 23.)

binds to the deoxy- form of haemoglobin in the space between the β chains [19] (Fig. 8.5), and is expelled from the molecule as this space closes up when the change to the oxy- form takes place. Thus the bonds binding 2,3-DPG tend to maintain the haemoglobin molecule in the deoxy- form of haemoglobin, lowering its oxygen affinity. Changes in pH will either strengthen or weaken the salt linkages between chains present only in the deoxy- form of haemoglobin and thus affect the equilibrium between the two forms of haemoglobin. In this way a rise in pH increases the oxygen affinity and *vice versa*. For a detailed discussion of the relationship of the changes in structure of haemoglobin to its function, see the various papers by Perutz, referred to on page 324.

Function of haemoglobin

The function of haemoglobin is to carry oxygen to the tissues. Several factors affect the amount of oxygen which the blood can deliver in a given time to the tissues:

1 the haemoglobin level;
2 the oxygen affinity of the blood;
3 the blood flow through the tissues;
4 arterial Po_2;
5 venous Po_2.

The way in which the haemoglobin level and blood flow affect oxygen delivery to the tissues is self-evident. For example, for a given haemoglobin level, doubling blood flow will double the amount of oxygen carried to

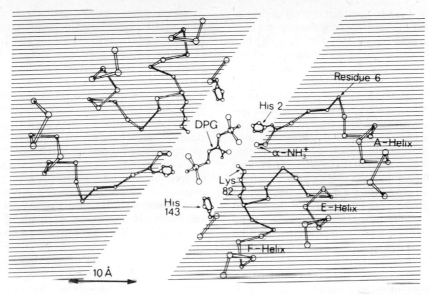

Fig. 8.5. Diagrammatic representation of the binding site of 2,3-DPG to human deoxyhaemoglobin A. (From Ref. 19.)

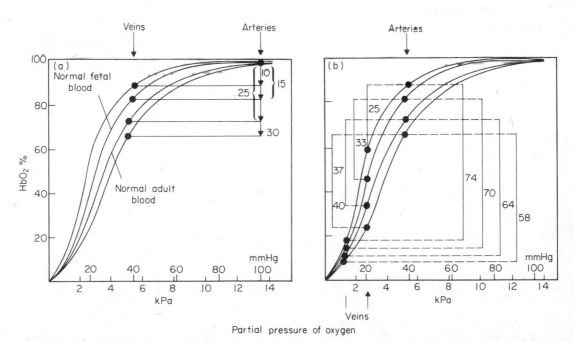

Fig. 8.6. Oxygen dissociation curves of human blood. (a) Normal adult and normal fetal blood and the effect of changing the oxygen affinity with normal partial pressures of oxygen in the arteries and veins, $Pa_{,O_2}$ and $Pv_{,O_2}$. It can be seen that lowering the oxygen affinity releases more oxygen to the tissues. (b) Effect of changing the oxygen affinity when there is a very low arterial Po_2 (40 mmHg). It can be seen that if the mean venous Po_2 is about 20 mmHg then lowering the oxygen affinity increases release. In contrast, with a lower mean venous Po_2 less oxygen is released to the tissues as the curve shifts to the right.

The SI units kPa have been indicated; 1.0 mmHg $= 0.133$ kPa. (From Ref. 23.)

the tissues. Thus it can be seen that control of cardiac output and blood flow are very important when considering tissue oxygen supply. However, these two factors are outside the scope of this chapter, and the reader is referred to text books on cardiovascular physiology. The level of haemoglobin in the blood determines the total amount of oxygen which can be carried by the blood. Each gram of haemoglobin can carry 1·34 ml of oxygen and the 'oxygen-carrying capacity' of the blood is about 20 ml of oxygen per 100 ml of blood. Of course it is not sufficient to have enough oxygen-carrying capacity, but the oxygen affinity must be such that all haemoglobin molecules will pick up oxygen in the lungs and release a large proportion as they pass through the tissues. In Figure 8.6, the oxygen dissociation curve of normal blood is shown. It can be seen that at arterial oxygen tensions, blood will be virtually fully saturated with oxygen provided there is time for equilibration to take place. The time scale of the combination of oxygen with haemoglobin is such that this is not the limiting step. However, diffusion of oxygen through the lungs, etc., until it reaches the haemoglobin in the red cells, is crucial. This is, of

course, facilitated by the anatomical arrangement of pulmonary blood flow in relation to the alveoli. Because the curve is flat at the top end, high degrees of saturation are achieved over quite a wide range of arterial Po_2. In the tissues, on the other hand, the object is to maximize oxygen release. From Figure 8.6 it can be seen that the sigmoid shape of the oxygen dissociation curve, due to the haem–haem interactions already discussed, does just this, and as blood passes from the lungs to the tissues, approximately 30% of the oxygen carried is given up, but here a small fall in Po_2 causes a relatively large release of oxygen. It can also be seen that lowering the oxygen affinity increases the amount of oxygen released at a given mean venous Po_2. During normal delivery of oxygen to the tissues, the lower pH and higher Pco_2 found in the tissues (compared to the lungs) will cause a small, but significant, increase in oxygen release. Other factors which alter the position of the oxygen dissociation curve are temperature [24, 25] and 2,3-DPG. The effect of temperature on the oxygen dissociation curve is significant in two conditions, pyrexia and exercise. Thus, during exercise the fall in pH and rise of tissue CO_2, as well as

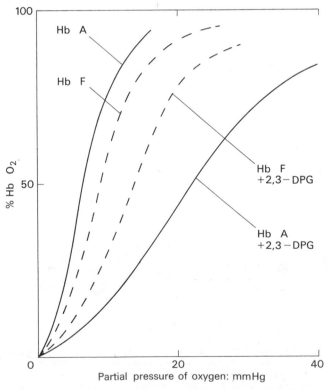

Fig. 8.7. Oxygen dissociation curves of purified Hb A and Hb F in a 0·05 M bis tris buffer, pH 7·0 with and without the addition of 2,3-DPG (two moles 2,3-DPG/mole Hb). (From Ref. 30.)

any increase in temperature, will decrease oxygen affinity and increase oxygen release.

The control of oxygen affinity by 2,3-DPG

The glycolytic intermediate 2,3-DPG occurs in very high concentration in human red cells compared to other tissues, and it is now known that its function is to modulate the oxygen affinity of the haemoglobin in the red cell [26–30]. 2,3-DPG lowers the oxygen affinity of haemoglobin (Fig. 8.7) by binding to a specific site only available in the deoxy- form as already discussed (p. 330). In the red cell, the concentration of 2,3-DPG (3·8–4·5 μM/ml RBC) is approximately the same as that of haemoglobin (on a molar basis), and changes in the concentration of 2,3-DPG cause significant shifts in the oxygen dissociation curve, an increase of 2,3-DPG of 1 μM/g Hb reducing oxygen affinity by about 0·7 mmHg. Other phosphates in the cell have a similar action on oxygen affinity; the effect of ATP is quantitatively similar to that of 2,3-DPG on a molar basis, but that of other phosphates is much less [21]. As 2,3-DPG has about five times the concentration of ATP and also because it can be specifically varied, it is the most important substance in the control of oxygen affinity in the cell. However, it is important to remember that other phosphates must account for about a quarter of the reduction of oxygen affinity between phosphate-free cells and normal red cells.

The level of 2,3-DPG in the red cell is maintained by a balance of its production from 1,3-DPG by DPG mutase and its destruction by DPG phosphatase. Important factors affecting this balance are the rate of glycolysis, the level of free 2,3-DPG and the red-cell pH; levels of other phosphate intermediates, such as ADP, 3PG, etc., also play a part (these interactions and the full chemical names for the abbreviations for phosphate intermediates described here are considered in Chapter 7, page 227).

A change in pH affects the red-cell 2,3-DPG in several ways. First, it affects the rate of glycolysis; a fall in pH reduces glycolysis so tending to reduce the 2,3-DPG level. Secondly, the pH dependence of the DPG phosphatase is such that small changes in pH cause relatively large changes in activity, a fall in pH causing increased enzyme activity, again tending to reduce 2,3-DPG. The level of free 2,3-DPG acts by product inhibition of DPG mutase and also by inhibition of some enzymes earlier in the glycolytic pathway (see Chapter 7, p. 226). 2,3-DPG is also a co-factor in the phosphoglyceromutase reaction which converts 3PG to 2PG. This reaction is indirectly involved in the control of 2,3-DPG as 3PG tends to inhibit DPG phosphatase and 2PG tends to stimulate it. Because more 2,3-DPG is bound to deoxy- than to oxygenated

haemoglobin, any increase in the average amount of deoxyhaemoglobin in the cells leads to increased binding of 2,3-DPG, reduction of free 2,3-DPG and increased synthesis of the compound by release of DPG mutase.

As ADP stimulates the conversion of 1-DPG to 3-PG by phosphoglycerate kinase with the formation of ATP; a high cell ADP tends to reduce the formation of 2,3-DPG. Thus the level of DPG in the cell is controlled by a complex series of interactions which in turn affect oxygen affinity.

The main conditions affecting 2,3-DPG level in the cell appear to be a change in pH and hypoxia, a change in pH acting on the rate of glycolysis and 2,3-DPG phosphatase while hypoxia will tend to increase 2,3-DPG in two ways, by increasing 2,3-DPG binding by haemoglobin and by the rise in intracellular pH, both of which are due to the increased average deoxyhaemoglobin in the cell. Various aspects of the biochemical control of the red-cell 2,3-DPG level are discussed by Rapoport [31, 32], Minakami [33] and Rorth [34]. In this connection it is of interest that the same function is carried out by inositol hexaphosphate in birds [26] and ATP in fishes [35].

It should be noted that the haemoglobins which do not interact with DPG have an intrinsic low oxygen affinity. It appears that the substitution of the hydrophilic histidine at β_2 (NA2) by a large hydrophobic residue, for example methionine in cow or sheep haemoglobin, prevents DPG binding and also causes the low oxygen affinity [22].

OXYGEN AFFINITY CHANGES IN DISEASE
From the above discussion it may appear that lowering the oxygen affinity will always increase oxygen delivery to the tissues. This is not so when the loading and unloading oxygen tensions are extremely low, and this is illustrated in Figure 8.6. With arterial oxygen tensions of 40 mmHg and a venous tension of 20 mmHg, most oxygen is still released to the tissues with the dissociation with the lowest oxygen affinity illustrated. However, with the same arterial (loading) oxygen tension and a venous tension of 10 mmHg, the greatest release of oxygen is with the dissociation curve with the highest oxygen affinity illustrated. From the practical point of view, such low oxygen tensions are only rarely present, and a right-shifted curve is almost always beneficial to oxygen delivery. This point may become of some importance in the management of severely hypoxic patients with acidosis when it becomes therapeutically possible to alter the oxygen affinity (see below), as well as in embryos before the placenta is functional. At that time in development, such low oxygen tensions may be commonplace and in embryonic red cells containing haemoglobins Gower 1

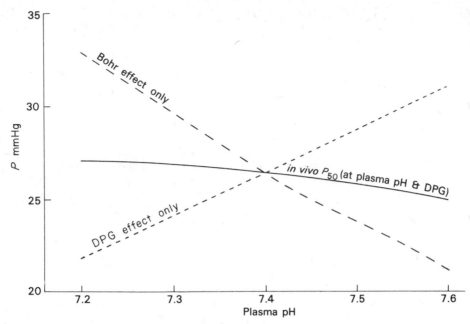

Fig. 8.8. Change in P_{50} as a function of plasma pH when only the Bohr-effect correction is made (2,3-DPG assumed constant), when the 2,3-DPG varies but pH is held at 7·4, and when both pH and 2,3-DPG (*in-vivo* condition) are taken into account. (From Ref. 49.)

and Gower 2 (p. 341) the Bohr shift below pH 7·0 is absent or reversed, preventing the oxygen affinity of embryonic blood in acidotic conditions becoming so low that oxygen delivery to the tissues is endangered.

Hypoxia
It has been known for a long time that in various anaemias there is a lower oxygen affinity of the red cells than in normal individuals [36–38], and this is due to an increased level of 2,3-DPG [39–42]. This shift of the oxygen dissociation curve is clearly detectable at a haemoglobin of about 10 g/dl and then gradually increases and makes an important contribution to oxygen delivery to the tissues. In anaemia of 7·5 g/dl the shift of the curve will increase oxygen release in the tissues by about 25%; further compensation is achieved by a reduction of the mean venous oxygen tension. In this way, the increase of cardiac output necessary to compensate for a given degree of anaemia is minimized and some leeway for exercise remains. However, in severe anaemia, shifting the oxygen dissociation curve and lowering the tissue oxygen tension are inadequate and during exercise the cardiac output has to rise sharply. This fits in well with the clinical features of anaemia, adequate compensation at rest and moderate activity without symptoms, while there is a markedly lowered exercise tolerance. Other causes of tissue hypoxia, such as heart disease [28, 43] and

thyrotoxicosis [44], are associated with an increase in red-cell 2,3-DPG and a lowered oxygen affinity. In hypothyroidism, a raised or normal oxygen affinity has been reported [45] (see Chapter 33).

Acid–base disturbances
As well as hypoxia, pH has been known for many years to affect the level of red-cell 2,3-DPG [46]. In acidosis, there is a reduction of 2,3-DPG. However, the change in oxygen affinity of whole blood is minimal. This is because the 2,3-DPG changes are such that they just balance the Bohr effect and thus *in-vivo* oxygen affinity remains normal (Fig. 8.8) [47, 48]. This picture is only true when there has not been any recent change of pH, as the Bohr effect is immediate, while the change of 2,3-DPG level is delayed for some hours. These changes are important in the management of patients with acidosis. As the half-time required for changes in red-cell 2,3-DPG are of the order of eight hours, any sudden correction of an established acidosis may cause a sharp rise in oxygen affinity through the Bohr effect and hence considerably impair tissue oxygenation in an already ill patient [48]. These considerations (as well as others) indicate that acidosis should be corrected slowly so that red-cell 2,3-DPG has time to adjust accordingly.

Similarly considerations apply to neonates, particularly prematures, with adjustment of the red-cell

2,3-DPG leading to gross changes in oxygen affinity. The situation is often made worse by the presence of a low arterial oxygen tension and anaemia. Some authors [50, 51] have suggested that exchange transfusion, replacing the Hb-F-containing cells with Hb-A cells, is of itself beneficial, but as their 2,3-DPG level will be modified by the neonatal environment this appears unlikely. Nevertheless transfusion for the correction of anaemia is of paramount importance as our own data clearly shows [52].

Mixed syndromes
There are a number of conditions in which hypoxia occurs alongside acid-base disturbances; these include renal and respiratory disease. In chronic renal disease, several factors determine the final blood oxygen affinity. The anaemia (and hyperphosphataemia, when present) [53] tends to raise the 2,3-DPG, while any acidosis present tends to reduce it. The final oxygen affinity of the blood reflects not only any change in 2,3-DPG but also the direct effect of the change in pH, the total shift of the curve being of the same magnitude as that found in anaemia of similar severity due to 2,3-DPG alone. At the present time very few data are available [54] to support this hypothesis. Similar arguments apply to respiratory disease with acidosis. Again, the change in 2,3-DPG found will be less than that expected for the degree of hypoxia [42]. However, the 2,3-DPG and Bohr effects will, in this case, both lower the oxygen affinity, and the resultant curve shows a similar degree of shift as would be expected from the hypoxia present.

Red-cell enzyme defects (see also Chapter 7)
In pyruvate-kinase deficiency, the 2,3-DPG in the red cells is two to three times higher than normal, and, as expected, this is associated with a low oxygen affinity. Typical changes are red-cell 2,3-DPG levels of 30–40 μM/g Hb (normal 13·5–15·5 μM/g Hb) with a low blood oxygen affinity, P_{50} c. 38 mmHg (normal c. 26 mmHg at pH 7·4) [55–57]. In contrast to this condition, in diphosphoglycerate mutase [58], hexokinase [59], phosphofructose-kinase deficiency [60], etc., a low 2,3-DPG with a raised oxygen affinity is found. Similar changes are found in other red-cell enzyme abnormalities, and the 2,3-DPG level and oxygen affinity may be helpful in the diagnosis of these conditions. In those cases where a raised 2,3-DPG is found, the defect is after 2,3-DPG in the glycolytic pathway, most commonly pyruvate-kinase deficiency, whilst if 2,3-DPG is low the defect is before 2,3-DPG. In defects of the pentose phosphate shunt (namely glucose-6-phosphate-dehydrogenase deficiency) no change in 2,3-DPG is found. Any changes in 2,3-DPG lead to the corresponding changes in oxygen affinity. As will be discussed later (p. 338) the oxygen affinity in haemolysis indirectly controls the red-cell mass. Thus, a raised 2,3-DPG is associated with a low oxygen affinity and a low packed cell volume and *vice versa*. In this way, the clinical picture of haemolysis due to a red-cell enzyme abnormality can indicate the possible site of the enzyme defect.

2,3-DPG in stored red cells (see also Chapter 35)
It has been known for a long time that storage of blood at 4°C in acid-citrate dextrose (ACD) leads to a gradual decrease in levels of organic phosphates in the red cells [61], 2,3-DPG decreasing rapidly during the first week of storage, while ATP falls more slowly. In 1954, Valtis & Kennedy [62] showed that blood stored for more than seven days had a higher oxygen affinity than normal blood. The *in-vivo* restoration of 2,3-DPG and ATP levels in transfused cells has also been studied, and the results show that these reach 50% of the normal levels in approximately eight hours and repletion is complete within 24 hours [63], which corresponds to the finding that at this time the oxygen dissociation curve of transfused cells is normal [62]. These results indicate that the high oxygen affinity of stored cells is not of importance in most transfusions carried out. However, when large amounts of blood are given, as in exchange transfusions or during cardiac surgery, the raised oxygen affinity may lead to tissue hypoxia and therefore in these cases fresh blood should be used for this as well as for other reasons.

Recently, it has been shown that storage of blood in citrate-phosphate dextrose (CPD) [64] results in better maintenance of 2,3-DPG levels and hence an oxygen affinity nearer normal for the first two weeks. As there are no contraindications to CPD on other grounds, it and it is now widely used for blood storage. It has also been shown that it is possible to replete red-cell 2,3-DPG of stored blood *in vitro* by incubation with inosine, etc. However, these agents are too toxic for clinical use.

Therapeutic changes in oxygen affinity
Finally I want to consider whether it would be useful to change the oxygen affinity in certain clinical situations such as lung disease, angina pectoris, sickle-cell disease, etc. In this connection it has to be remembered that with an increased oxygen affinity the proportion of oxygen released from the red cells will be decreased, consequently the erythropoietin drive to the marrow will increase and the haemoglobin level will rise. Conversely with a decreased oxygen affinity the haemoglobin level in the blood will fall. Using these ideas one can attempt to predict what the effect of altering the oxygen affinity would be in various clinical conditions to see if these would be beneficial.

The inherited red-cell defects with a low oxygen affinity, such as PK deficiency and some abnormal haemoglobins, for example Hb Hammersmith, would benefit by an increase in O_2 affinity. In these the return to a normal oxygen affinity would increase the erythropoietin drive to the marrow and thus increase the red-cell mass. This group also contains sickle-cell disease. As the polymerization of Hb S leading to sickling is dependent on the production of a sufficient concentration of deoxyHb S in the cell, a shift of the oxygen dissociation curve to the left (increase in oxygen affinity) will reduce sickling by decreasing the deoxygenation of the red cells at tissue Po_2. However, the increase in packed cell volume which is known to occur would increase the viscosity problems if sickling did occur.

In angina or intermittent claudication a lowering of the oxygen affinity might be beneficial in that the proportion of oxygen released from the blood would be increased, thus improving the amount of exercise possible before the onset of symptoms. Unfortunately lowering of the oxygen affinity will reduce erythropoietin production and lower the haematocrit. The end result after two or three weeks would be a return of oxygen delivery to the pretreatment value. The only long-term advantage might be that the lower haematocrit would minimize any viscosity problems which were contributing to the clinical symptoms. In a patient with a haemoglobin of, for example, 16 g/dl a lowering to 12 g/dl with the same oxygen release to the tissues might be of some benefit.

The situation in obstructive airways disease, chronic renal disease and in neonatal problems of oxygen delivery is not clear. In respiratory disease a case could be made out of raising the oxygen affinity to increase oxygen loading in the lungs but this may reduce release in the capillaries. However, careful analyses, taking into account the arterial and venous oxygen tension in relation to the position of the *in-vivo* oxygen dissociation curve as already discussed, are necessary. The optimum position for each patient could be calculated and perhaps aimed for with appropriate treatment when this becomes available. In chronic renal disease a further lowering of oxygen affinity may be of benefit, providing that this does not lead to further anaemia due to suppression of the erythropoietin drive to the marrow.

Physiological roles of 2,3-DPG

Developmental changes
One of the problems in understanding the relatively high oxygen affinity of fetal as compared to adult red cells is that the oxygen dissociation of the corresponding haemolysates is similar, and studies of purified fetal

haemoglobin show that it has a *lower* affinity than purified Hb A. Recent work on the interaction of 2,3-DPG with Hb F has clarified the situation. Studies have shown that while the addition of small amounts of 2,3-DPG greatly reduces the oxygen affinity of Hb A, the effect on Hb F is relatively small (Fig. 8.7) [65]. As the concentrations of haemoglobin and 2,3-DPG in fetal and adult red cells are similar, fetal red cells end up with a higher oxygen affinity than adult red cells.

Altitude adaptation
One of the ways in which man adapts to altitude is by lowering the oxygen affinity of his red cells, thereby increasing the amount of oxygen released to the tissues by the circulating haemoglobin. In this condition, there is hypoxia and a respiratory alkalosis; both conditions tend to raise the level of 2,3-DPG, thus lowering the oxygen affinity of the red cells. *In vivo*, when allowance is made for the Bohr effect, the decrease in oxygen affinity is not so marked. Studies carried out at 5000 metres above sea level indicate that measurable changes of red-cell 2,3-DPG and oxygen affinity occur within a few hours and are maximal within 24–36 hours; on return to sea level, the changes are reversed [66].

Exercise
Although it has been postulated that 2,3-DPG plays a role in adaptation to exercise, the available data [67] suggest that it is not involved. In acute exercise no change in red-cell 2,3-DPG was observed, and this fits in well with the slow response of DPG to the changed physiological conditions already mentioned. A small rise in 2,3-DPG was seen after several weeks' training, but the effect of this was small compared to the Bohr and temperature effects which lower the oxygen affinity during exercise. There are no studies on 2,3-DPG changes during prolonged exercise.

Synthesis of haemoglobin
The synthesis of a complex protein like haemoglobin has a number of separable stages:
1 synthesis of messenger RNA (mRNA) in the nucleus (Chapter 9);
2 combination of the mRNA with the ribosomes, and the assembly of the polypeptide chains (Chapter 9);
3 synthesis of the haem group (Chapters 13 and 14);
4 assembly of the various types of polypeptide chains with the haem groups into the tetramer haemoglobin molecule.

The developmental changes in haemoglobins referred to in Chapter 3 and later in this chapter are (probably) due to switching on and off the production of the corresponding mRNA. For example, the synthesis of the ε chains of the embryonic haemoglobins is directed by the production of a specific mRNA. Synthesis of this chain virtually ceases at the 35 mm CR stage of development and presumably this is due to cessation of the production of the appropriate messenger, gamma-chain mRNA being produced instead. Similarly, the synthesis of γ chains ceases when no more γ mRNA is produced and the synthesis of β mRNA leads to the synthesis of β chains. The way in which the synthesis of the various mRNAs is controlled is not known, but it has been postulated that, as in bacteria, controller genes, associated with each structural gene, carry out this function. If such controller genes exist, an important question is what activates them. Several possible hypotheses can be advanced, and there are data to refute some of them. One possibility is that the site of erythropoiesis is important. The finding that Hb A can be produced by erythropoiesis in the liver and spleen and that bone-marrow cells can synthesize Hb F makes this idea unlikely. Another hypothesis is that the environment 'turns on' the relevant genes. Experiments attempting to control Hb F synthesis in bone-marrow culture by altering the environment have also been unsuccessful [68]. It is now known that when red-cell progenitor cells (BFU-E) (see Chapter 2) in adult bone marrow are cultured, Hb F synthesis is activated [69, 70]. How this is brought about is not understood at present. Another idea is that there is a 'time clock' which governs these changes and some support for this comes from studies of premature babies. These show that the change from Hb F to Hb A production is not influenced by the time of delivery but is related to the normal 40-week gestation period [71]. In this connection, it is of interest that in certain sheep the synthesis of a specific haemoglobin chain occurs when the marrow is stimulated with erythropoietin [72, 73]. From the clinical point of view the reactivation of Hb F production is important because this is one of the theoretical forms of treatment for sickle-cell disease and β thalassaemia major.

The initiation and assembly of the polypeptide chains on the ribosomes is described in detail in Chapter 9. In outline, the ribosome attaches itself to the mRNA at the end which codes for the N-terminal part of the polypeptide chain, a step called initiation. The correct amino-acid is delivered to the ribosome on the corresponding amino-acid transfer RNA (tRNA). This tRNA has a base sequence which matches that on the mRNA. As each amino acid is delivered to the ribosome the ribosome moves along the mRNA ready to receive the next amino acid. Each amino acid is cleaved from its tRNA and peptide bonded to the previous amino acid, thus assembling the polypeptide chain. Completion of the polypeptide chain is signalled by a terminating codon on the mRNA and the completed chain is then released from the ribosome.

From the above it can be seen that there are several ways in which the amount of polypeptide chain synthesized can be increased or decreased. The first has already been mentioned and is by altering the amount of functional mRNA made in the nucleus, and this is used to bring about the changes seen in development, and is also the probable site of the defect in thalassaemia (see Chapter 9). The number of chains made can also be influenced by adjusting the rate of initiation, the rate of assembly or the rate of release of polypeptide synthesis. There is some evidence that either iron or haem (or both) promote peptide chain initiation and polysome formation, in this way increasing globin synthesis [74–76]. Thus, in iron deficiency, the total number of polypeptide chains synthesized would be slowed down by reduced initiation. The rate of assembly of any particular polypeptide chain, once initiation has taken place, is probably constant and when they are complete they are released from the ribosomes. The rate of assembly of α chains is slightly faster than that of β chains [77]. It has been suggested that control of the release step alters the rate of chain production, but this has not been confirmed. One idea was that combination with haem was necessary for accelerated release of completed chains, but it appears that globin chains are released from the ribosomes [78, 79]. Another suggestion was that free β chains promoted the release of α chains or vice versa [80], but this appears unlikely because both α chains and β chains can be released from the ribosomes without combination with their partner chains [81, 82].

The haem group is synthesized by a number of enzymic steps from glycine and succinyl-CoA [83, 84] (see Chapters 13 and 14). Inherited abnormalities of haem synthesis do not result in deficiency of haem production and anaemia but cause disease because of the abnormal porphyrins produced. Formation of δ-aminolaevulinic acid (δ-ALA) by the enzyme δ-ALA synthetase is strongly inhibited by any uncombined haem present in the cell [85–88] and in thalassaemia, when globin synthesis is inhibited, excess accumulation of haem is prevented by this feedback mechanism.

Once all the constituent parts of haemoglobin have been synthesized, the tetramer haem-containing molecule can be assembled. The amino-acid sequence of each polypeptide chain is such that once synthesis is complete it takes up the conformation of the corresponding subunit [79]. This automatically generates the binding site for the haem group and the sites which cause α chains to combine with β chains. In the absence of haem, an $\alpha\beta$-globin dimer is formed and this is converted to the tetramer by combination with haem [90]. Thus, the addition of haem alters the conformation of globin, generating the correct structure at the α_1-β_2 contact. The α chains have a higher affinity for haem than the β chains. Thus, a half haem-containing molecule can be formed, $\alpha_2^{haem}\beta_2^0$, and this is already a tetramer [91]. The presence of haem and the partner polypeptide chain greatly stabilizes the molecule; thus α and β chains are less stable than $\alpha\beta$ globin, which is much less stable than the haem-containing tetramer. The separated haem-containing globins, Hb α or Hb β_4, are also much less stable than the complete tetramer and the α subunit is much less stable than the β subunit.

In the completed red cell, the number of α chains equals the number of β chains. This is largely achieved by the production of the right amount of mRNA of both types by the nucleus. However, a slight excess of α chains is synthesized and, as this chain is very unstable, any left over are destroyed. The integration of synthesis of the various parts of the haemoglobin molecule has been reviewed by several workers [92–94].

From the preceding paragraphs it can be seen that, although the constituent parts of the haemoglobin molecule, the α chain, the β chain and the haem groups, are synthesized separately, control mechanisms ensure that equal amounts of each are available. When haem is deficient, globin synthesis is slowed down by decreasing initiation of synthesis on the ribosomes while, when globin synthesis is deficient, as in thalassaemia, haem synthesis is slowed down by feedback inhibition of ALA synthase. The number of α and β chains are kept equal by destruction of the slight excess of α chains normally synthesized. When an excess of non-α chains is made these chains, although somewhat unstable, combine with haem groups to form haemoglobin tetramers without α chains, Hb β_4 (Hb H) or Hb γ_4 (Hb Bart's).

The genetic control of haemoglobin

Since the original work on the inheritance of haemoglobin S by Pauling and his colleagues [95] and by Beet [96] and Neel [97], many of the details of the genetic control of haemoglobin synthesis have been worked out. However, recent investigations show that the full

story is not yet known. In the forties, the dictum 'one protein one gene' was elaborated, but this is now known to be an over-simplification. We now know that there is one 'structural gene' for each polypeptide chain; associated with this is one (or more) controller gene, and if the protein has a prosthetic group, like the haem group in haemoglobin, a further set of genes would regulate its enzymic synthesis. For haemoglobin, very little is known about controller genes, and genetic abnormalities of haem synthesis give rise to the porphyrias and will not be dealt with here (see Chapters 9, 13 and 14). The present dicussions will, therefore, be largely limited to consideration of the structural loci for each of the polypeptide chains.

The original work on the abnormal haemoglobins showed allelism between the genes determining Hb S and Hb C [98], as well as Hb D, Hb E and Hb G [99], now all known to be variants with abnormal β chains. In contrast to these findings, the locus controlling the synthesis of Hb Hopkins-2, now known to have abnormal α chains, segregates independently [100, 101]. Thus there are independent loci controlling the synthesis of α and β chains of Hb A, and recent work has shown that the structural loci for the α chains are situated on chromosome 16 [102], while those for the β chains are on chromosome 11 [103].

The finding in a Hungarian family that some individuals synthesize three types of α chains indicates that there are two loci coding for α chains [104] (Fig. 8.9) and this has recently been confirmed by gene-mapping experiments [105] (see Chapter 9). In some other families [106–108] only one α locus is found because homozygotes for the α-chain abnormality, Hb Tongariki, do not make any normal α^A chains. This is likely to be due to deletion of one of the α chain loci rather than failure of the α-chain duplication to spread to the involved populations because the α-chain loci are also duplicated in many primates and other mammals [109–111]; and also the red cells of the carriers and homozygotes of Hb Tongariki have the stigmata of thalassaemia

Fig. 8.9. The genetic control of the synthesis of haemoglobin in an individual heterozygous for Hb J_α trait at one α and Hb G_α at the other α locus in one of the individuals reported from Hungary [104]. Three haemoglobins are found, Hb J_α and Hb G_α, the two α-chain variants, and Hb A. The amount of Hb A found was approximately twice that of each variant haemoglobin, consistent with its formation being due to two α genes.

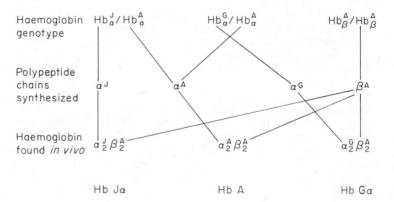

Haemoglobin genotype	Hb_α^J/Hb_α^A	Hb_α^G/Hb_α^A	Hb_β^A/Hb_β^A
Polypeptide chains synthesized	α^J α^A	α^G	β^A
Haemoglobin found *in vivo*	$\alpha_2^J\beta_2^A$	$\alpha_2^A\beta_2^A$	$\alpha_2^G\beta_2^A$
	Hb Jα	Hb A	Hb Gα

minor [108] (see also Chapter 9, p. 435). The finding that homozygotes for β-chain abnormalities, for example Hb S or Hb C, only make abnormal β chains, indicates that there is only one structural locus coding for β chains.

As each gene at each locus controls the synthesis of its own polypeptide chain, individuals who inherit one abnormal gene make two haemoglobins, Hb A and one containing the mutant chain involved. The demonstration of two α-chain structural loci leading to the synthesis of identical α chains is the reason that heterozygotes for α-chain variants, for example Hb_α^A/Hb_α^A, Hb_α^A/Hb_α^K, make only about 25% abnormal haemoglobin, the 75% Hb A formed being due to the presence of the three normal α^A genes [112, 113]. In individuals who have an α-chain variant with the second α locus on the same chromosome deleted, the amount of α-chain variant will be close to 50% as in Hb Tongariki [106–108] or Hb G Philadelphia heterozygotes [114]. As there is only one β-chain locus, the heterozygotes for β-chain variants therefore make close to 50% abnormal haemoglobin except when they are unstable [113] or in the presence of an α-thalassaemia gene (p. 436).

If a person inherits two abnormal genes, several situations can arise.

1 A person can inherit two abnormal genes of the same type as, for example, in the genotype Hb_α^A/Hb_α^A, Hb_β^C/Hb_β^C. In these subjects, only α^A and β^C chains are formed, and only Hb C ($\alpha_2^A\beta_2^C$) is found in the red cells.

2 When two different abnormal genes occur at the β locus, as, for example, in the genotype Hb_α^A/Hb_α^A, Hb_β^S/Hb_β^C, then α^A, β^S, and β^C chains are made, leading to the formation of only Hb S and Hb C.

3 If two different mutations occur, one at an α locus and one at the β locus, four different polypeptide chains are synthesized, leading to the formation of four haemoglobin species [114] (Fig. 8.10). In this connection, it is of interest that individuals with clinically severe sickle-cell anaemia have been reported who carry two abnormal haemoglobins [115, 116]. In these individuals there is homozygosity at the Hb_β locus for the β^S gene but heterozygosity at the Hb_α locus, giving the genotype Hb_α^A/Hb_α^G, Hb_β^S/Hb_β^S. Clearly, two haemoglobins, Hb S ($\alpha_2^A\beta_2^S$) and Hb G/S ($\alpha_2^G\beta_2^S$) will be made and, as both contain β^S chains, the patient has sickle-cell disease.

4 If the two mutations occur one on each α locus, two α-chain variants and Hb A will be formed [104].

HAEMOGLOBINS A₂ AND F AND THE EMBRYONIC HAEMOGLOBINS

The genetic control of synthesis of Hb A₂ and Hb F follows the same general pattern as that of Hb A. The α chains of normal human haemoglobins are all identical, arising from a common metabolic pool and thus are controlled by the same genetic locus (Fig. 8.11). Thus, abnormalities of α-chain synthesis affect not only Hb A, but also Hb A₂ and Hb F. Studies of several individuals synthesizing abnormal α chains have, in fact, shown that they carry not only the corresponding variant of Hb A but also those of Hb A₂, for example Hb G₂ ($\alpha_2^G\delta_2$) [117], and Hb F, for example Hb G/F ($\alpha_2^G\gamma_2$) [118] (Fig. 8.12). Thus any disease caused by abnormal α-chain synthesis, either α-thalassaemia or an α-chain mutant haemoglobin, will be manifest at birth, whereas disease arising due to β-chain abnormality will not be manifest at birth but develop after the first three months of life.

The non-α chain of Hb A₂, the δ chain, is controlled by its own genetic locus, and only 10 mutant haemoglobins affecting this polypeptide chain have been de-

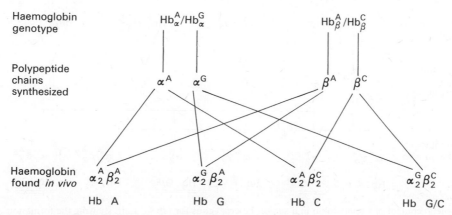

Fig. 8.10. The genetic control of the synthesis of haemoglobin in an individual heterozygous for the Hb C trait and the Hb G$_\alpha$ trait. The second normal α locus has been omitted for simplicity.

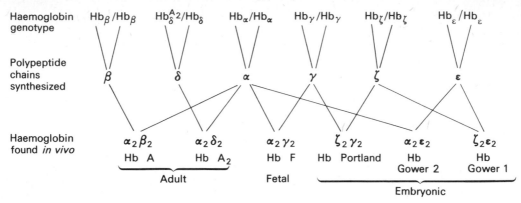

Fig. 8.11. The genetic control of the synthesis of normal adult haemoglobins, fetal haemoglobins, and the embryonic haemoglobins. The second normal α and γ loci have been omitted for simplicity.

scribed, and these are listed in Ref. 119. Some of them are quite common. Hb A_2' ($\alpha_2\delta_2^{16Gly\rightarrow Arg}$) [120] occurs in about two per cent of Negroes from certain regions of West Africa, while Hb Babinga ($\alpha_2\delta_2^{121Gly\rightarrow Asp}$) [121] occurs in about one per cent of Babinga Pygmies.

The reasons for the frequency of these variants are unknown.

Structural work on certain γ chain variants and on normal fetal haemoglobin from various sources has shown that there are two types of γ chains. These are similar, except for one amino-acid difference at position 136, one chain having a glycine residue while the other has alanine, and are called γ^{Gly} and γ^{Ala} chains. The reasons that these are not mutant haemoglobins but are caused by a duplication of the Hb γ locus are two-fold. First, analysis of normal Hb F reveals the presence of both alanine and glycine at position 136 in all samples. If this were an ordinary mutant, some homozygotes showing either alanine or glycine only

should be found. Secondly, mutant γ-chain haemoglobins show either alanine or glycine at position 136, indicating that they are mutations of either the γ^{Ala} or γ^{Gly} chains [122, 125]. The presence of two loci controlling γ-chain synthesis on chromosome 11 linked to the β locus has recently been confirmed by gene mapping (Fig. 8.13) (see p. 405). There are 16 known γ-chain variants equally distributed between the two types of chains [126]. From the structural point of view some might have abnormal oxygen dissociation properties, but these have not been studied. One cause of haemolytic disease of newborn is the presence of unstable γ-chain variants giving rise to haemolysis *in utero*, for example Hb F Poole ($^{G}\gamma^{Try\rightarrow Gly}$) [126a]. The presence of two loci controlling γ-chain synthesis explains the observation that γ-chain variants always occur at a proportion of less than 25% of total haemoglobin, there being three normal γ genes and one mutant gene.

Very little is known about the genetics of the

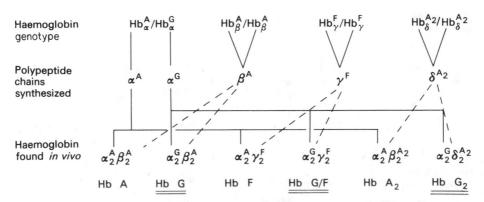

Fig. 8.12. The genetic control of haemoglobin in a subject heterozygous for Hb G_α trait, showing the formation of the three normal haemoglobins Hb A, Hb F and Hb A_2, as well as the corresponding α-chain variants Hb G, Hb G/F and Hb G_2. The second normal α and γ loci have been omitted for simplicity.

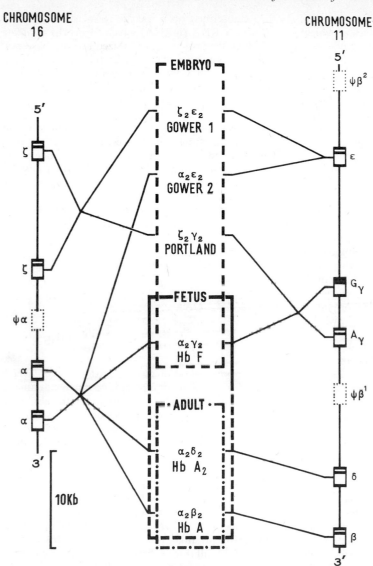

Fig. 8.13. Genetic control of globin-chain synthesis. The order of genes and distances between genes on each chromosome are as given in the literature (see Chapter 9). The dark stripes on each gene represent the DNA sequences coding for amino-acid sequences, the white part representing the non-coding inserts. (Data from Refs 102, 103, 105 and 128.) Recent studies indicate that the 'downstream' ζ locus is non-functional.

embryonic haemoglobins. The embryonic α-like chain, the ζ chain, has two structural loci closely linked to the α loci [105]. It is not known whether both are functional. The embryonic β-like chain, the ε chain, has a single structural locus closely linked to the γ- δ- β-gene cluster [128] (Fig. 8.13).

LINKAGE RELATIONSHIPS OF THE LOCI CONTROLLING HAEMOGLOBIN SYNTHESIS

Hb_α and Hb_β loci

Studies (see Ref. 129) of several families in which both α- and β-chain variants of Hb A are segregating show

that the locus controlling the synthesis of the α chains is not linked to that of the β chains. It has also been shown that neither locus is closely linked to genetic loci controlling certain blood or serum groups [130, 131].

Hb_β and Hb_δ loci

There are several families in which a Hb A_2 variant with abnormal δ chains segregates with a β-chain variant and no cross-overs have been detected, though this could have taken place in 61 opportunities [129, 131]. These family studies thus indicate that the locus controlling the synthesis of the δ chain is closely linked to that for the β chain.

Hb$_\beta$ and Hb$_\gamma$ loci

At the present time, no studies of families in which variants of both the γ and β chains occur have been reported. However, studies of families in which the β-chain variants Hb S or Hb C are segregating with a gene causing persistence of fetal haemoglobin, the so-called 'high-F gene', indicate that this gene is closely linked to the γ-chain locus [132, 133]. Further evidence for close linkage of the γ locus to the β locus comes from the occurrence of a 'fusion haemoglobin', Hb Kenya [134] with N-terminal γ-chain sequence and C-terminal β sequence. The results of these studies suggest that the order of genes on the chromosome is $^G\gamma$, $^A\gamma$, δ, β.

Chromosomal linkage of the Hb loci

Molecular genetic studies (see Chapter 9) have recently shown that the clusters of α-like genes are situated on chromosome 16 [102] while the cluster of β-like genes is on chromosome 11 [103]. Recent technical advances have made it possible to isolate each of the globin genes and study their structure and chromosomal organization, and Figure 8.13 outlines the present knowledge (see Chapter 9 for details).

During development, the synthesis of embryonic haemoglobin is succeeded by the synthesis of fetal haemoglobin which, in turn, is replaced by the adult haemoglobins, Hb A and Hb A$_2$, shortly after birth. This can be explained in terms of regulatory genes which control the rates of synthesis of various polypeptide chains, a concept derived from work in bacterial genetics. A mutation at one of these controller loci might result in changes in the rate of synthesis of a polypeptide chain without any alteration in its structure and it has been suggested that 'the hereditary persistence of fetal haemoglobin' and 'thalassaemia' are of this type (see Chapters 3 and 9). In this connection, it is of interest that arrangement of genes on the chromosome is in order of their appearance during development, the embryonic genes on the 5' side of the DNA, while the adult genes are nearer the 3' end, with the γ genes (fetal) in between (Fig. 8.13). The function of the pseudo [4] α and β chains is not known but may be related to the switch in mRNA production which occurs during haemoglobin development.

THE ABNORMAL HAEMOGLOBINS AND THE GENETIC CODE

In the genetic control of protein synthesis it is postulated that the amino-acid sequence of any protein is represented on the chromosome by a definite sequence of bases in the DNA. Each amino acid is coded for by three bases, and each 'code word' is specific for one amino acid, although there is often more than one 'code word' for each amino acid. This DNA code is then transcribed on a specific form of RNA called messenger RNA (mRNA) which forms the template on which the protein is synthesized by the ribosomes. There are a number of changes in the DNA which can give rise to abnormal haemoglobins, and virtually all postulated types of abnormality have been described.

Point mutations. These are the cause of most of the abnormal haemoglobins. In these there is a change of a single nucleotide base in the three-letter code word, and this results in a new code word at that position in the DNA, giving rise, in most cases, to a different amino acid in the polypeptide chain. The two substitutions at position 6 of the β chain: Glu→Val in Hb S and Glu→Lys in Hb C are typical examples of this:

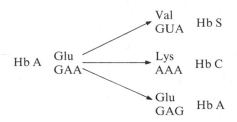

If the point mutation gives rise to a code word which codes for the same amino acid, no change in amino-acid sequence will, of course, result. In the abnormal haemoglobins all the differences described so far are single mutations of this type. Base changes can be of two types: purines (adenine, guanine) to pyrimidines (cytosine or thymidine), called transversions, or purine to purine and pyrimidine to pyrimidine, called transitions. In the abnormal haemoglobins there are more transitions than transversions [135].

There are three abnormal haemoglobins in which the valine $\beta67$ (E11) is substituted: Hb Sydney (Ala) [136], Hb Milwaukee (Glu) [137] and Hb Bristol (Asp) [138]. While all three substitutions can arise by single-step mutations from code words for valine, it is not possible to obtain codons for glutamic acid and aspartic acid starting from the same code word for valine. These (confirmed) findings can only be explained by the assumption, either that this is an example of a two-step base change or, more intriguingly, that there is polymorphism of this valyl codon [138].

Several haemoglobins with more than one point mutation have been described. In four of these, one is that of Hb S, namely $\beta6$, Glu→Val, while the second is $\beta73$ Asp→Asn in Hb C Harlem [139, 140], $\beta58$ Pro→Arg in Hb C Ziguinchor [14] and $\beta142$ Ala→Val in Hb S Travis [142], which also has a raised oxygen affinity. In Hb J Singapore the two substitutions are $\alpha78$ Asn→Asp and $\alpha79$ Ala→Gly [143], and in Hb

Table 8.2. Abnormal haemoglobins due to deletions; all are unstable

Leiden [145]	$\beta6$ (NA3) Glu deleted, high O_2 affinity
Lyon [146]	$\beta17$–18 (A14–15) Lys-Val deleted, high O_2 affinity
Freiburg [147]	$\beta23$ (B5) Gly deleted, high O_2 affinity
Niteroi [148]	$\beta42$–44 (CD1–CD3) Phe-Glu-Ser deleted, low O_2 affinity
Togichi [149]	$\beta56$–59 (D7–E3) Gly-Asn-Pro-Lys deleted
St Antoine [150]	$\beta74$–75 (E18–E19) Gly-Leu deleted, normal O_2 affinity
Tours [150]	$\beta87$ (F3) Thr deleted, high O_2 affinity
Gun Hill [151]	$\beta91$–95 (F7–FG2) Leu-His-Cys-Asp-Lys deleted, does not bind haem, high O_2 affinity
Leslie [152]	$\beta131$ (H9) Gln deleted, normal O_2 affinity
Coventry [153]	$\beta141$ (H19) Leu deleted
Mckees Rocks [650]	$\beta145$–146 (HC2–3) Tyr-His deleted

Arlington Park [144] they are $\beta6$ Val→Lys and $\beta95$ Lys→Glu.

Deletions and additions. Several abnormal haemoglobins have been described which are due to deletions (Table 8.2). All these are unstable and several have a raised oxygen affinity.

Several haemoglobins have been described with additions at the C-terminal end. Three of these, Hb Constant Spring [154], Hb Icaria [155] and Hb Koya Dora [156] are due to point mutations of the terminator codon of the α chain, give rise to α thalassaemia and are common (see Chapter 9, p. 435). Hb Wayne [157] is due to a deletion of a single nucleotide of codon 139, giving rise to an altered and extended sequence of the α chain. Hb Tak [158] is an addition to the β chain with a raised oxygen affinity, and Hb Cranston [159] has two altered C-terminal amino acids and an extended chain; it is unstable.

Hb Grady [160] is due to an insertion of three amino acids, Glu–Phe–Thr, between amino acids 118 and 119 of the α chain; it is unstable and has a raised oxygen affinity.

Unequal crossing over. The Lepore-type haemoglobins consist of the N-terminal part of the δ chain joined to the C-terminal part of the β chain, the total length of the Lepore chain (or $\delta\beta$ chain) being 146 amino acids, like the β chain (see also Chapter 9). Three types of Hb Lepore have been reported with different δ- and β-chain content, and all give rise to a form of β-thalas-

saemia trait [161–163]. These abnormal haemoglobins are thought to be due to a non-homologous crossing over between chromosomes (Fig. 8.14). On this hypothesis one should also find the so-called 'anti-Lepore' haemoglobins; Hb P [164], Hb Miyada [165] and Hb P Nilotic [166] are of this type. The family with Hb P reported by Dherte *et al.* [167] had one individual who carried both Hb A and Hb S as well as Hb P. This individual, therefore, showed the extra β locus expected with an anti-Lepore type haemoglobin (see Fig. 8.14).

A cross-over between the β and γ (Ala) loci has also been described [168]. This leads to the formation of Hb Kenya. These types of mutations are discussed further in Chapter 9, p. 425.

Developmental changes in haemoglobins

In development there are three phases during which the conditions of loading and unloading of oxygen from haemoglobin vary. From birth onwards oxygen is transported by the red cells from the lungs to the tissues; in the fetus the uptake of oxygen is via the placenta, whilst in the embryo, before the placenta is fully functional, oxygen is obtained from the maternal interstitial fluid. Studies of the haemoglobin found in these three stages of development have shown that each stage is associated with its own type of pigments. Thus, during early development embryonic haemoglobins are found; these are then replaced by fetal haemoglobin (Hb F). After birth, Hb F is replaced by the

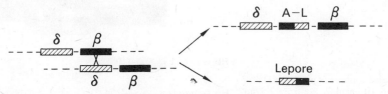

Fig. 8.14. Schematic representation of the postulated non-homologous cross-over leading to the formation of the Lepore and anti-Lepore (A-L) genes. (Modified from Ref. 161.)

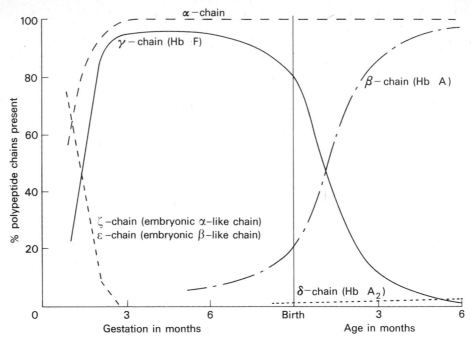

Fig. 8.15. The developmental changes in human haemoglobin chains.

adult pigments, Hb A and Hb A$_2$ (Fig. 8.15). (For review see Ref. 169.)

THE EMBRYONIC HAEMOGLOBINS

There are three embryonic haemoglobins: Hb Gower 1, Hb Gower 2 and Hb Portland 1 (Fig. 8.16). Hb Gower 1 and 2 are replaced by Hb F by the 10th week of pregnancy. Hb Portland 1 migrates on electrophoresis slightly anodally to Hb A, and there is some difficulty in separating these two pigments. In all samples so far studied, Hb F has also been found but in the smallest embryo (1·6 cm CR) this amounted to only about 20% of total haemoglobin. Beta-chain (i.e. Hb A) synthesis can be detected at six weeks' gestation

[170] and the presence of Hb A in the very large embryonic red cells of presumed yolk-sac origin has been shown immunologically [171].

Structure of the embryonic haemoglobins. There are two polypeptide chains specific to the embryonic period, the ε chains and the ζ chains; α chains and γ chains are also found. Hb Gower 2 has the structure $\alpha_2\varepsilon_2$ [172]; Hb Portland, $\zeta_2\gamma_2$ [173] and Hb Gower 1, $\zeta_2\varepsilon_2$ [174]. It is therefore clear that the ζ chain is the embryonic α-like chain, while the ε chain is the embryonic β-like chain. The sequence of the ε chain [174, 175] shows that it differs from the β chain at about 32 positions and from the γ chain by about 25

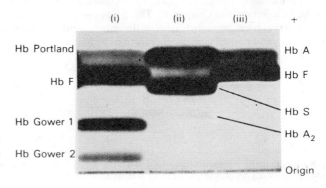

Fig. 8.16. Starch-gel electrophoresis in a tris-EDTA-borate buffer, pH 8·6: (i) haemolysate from 3·5 cm (CR) human embryo; (ii) Hb A + S marker; (iii) normal cord blood. (From Ref. 129.)

residues. Most of the changes are conservative and the ε chain is neither more β- or γ-like; it contains two fewer histidines, ε77 (E20) is Asn, ε116 (G18) is Thr and there is an extra lysine at ε87 (F3). The 2,3-DPG-binding site is β-like and the Bohr residues, Val 1 (NA1), His 2 (NA2), His 143 (H21) and His 146 (HC3), are preserved.

The ζ chains differ from the α chains by 50–60 residues [176], containing four more arginines and three less histidines than the α chains. The N terminal is acetylated, presumably affecting the Bohr shift, while His ζ122 (H5) is present.

Oxygen dissociation studies on red cells containing the embryonic haemoglobin suspended in isotonic phosphate buffer, pH 7·1, showed a similar oxygen affinity to cord-blood red cells; the Bohr shift and haem–haem interactions were normal [177]. However, studies of animal embryonic red cells and haemolysates [178, 179] suggested that the Bohr shift below pH 7·0 differed from that of adult or fetal red cells and studies on Hb Portland were consistent with this [180]. Studies on human embryonic red cells suggest that between pH 7·0 and pH 6·7 there is very little change in oxygen affinity or a weak *reversed* Bohr shift [181]. As has already been discussed (p. 336), the low arterial and tissue partial pressures of oxygen which can be assumed in the embryo before the placenta is functional, together with a low oxygen affinity, would give less delivery of oxygen than when a higher oxygen affinity is present. This reversed Bohr shift at pH 7·0 would prevent the oxygen affinity falling to extremely low levels. It also implies that perhaps the prevailing pH in the embryo is lower than in the mother or in the fetus when the placenta is functional.

FETAL HAEMOGLOBIN

Structure of fetal haemoglobin

The structure of fetal haemoglobin, or Hb F, is $\alpha_2\gamma_2$, the α chains being identical to those of Hb A. As mentioned earlier, there are two types of γ chain: one with Gly at position 136, the other with Ala. The γ chain differs from the β chain in 39 amino-acid residues (Table 8.1). The reason for most of these is not clear, and many are conservative or minor (i.e. the exchange of one amino acid for another of similar type) but include the substitution of the Tyr at 130 (H8) by Try, which accounts for the different spectral properties of Hb F. There are four differences in the $\alpha_1\beta_2$ contact. These presumably account for the lower affinity of γ chains compared to β chains for α chains [127].

Haemoglobin F₁. When haemolysates containing Hb F are examined by chromatography on IRC 50, a component called Hb F₁, amounting to about 10% of the total Hb, is regularly resolved [182], and this differs from Hb F in that the terminal amino groups of its γ chains are blocked by an acetyl group [183]. The functions of these haemoglobins with blocked terminal NH_2 groups are not known, but may be related to the carriage of CO_2 and reduction of the binding of 2,3-DPG [184, 19].

Haemoglobin γ₄ (see also Chapter 9, pp. 429 and 430) Haemoglobin γ₄, also called 'fast fetal haemoglobin' or Hb Barts, consists of the four normal γ chains of Hb F, each containing a single haem group [185, 186]. It is easily detected by electrophoresis and migrates more rapidly to the anode than either Hb A or Hb F, to a position behind Hb H (Hb β_4) (Fig. 8.17). In normal cord bloods at term, 0·2–0·3% of total haemoglobin is Hb γ₄. In early fetal and embryonic life, one to three per cent of Hb γ₄ is often found, but the amounts are very variable. Increased amounts of Hb γ₄ in cord blood are due to α thalassaemia. Oxygen dissociation studies [187] of Hb γ₄ show that it has a very high oxygen affinity, $P_{50} \simeq 3$ mmHg, in 0·1 M phosphate buffer pH 7·0, with absent haem–haem interactions ($n = 1·08$) and Bohr effect. In the red cell, Hb γ₄ oxygenates independently from Hb A or Hb F [188].

Function of fetal haemoglobin

Fetal red cells transport oxygen from the placenta to the fetal tissues. The higher oxygen affinity of fetal blood compared to maternal blood helps the transport of oxygen across the placenta. This difference in oxygen affinity is accentuated by the changes in pH which occur in the blood of the mother and fetus during gas exchange. As the maternal blood becomes more acid, its oxygen affinity decreases, thus releasing more oxygen, while the fetal blood becomes more alkaline with an increase in oxygen affinity. At the same time, the reverse is true for CO_2, and this is transferred from the fetus to the mother. The difference in oxygen affinity, although advantageous to the fetus, is not essential to its survival, as intra-uterine transfusion is a successful treatment for severe intra-uterine haemolytic disease due to rhesus antibodies.

The P_{O_2} of the blood leaving the placenta in the fetal vein is about 30–40 mmHg, and the P_{O_2} in the fetal tissues can be as low as 15 mmHg. These values correspond to oxygen saturations in the region of 80 and 30% respectively, indicating that over half the bound oxygen can be abstracted from the blood. Taking the high haemoglobin values of fetal blood into consideration, these figures imply that the amount of oxygen which can be delivered to the tissues by each ml of blood is about twice that achieved in the adult. For a detailed review of placental oxygen transport see Refs 189 and 190.

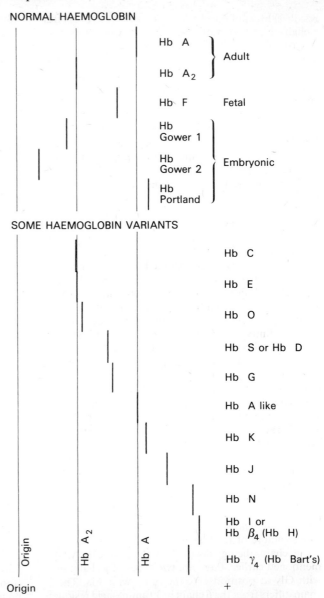

Fig. 8.17. Relative electrophoretic mobility of human haemoglobins on starch-gel electrophoresis in tris-EDTA-borate buffer, pH 8·6. Note that Hb S runs half-way between Hb A and Hb A₂, and Hb J is ahead of Hb A by approximately the same amount as Hb S is behind.

The higher oxygen affinity of fetal blood compared to that of adult blood is due to a difference in interaction of 2,3-DPG with Hb F compared to that with Hb A. 2,3-DPG binds less strongly to Hb F than Hb A [191]. This difference in 2,3-DPG binding is due to the substitution of histidine $\beta143$ (H21) present in Hb A by serine in Hb F. For this reason the effect on oxygen affinity of equal amounts of 2,3-DPG is much less marked with Hb F than with Hb A. Hb F without 2,3-DPG has a lower oxygen affinity than Hb A [192, 193]. The addition of small amounts of 2,3-DPG

greatly reduces the oxygen affinity of Hb A, whilst the effect on Hb F is relatively small (Fig. 8.17) [65]. As the concentrations of haemoglobin and 2,3-DPG in fetal and adult red cells are similar fetal red cells have a higher oxygen affinity than adult red cells.

Other properties of Hb F distinguishing it from Hb A

Resistance to alkali. The most familiar property of Hb F which distinguishes it from Hb A is its higher resistance to denaturation by alkali, and this led to its discovery by Körber in 1866. Many workers have used this property for the measurement of Hb F in blood as it is almost 100% specific [194, 195]. Two abnormal haemoglobins, Hb Cyprus 2 [196] and Hb Rainier [197], are more resistant to alkali than Hb A; carbonmonoxyhaemoglobin is also alkali resistant.

Spectroscopy. The parts of the spectra of Hb A and Hb F due entirely to the haem groups, i.e. from about 350 to 650 nm, are identical [198]. In the ultraviolet region of the spectrum the tryptophan fine structure band at about 290 nm is resolved in Hb F while in Hb A it is an unresolved inflection.

Electrophoresis. Hb F is difficult to separate from Hb A on paper and moving-boundary electrophoresis, but satisfactory separation can be achieved on starch or agar gel [199]. On starch-gel electrophoresis, satisfactory resolution can be achieved using a tris-EDTA-borate buffer system (Fig. 8.18).

Chromatograpy. Hb F can be satisfactorily resolved by various forms of ion-exchange chromatography: DEAE-Sephadex A50 [200], IRC 50 [182] and CM-Sephadex [201, 202].

Separation of the α and γ chains of Hb F. The best method of separating the α- and γ-globin chains of Hb F is by chromatography on CM cellulose [204] or CM Sepharose 6B [205], which also resolve the γ from the β chains. These systems are used in the antenatal diag-nosis of thalassaemia or sickle-cell disease (see p. 440 and Chapter 9). The $^{Gly}\gamma$- and $^{Ala}\gamma$-globin chains can be separated by polyacrylamide electrophoresis. This system also resolves α, β, ζ and ε chains [206].

The detection of intracellular Hb F. In 1957, Kleihauer and his colleagues [207] showed that Hb F was eluted much more slowly than Hb A from fixed blood films, using citrate buffers at pH 3·2, and this has made possible the detection and measurement of Hb F in individual cells. Hb F can also be detected by immunofluorescence using an anti-γ-globin antibody [208]. This method is more sensitive than the elution technique and up to five per cent of cells in normal adults are positive. At low levels the percentage Hb F correlates with the number of 'F' cells.

Disappearance of Hb F

The proportion of Hb F in fetal blood reaches a maximum of about 95% of total haemoglobin during the second three months of pregnancy and begins to fall from about 34 weeks' gestational age. In cord blood of full-term infants it forms 70–90% of total haemoglobin. After birth, Hb F continues to fall and has virtually disappeared from the red cells within 12 months of birth (Fig. 8.19 and Table 8.3).

The Hb F percentage at birth is closely related to time of gestation, those neonates with more Hb F being more premature and vice versa [52]. After 40 weeks' gestation the fall of Hb F is relatively rapid and follow-up of individual children shows the curves to be

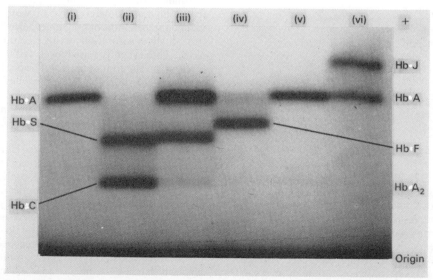

Fig. 8.18. Starch-gel electrophoresis in a tris-EDTA-borate buffer, pH 8·6: (i) normal adult haemolysate; (ii) Hb S + C; (iii) Hb A + S; (iv) normal cord haemolysate; (v) normal adult haemolysate; (vi) Hb A + J. (From Ref. 203.)

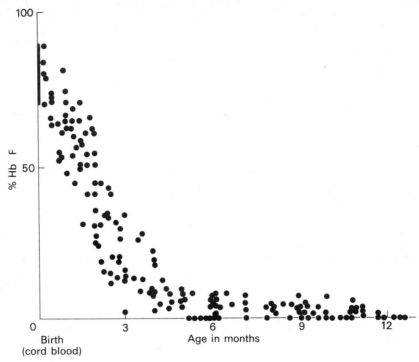

Fig. 8.19. Amounts of Hb F in the blood of normal infants of various ages to show the wide variation of levels found. (From Ref. 169.)

Table 8.3. Proportion of Hb F found at various ages

Age	Hb F (%)
Birth	70–90
1 month	50–75
2 months	25–60
3 months	10–35
4 months	5–20
6 months	<8
9 months	<5
1 year	<2
Adults	not detectable (<0·4)

detected by the usual methods; trace amounts can be demonstrated by immunological techniques [208] but these rarely exceed 0·4% of total haemoglobin [209].

Small amounts of fetal haemoglobin have also been found in approximately 10% of women during the second three months of pregnancy, using either a sensitive alkali denaturation or an immunological technique. These slightly raised levels fall to normal adult levels in the last trimester [210]. The occasional finding of high Hb F levels in late pregnancy may indicate transplacental fetal haemorrhage, but this is best detected by looking for fetal red cells in the maternal circulation by the acid elution technique.

Fetal haemoglobin in disease (see also Chapter 9, p. 444) The occurrence of Hb F in disease can be due to either the delayed disappearance of Hb F or the re-activation of γ-chain synthesis. Delayed disappearance is seen in all haemoglobinopathies affecting the synthesis of the β chains. With the non-pathological abnormal haemoglobins in the heterozygous state this is minor, and levels of less than two per cent are reached by the age of two to three years [211]. With the unstable haemoglobins, which cause haemolytic anaemia in the heterozygous state, small amounts (two to three per cent) of Hb F can still be detected in most affected adults (author's

parallel. The fall off in Hb F in premature babies is the same as would have occurred if the pregnancy had continued to full term [52].

In normal infants most of the Hb F present in the blood disappears by about six months but small amounts may be found up to one year of age. After this age. Hb F is difficult to detect, although in a small proportion of apparently normal children more than one per cent is found [20]. In adults, Hb F cannot be unpublished observations). In the homozygous hae-moglobinopathies, Hb F is often found in adults, par-ticularly in sickle-cell disease. In β thalassaemia, Hb F disappears much more slowly than in normal infants, but the final level attained in the affected adult depends on the particular type of genes involved; and this is discussed in Chapter 9.

Other inherited conditions are the so called 'high Hb F genes' which do not cause any disease (see also Chapter 9, p. 425). In one of these conditions, the 'Negro-type high Hb F gene', Hb F amounts to about 20–30% of total haemoglobin in the heterozygous form [133, 212, 213]. In this condition the fetal haemoglobin is uniformly distributed in the red cells [130, 214]. This contrasts with the finding of uneven Hb F distribution in the red cells in the other conditions mentioned above, such as sickle-cell anaemia [215] or thalassae-mia [216] where the persistence of Hb F is not the direct result of the genetic abnormality. The homozygous condition of the 'Negro-type high Hb F gene' leads to 100% Hb F in the red cells with only minor haemato-logical abnormality [217–219].

Two other types of inherited persistence of fetal haemoglobin have been described. One occurs in 0·25% of Greeks [220] and these individuals carry 11–18% Hb F without any other haematological ab-normalities; the Hb F is evenly distributed in the red cells. The other occurs in about one per cent of the population of southern Switzerland and here only two to three per cent Hb F is found without any other clinical or haematological abnormality [221, 222].

There is also a delay in the disappearance of Hb F in some chromosomal abnormalities [223–225] as well as in some congenital haemolytic anaemias not asso-ciated with haemoglobinopathy. In the latter condi-tions, the amount of Hb F found after the first year of life does not often exceed five per cent and only trace amounts are found in adults [209].

The reappearance of Hb F occurs in chronic granu-locytic leukaemia in children under the age of five years and may amount to 50% of total haemoglobin [226, 227]. In adult patients with leukaemia, small increases in Hb F are occasionally found, which presumably indicates that the red-cell precursors, as well as the white-cell series, are involved in the malignant process. Bromberg and colleagues [228] report a significantly raised Hb F in four patients with a molar pregnancy. A raised Hb F has also been reported in aplastic anaemia [229]. In all these patients, Hb F is unevenly distributed in the red cells. In pernicious anaemia, Hb F is present in small amounts (one to two per cent) in approxi-mately half the patients examined, and the proportion of this pigment often rises shortly after the commence-ment of treatment with vitamin B_{12} [209].

Iron deficiency, acquired haemolytic anaemias, and congenital cyanotic heart disease [230, 231a] are not associated with a raised Hb F (see also Chapter 9, p. 444).

ADULT HAEMOGLOBINS

As Hb F disappears from the red cells after birth, its place is taken by the adult haemoglobins Hb A and the minor component Hb A_2. Hb A has the structure $\alpha_2\beta_2$, and the amino-acid sequence of these chains is given in Table 8.1.

Haemoglobin A_2 (Hb A_2) occurs in every (normal) individual and amounts to 1·5–3·2% of total haemo-globin [231b–234]. The structure of Hb A_2 is $\alpha_2\delta_2$, the α chains being identical to those in Hb A [95]; the δ chain contains 146 amino acids and differs by only 10 amino acids from the β chain (Table 12.1). The level of Hb A_2 is increased in β thalassaemia (Chapter 9, p. 421), malaria [235], pernicious anaemia in relapse [236], and with some unstable haemoglobins [237]. In some con-ditions, like aplastic anaemia or erythroleukaemia, Hb A_2 may occasionally be raised or diminished [238]. In iron deficiency, Hb A_2 is lower than normal [239, 240]; low levels are also found in association with 'heredi-tary persistence of Hb F' (p. 444) and α thalassaemia (Chapter 9, p. 435). The function of Hb A_2 is not known; its oxygen dissociation properties are similar to those of Hb A [241]. It is easily separated from Hb A and Hb F by electrophoresis (Fig. 8.17). It is estimated by either electrophoresis on cellulose acetate [241a] or column chromatography [241b].

THE HAEMOGLOBINOPATHIES

The haemoglobinopathies which are caused by struc-tural abnormalities of haemoglobin comprise the fol-lowing:
1 sickle-cell disease;
2 the homozygous haemoglobinopathies: Hb C dis-ease, Hb E disease;
3 haemoglobins with abnormal functions: increased oxygen affinity, decreased oxygen affinity, Hb M; and
4 unstable haemoglobins (some with abnormal oxygen dissociation).

There are also many abnormal haemoglobins which are not associated with any disease [242]. Most of these have only been seen in the heterozygous state and whether they would cause disease in homozygotes is not known. Besides these inherited conditions there are also a few acquired abnormalities, such as methae-moglobinaemia, sulphaemoglobinaemia, and carbon-monoxy (CO) haemoglobinaemia.

Sickle-cell disease

Sickle-cell disease is a severe haemolytic disorder caused by the homozygous occurrence of the abnormal haemoglobin, Hb S.

General description

The haemolytic process is associated with repeated vaso-occlusive episodes leading to infarcts which give rise to painful crises and to the chronic degenerative changes seen as the disease progresses. As Hb S has abnormal β chains, the disease is not present at birth but appears only three to six months later as γ-chain (Hb F) synthesis is replaced by β-chain synthesis, in this case β^S chains. Once the disease is established, haemolysis due to the sickling process is present constantly and gives rise to chronic anaemia. Life expectancy in sickle-cell disease is definitely shortened. In primitive conditions in Africa most homozygous sicklers die in infancy, but with medical care and improved social conditions many now survive to adult life, and in the West Indies, North America and England patients in their thirties and forties or even older are often encountered. The commonest cause of death at all ages is infection.

Haematological findings. In the steady state, the haemoglobin level is approximately 7–8 g/dl with a normal MCHC; reticulocytes usually amount to 10%. The blood film shows some variation in size and shape of the red cells, with some sickle forms. The white-cell count is usually normal or slightly raised but there may be occasional normoblasts in the peripheral blood. The platelet count is normal or elevated, although it may fall during a crisis. The red-cell survival is variable but significantly shortened, the ^{51}Cr-labelled red-cell $T_{\frac{1}{2}}$ being around 10 days.

As in all haemolytic states, the haemoglobin level may fall due to depression of the bone marrow by intercurrent minor infections, but rapidly regains the steady-state level. At this time, the reticulocyte count is very much increased. The bone marrow is expanded to keep pace with the haemolysis, and bossing of the skull due to widening of the diploic spaces by invasion with erythropoietic bone marrow is sometimes seen. More severe anaemia may also be due to the usual causes of anaemia—haemorrhage, iron deficiency, malignancies, renal failure and other chronic diseases.

The diagnosis is made by demonstrating sickling of the red cells after reduction of the haemoglobin (Fig. 8.20). This test is prone to false negatives [244], and a more reliable demonstration of sickle haemoglobin is made by showing the insolubility of the deoxygenated haemoglobin in certain phosphate butters. This can now be done quickly and reliably using either commercially available kits, such as the 'Sickledex' test (Ortho) or more cheaply by making one's own [245, 246]. Neither the sickling test nor the solubility test differentiates between the different forms of sickling, and for

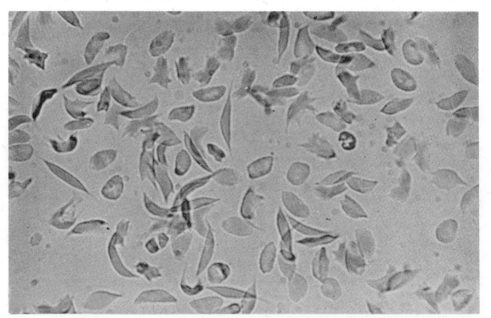

Fig. 8.20. Homozygous sickle-cell disease, deoxygenated blood showing sickled cells.

this starch-gel (or some other form of) electrophoresis should be carried out. In sickle-cell disease the major haemoglobin is Hb S; no Hb A is present and the amount of Hb A_2 is normal. All cases of sickle-cell disease carry some Hb F, and this can vary from two to 25% of total haemoglobin with the high levels usually being present in young patients.

Distribution of the sickling gene

The distribution of the sickle gene is shown in Figure 8.21. It can be seen that sickling occurs in tropical Africa, with a lower incidence in the Mediterranean region, southern Arabia and India. The incidence of the gene varies enormously, reaching a maximum of 40% in Amba on the slopes of Mount Ruwenzori in Uganda. It also occurs in emigré populations such as the American and West Indian Negroes.

It has been postulated that sickle-cell trait protects against death from falciparum malaria and in general the distribution of the trait with malaria fits this hypothesis. Because sickle-cell disease causes death in childhood under primitive conditions, it would be expected that considerable protection against death from malaria would be needed to balance the loss of sickle-cell genes. Although such studies are very difficult to carry out, the collected results of a number of investigators lend strong support to the malaria hypothesis. These show that among patients dead from cerebral malaria only one with sickle-cell trait was found, whereas 23 patients with this trait were expected, a highly significant finding ($\chi^2 = 20.5$; $p < 0.001$) [248].

The way in which sickle-cell trait protects against malaria is not known, but it is suggested that parasitation of the red cells containing Hb S causes them to sickle and leads to their destruction. In this way the life cycle of the parasite is cut short, and hyperinfection, necessary for the development of the fatal complications of malaria (i.e. cerebral malaria), is prevented [249]. More detailed studies of the mechanism involved have recently been reported [250].

The sickling process

The molecular abnormality causing sickling is in the β chains of adult haemoglobin, the glutamic acid which occurs in the sixth position from the N terminus being replaced by a valine. The structural formula of Hb S can be written Hb $\alpha_2^A \beta_2^{6 \text{ Val}}$ [251]. This amino-acid side chain occurs on the surface of the molecule, one on each of the β chains. Because of the symmetry of the molecule these side chains are on opposite sides of the molecule.

Sickling of the red cells is caused by the aggregation of deoxy Hb S molecules into long, straight fibres, which deform the red cell. Many aspects of the structure of these fibres are now understood from various

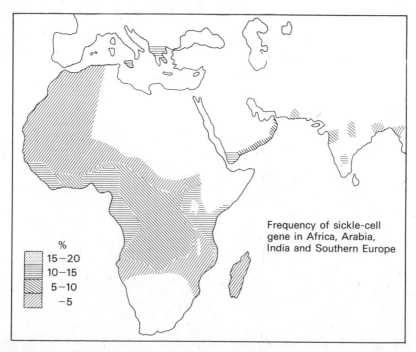

%
15–20
10–15
5–10
–5

Frequency of sickle-cell gene in Africa, Arabia, India and Southern Europe

Fig. 8.21. Frequency of the sickle-cell gene Hb$_{\beta^S}$ in various parts of the Old World. (From Ref. 247.)

electron-microscopic [252] and X-ray diffraction [253, 254] studies; it has also been shown that the structure of the fibre in the red cell corresponds closely to that derived from the other studies [255]. The sickle fibre (Fig. 8.22) consists of seven filaments twisted together. Each filament is made up of two linear threads of molecules. The details of some of the contacts between molecules are known from the X-ray diffraction studies and correspond closely to the results obtained

from gelling studies of Hb S in the presence of other haemoglobins [256, 257]. It is of interest that in the build up of the fibre, only one of the two $\beta6$ valines, the sickle amino-acid substitution, is involved in a contact. These fibres of deoxy Hb S become orientated in the same direction in the cell, several of them joining together to form sheets or bundles which deform the red cell to give it its sickle-shaped appearance. When sickle haemoglobin is oxygenated and the molecules take up

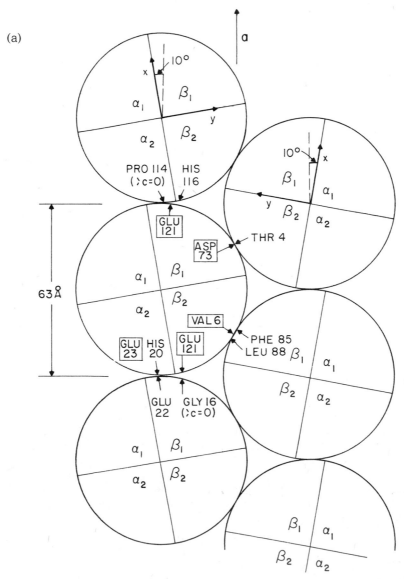

Fig. 8.22. The structure of the sickle fibre. The sickle fibre consists of seven filaments twisted together, each filament being made up of two linear threads of haemoglobin molecules. (a) The contacts between molecules in the filaments. (From Ref. 253.)

the oxy-conformation, the fit between molecules is destroyed and the filaments and fibres break up.

The way in which polymerization takes place is of importance in understanding the sickling process and has some bearing on the management of the disease. In order for polymerization to take place, the deoxy Hb S concentration must exceed a certain minimum; below this the sickle fibres do not form and sickling in red cells does not occur. In *in-vitro* experiments the minimum gelling concentration is about 17 g/dl at 37°C in the standard conditions used in our laboratory [260]. When the concentration of deoxy Hb S exceeds the minimum gelling concentration, polymer formation takes place. The formation of the polymer only starts at a finite time after deoxygenation has taken place, but then is rapidly completed [261]. The occurrence of this so-called lag phase, measured by the delay time, is thought to be due to the formation of small aggregates of deoxy Hb S molecules until these exceed a certain concentration, when rapid fibre formation and sickling

takes place. The length of the delay time (lag phase) is an important parameter in determining the propensity of a solution of deoxy Hb S to gel. This is greatly affected by the concentration of deoxy Hb S; the higher this is, the shorter the lag phase, and increase in deoxy Hb S concentration from 34 to 35 g/dl halves the lag phase. This, of course, will make sickling of the red cell take place more quickly. *In vivo*, the rate of sickling is clearly important in determining whether infarction will take place, because if cells can complete their circulation in less than the delay time, they cannot sickle, as they are reoxygenated in the lungs. Obviously any increase in circulation time due to stasis, for example in the spleen, will make sickling more likely.

The concentration of deoxy Hb S also increases the strength of the final gel or the rigidity of the sickle cell [262]. This is because the concentration of haemoglobin in the polymer is very high, about 53 g/dl [256] and as polymer is formed, the concentration of the soluble haemoglobin is reduced until its reaches the minimum

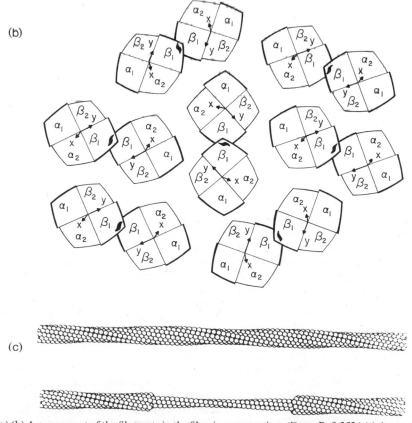

Fig. 8.22 (*cont.*) (b) Arrangement of the filaments in the fibre in cross section. (From Ref. 252.) (c) Arrangement of the fibre, top: complete, bottom: with the outer filaments stripped away to show the core. (From Ref. 252.)

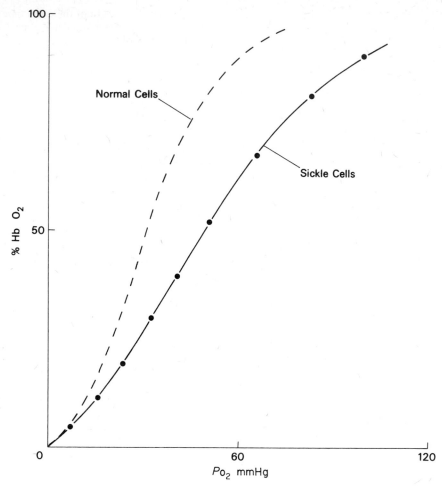

Fig. 8.23. Oxygen dissociation of red cells from a patient with homozygous sickle-cell disease, isotonic phosphate buffer, pH 7·1, 37°C.

gelling concentration, when no further polymer can form. Clearly if the MGC is 17 g/dl, more polymer will form when the deoxy Hb S concentration is, say, 30 g/dl, than when it is only 22 g/dl. Changes in the MGC will also affect the final concentration of polymer.

Factors which affect polymer formation are pH and temperature. A reduction in pH of 0·3 units will decrease the delay time by half [261, 263] and also reduce the minimum gelling concentration. Small increases in temperature act similarly: an increase in temperature from 37°C to 38·5°C halves the delay time. *In vivo*, besides these direct effects on polymer formation by pH and temperature, the associated lowering of oxygen affinity would increase the concentration of deoxy Hb S in the cells, further enhancing sickling.

One factor which reduces sickle polymer formation is the presence of another haemoglobin. However, all

haemoglobins do not act equally, as their ability to take part in polymer formation with Hb S varies. All haemoglobins in the oxy (R) conformation are virtually excluded from the polymer [264]. Neither does Hb A$_2$ take part in polymer formation [260, 265], while deoxy Hb F can be included in the polymer to some extent, and Hb A is included to a somewhat greater extent [260, 266, 267]. In the red cell, equal amounts of these haemoglobins would all inhibit sickling but Hb A$_2$ would be the most effective, followed by Hb F and then Hb A.

For this reason, the presence of Hb F in the red cells causes a significantly milder disease [268]. Also, as the Hb F distribution in the cells is not uniform, the sickle red cells with the most Hb F have the longest survival [269]. The reason that the presence of Hbs S and C in the red cells gives rise to a mild form of sickle-cell disease (p. 361), while Hbs A and S (sickle-cell trait) does not (p. 364) is because the hybrid $\alpha_2\beta^S\beta^C$ is incorporated in the polymer to the same extent as Hb S itself while the hybrid $\alpha_2\beta^A\beta^S$ is intermediate between Hb S and Hb A [260, 265].

The different degree various haemoglobins are incorporated into the polymer is related to the position of the amino-acid differences from Hb S and the contact regions between molecules in the polymer. This area has recently been reviewed [257]. With Hb O Arab $\beta^{(121\ Lys)}$ and Hb D Punjab $\beta^{(121\ Gln)}$, the substitution is at such a contact, but in these cases polymer formation is enhanced; the double heterozygotes Hb S+O [270, 271] and Hb S+D [325, 327] have a severe form of sickling. On the other hand, the presence of a second amino substitution in the β^S chain at β^{73} as in Hb C Harlem $\beta^{(73\ Asn)}$ or on the α chains as in Hb Memphis $\alpha^{(23\ Gln)}$ [272, 273] lead to milder forms of sickle-cell disease. Silent (uncharged) amino-acid difference may also occur, but have not so far been described.

Sickling in the red cell

From the above, it can be deduced that sickling *in vivo* can be facilitated by several mechanisms. Dehydration contributes by increasing the intracellular Hb S concentration, increasing the deoxy Hb S concentration at any given Po_2, lowering oxygen affinity and shortening the delay time. In addition, the red cells are closer together in the blood and therefore more likely, when sickled, to occlude small vessels. The roles of acidosis and temperature have already been discussed. The effects of the presence of another haemoglobin in the cells was also mentioned earlier. In this connection it has been suggested that the presence of carbonmonoxy haemoglobin [274] or of methaemoglobin [275] might inhibit sickling *in vivo*. However, from *in-vitro* studies, it can be calculated that 25% and 40% of altered haemoglobin respectively must be present in the cell to reduce sickling to the level which occurs in sickle-cell trait [264].

The low oxygen affinity of sickle red cells

The cause of the low oxygen affinity [276, 277] of the red cells in sickle-cell disease (Fig. 8.23) is also directly related to the molecular interaction taking place. Recent studies have shown that the low oxygen affinity of sickle cells is present in cells depleted of 2,3-DPG and that the oxygen affinity is markedly concentration-dependent [278], as would be expected of a protein–protein interaction. Thus, the molecular interaction in sickle-cell disease, which only takes place in the deoxy-conformation, tends to maintain the haemoglobin molecules in this low-affinity state and reduces the oxygen affinity of the red cells. Thus the difference in oxygen affinity of sickle cells from normal is a measure

of the propensity to polymer formation and thus indirectly of the sickling process. These results also explain the discrepancy between the low oxygen affinity seen in red cells and the normal oxygen affinity of haemolysates [279].

The haemolytic process

The increased destruction of the red cells is directly due to the sickling process [280]. However, there are several ways in which this may occur. As sickling only takes place when the blood is deoxygenated, most sickle cells are found on the venous side of the circulation, the cells unsickling again as they become fully oxygenated in the lungs. Any cells which remain sickled are unlikely to be able to pass through the capillary bed because of the rigidity of the cells and thus some are destroyed. The rigid, thin projections of sickled cells are liable to break off and this causes the increased mechanical fragility of the cells [281, 282]. This process may cause the immediate lysis of the cell or damage to the cell membrane. This damage to the cell membrane occurs invariably as the cell sickles and unsickles a number of times and leads to the formation of 'irreversibly sickled cells', often referred to as ISCs [283–285]. Another way the cell membrane is damaged is by the precipitation of Hb S on its internal surface [286]. The ISCs are rapidly haemolysed [287], particularly in the spleen if still present, and are a major cause of the short red-cell survival. The time taken for cells to become ISCs after release from the marrow is not known, but cells with more Hb S (or less Hb F or other haemoglobin) will be more liable to repeated sickling and quicker ISC conversion and consequently have a shorter survival [215, 287]. The haemoglobin in the ISCs can still oxygenate and deoxygenate and, as expected, the oxygenated cell does not contain any tactoids, the abnormal shape of the cells being due to rigidity of the cell membrane [288, 289]. Another feature of these cells is that they have a high MCHC and hence a very low oxygen affinity [290]. The proportion of ISCs in the blood is of some clinical importance because their number is related to the severity of the haemolytic process in sickle-cell disease in patients who no longer have a spleen [291, 292]. When the spleen is still present, ISCs, once formed, are rapidly destroyed in it and are only seen to a limited extent in the blood. For this reason there is often considerable splenic uptake of ^{51}Cr-labelled cells in sickle-cell patients with a palpable spleen. However, splenectomy does not improve the disease as the survival of ISCs once formed is very short even in the absence of the spleen.

The severity of the anaemia in sickle-cell disease

The severity of the anaemia in the various haemoglobinopathies does not correlate well with the degree of haemolysis as measured by the ^{51}Cr-labelled red-cell survival. It must therefore depend on the response of the marrow to increased red-cell destruction. Within very wide limits the bone marrow can expand many times as a result of erythropoietin stimulation. Erythropoietin production is geared to the oxygen supply to the tissues which in turn is controlled by the haemoglobin level and oxygen affinity (see p. 334), but is independent of cardiac output. As discussed above, the oxygen affinity of sickle-cell-disease blood is very much lower than normal (see p. 357), increasing the release of oxygen to the tissues per gram of haemoglobin, and thus decreasing the erythropoietin drive to the bone marrow. This accounts for the low haemoglobin level always found in sickle-cell disease. Conversely, the low oxygen affinity prevents the tissue hypoxia which the degree of anaemia present would imply, and stunted growth due to tissue hypoxia is not seen.

The degree of anaemia can be made worse by either increased haemolysis or decreased marrow compensation. A sudden increase in haemolysis of sufficient magnitude to increase anaemia occasionally accompanies the occurrence of an infarctive episode, but more frequently, increase in anaemia is caused by relative marrow depression. In order to maintain the red-cell mass at the steady-state level, the marrow output of red cells in sickle-cell anaemia must be about 10 times that of a normal person. Anything, such as intercurrent disease, which depresses the marrow output will make the anaemia worse. In this connection, it is important to remember that erythropoiesis which is increased compared to normal may be grossly depressed when compared to the rate of erythropoiesis usually present in the same patient. The shortened cell survival will also cause the quicker appearance of (more severe) anaemia than in the normal person. Thus an acute infection will not cause anaemia in a normal person, even if some short-term marrow depression occurs, but may cause significant reduction of haemoglobin level in patients with haemolysis. The haemoglobin level found in sickle-cell anaemia (as in other haemolytic conditions) is therefore much more variable than in the normal. Another cause of relative bone-marrow depression may be folate or iron deficiency. The latter may be more common that is realized, particularly in children from poor homes. In these children the haemoglobin is lower than the usual for sickle-cell disease and the spleen is found to be larger than expected. After iron therapy, the haemoglobin level goes up and the spleen decreases in size.

Natural history

The clinical pattern of sickle-cell disease evolves over the life of affected individuals. At birth, the children are normal because the main haemoglobin is the un-

affected Hb F. However, it is easy to make the diagnosis by electrophoresis using a citrate agar gel system at pH 6·0 [199] which separates Hb A and Hb S from Hb F and from each other. Hb C is also clearly separated. This electrophoretic system also distinguishes Hb D from Hb S and Hb E from Hb C, both Hb D and Hb E migrating with Hb A (while they are clearly separated from Hb A in conventional systems at pH 8·6).

The earliest sign of the disease is the onset of haemolysis and anaemia which can be detected at two to three months of age. The first presenting sign is often infarction of a metacarpal (tarsal) or phalangeal bone, and leads to the 'hand-foot syndrome'. The back of the affected hand or foot is swollen, warm and tender. After a few days the affected bone can be seen to be infarcted on X-ray. New bone formation eventually takes place as the lesion resolves. However, frequently the affected bone ceases to grow and a shortened finger results [293]. At this stage the spleen is found to be enlarged but it does not function normally [294]. Due to repeated infarction, the spleen regresses and is not usually palpable after the age of 10 years. During the first five years children are very prone to acute pneumococcal or other septicaemias [179, 295–297]. In some cases the spleen suddenly enlarges. This reflects trapping of the red cells in the organ which may lead to severe anaemia. The increased susceptibility to infection may be related to the loss of splenic function even though the spleen is enlarged, and it may be comparable to the proneness to septicaemia after splenectomy, particularly in young children. Abnormalities of the alternate pathway of complement have been described [298]. From the data now being collected, it appears that even in developed countries up to 20% of children with sickle-cell disease may die in the first five years of life from infection [299]. For these reasons, prophylactic oral penicillin and/or pneumococcal vaccine may be used in an attempt to prevent pneumococcal or other septicaemia, but there are no proper studies showing their efficacy. Indeed real evidence suggests that pneumococcal vaccines are not as effective as had been proposed [300].

After the age of five years, the main complication is the painful crises and complications due to tissue damage (see p. 359). However, it has to be remembered that the severity of each case is very variable, some having very few or even no episodes which bring them to the doctor, while in others the painful crises and other complications are much more common. Furthermore, a patient may have series of painful crises and then have several years without any attacks. When talking about the severity of sickle-cell disease, it is important to remember that the hospital doctor only sees the ill patient, and the disease may appear more severe than it is.

Later in life, the effects of tissue damage such as renal failure or loss of vision become particularly important. Renal failure [273] is an important cause of death in the middle-aged sickler. Having said this, there are many sicklers alive at the age of 60 or 70 years, particularly those with the milder double heterozygous sickle-cell syndromes (see p. 361).

Development

Good data on the development of patients with sickle-cell disease are at present not available and it is likely that one's views are based on description of a limited number of exceptional cases. Many children die in the first few years of life, particularly in a bad social environment. Thus, at one time virtually no homozygous sickle-cell disease cases reached maturity. Of the children who survive, many grow at a normal rate, slowing up only if complications, such as have been mentioned, occur. At puberty, there is often delayed development of the secondary sexual characteristics and the menarche, and this may be due to subclinical folate deficiency. There may also be delayed closure of the epiphyses of the long bones, leading to tall adults with relatively long limbs. Once adult life has been reached, the disease appears to get milder from the point of view of complications.

COMPLICATIONS

Painful crises

The most common complication of sickle-cell disease is the 'painful crisis' [301]. These episodes are characterized by the sudden onset of pain which can occur in any part of the body, but joints and muscles of the legs or arms, and the back, are the most commonly affected. The cause of these episodes is uncertain but they probably reflect the occurrence of multiple small infarcts in the muscles or bones. The attacks are first noticed in infancy or childhood although occasionally a first crisis may occur later in life. The frequency of the episodes becomes less with increasing age however. Usually no precipitating cause can be found, but the attacks are known to be more common during cold weather, pregnancy and menstruation; fever and even minor sepsis may precipitate them. Since it seems likely that the attacks result from intravascular sickling in the microcirculation it is clear that anything which will decrease the oxygenation of the blood will increase the risk of a painful crisis.

Because of the bizarre distribution of the pain in these episodes affected patients may present considerable diagnostic problems particularly to clinicians who are not used to treating sickle-cell anaemia and who may feel that there is a large functional element to the clinical picture. In some cases there may be marked abdominal pain which leads to a misdiagnosis of an acute abdomen. It is not uncommon for young children with this type of clinical picture to develop abdominal swelling with quiet bowel sounds and hence a picture very similar to that of an ileus. This may result from sickling in the mesenteric vessels. If the picture is not recognized as part of the sickling crisis unnecessary abdominal surgery may follow. Quite often the temperature may be normal at the onset of a crisis, only to rise after a few days following tissue infarction.

Two other unusual forms of crisis which seem to be related to the painful crisis are known as the 'lung' and 'cerebral' syndromes; these are discussed later.

Larger infarcts

Larger infarcts may produce localizing signs wherever they occur. A common site is the spleen and, as was mentioned earlier, splenic infarction leads to gradual fibrosis and autosplenectomy. Bone infarcts are also common [302, 303] and may give a clinical picture very similar to osteomyelitis. Indeed it is quite common during a painful crisis to find a localized area of bony tenderness. Bone infarction may also involve the bone marrow and aspiration over a painful site has revealed extensive marrow infarction. Rarely, this may lead to bone-marrow embolism to the lung. Although uncommon, cerebral infarcts are extremely important [304] and produce a variety of neurological syndromes and epileptic fits (the 'cerebral' syndrome). Once they have occurred there is a tendency for repeated episodes. Myocardial infarction has also been described [305].

Infarction of bone may have important and incapacitating sequelae. Aseptic necrosis of the femoral and humeral heads is a relatively common complication of all the serious sickling disorders [306]. Once this process has started it is often progressive and may lead to extreme deformity of the hip joint. Large bone infarcts may also become secondarily infected resulting in osteomyelitis due to a variety of different types of bacteria including *S. typhosa*. In addition to these post-infarctive changes small sclerotic changes are often present in various parts of the skeleton [307].

Acute haematological changes

In any painful crisis, particularly if there is underlying infection, the rate of haemolysis may increase and there may be a drop in haemoglobin level associated with a climbing reticulocyte count. Such haemolytic crises may require blood transfusion.

An acute exacerbation of the anaemia due to sequestration of a large number of sickled erythrocytes in the spleen, or occasionally the liver, has been alluded to earlier. Such sequestration crises occur commonly in infancy and early childhood and a very large proportion of the circulating red-cell mass may be sequestered in the organ within hours. This is a common cause of death in infancy at which time any significant increase in the size of the liver or spleen should suggest this diagnosis.

Finally, during infective episodes there may be a sudden onset of bone-marrow failure. Such aplastic crises are characterized by rapid drop in haemoglobin level associated with a reduced reticulocyte response. Since these episodes occur quite often within sibships with sickle-cell anaemia it seems very likely that they have an infective basis, probably viral. It should be remembered that during the increased haemolysis which occurs in many forms of sickling crisis, folic-acid requirements are markedly increased and acute folate deficiency with anaemia, a drop in the reticulocyte count and megaloblastic erythropoiesis may occur.

Priapism

This is another common, painful, very distressing complication of sickle-cell disease. In this condition, the trigger causing sickling of the blood in the penis is presumably the stasis associated with a normal erection but why sometimes this should lead to priapism is not known. Treatment in the first instance is symptomatic as often the condition subsides spontaneously. If this does not occur after two ot three days surgical treatment is usually undertaken. One of the problems is that priapism tends to recur and this gradually leads to impotence, although the sexual urge remains fully active.

Leg ulcers

These occur at one time or another in almost all cases of sickle-cell disease. The first sign is a painful inflammatory lesion under the skin, presumably due to a small sickle infarct. The skin later breaks and chronic ulceration occurs. Trauma to the leg and inadequate hygiene may be predisposing factors, and they certainly make any ulcer worse and delay healing. Treatment of these ulcers is similar to that of varicose ulcers, but healing may take several months. Serjeant and his colleagues [308] have suggested that oral zinc sulphate may be beneficial in these cases.

Renal lesions [273, 309–311]

A constant finding in sickle-cell disease is inability to concentrate the urine. During childhood the replacement of sickle cells with normal red cells by transfusion returns renal function to normal. However as the patient becomes older the tubular defect becomes permanent. Another common complication is haematuria. Both of these are due to abnormalities of the medullary circulation. Apparently the hyperosmolar-

ity in the medulla (during relative water deprivation) increases the sickling tendency of the cells in the vasa recta and these progressively become blocked. Thus the nephrons associated with the long loops of Henle disappear. In due course the medullary fibrosis seen in sickle-cell disease develops. Haematuria also commonly occurs and is probably due to infarction in the papilla or rupture of an anastomosis which has developed because of the obliteration of the vasa recta [312, 313]. These changes in the kidney may account for the increased incidence of pyelonephritis in sicklers. Besides the tubular damage there may also be glomerular congestion and enlargement with focal thickening of the basement membrane.

Eyes

A history of blurring of vision in one eye occurs in a proportion of cases of sickle-cell disease and this is usually due to vitreous haemorrhage. This usually clears over a period of a few weeks and only a few patients have a reduced visual acuity due to sickle-cell disease. Examination of the eyes shows conjunctival vascular abnormality in many cases, while the fundi often show various degrees of abnormality. There may only be whitening at the extreme periphery of the retina, while other patients show proliferative lesions called descriptively 'black sunbursts' and 'sea-fan lesions'. Vascular lesions such as tortuosity and occasional micro-aneurysms are also seen; silvery white occluded arterioles or retinal haemorrhages are sometimes present. For a description of the ocular lesions, see Refs 314 and 315.

Cardiovascular lesions

Cardiovascular complications of sickle-cell disease are those associated with chronic anaemia. Thus, cardiac enlargement due to left-ventricular hypertrophy and apical mid-systolic murmurs are found in many cases of sickle-cell disease. Of course, if the anaemia becomes severe, due to any intercurrent disease, cardiac failure may occur, but it is not as common a complication as might be expected from the degree of anaemia seen. Iron deposition may also occur when there is iron overload.

Pulmonary lesions

Patients with sickle-cell disease not uncommonly suffer from pulmonary infarction and pneumonia, the so-called 'lung syndrome' [316]. The clinical picture is characterized by fever, pleuritic chest pain, dyspnoea, cough and haemoptysis. The X-ray changes are often difficult to interpret and may resemble either pneumonia or infarction; possibly both may be present simultaneously.

Pregnancy

Pregnancy is associated with increased occurrence of the usual complications [317–319], such as abortion, premature labour, concealed accidental haemorrhage, etc. During pregnancy and labour, infarctive complications are also more common than usual in sickle-cell disease. Thus, fetal loss is a fairly frequent occurrence and the maternal mortality is higher than in normal women. Unfortunately data on the relative frequency of maternal mortality, etc., in sickle-cell disease are only available to a limited extent.

The mixed sickle-cell syndromes

The mixed sickle-cell syndromes arise in individuals who inherit one gene at the Hb$_\beta$ locus determining β^S-chain (Hb S) production together with another abnormal gene affecting the Hb$_\beta$ gene on the other chromosome. This may either be a β-thalassaemia gene, giving rise to sickle-cell β thalassaemia, or a haemoglobin with abnormal β chains, most commonly Hb C, giving rise to sickle-cell haemoglobin-C disease. The interactions with Hb D$_\beta$, Hb J$_\beta$, Hb O$_\beta$ and Hb E have also been described.

SICKLE-CELL β THALASSAEMIA
(see also Chapter 9)

Sickle-cell β thalassaemia arises from the interaction of a β-thalassaemia gene with an Hb β^S gene. As explained elsewhere (see Chapter 9, p. 414), there are a number of β-thalassaemia genes, suppressing β-chain synthesis to different degrees, and as a result three (main) forms of Hb S β-thalassaemia disease exist according to the amount of Hb A present in the cells. In the most severe form, no Hb A is synthesized. In the remaining cases, some Hb A is synthesized and patients appear to fall into two groups: those with 10–15% Hb A and those with 20–30% Hb A, the least severe form [320, 321].

The patients without any Hb A have a severe form of sickle-cell disease which, on clinical grounds, is not distinguishable from homozygous sickle-cell disease since the haemoglobin level, reticulocyte count and incidence of complications in the two conditions are very similar. Although as a group they may have a slightly milder disease, the overlap with the homozygous condition is such that in any individual case the two conditions cannot be distinguished. The diagnosis can therefore only be established by family or haemoglobin studies. Haemoglobin analysis usually shows mainly Hb S and no Hb A; Hb A$_2$ is raised and this differentiates it from the homozygous condition. Measurement of Hb F does not help to distinguish the two conditions as ranges obtained in genetically proven cases are similar [322]. In some forms of β thalassaemia, the Hb A$_2$ is not raised, and the haemo-

globin pattern does not help in establishing sickle-cell β-thalassaemia disease. In these cases, the diagnosis is best established by family studies. The blood count may also be helpful as the cells in the double heterozygotes tend to be smaller than in the homozygous condition, leading to a difference in MCH, the former (Hb S/β thal) having a level of less than about 23 pg and the latter (homozygous S) $30.2 \pm$ s.d. 2.0 pg (author's unpublished observations).

The group of patients with a low Hb A level also have a severe clinical course but are clearly distinguished by the presence of Hb A; the Hb A$_2$ level is also usually raised. It is important to remember that the presence of transfused cells will make the diagnosis of this group impossible. The haemoglobin level is similar to that in the homozygous condition, although complications are less frequent.

The group of patients with about 25% Hb A have a distinctly milder disease with a higher haemoglobin level, c. 10–11 g/dl, and lower reticulocyte counts; the MCH is also higher. There are fewer complications, such as painful crises and larger infarcts. However, retinal abnormalities are more common in this group than in homozygous sickle-cell disease [315]. This may be related to the higher haemoglobin level and consequently increased blood viscosity, which may be just wrong for the retinal arterioles, predisposing them to blockage.

One other clinical point is that splenomegaly more often persists into adult life in Hb S/β-thalassaemia disease than in the homozygous condition, being most frequent in the high Hb A group. Occasionally hypersplenism occurs or the plasma volume increases, both making the patient more anaemic; in these patients splenectomy may be of benefit. Otherwise the treatment and management are similar to those of the homozygous condition, bearing in mind the often milder course of the disease.

SICKLE-CELL HAEMOGLOBIN C DISEASE

This condition arises due to the inheritance of a gene determining Hb C formation as well as one for Hb S formation. As only β^C and β^S chains and no β^A chains are synthesized, only Hb S and Hb C, in approximately equal quantities, are found in the cell. There is also a normal amount of Hb A$_2$, but this does not separate from Hb C by electrophoresis. Although small amounts (1–2%) of Hb F are present, increased Hb F is not a feature of this syndrome. The Hb C haemoglobin crystals are present in the cells in this condition [323].

Clinically, this is a mild variant of sickle-cell disease, with haemoglobin levels of 11–12 g/dl and three to five per cent reticulocytes [324]. There are also fewer complications. However, as in the mildest form of Hb S/β

thalassaemia, ocular complications are more common than in the homozygous disease [314]. The spleen is usually palpable, even in adult life. One of the dangers of this condition is its mildness. Many patients have normal or near-normal haemoglobin levels and are unaware of the disease. If it is not picked up pre-operatively by specific screening procedures the patient may run into severe sickle-cell crises during operations or labour. Another complication is that in some patients the haemoglobin level rises gradually, not by increased red-cell mass but by decreased plasma volume. The viscosity problems of a high packed cell volume and liability to sickling lead to increased ocular complications and possibly severe and even fatal sickle-cell crises. It would definitely be better if these patients were kept anaemic with a haemoglobin level of 11 g/dl but it is difficult to achieve this in a controlled manner. Again, the general treatment and management are the same as in sickle-cell disease, bearing in mind the relative mildness of the clinical picture.

OTHER MIXED SICKLE-CELL SYNDROMES

Sickle-cell haemoglobin D_β disease [325–327], sickle-cell haemoglobin J disease [328], sickle-cell haemoglobin E disease [329] and disease caused by interaction with the Negro-type 'high fetal' gene [330, 331] are similar to Hb S+C disease. Sickle-cell haemoglobin $O_{(\beta)}$ disease [270] occurs rarely but is much more severe than the other mixed syndromes, giving a picture similar to homozygous sickle-cell disease.

The interaction of sickle-cell haemoglobin with α-chain abnormal haemoglobins has also been reported. In general, the severity of these syndromes is controlled by the type of β genes present, that is, if there is homozygosity for β^S, then homozygous sickle-cell disease results. An exception is Hb Memphis [273], which leads to a somewhat milder disease. The interaction of sickle-cell disease with genes determining α thalassaemia [332–334] also leads to a milder disease, presumably because of a low MCHC. The MCH is low but, suprisingly, the Hb A_2 is raised [334a].

TREATMENT OF SICKLE-CELL DISEASE

At the present time, there is no specific treatment of sickle-cell disease. The obvious approach is to prevent the occurrence of complications of the disease by reducing the propensity of the cells to sickle. It is known that sickling is exacerbated by hypoxia, acidosis, pyrexia and dehydration, and these should be avoided. Other factors precipitating crises are infection, fever and malaria, and it has been shown that patients are improved by long-term antibiotics and antimalarials [335]. Considering the situation theoretically, sickling can be reduced by raising the tissue oxygen tension, raising the oxygen affinity, lowering the concentration of Hb S in the cells and finally by preventing the sickling interaction from taking place. Raising the tissue P_{O_2} by allowing the patient to breathe pure oxygen is only possible as a short-term measure and therefore cannot be used to prevent the occurrence of crises. Experience has also shown that once a crisis is fully established, oxygen has little effect, as explained later. It is not known, however, whether treatment with oxygen as soon as symptoms of a crisis appear will abort it. Raising the oxygen affinity would reduce the amount of deoxy-Hb S in the cells at tissue P_{O_2} thus reducing *in-vivo* sickling, and several attempts have been made to achieve this. Alkalinization [336], taking advantage of the Bohr effect, has been tried but has not been successful, presumably because the change in oxygen affinity achieved is not great enough to reduce *in-vivo* sickling. Another way in which the pH of the red cell might be raised is by carbonic-anhydrase inhibitors [337]. In this case, the CO_2 effect on oxygen affinity is probably balanced by the decrease in intracellular pH and therefore does not affect the sickling process. 2,3-DPG is an important regulator of red-cell oxygen affinity (p. 335) and a decrease in 2,3-DPG would increase the oxygen affinity and reduce sickling. In this way, specific inhibition of 2,3-DPG synthesis may help patients with sickle-cell disease [338].

Carbamylation of haemoglobin by cyanate increases its oxygen affinity [338], and Cerami & Manning [339] have suggested that it might be a possible treatment for sickle-cell disease. After *in-vitro* reaction of sickle cells with cyanate, the ^{51}Cr-labelled red-cell survival improves [340–343] and becomes normal when the oxygen affinity is slightly higher than normal and about 30–40% of the free N-terminal amino groups have been carbamylated. Preliminary clinical trials of oral cyanate for a period of several months in a number of sicklers show promising results in that the red-cell survival is considerably lengthened and the haemoglobin and packed cell volumes are improved [344].

However, peripheral neuritis or cataract occurred in some patients after about 12 months of treatment, presumably due to carbamylation of other tissue proteins as had been shown experimentally [345, 346].

Another way in which the sickling process could be inhibited is by reducing the intracellular concentration of Hb S, and those patients with a low MCHC due to the presence of either α or β thalassaemia tend to have a milder course. The cellular concentration of Hb S may also be reduced by the presence of other haemoglobins (Hb F, Hb A, Hb C, etc.) in the cell, and these patients again have a milder disease. Thus the reactivation of Hb F production would be a useful form of treatment for this disease.

Another way that sickling could be prevented would

be by the prevention of polymer formation. Urea has been suggested as a possible agent but concentrations which can be achieved *in vivo* are ineffective [347, 348]. Attempts to abort the crisis by raising the tissue Po_2 by breathing pure oxygen or, more recently, hyperbaric oxygen [349, 350] have not been successful, presumably because by the time the patient is in hospital the micro-infarcts have already led to fibrin formation and cannot be reversed. Attempts to prevent this with anticoagulants or anti-platelet drugs have also been unsuccessful [351]. Other forms of treatment, such as infusion of magnesium glutamate together with alkalinization [336] or acetolazamide [352] also have no effect on the course of the disease. The present work on the development of inhibitors of sickling has been the subject of a recent symposium [353] and review [262], but no specific drugs are on the horizon.

Thus, the treatment of sickle-cell disease consists essentially of prevention of the following predisposing factors:

1 *Hypoxia* is particularly important during surgery and postoperatively.

2 *Dehydration* is probably the most important factor in initiating crises. It is particularly prone to occur in sicklers as they are unable to concentrate their urine and is (almost) invariably present in individuals admitted in crises. We treat all our sicklers with crises with intravenous fluid and in the cooperative urea trials [348] fluid replacement was found to be important in terminating crises.

3 *Infection* should be looked for in every crisis and treated appropriately. The possibility of osteomyelitis should be at the back of one's mind if localized pain persists or swelling is unusually severe.

4 *Acidosis*, when present, should be actively treated and is clearly important postoperatively.

5 *Pyrexia*: drugs such as aspirin are not only of use for pain relief but may also help by their antipyretic effect.

General management of the sickling crisis

Most painful crises should be managed in hospital. Careful clinical examination should be carried out to try to exclude precipitating causes such as infection. The patient should be kept under careful surveillance and have regular estimations of the haemoglobin level or packed cell volume, reticulocyte count, electrolyte levels and acid-base status. As part of the infection screen, the urine should be examined and blood cultures and throat swabs taken.

The main lines of treatment of painful crisis are rest, hydration, analgesia and oxygen therapy although the real value of the latter is uncertain. For mild pain, first-line analgesics such as aspirin, paracetamol or codeine are used. If this is not sufficient, pentazocine (Fortral), dihydrocodeine or pethidine are useful according to the severity of the pain. While addicting drugs should be used with caution it is important to realize that the pain of a sickling crisis may be very severe and they should not be withheld in particularly bad attacks. The latter usually only last for a few days and provided they are used sensibly these drugs are of great value. It is often difficult to persuade these patients to take adequate oral fluids and in all but the mildest crisis an intravenous line should be set up and adequate hydration restored with glucose/saline infusions. If there is evidence of infection it should be treated with appropriate antibiotics.

A straightforward painful crisis without evidence of a falling haemoglobin level does not require transfusion (see next section). However, if there is evidence of a sequestration crisis with enlargement of the spleen and liver and a falling haemoglobin level a transfusion should be administered urgently. Similarly, if there is a falling haemoglobin level with a coincident drop in the reticulocyte count, suggesting a hypoplastic crisis, transfusion is required as these patients may become profoundly anaemic over a period of a few hours.

Because the cerebral and lung syndromes tend to recur they should be managed by a long-term transfusion programme, as described in the following section.

Blood transfusion in sickle-cell disease

Another standby is blood transfusion, and we use this in patients who have repeated painful crises particularly if they start in a similar manner. In these cases we argue that before the damage from the micro-infarcts of one crisis have healed properly a second one starts. By replacing the sickle cells with normal red cells we hope to break the presumed vicious circle by using partial exchange and repeated transfusion until over 60% of the cells are normal and then maintaining this for varying amounts of time, usually three to six months. This kind of regimen is of course important if there are severe complications such as osteomyelitis so that any operative procedures can be carried out with minimum risk. We also use it when there are severe infarctive complications such as cerebral or myocardial infarcts or aseptic necrosis of the head of femur. In all these cases this is to allow maximum healing of the lesion.

Management of sickle-cell disease during pregnancy and anaesthesia

Patients with one of the sickle-cell syndromes present a special problem during pregnancy and surgery. The condition should be screened for by a reliable form of sickling test or by electrophoresis in persons of Negro extraction. If a positive sickling test is found, the condition should be further investigated by electrophoresis of haemoglobin and a full blood count (including reticulocytes) in order to diagnose the exact syndrome present.

Abortion, premature labour and other complications in pregnancy are more common than in normal women [317–319]. The children tend to be 'small for dates' at delivery. Although there are many patients with sickle-cell disease who have had no complications, the outcome in any individual case is always in doubt. The only consistently successful way of reducing the incidence of complications is by regular blood transfusion of the affected patients approximately every six weeks, so that the proportion of Hb A cells is about 60–70% of the total. Three to four units should be given at each transfusion. This regime has two effects. It raises the patient's haemoglobin level to near normal and considerably reduces complications due to the presence of sickle cells. The higher haemoglobin level reduces the erythropoietin drive to the marrow and thus the number of (sickle) cells made. As sickle cells are more rapidly destroyed than the transfused normal cells, each transfusion lasts longer in terms of replacing sickle cells than might otherwise be expected. In patients with sickle-cell trait, no special therapy is indicated, but special care should be taken not to allow them to become anoxic during labour.

The management of sickle-cell disease and its variants during surgery and anaesthesia [354, 355] is similar to that of pregnancy. Again, pre-operative transfusion so as to have 60–70% of normal cells is given. This can be achieved by two transfusions, one a week before and the other the day before the operation. If there is more urgency, then an exchange transfusion regime may be used. During anaesthesia it is again important to avoid anoxia of the tissues as well as acidosis and dehydration, as these will make the patient's own remaining cells more liable to sickle.

In this respect, the postoperative period is most important, and one has to make sure that the patient does not become anoxic during this period. Some workers recommend that the patient is initially nursed postoperatively in an intensive care unit.

No special preparation by transfusion is necessary in the management of sickle-cell trait during pregnancy and anaesthesia, *except for procedures likely to involve anoxia of parts of the body*, and the author has seen two cases of sickle-cell trait who died as a result of massive sickling occurring during cardiac surgery.

Sickle-cell disease and the contraceptive pill

As there is some risk of thrombosis from using the oestrogen-containing contraceptive pill, it has been suggested that the risk of this might be increased in sickle-cell disease. There is, at present, no evidence on this point. My own view is that the increased theoretical risk of the pill in sicklers is balanced by the known increased risks of unwanted pregnancy. The contraceptive pill, therefore, would not be contraindicated. In the small number of women with sickle-cell disease who are on the pill, no increased number of crises has been noted.

Sickle-cell disease and flying

Finally, one of the hazards of modern life is hypoxia during aircraft flight. Patients with one of the sickle-cell syndromes which cause haemolysis clearly have some degree of sickling at sea level, and the reduced Po_2 on flying in pressurized or unpressurized aircraft is liable to increase the sickling of the cells and thus precipitate a crisis or an infarct. In this connection it is important to remember that in pressurized aircraft the Po_2 corresponds to that present at 1500–2000 metres, which leads to a reduction of arterial Po_2 from 95 mmHg at sea level to 65–70 mmHg at 1750 metres. The risk incurred by any individual patient depends, of course, on whether they have homozygous sickle-cell disease or severe (without any Hb A) sickle-cell β thalassaemia, when the risk is greatest, or mild (with Hb A) sickle-cell β thalassaemia or Hb S + C disease, when it is smaller. In all of them, the risk of a crisis occurring is quite small and flying in pressurized aircraft is not contraindicated, but the risks should be explained to the patient. The patient is also advised not to get dehydrated and to avoid stasis of the blood flow in the limbs which would predispose to sickling. Unpressurized aircraft should be avoided, and when convenient surface transport is available this is preferred. If a crisis commences in flight, then attempts to abort it with oxygen, if available, should be carried out, but it is not known whether this will be effective. In patients who have experienced crises in previous flights the risk of recurrence is not known, but presumably is (slightly) greater than in other patients. In all patients, flying is best avoided during infection or fever as these in themselves predispose to crises. In sickle-cell trait, the risk of a crisis occurring during flight in a pressurized aircraft is extremely small indeed. The flying, as passengers, of individuals with various sickle-cell syndromes is, therefore, not contraindicated.

Sickle-cell trait

Sickle-cell trait is important because of its high frequency in certain peoples of the world (Fig. 8.22) and, as already mentioned, the homozygous state gives rise to a severe haemolytic–embolic disease. Diagnosis of the trait is important in genetic counselling. Furthermore, in certain situations the trait itself may give rise to pathology [356].

The diagnosis of sickle-cell trait is made by a positive haemoglobin solubility [244–246] (or 'Sickledex') test followed by starch-gel electrophoresis, demonstrating the presence of both Hb A and Hb S, with Hb A clearly in excess. Further confirmation that one is dealing with sickle-cell trait is obtained by the demonstration of a normal haemoglobin level and other red-cell parameters, including a reticulocyte count. The sickling test is not reliable enough for use as a screening procedure for sickle-cell trait as too many false negatives occur; nor is it enough to rely on a positive solubility test with a normal haemoglobin as this combination can occur in some of the other sickle-cell syndromes. The proportion of Hb S in the cells is $40 \pm$ s.d. five per cent [357, 358]. Family studies have shown that the proportion of Hb S varies between families [359]. The concomitant inheritance of an α-thalassaemia gene leads to a low proportion of Hb S in the cells with a low MCH [322, 323]; other causes of a relatively low Hb S level in the trait form are iron deficiency [360] and megaloblastic anaemia [361].

Consideration of the sickling process indicates that Hb S polymer formation takes place when the concentration of deoxy Hb S in the cell exceeds a given, as yet undetermined, value. The concentration of deoxy Hb S in the cell at given oxygen tensions depends on both the concentration of Hb S in the cell and the position of the oxygen dissociation curve. Thus, the severity of the sickling process diminishes from homozygous sickle-cell disease, with almost all Hb S, through the mixed syndromes down to sickle trait. In this condition, the concentration of Hb S in the cell and the oxygen affinity are such that a Po_2 of less than 15 mmHg is needed to cause sickling of the red cells. Furthermore, as the sickling process takes about two minutes to complete, it can be deduced that normally practically no *in-vivo* sickling will occur, and this agrees with the *general innocuous nature* of sickle-cell trait [362]. The expectation of life appears similar to that of the non-sickle-cell-trait population. However, as sufficient hypoxia of the red cells will cause sickling it is to be expected that in certain conditions *in-vivo* sickling will occur. As has already been mentioned, the concentration of Hb S in the cells is one factor which determines the liability of the cells to sickle, and those individuals with higher Hb S levels, near to 50% of total haemoglobin, will be more liable to sickling episodes than those with low levels, and the reported cases of sickle-cell trait with complications tend to have a higher proportion of Hb S than is usual.

It is accepted that most individuals with sickle-cell trait have partial loss of concentrating ability due to loss of tubular function associated with the long loops of Henle and the vasa recta; haematuria also occurs in a proportion of patients with sickle-cell trait [312] and it has been suggested that this could be treated with ε-amino-caproic acid [313]. In pregnancy there is an increased incidence of urinary infection [363], and this may be related to the above changes. It has also been suggested that there is an increased perinatal mortality in children born to mothers with sickle-cell trait [364]. The management of sickle-cell trait during pregnancy and surgery has already been referred to (p. 363).

There are some case reports of the complications of sickle-cell disease occurring in sickle-cell trait. As sickle-cell trait is very common these reports must represent a very low incidence indeed. Most of these complications also occur occasionally in patients without sickle-cell trait and it is impossible to be sure that they are directly related to the trait without the necessary statistical data comparing the incidence of such complications in the sickling and non-sickling populations; the only such study is by Heller & Moneer [365]. Several such studies are now under way, and it is hoped to have real knowledge of the pathology of sickle-cell trait. However, in the meantime it should be remembered that, except for the special circumstances mentioned, the trait is of no significance.

Genetic counselling in sickle-cell trait

As sickle-cell trait is common only in the black and certain other populations of the world and is easy to detect, the incidence of sickle-cell disease could be reduced by pre-marital screening and the avoidance of marriages where both partners carry the sickling gene. At the present time there is a great deal of debate as to whether the affected population groups should be screened for sickle-cell trait and whether to use such information in genetic counselling. This approach is used in some parts of the United States, but the danger is that, because the general innocuous nature of the trait is not generally understood, this may lead to discrimination against Hb A + S carriers. At present, therefore, we only screen for the sickling trait if requested by the individual concerned (or on admission to hospital). This service should be easily available, but a positive result should be accompanied by adequate reassurance of the benign nature of the condition as well as an explanation of the genetic risks involved. Again, on request, a potential spouse should also be screened and, in this instance, not only should sickle-cell trait be looked for, but also β-thalassaemia trait and other abnormal haemoglobins, and advice given according to the result.

It is possible to diagnose sickle-cell disease antenatally using either haemoglobin synthesis studies on fetal blood obtained by fetoscopy [366] or by restriction enzyme analysis of the DNA of amniotic-fluid fetal fibroblasts [367]. Using termination of pregnancy of affected fetuses, it would be possible to prevent the occurrence of sickle-cell disease. This is an accepted form of management in thalassaemia (see p. 440). However, sickle-cell disease is much milder, and at present antenatal diagnosis is only recommended if there is an affected member in the family already, or at the request of an informed couple at risk.

THE HOMOZYGOUS HAEMOGLOBINOPATHIES

Haemoglobin C

Haemoglobin C is relatively common in West Africa and people of West African extraction and has the amino-acid substitution $\alpha_2\beta_2^{6 \; Glu\rightarrow Lys}$, the same glutamic-acid residue as in Hb S being involved [368]. This amino-acid side chain is on the surface of the molecule. Oxygen dissociation studies show normal function in solution and in the cells [55, 369]. It is found in the heterozygous and homozygous states and interacting with β thalassaemia (Chapter 9, p. 428) or Hb S (p. 361).

THE HETEROZYGOUS STATE

This is of no pathological significance, and both Hb A and Hb C are found in the red cells, Hb C amounting to 30–40% of total haemoglobin. The presence of α thalassaemia reduces the proportion of Hb C in the cells [370, 371].

HOMOZYGOUS HB C DISEASE

This is a mild haemolytic disease occurring in individuals of West African extraction [372, 373]. The clinical features are non-specific; the spleen may be palpable. Haematologically, there is a mild to moderate anaemia, with a haemoglobin level of 8–12 g/dl, some hypochromia and variation in size and shape of the red cells, as well as some targetting. Intraerythrocytic haemoglobin crystals [323] can sometimes be seen in a small proportion of the red cells in the blood smear and it is thought that the increased rigidity of the cell caused by these crystals leads to increased red-cell destruction [374]. The osmotic fragility may be slightly reduced. A mild reticulocytosis compatible with the slightly shortened red-cell survival, $T_{\frac{1}{2}}$ of ^{51}Cr-labelled red cells of about 19 days, is present. This disease is of no further clinical importance and patients have a normal lifespan. No specific treatment is indicated.

Haemoglobin E

Haemoglobin E is the second most common abnormal haemoglobin in the world, occurring in people of Southeast Asian extraction. The abnormal haemoglobin has an electrophoretic mobility slightly faster (anodally) than Hb C and similar to that of Hb A$_2$ (Fig. 8.17). Hb E has the structure $\alpha_2\beta_2^{26 \; Glu\rightarrow Lys}$ [375]. Oxygen-dissociation properties of purified Hb E in solution are normal as is also its interaction with 2,3-DPG; while there is a lowered oxygen affinity in red cells containing only Hb E (Hb E homozygotes and Hb E β thalassaemia), cells containing Hb A + E have a normal oxygen affinity [376]. The low oxygen affinity in homozygous Hb E is due to an increase of 2,3-DPG in the cells [376]. Clinically only homozygous Hb E and its interaction with β thalassaemia (Chapter 9, p. 428) are important.

HAEMOGLOBINE E TRAIT

This occurs commonly in Southeast Asia (Fig. 8.24), with the red cells containing 25–30% Hb E. It is of no (known) clinical or pathological significance. The pro-

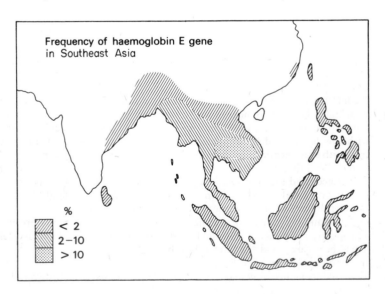

Fig. 8.24. Distribution of haemoglobin E. (From Ref. 248.)

portion of Hb E found in this trait is reduced by the concomitant inheritance of α thalassaemia [377]. The inheritance of one α-thalassaemia gene (see p. 436) leads to the presence of only 17–25% Hb E and with two α-thalassaemia genes (equivalent to Hb H disease in the absence of Hb E) even less, *c.* 14% Hb E is found; some Hb γ_4 is also present (see Chapter 9, p. 436).

HOMOZYGOUS HAEMOGLOBIN E DISEASE [378–380]
This is characterized by a mild anaemia. The red-cell count is raised because there is always some micro-cyosis, but changes in the blood film may be minimal. The red-cell survival is only slightly shortened. On clinical examination often nothing abnormal is found, while in other patients there is slight splenomegaly and sometimes mild jaundice. The expectation of life is normal. Homozygous Hb E with α thalassaemia in some cases gives rise to an intermediate form of thalas-saemia [381] (see Chapter 9, p. 437).

Several other abnormal haemoglobins have been found in the homozygous state. In some of these a mild Hb C disease-like picture has been seen, Hb D Punjab [382, 383]. Hb O Arab [384], while in others, no patho-logy was present: Hb G Accra [385], Hb G αIbadan [386], Hb J Tonghariki [106, 107]. Most other haemo-globins have been seen only in the heterozygous state and do not cause any pathology except those described below.

HAEMOGLOBINS WITH ABNORMAL FUNCTION

The oxygen affinity of haemoglobin in the red cell is determined by the equilibrium between the high-affinity and low-affinity forms of haemoglobin (see p. 332), and any structural change in the haemoglobins may affect this. For example, in Hb Kempsey which has a high oxygen affinity, this equilibrium is disturbed because the low-affinity form of haemoglobin is main-tained by one pair of hydrogen bonds fewer than in Hb A [6]. Consequently, the equilibrium is shifted to the high-affinity form and a high oxygen affinity results. In Hb Kansas the converse happens, and a low oxygen affinity results. Another way in which the equi-librium between the two forms of haemoglobin can be affected is by the introduction of new bonds, as occurs in the deoxy form of Hb S (see p. 357). Amino-acid substitutions affecting the residues involved in 2,3-DPG binding would indirectly also cause a raised oxygen affinity (see p. 331). References to individual haemoglobins are given in the tables and figures.

HAEMOGLOBINS WITH AN INCREASED OXYGEN AFFINITY
In the family carrying Hb Chesapeake [387] it was noticed that the heterozygotes for the abnormal hae-moglobins also had a raised packed cell volume. Further investigation showed that this was caused by the high oxygen affinity of the red cells due to the abnormal haemoglobin. Several other abnormal hae-moglobins with a raised oxygen affinity leading to polycythaemia have since been reported. Consider-ation of the oxygen dissociation curves of the blood from these patients (Fig. 8.25) shows that for normal oxygen delivery to the tissues there must either be a raised haemoglobin level, a low tissue oxygen tension or an increased cardiac output. At normal haemo-globin levels the situation is similar to anaemia in the otherwise normal person. The result would be a low tissue P_{O_2} and/or increased cardiac output. This situa-tion would lead to increased production of erythro-poietin resulting in increased erythropoiesis and red-cell mass. This process continues until the whole system is in balance. At this time, the haemoglobin level is such that the oxygen delivery to the tissues is (near) normal at (near) normal mean venous P_{O_2}, and the erythropoietin production will have fallen to a level just sufficient to maintain the balance of red-cell des-truction and production. As the number of red cells needed for this is only moderately above normal, only high normal levels of erythropoietin are found in the steady state. Thus, in this disease the cardiac output and tissue oxygen tension will be normal as long as the red-cell mass is raised. However, if it falls these patients are, in effect, anaemic at normal haemoglobin levels. A more detailed review has been published by Stamatoyannopoulos and his colleagues [388].

Although it has been suggested that the high oxygen affinity of maternal blood would be detrimental to oxygen transport to the fetus, this is not so as long as the maternal haemoglobin remains high. However, should the maternal haemoglobin fall to anaemic levels due to iron or folate deficiency, the situation is much more serious than in the otherwise normal preg-nant woman. In those cases who have an abnormal α-chain haemoglobin, for example in Hb Chesapeake, the person must have been affected *in utero* since he would have carried the corresponding α-chain variant of Hb F; this presumably would also have had a high oxygen affinity. If control of the level of haemoglobin in the fetus is the same as in adults then these fetuses might have a very high packed cell volume and get into difficulty because of the increased blood viscosity.

So far, most of the reported cases with polycythae-mia due to abnormal haemoglobins have been recog-nized because the abnormal haemoglobin was detected by either haemoglobin electrophoresis or the alkali denaturation test. However, the red-cell oxygen affinity should be measured in all cases, as neutral amino-acid substitutions can cause a similar change.

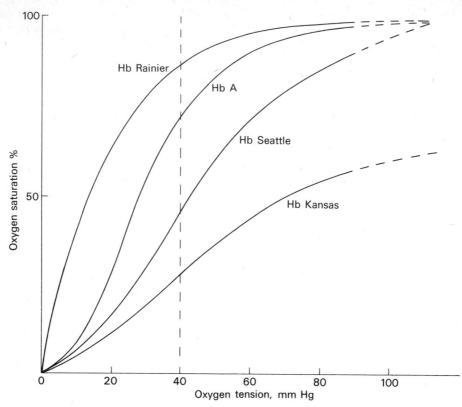

Fig. 8.25. Oxygen dissociation curves of some abnormal haemoglobins (whole blood, pH 7·4, 37°C). It can be seen that for Hb Rainier the amount of oxygen given up per gram of haemoglobin, as blood passes from the lungs to the tissues, is decreased, while for Hb Seattle it is increased. With Hb Kansas, despite some arterial desaturation, the delivery of oxygen per gram of haemoglobin is still greater than normal. (From Ref. 423.)

Some patients complain of headache and a feeling of fullness in the head which is relieved by venesection. Studies in polycythaemia from other causes have shown impaired cerebral blood flow at high packed cell volumes, and this may be the cause of the symptoms in these patients. Unfortunately, none of the patients with polycythaemia due to high-affinity haemoglobins have been studied adequately to determine the haemoglobin level at which oxygen delivery to the brain would be optimal.

HAEMOGLOBINS WITH A LOW OXYGEN AFFINITY
Only a few stable haemoglobins with a low oxygen affinity have been described. A low oxygen affinity of the blood will cause mild anaemia for the same reason that a high oxygen affinity causes polycythaemia. As mild anaemia from other causes is common and is, in any case, associated with a shift in the oxygen dissociation curve due to the 2,3-DPG mechanism, this type of haemoglobinopathy presents considerable difficulty in diagnosis, but presumably detailed investigation

(oxygen dissociation studies and red-cell 2,3-DPG measurement) will bring further cases to light. Haemoglobins with a low oxygen affinity are therefore discovered because of some other symptom or sign besides anaemia. This may be cyanosis or concomitant haemolysis due to haemoglobin instability. The latter is discussed in the next section. Hb Kansas was diagnosed because the patient had suffered from cyanosis since infancy, and this was caused by the very low oxygen affinity of his haemoglobin. There were no other clinical or haematological abnormalities. The finding of a normal haemoglobin level in the blood of this patient rather than the postulated anaemia is explained by the arterial desaturation of Hb Kansas. Other haemoglobins with a low oxygen affinity have been discovered because detailed investigations were carried out on purified haemoglobin solutions from previously undescribed variants. In these cases there was no oxygen dissociation abnormality present in red cells from the affected individuals who carried Hb A as well as the variant and, as the homozygous state has not been seen, it is not known what this would show. These findings are not of clinical importance but help us to understand the function of various residues in the haemoglobin molecule.

Again, the occurrence of a low oxygen affinity of the red cells is not of great clinical importance even if some cyanosis (as with Hb Kansas) is present. However, if for any reason the arterial Po_2 should fall, the situation would be correspondingly worse than with Hb A. At the present time there is no way in which the oxygen affinity of the red cells can be increased and no treatment is possible.

THE HAEMOGLOBINS M

The haemoglobins M are a rare, benign cause of congenital cyanosis. The differentiation of the biochemical causes of congenital cyanosis from cyanosis due to congenital heart disease is important. There are three such conditions. The first is congenital methaemoglo-

binaemia. In these patients there is reduced activity of the enzyme methaemoglobin reductase, and the pigment in the red cells has the spectral characteristics of normal methaemoglobin with an absorption maximum at 632 nm (Fig. 8.26) (see Chapter 7, p. 275). Measurement of the enzyme will confirm the diagnosis. The second type of biochemical congenital cyanosis is caused by the presence of Hb M. In these patients the pigment present has a different absorption spectrum from methaemoglobin with the absence of the maximum at 632 nm (Fig. 8.26). Spectral studies of the haemolysate show an abnormal peak at about 600 nm. The diagnosis can be confirmed by electrophoresis, in phosphate buffer pH 7.0, of the haemolysate after complete conversion to the acid methaemoglobin derivative. Under these conditions, the M haemoglobins migrate nearer to the anode than Hb A and are characterized by their unusual grey-green colour. The third cause of congenital biochemical cyanosis is the pres-

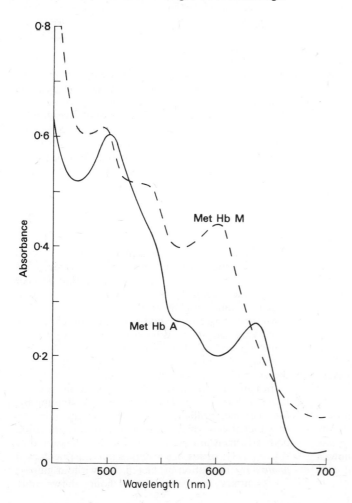

Fig. 8.26. Absorption spectra at pH 7.0 of methaemoglobin A, compared with methaemoglobin M Saskatoon. (From Ref. 652.)

ence of the low-oxygen-affinity haemoglobins already referred to.

The M haemoglobins were the first abnormal haemoglobins in which it was shown that the abnormality lay in the globin part of the molecule [389, 390]. In each of the four described types one of the two histidines in contact with the haem group in either the α or β chain is replaced by tyrosine, and the tyrosine forms an ionic bond with the ferric ion of methaemoglobin, preventing its reduction by methaemoglobin reductase. Although the affected subunit of Hb M cannot carry oxygen, the normal partner chain can, and the presence of these amino-acid substitutions has a marked systematic effect on their oxygen affinity, depending on whether the α or β chain is abnormal. In the two haemoglobins with affected α chains (Hb M Boston, $\alpha_2^{(58\ Tyr)}\beta_2^A$ [137], Hb M Iwate $\alpha_2^{(8\cdot7\ Tyr)}\beta_2^A$ [523]) there is a low oxygen affinity with grossly reduced subunit interactions and Bohr effect, while in the two haemoglobins with abnormal β chains (Hb M Saskatoon, $\alpha_2^A\beta_2^{(63\ Tyr)}$, Hb M Hyde Park, $\alpha_2^A\beta_2^{(92\ Tyr)}$) there is a raised oxygen affinity and reduced subunit interactions with a normal Bohr effect. Some instability of the haemoglobin molecule is also sometimes present, leading to mild haemolysis. Otherwise the condition is a benign form of congenital cyanosis and no treatment is required (or known).

THE UNSTABLE HAEMOGLOBINS

Clinical features
The unstable haemoglobins are one cause of the 'congenital non-spherocytic haemolytic anaemias', and their molecular and clinical features have recently been reviewed [327, 391–393]. In these conditions, various types of molecular abnormality lead to instability of the haemoglobin molecule and to haemolytic anaemia. Depending on whether the α or β chain is affected, the disease may either be present at birth or start a few months later. The clinical picture varies from patient to patient, some having only slight shortening of red-cell lifespan, whilst in others the degree of haemolysis is much more severe. In the more severely affected patients, there is usually pallor and jaundice as well as splenic enlargement. There is commonly a history of haemolytic crises associated with the ingestion of certain drugs (see later) or with infection. As the disease in these patients occurs in the heterozygous condition, its occurrence in several generations of the same family may be helpful in distinguishing it from haemolytic disease due to an enzyme deficiency, which usually occurs in the homozygous (or hemizygous in the case of G6PD) state. Haematological examination shows a variable anaemia and reticulocytosis; the red cells show variation in size and shape and are usually

hypochromic with a low MCHC. In the mildest cases, such as Hb Seattle, the blood film may be normal. Inclusion (Heinz) bodies can occasionally be seen in the film but are usually demonstrated by supravital stain, and this was the main feature of the first case, described by Cathie [394]. Often they are found only after incubation without glucose for 24 hours or after splenectomy. Dark urine is found in some cases due to the excretion of dipyrroles of the bilifuscin-mesobilifuscin type [395, 396]. Occasionally, cyanosis is present due to either a low oxygen affinity, as in Hb Hammersmith, or the formation of methaemoglobin. There are no specific physical or haematological signs, and the diagnosis rests on the demonstration of the unstable, abnormal pigment. As most of the known abnormal haemoglobins do not cause any haemolytic anaemia in the heterozygous state, other possible causes of haemolysis should be carefully excluded. In this connection, examination of other family members is particularly useful as the haemoglobin may be found without haemolysis, as we have seen in one case, or *vice versa*.

Detection of the unstable haemoglobins
One of the reasons why the presence of unstable haemoglobins has often been missed is that they are usually not detected by paper electrophoresis. The diagnosis depends on more sensitive electrophoretic techniques and on demonstrating haemoglobin instability. The demonstration of an abnormal oxygen affinity may be helpful in some cases. Electrophoresis on starch gel, Cellogel or acrylamide gel, is a suitably sensitive method, particularly if several different buffer systems at different pH values are used; these supporting media will also separate aggregated haemoglobin molecules. As some haemoglobins separate only in the met- form, this derivative should also be used. Free α chains should be looked for as they are present in small amounts in some cases. Fresh haemolysates from some cases contain small amounts, usually less than five per cent, of met-haemoglobin or haemochromogen; occasionally sulphaemoglobin is present.

Methods based on stability of the haemoglobin are demonstration of inclusion bodies in the cells, heat denaturation of the haemoglobin, para-mercuribenzoate (PCMB) precipitation of haemoglobin and the isopropanol precipitation test. Inclusion-body formation is due to intracellular haemoglobin precipitation and is demonstrated by supravital staining by, for example, brilliant cresyl blue. As the reticuloendothelial cells of the spleen remove any inclusion bodies formed *in vivo*, they are often only seen after splenectomy, or further precipitation must be caused *in vitro* by incubation of the red cells without glucose for 24 hours. Incubation for 24 hours shows more rapid methaemoglobin formation than with Hb A; GSH is also more rapidly reduced.

Another feature of the unstable haemoglobins is their more rapid precipitation than Hb A on heating of the haemolysate. This was first shown for Hb H by Betke and his colleagues [397] and then applied to the detection of the unstable haemoglobins [398, 399]. Again this test has its drawbacks; if the abnormal haemoglobin is present in only small amounts, or is only mildly unstable, differentiation from the normal may be difficult. We use a dilute haemoglobin solution (*c.* 0·15 g/dl) in phosphate buffer pH 6·5, divide this into test and control, incubate at 60°C for half an hour, then add an equal volume of Drabkin's solution and read in a spectrophotometer against suitable diluted Drabkin's reagent. Besides this quantitative measure of the amount of haemoglobin lost, a visual estimate of the precipitate should also be made as some of these variants do not carry a haem group on the affected chain. In the original method [398] 50°C was used but at this temperature some of the relatively stable 'unstable haemoglobins' would not be detected. In this test both the abnormal and the partner normal chain are precipitated [400].

Reaction of Hb A with excess parachloromercuribenzoate (PCMB) causes dissociation into the individual α and β chains which can then be separated by starch-gel electrophoresis [401]. By using strictly controlled conditions [10], specific precipitation of the abnormal chain of some unstable haemoglobins occurs, and this may be useful in diagnosis and for the isolation of the abnormal chain. With some electrophoretically inseparable haemoglobins the dissociated abnormal chain may be seen on electrophoresis. Still other haemoglobins may differ in their dissociation properties, either showing rapid dissociation into subunits, as in Hb Philly or failing to dissociate (completely) under the usual conditions. This technique is useful in scanning for unstable haemoglobins but, like all other methods, fails to detect some. More recently, Carrell & Kay [402] have described a simple, and perhaps more sensitive, test for unstable haemoglobins. Haemolysate (0·2 ml) is incubated in 2 ml of 17% iso-propanol in 0·1 M tris buffer pH 7·4 at 37°C for 30 minutes and precipitation looked for.

Finally, a number of the unstable haemoglobins have abnormal oxygen dissociation properties, and the finding of a high or low red-cell oxygen affinity without the corresponding shift in 2,3-DPG may point to a haemoglobin abnormality.

Molecular pathology of the unstable haemoglobins
There are three ways in which the haemoglobin molecule can become unstable. The first is by loss of the haem group [403–405], the second by dissociation of the molecule into its separate α and β chains [406], and thirdly, but equally important, by distortion and weakening of the structure of the affected subunit. In many cases of all three mechanisms are operative, although usually one is predominant. The instability of the molecule is associated with oxidative changes [407] in the molecule involving methaemoglobin formation, already referred to above, hemichrome formation [408] and blockage of the free sulphydryl groups forming mixed disulphides with GSH [403, 409], and leads to intracellular precipitation and formation of Heinz bodies.

Decreased haem binding is usually due to amino-acid substitutions involving one of the residues in contact with the haem group, but may also be caused by general distortion of the affected subunit. Methaemoglobin formation also leads to increased haem loss. In a number of cases the affected subunit does not bind haem at all. It is not surprising that loss of haem leads to molecular instability considering the well-documented instability of globin.

Increased dissociation into the individual α and β subunits is seen in many abnormal haemoglobins, usually due to general distortion of the affected subunit. In these cases, traces of free α-chain haemoglobin or Hb β_4 may be found in the fresh haemolysate. In substitutions affecting the $\alpha_1\beta_1$ contact, such as Hb Philly, dissociation of the molecule is a primary feature of the denaturing process and larger amounts of free chains may be found. The instability of the separated subunit even with their haem group is well known, the α chain being less stable than the β chain [410]. In this connection it is of interest to note that substitutions involving the $\alpha_1\beta_2$ contact do not cause instability, and this is because haemoglobin is normally partially dissociated at this contact.

Instability of one of the subunits itself may be caused in various ways. First, the new amino acid may be too large to be accommodated in the interior of a subunit, a kind of molecular 'space-occupying lesion'. The interior of each subunit consists of apolar or hydrophobic amino-acid side chains and the introduction of a polar (charged) amino acid is not possible without distortion of the structure as the hydrophilic group tries to reach the surface of the molecule or draws an oppositely charged side chain near it. A good example of this is Hb Wien. Another way in which the subunit structure may be broken up is the replacement of a helical residue by a prolyl residue. Proline can only be accommodated between helices and at the beginning and end of a helix. Several such substitutions are known (Table 8.5), all associated with haemoglobin instability and haemolysis. Finally, the subunit structure is held together by a number of bonds between helices; loss of some of these can lead to instability as, for example, in Hb Hopkins II. The changes described above can lead to instability of the haemoglobin molecule and precipitation of the haemoglobin in the red cell. This process is often associated with methaemoglobin formation, the formation of hemichromes and the blockage of the free sulphydryl groups, as has already been mentioned.

The precipitated haemoglobin is removed from the red cell by the pitting phenomenon in the spleen, as has been demonstrated by electron microscopy [411–413]. Consistent with this is the finding that inclusion bodies are more easily demonstrated after splenectomy. In some cases the abnormal chain is so unstable that a proportion of the abnormal chains made is precipitated shortly after synthesis and the precipitated haemoglobin is presumably removed by the reticuloendothelial cells of the marrow [414]. In many cases the amino-acid substitution leads not only to instability of the molecule but also to changes in oxygen affinity, resulting in important physiological consequences, discussed below.

The degree of haemolysis in these diseases is clearly related to the degree of instability of the haemoglobin involved. Recent studies of a number of unstable β-chain variants have shown that the rate of synthesis of the abnormal chains is nearly always the same as that of the corresponding normal chain [414]. The amount of abnormal haemoglobin found in the cells is then related to the amount which has already been precipitated. As precipitation followed by pitting causes damage to the red-cell membrane [285, 413, 415, 416], it follows that the less abnormal haemoglobin there is in the cell and the more cell-membrane damage there is, the greater the degree of haemolysis found. Analysis of the published data shows that there is a significant correlation between cell survival and the relative amount of abnormal haemoglobin, a small amount of abnormal haemoglobin (i.e. most precipitation and cell damage) being associated with the shortest cell survival [417]. Rather surprisingly, there is little correlation between the red-cell survival and the packed cell volume or haemoglobin level [417]. If the degree of red-cell destruction is not the main determinant of the blood haemoglobin level, then this must be controlled by the erythropoietic response of the marrow. As has already been pointed out (p. 367), in patients with red cells with an abnormal oxygen affinity, the red-cell mass is determined by the erythropoietin-mediated marrow response, a high oxygen affinity leading to greater erythropoietin production because of the relatively low release of oxygen per gram of haemoglobin and thus to polycythaemia, while the reverse happens with a low oxygen affinity. Applying similarly arguments to the haemolytic states it is found that there is a close correlation between

oxygen affinity of the red cells and the PCV of the peripheral blood [418]. This relationship applies not only to the unstable haemoglobins but also to the sickle-cell syndromes and the enzymopathies. In patients where this relationship between packed cell volume and oxygen affinity deviates from that expected, further investigations should be carried out. If the packed cell volume is too low, then the marrow response is lower than expected and some other complicating factor, such as increasing haemolysis, folate deficiency, etc., should be looked for. In one patient with Hb S + C disease whose packed cell volume was too high for the oxygen affinity, further studies showed, as expected, a low red-cell mass, the high PCV being due to a low plasma volume.

The finding that the packed cell volume (i.e. red-cell mass) is closely geared to the oxygen affinity of the red cells means that in haemolytic diseases in the steady state the oxygen-delivery capacity of the blood is the same regardless of whether there is a high or low level of haemoglobin present, and this conclusion accounts for the normal development of many of these patients and the mild nature of the disease. However, it should be noted that although this is undoubtedly true in the uncomplicated disease, in conditions of stress, such as strenuous exercise, increased anaemia, etc., when the tissue oxygen tensions tend to be lower than normal, patients with a high oxygen affinity and a high PCV are at a distinct advantage compared to those with a low oxygen affinity and a low PCV. This results in part from the position and shape of the oxygen dissociation curve as well as from the higher oxygen capacity of the blood of patients with a high PCV. Another advantage of high oxygen affinity is that the arterial oxygen content is protected against any fall in arterial Po_2 due, for example, to respiratory disease. These considerations may explain the finding that among the patients who are heterozygous for an abnormal haemoglobin a raised blood oxygen affinity is seen more frequently than a low affinity, and thus account for the relative frequency of Hb Köln. All these factors must be taken into account in the management of these diseases.

Treatment of diseases due to the unstable haemoglobins
There is no specific treatment for these diseases, but splenectomy is sometimes helpful in patients with severe haemolysis [419], while in others no improvement can be shown [394]. Each case must therefore be individually assessed by determining the degree of splenic red-cell destruction. In patients who have no symptoms, as occurs in most cases with Hb Köln, splenectomy is contraindicated. The increased liability to oxidation of the haemoglobin molecules often makes these patients sensitive to the same group of drugs that may cause crises in glucose-6-phosphate

dehydrogenase (G6PD) deficiency [470]. In the unstable haemoglobins the molecule is more easily oxidized, while in G6PD deficiency the reductive potential of the cell is reduced. In either case, haemoglobin precipitates in the cell and may lead to haemolytic crises. These drugs (see Chapter 7, p. 273) should therefore be avoided. Another possible line of treatment is by blood transfusions, but these are only occasionally indicated to tide the patient over intercurrent disease. In assessing the severity of the disease, not only the degree of anaemia but also the oxygen affinity of the red cells should be taken into account (see previous section).

The molecular pathology of the abnormal haemoglobins

The effect of any structural abnormality of haemoglobin is determined by the type of amino-acid difference and its position in the molecule. The present results are summarized below. The detailed atomic interactions occurring in those abnormal haemoglobins are given in Refs 242 and 421 or in the individual papers quoted.

Substitutions on the outside of the molecule (Table 8.4). Most of these substitutions are relatively benign; pathological effects only arise if new deleterious inter-actions occur, such as in sickle-cell disease, or if important stabilizing bonds are broken.

Substitutions on the interior of a subunit (Table 8.5). So far all substitutions described on the interior of a subunit have caused instability of the molecule due to their size or polar character, or because they involve the insertion of a proline into a helical part of the polypeptide chain.

Substitutions around the haem groups (Figs 8.27 and 8.28). Almost all these cause instability of the molecule due to reduced haem binding by the globin part of the molecule. The oxygen affinity is usually altered. The haemoglobins M form a special subgroup (see p. 369).

Substitutions in the $\alpha_1\beta_1$ intersubunit contact (Fig. 8.29). These substitutions are often benign but may give rise to instability if they cause increased dissociation at this contact. Some cause alteration in the oxygen affinity.

Substitutions in the $\alpha_1\beta_2$ intersubunit contact (Fig. 8.30). The substitutions at this contact do not cause instability because dissociation normally takes place here. As this contact is important in the change from the oxy- to the deoxy- form of haemoglobin, a change of oxygen affinity and subunit (haem–haem) interactions

Table 8.4. Effect of abnormal haemoglobins due to replacements at the surface of the molecule

---

A More than 100 (53α and 49β) are known without clinical or physiological abnormality: detailed stability and oxygen dissociation studies are not available on most. For reference see [243a].
B Disease in the homozygote.
   Hb S, Hb C, Hb E, Hb D Punjab. See text.
C Altered function.
  (i) Raised oxygen affinity:
     Sawara [455, 456] α6(A4) Asp→Ala; Asp forms salt bridge to 127 (H10)Lys same α chain.
     Porte Alegre [457] β9(A6) Ser→Cys; *in-vitro* polymerization by disulphide-bond formation; no disease.
     Olympia [458] β20(β2) Val→Met; normal Bohr.
     Hiroshima [459–462] β146(HC3) His→Asp. 'n' = 2, Bohr absent. C-terminal amino acid concerned with Bohr effect.
     G Hsi Tsou [463, 464] β79(EF3) Asp→Gly; Salt bridge to β8(A5) Lys same β chain in deoxy- form broken.
     D Punjab (see text) β121(GH4) Glu→Gln; Gln forms salt bridge to β17(A14) Lys same β chain.
     Andrew-Minneapolis [465] β144(HC1) Lys→Asn interfered with movement of βHC2 Tyr.
  (ii) Lowered oxygen affinity:
     Vancouver [466] β73(E17) Asp→Tyr.
     Mobile [467] β73(E17) Asp→Val.
     Agenogi [468, 469] β90(F6) Glu→Lys; Lys could form salt bridge with C-terminal —COOH of same chain.
  (iii) Unstable haemoglobins:
     Hasharon [470, 471] α47(CE5) Asp→HIS ⎫ cause of instability not clear.
     Arya [472] α47(CE5) Asp→Asn ⎭
     Hopkins II [100, 101, 473, 474] α112(G19) His→Asp surface residue stabilizing B and G helices.
     G Ferrara [475] β57 (E1) Asn→Lys.
     Duarte [476] β62(E6) Ala→Pro: raised oxygen affinity.
                      Proline residue not allowed in helix.
     Shepherd's Bush [471, 478] β74(E18) Gly→Asp; raised O_2 affinity, low DPG interaction. Larger polar residue intrudes into haem pocket.

Table 8.5. Haemoglobins due to replacements in the interior of a subunit

A   The insertion of a proline into a helix leads to its gross distortion and molecular instability

Port Phillip	[479]	α91(FG3)		
Bibba	[480]	α136(H19)	O₂ affinity raised	
Saki	[481, 482]	β14 (A11)		
Genova	[483, 484]	β28(B10)	O₂ affinity raised	
Perth	[485, 486]	β32(B14)	O₂ affinity raised	
Mizuho	[487]	β68(E12)		Leu→Pro
Atlanta	[488]	β75(E19)		
Santa Ana	[489–491]	β88(F4)		
Sabine	[492]	β91(F7)		
Southampton	[493, 494]	β106(G8)	O₂ affinity raised	
Madrid	[495]	β115(G17)		Ala→Pro
Bicêtre	[496]	β63(E7)		His→Pro
Newcastle	[497]	β92(F8)		His→Pro

B   The replacement of either a non-polar by a polar residue in the hydrophilic interior or a small by a larger residue leading to instability

Etobicoke	[498]	α84(F5)	Ser→Arg	O₂ affinity raised
Belfast	[499, 500]	β15(A12)	Trp→Arg	O₂ affinity raised
Strasbourg	[501]	β23(B5)	Val→Asp	
Riverdale-Bronx	[502]	β23(B5)	Val→Arg	
Savannah	[503]	β24(B6)	Gly→Val	increased subunit dissociation
Moscva	[504]	β24(B6)	Gly→Asp	low O₂ affinity
Volga	[505, 506]	β27(B9)	Ala→Asp	
St Louis	[507]	β28(B10)	Leu→Gln	O₂ affinity raised met haemoglobin
Castilla	[508]	β32(B14)	Leu→Arg	
Okaloosa	[509]	β48(CD7)	Leu→Arg	low O₂ affinity
J. Calabria	[510]	β64(E8)	Gly→Asp	
Baylor	[651]	β81(EF5)	Leu→Arg	raised O₂ affinity
Bryn Mawr	[511, 512]	β85(F1)	Phe→Ser	raised O₂ affinity
Peterborough	[513]	β111(G13)	Val→Phe	low O₂ affinity
Wien	[514, 515]	β130(H8)	Tyr→Asp	
North Shore	[516, 517]	β134(H12)	Val→Glu	normal O₂ affinity

C   Substitutions leading to increased oxygen affinity

Creteil	[518]	β89(F5)	Ser→Asn	
Vanderbilt	[519]	β89(F5)	Ser→Arg	

occurs in almost all abnormal haemoglobins affecting this contact.

Substitutions in the central cavity and at the β–β intersubunit contact (Table 8.6). Substitutions in this area may affect oxygen affinity by altering DPG binding (as, for example, in Hb ShB which indirectly affects lysine $β^{82}$) or by breaking some of the salt bridges maintaining the oxy structure of haemoglobin. Replacement of histidine $β^{146}$ reduces the Bohr effect (see also Fig. 8.30), but in Hb Cochin, $β^{(146 \; (HC3) \; His→Arg)}$ oxygen dissociation is normal [422]. Presumably the new arginyl residue is similar to the histidyl residue replaced. Amino-acid deletions and insertions (Table 8.2) have already been discussed on page 345.

Conclusion. Overall there is a very significant difference between the number of α-chain and β-chain variants described, about 90–170 respectively. Comparison of the distribution of the variants shows that the number of non-pathological variants at the surface of the molecule is approximately equal, 53α to 49β (Table 8.4), while there are 40 pathological haemoglobins in the α chains and 123 in the β chains (Tables 8.2, 8.4, 8.5, 8.6 and Figs 8.27, 8.28, 8.29, 8.30). These differences become even more significant if it is remembered that there are two α loci and only a single β locus. There is, therefore, double the opportunity for mutation to occur in the α chains compared to the β chains. This difference presumably reflects the more stringent selection of changes in haemoglobin struc-

Position	Amino acid		
32 (B13)	Met		
39 (C4)	Thr		
42 (C7)	Tyr		
43 (CD1)	Phe $\to$ Leu	Hirosaki, unstable [520]	
	$\to$ Val	Torino, unstable, low O_2 affinity [521]	
45 (CD3)	His $\to$ Arg	Fort de France, raised O_2 affinity [522]	
46 (CD4)	Phe		
58 (E7)	His $\to$ Tyr	M Boston, low O_2 affinity, subunit interactions and Bohr effect reduced [137, 523]	
61 (E10)	Lys $\to$ Asn	J Buda, low O_2 affinity, slight instability [524]	
62 (E11)	Val		
83 (F4)	Leu		
86 (F7)	Leu $\to$ Arg	Moabit, low O_2 affinity, unstable [525]	
87 (F8)	His $\to$ Tyr	M Iwate, low O_2 affinity, unstable, subunit interaction and Bohr effect absent [526–529]	
91 (FG3)	Leu		
93 (FG5)	Val		
97 (G4)	Asn		
98 (G5)	Phe		
101 (G8)	Leu		
129 (H12)	Leu		
132 (H15)	Val		
136 (H19)	Leu $\to$ Pro	Bibba, unstable [480]	

Fig. 8.27. Amino-acid substitutions of haem contacts of the α chain.

ture occurring during embryonic and fetal development when α chains form part of one of the main embryonic haemoglobin, Hb Gower 2, $\alpha_2 \varepsilon_2$ and of both fetal haemoglobins, $\alpha_2{}^A \gamma_2$ and $\alpha_2{}^C \gamma_2$ (see p. 341). That there are only relatively few γ-chain variants may either be because fewer cord-blood samples have been tested or may reflect the more stringent selection occurring during fetal life. Only one of these has been found because the abnormality was suspected clinically at birth [126a]. The others were found during cord-blood surveys.

Using hindsight I have seen one ε chain variant (out of approximately 40 embryonic samples examined); on electrophoresis both Hb Gower 2 and Hb Gower 1 were accompanied by a 'fast' (i.e. anodal) band amounting to *c.* 30% of each main band.

ACQUIRED HAEMOGLOBIN ABNORMALITIES

Methaemoglobinaemia (see also Chapter 7)
In the red cell, methaemoglobin forms slowly at the rate of about three per cent of total haemoglobin per day [423], its accumulation is prevented by certain enzyme systems and their relative contributions are [424–426]:

NADH methaemoglobin reductase I	61
Ascorbic acid (non-enzymic)	16
GSH (non-enzymic)	12
NADH methaemoglobin reductase II	6
NADPH methaemoglobin reductase	5

Thus, in the normal cell, methaemoglobin does not exceed 0·5% of total haemoglobin.

ACQUIRED METHAEMOGLOBINAEMIA
Increased methaemoglobin production in the cell may be due to the action of certain chemicals or drugs (Table 8.7) [427]. High doses of the offending chemical will produce methaemoglobin in most individuals, but some are much more sensitive to these drugs. The reason for this in any individual case is not usually known. The enzyme mechanism for methaemoglobin reduction may be deficient and thus the trait form of methaemoglobin-reductase deficiency, or deficiency of one of the other enzyme systems, may make an individual more sensitive. Another way in which the red cell prevents methaemoglobin formation is by removing 'oxidizing influences'. This consists of the removal of peroxides and drug detoxification by glutathione peroxidase [529] and catalase. Maintenance of reduced glutathione by glutathione reductase, glucose-6-P and 6P gluconate dehydrogenases and glutathione synthetase is essential for the normal functioning of this mechanism. Finally, the maintenance of ascorbic acid is important and this is also linked to the GSH system. These enzymic systems are discussed in detail in Chapter 7. Thus, if one of these systems is deficient, then the affected red cell is more liable to methaemoglobin formation than normal.

During the first few months babies are much more prone to develop methaemoglobinaemia than later in

Position	Amino acid	
31 (B13)	Leu	
38 (C4)	Thr	
41 (C7)	Phe→Tyr	Mequon, unstable, O_2 affinity normal [530]
42 (CD1)	Phe⟨Ser	Hammersmith, unstable, low O_2 affinity, slightly low subunit interaction [398, 399, 421, 531]
	Leu	Louisville/Bucaresti, unstable, low O_2 affinity [532]
44 (CD3)	Ser	
45 (CD4)	Phe	
63 (E7)	His⟨Arg	Zürich, unstable, high O_2 affinity, normal Bohr effect, reduced subunit interaction [420, 533–537]
	Tyr	M Saskatoon, unstable, high O_2 affinity, reduced subunit interactions, normal Bohr effect [137, 538, 539]
66 (E10)	Lys→Glu	Toulouse, unstable, normal O_2 dissociation, linked to propionic side chain of haem [540]
67 (E11)	Val⟨Asp	M Milwaukee, unstable, low O_2 affinity, normal Bohr effect, reduced subunit interactions [137, 541–543]
	Ala	Sydney, unstable [242, 544]
	Glu	Bristol, unstable, low O_2 affinity, normal Bohr effect, slightly decreased subunit interactions [138, 394]
70 (E14)	Ala→Asp	Seattle, unstable, low O_2 affinity, normal haem–haem interactions and Bohr effect [545–547]
71 (E15)	Phe→Ser	Christchurch, unstable [548]
74 (E18)	Gly→Asp	Shepherd's Bush, unstable, high O_2 affinity, normal Bohr effect, decreased subunit interaction, low 2,3-DPG effect [477, 478]
88 (F4)	Leu⟨Pro	Santa Ana, unstable, no haem group [489–491]
	Arg	Boras, unstable, high O_2 affinity [549, 550]
91 (F7)	Leu→Pro	Sabine, unstable, no haem group [492]
92 (F8)	His⟨Gln	St Etienne, unstable, high O_2 affinity [551, 552]
	Tyr	M Hyde Park, unstable, high O_2 affinity, low subunit interaction, normal Bohr shift [553–555]
	Asp	J Altgeld, normal O_2 affinity [556]
	Pro	Newcastle, unstable [497]
96 (FG3)	Leu	
98 (FG5)	Val⟨Ala	Djela, unstable, high O_2 affinity [557]
	Met	Köln, unstable, high O_2 affinity, low subunit interaction, normal Bohr effect (also in $\alpha^1\beta^2$ contact) [138, 558]
	Gly	Nottingham, similar to Köln [559]
103 (G5)	Phe	
106 (G8)	Leu→Pro	Casper, unstable, haem loss [494]
137 (H15)	Val	
141 (H19)	Leu→Arg	Olmstead, unstable [560]
85 (F1)	Phe→Ser	Bryn Mawr, unstable, high O_2 affinity [511]

Fig. 8.28. Amino-acid substitutions of haem contacts of the β chain.

life; this is because of the low level of methaemoglobin reductase in the red cells at this time [428, 429]. This may be precipitated by the ingestion of nitrite, derived from nitrate, present in water [430, 431] or in some vegetable purées particularly spinach or carrots [432, 433]. Contaminated milk has also been incriminated [434]. Another cause is the absorption of dyes used for marking nappies [435, 436].

The presence of methaemoglobin in the blood is only harmful in that it does not carry oxygen. Thus the presence of small amounts of the abnormal pigments will cause only a small reduction in the oxygen-carrying capacity of the blood and requires no specific treatment except for removing the chemical cause. The

methaemoglobin then disappears over the next 24–48 hours. If more than, say, 20% is present, then reduction can be speeded up by treatment with methylene blue as this stimulates reduction by the NADPH-dependent enzymes. Ascorbic acid is usually ineffective in these cases. In very severe cases exchange transfusion may be necessary.

CONGENITAL METHAEMOGLOBINAEMIA
(see also Chapter 7)
Congenital methaemoglobin is due to deficiency of the NADH-dependent methaemoglobin reductase (dia-phorase) in the red cell occurring in the homozygous form and is characterized by the presence of 10–20%

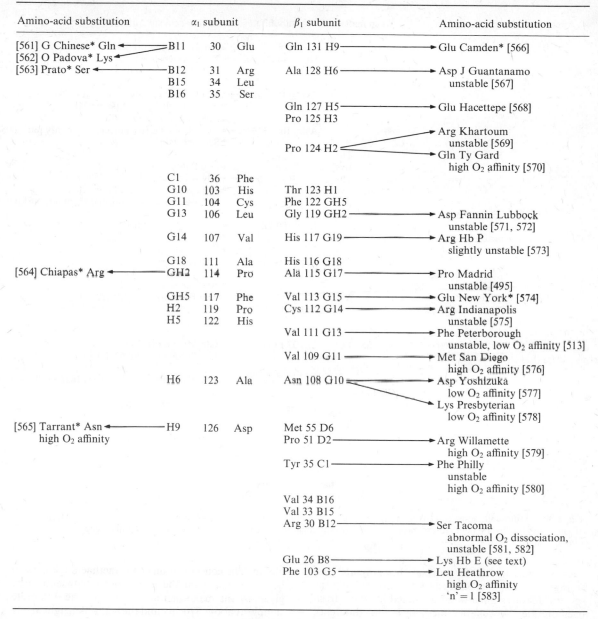

Amino-acid substitution		α_1 subunit		β_1 subunit	Amino-acid substitution
[561] G Chinese* Gln	B11	30	Glu	Gln 131 H9	Glu Camden* [566]
[562] O Padova* Lys					
[563] Prato* Ser	B12	31	Arg	Ala 128 H6	Asp J Guantanamo unstable [567]
	B15	34	Leu		
	B16	35	Ser		
				Gln 127 H5	Glu Hacettepe [568]
				Pro 125 H3	
				Pro 124 H2	Arg Khartoum unstable [569]
					Gln Ty Gard high O_2 affinity [570]
	C1	36	Phe		
	G10	103	His	Thr 123 H1	
	G11	104	Cys	Phe 122 GH5	
	G13	106	Leu	Gly 119 GH2	Asp Fannin Lubbock unstable [571, 572]
	G14	107	Val	His 117 G19	Arg Hb P slightly unstable [573]
	G18	111	Ala	His 116 G18	
[564] Chiapas* Arg	GH2	114	Pro	Ala 115 G17	Pro Madrid unstable [495]
	GH5	117	Phe	Val 113 G15	Glu New York* [574]
	H2	119	Pro	Cys 112 G14	Arg Indianapolis unstable [575]
	H5	122	His	Val 111 G13	Phe Peterborough unstable, low O_2 affinity [513]
				Val 109 G11	Met San Diego high O_2 affinity [576]
	H6	123	Ala	Asn 108 G10	Asp Yoshizuka low O_2 affinity [577]
					Lys Presbyterian low O_2 affinity [578]
[565] Tarrant* Asn high O_2 affinity	H9	126	Asp	Met 55 D6	
				Pro 51 D2	Arg Willamette high O_2 affinity [579]
				Tyr 35 C1	Phe Philly unstable high O_2 affinity [580]
				Val 34 B16	
				Val 33 B15	
				Arg 30 B12	Ser Tacoma abnormal O_2 dissociation, unstable [581, 582]
				Glu 26 B8	Lys Hb E (see text)
				Phe 103 G5	Leu Heathrow high O_2 affinity 'n' = 1 [583]

* No abnormal properties

Fig. 8.29. Amino-acid substitutions in the $\alpha_1\beta_1$ contact: α-chain residues on left, β-chain residues on right.

methaemoglobin in the red cells from birth [437]. Clinical examination of the patient reveals no abnormal physical signs except cyanosis. In about half the reported cases, mental deficiency is also present, and these patients often become institutionalized [437]. Except for mental deficiency and cyanosis, the disease itself causes no specific symptoms. Laboratory examination shows the presence of 10–20% methaemoglobin and this is distinguished from Hb M, sulphaemoglobin and haemochromogen in the red cells by examination of the spectrum, and by showing that the α-absorption band is at 632 nm. As met-

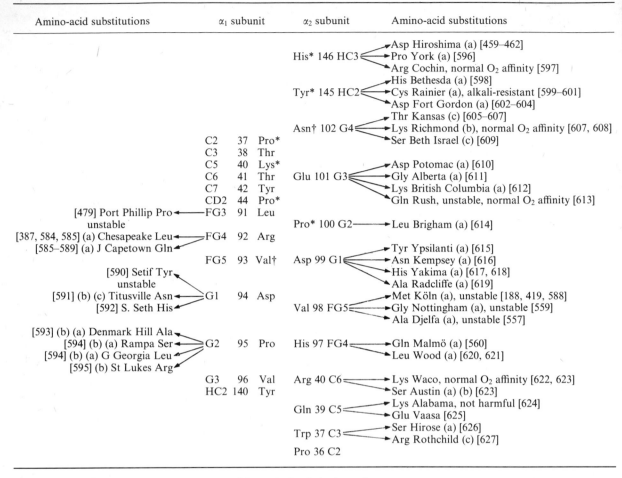

Amino-acid substitutions	α_1 subunit			α_2 subunit	Amino-acid substitutions
				His* 146 HC3	Asp Hiroshima (a) [459–462]
					Pro York (a) [596]
					Arg Cochin, normal O_2 affinity [597]
				Tyr* 145 HC2	His Bethesda (a) [598]
					Cys Rainier (a), alkali-resistant [599–601]
					Asp Fort Gordon (a) [602–604]
				Asn† 102 G4	Thr Kansas (c) [605–607]
	C2	37	Pro*		Lys Richmond (b), normal O_2 affinity [607, 608]
	C3	38	Thr		Ser Beth Israel (c) [609]
	C5	40	Lys*		
	C6	41	Thr	Glu 101 G3	Asp Potomac (a) [610]
	C7	42	Tyr		Gly Alberta (a) [611]
	CD2	44	Pro*		Lys British Columbia (a) [612]
[479] Port Phillip Pro	FG3	91	Leu		Gln Rush, unstable, normal O_2 affinity [613]
unstable				Pro* 100 G2	Leu Brigham (a) [614]
[387, 584, 585] (a) Chesapeake Leu	FG4	92	Arg		
[585–589] (a) J Capetown Gln				Asp 99 G1	Tyr Ypsilanti (a) [615]
	FG5	93	Val†		Asn Kempsey (a) [616]
					His Yakima (a) [617, 618]
[590] Setif Tyr					Ala Radcliffe (a) [619]
unstable				Val 98 FG5	Met Köln (a), unstable [188, 419, 588]
[591] (b) (c) Titusville Asn	G1	94	Asp		Gly Nottingham (a), unstable [559]
[592] S. Seth His					Ala Djelfa (a), unstable [557]
[593] (b) (a) Denmark Hill Ala				His 97 FG4	Gln Malmö (a) [560]
[594] (b) (a) Rampa Ser	G2	95	Pro		Leu Wood (a) [620, 621]
[594] (b) (a) G Georgia Leu					
[595] (b) St Lukes Arg				Arg 40 C6	Lys Waco, normal O_2 affinity [622, 623]
	G3	96	Val		Ser Austin (a) (b) [623]
	HC2	140	Tyr	Gln 39 C5	Lys Alabama, not harmful [624]
					Glu Vaasa [625]
				Trp 37 C3	Ser Hirose (a) [626]
					Arg Rothchild (c) [627]
				Pro 36 C2	

* In contact only in deoxy-form
† In contact only in oxy-form

Fig. 8.30. Amino-acid substitutions in the $\alpha_1\beta_2$ contact: α-chain residues on left, β-chain residues on right. (a): High oxygen affinity, very low haem–haem interactions; (b) abnormal dissociation into subunits; (c) low oxygen affinity, very low haem–haem interactions.

haemoglobin forms in normal haemolysates on storage or manipulation it cannot be isolated and the spectral features have to be identified in whole fresh haemolysate. A reliable method is the difference method described by West and her colleagues [438]. In this, dilute haemolysate is divided into two aliquots; to one is added a small amount of solid dithionite to reduce any methaemoglobin present. Both samples are then treated with carbon monoxide and their spectra and difference spectrum recorded, using, if necessary, an expanded scale to visualize the peak at 632 nm. A base line is drawn using the dithionite-treated solution in both cuvettes. The presence of the peak at 632 nm indicates that one is dealing with normal methaemo-globin. The concentration of the methaemoglobin can be calculated from the haemoglobin concentration, given by the maximum absorbance of the dithionite sample at about 570 nm, and the net peak height at 632 nm. This method is simpler and has a greater sensitivity than previously reported methods. The diagnosis can be confirmed by measuring the activity of the level of the NADH methaemoglobin reductase in the haemolysate [439]. Another test is to measure the rate of reduction in whole red cells after conversion to methaemoglobin. Normal red cells will reduce most of the methaemoglobin present during 24 hours' incubation while deficient cells show almost no reduction [440]. In both these tests the homozygous condition is clearly

Table 8.6. Abnormal haemoglobins in the central cavity and between like chains

Manitoba	[242, 628]	α102(G9)	Ser→Arg	slight instability
St Claude	[629]	α127(H10)	Lys→Thr	
Jackson	[630]	α127(H10)	Lys→Asn	
Singapore	[569]	α141(HC3)	Arg→Pro	
Surenes	[631]	α141(HC3)	Arg→His	high O_2 affinity
J. Cubujaqui	[632]	α141(HC3)	Arg→Ser	
Iregnano	[633]	α141(HC3)	Arg→Leu	high O_2 affinity
J. Camagüey	[634]	α141(HC3)	Arg→Gly	
Raleigh	[635]	β1(NA1)*	Val→Ac-Ala	low O_2 affinity†
Deer Lodge	[636]	β2(NA2)*	His→Arg	high O_2 affinity†
Hsi-Tsou	[463, 464]	β79(EF3)	Asp→Gly	high O_2 affinity†, SB‡ to β8(A5) Lys same β chains broken
Szuhu	[637, 638]	β80(EF4)	Asn→Lys	high O_2 affinity†
Helsinki	[639]	β82(EF6)*	Lys→Met	low O_2 affinity, low Bohr effect
Providence	[640, 641]	β82(EF6)*	Lys→Asn	low O_2 affinity, low Bohr effect†
Rehere	[642]	β82(EF6)*	Lys→Thr	high O_2 affinity, low Bohr effect†
Altdorf	[643]	β135(H13)	Ala→Pro	unstable, high O_2 affinity
Hope	[644]	β136(H14)	Gly→Asp	unstable, low O_2 affinity, low Bohr effect
Syracuse	[645]	β143(H21)*	His→Pro	high O_2 affinity, low Bohr effect†
Abruzzo	[646]	β143(H21)*	His→Arg	high O_2 affinity, low Bohr effect†
Little Rock	[647]	β143(H21)*	His→Gln	high O_2 affinity, low Bohr effect†

* These residues bind 2,3-DPG
† Discussed in Ref. 648
‡ SB: salt bridge

distinguished from the normal. The trait form usually gives intermediate values. However, the overlap with the normal range is such that they are often difficult to distinguish.

Recent studies suggest that in most cases congenital methaemoglobinaemia is due to the synthesis of an abnormal enzyme [438] and there are many different variants which can be distinguished by detailed studies of the enzymic and electrophoretic properties of the proteins concerned. In some cases the variant enzyme can be used to diagnose the heterozygous state. It is now known that the mitochondrial enzyme, cytochrome B5 reductase, is the same protein as red-cell diaphorase [441]. This explains the occurrence of mental deficiency in some cases if it is postulated that with some variants the enzyme is only unstable in solution and that it is stabilized by attachment to the mitochondrial membrane. In this case no mental deficiency occurs. If proper placing in the mitochondria is also not possible, mental deficiency results.

The presence of methaemoglobin in the red cells causes an increased oxygen affinity and reduced haem–haem interactions [442–444] and these patients usually have higher than normal haemoglobin levels. There is no treatment for any mental deficiency present, but the cyanosis can be relieved by treatment with large doses of vitamin C, 500 mg/day [445, 446], or methylene blue, 1–2 mg/kg body weight [447]. The latter acts by stimulating the NADPH methaemoglobin reductases, but has the drawback that it makes the urine blue.

Sulphaemoglobin

This is sometimes found in the blood after administration of drugs such as phenacetin, sulphonamides, etc., but rarely exceeds 10% of total haemoglobin. It is thought that methaemoglobin formation precedes sulphaemoglobin but the exact mechanism is not known,

Table 8.7. Compounds liable to cause methaemoglobin formation

Chlorate	Nitrates in water if reduced to nitrites	Phenacetin
Quinones, naphthoquinones	Nitrites, amyl nitrite	Nitrobenzene
Vitamin K	Prilocaine	Nitrotoluenes
Isoquinolines, codeine	Analine	Sulphonamides, dapsone
Methylene blue in large doses	Acetophenetidine	

nor is it known why some patients develop met- while others show sulphaemoglobin. Again, the only symptom is cyanosis after taking the offending drug. The diagnosis is made by demonstrating the spectrum of sulphaemoglobin with a maximum at 622 nm [448]. This condition is usually benign, but the sulphaemoglobin cannot be reduced by the cell and disappears only as the cells are destroyed. Usually there is no haemolysis. One other feature is that red cells containing sulphaemoglobin have a low oxygen affinity [449], in contrast to methaemoglobin, which causes a raised oxygen affinity. There is no treatment except for stopping the offending drug.

Carbonmonoxyhaemoglobin

Haemoglobin has a much greater affinity for carbon moxonide than for oxygen. Thus, even a small amount of CO in the inspired air will displace oxygen from haemoglobin, thus reducing oxygen delivery to the tissues. Carbon monoxide is found in coal gas (but not natural gas), exhaust fumes of petrol engines and tobacco (and other) smoke, especially from cigars. Carbon monoxide poisoning occurs essentially in two forms, acute and chronic. The acute form gives rise to headache, and the blood and face take on a distinctive purple-pink colour. It is usually due to a suicide attempt; other causes are the accidental breathing of exhaust fumes from a vehicle run in an enclosed space or smoke breathed by victims of fires. Diagnosis is made on the history, and treatment with oxygen to displace the CO from the haemoglobin is begun as quickly as possible. Exchange transfusion is a possible form of treatment but it is unlikely that it can be given quickly enough to do any good.

The proportion of CO haemoglobin in the blood can be measured with a Hartridge reversion spectroscope by comparing the difference between the α-absorption bands of oxyhaemoglobin and CO haemoglobin, namely 578 nm and 568 nm respectively. In any specimen, the shift in position of the band is proportional to the concentration of CO haemoglobin in the blood [450]. Alternatively, the absorbance ratio 576/560 nm is used: this is 1·72 for oxyhaemoglobin and 0·875 for CO haemoglobin [451]. The stability of CO haemoglobin to heat precipitation is also used [452].

Chronic carbon monoxide poisoning occur in garage workers and tobacco smokers. Faulty exhausts in cars can cause repeated formation of CO haemoglobin. The diagnosis of CO poisoning is often difficult to make as by the time blood tests are taken any CO bound by haemoglobin has been blown off and confirmation depends to a large extent on careful history-taking. The presence of CO haemoglobin in blood causes a rise in oxygen affinity and, in some cases, particularly cigar smokers, this leads to mild poly-

cythaemia. The increased blood viscosity and reduced oxygen delivery caused by these changes would be deleterious to patients suffering from ischaemic heart disease.

Glycosylated haemoglobin, Hb AIc

Besides the genetic control of the amino-acid sequence of the globin chains of haemoglobin already referred to (p. 840) there are also post-translational modifications of the haemoglobin chains, for example the γ chain in Hb F is acetylated at the N terminus to form Hb F_1 (p. 347). Similarly, several minor haemoglobins are present in adult cells which are not inherited variants but are due to post-translational modification [182, 453, 454, 653] and Rhabar in 1968 [654] pointed out that one of these, Hb AIc, was increased in diabetes mellitus. This compound is formed by the non-enzymic combination of glucose with the N terminus of the β chain forming first a Schiff base which then undergoes an Amadori rearrangement to form a stable ketoamine [655, 656].

There is considerable evidence that haemoglobin AIc is raised in diabetes and the level found is related to the blood sugar levels over the previous few weeks [657]. In many diabetic clinics the Hb AIc level is used to monitor control of the disease, attempts being made to keep the level near normal. However, the discovery of rapidly changing levels of Hb AIc has thrown some doubt on the interpretation and usefulness of this estimation [658]. Hb AIc has a reduced interaction with 2,3-DPG and a raised oxygen affinity of red cells would be expected, however in diabetes the whole blood oxygen dissociation curve under *in-vivo* conditions is normal [659]. Quantification of Hb AIc is technically difficult and with most of the the simpler techniques Hb AIc is measured together with some other 'fast' haemoglobins, such as Hb AIa and Hb AIb. These are also glycosylated haemoglobins but do not vary significantly in diabetes and their carbohydrate group(s) have not been identified. Another factor causing variation in the measured level is the presence of variable amounts of the labile Schiff base derivative. However, this variation can be overcome by dialysis of the samples to remove it or by rapid analysis minimizing its loss. Various ways of measuring Hb AIc used are: rapid micro-column chromatography [660, 661], electrophoresis on agar gel at pH 6·5 [662], isoelectric focusing [663]; a calorimetric method has also been proposed [664]. The measurement of Hb AIc separately from other fast components can be carried out by column chromatography [665] but this takes too long for clinical use. There is also an immunologic assay [665]. It is therefore important that the results obtained from any one laboratory are compared with the normal values obtained by the same technique locally. This area has recently been reviewed in detail [258].

Other haemoglobins besides Hb A are also glycosylated and glycosylated Hb F has been looked for in newborns from diabetic mothers as a reflection of the fetal blood glucose level *in utero* [667]. In this connection it is of interest that in mothers of large babies Hb AI(a + b + c) was significantly higher just after delivery than in controls and may identify some gestational diabetics [668].

Although Hb AIc is the main glycosylated component with the reaction of the terminal amino group, glucose can also combine with some of the lysyl groups but these derivatives do not separate from ordinary Hb A [669]. Their level has been measured and parallels that of Hb AIc in diabetes.

Finally, it is clear from *in-vitro* work that not only can haemoglobin be glycosylated but other proteins are also affected and this undoubtedly occurs *in vivo* in diabetes. The formation of other glycosylated proteins in diabetes may be one biochemical mechanism connecting the high blood glucose level to the long-term sequelae of the disease. For example, cataract and peripheral neuritis may be due to the glycosylation of specific proteins in the tissues concerned, while small vessel damage and renal effects may be secondary phenomena due to the precipitation of glycosylated plasma proteins. This is therefore an important area of research in diabetes.

REFERENCES

1 PERUTZ M.F., MUIRHEAD H., COX J.M. & GOAMAN L.C.G. (1968) Three-dimensional Fourier synthesis of horse oxyhaemoglobin at 2·8 Å resolution. II. The atomic model. *Nature (London)*, **219**, 131.

2 MUIRHEAD H. & GREER J. (1970) Three-dimensional Fourier synthesis of human deoxyhaemoglobin at 3·5 Å resolution. *Nature (London)*, **228**, 516.

3 BOLTON W. & PERUTZ M.F. (1970) Three-dimensional Fourier synthesis of horse deoxyhaemoglobin at 2·8 Å resolution. *Nature (London)*, **228**, 551.

4 PERUTZ M.F., MUIRHEAD H., MAZZARELLA L., CROWTHER R.A., GREER J. & KILMARTIN J.V. (1969) Identification of residues responsible for the alkaline Bohr effect in haemoglobin. *Nature (London)*, **222**, 1240.

5 PERUTZ M.F. (1971) Haemoglobin: the molecular lung. *New Scientist & Science Journal*, **50**, 676.

6 PERUTZ M.F. (1971) Haemoglobin: genetic abnormalities. *New Scientist & Science Journal*, **50**, 676 & 762.

7 FERMI G. (1975) Three-dimensional Fourier synthesis of human deoxyhaemoglobin at 2·5 Å resolution: refinement of the atomic model. *Journal of Molecular Biology*, **97**, 237.

8 BALDWIN J.M. & CHOTHIA C. (1979) Haemoglobin: the structural changes related to ligand binding and its allosteric mechanism. *Journal of Molecular Biology*, **129**, 175.

9 PERUTZ M.F. & TENEYCK L.F. (1971) Stereochemistry of cooperative effects in hemoglobin. *Cold Spring Harbor Symposia on Quantitative Biology*, **36**, 295.

10 ROSEMEYER M.A. & HUEHNS E.R. (1967) On the mechanism of the dissociation of haemoglobin. *Journal of Molecular Biology*, **25**, 253.

11 HUEHNS E.R. (1973) Diseases of haemoglobin synthesis. *Recent Advances in Medicine*, **16**, 365.

12 BRAUNITZER G., GEHRING-MULLER G., HILSCHMANN N., HILSE K., HOBOM G., RUDLOFF U. & WITTMAN-LIEBOLD B. (1961) Die Konstitution des normalen adulten Humanhämoglobins. *Hoppe-Seyler's Zeitschrift für physiologische Chemie*, **325**, 283.

13 KÖNIGSBERG W. & HILL R.J. (1962) The structure of human hemoglobin. III. The sequence of amino acids in the tryptic peptides of the α-chain. *Journal of Biological Chemistry*, **237**, 2547.

14 SCHROEDER W.A., SHELTON J.R., SHELTON J.B. & CORNICH J. (1962) Further sequences in the γ-chain of human fetal hemoglobin. *Proceedings of the National Academy of Sciences, USA*, **48**, 284.

15 SCHROEDER W.A. (1963) The hemoglobins. *Annual Review of Biochemistry*, **32**, 301.

16 JONES R.T. (1964) Structural studies of amino-ethylated hemoglobins by automatic peptide chromatography. *Cold Spring Harbor Symposia on Quantitative Biology*, **29**, 297.

17 PERUTZ M.F. (1970) Stereochemistry of cooperative effects in haemoglobin. *Nature (London)*, **228**, 724.

18 PERUTZ M.F. (1972) Nature of the haem–haem interactions. *Nature (London)*, **237**, 495.

19 ARNONE A. (1972) X-ray diffraction study of binding of 2,3-diphosphoglycerate to human deoxyhaemoglobin. *Nature (London)*, **237**, 146.

20 PERUTZ M.F. (1980) Stereochemical mechanism of oxygen transport by haemoglobin. *Proceedings of the Royal Society, London, B*, **208**, 135.

21 PERUTZ M.F., KILMARTIN J.V., NISHIKURA K., FOGG J.H., BUTLER P.J.G. & ROLLEMA H.S. (1980) Identification of residues contributing to the Bohr effect of human haemoglobin. *Journal of Molecular Biology*, **138**, 649.

22 PERUTZ M.F. & IMAI K. (1980) Regulation of oxygen affinity of mammalian haemoglobins. *Journal of Molecular Biology*, **136**, 183.

23 HUEHNS E.R. (1979) Oxygen delivery to the tissues. *Lab-Lore*, **8**, 587.

24 SEVERINGHAUS J.W. (1958) Oxyhemoglobin dissociation curve correction for temperature and pH variation in human blood. *Journal of Applied Physiology*, **12**, 485.

25 SEVERINGHAUS J.W. (1966) Blood gas calculator. *Journal of Applied Physiology*, **21**, 1108.

26 BENESCH R. & BENESCH R.E. (1967) The effect of organic phosphates from the human erythrocyte on the allosteric properties of haemoglobin. *Biochemical and Biophysical Research Communications*, **26**, 162.

27 CHANUTIN A. & CURNISH R.R. (1967) Effect of organic and inorganic phosphates on the oxygen equilibrium of human erythrocytes. *Archives of Biochemistry and Biophysics*, **121**, 96.

28 OSKI F.A., GOTTLIEB A.J., DELIVORIA-PAPADOPOULOS M. & MILLER W.W. (1970) The effects of deoxygenation

of adult and fetal hemoglobin on the synthesis of red cell 2,3-diphosphoglycerate and its *in vivo* consequences. *Journal of Clinical Investigation*, 49, 400.

29 OSKI F.A. & GOTTLIEB A.J. (1971) The interrelationship between red blood cell metabolites, hemoglobin and the oxygen-equilibrium curve. *Progress in Hematology*, VII, 33.

30 HUEHNS E.R. (1971) Biochemical compensation in anaemia. *Scientific Basis of Medicine Annual Reviews*, p. 216.

31 RAPOPORT S. (1968) The regulation of glycolysis in mammalian erythrocytes. *Essays in Biochemistry*, 4, 69.

32 RAPOPORT S. (1969) Regulation of concentration of DPG and ATP in red blood cells. *Försvarsmedicin*, 5, 168.

33 MINAKAMI S. (1968) Regulation of glycolysis in human red cells—application of 'cross over' theorem. In: *Metabolism and Membrane Permeability of Erythrocytes and Thrombocytes. 1st International Symposium* (ed. Deutsch E., Gerlach E. & Moser K.), p. 10. George Thieme, Stuttgart.

34 RORTH M. (1970) Dependence of oxyhaemoglobin dissociation and intraerythrocytic 2,3-DPG on acid–base status of blood. I. *In vitro* studies on reduced and oxygenated blood. *Advances in Experimental Medical Biology*, 6, 57.

35 GILLEN R.G. & RIGGS A. (1971) The hemoglobins of a fresh-water teleost, chichlasma cyanoguttarum (Baird and Girard). I. The effects of phosphorylated organic compounds upon the oxygen equilibria. *Comparative Biochemistry and Physiology*, 38B, 585.

36 RODMAN T., CLOSE H.P. & PURCELL M.K. (1960) The oxyhemoglobin dissociation curve in anemia. *Annals of Internal Medicine*, 52, 295.

37 TORRANCE J., JACOBS P., LENFANT C.K. & FINCH C. (1970) Intraerythrocytic adaptation to anaemia. *New England Journal of Medicine*, 283, 165.

38 KENNEDY A.C. & VALTIS D.J. (1954) The oxygen dissociation curve in anemia of various types. *Journal of Clinical Investigation*, 33, 1372.

39 EATON J.W. & BREWER G.J. (1968) The relationship between red cell 2,3-diphosphoglycerate and levels of hemoglobin in the human. *Proceedings of the National Academy of Sciences, USA*, 61, 760.

40 HJELM M. (1969) The content of 2,3-diphosphoglycerate and some other phosphocompounds in human erythrocytes from healthy adults and subjects with different types of anaemia. *Försvarsmedicin*, 5, 219.

41 VALERI C.R., FORTIER N.L. & FRENCH M.J. (1970) Red cell 2,3-diphosphoglycerate (2,3-DPG) and creatine levels in patients with red cell mass deficits or with cardiopulmonary insufficiency. *New England Journal of Medicine*, 281, 1452.

42 OSKI F.A., GOTTLIEB A.J., DELIVORIA-PAPADOPOULOS M. & MILLER W.W. (1969) Red cell 2,3-diphosphoglycerate levels in subjects with chronic hypoxemia. *New England Journal of Medicine*, 280, 1165.

43 WOODSON R.D., TORRANCE J.D., SHAPPELL S.D. & LENFANT C. (1970) The effect of cardiac disease on hemoglobin-oxygen binding. *Journal of Clinical Investigation*, 49, 1349.

44 GAHLENBECK H. & BARTELS H. (1968) Veränderung der Sauerstoffbindungskurven des Blutes bei Hyperthy-reosen und nach Gabe von Trijodthyronin bei Gesunden und bei Ratten. *Klinische Wochenschrift*, 46, 547.

45 GROSZ H.J. & FARMER B.B. (1969) Reduction-oxidation potential of blood determined by oxygen releasing factor in thyroid disorders. *Nature (London)*, 222, 313.

46 GUEST G.M. & RAPOPORT S. (1941) Organic acid-soluble phosphorus compounds of the blood. *Physiological Reviews*, 21, 410.

47 BELLINGHAM A.J., DETTER J.C. & LENFANT C. (1970) The role of haemoglobin affinity for oxygen and red-cell 2,3-DPG in the management of diabetic ketoacidosis. *Transactions of the Association of American Physicians*, 83, 113.

48 BELLINGHAM A.J., DETTER J.C. & LENFANT C. (1971) Regulatory mechanisms of hemoglobin oxygen affinity in acidosis and alkalosis. *Journal of Clinical Investigation*, 50, 700.

49 LENFANT C., BELLINGHAM A.J. & DETTER J.C. (1972) Physiological factors influencing the hemoglobin affinity for oxygen. In: *Oxygen Affinity of Hemoglobin and Red Cell Acid Base Status*. Proceedings A Benzon Symposium IV (ed. Rorth M. & Astrup P.), p. 736. Munksgaard, Copenhagen.

50 OSKI F.A. & DELIVORIA-PAPADOPOULOS M. (1970) The red cell, 2,3-diphosphoglycerate, and tissue oxygen release. *Journal of Paediatrics*, 77, 941.

51 OSKI F.A. & NAIMAN J.L. (1972). In: *Hematologic Problems in the Newborn*, p. 141. Saunders, Philadelphia.

52 WIMBERLEY P. & HUEHNS E.R. Unpublished.

53 LICHTMAN M.A. & MILLER D.R. (1970) Erythrocyte glycolysis, 2,3-diphosphoglycerate and adenosine triphosphate concentration in uremic subjects. *Journal of Laboratory and Clinical Medicine*, 76, 267.

54 MITCHELL T.R. & PEGRUM G.D. (1971) The oxygen affinity of haemoglobin in chronic renal failure. *British Journal of Haematology*, 21, 463.

55 BELLINGHAM A.J. & HUEHNS E.R. (1968) Compensatory mechanisms in haemolytic anaemias. *Proceedings of the Royal Society of Medicine*, 61, 1315.

56 MOURDJINIS A., WALTERS C., EDWARDS M.J., KOLER R.D., VAN DER HEIDER B. & METCALFE J. (1969) Improved oxygen delivery in pyruvate kinase deficiency. *Clinical Research*, 17, 153.

57 DELIVORIA-PAPADOPOULOS M., OSKI F.A. & GOTTLIEB A.J. (1969) Oxygen-hemoglobin dissociation curves. Effect of inherited enzyme defects of the red cell. *Science*, 165, 601.

58 LABIE D., LEROUX J.P., NAJMAN A. & REYROLLE C. (1970) Familial DPG mutase deficiency. Influence on the oxygen affinity curves of haemoglobin. *FEBS Letters*, 9, 37.

59 KEITT A.S. (1968) Hemolytic anemia with impaired hexokinase activity. *Journal of Clinical Investigation*, 48, 1997.

60 WATERBURY L. & FRENKEL E.R. (1972) Hereditary nonspherocytic hemolysis with erythrocyte phosphofructosekinase deficiency. *Blood*, 39, 415.

61 RAPOPORT S. (1947) Dimensional osmotic and chemical changes of erythrocytes in stored blood. I. Blood preserved in sodium citrate, neutral, and acid citrate-glucose (ACD) mixtures. *Journal of Clinical Investigation*, 26, 591.

62 VALTIS D.J. & KENNEDY A.C. (1954) Defective gas-

transport function of stored red blood cells. *Lancet*, **i**, 119.

63 VALERI C.R. & HIRSCH N.M. (1969) Restoration *in vivo* of erythrocyte adenosine triphosphate, 2,3-diphosphoglycerate, potassium ion and sodium ion concentrations following the transfusion of acid-citrate-dextrose-stored human red blood cells. *Journal of Laboratory and Clinical Medicine*, **73**, 722.

64 DAWSON R.B. & ELLIS T.J. (1970) Hemoglobin function of blood stored at 4°C in ACD and CPD with adenine and inosine. *Transfusion (Basel)*, **10**, 113.

65 TIYUMA I. & SHIMIZU K. (1969) Different responses to organic phosphates of human fetal and adult hemoglobins. *Archives of Biochemistry and Biophysics*, **129**, 404.

66 LENFANT C., TORRANCE J., ENGLISH E., FINCH C.A., REYNAFARJE C., RAMOS J. & FAURA J. (1968) Effect of altitude on oxygen binding by haemoglobin and on organic phosphate levels. *Journal of Clinical Investigation*, **47**, 2652.

67 SHAPPELL S.D., MURRAY J.A., BELLINGHAM A.J., WOODSON R.D., DETTER J.C. & LENFANT C. (1971) Adaptation to exercise: role of hemoglobin affinity for oxygen and 2,3-diphosphoglycerate. *Journal of Applied Physiology*, **30**, 827.

68 WOOD W., WHITTAKER J.A., CLEGG J.B. & WEATHERALL D.J. (1971) Haemoglobin synthesis in human marrow maintained in tissue culture. *British Journal of Haematology*, **21**, 356.

69 PAPAYANNOPOULOU TH., BRICE M. & STAMATOYANNOPOULOS G. (1977) Hemoglobin F synthesis *in vitro*: Evidence for control at the level of primitive erythroid stem cells. *Proceedings of the National Academy of Sciences, USA*, **74**, 2923.

70 KIDOGUCHI K., OGAWA M., KARAM J.D. & MARTIN A.G. (1978) Augmentation of fetal haemoglobin (Hb-F) synthesis in culture by human erythropoietic precursors in the marrow and peripheral blood: studies in sickle cell anaemia and nonhemoglobinopathic adults. *Blood*, **52**, 1115.

71 BARD H. (1973) Postnatal fetal and adult hemoglobin synthesis in early preterm newborn infants. *Journal of Clinical Investigation*, **52**, 1789.

72 VAN VLIET G. & HUISMAN T.H.J. (1964) Changes in the haemoglobin types of sheep as a response to anaemia. *Biochemical Journal*, **93**, 401.

73 GABUZDA T.G., SCHUMAN M.A., SILVER R.R. & LEWIS H.B. (1968) Erythropoietic kinetics in sheep studied by means of induced changes in haemoglobin phenotype. *Journal of Clinical Investigation*, **47**, 1895.

74 RABINOVITZ M., FREEDMAN M.L., FISHER J.M. & MAXWELL C.R. (1969) Translational control of haemoglobin synthesis. *Cold Spring Harbor Symposia on Quantitative Biology*, **34**, 567.

75 ZUCKER W.V. & SCHULMAN H.M. (1968) Stimulation of globin-chain initiation by hemin in the reticulocyte cell free system. *Proceedings of National Academy of Sciences, USA*, **59**, 582.

76 HUNT T., VANDERHOFF G. & LONDON I.M. (1972) Control of globin synthesis. The role of heme. *Journal of Molecular Biology*, **66**, 471.

77 HUNT T., HUNTER T. & MUNRO A. (1969) Control of haemoglobin synthesis: rate of translation of the messenger for α- and β-chains. *Journal of Molecular Biology*, **43**, 123.

78 HUEHNS E.R., JACOBS M. & YATES A. (1966) The assembly of the haemoglobin molecule. *International Symposium on Comparative Haemoglobin Structure*, Thessaloniki, p. 68.

79 WINTERHALTER K.H., HEYWOOD J.D., HUEHNS E.R. & FINCH C.A. (1969) The free globin in human erythrocytes. *British Journal of Haematology*, **16**, 523.

80 HUEHNS E.R. & SHOOTER E.M. (1962) Reaction of haemoglobin α^A with haemoglobin H. *Nature (London)*, **193**, 1083.

81 HUEHNS E.R. & McLOUGHLIN C.B. (1966) Haemoglobin synthesis in β-thalassaemia. *Proceedings of the XIth Congress of the International Society of Haematology*, Sydney, Abstracts, p. 264.

82 BAGLIONI C. & CAMPANA T. (1967) Alpha chain and globin: intermediates in the synthesis of rabbit hemoglobin. *European Journal of Biochemistry*, **2**, 480.

83 RIMINGTON C. (1959) Biosynthesis of haemoglobin. *British Medical Bulletin*, **15**, 19.

84 GRANICK S. & LEVERE R.D. (1964) Heme synthesis in erythroid cells. *Progress in Hematology*, **4**, 1.

85 LASCELLES J. (1960) The synthesis of enzymes concerned in bacterio-chlorophyll formation in growing cultures of *Rhodopseudomonas spheroides*. *Journal of General Microbiology*, **23**, 487.

86 BRUNS G.P. & LONDON I.M. (1965) The effect of hemin on the synthesis of globin. *Biochemical and Biophysical Research Communications*, **18**, 236.

87 BURNHAM B.F. & LASCELLES J. (1964) Control of porphyrin biosynthesis through a negative-feedback mechanism. Studies with preparations of δ-aminolaevulate synthetase and δ-aminolaevulate dehydratase from *Rhodopseudomonas spheroides*. *Biochemical Journal*, **87**, 462.

88 GRAYZEL A.I., HÖRSHNER P. & LONDON I.M. (1966) Stimulation of globin synthesis by heme. *Proceedings of the National Academy of Sciences, USA*, **55**, 650.

89 ANFINSEN C.B. (1962) The tertiary structure of ribonuclease. *Brookhaven Symposium of Biology*, **15**, 184.

90 WINTERHALTER K.H. & HUEHNS E.R. (1964) Preparation, properties and specific recombination of αβ globin subunits. *Journal of Biological Chemistry*, **239**, 3699.

91 WINTERHALTER K.H. & DERANLEAU D.A. (1967) The structure of a hemoglobin carrying only two hemes. *Biochemistry*, **6**, 3136.

92 TAVELL A.S., GRAYZEL A.I., VANDERHOFF G.A. & LONDON I.M. (1967) The control of hemoglobin synthesis. *Transactions of the Association of American Physiologists*, **80**, 305.

93 LONDON I.M., TAVELL A.S., VANDERHOFF G.A., HUNT T. & GRAYZEL A.I. (1967) Erythroid cell differentiation and the synthesis and assembly of hemoglobin. *Developmental Biology*, (Suppl. 1), 227.

94 HUNTER A.R. & JACKSON R.J. (1972) Control of haemoglobin synthesis: Coordination of α- and β-chain synthesis. *Hämatologie & Bluttranfusion*, **10**, 95.

95 PAULING L., ITANO H.A., SINGER S.J. & WELLS I.C. (1949) Sickle cell anemia, molecular disease. *Science*, **110**, 543.

96 BEET E.A. (1949) Genetics of the sickle-cell trait in a Bantu tribe. *Annals of Eugenics (London)*, **14**, 279.

97 NEEL J.V. (1949) The inheritance of sickle-cell anemia. *Science*, **110**, 64.

98 RANNEY H.M. (1954) Observations on the inheritance of sickle cell hemoglobin and hemoglobin C. *Journal of Clinical Investigation*, **33**, 1634.

99 NEEL J.V. (1956) The genetics of human haemoglobin differences: problems and perspectives. *Annals of Human Genetics*, **21**, 154.

100 SMITH E.W. & TORBERT J.V. (1958) Study of two abnormal hemoglobins with evidence for a new genetic locus for hemoglobin formation. *Bulletin of the Johns Hopkins Hospital*, **101**, 38.

101 ITANO H.A., SINGER S.J. & ROBINSON E. (1959) Chemical and genetical units of the haemoglobin molecule. *Ciba Foundation Symposia Biochemistry of Human Genetics* (ed. Wolstenholme G.E.W. & O'Connor C.M.), p. 96. Churchill, London.

102 DEISSEROTH A., NIENHUIS A., TURNER P., VELEZ R., ANDERSON W.F., RUDDLE R., LAWRENCE J., CREAGAN R. & KUCHERLAPATI R. (1977) Localization of the human α-globin structural gene to chromosome 16 in somatic cell hybrids by molecular hybridization assay. *Cell*, **12**, 205.

103 DEISSEROTH A., NIENHUIS A., LAWRENCE J., GILES R., TURNER P. & TUDDLE F. (1978) Chromosomal localization of human β-globin gene on human chromosome 11 in somatic cell hybrids. *Proceedings of the National Academy of Sciences, USA*, **75**, 1456.

104 HOLLAN S.R., SZELENYI J.G., BRIMHALL B., DUERST M., JONES R.T., KOLER R.D. & STOCKLEN Z. (1972) Multiple alpha chain loci for human haemoglobins: Hb-J Buda and Hb-G Pest. *Nature (London)*, **235**, 47.

105 LAUER J., SHEN C.-K.J. & MANIATIS T. (1980) The chromosomal arrangement of human α-like globin genes: sequence homology and α-globin gene deletions. *Cell*, **20**, 119.

106 ABRAMSON R.K., RUCKNAGEL D.L., SCHREFFLER D.C. & SAAVE J.J. (1970) Homozygous hemoglobin J. Evidence for only one alpha structural locus. *Science*, **169**, 194.

107 BEAVEN G.H., HORNABROOK R.W., FOX R.H. & HUEHNS E.R. (1972) The occurrence of heterozygotes and homozygotes for the α-chain haemoglobin variant Hb-J (Tongariki) in New Guinea. *Nature (London)*, **235**, 46.

108 OLD J.M., CLEGG J.B., WEATHERALL D.J. & BOOTH P.B. (1978) Haemoglobin J Tongariki is associated with α-thalassaemia. *Nature (London)*, **273**, 319.

109 WADE P.T., BARNICOT N.A. & HUEHNS E.R. (1967) Possible duplication of haemoglobin α-chain locus in the irus macaque. *Nature (London)*, **215**, 1485.

110 KILMARTIN J.V. & CLEGG J.B. (1967) Amino acid replacement in horse haemoglobin. *Nature (London)*, **213**, 269.

111 KITCHEN H. (1974) Animal hemoglobin heterogeneity. *Annals of the New York Academy of Sciences*, **241**, 12.

112 LEHMANN H. & CARRELL R.W. (1968) Differences between α- and β-chain mutants of human haemoglobin and between α- and β-thalassaemia. Possible duplication of the α-chain gene. *British Medical Journal*, **iv**, 748.

113 HUEHNS E.R. (1974) Genetic control of haemoglobin α-chain synthesis. *Haematologia*, **8**, 61.

114 RAPER A.B., GAMMACK D.B., HUEHNS E.R. & SHOOTER E.M. (1960) Four haemoglobins in one individual. A study of the genetic interaction of Hb-G and Hb-C. *British Medical Journal*, **ii**, 1257.

115 PUGH R.P., MONICAL T.V. & MINNICH V. (1964) Sickle cell anemia with two adult hemoglobins, Hb-S and Hb-G$_{Philadelphia}$/S. *Blood*, **23**, 206.

116 HALL-CRAGGS M., MARSDEN P.D., RAPER A.B., LEHMANN H. & BEALE D. (1964) Homozygous sickle cell anaemia arising from two different haemoglobins S. Interaction of haemoglobin S and Stanleyville-II. *British Medical Journal*, **ii**, 87.

117 HUEHNS E.R. & SHOOTER E.M. (1961) The polypeptide chains of haemoglobin A$_2$ and haemoglobin G$_2$. *Journal of Molecular Biology*, **3**, 257.

118 WEATHERALL D.J. & BOYER S.H. (1962) Evidence for the genetic identity of alpha chain determinants of hemoglobins A, A$_2$ and F. *Bulletin of the Johns Hopkins Hospital*, **110**, 8.

119 INTERNATIONAL HEMOGLOBIN INFORMATION CENTER (1979) Variants of the δ-chain. *Hemoglobin*, **3**, 110.

120 BALL E.W., MEYNELL M.J., BEALE D., DYNOCH P., LEHMANN H. & STRETTON A.O.W. (1966) Haemoglobin A$_2$, $\alpha_2 \delta_2^{16\,Glycine-arginine}$. *Nature (London)*, **209**, 1217.

121 DE JONG W.W.W. & BERNINI L.F. (1968) Haemoglobin Babinga (δ136 Glycine-Aspartic acid). A new delta chain variant. *Nature (London)*, **219**, 1360.

122 SCHROEDER W.A., HUISMAN T.H.J., SHELTON J.R., SHELTON J.B., KLEIHAUER E.F., DOZY A.M., ROBBERSON B. (1968) Evidence for multiple structural genes for the γ-chain of human fetal hemoglobin. *Proceedings of the National Academy of Sciences, USA*, **60**, 537.

123 SCHROEDER W.A., HUISMAN T.H.J., BROWN A.K. *et al.* (1971) Postnatal changes in the chemical heterogeneity of fetal hemoglobin. *Pediatric Research*, **5**, 493.

124 HUISMAN T.H.J., SCHROEDER W.A., DOZY A.M., SHELTON J.R., SHELTON J.B., BOYD E.M. & APELL G. (1969) Evidence for multiple structural genes for the γ-chain of human fetal hemoglobin in hereditary persistence of fetal hemoglobin. *Annals of the New York Academy of Sciences*, **165**, 320.

125 CAUCHI M.N., CLEGG J.B. & WEATHERALL D.J. (1969) Haemoglobin F (Malta), a new foetal haemoglobin variant with a high incidence in Maltese infants. *Nature (London)*, **223**, 311.

126 INTERNATIONAL HEMOGLOBIN INFORMATION CENTER (1979) Variants of the γ-chains. *Hemoglobin*, **3**, 110.

126a LEE-POTTER J.P., DEACON-SMITH R.A., SOIPKISS M.J., KANUZORA H. & LEHMAN H. (1975) A new cause of haemolytic anaemia in the newborn. A description of an unstable fetal haemoglobin: F Poole $\alpha_2^9\gamma_2$ 130 tryptophan→glycine. *Journal of Clinical Pathology*, **28**, 317.

127 HUEHNS E.R., BEAVEN G.H. & STEVENS B.L. (1964) Reaction of haemoglobin α^A with haemoglobins β$_4^A$, γ$_4^F$ and δ$_2^A$. *Biochemical Journal*, **92**, 444.

128 FRITSCH E.F., LAWN R.M. & MANIATIS T. (1980) Molecular cloning and characterization of the human β-like globin gene cluster. *Cell*, **19**, 959.

129 HUEHNS E.R. & SHOOTER E.M. (1965) Review article: Human haemoglobins. *Journal of Medical Genetics*, **2**, 48.

130 BRADLEY T.B., BRAWNER J.N. & CONLEY C.L. (1961) Further observation on an inherited anomaly characterized by persistence of fetal hemoglobin. *Bulletin of the Johns Hopkins Hospital*, **108**, 242.

131 NANCE W.E., CONNEALLY M., WONKANG K., REED T., SCHROEDER J. & ROSE S. (1970) Genetic linkage analysis of human hemoglobin variants. *American Journal of Human Genetics*, **22**, 453.

132 RUCKNAGEL D.L. & NEEL J.V. (1961) The hemoglo-

binopathies. In: *Progress in Medical Genetics 1* (ed. Steinberg A.G.), p. 158. Grune and Stratton, New York.

133 CONLEY C.L., WEATHERALL D.J., RICHARDSON S.N., SHEPARD M.K. & CHARACHE S. (1963) Hereditary persistence of fetal hemoglobin. A study of 79 affected persons in 15 Negro families in Baltimore. *Blood*, **21**, 261.

134 HUISMAN T.H.J., SCHROEDER A.A. & KENDALL A.G. (1972) Hemoglobin Kenya. The product of non-homologous crossing over of γ and β genes. *Blood*, **40**, 947.

135 BUNN H.F., BRADLEY J.B., DAVIS W.E., DRYSDALE J.W., BURTLE J.F., BECK W.S. & LAVER M.B. (1972) Structural and functional studies in haemoglobin Bethesda ($\alpha_2\beta_2^{145\,His}$), a variant associated with compensatory erythrocytosis. *Journal of Clinical Investigation*, **51**, 2299.

136 CARRELL R.W., LEHMANN H., LORKIN A.P., RAIK E. & HUNTER E. (1967) Hb-Sydney: β67 (E11) Valine→Alanine: an emerging pattern of unstable haemoglobin. *Nature (London)*, **215**, 626.

137 GERALD P.S. & EFRON M.L., (1961) Chemical studies of several varieties of Hb-M. *Proceedings of the National Academy of Sciences, USA*, **47**, 1758.

138 STEADMAN J.H., YATES A. & HUEHNS E.R. (1970) Idiopathic Heinz body anaemia, Hb-Bristol β67 (E11) Val→Asp. *British Journal of Haematology*, **18**, 435.

139 BOOKCHIN R.M., NAGEL R.L. & RANNEY H.M. (1967) Structure and properties of Hemoglobin C Harlem, a human hemoglobin variant with amino-acid substitutions in two residues of the β-polypeptide chain. *Journal of Biological Chemistry*, **242**, 248.

140 LANG A., LEHMANN H., McCURDY P.R. & PIERCE L. (1972) Identification of Haemoglobin C Georgetown. *Biochimica et Biophysica Acta*, **278**, 57.

141 GOOSSENS M., GAREL M.C., AUVINET J., BASSET P., GOMES P.F. & ROSA J. (1975) Hemoglobin C Ziguinchor $\alpha_2^A\beta_2 6(A3)$ Glu→Val β58 (E2) Pro→Arg: The second sickling variant with amino-acid substitutions in two residues of the β polypeptide chain. *FEBS Letters*, **58**, 149.

142 MOO-PENN W.F., SCHMIDT R.M., JUE D.L., BECHTEL K.C., WRIGHT J.M., HORNE M.K. III, HAYCRAFT G.L., ROTH E.F. & NAGEL R.L. (1977) Hemoglobin S Travis. A sickling hemoglobin with two amino-acid substitutions [β6(A3) Glutamic acid→Valine and β142 (H20) Alanine→Valine]. *European Journal of Biochemistry*, **77**, 561.

143 BLACKWELL R.Q., WONG HOCK BOON, LIU, C.-S. & WENG, M.I. (1972) Hemoglobin J Singapore: α78 Asn→Asp: α79 Ala→Gly. *Biochimica et Biophysica Acta*, **278**, 482.

144 ADAMS J.G. & HELLER P. (1973) Hemoglobin Arlington Park (β6 Glu→Lys 95 Lys→Glu): electrophoretically 'silent' hemoglobin variant with two amino-acid substitutions in the same polypeptide chain. *Blood*, **42**, 990.

145 DE JONG W.W.W., WENT L.N. & BERNINI L.F. (1968) Haemoglobin Leiden, deletion of β6 or 7 glutamic acid. *Nature (London)*, **220**, 788.

146 COHEN-SOLAL M., BLOUQUIT Y., GAREL M.C., THILLET J., GAILLARD L., CREYSSEL R., GIBAUD A. & ROSA J. (1974) Haemoglobin Lyon (β17–18(A14–15) Lys-Val→0) determination of sequenator analysis. *Biochimica et Biophysica Acta*, **351**, 306.

147 JONES R.T., BRIMHALL B., HUISMAN T.H.J., KLEIHAUER E. & BETKE K. (1966) Hemoglobin Freiburg: abnormal hemoglobin due to deletion of a single amino acid residue. *Science*, **154**, 1024.

148 WILTSHIRE B., PRAXEDES H. & LEHMANN H. (1972) Hb-Rio de Janeiro. *Proceedings XIVth International Congress of Haematology*.

149 SHIBATA S., MIYAJI T., UEDA S., MATSVOKA M., IUCHI I., YAMADA K. & SHINKAI N. (1970) Haemoglobin Tochigi (beta 56–59 deleted). A new unstable hemoglobin discovered in a Japanese family. *Proceedings of the Japanese Academy*, **46**, 440.

150 WAJCMAN H., LABIE D. & SCHAPIRA G. (1973) Two new hemoglobin variants with deletion. Hemoglobin Tours: Thr β87(F3) deleted and Hemoglobin St Antoine: Gly→Leu 74–75 (E18–19) deleted. Consequences for oxygen affinity and protein stability. *Biochimica et Biophysica Acta*, **295**, 495.

151 BRADLEY T.B., WOHL R.C. & RIEDER R.F. (1965) Hemoglobin Gun Hill: a beta chain abnormality associated with a haemolytic state. *Blood*, **28**, 975.

152 LUTCHER C.L., WILSON J.B., GRAVELY M.E., STEVENS P.D., CHEN C.J., LINDERMAN J.G., WONG S.C., MILLER A., GOTTLIEB M. & HUISMAN T.H.J. (1976) Hb Leslie, an unstable hemoglobin due to deletion of Glutaminyl residue S131(H9) occurring in association with β^0-thalassaemia, Hb-C, and Hb-S. *Blood*, **47**, 99.

153 CASEY R., LANG A., LEHMANN H. & SHINTON N.K. (1976) Double heterozygosity for two unstable haemoglobins: Hb Sydney (β67 E11) (Val→Ala) and Hb Coventry (β141 (H19) Leu deleted). *British Journal of Haematology*, **33**, 143.

154 MILNER P.F., CLEGG J.B. & WEATHERALL D.J. (1971) Haemoglobin H disease due to a unique haemoglobin variant with an elongated α-chain. *Lancet*, **i**, 729.

155 CLEGG J.B., WEATHERALL D.J., CONTOPOLOU-GRIVA I., CAROUTSOS K., POUNGOURAS P. & TSEVRENIS H. (1974) Haemoglobin Icaria, a new chain-termination mutant which causes α thalassaemia. *Nature (London)*, **251**, 245.

156 DE JONG W.W.W., MEERA KHAN P. & BERNINI L.F. (1975) Hemoglobin Koya Dora: High frequency of a chain termination mutant. *American Journal of Human Genetics*, **27**, 81.

157 MEHDI SEID-AKHAVEN, WINTER W.P., ABRAMSON R.K. & RUCKNAGEL D.L. (1972) Hemoglobin Wayne: A frameshift variant occurring in two distinct forms. *Blood*, **40**, 927.

158 LEHMANN H., CASEY R., LANG A., STATHOPOULOU R., IMAI K., TUCHINDA S., VINAI P. & FLATZ G. (1975) Haemoglobin Tak: A β-chain elongation. *British Journal of Haematology*, **31**, 119.

159 BUNN H.F., SCHMIDT G.J., HANEY D.N. & DLUHY R.G. (1975) Hemoglobin Cranston, an unstable variant having an elongated β chain due to non-homologous crossover between two normal β chain genes. *Proceedings of the National Academy of Sciences, USA*, **72**, 3609.

160 HUISMAN T.H.J., WILSON J.B., GRAVELY M. & HUBBARD M. (1974) Hemoglobin Grady: The first example of a variant with elongated chains due to an insertion of residues. *Proceedings of the National Academy of Sciences, USA*, **71**, 3270.

161 BAGLIONI C. (1962) The fusion of two peptide chains in hemoglobin Lepore and its interpretation as a genetic deletion. *Proceedings of the National Academy of Sciences, USA*, **48**, 1880.

162 BARNABAS J. & MULLER C.J. (1962) Haemoglobin Lepore_Hollandia. *Nature (London)*, **194**, 931.

163 OSTERTAG W. & SMITH E.W. (1969) Hemoglobin Lepore Baltimore: a third type of $\delta\beta$ crossover ($\delta^{50}\beta^{86}$). *European Journal of Biochemistry*, **10**, 371.

164 LEHMANN H. & CHARLESWORTH D. (1970) Observation on Hb-P (Congo type). *Biochemical Journal*, **119**, 43P.

165 OHTA Y., YAMAOKA K., SUMIDA I. & YANASE T. (1971) Haemoglobin Miyada, a β-δ fusion peptide (anti-Lepore) type discovered in a Japanese family. *Nature (New Biology)*, **234**, 218.

166 BADR F.M., LORKIN P.A. & LEHMANN H. (1973) Haemoglobin P-Nilotic containing a β-δ-chain. *Nature (New Biology)*, **242**, 107.

167 DHERTE P., LEHMANN H. & VANDEPITTE J. (1959) Haemoglobin P in a family in the Belgium Congo. *Nature (London)*, **184**, 1133.

168 HUISMAN T.H.J., WRIGHTSTONE R.N., WILSON J.B., SCHROEDER W.A. & KENDALL A.G. (1972) Hemoglobin Kenya, the product of fusion of γ and β polypeptide chains. *Archives of Biochemistry and Biophysics*, **153**, 850.

169 HUEHNS E.R. & BEAVEN G.H. (1971) Developmental changes in human haemoglobins. *Clinics in Developmental Medicine*, **37**, 175.

170 WOOD W.G. (1976) Haemoglobin synthesis during fetal development. *British Medical Bulletin*, **32**, 282.

171 JACOBS L. & HUEHNS E.R. Unpublished.

172 HUEHNS E.R., DANCE N., BEAVEN G.H., KEIL J.V., HECHT F. & MOTULSKY A.G. (1964) Human embryonic haemoglobins. *Nature (London)*, **201**, 1095.

173 CAPP G.L., RIGAS D.A. & JONES R.T. (1967) Hemoglobin Portland I: a new human hemoglobin unique in structure. *Science*, **117**, 65.

174 GALE R.E., CLEGG J.B. & HUEHNS E.R. (1979) Human embryonic haemoglobins Gower 1 and Gower 2. *Nature (London)*, **280**, 162.

175 CLEGG J.B. Unpublished.

176 FAROOQUI A.M. & HUEHNS E.R. (1970) Oxygen dissociation studies of red cells from very small human and chicken embryos. *Abhandlungen der Deutschen Akademie der Wissenschaften zu Berlin. VI. Internationales Symposium über Struktur und Funktion der Erythrocyten*, p. 217.

177 HUEHNS E.R. & FAROOQUI A.M. (1975) Oxygen dissociation properties of human embryonic red cells. *Nature (London)*, **254**, 335.

178 BAUER C., TAMM R., PETSCHOW D., BARTELS R. & BARTELS H. (1975) Oxygen affinity and allosteric effects of embryonic mouse haemoglobins. *Nature (London)*, **257**, 924.

179 DAVIS L.R. (1976) Changing blood picture in sickle-cell anaemia from shortly after birth to adolescence. *Journal of Clinical Pathology*, **29**, 898.

180 TUCHINDA S., NAGAI K. & LEHMANN H. (1975) Oxygen dissociation curve of haemoglobin Portland. *FEBS Letters*, **49**, 2957.

181 GALE R.E. & HUEHNS E.R. Unpublished.

182 ALLEN D.W., SCHROEDER W.A. & BALOG J. (1958) Observation on the chromatographic heterogeneity of normal adult and fetal hemoglobin. A study of the effect of crystallization and chromatography and isoleucine content. *Journal of the American Chemical Society*, **80**, 1628.

183 SCHROEDER W.A., CUA J.T., MATSUDA G. & FENNINGER W.D. (1962) Hemoglobin F1, an acetyl-containing hemoglobin. *Biochimica et Biophysica Acta*, **63**, 532.

184 KILMARTIN J.V. & ROSSI-BERNARDI L. (1969) Inhibition of CO_2 combination and reduction of the Bohr effect in haemoglobin chemically modified at its α amino groups. *Nature (London)*, **222**, 1243.

185 HUNT J.A. & LEHMANN H. (1959) Haemoglobin Bart's: a foetal haemoglobin without α-chains. *Nature (London)*, **184**, 872.

186 KEKWICK R.A. & LEHMANN H. (1960) Sedimentation characteristics of the γ-chain haemoglobin (haemoglobin 'Bart's'). *Nature (London)*, **187**, 158.

187 HORTON B.F., THOMPSON R.B., DOZY A.M., NECHTMAN C.M., NICHOLS E. & HUISMAN T.H.J. (1962) Inhomogeneity of hemoglobin. VI. The minor hemoglobin components of cord blood. *Blood*, **20**, 302.

188 BELLINGHAM A.J. & HUEHNS E.R. (1968) Compensation in haemolytic anaemias caused by abnormal haemoglobins. *Nature (London)*, **218**, 924.

189 BARTLES H. (1966) Carriage of oxygen in the blood of the foetus. *Ciba Foundation Symposium on Development of the Lung* (ed. de Reack A.V.S. & Porter R.), p. 276. Churchill, London.

190 DAWES G.S. (1967) New views on O_2 transfer across the placenta. *The Scientific Basis of Medicine Annual Reviews*, p. 74. British Postgraduate Medical Federation, University of London, Athlone Press.

191 DE VERDIER C.H. & GARBY L. (1969) Low binding of 2,3-diphosphoglycerate to haemoglobin F. A contribution to the knowledge of the binding site and an explanation for the high oxygen affinity of foetal blood. *Scandinavian Journal of Clinical and Laboratory Investigation*, **23**, 149.

192 MCCARTHY E.F. (1943) The oxygen affinity of human maternal and foetal haemoglobin. *Journal of Physiology*, **102**, 55.

193 ALLEN D.W., WYMAN J. & SMITH C.A. (1953) The oxygen equilibrium of fetal and adult human hemoglobin. *Journal of Biological Chemistry*, **203**, 81.

194 SINGER K., CHERNOFF A.I. & SINGER L. (1951) Studies on abnormal haemoglobins. I. Their demonstration in sickle-cell anemia and other hematologic disorders by means of alkali denaturation. *Blood*, **6**, 413.

195 BETKE K., MARTI H.R. & SCHLICHT I. (1959) Estimation of small percentages of foetal haemoglobin. *Nature (London)*, **181**, 1877.

196 GILLESPIE J.E.O'N., WHITE J.C., ELLIS M.J., BEAVEN G.H., GRATZER W.B., SHOOTER E.M. & PARKHOUSE R.M.E. (1959) A haemoglobin with unusual alkaline-denaturation properties in a Turkish-Cypriot woman. *Nature (London)*, **184**, 1876.

197 STAMATOYANNOPOULOS G., YOSHIDA A., ADAMSON J. & HEINENBERG S. (1968) Hemoglobin Rainier (β^{145} Tyr$\rightarrow$His): alkali-resistant hemoglobin with increased oxygen affinity. *Science*, **159**, 741.

198 BEAVEN G.H., HOCH H. & HOLIDAY E.R. (1951) The haemoglobins of the foetus and infant. Electrophoretic and spectroscopic differentiation of adult and foetal types. *Biochemical Journal*, **49**, 374.

199 ROBINSON A.R., ROBSON M., HARRISON A.P. & ZUELZER W.W. (1957) A new technique for differentiation of hemoglobin. *Journal of Laboratory and Clinical Medicine*, **50**, 745.

200 HUISMAN T.H.J. & DOZY A.M. (1965) Studies on the heterogeneity of hemoglobin. IX. The use of tris (hydroxymethyl) aminomethane-HCl buffers in the anion exchange chromatography of hemoglobins. *Journal of Chromatography*, **19**, 160.

201 ZADE-OPPEN A.M.M. (1963) Separation of hemoglobin A and F by cation exchange dextran gels. *Scandinavian Journal of Clinical and Laboratory Investigation*, **15**, 491.

202 HONIG G.R. (1967) Inhibition of synthesis of fetal hemoglobin by an isoleucine analogue. *Journal of Clinical Investigation*, **46**, 1778.

203 HUEHNS E.R. & SHOOTER E.M. (1964) Haemoglobin. *Science Progress*, **52**, 353.

204 CLEGG J.B., NAUGHTON M.A. & WEATHERALL D.J. (1966) Abnormal human hemoglobins. Separation and characterization of the α- and β-chains by chromatography, and the determination of two new variants, Hb-Chesapeake and Hb-J (Bangkok). *Journal of Molecular Biology*, **19**, 91.

205 SPARHAM S.J. & HUEHNS E.R. (1979) The separation of human globin chains by ion-exchange chromatography on sepharose CL-6B. *Hemoglobin*, **3**, 13.

206 ALTER B.P., GOFF S.C., EFREMOV G.D., GRAVELY M.E. & HUISMAN T.H.J. (1979) Globin chain electrophoresis: a new approach to the determination of the G_γ/A_γ ratio in fetal haemoglobin and to studies of globin synthesis. *British Journal of Haematology*, **44**, 527.

207 KLEIHAUER E., BRAUN H. & BETKE K. (1957) Demonstration von fetalen Hämoglobin in den Erythrocyten eines Blutanstrichs. *Klinische Wochenschrift*, **35**, 637.

208 WOOD W.G., STAMATOYANNOPOULOS G., LIM G. & NUTE P.E. (1975) F-cells in the adult: normal values and levels in individuals with hereditary and acquired elevations of Hb-F. *Blood*, **46**, 671.

209 BEAVEN G.H., ELLIS M.J. & WHITE J.C. (1960) Studies on foetal haemoglobin. II. Foetal haemoglobin levels in healthy children and adults and in certain haematological disorders. *British Journal of Haematology*, **6**, 201.

210 RUCKNAGEL D.L. & CHERNOFF A.I. (1955) Immunologic studies of hemoglobins. III. Fetal hemoglobin changes in the circulation of pregnant women. *Blood*, **10**, 1092.

211 BEAVEN G.H., ELLIS M.J. & WHITE J.C. (1961) Studies on human foetal haemoglobin. III. The hereditary haemoglobinopathies and thalassaemias. *British Journal of Haematology*, **7**, 169.

212 EDINGTON G.W. & LEHMANN H. (1955) Expression of the sickle-cell gene in Africa. *British Medical Journal*, **i**, 1308.

213 EDINGTON G.W. & LEHMANN H. (1955) Expression of the sickle-cell gene in Africa. *British Medical Journal*, **ii**, 1328.

214 THOMPSON R.B., MITCHENER J.W. & HUISMAN T.H.J. (1961) Studies on the fetal hemoglobin in the persistent high Hb-F anomaly. *Blood*, **18**, 267.

215 SINGER K. & FISHER B. (1952) Studies on abnormal hemoglobins. V. The distribution of type S (sickle cell) hemoglobin and type F (alkali resistant) hemoglobin within the red cell population in sickle cell anemia. *Blood*, **7**, 1216.

216 SHEPARD M.K., WEATHERALL D.J. & CONLEY C.L. (1962) Semi-quantitative estimations of the distributions of fetal hemoglobin in red cell populations. *Bulletin of the Johns Hopkins Hospital*, **110**, 293.

217 WHEELER J.T. & KREVANS J.R. (1961) The homozygous state of persistent fetal hemoglobin and the interaction of persistent fetal hemoglobin with thalassemia. *Bulletin of the Johns Hopkins Hospital*, **109**, 215.

218 BAGLIONI C. (1963) A child homozygous for persistence of foetal haemoglobin. *Nature (London)*, **198**, 1177.

219 SIEGEL W., COX R., SCHROEDER W., HUISMAN T.H.J., PENNER O. & ROWLEY P.T. (1970) An adult homozygous for persistent fetal hemoglobin. *Annals of Internal Medicine*, **72**, 533.

220 FESSAS P. & STAMATOYANNOPOULOS G. (1964) Hereditary persistence of fetal hemoglobin in Greece. A study and a comparison. *Blood*, **24**, 223.

221 MARTI H.R. & BUETLER R. (1961) Hemoglobin F and hemoglobin A_2 increase in the Swiss population. *Acta Haematologica (Basel)*, **26**, 65.

222 MARTI H.R. (1963) *Normale und anomale Menschliche Hämoglobine*, p. 85. Springer-Verlag, Basle.

223 HUEHNS E.R., HECHT F., KEIL J.V. & MOTULSKY A.G. (1964) Developmental hemoglobin anomalies in a chromosomal triplication: D_1 trisomy syndrome. *Proceedings of the National Academy of Sciences, USA*, **51**, 89.

224 POWARS D., ROHDE R. & GRAVES D. (1964) Foetal haemoglobin and neutrophil anomaly in the D_1 trisomy syndrome. *Lancet*, **i**, 1363.

225 BARD H. (1972) Postnatal fetal and adult hemoglobin synthesis in D_1 trisomy syndrome. *Blood*, **40**, 523.

226 BEAVEN G.H. & WHITE J.C. (1963) The occurrence of Hb-F or Hb-H in the leukaemic state. *Proceedings of the Congress of the European Society of Haematology, Lisbon, 1963*, p. 543.

227 HARDISTY R.M., SPEED D.E. & TILL M. (1964) Granulocytic leukaemia in childhood. *British Journal of Haematology*, **10**, 551.

228 BROMBERG Y.M., SALZBERGER M. & ABRAHAMOV A. (1957) Alkali resistant type of hemoglobin in women with molar pregnancy. *Blood*, **12**, 1122.

229 JONES J.H. (1961) Foetal haemoglobin in Fanconi type anaemia. *Nature (London)*, **192**, 982.

230 COOK C.D., BRODIE H.R. & ALLEN D.W. (1957) Measurement of fetal hemoglobin in newborn infants. Correlation with gestational age and intrauterine hypoxia. *Pediatrics*, **20**, 272.

231a FARRAR J.F. & BLOMFIELD J. (1963) Alkali resistant haemoglobin content of blood in congenital heart disease. *British Journal of Haematology*, **9**, 278.

231b KUNKEL H.G., CEPPELLINI R., MULLER-EBERHARD U. & WOLF J. (1957) Observations on the minor basic hemoglobin component in the blood of normal individuals and patients with thalassemia. *Journal of Clinical Investigation*, **36**, 1615.

232 GERALD P.S. & DIAMOND L.K. (1958) The diagnosis of thalassemia by starch block electrophoresis of hemoglobin. *Blood*, **13**, 61.

233 SILVESTRONI E. & BIANCO I. (1963) *Le Emoglobine Umane*, Edizioni dell'istitute 'Gregorio Mendel', Rome.

234 WEATHERALL D.J., GILLES H.M., CLEGG J.B., BLANKSON J.A., MUSTAFA D. & BOI-DOKU F.S. (1971) Preliminary surveys for the incidence of the thalassaemia genes in some African populations. *Annals of Tropical Medicine and Parasitology*, **65**, 253.

235 ARENDS T. (1967) High concentrations of haemoglobin A_2 in malaria patients. *Nature (London)*, **215**, 1517.

236 JOSEPHSON A.N., MASRI M.S., SINGER L., DWORKIN D.

& SINGER K. (1958) Starch block electrophoretic studies of human hemoglobin solutions. II. Results in cord blood, thalassemia and other hematologic disorders. Comparison with Tiselius electrophoresis. *Blood*, **13**, 543.

237 WHITE J.M. & DACIE J.V. (1971) The unstable haemoglobins, molecular and clinical features. *Progress in Haematology*, **7**, 69.

238 AKSOY M. & ERDEM S. (1967) Decrease in the concentration of haemoglobin A_2 during erythroleukaemia. *Nature (London)*, **213**, 522.

239 STEINER J., MARTI H.R. & DEAN H.D. (1971) Decreased haemoglobin A_2 concentration in iron deficiency anaemia. *Acta Haematologica*, **45**, 77.

240 WASI P., DISTHASONGCHAN P. & NA-NAKORN S. (1968) The effect of iron deficiency on the levels of haemoglobin A_2 and E. *Journal of Laboratory and Clinical Medicine*, **71**, 85.

241 EDISON G.G., BRIEHL R.W. & RANNEY H.M. (1964) Oxygen equilibria of hemoglobin A_2 and hemoglobin Lepore. *Journal of Clinical Investigation*, **43**, 2323.

242 PERUTZ M.F. & LEHMANN H. (1968) Molecular pathology of human haemoglobin. *Nature (London)*, **219**, 902.

243 INTERNATIONAL HEMOGLOBIN INFORMATION CENTER (1979) Listing of α-chain variants. *Hemoglobin*, **3**, 384.

243a INTERNATIONAL HEMOGLOBIN INFORMATION CENTER (1979) Listing of β-chain variants. *Hemoglobin*, **3**, 492.

244 SCHNEIDER R.G., ALPERIN J.B. & LEHMANN H. (1967) Sickling test. Pitfalls in performance and interpretation. *Journal of the American Medical Association*, **202**, 419.

245 CANNING D.M. & HUNTSMAN R.G. (1970) An assessment of Sickledex as an alternative to the sickling test. *Journal of Clinical Pathology*, **23**, 736.

246 HUNTSMAN R.G., BARCLAY G.P.T., CANNING D.M. & YAWSON G.I. (1970) A rapid whole blood solubility test to differentiate the sickle cell trait from sickle cell anaemia. *Journal of Clinical Pathology*, **23**, 781.

247 ALLISON A.C. (1961) Abnormal haemoglobin and erythrocyte enzyme deficiency traits. In: *Genetical Variation in Human Populations* (ed. Harrison G.A.), p. 16. Pergamon Press, Oxford.

248 MOTULSKY A.G. (1964) Hereditary red cell traits and malaria. *American Journal of Tropical Medicine and Hygiene*, **13**, No. 1, Pt. 2, p. 147.

249 LUZATTO L., NWACHUKU JARRETT E.S. & REDDY S. (1970) Increased sickling of parasitised erythrocytes as mechanism of resistance against malaria in the sickle cell trait. *Lancet*, **i**, 319.

250 PASVOL G. (1980) The interaction between sickle haemoglobin and the malarial parasite. *Plasmodium falciparum. Transactions of the Royal Society of Tropical Medicine & Hygiene*, **74**, 701.

251 INGRAM V.M. (1958) Abnormal human haemoglobins. I. The comparison of normal human and sickle-cell haemoglobins by finger-printing. *Biochimica et Biophysica Acta*, **28**, 539.

252 DYKES G.W., CREPEAU R.H. & EDELSTEIN S.J. (1979) Three dimensional reconstruction of the 14-filament fibers of hemoglobin S. *Journal of Molecular Biology*, **130**, 451.

253 WISHNER B.C., WARD K.B., LATTMAN E.E. & LOVE W.E. (1978) Crystal structure of sickle-cell deoxyhemoglobin at 5 Å resolution. *Journal of Molecular Biology*, **98**, 179.

254 LOVE W.E., FITZGERALD P.M.D., HANSON J.C. & ROYER W.E. (1979) Intermolecular interactions in crystals of human deoxy hemoglobin A, C, F and S. In: *Development of Therapeutic Agents for Sickle Cell Disease. INSERM Symposium No. 9* (ed. Rosa J., Beuzard Y. & Hercules J.), p. 65. Elsevier/North-Holland, Amsterdam.

255 MAGDOFF-FAIRCHILD M.B., CHIU C.C. & BERTLES J.F. (1979) The structure of fibers in sickled erythrocytes. In: *Development of Therapeutic Agents for Sickle Cell Disease. INSERM Symposium No. 9* (ed. Rosa J., Beuzard Y. & Hercules J.), p. 57. Elsevier/North-Holland, Amsterdam.

256 NAGEL R.M., JOHNSON J., BOOKCHIN R.M. *et al.* (1980) β-chain contact sites in the haemoglobin S polymer. *Nature (London)*, **283**, 832.

257 BENESCH R.E., KWONG S., BENESCH R. & EDALJI R. (1977) Location and bone type of intermolecular contacts in the polymerisation of haemoglobin S. *Nature (London)*, **269**, 772.

258 BUNN H.F. (1981) Evaluation of glycosylated hemoglobin in diabetic patients. *Diabetes*, **30**, 613.

259 CHEETHAM R.C., HUEHNS E.R. & ROSEMEYER M.A. (1979) Participation of haemoglobins A, F, A_2 and C in polymerization of haemoglobins S. *Journal of Molecular Biology*, **129**, 45.

260 HOFRICHTER J., ROSS P.D. & EATON W.A. (1974) Kinetics and mechanism of deoxyhaemoglobin S gelation: a new approach to understanding sickle cell disease. *Proceedings of the National Academy of Sciences, USA*, **71**, 4864.

261 HARRIS J.W. & BENSUSAN H.B. (1975) Demonstration of lag phase in the sol-gel transformation of deoxygenated S Hemoglobin without temperature alteration. *Proceedings of the National Academy of Sciences, USA*, **71**, 4864.

262 FRANKLIN I.M. & HUEHNS E.R. (1980) The molecular basis of antisickling agents. *Transactions of the Royal Society of Tropical Medicine and Hygiene*, **74**, 695.

263 EATON W.A., HOFRICHTER J. & ROSS P.D. (1976) Delay time of gelation: a possible determinant of clinical severity in sickle cell disease. *Blood*, **47**, 621.

264 FRANKLIN I.M., HUEHNS E.R. & ROSEMEYER M.A. (1980) The role of liganded haemoglobins in preventing polymerization of deoxyhaemoglobin S. *Proceedings of the 18th Congress of the International Society of Hematology, Montreal 1980*, Abstract No. 1615.

265 CHEETHAM R.C., HUEHNS E.R. & ROSEMEYER M.A. (1979) The interaction of Hb-A, Hb-A_2, Hb-F and Hb-C with Hb-S. In: *Development of Therapeutic Agents for Sickle Cell Disease, INSERM Symposium No. 9* (ed. Rosa J., Beuzard Y. & Hercules J.), p. 99. Elsevier/North-Holland, Amsterdam.

266 BOOKCHIN R.M., NAGEL R.L. & BALAZS T. (1975) Role of hybrid tetramer formation in gelation of haemoglobin S. *Nature (London)*, **256**, 667.

267 GOLDBERG M.A., HUSSON M.A. & BUNN H.F. (1977) Participation of hemoglobins A and F in polymerization of sickle hemoglobin. *Journal of Biological Chemistry*, **252**, 3413.

268 PERRINE R.P., BROWN M.J., CLEGG J.B., WEATHERALL D.J. & MAY A. (1972) Benign sickle-cell anaemia. *Lancet*, **ii**, 1163.

269 SINGER K. & FISHER B. (1952) Studies on abnormal hemoglobins. V. The distribution of type S (sickle cell)

hemoglobin and type F (alkali resistant) hemoglobin within the red cell population in sickle cell anaemia. *Blood*, **7,** 1216.

270 RAMOT B., FISHER S., REMEZ D., SCHNEERSON R., KAHANE D., AGER J.A.M. & LEHMANN H. (1960) Haemoglobin O in an Arab family: sickle-cell haemoglobin O trait. *British Medical Journal*, **ii,** 1262.

271 MILNER P.F., MILLER C., GRAY R., SEAKINS M., DE JONG W.W. & WENT L.W. (1970) Haemoglobin O$_{Arab}$ in 4 negro families and its interaction with haemoglobin S and haemoglobin C. *New England Journal of Medicine*, **283,** 1417.

272 KRAUS A.P., MIYAJI T., IUCHI I. & KRAUS L.M. (1967) Hemoglobin Memphis/S. A new variant of sickle cell anemia. *Transactions of the Association of American Physicians*, **80,** 297.

273 KRAUS L.M., MIYAJI T., IUCHI I. & KRAUS A.P. (1966) Characterization of α23 Gln in hemoglobin Memphis. Hemoglobin Memphis/S, a new variant of molecular disease. *Biochemistry*, **5,** 3701.

274 SIRS J.A. (1963) The use of carbon monoxide to prevent sickle cell formation. *Lancet*, **i,** 971.

275 BEUTLER E. & MIKUS B.J. (1961) The effect of methemoglobin formation in sickle cell disease. *Journal of Clinical Investigation*, **40,** 1856.

276 BECKLAKE M.R., GRIFFITHS S.B., McGREGOR M., GOLDMAN H.I. & SCHREVE J.P. (1955) Oxygen dissociation curves in sickle cell anemia and in subjects with the sickle cell trait. *Journal of Clinical Investigation*, **34,** 751.

277 BROMBERG P.A., JENSEN W.N. & McDONOUGH M. (1967) Blood oxygen dissociation curves in sickle cell disease. *Journal of Laboratory and Clinical Medicine*, **70,** 480.

278 MAY A. & HUEHNS E.R. (1972) The mechanism of the low oxygen affinity of red cells in sickle cell disease. *Hämatologie & Bluttransfusion*, **10,** 279.

279 WYMAN J. & ALLEN D.W. (1951) Heme interactions in hemoglobin and the basis of the Bohr effect. *Journal of Polymer Science*, **7,** 499.

280 GREENBERG M.S., KASS E.H. & CASTLE W.B. (1957) Studies on the destruction of red blood cells. XII. Factors influencing the role of S hemoglobin in the pathologic physiology of sickle cell anemia and related disorders. *Journal of Clinical Investigation*, **36,** 833.

281 JENSEN W.N. (1969) Fragmentation and the 'Freakish Poikilocyte'. *American Journal of Medical Sciences*, **257,** 355.

282 LANGE R.D., MINNICH V. & MOORE C.V. (1951) Effect of oxygen tension and of pH on the sickling and mechanical fragility of erythrocytes from patients with sickle cell anemia and sickle cell trait. *Journal of Laboratory and Clinical Medicine*, **37,** 789.

283 DIGGS L.W. & BIBB J. (1939) The erythrocyte in sickle cell anemia. *Journal of the American Medical Association*, **112,** 695.

284 PADILLA F., BROMBERG P.A. & JENSEN W.N. (1968) The sickle-unsickle cycle: A cause of cell fragmentation. *Journal of Laboratory and Clinical Medicine*, **72,** 1000.

285 JENSEN W.N. & LESSIN L.S. (1970) Membrane alterations associated with hemoglobinopathies. *Seminars in Hematology*, **7,** 409.

286 BANK A., MEARS G., WEISS R., O'DONNELL J.V. & NATTA C.L. (1974) Preferential binding of β^S globin chains associated with stroma in sickle cell disorders. *Journal of Clinical Investigation*, **54,** 805.

287 BERTLES J.F. & MILNER P.F.A. (1968) Irreversibly sickled erythrocytes: a consequence of the heterogenous distribution of hemoglobin types in sickle cell anemia. *Journal of Clinical Investigation*, **47,** 1731.

288 BERTLES J.F. & DÖBLER J. (1969) Reversible and irreversible sickling: a destruction by electron microscopy. *Blood*, **33,** 884.

289 DÖBLER J. & BERTLES J.F. (1968) Physical state of hemoglobin in sickle-cell anemia erythrocytes *in vivo*. *Journal of Experimental Medicine*, **127,** 711.

290 SEAKINS M., GIBBS W.N., MILNER P.F. & BERTLES J.F. (1973) Erythrocyte hemoglobin S concentration, an important factor in the low oxygen affinity of blood in sickle cell anaemia. *Journal of Clinical Investigation*, **52,** 422.

291 SERJEANT G.R., SERJEANT J. & MILNER P.F. (1969) The irreversibly sickled cell: a determinant of haemolysis in sickle cell anaemia. *British Journal of Haematology*, **17,** 527.

292 SERJEANT G.R. (1970) Irreversibly sickled cells and splenomegaly in sickle cell anaemia. *British Journal of Haematology*, **19,** 635.

293 SERJEANT G.R. & ASHCROFT M.T. (1971) Shortening of the digits in sickle cell anaemia. A sequela of the hand-foot syndrome. *Tropical and Geographical Medicine*, **23,** 341.

294 PEARSON H.A., McINTOSH S., RITCHEY A.K., LOBEL J.S., ROOKS Y. & JOHNSTON D. (1979) Developmental aspects of splenic function in sickle cell diseases. *Blood*, **53,** 358.

295 ROBINSON M.G. & WATSON R.J. (1966) Pneumococcal meningitis in sickle-cell anemia. *New England Journal of Medicine*, **274,** 1006.

296a POWARD D.R. (1975) Natural history of sickle cell disease —the first ten years. *Seminars in Hematology*, **12,** 267.

296b MANN J.R. (1981) Sickle cell haemoglobinopathies in England. *Archives of Diseases in Childhood*, **56,** 676.

297 BARRETT-CONNOR E. (1971) Bacterial infection and sickle cell anaemia: an analysis of 250 infections in 166 patients and a review of the literature. *Medicine (Baltimore)*, **50,** 97.

298 HAND W.L. & KING N.L. (1978) Serum opsonization of salmonella in sickle cell disease. *Americal Journal of Medicine*, **64,** 388.

299 LEADING ARTICLE (1978) Sickle cell anaemia in infancy. *British Medical Journal*, **i,** 1439.

300 AHONKHAI V.I., LANDESMAN S.H., FIKRIG S.M., SCHMALZER E.A., BROWN A.K., CHERUBIN C.E. & SCHIFFMAN G. (1979) Failure of pneumococcal vaccine in children with sickle cell disease. *New England Journal of Medicine*, **301,** 26.

301 DIGGS L.W. (1965) Sickle cell crises. *American Journal of Clinical Pathology*, **44,** 1.

302 DIGGS L.W., PULLIAM H.W. & KING J.C. (1937) The bone changes in sickle cell anaemia. *Southern Medical Journal*, **30,** 249.

303 MIDDLEMISS J.H. & RAPER A.B. (1966) Skeletal changes in the haemoglobinopathies. *Journal of Bone and Joint Surgery*, **48B,** 693.

304a BOROS L., THOMA C. & WEINER W.J. (1976) Large cerebral vessel infarct in sickle cell anaemia. *Journal of Neurology, Neurosurgery and Psychiatry*, **39,** 1236.

304b RUSSELL M.O., BOLDBERG H.I., REIS L., FRIEDMAN S., SLATER R., REIVICH M. & SWARTZ E. (1976) Transfusion therapy for cerebrovascular abnormalities in sickle cell disease. *Journal of Paediatrics*, **88**, 382.

305 LINDSAY J., MESHEL J.C. & PATTERSON R.H. (1974) The cardiovascular manifestations of sickle cell disease. *Archives of Internal Medicine*, **133**, 634.

306 TANAKA K.R., CLIFFORD G.O. & AXELROD A.R. (1956) Sickle cell anemia (homozygous S) with aseptic necroses of femoral head. *Blood*, **11**, 998.

307 GOLDING J.S.R., MACIVER J.E. & WENT L.N. (1959) The bone changes in sickle cell anaemia and its genetic variants. *Journal of Bone and Joint Surgery*, **41B**, 711.

308 SERJEANT G.R., GALLOWAY R.E. & GUERI C.G. (1970) Oral zinc sulphate in sickle cell ulcers. *Lancet*, **ii**, 891.

309 BERNSTEIN J. & WHITTEN C.F. (1960) Histologic appraisal of the kidney in sickle cell anemia. *Archives of Pathology*, **70**, 407.

310 PERILLE P.E. & EPSTEIN F.H. (1963) Sickling phenomenon produced by hypertonic solutions. Possible explanation for hyposthemuria of sicklemia. *Journal of Clinical Investigation*, **42**, 570.

311 McCOY R.C. (1969) Ultrastructural alteration in the kidney of patients with sickle cell disease and nephrotic syndrome. *Laboratory Investigation*, **21**, 87.

312 MOSTOFI F.K., VORDER BRUEGGE C.F. & DIGGS L.W. (1957) Lesions in kidneys removed for unilateral hematuria in sickle cell disease. *Archives of Pathology*, **63**, 336.

313 VEGA R., SHANBERG A.M. & MALLOY T.R. (1971) The use of epsilon amino caproic acid in sickle cell trait hematuria. *Journal of Urology*, **105**, 552.

314 GOLDBERG M.F. (1971) Natural history of untreated proliferative sickle retinopathy. *Archives of Ophthalmology*, **85**, 428.

315 CONDON P.I. & SERJEANT G.R. (1972) Ocular findings in sickle cell thalassemia in Jamaica. *American Journal of Ophthalmology*, **74**, 1105.

316 OPPENHEIMER E.H. & ESTERLY J.R. (1971) Pulmonary changes in sickle cell disease. *American Review of Respiratory Diseases*, **103**, 858.

317 ANDERSON M., WENT L.N., MACIVER J.E. & DIXON H.G. (1960) Sickle cell disease in pregnancy. *Lancet*, **ii**, 516.

318 McCURDY P. (1964) Abnormal hemoglobins in pregnancy. *American Journal of Obstetrics and Gynecology*, **90**, 891.

319 FORT A.T., MORRISON J.C., BERRERAS L., DIGGS L.E. & FISH S.A. (1971) High risks of pregnancy in sickle cell anaemia. *Gynaecology*, **111**, 324.

320 MONTI A., FELDHAKE C. & SCHWARTZ S.O. (1964) The S-thalassemia syndrome. *Annals of the New York Academy of Sciences*, **119**, 474.

321 SERJEANT G.R., ASHCROFT M.T., SERJEANT B.T. & MILNER P.F. (1973) Sickle cell β-thalassaemia in Jamaica. *British Journal of Haematology*, **24**, 19.

322 HUEHNS E.R. (1965) Thalassaemia. *Postgraduate Medical Journal*, **41**, 718.

323 DIGGS L.W. & BELL A. (1965) Intraerythrocytic hemoglobin crystals in sickle cell-hemoglobin C disease. *Blood*, **25**, 218.

324 TUTTLE A.H. & KOCH B. (1960) Clinical and hematologic manifestations of hemoglobin CS disease in children. *Journal of Paediatrics*, **56**, 331.

325 CAWEIN M.J., LAPPAT E.J., BRANGLE R.W. & FARLEY C.H. (1966) Hemoglobin S-D disease. *Annals of Internal Medicine*, **64**, 62.

326 RINGELHANN B., LEWIS R.A., LORKIN P.A., KYNOCH P.A.M. & LEHMANN H. (1967) Sickle cell haemoglobin D Punjab disease: S from Ghana and D from England. *Acta Haematologica*, **38**, 324.

327 STURGEON P., ITANO H.A. & BERGREN W.R. (1955) Clinical manifestations of inherited abnormal hemoglobins. I. The interaction of hemoglobin S with hemoglobin D. II. The interaction of hemoglobin E and thalassemia trait. *Blood*, **10**, 389.

328 CHARACHE S. & CONLEY C.L. (1964) Rate of sickling of red cells during deoxygenation of blood from persons with various sickling disorders. *Blood*, **24**, 25.

329 AKSOY M. & LEHMANN H. (1957) The first observation on sickle-cell haemoglobin E disease. *Nature (London)*, **179**, 1248.

330 JACOB G.F. & RAPER A.B. (1958) Hereditary persistence of foetal haemoglobin production, and its interaction with the sickle-cell trait. *British Journal of Haematology*, **4**, 138.

331 HERMAN E.C. & CONLEY C.C. (1960) Hereditary persistence of fetal hemoglobin. A family study. *American Journal of Medicine*, **29**, 9.

332 AKSOY M. (1963) The first observation of homozygous hemoglobin-S-alpha-thalassemia disease and two types of sickle cell thalassemia disease: (a) Sickle cell alpha-thalassemia disease; (b) Sickle cell beta-thalassemia disease. *Blood*, **22**, 757.

333 WEATHERALL D.J., CLEGG J.B., BLANKSON J. & McNIEL J.R. (1969) A new sickling disorder resulting from interaction of the genes for haemoglobin S and α-thalassaemia. *British Journal of Haematology*, **17**, 517.

334 VAN ENK A., LANG A., WHITE J.M. & LEHMANN H. (1972) Benign obstetric history in women with sickle-cell anaemia associated with α-thalassaemia. *British Medical Journal*, **iv**, 524.

334a SERJEANT G.R., HIGGS D.R., ALDRIDGE B., HAYES R.J. & WEATHERALL D.J. (1981) α-thalassaemia and homozygous sickle cell disease. *Progress in Clinical and Biological Research*, **55**, 781.

335 WARLEY M.A., HAMILTON P.J.S., MARSDEN P.D., BROWN R.F., MARSELIS J.G. & WILKS N. (1965) Chemoprophylaxis of homozygous sicklers with antimalarials and long acting penicilin. *British Medical Journal*, **ii**, 86.

336 HUGH-JONES K., LEHMANN H. & McALISTER J.M. (1964) Some experiences in managing sickle-cell anaemia in children and young adults using alkalis and magnesium. *British Medical Journal*, **ii**, 226.

337 FINNEY R.A. & HATCH F.E. (1965) Effect of carbonic anhydrase inhibitor (dichlorphenamide) on sickle cell anemia. *American Journal of Medical Sciences*, **250**, 154.

338 JENSEN M. & NATHAN D.G. (1972) The relationship between the intracellular 2,3-DPG concentration and the sickling of hemoglobin S (Hb-S) erythrocytes *in vitro*. *Blood*, **40**, 929.

339 CERAMI A. & MANNING J.M. (1971) Potassium cyanate as an inhibitor of sickling of erythrocytes *in vitro*. *Proceedings of the National Academy of Sciences, USA*, **68**, 1180.

340 GILETTE P.N., MANNING J.M. & CERAMI A. (1971) Increased survival of sickle-cell erythrocytes after treat-

ment *in vitro* with sodium cyanate. *Proceedings of the National Academy of Sciences, USA*, **68**, 2791.

341 MAY A., BELLINGHAM A.J., HUEHNS E.R. & BEAVEN G.H. (1972) Effect of cyanate on sickling. *Lancet*, **i**, 658.

342 SEGEL G.B., FEIG S.A., MENTZER W.C., McCAFFREY R.P., WELLS R., BUNN H.F., SHOHET S.B. & NATHAN D.G. (1972) Effects of urea and cyanate on sickling *in vitro*. *New England Journal of Medicine*, **287**, 59.

343 DE FURIA F.G., MILLER D.R., CERAMI A. & MANNING J.H. (1972) The effects of cyanate *in vitro* on red blood cell metabolism and function in sickle cell anemia. *Journal of Clinical Investigation*, **51**, 566.

344 GILLETTE P.N., PETERSON C.M., MANNING J.M. & CERAMI A. (1972) Preliminary Clinical Trials. *Red Cell Metabolism and Function*. Conference at Ann Arbor, Michigan. April, 1972.

345a HARKNESS D.R. & ROTH S. (1975) Clinical evaluation of cyanate in sickle cell anaemia. *Progress in Haematology*, **9**, 157.

345b OHNISHI A., PETERSON C.M. & DYCK P.J. (1975) Axonal degeneration in sodium cyanate-induced neuropathy. *Archives of Neurology*, **32**, 530.

346 NICHOLSON D.H., HARKNESS D.R., BENSON W.E. & PETERSON C.M. (1976) Cyanate induced cataracts in patients with sickle-cell haemoglobinopathies. *Archives of Ophthalmology*, **94**, 927.

347 NALBANDIAN R.M., HENRY R., NICHOLS B., KESSLER D.L., CAMP F.R. & VINING K.K. (1970) Sickling crises treated successfully by urea and invert sugar. *Annals of Internal Medicine*, **72**, 795.

348 COOPERATIVE UREA TRIALS (1974) *Journal of the American Medical Association*, **228**, 1120.

349 LASZLO J., OBENOUR W. & SALTZMAN H.A. (1969) Effects of hyperbaric oxygenation on sickle syndromes. *Southern Medical Journal*, **62**, 453.

350 REYNOLDS J.D.H. (1971) Painful sickle cell crisis: successful treatment with hyperbaric oxygen therapy. *Journal of the American Medical Association*, **216**, 1977.

351 SALVAGGIO J.E., ARNOLD G.A. & BANOV C.H. (1963) Long term anticoagulation in sickle cell disease: a clinical study. *New England Journal of Medicine*, **269**, 182.

352 HILKOVITZ G. (1957) Sickle cell disease. New method of treatment (preliminary report). *British Medical Journal*, **ii**, 266.

353 ROSA J., BEUZARD Y. & HERCULES J. (ed.) (1979) *Developments of Therapeutic Agents for Sickle Cell Disease, INSERM Symp. No. 9*. North-Holland, Amsterdam.

354 HOWELLS T.H., HUNTSMAN R.G., BOYS J.F. & MAHMOOD A. (1972) Anaesthesia and sickle-cell haemoglobin. *British Journal of Anaesthesia*, **44**, 975.

355 SEARLE J.F. (1973) Anaesthesia in sickle cell states: A review. *Anaesthesia*, **28**, 48.

356 LEVIN W.C. (1958) Asymptomatic sickle cell trait. *Blood*, **13**, 904.

357 WELLS I.C. & ITANO H.A. (1951) Ratio of sickle cell anemia hemoglobin to normal hemoglobin in sicklemics. *Journal of Biological Chemistry*, **188**, 65.

358 WRIGHTSTONE R.N., HUISMAN T.H.J. & VAN DER SAR (1968) Qualitative and quantitative studies of sickle cell hemoglobin in homozygotes and heterozygotes. *Clinica Chimica Acta*, **22**, 593.

359 NEEL J.V., WELLS I.C. & ITANO H.A. (1951) Familial differences in the proportion of abnormal hemoglobin present in sickle cell trait. *Journal of Clinical Investigation*, **30**, 1120.

360 LEVERE R.D., LICHTMAN H.C. & LEVINE J. (1964) Effects of iron deficiency anaemia on the metabolism of the heterogenic haemoglobins in sickle cell trait. *Nature (London)*, **202**, 499.

361 HELLER P., YAKULIS V.J., EPSTEIN R.B. & FRIEDLAND S. (1963) Variation in the amount of hemoglobin S in a patient with sickle cell trait and megaloblastic anemia. *Blood*, **21**, 479.

362 ASHCROFT M.T., MIALL W.E. & MILNER P.F. (1969) A comparison between the characteristics of Jamaican adults with normal hemoglobin and those with sickle cell trait. *American Journal of Epidemiology*, **90**, 236.

363 WHALLEY P.J., MARTIN F.G. & PRITCHARD J.A. (1964) Sickle cell trait and urinary trait infection during pregnancy. *Journal of the American Medical Association*, **189**, 903.

364 PLATT H.S. (1971) Effect of maternal sickle-cell trait on perinatal mortality. *British Medical Journal*, **iv**, 334.

365 HELLER P, & MONIER Y. (1971) Clinical problems: the usual and unusual. In: *Sickle Cell Disease: Diagnosis, Management, Education and Research* (ed. Abranson H., Bertles J.F. & Wethers D.L.), p. 39. Mosby, St. Louis.

366a LEADER (1977) Prenatal Diagnosis of the Haemoglobinopathies. *British Medical Journal*, **i**, 531.

366b ALTER B.P., MODELL C.B., FAIRWEATHER D., HOBBINS J.C., MAHONEY M.J., FRIGOLETTO F.D., SHERMAN A.S. & NATHAN D.G. (1976) Prenatal Diagnosis of Hemoglobinopathies. *New England of Medicine*, **295**, 1437.

366c KAN Y.W., GOLBUS M.S., TRECARTIN R.F. & FILLY R.A. (1977) Prenatal diagnosis of β-thalassaemia and sickle-cell anaemia. *Lancet*, **i**, 269.

367 KAN Y.W. & DOZY A.M. (1978) Antenatal diagnosis of sickle-cell anaemia by DNA analysis of amniotic-fluid cells. *Lancet*, **ii**, 910.

368 HUNT J.A. & INGRAM V.M. (1960) Abnormal human haemoglobins. IV. The chemical difference between normal human haemoglobin and haemoglobin C. *Biochimica et Biophysica Acta*, **42**, 409.

369 RANNEY H.M., BENESCH R.E., BENESCH R. & JACOBS A.S. (1963) Hybridization of deoxygenated human haemoglobin. *Biochimica et Biophysica Acta*, **74**, 544.

370 ZUELZER W.W. & KAPLAN E. (1954) Thalassemia-hemoglobin C disease. A new syndrome presumably due to the combination of thalassemia and hemoglobin C. *Blood*, **9**, 1047.

371 WEATHERALL D.J. (1963) Abnormal haemoglobins in the neonatal period and their relationships to thalassaemia. *British Journal of Haematology*, **9**, 265.

372 SPAET T.H., ALWAY R.H. & WARD G. (1953) Homozygous type 'C' hemoglobin. *Pediatrics*, **12**, 483.

373 SMITH E.W. & KREVANS J.R. (1959) Clinical manifestations of hemoglobin C disorders. *Bulletin of the Johns Hopkins Hospital*, **104**, 17.

374 CHARACHE S., CONLEY C.L., WAUGH D.E., UGORETZ R.J. & SPURRELL J.R. (1967) Pathogenesis of hemolytic anemia in homozygous hemoglobin C disease. *Journal of Clinical Investigation*, **46**, 1795.

375 HUNT J.A. & INGRAM V.M. (1961) Abnormal human haemoglobins. VI. The chemical difference between haemoglobins A and E. *Biochimica et Biophysica Acta*, **49**, 520.

376 MAY A. & HUEHNS E.R. (1975) The oxygen affinity of haemoglobin E. *British Journal of Haematology*, **30**, 177.

377 TUCHINDA S., RUCKNAGEL D.L., MINNICH V., BOONYA-PRAKOB U., BALANKURA K. & SUVATEE V. (1964) The

coexistence of genes of hemoglobin E and α-thalassemia in Thais, with resultant suppression of hemoglobin E synthesis. *American Journal of Human Genetics*, **16**, 311.

378 CHERNOFF A.I., MINNICH V., NA-NAKORN S., TUCHINDA S., KASHEMSANT C. & CHERNOFF R.R. (1956) Studies on hemoglobin E. 1. The clinical, hematologic and genetic characteristics of hemoglobin E syndromes. *Journal of Laboratory and Clinical Medicine*, **47**, 455.

379 LEHMANN H., STORY P. & THEIN H. (1956) Haemoglobin E in Burmese. Two cases of haemoglobin E disease. *British Medical Journal*, **i**, 544.

380 NA-NAKORN S. & MINNICH V. (1957) Studies on hemoglobin E. III. Homozygous hemoglobin E and variants of thalassemia and hemoglobin E. A family study. *Blood*, **12**, 529.

381 WASI P., NA-NAKORN S., POOTRAKUL S., SOOKANEK M., DISTHASONGCHAN P., PORNPATKUL M. & PANICH V. (1969) Alpha and beta-thalassaemia in Thailand. *Annals of the New York Academy of Sciences*, **165**, 60.

382 CHERNOFF A.I. (1958) The hemoglobin D syndromes. *Blood*, **13**, 116.

383 BIRD G.W.G. & LEHMANN H. (1956) Haemoglobin D in India. *British Medical Journal*, **i**, 514.

384 KOUZMANOVA P. (1970) Homozygous hemoglobin O. *Sovetskaya Meditsina*, **21**, 20.

385 LEHMANN H., BEALE D. & BOI-DOKU F.S. (1964) Haemoglobin G Accra. *Nature (London)*, **203**, 363.

386 SHOOTER E.M., SKINNER E.R., GARLICK J.P. & BARNICOT N.A. (1960) The electrophoretic characterization of haemoglobin G and a new minor haemoglobin, G2. *British Journal of Haematology*, **6**, 140.

387 CHARACHE S., WEATHERALL D.J. & CLEGG J.B. (1966) Polycythaemia associated with a haemoglobinopathy. *Journal of Clinical Investigation*, **45**, 813.

388 STAMATOYANNOPOULOS G., BELLINGHAM A.J., LENFANT C. & FINCH C.A. (1971) Abnormal haemoglobins with a high and low oxygen affinity. *Annual Review of Medicine*, **22**, 221.

389 HÖRLEIN H. & WEBER G. (1948) Methämoglobinämie und eine neue Modifikation des Methämoglobins. *Deutsche Medizinische Wochenschrift*, **73**, 476.

390 HÖRLEIN H. & WEBER G. (1957) Chronische familiäre Methämoglobinämie. *Zeitschrift für die gesamte innere Medizin und ihre Grenzgebiete*, **6**, 197.

391 HELLER P. (1966) Hemoglobinopathic dysfunction of red cell. *American Journal of Medicine*, **41**, 799.

392 CARRELL R.W. & LEHMANN H. (1969) The unstable haemoglobins. *Seminars in Haematology*, **6**, 116.

393 HUEHNS E.R. (1970) The unstable haemoglobins. *Bulletin de la Société de Chimie Biologique*, **52**, 1131.

394 CATHIE I.A.B. (1952) Apparent idiopathic Heinz body anaemia. *Great Ormond Street Journal*, **2**, 43.

395 SCHMID R., BRECHER G. & CLEMENS T. (1959) Familial hemolytic anemia with erythrocyte inclusion bodies and a defect in pigment metabolism. *Blood*, **14**, 991.

396 KREIMER-BIRNBAUM M., PINKERTON P.H., BANNERMAN R.M. & HUTCHISON H.E. (1966) Dipyrrolic urinary pigments in congenital Heinz body anaemia due to Hb-Köln and thalassaemia. *British Medical Journal*, **ii**, 396.

397 BETKE K., MARTI H.R., KLEIHAUER E. & BÜTIKOFER E. (1960) Hitzelabilität und Saurestabilität von Hämoglobin H. *Klinische Wochenschrift*, **38**, 529.

398 GRIMES A.J., MEISLER A. & DACIE J.V. (1964) Congenital Heinz body anaemia: further evidence on the cause of Heinz body production in red cells. *British Journal of Haematology*, **10**, 281.

399 GRIMES A.J. & MEISLER A. (1962) Possible cause of Heinz bodies in congenital Heinz body anaemia. *Nature (London)*, **194**, 190.

400 WINTERBOURNE C. & CARRELL R.W. (1972) Characterization of Heinz bodies in unstable haemoglobin haemolytic anaemia. *Nature (London)*, **240**, 150.

401 BUCCI E. & FRONTICELLI C. (1965) A new method for the preparation of α and β subunits of human hemoglobin. *Journal of Biological Chemistry*, **240**, 551.

402 CARRELL R.W. & KAY R. (1972) A simple method for the detection of unstable haemoglobins. *British Journal of Haematology*, **23**, 605.

403 JACOB H.S., BRAIN M.C., DACIE J.V., CARRELL R.W. & LEHMANN H. (1968) Abnormal haem binding and globin SH group blockade in unstable haemoglobins. *Nature (London)*, **218**, 1214.

404 JACOB H.S. & WINTERHALTER K.H. (1970) The role of heme loss in Heinz body formation. Studies with a partially heme-deficient hemoglobin and with genetically unstable hemoglobins. *Journal of Clinical Investigation*, **49**, 2008.

405 JACOB H.S. & WINTERHALTER K.H. (1970) Unstable hemoglobins: the role of heme loss in Heinz body formation. *Proceedings of the National Academy of Sciences, USA*, **65**, 697.

406 HUEHNS E.R. & SHOOTER E.M. (1966) Further studies on the isolation and properties of α-chain subunits of haemoglobin. *Biochemical Journal*, **101**, 843.

407 RIEDER R.F. (1970) Hemoglobin stability. Observations on the denaturation of normal and abnormal hemoglobins by oxidant dyes, heat and alkali. *Journal of Clinical Investigation*, **49**, 2369.

408 RACHMILEWITZ E.A. & HARARI E. (1972) Intermediate hemichrome formation after oxidation of three unstable haemoglobins (Freiburg, Riverdale-Bronx and Köln). *Hämatologie & Bluttransfusion*, **10**, 241.

409 JACOB H.S., BRAIN M.C. & DACIE J.V. (1968) Altered sulphydryl reactivity of hemoglobins and red blood cell membranes in congenital Heinz body hemolytic anemia. *Journal of Clinical Investigation*, **47**, 2664.

410 HUEHNS E.R., SHOOTER E.M., DANCE N., BEAVEN G.H. & SHOOTER K.V. (1961) Haemoglobin α^A. *Nature (London)*, **192**, 1057.

411 KOYAMA S., AOKI S. & DEGUCHI K. (1964) Electron microscopic observations of the splenic red pulp with special reference to the pitting function. *Mie Medical Journal*, **14**, 143.

412 WENNBERG E. & WEISS L. (1968) Splenic erythroclasia: an electron microscopic study of hemoglobin H disease. *Blood*, **31**, 778.

413 RIFKIN R.A. (1965) Heinz body anemia: an ultrastructural study. II. Red cell sequestration and destruction. *Blood*, **26**, 433.

414 HUEHNS E.R. (1970) Diseases due to abnormalities of hemoglobin structure. *Annual Review of Medicine*, **21**, 157.

415 JACOB H.S. (1970) Mechanisms of Heinz body formation and attachment to red cell membrane. *Seminars in Hematology*, **7**, 341.

416 RIFKIND R.A. & DANON D. (1965) Heinz body anemia: an ultrastructural study. I. Heinz body formation. *Blood*, **25**, 885.

417 HUEHNS E.R. (1974) The structure and function of haemoglobin. In: *Blood and its Disorders* (ed. Hardisty R.M. & Weatherall D.J.) 1st Edn, p. 526. Blackwell Scientific Publications, Oxford.

418 HUEHNS E.R. & BELLINGHAM A.J. (1969) Disease of function and stability of haemoglobin. *British Journal of Haematology*, **17**, 1.

419 HUTCHISON H.E., PINKERTON P.H., WATERS P., DOUGLAS A.S., LEHMANN H. & BEALE D. (1964) Hereditary Heinz body anaemia, thrombocytopenia, and haemoglobinopathy (Hb-Köln) in a Glasgow family. *British Medical Journal*, **ii**, 1099.

420 FRICK P.G., HITZIG W.H. & BETKE K. (1962) Hemoglobin Zurich. I. A new hemoglobin anomaly associated with acute hemolytic episodes with inclusion bodies after sulfonamide therapy. *Blood*, **20**, 261.

421 MORIMOTO H., LEHMANN H. & PERUTZ M.F. (1971) Molecular pathology of human haemoglobin. Stereochemical interpretation of abnormal oxygen affinities. *Nature (London)*, **232**, 408.

422 WAJCMAN H., KILMARTIN J.V., NAJMAN A. & LABIE D. (1975) Hemoglobin Cochin-Port-Royal—consequences of the replacement of the β chain C-terminal by an arginine. *Biochimica et Biophysica Acta*, **400**, 354.

423 KEITT A.S., SMITH T.W. & JANDL J.H. (1966) Red-cell 'pseudomosaicism' in congenital methemoglobinemia. *New England Journal of Medicine*, **275**, 397.

424 SCOTT E.M., DUNCAN I.W. & EKSTRAND V. (1965) The reduced pyridine nucleotide dehydrogenases of human erythrocytes. *Journal of Biological Chemistry*, **240**, 481.

425 JAFFE E.R. (1966) Hereditary methemoglobinemias associated with abnormalities in the metabolism of erythrocytes. *American Journal of Medicine*, **41**, 786.

426 JAFFE E.R. & HELLER P. (1964) Methemoglobinemia in man. *Progress in Hematology*, **4** (ed. Moore C. & Brown E.). Grune & Stratton, New York.

427 SMITH R.P. & OLSON M.V. (1973) Drug-induced methemoglobinemia. *Seminars in Hematology*, **10**, 253.

428 LIE-INGO LUAN ENG, MAY LOO & FOO KON FAH (1973) Diaphorase activity and variants in normal adults and newborns. *British Journal of Haematology*, **23**, 419.

429 ROSS J.D. (1963) Deficient activity of DPNH dependent methemoglobin diaphorase in cord blood erythrocytes. *Blood*, **21**, 51.

430 WINDLE TAYLOR E. (1970) *44th Report on the Results of Examination of the London Waters for 1969–70*. Metropolitan Waterboard, London.

431 COMLY H.H. (1945) Cyanosis in infants caused by nitrates in well water. *Journal of the American Medical Association*, **129**, 112.

432 KEATING J.P., LELL M.E., STRAUSS A.W., ZARKOWSKY H. & SMITH G.E. (1973) Infantile methemoglobinemia caused by carrot juice. *New England Journal of Medicine*, **288**, 824.

433 COMMITTEE ON NUTRITION (CHAIRMAN: FILER, L.J.) (1970) Infant methemoglobinemia; the role of dietary nitrate. *Pediatrics*, **46**, 475.

434 KNOTEK Z. & SCHMIDT P. (1964) Pathogenesis, incidence and possibilities of preventing alimentary nitrate methemoglobinemia in infants. *Pediatrics*, **34**, 78.

435 RODECK H. & WESTHAUS H. (1952) Die Anilinvergiftung durch Wäschetinten und Stempelfarben bei Säuglingen. *Archiev Kinderheilkunde*, **145**, 77.

436 GRAUBARTH J., BLOOM C.J., COLEMAN F.C. & SOLOMON H.N. (1945) Dye poisoning in the nursery. A review of seventeen cases. *Journal of the American Medical Association*, **128**, 1155.

437 JAFFE E.R., NEUMANN G., ROTHBERG H., WILSON T., WEBSTER R.M. & WOLFF J.A. (1966) Hereditary methemoglobin with and without mental retardation. *American Journal of Medicine*, **41**, 42.

438 WEST C.A., GOMPERTZ B.D., HUEHNS E.R., KESSEL I. & ASHBY J.R. (1967) Demonstration of an enzyme variant in a case of congenital methaemoglobinaemia. *British Medical Journal*, **iv**, 212.

439 SCOTT E.M. (1960) The relation of diaphorase of human erythrocytes to inheritance of methemoglobinemia. *Journal of Clinical Investigation*, **39**, 1176.

440 JAFFE E.R. (1959) The reduction of methemoglobin in erythrocytes incubated with purine nucleosides. *Journal of Clinical Investigation*, **38**, 1555.

441 KAPLAN J.C., LEROUX A. & BEAUVAIS P. (1979) Formes cliniques et biologiques du déficit en cytochrome B5 réductase. *C.R. Society of Biology* (Paris), **173**, 368.

442 BAIKIE A.G. & VALTIS D.J. (1954) Gas transport function of the blood in congenital familial methaemoglobinaemia. *British Medical Journal*, **ii**, 73.

443 CAWEIN M., BEHLEN C.H., LAPPAT E.J. & COHN J.E. (1964) Hereditary diaphorase deficiency and methemoglobinemia. *Archives of Internal Medicine*, **113**, 578.

444 DARLING R.C. & ROUGHTON F.J.W. (1942) Effect of methemoglobin on equilibrium between oxygen and hemoglobin. *American Journal of Physiology*, **137**, 56.

445 GIBSON Q.H. & HARRISON D.C. (1947) Familial idiopathic methaemoglobinaemia: Five cases in one family. *Lancet*, **ii**, 941.

446 GIBSON Q.H. (1948) Reduction in methaemoglobin in red cells and studies on the cause of idiopathic methaemoglobinaemia. *Biochemical Journal*, **42**, 13.

447 WILLIAMS J.R. & CHALLIS F.E. (1933) Methylene Blue as antidote for anilin dye poisoning: case report with confirmatory experimental study. *Journal of Laboratory and Clinical Medicine*, **19**, 166.

448 EVELYN K.A. & MALLOY H.T. (1938) Microdetermination of oxyhemoglobin: methemoglobin and sulphemoglobin in a single blood sample. *Journal of Biological Chemistry*, **126**, 655.

449 MAY A. & HUEHNS E.R. Unpublished.

450 GREEN D.E. (1934) The oxidation-reduction potentials of Cytochrome C. *Proceedings of the Royal Society, London, Series B*, **114**, 423.

451 HEILMEYER L. (1943) *Spectrophotometry in Medicine*, Hilger, London.

452 WHITEHEAD T.P. & WORTHINGTON S. (1961) The determination of carbonmonoxy hemoglobin. *Clinica Chimica Acta*, **6**, 356.

453 HORTON B.F. & HUISMAN T.H.J. (1965) Studies on the heterogeneity of haemoglobin VII minor haemoglobin components in haematological diseases. *British Journal of Haematology*, **11**, 296.

454 SRIVASTAVA S.K., VAN LOON C. & BEUTLER E. (1972) Characterization of a previously unidentified hemoglobin fraction. *Biochimica et Biophysica Acta*, **278**, 617.

455 SUMIDA I., OHTA Y., IMAMURA T. & YANASE T. (1973) Hemoglobin Sawara: α6 (A4) aspartic acid→alanine. *Biochimica et Biophysica Acta*, **322**, 23.

456 SASAKI J., IMAMURA T., SUMIDA I., YANASE T. & OHYA M. (1977) Increased oxygen affinity for hemoglobin

Sawara: αA4(6) aspartic acid→alanine. *Biochimica et Biophysica Acta*, **495,** 183.

457 BONAVENTURA J. & RIGGS A. (1967) Hemoglobin Porto Alegre: polymerization of hemoglobin of mouse and man structural basis. *Science*, **158,** 800.

458 STAMATOYANNOPOULOS G., NUTE P.E., ADAMSON J.W., BELLINGHAM A.J., FUNK D. & HORNUNG S. (1973) Hemoglobin Olympia (β20 Val→Met): an electrophoretically silent variant associated with high oxygen affinity and erythrocytosis. *Journal of Clinical Investigation*, **52,** 342.

459 HAMILTON H.B., IUCHI I., MIYAJI T. & SHIBATA S. (1969) Haemoglobin Hiroshima (β^{143} histidine→aspartic acid): a newly identified fast moving beta chain variant associated with increased oxygen affinity and compensatory erythrocytosis. *Journal of Clinical Investigation*, **48,** 525.

460 IMAI K. (1968) Oxygen equilibrium characteristics of abnormal hemoglobin Hiroshima, $\alpha_2 \beta_2^{143\,Asp}$. *Archives of Biochemistry*, **127,** 543.

461 PERUTZ M.F. (1969) Suggested interpretation of diminished Bohr effect in haemoglobin Hiroshima. *Nature (London)*, **224,** 269.

462 PERUTZ M.F., PULSINELLI P. DEL, TEN EYCK L., KILMARTIN J.V., SHIBATA S., IUCHI I., MIYAJI T. & HAMILTON H.B. (1971) Haemoglobin Hiroshima and the mechanism of the alkaline Bohr effect. *Nature (New Biology)*, **232,** 147.

463 BLACKWELL R.Q., SHIH T.-B., WANG C.-L. & LIU C.-S. (1972) Hemoglobin C-Hsi-Tsou: β79 Asp→Gly. *Biochimica et Biophysica Acta*, **257,** 49.

464 BENESCH R., EDILJI R. & BENESCH R.E. (1975) Oxygenation properties of hemoglobin variants with substitutions near the polyphosphate binding site. *Biochimica et Biophysica Acta*, **393,** 368.

465 ZAK S.J., BRIMHALL B., JONES R.T. & KAPLAN M.E. (1974) Hemoglobin Andrew-Minneapolis α2Aβ2 144 Lys→Asn: A new high-oxygen-affinity mutant human hemoglobin. *Blood*, **44,** 543.

466 JONES R.T., BRIMHALL B., POOTRAKUL S. & GRAY G. (1976) Hemoglobin Vancouver [$\alpha_2\beta_2$ 73(E17) Asp→Tyr]: Its structure and function. *Journal of Molecular Evolution*, **9,** 37.

467 SCHNEIDER R.G., HOSTY T.S., TOMLIN G., ATKINS R., BRIMHALL B. & JONES R.T. (1975) Hb Mobile [α2β2 73(E17) Asp→Val]: A new variant. *Biochemical Genetics*, **13,** 411.

468 MIYAJI T., SUZUKI H., OHTA Y. & SHIBATA S. (1966) Haemoglobin Agenogi ($\alpha_2\beta_2^{90\,Lys}$). A slow moving haemoglobin of a Japanese family resembling Hb-E. *Clinica Chimica Acta*, **14,** 624.

469 IMAI K., MORIMOTO H., KOLANI M., SHIBATA S., MIYAJI T. & MATSUMOTO K. (1970) Studies on the function of abnormal haemoglobins. II. Oxygen equilibrium of abnormal haemoglobins Shimonoseki, Ubell, Hikari, Gigu and Agenogi. *Biochimica et Biophysica Acta*, **200,** 197.

470 HALBRECHT I., ISAACS W.A., LEHMANN H. & BEN-PORAT J. (1967) Hemoglobin Hasheron (α^{47} aspartic acid→histidine). *Israel Journal of Medical Sciences*, **3,** 827.

471 CHARACHE S., MONDZAI A.M. & GESSNER U. (1969) Hemoglobin Hasharon ($\alpha_2^{47\,His}$ (CD5) β_2): A hemoglobin found in low concentration. *Journal of Clinical Investigation*, **48,** 834.

472 RAHBAR S., MAHDAVI N., NOWZARI G. & MOSTAFAVI I. (1975) Hemoglobin Arya: α_2 47(CD5) Aspartic acid→Asparagine. *Biochimica et Biophysica Acta*, **386,** 525.

473 CHARACHE S. & OSTERTAG W. (1970) Hemoglobin Hopkins-2 [(α112 Asp)₂β₂]: 'Low output' protects from potentially harmful effects. *Blood*, **36,** 852.

474 CHARACHE S., OSTERTAG W. & VON EHRENSTEIN G. (1972) Clinical studies and physiological properties of Hopkins-2 haemoglobin. *Nature (London)*, **234,** 248.

475 GIARDINA B., BRUNORI M., ANTONINI E. & TENTORI L. (1978) Properties of hemoglobin G Ferrara (β_{57}(E1) Asn→Lys). *Biochimica et Biophysica Acta*, **534,** 1.

476 BEUTLER E., LANG A. & LEHMANN H. (1974) Hemoglobin Duarte: α2β2 62(E6) Ala→Pro: A new unstable hemoglobin with increased oxygen affinity. *Blood*, **43,** 527.

477 WHITE J.M., BRAIN M.C., LORKIN P.A., LEHMANN H. & SMITH M. (1970) Mild 'unstable haemoglobin haemolytic anaemia' caused by haemoglobin Shepherd's Bush (β74 (E18) Gly→Asp). *Nature (London)*, **225,** 941.

478 MAY A. & HUEHNS E.R. (1972) The control of oxygen affinity of red cells with Hb-Shepherd's Bush. *British Journal of Haematology*, **22,** 599.

479 BRENNAN S.O., TAURO G.P., MELROSE W. & CARRELL R.W. (1977) Haemoglobin Port Phillip α91 (FG3) Leu→Pro. A new unstable haemoglobin. *FEBS Letters*, **81,** 115.

480 KLEIHAUER E.F., REYNOLDS C.A., DOZY A.M., WILSON J.B., MOORES R.R., BERENSON M.P., WRIGHT C.S. & HUISMAN T.H.J. (1968) Hemoglobin Bibba or $\alpha_2^{136\,Pro}\beta_2$, an unstable α-chain abnormal hemoglobin. *Biochimica et Biophysica Acta*, **154,** 220.

481 BEUZARD Y., BASSET P., BRACONNIER F., EL GAMMAL H., MARTIN L., OUDARD J.L. & THILLET J. (1975) Haemoglobin Saki α2β2 14 Leu→Pro (A11) structure and function. *Biochimica et Biophysica Acta*, **393,** 182.

482 MILNER P.F., CORLEY C.C., POMEROY W.L., WILSON J.B., GRAVELY M. & HUISMAN T.H.J. (1976) Thalassemia intermedia caused by heterozygosity for both β-thalassemia and Hemoglobin Saki (β14 (A11) Leu→Pro). *American Journal of Hematology*, **1,** 283.

483 SANSONE G. & PIK E. (1965) Familial haemolytic anaemia with erythrocyte inclusion bodies, bilifuscinuria and abnormal haemoglobin (haemoglobin Galliera Genova). *British Journal of Haematology*, **11,** 511.

484 SANSONE G., CARRELL R.W. & LEHMANN H. (1967) Haemoglobin Genova: β28 (B10) Leucine→Proline. *Nature (London)*, **214,** 877.

485 JACKSON J.M., YATES A. & HUEHNS E.R. (1973) Haemoglobin Perth: β32(B14) Leu→Pro. An unstable haemoglobin causing haemolysis. *British Journal of Haematology*, **25,** 607.

486 HONIG G.R., GREEN D., SHAMSUDDIN M., VIDA L.N., MASON R.G., GNARRA D.J. & MAURER H.S. (1973) Hemoglobin Abraham Lincoln, β32(B14) Leucine→Proline. An unstable variant producing severe hemolytic disease. *Journal of Clinical Investigation*, **52,** 1746.

487 OHBA Y., MIYAJI T., MATSUOKA M., SUGIYAMA K., SUZUKI T. & SUGIURA T. (1977) Hemoglobin Mizulo or beta 68(E12) Leucine→Proline, a new unstable variant associated with severe hemolytic anemia. *Hemoglobin*, **1,** 467.

488 HUBBARD M., WINTON E.F., LINDEMAN J.G., DESSAUER P.L., WILSON J.B., WRIGHTSTONE R.N. & HUISMAN

T.H.J. (1975) Hemoglobin Atlanta or $\alpha 2\beta 2$ 75 Leu→Pro (E19): an unstable variant found in several members of a Caucasian family. *Biochimica et Biophysica Acta*, **386**, 538.

489 OPFELL R.W., LORKIN P.A. & LEHMANN H. (1968) Hereditary non-spherocytic haemolytic anaemia with post-splenectomy inclusion bodies and pigmenturia caused by an unstable haemoglobin, Santa Ana $\beta 88$ (F4). *Journal of Medical Genetics*, **5**, 292.

490 FAIRBANKS V.F., OPFELL R.W. & BURGERT E.O. (1971) Three families with unstable hemoglobinopathies (Köln, Olmstead and Santa Ana) causing hemolytic anemia with inclusion bodies and pigmenturia. *American Journal of Medicine*, **46**, 344.

491 HOLLAN S.R., SZELÉNYI J.G., MILTÉNYI M., CHARLESWORTH O., LORKIN P.A. & LEHMANN H. (1970) Unstable haemoglobin disease caused by Hb-Santa Ana $\beta 88$ (F4) Leu→Pro. *Haematologia*, **4**, 141.

492 SCHNEIDER R.G., UEDA S., ALPERIN J.B., BRIMHALL B. & JONES R.T. (1969) Haemoglobin Sabine, beta 91 (F7) Leu→Pro. An unstable variant causing severe anaemia with inclusion bodies. *New England Journal of Medicine*, **280**, 739.

493 HYDE R.D., HALL M.D. WILTSHIRE B.G. & LEHMANN H. (1975) Haemoglobin Southampton, $\beta 106$(G8) Leu→Pro: An unstable variant producing severe haemolysis. *Lancet*, **ii**, 1170.

494 KOLER R.D., JONES R.T., BIGLEY R.H., LITT M., LOVRIEN E., BROOKS R., LAHEY M.E. & FOWLER R. (1973) Hemoglobin Casper: $\beta 106$(G8) Leu→Pro, a contemporary mutation. *American Journal of Medicine*, **55**, 549.

495 OUTEIRINO J., CASEY R., WHITE J.M. & LEHMANN H. (1974) Haemoglobin Madrid, $\beta 115$(G17) Alanine→Proline: An unstable variant associated with haemolytic anaemia. *Acta Haematologica*, **52**, 53.

496 WAJCMAN H., KRISHNAMOORTHY R., GACON G., ELION J., ALLARD C. & LABIE D. (1976) A new hemoglobin variant involving the distal histidine: Hb Bicêtre ($\beta 63$(E7) His→Pro). *Journal of Molecular Medicine*, **1**, 187.

497 FINNEY R., CASEY R., LEHMANN H. & WALKER W. (1975) Hb Newcastle: $\beta 92$(F8) His→Pro. *FEBS Letters*, **60**, 435.

498 CROOKSTON J.H., FARQUHARSON H.H., BEALE D. & LEHMANN H. (1969) Haemoglobin Etobicoke: $\beta 84$ (F5) serum replaced by arginine. *Canadian Journal of Biochemistry*, **47**, 143.

499 KENNEDY C.C., BLUNDELL G., LORKIN P.A., LANG A. & LEHMANN H. (1974) Haemoglobin Belfast 15(A12) Tryptophan→Arginine: A new unstable haemoglobin variant. *British Medical Journal*, **iv**, 324.

500 GACON G., WAJCMAN H., LABIE D., VARET B. & CHRISTOFOROV B. (1976) A second case of Haemoglobin Belfast (β^{15} [A12]Trp→Arg) observed in a French patient. *Acta Haematologica*, **55**, 313.

501 GAREL M.C., BLOUQUIT Y., AROUS N. & ROSA J. (1976) Hb Strasbourg $\alpha_2\beta_2 20$(B2) Val→Asp: A variant at the same locus as Hb Olympia β^{20} Val→Met. *FEBS Letters*, **72**, 1.

502 RANNEY H.M., JACOBS A.S., UDEM L. & ZALUNSKY R. (1968) Hemoglobin Riverdale-Bronx, an unstable hemoglobin resulting from the substitution of arginine for glycine or helical residue $\beta 6$ of the β polypeptide chain. *Biochemical and Biophysical Research Communications*, **33**, 1004.

503 HUISMAN T.H.J.., BROWN A.K., EFREMOV G.D., WILSON J.B., REYNOLDS C.R., VY R. & SMITH L.L. (1971) Hemoglobin Savannah (B6(24) δ glycine→valine): an unstable variant causing anemia with inclusion bodies. *Journal of Clinical Investigation*, **50**, 650.

504 IDELSON L.I., DIDKOVSKY N.A., CASEY R., LORKIN P.A. & LEHMANN H. (1974) New unstable haemoglobin (Hb Moscva, $\beta 24$(B6) Gly→Asp) found in the USSR. *Nature (London)*, **249**, 768.

505 IDELSON L.I., DIDKOVSKY N.A., FILIPPOVA A.V., CASEY R., KYNOCH P.A.M. & LEHMANN H. (1975) Haemoglobin Volga, $\beta 27$ (B9) Ala→Asp, a new highly unstable haemoglobin with a suppressed charge. *FEBS Letters*, **58**, 122.

506 KUIS-REERINK J.D., JONXIS J.H.P., NIAZI G.A., WILSON J.B., BOLCH K.C., GRAVELY M. & HUISMAN T.H.J. (1976) Hb Volga or $\alpha_2\beta_2$ 27(B9) Ala→Asp: An unstable hemoglobin variant in three generations of a Dutch family. *Biochimica et Biophysica Acta*, **439**, 63.

507 THILLET J., COHEN-SOLAL M., SELIGMANN M. & ROSA J. (1976) Functional and physicochemical studies of Hemoglobin St. Louis β^{28} (B10) Leu→Gln. *Journal of Clinical Investigation*, **58**, 1098.

508 GAREL M.C., BLOUQUIT Y. & ROSA J. (1975) Hemoglobin Castilla $\beta 32$(B14) Leu→Arg: A new unstable variant producing severe hemolytic disease. *FEBS Letters*, **58**, 145.

509 CHARACHE S., BRIMHALL B., MILNER P. & COBB L. (1973) Hemoglobin Okaloosa ($\beta 48$(CD7) Leucine→Arginine. An unstable hemoglobin with decreased oxygen affinity. *Journal of Clinical Investigation*, **52**, 2858.

510 TENTORI L. (1973) Three examples of double heterozygosis beta-thalassemia and rare hemoglobin variants. *International Symposium on Abnormal Hemoglobin and Thalassemia*, p. 53. Istanbul, Turkey, Abstract 68.

511 BRADLEY T.B., WOHL R.C., MURPHY S.B., OSKI F.A. & BUNN F. (1972) Properties of hemoglobin Bryn Mawr $\beta^{85 Phe→Ser}$. A new spontaneous mutation producing an unstable hemoglobin with high oxygen affinity. *Blood*, **40**, 947.

512 DE WEINSTEIN B.I., WHITE J.M., WILTSHIRE B.G. & LEHMANN H. (1973) A new unstable haemoglobin: Hb Buenos Aires, $\beta 85$(F1) Phe→Ser. *Acta Haematologica*, **50**, 357.

513 KING M.A.R., WILTSHIRE B.G., LEHMANN H. & MORIMOTO H. (1972) An unstable haemoglobin with reduced oxygen affinity, haemoglobin Peterborough, $\beta 111$ (G13) Valine→Phenylalanine, its interaction with normal haemoglobin and haemoglobin Lepore. *British Journal of Haematology*, **22**, 125.

514 KLEIHAUER E. & BETKE K. (1972) Eigenschaften des instabilen Hb-Wien. *Klinische Wochenschrift*, **50**, 907.

515 BRAUNSTEINER H., DIENSTL F., SAILER S. & SANDHOFER F. (1964) Angeborene hämolytische Anämie mit Mesobilifuscinurie und Innenkörperbildung nach Splenektomie. *Acta Haematologica (Basel)*, **32**, 314.

516 ARENDS T., LEHMANN H., PLOWMAN D. & STATHOPOULOU R. (1977) Haemoglobin North Shore-Caracas $\beta 134$ (H12) Valine→Glutamic acid. *FEBS Letters*, **80**, 261.

517 BRENNAN S.O., ARNOLD B., FLEMING P. & CARRELL R.W. (1977) A new unstable haemoglobin, $\beta 134$

Val→Glu. *Proceedings of the New Zealand Medical Journal*, **85**, 398.

518 THILLET J., BLOUQUIT Y., GAREL M.C., DREYFUS B., REYES F., COHEN-SOLAL M., BEUZARD Y. & ROSA J. (1976) Hemoglobin Creteil β89(F5) Ser→Asn: High oxygen affinity variant of hemoglobin frozen in a quaternary R-structure. *Journal of Molecular Medicine*, **1**, 135.

519 PANIKER N.V., KUANG-TZU DAVIS LIN, KRANTZ S.B., FLEXNER J.M., WASSERMAN B.K. & PUETT D. (1978) Haemoglobin Vanderbilt ($\alpha_2\beta_2$ 89 Ser→Arg): A new haemoglobin with high oxygen affinity and compensatory erythrocytosis. *British Journal of Haematology*, **39**, 249.

520 OHBA Y., MIYAJI T., MATSUOKA M., YOKOYAMA M., NUMAKURA H., NAGATA K., TAKEBE Y., IZUMI Y. & SHIBATA S. (1975) Hemoglobin Hirosaki (α43 [CE 1] Phe→Leu), a new unstable variant. *Biochimica et Biophysica Acta*, **405**, 155.

521 PRATO V., GALLO E., RICCO G., MAZZA U., BIANCO G. & LEHMANN H. (1970) Haemolytic anaemia due to haemoglobin Torino. *British Journal of Haematology*, **19**, 105.

522 BRACONNIER F., GACON G., THILLET J., WAJCMAN H., SORIA J., MAIGRET P., LABIE D. & ROSA J. (1977) Hemoglobin Fort de France (α_2^{45} (CD3) His→Arg β_2) a new variant with increased oxygen affinity. *Biochimica et Biophysica Acta*, **493**, 228.

523 SUZUKI T., HAYASHI A., YAMAMURA Y., ENOKI Y. & TYUMA I. (1965) Functional Abnormality of Hemoglobin M-Osaka. *Biochemical and Biophysical Research Communications*, **19**, 691.

524 BRIMHALL B., DUERST M., HOLLAN S.R., STENZEL P., SZELENYI J. & JONES R.T. (1974) Structural characterizations of Hemoglobins-J Buda (α61 (E10) Lys→Asn) and G Pest (α74 (EF3) Asp→Asn). *Biochimica et Biophysica Acta*, **336**, 344.

525 KNUTH A., PRIBILLA W., MARTI H.R. & WINTERHALTER K.H. (1974) Hemoglobin Moabit: Alpha 86 (F7) Leu→Arg. A new unstable abnormal hemoglobin. *Acta Haematologica*, **61**, 121.

526 MIYAJI T., IUCHI I., SHIBATA S., TAKEDA I. & TAMURA A. (1963) Possible amino acid substitution in the α-chain ($\alpha^{87\,\text{Tyr}}$) of Hb-M$_{\text{Iwate}}$. *Acta Haematologica Japonica*, **26**, 538.

527 JONES R.T., COLEMAN R.D. & HELLER P. (1964) The chemical structure of hemoglobin M$_{\text{Iwate}}$ (M$_{\text{Kankakee}}$). *Federation Proceedings. Federation of American Societies for Experimental Biology*, **23**, 173.

528 HAYASHI N., MOLOKAWA Y. & KIKUCHI G. (1966) Studies on relationships between structure and function of hemoglobin M$_{\text{Iwate}}$. *Journal of Biological Chemistry*, **241**, 79.

529 KIKUCHI G., HAYASHI N. & TAMURA A. (1964) Oxygen equilibrium of hemoglobin M$_{\text{Iwate}}$. *Biochimica et Biophysica Acta*, **90**, 199.

530 BURKETT L.B., SHARMA V.S., PISCIOTTA A.V., RANNEY H.M. & BRUCKHEIMER S. (1976) Hemoglobin Mequon β41 (C7) Phenylalanine→Tyrosine. *Blood*, **48**, 645.

531 DACIE J.V., SHINTON N.K., GAFFNEY P.J., CARRELL R.W. & LEHMANN H. (1967) Haemoglobin Hammersmith (β42(CDI) Phe→Ser). *Nature (London)*, **216**, 663.

532 BRATU V., LORKIN P.A., LEHMANN H. & PREDESCU C. (1971) Haemoglobin Bucuresti β42 (CDI) Phe→Leu. A

cause of unstable haemolytic anaemia. *Biochimica et Biophysica Acta*, **229**, 343.

533 BACKMANN F. & MARTI H. (1962) Hemoglobin Zürich. II. Physicochemical properties of the abnormal hemoglobin. *Blood*, **20**, 272.

534 MULLER C.J. & KINGMA S. (1961) Hemoglobin Zürich, $\alpha_2^A\beta_2^{63\,\text{Arg}}$. *Biochimica et Biophysica Acta*, **50**, 595.

535 RIEDER R.F., ZINKHAM W.H. & HOLTZMAN N.A. (1965) Hemoglobin Zürich. Clinical, chemical and kinetic studies. *American Journal of Medicine*, **39**, 4.

536 MOORE W.M.O., BATTAGLIA F.C. & HELLEGERS A.F. (1967) Whole blood oxygen affinities of women with various hemoglobinopathies. *American Journal of Obstetrics and Gynecology*, **97**, 63.

537 WINTERHALTER K.H., ANDERSON N.M., AMICONI G., ANTONINI E. & BRUNORI M. (1969) Functional properties of Hemoglobin Zürich. *European Journal of Biochemistry*, **11**, 435.

538 MURAWSKI E., CARTA S., SORCINI M., TENTORI L., VIVALDI G., ANTONINI E., BRIMORI M., WYMAN J., BUCCI E., ROSSI-FANELLI A. (1965) Observation on the structure and behaviour of hemoglobin M$_{\text{Radom}}$. *Archives of Biochemistry and Biophysics*, **111**, 197.

539 SUZUKI T., HAYASHI A., SHIMIZU A. & YAMAMURA Y. (1966) The oxygen equilibrium of hemoglobin M$_{\text{Saskatoon}}$. *Biochimica et Biophysica Acta*, **127**, 280.

540 ROSA J., LABIE D., WAJCMAN H., BOIGNE J.M., CABANNES R., BIERME R. & RUFFIE J. (1969) Haemoglobin I Toulouse β66(E10) Lys→Glu: a new abnormal haemoglobin with a mutation localized on the E10 porphyrin surrounding zone. *Nature (London)*, **223**, 190.

541 UDEM L., RANNEY H.M., BUAN H.F. & PISCIOTTA A. (1970) Some observations on the properties of hemoglobin M Milwaukee 1. *Journal of Molecular Biology*, **48**, 487.

542 PERUTZ M.F., PULSINELLI P. DEL & RANNEY H.M. (1972) Structure and subunit interaction of haemoglobin M Milwaukee. *Nature (London)*, **237**, 259.

543 LINDSTROM T.R., CHILIS H.O. & PISCIOTTA A.V. (1972) Nuclear magnetic resonance studies of haemoglobin M Milwaukee. *Nature (London)*, **237**, 263.

544 RAIK E. & HUNTER E.G. (1967) Compensated hereditary haemolytic disease resulting from an unstable haemoglobin fraction. *Medical Journal of Australia*, **1**, 955.

545 STAMATOYANNOPOULOS G., PARER J.T. & FINCH C.A. (1969) Physiologic implications of a hemoglobin with decreased oxygen affinity (Hemoglobin Seattle). *New England Journal of Medicine*, **281**, 915.

546 HUEHNS E.R., HECHT F., YOSHIDA A., STAMATOYANNOPOULOS G., HARTMAN J. & MOTULSKY A.G. (1970) An unstable hemoglobin causing chronic hemolytic anemia. *Blood*, **36**, 209.

547 ANDERSON N.L., PERUTZ M.F. & STAMATOYANNOPOULOS G. (1973) Site of the amino acid substitution in haemoglobin Seattle ($\alpha_2^A\beta_2^{70\,\text{Asp}}$). *Nature (New Biology)*, **243**, 274.

548 CARRELL R.W. & OWEN M.C. (1971) A new approach to hemoglobin variant identification. Hemoglobin Christchurch β71(E15) Phenylalanine→Serine. *Biochimica et Biophysica Acta*, **236**, 507.

549 SVENSSON B. & STRAND L. (1967) A Swedish family with haemolytic anaemia, Heinz bodies and abnormal hae-

moglobin. *Scandinavian Journal of Haematology,* **4,** 241.

550 HOLLENDER A., LORKIN P.A., LEHMANN H. & SVENSON B. (1969) New unstable haemoglobin Borås, β88 (F4) Leucine→Arginine. *Nature (London),* **222,** 953.

551 BEUZARD Y., COURVALIN J.C., COHEN SOLAL M., GAREL M.C. & ROSA J. (1972) Structural studies of Hb-St. Etienne, β92 (F8) His→Gln. A new abnormal hemoglobin with loss of β-proximal His and absence of heme on the β-chains. *FEBS Letters,* **27,** 76.

552 COHEN SOLAL M., THILLET J., GAILLARDON J. & ROSA J. (1972) Functional properties of hemoglobin Saint Etienne: A variant carrying heme only on α-chains. *Revue Européenne d'Etudes Cliniques et Biologiques,* **17,** 988.

553 HELLER R., COLEMAN R.D. & YAKULIS V.J. (1966) Hemoglobin M Hyde Park: A new variant of abnormal methemoglobin. *Journal of Clinical Investigation,* **45,** 1021.

554 HAYASHI A., SUZUKI T., SHIMIZU A., IMAI K., MORI-MOTO H., MIYAJI T. & SHIBATA S. (1968) Some observations on the physicochemical properties of haemoglobin M Hyde Park. *Archives of Biochemistry and Biophysics,* **125,** 895.

555 GREER J. (1971) Three-dimensional structure of abnormal human haemoglobins, M Hyde Park and M Iwate. *Journal of Molecular Biology,* **59,** 107.

556 ADAMS J.G. III, PRZYWARA K.P., SHAMSUDDIN M. & HELLER P. (1975) Hemoglobin J Altgeld Gardens (β92(F8) His→Asp): A new hemoglobin variant involving a substitution of the proximal histidine. *American Society of Hematology 18th Annual Meeting,* Dallas, Texas.

557 GACON G., WAJCMAN H. & LABIE D. (1975) A new unstable hemoglobin mutated in β98(FG5) Val→Ala: Hb Djelfa. *FEBS Letters,* **58,** 238.

558 CARRELL R.W., LEHMANN H. & HUTCHISON H.E. (1966) Haemoglobin Köln (β98 Valine→Methionine). An unstable protein causing inclusion body anaemia. *Nature (London),* **210,** 915.

559 GORDON SMITH E.C., BLECHER T.E., WILTSHIRE B.G. & LEHMANN H. (1973) Haemoglobin Nottingham βFG5 (98) Val→Gly: A new unstable haemoglobin producing severe haemolysis. *Proceedings of the Royal Society of Medicine,* **66,** 507.

560 LORKIN P.A., LEHMANN H., FAIRBANKS V.F., BERG-LUND G. & LEONHARDT T. (1975) Two new pathological haemoglobins: Olmsted β141 (H19) Leu→Arg and Malmö: β97(FG4) His→Gln. *Biochemical Journal,* **119,** 68.

561 SWENSON R.T., HILL R.L., LEHMANN H. & JIM R.T.S. (1962) A chemical abnormality in hemoglobin G from Chinese individuals. *Journal of Biological Chemistry,* **237,** 1517.

562 VETTORE L., DESANDRE G., DILORIO E.E., WINTER-HALTER K.H., LANG A. & LEHMANN H. (1974) A new abnormal hemoglobin O Padova, α30 (B11) Glu→Lys and a dyserythropoietic anemia with erythroblastic multinuclearity co-existing in the same patient. *Blood,* **44,** 869.

563 MARINUCCI M., MAVILIO F., MASSA A., GABBIANELLI M., TENTORI L. & IGNESTI C. (1978) Haemoglobin Prato: A new amino acid substitution (α31(B12) Arg→Ser). *IRCS Medical Science,* **6,** 234.

564 JONES R.T., BRIMHALL B. & LISKER R. (1967) Chemical characterization of hemoglobin Mexico and hemoglobin Chiapas. *Biochimica et Biophysica Acta,* **154,** 488.

565 MOO-PENN W.F., JUE D.L., JOHNSON M.H., WILSON S.M., THERREL B. JR & SCHMIDT R.M. (1977) Hemoglobin Tarrant: α126 (H9) Asp→Asn. A new hemoglobin variant in the $\alpha_1\beta_1$ contact region showing high oxygen affinity and reduced cooperativity. *Biochimica et Biophysica Acta,* **490,** 443.

566 WADE COHEN P.T., YATES A., BELLINGHAM A.J. & HUEHNS E.R. (1973) Amino-acid substitution on the α1β1 intersubunit contact of Haemoglobin Camden β131 (H9) Gln→Glu. *Nature (New Biology),* **243,** 467.

567 MARTINEZ G., LIMA F. & COLOMBO B. (1977) Hemoglobin J Guantanamo ($\alpha_2\beta_2$ 128 (H6) Ala→Asp). A new fast unstable hemoglobin found in a Cuban family. *Biochimica et Biophysica Acta,* **491,** 1.

568 ALTAY C., ALTINÖZ N., WILSON J.B., BOLCH K.C. & HUISMAN T.H.J. (1976) Hemoglobin Hacettepe or α2β2 127 (H5) Gln→Glu. *Biochimica et Biophysica Acta,* **434,** 1.

569 CLEGG J.B., WEATHERALL D.J., WONG HOCK BOON & MUSTAFA D. (1969) Two new haemoglobin variants involving proline substitutions. *Nature (London),* **222,** 379.

570 BURSAUX E., BLOUQUIT Y., POYART C., ROSA J., AROUS N. & BOHN B. (1978) Hemoglobin Ty Gard ($\alpha_2{}^A\beta_2$ 124(H$_2$) Pro→Gln). A stable high O_2 affinity variant at the $\alpha_1\beta_1$ contact. *FEBS Letters,* **88,** 155.

571 SCHNEIDER R.G., BERKMAN N.L., BRIMHALL B. & JONES R.T. (1976) Hemoglobin Fannin-Lubbock [$\alpha_2\beta_2{}^{119}$ (GH2) Gly→Asp]: A slightly unstable mutant. *Biochimica et Biophysica Acta,* **453,** 478.

572 MOO-PENN W.F., BECHTEL K.C., JOHNSON M.H., JUE D.L., THERRELL B.L. JR, MORRISON B.Y. & SCHMIDT R.M. (1976) Hemoglobin Fannin-Lubbock [$\alpha_2\beta_2{}^{119}$ (GH2) Gly→Asp]: A new hemoglobin variant at the $\alpha_1\beta_1$ contact. *Biochimica et Biophysica Acta,* **453,** 472.

573 SCHNEIDER R.G., ALPERIN J.B., BRIMHALL B. & JONES R.T. (1969) Hemoglobin P ($\alpha_2\beta_2{}^{117\,\text{Arg}}$): structure and properties. *Journal of Laboratory and Clinical Medicine,* **73,** 616.

574 RANNEY H.M., JACOBS A.S. & NAGEL R.L. (1967) Hemoglobin New York. *Nature (London),* **213,** 876.

575 ADAMS J.G., BOXER L.A., BAEHNER R.L., FORGET B.G., TSISTROKIS G.A. & STEINBERG M.H. (1978) Hemoglobin Indianapolis: Post-translational degradation of an unstable β-chain variant producing a phenotype of severe heterozygous β-thalassemia. *Clinical Research,* **26,** 501A.

576 NUTE P.E., STAMATOYANNOPOULOS G., HERMODSON M.A., ROTH D. & HORNUNG S. (1974) Hemoglobinopathic erythrocytosis due to a new electrophoretically silent variant, Hemoglobin San Diego (β109(G11) Val→Met). *Journal of Clinical Investigation,* **53,** 320.

577 IMAMURA T., FUJITA S., OHTA Y., HANADA M. & YANASE T. (1969) Hemoglobin Yoshizuka (G10(108)β Asn→Asp acid): a new variant with a reduced oxygen affinity from a Japanese family. *Journal of Clinical Investigation,* **48,** 2341.

578 MOO-PENN W.F., WOLFF J.A., SIMON G., VAČEK M., JUE D.L. & JOHNSON M.H. (1978) Hemoglobin Presbyterian: β108(G10) Asparagine→Lysine. A hemoglobin variant with low oxygen affinity. *FEBS Letters,* **92,** 53.

579 JONES R.T., KOLER R.D., DUERST M.L. & DHINDSA D.S.

(1976) Hemoglobin Willamette [α2β2 51 Pro→Arg (D2)] a new abnormal human hemoglobin. *Hemoglobin*, **1**, 45.

580 RIEDER R.F., OSKI F.A. & CLEGG J.B. (1969) Hemoglobin Philly (β35 tyrosine→phenylalanine): studies in molecular pathology of hemoglobin. *Journal of Clinical Investigation*, **48**, 1627.

581 BAUER E.W. & MOTULSKY A.G. (1965) Hemoglobin Tacoma. A β-chain variant associated with increased Hb-A₂. *Humangenetik*, **1**, 621.

582 BRIMHALL B., JONES R.T., BAUR E.W. & MOTULSKY A.G. (1969) Structural characterization of hemoglobin Tacoma. *Biochemistry*, **8**, 212.

583 WHITE J.M., SZUR L., GILLIES I.D.S., LORKIN P.A. & LEHMANN H. (1973) Familial polycythaemia caused by a new haemoglobin variant. Hb Heathrow β103(G5) Phenylalanine→Leucine. *British Medical Journal*, **iii**, 665.

584 NAGEL R.L., GIBSON Q.H. & CHARACHE S. (1967) Relation between structure and function in hemoglobin Chesapeake. *Biochemistry*, **6**, 2395.

585 GREER J. (1971) Three-dimensional structure of abnormal human haemoglobins Chesapeake and J Capetown. *Journal of Molecular Biology*, **62**, 241.

586 BOTHA M.C., BEALE D., ISAACS W.A. & LEHMANN H. (1966) Haemoglobin J Capetown α₂ 92 Arginine→Glutamine β₂. *Nature (London)*, **212**, 792.

587 LINES J.G. & McINTOSH R. (1967) Oxygen binding by haemoglobin J Capetown (α₂ 92 Arg→Glu). *Nature (London)*, **215**, 297.

588 JENKINS T., STEVENS K., GALLO E. & LEHMANN H. (1968) A second family possessing haemoglobin Jα Capetown. *South African Medical Journal*, **42**, 1151.

589 CHARACHE S., JENKINS T. & WILDER M.F. (1971) Oxygen equilibrium of hemoglobin J Capetown. *Journal of Clinical Investigation*, **50**, 1554.

590 WAJCMAN H., BELKHODJA O. & LABIE D. (1972) Hb Setif: G1 (94) αAsp→Tyr. A new α chain hemoglobin variant with substitution of the residue involved in a hydrogen bond between unlike subunits. *FEBS Letters*, **27**, 298.

591 SCHNEIDER R.G., ATKINS R.J., HOSTY T.S., TOMLIN G., CASEY R., LEHMANN H., LORKIN P.A. & NAGAI K. (1975) Haemoglobin Titusville: α94 Asp→Asn, a new haemoglobin with a lowered affinity for oxygen. *Biochimica et Biophysica Acta*, **400**, 365.

592 SCHROEDER W.A., SHELTON J.B., SHELTON J.R. & POWARS D. (1978) Hemoglobin Sunshine Seth—α₂ (94(G1) Asp→His) β₂. *Hemoglobin*, **3**, 145.

593 WILTSHIRE B.G., CLARK K.G.H., LORKIN P.A. & LEHMANN H. (1972) Hemoglobin Denmark Hill α95 (G2) Pro→Ala, a variant with unusual electrophoretic and oxygen-binding properties. *Biochimica et Biophysica Acta*, **278**, 459.

594 SMITH L.L., PLESE C.F., BOSTON B.P., CHARACHE S., WILSON T.B. & HUISMAN T.H.J. (1972) Sub-unit dissociation of the abnormal hemoglobins G. Georgia (α95 leu (G2)₂β₂) and Rampa (α95 ser (G2)₂β₂). *Journal of Biological Chemistry*, **247**, 1433.

595 BANNISTER W.H., GRECH J.L., PLESE C.F., SMITH L.L., BARTON B.P., WILSON J.B., REYNOLDS C.A. & HUISMAN T.H.J. (1972) Hemoglobin St. Luke's or α2 95 Arg (G2) β2. *European Journal of Biochemistry*, **29**, 301.

596 BAREM G.H., BROMBERG P.A., ALBEN J.O., BRIMHALL B., JONES R.T., MINTZ S. & ROTHER I. (1976) Altered C-terminal salt bridges in Haemoglobin York, cause: high oxygen affinity. *Nature (London)*, **259**, 155.

597 WAJCMAN H., KILMARTIN J.V., NAJMAN A. & LABIE D. (1975) Hemoglobin Cochin-Port-Royal—consequences of the replacement of the β chain C-terminal by an arginine. *Biochimica et Biophysica Acta*, **400**, 354.

598 HAYASHI A., STAMATOYANNOPOULOS G., YOSHIDA A. & ADAMSON J. (1971) Haemoglobin Rainier: β145 (HC2) tyrosine→cysteine and haemoglobin Bethesda: β145. (HC2) tyrosine→histidine. *Nature (New Biology)*, **230**, 264.

599 ADAMSON J.W., PARER J.T., STAMATOYANNOPOULOS G. & HEINENBERG S. (1969) Erythrocytosis associated with hemoglobin Rainier: oxygen equilibria and marrow regulation. *Journal of Clinical Investigation*, **48**, 1376.

600 GREER J. & PERUTZ M.F. (1971) Three dimensional structure of haemoglobin Rainier. *Nature (New Biology)*, **230**, 261.

601 AMICONI G., WINTERHALTER K.H., ANTONINI E. & BRUNORI M. (1972) Functional properties of hemoglobin Rainier. *FEBS Letters*, **21**, 341.

602 KLECKNER H.B., WILSON J.B., LINDEMAN J.G., STEVENS P.D., NIAZI G., HUNTER E., CHEN C.J. & HUISMAN T.H.J. (1975) Hemoglobin Fort Gordon or α2β2 145 Tyr→Asp, a new high-oxygen-affinity-hemoglobin variant. *Biochimica et Biophysica Acta*, **400**, 343.

603 CHARACHE S., BRIMHALL B. & JONES R.T. (1975) Polycythemia produced by Hemoglobin Osler (β145(HC2) Tyr→Asp). *Johns Hopkins Medical Journal*, **136**, 132.

604 GACON G., WAJCMAN H. & LABIE D. (1975) Structural and functional study of Hb Nancy β145 (HC2) Tyr→Asp: A high oxygen affinity hemoglobin. *FEBS Letters*, **56**, 39.

605 REISSMANN K.R., RUTH W.E. & NAMURA T. (1961) A human hemoglobin with lowered oxygen affinity and impaired heme-heme interactions. *Journal of Clinical Investigation*, **40**, 1826.

606 BONAVENTURA J. & RIGGS A. (1968) Hemoglobin Kansas, a human hemoglobin with a neutral amino acid substitution and an abnormal oxygen equilibrium. *Journal of Biological Chemistry*, **243**, 980.

607 GREER J. (1971) Three-dimensional structure of abnormal human haemoglobins Kansas and Richmond. *Journal of Molecular Biology*, **59**, 99.

608 EFREMOV G.D., HUISMAN T.H.J., SMITH L.L., WILSON J.B., KITCHENS J.L., WRIGHTSTONE R.N. & ADAMS H.R. (1969) Hemoglobin Richmond. A human hemoglobin which forms asymmetric hybrids with other hemoglobins. *Journal of Biological Chemistry*, **244**, 6105.

609 NAGEL R.L., JOSHUA L., JOHNSON J., LANDAU L., BOOKCHIN R.M. & HARRIS M.B. (1976) Hemoglobin Beth Israel: A mutant causing clinically apparent cyanosis. *New England Journal of Medicine*, **295**, 125.

610 CHARACHE S., JACOBSON R., BRIMHALL B., MURPHY E.A., HATHAWAY P., WINSLOW R., JONES R., RATH C. & SIMKOVICH J. (1978) Hb Potomac (β101 Glu→Asp): Speculations on placental oxygen transport in carriers of high-affinity hemoglobins. *Blood*, **51**, 331.

611 MANT M.J., SALKIE M.L., COPE N., APPLING F., BOLCH K., JAYALAKSHMI M., GRAVELY M., WILSON J.B. & HUISMAN T.H.J. (1977) Hb Alberta or α2β2 (101(G3)

Glu→Gly), a new high-oxygen-affinity hemoglobin variant causing erythrocytosis. *Hemoglobin*, **1**, 183.

612 JONES R.T., BRIMHALL B. & GRAY G. (1976) Hemoglobin British Columbia [α2β2 101(G3) Glu→Lys]: A new variant with high oxygen affinity. *Hemoglobin*, **1**, 171.

613 ADAMS J.B., WINTER W.P., TAUSK K. & HELLER P. (1974) Hemoglobin Rush [(β-101(G3) Glutamine)]: A new unstable hemoglobin causing mild hemolytic anemia. *Blood*, **45**, 261.

614 LOKICH J.J., MAHONEY C.W., BUNN H.F., BRUCKHEINER S.M. & RANNEY H.M. (1973) Hemoglobin Brigham (α2Aβ2 100 Pro→Leu). Hemoglobin variant associated with familial erythrocytosis. *Journal of Clinical Investigation*, **52**, 2060.

615 GLYNN K.P., PENNER J.A., SMITH J.R. & RUCKNAGEL D.L. (1968) Familial erythrocytosis. A description of three families, one with Hb-Ypsilanti. *Annals of Internal Medicine*, **69**, 769.

616 REED C.S., HAMPSON R., GORDON S., JONES R.T., NOVY M.J., BRIMHALL B., EDWARDS M.J. & KOLER R.D. (1968) Erythrocytosis secondary to increased oxygen affinity of a mutant hemoglobin, hemoglobin Kempsey. *Blood*, **31**, 623.

617 JONES R.T., OSGOOD E.E., BRIMHALL B. & KOLER R.D. (1967) Hemoglobin Yakima: I. Clinical and biochemical studies. *Journal of Clinical Investigation*, **46**, 1840.

618 NOVY M.J., EDWARDS M.J. & METCALFE J. (1967) Hemoglobin Yakima: II. High blood oxygen affinity associated with compensatory erythrocytosis and normal hemodynamics. *Journal of Clinical Investigation*, **46**, 1848.

619 WEATHERALL D.J., CLEGG J.B., CALLENDER S.T., WELLS R.M.G., GALE R.E., HUEHNS E.R., PERUTZ M.F., VIGGIANO G. & HO C. (1977) Haemoglobin Radcliffe (α2β2 99(G1)Ala): A high oxygen-affinity variant causing familial polycythaemia. *British Journal of Haematology*, **35**, 177.

620 TAKETA F., HUANG Y.P., LIBNOCH J.A. & DESSEL B.H. (1975) Hemoglobin Wood β97(FG4) His→Leu: A new high-oxygen-affinity hemoglobin associated with familial erythrocytosis. *Biochimica et Biophysica Acta*, **400**, 348.

621 TAKETA F., ANTHOLINE W.E., MAUK A.G. & LIBNOCH J.A. (1975) Nitrosylhemoglobin Wood: Effects of inositol hexaphosphate on thiol reactivity and electron paramagnetic resonance spectrum. *Biochemistry*, **14**, 3229.

622 BROWN W.J., NIAZI G.A., JAYALAKSHMI M., ABRAHAM E.C. & HUISMAN T.H.J. (1976) Hemoglobin Athens-Georgia, or α2β2 40(C6) Arg→Lys, a hemoglobin variant with an increased oxygen affinity. *Biochimica et Biophysica Acta*, **439**, 70.

623 MOO-PENN W.F., JOHNSON M.H., BECHTEL K.C., JUE D.L., THERRELL B.L. & SCHMIDT R.M. (1977) Hemoglobin Austin and Waco: two hemoglobins with substitutions in the α1β2 contact region. *Archives of Biochemistry and Biophysics*, **179**, 86.

624 BRIMHALL B., JONES R.T., SCHNEIDER R.G., HOSTY T.S., TOMLIN G. & ATKINS R. (1975) Two new hemoglobins: Hemoglobin Alabama (β39(C5) Gln→Lys) and Hemoglobin Montgomery (α48(CD6) Leu→Arg). *Biochimica et Biophysica Acta*, **379**, 28.

625 KENDALL A.G., PAS A.T., WILSON B.J., COPE N., BOLCH K. & HUISMAN T.H.J. (1977) Hb Vaasa or α2β2 (39(C5)

Gln→Glu), a mildly unstable variant found in a Finnish family. *Hemoglobin*, **1**, 292.

626 YAMAOKA K. (1971) Hemoglobin Hirose: α1β2 37(C3) Tryptophan yielding Serine. *Blood*, **38**, 730.

627 GACON G., BELKHODJA O., WAJCMAN H. & LABIE D. (1977) Structural and functional studies of Hb Rothschild β37(C3) Trp→Arg. A new variant of the α1β2 contact. *FEBS Letters*, **82**, 243.

628 CROOKSTON J.H., FARQUHARSON H., KINDERLEHRER J. & LEHMANN H. (1970) Hemoglobin Manitoba: α102 (G9) serine replaced by arginine. *Canadian Journal of Biochemistry*, **48**, 911.

629 VELLA F., GALBRAITH P., WILSON J.B., WONG S.C., FOLGER G.C. & HUISMAN T.H.J. (1974) Hemoglobin St. Claude or α2 127 (H10) Lys→Thr β2. *Biochimica et Biophysica Acta*, **365**, 318.

630 MOO-PENN W.F., BECHTEL K.C., JOHNSON M.H., JUE D.L., HOLLAND S., HUFF C. & SCHMIDT R.M. (1976) Hemoglobin Jackson, α127 (H10) Lys→Asn. *American Journal of Clinical Pathology*, **66**, 453.

631 POYART C., KRISHNAMOORTHY R., BURSAUX E., GACON G. & LABIE D. (1976) Structural and functional studies of Haemoglobin Suresnes or α2141 (HC3) Arg→His β2, a new high oxygen affinity mutant. *FEBS Letters*, **69**, 103.

632 SAENZ G.F., ELIZONDO J., ALVARADO M.A., ATMETLLA F., ARROYS G., MARTINEZ G., LIMA F. & COLOMBO B. (1977) Chemical characterization of a new haemoglobin variant Haemoglobin J Cubujuqui (α2141(HC3) Arg→Ser β2). *Biochimica et Biophysica Acta*, **494**, 48.

633 MAVILIO F., MARINUCCI M., TENTORI L., FONTANAROSA P.P., ROSSI U. & BIAGIOTTI S. (1978) Hemoglobin Legnano (α2 141 (HC3) Arg Leu β2): A new abnormal human hemoglobin with high oxygen affinity. *Hemoglobin*, **2**, 249.

634 MARTINEZ G., LIMA F., RESIDENTI C. & COLOMBO B. (1978) Hb J Camagüey α2 141 (HC3) Arg→Gly β2. A new abnormal human hemoglobin. *Hemoglobin*, **2**, 47.

635 MOO-PENN W.F., BECHTEL K.C., SCHMIDT R.M., JOHNSON M.H., JUE D.L., SCHMIDT D.E. jr, DUNLAP W.M., OPELLA S.J., BONAVENTURA J. & BONAVENTURA C. (1977) Hemoglobin Raleigh (β1 Valine→Acetylalanine). Structural and functional characterization. *Biochemistry*, **16**, 4872.

636 LABOSSIERE A., VELLA F., HIEBERT J. & GALBRAITH P. (1972) Hemoglobin Deer Lodge: α2β2 2 His→Arg. *Clinical Biochemistry*, **5**, 46.

637 BLACKWELL R.Q., YANG H.T. & WANG C.C. (1969) Hemoglobin G Szuhu: β80 Asn→Lys. *Biochimica et Biophysica Acta*, **188**, 59.

638 IMAI K., MORIMOTO H., KOTANI M., SHIBATA S., MIYAJI T. & MASUTOMO K. (1970) Studies on the function of abnormal hemoglobins. II. Oxygen equilibrium of abnormal hemoglobins: Shimonoseki, Ube II, Hikari, Gifu, and Agenogi. *Biochimica et Biophysica Acta*, **200**, 197.

639 IKKALA E., KOSKELA J., PIKKARAINEN P. RAHIALA E.-L. EL-HAZMI M.A.F., NAGAI K., LANG A. & LEHMANN H. (1976) Hb Helsinki: A variant with a high oxygen affinity and a substitution at a 2,3-DPG binding site (β82[EF6] Lys→Met). *Acta Haematologica*, **56**, 257.

640 MOO-PENN W.F., JUE D.L., BECHTEL K.C., JOHNSON M.H., SCHMIDT R.M., MCCURDY P.R., FOX J., BONAVENTURA J., SULLIVAN B. & BONAVENTURA C. (1976)

Hemoglobin Providence. A human hemoglobin variant occurring in two forms *in vivo*. *Journal of Biological Chemistry*, **251**, 7557.

641 BONAVENTURA J., BONAVENTURA C., SULLIVAN B., FERRUZZI G., McCURDY P.R., FOX J. & MOO-PENN W.F. (1976) Hemoglobin Providence. Functional consequences of two alterations of the 2,3-diphosphoglycerate binding site at position β82. *Journal of Biological Chemistry*, **251**,7563.

642 LORKIN P.A., STEPHENS A.D., BEARD M.E.J., WRIGLEY P.F.M., ADAMS L. & LEHMANN H. (1975) Haemoglobin Rahere (β82 Lys→Thr): A new high affinity haemoglobin associated with decreased 2,3-diphosphoglycerate binding and relative polycythaemia. *British Medical Journal*, **iv**, 200.

643 MARTI H.R., WINTERHALTER K.H., DI IORIO E.E., LORKIN P.A. & LEHMANN H. (1976) Hb Altdorf α2β2 135(H13) Ala→Pro: A new electrophoretically silent unstable haemoglobin variant from Switzerland. *FEBS Letters*, **63**, 193.

644 MINNICH V., HILL R.J., KHURI P.D. & ANDERSON M.E. (1965) Hemoglobin Hope: A beta chain variant. *Blood*, **25**, 830.

645 JENSEN M., OSKI F.A., NATHAN D.G. & BUNN H.F. (1975) Hemoglobin Syracuse (α2β2 143 (H21) His→Pro), a new high-affinity variant detected by special electrophoretic methods. *Journal of Clinical Investigation*, **55**, 469.

646 TENTORI L., CARTA SORCINI M. & BUCCELLA C. (1972) Hemoglobin Abruzzo: beta 143 (H21) His→Arg. *Clinica Chimica Acta*, **38**, 258.

647 BROMBERG P.A., ALBEN J.O., BARE G.H., BALCERZAK S.P., JONES R.T., BRIMHALL B. & PADILLA F. (1973) Hemoglobin Little Rock (β143 His→Gln: (H21)). A high oxygen affinity haemoglobin variant with unique properties. *Nature (New Biology)*, **243**, 177.

648 PERUTZ M.F., KILMARTIN J.V., NISHIKURA K., FOGG J.H., BUTLER P.J.G. & ROLLEMA H.S. (1980) Identification of residues contributing to the Bohr effect of human haemoglobin. *Journal of Molecular Biology*, **138**, 649.

649 LEE-POTTER J.P., DEACON-SMITH R.A., SIMPKISS M.J., KAMUZORA H. & LEHMANN H. (1975) A new cause of haemolytic anaemia in the newborn. A description of an unstable fetal haemoglobin: F Poole, α2Gγ2 130 Tryptophan→Glycine. *Journal of Clinical Pathology*, **28**, 317.

650 WINSLOW R.M., SWENBERG M-L., GROSS E., CHERVENICK P.A., BUCHMAN R.R. & ANDERSON W.F. (1976) Hemoglobin Mckees Rocks (α2β2 145 Tyr→Term): A human 'nonsense' mutation leading to a shortened β-chain. *Journal of Clinical Investigation*, **57**, 772.

651 SCHNEIDER R.G., HETTIG R.A., BILUNOS M. & BRIMHALL B. (1976) Hemoglobin Baylor [α2β2 81 (EF5) Leu→Arg]—an unstable mutant with high oxygen affinity. *Hemoglobin*, **1**, 85.

652 GERALD P.S. & GEORGE P. (1959) Second spectroscopically abnormal methemoglobin associated with hereditary cyanosis. *Science*, **129**, 393.

653 SCHNEK A.G. & SCHROEDER W.A. (1961) The relation between the minor components of whole normal human adult hemoglobin as isolated by chromatography and starch block electrophoresis. *Journal of the American Chemical Society*, **83**, 1472.

654 RHABAR S. (1968) An abnormal haemoglobin in red cells of diabetics. *Clinica Chimica Acta*, **22**, 296.

655 BUNN H.F., HANEY D.N., GABBAY K.H. & GALLOP P.M. (1975) Further identification of the nature and linkage of the carbohydrate in hemoglobin AIc. *Biochemical and Biophysical Research Communications*, **67**, 103.

656 KOENIG R.J., BLOBSTEIN S.H. & CERAMI A. (1977) Structure of carbohydrate of hemoglobin AIc. *Journal of Biological Chemistry*, **252**, 2992.

657 LEADING ARTICLE (1976) Glycosylated hemoglobin and diabetic control. *New England Journal of Medicine*, **295**, 443.

658 WIDENSS J.S., ROGIER-BROWN T.L., McCORMICK K.L., PETZOLD K.S., SUSA J.B., SCHWARTZ H.C. & SCHWARTZ R. (1980) Rapid fluctuations in glycohemoglobins (Hb AIc) related to acute changes in glucose. *Journal of Laboratory and Clinical Medicine*, **95**, 386.

659 ARTURSON G., GARBY L., ROBERT M. & ZAAR B. (1974) Oxygen affinity of whole blood *in vivo* and under standard conditions in subjects with diabetes mellitus. *Scandinavian Journal of Clinical and Laboratory Investigation*, **34**, 19.

660 KYNOCK P.A.M. & LEHMANN H. (1977) Rapid estimation (2 hours) of glycosylated haemoglobin for routine purposes. *Lancet*, **ii**, 16.

661 WELCH S.G. & BOUCHER B.J. (1978) A rapid microscale method for the measurement of Hb 1(a+b+c). *Diabetologia*, **14**, 209.

662 ALLEN R.C., STASTNY M., HALLETT D. & SIMMONS M.A. (1980). A comparison of isoelectric focusing and electrochromatography for the separation and quantification of hemoglobin AIc. In: *Electrophoresis* (ed. Radola B.J.), p. 663. de Gruyter, Berlin.

663 SPICER K.M., ALLEN R.C. & BUSE M.G. (1978) A simplified assay of hemoglobin AIc in diabetic patients by use of isoelectric focusing and quantitative microdensitometry. *Diabetes*, **27**, 384.

664 FISCHER R.W., DE JONG C., VOIGT E., BERGER W. & WINTERHALTER K.H. (1980) The colorimetric determination of Hb-AIc in normal and diabetic subjects. *Clinical and Laboratory Haematology*, **2**, 129.

665 McDONALD M.J., SHAPIRO R., BLEICHMAN M., SOLWAY J. & BUNN H.F. (1978) Glycosylated minor components of human adult hemoglobin. *Journal of Biological Chemistry*, **253**, 2327.

666 JAVID J., PETTIS P.K., KOENIG R.J. & CERAMI A. (1978) Immunologic characterization and quantification of haemoglobin AIc. *British Journal of Haematology*, **38**, 329.

667 POON P., TURNER R.C. & GILLMER M.D.G. (1981) Glycoslyated fetal haemoglobin. *British Medical Journal*, **283**, 469.

668 STEEL J.M., THOMPSON P., JOHNSTONE F. & SMITH A.F. (1981) Glycosylated haemoglobin concentrations in mothers of large babies. *British Medical Journal*, **282**, 1357.

669 BUNN H.F., McDONALD M.J., COLE R. & SHAPIRO R. (1981) Chromatographic analysis of glycosylated hemoglobin, In: *Advances in Hemoglobin Analysis* (ed. Hanash S.M. & Brewer G.J.), p. 83. *Progress in Clinical and Biological Research*, *Vol.60*. Alan R. Liss, Inc., New York.

Chapter 9
The molecular genetics of haemoglobin:
the thalassaemia syndromes

D. J. WEATHERALL AND J. B. CLEGG

INTRODUCTION

In 1925 Cooley and Lee described a severe form of anaemia occurring early in life and associated with splenomegaly and bone changes [1]. With the subsequent description of further cases and the realization that many of these patients were of Mediterranean origin, the condition became known as thalassaemia from 'Θαλασσα', the sea [2]. However, it was only in the period after 1940 that the true genetic character of this disorder was fully appreciated. It gradually became clear that the disease described by Cooley was the homozygous state for a partially dominant autosomal gene and that the heterozygous state is associated with a much milder haematological condition. The homozygous state became known as thalassaemia major and the heterozygous state as thalassaemia minor or minima [3–5].

The rapid increase in knowledge about the genetic control of the structure and synthesis of haemoglobin and the definition of the haemoglobinopathies, as described in the previous chapter, caused a renewal of interest in thalassaemia in the period after 1950. Since then it has become clear that 'thalassaemia' is not a single condition but a group of genetically determined disorders of haemoglobin synthesis, each characterized by either partial or total suppression of the synthesis of one or more of the globin chains of haemoglobin [6–8]. Furthermore, it has become clear that the condition is not confined to the Mediterranean region but has a widespread occurrence throughout the Middle East and Southeast Asia where it constitutes a major public health problem. Indeed, the thalassaemias are probably the most common group of single gene disorders among the world population.

In the last 5–10 years a great deal has been learnt about the molecular pathology of the thalassaemias. Much of this information has come from the application of the techniques of molecular biology to the analysis of human haemoglobin synthesis in health and disease and from direct structural study of the haemoglobin genome. In this chapter we shall review the different thalassaemia syndromes. Before doing this, however, it is necessary to describe briefly the molecular genetics of human haemoglobin and to outline some of the techniques which have elicited this information. The more formal genetics of the structure of human haemoglobin were described in the previous chapter. Here we take up the story at the level of the globin genes themselves.

Since the thalassaemia field has moved so rapidly over the last few years, and since much of the recent work is based on the newer techniques and advances in molecular biology, the field has become extremely complicated and far-ranging. In the space available, we can only give a brief outline of the subject; for more extensive coverage the reader is referred to a recent monograph which deals with it in greater detail [9].

THE GENETIC CONTROL OF HAEMOGLOBIN SYNTHESIS

All the normal human haemoglobins have a tetrameric structure (see previous chapter). Adult and fetal haemoglobins have α chains associated with β (Hb A, $\alpha_2\beta_2$), δ (Hb A$_2$, $\alpha_2\delta_2$) or γ (Hb F, $\alpha_2\gamma_2$) chains whereas in the embryo ζ chains combine with γ (Hb Portland, $\zeta_2\gamma_2$) or ε chains (Hb Gower 1, $\zeta_2\varepsilon_2$) and α and ε chains combine to form Hb Gower 2 ($\alpha_2\varepsilon_2$). The ζ and ε chains are the embryonic counterparts of the adult α and β, γ or δ chains respectively. Haemoglobin F in normal individuals is a mixture of two molecular species in which the γ chains have either glycine ($^G\gamma$) or alanine ($^A\gamma$) at position 136. Analysis of infants with abnormal fetal haemoglobin variants has provided evidence that the $^G\gamma$ and $^A\gamma$ chains are the products of distinct structural loci [10].

Clearly there must be at least seven different structural genes coding for globin. Indeed there is ample evidence from genetic analysis of families in which abnormal haemoglobin variants are segregating that the α, β, γ and δ chains are controlled by separate gene loci, and although similar information about the ζ and ε chains is lacking, more direct evidence, which we shall discuss later, indicates that the same is true for these globins also. In the previous chapter the general organization of the globin genes was described. It was established some years ago that the α and non-α genes lie in clusters on separate chromosomes. There is now good genetic evidence that there are two α genes per haploid genome making a total of four in all. Structural analysis of the DNA adjacent to these genes, which is described in greater detail later in this section, indicates that there are two ζ genes linked to the α-chain loci. The non-α-globin genes lie in a cluster in the order $^G\gamma$–$^A\gamma$–δ–β and again structural analysis of this region of the genome indicates that the ε genes lie 'upstream' from this cluster. Recent somatic cell fusion analysis has indicated that the α-globin genes lie on chromosome 16 and that the γ, δ, β cluster is on chromosome 11 [11, 12]. The general arrangement of the globin genes is shown in Figure 9.1.

During the last few years DNA hybridization and molecular cloning techniques have been applied to the analysis of the α-globin and non-α-globin gene clusters and hence detailed structural maps of these regions of the genome are now available. Before describing these in detail it seems appropriate to digress briefly to describe some of the basic principles and techniques which have made this work possible. These advances in the technology of molecular biology are of particular importance because they have also been applied to the analysis of the molecular pathology of many of the thalassaemia syndromes.

Molecular hybridization

The feasibility of using nucleic-acid hybridization to examine genetic homologies was recognized by Doty *et al.* [13] following their demonstration that the two strands in native DNA can be dissociated and reassociated *in vitro* by heating and subsequent cooling. They showed that hybrid DNA molecules could be made from the DNAs of different viruses or bacteria, and others extended the approach to the formation of double-stranded DNA/RNA molecules [14].

It was quickly realized that the annealing reactions were highly specific and thus provided a means of studying the relationship among the genomes of various organisms, including mammals. Techniques were developed for the immobilization of single-stranded DNA in various media and on nitrocellulose filters, so that it became possible to assay the reassociation of labelled single-stranded RNA or DNA molecules with the immobilized DNA. Among the surprises of this work was the finding of repeated sequences, hundreds of thousands of copies in some cases, in the DNA of higher organisms [15]. And one of the encouraging results was the ability to detect unique single-copy DNA sequences in mammalian genomes.

Quantitative hybridization of globin RNA and DNA

A decade of experience with hybridization methods was thus ready to exploit the discovery in 1970 of an enzyme in certain RNA tumour viruses capable of

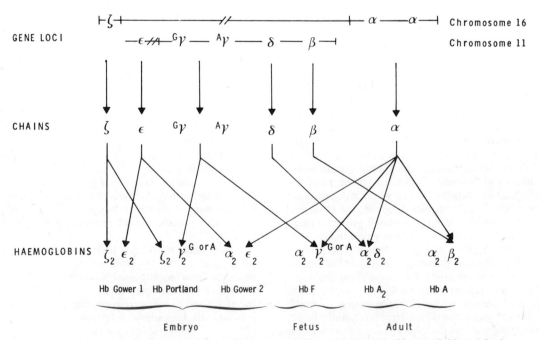

Fig. 9.1. The general arrangement of the globin genes and the genetic control of haemoglobin synthesis.

synthesizing a DNA molecule from an RNA template [16, 17]. The impact of this was immediate, for it was obvious, at least in theory, that if, for example, a globin messenger RNA could be used as a template, the enzyme would synthesize a DNA copy (cDNA) with a nucleotide sequence complementary to that of the mRNA template, and this would be identical to the sequence of one of the two strands of the DNA from which the mRNA was originally transcribed (Fig. 9.2). Moreover, the synthesized DNA copy could be made radioactive, and thus used as a hybridization probe for the presence of complementary sequences in genomic DNA, or in cellular RNA. It transpired that before it would work the enzyme (now called 'reverse transcriptase') needed a 'primer' to initiate synthesis, so use was made of polyadenylic acid (poly A) residues at the mRNA's 3' end (Fig. 9.2). By using polythymidilic acid (poly T), which binds to the poly A by the normal DNA base-pairing rules, as primer, highly labelled DNAs were synthesized from rabbit and human globin mRNAs [18–20]. It was shown that under the appropriate conditions these cDNAs hybridized in a highly specific manner to the respective DNAs or RNAs. Hence it became possible not only to test for the presence of a complementary RNA or DNA sequence, but actually to quantify it. For example, the ratios of human α- and β-globin mRNAs in cellular RNA can be determined by experiments in which increasing amounts of the test RNA are added to a fixed amount of radioactive cDNA probe and the mixtures incu-

bated under conditions favouring the formation of double-stranded cDNA/RNA hybrid molecules. As the RNA input increases, progressively more double-stranded molecules are formed, until a point is reached when the RNA concentration is high enough to ensure complete hybridization of the cDNA with the mRNA complementary strands. By comparing the amount of hybrid formation with either the α- or β-cDNA probes at particular concentrations of added cellular mRNA, the concentration of α and β sequences in the unknown mixed mRNAs sample can be calculated.

Similar approaches can be used to estimate the number of globin genes present in DNA by measuring either the rate or extent of hybridization. In the former method the kinetics of reannealing the excess DNA in the presence of labelled cDNA are studied. DNA is first denatured (by heating, or alkali treatment) to separate the two complementary strands, and then mixed with the labelled probe and allowed to reanneal under conditions favouring strand reassociation. Samples are withdrawn at various time intervals and the extent of hybridization assessed (for the bulk of the DNA by following the change in optical density; for the cDNA/DNA hybrids by following the amount of radioactivity associated with double-stranded DNA). The rate of hybridization is proportional to the concentration of DNA and increases with time. If the DNA concentration (as nucleotides) is expressed as C_0 moles/l and the time (t) in seconds, then the percentage hybridization is a function of log C_0t, and the values of

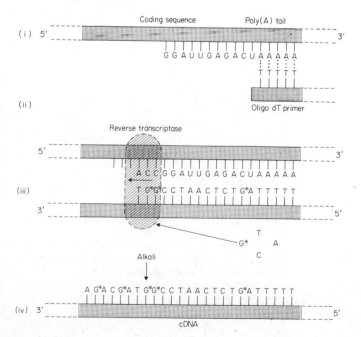

Fig. 9.2. Schematic representation of cDNA production. (From Ref. 9).

C_0t at which there is 50% hybridization ($C_0t_{\frac{1}{2}}$) can be used as a measure of the concentration of the sequences in question. This type of experiment was used to show that α-chain genes are deleted in some forms of α thalassaemia (see page 430).

A variation of this method uses the opposite strategy: a fixed amount of cDNA (in excess of the estimated globin gene DNA content of the total DNA) is hybridized for a fixed time to increasing amounts of the DNA under the study, to the point where a plateau is reached and the cDNA is 'saturated' by sequences present in the test DNA; in other words a form of titration. From the DNA input required to saturate the cDNA the number of copies of globin genes in the test DNA can be calculated.

Gene mapping

The above techniques rely on hybridization reactions that take place in solution. These give quantitative information about the globin sequences present in DNA, but tell one nothing about the physical arrangement of the genes in the chromosomal DNA. In 1975 Southern [23] introduced a method of hybridization in which one of the components in the reaction (the DNA under study) was immobilized on a cellulose nitrate filter. The real advantage of this lay in the fact that it became possible to transfer DNA from gel electrophoresis runs to these filters by blotting. Hence fragments of DNA separated on the basis of size by electrophoresis could be assayed for the presence or absence of specific genes.

Early experiments relied on reverse-copied mRNAs for the manufacture of radioactive gene probes. Availability of suitable mRNAs and the necessity to purify the cDNAs produced, so that cross-hybridization was minimized, had considerable disadvantages for many purposes, especially for ^{32}P-labelled probes with their limited half-lives. The advent of recombinant DNA techniques made things considerably simpler, since it became possible to 'clone' (i.e. selectively purify and amplify) a chosen DNA sequence. These methods have now become extraordinarily sophisticated, to the point that whole 'libraries' of cloned DNA fragments representing the entire human genome are available for study [24, 25].

Appropriate fragments of chromosomal DNA are most commonly produced by digestion with one or more restriction endonucleases. These bacterial enzymes cleave DNA at a small number of reproducible sites (typically of the order of one cleavage per few thousand base pairs). Thus by using one or more enzymes, or combinations of them, overlapping DNA fragments can be produced which can be aligned to give their physical arrangement in the original DNA.

Structure of human globin genome

Coupled with the ability to detect a gene, or genes, by hybridization to filters which have been blotted from gel electrophoresis separations of restriction endonuclease digests of DNA, one can thus build up a picture (gene map) of the physical organization and linkage of genes in the chromosomes. Using this general approach a detailed map of the order and linkage of the globin genes has been constructed over the last two or three years (Fig. 9.3) [26–33]. These studies provide direct physical evidence confirming gene arrangements tentatively deduced by more orothodox genetic studies.

The α-globin genes are separated from the ζ genes by an inactive α-like gene, $\psi\alpha$; the arrangement of these loci is 5'–ζ–ζ–$\psi\alpha$–α–α–3'. Similarly the embryonic non-α gene, the ε gene, lies 'upstream' from the γ, δ and β genes; the order is 5'–ε–$^G\gamma$–$^A\gamma$–δ–β–3'. The distances between these different gene loci are shown in Figure 9.3.

The two α-chain genes are closely linked together within a single Bam H1 restriction endonuclease fragment, and it is clear from detailed mapping of the restriction endonuclease sites in the two genes that many of them are repeated in the same position in each gene, further reinforcing the idea that two genes arose by duplication of an ancestral α gene. Similar conclusions may be drawn from the map of endonuclease cleavage sites surrounding the γ, δ and β genes, in which the two γ genes, and the δ and β genes share many sites in common.

Most of the information in Figure 9.3 was derived from the DNA of only one or two individuals and the question arises—how representative of humans in general is this? Jeffreys [35] has made a preliminary attempt to assess the extent of any variation by examining DNA from 60 individuals with eight different restriction endonucleases.

One δ-gene variant was found, but interestingly a Hind III cleavage site polymorphism was observed in both $^G\gamma$ and $^A\gamma$ genes in a number of individuals. As Jeffreys points out, his limited survey examined only 50 or so cleavage sites representing about 300 base pairs of DNA sequence, and three of the sites were polymorphic. If this one per cent is representative of the genome as a whole, then with a haploid genome size of 3×10^9 base pairs we might expect to find 3×10^7 variants at the DNA level, which would represent an enormous pool of genetic variability.

It has become clear recently that many mammalian genes, including those for haemoglobin, have one or more non-coding (in the sense that they are not found in the mature messenger RNA—*vide infra*) inserts or intervening sequences. Thus the β, γ, δ and ε genes each contain two inserts (introns) of approximately 100 and 700–800 base pairs between codons 30 and 31 and

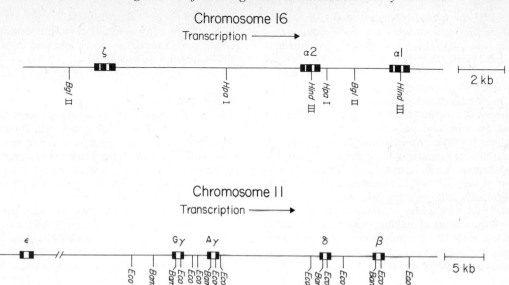

Fig. 9.3. Restriction endonuclease maps of the human α- and β-globin gene clusters on chromosomes 16 and 11.

codons 104 and 105 [34]. The α-globin genes also contain introns, although considerably smaller.

The functional significance of these non-coding regions is unknown, but the fact that they occur in identical positions in the human β, γ, δ and ε, and mouse and rabbit β genes suggests that they play a crucial role in gene expression, which has remained unchanged through millions of years of evolution. Interestingly, there appears to be little overall homology in the nucleotide sequences of these inserts, apart from the 'splicing regions' where the coding and non-coding sequences join [36]. It is clear from Figure 9.3 that the coding sequences represent only a small proportion of the total globin genome. Conceivably, the presence of many non-homologous intervening non-coding sequences may help to prevent inadvertent chromosomal misalignment leading to unequal crossing over at meiosis. However, it seems clear that much of the DNA not present in structural genes includes sequences important for the regulation of their expression.

Chromatin structure
As described earlier, there are the 'unique' sequences in DNA, present in only one or a few copies, for example the globin genes, and which account for approximately 60% of the total DNA. 10% of the total is found as highly repetitive DNA which contain non-transcribed sequences repeated many thousands of times. Finally, about 30% of the DNA is present as moderately repetitive sequences which are repeated, on average, a few

hundred times. These sequences are spaced throughout the genome, alternating with unique-sequence DNA [37]. Indeed, in many cases they lie adjacent to structural genes, prompting speculation that they may in some way be involved in the regulation of gene activity, perhaps by coordinating the activity of sets of related genes, as suggested by Davidson & Britten [38].

It must be remembered, of course, that the genes in mammalian cells are present, not as simple strands of DNA, but complexed with histones and other proteins in chromatin. One of the consequences of this is that the transcriptional activity of the total DNA can be quite limited, such that in erythroid cells, for example, only a few per cent of the total DNA sequences are transcribed and among them are a high proportion of globin genes. Some of this selectivity is achieved by gross alterations in chromatin structure.

Chromatin is composed of repeating subunits called nucleosomes which consist of eight histone molecules, two each of histones H2a, H2b, H3 and H4, associated with about 200 base pairs of DNA. Of this, 140 base pairs are wrapped around the histone core, with the remaining 'spacer' DNA being associated with histone H1. Almost all the DNA is present in nucleosomes, which are thus the basic chromosomal structural units of higher organisms.

Limited digestion of nuclei with DNAases has been used as a probe of chromatin structure. For example, when the nuclei from chicken erythroid cells are digested with pancreatic DNAase all the adult globin genes are selectively destroyed, even though only a few per cent of the total DNA is digested [39]. Oviduct nuclei similarly treated lose their ovalbumin, but not globin, genes [40]. These and other experiments have provided evidence for the idea that one of the basic controls of gene activity may be modulated by chromatin structure. Superimposed on this may be a hierarchy of more subtle regulators, most probably involving the interaction of these accessible DNA regions with non-histone proteins, and possibly RNA [41]. However, there is as yet little firm evidence for these concepts. The validity of reconstitution experiments aimed at demonstrating transcriptional specificity of non-histone proteins [42–44] has been questioned on technical grounds, although the introduction of recombinant DNA technology into this area of research offers the possibility of making 'minichromosomes', in which regions of the genome of interest may be studied in isolation from the background activity of hundreds or thousands of other genes.

BIOSYNTHESIS OF HAEMOGLOBIN

The general mechanism of eukaryotic protein synthesis is now well known (Fig. 9.4). The information content of the gene in nuclear DNA is first transcribed into an RNA copy which, after various modifications, is transported to the cytoplasm and then translated by ribosomes into protein [45].

Transcription

The initial process is thus the production of the RNA transcript of the DNA coding sequence. Three types of RNA polymerase have been identified in mammalian cells, two of which (types I and III respectively) are involved in the transcription of the genes for various cytoplasmic RNAs—18S and 28S RNA of ribosomes, and the 5S ribosomal and transfer RNAs. Type-II RNA polymerase transcribes the unique-sequence DNAs such as globin genes [46, 47]. All these enzymes are complex multimeric molecules which require additional cofactors for correct functioning [47]. To date, however, there is no evidence for the mammalian equivalents of the bacterial sigma and rho factors which promote the initiation and release of bacterial RNA polymerase at specific signal sequences in the DNA. Nevertheless, there is evidence that mammalian DNA synthesis follows essentially the same patterns as that seen in micro-organisms and that, *in vivo*, only one

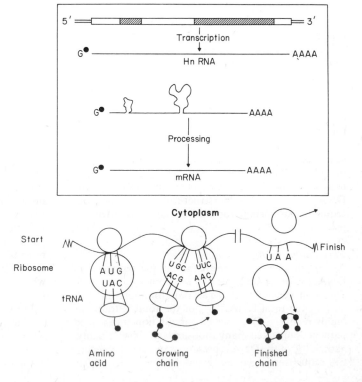

Fig. 9.4. Schematic representation of the steps involved in protein synthesis. (From Ref. 9.)

strand of the DNA (the sense strand) is transcribed into RNA.

Processing of the primary transcript

As we have seen, the genes coding for globin (and most other proteins studied) are interrupted by a number of non-coding DNA sequences. The first step in the production of mRNA is the transcription of the entire unit, coding and non-coding sequences included, in the form of a giant RNA precursor molecule (which may be 2–3 times the length of the mature mRNA molecule which finally reaches the cytoplasm [48, 49]) belonging to the general class of RNAs called heterogeneous nuclear RNA (HnRNA). This initial precursor is then chemically modified at the 5′ end by establishing a 5′ppp5′ linkage through GTP to form the so-called CAP structure (see below), and at the 3′ end by attaching a string of adenylic acid residues (poly A). One of the functions of this poly-A tail may be to stabilize the mature RNA. The non-coding intervening sequences are then removed by successive excision and ligation reactions (splicing) to form the mature mRNA [50, 51].

It is quite likely that during its time in the nucleus and for much of its time in the cytoplasm the HnRNA and mRNA is associated with various protein molecules, which may serve to stabilize and protect the RNAs from nuclease attack. It is conceivable, though not yet established, that the interaction of these proteins with RNA may be of importance in the regulation of RNA metabolism.

The globin messenger RNAs

The general structure of globin mRNA is shown in Figure 9.5 illustrating the features of human β-globin mRNA elucidated by Forget, Proudfoot, Kan and co-workers [52–56]. All globin mRNAs contain the modified 5′-end CAP structure and the 3′ poly-A tail. In addition there are non-coding sequences at the 5′ and 3′ ends. For example β globin has 53 nucleotides before the AUG initiation codon, and a further 132 nucleotides between the termination codon and the poly A. Thus, although the β chain has 146 amino acids (which require $3 \times 146 = 438$ nucleotides to code for them, in addition to the AUG initiator and UAA terminator, a total of 444 nucleotides in all), the β-globin mRNA is approximately 650–750 nucleotides long, depending on the exact size of the poly-A tail.

It is now established that many animal and viral mRNAs have a 5′ end structure containing methylated nucleotides [57]. Two versions, CAP-1 and CAP-2 have been found. CAP-2 is present on all globin mRNAs and in general appears to be present only on cytoplasmic mRNAs. CAP-1 is found in both the HnRNA and cytoplasmic mRNA and it is probable that CAP-2 is derived from CAP-1.

The enzymic removal of the CAP reduces the translational efficiency of globin mRNA in cell-free systems [58, 59], and CAP analogues inhibit its translation. Thus it is likely that CAP is necessary for the maximum translational efficiency of globin mRNA. There is some evidence for a direct interaction between the CAP and a reticulocyte initiation factor [60], although whether it is truly involved in the regulation of chain initiation is not yet known.

A string of adenylic acid residues at the 3′ end of mRNA has been found in all globin mRNAs studied [61, 62]. The exact length seems to vary with the age of the mRNA, being longest in newly synthesized RNA and shortest in mRNA isolated from 'old' reticulocytes. One of the main functions of poly A is probably to stabilize the mRNA. Although deadenylated mRNA will function in a cell-free system, its lifetime is much shorter than poly-A-containing mRNA when it is incubated in *Xenopus* oocytes over a period of several days [63, 64].

The nucleotide sequences of the human α, β and γ messenger RNAs (and by extrapolation from the DNA sequences of the cloned genes, those of δ and ε mRNA) are now known in considerable detail [52–56, 65, 66]. As we noted they have non-coding sequences at the 5′ and 3′ ends, as well as the 3′ poly-A tail. There is little overall homology in the non-coding sequences, although certain features such as the CUUPyUG sequence found near to the 5′ CAP and which may be involved in ribosome recognition, and the AAUAA sequence found in all eukaryotic messengers about 20 bases from the poly-A addition site, recur. The function of these non-coding regions is not clear. Obviously those at the 5′ end include the ribosome-binding site, and the differences between α and β 5′ non-coding sequences presumably account, at least in part, for the fact that α chains are initiated more slowly than β chains on these messengers. It may also be relevant that the potential exists for forming hairpin-loop struc-

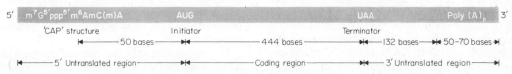

Fig. 9.5. The primary structure of human β messenger RNA (mRNA) showing the 5′ and 3′ untranslated regions, coding region and CAP structure.

tures in parts of these non-coding regions, and these may help to stabilize the molecules by preventing degradation by exonucleases.

Globin synthesis [45]

Globin chains are synthesized in the cytoplasm by the interaction of messenger RNA, ribosomes, transfer RNAs and various cofactors in a series of reactions proceeding through three separate phases. The initial step involves the formation of a tertiary complex between the initiation factor IEF-2, GTP and the initiation transfer RNA, $tRNA^{met}_{f}$, which then subsequently binds to the small 40S ribosomal subunit. With the help of other initiation factors, globin mRNA and the large ribosomal subunit are added to this complex so that in its final configuration the mRNA is aligned with the ribosome with the AUG initiation codon opposite the UAC anticodon of the $tRNA^{met}_{f}$. Once translation is started, the initiation factors dissociate to participate in another initiation cycle.

Protein synthesis then proceeds by stepwise addition of amino acids from the N-terminal end to form the growing peptide chain [67]. This cycle involves at least three distinct stages. The first is a codon-directed binding of aminoacyl-tRNA to a ribosome site next to that occupied by the initiator or peptidyl-tRNA. Peptide transfer then takes place between the newly bound aminoacyl-tRNA and the $tRNA^{met}_{f}$ or peptidyl-tRNA. Lastly, the newly made peptidyl-tRNA and the mRNA are both shifted from the acceptor to the donor site on the ribosome. In this way, the acceptor site is freed and the process can be repeated. At the same time the tRNA that donated the growing peptide chain is released. Two protein factors, EF-1, EF-2 are involved in the elongation process. EF-1 participates in the GTP-dependent reaction by which aminoacyl-tRNAs bind to ribosomes, while EF-2, or translocase, catalyses the translocation step in another GTP-dependent reaction. The N-terminal methionine incorporated during initiation is removed enzymatically from the globin chain after the addition of about 20 amino acids.

Most messenger RNAs are long enough to support a number of ribosomes active in synthesis along their length. Once a ribosome has moved away from the initiation site another ribosome can bind and start synthesis, thus forming polyribosome complexes. Finally, globin synthesis stops when the ribosome reaches a chain-termination codon (UAA, UAG, UGA) in the message. At this point the polypeptide chain is split from the tRNA in another GTP-dependent hydrolytic reaction which involves at least one protein cofactor. The ribosome is released from the mRNA and the ribosomes dissociate into subunits, which are then free to participate in another round of synthesis.

The regulation of globin synthesis

The processes of transcription and translation of the genetic information of DNA into protein are now understood in some detail. There is much less information available about how these processes are regulated, even for haemoglobin which is one of the most intensively studied model systems for mammalian protein synthesis.

It is useful to consider protein synthesis in two phases—nuclear and cytoplasmic. The latter has been exhaustively studied over many years, and is, indeed, quite well understood. In the case of haemoglobin, what has emerged is a detailed picture of the processes involved in the differential regulation of α- and β-chain synthesis, and the realization that at the cytoplasmic level, this only amounts to the fine-tuning of an essentially predetermined programme.

By inference and default, most of the real regulation must take place in the nucleus, in the determination of the relative amounts of α- and β-globin messenger RNAs which find their way into the cytoplasm. Unfortunately, very little if anything is known of how this is done, although one can speculate endlessly about regulation of transcription and messenger RNA processing and transport. On the optimistic side, techniques are becoming available for studying mRNA synthesis and nuclear RNA processing, so that one can look forward to a better understanding of these processes in the next few years.

It is now clear that chain initiation is the rate-limiting step in globin-chain synthesis [58] and that β mRNA is a more efficient initiator than α by a factor of about $1·5/1$. In order to compensate for this imbalance there is more α-globin mRNA than β mRNA in red-cell precursors. The net effect is that the numbers of α and β chains synthesized are almost, but not quite, equal; there is usually a slight overproduction of α chains and these are disposed of proteolytically to achieve the final balance.

The differential regulation of globin synthesis is thus achieved against a background of predetermined cytoplasmic mRNA levels. On the other hand, the overall level of protein synthesis in red-cell precursors is determined to a considerable extent by haem, which is a powerful stimulator of globin synthesis. In conditions of haem deficiency, a protein kinase specifically phosphorylates, and thereby inactivates, the initiation factor IEF-2.

It is interesting that the effect of haem, which is a ubiquitous compound, is not limited to erythroid cells but common to all cells, although it has perhaps become an especially important factor in red-cell precursors, being utilized to maintain the balance between haem and globin synthesis (see below).

Haem synthesis [68]

The structure of haem was described in Chapter 8 and its synthesis is described in greater detail in Chapters 13 and 14.

The biosynthesis of haem in red-cell precursors takes place in a series of enzyme-controlled steps, beginning with the condensation of glycine and succinyl-CoA to form α-amino β-keto adipic acid, which is then rapidly decarboxylated to form δ-amino laevulinic acid (ALA). This reaction, which is catalysed by the enzyme ALA synthase and requires pyridoxal phosphate and ferrous ions as cofactors, is the only step in the whole chain which requires energy (to convert succinate to succinyl-CoA), all the rest being essentially irreversible (with the possible exception of the formation of uroporphyrinogen III). Next, two molecules of ALA combine to form the mono-pyrrole porphobilinogen under the action of the enzyme ALA dehydratase, and then four of these por-phobilinogen molecules are condensed to form the basic tetrapyrrole ring, uroporphyrinogen. After side-chain modifications this is converted to protoporphyr-inogen which, on oxidation by oxygen in the presence of coproporphyrinogen oxidase, is finally converted to the red protoporphyrinogen molecule. Iron is then inserted by the enzyme haem synthetase to form haem.

The first and last two enzymes of this pathway are present in the mitochondria, while the rest are found in the cell cytoplasm, and it is interesting to note that both oxidation steps take place in the mitochondria.

Assembly of haemoglobin

Although the overall rates of synthesis of α and β chains are equal in maturing red-cell precursors, there is usually a small pool of excess α chains present in the cell cytoplasm [69, 70]. It has been suggested that free α chains from this pool associate with β chains on the ribosomes to aid their release as the α/β dimer [71]. While these may be true intermediates in haemoglobin assembly, and kinetic studies indicate that this is probably the case, it seems unlikely that their formation on ribosomes is obligatory, since in certain conditions such as haemoglobin H disease, β chains can be freely released from ribosomes into the cell cytoplasm.

Haem is probably incorporated into the α and β chains after their release into the cytoplasm [72] and tetramer formation follows immediately after their association into dimers [73].

It is often found that the levels of haemoglobin β-chain variants in heterozygotes depart considerably from the expected 50% (see Chapter 8, page 366). For example, haemoglobin S usually comprises about 35–40% of the total haemoglobin in sickle-cell carriers and this must be due to the base substitution on DNA leading to the Glu–Val change in the β^S chain. Many of the unstable variants are found in even lower amounts (see Chapter 8, page 370); on the other hand haemo-globins that do not show any functional abnormalities tend to be present in relatively higher proportions.

It is possible for the ratios of two like chains to differ considerably in the erythrocyte, even though the affinities of the two chains for their mutual partner or haem could lead to an accumulation of the chain of lower affinity which would then be destroyed by proteolysis. There is some evidence that something of this sort happens in some cases. For example, in double hetero-zygotes for haemoglobin S or E and α thalassaemia, the levels of haemoglobins S and E are much lower than in simple heterozygotes (see page 436), suggesting that when α chains are in short supply they tend to combine with β^A chains rather than β^S or β^E chains. Similarly it has been shown that most of the unstable β chains in haemoglobin Köln are rapidly destroyed after syn-thesis [74]. Direct evidence for the preferential com-bination of α chains with β^A rather than β^S chains has been obtained by DeSimone and his colleagues [75].

Although few experiments along these lines have been done, what evidence there is suggests that little if any regulation other than proteolytic removal of excess chains takes place. Indeed it seems unlikely that any compensatory mechanism at the transcriptional level is involved, otherwise individuals with unstable haemoglobins might not find themselves in the posi-tion of having to dispose of large quantities of useless and unwanted globin chains to the detriment of their red cells and themselves.

The principal control of the coordination of globin-chain synthesis therefore seems to be at the level of mRNA synthesis. Minor regulation may take place at chain initiation, and the final overall balance is achieved by proteolysis.

Developmental changes in haemoglobin production

The changes in haemoglobin constitution during nor-mal human development are considered in Chapters 3 and 8. The switchover from Hb F to Hb A and A_2 production occurs mainly at about 34–36 weeks' ges-tation, and at term normal infants synthesize about 50% Hb F in their cord bloods. There is then a rapid decline in Hb F synthesis and by the end of the first year of life Hb F makes up about 1–2% of total hae-moglobin. There is a further reduction in Hb F produc-tion over the first year of life although the normal adult level of less than 1% Hb F may not be reached until later in childhood. Although much has been written about how the switch from Hb F to Hb A production is regulated, virtually nothing is known about this mechanism (see Ref. 9).

In normal adults Hb F is confined to a few red cells called 'F cells'. Their number is remarkably consistent in the same individual and seems to be under genetic control. The $^{G}\gamma/^{A}\gamma$ ratio changes during the transition from fetal to adult life; the significance of this is not clear. It is interesting to note that the appearance of the different globin chains during development reflects their chromosomal arrangement, i.e. $\varepsilon \rightarrow ^{G}\gamma \rightarrow ^{A}\gamma \rightarrow \delta \rightarrow \beta$, and this order of gene activation may also occur during normal erythropoiesis. At the present time we have no idea how this gene cluster is regulated. As we shall see later, major deletions of the complex have profound differences on the haemoglobin pattern in adult life.

THE THALASSAEMIAS

The genetic disorders of haemoglobin fall into four overlapping groups (see Chapter 8). First, there are the structural haemoglobin variants, most of which are synthesized at the same rate as normal adult haemoglobin but may cause disease if they alter the shape, stability or function of the molecule. The second group, the thalassaemias, are characterized by a reduced rate of synthesis of one or other of the globin chains of haemoglobin. This leads to an overall reduction in the amount of haemoglobin synthesized and, even more importantly, to imbalanced globin-chain synthesis with precipitation of those chains which are produced in excess. The intracellular inclusions formed in this way are responsible for the defective erythroid maturation and survival common to all the thalassaemias. The third group is made up of structural haemoglobin variants which are synthesized at a reduced rate and hence are associated with globin-chain imbalance and the same phenotypes as the thalassaemias. Finally, there are the diverse conditions which are characterized by a failure of the normal neonatal switch from fetal to adult haemoglobin production in the absence of marked haematological changes. These have the general title of hereditary persistence of fetal haemoglobin (HPFH). However, it is becoming clear that many of them are simply mild types of thalassaemia, in which there is almost complete compensation for the lack of adult haemoglobin production by persistent synthesis of haemoglobin F.

Clearly, then, the thalassaemia syndromes are a diverse series of genetic disorders of haemoglobin synthesis which have in common a reduced output of one or more of the globin chains and an overall imbalance of globin chain production [9] (Table 9.1). They can be classified according to their clinical

Table 9.1. The thalassaemias

Clinical classification	Molecular classification
Thalassaemia major	α thalassaemia
Thalassaemia intermedia	β thalassaemia
Thalassaemia minor	$\delta\beta$ thalassaemia
	δ thalassaemia
	$\gamma\delta\beta$ thalassaemia

phenotypes into the severe or major forms of the illness, less severe but symptomatic forms called thalassaemia intermedia, and the asymptomatic carrier states, thalassaemia minor or trait. It is also possible to classify the thalassaemias according to which particular globin chain is synthesized ineffectively, i.e. into α, β, $\delta\beta$, δ and $\gamma\delta\beta$ thalassaemias. The clinical and molecular classifications are combined, when possible. Thus the severe transfusion-dependent form of β thalassaemia is called β thalassaemia major and the heterozygous carrier form β thalassaemia trait; the forms of intermediate severity are called the β thalassaemia intermedias.

Recent work indicates that there is a remarkable degree of genetic and molecular heterogeneity of each of the different forms of thalassaemia and there is increasing evidence that the phenotypic expression of the different molecular varieties may be different [9]. Furthermore, in many populations there are high gene frequencies for more than one form of thalassaemia and for structural haemoglobin variants. Hence in any one individual it is possible to find two or even more different genetic defects of haemoglobin synthesis and the resulting clinical phenotypes are endless in their variability. In Thailand, for example, over 50 different genetic combinations of haemoglobin disorders have been defined [76].

In the sections which follow we shall attempt to define the main clinical and haematological characteristics of the common types of thalassaemias. For a more extensive review the reader is referred to the monograph of Weatherall and Clegg [9].

THE β THALASSAEMIAS

There are two main types of β thalassaemia, β^+ and β^0 thalassaemia, in which there is, respectively a reduction in and total absence of β-chain production. Beta thalassaemia major usually results from the homozygous state for either β^+ or β^0 thalassaemia, or occasionally from the compound heterozygous state for both β^+ and β^0 thalassaemia. However, it should be remembered that even those patients who appear to be homozygous for either β^+ or β^0 thalassaemia may in

Table 9.2. The β thalassaemias. Each group is undoubtedly heterogeneous at the molecular level

Type	Homozygote	Heterozygote	Molecular defect
β^0	Thalassaemia major No Hb A 98% Hb F	Thalassaemia minor 5% Hb A_2	Heterogeneous Some undefined β-globin gene deletion
β^+ (Mediterranean)	Thalassaemia major 10–20% Hb A 70–80% Hb F	Thalassaemia minor 5% Hb A_2	Premature chain termination ? mRNA processing defect in some cases
β^+ (Negro)	Thalassaemia intermedia 30–50% Hb A 50–70% Hb F	Thalassaemia minor 5% Hb A_2	? mRNA processing defect in some cases
Normal Hb A_2 (type 1) ('silent')	Mild thalassaemia intermedia 10–30% Hb F Elevated Hb A_2 level	Minor red-cell changes Normal Hb A_2 level	Not defined
Normal Hb A_2 (type 2)	Not described	Thalassaemia minor Normal Hb A_2 level	Not defined

fact be compound heterozygotes for different molecular varieties of what appear to be the same condition (e.g. two different forms of β^0 thalassaemia) (Table 9.2).

The disorders produced by the homozygous states for β^+ and β^0 thalassaemia are very similar and hence we shall consider the clinical features of the homozygous states for the β thalassaemias together. What little is known about the expression of the different genetic varieties of β thalassaemia will be reviewed in a later section. Similarly the milder forms of β thalassaemia, i.e. β thalassaemia intermedia, will also be considered separately.

Molecular pathology

The basic defect in many of the β thalassaemias, i.e. the reason for defective β-chain synthesis, is still not fully understood. Recent globin-gene mapping analysis has shown that in the majority of β thalassaemias, the β-globin genes show no detectable abnormality. There is a small group of Afro-Asian β^0 thalassaemics in which there is a deletion of part of the 3′ end of the β-globin gene [77, 78] but this is the only variety of β^0 thalassaemia that has been shown to follow a major structural alteration in the β-globin genes.

There is increasing evidence that the β^0 thalassaemias are heterogeneous at the molecular level. In some cases no β-globin mRNA is produced [79–84] while in others some mRNA is transcribed but not translated. In the latter group the β-globin mRNA may be structurally abnormal or apparently full length but nonfunctional [83, 84]. In one case, structural analysis of inactive β-globin mRNA has shown that the AAG codon for lysine at position $\beta17$ has changed to UAG which is a chain-termination codon [85]. This leads to

premature chain termination with the production of a short 16 residue N-terminal fragment of the β chain [85, 86]. It may well be that other β^0 thalassaemias result from a similar molecular defect or from base substitutions at other critical areas such as the chain-initiation codon [83] or splicing sites [271, 272]. However, such predictions must remain speculative until structural analysis has been carried out. In β^0 thalassaemics from Ferrara there appears to be a unique defect in which their β-globin-chain synthesis can be induced by a soluble supernatant fraction from normal red cells or indeed by blood transfusion [87]. The molecular basis for this fascinating condition has yet to be determined.

Similarly, nothing is known about the molecular pathology of the β^+ thalassaemias. They all seem to result from a reduced production of β-globin mRNA but the reasons for this have yet to be determined. There is recent evidence that in some cases there is a defect in processing the large molecular weight β-globin mRNA precursor in the nucleus of the erythroblasts [88, 270].

Distribution

The β thalassaemias have a world-wide distribution [9]. They are particularly common in the Mediterranean region, parts of the Middle East, India and Pakistan and in Southeast Asia. The condition is rarer in Africa but occurs sporadically in practically every racial group. In the high-incidence areas, carrier rates ranging from 5 to 25% may be encountered.

There is only limited information about the distribution of the different types of β thalassaemia in world populations. It is clear, for example, that in Cyprus β^+ thalassaemia predominates over β^0 thalassaemia whereas in Greece both types occur. On the other hand, in Southeast Asia β^0 thalassaemia is much commoner. There may be differences in the distribution of the different β-thalassaemia types even within the same country. For example, in Italy β^0 thalassaemia is particularly common in the Ferrara region, whereas in other parts β^+ thalassaemia occurs frequently.

The reason for the high incidence of the β-thalassaemia genes in some populations is not fully understood although there is some convincing epidemiological evidence that carriers are more resistant to *P. falciparum* malaria infection. The cellular mechanism for this fascinating finding remains to be determined [9].

β thalassaemia major

The term β thalassaemia major is a clinical description of a condition which usually results from the homozygous state for either β^+ or β^0 thalassaemia or the compound heterozygous state for both determinants. It may also result from other interactions.

Clinical features

The classical textbook picture of homozygous β thalassaemia or Cooley's anaemia describes the condition as it occurred (and still occurs, unfortunately) in children who have not been transfused or else been given an inadequate transfusion regime. If children with this disorder are adequately transfused from early life they grow and develop almost normally and it is only when they reach the second decade that they start to develop complications due to the effect of iron loading. Hence in describing this disorder we have to consider the course and complications in early life in the context of the untransfused child and then deal with the later complications which occur in those children who have received adequate transfusion therapy.

The majority of infants with β thalassaemia major present in the first year of life. A later onset raises the possibility that the child has an intermediate form of the disorder [9]. Affected infants fail to thrive and gain weight normally and become progressively pale. Feeding problems, diarrhoea, irritability, recurrent bouts of fever and progressive enlargement of the abdomen due to splenomegaly, or failure to recover fully from an infective episode, are common presenting symptoms. At this stage of the illness the infant may look pale but otherwise may have no abnormal signs. On the other hand splenomegaly may already be present.

The untransfused thalassaemic child has chronic and progressive anaemia throughout infancy and childhood together with a variety of complications. Some children are growth retarded from early in life although, in general, slowing of growth is more marked as puberty approaches. There is pallor of the mucous membranes with a variable degree of icterus.

The skin colour may also show a grey-brown pigmentation related to iron loading. The inadequately transfused children fail to thrive and show features of a hypermetabolic state which include poor musculature, reduction of body fat, recurrent fever, poor appetite and lethargy. Indeed the neglected β thalassaemic with its protuberent abdomen, poor musculo-skeletal development and spindly legs looks very much like a child with malignant disease. There is a variable degree of hepatosplenomegaly and striking skeletal changes may develop. These include a characteristic facial appearance with bossing of the skull, hypertrophy of the maxillae which tend to expose the upper teeth, prominent malar eminences with depression of the bridge of the nose, puffiness of the eyelids and a tendency to a Mongoloid slant of the eyes (Fig. 9.6). The skeletal changes are associated with radiological alterations of the skull, long bones and hands. There is

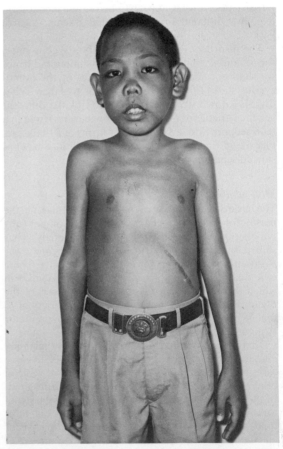

Fig. 9.6. Homozygous β thalassaemia. A child showing the typical thalassaemic facies and splenectomy scar.

dilatation of the diploic spaces and subperiostial bone grows in a series of radiating striations giving a typical 'hair on end' appearance (Fig. 9.7). There is cortical thickening of the long bones with porous rarefraction. Leg ulceration may occur at any time throughout childhood.

The poorly transfused thalassaemic child may develop a series of complications during childhood but if it survives until puberty it is prone to the same complications as the well-transfused child, i.e. the effects of progressive iron loading.

Well-transfused thalassaemic children remain asymptomatic until the age of about 10–12 years [89]. They then develop hepatic, cardiac and endocrine complications. Often the first indication of the latter is

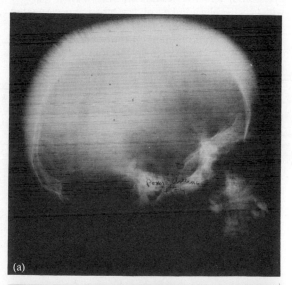

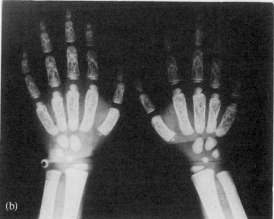

Fig. 9.7. X-ray changes in homozygous β thalassaemia. (a) Skull; (b) hands.

a failure or reduction of the pubertal growth spurt and this is usually associated with a failure of sexual maturation [89]. Throughout their teenage life these children have a variety of complications due to endocrine deficiency and nearly all develop cardiac symptoms in the latter half of the second decade.

The precise prognosis for a transfusion-dependent homozygous β thalassaemic is rather uncertain and depends on many factors including their transfusion status and whether they have received chelation therapy or not. However, at the time of writing it is clear that the majority of transfusion-dependent thalassaemics who have been maintained at an adequate haemoglobin level die towards the end of the second decade or during the third decade, usually from the effects of iron loading on the myocardium. On the other hand, children who have been inadequately transfused die early, usually of the combined effects of anaemia and infection [89, 90]. Recent analysis of patients maintained with or without chelation therapy for several years indicates that regular removal of iron may prolong life.

Complications

There are many complications of homozygous β thalassaemia and their form depends to some extent on whether the child has received an adequate transfusion regime. If so, the majority of complications are related to iron loading. We shall consider first the complications which occur most frequently in children who have been inadequately transfused.

Progressive enlargement of the spleen may lead to a variety of complications associated with hypersplenism. These include physical discomfort due to the size of the organ, an increasing transfusion requirement due to trapping of red cells in the enlarged spleen, severe thrombocytopenia with associated bleeding, and a variable degree of neutropenia which may be a factor in the increased susceptibility to infection which characterizes this disorder. Hypersplenism is often associated with a marked increase in the plasma volume which may be an important factor in producing the anaemia of hypersplenism [91].

Because of the rapid turnover of erythroid precursors, folic-acid deficiency is relatively common [92]. The skeletal changes already mentioned may cause a variety of complications including spontaneous fracture, gross facial deformity and severe dental problems, particularly malocclusion. In some populations a myopathic syndrome with proximal muscle weakness has been observed [93]. There is an increased proneness to infection in the poorly transfused thalassaemic child and although this seems to be more marked in children who have been splenectomized there is an increased incidence of infective episodes in children with intact spleens. The commonest organisms are the pneumococcus and streptococcus [94]. There is an increased occurrence of pericarditis and although in Thailand this may be associated with streptococcal infection [95] this does not appear to be the case in other parts of the world. The precise mechanism for the proneness to infection is unknown [9].

There are several metabolic complications which occur in poorly transfused thalassaemic children which include an increased incidence of gall stones, secondary gout, and vitamin deficiencies, particularly vitamin E [96]. Some affected children have a tendency to recurrent nose bleeds or other haemorrhagic phenomena and again although these are sometimes associated with thrombocytopenia there is often no obvious cause. Some children develop large tumour masses due to extramedullary bone-marrow expansion; particularly important sites are the chest, inner tables of the skull and vertebrae. The latter may provide a variety of neurological disorders [97].

Iron loading occurs in all homozygous β thalassaemics whether adequately transfused or not. In the latter group the loading occurs from a combination of both blood transfusion and increased iron absorption whereas in the well-transfused child it is mainly derived from blood transfusion. Modell [90] has estimated that by the time children maintained on high transfusion regimes reach the age of 11 years, they will have accumulated at least 30 g of iron. At about this level of iron loading, patients begin to show signs of hepatic, cardiac and endocrine disturbance. The iron deposition in the liver results in fibrosis and a varying degree of hepatic cirrhosis but liver failure is relatively uncommon except in those populations where there is high incidence of viral hepatitis derived from blood transfusion. A variety of endocrine deficiencies may occur (reviewed in detail by Weatherall and Clegg [9]). The commonest is pancreatic insufficiency with the development of frank diabetes mellitus. Most large series show some evidence of pituitary insufficiency although, curiously, growth-hormone levels are usually normal. Similarly there may be mild degrees of adrenal insufficiency and in heavily transfused children there is frequently failure of sexual development [89, 94]. Many affected children have biochemical evidence of hypoparathyroidism although clinical manifestations of parathyroid deficiency are thought to be unusual [98]; this requires further study.

The most serious complication of iron loading is cardiac failure. This may either take the form of long, drawn out, intractable, congestive cardiac failure or sudden death due to cardiac arrthymia [99]. It is difficult to predict this type of episode and the electrocardiogram may be normal immediately before a sudden fatal dysrhythmia. It has been suggested recently that more sophisticated studies such as echocardiography and radionuclide scanning techniques may be able to provide evidence of myocardial dysfunction in patients with iron loading before the disorder becomes obvious clinically [100].

Haematological changes

In the untransfused child there is always a severe degree of anaemia which is typically hypochromic and microcytic with a low MCH and MCV. The red cells show anisocytosis and poikilocytosis with many misshapen microcytes, occasional macrocytes and a variable number of target cells (Fig. 9.8). In addition there may be some well-haemoglobinized normocytes or macrocytes, almost transparent hypochromic elliptocytes, small spherocytes and spiculated cells, together with a variable number of tear-drop and elongated forms and a great assortment of bizarre poikilocytes and distorted cell remnants. Erythroblasts are almost always present and after splenectomy are found in large numbers. The morphology of the red cells varies depending on whether the spleen is present or not.

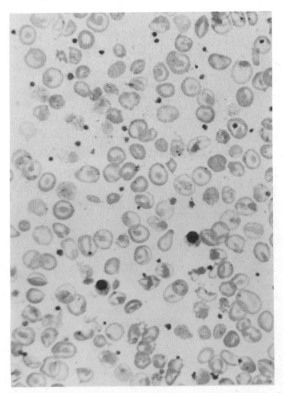

Fig. 9.8. The peripheral blood film in homozygous β thalassaemia (MGG stain, $\times 600$).

After splenectomy, large hypochromic cells are found together with small 'piscine' forms which are really no more than remnants of fragments of stroma.

After splenectomy, staining of the peripheral blood with methyl violet shows the presence of ragged inclusion bodies in the cytoplasm of both nucleated and non-nucleated red cells [101] (Fig. 9.9). Electron microscopic analysis (Fig. 9.9) indicates that these inclusions, although they resemble Heinz bodies, are not attached to the red-cell membrane [102].

The absolute reticulocyte count is usually slightly elevated and increases after splenectomy but never reaches a very high level even in the presence of severe anaemia.

In well-transfused patients the blood picture may look surprisingly normal with only an occasional abnormal cell. These findings indicate an almost complete suppression of endogenous erythropoiesis by repeated high-load transfusion.

There are no characteristic changes of the white cells and platelets in this disorder except that after splenectomy when there is often a persistent leucocytosis and thrombocytosis.

Bone marrow

In an anaemic patient the bone marrow is extremely cellular with marked erythroid hyperplasia. The red-cell precursors show defective haemoglobinization and many contain abundant amounts of iron which are distributed throughout the cytoplasm; ring sidero-blasts are not a feature of this disorder. On incubation of the marrow cells with methyl violet, many show ragged inclusion bodies [101]. These may result from precipitation of excess α chains during erythroid maturation. On electron-microscopic analysis the α-chain precipitates appear as foci of amorphous material whose electron density is higher than that of the cell cytoplasm [103, 104]. Their frequency increases with maturity of the precursors and they are found in virtually all the circulating late polychromatic erythroblasts (Fig. 9.10). Alpha-chain precipitates are also present in the nuclei [105]. It is not clear why this occurs although it has been suggested that they represent intracytoplasmic α-chain precipitates which have been trapped within nuclear territory during mitosis, or that they enter the interphase nucleus through a defect in the nuclear membrane; both mechanisms may occur.

In addition to the abnormalities of iron and globin precipitation the red-cell precursors of some patients with homozygous β thalassaemia contain considerable amounts of periodic-acid-Schiff (PAS) positive material [106]. It has been suggested that this represents an accumulation of glycogen due to unutilized energy in the erythroblasts which are blocked in the G1 phase of the cell cycle [107] (see below). In addition, the presence of large foamy cells resembling Gaucher cells has been demonstrated both in the bone marrow and in the spleen of patients with this disorder [108].

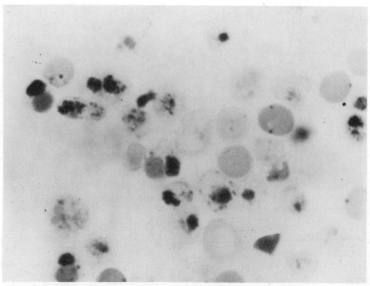

Fig. 9.9. The red-cell inclusions in the peripheral blood of a post-splenectomized thalassaemic patient (methyl violet stain, × 800).

(a)

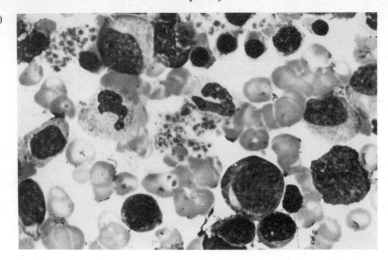

(b)

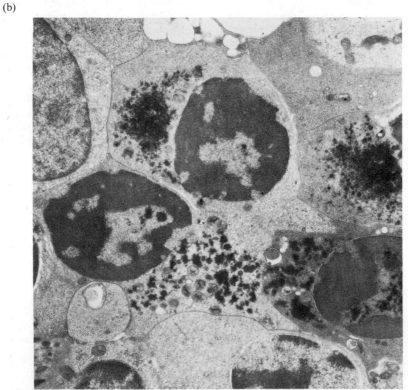

Fig. 9.10. The bone marrow in homozygous β thalassaemia. (a) Light microscopy (MGG stain, $\times 1000$) and (b) electron microscopy showing dense inclusion bodies ($\times 15\,000$)

The kinetics of cellular proliferation

In-vitro studies of cellular proliferation in the bone marrow of patients with β thalassaemia major have shown several abnormalities [109]. These include a slight increase in the proportion of basophilic erythro-poietic cells in S, and a corresponding decrease in the proportion of cells in G1.* In addition there is a marked increase in the proportion of early polychro-

* The various phases of the cell cycle are defined in Chapter 2.

matophilic erythroblasts in S with a concomitant increase in the proportion in G1 and there is a decrease in the ratio of the number of early polychromatophilic cells in S to a number of these cells in G2. It has been suggested that these abnormalities may be due to damage to red-cell precursors from the effects of precipitated α chains [109].

Red-cell survival, ferrokinetics and erythrokinetics
These aspects of homozygous β thalassaemia are considered in detail in Ref. 9. Red-cell survival is shortened and there is evidence for heterogeneity of cell populations and the existence of some very short-lived cells [110]. Iron absorption is increased in children maintained on an inadequate transfusion programme [111]. Combined ferrokinetic and erythrokinetic measurements indicate that there is a gross degree of ineffective erythropoiesis [112].

Haemoglobin pattern
There is nearly always a marked elevation in the relative amount of haemoglobin F in the peripheral blood of patients with β thalassaemia major [9]. β^0-thalassaemia homozygotes have only haemoglobins F and A_2. In β^+-thalassaemia homozygotes the level of haemoglobin F is variable but is nearly always in excess of 50–60% of the total haemoglobin if the patients are examined before transfusion. It should be remembered that in heavily transfused patients, erythropoiesis is markedly depressed and even several weeks after a transfusion there may only be relatively small amounts of haemoglobin F. The haemoglobin F is heterogeneously distributed among the red cells [113].

The haemoglobin-A_2 level is very variable in this condition, and of no diagnostic help. It tends to be low or normal in β^0-thalassaemia homozygotes and elevated in the milder forms of the condition, for example β^+-thalassaemia homozygotes in Negro populations. Under suitable conditions small quantities of free α chains can be demonstrated on haemoglobin electrophoresis in all types of severe homozygous β thalassaemia [114].

Other biochemical changes
The haemolytic component of β thalassaemia major is reflected by a mild elevation of a conjugated bilirubin, low levels or absence of haptoglobin and haemopexin, a raised plasma haemoglobin and, sometimes, by detectable levels of methaemalbumin. There is an increase in urobilinogen in the faeces.

Increased nuclear protein turnover results in increased levels of urates in the urine and the serum uric-acid levels are higher than in normal controls; clinical gout may sometimes occur [115]. Increased nuclear protein catabolism also results in the excretion of large amounts of β-amino isobutyric acid in the urine [116], and other catabolic products which are found in this condition probably result from a breakdown of haem in the bone marrow. Frequently, thalassaemic patients pass dark brown urine and this has been attributed to the presence of mesobilifucin and other dipyrroles [117].

Although there have been relatively few studies of erythropoietin metabolism in this condition those which have been carried out indicate that anaemic patients with this disorder have significantly elevated levels of erythropoietin in the blood and urine [118].

A variety of other biochemical changes have been observed. Leucocyte ascorbic-acid concentrations are significantly reduced [119]. This is probably secondary to iron loading. Vitamin-E deficiency is also common [96]. It has been suggested that this is the result of the continual process of peroxidation of thalassaemic red-cell membranes which may lead to excessive consumption of vitamin E as an antioxidant. There have been conflicting reports about the levels of certain trace metals in the blood. Several workers have observed increased serum copper levels and others have found decreased magnesium values. Furthermore, at least two studies have reported a deficiency of serum zinc. The problem of trace metals in thalassaemia is reviewed in detail in Ref. 9.

In-vitro haemoglobin synthesis
Haemoglobin synthesis has been examined *in vitro* in β-thalassaemic marrow or reticulocytes by following the incorporation of radioactive amino acids into the various globin fractions in short-term incubation experiments [120–124]. In all forms of β thalassaemia there is an imbalance of globin-chain production resulting in an excess of α as compared with β and γ chains (Fig. 9.11). The uncombined α chains are unstable and rapidly precipitate in the red-cell precursors. There is evidence that this material is subject to degradation by proteolytic enzymes and a variable amount may be destroyed within the red-cell precursors in this way [70].

The pathophysiology of the anaemia
Evidence from such sources as erythrokinetics, red-cell survival data, *in-vitro* haemoglobin synthesis experiments, and examination of the urine of patients with β thalassaemia has provided a fairly clear picture of the pathophysiology of this disorder [9, 125]. A schematic representation of the factors involved in the production of the anaemia of β thalassaemia is shown in Figure 9.12. The one finding common to all the β thalassaemias is globin-chain imbalance with the production of an excess of α chains. This phenomenon occurs throughout the red-cell precursor series in both

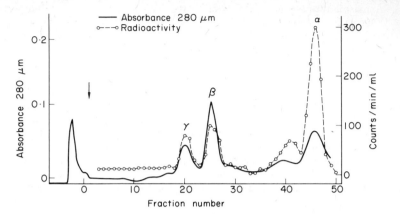

Fig. 9.11. Haemoglobin synthesis in homozygous β thalassaemia. The peripheral blood cells were incubated together with radioactive leucine for 30 min and then the globin chains were separated. The broken line represents radioactivity incorporated into α, β and γ chains; it is clear that there is a marked excess of α-chain synthesis.

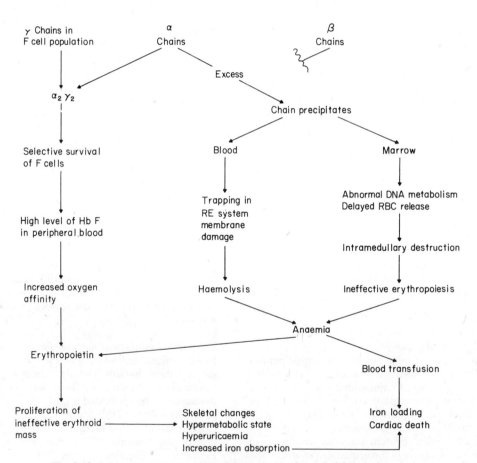

Fig. 9.12. Schematic representation of the pathophysiology of β thalassaemia.

the bone marrow and peripheral reticulocytes. Most of the haematological and erythrokinetic findings which characterize this disorder can be related to this basic imbalance of globin-chain synthesis.

The other factor which is of critical importance in current ideas regarding the pathogenesis of the anaemia of β thalassaemia is the observation that γ-chain production does not occur in a uniform way throughout the red-cell population, but is quite heterogeneously distributed; some precursors make relatively large amounts and others very little. Hence the magnitude of the excess of α chains in any particular red-cell precursor will depend on the number of γ chains which are synthesized. In those precursors where there is a relatively large amount of γ-chain production the overall excess of α chains will be less since they will combine with γ chains to produce fetal haemoglobin. Thus the cells with the largest amount of fetal haemoglobin have the smallest excess of free α chain. There is good evidence that excess α chain precipitates early in the life cycle of the erythroid precursor and that the cells with large α-chain precipitates are sequestered within the bone marrow and never appear in the peripheral blood. It seems very likely that the intramedullary destruction of these cells results in the marked increase in 'early labelled' bilirubin and urinary dipyrrole excretion which has been described in β thalassaemia [114]. This mechanism is presumably the basis for the gross degree of ineffective erythropoiesis in this condition.

The exact mechanism whereby the presence of α-chain inclusion bodies causes premature destruction of the red cells in the marrow is uncertain, but it seems likely that it is a mechanical effect mediated through the rigid inclusion body which prevents the normal passage of the red cells through the marrow sinusoids into the circulation. They may also have a direct effect on DNA metabolism and hence on cell division [9].

Since many of the peripheral red cells contain α-chain inclusions after splenectomy it seems likely that the spleen is a major site of the removal of these inclusions. It also seems likely that the shortened red-cell survival is the result of mechanical damage to cells containing rigid inclusions as they pass through the splenic sinusoids and probably other parts of the reticulo-endothelial system. This mechanism probably accounts for the very short-lived population seen on red-cell survival studies [110]. Those cells with the largest amount of fetal haemoglobin and therefore less free α chain, will have the longest survival. This also explains the longer-lived cell populations observed in ^{51}Cr-survival studies and also the observation that the turnover of fetal haemoglobin is slower than that of Hb A in β-thalassaemia homozygotes [126]. It also accounts for the results of *in-vitro* globin-chain syn-

thesis studies which show that during erythroid maturation there is a progressive increase in the amount of γ-chain relative to β-chain synthesis.

The severe anaemia stimulates erythropoietin production. Since many of the peripheral blood cells contain large amounts of Hb F, and since cells of this type have a high oxygen affinity, relatively less oxygen is given up to the tissues and this may be another factor in determining the very high output of erythropoietin in β thalassaemia. Certainly the erythroid stimulation and subsequent skeletal deformities are more marked in this disorder than in most of the other congenital haemolytic anaemias.

The primary defect in globin production is responsible for a series of abnormalities of erythrocyte metabolism. Due to the reduction in the amount of globin produced there is a secondary defect in haem synthesis and iron tends to accumulate within the red-cell precursors. There is also an increased rate of cation flux across the membrane, possibly due to mechanical damage caused by the removal of rigid inclusion bodies in the marrow, spleen and other parts of the reticulo-endothelial system. Certainly these changes are more marked in the young cell population which contains rigid inclusions [130].

There has been considerable interest recently in other possible mechanisms of shortened red-cell survival in β thalassaemia. During the precipitation of excess α chains, haemichromes are formed (see Chapter 8, page 371). During this process various activated forms of oxygen are generated which may directly damage the red-cell membrane by causing lipid peroxidation [131]. The oxidant stress to the thalassaemic red cell may be magnified by its low level of haemoglobin and high iron content. It has been suggested that the reduced levels of vitamin E are the result of its constant utilization as an intracellular antioxidant. These complicated interactions have been the subject of several extensive reviews [132, 133]. While it seems likely that they are of some importance there is no doubt that the haemolytic component of the anaemia of homozygous β thalassaemia is due mainly to mechanical damage to the red cells and that it is relatively unimportant as compared with the gross degree of ineffective erythropoiesis which occurs in this disorder.

In addition to these intracellular abnormalities there is a variable extracellular component to the pathogenesis of the anaemia which results from progressive enlargement of the spleen. This causes sequestration of a large fraction of the circulating red-cell mass. Furthermore, the total blood volume is increased, partly due to hypersplenism and also as a result of marrow expansion. Presumably it is the latter, with a massive turnover of red-cell precursors, that causes the hypermetabolic state, fever, weight loss, increased iron absorption and gross skeletal deformity.

All these factors combine together to produce an anaemia of extremely complex pathophysiology (Fig. 9.12) but it is clear that most of the components can be traced back to the basic defect, i.e. imbalanced globin-chain synthesis.

Heterozygous β thalassaemia

Although the older descriptions of the carrier states for β thalassaemia suggest that they show a broad clinical spectrum ranging from completely symptomless conditions to disorders associated with anaemia, jaundice and splenomegaly, more recent work has indicated that this is probably not true [9]. It is now clear that the true heterozygous carrier states for the β thalassaemias are characterized by a very mild anaemia and that splenomegaly is extremely uncommon. Indeed when the clinical and haematological features of several large series of β-thalassaemia heterozygotes from different racial groups are compared it is clear that it is a remarkably homogeneous and extremely mild disorder (see Ref. 9). The more severe forms of what appear to be heterozygous β thalassaemia are in fact due to the interaction of more than one β-thalassaemia gene or to an acquired disorder exacerbating the anaemia of heterozygous β thalassaemia. We shall discuss these conditions in a later section dealing with thalassaemia intermedia.

Clinical features

Heterozygous β thalassaemia is not associated with any symptoms or physical signs. Patients may develop a symptomatic anaemia during periods of stress such as pregnancy or infection. Increased folic acid demands may result in a secondary megaloblastic anaemia during these episodes. Some patients give a long history of tiredness, pallor or other vague symptoms and may have received iron or a variety of other medications from their practitioners for many years if the diagnosis has not been suspected [134].

Haematological changes

There is a mild anaemia with haemoglobin values in the 9–11 g/dl range. The red-cell indices are extremely useful in differentiating this condition from normal or from other forms of hypochromic anaemia [9]. The most characteristic finding is a relatively high red-cell count with a marked reduction in the MCH and MCV. The mean cell haemoglobin concentration (MCHC) is often within the normal range. The reticulocyte count is rarely elevated. The stained peripheral blood film usually shows a moderate degree of hypochromia with variation in the shape and size of the red cells, basophilic stippling and a variable number of target cells (Fig. 9.13). The latter finding is by no means constant, however. The bone marrow shows moderate erythroid hyperplasia.

The red-cell osmotic fragility is usually decreased and this is even more marked after sterile incubation of

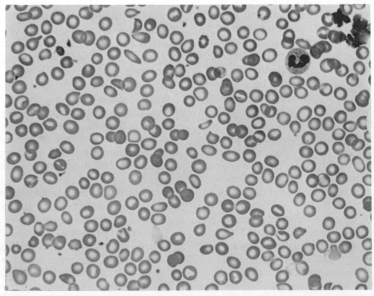

Fig. 9.13. The peripheral blood appearances in heterozygous β thalassaemia (MGG stain, × 800).

the blood for 24 hours. Autohaemolysis is usually normal or slightly increased.

Erythrokinetics and red-cell survival

Erythro- and ferrokinetic studies indicate that there is a moderate degree of ineffective erythropoiesis; ^{51}Cr half-life times are slightly short [135]. The results of iron absorption studies have been inconsistent. Plasma iron levels are usually normal unless the patient has received iron medication for a long period. Serum iron or plasma ferritin levels are useful in distinguishing the condition from iron-deficiency anaemia [9].

Haemoglobin constitution

Haemoglobin electrophoresis on conventional media usually reveals no abnormality. However the Hb A_2 level is always elevated in the range 3·5–6·5% [9]. If there is co-existent iron-deficiency anaemia the haemoglobin A_2 value may fall but is restored to its previous level by iron therapy. The fetal haemoglobin level is slightly elevated, in the 1–3% range, in about 50% of cases [9].

Haemoglobin synthesis

In the peripheral blood of heterozygous β thalassaemics there is an imbalance of globin-chain synthesis with α/β-synthesis ratios of approximately 2:1. When similar experiments have been carried out in the bone marrow of individuals with this disorder the degree of chain imbalance appears to be less [136]. However, this is probably an artefact due to the fact that the red-cell precursors have an extremely active proteolytic enzyme system capable of degrading newly made α chains if they are not paired with β chains. Thus, during these *in-vitro* biosynthesis experiments any excess α chains in the bone marrow will be rapidly destroyed by proteolysis [70]. It appears that it is only when the degree of α-chain excess exceeds the cells' proteolytic capacity that significant inclusion body formation occurs. In fact electron-microscopic analysis has indicated that inclusion body formation does occur in the bone-marrow cells of heterozygous β thalassaemics [137].

The inheritance of the β thalassaemias

The usual pattern of inheritance is to find heterozygous β thalassaemia in both parents of a child with β thalassaemia major. However, it should be remembered that many apparent β-thalassaemia homozygotes are really compound heterozygotes for different β-thalassaemia determinants, β^0 and β^+ thalassaemia or different molecular forms of β^0 thalassaemia, for example. Furthermore, other genes can interact with β^+ or β^0 thalassaemia to produce the clinical picture of Cooley's anaemia; some of these are mentioned in sub-sequent sections. No evidence for genetic linkage between the β-thalassaemia determinants and other genetic markers has been established. The β-thalassaemia determinants appear to be alleles of, or very closely linked to, the β and δ structural genes [9].

Other types of β thalassaemia

In addition to the well-characterized varieties of β thalassaemia described above there are some less common types [9] (Table 9.2). These are of particular importance when considering genetic counselling with a view to antenatal diagnosis (see page 439).

Normal A_2 β thalassaemia

There are two varieties of β thalassaemia in which the Hb A_2 level is not elevated. In one type, sometimes called 'silent β thalassaemia', there are virtually no haematological abnormalities but there is mild globin-chain imbalance [138]. When this condition interacts with true β thalassaemia it produces a mild form of β thalassaemia intermedia. There is another form of the condition in which the haematological changes are identical to those of heterozygous β thalassaemia [139]. This disorder may well represent the compound heterozygous state for both δ thalassaemia and β thalassaemia [139, 140]. The importance of recognizing it is that when it interacts with β thalassaemia with an elevated level of Hb A_2 it can produce a severe transfusion-dependent disorder [139, 140]. Finally, it should be remembered that the rare condition γ–δ–β thalassaemia also presents as a thalassaemic disorder with normal Hb A_2 levels in adult heterozygotes.

β thalassaemia with unusually high levels of haemoglobin F in heterozygotes

This condition, sometimes called the Dutch form of β thalassaemia, is not yet fully defined and has been described in only one family [141]. Heterozygotes carry about 10% haemoglobin F and homozygotes run a mild course and have over 90% Hb F. It is not absolutely certain whether this is a true entity or represents the heterozygous states for both β thalassaemia and Swiss hereditary persistence of fetal haemoglobin (see page 427).

Isolated elevated haemoglobin A_2

This condition is what it says, i.e. a normal haematological picture with an elevated Hb A_2 level. Its molecular basis is not understood but this genetic determinant can interact with true β thalassaemia and produce an intermediate form of the disorder (see Ref. 9).

Slightly elevated haemoglobin A_2 levels

A condition characterized by almost normal haematological findings and a slightly elevated haemoglobin A_2 has been reported in Greece. This may be a variant of silent β thalassaemia as it can interact with true β thalassaemia to produce a β-thalassaemia intermedia [142]:

'Heterozygous' β thalassaemia with an unusually severe course

As mentioned earlier, an occasional case of a thalassaemia-like disorder with anaemia, jaundice, splenomegaly and typical thalassaemic blood changes with an elevated haemoglobin A_2 level is encountered, in which there appears to be a heterozygous form of inheritance. This is a very heterogeneous group of conditions [9]. In some cases more careful genetic analysis indicates that such patients are heterozygous carriers of more than one β-thalassaemia determinant (see above). Others seem to result from the inheritance of highly unstable β-chain haemoglobin variants—for example haemoglobin Indianapolis [143]. There are still some disorders of this type in which the molecular basis has not been determined [144, 145]. However, it is most important to carry out detailed genetic and haemoglobin-synthesis analysis in a patient of this type since it is becoming clear that these disorders usually result from the interaction of more than one genetic determinant.

THE $\delta\beta$ THALASSAEMIAS

The $\delta\beta$ thalassaemias are a group of disorders characterized by a complete absence of β- and δ-chain synthesis in the homozygous state (Table 9.3). Because γ-chain synthesis is usually more efficient than is the case in the β thalassaemias, these conditions are usually associated with less globin-chain imbalance than in the β thalassaemias and hence they are, in general, milder disorders which in the homozygous state show the phenotype of thalassaemia intermedia. It has been possible to classify them according to the structure of the haemoglobin F which is produced into ${}^{G}\gamma{}^{A}\gamma$ and ${}^{G}\gamma$ $\delta\beta$ thalassaemias. The Hb Lepore thalassaemias also result from defective δ- and β-chain synthesis; they are considered in a later section (page 423).

Distribution

The $\delta\beta$ thalassaemias are less common than the β thalassaemias, but they have been encountered sporadically in many racial groups. What is known about their distribution has been fully discussed in two recent reviews of the condition [9, 146].

Molecular pathology

Both ${}^{G}\gamma$ and ${}^{G}\gamma{}^{A}\gamma$ $\delta\beta$ thalassaemia are heterogeneous at

Table 9.3. Inherited disorders of δ- and β-chain production. Hereditary persistence of fetal haemoglobin is included because it is a mild form of $\delta\beta$ thalassaemia. The whole group of $\delta\beta$-chain production defects form a continuum of conditions, the clinical severity of which seem to depend mainly on the degree of compensation by γ-chain synthesis

---

Haemoglobin Lepore
  Hb Lepore Boston $(\delta\beta)^+$
  Hb Lepore Baltimore $(\delta\beta)^+$
  Hb Lepore Hollandia $(\delta\beta)^+$
  ? Others with same charge as Hbs A or A_2

$\delta\beta$ *thalassaemia*
  ${}^{G}\gamma{}^{A}\gamma$ $(\delta\beta)^0$ thalassaemia
  ${}^{G}\gamma{}^{A}\gamma$ $(\delta\beta)^0$ thalassaemia (Sardinian type)
  ${}^{G}\gamma$ $(\delta\beta)^0$ thalassaemia
  ? Other $\delta\beta$ or $\gamma\delta\beta$ thalassaemias with partial or total suppression of $\delta\beta$-chain synthesis without increased Hb F

${}^{G}\gamma{}^{A}\gamma$ *and* ${}^{G}\gamma$ *hereditary persistence of fetal haemoglobin*
  Classified in detail in Table 9.4

---

the molecular level. The cases analysed so far have resulted from gene deletions in which the δ- and β-globin genes have been partially or completely lost together with a variable proportion of the DNA which lies between the ${}^{A}\gamma$- and δ-globin genes. In the case of ${}^{G}\gamma$ $\delta\beta$ thalassaemia the deletion also involves the ${}^{A}\gamma$-globin genes [28, 147a and b, 175].

Homozygous $\delta\beta$ thalassaemia

Clinical features. In the few reported cases of homozygous $\delta\beta$ thalassaemia [9] the clinical features have been milder than those of homozygous β thalassaemia. Many of the patients have been adults who have required either no blood transfusion or only occasional transfusion at the time of infection. The symptoms and signs are those of β thalassaemia intermedia.

Haematological findings. There is variable anaemia with reported haemoglobin values in the 8–11 g/dl range. The peripheral film is characterized by typical thalassaemic changes. Inclusion bodies have been observed, both in the bone marrow and peripheral blood.

Haemoglobin constitution. The haemoglobin is entirely of the fetal type; Hbs A and A_2 are absent. This observation provides strong evidence that $\delta\beta$ thalassaemia results from a complete absence of δ- and β-chain synthesis; this has been confirmed by globin-chain synthesis analysis. The fetal haemoglobin is either of the ${}^{G}\gamma$ or ${}^{G}\gamma$ and ${}^{A}\gamma$ varieties.

Heterozygous δβ thalassaemia

The clinical and haematological changes and red-cell indices in this disorder are similar to those of heterozygous β thalassaemia.

The characteristic finding is an elevated level of Hb F in the 5–20% range and normal or just subnormal levels of Hb A_2. The Hb F is heterogeneously distributed among the red cells.

The heterozygous state for β and δβ thalassaemia [9]

This clinical disorder has now been well-defined in many patients of Mediterranean background. The clinical findings are typical of β-thalassaemia intermedia. There are variable skeletal changes and hepatosplenomegaly. The peripheral blood findings are similar to those of homozygous β thalassaemia with relatively higher haemoglobin levels.

The haemoglobin pattern in this disorder is characterized by very high levels of Hb F in the 90–95% range with normal levels of Hb A_2. Occasionally, small quantities of Hb A have been found. The presence or absence of Hb A depends on whether the associated β-thalassaemia gene is of the $β^0$ or $β^+$ variety.

This condition is diagnosed by the finding of thalassaemia intermedia and a family study in which one parent has typical β-thalassaemia trait and the other δβ-thalassaemia trait.

The combination of δβ thalassaemia with structural haemoglobin variants is considered in a later section (page 428).

γδβ thalassaemia

This condition, which results from a deletion of the γ-globin genes and a variable portion of the remainder of the γδβ gene complex, is associated with neonatal haemolysis associated with a thalassaemic blood picture. Adult heterozygotes have a thalassaemic blood picture with normal levels of Hb A_2 (see Ref. 9).

Haemoglobin Lepore thalassaemia

In 1958 Gerald & Diamond [148] noted that one parent of a child with Cooley's anaemia, instead of showing the usual picture of heterozygous β thalassaemia, had a thalassaemic blood picture associated with a haemoglobin variant which migrated in the position of Hb S. This component, which made up about eight per cent of the total haemoglobin, was named Lepore after the family name of the patient. With the subsequent finding of other Lepore-like haemoglobins, in association with thalassaemia, this first variant was called haemoglobin Lepore Washington [149]. Other chemically distinct haemoglobins of this type have been found in Indonesians (Hb Lepore Hollandia) [150] and Africans (Hb Lepore Baltimore) [151] (Fig. 9.14).

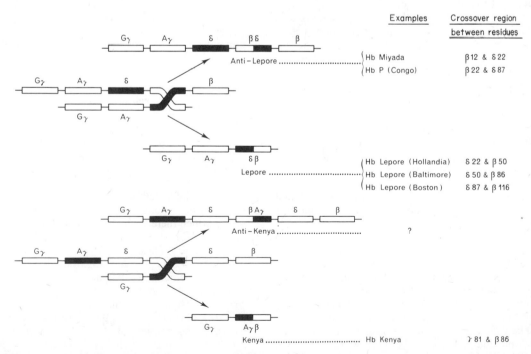

Fig. 9.14. The human crossover haemoglobin variants. The diagram represents the crossover events which generate the Lepore and anti-Lepore haemoglobins and haemoglobin Kenya.

The Hb Lepore disorders have been described in the homozygous and heterozygous state either alone or in association with β thalassaemia or Hbs S or C.

Distribution
The Lepore haemoglobins have been found sporadically in many racial groups [9, 152]. The common form, haemoglobin Lepore Washington, occurs most frequently in parts of Italy and Yugoslavia.

The chemistry and molecular pathology of the Lepore haemoglobins
Structural analysis has revealed that Hb Lepore has normal α chains combined with a pair of chains which are made up of the N-terminal residues of the δ chain fused to the C-terminal residues of the β chain [149, 153]. The composite $\delta\beta$ fusion chain of Hb Lepore is shown in Figure 9.14. The differences between the three Lepore haemoglobins are in the position of fusion between the δ- and β-chain components (Fig. 9.14). The composite $\delta\beta$ gene which directs the syntehsis of the $\delta\beta$ chain of the Lepore haemoglobins is thought to have arisen by chromosomal misalignment and unequal crossing over at the $\delta\beta$ gene complex [149, 153]. This type of mechanism is also thought to be the basis for the structure of the α chain of human haptoglobin and has been observed frequently in *Drosophilia* genetics. If this is indeed the way in which the Lepore haemoglobins have arisen, this type of genetic accident should have also resulted in the production of a chromosome which contains a normal δ- and β-chain gene together with a composite $\beta\delta$ chain of exactly opposite the constitution of the Lepore chain, i.e. an anti-Lepore haemoglobin (Fig. 9.14). Several examples of this type of haemoglobin have now been found and this observation adds considerable weight to the hypothesis outlined above for the production of the Lepore haemoglobins.

The notion that the $\delta\beta$ chain of Hb Lepore is the product of a $\delta\beta$ fusion gene has been confirmed by gene mapping analysis [26, 28]. The reason why the $\delta\beta$ chain is synthesized inefficiently is not known; it appears that the $\delta\beta$-globin messenger RNA is relatively unstable [154].

Homozygous state
In the few reported cases, the clinical condition has been similar to homozygous β thalassaemia; the haematological findings are also identical. However, as a group these cases are slightly less severe than the latter condition and at least a few cases have been characterized by a clinical course of intermediate severity. Haemoglobin analysis reveals about 80% Hb F with about 10–20% Hb Lepore. There is a complete absence of Hbs A and A$_2$, indicating that there is no normal β- or

δ-chain synthesis directed by the chromosome which carries the Hb Lepore determinant.

Heterozygous state
The clinical and haematological features are identical to heterozygous β thalassaemia. However, on haemoglobin electrophoresis, in addition to Hb A, there is approximately 10% Hb Lepore and slightly reduced levels of Hb A$_2$. All the Lepore haemoglobins reported to date migrate in the general position of Hb S at an alkaline pH. As a group there is a slightly higher Hb F level than is found in heterozygous β thalassaemia [9].

Heterozygous state for haemoglobin Lepore with β thalassaemia or haemoglobin S
The interaction of the genes for Hb Lepore and β thalassaemia produces a clinical picture very like Cooley's anaemia with very similar haematological features [152]. Some cases run a less severe course. The electrophoretic pattern is characterized by a preponderance of Hb F with about 10% Hb Lepore and a low level of Hb A$_2$. Haemoglobin A may be present if the β-thalassaemia gene is of the β^+ type.

Hb Lepore has occasionally been encountered in association with the sickle-cell gene [155]. The clinical disorder is similar to sickle-cell anaemia and the haemoglobin consists mainly of Hb S with an increased level of Hb F and a low level of Hb A$_2$. Since Hbs Lepore and S migrate in the same position on conventional electrophoretic media, techniques such as column chromatography or two-dimensional electrophoresis are required to diagnose this disorder.

Other Lepore variants and the anti-Lepore haemoglobins and their relationship to thalassaemia
All the Lepore haemoglobins described to date have been identified because they produce a haemoglobin variant with a different charge to haemoglobins A and A$_2$. However, as shown in Table 9.3, some sites of unequal crossing over would lead to gene products which would be indistinguishable from the δ chains of Hb A$_2$ or the β chains of Hb A. A mechanism of this type may be responsible for some forms of β thalassaemia in which there are high levels of Hb A$_2$ and no Hb A production. This hypothesis has yet to be verified by experimental studies.

Several anti-Lepore haemoglobins have now been identified including Hbs Miyada, P Nilotic and Arlington Park [9, 152]. As mentioned in the previous section the chromosome containing an anti-Lepore gene also carries a normal β- and δ-globin gene. Hence individuals, heterozygous for the anti-Lepore variants, should show no globin-chain imbalance or haematological changes and this is in fact the case. However, there is some extremely interesting evidence that suggests that if an individual inherits an anti-Lepore variant from one parent and a β-thalassaemia gene from the other, the two determinants can interact to produce an intermediate form of β thalassaemia [156]. This intriguing finding suggests that when a chromosome carries a $\beta\delta$ fusion gene between the δ and β loci it is not possible for that chromosome to increase the output of its β- or δ-globin genes, as usually occurs in response to a β-thalassaemia gene on the opposite pair of homologous chromosomes. The presence of an anti-Lepore variant with a charge similar to haemoglobin A_2 has been the underlying mechanism suggested for some forms of β thalassaemia with unusually high Hb A_2 levels [157].

HEREDITARY PERSISTENCE OF FETAL HAEMOGLOBIN

The term hereditary persistence of fetal haemoglobin (HPFH) was first used to describe a series of African individuals who had elevated levels of Hb F in the absence of any major haematological abnormalities [158–160]. As knowledge about this fascinating group of conditions has increased it has become clear that they are remarkably heterogeneous and that at least some of them have much in common with the $\delta\beta$ thalassaemias.

At the time of writing there is considerable confusion about how HPFH should be classified and about its true relationship to thalassaemia. It was pointed out recently that these disorders fall into two main subdivisions which can be identified by the intercellular distribution of Hb F [161] (Table 9.4). One group is characterized by a more-or-less homogeneous distribution and hence is called pancellular HPFH. In the other, the level of Hb F tends to be lower and it is more heterogeneously distributed; hence the term heterocellular HPFH has been used to describe this group. It is not yet clear whether this classification has any real biological significance although studies of the molecular genetics of these conditions suggest that at least some types of pancellular HPFH are caused by gene deletions whereas heterocellular HPFH is not and may result from a regulatory-gene mutation [9].

Pancellular HPFH
Pancellular HPFH has been most extensively studied in African Negro populations although it occurs frequently in Greeks and sporadically in many other racial groups (see Ref. 9). It has been further subclassified according to the structure of the associated haemoglobin F into $^G\gamma^A\gamma$, $^G\gamma$ and predominantly $^A\gamma$ forms [162–164].

The $^G\gamma^A\gamma$ form of HPFH has been extensively analysed in African Negro populations [165]. Based on the relative $^G\gamma^A\gamma$-chain ratios and levels of Hb F in heterozygotes, several subgroups have been defined although whether they are distinct genetic entities remains to be determined. In the common type, heterozygotes have between 15 and 25% Hb F while homozygotes have 100% Hb F and no Hb A or A_2. The latter have some degree of globin-chain imbalance and haematological changes typical of β thalassaemia. For this reason it appears that the $^G\gamma^A\gamma$ HPFH group can be looked upon as an extremely well-compensated form of $\delta\beta$

Table 9.4. Hereditary persistence of fetal haemoglobin. The nomenclature of the pancellular forms describes the $^G\gamma^A\gamma$ structure of the haemoglobin F and the + or 0 signs describe the output of the δ and β genes *cis* to the HPFH determinant. Apart from Swiss HPFH the heterocellular forms have been reported in single families only. They differ by the $^G\gamma^A\gamma$ composition of the haemoglobin F (see Ref. 9)

Type	Homozygote	Heterozygote	Molecular defect
Pancellular			
Negro $^G\gamma^A\gamma$ $(\delta\beta)^0$	100% Hb F	15–30% Hb F	Deletion of δ and β genes
Negro $^G\gamma$ β^+	—	$\sim$20% Hb F	
		Hb A present in compound heterozygotes for Hbs S or C	
Negro $^G\gamma$ (Hb Kenya)	—	5–15% Hb F	$\gamma\beta$ fusion gene
		5–10% Hb Kenya	Deletion of parts of $^A\gamma$ and β genes
Negro $^G\gamma$ $(\delta\beta)^0$	—	15–25% Hb F	—
Heterocellular			
British	19–21% Hb F	4–12% Hb F	—
Swiss	—	1–5% Hb F	—
Atlanta	—	2–4% Hb F	—
Seattle	—	3–8% Hb F	—

thalassaemia in which γ-chain synthesis almost, but not entirely, compensates for the absence of β- and δ-chain production [142]. There are no haematological abnormalities in heterozygotes who have almost balanced globin-chain synthesis. Heterozygous HPFH of this type can be distinguished from $\delta\beta$ thalassaemia by the lack of haematological changes and more even distribution of haemoglobin F among the red cells (Fig. 9.15).

When the genetic determinants for $^{G}\gamma^{A}\gamma$ HPFH interact with those for β thalassaemia, an extremely mild thalassaemic disorder results which is associated with a peripheral blood picture similar to that of heterozygous β thalassaemia, but in which there are large amounts of Hb F in the 60–70% range. The genetic determinants for HPFH have also been found in association with the genes for Hbs S and C. The Hb S/HPFH and Hb C/HPFH compound heterozygous states are associated with no clinical abnormalities and the haemoglobin patterns consist of Hbs S and

(a)

(b)

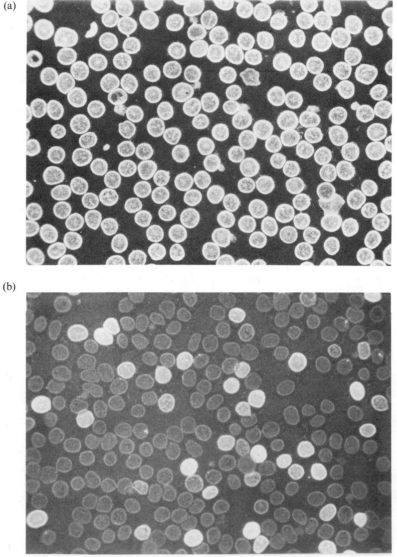

Fig. 9.15. The distribution of haemoglobin F in HPFH compared with $\delta\beta$ thalassaemia. (a) HPFH; (b) $\delta\beta$ thalassaemia (fluorescent anti-Hb F antibody preparation).

F or Hbs C and F respectively; the Hb F level ranges from 25 to 35% and it is uniformly distributed among the red cells [165].

Other rarer forms of HPFH have been observed in the Negro population. These include $^G\gamma$ β^+ HPFH which, in heterozygotes, is characterized by a normal haematological picture associated with approximately 20% $^G\gamma$ Hb F [166, 167]. The haemoglobin pattern in compound heterozygotes for this form of HPFH and the sickle-cell gene is made up of Hbs S and F with small amounts of Hb A. This indicates that the chromosome carrying the genetic determinant for this form of HPFH directs the synthesis of some β chains.

Another extremely interesting but uncommon form of HPFH is that associated with Hb Kenya [168, 169]. The latter has normal α chains combined with non-α chains which consist of part γ and part β chain. It has arisen in the same way as Hb Lepore (Fig. 9.14) by unequal crossing over with the production of a $\gamma\beta$ fusion gene. The presence of this determinant is associated with persistent $^G\gamma$-chain synthesis and hence Hb Kenya heterozygotes have elevated levels of $^G\gamma$ Hb F in the region of 10% together with Hbs A and Kenya.

In the Greek form of HPFH, heterozygotes have lower levels of Hb F than in the common Negro form, usually in the region of 15% [170]. When the determinant for this form of HPFH interacts with β thalassaemia in the Greek population a mild thalassae-mic disorder results which is associated with a haemo-globin pattern consisting of about 40% Hb F, the remainder being Hbs A and A$_2$. These findings suggest but do not prove that the chromosome carrying the Greek HPFH determinant produces some β chains. The Hb F in this disorder consists mainly of the $^A\gamma$

form but there are small but significant amounts of $^G\gamma$ chain synthesized as well [171].

Recent evidence indicates that at least some of the Negro forms of $^G\gamma^A\gamma$ HPFH and Hb Kenya have arisen by deletions involving a variable portion of the $\gamma\delta\beta$-globin gene cluster [147b, 172–175, 269]. For example $^G\gamma^A\gamma$ HPFH results from a deletion involving the δ- and β-globin genes and a part of the intergenic region between the δ and $^A\gamma$ genes. The crossover which resulted in the production of Hb Kenya has removed part of the $^A\gamma$ gene, the whole of the δ gene and part of the β gene. Clearly these deletions are similar to those which cause some forms of $\delta\beta$ thalassaemia (Fig. 9.16) and the reason for the differ-ence in phenotypes between the two conditions, i.e. the higher output of γ chains associated with the HPFH deletion, is not yet understood.

Heterocellular HPFH

Again, this form of HPFH is remarkably diverse. It was originally described in a Swiss army population [176] in whom it was shown that a proportion of individuals had slightly elevated levels of Hb F in the 1–3% range which was genetically determined. In recent years there has been great interest in the properties of the red cells of normal adults which contain Hb F, i.e. F cells [177]. It is clear that the level of F cells has a strong genetic component [178]. Indeed the Swiss form of HPFH can be considered as a genetically determined increase in the numbers of F cells. Unfortunately it is difficult to draw a dividing line between the upper limit of normal values for F cells and for this reason the genetic transmission of Swiss HPFH is very difficult to define. It is clear, however,

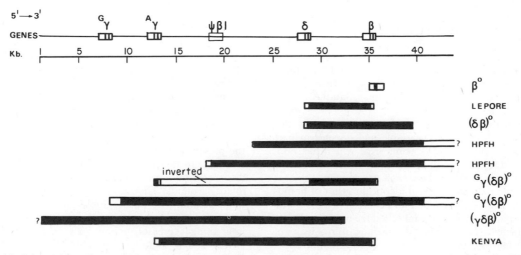

Fig. 9.16. Schematic representation of the various deletions which produce HPFH and $\delta\beta$ thalassaemia $(\delta\beta)^0 = {}^G\gamma$ $^A\gamma\delta\beta$ thalassaemia.

that individuals who inherit a gene for heterocellular HPFH and one for β thalassaemia have unusually high levels of Hb F [179, 180]. Similarly, individuals with sickle-cell anaemia who inherit an HPFH gene have higher levels of Hb F than is usually found in sickle-cell anaemia alone [181].

To complicate matters there have been reports of families in which there are several members with higher levels of Hb F than those which characterize Swiss HPFH. For example, a British family has been studied in which heterozygotes carry about 8% Hb F heterogeneously distributed among the red cells, and homozygotes have about 20% Hb F with a similar intercellular distribution [182]. There are no haematological abnormalities or globin-chain imbalance and it is quite clear that both the γ- and β-globin genes are active, unlike the situation in most forms of pancellular HPFH. Studies of this type suggest that at least some forms of heterocellular HPFH may result from regulatory-gene mutations although nothing is known of the molecular basis of these fascinating genetic variants.

β THALASSAEMIA AND ITS VARIANTS IN ASSOCIATION WITH STRUCTURAL HAEMOGLOBIN VARIANTS

In populations in which there is a high incidence of both β thalassaemia and β-chain haemoglobin variants, it is not uncommon to find patients doubly affected with both genes. The commonest combinations are sickle-cell thalassaemia, Hb C thalassaemia and Hb E thalassaemia. β thalassaemia has also been found in association with rare β-chain variants such as Hbs D, G, J, Norfolk and many others (see Ref. 9).

Sickle-cell thalassaemia [9, 183, 184]
This disorder is found most frequently in Africans but it also occurs in Greeks, Turks, Indians, North Africans and Rumanians. It has also been noted sporadically in individuals from other racial backgrounds including Cypriots, Lebanese, Saudi Arabians and Sudanese [9].

The clinical and haematological findings in this disorder are extremely variable and depend in part upon the type of thalassaemia gene which has been inherited together with the sickle-cell gene. In patients who inherit the $β^0$-thalassaemia determinant the haemoglobin pattern is almost identical to that of homozygous sickle-cell anaemia and consists of Hbs S and A_2. In patients who have inherited the mild $β^+$-thalassaemia gene (Negro type), the haemoglobin consists of about 60–70% Hb S and 25–30% Hb A, while those who have received the more severe type of $β^+$ thalassaemia (Mediterranean type) have lower levels of Hb A

in the 5–10% range. The Negro form of sickle-cell $β^+$ thalassaemia is generally milder than the types of sickle-cell thalassaemia in which no or low amounts of Hb A are produced.

Thus the clinical manifestations of sickle-cell thalassaemia are very variable. In some forms they are similar to those of sickle-cell anaemia with chronic haemolytic anaemia interspersed with crises of the type which have been described in the previous chapter. On the other hand some Negroes with sickle-cell $β^+$ thalassaemia are completely asymptomatic. The physical signs are also similar to sickle-cell anaemia except that in the milder cases persistent splenomegaly is not uncommon.

The haematological changes are similar to those of sickle-cell anaemia in the more severe cases although the red cells show more hypochromia. In the milder cases of sickle-cell $β^+$ thalassaemia the haematological findings are similar to β thalassaemia minor.

The haemoglobin electrophoretic findings are variable. In the Negro form of $β^+$ thalassaemia there is 15–25% Hb A with about 65–85% Hb S, a slight increase in Hb F and an elevated Hb A_2 level. Lower levels of Hb A are found when the $β^+$-thalassaemia gene is the more severe Mediterranean type. In the $β^0$-thalassaemia interaction the pattern is identical to the sickle-cell anaemia except that the Hb A_2 level is elevated.

Family studies reveal the sickle-cell trait in one parent and the β-thalassaemia trait in the other.

The combination of the sickle-cell gene with that for δβ thalassaemia produces a very mild clinical disorder, presumably because the relatively high level of Hb F protects against sickling. Affected individuals have about 20% Hb F with no Hb A and normal levels of Hb A_2.

Haemoglobin C thalassaemia
The disorder is found mainly in Negro populations although sporadic cases have been reported in North Africans and Italians [9].

The condition is usually symptomless. The haematological findings are those of a very mild haemolytic anaemia with the haemoglobin values in the 9–11 g/dl range. The peripheral blood film is characterized by the presence of many target cells and variable hypochromia. In fact it is not possible to distinguish the disorder from homozygous Hb C disease on morphological grounds. The red-cell indices are typical of β thalassaemia. The haemoglobin electrophoretic pattern varies; in cases where the $β^+$ thalassaemia is interacting it consists of about 70% Hb C with 20–30% Hb A and a slight elevation of Hb F; where the $β^0$-thalassaemia gene is involved the haemoglobin consists almost entirely of Hb C with 5–15% Hb F. It is not possible to estimate the level of Hb A_2 in the presence of Hb C.

Haemoglobin E thalassaemia

This disorder is frequently encountered in Southeast Asia and in parts of Burma, India and Pakistan [9, 76, 185].

The clinical findings may be similar to those of β thalassaemia major with marked anaemia, skeletal changes, retardation of growth, hepatosplenomegaly and severe iron loading with the related complications. Some cases are transfusion-dependent, others follow the course of a severe intermediate form of thalassaemia while others are much milder. The reasons for this remarkable variability in clinical course are not known. Some patients may also have inherited α-thalassaemia determinants which may modify the clinical findings (see page 436).

The blood picture is similar to homozygous β thalassaemia with severe anaemia, morphological changes of the red cells, erythroid hyperplasia of the bone marrow and the presence of inclusion bodies in the marrow and in the peripheral blood after splenectomy.

The haemoglobin pattern usually consists of Hbs E and F with Hb F values in the 10–50% range. Occasionally Hb A is found if there is an interacting β^+-thalassaemia determinant.

The severity of this condition is still not fully explained. Homozygous Hb E disease is a very mild condition (see Chapter 8, page 366) and it is not clear why Hb E and β thalassaemia can interact to produce a disorder not unlike β thalassaemia major. Recent work suggests that β^E chains may be synthesized less efficiently than β^A chains [186, 187], and that Hb E homozygotes and heterozygotes have a mild form of β thalassaemia; they have low MCH and MCV values [186]. Certainly this would explain the severity of the Hb E/β-thalassaemia interactions.

THE α THALASSAEMIAS

Although several well-defined clinical phenotypes resulting from genetic disorders of α-chain synthesis have been recognized for many years, it is only very recently that we have obtained some real understanding of the genetic transmission of these disorders. The major difficulty in this field is that the various heterozygous carrier states are extremely difficult to define by conventional haematological techniques or by haemoglobin analysis and hence it is only possible to clarify the inheritance of the α thalassaemias by resorting to sophisticated techniques such as globin gene mapping. This approach has provided a vast amount of information in the last few years; indeed

new molecular mechanisms have turned up so fast that there is no adequate nomenclature to describe them and it is very difficult to write about the α thalassaemias at the moment! What is clear is that there is a remarkably heterogeneous series of molecular defects which can given rise to similar phenotypes.

The important clinical disorders which result from α thalassaemia are the haemoglobin Bart's hydrops fetalis syndrome and haemoglobin H disease. These conditions result from the interaction of two main varieties of α-thalassaemia determinant.* The first, which is called α^0 thalassaemia or α thalassaemia 1, is characterized by a complete absence of α-chain synthesis from the chromosome carrying the α-thalassaemia determinant, and it is recognizable in the heterozygous state by a haematological picture rather similar to that of heterozygous β thalassaemia. The second, α^+ thalassaemia or α thalassaemia 2, is characterized by a reduced output of α-globin-chain synthesis directed by the chromosome which carries the α-thalassaemia gene; this condition may or may not be recognizable in the carrier state and in some cases there are no haematological abnormalities. It is now clear that both α thalassaemia 1 and α thalassaemia 2 are remarkably heterogeneous at the molecular level.

The homozygous state for the various α^0-thalassaemia determinants results in the haemoglobin Bart's hydrops fetalis syndrome and the compound heterozygous state for α^0 thalassaemia and α^+ thalassaemia results in Hb H disease. The difficulty arises because many different molecular defects can produce both α thalassaemia 1 and 2 phenotypes, and at the time of writing it is not clear whether the clinical (or phenotypic) expression of the different interactions of these various forms of α-thalassaemia determinants are distinguishable one from another.

The real problem for the haematologist is that it is still not possible to identify accurately the α-thalassaemia carrier states by any of the standard laboratory methods. Thus it is easy to make a diagnosis of haemoglobin Bart's hydrops fetalis syndrome or haemoglobin H disease but it is only possible to make an approximate guess at the likely genotype of any particular α-thalassaemia carrier.

A tentative classification of α thalassaemia is shown in Table 9.5.

Distribution

The haemoglobin Bart's hydrops syndrome occurs most frequently in Southeast Asia, particularly in Thailand, down the Malay peninsular and in Indone-

---

* Although the terms α thalassaemia 1 and 2 can still be used in the phenotype sense, we shall use the more precise forms, α^0 and α^+ thalassaemia in describing the α-thalassaemia genotypes.

Table 9.5. General classification of the α thalassaemias

Genetic determinants			
Designation	Haplotype	Heterozygous state	Homozygous state
α^0 *thalassaemia*			
α thalassaemia 1*	$--/$	5–10% Hb Bart's at birth Low MCH and MCV	Hb Bart's hydrops
Dysfunctional α thalassaemia	$-\alpha^0/$	? As above	?
a^+ *thalassaemia*			
α thalassaemia 2*	$-\alpha/$	0–2% Hb Bart's at birth Minimal haematological change	As for heterozygous α thalassaemia 1
Non-deletion α thalassaemia†	$\alpha\alpha/$	May be similar to above but haematological changes may be more severe	Hb H disease in some cases
Hb Constant Spring (CS) α 142 Gln	UAA→CAA	0–2% Hb Bart's at birth 0·5–1% Hb CS	Phenotype similar to hetero- zygous α thalassaemia 1 5–6% Hb CS
Hb Icaria α 142 Lys	UAA→AAA	As for Hb CS 0·5–1% Hb Icaria	?
Hb Koya Dora α 142 Ser	UAA→UCA	As for Hb CS 0·5–1% Hb Koya Dora	?
Hb Seal Rock α 142 Glu	UAA→GAA	As for Hb CS 0·5–1% Hb Seal Rock	?

Genetic interactions		
Interaction	Genotype	Disorder
α^0 thalassaemia/α^+ thalassaemia	$--/-\alpha$	Hb H disease
α^0 thalassaemia/non-deletion α thalassaemia	$--/\alpha\alpha$	Hb H disease
Non-deletion α thalassaemia/non-deletion α thalassaemia	$\alpha\alpha/\alpha\alpha$	Hb H disease
Dysfunctional α thalassaemia/α^+ thalassaemia	$-\alpha^0/-\alpha$	Hb H disease
α^0 thalassaemia/Hb CS	$--/\alpha\alpha^{CS}$	Hb CS-H disease
α^0 thalassaemia/Hb Q	$--/-\alpha^Q$	Hb Q-H disease
α^0 thalassaemia/Hb G (Phil)	$--/-\alpha^G$	Hb G-H disease
α^0 thalassaemia/Hb Hasharon	$--/-\alpha^{Hash}$	Hb Hasharon-H disease

* The terms α thalassaemia 1 and 2 are used in the phenotypic sense as in the original genetic analysis of the oriental α thalassaemias.

† Several different non-deletion α thalassaemias are known. A full explanation of the different types of α thalassaemia determinant and their interactions is given in appropriate sections of this chapter.

sia [9, 76]. There is a high frequency of haemoglobin H disease in the same region. The syndrome has been reported sporadically in Mediterranean populations, and Hb H disease occurs widely in this region and in parts of the Middle East. There is a very high incidence of the milder forms of α thalassaemia in African populations, although the haemoglobin Bart's hydrops syndrome has not been reported and Hb H disease is rare. Sporadic cases of haemoglobin H disease and various α-thalassaemia carrier states have been reported in practically every racial group.

The molecular basis of α thalassaemia

As mentioned earlier in the chapter there are two α-globin genes per haploid genome, i.e. four in all. The detailed arrangement of the α-globin genes on chromo-

some 16 is now known. The two embryonic α-like globin genes, the ζ genes, lie upstream (to the left) from the two α-globin genes and are separated from them by an inactive α-like gene called the $\psi\alpha$ gene (Fig. 9.3).

Many of the α^0-thalassaemia disorders result from deletions of both of the α-globin genes [21, 22], although the sizes of these deletions vary. For example, in Southeast Asia the deletion involves both α-globin genes, but both ζ genes are intact; whereas in some Mediterranean cases the deletion involves both α-globin genes and the 3′ ζ-globin gene [188–190]. Another deletion which has a widespread occurrence involves part of the 3′ α-globin gene, the whole of the 5′ gene and probably extends right through both ζ genes [191, 192] (Fig. 9.17). A similar but smaller deletion has recently been described [273].

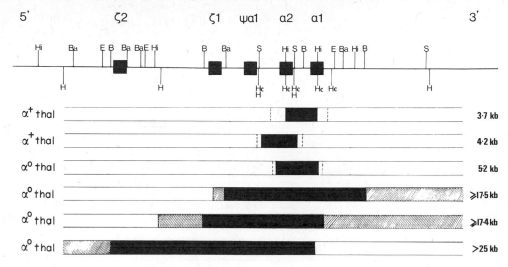

Fig. 9.17. A schematic representation of the deletions responsible for the various forms of α thalassaemia.

Alpha⁺-thalassaemia determinants result from deletions of one of the linked α-globin genes [193–196]. It seems likely that these have resulted from chromosomal misalignment with unequal crossing over, much in the same way as produced the Lepore haemoglobins. Gene-mapping analysis indicates that several different abnormal crossover events produced the α⁺-thalassaemia determinants [195–198]. Such an event would produce one chromosome containing a single α gene and another with three α-globin genes; the latter arrangement has been observed [199, 200].

One group of α-thalassaemia determinants is not associated with a detectable α-globin gene deletion (non-deletion α thalassaemia); the mechanism for the variable defect in α-chain production from a chromosome in which the α genes are intact remains to be determined [201]. In Saudi Arabia the non-deletion α-thalassaemia determinant is relatively severe and produces Hb H disease in the homozygous state [214].

Finally, some α-thalassaemia 2 phenotypes result from the inheritance of a chain-termination mutant haemoglobin such as Hb Constant Spring [202, 203]. These variants result from a single base mutations in the chain-termination codon such that codons at the 3′ end of the α-globin mRNA which are not normally translated are utilized with the production of elongated α-chain variants. These are produced at a very low rate, probably because the globin mRNA is unstable; hence they produce the clinical phenotype of α thalassaemia (Fig. 9.18).

The haemoglobin Bart's hydrops fetalis syndrome
This disorder is a frequent cause of stillbirth in Southeast Asia [204, 205]. Affected infants are either stillborn between 25 and 40 weeks' gestation or are live-born but die within the first few hours. There is pallor, oedema and hepatosplenomegaly and the clinical picture resembles that of hydrops fetalis due to rhesus blood group incompatibility. At autopsy, there is massive extramedullary haematopoiesis, hepatomegaly and enlargement of the placenta. The blood film is that of a severe thalassaemia with many nucleated red cells.

The haemoglobin in this disorder is comprised mainly of Hb Bart's with small amounts of Hbs H and Portland ($\zeta_2\gamma_2$). There is no Hb A or F and biosynthetic studies have confirmed a total absence of α-chain synthesis in these babies [206]. It is assumed that, since Hb Bart's is useless as an oxygen carrier, these infants survive to term because they continue to produce the embryonic haemoglobin, Hb Portland.

Examination of the parents shows a thalassaemic blood picture with low MCH and MCV values and a normal haemoglobin electrophoresis. Biosynthetic studies indicate that they have a significant reduction in α-chain synthesis with α/β production ratios of approximately 0·7. These findings are compatible with the carrier state for the α⁰-thalassaemia determinant.

Haemoglobin H disease
Haemoglobin H disease is extremely common in Southeast Asia, parts of the Middle East and the Mediterranean region, and has been found sporadically in practically every racial group [9, 205]. The disorder shows remarkable clinical variability; at one end of the scale there are patients with a clinical picture typical of Cooley's anaemia, while in others the condition may be compatible with a completely nor-

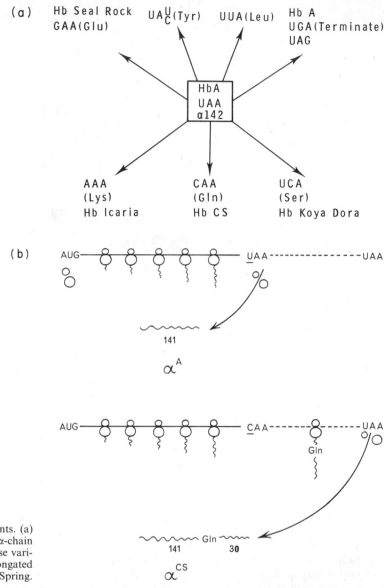

Fig. 9.18. The α-chain termination mutants. (a) The various base substitutions in the α-chain termination codan which give rise to these variants. (b) The molecular basis for the elongated α-chain variant, haemoglobuin Constant Spring.

mal life with haemoglobin values in the 10–11 g/dl range.

Clinical features

There are no specific symptoms and signs attributable to this disorder. In the more severe cases the clinical condition may resemble the more severe forms of β thalassaemia with anaemia from early life and the typical skeletal and developmental changes of those disorders. In the milder cases, moderate splenomegaly may be the only clinical finding. Radiological changes of the bones are only found in the more severe cases. In addition to these findings patients may give a history of haemolytic episodes particularly associated with infection or the use of oxidant drugs such as sulphonamides.

Haematological changes

Haemoglobin values range from 7 to 11 g/dl. The blood film shows hypochromia and aniso-poikilocytosis. The reticulocyte count is moderately elevated. Incubation of the red cells with brilliant cresyl blue results in the generation of ragged inclusion bodies in many of the cells. After splenectomy large single Heinz bodies are found in some of the red cells. These are formed by the precipitation of Hb H *in vitro* and only appear in the blood after splenectomy (Fig. 9.19). The inclusions which form on incubation with brilliant cresyl blue are due to precipitation of Hb H *in vitro* as the result of the redox action of the dye on the variant.

The bone marrow shows a variable degree of erythroid hyperplasia and some of the precursors contain precipitated Hb H.

Serum iron and ferritin levels are usually normal; the degree of iron loading is less than in the β thalassaemias, probably because there is relatively less ineffective erythropoiesis.

Haemoglobin constitution (Fig. 9.20)

The haemoglobin pattern in Hb H disease is variable. Haemoglobin A always constitutes the major component, while the level of Hb H varies from 5 to 40%. In addition there is nearly always a small amount of haemoglobin Bart's and a component consisting entirely of the δ chains of Hb A_2. The level of the latter is usually reduced. Haemoglobins H and Bart's are unique among the haemoglobin variants in that they migrate anodally at pH 6·5–7·0 and therefore are easily identified. In many cases of Hb H disease in Southeast Asia, trace amounts of haemoglobin Constant Spring can be observed on alkaline starch gel electrophoresis [202, 203].

Haemoglobin synthesis

In-vitro studies [9] have shown that β chains are synthesized about 2–3 times faster than α chains in this condition. The excess β chains, in addition to forming Hb H, produce a relatively large intracellular pool capable of combining with newly made α chains. These experiments have also confirmed that Hb H is prematurely destroyed within the circulation. The reduced level of α-chain production is reflected by an appropriate deficiency of α-globin mRNA.

Red-cell metabolism

The metabolic properties of the red cells in Hb H disease have been studied both in whole blood and in 'young and old' cell populations obtained by differential centrifugation [9, 130, 207–209]. The rates of glucose utilization and lactate formation are increased, a finding which must in part reflect an overall young cell population. Both young and old cells have increased cation permeability, the most marked changes being in the older population which contains single inclusion bodies in splenectomized individuals. It seems likely that the rapid rate of glucose utilization is partly due to the stimulation of the cation pump resulting from these changes in membrane permeability. Red-cell ATP levels are normal or slightly reduced. Haemoglobin H cells also have an increased rate of methaemoglobin production and high levels of glutathione peroxidase. Reduced glutathione levels are lower in the old cell population. Furthermore, hexosemonophosphate shunt activity is more marked in the older cells. It has been suggested that because Hb H is particularly sensitive to oxidative precipitation, its

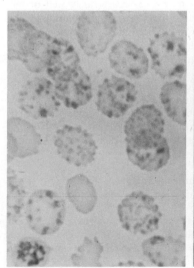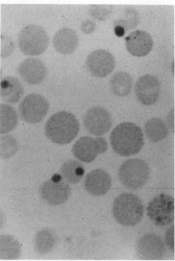

Fig. 9.19. Haemoglobin H inclusions: (left) after incubation of red cells with brilliant cresyl blue; (right) post-splenectomy showing large single inclusions stained with methyl violet.

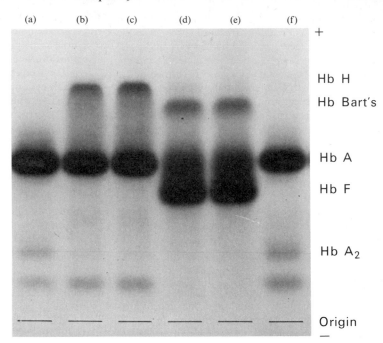

Fig. 9.20. The electrophoretic characteristics of haemoglobins H and Bart's (starch gel electrophoresis, tris EDTA borate system, pH 8·6, protein stain). Left to right (a) normal adult, (b) and (c) adult with Hb H disease, (d) and (e) cord bloods showing increased levels of Hb Bart's and (f) normal adult.

reactive thiols may participate in cellular reduction reactions and thus substitute for glutathione.

Pathophysiology [9, 130, 207–210]

There is now a considerable body of evidence that Hb H tends to precipitate as erythrocytes age and that the older cell populations contain large single inclusions resulting from this process. Thus centrifugation of cells from splenectomized patients produces heterogeneous populations; the upper (young) population contains very few preformed inclusions but shows variable amounts of Hb H on electrophoresis while the older population contains no Hb H but shows many cells with single inclusions [210].

It seems likely therefore that newly synthesized erythrocytes contain variable amounts of Hb H. During the lifespan of the red cell this tends to precipitate and form a rigid Heinz body. These bodies are pulled out of the red cells during their passage through the splenic sinusoids or other parts of the reticulo-endothelial system. It is the mechanical trauma which results from this process which is mainly responsible for the shortened red-cell survival in Hb H disease. Presumably the mechanical damage to the red-cell membrane is responsible for the changes in membrane function and permeability which were summarized in the previous section. Electron-microscopy studies [211] have provided a clear picture of the way in which Heinz bodies are removed from the spleen.

Although this general model of the progressive precipitation of Hb H in Hb H disease is probably correct there is no doubt that some precipitation starts early in the cell's lifespan and indeed inclusion bodies can be seen in the bone marrow in this disorder [212, 213]. The reason for this heterogeneity of cellular precipitation is uncertain, but it suggests that factors other than cell age are involved.

Inheritance

The genetics of Hb H disease are fairly well understood, at least for the oriental populations. The disorder results from two genetic combinations: either the compound heterozygous state for α^0 thalassaemia and α^+ thalassaemia, or the heterozygous state for α^0 thalassaemia and the Hb Constant Spring gene [202, 203]. Thus the overall deficit of α chains produced by the α^+-thalassaemia or Hb Constant Spring genes is similar. In Southeast Asia the α thalassaemia/Hb Constant Spring combination makes up about 40% of the cases of Hb H disease. The direct transmission of Hb H disease from one generation to the next is well documented.

This could occur if the various α-thalassaemia genes are not alleles and segregate independently or if a patient with Hb H disease was mated to an α^0 thalassaemia or α^+ thalassaemia carrier. Recent studies on the molecular basis of these α-thalassaemia disorders suggest that the second explanation is the correct one.

As described earlier, it is clear that the Hb H disease is very heterogeneous at the molecular level. Indeed, recent work suggests that it may sometimes result from the homozygous state for a α-thalassaemia determinant which has a phenotypic expression intermediate between that of the oriental α^0-thalassaemia and α^+-thalassaemia determinants [214]. It can also result from the inheritance of a non-deletion variant and a deletion form of α^0 thalassaemia.

α^0-thalassaemia and α^+-thalassaemia traits [9, 76, 215, 216]

The α^0-thalassaemia trait is characterized by the presence of 5–15% Hb Bart's at birth. The latter disappears during maturation and is not replaced by a similar amount of Hb H although α^0-thalassaemia heterozygotes may show an occasional cell with Hb H bodies after incubation with brilliant cresyl blue. The latter phenomenon is often used as a diagnostic test for α-thalassaemia trait. However, it is difficult to standardize and needs much experience to be useful; indeed it is far from certain just how reliable it is. In adult life, heterozygotes have morphological changes similar to heterozygous β thalassaemia with low MCH and MCV values. The electrophoretic pattern is normal but globin synthesis studies indicate a significant deficit of α-chain production with an α/β production ratio of approximately 0·7 [216, 217]. Similarly there is a significant deficit of α-globin mRNA [218].

The α^+-thalassaemia trait is characterized by a slight elevation of haemoglobin Bart's at birth in some but not all cases [216]. Haematological findings are very mild or absent and there is slight deficit of α-chain synthesis.

Although it is usually possible to recognize the α^0-thalassaemia trait, in any particular case it is not possible to distinguish it from the α^+-thalassaemia trait or, indeed, to distinguish the latter from normal, using haematological data or haemoglobin synthesis studies. The different α-thalassaemia traits can only be identified with certainty by mRNA or gene analysis.

Haemoglobin Constant Spring

Haemoglobin Constant Spring is an α-chain variant which has an elongated α chain with 31 extra residues attached to its C-terminal end [202, 203]. It is synthesized inefficiently and produces the clinical picture of α thalassaemia.

In the homozygous state for Hb Constant Spring, the blood picture is that of a mild thalassaemic disorder with small red cells [219]. The haemoglobin pattern is made up of about 5–6% Hb Constant Spring with normal levels of Hb A_2 and trace amounts of Hb Bart's.

The heterozygous state for Hb Constant Spring shows no haematological abnormality. The haemoglobin pattern is made up of normal levels of Hbs A and A_2 with approximately 0·5% Hb Constant Spring. The latter can be observed on alkaline starch gel electrophoresis as a faint band migrating between Hb A_2 and the origin. It is seen best on heavily loaded starch gels and is easily missed if other electrophoretic techniques are used (Fig. 9.20).

As mentioned in the previous section the genetic combination of α^0 thalassaemia and Hb Constant Spring is responsible for about 40% of cases of Hb H disease in Thailand and probably a similar number in Malaysia, at least in some ethnic groups [220]. This combination has also been observed in Greece but not as yet in other parts of the world [221]. The incidence of Hb Constant Spring in the oriental populations is not yet certain but it has been estimated that it occurs in about 4% of the total population of Thailand and has a high incidence down the Malay peninsula [76, 220].

The related elongated α-chain haemoglobin variants Icaria [222] and Koya Dora [223] are also associated with a clinical picture of α thalassaemia and the latter has been found, in combination with α^0 thalassaemia, to produce Hb H disease. The molecular mechanisms for the production of these elongated α-chain haemoglobin variants were considered in an earlier section.

α thalassaemia in association with structural haemoglobin variants

Alpha thalassaemia has been found in association with α-chain variants or β-chain variants.

α thalassaemia with α-chain variants

The commonest interaction between α thalassaemia and α-chain variants is the disorder called Hb Q-H disease or Hb Q-α thalassaemia [9, 224]. The clinical picture is identical to that of Hb H disease and the haemoglobin is made up of Hbs Q ($\alpha_2^Q\beta_2$), Q_2 ($\alpha_2^Q\delta_2$), H and Bart's; Hb A is absent. Recent gene-mapping analysis indicates that the chromosome which carries the α^Q-mutation only has a single α-chain gene ($-\alpha^Q$). When this is inherited together with a chromosome containing no α-chain genes, i.e. α^0 thalassaemia ($--$), the affected individual has only a single functional α-globin gene which carries the Hb Q mutation ($-\alpha^Q--$). Thus they have an identical disorder to Hb H disease except that instead of making haemoglobin A they make haemoglobin Q [225, 226].

Other interactions between α thalassaemia and α-chain variants have been reported, either as single cases or as small series in particular population groups. Reported interactions include those with Hbs I, J Mexico and Cape Town. They are fully reviewed in the monograph of Weatherall & Clegg [9].

The interactions with α thalassaemia and the α-

globin-chain termination mutants such as haemoglobin Constant Spring were discussed in a previous
section.

The combination of the sickle-cell gene with α
thalassaemia is found frequently in Negro populations. Because the latter do not have the α^0-thalassae-
mia determinant, i.e. individuals lacking both α-
globin genes on one chromosome, the interactions
which have been defined involve either the heterozygous or homozygous state for the sickle-cell gene with
either the heterozygous or homozygous states for the
deletion form of α^+ thalassaemia. These conditions
have recently been fully defined [195, 196].

Individuals with sickle-cell anaemia who are homozygous for α^+ thalassaemia have small red cells with
reduced MCH and MCV values, slightly elevated Hb
A_2 levels and imbalanced globin-chain synthesis.
Similarly, sickle-cell heterozygotes who are homozygous for α^+ thalassaemia have typical thalassaemic
indices and unusually low levels of Hb S for sickle-cell
carriers. The interactions of the sickle-cell genes with
the heterozygous state for α^+ thalassaemia are much
harder to define and since they are associated with mild
haematological changes can only be determined with
certainty by globin-gene mapping. Several Saudi
Arabians have been identified who have sickle-cell trait
or disease in association with the genotype of Hb H
disease; they produce Hb Bart's and not β_4^S molecules
[227] and have a clinical disorder similar to Hb H
disease.

Alpha thalassaemia has also been observed in
individuals with haemoglobin C trait [9, 228] and the
interaction produces a thalassaemic blood picture
associated with lower levels of Hb C than are usually
observed in simple heterozygotes for that variant [9].

β-chain variants

In populations such as those in Southeast Asia and
Africa where the genes for α thalassaemia and β-chain
haemoglobin variants are common, a series of disorders have been defined which result from the
inheritance of different combinations of these genes.
The interactions between α thalassaemia and Hbs E or
S have been well-defined.

The clinical disorders which result from the interaction of the genes for Hb E and α thalassaemia are
extremely common in Southeast Asia, particularly in
Thailand [76, 229, 230]. By far the commonest clinical
disorder is the heterozygous state for Hb E in association with both α^0 thalassaemia and α^+ thalassaemia.
Affected patients have the clinical picture of thalassaemia intermedia with haemoglobin values in the
6–10 g/dl range, skeletal changes, splenomegaly and, in
some cases, regular transfusion requirements. The
haemoglobin consists of Hbs A, E and Bart's. The level

of Hb E, which in uncomplicated Hb E heterozygotes
is approximately 25–30%, is markedly reduced in the
15% range. The interaction between Hb E and either α^0
thalassaemia or α^+ thalassaemia alone produces a less
severe disorder characterized by a thalassaemic blood
picture in association with unusually low levels of Hb
E, i.e. in the range 18–25%.

Clearly in any patient with an unusually low level of
Hb E and in whom the blood picture is more severe
than that usually observed in Hb E carriers the
presence of one or more α-thalassaemia genes should
be suspected. The true genotype can only be determined with certainty by a detailed family study.

**A summary of the different α-thalassaemia determinants
and their genetic inheritance**

Because of the confusing nature of the genetics of α
thalassaemia it might be helpful for the reader to
summarize briefly the relationship between molecular
forms of α thalassaemia and the clinical disorders
which we have described. The story is incomplete at the
time of writing but at least some sense can now be
made of this difficult field (Fig. 9.21).

The α^0-thalassaemia determinants, which result

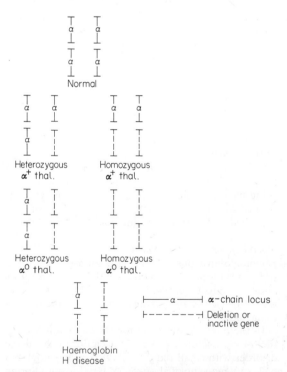

Fig. 9.21. The 'prototype' α thalassaemias. Hb H disease and
the Hb Bart's hydrops syndrome usually only occur in
populations in which there is a chromosome which carries
neither α-chain locus.

from several different deletions involving both the haploid α-globin genes interact in the homozygous state to cause a complete absence of α-globin synthesis and the Hb Bart's hydrops syndrome. It is presumed that the homozygous state for the α-thalassaemia determinants which result from more extensive deletions involving the ζ-globin genes will not be compatible with fetal survival, since infants with the Hb Bart's hydrops syndrome only survive until term because they synthesize Hb Portland ($\zeta_2\gamma_2$) [214]. It is of great interest that deletions involving the α-globin genes allow persistent ζ-chain synthesis; the situation is similar to that which occurs in $\delta\beta$ thalassaemia and hereditary persistence of fetal haemoglobin in which deletions of the δ- and β-globin genes are associated with persistent γ-chain synthesis.

Haemoglobin H disease results from the inheritance of one or other type of α^0-thalassaemia determinant together with an α^+ thalassaemia or a non-deletion α-thalassaemia determinant. It also occurs when α^0 thalassaemia interacts with one of several α globin-chain termination mutants. Finally, Hb H disease can be inherited as the homozygous state for a non-deletion α^+-thalassaemia determinant which is associated with a marked reduction of α-chain synthesis from the affected chromosome [214]. Clearly Hb H disease is remarkably heterogeneous at the molecular level.

The observations outlined above allow certain predictions to be made. Unless there is an α^0-thalassaemia determinant in the population it is unlikely that the Hb Bart's hydrops syndrome will occur and Hb H disease should be equally uncommon unless it results from the homozygous state for the non-deletion determinant. This prediction is borne out in studies of the Negro and Saudi Arabian populations. It has been known for many years that quite a high proportion of African Negroes have the clinical phenotype of α^0 thalassaemia yet the Hb Bart's hydrops syndrome has not been found and Hb H disease is very rare. It turns out that about 25–30% of African Negroes are heterozygous for the deletion form of α^+ thalassaemia and about 2% are homozygous for this variant [194–196]. Since individuals homozygous for α^+ thalassaemia only have two α-globin genes they have exactly the same phenotype as individuals heterozygous for α^0 thalassaemia, i.e. the phenotypic results of having two α-globin genes are the same whether the genes are on one chromosome or on opposite pairs of homologous chromosomes. Gene-mapping analysis of newborn infants in the African populations have provided clear evidence that babies with 5–15% Hb Bart's are homozygous for α^+ thalassaemia, whereas babies who are heterozygous for this variant may or may not show increased levels of Hb Bart's at birth [216]. Hence it is only possible to obtain an approximate estimate of the gene frequency for α thalassaemia by studying the haemoglobin pattern of newborn infants.

The Hb Bart's hydrops syndrome is rare in Saudi Arabia and yet Hb H disease occurs quite frequently. Again the α^0-thalassaemia determinant is rare but there appears to be a relatively high frequency of a severe non-deletion form of α^+ thalassaemia which, in the homozygous state, produces Hb H disease.

Finally, it is clear that some α-chain variants such as Hb Q occur on a chromosome which only contains a single α-globin gene. Hence if these are inherited together with a chromosome containing no α-chain genes the resulting disorder will resemble Hb H disease except that there will be no Hb A but only the α-chain variant and the variant Hb A_2 together with Hb H, for example in Hb Q-H disease the haemoglobins consist of H (β_4, Q ($\alpha_2^Q\beta_2$) and Q_2 ($\alpha_2^Q\delta_2$).

THALASSAEMIA INTERMEDIA

Thalassaemia intermedia is an ill-defined term used to describe those forms of the thalassaemia syndromes which, though more severe than the heterozygous carrier states, are not associated with such a marked degree of anaemia as to warrant regular blood transfusion. Clearly, the term means different things to different clinicians. As we saw in an earlier section the heterozygous carrier states for α or β thalassaemia are characterized by extremely mild anaemia and the absence of splenomegaly. If the degree of anaemia is more severe and if there is splenomegaly, then a thalassaemic disorder is described appropriately as being of an intermediate type. It is at the other end of the spectrum, where a child may be able to survive with a haemoglobin value in the 5–7 g/dl range, but in whom growth and development is retarded, skeletal changes are severe and the general state of health is poor, that the disorder becomes particularly difficult to define. Some children can grow and develop quite well at these low haemoglobin levels and the condition is then properly called thalassaemia intermedia. Others develop gross skeletal abnormalities and have continual poor general health and should be transfused; they are then classified as having thalassaemia major. Perhaps it is reasonable to define any thalassaemic disorder which is associated with a haemoglobin value compatible with survival as being a form of thalassaemia intermedia, always realizing that some of these patients are better maintained on blood transfusion.

Clearly many of the conditions that have been described earlier in this chapter are forms of thalassaemia intermedia (Table 9.6). These include the different interactions of the β thalassaemias with structural

Table 9.6. Some genetic combinations which can cause thalassaemia intermedia

---

Homozygous mild β thalassaemia (Negro form)
Homozygous β^+ or β^0 thalassaemia and α^0 or α^+ thalassaemia*
Homozygous β^+ or β^0 thalassaemia and pancellular HPFH
Heterozygous β^+ or β^0 thalassaemia and $\delta\beta$ thalasaemia
Heterozygous β thalassaemia and 'silent' β thalassaemia
Homozygous 'silent' β thalassaemia
Homozygous $\delta\beta$ thalassaemia
Heterozygous β^+ or β^0 thalassaemia and HPFH
Homozygous Hb Lepore†
Combinations of Hb Lepore with β or $\delta\beta$ thalassaemia
β^+ or β^0 thalassaemia with structural Hb variants, e.g. Hbs S, C or E
Heterozygous β thalassaemia with an acquired disorder, e.g. folate deficiency
Haemoglobin H disease
α thalassaemia with Hb variant

---

* The precise α-thalassaemia genotypes which modify homozygous β thalassaemia are not known.
† In some cases.

haemoglobin variants, the $\delta\beta$ thalassaemias and their various interactions, some of the Hb Lepore syndromes, interactions of β thalassaemia with hereditary persistence of fetal haemoglobin, and some of the α-thalassaemia syndromes, in particular Hb H disease. However, when these disorders have been excluded, patients are encountered from time to time who are apparently homozygous for β thalassaemia but who run a much milder clinical course. This condition can be designated homozygous β thalassaemia intermedia. In the sections which follow we shall briefly review the possible underlying cause for this disorder, its clinical manifestations and its complications. This problem has recently been reviewed in greater detail [9].

Molecular basis
At the present time there is only very scanty information about the factors which may reduce the severity of the homozygous state for β^+ or β^0 thalassaemia. There is some evidence that one genetic interaction which is capable of producing this effect is the inheritance of one or more α-thalassaemia genes [209, 231–233]. In a β-thalassaemia homozygote who has inherited an α-thalassaemia determinant the overall degree of globin-chain imbalance is reduced, the amount of ineffective erythropoiesis is less, and hence the degree of anaemia and expansion of the bone marrow is less marked. So far there is no good information about the types of α-thalassaemia determinant which are required to reduced the severity of homozygous β thalassaemia. For example, it is not clear whether a single α^+-thalassaemia determinant can 'change' homozygous β^+ or β^0 thalassaemia major into thalassaemia intermedia (Table 9.6).

Another possible interaction which may modify the course of β thalassaemia is the inheritance of a gene for heterocellular HPFH [179, 180, 234–236]. It is possible that the inheritance of a determinant of this type can elevate the level of γ-chain output and therefore decrease the severity of β thalassaemia.

In some populations, particularly those of the Middle East, homozygous β^0 thalassaemia intermedia occurs and there is no obvious reason why the condition is relatively mild. It is possible that there is a genetically determined ability to increase the output of γ chains to a more efficient degree than occurs in other populations but there is no real evidence in favour of this hypothesis [9].

Clinical and haematological findings
The clinical findings in thalassaemia intermedia are extremely variable. Some patients have a moderate degree of anaemia and splenomegaly and are otherwise unaffected. In other cases there may be a more severe degree of anaemia and splenomegaly associated with severe bone changes and skeletal deformity (Fig. 9.22). Tumour masses of extramedullary erythropoietic tissue are particularly common in this group. Recent studies indicate that these patients may have a marked increase in gastrointestinal iron absorption and as they grow older they may develop complications of iron loading including cirrhosis, endocrine deficiency, particularly diabetes mellitus, and skin pigmentation [237, 238]. So far there is no evidence that cardiac complications occur in this group and it is possible that iron derived from the gastrointestinal tract is less likely to cause damage to the myocardium than transfused iron [237].

From what little is known about the natural history of thalassaemia intermedia it appears that although affected patients develop progressive iron loading at approximately one-third of the rate of transfusion-dependent thalassaemics [9] they do not suffer such serious complications as the transfusion-dependent group. Diabetes and liver disease have been the two most commonly encountered by the present authors. The other distressing long-term complication is progressive bone and joint disease with severe bone pain and deformity, presumably due to massive and long-standing marrow expansion.

Many patients in this group develop hypersplenism and require splenectomy. As a group they are also prone to foliate deficiency and megaloblastic anaemia.

The haematological picture is characterized by a variable degree of anaemia and morphological changes of the red cells similar to those observed in

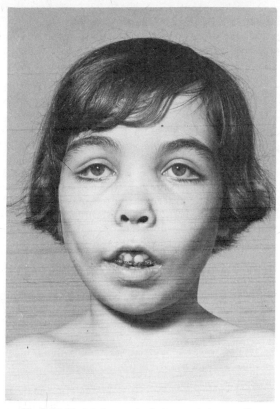

Fig. 9.22. Facial changes in thalassaemia intermedia.

thalassaemia major. There is marked hyperplasia of the red-cell precursors, many of which contain inclusions of precipitated α chains.

Haemoglobin constitution
The haemoglobin constitution is extremely variable in the intermediate forms of thalassaemia [9]. In patients of Mediterranean and African background the condition usually represents the homozygous state for β^+ thalassaemia and there is an increase in Hb F levels in the 20–70% range. Haemoglobin A_2 values may be normal or elevated. There appears to be a small subgroup in the Mediterranean region with unusually low levels of Hb F in the 5–15% range [9]. In homozygous β^0 thalassaemia intermedia there is no Hb A production and Hb A_2 levels tend to be normal or reduced. Globin-chain synthesis studies in this group have shown marked imbalance of globin-chain production but generally less than that observed in homozygous β thalassaemia major.

Family findings
Both parents show the picture of heterozygous β

thalassaemia with elevated levels of Hb A_2. In some families one or other of these parents is also a carrier for α thalassaemia. However, the combination of the α- and β-thalassaemia traits produces no change in the haemoglobin pattern from that found in the β-thalassaemia trait alone and the condition can only be diagnosed by globin-chain synthesis analysis which, instead of giving the usual α/β ratio of about 2/1 characteristic of β-thalassaemia heterozygotes, shows more balanced globin-chain production. However, it is extremely difficult to determine which form of α-thalassaemia determinant is present and this can only be achieved by globin-gene mapping analysis. If the latter cannot be carried out one useful approach is to examine the lateral relatives of the parents to see if there is in individual who has the α-thalassaemia trait without the β-thalassaemia trait, i.e. a person with a thalassaemic blood picture with a normal level of Hb A_2. What is known about these complicated interactions between α and β thalassaemia at the clinical and phenotypic level has been reviewed in detail recently [9] and is summarized in Table 9.6.

THE PREVENTION AND TREATMENT OF THALASSAEMIA

Unfortunately there is still no specific therapy for the thalassaemia syndromes and even as the basic molecular defects are worked out the possibilities of correcting them do not seem to come any nearer. However, there have been significant advances in the prevention of these disorders, particularly with the development of methods for antenatal diagnosis. Furthermore, a much clearer picture of the best methods for the conservative management of established cases has now emerged and there is some indication that given adequate medical resources many transfusion-dependent children with the disorder may lead long and useful lives.

Prevention
Since most of the important forms of thalassaemia can be diagnosed easily in the heterozygous state they should be preventable. Although many countries are now embarking on screening programmes to identify heterozygous carriers, it seems unlikely that these will have a great effect on the marital patterns within these communities [9]. For this reason, many centres have now set up programmes for screening pregnant women and when heterozygous carriers are found, for examining their husbands for the presence of thalassaemia genes. Couples at risk for carrying a homozygous fetus can then be offered the possibility of antenatal diagnosis and, where appropriate, therapeutic abortion.

The various methods available for antenatal diagnosis of thalassaemia have been reviewed in detail recently [239–242] and need only be described in outline here. Since the α thalassaemias cause either intrauterine death or a relatively mild disorder in adult life, they are of relatively little importance in this context. It is in the prevention of β thalassaemia that antenatal diagnosis has its main role. Since β-globin-chain synthesis occurs at a low level from early in fetal life, and the β-thalassaemia genes are expressed during early development, it is possible, by obtaining a fetal blood sample and measuring the relative rates of globin-chain synthesis, to diagnose the homozygous state for β^0 or β^+ thalassaemia at a time when therapeutic abortion is possible.

Once a couple have been identified as being at risk for carrying a fetus with homozygous β thalassaemia, the possibility of antenatal diagnosis and therapeutic abortion and its risks is explained to them in great detail. If they accept the procedure, a fetal blood sample is obtained by either placental puncture or fetoscopy. The relative number of fetal cells in the sample is determined by the acid elution technique, or by sizing the cell population automatically. Ideally the diagnosis is made on samples containing approximately 100% fetal cells although by a variety of techniques designed to concentrate the fetal red cells from a mixture of fetal and maternal cells it is possible to make a diagnosis with samples which are heavily contaminated with maternal blood. The sample is then incubated with radioactive amino acids and the relative rates of γ- and β-chain synthesis determined. In normal fetuses at about 18–20 weeks' gestation the β/γ globin-chain synthesis ratio is approximately 0·10. In infants homozygous for β^0 thalassaemia no β-chain synthesis is found and in infants homozygous for β^+ thalassaemia only 1–2% β-chain synthesis is found at this time. If this is the case the mother is told and offered a therapeutic abortion.

Despite the technical difficulties of this approach wide experience has indicated that in good hands there is only a 5% fetal loss and that the diagnosis can be made with a high degree of accuracy. The major difficulties are in obtaining an adequate fetal blood sample and in the interpretation of the globin-chain synthesis results.

Currently, techniques are being developed to attempt antenatal diagnosis by gene mapping of DNA obtained from amniotic fluid cells. This approach is relatively easy if the thalassaemia results from a gene deletion but unfortunately this is not the case for most types of β thalassaemia. However, it may be possible to use DNA polymorphisms outside the structural genes for β globin [243, 244] or related loci such as the γ-chain genes [245]. The Hb Bart's hydrops syndrome is easily diagnosed by gene mapping [246]; since this condition is associated with toxaemia of pregnancy and post-partum bleeding there may be a case for this approach in at-risk pregnancies.

Symptomatic treatment

A great deal can be done for β-thalassaemia homozygotes and it is essential that they are treated in a centre with experience of the condition. As soon as the disorder is first diagnosed the haemoglobin level should be carefully monitored and treatment only started if the latter falls to a level at which the child requires transfusion. It is often possible to make this decision from observations of the way in which the infant is thriving, its feeding and sleeping habits, and from a weight chart. It is bad practice to start transfusion too early because in this way children with thalassaemia intermedia may receive unnecessary transfusions, but in general if the haemoglobin level drops below 6–7 g/dl, transfusion will be necessary. If this is the case a detailed explanation of the general nature of the condition should be given to the parents and a very careful programme for the child's future outlined in great detail. It is vitally important to assure the parents that the child's condition is no fault of theirs and to try to make sure that both of them become involved in the child's hospital visits so that the burden of looking after a chronically sick child does not fall on one or other parent. A detailed analysis of the pastoral problems in managing these chronically sick children has been given in several recent reviews [9, 94, 247].

The principles of treatment include regular transfusion, the judicial use of splenectomy, iron chelation therapy, and the management and prevention of the many complications which may occur during the course of the illness.

Transfusion. It has now been established quite unequivocally that homozygous β-thalassaemic children grow better and develop far fewer complications if their haemoglobin level is maintained as close to normal as possible. Thus the object should be to maintain the haemoglobin between 10 and 14 g/dl and to try not to let the child become anaemic at any time.

Immediately after diagnosis a full blood group genotype should be obtained and once a steady-state haemoglobin level has been reached which requires transfusion, the child should be started on a regular transfusion regime. The transfusion sessions must run smoothly and veins must be conserved at all costs. Details of the methods of transfusion have been outlined in several recent accounts of the management of this disorder [9, 94, 247, 248]. In summary, it is very important that these children should be transfused with relatively fresh blood and that they should receive packed washed cells and not whole blood. They do not require plasma and during the washing process as many of the white cells should be removed as possible. Frozen blood is useful when available, largely because it is poor in white cells. However, adequately washed red cells are quite as good and techniques for preparing blood in this way have been recently reviewed [9].

A variety of complications may result from regular blood transfusion. The problem of iron loading will be dealt with in a later section. Sensitization to one or more blood-group antigens is all too common. When this occurs it is essential to find a compatible donor. If this is not possible it may still be possible to transfuse these patients if the sessions are covered with corticosteroid drugs. In tropical countries it is most important to screen all blood donors for malaria, and in any population children should only receive blood from donors screened for the Australia antigen. The causes of the rare hyperpyrexial reactions associated with convulsions which have been reported from Thailand and which affect children who have been transfused up to a high haemoglobin level before splenectomy are not known [249].

Splenectomy. The indications for splenectomy have been the subject of many discussions as have the results of the operation [9, 94, 248, 250]. Modell [94] has described a simple method whereby standard curves for blood requirements can be drawn for a thalassaemic child. If the requirements exceed the calculated amount it is likely that there is some degree of hypersplenism and the spleen should be removed. The indications for splenectomy are thus an increase in transfusion requirements, other evidence of hypersplenism such as neutropenia or thrombocytopenia, or physical discomfort from a large spleen. It seems likely that the incidence of hypersplenism is reduced if a child has been maintained on a high transfusion regime. Furthermore, the results of surgery are good if the child receives an adequate transfusion regime after the operation [94]; if not, there may be progressive hepatomegaly and little benefit from the operation.

There is good evidence that young children are more prone to serious infections after splenectomy [9, 94, 252] and the operation should be avoided in the first five years of life. Children should be maintained on oral penicillin after surgery and the parents warned about the danger of serious and overwhelming infection. The problems of splenectomy in children with thalassaemia intermedia will be considered later in the chapter.

Chelating agents. After many early disappointments it has been recently demonstrated that it may be possible to maintain children in iron balance even if they are on high transfusion regimes. The impetus to this work came from a trial which showed that children given chelation therapy developed less liver fibrosis than those who received transfusion alone [253].

The only chelating agent which has been found to be of real value in thalassaemic patients is desferrioxamine (Desferal, Ciba). Although early experience with this drug when used by intramuscular bolus indicated that it was not possible to maintain affected children in iron balance, and that significant iron excretion could only be obtained in patients already heavily iron loaded, more recent studies have shown that if the drug is given by a subcutaneous infusion or by continuous intravenous infusion it is possible to achieve a significant amount of iron excretion in the urine [254–258]. Furthermore, since a considerable amount of the iron is also excreted in the stools, the total amount of iron which can be removed by using desferrioxamine in this way is very considerable.

Details of the use of desferrioxamine by subcutaneous infusion have been reported in several reviews [9, 258, 259]. The drug is infused through a small-gauge needle placed in the subcutaneous tissue of the anterior abdominal wall by means of a small clockwork or electrical pump. The precise dose to be administered has to be worked out for each individual child [258]. To do this, a dose–response curve is set up. Starting at a dose of about 0·5 g desferrioxamine the infusion dose is increased in 0·5 g increments, and the urinary output for 24 hours after the 12-hour infusion is determined. In some children there is a linear dose–response curve while in others, after reaching doses of 1–2 g of the drug, there is no further increase in iron excretion. The dose at which maximal iron excretion is achieved is used. The drug is dissolved in an appropriate volume of distilled water and is infused over an 8–12 hour period, usually while the child is asleep. This can be carried out for five nights of the week and the child can have a rest at weekends. The child should be maintained on ascorbic acid, 100–200 mg daily; because of the possibility of cardiac toxicity this dose should not be exceeded.

To date there have been relatively few reported side effects following the use of Desferal by infusion. Some children develop soreness and irritation of the site of the infusion but this is usually a transient phenomenon and if care is taken to make sure that the needle is properly placed subcutaneously such reactions do not present a serious problem. There have been a few reported cases of what appears to be genuine allergy to the drug with fevers, rigors and generalized irritation [94]. From work in animals it has been established that desferrioxamine can cause cataracts if used in very large doses and there has been one well-documented report of this occurrence in a thalassaemic child [94]. For this reason children being treated in this way should have regular ophthalmological surveillance.

There is some promising evidence that it is possible to obtain a negative iron balance in patients receiving desferrioxamine by subcutaneous infusion even if the drug is started in the first few years of life [260]. Preliminary follow-up data indicate that there is minimal tachyphylaxis and that as judged by serum ferritin levels there is improvement in liver function in children treated in this way [261]. However, it is too early to say whether the effects of cardiac iron loading will be reduced although this seems likely.

Desferrioxamine therapy by continuous infusion is unpleasant and in many countries the compliance rate is low. The drug is expensive as are the pumps required for its administration and this is far from an ideal form of therapy for these children. However, until an adequate oral chelating agent is developed this regime is by far the best hope for maintaining thalassaemic children in negative iron balance. If it is impossible to use the drug in this way at least some benefit can be obtained by the use of daily intramuscular injections at a dose regime outlined in Table 9.7.

Table 9.7. Approximate dose range (about 25 mg/kg) and method of administration for Desferrioxamine (I.M.) at different ages (from Ref. 89)

Weight range (kg)	Age (years)	Dose (mg)	Distilled water (ml)
15–25	3–6	500	1·5–2
25–35	7–12	750	2
35–45	13–puberty	1000	2–3
45–65	Post-pubertal	1500	4

Other chelating agents have been developed and tested. These include dihydroxybenzoic acid and rhodotorulic acid and their pharmacology and iron-chelating properties have been fully reviewed [262, 263]. At the time of writing they seem to have little place to play in the management of thalassaemia.

General management
Thalassaemic children should be looked after by a good general paediatrician with a special interest in the disease. They develop all the common childhood complaints, any of which may exacerbate their anaemia. They are particularly prone to infection although the precise reason for this is still far from clear [9]. The patterns of infection vary in different parts of the world. For example, streptococcal infections seem to be particularly common in Thailand whereas in the

United Kingdom infection with *Diplococcus pneumonia* or *Haemophilus influenzae* seems to be a particular danger, especially in the splenectomized child. Since all infective episodes are associated with a worsening of the anaemia they should be treated energetically with the appropriate antibiotic.

Endocrine dysfunction must be anticipated in any child over the age of 10 years. Diabetes mellitus is common and should be treated with insulin at the appropriate dosage. Other hormone-replacement therapy is not usually required although some children are treated with androgens to potentiate their sexual development. This should only be carried out with extreme care because of the problems of premature fusion of the epiphyses.

The cardiological complications of thalassaemia are extremely difficult to manage [264]. Recurrent pericarditis is seen in all populations and although there is some evidence that it is related to streptococcal infection in the Far East, this does not seem to be the case elsewhere. It has been variously ascribed to iron loading or to splenectomy but the whole field is extremely unsatisfactory and the underlying mechanism is far from clear. It should be treated symptomatically with analgesia and rest. When affected children develop arrythmias or cardiac failure they should be treated symptomatically, although once this occurs the prognosis is extremely poor.

In those children who have been poorly transfused and who have developed gross bone changes, a variety of problems may occur. Recurrent pathological fractures should be managed by the usual orthopaedic methods of immobilization and affected children should be placed on a high transfusion regime. Similarly, if deformities of the face lead to complications such as recurrent sinus and middle ear infection the child should be treated with appropriate antibiotics and maintained on an adequate transfusion regime. A variety of surgical procedures have been described for attempting to correct some of the frightful facial deformities which may occur in a poorly transfused child [265].

Thalassaemia intermedia
This disorder presents a particular challenge to the clinician. Should these children be transfused and how should their complications be managed? The real problem is that the condition is so heterogeneous and the clinical course so variable. In general, children with haemoglobin levels below 6–7 g/dl will develop poorly and have increasing deformity of their skeleton and are better transfused and placed on an iron-chelation regime. At higher haemoglobin levels they can be followed and if hypersplenism develops, splenectomy

can be carried out later in childhood. They require regular folate supplementation and management of infection and other complications as mentioned in the previous section.

There is no doubt that some of these patients become iron loaded due to increased gastrointestinal absorption of iron [238]. They should have regular checks of their serum iron and ferritin levels and if they are becoming iron loaded they should be treated with desferrioxamine accordingly. At the time of writing several groups are engaged in attempting to work out methods of reducing gastrointestinal iron loading in these patients. It would seem sensible to put them on to a vegetarian diet so as to reduce iron intake to a minimum. At the time of writing no one method for reducing gastrointestinal iron absorption seems to be entirely satisfactory.

THE DIAGNOSIS OF THE THALASSAEMIA SYNDROMES

The steps in the diagnosis of the different forms of thalassaemia include the initial recognition of the disease as a thalassaemic disorder, its further definition by appropriate haematological and haemoglobin analytical procedures and its differentiation from other congenital and acquired disorders of haemoglobin synthesis which can mimic the thalassaemia syndromes. It is beyond the scope of this chapter to describe the laboratory methods in detail and the reader is referred to several monographs which cover this topic [9, 266].

Haematological studies

The haematological features of the thalassaemias have been reviewed in previous sections. It is most important to examine a well-stained blood film and to obtain accurate values for red-cell indices, particularly the MCH and MCV. Brilliant cresyl blue preparations should be set up to look for Hb H inclusions and the peripheral blood and marrow should be stained with methyl violet where β thalassaemia is suspected. Inclusions with the staining properties of Heinz bodies can usually be observed in the bone marrow in the homozygous form of the disease and also in the peripheral blood after splenectomy. Additional investigations which are useful include the reticulocyte count, serum iron and total iron-binding capacities together with serum ferritin levels and investigations to assess the degree of haemolysis including serum bilirubin and haptoglobin levels and, in some cases, chromium-labelled red-cell survival studies combined with external scanning to determine the major sites of red-cell destruction.

Haemoglobin analysis

The haemoglobin constitution should be determined by electrophoresis on either cellulose acetate, starch gel or agar gel. The level of Hb F should be determined by one of the alkali denaturation techniques, and its intracellular distribution examined by the acid elution method. Methods for Hb A_2 estimation which depend on visualization of electrophoretic strips are unreliable and a quantitative estimation should be carried out using either cellulose acetate or starch block electrophoresis or chromatography on small DEAE-cellulose columns. Where Hb H disease is suspected, electrophoresis should be performed using a phosphate buffer system, pH 6·5–7·0, on either cellulose acetate or starch gel. Haemoglobins H and Bart's are the only haemoglobin variants which migrate towards the anode under these conditions.

The haemoglobin constitution in the α and β thalassaemias is summarized in Tables 9.2 and 9.3 respectively.

Differential diagnosis

There are a variety of congenital and acquired disorders of haemoglobin synthesis which can mimic thalassaemia.

The congenital haemolytic anaemias due to enzyme defects or other metabolic abnormalities of the red cell do not often pose a problem since they are usually associated with normochromic red cells. Although some of the unstable haemoglobin disorders may resemble thalassaemia there is usually a positive heat precipitation test or the presence of an abnormal haemoglobin on electrophoresis. Congenital sideroblastic anaemia may superficially resemble thalassaemia but it is usually inherited in a sex-linked fashion and thus males are affected. Furthermore, although there are some hypochromic cells the red-cell appearances are usually dimorphic with a normochromic population as well. The Hbs A_2 and F values are normal in this condition. The congenital dyserythropoietic anaemias are distinguished from thalassaemia by the morphological appearances of the marrow and normal levels of Hb A_2.

Of the acquired disorders which may mimic thalassaemia, easily the commonest is simple iron deficiency. On morphological grounds it may not be possible to distinguish this from thalassaemia trait, but in the latter the serum iron is usually normal and there is stainable iron in the bone marrow. Furthermore, the Hb A_2 value is elevated in β thalassaemia while it tends to be low in iron-deficiency anaemia. In patients with β thalassaemia who are also iron deficient the Hb A_2 value may fall and return to its abnormally high level after iron therapy [267]. The acquired sideroblastic anaemias can be clearly distinguished from the thalassaemias by the finding of normal levels of Hb A_2 and the presence of increased numbers of 'ring' sideroblasts in the bone marrow, which do not occur in thalassaemia.

There are a variety of acquired disorders which may occasionally alter the relative amounts of Hbs A and A_2 or produce increased levels of fetal haemoglobin in adult life. Some of these conditions are summarized in Table 9.8. They can be clearly distinguished from

Table 9.8. Some acquired changes of haemoglobin production or structure

---

Increased levels of haemoglobin F
  Juvenile chronic myeloid leukaemia
  Other forms of leukaemia
  Aplastic anaemia and PNH
  Rapid marrow regeneration after marrow
    transplantation or transient erythroblastopenia
  Myeloblastic anaemia
  Pregnancy
  Choriocarcinoma
  Other neoplastic disorders

Reduced levels of haemoglobin A_2
  Iron-deficiency anaemia
  Juvenile chronic myeloid leukaemia

Acquired haemoglobin H disease
  Leukaemia and myeloproliferative disorders

Post-synthetic modifications
  Diabetes mellitus
  Lead poisoning

---

thalassaemia on morphological grounds and on the absence of any family history. Haemoglobin H has been observed in elderly patients with leukaemia or preleukaemic states [268]. These patients have no family history of findings of thalassaemia, have a dimorphic blood film with normochromic and hypochromic cells, and show a more severe deficit of α-chain production than in the genetic form of the disease.

Occasionally in clinical practice a thalassaemia-like disorder can be recognized which does not fit into any of the criteria outlined in this chapter. In such cases it is important to study as many family members as possible since the finding of a more typical form of thalassaemia in a near relative may give some indication as to the genotype of the affected patient. For example the inheritance of both α and β thalassaemia can produce a bizarre clinical disorder with normal levels of Hbs A_2 and F. The condition can only be diagnosed by the finding of either α- or β-thalassae-

mia trait in other members of the family (see Table 9.6).

REFERENCES

1 COOLEY T.B. & LEE P. (1925) A series of cases of splenomegaly in children with anemia and peculiar bone changes. *Transactions of the American Pediatric Society*, **37**, 29.

2 WHIPPLE G.H. & BRADFORD W.L. (1936) Mediterranean disease-thalassemia (erythroblastic anemia of Cooley); associated pigment abnormalities simulating hemochromatosis. *Journal of Pediatrics*, **9**, 279.

3 CHINI V. & VALERI C.M. (1949) Mediterranean hemopathic syndromes. *Blood*, **4**, 989.

4 BANNERMAN R.M. (1961) *Thalassemia. A Survey of Some Aspects.* Grune & Stratton, New York.

5 WEATHERALL D.J. (1980) Toward an understanding of the molecular biology of some common inherited anemias: the story of thalassemia. In *Blood, Pure and Eloquent* (ed. Wintrobe M.M.), p. 373. McGraw-Hill, New York.

6 PAULING L. (1954) Abnormality of hemoglobin molecules in hereditary hemolytic anemias. *The Harvey Lectures 1954–55.* Academic Press, New York.

7 ITANO H.A. (1957) The human hemoglobins: their properties and genetic control. *Advances in Protein Chemistry*, **12**, 216.

8 INGRAM V.M. & STRETTON A.O.W. (1959) Genetic basis of the thalassaemia diseases. *Nature (London)*, **184**, 1903.

9 WEATHERALL D.J. & CLEGG J.B. (1981) *The Thalassaemia Syndromes*, 3rd edn. Blackwell Scientific Publications, Oxford.

10 SCHROEDER W.A., HUISMAN T.H.J., SHELTON R., SHELTON J.B., KLEIHAUER E.F., DOZY A.M. & ROBBERSON B. (1968) Evidence for multiple structural genes for the γ-chain of human fetal hemoglobin. *Proceedings of the National Academy of Sciences, USA*, **60**, 537.

11 DEISSEROTH A., NIENHUIS A., TURNER P., VELEZ R., ANDERSON W.F., RUDDLE F., LAWRENCE J., CREAGAN R. & KUCHERLAPATI R. (1977) Localization of the human α-globin structural gene to chromosome 16 in somatic cell hybrids by molecular hybridization. *Cell*, **12**, 205.

12 DEISSEROTH A., NIENHUIS A., LAWRENCE J., RILES R., TURNER P. & RUDDLE F. (1978) Chromosomal localization of human β globin gene on chromosome 11 in somatic cell hybrids. *Proceedings of the National Academy of Sciences, USA*, **75**, 1456.

13 DOTY P., MARMUR J., EIGNER J. & SCHILDKRAUT, C. (1960) Strand separation and specific recombination in deoxyribunucleic acids: physical chemical studies. *Proceedings of the National Academy of Sciences, USA*, **46**, 461.

14 HALL B.D. & SPIEGELMAN S. (1960) Sequence complimentary of T2 DNA and T2-specific RNA. *Proceedings of the National Academy of Sciences, USA*, **47**, 137.

15 BRITTEN R.J. & KOHNE D.E. (1968) Repeated sequences in DNA. *Science*, **161**, 529.

16 TEMIN H.M. & MIZUTANI S. (1970) RNA-dependent

DNA polymerase in virions of Rous sarcoma virus. *Nature (London)*, **226**, 1211.

17 BALTIMORE D. (1970) RNA-dependent polymerase in virions of RNA tumor viruses. *Nature (London)*, **226**, 1209.

18 KACIAN D.L., SPIEGELMAN S., BANK A., TERADA M., METAFORA S., DOW L.W. & MARKS P.A. (1972) *In vitro* synthesis of DNA components of human genes for globin. *Nature (New Biology)*, **235**, 167.

19 ROSS J., AVIV H., SCOLNICK E. & LEDER P. (1972) *In vitro* synthesis of DNA complementary to purified rabbit globin mRNA. *Proceedings of the National Academy of Sciences, USA*, **69**, 264.

20 VERMA I.M., TEMPLE G.F., FAN H. & BALTIMORE D. (1972) *In vitro* synthesis of DNA complementary to rabbit reticulocyte 10S RNA. *Nature (New Biology)*, **235**, 163.

21 TAYLOR J.M., DOZY A., KAN Y.W., VARMUS H.E., LIE-INJO L.E., GANESON J, & TODD D. (1974) Genetic lesion in homozygous α thalassaemia (hydrops fetalis). *Nature (London)*, **251**, 392.

22 OTTOLENGHI S., LANYON W.G., PAUL J., WILLIAMSON R., WEATHERALL D.J., CLEGG J.B., PRITCHARD J., POOTRAKUL S. & WONG H.B. (1974) The severe form of α thalassaemia is caused by a haemoglobin gene deletion. *Nature (London)*, **251**, 389.

23 SOUTHERN E.M. (1975) Detection of specific sequences among DNA fragments separated by gel electrophoresis. *Journal of Molecular Biology*, **98**, 503.

24 MANIATIS T., HARDISON R.C., LACY E., LAUER J., O'CONNELL C., QUON D., SIM G.K. & EFSTRATIADIS A. (1978) The isolation of structural genes from libraries of eukaryotic DNA. *Cell*, **15**, 687.

25 LAWN R.M., FRITSCH E.F., PORTER R.C., BLAKE G. & MANIATIS T. (1978) The isolation and characterisation of linked δ- and β-globin genes from a cloned library of human DNA. *Cell*, **15**, 1157.

26 FLAVELL R.A., KOOTER J.M., DE BOER E., LITTLE P.F.R. & WILLIAMSON R. (1978) Analysis of the β-δ-globin gene loci in normal and Hb Lepore DNA: Direct determination of gene linkage and intergene distance. *Cell*, **15**, 25.

27 MEARS J.G., RAMIREZ F., LEIBOWITZ D. & BANK A. (1978) Organization of human δ- and β-globin genes in cellular DNA and the presence of intragenic inserts. *Cell*, **15**, 15.

28 MEARS J.G., RAMIREZ F., LIEBOWTIZ D., NAKAURA F., BLOOM A., KONOTEY-AHULU F.I.D. & BANK A. (1978) Changes in restricted human cellular DNA fragments containing globin gene sequences in thalassemias and related disorders. *Proceedings of the National Academy of Sciences, USA*, **75**, 1222.

29 SMITHIES O., BLECHL A.E., DENNISTON-THOMPSON K., NEWELL N., RICHARDS J.E., SLIGHTOM J.L., TUCKER P.W. & BLATTNER F.R. (1978) Cloning human fetal γ globin and mouse α-type globin DNA: characterization and partial sequencing. *Science*, **202**, 1284.

30 BERNARDS R., LITTLE P.F.R., ANNISON G., WILLIAMSON R. & FLAVELL R.A. (1979) Structure of the human $^G\gamma$-$^A\gamma$-δ-β-globin gene locus. *Proceedings of the National Academy of Sciences, USA*, **76**, 4827.

31 LITTLE P.F.R., FLAVELL R.A., KOOTER J.M., ANNISON G. & WILLIAMSON R. (1979) Structure of the human fetal globin gene locus. *Nature (London)*, **278**, 227.

32 PROUDFOOT N.J. & BARALLE F.E. (1979) Molecular cloning of the human ε-globin gene. *Proceedings of the National Academy of Sciences, USA*, **76**, 5435.

33 LAUER J., SHEN C.-K.J. & MANIATIS T. (1980) The chromosomal arrangement of human α-like globin genes: Sequence homology and α-globin gene deletions. *Cell*, **20**, 119.

34 LEDER P. (1978) Discontinuous genes. *New England Journal of Medicine*, **298**, 1079.

35 JEFFREYS A.J. (1979) DNA sequence variants in the $^G\gamma$-, $^A\gamma$-, δ- and β-globin genes of man. *Cell*, **18**, 1.

36 MILLER H.I., KONKEL D.A. & LEDER P. (1978) An intervening sequence of the mouse β-globin major gene shares extensive homology only with β-globin genes. *Nature (London)*, **275**, 772.

37 SCHMID C.W. & DEININGER P.L. (1975) Sequence organisation of the human genome. *Cell*, **6**, 345.

38 DAVIDSON E.H. & BRITTEN R.J. (1973) Organization, transcription and regulation of the animal genome. *Quarterly Review of Biology*, **48**, 565.

39 WEINTRAUB H. & GROUNDLINE M. (1976) Chromosomal subunits in active genes have an altered conformation. *Science*, **193**, 848.

40 GAREL A. & AXEL R. (1976) Selective digestion of transcriptionally active ovalbumin genes from oviduct nuclei. *Proceedings of the National Academy of Sciences, USA*, **73**, 3966.

41 BRITTEN R.J. & DAVIDSON E.H. (1969) Gene regulation for higher cells: A theory. *Science*, **165**, 349.

42 WILSON G.N., STEGGLES A.W. & KANTOR J.A. (1975) Cell-free transcription of mammalian chromatin: quantitative measurement of newly synthesised globin messenger RNA sequences. *Journal of Biological Chemistry*, **250**, 8604.

43 PAUL J., GILMOUR R.S., AFFARA N., BIRNIE G., HARRISON P., HELL A., HUMPHRIES S.M., WINDASS J. & YOUNG B. (1973) The globin genes: structure and expression. *Cold Spring Harbor Symposium on Quantitative Biology*, **38**, 885.

44 GILMOUR R.S. & PAUL J. (1973) Tissue-specific transcription of the globin gene in isolated chromatin. *Proceedings of the National Academy of Sciences, USA*, **70**, 3440.

45 NIENHUIS A.W. & BENZ E.J. (1977) Regulation of hemoglobin synthesis during the development of the red cell. Parts 1, 2 and 3, *New England Journal of Medicine*, **297**, 1313, 1371 and 1430.

46 CHAMBON P. (1975) Eukaryotic nuclear RNA polymerases. *Annual Review of Biochemistry*, **44**, 613.

47 ROEDER R.G. (1976) *Eukaryotic nuclear RNA polymerases, RNA polymerase* (ed. Lossick R. & Chamberlain M.), p. 285. Cold Spring Harbor Monograph Series.

48 ROSS J. (1976) A precursor of globin messenger RNA. *Journal of Molecular Biology*, **106**, 403.

49 HAYNES J.R., KALB F., ROSTEK P. & LINGREL J.B. (1978) The absence of a precursor larger than 16S to globin messenger RNA. *FEBS Letters*, **91**, 173.

50 BASTOS R.N. & AVIV H. (1977) Globin RNA precursor molecules: biosynthesis and processing in erythroid cells. *Cell*, **11**, 641.

51 KINNIBURGH A.J. & ROSS J. (1979) Processing of the mouse β-globin mRNA precursor: at least two cleavage-

ligation reactions are necessary to excise the larger intervening sequence. *Cell*, **17**, 915.

52 FORGET B.G. (1977) Nucleotide sequence of human β-globin messenger RNA. *Hemoglobin*, **1**, 879.

53 PROUDFOOT N.J. & LONGLEY J.I. (1976) The 3′ terminal sequences of human α- and β-globin messenger RNAs: comparison with rabbit globin messenger RNA. *Cell*, **9**, 733.

54 CHANG J.G., TEMPLE G.F., POON R., NEUMAN K.H. & KAN Y.W. (1977) The nucleotide sequences of the untranslated 5′ region of human α- and β-globin mRNAs. *Proceedings of the National Academy of Sciences, USA*, **74**, 5145.

55 MAROTTA C.A., WILSON J.T., FORGET B.G. & WEISSMAN S.M. (1977) Human β-chain messenger RNA. II. Nucleotide sequences derived from complementary DNA. *Journal of Biological Chemistry*, **252**, 5040.

56 PROUDFOOT N.J. (1977) Complete 3′ non-coding region sequences of rabbit and human β-globin messenger RNAs. *Cell*, **10**, 559.

57 SHATKIN A.J. (1976) Capping of eukaryotic mRNAs. *Cell*, **9**, 645.

58 LODISH H.F. (1976) Translational control of protein synthesis. *Annual Review of Biochemistry*, **45**, 39.

59 REVEL M. & GRONER Y. (1978) Post-transcriptional and translational controls of gene expression in eukaryotes. *Annual Review of Biochemistry*, **47**, 1079.

60 SHAFRITZ D.A., WEINSTEIN J.A., SOFER B., MERRICK W.C., WEBER L.A., HICKEY E.D. & BAGLIONI C. (1976) Evidence for role of $m^7G^{5'}$-phosphate group in recognition of eukaryotic mRNA by initiation factor IF-M₃. *Nature (London)*, **261**, 291.

61 LIM L. & CANELLAKIS E.S. (1970) Adenine-rich polymer associated with rabbit reticulocyte messenger RNA. *Nature (London)*, **227**, 710.

62 BURR H. & LINGREL J.B. (1971) Poly A sequences at the 3′ termini or rabbit globin mRNAS. *Nature (New Biology)*, **233**, 41.

63 MARBAIX G., HUEZ G. & BURNY A. (1975) Absence of polyadenylate segment in globin messenger RNA accelerates its degradation in *Xenopus* oocytes. *Proceedings of the National Academy of Sciences, USA*, **72**, 3065.

64 MANIATIS G.M., RAMIREZ F., CANN A., MARKS P.A. & BANK A. (1976) Translation and stability of human globin mRNA in *Xenopus* oocytes. *Journal of Clinical Investigation*, **58**, 1419.

65 PROUDFOOT N.J. & BROWNLEE G.G. (1976) Nucleotide sequences of globin messenger RNA. *British Medical Bulletin*, **32**, 251.

66 PROUDFOOT N.J., GILLAM S., SMITH M. & LONGLEY J.I. (1971) Nucleotide sequence of the 3′ terminal third of rabbit α-globin messenger RNA: comparison with human α-globin messenger RNA. *Cell*, **11**, 807.

67 DINTZIS H.M. (1961) Assembly of the peptide chains of hemoglobin. *Proceedings of the National Academy of Sciences, USA*, **47**, 247.

68 GRANICK S. & LEVERE R.D. (1964) Heme synthesis in erythroid cells. *Progress in Hematology*, **IV**, 1.

69 BAGLIONI C. & COLOMBO B. (1964) Control of hemoglobin synthesis. *Cold Spring Harbor Symposium on Quantitative Biology*, **29**, 347.

70 CLEGG J.B. & WEATHERALL D.J. (1972) Haemoglobin synthesis during erythroid maturation in β thalassaemia. *Nature (London)*, **240**, 190.

71 BAGLIONI C. & CAMPANA T. (1967) α chain and globin: intermediates in the synthesis of rabbit globin. *European Journal of Biochemistry*, **2**, 480.

72 FELICETTI L., COLOMBO B. & BAGLIONI C. (1966) Assembly of haemoglobin. *Biochimica et Biophysica Acta*, **129**, 380.

73 WINTERHALTER K.H. & HUEHNS E.R. (1964) Preparation, properties and specific recombination of αβ-globin subunits. *Journal of Biological Chemistry*, **239**, 3699.

74 HUEHNS E.R. (1970) The unstable haemoglobins. *Bulletin de la Societe de Chimie Biologique*, **52**, 1131.

75 deSIMONE J., KLEVE L., LONGLEY M.A. & SHAEFFER J. (1974) Rapid turnover of newly synthesised $β^S$ chains in reticulocytes from individuals with sickle-cell trait. *Biochemical and Biophysical Research Communications*, **57**, 248.

76 WASI P., NA-NAKORN S., POOTRAKUL S., SOOKANEK M., DISTHASONGCHAN P., PORNPATKUL M. & PANICH V. (1969) Alpha- and β-thalassemia in Thailand. *Annals of the New York Academy of Sciences*, **165**, 60.

77 ORKIN S.H., OLD J.M., WEATHERALL D.J. & NATHAN D.G. (1979) Partial deletion of β-globin gene DNA in certain patients with $β^0$ thalassemia. *Proceedings of the National Academy of Sciences, USA*, **76**, 2400.

78 ORKIN S.H., KOLONDER R., MICHELSON A. & HUSSON R. (1980) Cloning and direct examination of a structurally abnormal human $β^0$-thalassemia globin gene. *Proceedings of the National Academy of Sciences, USA*, **77**, 3586.

79 FORGET B.G., BALTIMORE D., BENZ E.J., HOUSMAN D., LEBOWITZ P., MAROTTA C.A., McCAFFREY R.P., SKOULTCHI A., SWERDLOW P.S., VERNON I.M. & WEISSMAN S.M. (1974) Globin messenger RNA in the thalassemia syndromes. *Annals of the New York Academy of Sciences*, **232**, 76.

80 FORGET B.G., HILLMAN D.G., COHEN-SOLAL M. & PRENSKY W. (1976) Beta-globin messenger RNA in $β^0$ thalassemia. *Blood*, **48**, 998.

81 HOUSMAN D., FORGET B.G., SKOULTCHI A. & BENZ E.J. (1973) Quantitative deficiency of chain-specific messenger ribonucleic acids in the thalassemia syndromes. *Proceedings of the National Academy of Sciences, USA*, **70**, 1809.

82 TOLSTOSHEV P., MITCHELL J., LANYON G., WILLIAMSON R., OTTOLENGHI S., COMI P., GIGLIONI B., MASERA G., MODELL B., WEATHERALL D.J. & CLEGG J.B. (1976) Presence of gene for β globin in homozygous $β^0$ thalassaemia. *Nature (London)*, **260**, 95.

83 OLD J.M., PROUDFOOT N.J., WOOD W.G., LONGLEY J.I., CLEGG J.B. & WEATHERALL D.J. (1978) Characterization of β-globin mRNA in the $β^0$ thalassemias. *Cell*, **14**, 289.

84 BENZ E.J., FORGET B.G., HILLMAN D.G., COHEN-SOLAL M., PRITCHARD J. & CAVALLESCO C. (1978) Variability in the amount of β-globin mRNA in $β^0$ thalassemia. *Cell*, **14**, 299.

85 CHANG J.C. & KAN Y.W. (1979) $β^0$ thalassemia, a nonsense mutation in man. *Proceedings of the National Academy of Sciences, USA*, **76**, 2886.

86 CHANG J.C., TEMPLE G.F., TRECARTIN R.F. & KAN

Y.W. (1979) Suppression of the nonsense mutation in homozygous β^0 thalassaemia. *Nature (London)*, **281**, 602.

87 CONCONI F., ROWLEY P.T., DEL SENNO L., PONTREMOLI S. & VOLPATO S. (1972) Induction of β-globin synthesis in the β thalassaemia of Ferrara. *Nature (New Biology)*, **238**, 83.

88 NIENHUIS A.W., TURNER P., & BENZ E.J. (1977) Relative stability of α- and β-globin messenger RNAs in homozygous β^+ thalassemia. *Proceedings of the National Academy of Sciences, USA*, **74**, 3960.

89 MODELL C.B. (1976) Management of thalassaemia major. *British Medical Bulletin*, **32**, 270.

90 MODELL C.B. *et al.* (1981) In preparation.

91 BLENDIS L.M., MODELL C.B., BOWDLER A.J. & WILLIAMS R. (1974) Some effects of splenectomy in thalassaemia major. *British Journal of Haematology*, **28**, 77.

92 LUHBY A.L. & COOPERMAN J.M. (1961) Folic-acid deficiency in thalassaemia major. *Lancet*, **ii**, 490.

93 LOGOTHETIS J., CONSTANTOULAKIS M., ECONOMIDOU J., STEFANIS C., HAKAS P., AUGOUSTAKI O., SOFRONIADOU K., LOEWENSON R. & BILEK M. (1972) Thalassemia major (homozygous β-thalassaemia): a survey of 138 cases with emphasis on neurological and muscular aspects. *Neurology*, **22**, 294.

94 MODELL C.B. (1977) Total management in thalassaemia major. *Archives of Diseases of Childhood*, **52**, 489.

95 WASI P. (1971) Streptococcal infection leading to cardiac and renal involvement in thalassaemia. *Lancet*, **i**, 949.

96 HYMAN C.B., LANDING B., ALFIN-SLATER R., KOZAK L., WEITZMAN J. & ORTEGA J.A. (1974) Dl-α-tocopherol, iron and lipofuscin in thalassemia. *Annals of the New York Academy of Sciences*, **232**, 211.

97 CROSS J.N., MORGAN O.S., GIBBS W.N. & CHERUVANKY I. (1977) Spinal cord compression in thalassaemia. *Journal of Neurology, Neurosurgery and Psychiatry*, **40**, 1120.

98 MCINTOSH N. (1976) Endocrinopathy in thalassaemia major. *Archives of Disease of Childhood*, **51**, 195.

99 EAGLE M.A. (1964) Cardiac involvement in Cooley's anemia. *Annals of the New York Academy of Sciences*, **119**, 694.

100 HENRY W.L., NIENHUIS A.W., WIENER M., MILLER D.R., CANALE V.C. & PIOMELLI S. (1978) Echocardiographic abnormalities in patients with transfusion-dependent anemia and secondary myocardial iron deposition. *American Journal of Medicine*, **64**, 547.

101 FESSAS P. (1963) Inclusions of hemoglobin in erythroblasts and erythrocytes of thalassemia. *Blood*, **21**, 21.

102 POLLIACK A. & RACHMILEWITZ E.A. (1973) Ultrastructural studies in β thalassaemia major. *British Journal of Haematology*, **24**, 319.

103 POLLIACK A., YATAGANAS X. & RACHMILEWITZ E.A. (1975) Ultrastructure of the inclusion bodies and nuclear abnormalities in β-thalassemic erythroblasts. *Annals of the New York Academy of Sciences*, **232**, 261.

104 WICKRAMASINGHE S.N. & BUSH V. (1975) Observations on the ultrastructure of erythropoietic cells and reticulum cells in the bone marrow of patients with homozygous β thalassaemia. *British Journal of Haematology*, **30**, 395.

105 WICKRAMASINGHE S.N. (1976) The morphology and kinetics of erythropoiesis in homozygous β-thalassaemia. *Congenital Disorders of Erythropoiesis*, Ciba Foundation Symposium, p. 221. North-Holland, Amsterdam.

106 ASTALDI G., RONDANELLI E.G., BERNADELLI E. & STROSSELLI E. (1954) An abnormal substance present in the erythroblasts of thalassaemia major. Cytochemical investigations. *Acta Haematologica*, **12**, 145.

107 YATAGANAS X., GAHRTON G., FESSAS P., KESSE-ELIAS M. & THORELL B. (1973) Proliferative activity and glycogen accumulation of erythroblasts in β-thalassaemia. *British Journal of Haematology*, **24**, 651.

108 ZAINO E.C. & ROSSI M.B. (1974) Ultrastructure of the erythrocytes in β-thalassemia. *Annals of the New York Academy of Sciences*, **232**, 238.

109 WICKRAMASINGHE S.N., MCELWAIN T.J., COOPER E.H. & HARDISTY R.M. (1970) Proliferation of erythroblasts in β-thalassaemia. *British Journal of Haematology*, **19**, 719.

110 HILLCOAT B.L. & WATERS A.H. (1962) The survival of ^{51}Cr-labelled autotransfused red cells in a patient with thalassaemia. *Australian Medical Journal*, **11**, 55.

111 HEINRICH H.C., GABBE E.E., OPPITZ K.H., WHANG D.H., BENDER-GOTZE C., SCHAFER K.H., SCHROTER W. & PFAU A.A. (1973) Absorption of inorganic and food iron in children with heterozygous and homozygous β-thalassemia. *Zeitschrift für Kinderheilkunde*, **115**, 1.

112 FINCH C.A., DEUBELBEISS, K., COOK J.D., ESCHBACH J.W., HARKNER L.A., FUNK D.D., MARSAGLIA G., HILLMAN R.S., SLICHTER S., ADAMSON J.W., GANZONI A. & GILBETT E.R. (1970) Ferrokinetics in man. *Medicine*, **49**, 17.

113 SHEPARD M.K., WEATHERALL D.J. & CONLEY C.L. (1962) Semi-quantitative estimation of the distribution of fetal hemoglobin in red-cell populations. *Bulletin of the Johns Hopkins Hospital*, **110**, 293.

114 FESSAS P. & LOUKOPOULOS D. (1964) Alpha-chain of human hemoglobin: occurrence *in vivo*. *Science*, **143**, 590.

115 FESSAS P. & LOUKOPOULOS D. (1974) The β thalassaemias. *Clinics in Haematology*, **3**, 411.

116 FESSAS P., KONIAVITIS A. & ZEIS P.M. (1969) Urinary β-aminoisobutyric acid excretion in thalassaemia. *Journal of Clinical Pathology*, **22**, 154.

117 KREIMER-BIRNBAUM M., RUSNAK P.A., BANNERMAN R.M. & GLASS U. (1974) Urinary pyrrole pigments in thalassemia and unstable hemoglobin diseases. *Annals of the New York Academy of Sciences*, **232**, 283.

118 HAMMOND G.D., ISHIKAWA A. & KEIGHLEY G. (1962) Relationship between erythropoietin and severity of anemia in hypoplastic and hemolytic states. In *Erythropoiesis* (ed. Jacobson L.O. & Doyle M.), p. 351. Grune & Stratton, New York.

119 MODELL C.B. & BECK J. (1974) Long-term desferrioxamine therapy in thalassemia. *Annals of the New York Academy of Sciences*, **232**, 201.

120 WEATHERALL D.J., CLEGG J.B., & NAUGHTON M.A. (1965) Globin synthesis in thalassaemia: an *in vitro* study. *Nature (London)*, **208**, 1061.

121 WEATHERALL D.J., CLEGG J.B., NA-NAKORN S. & WASI P. (1969) The pattern of disordered haemoglobin synthesis in homozygous and heterozygous β-thalassaemia. *British Journal of Haematology*, **16**, 251.

122 BANK A. & MARKS P.A. (1966) Excess α-chain synthesis relative to β-chain synthesis in thalassaemia major and minor. *Nature (London)*, **212**, 1198.

123 BARGELLESI A., PONTREMOLI S. & CONCONI F. (1967) Absence of β-globin synthesis and excess α-globin synthesis in homozygous β thalassemia. *European Journal of Biochemistry*, **1**, 73.

124 MODELL C.B., LATTER A., STEADMAN J.H. & HUEHNS E.R. (1968) Haemoglobin synthesis in β thalassaemia. *British Journal of Haematology*, **17**, 485.

125 NATHAN D.G. & GUNN R.B. (1966) Thalassemia: the consequences of unbalanced hemoglobin synthesis. *American Journal of Medicine*, **41**, 815.

126 GABUZDA T.G., NATHAN D.G. & GARDNER F.H. (1963) The turnover of hemoglobins A, F and A₂ in the peripheral blood of three patients with thalassemia. *Journal of Clinical Investigation*, **42**, 1678.

127 BRAVERMAN A.S. & BANK A. (1969) Changing rates of globin-chain synthesis during erythroid cell maturation in thalassemia. *Journal of Molecular Biology*, **42**, 57.

128 WEATHERALL D.J., CLEGG J.B., ROBERTS A.V. & KNOX-MACAULAY H.H.M. (1974) The clinical and chemical heterogeneity of the β thalassemias. *Annals of the New York Academy of Sciences*, **232**, 88.

129 NATHAN D.G. & BENZ E.J. (1976) Pathophysiology of the anaemia of thalassaemia. *Congenital Disorders of Erythropoiesis*, Ciba Foundation Symposium, p. 25. North-Holland, Amsterdam.

130 NATHAN D.G., STOSSEL T.B., GUNN R.B., ZARKOWSKY H.S. & LAFORET M.T. (1969) Influence of hemoglobin precipitation on erythrocyte metabolism in α and β thalassemia. *Journal of Clinical Investigation*, **48**, 33.

131 CARRELL R.W., WINTERBOURN C.C. & RACHMILEWITZ E.A. (1975) Annotation—Activated oxygen and haemolysis. *British Journal of Haematology*, **30**, 259.

132 RACHMILEWITZ E.A. (1974) Denaturation of the normal and abnormal hemoglobin molecule. *Seminars in Hematology*, **11**, 441.

133 RACHMILEWITZ E.A. (1976) Role of Heinz bodies in hemolysis of red blood cell (RBC) in thalassemia: the need for alternative concepts. *Birth Defects: Original Article Series*, **12**, 123.

134 KNOX-MACAULAY H.H.M. & WEATHERALL D.J. (1974) Studies of red-cell membrane function in heterozygous β thalassaemia and other hypochromic anaemias. *British Journal of Haematology*, **28**, 277.

135 CAZZOLA M., ALESSANDRINO P., BAROSI G., MORANDI S. & STEFANELLI M. (1979) Quantitative evaluation of the mechanisms of the anaemia in heterozygous β thalassaemia. *Scandinavian Journal of Haematology*, **23**, 107.

136 SCHWARTZ E. (1970) Heterozygous β thalassaemia: balanced globin synthesis in bone-marrow cells. *Science*, **167**, 1513.

137 WICKRAMASINGHE S.N., HUGHES M., HIGGS D.R. & WEATHERALL D.J. (1981) Ultrastructure of red cells containing haemoglobin H inclusions induced by redox dyes. *Clinical and Laboratory Haematology*, **3**, 51.

138 SCHWARTZ E. (1969) The silent carrier of β thalassaemia. *New England Journal of Medicine*, **281**, 1327.

139 KATTAMIS C., MATAXATOU-MAVROMATI A., WOOD W.G., NASH J.R. & WEATHERALL D.J. (1979) The heterogeneity of normal Hb A₂-β thalassaemia in Greece. *British Journal of Haematology*, **42**, 109.

140 BIANCO I., GRAZIANI B. & CARBONI C. (1977) Genetic patterns in thalassemia intermedia (constitutional microcytic anemia). Familial, hematologic and biosynthetic studies. *Human Heredity*, **27**, 257.

141 SCHOKKER R.C., WENT L.N. & BOK J. (1966) A new genetic variant of β thalassaemia. *Nature (London)*, **209**, 44.

142 FESSAS P. (1980) Personal communication.

143 ADAMS J.G., BOXER L.A., BAEHNER R.L., FORGET B.G., TSISTRAKIS G.A. & STEINBERG M.H. (1979) Hemoglobin Indianapolis (β112[G14]arginine). An unstable β-chain variant producing the phenotype of severe β thalassemia. *Journal of Clinical Investigation*, **63**, 931.

144 WEATHERALL D.J., CLEGG J.B., KNOX-MACAULAY H.H.M., BUNCH C., HOPKINS C.R. & TEMPERLEY I.J. (1973) A genetically determined disorder with features both of thalassaemia and congenital dyserythropoietic anaemia. *British Journal of Haematology*, **24**, 679.

145 STAMATOYANNOPOULOS G., PAPAYANNOPOULOU T., WOODSON R., HEYWOOD D. & KURACHI S. (1974) A new form of β-thalassemia trait. *Annals of the New York Academy of Sciences*, **232**, 159.

146 WOOD W.G., CLEGG J.B. & WEATHERALL D.J. (1979) Annotation—Hereditary persistence of fetal haemoglobin (HPFH) and δβ thalassaemia. *British Journal of Haematology*, **43**, 509.

147a ORKIN S.H., ALTER B.P. & ALTAY C. (1979) Deletion of the ᴬγ-globin gene in ᴳγ δβ-thalassemia. *Journal of Clinical Investigation*, **64**, 866.

147b FRITSCH E.F., LAWN R.M. & MANIATIS T. (1979) Characterisation of deletions which affect the expression of fetal globin genes in man. *Nature (London)*, **279**, 598.

148 GERALD P.S. & DIAMOND L.K. (1958) The diagnosis of thalassemia trait by starch block electrophoresis of the hemoglobin. *Blood*, **13**, 61.

149 BAGLIONI C. (1962) The fusion of two peptide chains in hemoglobin Lepore and its interpretation as a genetic deletion. *Proceedings of the National Academy of Sciences, USA*, **48**, 1880.

150 NEEB H., BEIBOER J.L., JONXIS J.H.P., SIJPESTEIJN J.A.K. & MULLER C.J. (1961) Homozygous Lepore haemoglobin disease appearing as thalassaemia major in two Papuan siblings. *Tropical and Geographic Medicine*, **13**, 207.

151 OSTERTAG W. & SMITH E.W. (1969) Hemoglobin Lepore Baltimore, a third type of δβ crossover (δ^{50}, β^{86}). *European Journal of Biochemistry*, **10**, 371.

152 EFREMOV G.D. (1978) Hemoglobin Lepore and anti-Lepore. *Hemoglobin*, **2**, 197.

153 LABIE D., SCHROEDER W.A. & HUISMAN T.H.J. (1966) The amino acid sequence of the δ-β chains of haemoglobin Lepore_Augusta = Lepore_Washington. *Biochimica et Biophysica Acta*, **127**, 428.

154 WOOD W.G., OLD J.M., ROBERTS A.V.S., CLEGG J.B., WEATHERALL D.J. & QUATTRIN N. (1978) Human globin gene expression: control of β-, δ- and δβ-chain production. *Cell*, **15**, 437.

155 STAMATOYANNOPOULOS G. & FESSAS P. (1963) Observations of hemoglobin 'Pylos': the hemoglobin Pylos-hemoglobin S combination. *Journal of Laboratory and Clinical Medicine*, **62**, 193.

156 ABU-SIN A., FELICE A.E., GRAVELY M.E., WILSON J.B.,

REESE A.L., LAM H., MILLER A. & HUISMAN T.H.J. (1979) Hb P-Nilotic in association with β^0-thalassemia: *cis*-mutation of a hemoglobin β^A-chain regulatory determinant. *Journal of Laboratory and Clinical Medicine*, **93**, 973.

157 SCHROEDER W.A., HUISMAN T.H.J., HYMAN C., SHELTON J.R. & APELL G. (1973) An individual with 'Miyada'- like hemoglobin indistinguishable from hemoglobin A$_2$. *Biochemical Genetics*, **10**, 135.

158 EDINGTON G.M. & LEHMANN H. (1955) Expression of the sickle-cell gene in Africa. *British Medical Journal*, **i**, 1308.

159 EDINGTON G.M. & LEHMANN H. (1955) Expression of the sickle-cell gene in Africa. *British Medical Journal*, **ii**, 1328.

160 JACOB G.F. & RAPER A.B. (1958) Hereditary persistence of foetal haemoglobin production, and its interaction with the sickle-cell trait. *British Journal of Haematology*, **4**, 138.

161 BOYER S.H., MARGOLET L., BOYER M.L., HUISMAN T.H.J., SCHROEDER W.A., WOOD W.G., WEATHERALL D.J., CLEGG J.B. & CARTNER R. (1977) Inheritance of F-cell frequency in heterocellular hereditary persistence of fetal hemoglobin: An example of allelic exclusion. *American Journal of Human Genetics*, **29**, 256.

162 HUISMAN T.H.J., MILLER A., COOK L., GORDON S. & SCHROEDER W.A. (1975) The molecular heterogeneity of some types of hereditary persistence of fetal hemoglobin (HPFH). *International Istanbul Symposium on Abnormal Hemoglobins and Thalassemia* (ed. Aksoy M.), p. 95.

163 HUISMAN T.H.J., SCHROEDER W.A., STAMATOYANNOPOULOS G., BOUVER N., SHELTON J.R., SHELTON J.B. & APELL G. (1970) Nature of fetal hemoglobin in the Greek type of hereditary persistence of fetal hemoglobin with and without concurrent β thalassaemia. *Journal of Clinical Investigation*, **49**, 1035.

164 HUISMAN T.H.J., SCHROEDER W.A., EFREMOV G.D., DUMA H., MLADENOVSKY B., HYMAN C.B., RACHMILEWITZ E.A., BOUVER N., MILLER A., BRODIE A., SHELTON J.R., SHELTON J.B. & APELL G. (1974) The present status of the heterogeneity of fetal hemoglobin in β thalassaemia; an attempt to unify some observations in thalassaemia and related conditions. *Annals of the New York Academy of Sciences*, **232**, 107.

165 CONLEY C.L., WEATHERALL D.J., RICHARDSON S.N., SHEPARD M.K. & CHARACHE S. (1963) Hereditary persistence of fetal hemoglobin: a study of 79 affected persons in 15 Negro families in Baltimore. *Blood*, **21**, 261.

166 HUISMAN T.H.J., MILLER A. & SCHROEDER W.A. (1975) A $^{G}\gamma$ type of the hereditary persistence of fetal hemoglobin with β-chain production in cis. *American Journal of Human Genetics*, **27**, 765.

167 HIGGS D.R., CLEGG J.B., WOOD W.G. & WEATHERALL D.J. (1979) $^{G}\gamma\beta^+$ type of hereditary persistence of fetal haemoglobin in association with Hb C. *Journal of Medical Genetics*, **16**, 288.

168 HUISMAN T.H.J., WRIGHSTONE R.N., WILSON J.B., SCHROEDER W.A. & KENDALL A.G. (1972) Hemoglobin Kenya, the product of fusion of γ and β polypeptide chains. *Archives of Biochemistry and Biophysics*, **153**, 850.

169 SMITH D.H., CLEGG J.B., WEATHERALL D.J. & GILLES H.M. (1973) Hereditary persistence of foetal haemoglobin associated with a $\gamma\beta$-fusion variant, Haemoglobin Kenya. *Nature (New Biology)*, **246**, 184.

170 FESSAS P. & STAMATOYANNOPOULOS G. (1964) Hereditary persistence of fetal hemoglobin in Greece. A study and a comparison. *Blood*, **24**, 223.

171 CLEGG J.B., METAXATOU-MAVROMATI A., KATTAMIS C., SOFRONIADOU K., WOOD W.G. & WEATHERALL D.J. (1979) Occurrence of $^{G}\gamma$ Hb F in Greek HPFH: Analysis of heterozygotes and compound heterozygotes with β thalassaemia. *British Journal of Haematology*, **43**, 531.

172 KAN Y.W., HOLLAND J.P., DOZY A.M., CHARACHE S. & KAZAZIAN H.H. (1975) Deletion of β-globin structural gene in hereditary persistence of foetal haemoglobin. *Nature (London)*, **258**, 162.

173 FORGET B.G., HILLMAN D.G., LAZARUS H., BARELL E.F., BENZ E.J., CASKEY C.T., HUISMAN T.H.J., SCHROEDER W.A. & HOUSMAN D. (1976) Absence of messenger RNA and gene DNA for β-globin chains in hereditary persistence of fetal hemoglobin. *Cell*, **7**, 323.

174 OTTOLENGHI S., GIGLIONI B., COMI P., GIANNI A.M., POLLI E., ACQUAYE C.T.A., OLDHAM J.H. & MASERA G. (1979) Globin gene deletion in HPFH, $\delta^0\beta^0$ thalassaemia and Hb Lepore disease. *Nature (London)*, **278**, 654.

175 OTTOLENGHI S., COMI P., GIGLIONI B., TOLSTOSHEV P., LANYON W.G., MITCHELL G.J., WILLIAMSON R., RUSSO G., MUSUMECI S., SCHILIRO G., TSISTRAKIS G.A., CHARACHE S., WOOD W.G., CLEGG J.B. AND WEATHERALL D.J. (1976) $\delta\beta$ thalassaemia is due to a gene deletion. *Cell*, **9**, 71.

176 MARTI H.R. (1963) *Normale und Anormale Menschliche Hamoglobine*, p. 81. Springer, Berlin.

177 WOOD W.G., STAMATOYANNOPOULOS G., LIM G. & NUTE P.E. (1975) F cells in the adult: normal values and levels in individuals with hereditary and acquired elevations of Hb F. *Blood*, **46**, 671.

178 ZAGO M.A., WOOD W.G., CLEGG J.B., WEATHERALL D.J., O'SULLIVAN M. & GUNSON H. (1979) Genetic control of F cells in human adults. *Blood*, **53**, 977.

179 WOOD W.G., WEATHERALL D.J., CLEGG J.B., HAMBLIN T.J., EDWARDS J.H. & BARLOW A.M. (1977) Heterocellular hereditary persistence of fetal haemoglobin (heterocellular HPFH) and its interactions with β thalassaemia. *British Journal of Haematology*, **36**, 461.

180 WOOD W.G., WEATHERALL D.J. & CLEGG J.B. (1976) Interaction of heterocellular hereditary persistence of foetal haemoglobin with β thalassaemia and sickle-cell anaemia. *Nature (London)*, **264**, 247.

181 SERJEANT G.R., SERJEANT B.E. & MASON K. (1977) Heterocellular hereditary persistence of fetal haemoglobin and homozygous sickle-cell disease. *Lancet*, **i**, 795.

182 WEATHERALL D.J., CARTNER R., CLEGG J.B., WOOD W.G., MACRAE I.A. & MACKENZIE A. (1975) A form of hereditary persistence of fetal haemoglobin characterised by uneven cellular distribution of haemoglobin F and the production of haemoglobins A and A$_2$ in homozygotes. *British Journal of Haematology*, **29**, 205.

183 SILVESTRONI E. & BIANCO I. (1955) *La Malattia Microdrepanocitica. Il Pensiero Scientifico*, Editore, Roma.

184 SERJEANT G.R., ASHCROFT M.T., SERJEANT B.E. & MILNER P.F. (1973) The clinical features of sickle-cell β thalassaemia in Jamaica. *British Journal of Haematology*, **24**, 19.

450 *Chapter 9*

185 CHERNOFF A.I., MINNICH V., NA-NAKORN S., TUCHINDA S., KASHAMSANT C. & CHERNOFF R.R. (1956) Studies on hemoglobin E: I. The clinical, hematologic, and genetic characteristics of the hemoglobin E syndromes. *Journal of Laboratory and Clinical Medicine*, **47**, 455 and 490.

186 FAIRBANKS V.F., GILCHRIST G.S., BRIMHALL B., JEREB J.A. & GOLDSTON E.C. (1979) Hemoglobin E trait re-examined: A cause of microcytosis and erythrocytosis. *Blood*, **53**, 109.

187 TRAEGER J., WOOD W.G., CLEGG J.B., WEATHERALL D.J. & WASI P. (1980) Defective synthesis of Hb E is due to reduced levels of β^E mRNA. *Nature (London)*, **288**, 497.

188 PRESSLEY L., HIGGS D.R., CLEGG J.B. & WEATHERALL D.J. (1980) Gene deletions in α thalassaemia prove that the 5′ ζ-locus is functional. *Proceedings of the National Academy of Sciences, USA*, **77**, 3586.

189 KATTAKIS C., METAXATOU-MAVROMATI A., TSIARTA E., METAXATOU C., WASI P., WOOD W.G., PRESSLEY L., HIGGS D.R., CLEGG J.B. & WEATHERALL D.J. (1980) The haemoglobin Bart's hydrops syndrome in Greece. *British Medical Journal*, **iii**, 268.

190 SOPHOCLEOUS T., HIGGS D.R., ALDRIDGE B., TRENT R.J., PRESSLEY L., CLEGG J.B. & WEATHERALL D.J. (1981) The molecular basis for the haemoglobin Bart's hydrops fetalis syndrome in Cyprus. *British Journal of Haematology*, **47**, 153.

191 ORKIN S.H., OLD J., LAZARUS H., ALTAY C., GURGEY A., WEATHERALL D.J. & NATHAN D.G. (1979) The molecular basis of α thalassemias: Frequent occurrence of dysfunctional α loci among non-Asians with Hb H disease. *Cell*, **17**, 33.

192 ORKIN S.H. & MICHAELSON A. (1980) Partial deletion of the α-globin structural gene in human α thalassaemia. *Nature (London)*, **286**, 538.

193 HIGGS D.R., PRESSLEY L., OLD J.M., HUNT D.M., CLEGG J.B., WEATHERALL D.J. & SERJEANT G.R. (1979) Negro α thalassaemia is caused by a deletion of a single α gene. *Lancet*, **ii**, 272.

194 DOZY A.M., KAN Y.W., EMBURY S.H., MENTZER W.C., WANG W.C., LUBIN D., DAVIS J.R. & KOENIG H.M. (1979) Alpha-globin gene organization in Blacks precludes the severe form of α thalassaemia. *Nature (London)*, **280**, 605.

195 HIGGS D.R., PRESSLEY L., SERJEANT G.R., CLEGG J.B. & WEATHERALL D.J. (1980) The genetics and molecular basis of α thalassaemia in association with HbS in Jamaican Negroes. *British Journal of Haematology*, **47**, 43.

196 HIGGS D.R., PRESSLEY L., CLEGG J.B., WEATHERALL D.J. & SERJEANT G.R. (1980) Alpha thalassemia in Black populations. *Johns Hopkins Medical Journal*, **146**, 300.

197 PHILLIPS J.A., SCOTT A.F., SMITH K.D., YOUNG K.D., LIGHTBODY K.L., JIJI R.M. & KAZAZIAN H.H. (1979) A molecular basis for hemoglobin-H disease in American Blacks. *Blood*, **54**, 1439.

198 KAN Y.W., DOZY A.M., STAMATOYANNOPOULOS G., HADJIMINAS M.G., ZACHARIADES Z., FURBETTA M. & CAO A. (1979) Molecular basis of hemoglobin-H disease in the Mediterranean. *Blood*, **54**, 1434.

199 GOOSSENS M., DOZY A.M., EMBURY S.H., ZACHARIADES

Z., HADJIMINAS M.G., STAMATOYANNOPOULOS G. & KAN Y.W. (1980) Triplicated α-globin loci in humans. *Proceedings of the National Academy of Sciences, USA*, **77**, 518.

200 HIGGS D.R., OLD J.M., PRESSLEY L., CLEGG J.B. & WEATHERALL D.J. (1980) A novel α globin gene arrangement in Man. *Nature (London)*, **284**, 632.

201 KAN Y.W., DOZY A.M., TRECARTIN R. & TODD D. (1977) Identification of a non-deletion defect in α thalassemia. *New England Journal of Medicine*, **297**, 1081.

202 MILNER P.F., CLEGG J.B. & WEATHERALL D.J. (1971) Haemoglobin H disease due to a unique haemoglobin variant with an elongated α chain. *Lancet*, **i**, 729.

203 CLEGG J.B., WEATHERALL D.J. & MILNER P.F. (1971) Haemoglobin Constant Spring—A chain termination mutant? *Nature (London)*, **234**, 337.

204 LIE-INJO L.E. & JO B.H. (1960) A fast-moving haemoglobin in hydrops foetalis. *Nature (London)*, **185**, 698.

205 WASI P., NA-NAKORN S. & POOTRAKUL S. (1974) The α thalassaemias. *Clinics in Haematology*, **3**, 383.

206 WEATHERALL D.J., CLEGG J.B. & WONG H.B. (1970) The haemoglobin constitution of infants with the haemoglobin Bart's hydrops foetalis syndrome. *British Journal of Haematology*, **18**, 357.

207 GABUZDA T.G. (1966) Hemoglobin H and the red cell. *Blood*, **27**, 568.

208 SCOTT G.L., RASBRIDGE M.R. & GRIMES A.J. (1970) *In vitro* studies of red-cell metabolism in haemoglobin H disease. *British Journal of Haematology*, **18**, 13.

209 KNOX-MACAULAY H.H.M., WEATHERALL D.J., CLEGG J.B., BRADLEY J. & BROWN M.J. (1972) Clinical and biosynthetic characterization of αβ thalassaemia. *British Journal of Haematology*, **22**, 497.

210 RIGAS D.A., KOLER R.D. & OSGOOD E.E. (1955) New hemoglobin possessing a higher electrophoretic mobility than normal adult hemoglobin. *Science*, **121**, 372.

211 WENNBERG E. & WEISS L. (1968) Splenic-erythroclasia: An electron microscopic study of hemoglobin H disease. *Blood*, **31**, 778.

212 FESSAS P. & YATAGANAS X. (1968) Intraerythroblastic instability of hemoglobin β_4 (Hgb H). *Blood*, **31**, 323.

213 WICKRAMASINGHE S.N. *et al.* (1980) In press.

214 PRESSLEY L., HIGGS D.R., CLEGGS J.B., PERRINE R.P., PEMBREY M.E. & WEATHERALL D.J. (1980) A new genetic basis for hemoglobin-H disease. *New England Journal of Medicine*, **303**, 1383.

215 WEATHERALL D.J. (1963) Abnormal haemoglobins in the neonatal period and their relationship to thalassaemia. *British Journal of Haematology*, **46**, 39.

216 HIGGS D.R., PRESSLEY L., CLEGG J.B., WEATHERALL D.J., SERJEANT G.R., HIGGS S. & CAREY P. (1980) Detection of α thalassaemia in Negro infants. *British Journal of Haematology*, **46**, 39.

217 SCHWARTZ E., KAN Y.W. & NATHAN D.G. (1969) Unbalanced globin-chain synthesis in α-thalassemia heterozygotes. *Annals of the New York Academy of Sciences*, **165**, 288.

218 HUNT D.M., HIGGS D.R., OLD J.M., CLEGG J.B., WEATHERALL D.J. & MARSH G.W. (1980) Determination of α-thalassemia phenotypes by messenger RNA analysis. *British Journal of Haematology*, **45**, 53.

219 LIE-INJO L.E., GANESAN J., CLEGG J.B. & WEATHERALL

D.J. (1974) Homozygous state for Hb Constant Spring (slow-moving Hb X components). *Blood*, **43**, 251.

220 LIE-INJO L.E., GANESAN J. & LOPEZ C.G. (1975) The clinical, hematological, and biochemical expression of hemoglobin Constant Spring and its distribution. *Abnormal Haemoglobins and Thalassaemia* (ed. Schmidt R.M.), p. 275. Academic Press, New York.

221 FESSAS P., LIE-INJO L.E., NA-NAKORN S., TODD D., CLEGG J.B. & WEATHERALL D.J. (1972) Identification of slow-moving haemoglobins in haemoglobin H disease from different racial groups. *Lancet*, **i**, 1308.

222 CLEGG J.B., WEATHERALL D.J., CONTOPOLOU-GRIVA I., CAROUTSOS K., POUNGOURAS P. & TSEVRENIS H. (1974) Haemoglobin Icaria, a new chain-termination mutant which causes α thalassaemia. *Nature (London)*, **251**, 245.

223 DE JONG W.W., KHAN P.M. & BERNINI L.F. (1975) Hemoglobin Koya Dora: high frequency of a chain-termination mutant. *American Journal of Human Genetics*, **27**, 81.

224 VELLA F., WELLS R.H.C., AGER J.A.M. & LEHMANN H. (1958) A haemoglobinopathy involving haemoglobin H and a new (Q) haemoglobin. *British Medical Journal*, **i**, 752.

225 LIE-INJO L.E., DOZY A.M., KAN Y.W., LOPES M. & TODD D. (1979) The α-globin gene adjacent to the gene for Hb Q-α 74 Asp→His is deleted, but not that adjacent to the gene for Hb G-α 30 Glu→Gln; three fourths of the α-globin genes are deleted in Hb Q-α thalassaemia. *Blood*, **54**, 1407.

226 HIGGS D.R., HUNT D.M., DRYSDALE C.D., CLEGG J.B., PRESSLEY L. & WEATHERALL D.J. (1980) The genetic basis of Hb Q-H disease. *British Journal of Haematology*, **46**, 387.

227 WEATHERALL D.J., CLEGG J.B., BLANKSON J. & MCNIEL J.R. (1969) A new sickling disorder resulting from interaction of the genes for haemoglobin S and α-thalassaemia. *British Journal of Haematology*, **17**, 517.

228 STEINBERG M.H. (1975) Haemoglobin C/α thalassaemia: haematological and biosynthetic studies. *British Journal of Haematology*, **30**, 337.

229 WASI P., SOOKANEK M., POOTRAKUL S., NA-NAKORN S. & SUINGDUMRONG A. (1967) Haemoglobin E and α-thalassaemia. *British Medical Journal*, **iv**, 29.

230 WASI P., NA-NAKORN S., POOTRAKUL S., PORNPATKUL M. & SUINGDUMRONG A. (1968) Haemoglobin H—an α-thalassaemia$_1$/α-thalassaemia$_2$ disease. *Proceedings of the XIIth Congress of the International Society of Haematology, New York*, p. 59.

231 KAN Y.W. & NATHAN D.G. (1970) Mild thalassemia: the result of interactions of α- and β-thalassemia genes. *Journal of Clinical Investigation*, **49**, 635.

232 LOUKOPOULOS D., LOUTRADI A. & FESSAS P. (1978) A unique thalassaemia syndrome: Homozygous α thalassaemia + homozygous β thalassaemia. *British Journal of Haematology*, **39**, 377.

233 MUSUMECI S., SCHILIRO G., PIZZARELLI G., FISCHER A. & RUSSO G. (1978) Thalassaemia of intermediate severity resulting from the interaction between α and β thalassaemia. *Journal of Medical Genetics*, **15**, 448.

234 KNOX-MACAULAY H.H.M., WEATHERALL D.J., CLEGG J.B. & PEMBREY M.E. (1973) Thalassaemia in the British. *British Medical Journal*, **iii**, 150.

235 WEATHERALL D.J., CLEGG J.B., WOOD W.G., OLD J.M., HIGGS D.R., PRESSLEY L. & DARBRE P.D. (1980) The clinical and molecular heterogeneity of the thalassemia syndromes. *Annals of the New York Academy of Sciences*, **344**, 83.

236 CAPPELLINI M.D., FIORELLI G. & BERNINI L.F. (1981) Interaction between homozygous $β^0$ thalassaemia and the Swiss type of hereditary persistence of fetal haemoglobin. *British Journal of Haematology*, **48**, 561.

237 BHAMARAPRAVATI N., NA-NAKORN S., WASI P. & TUCHINDA S. (1967) Pathology of abnormal hemoglobin diseases seen in Thailand. I. Pathology of β-thalassemia hemoglobin E disease. *American Journal of Clinical Pathology*, **47**, 745.

238 PIPPARD M.J., CALLENDER S.T., WARNER G.T. & WEATHERALL D.J. (1979) Iron absorption and loading in β thalassaemia intermedia. *Lancet*, **ii**, 819.

239 KAN Y.W. (1977) Prenatal diagnosis of hemoglobin disorders. *Progress in Hematology*, **10**, 91.

240 ALTER B.P. (1979) Prenatal diagnosis of hemoglobinopathies and other hematologic diseases. *Journal of Pediatrics*, **95**, 501.

241 ALTER B.P., ORKIN S.H., FORGET B.G. & NATHAN D.G. (1980) Prenatal diagnosis of hemoglobinopathies. The New England approach. *Annals of the New York Academy of Sciences*, **344**, 151.

242 ALTER B.P., ORKIN S.H. & NATHAN D.G. (1979) Prenatal diagnosis of the hemoglobinopathies. In: *Laboratory Investigation of Fetal Disease* (ed. Barson A.J.). Wright & Sons, London.

243 KAN Y.W. & DOZY A.M. (1978) Antenatal diagnosis of sickle-cell anaemia by DNA analysis of amniotic-fluid cells. *Lancet*, **ii**, 910.

244 KAN Y.W. & DOZY A.M. (1978) Polymorphisms of DNA sequence adjacent to human β-globin structural gene: relation to sickle mutation. *Proceedings of the National Academy of Sciences, USA*, **75**, 5631.

245 LITTLE P.F.R., ANNISON G., DARLING S., WILLIAMSON R., CAMBA L. & MODELL B. (1980) Model for antenatal diagnosis of β thalassaemia and other monogenic disorders by molecular analysis of linked DNA polymorphisms. *Nature (London)*, **285**, 144.

246 ORKIN S.H., ALTER B.P., ALTAY C., MAHONEY M.J., LAZARUS H., HOBBINS J.C. & NATHAN D.G. (1978) Application of endonuclease mapping to the analysis and prenatal diagnosis of thalassemias caused by globin-gene deletion. *New England Journal of Medicine*, **299**, 166.

247 MODELL C.B. & MATTHEWS R. (1976) Thalassaemia in Britain and Australia. In: *Birth Defects: Original Article Series*, XII (ed. Bergsma D., Cerami A., Peterson C.H. & Graziano J.H.), p. 13. Liss, New York.

248 MODELL C.B & BERDOUKAS V.A. (1981) *The Clinical Approach to Thalassemia*. Grune & Stratton, New York.

249 WASI P., NA-NAKORN S., POOTRAKUL P., SONAKUL D., PIANKIJAGUM A. & PACHAREE P. (1978) A syndrome of hypertensions, convulsions, and cerebral haemorrhage in thalassaemic patients after multiple blood transfusions. *Lancet*, **ii**, 602.

250 SMITH C.H., SCHULMAN I., ANDO R.E. & STERN G. (1955) Studies in Mediterranean (Cooley's) anemia. II.

The suppression of hematopoiesis by transfusions. *Blood*, **10**, 707.

251 ENGELHARD D., CIVIDALLI G. & RACHMILEWITZ E.A. (1975) Splenectomy in homozygous β thalassaemia: a retrospective study of 30 patients. *British Journal of Haematology*, **31**, 39.

252 SMITH C.H., ERLANDSON M.E., STERN G. & HILGARTNER H. (1964) Postsplenectomy infection in Cooley's anemia. *Annals of the New York Academy of Sciences*, **119**, 748.

253 BARRY M., FLYNN D.M., LETSKY E.A. & RISDON R.A. (1974) Long-term chelation therapy in thalassaemia major: effect on liver iron concentration, liver histology and clinical progress. *British Medical Journal*, **i**, 16.

254 PROPPER R.D., SHURIN S.B. & NATHAN D.G. (1976) Reassessment of the use of desferrioxamine B in iron overload. *New England Journal of Medicine*, **294**, 1421.

255 PROPPER R.D., COOPER B., RUFO R.R., NIENHUIS A.W., ANDERSON W.F., BUNN H.F., ROSENTHAL A. & NATHAN D.G. (1977) Continuous subcutaneous administration of deferrioxamine in patients with iron overload. *New England Journal of Medicine*, **297**, 418.

256 HUSSAIN M.A.M., GREEN N., FLYNN D.M., HUSSEIN S. & HOFFBRAND A.V. (1976) Subcutaneous infusion and intramuscular injection of desferrioxamine in patients with transfusional iron overload. *Lancet*, **ii**, 1278.

257 HUSSAIN M.A.M., GREEN N., FLYNN D.M. & HOFFBRAND A.V. (1977) Effect of dose, time and ascorbate in iron excretion after subcutaneous desferrioxamine. *Lancet*, **i**, 977.

258 PIPPARD M.J., CALLENDER S.T. & WEATHERALL D.J. (1978) Intensive iron chelation therapy with desferrioxamine in iron loading anaemias. *Clinical Science and Molecular Medicine*, **54**, 99.

259 MODELL C.B. (1979) Advances in the use of chelating agents for the treatment of iron loading. *Progress in Hematology*, **11**, 267.

260 PIPPARD M.J., CALLENDER S.T., LETSKY E.A. & WEATHERALL D.J. (1978) Prevention of iron loading in transfusion-dependent thalassaemia. *Lancet*, **i**, 1178.

261 HOFFBRAND A.V., GORMAN A., LAULICHT M., GARIDI M., ECONOMIDOU J., GEORGIPOULOU P., HUSSAIN M.A.M. & FLYNN D.M. (1979) Improvement in iron status and liver function in patients with transfusional iron overload with long-term subcutaneous desferrioxamine. *Lancet*, **i**, 947.

262 GRADY R.W., GRAZIANO J.H., AKERS H.A. & CERAMI A. (1976) The development of new iron chelating drugs. *Journal of Pharmacology and Experimental Therapeutics*, **196**, 478.

263 GRADY R.W., PETERSON C.M., JONES R.L., GRAZIANO J.H., BHARGAVA K.K., BERDOUKAS V.A., KOKKINI G., LOUKOPOULOS D. & CERAMI A. (1979) Rhodotorulic acid: investigation of its potential as an iron chelating drug. *Journal of Pharmacology and Experimental Therapeutics*, **209**, 343.

264 NIENHUIS A.W., PETERSON D.T. & HENRY W. (1977) Evaluation of endocrine and cardiac function in patients with iron overload on chelation therapy. *Chelation Therapy in Chronic Iron Overload* (ed. Zaino E.C. & Roberts R.H.). Ciba Medical Horizons Symposium. Symposia Specialists, Miami, Florida.

265 JURKIEWICZ M.J., PEARSON H.A. & FURLOW L.T. (1969) Reconstruction of the maxilla in thalassemia. *Annals of the New York Academy of Sciences*, **165**, 437.

266 HUISMAN T.H.J. & JONXIS J.H.P. (1977) *The Hemoglobinopathies: Techniques of Identification*. Marcel Dekker Inc., New York.

267 WASI P., DISTHASONGCHAN P. & NA-NAKORN S. (1968) The effect of iron deficiency on the levels of hemoglobins A_2 and E. *Journal of Laboratory and Clinical Medicine*, **71**, 85.

268 WEATHERALL D.J., OLD J., LONGLEY J., WOOD W.G., CLEGG J.B., POLLOCK A. & LEWIS M.J. (1978) Acquired haemoglobin H disease in leukaemia: pathophysiology and molecular basis. *British Journal of Haematology*, **38**, 305.

269 BERNARDS R. & FLAVELL R.A. (1980) Physical mapping of the globin-gene deletion in hereditary persistence of foetal haemoglobin (HPFH). *Nucleic Acids Research*, **8**, 1521.

270 MAQUAT L.E., KINNIBURGH A.J., BEACH L.R., HONIG G.R., LAZERSON J., ERSHLER W.B. & ROSS J. (1980) Processing of human β-globin mRNA precursors to mRNA is defective in three patients with β^+ thalassaemia. *Proceedings of the National Academy of Sciences, USA*, **77**, 4287.

271 WESTWAY D. & WILLIAMSON R. (1981) An intron nucleotide sequence variant in cloned β^+-thalassaemia globin gene. *Nucleic Acids Research*, **9**, 177.

272 SPRITZ R.A., JAGADEESWARAN P., CHOUDARY D., BIRO P.A., ELDER J.T., DERIEL J.K., MANLEY J.L., GEFTER M.L., FORGET B.G. & WEISSMAN S.M. (1981) Base substitution in an intervening sequence of a β^+ thalassemia human globin gene. *Proceedings of the National Academy of Sciences, USA*, **78**, 2455.

273 PRESSLEY L., HIGGS D.R., ALTRIDGE B., METAXATOU-MAVROMATI A., CLEGG J.B. & WEATHERALL D.J. (1980) Characterization of a new α thalassaemia 1 defect due to a partial deletion of the α globin gene complex. *Nucleic Acids Research*, **9**, 4899.

Chapter 10
The red-cell membrane: disorders of membrane function

M. C. BRAIN

The composition, structure and function of the red-cell membrane has been the subject of intensive study both in man, in health and disease, and in many animal species. The principal functions and properties of the red-cell membrane will be defined in general terms before discussing how the present state of knowledge has been derived from the many and varied biochemical, physiological and ultrastructural techniques employed, and how such knowledge has led to an understanding of haemolytic anaemia in man.

1 The membrane determines the discoid shape of the resting red cell and permits great deformability enabling the red cell to pass repeatedly through the microcirculation.

2 The red-cell membrane maintains the osmotic equilibrium between the cell and the plasma despite the osmotic effect of the high concentration of haemoglobin within the cell and the difference in cation composition between the cell and the plasma. Osmotic equilibrium is achieved by: (a) the membrane barrier to passive diffusion of cations; and (b) the presence of energy-dependent active transport systems within the membrane which transfer cations across the membrane against their concentration gradients. Other transport systems facilitate the uptake of metabolizable substrates.

3 The lipids and proteins of the membrane are responsible for the structural organization and determine the fundamental properties of the membrane such as passive permeability, and constitute membrane enzymes and transport systems. The carbohydrates of the membrane confer the negative surface charge due to sialic acid, whilst subtle differences in the terminal sugar residues of the glycolipids determine the highly specific red-cell surface antigens.

Normal membrane function is essential to the survival of the red cell in the circulation. Indeed it can be argued that a disorder of membrane function by virtue of the role of the membrane in determining cell size, shape and deformability underlies all disorders which lead to diminished red-cell survival. These disorders may be a direct consequence of a change of membrane structure or composition, or be an indirect consequence of loss of cell shape or deformability due to ATP depletion, or a change in haemoglobin solubility in the cell and the influence that this has on the deformability and rheological properties of the cell. How can a membrane, comprising a complex mixture of lipid, protein and carbohydrate approximately 75 Å in thickness, have the properties and fulfil the functions which it is known to possess? Until quite recently it was difficult to relate the properties of the membrane to specific structural features and overall organization. However, the past decade has seen a rapid expansion of knowledge of red-cell-membrane structure and organization, which has greatly furthered our understanding of the causes of haemolytic anaemia associated with red-cell-membrane disorders.

THE STRUCTURE AND ORGANIZATION OF THE RED-CELL MEMBRANE

An acceptable model of red-cell-membrane ultrastructure and molecular architecture must fulfil a number of criteria. The model must be compatible with the known proportions of proteins, lipids and carbohydrates in the membrane. It must take into account both the wide variations in molecular size of the proteins and the various classes of lipid present in red-cell membranes of any one species, and for the widely varying proportions of lipids in membranes of different species. The model must provide an appropriate environment for lipid–protein interaction bearing in mind that the membrane, by virtue of the lipid it contains, is a predominantly hydrophobic structure forming a barrier between the aqueous environments of the plasma and cytoplasm. The model must provide for the highly selective properties of the membrane, such as the million-fold difference in permeability to small hydrophilic anions and cations, and for the possession of highly specific active-transport functions, within a structure of relative unformity as seen in electron-microscopic sections.

MODELS OF MEMBRANE STRUCTURE

Gorter & Grendel [1] in 1925 first proposed that the basic structure of red-cell membranes was that of a lipid bilayer; a conclusion based on the measurement of the red-cell lipids and red-cell surface area. The lipid-bilayer concept of membrane structure was further elaborated by Davson & Danielli [2], who proposed that cell membranes comprised a sandwich-like structure in which the phospholipids were in an orderly array with the hydrophilic polar-head groups on the two surfaces and the long-chain fatty acids of the phospholipids formed the hydrophobic centre of the 'sandwich'. Davson & Danielli suggested that the membrane protein was present on the surface of the lipid bilayer attached to the hydrophilic polar groups of the phospholipid. The Davson–Danielli model of membrane structure was modified and extended by Robertson [3] who suggested that the surface protein was present as a monolayer in configuration. Robertson proposed that such a model might represent a universal structure for all cellular membranes [4]. The Davson–Danielli–Robertson model of membrane structure has received support from the demonstration by electron microscopy of a triple-layered structure in osmium-fixed red-cell membranes [3, 4], and by the presence of a lipid bilayer in red-cell membranes by X-ray-diffraction analysis [5].

Although the presence of a lipid bilayer as a major component of membrane organization in red cells and other cell membranes is widely accepted, the relationship of membrane protein to the lipid bilayer is still uncertain, and alternative models of membrane structure have been proposed [6–8]. Singer [8] has pointed out that the Davson–Danielli–Robertson model is incompatible with the known amounts, size and properties of the large-molecular-weight proteins which can be extracted from red-cell membranes. He argued that an acceptable model of membrane ultra-structure must take into account the thermodynamic requirements of a stable hydrophobic lipid–protein structure. He drew attention to the fact that analysis of membrane proteins has revealed a relative increase in the proportion of hydrophobic residues to polar or ionic residues compared with other proteins of comparable molecular weight. This finding would be more compatible with the concept that the proteins were an integral component of the hydrophobic lipid bilayer than with surface distribution. On the basis of further evidence on the stability of membrane proteins in the presence of media at increasing ionic strength, on the effects of removal of 60–70% of the polar heads of the membrane phospholipids on membrane-protein conformation, and the lack of solubility of lipid-depleted membrane proteins in aqueous solutions at neutral pH, Singer concluded that hydrophilic and hydro-phobic interactions are of predominant importance in the stabilization and organization of membranes. Singer thus asserted that the membrane proteins must form an integral component of the membrane, and that the 'function of the lipid appears to disperse and *solubilize* membrane proteins by a kind of detergent action, in which the hydrophobic portions of the lipids and proteins interact with one another'.

This concept of membrane organization has been confirmed by the detailed analysis and assignment of function to integral membrane proteins, through the elucidation of the nature of the interaction between specific classes of phospholipids on the inner aspect of the membrane and the cytoskeleton [9–11], and the evidence that modification of these interactions can profoundly influence the lateral mobility of integral membrane proteins within the lipid bilayer [12–14]. The model of membrane structure that has emerged is of a fluid mosaic lipid bilayer, containing intrinisc proteins, which is constrained by the linkages between integral membrane proteins and certain phospholipids on the inner surface to an underlying cytoskeletal protein network (Figs 10.1 and 10.2). Since both the nature and function of the lipid bilayer and the sub-membrane protein network are susceptible to changes in lipid composition, to modification by intracellular enzymes by changes in intracellular calcium and by the formation of disulphide bonds, in part the consequence of altered cell metabolism, maintenance of normal membrane structure and function and its influence of red-cell shape and survival is the outcome of dynamic rather than static influences. The following sections which describe the protein, lipid and carbohydrate components of the membrane will endeavour to emphasize the dynamic relationship of these components to each other, and will give less emphasis to the detailed analysis of membrane composition upon which knowledge of the more complex organizational arrangement of these components in the membrane is based.

Membrane proteins

Protein constitutes approximately 50% of the dry weight of red-cell membranes. The individual proteins have been separated and assigned identifying numbers on the basis of their electrophoretic migration in polyacrylamide gels after solubilization of the membrane by sodium dodecylsulphate (SDS) [15–17]. The staining of such gels with a protein stain reveals the principal proteins illustrated in Figure 10.3. Staining of the same gels by the periodic-acid-Schiff (PAS) method reveals additional proteins, principally glycophorins and sialoglycoproteins, the carbohydrate component of which stain with PAS, but which stain poorly with protein stains. Electrophoresis of proteins

FLUID MOSAIC STRUCTURE

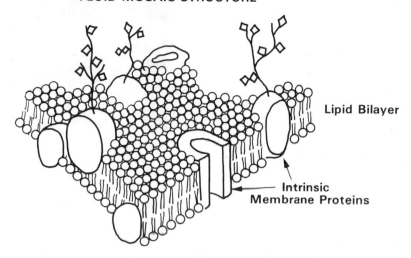

Fig. 10.1. Diagram of fluid mosaic structure of the red-cell membrane.

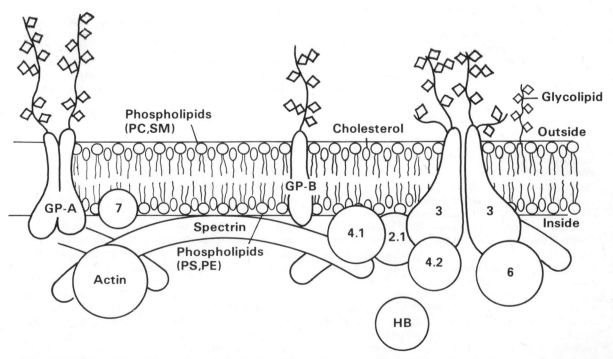

Fig. 10.2. Diagram of membrane (not to scale) showing relation of integral and internal membrane proteins to the lipid bilayer. The numbers refer to individual membrane proteins (see Fig. 10.4); GPA and GPB are glycophorins A and B; PC: phosphatidyl choline; SM: sphingomyelin; PS: phosphatidylserine; PE: phosphatidylethanolamine.

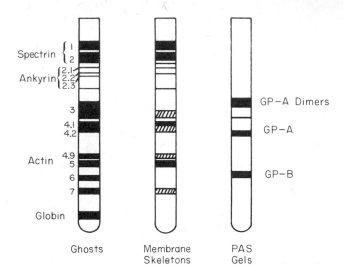

Fig. 10.3. Diagram of proteins identified by PAGE-SDS-gels from red-cell ghosts, lipid-depleted membrane skeletons stained with protein stains (left and centre) and red-cell-ghost proteins stained by PAS (right).

from isolated membranes after extraction with the non-ionic detergent Triton X-100 reveals those proteins which are not integral to the lipid component of the membrane and represent protein constituents of the sub-membrane protein network which forms the cytoskeleton of the membrane (Fig. 10.3). The proteins recovered after lipid extraction comprise about 60% of the total membrane protein, and include all of the spectrin (bands 1 and 2), actin (band 5), ankyrin (band 2.1), bands 2.2, 2.3, 2.6 and 4.1; and a proportion of the protein designated 3, 4.2, 4.9 and 7.3. Spectrin, actin and bands 4.1 and 4.9 form the basic constituents of the cytoskeleton as the other components can be eluted without loss of the discoid shape of the cytoskeleton, whereas removal of spectrin or actin results in loss of shape and integrity of the cytoskeleton [18].

Spectrin (bands 1 and 2) consists of large molecules (MW 240 000 and 220 000 daltons respectively) which probably are present as a tetramer in the intact cell [19]. The molecular shape of the spectrin dimers has been shown by the platinum–carbon replicas, formed by low-angle shadowing, to consist of long (approximately 1000 Å), slender (less than 50 Å diameter), tortuous molecules in which the two subunits are aligned in parallel and are variably coiled around each other [20] (Fig. 10.4). These molecules form a complex network in which two dimers are linked together as a tetramer in association with band 4.1, other portions of the molecule being linked by ankyrin to receptor sites on the cytoplasmic portion of the integral membrane-protein band 3 [21] (see Fig. 10.4). In addition to the specific binding of the spectrin network by ankyrin to the band-3 protein there is evidence of a less specific

attachment of the spectrin molecule to the serine groups of the phospholipid phosphatidylserine on the inner aspect of the membrane.

Evidence of the importance of the integrity and normal functions of the spectrin–actin network and its close association with the lipid bilayer of the membrane has come from a number of observations. It has been shown that in mice with genetic spherocytosis the red cells are deficient in spectrin, and that the osmotic stability of these cells can be improved by incorporation of spectrin into the deficient resealed ghost cells [22]. Furthermore, the spectrin-deficient mouse erythrocyte has a strikingly increased mobility in the lipid bilayer of fluorescent-labelled integral membrane proteins [23]. Thus, absence of spectrin is accompanied by inherent instability of the membrane and greatly increased freedom of integral membrane proteins to move laterally in the bilayer. The biochemical state of spectrin—as shown by diminished extractability of spectrin from red-cell ghosts—may be altered in at least two ways. The entry of calcium into the cell is accompanied by activation of a cytoplasmic transglutaminase resulting in the formation of spectrin polymers due to the formation of γ-glutamyl-ε-lysine side-chain bridges [24, 25]. The formation of such cross-links between the membrane proteins is prevented by the addition of histamine and related compounds which competitively inhibit the enzyme, and permits reversal of the calcium-induced shape change of red cells from discocytes to echinocytes [24, 25]. This observation suggests that the irreversible shape changes which take place in stored red cells and in sickle cells may be related to the effects of calcium-

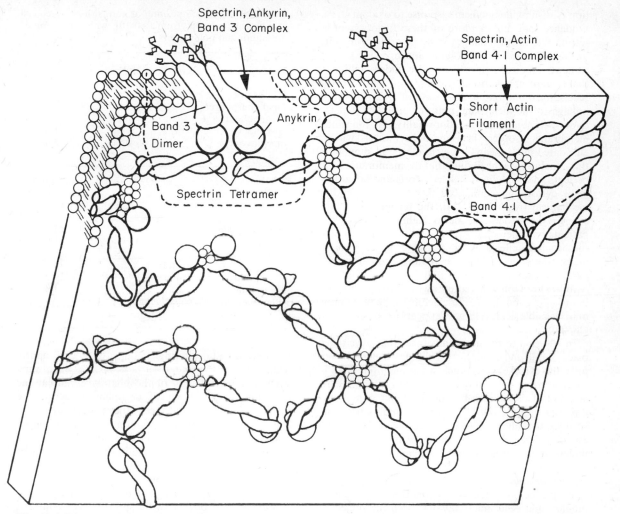

Fig. 10.4. Diagram of the inner surface of the membrane to show relationship of cytoskeleton to membrane (not to scale). Redrawn from Lux [20].

mediated formation of membrane-protein polymers [26, 27]. A further cause of membrane-protein polymerization is the formation of disulphide bridges which form on reduction of intracellular glutathione upon oxidant stress [28–30]. Spectrin is a principal substrate for phosphorylation of membrane proteins by ATP through the activity of membrane-located protein kinases [31]. The physiological consequences of spectrin phosphorylation or dephosphorylation are not yet fully understood. Nevertheless, there is evidence that modification of spectrin phosphorylation may be accompanied by disc–sphere transformation, and by reduced membrane deformability [31]. It has further been suggested that the shape change of red blood cells which can be induced by low-density

lipoproteins may be mediated through activation of an endogenous phosphatase capable of dephosphorylating spectrin [32].

The sub-membrane protein network which forms the cytoskeleton of the red blood cell is a major determinant of red-cell shape, and through its attachments to integral membrane proteins, notably band 3, profoundly influences the stability of the lipid bilayer. It seems probable that factors which influence the shape or the deformability of the red cell are mediated through changes in the biochemical and biophysical state of spectrin, and include modifications in the composition of the phospholipid and cholesterol in the membrane, changes in intracellular ATP concentration, increases in intracellular calcium, and the formation of disulphide bonds in response to oxidant stress. Evidence that one or more of these factors may be responsible for the changes in shape or deformability of blood cells in haemolytic anaemia is, as yet, somewhat indirect. Nevertheless, an understanding of the role of the various factors that influence the biochemical and biophysical state of spectrin and its linkage to the membrane make it probable that the underlying biochemical abnormality in congenital membrane disorders leading to haemolysis will be elucidated in the near future. Evidence in support of this conclusion is the finding that the membranes from patients with hereditary spherocytosis and hereditary elliptocytosis show enhanced thermal lability and/or mechanical fragility [33, 34], the recognition of the changes that underlie the thermal lability of red cells in patients with hereditary pyropoikilocytosis [35], and the beneficial effects of cross-linking reagents on the membrane abnormality in hereditary stomatocytosis [36, 37]. Likewise, an abnormality in membrane proteins has been found in patients with march haemoglobinuria [38], and the role of calcium in the production of irreversible sickle cells now appears to be established [26, 27].

In addition to the major advances that have taken place in our understanding of the proteins that comprise the cytoskeleton, much work has been done in characterizing the nature and function of band 3 [39, 40], and of the antigen-bearing proteins, notably the glycophorins [41, 42]. The information obtained from such studies, although of considerable intrinsic interest, is not at present of immediate relevance to our understanding of haemolytic anaemia in man.

Membrane lipids
The lipid composition of the red-cell membrane of humans and other mammals has been the subject of intensive study [9–11, 43]. Lipids comprise approximately 40% of the red-cell membrane by weight. Phospholipid amounts to 70% of the total membrane lipid, much of the residual 30% being made up of cholesterol with small proportions of glycolipid and free fatty acids. The lipid composition of the normal red-cell membrane is shown in Table 10.1. The significance of the proportions of the phospholipids is uncertain as they are strikingly different in the red cells of various mammalian species both with respect to the class of phospholipid present and of the fatty acids within particular classes of phospholipid. Furthermore, no less than 20 different molecular types of lecithin (phosphatidyl choline) varying with respect to fatty-acid chain length and saturation are present in human red cells [44]. Nevertheless, it is now known that the various classes of phospholipid are asymmetrically distributed between the inner and outer layers of

Table 10.1. Lipid composition of normal human red cell membranes (reprinted from Ref. 101, with permission of the author and publishers)

	$\mu g/10^8$ cells	$\mu mol/10^{11}$ cells
Cholesterol	12·67	32·8
Lipid phosphorus	1·23	39·7
Phospholipid	30·72	39·7
Glycolipid	1·12	1·0
Free fatty acid	0·81	2·6

	Total phospholipid (%)
Sphingomyelin	25·2
Lecithin	31·0
Phosphatidyl serine (+phosphatidyl inositol)	13·5
Phosphatidyl ethanolamine	27·3
Lysolecithin	1·3
Other (polyglycerol phosphatide, phosphatidic acid)	1·7

the bilayer. Phosphatidyl choline is predominantly localized on the outer surface of the membrane whereas at least 70–90% of phosphatidyl ethanolamine (PE) and nearly 100% of phosphatidyl serine are localized on the inner surface of the membrane [10, 11]. This asymmetrical distribution of phospholipid appears to be determined by the specific association of certain classes of phospholipid in specific domains of the membrane, probably due to interaction between subclasses of phospholipid, between phospholipids and integral membrane proteins, and on the inner aspect of the bilayer with spectrin. By contrast, cholesterol, which normally comprises more than 99% of the neutral lipid in the red-cell membrane, has been found to exchange freely between both the inner and outer layers of the bilayer, and is in equilibrium with free (non-esterified) cholesterol attached to the plasma lipoproteins [45, 46]. Thus, the cholesterol content of the red cells may be profoundly influenced by the amount of free cholesterol in the plasma, which is determined both by the levels of α and β lipoproteins, and by the rate of esterification of free cholesterol by lechithin-cholesterol acyltransferase (LCAT). Murphy [49] demonstrated that the increase in osmotic fragility which follows sterile incubation of normal red cells is in large part due to reduction in membrane surface area following the loss of cholesterol through a fall in serum-free cholesterol upon esterification by LCAT. Although cholesterol appears to be freely exchangeable between both components of the membrane, there is evidence of specific interaction between cholesterol and the band-3 protein of the membrane [48, 49].

Mature red cells are unable to synthesize the fatty acids of phospholipids *de novo* from acetate, although lengthening of the fatty-acid chain can taken place [50]. Plasma-free fatty acids rapidly exchange with a free-fatty-acid pool of the red-cell membrane and a proportion is actively incorporated into lyso-phosphatide, usually in the 2 position of glycerol utilizing ATP and coenzyme A [51, 52]. Shohet and co-workers [52, 53] calculated that approximately five per cent of the ATP derived from glycolysis would be utilized in the acylation of fatty acids by normal red cells. Apart from this energy-dependent process, change in phospholipid comes about through the dismutation of lysolecithin resulting in the generation of lecithin and glycerophosphorylcholine [53] and by direct exchange of intact phospholipid molecules in the membrane with the identical molecule in the plasma [54].

Despite the exchange between plasma cholesterol, free fatty acids and phospholipids and these components in the red-cell membrane, there are only slow and minor changes in fatty-acid composition of red-cell-membrane phospholipids in man consequent on changes in the fatty-acid composition of the diet [55]. More marked changes in cholesterol and phospholipid composition take place in various disease states (*vide infra*).

Membrane carbohydrate

Carbohydrate makes up approximately eight per cent of the dry weight of the red-cell membrane. It is all located on the outer surface of the membrane, the complex branched oligosaccharide chains forming a network over the surface of the membrane of considerably greater thickness than the lipid bilayer. The carbohydrates are attached to integral membrane proteins and to specific subclasses of lipids: the glycolipids. All integral membrane proteins located on the outer surface of the lipid bilayer have varying amounts of carbohydrate attached to them. A subclass of these glycoproteins differs in the length and complexity of the oligosaccharide chains and the proportion of the sialic-acid residues attached to them. These sialoglycoproteins, the glycophorins, can only be detected by staining SDS polyacrylamide gels by the PAS reaction. The glycophorins have been well characterized and their amino-acid and carbohydrate compositions have been determined [41, 42]. It is now recognized that there are four unique sialoglycoprotein components (α, β, γ and δ), some of which form dimers ($\alpha 2$, α/δ and $\delta 2$) to give rise to seven separately identifiable fractions ($\alpha 2$, α/δ, $\delta 2$, α (glycophorin A), β, γ and δ (glycophorin B)). Glycophorin A carries the MN antigens and has been extensively studied; it exists

in both monomeric and dimeric forms (Fig. 10.3). Glycophorin B carries the Ss blood group activity, and also has N-antigen activity, denoted as 'N', as it is detectable independently of the MN genotype of the cells. The presence of 'N' activity on glycophorin B accounts for the residual N activity of MM erythrocytes.

The biological significance of the glycophorins is as yet unknown. Complete absence of the α component of the glycophorins has been found in En(a$-$) erythrocytes, which lack MN antigens and have a greatly reduced sialic-acid content [56]. Although the antigenic activity of En(a$-$) cells is altered, presumably due to the reduced amount of sialic acid present which results in enhanced agglutinability by plant lectins and by incomplete anti-D sera, there is no evidence that loss of the major sialoglycoprotein is accompanied by altered morphology, osmotic fragility or shortened red-cell survival [50]. Nevertheless, it is of interest that absence of glycophorin A which characterizes the En(a$-$) cells, and of other cells with major deficiencies of the sialoglycoproteins, is accompanied by an increase in the carbohydrate content of band-3 protein [50]. Thus, loss of normal sialoglycoprotein is seemingly compensated for by an increase in the carbohydrate content of the residual glycoproteins of the membrane. Tanner [42] has suggested that the surface coating of carbohydrate on red cells may provide a protective function to the surface of the cell against the physical trauma it sustains in the circulation, thereby preventing the lipid bilayer from disruption or potential fusion with adjacent cells. The presence in the oligosaccharide chains of numerous analogous repeating sequences and of the many sialic-acid residues may permit close interaction between adjacent molecules by hydrogen bonding and through the formation of calcium bridges. In this regard it is of interest that in sialoglycoprotein-deficient cells, the additional carbohydrate present on band 3 and other glycoproteins may compensate for the potential adverse effects of depletion of carbohydrate on the surface of these abnormal cells [56].

It is well recognized that red-cell ageing *in vivo* is accompanied by loss of sialic acid but it is not as yet certain whether this is due primarily to loss of carbohydrate from the surface of the cell or to loss of units of cell membrane by exocytosis during the lifespan of the erythrocyte [57, 58].

The glycolipids, and the glycosphingolipids in particular, are of interest because the oligosaccharide sequences attached to the sphingolipids carry important blood-group determinants. Whereas the glycosphingolipids determining A, B and O blood groups are integral parts of the cell membrane and are synthesized by the cells in which they are found, the

Lewis (La^a and Le^b) glycosphingolipids are taken up by the membrane from the serum, having been synthesized elsewhere in the body [59]. In the ABO system, although almost all the antigen on the red cells is synthesized by the red-cell precursors, there is some uptake of antigen from the plasma. This process is not easy to demonstrate except in AB individuals whose circulation contains group O acquired by graft or by transfusion. The expression of the A, B, O and Lewis blood groups is governed by the presence or absence of four glycosyltransferases responsible for the synthesis of the characteristic blood-group-determining oligosaccharide residues. The step-wise synthesis of the carbohydrate provides a molecular basis for the differences in the ABO groups, and can also account for gene interactions, in which an antigen such as Le^b may appear in a hybrid, although absent in both homozygous parents [59]. Furthermore, incomplete synthesis of oligosaccharide chains may account for the multiple blood-group specificities found in individual sialoglycoproteins or sialoglycolipids (see Chapter 34).

The role of glycolipids in cell-membrane function is not understood, but may be related to antigen recognition and immune responsiveness. Of interest in relation to this hypothesis is the absence of glucose residues from animal glycolipids except in immediate proximity to the lipid moiety of the glycolipid, a finding characteristic only of those animals in which glucose is widely distributed in body fluids. The absence of glucose from the antigen-determining oligosaccharide sequences may have an evolutionary significance [60].

PASSIVE PERMEABILITY

The red-cell membrane confers a remarkable degree of discrimination in its relative permeability to cations and anions. The membrane is freely permeable to hydrophilic anions such as Cl$^-$ and HCO$_3^-$ but is a million times less permeable to small hydrophilic cations, Na$^+$ and K$^+$. Initially it was thought that this selective permeability was conferred by the fixed charge within the pore of the transmembrane protein of band 3, but recent studies have demonstrated that the selective permeability to Cl$^-$ is conferred by a small portion of the external part of the intramembranous component band 3. Careful kinetic studies in the presence or absence of specific inhibitors of Cl$^-$ transport have clearly defined the site and nature of the anion transport process [61]. The most acceptable model is of a protein channel in band 3 which has located at the outer surface a mobile carrier which functions as a gate. When loaded with an anion the carrier moves freely across the diffusion barrier in either direction. Adjacent to this carrier-like gate there is a modifier on the external surface which when occupied by an anion inhibits or reduces the rate of

transport [61]. The role and further characterization of this exceedingly rapid, non-energy-dependent transport mechanism for anions may be important for our understanding of the regulation of a much broader range of transport processes.

ACTIVE TRANSPORT

There has been an enormous advance in the elucidation of the energy-dependent membrane transport systems. Much of the work has been carried out on red cells because of their ready availability, and has been confirmed and extended in other cells, notably the squid nerve axon. Only a summary of the present state of knowledge will be presented as the subject has been reviewed in detail [62, 63].

The red-cell membrane possesses an ATP-dependent transport system by which the hydrolysis of a molecule of ATP results in the linked movements of three Na$^+$ ions from the cell and two K$^+$ ions into a cell. This active transport process is dependent upon the appropriate concentrations of Na$^+$ and K$^+$ on the inside and outside of the cell membrane and is specifically inhibited by low concentrations of cardiac glycosides. The partially purified Na$^+$, K$^+$ ATPase activity of red-cell membranes has a K_m of 20 mM for Na$^+$ and 2 mM for K$^+$, figures which correspond closely to the concentrations which produce half-maximal transport activity into and out of the intact red cell or red-cell ghost. The exact relationship between the ATPase activity and the mechanism which results in the transport of Na$^+$ and K$^+$ across the membrane is incompletely understood. There is evidence for the formation of a phosphorylated protein intermediate in the membranes of red cells and other cells [64]. Furthermore, the extraction of phospholipids reduces Na$^+$, K$^+$ ATPase activity which can be restored upon the addition of certain phospholipids to the partially purified ATPase.

Thus, it seems that the Na$^+$, K$^+$ transport system represents a complex protein–lipid moiety appropriately oriented within the membrane. The number of Na$^+$, K$^+$ transport sites in the red cell has been calculated from kinetic data and from the binding of tritium-labelled ouabain and is approximately 200 per cell [65]. The finding in low-potassium sheep red cells that the number of active cation transport sites in the membrane can be doubled by the action of blood-group specific antibodies on these cells has raised intriguing problems regarding the functional state of the transport mechanisms and their relationship to cell-surface antigens [66, 67].

The red-cell membrane possesses a Ca^{2+}, Mg^{2+} ATPase linked to a calcium pump [68–71], the activity of which has been shown to be influenced by calmodulin [72]. There is considerable evidence that much of the

Ca^{2+} in the red cell is attached to either the outer or inner surface of the membrane [73]. Recent evidence suggests that there is a relatively slow exchange between radioactive calcium in the cytosol and membrane-associated calcium. Accumulation of Ca^{2+} in the red cell is known to be accompanied by the formation of echinocytes, a process which is initially reversible when excess Ca^{2+} is actively transported out of the cell, but becomes irreversible through the formation of peptide linkages between the molecules of spectrin of the sub-membrane cytoskeleton [24, 25]. Of considerable interest has been the recognition that there is an increase in the membrane-associated Ca^{2+} in the red cells of patients with sickle-cell anaemia [26, 27], and that the accumulation of calcium may, in part, account for the irreversible sickle cell. The precise mechanism for the increased accumulation of Ca^{2+} in sickle cells is not as yet understood. There is evidence that the Ca^{2+} pump in sickle-cell erythrocytes does not respond normally, particularly after sickling has been induced [74], although this does not appear to be due to a reduction in calmodulin. At present it appears likely that the sickling process results in an abnormal accumulation of Ca^{2+} in the sickle cell, and that the Ca^{2+} bound to the membrane is less available for extrusion.

SUGAR AND AMINO-ACID TRANSPORT

The red-cell membrane possesses active transport systems for monosaccharides, and amino-acid transport has been demonstrated in avian erythrocytes. The transport mechanisms for monosaccharides has been studied in great detail and the transport protein has been partially purified [75]. Recent reviews [76, 77] give detailed accounts of the mechanisms of these active transport systems and their inhibitors.

MEMBRANE STRUCTURE AND RED-CELL SHAPE

The discoid shape of the red cell is determined by the membrane, and is a consequence of the excess of membrane area relative to cell volume and of the physical forces in the membrane. Although the red cell is highly deformable and readily alters shape at constant surface area, the membrane is highly resistant to dilation thereby accounting for the degree of resistance to hypotonic osmotic lysis [78, 79]. Indeed, the susceptibility of the phospholipids to the action of phospholipases suggests that the phospholipids in the membrane are under considerable lateral pressure due to the links between integral membrane proteins and the cytoskeleton [11]. The cytoskeleton retains its discoid shape after removal of lipids, a finding which

suggests that the cytoskeleton may be the primary determinant of cell shape [18]. This conclusion is supported by the observation that in hereditary elliptocytosis the lipid-extracted skeletons are elliptical in shape and also have increased mechanical fragility [80]. This suggests that the shape of the elliptocyte is due to an as yet undetermined disorder of the cytoskeleton. Although the cytoskeleton would seem to be the primary determinant of cell shape, the cell is also influenced by changes in the composition of the phospholipid bilayer. The incorporation of anionic and cationic amphiphatic compounds into the membrane results in echinocyte or stomatocyte formation [81]. The observation that lysophosphatyl choline incorporation into the outer layer of the bilayer causes echinocytosis, and into the inner layer stomatocytosis, has led to the suggestion that these shape changes may be due to bending forces through expansion of either of the two layers of the bilayer. More recently the extent to which amphiphatic compounds enter the bilayer has been questioned and may necessitate reconsideration of these observations [82].

One of the effects of Ca^{2+} accumulation is the activation of the enzyme phosphodiesterase which causes the dephosphorylation of phosphatidylinositols and the accumulation of diacylglyerol. It was suggested that the accumulation of diacylglycerol might be responsible for echinocyte formation [83], but this now appears unlikely [84]. Nevertheless, Ca^{2+}-induced changes in the phospholipid composition or reactivity of the inner layer of the bilayer may have an important role in governing transformations in red-cell shape.

The ease of deformability of the discoid red cell accounts for the low viscosity of blood under conditions of rapid flow and high shear rates [85]. The red cell does not behave as a solid particle but as a fluid drop. The fluid interior of the cell is influenced by the forces applied through the membrane under conditions of high shear, the cell being readily and reversibly transformed from a discoid shape to that of a prolate ellipsoid [86]. Under these conditions the membrane rotates around the cell like a 'tank-track' in response to movements resulting from the gradient of shear forces across the cell [87].

The remarkable deformability of the discoid red cell is evident in the changes in shape observed in the microcirculation. When flowing down a capillary of 7 μm in diameter the cell assumes a parachute-like shape [88, 89], a change which is more marked in smaller capillaries. Such immediately reversible changes in shape are not accompanied by a change in membrane surface area, the parachute-like appearance being due to redistribution of haemoglobin within the cell and not due to invagination of the membrane.

The ability of the red cell to deform permits repeated passage through the microcirculation in which many capillaries are smaller in diameter than the resting discoid cell, and has important influences on the ability of normal red cells to pass through the $3\cdot5$ μm slits between the Billroth cords and the splenic sinuses of the spleen (see Chapter 20).

CHANGES IN THE RED-CELL MEMBRANE IN DISEASE

EFFECT OF HAEMOGLOBIN ON RED-CELL DEFORMABILITY AND BLOOD VISCOSITY

Changes in the solubility of haemoglobin within the red cell profoundly influence red-cell deformability and membrane function [90]. Thus, blood containing haemoglobins S and C has an increased viscosity and the red cells show diminished filterability, properties which are exacerbated by deoxygenation and hyperosmolarity respectively [91–95]. The changes in the membrane which accompany sickling have recently been shown to be due, in part, to the influence of increased membrane-bound calcium, and the inability of the sickle cell to actively transport excess calcium from the cell [26, 27]. The reduction in red-cell deformability due to the formation of sickle cells is responsible for the ischaemia and infarction which accompanies sickling crisis (see Chapter 8).

Blood viscosity is increased by the formation of Heinz bodies [90]. The presence of Heinz bodies and haemoglobin H inclusions, by altering membrane deformability, results in the removal of these inclusions by the spleen [96, 97]. The reduction of glutathione which accompanies oxidative denaturation of haemoglobin results in the formation of disulphide bonds and the polymerization of spectrin which may further contribute to the altered membrane properties observed in oxidative haemolysis [28–30].

The mechanisms involved in red-cell destruction due to haemoglobin variants and Heinz bodies are discussed in detail in Chapters 8 and 9.

Factors influencing red-cell shape

Changes in shape may be brought about by either an increase or decrease in the membrane surface area, or by changes which influence the volume of the cell. Kwant & Seeman [98] showed that the haemoglobin-free, resealed red-cell ghost behaves as a perfect osmometer, changing in volume in relation to the osmotic pressure of the medium in which it is suspended. The intact red cell does not behave as a perfect osmometer as changes in the concentration of haemoglobin which take place when the cell shrinks or swells influence the charge on the surface of the molecule,

resulting in a change in the chloride content of the cell, thus influencing cell hydration and modifying the osmotic equilibrium.

CHANGES IN MEMBRANE LIPIDS

Influence of cholesterol

Free cholesterol in the plasma, in contrast to esterified cholesterol, is freely exchangeable with the cholesterol in both the outer and inner layers of membrane bilayer [45, 46]. A rise in membrane cholesterol is accompanied by an increase in the surface area and gives rise to target cells and increases the resistance to osmotic lysis (reflecting the increase in the ratio of surface area to volume of the cell). This mechanism accounts for the target cells observed in patients with inherited deficiency of the serum enzyme cholesterol:lecithin acyl transferase (LCAT) in whom diminished esterification of cholesterol results in an increase in the ratio of free to esterified cholesterol in the plasma and an accompanying increase in red-cell membrane cholesterol [99, 100].

Target cells of liver disease

The target cells in patients with liver disease have been found to have an increase in both cholesterol and phospholipids. The increase in cholesterol is greater than that of the phospholipid which is due to a rise in phosphatidyl choline [101, 102]. The exact mechanism of target-cell formation in liver disease is incompletely understood, as in addition to rises in serum cholesterol and phospholipids there is a reduction in serum LCAT activity. Bile-salt retention, due to obstructive jaundice, may enhance target-cell formation through inhibition of LCAT activity [102]. More recently it has been shown that lipoprotein X, a low-density lipoprotein composed predominantly of cholesterol and phosphatidyl choline, may cause the adherence of vesicle-like liposomes to a surface of the membrane, which can subsequently become incorporated into the membrane, forming islands of altered lipid and thereby disturbing the normal heterogeneous dispersion of the particles due to intrinsic membrane proteins in the membrane [11].

The target cells of liver disease are not necessarily associated with shortened red-cell survival. However, transient episodes of haemolytic anaemia have been reported in patients with hepatic cirrhosis often following an episode of acute alcoholism. Such patients have gross elevation of plasma triglycerides and a fatty liver, and these features when combined with acute haemolytic anaemia have been termed Zieve's syndrome [103]. The mechanism of haemolysis is not understood as the lipid content of the red cells does not differ from that of other patients with liver disease without evidence of frank haemolysis [105].

The anaemia accompanying liver disease is further considered in Chapter 33.

Spur cells of liver disease

In a small proportion of patients with severe hepato-cellular liver disease the red cells are found to be irregular in shape and spiculated, resembling acanthocytes. This has led to their designation as spur cells by Cooper [105]. Spur cells have a very marked increase in cholesterol, the cholesterol/phospholipid ratio being increased by as much as 75% above the normal value. Cooper and co-workers [106] suggested that the retention of the lithocholic acid due to aberrant bile-acid metabolism may be responsible for the remarkable accumulation of cholesterol in the spur red cell. The initial and expected increase in membrane surface area is masked by the loss of membrane from the surface of the cell, probably due to the action of the spleen, and leads to the presence of a proportion of osmotically fragile cells [105]. The spur cells also demonstrate greatly diminished filterability due to loss of membrane deformability. The gross changes in membrane lipid composition found in spur cells probably have many other effects on membrane function including altered cation transport [107].

Non-spherocytic haemolytic anaemia due to abnormal membrane lipids

Jaffé & Gottfried [108] described a large family in whom eight members had a non-spherocytic haemolytic anaemia associated with an increase in phosphatidyl choline (PC) content of the red-cell membrane. No abnormality could be found in red-cell glycolytic enzymes, in haemoglobin or in plasma lipids. The haemolytic anaemia and raised PC in the red cells were inherited as an autosomal dominant. Further studies on the disorder of lipid metabolism in the red cells of this family have been reported by Shohet and co-workers [109]. In addition to raised PC, the level of phosphatidyl ethanolamine (PE) was found to be reduced. The studies with labelled fatty acids revealed an increased incorporation into PC but a failure of transfer of fatty acids from PC to PE, an important pathway in PE synthesis. The imbalance in the ratio of these two important phospholipids which could result in an imbalance in the proportions of the two phospholipids between the outer and inner layers of the bilayer (PC being predominantly located in the outer, and PE in the inner layer), would appear to influence membrane function as these abnormal red cells were found to have abnormal cation content and increased cation transport.

Acanthocytosis (a-β-lipoproteinaemia)

In 1950, Bassen & Kornzweigh [110] reported two patients with an atypical retinitis pigmentosa in which the majority of the red cells were irregularly crenated. Singer and co-workers [111] described a further case and termed the red cells 'acanthrocytes' after the Greek word akantha—a spine or thorn. Subsequent workers have shortened the word to acanthocyte and this term has become universally adopted. The finding of low levels of blood cholesterol was followed in 1960 by the recognition of the absence of the β lipoproteins in the serum of these patients [112], and led to the term a-β-lipoproteinaemia, to described the association of neurological disease and acanthocytosis. This disorder has been reviewed by Herbert *et al.* [113] and is further considered in Chapter 33.

The red-cell-membrane cholesterol is either normal or slightly increased, whilst the phospholipid content is normal or slightly diminished, the cholesterol/phospholipid ratio tending to be increased. There is a reduction in red-cell PC and the ratio of cholesterol to PC is increased to values seen in the spur cells of liver disease [109]. The red cells exhibit increased auto-haemolysis and peroxidative haemolysis, features which are corrected by the addition of vitamin E (α tocopherol) *in vitro* and *in vivo* [114] but vitamin-E administration does not correct the morphological abnormalities [115].

VITAMIN E

The exact role of vitamin E in protecting the red-cell membrane is uncertain. Vitamin E is generally considered to act as a lipid antioxidant although this action has been questioned. The deficiency of vitamin E renders the unsaturated fatty acids of phospholipids liable to oxidation with the formation of lipid peroxides [114]. Red cells deficient in vitamin E undergo lysis *in vitro* on exposure to hydrogen peroxide either by direct addition [116] or through its intracellular generation [117]. Lipid peroxides have been observed to increase *in vitro* and *in vivo* after oxidant stress [119], a process accompanied by loss of phosphatidyl ethanolamine and by a reduction in membrane sulphydryl groups [117]. Furthermore, blockade of membrane sulphydryl groups increased the haemolysis on oxidative stress [117]. Thus, it seems that deficiency of vitamin E may render critical lipid–protein interactions within the membrane liable to oxidative disruption [118].

Deficiency of vitamin E has been observed in patients with persistent steatorrhoea, some of whom have shortened survival of their red cells [119]. Low levels of vitamin E have been found in premature infants with haemolytic anaemia and pyknotic red cells [120]. Treatment of such infants with vitamin E has lessened the haemolysis. Deficiency of vitamin E has also been observed in a-β-lipoproteinaemia (see above). Haemolysis has been produced in vitamin-E-deficient men and animals upon exposure to hyperbaric oxygen [117, 121]. More recently it has been observed that the treatment of patients with high doses of vitamin E (800 iu/day) improved red-cell survival in patients with glutathione-synthetase deficiency [122] and in patients with chronic haemolytic anaemia due to Mediterranean glucose-6-phosphate-dehydrogenase (G6PD) deficiency [123]. The mechanism in both these disorders is presumptively to reduce the susceptibility of the membrane to oxidative damage in red cells which are ineffective in guarding against minor degrees of oxidative stress. Although the benefits were slight the treatment with vitamin E may help in ameliorating haemolytic crises, but this conclusion requires well-controlled, prospective clinical trials. It has also been claimed that vitamin-E supplementation of the diet by the administration of 450 iu of vitamin E per day for six to 36 weeks caused a substantial reduction in the number of irreversible sickle cells in patients with sickle-cell anaemia [124]. The mechanism of this effect, which requires confirmation, is less obvious.

LOSS OF SURFACE AREA
Loss of membrane without an accompanying loss of cell content will reduce the surface area/volume ratio and results in the formation of a spherocyte. The development of a true spherocyte implies loss of membrane and must be distinguished from the transformation of the disc-shaped red cell to a crenated sphere [125] or echinocyte [126] in which no loss of membrane has taken place.

Loss of membrane reflecting loss of equal proportions of cholesterol and phospholipid occurs in hereditary spherocytic red cells on prolonged incubation [127]. Weed & Reed [128] suggested that this reduction in lipid was the result of loss of membrane fragments, although Langley & Axell [129] could not demonstrate loss of membrane protein. Although Jacob [130] suggested that lipid loss might be related to increased membrane transport, Cooper & Jandl [131] suggested that it was solely due to metabolic depletion.

Loss of membrane results from partial phagocytosis of red cells which have been coated with immunoglobulins [132, 133] and may also be brought about by mechanical trauma to cells within the circulation due to interaction with abnormal surfaces such as prosthetic heart valves (cardiac haemolytic anaemia) or within the microcirculation (microangiopathic haemolytic anaemia) (see Chapter 12).

Mechanical trauma results in the formation of both spherocytes and abnormally shaped red-cell fragments. The formation of a distorted fragment instead of an even sphere may reflect the nature and localization of the membrane damage which is such as to prevent the formation of a spheroidal shape after loss of a portion of red-cell membrane.

Change in red-cell shape through alteration in the solubility of haemoglobin within the cell, through changes in the composition of the lipids of the red-cell membrane or by loss of membrane lipids of fragments of membrane, may influence the deformability of the red cell and predispose to accelerated destruction and splenic sequestration [134].

MEMBRANE STRUCTURE AND FUNCTION AND ALTERED CATION COMPOSITION OF THE RED CELLS
The normal cation composition of the red cell is dependent upon maintaining an appropriate balance between passive permeability and active transport. Excessive gain in red-cell Na^+ and concomitant influx of water results in cell swelling or 'hydrocytosis', whilst excessive loss of K^+ and concomitant loss of water results in cell shrinkage or 'desiccytosis' [135]. Changes in cation and water composition of red cells is associated with a variety of haemolytic disorders [136]. However, the relationship between these changes and red-cell survival is not entirely clear. Thus, although there have been extensive studies of Na^+ transport in hereditary spherocytic cells following the observation of Harris & Prankerd [137] of increased Na^+ permeability in this disorder, it seems that this is a reflection of abnormal membrane function and plays only a minor role in the diminished survival of these cells [135]. This conclusion is supported by the finding of much more severe disturbances of red-cell cations in the absence of spherocytosis in patients with hereditary stomatocytosis [138–140] (*vide infra*). Increase in red-cell Na^+ due to failure of the red-cell Na^+,K^+ ATPase to respond normally to the rise in intracellular Na^+ has been observed in a variety of miscellaneous disorders: uraemia and carcinoma [141, 142], malaria [143], hyperthyroidism [144], and in Liddle's syndrome [146] (see Chapter 33).

Loss of K^+ from red cells with an accompanying loss of water causes an increase in cell viscosity and may have a more significant effect on red-cell survival than gain in Na^+ [135]. Loss of K^+ takes place from red cells deficient in pyruvate kinase (PK) [146]. Mentzer *et al.* [147] have shown that massive K^+ loss can be induced from PK-deficient red cells by the addition of cyanide. Since the PK-deficient red cell is dependent for ATP generation on oxidative phosphorylation by mitochondria [148], the effect of cyanide is to produce a rapid ATP depletion (see also Chapter 7, p. 289). Mentzer *et al.* [147] found that the falling ATP was accompanied by a rise in red-cell Ca^{2+}. The benefit of splenectomy in PK deficiency may in part reflect the exclusion of PK reticulocytes from the hypoxic environment of the spleen where a reduction in oxygen tension may impair oxidative phosphorylation upon which the deficient cell is dependent [147].

Entry of Ca^{2+} into red cells is accompanied by loss of K^+, the so-called Gardos effect [149]. This probably accounts for the K^+ loss from sickle cells following sickling [150]. Extreme microcytosis has also been described in association with increased K^+ influx in a child with a congenital haemolytic anaemia whose red cells were shown to have an increased Ca^{2+} leak [151]. Increased loss of K^+ *in vitro* has been observed from red cells containing Heinz bodies due to haemoglobin Köln [152] and in thalassaemia major [153] (see Chapters 8 and 9).

Of considerable general medical and genetic interest has been the reported finding of altered K^+ and Li^+ transport from the red cells of patients with essential hypertension [154, 155]. It would appear that the altered K^+ and Li^+ transport in red cells in such patients and a proportion of the members of their immediate families may be an example of the phenotypic expression of a more generalized cell-membrane disorder which may predispose to the development of essential hypertension in later life.

The red cells of patients with obesity have been found to have reduced Na^+, K^+ ATPase activity and a raised Na^+ level when compared with non-obese controls [213]. If this alteration in the membrane of red cells is indicative of altered cell metabolism the reduced energy requirements may contribute to obesity.

EFFECT OF ANTIBODIES ON MEMBRANE STRUCTURE AND FUNCTION

The binding of IgG antibodies to the red cell predisposes the cell to phagocytosis by macrophages which may result in membrane loss with the formation of spherocytes [132, 133]. The destruction of erythrocytes sensitized with IgG antibodies by macrophages is determined by the number of IgG molecules on the cell surface and whether or not the IgG molecule interacts with the Fc receptors on the phagocytic cell [156] (see Chapter 11). Overt haemolysis is seen less frequently when the antibody is of the IgG2 or IgG4 class of immunoglobulin than with IgG1 and IgG3 autoantibodies [157]. Anti-D, or its IgG fraction, reduces ATP synthesis by D-positive red-cell membrane although the mechanism is incompletely understood [157]. Palek and co-workers [158] have demonstrated diminished ATP synthesis in red cells treated with isoimmune anti-A antisera; the red-cell membranes from the antibody-treated cells showed an increase in Na^+, K^+ ATPase activity. By contrast a reduction in Na^+, K^+ ATPase activity was observed in red cells treated with rabbit anti-human red-cell antibodies [159].

Detailed studies of the effects of antibodies on red-cell-membrane function have been carried out on low-K^+ (LK) sheep red cells. The incubation of LK sheep red cells with antibodies prepared in high-K^+ (HK) sheep or with antibodies reacting specifically with LK cells results in a four- to fivefold increase in active transport of K^+ into LK cells [66] and a twofold increase in active transport sites [67].

The activation of complement by IgM antibodies on the red-cell membrane can result in the production of holes through the membrane thereby bringing about lysis. The red cells of patients with paroxysmal nocturnal haemoglobinuria are characterized by enhanced susceptibility to complement lysis, the numbers of complement-produced holes in the membrane being much greater in number than with normal red-cell membranes [160]. The mechanism of complement action in membrane disruption has been reviewed by Rosse [160] and is discussed in detail in Chapter 12.

CONDITIONS WHICH MAY RESULT FROM SPECIFIC RED-CELL-MEMBRANE DEFECTS

HEREDITARY SPHEROCYTOSIS (HS)

Familial jaundice with mild anaemia associated with the presence of small spherocytic red cells in the blood was first recognized towards the end of the nineteenth century. Dacie [161] has reviewed in detail the early descriptions of the disorder and the recognition of the inheritance. Subsequent studies have confirmed the autosomal-dominant nature of inheritance with nearly 50% expression in family members and an incidence of 200–300/million of the population in the United States and Great Britain [162]. Studies of a family with an 8/12 chromosomal translocation has suggested that the HS locus is located on or near the short arm of either chromosome 8 or chromosome 12 [163]. Further studies of this and other families with HS showed a lack of linkage with all marker loci except for Gm(IgG) and Pi (α-1-antitrypsin). It is probable, but not proven, that the Gm-Pi loci are on the short arm of chromosome 12, suggesting that the gene for HS is also in this region. This conclusion is supported by the report of an interesting family segregating for 50% glyceraldehyde-3-phosphate-dehydrogenase (G3PD) deficiency and HS [164]; the G3PD has been mapped on the short arm of chromosome 12.

Not uncommonly, classical examples of HS have been reported in patients in whom family studies have been entirely negative, suggesting that they have resulted from mutation; in other families the variation in the severity of the haemolysis and the degree of spherocytosis has suggested heterogeneity in expression of the gene [165].

Clinical features

Hereditary spherocytosis commonly presents in childhood and may be preceded by an unexplained episode of neonatal jaundice. The cardinal features are of mild jaundice, with absence of bile in the urine, mild anaemia (haemoglobin 8–12 g/dl), evidence of haemolytic anaemia (reticulocytosis, erythroid hyperplasia of the bone marrow, and shortened red-cell survival), splenomegaly, and the response of the anaemia and jaundice to splenectomy. Increased bile-pigment metabolism can lead to the formation of pigmented biliary calculi and, rarely, cholecystitis and biliary colic may be the presenting features in an otherwise symptomless adult. Family studies not infrequently reveal the presence of mild jaundice, anaemia or biliary calculi in otherwise symptomless members of the family in whom examination of the blood confirms the inheritance of the disorder.

The depth of jaundice and the degree of anaemia is variable and episodes of jaundice and pallor may complicate infective illnesses in childhood. Such episodes probably reflect a temporary increase in the rate of haemolysis or a reduction in erythropoiesis or more commonly a combination of the two mechanisms, secondary to the infection. Occasionally such episodes are of such severity as to constitute a 'haemolytic crisis' or 'aplastic crisis' with the sudden onset of severe anaemia.

The spleen is usually, but not invariably, enlarged clinically, or is found to be increased in size and weight when removed surgically. A rare complication in adults who have not undergone splenectomy is the development of intractable ulceration of the skin of either one or both legs above the ankle. The ulcers result from ischaemia of the skin probably due to impaired blood flow through small cutaneous blood vessels due to the increased viscosity and diminished deformability of the spherocytic red cells associated with the impaired blood flow in the superficial tissues of the lower leg. The ulcers resemble those seen in sickle-cell disease, but differ in that the condition normally improves after splenectomy.

Radiological investigations may reveal the presence of multiple small radiotranslucent calculi, whilst barium studies of the gastro-intestinal tract may reveal or confirm the enlargement of the spleen. Both of these investigations are now more readily carried out by ultra-sound imaging.

Laboratory investigation of patients before splenectomy usually reveals a mild anaemia (haemoglobin 8–12 g/dl), with a corresponding reduction in red-cell count, although the MCHC is often slightly raised, and an elevated reticulocyte count. Examination of the stained blood film or diluted wet preparations of blood reveals the presence of a variable proportion of red cells which although of regular outline are smaller and denser in colour, and which lack the pale centre of the normal disc-shaped red cell (Fig. 10.5). Measurements of red-cell size distribution, either visually or electronically, confirm the presence of a population of red cells

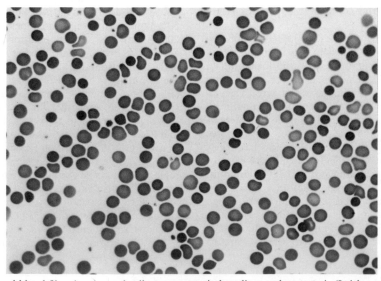

Fig. 10.5. Peripheral blood film showing red-cell appearances in hereditary spherocytosis (Leishmann's stain, × 440).

with a lower MCV. The white-cell count and platelet count are usually within normal limits. Examination of bone-marrow aspirations reveals normoblastic hyperplasia with normal granulopoiesis and thrombopoiesis.

The red-cell osmotic fragility is usually increased. The fragility curve (Fig. 10.6) shows a variety of forms—in some cases the whole curve is 'shifted to the right', indicating that the majority of cells are more susceptible to osmotic lysis than normal while, in others, the bulk of the curve may lie in the normal range with a 'tail' of unusually fragile cells making up 10–20% of the total population. The latter type of curve is more common but intermediate forms are also observed [161]. The increase in osmotic fragility is more marked after 24 hours' sterile incubation of the red cells, although it is uncertain whether this will distinguish very mild cases of hereditary spherocytosis from normal individuals [161]. The rate of autohaemolysis (see Chapter 7, p. 281) is usually increased and, like normal cells, this is reduced by the addition of glucose.

The level of serum bilirubin is usually only moderately raised, the plasma bilirubin in children and adults rarely being above 2 mg/dl, the major portion being unconjugated, unless there is liver or biliary disease. The neonatal jaundice may be of sufficient severity to be confused with the jaundice of feto-maternal ABO incompatibility and may warrant exchange transfusion [166].

The survival of autologous red cells in hereditary spherocytosis is shortened and surface counting over the spleen and liver reveals progressive splenic sequestration of the patient's cells. The survival of red cells after splenectomy is usually normal or only minimally reduced.

The survival of red cells from a patient with hereditary spherocytosis in a normal recipient lacking a spleen is normal or nearly so [167], whereas survival in normal subjects in whom the spleen has not been removed is reduced [168]. The role of the spleen in shortening the survival of red cells in hereditary spherocytosis is discussed more fully below.

The red-cell defect in hereditary spherocytosis (HS)
Hereditary spherocytosis (HS) red cells have lost surface area relative to volume, thus accounting for the characteristic increase in osmotic fragility of these cells. In addition to a shift in the median fragility there is frequently a small proportion of osmotically more sensitive cells reflecting the presence of small microspherocytes. As mentioned above, the osmotic fragility of HS red cells is strikingly increased by sterile incubation for 24 hours [169, 170]; on 48 hours' incubation autohaemolysis takes place and can be lessened by the initial addition of glucose [171, 172]. The latter observations suggested that there might be a metabolic disorder in HS red cells. However, subsequent studies revealed normal levels of ATP and of other phosphorylated glycolytic intermediates, and that glucose metabolism was either normal [172–174] or increased [175, 176]. In the absence of glucose,

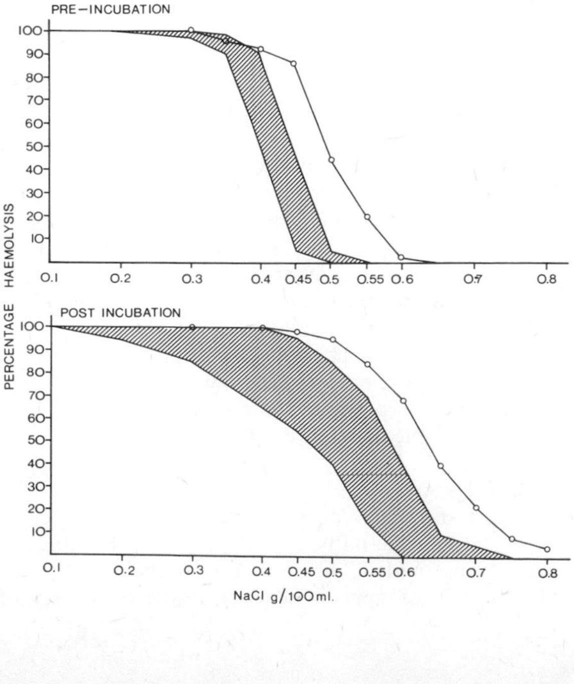

Fig. 10.6. Osmotic-fragility curves of hereditary spherocytosis. Top: a non-incubated fragility curve showing the marked increase in osmotic fragility as compared with the normal range which is shown by the shaded area. Bottom: incubated fragility; again normal range shown by shaded area.

incubation of HS red cells resulted in a rapid fall in ATP and 2,3-diphosphoglycerate [176–178]. The rapid utilization of ATP and increased glycolysis has been shown to be due to increased activity of the Na$^+$,K$^+$ ATPase pump since it is inhibited by the cardiac glycoside ouabain [175, 176]. This confirmed the previous finding of increased sodium influx and efflux [137, 179]. The increase in Na$^+$ permeability and Na$^+$, K$^+$ ATPase activity is improved or corrected by splenectomy [180, 181]. Although some workers have found an increase in calcium concentrations in HS red cells [182], others could not confirm this finding [183].

The increase in cation permeability would appear to be a manifestation of the membrane defect in HS but does not itself contribute to the disorder of membrane structure or function. Although an increase in phospholipid metabolism in the membranes of HS cells has been described [184] this has also been disputed [54].

Prolonged incubation of HS red cells results in loss of equal proportions of membrane phospholipid and cholesterol, an effect which was lessened by the provision of glucose [127]. Weed & Reed [128] suggested that this symmetrical loss of membrane lipid was due to loss of membrane fragments, but Langley & Axell [129] failed to demonstrate comparable loss of membrane protein. Nevertheless, an increase in membrane lipids improves HS-red-cell survival as was shown by Cooper & Jandl [131] who demonstrated enhanced survival when HS red cells were transfused into patients with target cells due to obstructive jaundice. They suggested that the accumulation of lipid in the membrane of the HS red cell might, by increasing the surface area of the cell, ameliorate the effects of membrane loss. Although intact HS red cells have been shown to have diminished deformability, the deformability of HS ghost cells is normal [185], suggesting that the loss of deformability is more closely related to changes in the ratio of surface area to volume than to an inherent disorder of the membrane cytoskeleton. Nevertheless, much attention has been directed to endeavouring to elucidate a presumptive disorder in the cytoskeleton proteins of the HS membrane. Initially, it was thought that HS-red-cell membrane had diminished phosphorylation of spectrin and of band 3. However, this observation could not be confirmed in intact cells.

Indirect evidence for an abnormality in the membrane proteins of HS cells has been provided by the finding by Jacob and co-workers that many of the characteristics of HS cells could be induced in normal red cells by treatment with vinblastine and colchicine [186]. These effects were blocked by cyclic nucleotides such as cAMP or cGMP [187]. Endeavours to detect an abnormality in the relative amounts or mobility of membrane proteins on electrophoresis have proved inconsistent, possibly because of the size and complexity of molecules thought to be involved, such as spectrin. The evidence that the spectrin-deficient mouse cell is markedly spherocytic [23], and is accompanied by profound alterations in the stability of the membrane, supports the potential importance of membrane-spectrin interaction for maintenance of normal membrane function and structure. This conclusion is further supported by the finding that lipid-extracted HS membranes have reduced stability [80]. It seems likely that in the near future techniques for analysing the interaction of spectrin or akyrin, or spectrin–actin interactions may reveal the nature of the primary defect in HS red cells [188].

The spleen in hereditary spherocytosis (HS)
Correction of the anaemia, jaundice and red-cell survival invariably follows removal of the spleen in patients with classical HS. Studies of HS red cells obtained from the splenic pulp immediately after surgical removal of the spleen have demonstrated an increased proportion of osmotically fragile cells [167, 169, 170]. Thus, the spleen in addition to selectively removing HS red cells from the circulation also enhances the degree of membrane loss, and thereby increases the degree of sphering of HS red cells [189]. The trapping of HS red cells relates to the diminished deformability of spherocytes when attempting to traverse the filter-like splenic circulation between the Bilroth cords and splenic sinuses, and reflects the diminished filterability of spherocytic red cells *in vitro* [190].

The mechanism by which the spleen enhances membrane loss from HS red cells is probably analogous to the loss of membrane which takes place on prolonged sterile incubation *in vitro*, in which there is both metabolic depletion and fall in pH from lactic-acid formation. The HS red cells from the spleen have higher levels of Na$^+$ and lower levels of ATP [177], whilst the level of glucose in the spleen is lower than that of the peripheral blood and falls more rapidly [191]. Furthermore, the HS red cell shows increased susceptibility to fall in pH [192], a further probable consequence of splenic engorgement. Thus, the spleen provides a uniquely adverse environment for the metabolism of the HS red cell and predisposes to the loss of membrane components, which in producing a greater degree of spherocytic shape will further predispose to splenic sequestration.

Management
There is no doubt that except in the mildest cases splenectomy should be carried out once the diagnosis has been made. There is the continuous risk of haemolytic or aplastic crises, and the possibility of

obstructive jaundice due to pigment stones increases with time. Furthermore, in cases with active haemolysis there is increased iron absorption which may lead to haemochromatosis with liver damage leading to liver failure [193]. Very mild cases found during family studies can be kept under surveillance. It is advisable to delay splenectomy until after the age of five years because of the risk of infection (see Chapter 20). The risk of pneumococcal sepsis following splenectomy may be reduced by the administration of polyvalent pneumococcal vaccine [194]. There have been occasional reports of relapses due to hypertrophy of accessory spleens (see Chapter 20) but otherwise the results of surgery are excellent.

STOMATOCYTOSIS

The term 'stomatocyte' has been employed to describe red cells which have a longitudinal mouth-like depression, in contrast to the central circular depression of the normal discoid red cell (Fig. 10.7). Stomatocytes have been described in normal blood films [195] and in association with a wide variety of disorders: acute alcoholism and alcoholic cirrhosis [196, 197], glutathione-peroxidase deficiency [140], HS [196], infectious mononucleosis [198], lead poisoning [195], thalassaemia minor [196], and in malignant disease of children and adults [141]. The significance of stomatocytosis in these disorders is uncertain.

In contrast there is now a well-recognized association between the presence of many (10–40%) stomatocytic red cells and hereditary haemolytic anaemia; hereditary stomatocytosis [135, 138–140, 199–201]. The patients have anaemia and reticulocytosis (up to 40%) and shortened red-cell survival. Recently the red cells of such patients have been the subject of detailed metabolic studies [135, 138–140]. The single most striking abnormality has been the finding of altered cation content and transport.

In a three-and-a-half-year-old boy described by Zarkowsky *et al.* [138], red-cell sodium was increased about ninefold and potassium reduced by about 50%. The red cells show a comparable increase in water content and increased osmotic fragility. Sodium efflux was increased, accompanied by an increase in glycolysis, but the efficiency of sodium transport was less than that of normal cells. Subsequent reports have described similar disorders of red-cell cation composition and transport, although the levels of sodium have been lower than those described by Zarkowsky *et al.* [138]. In one such patient the increase in the requirement for ATP for membrane transport was thought to account for an associated low level of 2,3-DPG [151]. Miller *et al.* [140] described detailed studies of an affected child of consanguineous parents. The propositus and two siblings had haemolytic anaemia with stomatocytosis (16–35%), and approximately a twice-normal red-cell sodium content with increased sodium efflux, and were regarded as being homozygous for the disorder. The parents, four siblings, and 44 other affected members of the family showed less marked stomatocytosis (1–25%) and mild reticulocytosis but were not anaemic and were considered to be heterozy-

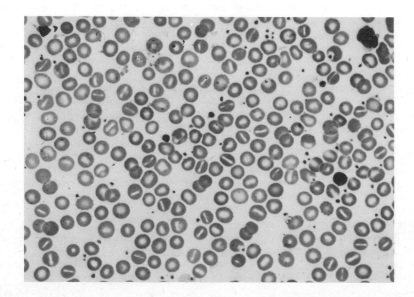

Fig. 10.7. The red cells of a patient with stomatocytosis. The slit-like appearance in the centre of the red cells is well shown (Leishmann's stain, ×440).

gous for the disorder. In contrast to other reports, the osmotic fragility of the red cells of both the homozygous and heterozygous members of the family was decreased.

The nature of the membrane abnormality which results in stomatocytic red cells and the disorder of red-cell cation permeability remains to be elucidated. No abnormalities of red-cell enzymes, red-cell-membrane lipid composition, of incorporation of fatty acids into membrane lipids, or of anion permeability have been found [139, 140]. Changes in membrane proteins have been found. Thus Beinzle *et al.* [202] have tentatively identified an abnormal membrane protein with an approximate MW of 25 000 daltons in the red cells from one patient. Mentzer *et al.* [37] have also noted a diminution in band 7. The latter workers have shown that incubation of stomatocytic red cells *in vitro* with a bifunctional cross-linking reagent, dimethyl adipimidate (DMA), corrects the morphological abnormality and is accompanied by marked improvement in cation composition. The DMA improves the cation permeability of stomatocytes at very low concentrations (1·0 mM) that result in barely detectable cross-linking of aminophospholipids or proteins. This finding has led Mentzer *et al.* [37] to suggest that the benefit arises from cross-linking of either a minor component present in only small quantities, or is due to intra-molecular rather than inter-molecular cross-linking. The further elucidation of the effects of DMA on specific membrane components may greatly assist in the elucidation of the defect and may throw important light on properties of normal red-cell membrane.

HEREDITARY ELLIPTOCYTOSIS (HE)
This disorder, characterized by the regular elliptical shape of the red cells (Fig 10.8), is inherited as an autosomal dominant [203]. It probably results from several different genetic determinants, one of which is linked to the Rh blood-group loci [204, 205]. Homozygous HE is associated with severe, and sometimes fatal, haemolytic anaemia in infancy. The red cells of HE homozygotes are longer than those of heterozygous carriers [205]. There is much greater variation in the haematological findings in heterozygotes; in many subjects there is no anaemia or evidence of haemolysis. Occasionally there may be relatively severe haemolytic anaemia with splenomegaly and this clinical presentation is observed in all affected family members. It seems likely that this clinical variability reflects underlying genetic heterogeneity. Evidence in favour of this has come from family studies by Bannerman & Renwick [206], who noted that the HE gene which is linked to the Rh locus is not usually associated with haemolytic anaemia. In contrast, patients in whom HE

segregates independently from the Rh gene have haemolytic anaemia and splenomegaly. The jaundice and haemolysis in HE is improved by splenectomy although the morphological abnormality of the red cells persists [207].

The nature of the red-cell abnormality in HE has yet to be fully elucidated. The lipid-extracted cytoskeletons of HE cells are elliptical in shape and have been found to have an increased membrane fragility when compared with the cytoskeletons of normal red-cell ghosts similarly prepared [81]. Furthermore, HE red cells show increased Na^+ efflux [208].

HEREDITARY PYROPOIKILOCYTOSIS (HP)
Zarkowsky *et al.* [35] described three children in whom congenital haemolytic anaemia was accompanied by striking microspherocytosis and cells with blunted projections or cells triangular in shape (Fig 10.9). The knowledge that normal red cells undergo fragmentation and microspherocyte formation on exposure to heat led these workers to investigate the susceptibility of the abnormal cells to the effects of temperature. They observed that the red cells from their patients underwent fragmentation at a temperature of 45°C, whereas normal cells did not undergo such changes until the temperature reached 49°C. They found that the heat-induced transformation of the patients' cells was accompanied by an increase in the membrane cholesterol/phospholipid and cholesterol/protein ratios, a finding suggestive of a selective loss of membrane components. The splenectomy lessened the haemolytic process which led the authors to suggest that the altered red-cell morphology was the result of *in-vivo* fragmentation and that the spleen was the major site of destruction of the abnormal cells. More recently Chang *et al.* [209] have shown from measurements of the circular dichromism of spectrin that this component of the membrane undergoes denaturation at lower temperatures than spectrin derived from normal red cells.

The property of increased susceptibility to temperature—implied by the name ('pyropoikilocytosis') coined by Zarkowsky *et al.* [35]—does not appear to be unique to this disorder as enhanced heat-induced fragmentation has also been observed in a patient with neonatal elliptocytosis [34]. Thus, although the precise biochemical abnormality in both hereditary elliptocytosis and pyropoikilocytosis has yet to be defined, both disorders would appear to reflect an inherent instability of the membrane cytoskeleton.

MARCH HAEMOGLOBINURIA
(See also Chapter 12)
The association of haemoglobinuria with a variety of physical activities, including running on hard surfaces

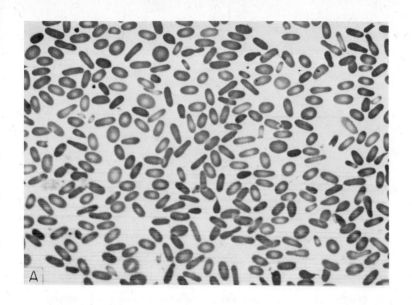

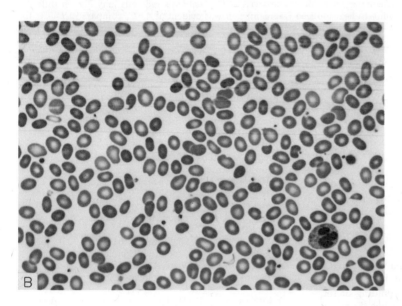

Fig. 10.8. The peripheral blood appearances in hereditary elliptocytosis. A, the findings in a more severely affected individual; B, the extremely mild oval cell deformity which may be found in the elliptocytosis trait (Leishmann's stain, × 440).

[210], karate [211], and the trauma associated with playing conga drums [212], led to the generally accepted view that normal red cells may undergo haemolysis within the circulation in response to externally applied physical forces. This view was put forward by Walker [210] who first demonstrated that the nature of the surface upon which the running took place and modification of the footwear could ameliorate the disorder. More recently Banga *et al.* [38] observed an absence of a 29 000 dalton band from the red-cell-membrane proteins of patients with march haemoglobinuria. It is of interest that there is no morphological accompaniment to the disorder and that increased haemolysis only takes place under unusual circumstances. Family studies have yet to be reported upon this presumably inherited abnormality.

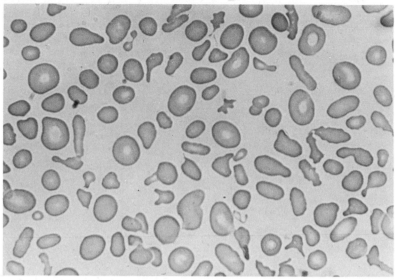

Fig. 10.9. The red cells of a patient with congenital poikilocytic haemolytic anaemia who failed to respond to splenectomy. The appearances are similar to those seen in hereditary pyropoikilocytosis (HP). This patient's red cells may have a different membrane defect as the increased susceptibility to heat-induced fragmentation was evident at 47°C, compared to 49°C for normal cells (a less marked abnormality than that reported in HP). The extracted spectrin was heat stable, and the patient's son had mild elliptocytosis. (Illustration by courtesy of Dr David Chui.)

CONCLUSION

Our understanding of disorders of the red-cell membrane in congenital and acquired haemolytic anaemia has in recent years progressed from the recognition of distinct clinical disorders to the characterization of defined disturbances of physiological function and biochemical composition. The complexity of the ultrastructure of cell membranes, including that of the red cell, has made it difficult, as yet, to relate disorders of function or of biochemical composition to molecular structure and organization. However, the pace of advance of knowledge makes it seem likely that in due course the characterization of abnormalities of structure of the red-cell membrane in haemolytic anaemia will contribute as much to our understanding of the molecular biology of cell membranes as has the study of abnormal haemoglobin to structure and function of the haemoglobin molecule.

REFERENCES

1 GORTER E. & GRENDEL F. (1925) On the biomolecular layers of lipids on the chromocytes of the blood. *Journal of Experimental Medicine*, **41**, 439.

2 DAVSON H. & DANIELLI J.F. (1943) *The Permeability of Natural Membranes.* Cambridge University Press, Cambridge.

3 ROBERTSON J.D. (1959) The ultrastructure of cell membranes and their derivatives. *Biochemical Society Symposia*, **16**, 3.

4 ROBERTSON J.D. (1964) Unit membranes. A review with recent new studies of experimental alterations and a new sub-unit structure in synaptic membranes. In: *Cellular Membranes in Development* (ed. Locke E.), p. 1. Academic Press, New York.

5 WILKINS M.H.F., BLAUROCK A.E. & ENGLEMAN D.M. (1971) Bilayer structure in membranes. *Nature (New Biology)*, **23**, 72.

6 STOECKENHUIS W. & ENGELMAN D.M. (1969) Current models for the structure of biological membranes. *Journal of Cell Biology*, **42**, 613.

7 HENDLER R.W. (1971) Biological membrane ultrastructure. *Physiological Reviews*, **51**, 66.

8 SINGER S.J. (1971) The molecular organization of biological membranes. In: *Structure and Function of Biological Membranes* (ed. Rothfield L.I.), p. 146. Academic Press, New York.

9 MARINETTI G.V. & CRAIN R.C. (1978) Topology of amino-phospholipids in red cell membranes. *Journal of Supramolecular Structure*, **8**, 191.

10 VAN DEENEN L.L.M. (1979) Structural organization and dynamics of phospholipids in red cell membranes. *Progress in Clinical and Biological Research*, **30**, 451.

11 VAN DEENEN L.L.M., DE GRIER J., VAN GOLDE L.M.G., NAUTA I.L.D., RENOOY W., VERKLEIJ A.J. & ZWAAL R.F.A. (1976) Some topological and dynamic aspects of

lipids in the erythrocyte membrane. In: *Structure of Biological Membranes* (ed. Abrahmsson S. & Pascher I.), p. 107. Plenum, New York.

12 GOODMAN S.R. & BRANTON D. (1978) Spectrin binding and the control of membrane protein mobility. *Journal of Supramolecular Structure*, **8**, 455.

13 GOLAN D.E. & VEATCH W. (1979) Lateral mobility of band 3 in the human erythrocyte membrane studied by fluorescence photobleaching recovery; evidence for control by cytoskeletal interactions. *Proceedings of the National Academy of Sciences, USA*, **77**, 2537.

14 SCHNIDLER M., KEPPELL D.E. & SHEETZ M.P. (1980) Modulation of membrane protein lateral mobility by polyphosphates and polyamines. *Proceedings of the National Academy of Sciences, USA*, **77**, 1457.

15 FAIRBANKS G., STECK T.L. & WALLACH D.F. (1971) Electrophoretic analysis of the major polypeptides of the human erythrocyte membrane. *Biochemistry*, **10**, 2606.

16 TRAYER H.R., NOZAKI Y., REYNOLDS J.A. & TANFORD C. (1971) Polypeptide chains from human red blood cell membranes. *Journal of Biological Chemistry*, **246**, 4485.

17 MARCHESI V.T, (1979) Functional proteins of the human red blood cell membranes. *Seminars in Hematology*, **16**, 3.

18 SHEETZ M. & SAWYER D. (1978) Triton shells of intact erythrocytes. *Journal of Supramolecular Structure*, **8**, 399.

19 JI T.H., KIEHM D.J. & MIDDAUGH C.R. (1980) The presence of spectrin tetramer in the erythrocyte membrane. *Journal of Biological Chemistry*, **255**, 2990.

20 LUX S.E. (1979) Dissecting the red cell membrane skeleton. *Nature (London)*, **281**, 426.

21 BENNET V. & STENBUCK P.J. (1980) Human erythrocyte ankyrin. *Journal of Biological Chemistry*, **255**, 2540.

22 SHOHET S.B. (1979) Reconstitution of spectrin-deficient spherocytic mouse erythrocyte membranes. *Journal of Clinical Investigation*, **64**, 483.

23 SHEETZ M.P., SCHINDLER M. & KOPPEL D.E. (1980) Lateral mobility of integral membrane proteins is increased in spherocytosis. *Nature (London)*, **285**, 510.

24 LORAND L., SIEFRING G.E. JR & LOWE-KRENTZ L. (1978) Formation of γ-glutamyl-ε-lysine bridges between membrane proteins by a Ca^{2+}-regulated enzyme in intact erythrocytes. *Journal of Supramolecular Structure*, **9**, 427.

25 LORAND L., SIEFRING G.E. JR & LOWE-KRENTZ L. (1979) Enzymatic basis of membrane stiffening in human eythrocytes. *Seminars in Hematology*, **16**, 65.

26 EATON J.W., JACOB H.S. & WHITE J.G. (1979) Membrane abnormalities of irreversibly sickled cells. *Seminars in Hematology*, **16**, 52.

27 PALEK J. & LIU S.-C. (1979) Dependence of spectrin organization in red blood cell membranes on cell metabolism: implications for control of red cell shape, deformability and surface area. *Seminars in Hematology*, **16**, 75.

28 FISCHER T.M., HAEST C.W.M., STOHR M., KAMP D. & DEUTICKE B. (1978) Selective alteration of erythrocyte deformability of SH-reagents. Evidence for an involvement of spectrin in membrane shear elasticity. *Biochimica et Biophysica Acta*, **510**, 270.

29 HAEST C.W.M., KAMP D. & DEUTICKE B. (1979) Formation of disulphide bonds between glutathione and membrane SH groups in human erythrocytes. *Biochimica et Biophysica Acta*, **557**, 363.

30 LIU S.C. & PALEK J. (1979) Metabolic dependence of protein arrangement in human erythrocyte membranes. II. Cross linking of major proteins in ghosts from fresh and ATP-depleted red cells. *Blood*, **54**, 1117.

31 FAIRBANKS G., AVRUCH J., DINO J.E. & PATEL V.P. (1978) Phosphorylation and de-phosphorylation of spectrin. *Journal of Supramolecular Structure*, **9**, 97.

32 HUI D.Y. & HARMONY J.A.K. (1979) Erythrocyte spectrin alteration induced by low-density lipoprotein. *Journal of Supramolecular Structure*, **10**, 253.

33 LUX S.E., PEASE B., TOMASELLI M.B., JOHN K.M. & BERNSTEIN S.E. (1979) Hemolytic anemias associated with deficient or dysfunctional spectrin. *Progress in Clinical and Biological Research*, **30**, 463.

34 ZARKOWSKY H.S. (1979) Heat-induced erythrocyte fragmentation in neonatal elliptocytosis. *British Journal of Haematology*, **41**, 515.

35 ZARKOWSKY H.S., MOHANDAS N., SPEAKER C.B. & SHOHET S.B. (1975) A congenital haemolytic anaemia with thermal sensitivity of the erythrocyte membrane. *British Journal of Haematology*, **29**, 537.

36 MENTZER W.C., LAM G.K.H., LUBIN B.H., GREENQUIST A., SCHRIER S.L. & LANDE W. (1978) Membrane effects of imidoesters in hereditary stomatocytosis. *Journal of Supramolecular Structure*, **9**, 275.

37 MENTZER W.C. & LUBIN B.H. (1979) The effect of crosslinking reagents on red-cell shape. *Seminars in Hematology*, **16**, 115.

38 BANGA J.P., PINDER J.C., GRATZER W.B., LINCH D.C. & HUEHNS E.R. (1979) An erythrocyte membrane-protein anomaly in march haemoglobinuria. *Lancet*, **ii**, 1048.

39 STECK T.L. (1978) The band 3 protein of the human red cell membrane: a review. *Journal of Supramolecular Structure*, **8**, 311.

40 KNAUF P.A. (1979) Erythrocyte anion exchange and the band 3 protein: transport kinetics and molecular structure. *Current Topics in Membranes and Transport*, **12**, 251.

41 FURTHMAYR H. (1977) Structural analysis of a membrane glycoprotein: glycophorin A. *Journal of Supramolecular Structure*, **7**, 121.

42 TANNER M.J.A. (1979) Erythrocyte glycoproteins. *Current Topics in Membranes and Transport*, **11**, 279.

43 COOPER R.A. (1970) Lipids of the human red cell membrane: normal composition and variability in disease. *Seminars in Hematology*, **7**, 296.

44 VAN DEENEN L.L.M. (1969) Membrane lipids and lipophilic proteins. In: *The Molecular Basis of Membrane Function* (ed. Toteson D.C.), p. 47. Prentice Hall, New Jersey.

45 BLAU L. & BITTMAN R. (1978) Cholesterol distribution between the two halves of the lipid bilayer of human erythrocyte ghost membranes. *Journal of Biological Chemistry*, **253**, 8366.

46 LANGE Y. & D'ALESSANDRO J.S. (1978) The exchangeability of human erythrocyte membrane cholesterol. *Journal of Supramolecular Structure*, **8**, 391.

47 MURPHY J.R. (1962) Erythrocyte metabolism. III. Relationship of energy metabolism and serum factors to

osmotic fragility after incubation. *Journal of Laboratory and Clinical Medicine*, **60**, 86.

48 Borochov H., Abbott R.E., Schachter D. & Shinitsky M. (1979) Modulation of erythrocyte membrane proteins by membrane cholesterol and lipid fluidity. *Biochemistry*, **18**, 251.

49 Klappauf E. & Schubert D. (1979) Interactions of band 3-protein from human erythrocyte membranes with cholesterol and cholesterol analogues. *Hoppe Seylers Zeitschrift für Physiologische Chemie*, **306**, 1225.

50 Pittman J.G. & Martin D.B. (1966) Fatty acid biosynthesis in human erythrocytes; evidence in mature erythrocytes for an incomplete long-chain fatty acid synthesizing system. *Journal of Clinical Investigation*, **45**, 165.

51 Shohet S.B., Nathan D.G. & Karnovsky M.L. (1968) Stages in the incorporation of fatty acids into red blood cells. *Journal of Clinical Investigation*, **47**, 1096.

52 Shohet S.B. (1970) Release of phospholipid fatty acid from human erythrocytes. *Journal of Clinical Investigation*, **49**, 1668.

53 Mulder E., Vandenberg J.W.O. & van Deenen L.L.M. (1965) Metabolism of red cell lipids. II. Conversion of lysophosphoglycerides. *Biochimica et Biophysica Acta*, **106**, 118.

54 Reed C.F. (1968) Phospholipid exchange between plasma and erythrocytes in man and the dog. *Journal of Clinical Investigation*, **47**, 749.

55 Farquhar J.W. & Ahrens E.H. jr (1963) Effects of dietary fats on human erythrocyte fatty acid patterns. *Journal of Clinical Investigation*, **42**, 675.

56 Anstee D.J. (1980) Blood group MNSs-active sialoglycoproteins of the human erythrocyte membrane. In: *Immunobiology of the Erythrocyte* (ed. Sandler S.G., Nusbacher J. & Schanfield M.S.), p. 67. Alan R. Liss Inc., New York.

57 Baxter A. & Beeley J.G. (1978) Surface carbohydrates of aged erythrocytes. *Biochemical and Biophysical Research Communications*, **83**, 466.

58 Greenwalt T.J., Steane E.A., Lau F.O. & Sweeney-Hammond K. (1980) Aging of the human erythrocyte. In: *Immunobiology of the Erythrocyte* (ed. Sandler S.G., Nusbacher J. & Schanfield M. S.), p. 195. Allen R. Liss Inc., New York.

59 Crookston M.C. (1980) Blood group antigens acquired from the plasma. In: *Immunobiology of the Erythrocyte* (ed. Sandler S.G., Nusbacher J. & Schanfield M.S.), p. 99. Alan R. Liss Inc., New York.

60 Ginsburg V. & Kobata A. (1971) Structure and function of surface components of mammalian cells. In: *Structure and Function of Biological Membranes* (ed. Rothfield L.I.), p. 439. Academic Press, New York.

61 Rothstein A., Knauf P.A., Grinstein S. & Shami Y. (1979) A model for the action of the anion exchange protein of the red blood cell. *Progress in Clinical and Biological Research*, **30**, 483.

62 Glynn I.M. & Karlish S.J.D. (1974) The association of biochemical events and cation measurements in $(Na^+ + K^+)$-dependent adenosine triphosphatase activity. In: *Membrane Adenosine Triphosphatase and Transport Processes* (ed. Brock J.R.), p. 145. Biochemical Society, London.

63 Whittam R. (1975) Enzymic aspects of sodium pump across membranes. In: *Biological Membranes* (ed. Parsons D.S.), p. 158. Clarendon Press, Oxford.

64 Blotstein R. (1970) Sodium-activated adenosine triphosphatase activity of the erythrocyte membrane. *Journal of Biological Chemistry*, **245**, 270.

65 Hoffman J.F. (1966) The red cell membrane and the transport of sodium and potassium. *American Journal of Medicine*, **41**, 666.

66 Ellory I.C. & Tucker E.M. (1969) Stimulation of the potassium transport system in low potassium type sheep red blood cells by a specific antigen-antibody reaction. *Nature (London)*, **222**, 477.

67 Lauf P.K., Rasmussen B.A., Hoffman P.G., Dunhman P.B., Cook P., Parmelee M.L. & Tosteson D.C. (1970) Stimulation of active potassium transport in L.K. sheep red cells by blood group-L-antiserum. *Journal of Membrane Biology*, **3**, 1.

68 Lee K.S. & Shin B.C. (1969) Studies on the active transport of Ca^{++} in human red cells. *Journal of General Physiology*, **54**, 713.

69 Olson E.J. & Cazort R.J. (1969) Studies on the transport of Ca^{++} in human red cells. *Journal of General Physiology*, **53**, 311.

70 Schatzman H.J. & Vincenzi F.F. (1969) Calcium movements across the membrane of human red cells. *Journal of Physiology*, **201**, 369.

71 Rosenthal A.S., Kregenow F.M. & Moses H.L. (1970) Some characteristics of a Ca^{++} dependent ATPase activity associated with a group of erythrocyte membrane proteins which form fibrils. *Biochimica et Biophysica Acta*, **196**, 254.

72 Cheung W.Y. (1980) Calmodulin plays a pivotal role in cellular regulation. *Science*, **207**, 19.

73 Schrier S.L., Johnson M., Junga I. & Krueger J. (1980) Calcium distribution within human erythrocytes. *Blood*, **56**, 667.

74 Palek J. & Liu S.C. (1979) Membrane protein organization in ATP-depleted and irreversibly sickled cells. *Journal of Supramolecular Structure*, **10**, 79.

75 Sogin D.C. & Hinkle P.C. (1978) Characterization of the glucose transporter from human erythrocytes. *Journal of Supramolecular Structure*, **8**, 447.

76 Lin E.C.C. (1971) The molecular basis of membrane transport systems. In: *Structure and Function of Biological Membranes* (ed. Rothfield L.I.), p. 286. Academic Press, New York.

77 Jung C.Y. (1975) Carrier-mediated glucose transport across human red cell membranes. In: *The Red Blood Cell* (ed. Surgenor D.M.), p. 706. Academic Press, New York.

78 Evans E.A. (1973) A new material concept for the red cell membrane. *Biophysical Journal*, **13**, 926.

79 Evans E.A. & Lacelle P. (1975) Intrinsic material properties of the erythrocyte membrane indicated by mechanical analysis of deformation. *Blood*, **45**, 29.

80 Liu S.C. & Palek J. (1980) Spectrin tetramer to dimer dissociation and cytoskeleton instability in abnormal erythrocytes. *International Society of Hematology and International Society of Blood Transfusion* (abstract), **383**, 87.

81 Mohandas N., Greenquist A.C. & Shohet S.B. (1978) Bilayer balance and regulation of red cell shape changes. *Journal of Supramolecular Structure*, **9**, 453.

82 CONRAD M.J. & SINGER S.J. (1979) Evidence for a large internal pressure in biological membranes. *Proceedings of the National Academy of Sciences, USA*, **76**, 5202.

83 ALLAN D. & MITCHELL R.H. (1975) Accumulation of 1,2 diacylglycerol in the plasma membrane may lead to echinocyte transformation of erythrocytes. *Nature (London)*, **258**, 218.

84 BURRIS S.M., EATON J.W. & WHITE J.G. (1980) Evaluation of the role of diacylgylcerol in calcium-induced erythrocyte shape change and rigidity. *Journal of Laboratory and Clinical Medicine*, **96**, 749.

85 CHIEN S. (1975) Biophysical behaviour of red cells in suspension. In: *The Red Blood Cell* (ed. Surgenor D.M.), p. 1032. Academic Press, New York.

86 SCHMID-SCHONBEIN H. & WELLS R. (1969) Fluid-drop-like transition of erythrocytes under shear. *Science*, **165**, 288.

87 FISHCER T.M., STOHR-LIESSEN M. & SCHMID-SCHONBEIN H. (1978) The red cell as a fluid droplet: tank tread-like motion of the human erythrocyte membrane in shear flow. *Science*, **202**, 894.

88 BRANEMARK P.I. & LINDSTROM J. (1963) Shape of circulating blood corpuscles. *Biorheology*, **1**, 139.

89 GUEST M.M., BOND T.P., COOPER R.G. & DERRICK J.R. (1963) Red blood cells: change in capillaries. *Science*, **142**, 1319.

90 JENSEN W.N. & LESSIN L.S. (1970) Membrane alterations associated with hemoglobinopathies. *Seminars in Hematology*, **7**, 409.

91 HARRIS J.W., BREWSTER H.A., HAM T.H. & CASTLE W.B. (1956) Studies on the destruction of red blood cells. X. The biophysics and biology of sickle-cell disease. *Archives of Internal Medicine*, **97**, 145.

92 DINTENFASS L. (1964) Rheology of the packed red blood cells containing hemoglobins A—A, S—A and S—S. *Journal of Laboratory and Clinical Medicine*, **64**, 594.

93 CHARACHE S., CONLEY C.L., WAUGH D.F., UGORETZ R.J. & SPURRELL J.R. (1967) Pathogenesis of hemolytic anemia in homozygous hemoglobin C disease. *Journal of Clinical Investigation*, **46**, 1795.

94 HAMM T.H., DUNN R.F., SAYRE R.W. & MURPHY J.R. (1968) Physical properties of red cells as related to effects *in vivo*. I. Increased rigidity of erythrocytes as measured by viscosity of cells altered by chemical fixation, sickling and hypertonicity. *Blood*, **32**, 847.

95 MURPHY J.R. (1968) Hemoglobin CC disease: rheological properties of erythrocytes and abnormalities in cell water. *Journal of Clinical Investigation*, **47**, 1483.

96 WEED R.I. & WEISS L. (1966) The relationship of red cell fragmentation occurring in the spleen to cell destruction. *Transactions of the Association of American Physicians*, **79**, 426.

97 WENNBERG E. & WEISS L. (1968) Splenic erythroclasia: an electron microscopic study of haemoglobin H disease. *Blood*, **31**, 779.

98 KWANT O.W. & SEEMAN P. (1970) The erythrocyte ghost as a perfect osmometer. *Journal of General Physiology*, **55**, 208.

99 NORUM K.R. & GJONE E. (1967) Familial plasma: lecithin acyl transferase deficiency. Biochemical study of a new inborn error of metabolism. *Scandinavian Journal of Clinical and Laboratory Investigation*, **20**, 231.

100 GJONE E., TORSVIK H. & NORUM K.R. (1958) Familial plasma cholesterol ester deficiency. A study of erythrocytes. *Scandinavian Journal of Clinical and Laboratory Investigation*, **21**, 327.

101 COOPER R.A. (1977) Abnormalities of cell membrane fluidity in the pathogenesis of disease. *New England Journal of Medicine*, **297**, 371.

102 COOPER R.A. & JANDL J.H. (1958) Bile salts and cholesterol in the pathogenesis of target cells in obstructive jaundice. *Journal of Clinical Investigation*, **47**, 809.

103 ZIEVE L. (1958) Jaundice, hyperlipemia and hemolytic anemia: a heretofore unrecognized syndrome associated with alcoholic fatty liver and cirrhosis. *Annals of Internal Medicine*, **48**, 471.

104 WESTERMAN M.P., BALCERZAK S.P. & HEINLE E.W. JR (1958) Red cell lipids in Zieve's syndrome: their relation to hemolysis and red cell osmotic fragility. *Journal of Laboratory and Clinical Medicine*, **72**, 663.

105 COOPER R.A. (1969) Anemia with spur cells: a red cell defect acquired in serum and modified in the circulation. *Journal of Clinical Investigation*, **48**, 1820.

106 COOPER R.A., ADMIRAND W.H., GARCIA F. & TREY C. (1970) The role of lithocholic acid in the pathogenesis of spur red cells and hemolytic anemia. *Journal of Clinical Investigation*, **48**, 18a.

107 WILEY S.S. & COOPER R.A. (1975) Inhibition of cation cotransport by cholesterol enrichment of human red cell membranes. *Biochimica et Biophysica Acta*, **413**, 425.

108 JAFFÉ E.R. & GOTTFRIED E.L. (1958) Hereditary non-spherocytic hemolytic disease associated with an altered phospholipid composition of erythrocytes. *Journal of Clinical Investigation*, **47**, 1375.

109 SHOHET S.B., LIVERMORE B.M., NATHAN D.G. & JAFFE E.R. (1971) Hereditary hemolytic anemia associated with abnormal membrane lipids: mechanism of accumulation of phosphatidyl choline. *Blood*, **38**, 445.

110 BASSEN F.A. & KORNZWEIG A.L. (1950) Malformation of the erythrocytes in a case of atypical retinitis pigmentosa. *Blood*, **5**, 381.

111 SINGER K., FISHER B. & PERLSTEIN M.A. (1952) Acanthrocytosis, a genetic erythrocytic malformation. *Blood*, **7**, 577.

112 SALT H.B., WOLFF O.H., LLOYD J.K., FOSBROOKE A.S., CAMERON A.H. & HUBBLE D.V. (1960) On having no beta-lipoprotein. A syndrome comprising a-beta-lipoproteinaemia, acanthocytosis and steatorrhoea. *Lancet*, **ii**, 325.

113 HERBERT P.N., GOTTO A.M. & FREDRICKSON D.S. (1978) Familial lipoprotein deficiency (abetalipoproteinemia, hypobetalipoproteinemia, and Tangier disease). In: *The Metabolic Basis of Inherited Disease*, 4th edn. (ed. Stanbury J.B., Wyngaarden J.B. & Frederickson D.S.), p. 544. McGraw-Hill, New York.

114 DODGE J.T., COHEN G., KAYDEN H.J. & PHILLIPS G.B. (1967) Peroxidative hemolysis of red blood cells from patients with a-beta-lipoproteinemia (acanthocytosis). *Journal of Clinical Investigation*, **46**, 357.

115 SIMON E.R. & WAYS P. (1964) Incubation hemolysis and red cell metabolism in acanthocytosis. *Journal of Clinical Investigation*, **43**, 1311.

116 ROSE C.S. & GYORGI P. (1952) Specificity of hemolytic reaction in Vitamin E deficient erythrocytes. *American Journal of Physiology*, **168**, 414.

117 JACOB H.S. & LUX S.E.V. (1958) Degradation of

membrane phospholipids and thiols in peroxide hemolysis: studies in Vitamin E deficiency. *Blood*, **32**, 549.

118 ROBINSON J.D. (1966) Interaction between protein
sulphydryl groups and lipid double bands of the
membrane. *Nature (London)*, **212**, 199.

119 BINDER J.H., HERTWIG D.C., HURST V. & FINCH S.C.
(1965) Tocopherol deficiency in man. *New England
Journal of Medicine*, **273**, 1289.

120 OSKI F.A. & BARNESS L.A. (1967) Vitamin E deficiency:
a previously unrecognized cause of hemolytic anemia in
premature infants. *Journal of Pediatrics*, **70**, 211.

121 MENGEL C.E., KANN H.E. JR, HEYMAN A. & METZ E.
(1965) Effects of *in vivo* hyperoxia on erythrocytes. II.
Hemolysis in a human after exposure to oxygen under
high pressure. *Blood*, **25**, 822.

122 SPEILBERG S.P., BOXER L.A., CORASH L.M. & SCHUL-
MAN J.D. (1979) Improved erythrocyte survival with
high-dose vitamin E in chronic hemolyzing G6PD and
glutathione synthetase deficiencies. *Annals of Internal
Medicine*, **90**, 53.

123 CORASH L., SPIELBERG S., BARTSOCAS C., BOXER L.,
STEINHERZ R., SHEETZ M., EGAN M., SCHLESSLEMAN J.
& SCHULMAN J.D. (1980) Reduced chronic hemolysis
during high-dose Vitamin E administration in Mediter-
ranean-type glucose-6-phosphate dehydrogenase deficiency. *New England Journal of Medicine*, **303**, 416.

124 NATTA C.L., MACHLIN L.J. & BRIN M. (1980) A
decrease in irreversibly sickled erythrocytes in sickle cell
anemia patients given vitamin E. *American Journal of
Clinical Nutrition*, **33**, 968.

125 PONDER E. (1948) *Haemolysis and Related Phenomena*,
p. 26. Grune & Stratton, New York.

126 BESSIS M. & LESSIN L.S. (1970) The discocyte-echinocyte
equilibrium of the normal and pathologic red cell.
Blood, **36**, 399.

127 REED C.F. & SWISHER S.N. (1966) Erythrocyte lipid loss
in hereditary spherocytosis. *Journal of Clinical Investigation*, **45**, 777.

128 WEED R.I. & REED C.F. (1966) Membrane alterations
leading to red cell destruction. *American Journal of
Medicine*, **41**, 681.

129 LANGLEY G.R. & AXELL M. (1968) Changes in erythrocyte membrane and autohaemolysis during *in vitro*
incubation. *British Journal of Haematology*, **14**, 593.

130 JACOB H.S. (1967) Membrane lipid depletion in hyper-
permeable red blood cells: its role in the genesis of
spherocytes in hereditary spherocytosis. *Journal of
Clinical Investigation*, **46**, 2083.

131 COOPER R.A. & JANDL J.H. (1959) The role of membrane lipids in the survival of red cells in hereditary
spherocytosis. *Journal of Clinical Investigation*, **48**, 736.

132 BESSIS M. & DE BOISFLEURY A. (1970) Étude des
differentes etapes de l'érythro-phagocytose par micro-
cinémato-graphic et microscopie électronique à
balayage. *Nouvelle Revue française d'Hématologie*, **10**,
223.

133 COOPER R.A. (1971) Loss of membrane components in
the pathogenesis of antibody-induced spherocytosis.
Journal of Clinical Investigation, **51**, 16.

134 LACELLE P.L. (1970) Alteration of membrane deformability. *Seminars in Hematology*, **7**, 355.

135 NATHAN D.G. & SHOHET S.B. (1970) Erythrocyte ion
transport defects and haemolytic anaemia: 'hydrocy-

tosis' and 'desiccytosis'. *Seminars in Hematology*, **7**, 381.

136 JANDL J.H. (1965) Leaky red cells. *Blood*, **26**, 367.

137 HARRIS E.J. & PRANKERD J.A. (1953) The rate of sodium
extrusion from human erythrocytes. *Journal of Physiology (London)*, **121**, 470.

138 ZARKOWSKY H.S., OSKI F.A., SHA'AFI R., SHOHET S.B.
& NATHAN D.G. (1958) Congenital hemolytic anemia
with high sodium, low potassium red cells. I. Studies of
membrane permeability. *New England Journal of Medicine*, **278**, 573.

139 OSKI F.A., NAIMAN J.L., BLUM S.F., ZARKOWSKY H.S.,
WHAUN J., SHOHET S.B., GREEN A. & NATHAN D.G.
(1969) Congenital hemolytic anemia with high sodium,
low potassium red cells. Studies of three generations of a
family with a new variant. *New England Journal of
Medicine*, **280**, 909.

140 MILLER D.R., RICKLES F.R., LICHTMAN M.A., LACELLE
P.L., BATES J. & WEED R.I. (1971) A new variant of
hereditary hemolytic anemia with stomatocytosis and
erythrocyte cation abnormality. *Blood*, **38**, 184.

141 WELT L.G., SACHS J.R. & MCMANUS T.J. (1964) An ion
transport defect in erythrocytes from uremic patients.
Transactions of the Association of American Physicians,
77, 169.

142 WELT L.G., SMITH E.K.M., DUNN M.J., CZERWINSKI
A., PROCTOR H., COLE C., BALFE J.W. & GITELMAN H.J.
(1967) Membrane transport defect: the sick cell. *Transactions of the Association of American Physicians*, **80**,
217.

143 DUNN M.J. (1969) Alterations of red blood cell sodium
transport during malarial infection. *Journal of Clinical
Investigation*, **48**, 674.

144 SMITH E.K.M. & SAMUEL P.D. (1970) Abnormalities in
the sodium pump of erythrocytes from patients with
hyperthyroidism. *Clinical Science*, **38**, 49.

145 GARDNER J.D., LAPEY A., SIMOPOULOS A.P. & BRAVO
E.L. (1971) Abnormal membrane sodium transport in
Liddle's syndrome. *Journal of Clinical Investigation*, **50**,
2253.

146 NATHAN D.G., OSKI F.A., SIDEL V.W. & DIAMOND L.K.
(1965) Extreme hemolysis and red cell distortion in
erythrocyte pyruvate kinase deficiency. II. Measurements of erythrocyte glucose consumption, potassium
flux and adenosine triphosphate stability. *New England
Journal of Medicine*, **272**, 118.

147 MENTZER W.C. JR, BAEHNER R.L., SCHMIDT-SCHONBEIN
H., ROBINSON S.H. & NATHAN D.G. (1971) Selective
reticulocyte destruction in erythrocyte pyruvate kinase
deficiency. *Journal of Clinical Investigation*, **50**, 688.

148 KEITT A.S. (1966) Pyruvate kinase deficiency and
related disorders of red cell glycolysis. *American Journal
of Medicine*, **41**, 762.

149 GARDOS G. (1959) The role of calcium in the potassium
permeability of human erythrocytes. *Acta Physiologica
Academiae Scientarium Hungaricae*, **15**, 121.

150 TOSTESON D.C., CARLSEN E. & DUNHAM E.T. (1955)
Effects of sickling on ion transport. I. Effect of sickling
on potassium transport. *Journal of General Physiology*,
39, 31.

151 WILEY J.S., COOPER R.A., ADACHI K. & ASAKURA T.
(1979) Hereditary stomatocytosis: association of low
2,3-diphosphoglycerate with increased cation pumping
by the red cell. *British Journal of Haematology*, **41**, 133.

152 JACOB H.S., BRAIN M.C. & DACIE J.V. (1968) Altered sulfhydryl reactivity of hemoglobins and red blood cell membranes in congenital Heinz body hemolytic anemia. *Journal of Clinical Investigation*, **47**, 2664.

153 CIVIDALLI G., LOCKER H. & RUSSELL A. (1971) Increased permeability of erythrocyte membrane in thalassemia. *Blood*, **37**, 716.

154 CANESSA M., ADRAGNA N., SOLOMON H.S., CONNOLLY T.M. & TOSTESON D.C. (1980) Increased sodium-lithium counter transport in red cells of patients with essential hypertension. *New England Journal of Medicine*, **302**, 772.

155 GARAY R.P., ELGHOZI J.-L., DAGHER G. & MEYER P. (1980) Laboratory distinction between essential and secondary hypertension by measurement of erythrocyte cation fluxes. *New England Journal of Medicine*, **302**, 769.

156 ENGELFRIET C.P., VON DEM BORNE A.E.G. KR., FLEER A., VAN DER MEULEN F.W. & ROOS D. (1980) *In vivo* destruction of erythrocytes by complement-binding and non-complement-binding antibodies. In: *Immunobiology of the Erythrocyte* (ed. Sandler S.G., Nusbacher J. & Schanfield M.S.), p. 213. Allen R. Liss Inc., New York.

157 SCHRIER S.L., MOORE L.D. & CHIAPELLA A.P. (1968) Inhibition of human erythrocyte membrane-mediated ATP synthesis by anti-D antibody. *American Journal of Medical Science*, **256**, 340.

158 PALEK J., MIRCEVOVA L., BRABEC V., FRIEDMAN B. & MAJSKY A. (1968) The effect of anti-A antibody on red cell organic phosphates and adenosine triphosphatase activity *in vitro*. *Scandinavian Journal of Haematology*, **5**, 191.

159 AVERDUNK R., GUNTERH T., DORN F. & ZIMMERMAN U. (1969) Über die Wirking von Antikorpen auf die ATPase-Aktivat und den aktiven Na-K-Transport von *E. coli* und Menschen-Erythrozyten. *Zeitschrift für Naturforschung: Teil B.*, **24**, 693.

160 ROSSE W.F. (1979) Interactions of complement with the red cell membrane. *Seminars in Hematology*, **16**, 128.

161 DACIE J.V. (1960) *The Haemolytic Anaemias, Congenital and Acquired. Part 1. The Congenital Anaemias*, p. 83. Churchill, London.

162 MORTON N.E., MACKINNEY A.A., KOSOWER N., SCHILLING R.F. & GRAY M.P. (1962) Genetics of spherocytosis. *American Journal of Human Genetics*, **14**, 170.

163 KIMBERLING W.J., TAYLOR R.A., CHAPMAN R.G. & LUBS H.A. (1978) Linkage and gene localization of hereditary spherocytosis (HS). *Blood*, **52**, 859.

164 MCCANN S.R., FINKEL B., CODMAN S. & ALLEN D.W. (1976) Study of a kindred with hereditary spherocytosis and glyceraldehyde-3-phosphate dehydrogenase deficiency. *Blood*, **47**, 171.

165 YOUNG L.E. (1955) Observations on the inheritance and heterogeneity of chronic spherocytosis. *Transactions of the Association of American Physicians*, **68**, 141.

166 STAMEY C.C. & DIAMOND L.K. (1957) Congenital hemolytic anemia in the newborn. Relationship to kernicterus. *American Journal of Diseases of Childhood*, **94**, 616.

167 EMERSON C.P. JR, SHEN S.C., HAM T.H., FLEMING E.M. & CASTLE W.B. (1956) Studies on the destruction of red blood cells. IX. Quantitative methods for determining the osmotic and mechanical fragility of red cells in the peripheral blood and splenic pulp, the mechanism of increased hemolysis in hereditary spherocytosis (congenital hemolytic jaundice as related to the functions of the spleen). *Archives of Internal Medicine*, **97**, 1.

168 WEISMAN R. JR, HAM T.H., HINZ C.F. & HARRIS J.W. (1955) Studies on the role of the spleen in the destruction of erythrocytes. *Transactions of the Association of American Physicians*, **68**, 131.

169 HAM T.H. & CASTLE W.B. (1940) Relation of increased hypotonic fragility and of erythrostasis to the mechanism of hemolysis in certain anemias. *Transactions of the Association of American Physicians*, **55**, 127.

170 EMERSON C.P. JR, SHEN S.C., HAM T.H. & CASTLE W.B. (1947) The mechanism of blood destruction in congenital hemolytic jaundice. *Journal of Clinical Investigation*, **26**, 1180.

171 DACIE J.V. (1941) Observations on autohaemolysis in familial acholuric jaundice. *Journal of Pathology and Bacteriology*, **52**, 331.

172 SELWYN J.G. & DACIE J.V. (1954) Autohemolysis and other changes resulting from the incubation *in vitro* of red cells from patients with congenital hemolytic anemia. *Blood*, **9**, 414.

173 DUNN I., IBSEN K.H., COE E.L., SCHNEIDER A.S. & WEINSTEIN I.M. (1963) Erythrocyte carbohydrate metabolism in hereditary spherocytosis. *Journal of Clinical Investigation*, **42**, 1535.

174 REED C.F. & YOUNG L.E. (1967) Erythrocyte energy metabolism in hereditary spherocytosis. *Journal of Clinical Investigation*, **46**, 1196.

175 JACOB H.S. & JANDL J.H. (1964) Increased cell membrane permeability in the pathogenesis of hereditary spherocytosis. *Journal of Clinical Investigation*, **43**, 1704.

176 MOHLER D.N. (1965) Adenosine triphosphate metabolism in hereditary spherocytosis. *Journal of Clinical Investigation*, **44**, 1417.

177 PRANKERD T.A.J. (1960) Studies on the pathogenesis of haemolysis in hereditary spherocytosis. *Quarterly Journal of Medicine*, **29**, 199.

178 PALEK J., MIRCEVOVA L. & BRABEC V. (1969) 2,3-diphosphoglycerate metabolism in hereditary spherocytosis. *British Journal of Haematology*, **17**, 59.

179 BERTLES J.F. (1957) Sodium transport across the surface membrane of red blood cells in hereditary spherocytosis. *Journal of Clinical Investigation*, **36**, 816.

180 WILEY J.S. (1969) Inheritance of increased Na pump in human red cells. *Nature (London)*, **221**, 1222.

181 WILEY J.W. & FIRKIN B.G. (1970) An unusual variant of hereditary spherocytosis. *American Journal of Medicine*, **48**, 63.

182 FEIG S.A. & BASSILAN S. (1975) Increased erythrocyte Ca^{2+} constant in hereditary spherocytosis. *Pediatric Research*, **9**, 928.

183 ZAIL S.S. & VAN DEN HOEK A.K. (1976) Studies on calcium transport and calcium-dependent adenosine triphosphatase activity of eyrthrocyte membranes in hereditary spherocytosis. *British Journal of Haematology*, **34**, 605.

184 JACOB H.S. & KARNOVSKY M.L. (1967) Concomitant

alterations of sodium flux and membrane phospholipid metabolism in red blood cells: studies in hereditary spherocytosis. *Journal of Clinical Investigation*, **46**, 173.

185 NAKASHIMA K. & BEUTLER E. (1979) Erythrocyte cellular and membrane deformability in hereditary spherocytosis. *Blood*, **53**, 481.

186 JACOB H., AMSDEN T. & WHITE J. (1972) Membrane microfilaments of erythrocytes: alteration in intact cells reproduced the hereditary spherocytosis syndrome. *Proceedings of the National Academy of Sciences, USA*, **69**, 471.

187 JACOB H.S., YAWATA Y., MATSUMOTO N., ABMAN S. & WHITE J. (1975) Cyclic nucleotide-membrane proteins interaction in the regulation of erythrocyte shape and survival: defect in hereditary spherocytosis. In: *Erythrocyte Structure and Function* (ed. Brewer, G.J.), p. 235. Alan R. Liss Inc., New York.

188 LUX S.E. (1979) Spectrin-actin membrane skeleton of normal and abnormal red blood cells. *Seminars in Hematology*, **16**, 21.

189 YOUNG L.E., PLATZER R.F., ERVIN D.M. & IZZO M.J. (1951) Hereditary spherocytosis. II. Observations on the role of the spleen. *Blood*, **6**, 1099.

190 JANDL J.H., SIMMONS R.C. & CASTLE W.B. (1961) Red cell filtration and the pathogenesis of certain hemolytic anemias. *Blood*, **18**, 133.

191 JANDL J.H. & ASTER R.H. (1967) Increased splenic pooling and the pathogenesis of hypersplenism. *American Journal of Medical Science*, **253**, 383.

192 MURPHY J.R. (1967) The influence of pH and temperature on some physical properties of normal erythrocytes and erythrocytes from patients with hereditary spherocytosis. *Journal of Laboratory and Clinical Medicine*, **69**, 758.

193 BARRY M., SCHEUER P.J., SHERLOCK S., ROSS C.F. & WILLIAMS R. (1968) Hereditary spherocytosis with secondary haemochromatosis. *Lancet*, **ii**, 481.

194 AMMANN A.J., ADDIEGO J., WARA D.W., LUBIN B., SMITH W.B. & MENTZER W.C. (1977) Pneumococcal immunization in sickle-cell anemia and asplenia. *New England Journal of Medicine*, **297**, 897.

195 BESSIS M. & DE BOISFLEURY A. (1970) Étude sur les poikilocytes au microscope à balayage en particulier dans la thalassémie. *Nouvelle Revue française Hématologies*, **10**, 515.

196 DUCROU W. & KIMBER R.J. (1969) Stomatocytes, haemolytic anaemia and abdominal pain in a Mediterranean migrant: some examples of a new syndrome. *Medical Journal of Australia*, **2**, 1087.

197 DOUGLASS C.C. & TWOMEY J.J. (1970) Transient stomatocytosis with hemolysis: a previously unrecognized complication of alcoholism. *Annals of Internal Medicine*, **72**, 159.

198 LO S.S., HITZIG W.H. & MARTI H.R. (1970) Stomatozy-tose. *Schweizerische Medizinische Wochenschrift*, **100**, 1977.

199 LOCK S.P., SMITH R.S., & HARDISTY R.M. (1961) Stomatocytosis. A hereditary red cell anomaly associated with haemolytic anaemia. *British Journal of Haematology*, **7**, 303.

200 MILLER G., TOWNES P.L., MACWHINNEY J.B. (1965) A new congenital hemolytic anemia with deformed erythrocytes (? 'stomatocytes') and remarkable susceptibility of erythrocytes to cold hemolysis *in vitro*. I. Clinical and hematologic studies. *Pediatrics*, **35**, 906.

201 WILEY J.S., ELLORY J.C., SHUMAN M.A., SHALLER C.C. & COOPER R.A. (1975) Characteristics of the membrane defect in hereditary stomatocytosis syndrome. *Blood*, **46**, 337.

202 BIENZLE U., BHADKI S., KNUFERMANN H., NIETHAMMER D. & KLEIHAUER E. (1977) Abnormality of erythrocyte membrane protein in a case of congenital stomatocytosis. *Klinische Wochenschrift*, **55**, 569.

203 WYANDT H., BANCROFT P.M. & WHINSHIP T.O. (1941) Elliptic erythrocyte in man. *Archives of Internal Medicine*, **68**, 1043.

204 CHALMERS J.N.M. & LAWLER S.D. (1952) Data on linkage in man; elliptocytosis and blood groups. I. Families 1 and 2. *Annals of Eugenics (London)*, **17**, 267.

205 NIELSEN J.A. & STRUNK K.W. (1968) Homozygous hereditary elliptocytosis as the cause of haemolytic anaemia in infancy. *Scandinavian Journal of Haematology*, **5**, 486.

206 BANNERMAN R.M. & RENWICK J.H. (1962) The hereditary elliptocytosis: clinical and linkage data. *Annals of Human Genetics*, **26**, 23.

207 GRECH J.L., CACHAIA E.A., CALLEJA F. & PULLICIANO F. (1961) Hereditary elliptocytosis in two Maltese families. *Journal of Clinical Pathology*, **14**, 365.

208 PETERS J.C., ROWLAND M., ISRAELS L.G. & ZIPURSKY A. (1966) Erythrocyte sodium transport in hereditary elliptocytosis. *Canadian Journal of Physiology & Pharmacology*, **44**, 817.

209 CHANG K., WILLIAMSON J.R. & ZARKOWSKY H.S. (1979) Effect of heat on the circular dichromism of spectrin in hereditary pyropoikilocytosis. *Journal of Clinical Investigation*, **64**, 326.

210 DAVIDSON R.J.L. (1979) March or exertional hemoglobinuria. *Seminars in Hematology*, **6**, 150.

211 STREETON J.A. (1967) Traumatic haemoglobinuria caused by karate exercises. *Lancet*, **ii**, 191.

212 KADEN W.S. (1970) Traumatic haemoglobinuria in conga-drum players. *Lancet*, **i**, 1341.

213 DE LUISE M., BLACKBURN G.L. & FLIER J.S. (1980) Reduced activity of the red cell–sodium–potassium pump in human obesity. *New England Journal of Medicine*, **303**, 1017.

Chapter 11
Immune haemolytic anaemias

SHEILA WORLLEDGE*

REVISED BY NEVIN C. HUGHES JONES AND BARBARA BAIN

As the name of this chapter implies, the increased destruction of the red cells in this group of haemolytic anaemias is thought to be a direct consequence of the absorption of antibody on to the red-cell surface. The rate of destruction, and consequently the symptoms, will depend on the immunoglobulin class and the thermal range of the antibody and whether or not it is capable of activating the complement sequence. The details of these mechanisms are discussed on page 504 under the heading 'Pathogenesis'.

Either the antibody or the red cells can be transferred from another person or made by the patient. Transfer of antibody or incompatible red cells by transfusion is discussed in Chapter 35. Transfer of antibody made by the mother through the placenta is the cause of haemolytic disease of the newborn. Antibody made by the patient, that affects his own red cells, may be either apparently directed against his own intrinsic antigens (autoimmune or autoallergic) or directed against drugs (immune or allergic). In this chapter haemolytic disease of the newborn will be discussed first, and this will be followed by accounts of autoimmune haemolytic anaemia not apparently provoked by drugs, and the immune haemolytic anaemias associated with drug therapy.

HAEMOLYTIC DISEASE OF THE NEWBORN

Haemolytic disease of the newborn (HDN) results from the passage of maternal IgG antibodies into the fetal circulation where they react with their specific antigens on the fetal red cells. Other immunoglobulins do not pass the placental barrier in significant amounts and it seems that there is an active mechanism for this IgG transfer.

The condition has been called by other names and until recently the term erythroblastosis fetalis was used to describe the whole clinical syndrome, although strictly it should be applied to the characteristic find-

* Dr Worlledge died while the second edition of this book was in preparation (see Preface).

ings of nucleated red cells in the peripheral blood and extramedullary haemopoiesis. Moreover, the clinical state of the newborn child was given various names which only comparatively recently have been recognized as variants of the same disease.

Clinical features of untreated haemolytic disease

Hydrops fetalis
This is the severest form of the disease and, as the name implies, the fetus has gross oedema and ascites. The placenta is also oedematous with swollen, friable cotyledons. This accumulation of fluid was thought to be due mainly to heart failure caused by the extreme anaemia and this probably is an important cause. Occasionally, however, infants with similar degrees of anaemia due to other causes are not hydropic, and the marked hypoproteinaemia which is present in the hydropic cases may be another important cause. The reasons for the hypoproteinaemia is uncertain: it may possibly be due to liver failure caused by the massive replacement of normal liver tissue by haemopoietic tissue. Haemopoietic tissue is also found in the spleen and both organs are grossly enlarged.

The fetus affected by hydrops has a very poor chance of survival and even intrauterine transfusion does little to improve the prognosis. The diagnosis of hydrops fetalis *in utero* is discussed by Gordon [1]. Most hydropic infants are born dead, often prematurely, and in those that are live-born the overall survival rate, even with modern treatment, is of the order of 14% [2].

Icterus gravis neonatorum
In this disorder, the infant is born superficially normal, but becomes grossly jaundiced within a few hours of birth. The infant's liver and spleen are always enlarged and increased red-cell destruction may be suspected from the yellow colouring of the amniotic fluid and the vernix caseosa. This jaundice can lead to neurological complications called kernicterus which may cause the death of the infant, or, if the infant survives the neonatal period, lead to permanent damage to the brain with spasticity, mental deficiency and deafness.

In normal newborn infants the formation of bilirubin is increased, while the capacity to excrete it is diminished. *In utero*, there is a transfer of bilirubin from the fetus to the mother, but even so, the level of bilirubin at birth is raised (up to 50 μmol/l) compared with levels in adult life. In every infant there is a rise of serum bilirubin during the first few days of life and in premature infants this will be more severe and prolonged.

Until recently it was thought that this rise in serum bilirubin was due mainly to immaturity of the liver enzyme, glucuronyl transferase, which conjugates bilirubin with glucuronic acid and renders it water-soluble. However, recent research has suggested other factors that may also be important: first, the hepatic uptake may be impaired by a temporary deficiency of 'carrier' proteins; secondly, a relative inability to excrete conjugated bilirubin may, through a feedback mechanism, result in accumulation of unconjugated bilirubin in the blood and thirdly, bilirubin may be reabsorbed from the intestine.

Anaemia neonatorum

Profound anaemia sometimes develops shortly after birth in infants that do not become grossly jaundiced, but this is just a rather rare variant of the severe disease. In the mildest form of the disease the infant appears normal at birth and jaundice is only slight, but the increased haemolysis may lead to late anaemia, which develops at about 30 days.

All these clinical states may be due to conditions other than haemolytic disease of the newborn, but this disorder is by far the commonest cause. Most IgG antibodies leading to this disease belong to the Rh and ABO blood-group systems. Severe symptoms are almost entirely due to Rh haemolytic disease, which will be described below. ABO haemolytic disease is usually mild and will be described in a later section. The rare cases of haemolytic disease due to antibodies in other blood-group systems will also be mentioned.

Rh haemolytic disease of the newborn

Immunization by the D antigen is much commoner than immunization by other Rh antigens. Giblett [3] found that in 93% of cases the antibodies were either anti-D or -CD. Approximately 6% were still within the Rh system and were usually anti-C, anti-E or anti-Ce. The remaining 1% were outside the Rh system, the commonest being in the Kidd, Kell, Duffy and S systems. In theory, any IgG antibody can cross the placenta and this should be kept in mind when investigating any case of HDN of obscure aetiology. Occasionally, the infants of women with variants of the D antigen, particularly that called Category VI (sometimes called D^B), are found to be affected with haemolytic disease due to an anti-D which reacts with their own and almost all Rh-positive cells but not those of their mother or other Category-VI red cells [4].

The development of Rh antibodies

Nowadays, the development of Rh antibodies in Rh-negative women of childbearing age is almost always the result of previous pregnancies. It can be calculated that about 60% of pregnant Rh-negative women will be carrying at least their first Rh-positive fetus and that 47% will be carrying their second [5]. Although fetal red cells may get into the mother's circulation at almost any time during pregnancy, they occur more frequently at the time of delivery [6]. Rh antibodies take time to appear and are only rarely found in the serum of an Rh-negative woman during the first pregnancy unless she has had a previous transfusion. However, one pregnancy with a full-term ABO-compatible, Rh-incompatible infant will immunize about 17% of Rh-negative women; about half will have antibodies detectable six months after delivery, and half will have antibodies detectable by the end of the second Rh-positive pregnancy [7]. If no antibodies have developed after two Rh-incompatible fetuses, the chance of developing antibodies with the third or subsequent children become much lower. This arises from the fact that about 30% of all women are apparently unable to form anti-D at all in response to the presence of Rh-positive red cells. The reason for this is not known [5]. If the infant is ABO-incompatible, e.g. a group A infant born to a group O mother, it is much less likely to cause Rh immunization. The probable explanation is that the A cells of the infant are immediately destroyed in the mother's circulation by her anti-A before a primary immunization to Rh can be initiated. Once the primary immunization has occurred, ABO-incompatibility does not give any protection against Rh haemolytic disease.

Incidence of Rh haemolytic disease of the newborn

Before prophylactic treatment became a routine procedure, the incidence of Rh haemolytic disease was about 1 in 180 births. When only the 'failures' remain the incidence can be expected to fall to 1 in 2000 births even if the present results are not improved.

Antenatal assessment

If IgG anti-Rh antibodies are formed by the mother, about 16% of the infants are born dead or dying if no intrauterine treatment is given and over half need treatment, often urgently, during the neonatal period [8, 9]. It is thus important to detect the antibodies in the mother's serum during pregnancy (a suitable scheme of tests is given in a later section, p. 506).

Infants with HDN who are born alive have a very

good chance of surviving; thus one of the main problems in treatment is to predict at an early stage those infants who will die *in utero* so that premature induction can be performed. This prediction is partly based on past history and partly on the results of amniocentesis. As far as past history is concerned, the relevant factor is whether there was a previous sibling with HDN and the extent of the disease in that infant. As can be seen from Table 11.1, the more severely affected the previous infant, the greater the likelihood of stillbirth in the succeeding child.

Table 11.1. The incidence of stillbirth due to HDN in relationship to the previous history (Walker *et al.* [8])

	Risk of stillbirth in present pregnancy (%)
No previously affected infant	7
Previous mildly affected infant	2
Previous moderately or severely affected infant	20
Previous very severely affected infant (cord Hb less than 9 g/dl)	55
One previous stillbirth	70
More than one previous stillbirth	80

The purpose of amniocentesis is to obtain evidence of the extent of haemolysis in the child by measuring the concentration of bilirubin in the amniotic fluid. Amniocentesis is not without risk and therefore some other means of prediction is also required in order to give some indication as to whether amniocentesis is justified. Maternal antibody titres are used for this purpose and wherever possible these should be carried out by automatic machines, such as the autoanalyser, since manual titrations can be considerably in error. Morley [10] has found that the phenotype of the father must be taken into account in assessing anti-D titres, since R_2r children are more severely affected than R_1r. Morley [10] found that a correct prediction of the need for amniocentesis was given in 85% of cases when maternal concentrations were above 2·4 μmol/l if the infant was R_1r and above 1·25 μmol/l for R_2r infants. These values are higher than those given by Rosenfield [11], who gave a figure of 0·34 μmol/l as the critical level which indicated the need for amniocentesis.

Amniotic-fluid analysis

Normally, the amniotic fluid is colourless or straw-coloured, but when the infant is suffering from haemolytic disease of the newborn it may be bright yellow. It is difficult to estimate the bilirubin by standard chemical methods, but in 1956, Bevis [12] showed that spectroscopic analysis of the fluid could be used to measure total bile pigments and the amount of these could be related to the severity of the haemolytic process. The optical density is measured at different wavelengths over the range 350–650 nm. When the results of a normal amniotic fluid are plotted on semi-logarithmic graph paper against the wavelength, an almost straight line is obtained. When the results of a fluid from an infant with severe haemolytic disease are plotted, a curve similar to that shown in Figure 11.1 is obtained. This shows a marked bulge with a peak at about 450 nm and the increase in density of this peak can be estimated by joining the reading at 350 nm and the reading at 550 nm with a straight line and taking the reading at which this line crosses 450 nm away from the total optical density of the peak at the same wavelength. In the case illustrated in Figure 11.1 the increase in optical density at 450 nm is 0·40.

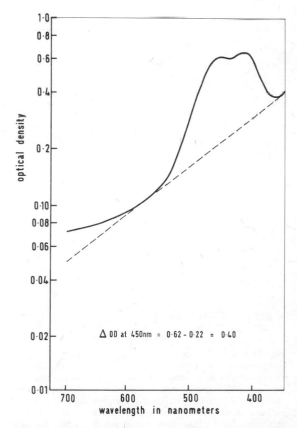

Fig. 11.1. The optical density readings of the amniotic fluid from an Rh-immunized woman at the 26th week of pregnancy. Reproduced from *Haematology* (ed. Hoffbrand A.V. & Lewis S.M.), William Heinemann Medical Books Ltd., London, with kind permission.

Normal amniotic fluid may show a slight increase in optical density at 450 nm which varies with the length of gestation, and in 1961 Liley [13] published a chart which related the increased optical density of the amniotic fluid in the mother at various stages of pregnancy to the predicted severity of the haemolytic process in the infant. Since then there has been ample confirmation of the usefulness of this chart, but considerable discussion as to the details. Nowadays, it is not usual to accept one reading of the increased density, but rather to repeat the test at suitable intervals and determine whether or not the quantity of the total bile pigments is falling or rising. A modification of Liley's chart is shown in Figure 11.2 and the increased optical density obtained in Figure 11.1 is plotted on it.

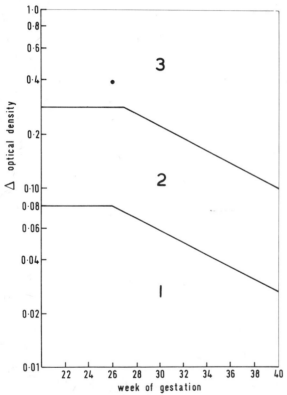

Fig. 11.2. Graph according to Liley [18] adapted for the earlier weeks of pregnancy, on which the optical-density increment can be plotted according to gestational age. An increment falling into area 1 indicates an Rh-negative or unaffected Rh-positive child; an increment falling into area 2 indicates haemolytic disease of intermediate severity; and an increment falling into area 3 indicates a severely affected infant and impending fetal death. The solid dot marks the optical-density increment from Figure 11.1. Reproduced from *Haematology* (ed. Hoffbrand A.V. & Lewis S.M.), William Heinemann Medical Books Ltd., London, with kind permission.

Amniocentesis carries a small, but definite, risk of immunizing an Rh-negative woman who has not developed antibodies. If this procedure must be done in such a woman, it is advisable to examine the mother's blood after the operation and, if fetal red cells are present, to give prophylactic anti-D, provided it is certain that the fetus is Rh-negative. The other risks of amniocentesis are small and are discussed by Robertson [14].

Assessment of the infant at birth

This is done to determine the need for immediate exchange blood transfusion. The criteria for this operation are becoming much less strict than previously and it is difficult to give absolute indications. However, after assessing the child clinically and determining the maturity, the results of the direct antiglobulin test and the cord blood haemoglobin and bilirubin levels must also be considered.

The direct antiglobulin test is very useful in the diagnosis of Rh haemolytic disease. Provided the test is done properly, and provided the infant has not been treated with intrauterine transfusion, it will always be positive. However, the strength of the reaction is not very useful in assessing the severity of the disease. All severely affected infants will give a strong positive test, but quite mildly affected infants can give equally strong results. When an infant has received intrauterine transfusions, the test may be negative or only weakly positive, in which case the cord blood will contain mainly adult blood of the donor's blood group.

It is important that the haemoglobin levels for the assessment of the severity of HDN should be measured on the cord blood sample: venous samples taken from an infant on the first day of life can be up to 1–3 g higher than the cord blood sample and skin-prick samples can be up to 6 g higher and are far less useful.

The assessment of severity of the disease centres around the question of whether to carry out exchange transfusion or not. The best indicators are the cord haemoglobin level and plasma bilirubin concentrations. The cord haemoglobin level is the best single indicator of severity. It can be seen from Figure 11.3 that the relationship between haemoglobin level and severity depends on maturity; in mature infants, the chances of survival falls considerably once the cord haemoglobin level falls below 12 g/dl and is appreciable even at 14 g/dl. If accurate and repeated serum bilirubin concentrations are not available, then it has been advised that all infants with haemoglobin levels below 14 g/dl should be transfused. If accurate serum bilirubin concentrations can be obtained then an expectant course can be followed. The criterion for exchange transfusion will then depend on bilirubin

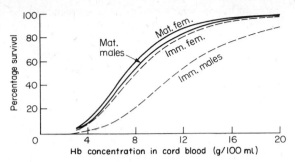

Fig. 11.3. The relationship between the Hb concentration of cord blood and the chance of survival in mature (Mat.) and immature (Imm.) infants not treated by exchange transfusion (after Armitage & Mollison [218]).

concentration, based on the knowledge that kernicterus becomes increasingly common once the plasma bilirubin exceeds 350 μmol/l. Allen & Diamond [15] give values which vary with the age of the infant; at 12 hours, exchange transfusion is carried out when the bilirubin concentration exceeds 200 μmol/l, at 24 hours when it exceeds 275 μmol/l.

Treatment of Rh haemolytic disease of the newborn

Treatment given to the mother. Attempts have been made to reduce the amount of antibody in the mother's serum by plasmapheresis or by administering large doses of corticosteroids, but in most cases without obvious benefit to the fetus [16]. Phenobarbitone, which induces an increased formation of liver enzymes, has been given to the mothers during the last trimester of pregnancy with some evidence of diminished formation of bilirubin in the newborn infant after birth [17]. This drug can also be given to the infant after birth but it has a smaller effect [18].

Premature delivery of the infant. The hazards of prematurity are so great that it is not justifiable to consider deliberate induction of labour before 34–36 weeks' gestation. Infants with evidence of mild or moderate haemolysis should not be delivered prematurely as there is no evidence that the disease will be worse at term.

Intrauterine transfusion. This method of treatment has obvious dangers, not only for the fetus, but also for the mother, and these are discussed by Friesen [19]. According to Bowes [20], the risk of this procedure causing death *in utero* to a non-hydropic fetus is about 6–24%, and 30% of the pregnancies so treated will end in premature labour before the 35th week of pregnancy, with a subsequent neonatal loss of about 15%.

There is probably no improvement in the survival rate when compared with babies who have a similar degree of severity of the disease but who are not treated with intrauterine transfusion [21].

Exchange transfusion. Immediate transfusions to combat severe anaemia and given in the delivery room are usually of small volume (about 100 ml), but an exchange of blood should be done instead of a simple transfusion because of the danger of heart failure. They should be accompanied by other resuscitative measures [22]. Later exchange transfusions to prevent or lower a high bilirubin concentration are usually of 1 unit. Suitable blood for this procedure is discussed in the practical section. The hazards of these transfusions are discussed by Mollison [5].

Subsequent exchange transfusion will be related to dangerous bilirubin concentrations (i.e. over 250–350 μmol/l). The bilirubin level can be expected to rise for about 3 days in full-term infants and for up to 6–7 days in premature infants. The steepness of the rise rather than the actual figure will determine the course to be taken.

Occasionally, later anaemia may require simple transfusion, but usually the infant's haemoglobin level falls to about 6–7 g/dl at 30–40 days and then rises spontaneously without treatment.

Phototherapy. Light from the blue-green visible spectrum decomposes bilirubin to biliverdin which is water-soluble and harmless. Exposure of infants to such light may be useful when the bilirubin is rising slowly and may prevent the necessity for a second or subsequent exchange transfusion. It is of no use in preventing rapid rises of serum bilirubin and is no substitute for exchange transfusion if the indications are already present [22].

The prevention of Rh haemolytic disease

It is now well established that the intramuscular injection of IgG anti-D into an unimmunized Rh-negative woman soon after delivery of an Rh-positive infant can prevent the development of Rh antibodies in about 90% of cases. Using this method, the incidence of failures in women who have ABO-compatible infants is about 10%; about half of these failures will have antibodies detectable six months after delivery and the remainder at the end of the second Rh-positive pregnancy [5].

There are probably two main reasons for the failure of administered anti-D to suppress immunization in a small number of cases. First, anti-D may have been given in insufficient amounts. It is thought that it is necessary to give 25 μg of anti-D for each millilitre of fetal red cells in the circulation in order to get complete suppression. Thus a 100 μg dose of anti-D is only sufficient for 4 ml of red cells. However, about 0·5% of women have more than 4 ml of fetal cells present after parturition and these women will not be fully protected. It is thus important to assess the degree of feto-maternal haemorrhage by examining maternal blood films after delivery. The most frequently used method of examination is the 'acid-elution' technique of Kleihauer, Braun & Betke [23] although many modifications of the test have been proposed. It depends on the fact that fetal haemoglobin is more resistant to elution in an acid medium than adult haemoglobin. Thus, after elution, the fetal red cells will stain darkly with the counterstain and the adult red cells will be colourless. If more than about nine fetal red cells are seen on scanning five low-power fields the actual number should be determined, the size of the bleed calculated and more anti-D given, if necessary.

Secondly, failure may be due to the woman being immunized by a previous abortion or by immunization during the course of the first pregnancy. Approximately 3% of Rh-negative women are immunized following abortion and hence anti-D should be given to all Rh-negative women after an abortion. The incidence of primary immunization during the first full-term pregnancy is thought to be about 0·5–1% and this process cannot be reversed by injection of anti-D after labour. In order to overcome this, trials have been carried out to determine the effect of giving anti-D at 28 and 34 weeks of pregnancy, with an additional dose after delivery. The trials are not yet completed but the preliminary evidence would suggest that the incidence of immunization is reduced to about one-quarter of that seen when only post-partum injections are given [24].

It is not known how IgG anti-D protects against immunization with the D antigen. The administration of this antibody leads to a rapid clearance of injected Rh-positive blood from the circulation of Rh-negative volunteers. Protection occurs with very small amounts of antibody and can even occur with quantities that can be calculated to cover not more than 5–10% of the D-antigen sites [25]. The simplest explanation is that the destruction of the red cells in the spleen brings about the rapid destruction of the Rh antigen and thus prevents primary immunization. This view is supported by the finding that Rh-positive red cells which are destroyed by an antibody of a different blood-group system (anti-Kell) do not bring about immunization to the D-antigen [26].

ABO haemolytic disease

Serological results are not so helpful in the diagnosis of ABO haemolytic disease and positive results can be found in infants who have no clinical evidence of the disorder.

Incidence

Only group O persons form IgG anti-A or anti-B at all regularly, so almost all mothers of infants with ABO haemolytic disease are group O. The combination of a group O mother carrying an A or B fetus will occur in about 15% of pregnancies in Britain. However, although some laboratory evidence of a very mild haemolytic process may occur in 3% of infants, severe haemolytic disease is very uncommon. In Dr Worledge's experience, only 29 infants who had laboratory evidence of ABO haemolytic disease, out of approximately 22 000 births, had a hyperbilirubinaemia of 250 μmol/l or more, and only six of these were treated by exchange blood transfusion (an incidence of 0·03%).

It appears that A_2 infants as well as A_1 and A_1B may be affected by ABO haemolytic disease and they are commonly secretors. This may reflect the fact that soluble antigen can stimulate antibody production. There is some evidence that group B infants are not quite so often affected as A infants [27].

Since it is common for group O persons to have IgG anti-A in their plasma, the disease is seen in the first ABO-incompatible pregnancy, approximately 50% of cases being seen in the first infant at risk. If the first infant is only mildly affected, subsequent infants may be unaffected. A severely affected infant is usually followed by further affected infants.

The reason why most cases of ABO haemolytic disease are so mild is that the A and B antigens are widely distributed on all tissues and thus divert any antibody that crosses the placenta away from the red cells.

Antenatal assessment

Since it is doubtful if ABO haemolytic disease ever causes intrauterine death (at least in late pregnancy) or a hydropic fetus, it is not worthwhile testing the serum of all group O mothers routinely during pregnancy. Tests are normally done only if the infant develops clinical evidence of a haemolytic process and antenatal tests should be reserved for women who give a history of previously affected infants.

Tests on the mother's serum

The presence of IgM anti-A or anti-B hampers the detection of IgG antibodies of the same specificity and many procedures have been devised to separate them. Some are discussed in a latter section (p. 505). Group O persons may have some IgG anti-A or anti-B before obvious immunization and titres of less than 64 are of little clinical significance: the mothers of infants with

ABO haemolytic disease will usually have titres of 1000 or more with adult A_1 or B red cells.

Tests on the infant's blood
The direct antiglobulin test is usually negative in affected infants; this is because the manual method, as carried out routinely, is insufficiently sensitive. If the manual test is modified to improve sensitivity or if the autoanalyser is used, then a positive antiglobulin test is frequently found. The autoanalyser is so sensitive that Hsu *et al.* [28] were able to find a small amount (8–85 molecules) of anti-A or anti-B on red cells of all A and B infants born to group O mothers, although all the infants were clinically unaffected. Romano *et al.* [29] found between 90 and 1320 molecules per cell in clinically affected babies. These values also explain why the direct antiglobulin test is so frequently negative, since it requires about 500 molecules of IgG antibody per cell to obtain a visible agglutination.

The cord blood of infants with ABO haemolytic disease may sometimes show spontaneous agglutination if it is spread on a glass slide. Free antibody is detectable in the cord blood serum; sometimes this will agglutinate the appropriate adult cells suspended in saline, but more often it is only detectable using enzyme-treated red cells or by the indirect antiglobulin test.

It is often useful to examine a film of the cord blood of infants suspected of having ABO haemolytic disease because in this disorder, unlike most cases of Rh HDN, the red cells are often spherocytic. This spherocytosis is associated with an increased fragility of the red cells in hypotonic NaCl solutions.

Treatment
Blood transfusion is seldom required. If necessary, the infant is transfused with fresh group O blood that has been tested to ensure that it does not come from a 'dangerous universal donor' (see Chapter 35). The Rh (D) group should be the same as that of the child.

Haemolytic disease of the newborn due to antibodies other than Rh or ABO
Antibodies against antigens in almost all the blood-group systems and against the so-called 'public' and 'private' antigens have been described as IgG and many have been reported to cause HDN. However, most of these antibodies are very rare except for anti-c, anti-E and anti-Kell. The disorder in the infant is very similar to Rh haemolytic disease and blood that lacks the appropriate antigen must be used for treatment.

AUTOIMMUNE HAEMOLYTIC ANAEMIA (AIHA)

Why a person should suddenly produce antibodies apparently directed against his own inherited antigens is entirely unknown and some speculations are discussed at the end of this section under the heading 'Aetiology'. The incidence of this disease is difficult to assess, but it appears to be relatively high. Apparently normal persons with a positive direct antiglobulin test can perhaps be regarded as the substratum from which patients with AIHA come and, according to Weiner [30], one such person occurs in about 4000 blood donors. If the ratio of patients with only a positive direct antiglobulin test to patients with overt haemolysis is much the same as in the disorder induced by methyldopa (20:1), the incidence of AIHA would be one in 80 000 of the population and this is the figure given by Pirofsky (Ref. 31, p. 21) for this disease.

It is useful to separate the AIHAs into three groups, depending on the *in-vitro* properties of the autoantibodies, because this correlates with distinct clinical syndromes *in vivo*. These are:
1 warm AIHA with autoantibodies that react with the red cells at 37°C;
2 cold haemagglutinin disease (CHAD) with autoantibodies that react with the red cells to a high titre at 4°C, but will not react at 37°C;
3 paroxysmal cold haemoglobinuria (PCH) with the characteristic Donath–Landsteiner antibody. These three clinical syndromes will be discussed separately.

AIHA associated with warm reactive autoantibodies

Clinical features
Warm AIHA occurs in both sexes but most authors agree that the incidence is higher in females than males. In an unpublished series studied by Worlledge (see Table 11.2), the incidence of males to females was two to three. It can occur at any age although it is more frequent in females over 40 and males over 50 years of age. The diagnosis of this disease before the age of 2–3 months is difficult because rare types of haemolytic disease of the newborn, such as those due to 'private' antigens, have to be excluded and because the newborn infant would not normally be expected to manufacture significant amounts of IgG antibody before that date.

The mode of presentation is extremely variable. In some cases the haemolysis can develop very insidiously and it may be many months before the patients' symptoms bring them to the doctor. In other cases there may be a very rapid development of anaemia with extreme prostration and jaundice occurring over a period of a few days. On examination, the patient will show a variable degree of pallor and jaundice and often a slightly enlarged spleen. Considerable enlargement of the spleen is not common and suggests an underlying lymphoma.

AIHA may occur in association with various well-defined disorders, in which case there will also be the signs and symptoms of the other condition. In the series shown in Table 11.2 about 56% were thought to

Table 11.2. The clinical classification and sex of 187 patients with warm AIHA studied at the Royal Postgraduate Medical School, London, during the years 1964–72

Clinical classification	Sex		Totals	%
	M	F		
'Idiopathic'	43	62	105	56
Associated with:				
Lymphoma	13	15	28	15
SLE	0	16	16 ⎫	
Other autoimmune disease	11	18	19 ⎭	24
Miscellaneous	6	3	9	5
Totals	73	114	187	100

have the 'idiopathic' form of the disease, where the AIHA with or without thrombocytopenia was unaccompanied by definite signs of another disease. This ratio of 'idiopathic' to so-called 'secondary' cases will, of course, vary with the clinical interests of the investigator and his colleagues and an extreme example of the differences that can arise is seen in Pirofsky's series of 234 cases of warm AIHA in which only 18% were thought to be 'idiopathic' and 82% occurred in association with some other disease (Ref. 31, p. 25). One of the main reasons for this was the very high incidence of lymphoma complicated by AIHA, which formed 49% of his series. Pirofsky estimates that about 25% of his patients with chronic lymphocytic leukaemia will eventually develop warm AIHA. This high incidence may perhaps be due to differences in defining AIHA, and Leddy & Swisher [32] think that the incidence of overt haemolysis in chronic lymphocytic leukaemia is probably less than 5%. However, up to 25–50% of these patients develop a positive direct antiglobulin test at some time in their illness.

It is of interest from an aetiological standpoint that although AIHA is often associated with lymphoma it is an uncommon complication of carcinoma. Amongst the miscellaneous group shown in Table 11.2, there were only three patients with malignant tumours: one with carcinoma of the breast, one with a carcinoid tumour of the small intestine and one with a teratoma of the ovary. The last association is rare, but well documented in the literature, and in this patient, like

the majority of recorded patients, all evidence of AIHA disappeared several months after the surgical removal of the tumour and had not reappeared five years later (see Baker et al. [33] for a review of the previous literature).

The association of AIHA with SLE and other autoimmune diseases is well known. The other autoimmune disorders shown in Table 11.2 included thyrotoxicosis, Hashimoto's thyroiditis, myasthenia gravis, autoimmune hepatitis, ulcerative colitis, rheumatoid arthritis and pernicious anaemia.

Blood picture
In haemolytic conditions, the bone marrow of a previously normal person can increase red-cell production about sixfold and so quite a marked reduction in red-cell lifespan may be associated with little or no anaemia, although there will be a moderate but persistently raised reticulocyte count. If the red-cell destruction is more severe, the haemoglobin level may be very low with a markedly raised reticulocyte count. The red cells in these severe cases often show a characteristic appearance on the peripheral blood film: the mature cells are grossly sphered and contrast markedly with numerous large polychromatic reticulocytes and nucleated red cells. This spherocytosis can often be differentiated from that due to hereditary spherocytosis because small agglutinates are seen in the thicker parts of the film. The leucocyte count is usually raised $(10–30 \times 10^9/l)$; this is mainly due to an increase in neutrophils, but early myeloid forms are often seen. When the red cells are coated with very large amounts of antibody, erythrophagocytosis may be seen, usually confined to the monocytes. The platelet count may be raised, normal or lowered.

Occasionally, a high reticulocyte count is not seen even with a low haemoglobin. This may occur just after a massive haemolytic episode when there is often a slight delay in reticulocyte increase, or it may occur in patients suffering from chronic haemolysis, in whom it is usually due to folic-acid deficiency. In this case the white-cell and platelet count may also be decreased and the bone marrow will show characteristic megaloblastic changes.

Chronic leucopenia is unusual in warm AIHA, but occasionally occurs. Thrombocytopenia is not uncommon. It occurred at some time during the course of the disease in 20% of the series of patients suffering from so-called 'idiopathic' warm AIHA (Table 11.2) although the low platelet counts did not necessarily coincide with the time of maximum haemolysis.

In severe haemolysis the bone marrow is grossly hyperplastic, the red-cell precursors are the predominant cells and development is normally macronormoblastic. Of course, if the AIHA is associated with a lymphoma the signs of this disease will complicate the blood picture and the reticulocyte response may not be so marked as the degree of anaemia would suggest.

Other laboratory findings

The urine usually shows an increase in urobilinogen and, when the haemolytic process is very severe, in bile pigments. Haemoglobinuria is uncommon and is usually associated with the mechanical fragility of the grossly spherocytic red cells rather than a lysin which gives *in-vitro* haemolysis of red cells at 37°C. This last type of antibody is extremely uncommon, but when it does occur gives rise to very severe haemolysis.

Measurement of the red-cell lifespan is seldom necessary for the diagnosis of AIHA unless the patient has a compensated haemolytic process. It may sometimes be useful in deciding what course of treatment to follow and is discussed again on page 491.

Serology

Direct antiglobulin test (DAT). Almost all patients suffering from warm AIHA have a positive direct antiglobulin test, at least at the time of the haemolysis. However, occasionally patients are seen with an acquired haemolytic anaemia and a negative DAT. Worlledge & Blajchman [34] reported 10 cases in their series of 333 patients. In eight of these cases, survival of compatible normal red cells was shortened. Chaplin [35] found that 2–4% of all patients with AIHA have a negative antiglobulin reaction.

In almost all cases, the reason for the negative antiglobulin test is that the number of IgG molecules present on the red cells is too low to be detected by the test as it is normally carried out but they can be detected with more sensitive methods. The direct antiglobulin test carried out manually with reliable reagents will probably detect 500 IgG molecules per red cell. Gilliland *et al.* [36, 3] used the far more sensitive complement-fixing antibody test and found the red cells from these patients with negative manual antiglobulin tests had between 70 and 434 molecules per cell. They were also able to elute antibody from the cells provided they used a large volume of cells for the procedure. Most of the antibodies had a specificity within the Rh system. Only one patient had IgG on the red cells within the normal range (< 35 molecules/cell). Rosse [38] has made similar findings. Parker *et al.* [39] have also shown that antibodies are present when the manual DAT is negative; they used the method of phagocytosis by mouse macrophages. Worlledge (unpublished results) has seen 10 patients who, in spite of a negative DAT and no autoantibodies in the serum, were tentatively diagnosed as suffering from warm AIHA (during the same period 187 patients with a positive DAT were similarly diagnosed).

The use of antiglobulin sera reactive with the heavy chains of immunoglobulins or with separate complement components has provided interesting information on the type of protein coating the red cells in warm AIHA (see Table 11.3). IgG and complement (C) were the most commonly found proteins. Over 86% of the red-cell samples were agglutinated by anti-IgG and 48% were agglutinated by anti-C. IgM and IgA are comparatively uncommon proteins and about 10% of the red-cell samples are agglutinated by these antisera. 10% of the patients' red cells were coated with complement without any detectable immunoglobulins. Engel-

Table 11.3. The types of positive antiglobulin reactions seen with red cells of 291 patients with warm AIHA (Worlledge [61])

Reactions with antisera K				Clinical classification with					
IgG	IgA	IgM	C	Idiopathic	Lymphoma	SLE	Other AID	Misc.	Total
+	−	−	−	64	10	0	17	3	94
−	+	−	−	2	1	0	0	0	3
+	+	−	−	5	0	0	0	0	5
+	−	+	−	0	1	0	0	0	1
+	+	+	−	0	1	0	0	0	1
+	−	−	+	68	26	19	12	5	130
+	+	−	+	2	0	0	0	0	2
+	+	+	+	1	0	2	0	0	3
+	−	+	+	8	1	4	1	0	14
−	−	−	+	17	5	0	3	2	27
−	−	−	−	11	0	0	0	0	11
Totals				178	45	25	33	10	291

friet gives a similar incidence for the different proteins [40].

It was hoped that the use of specific antisera might enable the clinician to decide whether the disease was 'idiopathic' or 'secondary'. Unfortunately this has not proved to be so and it will be seen from Table 11.3 that all types of reactions can be found, either with the red cells of patients who have 'idiopathic' disease or with the red cells of patients whose disease is associated with some other well-defined condition. Only in SLE does there seem to be any sort of pattern: patients suffering from SLE and haemolytic anaemia have IgG and complement with or without IgM on the surface of their red cells and as the haemolysis subsides the IgG component disappears.

Antibodies in the serum. The autoantibodies in warm AIHA are almost always 'incomplete', that is to say they will not agglutinate suitable red cells suspended in saline. They are best detected using enzyme-treated red cells and by the indirect antiglobulin test. They are nearly always present in the serum of a patient who is actively haemolysing, but may disappear from the serum even when the haemolytic episode is controlled, though the direct antiglobulin test remains strongly positive.

Enzyme-treated red cells not only enhance the detection of autoantibodies with the same properties and specificity as those bound to the red cells, but will also detect additional autoantibodies which are not necessarily represented in the direct antiglobulin reaction. These are most easily distinguished from other agglutinating autoantibodies when they are present as haemolysins. These haemolysins cannot be absorbed *in vitro* with the patient's own or normal untreated red cells, but will bring about lysis *in vitro* of all enzyme-treated red cells, including those of the patient. They appear to be almost always IgM even when they occur with IgG incomplete antibodies [49] and are found much more frequently in the sera of patients with complement on the surface of the red cells than in the sera of patients with only immunoglobulins on the surface of the red cells [34]. Their significance is not well understood: according to Engelfriet [40] they result in a moderate decrease of the survival time of red cells *in vivo* but, occasionally, they may be found in low titre in the sera of apparently normal persons.

The cold agglutinin titre is usually normal, that is to say under 32 at 4°C, but occasionally may be slightly raised (range 32–128). Autoagglutination occurring at 20°C is sometimes seen, particularly in patients who are suffering from SLE or other autoimmune disorders, but the titre at this temperature is low and the antibody does not react at 30°C.

The development of isoantibodies after transfusion appears to be more common in patients with warm AIHA than in other patients having multiple transfusions. Occasionally, isoantibodies may be found that are unlikely to have been provoked by transfusion [50]. Moreover, the titres of anti-A and anti-B may be increased above the average, suggesting a heightened immune response in general [50].

Specificity of the autoantibodies. Tests for specificity are easier to do with the autoantibodies eluted from the red cells because these tend to be of a higher titre than the autoantibodies present in the serum and the additional presence of isoantibodies in the serum may complicate the picture. IgA and IgG autoantibodies are easy to elute off the surface of the red cells, but Worlledge (unpublished observations) and Engelfriet [40], unlike others [47, 51–53], were unable to elute IgM or complement. Some writers have claimed that eluates may contain isoantibody as well as autoantibody and this has been called the Matuhasi–Ogata phenomenon [54–56]. However, Worlledge did not experience any difficulty that could be attributed to this phenomenon when the red cells were washed and eluted at 37°C.

Since the first report, in 1953, of a patient with autoantibodies of e-specificity [57], many of the autoantibodies have been shown to have specificity within the Rh system, the incidence depending on the genotype of the red cells used for the tests. When cells of common Rh genotype are used some specificity can be demonstrated in about one-third of the eluates and anti-e is much the most frequent antibody. When Rh_{null} cells are included and extensive absorption studies are carried out, the incidence rises to over 70% [58]. Table 11.4 shows the results of testing eluates from 93 patients correlated with the type of direct antiglobulin reaction found on the red cells from which the eluates came: when only IgG could be detected nearly 90% of the eluates showed Rh specificity; when both IgG and complement could be detected under 30% of the eluates showed Rh specificity.

Rh_{null} cells not only lack all CDE antigens, but also lack the LW antigen and, in most cases, give false negative reactions with anti-S and anti-U by the indirect antiglobulin test. It is possible that if the test cells were chosen only for their Rh genotype, some of the eluates that did not react with Rh_{null} cells might have anti-LW or anti-U specificity. No such specificity was demonstrated in the series shown in Table 11.4 but no absorption studies were done with the U-negative or LW-negative red cells. Autoantibodies with U and LW specificity have been described by other authors [59, 60].

One-third of the eluates shown in Table 11.4 reacted equally well or more strongly with Rh_{null} cells than they did with other red cells. These eluates had either Eu[a] or

Table 11.4. Specificity of the eluates from 93 patients with warm AIHA correlated with the type of direct antiglobulin reaction

Direct antiglobulin reaction	Rh specificity		No specificity	Totals	Percentage Rh specificity
	With cells of ordinary Rh genotype	Rh$_{null}$ cells only			
IgG only	25	28	8	61	87
IgG+IgA	0	1	2	3 ⎫	
IgA only	2	0	1	3 ⎬	50
IgG+C	2	5	19	26	27
Totals	29	34	30	93	69

Wr[b] specificity or a non-specific antibody, or a mixture of these with Rh specificity [61].

The specificity of the autoantibodies in the serum is usually similar to the specificity of eluted antibody. IgM autoantibody, however, cannot be eluted and the haemolysins against enzyme-treated red cells may occasionally show specificity within the I/i system [40], but usually they lyse all enzyme-treated red cells.

Other immunological abnormalities

Low serum complement titres have occasionally been reported in patients suffering from warm AIHA, particularly when complement is detectable on the red-cell surface, and studies with radioactive iodine-labelled C3 have confirmed the participation of serum complement in these reactions *in vivo* [62].

The appropriate organ-specific and non-organ-specific autoantibodies are found in the serum of patients suffering from AIHA associated with another autoimmune disease. However, patients whose disease is thought to be 'idiopathic' may have antinuclear antibodies (ANA) and anti-mitochondrial antibodies (15% and 5% respectively, in one series [63]). The significance of these findings is obscure. The antinuclear antibodies are generally of low titre and are present for many years without the development of any evidence of SLE. They may perhaps signify a generalized increase in immunological reactivity.

Abnormalities of the serum immunoglobulins are frequently found in patients with warm AIHA. Approximately half the patients whose disorder was thought to be 'idiopathic' had low levels of one or more classes of immunoglobulin in one series [64]. IgA was the immunoglobulin most frequently affected and the results were the same in patients whose AIHA was associated with lymphoma or other autoimmune diseases. The association of a low serum IgA and autoimmune disease in general has been noted by several authors and is the subject of an editorial by Fudenberg [65].

Mode of red-cell destruction

In almost all patients with haemolytic anaemia due to IgG autoantibodies, the haemolysis is extravascular. Haemolysins capable of bringing about *in-vitro* haemolysis and intravascular haemolysis *in vivo* are very rare, Engelfriet *et al.* [41] only finding two in 500 cases of AIHA.

Extravascular haemolysis takes place either in the liver or the spleen [5]. The spleen is a very efficient organ for removing IgG-coated red cells; Mollison *et al.* [42] found that as few as 10 molecules of anti-D per red cell would bring about destruction with a half-time of about four days. This finding explains why haemolysis can occur even when the manual antiglobulin test is negative. Despite this efficiency, the ability of autoantibodies to bring about destruction of red cells varies from one patient to another. On the one hand, destruction has been observed in AIHA with as few as 70 molecules per cell [36], and on the other hand, a positive antiglobulin test (probably indicating several thousand molecules per red cell) is occasionally found in apparently normal people with no evidence of haemolysis [43]. One explanation for this variation is that the subclasses of IgG show very different activities in this respect, although it does not fully explain differences between patients. Thus Engelfriet *et al.* [41] found no haemolysis in patients when antibody on the red-cell surface was of the IgG2 or IgG4 subclass. Only classes IgG1 and IgG3 brought about overt haemolysis, IgG3 almost always bringing about destruction, but IgG1 in only three-quarters of the cases. The reason why IgG1 and IgG3 subclasses are active is that macrophages only have receptors for these subclasses, and not for IgG2 and IgG4.

In those cases where the complement system is activated and C3 becomes attached to the surface, removal of red cells from the circulation occurs by binding to the C3 receptors on macrophages. The C3 receptor only attaches to the active form of C3, namely C3b. Attachment to the macrophages can thus only occur during the initial stages of C3 deposition, since C3b is rapidly split to C3c and C3d. Although C3d remains on the cell surface, it does not bind to the macrophage receptor. Hence, attachment of red cells to the macrophage takes place when C3b is on the cell surface, but if this is not rapidly followed by phagocytosis, the C3b is destroyed and the red cells released again into the circulation [44]. Cells coated with C3d survive normally [45].

The mechanism by which IgG autoantibody results in complement deposition on the cell surface is not at all clear. Most of these autoantibodies have Rh specificity and yet it is well established that IgG anti-Rh antibodies cannot activate the complement system. Engelfriet *et al.* [41] were not able to activate complement using antibody eluted from patients' cells and concluded that these autoantibodies are not capable of activating complement through the classical pathway by C1 activation. However, it has been reported that complement components can be bound when several Rh antibodies of different specificity react with the same red cells [46], and some authors suggest that complement is bound in warm AIHA by IgG autoantibodies of multiple specificity [47, 48].

Binding of red cells to macrophages through IgG receptors may not however be the only method of destruction, since haemolysis occurs when IgA is the only antibody demonstrable on the red-cell surface, despite the fact that no receptor for IgA has been demonstrated.

The class of protein found on the surface of the red cells usually remains unchanged over many years. However, changes may occur with treatment: the disappearance of IgG from the surface of the red cells of patients with SLE on the cessation of haemolysis has already been mentioned and occasionally new classes may appear. Although different patients with apparently the same amount of antibody protein on the red-cell surface may show very different rates of red-cell destruction, in an individual patient increases or decreases of the amount of antibody will correlate well with an increased or decreased rate of destruction and therefore with clinical improvement or relapse.

Prognosis

The clinical course of this disease is as variable as its mode of presentation. When it is associated with another disease the ultimate prognosis may be dominated by the other disease, although the haemolytic process is treated in much the same way as when it occurs alone. Occasionally 'idiopathic' AIHA may be a transient disease and perhaps this is more common in childhood. More often the disorder is a very prolonged one with a gradual waning of the haemolysis. Sometimes the patient suffers a series of exacerbations often associated with 'stressful' conditions such as infections, pregnancy or trauma, but at other times without obvious cause. In between relapses the patient may remain in relatively good health, but the direct antiglobulin test is usually positive. However, in certain patients the disease will eventually disappear as mysteriously as it came and the aim of treatment is to control the haemolysis until this happens. How often this occurs is difficult to say because the patient's red cells may still give a positive direct antiglobulin reaction for many years after all clinical or haematological evidence of haemolysis has ceased. In a series of patients suffering from 'idiopathic' disease studied at the Royal Postgraduate Medical School over a 10-year period, about 20% were thought to be clinically 'cured'.

Treatment

Adult patients with obvious haemolysis are treated with corticosteroids in doses equivalent to 40–100 mg of prednisone or prednisolone per day, with proportionally lower doses for children. If the patient is severely ill with rapid haemolysis, intravenous hydrocortisone in doses of 100 mg every six hours by infusion may be used until oral treatment can be given. Blood transfusion should not be withheld because of difficulties with the compatibility tests if the haemoglobin falls to critical levels (see practical section). About 90% of the patients will respond to this treatment within three weeks and will show a rise in haemoglobin and a fall in reticulocyte count. As the haemolysis lessens, the prednisone should be gradually reduced to about 10–20 mg/day depending on the haemoglobin level and the reticulocyte count. Even if both these values return to normal, it is advisable to continue to treat the patient with small doses of corticosteroids for a minimum of 3–4 months after the haemolytic episode. Most patients will need continuous treatment over a much longer period and alternate-day treatment may be a satisfactory method of administration, particularly for children. Prednisone probably exerts its effect by inhibiting the reaction between coated red cells and phagocytic cells [66]. In the long term, the drug may also lead to a reduction in the amount of autoantibody produced.

Five to 10% of patients fail to respond to corticosteroids in these doses. In such patients splenectomy is often done as an emergency operation, and it may also be considered for patients who after about six months' treatment still need prednisone in doses of 20 mg or more to control their haemolysis. Excessive accumulation in the spleen of the patient's red cells tagged with ^{51}Cr usually indicates that a good result will ensue from the operation, but good results also follow in patients whose surface counts indicate excessive accumulation in both the liver and spleen. Articles on the difficulties of interpretation of such data include those by Szur [67] and Ahuja *et al.* [67a]. After splenectomy it is usual for the patients still to require corticosteroids or cytotoxic drugs, but normally the dose is much smaller than before the operation. Patients who do not respond to corticosteroids before splenectomy may respond after the operation (see Fig. 11.4).

Cytotoxic drugs, such as 6-mercaptopurine, azathioprine and thioguanine have also been used in the treatment of warm AIHA [68, 69]. It is very difficult to assess the effectiveness of this treatment because of the small numbers of patients involved and the extreme variability of the natural course of the disease. The results of treating 15 patients who were thought to have 'idiopathic' warm AIHA are shown in Table 11.5. Azathioprine was used in doses of 75–200 mg/day for

Table 11.5. Results of treatment of 15 patients suffering from warm AIHA with cytotoxic drugs (all but one treated with azathioprine)

Response	No. of patients	Length of time treated
Good	6	4 mth–6 yr
Partial	2*	1–2 yr
None	6	3 mth–1½ yr
Good, but ended in malignancy	1	2½ yr
Total	15	

* 1 patient treated with cyclophosphamide.

all the patients except one, who was treated with cyclophosphamide. It will be seen that six patients had a good response to this treatment, that is to say, they developed normal haemoglobin levels and reticulocyte counts and maintained them even when the corticosteroids were withdrawn altogether. Another patient,

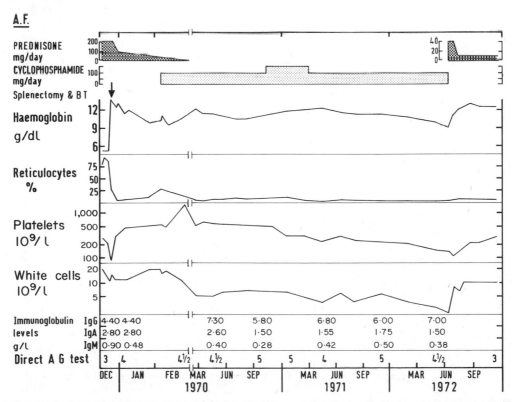

Fig. 11.4. Haematological and serological observations on A.F., a 53-year-old woman, suffering from warm AIHA, who failed to respond to 200 mg of prednisone a day and was treated by splenectomy and later by cyclophosphamide, and who 2½ years after the operation responded well to 40 mg of prednisone.

whose chart is shown in Figure 11.5, had a good initial response to azathioprine but after about two and a half years on this drug developed the signs and symptoms of Hodgkin's disease of which he died in about six months. The unwanted effects of these drugs are discussed in other sections of this book (Chapters 23 and 24). Only one of our series of patients developed leucopenia, but recovered quickly when the drug was discontinued; no patient developed thrombocytopenia. The most worrying problem related to the use of cytotoxic drugs is the potential risk of neoplasia. The incidence of *de-novo* tumours arising in immunosuppressed patients after organ transplants seems to be approximately 80 times greater than in a normal population of comparable age [70]. The risk to patients without a transplant is not yet known and, of course,

lymphoma may well be associated with AIHA in patients who have not had therapy with cytotoxic drugs. The problem is discussed in an article by Steinberg *et al.* [71].

Thymectomy may occasionally be useful, at least in the case of children under one year of age. Four such children are reported in the literature and an apparently complete 'cure' followed this operation in three of them [72–74]. One child failed to respond [75]. The long-term effects of this operation have yet to be assessed, but all these children were seriously ill with a disease that was unresponsive to prednisone and three had undergone splenectomy without benefit. One older child aged 11 years at the time of operation, who had had AIHA diagnosed when two years old, did not respond to thymectomy. It has also been carried out

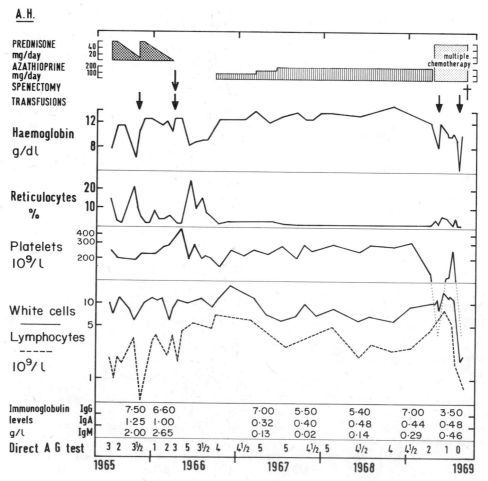

Fig. 11.5. Haematological and serological observations on A.H., a 58-year-old man, diagnosed originally as suffering from 'idiopathic' warm AIHA, who after 2½ years' treatment with azathioprine developed Hodgkin's disease from which he died despite multiple chemotherapy.

without success in teenagers and young adults with SLE [76].

Cold haemagglutinin disease (CHAD)

Like warm AIHA, CHAD can be 'idiopathic' or associated with well-defined disorders. The associated disorders are lymphoma, most often reticulum-cell sarcoma, and various infections, particularly atypical pneumonia, usually due to an infection with *Mycoplasma pneumoniae*, and very occasionally, infectious mononucleosis. CHAD associated with infections is an acute transient disorder. Idiopathic CHAD and CHAD associated with lymphomas is a chronic, very slowly progressive disease.

Acute transient cold haemagglutinin disease

Mycoplasma pneumoniae infection is followed by a rise in titre of the normal cold autoagglutinins in plasma in at least 50% of the cases and occasionally the titre and thermal range of the autoantibodies may be sufficient to give rise to acute haemolysis. The patient usually presents with symptoms of rapidly developing anaemia occurring about 10–20 days after the onset of the respiratory infection. Haemoglobinuria may also occur, but Raynaud's phenomenon is not often seen.

The cold agglutinin titre usually remains high for about a week after the onset of the anaemia but then falls gradually to normal so that 2–3 months later it is within normal limits. The patient's anaemia recovers spontaneously as the cold agglutinin titre falls and usually the patient needs no treatment apart from bedrest and warmth. Occasionally the anaemia may be very severe and blood transfusion may be necessary.

The autoantibody has the same specificity as the cold autoantibody present in almost all human sera and is designated as anti-I. It is almost always an IgM antibody and is associated with diffuse increase in the IgM band on serum electrophoresis. It can often be demonstrated that the cold autoantibodies are made up of both κ and λ light chains, although there is an overrepresentation of κ light chains [77].

Infectious mononucleosis is accompanied by a rise in titre of cold autoantibodies in about 50% of the cases, at least, in some series [78]. This autoantibody has the specificity of anti-i and it might be thought that it would be unlikely to affect adult I red cells. However, even adult I red cells will agglutinate to some extent with anti-i and I red cells can be shown to absorb the antibody well. It is rare for the cold autoantibody to be of sufficient titre and thermal range to cause acute haemolysis, but when it does, it gives rise to an illness exactly similar to that following *Mycoplasma pneumoniae* infection.

Chronic cold haemagglutinin disease

Clinical features. Chronic CHAD is a disorder of elderly people, both men and women, and the average age at presentation of the 'idiopathic' form of the disease is about 60 years. The patients usually present with a gradually developing anaemia which is much worse in cold weather and shows two features in addition to the anaemia and mild jaundice: namely, Raynaud's phenomenon and haemoglobinuria. As well as 'idiopathic' cases, about 16% of the patients will be shown to be suffering from a malignant lymphoma which may be diagnosed before, at the same time as, or after the diagnosis of CHAD is made (see Table 11.6). The autoantibody is often of the same specificity whether the disease is 'idiopathic' or 'secondary', and the serology will not be described separately.

Table 11.6. The clinical classification and sex of 58 patients with CHAD studied at the Royal Postgraduate Medical School, London, during the years 1964–72

Clinical classification	Sex		Totals
	M	F	
Acute:			
Associated with:			
Pneumonia	4	13	17
Infectious mononucleosis	1	2	3
Chronic:			
Idiopathic	16	16	32
Associated with lymphoma	4	2	6
Totals	25	33	58

Blood picture. The appearances of the peripheral blood are characteristic. Gross agglutination is seen at room temperature and the films are very difficult to spread. If the specimen is put in a refrigerator or if the room temperature is cold the red cells may be in one single mass and the tyro may think that the sample has clotted. However, if the specimen is warmed to 37°C and blood films are made on slides heated to 37°C, the cells will usually appear to be relatively normal, although there may be some polychromasia and a moderate increase in the reticulocyte count. Occasionally, in severe cases, the red cells may appear to be spherocytic and sometimes agglutination of the white cells is seen. A blood count made by automatic methods (such as the Coulter S counter) commonly shows a spurious elevation of the mean cell volume and reduction in red-cell numbers due to agglutination.

Other laboratory findings. Haemoglobinuria is common at the onset of the illness in the transient forms of the disease that may follow *Mycoplasma pneumoniae* infection or, rarely, infectious mononucleosis. This is probably due to the rapid increase in complement-binding autoantibody in a patient with normal complement levels. Haemosiderinuria is a more constant feature.

Direct antiglobulin test. The direct antiglobulin test is positive even though the red cells are taken into a warm syringe and warm container and washed at 37°C. This is because the autoantibody has reacted with the red-cell antigens and bound complement to the red cells at temperatures below 37°C *in vivo* (for instance, in the blood vessels of the exposed skin). At 37°C, the autoantibody will elute from the red cells and the positive direct antiglobulin reaction will be found to be due entirely to complement components (which do not elute at 37°C). Tests with antibodies against specific components and their breakdown products will show that the complement is mainly present as C3d and C4d, similar to the complement in warm AIHA. C3d is a non-haemolytic end-stage of the complement sequence and when present on the red-cell surface prevents further binding by physiologically active components. C3d on the cell surface probably protects the cell from haemolysis. Thus, Evans *et al.* [79] showed that when radio-labelled normal red cells were transfused to such patients, about half were destroyed at once, but when the same cells had been pre-treated with anti-I and sublytic doses of complement resulting in C3d deposition, the destruction was reduced to 0–20%.

Antibodies in the serum. The autoantibodies are 'complete'; that is to say they lead to agglutination of suitable red cells in a saline medium and are characteristically present in large amounts in the sera. At 4°C they agglutinate normal adult red cells to titres that are always 1000 or above and may be more than 64 000. Normally these titres are enhanced if enzyme-treated red cells are used.

These autoantibodies can be shown to fix complement *in vitro* and visible haemolysis of normal adult red cells can often be obtained at temperatures between 15 and 32°C, particularly if the pH of the cell-serum mixture is lowered to within the range pH 6·5–7·0. Enzyme-treated red cells are usually more sensitive to *in-vitro* haemolysis, and the titre of the haemolysin with these cells seems to parallel the degree of anaemia more closely than that with untreated red cells [80].

These antibodies are almost always IgM, although IgA cold autoagglutinins have been described [81, 82]. They are monoclonal proteins made from chains which show a remarkable restriction in variety, similar to myeloma proteins. Most belong to one μ-subgroup [83], and almost all have only κ light chains [84] many of which belong to the subclass $V_{\kappa11}$ [85]. However, κ light chains are not essential for anti-I specificity because autoagglutinins with similar specificity have occasionally been reported to have light chains which are λ in type [86].

These autoagglutinins often form an abnormal peak in the β–γ region if the sera are submitted to electrophoresis. On presentation, the average serum level of IgM is about 6·0 g/l and it is rarely more than 15 g/l. The other immunoglobulins are usually present in the normal amounts and if the serum is absorbed with adult red cells until it no longer agglutinates them at 4°C, the residual IgM level can usually be shown to be normal [80].

Specificity of the cold autoagglutinins. Red cells were designated I-positive or I-negative because they were or were not agglutinated at 20°C by the serum of a patient suffering from chronic CHAD and the autoantibody was called anti-I [87]. The I antigen is apparently only weakly developed at birth and normal adult status is not reached until about two years of age [88]. Red cells taken from the umbilical cord are designated as i-cord. Occasionally, adult persons may be found who apparently have very little I antigen and are designated as i-adult. Anti-i will, of course, agglutinate cord and i-adult red cells very strongly and only weakly agglutinate I-adult red cells. The specificity of the autoantibodies in a series of patients studied at the Royal Postgraduate Medical School is shown in Table 11.7. It would seem that anti-i occurring in the chronic form of the disease is often associated with malignant lymphoma. Occasionally, a few sera contain autoantibodies that agglutinate all human red-cell samples indiscriminately, but react very poorly with the same samples after they have been treated with enzymes. These antibodies have been called anti-'not I' or anti-Sp$_1$ by Jenkins & Marsh [89, 90] and anti-Pr$_1$ by Roelcke [91].

It is interesting that the patient's own red cells are less agglutinable and more resistant to lysis by their own high-titre autoantibody than normal adult red cells [91, 79]. However, normal red cells can be made to resemble the patient's red cells by treatment with the cold autoantibody and complement at a suitable temperature and pH, at which the complement components will be bound but no lysis will occur. It would seem as if these complement components in some way interfere with the subsequent agglutination of the red cells by the same antibody and, perhaps because they are rapidly broken down to inactive forms, prevent the subsequent binding of active complement fractions.

Table 11.7. Specificity of the high-titre cold agglutinins present at 20°C in the sera of 58 patients suffering from CHAD

Clinical classification	Specificity of the cold agglutinins			
	Anti-I	Anti-i	Anti-Sp₁	Total
Acute:				
Following atypical pneumonia	17	0	0	17
Following infectious mononucleosis	0	3	0	3
Chronic:				
Idiopathic	30	0	2	32
Associated with lymphoma	4	2	0	6
Totals	51	5	2	58

Other immunological abnormalities. The total haemolytic activity of the serum is often extremely low and may show no activity, particularly in those patients who have recently suffered from haemoglobinuria. These low total complement levels and the increased resistance of the red cells to further complement activity, probably protect the patient from the worst effects of his illness.

Progress. The disease is very gradually progressive and the serum IgM gradually rises (see Fig. 11.6). However, it may not lead to very severe symptoms and the symptoms can be alleviated by keeping warm.

Treatment. Most patients will not require treatment other than warmth and restriction of their outdoor

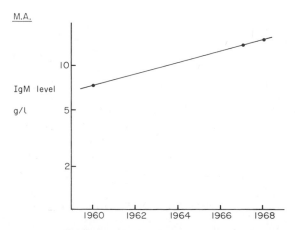

Fig. 11.6. The IgM levels over eight years of M.A., aged 79 in 1960 who was suffering from CHAD. She needed no treatment except warmth and restriction of her activities in cold weather.

activities in cold weather. Other more active patients may require especially warm clothing, particularly socks, gloves and ear-muffs. Others may feel too conspicuous in this clothing which is also rather cumbersome.

Splenectomy is not a useful form of treatment for patients suffering from CHAD, while prednisone is only of doubtful benefit and is not normally used because of the danger of masking infections. Sometimes the patient's abnormal serum IgM level will fall when chlorambucil is administered in doses of 2–4 mg/day and this may lead to a subsequent reduction in the symptoms. These cytotoxic drugs should probably not be continued indefinitely because many of the patients who respond at first seem to become unresponsive as the treatment is continued, and intermittent therapy may be more effective. The results of treating 15 patients with chlorambucil or similar cytotoxic drugs are shown in Table 11.8. The haematology chart of one patient on intermittent treatment is shown in Figure 11.7. The side-effects of these drugs have been discussed already (see p. 492). It will be seen from Table 11.8 that one patient developed a malignant lymphoma (Hodgkin's disease) after a year's treatment with chlorambucil.

Paroxysmal cold haemoglobinuria (PCH)

That PCH is the rarest of the AIHAs can be seen from the number of patients with this disease (see Table 11.9) compared with the number of patients in Tables 11.2 and 11.6, all of whom were studied during the same period of time. Classically it was associated with congenital syphilis, but now it is recognized that both 'idiopathic' and secondary cases occur and that, like CHAD, both groups can result in either an acute transient episode or a more chronic disorder.

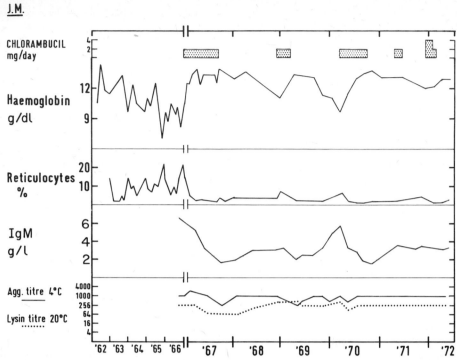

Fig. 11.7. Haematological and serological observations on J.M., a 55-year-old man, suffering from CHAD. He has been treated with small doses of chlorambucil intermittently over 5½ years, each time with a fall in his IgM level and reticulocyte count, and a rise in haemoglobin level.

Acute transient PCH

This disorder usually occurs in children and presents as haemoglobinuria lasting for one or two days. It is sometimes associated with an episode of exposure to cold but, in other cases, particularly those associated with virus infections, such as measles and mumps, it may occur even when the child is not exposed to cold. Most patients will start to recover spontaneously in a few days with rest and warmth. Sometimes the acute intravascular haemolysis may lead to a dangerous degree of anaemia and blood transfusion may be needed. As the child recovers, the titre and thermal range of the autoantibody (the Donath–Landsteiner antibody, see below) fall rapidly, so that 2–3 months later it is no longer detectable in the serum.

Chronic PCH

This disorder presents with episodes of haemoglobinuria occurring only when the weather is cold and which may persist for many years. The degree of cold

Table 11.8. Results of treatment of 11 patients suffering from chronic CHAD with chlorambucil

Response	No. of patients	Length of time treated
Good	3	1–6 yr
Good then none	2	4–5 yr
None	5	3 mth–2 yr
Good, but ended in malignancy	1	1 yr
Total	11	

Table 11.9. The clinical classification and sex of eight patients suffering from PCH studied at the Royal Postgraduate Medical School, London, during the years 1964–72

| Clinical classification | Sex | | Total |
	M	F	
Acute:			
Measles, mumps, 'flu, etc.	3	1	4
Idiopathic	2	1	3
Chronic:			
Idiopathic	1	0	1
Total	6	2	8

that provokes the symptoms is always more severe than in CHAD and the condition needs no treatment because once the diagnosis is made most patients can easily avoid such extreme chilling.

Direct antiglobulin test. The patient's red cells, if taken and washed at 37°C at the time, or soon after, an attack of haemoglobinuria, will give a positive reaction which can be shown to be due to complement components on the red-cell surface. If the red cells are cooled in the patient's serum some IgG may be detected as well. Between attacks the direct antiglobulin test will be negative.

Donath–Landsteiner antibody. All the patients, whether suffering from the acute or chronic form of PCH, seem to have a similar type of autoantibody in their serum. It has an extraordinary ability to bind complement components even though it is, in fact, an IgG antibody. It is sometimes called a biphasic cold antibody because it is often necessary to chill the patient's cells and serum to 0–4°C and then warm them to 37°C before demonstrating the haemolysis *in vitro*. However, the haemolysis can sometimes be demonstrated at room temperature and the cold–warm procedure is only necessary because of the low thermal range of the antibody. The upper limit of reaction may be as low as 15°C in patients with the chronic disease or in patients who are recovering from an acute episode.

Specificity. Most examples of the D–L antibody have the specificity of anti-P which reacts with both P_1 and P_2 red cells [92, 93]. The red cells of the patients group as P_1 or P_2. Occasionally other specificities have been described [40].

Aetiology of autoimmune haemolytic anaemia

If it was known exactly how responses to known antigens occurred and why antibody responses to self-antigens did not occur in most people, the aetiology of autoimmune disorders might be well understood. For the moment, one can only put forward some evidence, first on the induction of tolerance in general and secondly, on AIHA in particular.

It is by now well established that the *in-vivo* response to many antigens is dependent on collaboration between T and B lymphocytes and any theories of autoantibody production must include both types of cell. However, from experiments with suitably reconstituted irradiated animals it has been found that while tolerance is readily induced in T cells, it is much harder to induce in B cells [94]. Therefore, it is postulated that *in-vivo* tolerance to normal self-antigens is dependent largely or wholly on T cells and if in some way the

self-antigen is altered so that other T cells can cooperate with B cells, autoantibody will be produced.

An animal can be made to produce autoantibodies in response to self-antigens by injecting the antigen together with Freund's complete adjuvant or by sensitizing the animal to a hapten and then injecting the antigen coupled to the hapten [95]. Allison and his colleagues [95] have postulated that, in the first case, the adjuvant leads to a non-specific stimulation of the T cells and, in the second case, T cells already sensitive to the hapten are available, so that, in both cases, co-operation with B cells is possible. The second hypothesis has been used by the same authors to explain the autoantibody that may occur in patients taking methyldopa (see page 502).

The part played by virus infections in warm AIHA is unknown. Virus antigen can certainly be found on the surface of host cells and host antigens can be incorporated into virus envelopes. Allison and his colleagues also postulate that T-cell reactivity against the virus stimulates co-operation with B cells and autoantibody is produced in a manner analogous to that postulated for a hapten. It has been suggested that virus infections play an important role in the AIHA of NZB mice. Certainly, many of these mice are congenitally and chronically infected with Gross leukaemia viruses. However, they are not tolerant to this infection and form antibodies against antigens in the G system, and this may possibly indicate an abnormal, rather than normal, immune response [96]. Zuelzer and his colleagues [97] suggest that warm AIHA in children is often due to CMV or other virus infections in addition to an underlying immunological handicap. However, secondary infection with CMV is common in severely ill children and the matter remains uncertain.

Genetic factors are obviously important in the development of AIHA in NZB mice and sufficient cases of warm AIHA in families have been reported to make it unlikely that this occurs by chance [74]. It is now well known that genetic factors also play a part in the normal response to foreign antigens.

The association of warm AIHA with lymphomas has given rise to the hypothesis that 'forbidden clones' of cells elaborating autoantibody might arise by the same or similar mechanism to that responsible for the development of malignant clones of cells [98]. The idea that malignant tumours may arise because of lack of immunological surveillance has been supported by the association between immunosuppression and malignant neoplasms [63]. Warm AIHA is occasionally associated with congenital deficiency of immunoglobulins and this may support the idea that humoral antibody plays a role in this surveillance [99]. Deficiencies of one or more of the main immunoglobulins in the serum are quite common in warm AIHA, but these may return towards normal as the patient's haemolysis subsides.

The association of warm AIHA with other auto-immune disorders has led Pirofsky [31] to stress the idea that the haemolytic anaemia is only one part of a generalized 'immunologic disease'.

The AIHAs that are associated with cold-reactive antibodies (CHAD and PCH) would seem to be produced by a different mechanism. In these disorders the antibody will not react with the red-cell antigens at 37°C and so it would seem more likely that they are, in reality, cross-reacting antibodies and not the result of stimulation with red-cell antigens. The part played by viruses and bacteria (e.g. measles and mumps virus and *Treponema pallidum* in PCH and perhaps by the E–B virus and *Mycoplasma pneumoniae* in CHAD) is not at all clear. The antibodies giving rise to positive tests with cardiolipid or to the positive Paul–Bunnell test are easily separable from the D–L antibody and the cold autoagglutinin.

Chronic CHAD would appear to be a variety of macroglobulinaemia. Why the macroglobulin should have the specificity of anti-I, a cold autoantibody that is normally present in most sera in small amounts, is completely unknown.

IMMUNE DRUG-INDUCED HAEMOLYTIC ANAEMIAS

It is useful to classify the immune drug-induced haemolytic anaemias into two groups:
1 drug-induced 'immune' haemolytic anaemias in which the patient's serum does not react with normal red cells unless the offending drug is also present and
2 drug-induced 'autoimmune' haemolytic anaemias in which the drug provokes the development of autoantibodies very similar to those seen in warm AIHA; the drug is not involved in the reaction of these autoantibodies with normal red cells in any way.

Drug-induced 'immune' haemolytic anaemia

The drugs that have been reported to lead to 'immune' haemolytic anaemia are listed in Table 11.10. It will be seen from the table that this type of haemolytic anaemia occurs only infrequently with all these drugs and with several of them only one patient has been reported to have 'immune' haemolytic anaemia. It is useful to subdivide these anaemias into two groups on clinical grounds because the mechanism of haemolysis is different:
1 those who present with acute intravascular haemolysis, as exemplified by the case of stibophen-induced haemolytic anaemia which was described by Harris [100] in 1954; and

Table 11.10. Drugs which have been reported to provoke an 'immune' haemolytic anaemia; closely related drugs are grouped together

Drug	Year first described	No. of patients reported	
Stibophen [100–103]	1954	3	
Quinidine [104,–108] and quinine [109, 110]	1954	5 +2 }	7
Para-amino-salicylic acid [103, 111–113]	1958	6	
Phenacetin (acetophenetidin) [103, 110, 113]	1958	5	} 9
and paracetamol (acetamino-phen) [114–117]		+4	
*Penicillin [103, 110, 118–127]	1959	>20	
Insecticides [103]	1959	1	
Antazoline (Antistine) [103, 128]	1960	2	
Sulphonamides and derivatives:			
Sulphonamides [103]	1960	3	
Salicylazosulphapyridine (Salazopyrin) [103, 129]	1960	5	
Sulphonylureas:			
Chlorpropamide [110, 130]	(1970)	2	} 14
*Tolbutamide [131, 132]	(1972)	2	
Thiazide diuretics-hydrochlor-thiazide [110, 133]	(1976)	2	
Isonicotinic acid hydrazide (INAH) [103, 134]	1960	4	
Chlorpromazine [103]	1961	1	
Aminopyrine (Pyramidon) [103]	1961	1	
*Tetracycline [135]	1963	2	
Dipyrone [103]	1966	1	
*Melphalan [136]	1967	1	
Amphotericin [137]	1968	1	
*Cephalosporins:			
Cephaloridine [138]	1968	1	} 10
Cephalothin [139–143]	(1971)	6	
Cephalexin [144]	(1972)	2	
Cefazolin [145]	(1978)	1	
*Insulin [146]	1970	1	
Rifampicin [110, 147–152]	1971	>10	
Glafenine [153]	1974	1	
Hydralazine [154]	1977	1	
*Streptomycin [155, 156]	1977	2	
Triamterene [157]	1979	1	
Nomifensine [158]	1979	1	
Probenecid [110]	1979	1	
*Cisplatinum [159]	1980	1	

* Drugs which bind, at least to some extent, to the red-cell membrane (earlier reports not referenced individually are found in Ref. 103).

2 those who present with a gradually developing anaemia as exemplified by penicillin-induced haemolytic anaemia. The former occurs when a drug and an antibody directed against it form a complex which is pass-

ively attached to the red-cell membrane. Complement is then bound by the complex causing destruction of the red cell. These antibodies are usually detected *in vitro* by the complement they bind. In the latter case the drug binds firmly to the red-cell membrane and antibody directed against the drug complexes with the cell-bound drug. These antibodies are usually IgG and non-complement binding. A drug may cause an immune haemolytic anaemia by more than one mechanism as may be seen for penicillin [118, 120–122, 124].

Stibophen-induced immune haemolytic anaemia

Harris [100] reported the first well-authenticated case of drug-induced immune haemolytic anaemia. The patient was a young man who suddenly became anaemic with haemoglobinuria and haemoglobinaemia during a second course of injections with the drug stibophen, given for the treatment of schistosomiasis. At the time of haemolysis, the patient's red cells gave a positive direct antiglobulin reaction and his serum was found to contain an antibody which, in the presence of the drug but not in its absence, agglutinated normal red cells and sensitized them to antiglobulin serum. The drug was stopped and the patient's haemoglobin level returned to normal within 20 days. Thereafter, the direct antiglobulin reaction gradually became weaker and was negative about 60 days after the onset of the haemolytic episode [101]. In most of the published reports (except those referring to penicillin or the other drugs which are specifically mentioned below) the drug was being administered by mouth or parenterally in small or normal doses and for the second or subsequent time. The anaemia developed rapidly and haemoglobinaemia and haemoglobinuria were frequently observed. Within a few days of the onset of haemolysis there was an increase in the reticulocyte count. Spherocytosis was frequently seen on the stained blood film. In one patient the clinical course was complicated by disseminated intravascular coagulation [102] and several deaths occurred [102, 109] but, in general, cessation of the drug led to rapid improvement in the clinical state.

Many of the drugs which induce an immune haemolytic anaemia may also induce thrombocytopenia or agranulocytosis in other patients. Occasionally thrombocytopenia is observed in association with haemolytic anaemia [104, 105, 108, 117, 128, 159].

Direct antiglobulin test. In the majority of patients the direct antiglobulin reaction was found to be positive and when this reaction was characterized further it was shown to be due to complement components on the red-cell surface. The negative direct antiglobulin tests (DAGT) in some of the early reports may be attribu-

table to antisera which lacked anticomplement activity [103]. A negative DAGT may also occur if virtually all the sensitized cells have been destroyed [110]. The complement-fixing antibody may be of the IgG or IgM class.

Antibodies in the serum. The sera of all fully investigated patients were shown to contain an antibody which would not react with normal red cells unless the drug was also present. In the presence of the drug the antibodies sensitized the red cells to anti-complement sera, showing potential haemolytic activity. The use of fresh serum as a source of complement is important in these tests. All the antibodies had a well-defined specificity for the appropriate drug and sometimes for closely related drugs. Thus antibodies to phenacetin may cross-react with paracetamol and one patient with such a cross-reacting antibody suffered haemolysis both with phenacetin and with paracetamol [113, 114]. Antibodies to para-aminosalicylic acid may cross-react with sodium salicylate [113], those to triamterene with methotrexate [157] and those to tolbutamide with chlorpropamide and other sulphonylureas [131, 132]. Complement consumption may be demonstrated when the responsible drug is added to the patient's serum [128] and the patient's serum may opsonize normal red cells in the presence of the drug so that ingestion by monocytes occurs [108]. Serum complement levels are occasionally reduced [128, 149]. Occasionally antibody has been detected by the use of drug-treated red cells but this method is not ideal since drugs which are loosely bound to the red-cell surface may be lost during washing. Coating of a drug-albumin complex on to chromic chloride-treated cells has also been used [154].

Possible mechanisms of the haemolysis. There are two questions to be answered:
1 how does the drug provoke the production of antibodies? and
2 if the antibodies react mainly against the drug, why do they lead to haemolysis?

Neither question can be answered in detail, but it is assumed that the drug, because of its low molecular weight, acts as a hapten and must combine in the body with a macromolecule before it becomes antigenic. This macromolecule is thought to be a protein and could be present in the serum or on the red cells. However, there is no evidence that the drug can combine with the red-cell surface in this type of 'immune' haemolytic anaemia and most authors favour the theories that have evolved from the work of Miesher and his colleagues on platelets and immune complexes [160] and the elegant work of Shulman on stibophen, phenacetin, quinidine and quinine-provoked antibodies [161, 162]. Shulman reported that these anti-bodies had a high affinity for their drug and a low affinity for the red cells or platelets in the absence of the drug. However, when the drug was added to the mixture of serum and cells the resulting drug–anti-drug complex had a high affinity for the cells [161]. It has been known for about 50 years that immune complexes can be adsorbed on to red cells and it has been assumed that this adsorption is not associated with any specific antigenic properties of the red cells. The patient reported by Sosler *et al.* [110] suggests that the situation may be more complex; this patient had an acute chlorpropamide-induced haemolytic anaemia due to an autoanti-Jk^a which reacted with $Jk(a+)$ cells in the presence of chlorpropamide but not with $Jk(a-)$ cells. The antigen–antibody complexes are thought to bind complement components and lead to intravascular destruction of the red cells. The complement components C3 and C4 are detectable on the unlysed cells by the antiglobulin test. An antibody which causes complement binding to red-cell surfaces with activation of the complement sequence as far as C3 will sensitize red cells to phagocytosis and will cause extravascular haemolysis with cells being cleared by the liver as well as the spleen. If complement activation proceeds as far as C8 and C9, intravascular haemolysis occurs. This postulated mechanism has been described as the 'innocent-bystander' or immune-complex mechanism.

Other suspect drugs
In addition to the well-substantiated case reports tabulated in Table 11.10, there are reports suggesting a stibophen-type of haemolytic anaemia in association with other drugs, but details are insufficient for certainty or some features are inconsistent. This applies to one report in relation to nalidixic acid [163], one report in relation to thioridazine [164], and two reports in relation to ibuprofen [165, 166]. A third case report in relation to ibuprofen was more typical of an idiopathic or alphamethyldopa type of AIHA [167]. The precise nature of the immune haemolytic anaemia associated with chlorpromazine described by Hadnagy [168] is not clear; like the two cases described by Miesher & Jackson [103] it may have been a drug-induced AIHA.

Penicillin-induced haemolytic anaemia
The drugs that have been reported to cause a more slowly developing anaemia without sign of intravascular haemolysis are penicillin and perhaps melphalan [136], insulin [146], the cephalosporins [139, 141, 143] and several other drugs. The mechanism of haemolysis has been much more clearly elucidated for penicillin than for the other drugs, which have very rarely caused haemolysis. In most of the recorded cases of penicillin-induced haemolytic anaemia the drug was being administered for the second or subsequent time in very large doses (10–20 mega units a day by intravenous injection). Haemolytic anaemia was diagnosed by demonstrating a falling haemoglobin level despite a rising reticulocyte count and without evidence of bleeding. Typically the patients showed no evidence of intravascular haemolysis and red-cell survival studies in one patient showed sequestration of the patient's red cells in the spleen in a manner analogous to that seen in warm AIHA [10]. Haemolytic anaemia was sometimes accompanied by a moderate or marked granulocytopenia [127]. One patient died while severely anaemic [126] but in general there was rapid subsidence of all evidence of haemolysis when the drug was withdrawn.

Direct antiglobulin test. The red cells of all the patients gave a strongly positive direct antiglobulin reaction at the time the haemolytic anaemia was diagnosed and when the reaction was characterized further it was found to be due mainly to IgG on the red-cell surface. This protein has been eluted from the red cells of several patients and has been shown to be an antibody that reacted with normal red cells in the presence of the drug.

Antibodies in the serum. All the patients had an antibody in their serum that would only give a positive reaction with normal red cells in the presence of the offending drug. The antibody was almost entirely IgG and it bound negligible amounts of complement. Penicillin-coated and cephalosporin-coated red cells can be prepared *in vitro* by incubating large concentrations of the drug with normal red cells and the cells can then be washed and used to detect the antibody.

Mechanism of the haemolysis. It can easily be demonstrated that penicillin can combine firmly with the red-cell surface *in vivo* in persons taking large doses of the drug. However, the combination of the drug with the red cell is not, by itself, injurious and the patient must also have made IgG anti-penicillin antibody; it is the combination of this antibody with the penicillin on the red-cell surface that leads to premature destruction of the red cells.

It is well-known that penicillin or its breakdown products are antigenic and it is presumed that they act as haptens and combine with macromolecules in the body. There has been some discussion in the past about the exact specificity of the antibodies causing penicillin-induced haemolytic anaemia. However, Levine & Redmond [169] appear to have shown that they have specificity for derivatives which have benzylpenadoyl groups and that they can be completely neutralized by crude preparations of benzylpenadoylpropylamine.

The postulated mechanism has been described as the 'cell-hapten mechanism'. The great majority of penicillin-induced immune haemolytic anaemias are due to high-titre non-complement-fixing IgG antibodies, with haemolysis being induced by a long course of penicillin at high dosage. However, other mechanisms may also operate. Kerr *et al.* [119] described a patient with IgG complement-fixing antibodies in whom isologous cells also had a shortened survival although no penicillin was detectable in the serum; he postulated that in the presence of autologous cells coated with Ig and complement, complement was also being bound to isologous cells. Bird *et al.* [120] described an acute haemolytic anaemia associated with a normal dose of penicillin and due to an IgM complement-fixing antibody; spherocytes were prominent whereas in the classical penicillin-induced haemolytic anaemia they are a minor feature. Subsequently Bird *et al.* [121] described an acute intravascular haemolysis on standard penicillin dosage due to IgM and IgA antibodies; complement was also bound to the red cell, presumably by the IgM antibody. Dove *et al.* [122] also reported an IgM penicillin antibody causing haemolysis with standard dosage, while Ries *et al.* [124] described an IgG antibody which was complement-binding and caused massive intravascular haemolysis in a patient who had recently received high-dose penicillin.

Cephalosporins and other drugs
The cephalosporins are closely related to penicillin, and cephalothin and cephaloridine-coated red cells can be prepared in a similar way to penicillin-coated cells. The antibody in the sera of patients suffering from penicillin-induced haemolytic anaemia will also react with cells coated with cephalosporins although the titres will be less than with penicillin-coated red cells. This cross-reacting antibody can be completely absorbed out by penicillin-coated red cells, but some patients who develop haemolytic anaemia during exposure to cephalosporins have antibodies which can only be completely absorbed by cephalosporin-coated red cells [139, 143]; specific anti-penicillin antibodies may coexist with anti-cephalosporin antibodies [143]. Immune haemolytic anaemia has been reported in association with cephaloridine [138], cephalothin [139–143], cephalexin [144] and cefazolin [145]. Patients who suffer haemolysis on exposure to one cephalosporin may be similarly susceptible to another [145]. The mechanism of cephalosporin-induced haemolytic anaemia may be the same as the classical mechanism for penicillin-induced haemolytic anaemia, in that there is an IgG non-complement-binding antibody [139, 143]. However, in other patients the antibody is complement-binding [141, 145] and intravascular haemolysis has also been reported [140, 144].

It is of interest that three of the patients who suffered haemolysis on exposure to cephalosporins had a past history of penicillin allergy [138, 139, 145]. When haemolysis occurs within hours of first exposure to a cephalosporin it seems likely that sensitization by previous penicillin exposure is responsible [145]. One patient with cephalothin-induced haemolytic anaemia recovered slowly when changed to nafcillin [143].

Specific binding sites for insulin occur on red cells [170], and in the patient with insulin-induced haemolytic anaemia the antibody appeared to be entirely directed against insulin [146]. The patient with melphalan-induced haemolytic anaemia can be considered likely to have had a penicillin-like mechanism on the basis of the clinical features and the finding of an IgG antibody [136]. In several other instances with a number of drugs only IgG has been found on the red cells and the anaemia has developed more closely than the classical stibophen type of immune haemolysis. Thus a quinidine-related anaemia developed after 10 months [106], a tolbutamide-related anaemia after one year [132] and a hydralazine-related anaemia after three and a half years [154]. There is evidence that in occasional patients drugs which have a limited ability to bind to the red-cell membrane have induced an immune haemolytic anaemia due to non-complement-binding antibody. Such cases have occurred with quinidine [106], tolbutamide [131, 132], tetracycline [135] and cisplatinum [159]. It appears likely that antibody is complexing with cell-bound drug and the mechanism thus resembles penicillin-induced haemolytic anaemia.

Serological abnormalities without haemolysis provoked by drugs
A positive direct antiglobulin reaction has also been reported with the red cells of patients taking carbromal [171] and it is thought that the mechanism of production of this positive test is similar to that seen in penicillin-induced haemolytic anaemia. Over 50% of patients taking rifampicin in doses of 1200 mg per week develop drug-dependent antibodies [172] and yet drug-induced immune haemolytic anaemia is uncommon [110, 147–152]. This finding suggests that in patients taking drugs the development of antibodies may not be uncommon and perhaps haemolytic anaemia only results when the ratio of antigen to antibody is within fairly closely defined limits.

In early studies it was reported that 40–75% of patients taking cephalothin or cephaloridine had positive direct antiglobulin tests [173, 174]. This reaction differs in nature from the strongly positive test seen in the small number of patients suffering from cephalothin-induced haemolytic anaemia. It is not provoked by an immunological mechanism but is due to non-specific absorption of plasma proteins. Albumin, α_1-antitrypsin, α_2-macroglobulin and fibrinogen are adsorbed in addition to complement components and immunoglobulins. Later studies [176, 177] found a much lower incidence of positive DAGT in patients on cephalosporins; the presence of anti-albumin activity in some antiglobulin antisera is one possible explanation of the higher incidence initially reported. There have been conflicting reports of the frequency of a positive DAGT in patients on methadone. Sivamurthy *et al.* [178] reported that in 80 narcotic addicts commenced on methadone the percentage of positive tests rose from 8·9% to 85% during therapy, the positivity being due to IgG, complement or both. On the other hand, Sherwood *et al.* [179] found no positive tests among 67 patients on long-term methadone.

Drug-induced 'autoimmune' haemolytic anaemia

In 1966 Carstairs *et al.* reported a positive DAGT and an apparent autoimmune haemolytic anaemia in association with methyldopa [180, 181]. Other drugs which have been reported to provoke autoantibodies and lead to the development of autoimmune haemolytic anaemia are tabulated in Table 11.11 and include mefenamic acid [196–200], flufenamic acid [201] and L-dopa [202–206]. Since the autoantibodies developed are not distinguishable from those of idiopathic warm AIHA the evidence linking a drug with AIHA must be epidemiological rather than serological. It is thus difficult to establish the place of those drugs whose administration has been associated with the development of AIHA in only one or two patients and which are not chemically related to drugs already incriminated. Before that can be done, it must be shown that taking the drug regularly leads to the development of autoantibodies in a proportion of patients and that stopping the drug leads to cessation of the haemolysis and the gradual disappearance of the autoantibodies. The serological findings seem to be similar whether methyldopa, L-dopa or mefenamic acid is the provoking cause and they will all be described under the heading of methyldopa-induced haemolytic anaemia. The number of patients with methyldopa-induced autoimmune haemolytic anaemia far outweighs the number with AIHA induced by other drugs.

Methyldopa-induced haemolytic anaemia

Incidence of red-cell autoantibodies. About 15–20% of patients taking methyldopa develop a positive direct antiglobulin test. The incidence appears to be much less in Chinese and Negroes than Caucasians [177]. This reaction takes at least 3–4 months to develop and the incidence appears to be related to the dose of the drug. The reaction is entirely due to IgG autoantibody

on the red cells and is always associated with serum autoantibodies which are often detectable only with enzyme-treated red cells.

Evidence of overt haemolysis. Less than 1% of patients taking this drug develop overt evidence of haemolysis. In all these cases the direct antiglobulin test is strongly positive and of the same type as that found in non-anaemic patients and the autoantibodies in the serum can be detected not only with enzyme-treated red cells but also by the indirect antiglobulin test. It can be shown that these patients have developed more autoantibody than the non-anaemic patients [67].

Clinical and haematological features. Haemolytic anaemia has been diagnosed as early as 18 weeks [184] and as late as four years [185] after the onset of treatment. The patients presented with clinical and haematological findings that were identical to those seen in patients suffering from 'idiopathic' AIHA due to warm-reactive antibodies. Haemolysis is predominantly extravascular but in one patient a more acute intravascular haemolysis was reported [186].

Serology. The autoantibodies eluted from the red cells and those present in the serum are incomplete antibodies and can be shown to be IgG. No enhancement of the reaction of these autoantibodies with appropriate red cells is seen when methyldopa or closely related substances are added to the mixture [189]. They generally show Rh specificity: in the experience of Dr Worlledge about 50% of the eluates showed some specificity on titration with cells of ordinary Rh genotype (most commonly anti-e) and gave negative or weak results with Rh_{null} cells. When reactions were very strong an initial absorption with Rh_{null} cells was sometimes necessary to reveal the Rh specificity. Antibodies may also be directed against En^a and Wr^b [183] and patients have been reported with activity against U [187], LW and Jk^a antigens [188].

Other immunological abnormalities. An increased incidence (15%) of antinuclear activity (ANA) and of LE cells is found in patients taking methyldopa, occasionally in association with clinical features suggestive of systemic lupus erythematosus [190–192]. Other autoantibodies which may be induced by methyldopa include rheumatoid factor, platelet antibodies, leucoagglutinins, parietal-cell antibodies and hepatocyte antibodies [193]. Breckenridge *et al.* [190] did not find any relationship between antinuclear activity and a positive antiglobulin test, but two patients have been reported with autoimmune haemolytic anaemia, positive antinuclear activity and LE cells [194] and one with autoimmune haemolytic anaemia, cirrhosis and a positive antinuclear activity [195]. Serum immunoglobulin levels in most patients with methyldopa-induced haemolytic anaemia appear to be within normal limits [57].

Prognosis and treatment. Most patients recover completely once the drug is withdrawn and this may be the only treatment that is required. It is difficult to withhold corticosteroids from patients who are severely anaemic, particularly as they will only be needed for a short period of time and blood transfusion may be necessary for patients whose anaemia is life-threatening. If it is decided that the methyldopa must be continued, the patient's haemolytic anaemia can be treated with prednisone in a similar manner to warm AIHA and the clinical and haematological signs may resolve even though the serological findings remain. It is not necessary to withdraw methyldopa in patients who have a possible DAGT but no signs of haemolysis. The red cells continue to give a positive direct antiglobulin reaction for some time after the drugs are stopped, even in the non-anaemic patients, and this test may only become negative 1–24 months later, the length of time depending on the strength of the test at the time the drug was discontinued. In patients who have had haemolytic anaemia this test takes from seven months to over two years to become completely negative. The autoantibodies in the serum also gradually disappear as the direct antiglobulin test becomes weaker.

Possible mechanisms of the haemolysis. Methyldopa (α-methyl-3,4-dihydroxy-L-phenylalanine) and L-dopa bear no chemical resemblance to mefenamic acid (N-2,3-xylyl anthranilic acid) and flufenamic acid and yet all can cause a haemolytic anaemia identical to that seen in 'idiopathic' warm AIHA. The mechanism by which this drug-provoked haemolytic anaemia occurs has obvious relevance to the development of AIHA in general. Various hypotheses have been made [114]. A defect of suppressor T lymphocytes now appears most likely. Kirtland *et al.* [193] have shown that B lymphocytes from patients on methyldopa with a positive DAGT synthesize an increased amount of immunoglobulin only when co-cultured with autologous T lymphocytes. Their T cells were unable to generate suppressor activity and in one patient who stopped methyldopa because of autoimmune haemolytic anaemia the decreased suppressor activity persisted for four months. The effect may have been mediated by increased cellular levels of cAMP. Kruger *et al.* [207] had suggested that patients with idiopathic autoimmune haemolytic anaemia have reduced numbers of suppressor T cells and the preliminary findings of Kirtland *et al.* [193] on patients on alpha-

methyldopa with a positive DAGT are similar. Thus it appears likely that the production of autoantibodies in these patients is consequent on a decrease of the number or activity of suppressor T lymphocytes. An abnormal distribution of HLA tissue types in patients with methyldopa-induced haemolytic anaemia suggests that a genetic predisposition may play a role [193]. Furthermore, 18 of 21 patients with methyldopa-induced AIHA reported to the Swedish Adverse Drug Committee were women [182]; this female preponderance is greater than that observed in idiopathic AIHA [208] and, if observed in other series, needs to be taken into account in developing hypotheses as to aetiology.

Drugs other than methyldopa (Table 11.11). Seven cases of AIHA have now been reported in association with mefenamic acid [196–200]. Despite this a positive DAGT is uncommon in patients taking this drug; Scott *et al.* found only one positive test among 36 patients who had taken the drug for at least three months [196] and Worlledge [177] observed only occasional positives.

Levodopa (L-dopa) causes a positive DAGT in approximately 9% of patients and may also provoke antinuclear and rheumatoid activity [103]. Five patients have been reported with warm AIHA [110, 202–206]. A difficult clinical situation occurs when AIHA develops in patients with Parkinson's disease when the symptoms are incapacitating if L-dopa is withheld. It has been suggested that it may be possible to resume L-dopa in a lower dose if a peripheral decarboxylase inhibitor is also given [205] but this manoeuvre leads to similar blood levels of L-dopa to standard dosage and, when tried in another patient, was not successful [206]. An alternative approach is to continue L-dopa and suppress the AIHA with corticosteroids [206].

There have been isolated case reports of an association of AIHA with a variety of other drugs. The association is most convincing when the AIHA is accompanied by other recognized adverse reactions to the drug, or when the drug is known to cause other autoimmune phenomena. Thus a patient with AIHA

Table 11.11. Drugs which have been reported to provoke a warm 'autoimmune' haemolytic anaemia

Drug	Year first described	No. of patients
Methyldopa [180–195]	1966	< 100
Mefenamic acid [196–200]	1968	7
Flufenamic acid [201]	1969	1
Levodopa (L-dopa) [110, 202–206]	1973	6

associated with methysergide also had retroperitoneal fibrosis [103] and three of the four mesantoin-associated cases and a phenytoin-associated case had a pseudolymphomatous syndrome [209, 210] or other evidence of drug hypersensitivity [210, 211]. Procainamide is known to induce antinuclear activity and the development of LE cells, so the single report of its association with AIHA may be significant [212]. In other patients the reported association between a drug and AIHA may well have been coincidental; this applies to fenfluramine [213, 214], gold [215], tetracycline [216], chlorpromazine [103, 168], thioridazine [164], indomethacin [201] and chlordiazepoxide [201].

The patient reported by Rotoli *et al.* [217] appears unique in that an acute autoimmune haemolytic anaemia was induced on two occasions by cimetidine. The DAGT and IAGT were both positive and an anti-I specificity was found.

PATHOGENESIS OF THE AUTOIMMUNE HAEMOLYTIC ANAEMIAS

The addition of antibody, without complement, does not appear to have a very harmful effect on the red-cell surface *in vitro*. Agglutination may occur, but it is not known whether or not this affects the survival of the red cells, although it would be expected to hamper their passage through the sinusoids of the liver and spleen. However, it is well known that when IgG antibody is added to the appropriate red cells *in vivo* there is a rapid disappearance of these cells from the circulation (Ref. 6, p. 479). The rate of disappearance and the site of sequestration of the red cells is dependent largely on the concentration of the antibody on the cell surface; when the amount of antibody is small the cells are selectively removed by the spleen and when the amount of antibody is large the cells are removed both by the liver and spleen (Ref. 6, p. 544).

It was suggested by Ham & Castle [220] that the splenic sequestration was due to agglutination of the red cells coated with 'incomplete' antibodies in the high-protein environment of the spleen, with subsequent stasis and destruction. However, it now seems likely that an equal or more important role is played by macrophages which appear to have receptors for immunoglobulins on their surface [221]. *In vitro* at least, these receptors are specific only for IgG1 and IgG3 subclasses [222] and red cells coated with suitable antibody adhere to these cells under appropriate conditions. IgG3 seems to be more rapidly phagocytosed than IgG1 and Rh antibodies which are mainly IgG1 and IgG3 and are very suitable for these experiments. If large amounts of antibody are coating the red cells (i.e. 1000 molecules of IgG/cell or more) erythro-

phagocytosis may occur. Free IgG1 and IgG3 in the serum inhibit this adherence, but can be overcome by:
1 increasing the concentration of sensitized red cells or
2 increasing the amount of antibody on the red-cell surface.

Marked haemoconcentration occurs in the spleen and this may account for the fact that red cells coated with low concentrations of IgG antibody are sequestered predominantly in this organ. The fact that other subclasses of IgG are not adherent to macrophages may explain the very mild haemolysis found in a patient with a strongly positive direct antiglobulin test which was largely due to IgG4 on the red-cell surface [32].

Receptors for IgA and IgM do not seem to be present on macrophages. Rare patients with AIHA are found who appear to have only IgA on their red-cell surface. Red-cell survival studies in one of these patients showed a rapid removal of the red cells from the circulation and a predominantly splenic sequestration (Parker-Williams, personal communication). It may be that there was some IgG present in addition to IgA antibody because Abramson & Schur have shown in their *in-vitro* experiments that coating of the red cells with IgA and IgG3, admittedly by the use of chromic chloride, greatly enhanced the adherence to macrophages [223].

Most IgM auto- and isoantibodies fix complement components and if the whole complement sequence is completed, defects will appear in the red-cell membrane and intravascular haemolysis will follow. The Donath–Landsteiner antibody is an exceptional IgG autoantibody which also fixes the whole of the complement sequence. Many IgM auto- and isoantibodies and some IgG isoantibodies and, perhaps, IgG autoantibodies fix only part of the complement sequence and do not give rise to intravascular haemolysis. Cells coated with this type of antibody seem to be removed from the circulation more quickly than cells coated with a comparable amount of IgM or IgG antibody that does not fix complement (Ref. 5, p. 492). Moreover, studies with such cells tagged with radioactive chromium show a rapid accumulation of ^{51}Cr in the whole of the reticulo-endothelial system and, because of its larger blood supply, the liver appears to be the predominant organ of red-cell destruction.

It appears that macrophages, and perhaps other cells also, have separate receptors specific for active complement components. These receptors, which may be sensitive to active C3 only, are not inhibited by normal serum which does not contain significant amounts of activated complement components [44]. Cells coated with activated C3 can therefore adhere to and, if sufficient quantities are present, be phagocytosed by the macrophages in the whole of the reticulo-endothelial system. However, activated C3 has a very short half-life *in vitro* and *in vivo* and an inactivator is present in the serum which breaks down active C3 on the red-cell surface to the inactive form, C3d, to which the macrophage receptors appear insensitive [44].

The spherocytosis that is found in peripheral blood films of patients suffering from warm AIHA may also be due to this adherence. Electron microscopy of the interphase between the adherent red cells and the macrophage, at least in the case of cells coated with active C3, shows marked interdigitation between the membranes of the two cells, and if the red cell should break away from the macrophage it appears that part of the membrane is lost and a more spherocytic cell is formed [224]. Spherocytosis is not usual in the peripheral blood films of infants with Rh HDN, although it occurs characteristically in the peripheral blood films of infants with ABO HDN. The reason for this difference is not known, but it may possibly be due to differences in the IgG subclass of the two antibodies.

Spherical red cells are more rigid that normal red cells and this lack of deformability leads to sequestration, particularly in the spleen where the cells have to pass through holes 0·5–5 μm in diameter in the basement membrane separating the splenic cord from the adjacent sinuses [225].

The capacity of the reticulo-endothelial system to remove red cells is limited. From an experiment reported by Mohn *et al.* [226] in which a large volume of a potent Rh antibody was injected into an Rh-positive volunteer, it could be calculated that the average rate of red-cell destruction was about 0·15 ml/kg/hr. In chronic AIHA, the sequestration capacity of the reticulo-endothelial system hypertrophies and the splenic blood supply may increase up to 3–6 times above normal [227]. However, the volume of sensitized red cells is such that the ^{51}Cr half-life of the patient's own cells is measured in days while the ^{51}Cr half-life of small volumes of incompatible red cells injected into normal persons is measured in minutes.

SOME PRACTICAL ASPECTS OF THE DIAGNOSIS OF IMMUNE AND AUTOIMMUNE HAEMOLYTIC ANAEMIA

Direct antiglobulin tests

It is essential to have suitable control cells sensitized with the various immunoglobulins and complement components to ensure that the antiglobulin serum contains the appropriate antibodies and is being used at a suitable dilution. It is easy to prepare red cells coated with IgG because most 'incomplete' blood group isoantibodies are of this type. However, it is important to prepare red cells sensitized with 'incomplete' antibodies of specificity other than Rh, as well as Rh-sensitized red cells, because the optimum dilution of the antisera used to detect these other IgG antibodies on the red-cell surface is often not the same as that used to detect Rh antibody. Red cells coated with IgM can be prepared by incubating selected anti-Lewis sera (those that will give lysis *in vitro* of untreated Lewis-positive red cells) treated with EDTA with the appropriate Lewis-positive red cells. Red cells coated with only IgA are prepared by coupling purified IgA to group O red cells by the use of chromic chloride [135]. The same method can be used to couple IgG, IgM or purified IgG myeloma proteins of suitable subclasses to the red cells.

Complement-coated red cells can also be prepared. Normal whole blood incubated in low-ionic strength saline (0·15% NaCl in 6% sucrose) results in red cells coated with at least C4 and small amounts of active C3 and C3d components. Group O cells incubated with normal fresh serum at 4°C have mainly C4 on their surface. The appropriate red cells incubated with suitable anti-Lewis sera in the presence of complement have at least C4 and active C3 and C3d on their surface. Red cells from a patient with chronic CHAD taken and washed at 37°C have mainly C3d on their surface.

The red cells must be well washed to remove all traces of serum which would neutralize the antiglobulin serum. Since it is assumed the proteins that are detected by the direct antiglobulin test were bound *in vivo* it is important not to allow *in-vitro* antigen–antibody reactions to occur. Thus, the red cells are taken and washed at 37°C. However, antibody can dissociate rapidly at this temperature and after the first two washes in warm saline (which should be done as quickly as possible) subsequent washes may be done at room temperature. It is advisable to read the test by the tile method because

1 several tests can be read side by side and easily compared;
2 the rate at which the reactions develop can be seen. At least two dilutions of antiglobulin sera (one optimal for detecting immunoglobulins and one optimal for detecting complement) should be used if specially blended antisera are not available. The interpretation of positive direct antiglobulin tests has been discussed in detail by Worlledge [219].

Elution techniques

For patients suffering from warm AIHA and Rhesus haemolytic disease, a very satisfactory method for routine elution of antibodies from red cells is Rubin's modification [229] of Vos & Kelsall's method [230]. The technique of Landsteiner & Miller [231] is more satisfactory for the red cells of infants suffering from ABO haemolytic disease. The method of Kochwa & Rosenfield [232] is a very good one for the red cells of patients with warm AIHA and has the advantage that the eluate is free of haemoglobin and can be concentrated by various methods; its disadvantage is the time required for preparation.

Antibodies in the serum

Autoantibodies are tested for by standard serological techniques. It is important that the tests should be done at various temperatures and that the cells and serum should be brought to the temperature of the test before being mixed together. Moreover, both the antibody and complement may be very sensitive to changes in pH and tests should be performed not only at the pH of serum (usually about pH 7·8) but also after the serum and cell mixture have been adjusted to between pH 6·5–7·0. Patients with AIHA are frequently deficient in complement and the tests should also be done with added complement in the form of fresh compatible normal serum. Enzyme-treated red cells are especially valuable for detecting autoantibodies and should always be included.

Specificity tests should be done by standard techniques against red cells whose blood groups are known as completely as possible. It is frequently necessary to titrate an eluate or serum from a patient with warm AIHA to demonstrate relative specificity and absorption studies may also be done. Sera from patients with CHAD are also titrated at suitable temperatures and cord blood cells should always be available for the tests.

Blood grouping tests

It is often impossible to determine the blood group of a person with a positive direct antiglobulin test with 'incomplete' antisera. This is because the additive (albumin or enzymes) will make the patient's red cells agglutinate spontaneously and 'complete' antisera should always be used for such tests. The ABO group should be easy to determine: the tests should be done at 37°C with the red cells and serum of patients suffering from CHAD, but for other patients, tests at room temperature are usually satisfactory.

The red cells of an infant suffering from Rh haemolytic disease may not agglutinate with 'complete' anti-D if they are heavily coated with 'incomplete' anti-D. If the mother's serum contains this antibody it can be assumed that the child with a strongly positive DAT is Rh positive. If more exact tests are needed an eluate can be made and the eluted antibody identified. Moreover, after elution by Landsteiner & Miller's method [231], the red cells will sometimes agglutinate with 'complete' anti-D.

It is useful to determine the probable Rh genotype of patients with warm AIHA and the author has never seen absence of agglutination with 'complete' antisera that could be ascribed to specific autoantibodies. If it is thought that isoantibodies are present in the serum of patients with AIHA the red cells should be tested to demonstrate that the antigen is absent.

Compatibility tests

Infants with haemolytic disease of the newborn are given blood that lacks the antigen against which the antibody has developed in the mother. Compatibility tests are normally done with the mother's serum and infants with ABO haemolytic disease are given group O blood of the same Rh(D) group as the child. Infants with Rh haemolytic disease of the newborn are given blood of an ABO group which is compatible with both the mother and child. Group O blood is often used for intrauterine transfusions. However, blood of the same ABO group as the mother could be used, or an attempt could be made to determine the ABO group of the child from desquamated cells in the amniotic fluid.

Blood for intrauterine or exchange transfusions should be given within four days of taking and, if the blood has been taken into ACD solution, it should be 'converted' to heparinized blood by adding 5 ml of 10% calcium gluconate solution and 1500 i.u. of heparin and aspirating half the plasma.

Compatibility tests for patients with cold haemagglutinin disease will usually be negative if they are done strictly at 37°C. Compatibility tests for patients with warm AIHA are often grossly abnormal. It is useful to have tested the patient's serum to determine whether or not isoantibodies are present and blood should be selected lacking such antigens. If isoantibodies are not present and the autoantibodies appear to show specificity, blood lacking the antigens against which the autoantibodies are directed will often survive much better than blood of the patient's own group. If blood is needed urgently it may be sufficient to select such bottles of the same ABO and Rh(D) group as the patient that appear to be less, or no more incompatible than the patient's own red cells and serum tested at the same time. Although the survival of such blood may well be very short, the patient seldom comes to any harm.

Tests on the mother of infants with possible HDN

Antenatal tests for Rh and other antibodies (except anti-A and anti-B)

All mothers should have their ABO and Rh(D) groups determined as soon as possible after pregnancy has been diagnosed and their serum should be tested for antibodies outside the ABO group system. One suitable method is to test them at 37°C with pooled enzyme-treated red cells taken from not more than three donors who between them carry all the common antigens except A and B. Properly done, this is a very sensitive method of detecting Rh antibodies. However, since other antibodies may have equal importance and since some of the antigens against which they react are destroyed by enzyme-treatment of the red cells, at least selected sera should be tested with the same untreated red cells by the indirect antiglobulin test. This selection should include the sera of all Rh-negative mothers and all mothers who give a history of past transfusions or unexplained stillborn, jaundiced or anaemic infants.

If nothing is found from these tests, the sera of Rh (D)-positive mothers who have had no transfusions, and give no history suggestive of HDN, need not be reinvestigated unless the infant shows signs of HDN, in which case samples from both the mother and the baby must be tested immediately. Rh-negative mothers in their first pregnancy, who have had no transfusions, are unlikely to make detectable antibodies until after delivery and their sera probably only need to be retested at 30–34 weeks of pregnancy and at delivery if anti-D is to be given. Rh-negative multigravidae and all mothers, whether Rh-negative or Rh-positive, who have had previous transfusions or give a history suggestive of infants with HDN, should be retested more frequently during pregnancy. Suitable times for these tests are at 20–24 weeks and at least three times during the third trimester of pregnancy. When a woman gives a history suggestive of infants with HDN and no antibodies can be found with the usual panel of cells, it is advisable to test her serum with her husband's red cells to exclude HDN due to antibodies against 'private' antigens.

If the preliminary tests are positive or if positive results are found in any of the subsequent tests, further investigations will depend on the specificity of the antibodies. Some antibodies, such as anti-Lewis and anti-P_1 are almost always IgM and as such will not lead to haemolytic disease of the newborn. Their presence should be recorded because they make subsequent compatibility tests more difficult, but they need not be titrated. Other antibodies, such as Rh antibodies, anti-Kell, anti-Duffy, etc., are often IgG and if they react by the indirect antiglobulin test they should be titrated against suitable red cells.

Tests for IgG anti-A and anti-B

The mother's serum always contains IgM antibody of the same specificity and this must first be inactivated or inhibited. A simple method of inactivating IgM antibody is to incubate equal volumes of the serum with 0·1 M 2-mercaptoethanol in phosphate buffer pH 7·4 for two hours at 37°C and then titrate it against A_1 or B

cells employing the indirect antiglobulin method. A titre of IgG anti-A and/or anti-B of less than 64 is of no clinical importance and the mothers of infants that require exchange transfusion for ABO-incompatibility will usually have titres of 1000 or more. Other methods of inhibition include the use of A or B saliva or the test described by Polley *et al.* [233] in which IgG anti-A is looked for by titrating the mother's serum against pooled A whole blood and reading the results by the indirect antiglobulin test (the A substance in the plasma of A whole blood will neutralize the diluted IgM anti-A).

REFERENCES

1 GORDON H. (1971) The diagnosis of hydrops fetalis. The Rh problem. *Clinical Obstetrics and Gynecology*, **14**, 548.

2 PARKIN J.M. & WALKER W. (1968) Peritoneal dialysis in severe *hydrops fetalis* (letter). *Lancet*, **ii**, 283.

3 GIBLETT E.R. (1968) Blood group antibodies causing hemolytic disease of the newborn. *Clinical Obstetrics and Gynecology*, **7**, 1044.

4 RACE R.R. & SANGER R. (1968) *Blood Groups in Man*, 5th edn, p. 187. Blackwell Scientific Publications, Oxford.

5 MOLLISON P.L. (1979) *Blood Transfusion in Clinical Medicine*, 6th edn, Blackwell Scientific Publications, Oxford.

6 WOODROW J.C. & FINN R. (1966) Transplacental haemorrhage. *British Journal of Haematology*, **12**, 297.

7 WOODROW J.C. (1970) Rh immunization and its prevention. *Series Haematologica*, **3**, No. 3.

8 WALKER W., MURRAY S. & RUSSELL J.K. (1957) Stillbirth due to haemolytic disease of the newborn. *Journal of Obstetrics and Gynaecology in the British Empire*, **64**, 573.

9 WALKER W. (1958) The changing pattern of haemolytic disease of the newborn (1948–1957). *Vox Sanguinis*, **3**, 225, 336.

10 MORLEY G. (1978) Relationship between maternal anti-D levels, fetal phenotype and haemolytic disease of the newborn. *Vox Sanguinis*, **35**, 324.

11 ROSENFIELD R.E. (1969) The current status of some human blood group problems. In: *Textbook of Immunopathology*, Vol. II (ed. Miescher P.A. & Müller-Eberhard H.J.), p. 441. Grune & Stratton, New York.

12 BEVIS D.C.A. (1956) Blood pigments in haemolytic disease of the newborn. *Journal of Obstetrics and Gynaecology of the British Empire*, **63**, 68.

13 LILEY A.W. (1961) Liquor amnii analysis in the management of pregnancy complicated by Rhesus sensitisation. *American Journal of Obstetrics and Gynecology*, **82**, 1359.

14 ROBERTSON J.H. (1971) Diagnosis and management of the Rh-immunized patient. The Rh problem. *Clinical Obstetrics and Gynecology*, **14**, 494.

15 ALLEN F.H. JR. & DIAMOND L.K. (1958) *Erythroblastosis fetalis*. Little, Brown & Co., Boston.

16 POWELL L.C. JR. (1968) Intense plasmapheresis in the pregnant Rh-sensitized woman. *American Journal of Obstetrics and Gynecology*, **101,** 153.

17 RAMBOER C., THOMPSON R.P.H. & WILLIAMS R. (1969) Controlled trials of phenobarbitone therapy in neonatal jaundice. *Lancet*, **i**, 966.

18 MCMULLIN G.P., HAYES M.F. & ARORA S.C. (1970) Phenobarbitone in Rhesus haemolytic disease. A controlled trial. *Lancet*, **ii**, 949.

19 FRIESEN R.F. (1971) Complications of intrauterine transfusion. The Rhesus problem. *Clinical Obstetrics and Gynecology*, **14,** 572.

20 BOWES W.A. JR. (1971) Intrauterine transfusion: indications and results. The Rh problem. *Clinical Obstetrics and Gynecology*, **14,** 561.

21 ROBERTSON E.G., BROWN A., ELLIS M.I. & WALKER W. (1976) Intrauterine transfusion in the management of severe rhesus isoimmunization. *British Journal of Obstetrics and Gynaecology*, **83,** 694.

22 DAVIES P.A., ROBINSON R.J., SCOPES J.W., TIZARD J.P.M. & WIGGLESWORTH J.S. (1972) *Medical Care of Newborn Infants*, p. 65. William Heinemann Medical Books Ltd., London.

23 KLEIHAUER E., BRAUN H. & BETKE K. (1957) Demonstration von fetalem Hämoglobin in den Erythrocyten eines Blutausstrichs. *Klinische Wochenschrift*, **35,** 637.

24 DAVEY M.G. & ZIPURSKY A. (1979) Report on McMaster Conference on prevention of Rh immunization. *Vox Sanguinis*, **36,** 50.

25 HUGHES-JONES N.C. & MOLLISON P.L. (1968) Failure of a relatively small dose of passively administered anti-Rh to suppress primary immunization by a relatively large dose of Rh-positive red cells. *British Medical Journal*, **i**, 150.

26 WOODROW J.C., CLARKE C.A., DONOHOE W.T.A., FINN R., MCCONNELL R.B., SHEPPARD P.M., LEHANE D., ROBERTS F.M. & GIMLETTE T.M.D. (1975) Mechanism of Rh prophylaxis: an experimental study on specificity of immunosuppression. *British Medical Journal*, **ii**, 57.

27 ROSENFIELD R.E. & OHNO G. (1955) A–B hemolytic disease of the newborn. *Revue d'Hématologie*, **10,** 231.

28 HSU T.C.S., ROSENFIELD R.E. & RUBINSTEIN P. (1974) Instrumented PVP-augmented antiglobulin tests. III. IgG-coated cells in ABO incompatible babies. *Vox Sanguinis*, **26,** 326.

29 ROMANO E.L., HUGHES-JONES N.C. & MOLLISON P.L. (1973) Direct antiglobulin test in ABO-haemolytic disease of the newborn. *British Medical Journal*, **i**, 524.

30 WEINER W. (1965) 'Coombs positive' 'normal' people. *Proceedings of the 10th Congress of International Society of Blood Transfusion*, Stockholm, 1964, Fasc. 23, part I, *Bibliotheca Haematologica*, p. 35. Karger, Basel.

31 PIROFSKY B. (1969) *Autoimmunization and the Autoimmune Hemolytic Anemias*. Williams & Wilkins, Baltimore.

32 LEDDY J.P. & SWISHER S.N. (1971) Acquired immune hemolytic disorders. In: *Immunological Diseases*, Vol. II, 2nd edn (ed. Samter M.), p. 1083. Little, Brown & Co., Boston.

33 BAKER L.R.I., BRAIN M.C., AZZOPARDI J.C. & WORLLEDGE S.M. (1968) Autoimmune haemolytic anaemia associated with ovarian dermoid cyst. *Journal of Clinical Pathology*, **21,** 626.

34 WORLLEDGE S.M. & BLAJCHMAN M.A. (1972) The autoimmune haemolytic anaemias. *British Journal of Haematology*, **23,** Supplement, 61.

35 CHAPLIN H., JR. (1973) Clinical usefulness of specific antiglobulin reagents in autoimmune haemolytic anaemias. *Progress in Haematology*, **7,** 25.

36 GILLILAND B.C., BAXTER E. & EVANS R.S. (1971) Red-cell antibodies in acquired hemolytic anemia with negative antiglobulin serum tests. *New England Journal of Medicine*, **285,** 252.

37 GILLILAND B.C. (1976) Coombs-negative immune hemolytic anaemia. *Seminars in Hematology*, **13,** 267.

38 ROSSE W.F. (1974) The detection of small amounts of antibody on the red cell in autoimmune haemolytic anaemia. *Series Haematologica*, **7,** 358.

39 PARKER A.C., HABESHAW J. & CLELAND J.F. (1972) The demonstration of a 'plasmatic factor' in a case of Coombs' negative haemolytic anaemia. *Scandinavian Journal of Haematology*, **9,** 318.

40 ENGELFRIET C.P., VON DEM BORNE A.E.G. & BECKERS D. (1974) Autoimmune haemolytic anaemia. *Series Haematologica*, **7,** 328.

41 ENGELFRIET C.P., VON DEM BORNE A.E.G., BECKERS D. & VAN LOGHEM J.J. (1974) Autoimmune haemolytic anaemia: serological and immunochemical characteristics of the autoantibodies: mechanisms of cell destruction. *Series Haematologica*, **7,** 328.

42 MOLLISON P.L. & HUGHES-JONES N.C. (1967) Clearance of Rh-positive cells by low concentrations of Rh antibody. *Immunology*, **12,** 63.

43 GORST D.W., RAWLINSON V.I., MERRY A.H. & STRATTON F. (1980) Positive direct antiglobulin test in normal individuals. *Vox Sanguinis*, **38,** 99.

44 BROWN D.L., LACHMANN P.L. & DACIE J.V. (1970) The *in vivo* behaviour of complement-coated red cells: studies in C6-deficient, C3-depleted and normal rabbits. *Clinical and Experimental Immunology*, **7,** 401.

45 MOLLISON P.L. (1965) The role of complement in haemolytic processes *in vivo*. In: *Ciba Foundation Symposium on Complement* (ed. Wolstenholme G.E.W. & Knight J.), p. 323. Churchill, London.

46 ROSSE W.F. (1968) Fixation of the first component of complement (C'1a) by human antibodies. *Journal of Clinical Investigation*, **47,** 2430.

47 VOS G.H., PETZ L. & FUDENBERG H.H. (1970) Specificity of acquired haemolytic anaemia autoantibodies and their serological characteristics. *British Journal of Haematology*, **19,** 57.

48 EYSTER M.E. & JENKINS D.E. (1970) γ G erythrocyte autoantibodies: comparison of *in vivo* complement coating and *in vitro* 'Rh' specificity. *Journal of Immunology*, **105,** 221.

49 VON DEM BORNE A.E.G. ENGELFRIET C.P., BECKERS D., VAN DER KORT-HENKES, G., VAN DER GIESSEN M. & VAN LOGHEM J.J. (1969) Autoimmune haemolytic anaemias. II: Warm haemolysins—serological and immunochemical investigations and ^{51}Cr studies. *Clinical and Experimental Immunology*, **4,** 333.

50 SALMON C. & HOMBERG J.C. (1970) La formation des anticorps au cours des anémies hémolytiques autoimmunes. Quelques données récentes. *Annales de l'Institute Pasteur*, **118,** 459.

51 LEDDY J.P., BAKEMEIER R.F. & VAUGHAN J.H. (1965)

Fixation of complement components to autoantibody eluted from human RBC. *Journal of Clinical Investigation*, **44**, 1066.

52 EYSTER M.E., JENKINS D.E. JR & MOORE W.H. (1967) Antibody eluates in patients with positive antiglobulin reactions (abstract). *Clinical Research*, **15**, 275.

53 JENKINS D.E. JR & EYSTER M.E. (1968) Immunological studies in patients with positive direct antiglobulin reactions (abstract). *Clinical Research*, **16**, 82.

54 MATUHASI T. (1959) Plasmaprotein and antibody fractions observed from the serological point of view. *Proceedings of the 15th General Assembly of the Japanese Medical Congress*, 1959, Tokyo, **4**, 80.

55 OGATA T. & MATUHASI T. (1962) Problems of specific and cross reactivity of blood group antibodies. *Proceedings of the 8th Congress of the International Society of Blood Transfusion*, Tokyo, 1960. Fasc. 13, *Bibliotheca Haematologica*, p. 208. Karger, Basel.

56 ALLEN F.H., ISSITT P.D., DEGNAN T.J., JACKSON V.A., REIHART J.K., KNOWLIN R.J. & ADEBAHR M.F. (1969) Further observations of the Matuhasi–Ogata phenomenon. *Vox Sanguinis*, **16**, 47.

57 WEINER W., BATTEY D.A., CLEGHORN T.E., MARSON F.G.W. & MEYNELL M.J. (1953) Serological findings in a case of haemolytic anaemia with some general observations on the pathogenesis of this syndrome. *British Medical Journal*, **ii**, 125.

58 WEINER W. & VOS G.H. (1963) Serology of acquired hemolytic anemias. *Blood*, **22**, 606.

59 CELANO M.J. & LEVINE P. (1967) Anti-LW specificity in autoimmune acquired hemolytic anemia. *Transfusion (Philadelphia)*, **7**, 265.

60 MARSH W.L., REID M.E. & SCOTT E.P. (1972) Autoantibodies of U blood group specificity in autoimmune haemolytic anaemia. *British Journal of Haematology*, **22**, 625.

61 WORLLEDGE S. (1979) Tissue-specific autoantibodies in haemolytic anaemia. *Journal of Clinical Pathology*, **32**, Supplement 13, 90.

62 PETZ L.D., FINK D.J., LETSKY E.A., FUDENBERG H.H. & MÜLLER-EBERHARD H.J. (1968) *In vivo* metabolism of complement. 1. Metabolism of the third component (C′3) in acquired hemolytic anemia. *Journal of Clinical Investigation*, **47**, 2469.

63 BLAJCHMAN M.A. (1971) Tissue antibodies in idiopathic autoimmune haemolytic anaemia. *Clinical and Experimental Immunology*, **8**, 741.

64 BLAJCHMAN M.A., DACIE J.V., HOBBS J.R., PETTIT J.E. & WORLLEDGE S.M. (1969) Immunoglobulins in warm-type autoimmune haemolytic anaemia. *Lancet*, **ii**, 340.

65 FUDENBERG H.H. (1971) Genetically determined immune deficiency as the predisposing cause of 'autoimmunity' and lymphoid neoplasia. *American Journal of Medicine*, **51**, 295.

66 SCHREIBER A.D., PARSONS S.J., MCDERMOTT P. & COOPER R.A. (1975) Effect of corticosteroids on the human monocyte IgG and complement receptor. *Journal of Clinical Investigation*, **56**, 1189.

67 SZUR L. (1970) Surface counting in the assessment of sites of red cell destruction (annotation). *British Journal of Haematology*, **18**, 591.

67a AHUJA S., LEWIS S.M. & SZUR L. (1972) Value of surface counting in predicting response to splenectomy in haemolytic anaemia. *Journal of Clinical Pathology*, **25**, 467.

68 SCHWARTZ R.S. & DAMESHEK W. (1962) The treatment of autoimmune hemolytic anemia with 6-mercaptopurine and thioguanine. *Blood*, **19**, 483.

69 SWANSON M.A. & SCHWARTZ R.S. (1967) Immunosuppressive therapy: the relation between clinical response and immunologic competence. *New England Journal of Medicine*, **277**, 163.

70 PENN I. & STARZL T.E. (1972) Malignant tumours arising de novo in immunosuppressed organ transplant recipients. *Transplantation*, **14**, 407.

71 STEINBERG A.D., PLOTZ P.H., SHELDON M.W., WONG V.G., AGUS S.G., & DECKER J.L. (1972) Cytotoxic drugs in treatment of non-malignant disorders. *Annals of Internal Medicine*, **76**, 619.

72 WILMERS M.J. & RUSSELL P.A. (1963) Autoimmune haemolytic anaemia in an infant treated by thymectomy. *Lancet*, **ii**, 915.

73 KARAKALIS A., VALAES T., PANTELAKIS S.N. & DOXIADIS S.A. (1964) Thymectomy in an infant with autoimmune haemolytic anaemia. *Lancet*, **ii**, 778.

74 DACIE J.V. & WORLLEDGE S.M. (1969) Autoimmune hemolytic anemias. In: *Progress in Hematology*, Vol. VI (ed. Brown E.B. & Moore C.V.), p. 82. Grune & Stratton, New York.

75 OSKI F.A. & ABELSON N.M. (1965) Autoimmune hemolytic anemia in an infant. Report of a case treated unsuccessfully with thymectomy. *Journal of Pediatrics*, **67**, 752.

76 MACKAY I.R. & SMALLY M. (1966) Results of thymectomy in systemic lupus erythematosus: observations on clinical course and serological reactions. *Clinical and Experimental Immunology*, **1**, 129.

77 HARBOE M. & LIND K. (1966) Light chain types of transiently occurring cold haemagglutinins. *Scandinavian Journal of Haematology*, **3**, 269.

78 WORLLEDGE S.M. & DACIE J.V. (1969) Haemolytic and other anaemias in infectious mononucleosis. In: *Infectious Mononucleosis* (ed. Carter R.L. & Penman H.G.), p. 87. Blackwell Scientific Publications, Oxford.

79 EVANS R.S., TURNER E. & BINGHAM M. (1967) Chronic hemolytic anemia due to cold agglutinins: the mechanism of resistance of red cells to C′ hemolysis by cold agglutinins. *Journal of Clinical Investigation*, **46**, 1461.

80 COOPER A.G. & HOBBS J.R. (1970) Immunoglobulins in chronic cold haemagglutinin disease. *British Journal of Haematology*, **19**, 383.

81 ANGEVINE C.D., ANDERSON B.R. & BARNETT E.V. (1966) A cold agglutinin of the IgA class. *Journal of Immunology*, **96**, 578.

82 ROELCKE D. & DOROW W. (1968) Besonderheiten der Reaktionsweise eines mit Plasmocytom — γA — Paraprotein indentischen Kalteagglutinins. *Klinische Wochenschrift*, **46**, 126.

83 COOPER A.G., CHAVIN S.I. & FRANKLIN E.C. (1970) Predominance of a single μ chain subclass in cold agglutinin heavy chains. *Immunochemistry*, **7**, 479.

84 FRANKLIN E.C. & FUDENBERG H.H. (1964) Antigenic heterogeneity of human Rh antibodies, rheumatoid factors, and cold agglutinins. *Archives of Biochemistry and Biophysics*, **104**, 433.

85 COHEN S. & COOPER A.G. (1968) Chemical differences between individual cold agglutinins. *Immunology*, **15**, 93.

86 FEIZI T. (1967) Lambda chains in cold agglutinins. *Science*, **156**, 1111.

87 WEINER A.S., UNGER L.J., COHEN L. & FELDMAN J. (1956) Type-specific cold auto-antibodies as a cause of acquired hemolytic anemia and hemolytic transfusion reactions: biological test with bovine red cells. *Annals of Internal Medicine*, **44**, 221.

88 MARSH W.L. (1961) Anti-i: a cold antibody defining the Ii relationship in human red cells. *British Journal of Haematology*, **7**, 200.

89 MARSH W.L. & JENKINS W.J. (1968) Anti-Sp₁: the recognition of a new cold autoantibody. *Vox Sanguinis*, **15**, 177.

90 ROELCKE D. (1974) A review: cold agglutinin. Antibodies and antigens. *Clinical Immunology and Immunopathology*, **2**, 266.

91 BOYER J.T. (1967) Complement and cold agglutinins. II. Interactions of the components of complement and antibody within the haemolytic process. *Clinical and Experimental Immunology*, **2**, 241.

92 LEVINE P., CELANO M.J. & FALKOWSKI F. (1963) The specificity of the antibody in paroxysmal cold haemoglobinuria (PCH). *Transfusion (Philadelphia)*, **3**, 278.

93 WORLLEDGE S.M. & ROUSSO C. (1965) Studies of the serology of paroxysmal cold haemoglobinuria (PCH), with special reference to its relationship with the P blood group system. *Vox Sanguinis*, **10**, 293.

94 NOSSAL G.J.V. (1971) Recent advance in immunological tolerance. *Progress in Immunology* (ed. Amos B.), p. 665. Academic Press, New York.

95 ALLISON A.C., DENMAN A.M. & BARNES R.D. (1971) Cooperating and controlling function of thymus-derived lymphocytes in relation to autoimmunity. *Lancet*, **ii**, 135.

96 MELLORS R.C. (1971) Wild-type Gross leukemia virus and heritable autoimmune disease of New Zealand mice. *American Journal of Clinical Pathology*, **56**, 270.

97 ZUELZER W.W., MASTRANGELO R., STULBERG C.S., POULIK M.D., PAGE R.H. & THOMPSON R.I. (1970) Autoimmune hemolytic anemia. Natural history and viral-immunologic interaction in childhood. *American Journal of Medicine*, **49**, 80.

98 DACIE J.V. (1971) Aetiology of the autoimmune haemolytic anaemias. *Haematologica*, **5**, 351.

99 HILL L.E. (1971) Clinical features of hypogammaglobulinaemia. *Hypogammaglobulinaemia in the United Kingdom*. MRC working party on hypogammaglobulinaemia, p. 21. HMSO, London.

100 HARRIS J.W. (1954) Studies on the mechanism of a drug-induced hemolytic anemia. *Journal of Laboratory and Clinical Medicine*, **44**, 809.

101 HARRIS J.W. (1956) Studies on the mechanism of a drug-induced hemolytic anemia. *Journal of Laboratory and Clinical Medicine*, **47**, 760.

102 WEISS H.J., BERGER R.E. & TICE E.D. (1972) Fatal disseminated intravascular coagulation and hemolytic anemia following stibophen therapy; a study of basic mechanisms. *American Journal of Medical Science*, **264**, 375.

103 WORLLEDGE S.M. (1973) Immune drug-induced hemolytic anemias. *Seminars in Hematology*, **10**, 327.

104 WEISFUSE L., SPEAR P.W. & SASS M. (1954) Quinidine-induced thrombocytopenic purpura. *American Journal of Medicine*, **17**, 414.

105 FREEDMAN A.L., BARR P.S. & BRODY E.A. (1956) Hemolytic anemia due to quinidine: observations on its mechanism. *American Journal of Medicine*, **20**, 806.

106 BELL C.A., ZWICKER H., LEE S. & ALPERN H. (1973) Quinidine hemolytic anemia in the absence of thrombocytopenia in a patient with hemoglobin D. *Transfusion*, **13**, 100.

107 BALLAS S.K., CARE J.F. & MIGUEL O. (1978) Quinidine-induced hemolytic anemia: immunohematologic characterization. *Transfusion*, **18**, 215.

108 ZEIGLER Z., SHADDUCK R.K., WINKELSTEIN A. & STROUPE T.K. (1979) Immune haemolytic anemia and thrombocytopenia secondary to quinidine: *In vitro* studies of the quinidine-dependent red-cell and platelet antibodies. *Blood*, **53**, 396.

109 MUIRHEAD E.E., HALDEN E.R. & GROVES M. (1958) Drug-dependent Coombs (antiglobulin) test and anemia. Observations on quinine and acetophenetidin (phenacetin). *Archives of Internal Medicine*, **101**, 87.

110 GARRATTY G. (with PETZ L.D.) (1979) Laboratory investigation of drug-induced immune hemolytic anemia. Presented at the *32nd Annual Meeting of the American Association of Blood Banks*, Las Vegas, Nevada, 1979.

111 VERAN P., GUIMBRETIÈRE J., MOIGNETEAU C., COTTIN S. & CREQUET R. (1962) Découverte d'anticorps circulants spécifiques au cours de chocs au P.A.S. (Circonstance clinique et intérêt thérapeutique). *Revue de la Tuberculose* (Paris), **26**, 829.

112 MUELLER-ECKHARDT CH., KRETSCHMER V. & COBURG K.-H. (1972) Allergische, immunhämolytische Anämie durch para-Amino-salicylsäure (PAS). *Deutsche Medizinische Wochenschrift*, **97**, 234.

113 MacGIBBON B.H., LOUGHBRIDGE L.W., HOURIHANE D.O'B. & BOYD D.W. (1960) Autoimmune haemolytic anaemia with acute renal failure due to phenacetin and p-aminosalicylic acid. *Lancet*, **i**, 7.

114 WORLLEDGE S.M. (1969) Immune drug-induced hemolytic anemias. *Seminars in Hematology*, **6**, 181.

115 MEHROTRA T.N. & GUPTA S.K. (1973) Paracetamol-induced hemolytic anaemia. *Indian Journal of Medical Science*, **27**, 548.

116 MANOR E., MARMOR A., KAUFMAN S. & LEIBA H. (1971) Massive hemolysis caused by acetaminophen-positive determination by direct Coombs' test. *Journal of the American Medical Association*, **236**, 2777.

117 KORNBERG A. & POLLIACK A. (1978) Paracetamol-induced thromboyctopenia and haemolytic anaemia. *Lancet*, **ii**, 1159.

118 WHITE J.M., BROWN D.L., HEPNER G.W. & WORLLEDGE S.M. (1968) Penicillin-induced haemolytic anaemia. *British Medical Journal*, **iii**, 26.

119 KERR R.O., CARDAMONE J., DALMASSO A.P. & KAPLAN M.E. (1972) Two mechanisms of erythrocyte destruction in penicillin-induced hemolytic anemia. *New England Journal of Medicine*, **287**, 1322.

120 BIRD G.W.G., McEVOY M.W. & WINGHAM J. (1975) Acute haemolytic anaemia due to IgM penicillin anti-

body in a three-year-old child, a sequel to oral penicillin. *Journal of Clinical Pathology*, **28**, 321.

121 BIRD G.W.G., WINGHAM J., GUNSTONE R.F. & SMITH A.J. (1975) Acute haemolytic anaemia due to IgM and IgA penicillin antibody. *Lancet*, **ii**, 462.

122 DOVE A.F., THOMAS D.J.B., ARONSTAM A. & CHANT R.D. (1975) Haemolytic anaemia due to penicillin. *British Medical Journal*, **iii**, 684.

123 NESMITH L.W. & DAVIS J.W. (1968) Hemolytic anemia caused by penicillin. *Journal of the American Medical Association*, **203**, 27.

124 RIES C.A., ROSENBAUM T.J., GARRATTY G., PETZ L.D. & FUDENBERG H.H. (1975) Penicillin-induced immune hemolytic anemia—occurrence of massive intravascular hemolysis. *Journal of the American Medical Association*, **233**, 27.

125 FUNICELLA T., WEINGER R.S., MOAKE J.L., SPRUELL M. & ROSSEN R.D. (1977) Penicillin-induced immuno-hemolytic anemia associated with circulating immune complexes. *American Journal of Haematology*, **3**, 219.

126 JACKSON F.N. & JAFFE J.P. (1979) Fatal penicillin-induced hemolytic anemia. *Journal of the American Medical Association*, **242**, 2286.

127 PETZ L.D. & FUDENBERG H.H. (1966) Coombs-positive hemolytic anemia caused by penicillin administration. *New England Journal of Medicine*, **274**, 171.

128 BENGTSSON U., AHLSTEDT S., CURELL M. & KAIJSER B. (1975) Antazoline-induced immune hemolytic anemia, hemoglobinuria, and acute renal failure. *Acta Medica Scandinavica*, **198**, 223.

129 FISHMAN F.L., BARON J.M. & ORLINA A. (1973) Non-oxidative hemolysis due to salicylazosulfapyridine. Evidence for an immune mechanism. *Gastroenterology*, **64**, 727.

130 LOGUE G.L., BOYD A.E. & ROSSE W.F. (1970) Chlorpropamide-induced immune hemolytic anemia. *New England Journal of Medicine*, **283**, 900.

131 BIRD G.W.G., EELES G.H., LITCHFIELD J.A., RAHMAN M. & WINGHAM J. (1972) Haemolytic anaemia with antibodies to tolbutamide and phenacetin. *British Medical Journal*, **i**, 728.

132 MALACARNE P., CASTALDI G., BERTUSI M. & ZAVAGLI G. (1977) Tolbutamide-induced hemolytic anemia. *Diabetes*, **26**, 156.

133 VILA J.M., BLUM L. & DOSIK H. (1976) Thiazide-induced immune hemolytic anemia. *Journal of the American Medical Association*, **236**, 1723.

134 FREEDMAN J. & LIM F.C. (1978) An immunohematologic complication of isoniazid. *Vox Sanguinis*, **35**, 126.

135 WENZ B., KLEIN R.L. & LALEZARI P. (1974) Tetracycline-induced immune hemolytic anemia. *Transfusion*, **14**, 265.

136 EYSTER M.E. (1967) Melphalan (alkeran) erythrocyte agglutinin and hemolytic anemia. *Annals of Internal Medicine*, **66**, 573.

137 BOHNEN R.F., ULTMANN J.E., GORMAN J.G., FARHANGI M. & SCUDDER J. (1968) The direct Coombs' Test: Its clinical significance. *Annals of Internal Medicine*, **68**, 19.

138 KAPLAN K., REISBERG B. & WEINSTEIN L. (1968) Cephaloridine—studies of therapeutic activity and untoward effects. *Archives of Internal Medicine*, **121**, 17.

139 GRALNICK H.R., MCGINNISS M.H., ELTON W. & MCCURDY P. (1971) Hemolytic anemia associated with cephalothin. *Journal of the American Medical Association*, **217**, 1193.

140 LEMOLE G.M., FADALI A.M.A. & MOLTHAM L. (1972) Cephalothin-induced tachycardia following aortic valve replacement. *Journal of the American Medical Association*, **221**, 593.

141 JEANNET M., BLOCK A., DAYER J.M., FARQUET J.J., GERARD J.P. & CRUCHAUD A. (1976) Cephalothin-induced immune hemolytic anemia. *Acta Haematologica*, **55**, 109.

142 GREUL W., MERTELSMANN R. & SCHASSAN H.H. (1976) Hemolytische Anämie und akutes Nierenversagen unter Therapie mit Cephalotin und Furosemid. *Medizinische Klinik*, **71**, 1293.

143 RUBIN R.N. & BURKA E.R. (1977) Anticephalothin antibody and Coombs' positive hemolytic anemia. *Annals of Internal Medicine*, **86**, 64.

144 FORBES C.D., MITCHELL R., CRAIG J.H. & MCNICOL G.P. (1972) Acute intravascular haemolysis associated with cephalexin therapy. *Postgraduate Medical Journal*, **48**, 186.

145 MOAKE J.L., BUTLER C.F., HEWELL G.M., CHEEK J. & SPRUELL M.A. (1978) Hemolysis induced by cefazolin and cephalothin in a patient with penicillin sensitivity. *Transfusion*, **18**, 369.

146 FAULK W.P., TOMSOVIC E.J. & FUDENBERG H.H. (1970) Insulin resistance in juvenile diabetes mellitus. Immunologic studies. *American Journal of Medicine*, **49**, 133.

147 HASSE W., PHOLE H.D., WARNECKE F. & WIEK K. (1971) Hämolytische Krise durch Rifampicin. *Praxis der Pneumologie*, **25**, 466.

148 SORS C., SARRAZIN A. & HOMBERG J.C. (1972) Accidents hémolytiques récidivants d'origine immuno-allergique au cours d'un traitement intermittent par la rifampicine. *Revue de Tuberculose et de Pneumologie*, **36**, 406.

149 LAKSHMINARAYAN S., SAHN S.A. & HUDSON L.D. (1973) Massive haemolysis caused by rifampicin. *British Medical Journal*, **ii**, 282.

150 LEBACQ E. & TAMINAU E. (1974) Anomalies hématologiques au cours des traitements à la rifampicine. *Lille Médical*, **19**, 269.

151 CRIEL A. & VERWILGHEN R.L. (1980) Intravascular haemolysis and renal failure caused by intermittent rifampicin treatment. *Blut*, **40**, 147.

152 GANGUIN H.-G. (1971) Thrombozytopenische purpura under rifampicin. Symposium on rifampicin. Prague. Quoted by Swanson M. & Cook R. (1977) *Drugs, Chemicals and Blood Dyscrasias*. Drug Intelligence Publications, Inc., Hamilton, Illinois.

153 CHIVRAC D., MARTI R., FOURNIER A.F.N., FAILLE N., MESSERSCHMITT J. & LORRIAUX A. (1974) Hémolyse immuno-allergique compliquée d'insuffisance rénale aiguë après ingestion de glaférine. *La Nouvelle Presse Medicale*, **3**, 2578.

154 ORENSTEIN A.A., YAKULIS V., EIPE J. & COSTEA N. (1977) Immune hemolysis due to hydralazine. *Annals of Internal Medicine*, **86**, 450.

155 LETIONA J.M.L., BARBOLLA L., FRIEYRO E., BOUZA E., GILSANZ F. & FERNÁNDEZ M.N. (1977) Immune haemolytic anaemia and renal failure induced by streptomycin. *British Journal of Haematology*, **35**, 561.

156 PLA R.P., MARTIN C., ODRIOZOLA J., ARMENDOL R. & TRIGINER J. (1976) Anémie hémolytique immuno-aller-

gique liée à la streptomycine. *Revue française de Transfusion et Immunohématologie*, **19**, 379.

157 TAKAHASHI H. & TSUKADA T. (1979) Triamterene-induced immune haemolytic anaemia with acute intravascular haemolysis and acute renal failure. *Scandinavian Journal of Haematology*, **23**, 169.

158 BOURNERIAS F. & HABIBI B. (1979) Nomifensine-induced immune haemolytic anaemia and impaired renal function. *Lancet*, **ii**, 95.

159 GETAZ E.P., BECKLEY S., FITZPATRICK J. & DOZIER A. (1980) Cisplatin-induced hemolysis. *New England Journal of Medicine*, **302**, 334.

160 MIESCHER P. & STRAESSLE R. (1956) Experimentelle Studien über den Mechanismus der Thromcyten-Schädigung durch Antigen-Antikörper-Reaktionen. *Vox Sanguinis*, **1**, 83.

161 SHULMAN N.R. (1963) Mechanism of blood cell damage by absorption of antigen–antibody complexes. *Immunopathology, 3rd International Symposium*, La Jolla, California, p. 338. Schwabe, Basel.

162 SHULMAN N.R. (1964) A mechanism of cell destruction in individuals sensitized to foreign antigens and its implications in auto-immunity. *Annals of Internal Medicine*, **60**, 506.

163 GILBERTSON C. & ROWLEY JONES D. (1972) Haemolytic anaemia with nalidixic acid. *British Medical Journal*, **iv**, 493.

164 COOPER J.W. & PESNELL L.H. (1978) Thioridazine-associated immune hemolytic anemia. *Southern Medical Journal*, **71**, 1443.

165 LAW I.P., WICKMAN C.J. & HARRISON B.R. (1979) Coombs' positive hemolytic anemia and ibuprofen. *Southern Medical Journal*, **72**, 707.

166 GUIDRY J.B., OGBURN C.L. & GRIFFIN F.M. (1979) Fatal autoimmune hemolytic anemia associated with ibuprofen. *Journal of the American Medical Association*, **242**, 68.

167 KORSAGER S. (1978) Haemolysis complicating ibuprofen treatment. *British Medical Journal*, **i**, 79.

168 HADNAGY C. (1976) Coombs-positive haemolytic anaemia provoked by chlorpromazine. *Lancet*, **i**, 423.

169 LEVINE B.B. & REDMOND A.P. (1967) Immune mechanisms of penicillin-induced Coombs positivity in man (abstract). *Journal of Clinical Investigation*, **46**, 1085.

170 HAUGAARD N., HAUGAARD E.S. & STADIE W.C. (1954) Combination of insulin with cells. *Journal of Biological Chemistry*, **211**, 289.

171 STEFANINI M. & JOHNSON N.L. (1970) Positive antihuman globulin test in patients receiving Carbromal. *American Journal of the Medical Sciences*, **259**, 49.

172 POOLE G., STRADLING P. & WORLLEDGE S. (1971) Potentially serious side-effects of high-dose twice-weekly rifampicin. *British Medical Journal*, **iii**, 343.

173 GRALNICK H.R., WRIGHT L.D. & McGINNIS M.H. (1967) Coombs' positive reactions associated with sodium cephalothin therapy. *Journal of the American Medical Association*, **199**, 725.

174 MOLTHAN L., REIDENBERG M.M. & EICHMAN M.F. (1967) Positive direct Coombs tests due to cephalothin. *New England Journal of Medicine*, **277**, 123.

175 GARRATTY G. & PETZ L.D. (1975) Drug-induced hemolytic anemia. *The American Journal of Medicine*, **58**, 398.

176 SPATH P., GARRATTY G. & PETZ L.D. (1971) Studies on the immune response to penicillin and cephalothin in humans. II. Immunohematologic reactions to cephalothin administration. *Journal of Immunology*, **107**, 860.

177 WORLLEDGE S.M. (1973) Immune drug-induced haemolytic anaemias. In *Blood Disorders Due to Drugs and Other Agents* (ed. Girdwood R.H.). Excerpta Medica, Amsterdam.

178 SIVAMURTHY S., FRANKFURT E. & LEVINE M.E. (1973) Positive antiglobulin test in patients maintained on methadone. *Transfusion*, **13**, 418.

179 SHERWOOD G.K., McGINNISS M.H., KATON R.N., DUPONT R.L. & WEBSTER J.B. (1972) Negative direct Coombs' tests in narcotic addicts receiving maintenance doses of methadone. *Blood*, **40**, 902.

180 CARSTAIRS K.C., BRECKENRIDGE A., DOLLERY C.T. & WORLLEDGE S. (1966) Incidence of a positive direct Coombs test in patients on α-methyldopa. *Lancet*, **ii**, 133.

181 WORLLEDGE S.M., CARSTAIRS K.C. & DACIE J.V. (1966) Autoimmune haemolytic anaemia associated with α-methyldopa therapy. *Lancet*, **ii**, 135.

182 BOTTIGER L.E. & WESTERHOLM B. (1973) Acquired haemolytic anaemia. II. Drug-induced haemolytic anaemia. *Acta Medica Scandinavica*, **193**, 227.

183 ISSITT P.D., PAVONE B.G., GOLDFINGER D., ZWICKER H., ISSITT C.H., TESSELL J.A., KROOVAND S.W. & BELL C.A. (1976) Anti-Wr^b and other autoantibodies responsible for positive direct antiglobulin tests in 150 individuals. *British Journal of Haematology*, **34**, 5.

184 BUCHANAN J.G., RUSH B. & DE GRUCHY G.C. (1966) Methyldopa and acquired haemolytic anaemia. *Medical Journal of Australia*, **2**, 700.

185 EWING D.J., HUGHES C.J. & WARDLE D.F. (1968) Methyldopa-induced autoimmune haemolytic anaemia—a report of two further cases. *Guy's Hospital Reports*, **117**, 111.

186 NELSON R.B. JR. & NELSON R.B. III (1977) Methyldopa associated intravascular hemolysis. *Archives of Internal Medicine*, **137**, 1260.

187 KESSEY E.C., PIERCE S., BECK M.L. & BAYER W.L. (1973) Alphamethyldopa-induced hemolytic anemia involving autoantibody with U specificity. *Transfusion*, **13**, 360.

188 PATTEN E., BECK C.E., SCHOLL C., STROOPE R.A. & WUKASCH C. (1977) Autoimmune hemolytic anemia with anti Jk^a specificity in a patient taking Aldomet. *Transfusion*, **16**, 517.

189 LOBUGLIO A.F. & JANDL J.H. (1967) The nature of the α-methyldopa red-cell antibody. *New England Journal of Medicine*, **276**, 658.

190 BRECKENRIDGE A., DOLLERY C.T., WORLLEDGE S.M., HOLBOROW E.J. & JOHNSON G.D. (1967) Positive direct Coombs tests and antinuclear factor in patients treated with methyldopa. *Lancet*, **ii**, 1265.

191 FELTKAMP T.E.W., ENGELFRIET C.P. & VAN LOGHEM J.J. (1968) Autoantibodies and methyldopa. *Lancet*, **i**, 644.

192 ELIASTAM M. & HOLMES A.W. (1971) Hepatitis, arthritis and lupus cell phenomena caused by methyldopa. *Digestive Diseases*, **16**, 1014.

193 KIRTLAND H.H., MOHLER D.N. & HORWITZ, D.A. (1980) Methyldopa inhibition of suppressor-lymphocyte function. *New England Journal of Medicine*, **302**, 825.

194 SHERMAN J.D., LOVE D.E. & HARRINGTON J.F. (1967) Anemia, positive lupus and rheumatoid factors with

methyldopa. *Archives of Internal Medicine*, **120**, 321.

195 HYER S.L. & KNELL A.J. (1977) Cirrhosis and haemolysis complicating methyldopa treatment. *British Medical Journal*, **1**, 879.

196 SCOTT G.L., MYLES A.B. & BACON P.A. (1968) Autoimmune haemolytic anaemia and mefenamic acid therapy. *British Medical Journal*, **iii**, 534.

197 ROBERTSON J.H., KENNEDY C.C. & HILL C.M. (1971) Haemolytic anaemia associated with mefenamic acid. *Irish Journal of Medical Science*, **140**, 226.

198 FARID N.R., JOHNSON R.J. & LOW W.T. (1971) Haemolytic reaction to mefenamic acid. *Lancet*, **ii**, 382.

199 FARQUET J.J., DAYER J.M. & MIESCHER P.A. (1978) Anémie auto-immunohémalytique induite par l'acide méfénamique. *Schweizerische Medizinische Wochenschrift*, **108**, 1510.

200 SAKAI C., AKIHAMA T., MIURA A.B., KOMATSU K. & SHIBATA A. (1978) A case of mefenamic acid-induced autoimmune hemolytic anaemia. *Rinsho Ketsueki*, **19**, 1575.

201 DACIE J.V. & WORLLEDGE S.M. (1969) Autoimmune haemolytic anaemias. In: *Progress in Haematology* (ed. Brown E.), **6**, 82.

202 GABOR E.P. & GOLDBERG L.S. (1973) Levodopa-induced Coombs positive haemolytic anaemia. *Scandinavian Journal of Haematology*, **11**, 201.

203 TERRITO M.C., PETERS R.W. & TANAKA K.R. (1973) Autoimmune hemolytic anemia due to levodopa therapy. *Journal of the American Medical Association*, **226**, 1347.

204 HOORNTJE S.J. & PANDERS J.T. (1976) Hemolytische Anemie en levodopa. *Ned Tijdschr Geneeskunde*, **120**, 204.

205 LINDSTRÖM F.D., LIEDEN G. & ENGSTRÖM M.S. (1977) Dose-related levodopa-induced haemolytic anemia. *Annals of Internal Medicine*, **86**, 298.

206 BERSTEIN R.M. (1979) Reversible haemolytic anaemia after levodopa-carbidopa. *British Medical Journal*, **i**, 1461.

207 KRÜGER J., RAHMAN A., MOGK K.-U. & MUELLER-ECKHARDT C. (1976) T-cell deficiency in patients with autoimmune hemolytic anemia ('Warm Type'). *Vox Sanguinis*, **31**, 1.

208 DAUSSET J. & COLOMBANI J. (1959) The serology and the prognosis of 128 cases of autoimmune hemolytic anemia. *Blood*, **14**, 1280.

209 DOYLE A.P. & HELLSTROM H.R. (1963) Mesantoin lymphadenopathy morphologically simulating Hodgkin's disease. *Annals of Internal Medicine*, **59**, 363.

210 SWANSON M. & COOK R. (1977) *Drugs, Chemicals and Blood Dyscrasias*. Drug Intelligence Publications Inc., Hamilton, Illinois.

211 SNAPPER I., MARKS D., SCHWARTZ L. & HOLLANDER L. (1953) Hemolytic anaemia secondary to mesantoin. *Annals of Internal Medicine*, **39**, 619.

212 JONES G.W., GEORGE T.L. & BRADLEY R.D. (1978) Procainamide-induced haemolytic anemia. *Transfusion*, **18**, 224.

213 NUSSEY A.M. (1973) Fenfluramine and haemolytic anaemia. *British Medical Journal*, **i**, 177.

214 WALSHE A.M. (1972) Fenfluramine and propranalol. *British Medical Journal*, **iii**, 821.

215 HUNZIKER H. (1978) Goldinduzierte autoimmunhämolytische anämie? *Praxis*, **67**, 702.

216 NAWROT D. & PRYTEL-DABROWSKA T. (1977) Ostra polekowa niedokrwistosc autoimmunohemolytyczna. *Wiadomosci Lekarskie*, **30**, 379.

217 ROTOLI B., FORMISANO S. & ALFINITO F. (1979) Autoimmune haemolytic anaemia associated with cimetidine. *Lancet*, **ii**, 583.

218 ARMITAGE P. & MOLLINSON P.L. (1953) Further analysis of controlled trials of treatment of haemolytic disease of the newborn. *Journal of Obstetrics and Gynaecology of the British Empire*, **60**, 605.

219 WORLLEDGE S. (1978) The interpretation of a positive direct antiglobulin test. *British Journal of Haematology*, **39**, 157.

220 HAM T.H. & CASTLE W.B. (1940) Mechanism of hemolysis in certain anemias: significance of increased hypotonic fragility and of erythrostosis. *Journal of Clinical Investigation*, **19**, 788.

221 LoBUGLIO A.F., COTRAN R.S. & JANDL J.H. (1967) Red cells coated with immunoglobulin G: binding and sphering by mononuclear cells in man. *Science*, **158**, 1582.

222 HUBER H. & FUDENBERG H.H. (1968) Receptor sites of human monocytes for IgG. *International Archives of Allergy and Applied Immunology*, **34**, 18.

223 ABRAMSON N. & SCHUR P.H. (1972) The IgG subclasses of red-cell antibodies and relationship to monocyte binding. *Blood*, **40**, 500.

224 BROWN D.L. & NELSON D.A. (1973) Surface microfragmentation of red cells as a mechanism for complement-mediated immune spherocytosis. *British Journal of Haematology*, **24**, 301.

225 WEISS L. (1957) A study of the structure of splenic sinuses in man and in the albino rat with the light microscope and the electron microscope. *Journal of Biophysical and Biochemical Cytology*, **3**, 599.

226 MOHN J.F., LAMBERT R.M., BOWMAN H.S. & BRASON F.W. (1961) Experimental transfusion of donor plasma containing blood-group antibodies into incompatible normal human recipients. 1. Absence of destruction of red-cell mass with anti-Rh, anti-Kell and anti-M. *British Journal of Haematology*, **7**, 112.

227 JANDL J.H. (1965) Mechanisms of antibody-induced red-cell destruction. *Series Haematologica*, **9**, 35.

228 GOLD E.R. & FUDENBERG H.H. (1967) Chromic chloride: a coupling reagent for passive hemagglutination reactions. *Journal of Immunology*, **99**, 859.

229 RUBIN H. (1963) Antibody elution from red blood cells. *Journal of Clinical Pathology*, **16**, 70.

230 VOS G.H. & KELSALL G.A. (1956) A new elution technique for the preparation of specific immune anti-Rh serum. *British Journal of Haematology*, **2**, 342.

231 LANDSTEINER K. & MILLER C.P. JR. (1925) Serological studies on the blood of primates: II. The blood groups in anthropoid apes. *Journal of Experimental Medicine*, **42**, 853.

232 KOCHWA S. & ROSENFIELD R.E. (1964) Immunochemical studies of the Rh system: I. Isolation and characterization of antibodies. *Journal of Immunology*, **92**, 682.

233 POLLEY M.J., MOLLISON P.L., ROSE J. & WALKER W. (1965) A simple serological test for antibodies causing ABO—haemolytic disease of the newborn. *Lancet*, **i**, 291.

Chapter 12
The non-immune acquired haemolytic anaemias

E. C. GORDON-SMITH

Changes in the red-cell membrane, metabolism or content nearly always lead to an increased rate of destruction of the cells, so that minor degrees of haemolysis are seen in most anaemias, such as iron deficiency [1], aplastic anaemia [2] and megaloblastic anaemia [3]. The haemolysis in these disorders is unimportant compared with the main cause of the anaemia, namely the failure of red-cell or haemoglobin production. Haemolysis, on the other hand, is produced by a wide variety of unrelated diseases which have the common effect of altering the properties of the red-cell membrane or its deformability in such a way that destruction of the cells is greatly accelerated either in the reticulo-endothelial system or intravascularly.

These disorders may be grouped into four main categories for clinical convenience, though the underlying mechanisms of haemolysis may overlap in different groups. The four categories considered here are:
1 infection;
2 chemical and physical agents;
3 mechanical disorders; and
4 acquired defects of the red-cell membrane.

HAEMOLYTIC ANAEMIAS CAUSED BY INFECTIONS

MALARIA
(see also Chapter 33)
Malaria is caused by infection with protozoal parasites of the genus *Plasmodium*, which are transmitted in nature, from host to host, by the Anopheles mosquito. In man, disease is caused by the species *P. malariae*, *P. vivax*, *P. ovale* with *P. falciparum* (producing 'subtertian', 'malignant tertian' or 'aestivo-autumnal' malaria) the most virulent. Infection with *P. falciparum* is that most commonly associated with severe haemolytic anaemia though mixed infections are sometimes responsible.

Despite some early successful eradication programmes by the World Health Organization in circumscribed areas, malaria remains one of the commonest infections of the world [4, 5]. Rapid worldwide travel means that more people who live in non-malarial areas may become infected [6] particularly since effective anti-malarial prophylaxis is frequently ignored by transient visitors. Malaria may for the same reason develop unexpectedly in regions where it does not exist naturally and lead to problems of diagnosis.

The parasites may be transferred in other ways than by the natural vector. Blood used for transfusion is a common mode of transmission in malarial areas and chloroquine is often given to recipients of blood routinely. In non-malarial regions it may occasionally be spread via infected blood collected from donors recently returned from malarial areas. It has been recommended that donors who have visited malarial areas should not give blood for six months after their return even when prophylaxis has apparently been rigorous. Immigrants and residents from malarial areas probably should not give blood for three years following entry to non-malarial regions. This will eliminate all chance of serious malarial illness being transmitted [7]. The only exception is *P. malariae* (causing quartan malaria) which may persist for up to 50 years in the host [8]. Transmission from the use of a common syringe amongst drug addicts is reported [9], and rarely transmission occurs from mother to fetus [10, 11].

Haemolytic anaemia in malaria
Anaemia is common in malaria [12] particularly falciparum and is probably related to the degree of parasitaemia [13, 14]. Haemolysis is mainly responsible for the anaemia though there is usually some suppression of marrow activity manifest by the relatively low reticulocyte counts seen during acute attacks [15, 16]. It may also be that the reticulocytopenia is in part due to preferential invasion of young red cells by *P. falciparum* [17, 18] with consequent disappearance of this population. Blackwater fever is the most dramatic type of haemolysis seen in falciparum malaria, though it is now rare, but haemolysis accompanies most forms of severe falciparum malaria particularly when there is cerebral and/or respiratory involvement.

Fulminant falciparum malaria

This is occasionally seen in travellers returned from malarial areas. The severity depends on the delay in diagnosis. The clinical features include cerebral involvement with increasing coma, renal failure, thrombocytopenia and marked haemolytic anaemia with both intravascular and extravascular components. Pulmonary involvement with respiratory failure carries a particularly grave prognosis [19, 20]. There is often a very marked parasitaemia [21] but, depending on previous immunity, parasites may be difficult to find in some severely affected individuals. The association of intravascular haemolysis with low platelet counts have led to the suggestion that diffuse intravascular coagulation is an important mechanism of haemolysis in these patients [20–22], though the common finding that fibrinogen is normal and fibrin degradation products (FDP) are not present in increased amounts led some workers to conclude that coagulation was not involved [23]. This conclusion has been challenged on the grounds that these severe malarial infections usually produce a high fibrinogen level, and that normal levels represent a decrease in fibrinogen in this circumstance [24]. Certainly, the fibrinogen levels do fall as the disease progresses. Even when there is evidence of consumption coagulopathy, fibrin deposition in small blood vessels is difficult to demonstrate in post-mortem examinations [19, 20].

Treatment of the fulminant case relies mainly on the use of intravenous anti-malarials, chloroquine for most patients or quinine when chloroquine resistance is suspected, and supportive care. Transfusion may be necessary to correct anaemia. Heparin has been advocated, particularly when there is good evidence for diffuse intravascular coagulation (DIC), though some have challenged its usefulness [23]. Replacement therapy with platelets and fresh frozen plasma (FFP) should be given if heparin is used. Exchange transfusion has been used to reduce the parasitaemia in severely ill patients with survival in each reported case [19, 21, 25], and with avoidance of renal failure in one of them [21]. The mortality of this stage of malaria is of the order of 30% [19] though it may be even higher when respiratory failure is present [20].

Blackwater fever

This is the name given to a form of falciparum malaria characterized by extensive intravascular haemolysis and haemoglobinuria. Death frequently occurs as a result of oliguric renal failure, resulting from acute tubular necrosis caused by the hypovolaemia and electrolyte depletion which complicate the haemolysis [26–28]. It used to be thought that the disease was confined to Europeans and it seemed to be related to irregular treatment with quinine. Blackwater fever declined with the introduction of adequate prophylaxis and chemotherapy. Blackwater fever now occurs mainly in indigenous populations who live in areas where malaria eradication has been relatively successful [28, 29]. It seems possible that the disease depends upon incomplete immunity to the parasite and, except in rare cases, is not caused by drug-induced antibodies, nor by G6PD deficiency [28], though these must be excluded as causes of intravascular haemolysis. Parasitaemia is high in about 50% of the cases but in others parasites are not found. This may be a function of the time of sampling in relation to the haemolysis and emphasizes the importance of early examination of films for parasites in suspected cases [26]. Haemolysis is very rapid, the plasma haemoglobin may rise above 350 mg/dl and the haemoglobinuria be so profuse that the urine appears black. There are no specific morphological changes in the red cells of the peripheral blood but reticulocytosis may be delayed. Evidence of DIC is not found in these patients. The red-cell count may fall below $1 \times 10^{12}/l$ in 24 hours, neutropenia may develop but thrombocytopenia is rare.

Treatment is directed to the urgent correction of the fluid and electrolyte disorders, and preventing death from anaemia. Renal dialysis may be essential and may have to be continued for a month or more. It is therefore necessary to transfer these patients as early as possible to a centre equipped for dialysis [26]. Since Blackwater fever tends to recur in subsequent attacks of falciparum malaria, careful prophylaxis must be instituted from the time of the first attack.

Haemolytic mechanisms in malaria

There are probably many contributory factors in the development of haemolytic anaemia in falciparum malaria [12]. These may be divided into effects produced by invasion of red cells by the parasite and effects produced by the body's reaction to the infection. Shortening of red-cell survival occurs in both parasitized and non-parasitized cells, though it is greater in the former.

Invasion of the red cells by the plasmodium. This is followed by a period of growth and development of the parasite at the end of which intravascular rupture of the cells occurs with release of merozoites. The rate of haemolysis is proportional to the parasitaemia. Experimentally, using *P. berghei*-infected erythrocytes in rats, it has been shown that infected erythrocytes are cleared more quickly than uninfected and that this clearance is even greater in immune rats [30]. The clearance is mainly by the spleen. It is suggested that there is a decrease in the deformability of the infected red cells which contributes to their destruction. Electron-microscope studies show that the surface of red cells parasitized by *P. falciparum* have defects which may contribute to lack of deformability. Similar defects may be seen in unparasitized cells which may indicate abortive attack by parasites, nevertheless rendering the cell liable to destruction [31].

Immune reactions. These have been thought to be important in the destruction of red cells. Antibodies directed against parasites and against drugs used in therapy have been demonstrated. Drug-induced immune haemolytic anaemia generated by antibodies against quinine certainly occurs, but is rare. Antibodies against various malarial antigens have been demonstrated sometimes in high titre but have not been shown to be haemolytic [32, 33]. On the other hand, IgM antibodies directed against red cells do appear in *P. falciparum* infection [34], and are accompanied by a general rise in IgM and fall in C3. The changes are most marked in the most anaemic patients.

Diffuse intravascular coagulation (DIC). This has been discussed above in relation to fulminant falciparum malaria. Undoubtedly it does occur but many studies have demonstrated thrombocytopenia, often with falling fibrinogen levels, in most patients with malaria [23, 35, 36]. In one study, falling platelet counts coincided with a rise in total serum IgM, and recovery of platelets occurred as the IgM fell again [35]. In these patients, clotting abnormalities are not present and haemolytic anaemia is not marked. Probably, platelets are sequestered or destroyed in the reticulo-endothelial system in the same way as red cells. These findings have led to confusion and argument about DIC in malaria and to the role of anti-coagulants. It seems that true DIC only occurs in the fulminant disease.

Increased activity of the reticulo-endothelial (RE) system. This also plays a part in haemolysis [33]. Even when antibodies against red cells cannot be demonstrated, there may be increased splenic uptake of non-parasitized cells (37).

Relationship between haemoglobinopathies, G6PD deficiency and falciparum malaria
For many years it has been recognized that the geographical distribution of the haemoglobin S (Hb S) is similar to the distribution of malaria [38, 39] and it was suggested that the Hb S confers a selective advantage in the protection against the lethal effects of falciparum malaria [40, 41], an example of balanced polymorphism. Children with the sickle-cell trait are less likely to have massive parasitaemia from *P. falciparum* than normal children [40, 42, 43], and a possible mechanism for this finding has been suggested by workers in Ibadan who demonstrated that, when

red blood cells from individuals with the sickle trait with severe falciparum infections were incubated anaerobically, the sickling rate was two to eight times faster than in uninfected sickle-cell carriers [44]. Sickled cells are removed by the RE system which supports earlier concepts that parasitized cells containing Hb S are phagocytosed more rapidly than Hb A containing cells following sickling [45].

Further work confirmed that parasitized cells of A/S patients sickled more readily, but that this occurred only at oxygen tensions unlikely to be encountered in life [46]. An alternative mechanism has been suggested by the finding that, at low oxygen tension, cells containing Hb S have an increased resistance to invasion by *P. falciparum in vitro* [47], and that growth of the parasite is slowed at low Po_2 in these cells [47, 48]. In this model, the protection is afforded by the specific effect of Hb S and not by the sickling process.

The role of G6PD deficiency in protection against falciparum malaria is less certain; clinical investigation suggests that the deficiency offers some protection against massive parasitaemia [42], though not necessarily against mortality [49]. It is possible that the G6PD variants found in West Africa, A and A −, may provide protection against falciparum infection, heterozygous females of genotype A −/B and hemizygous A males having significantly lower parasite counts than other genotypes [50] (see Chapter 7, p. 299).

P. falciparum does not itself contain G6PD in its cytoplasm [51]. *P. berghei* in the mouse erythrocyte is dependent upon the host cell for a supply of NADPH [52]. Furthermore, in this experimental situation vitamin-E deficiency apparently protects against invasion [53].

Diagnosis and treatment
The diagnosis of malaria is made from the discovery of parasites in the peripheral blood. With the development of chloroquine-resistant *P. falciparum*, identification of the type of malarial parasite has once again become important. *P. falciparum* may be recognized from its ring forms, which may have two chromatin dots, and from the occurrence of more than one parasite in a single cell (Fig. 12.1) and the crescent-shaped gametocyte (see also Chapter 33).

The main lines of treatment for the acute malarial attack are chloroquine, to destroy the erythrocytic stage, and primaquine, to remove exoerythrocytic organisms. *P. falciparum* has no identifiable exoerythrocytic stage and chloroquine alone is sufficient for sensitive *P. falciparum* infections. Treatment has had to be devised to deal with the increasing occurrence of resistant forms; combination therapy with quinine, antifolate derivatives and sulphones or sulphonamides

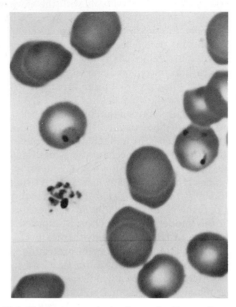

Fig. 12.1. Falciparum malaria. One red cell contains two *P. falciparum* trophozoites and some ring forms have two chromatin dots (× 1200).

is the favoured regime. The concentration of chloroquine at acid pH in lysosomes by the parasite has been suggested as a basis for chloroquine sensitivity and deficiency of this mechanism may account for resistance to the drug [54]. Chloroquine resistance is becoming a major public-health hazard worldwide [6].

Splenectomy is hazardous for people in malarial regions since the spleen is mainly responsible, together with macrophages of the liver and other sites, for destruction of merozoites released into the blood after asexual maturation of the trophozoites. Patients who have had a splenectomy should be particularly scrupulous about malarial prophylaxis when visiting possible endemic areas.

The haematological changes in malaria are considered further in Chapter 33.

TOXOPLASMOSIS

The manifestations of infection with *Toxoplasma gondii* are varied and depend particularly on the host resistance [55]. In most normal people, infection, as determined by serological testing, is asymptomatic, but an 'infectious-mononucleosis-like' syndrome or generalized lymphadenopathy occasionally develops. Toxoplasma may be identified from lymph-node biopsy in these patients but this does not indicate a necessarily recent infection [55]. In the immunologically compromised host, especially with haematological malignancies, a severe generalized disease involving

particularly the central nervous system may occur, and is usually fatal [56–58]. It may be transmitted by blood transfusion from infected hosts. Rarely toxoplasmosis causes an acute [59] or chronic [60] haemolytic anaemia with destruction within the reticulo-endothelial system.

Congenital toxoplasmosis
This, following infection of the fetus *in utero*, leads to severe disease; abortion, stillbirth or premature labour may occur. The dead fetus has a hydropic appearance similar to that seen in haemolytic disease of the newborn. Live infants who have overt signs of toxoplasma infection, again usually involving the central nervous system, often show an acute haemolytic anaemia which may require exchange or simple transfusion [61, 62]. The peripheral blood shows marked reticulocytosis and erythroblastosis. The subject is considered further in Chapter 33.

BACTERIAL INFECTIONS

The anaemia which commonly accompanies acute or chronic bacterial infections is usually the result of depression of erythropoiesis rather than haemolysis (see Chapter 33). However, some degree of shortened red-cell lifespan is often present and, in a few instances, haemolysis is the main cause of anaemia. Haemolysis may be brought about by the direct action of bacterial toxins on the red cell, by parasitization of the red cell or by immune interactions between the patients' red cells and the infecting bacteria [3]. Intravascular coagulation also plays an important part in the pathology of bacterial infections, particularly Gram-negative septicaemias associated with shock [63], and meningococcal septicaemias [64, 65]. Microangiopathic haemolytic anaemia may be present in these patients; this is discussed further in a later section (see p. 526).

Clostridium welchii

Infection with *Cl. welchii*, particularly following abortion or childbirth, is frequently accompanied by marked intravascular haemolytic anaemia. The haemolysis develops rapidly, the patient becomes deeply jaundiced, and purpura and bleeding may occur [66]. Haemoglobinuria is marked until anuria—a common complication—develops. The peripheral blood film shows intense microspherocytosis [67] and thrombocytopenia.

The haemolytic α and θ toxins of *Cl. welchii* have a lecithinase-like action which may account for the microspherocytosis of *Cl. welchii* septicaemia, though proteolytic toxins have also been implicated [68].

Intravascular coagulation may contribute to the renal failure.

The treatment of this highly lethal septicaemia is by eradication of the source of infection, if necessary by hysterectomy, antibiotics and supportive measures for the renal failure [69].

Bartonella bacilliformis

Bartonellosis, which occurs only in western South America, is caused by the organism *Bartonella bacilliformis*. The disease may present as 'Oroya fever', with fever, chills, severe pains in the bones, joints and muscles, generalized lymphadenopathy and a rapidly progressive haemolytic anaemia [70]. There is excessive phagocytosis of red cells by the reticulo-endothelial system [71], possibly due to the presence of the organism on or just within the surface of the red cell [72] (Fig. 12.2). The disease has a high mortality when untreated [73], but dramatic recovery may occur even

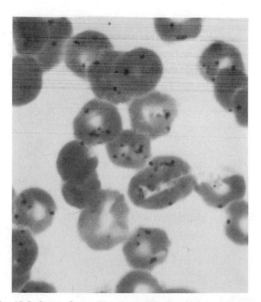

Fig. 12.2. Oroya fever. The *Bartonella bacilliformis* lies on or near the surface of the red cell. The organisms stain red with Romanowsky stain (× 1200).

when the red-cell count has fallen as low as $0.5 \times 10^{12}/l$. A second manifestation of the disease is the warty eruption of verruga peruana, which may occur with or without the prodrome of Oroya fever [70]. The common cause for these two diseases was demonstrated in 1870 by the dramatic self-experiment of the medical student David Carrion, who inoculated himself with material from verruga peruana and died from Oroya

fever [74]. Penicillin is an effective treatment for this disease [75].

CHEMICALLY INDUCED HAEMOLYSIS

A variety of drugs and chemicals produce haemolytic anaemia because of a direct chemical action on the red cell. Often the cause of the haemolysis is unsuspected and a diligent search for industrial contact or self-administration is necessary before the diagnosis can be confirmed. An understanding of the pathogenesis of haemolysis and a knowledge of the clinical syndromes produced by these compounds greatly increases the chances of arriving at the correct conclusion.

PATHOGENESIS

Haemolysis is usually produced by the oxidant action of drugs or chemicals upon the red cells [76, 77]. The red cell is susceptible to oxidant stress in a number of ways which impair its function or reduce its lifespan. Oxidation causes alterations in the red-cell membrane with auto-oxidation of lipids and the production of disulphide bonds, each of which decreases the deformability of the membrane. Oxidation of haemoglobin leads to methaemoglobin formation and precipitation of globin chains as Heinz bodies. Heinz bodies tend to form mixed disulphide bonds with the —SH groups on the inside of the red-cell membrane also leading to a loss of deformability of the cell, and even to its intravascular disruption [18]. Thus oxidative damage may lead to methaemoglobinaemia, Heinz-body formation and intravascular or extravascular haemolysis. Which of these features predominates depends upon the nature of the oxidative stress and the host response to the stress, particularly the host ability to generate reducing power.

Damage to the red cells will occur in three circumstances:

1 if an abnormally increased oxidant stress exceeds the normal sources of reducing power;

2 if there are structural abnormalities of the red cell or haemoglobin which render them more susceptible to oxidant stress despite normal sources of reducing power; or

3 if there is a deficiency of reducing power in the red cell so that it cannot counteract 'normally increased' oxidant stress.

Apart from drugs and chemicals, the red cell may be subjected to varying oxidant stress from a number of natural sources including absorption of oxidant compounds from the gastro-intestinal tract and the oxidizing substances produced by infection. All these observations indicate the marked individuality in host response to oxidant stress.

INDIVIDUAL VARIABILITY TO OXIDANT STRESS

Generation of reducing power
(see also Chapter 7, p. 278)
The major pathways by which reducing power is generated in the form of reduced glutathione (GSH) and NADPH and produced in the red cell, have been described in Chapter 7. These substances are mainly responsible for counteracting oxidant effects on the globin chains and red-cell membrane. The reduction of methaemoglobin, which occurs normally at the rate of three per cent per day [79] depends upon a supply of NADH produced by the glycolytic pathway and the integrity of the enzyme, NADH methaemoglobin

reductase. Many hereditary variants of the enzymes required for the generation of reducing power, particularly G6PD, have been described. Many of these variants are deficient in enzyme activity and hence affected individuals have increased susceptibility to oxidative stress (Table 12.1).

Inhibition of normal enzyme activity by drugs is another variable which may reduce resistance to oxidant stress. Salicylates inhibit pyruvate kinase [80] as well as G6PD activity [81, 82], though by itself this effect, at doses likely to be encountered, is insufficient to cause oxidant damage. However, it will allow damage to be produced by a lower dose of another oxidant agent. Oral contraceptives induce transketo-

Table 12.1. Chemically induced haemolysis in normal subjects

Drug or chemical	Probable haemolytic substance	Remarks	References
Phenacetin	2-hydroxy phenetidin	Cyanosis and HB* haemolysis, renal papillary necrosis	113–116
Sulphonamides	Hydroxy-amino derivatives	Acute haemolysis: hypersensitivity or G6PD deficiency. Chronic haemolysis: rare	77
Sulphones	4, hydroxylamino derivatives	HB haemolysis, dose-related	123, 129
Salicylazosulphapyridine	Sulphapyridine	HB haemolysis, dose-related	87, 118
Phenothiazine	?	Overdose produces HB haemolysis	110
Phenazopyridine	?	Methaemoglobinaemia common. Haemolytic HB anaemia may occur	77, 194
Para amino-salicylic acid	m-aminophenol	Solutions of PAS stored in warm become brown—m-NH_2 phenol	195, 196
Phenylhydrazine and acetyl phenylhydrazine	Phenylhydrazine	No longer used in treatment of polycythaemia vera. Self-administration may occur. Used as experimental oxidizing agent	110
Water-soluble vitamin-K analogues	2-methyl-14-napthoquinone	Premature infants at risk	110, 120, 121
Sodium or potassium chlorate	ClO_4^-	Weed killer: DIC† as well as HB haemolysis and methaemoglobinaemia (see text)	108, 133, 134
Naphthalene, naphthol	Naphthol	Moth balls, nappy sterilizer. May be absorbed through skin by infants	197
Wax crayons (red and red-orange)	p-nitroaniline	Not permitted now in most countries. Children and infants at risk	198
Well-water nitrates	Nitrite	Methaemoglobinaemia in infants. Haemolysis may occur	77, 130–132
Nitrobenzene derivatives Nitrotoluene TNT	Aromatic nitro groups	Industrial workers, especially in munitions, at risk	136, 137
Arsine	Arsine	Metal smelters at risk	109, 110, 138

* HB: Heinz body.
† DIC: Disseminated intravascular coagulation.

lase deficiency and may also increase susceptibility to oxidation.

Variability in drug metabolism

In many instances, it is a drug metabolite and not the drug itself which causes oxidation. Only certain sulphonamides cause methaemoglobinaemia and haemolysis and most of these only after metabolism in the liver. Variation in drug metabolism is detected in a number of ways, of which measurement of acetylating ability is the best known. Dapsone is an oxidant drug which is acetylated, and slow acetylators demonstrate a greater degree of toxicity from this agent [83]. The oxidant metabolite of phenacetin is 2-OH phenetidin which in most people forms only a small fraction of the breakdown products. Some subjects who develop chronic intravascular haemolysis or renal damage have a much higher proportion of phenacetin metabolized by this route [84].

Additional sources of oxidant stress

The effect of more than one source of oxidation is additive. Hence a potent second source of oxidation will reduce the dose of drug needed to cause oxidant lysis. Superoxide and hydrogen peroxide are produced during killing of bacteria by neutrophils and macrophages [85]. Infections by themselves may cause haemolysis in sufferers from favism [86]. *In vitro*, a combination of hydrogen peroxide and aspirin will produce lysis where neither will alone [87], and *in-vitro* stimulation of superoxide and H_2O_2 formation by polymorphs will cause lysis of red cells [88, 89].

Variability in absorption

Individual variation in absorption rates for drugs occurs but more important are differences produced by disease and by alteration in bowel flora. Partial gastrectomy in adults and physiological changes in the gastric acidity of neonates may encourage overgrowth of bowel flora which in turn may increase oxidant metabolites. Dapsone and salazopyrin (salazosulphapyridine) are both oxidant drugs which are used in conditions affecting the gastro-intestinal tract. Major changes in their absorption, and hence toxicity, may occur in the same individual at different times.

Variability in excretion

Renal and hepatic function mainly determine the rate of disappearance of oxidant drugs or metabolites. Renal failure particularly may aggravate toxic effects of oxidant drugs.

Structural abnormalities of haemoglobin
(see Chapter 8)

Probably all unstable haemoglobins are more suscep-

tible to oxidant stress than normal Hb A [90, 91]. Patients with Hb Zürich, $\beta63$ (E7) His→Arg develop acute intravascular haemolysis with Heinz-body formation on exposure to oxidant drugs, though there is little haemolysis in the absence of oxidant stress [92, 93]. The haemoglobins M are also unstable in the presence of excess oxidant stress [83]. Hb Hashoran, $\alpha47$ (CD5) Asp→His is unstable in the presence of sulphonamides. The chemical structure of the oxidizing compound, as well as its oxidation–reduction potential, is probably important in these interactions with abnormal haemoglobins [94]. Increased lysis has been described in patients with Hb H disease treated with hexachloropanoxylol for *Clonorchis sinensis* [95] and Hb F has been considered to increase sensitivity to other oxidative drugs [96].

Susceptibility of neonates and infants to oxidant stress
(see Chapters 3 and 7)

Methaemoglobinaemia with or without haemolysis in response to oxidant stress is more common in neonates than in older children or adults. There are many reasons for this. Neonates have a relative deficiency of reducing power because of lowered activity in the enzymes NADH-methaemoglobin reductase, catalase and glutathione peroxidase [97]. Vitamin-E deficiency is only likely to occur in neonates and bottle-fed infants and may by itself produce haemolytic anaemia [98]. The role of vitamin E in preventing haemolysis has been reviewed by Gross [99]. The relative immaturity of the liver in neonates delays metabolism of oxidizing drugs [100]. Hb F is more readily oxidized by nitrites than Hb A [101] and infants are more likely to be exposed to toxic levels of nitrites than adults (see below). The small size of infants means that toxic levels of oxidizing substances are more readily obtained anyway than in adults. Some substances which particularly cause oxidant problems in this group are listed in Table 12.1.

SYNDROMES OF OXIDATIVE DRUG DAMAGE

Methaemoglobinaemia with minimal or no haemolysis

This syndrome occurs mainly in neonates exposed to excessive concentrations of nitrates in well water contaminated with fertilizer [102]. Spinach [103] and carrot juice [104] may also accumulate nitrates. Bacteria within the gut convert nitrates to nitrites which actually produce the methaemoglobin [102]. Nitrite itself is a food preservative and may occasionally cause poisoning and gross cyanosis from methaemoglobinaemia [105]. In adults, overgrowth of bacterial flora have been considered a cause of cyanosis—'enterogenous cyanosis' [3]. In this syndrome, the cyanosis is the most striking feature and must be distinguished from cyanosis produced by respiratory or cardiac disease and from methaemoglobin-reductase deficiency. In severe cases, death may result from failure to deliver oxygen. This mainly occurs in infants but bizarre abuse of nitrite drugs, amylnitrite and butylnitrite, has been fatal in adults [106, 107].

Methaemoglobinaemia with chronic intravascular haemolysis

This condition occurs mainly in patients with normal reducing systems exposed to oxidant substances in fast toxic doses over a prolonged period. It was first recognized in aniline-dye workers who were called 'blue boys' because of the cyanosis. The haemolysis is intravascular and haemosiderin is found in the urine. The red cells in the peripheral blood have a characteristic range of shapes including helmet cells, cells with the haemoglobin contracted away from the membrane, and cells which look as if a piece has been torn from them [3] (Fig. 12.3). These changes are probably the result of Heinz-body formation though Heinz bodies may not be prominent in the peripheral blood if the splenic function is normal. Dapsone, salazopyrine and phenacetin are the prime causes of this type of oxidative damage. If splenic function is reduced, as it often is in dermatitis herpetiformis for which dapsone is given, Heinz bodies will be prominent (Fig. 12.4).

The condition is normally harmless and adjustment of therapy is not often required.

Acute intravascular haemolysis with or without methaemoglobinaemia

This syndrome occurs mainly in patients with a deficient reducing system. Favism is the most dramatic form of this syndrome. Methaemoglobinaemia is not prominent and is rarely clinically significant. Despite massive haemoglobinaemia and haemoglobinuria, renal failure is rare unless anaemia and/or hypotension occur at the same time. Treatment is straightforward—high fluid intake to maintain glomerular filtration rate and transfusion if necessary.

Acute intravascular haemolysis, methaemoglobinaemia, intravascular coagulation and renal failure

This is a severe and frequently fatal syndrome caused by ingestion or infusion of very strong oxidizing substances such as chlorate [108] or arsine [109]. Here the blood film presents an amazing appearance, the plasma the same colour as the whole blood, gross methaemoglobinaemia, fragmented and ghost cells together with evidence of intravascular coagulation [108]. The fall of haemoglobin is very rapid and, once it starts, renal failure is usual. Treatment is difficult and relies mainly on exchange transfusion and supportive measures for renal failure. Methylene blue should not be used to reverse methaemoglobinaemia in this condition.

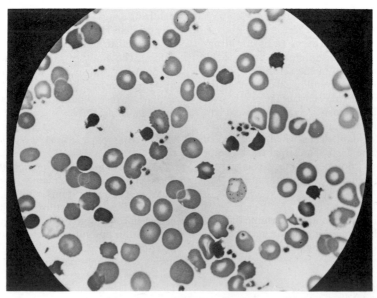

Fig. 12.3. Intravascular haemolysis induced by phenacetin. Cells with contracted haemoglobin and also some basophilic stippling indicating marked marrow stress (× 7300).

DRUGS WHICH CAUSE HAEMOLYSIS

Several reviews list the drugs and chemicals which have been implicated in oxidative haemolysis [77, 110–112], and it is not proposed to give an exhaustive list here. Some of the more commonly involved chemicals which cause haemolysis in normal individuals are listed in Table 12.1 (p. 520).

PHENACETIN

Phenacetin (acetophenotidin) used to be widely used as an analgesic but its toxicity, particularly nephrotoxicity, led to its withdrawal from the market in most countries. Its haematological toxicity was carefully observed and the mechanisms by which various syndromes of haemolytic anaemia were produced apply to many other currently used drugs. Chronic haemolytic anaemia with methaemoglobinaemia, sulphaemoglobinaemia and Heinz bodies, together with the appearance of a chemically induced haemolysis in the blood film, may be produced by continued doses of phenacetin as low as 1–2 g/day. Shahidi and his colleagues

observed that some patients who developed haemolysis on low doses had an excess of the metabolite 2-hydroxyphenetidin in the urine and that this compound caused oxidation of red cells *in vitro* [113, 114]. In patients with an intact spleen, the degree of Heinz-body formation may be very low but it has also been shown that most normal patients who have had splenectomy show some degree of Heinz-body production [115]. Methaemoglobinaemia is variable. Several patients with phenacetin-induced haemolysis have had previous gastrectomies but the aetiological role of this is uncertain [116]. As the dangers of phenacetin become accepted and the drug becomes less readily available, the incidence of haemolysis from this cause is likely to fall, but where the drug is freely available it is probably the commonest cause of chemically induced haemolysis.

Salazopyrin

Salazopyrin (salicylazosulphapyridine) is used in the treatment of ulcerative colitis and other inflammations of the bowel; that it may cause Heinz-body haemolytic anaemia was recognized early [117] (see Chapter 33).

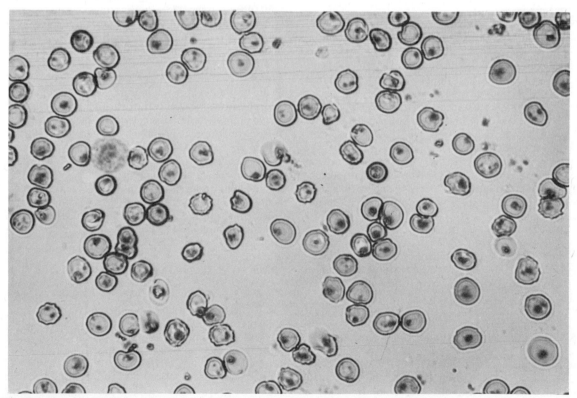

Fig. 12.4. Heinz bodies in the red cells from a patient treated with Dapsone. Vital staining with methyl violet (× 630).

The amount of haemolysis is related to the concentration of the metabolite sulphapyridine [118] which is higher in slow acetylators than in fast acetylators [119]. The number of cells containing Heinz bodies may be very high and these may appear before anaemia becomes apparent, so that the blood of patients receiving salazopyrin should be screened regularly for their presence. It seems probable that all people who receive salazopyrin for a sufficient length of time will develop Heinz-body anaemia.

Vitamin-K analogues
The water-soluble analogues for vitamin K may cause severe haemolytic anaemia if given in large doses to neonatal infants, especially premature infants [111, 120, 121]. Haemolysis is produced by 5–10 mg Synkavit daily [110], and a dose not exceeding 1 mg/day is recommended for premature infants [111]. This dose should be used with caution for infants with Mediterranean G6PD deficiency [91]. The effect of water-soluble vitamin-K analogues in rats is increased by vitamin-E deficiency [122], and it may be that deficiency of this vitamin plays a part in the Synkavit-induced haemolysis of the newborn.

Sulphones
The sulphone derivatives used in the treatment of leprosy and dermatitis herpetiformis, dapsone, sulfoxone and promin, induce Heinz-body haemolytic anaemia if given in sufficient dosage to normal patients [123–126]. As little as 50 mg/day for one month has produced haemolytic anaemia [123]. As with salazopyrin, Heinz bodies appear before anaemia develops and routine examination of the blood for Heinz bodies is necessary in patients receiving these drugs. Rasbridge & Scott [127–129] have demonstrated that the 4–hydroxylamino derivatives of dapsone have an oxidant effect on red cells *in vitro*, and that red cells from patients treated with dapsone show evidence of oxidative stress, both in their metabolism and membrane function.

Nitrites and nitrates
In infancy, absorption of nitrites from the ingestion of fertilizer-contaminated well water [130–132], spinach [103] or carrot juice [104] may cause severe cyanosis due to methaemoglobinaemia.

Chlorate poisoning
Sodium chlorate is a readily available weedkiller and several cases of accidental or deliberate self-administration have been recorded [108, 133]. In Germany, cases of accidental administration of intravenous sodium chlorate instead of sodium chloride have been recorded [134]. Following ingestion of the weedkiller

there is a delay of some hours before cyanosis develops due to the formation of methaemoglobin under the very strong oxidizing action of the chlorate ion. Massive intravascular haemolysis occurs and in addition to the oxidative damage to the red cells there is also damage to the kidney and other organs by DIC and oliguria usually develops. Treatment is by haemodialysis with exchange transfusion if necessary and an adequate fluid intake should be maintained as far as possible. Ascorbic acid may be used to combat methaemoglobinaemia, but under no circumstances should methylene blue be used since this converts the chlorate to hypochlorite, an even more toxic compound [135]. Heparin has been used to counteract DIC with apparent success [108].

Industrial chemicals
Chemically induced haemolysis with methaemoglobinaemia is a recognized hazard of several industrial processes in which aniline or nitrobenzene derivatives are used [136, 137]. Arsine (AsH_3) is a gas which may be produced accidentally in the smelting of various metal ores. Inhalation leads to a severe haemolytic anaemia with haemoglobinuria, frequently followed by anuria and death [110], though renal failure does not always occur [138]. Prevention is clearly the most important consideration, but if poisoning does occur treatment is directed towards correction of the anaemia and management of renal failure.

Lead
The harmful effects of chronic lead poisoning on porphyrin synthesis and the formation of haemoglobin have been often described [139] and the similarities to acute, intermittent porphyria pointed out [140] (see Chapters 17 and 18).

Haemolysis is a minor feature of chronic poisoning with only slight shortening of the $^{51}Cr\ T_{\frac{1}{2}}$ [139, 141]. Acute high-dosage lead poisoning, on the other hand, may produce rapid intravascular haemolysis with distortion and indentation of the red cells typical of chemically induced haemolysis [142].

THE MECHANICAL HAEMOLYTIC ANAEMIAS

Red cells may be destroyed within the vascular system when there is an obstruction to the normal laminar flow of the blood. Conditions which lead to intravascular destruction of red cells in this way arise in two circumstances: first when there are abnormalities of the vessel walls associated with turbulent flow in high pressure systems such as the left ventricle and the major blood vessels, and secondly when there are abnormalities of small blood vessels which impede, but do not prevent, the circulation of red cells. The first situation occurs most commonly following the insertion of artificial valves and patches at open-heart surgery and may be referred to as 'cardiac haemolysis' [143]. The second situation arises in a variety of disorders which collectively have been called the 'microangiopathic haemolytic anaemias' [144].

Mechanical haemolysis from any cause produces characteristic changes in the peripheral blood, with distortion and fragmentation of the red cells (Fig. 16.3, p. 635) [110, 145] the proportion of fragmented red cells usually being related to the severity of haemolysis [110].

CARDIAC HAEMOLYSIS
The realization that the repair of cardiac lesions with artificial materials may produce haemolytic anaemia came soon after the development of these techniques [146, 147]. The first detailed study of this type of haemolytic anaemia [148] established the typical pattern of fragmentation and failure of transfused red cells to survive better than those of the patient [110, 143]. Mechanical cardiac haemolytic anaemia is particularly likely to develop in situations where there is a foreign surface in association with high-pressure, turbulent blood flow, but severe mechanical haemolytic anaemia may follow surgical procedures on the heart where foreign material is not used. Furthermore the typical fragmented red cells may not be obvious. Such exceptions to the normal pattern have led to delay in diagnosis. Haemolytic anaemia, with negative Coombs test, following cardiac surgery is virtually always due to a malfunctioning of the surgical procedure.

Patch repairs
Mechanical haemolysis, following repair of atrial and ventricular septal defects with teflon patches has been described [148–150]. At re-operation the patch has been found to be bare of epithelium [110, 148] or associated with a regurgitant jet of blood through the mitral valve [149] and correction of these defects has led to a decrease in haemolysis.

Aortic-valve replacement
Haemolysis has been described following replacement of diseased aortic valves with most types of prosthesis [146, 147–155] except homografts [156]. In most cases, re-operation or post-mortem examination revealed abnormalities of the prosthesis or its attachment which would be expected to produce turbulent or regurgitant flow. The amount of haemolysis is influenced in part by the type of prosthetic material used [157] and in part by deformation of the prosthesis itself [152, 158].

The incidence of haemolytic anaemia following the insertion of a prosthetic aortic valve varies between five and 12% in different series [153, 159, 160]. A shortening of the red-cell lifespan without production of anaemia has been reported in up to 60% of patients with prosthetic valves [157, 160], though in other surgical centres there has been a much lower incidence of subclinical haemolysis in patients with normally functioning prosthetic devices [159].

Mitral-valve replacement and repair
Haemolysis following replacement of the mitral valve with a prosthetic device is less common than with aortic-valve replacement [159, 161, 162]. Regurgitation of blood through the prosthesis has been described in all reported cases where haemolytic anaemia occurred [148, 163]. A particularly severe form of cardiac haemolysis occurs when there is regurgitation of blood along a track at the side of the repair [164] or prosthesis [165], i.e. with a paravalvular or paraprosthetic leak. Possibly, the suture material which usually provides the site of the track or the inflammatory response in the wall provides the foreign surface. The severity of the haemolysis in these paraprosthetic leaks is much greater than the haemodynamic effects, which may be trivial. Haemolytic anaemia in double or triple valve replacements is common and may occur to a marked extent even with xenografts [166].

Cardiac haemolysis in unoperated patients
Anaemia due to mechanical destruction of red cells is uncommon in patients with aortic stenosis and regurgitation, even in severely affected patients [167], though there may be subclinical haemolysis. Intravascular haemolysis with anaemia has been described in a patient with calcification of both the mitral and aortic valves producing severe haemodynamic disease [168], and in a patient with a mitral valve further damaged by valvotomy [169]. In the latter case, replacement of the valve with a well-functioning prosthetic device cured the anaemia.

Haematological features of cardiac haemolytic anaemia
The typical finding in cardiac haemolysis is the presence of contracted and distorted red cells and intravascular haemolysis with raised plasma haemoglobin, low serum haptoglobins, raised heat-stable LDH, slight to moderate hyperbilirubinaemia, haemosiderinuria and, occasionally, frank haemoglobinuria. The degree of haemolysis is variable, but may be very severe [150]. The platelet count may fall in the immediate post-operative period, but usually rises again to normal levels though persistent thrombocytopenia has been recorded [110]. Iron deficiency may

result from the haemosiderinuria [148] and some improvement in haemoglobin level and cardiac state may be derived from iron therapy [149, 170–172]. The survival of red cells from both the patient and isologous donors is reduced but there is no excess uptake of ^{51}Cr by the spleen except in rare cases [150]. Splenectomy is of no value in the correction of haemolysis in this condition [154]. As emphasized above, atypical presentations with minimal or absent fragmentation may lead to difficulties in diagnosis.

Pathogenesis of cardiac haemolytic anaemia
The available evidence suggests that red cells are destroyed at the site of the prosthetic material and that destruction is brought about by contact of the red cells in a turbulent jet of blood with a roughened or foreign surface. Attempts have been made to measure *in vitro* the shearing stress necessary to disrupt red cells and to relate this to forces present *in vivo* [148]. However, these experiments were carried out in a cone vis-cometer so that the red cells came into contact with a foreign surface, and it has been shown that a much higher shear stress is necessary to disrupt red cells in the absence of such contact [173, 174].

That haemodynamic factors are important in the production of mechanical haemolysis is suggested by the finding that cardiac haemolysis is increased by exercise [175, 176]. The influence of changes in the wall of the vessels in the production of haemolysis is less well characterized. Fibrin deposition is common on artificial valves and the possible importance of calci-fied excrescences [168] has been mentioned but it is not clear whether the presence of an artificial material in the circulation causes mechanical destruction by itself. Thus, it has been found that insertion of a lucite tube in the aorta of dogs does not cause haemolysis, whereas a ball of this material does [177]. It seems, therefore, that turbulence is a necessary cofactor in the production of mechanical haemolysis, but whether this is because laminar flow is interrupted and so red cells are brought into contact with the foreign surface, or whether it is the shear stress induced in the turbulence which is important, is not clear.

MICROANGIOPATHIC HAEMOLYTIC ANAEMIA
The term 'microangiopathic haemolytic anaemia' [178] was adapted by Brain *et al.* [144] to provide a unifying concept for the aetiology of intravascular haemolysis with fragmentation and destruction of red cells secondary to disease of small vessels. Microangio-pathic haemolytic anaemia develops in a variety of disorders with different pathological changes in small vessels, of which microthrombi in capillaries and arteries, fibrinoid necrosis, necrotizing arteritis and invasion of capillary walls by carcinoma deposits are the most commonly reported features. Many of the disorders which produce microangiopathic haemolytic anaemia are associated with DIC and it has been suggested that the microthrombi are the cause of haemolysis, the red cells being fragmented by passage through the fibrin clots [179, 180]. Diffuse intravascu-lar coagulation (DIC) is considered in detail in Chapter 29 and will not be described here except where it is relevant to the diseases discussed. Some of the disorders which may be associated with microangio-pathic haemolytic anaemia are listed in Table 12.2. The relationship between this form of anaemia and car-cinoma is considered in Chapter 33.

The haemolytic uraemic syndromes
(see also Chapter 29)
'Haemolytic uraemic syndrome' was the name used by Gasser and his colleagues to describe the association of acute haemolytic anaemia with renal failure in five children [181]. Since then many cases have been reported from different parts of the world [182–190] and there have been several reviews of the subject [191–193]. It is clear that the association of intravascu-lar haemolytic anaemia with fragmentation of red-cell type, thrombocytopenia due to platelet destruction and a microangiopathy of the renal vessels is a syndrome which may arise in a number of different circumstances and with different associated disorders [193]. Three broad subdivisions of the syndrome may be recognized, the haemolytic uraemic syndrome of childhood, haemolytic uraemic syndrome associated with infections and thrombotic thrombocytopenic purpura of adults. The distinctions between these syndromes may be artificial and represent differences in host response as well as aetiology.

The haemostatic aspects of this condition are con-sidered in greater detail in Chapter 29.

Haemolytic uraemic syndrome of childhood

Clinical features. Both sexes are affected equally. Infants are more likely to develop the disease than older children though the peak incidence varies in different parts of the world being younger in the Argentine (at about 13 months [199]) than in Califor-nia (where the mean age is about four-and-a-half years [187]). There is a seasonal incidence in the syndrome, being most common in the northern hemisphere in the late spring and early summer months [187, 188]. There are reports of more than one member of a family being affected [200, 201], and of several cases occurring at the same time and place [188, 199, 202].

The syndrome usually develops following a febrile illness accompanied by diarrhoea and vomiting in previously healthy children. The gastro-intestinal

Table 12.2. Causes of microangiopathic haemolytic anaemias

Disease	Microangiopathy	References
Haemolytic/uraemic syndrome of childhood	Endothelial-cell swelling; microthrombi in renal arterioles	3, 183, 191, 192, 212, 213
Haemolytic/uraemic syndrome with bacterial infection	Endotoxaemia; microthrombi in renal arterioles	3, 225–227
Thrombotic thrombocytopenic purpura	Widespread microthrombi; microaneurysm and arteriolitis	3, 229, 235
Renal cortical necrosis	Necrotizing arteritis	144
Acute glomerular nephritis		144
Pre-eclampsia	Fibrinoid necrosis	144, 258, 259
Vasculitis	Arteritis	
Polyarteritis nodosa		144
Wegener's granulomatosis		260
Systemic lupus		144
Homograft rejection	Microthrombi in transplanted organ	261, 262
Meningococcal septicaemia	Endotoxaemia; diffuse intravascular coagulation	3
Carcinomatosis	Abnormal tumour vessels. Intravascular coagulation in tumour or disseminated	263–266
Primary pulmonary hypertension	Abnormal vasculature	267, 268
Cavernous haemangiona	Local vascular or thrombosis	269
Purpura fulminans	Microthrombi in skin (?)	270
Interferon induction by polycarbocylate	Intravascular coagulation	271

symptoms may be severe with bloody diarrhoea and marked abdominal pain [189, 190, 203] requiring differentiation from other acute abdominal emergencies. Occasionally, vaccination or inoculation of infants or children has preceded the syndrome [204–206]. Evidence of acute intravascular haemolysis with rapidly developing anaemia develops during, or shortly after, the prodromal illness and may precede or accompany the onset of oliguria. Further episodes of fever and abdominal pain may develop during haemolysis. Purpura and bleeding may occur during the acute phase. Drowsiness, convulsions and coma may develop in the absence of raised blood pressure or high fever [189] and suggest that there may sometimes be direct damage to the central nervous system. Death may occur during the acute phase from uncontrollable anaemia, haemorrhage or hypertension. About a third of the patients do not develop oliguria, about a third have up to 10 days' and the final third 10 days' to four weeks' oliguria. Nearly all patients without oliguria recover completely without treatment other than supportive care. In general, the longer the period of oliguria the more likely is chronic renal failure [187]. There is some evidence that patients with a well-defined gastro-enterological prodrome have a better

prognosis than those without [189]. The overall death rate of haemolytic anaemia syndrome varies from about two per cent [189, 206], with most series having about 10% [190]. In most patients who recover, haemolysis and thrombocytopenia cease after five to seven days. Widespread differences in prognosis between southern [182, 184, 199] and northern hemispheres [187–189] may reflect differences in aetiology, health care and support in these areas.

Laboratory investigations. The peripheral-blood film shows fragmentation and distortion of red cells, with occasional spherocytes and polychromasia [3]. In contrast to the cardiac haemolytic anaemias, thrombocytopenia is usual, though not invariable. Leucocytosis is common, sometimes with a marked shift to the left. There is evidence of intravascular haemolysis, with raised plasma haemoglobin, methaemalbumin, low serum haptoglobins and moderate hyperbilirubinaemia. The bone marrow is hyperplastic, with a predominance of red-cell precursors and sections of the aspirated marrow may show the presence of hyaline thrombi in capillaries [207]. Tests for clotting function have produced conflicting results in different series. Occasional reports of low fibrinogen levels

[208], reduced levels of other clotting factors [209], and the presence of fibrin degradation products (FDP) suggests that intravascular coagulation with consumption of clotting factors occurs in the haemolytic uraemic syndrome. Other authors have been unable to obtain evidence for consumption coagulopathy but have found increased fibrinolysis and a 'hypercoagulable state' with raised fibrinogen and shortened PTTK [210]. It may be that the different results obtained depend upon the time when the investigations were carried out in relation to the onset of the disease [211], the depletion in clotting factors being found early in the disorder.

Proteinuria is a constant finding in the haemolytic uraemic syndrome [182, 206], and hypoalbuminaemia may result. The blood urea is elevated and the rate of rise may be very rapid in the early stages [191]. There may be frank haemoglobinuria and the urine may also contain cells and granular casts. Haemosiderinuria is not usually present unless the condition becomes chronic. Virological studies, particularly a search for viruses of the herpes group, is an important part of the investigation of these patients.

Pathology. Renal biopsy and post-mortem studies from the acute phase of the disease reveal that the endothelial cells of the glomerular capillaries are swollen and separated from the basement membrane by accumulation of material in the subendothelial space [212]. In the renal arterioles, endothelial swelling is accompanied by deposition of hyaline material which stains as fibrin, with fluorescent stains indicating the presence of microthrombi [183, 212, 213]. Immunofluorescent studies with specific antiglobulin or anticomplement sera have consistently failed to demonstrate any evidence for immune-complex involvement in this syndrome.

The occurrence of microthrombi in the bone marrow has already been mentioned [207], and microthrombi may be found in other organs, including brain, lungs, liver, intestine and lymph nodes. When the vascular lesions are widespread, the distinction between haemolytic uraemic syndrome and thrombotic thrombocytopenia purpura becomes very blurred (see p. 529) and until the factors which determine the distribution of vascular lesions are known, the classification in individual cases is likely to remain arbitrary.

Aetiology and pathogenesis. The cause of the haemolytic uraemic syndrome is unknown. The development of the syndrome after a febrile illness, its occurrence in small epidemics and its seasonal variation suggest that an infective agent is responsible [188]. Viruses [199, 213, 214], rickettsiae [215] and bacteria [216] have each

been detected in individual cases and have been thought to be important in the pathogenesis of the syndrome but in the majority of patients no organism can be found [206]. The delay between the febrile illness and the onset of haemolysis has led some authors to doubt whether there is a direct cause-and-effect relationship between the presumed infection and the onset of haemolysis, and to suggest that the immune response to the infecting organism triggers intravascular coagulation [191, 199]. As mentioned above, it has been consistently impossible to detect any evidence for immune-complex deposition in the microangiopathic lesions of these patients. It seems most likely that there is primary damage to the vascular endothelium of the renal arterioles and glomerular capillaries with secondary deposition of fibrin, particularly in the former. The opposite view, that the swelling of the endothelial cells is secondary to the phagocytosis of fibrin products, has also been advocated [217]. Prevention of intravascular coagulation in experimentally induced nephritis prevents the endothelial changes without affecting the basic renal lesion.

Treatment. The mainstay of treatment is supportive care, transfusion, hydration, control of hypertension and, if necessary, dialysis. Most patients will recover with these measures alone. Extensive haemorrhage is one indication for more active intervention. The finding of microthrombi in the renal lesions and the assumption that intravascular coagulation was responsible for the low platelet count led to the use of heparin for treatment [209, 216, 218–220], but the effects of this treatment are difficult to assess and side-effects in the form of further haemorrhage are common. If heparin is used because of clear-cut evidence of intravascular coagulation from coagulation studies, then massive replacement therapy with platelets and clotting factors should be given at the same time. Fibrinolytic therapy has been given to patients with oliguria and the patients recovered. Streptokinase and heparin were used [221]. The risks of haemorrhage with this treatment are high. An alternative theory of pathogenesis suggests that endothelial damage leads to increased sticking of platelets, possibly because of a failure of prostacyclin production [222]. Success has been claimed for the management of haemolytic uraemic syndrome with inhibitors of platelet function [223] and with synthetic prostacyclin [222]. The numbers so treated are very small and no conclusion may yet be drawn from these observations. Antiplatelet drugs seem to be less toxic. Corticosteroids and ACTH do not seem to have an important part in the therapy of the disease and may theoretically make it worse [224].

Haemolytic uraemic syndrome with bacterial infections
A number of bacterial infections are associated with intravascular haemolysis with fragmentation of red cells, consumption coagulopathy with thrombocytopenia and a microangiopathy of the renal vessels. Some of these infections (e.g. meningococcal septicaemia) are particularly well identified, others are less well known and may be readily confused with a haemolytic uraemia syndrome in children or with thrombotic thrombocytopenia in adults. The tragedy is that many of these infections are amenable to treatment. Shigellosis is one bacterial infection in which the haemolytic uraemic syndrome develops commonly. In Bangladesh, about 10% of children with shigellosis developed acute haemolytic anaemia, leukaemoid reaction, thrombocytopenia and oliguria [225]. Those who had this syndrome had evidence for endotoxaemia. Other bacterial infections include *H. influenzae* [226] and the pneumococci [227].

Thrombotic thrombocytopenic purpura
Thrombotic thrombocytopenic purpura, Moschowitz's syndrome [228], is another disorder associated with the presence of microthrombi in small blood vessels. Since the aetiology is unknown the diagnosis is made only on clinical and pathological grounds so that overlap with other disorders of widespread microangiopathy, particularly the haemolytic uraemic syndrome [191] and systemic lupus erythromatosus [229], is inevitable.

The haemostatic aspects of this disorder are considered further in Chapter 29.

Clinical features. The features of thrombotic thrombocytopenic purpura are pyrexia, anaemia, thrombocytopenic purpura, neurological disorders and renal abnormalities [230]. Both sexes are affected equally and the disease may occur at any age, with a peak incidence in young adults. The onset is often sudden, with the development of a high fever and signs of neurological damage. The commonest neurological disorders are convulsions, coma, transient or permanent paralysis and bizarre psychiatric disturbances, sometimes with hallucinations [231]. Purpura may accompany or follow the neurological signs and sometimes there is more serious bleeding. Anaemia is not usually severe, although occasionally there is evidence of dramatic haemolysis with haemoglobinuria. The acute illness runs a fluctuating course of days or weeks but the outcome is usually fatal. Rarely, there may be a series of acute episodes with apparent recovery in between [229, 232–234]. Recurrent thrombotic thrombocytopenic purpura is considered below. In some patients, there is a short period of malaise and fever before the abrupt onset of neurological signs.

More rarely, there is a history of recurrent neurological or psychiatric disturbance going back for months or years before onset of the acute disease. Purpura and haemolysis have not been recorded during these episodes.

Laboratory investigations. The main haematological features in this disorder are a mild to severe haemolytic anaemia with fragmentation and contraction of cells and thrombocytopenia (Fig. 12.5). Haemolysis may be

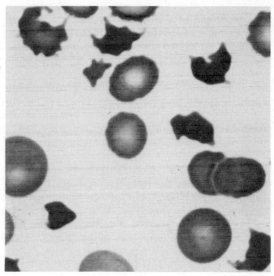

Fig. 12.5. Microangiopathic haemolytic anaemia from a patient with thrombotic thrombocytopenic purpura. Fragments, contracted cells and helmet cells are present (× 1200).

minimal and occasionally patients are seen with clinical and pathological evidence of thrombotic thrombocytopenic purpura in which there is no anaemia, and fragmentation of red cells is not present. The bone marrow is active and cellular, and megakaryocytes, which are present in increased numbers, have normal morphology. A neutrophil leucocytosis is usual but not inevitable. Coagulation studies may show evidence for a consumption coagulopathy with reduced fibrinogen levels, low factor VIII and the presence of fibrin/fibrinogen degradation products (see Chapters 25 and 29).

Some degree of proteinuria is almost inevitable and there is usually further evidence of renal damage in the form of raised blood urea or reduced creatinine clearance. The results of other investigations depend upon which organs are involved in the thrombotic process, liver, pancreas, heart, lungs and brain being variably affected. In a proportion of cases there may be some of the features of systemic lupus erythomatosus, including a false positive WR [229].

Pathology. The typical manifestations of thrombotic thrombocytopenic purpura include the presence of hyaline material within the lumen of small vessels, endothelial proliferation and aneurysmal dilatation of small vessels [229, 235].

The first two manifestations are the features of intravascular coagulation whereas the aneurysmal dilatation of small vessels is also seen in polyarteritis nodosa and systemic lupus erythromatosus. In addition, some patients with thrombotic thrombocytopenic purpura have other pathological changes more commonly associated with systemic lupus erythromatosus, including periarteriolar fibrosis in the spleen, thickening of the glomerular basement membrane with the appearance of 'wire loops', atypical verrucous endocarditis and positive LE preparations [229]. It is clear that until specific diagnostic criteria or the aetiologies of these disorders are defined, there is bound to be some confusion in classifying a proportion of cases.

A recent upsurge of interest in thrombotic thrombocytopenic purpura has followed the suggestion, supported by some laboratory evidence, that an increase in platelet adhesion caused by a failure of prostacyclin production by the vascular endothelium is the basic lesion in the disease. It has been shown that in some of these patients there is a lack of a factor in the serum which allows the renewal of prostacyclin production as measured by rabbit aorta *in vitro* [236]. Furthermore, in some patients with TTP there is a decrease in excretion of the metabolite of prostacyclin 6-keto-$PGF_{1\alpha}$ [237]. The recovery of a few patients following plasma infusion has also supported the idea that there may be a lack of specific factor in these patients (see below). In a proportion of patients immunological factors including circulating immune complexes may play a part in pathogenesis [238, 239], though laboratory or histological evidence for this is poor.

Treatment. The treatment of thrombotic thrombocytopenic purpura has undergone a great change with the idea that prostacyclin production may be defective in some of these patients and the empirical observation that plasmapheresis and exchange transfusion may be of benefit in some cases. The general applicability of both the theory and the therapy has yet to be proven. The mainstay of treatment remains support for the patient. Recovery may occur even after several weeks of coma and renal failure, even when specific treatment has apparently failed. Heparin, given to prevent intravascular coagulation, was the first such specific

treatment and some apparent success was achieved in a few patients [229, 231, 240], but the eventual outcome was still often fatal [229]. The spleen has been removed from many patients with this disease, often with apparent remission [229, 241–243]. The theoretical basis for splenectomy is shaky and includes suggestions that the spleen may be a major source of destruction of platelets which have been damaged by the process of adhesion [244]. If splenectomy is contemplated for these patients it should be carried out early in the disease before such organs as the heart have suffered damage from microthrombi. Antiplatelet-aggregating drugs—dipyridamole, aspirin and dextran 70—have all been tried in TTP with apparent success [245, 246]. However, many reports on the efficacy of other forms of therapy question the value of these agents. The most recent approaches to treatment concern the removal from, or addition to, the blood of various undefined substances which may be important in the pathogenesis of TTP [230, 247]. Historically, exchange transfusion was found to benefit some patients before such theories developed [248]. Plasmapheresis is simpler and quicker to perform and appears to work in the same proportion of patients as exchange transfusion [249] though the latter is still advocated [250]. Plasmapheresis has proved useful in some cases of TTP associated with pregnancy [251], though in others it was only partially successful [252]. In 1977, it was noted that fresh frozen plasma (FFP) by itself might lead to remission in TTP without the use of plasma exchange [253], possibly by replacing a missing prostacyclin-stimulating factor [236]. Such a factor would, of course, also be replaced by the blood products used in plasmapheresis. In at least one responder, 6-keto-$PGF_{1\alpha}$ levels rose after remission was obtained using plasmapheresis [254]. However, in another patient plasmapheresis was only partially successful whereas plasma infusion led to remission [252]. Whatever the pathogenesis eventually turns out to be, and it seems most likely that there will be several mechanisms leading to the same end point, some plan of therapy is necessary for each case. At present, it would seem reasonable to start patients on antiplatelet drugs once infection or another underlying cause has been excluded. If there is no response, plasma exchange should be initiated within 24 hours. If the patient responds to treatment with a rise in platelet count and cessation of haemolysis, plasma infusion alone may be given with reintroduction of plasma exchange if infusion alone fails [255]. If there is no response to either of these measures within a period of three to five days, splenectomy should be undertaken. Throughout, total support is necessary. With these measures the mortality of TTP will be of the order of 30%.

Thrombotic thrombocytopenic purpura in pregnancy
Thrombotic thrombocytopenic purpura seems to occur more commonly during pregnancy or in the post-partum period and probably accounts for the excess of young women affected by this disease [256]. In most cases, the dramatic problems presented by the disease lead to termination of pregnancy either deliberately or through miscarriage. Removal of the fetus does not always lead to remission, however, and there are occasional reports of successful therapy to both mother and fetus by plasmapheresis or plasma infusions [252, 257]. Clearly, this is a reasonable first approach to therapy in this circumstance.

Chronic relapsing and familial TTP
There appears to be a subgroup of patients with a TTP-like illness who have a long history of relapse going back to childhood, again with a syndrome like haemolytic uraemic syndrome when young [229]. Some of these patients respond repeatedly and predictably to plasma infusion [234] and it may be that these patients have abnormal prostacyclin control mechanisms.

MARCH HAEMOGLOBINURIA
Haemoglobinuria following exercise has been recognized as a syndrome since the nineteenth century, but the studies of Davidson [272] first established that the haemolysis in this disorder is mechanical in origin.

Clinical features
Young men are much more commonly diagnosed as having the condition than females, though the phenomenon probably goes unremarked in numerous individuals [273]. Typically, there is haemoglobinuria lasting a few hours after running or walking on a hard surface. Occasionally the haemoglobinuria is accompanied by nausea, abdominal cramps and aching legs [273].

Splenomegaly has been reported in a few cases and there may be slight icterus, but physical examination usually reveals no abnormality apart from lumbar lordosis—the significance of which is obscure [273].

Laboratory findings
Apart from transient haemoglobinuria and haemoglobinaemia following exercise, there are no diagnostic findings. Anaemia is uncommon and the peripheral-blood film does not show evidence of microangiopathic haemolysis.

Pathogenesis
Intravascular haemolysis is produced by mechanical trauma resulting from a hard surface and the gait of the patient [272]. There is no definite evidence for an intrinsic defect in the red cells of these patients (see Chapter 10, p. 470 for recent studies of the red-cell membrane in this disorder). Modification of running shoes or training on grass as opposed to road surfaces prevents symptoms recurring in affected athletes.

ACQUIRED DISORDERS OF THE RED-CELL MEMBRANE

The mature red cell has no capacity for the *de-novo* synthesis of lipids or proteins. Once the cell is formed, therefore, there is no way in which lost membrane can be replaced. There is, however, a dynamic equilibrium of some membrane lipids with those in the plasma and some chemical rearrangement is possible in the mature red-cell membrane [274]. The lipid content of the plasma, and particularly the free cholesterol and phospholipids, may therefore affect the lipid content of the cell and may alter the shape and osmotic fragility of the cell by affecting changes in its surface-area to volume ratio [274]. In addition to such passive changes, red-cell lipids are subject to autoxidation of unsaturated fatty-acid side chains which alter the properties of the cell so that haemolysis may develop [275]. Haemolytic anaemia may develop in a variety of diseases as a result of these changes, particularly through changes in red-cell deformability [276] (see also Chapter 10).

In addition to such 'passive' alterations of the red-cell membrane, changes may occur at the stem-cell level which produce specific defects of the red-cell membrane, as in paroxysmal nocturnal haemoglobinuria (PNH) or non-specific defects associated with disordered maturation of the cell as in megaloblastic anaemias or leukaemias. Since the non-specific changes do not produce significant haemolysis they will not be considered here except with reference to PNH.

LIPID DISORDERS

Liver disease
Some haemolysis probably occurs in a majority of patients with acute hepatitis, cirrhosis [3] and even Gilbert's disease [3, 277] though the patients are not necessarily anaemic (see also Chapter 33).

Target cells are usually present in chronic biliary obstruction and mild to moderate hepatocellular disease and their development may be related to the presence of bile salts and an increase in plasma lipids with a fall in the free cholesterol to lecithin ratio [278]. These patients do not usually have haemolytic anaemia but in severe hepatocellular disease and alcoholic cirrhosis, spur cells or acanthocytes (Fig. 12.6) may

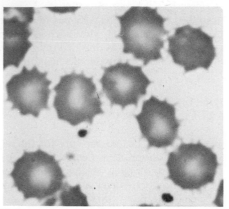

Fig. 12.6. Acanthocytosis in an unsplenectomized patient in coma resulting from rapidly fatal infectious hepatitis (× 1200).

appear and haemolysis may be marked [280]. In these patients the cholesterol/lecithin ratio in the plasma is increased [274]. When the normal cells are transfused they develop the abnormal shape and are destroyed as rapidly as autologous cells, whereas the reverse occurs when the acanthocytes are transfused into a normal circulation [278].

Zieve's syndrome [281] refers to acute abdominal pain and haemolytic anaemia occurring in chronic alcoholics with cirrhosis, hyperlipidaemia and jaundice. The unusual feature in these cases is the presence of spherocytes and increased osmotic fragility, whereas the usual change in liver disease is a decrease in osmotic fragility. However, it is unlikely that there is any special feature in these patients which leads to a decreased red-cell survival, other than passive changes in the red-cell membrane.

A-β-lipoproteinaemia (hereditary acanthocytosis)
In this rare inherited deficiency of low-density lipoproteins there is a low plasma cholesterol and phospholipid with an increase in the ratio of cholesterol to phospholipid [274]. Acanthocytes appear, probably reflecting the lipid changes [282]. In addition to haemolytic anaemia, the condition is characterized by retinitis pigmentosa, steatorrhoea, ataxia and mental deficiency (see also Chapter 33).

Vitamin-E deficiency
Vitamin E (tocopherol) is a powerful anti-oxidant which is necessary for the prevention of autoxidation of unsaturated fatty-acid side chains in the red-cell membrane [275, 283]. Haemolysis with acanthocytosis and thrombocytosis in infants has been attributed to vitamin-E deficiency and a diet rich in polyunsaturated fats [284, 285]. The hydrogen peroxide haemolysis test, which was originally devised as a test for tocopherol deficiency, is not specific for this condition [260, 286], but is a useful screening test in infants with acanthocytosis and haemolysis to detect excessive sensitivity to oxidant stress.

HAEMOPHAGOCYTIC SYNDROME
Excessive phagocytosis of haemopoietic cells and mature blood cells by bone-marrow histiocytes may occur in a number of infections, especially virus infections [287]. Pancytopenia with varying evidence of haemolysis is usually present. The disease is most common in immunodepressed patients with lymphoid malignancies or after renal transplantation, but may occur without underlying disease, particularly in children [287]. The difficulty is to distinguish this disease from histiocytic medullary reticulo-endotheliosis, a malignant condition [287, 288]. An intensive search for possible viral agents should be carried out, particularly for herpes-group viruses. Management is supportive with withdrawal of immunosuppressive agents if possible.

PAROXYSMAL NOCTURNAL HAEMOGLOBINURIA
Paroxysmal nocturnal haemoglobinuria (PNH) in its characteristic form with haemoglobinuria occurring after sleep is a dramatic haemolytic disease which, not surprisingly, was recognized relatively early in the history of modern haematology and which has acquired many synonyms and eponyms of which 'Machiafava–Micheli' syndrome is perhaps the most well known [289]. The condition results from an acquired disorder of the red-cell membrane which renders the cell especially liable to lysis by activated complement components. There are many extensive reviews of this interesting, though rare, disorder [110, 290–292].

The red cell in PNH
The red cell in PNH shows a number of abnormalities, of which increased sensitivity to lysis by complement is the most specific and which forms the basis for the diagnostic tests for this disorder. In addition, there are non-specific abnormalities of the red-cell membrane which may be seen in other disordered states of red-cell production, namely an increase in I- and i-antigen expression and a reduction in membrane acetylcholinesterase activity. The basic defect in PNH remains unknown, though some of the pathogenetic pathways are becoming a little more clear.

In 1973, Rosse demonstrated that there were at least two different types of red cell, apart from remaining normal cells, which could be demonstrated in patients with PNH, and that various combinations of cells might be found in different patients—whom he divided into four groups [293]. The different types of cells were identified by their sensitivity to lysis by complement activated via the classical pathway by standard anti-I preparations. Type-I cells were normal, type II (PNH-II) were three to five times more sensitive and type III (PNH-III) were 10–15 times more sensitive to complement lysis than type I. The sensitivity was calculated from the number of activated C3 molecules which caused lysis [293]. The four groups of patients were identified by those having:

1 normal and PNH-III cells;
2 PNH-II and PNH-III cells;
3 normal, PNH-II and PNH-III; and
4 PNH-II cells only.

Patients have since been found who have PNH-III cells only [294]. Both PNH-II and PNH-III cells bind C1 and C4 normally but bind excessive amounts of C3 for a given amount of C4 binding [295]. However, only PNH-III cells are extra-sensitive to lysis for a given amount of C3 binding. This appears to be due to an increased susceptibility to bind the late products of the activated complement pathway, C8/C9 [294]. The additional binding sites present on the PNH-III cell after the attachment of the complement components C5, 6, 7 (PNH-III C567) appear to be rendered labile by the addition of C8 so that, at least *in vitro*, simultaneous addition of C8 and C9 produces greater lysis than when C8 is added before C9 [296]. These findings indicate an abnormality in the binding of activated C3 to the PNH membrane which is common to all PNH cells. The proportion of PNH-II and PNH-III cells does not remain constant throughout an individual patient's illness [295]. An increase in PNH-III cells leads to an increase in intravascular haemolysis. On the other hand, after a period of increased haemolysis PNH-III cells are reduced in number. An increase in red-cell production, for example following correction of iron deficiency, leads to an increase in PNH-III cells and increased intravascular haemolysis. Finally, disappearance of PNH-III cells during the course of the illness is associated with clinical recovery despite persistence of PNH-II cells.

The origin of the PNH cell has been the subject of much debate. One theory suggested that it might arise from a somatic mutation which produced a stable clone of cells having a relative survival value over normal cells in the milieu of the marrow [297]. The clonal nature of the PNH cells is supported by the finding that in a patient heterozygous for two types of G6PD, only one type was present in complement-sensitive cells [298]. This is not incompatible with the observation that there are at least two types of PNH cell, since the additional sensitivity of PNH-III cells to lysis by C8/C9 could be a post-translational modification of PNH-II cell membrane.

Neutrophils and platelets in PNH

That the defect in PNH affects more primitive precursor cells than those of the red-cell series alone is demonstrated by the finding that both platelets and neutrophils are abnormal in this disease and that the defect is similar or identical to that seen in the red cell. Increased complement-mediated lysis of PNH platelets and granulocytes occurs *in vitro* [299]. In the PNH platelet, following activation of complement, more C3 is bound to PNH platelets than normal, C3 binding to PNH platelets (but not to normal platelets) is followed by serotonin release, which does not require further activation of the later steps of the complement pathway [300]. This phenomenon may account for the increased risk of venous thrombosis in PNH (see below). There is an abnormal neutrophil population which has an increased sensitivity to complement-mediated lysis following the binding of anti-I antibody [301].

Clinical features

PNH exists in two major forms with all variations in between. On the one hand there is classical PNH in which intravascular haemolysis and morning haemoglobinuria dominate the clinical picture, while on the other hand there are patients who have a failure of bone-marrow function in whom a clinically unimportant PNH defect is detected in the laboratory. The association of PNH with bone-marrow disorders accounts for the delay in diagnosis so often encountered in this disease [110].

Classical PNH may present at any age with a peak incidence at 25–35 years. It is rare in childhood and females are slightly more frequently affected than males. The condition may present in a number of ways. Symptoms produced by intravascular haemolysis are perhaps commonest, including the effects of anaemia and the passage of red urine, particularly when awakening from sleep. The association of haemoglobinuria with sleep is striking and has lead to a number of explanations for this phenomenon. The original suggestions included the effects of a fall in pH due to retention of CO_2 during sleep, but artificial elevation of the arterial CO_2 does not lead to increased lysis. Another possibility is that during sleep there is a relative inefficiency of the reticulo-endothelial cells, particularly in the liver, and that clearing of endotoxin from the gut may be impaired, hence leading to an increased activation of complement. The typical pattern is not observed in all patients and the haemolysis may be variable both in time and amount. The loss of iron in the urine, both as free haemoglobin and as haemosiderin, often produces iron deficiency in these patients, which increases the anaemia and symptoms of general weakness.

The other major presentation of PNH is caused by its most dangerous complication, i.e. venous thrombosis. Recurrent attacks of abdominal pain are thought to be due to thrombosis of venules of the mesenteric veins. Micro-infarcts may occur. Larger areas of infarction and obstruction have been described [302] with surgical intervention required. Hepatic-vein thrombosis (Budd–Chiari syndrome) is another severe thrombotic complication of PNH [303], which may be the mode of presentation. The onset is usually abrupt with pain over the swiftly enlarging liver, the development of ascites and, usually, death either from haemorrhage from oesophageal or gastric varices, or from liver failure. Hepatic-vein thrombosis may occur during the course of PNH and sometimes a more chronic piecemeal thrombosis of hepatic veins occurs. Femoral- and iliac-vein thromboses are also seen in PNH and may lead to pulmonary emboli.

It has been found that incubation of PNH red cells *in vitro* releases a powerful thromboplastin into the serum [304], a finding in many types of haemolytic anaemia and not peculiar to PNH [276]. It seems more likely that the intrinsic defect of the platelets in PNH is the major contributory factor [300]. Whatever the mechanism may be, it is important to remember that venous thrombosis may occur in PNH even in the presence of a reduced platelet count.

Paroxysmal nocturnal haemoglobinuria and disorders of the bone marrow

The commonest association of PNH is with hypoplasia of the bone marrow [292, 305]. The depression of bone-marrow function may precede the appearance of PNH cells by many years or the PNH clone may be present from the start. Frequently, the PNH cells seem to form only a small proportion of the remaining red cells and their presence is clinically unimportant. Occasionally, the reverse is true and PNH with a marked haemolytic component may follow apparent recovery from aplastic anaemia. The PNH clone may be transient, lasting only a few weeks or months and sometimes the disappearance of the PNH clone heralds the development of acute leukaemia.

Myeloproliferative disorders may also be associated with PNH. Typical myelosclerosis and PNH have been described together [306] as have the associations of PNH with Philadelphia-chromosome-negative chronic myelogenous leukaemia [307–309] and erythremic myelosis [310]. Occasionally, the PNH syndrome may terminate in acute myeloid or myelomonocytic leukaemia [292]. In all these associations the temporal relationship between PNH and the marrow disorder is unpredictable, but the most common sequence is the presence of PNH with a major haemolytic component for a variable period of time, followed by disappearance of the PNH clone as the more malignant disorder develops.

Physical signs

There are usually few clinical signs. Pallor and jaundice depend upon the degree of anaemia and haemolysis. The urine is usually positive for blood or haemoglobin testing, but red cells are absent from the sample. The spleen is not usually enlarged—its presence should raise the possibility of an underlying myeloproliferative disorder. Occasionally, the spleen enlarges in patients who have received many transfusions and may contribute to increased transfusion requirements and pancytopenia. An enlarged liver, particularly if tender, raises the possibility of hepatic-vein thrombosis. Purpura and infections develop as bone-marrow failure increases. The smooth tongue and koilonychia of iron deficiency may be present.

Laboratory findings

The peripheral-blood film. This does not show any characteristic features. Normally there is anisocytosis with some macrocytosis. Poikilocytosis with tear-drop formation may be conspicuous. There is a variable reticulocytosis which is frequently less than would be expected for the degree of anaemia [305]. Platelet counts of less than $100 \times 10^9/l$ are common and there may be neutropenia, the neutrophils having a low neutrophil-alkaline-phosphatase (NAP) score. A rise in the NAP score in a patient wih PNH may presage the development of frank aplastic anaemia. More marked deviations of the peripheral blood from normal will be seen when PNH is associated with other bone-marrow disorders. Haemoglobinaemia may be obvious to the naked eye and methaemalbumin can normally be detected spectroscopically; the Schumm's test is positive and haptoglobulins are absent. The level of Hb F may be increased but the fetal Hb is uniformly distributed between normal and PNH cells [311].

The bone marrow. In PNH this is very variable. In the typical haemolytic case the marrow is very active, even when there is a degree of pancytopenia. In the less typical cases the marrow will show the features of the underlying marrow disease.

The urine. This may show free haemoglobin, typically after sleep. During quiescent phases of the disorder and in mild cases no free haemoglobin may be seen, but haemosiderinuria is a constant finding. The daily loss of iron may be sufficient to cause iron deficiency. Despite the haemoglobinuria and haemosiderosis of the kidney, impairment of renal function is rare, although a few cases have been reported.

Diagnosis

The diagnosis depends upon the demonstration of increased sensitivity of the patient's red cells to lysis by complement. The acidified serum lysis test (Ham's test) [312] is the definitive investigation. It depends for its effect on the activation of the alternative pathway of complement activation by increased hydrogen ion concentration. The diagnosis of PNH is made if the test is positive using both an ABO-compatible fresh serum as a source of complement and the patient's own serum, and is negative when the serum is heated to 56°C to destroy complement. The acidified serum lysis test is also positive in congenital dyserythropoietic anaemia (CDA-type II) but only when compatible serum is used, not the patient's own serum [313] (see p. 533). The sugar-water lysis test [314] is a sensitive test for PNH but is less specific [315]. The same is true of the cold-antibody lysis test [316] where small amounts of lysis may occur in cases of bone-marrow failure without PNH. This test and the thrombin test of Crosby [317] both owe their action to the activation of complement by the classical pathway.

Treatment and prognosis

The mainstay of treatment for PNH is transfusion of red blood cells. Patients may require transfusions over many years and febrile hypersensitivity reactions are common. For this reason, washed [319] or sedimented red cells [290], freed from white cells and platelets, should be used. Since iron is lost as haemosiderin in urine, iron overload from transfusion is uncommon; indeed iron deficiency may become a problem [110]. Intramuscular iron has been thought to provoke haemolysis [293, 320]. It has been recommended that oral iron should be given to patients with PNH [290, 321] who have iron deficiency demonstrated by changes in the peripheral blood and absence of iron stores in the bone marrow.

Androgens have been recommended in an attempt to expand the red-cell-precursor pool in PNH [322]. The degree of marrow depression may determine whether androgens should be used, but if therapy is started it should be continued in high dosage for at least three months before the response can be assessed [297, 323]. There may be some increase in haemolysis following the introduction of androgens [321], but some rise in total haemoglobin usually occurs [290].

Bone-marrow transplantation from an allogeneic, HLA-compatible sibling donor has been successful in the treatment of PNH associated with an aplastic marrow [324]. More remarkably, two cases of PNH have been described where infusion of syngeneic marrow from identical twins without prior immuno-suppression treatment has resulted in a cure of the pancytopenia and disappearance of the PNH clone [325, 326]. The relationship of the disappearance of the PNH clone to marrow infusion is not entirely clear however. In the Seattle case [325] the acidified-serum lysis test apparently remained positive for about a year post marrow infusion and in the UCLA case [326] the Ham's test had become negative prior to infusion, though the sugar-water lysis test was still positive.

The prognosis in PNH is variable. Venous thrombosis is the major serious complication and some patients may die as a result of pulmonary embolism or hepatic venous thrombosis. In a few patients, the PNH defect may disappear and the patient recovers completely. Where PNH develops in association with aplasia or myeloproliferative disease, the prognosis is dependent upon the bone-marrow defect rather than haemolysis. The overall median survival in PNH is about 10 years [323]. It is not yet clear whether the use of anticoagulants is really effective in reducing the number of thromboembolic incidents but they certainly should be given to any patient with PNH who has had such a thrombotic episode and in whom there is a marked degree of haemolysis, and should be continued whilst the PNH is active.

REFERENCES

1 LAYRISSE M., LINARES J. & ROCHE M. (1965) Excess haemolysis in subjects with severe iron deficiency anemia associated and non-associated with hookworm infection. *Blood*, **25**, 73.

2 LEWIS S.M. (1962) Red cell abnormalities and haemolysis in aplastic anaemia. *British Journal of Haematology*, **8**, 322.

3 DACIE J.V. (1967) *The Haemolytic Anaemias, Congenital and Acquired.* III. Secondary or symptomatic haemolytic anaemias. Churchill, London.

4 WORLD HEALTH ORGANIZATION (1967) Third report on the world health situation. *Official Record 155*, WHO, Geneva.

5 BRUCE-CHWATT L.J. (1969) Malaria eradication at the crossroads. *Bulletin of the New York Academy of Medicine*, **45**, 999.

6 EDITORIAL (1979) Malaria, the phoenix with drug resistance. *Lancet*, **i**, 1328.

7 HUESTIS D.W. (1970) Correspondence. *Transfusion*, **13**, 253.

8 SHUTE P.G. & MARYON M. (1969) Imported malaria in the United Kingdom. *British Medical Journal*, **ii**, 781.

9 BICK R.L. & ANHALT J.E. (1971) Malaria transmission among narcotic addicts. A report of 10 cases and review of the literature. *California Medicine*, **115**, 51.

10 ECKSTEIN A. & NIXON W.C.W. (1946) Congenital malaria. *British Medical Journal*, **i**, 432.

11 MCQUAY R.M., SILBERMAN S., MUDRIK P. & KEITH L.E. (1967) Congenital malaria in Chicago. A case

report and a review of published reports (USA). *American Journal of Tropical Medicine and Hygiene*, **16**, 258.

12 ESSAN G.J.F. (1975) Haematological aspects of malaria. *Clinics in Haematology*, **4**, 247.

13 CANFIELD C.J. (1969) Renal and hematologic complications of falciparum malaria in Vietnam. *Bulletin of the New York Academy of Medicine*, **45**, 1043.

14 CONRAD M.E. (1971) Hematologic manifestations of parasitic infections. *Seminars in Hematology*, **8**, 267.

15 SRICHAIKUL T., PANIKTUR N. & JEUMTRAKUL P. (1967) Bone marrow changes in human malaria. *Annals of Tropical Medicine and Parasitology*, **61**, 40.

16 SRICHAIKUL T. (1969) Ferrokinetic studies and erythropoiesis in malaria. *Archives of Internal Medicine*, **124**, 623.

17 LUZZATTO L., USANEA E.A. & REDDY S. (1969) Glucose-6-phosphate dehydrogenase deficiency red cells: resistance to infection by malarial parasites. *Science*, **164**, 839.

18 PASVOL E., WEATHERALL D.J., WILSON R.J.M., SMITH D.H. & GILLES H.M. (1976) Fetal haemoglobin and malaria. *Lancet*, **i**, 1269.

19 STONE W.J., HANCHETT J.E. & KNEPSHIELD J.H. (1972) Acute renal insufficiency due to falciparum malaria: review of 42 cases. *Archives of Internal Medicine*, **129**, 620.

20 PUNYAGUPTA S., SRICHAIKUL T., NITIYANANT P.O. & PETCHCLAI B. (1974) Acute pulmonary insufficiency in falciparum malaria: summary of 12 cases with evidence of DIC. *American Journal of Tropical Medicine and Hygiene*, **23**, 551.

21 GYR K., SPECK B., RITZ R., CORNU P. & BUCKNER C.D. (1974) Zerebrale Malaria Tropica mit Schwarzwasserfieber: ein aktuelles diaprostischer und therapeutisches Problem. *Schweizerische Medizinische Wochenschrift*, **104**, 1628.

22 NIELSEN R.L., KOHLER R.B., CHIN W., McCARTHY L.S. & LUFT F.C. (1979) The use of exchange transfusions: a potentially useful adjunct in the treatment of fulminant falciparum malaria. *American Journal of Medical Science*, **277**, 325.

23 FREEKEN J. & CREMER-COTTE Th.M. (1978) Haemostatic defect in non-immune patients with falciparum malaria: no evidence of DIC. *British Medical Journal*, **ii**, 533.

24 STUART J. (1978) Intravascular coagulation in falciparum malaria. *British Medical Journal*, **ii**, 774.

25 RONCORONI A.J. & MARTINO O.A. (1975) Therapeutic use of exchange transfusion in malaria. *American Journal of Tropical Medicine and Hygiene*, **28**, 440.

26 JACKSON R.C. & WOODRUFF A.W. (1962) The artificial kidney in malaria and blackwater fever. *British Medical Journal*, **i**, 1367.

27 ROSEN S., HANO J.E., INMAN M.M., GILLILAND P.F. & BARY K.G. (1968) The kidney in blackwater fever. *American Journal of Clinical Pathology*, **49**, 358.

28 DUKES D.C., SEALEY B.J. & FORBES J.I. (1968) Oliguric renal failure in blackwater fever. *American Journal of Medicine*, **45**, 899.

29 LEADING ARTICLE (1969) More Blackwater fever. *British Medical Journal*, **iii**, 372.

30 QUINN T.C. & WYLER D.J. (1979) Intravascular clearance of parasitised erythrocytes in rodent malaria. *Journal of Clinical Investigation*, **63**, 1187.

31 BALCERZAK S.P., ARNOLD J.D. & MARTIN D.C. (1972) Anatomy of red cell damage by *P. falciparum* in man. *Blood*, **40**, 98.

32 BROWN I.N. (1969) Immunological aspects of malarial infection. *Advances in Immunology*, **11**, 138.

33 NEVA F.A., SHULMAN N.R., SHEAGDEN J.N. & CANFORD C.J. (1970) Malaria: host defence mechanisms and complications. *Annals of Internal Medicine*, **43**, 255.

34 ROSENBERG E.B., STRICKLAN G.T., YANE S.L. & WHALE W.G.E. (1973) IgM antibodies to red cells and autoimmune anaemia in patients with malaria. *American Journal of Tropical Medicine and Hygiene*, **22**, 146.

35 BEALE B.J., CORMACK J.D. & OLDREY T.B.N. (1972) Thrombocytopenia in malaria with immunoglobulin (IgM) changes. *British Medical Journal*, **i**, 345.

36 BUTLER T., TONG M.T., FLETCHER J.N., DOSTALEK R.J. & ROBBINS T.O. (1973) Blood coagulation studies in *Plasmodium falciparum* malaria. *American Journal of Medical Science*, **265**, 63.

37 GREENWOOD B.M., STRATTON D & WILLIAMSON W.A. (1978) A study of the role of immunological factors in the pathogenesis of acute malaria. *Transactions of the Royal Society of Tropical Medicine and Hygiene*, **72**, 378.

38 BEET E.A. (1946) Sickle cell diseases in Balovale District of Northern Rhodesia. *East African Medical Journal*, **23**, 75.

39 BRIAN P. (1952) The sickle cell trait. Its clinical significance. *South African Medical Journal*, **26**, 925.

40 ALLISON A.C. (1954) Protection afforded by sickle cell trait against subtertian malarial infection. *British Medical Journal*, **i**, 290.

41 RAPER A.B. (1949) Incidence of sicklaemia. *East African Medical Journal*, **26**, 281.

42 GILLES H.M., FLETCHER K.A., HENDRICKSE R.G., LINDER R., REDDY S. & ALLAN N. (1967) Glucose-6-phosphate-dehydrogenase deficiency, sickling and malaria in African children in South Western Nigeria. *Lancet*, **i**, 138.

43 HENDRICKSE R.G., HASAN A.H., OLUMIDE L.O. & AKINKUNMI A. (1971) Malaria in early childhood. An investigation of 500 seriously ill children in whom a clinical diagnosis of malaria was made on admission to the children emergency room at University College, Ibadan. *Annals of Tropical Medicine and Parasitology*, **65**, 1.

44 LUZZATTO L., NWACHUKU-JARRETT E.S. & REDDY S. (1970) Increased sickling of parasitized erythrocytes as a mechanism of resistance against malaria in the sickle-cell trait. *Lancet*, **i**, 319.

45 MACKEY J.P. & VIVARELLI F. (1954) Sickle cell anaemia. *British Medical Journal*, **i**, 276.

46 RUTH E.F., FRIEDMAN M., UEDA Y., TELLEZ I., TRAGER W. & NAGEL R.L. (1978) Sickling rates of human AS red cells infected *in vitro* with *Plasmodium falciparum* malaria. *Science*, **202**, 650.

47 PASVOL G., WEATHERALL D.J. & WILSON R.J.M. (1977) Cellular mechanism for the protective effect of Hb S against *P. falciparum* malaria. *Nature (London)*, **274**, 701.

48 FRIEDMAN M.J. (1978) Erythrocytic mechanism of

sickler resistance to malaria. *Proceedings of the National Academy of Sciences, USA*, **75**, 1994.

49 KRUATRACHUE M., SADUDEE N. & SRIRIPANICH B. (1970) Glucose-6-phosphate-dehydrogenase deficiency and malaria in Thailand: the comparison of parasite densities and mortality rates. *Annals of Tropical Medicine and Parasitology*, **64**, 11.

50 BIENZLE U., AYENI O., LUCAS A.O. & LUZZATTO L. (1972) Glucose-6-phosphate dehydrogenase and malaria. *Lancet*, **i**, 10.

51 THEAKSTON R.D.G., FLETCHER K.A. & MOORE G.A. (1976) Glucose-6-phosphate and 6-phosphogluconate dehydrogenase activities in human erythrocytes infected with *P. falciparum. Annals of Tropical Medicine and Hygiene*, **70**, 125.

52 ECKMAN J.R. & EATON J.W. (1979) Dependence of plasmodial glutathione metabolism on the host cell. *Nature (London)*, **278**, 754.

53 EATON J.W., ECKMAN J.R., BERGER E. & JACOB H.S. (1976) Suppression of malaria infection by oxidant sensitive host erythrocytes. *Nature (London)*, **264**, 758.

54 HOMEWOOD C.A., WARHURST D.C., PETERS W. & BAGGELEY V.C. (1972) Malaria—lysosomes, pH and the action of chloroquine. *Nature (London)*, **235**, 50.

55 KRICK J.A. & REMINGTON J.S. (1978) Toxoplasmosis in the adult—an overview. *New England Journal of Medicine*, **298**, 550.

56 VIETZKE W.M., GELDERMAN A.H., GRIMLEY P.M. & VALSAMIS M.P. (1968) Toxoplasmosis complicating malignancy. *Cancer*, **21**, 816.

57 COHEN S.N. (1970) Toxoplasmosis in patients receiving immunosuppressive therapy. *Journal of the American Medical Association*, **211**, 657.

58 RUSKIN J. & REMINGTON J.S. (1976) Toxoplasmosis in the compromised host. *Annals of Internal Medicine*, **84**, 193.

59 HOPPELLER A., BRISOU J., PAPILLON A. & CHARDAC R. (1960) Anémie hémolytique aiguë chez un enfant de cinq ans: découverte de toxoplasmes dans le sang circulant. *Archives françaises de Pédiatrie*, **17**, 1250.

60 KALDERON A.E., KIKKAWA Y. & BERNSTEIN J. (1954) Chronic toxoplasmosis associated with severe hemolytic anemia: case report and electron microscopic studies. *Archives of Internal Medicine*, **114**, 95.

61 MILLER L.H., REIFSNYDER D.N. & MARTINEZ S.A. (1971) Late onset of disease in congenital toxoplasmosis. *Clinical Pediatrics* (Philadelphia), **10**, 78.

62 ARNAUD J.P., GRISELL C., COUVREUR J. & DESMONTS G. (1975) Anomalies hématologiques et immunologiques de la toxoplasmose congénitale. *Nouvelle Revue française d'Hématologie*, **15**, 496.

63 CORRIGAN J.J., WALKER L.R. & MAY N. (1968) Changes in the blood coagulation system associated with septicemia. *New England Journal of Medicine*, **279**, 851.

64 McGEHEE W.G., RAPAPORT S.I. & HJORT P.F. (1967) Intravascular coagulation in fulminant meningococcemia. *Annals of Internal Medicine*, **67**, 250.

65 WINKELSTEIN A., SONGSTER C.L., CARAS T.S., BERMAN H.H. & WEST W.L. (1969) Fulminant meningococcemia and disseminated intravascular coagulation. *Archives of Internal Medicine*, **124**, 55.

66 MAHN H.E. & DANTUONO L.M. (1955) Post abortal septico-toxemia due to *Clostridium welchii*: seventy-five cases from the Maternity Hospital, Santiago, Chile. *American Journal of Obstetrics and Gynecology*, **70**, 604.

67 HADLEY G.C. & EKROTH R.D. (1954) Spherocytosis as a manifestation of postabortal *Clostridium welchii* infections. *American Journal of Obstetrics and Gynecology*, **67**, 691.

68 TAY S. & PANKO E. (1971) Structural and compositional changes in the red cell membrane during *Clostridium welchii* infection. *British Journal of Haematology*, **21**, 173.

69 EATON C.J. & PETERSON E.P. (1971) Diagnosis and acute management of patients with advanced clostridial sepsis complicating abortion. *American Journal of Obstetrics and Gynecology*, **109**, 1162.

70 RICKETTS W.E. (1949) Clinical manifestations of Carrion's disease. *Archives of Internal Medicine*, **84**, 751.

71 REYNAFARJE C. & RAMOS J. (1961) The hemolytic anemia of human bartonellosis. *Blood*, **17**, 562.

72 CUADRA M. & TAKANO J. (1969) Relationship of *Bartonella bacilliformis* to the red blood cell as revealed by electron microscopy. *Blood*, **33**, 708.

73 RICKETTS W.E. (1948) *Bartonella bacilliformis* fever (Oroya fever): a study of thirty cases. *Blood*, **3**, 1025.

74 SCHULTZ M.G. (1968) David Carrion's experiment. *New England Journal of Medicine*, **278**, 1323.

75 MERINO C. (1945) Penicillin therapy in human bartonellosis (Carrion's disease). *Journal of Laboratory and Clinical Medicine*, **30**, 1021.

76 EMERSON C.P., HAM T.H. & CASTLE W.B. (1941) Hemolytic action of certain organic oxidants derived from sulfanilamide, phenylhydrazine and hydroquinone. *Journal of Clinical Investigation*, **20**, 451.

77 GORDON-SMITH E.C. (1980) Drug-induced oxidative haemolysis. *Clinics in Haematology*, **9**, 557.

78 AMARE M., LAWSON B. & LARSEN W.E. (1972) Active extrusion of Heinz bodies in drug-induced haemolytic anaemia. *British Journal of Haematology*, **23**, 215.

79 KEITT A.S., SMITH T.W. & JANDL J.H. (1966) Red cell 'pseudomosaicism' in congenital methemoglobinemia. *New England Journal of Medicine*, **275**, 399.

80 GLADER B.E. (1976) Salicylate-induced injury of pyruvate kinase deficient erythrocyte. *New England Journal of Medicine*, **294**, 916.

81 WORATHUMRONG N. & GRIMES A.J. (1975) The effect of o-salicylate upon the pentose phosphate pathway activity in normal and G6PD-deficient red cells. *British Journal of Haematology*, **30**, 225.

82 GLADER B.E. (1976) Evaluation of hemolytic role of aspirin in glucose-6-phosphate-dehydrogenase deficiency. *Journal of Pediatrics*, **89**, 1027.

83 VESSEL E.S. (1972) Drug therapy: pharmacogenetics. *New England Journal Medicine*, **287**, 904.

84 SHAHIDI N.T. (1968) Acetophenetidin-induced methemoglobinemia. *Annals of the New York Academy of Sciences*, **151**, 822.

85 LEVINE P.H., WEINGER R.S., SIMON J., SCOON K.L. & KRINSKY N.I. (1976) Leukocyte–platelet interaction. Release of hydrogen peroxide by granulocytes as a modulator of platelet reactions. *Journal of Clinical Investigation*, **57**, 955.

86 BACHNER R.L., NATHAN D.G. & CASTLE W.B. (1971) Oxidant injury of caucasian glucose-6-phosphate-

dehydrogenase-deficient red cells by phagocytosing leukocytes during infection. *Journal of Clinical Investigation*, **50**, 2466.

87 STOCKMAN J.A., LUBIN B. & OSKI F.A. (1978) Aspirin induced hemolysis. The role of concomitant oxidant (H$_2$O$_2$) challenge. *Pediatric Research*, **12**, 927.

88 KELLOGG F.W. & FRIDOVICH I. (1979) Liposome oxidation and erythrocyte lysis by enzymatically generated superoxide and hydrogen peroxide. *Journal of Biological Chemistry*, **252**, 6721.

89 WEISS S.J. & LOBUGLIO A.F. (1980) An oxygen dependent mechanism of neutrophil mediated cytotoxicity. *Blood*, **55**, 1020.

90 WHITE J.M. (1974) The unstable haemoglobin disorders. *Clinics in Haematology*, **8**, 333.

91 ZINKMAN W.H. (1977) Unstable hemoglobins and the selective hemolytic action of sulfonamides. *Archives of Internal Medicine*, **137**, 1356.

92 FRICK P.G., HITZIG W.H. & BETKE K. (1962) Hemoglobin Zürich. A new hemoglobin anomaly associated with acute hemolytic episodes with inclusion bodies after sulfonamide therapy. *Blood*, **20**, 261.

93 RIEDLER R.F., ZINKMAN W.H. & HOLTZMAN N.A. (1965) Hemoglobin Zürich. Clinical, chemical and kinetic studies. *American Journal of Medicine*, **39**, 4.

94 HARVEY J.W. & KANEKO J.J. (1976) Oxidation of human and animal haemoglobins with ascorbate, acetylphenylhydrazine nitrite and hydrogen peroxide. *British Journal of Haematology*, **32**, 195.

95 LIU J., XUEYUNG Y., WENGAN T. & JITAO T. (1979) Hexachloroparaxylol induced haemolysis. *Chinese Medical Journal*, **92**, 286.

96 ROWLEY P.T. (1973) Drug sensitive hemoglobinopathies. *New England Journal of Medicine*, **288**, 374.

97 HERTZOG P. & FEIG S.A. (1978) Methaemoglobinaemia in the newborn infant. *Clinics in Haematology*, **7**, 75.

98 OSKI F.A. & BARNESS L.A. (1967) Vitamin E deficiency: a previously unrecognised cause of hemolytic anemia in premature infants. *Journal of Pediatrics*, **70**, 211.

99 GROSS S. (1976) Hemolytic anemia in premature infants: relationship to vitamin E, selenium, glutathione peroxidase and erythrocyte lipids. *Seminars in Hematology*, **13**, 187.

100 VEST M.F. & SALZBERG R. (1965) Conjugation reactions in the new born infant: the metabolism of para-aminobenzoic acid. *Archives of Diseases in Childhood*, **40**, 97.

101 MARTIN H. & HUISMAN T.H.J. (1963) Formation of ferrihaemoglobin of isolated human haemoglobin types by sodium nitrite. *Nature (London)*, **200**, 898.

102 MILLER L.W. (1971) Methemoglobinemia associated with well water. *Journal of the American Medical Association*, **216**, 1642.

103 HÖLSCHER P.M. & NATSCHKA J. (1964) Methämoglobinäemie bei jungen Sänglingen durch nitrathaltigen Spinat. *Deutsche Medizinische Wochenschrift*, **89**, 1751.

104 KEATING J.P., LELL M.E., STRAUSS A.W., ZARKOWSKY H. & SMITH G.E. (1973) Infantile methemoglobinemia caused by carrot juice. *New England Journal of Medicine*, **288**, 824.

105 SINGLEY T.L. (1962) Secondary methemoglobinemia due to adulteration of fish with sodium nitrite. *Annals of Internal Medicine*, **57**, 800.

106 HORNE M.K., WATERMAN M.R., SIMON L.M., BARRIOTT J.C. & FOERSTER E.H. (1979) Methemoglobinemia from sniffing butyl nitrite. *Annals of Internal Medicine*, **91**, 417.

107 SHESSER R., DIXON D., ALLEN Y., MITCHELL J. & EDELSTEIN S. (1980) Fatal methemoglobinemia from butyl nitrite ingestion. *Annals of Internal Medicine*, **92**, 131.

108 LEE D.B.N., BROWN D.L., BAKER L.R.I., LITTLEJOHNS D.W. & ROBERTS P.D. (1970) Haematological complication of chlorate poisoning. *British Medical Journal*, **ii**, 31.

109 PARISH G.G., GLASS R. & KIMBRUGH R. (1979) Acute arsine poisoning in two workers cleaning a clogged drain. *Archives of Environmental Health*, **34**, 224.

110 DACIE J.V. (1967) *The Haemolytic Anaemias. Congenital and Acquired*. IV. Drug-induced haemolytic anaemias, paroxysmal nocturnal haemoglobinuria, haemolytic disease of the newborn. Churchill, London.

111 GASSER C. (1959) Heinz-body anemia and related phenomena. *Journal of Pediatrics*, **54**, 673.

112 DE LEEUW N.K.M., SHAPIRO L. & LOWENSTEIN L. (1963) Drug induced hemolytic anemia. *Annals of Internal Medicine*, **58**, 592.

113 SHAHIDI N.T. (1968) Acetophenatidin-induced methemoglobinemia. *Annals of the New York Academy of Sciences*, **151**, 822.

114 SHAHIDI N.T. & NEMAIDAN A. (1969) Acetophenacetin-induced methemoglobinemia and its relation to the excretion of diazotizable amines. *Journal of Laboratory and Clinical Medicine*, **74**, 581.

115 SELWYN J.G. (1955) Heinz bodies in red cells after splenectomy and after phenacetin administration. *British Journal of Haematology*, **1**, 173.

116 HUTCHINSON H.E., JACKSON J.M. & CASSIDY P. (1962) Phenacetin induced haemolytic anaemia. *Lancet*, **ii**, 1022.

117 TRUELOVE S.C. (1958) Heinz body anaemia due to salicylazo-sulphapyridine. *Lancet*, **i**, 1039.

118 GOODACRE R.L., ALI M.A., VANDERLINDEN B., HAMILTON J.D., CASTELIR M. & SEATON T. (1978) Hemolytic anemia in patients receiving sulfasalazine. *Digestion*, **17**, 503.

119 DAS K.M. & STEMLIEB I. (1975) Salicylazosulfapyridine in inflammatory bowel disease. *American Journal of Digestive Diseases*, **20**, 971.

120 MEYER T.C. & ANGUS J. (1956) The effect of large doses of 'Synkavit' in the newborn. *Archives of Diseases in Childhood*, **31**, 212.

121 ALLISON A.C. (1955) Danger of vitamin K to the newborn. *Lancet*, **i**, 669.

122 HARLEY J.D. (1961) Acute haemolytic anaemia in Mediterranean children with glucose-6-phosphate-dehydrogenase-deficient erythrocytes. *Australasian Annals of Medicine*, **10**, 192.

123 SMITH R.S. & ALEXANDER S. (1959) Heinz body anaemia due to dapsone. *British Medical Journal*, **i**, 625.

124 DESFORGES J.F., THAYER W.W. & DAWSON J.P. (1959) Hemolytic anemia induced by sulfoxone therapy with investigation into the mechanisms of its production. *American Journal of Medicine*, **21**, 132.

125 PENGELLY C.D.R. (1963) Dapsone-induced haemolysis. *British Medical Journal*, **ii**, 262.

126 COOKE T.J.L. (1970) Dapsone poisoning. *Medical Journal of Australia*, **1**, 1158.

127 SCOTT G.L. & RASBRIDGE M.R. (1973) The *in vitro* action of dapsone and its derivatives on normal and G6PD-deficient red cells. *British Journal of Haematology*, **24**, 307.

128 RASBRIDGE M.R. & SCOTT G.L. (1973) The haemolytic action of dapsone: the effect on red-cell glycolysis. *British Journal of Haematology*, **24**, 169.

129 RASHBRIDGE M.R. & SCOTT G.L. (1973) The haemolytic action of dapsone: changes in the red cell membrane. *British Journal of Haematology*, **24**, 183.

130 COMY H.H. (1945) Cyanosis in infants due to ingestion of nitrates in well water. *Journal of the American Medical Association*, **129**, 112.

131 WALTON G. (1951) Survey of literature relating to infant methemoglobinemia due to nitrate contaminated well water. *American Journal of Public Health*, **41**, 986.

132 MILLER L.W. (1971) Methemoglobinemia associated with well water. *Journal of the American Medical Association*, **216**, 1642.

133 JACKSON R.C., ELDER W.J. & McDONNELL H. (1961) Sodium chlorate poisoning complicated by acute renal failure. *Lancet*, **ii**, 1381.

134 EHRHARDT L. (1952) Tödliche Natriumchloratvergiftung zweier Säuglinge. *Deutsche Zeitschrift für die gesamte gerichtliche Medizin*, **41**, 96.

135 MOESCHLIN S. (1964) *Poisoning*, 4th edn. Grune & Stratton, New York.

136 MINOT G.R. (1919) Blood examinations of trinitrotoluene workers. *Journal of Industrial Hygiene*, **1**, 307.

137 LUBASH G.D., BONSNES R.M., PHILLIPS R.E. & SHIELDS J.D. III (1964) Acute aniline poisoning treated by hemodialysis. *Archives of Internal Medicine*, **114**, 530.

138 JENKINS G.C., IND J.E., KAZATZIS G. & OWEN R. (1965) Arsine poisoning: massive haemolysis with minimal impairment of renal function. *British Medical Journal*, **ii**, 78.

139 WALDRON H.A. (1966) The anaemia of lead poisoning: a review. *British Journal of Industrial Medicine*, **23**, 83.

140 SMITH J. (1965) Relationship between lead poisoning and acute intermittent porphyria. *Quarterly Journal of Medicine*, **23**, 83.

141 GRIGGS R.C. & HARRIS J.W. (1958) Erythrocyte survival and heme synthesis in lead poisoning. *Clinical Research*, **6**, 188.

142 BROOKFIELD R.W. (1928) Blood changes occurring during the course of treatment of malignant disease by lead, with special reference to punctate basophilia and the platelets. *Journal of Pathology and Bacteriology*, **31**, 277.

143 MARSH G.W. & LEWIS S.M. (1969) Cardiac hemolytic anemia. *Seminars in Hematology*, **6**, 133.

144 BRAIN M.C., DACIE J.V. & HOURIHANE D.O'B. (1962) Microangiopathic haemolytic anaemia: the possible role of vascular lesions in pathogenesis. *British Journal of Haematology*, **8**, 358.

145 LOCK S.P. & DORMANDY K.M. (1961) Red cell fragmentation syndrome. A condition of multiple aetiology. *Lancet*, **i**, 1020.

146 ROSE J.C., HUENAGEL C.A., FREIS E.D., HARVEY W.P. & PARTENOPE E.A. (1954) The hemodynamic alterations produced by a plastic valvular prosthesis for severe aortic insufficiency in man. *Journal of Clinical Investigation*, **33**, 891.

147 SARNOFF S.J. & CASE R.B. (1955) Physiologic considerations relating to the Hugnagel operation with special reference to postoperative anemia. In: *Henry Ford Hospital International Symposium on Cardiology Surgery* (ed. Lam C.R.), p. 328. W. B. Saunders, Philadelphia.

148 REED W.A. & DUNN M. (1964) Fatal hemolysis following ball valve replacement of the aortic valve. *Journal of Thoracic and Cardiovascular Surgery*, **48**, 431.

150 WESTRING D.W. (1966) Aortic valve disease and hemolytic anemia. *Annals of Internal Medicine*, **65**, 20.

151 McGARVEY J.F.X., SPITZER S., SEGAL B.L. & BRODSKY I. (1966) Hemolytic anemia with aortic ball valve prosthesis. *Diseases of the Chest*, **50**, 203.

152 GARCIA M.C., CLAYRISSE A.M., ALEXANDER C.S., SAKO Y. & SWAIM W.R. (1968) Hemolytic anemia due to progressive enlargement of plastic ball component of aortic prosthesis. *Circulation*, **38**, 505.

153 MARSH G.W. (1964) Intravascular haemolytic anaemia after aortic valve replacement. *Lancet*, **ii**, 986.

154 VINER E.D. & FROST J.W. (1965) Hemolytic anemia due to a defective teflon aortic valve prosthesis. *Annals of Internal Medicine*, **63**, 295.

155 YEH T.J., ELLISON R.G. & WRIGHT C.S. (1965) Hemolytic anemia due to ruptured prosthetic aortic cusp. *Journal of Thoracic and Cardiovascular Surgery*, **49**, 693.

156 RABINOWITZ M.J., ROWE G.G., YOUNG W.P., AZEN E.A. & CLATANOFF D.V. (1970) Studies for hemolysis following aortic homograft surgery. *Journal of Thoracic and Cardiovascular Surgery*, **9**, 668.

157 CREXELLES C., AERICHIDE N., BONNY Y., LEPAGE G. & CAMPEAU L. (1972) Factors influencing hemolysis in valve prosthesis. *American Heart Journal*, **84**, 161.

158 EYSTER E. (1969) Traumatic hemolysis with hemoglobinuria due to ball variance. *Blood*, **33**, 391.

159 YACOUB M.H. & KEELING D.H. (1968) Chronic haemolysis following insertion of ball valve prosthesis. *British Heart Journal*, **30**, 1676.

160 BRODEUR M.T.H., SUTHERLAND D.W., KOLER R.D., STARR A., KIMSEY J.A. & GRISWOLD H.E. (1965) Red blood cell survival in patients with aortic valvular disease and ball valve prosthesis. *Circulation*, **32**, 570.

161 ANDERSON M.N., GABRIELLI E. & ZIZZI J.A. (1965) Chronic hemolysis in patients with ball valve prosthesis. *Journal of Thoracic and Cardiovascular Surgery*, **50**, 501.

162 MARSH G.W. (1966) Mechanical haemolytic anaemia after mitral valve replacement. *British Medical Journal*, **ii**, 31.

163 WALINSKY P., SPITZER S., BRODSIL I., KASPARIAN H. & MASON D. (1967) Hemolytic anemia with a Cross–Jones prosthesis. *American Journal of Medical Sciences*, **254**, 831.

164 NARNES C., HONEY M., BROOKS N., DAVIES J., GORMAN A. & PARKER N. (1980) Mechanical haemolytic anaemia after valve repair operations for non-rheumatic mitral regurgitation. *British Journal of Haematology*, **44**, 581.

165 SOORAE A.S. (1979) Massive intravascular haemolysis due to mitral Bjork–Shiley paraprosthetic regurgitation. *Thorax*, **34**, 686.

166 MAGILLIGAN D.J., FISHER E. & ALAM M. (1980) Hemolytic anemia with porcine xenograft aortic and mitral

valves. *Journal of Thoracic and Cardiovascular Surgery*, **79** (Suppl. 4), 628.

167 YACOUB M.H., ROGER I. & TAYLOR P.C. (1965) Red cell survival in patients with aortic valve disease. *Thorax*, **20**, 307.

168 DAMESHEK W. (1964) Case records of the Massachusetts General Hospital. Case 52—1964. *New England Journal of Medicine*, **271**, 898.

169 ZIPEROVICH S. & PALEY H.W. (1966) Severe mechanical hemolytic anemia due to valvular heart disease without prosthesis. *Annals of Internal Medicine*, **65**, 342.

170 WALSH J.R., BRODEUR M.T.H., RITZMAN L.W., SUTHERLAND D.W. & STARR A. (1966) Urinary iron excretion in patients with prosthetic heart valves. *Journal of the American Medical Association*, **198**, 91.

171 SANYL S.K., POLESKY H.F., HUME M. & BROWNE M.J. (1964) Spontaneous partial remission of postoperative hemolytic anemia in a case with ostium-primium defect. *Circulation*, **30**, 803.

172 REYNOLDS R.D., COLTMAN C.A. & BELLER B.M. (1967) Iron treatment in sideropenic intravascular hemolysis due to insufficiency of Starr–Edwards valve prosthesis. *Annals of Internal Medicine*, **66**, 659.

173 BLACKSHEAR P.L. JR, DORMAN F.D. & STEINBACH J.H. (1965) Some mechanical effects that influence hemolysis. *Transactions of the American Society for Artificial Internal Organs*, **11**, 112.

174 BLACKSHEAR P.L. JR, DORMAN F.D., STEINBACH J.H., MAYBACH E.J., SINGH A. & COLLINGHAM R.E. (1966) Shear, wall interaction and hemolysis. *Transactions of the American Society for Artificial Internal Organs*, **12**, 113.

175 SEARS D.A. & CROSBY W.H. (1965) Intravascular hemolysis due to intracardiac prosthetic devices. Diurnal variations related to activity. *American Journal of Medicine*, **39**, 341

176 MILLER D.S., MENGEL C.E., KREMER W.B., GUTTERMAN J. & SENNINGEN R. (1966) Intravascular hemolysis in a patient with valvular heart disease. *Annals of Internal Medicine*, **65**, 210.

177 STOHLMAN F. JR, SARNOFF S.J., CASE R.B. & NESS A.T. (1956) Hemolytic syndrome following the insertion of a lucite ball valve prosthesis into the cardiovascular system. *Circulation*, **13**, 586.

178 SYMMERS W.S.C. (1952) Thrombotic microangiopathic haemolytic anaemia (thrombotic microangiopathy). *British Medical Journal*, **ii**, 897.

179 BRAIN M.C. & BECK E.A. (1965) Relationship of intravascular coagulation to intravascular haemolysis. *Clinical Research*, **13**, 268.

180 BRAIN M.C., ESTERLY J.R. & BECK E.A. (1967) Intravascular haemolysis with experimentally produced vascular thrombi. *British Journal of Haematology*, **13**, 135.

181 GASSER W.C., GAUTIER E., STECK A., SIEBENMANN R.E. & OECHSLIN R. (1955) Hämolytischurämische Syndrome: bilaterale Nierenvidennekorsen bei akuten erwobenen hämolytischen Anämien. *Schweizerische Medizinische Wochenschrift*, **85**, 905.

182 GIANANTONIO C.A., VITACCIO M., MENDILAHARZU F. & GALLO G. (1968) The hemolytic-uremic syndrome: renal status of 76 patients at long term follow up. *Journal of Pediatrics*, **72**, 757.

183 HABIB R., COURTECUISSE V., LECLERC F., MATHIEU H. &

ROYER P. (1969) Etude anatamopathologique de 35 observations de syndrome hémolytique et urémique de l'enfant. *Archives françaises de Pediatrie*, **26**, 391.

184 KAPLAN B.S., KATZ J., KRAWITZ S. & LURIE A. (1971) An analysis of the results of therapy in 67 cases of hemolytic-uremic syndrome. *Journal of Pediatrics*, **78**, 420.

185 KIBEL M.A. & BARNARD P.J. (1968) The haemolytic-uraemic syndrome: a survey in southern Africa. *South African Medical Journal*, **42**, 692.

186 GIANANTONIO C., VITACCO M. & MENDILAHARZU F. (1973) The hemolytic uremic syndrome. *Nephrone*, **II**, 174.

187 TUNE B.M., LEVITT T.S. & GRIBBLE T.S. (1973) The hemolytic uremic syndrome in California: A review of 28 non-heparinised cases with long term follow up. *Journal of Pediatrics*, **82**, 304.

188 VAN WIERINGEN P.M.V., MONNENS L.A.H., SCHRETLEN E.D.A.M. (1974) Hemolytic uremic syndrome—epidemiological and clinical study. *Archives of Diseases in Children*, **49**, 432.

189 DOLISLAGER D. & TUNE B. (1978) The hemolytic-uremic syndrome: spectrum of severity and significance of prodrome. *American Journal of Diseases of Children*, **132**, 55.

190 SORRENTI L.Y. & LEVY P.R. (1978) The hemolytic uremic syndrome: experience at a centre in the Mid West. *American Journal of Diseases in Children*, **132**, 59.

191 BRAIN M.C. (1969) The hemolytic uremic syndrome. *Seminars in Hematology*, **6**, 162.

192 LIEBERMAN E. (1972) Hemolytic-uremic syndrome. *Journal of Pediatrics*, **80**, 1.

193 KAPLAN B.S. & DRUMMON K.V. (1978) The hemolytic-uremic syndrome as a syndrome. *New England Journal of Medicine*, **298**, 964.

194 NATHAN D.M., SIEGEL A.J. & BUNN F. (1977) Acute methemoglobinemia and hemolytic anemia with phenazopyridine. *Archives of Internal Medicine*, **137**, 1636.

195 CLAPS F.X. (1957) Two cases of methemoglobinemia and acute hemolytic anemia with death following the ingestion of a solution of paraminosalicylic acid. *American Review of Tuberculosis*, **76**, 862.

196 MUNROE W.D., LAWSON W.J. & HOLCOMB T.M. (1964) Hemolytic anemia due to aminosalicylic acid. Anemia with methemoglobinemia. *American Journal of Diseases of Children*, **108**, 425.

197 ANZIULEWICZ Y.A., DICK H.J. & CHIARULLI E.E. (1959) Transplacental naphthalene poisoning. *American Journal of Obstetrics and Gynecology*, **78**, 519.

198 CLARK B.B. (1945) Poisoning due to ingestion of wax crayons. *Journal of the American Medical Association*, **135**, 917.

199 GIANANTONIO C., VITACCIO M., MENDILAHARZU F., MENDILAHARZU J. & RUTTY A. (1964) The hemolytic uremic syndrome. *Journal of Pediatrics*, **64**, 478.

200 ANTHONY P.P. & KAPLAN A.B. (1968) Fatal haemolytic uraemic syndrome in two siblings. *Archives of Diseases in Childhood*, **43**, 316.

201 HAGGE W.W., HOLLEY K.E., BURKE E.C. & STICKLER G.B. (1967) Hemolytic uremic syndrome in two siblings. *New England Journal of Medicine*, **277**, 138.

202 McCLEAN M.M., JONES C.H. & SUTHERLAND D.A.

(1966) Haemolytic uraemic syndrome. A report of an outbreak. *Archives of Diseases in Childhood*, **41**, 76.

203 WHITINGTON P.F., FRIEDMAN A.L. & CHESNEY R.W. (1979) Gastrointestinal disease in the hemolytic-uremic syndrome. *Gastroenterology*, **76**, 728.

204 HABIB R., MATHIEU H. & ROYER P. (1967) Le syndrome hémolytique et urémique de l'enfant: aspects cliniques et anatomiques dans 27 observations. *Nephron*, **277**, 138.

205 MOORHEAD J.F., EDWARDS E.C. & GOLDSMITH H.J. (1965) Haemodialysis of three children and one infant with haemolytic uraemic syndrome. *Lancet*, **ii**, 570.

206 MATHIEU H., LECLERC F., HABIB R. & ROYER P. (1969) Étude clinique et biologique de 37 observations de syndrome hémolytique et urémique. *Archives françaises de Pediatrie*, **26**, 369.

207 BLECHER T.R. & RAPER A.B. (1967) Early diagnosis of thrombotic microangiopathy by paraffin section of aspirated bone marrow. *Archives of Diseases in Childhood*, **42**, 158.

208 BUKOWSKI J. & KOBLENZER P.J. (1962) Thrombotic-thrombocytopenic purpura: report of a case with unusual features of hypofibrinogenemia and leukopenia. *Journal of Pediatrics*, **60**, 84.

209 MONNENS L. & SCHRETLEN E. (1967) Intravascular coagulation in an infant with the haemolytic-uraemic syndrome. *Acta Paediatrica Scandinavica*, **56**, 436.

210 AVALOS J.S., VITACCO M., MOLINAS F., PENALVER J. & GIANANTONIO C. (1970) Coagulation studies in the hemolytic uremic syndrome. *Journal of Pediatrics*, **76**, 538.

211 METZ J. (1972) Observations on the mechanism of the haematological changes: in the haemolytic uraemic syndrome of infancy. *British Journal of Haematology*, **23** (Suppl.), 53.

212 GERVAIS M., RICHARDSON J.B., CHIU J. & DRUMMOND K.N. (1971) Immunofluorescent and histologic findings in the hemolytic uremic syndrome. *Pediatrics*, **47**, 352.

213 ROSEN S. & SCHEIN P.S. (1970) Hemolytic uremic syndrome in an adult: light and electron microscopic observations. *American Journal of Clinical Pathology*, **54**, 33.

214 RAY C.E., TUCKER V.L., HARRIS D.J., CUPPAGE F.E. & CHINT D.Y. (1970) Enteroviruses associated with the hemolytic-uremic syndrome. *Pediatrics*, **46**, 378.

215 METTLER N.E. (1969) Isolation of a microtatobiote from patients with hemolytic-uremic syndrome and thrombotic thrombocytopenic purpura and from mites in the United States. *New England Journal of Medicine*, **281**, 1023.

216 SHARPSTONE P., EVANS R.G., O'SHEA M., ALEXANDER L. & LEE H.A. (1968) Haemolytic uraemic syndrome: survival after prolonged oliguria. *Archives of Diseases in Childhood*, **43**, 711.

217 COURTECUISSE V., HABIB R. & MONNER C. (1967) Non-lethal hemolytic and uremic syndrome in children: an electron microscopic study of renal biopsies from six cases. *Experimental and Molecular Pathology*, **7**, 327.

218 BRAIN M.C., BAKER L.R.I., McBRIDE J.A. & RUBENBERG M. (1967) Heparin therapy in the haemolytic-uraemic syndrome. *Quarterly Journal of Medicine*, **36**, 608.

219 BRAIN M.C., BAKER L.R.I., McBRIDE J.A., RUBENGERG M.L. & DACIE J.V. (1968) Treatment of patients with microangiopathic haemolytic anaemia with heparin. *British Journal of Haematology*, **15**, 603.

220 KIBEL M.A. & BARNARD P.J. (1964) Treatment of acute haemolytic-uraemic syndrome with heparin. *Lancet*, **ii**, 25.

221 BERGSTEIN J.M., EDSON J.R. & MICHAEL A.F. (1972) Fibrinolytic treatment of the haemolytic uraemic syndrome. *Lancet*, **i**, 448.

222 WEBSTER J., REES A.J., LEWIS P.J. & HENSBY C.N. Prostacyclin deficiency in haemolytic-uraemic syndrome. *British Medical Journal*, **ii**, 271.

223 THORSEN C.A., ROSSI E.C., GREEN D. & CARONE F.A. (1979) The treatment of hemolytic uremic syndrome with inhibitors of platelet function. *American Journal of Medicine*, **66**, 711.

224 BLIX S. & JACOBSEN C.D. (1966) Intravascular coagulation: a possible accelerating effect of prednisone. *Acta Medica Scandinavica*, **180**, 723.

225 KOSTER F., LEVIN J., WALKER L., TUNG K.S.K., GILMAN R.H., RAHMAN M.M., MAJID A., ISLAM S. & WILLIAMS R.C. (1978) Hemolytic uremic syndrome after shigellosis. Relation to endotoxemia and circulating immune complexes. *New England Journal of Medicine*, **298**, 927.

226 ADELMAN R.D., HALSTED C.C. & SHEIKHOLISHLAM B.M. (1980) Hemolytic uremic syndrome: associated conditions. *Journal of Pediatrics*, **97**, 161.

227 MOORTHY C. & MAKKER S.P. (1979) Hemolytic uremic syndrome associated with pneumococcal sepsis. *Journal of Pediatrics*, **95**, 558.

228 MOSCHOWITZ E. (1925) Acute febrile pleiochromic anemia with hyaline thrombosis of terminal arterioles and capillaries: undescribed disease. *Archives of Internal Medicine*, **36**, 89.

229 LEVINE S. & SHEARN M.A. (1964) Thrombotic thrombocytopenic purpura and systemic lupus erythematosus. *Archives of Internal Medicine*, **113**, 826.

230 MAILLARD J. (1961) Thrombotic thrombocytopenic purpura—clinical and pathological findings in 49 cases. *Blood*, **17**, 366.

231 SILVERSTEIN A. (1968) Thrombotic thrombocytopenic purpura. The initial clinical manifestations. *Archives of Neurology*, **18**, 358.

232 DRUKKER A., WINTERBORN M., BENNETT B., CHURG J., SPITZER A. & GREIFER I. (1975) Recurrent haemolytic-uraemic syndrome: a case report. *Clinical Nephrology*, **4**, 68.

233 SPIRER Z., KNOBEL B., EARON J., HEYMAN I. & BOGAR N. (1977) Recurrent hemolytic uremic syndrome. A report of 2 cases. *Helvetica Paediatrica Acta*, **32**, 165.

234 BATEMAN S.M., HILGARD P. & GORDON-SMITH E.C. (1979) Thrombotic thrombocytopenic purpura: a possible plasma factor deficiency. *British Journal of Haematology*, **43**, 498.

235 ORBISON J.L. (1962) Morphology of thrombotic thrombocytopenic purpura with demonstration of aneurysms. *American Journal of Pathology*, **28**, 129.

236 REMUZZI G., MISIANI R.M., MARCHESI D., LIVIO M., MECLA G. & DE GAETANO G. (1978) Haemolytic uraemic syndrome: deficiency of plasma factor(s) regulating prostacyclin activity? *Lancet*, **ii**, 871.

237 HENSBY C.N., LEWIS P.J., HILGARD P., MUFTI G.J., HOWS J. & WEBSTER J. (1979) Prostacyclin deficiency in thrombotic thrombocytopenic purpura. *Lancet*, **ii**, 748.

238 ASTER R.H. (1977) TTP: New clues to the etiology of an enzymatic disease. *New England Journal of Medicine*, **197**, 1400.

239 EDITORIAL (1979) Plasma exchange in thrombotic thrombocytopenic purpura. *Lancet*, **i**, 1065.

240 DAMESHEK W.D. (1966) Heparin in thrombotic microangiopathy. *Lancet*, **i**, 1033.

241 SCHWARTZ J., ROSENBERG A. & COOPERBERG A.A. (1972) Thrombotic thrombocytopenic purpura: successful treatment of two cases. *Canadian Medical Association Journal*, **106**, 1200.

242 REYNOLDS P.M., JACKSON J.M., BRINE J.A.S. & VIVIAN A.B. (1976) Thrombotic thrombocytopenic purpura—a remission following splenectomy. *American Journal of Medicine*, **64**, 439.

243 RUTKOW I.M. (1978) Thrombotic thrombocytopenic purpura (TTP) and splenectomy: a current appraisal. *Annals of Surgery*, **188**, 701.

244 KADRI A., MOINUDDIN M. & LEEUW N.M. (1975) Phagocytosis of blood cells by macrophages in thrombotic thrombocytopenic purpura. *Annals of Internal Medicine*, **82**, 799.

245 ZACHARSKI L.R., WALWORTH C. & McINTYRE O.R. (1971) Antiplatelet therapy for thrombotic thrombocytopenic purpura. *New England Journal of Medicine*, **285**, 408.

246 AMOROSI E.L. & KARPATKIN S. (1977) Antiplatelet treatment of thrombotic thrombocytopenic purpura. *Annals of Internal Medicine*, **86**, 102.

247 LIAN E.C. (1979) Presence of a platelet aggregating factor in the plasma of patients with thrombotic thrombocytopenic purpura (TTP) and its inhibition by normal plasma. *Blood*, **53**, 333.

248 BUKOWSKI R.M., HEWLETT J.S., HARRIS J.W., HOFFMAN G.C., BATTLE J.D., SILVERBLATT E. & YAORG I.-Y. (1976) Exchange transfusions in the treatment of thrombotic thrombocytopenic purpura. *Seminars in Hematology*, **13**, 219.

249 BUKOWSKI R.M., KING J.W. & HEWLETT J.S. (1977) Plasmapheresis in the treatment of thrombotic thrombocytopenic purpura. *Blood*, **50**, 413.

250 PISCIOTTA A.V., GARTHWAITE T., DARIN J. & ASTER R.H. (1977) Treatment of thrombotic thrombocytopenic purpura by exchange transfusion. *American Journal of Hematology*, **3**, 73.

251 YANG C., MUSSBAUM M. & PARK H. (1979) Thrombotic thrombocytopenic purpura in early pregnancy. Remission after plasma exchange. *Acta Haematologica*, **62**, 112.

252 WALKER B.K., BALLAS S.K. & MARTINEZ J. (1980) Plasma infusion for thrombotic thrombocytopenic purpura during pregnancy. *Archives of Internal Medicine*, **140**, 981.

253 BYRNES J.J. & KHURANA M. (1977) Treatment of thrombotic thrombocytopenic purpura with plasma. *New England Journal of Medicine*, **297**, 1386.

254 MACHIN S.J., DEFREYN G., CHAMONE D.A.F. & VERMYLEN J. (1980) Plasma 6-keto-PGF$_{1\alpha}$ levels after plasma exchange in thrombotic thrombocytopenic purpura. *Lancet*, **i**, 661.

255 ANSELL J. (1978) Thrombotic thrombocytopenic purpura fails to respond to fresh frozen plasma infusions. *Annals of Internal Medicine*, **89**, 647.

256 MAY H.V., HARBERT G.M. & THRONTON W.V. (1976) Thrombotic thrombocytopenic purpura associated with pregnancy. *American Journal of Obstetrics and Gynaecology*, **126**, 452.

257 FITZGIBBONS J.F., GOODNIGHT S.H. & BURKHARDT J.H. (1977) Survival following thrombotic thrombocytopenic purpura in pregnancy. *Journal of Obstetrics and Gynaecology*, **50** (Suppl. 1), 66.

258 HUTCHINSON H.E., LAWSON D.H., LEVER A.F., MACADAM R.F., McNICOL G.P. & ROBERTSON J.I.S. (1969) Microangiopathic haemolytic anaemia and the pathogenesis of malignant hypertension. *Lancet*, **i**, 1277.

259 BAKER L.R.I., SEVITT L.H. & WRONG O.M. (1969) Vascular lesions in malignant hypertension. *Lancet*, **ii**, 59.

260 CRUMMY C.S., PERLIN E. & MOQUIN R.B. (1971) Microangiopathic hemolytic anemia in Wegener's granulomatosis. *American Journal of Medicine*, **51**, 544.

261 LICHTMAN M.A., HOYER L.W. & SEARS D.A. (1968) Erythrocyte deformation and hemolytic anemia coincident with the microvascular disease of rejecting renal transplants. *American Journal of Medical Sciences*, **256**, 239.

262 FLUTE P.T., RAKE M.O., WILLIAMS R., SEAMAN M.J. & CALNE R.Y. (1969) Liver transplant in man. IV. Haemorrhage and thrombosis. *British Medical Journal*, **i**, 20.

263 BRAIN M.C., AZZOPARDI J.G., BAKER L.R.I., PINEO G.N., ROBERTS P. & DACIE J.V. (1970) Microangiopathic haemolytic anaemia and mucin-forming adenocarcinoma. *British Journal of Haematology*, **18**, 183.

264 LOHRMANN H.P., ADAM W., HEYMER B. & KUBANEK B. (1973) Microangiopathic hemolytic anemia in metastatic carcinoma. *Annals of Internal Medicine*, **79**, 368.

265 ANTMAN K.H., SKARIN A.T., MAYER R.J., HARGREAVES H.K. & CANELLOS G.P. (1979) Microangiopathic hemolytic anemia and cancer: a review. *Medicine* (Baltimore), **58**, 377.

266 HILGARD P. & GORDON-SMITH E.C. (1974) Microangiopathic haemolytic anaemia and experimental tumour cell embolism. *British Journal of Haematology*, **26**, 651.

267 WANG Y., FROM A.H.L. & KRIVIT A. (1965) Disseminated pulmonary arterial thrombosis associated with thrombocytopenic occurrence in identical twins. *Circulation*, **31** (Suppl. 2), 215.

268 STUARD I.D., HEUSINKVELD R.S. & MOSS A. (1972) Microangiopathic hemolytic anemia and thrombocytopenia in primary pulmonary hypertension. *New England Journal of Medicine*, **287**, 869.

269 PROPP R.P. & SCHARFMAN W.B. (1966) Hemangioma-thrombocytopenia syndrome associated with microangiopathic anemia. *Blood*, **28**, 623.

270 HOLLINGSWORTH J.H. & MOHLER D.N. (1968) Microangiopathic hemolytic anemia caused by purpura fulminans. *Annals of Internal Medicine*, **68**, 1310.

271 LEAVITT T.J., MERIGAN R.C. & FREEMAN J.M. (1971) Hemolytic-uremic-like syndrome following polycarboxyl interferon induction. Treatment of Dawson's inclusion body encephalitis. *American Journal of Disease in Childhood*, **121**, 43.

272 DAVIDSON R.J.L. (1964) Exertional haemoglobinuria: a report on three cases with studies on the haemolytic mechanism. *Journal of Clinical Pathology*, **17**, 536.

273 DAVIDSON R.J.L. (1969) March or exertional hemoglobinuria. *Seminars in Hematology*, **6**, 150.

274 COOPER R.A. (1970) Lipids of human red cell membrane: normal composition and variability in disease. *Seminars in Hematology*, **7**, 296.

275 DORMANDY T.L. (1971) Annotation: the autoxidation of red cells. *British Journal of Haematology*, **20**, 457.

276 MOHANDAS N., PHILLIPS W.M. & BESSIS M. (1979) Red blood cell deformability and hemolytic anemias. *Seminars in Hematology*, **16**, 95.

277 PITCHER C.S. & WILLIAMS R. (1963) Reduced red cell survival in jaundice and its relation to abnormal glutathione metabolism. *Clinical Science*, **24**, 235.

278 COOPER R.A. & JANDL J.H. (1968) Bile salts and cholesterol in the pathogenesis of target cells in obstructive jaundice. *Journal of Clinical Investigation*, **47**, 809.

279 COOPER R.A., KIMBALL D.B. & DUROCHER J.R. (1974) Role of the spleen in membrane conditioning and hemolysis of spur cells in liver disease. *New England Journal of Medicine*, **290**, 1279.

280 SMITH J.A., LONERGAN E.T. & STERLING K. (1964) Spur cell anemia: hemolytic anemia with red cells resembling acanthocytes in alcoholic cirrhosis. *New England Journal of Medicine*, **271**, 396.

281 ZIEVE L. (1958) Jaundice, hyperlipemia and hemolytic anemia: a heretofore unrecognized syndrome associated with alcoholic fatty liver and cirrhosis. *Annals of Internal Medicine*, **48**, 471.

282 WAYS P., REED C.F. & HANAHAN D.J. (1963) Red-cell and plasma lipids in acanthocytosis. *Journal of Clinical Investigation*, **42**, 1248.

283 DODGE J.T. & PHILLIPS G.B. (1966) Autoxidation as a cause of altered lipid distribution in extracts from human cells. *Journal of Lipid Research*, **7**, 387.

284 OSKI F.A. & BARNESS L.A. (1967) Vitamin E deficiency: a previously unrecognized cause of hemolytic anemia in the premature infant. *Journal of Pediatrics*, **70**, 211.

285 RITCHIE J.H., FISH M.B., MCMASTERS V. & GROSSMAN M. (1968) Edema and hemolytic anemia in premature infants. *New England Journal of Medicine*, **279**, 1185.

286 MELHORN D.K., GROSS S., LAKE G.A. & DEU J.A. (1971) The hydrogen peroxide fragility test and serum tocopherol level in anemias of various etiologies. *Blood*, **37**, 438.

287 RISDALL R.J., MCKENNA R.W., NESBIT M.E., KRIVIT W., BALFOUR H., SIMMONS R.L. & BRUNNER D. (1979) Virus associated hemophagocytic syndrome: a benign histiocytic proliferation distinct from malignant histiocytosis. *Cancer*, **44**, 993.

288 MANOHARAN A., CATOVSKY D., LAMPERT I.A., AL-MASHADHANI, GORDON-SMITH E.C. & GALTON D.A.G. (1981) Histiocytic medullary reticulosis complicating lymphocytic leukaemia: malignant or reactive? *Scandinavian Journal of Haematology*, **26**, 5.

289 DACIE J.V. (1980) The lifespan of the red blood cell and circumstances of its premature death. In: *Blood, Pure and Eloquent* (ed. Wintrobe M.M.), p. 211. McGraw Hill, New York.

290 GARDNER F.H. & BLUM S.F. (1967) Aplastic anemia in paroxysmal noctural hemoglobinuria. Mechanisms and therapy. *Seminars in Hematology*, **4**, 250.

291 SYMPOSIUM (1972) Paroxysmal nocturnal haemoglobinuria. *Series Haematologica*, **3**, 1.

292 ROSSE W.E. (1978) Paroxysmal nocturnal haemoglobinuria in aplastic anaemia. *Clinics in Haematology*, **7**, 541.

293 ROSSE W.F. (1973) Variations in the red cells in paroxysmal nocturnal haemoglobinuria. *British Journal of Haematology*, **24**, 327.

294 PACKMAN C.H., ROSENFELD S.I., JENKINS D.E., THIEM P.A. & LEDDY J.P. (1977) Complement lysis of human erythrocytes. Differing susceptibility of two types of paroxysmal nocturnal hemoglobinuria cells to C5b-9. *Journal of Clinical Investigation*, **64**, 428.

295 ROSSE W.F., ADAMS J.P. & THORPE A.M. (1974) The population of cells in paroxysmal nocturnal haemoglobinuria of intermittent sensitivity to complement lysis. *British Journal of Haematology*, **28**, 181.

296 PACKMAN C.H., ROSENFELD S.T., JENKINS D.E. & LEDDY J.P. (1980) Complement lysis of human erythrocytes. II. A unique interaction of human C8 and C9 with paroxysmal nocturnal haemoglobinuria erythrocytes. *Journal of Immunology*, **124**, 2818.

297 ROSSE W.F. & DACIE J.V. (1966) Immune lysis of normal human and paroxysmal nocturnal hemoglobinurla (PNH) red blood cells. I. The sensitivity of PNH cells to lysis by complement and specific antibody. *Journal of Clinical Investigation*, **45**, 736.

298 ONI S.B., OSUNKOYA B.O. & LUZZATTO L. (1970) Paroxysmal nocturnal hemoglobinuria: evidence for monoclonal origin of abnormal red cells. *Blood*, **36**, 14.

299 ASTER R.H. & ENRIGHT S.E. (1969) A platelet and granulocyte membrane defect in paroxysmal nocturnal haemoglobinuria: usefulness for detecting platelet antibodies. *Journal of Clinical Investigation*, **48**, 1199.

300 DIXON R.H. & ROSSE W.F. (1977) Mechanism of complement mediated activation of human blood platelets *in vitro*: comparison of paroxysmal nocturnal hemoglobinuria platelets. *Journal of Clinical Investigation*, **59**, 360.

301 STERN M. & ROSSE W.E. (1979) Two populations of granulocytes in paroxysmal nocturnal hemoglobinuria. *Blood*, **53**, 928.

302 BLUM S.F. & GARDNER F.H. (1966) Intestinal infarction in paroxysmal nocturnal hemoglobinuria. *New England Journal of Medicine*, **274**, 1137.

303 PEYTREMANN R., RHODES R.S. & HARTMANN R.C. (1972) Thrombosis in paroxysmal nocturnal hemoglobinuria (PNH) with particular reference to progressive, diffuse hepatic vein thrombosis. *Series Haematologica*, **3**, 115.

304 MCKELLER M. & DACIE J.V. (1958) Thromboplastic activity of the plasma in paroxysmal nocturnal haemoglobinuria. *British Journal of Haematology*, **4**, 404.

305 DACIE J.V. & LEWIS S.M. (1961) Paroxysmal nocturnal haemoglobinuria: variation in chemical severity and association with bone marrow hypoplasia. *British Journal of Haematology*, **7**, 442.

306 HANSEN N.E. & KILLMAN S.A. (1970) Paroxysmal nocturnal hemoglobinuria in myelofibrosis. *Blood*, **36**, 428.

307 TSO S.C. & CHAN T.K. (1973) PNH and chronic myeloid leukaemia in the same patient. *Scandinavian Journal of Haematology*, **10**, 384.

308 COWALL D.E., PASQUALE D.N. & DIKKER P. (1979)

Paroxysmal nocturnal hemoglobinuria terminating as erythroleukemia. *Cancer*, **45**, 1914.

309 CARMEL R., COLTMAN C.A., YATTEAN R.F. & COSTANZI J.S. (1970) Association of PNH with erythroleukemia. *New England Journal of Medicine*, **283**, 1329.

310 LUZZATTO L. (1979) The PNH abnormality in myeloproliferative disorders: association of PNH and acute erythemic myelosis in two children. *Haematologica* (Paris), **64**, 13.

311 PAPAYANNOPOULOU T., ROSSE W. & STAMATOYANNOPOULOS G. (1978) Fetal hemoglobin in paroxysmal nocturnal hemoglobinuria (PNH): evidence for derivation of HbF-containing erythrocytes (F cells) from PNH clone as well as from normal hemopoietic stem cell lines. *Blood*, **52**, 740.

312 HAM T.H. & DINGLE J.H. (1939) Studies on the destruction of red blood cells. II. Chronic hemolytic anemia with paroxysmal nocturnal hemoglobinuria: certain immunological aspects of the hemolytic mechanism with special reference to serum complement. *Journal of Clinical Investigation*, **96**, 574.

313 ROSSE W.F., LOGUE G.L., ADAMS J. & CROOKSTON J.H. (1974) Mechanism of immune lysis of the red cells in hereditary multinuclearity with a positive acidified serum lysis test and paroxysmal nocturnal hemoglobinuria. *Journal of Clinical Investigation*, **53**, 31.

314 HARTMANN R.C. & JENKINS D.R. JR (1960) The 'sugar-water' test for paroxysmal nocturnal hemoglobinuria. *New England Journal of Medicine*, **275**, 155.

315 SIRCHIA G., MARUBINI E., MERCURIALI F. & FERRONE S. (1975) Study of two *in vitro* diagnostic tests for paroxysmal nocturnal haemoglobinuria. *British Journal of Haematology*, **24**, 751.

316 DACIE J.V., LEWIS S.M. & TILLS D. (1960) Comparative sensitivity of erythrocytes in paroxysmal nocturnal haemoglobinuria to haemolysis by acidified normal serum and by high titre cold antibody. *British Journal of Haematology*, **6**, 362.

317 CROSBY W.H. (1950) Paroxysmal nocturnal hemoglobinuria. A specific test for this disease based on the ability of thrombin to activate the hemolytic factor. *Blood*, **5**, 843.

319 DACIE J.V. (1948) Transfusion of saline washed red cells in nocturnal haemoglobinuria. *Clinical Science*, **7**, 65.

320 MENGEL C.E., KANN H.E. JR & O'MALLEY B.W. (1965) Increased hemolysis after intramuscular iron administration in patients with paroxysmal nocturnal hemoglobinuria. *Blood*, **20**, 74.

321 HARTMANN R.C., JENKINS D.E.J., McKEE C. & HEYSSEL R.M. (1966) Paroxysmal nocturnal hemoglobinuria: clinical and laboratory studies relating to iron metabolism and therapy with androgen and iron. *Medicine*, **45**, 331.

322 GORDON-SMITH E.C. & LEWIS S.M. (1972) Treatment of aplastic anaemia and allied disorders with oxymetholone. In: *Steroids in Modern Medicine*, p. 8. Excerpta Medica, Amsterdam.

323 DACIE J.V. & LEWIS S.M. (1972) Clinical presentation and natural course of paroxysmal nocturnal haemoglobinuria. *Series Haematologica*, **3**, 3.

324 STORB R., EVANS R.S., THOMAS E.D., BUCKNER C.D., CLIFT R.A., FEFER A., NEIMAN P. & WRIGHT S.E. (1975) Paroxysmal nocturnal haemoglobinuria and refractory marrow failure treated by marrow transplantation. *British Journal of Haematology*, **24**, 743.

325 FEFER A., FREEMAN H., STORB R., HILL J., SINEER J., EDWARDS A. & THOMAS E. (1976) Paroxysmal nocturnal hemoglobinuria and marrow failure treated by infusion of marrow from an identical twin. *Annals of Internal Medicine*, **84**, 892.

326 HERSHKO C., EAGLE R.P., HO N.G. & CLINE M.J. (1979) Case of aplastic anaemia in paroxysmal nocturnal haemoglobinuria by marrow transfusion from identical twin: failure of peripheral leukocyte transfusion to correct marrow aplasia. *Lancet*, **i**, 945.

Chapter 13
Haem and pyridoxine metabolism: the sideroblastic and related refractory anaemias

J. M. WHITE AND D.C. NICHOLSON

Refractory anaemia, associated with a hyperplastic bone marrow, has been recognized for many years, and recently some progress has been made in the further classification of this heterogeneous group of disorders. At least one fairly well-defined group, the sideroblastic anaemias, can now be separated off by virtue of the morphological appearances of, and distribution of iron in, the sideroblasts.

The sideroblastic anaemias are a class of disorders characterized by defective haemoglobinization of a population of red cells, dyshaemopoietic erythropoiesis and an abnormal accumulation of iron in the maturing erythroblasts. The iron in the latter is distributed characteristically in the form of a perinuclear ring. This type of anaemia may be inherited or acquired and the latter variety may have no obvious cause or may result from the action of specific metabolic inhibitors or non-specific cellular toxins. There is increasing evidence that anaemias of this class have in common an inability of the erythroblasts to synthesize haem. However, in the majority of instances, the precise molecular defect in the haem-synthetic pathway is unknown and, indeed, it is by no means certain that abnormal haem production is the *primary* abnormality.

The sideroblastic anaemias have already been the subject of several reviews [1–8]. The earlier accounts dealt largely with the classification, morphological features and diagnosis of these anaemias, but later ones have concentrated on biochemical abnormalities as these have been elucidated. In addition to a brief consideration of haem and pyridoxine metabolism, this chapter will cover three main aspects of sideroblastic anaemia. First, the biochemical abnormalities associated with haem synthesis, pyridoxine metabolism and iron metabolism; secondly, the clinical classification and haematological manifestations of these anaemias and their treatment and prognosis; and finally, the related conditions which are also characterized by dyshaemopoietic anaemia.

HAEM AND PYRIDOXINE METABOLISM

The genetic control of haemoglobin production is considered in Chapter 8 and protein synthesis in general and globin synthesis in particular are described in Chapter 9. The account which follows deals mainly with haem synthesis and should be read in conjunction with these previous sections (pp. 339 and 409), and with the description of porphyrin metabolism in Chapter 14. The normal red cell develops from its early-committed progenitors by a process of mitotic division (three to four divisions in four to six days). The final product is the anucleated reticulocyte which is extruded from the marrow sinusoids into the vascular circulation. As the red cell matures, concurrent with a reduction in volume, there is a linear accumulation of haemoglobin. Haemoglobin begins to be synthesized in a basophilic normoblast (90 hours); its synthesis is maximal in the intermediate normoblast (140 hours), and thereafter it declines. At the reticulocyte stage (180 hours), the cell has acquired 90% of its haemoglobin (see Chapter 4) [9]. The synthesis of haemoglobin is not only synchronized with the maturation of the red cell, but also with respect to the amount of haem and globin produced and the amount of iron incorporated into the erythroid precursor. As a result, under normal circumstances, little excess of these intermediates is present in the mature red cells [10].

The way in which these synthetic steps are regulated is not yet fully understood (see also p. 409). There is increasing evidence that haem plays an important role, however. Haem can probably control its own rate of synthesis by end-product inhibition or repression of δ-aminolaevulinic-acid synthase, the rate-limiting enzyme in the haem pathway [11] (*vide infra*). This enzyme is induced by several naturally occurring steroids [12, 13], a possible mechanism for the regulation of haemoglobin synthesis during red-cell maturation. Haem also regulates the rate of globin-chain production, at least in *in-vitro* reticulocyte and bone-marrow experiments, although there is considerable controversy about how such control is mediated [14, 18] (see Chapter 9, p. 339). In addition, there is some evidence, again from *in-vitro* studies, that the level of haem may regulate the rate of movement of iron across the red-cell membrane [19]. Certainly a model which attributes such a central controlling role to a small-molecular-weight molecule like haem is attractive and, although still highly speculative, is compatible with many of the observed biochemical abnormalities associated with a deficiency of haem in the red cell.

HAEM SYNTHESIS (see also page 577)

Haem is a tetrapyrrole which consists of an iron atom coordinated to four pyrrole rings through their respective nitrogen atoms (the structure is shown in Fig. 8.1, p. 323). The α positions of the pyrrole rings are joined to each other through methene bridges and these, together with the pyrrole rings, form an extended conjugated ring structure. The iron atom is bound in coordination with each of the pyrrole rings leaving two other ligand-binding sites. One of these is bound to a histidine residue of a globin chain (see Chapter 8, p. 329) while the other is the binding site for oxygen in the oxyhaemoglobin form.

The synthesis of haem in the red-cell precursors takes place mainly in the mitochondria but some intermediates are formed in the cytoplasm (Fig. 13.1) (see also Chapter 14, p. 577). The initial reaction involves the condensation of glycine and succinyl coenzyme A (from the citric-acid cycle) to form δ-aminolaevulinic acid (ALA) through the action of δ-aminolaevulinic-acid synthase; α-amino-β-keto-adipic acid may be an unstable intermediate which is rapidly decarboxylated. Pyridoxal phosphate is the only established cofactor for this reaction [20] in which it probably forms a Schiff's base linkage with glycine. ALA synthase is highly unstable and is believed to be the rate-limiting enzyme for haem synthesis in all systems [21–23]. Two molecules of ALA are condensed to the monopyrrole, porphobilinogen (PBG), by ALA dehydratase. The ALA leaves the mitochondria and is converted to porphobilinogen by cytosolic ALA dehydratase. Still within the cytoplasm, four molecules of porphobilinogen are polymerized to the tetrapyrro-lic uroporphyrinogen III. Two enzymes are required, uroporphyrinogen I synthase and uroporphyrinogen co-synthase [23, 24]. The exact steps in the reaction are not fully understood but it is believed that three molecules of porphobilinogen condense to form a tripyrrylmethane; this is then broken enzymatically

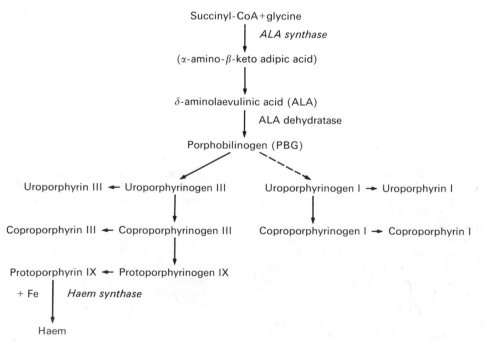

Fig. 13.1. The biochemical pathway for the synthesis of haem. Only those enzymes of clinical interest are included. The enzymes in italics are found in the mitochondria, while the others are cytoplasmic.

into a dipyrrylmethane and a monopyrrole. Two types of dipyrroles (A and B) are formed, depending on where the break takes place (see Chapter 14, p. 577). The condensation of two type A molecules will result in the tetrapyrrole uroporphyrinogen I, and if one A and one B condense, uroporphyrinogen III will be formed. Recent studies by Battersby *et al.* have shown uroporphyrinogen-I-synthase and uroporphyrinogen cosynthase to act separately in haem biosynthesis. The synthase catalyses the polymerization of porphobilinogen to an open-chain tetrapyrrole analogous to that hypothetically derived by opening the uroporphyrinogen-I molecule. This linear structure is the substrate for the cosynthase and contains a pyrrole ring which is inverted with consequent reversal of the acetic and propionic-β substituents. A type-III structure results and macro-ring closure produces uroporphyrinogen III [224]. Coproporphyrinogen III (and I) is formed by decarboxylation. During these last two stages the I isomers of both compounds are formed, which undergo autoxidation to uroporphyrin I and coproporphyrin I. These are not utilized by the cell. In the mitochondria, coproporphyrinogen III is converted to protoporphyrin IX by a complex reaction involving at least two enzymes, a decarboxylase and a dehydrogenase [25]. The final step is the insertion of Fe^{2+} into protoporphyrin IX to form haem. This reaction is catalysed by ferrochelatase. *In vitro*, this reaction is inhibited by oxidation and is enhanced by such reducing agents as glutathione and vitamin C. Their importance *in vivo* has yet to be assessed, however.

The synthesis of haem is therefore a complex reaction and subject to many chemical and physical variables (for reviews see Refs 25 and 26). One relevant aspect is its dependence on the integrity of the mitochondria and it is likely that any non-specific damage to the mitochondria may seriously impair haem synthesis (see p. 550).

The main control steps in this complex pathway are reviewed briefly in Chapter 14, p. 577. End-product inhibition is well documented in the rabbit reticulocyte and bacterial systems and it seems likely that this is achieved by the inhibition of ALA synthase [11, 21]. It appears that this reaction is reversible, and is not related to the concentration of glycine, pyridoxal phosphate or succinyl-CoA. Thus ALA synthase appears to be the rate-limiting enzyme in the haem pathway and a model has been proposed in which the genetic locus for the enzyme forms part of an operon [22]. In this system, haem reduces the rate of ALA-synthase production by forming a repressor complex with the aporepressor product of the repressor locus. It is known that certain naturally occurring steroids will induce ALA-synthase production [14, 15]

(see Chapter 14, p. 577) and these may act by blocking the combination of haem with the aporepressor, so derepressing the structural gene for ALA synthase.

The relationship between haem and globin synthesis is described in Chapter 9 (p. 409), and has been the subject of several reviews [14, 16, 18].

Haemoglobin synthesis in the presence of haem deficiency

In two disorders in which the synthesis of haem is defective, iron deficiency and lead poisoning, there are characteristic alterations of both porphyrin metabolism and globin-chain synthesis. In iron deficiency there is an abnormal accumulation of both free coproporphyrin and protoporphyrin within the cell, presumably due to the increased activity of ALA synthase. The normal balance between haem and globin production is disturbed, resulting in a relative excess of the latter. Thus a large proportion of the α and β chains synthesized are not converted into haemoglobin but are free in the cell as $\alpha\beta$ dimers [27]. The same changes have been found in the red cells and reticulocytes of patients with lead poisoning, namely an accumulation of porphyrins (see p. 592) and free α- and β-globin chains [28]. It is noteworthy that in this condition ring sideroblasts can be seen in the bone marrow. It will be shown later that these abnormalities of globin synthesis associated with the haem-deficiency states are also found in the reticulocytes of patients with sideroblastic anaemia; this provides evidence, albeit indirect, that the molecular defect responsible for this condition is an inability of the erythroblast to synthesize haem.

PYRIDOXINE (VITAMIN B6) METABOLISM

There is much evidence which associates deficiency or abnormal metabolism of pyridoxine with sideroblastic anaemia. Approximately 30% of patients with all types of sideroblastic anaemia have evidence of disturbed pyridoxine metabolism and about the same proportion show some haematological improvement when treated with pyridoxine [8]. Furthermore, several known inhibitors of pyridoxine metabolism, antituberculous drugs and alcohol, for example, cause a secondary sideroblastic anaemia in some patients, and animals made pyridoxine deficient develop a microcytic, hypochromic anaemia with abnormal sideroblasts in the bone marrow.

Pyridoxine has several well-documented functions in normal cellular chemistry. In amino-acid metabolism it is required as a co-enzyme in such reactions as decarboxylation, deamination, transamination, transulphuration and desulphuration. It is also required for the normal cellular transport of amino acids and for the activity of the enzyme kynurenase required for tryptophan metabolism. With regard to the synthesis of haem, it is essential as a co-enzyme for the formation of δ-aminolaevulinic acid.

Pyridoxine exists in nature in three biologically active forms; pyridoxine (from fruit, vegetables and cereals), pyridoxamine and pyridoxal (from meat and animal products). The daily requirement in man is about 0·5–2 mg and signs of deficiency will result with intakes of 0·1 mg/day or less [29, 30].

Anderson *et al.* [31] have partly clarified the mechanism for conversion of pyridoxine to the metabolically active form, pyridoxal, in mature red cells (Fig. 13.2). They have also made the important observation that the mature cell may be the only major site for this conversion. It will be stressed later that in some types of sideroblastic anaemia specific defects in this pathway have been detected.

Nutritional pyridoxine deficiency in man is rare. It is manifest by glossitis, dermatitis and neurological abnormalities; anaemia, however, is not common. Mice maintained on a pyridoxine-deficient diet develop a hypochromic anaemia and abnormal sideroblasts in the bone marrow after six weeks. Typical ring

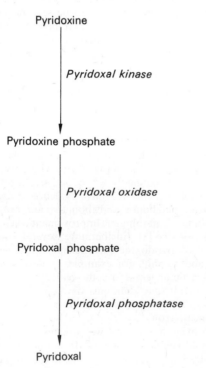

Pyridoxine

Pyridoxal kinase

Pyridoxine phosphate

Pyridoxal oxidase

Pyridoxal phosphate

Pyridoxal phosphatase

Pyridoxal

Fig. 13.2. The conversion of pyridoxine to pyridoxal within the mature red cell according to Anderson *et al.* [31].

sideroblasts are usually absent, but they can be produced if the animals are given additional iron or the pyridoxine antagonists cycloserine and isoniazid [32]. In swine, experimental pyridoxine deficiency results in a microcytic, hypochromic anaemia, a raised serum iron and saturated TIBC [32]. The bone marrow shows an increase in sideroblasts. However, the blood film is not dimorphic and basophilic stippling is absent. In man, the effects of pyridoxine deficiency vary between different subjects. This is well illustrated by the reports of two pairs of brothers who were deficient in pyridoxine. In each case, one of the brothers developed neurological abnormalities whilst the other became anaemic [33, 34].

The exact relationship between disturbances in pyridoxine metabolism and sideroblastic anaemia is still unclear. Is a disturbance of pyridoxine metabolism a primary cause of the disease or is it a secondary manifestation? Bishop & Bethnell [35] considered that it was secondary to the damage caused by iron to the mitochondria. There is no direct evidence for this, but it is supported by two observations: first, that the dose of pyridoxine required to treat sideroblastic anaemia is 100 times greater than the physiological requirements; secondly, that patients may not show disturbances in pyridoxine metabolism until late in the disease [5]. The red-cell metabolism of pyridoxine in sideroblastic anaemia has been studied *in vitro* by Anderson *et al.* [30a]. In 28 patients with sideroblastic anaemia, 11 primary, four inherited (one pyridoxine responsive) and 13 secondary, it was found that the conversion rate of pyridoxine to pyridoxal and pyridoxal phosphate was normal or increased, even if the patient responded to pyridoxine. It is thought that the normal or high rate of conversion is due to a compensatory mechanism, as is seen in iron deficiency and megaloblastic anaemia. Nevertheless, in several types of secondary acquired sideroblastic anaemia caused by lead, isoniazid, cycloserine and pyrazinamide, disorders of pyridoxine metabolism have been shown.

At present the most convenient (though indirect) way of detecting pyridoxine deficiency depends on the abnormal metabolism of tryptophan. For tryptophan to be converted to kynurenine requires kynurenase and this enzyme uses pyridoxine as a cofactor; if it is deficient, tryptophan is converted to xanthurenic acid which is excreted in the urine.

THE IRON STATUS OF THE ERYTHROBLAST

THE NORMAL SIDEROCYTE AND SIDEROBLAST

The iron content of the normal maturing erythroblast is unknown. Iron can be demonstrated in normal or iron-loaded red-cell precursors by staining bone-marrow preparations with Prussian-blue dye, when the iron stains blue. Grüneberg [36, 37] first reported that red cells of animals and humans contained small amounts of stainable iron. Doniach *et al.* [38] observed these cells in the blood of splenectomized patients and iron granules were later observed in mature red cells and erythroblasts of patients with a variety of anaemias [39–41]. These cells were at first thought to be associated only with pathological states but, subsequently, they were found in the circulating blood [40] and in bone-marrow preparations [42, 43] of normal subjects. However, in patients with haematological disorders they were always found in greater numbers. Douglas & Dacie [42] noted that in the marrow preparations of normal subjects the iron granules within siderocytes were always difficult to see—they varied in size and were evenly distributed throughout the cytoplasm. In iron deficiency they were absent. By light microscopy, the number of granules rarely exceeds four. However, by electron microscopy virtually all the normoblasts contain iron in the form of ferritin molecules [44]. Under electron microscopy, the iron-containing granules are within the cytoplasm and not associated with the mitochondria [44a] or cytoplasmic organelles. They appear to be membrane-free aggregates of ferritin. During erythropoiesis the aggregation of ferritin increases with maturation and this is visible in the late normoblast by light microscopy. Ferritin is removed progressively from the red cell as it matures. The process appears to be ATP dependent but the mechanism is not understood. When the nucleus of the normoblast is extruded from the marrow the remaining ferritin granules are retained.

The proportion of the total erythroblasts which contain iron granules of this type in normal subjects varies between 20 and 90%. It is now generally accepted that these ferritin molecules represent iron which has not been utilized for the formation of haem. It is not known whether it represents iron in excess of the requirements of the cell or if it is still to be utilized. The finding of increased numbers of siderocytes in the blood of splenectomized patients indicates that the spleen has a function in the removal of iron from the reticulocyte. It has been suggested that during the period in which the reticulocyte remains in the spleen, before its release into the circulation, the iron is utilized for making haemoglobin [5]. However, there is no evidence to support this and excess iron may be removed by other processes along with the redundant ribonuclear material.

THE ABNORMAL SIDEROBLASTS

In many pathological states the numbers of siderocytes and sideroblasts, and the quantity of iron they contain, increase markedly. Electron microscopy indicates a dense accumulation of iron (Fig. 13.3) in the cristae of the mitochondria. At higher resolution there is no ultrastructural pattern of ferritin and the electron-microscopic appearance of the mitochondria is grossly distorted. Such granules are seen in conditions such as thalassaemia major or haemolytic anaemia. Two types of abnormal sideroblasts are recognized [4]. The first is the sideroblast associated with dyshaemopoiesis but with normal haemoglobin synthesis. In these cells the granules, though they are more numerous and coarser than normal, are still evenly distributed throughout the cytoplasm. This type of sideroblast is associated particularly with conditions such as haemolytic anaemia, megaloblastic anaemia, haemochromatosis and transfusion siderosis. In these disorders, the iron-binding capacity of the plasma is reduced or saturated and the number of abnormal sideroblasts seen is proportional to the degree of saturation [45]. The second type is the pathological sideroblast associated either with disorders of globin synthesis (the thalassaemias) or with disorders of haem synthesis (the sideroblastic anaemias). In these cells the granules are larger, coarser and more numerous. The majority of erythroblasts show siderotic granulations and there is no correlation between the numbers of granules, the

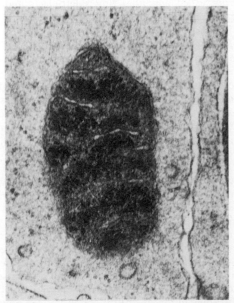

Fig. 13.3. EM photograph (× 66 400) of iron-laden mitchondria within an erythroblast of a patient with sideroblastic anaemia. The authors are grateful to Professor S. N. Wickramasinghe for this photomicrograph.

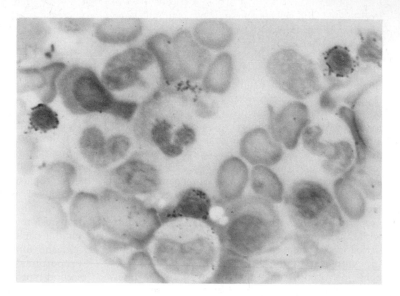

Fig. 13.4. Photomicrograph of bone-marrow preparation of patient suffering from idiopathic acquired sideroblastic anaemia. Ring sideroblasts are present. (Perl's stain, × 1300.)

proportion of sideroblasts, and the degree of saturation of the plasma transferrin [1, 45]. The major difference between the abnormal sideroblasts associated with thalassaemia and sideroblastic anaemia is that in the latter the granules are clustered around the nucleus in the form of a ring or collar (Fig. 13.4). These cells are called abnormal ring sideroblasts and are diagnostic of a sideroblastic anaemia.

THE ABNORMAL RING SIDEROBLAST

In the abnormal ring sideroblast, the iron within the cell is found to be almost entirely attached to perinuclear mitochondria [46, 53, 54]. The reason for this unusual distribution is not known. It has been suggested that the granules represent dead mitochondria which persist in their perinuclear arrangement during the maturation of the cell [14, 51, 56]. With light microscopy they are rarely found on the nucleus. The size of the granules varies. In the ring sideroblasts associated with primary sideroblastic anaemia or with chloramphenicol toxicity, they measure 3–4 μm across. In less severe conditions, porphyria cutanea tarda for example, they are much smaller, 0·3–0·4 μm [48]. The granules lie within the mitochondria, between the cristae, and often there is a marked disturbance of mitochondrial structure. The internal structure is disrupted with swelling and displacement of cristae, vacuolation and a complete loss of internal structure and, in some instances, the mitochondria can only be recognized because of the accumulated iron [4].

The type of erythroblast affected appears to depend on the type of sideroblastic anaemia, but not necessarily on the severity of the anaemia [55]. Usually all erythroblasts contain siderotic granules; in young forms they are fine, but become coarser and larger as the cell matures. Hines & Grasso [4] noted that in the secondary sideroblastic anaemias it was only the intermediate or late normoblasts which were particularly affected.

It is reasonable to assume that the metabolism of such mitochondria must also be abnormal, resulting in a vicious circle, namely haem deficiency—iron accumulation—distortion of mitochondria—abnormal function—haem deficiency. It has been suggested that the accumulation of iron on the mitchondria may be the primary cause of haem deficiency [35]. However, against this is the observation that if iron deficiency co-exists with sideroblastic anaemia, ring sideroblasts are not seen [56, 57]. Cartwright & Deiss [44a] have investigated the formation of ringed sideroblasts. The form of iron (i.e. ferric or ferrous) which is presented to the mitochondria is not known. There is evidence that iron is accumulated by an ATP-dependent pathway or by passive absorption. There appears to be a small free-iron pool within the mitochondria which may be available for haem synthesis (Fig. 13.5).

Other inclusion bodies can be seen by electron microscopy in the erythroblasts of patients with sideroblastic anaemia. Several workers have noted free ferritin granules in the cytoplasm [46–50, 52], but this has been questioned [5]. Another feature is the iron-laden spherical vesicles, 0·6–0·8 μm in diameter, which have been termed siderosomes [58, 59]. They have been observed in normal proerythroblasts [46], and it has

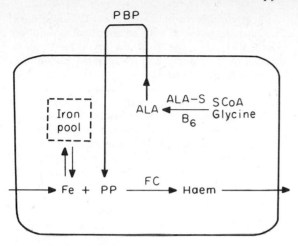

Fig. 13.5. Diagrammatic representation of intramitochrondrial iron pathways. Fe: iron; PP: protoporphyrin; Fc: ferrochelatase; ScoA: succinyl CoA; ALA: aminolaevulinic acid; ALA-S: aminolaevulinic-acid synthase; B_6: pyridoxal-5′-phosphate; and PBP: porphyrin biosynthetic pathway. (Reproduced with permission of Cartwright & Deiss [44a].)

been suggested that they are lysosomes [4]. Glycogen granules have also been observed [47].

THE BIOCHEMICAL DEFECT IN SIDEROBLASTIC ANAEMIA

The specific biochemical abnormalities of the erythroblast which cause sideroblastic anaemia and the morphological changes outlined above are still not clear. From the experimental evidence which has been reported it has been concluded that it is defective synthesis of haem. It could be argued, however, that much of this evidence is indirect. Nevertheless, when it is examined in terms of the normal synthesis of haemoglobin, and especially when it is compared with the biochemical findings associated with the known haem-deficiency states, which have already been discussed (see p. 547), this conclusion becomes more acceptable.

HAEMOGLOBIN SYNTHESIS IN SIDEROBLASTIC ANAEMIA

The experimental studies reported on the synthesis of haemoglobin in patients suffering from a sideroblastic anaemia have indicated that the disturbances in porphyrin metabolism and globin synthesis outlined above are also present.

Disturbances in porphyrin metabolism have been

reported to be associated with all types of sideroblastic anaemia. These are mainly an increase in the levels of coproporphyrin and a decrease in the levels of protoporphyrin, or *vice versa*. With respect to haem and globin synthesis, initial studies on the *in-vitro* incorporation of radioactive glycine and valine into bone-marrow precursors indicated that less haem was synthesized than globin [60–62]. Later it was shown that in the reticulocytes of these patients a large proportion of the α- and β-globin chains synthesized were not associated with haemoglobin but were free within the cell as αβ dimers (Fig. 13.6). This suggests that the defect in haemoglobin synthesis must be due to a deficiency of haem; the same pattern is seen in iron deficiency and lead poisoning. This was confirmed when it was shown that the addition of haem to the reticulocytes not only stimulated globin synthesis but also removed the free chains with the formation of haemoglobin [63] (Fig. 13.7). Collectively, therefore, this evidence indicates that the basic molecular abnormality is a defective synthesis of haem in the erythroblasts. The problem has been to locate the block in haem synthesis. Specific defects of some enzymes in the haem pathway (e.g. ALA synthase, uroporphyrinogen decarboxylase and ferrochelatase) have been reported in isolated cases [61, 64, 65]. However, in the largest study [66], on the reticulocytes of 13 patients, the

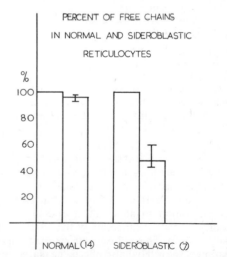

Fig. 13.6. Percentage of free newly synthesized α- and β-globin chains within reticulocytes of patients suffering from sideroblastic anaemia, compared to normal reticulocytes. Thirty to 50% of the α and β chains synthesized within the sideroblastic reticulocyte are *not* associated with haemoglobin (haem-free) but are free within the cell as αβ dimers. In each pair, the left-hand box represents *total* globin in the cell, that on the right, globin combined as haemoglobin.

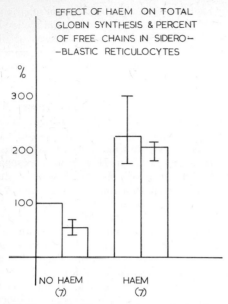

EFFECT OF HAEM ON TOTAL GLOBIN SYNTHESIS & PERCENT OF FREE CHAINS IN SIDERO—BLASTIC RETICULOCYTES

Fig. 13.7. The effect of haem on the synthesis of α- and β-globin chains *in vitro*. The addition of haem not only stimulates the total synthesis of the globin chains, but also converts most of the chains into haemoglobin, thus removing the free αβ-dimer pool (cf. Fig. 13.6).

activity of all the enzymes in the haem pathway, with the exception of ALA synthase (not measured), was found to be normal.

There are two possible explanations for these discrepancies. First, the activity of the enzymes in the reticulocytes may not reflect their activity in bone-marrow precursors; secondly, the iron-laden mitochondria may be too severely damaged to be useful in the detection of subtle changes in haem synthesis.

THE CLINICAL AND HAEMATOLOGICAL CONSEQUENCES OF DEFECTIVE HAEM SYNTHESIS

Although the sideroblastic anaemias are a diverse group, there are certain clinical and haematological features common to all of them due to the basic pathology, namely the inability of the erythroblast to synthesize haem. This not only affects the haemoglobinization of the cell but also affects the maturation of red cells and their delivery to the peripheral blood, resulting in an uncompensated anaemia. This, in turn, leads to an excessive absorption and accumulation of iron resulting eventually in a secondary haemosiderosis.

The anaemia associated with sideroblastic anaemia is dyshaemopoietic. Marked erythroid hyperplasia is found in the bone marrow, with a lowering or reversal of the myeloid/erythroid ratio. Many cells also show the features associated with an abnormal maturation (see p. 123). The nuclei of the erythroblasts have megaloblastic features and binucleated and multinucleated forms may be obvious. The intermediate and late normoblasts are often macrocytic and the cytoplasm, as well as being poorly haemoglobinized, is ragged and contains several perinuclear vacuoles. The latter represent areas which contain iron-laden mitochondria. Reticulum cells are seen in increased numbers and are often observed actively phagocytosing degenerate normoblasts. The factors responsible for the dyshaemopoiesis are unknown; it is not confined to the sideroblastic anaemias, but is associated with any anaemia in which haemoglobinization of the cell is defective (even iron deficiency: R. Hill, personal communication). It would appear that the normal synthesis of haemoglobin in the maturing cell must influence its maturation and division, but there is no evidence as to how this takes place.

The dyshaemopoiesis is reflected by an inappropriate reticulocyte response in the presence of severe anaemia and is largely responsible for the increased bilirubin levels and the increased production of 'early-labelled' bile pigment [67] found in some patients (see Chapter 4, p. 131). Curiously, however, the levels of serum lactate dehydrogenase, a sensitive index of dyshaemopoiesis, have been found to be normal [68, 69]. Nevertheless, other more sensitive indices, such as the production of carbon monoxide [70] and the *in-vivo* utilization of injected ^{59}Fe, have confirmed that marked intramedullary destruction of red cells is occurring [71, 72]. The clinical features associated with dyshaemopoiesis, namely expansion of the bone-marrow spaces resulting in frontal bossing, etc., are not usually seen in patients with sideroblastic anaemia, probably because of the late onset of the anaemia. However, other features such as hepatosplenomegaly are usually present to a moderate degree in the hereditary variety. Retardation of growth, however, is exceptional. Five patients with hereditary sideroblastic anaemia whom we have studied have not shown any disturbances in endocrine function, nor have any been reported.

THE SIDEROBLASTIC ANAEMIAS

Any classification of the sideroblastic anaemias is at present unsatisfactory. However, it is convenient to categorize them depending on whether the condition is inherited or acquired, secondary to drugs or systemic disease, and whether the anaemia responds to pyridoxine. The classification presented here (Table 13.1) has been adapted from that of Kushner *et al.* [73]. It may be artificial and undoubtedly will have to be modified as

Table 13.1. Classification of the sideroblastic anaemias

Type	Possible aetiology
1 *Hereditary*	
A X-linked	
(i) Pyridoxine-responsive	Inborn errors of metabolism, probably due to abnormal structure or
(ii) Pyridoxine-refractory	synthesis of one of the enzymes in the haem pathway. Relationships
(a) Anaemia hypochromica	with pyridoxine metabolism uncertain
Sideroblastica	
Hereditaria	
(b) Others	
B Autosomal	
(i) Pyridoxine-responsive	
2 *Acquired*	
A Primary idiopathic	? Somatic mutation of clone of erythroblasts. Abnormality expressed
(i) Pyridoxine-refractory	as defective haem synthesis. Separation of groups ? artificial
(ii) Pyridoxine-responsive	
B Secondary	
(i) Specific:	
Malabsorption	? True pyridoxine deficiency
Haemolysis	
Alcohol	? Defective phosphorylation of pyridoxine→pyridoxal
Antituberculous drugs	Chemical inhibitors of pyridoxine metabolism. Sensitive population
Lead	Inhibitors of enzymes in haem pathway. Chelates with —SH groups
Chloramphenicol	Mitochondrial toxin, inhibits protein synthesis; sensitive population
(ii) Non-specific:	
Myeloproliferative disorders	Unknown
Leukaemia	
Secondary malignancy	

more biochemical data become available. Recently, Bottomley [8] has classified these disorders into 'reversible' and 'irreversible' types, which may be a more realistic clinical approach.

The first group is the hereditary sideroblastic anaemias in which the abnormality is usually inherited in an X-linked recessive fashion. It can be further subdivided into those patients who respond to pyridoxine and those who are refractory.

The second, and larger, group is made up of the acquired sideroblastic anaemias and is subdivided into those in which no cause is apparent, idiopathic acquired, and those in which the condition is associated with specific toxins or systemic disease, secondary acquired. Each subgroup can be further classified depending on the response to pyridoxine. They will be considered separately as regards the clinical features, haematological and biochemical findings and pathogenesis. The treatment, complications and prognosis of each group will be considered collectively.

HEREDITARY SIDEROBLASTIC ANAEMIA
Probable cases of hereditary sideroblastic anaemia were reported in 1945 and 1946 [77, 78] but the familial nature of the disease was not confirmed until 1965 [71, 79]. In the literature there are reports of four families which clearly demonstrate the X-linkage of this abnormality [80–83]. In two of these families, X-linkage was strongly supported by a concomitant inheritance with the Xg^A antigen [81] and G6PD deficiency [83] although subsequent studies [87] did not confirm the Xg^A association. Reports of other families lack precise data but are probably further examples [2, 35, 80–84]. In most of these families there is a preponderance of severely affected males. It is interesting that in the family reported by Cottom & Harris [89], the inheritance was consistent with an autosomal gene. Amongst the X-linked variety three other subgroups can be found, but it is not clear whether or not the distinction is real. The first group consists of those patients who respond to pyridoxine [2, 35, 83, 86]; the second group are those who are refractory [81, 84, 85, 87]; and the third group are patients who have increased levels of coproporphyrin and decreased levels of protoporphyrin [84, 85] in contrast to the findings in the majority of patients with hereditary sideroblastic anaemia. This type has been termed 'anaemia hypochromica sideroblastica hereditaria'.

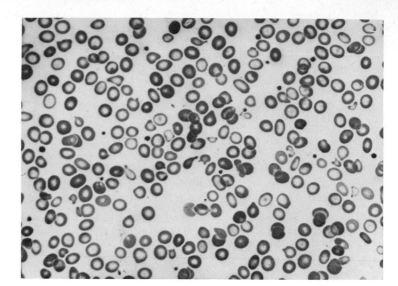

Fig. 13.8. Photograph of peripheral blood of a patient suffering from hereditary sideroblastic anaemia. (May–Grünwald–Giemsa stain, × 570.) The red cells are largely hypochromic but some normochromic cells are present.

The age of onset of the anaemia varies from the first year of life to after the third decade [5]. Presentation at birth is extremely rare but not unknown.

Apart from anaemia, there are no specific physical signs. However, growth retardation may be apparent, but is not common, as is mild or moderate spleno-megaly; other features such as frontal bossing are uncommon.

The haematological findings are quite characteristic. The MCH is usually 20–24 pg or lower, and the MCV is between 74–85 fl. These values are never increased, in contrast to the primary acquired sideroblastic anaemias. Also, in family members who do not appear to be affected these values are significantly reduced. The circulating red cells are predominantly hypochromic but variable numbers of normochromic cells are always seen (Figs 13.8 and 13.9). Basophilic stippling of the red cells may be a prominent feature and a few normoblasts are usually seen. Siderocytes are rarely numerous unless the spleen has been removed. The leucocyte and platelet counts are normal or slightly reduced and the reticulocyte count is also usually normal, but occasionally it can be raised in the five per cent range. Bone-marrow preparations show a reduction in the myeloid/erythroid ratio. The maturation of red-cell precursors is usually normoblastic, but vacuo-

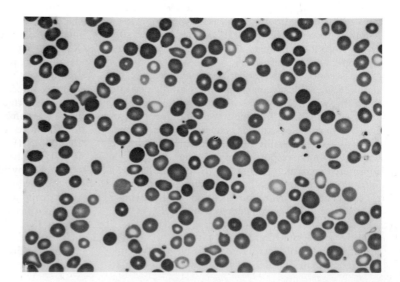

Fig. 13.9. Photomicrograph of peripheral blood of patient suffering from hereditary sideroblastic anaemia. (May–Grünwald–Giemsa stain, × 570.) The cells are mainly normochromic but some hypochromic cells are present. The morphology differs from that of the patient shown in Figure 13.8.

lation of the cytoplasm is often present, especially in the later forms. Iron staining shows that the majority of late red-cell precursors are ring sideroblasts (Fig. 13.10). Iron-laden mitochondria are only seen in the late normoblasts [75]. This might explain why, in the congenital form, the mature red cell is very hypochromic. Wickramasinghe [76] has also demonstrated that ineffective haemoglobinization is the major defect rather than defective division of erythroblasts.

The serum iron is usually raised and the plasma transferrin, though normal in amount, is usually saturated. The clearance of ^{59}Fe is greatly increased but the iron utilization is depressed. The ^{51}Cr I$_{\frac{1}{2}}$ is usually only slightly reduced. The level of Hb F is not increased, while that of Hb A$_2$ is usually reduced [5]; there is increased 'i' antigen on the red-cell membrane [48, 90].

The diagnosis is usually not difficult and is made by the combination of anaemia, ring sideroblasts in the bone marrow, and the finding of affected family members. The usual problem is to find a severely affected male whose mother, though not anaemic, shows a small population of hypochromic cells. Occasionally, severely affected females are encountered. The differential diagnosis rests between other causes of inherited hypochromic anaemia (e.g. thalassaemia), or congenital dyserythropoietic anaemia (see p. 569 and Chapter 31). The former can usually be excluded by the elevated levels of Hb A$_2$ and/or Hb F and the absence of ring sideroblasts in the marrow. Congenital dyserythropoietic anaemia can be excluded by the absence of multinucleation of erythroblasts and internuclear or intercytoplasmic bridges.

The finding of a positive family history is important but it is not essential. Not infrequently, cases arise *de novo*.

The biochemical abnormality
No conclusive abnormalities of haem synthesis have been found in these patients. However, porphyrin metabolism within the red cells is usually disturbed. The most consistent defect is that of raised levels of coporporphyrin and normal or reduced levels of protoporphyrin [59, 86]. Vogler & Mingioli [86] found that there was a marked decrease of glycine-2-^{14}C incorporation into haem with a slight reduction of incorporation of ALA into the marrow precursors of three affected patients.

Studies on three patients—two of whom were siblings—showed that in the siblings the levels of free protoporphyrin IX were decreased, whilst in the other patient they were increased. Red-cell coproporphyrin levels were not measured. In the reticulocytes of the brothers, globin-chain synthesis was stimulated *in vitro* by the addition of ALA as well as by haem, whilst in the other child only haem was effective [91] (Fig. 13.11). It was inferred from these findings that the brothers had a block in haem synthesis at or above the level of ALA, whilst in the other patient the block was at the level of the ferrochelatase. It is noteworthy that these patients differed in their age of presentation and in the morphology of their peripheral bloods (Figs 13.8 and 13.9). One possible explanation for these findings is that in the siblings with decreased levels of protoporphyrin IX there was a secondary defect of coproporphyrinogenase. In the other patient with an increased

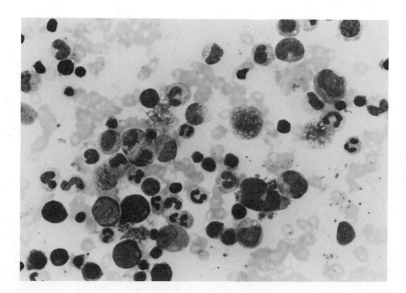

Fig. 13.10. Photomicrograph of bone marrow of patient suffering from hereditary sideroblastic anaemia. (May–Grünwald–Giemsa stain, × 570.) Increased numbers of erythroblasts are seen, the maturation of which is abnormal. Note the degeneration of cytoplasm of the later normoblasts.

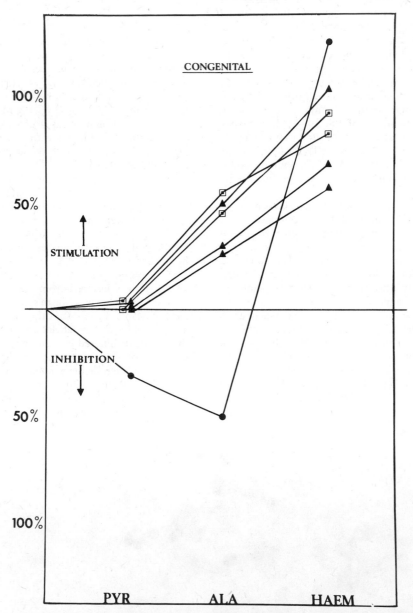

Fig. 13.11. Effect of: pyridoxine (PYR); δ aminolaevulinic acid (ALA); and haematin hydrochloride (haemin) on the *in-vitro* synthesis of globin by reticulocytes of three patients with hereditary sideroblastic anaemia. Patients ▲ and □ were siblings in which globin synthesis was stimulated by ALA and haemin, whereas in the other patient, ●, only haem was effective.

level of protoporphyrin IX the defect may have been due to a deficiency of protoporphyrin oxidase or of ferrochelatase, or a reduced negative feedback inhibiting ALA synthase.

In some patients the erythrocyte glycine and glutamate levels were increased, indicating a reduction in the condensation of succinyl Co-A and glycine for ALA formation [76a]. A marked reduction of ALA synthase has been reported in several cases [93–95].

It is apparent that amongst patients with congenital sideroblastic anaemia there is marked heterogeneity, not only in the clinical presentation of the condition but also in the biochemical defects. The condition represents a very broad spectrum of biochemical defects. As suggested by Bottomley [8], at present there are no data to discount a primary defect of the mitochondria or iron transport.

At present, one can only infer that patients with hereditary sideroblastic anaemia have an abnormality of one of the enzymes associated with porphyrin or haem synthesis. However, until better techniques are available to determine the activity of these enzymes, this problem will not be settled.

PRIMARY (IDIOPATHIC) SIDEROBLASTIC ANAEMIA

Clinical features

Primary sideroblastic anaemia probably reflects a mutation of stem cells and is considered by many to be a 'pre-leukaemic' disorder. There is very good evidence that it is due to a defect of haem synthesis (see p. 551). This condition is characterized by an onset late in life, lack of affected family members and no history of drug exposure or systemic disease. It occurs equally in males and females. Patients with this disorder have been subdivided by some workers into those who respond to pyridoxine and those who are refractory to this agent [4, 73]. Pyridoxine-responsive anaemias will be considered separately.

The first cases of primary acquired sideroblastic anaemia were reported by Bjorkman in 1963 [92] and since then it has become recognized as a distinct, and not uncommon, clinical entity. (For reviews see Refs 5, 73, 96, 97 and 104.) Kushner *et al.* [73] have suggested that this diagnosis should be confined to those patients who fulfil all of the following criteria: chronic anaemia; ring sideroblasts in the marrow; lack of family history; no history of other systemic diseases, nutritional deficiency or drug exposure; and, finally, a failure to respond to haematinics, in particular to large doses of pyridoxine. They found that 80% of 97 cases reported as examples of primary idiopathic sideroblastic anaemia fulfilled all these criteria.

The age of onset of the disease is usually during or after the fifth decade but often long histories of anaemia can be elicited. The red-cell indices contrast with those found in the inherited variety. The MCHC is usually normal, 30–34%, and the MCV is increased to 100–120 fl. The morphological picture of the red cells is usually normochromic and macrocytic but some hypochromic cells are always seen (Fig. 13.12). Rarely, the red cells may be very hypochromic [56]. Anisocytosis and poikilocytosis may be marked and stippled cells and normoblasts are often evident. The reticulocyte count is usually normal or slightly elevated.

The leucocyte count is usually normal but approximately 30% of cases are reported to have developed leucopenia at some time. The platelet count is usually normal but thrombocytopenia has been observed on occasions in 20% of cases; thrombocytosis has also been described.

The differential leucocyte count is usually normal but both eosinophilia (13%) and monocytosis (18%) have been reported. A monocytosis has been regarded as a pre-terminal finding [56], but in some patients it has been reported as a persistent feature [73]. In nearly 50% of the reported cases the leucocyte alkaline-phosphatase score was low; in 43% it was normal and in three per cent it was elevated.

Bone-marrow preparations show marked erythroid hyperplasia; the mean myeloid/erythroid ratio is 1:1 [73]. The maturation of the red-cell precursors contrasts with that associated with hereditary sideroblastic anaemia. It is usually macronormoblastic, the late precursors having abundant cytoplasm which is often vacuolated [5] (Fig. 13.13). Megaloblastic changes have been found in 20% of reported cases. Reduced folate levels have been found in some patients, but in the majority the level is normal, as is the deoxyuridine suppression test.

On iron staining, many of the precursors are abnormal ring sideroblasts. Their numbers vary and range from 50 to 100%.

The degree of periodic-acid-Schiff (PAS) positivity of the marrow cells is usually normal [73, 99, 100], but Barry & Day [56] found high levels in two patients. This is an important investigation in the differentiation of this condition from Di Guglielmo's disease.

At the time of diagnosis, 50% of patients have increased serum iron levels and reduced iron-binding capacity. Rarely, however, this may be normal. The plasma turnover is increased but the marrow transit time is prolonged and iron incorporation is reduced. These studies indicate active erythropoiesis associated with intramedullary death and recycling of iron in the marrow. A common change in iron kinetics during the progression of the disorder is initially a reduction of iron utilization, then the picture of ineffective erythropoiesis and, finally, in some patients a pattern of aplastic anaemia [101]. Bottomley [102] has shown, *in*

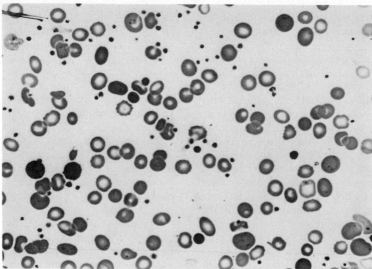

Fig.13.12. Photomicrograph of peripheral blood of patient suffering from idiopathic acquired sideroblastic anaemia. The spleen has been removed. (May–Grünwald–Giemsa stain, × 570.) The cells are macrocytic and dimorphic. Many siderocytes are seen.

vitro, an abnormal uptake of iron by erythroblasts, with an increased uptake by mitochondria. Also, Riedler & Straub [103] have shown that the hypochromic population of red cells has a reduced uptake of iron and a decreased red-cell survival compared with a moderate reduction of both of these measurements in the normochromic cells.

Cellular, genetic and biochemical abnormalities
A question of major importance in relationship to the

diagnosis and therapy of the acquired sideroblastic anaemias is whether they are clonal disorders. The observation that the red cells and all the white-cell series, including the lymphocytes, of a Negro female with sideroblastic anaemia who was also heterozygous for both A and B glucose-6-phosphate dehydrogenase isozymes were of a single type provides strong evidence for the clonal origin of this disorder [103a]. This observation is of particular interest because it suggests that the underlying cellular transformation which was

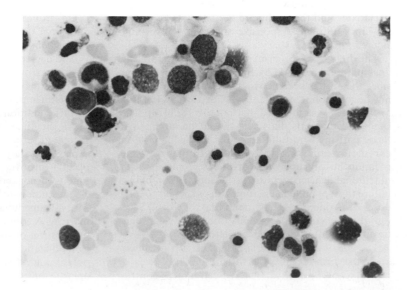

Fig. 13.13. Photomicrograph of bone-marrow preparation of patient suffering from idiopathic acquired sideroblastic anaemia. (May–Grünwald–Giemsa stain, × 570.) Erythropoiesis shows macronormoblastic maturation, with vacuolation of the cytoplasm of normoblasts.

responsible for this sideroblastic anaemia must have occurred in an early stem-cell population which still had the potential to differentiate both down the erythroid, granulocyte and lymphoid lines. Further evidence for the clonal origin of primary acquired sideroblastic anaemia is reviewed by Bottomley [8]. She points out that there is often an associated defect in the lymphoid/macrophage system in this disorder. Thus sideroblastic anaemia is frequently associated with other autoimmune disorders such as rheumatoid arthritis [104], lupus erythematosus [105], malignant lymphoma [105a], immunosuppressive therapy [107] and autoimmune haemolytic anaemia [106]. Chromosomal defects are found in about 50% of cases. These usually are characterized by trisomy 8 but other random defects have been reported.

As stated previously, the two red-cell lines have different functional characteristics in terms of the uptake of iron and *in-vivo* survival. If the evidence is correct, primary acquired sideroblastic anaemia can be considered as a clonal disorder in which the basic biochemical defect in the abnormal red-cell progenitor is at the stage of haem synthesis (cf. PNH, p. 532). Changes in red-cell differentiation have been reported by Wickramasinghe [76] and Wickramasinghe & Hughes [108]. There is an arrest of DNA synthesis and delayed entry of G_2 cells into mitosis in early polychromatic erythroblasts. Also, there is a reduction of thymidine uptake into DNA and reduced RNA and protein synthesis. All these abnormalities are correlated with the degree of iron deposition in the mitochrondria. Lourenco *et al.* [109] found that the incorporation of uridine was reduced. It is still unclear whether the nuclear dysfunction is secondary to the mitochondrial abnormality.

The biochemical abnormality has yet to be clearly defined. The most consistent abnormality associated with porphyrin metabolism is an *increase* in the free red-cell protoporphyrin. Heilmeyer [5a] found raised levels in 18 patients, and Kushner *et al.* [73] found raised levels in 16 out of 17 patients. However, Dacie *et al.* [96] found it to be raised in only one out of six patients. The levels of free coproporphyrin reported have also been inconsistent. Seventeen out of the 18 patients reported by Heilmeyer [59] had increased levels, whereas in the 17 patients reported by Kushner *et al.* [73] they were normal or decreased. The activity of ferrochelatase has been found to be normal in 24 patients [66, 73]. Indeed, Vavra & Poff in their study on 13 patients found that the activity of all the enzymes in the haem pathway, with the exception of ALA synthase (not measured), was normal in circulating reticulocytes [66]. However, Waltuch *et al.* [110], suggested that the pattern of incorporation of radioactive glycine and valine into haem and globin by marrow cells in three patients indicated that the synthesis of haem was reduced.

Our own studies on eight patients showed that in mature red cells, free erythrocyte protoporphyrin levels were increased. It was also shown that globin synthesis in the reticulocytes could be stimulated by the addition of haem. Other haem intermediates, pyridoxine and ALA, had no effect (Fig. 13.14). There is no doubt that there is a defect in the synthesis of haem. Most patients have increased levels of erythrocyte protoporphyrin and a reduced incorporation of glycine and ALA into haem. In the majority, there is a defect of ALA synthase and ferrochelatase activity; however, there are exceptions [95, 111]. It is still unresolved as to whether the defects which have been detected are primary, or secondary due to mitochondrial damage caused by excess iron.

It has been reported that a primary enzyme defect can result in excessive accumulation of iron in the mitochondria [112] associated with a reduced ALA synthase activity. Bottomley *et al.* [113] found that patients with hereditary protoporphyria showed a reduced activity of ferrochelatase. Also, the reported reduction of RNA and protein synthesis may be due to an impairment of mitochondrial enzymes. Bottomley [8] has considered the arguments that idiopathic sideroblastic anaemia may be due to a primary defect in iron metabolism. Hunter *et al.* [114], Brown [115] and Morrow *et al.* [116] reported that excessive loading of the mitochondria with iron can impair overall enzyme activity, specifically ALA synthase. This argument is supported by the beneficial effects of removal of total body iron, but the evidence is not convincing (see Hines [116a]). Bottomley [8] has rightly suggested that this problem will only be resolved by investigating the enzyme activity of the early differentiated erythroblasts.

There is much evidence that a normal haem synthesis pathway is required for normal red-cell maturation *in vitro* [117, 118]. This is supported by studies on chloramphenicol by Stathakis *et al.* [120] (see p. 564).

Other intracellular defects in sideroblastic anaemia include an impairment of globin synthesis and iron metabolism. The former is characterized by a reduction of α-chain synthesis [121–123]. Hb H (β_4) has been reported in two patients [124, 125]. With respect to iron metabolism, iron absorption is increased, and during the course of the disease total body iron stores are increased (irrespective of transfusion). The pattern of iron utilization and turnover is compatible with ineffective erythropoiesis [101, 126]. Bottomley [102] has shown an altered uptake of iron by marrow cells and an abnormal distribution of iron in the red-cell precursors.

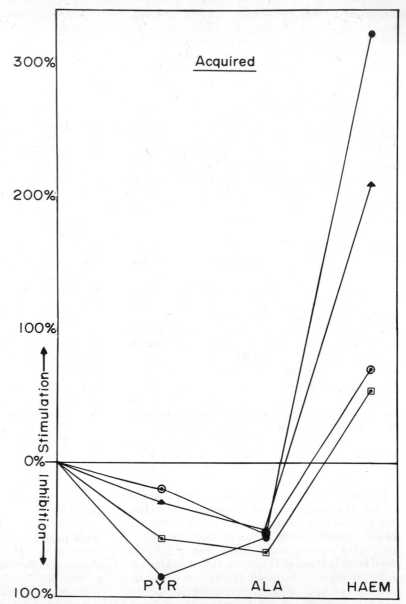

Fig. 13.14. Effect of pyridoxine, δ aminolaevulinic acid and haemin on the synthesis of globin in the reticulocytes of four patients suffering from idiopathic acquired sideroblastic anaemia. Only haemin was effective in stimulating globin synthesis.

From the work of Hrinda & Goldwasser [127] and Storing & Faith [128], it appears that so-far uncharacterized iron-containing factors are required for RNA and protein synthesis in red-cell precursors in response to erythropoietin. Also, storage of iron is maximal during the latter stages of erythrocyte development [129]. It would appear that these two processes can be modified by the iron content of the erythroblast [130, 131]. The intracellular release of iron *in vitro* requires an intact mitochondrial system. Other factors involved

include a low-molecular-weight carrier [128, 132, 133], transferrin [134, 135] and ferritin [136–139]. Also, the normal synthesis of haem appears to be closely linked to iron metabolism in that the presence of an adequate amount of haem is required for the availability of intracellular iron [135, 140]. It is also recognized that it is required for the normal uptake of iron by mitochondria [132, 134]. Within the mitochondria, reduction systems are essential for iron utilization [141–143] and there is some evidence that these require a normal haem synthetic pathway. The sideroblastic anaemias could result from any one of a series of potential defects involving their complex interactions.

In summary, the defect causing primary acquired sideroblastic anaemia may lie at several levels; namely, a defect of transferrin, a defect of the red-cell membrane, cytosolic iron binding, a defect of mitochondrial components or mitochondrial activity.

Thus, it is evident that the aetiology of idiopathic primary sideroblastic anaemia is still unknown. It is undoubtedly an acquired disorder, and progressive, but it is not clear whether one or more aetiological factors are responsible. Kushner *et al.* [73] consider that there are four possible explanations:

1 neoplasia;
2 nutritional deficiency;
3 toxic reaction; and
4 somatic mutation.

They conclude that although each of these mechanisms is possible, somatic mutation is the most likely. The association between sideroblastic anaemia and leukaemia will be considered separately (p. 565). Attention was first drawn to this by Dameshek [144], but his early prediction that all types of sideroblastic anaemia are related to leukaemia has not been borne out.

In favour of nutritional deficiency is the fact that sideroblastic anaemia can result from an acquired deficiency of vitamin B_6 and also that the abnormal maturation of the red cells is not dissimilar to that associated with vitamin-B_{12} or folic-acid deficiency. However, although the metabolism of these compounds may be abnormal in such patients, it is not a consistent finding and haematological remission is never seen when they are given.

Several metabolic inhibitors and cellular toxins are known to cause sideroblastic anaemia and these will be reviewed separately. However, there is no evidence that any of these or related compounds is active in idiopathic acquired sideroblastic anaemia.

The most fashionable explanation at present is that sideroblastic anaemia arises from a somatic (clonal) mutation of an erythroid stem cell (reviewed by Bottomley [8]). In support of this concept is the enzymological, morphological and kinetic evidence of two cell lines, the age of onset of the disease, and the frequency with which leukaemia occurs after a number of years. The rare association of thrombocytopenia and leucopenia has been proposed as further evidence that it could arise from the somatic mutation of a non-committed stem cell [73].

PYRIDOXINE-RESPONSIVE ANAEMIA

Hines & Grasso [4], in their classification of sideroblas-

tic anaemias, chose to separate a group of patients who showed several differences from the majority of patients with primary acquired sideroblastic anaemia, the main difference being that their anaemia remitted on pyridoxine therapy. They stressed other differences, however. The patients are usually young or middle-aged, the anaemia is usually hypochromic, the red-cell maturation is normoblastic and the leucocyte and the platelet counts are normal. However, Mollin & Dacie [145] consider that this separation is artificial. There is evidence for and against both arguments but it will only be settled by a better understanding of the underlying biochemical abnormalities.

The evidence for the role of vitamin B_6 in 'causing' primary acquired sideroblastic anaemia is difficult to evaluate. Some patients, probably about 10%, respond to pharmacological doses (or physiological doses) of vitamin B_6 [95, 146]. Some patients, who do not respond to pyridoxine, respond to pyridoxal phosphate (PLP) [111, 147, 148]. The effectiveness of pyridoxine or PLP has been shown to result from enhancement of the activity of ALA synthase in marrow *in vitro* and *in vivo* [95, 111]. However, although the haematological and bone-marrow abnormalities improve, they never return to normal. It is significant that if either the vitamin or its intermediates are withdrawn the patient relapses. However, the improvement is always accompanied by an increase of erythrocyte protoporphyrin, which has led Bottomley [111], Konopka & Hoffbrand [95] and Solomon & Hillman [149] to conclude that the activity of ferrochelatase (haem synthetase) is defective, or that the supply of ferrous iron is rate limiting.

There is no correlation between the severity of the disorder and its responsiveness to pyridoxine or PLP (see p. 566). However, Bottomley [8] has suggested that it may be an index of the 'supply' of pyridoxine or PLP to the erythron or, specifically, the mitochondria. Also, the activity of ALA synthase may be enhanced. However, overall there is no consistent pattern of defects of pyridoxine metabolism apart from a very few isolated cases. In summary, although pyridoxine may be of value in approximately 30% of cases, the biochemical pharmacology of this vitamin in relation to the disease is poorly understood.

The majority of these patients achieve normal haemoglobin levels after pyridoxine therapy and withdrawal of the vitamin usually results in a relapse in two to three months. Other haematinics are usually of no value. Doses of pyridoxine of the order of 25–200 mg/day are required for remission, but even when the haemoglobin levels become normal, sideroblasts still remain in the bone marrow and the haematological picture remains slightly abnormal [5]. The serum iron values have been reported to return to normal. Nevertheless, the patients eventually manifest the signs and symptoms of haemosiderosis [5].

These patients cannot yet be distinguished from those who are refractory to pyridoxine therapy since the clinical and biochemical features are similar. Moreover, there is no evidence for defective haem synthesis, nor for pyridoxine deficiency, although 80% of the patients have evidence of abnormal tryptophan metabolism [146].

Some insight into the pathogenesis of this type of sideroblastic anaemia has been obtained by Hines & Grasso [4]. Detailed studies on one patient showed that $19\frac{1}{2}$ months after withdrawal of pyridoxine the patient's packed cell volume fell to 32%, the serum iron rose, and he manifested the full clinical and haematological picture of sideroblastic anaemia. Sequential biochemical studies over this period showed that the serum and red-cell folate levels decreased, as did the levels of pyridoxal phosphate. The patient was treated with 0·1–1·0 mg of pyridoxine, following which the packed cell volume rose to 46%, the iron-binding capacity fell to 35%, the PLP level rose to 29–36 ng/ml, and the red-cell folate became normal. The morphology of the marrow at this time was not reported. These authors postulated that in this group of patients the defect lies in the conversion of pyridoxine to PLP and that the disorder is due to a deficiency of the latter. This receives some support from Gehrmann [33] who showed that three similar patients responded better to PLP than to pyridoxine.

THE SECONDARY SIDEROBLASTIC ANAEMIA

These are the commonest sideroblastic anaemias. At present they are best divided into those resulting from:

1 defective pyridoxine metabolism;
2 defects of enzymes in the haem pathway;
3 mitochondrial poisons;
4 systemic disease, in which cases the cause of sideroblastic anaemia is unknown.

The degree of anaemia and morphological abnormality associated with these types of sideroblastic anaemia is extremely variable; it may be severe on occasions. However, the degree of sideroblastic change in the bone marrow is rarely gross. The anaemia does not usually respond to treatment but follows the progress of the primary disease; removal of the offending agent often results in remission.

DISORDERS OF PYRIDOXINE METABOLISM

Pyridoxine (vitamin B_6) deficiency
Sideroblastic anaemia resulting from a deficiency of pyridoxine has yet to be documented in man. How-

ever, there are several instances where such a deficiency can be incriminated indirectly. Intestinal disease resulting in malabsorption should, in theory, result in pyridoxine deficiency, but the association of malabsorption and sideroblastic anaemia is rare. Mollin & Hoffbrand [5] reported that they had seen such cases, all of whom also had nutritional megaloblastic anaemia. When these patients were treated with folic acid and given normal hospital diets, the sideroblastic change remitted [5]. Dawson *et al.* [150] reported a case of sideroblastic anaemia associated with gluten-sensitive coeliac disease. Both the sideroblastic change and the steatorrhoea remitted on a gluten-free diet. Possible reasons for the apparent rarity of this association include lack of attention to marrow morphology and concomitant iron deficiency [150].

We have recently seen three patients with chronic haemolysis and sideroblastic anaemia. All were shown to have abnormal tryptophan metabolism, and in each case the anaemia responded to oral pyridoxine [151]. None of the patients was deficient in folic acid, but all were ill and sustained on poor diets. It is possible that in times of chronic marrow stress, the requirements for pyridoxine may increase. Petz & Goodman [51] have described two similar patients with chronic haemolysis who developed sideroblastic change. They concluded, however, that it was due to the hyperferraemic state of these individuals.

Defects in the conversion of pyridoxine to pyridoxal-5'-phosphate
The pathway for the conversion of pyridoxine to pyridoxal has already been discussed (p. 548). There is now growing evidence to incriminate abnormalities in this pathway as a cause of sideroblastic anaemia. Such cases are those caused by alcohol and antituberculous drugs, and recent evidence indicates that defective conversion of pyridoxine to its active form, pyridoxal phosphate (PLP), may be responsible for some cases of idiopathic acquired sideroblastic anaemia and pyridoxine-responsive sideroblastic anaemia.

Alcohol intoxication appears to be the most common cause of sideroblastic anaemia—at least in the USA [4, 152]. The anaemia is dimorphic and associated with both sideroblastic and megaloblastic changes in the bone marrow. Patients are nearly always deficient in folic acid, magnesium and potassium. The condition is easily reversible in hours, after withdrawal of alcohol [48, 153], and the degree of iron overloading of the red-cell precursors is less than in idiopathic sideroblastic anaemia [14]. Hines & Gowan [154] induced sideroblastic anaemia in two out of three volunteers maintained on excessive alcohol intake and a folate-deficient diet. All three showed the biochemical abnormalities of alcohol intoxication and also the conversion of pyridoxine to pyridoxal phosphate was found to be defective. The sideroblastic change did not remit following treatment with pyridoxine or folic acid, but remitted rapidly with parenteral PLP. The association between this condition and folic-acid deficiency is not certain: it is nearly always present but on occasions the level of serum folate may be normal [4]. Low erythrocyte and plasma PLP levels have been reported [116, 148, 155, 156]. Others, however, found that the intracellular levels were normal [149, 157]. The conversion of infused pyridoxine to PLP has been found to be reduced, as has the activity of pyridoxal kinase [154]. However, the exact biochemical explanation is still unclear.

More recently, evidence has been reported that defective conversion of pyridoxine to pyridoxal is also present in patients with idiopathic acquired sideroblastic anaemia refractory to pyridoxine [4], and also in patients who are responsive [33]. However, these findings have yet to be confirmed.

The antituberculous drugs isoniazid, cycloserine and pyrazinamide, given either alone or in combination, are well recognized as causing secondary sideroblastic anaemia [82, 158]. The incidence of sideroblastic anaemia in patients receiving these drugs is low, which would indicate that there is a 'high-risk' population. The highest incidence is reported by Roberts *et al.* [159] who found increased numbers of abnormal sideroblasts in 16 out of 28 non-anaemic tuberculous patients taking isoniazid (INH) or para-aminosalicylic acid (PAS) for six months or more; INH alone or with PAS rarely causes anaemia, but after several months sideroblastic changes in the bone marrow are often detected [160–163]. In contrast, cycloserine and pyrazinamide readily produce anaemia [32, 163].

The exact action of these drugs *in vivo* is unknown and appears to be multifactorial. Isoniazid (INH) has been the most studied drug and several defects in the haem synthetic pathway have been reported; the formation of a hydrozone complex with PLP, inhibition of pyridoxine kinase, enhanced urinary excretion of pyridoxine [164–166], decreased ALA synthase in the bone marrow corrected by PLP [95], decreased ALA synthase activity [167], and increased uptake of iron into reticulocytes [132].

The action of cycloserine or pyrazinamide has not been well studied. However, cycloserine inhibits PLP-dependent enzymes and also inactivates PLP [82, 164].

SPECIFIC INHIBITORS OF ENZYMES IN THE HAEM PATHWAY: LEAD

Effects of lead on red-cell metabolism (see also p.592)
Lead is the only common agent known to inhibit enzymes in the haem pathway and thus to cause a

sideroblastic anaemia [1, 59, 169]. However, marked erythroblastic changes are rare [8, 170]. Lead affects all enzymes of the haem pathway but to a varying degree [102]. The mechanism is probably due to chelation with the —SH groups of the enzymes. ALA dehydratase is the most sensitive, followed by haem synthase, coproporphyrin oxidase and uroporphyrin-I synthase respectively. ALA synthase, in contrast to earlier reports, is stimulated, probably due to a decrease in the availability of haem [171, 172].

Bottomley [8] has pointed out the variation between the *in-vitro* effects of lead and the degree of disordered metabolism found *in vivo*, and has suggested that they may be explained by the defects of iron and/or copper metabolism *in vivo*. For example, iron decreases lead absorption and thus iron deficiency would enhance it. Also, iron inhibits lead uptake by red cells [173] and, conversely, lead decreases, by competitive binding to the active site of iron uptake, the transport of iron across the membrane. Williams *et al.* [143] have suggested that the pattern of iron metabolism caused by lead toxicity is similar to that caused by copper deficiency, and that the effects of lead upon iron may be indirectly due to a defect in copper metabolism. Copper deficiency potentiates the anaemia of lead toxicity and stimulates ferrochelatase [174]. Another explanation is that the effect of lead is mainly upon cytochrome oxidase, thus inhibiting the reduction of iron to the ferrous form.

Therefore, in spite of the known effects of lead on haem synthesis, the apparent lack of sideroblastic changes may be due, either directly or via disturbed copper metabolism, to iron metabolism. There is usually a marked increased in the excretion of urinary coproporphyrin which may exceed 1 mg/day and urinary ALA levels may be as high as 40 mg/day. There is an increased urinary porphobilinogen and a high proportion of patients show fluorescence of their erythrocytes; there is a marked increase in erythrocyte protoporphyrin zinc. In addition, lead causes an abnormal accumulation of iron in the red-cell precursors and may shorten the red-cell lifespan by a direct action on the membrane cationic pumps [175]. It also causes a retardation of globin synthesis; the associated basophilic stippling is produced by aggregations of altered ribosomes.

Lead poisoning
Lead poisoning in adults occurs as the result of either industrial exposure or, occasionally, improper storage or transport of water. In young children, the most common cause is pica, although outbreaks due to contaminated water supplies are still reported occasionally in the younger age groups. Plumbism occurs in two main forms: an acute encephalopathy, or a more

chronic disorder associated either with intermittent abdominal colic or a peripheral neuropathy. The gastro-intestinal syndrome is, in general, more common than the encephalitic and this is particularly the case in adults who have inhaled organic lead dust. The encephalitic form is seen mainly in children or after tetraethyl lead poisoning. In children the condition, which has a distinct seasonal peak incidence in the summer months, is characterized by irritability, anorexia, failure to gain weight, behavioural disturbances and, if untreated, a progression to convulsions, mania and coma. The physical signs are variable. In mild cases there may be pallor and sometimes a lead line on the gums. In cases with more severe neurological involvement there may be evidence of meningeal irritation, optic atrophy, and raised intracranial pressure. Adults with the more chronic form of lead poisoning complain either of intermittent attacks of colic associated with constipation, irritability, depression and anorexia or weakness of the limbs. Diarrhoea and epileptiform attacks have been described. There is an increased incidence of gout. A lead line may be seen on the gums and there may be evidence of peripheral neuropathy, particularly wrist or foot drop. The relationship between these clinical changes and the associated abnormalities of porphyrin metabolism is uncertain [176]. The long-term complications include mental deficiency in affected children [177, 178]. Thus, in a survey of 425 children who had survived lead poisoning, 61% had no sequelae, 22% were mentally retarded, 20% had seizures, one per cent had optic atrophy and two per cent had cerebral palsy. There is also a possibility of chronic renal damage in patients who have had severe lead poisoning.

The haematological changes in lead poisoning are extremely variable. In the more severe cases, there is usually a moderate degree of anaemia with a slightly elevated reticulocyte count, polychromasia, punctate basophilia, and an increased red-cell osmotic fragility. There is a shortened red-cell survival and the red cells have a shorter life than normal when transfused into a normal recipient. These changes may result from the toxic effects of lead on the membrane pumps. The bone marrow shows erythroid hyperplasia and variable numbers of ring sideroblasts. The plasma clearance rate for ^{59}Fe is often slow and there is a reduced amount of incorporation into haemoglobin; these changes are reversible, however. Children with lead poisoning very frequently have an associated iron deficiency and, in such cases, haemoglobin electrophoresis may show a rapidly migrating haemoglobin component in the general region of haemoglobin A_3 (see Chapter 8). The plasma iron level is often elevated in adults with lead poisoning.

The diagnosis of lead poisoning cannot be made by any single parameter and requires such evidence as a history of exposure, the finding of basophilic stippling of the red cells, the haematological changes already described, the presence of increased lead in the urine, or an increased blood level of lead together with changes in porphyrins outlined above. The degree of basophilic stippling is a poor indicator of the degree of lead poisoning and does not correlate well with the clinical severity; it is more marked in marrow than peripheral blood [179]. Some of these diagnostic features are summarized in Table 13.2. Although clinical lead poisoning is usually seen with blood lead levels above 80 μg/100 ml, haem synthesis may be inhibited by levels as low as 20 μg/100 ml. The importance of such subclinical lead poisoning is not yet worked out [180]. The management of lead poisoning is reviewed on page 567.

Table 13.2. The laboratory diagnosis of lead poisoning

Haematological changes
  Anaemia
  Basophilic stippling
  Reticulocytosis
  Ring sideroblasts in the marrow
  Raised serum iron (in adults)
  'Fast' haemoglobin (in children with associated iron
    deficiency)

Lead determinations
  Increased blood lead*
  Increased urinary lead
  Increased urinary lead after EDTA

Porphyrin changes
  Increased urinary ALA
  Increased urinary porphobilinogen (rarely)
  Increased urinary coproporphyrin III
  Increased erythrocyte protoporphyrin

* The problem of relating levels of lead in the blood to the clinical manifestations of lead poisoning is considered in the text.

MITOCHONDRIAL TOXINS
Chloramphenicol in therapeutic doses can cause a reversible sideroblastic anaemia in some patients [182, 183]. The mechanism of action is not clear, but it would appear that there is a sensitive population of individuals. Beck & Gabathuler [183] showed that in patients who were not sensitive, chloramphenicol would not cause depression of haem synthesis *in vitro*, whereas in three sensitive patients a 37% reduction of haem synthesis was demonstrated. One explanation is that chloramphenicol is known to inhibit mitochondrial protein synthesis. Damage to the mitochondria can be seen on electron microscopy as swelling and

dissolution of the matrix [184, 185]. The reduction of protein synthesis is probably due to the inhibition of cytochromes, specifically cytochrome oxidase [186, 187], and thus the defect of haem synthesis is secondary, since neither haem synthetase or ALA synthase is synthesized on the mitochondria [188, 189].

Other drugs such as phenacetin and paracetamol have been reported as causing sideroblastic anaemia in a few patients. In these cases, however, it is usually associated with malabsorption, haemolytic anaemia and folic-acid deficiency [5].

SIDEROBLASTIC ANAEMIA SECONDARY TO SYSTEMIC DISEASES

Sideroblastic anaemia has been reported as a secondary complication of a diverse group of systemic diseases. These disorders can be divided into non-haematological and primary haematological. Amongst the group of non-haematological disorders are conditions such as infections, hypothyroidism, rheumatoid arthritis, porphyria cutanea tarda, erythropoietic porphyria and polyarteritis nodosa [1, 48, 59, 97, 144, 190–193]. In the majority of cases, the sideroblastic changes are minimal but occasionally they are the major cause of the anaemia [5]. The aetiology of the sideroblastic anaemia in these conditions is obscure. MacGibbon & Mollin [97] have found that 80% of the patients in their series of 35 (which also included three with haematological abnormalities) had evidence of folic-acid deficiency. Fifty per cent of these patients also had an abnormal xanthurenic-acid excretion test which correlated well with the number who responded to pyridoxine therapy. Lee *et al.* [194] found that in a patient with prostatic carcinoma, although no defect of the haem pathway could be demonstrated in mature red cells *in vitro*, small amounts of pyridoxine caused a marked elevation of the red-cell protoporphyrin levels.

The haematological disorders which have been associated with secondary sideroblastic anaemia are haemolytic anaemia, pernicious anaemia, erythraemic myelosis, leukaemia, myeloma, lymphoma and the myeloproliferative disorders [1, 48, 51, 59, 73, 97, 144, 195, 196]. Its association with haemolytic anaemia has been discussed and its rare association with pernicious anaemia is not understood.

Its association with leukaemia deserves separate consideration. Attention was first drawn to this by Dameshek [197] who suggested that primary acquired sideroblastic anaemia is an early phase of erythraemic myelosis, and reported that half the cases which he followed terminated in this way. However, this has not been the experience of others. Nevertheless, leukaemia

is more common (seven per cent) in patients with acquired idiopathic sideroblastic anaemia than in the general population. Many cases have been reported [5, 56, 73, 97, 195, 198–203]. The most common type is acute myeloblastic leukaemia, but chronic granulocytic leukaemia has been reported [195, 203]. Leukaemia has not been described in cases with inherited sideroblastic anaemia. Several authors have noted changes in the granulocytes without an overt leukaemic state. These include abnormalities of nuclear and cytoplasmic maturation, abnormal configuration of the primary cytoplasmic granules resembling Auer rods, Pelger-like abnormalities, agranular neutrophils, and low LAP scores [47, 56, 96, 195, 202]. The association with myeloma has been reported several times [1, 97, 195].

Sideroblastic anaemia has been more frequently associated with the myeloproliferative syndromes, polycythaemia rubra vera and myelofibrosis.

The reason for the association between these abnormalities of haemopoiesis and sideroblastic anaemia is not clear, but the most likely explanation has been postulated by Catovsky *et al.* [195]. They suggest that it represents a mutation in a clone of cells which predisposes either to sideroblastic change or to leukaemia. In several instances, one change might precede the other; this would explain the onset of sideroblastic anaemia several years before the leukaemic changes.

THE TREATMENT OF SIDEROBLASTIC ANAEMIA

The treatment of sideroblastic anaemia can be considered under two headings, namely, the treatment of the anaemia and the treatment of the secondary haemosiderosis. The latter reflects therapeutic failure. The only real success is seen with the treatment of the secondary acquired type; treatment of the primary type, hereditary or idiopathic, is disappointing.

PRIMARY SIDEROBLASTIC ANAEMIA
At the present time there is little rationale for the treatment of the primary sideroblastic anaemias. It should also be stressed that even though a drug, or combination of drugs, results in a haematological remission as judged by a rise in the haemoglobin level, this is not accompanied by a *complete* reversal of the morphological abnormalities.

The drugs which have been used successfully, either alone or in combination, are pyridoxine, folic acid, vitamin C, crude liver extract, and androgens. Others have been used, but so rarely that they merit little consideration. The effectiveness of each of these drugs will be considered but it should be stressed that no reliance can be placed on the biochemical investigations to determine, before treatment, if patients are deficient in pyridoxine or folic acid. They should always be given a trial of these drugs, on the possibility of improving the haemoglobin level.

Pyridoxine

As already discussed, there is much evidence to associate a deficiency or an abnormal metabolism of pyridoxine with sideroblastic anaemia. MacGibbon & Mollin found that 50% of all patients with sideroblastic anaemia have low levels of pyridoxal phosphate and a similar number show disturbances in pyridoxine metabolism [104]. This has been sustained by Hines & Grasso [4] and Gehrmann [33], who also found low levels of pyridoxal phosphate in their patients. Moreover, they also showed that a haematological response to pyridoxal phosphate was better than with pyridoxine. Pyridoxine or its derivatives are the single most effective form of therapy at the present time. Amongst the patients studied by MacGibbon & Mollin [104], 40% were found to respond to large doses of pyridoxine (25–100 mg/day). The response, however, was variable and did not correlate with the findings of the xanthurenic-acid excretion test. The best response is seen in patients with hereditary sideroblastic anaemia; it may be dramatic or slowly progressive over several months. Normal haemoglobin levels are sometimes reached [35, 71, 79, 104, 196], but even in these patients some abnormality of the peripheral blood persists, as do the abnormal ring sideroblasts in the bone marrow.

The doses of pyridoxine required are of the order of 25–100 mg t.d.s., but even higher doses may be needed and it should be given for several months before it is abandoned. there is no clear explanation why such large doses are required but Gehrmann [33] has postulated that if there is a block at one of the steps in the conversion pathway, this might increase the substrate requirement of the enzyme. Alternatively, large doses of pyridoxine may allow synthesis of another biologically active oxidative product, isopyridoxal [204].

Folic acid

Twenty to 30% of all patients with sideroblastic anaemia have reduced folate levels. Amongst the primary acquired groups the figure is even higher; 80% have low serum folates and a similar number have a positive Figlu test. The morphology of the red-cell precursors may not indicate whether patients are deficient in folic acid or if they will respond to treatment. Mollin & Hoffbrand [5] stress that folic-acid deficiency is rarely a cause of sideroblastic anaemia. Approximately 30% of patients will respond to folic-acid therapy, but usually to a slight degree [97,

145]. However, dramatic responses have been reported on a few occasions [97, 145, 205].

Vitamin C

This has been found to induce a partial response in some patients [104, 206, 207]. Goldberg [208] has suggested that vitamin C may act as a co-enzyme for ferrochelatase by protecting the —SH groups of the enzyme from oxidation. In general, responses to vitamin C have been disappointing [73, 96, 98]. The findings of Wapnick *et al.* [209] that ascorbic-acid metabolism is abnormal in patients with iron-overload states, and that the chelating effect of desferrioxamine is greatly enhanced by the administration of vitamin C, may prove extremely important.

Androgen therapy

There is little evidence that androgens have any real place in the treatment of primary sideroblastic anaemia. The number of reported successes (and failures) has been small. Vavra & Poff [66] achieved a complete remission in one patient with testosterone enanthate. Kushner *et al.* [73] treated nine patients either with oxymetholone (50–150 mg/day) or testosterone enanthate, singly or in combination, for three months. Three patients showed a rise in packed cell volume, a fall in the transfusion requirements and a fall in the free erythroctye protoporphyrin levels. Two of these patients, however, became refractory to treatment. Barry & Day [56] state that in their experience androgen therapy has been unsuccessful, but types of drug, doses, and duration of therapy were not given.

Miscellaneous drugs

Isolated instances of remissions have been reported with the use of crude liver extract [104, 145, 210], histidine [154], and a combination of riboflavin, niacin and pyridoxine [211]. However, the numbers are too few to permit any conclusions as to their importance.

Blood transfusion

This is in many cases the only effective therapy which permits the patient to lead a normal life. It should be stressed, however, that the decision to transfuse should not be made lightly. Patients can often lead a relatively normal life even with low haemoglobin levels, but once transfused they may soon become dependent on the higher haemoglobin level. With each 500 ml of transfused blood, the patients acquires 250 mg of iron which will add to his already iron-overloaded state. If transfusion is essential, it should be combined with attempts to remove the added iron (see p. 567).

Splenectomy

Removal of the spleen appears to be of no value and

may be harmful in predisposing patients to the risk of thromboembolism associated with thrombocytosis [212, 213].

Treatment of the haemosiderosis
Haemosiderosis is the most common complication associated with sideroblastic anaemia. The evidence of excess iron deposition in these patients is unquestionable. The iron comes from three main sources:
1 oral iron given mistakenly to treat an undiagnosed hypochromic anaemia (often for many years);
2 a normal or increased intestinal absorption;
3 multiple blood transfusions.

The most important harmful effects of iron result from its deposition in liver and myocardium and effects should be made at an early stage in the treatment of the disease to limit iron intake and to remove that already present.

Limiting intake. At the present time, the value of oral chelating agents is uncertain and in practice it is difficult to construct a diet low in iron. Furthermore, the amount of iron absorbed from the diet will, at most, be 1 mg/day (often much less) and if the patient is receiving regular transfusions this amount is negligible.

Removal of iron. The most effective method is venesection, but for obvious reasons that can only be done in patients with high haemoglobin levels. The beneficial effect on the anaemia has already been discussed, and it is felt that in any case of sideroblastic anaemia, all attempts should be made to remove the iron in this way if the anaemia is not too severe. The most effective method is that used for the treatment of patients with thalassaemia major; namely, 1–2 gm of desferrioxamine daily, given subcutaneously over 12 hours using a constant infusion pump, and vitamin C, 200 mg daily (see Chapter 9, p. 441).

The treatment of secondary sideroblastic anaemia
In most cases the treatment of secondary sideroblastic anaemia must be directed towards the underlying blood disorder or drug toxicity. Removal of the offending drug or toxic agent usually results in a complete reversion to normal marrow appearances, although this may take a considerable length of time. The treatment of sideroblastic anaemia secondary to lead poisoning requires special mention, however,

Symptomatic lead poisoning in childhood is always potentially serious and affected children should be admitted to hospital, at least in the first instance. Where there is a history of recent exposure it is important to X-ray the bowel to make sure that there is no lead remaining in the gut, since the institution of treatment may cause a rapid absorption of the lead with the production of encephalopathy. The main drugs used either singly or in combination for the treatment of this disorder are calcium sodium versenate (EDTA) and penicillamine. For affected children, EDTA should be given in a dosage of approximately 50 mg/kg, either intramuscularly or intravenously. For intramuscular injection it is necessary to mix a local anaesthetic with the EDTA since the injections are painful. For i.v. infusion, EDTA should be made up in five per cent glucose and infused slowly over about 12 hours. The initial course of treatment is usually carried out for about five to 10 days, and the blood and urinary lead levels are monitored during and after treatment. Penicillamine can also be used in a dosage of 20–25 mg/kg for four weeks. This has the advantage that it can be given by mouth. The return of symptoms, failure of haematological improvement or a rising blood or urinary lead level are indications for further treatment. Renal function should be monitored regularly.

For an adult with moderately severe lead poisoning, a regime using EDTA, 500 mg in 250–500 ml of five per cent glucose given every 12 hours for 10 days, would be an adequate schedule. Oral penicillamine is the drug of choice for mild cases. Lead encephalopathy requires urgent hospital treatment. Measures to reduce intracranial pressure by the infusion of 30% urea, mannitol or corticosteroids should be used together with an active chelating regime. If there are associated attacks of lead colic they can usually be controlled with i.v. 10% calcium gluconate. Adequate analgesia is also required.

In cases where there has been exposure to lead and there is a moderately elevated blood level but no symptoms or haematological changes, it is reasonable to monitor the blood levels together with urinary coproporphyrin and ALA levels, without active treatment.

COMPLICATIONS AND PROGNOSIS OF SIDEROBLASTIC ANAEMIA

Complications
The most common complication of this disease is secondary haemosiderosis. There are not enough data in the literature to evaluate how often this occurs, in what way it manifests itself and how often it directly results in death.

Tissue iron stores (liver, spleen and bone marrow) are invariably increased. In some cases, the increase is due to previous iron therapy or blood transfusions, but in others the degree of iron loading cannot be explained on these grounds [71]. The most likely explanation is an increase in the absorption of dietary iron associated with dyshaemopoiesis. This has been demonstrated [71, 72] but in the 10 patients studied by Brain & Herdan [214] only one showed an increased absorption, although in the other nine, despite the body iron being loaded, absorption remained at a normal rate.

It is interesting that haemosiderosis is particularly frequent amongst those patients who are responsive to pyridoxine [215]. Hathaway *et al.* [215] showed that as many as 30% of their patients had evidence of liver damage (i.e. excessive iron deposition, portal fibrosis and disordered liver architecture). Mollin & Hoff-brand [5] have suggested that the explanation for the excessive iron storage in those who respond to pyridoxine may be that pyridoxine deficiency is a late manifestation of the disease resulting from a disturbed metabolism in the liver. These authors also suggested that the liver damage may reflect the deficiency of pyridoxine. They noted that in some patients the pathological findings in the liver resembled those of animals made pyridoxine deficient [216]. On the other hand, different workers, although confirming the haemosiderosis, have failed to find much evidence for liver damage [73, 96]. In the 13 patients examined by Brain & Herdan [214], nine had evidence of portal fibrosis, two had hepatic cirrhosis, six had iron in biliary epithelium and four had diabetic-like glucose-tolerance tests.

Disturbances in liver function have not been reported frequently but diabetes seems to be fairly common. Data on iron deposition in the myocardium and myocardial abnormalities are not available. The authors have seen two patients in whom this was a terminal event. The initial manifestations of myocardial damage were conduction defects progressing to cardiac failure after months.

Prognosis

Hereditary sideroblastic anaemia. It is unfortunate that there are not enough data in the literature to evaluate the prognosis in this condition. It appears that a spectrum of severity is seen, from death in the first decade to long-term survival. It is unknown whether or not response to treatment and/or removal of the body iron have any beneficial effect on the long-term survival.

Idiopathic acquired sideroblastic anaemia. The data on the prognosis of these patients have been well reviewed by Kushner *et al.* [73]. These authors stressed that this disease was relatively benign with a median survival of 10 years. They emphasized the obvious fact that median survival for non-transfused patients was 15 years, whilst that of the transfused was 8·4 years. Of 24

deaths reported [56, 73, 96, 110], 10 were due to haematological causes: myeloblastic leukaemia, chronic granulocytic leukaemia, aplasia and 'anaemia'. Other causes were pneumonia, cerebrovascular accident and myocardial infarction, and uraemia.

REFRACTORY ANAEMIA WITH HYPERPLASTIC BONE MARROW

It is not uncommon to encounter patients with a variable degree of anaemia associated with a hyperplastic bone marrow who fail to respond to all the standard haematinic preparations. These patients have in common marked hyperplasia and morphological abnormalities of the red-cell precursors, erythrokinetic and ferrokinetic evidence of ineffective erythropoiesis and often quantitative or qualitative changes in the leucocytes and platelets. The morphological features of this group of anaemias, and the factors which distinguish them from the aplastic anaemias, are considered in detail in Chapter 31.

Although at the moment many of these disorders can only be classified at a descriptive morphological level it is clear that they fall into two main groups: those which appear to be congenital, probably with an inherited basis, and those which are acquired later in life (Table 13.3).

Table 13.3. Refractory anaemia with hyperplastic bone marrow

---

1 *Congenital*
    Thalassaemia syndromes
    Sideroblastic anaemia
    Refractory megaloblastic anaemia, e.g. orotic aciduria
    Dyserythropoietic anaemia, types 1, 2 and 3
    Hypoplastic anaemia*

2 *Acquired*
    Sideroblastic anaemia
    Myeloproliferative disorders
    Refractory anaemia with pancytopenia syndrome
    Hypoplastic anaemia*

---

* It is not uncommon to encounter a random hyperplastic sample of marrow in a patient with hypoplastic anaemia.

Congenital refractory anaemia with hyperplastic marrow
This clinical picture can be produced by several conditions which have been described elsewhere in this book: the thalassaemias (Chapter 9), sideroblastic anaemias (described earlier in this chapter) and the refractory megaloblastic anaemias (Chapter 6). Furthermore, it may be encountered in children with

congenital hypoplastic anaemia if the bone-marrow biopsy happens to sample a hyperplastic area (see Chapter 31).

Recently a further group of anaemias of this type has been classified as the 'congenital dyserythropoietic anaemias' [217–222]. Based on red-cell-precursor morphology and serological tests three main types have been recognized: type 1, in which there are megaloblastoid erythroblasts with marked erythroblastic internuclear chromatin bridges; type 2, which is characterized by erythroblastic multinuclearity and a positive acid-serum lysis test using the sera of some but not all individuals, and not (in contrast to PNH) when using the patient's serum (this disorder has been called HEMPAS, i.e. hereditary erythroblastic multinuclearity with positive acid-serum lysis); and type 3, which is characterized by erythroblastic multinuclearity with large abnormal erythroblasts termed gigantoblasts. At the time of writing the mode of genetic transmission and underlying metabolic defect of this group of disorders is not clear and they can only be defined on morphological or serological grounds associated, in some cases, with a family history. Recent studies in HEMPAS suggest an autosomal-recessive transmission [218]. These conditions are considered further in Chapter 31.

It is not certain whether all the described cases are indeed congenital or whether the morphological groups represent distinct clinical entities. Furthermore, there is some overlap in morphological features and there may be variants of each type.

Acquired refractory anaemia with hyperplastic bone marrow (see also Chapter 32)

It is possible by studying the morphological appearances and distribution of iron in the red-cell precursors to distinguish clearly the sideroblastic anaemias in the group. Furthermore, some patients with atypical myelosclerosis may present with the clinical picture of refractory anaemia and hyperplastic bone marrow, but usually the bone-marrow-biopsy appearances allow the diagnosis to be made (see Chapter 32). Like the childhood form of the condition, aplastic anaemia acquired in adult life may occasionally present difficulties in that a hyperplastic sample of marrow may be obtained (see Chapter 31).

When these conditions have been excluded there remains a group of disorders which are ill-defined and can best be described as the syndrome of refractory anaemia with pancytopenia [223]. These disorders are more common in the older age groups although they may be seen at any time of life. Typically affected patients present with the symptoms and signs of anaemia and the peripheral-blood picture shows a pancytopenia with some variation in the shape and size

of the red cells. The reticulocyte count is usually normal or only slightly elevated. The bone marrow is hyperplastic and the red-cell precursors show nuclear abnormalities. There are often associated changes in the white-cell precursors and megakaryocytes. Thus there may be a 'shift-to-the-left' in the myeloid series with abnormal granulation. Sometimes the term 'maturation arrest' is applied to this type of marrow although this is probably an incorrect concept. Ferrokinetic and erythrokinetic studies indicate a variable degree of ineffective erythropoiesis. There is often an increase in the antigen on the red cells and the level of haemoglobin F is increased. Although there may be stainable iron in the marrow there are few abnormal sideroblasts. In some patients with this type of condition, the clinical picture remains relatively unchanged for a considerable period of time and repeated blood transfusions are required. A trial of corticosteroid or androgen therapy is indicated, although there are some reported data which indicate that leukaemic transformation may occur in this type of patient following treatment with oxymetholone. There have been some reports of improvement after splenectomy.

There are several disorders which may present with clinical and haematological findings very similar to those described above. Thus a similar clinical picture may precede the development of myeloid or monocytic leukaemia by several months and the condition may also resemble the more chronic forms of the di Guglielmo syndrome or erythraemic myelosis (see Chapter 22). Indeed the dividing line between chronic erythraemic myelosis and the syndrome of pancytopenia with a cellular marrow is incomplete. Two other variants of this type of disorder are described in Chapter 31. One of these, refractory anaemia with medullary myeloblastosis, is a condition of old people characterized by pancytopenia, dyserythropoiesis and a marked proliferation of the granulocyte series with increased numbers of myeloblasts. This must be considered to be a preleukaemic state although many of these patients go on for years suffering from the symptoms of pancytopenia. The other condition, termed 'refractory anaemia with proliferative dysplasia', which is probably related to the myeloproliferative disorders, is also described in Chapter 31.

These conditions belong to a spectrum and it may be difficult to distinguish one from another when the patient is first seen. Studies of haematology, bone-marrow biopsies, ferrokinetics, etc., will help to categorize the condition in some cases. Where this is impossible the patient must be managed symptomatically with blood transfusions, a cautious trial of androgen or oxymetholone therapy, and symptomatic treatment for such complications as infection and thrombocytopenia.

REFERENCES

1 DACIE J.C. & MOLLIN D.L. (1966) Siderocytes, sideroblasts and sideroblastic anemia. *Acta Medica Scandinavica*, **445** (Suppl.), 237.

2 HARRIS J.W. & HORRIGAN D.L. (1964) Pyridoxine-responsive anaemia. The prototype and variations on the theme. Analysis of 72 patients. *Vitamins and Hormones* (New York), **22**, 721.

3 HEILMEYER L. (1963) Symposium on sideroachrestic anaemias. *Proceedings of the IX Congress of the European Society of Haematology, Lisbon*, p. 240. Karger, Basel.

4 HINES J.D. & GRASSO J.A. (1970) The sideroblastic anaemias. *Seminars in Haematology*, **7**, 86.

5 MOLLIN D.L. & HOFFBRAND A.V. (1968) Sideroblastic anaemia. *Recent Advances in Clinical Pathology*, Series V, p. 293. Churchill, London.

6 MORROW J.J. & GOLDBERG A. (1965) The sideroblastic anaemias. *Postgraduate Medical Journal*, **41**, 740.

7 VERLOOP M.C. (1967) In: *Progrès en Hématologie*, Editairs Medicales (ed. Dreyfus B.). Flammarias, Paris.

8 BOTTOMLEY S.S. (1980) Sideroblastic anaemia. *Iron metabolism in biochemistry and medicine II*, 11, p. 363. Academic Press, London.

9 GRANICK S. & LEVERE R. (1968) Controls of haemoglobin synthesis. *Proceedings of the XII Congress of the International Society of Haematology*, p. 274. New York.

10 WINTERHALTER K.H., HEYWOOD J.D., HUEHNS E.R. & FINCH C.A. (1969) The free globin in human erythrocytes. I. *British Journal of Haematology*, **16**, 523.

11 HORIBAN D. & LONDON I.M. (1965) Control of heme synthesis by feed-back inhibition. *Biochemical and Biophysical Research Communications*, **18**, 2413.

12 GRANICK S. & KAPPAS A. (1967) Steroid induction of porphyrin synthesis in liver cell culture. I. Structural basis and possible physiological role in the control of heme formation *Journal of Biological Chemistry*, **24**, 4587.

13 KAPPAS A. & GRANICK S. (1968) Steroid induction of porphyrin synthesis in liver cell culture. II. The effects of heme uridine diphosphate glucuronic acid and inhibitors of nucleic acid and protein synthesis on the induction process. *Journal of Biological Chemistry*, **243**, 346.

14 GRAYZEL A.I., HÖRSCHER P. & LONDON I.M. (1966) The stimulation of globin synthesis by heme. *Proceedings of the National Academy of Sciences, USA*, **55**, 650.

15 WAXMAN H.S. & RABINOVITZ M. (1966) Control of reticulocyte polyribosomes content and hemoglobin synthesis of heme. *Biochimica et Biophysica Acta*, **129**, 369.

16 ZUCKER W.V. & SCHULMAN H.M. (1968) Stimulation of globin chain initiation by haem in the reticulocyte cell-free system. *Proceedings of the National Academy of Sciences, USA*, **59**, 582.

17 TAVILL A.S., GRAYZELL A.I., LONDON I.M., WILLIAMS M.K. & VANDERHOFF G.A. (1968) The role of heme in the synthesis and assembly of hemoglobin. *Journal of Biological Chemistry*, **243**, 4987.

18 MAXWELL C.R. & RABINOVITZ M. (1969) Evidence of an inhibitor in the control of globin synthesis by hemin in a reticulocyte lysate. *Biochemical and Biophysical Research Communications*, **35**, 79.

19 PONKA P. & NEUWIRT J. (1971) Iron uptake by reticulocytes with various rates of haem and globin synthesis. In: *The Regulation of Erythropoiesis and Haemoglobin Synthesis* (ed. Travnicek T. & Neuwirt J.), p. 326. Universita Karlova, Prague.

20 KIKUCHI G., KUMAR A., TALRIADGE P. & SHEMUS D. (1958) The enzymatic synthesis of delta-aminolevulinic acid. *Journal of Biological Chemistry*, **233**, 1214.

21 BURNHAM B.F. & LASCELLES J. (1963) Control of porphyrin biosynthesis through negative feed-back mechanism. Studies with preparations of delta-aminolaevulate synthetase and delta-aminolaevulic dehydratase from *Rhodopseudomonas spheroids*. *Biochemical Journal*, **87**, 462.

22 KAPLAN B.H. (1970) Control of heme synthesis. In: *Regulation of Hematopoiesis*, Vol. 1 (ed. Gordon A.S.), p. 677. Appleton-Century-Crofts, New York.

23 BOGARAD L. (1958) The enzymatic synthesis of porphyrins from porphobilinogen. I. Uroporphyrin I. *Journal of Biological Chemistry*, **233**, 501.

24 BOGARAD L. & GRANICK S. (1953) The enzymatic synthesis of porphyrins from porphobilinogen. *Proceedings of the National Academy of Sciences, USA*, **39**, 1176,

25 BURNHAM B.F. (1968) The chemistry of the porphyrins. *Seminars in Haematology*, **5**, 296.

26 KAPPAS A., LEVERE R.S. & GRANICK S. (1968) The regulation of porphyrin and heme synthesis. *Seminars in Hematology*, **5**, 323.

27 BARR R.B., HOFFBRAND A.V. & WHITE J.M. (1972) Globin chain synthesis by marrow precursors in iron deficiency. *Nature (London)*, **2**, 261.

28 WHITE J.M. & HARVEY R.S. (1972) Globin synthesis in lead poisoning. *Nature (London)*, **237**, 71.

29 BABCOCK M.J., BRUSH M. & SOSTMAN E. (1960) Evaluation of vitamin B_6 nutrition. *Journal of Nutrition*, **70**, 369.

30 HARDING R.S., PLOUGH I.C. & FRIEDEMANN T.E. (1959) The effect of storage on the vitamin B_6 content of a packaged army ration, with a note on the human requirement for the vitamin. *Journal of Nutrition*, **68**, 323.

30a ANDERSON B.B., MOLLIN D.L., CHILD J.A., MODELL C.B. & PERRY G.M. (1975). Red cell metabolism of pyridoxine in sideroblastic anaemia and thalassaemia. In: *Iron Metabolism and its Disorders* (ed. Kief H. *et al.*), 366, 241. Excerpta Medica, Amsterdam.

31 ANDERSON B.B., FULFORD-JONDS C.E., CHILD J.A., BEARD M.E.J. & BATEMAN C.J.T. (1971) Conversion of vitamin B_6 compounds to active forms in the red blood cells. *Journal of Clinical Investigations*, **50**, 1901.

32 HARRIS E.B., MacGIBBON B.H. & MOLLIN D.L. (1965) Experimental sideroblastic anaemia. *British Journal of Haematology*, **11**, 99.

33 GEHRMANN G. (1965) Pyridoxine-responsive anaemias. *British Journal of Haematology*, **11**, 86.

34 SNYDERMAN S.E., HOLT L.E. JR, CARRETERO R. & JACOBS K.G. (1953) Pyridoxine deficiency in the human infant. *American Journal of Clinical Nutrition*, **1**, 200.

35 BISHOP R.C. & BETHNELL F.H. (1959) Hereditary hypochromic anemia with transfusion siderosis treated

with pyridoxine. *New England Journal of Medicine*, **261**, 486.

36 GRÜNEBERG H. (1941) Siderocytes: a new kind of erythrocyte. *Nature (London)*, **148**, 114.

37 GRÜNBERG H. (1941) Siderocytes in man. *Nature (London)*, **148**, 114.

38 DONIACH I., GRÜNEBERG H. & PEARSON J.E.G. (1943) The occurrence of siderocytes in adult human blood. *Journal of Pathology and Bacteriology*, **55**, 23.

39 DACIE J.V. & DONIACH I. (1947) The basophilic property of the iron-containing granules in siderocytes. *Journal of Pathology and Bacteriology*, **59**, 687.

40 McFADZEAN A.J.S. & DAVIS L.J. (1947) Iron staining erythrocyte inclusions with special reference to acquired haemolytic anaemia. *Glasgow Medical Journal*, **28**, 237.

41 McFADZEAN A.J.S. & DAVIS L.J. (1947) On the nature and significance of stippling in lead poisoning with reference to the effect of splenectomy. *Quarterly Journal of Medicine*, **18**, 57.

42 DOUGLAS A.S. & DACIE J.V. (1953) The incidence and significance of iron-containing human erythroctyes. *Journal of Clinical Pathology*, **6**, 307.

43 KAPLAN E., ZUELZER W.W. & MOURIQUAND C. (1954) Sideroblasts. A study of stainable non-hemoglobin iron in marrow normoblasts. *Blood*, **9**, 203.

44 WINTRAUB L.R. (1970) The continuing saga of the sideroblast. *New England Journal of Medicine*, **283**, 486.

44a CARTWRIGHT G.E. & DEISS A. (1975) Sideroblasts, siderocytes and sideroblastic anaemia. *New England Journal of Medicine*, **292**, 185.

45 BAINTON D.F. & FINCH C.A. (1964) The diagnosis of iron deficiency anaemia. *American Journal of Medicine*, **37**, 62.

46 BESSIS M.C. & BRETON-GORIUS J. (1962) Iron metabolism in the bone marrow as seen by electron microscopy: a critical review. *Blood*, **19**, 635.

47 BESSIS M., DREYFUS B., BRETON-GORIUS J. & SULTAN C. (1969) Étude au microscope électronique de onze cas d'anémies refractaires avec enzymopathies multiples. *Nouvelle Revue française d'Hématologie*, **9**, 87.

48 GOODMAN J.R. & HALL S.G. (1967) Accumulation of iron in mitochondria of erythroblasts. *British Journal of Haematology*, **13**, 355.

49 GRASSO J.A. & HINES J.D. (1969) A comparative electron microscopic study of refractory and alcoholic sideroblastic anaemia. *British Journal of Haematology*, **17**, 34.

50 LARIZZA P. & OILANDI F. (1964) Electron microscopic observations on bone marrow and liver tissue in non-hereditary refractory sideroblastic anaemia. *Acta Haematologica*, **31**, 1964.

51 PETZ L.D., GOODMAN J.R., HALL S.G. & FINK D. (1966) Refractory normoblastic (sideroblastic) anemia. *American Journal of Clinical Pathology*, **45**, 581.

52 SORENSON G.D. (1962) Electron microscopic observations of bone marrow from patients with sideroblastic anemia. *American Journal of Clinical Pathology*, **40**, 2971.

53 TANAKA Y., BUCHER G. & BULL B. (1966) Ferritin localisation on the erythroblast cell membrane and ropheocytosis in hyper-siderotic human bone marrow. *Blood*, **28**, 758.

54 BESSIS M. & JENSEN W.N. (1965) Sideroblastic anaemia, mitochondria and erythroblast iron. *British Journal of Haematology*, **11**, 49.

55 BATEMAN C.J.T. & MOLLIN D.L. (1970) Sideroblastic anaemia. *British Journal of Hospital Medicine*, **4**, 3, 371.

56 BARRY W.E. & DAY H.J. (1964) Refractory sideroblastic anaemia. *Annals of Internal Medicine*, **61**, 1029.

57 BJORKMAN S. (1956) Chronic refractory anemia with sideroblastic bone marrow. A study of four cases. *Blood*, **11**, 250.

58 HAGASAKI R. (1966) Pathophysiological studies on iron metabolism, clinical and electron microscopic studies on sideroblasts. *Journal of the Kyushu Haematological Society*, **16**, 223.

59 HEILMEYER L. (1966) *Disturbances in Heme Synthesis: Special Consideration of the Sideroachrestic Anemias and Erythropoietic Porphyrias*, p. 103. C. C. Thomas, Springfield, Illinois.

60 BOUSSER J., GAJDOS A., GAJDOS-TOROK M., BILSKI-PASQUIER G. & ZIHOUN R. (1967) Anemie sideroblastique idiopathique acquise: incorporation de la glycine-2-C^{14} dans l'héme et la globin des erythroblastes medullares *in vitro*. *Nouvelle Revue française de Hématologie*, **7**, 847.

61 HEILMEYER L. (1967) In-vitro testing B$_6$ Sensibler Anaemien. *Blut*, **16**, 1.

62 KRAMER S., VILJOEN E., BECKER D., ZAIL S.S. & METZ J. (1969) The relationship between haem and globin synthesis by erythroid precursors in refractory normoblastic anaemia. *Scandinavian Journal of Haematology*, **6**, 293.

63 WHITE J.M., BRAIN M.C. & ALI M.A.M. (1971) Globin synthesis in sideroblastic anaemia. 1. α and β peptide chain synthesis. *British Journal of Haematology*, **20**, 263.

64 ROTHSTEIN G., LEE G.R. & CARTWRIGHT G.E. (1968) Refractory sideroblastic anaemia associated with reduced heme synthetase activity in the reticulocytes (Abstract). *Abstracts XII Congress of the International Society of Haematology, New York*, p. 65. Grune & Stratton, New York.

65 VOLGER W.R. & MINGIOLI E.S. (1965) Heme synthesis in pyridoxine-responsive anaemia. *New England Journal of Medicine*, **273**, 397.

66 VAVRA J.D. & POFF S.A. (1967) Heme and porphyrin synthesis in sideroblastic anaemia. *Journal of Laboratory and Clinical Medicine*, **69**, 904.

67 BARRETT P.V.D., CLINE M.J. & BERLIN N. (1966) The association of the urobilin 'early peak' and erythropoiesis in man. *Journal of Clinical Investigations*, **45**, 1657.

68 HOFFBRAND A.V., KREMENCHUZKY S. & BUTTERWORTH P.J. (1966) Serum lactic dehydrogenase activity and folate deficiency in myelosclerosis and other haematological disorders. *British Medical Journal*, **i**, 577.

69 ROSENTHAL D.S., SKARIN A.T. & MALONEY W.C. (1968) Serum lactic dehydrogenase in refractory anaemia. *Acta Haematologica*, **40**, 187.

70 WHITE P., COBURN R.F. & WILLIAMS W.J. (1967) Carbon monoxide production associated with ineffective erythropoiesis. *Journal of Clinical Investigation*, **46**, 1486.

71 LOSOWSKY M.S. & HALL R. (1965) Hereditary sideroblastic anaemia. *British Journal of Haematology*, **11**, 70.

72 VERLOOP M.C., PLOEM J.E. & LEUNIS I. (1964) Heredi-

tary hypochromic hypersideraemic anaemia. In: *Iron Metabolism* (ed. Dreyfus B. & Schapiro S.), p. 376. Springer-Verlag, Berlin.

73 KUSHNER J.P., LEE G.T., WINTROBE M.M. & CARTWRIGHT G.E. (1971) Idiopathic refractory sideroblastic anemia. Clinical and laboratory investigation of 16 patients and review of the literature. *Medicine*, **50**, 139.

74 VON LUKL P., WIEDERMAN B. & BARBORIK. Hereditäre Leptocyten-Anämie bei Männern. *Folia Haematologica*, Neue Folge, Bd. **3**, 17.

75 WICKRAMASINGHE S.N., FULKER M.J., LOSOWSKY M.S. & HALL R. Microspectrophotometric and electron microscopic studies of bone marrow in hereditary sideroblastic anaemia. *Acta Haematologica* (Basel), **45**, 236.

76 WICKRAMASINGHE S.N. (1975) *Human Bone Marrow*, p. 339. Blackwell Scientific Publications, Oxford.

76a SEIP M., GJESSING L.R. & LIE S.O. (1971) Congenital sideroblastic anaemia in a girl. *Scandinavian Journal of Haematology*, **8**, 505.

77 COOLEY T.B. (1945) A severe type of hereditary anemia with elliptocytosis. Interesting sequence of splenectomy. *American Journal of Medical Sciences*, **209**, 561.

78 RUNDLES R.W. & FALLS H.F. (1946) Hereditary (? sex-linked) anemia. *American Journal of Medical Sciences*, **211**, 691.

79 BOURNE M.S., ELVES M.W. & ISRAELS M.C.G. (1965) Familial pyridoxine-responsive anaemia. *British Journal of Haematology*, **11**, 1.

80 ELVES M.W., BOURNE M.S. & ISRAELS M.C.G. (1966) Pyridoxine-responsive anaemia determined by an X-linked gene. *Journal of Medical Genetics*, **3**, 1.

81 LEE G.R., MACDIARMID W.D., CARTWRIGHT G.E. & WINTROBE M.M. (1968) Heredity X-linked sidero-achrestic anemia. The isolation of two erythrocyte populations differing in Xg^a blood type and porphyrin content. *Blood*, **32**, 59.

82 MCCURDY P.R., DONOHOE R.F. & MCGOVERN M. (1966) Reversible sideroblastic anemia caused by pyruzinoic acid (pyrazinamide). *Annals of Internal Medicine*, **64**, 1280.

83 PRASAD A.S., TRACHIDA L., KONNO E.T., BERMAN L., ALBERT S., SING C.F. & BREWER G.J. (1968) Hereditary sideroblastic anemia and glucose-6-phosphate dehydrogenase deficiency in a Negro family. *Journal of Clinical Investigation*, **47**, 1415.

84 GARBY L.S., SJOLIN S. & BAHLQUIST B. (1957) Chronic refractory hypochromic anaemia with disturbed haem metabolism. *British Journal of Haematology*, **3**, 55.

85 HEILMEYER L., KEIDERLING W., MERKER H., CLOTTEN R. & SCHUBOTHE H. (1960) Die Anaemia Refracteria Sideroblastica und ihre Beiziehungen zur Lebersiderose und Haemochromatose. *Acta Haematologica* (Basel), **23**, 1.

86 VOLGER W.R. & MINGIOLI E.S. (1967) Prophyrin synthesis and heme synthetase activity in pyridoxine-responsive anemia. *Blood*, **30**, 366.

87 WEATHERALL D.J., PEMBREY M.E., HALL E.G., SANGER R., TIPPETT P. & GAVIN J. (1970) Familial sideroblastic anaemia: Problem of Xg and X chromosome inactivation. *Lancet*, **ii**, 744.

88 WINTRAUB L.R., CONRAD M.E. & CROSBY W.H. (1966) Iron loading anemia. Treatment with repeated phlebo-

tomies and pyridoxine. *New England Journal of Medicine*, **275**, 169.

89 COTTOM H.B. & HARRIS J.W. (1962) Familial pyridoxine-responsive anemia. *Journal of Clinical Investigation*, **41**, 1352.

90 COOPER A.G., HOFFBRAND A.V. & WORLLEDGE S.M. (1968) Increased agglutinability and megaloblastic anaemia. *British Journal of Haematology*, **15**, 381.

91 WHITE J.M., BRAIN M.C. & ALI M.A.M. (1969) α and β peptide chain synthesis in sideroblastic anaemia. *British Journal of Haematology*, **17**, 607.

92 BJORKMAN S.E. (1963) Prognosis and therapy of acquired form of sideroachrestic anaemia. *Proceedings of the 9th Congress of the European Society of Haematology*, Lisbon, Vol. 2, p. 273. Karger, New York.

93 AOKI Y., URATA G., WADA O. & TAKAKU F. (1974) Measurement of delta-aminolevulinic acid synthetase activity in human erythroblasts. *Journal of Clinical Investigations*, **53**, 1326.

94 BUCHANAN G.R., BOTTOMLEY S.S. & NITSCHKE R. (1980). Bone marrow delta aminolaevulinate synthase deficiency in a female with congenital sideroblastic anaemia. *Blood*, **55**, 109.

95 KONOPKA L., HOFFBRAND A.V. (1979) Haem synthesis in sideroblastic anaemia. *British Journal of Haematology*, **42**, 73.

96 DACIE J.V., SMITH M.D., WHITE J.C. & MOLLIN D.L. (1959) Refractory normoblastic anaemia: a clinical and haematological study of seven cases. *British Journal of Haematology*, **5**, 56.

97 MOLLIN B.L. (1965) Sideroblasts and sideroblastic anaemia. *British Journal of Haematology*, **11**, 41.

98 VERLOOP M.C., PANDERS J.T., PLOEM J.E. & BOS C.C. (1965) Sidero-achrestic anaemias. *Scandinavian Journal of Haematology*, Series Haematologica, **5**, 76.

99 HAYHOE F.G.J. & QUAGLINO D. (1960) Refractory sideroblastic anaemia and erythraemic myelosis: possible relationship and cytochemical observations. *British Journal of Haematology*, **6**, 381.

100 MERKEY H. (1963) The differentiation between anaemia sideroblastica refractoria and erythremic myelosis by cytochemical methods. *Proceedings of the 9th Congress of the European Society of Haematology*, Lisbon, Vol. 2, p. 290. Karger, New York.

101 SINGH A.K., SHINTON N.K. & WILLIAMS J.D. (1970) Ferrokinetic abnormalities and their significance in patients with sideroblastic anaemia. *British Journal of Haematology*, **18**, 67.

102 BOTTOMLEY S.S. (1977) Porphyrin and iron metabolism in sideroblastic anemia. *Seminars in Hematology*, **14**, 169.

103 RIEDLER G.F. & STRAUB P.W. (1972) Abnormal iron incorporation, survival protoporphyrin content and fluorescence of one red cell population in preleukemic sideroblastic anemia. *Blood*, **40**, 345.

103a PRCHAL J.T., THROCKMORTON D.W., CARROLL A.J., FUSON E.W. GAMS R.A. & PRCHAL J.F. (1978) A common progenitor for human myeloid and lymphoid cells. *Nature (London)*, **274**, 590.

104 MACGIBBON B.H. & MOLLIN D.L. (1965) Sideroblastic anaemia in man: observations on seventy cases. *British Journal of Haematology*, **11**, 59.

105 BALLAS S.K. (1973) Sideroblastic refractory anemia in a

patient with systemic erythematosus. *American Journal of Medical Sciences*, **265**, 225.

105a TRANCHIDA L., PATLUTKE M., POULIK M.D. & PRASAD A.S. (1973) Primary acquired sideroblastic anaemia preceding monoclonal gammopathy and malignant lymphoma. *American Journal of Medicine*, **55**, 559.

106 CELADA A., FARQUET J.J. & MULLER A.F. (1977) Refractory sideroblastic anemia secondary to auto-immune hemolytic anemia. *Acta Haematologica* (Basel), **58**, 213.

107 RITCHEY A.K., HOFFMAN R., DAINIAK N., McINTOSH S., WEININGER R. & PEARSON H.A. (1979) Antibody-mediated acquired sideroblastic anemia: response to cytotoxic therapy. *Blood*, **54**, 734.

108 WICKRAMASINGHE S.N. & HUGHES M. (1978) Capacity of ringed sideroblasts to synthesize nucleic acids and protein in patients with primary sideroblastic anaemia. *British Journal of Haematology*, **38**, 345.

109 LOURENCO G., EMBURY S., SCHRIER S.L. & KEDES L.G. (1978) Decreased ribosomal RNA content and *in-vitro* RNA synthesis in purified bone marrow erythroblasts of patients with idiopathic ineffective erythropoiesis and di Guglielmo disease. *American Journal of Hematology*, **5**, 169.

110 WALTUCH G., LANZAROTTI A.K. & SCHRIER S.L. (1968) Marrow defect in idiopathic ineffective erythropoiesis. *Annals of Internal Medicine*, **68**, 1005.

111 BOTTOMLEY S.S., TANAKA M. & SELF J. (1973) Delta-aminolevulinic acid synthetase activity in normal human bone marrow and in patients with idiopathic sideroblastic anemia. *Enzyme*, **16**, 138.

112 HAMMOND E., DEISS A., CARNES W.H. & CARTWRIGHT G.E. (1969) Ultrastructural characteristics of sidero-cytes in swine. *Laboratory Investigations*, **21**, 292.

113 BOTTOMLEY S.S., TANAKA M. & EVERETT M.A. (1975) Diminished erythroid ferrochelatase activity in proto-porphyria. *Journal of Laboratory and Clinical Medicine*, **86**, 126.

114 HUNTER F.E. JR, GEBICKI J.M., HOFFSTEN P.E., WEIN-STEIN J. & SCOTT A. (1963) Swelling and lysis of rat liver mitochondria induced by ferrous ions. *Journal of Biological Chemistry*, **238**, 828.

115 BROWN E.G. (1958) Evidence for the involvement of ferrous iron in the biosynthesis of δ-aminolaevulinic acid by chicken erythrocyte preparation. *Nature (London)*, **182**, 313.

116 MORROW J.J., URATA G. & GOLDBERG A. (1969) The effect of lead and ferrous and ferric iron on delta-amino-laevulic acid synthetase. *Clinical Science*, **37**, 533.

116a HINES J.D. (1976) Effect of pyridoxine plus chronic phlebotomy on the function and morphology of bone marrow and liver in pyridoxine-responsive sideroblastic anemia. *Seminars in Hematology*, **13**, 133.

117 FREEDMAN M.L., WILDMAN J.M., ROSMAN J., EISEN J. & GREENBLATT D.R. (1977) Benzene inhibition of in vitro rabbit reticulocyte haem synthesis at delta aminolaevu-linic acid synthetase: reversal of benzene toxicity by pyridoxine. *British Journal of Haematology*, **35**, 49.

118 PORTER P.N., MEINTZ R.H. & MESNER K. (1979) Enhancement of erythroid colony growth in culture by hemin. *Excerpta Haematologica*, **7**, 11.

120 STATHAKIS N.E., GIDARI A.S. & LEVERE R.D. (1977) Refractory anemia with hyperplastic bone marrow: subclassification based on responsiveness to erythro-poietin *in vitro*. *Acta Haematologica* (Basel), **58**, 34.

121 WHITE J.M., BRAIN M.C. & ALI M.A.M. (1971) Globin synthesis is sideroblastic anaemia. I. Alpha and beta peptide chain synthesis. *British Journal of Haematology*, **20**, 263.

122 WHITE J.M. & ALI M.A.M. (1973) Globin synthesis in sideroblastic anaemia. II. The effect of pyridoxine. *British Journal of Haematology*, **24**, 481.

123 ALI M.A.M. & QUINLAN A. (1977) Effect of lead synthesis *in vitro*. *American Journal of Clinical Pathology*, **67**, 77.

124 FREEDMAN M.L. & ROSMAN J. (1976) A rabbit reticulo-cyte model for the role of hemin-controlled repressor in hypochromic anemias. *Journal of Clinical Investigations*, **57**, 594.

125 BOEHME W.M., PIIRA T.A., KURNICH J.E. & BETHLEN-FALVAY N.C. (1978) Acquired hemoglobin H in refrac-tory sideroblastic anemia. A preleukemic marker. *Archives of Internal Medicine*, **138**, 603.

126 BAROSI G., GIAZZOLI M., MORANDI S., STEFANELLI M. & PERUGINI S. (1978) Estimation of ferrokinetic para-meters by a mathematical model in patient with primary acquired sideroblastic anaemia. *British Journal of Hae-matology*, **39**, 409.

127 HRINDA M.E. & GOLDWASSER E. (1969) On the mechanism of erythropoietin-induced differentiation. VI. Induced accumulation of iron by marrow cells. *Biochimica et Biophysica Acta*, **195**, 165.

128 STORRING P.L. & FAITH S. (1975) Erythropoietin effects on iron metabolism in rat bone marrow cells. *Biochi-mica et Biophysica Acta*, **392**, 26.

129 DENTON M.J., DELVES H.T. & ARNSTEIN H.R. (1974) The mobilisation of iron from the cell stroma during erythroid maturation. *Biochemical and Biophysical Research Communications*, **61**, 8.

130 GROSS M. & GOLDWASSER E. (1970) On the mechanism of erythropoietin-induced differentiation. VIII. The effect of iron on stimulated marrow cell functions. *Biochimica et Biophysica Acta*, **217**, 461.

131 KAILIS S.G. & MORGAN E.H. (1974) Transferrin and iron uptake by rabbit marrow cells *in vitro*. *British Journal of Haematology*, **28**, 37.

132 BOROVA J. PONKA P. & NEUWIRT J. (1973) Study of intracellular iron distribution in rabbit reticulocytes with normal and inhibited haem synthesis. *Biochimica et Biophysica Acta*, **320**, 143.

133 BATES G.W. & WORKMAN E.F. JR (1974) Siderochelin: a newly discovered cytoplasmic iron transport agent of rabbit reticulocytes. *Federation Proceedings*, **33**, 1395.

134 KOLLER M.E., PRANTE P.H., ULVAK R. & ROMSLO I. (1976) Effect of hemin and isotonic acid hydrazide on the uptake of iron from transferrin by isolated rat liver mitochondria. *Biochemical and Biophysical Research Communications*, **71**, 339.

135 PONKZ P., NEUWIRT J., BOROVA J. & FUCHS O. (1976) Control of iron delivery to haemoglobin in erythroid cells. *Ciba Foundation Symposium*, **51**, 167.

136 ULVIK R. & ROMSLO I. (1978) Studies on the utilization of ferritin iron in ferrochelatase reaction of isolated rat liver mitochondria. *Biochimica et Biophysica Acta*, **541**, 251.

137 NUNEZ M.T., GLASS J. & ROBINSON S.H. (1978) Mobili-

zation of iron from the plasma membrane of the murine reticulocyte. The role of ferritin. *Biochimica et Biophysica Acta*, **509**, 170.

138 SPEYER B.E. & FIELDING J. (1979) Ferritin as a cytosol iron transport intermediate in human reticulocytes. *British Journal of Haematology*, **42**, 255.

139 KONIJN A.M., HERSHKO C. & IZAK G. (1978) Ferritin synthesis in developing erythroid precursor cells. *Israeli Journal of Medical Sciences*, **14**, 1181.

140 KOLLER M.E. & ROMSLO I. (1977) Studies on the ferrochelatase activity of mitochrondria and submitochondrial particles with special reference to the regulatory function of the mitochondrial inner membrane. *Biochimica et Biophysica Acta*, **461**, 283.

141 BARNES R. & JONES O.T.G. (1973) The availability of iron for haem synthesis in red blood cells. *Biochimica et Biophysica Acta*, **304**, 304.

142 FLATMARK T. & ROMSLO I. (1975) Energy-dependent accumulation of iron by isolated rat liver mitochondria. Requirement of reducing equivalents and evidence for a unidirectional flux of Fe (II) across the inner membrane. *Journal of Biological Chemistry*, **250**, 6433.

143 WILLIAMS D.M., LOUKOPOULOS D., LEE G.R. & CARTWRIGHT G.E. (1976) Role of copper in mitochondrial iron metabolism. *Blood*, **48**, 77.

144 DAMESHEK W. (1965) Sideroblastic anaemia: is this a malignancy? *British Journal of Haematology*, **11**, 52.

145 MOLLIN D.L. & DACIE J.V. (1960) Further observations on refractory normoblastic anaemia. *Proceedings of the 7th Congress of the European Society of Haematology*, London, Vol. 2. Karger, Basel.

146 HARRIS J.W. & HORRIGAN D.L. (1968) Pyridoxine-responsive anemias in man. *Vitamins and Hormones*, **25**, 453.

147 MASON D.Y. & EMERSON P.M. Primary acquired sideroblastic anaemia: response to treatment with pyridoxal-5-phosphate. *British Medical Journal*, **i**, 389.

148 HINES J.D. & LOVE D. (1975) Abnormal vitamin B_6 metabolism in sideroblastic anemia: Effect of pyridoxal phosphate (PLP) therapy. *Clinical Research*, **23**, 403a.

149 SOLOMON L.R. & HILLMAN R.S. (1979) Vitamin B_6 metabolism in anaemia and alcoholic man. *British Journal of Haematology*, **41**, 343.

150 DAWSON A.M., HOLDSWORTH C.D. & PITCHER C.S. (1964) Sideroblastic anaemia in adult coeliac disease. *Gut*, **5**, 304.

151 SHAW R., WHITE J.M. & HOFFBRAND A.V. Haemolytic anaemia and sideroblastic erythropoiesis: association with vitamin B_6 deficiency. In press.

152 EICHNER R. & HILLMAN R.S. (1969) Intracellular iron defect in alcoholism. *Clinical Research*, **17**, 324.

153 HINES J.D. (1969) Reversible megaloblastic and sideroblastic abnormalities in alcoholic patients. *British Journal of Haematology*, **16**, 87.

154 HINES, J.D. & GOWAN D.H. (1970) Studies on the pathogenesis of alcohol-induced sideroblastic bone marrow abnormalities. *New England Journal of Medicine*, **283**, 441.

155 PIERCE H.I., McGUFFIN R.G. & HILLMAN R.S. (1976) Clinical studies in alcoholic sideroblastosis. *Archives of Internal Medicine*, **136**, 283.

156 LUMENG L. & LI T.K. (1974) Vitamin B_6 metabolism in chronic alcohol abuse. Pyridoxal phosphate levels in plasma and the effects of acetaldehyde on pyridoxal phosphate synthesis and degradation in human erythrocytes. *Journal of Clinical Investigations*, **53**, 693.

157 CHILLAR R.K., JOHNSON C.S. & BEUTLER E. (1976) Erythrocyte pyridoxine kinase levels in patients with sideroblastic anemia. *New England Journal of Medicine*, **295**, 881.

158 McCURDY P.R. & DONOHOE R. (1966) Pyridoxine responsive anemia conditioned by isonicotinic acid hydrazide. *Blood*, **27**, 352.

159 ROBERTS P.D., HOFFBRAND A.V. & MOLLIN D.L. (1966) Iron and folate metabolism in tuberculosis. *British Medical Journal*, **ii**, 198.

160 KOHN R., HEILMEYER L. & CLOTTEN R. (1962) Reversible pyridoxin-sensible symptomatische sideroachrestische Anamie unter Isoniazidberhandling bei einer kasigen Lymphknotentuberkulose mit Pleurtis Exsudativa. *Deutsche Medizinische Wochenschrift*, **87**, 1765.

161 McCURDY P.R. (1963) Isoniazid conditioned pyridoxine responsive anaemia. *Clinical Research*, **11**, 59.

162 REDLEAF P.F. (1962) Pyridoxine-responsive anaemia in a patient receiving isonizid. *Diseases of the Chest*, **42**, 222.

163 VERWILGHEN R., REYBROUCK G., COLLENS L. & COSEMANS J. (1965) Antituberculosis drugs and sideroblastic anaemia. *British Journal of Haematology*, **11**, 92.

163a LICHSTEIN H.C. (1956) Vitamin B_6 and protein synthesis. *Journal of Biological Chemistry*, **219**, 27.

164 BRAUNSTEIN A.F. (1964) Binding and reactions of the vitamin B_6 coenzyme in the catalytic center of aspartate transaminases. *Vitamins and Hormones*, **22**, 451.

165 McCORMICK D.B. & SNELL E.E. (1961) Pyridoxal phosphokinase. II Effect of inhibitor. *Journal of Biological Chemistry*, **236**, 2085.

166 VILTER R.W. (1964) The vitamin B_6-hydrazide relationship. *Vitamins and Hormones*, **22**, 797.

167 PONKA P. & NEUWIRT J. (1974) Haem synthesis and iron uptake by reticulocytes. *British Journal of Haematology*, **28**, 1.

168 McCORMICK D.B. & ESMOND E.S. (1974) Pyridoxal phosphokinases. II. Effects of inhibitors. *Journal of Biological Chemistry*, **236**, 2085.

169 JENSEN W.N., MORENO G. & BESSIS M.C. (1968) An electron microscopic description of basophilic stippling in red cells. *Blood*, **25**, 933.

170 BERK P.D., TSCHUDY D.P., SHEPLEY L.A., WAGGONER J.G. & BERLIN N.I. (1970) Hematological and biochemical studies in a case of lead poisoning. *American Journal of Medicine*, **48**, 137.

171 CAMPBELL B.C., BRODIE M.J., THOMPSON G.G., MEREDITH P.A., MOORE M.R. & GOLDBERG A. (1977) Alterations in the activity of enzymes of haem biosynthesis in lead poisoning and acute hepatic porphyria. *Clinical Science and Molecular Medicine*, **53**, 335.

172 LAMON J.M., FRYKHOLM B.S. & TSCHUDY D.P. (1979) Hematin administration to an adult with lead intoxication. *Blood*, **53**, 1007.

173 KAPLAN M.L., JONES A.G., DAVIS M.A. & KOPITO L. (1975) Inhibitory effect of iron on the uptake of lead by erythrocytes. *Life Sciences*, **16**, 1545.

174 SARDESAI V.M., MELCER I. & ORTEN J.M. (1974) The

effect of certain inorganic ions on *in vitro* porphyrin-heme formation. *Biochemistry in Medicine*, **7**, 405.

175 WHITE J.M. & SELHI H.S. (1975) Lead and the red cell. *British Journal of Haematology*, **30**, 133.

176 GOLDBERG A. (1968) Lead poisoning as a disorder of heme synthesis. *Seminars in Hematology*, **5**, 424.

177 PERLSTEIN M.A. & ATTALA R. (1966) Neurological sequelae of plumbism in children. *Clinical Pediatrics*, **5**, 292.

178 HENDERSON D.A. (1954) A follow up of cases of plumbism in children. *Australasian Annals of Medicine*, **3**, 219.

179 WALDRON H.A. (1966) The anaemia of lead poisoning: a review. *British Journal of Industrial Medicine*, **23**, 83.

180 LEADING ARTICLE (1973) Subclinical lead poisoning. *Lancet*, **i**, 87.

181 HINES J.D. & LOVE D.S. (1969) Determination of serum and blood pyridoxal phosphate concentrations with purified rabbit skeletal muscle phosphorylase. *Journal of Laboratory and Clinical Medicine*, **73**, 343.

182 BECK E.A. (1967) Reversible sideroachrestic disorder after treatment with chloramphenicol. *Helvetica Medica Acta*, **34** (Suppl.), 139.

183 BECK E.A. & GABATHULER M.B. (1971) Effect of chloramphenicol on heme synthesis by human marrow hemolysates. (Abstract.) *Abstracts XII Congress of the International Society of Haematology*, New York, p. 281. Grune & Stratton, New York.

184 SMITH U., SMITH D.S. & YUNIS A.A. (1970) Chloramphenicol-related changes in mitochondrial ultrastructure. *Journal of Cell Science*, **7**, 1970.

185 SKINNIDER L.F. & GHADIALLY F.N. (1976) Chloramphenicol-induced mitochondrial and ultrastructural changes in hemopoietic cells. *Archives of Pathology and Laboratory Medicine*, **100**, 601.

186 YUNIS A.A. (1973) Chloramphenicol-induced bone marrow suppression. *Seminars in Hematology*, **10**, 225.

187 FIRKIN F.C. (1972) Mitochondrial lesions in reversible erythropoietic depression due to chloramphenicol. *Journal of Clinical Investigations*, **51**, 2085.

188 MANYAN D.R., ARIMURA G.K. & YUNIS A.A. (1972) Chloramphenicol-induced erythroid suppression and bone marrow ferrochelatase activity in dogs. *Journal of Laboratory and Clinical Medicine*, **79**, 137.

189 ROSENBERG A. & MARCUS O. (1974) Effect of chloramphenicol on reticulocyte delta-aminolaevulinic acid synthetase in rabbits. *British Journal of Haematology*, **26**, 79.

190 BOWMAN W.C. (1967) Reversible sideroblastic anemia during infectious mononucleosis: report of a case. *Rocky Mountain Medical Journal*, **64**, 47.

191 DANIELI G., MASETTI G.P., SANGIORGI F. & PENSABENI L. (1964) Forma sideroachrestica dell'anemia in corso di uremia cronica. *Giornale di Clinica Medica*, **45**, 855.

192 GROSS S., SCHOENBERG M.D. & MUMAW V.R. (1965) Electron microscopy of the red cells in erythropoietic porphyria. *Blood*, **25**, 49.

193 RICHTER R., STABBE H. & MARX I. (1965) Zur Diagnostik idiopathischer und symptomatischer sideroblastischer Anaemien. *Folia Haematologica*, **89**, 295.

194 LEE G.R., CARTWRIGHT G.E. & WINTROBE M.M. (1966) The response of free erythrocyte protoporphyrin to

195 CATOVSKY D., SHAW M.T., HOFFBRAND A.V. & DACIE J.V. (1971) Sideroblastic anaemia and its association with leukaemia and myelomatosis. A report of five cases. *British Journal of Haematology*, **20**, 385.

196 HARRIS J.W., WHITTINGTON R.M., WEISMAN R. JR & HORRIGAN D.L. (1956) Pyridoxine-responsive anemia in the human adult. *Proceedings of the Society of Experimental and Biological Medicine*, **91**, 427.

197 DAMESEK W. (1969) The DiGuglielmo syndrome revisited. *Blood*, **34**, 567.

198 ANDRE R., DUHAMEL G. & NAJMAN A. (1970) Anémie sideroblastique refractaire acquise et leucémie aigue terminale. *Annales de Medicine Interne*, **121**, 223.

199 BROUN G.O. JR (1969) Chronic erythromonocytic leukemia. *American Journal of Medicine*, **47**, 785.

200 DREYFUS B., ROCHANT H. & SULTAN C.P. (1969) Anémies refractaires enzymopathies acquises des cellules souches hématopoietiques. *Nouvelle Revue française d'Hématologie*, **9**, 65.

201 FARRARAS-VALENTI P., ROZMAN C. & WAESSNER S. (1964). Anémies refractaires sideroblastiques préhypoplastiques. *Nouvelle Revue française d'Hématologie*, **4**, 519.

202 HEILMEYER L. (1959) The sideroachrestic anaemias. *German Medical Monthly*, **4**, 403.

203 VERLOOP M.C. & BOS C.C. (1963) Differential diagnosis between Bjorkmans anaemia refractoria sideroblastica and erythaemic myelosis (Di Guglielmo's disease). *Proceedings of the 9th Congress of the European Society of Haematology*, Lisbon, Vol. 2, p. 964. Karger, New York.

204 SNELL E.E. (1958) Chemical structure in relation to biological activities of vitamin B_6. *Vitamins and Hormones*, **16**, 77.

205 HINES J.D. & HARRIS J.W. (1964) Pyridoxine-responsive anemia. Description of three patients with megaloblastic erythropoiesis. *American Journal of Clinical Nutrition*, **14**, 137.

206 VERLOOP M.C. & RADEMAKER W. (1960) Anaemia due to pyridoxine deficiency in man. *British Journal of Haematology*, **6**, 66.

207 VUYBITEKE J., VERLOOP M.C. & DROGENDINK A.C. (1961) Favourable effect of pyridoxine and ascorbic acid in a patient with refractory sideroblastic anaemia and haemochromatosis. *Acta Medica Scandinavica*, **169**, 113.

208 GOLDBERG A. (1965) Sideroblastic anaemia: a commentary. *British Journal of Haematology*, **11**, 114.

209 WAPNICK A.A., LYNCH S.R., CHARLTON R.W. SEPTEL H.C. & BOTHWELL T.H. (1969) The effect of ascorbic acid deficiency on desferrioxamine induced urinary iron excretion. *British Journal of Haematology*, **17**, 563.

210 HORRIGAN D.L., WHITTINGTON R.M., WEISMAN R. JR & HARRIS J.W. (1957) Hypochromic anemia with hyperferricemia responding to oral crude liver extract. *American Journal of Medicine*, **22**, 99.

211 HADNAGY C.S. & HUSZAR I. (1966) Effect of pyridoxine, riboflavine and niacin on sideroachrestic anaemia. (Abstract.) *Proceedings of the XI International Congress of Haematology*, Sydney, p.349.

212 BYRD R.B. & COOPER T. (1961) Hereditary iron loading

anemia with secondary hemochromatosis. *Annals of Internal Medicine*, **55**, 103.

213 MILLS H. & LUCIA S.P. (1949) Familial hypochromic anemia associated with postsplenectomy erythrocytic inclusion bodies. *Blood*, **4**, 891.

213a KARABUS C.D. & FIELDING J. (1967) Desferrioxamine chelatable iron in haemolytic, megaloblastic and sideroblastic anaemias. *British Journal of Haematology*, **13**, 924.

214 BRAIN M.C. & HERDAN A. (1965) Tissue iron stores in sideroblastic anaemia. *British Journal of Haematology*, **11**, 107.

215 HATHAWAY D., HARRIS J.W. & STENGER R.J. (1967) Histopathology of the liver in pyridoxine responsive anemia. *Archives of Pathology*, **83**, 175.

216 WIZGIRD J.P., GREENBERG L.D. & MOON H.D. (1965) Hepatic lesions in pyridoxine deficient monkeys. *Archives of Pathology*, **79**, 317.

217 HEIMPEL H. & WENDT F. (1968) Congenital dyserythropoietic anaemia with karyorrhexis and multinuclearity of erythroblasts. *Helvetica Medica Acta*, **34**, 103.

218 CROOKSTON J.H., CROOKSTON M.C., BURNIE K.L., FRANCOMBE W.H., DACIE J.V., DAVIS J.A. & LEWIS S.M. (1969) Hereditary erythroblastic multinuclearity associated with a positive acidified serum test: a type of congenital dyserythropoietic anaemia. *British Journal of Haematology*, **17**, 11.

219 LEWIS S.M., NELSON D.A. & PITCHER C.S. (1972) Clinical and ultrastructural aspects of congenital dyserythropoietic anaemia Type I. *British Journal of Haematology*, **23**, 113.

220 HEIMPEL H., FORTEZA-VILA J., QUEISSER W. & SPIERTZ E. (1971) Electron and light microscopic study of the erythroblasts of patients with congenital dyserythropoietic anemia. *Blood*, **37**, 209.

221 HEIMPEL H., WENDT F., KLEMM D., SCHUBOTHE H. & HEILMEYER L. (1968) Kongenitale dyserythropoietische Anamie. *Archiv für Klinische Medizin*, **215**, 174.

222 GOUDSMIT R., DO BECKERS, DE BRUIJNE J.I., ENGELFRIET C.P., JAMES J., MORSELT A.F.W. & REYNIERSE E. (1972) Congenital dyserythropoietic anaemia Type III. *British Journal of Haematology*, **23**, 97.

223 VILTER R.W., WILL J.J. & JARROLD T. (1967) Refractory anemia with hyperplastic bone marrow (aregenerative anemia). *Seminars in Hematology*, **4**, 175.

224 BATTERSBY A.R., FOOKES C.J.R., MATCHAM G.W.J. & MCDONALD E. (1980) Biosynthesis of the pigments of life: formation of the macrocyte. *Nature (London)*, **285**, 17.

Chapter 14
Porphyrin metabolism and the porphyrias

K. E. L. McCOLL, M. R. MOORE AND A. GOLDBERG

The porphyrias are diseases resulting from hereditary abnormalities in the biochemical pathway of haem formation. Haem biosynthesis is one of the essential pathways of life in both plants and animals [1]. It occurs in all metabolically active human cells, but is most active in erythropoietic tissue where it is required for haemoglobin synthesis and in hepatic tissue where the haem forms the basis of haem-containing enzyme systems such as cytochrome P_{450}, cytochrome b, catalase, peroxidases and tryptophan pyrrolase [2].

THE PATHWAY OF HAEM BIOSYNTHESIS

The biosynthesis of haem is described in the previous chapter. Here we summarize briefly those features necessary for an understanding of the porphyrias.

The enzymes of haem biosynthesis and the functioning of the pathway are shown in Figure 14.1. At the commencement of the pathway, glycine as the activated pyridoxal-phosphate-Schiff base and succinyl CoA from the tricarboxylic-acid cycle condense under the aegis of the initial enzyme of the biosynthetic pathway δ-aminolaevulinic acid (ALA) synthase [3]. The next four stages of the biosynthetic pathway take place in the cytoplasm. The first of these is the condensation of two mol of ALA which has passed out of the mitochondrion to form the monopyrrole porphobilinogen (PBG) by the action of the enzyme ALA dehydratase. The next stage of the pathway requires the concerted action of two enzymes; uroporphyrinogen-I-synthase and uroporphyrinogen cosynthase to produce the asymmetrical octa-carboxylic uroporphyrinogen III. In circumstances where there is a deficiency of uroporphyrinogen cosynthase, uroporphyrinogen-I-synthase produces the symmetrical uroporphyrinogen I. Both of these forms of uroporphyrin may then be sequentially decarboxylated starting on the 'D' ring to form coproporphyrinogen I and III which have four carboxyl groups, although the series-I isomer is decarboxylated more slowly than the series-III isomer. Coproporphyrinogen I may not be metabolized further and is therefore excreted as copropor-

phyrin I. At this point the pathway re-enters the mitochondrion where, by oxidation and decarboxylation of two propionyl groups to vinyl groups, coproporphyrinogen III is converted to protoporphyrinogen IX by coproporphyrinogen oxidase. Protoporphyrin IX is oxidized to protoporphyrin IX by protoporphyrinogen oxidase and finally ferrous iron is inserted into the structure of protoporphyrin IX by ferrochelatase to form haem, the end-product of the pathway [4]. The rate of the synthesis is controlled by the initial enzyme ALA synthase which is under negative feedback control by haem. The haem results in repression and inhibition of ALA synthase at both transcriptional and translational cellular levels [5]. A secondary control mechanism at the level of uroporphyrinogen-I-synthase may be important when the inhibition of ALA synthase is removed [6].

Haem catabolism (see Chapter 4, p. 118) commences with the reductive cleavage by haem oxygenase, of the cyclic tetrapyrrole to a linear tetrapyrrole with loss of iron. These linear tetrapyrroles are the bile pigments and since there are four different ring positions at which cleavage may take place there are potentially four different biliverdins. In mammalian systems the cleavage generally produces biliverdin 9 α where cleavage has taken place between rings A and B. The products of the reaction are biliverdin, iron and carbon monoxide. The final stage of degradation is catalysed by biliverdin reductase which produces bilirubin. This toxic compound must then be conjugated with bilirubin glucuronide and excreted, usually in the faeces where it is transformed to compounds such as mesobilirubinogen, stercobilinogen, stercobilin and urobilinogen [7].

CLASSIFICATION OF THE PORPHYRIAS

Clinical classification
Clinically there are the *acute porphyrias*—acute intermittent porphyria, hereditary coproporphyria and variegate porphyria and the *non-acute porphyrias*—cutaneous hepatic porphyria, erythropoeitic protoporphyria and congenital porphyria (Table 14.1). The

acute porphyrias present with intermittent attacks of systemic illness characterized by abdominal pain and often with accompanying neuropathy and a neuro-psychiatric syndrome. Patients with variegate porphyria or hereditary coproporphyria may, in addition,

association with accumulation of porphyrin precursors.

Biochemical classification
The six different forms of porphyria are the result of

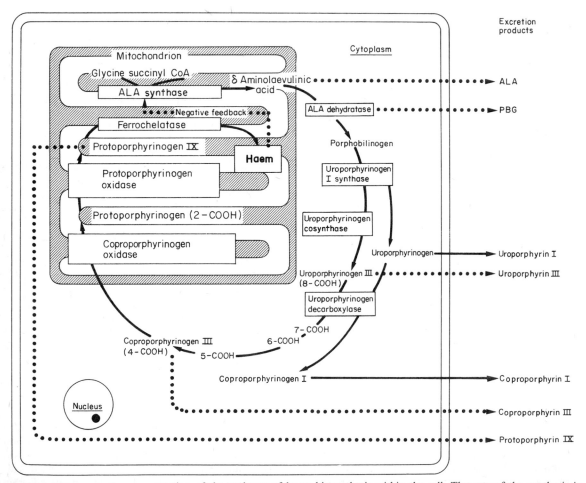

Fig. 14.1. Diagrammatic representation of the pathway of haem biosynthesis within the cell. The rate of the synthesis is controlled by the initial enzyme ALA synthase which is under negative feedback control by haem.

develop solar-photosensitive skin lesions. The non-acute porphyrias present solely with cutaneous manifestations. In the acute porphyrias there is increased excretion of the porphyrin precursors (ALA and PBG) and porphyrins. In the non-acute porphyrias there is increased excretion of porphyrins but normal excretion of the porphyrin precursors. The photosensitive skin lesions are seen where there is accumulation of formed porphyrins while acute attacks are seen in

partial deficiency of different enzymes in the pathway of haem biosynthesis [6]. As a result of the enzyme deficiency there is reduction in haem synthesis and, therefore, by negative feedback control, increased activity of the rate-controlling enzyme, ALA synthase, an increase which is found in all the porphyrias. The combination of increased activity of the initial enzyme ALA synthase and partial enzymatic block later in the pathway results in an accumulation of porphyrins and porphyrin precursors formed proximal to the block; these may appear in blood, urine and faeces. Each of the different types of porphyria, therefore, has a characteristic pattern of overproduction of porphyrins and precursors determined by the site of the enzymatic block.

The enzyme deficiency in acute intermittent porphyria is uroporphyrinogen-I-synthase, in hereditary coproporphyria, coproporphyrinogen oxidase, in porphyria variegata, proroporphyronogen oxidase, in

THE ACUTE PORPHYRIAS

Acute intermittent porphyria

This is the commonest and most severe form of the acute porphyrias. It is inherited in an autosomal-dominant fashion. Estimates of the prevalence of symptomatic acute intermittent porphyria vary considerably from country to country. The highest rate is probably in Lapland, where it is estimated as 1/1000

Table 14.1. Clinical classification of the porphyrias

The acute porphyrias

Acute intermittent porphyria
Hereditary coproporphyria ⎱ Acute attacks of neurodysfunction
Variegate porphyria

The non-acute porphyrias

Cutaneous hepatic porphyria
Erythropoietic protoporphyria   Photosensitive skin lesions
Congenital porphyria

cutaneous hepatic porphyria, uroporphyrinogen decarboxylase, in erythropoietic protoporphyria, ferrochelatase and in congenital porphyria, uroporphyrinogen cosynthetase. It has been reported that a further form of acute porphyria may exist which, in common with lead poisoning, presents with depressed activity of ALA dehydratase [9, 157]. The activity of the enzyme uroporphyrinogen-I-synthase is particularly important in determining the biochemical and clinical presentation of the porphyrias. In acute intermittent porphyria the activity of this enzyme is reduced, but in the other two acute porphyrias, it is normal. In each of the non-acute porphyrias it is increased. This enzyme is at the point in the pathway where porphyrin precursors are converted into porphyrins. It is probably the increased activity of uroporphyrinogen-I-synthase which prevents the accumulation of porphyrin precursors in the non-acute porphyrias [6] as illustrated in Figure 14.2. Further details of the biochemical disorder will be given under the discussion of individual types of porphyria.

[10]. In Western Australia, on the other hand, the prevalence (including latent cases) is only 3/100 000 [11]. Though the genetic trait is equally distributed between sexes the clinical disease is more commonly seen in females. This is probably due to the hormonal fluctuations in females increasing the incidence of clinical attacks.

Acute intermittent porphyria presents with attacks of neurological dysfunction, the patient usually enjoying good health between attacks. It is the one form of porphyria which is not associated with photosensitive skin lesions. The frequency and severity of attacks varies considerably from patient to patient. In a proportion of patients, the disease remains latent throughout life, even in the presence of precipitating factors. Other patients experience frequent and sometimes life-endangering attacks even in the absence of extrinsic precipitating factors. In spite of recent therapeutic advances an acute attack of porphyria with severe neurological involvement may have a fatal outcome.

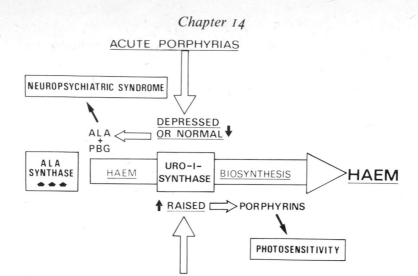

Fig. 14.2. In the acute porphyrias the activity of uroporphyrinogen (URO)-I-synthase is normal or reduced and there is overproduction of porphyrins and the porphyrin precursors ALA and PBG. In the non-acute porphyrias there is increased activity of uroporphyrinogen-I-synthase and accumulation of porphyrins but not of porphyrin precursors.

Underlying biochemical disorder

The basic defect in acute intermittent porphyria appears to be partial deficiency of the enzyme uroporphyrinogen-I-synthase [6]. This has been demonstrated in erythrocytes [12], skin fibroblast cultures [13] and amniotic cells [14]. As a result, there is excess formation and urinary excretion of the porphyrin precursors ALA and PBG [15]. There is also increased urinary and, to a lesser extent, faecal excretion of uroporphyrin. The excess uroporphyrin is probably not due to hepatic overproduction but merely the result of spontaneous polymerization of the excess PBG. An attack is always associated with increased urinary excretion of ALA and PBG though there is no close correlation between the magnitude of this and the severity of the attack. Most patients excrete excess porphyrin precursors during asymptomatic periods between attacks. A small proportion of patients have completely normal excretion profiles between attacks.

Patients with acute intermittent porphyria are also known to produce excess steroids of the 5β-H configuration [16]. This is due to deficiency of hepatic 5α reductase [17]. Some of the 5β-H steroids, which are found in excess, can induce ALA synthase in rat hepatic tissue and they may play a role in the precipitation or exacerbation of the acute attacks [18].

Features of the acute attack

The acute attacks of neurological dysfunction seen in acute intermittent porphyria are similar to those seen in hereditary coproporphyria and porphyria variegata. Attacks are rarely seen before puberty. The highest incidence of onset of symptoms is between puberty and 30 years of age and attacks are most common in the decade from 20–30 years [19]. It should be emphasized, however, that serious attacks may occur for the first time at any age. In one-third of reported cases there is no family history either prospectively or retrospectively, the condition presumably having remained latent for several generations [20].

Abdominal pain is the most frequent complaint, occurring in 95% of cases. The pain is often very severe and Patients frequently require parenteral narcotic analgesics. It may be either colicky or constant in nature. The pain may be localized to one region of the abdomen, but is more usually felt diffusely over the abdomen. patients are almost always constipated during an acute attack. About 10%, however, experience diarrhoea. Anorexia usually occurs and there is often associated nausea and vomiting. On abdominal examination there is usually mild generalized tenderness which often appears inappropriately mild for the degree of pain experienced by the patient. Muscle guarding is rarely seen and bowel sounds are normal. Patients presenting with their first attack may be misdiagnosed as having appendicitis, biliary or renal colic or small-intestinal obstruction, and if they are subjected to an unnecessary laparotomy their condition may be considerably aggravated.

Peripheral neuropathy may be the presenting feature of an acute attack and it complicates more than 50% of porphyric attacks. Ridley [21] found that in most of his cases the neuropathy began with motor symptoms consisting of muscle weakness often preceded by cramp-like pain and stiffness. The peripheral flexor muscles are often the first to be affected resulting in foot-drop and wrist-drop. The motor neuropathy may extend, sometimes rapidly, to involve other muscles. The tendon jerks become diminished or absent and, later, muscle wasting becomes evident. Patients may also complain of parasthaesiae, and sensory diminution may be found on testing. Varying combinations and degrees of motor and sensory involvement may be seen. Difficulty controlling micturition may be experienced. In severe cases with extensive neuropathy, the muscles of ventilation become involved. This is the most serious complication of the acute attack. It is often heralded by weakening of the voice. Cranial-nerve palsies are occasionally seen. Grand-mal convulsions may also occur and are commonest at the height of an attack.

Psychiatric manifestations are common. Waldenstrom [22] found pronounced mental symptoms in 55% of 233 patients with acute intermittent porphyria. Patients may be misdiagnosed as suffering from a purely psychiatric condition and admitted to psychiatric wards. In one study by Kaebling *et al.* [23], 2500 consecutive patients admitted to a mental hospital were screened for acute porphyria. Of the 35 positive tests obtained, the admitting diagnoses included schizophrenia, psychiatric depression, neuroses, personality disorders, alcoholism and acute and chronic brain syndromes. The psychiatric symptoms occasionally persist between attacks.

Tachycardia and hypertension are features of the vast majority of attacks. Sinus tachycardia of up to 160/minute may be seen. the hypertension may be severe and result in encephalopathy and cardiac failure. The hypertension tends to be labile. A substantial proportion of patients will be found to have postural hypotension sometimes resulting in syncope if the blood pressure is checked with the patient erect as well as supine. A percentage of patients remain hypertensive between attacks [24].

In some patients a low-grade pyrexia is noted during an attack. The urinary output is nearly always low during an attack. The urine itself is dark reddish-brown in colour and this becomes more pronounced if the urine is left standing.

Diagnosis of acute attack of porphyria

Any patient presenting with unexplained abdominal pain, neuropathy or psychiatric manifestations should be tested for acute porphyria (Fig. 14.3). All patients in acute attack excrete excess ALA and PBG in the urine.

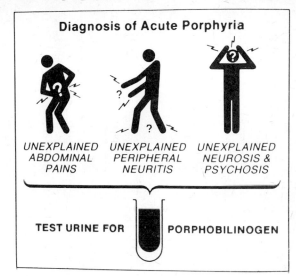

Fig. 14.3. Some presentations of acute porphyria.

The modified Watson–Schwartz test [25] provides a simple and rapid method of demonstrating excess urinary PBG. Two millilitres of fresh urine is added to a test tube. The addition of a further 2 ml of fresh Ehrlich's Aldehyde reagent will result in a red–pink discoloration in the presence of excess PBG or urobilinogen. These can be differentiated by the further addition of 4 ml of chloroform. If the discoloration is due to excess PBG it will remain only in the upper aqueous layer. In order to confirm the diagnosis, quantitative estimation of porphyrins and precursors should be performed on faeces, and 24-hour collection made. This also allows diagnosis of the particular type of acute porphyria. The normal values for porphyrins and their precursors and the alteration of porphyrin and precursor excretion characterizing the different forms of porphyria are shown in Table 14.2.

Other laboratory findings in acute attack

Haematology. The haemoglobin concentration usually remains normal during the acute attack. This is in some ways surprising in a disease due to a partial block in the pathway of haem biosynthesis. The white-cell count and erythrocyte sedimentation rate are also normal or occasionally slightly elevated.

Biochemistry. Electrolyte abnormalities are common in the acute attack [26]. Vomiting and inadequate fluid intake may result in hypokalaemia and varying degrees of uraemia. The creatinine clearance is reduced in a proportion of patients in attack [27]. Severe dilutional hyponatraemia may occur as a result of inappropriate

Table 14.2. Values for porphyrins and precursors in different types of porphyria, plus normal values

	Acute intermittent porphyria	Cutaneous hepatic porphyria	Porphyria variegata	Hereditary coproporphyria	Congenital porphyria	Erythropoetic protoporphyria
Erythrocyte protoporphyrin 0–657 nmol/l erythrocytes	Normal	Normal	Normal	Normal	Usually raised	Raised—usually very high
Erythrocyte coproporphyrin 0–64 nmol/l erythrocytes	Normal	Normal	Normal	Sometimes raised in attack	Usually raised	Sometimes slightly raised
Urinary δ-aminolaevulinic acid 0–40 μmol/24 hours	Raised—very high in attack	Usually normal	Raised in attack	Raised in attack	Usually normal	Normal
Urinary porphobilinogen 0–16 μmol/24 hours	Raised—very high in attack	Usually normal	Raised in attack	Raised in attack	Usually normal	Normal
Urinary uroporphyrin 0–49 nmol/24 hours	Usually raised	Raised—very high in attack	Sometimes raised	Sometimes raised in attack	Raised—isomer 1	Normal
Urinary coproporphyrin 1–432 nmol/24 hours	Sometimes raised	Slightly raised	Sometimes raised	Usually raised—always in attack	Raised—isomer1	Normal
Faecal X porphyrin 0–15 μg/g dry weight	Sometimes raised	Raised	Raised—very high in attack	Sometimes raised—especially with photosensitivity	Raised	Normal
Faecal protoporphyrin 0–200 nmol/g dry weight	Sometimes raised	Raised in remission	Raised	Usually normal	Sometimes raised	Usually raised
Faecal coproporphyrin 0–76 nmol/g dry weight	Sometimes raised	Raised in remission	Raised	Raised	Raised	Normal

secretion of antidiuretic hormone, possibly due to hypothalamic dysfunction [28]. The plasma albumin concentration is frequently low in severe or prolonged attacks, but there is little information available on the mechanisms responsible. A proportion of patients in acute attacks have increased serum concentrations of total thyroxine and tri-iodothyronine [29]. This may be at least partly explained by increased thyroid-binding globulin [30]. An elevation of serum asparate and alanine transaminases has been noted in a number of our patients during the acute attack. Glucose metabolism is deranged during the acute attack, the glucose tolerance frequently being diabetic in type [31]. There is delayed but excessive insulin secretion after a glucose load and this may result in hypoglycaemia several hours after glucose ingestion. Hypercholesterolaemia occurs in about 50% of patients during the acute attack [32]. Examination of CSF is usually normal but slight elevation of the protein is sometimes seen [33].

Electrophysiology. The electroencephalogram (EEG) is abnormal in the majority of patients experiencing an acute attack and in a proportion this persists during remission [34]. This usually takes the form of a generalized slowing of the record and, in addition, focal abnormalities may be evident. Peripheral-nerve-conduction studies in the presence of clinically established neuropathy show changes consistent with axonal injury predominantly of motor nerves [35]. Wochnik-Dyjas *et al.* found nerve-conduction abnormalities which were initially reversible and only sometimes proceeded to axonal degeneration [36].

Relationship between biochemical disorder and clinical features of the acute attack
All the clinical features of the acute attack of porphyria can be explained by neurological dysfunction, involving the central, peripheral and autonomic nervous system. Post-mortem examinations of patients who have died during an acute attack of porphyria have shown demyelination and axonal degeneration of peripheral nerves and autonomic tissue [37]. Changes including demyelination, chromatolysis and vacuolation have also been noted in the brain and spinal cord. The mechanism by which the abnormality of the pathway of haem biosynthesis results in the functional and structural alterations of nervous tissue remains to be elucidated. A number of hypotheses have been postulated [38]. There is some evidence for a neurotoxic [39] and neuropsychiatric [40] effect of ALA. The ALA is structurally similar to the neurotransmitter γ-aminobutyric acid (GABA) and has been shown to have GABA agonist effects in concentrations similar to those thought to occur in nervous tissue of patients with acute porphyrias [41]. The main argument against

the ALA theory is the poor correlation between plasma and urinary ALA concentrations and neurological manifestations. Unfortunately there are few data available regarding correlation between CSF concentrations of ALA and neurological signs [42]. The neuropathy may be the result of haem deficiency. There may be deficiency of haem synthesis within nerve cells for the formation of haemoproteins necessary for normal cellular function and structure. Deficient haem synthesis in the liver could result in altered hepatic metabolism resulting in deficient hepatic clearance of neurotoxic materials or in failure of hepatic synthesis of substance needed by the nervous tissue.

Factors which may precipitate acute attacks
A number of factors are capable of triggering off acute neurological attacks in patients with any of the acute porphyrias as shown in Table 14.3. All of these factors are known to result in or facilitate increased activity of ALA synthase in animal hepatic tissue and chicken-embryo culture preparations. The mechanism by which these factors cause increased ALA synthase activity has not been fully elucidated and several mechanisms probably operate.

Table 14.3. Factors which may precipitate attacks of porphyria

Certain drugs
Hormonal factors
Alcohol
Dieting or fasting
Acute infection and stress

Drugs. A considerable number of drugs are capable of precipitating acute attacks (Table 14.4). The barbiturates were among the first drugs to be so identified. The vast majority of these drugs are inducers of the mixed-function oxidase enzyme system and stimulate increased synthesis of the haemoprotein cytochrome P_{450}. The increased activity of ALA synthase due to these drugs is probably secondary to the utilization of haem for the formation of this cytochrome [43].

Alcohol. Acute alcohol ingestion may trigger off attacks in some subjects [44]. It has recently been shown that the consumption of moderate quantities of alcohol by normal subjects results in increased activity of ALA synthase and depression of several of the intermediate enzymes of the pathway [45].

Hormonal factors. Hormonal factors, especially steroid hormones, are also important in the development of acute attacks. Patients rarely experience attacks before puberty. Women experience attacks more commonly than men and attacks are most common pre-menstrually. Pregnancy and the contraceptive pill may also precipitate attacks. It has recently been shown that there is considerable fluctuation in the activity of ALA synthase throughout the menstrual cycle in normal females compared to normal males [46].

Dieting and fasting. A reduction in calorie intake may precipitate attacks in some patients [47].

Infection or stress. Attacks may also be precipitated by stress such as acute infection or trauma [44].

Management of an acute attack of porphyria

In patients presenting during an acute attack of porphyria it is important to identify and, where possible, remove any precipitating factors. Fluid and electrolyte balance should be monitored and corrected appropriately. The maintenance of adequate carbohydrate intake is essential. It is known that calorie restriction can precipitate attacks and also that the maintenance of a good carbohydrate intake reduces the incidence of attacks [48, 49]. Carbohydrates have been shown to block the induction of hepatic ALA synthase and many other enzymes and this has come to be known as the 'glucose effect' [50, 51]. Acute attacks are generally associated with nausea and vomiting and

Table 14.4. Effects of drugs on porphyria

Drugs believed to be unsafe in the acute porphyrias

Alphaxalone	Flufenamic acid	Oral contraceptives
Aluminium preparations	Flunitrazepam	Oxazolidinediones
Aminoglutethimide	Fluroxine	(Paramethadione and
Amitriptyline		Trimethadione)
Amphetamines	Glutethimide	Oestrogens
Apronalide	Gold preparations (Myocrisin)	Oxazepam
Azapropazone	Griseofulvin	
		Pancuronium
Barbiturates	Halothane	Pargyline
Bemegride	Hydantoins (Phenytoin,	Pentazocine
Busulphan	Ethotoin, Mephenytoin)	Pentylenetetrazol
	Hydrallazine	Phenoxybenzamine
Carbromal	Hydrochlorthiazide	Phenylbutazone
Carbamazepine	Hyoscine Butyl Bromide	Phenylhydrazine
Chlorambucil		Primidone
Chloramphenicol	Imipramine	Probenicid
Chlordiazepoxide	Isoniazid	Progesterone
Chlormezanone	Isopropylmeprobamate	Pyrazinamide
Chloroform		Pyrazolones
Chlormethiazole	Ketoprofen	(amidopyrine, antipyrine,
Chlorpropamide		isopropylantipyrine, dipyrone,
Cimetidine	Lignocaine	sodium phenyl dimethyl
Clonidine		pyrazolone)
Cocaine	Mefenamic acid	Pyrimethamine
Colistin	Mephenezine	
Cyclophosphamide	Meprobamate	Spironolactone
	Mercury preparations	Steroids
Danazol	Methoxyflurane	Succinimides (ethosuximide,
Dapsone	Methyldopa	methsuximide, phensuximide)
Dichoralphenazone	Methyprylone	Sulphonamides
Diethylpropion	Metoclopramide	Sulphonylureas
Dimenhydrinate	Metyrapone	Sulthiame
	Metronidazole	
Enflurane		Tetracyclines
Ergot preparations	Nalidixic Acid	Theophylline
Erythromycin	Nikethamide	Tolazamide
Ethanol	Nitrazepam	Tolbutamide
Ethchlorvynol	Nitrofurantoin	Tranylcypromine
Ethianamate	Novobiocin	Troxidone
Etomidate		
		Xylocaine

Table 14.4. (Cont.)

Drugs believed to be safe in the acute porphyrias

Acetazolamide	EDTA	Quinine
Adrenaline	Ether (Diethyl)	
Amethocaine		Paracetamol
Aspirin	Fentanyl	Penicillins
Atropine	Flurbiprofen	Penicillamine
		Pethidine
Biguanides (Phenformin,	Gentamycin	Phenoperidine
Metformin)	Glipizide	Prednisolone
Bromides	Guanethidine	Procaine
Bumetanide		Prilocaine
Bupivicaine	Heparin	Promethazine
Buprenorphine	Hyoscine	Propantheline Bromide
		Propanidid
Cephalexin	Ibuprofen	Primaquine
Cephalosporins	Indomethacin	Propoxyphen
Chloral hydrate	Insulin	Propranolol
Chlorpheniramine		Prostigmine
Chlorpromazine	Ketamine	
Chlorthiazides		Reserpine
Clofibrate	Labetalol	Resorcinol
Clonazepam	Lithium	
Codeine		Streptomycin
Colchicine		Succinylcholine
Corticosteroids	Mecamylamine	
Cyclizine	Meclozine	Thiouracils
	Mersalyl	Trifluoperazine
Dexamethasone	Methadone	Thiazides
Diamorphine	Methylphenidate	Tripelennamine
Diazepam	Morphine	Tubocurarine
Diazoxide		
Digitalis compounds	Naproxen	
Diphenhydramine	Neostigmine	
Dicoumarol anticoagulants	Nitrous oxide	
Droperidol	Nortriptyline	

thus reduced caloric intake, which almost certainly aggravates the attack. This cycle must be broken. Adequate caloric intake may be maintained orally using high-calorie drinks. Chlorpromazine or promazine may be helpful in alleviating the nausea and vomiting. Improved oral calorie intake may be achieved by slow, continuous infusion via a soft, thin nasogastric tube. The infusion of 20% laevulose (two litres per 24 hours) via a central venous line results in biochemical and clinical improvement in a proportion of patients [52].

Great care must be taken in order to ensure that the patient is not prescribed any of the contraindicated drugs. A list of drugs believed to be safe and others which are unsafe is shown in Table 14.4. Analgesics are usually required to relieve the abdominal pain. Aspirin, paracetamol, dihydrocodeine, pethidine, morphine or diamorphine may be used according to

the severity of the symptoms. The abdominal pain of acute porphyria is sometimes very refractory and some patients require large, frequent doses of intramuscular narcotic analgesics. Severe postural hypotension may result from the use of powerful narcotics, especially if combined with any of the phenothiazines. This can be treated by keeping the patient horizontal and if necessary elevating the foot of the bed. A fuller understanding of the mechanism of the abdominal pain might promote more effective treatment. It has been suggested that it is due to autonomic neuropathy leading to imbalance of the innervation of the gut, with resultant areas of spasm and dilatation [37]. Bowel spasms have been observed in patients with acute porphyria subjected to laparatomy [53]. The use of ganglion-blocking drugs and splanchnicectomy have been tried but with limited success [54]. The hypertension and tachycardia which frequently occur in an acute attack can be controlled by adequate doses of propranolol [55]. There is also some evidence that propranolol may have a beneficial effect on the abnormal porphyrin metabolism [56]. Severe agitation and other forms of psychiatric disturbance which may occur can be controlled with promazine or chlorpromazine. Diazepam may also be used. If long-term anticonvulsant therapy is required, sodium valproate may be safely used. Constipation is usually a problem and neostigmine may be required to alleviate this.

The main advance in the treatment of acute porphyria over the past decade has been the administration of haem in the form of intravenous haematin. This appears to be able to enter the mitochondria and there repress the activity of ALA synthase and thereby reduce the overproduction of porphyrins and precursors. In nearly all the patients treated to date the haematin therapy has lowered the plasma and urinary levels of porphyrin precursors [57, 58]. It has also been shown to repress the activity of ALA synthase which was monitored in peripheral leucocytes [59]. The clinical response has unfortunately not been as consistent as the biochemical one, only slightly over 50% of the patients showing definite objective evidence of clinical improvement. The haematin appears to be less effective in the presence of persistent inducing factors. It is more effective when given fairly early in the course of a severe attack rather than when administered after clinical neuropathy is established. The haematin is prepared from expired Hbs Ag negative blood [60]. It is administered by intravenous infusion over 20 minutes in a dosage of 4 mg/kg body weight. Daily or 12-hourly doses are usually given for several days. It is fairly irritant to small peripheral veins and is probably best given into a large vein or via a central venous line. It appears, to date, to be free of any serious side-effects when given in the above doses. One patient developed transitory renal failure after receiving the relatively large dose of 1000 mg by intravenous bolus injection [61]. Experience with haematin is still limited. The evidence available indicates that it may be used if a satisfactory response is not achieved by the removal of precipitating factors and administration of laevulose. Clinical evidence of developing neuropathy is an indication for early haematin therapy. The biochemical and clinical response of a patient who responded well to three courses of haematin therapy is shown in Figure 14.4.

Prevention of acute attacks of porphyria
Prophylaxis is important in the management of patients with acute porphyria. Time must be spent with the patients explaining the nature of the disease and informing them of the factors which may initiate an attack. A list of contra-indicated drugs should be given to each patient. They should also be told to inform any future medical attendants that they have acute porphyria. We advise all our patients to wear bracelets or necklaces stating that they suffer from the condition. Though pregnancy may precipitate attacks, acute porphyria is not a contraindication to pregnancy and if carefully managed there is little increase in mortality to mother or baby [62]. Patients with recurrent attacks, however, should be advised against pregnancy until they have been symptom-free for at least one year.

Screening of relatives
As the acute porphyrias are inherited in an autosomal-dominant fashion, it is important to investigate all the blood relatives of a new case. In this way, latent cases can be identified and advised regarding the prevention of attacks. Screening of all blood relatives should be performed initially by quantitative estimations of porphyrins and precursors in a random urine collection and 5 g faecal sample. If the results are negative this does not completely exclude the condition as patients may have normal porphyrin excretion when in remission. Recently it has been possible to detect latent cases by measuring the enzymes of haem biosynthesis in peripheral-blood cells. The measurement of porphyrins and precursors will allow the detection of only about 30% of latent cases whereas the enzyme tests will raise this to nearer 80% [63].

Porphyria variegata
Porphyria variegata is so-called because it presents with both acute attacks of neurological dysfunction, as seen in acute intermittent porphyria, and with photosensitive skin eruptions. It is inherited as a Mendelian autosomal-dominant trait. The disorder was described and named in South Africa by Dean & Barnes [64] who traced over a 1000 patients with porphyria variegata to a Dutch-Cape settler who married an orphan girl in 1688. The prevalence of the disorder varies from country to country and appears to be highest in the white population of South Africa where it is estimated to be 3:1000 [65]. Porphyria variegata may present in an identical fashion to acute intermittent porphyria with acute attacks of neurological dysfunction and no cutaneous manifestations [66]. More usually, patients in acute attack will show evidence of photosensitive skin eruptions. Patients may also present solely with the cutaneous manifestations. The prominence of the skin lesions is largely determined by the extent of exposure to sunlight.

Underlying biochemical disorder
The disease is probably the result of partial deficiency of the enzyme protoporphyrinogen oxidase [156], though previous workers have also noted a 50%,

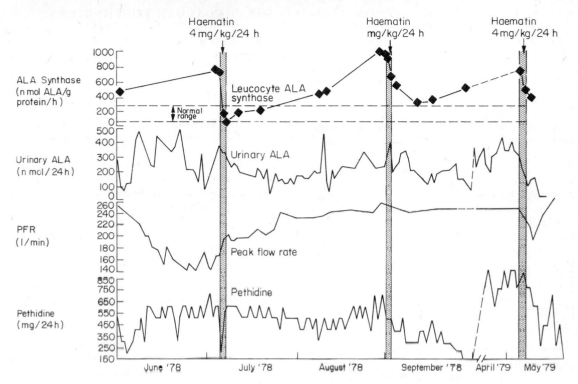

Fig. 14.4. Biochemical and clinical response to three courses of haematin therapy in a 29-year-old woman in a prolonged attack of acute intermittent porphyria. The haematin repressed the activity of ALA synthase, which was monitored in peripheral leucocytes, and reduced the urinary excretion of ALA. There was associated clinical improvement as reflected in rise in respiratory peak flow rate and drop in analgesic requirement.

deficiency of ferrochelatase activity in normoblasts [67] and in fibroblasts [8] of patients with the disease. Patients with porphyria variegata show markedly increased faecal excretion of protoporphyrin and, to a lesser extent, coproporphyrin [68]. There is also a considerable increase of the porphyrin peptide complex known as porphyrin X in the faeces [69, 70]. There may be increased urinary excretion of coproporphyrin and, to a lesser extent, uroporphyrin. During an acute attack there is markedly increased urinary excretion of ALA and PBG and also of uroporphyrin; the latter probably being due to non-specific conversion from PBG. In porphyria variegata there is a close correlation between the urinary excretion of ALA and PBG and the manifestations of acute neurological attacks [71].

Cutaneous manifestations
The skin lesions of porphyria variegata occur on the sun-exposed areas (back of the hands, lower arms, face and neck). The most important feature is increased

skin fragility, minimal trauma being sufficient to cause lesions even to unblemished areas of skin. Lesions usually start as erythema progressing to vesicles that become confluent to form bullae. Haemorrhage may occur into the bullae which heal, leaving scars. There may be local pitting oedema at the site of lesions. Hyperpigmentation may occur and hirsutism may be troublesome in women. Light-microscopy examination of the skin shows the presence of an amorphous material around the smaller blood vessels and capillaries which stain strongly with PAS [72, 73]. The bullae are commonly subdermal rather than intradermal in type [74].

The skin lesions in the porphyrias appear to be the result of interaction between porphyrin deposited in the skin and visible light [75]. Monochromator studies demonstrate that light of the same wavelength as that absorbed by the porphyrin molecule (400 nm) will cause skin lesions in the porphyric patient. Absorption of a suitable quantum of light is thought to convert the porphyrins into the so-called 'triplet state'. The porphyrins, in this excited and reactive state, then transfer their energy to oxygen, forming a molecule of excited oxygen. The cellular damage is probably the result of the excited oxygen forming oxidized products of biological substrates.

Treatment of porphyria variegata

The treatment and prevention of acute neurological attacks of porphyria variegata is the same as for acute intermittent porphyria. There is no specific treatment for the dermatological manifestations. Patients should avoid exposure of skin to sunlight or strong daylight. The wavelength of light which is most damaging to the skin is within the visible spectrum and therefore the ultraviolet barrier creams used to protect against sunburn are of little use. Creams filtering visible light would of necessity be opaque and therefore unacceptable for cosmetic reasons. There is evidence that β carotene may block the interaction of the light and porphyrin molecule and in this way offer a degree of protection [75].

Hereditary coproporphyria

Hereditary coproporphyria is the least common of the acute porphyrias. The disease was named in 1955 by Berger & Goldberg when they reported four cases in a Swiss family [76]. It is inherited as an autosomal-dominant and often remains clinically latent [77]. It presents with attacks of neurological dysfunction, which are similar to the attacks seen in acute intermittent porphyria though generally less severe. During an attack patients may develop photosensitive skin eruptions similar to that seen in porphyria variegata. The skin lesions in hereditary coproporphyria are rarely seen except in an attack [78].

Underlying biochemical disorder

Hereditary coproporphyria is thought to be due to a partial deficiency of the enzyme coproporphyrinogen oxidase. This was demonstrated in circulating leucocytes by Brodie *et al* in 1977 [79] and later in cultured skin fibroblasts [80] and lymphocytes [81]. Patients with hereditary coproporphyria excrete large amounts of coproporphyrin of the isomer-III type in faeces and, to a lesser extent, urine [82, 83]. As in the other forms of acute porphyria neurological attacks are associated with increased urinary excretion of ALA, PBG and uroporphyrin. As in acute intermittent porphyria, 17 oxosteroids are excreted in excess in this disease [84].

Treatment

Prevention and treatment of acute neurological attacks is as for acute intermittent porphyria. In addition patients should be advised to avoid overexposure to sunlight.

THE NON-ACUTE PORPHYRIAS

Cutaneous hepatic porphyria

(PORPHYRIA CUTANEA TARDA, SYMPTOMATIC PORPHYRIA)

This is the commonest form of porphyria seen in Europe and North America and presents with photosensitive skin lesions. There has been a considerable amount of discussion concerning the aetiology of this form of porphyria and both hereditary and exogenous factors seem to be important. The relative importance of these two factors vary from case to case. There is some evidence for two distinct forms of cutaneous hepatic porphyria: a hereditary form in which the trait is passed on in an autosomal-dominant fashion and a sporadic form mainly resulting from exogenous factors [85]. The cutaneous lesions are similar to those seen in porphyria variegata occurring on the light-exposed areas. They start as erythema, progressing to vesicles which become confluent-forming bullae. Haemorrhage into the bullae may occur which heal, leaving scars. Pruritis is often troublesome. Pitting oedema may occur locally at the site of the skin lesions. Increased fragility of the skin is an important feature and in less severe cases may be the only clinical sign. Hyperpigmentation is common. Female patients often complain of hirsutism involving the face, arm and legs.

There is an association between cutaneous hepatic porphyria and alcohol ingestion. Eighty per cent of patients eventually admit to chronic alcohol abuse [78]. Evidence of hepatocellular disease is also commonly found [86]. Liver biopsy usually shows changes of alcoholic damage of varying severity, and hepatic siderosis is an almost constant feature [87]. Hepatocellular disease of non-alcoholic aetiology, for example chronic active hepatitis, may also be seen. Berman *et al.* [88] reported a high incidence of hepatomas in their cirrhotic group of patients with cutaneous hepatic porphyria. There is also an increased incidence of diabetes mellitus [89].

Biochemical findings

In cutaneous hepatic porphyria, the liver forms excessive porphyrins which are normally excreted in the bile and pass into the faeces. With the progression of hepatic disease, this route of excretion becomes less common and porphyrins are deviated to the systemic circulation and excreted mainly as uroporphyrin. Thus the main abnormality in relapse is a high urinary excretion of uroporphyrin and heptacarboxylic porphyrin and to a lesser extent coproporphyrin, together with detectable amounts of plasma porphyrins [90] and X porphyrins in faeces [91]. In remission the urinary porphyrin excretion falls and faecal excretion of coproporphyrin and protoporphyrin rises. The urinary excretion of porphyrin precursors is normal as is the erythrocyte porphyrin concentrations. The characteristic pattern of porphyrin overproduction in cutaneous hepatic porphyria is consistent with the observation of reduced activity of uroporphyrinogen decarboxylase in the liver [92, 93].

Aetiology

Cutaneous hepatic porphyria is aetiologically heterogeneous, both hereditary and acquired factors being important. In a proportion of patients with this condition, there is a history of affected relatives. Studies of these families have shown a reduced activity of uroporphyrinogen decarboxylase in erythrocytes and this is inherited in an autosomal-dominant fashion [94, 95]. It is unlikely that in these families a deficiency of hepatic uroporphyrinogen decarboxylase activity will be likewise inherited and this is supported by the finding of increased urinary excretion of uroporphyrin in some asymptomatic relatives with the erythrocyte enzyme abnormality [96]. In most cases of cutaneous hepatic porphyria there is no family history and the erythrocyte uroporphyrinogen-decarboxylase activity is normal. Acquired factors are important in all cases of cutaneous hepatic porphyria including the familiar ones described above. Chronic alcohol abuse resulting in varying degrees of hepatic dysfunction seems to be the commonest precipitating agent [97]. The relative contribution of the alcohol, liver damage and the almost constantly associated hepatic siderosis to the biochemical disorder is not known. Oestrogen administration may also precipitate cutaneous hepatic porphyria. There have been a number of reports of cases developing in men receiving oestrogen therapy for prostratic cancer [98]. We have recently seen an increased incidence in young women on the contraceptive pill. A number of chemical agents can result in cutaneous hepatic porphyria. There was a famous outbreak in Turkey between 1956 and 1960 when several thousand new cases appeared and this was found to be the result of bread being contaminated with hexachlorobenzene which had been sprayed on to the wheat as a fungicide [65]. Cutaneous hepatic porphyria was also found in a survey of chemical workers in a 2,4-dichlorophenoxyacetic acid and 2,4,5-trichlorophenoxy acetic-acid plant [99]. Similar effects are likely to be associated with many halogenated hydrocarbons [100].

Treatment

Factors known to precipitate cutaneous hepatic porphyria such as alcohol, hormonal therapy or chemicals should be identified and avoided. This will result in biochemical and clinical improvement. Most cases are associated with hepatic siderosis and this is often reflected by increased plasma concentration of iron and ferritin. Removal of this iron by venesection accelerates the improvement [101]; 500 ml of blood should be removed every two weeks until clinical and chemical remission is achieved or the haemoglobin falls below 12 g/dl. The iron stores are usually increased by only 1–2 g and removal of 2–4 l of blood is usually adequate. There are some reports of the use of chloroquine in the treatment of cutaneous hepatic porphyria [102]. This initially results in a marked increase of urinary porphyrin excretion with significant side-effects. As most patients can be adequately controlled by removal of precipitating agents and venesection we would not recommend the use of this relatively toxic and poorly understood form of therapy.

Erythropoietic protoporphyria

Erythropoietic protoporphyria is inherited in a Mendelian autosomal-dominant fashion and may present at any age including infancy and childhood [103]. Patients present with photosensitive skin lesions (Fig. 14.5). Liver damage may also occur in some patients.

Underlying biochemical disorder

Erythropoietic protoporphyria appears to be the result of reduced activity of ferrochelatase, the final enzyme in the pathway of haem biosynthesis which inserts iron into protoporphyrin to form haem. Reduced activity of the enzyme has been noted in erythrocytes [104], leucocytes [105], cultured skin fibroblasts [106] and hepatocytes [107] of patients with erythropoietic protoporphyria. This results in overproduction and accumulation of protoporphyrin which is most marked in erythrocytes. In symptomatic cases the erythrocyte protoporphyrin concentration is considerably higher than occurs in iron-deficiency states or lead poisoning. There is also overproduction of protoporphyrin by the liver and increased excretion of this in the faeces. Erythropoiesis is normoblastic and white-cell and platelet series are normal. Unstained bone-marrow smears exhibit intense red fluorescence when examined in light of wavelength 380–420 nm emitted by an iodine quartz lamp. Porphyrin fluoresence can also be seen in liver-biopsy specimens [108]. Urinary porphyrin and precursor excretion is normal.

There is decreased activity of the enzyme ferrochelatase in both erythropoietic porphyria and porphyria variegata, though it is more marked in the former. It has been suggested that erythropoietic protoporphyria is due to a genetic mutation resulting in an unstable ferrochelatase whereas in porphyria variegata a dominantly inherited structural gene mutation results in an inactive ferrochelatase [8]. As in the other non-acute porphyrias the activity of uroporphyrino-

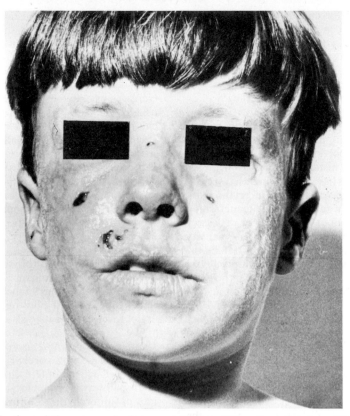

Fig. 14.5. Erythropoietic protoporphyria in an eight-year-old boy (by permission of Dr A. Lyell).

gen-I-synthase has been noted to be increased in erythrocytes of patients with erythropoietic protoporphyria whereas in porphyria variegata the activity of this enzyme is normal.

Clinical features

On exposure to sunlight, patients develop a pruritic urticarial swelling and reddening of the skin. The most distressing symptom is a burning sensation in the affected parts which may become so unbearable that the patient contemplates suicide. Magnus [74] describes how some patients have been known to sit on a chair in the rain for prolonged periods or even attempt to get themselves into a refrigerator. Some authors have described an eczematous type of skin reaction and scarring may take place especially in regions where sunlight is of great intensity. Monochromator tests show the greatest skin sensitivity to be in the 400–410 nm region but the reaction differs from that of hepatic cutaneous porphyria in that erythema and weal formation are the characteristic lesions produced. β carotene is useful in controlling the cutaneous manifestations of erythropoietic protoporphyria [75].

The excess protoporphyrin is excreted solely, and in high concentrations, in the bile. There may be deposition of protoporphyrin crystals in the biliary system and liver cells and this can result in cholestasis, hepatitis, cirrhosis and liver failure [109]. Once liver damage is initiated and cholestasis develops, the protoporphyrin cannot be excreted and there is consequently a rapid accumulation in the liver. The common history of patients with protoporphyria who have died of liver failure is that death occurred within a few months of the onset of jaundice. There is also an increased incidence of gall stones in erythropoietic protoporphyria [110].

Therapy for liver disease in erythropoietic protoporphyria should be directed at decreasing the overproduction of protoporphyrin and decreasing the amount the liver needs to handle. Iron deficiency and fasting both increase protoporphyrin production and should be avoided. Vitamin-E administration has been proposed as a means of lowering protoporphyrin production but clinical results have been inconsistent [111]. Reducing the amount of protoporphyrin the liver needs to handle can be done by interrupting the enterohepatic circulation of protoporphyrin with cholestyramine [112]. Kniffen [113] and Lischner [114] reported that cholestyramine therapy reversed the hepatic disease.

As liver disease in erythropoietic protoporphyria may be rapidly progressive, it is important to identify the small proportion of patients who are liable to develop it. Faecal protoporphyrin excretion does not appear to correlate with potential liver damage but red-cell protoporphyrin has been very high in patients who have developed liver damage. Liver biopsy should be performed on any patients who show even minimal alteration of liver-function tests and if this shows evidence of liver disease, appropriate cholestyramine therapy commenced [109].

Congenital (erythropoietic) porphyria
(GUNTHER'S PORPHYRIA)
This is the rarest form of porphyria and it is, therefore, curious that the first recorded case of porphyria which was reported by Schultz in 1874 [115] was probably of the congenital type. It is inherited in a Mendelian autosomal-recessive fashion [65]. It presents usually in early childhood with photosensitive skin lesions which are more severe than those seen in the other cutaneous porphyrias. Haematological abnormalities are also found.

Underlying biochemical disorder
In congenital porphyria there is deficiency of the haem enzyme uroporphyrinogen-III-cosynthase which has been measured in erythrocytes [116] and skin fibroblasts [117]. There is markedly increased excretion of uroporphyrin I in the urine and to a lesser extent in faeces. There is increased faecal excretion of coproporphyrin I. There is increased plasma and erythrocyte concentrations of uroporphyrin I, coproporphyrin I and protoporphyrin. Porphyrin-precursor excretion is normal.

Clinical features
Sensitivity of the skin to sunlight is the principal symptom of congenital porphyria. Pruritis and erythema are the initial features followed by vesicle and bullae formation. The bullae rupture leaving ulcers which frequently harbour secondary infection. Eventually healing with scar formation takes place. There is considerable variation in severity of the lesions but the results in some cases may be quite devastating. Dystrophic changes in the nails may cause them to curl and drop off. Scarring of the skin on the hand may cause a claw-shaped deformity. Lenticular scarring may lead to blindness. Hypertrichosis may be seen on the face, arms and legs. Pigmentation may be marked. A brownish-pink discoloration of the teeth due to their porphyrin content is an invariable finding. Congenital porphyria can thus result in marked disfigurement and extensive plastic surgery may be required.

Splenomegaly is a consistent finding in this form of porphyria. There is usually a normochromic, normocytic anaemia with polychromasia, anisocytosis and poikilocytosis. A moderate reticulocytosis is present and normoblasts may be present in peripheral blood. Leucopenia and thrombocytopenia may also occur as part of the picture of hypersplenism. The bone marrow usually shows normoblastic hyperplasia and porphyrin fluorescence can be demonstrated in the normoblasts. Erythrokinetic studies by Kramer *et al.* [118] suggested that the anaemia of congenital porphyria is due to ineffective erythropoiesis and shortened red-cell survival.

Management
As in the other forms of cutaneous porphyria, patients should be protected from the harmful effects of sunlight. Splenectomy has been done in several patients and in almost every case the anaemia has improved. Photosensitivity has also improved in about half the patients treated in this way. Splenectomy diminishes the haemolytic process and consequently the hyperactivity of the bone marrow. Thus, although the genetic defect persists, there is considerable reduction in the formation of porphyrins.

ABNORMAL PORPHYRIN METABOLISM IN DISEASES OTHER THAN PORPHYRIA

Altered porphyrin metabolism occurs in a number of conditions other than the porphyrias [119]. The most important of these are lead poisoning, iron-deficiency anaemia and alcohol ingestion.

Lead poisoning
It has been known for some time that in patients suffering from lead poisoning, there is accumulation of protoporphyrin in erythrocytes [120] and increased urinary excretion of ALA [121], coproporphyrin [122] and, rarely in severe cases, PBG [123]. This accumulation of porphyrins and precursors is now known to be the result of the lead inhibiting several of the enzymes of haem biosynthesis. In 1977, Campbell *et al.* [124] measured the activity of six of the enzymes of haem biosynthesis in peripheral-blood cells in patients with lead poisoning and found depression of ALA dehydratase, coproporphyrinogen oxidase and ferrochelatase and increased activity of the rate-controlling enzyme ALA synthase. It has been suggested that lead may inhibit the enzymes by binding to sulphydryl (—SH) groups near their active site [120].

Many of the clinical manifestations of lead poisoning may be the result of the alteration of haem biosynthesis. the anaemia of lead poisoning may be due to the depressant effect of the lead on haem biosynthesis though haemolysis and depression of globin synthesis may also be important [125]. Many of the clinical features of lead poisoning, for example abdominal pain, constipation and peripheral neuropathy, are also seen in acute attacks of hepatic porphyria. These manifestations can all be explained by neurodysfunction. Neuropathy seen in lead poisoning may also be the result of disordered haem biosynthesis and, as in the porphyrias, the mechanism remains to be elucidated.

Alterations in porphyrin metabolism have provided a useful means of detecting and assessing the severity of lead exposure and poisoning [126]. The activity of erythrocyte ALA dehydratase and erythrocyte protoporphyrin levels have aroused the greatest interest, although others such as urinary ALA and coproporphyrin have also been used. For screening purposes a portable spectrofluorimeter has been developed for the rapid determination of protoporphyrin in an untreated drop of blood [127].

Iron-deficiency anaemia

It has been recognized for some time that in iron-deficiency anaemia there is a marked accumulation of protoporphyrin in erythrocytes [128] through this rarely reaches the level seen in erythropoietic protoporphyria. There have been a number of conflicting reports regarding alterations of other porphyrins and precursors [129–131]. The measurement of the erythrocyte protoporphyrin is a useful diagnostic procedure in the investigation of anaemia. It may be raised in latent iron deficiency before changes appear in peripheral blood [132]. It is also helpful when serum iron and ferritin levels may be misleading as a result of patients having been commenced previously on iron therapy or due to the co-existence of inflammatory conditions [133]. The erythrocyte protoporphyrin may also be useful in distinguishing the microcytosis of iron deficiency from that of β thalassaemia, as it is normal in the latter [134].

Alcohol

The association between ethanol ingestion and alterations in porphyrin metabolism was first noted by Franke & Fikentscher in 1935 who found that after drinking one litre of beer or 90 ml of cognac, a subject generally doubled his urinary coproporphyrin excretion [135]. Orten *et al.* noted that chronic alcoholics had an increased urinary excretion of coproporphyrin, mainly isomer III, but normal urinary excretion of uroporphyrin, ALA and PBG [136]. The ratio of urinary excretion of coproporphyrin isomer I–III varies with drinking habit [100]. More recently, ethanol has been noted to cause marked alteration in activity of several of the enzymes of haem biosynthesis. Acute ethanol dosage results in depression of activity of ALA dehydratase and ferrochelatase [137] and increased activity of the rate-controlling enzyme of the pathway, ALA synthase [138], in rat hepatic tissue. In 1971, Moore *et al.* noted that acute ethanol ingestion markedly depressed the activity of ALA dehydratase in peripheral leucocytes [139]. We have recently monitored the activity of six of the enzymes of haem biosynthesis in peripheral-blood cells of eight healthy subjects following the consumption of 200 ml vodka (69·5° proof) [45]. The mitochondrial enzymes, ALA synthase, coproporphyrinogen oxidase and ferrochelatase were measured in leucocytes and the cytosolic enzymes ALA dehydratase, uroporphyrinogen-I-synthase and uroporphyrinogen decarboxylase in erythrocytes. The ethanol administration resulted in increased activity of ALA synthase and uroporphyrinogen-I-synthase, the two enzymes of the pathway which play a rate-controlling role, and depression of the activity of each of the other four enzymes studied. Ferrochelatase, the enzyme which inserts iron into protoporphyrin to form haem, showed the most marked depression. These ethanol-related alterations in haem biosynthesis may be relevant to ethanol-related sideroblastic anaemia. In this condition, there is accumulation of non-haem iron in the mitochondria of blood-cell precursors and also accumulation of protoporphyrin and coproporphyrin in erythrocytes [140]. The alcohol-related marked depression of ferrochelatase activity may explain both of these findings. Patients with ethanol-related sideroblastic anaemia have been noted to have increased activity of ALA synthase in bone marrow [141]. The depression of ferrochelatase activity may also be relevant to ethanol-related siderosis.

Miscellaneous

Minor alterations of haem biosynthesis have been reported in a variety of other haematological conditions including several forms of sideroblastic anaemia [142], megaloblastic anaemia [131], the anaemia of chronic renal failure [143, 144], haemolytic anaemias [145], sickle-cell anaemia [146], leukaemia [120] and polycythaemia [147]. In liver disease there may be increased urinary excretion of coproporphyrin of predominantly the isomer-I type [148, 149]. In the Dubin–Johnson syndrome there is increased urinary excretion of coproporphyrin isomer I and reduced excretion of coproporphyrin isomer III, possibly as a result of deficiency of hepatic uroporphyrinogen-III-isomerase [150]. In Rotor syndrome, urinary excretion of coproporphyrin I is increased with normal copro-porphyrin-III excretion and in Gilbert's disease there is increased urinary excretion of coproporphyrin-I and -III isomers [149]. A slight alteration of faecal porphyrin excretion may be seen in patients with malabsorption [151]. In hereditary tyrosinemia, there may be a marked increase in urinary excretion of ALA [152]. Increased urinary excretion of porphyrin-like substances has been found in a varying proportion of psychiatric patients not having porphyria [153, 154]. The association between this biochemical finding and the psychiatric disorder is not known, although the monopyrrole haemopyrrole lactam is excreted in excess in urine in both acute intermittent porphyria and schizophrenia [155].

REFERENCES

1 ROMEO G. (1977) Enzymatic defects of hereditary porphyria: an explanation of dominance at the molecular level. *Human Genetics*, **39,** 261.

2 MAINES M.D. (1979) Role of trace metals in regulation of cellular heme and hemoprotein metabolism: sensitizing effects of chronic iron treatment on acute gold toxicity. *Drug Metabolism Reviews*, **9,** 237.

3 BONKOWSKY H.L., SINCLAIR P.R. & SINCLAIR J.F. (1979) Hepatic heme metabolism and its control. *Yale Journal of Biology and Medicine*, **52,** 13.

4 MOORE M.R., McCOLL K.E.L. & GOLDBERG A. (1979) The porphyrias. *Journal of Diabetes and Metabolism*, **5,** 323.

5 GRANICK S. & SASSA S. (1971) Delta-aminolaevulinic acid synthetase and the control of haem and chlorophyll synthesis. In: *Metabolic Regulation* (ed. Vogel H.J.), p. 77. Academic Press, New York and London.

6 BRODIE M.J., MOORE M.R. & GOLDBERG A. (1977) The enzyme abnormalities in the porphyrias. *Lancet*, **ii,** 699.

7 TAIT G.M. (1978) The biosynthesis and biodegradation of heme. In: *Heme and Hemoproteins* (ed. De Matteis F. & Aldridge W.N.), p. 1. Springer-Verlag, Berlin.

8 VILJOEN D.J., CAYANIS E., BECKER D.A., KRAMER S., DAWSON B. & BERNSTEIN R. (1979) Reduced ferrochelatase activity in fibroblasts from patients with porphyria variegata. *American Journal of Hematology*, **6,** 185.

9 DOSS M., TIEPERMANN R.V. & SCHNEIDER J. (1980) Acute hepatic porphyria syndrome with porphobilinogen synthase defect. *International Journal of Biochemistry*, **12,** 823.

10 GOLDBERG A. & RIMINGTON C. (1962) *Diseases of Porphyrin Metabolism.* C.C. Thomas, Springfield, Illinois.

11 TSCHUDY D.P. (1974) Porphyrin metabolism and the porphyrias. In: *Duncan's Diseases of Metabolism* (ed. Bondy P.K. & Rosenberg L.E.), 7th edn, p. 775. W.B. Saunders, Philadelphia, London and Toronto.

12 MEYER U.A., STRAND L.J., DOSS M., REES A.C. & MARVER H.S. (1972) Intermittent acute porphyria—demonstration of a genetic defect in porphobilinogen metabolism. *New England Journal of Medicine*, **286,** 1277.

13 BONKOWSKY H.L., TSCHUDY D.P., WEINBACH E.C., EBERT P.S. & DOHERTY J.M. (1975) Porphyrin synthesis and mitochondrial respiration in acute intermittent porphyria; studies using cultured human fibroblasts. *Journal of Laboratory and Clinical Medicine*, **85,** 93.

14 SASSA S., SOLISH G., LEVERE R.D. & KAPPAS A. (1975) Studies in porphyria. IV. Expression of the gene defect of acute intermittent porphyria in cultured human skin fibroblasts and amniotic cells: prenatal diagnosis of the porphyric trait. *Journal of Experimental Medicine*, **142,** 722.

15 TSCHUDY D.P. (1965) Biochemical lesions in porphyria. *Journal of the American Medical Association*, **191,** 718.

16 GOLDBERG A., MOORE M.R., BEATTIE A.D., HALL P.E., McCALLUM J. & GRANT J.K. (1969) Excessive urinary excretion of certain porphyrinogenic steroids in human acute intermittent porphyria. *Lancet*, **i,** 115.

17 KAPPAS A., BRADLOW H.L., GILLETTE P.M. & GALLAGHER T.F. (1971) Abnormal steroid hormone metabolism in the genetic liver disease acute intermittent porphyria. *Annals of the New York Academy of Sciences*, **179,** 611.

18 MOORE M.R., PAXTON J.W., BEATTIE A.D. & GOLDBERG A. (1973) 17-oxosteroid control of porphyrin biosynthesis. *Enzyme*, **16,** 314.

19 WALDENSTROM J. & HAEGER-ARONSEN B. (1963) Different patterns of porphyria. *British Medical Journal*, **ii,** 272.

20 BEATTIE A.D. & GOLDBERG A. (1973) The porphyrias. *Medicine*, **12,** 774.

21 RIDLEY A. (1969) The neuropathy of acute intermittent porphyria. *Quarterly Journal of Medicine*, **38,** 307.

22 WALDENSTROM J. (1957) The porphyrias as inborn errors of metabolism. *American Journal of Medicine*, **22,** 758.

23 KAEBLING R., CRAIG J. & RUSUMANIK B. (1961) Urinary porphobilinogen. *Archives of General Psychiatry*, **5,** 494.

24 BEATTIE A.D. & GOLDBERG A. (1976) Acute intermittent porphyria. Natural history and prognosis. In: *Porphyrins in Human Diseases* (ed. Doss M.), p. 245. Karger, Basel.

25 WATSON C.J., BOSSENMAIER I. & CARDINAL R. (1961) Acute intermittent porphyria—urinary porphobilinogen and other Ehrlich reactors in the diagnosis. *Journal of the American Medical Association*, **175,** 1087.

26 EALES L. & DOWDLE F.B. (1969) Electrolyte abnormalities in porphyria. *Lancet*, **i,** 51.

27 EALES L., DOWDLE F.B. & SWEENEY G.D. (1971) The electrolyte disorder of the acute porphyric attack and the possible role of δ-aminolaevulinic acid. *South African Journal of Laboratory and Clinical Medicine* (special issue), **17,** 89.

28 LUDWIG G.D. & GOLDBERG A. (1963) Hyponatraemia in acute intermittent porphyria probably resulting from inappropriate secretion of anti-diuretic hormone. *Annals of the New York Academy of Sciences*, **104,** 710.

29 BRODIE M.J., GRAHAM D.J.M., GOLDBERG A., BEASTALL G.H., RATCLIFFE W.A., RATCLIFFE J.G. & YEO P.P.B. (1978) Thyroid function in acute intermittent porphyria: a neurogenic cause of hyperthyroidism. *Hormone and Metabolism Research*, **10,** 327.

30 HOLLANDER C.S., SCOTT R.L., TSCHUDY D.P., PERLROTH M.G., WAXMAN A & STERLING K. (1967) In-

creased protein-bound iodine and thyroxine-binding globulins in acute intermittent porphyria. *New England Journal of Medicine*, **277**, 995.

31 WAXMAN A., SCHALCH D.S., ODELL W.D. & TSCHUDY D.P. (1967) Abnormalities of carbohydrate metabolism in acute intermittent porphyria. *Journal of Clinical Investigation*, **46**, 1129.

32 TADDEINI L., NORSTROM K.L. & WATSON C.J. (1964) Hypercholesterolaemia in experimental and human hepatic porphyria. *Metabolism*, **13**, 691.

33 STEIN J.A. & TSCHUDY D.P. (1970) Acute intermittent porphyria: a clinical and biochemical study of 46 patients. *Medicine*, **49**, 1.

34 ALBERS J.W., ROBERTSON W.C. & DAUBE J.R. (1978) Electrodiagnostic findings in acute porphyric neuropathy. *Muscle and Nerve*, **1**, 292.

35 CAVANAGH J.B. & MELLICK R.S. (1965) On the nature of peripheral nerve lesions associated with acute intermittent porphyria. *Journal of Neurology, Neurosurgery and Psychiatry*, **28**, 320.

36 WOCHNIK-DYJAS D., NIEWIADOMSKA M. & KOSTRZEWSKA E. (1978) Porphyric polyneuropathy and its pathogenesis in the light of electrophysiological investigations. *Journal of the Neurological Sciences*, **35**, 243.

37 GIBSON J.B. & GOLDBERG A. (1956) The neuropathy of acute porphyria. *Journal of Pathology and Bacteriology*, **71**, 495.

38 LAMON J.M., FRYKHOLM B.C., HESS R.A. & TSCHUDY D.P. (1979) Hematin therapy for acute porphyria. *Medicine*, **58**, 252.

39 BECKER D.M. & KRAMER S. (1977) The neurological manifestations of porphyria: a review. *Medicine*, **56**, 411.

40 CUTLER M.G., MOORE M.R. & EWART F.G. (1979) Effects of δ-aminolaevulinic acid administration on social behaviour in the laboratory mouse. *Psychopharmacology*, **61**, 131.

41 MULLER W.E. & SNYDER S.H. (1977) Delta-aminolaevulinic acid: influences on synaptic GABA receptor binding may explain CNS symptoms of porphyria. *Annals of Neurology*, **2**, 340.

42 PERCY V.A. & SHANLEY B.C. (1977) Porphyrin precursors in blood, urine and cerebrospinal fluid in acute porphyria. *South African Medical Journal*, **52**, 219.

43 MCCOLL K.E.L., MOORE M.R., THOMPSON G.G. & GOLDBERG A. (1980) Induction of delta-aminolaevulinic acid synthase in leucocytes of patients on diphenylhydantoin therapy—comparison with changes in rat hepatic tissue. *British Journal of Clinical Pharmacology*, **9**, 327.

44 EALES L. (1971) Acute porphyria: the precipitating and aggravating factors. *South African Journal of Laboratory and Clinical Medicine* (special issue), **17**, 126.

45 MCCOLL K.E.L., THOMPSON G.G., MOORE M.R. & GOLDBERG A. (1980) Acute ethanol ingestion and haem biosynthesis in healthy subjects. *European Journal of Clinical Investigation*, **10**, 107.

46 MCCOLL K.E.L. (1979) Studies of activity of leucocyte δ-aminolaevulinic acid synthase throughout human menstrual cycle. (Personal communication.)

47 KNUDSEN K.B., SPARBERG M. & LECOCQ F. (1967) Porphyria precipitated by fasting. *New England Journal of Medicine*, **277**, 350.

48 WELLAND F.H., HELLMAN E.S., GADDIS E.M., COLLINS A., HUNTER G.W. JR & TSCHUDY D.P. (1964) Factors affecting the excretion of porphyrin precursors by patients with acute intermittent porphyria. I. The effect of lead. *Metabolism*, **13**, 232.

49 FELSCHER B.F. & REDEKER A.G. (1967) Acute intermittent porphyria: effect of diet and griseofulvin. *Medicine*, **46**, 217.

50 TSCHUDY D.P., WELLAND F.H., COLLINS A. & HUNTER G.W. JR (1964) The effect of carbohydrate feeding on the induction of δ-aminolaevulinic acid synthetase. *Metabolism*, **13**, 396.

51 GOLDBERG M.L. (1974) The glucose effect, carbohydrate repression of enzyme induction, RNA synthesis, and glucocorticoid activity—a role for cyclic AMP and cyclic GMP. *Life Sciences*, **17**, 1747.

52 BRODIE M.J., MOORE M.R., THOMPSON G.G. & GOLDBERG A. (1977) The treatment of acute intermittent porphyria with laevulose. *Clinical Science and Molecular Medicine*, **53**, 365.

53 MASON V.R., COURVILLE C. & ZISKIND E. (1933) The porphyrins in human disease. *Medicine*, **12**, 355.

54 WEHRMACHER W.H. (1952) New symptomatic treatment for acute intermittent porphyria. *Archives of Internal Medicine*, **89**, 111.

55 DOUER D., WEINBERGER A., PINKHAS J. & ATSMON A. (1978) Treatment of acute intermittent porphyria with large doses of propranolol. *Journal of the American Medical Association*, **240**, 766.

56 BLUM I. & ATSMON A. (1976) Reduction of porphyrin excretion in porphyria variegata by propranolol. *South African Medical Journal*, **50**, 898.

57 WATSON C.J., PIERACH C.A., BOSSENMAIER I. & CARDINAL R. (1978) Use of haematin in the acute attack of the 'inducible' hepatic porphyrias. *Advances in Internal Medicine*, **23**, 265.

58 LAMON J.M., FRYKHOLM B.C., HESS R.A. & TSCHUDY D.P. (1979) Haematin therapy for acute porphyria. *Medicine*, **58**, 252.

59 MCCOLL K.E.L., THOMPSON G.G., MOORE M.R. & GOLDBERG A. (1979) Haematin therapy and leucocyte δ-aminolaevulinic acid synthetase activity in prolonged attack of acute porphyria. *Lancet*, **i**, 133.

60 MCCOLL K.E.L., MOORE M.R., THOMPSON C.G. & GOLDBERG A. (1981) Treatment with haematin in acute hepatic porphyria. *Quarterly Journal of Medicine*, In press.

61 DHAR G.J., BOSSENMAIER I., CARDINAL R., PETRYKA Z.J. & WATSON C.J (1978) Transitory renal failure following rapid administration of a relatively large amount of haematin in a patient with acute intermittent porphyria in clinical remission. *Acta Medica Scandinavica*, **203**, 437.

62 BRODIE M.J., MOORE M.R., THOMPSON G.G., GOLDBERG A. & LOW R.A.L. (1977) Pregnancy and the acute porphyrias. *British Journal of Obstetrics and Gynaecology*, **84**, 726.

63 LAMON J.M., FRYKHOLM B.C. & TSCHUDY D.P. (1979) Family evaluations in acute intermittent porphyria using red-cell uroporphyrinogen-I-synthase. *Journal of Medical Genetics*, **16**, 134.

64 DEAN G. & BARNES H.D. (1955) The inheritance of porphyria. *British Medical Journal*, **ii**, 89.

65 DEAN G. (1971) *The Porphyrias—A Story of Inheritance and Environment.* 2nd edn. Pitman, London.

66 KRAMER S. (1980) *Variegate Porphyria in Clinics in Haematology* (ed. Goldberg A. & Moore M.R.), p. 303. W.B. Saunders, London.

67 BECKER D.M., VILJOEN J.D., KATZ J. & KRAMER S. (1977) Reduced ferrochelatase activity: a defect common to porphyria variegata and protoporphyria. *British Journal of Haematology*, **36**, 171.

68 BARNES H.D. (1958) Porphyria in South Africa: the faecal excretion of porphyria. *South African Medical Journal*, **32**, 680.

69 RIMINGTON C., LOCKWOOD W.H. & BELCHER R.V. (1968) The excretion of porphyrin-peptide conjugates in porphyria variegata. *Clinical Science*, **35**, 211.

70 EALES L., GROSSER Y. & SEARS W.G. (1975) The clinical biochemistry of the human hepatocutaneous porphyrias in the light of recent studies of newly identified intermediates and porphyrin derivatives. *Annals of the New York Academy of Sciences*, **244**, 441.

71 KRAMER S., BECKER D. & VILJOEN D. (1973) Significance of the porphyrin precursors δ-aminolaevulinic acid (ALA) and porphobilinogen (PBG) in the acute attack of porphyria. *South African Medical Journal*, **47**, 1735.

72 FINDLAY G.H., SCOTT F.P. & CRIPPS D.J. (1966) Porphyria and lipid proteinosis. A clinical histochemical and biochemical comparison of 19 South African cases. *British Journal of Dermatology*, **78**, 69.

73 VAN DER SAR A. & DEN OUDEN A. (1976) Porphyria variegata in a Curaçao negroid female. *Netherlands Journal of Medicine*, **19**, 19.

74 MAGNUS I.A. (1968) The cutaneous porphyrias. *Seminars in Hematology*, **5**, 380.

75 MAGNUS I.A. (1980) Cutaneous porphyria. In: *Clinics in Haematology* (ed. Goldberg A. & Moore M.R.), p. 273. W.B. Saunders, London.

76 BERGER H. & GOLDBERG A. (1955) Hereditary coproporphyria. *British Medical Journal*, **ii**, 85.

77 BRODIE M.J. & GOLDBERG A. (1980) The acute porphyrias. In: *Clinics in Haematology* (ed. Goldberg A. & Moore M.R.), p. 253. W.B. Saunders, London.

78 GOLDBERG A., BRODIE M.J. & MOORE M.R. (1978) Porphyrin metabolism and the porphyrias. In: *Price's Textbook of Medicine* (ed. Bodley-Scott R.) 12th edn, p. 420. Oxford University Press, Oxford and New York.

79 BRODIE M.J., THOMPSON G.G., MOORE M.R., BEATTIE A.D. & GOLDBERG A. (1977) Hereditary coproporphyria: demonstration of the abnormalities in haem biosynthesis in peripheral blood. *Quarterly Journal of Medicine*, **46**, 229.

80 EDLER G.H., EVANS J.O., THOMAS N., COX R., BRODIE M.J., MOORE M.R., GOLDBERG A. & NICHOLSON D.C. (1976) The primary enzyme defect in hereditary coproporphyria. *Lancet*, **ii**, 1217.

81 GRANDCHAMP B., PHUNG N., GRELIER M., DE VERNEUIL H., NOIRE J., OHNET J.P. & NORDMANN Y. (1978) Mise en evidence du deficit enzymatique hereditaire dans la coproporphyrie. *Nouvelle Press Medicale*, **6**, 1537.

82 MARVER H.S. & SCHMID R. (1972) In: *Metabolic Basis of Inherited Diseases* (ed. Stanbury J.B., Wyngaarden J.B. & Fredrickson D.S.) 3rd edn, p. 1087. McGraw-Hill, New York.

83 GOLDBERG A., RIMINGTON C. & LOCHHEAD A.C. (1967) Hereditary coproporphyria. *Lancet*, **i**, 636.

84 PAXTON J.W., MOORE M.R., BEATTIE A.D. & GOLDBERG A. (1975) Urinary excretion of 17-oxosteroids in hereditary coproporphyria. *Clinical Science and Molecular Medicine*, **49**, 441.

85 ELDER G.H., SHEPPARD D.M., DE SALAMANCA R.E. & OLMOS A. (1981) Identification of two types of porphyria cutanea tarda by measurement of red-cell uroporphyrinogen decarboxylase. *Clinical Science* (in press).

86 EALES L. (1963) Porphyria as seen in Cape Town. A survey of 250 patients and some recent studies. *South African Journal of Laboratory and Clinical Medicine*, **9**, 151.

87 LAMONT N.M. & HATHORN M. (1960) Increased plasma iron and liver pathology in Africans with porphyria. *South African Medical Journal*, **34**, 279.

88 BERMAN J. & BRAUN A. (1962) Incidence of hepatoma in porphyria cutanea tarda. *Review of Czechoslovak Medicine*, **8**, 290.

89 KEELEY K.H. (1963) Porphyria in Bantu subjects. *South African Journal of Laboratory and Clinical Medicine*, **9**, 309.

90 MOORE M.R., THOMPSON G.G., ALLAN B.R., HUNTER J.A.A. & PARKER S. (1973) Plasma porphyrin concentrations in porphyria cutanea tarda. *Clinical Science and Molecular Medicine*, **45**, 711.

91 MOORE M.R., THOMPSON G.G. & GOLDBERG A. (1972) Amounts of faecal porphyrin peptides—conjugates in the porphyrias. *Clinical Science*, **43**, 299.

92 KUSHNER J.P., BARBUTO A.J. & LEE G.R. (1976) An inherited enzyme defect in porphyria cutanea tarda: decreased uroporphyrinogen decarboxylase activity. *Journal of Clinical Investigation*, **58**, 1089.

93 ELDER G.H., LEE G.B. & TOVEY J.A. (1978) Decreased activity of hepatic uroporphyrinogen decarboxylase in sporadic porphyria cutanea tarda. *New England Journal of Medicine*, **299**, 274.

94 TIEPERMANN R., TOPI G., D'ALESSANDRO GANDOLFO L. & DOSS M. (1978) Uroporphyrinogen decarboxylase defect in erythrocytes in hereditary chronic hepatic porphyria. *Journal of Clinical Chemistry and Biochemistry*, **16**, 52.

95 VERNEUIL H., DE AITKEN G. & NORMANN Y. (1978) Familial and sporadic porphyria cutanea tarda: two different diseases. *Human Genetics*, **44**, 145.

96 BENDETTO A.V., KUSHNER J.P. & TAYLOR J.S. (1978) Porphyria cutanea tarda in three generations of a single family. *New England Journal of Medicine*, **298**, 358.

97 BRUNSTING L.A. (1954) Observations on porphyria cutanea tarda. *Archives of Dermatology and Syphilogy*, **70**, 551.

98 ROENIGK H.H. & GOTTLAB M.E. (1970) Oestrogen-induced porphyria cutanea tarda. *Archives of Dermatology*, **102**, 260.

99 POLAND A., SMITH D., METTER G. & POSSICK P. (1971) A health survey of workers in a 2,4-D and 2,4,5-T plant: with special attention to chloracne, porphyria cutanea tarda and psychologic parameters. *Archives of Environmental Health*, **22**, 316.

100 ELDER G.M. (1976) Acquired disorders of haem synthesis. *Essays in Medical Biochemistry*, **2**, 75.

101 LUNDVALL O. & WEINFIELD A. (1968) Studies of the clinical and metabolic effects of phlebotomy treatment in porphyria cutanea tarda. *Acta Medica Scandinavica*, **184**, 191.

102 SWANBECK G. & WENNERSTEN G. (1977) Treatment of porphyria cutanea tarda with chloroquine and phlebotomy. *British Journal of Dermatology*, **97**, 77.

103 LYNCH P.J. & MIEDLER L.J. (1965) Erythropoietic protoporphyria—report of a family and a critical review. *Archives of Dermatology*, **92**, 351.

104 DE GOEIJ A.F.P.M., SMIT S. & VAN STEVENINCK J. (1977) Porphyrin synthesis in blood cells of patient with erythropoietic protoporphyria. *Clinica Chimica Acta*, **74**, 27.

105 BRODIE M.J., MOORE M.R., THOMPSON G.G., GOLDBERG A. & HOLTI G. (1977) Haem biosynthesis in peripheral blood in erythropoietic protoporphyria. *Clinical and Experimental Dermatology*, **2**, 381.

106 BONKOWSKY H.L., BLOOMER J.R., EBERT P.S. & MAHONEY M.J. (1975) Haem synthetase deficiency in human protoporphyria. Demonstration of the deficit in liver and cultured skin fibroblasts. *Journal of Clinical Investigation*, **56**, 1139.

107 CRIPPS D.J. & McEACHERN W.N. (1971) Hepatic erythropoietic protoporphyria. *Archives of Pathology*, **91**, 497.

108 REDEKER A.G., BRONOW R.S. & STERLING R.E. (1963) Erythropoietic protoporphyria. *South African Journal of Laboratory and Clinical Medicine*, **9**, 235.

109 BLOOMER J.R. (1979) Pathogenesis and therapy of liver disease in protoporphyria. *Yale Journal of Biology and Medicine*, **52**, 39.

110 DELEO V.A., POH-FITZPATRICK M. & MATTHEWS-ROTH M. (1976) Erythropoietic protoporphyria. Ten years' experience. *American Journal of Medicine*, **60**, 8.

111 WATSON C.G., BOSSENMAIER I. & CARDINAL R. (1973) Lack of significant effect of vitamin E on porphyrin metabolism. Report of four patients with various forms of porphyria. *Archives of Internal Medicine*, **131**, 698.

112 STRATHERS G.M. (1966) Porphyrin-binding effect of cholestyramine. Results of *in vitro* and *in vivo* studies. *Lancet*, **ii**, 780.

113 KNIFFEN J.C. (1970) Protoporphyrin removal intrahepatic prophyrastasis. *Gastroenterology*, **58**, 1027.

114 LISCHNER H.W. (1966) Cholestyramine and porphyrinbinding. *Lancet*, **ii**, 1079.

115 SCHULTZ J.H. (1874) *Ein Fall von Pemphigus leprosus, complicirt durch Lepra visceralis.* Inaugural dissertation. Griefswold.

116 ROMEO G., GLENN B.L. & LEVIN E.Y. (1970) Uroporphyrinogen-III-cosynthetase in asymptomatic carriers of congenital erythropoietic porphyria. *Biochemical Genetics*, **4**, 719.

117 IPPEN H. & FUCHS T. (1980) Congenital porphyria: porphyria erythropoietica congenita, Gunther. In: *Clinics in Haematology* (ed. Goldberg A. & Moore M.R.), p. 323. W.B. Saunders, London.

118 KRAMER S., VILJOEN E., MEYER A.M. & METZ J. (1965) The anaemia of erythropoietic porphyria with the first description of the disease in an elderly patient. *British Journal of Haematology*, **11**, 666.

119 McCOLL K.E.L. & GOLDBERG A. (1980) Abnormal porphyrin metabolism in diseases other than porphyria.

In: *Clinics in Haematology* (ed. Goldberg A. & Moore M.R.), p. 427. W.B. Saunders, London, Philadelphia and Toronto.

120 MOORE M.R. & GOLDBERG A. (1974) Normal and abnormal haem biosynthesis. In: *Iron in Biochemistry and Medicine* (ed. Jacobs A. & Worwood M.), p. 115. Academic Press, London.

121 HAEGER-ARONSEN B. (1957) Increased content of δ-aminolaevulinic acid-like substance in urine from workers in lead industry. *Scandinavian Journal of Clinical and Laboratory Investigations*, **9**, 211.

122 GROTEPASS W. (1932) Zur Kenntnis des im harn auftretenden Porphyrins bei Blejvergiftung. *Hoppe Seyler's Zeitschrift für Physiologische Chemie*, **205**, 193.

123 GIBSON S.L.M., MacKENZIE J.C. & GOLDBERG A. (1968) The diagnosis of industrial lead poisoning. *British Journal of Industrial Medicine*, **25**, 40.

124 CAMPBELL B.C., BRODIE M.J., THOMPSON G.G., MEREDITH P.A., MOORE M.R. & GOLDBERG A. (1977) Alterations in the activity of enzymes of haem biosynthesis in lead poisoning and acute hepatic porphyria. *Clinical Science and Molecular Medicine*, **53**, 335.

125 MOORE M.R., MEREDITH P.A. & GOLDBERG A. (1979) Lead and haem biosynthesis. In: *Lead Toxicity* (ed. Singhal R.L. & Thomas J.A.), p. 79. Yrban and Schwartzeberg, Baltimore.

126 MEREDITH P.A., MOORE M.R. & GOLDBERG A. (1979) Erythrocyte δ-aminolaevulinic acid dehydratase activity and blood protoporphyrin levels as indices of lead exposure and altered haem biosynthesis. *Clinical Science*, **56**, 61.

127 BLUMBERG W.E., EISINGER J., LAMOLA A.A. & ZUCKERMAN D.M. (1977) The hematofluorimeter. *Clinical Chemistry*, **23**, 270.

128 PAGLIARDI E., PRATO V., GIANGRANDI E. & FIORINA L. (1959) Behaviour of the free erythrocyte protoporphyrin and of the erythrocyte copper in iron-deficiency anaemias. *British Journal of Haematology*, **5**, 217.

130 KANEKO K. (1970) Disturbances of haem synthesis in iron-deficiency anaemia. *Acta Haematologica Japonica*, **33**, 857.

131 CAMPBELL B.C., MEREDITH P.A., MOORE M.R. & GOLDBERG A. (1978) Erythrocyte δ-aminolaevulinic acid dehydratase activity and changes in δ-aminolaevulinic acid concentrations in various forms of aneamia. *British Journal of Haematology*, **40**, 397.

132 DAGG J.H., GOLDBERG A. & LOCHHEAD A. (1966) Value of erythrocyte protoporphyrin in the diagnosis of latent iron deficiency. *British Journal of Haematology*, **12**, 326.

133 THOMAS W.J., KOENIG H.M., LIGHTSEY A.L. & GREEN R. (1977) Free erythrocyte porphyrin: haemoglobin ratios, serum ferritin and transferrin saturation levels during treatment of infants with iron-deficiency anaemia. *Blood*, **49**, 455.

134 STOCKMAN J.A., WEINER L.S., SIMON G.E., STUART M.J. & OSKI F.A. (1975) The measurement of free erythrocyte porphyrins as a simple means of distinguishing iron deficiency from β-thalassaemia trait in subjects with microcytosis. *Journal of Laboratory and Clinical Medicine*, **85**, 113.

135 FRANKE K. & FIKENTSCHER R. (1935) Die Bedeutung der quantitativen Porphyrin bestimmung mix der Lumineszenzmessung für die prufund der Leberjunk-

tion und for Ernahrungsfrogen. *Munchener Medizinische Wochenschrift*, **82**, 171.

136 ORTEN J.M., DOEHR S.A., BOND C., JOHNSON H. & PAPPOS A. (1963) Urinary excretion of porphyrins and porphyrin intermediates in human alcoholics. *Quarterly Journal of Studies on Alcohol*, **24**, 598.

137 MOORE M.R. (1973) The effect of ethanol on haem biosynthesis. *Proceedings of the First International Symposium on Alcohol and Aldehyde Metabolizing Systems*, Stockholm, p. 21.

138 SHANLEY B.C., ZAIL S.S. & JOUBERT S.M. (1968) Effect of ethanol on liver δ-aminolaevulinic synthetase in rats. *Lancet*, **i**, 70.

139 MOORE M.R., BEATTIE A.D., THOMPSON G.G. & GOLDBERG A. (1971) Depression of δ-aminolaevulinic acid dehydratase activity by ethanol in man and rat. *Clinical Science*, **40**, 81.

140 ALI M.A.N. & SWEENEY G. (1974) Erythrocyte coproporphyrin and protoporphyrin in ethanol-induced sideroblastic erythropoiesis. *Blood*, **43**, 291.

141 FRASER M.B. & SCHACTER B.A. (1977) Increased bone marrow δ-aminolaevulinic acid synthetase activity in the acute reversible sideroblastic anaemia of alcoholics. *Blood*, **50** (Suppl. 1), 92.

142 BOTTOMLEY S.S. (1977) Porphyrin and iron metabolism in sideroblastic anaemia. In: *Iron Excess: Aberrations of Iron and Porphyrin Metabolism* (ed. Müller-Eberhard U., Miescher P.A. & Jaffé E.R.), p. 169. Academic Press, London.

143 VLASSAPOULOUS K., MELISSINOS K. & DRIVAS G. (1975) The erythrocyte protoporphyrin in chronic renal failure. *Clinica Chimica Acta*, **64**, 389.

144 LINKESCH W., STRUMMVOLL H.K., WOLF A. & MULLER M. (1978) Haem synthesis in anaemia of uraemic state. *Israel Journal of Medical Sciences*, **14**, 1173.

145 ANDERSON K.E., SASSA S., PETERSON C.M. & KAPPAS A. (1977) Increased erythrocyte uroporphyrinogen-I-synthetase, δ-aminolevulinic acid dehydratase and protoporphyrin in hemolytic anemias. *American Journal of Medicine*, **63**, 359.

146 NAUMANN H.N., DIGGS L.W., SCHLENKER F.S. & BARRERAS L. (1966) Increased urinary porphyrin excretion in sickle-cell crises. *Proceedings of the Society for Experimental Biology and Medicine*, **123**, 1.

147 POTHIER L., LIBBY P.R., GALLAGHER J.F., McGARRY M.P. & MIRAND E.A. (1979) δ-aminolaevulinic acid synthetase activity in spleens of mice infected by the polycythaemia-inducing Friend virus. *Experimental Haematology*, **7**, 36.

148 HOOFBAUER, F.W., WATSON C.J. & SCHWARTZ S. (1953) Urinary and faecel coproporphyrin excretion in rats. II. Results in experimental liver damage. *Proceedings of the Society for Experimental Biology and Medicine*, **83**, 232.

149 BENN-EZZER J., RIMINGTON C., SHANI M., SELIGSOHN U., SHEBA C.H. & SZEINBERG A. (1971) Abnormal excretion of the isomers of urinary coproporphyrin by patients with Dubin–Johnson syndrome in Israel. *Clinical Science*, **40**, 17.

150 WOLKOFF A.W., COHEN L.E. & ARIAS I.M. (1978) Inheritance of the Dubin–Johnson syndrome. *New England Journal of Medicine*, **288**, 113.

151 ENGLAND M.T., COTTON V. & FRENCH J.M. (1962) Faecal porphyrin excretion in normal subjects and in patients with the 'malabsorption syndrome', *Clinical Science*, **22**, 447.

152 GENTZ J., JOHANSSON S., LINDBLAD B., LINDSTEDT S. & ZETTERSTROM R. (1969) Excretion of δ-aminolaevulinic acid in hereditary tyrosinemia. *Clinical Chimica Acta*. **23**, 257.

153 IRVINE D.G. (1978) Pyrroles in neuropsychiatric and porphyric disorders: confirmation of a metabolite structure by synthesis. *Life Sciences*, **23**, 983.

154 GRAHAM D.J.M. (1978) Monopyrroles in porphyria and related disorders. Ph.D. thesis. Glasgow University.

155 MOORE M.R. & GRAHAM D.J.M. (1980) Monopyrroles in porphyria, psychosis and lead exposure. *International Journal of Biochemistry*, **12**, 827.

156 BRENNER D.A. & BLOOMER J.R. (1980) The enzymatic defect in variegate porphyria. *New England Journal of Medicine*, **302**, 765.

157 BIRD T.D., HAMERNYIK P., NUTTER J.Y. & LABBE R.F. (1979) Inherited deficiency of delta-aminolevulinic acid dehydratase. *American Journal of Human Genetics*, **31**, 662.

SECTION 3
THE WHITE CELLS AND RETICULOENDOTHELIAL SYSTEM AND THEIR DISORDERS

Chapter 15
Production and kinetics of the phagocytic leucocytes and their disorders

J. M. GOLDMAN

MYELOID STEM CELLS

In all mammalian species, blood cells arise from a common stem cell. By definition a stem cell has a choice of two options: it may either replicate itself or it may proliferate and differentiate into more mature progeny with limited capacity for further differentiation. A *pluripotent* stem cell can differentiate along one of a series of pathways and produce either mature granulocytes, erythrocytes or other blood cells; in contrast a *unipotent* stem cell can replicate itself but can differentiate along only a single pathway (see Chapter 2). The morphological nature of the putative haemopoietic stem cell has in the past been much debated [1], but the introduction in recent years of new techniques employing experimental animals and *in-vitro* culture systems has provided operational definitions of such stem cells and has bypassed the need for their recognition by conventional microscopy. In rodents at least, pluripotent haemopoietic stem cells are now known to be present in the marrow of the adult animal [2]. The study of animal and human haemopoietic cells by various *in-vitro* culture methods has also provided evidence for the existence of a series of *committed progenitor cells* which are presumed to be descended from a single pluripotent stem cell; the differentiation and proliferation of such progenitor cells *in vitro* appear to be regulated by corresponding humoral factors, such as 'colony-stimulating factor', and restrained by specific inhibitors, such as prostaglandins or lactoferrin, but the physiological relevance of such experimental findings remains to be established.

Historical
For many years, debate centred on the question of whether blood cells in the adult were derived from a single stem cell or whether there existed a series of stem cells giving rise to different mature cellular components of the blood. Proponents of the former theory, known as the 'monophyletic' or 'unitarian' school, believed that the lymphocyte of lymphatic tissue was a truly totipotential stem cell that could under appro-

priate conditions give rise to any other blood cell type [3], while supporters of the contrasting 'polyphyletic' school described a number of precursor 'blast' cells, each already committed to differentiation along specified cell lines. A proponent of the polyphyletic school was Naegeli, whose 'dualistic' theory distinguished between myeloblasts and lymphoblasts [4]. In fact Naegeli's theory incorporated three precursors of blood cells:

1 the lymphoblast, ancestor of the 'mature' lymphocyte;

2 the myeloblast, from which myelocytes and mature granulocytes were derived; and

3 the pronormoblast, whence came the red cells.

Schilling later modified this theory by asserting that monocytes were independent of granulocyte precursors and this variant was termed the 'trialistic' theory [5]. The 'complete' polyphyletic school of Sabin and her associates assumed the existence of a different stem cell for each of the cells of the blood [6]. In her scheme, the two precursors were the primitive reticulum cell and the endothelial cell: the former gave rise to free-moving multipotent stem cells which could in turn produce myeloblasts, lymphoblasts or monoblasts, while the latter gave birth to erythroid cells and also to macrophages or histiocytes.

Experimental data from rodents
In 1961 a new era opened in experimental haematology when Till & McCulloch showed that a mouse subjected to whole-body irradiation, that would otherwise prove lethal, could be rescued by an intravenous infusion of bone-marrow cells collected from a syngeneic animal [2]. Such bone-marrow cells repopulated the marrow of the recipient animal but also formed discrete aggregates or 'colonies' of haemopoietic cells in the recipient's spleen. These colonies contained differentiated cells of the erythroid, granulocytic and megakaryocytic lines; lymphoid elements were also sometimes present [7]. Subsequently cytogenetic studies with marker chromosomes showed that each colony had arisen from a single cell that had been designated 'colony-forming unit in spleen' (CFU-S) [8]. Analo-

gous colonies could be demonstrated in the spleens of rats but not of other species. These studies provided evidence for the existence, at least in rodents, of a pluripotent stem cell.

In 1966 workers in Israel and Australia were simultaneously able to grow haemopoietic cells of murine origin in semi-solid agar culture [9, 10]. Subsequently, methyl cellulose was found equivalent to agar in providing a support matrix necessary for cell proliferation [11]. In these systems, discrete colonies containing differentiated cells of the granulocyte and monocyte series became visible after incubation of the culture plates for seven to 10 days. The colonies ranged in size from 50 to several thousand cells and could readily be counted and characterized. Each colony was thought to derive from a single cell [9, 12] which was designated 'colony-forming unit in culture' (CFU-C) or, more recently, 'colony-forming unit-granulocyte/macrophage' (CFU-GM). Such studies provided evidence for a common committed progenitor-cell origin for both granulocyte and monocyte cell lines. Because the replicative capacity of the CFU-GM seemed to be limited, the cell could not truly be regarded as a stem cell.

Human CFU-GM

In 1970 the murine system was successfully adapted for culture of human CFU-GM *in vitro* [13]. In the adult, such cells are at highest concentration in the marrow, where about one of every 3000 nucleated cells is a CFU-GM; their concentration in the peripheral blood and spleen is lower (Table 15.1). *In-vitro* human colonies take longer to develop than their murine counterparts and their eventual size is smaller [14].

The properties of the CFU-GM have been characterized to a certain extent. Their buoyant density is about 1·07 g/ml and about 30% of them are in active DNA synthesis at any given time [15–17]: this observation indicates that virtually all of the CFU-GM are in proliferative cycle, in contrast to CFU-S. In highly purified populations of marrow from mouse or man, CFU-GM appears as a small cell with high nuclear/cytoplasmic ratio and morphological characteristics resembling that of the 'transitional' lymphocyte [1, 18].

Colony-stimulating factor(s)

The CFU-GM will proliferate *in vitro* to form macroscopically visible colonies only in the presence of a humoral material that has been designated *colony-stimulating factor* (CSF) or *colony-stimulating activity* (CSA). Material active in stimulating colony formation from human CFU-GM can be obtained from a variety of sources, including normal blood leucocytes, placenta and urine [19–21]. When purified from human urine, CSA appears to be a glycoprotein with a molecular weight of about 45 000 daltons [22, 23]. In the blood its principal source is monocytes and to a lesser extent lymphocytes; granulocytes produce no CSA [19, 24]. In the laboratory CSA can be obtained from a number of continuous cell lines derived from neoplastic tissues [25, 26]. In general, there is a sigmoid dose–response curve for the relationship between the CSA content of a given culture and the number of colonies stimulated [27]. It is assumed that these materials derived from the various human sources are variants of a single molecule, all capable of stimulating colony formation *in vitro*; one or more of such molecules may be equivalent to the physiological 'granulopoietin' that is believed to stimulate the production of granulocytes in the bone marrow. Proof of this assumption has not yet been obtained.

Inhibitory factors

Analogy with other biological systems suggests that granulopoiesis may be inhibited or restrained *in vivo* by a negative feedback mechanism. One possible source of such inhibitory influence is the mature granulocyte. Polymorphs and extracts of mature polymorphs introduced into the CFU-GM culture system inhibit the production of CSA from monocytes [28]. This inhibitory pathway is not yet fully defined but it may be mediated by the direct action of lactoferrin released from polymorphs and interacting with monocyte membrane receptors [29]. Granulocyte-specific chalones which may inhibit granulopoiesis *in vivo* have also been described [30]. Prostaglandins (PGE_1 and PGE_2) are also potent inhibitors of CFU-GM proliferation *in vitro* and their possible elaboration by monocytes and macrophages suggests a further possible pathway mediating physiological restraint of granulopoiesis [31].

Table 15.1. Average number of CFU-GM and cluster-forming cells in human tissues

	CFU-GM*	Clusters
Bone marrow		
per 10^5 nucleated cells	20–50	100–200
Spleen		
per 10^5 nucleated cells	5–50	30–200
Blood		
per 10^6 nucleated cells	3–20	10–50

* CFU-GM are defined as progenitor cells capable of giving rise *in vitro* to colonies containing 50 or more granulocytes or macrophages; smaller aggregates of cells are designated 'clusters'

Pluripotent stem cells in man

The finding of pluripotent stem cells in the bone marrow [2] and peripheral circulation in a number of animal species [32, 33] suggests that they may have the same distribution in man. Until an *in-vitro* assay is developed for such human cells, however, conclusions must be based on indirect evidence. For example, the observation that the Ph[1] chromosome that characterizes chronic granulocytic leukaemia, assumed to result from a mutation occurring in a single somatic cell, can be identified in cells of the granulocytic, erythroid, megakaryocytic and macrophagic lines [34, 35], is some evidence for the existence of a pluripotent stem cell in the marrow of adult man. On the other hand, the capacity of transplanted marrow to re-establish myeloid haemopoiesis in patients with aplastic anaemia or acute leukaemia does not unequivocally prove the existence of a pluripotent stem cell in adult marrow: the same result could be achieved by a series of unipotent progenitor cells with self-replicative capacity.

Further indirect evidence for the presence of a pluripotent stem cell in the human circulation comes from the observation in one study that human peripheral-blood leucocytes transfused from one identical twin to another appeared responsible for early marrow recovery after administration of cytotoxic drugs [36]. In another study, however, such blood cells were unable to induce regeneration of marrow function in a patient with aplastic anaemia, when subsequent marrow transplantation was successful [37].

GRANULOCYTE PRODUCTION

The system for producing granulocytes in the bone marrow has four sequentially linked components:

1 a *stem-cell compartment*;
2 a subsequent *mitotic pool* in which division and maturation both occur;
3 a non-mitotic pool in which only *maturation* takes place; and
4 a storage pool of mature cells designated the *marrow granulocyte reserve* (MGR) (Fig. 15.1).

The stem-cell compartment is not morphologically identifiable. The mitotic pool comprises three principal cell types: the earliest recognizable granulocyte precursor is the myeloblast, which divides and progresses to a promyelocyte and subsequently to a myelocyte. As the

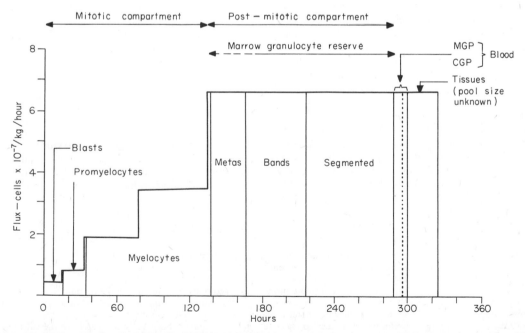

Fig. 15.1. Schematic representation of the flow of cells through granulopoiesis. The ordinate represents the flow of cells relative to the granulocyte turnover rate, and the abscissa the transit time for each compartment. The area shown for each compartment is proportional to the number of cells it contains. The scheme assumes that myeloblasts and promyelocytes each divide once and myelocytes twice. The depicted size of the tissue pool is speculative. (Scheme modified from Ref. 41 with permission.)

cells divide and progress through these several stages there are changes in the cell cytoplasm, with acquisition first of primary or non-specific granules and later of secondary or specific granules. After the myelocyte stage, the cell matures further but no further division takes place. In the marrow the non-mitotic pool consists of metamyelocytes, band neutrophils and mature segmented neutrophils. After release from the bone marrow, band forms and mature granulocytes enter the blood where they are distributed between a circulating granulocyte pool (CGP) and a pool of cells adherent along vessel walls, the marginal (or marginated) granulocyte pool (MGP). Together these constitute the total blood granulocyte pool (TBGP). Under normal steady-state conditions granulocytes leave the blood and enter the tissues by a process of apparently random migration. The details of this system have been studied extensively in the last 25 years and have recently been reviewed [38–43]. The terminology is summarized in Table 15.2.

Historical

The identification of leucocytes in the blood is usually attributed to William Hewson (1739–1774). He recognized colourless cells with nuclei (he used the term 'central particles') in blood and believed that they originated from lymph nodes or the thymus. He believed also that nucleated cells in lymphatic channels entered the blood and were transformed into red cells in the spleen. With only a microscope at his disposal, his conclusions were remarkable if not entirely accurate [44]. A hundred years later Neumann was able to show that at least in the adult animal the main site of blood formation was in fact the bone marrow [45]. By the end of the nineteenth century the relationship of the site of haemopoiesis to the development of the mammalian organism was established: haemopoiesis starts in the yolk sac, shifts to the liver during fetal development and is finally located in the bone marrow after birth. By 1925, Sabin was able to summarize the

essential relationships between the production, distribution, survival and disappearance of the leucocytes [46]. Further knowledge awaited the introduction of the newer techniques for labelling leucocytes.

TECHNIQUES FOR STUDYING GRANULOCYTE KINETICS

A variety of techniques has been used for the study of granulopoiesis and granulocyte kinetics.

Radionuclide labels

Valuable early studies were carried out by transfusion of granulocytes with morphologically identifiable abnormalities (Pelger–Huët anomaly), the survival of which could be followed in the recipient's circulation [47]. The first radioisotopic labels used in the study of granulocyte kinetics were isotopes that were incorporated into DNA. *Radiophosphorus* (^{32}P) was introduced in 1952 [48]: ^{32}P labels all cells but has the disadvantage that it is incorporated into cell constituents other than DNA, including phospholipids and phosphoproteins; it is also unsuitable for autoradiography. Radiophosphorus (^{32}P) was therefore soon replaced by *tritiated thymidine*, [^{3}H]thymidine, when this became available in 1958 [49]. [^{3}H]thymidine is selectively bound only to DNA, can label cells both *in vitro* and *in vivo* and is a weak beta-emitter ideal for autoradiography. Moreover, material not incorporated into DNA is rapidly degraded and the label is not re-utilized. [^{3}H]thymidine is thus an excellent label for cells in S-phase (cells synthesizing DNA) in the pool of mitotically active cells. Such cells retain their label when they pass into the maturation pool and can be identified subsequently in the blood.

Another label, di*iso*propylfluorophosphate (DFP) containing either ^{32}P or ^{3}H, was introduced in the late 1950s [50]. The DFP binds exclusively to granulocytes and not to other types of leucocyte. It binds both dividing and non-dividing cells; it does not elute from

Table 15.2. Definition of some of the terms used in evaluation of leucocyte kinetics

Compartment	Population of cells sharing at least one common feature
Pool	Subdivision of a compartment
Generation time	Time interval between successive mitoses
Doubling time	Time for entire cell population to undergo one division and double its numbers
Turnover rate	Number of cells entering or leaving a non-mitotic compartment in unit time
Turnover time	Time to replace a complete cohort of cells in a given compartment
Transit time	Mean time for a cell to traverse a given compartment, usually equivalent to the turnover time
Half-disappearance time ($T_{\frac{1}{2}}$)	Time for 50% of a given population of cells to leave a compartment assuming random removal of cells

the labelled cell and is not re-utilized like [³H]thymidine. It can be used as a granulocyte label both *in vitro* and *in vivo*; *in vitro*, DFP can be used to measure the total blood granulocyte pool, while administered intravenously it allows measurement of marrow transit times, granulocyte reserves and myelocyte turnover rates. Radioactive sulphate (^{35}S) has also been used to label granulocytes [51], and radiochromium (^{51}Cr) and radio-technetium (^{99}Te^m) have gained some favour as leucocyte labels [52, 53]. The use of ^{51}Cr permits external scanning of the patient, but the isotope labels other types of leucocyte and elutes rapidly from granulocytes. In the last few years radiolabelled indium-oxine (^{111}In-oxine) has been used to monitor platelet and lymphocyte kinetics [54, 55]; this gamma-emitting isotope binds tightly to cytoplasmic components and is suitable for external scanning. Preliminary reports of its use to label granulocytes suggest that it may prove to be a valuable agent for kinetic studies [56, 56a].

Granulocyte-depletion techniques
Large numbers of leucocytes can be removed from the body by cross-circulation of a donor with a leucopenic recipient [57] or by leucapheresis [58]. The latter technique (more correctly 'leucocytapheresis') involves removal of leucocytes from whole blood by centrifugation with return of leucocyte-depleted blood to the donor. The changes that occur in blood and marrow leucocyte numbers following such depletion procedures provide some information about granulocyte reserves.

Induced inflammation
Cutaneous lesions can be artificially induced by a number of methods. The skin-window technique involves denuding the skin down to the level of the capillaries; coverslips are applied to the lesion and the number and types of cell migrating to the lesion can be examined at intervals [59]. Alternatively the application to the skin of 'skin chambers' permits collection of larger numbers of cells and quantitation of cellular response [60].

GRANULOCYTE KINETICS IN THE MARROW
The kinetics of granulocyte production in the marrow and release into the blood have been studied by a number of workers using various different techniques. The subject has been reviewed recently by a number of writers [38–43, 61].

The mitotic compartment
Progenitor cells enter the marrow mitotic compartment from the stem-cell compartment. In the mitotic compartment, maturation is believed to proceed in the direction: myeloblast→promyelocyte→myelocyte. The number of divisions that occurs at each morphological stage is unknown. Analysis of the exponential decrease in radioactivity of the *in-vivo* curve for DF^{32}P suggests that there may be a single division in the myeloblast stage, a single division at the promyelocyte stage and three divisions at the myelocyte stage; this would suggest a total compartmental expansion factor of 32 [62]. Others have suggested that there may be only two divisions at the myelocyte stage [41, 63], or as many as five [64]. It is clear that the output of cells from the mitotic pool must equal the blood granulocyte turnover rate. Whether granulocyte production is actually greater than this in order to compensate for a proportion of cells that die prematurely in the marrow, tantamount to ineffective granulopoiesis, is unknown.

The myelocyte generation time has been estimated at 24–48 hours [65]. Data obtained from analysis of autoradiography of marrow smears have been interpreted as consistent with a total time spent in the myeloblast, promyelocyte and myelocyte pool (i.e. the mitotic-pool transit time) of 135 hours [42, 66].

Marrow granulocyte reserve (MGR)
When leucocytes are removed from the peripheral blood of dogs by leucapheresis, granulocytes are mobilized from the marrow to make up the deficit [67]. One must remove four or more times the total number of leucocytes present in the circulation over a relatively short period of time in order to produce granulocytopenia; that such granulocytes are mobilized from a storage pool, and have not been produced in response to the sudden increased demand, was demonstrated by the inability of radiation to prevent this mobilization of granulocytes from the marrow. Using radionuclides that label only dividing cells, one can show that the mean time for a cell labelled at its last division to traverse the marrow storage pool is six to eight days and that the minimal transit time is four to six days [68, 69] (Table 15.3). From a knowledge of the daily granulocyte production rate one can calculate that the

Table 15.3. Granulocyte kinetic data for normal man

	Mean value	Range
Marrow-granulocyte-reserve transit time	8 days	4–14 days
Granulocyte turnover rate	163×10^7 cells/kg/day	50–340×10^7 cells/kg/day
Blood half-disappearance time	6·7 hours	4–10 hours

Table compiled from data summarized in Refs 38 and 39.

Table 15.4. Data for granulocyte pool sizes in normal man

Pool	Cells × 10^{-7}/kg	Cells in 70 kg man (× 10^{-9})
Marrow granulocyte reserve	650–1300	630
Total blood granulocyte pool	70	49
Circulating granulocyte pool	31	22
Marginal granulocyte pool	39	27

Table compiled from results summarized in Ref. 39

size of the marrow granulocyte reserve must average $6.5–13 \times 10^9$ cells/kg in a normal man [39, 70] (Table 15.4).

Daily granulocyte production

The absolute number of granulocyte precursors in the marrow has been calculated on the basis of radio-iron measurements of erythroid-cell numbers in marrow-cell suspensions [70], or using marrow sections [69, 71]. The former method gives results slightly higher than those calculated from marrow sections, but total numbers range between 770 and 1140×10^7 cells/kg [41]. Similarly the rate of cell production can be calculated either from assessment of the size and transit time of the non-dividing pool [69], or from knowledge of the fractional myelocyte production and myelocyte numbers [63]; the respective values are 3·5 and $5·1 \times 10^7$ cells/kg/hour. Estimates for the transit time through the non-proliferating compartment range from 130 to 158 hours. Assuming a transit time through the mitotic pool of 135 hours, the total time from stem cell to mature granulocyte would be of the order of 265–293 hours or 11–12 days. These figures agree well with calculations for the number of granulocytes released daily into the blood (granulocyte turnover rate) using _in-vitro_ and _in-vivo_ DF^{32}P data, which give a value of 163×10^7 cells/kg/day [38] (Table 15.3).

GRANULOCYTE KINETICS IN THE BLOOD

Total blood granulocyte pool (TBGP)

The total blood granulocyte pool comprises all the granulocytes within the vascular space. Studies with granulocytes labelled _in vitro_ with DF^{32}P have led to the conclusion that the TBGP measures about 70×10^7 cells/kg [39] (Table 15.4). However, only 44% of the reinjected labelled granulocytes could be accounted for in the sampled blood [72]. This observation gave rise to the interpretation that the TBGP is divided into two

sub-pools, a pool of granulocytes that move freely in the circulation and another pool of cells that are temporarily sequestered in small blood vessels or adherent to the endothelial lining of larger ones; together this 'marginated granulocyte pool' (MGP) and the 'circulating granulocyte pool' (CGP) make up the TBGP. This conclusion is supported by the knowledge that exercise or injection of adrenaline immediately after the reinfusion of labelled granulocytes leads to increased recovery of labelled cells [73]. Because the measurement of TBGP during exercise or adrenaline-induced leucocytosis gives normal values, it is assumed that such measures lead to mobilization of granulocytes into the CGP from the MGP and that no input from the MGR is involved. In resting conditions there is probably rapid exchange of granulocytes between the two pools.

Half-disappearance times (T$_{\frac{1}{2}}$)

When the rate of disappearance of granulocytes from the blood of normal subjects is measured by following the rate of cells labelled _in vitro_ with DF^{32}P, granulocyte radioactivity decreases exponentially with a mean $T_{\frac{1}{2}}$ of 6·7 hours [73, 74]. This finding indicates that granulocytes leave the blood in a random manner; they thus do not have a specific survival time in the blood, in contrast to erythrocytes and platelets. Other studies using [^{3}H]thymidine gave a $T_{\frac{1}{2}}$ of 7·6 hours [69]. Calculations using ^{51}Cr-labelled cells gave relatively longer $T_{\frac{1}{2}}$ (16·1 hours) [75]; such results may in fact be over-estimates related in part to the lack of specificity of ^{51}Cr as a granulocyte label.

If the estimates of TBGP are approximately correct, and if one also accepts the assumption that granulocytes leave the blood mainly in a random fashion, one can easily calculate the blood granulocyte turnover rate (GTR) from the equation for first-order decay [39, 41, 76]:

$$GTR = \frac{\text{Log}_e 2 \times TBGP}{T_{\frac{1}{2}}}$$

$$GTR = \frac{0·693 \times TBGP}{T_{\frac{1}{2}}}$$

TISSUE PHASE

The manner in which granulocytes leave the blood in the absence of trauma or infection is not precisely known. It is assumed that there are some natural losses of cells into the bodily secretions (saliva, intestinal fluids, urine), and some cells may be removed by the reticulo-endothelial system as a result of senescence [38]. In contrast, the migration of granulocytes into artificially induced or naturally occurring inflammatory exudates has been studied extensively in man.

Following simple trauma, a few neutrophils can be found in the exudate that develops within 30 minutes and they become abundant by three hours [59, 77, 78]. If the trauma is not repeated, further migration of granulocytes ceases within 24 hours, and leucocytes that continue to migrate are mainly mononuclear cells. If, however, the inflammatory stimulus is continued, then migration of granulocytes to the site may persist for some days [38]. Boggs studied the accumulation of labelled granulocytes in the exudate of a spontaneously occurring empyema and found that the minimum blood-to-exudate transit time was 30 minutes [38]; there was a rapid turnover of cells in the exudate: the labelled cells had a $T_{\frac{1}{2}}$ of 24 hours. One may wonder whether granulocytes entering an exudate might accumulate from a pool of reserve granulocytes in the normal tissues other than blood or marrow: in fact there is general agreement that all the granulocytes entering the blood can be accounted for as coming from the marrow [67, 77], and those entering an exudate come only from the blood [79].

CONTROL OF GRANULOPOIESIS *IN VIVO*
At least three observations combine to suggest that the number of granulocytes in the circulation is controlled by a precise regulatory mechanism:
1 their numbers remain remarkably constant in the normal individual;
2 their numbers are increased by infection or drugs such as corticosteroids, aetiocholanolone or endotoxin, and reduced by leucapheresis or alkylating agents, in a predictable manner; and
3 the rates of return to normal after such perturbations are consistent [39].

There are a number of points at which the regulatory mechanism could exert its control:
1 by expanding the stem-cell compartment;
2 by governing the inflow from the stem-cell compartment to the mitotic pool;
3 by increasing the rate of production in the mitotic pool;
4 by increasing release from the marrow granulocyte reserve;
5 by altering the ratio between marginated and circulating pools; or
6 by affecting the egress of cells into the tissues.
Our knowledge of the specific details of this putative regulatory mechanism is very incomplete.

Oscillatory nature of granulocyte production
Cyclical oscillation of the peripheral-blood count may be observed in patients with cyclical neutropenia [80] and in some patients with chronic granulocytic leukaemia [81, 82]; it also occurs in grey collie dogs [83]. Though cycling is difficult to demonstrate in

normal man [84], these observations formed the basis of a speculative model simulating the control of granulopoiesis, in which blood granulocyte numbers are controlled by two feedback loops, one influencing the rate of production and the other controlling the rate of release of cells from the marrow [85, 86]. The model predicts that the concentration of granulocytes in the blood should rise and fall in sine-wave fashion with a cycle length of 14–23 days.

Factors controlling production and maturation
The possible role of *colony-stimulating factor* (CSF) in controlling granulopoiesis *in vivo* has been discussed above. An alternative material that may act to stimulate granulopoiesis *in vivo* has been designated *diffusible granulopoietic substance* (DGS). When normal bone marrow is placed in cell-tight millipore chambers (diffusion chambers) and implanted into the peritoneal cavities of rodents, the growth of neutrophils in the chamber can be enhanced if the host animal is made neutropenic by X-rays or cytotoxic drugs [87, 88]. The effect must be mediated by host-derived DGS entering the millipore chamber.

A variety of factors inhibiting cell growth or synthesis of DNA has been described. *Chalones* are tissue-specific, but species-non-specific, materials of low molecular weight originally demonstrated on the basis of their ability to inhibit incorporation of DNA into immature granulocytes [30]. Other materials of higher molecular weight, some lipoprotein in nature, inhibit granulopoiesis *in vitro* but their physiological relevance is unknown [89]. Interferon can also inhibit granulopoiesis *in vitro* [90], as can prostaglandins E_1 and E_2 [91].

Factors controlling release of granulocytes from marrow
A factor originally demonstrated in the plasma of dogs rendered neutropenic by myelotoxic agents or injections of endotoxin was designated *neutrophil-releasing factor* (NRF) [92, 93]. It can also be demonstrated in man [94] and apparently acts by inducing rapid efflux of mature band and segmented granulocytes from marrow to blood. A similar factor, that promotes movement of marrow granulocytes into the blood in rats rendered neutropenic by leucapheresis or endotoxin, has been termed *leucocytosis-inducing factor* (LIF) [95]; LIF may be identical with NRF.

EOSINOPHILS

In 1846, Jones described a 'coarse granular cell' in a report to the Royal Society in London. This may well have been the first description of an eosinophil [96]. In 1879, Ehrlich noted that the cytoplasmic granules in one type of granulocyte had an affinity for acidic dyes, and gave the cell the name 'eosinophil'. Though eosinophils are clearly related in some way to the pathogenesis of allergic disease, their precise function remains unknown; they have an ill-defined role in processing immune complexes and perhaps in limiting the inflammatory reaction [97, 98].

Eosinophil stem cells
The great majority of eosinophils are produced in the bone marrow. Whether they originate from the same pluripotent stem cell as the neutrophil granulocyte is uncertain. The finding in certain individuals of genetically determined selective absence of either eosinophil or neutrophil peroxidases, for example, suggests that the stem-cell origins of the two cell lines may be separate [99–101]. Moreover, children with congenital neutrophil agranulocytosis may have normal or elevated eosinophil production [102]. Data from *in-vitro* culture studies provide additional support for the separate development of the two lines: colonies presumed to be derived from single progenitor cells are composed either of neutrophilic or of eosinophilic granulocytes, but colonies of mixed eosinophilic/neutrophilic cells have not been identified [103]. One line of evidence does, however, suggest that eosinophils may, at least in some cases, share a stem cell with other cells in the myeloid series: it has recently been shown that eosinophilic precursors in patients with chronic granulocytic leukaemia carry the Ph[1] chromosome [104].

Production and maturation
The earliest identifiable eosinophil is the promyelocyte, which has several small eosinophilic granules in the cytoplasm. The later promyelocyte may have additional non-specific or azurophilic granules, but these have largely disappeared by the myelocyte stage. The eosinophilic metamyelocyte is smaller than the myelocyte and contains fewer cytoplasmic granules. The mature eosinophil typically has a bilobed nucleus and a cytoplasm densely packed with eosinophilic granules [97]. The biochemical nature of the granules is not precisely established, but they contain large quantities of an arginine-rich basic protein with a high content of extractable zinc [98, 105, 106].

Kinetics of eosinophils
The eosinophil arises from its unidentified precursor in the marrow and proceeds through several cell divisions before maturing and entering the blood stream. In the unstimulated rat, calculations have shown a mean cycle time of 22–30 hours and a total marrow transit time of 5·5 days [107, 108]. However, when stimulated by injection of *Trichinella spiralis* larvae, the total cell-cycle time was reduced to nine hours and the marrow

transit time to 3·6 days [108]. Other factors can also influence the rate of production of eosinophils: ACTH and corticosteroids inhibit their release from marrow and produce a blood eosinopenia [109, 110]; conversely, histamine increases the number of circulating eosinophils and also the marrow content of eosinophil precursors [111].

Only a very small proportion of the body's eosinophils are present in the blood. Hudson [112] has calculated that the marrow eosinophil reserve is perhaps 300 times greater than the number in the circulation and an equally large number may be present in the tissues. The post-mitotic eosinophil reserve has been calculated to be 14×10^7/cells/kg [113]. In dogs the $T_{\frac{1}{2}}$ has been calculated to be about 30 minutes [114], but studies in normal man and in rats suggest values of three to eight [115] and seven to 11 hours [116, 117] respectively, results which accord more closely with survival times for normal neutrophils. The survival of eosinophils in the tissues, however, is probably longer than that of neutrophils.

Tissue distribution
After passing through the circulation, eosinophils migrate to the tissues, whence few, if any, return to the blood. They localize particularly in areas exposed to the external environment, such as the skin, bronchial mucosa, gastro-intestinal tract, vagina and uterine wall [110, 118, 119]. The eventual fate of eosinophils is not well established: they may be shed into the lumen of a viscus, degenerate at a local site or be engulfed by macrophages.

BASOPHILS

The basophil in the blood was originally described by Ehrlich in 1897 [120] and its presence confirmed by Maximow in 1910 [121]. Initially, no clear distinction was made between basophils and tissue mast cells, which share many characteristics, but certain morphological differences are now recognized and tissue mast cells are not normally present in the blood. Blood basophils are presumed to derive from precursor cells in the marrow [122]. This conclusion is based on the observation of immature basophilic precursor cells in mitosis in the marrow [123]. Moreover, basophilic precursor cells are increased in the marrow when basophil numbers are increased in the blood, as in some myeloproliferative disorders. As with the eosinophil, the identity of the basophil stem cell is unknown. Again, however, the observation that basophil precursors in patients with chronic granulocytic leukaemia (CGL) carry a Ph[1] chromosome is some evidence that basophils may, at least in some circumstances, share a primitive pluripotent stem cell with other granulocytes, and perhaps even with cells of the lymphoid series [124].

The relatively small numbers of basophils in the blood and the lack of suitable techniques explain the paucity of knowledge of basophil kinetics. On the basis mainly of morphological observations, basophils are thought to be produced in the bone marrow, to be released into the circulation, where they remain for a short time, and then to migrate into tissues. Their numbers vary with age, being highest in the newborn and progressively falling throughout adult life [125]. Injections of ACTH cause a fall in circulating basophil numbers [126]. Their numbers are also low in thyrotoxicosis but return to normal when the patient becomes euthyroid [127].

MONOCYTES AND MACROPHAGES

Although the monocyte was originally thought to be a member of the lymphocytic series, its separate identity was established in 1910 by the work of Pappenheim & Ferrata [128]. It was later shown that large mononuclear phagocytes present in the circulation of all classes of vertebrates were capable of becoming 'macrophages similar to those found in connective tissue, liver, spleen and lymph nodes' [129, 130]. Thus the concept that the blood monocyte was in most cases the precursor of the tissue macrophage came to be accepted. It received further confirmation from studies in which monocytes were observed through transparent chambers in the ear of a rabbit: monocytes containing phagocytosed carbon particles or stained with supravital dyes could be seen migrating from blood vessels into adjacent connective tissues, where they transformed into cells indistinguishable from tissue macrophages [131]. The transformation of monocyte to macrophage is associated with a number of specific changes: the cell may become substantially larger, its granules may become bigger and more abundant and there is increased content of various cytoplasmic enzymes. The number of mitochondria may also increase and there is an increase in the rate of cell respiration. The majority of these changes can be demonstrated by manipulation of blood monocytes *in vitro* or *in vivo*; they are reviewed in various publications [132–135].

Monocyte stem cells
Several lines of evidence suggest that the monocyte shares a common progenitor with cells of the granulocytic series. For example, monocytes as well as granulocytes are apparently involved in the same neoplastic clone in some types of acute myeloid leukaemia

(AML) [136]. Moreover, studies of colonies presumed to have originated from single progenitor cells *in vitro* may show both granulocytes and monocytes in the same colony [137]. The observation that the Ph[1] chromosome can be found in dividing macrophages in patients with CGL adds further weight to the concept that granulocytes and monocytes are closely related in development [138]. The mechanism that determines whether a developing progenitor cell becomes a monocyte or a granulocyte is however largely unknown.

Monocytes in the marrow
That monocytes originate from the bone marrow was first demonstrated in irradiated animals whose blood monocyte and tissue macrophage numbers were restored only after transfusion of donor marrow cells [139–141]; studies with [3H]thymidine-labelled syngeneic bone-marrow cells infused into irradiated animals supported this conclusion [142]. Direct culture of bone-marrow cells also showed that a high proportion of mononuclear cells incorporate [3H]thymidine *in vitro*, thus indicating that a high proportion of the mononuclear cells in the marrow are capable of proliferating [143]. The earliest monocyte precursors are not identifiable in normal bone marrow, but presumably equivalent 'blast' cells ('monoblasts') are seen in monocytic leukaemia. Promonocytes can be identified in normal marrow [136]. They are relatively large (10–20 μm), have a high nuclear/cytoplasmic ratio, cytoplasmic peroxidase activity and the capacity to adhere to glass and incorporate [3H]thymidine [133, 134, 144]. In experiments with mice receiving [3H]-thymidine *in vivo*, the labelling index of monocytes rose during the first 24 hours to a maximum of about 33% [148]. These findings led to the conclusion that promonocytes are self-replicating cells which divide three or four times in the marrow and give rise to monocytes, which under steady-state conditions do not themselves divide. The average generation time of marrow promonocytes was computed to be 9·7 hours [145].

Monocytes in the blood
Like neutrophils, monocytes spend only a relatively short time in the blood on the pathway from their site of production to their site of ultimate function. Experiments in mice showed the appearance of labelled monocytes within two hours of injection of [3H]thymidine: this means that at least some monocytes leave the marrow very soon after their formation and the pool of mature monocytes in the marrow is consequently small [143]. Labelled monocytes appear to leave the circulation in a random fashion, as do neutrophils, and the $T_{\frac{1}{2}}$ in mice has been calculated at 22 hours [143]. Studies with human subjects, however, suggest a very much shorter $T_{\frac{1}{2}}$ of 8·4 hours [146]. In

man the total blood monocyte pool consists of a circulating pool and a marginated pool; the latter is about three times the size of the former [146]. The normal monocyte turnover rate averages about 7×10^6 cells/kg/hour [146].

Tissue macrophages

When the monocyte leaves the blood and enters the tissues it undergoes changes in morphology, in granule and enzyme content and in metabolism, as outlined above. In the tissues the cell is usually referred to as a 'macrophage' or 'histiocyte', and macrophages studied in different locations in the body have somewhat different characteristics [134].

Peritoneal macrophages. Macrophages in the peritoneal cavity are relatively easy to harvest and have been regarded as typical of the 'free' macrophages found in serous cavities, as distinct from the 'fixed' macrophages found in other organs. Experiments with transfusion of chromosomally marked cells have shown that they originate from precursors in bone marrow [139, 140]. In the resting state they have a turnover time calculated at 20–40 days [143], but this rate can be greatly increased by inflammation or by peritoneal dialysis.

Liver macrophages. Experiments with mice have shown that less than 1·5% of Kupffer cells in the liver are labelled within two hours of a pulse injection of [³H]thymidine [147, 148]. These and similar studies suggest that Kupffer cells divide very infrequently in the resting state—their turnover time has been calculated at about 60 days [133]. Like the macrophages in the peritoneal cavity, Kupffer cells originate from circulating monocytes which in turn are derived from precursor cells in the marrow [133].

Lung macrophages. The pulmonary alveolar macrophage plays an important role in defending the lung against damage by inhaled particulate matter [149]. Partly because it is located at an air–tissue interface, unlike other tissue macrophages, it has become specifically adapted in various ways. It is readily available for study in man as a result of the technique of bronchopulmonary lavage [149]. Direct evidence for the bone-marrow origin of the alveolar macrophage in man comes from observations of macrophages in patients who have received bone-marrow transplants from patients of the opposite sex [150]. When marrow from a male donor was transplanted into a female recipient, there was a progressive increase over time in the percentage of alveolar macrophages containing the fluorescent Y body (male marker); host macrophages

were entirely replaced within 100 days of transplantation.

In normal persons the [³H]thymidine labelling index ranges from 0·35 to 1·25%, which suggests that like the peritoneal macrophages only a small fraction of the alveolar macrophages are replicating [133, 151, 152]. However, in a patient receiving chemotherapy for acute leukaemia, pulmonary alveolar macrophage numbers were maintained even in the face of severe monocytopenia [153], showing that in man the alveolar macrophage population can sustain itself by replication in the lung. In summary, therefore, alveolar macrophages originate from precursors in bone marrow but maintain their numbers in part through local proliferation and in part by recruiting new monocytes from the circulation [133].

In material collected by lavage of human lung, three types of pulmonary alveolar macrophage can be identified [134, 149, 154]. These are designated types A, B and C. Type-A cells constitute the majority: 94–98%. They are large cells with a mean diameter of 25 μm and a dark cytoplasm containing dark-blue granules and often vacuoles; there may be large cytoplasmic inclusions and sometimes ingested red cells. Type-B macrophages comprise about five per cent of the cells harvested by lavage: they are about the same size as type-A cells (mean diameter 30 μm) but have a relatively much smaller nucleus and a prominent nucleolus. Type-C macrophages represent less than one per cent of cells collected from normal lungs: they are larger than either of the other types (mean diameter 40 μm) and their cytoplasm is packed with vacuoles; they are present in great numbers in material collected from the bronchial tree of patients with lipoid pneumonia.

DISORDERS OF GRANULOCYTE NUMBERS

The techniques that have been used for the evaluation of granulocyte kinetics in the normal subject have provided some information about the mechanisms underlying changes in granulocyte numbers that occur in response to pharmacological agents and in disease. Changes in the number of granulocytes in the circulation can in general result from alterations in the rates of production of granulocytes and of their release into the circulation, from changes in the rate of their destruction or utilization, or from changes in the distribution of granulocytes within the various compartments [155]. Thus, granulocytopenia may result from reduced granulocyte production and release, increased peripheral destruction, changes in distribution between circulating and marginated pool, or from some combination of these mechanisms; conversely granulocyte leucocytosis may be due to excessive production, alterations within the TBGP, reduced destruction or combinations of such changes.

NEUTROPENIA

Leucopenia is usually defined as a reduction in the number of leucocytes in the blood below $4.0 \times 10^9/l$. It may be due to a reduction of granulocyte numbers or of lymphocyte numbers or both. In practice, the commonest cause of leucopenia is a reduction in granulocyte numbers, correctly described as granulocytopenia, but often referred to as neutropenia. The causes of neutropenia are listed in Table 15.5.

Table 15.5. Causes of neutropenia

Drugs:
    Selective neutropenia
    Agranulocytosis
    (Aplastic anaemia)

Infections:
    Viral—including hepatitis, influenza, rubella
    Bacterial—typhoid fever, brucellosis,
       miliary tuberculosis
    Rickettsial and protozoal infections (sometimes)

Megaloblastic anaemia:
    Vitamin B_{12} or folate deficiency

Chronic neutropenia:
    Chronic idiopathic neutropenia
    Immune neutropenia
    Congenital neutropenias
    Cyclical neutropenia

Hypersplenism:
    Primary
    In association with cirrhosis, Felty's syndrome, etc.

Ionizing radiation and cytotoxic drugs:
    Radiotherapy
    Alkylating agents, antimetabolites, others

Malignant disease:
    Acute leukaemia
    Leuco-erythroblastic anaemia due to
       metastatic carcinoma, multiple myeloma or lymphoma

Miscellaneous conditions:
    Systemic lupus erythematosus, myxoedema,
       hypopituitarism, iron deficiency, anaphylactic shock

Drugs and irradiation

A number of agents, including toxic chemicals such as benzene, arsenic and the cytotoxic drugs used mainly in the treatment of malignant disease, cause depression of bone-marrow function with consequent neutropenia in a partially predictable manner. Thus alkylating agents (e.g. nitrogen mustard, chlorambucil and cyclophosphamide), antimetabolites (e.g. methotrexate and 6-mercaptopurine) and other anticancer drugs

(e.g. anthracyclines and nitrosoureas) are examples of cytotoxic drugs, the major toxicity of which is marrow depression; in many cases the factor limiting the dosage of such a drug is the acceptability of the level of marrow depression anticipated. Irradiation as administered in the treatment of malignant disease has a similar capacity to depress marrow function and induce neutropenia and thrombocytopenia; the extent of marrow depression induced by irradiation is related to the amount of irradiation administered and the functional reserve of normal marrow. If the marrow reserve is normal or near normal before treatment, neutropenia induced by cytotoxic drugs or by irradiation is reversed within a few weeks of completing treatment.

A wide variety of non-cytotoxic drugs in common use has been implicated in the induction of neutropenia (with or without associated thrombocytopenia) in some but not all recipients. The frequency with which these different agents induce neutropenia is, however, very variable. The mechanism in most cases is unknown; thus in some cases individual drugs are thought to suppress cell metabolism and to interfere with cell division while in other cases an immunological mechanism for destruction of immature granulocytes in the marrow or mature granulocytes in the circulation has been postulated. Some of the drugs incriminated in the sporadic production of neutropenia are listed in Table 15.6.

The term 'agranulocytosis' is usually reserved for a reasonably well-defined syndrome characterized by severe infection and marked neutropenia that is today regarded as due to one of a number of specific drugs [156]. In 1922, Schultz [157] described an illness seen mainly in middle-aged women and characterized by severe prostration, necrotic lesions in the mouth and throat, and total or near-total absence of granulocytes from the blood; many of the patients developed septicaemia and died. He regarded the syndrome as a clinical entity, the cause of which was then unknown. In retrospect many of his cases were probably due to ingestion of the analgesic drug, amidopyrine (aminopyrine) [158].

Schultz suggested the name *agranulocytosis* for this clinical picture of fever, sepsis and severe neutropenia. It is now believed that where amidopyrine is incriminated the mechanism of neutropenia is immunological and parallels quinidine-induced thrombocytopenia: circulating granulocytes, rather than platelets, are sensitized with drug–antibody complex and are then preferentially removed by the reticulo-endothelial system. The bone marrow is typically active in these cases but more-mature granulocyte precursors (myelocytes, metamyelocytes and bands) may be missing. This has in the past erroneously been described as a

Table 15.6. Drugs that may cause neutropenia*

Analgesics:
  Amidopyrine, colchicine, gold salts, indomethacin, oxyphenbutazone, phenylbutazone
Antimalarials:
  Amodiaquine, dapsone, hydroxychloroquine, pyrimethamine
Antimicrobials:
  Ampicillin, carbenicillin, cephalexin, chloramphenicol, gentamicin, griseofulvin, isoniazid, methicillin, metronidazole, penicillin, rifampicin, streptomycin
Anticonvulsants:
  Carbamazepine, diphenylhydantoin
Antihistamines:
  Chlorpheniramine, promethazine, mepyramine, etc.
Antithyroids:
  Thiouracil, propylthiouracil, carbimazole
Antidiabetic agents:
  Carbutamide, tolbutamide, chlorpropamide
Antiarrhythmic agents:
  Procainamide, propranolol, quinidine
Tranquillizers:
  Promazine, chlorpromazine, prochlorperazine, meprobamate, etc.
Miscellaneous agents:
  Allopurinol, cimetidine, barbiturates, chlorothiazides, levamisole, penicillamine, phenindione

* This list includes only commonly used drugs that may cause neutropenia. For a more complete list the reader is referred to Ref. 156.

'maturation arrest'; it is in fact a depletion phenomenon, since maturing cells have emerged from the marrow at the earliest opportunity or have been destroyed *in situ*.

Agranulocytosis may today be caused by a number of other drugs included in Table 15.7. Phenothiazines, for example, appear to cause agranulocytosis with an incidence of about one in 1200 [159, 160]. In suscep-

Table 15.7. Drugs and other agents especially likely to cause agranulocytosis

Amidopyrine
Sulphonamides
Chloramphenicol
Phenothiazines
Phenulbutazone
Gold salts
Benzene, arsenic, DDT, dinitrophenol
Any of the agents listed in Table 15.6

tible individuals the agranulocytosis appears to be dose-related and the marrow may be hypoplastic. The picture is therefore due more probably to direct 'idiosyncratic' myelosuppression than to an immune mechanism. Chloramphenicol may also inhibit marrow function in a dose-related manner. In such cases neutropenia and thrombocytopenia are the rule and the changes are reversed when the drug is withdrawn; these dose-related effects are probably distinct in pathogenesis from the rare, and usually severe, aplastic anaemia also attributable to chloramphenicol [161–163] (see Chapter 31).

Cyclical neutropenia
Cyclical (or periodic) neutropenia is a rare disorder described originally in 1910 [164]. The patient suffers from periodic episodes of neutropenia that occur at more or less regular intervals. The most commonly reported period of oscillation is 19–21 days but extremes of 14 and 35 days have been reported. There is a periodic reduction in the size of the granulocyte mitotic pool in the bone marrow, followed by the onset of neutropenia that may be so severe that granulocytes disappear completely from the blood; the degree of leucopenia is less intense and there may be a concomitant increase in circulating monocytes [165–169].

At the nadir of the granulocyte count, and especially if the count falls below 500×10^6/l, patients may develop fever, chills, oral ulceration and skin infections. These episodes usually subside as the granulocyte count rises but death from infection has occasionally been described. Other problems may co-exist, including splenomegaly, arthralgias or abdominal pain.

The disease usually starts in infancy but may be diagnosed at any age. There may be a history of similar disorders in other family members [167] and it may be inherited in an autosomal-dominant manner. Treatment is generally unsatisfactory; splenectomy appears to be of little value but haematological improvement following treatment with testosterone has been reported [168].

The occurrence of cyclical neutropenia in these patients, the observation that cyclical oscillation of granulocyte counts may be seen in some normal individuals, and consideration of a similar syndrome observed in grey collie dogs [83] suggested to King-Smith & Morley [85, 170] that granulopoiesis could be controlled in part by a negative-feedback mechanism with an inherent time delay (see p. 607). The postulated model contains two feedback loops whereby the concentration of granulocytes in the blood can control:
1 the production of granulocytes in the bone marrow; and

2 their rate of release from marrow storage compartments.

An undue sensitivity to inhibition of granulocyte production could, according to this model, result in the haematological features of cyclical neutropenia: such a mechanism might also underlie the oscillations seen in some patients with untreated CGL [40].

Chronic idiopathic neutropenia

This term has been applied to patients whose blood neutrophil counts remain below 2.0×10^9/l for long periods without obvious reason [170a]; there is no history of exposure to toxic agents, the spleen is not enlarged and no other systemic or marrow disease can be identified. In some cases the clinical picture may be difficult to distinguish from that associated with congenital neutropenias, which are considered separately below.

Though most reports describe single cases of chronic idiopathic neutropenia, a series of 29 patients has recently been reported [170b]. Twenty-two were females and their average age was 30. The majority had mean neutrophil counts below 1.0×10^9/l and in 17 there were less than 500×10^6/l for long periods. Infections in general were not severe and consisted of recurrent upper-respiratory-tract infections, occasional pneumonia, furunculosis and otitis media. Bone-marrow cellularity was usually normal, as was the marrow concentration of CFU-GM. No immunological cause for the neutropenia could be demonstrated in most cases. The natural history of the condition was benign: no patient developed leukaemia or aplastic anaemia. Antibiotics were used with benefit but corticosteroids, androgens, cytotoxic drugs and splenectomy were all considered unhelpful. The occasional patient with recurrent severe infections could, however, derive benefit from judicious use of steroids, e.g. 40–80 mg of prednisone on alternate days.

Neutropenia due to immunological mechanisms

The probable immunological cause of neutropenia associated with amidopyrine has been referred to above. The evidence that such mechanisms underlie the neutropenia associated with other drugs is less convincing [155]. Occasionally, however, patients are seen who have moderate or severe persistent neutropenia that cannot be attributed either to drugs or to alloantibodies due to previous pregnancy or blood transfusion. Factors capable of opsonizing or agglutinating neutrophils can sometimes be demonstrated in the patient's serum and the condition is then thought to represent 'autoimmune' neutropenia [171, 172]. In some cases antineutrophil antibody with anti-NA$_2$ specificity has been demonstrated [173, 174]. The patient's symptoms are variable and usually mild; he may have malaise, pharyngitis, cellulitis or mucosal ulceration. Treatment with corticosteroid drugs may produce transient or more long-lived elevation of the neutrophil count. Splenectomy is usually contraindicated because of the increased risk of infection after such surgery.

Neutropenia is occasionally seen in newborn infants whose mothers have been exposed to repeated alloantigenic stimulation in previous pregnancies. The condition is termed *neonatal isoimmune neutropenia* and is thought to be due to antibodies formed in the mother against neutrophil-specific or histocompatibility antigen on the fetal cells; these antibodies traverse the placenta and inhibit granulopoiesis or destroy granulocytes in the fetus [174–177]. The neonatal neutropenia may be severe and can last as long as 12 weeks or more; it carries a significant mortality from infection, for which antibiotic therapy may need to be supplemented by plasma exchange to lower the antibody titre.

Congenital neutropenias

A number of apparently distinct hereditary syndromes have been described involving congenital neutropenia either alone or in association with other defects. Some of these are essentially benign, and even symptomless, while others carry a high mortality.

Infantile genetic agranulocytosis. In 1956, Kostmann [178] described 14 children from a closely inbred community in northern Sweden, in whom very severe neutropenia was associated, during early infancy, with recurrent skin and umbilical sepsis, progressing to pneumonia, septicaemia and bacterial infections of various other organs, and almost uniformly fatal during infancy or early childhood. This condition is clearly inherited as an autosomal-recessive trait, though most of the similar cases subsequently reported have been without a family history.

Severe neutropenia (usually less than 0.3×10^9/l) is the rule, and is commonly associated with a monocytosis. Platelets are unaffected, but anaemia often results from the recurrent infections. The bone marrow is usually of normal cellularity, but contains a preponderance of promyelocytes and myelocytes with azurophilic granules, and lacks more mature granulocyte precursors [179]. Cytoplasmic vacuolation is prominent. Transfused granulocytes survive normally, but there is evidently a defect of granulocyte differentiation [179a]. An inhibitory factor in the marrow environment may suppress granulopoiesis *in vivo* [180, 181]. Infusion of normal plasma is without effect, as are corticosteroids. Life can be prolonged by the judicious and vigorous use of antibiotics, but no means have yet been found of stimulating granulopoiesis.

Familial benign neutropenia. This relatively benign condition, first described by Gänsslen in 1941 [183, 184], is inherited on an autosomal-dominant basis. Mild to moderate neutropenia $(1-4 \times 10^9/l)$ may be symptomless, or associated with recurrent periodontal disease or furunculosis. The cellularity of the marrow is normal but, as in Kostmann's neutropenia, the more mature granulocyte precursors may be deficient. No special treatment is needed. By extension, this condition may be regarded as identical with that seen in several large ethnic groups, notably African blacks [184a] and Yemenite Jews [184b], amongst whom the distribution of neutrophil counts is significantly lower than in other races. Recent evidence suggests that the asymptomatic neutropenia seen in a proportion of black Americans is due to a diminished bone-marrow granulocyte reserve [184c].

Familial severe neutropenia. In 1959, Hitzig [185] described a father and two children with severe neutropenia and hyper-γ-globulinaemia: the pattern of inheritance was evidently autosomal-dominant, and the patients suffered from severe infections, especially of the buccal cavity. Their blood showed severe neutropenia with monocytosis. In this family, as in other similar cases described subsequently, the condition was compatible with survival to adult life despite repeated infections. The bone marrow is characteristically normocellular with a deficiency of granulocytes later than the myelocyte stage.

Reticular dysgenesis (alymphocytic neutropenia). Babies with this condition (see also Chapter 18, p. 686) have a complete absence of lymphocytes in a hypoplastic thymus [186, 187], and myeloid precursor cells are absent from the bone marrow; there is consequently a virtually complete absence of leucocytes in the blood. Bacterial and viral infections are frequent and severe, and death usually occurs soon after birth. In milder cases, designated thymic alymphoplasia, survival may be longer but death still occurs early [188]. If a tissue-matched donor is available, bone-marrow transplantation offers the only hope of successful treatment.

Shwachman's syndrome [188a]. This is an autosomal-recessive trait comprising exocrine pancreatic insufficiency, neutropenia, metaphysial chondrodysplasia and growth retardation. Symptoms referable to the malabsorption first appear in infancy, and are typically associated with recurrent respiratory and skin infections. The neutrophils are defective in mobility (see Chapter 16, p. 636) as well as in number, and some degree of thrombocytopenia is usually also present. The neutrophil and platelet counts occasionally show a cyclical variation. The bone marrow tends to be somewhat hypoplastic. Treatment of the malabsorption with pancreatic extract does not affect the blood picture, but in some cases the neutropenia and thrombocytopenia have responded to low-dose corticosteroid therapy.

Neutropenia with cartilage-hair hypoplasia. Children with this disorder are short-limbed dwarfs with abnormally fine hair, neutropenia and lymphopenia (see Chapter 18, p. 683). Defective cellular immunity leads to increased susceptibility to severe varicella and other virus infections, and recurrent bacterial infections may also occur as a result of the neutropenia. Bone-marrow findings show that the neutropenia is due to a defect of granulocyte maturation [189].

Other congenital neutropenias. Neutropenia is a feature of the 'lazy leucocyte' syndrome and the Chediak–Higashi syndrome; both of these are primarily disorders of granulocytic function, and are therefore described in Chapter 16. Neutropenia is also commonly seen in children with hypo-γ-globulinaemia, particularly in association with raised levels of IgM (see Chapter 18, p. 679). Correction of the neutropenia, with accompanying healing of mouth ulcers, was achieved in three boys with this syndrome by replacement therapy with plasma and γ globulin [189a].

Neutropenia due to increased peripheral destruction
The spleen can influence haemopoiesis in a manner that is poorly defined and splenic pathology can lead to alterations in the blood picture. *Hypersplenism* is a vague concept (see Chapter 20), but a reasonable working definition is 'reduction of one or more of the cellular elements of the peripheral blood that is "usually" associated with splenomegaly and that is corrected by removal of the spleen' [155]. The enlargement of the spleen may be secondary to a variety of causes—for example chronic infection, thalassaemia, lymphoma or Gaucher's disease—but on rare occasions no cause can be identified.

Primary hypersplenic neutropenia. This is a disorder characterized by somewhat vague symptoms including lassitude, fever and pains in the limbs [190]. Patients have splenomegaly for which no cause can be discerned. The blood shows neutropenia and the patients may suffer from severe infections. The condition is apparently cured by splenectomy [190].

Neutropenia is a characteristic finding in patients with systemic lupus erythematosus (SLE) [191] and occurs less commonly in rheumatoid arthritis. In SLE, granulocyte production may be reduced and granulocyte survival may be impaired by an autoantibody; in both SLE and rheumatoid arthritis, splenomegaly may be associated with neutropenia.

Felty's syndrome. This involves malaise, weight loss, lymphadenopathy and increased susceptibility to infection, in conjunction with rheumatoid arthritis [192–195]. One or more of the cellular elements of the blood is reduced and the neutropenia may be severe. The bone marrow is usually hyperplastic. Felty's syndrome occurs in about one per cent of patients with rheumatoid arthritis. Splenectomy is commonly carried out as treatment and neutrophil numbers frequently show considerable increases post-operatively; in most cases, however, such improvement is not maintained [196].

Extracorporeal circulations. Severe neutropenia may occur within a short time of beginning haemodialysis in patients with renal failure. The neutrophil count usually returns to normal during the procedure and may show 'rebound' leucocytosis [197]. Similar blood changes have been seen during heart–lung bypass procedures and in normal subjects undergoing filtration leucopheresis for granulocyte donation [198]. The mechanism of neutropenia in these circumstances is poorly understood, but it is possible that contact of granulocytes with plastic and other foreign surfaces leads to release into the extracorporeal circuit of factors that promote margination and aggregation of neutrophils in the pulmonary capillary circulation. This change may be mediated by activation of complement [199].

NEUTROPHILIA

Leucocytosis is defined as an increase in the number of circulating leucocytes above the normal range, usually above $10–11 \times 10^9/l$. Such leucocytes may be of any cell type or of any level of maturity—when blasts predominate the diagnosis of acute leukaemia is suggested—but in practice leucocytosis is usually due to an increase in the number of neutrophilic granulocytes; the term 'neutrophilia' may then correctly be used. The term 'leukaemoid reaction' describes the less common leucocytosis in which the blood picture resembles that of leukaemia but is in fact due to another identifiable cause.

Neutrophilia can theoretically result from one or other of a number of mechanisms:

1 an increased production of neutrophils in the marrow;

2 an increased release of neutrophils from the marrow granulocyte reserve;

3 a reduced rate of egress of cells from the circulation; or

4 a shift in the distribution of neutrophils within the

circulation from the marginated to the circulating granulocyte pool [38, 155].

In general, acute changes in neutrophil numbers, occurring within minutes or hours of a specific 'stimulus' or event, are mainly due to release of granulocytes from marrow reserves and shifts from marginated to circulating pools [220]: in contrast, chronic or long-sustained neutrophilia is due in most cases to increased production of neutrophils from their precursors in the marrow [38].

Infections

The commonest cause of neutrophilia is bacterial infection (Table 15.8). Neutrophil increases may be

Table 15.8. Causes of neutrophilia

Acute infections:
Bacterial, viral, fungal, mycobacterial and rickettsial

Physical stimuli:
Trauma, electric shock, anoxia, pregnancy

Drugs and chemicals:
Corticosteroids, aetiocholanolone, adrenaline, lead, mercury poisoning, lithium

Haematological causes:
Acute haemorrhage, acute haemolysis, transfusion reactions, post-splenectomy, leukaemia and myeloproliferative disorders

Malignant diseases:
Carcinoma, especially of gastro-intestinal tract, liver or bone marrow

Miscellaneous conditions:
Certain dermatoses, hepatic necrosis, chronic idiopathic leucocytosis

moderate ($15–25 \times 10^9/l$) but much higher numbers (up to or exceeding $40 \times 10^9/l$) may occur, particularly in children and when the infection is due to pyogenic bacteria. Such infections may be localized in the form of abscesses or generalized, as in septicaemia. Neutrophilia may also occur with inflammation produced by toxins, neoplasms, burns or acute trauma [201]. It may also characterize acute haemorrhage. Usually in these circumstances the blood shows an increase mainly in mature neutrophils, but 'band' forms, metamyelocytes and myelocytes may also be present [202]. The cytoplasm often contains 'toxic granulations'. However, in certain infectious illnesses, leucocytosis does not occur in the absence of complications; its absence can then be of some diagnostic value. Thus neutrophilia is not a usual feature of uncomplicated typhoid fever, tuberculosis or viral infections such as measles, mumps and varicella.

Drugs

Certain pharmacological agents can induce neutrophilia. Corticosteroids often produce a prolonged increase in numbers of circulating neutrophils. In such patients the absolute turnover rate of blood neutrophils is apparently normal, but blood pool sizes may be increased as much as fivefold [73, 203]. In contrast, the administration of adrenaline or aetiocholanolone produces a short-lived neutrophilia, probably due mainly to shift of neutrophils from marginated to circulating pools [73, 204–206]; exercise can induce neutrophilia by the same mechanism [73]. It has recently been recognized that lithium salts used in the treatment of psychiatric disorders can produce prolonged neutrophilia [207]; since lithium stimulates the production of CSA *in vitro* [208, 209], it may act to enhance marrow granulocyte production by a similar mechanism *in vivo*; it appears also to have a direct stimulatory effect on the stem cell.

Leukaemoid reactions

Leukaemoid reactions can occur in a variety of conditions, including severe infection, intoxications and malignancy [155, 210]. The peripheral leucocyte count may exceed $50 \times 10^9/l$ and the presence in the blood of immature precursor cells raises the possibility of leukaemia. Leukaemoid reactions may be granulocytic or lymphoid, according to the variety of leukaemia simulated, but the former is the more common. The mature cells usually show toxic granulation and have a high cytoplasmic content of alkaline phosphatase. Döhle bodies may also be seen. The toxic granulation and the high alkaline phosphatase score are valuable in helping to exclude a diagnosis of leukaemia, but final proof of the non-neoplastic nature of the clinical picture depends on its resolution when the primary cause is removed. When the leucocyte count is extremely high but immature forms are absent from the blood, the term 'hyperleucocytosis' is probably preferable to leukaemoid reaction. The causes of the two reactions are identical (Table 15.9).

Leuco-erythroblastic anaemia

The term 'leuco-erythroblastic anaemia' (myelophthisic anaemia) is used to characterize a form of anaemia in which nucleated red cells and immature granulocytes are prominent in the blood [211]. There is often irregularity in size and shape of the red cells. The leucocyte count may be raised and a full spectrum of immature granulocytes including blast cells may be identified. The platelet count is normal or reduced. Leuco-erythroblastic anaemia is seen typically when the marrow is invaded by malignant disease. It may also be seen in myelosclerosis and in a minority of

Table 15.9. Causes of leukaemoid reactions or leuco-erythroblastic anaemia

---

Severe infections, especially in children:
  (a) Pneumonia, septicaemia, meningococcal meningitis
  (b) Infectious mononucleosis, pertussis
Intoxications:
  Eclampsia, severe burns, mercury poisoning
Neoplasia, especially with bone-marrow infiltration
Severe haemorrhage or haemolysis

---

patients with multiple myeloma. Other causes are listed in Table 15.9.

EOSINOPHILIA

Eosinophilia is the term usually applied to an increase in the total number of eosinophils above $440 \times 10^6/l$ in the peripheral blood. The increase is usually moderate but in some cases (e.g. bronchial asthma, parasitic diseases and occasionally in Hodgkin's disease), very great numbers (more than $40 \times 10^9/l$) of eosinophils are seen [97, 98]. The major causes of eosinophilia are listed in Table 15.10. Some of these are considered in greater detail below.

Allergic reactions

Eosinophil numbers are increased in the blood tissues and secretions of patients with various allergies and atopic states. Blood eosinophilia is very common in patients with asthma, although counts above $2.0 \times 10^9/l$ are rare [212–214]. Eosinophil numbers may also be raised in patients with urticaria and angioneurotic oedema. Treatment with corticosteroids in these conditions may or may not restore blood eosinophil numbers to normal or subnormal values [213, 214].

Parasitic infestation

The association of eosinophilia with metazoan parasitic infestation was first noted in 1891 in ankylostomiasis [215], and subsequently described in trichinosis [216]. In trichinosis, eosinophilia begins in the blood about one week after intake of infected food, may reach a maximum at three weeks and may persist for six months or longer [216, 217]. Eosinophilia is a prominent feature also of many other metazoan infestations in which tissue invasion occurs; these include filariasis, schistosomiasis, echinococcal disease and liver fluke (*Clonorchis sinensis*) [218]. Eosinophilia is far less commonly seen in protozoan infections: it is variably present in malaria [219] and is not a feature of trypanosomiasis or kala-azar. Parasites that inhabit the intestine cause eosinophilia infrequently: when present, it is usually an indication that some degree of

Table 15.10. Causes of eosinophilia

Allergic reactions:
Asthma, hay fever, urticaria, angioneurotic
oedema

Parasitic infestation:
Tissue parasites—trichinosis, filariasis,
visceral larva migrans, etc.
Intestinal parasites—*Ascaris, Taenia,* etc.
(less regularly)

Skin disorders:
Pemphigus, pemphigoid, eczema, psoriasis,
(dermatitis herpetiformis)

Drug hypersensitivity reactions:
Especially iodides, penicillin, allopurinol,
gold salts, tartrazine

Löffler's pulmonary syndrome and Löffler's
endomyocarditis

Tropical eosinophilia (probably filarial)

Malignant diseases:
Especially Hodgkin's disease, carcinoma of ovary,
lung, stomach, angio-immunoblastic lymphadenopathy

Following irradiation or splenectomy

Hypereosinophilic syndromes

Eosinophilic leukaemia

Miscellaneous conditions:
Polyarteritis nodosa, ulcerative colitis,
sarcoidosis, scarlet fever, pernicious anaemia,
chronic active hepatitis, eosinophilic granuloma,
familial eosinophilia

invasion of tissues has occurred. Thus, varying degrees of eosinophilia may be seen in patients with taenia, strongyloides or ascaris infestations [98].

Skin diseases
Pemphigus and pemphigoid are characteristically accompanied by eosinophilia in the blood and these cells are found also in fluid from bullae [220–222]. Atopic dermatitis may also be associated with eosinophilia, as may eczema not obviously of atopic origin. Urticaria is variably associated with eosinophilia, which is particularly likely to occur in acute urticarial reactions related to food or drug allergies or helminthic infections; it is not a feature of chronic urticaria. Dermatitis herpetiformis is often quoted as a major cause of blood eosinophilia, but the association may have been overemphasized, though undoubtedly eosinophils are often present in the vesicular skin lesions of this disease [223, 224].

Drugs
A large number of pharmacological agents are capable of inducing blood eosinophilia. Presumably after

ingestion the drug links with a large molecule and acts as a hapten [97, 98]. In most cases the only sign of drug allergy is the eosinophilia, but serum levels of IgE are sometimes raised [225], and there may occasionally be fever or a skin rash as further evidence of drug-induced allergic reaction [98].

Eosinophilia is a feature of sensitivity to penicillin. It may also be seen as part of an allergic response to potassium iodide [226]. Perhaps the most common cause of eosinophilia is hypersensitivity to gold, such as sodium aurothiomalate, used in the treatment of rheumatoid arthritis [227]; in one series eosinophilia greater than $400 \times 10^6/l$ was seen in 47% of patients receiving such treatment [228].

Pulmonary eosinophilic syndrome (Löffler's syndrome)
In 1936, Löffler [229] described a relatively mild clinical syndrome consisting of cough, eosinophil-containing sputum and blood eosinophilia. Chest X-rays showed transient 'fluffy' pulmonary infiltrates which appeared and disappeared. The disorder usually subsided within three or four weeks. The picture has been reported many times subsequently and probably has a variety of causes; these include drugs such as sulphonamides and chlorpropamide, environmental antigens and frequently helminthic infestations [230]. A more severe disease involving pulmonary infiltration, blood eosinophilia and high fever that may last for a number of weeks has been designated *pulmonary infiltration with eosinophilia* [231]. There may be a good clinical response to treatment with steroids but features often return when treatment is stopped. Most patients eventually recover completely [232, 232a, 233].

Eosinophilic myocardial disease (Löffler's endomyocarditis)
Also in 1936, Löffler described a specific form of heart disease progressing to cardiac failure that had some features suggestive of constrictive pericarditis. Autopsy examination revealed dense thickening of the endocardium and mural thrombi [234]. Subsequently a similar clinical picture was reported in Ugandan children, many of whom had blood eosinophilia [235]. Löffler's endomyocarditis has also since been described in eosinophilic leukaemia and hypereosinophilic syndromes (see below). It is likely that high and prolonged blood eosinophilia of any cause can damage the heart in a highly specific manner, leading to mural thrombus formation, marked thickening of the endocardium and degeneration of the subendocardial portion of the myocardium [236–238]. Patients sustaining such cardiac damage may have a large number of eosinophils in the circulation that show features of 'activation' or 'stimulation': the cells may have receptors for IgG and C3b, contain cytoplasmic vacuoles

and show partial degranulation [239]. They may thus have already released into the blood stream granule products which mediate the cardiac damage [240].

Tropical (filarial) eosinophilia
Tropical pulmonary eosinophilia is seen mainly in India, Southeast Asia and the South Pacific islands [241, 241a]. The pulmonary changes have in the past been confused with tuberculosis. The condition is more common in males than in females and Indians seem especially susceptible [241, 242]. Serum IgE levels may be extremely high [243]. It is due to filariasis and responds frequently to treatment with the antifilarial agent diethylcarbamazine [98, 241, 244].

Eosinophilia in association with malignant disease
Increased numbers of eosinophils in the blood have been reported in association with a number of malignant tumours [98]. In one series 11·4% of 140 patients with bronchogenic carcinoma had eosinophilia [245], but a figure of five per cent may be more typical [246]. Eosinophilia may also be seen in carcinomas of pancreas, colon, uterine cervix and even cerebral glioblastoma [98]. The mechanism underlying the eosinophilia is unclear. There may be neoantigen in the tumour that provokes an autoallergic response. Alternatively the tumour may secrete a polypeptide or other material with eosinophil-stimulating properties: this is the likely explanation for the eosinophilia seen in association with some leukaemias that are unquestionably of lymphoid-cell origin [247].

The incidence of blood eosinophilia in patients with Hodgkin's disease is probably about five per cent [98]. However, eosinophils may be prominent in the marrow and in histological material from lymph nodes and other involved tissues, even when normal numbers are present in the blood [248]. Conversely, extreme blood leucocytosis with high proportions of eosinophils is sometimes seen, especially when the involved lymph nodes show necrosis [249]. Patients with Hodgkin's disease who have blood eosinophilia usually have high serum IgE levels [250]. *Angioimmunoblastic lymphadenopathy* (see Chapter 24, p. 942) is a newly described clinical syndrome of unknown cause. There is sometimes a history of exposure to specific allergens. Patients have generalized lymphadenopathy and hepatosplenomegaly in association with variable fevers, rashes, pulmonary infiltrates and abnormalities in serum proteins [251–253]. About 30% of patients have blood, or blood and marrow, eosinophilia. In some cases, the disease responds poorly to treatment with steroids or cytotoxic drugs and runs an apparently malignant course; in other cases spontaneous regression or prolonged remission following minimal treatment has been reported [253].

Radiation-related eosinophilia
Eosinophilia may develop in patients receiving super-voltage radiotherapy for carcinoma. In one study 40% of patients treated by irradiation for intra-abdominal neoplasms showed eosinophilia at some point during treatment [254, 255].

Hypereosinophilic syndromes
The term hypereosinophilic syndrome (HES) was introduced by Hardy & Anderson [256] in 1968 to describe a spectrum of disease characterized by high levels of eosinophils in the blood with variable involvement of other organ systems. By 1975, 57 cases were recognized: features in addition to eosinophilia included weight loss, rash, various neurological abnormalities, hepatosplenomegaly, fever, oedema, signs of abdominal involvement and involvement of the heart and lungs [238]. The bone marrow also shows increased eosinophilic precursors but no other specific change. Cytogenetic abnormalities in the myeloid series are not seen. The cause of HES is unknown but some patients gain benefit from treatment with corticosteroids and hydroxyurea [257] or vincristine.

Eosinophilic leukaemia
The question of whether eosinophilic leukaemia can ever exist as a distinct entity has in the past been much debated [236, 238, 258]. Some feel that even when patients with high eosinophil counts have evidence of tissue invasion and ultimately die of their disease, there is never good evidence of a malignancy. In some cases, however, patients with high blood-eosinophil levels may show a Ph[1] chromosome when cytogenetic analysis of marrow is carried out [238, 259, 260]. These patients presumably have an eosinophilic variant of CGL. Yet there remains a small number of patients with blood eosinophilia, including immature forms, whose clinical course closely resembles that of a myeloid leukaemia: when a consistent cytogenetic abnormality (other than the Ph[1] chromosome) is demonstrated in myeloid cells [261, 262], or when agar cultures of blood or marrow resemble CGL [263], the diagnosis of eosinophilic leukaemia *sui generis* seems justified.

Miscellaneous causes of eosinophilia
Eosinophilia may be seen in a number of other clinical situations: occasionally in polyarteritis nodosa when there is lung involvement, in sarcoidosis [264], chronic active hepatitis [265] and perhaps pernicious anaemia [266]. A family has been reported in which 12 infants died of a disease of the reticulo-endothelial system in which eosinophilia was prominent [267]: the children had widespread skin eruptions with fever, lymphadenopathy and enlargement of liver and spleen. The

disease may have been a variant of severe combined immunodeficiency [268].

Basophil leucocytes normally number up to $100 \times 10^6/l$ in the blood. Young women usually have slightly higher basophil counts than other adults. A basophil leucocytosis is not normally an isolated finding but may occur in myxoedema [127, 269], and less commonly in chickenpox, smallpox and chronic ulcerative colitis [270]. Absolute numbers of basophils are frequently raised in myeloproliferative disorders, especially CGL and polycythaemia rubra vera.

DISORDERS OF MONOCYTE NUMBERS

In view of the probable common origin of monocytes and granulocytes it is not surprising to find in some circumstances that changes in the numbers of the two cell types occur *pari passu* in the blood. For example, monocyte and granulocyte production are suppressed similarly by cytotoxic drugs, and monocytes and granulocytes may both be involved in the leucocytosis that characterizes certain forms of myeloid leukaemia (see Chapter 22). In other circumstances changes in monocyte numbers appear to occur in isolation [133].

Monocytosis
The absolute number of monocytes in the blood varies between 285 and $500 \times 10^6/l$ in adults [134], and monocytosis is conveniently defined as an increase above $800 \times 10^6/l$. Monocytes are an important com-

Table 15.11. Causes of monocytosis

Chronic bacterial infections:
  Tuberculosis, subacute bacterial endocarditis, brucellosis

Other specific infections:
  Malaria, kala-azar, trypanosomiasis, typhus, Rocky Mountain spotted fever

Malignant diseases:
  Hodgkin's disease, carcinoma

Leukaemia:
  Acute myeloid leukaemia, chronic monocytic leukaemia

Neutropenias:
  Familial benign and severe neutropenia
  Cyclical neutropenia
  Chronic idiopathic neutropenia
  Drug-induced agranulocytosis

Miscellaneous:
  Cirrhosis, systemic lupus erythematosus, rheumatoid arthritis

---

ponent of the cellular reaction to mycobacteria in the tissue and blood and monocytosis is therefore a feature of tuberculosis. Monocytosis may also be a feature of other chronic infections [134, 271, 272] (Table 15.11), particularly those due to intracellular microorganisms or parasites, and is a regular and persistent feature of various neutropenic states. In subacute bacterial endocarditis, monocytosis may occur and in this disease some of the cells in the capillary circulation may have prominent vacuoles while others may show phagocytosis of erythrocytes or leucocytes [273]. Monocyte numbers are often increased in the blood of patients with Hodgkin's disease [274] and other neoplastic disease [275]. Increased numbers of circulating monocytes are found also in acute myeloid leukaemias and chronic monocytic leukaemia (see Chapters 22 and 23).

REFERENCES

1 DICKE K.A., VAN NOORD M.J., MAAT B., SCHAEFER U.W. & VAN BEKKUM D.W. (1973) Identification of cells in primate bone marrow resembling the hemopoietic stem cell in the mouse. *Blood*, **42**, 195.

2 TILL J.E. & McCULLOCH E.A. (1961) A direct measurement of the radiation sensitivity of normal mouse bone marrow cells. *Radiation Research*, **14**, 213.

3 MAXIMOW A.A. (1924) Relation of blood cells to connective tissues and endothelium. *Physiological Reviews*, **4**, 533.

4 NAEGELI O. (1931) *Blutkrankheiten und Blutdiagnostik*. Springer-Verlag, Berlin.

5 SCHILLING V. (1929) The blood picture and its clinical significance. (Trans. Gradwohl R.B.H.), 78th edn., Mosby, St Louis.

6 SABIN F., MILLER F.R., SMITHBURN K.C., THOMAS R.M. & HUMMEL L.E. (1936) Changes in the bone marrow and blood cells of developing rabbits. *Journal of Experimental Medicine*, **64**, 97.

7 WU A.M., TILL J.E., SIMINOVITCH L. & McCULLOCH E.A. (1968) Cytological evidence for a relationship between normal hematopoietic colony-forming cells and cells of the lymphoid system. *Journal of Experimental Medicine*, **127**, 455.

8 WU A.M., TILL J.E., SIMINOVITCH L. & McCULLOCH E.A. (1967) A cytological study of the capacity for differentiation of normal hemopoietic colony-forming cells. *Journal of Cellular and Comparative Physiology*, **69**, 177.

9 PLUZNIK D.H. & SACHS L. (1966) The induction of clones of normal mast cells by a substance from conditioned medium. *Experimental Cell Research*, **43**, 553.

10 BRADLEY T.R. & METCALF D. (1966) The growth of mouse bone marrow cells *in vitro*. *Australian Journal of Experimental Biology and Medical Science*, **44**, 287.

11 ISCOVE N.N., SENN J.S., TILL J.E. & McCULLOCH E.A. (1971) Colony formation by normal and leukemic

human marrow cells in cultures: effect of conditioned medium from human leukocytes. *Blood*, **37**, 1.

12 MOORE M.A.S., WILLIAMS N. & METCALF D. (1972) Purification and characterization of the in vitro colony-forming cell in monkey hemopoietic tissue. *Journal of Cellular Physiology*, **79**, 283.

13 PIKE B.L. & ROBINSON W.A. (1970) Human bone marrow colony growth in agar-gel. *Journal of Cellular Physiology*, **76**, 77.

14 CHERVENICK P.A. & BOGGS D.R. (1971) In vitro growth of granulocytic and mononuclear cell colonies from blood of normal individuals. *Blood*, **37**, 131.

15 HASKILL J.S., McNEILL T.A. & MOORE M.A.S. (1969) Density distribution analysis of in vivo and in vitro colony forming cells in bone marrow. *Journal of Cellular Physiology*, **75**, 167.

16 RICKARD K.A., SHADDUCK R.K., HOWARD D.E. & STOHLMAN F. (1970) A differential effect of hydroxyurea on hemopoietic stem cell colonies *in vitro* and *in vivo*. *Proceedings of the Society of Experimental Biology and Medicine*, **134**, 152.

17 LAJTHA L.G., POZZI L.V., SCHOFIELD R. & FOX M. (1969) Kinetic properties of haemopoietic stem cells. *Cell and Tissue Kinetics*, **2**, 39.

18 MOFFATT D.J. & YOFFEY J.M. (1967) Identity of the haemopoietic stem cell. *Lancet*, **ii**, 547.

19 CHERVENICK P.A. & LOBUGLIO A.F. (1972) Human blood monocytes: stimulators of granulocyte and mononuclear colony formation *in vitro*. *Science*, **178**, 164.

20 BURGESS A.W., WILSON E.C. & METCALF D. (1967) Stimulation by human placenta conditioned medium of hemopoietic colony formation by human marrow cells. *Blood*, **49**, 573.

21 STANLEY E.R., METCALF D., MARITZ J.S. & YEO G.F. (1972) Standardized bioassay for bone marrow colony stimulating factor in human urine: levels in normal man. *Journal of Laboratory and Clinical Medicine*, **79**, 657.

22 STANLEY E.R. & METCALF D. (1972) Purification and properties of human urinary colony stimulating factor (CSF). *Cell Differentiation*, **18**, 272.

23 STANLEY E.R. & METCALF D. (1971) The molecular weight of colony-stimulating factor (CSF). *Proceedings of the Society for Experimental Biology and Medicine*, **137**, 1029.

24 GOLDE D.W. & CLINE M.J. (1972) Identification of the colony-stimulating cell in human peripheral blood. *Journal of Clinical Investigation*, **51**, 2981.

25 DIPERSIO J.F., BRENNAN J.K., LICHTMAN M.A. & SPEISER B.L. (1978) Human cell lines that elaborate colony-stimulating factor for the marrow cells of man and other species. *Blood*, **51**, 507.

26 GOLDE D.W., QUAN S.G. & CLINE M.J. (1978) Human T lymphocyte cell line producing colony-stimulating activity. *Blood*, **52**, 1068.

27 METCALF D. (1977) Hemopoietic colonies. *Recent Results in Cancer Research*. No. 61 (ed. Rertchnick P), p. 71. Springer-Verlag, New York.

28 BROXMEYER H.E., MOORE M.A.S. & RALPH P. (1977) Cell-free granulocyte colony inhibiting activity derived from human polymorphonuclear neutrophils. *Experimental Hematology*, **5**, 77.

29 BROXMEYER H.E., SMITHYMAN A., EGER R.R., MEYERS P.A. & DE SOUSA M. (1978) Identification of lactoferrin as the granulocyte-derived inhibitor of colony-stimulating activity production. *Journal of Experimental Medicine*, **148**, 1052.

30 RYTOMAA T. & KIVINIEMI K. (1968) Control of granulocyte production. I. Chalone and antichalone, two specific humoral regulators. *Cell and Tissue Kinetics*, **1**, 329.

31 KURLAND H.I., BROXMEYER H.E., PELUS L.M., BOCKMAN R.S. & MOORE M.A.S. (1978) Role of monocyte-macrophage derived colony stimulating factor and prostaglandin E in the positive and negative feedback control of myeloid stem cell proliferation. *Blood*, **52**, 388.

32 KÖRBLING M., FLIEDNER T.M., CALVO W., ROSS W.M., NOTHDURFT W. & STEINBACH I. (1979) Albumin density gradient purification of canine hemopoietic blood stem cells (HBSC): long term allogeneic engraftment without GVH-reaction. *Experimental Hematology*, **7**, 277.

33 STORB R., GRAHAM T.C., EPSTEIN R.B., SALE G.E. & THOMAS E.D. (1977) Demonstration of hemopoietic stem cells in the peripheral blood of baboons by cross circulation. *Blood*, **50**, 537.

34 LAWLER S.D. (1977) The cytogenetics of chronic granulocytic leukaemia. *Clinics in Haematology*, **6**, 55.

35 GOLDE D.W., BURGALETA C., SPARKES R.S. & CLINE M.J. (1977) The Philadelphia chromosome in human macrophages. *Blood*, **49**, 367.

36 McCREDIE K.B., HERSH E.M. & FREIREICH E.J. (1971) Cells capable of colony formation in the peripheral blood of man. *Science*, **171**, 293.

37 HERSHKO C., GALE R.P., HO W.G. & CLINE M.J. (1979) Cure of aplastic anaemia in paroxysmal nocturnal haemoglobulinuria by marrow transfusion from identical twin: failure of peripheral leucocyte transfusion to correct marrow aplasia. *Lancet*, **i**, 945.

38 BOGGS D.R. (1967) The kinetics of neutrophilic leukocytes in health and disease. *Seminars in Hematology*, **4**, 359.

39 ATHENS J.W. (1970) Neutrophil granulocyte kinetics and granulocytopoiesis. In: *Regulation of Hematopoiesis, Vol. 2* (ed. Gordon A.S.), p. 1143. Appleton-Century-Crofts, New York.

40 ROBINSON W.A. & MANGALIK A. (1975) The kinetics and regulation of granulopoiesis. *Seminars in Hematology*, **12**, 7.

41 VINCENT P.C. (1977) Granulocyte kinetics in health and disease. *Clinics in Haematology*, **6**, 695.

42 CRONKITE E.P. (1979) Kinetics of granulocytopoiesis. *Clinics in Haematology*, **8**, 351.

43 CRADDOCK C.G. (1980) Defences of the body: the initiators of defense, the ready reserves and the scavengers. In: *Blood, Pure and Eloquent* (ed. Wintrobe M.M.), p. 417. McGraw-Hill, New York.

44 GULLIVER D. (ed.) (1846) *The Works of William Hewson FRS*. Sydenham Society, London.

45 NEUMANN E. (1868) Über die Bedeutung des Knochenmarkes für die Blutbildung. *Zentral Med Wissensch*, **6**, 689.

46 SABIN F.R., CUNNINGHAM R.S., DOAN C.A. & KINDWALL J.A. (1925) The normal rhythm of the white blood cells. *Bulletin of the Johns Hopkins Hosptial*, **37**, 14.

47 ROSSE W.F. & GURNEY C.W. (1959) Pelger–Huet ano-

maly in three families and its use in determining the disappearance of transfused neutrophils from the peripheral blood. *Blood*, **14**, 170.

48 OSGOOD E.E., TIVEY H., DAVISON K.B., SEAMAN A.J. & LI J.E. (1952) Relative rates of formation of new leukocytes in patients with acute and chronic leukemias measured by uptake of radioactive phosphorus in isolated DNA. *Cancer*, **5**, 331.

49 CRONKITE E.P., FLIEDNER T.M., RUBINI J.R., BOND V.P. & HUGHES W.L. (1958) Dynamics of proliferating cell systems studied with tritiated thymidine. *Journal of Clinical Investigation*, **37**, 887.

50 MAUER A.M., ATHENS J.W., WARNER H.R., ASHENBRUCKER H., CARTWRIGHT G.E. & WINTROBE M.M. (1959) An analysis of leukocyte radioactivity curves obtained with radioactive diisopropylfluorophosphate (DFP^{32}). In: *The Kinetics of Cellular Proliferation*. (ed. Stohlman F.), p. 231. Grune & Stratton, New York.

51 VODOPICK H.A., ATHENS J.W., WARNER H.R., BOGGS D.R., CARTWRIGHT G.E. & WINTROBE M.M. (1966) An evaluation of radiosulfate as a granulocyte label in the dog. *Journal of Laboratory and Clinical Medicine*, **68**, 47.

52 DRESCH C., NAJEAN Y. & BAUCHET J. (1971) In vitro ^{51}Cr and ^{32}P-DFP labelling of granulocytes in man. *Journal of Nuclear Medicine*, **12**, 774.

53 UCHIDA T. & KARRIYONE S. (1973) Organ distribution of ^{99}mTc-labelled white cells. *Acta Haematologica Japonica*, **36**, 78.

54 KLONIZAKIS I., PETERS A.M., FITZPATRICK M.L., KENSETT M.J., LEWIS S.M. & LAVENDER J.P. (1980) Radionuclide distribution following injection of ^{111}Indium-labelled platelets. *British Journal of Haematology*, **46**, 595.

55 LAVENDER J.P., GOLDMAN J.M., ARNOT R.N. & THAKUR M.L. (1977) Kinetics of indium-111 labelled lymphocytes in normal subjects and patients with Hodgkin's disease. *British Medical Journal*, **ii**, 797.

56 WEIBLEN B., FORSTROM L. & McCULLOUGH J. (1979) Studies of the kinetics of indium-111-labelled granulocytes. *Journal of Laboratory and Clinical Medicine*, **94**, 246.

56a DUTCHER J.P., SCHIFFER C.A. & JOHNSTON G.S. (1981) Rapid migration of ^{111}indium-labelled granulocytes to sites of infection. *New England Journal of Medicine*, **304**, 586.

57 THOMAS E.D., PLAIN G.L. & THOMAS D. (1965) Leucocyte kinetics in the dog studied by cross-circulation. *Journal of Laboratory and Clinical Medicine*, **66**, 64.

58 BIERMAN H.R., KELLY K.H., BYRON R.L. & MARSHALL G.J. (1961) Leucopheresis in man. I. Haematological observations following leucocyte withdrawal in patients with non-haematological disorders. *British Journal of Haematology*, **7**, 51.

59 REBUCK J.W. & CROWLEY J.H. (1955) A method for studying leukocytic functions *in vivo*. *Annals of the New York Academy of Science*, **59**, 757.

60 SENN H., HOLLAND J.F. & BANERJEE T. (1969) Kinetic and comparative studies on localized leukocyte mobilization in normal man. *Journal of Laboratory and Clinical Medicine*, **74**, 742.

61 CLINE M.J. (1975) Production, destruction and distribution of neutrophilic granulocytes. In: *The White Cell*, p. 22. Harvard University Press, Cambridge, Mass.

62 WARNER H.R. & ATHENS J.W. (1964) An analysis of granulocyte kinetics in blood and bone marrow. *Annals of the New York Academy of Sciences*, **113**, 523.

63 CRONKITE E.P. & VINCENT P.C. (1969) Granulocytopoiesis. *Series Hematologica II*, **4**, 3.

64 SIN Y.M. & SAINTE-MARIE G. (1965) Granulopoiesis in the rat thymus. II. *British Journal of Haematology*, **11**, 624.

65 STRYCKMANS P., CRONKITE E.P., FACHE J., FLIEDNER T.M. & RAMOS J. (1966) Deoxyribonucleic acid synthesis time of erythropoietic and granulopoietic cells in human beings. *Nature (London)*, **211**, 717.

66 FINCH C.A., HARKER L.A. & COOK J.D. (1977) Kinetics of the formed elements of human blood. *Blood*, **50**, 699.

67 CRADDOCK C.G., PERRY S. & LAWRENCE J.S. (1956) The dynamics of leukopoiesis and leukocytosis as studied by leukopheresis and isotopic techniques. *Journal of Clinical Investigation*, **35**, 285.

68 FLIEDNER T.M., CRONKITE E.P., KILLMAN S.A. & BOND V.P. (1964) Granulocytopoiesis. II. Emergence and pattern of labelling of neutrophilic granulocytes in humans. *Blood*, **24**, 683.

69 DANCEY J.T., DEUBELBEISS K.A., HARKER L.A. & FINCH C.A. (1976) Neutrophil kinetics in man. *Journal of Clinical Investigation*, **58**, 705.

70 DONOHUE D.M., REIFF R.H., HANSON M.L., BETSON Y. & FINCH C.A. (1958) Quantitative measurement of the erythrocytic and granulocytic cells of the marrow and blood. *Journal of Clinical Investigation*, **37**, 1571.

71 DEUBELBEISS K.A., DANCEY J.T., HARKER L.A. & FINCH C.A. (1975) Marrow erythroid and neutrophil cellularity in the dog. *Journal of Clinical Investigation*, **55**, 825.

72 MAUER A.M., ATHENS J.W., ASHENBRUCKER H., CARTWRIGHT G.E. & WINTROBE M.M. (1960) Leukokinetic studies. II. A method for labelling granulocytes *in vitro* with radioactive diisopropylfluorophosphate (DF^{32}P). *Journal of Clinical Investigation*, **39**, 1481.

73 ATHENS J.W., HAAB O.P., RAAB S.O., MAUER A.M., ASHENBRUCKER H., CARTWRIGHT G.E. & WINTROBE M.M. (1961) Leukokinetic studies. IV. The total blood, circulating and marginal granulocyte pools and the granulocyte turnover rate in normal subjects. *Journal of Clinical Investigation*, **40**, 989.

74 CARTWRIGHT G.E., ATHENS J.W. & WINTROBE M.M. (1964) The kinetics of granulopoiesis in normal man. *Blood*, **24**, 780.

75 DRESCH C., NAJEAN Y. & BAUCHET J. (1975) Kinetic studies of ^{51}Cr and DF^{32}P labelled granulocytes. *British Journal of Haematology*, **29**, 67.

76 GALBRAITH P.R., VALBERG L.S. & BROWN M. (1965) Patterns of granulocyte kinetics in health, infection and in carcinoma. *Blood*, **25**, 683.

77 GRANT L. (1965) The sticking and emigration of white blood cells in inflammation. In: *The Inflammatory Process* (ed. Zweifach B.E., Grant L. & McClusky R.J.), p. 197. Academic Press, New York.

78 BOGGS D.R. (1960) The cellular composition of inflammatory exudates in human leukemias. *Blood*, **15**, 466.

79 BOGGS D.R., ATHENS J.W., HAAB O.P., RAAB S.O., CARTWRIGHT G.E. & WINTROBE M.M. (1964) Leuko-

kinetic studies. VIII. A search for an extramedullary tissue pool of neutrophilic granulocytes. *Proceedings of the Society for Experimental Biology and Medicine*, **115**, 792.

80 REIMANN H.A. (1948) Periodic disease: a probable syndrome including periodic fever, benign paroxysmal peritonitis, cyclic neutropenia and intermittent arthralgia. *Journal of the American Medical Association*, **136**, 239.

81 MORLEY A.A., BAIKIE A.G. & GALTON D.A.G. (1967) Cyclic leucocytosis as evidence for retention of normal homeostatic control in chronic granulocytic leukaemia. *Lancet*, **ii**, 1320.

82 GATTI R.A., ROBINSON W.A., DEINARD A.S., NESBIT M., McCULLOUGH J.J., BALLOW M. & GOOD R.A. (1973) Cyclic leukocytosis in chronic myelogenous leukemia: new perspective on pathogenesis and therapy. *Blood*, **41**, 771.

83 DALE D.C., ALLING D.W. & WOLFF S.M. (1972) Cyclic hematopoiesis: the mechanism of cyclic neutropenia in grey collie dogs. *Journal of Clinical Investigation*, **51**, 2197.

84 MORLEY A.A. (1966) A neutrophil cycle in healthy individuals. *Lancet*, **ii**, 1220.

85 KING-SMITH E.A. & MORLEY A. (1970) Computer simulation of granulopoiesis: normal and impaired granulopoiesis. *Blood*, **35**, 751.

86 MORLEY A., KING-SMITH E.A. & STOHLMAN F. (1970) The oscillatory nature of hemopoiesis. In: *Hemopoietic Cellular Proliferation* (ed. Stohlman F.), p. 3. Grune & Stratton, New York.

87 ROTHSTEIN G., CHRISTENSEN R.D., HUGL E.H. & ATHENS J.W. (1971) Stimulation of granulopoiesis by a diffusable factor *in vivo*. *Journal of Clinical Investigation*, **50**, 200.

88 McVITTIE T. & MacCARTHY K. (1974) Increased proliferation of hematopoietic stem cells within diffusion chambers implanted into irradiated mice pretreated with cyclophosphamide. *Radiation Research*, **59**, 291.

89 CHAN S.H., METCALF D. & STANLEY E.R. (1971) Stimulation and inhibition by normal human serum of colony formation *in vitro* by bone marrow cells. *British Journal of Haematology*, **20**, 329.

90 McNEILL T.A., FLEMMING W.A. & McCANCE D.J. (1972) Interferon and haemopoietic colony inhibitor responses to poly I–poly C in rabbits and hamsters. *Immunology*, **22**, 711.

91 KURLAND J.I., BROXMEYER H.E., PELUS L.M., BOCKMAN R.S. & MOORE M.A.S. (1978) Role of monocyte-macrophage derived colony-stimulating factor and prostaglandin E in the positive and negative feedback control of myeloid stem cell proliferation. *Blood*, **52**, 388.

92 BOGGS D.R., CARTWRIGHT G.E. & WINTROBE M.M. (1966) Neutrophilia-inducing activity in plasma of dogs recovering from drug-induced myelotoxicity. *American Journal of Physiology*, **211**, 51.

93 BOGGS D.R. (1966) Homeostatic regulatory mechanisms of hematopoiesis. *Annual Review of Physiology*, **28**, 39.

94 BOGGS D.R., MARSH J.C., CHERVENICK P.A., CARTWRIGHT G.E. & WINTROBE M.M. (1968) Neutrophil-releasing activity in plasma of normal human subjects injected with endotoxin. *Proceedings of the Society for Experimental Biology and Medicine*, **127**, 689.

95 GORDON A.S., HANDLER E.S., SIEGEL C.D., DORNFEST B.S. & LOBUE J. (1964) Plasma factors influencing leukocyte release in rats. *Annals of the New York Academy of Sciences*, **113**, 766.

96 JONES T.W. (1846) The blood corpuscle considered in its different phases of development in the animal series. Memoir I. Vertebrata Phil. *Transactions of the Royal Society of London*, **136**, 63.

97 CLINE M.J. (1975) The eosinophil. In: *The White Cell*, p. 104, Harvard Unversity Press, Cambridge, Mass.

98 BEESON P.B. & BASS D.A. (1977) *Major Problems in Internal Medicine* (ed. Smith L.H.), p. 107. W. B. Saunders, London.

99 PRESENTEY B. (1969) Cytochemical characterization of eosinophils with respect to a newly discovered anomaly. *American Journal of Pathology*, **51**, 451.

100 PRESENTEY B. (1969) Hereditary deficiency of peroxidase and phospholipids in eosinophilic granulocytes. *Acta Haematologica*, **41**, 359.

101 SALMON S.E., CLINE M.J., SCHULTZ J. & LEHRER R.I. (1970) Myeloperoxidase deficiency: immunologic study of a genetic leukocyte defect. *New England Journal of Medicine*, **282**, 250.

102 GILMAN P.A. JACKSON D.P. & GUILD H.G. (1970) Congenital agranulocytosis: prolonged survival and terminal acute leukemia. *Blood*, **36**, 576.

103 DAO C., METCALF D. & BILSKI-PASQUIER G. (1977) Eosinophil and neutrophil colony-forming cells in culture. *Blood*, **50**, 833.

104 KOEFFLER H.P., LEVINE A.M., SPARKES M. & SPARKES R.S. (1980) Chronic myelocytic leukemia: eosinophils involved in the malignant clone. *Blood*, **55**, 1063.

105 GLEICH G.J., LOEGERING D.A. & MALDONADO J.E. (1976) Identification of a major basic protein in guinea pig eosinophil granules. *Journal of Experimental Medicine*, **137**, 1459.

106 GLEICH G.J., LOEGERING D.A., MANN K.G. & MALDONADO J.E. (1976) Comparative properties of the Charcot–Leyden crystal protein and the major basic protein from human eosinophils. *Journal of Clinical Investigation*, **57**, 633.

107 ALEXANDER P., MONETTE F.C., LOBUE J., GORDON A.S. & CHAN P.C. (1969) Mechanisms of leukocyte production and release. X. Eosinophil proliferation in rats of different ages. *Scandinavian Journal of Haematology*, **6**, 319.

108 SPRY C.J.F. (1971) Mechanism of eosinophilia. V. Kinetics of normal and accelerated eosinopoiesis. *Cell and Tissue Kinetics*, 4, 351.

109 HILLS A.G., FORSHAM P.H. & FINCH C.A. (1948) Changes in circulating leukocytes induced by the administration of pituitary adenocorticotrophic hormone (ACTH) in man. *Blood*, **3**, 755.

110 ARCHER R.K. (1957) The mechanism of eosinopenia produced by ACTH and corticoids in the horse. *Journal of Pathology and Bacteriology*, **74**, 387.

111 ARCHER R.K. (1970) Regulatory mechanisms in eosinophil leukocyte production, release and distribution. In: *Regulation of Hematopoiesis, Vol. 2* (ed. Gordon A.S.), p. 917. Appleton-Century-Crofts, New York.

112 HUDSON G. (1968) Quantitative study of the eosinophil granulocytes. *Seminars in Hematology*, **5**, 166.

113 WALLE A.J. & PARWARESCH M.R. (1979) Estimation of effective eosinopoiesis and bone marrow eosinophil reserve capacity in normal man. *Cell and Tissue Kinetics*, **12**, 249.

114 CARPER H.A. & HOFFMAN P.L. (1966) The intravascular survival of transfused canine Pelger–Huët cells and eosinophils. *Blood*, **27**, 739.

115 PARWARESCH H.R., WALLE A.J. & ARNDT T. (1976) The peripheral kinetics of human radiolabelled eosinophils. *Virchows Archiv (Cell Pathology)*, **21**, 57.

116 FOOT E.C. (1965) Eosinophil turnover in the normal rat. *British Journal of Haematology*, **11**, 439.

117 SPRY C.J.F. (1971) Mechanisms of eosinophilia. VI. Eosinophil mobilisation. *Cell and Tissue Kinetics*, **4**, 365.

118 TEIR H., WEGELIUS O., SUNDELL B., PAIRVARINNE I. & KUUSI T. (1955) Experimental alterations in the tissue eosinophilia of the glandular stomach of the rat. *Acta Medica Scandinavica*, **152**, 275.

119 RYTOMAA T. (1960) Organ distribution and histochemical properties of eosinophil granulocytes in the rat. *Acta Pathologica et Microbiologica Scandinavica*, **50** (Suppl. 140), 1.

120 EHRLICH P. (1879) Beiträge zur Kenntis der granulierten Bindegewebzellen und der eosinophilen Leukocyten. *Archives of Anatomy and Physiology*, **3**, 166.

121 MAXIMOW A. (1910) Untersuchungen über Blut und Bindegewebe. III. Die embryonale Histogenese des Knochenmarks der Saugetiere. *Archiv für Mikroskopische Anatomie*, **83**, 247.

122 PARWARESCH M.R., LEDER L.D. & DANNENBERG K.E.G. (1971) On the origin of human basophilic granulocytes. *Acta Haematologica*, **45**, 273.

123 JOLLY M. (1900) Recherches sur la division indirecte des cellules lymphatiques granuleuses de la moelle de os. *Archives d'Anatomie Microscopique et de Morphologie Experimentale*, **3**, 168.

124 DENEGRI J.F., NAIMAN S.C., GILLEN J. & THOMAS J.W. (1978) In vitro growth of basophils containing the Philadelphia chromosome in the acute phase of chronic myelogenous leukaemia. *British Journal of Haematology*, **40**, 351.

125 JAMES G.W., WRIGHT D.U., WILDERSON V. & SHELLENBERG R. (1955) Observations on the absolute basophil count in health and disease. *Clinical Research Proceedings*, **3**, 31.

126 BOSEILA A.W.A. & UHRBRAND H. (1958) Basophil-eosinophil relationship in human blood. Studies on the effect of corticotrophin. *Acta Endocrinologica*, **28**, 49.

127 MITCHELL R.G. (1958) Basophil leucocytes in children in health and disease. *Archives of Diseases in Childhood*, **33**, 193.

128 PAPPENHEIM A. & FERRATA A. (1910) Über die verschieden lymphoiden Sellformen des normalen und pathologischen Blutes mit speziellen Beruchsichtigung des grossen Mononucleären des Normalblutes und ihrer Beziehung zu Lymphozyten und myeloischen Lymphoidzellen am Meerschweinchen demonstriert. *Folia Haematologica*, **10**, 78.

129 LEWIS M.R. (1925) The formation of macrophages, epithelioid cells and giant cells from leukocytes in incubated blood. *American Journal of Pathology*, **1**, 91.

130 LEWIS M.R. & LEWIS W.H. (1926) Transformation of mononuclear blood cells into macrophages, epitheloid cells and giant cells in hanging drop cultures of lower vertebrates. Carnegie Institute, Washington. Publication 96, *Contributions in Embryology*, **18**, 95.

131 EBERT R.H. & FLOREY H.W. (1939) The extravascular development of the monocyte observed *in vitro*. *British Journal of Experimental Pathology*, **20**, 342.

132 LOBUGLIO A.F. (1970) Factors influencing monocyte development and function. In: *Regulation of Hematopoiesis, Vol. 2* (ed Gordon A.S.), p. 983. Appleton-Century-Crofts, New York.

133 VAN FURTH R. (1970) Origin and kinetics of monocytes and macrophages. *Seminars in Hematology*, **7**, 125.

134 CLINE M.J. (1975) Morphogenesis and production of monocytes and macrophages. In: *The White Cell*, p. 459. Harvard University Press, Cambridge, Mass.

135 CLINE M.J., LEHRER R.I., TERRITO C. & GOLDE D.W. (1978) Monocytes and macrophages: functions and diseases. *Annals of Internal Medicine*, **88**, 78.

136 BENNETT M.J., CATOVSKY D., DANIEL M.T., FLANDRIN G., GALTON D.A.G., GRALNICK H.R. & SULTAN C. (1976) Proposals for the classification of the acute leukaemias. *British Journal of Haematology*, **33**, 451.

137 METCALF D. (1971) Transformation of granulocytes to macrophages in bone marrow colonies *in vitro*. *Journal of Cellular Physiology*, **77**, 277.

138 GOLDE D.W., BURGALETA C., SPARKES R.S. & CLINE M.J. (1977) The Philadelphia chromosome in human macrophages. *Blood*, **49**, 367.

139 BALNER H. (1963) Identification of peritoneal macrophages in mouse radiation chimeras. *Transplantation*, **1**, 217.

140 GOODMAN J.W. (1964) On the origin of peritoneal fluid cells. *Blood*, **23**, 18.

141 VIROLAINEN M. (1968) Hematopoietic origin of macrophages as studied by chromosome markers in mice. *Journal of Experimental Medicine*, **127**, 943.

142 VOLMAN A. & GOWANS J.L. (1965) The origin of macrophages from bone marrow in the rat. *British Journal of Experimental Pathology*, **46**, 62.

143 VAN FURTH R. & COHN Z.A. (1968) The origin and kinetics of mononuclear phagocytes. *Journal of Experimental Medicine*, **128**, 415.

144 VAN FURTH R., RAEBURN J.A. & VAN ZWET T.L. (1979) Characteristics of human mononuclear phagocytes. *Blood*, **54**, 485.

145 VAN FURTH R. & DIESSELHOFF-DEN-DULK M.M.C. (1970) The kinetics of promonocytes and monocytes in the bone marrow. *Journal of Experimental Medicine*, **132**, 813.

146 MEURET B. & HOFFMAN G. (1973) Monocyte kinetic studies in normal and disease states. *British Journal of Haematology*, **24**, 275.

147 EDWARDS J.L. & KLEIN R.E. (1961) Cell renewal in adult mouse tissues. *American Journal of Pathology*, **38**, 437.

148 NORTH R.J. (1969) The mitotic potential of fixed phagocytes in the liver as revealed during development of cellular immunity. *Journal of Experimental Medicine*, **130**, 315.

149 HOCKING R.G. & GOLDE D.W. (1979) The pulmonary-alveolar macrophage. *New England Journal of Medicine*, **301**, 580.

150 THOMAS E.D., RAMBERG R.E., SALE G.E., PARKES R.S. & GOLDE D.W. (1976) Direct evidence for a bone marrow origin of the alveolar macrophage in man. *Science*, **192**, 1016.

151 SHORTER R.G., TITUS J.L. & DIVERTIE M.B. (1964) Cell turnover in the respiratory tract. *Diseases of the Chest*, **46**, 138.

152 BOWDEN D.H., ADAMSON I.Y.R., GRANTHAM W.G. & WYATT J.P. (1969) Origin of the lung macrophage. *Archives of Pathology*, **88**, 540.

153 GOLDE D.W., FINLEY T.N. & CLINE M.J. (1974) The pulmonary macrophage in acute leukemia. *New England Journal of Medicine*, **290**, 875.

154 COHEN A.B. & CLINE M.J. (1971) The human alveolar macrophage. Isolation, cultivation *in vitro* and studies of morphologic and functional characteristics. *Journal of Clinical Investigation*, **50**, 1390.

155 CLINE M.J. (1975) Abnormalities of neutrophil production, destruction and morphogenesis. In: *The White Cell*, p. 156. Harvard University Press, Cambridge, Mass.

156 YOUNG G.A.R. & VINCENT P.C. (1980) Drug-induced agranulocytosis. *Clinics in Haematology*, **9**, 483.

157 SCHULTZ W. (1922) Über eigenartige Halserkrankungen. *Deutsche Medizinische Wochenschrift*, **48**, 1495.

158 MADISON F.W. & SQUIER T.L. (1934) Etiology of primary granulocytopenia (agranulocytic angina). *Journal of the American Medical Association*, **102**, 755.

159 KINROSS-WRIGHT J. (1967) The current status of phenothiazines. *Journal of the American Medical Association*, **200**, 461.

160 PISCIOTTA A.V. (1969) Agranulocytosis induced by certain phenothiazine derivatives. *Journal of the American Medical Association*, **208**, 1862.

161 SCOTT J.L., CARTWRIGHT G.E. & WINTROBE M.M. (1965) Acquired aplastic anemia: analysis of thirty-nine cases and review of the pertinent literature. *New England Journal of Medicine*, **272**, 1137.

162 GUSSOFF B.D. & LEE S.L. (1966) Chloramphenicol-induced hematopoietic depression: a controlled comparison with tetracycline. *American Journal of Medical Sciences*, **251**, 8.

163 YUNIS A.A. & BLOOMBERG G.R. (1964) Chloramphenicol toxicity: clinical features and pathogenesis. In: *Progress in Hematology*, *Vol. 4* (ed. Moore C.V. & Brown E.B.), p. 138. Grune & Stratton, New York.

164 LEALE M. (1910) Recurrent furunculosis in an infant showing an unusual blood picture. *Journal of the American Medical Association*, **54**, 1854.

165 FULLERTON H.W. & DUGUID H.L.D. (1949) A case of cyclical agranulocytosis with marked improvement following splenectomy. *Blood*, **4**, 269.

166 PAGE A.R. & GOOD R.A. (1957) Studies on cyclic neutropenia: a clinical and experimental investigation. *American Journal of Diseases of Children*, **94**, 623.

167 HAHNEMAN B.M. & ALT H.L. (1958) Cyclic neutropenia in a father and daughter. *Journal of the American Medical Association*, **168**, 270.

168 BRODSKY I., REIMANN H.A. & DENNIS L.H. (1965) Treatment of cyclic neutropenia with testosterone. *American Journal of Medicine*, **38**, 802.

169 MORLEY A.A., CAREW J.P. & BAIKIE A.G. (1967) Familial cyclical neutropenia. *British Journal of Haematology*, **13**, 719.

170 MORLEY A. & STOHLMAN F. JR (1970) Cyclophosphamide-induced cyclical neutropenia: an animal model of a human periodic disease. *New England Journal of Medicine*, **282**, 643.

170a KYLE R.A. & LINMAN J.W. (1968) Chronic idiopathic neutropenia. A newly recognised entity? *New England Journal of Medicine*, **279**, 1045.

170b DALE D.C., GUERRY DU P., WEWERKA J.R., BULL J.M. & CHUSID M.J. (1979) Chronic neutropenia. *Medicine* (Baltimore), **58**, 128.

171 BOXER L.A. GREENBERG M.S., BOXER G.J. & STOSSEL T.P. (1975) Autoimmune neutropenia. *New England Journal of Medicine*, **293**, 748.

172 VERHEUGHT F.W.A., VON DEM BORNE A.E.G.KR, VAN NOORD-BOKHORST J.C. & ENGELFRIET C.P. (1978) Autoimmune granulocytopenia: the detection of granulocyte autoantibodies with the immunofluorescence test. *British Journal of Haematology*, **39**, 339.

173 LALEZARI P., JIANG A.-F., YEGEN L. & SANTORINEOU M. (1975) Chronic autoimmune neutropenia due to anti-NA₂ antibody. *New England Journal of Medicine*, **293**, 744.

174 WEETMAN R.M. & BOXER L.A. (1980) Childhood neutropenia. *Pediatric Clinics of North America*, **27**, 361.

175 BRAUN E.H., BUCKWOLD A.E., EMSON H.E. & RUSSELL A.V. (1960) Familial neonatal neutropenia with maternal leukocyte antibodies. *Blood*, **16**, 1745.

176 HALVORSEN K. (1965) Neonatal leucopenia due to fetomaternal leucocyte incompatibility. *Acta Paediatrica Scandinavica*, **54**, 86.

177 NYMAND G., HERON I., JENSEN K. & LUNDSGAARD A. (1971) Occurrence of cytotoxic antibodies during pregnancy. *Vox Sanguinis*, **21**, 21.

178 KOSTMANN R. (1956) Infantile genetic agranulocytosis (agranulocytosis infantilis hereditaria). A new recessive lethal disease in man. *Acta Paediatrica Scandinavica*, **45** (Suppl. 105), 1.

179 WRIEDT K., KAUDER E. & MAUER A.M. (1966) Failure of myeloid differentiation as a cause of congenital neutropenia. *Journal of Pediatrics*, **68**, 839.

179a WRIEDT K., KAUDER E. & MAUER A.M. (1970) Defective myelopoiesis in congenital neutropenia. *New England Journal of Medicine*, **283**, 1072.

180 AMATO D., FREEDMAN M.H. & SUNDERS E.F. (1976) Granulopoiesis in severe congenital neutropenia. *Blood*, **47**, 531.

181 CHUSID M.J., PISCIOTTA A.V., DUQUESNOY R.J., CAMITTA B.M. & TOMASULO P.A. (1980) Congenital neutropenia: studies of pathogenesis. *American Journal of Hematology*, **8**, 315.

182 LANG J.E. & CUTTING H.O. (1965) Infantile genetic agranulocytosis. *Pediatrics*, **35**, 596.

183 CUTTING H.O. & LANG J.E. (1964) Familial benign chronic neutropenia. *Annals of Internal Medicine*, **61**, 876.

184 GÄNSSLEN M. (1941) Konstitutionelle familiäre Leukopenie (Neutropenie). *Klinische Wochenschrift*, **20**, 922.

184a SHAPER A.G. & LEWIS P. (1971) Genetic neutropenia in people of African origin. *Lancet*, **ii**, 1021.

184b DJALDETTI M., JOSHUA H. & KALDERON M. (1961) Familial leukopenia-neutropenia in Yemenite Jews. *Bulletin of the Research Council of Israel*, **E9**, 24.

184c MASON B.A., LESSIN L. & SCHECHTER G.P. (1979) Marrow granulocyte reserves in black Americans. Hydrocortisone-induced granulocytosis in the 'benign' neutropenia of the black. *American Journal of Medicine*, **67**, 201.

185 HITZIG W.H. (1959) Familiäre Neutropenie mit dominantem Erbgang und Hypergammaglobulinämia. *Helvetica Medica Acta*, **26**, 779.

186 DE VAAL O.M. & SYNHAEVE V. (1969) Reticular dysgenesis. *Lancet*, **ii**, 1123.

187 GITLIN D., VAWTER G. & CRAIG J. (1964) Thymic alymphoplasia and congenital aleukocytosis. *Pediatrics*, **33**, 184.

188 FIREMAN P., JOHNSON H.A. & GITLIN D. (1966) Presence of plasma cells and Y_1M-globulin synthesis in a patient with thymic alymphoplasia. *Pediatrics*, **37**, 485.

188a SHWACHMAN H., DIAMOND L.K., OSKI F.A. & KHAW K.T. (1964) The syndrome of pancreatic insufficiency and bone marrow dysfunction. *Journal of Pediatrics*, **65**, 645.

189 LUX S.E., JOHNSTON R.B., AUGUST C.S., SAY B., PENCHAZADEH V.B., ROSEN F.S. & McKUSICK V.A. (1970) Chronic neutropenia and abnormal cellular immunity in cartilage-hair hypoplasia. *New England Journal of Medicine*, **282**, 231.

189a RIEGER C.H.L., MOOHR J.W. & ROTHBERG R.M. (1974) Correction of neutropenia associated with dysgammaglobulinemia. *Pediatrics*, **54**, 508.

190 WISEMAN B.K. & DOAN C.A. (1939) A newly recognised granulocytic syndrome caused by excessive leukolysis and successfully treated by splenectomy. *Journal of Clinical Investigation*, **18**, 473.

191 HARVEY A.M., SHULMAN L.E., TUMULTY P.A., CONLEY C.L. & SHOENRICH H.E. (1954) Systemic lupus erythematosus: a review of the literature and clinical analysis of 138 patients. *Medicine*, **33**, 291.

192 FELTY A.R. (1924) Chronic arthritis in the adult, associated with splenomegaly and leucopenia. *Bulletin of the Johns Hopkins Hospital*, **35**, 16.

193 DE GRUCHY G.C. & LANGLEY G.R. (1961) Felty's syndrome. *Australian Annals of Medicine*, **10**, 292.

194 COLLIER R.L. & BRUSH B.E. (1966) Hematologic disorder in Felty's syndrome. prolonged benefits of splenectomy. *American Journal of Surgery*, **112**, 869.

195 DANCEY J.T. & BRUBAKER L.H. (1979) Neutrophil marrow profiles in patients with rheumatoid arthritis and neutropenia. *British Journal of Haematology*, **43**, 607.

196 MOORE R.A., BRUNNER C.M. & SANDUSKY W.R. (1971) Felty's syndrome: long-term follow-up after splenectomy. *Annals of Internal Medicine*, **75**, 381.

197 BRUBAKER L.H. & NOLPH K.D. (1971) Mechanisms of recovery from neutropenia induced by hemodialysis. *Blood*, **36**, 623.

198 SCHIFFER C.A., AISNER A.J. & WIERNIK P.H. (1975) Transient neutropenia induced by transfusion of blood exposed to nylon fiber filters. *Blood*, **45**, 141.

199 HAMMERSCHMIDT D.E., CRADDOCK P.R., McCUL-LOUGH J., KRONENBERG R.S., DALMASSO A.P. & JACOB H.S. (1978) Complement activation and pulmonary leukostasis during nylon fiber filtration leukapheresis. *Blood*, **51**, 721.

200 PERRY S., WEINSTEIN I.M., CRADDOCK C.G. & LAWRENCE J.S. (1958) Rates of appearance and disappearance of white blood cells in normal and various disease states. *Journal of Laboratory and Clinical Medicine*, **51**, 101.

201 WINTROBE M.M. (1939) Diagnostic significance of changes in leukocytes. *Bulletin of the New York Academy of Sciences*, **15**, 223.

202 STEPHENS D.J. (1934) The occurrence of myelocytes in the peripheral blood in lobar pneumonia. *American Journal of Medical Sciences*, **188**, 332.

203 BOGGS D.R., ATHENS J.W., CARTWRIGHT G.E. & WINTROBE M.M. (1965) Leukokinetic studies. IX. Experimental evaluation of a model of granulopoiesis. *Journal of Clinical Investigation*, **44**, 643.

204 DALE D.C., FAUCI A.S., GUERRY D. & WOLFF S.M. (1975) Comparison of agents producing a neutrophil leukocytosis in man. *Journal of Clinical Investigation*, **56**, 808.

205 STEEL C.M., FRENCH E.B. & AITCHISON W.R.C. (1971) Studies on adrenaline-induced leucocytosis in man. I. The role of the spleen and of the thoracic duct. *British Journal of Haematology*, **21**, 413.

206 JOYCE R.A., BOGGS D.R., HASIBA U. & SRODES C.H. (1976) Marginal neutrophil pool size in normal subjects and neutropenic patients as measured by epinephrine infusion. *Journal of Laboratory and Clinical Medicine*, **88**, 614.

207 ROTHSTEIN G., CLARKSON D.R., LARSEN W., GROSSER B.I. & ATHENS J.W. (1978) Effects of lithium on neutrophil mass and production. *New England Journal of Medicine*, **298**, 178.

208 TISMAN G., HERBERT V. & ROSENBLATT S. (1973) Evidence that lithium induces human granulocyte proliferation: elevated serum B_{12} binding capacity *in vivo* and granulocyte colony proliferation *in vitro*. *British Journal of Haematology*, **24**, 767.

209 LEVITT L.J. & QUESENBERRY P.J. (1980) The effect of lithium on murine hematopoiesis. *New England Journal of Medicine*, **302**, 713.

210 ATHENS J.W. (1975) Disorders of neutrophil proliferation and circulation: a pathophysiological view. *Clinics in Haematology*, **4**, 533.

211 VAUGHAN J.M. (1936) Leucoerythroblastic leukaemia. *Journal of Pathology and Bacteriology*, **48**, 339.

212 LOWELL F.C. (1967) Clinical aspects of eosinophilia in atopic disease. *Journal of the American Medicial Association*, **202**, 109.

213 STRANG L.B. (1960) Eosinophilia in children with asthma and bronchiectasis. *British Medical Journal*, **i**, 167.

214 HORN B.R., ROBIN E.D., THEODORE J. & VAN KESSEL A. (1975) Total eosinophil counts in the management of bronchial asthma. *New England Journal of Medicine*, **292**, 1152.

215 MÜLLER H.F. & RIEDER H. (1891) Ueber verkommen und klinische Bedeutung der eosinophilen Zellen, Ehrlich, im circulirenden Blute des Menschen. *Deutsches Archiv für Klinische Medizin*, **48**, 96.

216 BROWN T.R. (1897) Studies in trichinosis. *Bulletin of the Johns Hopkins Hospital*, **8**, 79.

217 REIFENSTEIN E.C., ALLEN G.E. & ALLEN G.S. (1932) Trichiniasis. *American Journal of Clinical Science*, **183**, 668.

218 CONRAD M.E. (1971) Hematologic manifestations of parasitic infections. *Seminars in Hematology*, **8**, 267.

219 LOWE T.E. (1944) Eosinophilia in tropical disease. *Medical Journal of Australia*, **1**, 453.

220 SCHAMBERG J.F. & STRICKLER A. (1912) Report on eosinophilia in scabies, with a discussion on eosinophilia in various diseases of the skin. *Journal of Cutaneous Diseases*, **30**, 53.

221 GRACE A.W. (1934) Pemphigus. Evidence in support of a bacteremia as an explanation of certain terminal changes in the blood picture. *Archives of Dermatology and Syphilology*, **30**, 22.

222 EMMERSON R.W. & WILSON-JONES E. (1968) Eosinophilic spongiosus in pemphigus. *Archives of Dermatology*, **97**, 252.

223 ALEXANDER J.O'D. (1975) *Dermatitis Herpetiformis*, p. 233. W. B. Saunders, Philadelphia.

224 ENG A.M. & MONCADA B. (1974) Bullous pemphigoid and dermatitis herpetiformis. *Archives of Dermatology*, **110**, 51.

225 ZOLOV D.M. & LEVINE B.B. (1969) Correlation of blood eosinophilia with antibody classes. *International Archives of Allergy and Applied Immunology*, **35**, 179.

226 JACOB H.S., SIDD J.J., GREENBERG B.H. & LINDLEY J.F. (1964) Extreme eosinophilia with iodide hypersensitivity: report of a case with observations on the cellular composition of inflammatory exudates. *New England Journal of Medicine*, **271**, 1138.

227 DAVIS P. & HUGHES G.R.V. (1974) Significance of eosinophilia during gold therapy. *Arthritis and Rheumatism*, **17**, 964.

228 JESSOP J.D., DIPPY J., TURNBULL A. & BRIGHT M. (1974) Eosinophilia during gold therapy. *Rheumatology and Rehabilitation*, **13**, 75.

229 LÖFFLER W. (1936) Die fluchtigen Lungeninfiltrate mit Eosinophilie. *Schweizerische Medizinische Wochenschrift*, **17**, 1069.

230 PEPYS J. (1969) Hypersensitivity diseases of the lung due to fungi and organic dusts. *Monographs in Allergy, Vol. 5.* Karger, Basel.

231 REEDER W.H. & GOODRICH B.D. (1952) Pulmonary infiltration with eosinophilia (PIE syndrome). *Annals of Internal Medicine*, **36**, 1217.

232 CARRINGTON C., ADDINGTON, W., GOFF A., MADOFF I., MARKS A., SCHWABER J. & GAENSLER E. (1969) Chronic eosinophilic pneumonia. *New England Journal of Medicine*, **280**, 787.

232a SPRY C.J.F. (1982) Pulmonary eosinophilic syndromes. *Current Perspectives in Allergy*, **1**. (In press).

233 LIEBOW A.A. & CARRINGTON C.B. (1969) The eosinophilic pneumonias. *Medicine* (Baltimore), **48**, 251.

234 LÖFFLER W. (1936) Endocarditis parietalis fibroplastica mit Bluteosinophilie, ein eigenertiges Krankheitsbild. *Schweizerische Medizinische Wochenschrift*, **17**, 817.

235 DAVIS J.N.P. & BALL J.D. (1955) The pathology of endomyocardial fibrosis in Uganda. *British Heart Journal*, **17**, 337.

236 BENVENISTI D.S. & ULTMANN J.E. (1969) Eosinophilic leukemia: report of five cases and review of literature. *Annals of Internal Medicine*, **71**, 731.

237 YAM L.T., LI C.Y., NECHELES T.F. & KATAYAMA I. (1972) Pseudoeosinophilic endocarditis and eosinophilic leukemia. *American Journal of Medicine*, **53**, 193.

238 CHUSID J.M., DALE D.C., WEST B.C. & WOLFF S.M. (1975) The hypereosinophilic syndrome: analysis of fourteen cases with review of the literature. *Medicine* (Baltimore), **54**, 1.

239 SPRY C.J.F. & TAI P.C. (1976) Studies on blood eosinophils. II. Patients with Löffler's cardiomyopathy. *Clinical and Experimental Immunology*, **24**, 423.

240 OLSEN E.G.J. & SPRY C.J.F. (1979) The pathogenesis of Löffler's endomyocardial disease, and its relationship to endomyocardial fibrosis. *Progress in Cardiology*, **8**, 281.

241 DONOHUGH D.C. (1963) Tropical eosinophilia: an etiologic inquiry. *New England Journal of Medicine*, **269**, 1357.

241a NEVA F.A. & OTTESEN E.A. (1978) Current concepts in parasitology. Tropical (filarial) eosinophilia. *New England Journal of Medicine*, **298**, 1129.

242 GREWAL K.S., DIXIT R.P. & DUTTA B. (1965) Pulmonary eosinophilosis: a review of 139 cases. *Journal of the Indian Medical Association*, **44**, 53.

243 EZEOKE A., PERERA A.B.V. & HOBBS J.R. (1973) Serum IgE elevation with tropical eosinophilia. *Clinical Allergy*, **3**, 33.

244 WEBB J.K.G., JOB C.K. & GAULT E.W. (1960) Tropical eosinophilia: demonstration of microfilaria in lung, liver and lymph nodes. *Lancet*, **i**, 835.

245 HEALY T.M. (1974) Eosinophilia in bronchogenic carcinoma. (Letter.) *New England Journal of Medicine*, **291**, 794.

246 DELLON A.L., HUME R.B. & CRETEIN P.B. (1974) Eosinophilia in bronchogenic carcinoma. *New England Journal of Medicine*, **291**, 207.

247 CATOVSKY D., BERNASCONI C., VERDONCK P.J., POSTMA A., HOWS J., VAN DER DOES-VAN DEN BERG A., REES J.K.H., CASTELLI G., MORRA E. & GALTON D.A.G. (1980) The association of eosinophilia with lymphoblastic leukaemia or lymphoma: a study of seven patients. *British Journal of Haematology*, **45**, 523.

248 KASS L. & VOTAW M.L. (1975) Eosinophilia and plasmacytosis of the bone marrow in Hodgkin's disease. *American Journal of Clinical Pathology*, **64**, 248.

249 TAURO G.P. (1966) Hodgkin's disease associated with raised eosinophil counts. *Medical Journal of Australia*, **2**, 604.

250 WALDMANN T.A., POLMAR S.H., BALESTRA S.T., JOST M.C., BRUCE R.M. & TERRY W.D. (1972) Immunoglobulin E in immunologic deficiency diseases. II. Serum IgE concentration of patients with acquired hypogammaglubulinemia, thymoma and hypogammaglobulinema, myotonic dystrophy, intestinal lymphangiectasia and Wiskott–Aldrich syndrome. *Journal of Immunology*, **109**, 304.

251 LUKES R.J. & TINDLE B.H. (1975) Immunoblastic lymphadenopathy. A hyperimmune activity resembling Hodgkin's disease. *New England Journal of Medicine*, **292**, 1.

252 RAPPAPORT H. & MORAN E.M. (1975) Angio-

immunoblastic (immunoblastic) lymphadenopathy. *New England Journal of Medicine*, **292**, 42.

253 CULLEN M.H., LISTER T.A., BREARLEY M.I., SHAND W.S. & STANSFELD A.G. (1979) Angio-immunoblastic lymphadenopathy: report of ten cases and review of the literature. *Quarterly Journal of Medicine*, **48**, 151.

254 MUGGIA F.M., GHOSSEIN N.A. & WOHL H. (1973) Eosinophilia following radiation therapy. *Oncology*, **27**, 118.

255 GHOSSEIN N.A., BOSWORTH J.L., STACEY P., MUGGIA F.M. & KRISHNASWAMY V. (1975) Radiation related eosinophilia. *Radiology*, **117**, 413.

256 HARDY E.R. & ANDERSON R.E. (1968) The hypereosinophilic syndrome. *Annals of Internal Medicine*, **68**, 1220.

257 PARRILLO J.E., FAUCI A.S. & WOLFF S.M. (1978) Therapy of the hypereosinophilic syndrome. *Annals of Internal Medicine*, **89**, 167.

258 RICKLES F.R. & MILLER D.R. (1972) Eosinophilic leukemoid reaction. *Journal of Pediatrics*, **80**, 418.

259 GRUENWALD H., KIOSSOGLOU K.A., MITUS W.J. & DAMESHEK W. (1965) Philadelphia chromosome in eosinophilic leukemia. *American Journal of Medicine*, **39**, 1003.

260 ELVES M.W. & ISRAELS M.C.G. (1967) Cytogenetic studies in unusual forms of chronic myeloid leukaemia. *Acta Haematologica* (Basel), **38**, 129.

261 GOH K.-O., SWISHER S.N. & TROUP S.B. (1964) Submetacentric chromosome in chronic myelocyte leukemia. *Archives of Internal Medicine*, **114**, 439.

262 MITELMAN F., PANANI A. & BRANDT L. (1975) Isochromosome 17 in a case of eosinophilic leukaemia. An abnormality common to eosinophilic and neutrophilic cells. *Scandinavian Journal of Haematology*, **14**, 308.

263 GOLDMAN J.M., NAJFELD V. & TH'NG K.H. (1975) Agar culture and chromosome analysis of eosinophilic leukaemia. *Journal of Clinical Pathology*, **28**, 956.

264 MAYCOCK R.L., BERTRAND P., MORRISON C.E. & SCOTT J.H. (1963) Manifestations of sarcoidosis. *American Journal of Medicine*, **35**, 67.

265 WILLCOX R.G. & ISSELBACHER K.G. (1961) Chronic liver disease in young people. *American Journal of Medicine*, **30**, 185.

266 LEVINE S.A. & LADD W.S. (1921) Pernicious anemia: a clinical study of one hundred and fifty consecutive cases with special reference to gastric anacidity. *Bulletin of the Johns Hopkins Hospital*, **32**, 254.

267 OMENN G.S. (1965) Familial reticuloendotheliosis with eosinophilia. *New England Journal of Medicine*, **273**, 427.

268 OCHS H.D., DAVIS S.D., MICKELSON E., LERNER K.G. & WEDGWOOD R.J. (1974) Combined immunodeficiency and reticuloendotheliosis with eosinophilia. *Journal of Pediatrics*, **85**, 463.

269 INAGAKI S. (1957) The relationship between the level of circulating leukocytes and thyroid function. *Acta Endocrinologica*, **26**, 477.

270 JUHLIN L. (1961) Basophil leukocytes in ulcerative colitis. *Acta Medica Scandinavica*, **173**, 351.

271 MALDONADO J.E. & HANLON D.G. (1965) Monocytosis: a current appraisal. *Mayo Clinic Proceedings*, **40**, 248.

272 TERRITO M.C. & CLINE M.J. (1975) Mononuclear phagocytic proliferation, maturation and function. *Clinics in Haematology*, **4**, 685.

273 DALAND G.A., GOTTLIEB L., WALLERSTEIN O. & CASTLE W.B. (1956) Hematologic observations in bacterial endocarditis. *Journal of Laboratory and Clinical Medicine*, **48**, 827.

274 LEVINSON B., WALTER B.A., WINTROBE M.M. & CARTWRIGHT G.E. (1957) A clinical study in Hodgkin's disease. *Archives of Internal Medicine*, **99**, 519.

275 BARRETT O. (1970) Monocytosis in malignant disease. *Annals of Internal Medicine*, **73**, 991.

Chapter 16
Phagocyte function and its defects

J. F. SOOTHILL AND A. W. SEGAL

Phagocytosis is a function common to many cells, but the term 'phagocytes' is applied to those specialized for this function which were the first cells recognized, by Metchnikoff, to be of immunological importance. They maintain health, without the aid of adaptive immunity mechanisms, in such primitive forms as the coelenterates. It is therefore possible to consider the lymphocytes (T and B), antibody and complement merely as factors enhancing their effectiveness. In blood the most actively phagocytic cells are the polymorphonuclear leucocytes—neutrophil, eosinophil, and basophil—and the monocytes. It is likely that the tissue macrophages, which originate as circulating monocytes, are functionally the most important phagocytes of all, but the role of the circulating macrophage is less well established. The importance of neutrophil polymorphonuclear leucocytes (neutrophils) is clear from the severe symptoms associated with neutropenia (see Chapter 15), and from the considerable range of recently recognized primary and secondary disorders of neutrophil function, described in this chapter (for a recent comprehensive review see Ref. 1); we have much less information about functional disorders of monocytes, and none about those of eosinophils and basophils. All these cells move out of the blood compartment (see Chapter 15) and are probably functionally most effective at sites of inflammation in the tissues, but the blood constitutes a useful source for sampling for diagnostic purposes.

The functions of phagocytes are listed in Table 16.1. As with other immunity mechanisms, they may be defective because of primary or secondary disorders, or because of immaturity; they may also be refractory after previous phagocytosis. A number of factors leading to secondary defective mobility and killing are listed in Table 16.2. The capacity of a neutrophil to enter the circulation from the bone marrow and to leave the blood vessels or the marginating pool depends on its mobility and on its capacity to adhere to the endothelium. Movement occurs up a concentration gradient of a chemotactic agent (chemotaxis) or may be undirected; the latter may be accelerated by humoral factors (chemokinesis).

Mobility and later stages of neutrophil function are strongly influenced by humoral factors, especially antibody and complement, which are only briefly outlined here but are treated more fully in Chapter 17. Some properties of particles themselves contribute to the activity of phagocytes in ingesting them; these include spontaneous activation of complement by the alternative pathway (e.g. yeast), size, a hydrophobic surface, charge, surface sugars, etc.

After contact with the particle, adherence, endocytosis and killing (and/or digestion) occur. Though defects of the earlier phases probably exist, their diagnosis has been restricted by lack of suitable techniques. In some primary defects of neutrophil function, more than one of the functions listed in Table 16.1 may be defective.

The demonstration of defective bacterial killing in chronic granulomatous disease (CGD) by Quie et al. [2] (see p. 638), stimulated the sudden advance in identification of these defects, but in CGD and many other neutrophil function defects, the primary gene product is not yet clearly established, and diagnosis still depends on function tests which are not strictly quantitative and which vary from laboratory to laboratory. A local age-related 'normal range' must be established, but the considerable volume of blood required for some of the tests makes this difficult in children. All are open to considerable variation due to environmental factors, which include age, nutrition, metabolic diseases, anaesthesia and the effects of infection, so clinical judgement plays an important part in establishing such diagnoses and it is very desirable to demonstrate similar functional abnormality in the parents, to confirm that the defect is primary. Inevitably, the clinical associations of the different defects contribute to diagnosis, but the routine application of a series of immunity function tests (including selected neutrophil function tests) to all patients presenting with frequent infection [3] showed that our present assumptions of the clinical effects of these various abnormalities are too restricted. None the less, the following generalizations apply. Children with neutropenia (see Chapter 15)

Table 16.1. Functions of phagocytes

Intravascular distribution
Mobility
Adherence
Ingestion
Killing

---

have frequent bacterial infections, particularly of the respiratory tract and skin, and oral ulceration, and most patients with neutrophil function defects, as well as deficiency of antibody or of C3, have similar symptoms; the exception is CGD, which results in chronically discharging lesions of lymph nodes, liver, bone and chest and skin infections, due to certain bacteria and fungi.

The diagnosis of these defects is important, not only for genetic counselling but also for treatment. In many forms of immunodeficiency the symptoms are worst in infancy and early childhood, and if the child survives this without chronic damage, he often has a prospect of a much healthier life, even though the defect persists. Appropriate treatment of individual infections, and prophylactic cotrimoxazole, are probably important here [4], but some defects may be treatable themselves: reports on *in-vitro* and *in-vivo* benefit from large doses of ascorbic acid in Chediak–Higashi disease [5] and in neutrophil mobility defect with delayed cord separation [6] suggest that recent progress in this field may prove of real value.

MECHANISMS OF PHAGOCYTE FUNCTION

Mobility

Mobility of phagocytes, and also several other functions including endocytosis and degranulation, require contractile proteins and a cytoskeleton; these, the microfilaments and microtubules respectively, are components of all eukaryotic cells [7, 8]. They permit movement of the cell as a whole and of structures within the cell, which include in the neutrophil the proteins on its surface, phagocytic vesicles and cytoplasmic granules. The microtubules are straight hollow cylinders 24 nm in diameter which radiate from the centriole. The wall of the microtubule (5 nm thick) is composed of 13 helically wound protofilaments; these, the tubulins, are dimeric molecules of MW 115 000 daltons which are composed of α- and β-tubulin subunits [9]. The components of neutrophil microtubules are in a state of dynamic equilibrium between a structured polymerized form and a soluble subunit pool. They are assembled at microtubule organizing centres, the process being influenced by microtubule-associated proteins, nucleotides, divalent cations and the redox state [10].

The microfilaments (5–8 nm in diameter) are composed of two helically wound polymers of actin (MW of monomer about 43 000 daltons) and include bound calcium and magnesium and ATP [11]. The microfilaments are in equilibrium between the filamentous (F-actin) and soluble globular (G-actin) monomeric forms. Myosin, which is composed of two chains, binds to actin to become an active ATPase; this

Table 16.2. Secondary defects of neutrophil function due to some environmental factors

Mobility		Killing	
Factor	Reference	Factor	Reference
Immaturity	130	Immaturity	141
Malnutrition*	131, 132	Malnutrition	142
Infection†	102, 133	Infection	143
Anaesthetics	134	Iron deficiency	144
Burns	135	Burns	145
Diabetes	136	Irradiation	146
Renal failure	137		
Haemodialysis	138		
Ulcerative colitis	139		
Rheumatoid arthritis	140		

* ? Largely the effect of secondary infection.
† But see contradictory data [100].

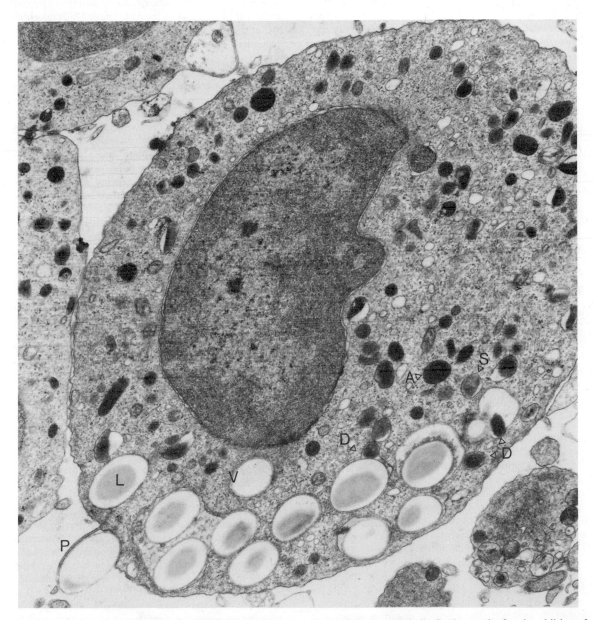

Fig. 16.1. A human neutrophil phagocytosing latex particles, opsonized with immunoglobulin G, 10 seconds after the addition of the particles (× 22 000, courtesy of Mr Jack Dorling). The particles (L) attach to the plasma membrane, which invaginates to form the wall of the phagocytic vacuole (V) as pseudopodia (P) surround it and then fuse. The specific (S) and azurophil (A) cytoplasmic granules then degranulate their contents into the vacuole by fusing their containing membranes with the wall of the vacuole (D). The microfilaments are seen as an electron-dense network just beneath the plasma membrane.

function provides the energy for the movement of these molecules in relation to each other. A range of associated proteins, such as cytoplasmic α-actinin, control the interaction of actin and myosin [12]. These microfilamentous proteins are most evident just beneath the plasma membrane. Dense accumulations of filaments are seen in areas of membrane perturbation and in protrusions such as pseudopodia (Fig. 16.1). A third category of filaments (10 nm diameter) is seen by electron microscopy, but they have not been characterized either biochemically or functionally.

Our understanding of the function of these structures depends largely on the effect of drugs known to inhibit their action. Thus random cell movement, change of surface shape, chemotaxis and phagocytosis are all reduced by cytochalasin B [13], whereas the extracellular release of granule proteins is enhanced [14]. These findings, the observation of condensation of microfilaments at areas of membrane translocation, and the separation of the cytoplasmic granules from the plasma membrane by filaments, suggest that the microfilaments are concerned with mechanical movement and membrane deformation. Colchicine-treated cells round up and their chemotactic movement and degranulation is reduced, but not their random movement or their phagocytosis [10]. Fluorescein-labelled concanavalin A is capped on colchicine-treated cells, but not on normal cells [15], suggesting that microtubules reduce the mobility of proteins in the plasma membrane.

Adherence, phagocytosis and degranulation
The neutrophil adheres to the particle to be phagocytosed; IgG and C3 receptors are important for this. Then pseudopodia are formed around the particle until the cell wall fuses, with the particle within a phagocytic vacuole or phagosome; this process is apparently dependent on receptors distributed all over the particle which result in a continuous and progressive binding to the cell surface—the zipper mechanism [16]. The process depends on the contractile proteins which are also involved in mobility.

Then neighbouring granules, azurophilic and specific, round up and burst into the phagosome [17] by merging with the plasma membrane, to form phagolysosomes, in which the released enzymes attack the phagocytosed particle. Where degranulation occurs before full endocytosis and closure of the phagosome, some of the enzymes may be released into the surrounding medium. Indigestible particles may be released from the neutrophil by a reversal of phagocytosis [18]. These effects may contribute to tissue injury.

Killing and digestion of phagocytosed particles
When a neutrophil engulfs a bacterium, there is a race between the cell killing the organism and the organism proliferating and killing the cell. The cell kills microbes by at least two different mechanisms, oxygen-dependent (aerobic) and oxygen-independent (anaerobic).

Oxygen-dependent microbial killing. Phagocytosis by neutrophils is associated with a burst of oxygen consumption [19], called the 'extra respiration of phagocytosis'. Phagocytosis will take place in anaerobic conditions [20], however, so it is not dependent on this respiratory burst, though the killing of some bacteria is. The respiratory burst takes place in the presence of cyanide [21], showing that it is not associated with the mitochondrial cytochrome system. Bacteria for which the respiratory burst is required for killing include *Staph. aureus, E. coli, Serratia marcescens, Klebsiella pneumoniae, Proteus vulgaris* and *S. typhimurium* [22]. The susceptibility of bacteria to anaerobic killing by neutrophils is apparently inversely related to the concentration of catalase they contain [23]. Since glucose utilization is increased during the respiratory burst and 2-deoxyglucose inhibits it [24], glucose is presumably a primary substrate. There are two main pathways of glucose utilization (Fig. 16.2): the Embden–Meyerhof pathway, which reduces NAD to NADH [25], and the hexose monophosphate (HMP) shunt, which regenerates NADPH from NADP. Studies of the metabolism of glucose labelled with ^{14}C on the sixth and first carbon atom respectively, provide a means of assessing the relative rates of glucose consumption through these two pathways, although it is difficult to assess the absolute throughput. Whereas the former is responsible for 95% of the glucose consumption of the resting neutrophil, the latter increases seven- to ten-fold during the respiratory burst [26]. These pathways are interlinked, since the pentose (ribulose 5-phosphate) produced by the hexose monophosphate shunt enters the Embden–Meyerhof pathway; the three-carbon fragments released by the Embden–Meyerhof pathway are metabolized by the citric-acid cycle. The ratios of both NADP to NADPH and NAD to NADH are elevated after phagocytosis [27, 28]. Thus either NADH or NADPH or both could be acting as the source of reducing equivalents for the oxidase system. The identity of the electron donor is uncertain, partly because transhydrogenases exist which can transfer electrons between these two pyridine nucleotides [31]. Other possible intermediates between glucose and oxygen include sulphydryl groups, which are consumed in stimulated cells [29]; ascorbic acid may play a role, since bacterial killing and the activity of the HMP

Metabolism by phagocytosing neutrophils

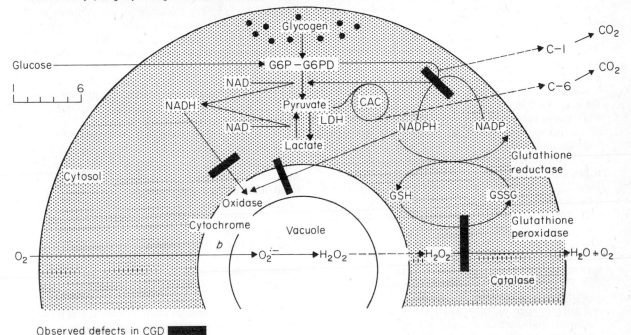

Fig. 16.2. The metabolic pathways involved in the respiratory burst. Glucose enters the cell and is phosphorylated to form glucose 6-phosphate (G6P) which is then used in two major pathways which can be distinguished by radiolabelling the carbon atoms in the one and six positions. The C-6 atom is metabolized by the Embden–Meyerhof pathway to pyruvate which can enter the citric-acid cycle (CAC) to release CO_2; this pathway generates NADH from NAD. The C-1 atom of glucose is oxidized to CO_2 in the hexose monophosphate (HMP) shunt which reduces NADP to NADPH. Oxygen is reduced to superoxide (O_2^-) and then to hydrogen peroxide (H_2O_2) and finally to water. The subsequent metabolism of NADH or NADPH is uncertain but involves a cytochrome *b* in the wall of the phagocytic vacuole. The reducing equivalents (i.e. electrons) probably originate mainly in the HMP shunt, the activity of which is greatly increased during phagocytosis. The HMP shunt also detoxifies H_2O_2 through the action of glutathione peroxidase which oxidizes glutathione (GSH). Defects of many of these enzymes (■■■) have been detected in cell from patients with CGD, but none have withstood critical appraisal as the primary gene product. These widespread abnormalities of oxidase activity could result from lack or defective function of the cytochrome *b*.

shunt have been reported as being depressed in scorbutic guinea-pigs [30].

During the respiratory burst which follows phagocytosis of IgG-coated latex particles, neutrophils increase their oxygen consumption 10-fold, to 4 fmols/cell/min. This burst may persist for a few minutes, but the consumption of oxygen within each phagocytic vacuole appears to be very brief and self-limiting, consuming a standard quantity of oxygen (0·2 fmols) [32].

Studies with radioactive O_2 indicate that most, if not all, of the oxygen is reduced to H_2O [33], probably sequentially by the addition of electrons, first to form the superoxide radical, then hydrogen peroxide and finally hydroxyl radicals. (Radicals are molecules which contain a single unpaired electron and so are unstable and seek to gain or lose an electron.) These reactions can take place as follows:

$$2O_2 + NADPH \text{ or } NADH \rightarrow 2O_2^- + NADP \text{ or } NAD$$

The addition of a third electron, possibly from another superoxide molecule, splits the hydrogen peroxide molecule to form a hydroxyl radical and a hydroxyl anion [34].

It has been suggested that these radicals may be

directly responsible for the killing of microbes [35, 36], but it is uncertain whether they are generated and released as such, or whether they are simply intermediates in a complex electron-transport system [37, 38]. It has also been suggested that hydrogen peroxide forms the substrate for myeloperoxidase, which oxidizes a halide such as iodide or chloride to iodine or a chloramine, and that these substances then react with the organism [36, 39]. However, as described below (p. 639), many subjects with myeloperoxidase deficiency do not get recurrent infections. Neutrophils emit light following phagocytosis [40]; this chemiluminescence may result from the reversion of singlet oxygen ($^1O_2$) to triplet oxygen (O_2), though myeloperoxidase may also play a part in this. Whatever its mechanism, it is quantitatively related to the respiratory burst.

It is likely that the electron donors for this reaction include NADH and NADPH. Enzymes have been described for their oxidation: NADH [41] and NADPH oxidases [42, 43]. NADH and NADPH are very reactive substances which will interact with many different 'diaphorase' systems in the cell, and the available assays are artificial. An alternative hypothesis for transfer of their electrons is an electron-transport chain, which includes a recently described cytochrome b located in the plasma membranes of the cell [38, 44], and possibly myeloperoxidase in the vacuole. It is also possible, however, that the primary role of the system is to regulate the intravacuolar pH, since pH-regulating systems are often associated with electron-transport mechanisms such as this [45, 98]. The efficient functioning of microbicidal processes might be dependent upon the pH changes generated by this cytochrome-b-related electron transport.

Oxygen-independent microbial killing. Neutrophils can kill some organisms in the absence of oxygen; these include *Staph. epidermidis*, enterococci, *Strep. viridans*, *Ps. aeruginosa* and a number of anaerobes [22]. The mechanism is unknown, but possibilities include sequestration within the vacuole and limitation of growth factors, acidity within the vacuole, and factors released from granules into the phagosome.

Neutrophils contain several different granules: the *specific granules* contain lactoferrin, lysozyme and a vitamin-B_{12}-binding protein; the *azurophil granules* contain myeloperoxidase and lysozyme; the *lysosomes* (possibly a distinct group of granules) contain acid hydrolases [46]. The granules also contain a large variety of cationic proteins [47]. Lysozyme, which is released from both specific and azurophilic granules, can kill some organisms (e.g. *Micrococcus lysodeikticus*) which have only loosely cross-linked tetrapeptides between the polysaccharide chains in the cell wall. Its killing effect can be enhanced by a variety of agents including acid, alkali, polymyxin, antibody and complement [48, 49]. Lactoferrin, which binds iron very strongly even at low pH, is bacteriostatic because it deprives the organism of it [50]. This may well be functionally important, but would not explain the rapid killing of organisms. Free iron could impair electron transport by the cytochrome-b oxidase system and lactoferrin might prevent this by chelating free iron. A number of bactericidal factors, including lysozyme and cationic proteins, are released from the neutrophils into the plasma and tissue fluid [51]. It is likely that many components interact in the process of killing, which is not fully understood. We know even less about the ability of these cells to digest phagocytosed material and the pathology that results from defective digestion.

HUMORAL FACTORS INFLUENCING PHAGOCYTIC FUNCTION

Following the classical demonstration by Wright & Douglas in 1903 [52] that serum, especially from immunized subjects, rendered bacteria appetizing for ingestion by neutrophils ('opsonization'), and following Dean's demonstration [52a] that there were two components involved, heat-stable and heat-labile, it was clear that antibody and complement were involved. Sera from unimmunized animals have some opsonizing capacity, however, and heat lability and other characteristics suggested that complement might play a part here too [53]. Purified C3 will bind to non-encapsulated pneumococci and will opsonize them provided it is activated to C3b [54]; the presence on them of C3 and later components, but not of C1, C4 or C2, suggest that the alternative pathway of complement is involved in opsonization in the absence of antibody. Support for the concept of antibody-independent opsonization comes from the observation that sera virtually devoid of immunoglobulin will opsonize certain organisms (e.g. yeasts) normally [55], though for most organisms antibody is much more efficient. The factor mainly involved is C3b but a complex of C5, 6 and 7 also plays a part. Possibly the method of opsonization influences the efficiency of *in-vitro* killing as well as the early stage of phagocytosis [56]. There are other opsonizing factors in serum: C-reactive protein [57] and an α_2 acid glycoprotein [58]. More work on the significance and interaction of these complicated mechanisms is needed.

Though antibody-mediated opsonization is greatly assisted by complement, IgG can lead to phagocytosis on its own. Mononuclear and polymorphonuclear phagocytes have IgG receptors [59, 60] which bind only IgG1 and IgG3 [61], and bind aggregated IgG better than native IgG. Antibody bound to the receptors (cytophilic antibody) arms them to attack cells which have the appropriate antigen on their surface.

Before opsonization can be effective, the phagocyte must get to the particle, and this is an important function of complement. The C5a is released into the surrounding fluid, which provides a chemotactic gradient [62] up which the phagocytes migrate; C3a may also contribute. The latter is also an important anaphylotoxin, rendering blood vessels leaky so that polymorphs and other components can get out of the vessels. Though any system of complement activation results in a chemotactic gradient, some substances (e.g. casein) are chemotactic in the absence of complement, while others, including proteins generally, increase the undirected polymorph mobility (chemokinesis); many *in-vitro* systems depend on this rather than chemotaxis. Other physiological chemotactic factors include lymphokines (factors released from activated lymphocytes) [63]; one of these has a specific effect on eosinophils [64]. There is therefore a powerful humoral system for summoning the phagocytes and for directing them precisely to react with the particle. What happens then depends on the functional capacity of the phagocyte itself.

DEFECTS OF NEUTROPHIL FUNCTION

As with other forms of immunodeficiency, these disorders may be classified as primary (genetic or cause unknown) or secondary. Secondary factors may be superimposed on a primary defect of function. They can also be classified by the nature of the abnormality, itself dependent on the limited tests available. Recognized diseases are confined to those with morphological abnormality and those with defective mobility and defective killing of organisms; presumably the latter are usually related to defects of the respiratory enzymes responsible for killing (see above), and the former two to defects of the cytoskeleton and contractile systems. All three types of abnormality may occur in the same disease. There are also less well defined defects of the earlier stages of interaction of phagocyte with the particle [65].

MORPHOLOGICAL ABNORMALITIES

Chediak–Higashi syndrome

This autosomal-recessive defect was described by Beguez Cesar in 1943 [66]. The diagnosis, and probably all the functional abnormalities, spring from the formation of abnormal granules, which are widespread in other tissues, as well as the circulating neutrophils (Fig. 16.3). These patients also have a range of abnormalities of pigment of skin, hair (leading to an unusual silvery appearance which may be patchy), and eyes (iris and retina), the last leading to photophobia and nystagmus.

These have the effects characteristic of defective neutrophil function—frequent bacterial infection of the upper and lower respiratory tract, and of the skin (pyoderma and subcutaneous abscesses). *Staph. aureus* predominates but *Strep. pyogenes*, *H. influenzae*, *Strep. pneumoniae* and a number of Gram-negative

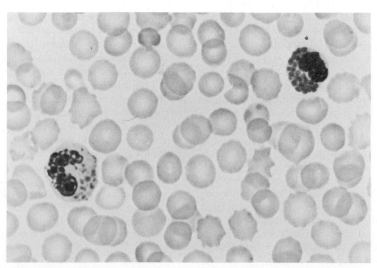

Fig. 16.3. Blood film from a patient with the Chediak–Higashi syndrome, showing a neutrophil and an eosinophil containing characteristic large granules.

organisms may also cause trouble [67]. Though fungal infections may occur, the common viral infections are handled normally.

During the earlier phase of the disease, the neutrophil count tends to be normal or rather low, though a neutrophil response can occur. Though earlier studies were negative, there is evidence of both defective mobility in response to chemotactic stimuli *in vitro* and *in vivo* [68] and defective killing of some bacteria, including *Staph. aureus*, though phagocytosis appears to be normal [69].

Initially, episodes of infection respond effectively to appropriate antibiotics, but later an 'accelerated phase' occurs with widespread lymphoid infiltration, which occasionally appears to be neoplastic [70]. Other manifestations at this stage include anaemia and neutropenia, with more refractory infections and haemorrhage associated with thrombocytopenia and defective platelet function (see Chapter 26). Hyperlipidaemia may occur. Besides obvious supportive measures which are effective in the early phases, steroids, cytotoxic drugs and splenectomy have all been tried in the accelerated phase [70], but with unsatisfactory results; these patients rarely reach adult life.

The observation of raised cyclic AMP levels in the polymorphs of one patient with the syndrome led to giving large doses of ascorbic acid, with apparent correction of this and the defect of mobility and bacterial killing function of the polymorphs *in vitro* and *in vivo* [5]. This clearly needs more study.

The assertion of autosomal-recessive inheritance is based on a number of large families, including instances of consanguinity [71]. This is supported by the observation of abnormal granules and cytoplasmic inclusions in a small proportion of blood lymphocytes of healthy heterozygotes [72–74] and abnormal cytoplasmic inclusions in their skin fibroblasts.

Mechanism of defect. The morphological and functional abnormalities seen in this disease and in similar diseases in several other species, including the beige mouse [75], are similar to those observed in colchicine-treated cells. Both have defective chemotaxis and lysosomal degranulation with normal phagocytosis and giant cytoplasmic granules; there are giant phagolysosomes which incorporate different types of granules [72, 76]. Fluorescent concanavalin A is spontaneously 'capped' by Chediak–Higashi cells; normal cells do this only after colchicine treatment [77]. The tubulin is normal, and the defect appears to lie in the mechanism controlling the equilibrium between its polymerization and depolymerization. Improved function following the addition of cholinergic agonists, ascorbic acid and cyclic GMP, supports the view

that the defect is in this mechanism, but the nature of the defective primary gene product is not known.

Other primary morphological abnormalities
There are other morphological abnormalities of neutrophils, both primary and secondary, besides those seen in the Chediak–Higashi syndrome and in granulocytic leukaemias (see Chapter 23). Large basophilic cytoplasmic inclusions are seen in the autosomal-recessive May–Hegglin anomaly, but although a minor functional abnormality has been described [78], this seems to have little clinical effect. The abnormal nuclear segmentation in the dominantly inherited Pelger–Huet anomaly is also associated with minor disturbance of function [78], perhaps partly because of limited nuclear deformability, but this also is of little clinical significance. Abnormal nuclear structure of neutrophils has been reported in Down's syndrome [79] and may be associated with defective function.

DEFECTS OF NEUTROPHIL MOBILITY
Neutrophil mobility may be measured *in vivo* by the skin-window technique [80, 81], or *in vitro* by passage through membranes [82], under gel [83], or in fluid media. Various media are used, with different activating agents, whether chemotactic or chemokinetic. In general, the different abnormalities may be diagnosed by any one of these methods, though there are exceptions. This function is particularly vulnerable to environmental factors including infection, and defects may occur as a secondary phenomenon (see below) or, in many diseases, may result from the presence of a humoral inhibitor; in such circumstances diagnosis of a primary cellular abnormality may be impossible. None the less, a number of isolated cases have been described in which susceptibility to frequent infections was ascribed to primary defective neutrophil mobility—lazy-leucocyte syndrome, Job's syndrome, etc., [84–87]. These patients sometimes have eczema and a very high IgE as well as frequent infections. Description of more than one affected member of the same family [88] strengthened the view that there were primary abnormalities of this type, but they remain heterogeneous and undefined (see below). Reports of benefit from ascorbic-acid treatment [5, 6] render diagnosis important. The identification of certain familial defects linked to diagnosable syndromes, and one possible primary gene product, is leading to increased confidence in this field, but the majority are in the miscellaneous group and may be fairly common. We describe the identifiable syndromes first.

Shwachman's syndrome
The syndrome of exocrine pancreatic insufficiency, neutropenia, metaphysial chondrodysplasia, growth

retardation and frequent infections was described by Shwachman *et al.* [89]. Because the upper and lower respiratory infections and septicaemia seemed more than the minor neutropenia and occasional immunoglobulin deficiency would explain, and because some forms of defective neutrophil mobility are associated with neutropenia [85], Aggett *et al.* [90] studied neutrophil mobility in 14 patients with this syndrome, and 13 of their parents. Both groups gave values significantly lower than appropriate controls; though the findings in the propositi could have been secondary, the intermediate values in the healthy heterozygotes provide strong evidence that defective mobility of morphologically normal neutrophils does occur as a primary genetic abnormality and supports the case for autosomal-recessive inheritance in this syndrome. Unlike many other conditions associated with defective neutrophil mobility, there is no obvious link with atopy. There is no coherent unifying hypothesis for the features of the syndrome. The recognition of the neutrophil function defect may contribute to the diagnosis and so to the early institution of specific treatment for other aspects of the syndrome, such as the malabsorption.

Actin dysfunction syndrome
Boxer *et al.* [91] described one infant with repeated staphylococcal skin infections and septicaemia in whom biopsies showed little pyogenic response. Both chemotactic mobility and phagocytosis were defective. Defective polymerization of the actin of the patient's neutrophils *in vitro* suggested that there might be a primary defect of the actomyosin system, presumably the primary gene product, though there is no evidence at present that this abnormality is inheritable, and the finding has yet to be confirmed in other patients.

Defective neutrophil mobility with delayed umbilical cord separation
Six members of two families had delayed (more than four weeks) separation of the umbilical cord, local and general skin infection and septicaemia. Neutrophil mobility was defective in the two affected members studied [6]; the parents' neutrophil mobility was normal. Following the observation of correction of the defect *in vitro* with ascorbic acid, it was given to the child with both correction of the defect *in vivo* and loss of symptoms. Other families with this association have been described by Bowen *et al.* [92], who noted that the neutrophils also failed to adhere to glass, and by P. G. Quie (personal communication).

Miscellaneous patients and families
The above associations establish the concept of primary neutrophil mobility defects, and strengthen the

considerable literature [1] of other associations. In patients who do not have one of these established syndromes, definite diagnosis of a primary defect probably depends on observing more than one affected member of a family or on showing that the parents have abnormal values [93]. These criteria are attainable in only some patients with primary defects, however, so these are likely to be underdiagnosed. The symptoms associated with these are likely to include recurrent infection and atopy, especially eczema and periodontal disease [94]. Some patients with frequent infection and eczema may have extremely high levels of IgE (the so-called hyper-IgE syndrome) [95] whereas other patients with primary defective mobility may have normal values. Hill & Quie [95] considered the possibility that the atopy caused the defective neutrophil mobility, since mobility is retarded by histamine. Mobility is normal in most atopics, however, so the association may be an example of the predisposition to atopy which results from defects of the antibody–complement–phagocyte system [96]. Patients with the hyper-IgE syndrome also have abnormal T-cell function which may reflect defective T-cell suppression [97], so the syndrome is certainly complicated.

Lazy-leucocyte syndrome.
In the first report of primary defective neutrophil mobility, Miller *et al.* [84] described two infants with frequent fever and mouth and ear infections; besides defective mobility, both directed and random, there was severe neutropenia, and low neutrophil migration into skin windows; other such patients have been described since. They used the attractive term 'lazy-leucocyte syndrome' but, because there are no characteristic diagnostic features, it is not possible to accept this as an established entity. The existence of other patients with defective neutrophil mobility but normal numbers raises some doubts about the view that the neutropenia resulted from failure of migration from marginated pools, though this effect could differ in different forms of mobility defect.

Job's syndrome.
This was initially described as recurrent cold subcutaneous staphylococcal abscesses and eczema in red-haired girls [85] and is associated with defective neutrophil mobility [86], but like the lazy-leucocyte syndrome, it falls short of a diagnosable entity. Other features, including occurrence in boys and high IgE, have subsequently been noted and have added to the complexity.

Though these were the first two examples of presumed primary neutrophil mobility defects, they probably cannot be clearly separated from the majority, and the particular characteristics described should not restrict the range of patients with frequent infection investigated for this defect. Since mobility is a property of many cells, it is possible that the abnormality involves other cells besides neutrophils. There has been little study of this, but lymphocyte mobility [99] may also be defective in some patients with primary defects of neutrophil mobility.

Secondary neutrophil mobility defects

Some of the very wide range of environmental factors and diseases associated with defective neutrophil mobility are listed in Table 16.2. Though they may contribute to the vulnerability to infection of some of these patients, the significance of this for their management has not yet been systematically studied. They are mainly important in the problems they present for diagnosis of primary defects, particularly the effect of infection, the usual presentation of the patients with primary defects. The literature here is contradictory, however, since Hill *et al.* [100] report that mobility may be enhanced with infection. The demonstration of return to normal of defective neutrophil function in a patient with periodontal infection when his teeth were removed, shows the importance of such secondary dysfunction [101]. It is possible that such environmental factors are especially damaging in patients with primary defects (e.g. anaesthesia in Shwachman's disease [90]). Further study should lead to a reduction of such risks.

Mechanisms of defective mobility

Defective mobility could result from defective receptors for stimulant factors, stiffness of the cell itself (due to nuclear rigidity or other reasons), defective energy metabolism, or defects of the contractile or skeletal system. Only examples of the last—actin dysfunction [91]—and lack of deformability [102] have been recognized so far. The varying results of different tests provide some indication of the heterogeneity. For instance, cells with defective mobility through membranes but normal mobility in fluid media, such as those of the Chediak–Higashi syndrome, have defective deformability [102]. The effect of ascorbic acid and glutathione on normal neutrophil mobility and respiration, and the effect of ascorbic acid on defective neutrophil mobility [5, 6, 103] suggest that metabolic factors controlled by cyclic AMP and cyclic GMP [104] may be relevant here.

DEFECTS OF KILLING OF MICRO-ORGANISMS

Chronic granulomatous disease

With the demonstration that the neutrophils of patients with a remarkable syndrome of infection, which had already been recognized, failed to kill certain bacteria which they phagocytosed normally [2], our knowledge of neutrophil function defects began.

Clinical features. The syndrome is of recurrent and chronic abscesses of lymph nodes (particularly neck and groin) and liver, osteomyelitis, and localized and diffuse lung disease. Eczema, skin infection and splenomegaly are also common. When the abscesses are drained they often result in chronic discharging sinuses. Other clinical features include diarrhoea, nausea, anorexia, abdominal pain, distension and failure to gain weight [105]. Inflammation and thickening of the wall of the gastro-intestinal tract may occur at any level and fistulae may develop. Granulomatous cystitis [106] and chorioretinal lesions may be seen [107]. Though the first patients diagnosed were very ill, and died in early childhood, several centres know of reasonably healthy adults with the disease. It is not yet sure whether this reflects natural history of improvement if early childhood is survived, improved management, or heterogeneity of the disease.

Histology. The lesions are chronic granulomata, with polymorphonuclear, lymphocytic, macrophage and plasma-cell infiltration. Occasional giant cells are seen, as are widespread macrophages containing a lipid pigment [108]. The failure of both neutrophils and monocytes [109] to kill phagocytosed organisms results in their being sequestered from humoral antibacterial factors including antibody and complement. Presumably the infected neutrophils are phagocytosed by the fixed macrophages, in which the bacteria also survive, so bacteria which usually elicit a pyogenic response elicit the response common to intracellular pathogens—the chronic granulomatous reaction—in the tissues containing many macrophages, especially lymph nodes, liver, bone marrow and lung.

Microbiology. The organisms cultured from the lesions in one characteristic series [110] included *Staph. aureus*, *E. coli*, *Klebsiella*, *Serratia marcescens*, salmonellae, and a range of fungi including *Candida albicans*, *Aspergillus fumigatus* and *Actinomyces israelii*. Unusual opportunist infections such as Nocardiasis may occur. Beta haemolytic streptococci, *Strep. pneumoniae*, *H. influenzae*, and viruses do not give special trouble, though mycoplasma pneumonia may occur. Dissemination of BCG infection [111] suggests that these patients are abnormally susceptible to mycobacteria, but the spurious deduction from the histology that the lesions are tuberculous should be avoided unless the organisms are detected. The fungal lesions are of lymph nodes, lung, etc., and not mucocutaneous candidiasis.

Within the cells, the bacteria are segregated from

most antibiotics [112] as well as the physiological humoral bactericidal systems, but rifampicin is apparently capable of gaining access to them [113].

Inheritance. The syndrome is clearly heterogeneous since, though the great majority of patients are boys, with a familial incidence suggestive of X-linked inheritance, it is also seen in girls, presumably with different metabolic abnormalities (see below). Probably most boy patients have the X-linked disease, but some have the autosomal-recessive form. We know of no systematic comparison of the different clinical manifestations in the two groups. The female carriers of the X-linked form have, as a group, low levels of bactericidal activity and of a range of the other diagnostic tests applied (see below), but there is a considerable scatter and exclusion of heterozygosity in female relatives is still not secure. Heterozygotes may have lupus erythematosus—discoid and sometimes systemic [110]—and excess infections. The inheritance has been further confused by the significant association in some boys with this disease, with certain antigens of the Kell blood-group system, which are not inherited on the X chromosome. Boys with CGD may lack the Kx antigen on their leucocytes, and sometimes on their erythrocytes too; patients with the autosomal-recessive form do not. This was noted following blood-transfusion reactions [114, 115]. It is suggested that a precursor of the particular blood-group substance may be inherited on the X chromosome, rather than the type itself.

Mechanism. The unifying biological abnormality of the cells in this syndrome is an absence of the sudden burst of respiratory activity that usually accompanies phagocytosis [116]. This malfunction has been ascribed to a defect of various 'oxidase enzymes', which have been variously identified as a NADH oxidase [41], a NADPH oxidase [42] and a D-amino-acid oxidase [117] and, in girls, as a glutathione peroxidase [118]. There is doubt whether any of these is the primary product of the defective gene; the recent description of an electron-transporting system containing a *b* type of cytochrome [38, 44] may provide an explanation of these findings, since it is lacking in X-linked CGD [119] and it is possible that the other enzyme abnormalities may be secondary to this defect. The patients with the autosomal-recessive form have normal amounts of this cytochrome *b*, but unlike that of normal subjects this is not reduced when the respiratory activity of their neutrophils is stimulated with phorbol myristate acetate. This suggests that these patients lack a proximal component of the electron-transport chain, or that there is some defect in the activation process [119].

Treatment. As with all immunodeficiency, individual infections should be treated with appropriate antibiotics (with bacterial antibiotic sensitivity testing) and surgery; the wounds do heal in the end. Rifampicin may have a special place in treating some staphylococcal infections in CGD [113], but always with another anti-staphylococcal antibiotic in view of the rapid development of bacterial resistance. It is not likely to be effective against many of the other organisms infecting these patients.

The wide use of Septrin (cotrimoxazole) prophylactically in CGD [4], though not established by a controlled trial, appears to result in a very considerable reduction in infections. It has been reported [121] that sulphafurazole (Sulfisoxazole) enhances the capacity of CGD neutrophils to kill bacteria which are resistant to it, and it therefore seems possible that the benefit from Septrin may be due to a similar effect of Sulphamethoxazole. However it works, Septrin prophylaxis appears to be of considerable value, though there remains a risk from organisms resistant to it.

Less common primary defects of bacterial killing

There are a number of other primary defects of bacterial killing, in some of which the syndrome may be similar to CGD, though in others it may be rather different. In some, the primary enzyme defect has been identified.

Myeloperoxidase deficiency. The first two siblings described with deficiency of the peroxidase of neutrophils and monocytes were healthy [122]. The use of automated differential leucocyte-counting techniques, in which the cells are identified by their peroxidase content and size, has resulted in the discovery of large numbers of asymptomatic myeloperoxidase-deficient individuals. However, Lehrer & Cline [123] described such a patient with extensive infection with *Candida albicans* whose neutrophils phagocytosed fungi and bacteria effectively, but failed to kill some, especially *Candida albicans*, *Staph. aureus*, *S. marcescens*, and *E. coli*. This range of organisms is similar to, but not identical with, those incriminated in CGD. Not only are the patients less severely ill, but the lesions of myeloperoxidase deficiency do not have the same characteristic sites and histological reactions. The peroxidase of the eosinophils is normal. The detection of the defect in siblings of both sexes and intermediate values of myeloperoxidase in the cells of the parents of patients [123] suggests autosomal-recessive inheritance. Management is as for CGD.

Myeloperoxidase has been reported to be deficient, apparently as a secondary phenomenon, in some patients with acute myeloid leukaemias and in a number of miscellaneous patients [1], including some forms of Batten's disease [124]. No leucocyte function defect has been described in the latter.

Glucose-6-phosphate-dehydrogenase (G6PD) deficiency. Profound deficiency of G6PD, with a residual activity less than five per cent of normal, may be associated with a mild CGD [125]. This provides support for NADPH as a natural substrate of the oxidase system, because G6PD generates NADPH by the hexose monophosphate shunt. A low intracellular concentration of NADPH could impair the function of the neutrophil in other ways. The NADPH maintains sulphydryl groups in a reduced state, which seems to be essential for normal cellular activity. The intracellular

concentrations of many redox compounds are kept fairly constant in relation to each other by transhydrogenase enzymes; thus a fall in the total intracellular reducing power will decrease the concentration of many reduced compounds including NADH [31], any of which could be the natural substrate of the oxidase system.

Glutathione-peroxidase (GP) deficiency. This enzyme catalyses the glutathione-dependent reduction of H_2O_2 to H_2O. It deficiency has been reported in a number of patients with non-X-linked CGD [118, 126]. It is not clear why GP deficiency should cause this syndrome, which is thought to be associated with defective generation of H_2O_2, since it is involved in its catab-

Table 16.3. Tests of neutrophil function

Functions	Function investigated	Basis of test	Reference
Circulating number	Production	Histological examination of bone marrow	
		Colony formation by bone-marrow cells in *in-vitro* culture	147
	Release and redistribution	Prednisolone or adrenaline effect on count	See Chapter 15
	Intravascular survival and distribution	Survival and distribution of radiolabelled cells	See Chapter 15
Mobility	Deformability	Pressure necessary to aspirate into micropipette	148
	Orientation	Effect of chemoattractant on cellular alignment	149
	Mobility	Chemotaxis and chemokinesis of cells through 3 μm pores in millipore filters or under agarose	82, 83, 90
	Accumulation at inflammatory sites	Arrival of cells at skin abrasions—qualitative (slide) or quantitative (chamber)	80, 81
	Microfilaments and tubules	Capping fluorescent concanavalin A	10
Adherence and ingestion	Adherence	Adherence to columns of nylon wool	150
	Surface receptors	Rosetting of immunoglobulin- and complement-coated particles	151
	Ingestion	Uptake of particles (e.g. bacteria, yeasts or stained lipid droplets)	152
Killing	Killing	Survival of intracellular organisms—bacterial count, radioactivity incorporation or fungal staining	2, 56, 125
	Degranulation	Electron microscopy and histochemistry	152
		Isolation of phagocytic vacuoles by flotation	153
		Secretion induced by 'frustrated phagocytosis'	51
	Secretion	Release of granule contents from stimulated cells into surrounding medium	154
	Respiratory burst	Oxygen consumption	32
		Hydrogen peroxide production	155
		Chemiluminescence	156
		Iodination	157
		Hexose monophosphate shunt activity	43
		Nitro-blue tetrazolium reduction	158, 159
	Digestion	Release of radioactivity from killed ingested organisms	160

olism. Possibly the assay may not be specifically measuring GP. The GP may be necessary to keep the oxidase system reduced.

Others. Defective bacterial killing has been reported with neutrophil pyruvate-kinase (PK) deficiency [127] and, much more commonly but of lesser severity and clinical relevance, in Down's syndrome and other chromosomal abnormalities [128]. Reports of other individual patients suggest that such defects will be found to be far more common and complex, involving a wider range of function than is recognized at present. In one such patient, the neutrophils failed to elicit a respiratory burst after engulfment of micro-organisms, though it occurred following contact with soluble stimuli [129]. Other defects are apparently related to the earlier phases of neutrophil function [65].

Secondary defects of bacterial killing

Some environmental factors and diseases which reduce bactericidal capacity of normal neutrophils are listed in Table 16.2. The mechanisms of these are largely unknown and their principal practical significance is that they complicate the diagnosis of primary defects.

TESTS OF NEUTROPHIL FUNCTION

Tests in use for diagnosis and others which may well have a place are listed in Table 16.3, classified according to the function to be measured. The usual indication is recurrent infection, and they are under-taken as part of the investigation of immunodeficiency [31, 161]. If possible, testing should be done while the patient is well; defective results should be repeated and, if possible, measured in the parents to reduce the likelihood that they are due to a secondary abnor-mality. Despite this, the diagnosis of defects of neutro-phil function, apart from the structural ones, is insecure, and tests should be carefully related to other clinical data.

At present, besides counting and inspection for morphological abnormalities, tests which are estab-lished are largely confined to defects of mobility and the killing of organisms. Though the direct test for the latter must be the final arbiter, a number of the other simpler tests are associated with such defects. Any of the nitro-blue tetrazolium tests, including the simple slide tests [158, 159], can be used to diagnose X-linked CGD; the slide tests are probably the best for diagnos-ing heterozygotes [159] and permit intrauterine diag-nosis [162], but they are normal in some other killing defects. Iodination and chemiluminescence parallel killing more widely, but their complete identity cannot be assumed. Where appropriate, tests for individual

enzyme activity are applied, and only then can a precise diagnosis be made.

This field is very new, still largely in an elementary stage based on function tests, and advancing rapidly. It is likely that, with improved techniques, a large field of defective phagocyte function, neutrophil and mononuclear, will be recognized.

REFERENCES

1 KLEBANOFF S.J. & CLARK R.A. (1978) *The Neutrophil: Function and Clinical Disorders.* North-Holland, Amsterdam.
2 QUIE P.G., WHITE J.G., HOLMES B. & GOOD R.A. (1967) In vitro bactericidal capacity of human polymor-phonuclear leucocytes; diminished activity in chronic granulomatous disease of childhood. *Journal of Clinical Investigation,* **46,** 668.
3 HOSKING C.S., FITZGERALD M.G. & SHELTON M.J. (1977) Results of immune function testing in children with recurrent infection. *Australian Paediatric Journal,* **13** (Suppl.), 61.
4 WORLD HEALTH ORGANIZATION (1978) Scientific group on immunodeficiency. *Technical Report Series 630.* WHO, Geneva.
5 BOXER L.A., WATANABE A.M., RISTER M., BESCH H.R., ALLEN J. & BAEHNER R.L. (1976) Correction of leuko-cyte function in Chediak–Higashi syndrome by ascor-bate. *New England Journal of Medicine,* **295,** 1041.
6 HAYWARD A.R., HARVEY B.A.M., LEONARD J., GREEN-WOOD M.C., WOOD C.B.S. & SOOTHILL J.F. (1979) Delayed separation of the umbilical cord, widespread infections and defective neutrophil mobility. *Lancet,* **i,** 1099.
7 BURNSIDE B. (1975) The form and arrangement of microtubules; an historical, primary morphological review. *Annals of the New York Academy of Sciences,* **253,** 14.
8 NICOLSON G.L. (1976) Transmembrane control of the receptors on normal and tumour cells. I. Cytoplasmic influence over surface components. *Biochimica et Bio-physica Acta,* **457,** 57.
9 SNYDER J.A. & MCINTOSH J.R. (1976) Biochemistry and physiology of microtubules. *Annual Review of Biochem-istry,* **45,** 699.
10 OLIVER J.M. (1978) Cell biology of leukocyte abnorma-lities—membrane and cytoskeletal function in normal and defective cells. *American Journal of Pathology,* **93,** 221.
11 CLARKE M. & SPUDICH J.A. (1977) Non-muscle con-tractile proteins; the role of actin and myosin in cell motility and shape determination. *Annual Review of Biochemistry,* **46,** 797.
12 STOSSEL T.P. & HARTWIG J.H. (1976) Interaction of actin, myosin, and a new actin-binding protein of rabbit pulmonary macrophages. *Journal of Cellular Biology,* **68,** 602.
13 ALLISON A.C., DAVIES P. & DE PETRIS S. (1971) Role of contractile microfilaments in macrophage movement and endocytosis. *Nature (New Biology),* **232,** 153.

14 DAVIES P., ALLISON A.C., FOX R.I., POLYZONIS M. & HASWELL A.D. (1972) The exocytosis of polymorpho-nuclear-leukocyte lysosomal enzymes induced by cytochalasin B. *Biochemical Journal*, **128**, 78.

15 BERLIN R.D. & OLIVER J.M. (1978) Analogous ultrastructure and surface properties during capping and phagocytosis in leukocytes. *Journal of Cellular Biology*, **77**, 789.

16 GRIFFIN F.M., GRIFFIN J.A. & SILVERSTEIN S.C. (1976) Studies on the mechanism of phagocytosis. II. The interaction of macrophages with anti-immunoglobulin IgG-coated-bone marrow-derived lymphocytes. *Journal of Experimental Medicine*, **144**, 788.

17 HIRSCH J.G. (1962) Cinemicrophotographic observations of granule lysis in polymorphonuclear leucocytes during phagocytosis. *Journal of Experimental Medicine*, **116**, 827.

18 HENSON P.M. (1971) Interaction of cells with immune complexes; adherence, release of constituents and tissue injury. *Journal of Experimental Medicine*, **134**, 1145.

19 BALDRIDGE C.W. & GERARD R.W. (1933) The extra respiration of phagocytosis. *American Journal of Physiology*, **103**, 235.

20 SELVARAJ R.J. & SBARRA A.J. (1966) Relationship of glycolytic and oxidative metabolism to particle entry and destruction in phagocytosing cells. *Nature (London)*, **211**, 1272.

21 SBARRA A.J. & KARNOVKSY M.L. (1959) The biochemical basis of phagocytosis. I. Metabolic changes during the ingestion of particles by polymorphonuclear leukocytes. *Journal of Biological Chemistry*, **234**, 1355.

22 MANDELL G.L. (1974) Bactericidal activity of aerobic and anaerobic polymorphonuclear neutrophils. *Infection and Immunology*, **9**, 337.

23 MANDELL G.L. (1975) Catalase, superoxide dismutase and virulence of *Staphylococcus aureus*: in vitro and in vivo studies with emphasis on staphylococcal-leukocyte interaction. *Journal of Clinical Investigation*, **55**, 561.

24 COHEN H.J. & CHOVANIEC M.E. (1978) Superoxide production by digitonin-stimulated guinea pig granulocytes. The effects of N-ethyl maleimide, divalent cations, and glycolytic and mitochondrial inhibitors on the activation of the superoxide generating system. *Journal of Clinical Investigation*, **61**, 1088.

25 LEHNINGER A.L. (1970) *Biochemistry*, Chapter 15. Worth, New York.

26 STJERNHOLM R.L. & MANAK R.C. (1970) Carbohydrate metabolism in leukocytes. XIV. Regulation of pentose cycle activity and glycogen metabolism during phagocytosis. *Journal of the Reticuloendothelial Society*, **8**, 550.

27 SELVARAJ R.J. & SBARRA A.J. (1967) The role of the phagocyte in host-parasite interactions. VII. Di- and triphosphopyridine nucleotide kinetics during phagocytosis. *Biochimica et Biophysica Acta*, **141**, 243.

28 AELLIG A., MAILLARD M., PHAVORIN A. & FRIE J. (1977) The energy metabolisms of the leukocyte. VIII. The determination of the concentration of the co-enzymes NAD, NADH, NADP and NADPH in polymorphonuclear leukocytes at rest and after incubation by enzymic cycling. *Enzyme*, **22**, 196.

29 REED P.W. (1969) Glutathione and the hexose monophosphate shunt in phagocytizing and hydrogen peroxide-treated rat leukocytes. *Journal of Biological Chemistry*, **244**, 2459.

30 SHILOTRI P. G. (1977) Glycolytic hexose monophosphate shunt and bactericidal activities of leukocytes in ascorbic acid deficient guinea pigs. *Journal of Nutrition*, **107**, 1507.

31 BAEHNER R.L., JOHNSTON R.B. & NATHAN D.G. (1972) Comparative study of the metabolic and bactericidal characteristics of severely glucose-6-phosphate dehydrogenase deficient polymorphonuclear leukocytes and leukocytes from children with chronic granulomatous disease. *Journal of the Reticuloendothelial Society*, **12**, 150.

32 SEGAL A.W. & COADE S.B. (1978) Kinetics of oxygen comsumption by phagocytosing human neutrophils. *Biochemical and Biophysical Research Communications*, **84**, 611.

33 SEGAL A.W., CLARK J. & ALLISON A.C. (1978) Tracing the fate of oxygen consumed during phagocytosis by human neutrophils with $^{15}O_2$. *Clinical Science and Molecular Medicine*, **55**, 413.

34 HABER F. & WEISS J. (1934) The catalytic decomposition of hydrogen peroxide by iron salts. *Proceedings of the Royal Society A.*, **147**, 332.

35 BABIOR B.M., CURNUTTE J.T. & KIPNES R.S. (1975) Biological defense mechanisms. Evidence for the participation of superoxide on bacterial killing by xanthine oxidase. *Journal of Laboratory and Clinical Medicine*, **85**, 235.

36 KLEBANOFF S.J. (1975) Antimicrobial mechanisms in neutrophilic polymorphonuclear leukocytes. *Seminars in Hematology*, **12**, 117.

37 SEGAL A.W. & MESHULAM T. (1979) Production of superoxide by neutrophils; a reappraisal. *FEBS Letters*, **100**, 27.

38 SEGAL A.W. & JONES O.T.G. (1978) A novel cytochrome *b* system in phagocytic vacuoles from human granulocytes. *Nature (London)*, **276**, 515.

39 KLEBANOFF S.J. (1967) Iodination of bacteria; a bactericidal mechanism. *Journal of Experimental Medicine*, **126**, 1063.

40 ALLEN R.C., STJERNHOLM R.L. & STEELE R.H. (1972) Evidence for the generation of an electronic excitation state in human polymorphonuclear leukocytes and its participation in bactericidal activity. *Biochemical and Biophysical Research Communications*, **47**, 679.

41 EVANS W.H. & KARNOVSKY M.L. (1961) A possible mechanism for the stimulation of some metabolic functions during phagocytosis. *Journal of Biological Chemistry*, **236**, 30.

42 IYER G.Y.N., ISLAM M.F. & QUASTEL J.H. (1961) Biochemical aspects of phagocytosis. *Nature (London)*, **192**, 535.

43 ROSSI F. & ZATTI M. (1964) Changes in the metabolic pattern of polymorphonuclear leukocytes during phagocytosis. *British Journal of Experimental Pathology*, **45**, 548.

44 SEGAL A.W. & JONES O.T.G. (1979) The subcellular distribution and some properties of the cytochrome *b* component of the microbicidal oxidase system of human neutrophils. *Biochemical Journal*, **180**, 33.

45 MITCHELL P. (1966) Chemiosmotic coupling in oxidative and photosynthetic phosphorylation. *Biological Reviews*, **41**, 445.

46 SEGAL A.W., DORLING J. & COADE S. (1980) Kinetics of fusion of the cytoplasmic granules with phagocytic vacuoles in human polymorphonuclear leukocytes. Biochemical and morphological studies. *Journal of Cellular Biology*, **84**, 42.

47 ODEBERG H. & OLSSON I. (1975) Antibacterial activity of cationic proteins from human granulocytes. *Journal of Clinical Investigation*, **56**, 1118.

48 AMANO T., INAI S., SEKI Y., KASHIBA S., FUJIKAWA K. & NISHIMURA S. (1954) Studies on the immune bacteriolysis. I. Accelerating effect on the immune bacteriolysis by lysozyme-like substance of leukocytes and egg-white lysozyme. *Medical Journal of Osaka University*, **4**, 401.

49 GLYNN A.A. (1969) The complement-lysozyme sequence in immune bacteriolysis. *Immunology*, **16**, 463.

50 MASSON P.L., HEREMANS J.F., PRIGNOT J.J. & WAUTERS G. (1966) Immunochemical localization and bacteriostatic properties of an iron-binding protein from bronchial mucus. *Thorax*, **21**, 538.

51 HENSON P.M. (1971) The immunologic release of constituents from neutrophil leukocytes. II. Mechanisms of release during phagocytosis, and adherence to non-phagocytosable surfaces. *Journal of Immunology*, **107**, 1547.

52 WRIGHT A.E. & DOUGLAS S.R. (1903) An experimental investigation of the role of the blood fluids in connection with phagocytosis. *Proceedings of the Royal Society*, **72**, 357.

52a DEAN G. (1905) An experimental enquiry into the nature of the substance in serum which influences phagocytosis. *Proceedings of the Royal Society, Series B*, **76**, 506.

53 SMITH M.R. & WOOD W.B. (1969) Heat labile opsonins to pneumococcus. I, Participation of complement. *Journal of Experimental Medicine*, **130**, 1209.

54 SHIN H.S., SMITH M.R. & WOOD W.B. (1969) Heat labile opsonins to pneumococcus. II. Involvement of C3 and C5. *Journal of Experimental Medicine*, **130**, 1229.

55 SOOTHILL J.F. & HARVEY B.A.M. (1976) Defective opsonisation; a common immunity deficiency. *Archives of Diseases of Childhood*, **51**, 91.

56 BRIDGES C.G., DASILVA G., YAMAMURA M. & VALDIMARSSON H. (1980) A radiometric assay for the combined measurement of phagocytosis and intracellular killing of *C. albicans*. *Clinical and Experimental Immunology*. (In press).

57 GANROT P.O. & KINDMARK C.O. (1969) C reactive protein. A phagocytosis promoting factor. *Scandinavian Journal of Clinical and Laboratory Investigation*, **24**, 215.

58 VAN SCOY R.E., HILL H.R., RITTS R.E. & QUIE P.G. (1975) Familial neutrophil chemotaxis defect, recurrent bacterial infections, mucocutaneous candidiasis and hyperimmunoglobulin E. *Annals of Internal Medicine*, **82**, 766.

59 HENSON P.M. (1969) The adherence of leukocytes and platelets induced by fixing IgG antibody or complement. *Immunology*, **16**, 107.

60 HUBER H. & FUDENBERG H.H. (1968) Receptor sites of human monocytes for IgG. *Internal Archives of Allergy*, **34**, 18.

61 OKAFOR G.O., TURNER M.W. & HAY F.C. (1974) Localisation of monocyte binding site of human immunoglobulin G. *Nature (London)*, **248**, 228.

62 SNYDERMAN R., SHIN H.S., PHILLIPS J.K., GEWURZ H. & MERGENHAGEN S.E. (1969) A neutrophil chemotactic factor derived from C5 upon interaction of guinea pig serum with endotoxin. *Journal of Immunology*, **103**, 413.

63 WARD P.A., REMOLD H.G. & DAVIES J.R. (1970) The production by antigen-stimulated lymphocytes of a leukotactic factor distinct from migration inhibitory factor. *Cellular Immunology*, **1**, 162.

64 KAY A.B., STECHSCHULTE D.J. & AUSTIN K.F. (1971) An eosinophil leukocyte chemotactic factor of anaphylaxis. *Journal of Experimental Medicine*, **133**, 602.

65 EDELSON P.J., STITES D.P., GOLD S. & FUDENBERG H.H. (1973) Disorders of neutrophil function. Defects in the early stages of the phagocytic process. *Clinical and Experimental Immunology*, **13**, 21.

66 BEGUEZ CESAR A. (1943) Neutropenia cronica maligna familiar con granulaciones atipicas de los leucocitos. *Sociedad Cubana de Pediatrica Boletin*, **15**, 900.

67 BLUME R.S. & WOLFF S.M. (1972) The Chediak–Higashi syndrome; studies of four patients and a review of the literature. *Medicine*, **51**, 247.

68 CLARK R.A. & KIMBALL H.R. (1971) Defective granulocyte chemotaxis in the Chediak–Higashi syndrome. *Journal of Clinical Investigation*, **50**, 2645.

69 ROOT R.K., ROSENTHAL A.S. & BALESTRA D.J. (1972) Abnormal bactericidal metabolic and lysosomal functions of Chediak–Higashi syndrome leukocytes. *Journal of Clinical Investigation*, **51**, 649.

70 DENT P.B., FISH L.A., WHITE J.G. & GOOD R.A. (1966) Chediak–Higashi syndrome. Observations on the nature of the associated malignancy. *Laboratory Investigation*, **15**, 1634.

71 SADEM N., YAFFE D., ROSENSZAJN L., ADAR H., SOROKER B. & EFRATI P. (1965) Cytochemical and genetic studies in four cases of Chediak–Higashi–Steinbrinck syndrome. *Acta Haematologica*, **34**, 20.

72 DOUGLAS S.D., BLUME R.S. & WOLFF S.M. (1969a) Fine structured studies of leukocytes from patients and heterozygotes with the Chediak–Higashi syndrome. *Blood*, **33**, 527.

73 DOUGLAS S.D., BLUME R.S., GLADE P.R., CHESSIN L.N. & WOLFF S.M. (1969) Fine structure of continuous long term lymphoid cell cultures from a Chediak–Higashi patient and heterozygote. *Laboratory Investigation*, **21**, 225.

74 DANES B.S. & BEARN A.G. (1967) Cell culture and the Chediak–Higashi syndrome. *Lancet*, **ii**, 65.

75 LUTZNER M.A., LOWRIE C.T. & JORDAN H.W. (1967) Giant granules in leukocytes of the beige mouse. *Journal of Heredity*, **58**, 299.

76 WHITE J.G. (1967) The Chediak–Higashi syndrome; cytoplasmic sequestration in circulating leukocytes. *Blood*, **29**, 435.

77 OLIVER J.M. (1978) Cell biology of leukocyte abnormalities—membrane and cytoskeletal function in normal and defective cells. *American Journal of Pathology*, **93**, 221.

78 REBUCK J.W., BARTH C.L. & PETZ A.J. (1963) New leukocytic dysfunction at the inflammatory sites in Hegglin's, Hurler's and Pelger–Huet anomalous states. *Federation Proceedings*, **22**, 427.

79 DJALDETTI M., BESSLER H., FISHMAN P., VAN DE LYN E. & JOSHUA H. (1974) Ultrastructural features of the

granulocytes in Down's syndrome. *Scandinavian Journal of Haematology*, **12**, 104.

80 REBUCK J.W. & CROWLEY J.H. (1955) A method of studying leukocyte function *in vivo*. *Annals of the New York Academy of Sciences*, **59**, 757.

81 SENN H.J. & JUNGI W.F. (1975) Neutrophil migration in health and disease. *Seminars in Hematology*, **12**, 27.

82 BOYDEN S. (1962) The chemotactic effect of mixtures of antibody and antigen on polymorphonuclear leukocytes. *Journal of Experimental Medicine*, **115**, 453.

83 NELSON R.D., QUIE P.G. & SIMMONS R.L. (1975) Chemotaxis under agarose. A new and simple method for measuring chemotaxis and spontaneous migration of human polymorphonuclear leukocytes and monocytes. *Journal of Immunology*, **115**, 1650.

84 MILLER M.E., OSKI F.A. & HARRIS M.B. (1971) Lazy leucocyte syndrome. A new disorder of neutrophil function. *Lancet*, **i**, 665.

85 DAVIS S.D., SCHALLER J. & WEDGWOOD R.J. (1966) Job's syndrome. Recurrent 'cold' staphylococcal abscesses. *Lancet*, **i**, 1013.

86 HILL H.R., OCHS H.D., QUIE P.G., CLARK R.A., PABST H.F., KLEBANOFF S.J. & WEDGWOOD R.J. (1974) Defect in neutrophil granulocyte chemotaxis in Job's syndrome of recurrent 'cold' staphylococcal abscesses. *Lancet*, **ii**, 617.

87 CLARK R.A., ROOT R.K., KIMBALL H.R. & KIRKPATRICK C.H. (1973) Defective neutrophil chemotaxis and cellular immunity in a child with recurrent infections. *Annals of Internal Medicine*, **78**, 515.

88 VAN SCOY R.E., HILL H.R., RITTS R.E. & QUIE P.G. (1975) Familial neutrophil chemotaxis defect, recurrent bacterial infections, mucocutaneous candidiasis and hyperimmunoglobulin E. *Annals of Internal Medicine*, **82**, 766.

89 SHWACHMAN H., DIAMOND L.K., OSKI F.A. & KHAW K.T. (1964) The syndrome of pancreatic insufficiency and bone marrow dysfunction. *Journal of Pediatrics*, **65**, 645.

90 AGGETT P.J., HARRIES J.T., HARVEY B.A.M. & SOOTHILL J.F. (1979) An inherited defect of neutrophil mobility in Shwachman syndrome. *Journal of Pediatrics*, **94**, 391.

91 BOXER L.A., HEDLEY-WHITE E.T. & STOSSEL T.P. (1976) Neutrophil actin dysfunction and abnormal neutrophil behaviour. *New England Journal of Medicine*, **291**, 1093.

92 BOWEN T., OCHS H.D. & WEDGWOOD R.J. (1979) Chemotaxis and umbilical separation. *Lancet*, **ii**, 302.

93 FARHOUDI A., HARVEY B.A.M. & SOOTHILL J.F. (1978) Clinicopathological findings in patients with primary and secondary defects of neutrophil mobility. *Archives of Diseases in Childhood*, **53**, 625.

94 CLARK R.A., PAGE R.C. & WILDE G. (1977) Defective neutrophil chemotaxis in juvenile periodontitis. *Infection and Immunology*, **18**, 694.

95 HILL H.R. & QUIE P.G. (1974) Raised serum-IgE levels and defective neutrophil chemotaxis in three children with eczema and recurrent bacterial infections. *Lancet*, **i**, 183.

96 SOOTHILL J.F. (1976) Some intrinsic and extrinsic factors predisposing to allergy. *Proceedings of the Royal Society of Medicine*, **69**, 439.

97 BUCKLEY R.H. & BECKER W.B. (1978) Abnormalities in the regulation of human IgE synthesis. *Immunology Review*, **41**, 288.

98 SEGAL A.W., GEISON M., GARCIA R., HARPER A. & MILLER R. (1981) The respiratory burst of phagocytic cells is associated with a rise in vacuolar pH. *Nature (London)*, **290**, 406.

99 SMOGORZEWSKA E., LAYWARD L. & SOOTHILL J.F. (1981) T lymphocyte mobility; defects and effects of ascorbic acid, histamine and complexed IgG. *Clinical and Experimental Immunology*, **43**, 174.

100 HILL H.R., GERRARD J.M., HOGAN N.A. & QUIE P.G. (1974) Hyperactivity of neutrophil leucocyte responses during active bacterial infection. *Journal of Clinical Investigation*, **53**, 996.

101 SURIN S.B., SOCRAWSKY S.S., SWEENEY E. & STOSSEL J.P. (1979) A neutrophil disorder induced by Capnocytophaga, a dental micro-organism. *New England Journal of Medicine*, **301**, 849.

102 MILLER M.E. (1975) Pathology of chemotaxis and random mobility. *Seminars in Hematology*, **12**, 59.

103 GOETZL E.J., WASSERMAN S.I., GIGLI I. & AUSTEN K.F. (1974) Enhancement of random migration and chemotactic response of human leucocytes by ascorbic acid. *Journal of Clinical Investigation*, **53**, 813.

104 HILL H.R., ESTENSEN R.D., QUIE P.G., HOGAN N.A. & GOLDBERG N.D. (1975) Modulation of human neutrophil chemotactic responses by cyclic $3'5'$ guanosine monophosphate and cyclic $3'5'$ adenosine monophosphate. *Metabolism*, **24**, 447.

105 AMENT M.E. & OCHS H.D. (1973) Gastrointestinal manifestations of chronic granulomatous disease. *New England Journal of Medicine*, **288**, 382.

106 KONTRAS S.B., BODENBENDER T.G., MCCLAVE C.R. & SMITH J.P. (1971) Interstitial cystitis in chronic granulomatous disease. *Journal of Urology (Baltimore)*, **105**, 575.

107 MARTYN L.J., LISCHNER H.W., PILEGGI A.J. & HARLEY R.D. (1972) Chorioretinal lesions in familial chronic granulomatous disease of childhood. *American Journal of Ophthalmology*, **73**, 403.

108 LANDING B.H. & SHIRKEY H.S. (1957) A syndrome of recurrent infection and infiltration of viscera by pigmented lipid histocytes. *Pediatrics*, **20**, 431.

109 DAVIS W.C., HUBER H., DOUGLAS S.D. & FUDENBERG H.H. (1968) A defect in circulating mononuclear phagocytes in chronic granulomatous disease of childhood. *Journal of Immunology*, **101**, 1093.

110 THOMPSON E.N. & SOOTHILL J.F. (1970) Chronic granulomatous disease; quantitative clinicopathological relationships. *Archives of Diseases in Childhood*, **45**, 24.

111 ESTERLY J.R., STURNER W.Q., ESTERLY N.B. & WINDHORST D.B. (1971) Disseminated BCG in twin boys with presumed chronic granulomatous disease of childhood. *Pediatrics*, **48**, 141.

112 ALEXANDER J.W. & GOOD R.A. (1968) Effect of antibiotics on the bactericidal activity of human leucocytes. *Journal of Laboratory and Clinical Medicine*, **71**, 971.

113 EZER G. & SOOTHILL J.F. (1974) Intracellular bactericidal effects of rifampicin in both normal and chronic granulomatous disease polymorphs. *Archives of Diseases in Childhood*, **49**, 463.

114 GIBLETT E.R., KLEBANOFF S.J., PINCUS S.H., SWANSON J., PARK B.H. & MCCULLOUGH J. (1971) Kell pheno-

types in chronic granulomatous disease; a potential transfusion hazard. *Lancet*, **i**, 1235.

115 MARSH W.L., OYEN R. & NICHOLS M.E. (1976) Kx antigen, the McLeod phenotype and chronic granulomatous disease. *Vox Sanguinis (Basel)*, **31**, 356.

116 HOLMES B., PAGE A.R. & GOOD R.A. (1967) Studies of the metabolic activity of leukocytes from patients with a genetic abnormality of phagocytic function. *Journal of Clinical Investigation*, **46**, 142.

117 CLINE M.J. & LEHRER R.I. (1969) D-amino acid oxidase in leukocytes; a possible D-amino acid-linked system. *Proceedings of the National Academy of Sciences, USA*, **62**, 756.

118 HOLMES B., PARK B.H., MALAWISTA S.E., QUIE P.G., NELSON D.L. & GOOD R.A. (1970) Chronic granulomatous disease in females. A deficiency of leukocyte glutathione peroxidase. *New England Journal of Medicine*, **283**, 217.

119 SEGAL A.W. & JONES O.T.G. (1980) Absence of cytochrome *b* reduction in stimulated neutrophils from both female and male patients with chronic granulomatous disease. *FEBS Letters*, **110**, 111.

121 JOHNSTON R.B., WILFERT C.M., BUCKLEY R.H., WEBB L.S., DE CHATELET L.R. & McCALL C.E. (1975) Enhanced bactericidal activity of phagocytes from patients with chronic granulomatous disease in the presence of sulphisoxazole. *Lancet*, **i**, 824.

122 GRIGNASCHI V.I., SPERPERATO A.M., ETCHEVERRY M.J. & MACARIOA J.L. (1963) Ma nuevo cuadro citoquimico; negatividad espontanea de las reacciones de peroxidasas, oxidasas y lipido en la progenic neutrofila y en los monocitos de dos hermanos. *Revista de la Asociación Paediatricia Argentina*, **77**, 218.

123 LEHRER R.J. & CLINE M.J. (1969) Leukocyte myeloperoxidase deficiency and disseminated candidiasis; the role of myeloperoxidase in resistance to Candida infection. *Journal of Clinical Investigation*, **48**, 1478.

124 ARMSTRONG D., DIMMITT S. & VAN WORMER D.E. (1974) Studies in Batten's disease. I. Peroxidase deficiency in granulocytes. *Archives of Neurology (Chicago)*, **30**, 144.

125 COOPER M.R., DE CHATELET L.R., McCALL C.E., LaVIA M.F., SPURR C.L. & BAEHNER R.L. (1972) Complete deficiency of leukocyte glucose-6-phosphate dehydrogenase with defective bactericidal activity. *Journal of Clinical Investigation*, **51**, 769.

126 MATSUDA I., OKA Y., TANIGUCHI N., FURUYAMA M., KODAMA S., ARASHIMA S. & MITSUYAMA T. (1976) Leukocyte glutathione peroxidase deficiency in a male patient with chronic granulomatous disease. *Journal of Pediatrics*, **88**, 581.

127 BURGE P.S., JOHNSON W.S. & HAYWARD A.R. (1976) Neutrophil pyruvate kinase deficiency with recurrent staphylococcal infections. First reported case. *British Medical Journal*, **i**, 742.

128 SEGER R., WILDFEUER A., BUCHINGER G., ROMEN W., CATTY D., DYBAS L., HAFERKAMP O. & STRODER J. (1976) Defects in granulocyte function in various chromosomal abnormalities. *Klinische Wochenschrift*, **54**, 177.

129 HARVATH L. & ANDERSEN B.R. (1979) Defective initiation of oxidative metabolism in polymorphonuclear leucocytes. *New England Journal of Medicine*, **300**, 1130.

130 MILLER M.E. (1971) Chemotactic function in the human neonate; humoral and cellular aspects. *Pediatric Research*, **5**, 487.

131 CHANDRA R.K., CHANDRA S. & GHAI O.P. (1976) Chemotaxis, random mobility and mobilization of polymorphonuclear leucocytes in malnutrition. *Journal of Clinical Pathology*, **29**, 224.

132 SCHOPFER K. & DOUGLAS S.K. (1976) Neutrophil function in children with kwashiorkor. *Journal of Laboratory and Clinical Medicine*, **88**, 450.

133 MOWAT A.G. & BAUM J. (1971a) Polymorphonuclear leucocyte chemotaxis in patients with bacterial infections. *British Medical Journal*, **iii**, 617.

134 BRUCE D.L. (1966) Effect of Halothane anaesthesia on extravascular mobilization of neutrophils. *Journal of Cellular Physiology*, **68**, 81.

135 ALEXANDER J.W. & WIXSON D. (1970) Neutrophil dysfunction and sepsis in burn injury. *Surgery, Gynecology and Obstetrics*, **130**, 431.

136 MOWAT A.G. & BAUM J. (1971) Chemotaxis of polymorphonuclear leucocytes from patients with diabetes mellitus. *New England Journal of Medicine*, **284**, 621.

137 BAUM J., CESTERO R.V.M. & FREEMAN R.B. (1975) Chemotaxis of the polymorphonuclear leukocytes and delayed hypersensitivity in uraemia. *Kidney International*, **7**, (Suppl.), 147.

138 HENDERSON L.W., MILLER M.E., HAMILTON R.W. & NORMAN M.E. (1975) Haemodialysis leukopenia and polymorph random mobility. A possible correlation. *Journal of Laboratory and Clinical Medicine*, **85**, 191.

139 BINDER V. & RIIS P. (1977) Leucocyte chemotactic function in patients with ulcerative colitis. *Scandinavian Journal of Gastroenteritis*, **12**, 141.

140 MOWAT A.G. & BAUM J. (1971) Chemotaxis of polymorphonuclear leukocytes from patients with rheumatoid arthritis. *Journal of Clinical Investigation*, **50**, 2541.

141 COEN R., GRUSH O. & KAUDER E. (1969) Studies of bactericidal activity and metabolism of the leukocyte in full-term neonates. *Journal of Pediatrics*, **75**, 400.

142 SETH V. & CHANDRA R.K. (1972) Opsonic activity, phagocytosis and bactericidal capacity of polymorphs in undernutrition. *Archives of Diseases in Childhood*, **47**, 282.

143 KOSTINA V.V. & KUDRYASHOVA K.I. (1968) Changes of the functional activity of phagocytes in protracted and chronic pneumonia. *Zhurnal microbiologii, épidemiologii i immunobiologii*, **11**, 59.

144 CHANDRA R.A. (1973) Reduced bactericidal capacity of polymorphs in iron deficiency. *Archives of Diseases in Childhood*, **48**, 864.

145 ALTMAN L.C., FURUKAWA C.T. & KLEBANOFF S.J. (1977) Defective polymorphonuclear leukocyte (PMN) function in thermally injured patients. *Clinical Research*, **25**, 117a.

146 BAEHNER R.L., NEWBURGER R.G., JOHNSON D.E. & MURRMANN S.M. (1973) Transient bactericidal defect of peripheral blood phagocytes from children with acute lymphoblastic leukemia receiving craniospinal irradiation. *New England Journal of Medicine*, **289**, 1209.

147 QUESENBERRY P. & LEVITT L. (1979) Hematopoietic stem cells. *New England Journal of Medicine*, **301**, 755.

148 LICHTMAN M.A. (1970) Cellular deformability during maturation of the myeloblast. Possible role in marrow egress. *New England Journal of Medicine*, **283**, 943.

149 ZIGMOND S.H. (1977) Ability of polymophonuclear leukocytes to orientate in gradients of chemotactic factors. *Journal of Cellular Biology*, **75,** 606.

150 MacGREGOR R.R., SPAGNUOLO P.J. & LENTNEK A.L. (1974) Inhibition of granulocyte adherence by ethanol, prednisone, and aspirin measured with an assay system. *New England Journal of Medicine*, **291,** 642.

151 MORETTA L., FERRARINI M., MINGARI K.C., MORETTA A. & WEBB S.R. (1976) Subpopulations of human T cells identified by receptors for immunoglobulins and nitrogen responsiveness. *Journal of Immunology*, **117,** 2171.

152 STOSSEL T.P. (1974) Phagocytosis. *New England Journal of Medicine*, **290,** 717.

153 SEGAL A.W., DORLING J. & COADE S. (1980) Kinetics of fusion of the cytoplasmic granules with phagocytic vacuoles in human polymorphonuclear leukocytes. Biochemical and morphological studies. *Journal of Cellular Biology*, **84,** 42.

154 WISEMAN G., SMOLEN J.E. & KORCHAK H.M. (1980) Release of inflammatory mediators from stimulated neutrophils. *New England Journal of Medicine*, **303,** 27.

155 ROOT R.K., METCALF J., OSHINO N. & CHANCE B. (1975) H_2O_2 release from human granulocytes during phagocytosis. I. Documentation, quantitation and some regulating factors. *Journal of Clinical Investigation*, **55,** 945.

156 ALLEN R.C., STJERNHOLM R.L. & STEELE R.H. (1972) Evidence for the generation of an electronic excitation state (s) in human polymorphonuclear leukocytes and its participation in bactericidal activity. *Biochemical and Biophysical Research Communications*, **47,** 679.

157 KLEBANOFF S.J. & WHITE L.R. (1969) Iodination defect in the leukocytes of a patient with chronic granulomatous disease of childhood. *New England Journal of Medicine*, **280,** 460.

158 PARK B.H., FIKRIG S.M. & SMITHWICK E.M. (1968) Infection and nitroblue-tetrazolium reduction by neutrophils. *Lancet*, **ii,** 532.

159 OCHS H.D. & IGO R.P. (1973) The NBT slide test. A simple screening method for detecting chronic granulomatous disease and female carriers. *Journal of Pediatrics*, **83,** 77.

160 COHN Z.A. (1963) The fate of bacteria within phagocytic cells. I. The degradation of isotopically labelled bacteria by polymorphonuclear leukocytes and macrophages. *Journal of Experimental Medicine*, **117,** 27.

161 HAYWARD A.R. Immunodeficiency. In: *Paediatric Clinical Immunology* (ed. Soothill J.F., Hayward A.R. & Wood C.B.S.). Blackwell Scientific Publications, London. (In press).

162 NEWBURGER P.E., COHEN H.J., ROTHSCHILD S.B., HOBBINS J.C., MALAWISTA S.E. & MAHONEY M.J. (1979) Prenatal diagnosis of chronic granulomatous disease. *New England Journal of Medicine*, **300,** 178.

Chapter 17
The lymphocytes: formation and function

I. C. M. MacLENNAN

During the last few years, knowledge of lymphoid cells has increased greatly. Identification of many functional types of lymphocyte has proceeded in parallel with advances in understanding of the way in which these interact to provide the basis for specific protective immunity. Studies of normal lymphocytes have gone hand in hand with investigation of lymphocytes in disease. This has now provided a rational basis for the classification of non-Hodgkin's lymphoma and leukaemia, identification of the cellular basis of immunodeficiency, and a more realistic approach to the understanding of inflammatory diseases with autoimmune phenomena. In a number of instances pathological description has pointed to subsequent physiological advance. Analysis of the characteristics of neoplastic cells in acute leukaemia provides an outstanding example of this pattern. Apart from recognition of lymphocyte subsets, there has been great progress in understanding of the regulation of immune responses. It has been realized that self-recognition plays an integral part in antigen recognition. Genetic aspects of individual variation in immune responsiveness have been probed and the genetic basis of immunological specificity is now beginning to be revealed. In this chapter the different types of lymphocyte will be classified systematically, the basis of immunological specificity will be discussed, and repeated reference will be made to the function of the immune system as a whole.

Morphological heterogeneity of lymphocytes
Blood films made from healthy donors show three broad types of mononuclear cell: small and large lymphocytes, and mononuclear phagocytes. Although it is common experience that there is morphological heterogeneity within the two groups of lymphocyte, these differences in general have failed to indicate clear differences in function. Also, small and large lymphocytes are not distinct classes of lymphocyte in the sense of being either T or B. Size is rather a reflection of state of activity and stage of differentiation. This is illustrated in Figure 17.1, in which large lymphocytes are seen to be in a state of mitotic activity, for they have

taken up tritiated thymidine *in vitro*. These large cells have arisen from small lymphocytes which have been activated by antigen. It is impossible to tell on simple morphological grounds if the large cells in Figure 17.1 are T or B blasts. Even transmission and scanning electron microscopy would not have been able to make this distinction reliably.

Heterogeneity of antigen reactivity of lymphocytes
Specific immune responses depend on recognition systems associated with lymphocytes. Current evidence strongly supports the concept that each lymphocyte is able to recognize only one antigenic structure. Also, in general, and possibly always, when a lymphocyte divides, its progeny recognize the same antigenic determinants as their parent. In other words the vast repertoire of antigens which can give rise to specific immune responses is matched by an equally large number of clones of lymphocytes, each of which can only recognize one antigenic structure.

Functional heterogeneity in lymphocytes
There are several different functional classes of lymphocyte (Table 17.1). The most easily defined of these is the *B-cell series* of antibody-producing cells and their precursors. This series also includes the poorly understood group of cells which comprise the main lymphocyte component of germinal centres. The second major class of lymphocytes is functionally highly diverse: these are the cells of the *T-cell series*. They derive their name from their relative, and in some cases absolute, requirement for the thymus in their development. The T-cell series includes:
1 lymphocytes which assist in the initiation of immune responses, known as helper cells;
2 lymphocytes which limit immune responses, referred to as suppressor cells; and
3 lymphocytes with effector functions, including cytolytic T cells.

There is a close interplay between T cells and macrophages: a number of T-cell-derived factors have been described which are able to activate macrophages for effector functions. Macrophages are also thought

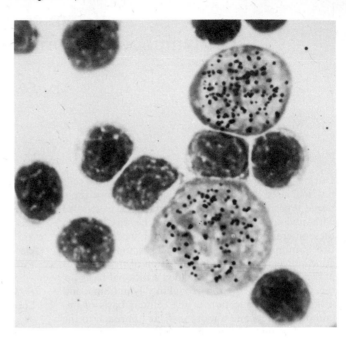

Fig. 17.1. Autoradiograph of rat thoracic-duct lymphocytes which had been incubated for one hour *in vitro* with [³H]thymidine. The nuclei of the two large lymphocytes are heavily labelled; the small lymphocytes are unlabelled. This typical field underlines the different rates of proliferation of large and small lymphocytes (× 2250). From Ref. 1, by permission of the author and publishers.

to play an important role in antigen presentation, and this function in turn may be regulated by T cells. A third group of lymphocytes has now been defined which has cytolytic capacity. These cells, which are known as *K cells*, do not kill targets by the direct recognition of antigens on their surface. They are triggered to kill by IgG-antibody bound to target-cell antigens. In this chapter the origins, distribution and functional diversity of the B-lymphocyte series will be considered first.

CLASSIFICATION OF FUNCTIONAL TYPES OF LYMPHOCYTE

The B-cell series

Definition of B cells
(Fig. 17.2)
The B cells are characterized by their capacity to synthesize immunoglobulin. The immunoglobulin which is produced may be confined to the cytoplasm,

Table 17.1. Functional types of lymphocyte

B-cell series:
Antibody-secreting cells and their precursors.
The major lymphocytic component of germinal centres are also B cells.

T-cell series:
(a) Regulator cells
    (1) T helper cells (i.e. cells which assist the activation of other lymphocytes by antigen).
    (2) T suppressor cells (i.e. cells which inhibit the activation of other lymphocytes by antigen).
(b) Effector cells
    (1) Cytolytic T cells.
    (2) Cells producing factors (not antibody) which either have direct mediator function or activate certain macrophages to
        effector functions.

K cells:
Lymphocytes which kill cells via IgG antibody bound to the surface of the victim.

NK cells:
Cells which show spontaneous cytolytic activity against certain types of abnormal cell, particularly transformed culture cell lines.

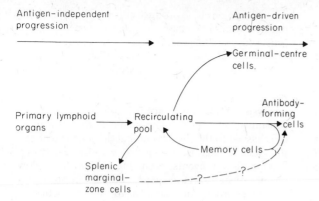

Fig. 17.2. A summary of the antigen-dependent and antigen-independent stages of B-cell maturation. Details of the different stages of maturation are given in the text.

expressed as surface-membrane immunoglobulin or secreted. It should be noted that many non-B cells have receptors which enable them to bind exogenous immunoglobulin in the form of aggregate or immune complex. These are found on monocytes [2, 3], some T cells [4], K cells [5] and B cells themselves [6].

B-cell development in primary lymphoid organs
The primary lymphoid organs in the case of the B-cell series are fetal liver, fetal spleen, and adult and fetal bone marrow. The first cells which are seen to produce immunoglobulin components are found in mouse fetal liver as early as 11 days post-conception [7]. At this stage the immunoglobulin is in the form of μ heavy chains without associated light chains. The μ chains are not expressed on the cell surface but are found in low concentrations in the cytoplasm. These cells are termed pre-B cells. This terminology was adopted as, historically, the earliest representative of the B-cell series was thought to have surface-membrane immunoglobulin. By the 13th day of fetal life in mice [8] and at nine weeks in the case of the human fetus [9], B

cells with surface membrane IgM appear in fetal liver. The surface-membrane IgM molecules have both heavy and light chains. This IgM is in monomeric form with paired heavy chains and light chains and two antigen-binding sites per molecule. IgM found in body fluids, on the other hand, is mainly in pentameric form, with 10 antigen-binding sites per molecule. Both pre-B cells and B cells are found in adult bone marrow. Studies in adult mice have shown that the pre-B cells are rapidly dividing while the B cells are not. When bone-marrow cells are labelled by infusion of tritiated thymidine into mice, 80% of pre-B cells are seen to have incorporated label into their DNA by 24 hours; B cells are unlabelled at this stage [10] (Fig. 17.3). If, however, the animals are examined at 48 and 72 hours after a one-day pulse of tritiated thymidine, many labelled B cells are seen. Experiments of this sort have been taken to indicate that a rapidly dividing precursor population (pre-B cells) is giving rise to non-dividing B cells [10, 11]. This, though indirect, is still probably the most convincing evidence that pre-B cells expressing cytoplasmic μ chains give rise to B cells.

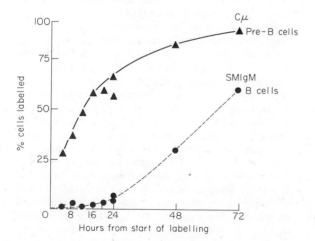

Fig. 17.3. Adult mouse bone-marrow cells were taken at various times after pulse labelling *in vivo* with tritiated thymidine. Labelled cells can be assumed to have gone through S phase during the period of pulse labelling. The experiment suggests:
1 that pre-B cells are showing rapid mitotic activity; and
2 that B cells are not in active mitosis but that over half the B cells in marrow have gone through S phase within the previous three days. Data derived from Ref. 10 by kind permission of Professor J. J. T. Owen.

Expression of surface-membrane immunoglobulin on B cells

Surface-membrane immunoglobulin provides B cells with their antigen-recognition receptors. Studies on cloned B-cell lines and neoplastic B cells strongly suggest that B cells are committed to produce immunoglobulin with a single antigen-binding structure (idiotype) [12]. This commitment appears to have been made by the time that B cells first synthesize immunoglobulin. As well as showing commitment in respect of antigen-recognizing capacity, B-cell clones are also committed to produce immunoglobulin with a single type of light chain, i.e. kappa or lambda, but not both [13]. Conversely, single B cells often produce immunoglobulin with more than one heavy-chain class [13, 14]. For example, B cells with both IgM and IgD on their surface are seen more often in blood than B cells with only one class of surface-membrane immunoglobulin.

Genetic aspects of immunoglobulin expression

The precise way in which the antigen-binding sequences of immunoglobulin heavy and light chains are generated is still not known. However, the reader may find it helpful to consider at this stage the genetic coding for immunoglobulins. It is known that there are three quite separate gene clusters in the genome which are concerned with coding for immunoglobulin variable regions. These gene clusters are linked respectively to the genes coding for heavy-chain constant regions, λ-light-chain constant region and κ-light-chain constant region (Fig. 17.4). Hybrid-DNA technology has shown that by the time B cells have started to produce immunoglobulin there is sorting and selection within the V region, so that a DNA sequence coding for a particular antigen-combining structure is selected. Within one clone of B cells it is clear that only one of the light-chain gene clusters is activated to the extent of giving rise to an RNA message in the cytoplasm, i.e.

   (1) κ-light-chain gene cluster:
       Variable κ——Constant κ
       Variable κ'——Constant κ'
   (2) λ-light-chain gene cluster:
       Variable λ——Constant λ
       Variable λ'——Constant λ'
   (3) Heavy-chain gene cluster:
       Variable heavy——Constant heavy
       Variable heavy'——Constant heavy'

Fig. 17.4. The three immunoglobulin gene clusters. B-cell clones produce light chains coded for by only one of the four chromosomes coding for light chains, i.e. κ, κ', λ or λ', and heavy chains coded for by one of the two chromosomes with genetic material coding for heavy chains, i.e. H or H'. This gives eight possible combinations: κH, κH', κ'H, κ'H', λH, λH', λ'H, λ'H', which can be used to code for immunoglobulins.

cells of a single clone produce either κ or λ light chains but not both. The heavy-chain gene cluster is always activated, but B-cell clones are not committed to the expression of one class of heavy chains. There is evidence that some antibody-secreting cells have lost DNA coding for some of the heavy-chain classes. This particularly applies to cells secreting γ or α chains. Analysis of the sequence of loss of heavy-chain constant-region gene material in antibody-secreting cells has led to the suggestion that the gene sequence in this gene cluster is: VH–μ–δ–γ–α–ε. Extremely rare recombination events occurring within the heavy-chain constant-region gene complex confirm this sequence order. In addition to the restriction of expression of B-cell clones to one light-chain class, the message coding for immunoglobulin structure is produced from only one of the paired chromosomes, i.e. immunoglobulin synthesis by a B-cell clone is allelically restricted. A concise and clear review of the organization and expression of immunoglobulin genes has been written by Adams [15].

Antigen-independent dispersal of B cells

Cells with surface-membrane immunoglobulin leave the bone marrow and other primary sites of B-cell development as immunologically competent small lymphocytes. The majority of these cells then enter a phase of constant non-random migration through the various lymphoid organs. Other virgin B cells, however, form a non-migrating B-cell sub-set which is located in the marginal zones of the splenic white pulp [16] (Fig. 17.14).

B-cell recirculation. The repeated migration of lymphocytes between secondary lymphoid organs and the blood is termed recirculation (reviewed in Ref. 17) (Fig. 17.5). Secondary lymphoid organs in this context are the spleen, lymph nodes, bone marrow and gut-associated lymphoid tissue (GALT). The GALT includes the tonsils and other components of Waldeyer's ring, appendix, Peyer's patches and numerous tiny accumulations of small lymphocytes found in the lamina propria along the length of the gut. In addition there is a small but significant traffic into the general tissues of the body. Tissue lymphocyte migration may be markedly increased in certain diseases: for example, the synovium takes on the appearance and organization of a secondary lymphoid organ in rheumatoid arthritis, and similar secondary lymphoid-tissue organization may be seen in the thyroid in Hashimoto's disease. Some lymphocytes leave the blood for the general tissues through capillaries and subsequently migrate to lymph nodes via afferent lymphatics. The majority of small lymphocytes entering lymph nodes and the GALT, however, come

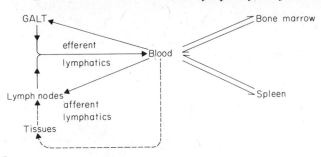

Fig. 17.5. Diagrammatic representation of the recirculation pathways of lymphocytes. Lines to and from the tissues are shown interrupted, to indicate that around 90% of lymphocytes arriving in lymph nodes do so by passing directly from the blood through the walls of high endothelial venules in the paracortex of the nodes. GALT = gut-associated lymphoid tissue.

directly from the blood via specialized venules with characteristic high endothelium. Return to the blood from these tissues is via the efferent lymphatic system. Lymphocyte migration to the spleen and bone marrow is directly from the blood and return is directly into the blood. Approximately five per cent of the body's lymphocytes are in the blood at any one time and the proportions of these cells migrating into the secondary lymphoid organs is approximately 45% to spleen, 35% to lymph nodes and GALT, 10% to the bone marrow and 10% to the other tissues. About 24–36 hours elapses between the time that B cells leave the blood for secondary lymphoid tissues and their return to the blood. The passage through the secondary lymphoid tissues is complex and will be considered later in conjunction with T-cell migration when the structure of lymphoid tissues is described. If one interrupts the recirculation cycle at any one point, for example by thoracic-duct drainage or placing a β-emitting ^{32}P-impregnated strip on the spleen, recirculating lymphocyte numbers diminish in all secondary lymphoid tissues [18]. Experiments of this sort indicate that the majority of recirculating B cells are not committed to visiting one type or regional group of secondary lymphoid tissues. On the other hand, alternative experiments, which compare migration of labelled B cells taken from various lymphoid organs, indicate that there may be relative if not absolute preference for lymphocyte migration through a particular type of lymphoid tissue. For discussion see Ref. 17.

Antigen-dependent B-cell maturation
(Fig. 17.6)
The life history of B cells which has been described so far relates to maturation which occurs in the absence of antigenic stimulus. Peripheral virgin B lymphocytes are poised to respond, by proliferation and further differentiation, to antigen presented in an appropriate way. The conditions which are required for antigenic stimulation are complex and will be considered later. At this stage it suffices to describe the events which occur following successful antigenic stimulation. Activation of B cells by antigen mainly occurs in secondary lymphoid tissues. It is clear that there is a phase immediately following encounter with antigen when B cells are selectively retained at the site of antigenic stimulation [19]. This retention lasts for a period of up to three days, after which the stimulated B cells leave the small-lymphocyte zones of the secondary lymphoid tissues and migrate via blood and/or lymph to sites of antibody production. The main sites of antibody production are normally the lamina propria of the gut, the bone marrow, the medulla of lymph nodes, the red pulp of the spleen, the bronchial mucosa, serous cavities such as the peritoneal space and some

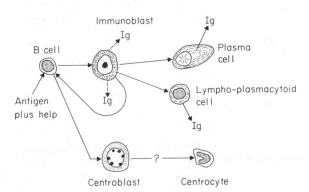

Fig. 17.6. Pathways of antigen-driven maturation of B cells. Ig indicates secreted immunoglobulin. The progression of centroblast to centrocyte is not established. However, the appearance of centroblasts in germinal centres does precede that of centrocytes by several days. The return line from immunoblast to small B cell indicates memory-B-cell formation.

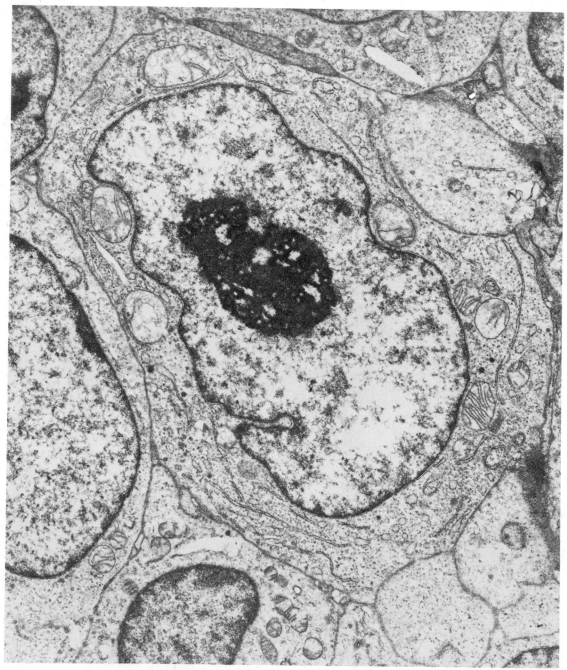

Fig. 17.7. Electron micrograph of an immunoblast from a patient with an immunoblastoma of gut origin (× 11 850). Although this is a neoplastic immunoblast it shows all the features of normal immunoblasts described in the text. (Courtesy of Dr E. L. Jones.)

sites of chronic inflammation. Activated B cells are morphologically distinct from small B lymphocytes (Fig. 17.1): they are large lymphoid cells, and are in mitotic cycle; they characteristically have a central nucleus with a single large nucleolus; their pyroninophilic cytoplasm is accounted for by the high density of single and polyribosomes; endoplasmic reticulum is not prominent (Fig. 17.7). Some of these cells can be shown to be actively secreting antibody [20]. The term for these cells preferred by the author is *immunoblast* rather than lymphoblast, which has sometimes been used, but is now firmly associated with early lymphocytes which are dividing under antigen-independent control. This preferred terminology fits in with current nomenclature for B-cell neoplasia [21]. It should be noted that on morphological grounds there is no clear difference between B and T immunoblasts. The migration of immunoblasts is far from random (reviewed in Ref. 22).

Antigenic stimulation in a lymph node results first in localized production of cells in the medulla of that node. Immunoblasts pass into the efferent lymph via the major lymphoid channels and blood and then localize to sites of antibody production adjacent to the site of antigenic stimulation. For example, immunoblasts from mesenteric lymph nodes preferentially migrate to the lamina propria of the gut, while splenic immunoblasts home to the splenic red pulp, though they also migrate in substantial numbers to bone marrow after secondary immunization [23].

Antibody-secreting cells. Although immunoblasts are capable of secreting some antibody, they are not in themselves thought to be end cells. After they have completed their journey they undergo metamorphosis into specialized antibody-secreting cells. Two forms of differentiated antibody-secreting cell are recognized. One of these is little larger than a small lymphocyte and can easily be overlooked in conventional haematoxylin and eosin sections: the nucleus is central and not clearly distinguishable from that of other small lymphocytes, but the scanty cytoplasm is strongly pyroninophilic and contains abundant endoplasmic reticulum; immuno-enzymatic techniques can easily demonstrate the cytoplasmic immunoglobulin in these cells. Small antibody-secreting cells of this sort are termed *lymphoplasmacytoid cells*. They can be found physiologically in lymph nodes and Askenazy nodules of bone marrow and associated with small lymphocytes in the GALT. Tumours of these cells are frequently associated with macroglobulinaemia but may produce other classes of immunoglobulin and may even be non-secreting [24]. Not all such tumours are pure lymphoplasmacytoid cells: sometimes monoclonal collections of lymphoplasmacytoid cells,

plasma cells, immunoblasts and intermediate forms are seen. The author has also seen two cases of myelomatosis in which islands of lymphoplasmacytoid cells were seen in a marrow where ipsiclonal plasma cells were scattered throughout normal myelopoietic tissues. Tumours of lymphoplasmacytoid cells are sometimes termed immunocytomas [21], although of course lymphoplasmacytoid cells are only one of the products of immunoblasts.

The second and more familiar type of antibody-secreting cell is the *plasma cell* (Fig. 17.8). These cells are much larger than small lymphocytes. The nucleus is eccentric with characteristic radial condensations of chromatin. The abundant cytoplasm is filled with extensive endoplasmic reticulum and the Golgi apparatus is prominent. The staining reaction of the cytoplasm is characteristically basophilic and pyroninophilic. As with lymphoplasmacytoid cells, immunohistological techniques can easily pick up cytoplasmic immunoglobulin (Fig. 17.9).

Antibody-forming cells are generally short-lived. In rodents, if immunoblasts are transferred without antigen to non-immune syngeneic recipients, the resulting plasma cells are detectable only for four to five days [25].

Memory B cells. A small proportion of immunoblasts isolated from the thoracic duct of animals can be shown to revert to small recirculating lymphocytes [26]. It seems reasonable to suppose that these cells represent an augmented pool of cells which will be able to bring about a more rapid immune response on secondary challenge with antigen.

Germinal-centre cells. Formation of germinal centres is highly dependent upon antigenic stimulation. They are absent in laboratory animals kept in germ-free conditions from birth [27]. However, around four days after antigenic challenge, when antibody formation has already started, foci of large pyroninophilic cells appear within follicles in the cortex of lymph nodes [28]. These are rapidly dividing cells and have B-cell surface characteristics. Over the next few days the number of cells in these foci increases. After the first week or so, smaller cells with characteristically irregular nuclear outline appear. These cells also have B-cell markers. Gradually, over a period of weeks, the germinal centres wane. The large B cells of germinal centres (*centroblasts*) characteristically have a large pale nucleus which contains several small nucleoli distributed near the nuclear membrane. The cytoplasm is evenly dispersed around the nucleus and contains abundant single ribosomes. Mitoses are frequently seen in these cells and cell kinetic studies indicate that over half the cells go through S phase every three

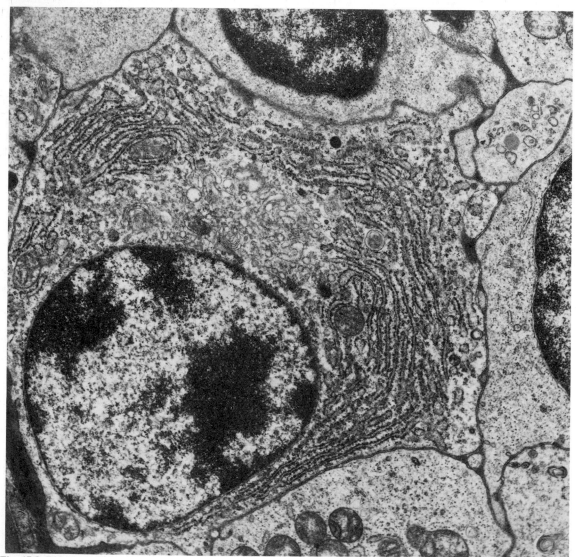

Fig. 17.8. Electron micrograph of a plasma cell from the medulla of an axillary lymph node. Note the eccentric nucleus with characteristic irregular condensations of chromatin. The cytoplasm is filled with endoplasmic reticulum which does not, however, extend into the Golgi region which is also prominent. (Courtesy of Dr E. L. Jones.)

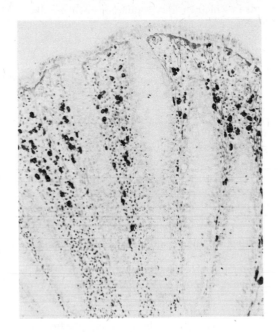

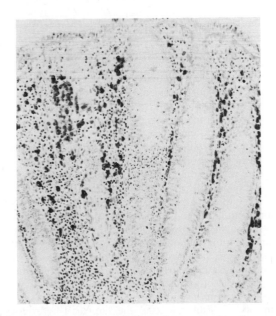

Fig. 17.9. Two serial 4 μm-thick sections stained by the PAP technique to reveal plasma cells containing either (a) κ light chains or (b) λ light chains. The sections are taken from a patient with chronic lymphocytic leukaemia and show normal numbers of plasma cells (large dark dots) in the lamina propria [24]. The small dark dots are the nuclei of small lymphocytes stained by the haematoxylin, which are present in abnormally high numbers.

hours. The small B cells from germinal centres (*centrocytes*), by contrast, are not dividing. The chromatin in their nucleus is relatively condensed while the cytoplasm is not strikingly pyroninophilic. Indirect evidence indicates that germinal-centre B cells are derived from the recirculating pool of small lymphocytes. However, it is by no means clear that centrocytes are the ultimate progeny of centroblasts. The function of germinal-centre B cells is still unknown. On the other hand, cells which resemble germinal-centre cells morphologically give rise to the single most common group of B-cell neoplasms, the follicle-centre cell tumours. Further discussion of germinal centres and their role in antigen presentation appears in the section on the structure of secondary lymphoid tissue (see pp. 661–3).

The T-cell series

Definition of T cells

The T cells are theoretically defined as cells which depend upon the thymus for their development. In practice, thymus dependency has often proved difficult to establish and evidence that a cell is of T-cell origin frequently has to be based upon surface-marker taxonomy. As a reasonable compromise the following definition may therefore be adopted for human T cells: T cells are non-B lymphocytes which share phenotypic characteristics with cells which require the thymus for their development. This must clearly be an interim definition, but it has the advantage of being honest and workable. In man, T cells by this definition are cells which form spontaneous rosettes with sheep red blood cells [29], and in mice, lymphocytes which bear the antigen Thy 1 or θ [30].

The origins of T cells

The thymus develops from fusion of tissue from ectoderm of the third and fourth branchial clefts and endoderm of the corresponding pharyngeal pouches. The fused tissues from both sides of the neck subsequently descend to their anterior and superior mediastinal position where they form the two distinct lobes of the thymus. The branchial-arch tissue forms the thymic stroma but does not give rise to lymphocytes. The lymphocytes migrate to the thymus during fetal life from the primary lymphoid organs which also give rise to B cells, namely the fetal liver, the bone marrow and the spleen. Cells capable of populating the thymus are also found in adult mouse bone marrow [31]. There is little in the way of direct evidence that T-cell commitment occurs before arrival in the thymus; indeed le Douarin [31a] has shown that in birds, primitive lymphocytes which have already migrated to the thymus can be induced to enter the bursa (primary B-cell organ of birds) and develop into B cells. The evidence put forward for pre-T cells in mammals is based upon the finding of cells with T-associated markers in fetal liver.

Lymphocytes in the thymus are classified by their location either in the cortex or the medulla. Cortical thymocytes are rapidly dividing cells and are highly sensitive, at least in rodents, to lysis by corticosteroids [32]. Their surface bears very little HLA-A, B or C locus-coded antigen, but antigens which are not associated with normal peripheral T cells are present. About 85% of thymic lymphocytes in young mammals, including man [33], are cortical thymocytes. The remaining 15% of thymocytes are located in the medulla: these cells are cortisone-resistant, possess HLA-A, B and C locus-coded antigens and are not rapidly dividing; they resemble peripheral T cells in their functional properties. The relation between cortical and medullary thymocytes is not clearly defined. It is tempting to conclude that the rapidly dividing cortical cells either die *in situ* or give rise to medullary cells which then leave the thymus as peripheral T cells. This sequence of events is simple and easy to understand, but repeated attempts to provide formal confirmation indicate that the system is far from fully understood. It seems likely that about 90% of cells generated in the thymic cortex die *in situ* [31].

CONCEPT OF THYMUS DEPENDENCY

T cells and regulation of immune responses
Observations by Miller [34, 35] and Parrott [36] show that neonatal thymectomy in mice gives rise after weaning to abnormal susceptibility to certain infections, deficient growth, defective allograft rejection and impaired capacity to mount effective antibody responses against certain antigens. These effects can be reversed by passive transfer of adult syngeneic lymphocytes [38]. Such observations gave rise to the concept of the thymus dependency of certain aspects of the immune system in rodents. It should be mentioned that early fetal thymectomy and depletion of residual lymphocytes with anti-lymphocyte serum fail to produce marked immunodeficiency in sheep [39]. Similarly, thymus dependency as defined in murine systems is not clearly established in man. Congenital thymic aplasia, as manifest in Di George's syndrome for example, gives rise to incomplete and frequently transient deficiency of immunological competence [40]. Despite these cautionary notes on thymus dependency in man, it is clear that humans possess a major population of lymphoid cells which are not B cells and which can be shown, at least *in vitro*, to function in a similar way to thymus-dependent cells of rodents.

T helper function. Claman *et al.* [41] described experiments in which various populations of lymphoid cells were used to reconstitute immune responsiveness in lethally irradiated mice. They found that immune responses to sheep red blood cells were poor in mice receiving either bone-marrow cells or thymocytes. However, mice which had received cells from both these sources responded to the antigen. Reconstitution experiments with spleen cells alone resulted in good restoration of the recipient's capacity to mount an immune response against sheep erythrocytes. It seemed likely from these experiments that two populations of cells were required to produce an antibody response against sheep red cells. One of these was found in the thymus, the other in bone marrow, while both cell types were found in the spleen. This sort of experiment was found to apply to many other antigens. However, some antigens were found to be capable of inducing normal antibody responses in the absence of the thymic component [42]. As a result of these experiments it became clear that there were both thymus-dependent and thymus-independent antigens with respect to antibody responses. Further analysis of the cellular aspects of antibody production confirmed that in no case were the antibody-producing cells derived from the thymus. Antibody production was a property of cells with surface-membrane immunoglobulin which were derived from the bone marrow and were found in the secondary lymphoid tissues, as described in the previous section. The thymus-dependent component was seen to provide a specific helper effect. Mitchison [43] analysed the nature of this effect using compound antigens. It had been known for many years that certain small chemical determinants, which are not in themselves antigenic, can become so if linked to protein-carrier molecules; such chemical determinants are commonly referred to as haptens. Clinically important haptens are skin-sensitizing agents such as dinitrochlorobenzene. Ovary & Benacerraf [44] had shown that if an animal is immunized with a hapten–carrier conjugate, then secondary exposure to that hapten on a different carrier will not result in an augmented secondary immune response but a further primary immune response. Challenge with the hapten on the same carrier molecule gives a full secondary immune response, characterized by a more rapid onset of antibody production, more prolonged antibody response and higher peak levels of serum antibody. Mitchison used the hapten 4-hydroxy-5-iodo-3-nitrophenoacetyl (NIP) linked to either ovalbumin or bovine serum albumin. He immunized mice with NIP–ovalbumin and then used the spleen cells from these mice to reconstitute lethally irradiated syngeneic mice. These recipient mice produced secondary-type anti-NIP responses if subsequently immunized with NIP–ovalbumin, but only mounted a primary response to NIP–bovine-serum-albumin. However, if the recipients were also given spleen cells from mice immunized with bovine serum albumin in the absence of NIP, they then produced a secondary anti-NIP immune response to NIP–bovine-serum-albumin (Fig. 17.10). The inference from these experiments was that helper cells recognizing bovine serum albumin had cooperated with memory B cells which had specificity for NIP. This interpretation received strong support when Raff [45] showed that the carrier-specific cells in experiments of this sort bore the surface antigen Thy-1 or θ which is found on thymus-dependent cells but not B cells in mice.

The existence of thymus-dependent helper cells is now firmly established. The use of systems which induce primary immune responses *in vitro* [46, 47] has greatly facilitated analyses of the cellular components involved in the triggering of B cells. Mosier and his colleagues [48, 49] were among the first to show that cooperation between I and B cells could be demonstrated *in vitro*, and that in addition macrophages were important ancillary cells in the induction reaction. Cooper & Lawton [50] showed that it was possible to study the differentiation of human blood B cells to antibody-forming cells in tissue culture. Their system involved the use of the lectin pokeweed mitogen, which is able to induce polyclonal differentiation of B cells to antibody-forming cells. However, activation of B cells

by this mitogen is in turn dependent on T help [51]. More recently, specific immune responses *in vitro* have been described using human blood lymphocytes [52, 53]. T help has not only been shown to be of importance in the triggering of B-cell responses but has been shown to have an equally important role in triggering effector T cells [54] and suppressor T cells [55, 56].

T-cell help: a function of a distinct subset of T cells. Helper T cells have been shown to be a distinct subset of T cells, distinguishable by a number of criteria from T effector cells or T suppressor cells. Apart from experiments showing functional dissociation of the appearance of the different types of T cells, surface properties of these cells allow them to be at least partially separated. This was first achieved in mice when it was shown that the Ly alloantigens could reveal functional subsets of T cells. Peripheral T cells bearing the Ly 1.2 antigen only were associated with helper properties, while those also bearing Ly 2.2 and Ly 3.2 had suppressor or cytotoxic functions [57]. These distinctions made on the basis of surface-marker expression are helpful, but identification by such means cannot be taken as absolute. More recently the development of techniques for making continuous hybrid clones of antibody-producing cells [58] has yielded antibodies which have the ability to identify a

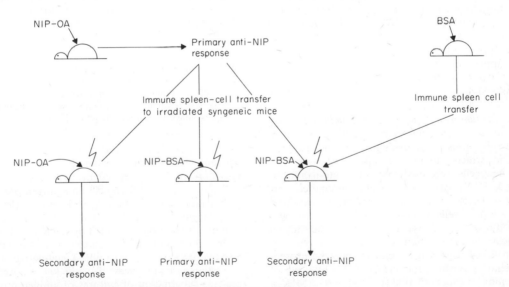

Fig. 17.10. A summary of Mitchison's [43] classical experiment showing:
1 that T help can be provided by cells recognizing antigenic determinants on carrier molecules in responses against haptens attached to those carriers;
2 that T-cell memory in this situation can be generated in the absence of hapten; and
3 that T-cell help is carrier-specific.
OA, ovalbumin; BSA, bovine serum albumin; ⚡, lethal total body irradiation given to destroy recipient's immune capacity.

large number of surface antigens in other species including man. Some of these seem able to identify T-cell subsets and are already commercially available. Among the best characterized of these are the OK series of monoclonal antibodies [59, 60]. The OKT4 monoclonal antibody appears to identify a subset of human non-B cells which can cooperate in the induction of B-cell differentiation by the polyclonal B-cell mitogen: pokeweed mitogen. Monoclonal antibody OKT8, on the other hand, identifies a different subset of non-B cells which is able to suppress the B-cell maturation and division signal provided by pokeweed mitogen and OKT4-positive cells. However, it appears that the OKT8 cells themselves require OKT4-positive cells to become active suppressors. The use of monoclonal antibodies is likely to replace the use of polyclonal alloantibody reagents which have been used to identify human T-cell subsets. Sera from some patients with Still's disease have been found to contain antibodies which react against approximately 30% of the human-blood lymphocytes which formed spontaneous rosettes with sheep red blood cells [61]. The T cells not reacting with these sera were able to provide help in polyclonal B-cell activation by pokeweed mitogen. Morretta *et al.* [62] showed that human T cells could also be divided into two groups on the basis of receptors for the Fc portion of different classes of immunoglobulin, i.e. cells which recognized Fc μ and cells which bound to Fc γ. There appears to be some correlation between these markers and helper and suppressor function in pokeweed-mitogen-induced B-cell proliferation [63]: Fc-μ-positive cell preparations provide help, while Fc-γ cells are associated with suppression. Similar conclusions have been reached from the analysis of antigen-induced B-cell responses [64].

Self-recognition as a requirement in T help. The early studies of thymocyte–bone-marrow-cell cooperation in immune responses by Claman's group included experiments in which mixtures of allogeneic and even xenogeneic cells were used to reconstitute irradiated mice [65, 66]. It was concluded that optimal cooperation was only seen when syngeneic bone marrow and thymus-derived cells were used. This observation was extended by Katz and his colleagues [67], who showed that successful cooperation between T and B lymphocytes in B-cell triggering depended upon the protagonists sharing certain products coded for by genes of the major histocompatibility complex (MHC). Further studies revealed that this requirement for identity in relation to certain MHC products extended to antigen presentation by macrophages and macrophage-like cells [68–70]. The use of congenic strains of mice and human family studies have proved invaluable

in identifying the products of the MHC which are important in T-cell help. In this way cells from donors which differ from each other only at one of the loci of the MHC can be used in cooperation experiments. Most readers will be familiar with the outline of the MHC in both man and mice, which is summarized in Figure 17.11. It now seems clear that the MHC products, which in some situations must be coincident if help is to take place in T-cell-dependent antibody responses, are located at or near the DR locus in man [64] and the I region in mice [72]. Help in particular seems to relate most closely to the I-A and I-C subregions of the mouse MHC [73].

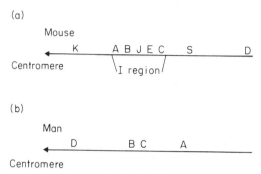

Fig. 17.11. Diagramatic representation of the major histocompatibility complex of (a) mouse and (b) man. The mouse system is known as the H2 system and is located on chromosome 17. The human system is known as the HLA system and is located on chromosome 6. The structures coded in the H2K and H2D region show homology with themselves and HLA-A, HLA-B and HLA-C-coded structures [71]. Ia antigens are coded within the mouse I region and are closely related to human D locus antigens. The term DR refers to human D locus products detected on human B cells by serological means. The D locus was defined originally using the mixed lymphocyte reaction [72].

T-cell-derived helper factors. So far three cellular reactants have been considered in relation to the initiation of T-cell-dependent antibody responses. These are helper T cells, B cells and antigen-presenting cells. In addition to antigen-specific recognition by the lymphocytes there is also a requirement for recognition of self components coded by the MHC. It is now clear that in addition to direct cell interactions there is also the participation of soluble T-cell-derived factors in certain circumstances. Taussig [74] showed that cell-free supernatant of cultures of antigen-primed T cells was able to replace T help specifically when pure B-cell preparations were transferred with supernatant plus antigen into irradiated syngeneic mice. These factors have now been described by a number of groups in both human [64] and murine systems [75]. In both cases the action of the factor is antigen-specific. However, the physical and antigenic characteristics of these factors indicate that they are not immunoglobulin. In addition to antigen-binding capacity they appear to react with antisera directed against I-region components of the MHC.

The way in which these factors, and the cellular components described above, interact with antigen to trigger B-cell proliferation and differentiation is not understood. Much of the analytical work on these systems has been carried out wholly or in part *in vitro*. Some of these interactions may be more significant as fine-tuning systems rather than absolute requirements to mount effective protective immunity *in vivo*.

T-cell suppression. It is now abundantly clear that, in addition to T-cell-specific help in the induction of lymphocyte differentiation by antigen, there are cells which can suppress lymphocyte triggering. In most cases these cells have been shown to be of T-cell origin, acting either directly or through macrophages. However, suppressor B cells have also been described, as have non-specific inhibitory effects, usually *in vitro*, of other cells, particularly macrophages.

The phenomenon of immunological tolerance has been recognized for many years and predates the more recent concept of suppressor cells. Tolerance in an immunological sense is the acquired inability of an individual to mount an immune response against a chemical structure which in normal circumstances is antigenic. Tolerance, by definition, is antigenically specific and an individual rendered incapable of responding to one antigen will still respond normally to other antigens. Specific immunological unresponsiveness may involve part or all of the immune system, i.e. an individual may be rendered unable to mount an antibody response against an antigen while still showing delayed hypersensitivity to that antigen. It is now clear that there are several mechanisms by which tolerance is mediated. In some circumstances there is deletion or inactivation of antigen-responsive clones [76]. In this case tolerance may be rapidly reversed when antigen is withdrawn, as the result of generation of new clones of immunologically competent cells. Reversal is also possible by the passive transfer of lymphocytes from a syngeneic donor. However, in tolerant animals the passive transfer of antigen-reactive cells does not always result in loss of specific immunological unresponsiveness [77–79]. Also in a number of instances passive transfer of specific unresponsiveness to normal syngeneic recipients has been achieved with lymphocyte preparations from tolerant donors [80, 81]. Gershon & Kondo [82, 83] studied the passive transfer of tolerance to sheep red blood cells in mice; they showed that tolerant mice possessed B cells which were able to respond to sheep red cells in the presence of active T help, and that specific unresponsiveness to sheep red cells could not be explained by loss of T help. It appeared that there were T cells which were specifically inhibiting the activation of B cells by antigen in the presence of T help. From these studies of immunological tolerance the concept arose that suppressor T cells might play an important physiological role in the regulation of antibody responses. It became clear that there are distinct subsets of T cells which are able to suppress the activation of both B and T cells by antigen. In mice these cells are seen to be particularly associated with the combined expression of Ly antigens, Ly 2.2 and Ly 3.2 [57]; in man the phenotype on peripheral lymphocytes of sheep red-cell-binding, Fc-γ positivity and OKT8 positivity is associated with cells which can inhibit human B-cell proliferation, despite the presence of T help and macrophages, in the pokeweed-mitogen system [60, 62, 63].

Analysis of T-cell-mediated suppression strongly indicates that this acts at the level of preventing B- or T-cell activation by antigen [84]; there is little evidence to suggest that these cells are able to inhibit the differentiation and proliferation of immunoblasts, i.e. antigen-activated lymphocytes. Plasma cells are short-lived cells (a matter of several hours to a few days [25]) and effector T cells require periodic restimulation by antigen if they are to retain activity [85]. One can conclude, therefore, that maintenance of immune responses requires the continued activation of antigen-sensitive lymphocytes and that regulation is to a large extent a matter of affecting the rate of lymphocyte activation.

Suppressor factors. Studies in both man and mice indicate that suppressor cells can produce biologically active and specific suppressor factors [64, 73]. This is a highly complex subject which is still far from fully worked out. In many ways some of the factors described resemble helper factors described above. They are non-immunoglobulin, T-cell-derived, antigen-specific macromolecules which bear antigens associated with the I region of the MHC. The I-region specificity in this case, however, is not generally associated with I-A or I-C coded structure but those associated with a third I-region locus, I-J (Fig. 17.11) [86, 87]. Although some degree of MHC restriction can be demonstrated in some suppressor systems, this is at best a partial restriction and in any case less rigorous than that already described in relation to T help [88].

T cells with effector function

So far we have discussed the way in which T cells control the activation of certain B cells. There are in

addition a number of T-cell-associated effector-cell functions. These fall into two main categories:
1 cytolytic T cells; and
2 effector T cells, which act by releasing factors which interact with macrophages to induce delayed-type hypersensitivity and allied reactions.
These two types of effector system are mediated and to some extent controlled by distinct cell systems.

Cytolytic T cells. Cytolytic T cells were first identified in mice which had received allografts or injections of allogeneic cells. Some days after immunization in this way, cytolytic cells can be recovered from the recipient which will kill cells sharing antigens with those used in immunization. Analysis of the effector cells in such systems often showed that they carried the T-cell-associated antigen Thy 1 (non-T cytolytic systems also exist, and will be discussed later). Such cytolytic T cells were shown to have a high level of specificity in their action. if strain-A mice are sensitized with strain-B cells, the effector cells derived will kill strain-B cells but not strain-A or strain-C cells. Furthermore, if strain-A effector cells sensitized against strain-B antigens are exposed to a mixture of strain-B and strain-C cells, only the strain-B cells are killed: i.e. effector cells kill target cells to which they are sensitized but in so doing do not release factors which are cytolytic to adjacent cells [85]. It was soon shown that it was possible to generate alloreactive cytolytic T cells *in vitro* [89, 90]. Unidirectional sensitization in these reactions is achieved by X-irradiation or mitomycin-C treatment of the sensitizing cell population. The use of sensitization *in vitro* has allowed extensive study of the generation of cytolytic T cells in man. Optimal sensitization requires the presence of both T-cell help and syngeneic macrophages. I-region compatibility between helper T cells, macrophages and cytolytic T cells may also be required [91].

More recently it has become clear that cytolytic T cells are able to kill autologous cells which have virus-coded antigens or other haptens on their surface. These studies have shown that killing often involves the recognition of self as well as hapten. Analysis of the self component involved has shown that this too is a product of MHC. However, in the case of the effector stage of cytolytic T cells, the self MHC component recognized is coded not from the I region, but from the D or K loci in mice [92] or the equivalent A, B and C loci in man [93] (Fig. 17.11). Individual clones of cytolytic T cells in mice recognize hapten plus either self D- or self K-associated products, but not both.

Analysis of the surface phenotype of cytolytic T cells in mice shows that they have the same Ly-antigen expression as suppressor T-cell activity, i.e. Ly $2.2 + 3.2$.

In man, Fc-γ receptors have been associated with cytolytic T-cell activity.

Very recent studies have shown that the precursors of cytolytic θ-positive cells are present in athymic mice [94]. They can be rendered cytolytic if T help is provided. It seems likely from these studies that while T help is thymus-dependent this may not be absolute in the case of the cytolytic effectors themselves.

T effector cells in delayed hypersensitivity reactions
Delayed hypersensitivity reactions are initiated by the interaction of T lymphocytes with antigen and the secondary recruitment of macrophages into the reaction by factors released from the T cells. As well as the classical skin reaction to tuberculin, this sort of reaction has been implicated in the rejection of some murine tumours [95, 96] and also appears to be closely related to certain manifestations of graft-versus-host disease. Studies of self-recognition requirements in these reactions suggest that where MHC restriction can be identified it relates to I-region rather than D- or K-locus products [97]. Therefore, although cytolytic T-cell generation and the capacity to mount a delayed-type hypersensitivity reaction may occur simultaneously, dissociation between these two phenomena can be made on the basis of MHC restriction. Also in a number of situations cytolytic T-cell activity can be separated from cells which induce graft-versus-host disease [98].

Lymphokines. This is the generic term that has been given to non-immunoglobulin factors produced by lymphocytes which directly or indirectly influence immune responses. The term as originally used [99] certainly included factors which would activate lymphocytes themselves, as well as factors influencing the activity of macrophages. Helper and suppressor factors elaborated by T lymphocytes have already been discussed. The way in which these may interact with macrophages and other lymphocytes in the activation of immunologically competent cells has also been described. In the context of delayed hypersensitivity we are concerned with factors which have direct or indirect effector function. A large number of these factors have been described. The true degree of heterogeneity remains unclear as precise chemical characterization has still not been achieved and specific antisera against these factors have not been made. Probably the best characterized factor is migration inhibition factor. This factor (or factors) can be shown to inhibit the migration of both guinea-pig peritoneal macrophages [100, 101] and human-blood leucocytes [102]. The inhibition of migration is immunologically specific: it results from the specific activation of lymphocytes by antigen. These lymphocytes then secrete factors which inhibit the outgrowth of macrophages or blood leucocytes from cells concentrated in capillary tubes. The factors themselves are not immunologically specific, it is the trigger for their secretion which is specific. The induction of secretion of migration inhibition factor by an antigen has been shown in laboratory animals to correlate well with the ability of the animal to mount a delayed-hypersensitivity reaction against that antigen [103, 104]. Other factors described include macrophage activation factor and macrophage chemotactic factor. It is plausible that these factors attract macrophages to antigen and then activate the macrophages, causing the cellular infiltrate and inflammatory reaction seen in delayed hypersensitivity. Evans & Alexander [95, 96] have described an interesting system in mice where lymphocytes from animals which had rejected tumour grafts were able to arm macrophages with a factor which allows them to become specifically cytotoxic to the tumour cells. In this system the triggering of cytotoxic activity in the armed macrophages requires direct contact with the tumour cells, but once activated the macrophages show indiscriminate cytotoxic activity. In this and other respects, the mechanism differs from that of cytolytic T cells.

The Evans–Alexander system is in many ways analogous to that described by Mackaness [105] as the basis for immunological protection in mice against infection with *Listeria monocytogenes*.

Immune-response genes

The systematic description of immunologically competent cells given above has emphasized the necessity for self-recognition in association with antigenic recognition, during cellular interactions involved in triggering lymphocytes. Studies of the immune responses produced by different strains of laboratory animals have shown marked differences in the quality and magnitude of the response to individual antigens between strains. Analysis of these differences has shown that one of the main factors responsible for them is coded within the MHC. It appears that the capacity to present different antigens is in part governed by the particular self MHC product which is being recognized in conjunction with antigen. In other words, in the induction of T help some I-A coded alleles appear to be more successful at presenting certain antigens than others. This linkage of immune responsiveness with the MHC provides a rational basis for looking for associations between the alleles expressed by an individual at the HLA loci and disease susceptibility. The reader will find a fuller account of immune-response genes in Ref. 106.

Antigen-presenting cells

Antigen presentation is a vital factor in the initiation and maintenance of immune responses. The role of macrophages has already been discussed in this context. However, not all macrophages can or are in a position to present antigen and some cells which are associated with the long-term persistence of antigen are highly specialized cells which bear only slight resemblance to conventional macrophages.

When antigen is presented *in vitro* to peritoneal macrophages, a sizeable proportion is rapidly ingested and degraded, but some persists for long periods. This residual antigen associated with macrophages is highly immunogenic *in vivo* [107]. After injection of antigen *in vivo*, localization to macrophages of the lymph-node medulla is associated with rapid breakdown of antigen. However, in an unprimed animal localization also occurs in specialized cells found in the intrafollicular areas and paracortex of lymph nodes. These are known as interdigitating cells, as they have dendritic processes interdigitating with other cells. These cells have typical elongated cytoplasmic granules, referred to as Birbeck granules [108], which are not characteristic of conventional macrophages and monocytes. Cells carrying antigen and containing Birbeck granules have been found in afferent lymph [109] and peripheral tissues. Cells of this sort found in the skin are known as Langerhans cells (reviewed in Ref. 110).

Long-term availability of antigen is likely to be necessary to maintain secondary immune responses over periods of weeks or even months. In this respect the localization of antigen in germinal centres is of particular interest. If antibody is present when antigen enters the body, then after a delay of several hours antigen–antibody complexes are found localized in germinal centres [111–113]. This antigen is associated with dendritic reticulum cells and persists on these for periods as long as some months. The role of this antigen in maintaining immune responses, however, remains to be established.

ORGANIZATION OF SECONDARY LYMPHOID TISSUE

The elements of the immune system have been described, and the distribution of these elements within the secondary lymphoid organs will now be considered. Much emphasis has been placed on the interaction between different types of lymphocyte and antigen-presenting cells, and the importance of continued stimulation of immunologically competent cells in order to maintain immune responses has also been stressed. The sites in the body where the necessary components of the immune system meet are therefore of considerable importance. These interaction sites for the most part are in secondary lymphoid tissue.

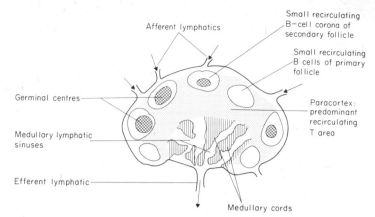

Fig. 17.12. Lymphoid areas and lymph flow through lymph nodes. Lymphatic flow is from the afferent lymphatics via the intrafollicular areas through the paracortex to the medullary sinuses: less than 10% of lymphocytes arriving at lymph nodes arrive via afferent lymph. All lymphocytes leaving the node do so via the efferent lymph.

Structure of lymph nodes

Lymph nodes represent collections of lymphoid cells, antigen-presenting cells and other components situated at intervals along lymph vessels. Figures 17.12 and 17.13 indicate the basic structure of lymph nodes. The node is depicted with respect to lymph passage in Figure 17.12. The afferent lymph filters into the cortex of the node, mainly through the interfollicular areas; it then continues through the paracortex and leaves the node via lymphatic sinuses in the medulla. These have clear vessel walls separating the sinuses from the tissues of the medulla. The lymphoid tissue of the node is mainly situated in the cortical and paracortical regions. There are spherical accumulations of lymphoid tissue known as the follicles in the cortex. These are of two types: primary follicles which are made up entirely of small lymphocytes, and secondary follicles which have an outer corona or mantle of small lymphocytes encircling a germinal centre. In the deeper layers of the cortex, the so-called paracortex, there are continuous sheets of small lymphocytes, and it is here that the high-endothelial venules, which have already been described, are found. The medullary tissue contains relatively fewer lymphocytes but large numbers of macrophages are located in this site. Mast cells are often a prominent feature of the medulla. After local antigenic challenge within the drainage area of a node, antibody-producing cells are prominent in the medulla of that node. Active lymph nodes, therefore, have large numbers of plasma cells and immunoblasts in the medulla. In addition, immunoblasts which are leaving the node are found in the lymphatic channels which pass through the medulla. They are also seen in the paracortex and interfollicular regions where antigenic stimulation is taking place, probably in conjunction with interdigitating cells.

Distribution and migration of lymphocytes through lymph nodes

The blood supply to lymph nodes is shown diagrammatically in Figure 17.13. It will be seen that the main artery and vein arrive and leave via the hilum of the node. The artery branches within the node and forms capillary networks around each follicle. These capillaries rejoin to form specialized vessels which have a characteristic high endothelium [114]. The high-

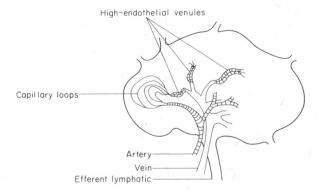

Fig. 17.13. Blood supply to lymph nodes. For simplicity only one capillary network is shown. 90% of all lymphocytes arriving at the node traffic through the high-endothelial venules. After antigenic challenge considerable increase occurs in the number of capillaries in the interfollicular areas and paracortex.

endothelial venules are only one cell thick and approximately 90% of the lymphocytes arrive in the node through these vessels [115]. The lymphocytes pass between the cells of the high-endothelial vessels to enter the paracortex. Both T and B lymphocytes enter via this route, but once in the paracortex T and B lymphocytes start to show distinct migration patterns [116]. The B cells move outwards to the follicles, where they form the predominant cell. Recirculating cells themselves, however, do not enter germinal centres in appreciable numbers, but remain in the small-lymphocyte zones of the follicles for some hours before returning via the paracortex to the efferent lymphatics. T lymphocytes, on the other hand, do not migrate to the follicles but remain in the paracortex until they too migrate to the efferent lymphatic channels. The site, therefore, where T cells and B cells come together in lymph nodes is the paracortex. Antigen-presenting cells in the form of interdigitating cells are also present at that site. It is unknown how or if antigen available in germinal centres is used to activate recirculating T and B cells. However, the double capillary system which takes lymphocytes through capillaries in the follicle before they pass out through the high-endothelial venules deserves further attention.

Structure of Peyer's patches and other gut-associated lymphoid tissue
These will not be discussed in detail, for the GALT has essentially the same basic structure as lymph nodes. Lymphocytes enter the tissue via high-endothelial venules, which are located in predominantly T-dependent areas. The GALT has primary and secondary follicles as in lymph nodes, and lymphocytes leave via lymphatics. This applies equally to appendix, Peyer's patches and tonsils.

Structure of the spleen considered as a secondary lymphoid organ
(Fig. 17.14)
The lymphoid tissue of human and rodent spleen is organized around the terminal arborizations of the

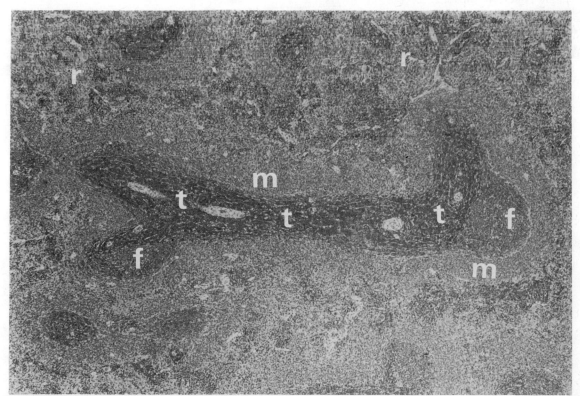

Fig. 17.14. Normal white pulp of a three-month-old rat spleen. This is essentially similar to the appearance of the spleen in human children and young adults; m = marginal zone; f = follicles; t = T-cell zone or periarteriolar lymphocytic zone; r = red pulp. The central arteriole is seen in several places in the T-cell zone. The marginal sinus is easily seen on the right of the photograph between a follicle and the marginal zone. The marginal sinus, however, is not an obvious feature of human spleens.

splenic artery to form the white pulp or Malpighian corpuscles. The white pulp consists of an inner zone containing mainly small lymphocytes closely packed around the central arterioles, surrounded by an outer marginal zone in which most of the cells are intermediate-sized lymphocytes [117, 118]. The cells of the marginal zone are arranged more loosely than the lymphocytes of the inner small-lymphocytic zone. The marginal zone comprises a massive vascular sinusoidal network which is fed by branches of the central arteriole [114]. These sinusoids are bounded on their inner aspect by the marginal sinus. This is lined by endothelium on the side adjacent to the small-lymphocytic zone, but communicates freely by numerous pores with the sinusoids of the marginal zone [119]. The marginal-zone sinusoids in turn feed the sinusoidal network of the red pulp, although there are also direct arterial connections with the red pulp.

Recirculating lymphocytes, both B and T, enter the splenic white pulp through the marginal-zone sinusoids [116]. At no time, however, do these cells in transit form a major component of the marginal-zone lymphocytes. The majority of cells is always the intermediate-sized lymphocytes, which are not part of the recirculating pool [119]. Recirculating B cells leave the marginal zone rapidly and move to the small-lymphocyte zone. The T cells remain in the periarteriolar region, while the B cells migrate through this region to primary and secondary follicles, which are located at intervals on the outer aspect of the T-cell area but within the marginal sinus. The T-cell-rich periarteriolar lymphocytic sheath can be easily demonstrated in sections from the spleens of rats which have been depleted of B lymphocytes by repeated injections of anti-μ antibody from birth (Fig. 17.15) [120]. This section also indicates that the follicles and marginal

zones, which are almost completely depleted of lymphocytes, are areas normally populated by B cells. Morphometric analysis of the spleen of rats shows that the largest single white-pulp area is the marginal zone. Approximately equal numbers of lymphocytes are found in the marginal zones and the small-lymphocytic zones. The static B cells of the marginal zone outnumber the recirculating B cells of the follicles by around threefold (Table 17.2) [119].

The site of triggering of immunologically competent cells in the spleen by antigen is uncertain. However, marginal-zone cells have Ia antigens, Fc receptors and receptors for C3 as well as their own surface-membrane immunoglobulin. They are ideally sited to pick up antigen from the blood and are in an area where recirculating T and B cells meet.

Non-B, thymus-independent cytolytic cells
These include K cells and NK cells. There is now considerable doubt, however, that the effector cells of T-cell-mediated cytolysis are themselves wholly thymus-dependent [94].

K cells
Experimental analysis of cell-mediated cytolysis against foreign cells in mice initially revealed that the main mechanism involved was antibody-independent. The effector system in this species appeared predominantly to involve cytolytic T cells or the indirect macrophage-mediated effect described above. Experiments in the guinea-pig [121], rat [122] and man [123], however, made it clear that there were lymphocytes which were capable of lysing cells whose surface antigens were complexed with IgG antibody. These cells with the capacity to kill antibody-coated cells are now referred to as K cells. The failure to demonstrate

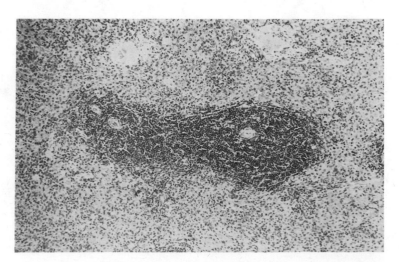

Fig. 17.15. Section of spleen from a three-month-old rat depleted of B cells by continued exposure to anti-μ antibody from birth. The B areas (i.e. follicles, marginal zone and germinal centres) contain few lymphoid cells. The T-cell zone is still apparent, however.

Table 17.2. Relative number of cells in the different white-cell compartments of rat spleen

	Marginal zones	Periarteriolar lymphocytic zone	Follicular zones*	Germinal centres
Percentage of all cells in white pulp	43	36	20	1

* Rats were three-month-old PVGc × Agus F_1 hybrids. Quantification was carried out as in Ref. 37. Follicular zones exclude germinal centres.

K-cell activity in early experiments reflects the apparent deficiency of this cell type in mice [124]. K cells are non-phagocytic cells which do not adhere spontaneously to glass or plastic as is characteristic of mononuclear phagocytes. They develop in congenitally athymic (nude) rats and are present in rats selectively depleted of T cells [125]. While clearly not thymus-dependent, K cells also do not express surface-membrane immunoglobulin and as such cannot be identified with the B-cell lineage. The origin of K cells is unknown: they are not found in significant numbers in bone marrow and are present in spleen before the stage at which the white pulp becomes populated with lymphocytes. Splenectomy, on the other hand, does not result in depletion of K cells from the blood.

The function of K cells in man extensively overlaps that of cytolytic T cells. They are able to kill allogeneic as well as syngeneic target cells [123, 126]. Several groups have demonstrated their capacity to lyse virus-infected cells sensitized with antibodies against virus-coded determinants [127–130]. Analysis of the mechanism of lysis mediated by K cells shows that it is similar, if not identical, to that of cytolytic T cells [131, 132]; by contrast, antibody-dependent cytolysis mediated by macrophages and neutrophils can easily be shown to be different.

NK cells

This is a term which has been adopted to describe cells with the capacity to kill certain target cells whose antigens have not apparently been encountered by the immune system. The range of target cells which are vulnerable to this sort of lysis is restricted. In general, normal tissue cells which have been freshly explanted are not vulnerable to lysis. Tissue-culture cell lines are frequently highly vulnerable to lysis by NK cells, as are certain freshly explanted tumour cells [133]. The possible role of NK cells in protection against tumour cells *in vivo* has aroused intense interest, but remains to be determined. It seems that there are at least two types of NK cell. One of these has the physical properties of K cells. Perlmann *et al.* [134] have argued that part of the spontaneous cytotoxicity shown against certain target cells by human blood lymphocytes is attributable to K cells. Here sensitization of the target cells results from antibody produced *in situ*, as described by MacLennan & Harding [135]. This does not explain all NK activity, particularly that seen in mice. There is a substantial component of NK activity which can be induced by stimulation *in vivo* with certain agents, including BCG and interferon, which is attributable to cells which do not bear Fc-γ receptors [136]. In common with K cells, NK activity has not been associated with either the T- or B-cell lineage. NK-cell activity has been described in both nude mice and nude rats.

QUANTIFICATION OF LYMPHOCYTES IN MAN

The principles of methods used to identify lymphocytes are given in this section. For precise details of these methods the reader is referred to Ref. 137.

Blood lymphocyte count

In most clinical situations the only readily available source of lymphocytes for assessment is the blood. Only about five per cent of the lymphocytes of the body are in the blood at any one time [138]. Some lymphocytes, such as those of the marginal zone of the spleen and germinal-centre lymphocytes, do not recirculate through the blood [117]. However, the recirculating pool of small lymphocytes is repeatedly passing between the blood and the secondary lymphoid tissues [17, 116]. In general, a good idea of the composition of the recirculating pool can be achieved by examination of the blood. Under certain circumstances, however, marked changes in the composition of the blood lymphocyte pool can occur without destruction of lymphocytes. A striking example of this occurs following the administration of corticosteroids: Clarke *et al.* [139] found that the injection of prednisolone caused an immediate fall in blood lymphocyte count from a

Fig. 17.16. Effect of steroids on total blood lymphocyte counts and T- and B-cell counts. Prednisone 40 mg was given intravenously at time 0, and 40 mg daily thereafter for seven days to the patients shown in (a); patients in (b) received placebo. Results at each point represent the geometric mean ± SE of values from 10 subjects. Reproduced from Ref. 139, with permission.

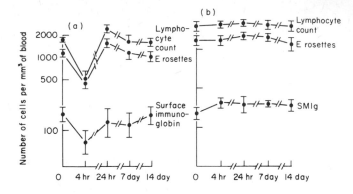

mean of $2 \times 10^9/l$ before injection to $0.5 \times 10^9/l$ four hours after injection; this effect was transient, however, and by 24 hours after injection, despite the continued administration of the drug, the blood lymphocyte counts had returned to supranormal levels (Fig. 17.16). While this effect was seen for both T and B cells, the time course of fluctuation of K-cell activity was totally different; it was normal four hours after prednisolone injection, but an almost tenfold reduction in activity was seen after 24 hours and persisted for several days. It is also possible to achieve marked changes in blood lymphocyte count following stress and exercise, which may well be causally related to changes in blood cortisol levels.

Blood lymphocyte counts vary greatly with age during childhood and adolescence [140], but are remarkably stable in relation to age during adult life [141]. There is relatively little alteration in the relative proportions of total T and B cells with age (Table 17.3).

Distinguishing lymphocytes from monocytes

Simple morphological identification of mononuclear phagocytes on standard blood films by experienced haematologists results in a consistent underestimate of their numbers. Objective identification should be used whenever possible. A reliable and convenient cytochemical means for testing monocytes in blood is the

Table 17.3. Percentages and absolute number (cells $\times 10^9/l$) of E-rosetting and SmIg positive cells and total lymphocytes in children of different ages (reproduced from Ref. 140, with permission)

Age	Number of Subjects	Percentage		Absolute Number*		
		E-Rosette	SmIg	E-Rosette	SmIg	Total lymphocytes
Newborn	7	59·7 ± 3·4†	14·0 ± 4·8‡	2·71 ± 1·42†	0·56 ± 0·16†	5·12 ± 2·57†
5 days	3	62·6 ± 9·2¶	11·6 ± 2·5¶	2·31 ± 0·61†	0·43 ± 0·09‡	3·80 ± 1·48†
1–3 months	27	60·2 ± 7·0†	14·1 ± 3·1‡	3·49 ± 1·16†	0·81 ± 0·27†	5·86 ± 1·72†
4–6 months	9	59·4 ± 8·1†	17·9 ± 5·3†	3·27 ± 1·29†	1·08 ± 0·58†	6·02 ± 1·52†
7–11 months	13	60·3 ± 6·5†	17·1 ± 5·3†	3·31 ± 1·18†	0·98 ± 0·67†	5·70 ± 1·90†
1–2 years	8	59·3 ± 6·4†	15·6 ± 4·0†	2·99 ± 1·15†	0·92 ± 0·36†	5·33 ± 2·13†
3–4 years	13	63·6 ± 7·6§	12·6 ± 2·7¶	2·03 ± 0·63†	0·48 ± 0·17†	2·94 ± 1·04†
5–6 years	16	62·8 ± 5·1‡	12·5 ± 2·7¶	1·92 ± 0·67†	0·37 ± 0·12†	3·04 ± 0·97†
7–8 years	7	67·0 ± 5·0¶	12·7 ± 3·6¶	1·50 ± 0·38¶	0·31 ± 0·12¶	2·39 ± 0·57¶
Adults	51	67·3 ± 5·5	12·0 ± 2·3	1·32 ± 0·46	0·24 ± 0·10	1·90 ± 0·70

Each value represents mean ± 1 s.d.
* Cells × $10^9/l$.
† Significantly different from adult values of the same column, $P < 0.001$.
‡ Significantly different from adult values of the same column, $P < 0.01$.
§ Significantly different from adult values of the same column, $P < 0.05$.
¶ Not significantly different from adult values of the same column, $P > 0.05$.

demonstration of α-naphthyl-acetate-esterase activity [142]: monocytes give a granular staining pattern throughout the cytosol, easily distinguishable from the polar punctate staining which is given by the majority of human T cells [143, 144]. The correlation between the numbers of cells with diffuse α-naphthyl-acetate-esterase activity and the number of cells which will phagocytose opsonized red cells is good, although there is usually a slightly higher proportion of cells detected by the histochemical method [145]. It is essential to identify blood monocytes if accurate quantification of lymphocyte subsets is required. This applies particularly where immunoglobulin is being detected or whole immunoglobulin is used in an assay, for monocytes have powerful receptors for the Fc portion of IgG [2, 3]. Monocytes also have receptors for the breakdown products of the third component of complement, C3b and C3d [2].

Identification of T cells

Rosettes with sheep red cells. The established marker assay for T cells is based on the finding that these cells have the capacity to form spontaneous rosettes with sheep red blood cells [29, 146]. This in general has proved a reliable assay in laboratories throughout the world. However, there is marked heterogeneity in the strength of red-cell binding. This has been exploited by Wybran who identifies active and ordinary rosettes [147].

Enzyme histochemistry. The use of enzyme histochemistry to identify the polar lysosomes of T cells has already been discussed in the previous section. In addition to α-naphthyl-acetate-esterase activity, acid phosphatase, β-glucuronidase, and N-acetyl β-glucosaminidase have also been used to identify T-cell lysosomes [148, 149]. One of the advantages of these enzyme histochemical techniques is that they can be used to identify positive and negative cells in tissue sections. The T-positive, B-negative pattern for these polar lysosomes broadly holds true in mice as well as in man [150]. This is not the case in rats where both T-dependent and B cells show polar positivity [151].

Fc receptors. The identification of T-cell subsets on the basis of possession of Fc receptors has been described earlier [62, 63]. As a broad generalization, Fc-μ cells are associated with helper activity and Fc-γ cells with suppressor activity. It is, however, far from clear that these receptors identify irrevocably distinct subsets of T cells: i.e. can T μ cells develop into T γ cells?

Measles-virus binding. Valdimarsson *et al.* [152] described binding of measles virus to T cells. There is

some evidence that the binding site for measles virus is closely linked or identical to that which binds sheep red cells, for measles virus is reported to inhibit sheep red-cell binding.

Antisera to T-cell antigens. These have already been discussed at length. All polyclonal antisera have the disadvantage of not being standard reagents and so far no clearly identifiable serological determinants have been described using such reagents. Monoclonal antibodies already appear to be showing the capacity to identify T-cell subsets [59, 60]. Developments in the next year or two promise to improve greatly our capacity to identify and quantify T-cell subsets. The extent to which this will be of clinical value remains to be seen; indirect evidence on the relative importance of loss of different classes of T cell to vulnerability to interstitial pneumonia and viral encephalitis indicates one area in which positive T-cell identification could be of considerable use [153]. Markers which distinguish suppressor from helper T-cell subsets, as assessed using the pokeweed-mitogen assay for polyclonal stimulation of B-cell antibody production, are shown in Table 17.4.

Table 17.4. Selective markers identifying human suppressor and helper T-cell subsets*

	Help	Suppression
OKT4 monoclonal	+	−
OKT8 monoclonal	−	+
Fc μ	+	−
Fc γ	−	+
Still's disease serum	−	?+

* Help and suppression in this table are defined in relation to antibody production induced *in vitro* by pokeweed mitogen.

Identification of immature T cells. Cortical thymocytes differ markedly in their surface marker phenotype from peripheral T cells (Table 17.5). Two monoclonal antibodies have been produced which are particularly discriminating in this respect [33]. While both cortical thymocytes and peripheral T cells have receptors for sheep red blood cells, cortical thymocytes lack surface antigens coded by the MHC loci HLA-A, HLA-B, and HLA-C. There is a common core structure to the molecules coded at each of these loci and this is detected by the monoclonal antibody W6-32 [154]. Peripheral T cells have abundant HLA-core antigen, as do medullary thymocytes. The second monoclonal,

Table 17.5. Human T-cell markers differentiating cortical thymocytes and peripheral T cells.

	Peripheral T cells	Cortical thymocytes
Spontaneous rosettes with sheep red cells	+ +	+ +
NA1/34 monoclonal [155]	−	+ +
HLA-A, B and C monoclonal W6-32 [154]	+ +	−

described by McMichael *et al.* [155], detects cortical thymocytes but does not pick up cells in the thymic medulla or peripheral T cells. In mice, peanut agglutinin acts as a marker for cortical thymocytes and not peripheral T cells [156]. It is, however, positive for some germinal-centre cells [157].

B-cell markers
Surface-membrane immunoglobulin remains the central component used in B-cell identification. The earliest B cells express surface-membrane IgM only. Subsequently many B cells express multiple heavy-chain isotypes: $\mu + \delta$ is the commonest isotype combination, but triple and single expressors are not uncommon. As indicated in the section on phagocytes, care must be taken when detecting cell-associated immunoglobulin that it is not passively absorbed through Fc receptors, or that serum antibodies directed against leucocyte-surface antigens are not giving false positive results. This question is discussed in more detail in Ref. 137.

Apart from the detection of polyclonal reduction or elevation of the total number of B cells, the single most important use of immunoglobulin isotype detection is to see if there is expansion of a single clone of B cells. In this respect assessment of the numbers of κ-bearing and λ-bearing cells is of particular importance. Figure 17.17 shows the κ/λ ratios in the blood of patients presenting to our department in whom the diagnosis of B-cell lymphoma of one type or another was suspected. It will be seen that many individuals with normal or near-normal blood lymphocyte counts showed clear evidence of gross deviation from the normal κ/λ ratio. In all of the cases outside the horizontal bars in Figure 17.17, subsequent tissue biopsy revealed the histological picture of non-Hodgkin lymphoma. The detection of heavy-chain isotypes is of less use in the diagnosis of B-cell neoplasia. Although detection of idiotypes can give strong evidence for the presence of a neoplastic clone of B cells, this is generally not a practical approach because of the difficulty of producing the reagents required.

Non-immunoglobulin B-cell markers. A number of

other surface markers are characteristically found on B cells or subsets of B cells. These include: DR locus antigens of the MHC; Fc-γ receptors [13]; and receptors for breakdown products of the third component of complement [158]. None of these antigens is exclusively found on B cells, however, and their diagnostic use is limited.

Spontaneous rosette formation with mouse red cells. Only a very small proportion of mouse red-cell-binding cells are found in normal human blood. Some neoplastic B-cell clones, however, do possess a large proportion of cells which form spontaneous rosettes with mouse red cells [159]. Although this was first described in relation to chronic lymphocytic leukaemia, the marker in our experience (Ling &

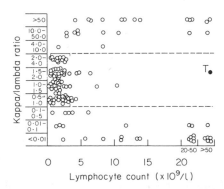

Fig. 17.17. The ratio of blood lymphocytes expressing surface κ to those expressing λ, plotted as a function of blood lymphocyte count. The values are from patients suspected of having non-Hodgkin lymphoma, tested over a six-month period. All the patients whose values fall outside the horizontal dotted lines, but only some of the other patients, had B-cell lymphoma at tissue biopsy. T = a patient with T-zone lymphoma. The patients with high counts had CLL but many of the patients with low counts and abnormal κ/λ ratios had other forms of non-Hodgkin lymphoma. In our experience about 50% of patients with follicle-centre cell tumour have B-cell leukaemia. Overt B-cell leukaemia diagnosable by this means is rare in myelomatosis and in patients with lymphoplasmacytoid tumours. The technique used is described in Ref. 14.

MacLennan, unpublished) is also present on neoplastic cells in the blood from a proportion of patients with other B-cell neoplasms, including follicle-centre cell tumour.

Epstein–Barr-virus receptors. See below.

Functional assays for lymphocytes

Cell-mediated cytolysis. Simple and standardized methods are available for determining cytolytic activity in human-blood lymphocytes. These are mostly based upon the principle that the proportion of target cells killed by lymphocytes is sigmoidally related to the log number of effector cells added to each culture. The cytolytic capacity of a lymphocyte preparation is generally expressed as the number of lymphocytes required to produce a given level of cytolysis. The number of target cells killed in these assays is assessed objectively by measuring the release of a radioactive isotope which has been incorporated into the target cells: $^{51}CrO_4^{--}$ is most often used for this purpose [137]. This sort of assay can be used for T-cell-mediated cytolysis, K-cell-mediated cytolysis, killing mediated by lymphocytes and induced by lectins and assessment of NK activity [160].

Production of antibody in vitro. The pokeweed-mitogen system has already been described. This is a complex system in which T-cell as well as B-cell function can be assessed. Immunoglobulin produced can be measured by a variety of sensitive techniques including radioimmunoassay and ELISA. Alternatively individual antibody-producing cells can be identified using the reverse-plaque technique [161, 162]. Other mitogens can be used to study B-cell function in isolation and in this context the Epstein–Barr (EB) virus is particularly useful [163]. This virus binds specifically to B cells and induces division and differentiation to antibody-producing cells. The EB-virus stimulation is T-cell-independent. It should be noted that although EB virus invades B cells exclusively in infectious mononucleosis, the characteristic large lymphocytes seen in this disease are not virus-infected cells, but T cells which are assumed to be reacting to virus-infected B cells [164]. As well as polyclonal antibody production induced by mitogens, specific primary immune responses to certain antigens by human-blood lymphocytes can be obtained *in vitro*.

T-cell mitogens. In addition to the mixed T-plus-B and B-selective mitogens, there are a number of agents which selectively bring about T-cell activation in the absence of equivalent B-cell stimulation. Among the best known of these are concanavalin-A and phyto-haemagglutinin. These agents have been shown to induce mitosis of T cells, cytolytic activity and factor production. These agents have been used extensively to assess T-cell function in both clinical and experimental situations [165].

REFERENCES

1 GOWANS J.L. (1962) The fate of parental strain small lymphocytes in F_1 hybrid rats. *Annals of the New York Academy of Sciences*, **99**, 432.

2 HUBER H., POLLEY M.J., LINSCOTT W.D., FUDENBERG H.H. & MULLER-EBERHARD H.J. (1968) Human monocytes: distinct receptor sites for the third component of complement and for immunoglobulin A. *Science*, **162**, 1281.

3 HUBER H., DOUGLAS S.D., NUSBACHER J., KOCHWA S. & ROSENFIELD R.E. (1971) IgG subclass specificity of human monocyte receptor sites. *Nature (London)*, **229**, 419.

4 FERRARINI M., MORETTA L., ABRILE R. & DURANTE M.L. (1975) Receptors for IgG molecules on human lymphocytes forming spontaneous rosettes with sheep red blood cells. *European Journal of Immunology*, **5**, 70.

5 MACLENNAN I.C.M. (1972) Antibody in the induction and inhibition of lymphocyte cytotoxicity. *Transplantation Reviews*, **13**, 67.

6 BASTEN A., MILLER J.F.A.P., SPRENT J. & PYE J. (1972) A receptor for antibody on B lymphocytes. I. Method of detection and functional significance. *Journal of Experimental Medicine*, **135**, 610.

7 RAFF M.C., MEGSON M., OWEN J.J.T. & COOPER M.D. (1976) Early production of intracellular IgM by B lymphocyte precursors in mouse. *Nature (London)*, **259**, 224.

8 ROSENBERG Y.J. & PARISH C.R. (1977) Ontogeny of the antibody-forming cell line in mice. IV. Appearance of cells bearing Fc receptors, complement receptors and surface immunoglobulin. *Journal of Immunology*, **118**, 612.

9 GATHINGS W.E., LAWTON A.R. & COOPER M.D. (1977) Immunofluorescence studies of the development of pre-B cells, B lymphocytes and immunoglobulin isotype diversity in humans. *European Journal of Immunology*, **7**, 804.

10 OWEN J.J.T., WRIGHT D.E., HABU S., RAFF M.C. & COOPER M.D. (1977) Studies on the generation of B lymphocytes in foetal liver and bone marrow. *Journal of Immunology*, **118**, 1067.

11 OSMOND D.G. & NOSSAL G.J.V. (1974) Differentiation of lymphocytes in mouse bone marrow. II. Kinetics of maturation and renewal of antiglobulin-binding cells studied by double labelling. *Cell Immunology*, **13**, 132.

12 FU S.M., WINCHESTER R.J. & KUNKEL H.G. (1975) Similar idiotypic specificity for the membrane IgD and IgM of human B lymphocytes. *Journal of Immunology*, **114**, 250.

13 KUNKEL H.G. (1976) Surface markers of human lymphocytes. *Behring Institute Mitteilungen* **59**, 1.

14 DHALIWAL H.S., LING N.R., BISHOP S. & CHAPEL H. (1978) Expression of immunoglobulin G on blood

lymphocytes in chronic lymphocytic leukaemia. *Clinical and Experimental Immunology*, **31**, 226.

15 ADAMS J.M. (1980) The organisation and expression of immunoglobulin genes. *Immunology Today*, **1**, 10.

16 KUMARARATNE D.S., BAZIN H. & MACLENNAN I.C.M. (1981) Marginal zones: the major B cell compartment of rat spleens. *European Journal of Immunology*. (In press.)

17 FORD W.L. (1975) Lymphocyte migration and immune responses. *Progress in Allergy*, **19**, 148.

18 FORD W.L. (1968) The mechanism of lymphopenia produced by chronic irradiation to the rat spleen. *British Journal of Experimental Pathology*, **409**, 502.

19 SPRENT J. (1980) Antigen-induced selective sequestration of T lymphocytes: role of the major histocompatibility complex. *Monograms in Allergy*, **16**, 233.

20 HUMMERLER K., HARRIS T.N., HARRIS S. & FARBER M.B. (1972) Studies on antibody producing cells. IV. Ultrastructure of plaque forming cells in rabbit lymph. *Journal of Experimental Medicine*, **135**, 491.

21 LENNERT K. (1978) *Malignant Lymphomas other than Hodgkin's Disease*. Springer-Verlag, Berlin.

22 SMITH E.M., MARTIN A.F. & FORD W.L. (1980) Migration of lymphoblasts in the rat. Preferential localisation of DNA-synthesising lymphocytes in particular lymph nodes and other sites. *Monograms in Allergy*, **16**, 203.

23 BENNER R. & VAN OUDENAREN A. (1977) Antibody formation in bone marrow. VI. The regulating influence of the spleen on the bone marrow plaque-forming cell response to *Escherichia coli* lipopolysaccharide. *Immunology*, **32**, 513.

24 LEONARD R.C.F., MACLENNAN I.C.M., SMART Y., VANHEGAN R.I. & CUZICK J. in conjunction with the Medical Research Council's Working Party for Leukaemia in Adults and the Oxford Lymphoma Group (1979) Light chain isotype-associated suppression of normal plasma cell numbers in patients with multiple myeloma. *International Journal of Cancer*, **24**, 385.

25 GAGNON R.F. & MACLENNAN I.C.M. In preparation.

26 HOWARD J.C. (1972) The life span of recirculating and marrow-derived small lymphocytes from rat thoracic duct. *Journal of Experimental Medicine*, **135**, 185.

27 THORBECKE G.J., GORDON H.A., WOSTMAN B.S., WAGNER M. & REYNIERS J.A. (1957) Lymphoid tissue and serum gamma globulin in young germ-free chickens. *Journal of Infectious Diseases*, **101**, 237.

28 LANGEVOORT H.L. (1963) The histophysiology of the antibody response. 1. Histogenesis of the plasma cell reaction in rabbit spleen. *Laboratory Investigation*, **12**, 106.

29 JONDAL M., HOLM G. & WIGZELL H. (1972) Surface markers on human T and B lymphocytes. A large population of lymphocytes forming non-immune rosettes with sheep red blood cells. *Journal of Experimental Medicine*, **136**, 207.

30 RAFF M.C. (1970) Two distinct populations of peripheral lymphocytes in mice distinguishable by immunofluorescence. *Immunology*, **19**, 637.

31 DAVIES A.J.S. (1969 The thymus and the cellular basis of immunity. *Transplantation Review*, **1**, 44.

31a LE DOUARIN N.M. (1978) Ontogeny of hematopoietic organs studied in avian embryo interspecies chimeras.

In: *Differentiation of Normal and Neoplastic Hematopoietic Cells* (ed. Clarkson B.), p. 5. Cold Spring Harbor Symposium.

32 CLAMAN H.N. (1972) Corticosteroids and lymphoid cells. *New England Journal of Medicine*, **287**, 388

33 BROWN G., BIBERFELD P., CHRISTENSEN B. & MASON D.Y. (1979) The distribution of HLA on human lymphoid bone marrow and peripheral blood cells. *European Journal of Immunology*, **9**, 272.

34 MILLER J.F.A.P. (1961) Immunological function of the thymus. *Lancet*, **ii**, 748.

35 MILLER J.F.A.P. (1961) Analysis of the thymus influence in leukaemogenesis. *Nature (London)*, **191**, 248.

36 PARROTT D.M.V. (1962) Strain variation in mortality and runt disease in mice thymectomised at birth. *Transplantation Bulletin*, **29**, 102.

37 KUMARARATNE D.S., GAGNON R.F. & SMART Y. (1980) Selective loss of large lymphocytes from the marginal zone of the white pulp in rat spleens following a single dose of cyclophosphamide. *Immunology*, **40**, 123.

38 MILLER J.F.A.P. (1962) Role of the thymus in transplantation immunity. *Annals of the New York Academy of Sciences*, **99**, 340.

39 MORRIS B. (1973) Effect of thymectomy on immunological responses in the sheep. In: *Contemporary Topics in Immunobiology* (ed. Davies A.J.S. & Carter R.L.), p. 39. Plenum Press, New York.

40 ASHERSON G.L. & WEBSTER A.D.B. (1980) *Diagnosis and Treatment of Immunodeficiency Diseases*. Blackwell Scientific Publications, Oxford.

41 CLAMAN H.N., CHAPTERON E.A. & TRIPLETT R.F. (1966) Thymus-marrow cell combinations. Synergism in antibody production. *Proceedings of the Society of Experimental Biology and Medicine*, **122**, 1167.

42 BASTEN A. & HOWARD J.G. (1973) Thymus independence. In: *Contemporary Topics in Immunobiology* (ed. Davies A.J.S. & Carter R.L.), p. 265. Plenum Press, New York.

43 MITCHISON N.A. (1967) Antigen recognition responsible for the induction *in vitro* of the secondary response. *Cold Spring Harbor Symposium of Quantitative Biology*, **32**, 431.

44 OVARY Z. & BENACERRAF B. (1963) Immunological specificity of the secondary response with dinitrophenylated proteins. *Proceedings of the Society for Experimental Biology and Medicine*, **14**, 72.

45 RAFF M.C. (1970) Role of thymus-derived lymphocytes in the secondary humoral immune response in mice. *Nature (London)*, **226**, 1257.

46 MISHELL R.I. & DUTTON R.W. (1967) Immunisation of dissociated spleen cell cultures from normal mice. *Journal of Experimental Medicine*, **126**, 423.

47 MARBROOK J. (1967) Primary immune response in cultures of spleen cells. *Lancet*, **ii**, 1279.

48 MOSIER D.E. & COPPLESON L.W. (1968) A three-cell interaction required for the induction of the primary immune response *in vitro*. *Proceedings of the National Academy of Sciences, USA*, **61**, 542.

49 MOSIER D.E., FITCH F.N., ROWLEY D.A. & DAVIES A.J.S. (1970) Cellular deficit in thymectomised mice. *Nature (London)*, **225**, 276.

50 COOPER M.D. & LAWTON A.R. (1971) Agammaglobu-

linaemia with B lymphocytes. Specific defect of plasma cell differentiation. *Lancet*, **ii**, 791.

51 JANOSSY G., GOMEZ DE LA CONCHA E., LUNQUETTI A., SNAJDR M.J., WAXDAL M.J. & PLATTS-MILLS T.A.E. (1977) T-cell regulation and immunoglobulin synthesis and proliferation in pokeweed (Pa-1)-stimulated human lymphocyte cultures. *Scandinavian Journal of Immunology*, **6**, 109.

52 WAGNER H. (1963) Synergy among T lymphocytes during *in vitro* cytotoxic allograft responses. *Science*, 1380.

53 DOSCH H.M. & GELFAND E.W. (1977) Generation of human plaque-forming cells in culture: tissue distribution antigenic and cellular requirements. *Journal of Immunology*, **118**, 302.

54 DELFRAISSY J.F., GALANAUD P., DORMONT J. & WALLON C. (1977) Primary *in vitro* antibody responses from human peripheral blood lymphocytes. *Journal of Immunology*, **118**, 630.

55 TADA T., TAKEMOR K., OKUMURA M., NONAKA M., TOKUHISA T. (1978) Two distinct types of helper T cells involved in secondary antibody responses: independent and synergistic effects of Ia⁻ and Ia⁺ helper T cells. *Journal of Experimental Medicine*, **147**, 446.

56 CANTOR H., HUGENBERGER J., McVAY-BONDREAU L., FANDLEY D.D., KEMP J., SHEN F.W. & GERSHON R.K. (1978) Immunoregulatory circuits among T-cell sets. Identification of a subpopulation of T helper cells that induces feedback inhibition. *Journal of Experimental Medicine*, **148**, 871.

57 CANTOR H. & GERSHON R.K. (1979) Immunological circuits: cellular composition. *Federation Proceedings*, **38**, 2058.

58 KOHLER G. & MILSTEIN C. (1975) Continuous cultures of fused cells secreting antibody of predefined specificity. *Nature (London)*, **256**, 496.

59 REINHERZ E.L., KUNG P.C., GOLDSTEIN G. & SCHLOSSMAN S.F. (1979) Further characterisation of human inducer T cell subsets defined by monoclonal antibody. *Journal of Immunology*, **123**, 2894.

60 THOMAS Y., SASMAN J., IRIGOYEN O., FRIEDMAN S., KUNG C., GOLDSTEIN G. & CHESS L. (1980) Functional analysis of human T cell subsets defined by monoclonal antibodies. I. Collaborative T–T interactions in the immunoregulation of B cell differentiation. *Journal of Immunology*, **125**, 2402.

61 SCHLOSSMAN S.F., EVANS R.L. & STRELKAUSKAS A.J. (1978) Human lymphocyte differentiation: its application. *Inserm Symposium 8* (ed. Serrou B. & Rosenfeld C.), p. 83. North-Holland, Amsterdam.

62 MORETTA L.S., FERRARINI M., MINGARI M.C., MARRETTA A. & WEBB S.R. (1976) Sub-populations of human T cells identified by receptors for immunoglobulin and mitogen responsiveness. *Journal of Immunology*, **117**, 2171.

63 MORETTA L.S., WEBB S.R., GROSSI C.E., LYDYARD P.M. & COOPER M.D. (1977) Functional analysis of two human T cell subpopulations: help and suppression of B cell responses by T cells bearing Fc receptors for IgM or IgG. *Journal of Experimental Medicine*, **146**, 184.

64 HEIJNEN C.J., UYTDE HAAG F. & BALLIEUX R.E. (1980) *In vitro* antibody response to human lymphocytes. *Springer Seminars in Immunopathology*, **3**, 63.

65 CLAMAN H.N., CHAPERON E.A. & SELNER J.C. (1968) Thymus-marrow immunocompetence. III. The requirement for living thymus cells. *Proceedings of the Society of Experimental Biology and Medicine*, **127**, 462.

66 CLAMAN H.N., CHAPERON E.A. & HAYES L.A. (1969) Thymus-marrow immunocompetence. IV. The growth and immunocompetence of transferred marrow, thymus and spleen cells in parent and F₁ hybrid mice. *Transplantation*, **7**, 87.

67 KATZ D.H., HAMAOKA T. & BENACERRAF B. (1973) Cell interactions between histoincompatible T and B lymphocytes. II. Failure of physiologic cooperative interactions between T and B lymphocytes from allogeneic donor strains in humoral responses to hapten-protein conjugates. *Journal of Experimental Medicine*, **137**, 1405.

68 ROSENTHAL A.S. & SHEVACH E.M. (1973) Function of macrophages in antigen recognition by guinea pig T lymphocytes. I. Requirement for histocompatible macrophages and lymphocytes. *Journal of Experimental Medicine*, **138**, 1194.

69 ERB P. & FELDMAN M. (1975) The role of macrophages in the generation of T-helper cells. II. The genetic control of the macrophage–T cell interaction for helper cell induction with soluble antigens. *Journal of Experimental Medicine*, **142**, 460.

70 KAPPLER J.W. & MARRACK P.C. (1976) The role of H-Z linked genes in helper T-cell function. IV. Importance of T-cell genotype and host environment In I-region and Ir gene expression. *Journal of Experimental Medicine*, **148**, 1510.

71 OWEN M.J. & CRUMPTON M.J. (1980) Biochemistry of major human histocompatibility antigens. *Immunology Today*, **1**, 117.

72 BACH F.H. & VAN ROOD J.J. (1976) The major histocompatibility complex—genetics and biology. *New England Journal of Medicine*, **295**, 806.

73 GERMAIN R.N. & BENACERRAF B. (1980) Helper and suppressor T cell factors. *Springer Seminars in Immunopathology*, **3**, 93.

74 TAUSSIG M.J. (1974) T cell factor which can replace the activity of T cells *in vitro*. *Nature (London)*, **248**, 234.

75 GERMAIN R.N. & BENACERRAF B. (1980) Helper and suppressor T cell factors. *Springer Seminars in Immunopathology*, **3**, 93.

76 HOWARD J.G. & MITCHISON N.A. (1975) Immunological tolerance. *Progress in Allergy*, **18**, 43.

77 ASHERSON G.L., ZEMBALA M. & BARNES R.M.R. (1971) The mechanism of immunological unresponsiveness to picryl chloride and the possible role of antibody mediated depression. *Clinical and Experimental Immunology*, **9**, 111.

78 TONG J.L. & BOOSE D. (1970) Immunosuppressive effect of serum from CBA mice made tolerant by the supernatant from ultracentrifuged bovine γ-globulin. *Journal of Immunology*, **105**, 426.

79 TERMAN D.S., MINDEN P. & CROWLE A.J. (1973) Resistance of neonatal tolerance in mice to abrogation by normal immunocytes. *Cellular Immunology*, **6**, 273.

80 CROWLE A.J. & HU C.C. (1969) Adoptive transfer of immunologic tolerance into normal mice. *Journal of Immunology*, **103**, 1242.

81 SHELLAM G.R. (1971) Mechanism of induction of

immunological tolerance. VII. Studies of adoptive tolerance to flagellin. *Internal Archives of Allergy*, **40**, 507.

82 GERSHON R.K. & KONDO K. (1970) Cell interactions in the induction of tolerance: the role of thymic lymphocytes. *Immunology*, **18**, 723.

83 GERSHON R.K. & KONDO K. (1971) Infectious immunological tolerance. *Immunology*, **21**, 903.

84 TADA T. & OKUMURA K. (1980) The role of antigen specific T cell factors in the immune response. *Advances in Immunology*, **28**, 1.

85 CERROTINI J.C. & BRUNNER T.K. (1974) Cell-mediated cytotoxicity allograft rejection and tumour immunity. *Advances in Immunology*, **18**, 67.

86 TANIGUCHI M. & MILLER J.F.A.P. (1977) Of specific suppressor T cells and characterisation of their surface markers. *Journal of Experimental Medicine*, **146**, 1450.

87 TANIGUCHI M. & MILLER J.F.A.P. (1978) Specific suppressive factors produced in hybridomas derived from fusion of enriched suppressor T cells and a T lymphoma cell line. *Journal of Experimental Medicine*, **148**, 373.

88 PIERRES A., BROMBERG J.S., SY M.S., BENACERRAF B. & GREEN M.I. (1980) Mechanisms of regulation of cell mediated immunity. IV. Antigen density dependence of the induction of genetically restricted suppressor cells. *Journal of Immunology*, **124**, 343.

89 HAYRY P. & DEFENDI V. (1970) Mixed lymphocyte cultures produce effector cells: model *in vitro* for allograft rejection. *Science*, **168**, 133.

90 WAGNER H. (1971) Cell-mediated immune response *in vitro*: independent differentiation of thymocytes into cytotoxic lymphocytes. *European Journal of Immunology*, **1**, 498.

91 VAN BOEHMER H. & HAAS W. (1979) Distinct Ir genes for helper and killer cells in the cytotoxic response to H-Y antigen. *Journal of Experimental Medicine*, **150**, 1134.

92 ZINKERNAGEL R.M. & DOHERTY P.C. (1974) Immunological surveillance against altered self components by sensitised T lymphocytes in lymphocytic choriomeningitis. *Nature (London)*, **251**, 547.

93 MCMICHAEL A.J. (1980) HLA restriction on human cytotoxic T cells. *Springer Seminars in Immunopathology*, **3**, 3.

94 MARYANSKI J.L. & CEROTTINI J.C. (1980) Limiting dilution analysis of cytolytic T lymphocyte precursor cells in nude mice. In: *Abstracts, IV International Congress of Immunology* (ed. Preud'homme J.L. & Hawken V.A.L.), No. 3.1.16. French Society for Immunology, Paris.

95 EVANS R. & ALEXANDER P. (1970) Cooperation of immune lymphoid cells with macrophages in tumour immunity. *Nature (London)*, **228**, 620.

96 EVANS B. & ALEXANDER P. (1972) Mechanism of immunologically specific killing of tumour cells by macrophages. *Nature (London)*, **236**, 168.

97 MILLER J.F.A.P., VADAS M.A., WHITELAW A. & GAMBLE J. (1975) H-2 gene complex restricts transfer of delayed-type hypersensitivity in mice. *Proceedings of the National Academy of Sciences, USA*, **72**, 5095.

98 CHISHOLM P.M. & FORD W.L. (1978) Selection of antigen-specific cells by adherence to allogeneic cell monolayers: cytolytic activity, graft vs. host activity and numbers of adherent and non-adherent cells. *European Journal of Immunology*, **8**, 438.

99 DUMONDE D.L., WOLSTENCROFT R.A., PANAYI G.S., MATHEW M., MORLEY J. & HOWSON W.T. (1969) Lymphokines—non-antibody mediators of cellular immunity generated by lymphocyte activation. *Nature (London)*, **224**, 38.

100 DAVID J.R. (1966) Delayed hypersensitivity *in vitro*: its mediation by cell-free substances formed by lymphoid cell-antigen interaction. *Proceedings of the National Academy of Sciences, USA*, **56**, 72.

101 BLOOM B.R., BENNETT B., OETTGEN H.F., MCLEAN E.P. & OLD L.J. (1969) Demonstration of delayed hypersensitivity to soluble antigens of chemically induced tumours by inhibition of macrophage migration. *Proceedings of the National Academy of Sciences, USA*, **64**, 1176.

102 SÖBORG M. & BENDIXEN G. (1967) Human lymphocyte migration as a parameter of hypersensitivity. *Acta Medica Scandinavica*, **181**, 247.

103 BLOOM B.R. (1971) *In vitro* approaches to the mechanism of cell-mediated immunity. *Advances in Immunology*, **13**, 205.

104 DAVID J.R. & DAVID R.R. (1972) Cellular hypersensitivity in immunity. *Progress in Allergy*, **16**, 300.

105 MACKANESS G.B. (1964) The immunological basis of acquired cellular resistance. *Journal of Experimental Medicine*, **120**, 105.

106 BENACERRAF B. & UNANUE E. (1979) *Textbook of Immunology*. Williams & Wilkins, Baltimore.

107 MITCHISON N.A. (1969) The immunogenic capacity of antigen taken up by peritoneal exudate cells. *Immunology*, **16**, 1.

108 BIRBECK M.S., BREATHNACH A.S. & EVERALL J.D. (1961) An electronmicroscopic study of basal melanocytes and high level clear cells (Langerhans cells) in vitiligo. *Journal of Investigative Dermatology*, **37**, 51.

109 SILBERBERG J., BAER R.L. & ROSENTHAL S.A. (1974) Circulating Langerhans cells in a dermal vessel. *Acta dermato-venereologica (Stockholm)*, **54**, 81.

110 SILVERBERG-SINAKIN I., BAER R.L. & THORBECKE G.J. (1978) Langerhans cells. *Progress in Allergy*, **24**, 268.

111 WHITE R.G. (1963) Functional recognition of immunologically competent cells by means of the fluorescent antibody technique. In: *Ciba Foundation Study Group 16. The Immunologically Competent Cell: Its Nature and Origin* (ed. Wolstenholme G.E.W. & Knight E.J.). Churchill, London.

112 BALFOUR B.M. & HUMPHREY J.H. (1967) Localisation of gammaglobulin and labelled antigen in germinal centres in relation to the immune response. In: *Germinal Centres in Immune Responses*, (ed. Cottier H., Odartchenko N., Schindler R. & Congdon C.C.), p. 131. Springer-Verlag, New York.

113 HANNA M.G. & SZAKAL A.K. (1968) Localisation of ^{125}I labelled antigen in germinal centres of mouse spleen. Histologic and ultrastructural autoradiographic studies of the secondary immune reaction. *Journal of Immunology*, **72**, 66.

114 HERMAN P.G. (1980) Microcirculation of lymphoid tissues. *Monographs in Allergy*, **16**, 126.

115 HALL J.G. & MORRIS B. (1965) The origin of the cells in

the efferent lymph from a single lymph node. *Journal of Experimental Medicine*, **121**, 901.

116 NIEUWENHUIS P. & FORD W.L. (1976) Comparative migration of B and T lymphocytes in the rat spleen and lymph nodes. *Cellular Immunology*, **23**, 254.

117 KRUMBHAAR E.B. (1948) Hematopoietic perifollicular envelope in rat spleen. *Blood*, **3**, 953.

118 VEERMAN A.J.P. & VAN EWIJK W. (1975) White pulp compartments in the spleen of rats and mice. Light and electronmicroscopic study of lymphoid and non-lymphoid cell types in T and B areas. *Cell Tissue Research*, **156**, 417.

119 KUMARARATNE D.S., BAZIN H. & MACLENNAN I.C.M. (1981) Marginal zone: the major B cell compartment of rat spleens. *European Journal of Immunology*. (In press.)

120 BAZIN H., PLATTEAU B., BECKERS A. & PAUWELS R. (1978) Differential effect of neonatal injection of anti-μ or anti-δ antibodies on the synthesis of IgM, IgD, IgE, IgA, IgG1, IgG2a, IgG2b, IgG2c immunoglobulin classes. *Journal of Immunology*, **121**, 2083.

121 PERLMANN P. & HOLM G. (1968) Studies on the mechanism of lymphocyte cytotoxicity. In: *Mechanisms of Inflammation Induced by Immune Reactions* (ed. Miescher P. & Graber P.), p. 325. Schabe & Co., Basel.

122 MACLENNAN I.C.M. & LOEWI G. (1968) The effect of specific antibody to target cells on their specific and non-specific interactions with lymphocytes. *Nature (London)*, **219**, 1069.

123 MACLENNAN I.C.M., LOEWI G. & HOWARD A. (1969) A human serum immunoglobulin with specificity for certain homologous target cells which induces target cell damage by normal human lymphocytes. *Immunology*, **17**, 887.

124 TADA M., HINUMA S., ABO T. & KUMAGAI K. (1980) Murine antibody-dependent cell mediated cytotoxicity: failure to detect effector cells equivalent to human K cells. *Journal of Immunology*, **124**, 1929.

125 MACLENNAN I.C.M. (1972) Antibody in the induction and inhibition of lymphocyte cytotoxicity. *Transplantation Reviews*, **13**, 67.

126 HERSEY P., CULLEN P. & MACLENNAN I.C.M. (1973) Lymphocyte dependent cytotoxic antibody activity against human transplantation antigens. *Transplantation*, **16**, 9.

127 ANDERSSON T., STEJSKAL V. & HARFAST B. (1975) An *in vitro* method for study of human lymphocyte cytotoxicity against mumps-virus infected target cells. *Journal of Immunology*, **114**, 237.

128 HARFAST B., ANDERSSON T. & PERLMANN P. (1975) Human lymphocyte cytotoxicity against mumps-virus infected target cells. Requirement for non-T cells. *Journal of Immunology*, **114**, 1820.

129 RUSSELL A.S., PERCY J.S. & KOVITHARONGS T. (1975) Cell-mediated immunity to herpes simplex in humans. Lymphocyte cytotoxicity measured by Cr^{51} release from infected cells. *Infectious Immunology*, **11**, 355.

130 JONDAL M. (1976) Antibody-dependent cellular cytotoxicity (ADCC) against Epstein–Barr virus-determined membrane antigens. I. Reactivity in sera from normal persons and from patients with acute infectious mononucleosis. *Clinical and Experimental Immunology*, **25**, 1.

131 GOLSTEIN P. & FEWTRELL C. (1975) Functional frac-
tionation of human cytotoxic cells using differences in their cation requirements. *Nature (London)*, **255**, 491.

132 MACLENNAN I.C.M. & GOLSTEIN P. (1978) Recognition by cytolytic T and K cells: identification in both systems of a divalent cation-independent cytochalasin A-sensitive step. *Journal of Immunology*, **121**, 2542.

133 HERBERMAN R.B. & HOLDEN H.T. (1978) Natural cell-mediated immunity. *Advances in Cancer Research*, **27**, 305.

134 PERLMANN P., TROYE M., PAPE G.R., HARFAST B. & ANDERSSON T. Natural cytotoxicity of human lymphocytes. Immunoglobulin dependent and independent systems. In: *Natural and Induced Cell-Mediated Cytotoxicity* (ed. Riethmuller G., Wernet P. & Cudkowicz G.), p. 29. Academic Press, New York.

135 MACLENNAN I.C.M. & HARDING B. (1970) The role of immunoglobulins in lymphocyte-mediated cell damage, *in vitro*. II. The mechanism of target cell damage by lymphoid cells from immunised rats. *Immunology*, **18**, 405.

136 TRINCHIERI G. & SANTOTI D. (1978) Anti-viral activity induced by culturing lymphocytes with tumours derived or virus-transformed cells. Enhancement of natural killer cell activity by interferon and antagonistic inhibition of susceptibility of target cells to lysis. *Journal of Experimental Medicine*, **147**, 1314.

137 MACLENNAN I.C.M. & LING N.R. (1981) Analysis of lymphocytes in blood and tissues. In: *Techniques in Clinical Immunology*, 2nd edn. (ed. Thompson R.A.), p. 222. Blackwell Scientific Publications, Oxford.

138 MEDICAL RESEARCH COUNCIL WORKING PARTY ON LEUKAEMIA IN CHILDHOOD (1978) Analysis of treatment in childhood leukaemia. IV. The critical association between dose fractionation and immunosuppression induced by cranial irradiation. *Cancer*, **41**, 108.

139 CLARKE J.R., GAGNON R.F., GOTCH F.M., HEYWORTH M., MACLENNAN I.C.M., TRUELOVE S.C. & WALLER C.A. (1977) The effect of prednisolone on leucocyte function in man: a double blind controlled study. *Clinical and Experimental Immunology*, **28**, 292.

140 FALCÃO R. (1980) Human blood lymphocyte subpopulations from birth to eight years. *Clinical and Experimental Immunology*, **39**, 203.

141 WALLER C.A. (1977) Studies on human lymphocytes. University of Oxford, D.Phil. thesis.

142 YAM L.T., LI C.Y. & CROSBY W.H. (1971) Cytochemical identification of monocytes and granulocytes. *American Journal of Clinical Pathology*, **55**, 283.

143 RANKI A., TOTTERMAN T.H. & HAYRY P. (1976) Identification of resting human T and B lymphocytes by acid alpha-naphthyl acetate esterase staining combined with rosette formation with staphylococcus aureus strain Cowan i. *Scandinavian Journal of Immunology*, **5**, 1129.

144 KULENKAMP H.J., JANOSSY G. & GREAVES M.F. (1977) Acid esterase in human lymphoid cells and leukaemic blasts—a marker for peripheral T-lymphocytes. *British Journal of Haematology*, **36**, 231.

145 GILL G., WALLER C.A. & MACLENNAN I.C.M. (1977) Relationship between different functional properties of human monocytes. *Immunology*, **33**, 873.

146 BRAIN P., GORDON J. & WILLETS R.A. (1970) Rosette formation by peripheral lymphocytes. *Clinical and Experimental Immunology*, **6**, 681.

147 WYBRAN J. & FUDENBERG H.H. (1976) T-cell rosettes in human cancer. In: *Clinical Tumour Immunology* (ed. Wybran J. & Stagnet M.J.), p. 31. Pergamon Press, Oxford.

148 TAMAOKI N. & ESNER E. (1969) Distribution of acid phosphatase, B-glucuronidase and N-acetyl-B-glucosaminidase activities in lymphocytes and lymphatic tissues of man and rodents. *Journal of Histochemistry and Cytochemistry*, **17**, 238.

149 SEYMOUR G.J., DOCKRELL H.M. & GREENSPAN J.G. (1978) Enzyme differentiation of lymphocyte sub-populations in sections of human lymph nodes, tonsils and peridontal disease. *Clinical and Experimental Immunology*, **32**, 169.

150 MUELLER J., BRUN DEL RE G., BUERKI H., KELLER H.U., HESS M.W. & COTTIER H. (1975) Non-specific acid esterase activity: a criterion for differentiation of T and B lymphocytes in mouse lymph nodes. *European Journal of Immunology*, **5**, 270.

151 KUMARARATNE D.S. (1979) Quantitation and interpretation of changes in lymphoid compartments of the spleen, with special reference to the marginal zone of the white pulp. University of Oxford, D.Phil. thesis.

152 VALDIMARSSON H., AGNARSDOTTIR G. & LACHMANN P.J. (1974) Cellular immunity in subacute sclerosing panencephalitis. *Proceedings of the Royal Society of Medicine*, **67**, 1125.

153 WALLER C.A., MACLENNAN I.C.M., CAMPBELL A.C., FESTENSTEIN M., KAY H.E.M. AND THE MEDICAL RESEARCH COUNCIL'S WORKING PARTY ON LEUKAEMIA IN CHILDHOOD (1977) Analysis of treatment in childhood leukaemia. III. Independence of lymphopenia induced by irradiation and by chemotherapy. *British Journal of Haematology*, **35**, 597.

154 BARNSTABLE C.J., BODMER W.F., BROWN G., GALFRE G., MILSTEIN C., WILLIAMS A.F. & ZIEGLER A. (1978) Production of monoclonal antibodies to group A erythrocytes, HLA and other human cell surface antigens—new tools for genetic analysis. *Cell*, **14**, 9.

155 MCMICHAEL A.J., PILCH J.R., GALFRE G., MASON D.Y., FABRE J. & MILSTEIN C. (1979) A human thymocyte antigen defined by a hybrid myeloma monoclonal antibody. *European Journal of Immunology*, **9**, 205.

156 REISNER Y., LINKER-ISRAELI M. & SHARON N. (1976) Separation of mouse thymocytes into two subpopulations by the use of peanut agglutinin. *Cellular Immunology*, **25**, 129.

157 ROSE M.L., BIRBECK M.S.C., WALLIS V.J., FORRESTER J.A. & DAVIES A.J.S. (1980) Peanut lectin binding properties of germinal centres of mouse lymphoid tissue. *Nature (London)*, **284**, 364.

158 BIANCO C., PATRICK R. & NUSSENZWEIG V. (1972) A population of lymphocytes bearing a receptor for antigen–antibody complement complexes. I. Separation and characterisation. *Journal of Experimental Medicine*, **132**, 702.

159 STATHOPOULOS G. & ELLIOT E.V. (1974) Formation of mouse or sheep red blood cell rosettes by lymphocytes from normal and leukaemic individuals. *Lancet*, **i**, 600.

160 MACLENNAN I.C.M., CAMPBELL A.C. & GALE D.G.L. (1976) Quantitation of K cells. *In vitro* methods. In: *Cell-mediated Immunity and Tumour Immunity* (ed. Bloom B. & David J.), Academic Press, New York.

161 FAUCI A. & PRATT K. (1976) Activation of human lymphocytes. I. Direct plaque forming assay for the measurement of polyclonal activation and antigenic stimulation of human B lymphocytes. *Journal of Experimental Medicine*, **144**, 674.

162 HAMMERSTROM A., BIRD A.G., BRITTON S. & SMITH C.I.E. (1979) Pokeweed mitogen-induced differentiation of human B cells: evaluation by a protein A haemolytic plaque assay. *Immunology*, **38**, 181.

163 BIRD A.G. & BRITTON S. (1979) A live human B-cell activator operating in isolation of other influences. *Scandinavian Journal of Immunology*, **9**, 507.

164 DENMAN A.M. & PELTON B.K. (1974) Control mechanisms in infectious mononucleosis. *Clinical and Experimental Immunology*, **18**, 13.

165 SCHECHTER B. (1980) Lymphocyte stimulation by non-specific mitogens. In: *Lymphocyte Stimulation* (ed. Castellani A.), Plenum Press, New York.

Chapter 18
Lymphocyte disorders

A. R. HAYWARD

This chapter is concerned with non-malignant disorders of lymphocytes. For convenience these are divided into abnormalities of blood lymphocyte count and disorders of lymphocyte function. There is overlap between these headings and the overall applicability of this approach has other limitations. One is that lymphocytes circulate through blood, tissues, lymph nodes and spleen so that only a small and possibly unrepresentative proportion is present in the blood at any one time. Another difficulty arises from the definition of a lymphocyte. Classically this is based on morphology in blood films but it is clear that not all cells with lymphocyte morphology contribute to adaptive immunity, and so fall within the immunologist's view of a lymphocyte (Chapter 17). The heterogeneity of the various lymphocyte populations and subpopulations is not apparent in a blood film but this information can be critical in the interpretation of alterations in number. For example, non-heterogeneous (monoclonal) increases in B cells (as in chronic lymphocytic leukaemia) or T cells (T-cell leukaemia and perhaps Sézary syndrome) are mostly malignant; these are described in Chapters 22–24.

DISORDERS OF LYMPHOCYTE NUMBER

LYMPHOCYTOSIS

A lymphocytosis is conventionally defined as a blood lymphocyte count above 4×10^9/l in adults or 9×10^9/l in infants and children; the most important causes are listed in Table 18.1 and some of these are further discussed below.

Infectious mononucleosis

Pathogenesis (see Chapter 33). Infectious mononucleosis is the result of a primary infection with the Epstein–Barr virus (EBV), a member of the herpes virus group [1]. The virus is easiest to grow in B lymphocytes but may also grow in pharyngeal epithelial cells; its spread is thought to be mostly oropharyngeal following salivary transfer. Transmission

through blood transfusion has occurred but is rare, probably because most blood donors have anti-EBV antibodies. The virus persists in the pharynx of up to 18% of adults, many years after infection. Virus entry into B lymphocytes is through a surface receptor close to or identical with the C3 receptor [2]. Epstein–Barr-virus-infected B cells proliferate and also differentiate, to some extent, into immunoglobulin-secreting plasmablasts. Infected B cells are relatively easy to keep in continuous culture and their proliferation ultimately resembles that of malignant cell lines; EBV carriage by B cells can be identified by an extractable nuclear antigen [3], by virus production and by hybridization. *In vivo*, the proliferation of infected cells is limited mainly by specifically reactive T cells, which constitute the atypical lymphocytes seen in blood films [4]. Like other herpes viruses, EBV tends to persist in the body and can be recovered from blood B cells or oropharyngeal washings. Rarer consequences of EBV infection include the X-linked lymphoproliferative syndrome (p. 690), Burkitt's lymphoma [5] and possibly anaplastic nasopharyngeal carcinoma [6].

Clinical features. The incubation period is probably in the range of five to seven weeks. Onset is with malaise, headache, fever and pharyngitis. Important physical findings are generalized lymphadenopathy, affecting especially the neck, splenomegaly, exudative tonsillitis or pharyngitis. Less common are abdominal pain, epistaxis, jaundice and hepatosplenomegaly; very rarely there is central or peripheral nervous-system involvement. The disease usually lasts two to four weeks.

Laboratory findings. The leucocyte count is usually in the range of 10–20×10^9/l, 50% or more being large blast cells. Red cells and platelets are normal except in rare patients who develop thrombocytopenia or autoimmune haemolytic anaemia. The diagnosis is most simply confirmed by an heterophil agglutinin test (or its monospot modification) which becomes positive during the acute phase in over 90% of patients. This test depends on the agglutination of horse erythrocytes

Table 18.1. Non-malignant causes of lymphocytosis

Virus infections
Infectious mononucleosis
Infectious lymphocytosis
Cytomegalovirus infection
Occasionally mumps, varicella, hepatitis, rubella, influenza

Bacterial infections
Pertussis
Occasionally cat-scratch fever, tuberculosis, syphilis,
    brucellosis

Protozoal infections
Toxoplasmosis
Occasionally malaria

Other rare causes
Hyperthyroidism, congenital adrenal hyperplasia

---

by IgM antibodies in the patient's serum which are absorbed out by ox red blood cells but not by guinea-pig kidney [7]. The sensitivity and specificity of the heterophil test is largely determined by the species of red cell used. IgM antibodies to the viral capsid antigen (VCA) are probably more specific and they appear rather earlier than the heterophil agglutinins. Virus isolation from the blood is evidence of past or present EBV infection.

Immunological aspects. The EBV is a polyclonal B-cell activator which does not require T-cell help [8]. In the early stages of the infection the B cells which are triggered by the virus differentiate at least partially, causing a rise in serum IgM levels and the appearance of a wide range of antibodies. The B-cell independence of T-cell control during polyclonal activation may partly explain the occasional production of autoantibodies, though the impairment of cell-mediated immunity which has been found during the first weeks of EBV infection could point to a wider interference with T-cell regulation [9]. The B-cell target for the T-cell response to infection is called a 'lymphocyte-detected membrane antigen' (LYDMA) and the number of cells bearing this falls rapidly during recovery, though a few persist for life.

Infectious lymphocytosis
Infectious lymphocytosis is a poorly defined condition thought to be caused by a virus infection, probably of the Coxsackie group [10]. It is characterized by a leucocytosis of up to $100 \times 10^9/l$ (more usually $20-30 \times 10^9/l$) which lasts three to five weeks. Most of the leucocytes are small lymphocytes without morphological abnormalities. Co-existent symptoms are mild or even absent, but may resemble those of infectious mononucleosis, with a morbilliform rash but without

anaemia or splenomegaly. The condition is commonest in children, occurs in epidemics with an incubation period of 12–21 days and resolves spontaneously. Heterophil agglutinins are not found, and the EBV is not implicated.

Cytomegalovirus infections
Cytomegalovirus is a herpes-group virus which can cause congenital infection (leading to mental retardation) and, in healthy adults, a clinical syndrome closely resembling infectious mononucleosis. The mechanism of spread is uncertain but can include blood transfusion [11]; the 'post-perfusion syndrome' (Chapter 35) is a common complication of cardiopulmonary bypass, with onset three to six weeks after operation, and the incidence increases with the number of units of blood transfused. Prominent symptoms at the onset include headache, low-grade fever, malaise and cough but there is little pharyngitis. Signs include lymphadenopathy, hepatosplenomegaly and, occasionally, jaundice. Laboratory findings are of an absolute lymphocytosis with large atypical lymphocytes and the liver-function tests are often abnormal. The heterophil agglutinin test is negative and the diagnosis is made by virus isolation from the urine or blood or by a rise in antibody titre. The illness subsides spontaneously within two to three weeks, but the splenomegaly may persist for longer.

It is likely that the majority of infections with cytomegalovirus are not formally diagnosed and that the virus persists in the host. It may become active in immunosuppressed patients causing widespread lung involvement which is often fatal. The diagnosis may be suspected in such cases through the observation of typical intranuclear inclusions in lung or liver-biopsy material.

Pertussis
Infection with *Bordetella pertussis* is accompanied by a lymphocytosis which is useful diagnostically. Leucocyte counts occasionally reach $90 \times 10^9/l$ but are more usually in the $20-40 \times 10^9/l$ range: most of these cells are small lymphocytes. Interference with lymphocyte recirculation probably accounts for the lymphocytosis, because mouse lymphocytes incubated *in vitro* with pertussis antigen fail to leave the circulation and enter the lymph nodes or spleen [12]. The effect on the lymphocytes is presumably reversible since the lymphocytosis disappears during convalescence without any long-term impairment of immunological memory.

Cat-scratch fever
Cat-scratch fever is caused by a chlamydia belonging to the same group of organisms as causes trachoma, lymphogranuloma venereum and psittacosis. Ten to

30 days after a peripheral inoculation through a cat or other scratch there is onset of headache, malaise and fever. The draining lymph nodes (most often axillary) enlarge and in about 25% of cases they suppurate. An absolute lymphocytosis occurs during this phase and some of the cells may be atypical. Spontaneous recovery in one to two months is the usual outcome. The diagnosis can be confirmed with a skin test [13] or by biopsy of the involved node.

Toxoplasmosis

Toxoplasma gondii is a protozoon which probably reaches man in the form of infective oocysts passed in the faeces of the domestic cat. Infection may be congenital or acquired. The former is important because it causes jaundice, hepatosplenomegaly, skin rashes, chorioretinitis and sometimes mental retardation and cerebral calcification. Adult infection resembles infectious mononucleosis even to the extent of pharyngitis, though the heterophil antibody test is negative: chorioretinitis occurs less often than in infants and is usually unilateral. The blood leucocyte count is raised, with an absolute lymphocytosis and some atypical lymphocytes. Diagnosis is based on antibody testing and treatment with co-trimoxazole is effective.

LYMPHOPENIA

Lymphopenia is defined as a blood lymphocyte count of less than $1.4 \times 10^9/l$ in infants or $1 \times 10^9/l$ in adults. The commonest primary causes are the congenital immunodeficiency syndromes described under functional disorders below. There are numerous secondary causes, the more important of which are listed in Table 18.2. Any cause of severe and prolonged lymphopenia is likely to lead to secondary immunodeficiency (p. 690). Many (perhaps most) blood lymphocytes are long-lived recirculating cells so it is unlikely that a failure of lymphocyte production would lead rapidly to lymphopenia. Thymectomy, for example, probably cuts off the supply of new T cells to the recirculating pool but it does not cause lymphopenia for many years, if ever [14]. Long-standing malnutrition, B_{12}, folate or zinc deficiency are all associated with lymphopenia but it is not certain that this is a direct effect, rather than a consequence of stress mediated through corticosteroids. Cortisol causes a rapid and reversible lymphopenia [15] which is thought to result largely from sequestration of T cells in the bone marrow [16] rather than lymphocyte destruction. In contrast, the effects of some cytotoxic drugs are clearly highly toxic to T cells [17] while anti-leukaemia treatment depletes both T and B cells [18]. The effect of infections is variable though a few, such as influenza [19] are reasonably well associated with lymphopenia.

Table 18.2. Causes of secondary lymphopenia

Loss
Mostly from gut as in intestinal lymphangiectasia, Whipple's disease and rarely Crohn's disease
Thoracic-duct fistula

Malnutrition
Primary, or secondary to gut disease
B_{12} or folate deficiency
Zinc deficiency

Pharmacological agents
Antilymphocyte globulin
Corticosteroids
Cytotoxic drugs

Infections
Severe septicaemias
Influenza, occasionally other virus infections
Colorado tick fever
Miliary tuberculosis

Other miscellaneous conditions
Collagen vascular diseases, especially SLE
Malignant disease
Other conditions with lymphocytotoxins
Radiotherapy
Graft-versus-host disease

DISORDERS OF LYMPHOCYTE FUNCTION

The main consequences of lymphocyte malfunction are an increased susceptibility to infection and autoimmune diseases; these two often occur together. A wider interpretation of functional abnormalities might include atopy; this relationship is outside the scope of this Chapter but is discussed in Ref. 20. The classification of the primary immunodeficiency syndromes is frequently revised but remains unsatisfactory; the system followed here (Table 18.3) is based on the World Health Organization Select Committee's guidelines [21] which primarily separate antibody deficiency from defects of cell-mediated immunity and combined immunodeficiency.

ANTIBODY-DEFICIENCY SYNDROMES

Pathogenesis

Most patients with antibody deficiency make at least some immunoglobulin, but their levels in serum and secretions are low. The commonest cellular correlate of hypogammaglobulinaemia is a failure of B-lymphocyte proliferation and differentiation into plasma cells following antigen stimulation. In most cases this appears to result from an intrinsic defect of the patient's B lymphocytes [22], though in a few cases plasma cells appear but fail to glycosylate their

Table 18.3. Simple classification of primary specific immuno-deficiency syndromes

---

Antibody-deficiency syndromes
Congenital X-linked agammaglobulinaemia
X-linked hypogammaglobulinaemia with IgM
Varied immunodeficiency affecting predominantly antibody
Transient hypogammaglobulinaemia
Selective immunoglobulin deficiencies
Selective IgA deficiency
Selective IgM deficiency
Selective IgE deficiency

Cell-mediated immunodeficiency syndromes
Purine nucleoside phosphorylase deficiency
Thymic hypoplasia (Di George's syndrome)
Cartilage-hair hypoplasia
Varied immunodeficiency affecting predominantly cell-mediated immunity

Combined immunodeficiency syndromes
Severe combined immunodeficiency
Adenosine deaminase deficiency
SCID with immunoglobulins
SCID with leucopenia
SCID with reticulo-endotheliosis

Miscellaneous syndromes affecting antibody and cell-mediated immunity
Ataxia telangiectasia
Wiskott–Aldrich syndrome
Thymoma
Lymphopenia with lymphocytotoxins
Transcobalamin-II deficiency

---

immunoglobulin for secretion [23]. There are no other direct clues as to the cause of the failure of B-cell differentiation and different patterns of inheritance indicate that several mechanisms may fail. Congenital X-linked agammaglobulinaemia presumably results from a single gene defect but which enzyme or structural protein is abnormal is not known; the consequence is a failure of B-cell development beyond the pre-B-cell stage [24] and few if any B cells are found in the blood. In the much commoner conditions of varied immunodeficiency and selective IgA deficiency the inheritance is unclear, though the occurrence of serum immunoglobulin abnormalities or autoimmune diseases in the patient's relatives suggests an underlying genetically determined immunoregulatory defect. There has been considerable interest in the possibility that hypogammaglobulinaemia might result from excessive suppression of the immune response by a specialized subclass of T cell [25]. Although suppressor cells are readily identified in the blood of some antibody-deficient patients, and some healthy donors too [26] it has not generally been possible to substantiate the view that these cells have a primary pathogenetic role. A lack of helper T cells would be expected

to cause antibody deficiency but the current impression is that cell-mediated immunity also fails, so that the clinical presentation is as combined immunodeficiency.

Congenital X-linked agammaglobulinaemia
Of all the antibody deficiency syndromes, this is the best defined so it is a convenient prototype. The diagnosis is based on panhypogammaglobulinaemia, found either by screening boys in an affected family or, more commonly, during the investigation of a boy with recurrent infections. Bruton's original case had repeated episodes of meningitis and pneumonia [27] before protein chemistry became sufficiently advanced for the γ-globulin deficiency to be recognized. The child's survival through these infections must have been due mainly to effective antibiotics. The infecting organisms were *H. influenzae*, *Strep. pneumoniae* and *N. meningitidis* and in general it is bacteria which are most troublesome in these patients. Fungal infections are rare except when they occur in structurally damaged lung. Recovery from virus infections such as measles or influenza is usually normal though some such as rotavirus can be more persistent [28].

The respiratory tract is by far the commonest site for infections and chronic lung damage leading to respiratory failure is a major cause of reduced life expectancy in immunodeficiency. Upper-respiratory-tract involvement (sinusitis, otitis media) is frequent and may permanently impair hearing. Other areas which are often infected include the skin (giving boils and cellulitis and delayed wound healing), the conjunctiva and the gut. Urinary-tract infections are rare.

Complications affecting the joints, gut or brain each occur in about 10% of patients. The arthritis most often affects the knees, followed by the ankles; occasionally multiple joints are involved [29]. Joint symptoms usually remit with adequate immunoglobulin replacement therapy and may reappear with cessation of treatment. Mycoplasmas have been isolated from a few patients' joint fluids and remission of the arthritis following treatment with tetracycline or erythromycin supports the view that these organisms may cause the arthritis [30]. Diarrhoea and failure to thrive are inconstant complications of antibody deficiency; the most severely affected patients have malabsorption with abnormal barium meals (even resembling Crohn's disease) and patchy partial villous atrophy in the jejunum [31]. The extent to which these abnormalities can be attributed to bacterial or protozoal overgrowth is uncertain because recognized pathogens such as *Giardia lamblia* [32] are only rarely recovered from small-intestinal aspirates or biopsies. A proportion of cases responds to metronidazole, which has anti-bacterial and anti-*Giardia* activity. Severe enteropathy in antibody-deficient patients can make effective immunoglobulin replacement difficult if protein is lost into the bowel.

Encephalitis is a particularly serious complication because it is often progressive. Clinical presentation is usually with ataxia, visual impairment due to optic atrophy or intellectual deterioration. The course, when progressive, may be over months or years while a few children have apparently isolated encephalitic episodes with subsequent stabilization. Polio and measles viruses have been incriminated but when a virus is isolated from the brain it is most often a member of the ECHO group [33, 34]. Transfer factor, injections of anti-ECHO virus antibodies and increased immunoglobulin replacement have all been tried as treatments without obvious success. X-linked hypogammaglobulinaemia was associated with isolated growth-hormone deficiency in a single family [34a].

Diagnosis. Evidence for X-linked transmission may be lacking if the family size is small, in which case more reliance has to be placed on the phenotype. Characteristic features are panhypogammaglobulinaemia, a lack of B lymphocytes with normal numbers of T lymphocytes in the blood, and the presence of pre-B but not B cells or plasma cells in the bone marrow.

Hypogammaglobulinaemia with IgM

If any immunoglobulin class is present in normal or high amounts in patients with antibody deficiency it is usually IgM. Perhaps the commonest form of this syndrome has an X-linked inheritance [35], while affected females in other families indicate that an autosomal-recessive inheritance is possible too; rare cases may be secondary to congenital rubella [36]. These patients' IgM often lacks useful antibody function as judged by lack of isohaemagglutinins and the absence of any correlation between the IgM levels and susceptibility to meningitis [37]. One observation which may be related to the production of large amounts of IgM is the presence of plasmacytoid cells in the patient's blood. These cells are 10–14 μm in diameter and have both surface and cytoplasmic IgM, which they synthesize and secrete *in vitro*. They lack C3 receptors and incorporate thymidine without requiring mitogen stimulation [38]. B lymphocytes with IgM and IgD on their surface are also present in the patients' blood, but they differ from normal B cells in that following pokeweed-mitogen stimulation they make only IgM and not IgG or IgA. The T-cell responses of this series of patients [38] were normal, but others have found low numbers of blood E-rosette-forming cells (E-RFC), low PHA responses and susceptibility to *Candida* or *Pneumocystis carinii* infections.

Clinical features. Infections in the X-linked recessive form of this syndrome usually start in infancy and mainly affect the respiratory tract. There is a marked susceptibility to septicaemia, particularly in patients with neutropenia. Presentation is sometimes with *Pneumocystis carinii* pneumonia, even when there is no obvious evidence for defective cell-mediated immunity [39].

It is the haematological complications which make this syndrome difficult to manage. Many of the patients have chronic neutropenia with reduced marrow granulopoiesis, and their neutrophil count may fall further during infections [40]. Thrombocytopenia occurs too, but is not usually sufficiently severe to cause bleeding. Other problems have included auto-immune haemolytic anaemia [41] and sensitization to IgA, both due to IgM antibodies.

Varied immunodeficiency affecting predominantly antibody

This is a provisional name for a group of syndromes incorporating those previously known as 'primary acquired agammaglobulinaemia' and dysgammaglobulinaemia, plus others awaiting better definition. Serum immunoglobulins are low or undetectable in serum and saliva; the immunoglobulin class which is most often spared is IgM but patients who make this immunoglobulin rarely make significant amounts of antibody in it. There is a spectrum of other immunoglobulin class deficiencies such as normal IgG levels with absent or very low IgA and IgM, or very rarely normal IgA with absent IgM and IgG. The pattern of deficiency has been used to classify different dysgammaglobulinaemias, but this approach is rarely used now because levels of individual immunoglobulin classes sometimes varied with time, and the lack of concordance between affected relatives suggested that these were secondary effects. Many patients with varied immunodeficiency syndromes have IgG subclass imbalances [42] which are thought to be another manifestation of their basic abnormality. The very rare patients with κ or λ light-chain deficiencies [43, 44] can also be included in the varied immunodeficiency group, at least until there is better evidence that these deficiencies are primary. Laboratory tests indicate that up to 50% of patients have defects of cell-mediated immunity in addition to their antibody deficiency; these may be severe enough to increase susceptibility to herpes virus and fungal infections. The frequent occurrence of allergic and autoimmune disease or serum immunoglobulin abnormalities in other family members suggests that the aetiology is at least partly genetically determined.

Clinical features. Presentation is most often with

respiratory tract or skin infections, occasionally with chronic diarrhoea or arthritis. Achlorhydria and a pernicious anaemia-like syndrome occur more often in adults than children. Vitamin-B_{12} absorption is reduced but tests for parietal-cell or intrinsic-factor antibodies are negative [45]. It seems likely that the parietal-cell destruction in these patients is caused by T lymphocytes. Reduced gastric acidity may allow increased bacterial overgrowth of the small intestine, resulting in malabsorption; *Giardia lamblia* has also been cited as a common cause of gut symptoms [31]. Associated morphological findings are partial villous atrophy, patchily distributed in the upper jejunum, and nodular lymphoid hyperplasia. The latter can occur throughout the intestine and gives characteristic radiographic changes; it is probably due to uncontrolled B-cell proliferation but is not thought to cause symptoms or to precede lymphoma [46].

Diagnosis. This depends on serum immunoglobulin measurement: rare patients may have relatively normal levels but have grossly impaired antibody responses [47].

Transient hypogammaglobulinaemia

Infants' serum IgG concentrations normally fall during the first three to four months of life, as maternal IgG is diluted and catabolized. IgG synthesis by the infant normally sustains adult IgG levels from about one year of age. The diagnosis of transient hypogammaglobulinaemia is applied to those infants who are slow to achieve adult IgG levels, although they eventually do so. Ascertainment artefact makes it difficult to arrive at any secure conclusions concerning the prevalence of transient hypogammaglobulinaemia or its prognosis. In one study [48] the outlook for the transiently immunodeficient siblings of patients with established immunodeficiency was better than that for patients without a family history. This difference may have arisen from the frequent infections which prompted immunoglobulin estimation in those without a family history. Practically, the most important questions are how to distinguish transient from other types of hypogammaglobulinaemia and which infants should receive IgG replacement injections. The differential diagnosis can sometimes be made by the presence of normal amounts of IgM in serum and IgG in saliva in those with transient hypogammaglobulinaemia and by their ability to make antibody. Replacement IgG could rationally be given to any hypogammaglobulinaemic infant with a severe infection as there is little evidence to suggest that this would interfere with diagnosis or subsequent development of normal immunity [49].

Treatment of antibody deficiency

Most antibody-deficient patients need immunoglobulin replacement, generally as weekly intramuscular injections of about 25 mg of human IgG per kilogram of body weight. Evidence that this significantly protects against infection is strong and it is the primary treatment of choice. Injections of 50 mg/kg give greater freedom from infection than the standard dose [50] but patients complain of pain because the volume of the injection is large. Subcutaneous infusion may be a convenient alternative [50a] Intravenous administration of IgG concentrate meant for intramuscular injection causes severe reactions, which is unfortunate because this route is relatively painless and much larger amounts of IgG could be given. Several types of aggregate-free human IgG specially prepared for intravenous use are currently being evaluated [51, 52] and it seems likely that they will be a major improvement over intramuscular injections.

Immunoglobulin reactions. About one-third of antibody-deficient patients who are treated with intramuscular IgG injections experience reactions at some time [53] though the overall frequency of reactions is low. Their onset is generally within 30 minutes of the injection and early symptoms are limb and backache, facial flushings and acute anxiety. Signs include shivering, tachycardia, fever, hypotension and shock. There have been a few fatalities. Treatment, as for other shock syndromes, is to ensure adequate oxygenation and an adequate venous return to the heart. Adrenaline is conventionally recommended but plasma expanders might be more effective; most reactions resolve spontaneously in two to three hours. Since the requirement for IgG replacement persists, it is important to provide the patient with sympathy and support during the acute phase of the reaction. Available evidence suggests that immunoglobulin reactions are due to IgG aggregates in the injected material entering the circulation too rapidly and their sporadic occurrence argues against an allergic aetiology. Why some patients, particularly boys with X-linked agammaglobulinaemia and others with secondary hypogammaglobulinaemia, should have reactions much more rarely than those with varied immunodeficiency syndromes, is unclear. Repeat treatment of a patient with an IgG batch which has previously caused a reaction does not usually cause a repetition of the reaction so there is no clear case for changing IgG batches or suppliers.

Intravenous immunoglobulin preparations stabilized with maltose cause few, if any, reactions [54].

Plasma infusions. Plasma contains about 1 g of IgG per 100 ml so relatively large volumes have to be given to treat hypogammaglobulinaemia; 15 ml/kg every three weeks is an effective regime in children [55]. The main advantage of plasma is that it can be given intravenously safely and that it is more readily available than intravenous IgG preparations. The danger of hepatitis usually means that only the patient's immediate family can safely be used as donors; this is simple when the volume requirements are small, as for infants, but can lead to difficulties for adults. Viral hepatitis has been responsible for the deaths of several patients treated with pooled or blood-bank plasma. Plasma contains much more IgA than IgG preparations for intramuscular use, so it is perhaps more likely to cause reactions in patients with selective IgA deficiency.

Other immunoglobulins. The half-lives of IgA (five days) and IgM (six days) are too short for replacement therapy to be practicable. It is also unlikely that IgA obtained from the serum and given intravenously would reach the secretions in significant amounts. Oral treatment with bovine colostrum was used for a boy with secretory component deficiency but has apparently not been tried in selective IgA deficiency.

SELECTIVE IMMUNOGLOBULIN DEFICIENCIES

Selective IgA deficiency

Pathology. Criteria for selective IgA deficiency are a serum IgA level of less than 5 mg/100 ml with normal IgG and IgM and normal cell-mediated immunity. The condition has a prevalence of 1:500–1:1200 in Caucasians, depending on the method of ascertainment, so it is the commonest primary defect of specific immunity. Familial cases occur [56] but there is no consistent pattern of inheritance and in one family the deficiency appeared to be HLA haplotype-associated [57]. There are few clues as to aetiology: almost all IgA-deficient patients have IgA-bearing B lymphocytes in their blood and in some cases these cells can be stimulated by pokeweed mitogen to make small amounts of IgA. Why there is failure of normal maturation into IgA-secreting plasma cells *in vivo* is unclear, though an intrinsic defect in the B cells appears most likely at present [58]. Other evidence has pointed to increased monocyte-mediated suppressor activity [59] and to mild degrees of T-cell abnormality. A small proportion of IgA-deficient patients have abnormalities of chromosome 18 [60], but this does not cause IgA deficiency through a structural gene deletion. Selective IgA deficiency can occur secondarily to congenital rubella [61] and to treatment with phenytoin [62]. There is an independent association between low levels of IgA and idiopathic epilepsy [63].

Clinical features. Population studies suggest that perhaps three out of four patients with selective IgA deficiency ultimately develop some of the symptoms described below. Why some should be spared is not known, though it is tempting to speculate that their ability to protect their mucosal surfaces with IgG or IgM might be responsible [64].

Infections: chronic sinusitis, otitis and bronchitis are common, while pneumonia is rare compared with patients with panhypogammaglobulinaemia. Diarrhoea is the main gastro-intestinal feature; about eight per cent have gluten-sensitive enteropathy [65] and rare patients have Crohn's disease or ulcerative colitis [66]. Some patients become chronic *Salmonella* carriers.

Allergy: both abnormally high and low serum IgA levels occur more commonly in allergic than in healthy people [67]. There is also a link between transient IgA deficiency in infancy and the subsequent development of eczema or asthma [68]. A failure of normal T-cell regulation could account for these associations.

Autoimmunity: antibodies to collagen, IgA, IgM, and DNA have been found in 16–40% of IgA-deficient patients [69] and a proportion develops thyroiditis, systemic lupus erythematosus, dermatomyositis or arthritis. There is no clear link between the presence of circulating immune complexes and susceptibility to autoimmune disease [70]. In general, the response to treatment is not different from patients with normal IgA. The anti-IgA antibodies are sometimes responsible for transfusion reactions [71] and for this reason avoidance of blood or plasma products has been recommended. However, some IgA-deficient patients develop anti-IgA antibodies without ever being exposed to heterologous human IgA.

Diagnosis. The diagnosis is made by serum immunoglobulin measurement. It is important to remember that healthy children do not reach adult serum IgA levels until 10–12 years of age, though they make secretory IgA (much of which is IgA_2) from infancy. Selective lack of secretory IgA has been described in one case of secretory component deficiency [72]. The child's symptomatology resembled that of selective IgA deficiency except that serum IgA levels were normal.

Treatment. There is no practical way of restoring IgA to mucosal surfaces, though the patient with secretory-component deficiency benefited from bovine colostrum. Those with recurrent respiratory-tract infections have been treated with antibiotics or, occasionally, with IgG injections. The rationale for the latter is based on the view that IgA-deficient patients make suboptimal antibody responses in other isotypes too.

IgG injections have also been condemned on the grounds that the trace amounts of IgA they contain may elicit the production of anti-IgA antibodies. There seem to be no satisfactory data to resolve this difference.

Selective IgM deficiency

Criteria proposed by Hobbs for primary cases [73] are a serum IgM level more than two standard deviations below the mean, with normal IgG, IgA and cell-mediated immunity. This combination is rare, and little is known of its pathogenesis: affected patients mostly have IgM-bearing B lymphocytes in their blood [73a] but few if any IgM-containing plasma cells in their bone marrow. There are reports of familial cases [74, 75] in which IgM levels have been lowest in males. This may in part reflect the tendency for males to have lower IgM levels than females [76].

Clinical features. Septicaemia with *Pseudomonas pyocyanea*, meningococci or other pyogenic bacteria has been common and often fatal in the patients who have had a splenectomy on account of splenomegaly [73]. Some IgM-deficient patients are neutropenic too [73], which probably considerably increases their susceptibility to infection.

Treatment. Prompt antibiotic treatment has been urged for these patients should they become ill, and splenectomy should probably be avoided [73]. It is possible that the resistance to pneumococcal or meningococcal septicaemia could be increased by immunization in those who made IgG antibody responses normally.

SELECTIVE DEFECTS OF CELL-MEDIATED IMMUNITY

Pathogenesis

Selective impairment of cell-mediated immunity in a patient with normal antibody responses is very rare. This is probably a result of the shared requirement for T lymphocytes for both antibody and cell-mediated immunity. Some separation may be possible because B-cell responses can be helped by relatively few T cells, and these do not have to divide [77], while the effector limb of cell-mediated immunity requires the division of responding T cells. Thymic hypoplasia (Di George's syndrome) has been widely cited as an example of a selective T-cell deficiency, but it now appears that many cases of purine nucleoside phosphorylase deficiency fit this category more closely. A complete lack of T lymphocytes would most likely cause severe combined immunodeficiency because those B cells which developed would be unlikely to respond to antigen stimulus in the absence of T-cell help.

Purine nucleoside phosphorylase (PNP) deficiency

The PNP converts adenosine, inosine, guanosine and their corresponding deoxy compounds to adenine, hypoxanthine and guanine respectively. The structural locus for PNP is on the long arm of chromosome 14 and deficiency is symptomatic only in homozygotes, so transmission is autosomal recessive [78]. About eight affected families have been identified, one of whom carried a gene for a functionally abnormal form of PNP. Interference with lymphocyte function in the absence of PNP probably results from intracellular accumulation of adenosine and guanosine and particularly deoxyguanosine triphosphate (dGTP). The feedback inhibition which this compound exerts on ribonucleotide reductase resembles that caused by dATP in adenosine-deaminase deficiency and as a result T-cell division is prevented. *In-vitro* tests on patients' lymphocytes suggest that T-cell suppressor function is relatively more impaired than helper function: this may account for the propensity to autoimmune haemolytic anaemia and, in two cases, monoclonal gammopathy.

Clinical features. Patients' ages at diagnosis have ranged from three months to seven years. The main problems have been anaemia, pneumonia and severe or fatal pox-virus infections. Several cases have had Coombs-positive haemolytic anaemias. Spasticity in some children may be due to hypoxanthine deficiency because PNP deficiency reduces the availability of substrate for hypoxanthine-guanine phosphoribosyl transferase, so causing a Lesch–Nyhan-like syndrome [78].

Diagnosis. This depends on demonstrating PNP deficiency either in red-cell lysates or in cultured fibroblasts. Measurement of urinary purines is another possibility but is technically demanding. Screening methods employing whole blood are in the stage of evaluation [79]. Affected patients have generally had low blood lymphocyte counts, absent delayed-hypersensitivity skin responses, low *in-vitro* response to PHA and normal serum and salivary immunoglobulins.

Treatment. There is a rational basis for oral or intravenous deoxycytosine since this may bypass the metabolic block [80], but the *in-vivo* effect has been slight. Additional measures have included thymosin, thymus grafts and infusions of irradiated red cells but none is of established benefit. It may be difficult to treat PNP deficiency by bone-marrow grafting because the patients have some residual immunity.

Thymic hypoplasia (Di George's syndrome)
The epithelial-cell component of the thymus is derived from the third and fourth pharyngeal pouches and it grows down into the mediastinum between six and seven weeks of gestation. The parathyroids have the same embryological origin and for unknown reasons they and the thymus sometimes fail to develop normally. Related structures are usually also affected, giving major cardiac defects and facial peculiarities such as a small mandible and a short philtrum. Familial cases are exceptional [81], so the aetiology is generally assumed to be intrauterine damage caused by an environmental agent, possibly a virus.

Clinical features. The main causes of presentation are neonatal hypocalcaemia and cardiac failure; sometimes the diagnosis is made during the course of cardiac surgery when no thymus is found in the anterior mediastinum. The hypocalcaemia is of variable severity and may become obvious only after incidental stress such as cardiac surgery. Even when it is not severe, the parathormone levels remain inappropriately low. The commonest cardiac defects are truncus arteriosus and interrupted aortic arch; difficulties in repairing those are probably the commonest causes of death in this syndrome. The fact that several children with the phenotypic features of thymic hypoplasia have received one or more units of unrelated blood during the course of cardiopulmonary bypass without subsequently developing graft-versus-host disease suggests that they may have had some immunity. Septicaemia has caused a few deaths but susceptibility to infection is usually limited to oral *Candida* or *Pneumocystis carinii* pneumonia.

Diagnosis. Because the cardiac, immunological and endocrine abnormalities are all independently variable, there are no generally accepted diagnostic criteria other than a lack of thymic tissue. The blood lymphocyte count has been normal or low and the percentage of T cells has ranged from less than five to 35. Affected infants have been too young for negative delayed-hypersensitivity skin tests to be meaningful, but the blood lymphocyte response to PHA is low or absent. Serum immunoglobulins are usually normal, antibody activity is detectable, but the response to immunization may be subnormal.

Treatment. Rapid restoration of the blood lymphocyte response to PHA following grafting with fetal thymus was reported in 1968 (reviewed in Ref. 82). This effect has been confirmed in a few subsequent cases but in others the results have been less clear-cut. In some patients a gradual improvement in the percentage of T cells in the blood and in PHA response without any treatment suggests that thymic epithelial tissue is quantitatively rather than qualitatively deficient.

Short-limbed dwarfism
This is a heterogeneous group of conditions, some of which are associated with immunodeficiency. The best established link is with cartilage-hair hypoplasia, while a small number of short-limbed dwarfs have severe combined immunodeficiency [83]. Some of the latter may have had adenosine-deaminase deficiency since this causes severe combined immunodeficiency, commonly with skeletal abnormalities [84]. Two of the 91 cases of immunodeficiency with short-limbed dwarfism reviewed by Ammann *et al.* [83] had selective antibody deficiency.

Cartilage-hair hypoplasia (CHH)
Cartilage-hair hypoplasia is characterized by short-limbed dwarfism, abnormally fine and sparse hair and hyperextensible joints. The syndrome was first identified in the Amish kindred and several of the original cases died of varicella [85]. Laboratory abnormalities include megaloblastic anaemia, lymphopenia, impaired PHA transformation and delayed hypersensitivity skin responses with normal immunoglobulins. Herpes- and pox-group viruses seem to cause the most severe infections in these patients. Chronic otitis media, sinusitis and pneumonia occur in some, perhaps as a result of neutropenia [86]. One patient who was grafted with tissue-matched sibling bone marrow achieved T-cell and erythrocyte chimaerism as well as clinical improvement [87]. Fetal thymus grafts and injections of thymus extracts have been less obviously successful [88]; anti-virus drugs may help with severe varicella.

Hyperimmunoglobulinaemia-E syndrome
This is characterized by eczema, impaired neutrophil mobility, very high serum IgE levels and impaired cell-mediated immunity. Many of the patients have had recurrent pyogenic skin infections [89] and two had coarse facies [90]. The pathogenesis of the condition is obscure and a family history is generally lacking. Failure of both neutrophil and lymphocyte function could result from intracellular cyclic-nucleotide disturbances since these regulate both lymphocyte triggering [91] and microtubule assembly in neutrophils [92]. The high levels of IgE may be due to deficient suppressor-T-cell function [93]. Response to treatment with levamisole [94] and transfer factor [95] have been linked to changes in cyclic-nucleotide metabolism.

Other primary defects of cell-mediated immunity
Most immunodeficiency clinics have a few patients

with low-to-normal blood lymphocyte counts, absent delayed hypersensitivity skin responses, low responses of blood lymphocytes to PHA but normal antibody responses. A few such cases in children have been published [96, 97]. Some of these patients may have had PNP deficiency and others probably have as yet undescribed metabolic defects. Their susceptibility to virus infections, especially with cytomegalovirus, Herpes and varicella, is similar to that seen with other deficiencies of cell-mediated immunity, but some patients have had recurrent bacterial infections too. Defective neutrophil mobility could contribute to the latter.

Treatment of selective defects of cell-mediated immunity

It is not possible to replace the effector limb of cell-mediated immunity with the same effectiveness as is possible for antibody deficiency. This reflects the requirement for cells, rather than soluble factors, to perform antigen-specific, cell-mediated functions. Consequently most treatments for deficient cell-mediated immunity have a theoretical basis which involves the expansion of specific lymphocyte populations or the induction of lymphocyte development.

Human fetal thymus grafts were originally used in thymic hypoplasia and following their insertion, usually into the rectus sheath, there were dramatic increases in blood lymphocyte counts, response to PHA and clearing of superficial candidiasis [82]. The recipients did not become lymphocyte chimaeras so improvement has been attributed to thymic humoral factors acting on the recipient's own precursors. Thymic hypoplasia is too rare, and the impression of therapeutic benefit is perhaps too strong, for any controlled trials to have been undertaken. However, spontaneous improvement in immunity has also taken place in patients with thymic hypoplasia, so the case for fetal thymus grafting is not entirely established. Patients with a range of other primary immunodeficiencies such as severe combined immunodeficiency, Wiskott–Aldrich syndrome, chronic mucocutaneous candidiasis and cartilage-hair hypoplasia have been grafted with fetal thymus, mostly with little lasting evidence of success and rarely with graft-versus-host disease (p. 691).

Thymus extracts. It seems likely that thymic factors are responsible for recruiting stem cells into the thymus and perhaps also for a post-thymic maturational step (see Chapter 17). Several laboratories have characterized different putative thymic factors which are supposed to cause lymphocyte maturation, and these have been somewhat haphazardly given to patients but no clear picture of their usefulness has emerged. There were increases in the number of E-rosetting blood lymphocytes and their mitogen-responsiveness in some patients [98].

Thymic epithelial-cell grafts. Small pieces (approximately 1 mm³) of human thymus cultured *in vitro* for two or more weeks gradually lose their lymphoid component, while epithelial cells remain. Such fragments have been used to treat patients with severe combined immunodeficiency who did not have compatible sibling donors [99], and a patient with thymic hypoplasia [100]. Preliminary results in both groups appear promising; this is surprising in the patients with combined immunodeficiency since one might not expect lymphocytes which had been educated in an allogeneic thymus to be able to recognize antigen presented with autologous histocompatibility antigens [101].

Levamisole. Levamisole is an anti-helminthic imidazole drug which can increase skin-test responsiveness in patients with impaired cell-mediated immunity [102]. The mechanism of this effect is unknown, but may be related to alterations in lymphocyte cyclic-nucleotide levels. The drug also increases neutrophil mobility in some patients with chemotaxis defects. Side effects have been few apart from neutropenia and nausea but the therapeutic role of Levamisole is not yet established [103].

COMBINED IMMUNODEFICIENCY SYNDROMES

Pathogenesis

This group of disorders is characterized by severe impairment of both antibody and cell-mediated immunity. Most cases are congenital and thus, presumably, genetically determined; autosomal- and X-linked recessive inheritance is recognized and there are minor clinical and laboratory differences between these two forms of the disease. Occasionally adults acquire defects of antibody and cell-mediated immunity as severe as those which occur in the primary form of the disease: this may be a severe form of varied immunodeficiency or it may occur with thymoma.

The dual failure of antibody and cell-mediated responses in congenital severe combined immunodeficiency (SCID) led to the view that the disease arose from the failure of a common lymphoid stem cell to develop during ontogeny. Tests for lymphocyte populations suggest that this is not generally so, since most infants with SCID have at least some B cells and a few have low numbers of T cells also. A minority lack pre-B cells, B cells and T cells and a failure of stem-cell development remains a possibility in them, though whether this might be due to an intrinsic defect or a failure of an inductive environment is unknown. The B cells of those patients that have them may secrete immunoglobulin when they are stimulated with mitogens in the presence of normal T cells [104]. It seems likely that a primary lack of T cells can, through failure of help to B cells, result in antibody deficiency as well as defective cell-mediated immunity. A clearer picture of the pathogenesis of SCID exists only in adenosine-deaminase deficiency (see below).

Clinical features
Affected infants usually develop infections during the first three months of life. The infecting organism depends on exposure: when infants were vaccinated against smallpox, those with SCID used to develop disseminated vaccinia [105]; now they sometimes present with progressive BCG infection [106]. The commonest presenting symptom of SCID is diarrhoea with failure to thrive; the gut disturbance is almost universal and it sometimes causes recurrent vomiting too. Dietary changes may give temporary improvement, even with weight gain, but relapse is usual. The transient appearance of skin rashes (of unknown aetiology) and sometimes of eosinophilia may strengthen the impression that the patient has food allergy. Gastro-intestinal investigations including X-rays, absorption tests or biopsy are not usually helpful, though a lack of lymphocytes in the mucosa could be a diagnostic clue. There is a clinical impression that babies with SCID who are exclusively breast-fed tend to remain in better health for the first few months of life than those who are artificially fed.

Skin or respiratory-tract infections predominate in some infants: a candida nappy rash is almost universal and oral candidiasis is common too. Pneumonias in the first few months of life may be caused by *Pneumocystis carinii* and later they are caused by pyogenic bacteria as well. Both usually respond well to the appropriate antibiotics. Without successful immunological reconstitution the clinical course is of progressive emaciation leading to death in one to two years. Even intensive antibiotic treatment rarely sustains life beyond this.

Varieties of severe combined immunodeficiency (see Table 18.4)

Adenosine-deaminase deficiency. This accounts for about 20% of cases of SCID. Occasionally the enzyme defect results in an apparently selective loss of cell-mediated immunity, which may be an antecedent of combined immunodeficiency. The clinical picture of ADA-deficient SCID differs little from that described above except that affected infants' lymphocytes may be normal at birth and they may make some immunoglobulin for the first few months of life [107]. The immunodeficiency tends to be progressive and at autopsy the thymus is small, with a few Hassall's corpuscles. Many ADA-deficient patients have had defects of ossification leading to typical, but probably not diagnostic, X-ray findings [84]. ADA and purine nucleoside phosphorylase (PNP) deficiency afford the clearest insight into the pathogenesis of any primary immunodeficiency, so their metabolic basis is described in detail (see also Ref. 107). ADA converts

Table 18.4. Types of SCID, listed in approximate order of incidence, which can be distinguished by family history, clinical features or laboratory tests

Name	Synonyms	Inheritance
SCID (unclassified)	Swiss-type gammaglobulinaemia, thymic alymphoplasia	Autosomal recessive or X-linked
Adenosine deaminase deficiency	—	Autosomal recessive
SCID with immunoglobulins	Nezelof syndrome	Autosomal recessive or X-linked
SCID with neutropenia	Reticular dysgenesis	?
SCID with reticulo-endotheliosis	—	?

adenosine and deoxyadenosine into inosine and deoxyinosine. The structural locus of the enzyme is on chromosome 20 and there are two alleles. Individuals who are homozygous for a null gene have to rely on other less specific enzymes, such as adenosine aminohydrolase, to deaminate adenosine, and these pathways require relatively higher substrate concentrations. The adenosine and deoxyadenosine which accumulate intracellularly are phosphorylated by adenosine kinases to ATP and dATP. Ribonucleotides diffuse poorly out of cells, so this phosphorylation results in trapping. DeoxyATP is the most toxic substrate to accumulate because it blocks ribonucleotide reductase at concentrations as low as 4 μM and so interferes with the synthesis of other ribonucleotides. The special vulnerability of T cells compared with other cells (such as B cells) to ADA deficiency probably results from their relatively higher concentrations of adenosine kinase and their lack of 5′ nucleotidase [108]. Ribonucleotide synthesis is not the only pathway which may fail because increased intracellular concentrations of adenosine can lead to the accumulation of S′-adenosylhomocysteine and deoxyadenosine blocks S-adenosylhomocysteine hydrolase [109]. Both of these effects would result in a failure of methylation reactions.

ADA is present in red cells and infusions of irradiated red cells are sometimes effective for treatment [110].

Severe combined immunodeficiency with immunoglobulins. This is a poorly defined group of patients who have been separately classified from others with SCID because they have some serum immunoglobulins [111]. Onset is usually with diarrhoea, malabsorption or recurrent chest infections and occurs at ages ranging from three months to seven years. Most patients die within two years unless it is possible to restore their immunity. Both X-linked and autosomal-recessive forms of transmission exist; some of those with autosomal-recessive transmission may have had ADA deficiency. There is a tendency for affected boys in families with an X-linked transmission to have high percentages of blood B cells, and these B cells appear immature because of multiple surface immunoglobulin isotypes. The relative constancy of laboratory and clinical findings in these boys may permit them to be classified separately.

Severe combined immunodeficiency with neutropenia. A few patients with SCID have neutropenia as well as lymphopenia. Whether or not they should be separately classified is still uncertain. The original cases were monozygotic twins [112], and they died within a few days of birth; blood counts in these and other patients are listed in Table 18.5. One of a pair of affected male siblings had a normal neutrophil count at birth but low numbers at 40 days of age; at necropsy, following death from pseudomonas septicaemia at 52 days, granulocyte precursors were lacking from the bone marrow. His sibling lacked granulocytes in the blood, but had normal numbers of blood lymphocytes, some of which made E rosettes although they did not respond to mitogens *in vitro*. The pathogenesis of SCID with neutropenia has been attributed to failure of a common haemopoietic stem cell: the sparse and variable results in children diagnosed as having this condition neither confirm nor refute this hypothesis.

Table 18.5. Severe combined immunodeficiency with neutropenia: blood counts and marrow studies

Ref.	Patient	Sex	Marrow myeloid cells	T cells	B cells	Neutrophils at weeks of age $\times 10^{-9}$/l					
						1	2	6	7	8	9–10
112*	1	M	Absent			0					
	2	M	Absent			0					
179†	1	F	Absent			15–20					
180†	1	F	Reduced								1100–1600
181‡	1	M	Reduced				3120	1216	20		
	2§	M	Absent	66%		0					
182‡	1	M	Reduced				770				
	2	M	Reduced	Low	0	792	45				
183	1	M	Reduced	Low		20	< 10	60		50	< 20

* The original patients were monozygotic twins.

† Both these patients received transfusions of fresh blood and may have developed graft-versus-host disease.

‡ Patients 1 and 2 were affected male siblings.

§ This patient had congenital cytomegalovirus infection.

Severe combined immunodeficiency with reticulo-endotheliosis. A minority of patients with an erythematous scaling-skin rash, lymphadenopathy and splenomegaly lack serum immunoglobulins and PHA-responsive lymphocytes. This group differs from patients with histiocytosis whose immunity is normal in the early stages of the disease. The skin and reticulo-endothelial changes may be due to graft-versus-host disease, but not all these patients have been transfused. Maternal lymphocytes acquired across the placenta have been considered as a possible source of foreign cells [112a]. The prognosis in this type of SCID appears bleak [113, 114].

Treatment of severe combined immunodeficiency

Bone-marrow transplantation. Infants with any form of SCID who are fortunate enough to have a sibling with the same major histocompatibility antigens have a 50% or better chance of cure with a bone-marrow graft. Adequate degrees of histocompatibility are generally only found between siblings who have identical HLA-A and B-locus antigens and it is HLA-D-locus identity (shown by non-reactivity in mixed-lymphocyte culture) which is of prime importance. Some idea of which siblings, if any, are likely to be HLA-D-identical with the patient can usually be obtained from A- and B-locus antigens because the MHC haplotypes on chromosome 6 segregate according to classical genetic principles; the chances of any two siblings being HLA-identical is 1:4 (Table 18.6). Rare successful grafts have been performed between other family members who were D-locus-identical with the patient although they may have differed at A or B loci. Compatibility of this sort is seen in inbred communities where antigens may be shared between parents, or it can result from chromosomal crossing over; it is relatively rare.

Special pathogen-free environments are generally not required for SCID patients who are to be grafted with compatible sibling bone marrow. This is because immunological reconstitution is usually rapid and no special immunosuppressive treatments are required to ensure acceptance of the graft. Marrow is aspirated from the donor's iliac crest until sufficient cells have been obtained to give the patient between 10^8 and 10^9/kg body weight. Since SCID patients are generally small, the volume of blood lost by the donor may be less than 40 ml, so transfusion replacement is rarely necessary. Immediate hazards of the marrow infusion to the recipient include volume overload and interference with the pulmonary circulation by clumps of cells or fat; both are minimized by giving the marrow slowly. The main late hazard is graft-versus-host disease, which is described on page 691.

Table 18.6. Tissue-typing evidence for donor selection for bone-marrow graft treatment of severe combined immunodeficiency

HLA A- and B-locus typing:

Mother	Father
A 1 B 8	A 2 B 27
A 2 B 12	A 28 B 35

Sib 1	Sib 2*	Sib 3 (patient)
A 1 B 8	A 2 B 12	A 2 B 12
A 28 B 35	A 2 B 27	A 2 B 27

Tritiated thymidine uptake in mixed lymphocyte cultures:

Responder	Stimulator	Counts/min
Sib 1	Patient	8630
Sib 2	Patient	242*
Control	Patient	10 110
Sib 1	Control	11 151
Sib 2	Control	9268
Patient	Control	180
Sib 1	Sib 1	260
Sib 2	Sib 2	241
Control	Control	292

* These results suggest that Sib 2 would be a suitable donor for the patient.

In countries where the family size is small, the majority of SCID patients do not have compatible related donors, and at present their outlook is poor. Possible lines of treatment include grafting with unrelated A-, B- and D-locus-identical marrow, but such grafts may fail to take or may be followed by chronic graft-versus-host disease [115]. Occasional patients have benefited from fetal liver [116] or fetal thymus grafts [114], but this is exceptional. Some success has been claimed for grafts of 'thymic epithelium' [99]. These comprise chopped pieces of human thymus, removed from donors undergoing cardiac surgery, which are kept in tissue culture for two to three weeks. Few lymphocytes remain in the tissue pieces after this time, although cells with epithelial morphology survive.

Red-cell transfusions. About half of infants with ADA deficiency have had increased blood lymphocyte counts, increased lymphocyte response to mitogens and rises in serum immunoglobulins following infusions of 15 ml/kg of irradiated packed red cells at four-week intervals [110]. This effect is attributed to the ADA which is present in the transfused red cells and the therapeutic benefit is greatest in those who have the most residual immunity at the time treatment is started. Sensitization to non-ABO antigens is a risk, so ADA trapped into the patient's own red-cell ghosts is being evaluated, but these ghosts have a shorter survival than donor RBC. Red-cell transfusions have been tried empirically in other types of SCID without success but there is certainly a case for this practice in patients who have no related bone-marrow donors.

Germ-free care and other supportive measures. Infants with SCID delivered into and maintained in germ-free conditions thrive [118]. The therapeutic relevance of such technical feats remains unestablished. Most successful sibling bone-marrow grafts for SCID have been done without germ-free care because immunological reconstitution is fast compared with the slow spontaneous decline which otherwise occurs. It could be argued that germ-free care would be useful for infants who lack sibling donors for whom more hazardous grafting procedures are planned. Possible benefits should perhaps be weighed against the risk that the attempts to reconstitute the patient may fail, so making it difficult to withdraw germ-free support.

Non-specific supporting measures such as attention to adequate nutrition and co-trimoxazole prophylaxis against *Pneumocystis carinii* may significantly prolong life. There is an impression that infants with SCID who are exclusively or largely breast-fed thrive better than those who are bottle-fed, at least for the first six months of life. Weekly intramuscular injections of human IgG seem to provide little protection from infection, but larger amounts, as can be given intravenously, may be more effective.

MISCELLANEOUS DISORDERS ASSOCIATED WITH DEFECTS OF ANTIBODY OR CELL-MEDIATED IMMUNITY

Ataxia telangiectasia

Ataxia telangiectasia is a complex syndrome characterized by ataxia, oculocutaneous telangiectasia and immunodeficiency. The predominant features of the latter are deficiency of IgE and IgA [119] and a small abnormal thymus; infections are mostly of the respiratory tract. The inheritance is autosomal and recessive and a progressive cerebellar ataxia is the usual presenting symptom [128]. The telangiectases may not become visible for months or years following the onset of the ataxia: they are most prominent on the bulbar conjunctivae, the bridge of the nose and the ears. The intellect is usually preserved until late in the course of the disease; immunity may also be unimpaired until late, and up to a third of patients may die without any clear evidence of immunodeficiency. Other abnormali-

ties which occur in this syndrome include raised α-fetoprotein levels, impaired glucose tolerance and infertility. No single hypothesis adequately explains all these defects but it is clear that immunodeficiency is only an inconstant part of the totality. Perhaps the most fundamental abnormality yet discovered is a failure of DNA repair [121], which may account for the increased incidence of malignancy in ataxia telangiectasia patients and their first-degree relatives [122].

Diagnosis depends primarily on the neurological features, supported by a family history or telangiectases of appropriate distribution. Presence or absence of IgA is not itself sufficient, nor are the T-cell abnormalities diagnostic.

Treatment is unsatisfactory. It is possible to improve cell-mediated immunity in some patients with injections of thymus extracts, transfer factor or fetal thymus grafts, but there is no evidence to suggest that these manipulations affect the progress of the neurological disease.

Wiskott–Aldrich syndrome

This syndrome is characterized by thrombocytopenia, eczema and immunodeficiency. It has an X-linked recessive inheritance but it is not known what the defective gene product is. Only the platelet abnormality has been detected in carriers [123], so this manifestation is presumably more closely related to the primary defect than the eczema or susceptibility to infection, which occur only in affected boys. The abnormal platelets are small and they fail to aggregate normally in response to ADP [124]. The immunological abnormalities are complex and tend to become increasingly severe as the child grows. Early defects include a failure to make antibody to polysaccharide antigens [125] and low serum IgM with high serum IgE. A generalized protein hypercatabolism is one factor which contributes to the reduced IgM, while IgG and IgA synthetic rates appear to keep up with the hypercatabolism [126]. Blood lymphocyte responses to mitogens (mostly PHA) are normal initially but may become diminished with time [124]; the number of blood T cells falls also. A lack of T-cell suppression may account for the raised IgE levels and perhaps also for some of the later complications such as monoclonal proteins [128] or autoimmune haemolytic anaemia [129].

Clinical features. Common presenting symptoms are bloody diarrhoea or stroke as a result of intracranial haemorrhage; both result from the thrombocytopenia. The eczema commonly appears in infancy and has the same distribution and appearance as atopic eczema.

Infections may be more obvious later; they involve the respiratory tract and the skin and are usually bacterial. Patients who cannot be successfully reconstituted usually die before the age of 12, mostly from intracranial haemorrhage, septicaemia or lymphoma.

Treatment. Grafting with tissue-matched sibling bone marrow appears to offer the best hope for affected boys [130], though how successful the grafts will be in the long term is not yet established. Bone-marrow grafting in Wiskott–Aldrich syndrome is more difficult than in severe combined immunodeficiency because the recipients do not completely lack cell-mediated immunity, so that graft rejection is a possibility. Recently the recipients have been pre-treated with anti-lymphocyte globulin and irradiation, and donor red-cell, granulocyte, platelet and lymphocyte populations were established [130].

Most Wiskott–Aldrich-syndrome patients do not have tissue-matched siblings, so alternative forms of treatment are required. Improvement in the eczema, with laboratory evidence for improved T-cell function, has been claimed for transfer-factor treatment. In a large uncontrolled trial about 50% of the patients benefited [131] and there was some reduction in bleeding. Immunoglobulin replacement therapy is probably not helpful because of the hypercatabolism, and splenectomy carries a high risk of subsequent septicaemia [132]; this can evidently be greatly reduced by continuous prophylaxis with antibiotics, however, and the corrective effect on the platelet count may make splenectomy worthwhile [132a].

Chronic mucocutaneous candidiasis

Pathology. Chronic mucocutaneous candidiasis (CMC) is characterized by recurrent superficial *Candida* infection of skin, mucous membranes (particularly oral) and nails. Some cases are familial, others are sporadic, and there are differences in associated features such as endocrinopathy and susceptibility to staphylococcal infection. It is therefore likely that CMC comprises a number of related syndromes with similar clinical manifestations but different underlying immunological defects. Most CMC patients have normal serum immunoglobulins and make large amounts of anti-candida antibodies [133] while a few have had varied immunodeficiency syndromes with low serum IgA [134]. The blood lymphocyte count is usually normal and the number of T cells and response to PHA may be normal or low. There is some suggestion that patients with defective lymphocyte migration-inhibition-factor (MIF) production are more likely to have a chronic granulomatous form of the disease [135] but the patients' abnormalities in

these and other lymphocyte-function tests are not always stable. The variability in test results may be due to the presence of serum factors such as the anti-candida antibodies, which can block candida killing [133], and candida-derived polysaccharide antigens which interfere with lymphocyte stimulation [136]. Some children with CMC have recurrent staphylococcal abscesses [137]; the basis of this complication is not known but neutrophil bacterial killing and mobility appears to be normal *in vitro*. Thyroid, adrenal, parathyroid and pituitary deficiencies sometimes occur, with autoantibody present in the serum. Whether the tendency to autoimmune disease is primary or secondary is unclear [138].

Clinical features. Onset is usually in childhood and the severity is variable, ranging from disfiguring to relatively minor nail and oral candidiasis. Children with pituitary deficiency tend to grow slowly and ovarian failure may delay menarche. There is an increased incidence of sudden death from unknown causes.

Treatment. Conventional treatment comprises topical and systemic anti-fungal drugs (miconazole and amphotericin B) with avulsion of affected nails, and oral or intravenous iron for those with iron deficiency [139]. The toxicity of the anti-fungal drugs prohibits their continuous systemic use, but with intermittent treatment the candidiasis can usually be cleared at least temporarily. About 50% of patients were found to benefit from transfer-factor treatment [140], with best results when this was given after chemotherapy.

Lymphocytotoxins and episodic lymphocytopenia

Complement-fixing lymphocytotoxins which are capable of lysing lymphocytes *in vitro* occur in some patients with systemic lupus erythematosus [141], in people over about 60 years of age [142], and following virus infections [143]. The lymphocytotoxins of patients with SLE sometimes have specificity for suppressor T cells, so it is conceivable that they are of primary pathological significance [144], while in other adults there is little evidence that the lymphocytotoxins are damaging. Antibody deficiency in one adult female was attributed to lymphocytotoxins with specificity for B cells [145], and removal of the antibody by plasmapheresis was followed by an increase in the number of circulating B cells.

A few children have been reported who had episodes of lymphopenia associated with the production of complement-fixing lymphocytotoxins [146]. Their antibody and cell-mediated immunity was impaired and one died with a reticulum-cell sarcoma.

The presence of lymphocytotoxins can confuse tests for T and B cells, since T cells coated with antibody (which is often IgM) will stain positively for surface immunoglobulin [147].

Thymoma

About 10% of patients with thymomas develop hypo-gammaglobulinaemia: most of these patients have spindle-cell tumours [148]. Usually all immunoglobu-lin classes are affected and their levels do not rise following removal of the thymoma. Thymoma patients with hypogammaglobulinaemia are unusual in that they lack B cells in their blood and pre-B cells in their bone marrow, while their cell-mediated immunity may be normal or impaired [149]. Other haematologi-cal associations are eosinopenia and red-cell aplasia (see Chapter 31). The pathogenesis of these acquired defects is unknown: one possibility is that the thy-moma produces an excess of suppressor T cells which limit pre-B and red-cell-precursor activity. Immuno-regulatory disturbances, as judged by autoantibody production, are common with other types of thymoma and they may cause haemolytic anaemia, myasthenia gravis, systemic lupus erythematosus and endocrine failure [150].

SECONDARY IMMUNODEFICIENCY

Secondary is very much more common than primary immunodeficiency. The great variety of agents which can interfere with specific immunity makes classifica-tion difficult, so only an empirical listing is given here (Table 18.7). The subject is reviewed in greater detail in Refs 21 and 151 and is discussed here only in relation to possible diagnostic confusion. Severe malnutrition bears a complex relation to immunodeficiency in that specific immunity is clearly depressed but the resulting

Table 18.7. Causes of secondary immunodeficiency

Malnutrition
Primary, dietary
Secondary to gut disease
Selective trace-element or vitamin deficiency

Loss, affecting:
Lymphocytes and protein from gut in intestinal lymphan-giectasia or other enteropathy
Protein in nephrotic syndrome
Protein in burns, with secondary effects on lymphocytes

Drugs
Steroids
Cytotoxic
Miscellaneous, including anaesthetics, phenytoin, penicilla-mine, phenothiazines

Infections
Protozoal (malaria)
Bacterial
Viral: measles and others

---

infections themselves interfere with nutrition. Serum immunoglobulins remain normal until late in primary malnutrition, after cell-mediated immunity and pri-mary antibody responses are impaired. Protein-losing enteropathy usually causes a non-selective loss of serum proteins so that the serum albumin is low, as well as IgG levels: diagnostic error can be avoided by measuring serum albumin on all patients with hypo-gammaglobulinaemia. Intestinal lymphangiectasia is one rare cause of protein-losing enteropathy which is important in that it can result in lymphopenia. Tests of cell-mediated immunity may be impaired and serum IgG levels are low; though these patients seem to have few infections in relation to the abnormality of their laboratory tests.

Fatal infection with opportunists such as herpes-group viruses or fungi have become a common complication of highly immunosuppressive drug regimes. Drugs given continuously are generally more immunosuppressive than those given intermittently [152] and the lymphoid system may take three months or more to recover after leukaemia remission main-tenance treatment [18]. Radiotherapy is very immuno-suppressive also and causes long-term alterations in blood lymphocyte populations [153].

Two drugs, phenytoin [63] and penicillamine [154], sometimes cause IgA deficiency. Probably fewer than 25% of patients taking phenytoin are affected and the effect is difficult to analyse because there is also an independent association between idiopathic epilepsy and IgA deficiency. However, some patients' IgA levels rise when the drug is discontinued. Patients with phenytoin-induced IgA deficiency continue to have IgA-bearing B cells in their blood: perhaps their failure to make IgA is due to interference with T-cell help since phenytoin has been found to interfere with T-cell proliferation and it sometimes causes widespread lymphadenopathy [62].

X-linked lymphoproliferative syndrome (Duncan's disease)

Duncan's disease was originally described as a rare and frequently fatal form of infectious mononucleosis which occurred in six of 18 boys in the Duncan kindred [155]. With the recognition of other affected families the heterogeneity of the syndrome has become appar-ent [156]; its features include massive lymphopro-liferation, non-tropical Burkitt's lymphoma, plasma-cytoma, aplastic anaemia and sometimes acquired hypogammaglobulinaemia. The outcome is com-monly fatal. Evidence for the association with Epstein–Barr virus is based partly on the presence of heterophile antibodies in the patients and, more securely, on the recovery of the EBV genome by hybridization. Tests for antibody to the EBV early antigen or the viral capsid antigen are usually negative. The defect which underlies these patients' inability to control their EBV infections is not known; possible candidates include an intrinsic defect of B cells or a failure to control the infection by T cells. The X-linked inheritance could perhaps be accounted for more readily by a B-cell surface-antigen defect, possibly analogous to the CBA/N defect in mice [157].

Transcobalamin-II deficiency (see also Chapter 6)
Transcobalamin II (TC II) is a serum protein which normally transports vitamin B_{12} from the gut epithelium to cells. It has a genetic polymorphism and rare individuals who are homozygous for a null gene lack detectable serum TC II. Only one of the few affected individuals to have been identified was immunodeficient [158]. The patient's parents were first cousins and Moroccan and he was delivered by Caesarean section into a sterile environment because two previous siblings in the family had died of infection in infancy. Antibody deficiency was diagnosed and was treated by replacement IgG injections from three months of age. At four months the boy developed severe diarrhoea and bronchopneumonia, followed by anaemia (macrocytic and megaloblastic), leucopenia and thrombocytopenia. There was a rapid haematological response to injections of 1 mg B_{12} and the serum IgM and IgA levels subsequently became normal. Recurrent lung infections persisted and at five years of age a defect of bacterial killing was found. This was corrected by treatment with formyl-tetrahydrofolic acid. A second affected family has recently been identified [158a].

Graft-versus-host disease
Graft-versus-host (GVH) disease results from giving foreign immunocompetent lymphocytes to patients with severely impaired cell-mediated immunity. The disease is initiated by the donor lymphocytes and is prevented if the donated lymphocytes are irradiated to 1000 rads or more [159]. Experimental work in inbred strains of mice suggests that the disease depends on the recognition of certain host histocompatibility antigens which are foreign to the donor, which stimulate the donor cells to proliferate and to attack host target cells [160]. The antigens responsible for the initial stimulation are coded for in the I region of the mouse histocompatibility complex while the targets for attack are coded for in the K and D regions. The human equivalents for these antigens would be the Ia (or possibly the DRw) antigens as stimulators and the A and B determinants as targets [161]. Graft-versus-host disease is also accompanied by the production of autoantibodies to a range of host antigens, resulting in Coombs-positive haemolytic anaemia [162] and immune-complex glomerulonephritis due to DNA–anti-

DNA antibody complexes [163]. The antibodies in these instances may be made by host plasma cells.

Grafts between members of an inbred strain do not generally result in GVH disease, and genetic disparity outside the major histocompatibility locus is only a weak stimulus to the disease. In man the situation is very different because only identical twins have the same degree of genetic identity as inbred mice; the random segregation of chromosomes during meiosis results in major differences between other siblings. Since each parent has two major histocompatibility loci (one from each parent, on chromosome 6) there are only four possible permutations amongst the offspring, so the chances that any one sibling will be HLA-compatible with another is 1:4. Grafts between HLA-matched siblings where the recipient has severe combined immunodeficiency or aplastic anaemia are commonly followed by transient mild to severe GVH which has conventionally been attributed to incompatibility at minor histocompatibility loci outside the HLA A, B, C and D regions, presumably on another chromosome. The recent observation of GVH-like syndromes in the recipients of grafts from identical twins [164] raises the possibility that GVH disease may sometimes be due to an imbalance between T-cell-helper and suppressor activities, resulting in an acute autoimmune syndrome [165].

In order for the recipient to become susceptible to GVH disease, his cell-mediated immunity has to be virtually absent, as in severe combined immunodeficiency, or to have been severely impaired by cytotoxic drugs and/or irradiation, as in antileukaemia treatment [166]. The danger of GVH disease is at least partly related to the degree of immunodeficiency and the number of foreign lymphocytes which are given; infants with severe combined immunodeficiency have died following transfusion of as little as 50 ml whole blood.

Clinical features. The first clinical finding is usually of an erythematous and then maculopapular rash which may be localized or generalized. It rarely appears earlier than five days after the giving of incompatible cells and may be delayed for several weeks, particularly if the number of cells given was small. The histology of the skin rash is helpful in diagnosis; characteristic features include a mild vasculitis with mononuclear-cell infiltration of the dermis. The basal-cell layer is disorganized with vacuolization and lymphocyte infiltration and the epidermal cells lose their polarity [167]. In severe GVH the rash progresses to an exfoliative dermatitis, and in milder cases it may become chronic and scaly or sclerodermatous [168]. In transient GVH the rash fades completely; this may be due to the development of tolerance [169] or to the loss of graft

function. The main extradermal manifestation of
GVH disease is diarrhoea and this may be accompanied by bleeding. The blood count varies: eosinophilia is often an early finding and if the disease progresses
there may be bone-marrow aplasia, neutropenia, haemolytic anaemia and, rarely, thrombocytopenia. The
number of small lymphocytes in the blood decreases,
to be replaced by large atypical or monocytoid cells.
Lymphadenopathy may accompany the skin rash,
especially if it becomes chronic, later there may be
splenomegaly and liver enlargement. Raised transaminases often give laboratory evidence of hepatitis.
Lung involvement is seen on X-ray as pulmonary
infiltrates and histologically as thickening and
mononuclear infiltration of alveolar septa.

Treatment. The treatment of established GVH is
unsatisfactory whether steroids, anti-lymphocyte
globulin or cytotoxic drugs are used [170]. Prevention,
by good matching, is best. Experimental preventive
measures include total lymphoid irradiation [171] and
treatment with cyclosporin A [172]. Other measures
such as post-grafting treatment with methotrexate
have some effect but tend to leave the recipient with
secondary immunodeficiency [173].

DIAGNOSIS OF IMMUNODEFICIENCY
Most immunity function tests are relatively crude, so
the diagnosis or exclusion of immunodeficiency
depends on clinical, as well as laboratory, evidence.
The most useful diagnostic clues come from the
history. A family history of recurrent infections
favours primary over secondary immunodeficiency
and if the inheritance is clear it may point directly to a
diagnosis. Many types of primary immunodeficiency
are commoner in boys than girls, but it should be
remembered that affected male siblings are compatible
with, but not diagnostic of, an X-linked inheritance.
Rare primary immunodeficiencies are usually first
identified in the offspring of consanguineous parents,
so it is worth asking whether any such relationship
exists. A family history of autoimmunity could be
informative in diagnosing adult-onset varied immunodeficiency, since this appears to be a complex immuno-
pathological disorder with polygenic inheritance.

Infections
Recurrent infections at a single site may be due to local
anatomical defects. Since it is the lungs which are most
often infected in immunodeficiency it is important to
exclude cystic fibrosis, tracheo-oesophageal fistula,
aspirated foreign body, saliva or α_1-antitrypsin deficiency. Tumours should be considered in adults. The
organism and type of infection can give useful clues
(Table 18.8), though co-existence of defects such as

cell-mediated immunity and neutrophil mobility may
affect this.

Age of onset
Apart from thymic hypoplasia and antibody deficiency due to congenital virus infection, most congenital immunodeficiency is genetically determined. Congenital antibody deficiency rarely causes an excess of
infections for the first four or five months of life while
maternal antibody persists. Exceptions to this generalization include infections by organisms to which the
mother lacked antibody, and a premature fall in
maternal IgG due to prematurity or to protein loss.
There is no significant passive transfer of specific
cell-mediated immunity or non-specific immunity, so
infants with severe combined immunodeficiency or
chronic granulomatous disease are at risk from the
time that they are colonized by environmental
organisms. Congenital immunodeficiencies in which
there is immunological attrition, such as ADA or PNP
deficiency or Wiskott–Aldrich syndrome, tend to
present after three or four months or later.

Physical and X-ray findings
Infants with most types of severe combined immunodeficiency lack palpable lymph nodes; exceptions are
those with reticulo-endotheliosis (p. 687) or GVH.
Antibody-deficient patients usually have small but
palpable nodes, but their tonsils are small and a lateral
X-ray view of the pharynx may show paucity of
adenoid and retropharyngeal lymphoid tissue. Chest
X-rays may provide evidence of previous lung damage
and one would not expect to see a thymus shadow in an
infant with thymic hypoplasia or severe combined
immunodeficiency. Lack of a thymus shadow is common in children with any long-standing illness.

Investigations
Selection amongst the tests listed in Table 18.9 should
be guided by the clinical features. More sophisticated
tests are best left to laboratories which have extensive
experience in their application, and sufficient control
data to permit interpretation. Some of the limitations
of the simpler tests are described next.

Antibody-mediated skin tests. Positive immediate
hypersensitivity skin responses to common antigens
such as pollen or cat fur indicate IgE production and a
possibility of allergy. A negative Schick test in a
diphtheria-immunized person indicates the presence of
antibody, but it is currently difficult to obtain Schick
antigen so this test is of limited application.

Delayed-hypersensitivity skin tests. A positive delayed-
hypersensitivity skin test is good evidence for normal

Table 18.8. Correlations between infecting agent and primary immunodeficiency

Organism	Associated immunodeficiency
Bacteria	
Staph. aureus	Antibody deficiency
	Chronic granulomatous disease
Other pyogenic bacteria	Antibody deficiency
	C3 deficiency
Neisseria (disseminated)	C5–9 deficiency
Mycobacteria:	
Progressive BCG	Chronic granulomatous disease
disseminated BCG	Severe combined immunodeficiency
Fungi	
Superficial *Candida*	Severe combined immunodeficiency
	Selective T-cell defects
	Chronic mucocutaneous candidiasis
Invasive aspergillosis	Chronic granulomatous disease
Protozoa	
Pneumocystis carinii	Severe combined immunodeficiency
Giardiasis	Antibody deficiency
Viruses	
Severe or progressive	Severe combined immunodeficiency
varicella	Defects of cell-mediated immunity
Disseminated vaccinia	Defects of cell-mediated immunity

cell-mediated immunity. The most useful test antigens are those to which most healthy people are likely to be sensitive; PPD has been extensively used in the past but tetanus toxoid, candida or trichophyton are probably preferable now [174].

Immunoglobulin measurement. Most patients with any form of antibody deficiency have an abnormality of serum immunoglobulin levels, so immunoglobulin measurement is a useful screening test. The reproducibility of radial immunodiffusion measurement should be within $\pm 10\%$ for IgG and IgA and $\pm 20\%$ for IgM. Automated nephelometry should be more accurate than this but is difficult to apply to lipaemic samples with low levels. Immunoglobulin measurements are calibrated against a reference serum and are best expressed as iu/ml by comparison with the WHO standard. International-unit values can be converted to mg/l [175] but the weight values may err considerably, especially in patients with monoclonal excesses. It is essential to use age-matched control data for interpreting results in children, since adult levels are not reached until nine months for IgM, two years for IgG and 12 years for IgA.

Antibody tests. These are most useful for evaluating patients who have the clinical features of an antibody-deficiency syndrome with significant amounts of serum immunoglobulins. The choice of antibody to test for should be determined by the antigen experience of the patient and by the facilities available. Isohaemagglutinins are a convenient IgM antibody to test for in patients over the age of one year, provided they are not blood group AB. Alternatives include *E. coli* agglutinins [176] and anti-*Salmonella* O antibodies. For IgG antibodies most laboratories can test for anti-streptolysin O and some activity (in the eight to 50 unit range) is generally detectable in adults. Patients who have been immunized can be tested for antibodies to tetanus toxoid, diphtheria toxoid, polio virus, rubella or measles. Patients with low antibody levels can safely be boosted with tetanus and diphtheria toxoids but endotoxin-containing antigens such as *Pertussis* or *Salmonella* (TAB) are probably best avoided if IgM levels are low, because of the risk of reactions. Certain antigens such as Øx 174 or flagellin have particular advantages for antibody tests [177] but facilities for these are not widely available.

Lymphocyte-population tests. Counts of T and B lymphocytes may be diagnostically useful for distinguishing between certain types of antibody deficiency and some types of severe combined immunodeficiency. They are much less useful in the diagnosis or management of the much commoner varied immunodeficiency syndromes. Most laboratories use

Table 18.9. Specific immunity function tests*

Test level	Function tested	
	Antibody immunity	Cell-mediated immunity
Simple clinical or lab test	Serum immunoglobulins, salivary IgA, isohaemagglutinins (IgM antibodies)	Delayed hypersensitivity skin tests with candida, trichophyton, tetanus toxoid, mumps, PPD
Special tests, first level	ASO, anti-diphtheria or tetanus antibodies (IgG), anti-virus antibodies	Whole blood PHA response
Special tests, second level	Antibody responses to defined antigens: KLH, Øx174 Immunoglobulin subclasses, κ/λ ratios, IEP for immunoglobulin heterogeneity. Blood B-cell numbers, bone marrow for B and pre-B cells. *In-vitro* B-cell differentiation	Blood T-cell numbers, T-cell subpopulations, lymphocyte response to other mitogens (Con A, PWM), response to antigens and in mixed-lymphocyte culture, mediator production

* For a description of laboratory methods see Refs 184 and 185.
Abbreviations: ASO, antistreptolysin O titre; Con A, concanavalin A; IEP, immunoelectrophoresis; PHA, phytohaemagglutinin; PWM, pokeweed mitogen; Øx 174, bacteriophage; KLH, keyhole limpet haemocyanin.

immunofluorescence for surface IgM to identify B cells, but the discrepancy between these results and the much higher percentages obtained by anti-globulin rosetting methods [178] are not yet resolved. Measurement of EAC-rosetting cells is not an adequate substitute for surface immunoglobulin measurement. The E-rosette test is the commonest test at present for T cells, but it is being replaced by immunofluorescence for T cells using monoclonal hybridoma antibodies [178a]. Currently available antibodies can distinguish between T-cell precursors, thymocytes, mature T cells and their helper-inducer and cytotoxic-suppressor subsets.

Lymphocyte-function tests. Measurement of the proliferative response of T lymphocytes to phytohaemagglutinin (PHA) is the most useful lymphocyte-function test, since low responses correlate with impaired or absent cell-mediated immunity. A screening method using whole blood is often more informative than a test using separated lymphocytes, and it requires only 0·2 ml of blood or less, which is an important consideration in testing infants. Many other mitogens will stimulate T cells but none is as clinically useful as PHA. Other tests for T-cell function include their proliferative response to antigen, help to B cells, cytotoxicity or mediator production. These are more valuable as research tools than as routine clinical tests.

REFERENCES

1 EPSTEIN M.A. & ACHONG B.G. (eds) (1979) *The Epstein–Barr Virus.* Springer-Verlag, Berlin.
2 YEVENOF E. & KLEIN G. (1977) Membrane receptor stripping confirms the association between EBV receptors and complement receptors on the surface of human B lymphoma lines. *International Journal of Cancer*, **20**, 347.
3 REEDMAN B.M. & KLEIN G. (1973) Cellular localization of an Epstein–Barr virus-associated complement-fixing antigen in producer and non-producer lymphoblastoid cell lines. *International Journal of Cancer*, **11**, 599.
4 WAELE M.D., THIELEMANS C. & VAN CAMP B.K.G. (1981) Characterization of immunoregulatory T cells in EBV-induced infectious mononucleosis by monoclonal antibodies. *New England Journal of Medicine*, **304**, 460.
5 EPSTEIN M.A. & ACHONG B.G. (1979) The relationship of the virus to Burkitt's lymphoma. In: *The Epstein–Barr Virus* (ed. Epstein M.A. & Achong B.G.), p. 322. Springer-Verlag, Berlin.
6 KLEIN G. (1972) Herpes viruses and oncogenesis, *Proceedings of the National Academy of Sciences, USA*, **69**, 1056.
7 DAVIDSOHN I. & LEE C.L. (1969) The clinical serology of infectious mononucleosis. In: *Infectious Mononucleosis* (ed. Carter R.L. & Penman H.G.), p. 177. Blackwell Scientific Publications, Oxford.
8 BIRD A.G. & BRITTON S. (1979) A new approach to the study of human B-lymphocyte function using an indirect plaque assay and a direct B-cell activator. *Immunological Reviews*, **45**, 41.

9 MANGI R.J., NIEDERMAN J.C., KELLEHER J.E., DWYER J.M., EVANS A.S. & KANTOR F.S. (1974) Depression of cell-mediated immunity during acute infectious mononucleosis. *New England Journal of Medicine*, **291**, 1149.

10 RILEY H.D. (1953) Acute infectious lymphocytosis. *New England Journal of Medicine*, **248**, 92.

11 KANTOR G.L. & GOLDBERG L.S. (1971) Cytomegalovirus-induced post-perfusion syndrome. *Seminars in Hematology*, **8**, 261.

12 TAUB R.N., ROSETT W., ADLER A. & MORSE S.I. (1972) Distribution of labelled lymph node cells in mice during the lymphocytosis induced by Bordetella pertussis. *Journal of Experimental Medicine*, **136**, 1581.

13 KALTER S.S., RODRIGUEZ A.R. & HEBERLING R.L. (1977) Cat-scratch disease skin-test antigen preparation. *Lancet*, **ii**, 606.

14 SCADDING G.K., THOMAS H.C. & HAVARD C.W.H. (1979) The immunological effects of thymectomy in myasthenia gravis. *Clinical and Experimental Immunology*, **36**, 205.

15 FAUCI A.S. & DALE D.C. (1974) The effect of *in vivo* hydrocortisone on subpopulations of human lymphocytes. *Journal of Clinical Investigation*, **53**, 240.

16 FAUCI A.S. (1975) Corticosteroids and circulating lymphocytes. *Transplantation Proceedings*, **7**, 37.

17 BACH J.F. (1975) *The Mode of Action of Immunosuppressive Agents*. North-Holland, Amsterdam.

18 PAOLUCCI P., HAYWARD A.R. & RAPSON N.T. (1979) Pre-B and B cells in children on leukaemia remission maintenance treatment. *Clinical and Experimental Immunology*, **37**, 259.

19 ZACHARSKI L.R. & LINMAN J.W. (1971) Lymphocytopenia: its causes and significance. *Mayo Clinic Proceedings*, **46**, 168.

20 SOOTHILL J.F., STOKES C.R., TURNER M.W., NORMAN A.P. & TAYLOR B. (1976) Predisposing factors and the development of reaginic allergy in infancy. *Clinical Allergy*, **6**, 305.

21 WORLD HEALTH ORGANIZATION (1978) Immunodeficiency. *Technical Report Series No. 630*, World Health Organization.

22 DE LA CONCHA E.G., OLDHAM G., WEBSTER A.D.B., ASHERSON G.L. & PLATTS-MILLS T.A.E. (1977) Quantitative measurements of T and B cell function in variable primary hypogammaglobulinaemia: evidence for a consistent B-cell defect. *Clinical and Experimental Immunology*, **27**, 208.

23 CICCIMARA F., ROSEN F.S., SCHNEEBERGER E. & MERLER E. (1976) Failure of heavy chain glycosylation of IgG in some patients with common variable agammaglobulinaemia. *Journal of Clinical Investigation*, **57**, 1386.

24 PEARL E.R., VOGLER L.B., OKOS A.J., CRIST W.M., LAWTON A.R. & COOPER M.D. (1978) B lymphocyte precursors in human bone marrow: an analysis of normal individuals and patients with antibody-deficiency states. *Journal of Immunology*, **120**, 1169.

25 WALDMANN T.A., DURM M., BRODER S., BLACKMAN M., BLAESE R.M. & STROBER W. (1974) Role of suppressor T cells in pathogenesis of common variable hypogammaglobulinaemia. *Lancet*, **ii**, 609.

26 SIEGAL F.P., SIEGAL M. & GOOD R.A. (1978) Role of helper, suppressor and B-cell defects in the pathogenesis of the hypogammaglobulinemias. *New England Journal of Medicine*, **299**, 172.

27 BRUTON O.C. (1952) Agammaglobulinemia. *Pediatrics*, **9**, 722.

28 SAULSBURY F.T., WINKELSTEIN J.A. & YOLKEN R.H. (1980) Chronic Rotavirus infection in immuno-deficiency. *Journal of Pediatrics*, **97**, 61.

29 LAWRENCE J.S. (1971) Rheumatic disease in hypogammaglobulinaemia. In: *Hypogammaglobulinaemia in the United Kingdom*, p. 35. Medical Research Council Special Report Series 310, HMSO, London.

30 WEBSTER A.D., TAYLOR-ROBINSON D., FURR P.M. & ASHERSON G. (1978) Mycoplasmal (ureaplasma) septic arthritis in hypogammaglobulinaemia. *British Medical Journal*, **i**, 478.

31 WEBSTER A.D.B. (1976) The gut and immunodeficiency disease. *Clinics in Gastroenterology*, **5**, 323.

32 AMENT M.E., OCHS H.D. & DAVIS S.D. (1973) Structure and function of the gastrointestinal tract in primary immunodeficiency syndromes: a study of 39 patients. *Medicine*, **52**, 227.

33 WEBSTER A.D.B., TRIPP J.H., HAYWARD A.R., DAYAN A.D., DOSHI R., MacINTYRE E.H. & TYRRELL D.A.J. (1978) Echovirus encephalitis and myositis in primary immunoglobulin deficiency. *Archives of Diseases of Childhood*, **53**, 33.

34 WILFERT C.M., BUCKLEY R.H., MOHANAKUMAR T., GRIFFITH J.W., KATZ S.L. WHISNANT J.K., EGGLESTON P.A., MOORE M., TREADWELL E., OXMAN M.N. & ROSEN F.S. (1977) Persistent and fatal central nervous system echovirus infections in patients with agammaglobulinemia. *New England Journal of Medicine*, **296**, 1485.

35 ROSEN F.S. & JANEWAY C.A. (1966) The gamma globulins. III. The antibody deficiency syndromes. *New England Journal of Medicine*, **275**, 709.

35a FLEISHER T.A., WHITE R.M., BRODER S., NISSLEY P., BLAESE R.M., MULVHILL J.J., OLIVE G. & WALDMANN T.A. (1980) X-linked hypogammaglobulinemia and isolated growth hormone deficiency. *New England Journal of Medicine*, **302**, 1429

36 SOOTHILL J.R., HAYES K. & DUDGEON J.A. (1966) The immunoglobulins in congenital rubella. *Lancet*, **i**, 1385.

37 MEDICAL RESEARCH COUNCIL (1971) *Hypogammaglobulinaemia in the United Kingdom*. Medical Research Council, p. 55. Special Report Series 310. HMSO, London.

38 GEHA R.S., HYSLOP N., ALAMI S., FARAD F., SCHNEEBERGER E.E. & ROSEN F.S. (1979) Hyperimmunoglobulin M immunodeficiency. *Journal of Clinical Investigation*, **64**, 385.

39 STIEHM E.R. & FUDENBERG H.H. (1966) Clinical and immunologic features of dysgammaglobulinemia type 1. *American Journal of Medicine*, **40**, 805.

40 HILL L.E. (1971) Clinical features of hypogammaglobulinaemia. In: *Hypogammaglobulinaemia in the United Kingdom*, p. 9. Medical Research Council Special Report Series 310. HMSO, London.

41 WOLF J.K. (1962) Primary acquired agammaglobulinemia with family history of collagen disease and hematologic disorders. *New England Journal of Medicine*, **266**, 473.

42 OXELIUS V.A. (1979) Quantitative and qualitative investigations of serum IgG subclasses in immunodeficiency diseases. *Clinical and Experimental Immunology*, **36**, 112.

43 BARANDUN S., MORELL A., SKVARIL F. & OBERDORFER A. (1976) Deficiency of κ or λ type immunoglobulins. *Blood*, **47**, 79.

44 BERNIER G.M., GUNDERMAN J.R. & RUYMANN F.B. (1972) Kappa chain deficiency. *Blood*, **40**, 795.

45 TWOMEY J.J., JORDAN P.H., LAUGHTER A.H., MEUWISSEN H.J. & GOOD R.A. (1970) The gastric disorder in immunoglobulin deficient patients. *Annals of Internal Medicine*, **72**, 499.

46 NAGURA H., KOHLER P.F. & BROWN W.R. (1979) Immunocytochemical characterization of the lymphocytes in nodular lymphoid hyperplasia of the bowel. *Laboratory Investigation*, **40**, 66.

47 GIEDION A. & SCHEIDEGGER J.J. (1957) Kongenitale immunoparese bei Fahlen Spezifischer β_2 globuline und normalen γ globulinen. *Helvetica Paediatrica Acta*, **12**, 241.

48 TILLER T.L. & BUCKLEY R.H. (1978) Transient hypogammaglobulinemia of infancy: review of the literature, clinical and immunologic features of 11 new cases, and long term follow-up. *Journal of Pediatrics*, **92**, 347.

49 OTT E., IBOTT F.A., O'BRIEN D. & KEMPE C.H. (1963) The effect of monthly gammaglobulin administration on morbidity and mortality from infection in premature infants during the first year of life. *Journal of Pediatrics*, **32**, 4.

50 HILL L.E. & MOLLISON P.L. (1971) *Hypogammaglobulinaemia in the United Kingdom*, p. 124. Medical Research Council Special Report Series 310. HMSO, London.

50a BERGER M., CUPPS T.R. & FAUCI A.S. (1980) Immunoglobulin replacement therapy by slow subcutaneous infusion. *Annals of Internal Medicine*, **93**, 55.

51 NOLTE M.T., PIROFSKY B., GERRITZ G.A. & GOLDING B.B. (1979) Intravenous immunoglobulin therapy for antibody deficiency. *Clinical and Experimental Immunology*, **36**, 237.

52 YAMANAKA T., ABO W., CHIBA S., NAKAO T., MASUHO Y., TOMIBE K. & NOGUCHI T. (1979) Clinical effect and metabolism of S-sulphonated immunoglobulin in seven patients with congenital humoral immunodeficiency. *Vox Sanguinis*, **37**, 14.

53 SOOTHILL J.F. (1971) Reactions to immunoglobulin. In: *Hypogammaglobulinaemia in the United Kingdom*, p. 106. Medical Council Special Report Series 310. HMSO, London.

54 OCHS H.D., BUCKLEY R.H., PIROFSKY B., FISCHER S.H., ROUSELL R.H., ANDERSON C.J. & WEDGWOOD R.J. (1980) Safety and patient acceptability of intravenous immune globulin in 10% maltose. *Lancet*, **ii**, 1158.

55 BUCKLEY R.H. (1977) Replacement therapy in immunodeficiency. In: *Recent Advances in Clinical Immunology 1* (ed. Thompson R.), p. 219, Churchill, London.

56 VAN LOGHEM E. (1974) Familial occurrence of isolated IgA deficiency associated with antibodies to IgA. Evidence against a structural gene defect. *European Journal of Immunology*, **4**, 57.

57 VAN THIEL D.H., SMITH W.I., RABIN B.S., FISHER S.E. & LESTER R. (1977) A syndrome of immunoglobulin A deficiency, diabetes mellitus, malabsorption and a common HLA haplotype. *Annals of Internal Medicine*, **86**, 10.

58 CASSIDY J.T., OLDHAM G. & PLATTS-MILLS T.A.E. (1979) Functional assessment of a B cell defect in patients with selective IgA deficiency. *Clinical and Experimental Immunology*, **35**, 296.

59 WALDMANN T.A., BRODER S., KRAKAUER R., DURM M., MEADE B. & GOLDMAN C. (1976) Defect in IgA secretion and in IgA specific suppressor cells in patients with selective IgA deficiency. *Transactions of the Association of American Physicians*, **89**, 215.

60 STEWART J., GO S., ELLIS E. & ROBINSON A. (1970) Absent IgA and deletions of chromosome 18. *Journal of Medical Genetics*, **7**, 11.

61 BUCKLEY R.H. (1975) Clinical and immunologic features of selective IgA deficiency. In: *Immunodeficiency in Man and Animals* (ed. Bergsma D., Good R.A. & Finstad J.), p. 134. Sinauer Press, Sunderland.

62 SORELL T.C. & FORBES I.J. (1975) Depression of immune competence by phenytoin and carbamazepine. *Clinical and Experimental Immunology*, **20**, 275.

63 SEAGER J., JAMISON D.L., WILSON J., HAYWARD A.R. & SOOTHILL J.R. (1975) IgA deficiency, epilepsy and phenytoin treatment. *Lancet*, **i**, 632.

64 OGRA P.A., COPPOLA P.R., MACGILLIVRAY M.H. & DZIERBA J.L. (1974) Mechanisms of mucosal immunity to viral infections in α-A-immunoglobulin deficiency syndromes. *Proceedings of the Society for Experimental Biology and Medicine*, **145**, 811.

65 AMMANN A.J. & HONG R. (1971) Selective IgA deficiency: presentation of 30 cases and a review of the literature. *Medicine*, **50**, 223.

66 CLAMAN H.N., MERRILL D.A., PEAKMAN D. & ROBINSON A. (1970) Isolated severe gamma A deficiency: immunoglobulin levels, clinical disorders and chromosome studies. *Journal of Laboratory and Clinical Medicine*, **75**, 307.

67 KAUFMAN H.S. & HOBBS J.R. (1970) Immunoglobulin deficiencies in an atopic population. *Lancet*, **ii**, 1061.

68 TAYLOR B., NORMAN A.P., ORGEL H.A., STOKES C.R., TURNER M.W. & SOOTHILL J.F. (1973) Transient IgA deficiency and pathogenesis of infantile atopy. *Lancet*, **ii**, 111.

69 AMMANN A.J. & HONG R. (1970) Selective IgA deficiency and autoimmunity. *Clinical and Experimental Immunology*, **7**, 833.

70 CUNNINGHAM-RUNDLES C., BRANDEIS W.E., GOOD R.A. & DAY N.K. (1978) Milk precipitins, circulating immune complexes and IgA deficiency. *Proceedings of the National Academy of Sciences, USA*, **75**, 3387.

71 VYAS G.N. & FUDENBERG H.H. (1970) Immunobiology of human anti-IgA: a serologic and immunogenetic study of immunization to IgA in transfusion and pregnancy. *Clinical Genetics*, **1**, 45.

72 STROBER W., KRAKAUER R., KLAEVEMAN H.L., REYNOLDS H.Y. & NELSON D.L. (1976) Secretory component deficiency. *New England Journal of Medicine*, **294**, 351.

73 HOBBS J.R. (1975) IgM deficiency. In: *Immunodeficiency in Man and Animals* (ed. Bergsma D., Good R.A. & Finstad J.), p. 112. Sinauer Press, Sunderland.

73a LEVITT D. & COOPER M.D. (1980) IgM production: normal development and selective deficiency. In: *Primary Immunodeficiencies* (ed. Seligmann M. & Hitzig W.H.), p. 3. Elsevier/North-Holland, Amsterdam

74 HOBBS J.R., MILNER R.D.G. & WATT P.J. (1967) Gamma-M deficiency predisposing to meningococcal septicaemia. *British Medical Journal*, iv, 583.

75 FAULK W.P., KIYASU W.S., COOPER M.D. & FUDENBERG H.H. (1971) Deficiency of IgM. *Pediatrics*, 47, 399.

76 BUCKLEY R.H. & DORSEY F.C. (1971) Serum immunoglobulin levels throughout the life span of healthy man. *Annals of Internal Medicine*, 75, 673.

77 FAUCI A.S. (1979) Human B cell function in a polyclonally induced plaque forming cell system. Cell triggering and immunoregulation. *Immunological Reviews*, 45, 93.

78 AMMANN A.J. (1979) Immunological aberrations in purine nucleoside phosphorylase deficiency. In: *Enzyme Defects and Immune Dysfunction*, p. 55. Ciba Foundation Symposium 68, Excerpta Medica, Amsterdam.

79 ITO K., SAKURA N., USUI T. & UCHINO H. (1977) Screening for primary immunodeficiencies associated with purine nucleoside phosphorylase or adenosine deaminase deficiency. *Journal of Laboratory and Clinical Medicine*, 90, 844.

80 ZEGERS B.J.M., STOOP J.W., STAAL G.E.J. & WADMAN S.K. (1979) An approach to the restoration of T cell function in a purine nucleoside phosphorylase deficient patient. In: *Enzyme Defects and Immune Dysfunction*, p. 231. Ciba Foundation Symposium 68, Excerpta Medica, Amsterdam.

81 STEELE R.W., LIMAS C., THURMAN G.B., SCHUELEIN M., BAUER H. & BELLANTI J.A. (1972) Familial thymic aplasia (attempted reconstitution with fetal thymus in a millipore diffusion chamber). *New England Journal of Medicine*, 287, 787.

82 CLEVELAND W.W. (1975) Immunological reconstitution in the Di George syndrome by fetal thymic transplant. In: *Immunodeficiency in Man and Animals* (ed. Bergsma D., Good R.A. & Finstad J.), p. 352. Sinauer Press, Sunderland.

83 AMMANN A.J., SUTLIFF W. & MILLINCHICK E. (1974) Antibody mediated immunodeficiency in short limbed dwarfism. *Journal of Pediatrics*, 84, 200.

84 WOLFSON J.T. & CROSS V.F. (1975) The radiographic findings in 49 patients with combined immunodeficiency. In: *Combined Immunodeficiency Disease and Adenosine Deaminase Deficiency* (ed. Meuwissen H.). Academic Press, New York.

85 MCKUSICK V.A. (1964) Metaphyseal dysostosis and thin hair: a new recessively inherited syndrome? *Lancet*, i, 832.

86 LUX S.W., JOHNSTON R.B., AUGUST C.S. SAY B., PENCHASZADEH V.B., ROSEN F.S. & MCKUSICK V.A. (1970) Chronic neutropenia and abnormal cell-mediated immunity in cartilage-hair hypoplasia. *New England Journal of Medicine*, 282, 231.

87 HONG R., AMMANN A.J., HUANG S.-W., LEVY R.L., DAVENPORT G., BACH M.L., BACH F.H., BORTIN M.M. & KAY H.E.M. (1972) Cartilage-hair hypoplasia: effect of thymus transplants. *Clinical Immunology and Immunopathology*, 1, 15.

88 STEELE R.W., BRITTON H.A., ANDERSON C.T. & KNIKER W.T. (1976) Severe combined immunodeficiency with cartilage-hair hypoplasia: *in vitro* response to thymosin and attempted reconstitution. *Pediatric Research*, 10, 1003.

89 HILL H.R. & QUIE P.G. (1974) Raised serum IgE levels and defective neutrophil chemotaxis in three children with eczema and recurrent bacterial infections. *Lancet*, i, 183.

90 BUCKLEY R.H., WRAY B.B. & BELMAKER E.Z. (1972) Extreme hyperimmunoglobulinemia E and undue susceptibility to infection. *Pediatrics*, 49, 59.

91 PARKER C.W. (1974) Cyclic AMP and the immune response. *Advances in Cyclic Nucleotide Research*, 4, 1.

92 GALLIN J.I., MALECH H.L., WRIGHT D.G., WHISNANT J.K. & KIRKPATRICK C.H. (1978) Recurrent severe infections in a child with abnormal leukocyte function: possible relationship to increased microtubule assembly. *Blood*, 51, 919.

93 BUCKLEY R.H. & BECKER W.G. (1978) Abnormalities in the regulation of human IgE synthesis. *Immunological Reviews*, 41, 288.

94 WRIGHT D.G., KIRKPATRICK C.H. & GALLIN J.I. (1977) Effects of levamisole on normal and abnormal leukocyte locomotion. *Journal of Clinical Investigation*, 59, 941.

95 KESARWALA H.H., PRASAD R.V.S.K., SZEP R., OLDMAN E., LANE S. & PAPAGEORGIOU P.S, (1979) Transfer factor therapy in hyperimmunoglobulinemia E syndrome. *Clinical and Experimental Immunology*, 36, 465.

96 BALLOW M. & GOOD R.A. (1975) Report of a patient with T cell deficiency and normal B cell function. *Cellular Immunology*, 19, 219.

97 REZZA E., AIUTI F., BUSINCO L. & CASTELLO M.A. (1974) Familial lymphopenia with T lymphocyte defect. *Journal of Pediatrics*, 84, 178.

98 AIUTI F., AMMIRATI P., FIORILLI M., D'AMELIO R., CALVANI M. & BUSINCO L. (1979) Immunologic and clinical investigation on a bovine thymic extract: therapeutic applications in primary immunodeficiencies. *Pediatric Research*, 13, 797.

99 HONG R., SANTOSHAM M., SCHULTE-WISSERMANN H., HOROWITZ S., HSU S.H. & WINKELSTEIN J.A. (1976) Reconstitution of T and B lymphocyte function in severe combined immunodeficiency disease after transplantation with thymic epithelium. *Lancet*, ii, 1270.

100 THONG Y.H., ROBERTSON E.F., RISCHBIETH H.G., SMITH G.J., BINNS G.F., CHENEY K. & POLLARD A.C. (1978) Successful restoration of immunity in the Di George syndrome with fetal thymic epithelial transplant. *Archives of Diseases of Childhood*, 53, 580.

101 ZINKERNAGEL R.M. (1978) Thymus function and reconstitution of immunodeficiency. *New England Journal of Medicine*, 298, 222.

102 VERHAEGEN H., DE CREE J., DE COCK W. & VERBRUGGEN F. (1977) Restoration by levamisole of low E-rosette-forming cells in patients suffering from various diseases. *Clinical and Experimental Immunology*, 27, 313.

103 EDITORIAL (1979) *Lancet*, ii, 291.

104 SEEGER R.C., ROBINS R.A., STEVENS R.H., KLEIN R.B., WALDMAN D.J., ZELTZER P.M. & KESSLER S.W. (1976) Severe combined immunodeficiency with B lymphocytes: *in vitro* correction of defective immunoglobulin

production by addition of normal T lymphocytes. *Clinical and Experimental Immunology*, **26**, 1.

105 FULGINITI V.A., KEMPE C.H., HATHAWAY W.E., PEARLMAN D.S., SIEBER O.F., ELLER J.J., JOYNER J.J. & ROBINSON A. (1968) Progressive vaccinia in immunologically deficient individuals. In: *Immunologic Deficiency Diseases in Man. Birth Defects. IV*. (ed. Bergsma D.), p. 129. National Foundation, March of Dimes, New York.

106 MATSANIOTIS N. & ECONOMOU-MAVROU C. (1968) Fatal generalized BCG infection: a result of immunologic deficiency. In: *Immunologic Deficiency Diseases in Man. Birth Defects. IV*. (ed. Bergsma D.), p. 124. National Foundation, March of Dimes, New York.

107 HIRSCHHORN R. (1979) Clinical delineation of adenosine deaminase deficiency. In: *Enzyme Defects and Immune Dysfunction*, p. 35. Ciba Foundation Symposium 68, Excerpta Medica, Amsterdam.

108 ROWE M., DE GAST C.G., PLATTS-MILLS T.A.E., ASHERSON G.L. & WEBSTER A.D.B. (1979) 5′ nucleotidase of B and T lymphocytes isolated from human peripheral blood. *Clinical and Experimental Immunology*, **36**, 97.

109 HERSCHFIELD M.S., KREDICH N.M., OWNBY D., OWNBY H. & BUCKLEY R. (1979) *In vitro* inactivation of erythrocyte S-adenosyl cysteine hydrolase by 2′-deoxy adenosine in adenosine deaminase deficient patients. *Journal of Clinical Investigation*, **63**, 807.

110 POLMAR S.H. (1979) Enzyme replacement and other biochemical approaches to the therapy of adenosine deaminase deficiency. In: *Enzyme Defects and Immune Dysfunction*, p. 213. Ciba Foundation Symposium 68, Excerpta Medica, Amsterdam.

111 LAWLOR G.J., AMMANN A.J., WRIGHT W.C., LAFRANCHI S.H., BILSTROM D. & STIEHM R. The syndrome of cellular immunodeficiency with immunoglobulins. *Journal of Pediatrics*, **84**, 183.

112 DE VAAL O.M. & SEYNAHAEVE V. (1959) Reticular dysgenesia. *Lancet*, **ii**, 1123.

112a CHURCH J.A. & UITTENBOGAART C. (1980) Partial immunologic reconstitution and hyperimmunoglobulinemia E in neonatally acquired graft versus host disease. *Annals of Allergy*, **44**, 212.

113 CEDERBAUM S.D., NIWAYAMA G., STIEHM E.R., NEERHOUT R.C., AMMANN A.J. & BERMAN W. (1974) Combined immunodeficiency presenting as the Letterer–Siwe syndrome. *Journal of Pediatrics*, **85**, 466.

114 OCHS H.D., DAVIS S.D., MICKELSON E., LERNER K.G., & WEDGWOOD R.J. (1974) Combined immunodeficiency and reticulo-endotheliosis with eosinophilia. *Journal of Pediatrics*, **85**, 463.

115 KENNY A.B. & HITZIG W.H. (1979) Bone marrow transplantation for severe combined immunodeficiency disease. *European Journal of Pediatrics*, **131**, 155.

116 BUCKLEY R.H., WHISNANT J.K., SCHIFF R.I., GILBERTSEN R.B., HUANG A.T. & PLATT M.S. (1976) Correction of severe combined immunodeficiency by fetal liver cells. *New England Journal of Medicine*, **294**, 1076.

117 RACHELEFSKY G.S., STIEHM E.R., AMMANN A.J., CEDERBAUM S.D., OPELZ G. & TERASAKI P.I. (1975) T cell reconstitution by thymus transplantation and transfer factor in severe combined immunodeficiency. *Pediatrics*, **55**, 114.

118 MUKHOPADHYAY N., RICHIE E., MACKLER B.F., MONTGOMERY J.R., WILSON R., FERNBACH D.J. & SOUTH M.A. (1978) A longitudinal study of T and B lymphocytes from a three year old patient with severe combined immunodeficiency in gnotobiotic protection. *Experimental Hematology*, **6**, 129.

119 POLMAR S.H., WALDMANN T.A. & TERRY W.D. (1972) IgE in immunodeficiency. *American Journal of Pathology*, **69**, 499.

120 BODER E. (1975) Ataxia telangiectasia: some historic, clinical and pathologic observations. In: *Immunodeficiency in Man and Animals* (ed. Bergsma D., Good R.A. & Finstad J.), p. 255. Sinauer Press, Sunderland.

121 HOAR D.I. & SARGENT P. (1976) Chemical mutagen hypersensitivity in ataxia telangiectasia. *Nature (London)*, **261**, 590.

122 SWIFT M., SHOLMAN L., PERRY M. & CHASE C. (1976) Malignant neoplasms in the families of patients with ataxia telangiectasia. *Cancer Research*, **36**, 209.

123 SHAPIRO R.S., GERRARD J.M., PERRY G.S., WHITE J.G., KRIVIT W. & KERSEY J.H. (1978) Wiskott–Aldrich syndrome: detection of carrier state by metabolic stress of platelets. *Lancet*, **i**, 121.

124 KURAMOTO A., STEINER M. & BALDINI M.G. (1970) Lack of platelet response to stimulation in the Wiskott–Aldrich syndrome. *New England Journal of Medicine*, **282**, 475.

125 COOPER M.D., CHASE H.P., LOWMAN J.T., KRIVIT W. & GOOD R.A. (1968) Immunologic defects in patients with Wiskott–Aldrich syndrome. In: *Immunologic Deficiency Diseases in Man. Birth Defects. IV*. (ed. Bergsma D.), p. 378, National Foundation, March of Dimes, New York.

126 BLAESE R.M., STROBER W., LEVY A.L. & WALDMANN T.A. (1971) Hypercatabolism of IgG, IgM and albumin in the Wiskott–Aldrich syndrome. *Journal of Clinical Investigation*, **50**, 2331.

127 OPPENHEIM J.J., BLAESE R.M. & WALDMANN T.A. (1970) Defective lymphocyte transformation and delayed hypersensitivity in Wiskott–Aldrich syndrome. *Journal of Immunology*, **104**, 835.

128 BRUCE R.M. & BLAESE R.M. (1974) Monoclonal gammopathy in the Wiskott–Aldrich syndrome. *Journal of Pediatrics*, **85**, 204.

129 BALLOW M., DUPONT B. & GOOD R.A. (1973) Autoimmune hemolytic anaemia in Wiskott–Aldrich syndrome during treatment with transfer factor. *Journal of Pediatrics*, **83**, 772.

130 PARKMAN R., RAPPAPORT J., GEHA R., BELLI J., CASSADY R., LEVEY R., NATHAN D.G. & ROSEN F.S. (1978) Complete correction of the Wiskott–Aldrich syndrome by allogeneic bone marrow transplantation. *New England Journal of Medicine*, **298**, 921.

131 SPITLER L.E. (1979) Transfer factor therapy in the Wiskott–Aldrich syndrome. Results of long term follow-up in 32 patients. *American Journal of Medicine*, **67**, 59.

132 HUNTLEY C.C. & DEES S.C. (1957) Eczema associated with thrombocytopenic purpura and purulent otitis media. Report of five fatal cases. *Pediatrics*, **19**, 351.

132a LUM L.G., TUBERGEN D.G., CORASH L. & BLAESE R.M. (1980) Splenectomy in the management of the thrombocytopenia of the Wiskott–Aldrich Syndrome. *New England Journal of Medicine*, **302**, 892.

133 KIRKPATRICK C.H., RICH R.R. & BENNETT J.E. (1971) Chronic mucocutaneous candidiasis: model building in cellular immunity. *Annals of Internal Medicine*, **74**, 955.

134 SCHLEGEL R.J., BERNIER G.M., BELLANTI J.A., MAYBEE D.A., OSBORNE G.B., STEWART J.L., PEARLMAN D.S., OVELETTE J. & BIEHUSEN F.C. (1970) Severe candidiasis associated with thymic dysplasia, IgA deficiency and plasma antilymphocyte effects. *Pediatrics*, **45**, 926.

135 VALDIMARSSON H., WOOD C.B.S., HOBBS J.R. & HOLT P.J.L. (1972) Immunological features in a case of chronic granulomatous candidiasis and its treatment with transfer factor. *Clinical and Experimental Immunology*, **11**, 151.

136 FISCHER A., BALLET J.J. & GRISCELLI C. (1978) Specific inhibition of *in-vitro* candida-induced lymphocyte proliferation by polysaccharide antigens present in the serum of patients with chronic mucocutaneous candidiasis. *Journal of Clinical Investigation*, **62**, 1005.

137 BUCKLEY R.H., LUCAS Z.J., HATTLER B.G., SMIJEWSKI C.M. & AMOS D.B. (1968) Defective cellular immunity associated with chronic mucocutaneous moniliasis and recurrent staphylococcal botryomycosis: immunological reconstitution by allogeneic bone marrow. *Clinical and Experimental Immunology*, **3**, 153.

138 ARULANANTHAM K., DWYER J.M. & GENEL M. (1979) Evidence for defective immunoregulation in the syndrome of familial candidiasis endocrinopathy. *New England Journal of Medicine*, **300**, 164.

139 HIGGS J.M. & WELLS R.S. (1972) Chronic mucocutaneous candidiasis, associated abnormalities in iron metabolism. *British Journal of Dermatology*, **86** (Suppl. 8), 88.

140 LITTMAN B.H., ROCKLIN R.E., PARKMAN R. & DAVID J.R. (1978) Transfer factor treatment of chronic mucocutaneous candidiasis: requirement for donor reactivity to candida antigen. *Clinical Immunology and Immunopathology*, **9**, 97.

141 WINFIELD J.B., WINCHESTER R.J., WERNET P., FU S.M. & KUNKEL H.G. (1975) Nature of cold reactive antibodies to lymphocyte surface determinants in systemic lupus erythematosus. *Arthritis and Rheumatism*, **18**, 1.

142 OOI B.S., ORLINA A.R., MASAITIS L., FIRST M.R., POLLAK V.E. & OOI Y.M. (1974) Lymphocytotoxins in aging. *Transplantation*, **18**, 190.

143 MOTTIRONI V.D. & TERASAKI P.I. (1970) Lymphocytotoxins in disease. In: *Histocompatibility Testing*, p. 301, Williams & Wilkins, Baltimore.

144 MILLER K.B. & SCHWARTZ R.S. (1979) Familial abnormalities of suppressor cell function in systemic lupus erythematosus. *New England Journal of Medicine*, **301**, 803.

145 TURSZ T., PREUD'HOMME J.-L., LABAUME S., MATUCHANSKY C. & SELIGMANN M. (1977) Autoantibodies to B lymphocytes in a patient with hypoimmunoglobulinaemia. *Journal of Clinical Investigation*, **60**, 405.

146 GELFAND E.W., PARKMAN R. & ROSEN F.S. (1975) Lymphocytotoxins and immunological unresponsiveness. In: *Immunodeficiency in Man and Animals* (ed. Bergsma D., Good R.A. & Finstad J.), p. 158. Sinauer Press, Sunderland.

147 BROUET J.-C. & PRIEUR A.M. (1974) Membrane markers on chronic lymphocytic leukemia cells. *Clinical Immunology and Immunopathology*, **2**, 481.

148 JEUNET F.S. & GOOD R.A. (1968) Thymoma, immunologic deficiencies and hematological abnormalities. In: *Immunologic Deficiency Diseases in Man. Birth Defects. IV.* (ed. Bergsma D.), p. 192. National Foundation, March of Dimes. New York.

149 SIEGAL F.P., SIEGAL M. & GOOD R.A. (1978) Role of helper, suppressor and B-cell defects in the pathogenesis of the hypogammaglobulinemias. *New England Journal of Medicine*, **299**, 172.

150 LITWIN S.D. (1979) Immunodeficiency with thymoma: failure to induce immunoglobulin production in immunodeficient lymphocytes co-cultured with normal T cells. *Journal of Immunology*, **122**, 728.

151 HAYWARD A.R. (1977) *Immunodeficiency.* Current Topics in Immunology 6. Edward Arnold, London.

152 BERENBAUM M.C. (1975) The clinical pharmacology of immunosuppressive agents. In: *Clinical Aspects of Immunology*, 3rd edn, (ed, Gell P., Coombs R. & Lachmann P.), p. 689. Blackwell Scientific Publications, Oxford.

153 PETRINI B., WASSERMAN J., BLOMGREN H., BARAL E., STRENDER L-E. & WALLGREN A. (1979) Blood lymphocyte subpopulations in breast cancer patients following post operative adjuvant chemotherapy or radio therapy. *Clinical and Experimental Immunology*, **38**, 361.

154 STANWORTH D.R., JOHNS P., WILLIAMSON N., SHADFORTH M., FELIX-DAVIS D. & THOMPSON R. (1977) Penicillamine-induced IgA deficiency. *Lancet*, **i**, 1001.

155 PURTILO D.T., CASSEL C.K., YANG J.P.S., HARPER R., STEPHENSON S.R., LANDING B.H. & VAWTER G.F. (1975) X-linked recessive progressive common variable immunodeficiency (Duncan's disease). *Lancet*, **i**, 935.

156 PURTILO D.T, DE FLORIO D., HUTT L.M., BHAWAN J., YANG J.P.S., OTTO R. & EDWARDS W. (1977) Variable phenotypic expression of an X-linked recessive lymphoproliferative syndrome. *New England Journal of Medicine*, **297**, 1077.

157 MOSIER D.E., SCHER I. & PAUL W.E. (1976) *In vitro* responses of CBA/N mice. Spleen cells of mice with an X-linked defect that precludes immune responses to several thymus independent antigens can respond to TNP-lipopolysaccharide. *Journal of Immunology*, **117**, 1363.

158 HITZIG W.H., FRATER-SCHRODER M. & SEGER R. (1979) Immunodeficiency due to transcobalamin II deficiency. In: *Enzyme Defects and Immune Dysfunction*, p. 77. Ciba Foundation Symposium 68, Excerpta Medica, Amsterdam.

158a FRATER-SCHRÖDER M., SACHER M. & HITZIG W.H. (1980) Inheritance of transcobalamin II (TC II) in two families with TC II deficiency and related immunodeficiency. In: *Primary Immunodeficiencies* (ed. Seligmann M. & Hitzig W.H.), p. 493. Elsevier/North-Holland, Amsterdam.

159 VAN BEKKUM D.W. (1972) Use and abuse of haemopoietic cell grafts in immune deficiency diseases. *Transplantation Reviews*, **9**, 3.

160 GREBE S.C. & STREILEIN J.W. (1976) Graft versus host reactions. A review. *Advances in Immunology*, **22**, 119.

161 VAN BEKKUM D.W. (1977) Bone marrow transplantation. *Transplantation Proceedings*, **9**, 147.

162 GLUCKSBERG H., STORB R., FEFER A., BUCKNER C.D., NEIMAN P.E., CLIFT R.A., LERNER K.G. & THOMAS E.D.

(1974) Clinical manifestation of graft versus host disease in human recipients of marrow from HLA-matched sibling donors. *Transplantation*, **18**, 295.

163 GLEICHMANN E. & GLEICHMANN H. (1972) Differential immunogenicity of D and K end antigens and its possible significance for HLA. *Transplantation*, **13**, 180.

164 RAPPAPORT J., MIHM M., REINHERZ E., LOPANSRI S. & PARKMAN R. (1979) Acute graft-versus-host disease in recipients of bone marrow transplants from identical twin donors. *Lancet*, **ii**, 717.

165 REINHERZ E.L., PARKMAN R., RAPPAPORT J., ROSEN F.S. & SCHLOSSMAN S.F. (1979) Abberations of suppressor T cells in human graft-versus-host disease. *New England Journal of Medicine*, **300**, 1061.

166 FORD J.M., LUCEY J.J., CULLEN M.H., TOBIAS J.S. & LISTER T.A. (1976) Fatal graft-versus-host disease following transfusions of granulocytes from normal donors. *Lancet*, **ii**, 1167.

167 LERNER K.G., KAO G.F., STORB R., BUCKNER C.D., CLIFT R.A. & THOMAS E.D. (1974) Histopathology of graft-versus-host reaction in human recipients of marrow from HL-A matched sibling donors. *Transplantation Proceedings*, **6**, 367.

168 VAN VLOTEN W.A., SCHEFFER E. & DOOREN L.J. (1977) Localized scleroderma like lesions after bone marrow transplantation in man. *British Journal of Dermatology*, **96**, 337.

169 JOSE D.G., KERSEY J.H., CHOI Y.S., BIGGAR W.D., GATTI R.A. & GOOD R.A. (1971) Humoral antagonism of cellular immunity in children with immune deficiency reconstituted by bone marrow transplantation. *Lancet*, **ii**, 841.

170 SANTOS G.W. (1974) Immunosuppression for clinical marrow transplantation. *Seminars in Hematology*, **11**, 341.

171 STROBER S., SLAVIN S., GOTTLIEB M., ZAN-BAR I., KING D.P., HOPPE R.T., FUKS Z., GRUMET F.C. & KAPLAN H.S. (1979) Allograft tolerance after total lymphoid irradiation. *Immunological Reviews*, **46**, 87.

172 POWLES R.L., BARRETT A.J., CLINK H., KAY H.E.M. SLOANE J. & McELWAIN T.J. (1978) Cyclosporin A for the treatment of graft-versus-host disease in man. *Lancet*, **ii**, 1327.

173 OTTERNESS I.G. & CHANG Y.-H. (1976) Comparative study of cyclophosphamide, GMP, azathioprine and methotrexate. Relative effects on the humoral and cellular immune response in mice. *Clinical and Experimental Immunology*, **26**, 346.

174 SPITLER L.E. (1976) Delayed hypersensitivity skin testing. In: *Manual of Clinical Immunology* (ed. Rose N.R. & Friedman H.), p. 53. American Society of Microbiology, Washington.

175 HUMPHREY J.H. & BATTY I. (1974) International reference preparation for human serum IgG, IgA and IgM. *Clinical and Experimental Immunology*, **17**, 708.

176 WEBSTER A.D.B., EFTER T. & ASHERSON G.L. (1974) *Escherichia coli* antibody: a screening test for immunodeficiency. *British Medical Journal*, **3**, 16.

177 WEDGWOOD R.A., OCHS H.D. & DAVIS S.D. (1975) The recognition and classification of immunodeficiency diseases with bacteriophage Ø × 174. In: *Immunodeficiency in Man and Animals*, (ed. Bergsma D., Good R.A. & Finstad J.), p. 331. Sinauer Press, Sunderland.

178 LING N.R., BISHOP S. & JEFFERIS R. (1977) Use of antibody coated red cells for the sensitive detection of antigen and in rosette tests for cells bearing surface immunoglobulins. *Journal of Immunological Methods*, **15**, 279.

178a REINHERZ E.L. & SCHLOSSMAN S.F. (1980) Regulation of the immune-response-induced and suppressor T lymphocyte subsets in human beings. *New England Journal of Medicine*, **303**, 370.

179 GITLIN D., VAWTER G. & CRAIG J.M. (1964) Thymic alymphoplasia and congenital aleukocytosis. *Pediatrics*, **33**, 184.

180 ALONSO K., DEW J.M. & STARKE W.R. (1972) Thymic alymphoplasia and congenital aleukocytosis (reticular dysgenesis). *Archives of Pathology*, **94**, 179.

181 OWNBY D.R., PIZZO S., BLACKMAN L., GALL S.A. & BUCKLEY R.H. (1976) Severe combined immunodeficiency with leukopenia (reticular dysgenesis) in siblings: immunologic and histopathologic findings. *Journal of Pediatrics*, **89**, 382.

182 ESPANOL T., COMPTE J., ALVAREZ C., TALLADA N., LAVERDE R. & PEGUERO G. (1979) Reticular dysgenesis: report of two brothers. *Clinical and Experimental Immunology*, **38**, 615.

183 HAAS R.J., NIETHAMMER D., GOLDMAN S.F., HEIT W., BIENZLE V. & KLEIHAUER E. (1977) Congenital immunodeficiency and agranulocytosis (reticular dysgenesis). *Acta Paediatrica Scandinavia*, **66**, 279.

184 ROSE N.R. & FRIEDMAN H. (1976) *Manual of Clinical Immunology*. American Society for Microbiology, Washington D.C..

185 THOMPSON R. (1978) *Methods in Clinical Immunology*. Blackwell Scientific Publications, Oxford.

Chapter 19
The paraproteinaemias

D. Y. MASON

Before considering clinical aspects of human paraproteinaemia it is necessary briefly to outline aspects of B
lymphoid cell maturation and immunoglobulin production which are of relevance to an understanding of
these disorders. For a fuller description of human
lymphoid physiology and immunochemistry, readers
should refer to Chapter 17. This introductory section
also deals with the nomenclature and classification of
human paraproteinaemia, and with the antigen-
binding activity of paraproteins.

B-CELL MATURATION AND
IMMUNOGLOBULIN PRODUCTION

The concept of lymphoid clones
The B lymphoid system is based upon the existence of a
very large number (in excess of 10^6) of independent cell
lines or 'clones', each of which derives from a single
lymphoid stem cell. The maturation steps through
which each clone passes as it differentiates towards a
mature plasma cell are shown in Figure 19.1. As
outlined below, the antigen-binding specificity of the
immunoglobulin produced by any individual clone
remains constant throughout its maturation.

Immunoglobulin structure
From an early stage in its development a B cell is
capable of immunoglobulin synthesis (Fig. 19.1). The
basic structure of immunoglobulin molecules (Fig.
19.2) comprises four polypeptide chains: two heavy
chains, each with a molecular weight of approximately
60 000; and two light chains of approximately 20 000
molecular weight. Both heavy and light chains are
made up of a 'constant' region and of a 'variable'
region. The variable region is so called because the
amino-acid sequence in this portion of the molecule
differs from clone to clone, no two clones sharing
precisely the same sequence. This leads, given the large
number of different B-cell clones, to a remarkable
degree of molecular heterogeneity for immunoglobulin. The explanation for this phenomenon (which is
unmatched by any other protein in the body) is that it

endows the B lymphoid system with a very wide
repertoire of antigen-binding specificities, since the
antigen-binding site of the immunoglobulin molecule
is formed by the apposition of the variable regions of
heavy and light chains.

In contrast to the variable regions, the constant
regions show much less heterogeneity, and can therefore be classified into a number of broad categories
(e.g. γ, μ, δ, and ε for heavy chains; κ and λ for light
chains—see Table 19.1) on the basis of structural
differences in the constant regions. Antigenic determinants conferred on the constant regions by these
structural differences provide a convenient means of
distinguishing the different heavy- and light-chain
classes (using specific antisera).

Immunoglobulin production
Immunoglobulin synthesized by immature or resting B
cells is incorporated into their surface membrane (Fig.
19.1), where it acts as an antigen receptor. Binding of
antigen to these molecules triggers differentiation of
the clone towards the terminal plasma-cell stage. In
following this sequence the B cell ceases production of
surface Ig (since its role as antigen receptor has been
fulfilled) and initiates synthesis of Ig for secretion. This
Ig accumulates in the cytoplasm prior to export, and its
demonstration by immunocytochemical means is of
practical value in identifying and classifying B-cell
lymphoproliferative disorders (see pp. 716–717).

In the context of human paraproteinaemia, an
important feature of immunoglobulin secretion by the
maturing B cell is that it is a function performed not
only by plasma cells but also by more immature cells
(e.g. lymphoplasmacytoid cells, germinal-centre cells,
immunoblasts) (see Fig. 19.1). In consequence, a
proliferative process involving any of these maturation
steps may lead to the appearance in the serum (and/or
urine) of secreted immunoglobulin (or 'paraprotein'—
see Table 19.2). This accounts for the fact that
paraproteins are found not only in cases of multiple
myeloma, but also in a proportion (albeit minor) of
non-myelomatous lymphoproliferative disorders (Fig.
19.3).

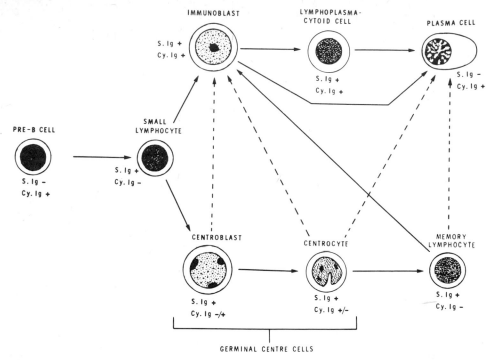

Fig. 19.1. Pathways of B-cell maturation (based upon the scheme proposed by Lennert *et al.*). The presence or absence of surface immunoglobulin (S.Ig.) and of cytoplasmic immunoglobulin (Cy.Ig.) at each maturation stage is indicated. Some of the developmental relationships (e.g. the ability of germinal-centre cells to differentiate directly into plasma cells) are not established with certainty (as indicated by dashed arrows).

A further features of B-cell immunoglobulin synthesis which is of relevance to human paraproteinaemia is that a single B-cell clone expresses, at successive stages in its maturation, the same heavy-chain variable-region amino-acid sequence linked to a number of different heavy-chain constant regions. Throughout this period the light chain synthesized by the cell remains the same. Thus, for example, a single clone may sequentially express surface IgMκ, surface IgDκ, cytoplasmic IgMκ, and cytoplasmic IgGκ. The

way in which this unusual molecular 'splicing' of the two heavy-chain regions takes place is poorly understood, but it has the important consequence that the same antigen-binding activity (and hence the same idiotype—see 'Cellular Aspects of Myeloma', p. 708) is maintained by the clone throughout its development.

A final important aspect of the cellular biosynthesis of immunoglobulin is that immunoglobulin-secreting cells synthesize heavy and light chains separately, the intact immunoglobulin molecule being assembled

Table 19.1. Categories of human immunoglobulin

Class	Heavy chain	Light chain	Number of units	Molecular formula	Serum concentration (mg/ml)
IgG	γ	κ or λ	Monomer	$\gamma_2\kappa_2$ or $\gamma_2\lambda_2$	8–16
IgA	α	κ or λ	Monomer, dimer or polymers	$(\alpha_2\kappa_2)$1-n or $(\alpha_2\lambda_2)$1-n	1·4–4·0
IgM	μ	κ or λ	Pentamer	$(\mu_2\kappa_2)$5 or $(\mu_2\lambda_2)$5	0·5–2·0
IgD	δ	κ or λ	Monomer	$\delta_2\kappa_2$ or $\delta_2\lambda_2$	<0·4
IgE	ε	κ or λ	Monomer	$\varepsilon_2\kappa_2$ or $\varepsilon_2\lambda_2$	0·02–0·45

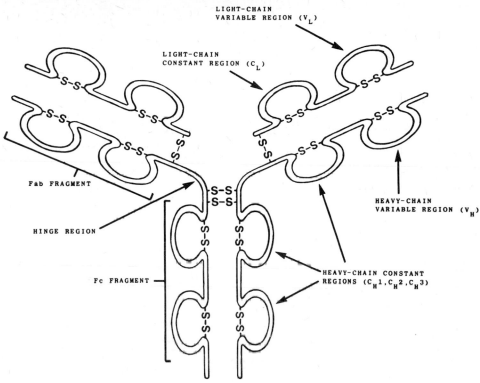

Fig. 19.2. The basic molecular structure of immunoglobulin. The molecular weight of the complete molecule is of the order of 160 000 daltons. The two heavy chains are of identical amino-acid sequence (approx. 450 amino acids each) as are the two light chains (approx. 214 amino acids each). In consequence, the molecule is symmetrical and the two antibody-combining sites formed by the heavy- and light-chain variable regions are of identical structure (and identical antigen-binding specificity). The molecular pattern shown represents the basic structure of IgG, IgD and IgE (although minor variations occur). IgA is found both in this form and also as dimers (the form in which IgA appears in secretions) or higher-molecular-weight polymers; IgM is almost all in the form of a 19S pentamer (Table 19.1).

from its constituent chains immediately before release from the cell. Neoplastic Ig-secreting cells not infrequently manifest an imbalance between the rates of synthesis of the two types of chain, with the consequence that free light chains are released by the cell (in addition to intact immunoglobulin). This abnormality (which is reminiscent of the imbalance in haemoglobin α- and β-chain synthesis encountered in some neoplastic erythroid cells) provides a convenient marker for neoplastic B cells, since urinary excretion of free light chains is very rarely encountered in benign states.

Polyclonal versus monoclonal proliferation

When a foreign antigen (e.g. bacterial polysaccharide) comes in contact with the lymphoid system a number of clones are 'switched on', each of which shows a greater or lesser ability to bind a determinant on the stimulating antigen. Since the immunoglobulin mole-

cule produced by each clone is unique in its variable-region sequences, its physico-chemical properties will also be unique. In consequence if these antibodies are analyzed by a technique such as electrophoresis, which reveals differences in molecular properties, a very heterogeneous picture is obtained (Fig. 19.4). This feature is even more marked when polyclonal antibodies against numerous different antigens are present (as is the case in normal human serum).

This 'polyclonal' electrophoretic pattern may be contrasted with the much more restricted mobility of 'monoclonal' immunoglobulin secreted by a single neoplastic clone of B cells (Fig. 19.4). This difference forms the basis on which paraproteins are detected in routine clinical practice. Further evidence for the monoclonal nature of a paraprotein can be obtained if necessary by demonstrating that it is of a single heavy- and light-chain class, and thus contrasts with the pattern of polyclonal immunoglobulin (see p. 718).

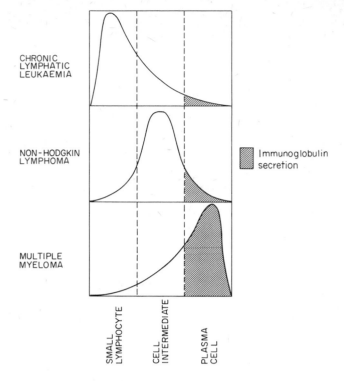

Fig. 19.3. Schematic representation of the fact that in different B lymphoproliferative disorders (which may behave clinically in very different ways) the neoplastic clone covers a spectrum of differentiation stages from the small lymphocyte to the mature plasma cell (see Fig. 19.1). Whether or not a paraprotein is detected depends largely upon the number of cells which are present in the final Ig-secreting compartment. In as many as 50% of non-Hodgkin lymphoma cases, however, immunocytochemical analysis of tissue biopsies reveals monoclonal Ig (i.e. of a single heavy- and light-chain class) in the cytoplasm of a proportion of the neoplastic cells, despite the fact that no serum paraprotein is detectable by electrophoresis. Furthermore, even when no Ig can be demonstrated by immunocytochemistry its synthesis and secretion in small amounts can be demonstrated in almost all cases of non-Hodgkin lymphoma by the use of sensitive biosynthetic radiolabelling techniques.

NOMENCLATURE OF PARAPROTEIN-AEMIA

The terminology currently used in relation to human paraproteinaemia is summarized and defined in Table 19.2. At first sight this nomenclature may appear complex and contradictory. However, this stems from the fact that this terminology has been introduced into the medical literature over a long period, during much of which little was known of the underlying nature of the paraproteinaemias. Even a point as fundamental as the plasma-cell origin of myeloma was not universally accepted until the 1940s (Table 19.2), whilst a further 20 years were to elapse before the immunochemical

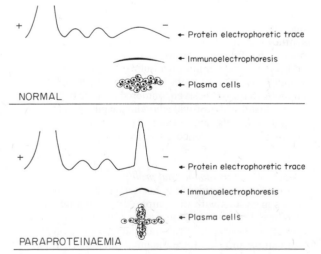

Fig. 19.4. Illustration of the difference between polyclonal and monoclonal plasma-cell proliferation. In normal subjects immunoglobulin is secreted by a number of plasma-cell clones and consequently shows a diffuse distribution on electrophoresis (polyclonal pattern). In contrast, a single plasma-cell clone predominates in paraproteinaemia patients and its secreted Ig product appears as a homogeneous 'spike' of restricted mobility on electrophoresis (monoclonal pattern). Immunoelectrophoresis against antiserum specific for the heavy or light chain of the paraprotein shows deformation or kinking in the region of the paraprotein.

Table 19.2. The nomenclature of paraproteinaemia

Term	Meaning
Bence Jones protein or Bence Jones light chain	This term refers to the immunoglobulin light chains found in the urine of many myeloma and amyloid patients (and less frequently of Waldenström's macroglobulinaemia and non-Hodgkin lymphoma patients). The name arises from the description in 1847 by Dr Henry Bence Jones of a patient whose urine, when heated, produced a coagulum which then redissolved on further heating (thus distinguishing it from the heat-insoluble precipitate of albumin observed when testing cases of Bright's disease). The original observation of this phenomenon was made and clearly described by Dr William MacIntyre, who then referred his patient for further investigation to Bence Jones. The original Bence Jones heat test has been superseded by electrophoretic and immunoelectrophoretic testing (see text). The eponym is still frequently used, however
'Bence Jones only' myeloma	This term refers to those cases of myeloma in which the only detectable paraprotein consists of urinary light chains. The term is synonymous with 'light-chain disease' (see Table 19.4)
Gammopathy	This term originates from the time when little was known of the nature or origin of immunoglobulins, and refers to the fact that many paraproteins migrate in the γ region on electrophoresis. The term is unsatisfactory since it cannot, strictly speaking, be applied to paraproteins which migrate in the β position (see Fig. 19.9). The alternative spelling 'gammapathy' is frequently encountered
Immunocytoma	The term 'immunocyte' refers to any cell capable of immunological response to an antigen (i.e. T or B lymphoid cells but not cells of the mononuclear phagocyte series) and 'immunocytoma' hence indicates a neoplasm of such cells. The term is a theoretical (rather than cytological) definition and confusion may arise when attempting to define 'immunocytic' or 'immunoblastic' tumours histologically
M protein	Synonymous with paraprotein. 'M' stands for monoclonal (and also, coincidentally, for myeloma and macroglobulinaemia)
Myeloma	Plasma-cell neoplasia. The terms refers to the origin of the process within the bone marrow, although tumours of identical histological appearance may arise outside the marrow. When the term was first coined in 1889 by Kahler (and for many years afterwards) the cellular origin of myeloma was unknown. It was generally believed in the early part of this century that any cell type in the bone marrow could give rise to a myeloma. This accounts for the use in the past of terms such as 'erythroblastic', 'myelocytic' and even 'megakaryocytic' myeloma; the belief is still echoed today by the tautologous term 'plasma-cell myeloma'. *Solitary myeloma* refers to a single plasma-cell tumour arising from bone marrow; *multiple myeloma* or *myelomatosis* to the more usual pattern of disseminated tumours
Paraprotein	Immunoglobulin secreted by a single clone of B cells
Paraproteinaemia	Generic name covering all conditions in which a paraprotein is produced. Cases in which the only detectable paraprotein consists of urinary light chains (e.g. light-chain disease, primary amyloidosis) are included in this category, though strictly it should only be applied to individuals found to have circulating paraproteins
Plasmacytoma	Synonymous with myeloma, except that it is not restricted to plasma-cell tumours arising in the marrow cavity

nature of paraproteins, and their identity with anti-bodies, was generally appreciated.

CLASSIFICATION OF PARAPROTEIN-AEMIAS

The following categories of paraproteinaemia are described in this chapter:
1 multiple myeloma;
2 Waldenström's (or primary) macroglobulinaemia;
3 primary amyloidosis;
4 heavy-chain diseases;
5 paraproteinaemia in lymphoma and leukaemia;
6 benign paraproteinaemia.

These disorders clearly have few clinical features in common, and it may thus be asked why they should be arbitrarily grouped together purely on the basis of a shared laboratory abnormality. This question becomes even more pertinent when it is realized that this categorization may also on occasion lead to the sub-division (into paraproteinaemic and non-paraproteinaemic sub-groups) of what appear, on clinical and histological criteria, to be homogeneous disease entities. The problems created by such sub-division are epitomized by Waldenström's macroglobulinaemia, the histological pattern of which ('lymphoplasmacytoid lymphoma') may also be found in patients in whom no IgM paraprotein is detectable. Such cases have been referred to as 'macroglobulinaemia without macroglobulinaemia' (a term reminiscent of 'aleukaemic leukaemia'). The occasional myeloma patient in whom no paraprotein can be detected ('non-secretory' myeloma) represents a further example of the unsatisfactory nature of the term 'paraproteinaemia', since such patients should not strictly, although cytologically and clinically typical of myeloma, be classified as paraproteinaemias.

A further objection to the use of the term 'paraproteinaemia' as a disease category is that the frequency with which paraproteins are detected is to some extent a function of the care and expertise with which they are sought. Paraproteins rarely escape detection in cases of myeloma (because of their high concentration); in disorders such as primary amyloidosis and heavy-chain disease, or in cases of lymphoma secreting minimal amounts of immunoglobulin, however, the paraprotein may be much harder to demonstrate.

These problems of nomenclature may be resolved if it is realized that the presence of a detectable paraprotein is a secondary phenomenon which may be found, with varying frequency, in most (if not all) B-cell lymphoproliferative disorders. It is now realized that the neoplastic B-cell clone in any individual patient (whether a case of myeloma, chronic lymphocytic leukaemia, non-Hodgkin lymphoma, etc.) may include cells covering the full maturation span from lymphoid stem cells to fully differentiated plasma cells. The particular stage at which cells 'pile up' is the feature governing the clinico-pathological diagnosis, whilst the number of cells which are in the mature (Ig-secreting) compartment decides whether or not a paraprotein will be found.

This unifying concept of the paraproteinaemias (schematically illustrated in Fig. 19.3) not only explains why paraproteins may be found in disorders which appear clinically and histologically very different from each other (e.g. chronic lymphocytic leukaemia and myeloma), but also accounts for the tendency of the predominant neoplastic cell type to change during the course of the disease (e.g. for anaplastic lymphoid neoplasms to develop in cases of myeloma—see p. 714). It may also be noted that the relationship between different B-cell lymphoproliferative disorders illustrated in Figure 19.3 is similar to that existing between different types of myeloid leukaemia. Acute myeloblastic leukaemia represents a predominance of immature myeloid cells but may be associated with the maturation of a few cells to the terminal neutrophil stage (as evidenced by abnormal neutrophil morphology or granule protein deficiencies) whilst in chronic myeloid leukaemia (CML) mature polymorphs predominate, but there is a 'tail-back' of small numbers of polymorph precursors, including myeloblasts. A further parallel with lymphoproliferative disorders may be found in the tendency of CML to de-differentiate into a more primitive neoplasm.

ANTIBODY ACTIVITY OF PARAPROTEINS

Since most paraproteins are indistinguishable in molecular structure from normal immunoglobulins they should be capable of binding antigenic determinants in exactly the same way as do normal antibodies. However, it might be predicted that the chances of identifying the antigenic specificity of individual paraproteins would be extremely low, given the large number of antigen-binding specificities expressed by normal B lymphoid cells. Thus it is at first sight surprising that antigen-binding activity has so frequently been detected in human paraproteins (Table 19.3) [1–6, 9–11].

One explanation may lie in animal experiments which suggest that much of the background serum polyclonal immunoglobulin (particularly IgM) in normal individuals is directed against self antigens (e.g. red-cell antigens, IgG) [7]. Thus, if monoclonal proliferation is a random event, equally likely to occur in any B-cell clone, it follows that many human parapro-

Table 19.3. Human monoclonal paraproteins exhibiting antigen-binding specificity*

Antigen	Ig class	Comment	Ref.
Autoantigens			
Red blood cell antigens (A, I, i, aged red cells)	IgM	A minority of patients develop symptoms (cold haemagglutinin disease).	1
IgG	IgM, IgG, IgA	Cryoglobulinaemia (occasionally symptomatic) may occur.	1
Lipoproteins	IgG, IgA	Hyperlipidaemia, with or without associated xanthoma formation, may be observed.	1
Gastric parietal cells	IgA		2
Actin	IgA		3
Transferrin	IgG	A single patient in whom a transferrin-binding paraprotein caused haemachromatosis has been described.	1
Fibrin monomer	IgG	The paraprotein may interfere with fibrin polymerization, although the clinical relevance and true antigen–antibody nature of the reaction is not always clear.	1
Microbiological antigens			
Streptococcal hyaluronidase	IgA		4
Streptolysin	IgG, IgD	Has been described in a patient with a long history of recurrent streptococcal skin infections.	5, 6
Rubella	IgG		1
Klebsiella	IgM		1
Miscellaneous antigens			
Flavin	IgG	Patient developed yellow skin and hair pigmentation.	9
Copper	IgG	Hypercupranaemia caused ocular deposition of copper.	10, 11
Horse α_2-macroglobulin	IgG	Patient had received horse-serum injections in the past.	1
Dinitrophenyl groups	IgG, IgM, IgA		1

* This table is not exhaustive and further reports of antigen-binding paraproteins may be found in the literature.

teins will express autoantibody activity. This not only simplifies the search for antigen-specific paraproteins (since many of them will be directed against well-recognized human antigens) but also means that the antibody activity of some paraproteins will give rise to clinical symptoms as a result of their interaction *in vivo* with self antigens. Chronic cold haemagglutinin disease due to anti-I activity, cryoglobulin-related symptoms due to rheumatoid-factor activity of paraproteins, haemochromatosis due to transferrin binding, and xanthoma formation due to paraprotein–lipoprotein complexing, are all examples in this category [1, 8]. Single cases of a flavin-binding myeloma paraprotein (causing unusual skin pigmentation) [9] and of a copper-binding paraprotein [10] (causing corneal deposition of copper) [11] may also be quoted in this context. The occurrence of peripheral neuropathy in a minority of paraproteinaemia patients may also represent the clinical consequences of paraprotein–antigen binding [12], although the finding in these patients of monoclonal immunoglobulin in peripheral-nerve biopsies may sometimes be secondary to nerve damage rather than its cause [13].

MYELOMA

DEFINITION

Myeloma may be defined as a moderately well-differentiated neoplastic disorder of B lymphoid cells, in which the predominant cell type is a plasma cell. The reason for defining it in this way, rather than simply as a plasma-cell neoplasm, is that the original mutation probably occurs in an immature B cell, rather than in a plasma cell. Furthermore the neoplasm is subsequently maintained by cell division occuring at a relatively primitive stage in B lymphoid maturation [14], the majority of plasma cells probably being incapable of cell division [15].

AETIOLOGY

Although myeloma is now clearly established as a B-cell neoplasm, there is little clue as to why the initial mutation giving rise to the malignancy occurs. It has been suggested that viruses may be responsible for transmission of the disease, but searches for 'clusters' of patients to support this hypothesis have usually proved negative [16, 17]. The risk of myeloma increased in survivors of the Nagasaki and Hiroshima atomic bombs [18], but there is little evidence that radiation plays a causative role in other cases of myeloma. In view of the fact that plasmacytomas can arise in BALB/c mice following induction of a chronic inflammatory state, it has been suggested that prior antigenic stimulation (e.g. by chronic infection) could provide the background for the development of myeloma in man [19, 20]. In particular, an association between IgA myeloma and a history of inflammatory disease, often affecting the biliary tract, has been reported [21]. However, a systematic search for activity against bacteria in a large number of myeloma paraproteins has yielded negative results [22].

It has also been suggested that myeloma may develop in genetically predisposed individuals. Families with a high incidence of paraproteinaemia have occasionally been reported [23–25], and abnormal serum immunoglobulin levels may be found in the families of myeloma patients [26]. However, the significance of such findings, and of alterations in the frequency of certain HLA groups in myeloma patients, remains uncertain [27, 28].

CELLULAR ASPECTS OF MYELOMA

As noted above, the neoplastic mutation in myeloma is thought to occur at an early stage in the B-cell maturation pathway. Evidence for this comes from the use of anti-idiotype antisera raised against individual patients' paraproteins. Extensive absorption with normal immunoglobulin renders these sera specific for antigenic determinants (idiotypes) unique to the variable region of the paraprotein. Immunofluorescent labelling with anti-idiotype antisera has shown that myeloma patients at the time of diagnosis frequently have a substantial percentage of circulating small lymphoid cells carrying the same idiotype as the paraprotein [29, 30]. Although some transitional forms between small lymphocytes and plasmacytoid cells can be demonstrated by optical and electron-microscopic examination the majority of these idiotype-positive cells show minimal differentiation towards plasma cells [31]. These results provide the major evidence for the concept (see p. 707) that the myeloma clone embraces a wide spectrum of cells ranging from a small early lymphoid cell through to the mature, fully differentiated plasma cell. The labelling index (as assessed by [3H]thymidine incorporation) of idiotype-bearing small lymphocytes is higher than that of idiotype-positive plasmacytoid cells [15]. As would be expected, treatment of myeloma leads to a reduction in the numbers of idiotype-positive peripheral lymphoid cells.

This reassessment of the cellular basis of myeloma has raised the question of how early in the B-cell maturation pathway the original mutation may occur. There is evidence that this event takes place prior to the pre-B-cell stage [30], but subsequent to the separation of the B- and T-cell maturation pathways, since idiotype-positive peripheral T cells have not been found (with one possible exception [32]) in cases of myeloma.

IMMUNOCHEMICAL CLASSES OF MYELOMA

Heavy- and light-chain production

Cases of myeloma may be classified on the basis of the heavy- and light-chain class of the paraprotein produced by the neoplastic cells (Table 19.4). The relative frequency of these different immunochemical classes of myeloma approximates to the frequency of plasma cells producing these heavy and light chains in non-neoplastic lymphoid tissue. Myeloma cells differ from normal plasma cells, however, in that in more than 50% of cases an excess of light chains (relative to heavy chains) is synthesized (Table 19.4). The light chains are filtered by the glomeruli and, when the tubular reabsorption capacity is exceeded, appear in the urine. For reasons which are not clear these light chains (especially when of γ class) tend to form disulphide-linked dimers. As discussed below, the detection of a homogeneous band of light chains on urinary electrophoresis (alias 'Bence Jones protein'—see Table 19.2) is of considerable importance in the diagnosis and investigation of myeloma and related disorders.

A further atypical feature of neoplastic plasma cells is that in approximately 20% of cases of myeloma no heavy chains are synthesized (Table 19.4). In the majority of cases of this type of myeloma (variously referred to as 'light-chain disease', 'Bence Jones only myeloma' and 'light-chain myeloma'), no serum paraprotein is detectable on routine electrophoresis (see p. 717), the only abnormality being found in the urine. In consequence cases may be overlooked if the urine is not examined.

Non-secretory myeloma

In a small percentage (approximately two per cent) of myeloma patients no paraprotein is found in the serum or urine, despite careful analysis [33–36]. Cases of 'non-secretory myeloma' are indistinguishable clinically from classical myeloma patients, except that

Table 19.4. Immunochemical classes of myeloma

Class of myeloma	Relative frequency (%)	Proportion of cases excreting light chains (%)*	κ/λ ratio
IgG	55–60	50–70	2:1
IgA	20–25	50–70	2:1
Light-chain disease	20	100	1·2:1
IgD	1	90	1:9
Other (IgM, biclonal, non-secretory)	1		

* The frequency with which light chains are detected is partly dependent upon technical factors (e.g. the degree to which the urine is concentrated before testing, the sensitivity of the electrophoresis procedure, etc.), hence the considerable variation between published reports.

phenomena directly attributable to the presence of a paraprotein are absent. In the majority of these cases the neoplastic cells' failure to produce immunoglobulin appears to be accounted for by a defect in excretion rather than in cell synthesis, since immunocytochemical staining usually reveals normal quantities of intracellular immunoglobulin [35].

Multiple paraproteins

In a minority of myeloma patients, more than one homogeneous protein band is seen on serum electrophoresis. In some cases this is artefactual, being accounted for by a single paraprotein which undergoes partial degradation, complexing or polymerization. In other cases, however, the patient's neoplastic plasma cells secrete two (or rarely more) separate paraproteins. Such patients account for approximately one per cent of all cases of myeloma. Although they have no clinical features to distinguish them from classical myeloma, these patients are of great theoretical interest [37] in view of the light which they can throw on the pattern of immunoglobulin production during B-cell maturation. Amino-acid sequence analysis and studies of idiotypic determinants commonly reveal that the two paraproteins in cases of 'biclonal' myeloma consist of identical light chains and identical heavy-chain variable regions associated with different heavy-chain constant regions (e.g. IgGκ and IgMκ). These findings are in keeping with the concept that a B-cell clone 'switches' the heavy-chain class of immunoglobulin which it synthesizes during its maturation (see p. 702). Not all biclonal paraproteinaemias conform to this pattern, however (e.g. two different light chains may be found), and a variety of alternative mechanisms must account for such cases [37, 38].

Structurally abnormal paraproteins

Although the neoplastic cells in the great majority of cases of myeloma produce normal intact immunoglobulin molecules and/or normal light chains, very occasionally cases characterized by the production of structurally abnormal molecules may be encountered. The commonest of these anomalies is a 'half-molecule' paraprotein in which one heavy chain is linked to one light chain [39–43]. Internal deletions in the heavy chain may also be present, although, in contrast to heavy-chain disease proteins (see pp. 736–7), this is usually in the Fc region of the molecule rather than in the Fab portion.

THE GROWTH OF MYELOMA

The concentration of serum paraprotein in an individual myeloma patient is closely related to the tumour-cell mass, a feature which enables the growth and regression of the neoplastic cell population to be monitored with a precision unmatched in any other class of human neoplasm [44]. Studies based upon observation of the rate of paraprotein increase in untreated patients suggested, by extrapolation, that surprisingly long periods (e.g. of the order of 33 years for IgG myeloma) might elapse between the initial neoplastic mutation and the emergence of clinical symptoms [45]. However, these estimates were based upon the assumption of a constant exponential growth rate. Subsequent extensive studies, involving analysis of paraprotein metabolic rates, *in-vitro* assay of the rate of immunoglobulin synthesis by myeloma cells and an agar cloning assay for myeloma stem cells, have shown that the rate of myeloma cell growth tends to diminish progressively as the tumour mass increases ('Gompertzian growth') [46], with the consequence that the tumour is growing much more slowly at the time of diagnosis (doubling time: three to six months), than immediately after the initial mutation (doubling time: three days) [47]. The fact that the labelling index of myeloma cells is inversely related to the neoplastic cell mass [48] provides further support for this concept, which gives a total period from the initial mutation to diagnosis of between one and three years [47].

INCIDENCE, AGE AND SEX RATIO

The annual incidence of multiple myeloma in Europe and in the United States is of the order of three cases per 100 000 members of the population, giving it a frequency comparable to that of Hodgkin's disease or chronic lymphocytic leukaemia. There is some suggestion that the incidence may be higher in blacks than in whites. It is most commonly seen in the age range of 50–80 years, cases under the age of 40 being rare. In the majority of reported series, male patients are slightly commoner than female patients (by up to 50%). However, for unexplained reasons, IgD myeloma, which accounts for only about two per cent of all cases of the disease, is characterized by a 3:1 preponderance of male patients [49, 50].

CLINICAL ASPECTS OF MYELOMA

The clinical features of myeloma, and the way in which they arise, are illustrated schematically in Figure 19.5 [51]. As will be seen, some of these phenomena are directly attributable to neoplastic cell growth (e.g. bone erosion), whilst other features can be ascribed to the effects of the monoclonal immunoglobulin synthesized by the myeloma cells. It should be noted, however, that some clinical aspects of myeloma fit into neither of these categories, being either multi-factorial in origin (e.g. anaemia), or arising through mechanisms which are not clearly understood (e.g. immune suppression).

In most cases of myeloma there is little relationship between immunochemical class (Table 19.4) and the frequency of the various clinical features discussed below. However, obvious exceptions are provided by light-chain disease and IgD myeloma. In the former type of myeloma, symptoms due to a circulating serum paraprotein (e.g. hyperviscosity) do not occur; whilst in IgD myeloma several features (notably the sex ratio and the frequency of extraosseous myeloma deposits and of light-chain nephropathy) are atypical [49, 50]. Furthermore the risk of renal failure is significantly higher in cases of myeloma in which the paraprotein is of the λ class [52, 53].

Bone pain

Bone pain is the cardinal clinical symptom in myeloma, being present at diagnosis in approximately three-quarters of patients. Although superficially the pain caused by multiple myeloma resembles that arising from skeletal carcinomatous metastases, the mechanism is different. Myeloma cells appear to cause bone erosion by stimulation of osteoclasts rather than by direct pressure upon the bone [54]. The process is therefore *per se* painless, and symptoms only arise when sites which are subjected to stress or weight-bearing are mechanically so weakened that they start to undergo deformation and incipient fractures ('infraction') [55].

This explains why the bone pain in myeloma shows certain clinical features which may help to distinguish it from the bone pain of carcinomatosis. Bone pain in myeloma is rare in areas which are not weight-bearing (e.g. the vault of the skull), even when there is extensive bone destruction. Bone pain in myeloma is frequently alleviated at night, only to return during the day when the patient starts to move again. It may also arise abruptly in a new site, presumably as the bones start to 'give'.

Pathological fractures and vertebral collapse

The weakened bones of myeloma patients are prone to

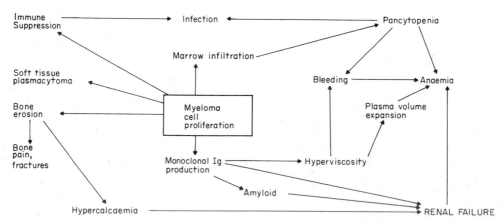

Fig. 19.5. Summary of the major clinical features of myeloma and the way in which they arise.

pathological fractures which may occur with minimal trauma, for example, whilst moving in bed. The vertebral column is commonly affected, causing both generalized shortening (which may lead to loss of several inches in height) and wedging of individual vertebral bodies. The next most frequently involved sites are the ribs and femurs, whilst other sites (mandible, humerus, pelvis, sternum, clavicle) are less commonly affected. Occasionally multiple rib fractures may cause a flail chest and respiratory embarrassment.

Non-specific symptoms

Weakness, fatigue and malaise are common complaints at presentation in myeloma patients. These symptoms may arise from a variety of different causes including anaemia, uraemia, hypercalcaemia and hyperviscosity. Anaemia is caused by several factors, the most important of which clinically is an increased plasma volume [56, 57]. This occurs in patients with raised serum viscosity, and presumably represents a physiological compensatory mechanism which lowers whole-blood viscosity by reducing the haematocrit level.

When hypercalcaemia is present the non-specific symptoms noted above may be accompanied by nausea, vomiting, constipation and dehydration.

Infection

Infections are an important clinical complication of myeloma which may be found in up to 50% of patients. They are usually bacterial, affecting most commonly the respiratory tract (classically pneumococcal) and urinary tract (commonly *E. coli*), although cutaneous eruptions due to herpes zoster and simplex are also not infrequently encountered [58]. Recently an increased tendency for myeloma patients to suffer from gram-negative infections has been noted, probably reflecting the general increase in this type of infection in hospitals [58, 59].

It is not possible to predict which myeloma patients will be susceptible to infection. There appears to be no clear correlation with the degree of neutropenia [60] or suppression of immunoglobulin levels [61], although there is some suggestion that severe anaemia may predispose to infection. Recent studies have suggested that the immune defect in myeloma may be at least partially accounted for by the over-activity of a suppressor mononuclear cell population (which inhibits the transformation of normal lymphocytes into plasma cells following antigenic stimulation [62–65]). Impaired neutrophil bacterial killing [66] and adherence [67, 68] (probably a direct effect of the circulating paraprotein) may also play a role in predisposing to infection.

Haemorrhagic tendency

Abnormal bleeding is noted in 10–20% of myeloma patients at the time of diagnosis. Epistaxes and/or cutaneous haemorrhages are seen most commonly, gastro-intestinal bleeding and haemorrhage from other sites occurring less frequently.

Numerous different factors have been implicated in this haemorrhagic state [69]. Thrombocytopenia and uraemia may contribute, but the most important cause is probably interference by the circulating paraprotein with platelet/capillary interaction and/or with clotting factors. The clinical pattern of bleeding (epistaxis, purpura) suggests that the former mechanism is probably more important. It may be noted that although coagulation tests on myeloma patients frequently reveal a wide range of abnormalities [69, 70], the severity of these defects shows little correlation with clinical episodes of bleeding [69]. Measurements of bleeding time and of platelet adhesiveness, on the other hand, correlate more closely with the degree of haemorrhage.

Thrombosis

Although bleeding is a common feature of myeloma patients, occasional cases are seen in whom thrombosis occurs [71, 72]. It has also been suggested that disseminated intravascular coagulation (DIC) in myeloma may occasionally be responsible for the development of acute renal failure (see p. 714) [73]. It is probable that many of the episodes of thrombosis are related to the physico-chemical properties of the circulating paraprotein.

Hyperviscosity syndrome

This syndrome provides a dramatic example of how the circulating paraprotein in myeloma patients can directly give rise to clinical manifestations [74–76]. These features include non-specific symptoms (tiredness, loss of appetite and possibly loss of weight), haemorrhage (see above), cardiac failure and neurological complications (headache, fits, hemiplegia, and clouding of consciousness progressing rarely to coma). On clinical examination, a striking finding is the presence of severe retinal changes, including irregular 'sausage-shaped' dilatation of the retinal veins, haemorrhages and sometimes papilloedema. Occasionally visible sludging in retinal veins may be visible. The ways in which these different clinical features arise is illustrated schematically in Figure 19.6.

It should be noted that several of the signs and symptoms traditionally attributed to hyperviscosity in myeloma are probably not directly caused by increased blood viscosity but rather by the presence of a circulating paraprotein, which has several independent effects of which increased viscosity—the easiest to

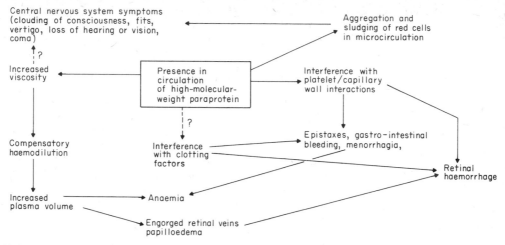

Fig. 19.6. Summary of the nature and origin of the clinical complications encountered in the hyperviscosity syndrome.

measure objectively in the laboratory—is only one. This is suggested by the fact that several of these clinical features are not encountered in other diseases associated with increased blood viscosity (e.g. polycythaemia rubra vera). The haemorrhagic tendency in myeloma (which constitutes the most commonly encountered sign of 'hyperviscosity') is probably due to abnormal platelet/capillary interaction (see p. 711) rather than to increased blood viscosity.

The hyperviscosity syndrome in paraproteinaemia was first recognized in IgG myeloma and in Waldenström's macroglobulinaemia (see p. 727). In IgG myeloma, aggregation of the paraprotein into a higher-molecular-weight complex frequently accounts for the syndrome [77–79], although occasionally symptoms may arise when very high levels of monomeric IgG paraprotein are present. More recently it has been recognized that hyperviscosity syndrome is a relatively common complication of IgA myeloma [74, 80–83]. This is associated with the presence of a paraprotein which is polymerized (probably before it is secreted by the cell [74, 81]). These polymers have a high intrinsic viscosity: they may be conveniently detected by immunoelectrophoretic analysis using anti-J-chain antisera, since monomeric IgA does not contain this polypeptide [84].

Renal failure
Renal failure is a major cause of early death in multiple myeloma [53], particularly since it has become possible to suppress many of the other features of the disease by cytotoxic therapy, antibiotic treatment, plasmapheresis, etc. A number of factors may contribute to impaired renal function in myeloma (e.g. pyelonephritis, amyloid deposition, hypercalcaemia, hyper-

uricaemia, plasma-cell infiltration), but in practice the major cause is damage to renal tubules secondary to light-chain excretion. As the concentration of the glomerular filtrate rises, and also probably as a result of changes in pH and salt concentration, the light chains form insoluble precipitates. These proteinaceous casts have a characteristic histological appearance, variously described as laminated, hyaline, concentric or fractured, and are the most characteristic feature of 'myeloma kidney' [85–87] (Fig. 19.7). They excite an inflammatory reaction in the tubular epithelium leading to giant-cell formation and tubular atrophy. Less frequently, nephrocalcinosis and focal interstitial myeloma-cell infiltration is detectable histologically [87].

It is important to note that light chains from different cases of myeloma differ markedly in their nephrotoxicity, presumably reflecting differences in their physico-chemical properties and ability to excite an inflammatory reaction. In consequence, at least half of the myeloma patients who excrete substantial amounts of light chains show no evidence of renal failure at presentation. Furthermore, renal damage is more frequently associated with λ-light-chain excretion than with κ-chain production, although this may be partly a reflection of the fact that λ chains tend to be excreted at a higher concentration than κ chains in myeloma.

Although the classical histological hallmark of myeloma kidney is the presence of tubular lesions, a minority of patients develop glomerular abnormalities [88–91]. These include amyloid deposition (which usually manifests itself by the presence of non-selective proteinuria), nodular lesions (resembling those seen in diabetes mellitus), mesangial sclerosis, proliferative

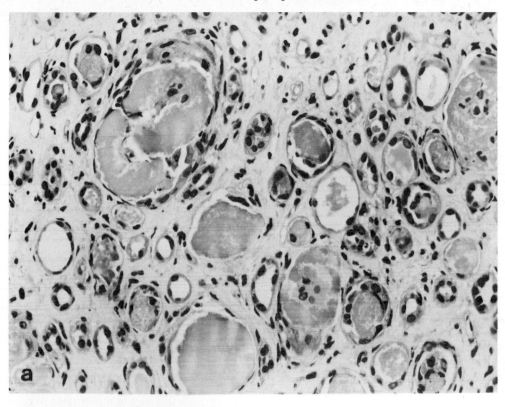

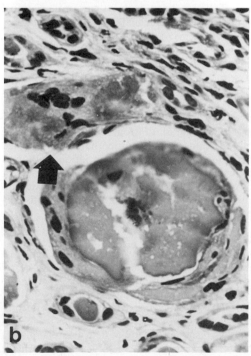

Fig. 19.7. Characteristic appearance of 'myeloma kidney'. Hyaline proteinaceous material (precipitated light chains) is present in many of the tubules. At higher magnification (b) a giant cell, characteristic of the cellular reaction induced by the light-chain precipitates, is indicated by an arrow (H & E).

glomerulopathy and ill-defined electron-dense sub-epithelial deposits.

Although renal failure in myeloma is usually a slowly progressive disorder, occasional cases of acute renal failure are encountered [92–96]. A notorious (though fortunately rare) cause is intravenous pyelography: in other cases hypercalcaemia, dehydration and possibly intravascular coagulation may play a role [73].

Finally, mention may be made of the rare cases of myeloma in which adult Fanconi syndrome develops. The cause of this complication is unknown but it is presumably related to interference by light chains with renal tubular transport [97, 98].

Extramedullary myeloma deposits

Although myeloma is classically confined within the bone marrow, soft-tissue deposits are seen in a minority of patients, and occasionally constitute the initial presenting complaint [99–101]. For reasons that remain obscure, IgD myeloma is particularly prone to spread in this way [49, 50, 102]. Extramedullary deposits may arise by direct extension through the cortical bone. Lesions of this sort account for a proportion of cases of spinal-cord compression in myeloma and probably for the majority of cases of pleural myelomatous involvement (which often leads to pleural effusions in which myeloma cells may be detected) [103–107]. In other patients, these soft-tissue deposits are not in continuity with the skeletal system and may involve almost any site in the body, including skin, subcutaneous tissues, lung, spleen, liver and pancreas [108, 109].

The clinical behaviour of cases showing extramedullary spread at the time of presentation is not clearly different from that of purely intraosseous cases [99]. In contrast, the development of myeloma deposits in soft tissues during the course of the disease is of more serious prognostic significance since it often heralds relapse [102, 110]. The histological appearance of extramedullary deposits, especially when they occur in a terminal phase, may be relatively primitive, reflecting the more anaplastic nature of these deposits [111, 112].

Primary extramedullary plasmacytoma

It is important to distinguish soft-tissue plasmacytomas arising as a result of extraosseous spread of multiple myeloma from cases of primary extramedullary plasmacytoma. The latter neoplasms frequently arise in association with the upper air passages and their clinical behaviour is quite different from that of multiple myeloma [113]. An obvious feature is their tendency to spread to other soft tissues; bony involvement is not uncommon but shows no predilection for regions containing active haemopoietic tissue and is rarely widespread. Prolonged survival is frequently achieved following radiotherapy and/or surgery for the local lesion. Furthermore, because of the rarity with which the bone marrow is involved, patients with disseminated disease can usually be treated with relatively large doses of chemotherapy.

Solitary myeloma of bone

In contrast to primary extramedullary plasmacytoma, solitary plasmacytic neoplasms of bone appear to be closely related to multiple myeloma [114–116]. In a number of patients bone-marrow examination at sites distant from the tumour reveals diffuse infiltration with plasma cells. In other patients, the tumour is apparently truly localized at first, but subsequently disseminates; cases in which this has occurred after many years have been reported [117]. Finally, there is a group of patients in whom the plasmacytoma remains localized throughout the period of observation.

Cutaneous manifestations

In a minority of myeloma patients generalized and persistent xanthomata of an eruptive maculopapular nodular nature are found [118–120]. These lesions are especially prominent in palmar creases and on extensor surfaces of the elbows and knees. Many of these patients have hyperlipidaemia [119–121], and in a proportion of cases this may be attributable to complexing of lipoproteins with a paraprotein (most commonly IgA) which exhibits autoantibody activity against lipoproteins (Table 19.3).

As noted above, cutaneous deposits of myeloma may occasionally be encountered [122], usually associated with generalized extraosseous spread of the disease [102, 110]. Cutaneous haemorrhage is not infrequent in myeloma, most commonly as a manifestation of the hyperviscosity syndrome (see above), cryoglobulinaemia or amyloid deposition. A wide variety of dermatological disorders have been reported as occurring occasionally in association with myeloma, including subcorneal pustulosis, annular erythema, pyoderma gangrenosum, pruritis, scleroderma-like disorders, erythema elevatum diutinum, cutis laxa and papular mucinosis [123–131].

Neurological complications

Approximately 10% of myeloma patients manifest evidence of spinal-cord compression due to vertebral collapse and/or to extradural extension of myeloma tissue from a vertebral body [58]. In view of the long-term benefit which may be obtained from decompressive laminectomy (see p. 725), this diagnosis should be considered in any patient complaining of numbness or weakness of the legs and/or urinary symptoms. Nerve-root compression, giving rise to a radicular pattern of pain associated with motor and/or sensory deficits, may also occur in myeloma patients.

A less commonly encountered neurological manifestation in myeloma is peripheral neuropathy, usually sensory in type. This complication, which can occur when only a solitary myeloma is present, may be due to amyloid deposition. However, in other patients the cause of the nerve damage remains obscure. It is also not clear why polyneuropathy should be frequent among the rare cases of myeloma in which bone X-rays reveal osteosclerosis [132–134].

DIAGNOSIS OF MYELOMA

A variety of laboratory and radiological abnormalities may be encountered in multiple myeloma (Table 19.5). From a practical diagnostic point of view the most important investigations are examination of a bone-marrow sample, analysis of serum and urine for evidence of paraproteins and immunoglobulin abnormalities, and radiological survey of the skull, thoracic cage, spine and pelvis. Other investigations (e.g. measurement of blood urea and calcium levels, immunochemical typing of the paraprotein and measurement of blood viscosity) are of secondary importance.

Haematological abnormalities

Blood count. The peripheral blood in myeloma usually shows a mild degree of anaemia. Modest depression of the neutrophil and platelet count is frequently seen, but severe neutropenia and thrombocytopenia are uncommon. Pancytopenia is most likely to occur in cases of plasma-cell leukaemia or in patients who, after a period of therapy, develop acute leukaemia (see p. 726).

A minority of myeloma patients have elevated platelet counts, a phenomenon possibly related to the thrombocytosis encountered in other types of malignant disease [135, 136]. However, when such a result is obtained using an automated platelet counter, the possibility should be raised that the result is a spurious one due to interference by the paraprotein [137]. Falsely high automated measurements of white-cell counts have also been reported in myelomatous cryoglobulinaemia [138].

Small numbers of myeloma cells are probably present in the circulation quite frequently without being recognized [31]. Occasionally, however, they are found in sufficient numbers to justify the diagnosis of 'plasma-cell leukaemia' [139–142]. The clinical pattern in such cases tends to differ from that of classical

Table 19.5. Common laboratory and radiological abnormalities in myeloma*

Haematological abnormalities
  Blood count
    Anaemia
    Raised ESR
    Rouleaux on film
  Bone marrow
    Infiltration with plasma cells

Immunochemical abnormalities
  Serum electrophoresis
    Serum M band of a single heavy- and light-chain class
    Reduction of background immunoglobulin
  Urine electrophoresis
    Light-chain band of a single light-chain class
  Serum immunoglobulins
    Elevation of IgG or IgA due to paraprotein (see Table 19.6)
    Suppression of other Ig classes

Biochemical abnormalities
  Hypercalcaemia
  Uraemia, raised creatinine, hyperuricaemia, hypoalbuminaemia

Radiological abnormalities
  Lytic lesions, pathological fractures, soft tissue masses

---

* In the great majority of cases of suspected myeloma the diagnosis may be confirmed (or confidently excluded) on the basis of bone-marrow aspiration, serum and protein electrophoresis and X-rays of skull, chest, vertebral column and pelvis.

myeloma. Patients are usually younger than average; have a lower incidence of bone pain but a higher frequency of severe pancytopenia; are more likely to show soft-tissue deposits and organomegaly; commonly excrete urinary light chains; and respond relatively poorly to therapy. However, there is considerable overlap between plasma-cell leukaemia and classical myeloma, and patients with circulating plasma cells should not automatically be assumed to have a poor prognosis.

In addition to patients who manifest plasma-cell leukaemia at the time of presentation, an approximately equal number develop this blood picture as they enter a terminal disseminated phase of the disease.

Additional haematological abnormalities which may be noted include phenomena directly attributable to the presence of a circulating paraprotein (e.g. a high ESR, marked rouleaux formation—which may lead to difficulty in cross-matching blood—and a bluish protein background on the blood film). Occasionally a dimorphic blood picture is seen indicating sideroblastic anaemia (frequently a pre-leukaemic phenomenon) [143].

Bone-marrow examination. The majority of marrow aspirates from myeloma patients at presentation show a clear increase in the number of plasma cells, although the percentage of neoplastic cells may vary widely from one case to another and between different samples taken from the same patient.

A number of cytological features may be of diagnostic value (Fig. 19.8). Myeloma cells are typically larger than normal plasma cells and the maturation of the nucleus is said to lag behind that of the cytoplasm

(nuclear–cytoplasmic asynchrony) [144]. This gives rise to a large nucleus with stippled, poorly condensed chromatin (and often a large nucleolus) lying eccentrically within abundant pale-blue cytoplasm. In contrast, reactive plasma cells have coarsely clumped chromatin and deeply basophilic cytoplasm. Areas of cytoplasmic eosinophilia (probably corresponding to dilated immunoglobulin-containing cisternae of endoplasmic reticulum) are sometimes seen. These 'flaming' cells or 'thesaurocytes' (storage cells) were once thought to be indicative of IgA myeloma, but have more recently been shown to occur in all classes of myeloma, including non-secretory myeloma [145]. Other cytoplasmic inclusions (Russell bodies, crystals) are occasionally seen in myeloma cells but may also be found in reactive plasma cells [146–148]. Binucleate plasma cells are also not uncommon in cases of reactive plasmacytosis. However, the presence of more than two nuclei (or nuclei of unequal sizes) is rare in non-neoplastic plasma cells, as is the finding of intranuclear inclusions [149–151].

When examination of a bone-marrow aspirate does not provide adequate diagnostic information it may be possible to recognize myelomatous infiltration in histological sections of the marrow sample [152]. Characteristic features include the presence of homogeneous nodules of plasma cells as well as more diffuse infiltrates.

A number of cytochemical techniques for identifying myeloma cells have been described. Although abnormal reactions for several enzymes (e.g. acid phosphatase) are said to be of diagnostic value, this approach has not been widely used [153, 154]. Immunofluorescent labelling of cytoplasmic immunoglobulin provides a more

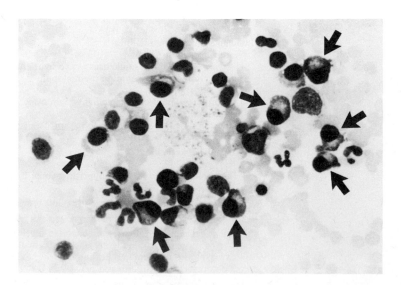

Fig. 19.8. Bone-marrow aspirate from a case of myelomatosis. Numerous atypical plasma cells (arrowed) are present, showing eccentric nuclei, a pale juxtanuclear 'hof' region in some of the cells, and basophilic cytoplasm (not appreciable in monochrome reproductions). (May–Grünwald–Giemsa.)

objective means of distinguishing between myeloma cells (which contain a single heavy- and light-chain class of Ig) and polyclonal reactive plasma cells (in which different classes of heavy and light chains will be found). A practical obstacle to the routine use of this technique, however, is the necessity for washing the aspirated bone-marrow cells (to remove serum immunoglobulin) before smearing, fixation and staining.

An alternative to immunofluorescent labelling of cell smears is provided by immunoperoxidase staining of myeloma cells in histological tissue sections [155–157]. This approach has the advantage that it can be applied retrospectively to routinely fixed and embedded tissues. Furthermore, sections stained in this way retain their label permanently and allow cell morphology to be visualized much more clearly than is possible following immunofluorescent labelling. However it should be pointed out that immunohistological analysis of myeloma samples is prone to a number of technical difficulties, and that both false-negative reactions (due to 'masking' of antigens), and false-positive reactions (due to extracellular immunoglobulin) may complicate the interpretation of sections stained in this way [158].

Karyotypic analyses of marrow aspirates from multiple-myeloma patients usually show no abnormality, probably because of the low mitotic rate of the neoplastic cells [159]. In the terminal accelerated phase of the disease, however, chromosomal changes are relatively frequent, the commonest abnormality being the appearance of a $14q^+$ marker [160]. This abnormality is also common in Burkitt's lymphoma and undifferentiated lymphoma.

Finally, it should be noted that in addition to the presence of neoplastic cells in aspirates from myeloma marrows, a variety of other abnormalities may be encountered, including dyserythropoietic and sideroblastic changes (which may, as noted above, herald the development of acute leukaemia), and also megaloblastic changes [143, 161–164].

Immunochemical investigations

Serum and urine electrophoresis. In approximately 80% of cases of myeloma, an M band in the γ or β region is visible on serum electrophoresis. When the myeloma cells secrete only light chains ('light-chain disease') a serum M band will not be visible unless failing renal function leads to high levels of free light chains in the serum [165]. It may be noted, however, that very occasionally monoclonal light chains form tetramers which (because of their higher molecular weight) are not filtered by the kidneys and consequently appear on serum electrophoresis [166, 167]. Serum electrophoresis frequently also shows evidence of reduction in normal serum immunoglobulin levels ('immune paresis') (Fig. 19.9).

Urine electrophoresis should be carried out in all suspected myeloma patients, and its superiority over older non-specific physico-chemical methods such as the 'Bence Jones' heat test or the Bradshaw ring test is clearly established. It should be noted, however, that the concentration of monoclonal light chains excreted in myeloma varies widely from case to case, some urine samples containing such high concentrations that a monoclonal band is visible on electrophoresis of unconcentrated urine, whilst other samples require concentration by a factor of more than 100-fold before light chains are detectable. The question therefore arises, when the clinical biochemistry laboratory reports the absence of urinary light chains, as to whether more assiduous analysis (e.g. by testing repeated urine samples or more highly concentrated urine) would yield a positive result. This problem may be put into perspective by emphasizing that in light-chain disease (the major category of myeloma in which the detection of monoclonal urinary light chains is of essential diagnostic importance), light chains are almost always present at easily detectable levels, presumably because the neoplastic cells do not produce heavy chains which can 'consume' light chains by forming intact Ig molecules. When low levels of light-chain excretion occur it is almost always in cases of IgG or IgA myeloma. Since light-chain excretion is not, *per se*, indicative of poor prognosis (see p. 723), and does not require different clinical management, its detection, when present in trace amounts, is of secondary importance. The only clinical setting in which the detection of trace amounts of urinary light chains may be diagnostically valuable is in distinguishing between an early case of myeloma and a benign paraproteinaemia, since free monoclonal light chains are strongly suggestive of plasma-cell malignancy.

The interpretation of serum and urinary protein electrophoretic patterns is usually straightforward [168, 169]. The presence of haemoglobin, fibrinogen or high levels of transferrin may occasionally mimic a paraprotein [170]. Conversely, paraproteins may escape detection when present at low levels. This is particularly common in cases of IgD myeloma due to the high turnover rate of this class of immunoglobulin (and in some cases to its tendency to degrade spontaneously on storage). The technical quality of the electrophoretic preparation is clearly of crucial importance in evaluating difficult cases, and it is worth noting that commercial electrophoretic 'kits', usually based upon electrophoresis in agarose, are now available and allow high-resolution electrophoresis to be simply and reproducibly performed.

Immunoelectrophoretic analysis of serum and

718

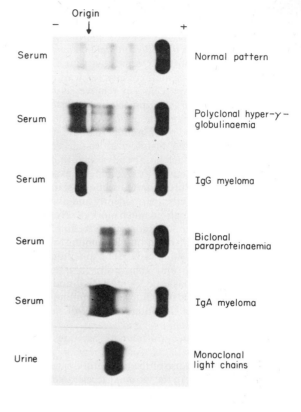

Fig. 19.9. Agarose electrophoresis of serum from a normal subject compared with polyclonal hyper-γ-globulinaemia and different types of paraproteinaemia. Note the contrast between the diffuse Ig increase characteristic of polyclonal hyper-γ-globulinaemia and the restricted mobility of the serum paraprotein in IgG myeloma (see also Fig. 19.4). Marked depression of background immunoglobulin is also seen in this sample. The IgA myeloma protein migrates in the β-globulin region, a feature typical of this class of paraprotein (although IgG and IgM paraproteins may also occasionally show similar mobility). Its relatively broad electrophoretic distribution (compared to that of the IgG myeloma paraprotein) may reflect paraprotein polymerization, a phenomenon found in approximately 50% of cases of IgA myeloma.

urinary paraproteins using antisera specific for heavy- and light-chain classes allows the immunochemical class of the paraprotein to be established on the basis of abnormalities in the position and/or shape of the precipitin arcs which are formed. The precipitin line commonly shows bowing, kinking or splitting in the region of the paraprotein. It may be noted, however, that the heavy-chain class of a circulating paraprotein is almost always apparent following quantification of serum immunoglobulin levels (see below), whilst the light-chain class of the paraprotein is of no diagnostic or prognostic importance for any individual patient. Immunoelectrophoresis is therefore of value in only a minority of cases of myeloma, for example, in diagnosing IgD myeloma, in detecting low levels of paraproteinaemia, and in investigating urine samples for light-chain excretion. In the context of IgD myeloma it may be noted that the paraprotein is often present at low concentration in the serum and the light chains in the paraprotein (usually of the λ class) may fail to react with anti-light-chain antisera [171]. As in the case of protein electrophoresis, the interpretation of immunoelectrophoretic results is dependent upon techni-

cal factors and the availability of commercial electrophoretic 'kits' is of value in this context.

Recently, alternatives to immunoelectrophoresis, which may have advantages in specific contexts (e.g. when a paraprotein is masked by normal polyclonal Ig), have been provided by 'immunofixation' and 'immunoselection' techniques, but the role of these procedures in a routine clinical context has yet to be clearly established [172–175].

Measurement of serum immunoglobulins. This is commonly performed by the radial immunodiffusion (Mancini) technique, in which the serum sample diffuses from a well into agar containing antiserum specific for human IgG, IgA or IgM. The concentration of each of these three classes of immunoglobulin is then calculated from the diameter of the precipitin ring which forms around the well. This technique has the advantage of simplicity, although it usually requires at least an overnight period of incubation (longer for IgM) before results can be read, and in some laboratories more rapid techniques (e.g. laser nephelometry or 'rocket' immunoelectrophoresis) are preferred.

Typical serum Ig patterns encountered in myeloma are given in Table 19.6. As will be seen, cases of IgG and IgA myeloma are characterized by a high reading for the appropriate class of immunoglobulin, associated with depression of the other two classes. The high reading represents detection of both the paraprotein and of residual normal polyclonal Ig of the same class. The dual nature of this reaction may sometimes be indicated by the formation of two concentric precipitin rings [176], although this phenomenon may also occasionally occur in non-paraprotein-containing samples. Paraproteins, since they lack the range of antigens found on normal polyclonal Ig, frequently give rise to spuriously large precipitin rings (relative to their true serum concentration) in Mancini plates [177]. In consequence, results obtained by this method (whilst they provide a convenient means of identifying the heavy-chain class of the paraprotein) provide an overestimate of the true concentration of the paraprotein. Densitometric scanning of electrophoretic strips is therefore preferable for quantification of paraprotein levels [178].

In cases of light-chain disease all three classes of immunoglobulin are frequently depressed (Table 19.6). A similar picture is seen in IgD myeloma and in non-secretory myeloma.

Table 19.6. Patterns of serum immunoglobulin levels in different immunochemical classes of myeloma

Myeloma class	Serum immunoglobulin levels		
	IgG	IgA	IgM
IgG	Raised	Low	Low
IgA	Low	Raised	Low
IgD	Low	Low	Low
Light-chain disease	Low	Low	Low

Biochemical investigations

Serum calcium. Between a quarter and a half of all myeloma patients have increased serum calcium levels at presentation. The frequency of this abnormality appears to be highest in cases of light-chain disease and in patients with advanced myelomatous skeletal destruction. In a minority of patients, marked hypercalcaemia may be present in the absence of any clinical symptoms, a discrepancy attributable to the fact that the paraprotein binds calcium, with the result that the ionized serum calcium level (upon which the development of symptoms depends) is lower than the total blood calcium level would suggest [179–182].

Blood urea, creatinine and uric acid. Evidence of renal failure is found in approximately 50% of myeloma patients at presentation, although in a proportion of less severely affected cases normal renal function is restored following correction of dehydration. Hyperuricaemia is found in approximately one-third of patients but is usually secondary to renal failure rather than its cause. Once a myeloma patient has been diagnosed and chemotherapy initiated it is standard practice to administer allopurinol, with the consequence that any possible rise in serum uric acid due to malignant cell destruction is prevented. In consequence, clinical manifestations of hyperuricaemia are rarely encountered in myeloma patients.

Serum alkaline phosphatase. The level of this enzyme is traditionally said to be normal in myeloma patients, even when marked hypercalcaemia and radiological evidence of bone destruction are present. This is a reflection of the lack of osteoblastic response to bone erosion, and may provide a simple means of distinguishing myeloma patients from cases of carcinomatous bone destruction. However, if myeloma patients are studied sequentially following the initiation of chemotherapy, a transient increase in the level of serum alkaline phosphatase is commonly seen after a few weeks, presumably representing a process of bone repair.

Serum sodium and the anion gap. In a minority of myeloma patients, a low serum sodium level and/or a reduced anion gap is noted [183–187]. These abnormalities are probably related to a decrease in plasma water secondary to increased total serum protein, and also to the retention of chloride and/or bicarbonate to compensate for a cationic paraprotein [188]. The importance of hyponatraemia is that it may lead to inappropriate electrolyte therapy, the risks of which are compounded by the tendency of myeloma patients to have an increased plasma volume.

Serum albumin levels. In the first MRC trial of myeloma chemotherapy it was noted that a low serum albumin level was an important prognostic indicator, patients with a serum albumin level of less than 30 g/l having a mortality risk (after correction for the influence of uraemia) more than twice that of patients with values above 40 g/l [53]. It has been suggested that this reflects the more rapid catabolism of albumin by aggressive myeloma cells, but this hypothesis remains to be confirmed.

Blood viscosity

Although more frequently of clinical relevance in the context of Waldenström's macroglobulinaemia (see p. 727), viscosity measurements are indicated in a minority

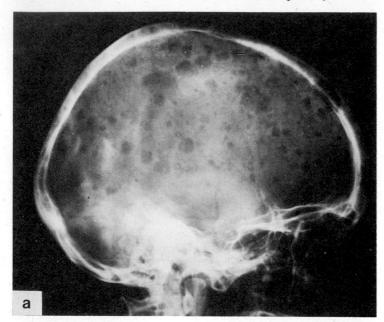

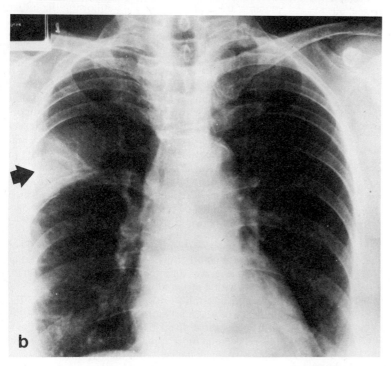

Fig. 19.10. Radiological abnormalities typical of multiple myeloma: (a) skull X-ray showing numerous radiolucent myeloma deposits in the cranial bones; (b) chest X-ray showing partial destruction of the sixth right rib associated with extraosseous spread, giving rise to a soft-tissue pleural plasmacytoma (arrowed); facing page, (c) X-ray of the pelvis showing erosive myeloma deposits in the right ischial ramus and the right lesser trochanter (arrowed).

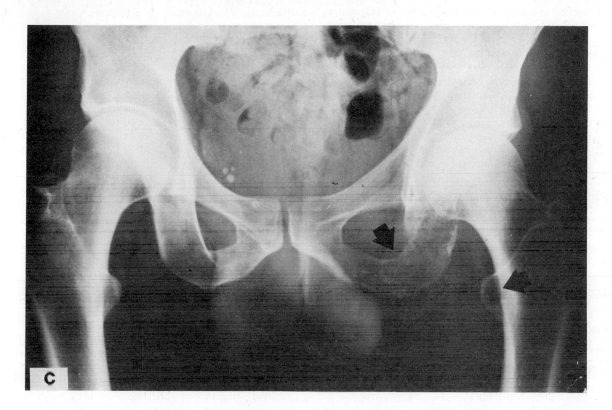

of myeloma patients. The Ostwald viscometer, which measures the time taken for the sample to flow from one chamber to another through a U-shaped capillary tube, has been widely used in the past for measuring blood and serum viscosity. Results are expressed as 'relative viscosity' values (flow time for sample divided by flow time for water) and normal serum gives values of approximately 1·5. Viscosity symptoms are usually only encountered when the relative viscosity rises above a value of 6·0. It may be noted, however, that the relative viscosity of normal serum shows little change as the sample is cooled, even when the temperature approaches 0°C. In contrast, hyperviscous paraprotein-containing sera often show a steep increase in viscosity as the temperature falls, and this may be of relevance to the development of cold-related symptoms.

A simple alternative to the Ostwald viscometer is provided by measuring the rate at which the serum runs out of a small bulb pipette under gravity, since the results correlate well with those obtained using the Ostwald instrument [189]. Recently, cone viscometers which enable serum viscosity to be measured at a number of different shear rates have been used, and it is claimed that these give results of more clinical rele-

vance. It may be noted that when using this instrument (as well as the Ostwald viscometer) whole blood viscosity can be calculated from the value for serum viscosity, using a formula which takes into account the haematocrit value [190, 191].

Radiological findings
In about 75% of myeloma patients radiological examination of the skull, thoracic cage, spine and pelvis shows evidence of bone disease (Fig. 19.10). The classical abnormality consists of scattered 'punched-out' osteolytic bone lesions, without evidence of a sclerotic reaction. These lesions are said to occur most commonly in cases of light-chain disease [192, 193]. The radiological picture may be indistinguishable from that seen in metastatic carcinoma, although the tendency for myeloma to extend from bone (especially from ribs and vertebral column) into adjacent soft tissue, and the fact that myelomatous infiltration usually spares the vertebral pedicles, may suggest the true diagnosis to the radiologist.

Less frequently, patients show diffuse osteoporosis rather than osteolytic lesions. Given the prevalence of osteoporosis in the age range in which myeloma occurs, this finding may be difficult to evaluate. A much rarer radiological pattern, occasionally encountered in myeloma, is that of osteosclerosis [194]. Less than 100 cases showing this appearance have been reported; it is of interest that there appears to be an association between osteosclerotic myeloma and peripheral neuropathy, and also possibly with IgE myeloma [132, 133, 195].

Radiological examination of the myeloma patient may also reveal secondary effects due to neoplastic cell proliferation (e.g. fractures, vertebral collapse, pleural and pulmonary infiltrates).

Difficulties in the diagnosis of myeloma

In practice, the major obstacle to the diagnosis of myeloma is not that the appropriate investigations yield equivocal results, but rather that myeloma is not included among the list of differential diagnoses. This is most likely to occur in the case of a patient who has few or no skeletal symptoms, and who presents with renal failure, sepsis, anaemia or soft-tissue plasmacytoma. As has been noted previously, the cell morphology of extramedullary plasmacytomas is often primitive, and the true origin of the growth may not be immediately apparent to the histologist.

A further problem is posed by the patient who presents at an early stage of the disease, or who is even found to have a paraprotein by chance when totally asymptomatic. Not only are these patients free of bone pain, but other diagnostic features of the disease (e.g. radiological and bone-marrow abnormalities, reduction of normal serum immunoglobulin levels) are often absent or equivocal. However, such cases will usually declare themselves as overt myeloma if observed over a period of a year or two. There is no evidence that delaying the initiation of therapy at such an early stage of the disease has any fundamental influence on the final outcome. It should also be noted that if chemotherapy is initiated before the diagnosis of myeloma is clearly established, there is a risk not only of mistakenly treating a benign paraproteinaemia, but also of prematurely exposing the patient to the mutagenic effect of chemotherapy. Once the diagnosis is clearly established, however, there should be no delay in initiating treatment, since it is well established that the prognosis is related to the extent of the disease at the time of commencing treatment.

In recent years a minority group of myeloma patients has been identified who follow an 'indolent' or 'smouldering' course in that they show clear evidence of early myeloma, but do not progress clinically, even though untreated, when observed over a period of months or years [114, 196–198]. A parallel may be drawn with the occasional case of acute leukaemia which remains spontaneously stable over a period.

CLINICAL MANAGEMENT OF MYELOMA

Chemotherapy

Melphalan and cyclophosphamide. Two alkylating agents, melphalan (L-phenylalanine mustard) and cyclophosphamide, have been extensively employed in the therapy of myeloma. Although these two drugs appear to be of comparable cytotoxic efficacy [199], melphalan has been far more extensively used. This drug is usually administered orally in intermittent dosage (0·15–0·25 mg/kg daily for four to seven days every four to six weeks) although the apparent superiority of this schedule over continuous melphalan therapy [200] may be due to faster symptomatic response rather than to a higher response rate or longer overall survival [201]. Moderate marrow suppression commonly occurs as a result of melphalan therapy but almost always recovers promptly during the gaps between courses. Various side effects (including pulmonary fibrotic, pneumonitic and hypersensitivity reactions) have been reported but are uncommon [202–205].

Prednisone (40 mg/day) is usually given in conjunction with intermittent courses of melphalan, and appears to increase the number of patients who respond [206]. The role of this drug is the subject of some debate, however, since it may not prolong overall survival, and indeed may shorten the survival of poor-risk patients [207] (see p. 723) and/or non-responding patients [208] especially if given in excessive dosage.

It was established by the early 1970s that intermittent melphalan and prednisone therapy produces a good response (defined as a reduction of the paraprotein level by at least 75%) in approximately 50% of patients, and an overall median survival of approximately two years [206, 209]. In about 30% of responding patients, serial radiological examination reveals evidence of bone repair [210].

These figures may not appear to represent a very striking improvement upon the projected untreated median survival of six months, but they conceal the fact that a number of patients now survive for very long periods, whilst other patients, even when achieving only partial remissions, may enjoy considerable alleviation of symptoms.

New chemotherapeutic schedules. The major limitations of melphalan/prednisone therapy are that a sizable proportion of patients do not respond to treatment, and that among responding patients a period of remission (during which paraprotein levels reach a 'plateau' level) is followed almost inevitably by relapse (and resistance to melphalan) [211–213]. There is evidence that there are two neoplastic-cell populations in myeloma patients (one sensitive to chemotherapy and the other resistant) and that it is regrowth of the latter population which accounts for the temporary nature of the initial response [214]. It should be noted, however, that myeloma-cell behaviour during the plateau phase is poorly understood. It has recently been suggested that this period is often cytokinetically quiescent (as assessed by measurements of labelling indices, agar culture and urinary polyamine production) [215], with the implication that maintenance therapy during remission is unnecessary. This is in keeping with clinical trials in which it has been shown that such treatment fails to prolong remission or survival (and indeed may entail a greater risk of complications due to marrow toxicity) [216–218].

These considerations have prompted a number of treatment centres to explore the use of alternative, more aggressive chemotherapeutic regimes [219], based upon drugs such as adriamycin (doxorubicin), BCNU (carmustine), bleomycin and vincristine, often given in multiple-drug schedules [211, 213, 218–226]. As well as seeking to increase the number of responding patients, these schedules have been aimed at achieving longer remission periods (by producing greater initial neoplastic-cell destruction), or even complete eradication of the disease. Several centres have also investigated the value of these regimes in treating patients who are resistant to melphalan (either initially or following relapse) [226].

Increased initial response rates, approaching 90%, have been reported using multiple drug combinations (e.g. melphalan, cyclophosphamide, BCNU, vincristine and prednisone) in most [218, 223, 225] (but not all [222]) studies. It has been suggested that the inclusion of vincristine may be an essential element in the greater efficacy of these regimes compared to melphalan and prednisone [218], although other explanations are possible [227]. In this context it may be noted that there is evidence that the growth fraction (and hence the number of cells susceptible to cycle-specific agents such as vincristine) is increased following initial nonspecific cytoreduction with alkylating agents [48, 228]. The role of vincristine in the treatment of myeloma remains to be more clearly established, however, and it has recently been pointed out that the increase in labelling indices is only transient and does not persist during the plateau phase of the disease [215].

Median survival of patients responding to multiple-drug regimes may be greater than that of patients treated with conventional prednisone/melphalan regimes [218, 223], although information on this aspect of these newer schedules is still limited. However, since the duration of remission in myeloma is related to the degree of maximal initial cell killing, there are at least theoretical grounds for hoping that newer chemotherapeutic regimes will be shown to produce longer survival.

Melphalan resistance remains a major problem in the management of myeloma. Some centres have reported good results with multiple chemotherapy regimes (e.g. melphalan, cyclophosphamide, BCNU and vincristine) or with high-dose cyclophosphamide [223, 224, 226, 229, 230]. However, other centres have reported less success when using such regimes [212, 213]. It may be noted that there is evidence that cessation of therapy during a period of remission may carry the benefit that the patient is more likely to respond subsequently to readministration of melphalan when relapse occurs [217].

Prognostic indicators and clinical staging

In the course of chemotherapy trials in both Europe and the United States, information has been gathered which allows a number of prognostic factors to be identified. Principal among these is the presence of renal failure [53, 220], the death rate in the first MRC myeloma trial for patients with a blood urea level at presentation of 80 mg/100 ml or greater being five times that of patients with urea levels of less than 40 mg/100 ml. Other factors at presentation indicating a poor prognosis include anaemia, the excretion of λ (rather than κ) light chains, hypercalcaemia, hypoalbuminaemia and extensive bony destruction [52, 53, 222, 231–233]. However, not all studies have been in agreement on the prognostic importance of these factors and in some instances the reported influence of one factor may have been due to its association with another (e.g. the poor prognosis of cases excreting λ light chains may be related to the fact that the level of urinary excretion is higher in this class of myeloma) [53].

An alternative to the identification of single factors as indicators of prognosis is provided by studies which have shown that survival is related to the magnitude of the neoplastic-cell population at presentation (i.e. to the clinical 'stage'). The background to these studies is to be found in the work of Salmon and his colleagues, who calculated tumour-cell mass in a number of patients from direct measurements of rates of paraprotein synthesis and turnover [46, 47]. By correlating the tumour-cell mass measured in this way with clinical, radiological and laboratory findings they identified four parameters (skeletal lesions, haemoglobin level, serum calcium and paraprotein concentration) which enable new patients to be assigned at presentation to one of three clinical stages (I, II and III) corresponding to low, intermediate or high neoplastic-cell loads [234] (Table 19.7). Each stage is further divided into

Table 19.7. Clinical myeloma staging system*

Stage	Criteria	Myeloma cell mass (10^{12} cells/m^2)
I (low cell mass)	All of the following: Hb > 10 g/dl Serum calcium (corrected) ⩽ 3·0 mmol/l X-rays: normal bone structure or solitary lesion only Low rate of paraprotein production: (a) IgG paraprotein < 50 g/l (b) IgA paraprotein < 30 g/l (c) Urinary light-chain excretion < 4 g/24 hours	< 0·6
II (intermediate cell mass)	Fitting neither stage I nor III	0·6–1·2
III (high cell mass)	Any of the following: Hb < 8·5 g/dl Serum calcium (corrected) > 3·0 mmol/l Advanced lytic bone lesions High paraprotein production rate (a) IgG paraprotein > 70 g/l (b) IgA paraprotein > 50 g/l (c) Urinary light-chain excretion > 12 g/24 hours	> 1·2

* Subclassification:
A: Serum creatinine < 2·0 mg/100 ml (or BUN < 30 mg/100 ml if creatinine not available);
B: Serum creatinine ⩾ 2·0 mg/100 ml.

two sub-categories (A or B) on the basis of renal function.

Retrospective analysis of large numbers of conventionally treated myeloma patients has shown that this staging system correlates with prognosis, in that patients with the highest mass (stage III) at presentation have the shortest median survival (reflecting shorter periods of remission in these patients rather than lower response rates) [217, 233, 235]. This inverse relation between indicators of advanced disease and median survival implies that it may be cell mass, rather than any intrinsic property of the individual neoplastic clone, which dictates the likelihood of inducing prolonged remissions. It has been suggested that this may reflect the greater probability that a high-cell-mass patient will harbour a sub-line of drug-resistant cells.

One further major prognostic indicator in myeloma which has emerged from therapeutic trials is to be found in the drug sensitivity of the neoplastic cells (as assessed from sequential measurements of paraprotein levels) during the first few months of chemotherapy [219, 227]. Not only do non-responsive patients have a predictably poor prognosis, but the length of remission appears to be directly related to the degree of maximal neoplastic-cell suppression, the longest survival being obtained in patients whose myeloma is suppressed to undetectable levels [209, 217, 233]. Some studies have also shown that the speed of the initial response to chemotherapy is of prognostic significance, in that rapidly responding patients relapse sooner than do slow responders [45, 233], although in at least one trial (of multiple chemotherapy) no difference of this sort was detectable [223].

Conclusions concerning chemotherapy
The increasing complexity of the treatment schedules currently being explored in the management of myeloma and the difficulty of comparing patient populations from different centres makes it impossible at this juncture to draw definitive conclusions concerning the optimal chemotherapeutic strategy for myeloma. These difficulties are likely to be compounded in the future by the fact that questions concerning long-term survival cannot, by their very nature, be answered before patients have been observed for prolonged periods. Furthermore, the fact that patients during the plateau phase of the disease may be either cytokinetically stable or unstable [215], and the identification of high- and low-risk patient groups on the basis of clinical staging and other parameters, provides further permutations to be taken into account when planning chemotherapy trials. In one recent study it was shown that a multiple-drug regime (melphalan, cyclophosphamide, BCNU and prednisone) produced longer

survival than a conventional intermittent melphalan/prednisone schedule only in high-cell-mass patients, whilst better prognosis (low-cell-mass) subjects had a shortened survival on this regime [221]. Future treatment trials will therefore probably stratify patients at entry into high- and low-risk groups and assign them to different drug regimes.

Against this complex background of current investigation into myeloma chemotherapy, the most generally acceptable strategy is to treat all patients initially with intermittent melphalan and prednisone, and to reserve multiple-drug regimes for patients who do not show a substantial response to this treatment, or who are in relapse [227]. Once maximal response has been achieved (usually well within one year) chemotherapy should be stopped.

Interferon therapy

Human leucocyte interferon has recently been reported as producing clinical response and reduction of paraprotein levels in a proportion of myeloma patients when administered in the absence of conventional chemotherapy [236, 237]. The efficacy of this agent is now being investigated in a number of centres; however, preliminary results from the United States do not indicate that it is strikingly superior to conventional chemotherapy and its role in the management of myeloma will only become apparent after further studies have been completed.

Ancillary treatment [238]

Renal failure. There has been an increasing trend in recent years, now that the benefits of chemotherapy in myeloma have been appreciated, to treat patients who present in renal failure more aggressively [239, 240]. Prompt rehydration and correction of hypercalcaemia (see below) may partially restore renal function [58]. Short-term haemodialysis may be required to treat acute renal failure, while longer-term haemodialysis and renal transplantation may have a role to play in the management of myeloma patients whose kidney function is irreversibly damaged, but whose neoplastic cells are responsive to chemotherapy [58, 240–242].

Hypercalcaemia. If this complication does not respond to prednisone (40–60 mg daily), the use of oral or intravenous phosphate [58] (up to 5 g daily), mithramycin (25 μg/kg intravenously as a single dose or four daily doses of 15 μg/kg) [243, 244], or calcitonin (200–400 MRC units, eight-hourly) [245] may be indicated. There is a theoretical risk following phosphate therapy of metastatic calcification in other tissues, but this is usually of little practical importance.

Surgical treatment. Cases of spinal-cord compression often respond well to decompressive laminectomy, usually followed by radiotherapy [246, 247]. Surgical treatment should not be delayed since there is a correlation between the duration of paraparesis before operation and the risk of subsequent paraplegia [248]. Myeloma patients often survive for prolonged periods following laminectomy, probably because these cases may represent a relatively early localized form of myeloma [114]. Additional surgical measures which may be indicated in myeloma patients include orthopaedic repair of fractured long bones.

Radiotherapy. Local radiotherapy is invaluable in palliating the severe pain arising from a site of skeletal erosion. Recently, more widespread bone pain due to drug-resistant advanced myeloma has been treated with whole-body irradiation (administered as two sequential half-body treatments) with encouraging results [249, 250].

Hyperviscosity. Plasmapheresis by means of a centrifugal cell separator may be indicated in the management of hyperviscosity [74, 251, 252]. The paraprotein in such cases is frequently of high molecular weight (because of polymerization or aggregation) and consequently tends to be confined to the circulation. This explains why plasmapheresis is more effective at reducing the level of circulating paraprotein than it would be in the case of monomeric immunoglobulin.

Plasmapheresis may also have a role to play in myeloma patients who develop acute renal failure [253]. It may also be noted that plasmapheresis appears to remove light chains from the circulation more efficiently than does peritoneal dialysis [254].

Infection, bone pain and anaemia. All myeloma patients and their physicians should be aware of the ever-present risk of infection, and antibiotics must be administered promptly if this complication is suspected [58]. Analgesia should also be provided in adequate amounts, especially in the early stages of chemotherapy before symptomatic improvement has been achieved. Bone healing may be encouraged by the administration of sodium fluoride supplemented with calcium carbonate. Objective evidence of increased bone density and mass has been provided in a trial of these agents in myeloma patients, the authors pointing out that the poor results previously obtained from the use of fluoride in myeloma were due to the omission of supplemental calcium [255].

Anaemic myeloma patients not infrequently require blood transfusion. However, it should be remembered that myeloma patients frequently have an increased plasma volume which not only causes a spurious anaemia but also increases the risk of circulatory overload following transfusion.

CAUSES OF DEATH IN MYELOMA

A proportion of myeloma patients die shortly after diagnosis, usually because of irreversible renal failure or because their disease proves resistant to all cytotoxic therapy. Most patients surviving this initial period subsequently die as a result of relapse of their disease. In some cases, the neoplastic cells secrete the same paraprotein during relapse as was present at diagnosis. However, in a substantial minority, the cells lose the ability in relapse to secrete heavy chains, giving rise to increasing urinary light-chain excretion unaccompanied by a rise in serum paraprotein levels ('Bence Jones escape') [256].

The neoplastic cells during relapse are often considerably more anaplastic in morphology than those present at diagnosis [111, 112], and tend to spread into the circulation (giving rise to a plasma-cell leukaemia) and/or to the soft tissues, where they may cause widespread tumour deposits. A clinical picture resembling that of acute leukaemia, characterized by fever and pancytopenia, has been described in approximately one-third of relapsing myeloma patients [257].

Among the other causes of death in myeloma, infection is the most important. A small proportion of myeloma patients (approximately four per cent) develop acute leukaemia [258, 259], almost always of the acute myeloblastic or myelomonocytic type, although a few instances of erythroleukaemia have been reported [161, 260–262]. The risk of this complication in a large population of treated myeloma patients has been estimated at approximately 50 times that of the normal population [263], although it may be noted that the risk appears to increase steadily with time [222]. The leukaemia probably represents a mutation induced by melphalan or cyclophosphamide therapy, since the same drugs may occasionally produce acute leukaemia in non-myelomatous patients. Furthermore, karyotypic analysis of bone-marrow samples during remission frequently shows evidence of chromosomal damage, presumably secondary to drug therapy [162]. When leukaemia develops, the chromosomal changes seen are similar to those characteristic of other presumed drug-induced leukaemias (in Hodgkin's disease and polycythaemia rubra vera) [264]. As noted previously (see p. 716), the development of acute leukaemia in myeloma is not uncommonly preceded by a period of dyserythropoietic or sideroblastic anaemia.

It may be noted that occasional patients have been reported in whom myeloma and acute leukaemia (usually myeloblastic) have occurred simultaneously [265, 266]. It is conceivable that such cases represent a mutation occurring in an undifferentiated stem cell common to both lymphoid and myeloid cells.

WALDENSTRÖM'S MACROGLOBULINAEMIA [267–269]

DEFINITION

Three major features distinguish this disease from myeloma. First, the neoplastic cells are pleomorphic in morphology, ranging from small lymphoid forms to mature plasma cells. Secondly, the neoplasm spreads diffusely through the lymphatic tissue, causing hepatosplenomegaly and lymphadenopathy in a way reminiscent of non-Hodgkin's lymphoma. Although the bone marrow is usually infiltrated, erosive bony lesions of the myelomatous type are exceptional. Finally, the neoplastic cells in Waldenström's macroglobulinaemia secrete an IgM paraprotein and the symptoms attributable to this paraprotein (principally hyperviscosity) usually dominate the clinical picture.

INCIDENCE, AGE AND SEX RATIO

The disease is approximately 10 times less frequent than myeloma. The mean age at presentation is in the early 60s; patients are rarely seen under the age of 40. There has been a modest preponderance of male patients in most reported series.

AETIOLOGY

As in the case of myeloma, the precipitating event in Waldenström's macroglobulinaemia is unknown. Abnormalities in serum immunoglobulins and autoimmune phenomena have been found in the families of macroglobulinaemia patients [270], and occasionally multiple cases of the disease occur within one family [271]. There is some suggestion that the disease develops against a background of chronic infection.

Cellular aspects of Waldenström's macroglobulinaemia

Waldenström's macroglobulinaemia and multiple myeloma are commonly thought of as neoplasms involving two successive steps in the maturation of Ig-secreting B cells, i.e. the lymphoplasmacytoid cell in the case of Waldenström's, the plasma cell in the case of myeloma. However, this view, which is based upon cell morphology in the two diseases and on the concept of a switch from IgM to IgG secretion during B-cell maturation, may be an oversimplifcation. It may be noted that myeloma cases never de-differentiate into IgM-secreting neoplasms, as might be expected if Waldenström's represented a precursor of myeloma. Furthermore, the benign clinical behaviour of Waldenström's, and its clearly distinguishable growth pattern, is not in keeping with its representing a less differentiated form of myeloma. Finally, although many of the neoplastic cells in Waldenström's are lymphoid or lymphoplasmacytoid in morphology, it is not in these cells that IgM synthesis occurs but rather in the mature plasmacytoid component [272].

However, whatever the true relationship between Waldenström's and myeloma, the two diseases share a similarity in that it is possible to demonstrate lymphoid cells in the circulation of Waldenström's patients which carry on their surface membrane Ig of the same light-chain type as the circulating paraprotein [272]. Hence, as in myeloma, the neoplastic clone probably arises from a mutant primitive lymphoid stem cell and the paraprotein is produced by the most differentiated members of this clone.

CLINICAL FEATURES [289]

The major presenting signs and symptoms in Waldenström's macroglobulinaemia are illustrated schematically in Figure 19.11.

Lassitude, weakness and weight loss

Although many patients are anaemic at presentation, the severity of non-specific symptoms is often out of proportion to the degree of anaemia. This may possibly represent an effect of increased blood viscosity on the CNS microcirculation. For unexplained reasons, weight loss is also relatively frequent in macroglobulinaemia patients.

Hyperviscosity syndrome

The clinical features of this complication are essentially identical to those seen in hyperviscous myeloma patients (p. 711). Abnormal bleeding (particularly epistaxes and purpura) is the commonest finding. Less

frequently, neurological manifestations attributable to hyperviscosity are encountered (e.g. headache, mental changes, depression of the level of consciousness— progressing in rare instances to 'coma paraproteinae-cum'—and sudden deafness) [273]. Visual disturbances may also occur, usually secondary to retinal haemorrhages and exudates. As in myeloma patients, hyperviscosity commonly produces increased plasma volume, causing sausage-like dilatation of the retinal veins.

Neurological manifestations

The term 'Bing–Neel syndrome' refers to the association between neurological symptoms and macroglobulinaemia. These complications may be found in as many as 25% of patients [274]. As outlined above, some of these phenomena are attributable to hyperviscosity. However, peripheral neuropathy, usually sensory or sensorimotor, is relatively frequent [275]. Other patterns (mononeuritis multiplex, cranial neuropathies, motor neuropathy, carpal-tunnel syndrome and Guillain–Barré syndrome) are also occasionally encountered [276–280]. The aetiology of peripheral neuropathy in Waldenström's macroglobulinaemia is obscure, although there is evidence that monoclonal IgM may show an affinity for nervous-tissue antigens, especially those in axonal and glial tissues [275, 280]. Furthermore, idiotypic cross-reactivity has recently been demonstrated between the paraproteins of Waldenström's patients suffering from polyneuropathy (but not between the paraproteins from non-neuropathic patients) [12]. This suggests that the neuropathy is directly related to the antibody-binding activity of the paraprotein. In addition to the neurological manifestations discussed above, occasional patients develop focal syndromes (e.g. strokes) which

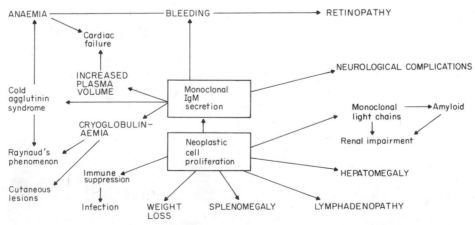

Fig. 19.11. Summary of the symptomatology of Waldenström's macroglobulinaemia. The more frequently encountered features are printed in capitals.

may be attributable to bleeding or thrombosis [274, 277].

Lymphadenopathy and splenomegaly

These features are present in a substantial minority of patients. Less frequently, soft-tissue infiltration (e.g. of lung, kidneys or spleen) is clinically manifest [281], although this is a much commoner feature at the microscopic level.

Rare complications

Infection, especially of the respiratory tract [281], occasionally occurs but is considerably rarer than in myeloma. This is in keeping with the much lower incidence of severe suppression of normal serum immunoglobulin levels. Symptoms related to cryoprecipitation of the serum paraprotein are sometimes encountered [282]: these include Raynaud's phenomenon, cold urticaria, cold sensitivity and, rarely, vascular occlusion leading to gangrene [8]. A circulating paraprotein may show specificity for red-cell antigens (most commonly the I antigen), giving rise to a cold-haemagglutinin syndrome. Other occasional complications of macroglobulinaemia include amyloidosis and cardiac failure.

LABORATORY FINDINGS

Haematological

Anaemia, due particularly to plasma-volume expansion, is a common finding. Iron deficiency, secondary to haemorrhage, may also contribute to this complication. Neutropenia and thrombocytopenia on the other hand are uncommon. Neoplastic cells are frequently present in the circulation, though they may be overlooked on a blood film because of their low numbers and nondescript lymphocytic morphology. Rouleaux formation is usually evident.

Bone-marrow aspiration reveals a high proportion of cells ranging in morphology from small lymphocytes to plasma cells (Fig. 19.12). Immunofluorescence reveals IgM of a single light-chain class (most frequently κ) in the cytoplasm of the plasmacytoid cells. The histology of biopsied lymph nodes characteristically shows diffuse replacement of the tissue with lymphoid cells, which frequently infiltrate through the capsule of the node into adjacent tissue. Features which allow the neoplasm to be distinguished from other types of non-Hodgkin lymphoma include the tendency to plasmacytoid differentiation, the rarity of mitotic figures, an increased number of mast cells and the presence of PAS-positive cytoplasmic and intranuclear inclusions [283]. Immunoperoxidase staining may be of diagnostic value in that IgM of a single light-chain class is found in the cytoplasm of many neoplastic cells (and often in the inclusion bodies) [155, 156].

Serum electrophoresis

The major diagnostic finding is the demonstration of

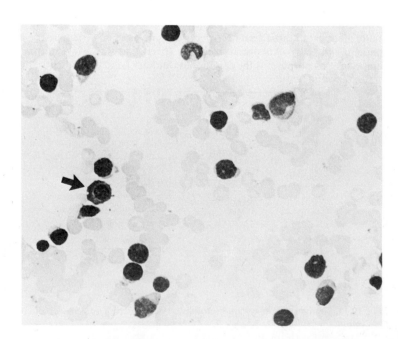

Fig. 19.12. Bone-marrow aspirate from a case of Waldenström's macroglobulinaemia. Numerous small lymphoid cells are present, together with occasional plasmacytoid cells (arrowed).

an IgM paraprotein, its concentration usually exceeding 10 g/l. Paraproteins of κ type are approximately two and a half times more frequent than λ paraproteins. Urinary monoclonal light-chain excretion is not uncommonly found, although renal impairment is considerably rarer than in cases of myeloma. This may reflect the rarity of hypercalcaemia in macroglobulinaemia, and also possibly the lower frequency of λ light-chain excretion. Biopsies from macroglobulinaemia patients frequently show evidence of glomerular damage, the most typical lesion consisting of PAS-positive eosinophilic subendothelial deposits [86, 87], probably related to hyperviscosity and/or to paraprotein precipitation, but clinical evidence of glomerular impairment is rare.

Serum viscosity
Viscosity is frequently raised [190, 191], a feature which may be visible with the naked eye when the tube containing the serum sample is inverted. The serum may gel completely at room temperature; alternatively a flocculent cryoprecipitate may separate out from the serum on standing. IgM paraproteins may also occasionally precipitate on heating ('pyroglobulin').

DIFFERENTIAL DIAGNOSIS AND RELATED DISORDERS
Although many patients in whom an IgM paraprotein is found manifest the typical clinical features of Waldenström's macroglobulinaemia, it is important to realize that IgM paraproteins may also be found in a number of other disorders. In particular, different types of non-Hodgkin lymphoma (including chronic lymphocytic leukaemia), which are histologically clearly distinct from the pattern seen in Waldenström's macroglobulinaemia, may be associated with an IgM paraprotein (see p. 738) [284]. Some authors prefer to group such cases together with classical Waldenström's disease into a single category of 'macroglobulinaemia', pointing out that the histological pattern in a single case may change with time from one category to the other, and claiming that the clinical response of IgM-paraprotein patients in whom a non-Waldenström's lymphoma is diagnosed does not differ from that of typical Waldenström's macroglobulinaemia [268].

IgM paraproteins may also be found in association with a wide variety of non-lymphoproliferative disorders, or in healthy subjects (see p. 739). A proportion of these patients may subsequently develop clinically overt lymphoproliferative disease and should consequently be followed up over a period of time.

It should also be noted that very occasionally IgM paraproteins are found in patients with the typical radiological and bone-marrow features of myeloma [285]. Conversely, rare patients have been described with cytologically typical features of Waldenström's macroglobulinaemia associated with an IgG or IgA, (or, in one case, IgE) paraprotein [286–288].

CLINICAL MANAGEMENT
There are two aspects to the management of Waldenström's macroglobulinaemia. First, symptoms which arise as a direct result of neoplastic cell growth (e.g. lymphadenopathy) require treatment by chemotherapy. Symptoms directly attributable to the effect of the circulating paraprotein (e.g. hyperviscosity), on the other hand, may also demand symptomatic treatment by plasmapheresis, in the period before chemotherapy has had a chance to be effective. It should also be appreciated that the disease shows considerable variation in its clinical severity from one patient to another. Consequently, the management of any individual case must take into account both the severity of symptoms and also their estimated rate of future progression [268].

Chemotherapy
If the disorder appears to be progressing rapidly, chemotherapy is indicated, chlorambucil being the most widely used drug [267, 269]. Some cases are resistant, however, and more aggressive multiple-drug regimes may then be substituted, although, as in other lymphoproliferative disorders, evidence that they offer substantial benefit is limited. It is frequently advisable to observe newly diagnosed patients over a period, so as to avoid exposing individuals in whom the disease is virtually static to the risks of chemotherapy.

Plasmapheresis
The efficacy of this therapy, although it has no influence on the growth of the neoplastic cell clone, stems from the fact that much of the IgM paraprotein is found within the circulation, with the consequence that a five-litre plasma exchange will remove 80% of the circulating load of paraprotein [289]. Furthermore, the slow growth of the underlying neoplasm (and the rarity with which it, rather than the paraprotein, causes symptoms) means that patients can often be treated effectively over long periods with an initial intensive course of plasmapheresis, followed at intervals by further plasmapheresis sessions [289].

PROGNOSIS
The median survival in Waldenström's macroglobulinaemia (approximately four years) is longer than that of myeloma patients [267]. However, there is considerable variation between patients, and survival for more than ten years is not uncommon. Death is most

frequently due to infection, severe anaemia, hyperviscosity and malignant cell growth. Occasionally (as in other lymphoid neoplasms), relatively benign cases transform into a rapidly progressive anaplastic disease [290].

A number of features associated with a good prognosis (e.g. intermediate levels of IgM paraprotein, absence of light-chain excretion or renal damage) have been identified by retrospective analysis of large numbers of Waldenström's macroglobulinaemia patients [291], although this information is of little value in the management of individual cases. As with myeloma, however, the initial response to chemotherapy provides some indication of the future course of the disease.

AMYLOIDOSIS

DEFINITION AND NATURE OF AMYLOID
The term 'amyloid' was initially coined in the nineteenth century in a botanical context to describe a normal constituent of plant tissue. The use of the term to describe human amyloid originates from Virchow, who believed it, on the basis of its iodine-staining reactions, to be related to starch or cellulose [292].

It is now known, however, that amyloid (regardless of its site or aetiology) is almost entirely composed of protein or polypeptide [292]. These constituents are laid down as felt-like deposits of linear, non-branching fibrils (approximately 1 nm in diameter). Low-angle X-ray diffraction analysis has revealed that the fibrils have a β-pleated-sheet structure. This molecular configuration, which is not found in such a pure state in any other constituent of mammalian tissue, probably accounts for the insolubility of amyloid and its resistance to enzymatic degradation, and thus explains the inexorable way in which (in the absence of effective physiological mechanisms for its removal), it accumu-lates in the tissues. The β-pleated-sheet structure also confers upon amyloid a diagnostically important property, in that molecules of dyes such as Congo Red bind to amyloid and orientate themselves parallel to the axial folds in the fibrils. This parallel alignment of the dye molecules is responsible for the characteristic green birefringence seen when Congo-Red-stained amyloid deposits in tissue sections are viewed by polarized microscopy.

Classification of amyloidosis
In the past, amyloidosis has been classified on the basis of its macroscopic and microscopic tissue distribution. Two distinctive patterns were recognized [293, 294]: one (sometimes referred to as 'pericollagen' or 'mesenchymal') involves principally the tongue, heart, gastro-intestinal tract, skeletal and smooth muscle, carpal ligaments, nerves and skin; whilst the other ('perireticulin' or 'parenchymal') typically involves liver, spleen, kidneys and adrenal glands. In practice, however, the distinction between these two categories is not clear-cut and patients showing a mixed distribution pattern are commonly encountered.

An alternative classification is based upon the clinical setting in which amyloid deposition occurs, and also distinguishes systemic from localized amyloidosis. This classification (see Table 19.8) is more satisfactory since the distinctions which it draws correlate well with the different immunochemical types of amyloid.

From a haematological point of view the only types of amyloid of relevance are those associated with monoclonal plasma-cell proliferation (referred to subsequently as 'immunocyte-related amyloid'). The proliferating cells may be clinically overt (i.e. the patient is diagnosed as having myeloma or, less frequently, Waldenström's macroglobulinaemia or lymphoma); or, in a roughly equal number of patients, their presence is not clinically manifest ('primary amyloid').

Table 19.8. Classification of amyloidosis*

Type of amyloidosis	Chemical nature of fibrils	Precursor
Immunocyte-related (e.g. primary amyloidosis or amyloid arising in association with myeloma, Waldenström's macroglobulinaemia or other lymphoproliferative disorders)	Ig light chains (whole or fragment)	Monoclonal Ig light chains
Secondary (e.g. to rheumatoid arthritis, TB, Hodgkin's disease) and some familial forms	A A protein	Serum A A protein
Localized endocrine	Hormones	Calcitonin, insulin, etc.
Senile	A S protein	?
Familial	AF$_P$ and other proteins	?

* A more extensive classification of amyloidosis along these lines is given by Glenner [292].

Immunochemical nature of amyloid [292]

In all patients with immunocyte-related amyloid, the fibrils are derived from monoclonal immunoglobulin light chains, themselves the product of the proliferating immunocytes. The light chains are usually incomplete, consisting of continuous sequences (average MW 14 000 daltons) running from the N-terminal end and hence including the variable region of the chain. However, in some amyloid deposits an admixture of intact light chains may be present in addition to the variable-region fragments.

It is probable that the fibrils are formed as a result of tissue proteolytic enzymes digesting circulating monoclonal light chains. Evidence for this mechanism is provided by the fact that fibrils with the typical ultrastructural and tinctorial properties of amyloid can be produced *in vitro* by digesting monoclonal light chains with leucocyte proteases (as well as with other proteolytic enzymes such as trypsin) [292]. Interestingly, the renal tubular light-chain casts typical of myeloma kidney may contain amyloid fibrils in patients in whom no other evidence of systemic amyloid deposition is present. Presumably, in these cases, the renal tubular lysosomal enzymes selectively cleave intratubular light chains to form amyloid.

Relationship of amyloidosis to myeloma

Only about 10% of all myeloma patients show evidence of amyloid deposition, despite the fact that a high proportion of myeloma patients excrete substantial quantities of monoclonal light chains. Conversely, patients suffering from primary amyloidosis (Table 19.8) develop amyloid deposition despite the fact that the population of monoclonal plasma cells is far less advanced than is typically found at diagnosis in myeloma, and the level of monoclonal light-chain production is correspondingly low.

The probable explanation for this lack of relationship between the presence and level of light-chain excretion on the one hand and the deposition of amyloid on the other, lies in inherent physico-chemical properties possessed by a minority of monoclonal light chains which render them 'amyloidogenic' [292]. An obvious analogy can be drawn with the idiosyncratic characteristics of other types of paraprotein (e.g. cryoprecipitability or tendency to polymer formation). However, the molecular features which explain this tendency to precipitate as amyloid fibrils remain obscure. Despite the fact that only a minority of monoclonal light chains give rise to amyloid fibrils *in vitro* when digested with proteolytic enzymes, this property does not correlate in individual cases with a tendency to cause amyloid deposition *in vivo*. Attempts to demonstrate antigenic determinants (reflecting shared amino-acid sequences) in amyloidogenic light

chains have been unsuccessful. However λ light chains are more likely to give rise, both *in vitro* and *in vivo*, to amyloid fibrils. There also appears to be a tendency for λ chains of a rare sub-group ($V_{\lambda VI}$) to be associated with *in-vivo* amyloid deposition [292].

A further unexplained feature of immunocyte-related amyloid is the fact that certain tissues (e.g. tongue, carpal ligament, nerves, kidneys) are particularly likely to be involved. This may reflect the presence in these tissues of constituents for which amyloidogenic light chains have a particular affinity, an explanation which finds some experimental support from studies showing binding of light chains from amyloid patients to cryostat sections of these tissues. However, there is considerable variation from one patient to another in the degree to which individual tissues or organs are involved, and it is not clear whether this reflects differences inherent in the patient or in the light chain.

INCIDENCE, SEX RATIO AND AGE IN IMMUNOCYTE-RELATED AMYLOIDOSIS

Accurate figures for the incidence of primary amyloidosis are not available, but its frequency is of the same order as that of primary macroglobulinaemia (i.e. new patients are seen approximately 10 times less frequently than new myeloma patients). Among myeloma patients, the incidence of cases giving rise to clinical symptoms is probably less than five per cent although careful post-mortem histological examination may reveal tissue amyloid deposition in a considerably higher percentage. Among macroglobulinaemia and lymphoma patients, amyloid is even less frequently encountered. Interestingly, amyloid may be relatively frequent in the rare γ and μ heavy-chain diseases.

The patterns of sex and age distribution of primary amyloid patients are essentially indistinguishable from those of classical myeloma, with a modest preponderance of males, and a peak frequency around the age of 60.

CLINICAL FEATURES OF IMMUNOCYTE-RELATED AMYLOIDOSIS

The clinical features of amyloid deposition are identical both in primary amyloidosis and in cases of amyloidosis associated with myeloma, macroglobulinaemia or lymphoma. In the latter category of diseases, however, clinical features directly attributable to the immunocytic neoplasm (e.g. skeletal destruction, hyperviscosity) are superimposed on the clinical manifestations of amyloid deposition.

The presenting symptoms and signs encountered in amyloid patients are listed in approximately decreasing order of frequency in Table 19.9 [293], and the

Table 19.9. Clinical features of primary amyloidosis

Symptoms*	Signs*	Syndromes
Fatigue	Hepatomegaly	Carpal-tunnel syndrome
Weight loss	Oedema	Cardiac failure
Dyspnoea	Purpura	Orthostatic hypotension
Paraesthesiae	Macroglossia	Nephrotic syndrome
'Hoarseness'	Splenomegaly	Peripheral neuropathy
	Skin lesions	

* The symptoms and signs are listed in decreasing order of frequency. When amyloidosis occurs in association with myeloma or other lymphoproliferative disorder the clinical features of both diseases will be encountered together.

relation between these clinical features and the sites of amyloid deposition are set out in Figure 19.13.

Many of the signs and symptoms listed in Table 19.9 are non-specific (e.g. there is little to distinguish amyloid-induced autonomic neuropathy from that associated with diabetes, or hepatomegaly due to amyloid from other causes of hepatic enlargement). This fact, together with the relative rarity of primary amyloid and its rapid and fatal clinical course in many patients, accounts for the frequency with which the diagnosis is overlooked in life.

Macroglossia

This is one of the most striking signs encountered in amyloid. The tongue is often irregularly indented, this moulding corresponding to the pattern of missing teeth (Fig. 19.14). Enlargement of submandibular structures by amyloid deposition may exacerbate the degree of macroglossia.

Purpura

This feature is attributable to the deposition of amyloid in cutaneous blood vessels, and tends to show

a predilection for the eyelids, where it can be elicited by pinching the skin. Bilateral periorbital purpura may be produced by vomiting, coughing, the Valsalva manoeuvre, proctoscopy ('PPPP = post-proctoscopic palpebral purpura') [293], and even renal biopsy [295]. An additional, although rare, cause of bleeding in amyloidosis is acquired deficiency of factor X, possibly attributable to absorption of this factor by amyloid deposits [69].

Neurological complications [296]

The three major neurological manifestations of immunocyte-related amyloid are peripheral neuropathy [297] (most frequently presenting as parasthesiae and/or pain, particularly in the legs); carpal-tunnel syndrome; and autonomic dysfunction (which may be the sole initial manifestation of amyloidosis, causing diarrhoea, lack of sweating, orthostatic hypotension, impotence and occasionally faecal or urinary retention or incontinence) [293].

Amyloid arthropathy [298, 299]

This complication clinically resembles rheumatoid arthritis, with symmetrical involvement of a number of joints (most commonly shoulders, followed by knees, wrists, metacarpophalangeal and proximal interphalangeal joints) and rheumatoid-like nodules in the vicinity of involved joints. However, amyloid arthropathy differs from typical rheumatoid disease in that there is no joint inflammation or tenderness, fever is absent, and the age of onset is relatively late. Periarticular swellings around the shoulder joints may be very striking, giving rise to the almost pathognomonic 'shoulder-pad' sign.

Renal failure

Amyloid deposition in renal glomeruli frequently leads to severe nephrotic syndrome. These deposits are usually readily recognized in renal biopsies by virtue of

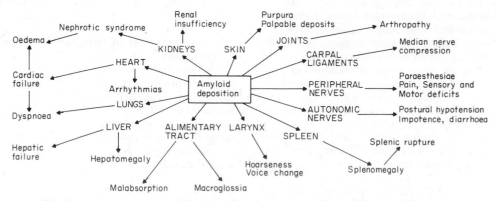

Fig. 19.13. Summary of the clinical manifestations of amyloid deposition in different sites.

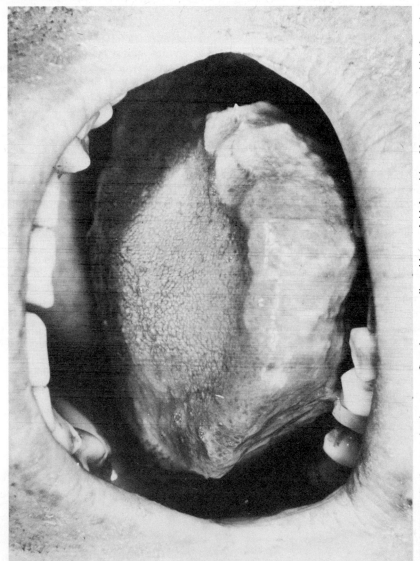

Fig. 19.14. Macroglossia occurring in a case of myeloma complicated by amyloid deposition. Note the way in which the enlarged tongue has moulded itself so as to show a negative impression of the upper and lower teeth.

their characteristic tinctorial and electron microscopic appearances (Fig. 19.15). However, it is noteworthy that a condition which mimics amyloid glomerulo-pathy has recently been recognized [300–302]. In these patients (in whom monoclonal urinary light-chain excretion occurs in the absence of overt evidence of immunocytic neoplasia) the glomerular deposits do not show any ultrastructural resemblance to amyloid. These patients appear to represent a rare form of occult plasma-cell dyscrasia in which (as in primary amyloidosis) monoclonal light chains precipitate in the tissues, but do so without being converted to amyloid.

Congestive cardiac failure

This complication is seen in more than a quarter of patients with immunocyte-related amyloidosis and accounts for the death of one-third of all patients. There is only minimal cardiomegaly to be seen on chest X-ray, electrocardiography reveals low-voltage tracings, conduction disturbances, arrhythmias and patterns that may simulate acute myocardial infarction. Amyloid cardiomyopathy responds poorly to digitalis, which may in some patients induce fatal arrythmias.

Changes in the voice

A minority of patients complain of hoarseness or an alteration in the voice producing a weakened, high-pitched sound. This is so characteristic that it should alert the physician to the possible diagnosis of amyloidosis.

LABORATORY INVESTIGATION

Tissue biopsy

This is an essential step in the diagnosis of amyloidosis. Ideally, a biopsy should be taken from a tissue suspected on clinical grounds of amyloid infiltration, although in some cases this may be impossible or dangerous (e.g. biopsy of heavily infiltrated liver tissue carries a risk of subsequent haemorrhage). Rectal biopsy is commonly resorted to as an alternative: this investigation has a high positivity rate (approximately 80%) provided that an adequate sample, including submucosal tissue, is obtained.

In haematoxylin and eosin-stained sections, amyloid has a characteristic hyaline eosinophilic appearance (Fig. 19.15). Staining with thioflavine-T induces strong fluorescence, but this reaction is not entirely specific and the characteristic apple-green birefringence in polarized light induced by Congo-Red staining should be demonstrated. In a minority of cases in which amyloid deposition is not visible by light microscopy, the characteristic irregularly arranged fibrils will be revealed by electron microscopy (Fig. 19.16).

Given the immunoglobulin origin of amyloid it might be expected that anti-light-chain antisera could be used to identify it in tissue sections. However, although some success with this approach has been reported [303], no routine diagnostic role for this investigation has been established. The tendency of amyloid deposits to bind proteins non-specifically, the

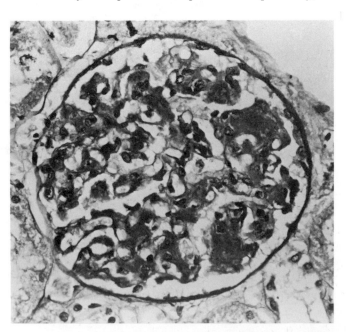

Fig. 19.15. Histological appearance of amyloid in a renal glomerulus, showing the amorphous hyaline nature of the deposits (H & E).

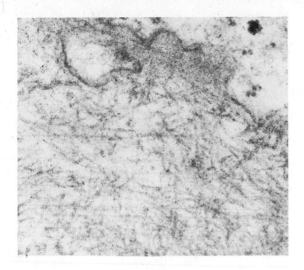

Fig. 19.16. Ultrastructural appearance of amyloid deposits. The irregularly arranged fibrils in the lower part of the figure are typical and may be seen even when light-microscopic examination reveals no abnormality.

fact that conventional anti-light-chain antisera are predominantly directed against constant-region determinants, and the possibility that fibril formation may mask light-chain antigenic determinants probably all account for the difficulties encountered in immuno-histochemical analysis of amyloid.

Haematological investigation

In cases of primary amyloidosis, the blood will show moderate anaemia in a proportion of patients, other values usually being normal. Marrow aspiration commonly reveals a slight increase in plasma cells, which are frequently atypical or immature in morphology. However, assessment of these cytological abnormalities is inevitably—given the low number of plasma cells—very subjective. More tangible evidence for the existence of a monoclonal plasma-cell population may therefore be sought by immunocytochemical staining of smears of washed marrow cells, or of paraffin-embedded marrow particles. These investigations often reveal a relative excess of plasma cells containing one or other light-chain class.

When amyloid is secondary to myeloma or macro-globulinaemia, blood examination and bone-marrow aspiration reveal the abnormalities characteristic of these conditions.

Electrophoretic analysis

A monoclonal paraprotein is frequently found on electrophoretic and immunoelectrophoretic analysis of the serum and urine from primary amyloid patients [294]. Light-chain excretion is relatively more common than in classical myeloma, whilst serum IgG, IgA or IgD paraproteins are found less frequently. The urinary light chains and serum paraproteins in im-

munocyte-related amyloidosis are more frequently of λ than κ class (in contrast to the 2:1 excess of κ paraproteins in cases of myeloma), and urinary light chains from primary amyloid patients tend to show greater mobility towards the anode on electrophoresis [293, 294, 304], most of them running in the β or α_2 regions. This fact, together with the frequent presence of serum proteins escaping into the urine via damaged glomeruli, may hinder the detection of monoclonal urinary light chains in many primary amyloid patients.

Serum immunoglobulins

The levels of normal polyclonal immunoglobulin in cases of primary amyloid are often low, reflecting the immunosuppressive effects of the proliferating immunocyte clone [304].

Biochemical investigations

A variety of biochemical abnormalities may be found in primary amyloidosis, depending upon the organs involved by the disease. Serum alkaline-phosphatase levels are increased in about 50% of patients, reflecting the frequency of liver damage. In these patients other liver function tests will also usually be abnormal. Hypoalbuminaemia is frequently present, a consequence of liver damage and/or nephrotic syndrome. A moderate increase in serum urea and creatinine levels may be encountered, but severe renal insufficiency is uncommon. This reflects the fact that renal damage in primary amyloidosis (unlike that in cases of light-chain-excreting myeloma) primarily affects glomeruli rather than tubules.

In patients in whom amyloid develops in association with multiple myeloma or macroglobulinaemia, the biochemical abnormalities due to amyloid are superimposed upon those attributable to the underlying immunocytic neoplasm.

TREATMENT OF IMMUNOCYTE-RELATED AMYLOIDOSIS

Amyloidosis carries a poor prognosis, cardiac and renal damage accounting for the majority of deaths. The median survival in primary amyloidosis is little more than a year, whilst that of patients suffering from amyloid associated with myeloma is even shorter. Experience of therapeutic measures is relatively limited, as a consequence of the rarity of amyloidosis. In the discussion below only the management of primary amyloidosis is considered, cases of amyloid associated with myeloma or macroglobulinaemia usually being treated as appropriate for those diseases.

Alkylating agents

Realization of the immunocytic nature of primary amyloidosis prompted the use of melphalan and prednisone for its treatment. Occasional cases show striking response to such therapy [305, 306]. In the majority of cases, however, there is little or no improvement in renal function or prolongation of survival [307]. These findings have been confirmed in a double-blind comparison of alkylating therapy with placebo [308].

It may be noted that cases of acute myeloid leukaemia have been reported following the treatment of primary amyloidosis with alkylating agents [309], and that there is some evidence that cytotoxic therapy may enhance rather than suppress amyloid deposition [310].

Renal dialysis and transplantation

A number of cases of primary amyloidosis, complicated by renal failure, have been treated by transplantation [311]. It has been concluded that, although the final outcome is inferior to that in other types of renal disease, this form of treatment may nevertheless be justified in selected patients. Haemodialysis may also be used when renal function fails.

Supportive measures

A variety of palliative measures may be required to treat the different complications of amyloidosis [292]. As noted previously, cardiac damage secondary to amyloid deposition is commonly associated with an increased risk of digitalis-induced arrhythmias. Diuretics must also be used with caution in view of the risks of cardiovascular collapse. Postural hypotension due to autonomic neuropathy may be helped by elastic stockings. Malabsorption may be ameliorated by the administration of broad-spectrum antibiotics. Additional therapeutic measures which may be considered

on occasion include tracheostomy (because of upper-respiratory obstruction due to macroglossia), bronchoscopy and curettage of bronchial amyloid deposits, and splenectomy (for factor-X deficiency).

HEAVY-CHAIN DISEASES

From the preceding accounts of myeloma, macroglobulinaemia and amyloidosis, it will be apparent that neoplastic Ig-secreting cells usually synthesize intact immunoglobulin, immunoglobulin plus light chains or light chains alone. However, in the group of disorders covered by the term 'heavy-chain disease', the neoplastic cells synthesize and secrete immunoglobulin heavy chains but appear in the majority of cases to be incapable of synthesizing light chains [312].

Three types of heavy-chain disease have been recognized, corresponding to the heavy chains present in the three major classes of immunoglobulin (γ, α and μ chains—see Table 19.1). The relative infrequency of IgD-and IgE-secreting cells in normal tissue presumably accounts for the fact that cases of δ and ε heavy-chain disease have yet to be reported.

GAMMA-CHAIN DISEASE [312]

Immunochemical characteristics

In most cases of γ heavy-chain disease the neoplastic cell product consists of two γ heavy chains linked together either covalently or non-covalently. The molecular weight of the individual heavy chains varies from case to case (mean value: 35 000 daltons) but is almost always less than that of normal γ heavy chains. This is accounted for by the presence of an internal deletion in the chain which may, at its most extensive, involve almost all of the variable region, and all of the first domain of the constant region (C_H1). The normal sequence of the chain usually resumes at the beginning of the hinge region (between C_H1 and C_H2), although a few cases in which the hinge region is involved in the deletion have been reported. In the majority of cases, the constant region of the heavy chain appears to be completely intact.

Why internal deletions should be found so frequently in cases of γ heavy-chain disease remains obscure, although it is probable that the way in which these deletions cease just before or after the hinge region and spare the constant region is related to the fact that non-contiguous DNA sequences code for variable and constant regions (see p. 702). As will be discussed below, the cell product in α-chain disease also contains an internal deletion. The inability of the neoplastic cells in γ heavy-chain disease to synthesize a light chain also remains unexplained.

Incidence, age and sex ratio

Gamma heavy-chain disease was first described in 1964 [313], and less than 100 further cases have been described since that time. The age distribution and sex ratio are essentially the same as those of the other paraproteinaemias, with a peak incidence in the 60s and a moderate preponderance of males.

Clinical presentation [312]

The clinical picture resembles that of a lymphoma. Lymphadenopathy, anaemia and fever are the commonest initial manifestations, often accompanied by malaise, weakness and hepatosplenomegaly. Lymphadenopathy tends to become generalized as the disease progresses, and involvement of Waldeyer's ring may lead to respiratory difficulties. Infections are common but erosive bone lesions very rare.

Haematological investigations

Anaemia is always present, often associated with a greater or lesser degree of neutropenia and thrombocytopenia. Eosinophilia is commonly present. Atypical lymphocytes and plasma cells may be found in the circulation and two cases of γ heavy-chain disease progressing to terminal plasma-cell leukaemia have been reported.

Marrow aspiration usually shows an increase in plasma cells and/or lymphocytoid cells, often associated with eosinophilia. However, cases in which marrow samples show no abnormality, or eosinophilia alone, have been reported.

Serum electrophoresis

A monoclonal 'spike' in the γ or β region is almost invariably present on serum electrophoresis, although it is typically rather broad in pattern and its concentration exceeds 20 g/l in only 50% of cases. On immunoelectrophoresis the protein reacts with antisera specific for IgG or γ chains but not with anti-light-chain antisera.

Treatment and prognosis

In view of the rarity of the disease very little information is available on response to treatment. Although survival for periods of more than five years has been reported in several cases, the disease not infrequently pursues an aggressive course leading to death from infection or generalized malignancy within a few months.

ALPHA-CHAIN DISEASE [314]

This disorder has a number of remarkable aspects, including its unique geographical distribution, its localization to the gastro-intestinal tract and, most intriguingly, its tendency to follow a biphasic course in which a period of relatively benign plasma-cell proliferation (responding in some instances to antibiotic therapy alone) is followed in many cases by the development of a frankly malignant lymphoma. Thus the disease (in common with disorders such as immunoblastic lymphadenopathy or Sjögren's syndrome) occupies the ill-defined area between reactive and neoplastic lymphoid proliferation.

Immunochemical features [315]

Alpha-chain disease resembles γ heavy-chain disease in that the cell product is an incomplete heavy chain. The molecular weight varies from case to case but lies in the range 29 000–34 000 daltons, indicating that between a quarter and a half of the chain is missing. Technical reasons (probably related to post-synthetic degradation of α chains causing N-terminal heterogeneity) have prevented analysis of the nature of this deletion by amino-acid sequencing. However, on the basis of antigenic and chemical analyses, it is known that the constant and hinge regions are intact, and that the C-terminal characteristic of normal α chains is present. Consequently, there appears to be an internal deletion, similar to that in γ heavy-chain disease, involving both the variable region and the first constant domain.

Incidence and geographic distribution

The majority of cases of α-chain disease have been diagnosed in patients of Near-Eastern or Mediterranean origin (principally from Tunisia, Algeria, Iran, Spain, Israel, southern Italy and Turkey) [315]. This distribution may partly reflect a genetic predisposition to the disease, probably associated with an Arabic genetic background. However, poor socio-economic conditions in these countries leading to chronic gastrointestinal infection and diarrhoea appears to be an important environmental factor, and it is noteworthy that the first reported series of cases of α heavy-chain disease included a European patient who had lived in Algeria for many years. Cases in the indigenous inhabitants of northern European countries or other Western 'developed' regions are very rare and tend to show a respiratory rather than gastro-intestinal pattern of neoplastic-cell proliferation [315, 316].

Clinical features [317]

Patients usually present with malabsorption syndrome, associated with severe steatorrhoea, abdominal pain, vomiting, marked weight loss and finger clubbing. The disease at this stage, however, may follow an intermittent course in which there are periods of more or less complete remission. Radiological investigation usually shows a malabsorption pattern in the small bowel, with mucosal-fold thickening and barium flocculation. If untreated, rapid deterioration occurs, frequently culminating in the development of one or more localized small-bowel lymphomata which may lead to obstruction, intussusception or perforation. However, even at this stage, spread outside the abdominal cavity is limited.

Laboratory investigations

The two major diagnostic investigations are peroral or open surgical biopsy of the small bowel, and immunochemical analysis of serum and urine samples.

Small bowel biopsy [318]. This investigation reveals diffuse infiltration of the lamina propria of the small bowel with plasmacytoid cells, almost invariably involving all of the duodenum and jejunum as well as extensive regions of more distal small bowel. The infiltrate causes wide separation of the crypts and may spread into the submucosa, but the epithelium and crypts themselves remain intact. Regional lymph nodes may be involved, but large bowel, stomach and non-gastro-intestinal tissues are rarely involved. Immunocytochemical staining reveals α chains unaccompanied by κ or λ chains in the majority of lamina-propria plasmacytoid cells, although infrequent κ- and λ-positive plasma cells (representing residual normal IgA plasma cells) are also seen.

The lymphoma which so frequently supervenes on this pre-malignant phase of the disease is usually a large-cell neoplasm most commonly classified as 'immunoblastic'. There is evidence, based on the identification of α chains in the lymphoma cells, that they represent a mutant clone derived from the α-chain-containing plasma-cell infiltrate [319–321]. It should be noted, however, that immunocytochemical analysis of both the pre-malignant and malignant phases of the disease is hampered by the fact that the cells do not (by definition) contain light chains (which provide a convenient indicator of monoclonality in other types of paraproteinaemia), and that the α chain is incomplete and does not therefore possess idiotypic determinants. Consequently, whilst it is generally considered that the proliferating cells in both phases of the disease are monoclonal in origin, direct immunochemical evidence for this belief is lacking.

Serum and urine electrophoresis. Serum electrophoresis reveals a broad band in the α_2 or β region in approximately 50% of patients; in the remainder no abnormality is detected. Protein migrating with the same mobility may also be found in the urine, but its concentration is usually low.

Immunoelectrophoresis of serum against anti-IgA antisera reveals a long precipitin line due to the α-chain protein, but no reactivity against anti-κ or anti-λ antisera. However, IgA myeloma paraproteins may on occasion be unreactive with commercial anti-light-chain antisera, and specialized techniques such as electrophoretic immunoselection in agar containing antibodies specific for Fabα [322–324], or polyacrylamide gel electrophoresis of the protein after reduction and alkylation, may be required to confirm the presence of free α chains.

Biochemical investigations. A biochemical abnormality which may be of diagnostic value is the presence of an increased serum alkaline-phosphatase level [317]. This finding is present in a proportion of patients and is accounted for by an increase in intestinal isoenzyme.

Treatment

Treatment of the pre-malignant phase of α-chain disease with broad-spectrum antibiotics has resulted in at least temporary regression in a number of patients [317, 325], providing evidence that the infiltrating plasma cells may be 'driven' by antigenic stimulation from bacteria in the small-bowel lumen. In a few patients this treatment has been followed by periods of remission lasting for several years. Cytotoxic therapy with chlorambucil or cyclophosphamide has been used in a few cases. The prognosis once lymphoma has developed is poor, however.

MU-CHAIN DISEASE [326, 327]

Less than 20 cases of μ-chain disease have been diagnosed. Most patients have been over the age of 40 and have either come from parasite-infected areas (e.g. the Ivory Coast) [328, 329], or have had a clinical picture of chronic lymphatic leukaemia or anaplastic lymphoma [330]. Splenic and hepatic enlargement is more marked than lymphadenopathy [329, 330]. A characteristic feature is the presence in the bone marrow of plasma cells containing one to three large cytoplasmic vacuoles [326, 331].

The disease resembles γ- and α-chain disease in that the μ heavy chains may contain deletions [328, 329, 332], but it differs from the former disease in that the neoplastic cells frequently produce light chain in addition to μ chain [326, 330–332]. However, these light chains do not link to the μ chains to produce intact IgM, and are excreted in the urine.

PARAPROTEINAEMIA IN LYMPHOMA AND LEUKAEMIA

As indicated in the introduction to this chapter, most, if not all, types of B lymphoproliferative disease may be associated with the presence of a paraprotein. In cases of chronic lymphocytic leukaemia and diffuse non-Hodgkin lymphoma, the frequency is of the order of six to seven per cent [284, 333]. In nodular lymphoma, however (and in hairy-cell leukaemia), paraproteins are much rarer. A small proportion of cases of lymphoma or leukaemia associated with paraproteinaemia reflect the background frequency of benign paraproteins in the normal population (see below). The majority, however, presumably represent limited terminal differentiation by the neoplastic lymphoid clone to an Ig-secreting stage (Fig. 19.3). Screening for serum paraproteins provides an underestimate of the true frequency of Ig-synthesizing lymphomas, since analysis of lymphoma tissue homogenates or immunohistological labelling of lymphoma tissue sections reveals monoclonal Ig in a much higher proportion of cases [158, 334].

The paraproteins found in cases of chronic lymphocytic leukaemia and diffuse non-Hodgkin lymphomas are of the IgM class in approximately 50% of cases, and the κ/λ ratio (2:1) is similar to that found in myeloma (and in normal serum immunoglobulins). Occasionally anaplastic lymphoid neoplasms synthesize light chains alone.

BENIGN PARAPROTEINAEMIA

This concluding section is concerned with cases of paraproteinaemia in whom no underlying lymphoproliferative disorder is detectable, and in whom the paraprotein level remains constant over a period of time [335]. This type of paraproteinaemia (also referred to as 'essential' or 'asymptomatic' paraproteinaemia) may be found both in healthy subjects (sometimes referred to as 'primary' benign paraproteinaemia), and in hospital patients suffering from non-lymphoproliferative disorders ('secondary' benign paraproteinaemia).

BENIGN PARAPROTEINAEMIA IN HOSPITAL PATIENTS
Benign paraproteins have been detected in patients suffering from a very wide variety of clinical disorders, and in at least some cases the association is fortuitous, reflecting both the frequency with which serum from hospital patients is analysed electrophoretically and also the fact that older individuals (who predominate among hospital patients) have the highest incidence of benign paraproteinaemia (see next section).

However, several types of disease appear to be associated particularly frequently with benign paraproteinaemia, suggesting a causal relationship. These disorders include chronic inflammatory states (particularly affecting the biliary tract), liver disease, connective-tissue disorders and neoplasia (especially of the colon, biliary system and lung) [20, 333, 336]. It

has been suggested that repeated antigenic stimulation of the lymphoreticular system (by either bacterial, viral, neoplasia-associated or autologous antigens) accounts for the emergence of the paraprotein-producing clone in such cases [20, 337]. Indirect evidence for this explanation is provided by the occasional case of 'transient' benign paraproteinaemia in whom the paraprotein disappears spontaneously, presumably when the causative antigenic stimulus is no longer present [338, 339]. It may be noted, however, that the majority of patients responding briskly to antigenic stimulation (as evidenced by polyclonal hyper-γ-globulinaemia) do not develop paraproteins, and furthermore that attempts to demonstrate binding of benign paraproteins to putative stimulating antigens (e.g. Australia antigen) almost always prove fruitless.

Paraproteins found in hospital patients may be of any heavy- or light-chain class, although about 20–25% of benign paraproteins found in cases of liver disease and connective tissue disorders are of the IgM class, contrasting with the relative rarity of this paraprotein among other types of benign paraproteinaemia [333, 340].

BENIGN PARAPROTEINAEMIA IN NORMAL SUBJECTS
As a result of systematic screening studies involving the electrophoretic analysis of many thousands of samples it is known that serum paraproteins are found in 0·1–1·0% of the normal adult population [341–343]. A few of these individuals represent early cases of lymphoproliferative diseases. In most cases, however, there is no change in serum paraprotein over a long period of time and these individuals remain asymptomatic [344, 345].

The frequency of benign paraproteinaemia in healthy subjects rises steeply with advancing age, being of the order of three per cent in subjects over the age of 70 [346, 347].

DIAGNOSIS OF BENIGN PARAPROTEINAEMIA
There is usually no difficulty (following clinical examination and laboratory investigation) in distinguishing between benign paraproteinaemia and a paraprotein associated with lymphoproliferative neoplasia. Occasionally, however, diagnostic difficulty may arise over a myeloma or Waldenström's patient whose paraprotein is detected early in the course of the disease (before the classical diagnostic features have emerged) or in a case of 'indolent' or 'smouldering' myeloma [197, 198]. In these circumstances, the presence of monoclonal urinary light chains is generally considered indicative of a malignant lymphoproliferative disorder [336, 337], although some authors have reported this abnormality in cases of apparently

benign paraproteinaemia (especially when highly concentrated urine samples are tested) [348]. It may be noted in this context that cases of 'benign Bence Jones proteinuria' are occasionally encountered in whom considerable amounts of monoclonal urinary light chains are excreted over a period of time without any evidence of lymphoreticular neoplasia [349].

Two further criteria which are widely (although not universally) accepted as indicative of lymphoproliferative malignancy are the presence of 'immune paresis' (suppression of normal serum immunoglobulin levels) and a serum paraprotein level greater than 20 g/l. With regard to the latter criterion it should be noted that, whilst benign paraproteins rarely exceed this threshold, it is not uncommon for myeloma proteins to be present at levels below this value. This is most frequent in cases of early myeloma, i.e. in just those cases which are most difficult to distinguish on other grounds from benign paraproteinaemia.

When doubt remains over the true diagnosis the most reliable discriminating feature is the behaviour of the patient's paraprotein over a period of time. However, occasional cases of benign paraproteinaemia are encountered who appear to 'transform' after a period of months or years into overt myeloma or Waldenström's macroglobulinaemia. In consequence, even when a constant level of paraprotein has been observed over a period of time the patient should continue to be reviewed at regular intervals.

CLINICAL PHENOMENA ATTRIBUTABLE TO A
BENIGN PARAPROTEIN

Although the plasma-cell clone secreting a benign paraprotein does not give rise directly to symptoms (e.g. due to bone erosion or lymphadenopathy), a variety of clinical phenomena may be encountered which are attributable to the effects of the paraprotein itself. These complications are a consequence either of the antibody activity of the paraprotein or of its physico-chemical characteristics. This distinction is not clear-cut, however, since in some syndromes (e.g. peripheral neuropathy [350] or acquired von Willebrand's syndrome [351]) the evidence for antibody–antigen binding is not conclusive, and the antigen is not identified with certainty. Papular mucinosis (lichen myxoedematosus) is also difficult to categorize [352, 353]. A slowly migrating IgG paraprotein (usually of λ type) is almost always present, without evidence of plasma-cell proliferation, but the reason for this association remains obscure. It has not been possible to demonstrate idiotypic cross-reactivity between the paraproteins from different cases of papular mucinosis [354] (in contrast to the idiotypic relatedness of IgM paraproteins in Waldenström's patients suffering from polyneuropathy [12]).

The antibody activity of paraproteins and their clinical consequences have been considered in the introduction to this chapter (Table 19.3). It may be noted, however, that in some syndromes, most notably cold-haemagglutinin disease due to the reactivity of the paraprotein against red cells, the clinical consequences may become manifest when the paraprotein is present at very low levels. In consequence the paraprotein may not be visible on serum electrophoresis and evidence for its monoclonality may only be obtained by immunochemical typing with specific anti-Ig heavy- and light-chain antisera. Furthermore, cases of apparently benign IgM paraproteinaemia causing chronic cold-haemagglutinin syndrome may subsequently develop overt Waldenström's macroglobulinaemia. In most cases this probably reflects the early stage at which the underlying neoplastic process was first detected, rather than the transformation of a truly benign paraproteinaemia into a progressive lymphoproliferative condition.

The syndrome most clearly attributable to the physico-chemical characteristics of a benign paraprotein is cryoglobulinaemia [8]. The paraprotein is usually IgG in class, and precipitates in the cold without interacting with other immunoglobulin (in contrast to mixed cryoglobulins due to paraproteins with anti-IgG activity). In practice, however, clinically significant cryoglobulinaemia due to a benign paraprotein is rare (presumably because of the low serum concentration of most benign paraproteins); most paraproteinaemia patients with symptomatic cryoglobulinaemia suffer from myeloma or Waldenström's macroglobulinaemia.

Primary amyloidosis (and the rare plasma-cell dyscrasia in which monoclonal light chains form non-amyloid deposits in the tissues) [300–302] should logically be included in the list of conditions due to the physico-chemical properties of a benign paraprotein. However, presumably because of the poor prognosis of primary amyloidosis (and its overlap with myeloma-associated amyloidosis), the disease is not normally classified as a benign paraproteinaemia.

REFERENCES

1 SELIGMANN M. & BROUET J.-C. (1973) Antibody activity of human myeloma globulins. *Seminars in Hematology*, **10,** 163.

2 MICOUIN C., RIVAT C., BENSA J.C., STOEBNER P., FAVRE M. & HUDRY E. (1977) A human immunoglobulin in a myeloma patient with anti-gastric parietal cell auto-antigen activity. *Clinical and Experimental Immunology*, **27,** 78.

3 TOH B.H., CEREDIG R., CORNELL F.N. & CLARKE F.M. (1977) Multiple myeloma and monoclonal IgA with

anti-actin reactivity. *Clinical and Experimental Immunology*, **30**, 379.

4 VIDEBÆK A., MANSA B. & KJEMS E. (1973) A human IgA myeloma protein with anti-streptococcal hyaluronidase (ASH) activity. *Scandinavian Journal of Haematology*, **10**, 181.

5 SWIERCZYNSKA Z., WOZNISCZKO-ORLOWSKA G. & MALDYK H. (1976) An IgD myeloma protein with anti-streptolysin O activity. *Immunochemistry*, **13**, 379.

6 KALLIOMÄKI J.L., GRANFORS K. & TIOVANEN A. (1978) An immunoglobulin G myeloma with antistreptolysin activity and a lifelong history of cutaneous streptococcal infection. *Clinical Immunology and Immunopathology*, **9**, 22.

7 CUNLIFFE D.A. & COX K.D. (1980) IgM autoantibodies against isologous erythroctyes also react with isologous IgG (Fc). *Nature (London)*, **286**, 720.

8 BROUET J.-C., CLAUVEL J.-P., DANON F., KLEIN M. & SELIGMANN M. (1974) Biological and clinical significance of cryoglobulins. *American Journal of Medicine*, **57**, 775.

9 FARHANGI M. & OSSERMAN E.F. (1976) Myeloma with xanthoderma due to an IgG λ monoclonal antiflavin antibody. *New England Journal of Medicine*, **294**, 177.

10 BAKER B.L. & HULTQUIST D.E. (1978) A copper-binding immunoglobulin from a myeloma patient. *Journal of Biological Chemistry*, **253**, 8444.

11 LEWIS R.A., FALLS H.F. & TROYER D.O. (1975) Ocular manifestations of hypercupranemia associated with multiple myeloma. *Archives of Ophthalmology*, **93**, 1050.

12 DELLAGI K., BROUET J.-C. & DANON F. (1979) Cross-idiotypic antigens among monoclonal immunoglobulin M from patients with Waldenström's macroglobulinaemia and polyneuropathy. *Journal of Clinical Investigation*, **64**, 1530.

13 SWASH M., PERRIN J. & SCHWARTZ M.S. (1979) Significance of immunoglobulin deposition in peripheral nerves in neuropathies associated with paraproteinaemia. *Journal of Neurology, Neurosurgery and Psychiatry*, **42**, 179.

14 HAMBERGER A. & SALMON S.E. (1977) Primary bioassay of human myeloma stem cells. *Journal of Clinical Investigation*, **60**, 846.

15 MELLSTEDT H., KILLANDER D. & PETTERSSON N.D. (1977) Bone marrow kinetic studies on three patients with myelomatosis. *Acta Medica Scandinavica*, **202**, 413.

16 KYLE R.A., FINKELSTEIN S., ELVEBACK L.R. & KURLAND L.T. (1972) Incidence of monoclonal proteins in a Minnesota community with a cluster of multiple myeloma. *Blood*, **40**, 719.

17 GUNZ F.W., GUNZ J.P. & LEIGH J. (1978) Contacts among patients with haematological malignancies. *Cancer*, **41**, 2379.

18 ISHIMARU T. & FINCH S.C. (1979) More on radiation exposure and multiple myeloma. *New England Journal of Medicine*, **301**, 439.

19 PENNY R. & HUGHES S. (1970) Repeated stimulation of the reticuloendothelial system and the development of plasma cell dyscrasias. *Lancet*, **i**, 77.

20 ISOBE T. & OSSERMAN E.F. (1971) Pathologic conditions associated with plasma cell dyscrazias. *Annals of the New York Academy of Sciences*, **190**, 507.

21 SCHAFER A.I. & MILLER J.B. (1979) Association of IgA multiple myeloma with pre-existing disease. *British Journal of Haematology*, **41**, 19.

22 PILLOT J., CREAU-GOLDBERG N. & GONZALES Y. (1976) Lack of antibody activity directed against the most common human bacteria in human myeloma protein. *Journal of Immunology*, **117**, 2042.

23 MEIJERS K.A.E., DE LEEUW B. & VOORMOLEN-KALOVA M. (1972) The multiple occurrence of myeloma and asymptomatic paraproteinaemia within one family. *Clinical and Experimental Immunology*, **12**, 185.

24 MALDONADO J.E. & KYLE R.A. (1974) Familial myeloma. *American Journal of Medicine*, **59**, 875.

25 ZAWADZKI Z.A., AIZAWA Y., KRAJ M.A., HARADIN A.R. & FISHER B. (1977) Familial immunopathies. *Cancer*, **40**, 2094.

26 FESTEN J.J.M., MARRINK J., DE WAARD-KUIPER E.H. & MANDEMA E. (1977) Immunoglobulins in families of myeloma patients. *Scandinavian Journal of Immunology*, **6**, 887.

27 MASON D.Y. & CULLEN P.R. (1975) HL-A antigen frequencies in myeloma. *Tissue Antigens*, **5**, 238.

28 SMITH G., WALFORD R.L., RISHKIN B., CARTER P.K. & TANAKA K. (1974) HLA phenotypes, immunoglobulins and K and L chains in multiple myeloma. *Tissue Antigens*, **4**, 374.

29 MELLSTEDT H., HAMMARSTRÖM S. & HOLM G. (1974) Monoclonal lymphocyte population in human plasma cell myeloma. *Clinical and Experimental Immunology*, **17**, 371.

30 KUBAGAWA H., VOGLER L.B., CAPRA J.D., CONRAD M.E., LAWTON A.R. & COOPER M.D. (1979) Studies on the clonal origin of myeloma. *Journal of Experimental Medicine*, **150**, 792.

31 BIBERFELD P., MELLSTEDT H. & PETTERSSON D. (1977) Ultrastructural and immunocytochemical characterisation of circulating mononuclear cells in patients with myelomatosis. *Acta Pathologica et Microbiologica Scandinavica (A)*, **85**, 611.

32 PREUD'HOMME J.-L., LABAUME S. & SELIGMANN M. (1977) Idiotype-bearing and antigen binding receptors produced by blood T-lymphocytes in a case of human myeloma. *European Journal of Immunology*, **7**, 840.

33 RIVER G.L., TEWKSBURY D.A. & FUDENBERG H.H. (1972) 'Non-secretory' multiple myeloma. *Blood*, **40**, 204.

34 TURESSON I. & GRUBB A. (1978) Non-secretory or low-secretory myeloma with intracellular kappa chains. *Acta Medica Scandinavica*, **204**, 445.

35 PREUD'HOMME J.-L., HUREZ D., DANON F., BROUET J.-C. & SELIGMANN M. (1976) Intracytoplasmic and surface-bound immunoglobulins in 'nonsecretory' and Bence Jones myeloma. *Clinical and Experimental Immunology*, **25**, 428.

36 MANCILLA R. & DAVIS G.L. (1977) Non-secretory multiple myeloma. *American Journal of Medicine*, **63**, 1015.

37 FAIR D.S. & KRUEGER R.G. (1979) Analysis of biclonal immunoglobulins and their contributions to understanding the developmental aspects of the antibody response. *Contemporary Topics in Molecular Immunology*, **7**, 51.

38 VAN CAMP B.G.K., SHUIT H.R.E., HIJMANS W. & RADL

J. (1977) The cellular basis of double paraproteinaemia in man. *Clinical Immunology and Immunopathology*, **9**, 111.

39 SELIGMANN M., MIHAESCO E., CHEVALIER A. & MIGLIERINA R. (1978) Immunochemical study of a human myeloma IgG1 half molecule. *Annales d'Immunologie*, **129C**, 855.

40 SPIEGELBERG H.L. (1975) Human myeloma IgG half-molecules. Catabolism and biological properties. *Journal of Clinical Investigation*, **56**, 588.

41 SPIEGELBERG H.L. & FISHKIN B.G. (1976) Human myeloma IgA half-molecules. *Journal of Clinical Investigation*, **58**, 1259.

42 SAKURABAYASHI I., KIN K. & TADASHI K. (1979) Human IgA₁ half-molecules: clinical and immunological features in a patient with multiple myeloma. *Blood*, **53**, 269.

43 HOBBS J.R. & JACOBS A. (1969) A half molecule GK plasmacytoma. *Clinical and Experimental Immunology*, **5**, 199.

44 HOBBS J.R. (1975) Monitoring myelomatosis. *Archives of Internal Medicine*, **135**, 125.

45 HOBBS J.R. (1969) Growth rates and responses to treatment in human myelomatosis. *British Journal of Haematology*, **16**, 607.

46 SALMON S.E. (1973) Immunoglobulin synthesis and tumor kinetics of multiple myeloma. *Seminars in Hematology*, **10**, 135.

47 SALMON S.E. & DURIE B.G.M. (1975) Cellular kinetics in multiple myeloma. *Archives of Internal Medicine*, **135**, 131.

48 SALMON S.E. (1975) Expansion of the growth fraction in multiple myeloma with alkylating agents. *Blood*, **45**, 119.

49 HOBBS J.R. & CORBETT A.A. (1969) Younger age of presentation and extraosseous tumours in IgD myelomatosis. *British Medical Journal*, **i**, 412.

50 JANCELEWITZ Z., TAKATSUKI K. & SUGAI S. (1975) IgD multiple myeloma. Review of 133 cases. *Archives of Internal Medicine*, **135**, 87.

51 KYLE R.A. (1975) Multiple myeloma: review of 869 cases. *Mayo Clinic Proceedings*, **50**, 29.

52 ACUTE LEUKAEMIA GROUP B (1975) Correlation of abnormal immunoglobulins with clinical features of myeloma. *Archives of Internal Medicine*, **135**, 46.

53 GALTON D.A.G. & PETO R. (1973) Report on the First Myelomatosis Trial. *British Journal of Haematology*, **24**, 123.

54 MUNDY G.R., RAISZ L.G., COOPER R.A., SCHECHTER G.P. & SALMON S.E. (1974) Evidence for the secretion of an osteoclast stimulating factor in myeloma. *New England Journal of Medicine*, **291**, 1041.

55 CHARKES N.D., DURANT J. & BARRY W.E. (1972) Bone pain in multiple myeloma. Studies with radioactive 87mSr. *Archives of Internal Medicine*, **130**, 53.

56 TUDDENHAM E.G.D. & BRADLEY J. (1974) Plasma volume expansion and increased serum viscosity in myeloma and macroglobulinaemia. *Clinical and Experimental Immunology*, **16**, 169.

57 ALEXANIAN R. (1977) Blood volume in monoclonal gammopathy. *Blood*, **49**, 301.

58 COHEN H.J. & RUNDLES R.W. (1975) Managing the complications of multiple myeloma. *Archives of Internal Medicine*, **135**, 177.

59 MEYERS B.R., HIRSCHMAN S.Z. & AXELROD J.A. (1972) Current patterns of infection in multiple myeloma. *American Journal of Medicine*, **52**, 87.

60 TWOMEY J.J. (1973) Infection complicating multiple myeloma and chronic lymphatic leukaemia. *Archives of Internal Medicine*, **132**, 562.

61 FATEH-MOGHADAM A., LAMERZ R., KNEDEL M. & BAUER B. (1973) Quantitative immunologische Bestimmung von Serumproteinen bei Paraproteinämien. *Deutsche Medizinische Wochenschrift*, **98**, 309.

62 KOLB J.-P., ARRIAN S. & ZOLLA-PAZNER D. (1977) Suppression of the humoral immune response by plasmacytomas: mediation by adherent mononuclear cells. *Journal of Immunology*, **118**, 702.

63 KRAKAUER R.S., STROBER W. & WALDMANN T. (1977) Hypogammaglobulinemia in experimental myeloma: the role of suppressor factors from mononuclear phagocytes. *Journal of Immunology*, **118**, 1385.

64 PAGLIERONI T. & MACKENZIE M.R. (1977) Studies on the pathogenesis of an immune defect in multiple myeloma. *Journal of Clinical Investigation*, **59**, 1120.

65 BRODER S., HUMPHREY R., DURM M., BLACKMAN M., MEADE B., GOLDMAN C., STROBER W. & WALDMANN T. (1975) Impaired synthesis of polyclonal (non-paraprotein) immunoglobulins by circulating lymphocytes from patients with multiple myeloma. *New England Journal of Medicine*, **293**, 887.

66 VAN EPPS D.E., REED K. & WILLIAMS R.C. (1978) Suppression of human PMN bactericidal activity by human IgA paraproteins. *Cellular Immunology*, **36**, 363.

67 SPITLER L.E., SPATH P., PETZ L., COOPER N. & FUDENBERG H.H. (1975) Phagocytes and C4 in paraproteinaemia. *British Journal of Haematology*, **29**, 279.

68 MACGREGOR R.R., NEGENDANK W.G. & SCHREIBER A.D. (1978) Impaired granulocyte adherence in multiple myeloma: relationship to complement system, granulocyte delivery and infection. *Blood*, **51**, 591.

69 LACKNER H. (1973) Hemostatic abnormalities associated with dysproteinemia. *Seminars in Hematology*, **10**, 125.

70 PERKINS H.A., MACKENZIE M.R. & FUDENBERG H.H. (1970) Hemostatic defects in dysproteinemias. *Blood*, **35**, 695.

71 CATOVSKY D., IKOKU N.B., PITNEY W.R. & GALTON D.A.G. (1970) Thromboembolic complications in myelomatosis. *British Medical Journal*, **iii**, 438.

72 MONTA L.E. & RAMANAN S.V. (1975) Recurrent pulmonary embolism. A sign of multiple myeloma. *Journal of the American Medical Association*, **233**, 1192.

73 PRESTON F.E. & WARD A.M. (1972) Acute renal failure in myelomatosis from intravascular coagulation. *British Medical Journal*, **i**, 604.

74 PRESTON F.E., COOKE K.B., FOSTER M.E., WINFIELD D.A. & LEE D. (1978) Myelomatosis and the hyperviscosity syndrome. *British Journal of Haematology*, **38**, 517.

75 BLOCH K.J. & MAKI D.K. (1973) Hyperviscosity syndrome associated with immunoglobulin abnormalities. *Seminars in Hematology*, **10**, 113.

76 LINDSLEY H., TELLER D., NOONAN B., PETERSON M. & MANNIK M. (1973) Hyperviscosity syndrome in multiple myeloma. *American Journal of Medicine*, **54**, 682.

77 CAPRA J.D. & KUNKEL H.G. (1970) Aggregation of gamma-G3 proteins: relevance to the hyperviscosity syndrome. *Journal of Clinical Investigation*, **46**, 610.

78 BENNINGER G.W. & KREPS S.I. (1971) Aggregation phenomenon in an IgG multiple myeloma resulting in the hyperviscosity syndrome. *American Journal of Medicine*, **51**, 287.

79 MACKENZIE M.R., FUDENBERG H.H. & O'REILLY R.A. (1970) The hyperviscosity syndrome in IgG myeloma. The role of protein concentration and molecular shape. *Journal of Clinical Investigation*, **49**, 15.

80 WHITTAKER J.A., TUDDENHAM E.G.D. & BRADLEY J. (1973) Hyperviscosity syndrome in IgA multiple myeloma. *Lancet*, **ii**, 572.

81 VIRELLA G., PRETO R.V. & GRACA F. (1975) Polymerised monoclonal IgA in two patients with myelomatosis and hyperviscosity syndrome. *British Journal of Haematology*, **30**, 479.

82 ROBERTS-THOMPSON P., MASON D.Y. & MACLENNAN I.C.M. (1976) Paraprotein polymerisation in IgA myelomatosis. *British Journal of Haematology*, **33**, 117.

83 TUDDENHAM E.G.C., WHITTAKER J.A., BRADLEY J., LILLEYMAN, J.S. & JAMES D.R. (1974) Hyperviscosity syndrome in IgA multiple myeloma. *British Journal of Haematology*, **27**, 65.

84 MESTECKY J., HAMMACK, W.J., KULHAVY R., WRIGHT G.P. & TOMANA M. (1977) Properties of IgA myeloma proteins isolated from sera of patients with hyperviscosity syndrome. *Journal of Laboratory and Clinical Medicine*, **89**, 919.

85 COHEN A.H. & BORDER W.A. (1980) Myeloma kidney. *Laboratory Investigation*, **42**, 248.

86 ZLOTNIK A. & ROSENMANN E. (1975) Renal pathological findings associated with monoclonal gammopathies. *Archives of Internal Medicine*, **135**, 40.

87 DUNNILL M.J. (1976) The kidney in multiple myelomatosis and cryoglobulinaemia. In: *Pathological Basis of Renal Disease*, p. 277. W. B. Saunders, London.

88 SØLLING K. & ASKJAER S.A. (1973) Multiple myeloma with urinary excretion of heavy chain components of IgG and nodular glomerulosclerosis. *Acta Medica Scandinavica*, **194**, 23.

89 SILVA F.G., MEYRIER A., MOREL-MAROGER L. & PIRANI C.L. (1980) Proliferative glomerulonephropathy in multiple myeloma. *Journal of Pathology*, **130**, 229.

90 DHAR S.K., SMITH E.C. & FRESCO R. (1977) Proliferative glomerulonephritis in monoclonal gammopathy. *Nephron*, **19**, 288.

91 TANGE T., KURUMADO K., NAKAZAWA M., IMAMURA Y., KOSAKA K. & KAWAOI A. (1978) Glomerular lesions in multiple myeloma. *Acta Pathologica Japonica*, **28**, 325.

92 KJELDSBERG C.R. & HOLMAN B.E. (1971) Acute renal failure in multiple myeloma. *Journal of Urology*, **105**, 21.

93 KRULL P., KÜHN K., ZOBL H. & STERZEL R.B. (1973) Akutes Nierenversagen bei Bence Jones-plasmozytom. *Deutsche Medizinische Wochenschrift*, **98**, 318.

94 SCHUBERT G.E., VEIGEL J. & LENNERT K. (1972) Structure and function of the kidney in multiple myeloma. *Virchow's Archiv. A: Pathological Anatomy*, **355**, 135.

95 DEFRONZO R.A., HUMPHREY R.L., WRIGHT J.R. & COOKE C.R. (1975) Acute renal failure in myeloma. *Medicine*, **54**, 209.

96 BOOTH L.J., MINIELLY J.A. & SMITH E.K.M. (1974) Acute renal failure in multiple myeloma. *Canadian Medical Association Journal*, **111**, 335.

97 LEE D.B.N., DRINKARD J.P., ROSEN V.J. & CONICK H.C. (1972) The adult Fanconi syndrome. *Medicine*, **51**, 107.

98 VON SCHEELE C. (1976) Light chain myeloma with features of the adult Fanconi syndrome: six years remission following one course of melphalan. *Acta Medica Scandinavica*, **199**, 533.

99 BEEVERS D.G. (1972) Cutaneous lesions in multiple myeloma. *British Medical Journal*, **iv**, 275.

100 EDWARDS G.H. & ZAWADSKI Z.A. (1967) Extraosseous lesions in plasma cell myeloma. *American Journal of Medicine*, **43**, 194.

101 OBERKIRCHER P.E., MILLER W.T. & ARGER P.H. (1972) Non-osseous presentation of plasma cell myeloma. *Radiology*, **104**, 515.

102 GOMEZ E.C., MARGUILIES M., RYWLIN A., CABELLO B. & DOMINGUEZ C. (1978) Cutaneous involvement in IgD myeloma. *Archives of Dermatology*, **114**, 1700.

103 GONDOS B., MILLER T.R. & KING E.B. (1978) Cytologic diagnosis of multiple myeloma and macroglobulinemia. *Annals of Clinical and Laboratory Science*, **8**, 11.

104 SHOENFELD Y., PICK A.I., WEINBERGER A., BEN-BESSAT M. & PINKHAS J. (1978) Pleural effusion—presenting sign in multiple myeloma. *Respiration*, **36**, 160.

105 KAPADIA S.B. (1977) Cytological diagnosis of malignant pleural effusion in myeloma. *Archives of Pathology and Laboratory Medicine*, **101**, 534.

106 BADRINAS F., RODRÍGUEZ-ROISIN R., RIVES A. & PICADO C. (1974) Multiple myeloma with pleural involvement. *American Review of Respiratory Diseases*, **110**, 82.

107 KINTZER J.S., ROSENOW E.C. & KYLE R.A. (1978) Thoracic and pulmonary abnormalities in multiple myeloma. *Archives of Internal Medicine*, **138**, 727.

108 BJÖRKHOLM M., HOLM G., MELLSTEDT H. & SJÖGREN A. (1976) Extensive nodular infiltration of extra-osseous tissues in human myelomatosis. *Acta Medica Scandinavica*, **200**, 139.

109 SIMON T.L., RUGHANI I.K., PIERSON D.J. & HEBARD D.W. (1978) Multiple plasmacytomas with thoracic and biliary involvement. *Archives of Internal Medicine*, **138**, 1165.

110 ALBERTS D.S. & LYNCH P. (1978) Cutaneous plasmacytomas in myeloma. *Archives of Dermatology*, **114**, 1784.

111 HOLT J.M. & ROBB-SMITH A.H.T. (1973) Multiple myeloma: development of plasma cell sarcoma during apparently successful chemotherapy. *Journal of Clinical Pathology*, **26**, 649.

112 PASMANTIER N.W. & AZAR H.A. (1969) Extraskeletal spread in multiple myeloma. *Cancer*, **23**, 167.

113 WILTSHAW E. (1976) The natural history of extramedullary plasmacytoma and its relation to solitary myeloma of bone and myelomatosis. *Medicine*, **55**, 217.

114 CONKLIN R. & ALEXANIAN R. (1975) Clinical classification of plasma cell myeloma. *Archives of Internal Medicine*, **135**, 139.

115 ALEXANIAN R. (1980) Localised and indolent myeloma. *Blood*, **56**, 521.

116 MEYER J.E. & SCHULTZ M.D. (1974) 'Solitary' myeloma of bone. A review of 12 cases. *Cancer*, **34**, 438.

117 PANKOVICH A.M. & GRIEM M.C. (1972) Plasma cell myeloma. A thirty year follow up. *Radiology*, **104**, 521.

118 TAYLOR J.S., LEWIS L.A., BATTLE J.D., BUTKUS A., ROBERTSON A.L., DEODHAR S. & ROENIGK H.H. (1978) Plane xanthoma and multiple myeloma with lipoprotein–paraprotein complexing. *Archives of Dermatology*, **114**, 425.

119 WILSON D.E., FLOWERS C.M., HERSHGOLD E.J. & EATON R.P. (1975) Multiple myeloma, cryoglobulinemia and xanthomatosis. *American Journal of Medicine*, **59**, 721.

120 MARIEN K.J.C. & SMEENK G. (1975) Plane xanthomata associated with multiple myeloma and hyperlipoproteinaemia. *British Journal of Dermatology*, **93**, 407.

121 ROBERTS-THOMPSON P.J., VENABLES G.S., ONITIRI A.C. & LEWIS B. (1975) Polymeric IgA myeloma hyperlipidaemia and xanthomatosis: a further case and review. *Postgraduate Medical Journal*, **51**, 44.

122 RODRIGUEZ J.M., LAM S. & SILBER R. (1977) Multiple myeloma with cutaneous involvement. *Journal of the American Medical Association*, **237**, 2625.

123 SCOTT M.A., KAUH Y.C. & LUSCOMBE H.A. (1976) Acquired cutis laxa associated with multiple myeloma. *Archives of Dermatology*, **112**, 853.

124 BEUTLER S.M. FRETZIN D.F., JAO W. & DESSER R. (1978) Xanthomatosis resembling sclerodema in multiple myeloma. *Archives of Pathology and Laboratory Medicine*, **102**, 567.

125 ERSKINE J.G., ROWAN R.M., ALEXANDER J.O'D. & SEKONI G.A. (1977) Pruritus as a presentation of myelomatosis. *British Medical Journal*, **i**, 687.

126 CREAM J.J., GRIMES S.M. & ROBERTS P.D. (1977) Subcorneal pustulosis and IgA myelomatosis. *British Medical Journal*, **i**, 550.

127 MÖLLER H., WALDENSTRÖM J.G. & ZETTERVALL O. (1978) Pyoderma gangraenosum (dermatitis ulcerosa) and monoclonal (IgA) globulin healed after melphalan treatment. *Acta Medica Scandinavica*, **203**, 293.

128 KROOK G. & WALDENSTRÖM J.G. (1978) Relapsing annular erythema and myeloma successfully treated with cyclophosphamide. *Acta Medica Scandinavica*, **203**, 289.

129 ARCHIMANDRITIS A.J., FERTAKIS A., ALEGAKIS G., BARTSOKAS S. & MELISSINOS K. (1977) Erythema elevatum diutinum and IgA myeloma: an interesting association. *British Medical Journal*, **ii**, 613.

130 BATAILLE R., ROSENBERG F., SANY J., SERR H., MEYNADIER J., GUILHOU J.J., BALDET P. & BARNEON G. (1978) Association d'une mucinose papuleuse et d'un myélome multiple IgG lambda. *Semaines des Hôpitaux de Paris*, **54**, 865.

131 JABLONSKA S. & STACHOW A. (1972) Scleroderma-like lesions in multiple myeloma. *Dermatologica*, **144**, 257.

132 RODRIGUES A.R., LUTCHER C.L. & COLEMAN F.W. (1976) Osteosclerotic myeloma. *Journal of the American Medical Association*, **236**, 1872.

133 WALDENSTRÖM J.G., ADNER A., GYDELL K. & ZETTERVALL O. (1978) Osteosclerotic 'plasmacytoma' with polyneuropathy, hypertrichosis and diabetes. *Acta Medica Scandinavica*, **203**, 297.

134 ROUSSEAU J.J., FRANCK G., GRISAR T., REZNIK M.,

HEYNEN G. & SALMON J. (1978) Osteosclerotic myeloma with polyneuropathy and ectopic secretion of calcitonin. *European Journal of Cancer*, **14**, 133.

135 ZIMELMAN A.P. (1973) Thrombocytosis in multiple myeloma. *Annals of Internal Medicine*, **78**, 970.

136 SELROOS O. & VAN ASSENDELFT A. (1977) Thrombocythaemia and multiple myeloma. *Acta Medica Scandinavica*, **201**, 243.

137 HALL P.C. & IBBOTSON R.M. (1974) The influence of paraproteinaemia on the Technicon automated platelet counter. *Journal of Clinical Pathology*, **27**, 583.

138 HAENEY M.R. (1976) Erroneous values for the total white cell count and ESR in patients with cryoglobulinaemia. *Journal of Clinical Pathology*, **29**, 894.

139 SHAW M.T., TWELE T.W. & NORDQUIST R.E. (1974) Plasma cell leukemia: detailed studies and response to therapy. *Cancer*, **33**, 619.

140 WOODRUFF F.R., MALPAS J.S., PAXTON A.M. & LISTER T.A. (1978) Plasma cell leukemia (PCL): a report on 15 patients. *Blood*, **52**, 839.

141 KYLE R.A., MALDONADO J.E. & BAYRD E.D. (1974) Plasma cell leukemia: report of 17 cases. *Archives of Internal Medicine*, **133**, 813.

142 PRUZANSKI W., PLATTS M.E. & OGRYZLO M.A. (1969) Leukemic form of immunocytic dyscrasia (plasma cell leukemia). A study of 10 cases and a review of the literature. *American Journal of Medicine*, **47**, 60.

143 PHADKE K.P., KWAN Y.L. & YOUNG S.G. (1978) Sideroblastic anaemia and leukaemia in multiple myeloma. *Australia and New Zealand Journal of Medicine*, **8**, 539.

144 BERNIER G.M. & GRAHAM R.C. (1976) Plasma cell asynchrony in myeloma: correlation of light and electron microscopy. *Seminars in Hematology*, **13**, 239.

145 HAYHOE F.G.J. & NEUMAN Z. (1976) Cytology of myeloma cells. *Journal of Clinical Pathology*, **29**, 916.

146 STAVEM P., HOVIG T., FRØLAND S. & SKREDE S. (1974) Immunoglobulin-containing inclusions in plasma cells in a case of IgG myeloma. *Scandinavian Journal of Haematology*, **13**, 266.

147 BLOM J., MANSA B. & WIIK A. (1976) Study of Russell bodies in human monoclonal plasma cells by means of immunofluorescence and electron microscopy. *Acta Pathologica et Microbiologica Scandinavica (A)*, **84**, 335.

148 BERNIER G.M., DEL DUCA V., BRERETON R. & GRAHAM R.C. (1975) Multiple myeloma with intramedullary masses of M-component. *Blood*, **46**, 931.

149 BRUNNING R.D. & PARKIN B.A. (1976) Intranuclear inclusions in plasma cells and lymphocytes from patients with monoclonal gammopathies. *American Journal of Pathology*, **66**, 10.

150 COHEN H.J. & LEFER L.G. (1975) Intranuclear inclusions in Bence-Jones lambda plasma cell myeloma. *Blood*, **45**, 131.

151 DJALDETTI M. & LEWINSKI U.H. (1978) Origin of intranuclear inclusions in myeloma cells. *Scandinavian Journal of Haematology*, **20**, 200.

152 CANALE D.D. & COLLINS R.D. (1974) Use of bone marrow particle sections in the diagnosis of multiple myeloma. *American Journal of Clinical Pathology*, **61**, 382.

153 CASSUTO J.P., HAMMOU J.C., PASTORELLI E., DUJARDIN

P. & MASSEYEFF R. (1977) Plasma cell acid phosphatase, a discriminative test for benign and malignant monoclonal gammopathies. *Biomedicine*, **27**, 197.

154 BATAILLE R., DURIE B.G.M., SANY J. & SALMON S.E. (1980) Myeloma bone marrow acid phosphatase staining: a correlative study of 38 patients. *Blood*, **55**, 802.

155 TAYLOR C.R. & MASON D.Y. (1974) The immunohistological detection of intracellular immunoglobulins in formalin paraffin sections from multiple myeloma and related conditions using the immunoperoxidase technique. *Clinical and Experimental Immunology*, **18**, 417.

156 PINKUS G.S. & SAID J.W. (1977) Specific identification of intracellular immunoglobulin in paraffin sections of multiple myeloma and macroglobulinemia using an immunoperoxidase technique. *American Journal of Pathology*, **87**, 47.

157 KNOWLES D.M., HALPER J.A., TROKEL S. & JAKOBIEC F.A. (1978) Immunofluorescent and immunoperoxidase characteristics of IgD λ myeloma involving the orbit. *American Journal of Ophthalmology*, **85**, 485.

158 MASON D.Y., BELL J.I., CHRISTENSSON B. & BIBERFELD P. (1980) An immunohistological study of human lymphoma. *Clinical and Experimental Immunology*, **40**, 235.

159 WURSTER-HILL D.H., MCINTYRE O.R. & CORNWELL G.G. (1978) Chromosome studies in myelomatosis. *Virchow's Archiv. B: Cellular Pathology*, **29**, 93.

160 LIANG W., HOPPER J.E. & ROWLEY J.D. (1979) Karyotypic abnormalities and clinical aspects of patients with multiple myeloma and related paraproteinemic disorders. *Cancer*, **44**, 630.

161 ZWAAN F.E., DEN OTTOLANDER G.J., BREDEROO P., VAN ZEWT TH.L., TE VELDE J. & WILLEMZE R. (1976) The morphology of dyserythropoiesis in a patient with acute erythroleukaemia associated with multiple myeloma. *Scandinavian Journal of Haematology*, **17**, 353.

162 DAHLKE M.B. & NOWELL P.C. (1975) Chromosomal abnormalities and dyserythropoiesis in the preleukaemic phase of multiple myeloma. *British Journal of Haematology*, **31**, 111.

163 KHALEELI M., KEANE W.M. & LEE G.R. (1973) Sideroblastic anemia in multiple myeloma—a preleukemic change. *Blood*, **41**, 17.

164 RENOUX M., BERNARD J.F., BEZEAU A., AMAR M. & BOIVIN P. (1978) Myelome multiple et leucémie aiguë. Evolution simultanée des clones plasmocytaires et myélomonocytaires. *Semaines des Hôpitaux de Paris*, **54**, 809.

165 ZINNEMAN H.H. & SEAL U.S. (1969) Double spike in myeloma serum due to retention of light chain. *Archives of Internal Medicine*, **124**, 77.

166 KOZURU M., BENOKI H., SUGIMOTO H., SAKAI K. & IBAYASHI H. (1977) A case of lambda type tetramer Bence-Jones proteinaemia. *Acta Haematologica*, **57**, 359.

167 CAGGIANO V., DOMINGUEZ G., OPFELL R.W., KOCHWA S. & WASSERMAN L.R. (1969) IgG myeloma with closed tetrameric Bence-Jones proteinuria. *American Journal of Medicine*, **47**, 978.

168 KOHN J. (1973) The laboratory investigation of paraproteinaemia. In: *Recent Advances in Clinical Pathology* (ed. Dyke S.C.), p. 363. Churchill Livingstone, Edinburgh.

169 JEPPSSON J.-O., LAURELL C.-B. & FRANZÉN B. (1979) Agarose gel electrophoresis. *Clinical Chemistry*, **25**, 629.

170 ZAWADZKI Z.A. & EDWARDS G.A. (1970) Pseudoparaproteinemia due to hypertransferrinemia. *American Journal of Clinical Pathology*, **54**, 802.

171 CEJKA J. & KITHIER K. (1979) IgD myeloma protein with 'unreactive' light chain determinants. *Clinical Chemistry*, **25**, 1495.

172 WHICHER J.T., HAWKINS L. & HIGGINSON J. (1980) Clinical applications of immunofixation: a more sensitive technique for the detection of Bence-Jones protein. *Journal of Clinical Pathology*, **33**, 779.

173 SUN T., LIEN Y.Y. & DEGNAN T. (1979) Study of gammopathies with immunofixation electrophoresis. *American Journal of Clinical Pathology*, **72**, 5.

174 KOHN J. & RICHES P.G. (1978) A cellulose acetate immunofixation technique. *Journal of Immunological Methods*, **20**, 325.

175 PEDERSEN N.S. & AXELSEN N.H. (1979) Detection of M-components by an easy immunofixation procedure: comparison with agarose gel electrophoresis and classical immunoelectrophoresis. *Journal of Immunological Methods*, **30**, 257.

176 MULDER J. & VERHAAR M.A.T. (1973) Multiple precipitations of sera containing monoclonal IgG proteins by radial immunodiffusion. *Clinica Chimica Acta*, **45**, 325.

177 MORELL A., SKARIL F. & BARANDUN S. (1973) Qualitative and quantitative investigations on the reaction of normal and monoclonal IgG with antisera to IgG. *Clinical and Experimental Immunology*, **13**, 293.

178 SMITH A.M. & THOMPSON R.A. (1978) Paraprotein estimation: a comparison of immunochemical and densitometric techniques. *Journal of Clinical Pathology*, **31**, 1156.

179 SPIRA G., SILVIAN I., TATARSKY I. & HAZANI A. (1980) A calcium-binding IgG myeloma protein. *Scandinavian Journal of Haematology*, **24**, 193.

180 LINDGARDE F. & ZETTERVAL O. (1973) Hypercalcaemia and normal ionised serum Ca in a case of myelomatosis. *Annals of Internal Medicine*, **78**, 396.

181 JAFFE J.P. & MOSHER D.F. (1979) Calcium binding by a myeloma protein. *American Journal of Medicine*, **67**, 343.

182 SORIA J., SORIA C., DAO C., JAMES J.-M., BOUSSIER J. & BILSKI-PASQUIER G. (1975) Immunoglobulin-bound calcium and ultrafiltrable serum calcium in myeloma. *British Journal of Haematology*, **34**, 343.

183 TARAIL R., BUCHWALD K.W., HOLLAND J.F. & SELAWRY O.S. (1962) Misleading reduction of serum sodium and chloride associated with hyperproteinemia in patients with multiple myeloma. *Proceedings of the Society for Experimental Biology and Medicine*, **110**, 145.

184 PALADINI G. & SALA P.G. (1979) Anion gap in multiple myeloma. *Acta Haematologica*, **62**, 148.

185 BLOTH B., CHRISTENSSON T. & MELLSTEDT H. (1978) Extreme hyponatraemia in patients with myelomatosis. *Acta Medica Scandinavica*, **203**, 273.

186 FRICK P.G., SCHMIDT J.R., KISTLER H.J. & HITZIG W.H. (1966) Hyponatraemia associated with hyperproteinaemia in multiple myeloma. *Helvetica Medica Acta*, **33**, 316.

187 MURRAY T., LONG W. & NARINS R.G. (1975) Multiple

myeloma and the anion gap. *New England Journal of Medicine*, **292**, 574.

188 SCHNUR M.J., APPEL G.B., KARP G. & OSSERMANN E.F. (1977) The anion gap in asymptomatic plasma cell dyscrasia. *Annals of Internal Medicine*, **86**, 304.

189 WRIGHT D.J. & JENKINS D.E. (1970) Simplified method for estimation of serum and plasma viscosity in multiple myeloma and related disorders. *Blood*, **36**, 516.

190 MANNIK M. (1974) Blood viscosity in Waldenström's macroglobulinemia. *Blood*, **44**, 87.

191 MacKENZIE M.R. & LEE T.K. (1979) Blood viscosity in Waldenström's macroglobulinemia. *Blood*, **49**, 507.

192 HOBBS J.R. (1969) Immunochemical classes of myelomatosis including data from a therapeutic trial conducted by a MRC working party. *British Journal of Haematology*, **16**, 599.

193 PRUZANSKI W. (1976) Clinical manifestations of multiple myeloma: relation to class and type of M component. *Canadian Medical Association Journal*, **114**, 896.

194 SHIN M.S., MOWRY R.W. & BODIE F.L. (1979) Osteosclerosis (punctate form) in multiple myeloma. *Southern Medical Journal*, **72**, 226.

195 ROGERS J.S., SPAHR J., JUDGE D.M., VARANO L.A. & EYSTER M.E. (1977) IgE myeloma with osteoblastic lesions. *Blood*, **49**, 295.

196 NØRGAARD O. (1971) Three cases of multiple myeloma in which the preclinical asymptomatic phases persisted throughout 15–24 years. *British Journal of Cancer*, **25**, 417.

197 KYLE R.A. & GREIPP P.R. (1980) Smouldering multiple myeloma. *New England Journal of Medicine*, **302**, 1347.

198 ALEXANIAN R. (1980) Localised and indolent myeloma. *Blood*, **56**, 521.

199 MEDICAL RESEARCH COUNCIL (1971) Myelomatosis: comparison of melphalan and cyclophosphamide therapy. *British Medical Journal*, **i**, 640.

200 GEORGE R.P., POTH J.L., GORDON D. & SCHRIER S.A. (1972) Multiple myeloma—intermittent combination chemotherapy compared to continuous therapy. *Cancer*, **29**, 1665.

201 BROOK J., BATEMAN J.R., GOCKA E.F., NAKAMURA E. & STAINFELD J.L. (1973) Long-term low dose melphalan treatment of multiple myeloma. *Archives of Internal Medicine*, **131**, 545.

202 WESTERFIELD B.T., MICHALSKI J.P., McCOMBS C. & LIGHT R.W. (1980) Reversible melphalan-induced lung damage. *American Journal of Medicine*, **68**, 767.

203 TAETLE R., DICKMAN P.S. & FELDMAN P.S. (1978) Pulmonary histopathologic changes associated with melphalan therapy. *Cancer*, **42**, 1239.

204 VON EYBEN F. & OLSEN T.S. (1978) Cytomegalovirus pneumonia after treatment with melphalan and prednisone. *Acta Medica Scandinavica*, **203**, 333.

205 CORNWELL G.G., PAJAK T.F. & McINTYRE O.R. (1979) Hypersensitivity reactions to i.v. melphalan during treatment of multiple myeloma. *Cancer Treatment Report*, **63**, 399.

206 ALEXANIAN R., HAUT A., KAHN A.U., LANE M., McKELVEY E.M., MIGLIORE P.J., STUCKEY W.J. & WILSON H.E. (1969) Treatment for multiple myeloma: combination chemotherapy with different melphalan dose regimens. *Journal of the American Medical Association*, **208**, 1680.

207 COSTA G., ENGLE R.L. JR, SCHILLING A., CARBONE P., KOCHWA S., NACHMAN R.L. & GLIDEWELL O. (1973) Melphalan and prednisolone: an effective combination for the treatment of multiple myeloma. *American Journal of Medicine*, **54**, 589.

208 HOOGSTRATEN B. (1975) Steroid therapy of multiple myeloma and macroglobulinemia. *Medical Clinics of North America*, **57**, 1321.

209 ALEXANIAN R., BONNET J., GEHAN E., HAUT A., HEWLETT J., LANE M., MONTO R. & WILSON H. (1972) Combination chemotherapy for multiple myeloma. *Cancer*, **30**, 382.

210 RODRIGUEZ L.H., FINKELSTEIN J.B., SHULLENBERGER C.C. & ALEXANIAN R. (1972) Bone healing in multiple myeloma with melphalan chemotherapy. *Annals of Internal Medicine*, **76**, 551.

211 BENNETT J.M., SILBER R., EZDINLI E., LEVITT M., OKEN M., BAKEMEIER R.F., BAILAR J.C. & CARBONE P.P. (1978) Phase II study of adriamycin and bleomycin in patients with myeloma. *Cancer Treatment Reports*, **62**, 1367.

212 KYLE R.A., SELIGMAN B.R., WALLACE H.J., SILVER R.T., GLIDEWELL O. & HOLLAND J.F. (1975) Multiple myeloma resistant to melphalan (NSC-8806) treated with cyclophosphamide (NSC-26271), prednisone (NSC-10023) and chloroquine (NSC-187208). *Cancer Chemotherapy Reports*, **59**, 557.

213 KYLE R.A., GAILANI S., SELIGMAN B.R., BLOM J., McINTYRE O.R., PAJAK T.F. & HOLLAND J.F. (1979) Multiple myeloma resistant to melphalan: treatment with cyclophosphamide, prednisone and BCNU. *Cancer Treatment Report*, **63**, 1265.

214 HOKANSON J.A., BROWN B.W., THOMPSON J.R., DREWINKO B. & ALEXANIAN R. (1977) Tumor growth patterns in multiple myeloma. *Cancer*, **39**, 1077.

215 DURIE B.G.M., RUSSELL D.H. & SALMON S.E. (1980) Reappraisal of plateau phase in myeloma. *Lancet*, **ii**, 65.

216 ALEXANIAN R., BALCERZAK S., HAUT A. HEWLETT J. & GEHAN E. (1975) Remission maintenance therapy for multiple myeloma. *Archives of Internal Medicine*, **135**, 147.

217 ALEXANIAN R., GEHAN E., HAUT A., SAIKI J. & WEICK J. (1978) Unmaintained remissions in multiple myeloma. *Blood*, **51**, 1005.

218 ALEXANIAN R., SALMON S., BONNET J., GEHAN E., HAUT A. & WEICK J. (1977) Combination therapy for multiple myeloma. *Cancer*, **40**, 2765.

219 McINTYRE O.R. (1979) Multiple myeloma. *New England Journal of Medicine*, **301**, 193.

220 COHEN H.J., SILBERMAN H.R., LARSEN W.E., JOHNSON L., BARTOLUCCI A.A. & DURRANT J.R. (1979) Combination chemotherapy with intermittent 1-3-Bis (2-chloroethyl) 1-nitrosourea (BCNU), cyclophosphamide and prednisone for multiple myeloma. *Blood*, **54**, 824.

221 HARLEY J.B., PAJAK T.F., McINTYRE O.R., KOCHWA S., COOPER M.R., COLEMAN M. & CUTTNER J. (1979) Improved survival of increased-risk myeloma patients on combined triple-alkylating-agent therapy: a study of the CALGB. *Blood*, **54**, 13.

222 BERGSAGEL D.E., BAILEY A.J., LANGLEY G.R., MAC-

DONALD R.N., WHITE D.F. & MILLER A.B. (1979) The chemotherapy of plasma cell myeloma and the incidence of acute leukemia. *New England Journal of Medicine*, **301**, 743.

223 CASE D.C., LEE B.J. & CLARKSON B.D. (1977) Improved survival times in multiple myeloma treated with melphalan, prednisone, cyclophosphamide, vincristine and BCNU. M-2 protocol. *American Journal of Medicine*, **63**, 897.

224 LEE B.J., SAHAKIAN G., CLARKSON B.D. & KRAKOFF I.H. (1974) Combination chemotherapy of multiple myeloma with alkeran, cytoxan, vincristine, prednisone and BCNU. *Cancer*, **33**, 533.

225 AZAM L. & DELAMORE I.W. (1974) Combination therapy for myelomatosis. *British Medical Journal*, **iv**, 560.

226 PRESANT C.A. & FLAHR C. (1978) Adriamycin, 1,3-Bis (2-chloro-ethyl)-1-nitrosourea (BCNU), cyclophosphamide plus prednisone in melphalan resistant multiple myeloma. *Cancer*, **42**, 1222.

227 MALPAS J.S. & PARKER D. (1978) Drugs for myeloma. *British Medical Journal*, **ii**, 563.

228 DREWINKO B., BROWN B.W., HUMPHREY R. & ALEXANIAN R. (1974) Effect of chemotherapy on the labelling index of myeloma cells. *Cancer*, **34**, 526.

229 BERGSAGEL D.E., COWAN D.H. & HASSELBACK R. (1972) Plasma cell myeloma: response of melphalan resistant patients to high dose intermittent cyclophosphamide. *Canadian Medical Association Journal*, **107**, 851.

230 ALBERTS D.S., DURIE B.G.M. & SALMON S.E. (1976) Doxorubicin/B.C.N.U. chemotherapy for multiple myeloma in relapse. *Lancet*, **i**, 926.

231 CORNELL C.J., McINTYRE O.R., KOCHWA S., WEKSLER B.B. & PAJAK T.F. (1979) Response to therapy in IgG myeloma patients excreting κ or λ light chains. *Blood*, **54**, 23.

232 SHUSTIK C., BERGSAGEL D.E. & PRUZANSKI W. (1976) κ and λ light chain disease: survival rates and clinical manifestations. *Blood*, **48**, 41.

233 ALEXANIAN R., BALCERZAK S., BONNET J.D., GEHAN E.A., HAUT A., HEWLETT J.S. & MONTO R.W. (1975) Prognostic factors in multiple myeloma. *Cancer*, **36**, 1192.

234 DURIE B.G.M. & SALMON S.E. (1975) A clinical staging system for multiple myeloma. *Cancer*, **36**, 842.

235 WOODRUFF R.K., WADSWORTH J., MALPAS J.S. & TOBIAS J.S. (1979) Clinical staging in multiple myeloma *British Journal of Haematology*, **42**, 199.

236 IDESTRÖM K., CANTELL K., KILLANDER D., NILSSON K., STRANDER H. & WILLEMS J. (1979) Interferon therapy in multiple myeloma. *Acta Medica Scandinavica*, **205**, 149.

237 MELLSTEDT H., BJÖRKHOLM M., AHRE A., HOLM G., JOHNSSON B. & STRANDER H. (1979) Interferon therapy in myelomatosis. *Lancet*, **i**, 245.

238 SCHILLING A. & FINKEL H.E. (1975) Ancillary measures in treatment of myeloma. *Archives of Internal Medicine*, **135**, 193.

239 JOHNSON W.J., KYLE R.A. & DAHLBERG P.J. (1980) Dialysis in the treatment of multiple myeloma. *Mayo Clinic Proceedings*, **55**, 65.

240 BROWN W.W., HEBERT L.A., PIERING W.F., PISCIOTTA A.V., LEMANN J. & GARANCIS J.C. (1979) Reversal of chronic end-stage renal failure due to myeloma kidney. *Annals of Internal Medicine*, **90**, 793.

241 SPENCE R.K., HILL G.S., GOLDWEIN M.I., GROSSMAN R.A., BARKER C.F. & PERLOFF L.J. (1979) Renal transplantation for end-stage myeloma kidney. *Archives of Surgery*, **114**, 950.

242 HUMPHREY R.L., WRIGHT J.R., ZACHARY J.B., STERIOFF S. & DEFRONZO R.A. (1975) Renal transplantation in multiple myeloma. *Annals of Internal Medicine*, **83**, 651.

243 SMITH L.E. & POWLES T.J. (1975) Mithramycin for hypercalcaemia associated with myeloma and other malignancies. *British Medical Journal*, **i**, 268.

244 STAMP T.C.B., CHILD J.A. & WALKER P.G. (1975) Treatment of osteolytic myelomatosis with mithramycin. *Lancet*, **i**, 719.

245 BEHN A.R. & WEST T.E.T. (1977) Emergency treatment with calcitonin of hypercalcaemia associated with multiple myeloma. *British Medical Journal*, **i**, 755.

246 UNANDER-SCHARIN L., WALDENSTRÖM J.G. & ZETTERVALL O. (1978) Surgical treatment of myelomatosis—a review of 18 cases. *Acta Medica Scandinavica*, **203**, 265.

247 HALL A.J. & MacKAY N.N.S. (1973) The results of laminectomy for compression of the cord and cauda equina by extradural malignant tumours. *Journal of Bone and Joint Surgery*, **558**, 497.

248 DAHLSTRÖM U., JÄRPE S. & LINDSTRÖM F.D. (1979) Paraplegia in myelomatosis—a study of 20 cases. *Acta Medica Scandinavica*, **205**, 173.

249 QASIM M.M. (1979) Techniques and results of half body irradiation (HBI) in metastatic carcinomas and myelomas. *Clinical Oncology*, **5**, 65.

250 JAFFE J.P., BOSCH A. & RAICH P.C. (1979) Sequential hemi-body radiotherapy in advanced multiple myeloma. *Cancer*, **43**, 124.

251 POWLES R., SMITH C., KOHN J. & HAMILTON-FAIRLEY G. (1971) Method of removing abnormal protein rapidly from patients with malignant paraproteinaemias. *British Medical Journal*, **iii**, 664.

252 ISBISTER J.P., BIGGS J.C. & PENNY R. (1978) Experience with large volume plasmapheresis in malignant paraproteinaemia and immune disorders. *Australian and New Zealand Journal of Medicine*, **8**, 154.

253 MISIANI R., REMUZZI G., BERTANI T., LICINI R., LEVONI P., CRIPPA A. & MECCA G. (1979) Plasmapheresis in the treatment of acute renal failure in multiple myeloma. *American Journal of Medicine*, **66**, 684.

254 RUSSELL J.A., FITZHARRIS B.M., CORRINGHAM R., DARCY D.A. & POWLES R.L. (1978) Plasma exchange versus peritoneal dialysis for removing Bence-Jones protein. *British Medical Journal*, **ii**, 1397.

255 KYLE R.A., JOWSEY J., KELLY P.J. & TAVES D.R. (1975) Multiple myeloma bone disease. *New England Journal of Medicine*, **293**, 1334.

256 HOBBS J.R. (1971) Modes of escape from therapeutic control in myelomatosis. *British Medical Journal*, **ii**, 235.

257 BERGSAGEL D.E. & PRUZANSKI W. (1975) Treatment of plasma cell myeloma with cytotoxic agents. *Archives of Internal Medicine*, **135**, 172.

258 ROSNER F. & GRUNWALD H. (1974) Multiple myeloma terminating in acute leukemia. *American Journal of Medicine*, **57**, 927.

259 KARCHMER R.K., AMARE M., LARSEN W.F., MALLOUK

A.G. & CALDWELL G.G. (1974) Alkylating agents as leukemogens in multiple myeloma. *Cancer*, **33**, 1103.

260 CARDAMONE J.M., KIMMERLE R.I. & MARSHALL E.Y. (1974) Development of acute erythroleukemia in B-cell immunoproliferative disorders after prolonged therapy with alkylating drugs. *American Journal of Medicine*, **57**, 836.

261 FISHMAN S.A. & RITZ N.D. (1975) Erythroleukemia following melphalan therapy for multiple myeloma. *New York State Journal of Medicine*, **75**, 2402.

262 MEYTES D., SELIGSOHN U. & RAMOT B. (1976) Multiple myeloma with terminal erythroleukaemia. *Acta Haematologica*, **55**, 358.

263 GONZALEZ F., TRUJILLO J.M. & ALEXANIAN R. (1977) Acute leukemia in multiple myeloma. *Annals of Internal Medicine*, **86**, 440.

264 HOSSFIELD D.K., HOLLAND J.F., COOPER R.G. & ELLISON R.R. (1975) Chromosome studies in acute leukemias developing in patients with multiple myeloma. *Cancer Research*, **35**, 2808.

265 TURSZ T., FLANDRIN G., BROUET J.-C., BRIERE J. & SELIGMANN M. (1974) Simultaneous occurrence of acute myeloblastic leukaemia and multiple myeloma without previous chemotherapy. *British Medical Journal*, **ii**, 642.

266 THIAGARAJAN P. (1979) Simultaneous presentation of multiple myeloma and acute leukemia in the absence of previous chemotherapy. *Mount Sinai Journal of Medicine*, **46**, 360.

267 KRAJNY M. & PRUZANSKI W. (1976) Waldenström's macroglobulinemia: review of 45 cases. *Canadian Medical Association Journal*, **114**, 899.

268 MACKENZIE M.R. & FUDENBERG H.H. (1972) Macroglobulinemia: an analysis of forty patients. *Blood*, **39**, 874.

269 MCCALLISTER B.D., BAYRD E.D., HARRISON E.G. & MCGUCKIN W.F. (1967) Primary macroglobulinemia. *American Journal of Medicine*, **43**, 394.

270 FINE J.M., LAMBIN P., VALENTIN L. & BLATRIX C. (1973) IgG monoclonal gammopathy in the sister of a patient with Waldenström's macroglobulinaemia. *Biomedicine Express*, **19**, 117.

271 BJÖRNSSON O.G., ARNASON A., GUDMUNDSSON S., JENSSON O., OLAFSSON S. & VALDIMARSSON H. (1978) Macroglobulinaemia in an Icelandic family. *Acta Medica Scandinavica*, **203**, 283.

272 PREUD'HOMME J-L. & SELIGMANN M. (1972) Immunoglobulins on the surface of lymphoid cells in Waldenström's macroglobulinemia. *Journal of Clinical Investigation*, **51**, 701.

273 WELLS M., MICHAELS L. & WELLS D.G. (1977) Otolaryngological disturbances in Waldenström's macroglobulinaemia. *Clinical Otolaryngology*, **2**, 327.

274 LOGOTHETIS J., SILVERSTEIN P. & CO J. (1960) Neurologic aspects of Waldenström's macroglobulinemia. *Archives of Neurology*, **3**, 964.

275 JULIEN J., VITAL C., VALLAT J.-M., LAGUENY A., DEMINIERE C. & DARRIET D. (1978) Polyneuropathy in Waldenström's macroglobulinaemia. Deposition of M components on myelin sheaths. *Archives of Neurology*, **35**, 43.

276 BAUER M., BERGSTRÖM R., RITTER B. & OLSSON Y. (1977) Macroglobulinaemia Waldenström's and motor neurone syndrome. *Acta Neurologica Scandinavica*, **55**, 245.

277 FRASER D.M., PARKER A.C., AMER S. & CAMPBELL I.W. (1976) Mononeuritis multiplex in a patient with macroglobulinaemia. *Journal of Neurology, Neurosurgery and Psychiatry*, **39**, 711.

278 IWASHITA H., ARGYRAKIS A., LOWITZSCH K. & SPAAP F-W. (1974) Polyneuropathy in Waldenström's macroglobulinemia. *Journal of Neurological Sciences*, **21**, 341.

279 MASSEY E.W., PLEET A.B. & BRANNON W.L. (1978) Waldenström's macroglobulinemia and mononeuritis multiplex. *Annals of Internal Medicine*, **88**, 360.

280 PROPP R.P., MEANS E., DEIBEL R., SHERER G. & BARRON K. (1975) Waldenström's macroglobulinemia and neuropathy. *Neurology*, **25**, 980.

281 BANHAM S.W. & BATESON M.C. (1977) Severe pulmonary disease and hyperviscosity in macroglobulinaemia. *Postgraduate Medical Journal*, **53**, 631.

282 KESHGEGIAN A.A. & SEVIN P. (1979) Waldenström's macroglobulinemia associated with a mixed cryoglobulin. *Archives of Pathology and Laboratory Medicine*, **103**, 270.

283 HARRISON C.V. (1972) The morphology of the lymph node in the macroglobulinaemia of Waldenström. *Journal of Clinical Pathology*, **25**, 12.

284 ALEXANIAN R. (1975) Monoclonal gammopathy in lymphoma. *Archives of Internal Medicine*, **135**, 62.

285 LEB L., GRIMES E.T., BALOGH K. & MERRITT J.A. (1977) Monoclonal macroglobulinemia with osteolytic lesions. *Cancer*, **39**, 227.

286 TURSZ T., BROUET J.-C., FLANDRIN G., DANON F., CLAUVEL J.-P. & SELIGMANN M. (1977) Clinical and pathological features of Waldenström's macroglobulinemia in seven patients with serum monoclonal IgG and IgA. *American Journal of Medicine*, **63**, 499.

287 HIJMANS W. (1975) Waldenström's disease with an IgA paraprotein. *Acta Medica Scandinavica*, **198**, 519.

288 SHIRAKURA T., TAKEKOSHI K., UMI M., KANAZAWA K., OKABE H., INOUE T. & IMAMURA Y. (1978) Waldenström's macroglobulinaemia with IgE M component. *Scandinavian Journal of Haematology*, **21**, 292.

289 BUSKARD N.A., GALTON D.A.G., GOLDMAN J.M., KOHNER E.M., GRINDLE C.F.J., NEWMAN D.L., TWINN K.W. & LOWENTHAL R.M. (1977) Plasma exchange in the long term management of Waldenström's macroglobulinaemia. *Canadian Medical Association Journal*, **117**, 135.

290 CHOI Y.J., YEH G., REINER L. & SPIELVOGEL A. (1979) Immunoblastic sarcoma following Waldenström's macroglobulinemia. *American Journal of Clinical Pathology*, **71**, 121.

291 CARTER P., KOVAL J.J. & HOBBS J.R. (1977) The relation of clinical and laboratory findings to the survival of patients with macroglobulinaemia. *Clinical and Experimental Immunology*, **28**, 241.

292 GLENNER G.G. (1980) Amyloid deposits and amyloidosis. *New England Journal of Medicine*, **302**, 1283.

293 KYLE R.A. & BAYRD E.D. (1975) Amyloidosis: review of 236 cases. *Medicine*, **54**, 271.

294 ISOBE T. & OSSERMAN E.F. (1974) Patterns of amyloidosis and their association with plasma cell dyscrasia,

monoclonal immunoglobulins and Bence-Jones proteins. *New England Journal of Medicine*, **290**, 473.

295 MILUTINOVICH J., WU W. & SAVORY J. (1979) Periorbital purpura after renal biopsy in primary amyloidosis. *Journal of the American Medical Association*, **242**, 2555.

296 FITTING J.W., BISCHOFF A., REGLI F. & CROUSAZ G. (1979) Neuropathy, amyloidosis and monoclonal gammopathy. *Journal of Neurology, Neurosurgery and Psychiatry*, **42**, 193.

297 BENSON M.D., COHEN A.S., BRANDT K.D. & CATCHART E.S. (1975) Neuropathy, M components and amyloid. *Lancet*, **i**, 10.

298 EDITORIAL (1973) Amyloid joint disease. *Lancet*, **i**, 474.

299 EDITORIAL (1974) Amyloid arthropathy. *British Medical Journal*, **i**, 297.

300 GALLO G.R., FEINER H.D., KATZ L.A., FELDMAN G.M., CORREA E.B., CHUBA J.V. & BUXBAUM J.N. (1980) Nodular glomerulopathy associated with nonamyloidotic kappa light chain deposits and excess immunoglobulin light chain synthesis. *American Journal of Pathology*, **99**, 621.

301 RANDALL R.E., WILLIAMSON W.C., MULLINAX F., TUNG M.Y. & STILL W.J.S. (1976) Manifestations of systemic light chain deposition. *American Journal of Medicine*, **60**, 293.

302 MALLICK N.P., DOSA S., ACHESON E.J., DELAMORE I.W., McFARLANE H., SENEVIRATNE C.J. & WILLIAMS G. (1978) Detection, significance and treatment of paraproteins in patients presenting with 'idiopathic' proteinuria without myeloma. *Quarterly Journal of Medicine*, **186**, 145.

303 CORNWELL G.G., HUSBY G., WESTERMARK P., NATVIG J.B., MICHAELSEN T.E. & SKEGER B. (1977) Identification and characterisation of different amyloid fibril proteins in tissue sections. *Scandinavian Journal of Immunology*, **6**, 1071.

304 PRUZANSKI W. & KATZ A. (1976) Clinical and laboratory findings in primary generalised and multiple myeloma-related amyloidosis. *Canadian Medical Association Journal*, **114**, 906.

305 COHEN H.J., LESSIN L.S., HALLAL J. & BURKHOLDER P. (1975) Resolution of primary amyloidosis during chemotherapy. *Annals of Internal Medicine*, **82**, 466.

306 JONES N.F., HILTON P.J., TIGHE J.R. & HOBBS J.R. (1972) Treatment of 'primary' renal amyloidosis with melphalan. *Lancet*, **iii**, 616.

307 COHEN H.J. (1978) Combination therapy for primary amyloidosis reconsidered. *Annals of Internal Medicine*, **89**, 572.

308 KYLE R.A. & GREIPP P.R. (1978) Primary systemic amyloidosis: comparison of melphalan and prednisolone versus placebo. *Blood*, **52**, 818.

309 KYLE R.A., PIERRE R.V. & BAYRD E.D. (1974) Primary amyloidosis and acute leukemia associated with melphalan therapy. *Blood*, **44**, 333.

310 ZILKO P.J. & DAWKINS L. (1975) Amyloidosis associated with dermatomyositis and features of multiple myeloma. *American Journal of Medicine*, **59**, 448.

311 KUHLBÄCK B., FALCK H., TÖRNROTH T., WALLENIUS M., LINDESTRÖM B.L. & PASTERNACK A. (1979) Renal transplantation in amyloidosis. *Acta Medica Scandinavica*, **205**, 169.

312 FRANGIONE B. & FRANKLIN E.C. (1973) Heavy chain diseases: clinical features and molecular significance of the disordered immunoglobulin structure. *Seminars in Hematology*, **10**, 53.

313 FRANKLIN E.C., LOWENSTEIN J., BIGELOW B. & MELTZER M. (1964) Heavy chain disease—a new disorder of serum γ-globulins. *American Journal of Medicine*, **37**, 332.

314 SELIGMANN M., DANON F., HUREZ D., MIHAESCO E. & PREUD'HOMME J.-L. (1968) Alpha-chain disease: a new immunoglobulin abnormality. *Science*, **162**, 1396.

315 SELIGMANN M. (1977) Immunobiology and pathogenesis of alpha-chain disease. *CIBA Foundation Symposium*, **46**, 263.

316 FLORIN-CHRISTENSEN A., DONIACH D. & NEWCOMB P.B. (1974) Alpha-chain disease with pulmonary manifestations. *British Medical Journal*, **ii**, 413.

317 RAMBAUD J.C., GALIAN A., MATUCHANSKY C., DANON F., PREUD'HOMME J.-L., BROUET J.-C. & SELIGMANN M. (1978) Natural history of alpha-chain disease and the so-called Mediterranean lymphoma. *Recent Results in Cancer Research*, **64**, 271.

318 GALIAN A., LECESTRE M.-J., SCOTTO J., BOGNEL G., MATUCHANSKY C. & RAMBAUD J.-C. (1977) Pathological study of alpha-chain disease with special emphasis on evolution. *Cancer*, **39**, 2081.

319 BROUET J.-C., MASON D.Y., DANON F., PREUD'HOMME J.-L., SELIGMANN M., REYES F., NAVAB F., GALIAN A., RENE E. & RAMBAUD J.-C. (1977) Alpha-chain disease: evidence for common clonal origin of intestinal immunoblastic lymphoma and plasmacytic proliferation. *Lancet*, **i**, 860.

320 RAMOT B., LAVANON M., HAHN Y., LAHAT N. & MOROZ C. (1977) The mutual clonal origin of the lymphoplasmacytic and lymphoma cell in alpha heavy chain disease. *Clinical and Experimental Immunology*, **27**, 440.

321 PANGALIS G.A. & RAPPAPORT H. (1977) Common clonal origin of lymphoplasmacytic proliferation and immunoblastic lymphoma in intestinal alpha-chain disease. *Lancet*, **ii**, 880.

322 DOE W.F., DANON F. & SELIGMANN M. (1979) Immunodiagnosis of alpha-chain disease. *Clinical and Experimental Immunology*, **36**, 189.

323 DOE W.F. & SPIEGELBERG H.L. (1979) Characterisation of an antiserum specific for the Fab_2 fragment. *Journal of Immunology*, **122**, 19.

324 AL-SALEEM T.I., AL-QADIRY W., ISSA F.S. & KING J. (1979) The immunoselection technique in laboratory diagnosis of alpha heavy-chain disease. *American Journal of Clinical Pathology*, **72**, 132.

325 MANOUSOS O.N., ECONOMIDOU J.C., GEORGIADOU D.E., PRATSIKA-DUGOURLOGLOU K.G., HADZIYANNIS S.J., MERIKAS G.E., HENRY K. & DOE W.F. (1974) Alpha-chain disease with clinical, immunological, and histological recovery. *British Medical Journal*, **ii**, 409.

326 FORTE F.A., PRELLI F., YOUNT W.J., JERRY M., KOCHWA S., FRANKLIN E.C. & KUNKEL H.G. (1970) Heavy chain disease of the μ (γM) type: report of the first case. *Blood*, **36**, 137.

327 BALLARD H.S., HAMILTON L.M., MARCUS A.J. & ILLES C.H. (1970) A new variant of heavy chain disease (μ-chain disease). *New England Journal of Medicine*, **282**, 1060.

328 BONHOMME J., SELIGMANN M., MIHAESCO C., CLAUVEL J.P., DANN F., BROUET J.-C., BOUVRY P., MARTINE J. & CLERC M. (1974) Mu-chain disease in an African patient. *Blood*, **43**, 485.

329 DANON F., MIHAESCO C., BOUVRY M., CLERC M. & SELIGMANN M. (1975) A new case of heavy mu-chain disease. *Scandinavian Journal of Haematology*, **15**, 5.

330 MAMMACCO F., BONOMO L. & FRANKLIN E.C. (1974) A new case of mu heavy chain disease: clinical and immunochemical studies. *Blood*, **43**, 713.

331 BROUET J.-C., SELIGMANN M., DANON F., BELPOMME D. & FINE J.-M. (1979) μ-chain disease. Report of two new cases. *Archives of Internal Medicine*, **139**, 672.

332 LEBRETON J.P., ROPARTZ C., ROUSSEAUX J., ROUSSEL P., DAUTREVAUX M. & BISERTE G. (1975) Immunochemical and biochemical study of a human Fcμ-like fragment (μ-chain disease). *European Journal of Immunology*, **5**, 179.

333 AMEIS A., KO H.S. & PRUZANSKI W. (1976) M components—a review of 1242 cases. *Canadian Medical Association Journal*, **114**, 889.

334 STEIN H., LENNERT K. & PARWARESCH M.R. (1972) Malignant lymphoma of B cell type. *Lancet*, **ii**, 855.

335 KOHN J. (1974) Benign paraproteinaemia. *Journal of Clinical Pathology*, **28** (Suppl. 6), 77.

336 COOKE K.B. (1969) Essential paraproteinaemia. *Proceeding of the Royal Society of Medicine*, **62**, 777.

337 RITZMANN S.E., LOUKAS D., SAKAI H., DANIELS J.C., LEVIN W.C. (1975) Idiopathic (asymptomatic) monoclonal gammopathies. *Archives of Internal Medicine*, **135**, 95.

338 DANON F. & SELIGMANN M. (1972) Transient human monoclonal immunoglobulins. *Scandinavian Journal of Immunology*, **1**, 323.

339 YOUNG V.H. (1969) Transient paraproteins. *Proceedings of the Royal Society of Medicine*, **62**, 778.

340 ABRAMSON N. & SHATTIL S.J. (1973) M components. *Journal of the American Medical Association*, **223**, 156.

341 KOHN J. & SRIVASTAVA P.C. (1973) Paraproteinaemia in blood donors and the aged: benign and malignant. In: *Protides of the Biological Fluids* (ed. Peters H.), p. 257. Pergamon Press, Oxford.

342 AXELSSON U., BACHMANN R. & HALLEN J. (1966) Frequency of pathological proteins (M-components) in 6995 sera from an adult population. *Acta Medica Scandinavica*, **179**, 235.

343 FINE J.M., LAMBIN P. & LEROUX P. (1972) Frequency of monoclonal gammopathy ('M components') in 13 400 sera from blood donors. *Vox Sanguinis*, **23**, 336.

344 AXELSSON U. (1977) An 11 year follow up on 64 subjects with M components. *Acta Medica Scandinavica*, **201**, 173.

345 FINE J.M., LAMBIN P. & MULLER J.Y. (1979) The evolution of asymptomatic monoclonal gammopathies. *Acta Medica Scandinavica*, **205**, 339.

346 DERYCKE C., FINE J.-M. & BOFFA G.A. (1965) Dysglobulinémies 'essentielles' chez les sujets agés. *Nouvelle Revue française d'Hématologie*, **5**, 729.

347 HÄLLÉN J. (1963) Frequence of 'abnormal' serum globulins (M-component) in the aged. *Acta Medica Scandinavica*, **173**, 737.

348 LINDSTROM F.D. & DAHLSTRÖM U. (1978) Multiple myeloma or benign monoclonal gammopathy? A study of differential diagnostic criteria in 44 cases. *Clinical Immunology and Immunopathology*, **10**, 168.

349 KYLE R.A., MALDONADO J.E. & BAYRD E.D. (1973) Idiopathic Bence-Jones proteinuria—a distinct entity. *American Journal of Medicine*, **55**, 222.

350 LATOV N., SHERMAN W.H., NEMNI R., GALASSI G., SHYONG J.S., PENN A.S., CHESS L., OLARTE M.R., ROWLAND L.P. & OSSERMAN E.F. (1980) Plasma cell dyscrasia and peripheral neuropathy with monoclonal antibody to peripheral-nerve myelin. *New England Journal of Medicine*, **303**, 618.

351 ROSSBOROUGH T.K. & SWAIM W.R. (1978) Acquired von Willebrand's disease, platelet-release defect and angiodysplasia. *American Journal of Medicine*, **65**, 96.

352 JAMES K., FUDENBERG H.H., EPSTEIN W.L. & SHUSTER J. (1967) Studies on a unique diagnostic serum globulin in papular mucinosis (lichen myxedematosus). *Clinical and Experimental Immunology*, **2**, 153.

353 DANBY F.W., DANBY C.W.E. & PRUZANSKI W. (1976) Papular mucinosis with IgG (K) M component. *Canadian Medical Association Journal*, **114**, 920.

354 WELLS J.V., FUDENBERG H.H. & EPSTEIN W.L. (1972) Idiotypic determinants on the monoclonal immunoglobulins associated with papular mucinosis. *Journal of Immunology*, **108**, 977.

Chapter 20
The spleen in disorders of the blood

A. J. BOWDLER

Disorders of the spleen frequently complicate diseases of the haemopoietic and monocyte–macrophage systems, and therapy related to the organ may significantly modify such conditions. The pathophysiological role of the spleen has been studied by clinical and pathological observation and by human and animal experiment, but much valid empirical information has still to be integrated satisfactorily with knowledge of splenic function at a cellular or molecular level.

Correlation of haematological investigations with critical morphological studies is still lacking for many conditions [1], and since the spleen shares its predominant cellular components with other lymphatic and reticulo-endothelial tissues, its specific contribution to the activity of these systems is often uncertain. Many long-standing assumptions concerning the spleen in man have lacked experimental support and remain difficult to translate into useful clinical concepts. However, the relevance of the spleen to many important fields, including the suppression of the immune response, transplantation theory, and aberrations of the immune state, has stimulated efforts towards a clearer understanding of splenic function.

THE NORMAL SPLEEN

The normal spleen in the adult is situated in the left hypochondrium, its long axis corresponding to the proximal half of the tenth rib. Its position posteriorly in the abdomen, under cover of the thoracic cage, prevents palpation of the normal adult spleen and percussion does not elicit dullness anterior to the left mid-axillary line. The convex surface of the spleen is applied principally to the diaphragm while the antero-medial (visceral) surface is in contact with the stomach, the left kidney and the left colic flexure, with the tail of the pancreas approaching the hilum of the spleen medially. Except at the hilum, the spleen is invested by peritoneum which forms a series of folds, notably the lienorenal ligament which carries the splenic vessels to the hilum, and the gastrosplenic ligament which carries branches of the splenic artery to the stomach.

The weight of the normal adult spleen is estimated from autopsy material to lie between 120 g and 200 g [2–5]. Boyd [6] has shown that spleen weight is not normally distributed and estimates within limited age groups show markedly skewed distributions: the 2·5 and 97·5 percentile values in the third decade were 96 and 364 g for men and 65 and 300 g for women. There is a significant secular trend, with the spleen weight declining with age: by the eighth decade the corresponding values were 66 and 234 g for men and 70 and 195 g for women.

Accessory spleens. These are found at autopsy in approximately 10% of individuals. They are found more frequently in younger subjects, probably due to the involutional effect of ageing on lymphatic tissues. The incidence is significantly higher in pathological circumstances [7, 8]. In 90% of cases, one accessory spleen only is present, but as many as 10 have been found in one subject; multiple accessory spleens may be associated with other congenital anomalies [9, 10]. The principal sites of occurrence are at the hilum of the spleen, in the lienorenal and gastrosplenic ligaments, in the tail of the pancreas [11], adjacent to the splenic artery, in the greater omentum and mesentery, in the wall of the jejunum [12], and associated with the ovary or testis, especially on the left side [13–15]. A rare form of the latter may be accompanied by other congenital anomalies, especially peromelus and micrognathia. Clinically, the significance of the accessory spleen is that it is usually, though not invariably, simultaneously involved in pathological processes affecting the spleen [12, 16]. Recurrence or relapse of disease following initial improvement by splenectomy has been shown to be due in many instances to a residual accessory spleen, especially in autoimmune haemolytic disease, hereditary spherocytosis and idiopathic thrombocytopenic purpura [7, 17–24].

THE ARCHITECTURE OF THE SPLEEN

The spleen consists of a connective tissue framework supporting a specialized vascular system. The *white pulp* consists of lymphatic tissue organized in relation to the arterial vessels; the greater part of the remainder of the parenchyma constitutes the vascular *red pulp*.

The capsule, trabeculae and the reticulum of the splenic pulp provide in continuity the connective tissue framework of the organ. Lying immediately beneath the peritoneal mesothelium, the capsule consists of dense connective tissue from which lace-like extensions, the trabeculae, extend into the splenic pulp, carrying blood vessels, lymphatic vessels and autonomic nerve fibres. In man, the capsule and trabeculae consist predominantly of collagen and elastin fibres, the latter especially well represented in the trabeculae and the deeper aspects of the capsule. Smooth muscle cells are sparse, indicating that active muscular contraction is unimportant in man in determining spleen size, which is principally dependent on passive adaptations to blood flow.

Capsular and trabecular collagen is in direct continuity with the fibrous component of the reticular meshwork, which supports the pulp vessels and forms the basement membranes of the arterial capillaries and splenic sinuses. Closely associated with the reticular fibres are moderately phagocytic reticular cells. Modifications of the reticular pattern conform to specific structural arrangements of the pulp, notably in relation to the white pulp, the marginal zones of the follicles, and the walls of the splenic sinuses [25, 26].

Blood vessels

The vascular organization of the spleen brings blood from the systemic circulation into a uniquely close relationship with lymphatic tissue and the tissue macrophages. With rare exceptions, lymphatic tissues elsewhere are principally perfused by lymph directed through lymphatic channels, whereas in the spleen, these are confined to the trabeculae and capsule, and are functionally unrelated to the splenic pulp (Figs. 20.1 and 20.2).

The splenic artery arises from the coeliac axis and follows a tortuous course to the left behind the upper margin of the pancreas and in the posterior wall of the lesser sac. After traversing the lienorenal ligament it enters the connective tissue external to the hilum and divides into a series of branches which enter the organ to form the trabecular arteries. Within the spleen the arterial supply conforms to an arborization pattern without significant interarterial connections, so that the intrasplenic vessels are functionally end-arteries [27, 28]. The trabecular arteries show progressive subdivision until small radicles are produced which enter the splenic pulp.

On leaving the trabeculae, the arteries develop a modified tunica adventitia consisting essentially of a lymphatic sheath, so that each artery is surrounded by a coaxial cylinder of lymphatic tissue, in continuity with more eccentrically placed lymphoid nodules. Arteriolar branches from the central arteries penetrate the surrounding lymphatic tissue to a variable extent, some ending in the white pulp while others reach the marginal zone and the red pulp. There is no accompanying venous component to the vasculature at this level; essentially, blood flow through the white pulp is centrifugally directed to the marginal zone, where circumferentially placed vessels present openings to

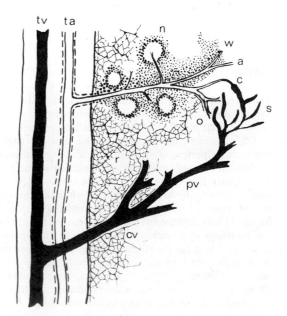

Fig. 20.1. Schematic diagram of the microstructure of the spleen: tv, trabecular vein; ta, trabecular artery; n, nodular white pulp; w, white pulp; a, artery of the pulp; c, direct vascular connection between arterial capillary and splenic sinus; O, 'open' vascular pathway from arterial capillary to splenic sinus; s, splenic sinuses; r, reticulum; pv, pulp vein; cv, collecting vein.

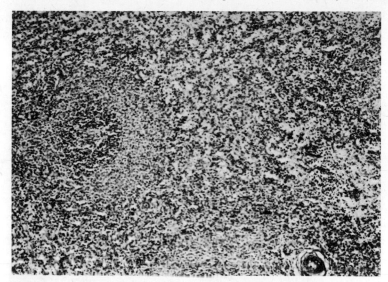

Fig. 20.2. Section of normal spleen (H & E). At the left is a small germinal centre with concentric layers of small and large lymphocytes. Surrounding this is the more loosely organized structure of the red pulp. (By courtesy of Dr C. Pichyangkura.)

the pulp adjacent to the lymphatic tissue [25]. Weiss [41] suggests that 'plasma skimming' occurs in the vessels of the white pulp, the marginal layer of plasma carrying leucocytes to the white pulp, while the concentrated axial stream of red cells is forwarded to the red pulp.

Arteries entering the red pulp divide further, losing the lymphatic sheath at a critical diameter of approximately 50 μm. Some form long, slender penicillate vessels, and when further reduced in diameter to approximately 15 μm a proportion of the blood vessels acquires small clusters of associated phagocytes or 'sheaths of Schweigger-Seidel', which are inconspicuous in the human spleen [30]. Muscular and adventitial coats become tenuous or lost, and the arterioles terminate either in direct continuity with splenic sinuses, or more frequently in free ampullary or funnel-shaped endings in the splenic cords.

The splenic cords are reticulum-lined spaces within the pulp, containing blood cells and macrophages. The splenic sinuses are irregular, elongated vessels of 20–40 μm diameter lined by longitudinally arranged endothelial (littoral) cells supported externally by a tenuous fenestrated basement membrane formed from circumferential reticular fibres [31, 32]. Slit-like openings between the endothelial cells are limited by these fibres. It is not clear whether these openings are normally patent or closed by a homogeneous membrane, but there is no doubt that normal blood cells easily penetrate the sinus wall. The splenic sinuses drain through the veins of the pulp to collecting and trabecular veins which enter the tributaries of the splenic vein [33]. The splenic vein leaves the hilum of the spleen to drain into the portal vein.

The arterio-venous connections. These are critical to the filtration function of the spleen, and have provided a continuing controversy, now largely clarified by scanning electron microscopy. The three principal concepts have been:

1 that the circulation is 'open' with blood passing from the arterial capillaries through the pulp cords to the sinuses [34, 35];
2 that the circulation is 'closed', blood flowing directly from the arterial capillaries to the sinuses through closed endothelium-lined channels [36]; and
3 that both routes are present [37].

The suggestion that cordal blood flow originates from the sinuses has not received confirmation [26, 38, 39]. Histological evidence for both 'open' and 'closed' pathways is unequivocal and functionally the 'open' circulation through the pulp cords is predominant [40–44]. The direct conduits between arterial capillaries and the venous sinuses are more easily demonstrable by scanning electron microscopy than in material examined by transmission microscopy [45–48].

The transit time required for passage through the pulp cords is variable; this is partly due to the presence of large pulp channels between some arterial endings and the sinuses [47, 48] and to variability in the proximity of arterial terminations to the recipient sinus wall [29]. Elements of the blood entering the 'open' pathway are potentially subject to widely varying experiences in transit, dependent both on structural variability within the pulp and on the incompletely explained lability of flow pattern through the cords [44]. Ultimately, the majority of blood cells destined to rejoin the general circulation must penetrate the sinus

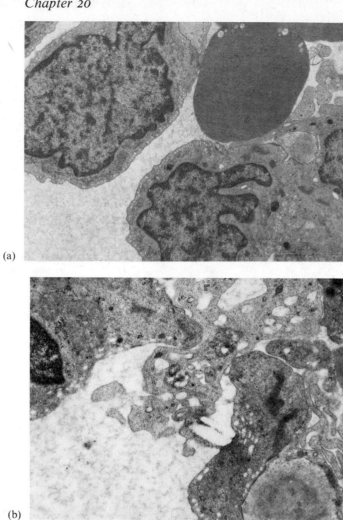

(a)

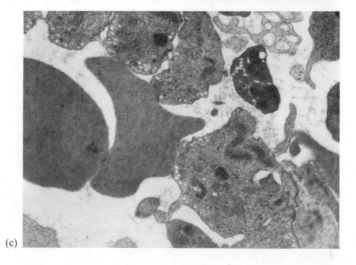

(b)

(c)

Fig. 20.3. Direct electron micrographs of the human spleen showing blood cells in relation to the slit-like spaces between the endothelial cells of the splenic sinuses (original magnification, ×3900). (a) Red cell apposed to the space between two littoral cells, on the pulp side of the sinus wall. Sinus lumen is below and to the left. (b) The tesselated leading edge of a leucocyte has entered the sinus lumen, which is below and to the left. (c) Platelet situated on pulp side of the sinus wall. Two red cells and another platelet are visible in the sinus lumen. (By courtesy of Dr Joan Mattson, Department of Pathology, Michigan State University.)

walls: this is shown in Figure 20.3. It is here that a potential barrier exists to the passage of abnormal cells.

Lymphatic tissue

Organized lymphatic tissue in the spleen is associated with the extratrabecular arterial system and constitutes the white pulp, which consists of the 'sheath-like' pulp and 'nodular' components: lymphocytes are also found in the red pulp. The 'sheath-like' pulp is the T-cell domain, which encloses the arteries in a cellular layer comprised predominantly of lymphocytes, but also including plasma cells, reticular cells, granulocytes and macrophages. It lacks the characteristically highly ordered structure of typical lymphatic tissue, but is continuous with the nodular pulp. The nodular pulp is composed of spheroidal follicles, the majority of which are eccentrically located with respect to the arteries; this constitutes the B-cell domain.

A typical nodule consists of a series of concentric cellular shells of differing composition. The 'germinal centre' is a lightly staining area, sometimes penetrated by a central artery, with two principal cellular components, reticular cells and large actively proliferating basophilic cells. In the larger centres these two cell types may be present in distinctive zones [49, 50]; in addition there may be small lymphocytes and 'tingible-body' macrophages containing phagocytosed nuclear remnants [51]. External to the germinal centre is a layer of small lymphocytes, beyond which appears the marginal zone ('perifollicular envelope') in which are lighter-staining cells with a high ratio of cytoplasmic to nuclear volume, and which is sometimes the site of capillary congestion. A zone of venous sinuses lies outside the marginal zone, although in man these seldom form the prominent marginal sinus seen in some mammals.

Variations are found in both the quantity and configuration of the white pulp; transitional areas with characteristics of both sheath-like and nodular lymphatic tissue are found, where T and B cells may interact. The germinal centres are also variable with respect to cellular content. In addition there are quite marked individual variations, related to age and the immune experience of the individual.

Free cells

In addition to cells comprising the fixed structures and organized formations of lymphatic tissue, the spleen has a significant population of free cells in both the white and the red pulp. These are principally derived from the blood and include erythrocytes, granulocytes, lymphocytes and plasma cells, platelets and free macrophages.

Nerve supply

The abundant autonomic nerve supply of the spleen is distributed in man predominantly to the smooth muscle coats of the blood vessels, and only to a minor extent to the few smooth muscle fibres of the capsule and trabeculae. Post-ganglionic fibres from the coeliac ganglia are distributed through the coeliac and splenic plexuses to the spleen. Parasympathetic fibres are mainly derived from the right vagus.

THE FUNCTIONS OF THE NORMAL SPLEEN

The spleen subserves a multiplicity of functions: the removal of the spleen from the normal adult individual in most cases appears to be well tolerated, with the exceptions of higher mortality from pneumonia and ischaemic heart disease [52, 53]. It is reasonable to assume that in normal subjects after splenectomy the function of the spleen is to a considerable extent compensated by the activity of other organs. Among the principal functions suggested for the spleen are:
1 the production, storage and destruction of blood cells;
2 the production of factors influencing haemopoiesis;
3 a role in the immune response;
4 the removal from the circulation of particulate material;
5 iron storage; and
6 the storage or synthesis of specific proteins.

Intrasplenic haemopoiesis

Splenic erythropoiesis, and to a lesser extent granulopoiesis, is most active antenatally between the second and the sixth months of gestation, although even at this stage the spleen is quantitatively less significant in this respect than the liver. At birth, extramedullary haemopoiesis may still be detected in the liver, spleen, lymph nodes, adrenals, mammary glands, testes and elsewhere, but these sites are normally inactive by the end of infancy [54]. In the adult it is doubtful whether the cytologically recognizable precursors of red cells and granulocytes exist normally in organs other than the bone marrow; if so, they must be extremely rare. The spleen retains the capacity to support haemopoiesis in abnormal circumstances, notably as a compensatory phenomenon in the presence of chronic haemolysis and in pathological conditions such as primary myeloid metaplasia. Despite this the involvement of the spleen in compensatory erythropoiesis is often surprisingly unimpressive, even when extensive masses of heterotopic haematopoietic tissue occur elsewhere, and long-standing haemolysis with anaemia, as in hereditary spherocytosis, may result in only a few small scattered foci of erythropoietic cells in the spleen [55–59]. Consequently, the contribution of haemopoietic cells to enlargement of the spleen is minimal in most cases, and alternative causes of enlargement are usually present, such as the development of a red-cell pool in the splenic pulp.

Lymphopoiesis

The spleen was classically regarded as a site of active lymphocyte production; splenic venous blood shows an excess of lymphocytes when compared with arterial blood, especially following an antigenic stimulus [60–62]. This view was based on:
1 the massive population of lymphocytes present;
2 the abundant mitotic activity of the germinal centres; and
3 the assumption that the lymphocyte is essentially a short-lived cell.

However, Flemming's concept [51] of the germinal centre as the site of origin of the surrounding lymphocytes has lacked confirmation [63–65], and a high proportion of splenic lymphocytes is in fact in process of transit between extrasplenic sites.

The lymphocyte population is heterogeneous with respect to lifespan [66] and the long-lived small lymphocytes of the periarteriolar sheaths belong to a population of T cells continually recirculating between the spleen, blood, lymph-node cortex and lymph, with an average stay in the spleen of four to six hours in both man and rat [67–76]. Such cells comprise between 30 and 50% of the lymphocyte population of the spleen.

The spleen also contains B lymphocytes produced in non-thymic lymphatic tissues, including the bone marrow and lymph nodes [70, 77]. Within the spleen, lymphoblasts are widely scattered through the red and white pulp, and probably constitute a self-sustaining pool of lymphocyte precursors, while other blast cells enter the spleen from the bone marrow [78, 79]. However, even with respect to the short-lived lymphocytes the splenic population is partly derived from the bone marrow, cells entering both the red and white pulp [80].

It thus appears that the spleen is a less active site of primary lymphopoiesis than was formerly assumed: splenectomy does not reduce circulating lymphocyte levels, and in germ-free animals there is little splenic lymphopoiesis, suggesting that lymphocyte production in the organ is principally secondary to antigenic stimulation.

Red-cell storage

Many mammals show significant red-cell storage in the spleen [4, 81–88], but in man there is no evidence for a significant splenic storage pool of mature red cells. The normal complement of red cells in the spleen is approximately 20–40 ml, which would be insignificant in augmenting the circulating red-cell mass [89–92]. The slight rise in venous haematocrit induced in man by adrenaline or exercise is not prevented by splenectomy, and is of lesser magnitude than that obtained in animals with storage spleens [93–96].

Although mature red cells are not normally pooled in the spleen, this is not true of reticulocytes [97–101]. Jandl showed that reticulocytes are less filtrable and have greater surface adhesiveness than mature red cells [102]. Furthermore, blood from the splenic pulp has a higher proportion of reticulocytes than peripheral blood [99, 101–106] and it is probable that the immature red cell completes its maturation within the spleen. Consequently, splenectomy is followed by an increase in circulating reticulocytes, which may persist despite the absence of significant post-operative changes in haemoglobin production and cell lifespan [98–100].

The pooling of platelets

In normal subjects the intravenous injection of normal platelets collected in acid-citrate-dextrose solution and labelled with [51Cr]chromate is followed within the first 10 minutes from injection by a fall in circulating radioactivity of 20–40%. Surface scanning shows high levels of radioactivity in the region of the spleen, and the ratios of activity at this site to the activity detectable over the liver and precordium are four to six times higher than those found following the injection of 51Cr-labelled red cells. This is consistent with the splenic pooling of 20–40% of the platelets available to the circulation [107–110]; consequently a significantly higher fraction of transfused platelets remains in the circulation after splenectomy.

The pooling of platelets may not be a random process; the spleen appears to select preferentially those platelets with higher adhesive properties. Ljungqvist found increased platelet adhesiveness of splenic-vein platelets of the dog when compared with arterial platelets, and has also shown that the temporary rise in platelet adhesiveness and aggregability which follows haemorrhage is abolished by splenectomy [111–113]. Platelet adhesiveness is increased after splenectomy in man [114, 115], the rabbit [116], and the dog [117], and Steiman *et al.* [118] have produced splenic extracts which inhibit the aggregation of platelets by ADP.

The spleen and the circulating granulocyte

The relationship of the spleen to the circulating granulocyte is still incompletely defined: splenic pooling of [51Cr]chromate-labelled granulocytes is not demonstrable in normal subjects although it is readily apparent in chronic granulocytic leukaemia [119–121].

The injection of adrenaline into the splenic artery initially releases leucocytes from the pulmonary vascular bed, and is followed after an interval of two to three minutes by a supplementary leucocytosis originating from the spleen and other splanchnic sites [122]. Surface counting following the injection of adrenaline in subjects with labelled leucocytes shows a fall in radioactivity in the splenic area and a rise at other sites, indicating a denser accumulation of granulocytes in the marginal pool in the spleen than is present elsewhere [119]. This is consistent with the finding that the total granulocyte pool is not increased by splenectomy: there occurs a shift of granulocytes from the marginal pool to the freely circulating population, which produces leucocytosis when the magnitude of the shift is sufficient [123].

The non-pathological destruction of blood cells

Despite extensive studies of the destruction of red cells in pathological circumstances, the terminal processes by which the normal red cell is destroyed are still incompletely understood. The spleen has long been regarded as one site in which such destruction is active, but the relative importance of intravascular lysis [121], cell fragmentation [91, 125] and erythrophagocytosis is controversial [124]. Electron microscopy has been directed to this problem in only a few species, and significant interspecies differences have been detected. Studies in the normal rat [126] and rabbit [127, 128] have demonstrated phagocytosis of red cells by macrophages in the splenic cords, the marginal zones and the periphery of the white pulp, but the endothelial cells of the sinuses are not involved. The red cells are apparently intact at the time of phagocytosis; processing within the phagosome is not identical in the two species studied but, in both species, granules of ferritin were shown to penetrate the wall of the phagosome to enter the cytoplasm of the macrophage. To a lesser degree, phagocytosis of leucocytes and platelets was also demonstrated [126, 128].

The spleen is neither unique nor indispensible to the normal destruction of the red cell in man, however; there is no evidence that splenectomy significantly alters the lifespan of the red cell in the normal subject [129–136] and it is probable that the removal of senescent cells is a function widely distributed throughout the reticulo-endothelial system. Similar findings have been made with respect to normal platelets, splenectomy leaving the platelet lifespan unaffected [137]. Platelet destruction is detectable in the spleen, liver and bone marrow; on a weight-related basis the spleen is 20 times as efficient as the liver in this respect. Splenectomy is followed by increased destruction at sites other than the spleen [138].

Humoral control of haemopoiesis

Quantitative changes following splenectomy may include persisting leucocytosis [139], reticulocytosis, and sustained megakaryocytosis and thrombocytosis without an increase in platelet lifespan [140, 141]. Such observations led to speculation that the spleen elaborates humoral inhibitors of the production or release of cells from the bone marrow; this concept was central to one view of the causation of hypersplenism [142]. No such humoral agents have been identified and most such observations are satisfactorily explained in terms of the removal of a site of cell destruction or pooling [143].

Despite its inadequacy as an explanation of hypersplenism, it is not entirely certain that no such effect exists [144]. Splenectomy has been claimed to lessen the inhibitory effect of irradiation on the bone marrow [145], and Wetherley-Mein *et al.* [146] found evidence of increased marrow uptake of iron after splenectomy in myeloid metaplasia. Reduction in the reticulocyte count following irradiation of the spleen in the rabbit has been interpreted as due to release of an inhibitory factor [147], and splenectomy leads to increased thymic release of lymphocytes into the blood [148]. It has further been found that feeding raw spleen inhibits the leucocytosis of the splenectomized rat [149]. Such findings are at least suggestive of servocontrol mechanisms, but the mediators remain unidentified.

The picture is complicated by experimental evidence of stimulatory factors released by the spleen. The emergence of early leucocyte forms from the marrow after whole body irradiation has been claimed to be inhibited by splenectomy and stimulated by a lipid-soluble splenic extract [145, 150, 151]. A factor in the serum and spleen of mice has been shown to stimulate mitosis in the surviving stem cells of the bone marrow of the sublethally irradiated animal, although no effect was obtained in intact mice [152]. The factor was detectable in non-cellular material from irradiated spleens, and is possibly related to an α globulin isolated from the ovine spleen which enhances the rate of regeneration of irradiated thymic and bone marrow tissue [153]. The physiological status and clinical relevance of such factors have not yet been defined.

The spleen and immunity

The route of administration affects the distribution of lymphatic sites maximally responsive to an immune challenge, the spleen being preferentially stimulated by intravenous antigen [154, 155]. The effect of splenectomy on immune responsiveness is often unremarkable, but Rowley [156] found that splenectomized human subjects showed subnormal production of haemolysin when challenged with xenotypic red cells.

It is still uncertain whether the spleen contains the

full complement of cells utilized in the primary response [157, 158]; in the rabbit, intravenous primary immunization stimulates the migration of lymphocytes to secondary lymphatic centres including the spleen [159–162]. There is, however, evidence that spleen cells in tissue culture have the capacity for primary antibody production [163–169], although there must always be some doubt with regard to possible prior exposure to cross-reactive antigen in preparations derived from animals not raised in a germ-free environment. Release of antibody and immunocompetent cells has been obtained from the isolated perfused spleen [170–172].

Phagocytosis

The spleen is characterized by the densest accumulation of phagocytic cells in the body; the unique vascular structure of the red pulp provides an exceptionally large population of phagocytic cells in contact with blood having potentially a very slow transit time [173]. The principal phagocytes are the fixed reticular cells in the marginal zones of the lymphoid follicles and the splenic cords, and the free macrophages of the cords and sinuses. The sinus endothelial cells are histologically distinct, have few lysosomes, appear relatively inactive in ingesting particulate material, and probably do not function as phagocytes in normal circumstances [174–177].

The primary function of the splenic macrophage is the clearance from the circulation of particulate material, including cells, micro-organisms, colloidal particles, immune complexes and fibrin monomers [178]. Subsequent processing involves the activity of lysosomally derived enzymes and follows kinetics distinct from those of blood clearance, neither the onset nor the ultimate catabolic rate being related to the initial rate of phagocytosis [179, 180]. The processing sequence may have significant secondary effects, both with regard to iron metabolism (see below) and antibody formation, especially against foreign cells [181].

Macrophages do not appear to be capable of antibody production [182], although there are reports of cells which show both antibody formation and phagocytosis [183, 184]. It has been suggested that preliminary processing by macrophages leads to a state of immunity, whereas primary contact of antigen with lymphocytes provokes tolerance [185], and interaction of macrophage and antigen appears necessary to the primary response [186]. The mechanism of the intermediary action of the macrophage is uncertain, but it may involve solubilization and storage of the antigen, or the synthesis of a coded carrier for the structural sequencing of antibody.

Iron metabolism

Iron in the spleen is derived from the destruction of red cells. An additional, normally minor, source of iron is the siderocyte from which siderotic nodules are removed during its passage through the spleen [187–189]. Erythrophagocytosis results in the enclosure of the red cell by a membrane-bound vacuole, and ferritin granules appear within the cell during its degradation. These come to line the wall of the vacuole and at a later stage enter the cytoplasm of the macrophage [126]. Splenic ferritin may be partially stored, the remainder releasing iron to plasma transferrin. Iron in the spleen constitutes a more labile store than hepatic iron; following the infusion of non-viable red cells containing isotopically labelled haemoglobin iron, splenic radioactivity falls more rapidly than activity related to the liver [190].

The storage of antihaemophilic globulin (factor VIII)

Factor VIII levels in the plasma rise following exercise, surgery, hypothalamic stimulation and adrenaline administration [191–195], suggesting the presence of readily available tissue stores. The post-operative rise does not occur following splenectomy or in splenectomized subjects [193, 196] and perfusion experiments of the normal spleen show increased effluent factor VIII levels [197–199]. Homotransplantation of the spleen to the haemophilic dog produces a rise in factor VIII levels [200–203], but this is of limited duration, and splenectomy in the normal animal does not reduce the circulating level of factor VIII. The increased synthesis of plasma factor VIII in bleeder swine following infusion of normal serum is comparable to the response in patients with von Willebrand's disease: it has been found to be unaffected by splenectomy [204]. The major site of factor VIII synthesis thus appears to be elsewhere—probably the liver—with the spleen acting as a store providing for short-term increases in circulating levels.

Protein synthesis

The spleen is an active site of protein synthesis, principally in relation to cell division and immunoglobulin production following immunization [205, 206]. Production of specific cell-coating IgG is also a function of the spleen; erythrophilic γ-globulin and leucokinin, a leucocyte-associated globulin necessary for phagocytic activity, are reduced in the serum of the dog for four to eight months following splenectomy, probably because the spleen is the primary site of synthesis, with other sites later providing compensatory synthesis following the removal of the organ [207].

PATHOPHYSIOLOGY OF THE SPLEEN

The pathological spleen may give rise to a series of abnormal phenomena, of which the most extensively investigated have been related to the filtration function, the destruction of blood cells, and the secondary consequences of splenic enlargement on the splanchnic circulation. The majority of such abnormalities are not confined to single aetiologically defined diseases, but reflect common functional derangements in diverse splenic conditions.

Red-cell pooling

Surface estimation of radioactivity at the site of the spleen following intravenous injection of [^{51}Cr]chromate-labelled red cells in normal subjects shows a single-phase rapid rise in activity with a half-time of approximately eight to 20 seconds. In many conditions with splenomegaly this is followed by a second phase with a half-time of rise between three and 40 minutes [208–210]. The secondary rise appears with abnormal red cells: cells from patients with hereditary spherocytosis, thalassemia major, autoimmune haemolytic disease and untreated pernicious anaemia accumulate in the spleen when injected into the circulation of normal subjects. In other cases, normal red cells will accumulate in the abnormal spleen, and the slow phase of accumulation of radioactivity appears related to abnormal intrasplenic circulatory pathways in conditions such as primary myeloid metaplasia, chronic myeloid leukaemia, primary hypersplenism, lymphomata and portal hypertension.

In normal subjects, estimates of the volume of distribution of labelled red cells at six and 45 minutes after injection differ by approximately one per cent [211]. In patients with splenomegaly in steady-state conditions, the difference is often considerably greater, commonly between five and 10%, and exceptionally reaching 50% of the total red-cell mass. It is clear that disappearance of cells from the circulation at such rates cannot be the result of red-cell destruction, and it has been shown that the pattern of accumulation in the spleen is compatible with the slow exchange of red cells between the greater circulating red-cell mass of the general circulation and a lesser pool of intrasplenic red cells [212]. Estimates of the parameters of the splenic pool are given in Table 20.1; despite high pooling volumes, the blood flow through the pool is insufficient to provide for the increased splenic blood flow which accompanies splenomegaly, which must therefore be predominantly through the fast pathway.

There is evidence, therefore, for two patterns of transit for red cells through the spleen: the fast pathway is predominant in the normal spleen, while a latent slow pathway immediately accepts abnormal cells, and will admit normal red cells in a structurally abnormal spleen. The anatomical location of the slow pathway is uncertain, but in hereditary spherocytosis and autoimmune haemolytic disease, which show marked red-cell pooling, the splenic cords show a gross excess of red cells [213]. In diseases with abnormal splenic architecture, such as primary myeloid metaplasia, chronic myeloid leukaemia and lymphomata, there is likewise an increased red-cell content in the cords [214] and the pool is presinusal.

Attempts to equate the fast and slow pathways with the anatomically defined 'closed' and 'open' routes imply a highly effective directional vector capable of distinguishing abnormal cells. Evidence for such a mechanism is lacking. A more acceptable hypothesis is that the majority of red cells are committed to the open pathway of the splenic cords, where characteristics of cell shape, deformability or adhesiveness lead to differential impedance to flow, either within the cordal

Table 20.1. Dimensions of the red-cell pool in man*

| | Number of subjects | Volume | | Flow | | Turnover time (min) |
		ml	Percentage of total red-cell mass	ml/min	Percentage of extrasplenic RBC/min	
Myeloproliferative disorders	15	50–710	3–26	2–31	0·1–1·6	11–39
Haemolytic† disorders	8	30–220	2–15	1–8	0·1–0·7	6–44
Polycythaemia vera	7	120–530	3–16	6–115	0·2–4·2	5–38
Miscellaneous	14	30–580	1–48	3–90	0·3–5·8	5–36

* Author's observations (1967).
† Hereditary spherocytosis and autoimmune haemolytic disease.

labyrinth or at the level of the sinus wall. In the structurally abnormal spleen, the flow may be non-selectively impaired by distortion of the pathway between the arteriolar terminations and the sinus wall.

The significance of the splenic pool in anaemic subjects is twofold:

1 the red cells are confined at high concentration in the proximity of cells of substantially higher metabolic rate, including leucocytes and reticular cells. In these circumstances the glucose concentration and pH fall [215–217] and contribute to the conditioning of the red cell for lysis. This has been especially studied with the red cells in hereditary spherocytosis, in which splenic erythrocytes are more fragile than those of the general circulation [218–222] and cross-transfusion studies have demonstrated the contribution of the spleen to the increase in red-cell osmotic fragility [89]; and

2 in subjects in whom erythropoiesis is impaired or already maximally stressed, the red cells in the pool may represent a significant fraction of the red-cell mass which is prevented from effectively contributing to the general circulation, and for which compensation by additional red-cell production is not available.

The whole-body haematocrit/venous haematocrit ratio

Measurement of the plasma volume and red-cell mass with labelled albumin and red cells allows calculation of the 'whole-body haematocrit', which is generally lower than the 'large-vessel haematocrit' of venous blood. The mean ratio of the whole-body haematocrit to venous haematocrit (H_b/H_v) in normal subjects has been found consistently to be in the range between 0·899 and 0·924, with standard deviations between 0·018 and 0·032 [211, 223–228]. Many patients with splenomegaly show raised H_b/H_v ratios [229–232] which are due to the plasma-poor state of the red cells in the splenic red-cell pool [211]. The ratio does not, however, provide a satisfactory index of the mass of pooled red cells; the fraction of the total red-cell mass present in the pool is not the main determinant of the raised ratio, which is more dependent on the increase in splenic pool haematocrit relative to venous haematocrit. This in turn has limits which are especially significant when the haematocrit is high: marked splenic pooling occurs in polycythaemia without a rise in H_b/H_v ratio.

Portal hypertension and splenic blood flow

Portal hypertension. This complicates a significant number of cases with splenomegaly due to blood dyscrasias, the evidence for which is most commonly the expansion of porto-systemic collateral vessels. In some cases it is a contributory cause of gastro-intestinal haemorrhage. Extrasplenic pathology provides an explanation for portal hypertension in many such cases, the lesions including splenic-vein thrombosis, portal-vein thrombosis and intrahepatic infiltration of the portal tracts [233]. There is a residuum of cases in which no extrasplenic structural cause can be found; in these the probability exists of hyperkinetic portal hypertension due to increased splenic blood flow into the portal circulation [234, 235]. This concept is supported by evidence of increased intrasplenic pressure in the presence of splenomegaly due to blood dyscrasias, and this correlates significantly with increased splenic blood flow, which may amount to 15% of the cardiac output when measured by the radioactive [133]xenon surface counting technique [236, 237].

The expansion of blood volume and dilutional anaemia

McFadzean *et al.* [238] demonstrated that patients with cryptogenic splenomegaly show increased plasma volumes which contribute to anaemia by dilution of the red cells in the circulation. Splenectomy was followed by a delayed, but significant, improvement in the anaemia provided that hepatic cirrhosis was not present [239]. Subsequent studies have shown expansion of plasma volume with dilutional anaemia in Gaucher's disease [240], primary myeloid metaplasia, chronic leukaemias, thalassaemia major, haemoglobinopathies with splenomegaly [241, 242], primary hypersplenism [243], Felty's syndrome [244] and tropical splenomegaly [245–247]. The total blood volume increases one to two per cent for every centimetre the spleen enlarges below the costal margin. Splenectomy usually reduces the plasma volume and raises the venous haematocrit, although the correction may be incomplete, especially in the presence of hepatic disease [241, 248]; later-developing hepatic enlargement may lead to relapse.

The cause of the expanded plasma volume is uncertain. In tropical splenomegaly it has been attributed to raised serum globulin levels [245], by analogy with the hypervolaemia of hyperglobulinaemic rabbits and mice [249] and Waldenström's macroglobulinaemia in man [250, 251]. However, the importance of the globulin concentration to blood volume changes in macroglobulinaemia has been questioned [252] and undoubtedly splenomegalic conditions with blood volume expansion occur without significant alterations in the plasma proteins.

Hess *et al.* [253] found increased forearm blood flow and venous capacitance in six patients with dilutional anaemia, and suggested an analogy to the chronic circulatory effects of bradykinin, with stimulation of the renin–angiotensin–aldosterone system, but were unable to demonstrate bradykinin activation in splenic-vein blood [248]. In addition, general expansion of extracellular fluid volume does not appear to accompany the plasma volume expansion of spleno-megaly due to blood dyscrasias [244].

There is some evidence that blood volume expansion is not confined to the plasma compartment; although plasma volume correlates closely with spleen size, there is also a lesser, but still significant, positive correlation in these patients between spleen size and red-cell mass [242, 244]. While it is possible that this could arise from haemodilution producing a secondary stimulus to erythropoiesis [254], it may alternatively reflect a primary expansion of blood volume in response to the increase in intravascular space generated by the pre-sence of the enlarged spleen. In some patients both red-cell mass and plasma volume increase propor-tionately, and no dilutional anaemia supervenes; it is reasonable to suppose that in patients with anaemia, red-cell production has been unable to respond ade-quately [255] so that the contribution of the plasma becomes disproportionately large.

The distribution of the increased volume is not confined to the spleen. Blendis *et al.* [244] could recover no more than 30% of the excess plasma volume from the excised organ. Furthermore, plasma volume con-traction following splenectomy continues slowly over many weeks, probably indicating the slow obliteration of vessels in the splenic bed [238]. It is most probable that a significant proportion of the volume expansion is the consequence of portal hypertension arising from hyperkinetic splenic blood flow, leading to dilation of splanchnic vessels other than those immediately related to the organ.

Haemolysis

Pathological destruction of red cells by the spleen is found in two broadly defined clinical circumstances.

1 *Overtly abnormal red cells* occur in conditions such as hereditary spherocytosis, hereditary elliptocytosis with haemolytic anaemia, and autoimmune haemoly-tic disease of warm-antibody type. In hereditary spherocytosis invariably, and in other conditions frequently, the spleen is the dominant organ of destruction, and the organ usually shows slight to moderate enlargement. Marked shortening of the red-cell lifespan beyond the compensatory capacity of the erythropoietic reserve leads to the classical findings of haemolytic anaemia.

2 In many conditions with *gross splenic enlargement*, including lymphomata, chronic leukaemias, primary myeloid metaplasia, hepatic cirrhosis and lipid storage diseases, a moderate reduction of red-cell survival is found, often to the range of one-quarter to one-half of normal. The red cells may show no overt abnormality beyond minor morphological changes, and there is commonly little evidence of haemolysis with the usual clinical tests. In the presence of a normally responsive bone marrow, no anaemia results. However, in many of these conditions the marrow is incompletely respon-sive and the shortened red-cell lifespan is then a contributory cause of anaemia [255, 256]. It is rare for a spleen showing red-cell pooling not to be associated with accelerated red-cell destruction, but in some cases the pooling and haemolysis are independent correlates of splenomegaly.

The capacity of the macrophage system to remove non-viable cells is high, but has limits estimated at between 20 and 40 times the normal rate of red-cell destruction [89, 190]. Acute loading in normal subjects provides evidence of the competitive removal of the more severely damaged cells [190], and retarded clear-ance occurs when the transfused load exceeds about five per cent of the normal red-cell mass [179]. In these circumstances, the fraction of the red cells cleared by the liver and spleen is proportional to blood flow, the spleen removing 12–15% of the total load [257].

Amongst the variables which may affect the effi-ciency of the pathological spleen in clearing abnormal cells from the circulation are the reactive increase in mass of the spleen in response to haemolysis [258], splenic blood flow, filtration pressure in the splenic pulp, and the saturation characteristics of the macro-phage system in the presence of chronic haemolysis [275]. Studies of the circulatory clearance of modified cells, usually heat-treated red cells, provide some measure of overall splenic clearing capacity [259–265], but do not identify the component factors or their relationship to the actual current load. In hepatic cirrhosis, clearance rates correlate well with the degree of splenic enlargement, but poorly with elevation of portal pressure [259]; in homozygous haemoglobin C disease, sickle-thalassaemia and sickle-cell disease, clearance rates may be normal or subnormal [264].

In the majority of severe haemolytic states there are demonstrable abnormalities of the red cell. Experi-mentally, splenic destruction is prominent with heredi-tary spherocytes, heat-induced spherocytes, lipid-depleted cells [266], cells coated with metallic cations [267] or treated with sulphydryl-blocking agents [268], thalassaemic cells [212, 266, 269] and sickle-cells [270]. Cells coated with incomplete isoantibodies [261, 271, 272] and autoimmune 'warm' antibodies are fre-quently subject to splenic localization. Quantitative factors are also involved: brief incubation of red cells at 50°C leads to sphering and uptake by the spleen while longer incubation leads to fragmentation and destruction in the liver [262]; exposure to low doses of sulphydryl inhibitors leads to cell destruction in the spleen, while higher doses produce predominantly extrasplenic destruction [260, 268]; very low degrees of sensitization with anti-B isoagglutinin produce splenic uptake, while higher levels produce hepatic uptake.

Similar dose-related patterns are found with non-complement-fixing IgG antibodies such as incomplete anti-D [273, 274]. In autoimmune haemolytic disease of warm-antibody type, Rosse [276] has shown that following splenectomy up to 10 times as much antibody must be present on the cell surface to produce the degree of haemolysis present before splenectomy. The role of the spleen in haemolysis is therefore characterized by the organ being sensitive to lesser degrees of cell abnormality than are other sites.

The mechanisms by which these widely differing abnormalities lead to red-cell trapping are incompletely defined. Impairment of flow through the splenic cords appears to be of primary importance, mediated by reduced deformability of the red cell [277]. The filtrability of red cells provides a measure of the difficulty with which they penetrate the microvasculature [278] and is principally dependent on cell rigidity, and possibly surface adhesiveness [279]. Red-cell rigidity is a function of the state of the cell contents, as in the sickled cell, of cell shape, especially sphering, and possibly of the intrinsic properties of the cell membrane. Decreased deformability has been demonstrated in hereditary spherocytosis, sickle-cell disease and trait, and homozygous haemoglobin C disease [278, 280–282], and is generated at the membrane level by conditions of metabolic deprivation with reduced intracellular ATP [283], low pH [281, 284] and low oxygen tension [277], all of which are characteristic of the environment provided by the splenic red-cell pool. These conditions also favour fragmentation of red cells, leading to the formation of rigid spheres, to which the trauma of passage through small diameter vessels also contributes [285].

The splenic vasculature appears to provide pathways of critically small diameter both in the cords and in the walls of the sinuses. The minimal diameter of a cylindrical channel penetrable by a red cell is approximately 3 μm, with somewhat smaller diameters passable where the channel length is short, as in the sinus wall [277, 283]. With impaired cellular deformability such pathways will become impassable, and potentially traumatic to the red cell. Splenectomy results in an increase in the minimal diameter in the general circulation to approximately 4 μm [286], permitting the continued circulation of cells which would otherwise fail to survive.

Inclusion bodies provide a special circumstance predisposing to the loss of cell membrane which is characteristic of fragmentation. They are found in thalassaemia major [287–289], haemoglobin H disease [290, 291] and Heinz-body anaemias, and are removed during circulation through the spleen with partial loss from the cell of membrane fragments [292].

It has been found difficult to reconcile the quantity of isotope desposited in the spleen from isotope-labelled red cells with the total cell loss from the circulation, even in conditions in which the spleen has been shown to be predominantly responsible for haemolysis [293]. One cause of this, demonstrable in hereditary spherocytosis, is the progressive conditioning of red cells in the spleen for haemolysis elsewhere, presumably as the result of partial fragmentation during successive passages through the organ. A second cause is the liberation of haemoglobin from cells destroyed by the spleen, and released to the plasma for uptake elsewhere: this has been found experimentally to accompany the extravascular haemolysis of Rh-sensitized cells [271] and to a minor extent phenylhydrazine haemolysis [288, 294]. It has also been found in severe autoimmune haemolytic anaemia [212].

Phagocytosis of red cells in the spleen is found to vary in prominence in various haemolytic diseases. The predominant cell involved is the monocytic macrophage, and erythrophagocytosis appears to provide a proliferative stimulus to the macrophage system [258]. Partial phagocytosis, with incomplete destruction of the cell, can occur [295] and morphological injury with sphering and fragmentation has been shown to result from the specific adhesion of IgG-coated red cells to the monocyte [296]. Phagocytosis is frequently regarded as a non-specific end-stage in the destruction of red cells subjected to widely varying types of injury; the *in-vitro* incubation of red cells permits their phagocytosis in the absence of antibody or complement [297]. Human monocytes will also phagocytose red cells sensitized with incomplete antibodies in the absence of complement [298] and have specific receptor sites for IgG and C3 which may function independently or cooperatively in inducing phagocytosis [299]; the possible role of such receptors in the particular circumstances of the splenic removal of sensitized red cells remains to be determined.

The spleen also contributes to autoimmune haemolysis by providing a site for antibody production [300]. The effect of splenectomy on autoimmune antibody titres is variable: occasional cases show marked falls in serum titre, which indicate the spleen to be the principal source of antibody in such cases. Possibly of greater importance is the potential of the splenic pulp to provide a site for the close approximation of antibody-forming cells to the target red cells, thereby facilitating the critical transfer of antibody to the red-cell surface.

Splenomegaly and the platelet

That the spleen is closely involved in the production of thrombocytopenia in certain pathological states is shown by the effectiveness of splenectomy in idiopathic thombocytopenic purpura (ITP), remission being induced in 60–90% of cases in various series [301–309]. There are three principal mechanisms whereby the spleen may contribute to thrombocytopenia:

1 by increasing the size of the splenic storage pool of platelets;
2 by destruction of platelets within the organ; and
3 by producing specific antiplatelet antibody.

While splenomegaly bears no necessary relationship to platelet lifespan, there is an approximate correlation between the size of the spleen and the fraction of the total platelet population which is in the splenic platelet pool [109, 110]; as many as 90% of the total platelets may be present in an enlarged spleen [108]. A reactive increase in platelet production provides partial compensation for the resulting thrombocytopenia, although this is seldom complete and does not reach the maximal levels of output obtained in response to platelet destruction [310].

The destruction of platelets by the spleen has been demonstrated by estimating platelet numbers in arterial and venous blood samples obtained at operation [311]. In ITP, the thrombocytopenia induced by the infusion of plasma from patients into normal recipients is greatly diminished in splenectomized recipients [312]. Further, the circulating lifespan of platelets in this condition has been shown to be shortened, and may return to normal after splenectomy [313, 314]. Surface counting techniques for identifying the sites of destruction of ^{51}Cr-labelled platelets have indicated excessive secondary accumulation of radioactivity exclusively or predominantly in the spleen in more than half the patients with ITP studied [315–320]; similar results have been obtained in onyalai [321]. Splenic destruction has also been demonstrated in some thrombocytopenic patients with hepatic cirrhosis, primary myeloid metaplasia, thalassaemia, primary hypersplenism [316] and Gaucher's disease [322]. As in the case of the red cell, there is a tendency for mildly damaged platelets to be subject to splenic destruction while more severely damaged platelets are destroyed by the liver [323, 324].

'Hypersplenism'

'Hyersplenism' denotes a syndrome comprising:
1 splenomegaly;
2 reduction in the circulating levels of one or more cell lines in the peripheral blood, producing anaemia, leucopenia, neutropenia and thrombocytopenia, but without the appearance of immature cells; and
3 a bone marrow which is normal or hypercellular, especially with respect to the cell lines depleted in the peripheral blood. Retrospectively, the term may be justified by the correction of the deficits by splenectomy.

The criteria for hypersplenism are met in a series of conditions, some of which are 'primary', in the sense that no other recognizable disease is present, while the remainder are 'secondary', with the pattern of hypersplenism superimposed on existing disease (Table 20.2). The primary conditions of hypersplenism are themselves syndromes [243, 325–330], distinguished principally by the pattern of deficits in the peripheral blood. There appear, however, to be no unequivocal pathological characteristics by which these various syndromes can be shown to differ, and provisionally the term 'primary hypersplenism' could reasonably be applied to any condition within the spectrum.

With the clearer definition of the pathogenesis of conditions such as hereditary spherocytosis and idiopathic thrombocytopenic purpura, these diseases have ceased to be regarded as instances of hypersplenism, so that the residuum of conditions to which the term is applied inevitably includes those for which the mechanisms involved are least well understood. Three principal concepts have been proposed to explain the cellular deficits of hypersplenism.

1 The spleen has been regarded as the source of inhibitors of maturation or release of precursor cells in the marrow [142, 331, 332]. As discussed previously, this proposal lacks experimental support, and the evidence for an influence by the spleen on haemopoiesis does not suggest a model relevant to the syndrome defined.

2 Cell destruction by the spleen was proposed by Doan [327] as the principal cause of hypersplenism. The importance of the spleen as a site of cell destruction has been shown in many conditions, but the general proposition that the enlargement of the spleen is in itself sufficient cause for the increased intrasplenic destruction of red cells, leucocytes and platelets is certainly not valid. There is evidence for the spleen in portal hypertension affecting the lifespan of normal red cells [333], but in most circumstances marked haemolysis is dependent on abnormalities of the red cell and the role of the spleen is essentially passive in removing the defective cells presented to it. The moderate shortening of red-cell survival commonly found in conditions with marked splenomegaly is not the sole cause of anaemia when present, and is not invariably corrected by splenectomy [240]. Histological evidence of splenic phagocytosis of peripheral blood cells may not be prominent in hypersplenism [334], and conditions with splenomegaly do not necessarily produce high clearance rates from the peripheral blood of cells damaged *in vitro* [264, 335, 336]. There is therefore little support for the concept of the cytopenias arising primarily from pathologically aggressive macrophage activity.

3 An autoimmune basis for hypersplenism has been

Table 20.2. Principal conditions associated with 'hypersplenism'

	References
A. Primary hypersplenism	330, 345
Primary splenic panhaematopenia*	327, 328
Primary splenic neutropenia	326
Primary hypersplenic pancytopenia*	329
Splenic anaemia of thrombocytopenic type	325
Non-tropical idiopathic splenomegaly	330
Simple splenic hyperplasia	345
B. Secondary hypersplenism	
1 Acute infections with splenomegaly	344
2 Chronic infections	
Splenic tuberculosis	349
Brucellosis	
Malaria	
Kala-azar	346
3 Inflammatory conditions and granulomata	
Felty's syndrome	347, 348, 353, 359
Sarcoidosis	360
4 Congestive splenomegaly	354, 355, 357
5 Storage diseases	
Gaucher's disease	322, 352
Hurler's syndrome	
6 Leukaemias and lymphomata	350, 351, 356
7 Miscellaneous	
Primary myeloid metaplasia	358
Thalassaemia major	
Splenic haemangioma	
Hypersplenism–hypogammaglobulinaemia syndrome	361, 362, 363, 364, 365
Hyperthyroidism	366
Splenic mastocytosis	384
Carcinomatosis	606

* Probably synonyms.

proposed [337], affecting both the spleen itself and the peripheral blood cells. This concept has not been exhaustively explored, but the direct red-cell antiglobulin reaction is positive in a proportion of patients with primary hypersplenism [330], and 'an abnormal immunological reaction to an infective agent' has been suggested to be present in tropical (idiopathic) splenomegaly [338].

Misunderstanding with respect to hypersplenism has arisen from three principal causes:

1 it has been regarded as a process and not a syndrome;

2 it has been felt necessary to find a single common explanation for the deficits in the peripheral blood which would apply to each of the cell lines affected; and

3 the postulated mechanisms have been assumed to depend upon an exaggeration of the normal functions of the organ, which are themselves incompletely understood.

However, the most predictable effects of splenic enlargement are expansion of blood volume and red-cell pooling, which are epiphenomena of splenomegaly and unrelated to normal splenic function. These, together with platelet pooling, contribute significantly to anaemia and thrombocytopenia, and other factors, such as shortened cell lifespan, are commonly present. It is clear that no single factor predictably accounts for the expression of the syndrome in every case.

Haemorrhagic disorders

The only haemorrhagic disorder commonly associated with isolated splenic disease is purpura secondary to thrombocytopenia. Haemangioma of the spleen has been a rare cause of the Kasabach–Merritt syndrome: thrombocytopenia, hypofibrinogenaemia, low normal levels of factors V and VIII, fibrin split products in the serum and reduced fibrinogen survival have been shown in one paediatric patient [339], and less complete but similar observations were made in another

[340]. A haemorrhagic disorder has been described in an adult with angiosarcoma of the spleen [341], but in this case the interpretation of the findings was complicated by concurrent corticosteroid therapy.

Hyperfibrinolysis has been found in Chinese patients with cryptogenic splenomegaly and was corrected by splenectomy [342]. A coagulation defect with thrombocytopenia, hypofibrinogenaemia and a low plasminogen level accompanied idiopathic splenome-galy in one reported case; the defects were corrected by splenectomy [343].

SPLENOMEGALY

Pathological processes contributing to enlargement of the spleen include:
1 acute, subacute and chronic inflammation;

Table 20.3. The principal causes of splenomegaly

A. Infection
1 *Acute:* septicaemias, virus hepatitis, infectious mono-nucleosis, typhoid, paratyphoid, brucellosis, typhus, plague, anthrax, relapsing fever, tularaemia
2 *Subacute and chronic:* subacute bacterial endocarditis, chronic meningococcal septicaemia, brucellosis, tuberculosis, histoplasmosis, malaria, leishmaniasis (visceral; infantile), syphilis (congenital; secondary; gummatous), bilharziasis (early; chronic), trypanosomiasis

B. Other inflammatory and granulomatous conditions
Rheumatoid disease; Felty's syndrome
Systemic lupus erythematosus
Acute rheumatism
Sarcoidosis
Berylliosis

C. Congestive splenomegaly
1 *Intrahepatic portal hypertension:* portal cirrhosis, post-necrotic cirrhosis, biliary cirrhosis, hepatolenticular degeneration, haemochromatosis, congenital hepatic fibrosis, hepatic venous occlusion, hepatic sarcoidosis

2 *Extrahepatic portal hypertension:*
(a) Portal vein: cavernous malformation, thrombosis, stenosis, atresia, arteriovenous aneurysm; lympha-denopathy, abscess or neoplastic deposits at porta hepatis
(b) Splenic vein: angiomatous malformation, thrombosis, stenosis, atresia, arteriovenous fistula; occlusion due to pancreatic cyst, carcinoma or aneurysm of splenic artery
3 *Cardiac:* congestive cardiac failure; constrictive pericarditis.

D. Haematological diseases
1 *Haemolytic diseases:*
Hereditary spherocytosis
Hereditary elliptocytosis with haemolytic anaemia
Autoimmune haemolytic disease ('warm' antibody type)
Erythroblastosis foetalis
2 *Malignancy:*
Acute leukaemia
Chronic myeloid leukaemia
Chronic lymphocytic leukaemia
Reticuloendotheliosis

Malignant lymphomata
Malignant histiocytosis
Histiocytic medullary reticulosis
3 *Haemoglobinopathies:*
Thalassaemia major
Haemoglobin SS disease
Haemoglobin SC disease
Sickle-thalassaemia
4 *Miscellaneous:*
Primary myeloid metaplasia
Erythroleukaemia
Polycythaemia vera
Idiopathic splenomegaly
Megaloblastic anaemias
Iron-deficiency anaemia
Myelomatosis

E. Storage diseases
Gaucher's disease
Niemann–Pick disease
Tay–Sachs' disease
Idiopathic histiocytosis
Tangier disease
Familial hyperlipoproteinaemia (type I)
Hurler's syndrome

F. Neoplastic diseases
1 *Benign:* haemangioma, lymphangioma, fibroma, hamar-toma
2 *Malignant:*
Primary: angiosarcoma, lymphosarcoma, fibrosarcoma, plasmacytoma.
Secondary: carcinoma, melanoma

G. Cysts
1 *Cysts:* echinococcus, cystic haemangioma, cystic lym-phangioma, dermoid
2 *Pseudocysts:* traumatic, post-infarction

H. Miscellaneous
Hyperthyroidism
Amyloidosis
Albers–Schönberg disease
Splenic mastocytosis
Congenital erythropoietic porphyria
Hereditary haemorrhagic telangiectasia

2 hyperplasia of the splenic reticulum;

3 granuloma formation;

4 amyloid infiltration;

5 lipid storage;

6 compensatory and metaplastic haemopoiesis;

7 congestive splenomegaly with raised splenic venous pressure;

8 red-cell pooling;

9 neoplasia; and

10 cyst formation.

Commonly, more than one process is present and a strictly satisfactory classification on a pathological or aetiological basis is not available. Table 20.3 provides a summary of the principal conditions associated with splenomegaly.

Massive splenomegaly in temperate climates is most commonly due to chronic myeloid leukaemia, primary myeloid metaplasia, Gaucher's disease and primary hypersplenism. Chronic lymphocytic leukaemia, lymphomata and congestive splenomegaly may also produce a grossly enlarged spleen, although in these conditions the degree of splenic enlargement is usually less conspicuous.

The clinical significance of splenomegaly is that when detected it implies, almost without exception, a pathological circumstance which must be pursued to the point of diagnosis. The relationship of the spleen to specific conditions is considered elsewhere in appropriate sections: some circumstances in which the spleen is especially prominent are outlined below.

IDIOPATHIC SPLENOMEGALY

In many parts of the world significant, and sometimes massive, splenomegaly occurs in the absence of clearly defined aetiological factors. Such syndromes are commonly distinguished by geographical terms such as Bengal, Algerian, Colombian or Egyptian splenomegaly. With the exception of Egyptian splenomegaly, in which bilharziasis appears frequently to be implicated, evidence of aetiology is scanty and it is uncertain to what extent the similarities in the syndromes represent merely the limited common expression of diverse processes leading to splenomegaly. The three syndromes to be described reflect significant attempts to make rational generalizations concerning the features of idiopathic splenomegaly in defined circumstances and are not inclusive of all the variants which may occur.

Primary hypersplenism has been studied by Dacie *et al.* [330] under the synonym 'non-tropical idiopathic splenomegaly'. Morphological findings in the spleen were compared with those of a matching series of apparently normal spleens removed during gastric or oesophageal surgery: there was no single unequivocal pattern common to all the abnormal spleens, but some showed loss of definition of the cellular shells of the lymphoid follicles, with greater intermixture of small and large lymphocytes, an increase in the mitotic figures in the follicles and an appreciable increase in follicular reticulin. Other features included dilatation of the venous sinuses, an increase in small lymphoid foci and macrophages, and erythrophagocytosis. Clinical findings included gross splenomegaly in all 10 patients, hepatomegaly without evidence of hepatic cirrhosis in seven, and anaemia in all patients, accompanied by minor changes in red-cell morphology and slight or moderate reticulocytosis, severe leukopenia and neutropenia, slight or moderate lymphopenia, and moderate thrombocytopenia. Positive direct red-cell antiglobulin reactions were found in five patients, and in two of three subjects in whom blood volumes were measured there was hypervolaemia, confirming a feature of the condition observed by others [241, 243]. Splenectomy led to haematological improvement 'in most instances', with neutropenia being the least responsive feature. The authors suggested that the condition might represent an autoimmune disease expressed by lymphoreticular proliferation rather than antibody production.

The tropical splenomegaly syndrome is found widely in West and East Africa and India, and has an especially high incidence in parts of New Guinea. It consists essentially of chronic, usually massive, splenomegaly in the absence of known causes of splenic enlargement, and diagnosis requires the exclusion of bilharziasis, leishmaniasis, hepatic cirrhosis, typhoid, brucellosis, primary myeloid metaplasia, lymphomata and haemoglobinopathies. Hepatomegaly is commonly present, with a smooth palpable border, and frequently the left lobe is disproportionately affected [338]. The spleen shows a marked reduction in the prominence of the white pulp, but Ugandan spleens may show foci of lymphocytic proliferation. In addition, there is dilatation of the venous sinuses, giant macrophages which may show erythro-leucophagocytosis, and sometimes foci of erythropoiesis. Fibrosis of the spleen and reticulin formation in the red pulp are not prominent. The liver shows dilatation of the sinusoids with patchy lymphocytic infiltration of the sinusoids and portal tracts and Kupffer-cell hyperplasia, often with evidence of phagocytosis [367–369]. Parenchymal hepatic lesions are minimal and hepatic architecture is preserved. The severity of the hepatic lesions does not closely parallel the degree of splenomegaly. Lymphocytosis and lymphocytic infiltration of the bone marrow have been described in Nigerian cases [370].

Anaemia is almost invariably present, and may be exacerbated during pregnancy; leucopenia and thrombocytopenia are common [371, 378]. The intensity of the anaemia correlates with the degree of spleno-megaly; there is shortening of the red-cell lifespan, sometimes with evidence of frank haemolysis, and red-cell pooling. A major factor is expansion of the blood volume, leading to dilutional anaemia, so that anaemia may be present despite a normal red-cell mass [246]. The peripheral-blood deficits are usually corrected by splenectomy [245]. Serological reactions may be abnormal: there is a high incidence of positive reactions for rheumatoid factor [372], cold agglutinins of anti-i specificity, and high titres of malarial antibody [373]. Serum IgM levels may be markedly raised [374, 375, 383]. No specific defect in humoral or cellular immunity was detected in a limited series of Ugandan patients [376], and phytohaemagglutinin-induced blastic transformation of lymphocytes is normal [383].

The aetiology of the condition remains conjectural despite much circumstantial evidence of a relationship with malaria: the areas where the condition is found are malarious; malarial antibody titres tend to be high in affected individuals; hepatic sinusoidal infiltration with lymphocytes is common in areas of high malaria incidence [377]; prolonged antimalarial therapy may lead to reduction in spleen size [370, 379]; *Plasmodium malariae* has been recovered from the blood in a high proportion of the cases in one series [371]; and sickle-cell trait has been reported absent from patients with the syndrome [380]. Since gross splenomegaly is a feature of the chronic malaria of childhood rather than adult life, it has been proposed that the tropical splenomegaly syndrome results from an abnormal immunological response to malaria leading to persistent splenic enlargement [338]. However, others have not confirmed the incidence of parasitaemia, and have suggested that the condition is a lymphoreticular proliferative disorder [376] possibly related to chronic lymphocytic leukaemia [370].

Despite the improvement in haematological parameters following splenectomy, it has been suggested that this should be considered only after prolonged trial of antimalarial therapy: mortality rates may be as high as 20% within a few months of operation [245] and death from cerebral malaria following splenectomy has been reported [370, 379].

Cryptogenic splenomegaly of Chinese subjects appears to differ in several respects from the tropical splenomegaly syndrome. Splenomegaly is associated with a remarkable degree of hyperplasia of the venous sinuses and efferent venous vessels, and there is variable fibrosis of the pulp, both peritrabecular and periarterial, which in some cases may be virtually obliterative. Splenic infarction is not uncommon and leads to pain and tenderness in the organ. There is a high incidence of hepatic parenchymal disease similar to post-necrotic scarring, approximately two-thirds of patients being affected [239, 381]. Lesser degrees of hepatic involvement are found in other cases. Portal hypertension is commonly found and there is a high incidence of portal-vein thrombosis. Anaemia, leucopenia and thrombocytopenia are frequently present: haemolysis and haemodilution contribute to the anaemia; splenectomy leads to reduced haemolysis [382] and correction of the dilutional anaemia in those cases in which hepatic involvement is not prominent [238, 239]. There is some evidence that splenectomy may slow the development of the hepatic lesions.

CONGESTIVE SPLENOMEGALY

Congestive splenomegaly is a condition of the spleen resulting from raised splenic venous pressure. The causes are diverse (Table 20.3), but the pathological changes in the spleen are similar regardless of the causal condition, although the more distant the site of venous obstruction is from the spleen, the less intense the lesions tend to be [385]. The duration of venous hypertension appears to be more important in the development of congestive splenomegaly than the height of venous pressure. The raised venous pressure is conducted to the splenic pulp and can be estimated manometrically from the intrasplenic pressure [386]. Total blood flow through the spleen tends to increase despite the venous obstruction [387].

Splenomegaly is common in portal hypertension whatever the cause, although it may be difficult to assess clinically in the presence of ascites. At autopsy, splenomegaly has been found in approximately 70% of cases of portal cirrhosis, although clinical estimates are lower [388], and there is a tendency for the largest spleens to be associated with the most advanced degrees of hepatic cirrhosis. The degree of enlargement varies considerably: in one series the splenic weight varied from 500 to 2700 g, with a mean of 878 g [389].

Two principal factors contribute to the splenomegaly: venous congestion itself may produce a threefold increase in spleen size, and cellular proliferation adds further to the enlargement. The capsule and trabeculae are thickened, and histologically there are periarterial and perifollicular haemorrhages, which become organized to form concentrically layered nodules of fibrous tissue. This may hyalinize, and in the presence of trapped iron-containing pigment, may produce siderotic nodules up to 0·5 mm in diameter. The haemorrhages tend to appear in the region of terminations of the penicillate vessels and apparently do not result from rupture of arteries or trabecular veins [389]. Widening of the splenic cords is usually present; there is macrophage and fibroblast proliferation and an increase in fibrous tissue, which varies inversely with the blood cell content of the cords [385]. The follicles may be reduced in size, mainly as the result of perifollicular fibrosis. The venous sinuses are prominent and their walls thickened and collagenized. Splenic veins show intimal thickening and tortuosity, and thrombosis may supervene on endophlebitis.

In the presence of hepatic cirrhosis, anaemia may result from haemorrhage, impaired erythropoiesis [256], haemodilution, folate deficiency and haemolysis in which the spleen frequently plays a major role [390]. Thrombocytopenia and leucopenia each appear in approximately 30% of cases of hepatic cirrhosis, with a reportedly higher incidence in bilharziasis [355]. The leucocytic response to haemorrhage may be suppressed. Thrombocytopenia and leucopenia are uncommon with congestive splenomegaly and only rarely of sufficient severity to warrant surgical intervention.

Porta-caval anastomoses have a variable effect on the haematological status: improvement has been reported in approximately one-third of cases [393–396], but some patients remain severely affected despite the shunt [397] and subsequent splenectomy may be required. Splenectomy commonly (but not invariably) corrects the thrombocytopenia and leucopenia of portal hypertension, but with the exception of cases of splenic-vein thrombosis this is not, in isolation, an optimal procedure: it does not correct portal hypertension [391, 392] and in patients showing recurrent haemorrhage the period free from haemorrhage is relatively short [354]. In addition, significant portal-systemic venous collaterals may be interrupted, and subsequent surgery compromised by obliteration of the splenic vein. With extrahepatic obstruction treated with a splenorenal anastomosis, splenectomy is part of the primary operation; in other circumstances in which splenectomy is considered for the correction of peripheral blood cell deficits, it may be advisable to combine this with a shunting procedure, provided that this is not contra-indicated on other grounds [355].

MONOCYTE-MACROPHAGE DISORDERS

There is a heterogeneous group of disorders, principally characterized by excessive proliferation within the macrophage system, which become of importance haematologically mainly because of secondary cytopenias and recognizable hepato-splenomegaly. They are diverse in aetiology and pathogenesis and are considered conveniently together because of the diagnostic problems which many of them present in common.

Hereditary storage disorders

These disorders arise from excessive storage within the macrophage system of diverse molecular forms, especially lipids and mucopolysaccharides. Extensive studies were undertaken in the past to determine whether the stored materials arise from excessive synthesis, the production of aberrant molecular forms, or defective catabolism. It is now clear that the central defect in most instances is deficient (though rarely absent) activity of an enzyme required for the catabolic degradation of the stored substance.

The *sphingolipidoses* provide examples of storage diseases due to inherited deficiencies in enzymes required for the lysosomal degradation of sphingolipids. Sphingolipids have an acylated sphingosine (ceramide) as a common structure, and the principal derivatives differ in the composition of an attached polysaccharide chain. Table 20.4 summarizes their structure; during catabolism, the glycosidic linkages of the carbohydrate must be broken sequentially before the ceramide can be hydrolysed. Consequently, when the enzyme activity required to degrade the polysaccharide is diminished, the residual molecule accumulates *in situ*. The globosides are found in all mammalian cell membranes, and consequently require catabolic degradation following the phagocytosis of cells, including leucocytes, platelets and erythrocytes. Gangliosides are acidic sphingolipids and are found predominantly in the central nervous sytem.

Other storage disorders arise from inherited defects in the catabolism of lipid and mucopolysaccharides, and in the synthesis of lipid transport proteins.

Acquired disorders

These disorders may simulate some aspects of the hereditary storage disorders. One mechanism is the pathologically excessive turnover of cells to a degree sufficient to exceed the maximum capacity of the catabolic pathways.

Idiopathic histiocytosis

This comprises a group of disorders of unknown aetiology in which there is histiocytic proliferation and granuloma formation. The extent of the tissue involvement is variable: it may be either solitary or multifocal in *eosinophilic granuloma of bone*, and is diffusely distributed in the *Lettere–Siwe syndrome*.

The principal features of representative forms of these conditions are outlined in the following sections:

Gaucher's disease (glucosyl ceramide lipidosis) is a familial sphingolipidosis due to deficient activity of β glucocerebrosidase [398, 399], which leads to excessive accumulation of glucosyl ceramide in tissues, erythrocytes and plasma. There are probably several different mutant forms of the enzyme and the pattern of inheritance is consistent with an autosomal-recessive character of variable penetrance [404]. Clinically, three principal forms are distinguished: in the *adult* form

Table 20.4. Sphingolipid storage diseases

Sphingomyelin

$$\text{CERAMIDE} \overset{(1)}{\text{------}} \text{phosphate} \text{------} \text{choline}$$

Globoside

$$\text{CERAMIDE} \overset{(5)}{\text{------}} \text{glucose} \overset{(4)}{\text{------}} \text{galactose} \overset{(3)}{\text{------}} \text{galactose} \overset{(2)}{\text{------}} \text{N. acetylgalactosamine}$$

Ganglioside

$$\text{N. acetylneuraminic acid}$$
$$|$$
$$\text{CERAMIDE} \overset{(9)}{\text{------}} \text{glucose} \overset{(8)}{\text{------}} \text{galactose} \overset{(7)}{\text{------}} \text{N. acetylgalactosamine} \overset{(6)}{\text{------}} \text{galactose}$$

Substrate	Enzyme	Deficiency disease
Sphingomyelin	1 Sphingomyelinase	Niemann–Pick disease
Globoside	2 Hexosaminidase A & B	Sandhoff's disease
	3 α-galactosidase	Fabry's disease
	4 β-galactosidase	Lactosyl ceramidosis
	5 β-glucosidase	Gaucher's disease
Ganglioside	6 β-galactosidase	Generalized gangliosidosis
	7 Hexosaminidase A	Tay–Sachs' disease
		Sandhoff's disease
	8 β-galactosidase	Lactosyl ceramidosis
	9 β-glucosidase	Gaucher's disease

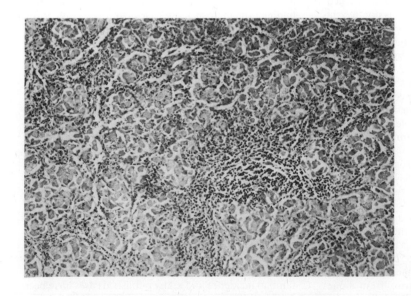

Fig. 20.4. Section of spleen in Gaucher's disease (H & E) showing extensive replacement of splenic pulp by nests of Gaucher cells. (By courtesy of Dr C. Pichyangkura.)

there is no neurological involvement, whereas in the rare *infantile* form, early and severe neurological involvement occurs. Findings are intermediate in the *juvenile* form. The adult form has a conspicuously high incidence in Ashkenazi Jews.

The predominant pathological finding is the Gaucher cell, resulting from the accumulation of glucosyl ceramide in the lysosomal membranes of tissue macrophages [400–403]. The typical Gaucher cell is 20–80 μm in diameter, with one or multiple small eccentric nuclei (Fig. 20.4). The abundant cytoplasm shows a finely wrinkled appearance due to fibrillae, which by electron microscopy appear as elongated membrane-bound inclusion bodies consisting of longitudinally oriented arrays of tubular fibrils [322, 405]. The glucosyl ceramide probably arises from ingested blood cells, of which the neutrophils, with their high turnover rate and high glycolipid content, are probably the major source [407]. Phagocytosed remnants of red cells [405–407], leucocytes [407, 408] and platelets [322] may be found in Gaucher cells, in addition to ferritin in some cases [410–412].

In the *adult* variant the principally affected organs are the spleen, liver, bone marrow and lymph nodes. With rare exceptions the spleen is enlarged [428], the average weight in adult cases being approximately 2·8 kg, and in children 780 g [414, 415], while spleen weights between six and eight kg have been recorded [415, 416]. There is extensive replacement of the splenic pulp with Gaucher cells, often in groups or nests, and haemorrhages, fibrosis and congestion with red cells occur.

Haematological findings include anaemia, leucopenia and thrombocytopenia. Anaemia is not invariably present, but tends to be slowly progressive after onset. Usually the red cells are normochromic, and may show microcytosis; a macrocytic anaemia has also been described [417]. The anaemia is commonly ascribed to replacement infiltration of the marrow with Gaucher cells [418], and in advanced cases this is supported by the presence of extramedullary haemopoiesis and leuco-erythroblastosis. Splenomegaly may result in dilutional anaemia [240]: this may be corrected by splenectomy, but later relapse has been observed, presumably because of progression of the disease with organomegaly elsewhere, especially of the liver. Haemorrhage secondary to thrombocytopenia may be a contributory factor. Moderate shortening of the red-cell lifespan is sometimes found [240, 409], and occasional cases show a frankly haemolytic anaemia with spherocytosis and reticulocytosis [416].

Thrombocytopenia is common [352] and may be accompanied by purpura. As with anaemia, thrombocytopenia has been assumed to arise from bone-marrow infiltration, but limited studies indicate that splenic destruction of platelets is sometimes a factor [322]. Splenectomy usually improves the thrombocytopenia [352, 419, 420], but the correction may be incomplete. Removal of the spleen may also be considered for relief of local pain and discomfort, dilutional anaemia and haemolysis; however, there is no evidence that splenectomy affects the underlying disease process, and the operation may be followed by extension of osseous and hepatic lesions [415, 420, 421]. In addition, following splenectomy there may be raised levels of plasma and erythrocyte glucosyl ceramide, which slowly decline about six months later, suggesting deposition in residual sites of the reticulo-endothelial system [457].

Other findings in Gaucher's disease include raised levels of plasma acid phosphatase, monocytosis and, in one instance, a haemorrhagic syndrome associated with hypofibrinogenaemia [422].

The *infantile* (acute) form of the disease appears in the first year of life with retarded development, multiple neurological defects, hepato-splenomegaly, more rapidly progressive haematological deficits, and an early fatal outcome. The Gaucher cells are found principally in the thymus, tonsils, lungs, adrenals and lymphatic tissue of the gastro-intestinal tract. The cerebral cortex shows vacuolated pyramidal cells [414], and the neurones are predominantly degenerative, rather than showing the 'ballooning' and distension found in other lipid storage disorders.

The *juvenile* (subacute) form is even less common: there is hepato-splenomegaly, Gaucher cells in the bone marrow, and neurological involvement developing later than in the acute form. The neurological findings distinguish these cases from the adult form, although a few cases have been described in which the expression of the neurological deficits was delayed until adult life.

Acquired Gaucher cells. Gaucher cells are not pathognomonic of Gaucher's disease; they may also be present in the bone marrow and spleen in chronic myeloid leukaemia in the absence of glucocerebrosidase deficiency [407, 408, 413]. It is probable that they arise as the result of saturation of the normal catabolic pathway for globoside degradation, in the face of an overwhelming excess of leucocytes presenting for destruction.

Niemann–Pick disease (sphingomyelin lipidosis). This is an autosomal recessive disorder resulting in deficiency of sphingomyelinase, the enzyme required for degrading sphingomyelin to ceramide and phosphoryl choline. As in Gaucher's disease, there is a high familial incidence and many published cases have been Jewish, although the condition is not confined to

Caucasians. The first manifestations usually appear before the age of six months, and death commonly supervenes within a few months, although occasional patients survive into adult life. The tissues have a high content of sphingomyelin and cholesterol, principally within 'foam histiocytes', which are lipid-containing macrophages and reticulum cells. These are 20–90 μm in diameter, single or multinucleate, and the cytoplasm contains fairly uniform lipid droplets. The lipid is principally sphingomyelin, and ceroid may also be found. Electron microscopy shows amorphous or lamellated pleomorphic cytoplasmic granules.

The liver tends to be affected early, and the spleen may be enlarged to more than five per cent of the body weight. Bone marrow, lymph nodes, skin, lung, tonsils, endocardium, intestinal wall and the central nervous system may be affected. Bone-marrow involvement is usually less extensive than in Gaucher's disease, but the splenic pulp may be virtually replaced by foam cells.

Haematological features are both qualitative and quantitative. Vacuolation of blood lymphocytes and monocytes can be found in nearly all patients by light microscopy [423–426], and lipid cytosomes are present in lymphocytes, monocytes, platelets and early eosinophils, differing morphologically from those present in visceral cells and cells of the central nervous system [426]. The bone marrow shows typical 'foam histiocytes'. However, anaemia was present in only five of 16 patients investigated by Crocker & Farber [425]; no close relationship was found between anaemia and spleen size. Moderately depressed platelet counts occur in patients with significant splenomegaly, and leucopenia may also be present. Occasionally, thrombocytopenia and leucopenia may be severe. Transient leucocytosis may occur in the absence of fever or infection.

Splenectomy in this condition has been performed for diagnostic purposes and for the correction of deficits in the peripheral blood: in anaemic patients there may be a subsequent slow rise in haemoglobin continuing over several months, and persistently high post-splenectomy leucocyte and platelet counts have been observed [425]. Respiratory and gastro-intestinal symptoms arising from splenomegaly may be relieved, but splenectomy does not conspicuously alter the course of the disease or the prognosis.

Wolman's disease (cholesteryl ester storage disease). This is an invariably fatal disorder in which the deficiency of lysosomal acid hydrolase activity leads to widespread tissue storage of cholesteryl esters and glycerides. The disease becomes apparent soon after birth, and clinically it resembles Niemann–Pick disease. Anaemia appears within a few weeks and is progressive. Bone-marrow aspirates show lipid-laden histiocytes, and hepato-splenomegaly is invariably present. A distinctive feature is calcification of the adrenal glands, and diminished responsiveness to adrenocorticotrophic stimulation.

Tay–Sachs' disease (ganglioside lipidosis). This is a genetically determined condition associated with tissue accumulation of ganglioside, due to deficiency of β hexosaminidase. It is an autosomal-recessive character, and the gene incidence has been estimated to be as high as 1:100 in Ashkenazi Jews. The condition is usually first manifest at about the age of six months, and the most significant effects arise from involvement of the central nervous system, with motor weakness leading to paralysis, dementia and amaurosis. Related syndromes occur later in life; late infantile, juvenile and adult forms are recognized.

Visceral involvement has been regarded as denying the diagnosis, but a few cases otherwise indistinguishable from Tay–Sachs' disease have been shown to have widely distributed foam-cell accumulations in extraneural tissues [429, 430]. Significant splenomegaly does not occur and in one case the organ was atrophic [430]. Microscopically, foam cells form large aggregates replacing the lymphoid follicles, and smaller groups of cells are present in the pulp. A small proportion of peripheral blood lymphocytes shows vacuolation [426].

Sandhoff's disease is clinically similar to Tay–Sachs' disease, and differs principally in that both isoenzymes of hexosaminidase are suppressed, whereas in Tay–Sachs' disease the deficiency is confined to the A-isoenzyme.

Fabry's disease (α-galactosidase A deficiency). This differs from other sphingolipidoses in being transmitted as an X-linked defect. The predominant lipid is a trihexosyl-ceramide, which is extensively stored in the walls of blood vessels, muscle cells, connective tissue cells, ganglion cells, and epithelial cells of the cornea and kidney. Progression is quite variable in the affected hemizygous male; among the manifestations, the cutaneous angiectases which form the basis for the *angiokeratoma corporis diffusum universale* need to be distinguished from other causes of telangiectasia. Foam cells may be found in the bone marrow, and anaemia with a low serum iron concentration and reticulocytosis has been described [431, 432].

Tangier disease (familial high-density lipoprotein deficiency). This is a rare familial disease characterized by a distinctive tonsillar enlargement, and an almost complete absence of high-density lipoprotein from the plasma [433]. The tonsils have a characteristic orange streaking *in vivo*, and a greyish-yellow coloration after removal. Other features include hepatomegaly, splenomegaly, and enlarged lymph nodes; a low plasma cholesterol level is accompanied by high triglyceride levels. Affected tissues have a high content of cholesterol esters present in foam cells, but no granulomatous changes occur. The condition appears to arise in homozygotes for an autosomal gene, the heterozygous state being detectable by demonstration of low plasma levels of high-density lipoprotein [434]. It is relatively benign and has been described in adults, who show the additional features of corneal infiltrates, and foam cells in the rectal mucosa on biopsy. Foam cells have also been demonstrated by liver and bone-marrow biopsies. Some subjects develop mononeuritis multiplex. One adult patient with splenomegaly showed red-cell anisocytosis, polychromasia, reticulocytosis, leucopenia and thrombocytopenia which were corrected by splenectomy [435]: the spleen had a high content of total lipids, especially with respect to esterified cholesterol and triglycerides, and the splenic pulp showed scattered cholesterol crystals and foam cells.

Familial hyperlipoproteinaemia (Type I). This is a rare familial disorder characterized by massive chylomicronaemia, which is corrected by a fat-free diet [436]. Its basis is believed to be a tissue deficiency of lipoprotein lipase, and foam cells are found in the bone marrow, spleen and liver. Clinically, there are eruptive xanthomata, lipaemia retinalis and usually splenic and hepatic enlargement. Abdominal pain is common, in some cases due to pancreatitis, and in others attributable to splenic infarction. In one case, the spleen was removed because of pain [437] and showed congestion and polymorphonuclear infiltration of the red pulp, foam cells, some of which were phagocytic, and diffuse lipid infiltration of blood vessel walls; the organ had a high total triglyceride content.

Hurler's syndrome. This is a familial, genetically determined mucopolysaccharidosis, characterized by skeletal abnormalities (dysostosis multiplex), mental retardation, corneal clouding and hepatosplenomegaly. The skeletal abnormalities include a shortened stature, gibbus formation, deformity of the skull and hypertelorism. Enlargement of the liver and spleen are usual, but exceptions occur. There appear to be two patterns of inheritance, one due to an autosomal recessive gene and the other X-linked. The basic deficiency is in the activity of a lysosomal hydrolase, α-L-iduronidase, which is required for the degradation of both heparan sulphate and dermatan, since both have iduronic acid residues. There are two abnormal

populations of cells in affected tissues [438], the predominant cells being large vacuoated 'clear cells' containing granular metachromatic material, while a lesser population of lipid-containing cells has also been demonstrated. The principal storage material consists of acid mucopolysaccharides. The spleen may be strikingly enlarged, hard and greyish in colour; vacuolated cells are frequent in the red pulp and in the walls of the venous sinuses, with occasional clear cells also present in the white pulp. Leucocytes of the peripheral blood may contain metachromatic granules ('Reilly bodies') especially in the granulocytes [439], and these may also be found in reticulum cells and lymphocytes in the bone marrow [440].

The syndrome of the sea-blue histiocyte. This is a systemic histiocytosis characterized by the presence in bone-marrow and splenic aspirates of histiocytes with variable, but often dense, granulation which produces sea-blue coloration with the Wright–Giemsa method. The staining method is not biochemically specific, but it appears that the affected tissues have a high lipid content, especially with respect to sphingolipids, and that the cells are PAS-positive [441].

The condition is found as a primary familial syndrome, affecting all ages between infancy and the ninth decade; however, the presentation is commonest in young adults. In many cases it proves to be only slowly progressive. Splenomegaly is almost invariable and may be massive: the architecture of the organ is little affected, but the characteristic cells are widely distributed throughout the red pulp and in the walls of the splenic sinuses. Foci of myeloid metaplasia are usually present [442]. Hepatomegaly is common, but the histological findings are variable. Lymph nodes may also be infiltrated with characteristic histiocytes, but are rarely prominent clinically.

Other clinical features have included ophthalmological abnormalities, especially a foveal ring, thrombocytopenia sometimes accompanied by purpura and other haemorrhagic manifestations [443], skin pigmentation, pulmonary infiltration and, in younger subjects, a neurological disorder [444].

The familial occurrence of the syndrome, especially with respect to its incidence within sibships, has suggested a genetically determined origin for the condition, possibly as an autosomal-recessive trait with variable expressivity. Studies of cultured fibroblasts from siblings affected by the syndrome showed subnormal sphingomyelinase activity, suggesting that a partial sphingomyelinase deficiency is a cause of at least one variant of the syndrome [445].

The syndrome also occurs in non-familial form, sometimes with marked splenomegaly, while in others it is limited to the finding of the characteristic cells in bone-marrow aspirates. The acquired form appears frequently to be secondary to other disorders, including idiopathic thrombocytopenic purpura [446], hyperlipaemia [447], chronic myeloid leukaemia, chronic granulomatous disease and Takayasu arteritis [448].

Idiopathic histiocytosis. This comprises a group of conditions of unknown aetiology (histiocytosis X, eosinophilic xanthomatous granuloma), characterized by lesions showing histiocytic proliferation, granuloma formation with eosinophil infiltration and giant cells, xanthoma formation with cholesterol-containing foam cells, and fibrosis [414, 427]. The lesions show mixed characteristics, or may predominantly express the proliferative process, eosinophilia, xanthoma formation or fibrosis. Progression tends to be more rapid and extensive when the onset occurs early in life. The xanthomatous lesions have a high content of cholesterol, but this is not reflected in the plasma cholesterol level, which is usually normal.

Extensive studies have failed to demonstrate infection or other factors as being implicated in the aetiology of the condition, although the diffuse form has some features suggestive of neoplastic proliferation. The clinical and pathological findings vary widely, but three principal forms can be usefully distinguished.

1 *Solitary eosinophilic granuloma* of bone is the least disseminated variant of the condition, and rarely involves more than a single circumscribed site in the skeleton. The lesions are benign and confined to bone, and the symptomatology is essentially related to the bone lesions and their sequelae, including fractures. The condition is found most commonly in adolescents and young adults.

2 *Chronic systemic histiocytosis* (Hand–Schuller–Christian disease) is usually of intermediate severity, and follows a chronic course after its onset in the child or young adult. The basic lesions are multifocal eosinophilic granulomata of bone, especially affecting the calvarium, sella turcica and orbit. This may produce the classical triad of membrane bone defects, diabetes insipidus and exophthalmos. However, the femora, ribs, vertebrae and long bones of the limbs are also involved in some cases. Although not part of the original syndrome, it would be arbitrary to exclude from the designation the frequently found generalized manifestations: skin lesions include petechiae and xanthoma disseminata; the pulmonary lesions include 'honeycomb' changes and diffuse fibrosis; enlargement of lymph nodes, spleen and liver; and central-nervous-system lesions. Anaemia may be present, presumably because of involvement of the bone marrow, and in some cases there is leucopenia and thrombocytopenia.

3 *Acute systemic histiocytosis* (Lettere–Siwe's disease) is an acute progressive form, usually appearing before the age of three years with fever, lymphadenopathy, hepato-splenomegaly, osteolytic bone lesions, cutaneous lesions, progressive anaemia and purpura. The lesions show little evidence of lipid formation or granuloma, which may reflect a necessary chronicity for such processes, which do not have time to develop during the rapid progression of the disorder.

INVESTIGATION OF THE SPLEEN

Enlargement of the spleen is a feature of widely diverse disorders (Table 20.3) and no stereotyped sequence of investigation is applicable in all circumstances. In the context of haematological disease, it is principally of importance to establish whether the spleen is enlarged, and if so, to determine its degree, to define its cause and to assess its contribution to the clinical condition of the patient. The principal methods of investigation directed towards the organ itself are:

1 clinical;
2 radiological;
3 radioisotopic scanning;
4 splenic puncture; and
5 special tests of abnormal activity.

CLINICAL METHODS

In the presence of very marked enlargement, the spleen may be detectable on inspection of the abdomen, and in cases of long standing, a cluster of thin white striae may be seen in the skin radiating from the region of the tip of the spleen. Palpation of the spleen is usually possible when the organ is approximately three times the normal size; the direction of enlargement may be predominantly medially into the epigastrium, infero-medially towards and beyond the umbilicus, or inferiorly towards the left iliac fossa. In extreme instances, enlargement may extend the organ into the pelvis and the right iliac fossa. Identification of the palpable mass is assisted by finding the characteristic notching of the smooth circumferential border, by establishing that the mass moves inferiorly on inspiration, and that it is not possible to define its upper limits by palpation beneath the costal margin.

Percussion between the left costal margin and the mid-axillary line may elicit abnormal dullness suggestive of splenic enlargement when the organ is not palpable. Placing the patient on the right side with the left arm drawn forward improves the detection of the spleen by percussion [449], and from this position, partial rotation of the left side of the trunk forwards may make the spleen more easily palpable. Auscultation sometimes detects soft systolic bruits over a vascular spleen, and a harsh friction rub in cases with splenic infarction or perisplenitis.

Clinical estimates of spleen size require the use of an arbitrary measurement; with moderate or marked enlargement, the distance from the midpoint of the left costal margin to the lowermost dextrad point on the splenic border provides a reasonably reproducible index for serial comparisons.

RADIOLOGICAL METHODS

Radiological methods have generally been underutilized in the detection and investigation of the abnormal spleen. They provide the means for detecting splenomegaly when this is not accessible to clinical examination and allow a more accurate estimate of spleen size [450, 451]. In blood disorders there are usually few specific qualitative changes to be demonstrated, other than splenic infarction or splenic vein thrombosis, but radiography may suggest the presence of incidental disease of the spleen, such as cystic changes, hamartomata or angiomata.

The methods available have been comprehensively reviewed [452, 453] and include the following:

Plane radiography of the abdomen

The spleen appears as a homogeneous shadow below the left hemidiaphragm, and in approximately half of normal subjects there is a visible lower pole. Disease may result in enlargement, an irregular outline, displacement or calcification. Estimates of spleen size may be made by simple axial measurements [452, 454–456], or by measurement of the area of projection of the spleen, which bears a relationship to body surface area [5]. Visualization of the spleen may be improved by air insufflation of the colon or stomach, and by retroperitoneal gas insufflation.

Computer tomography

Computer tomography (CT) scanning offers the most accurate method for assessing spleen size, but its principal clinical applications are:
1 in differentiating the enlarged spleen from other upper abdominal masses; and
2 in detecting focal splenic lesions, such as lymphomatous nodules.

It has the advantage of simultaneously detecting abnormalities in other sites, which is especially useful with respect to the posterior abdominal lymph nodes. The vascularity of the pulp makes enhancement by intravenous contrast infusions especially effective.

Ultrasonography

Although not a radiographic technique, ultrasonography is conveniently considered in parallel with CT scanning as both techniques provide similar information, though with differing precision. The normal spleen is difficult to demonstrate, but as enlargement progresses so the organ is more easily visualized. Some broad conclusions can be achieved as to the consistency of the enlarged spleen, and some focal lesions are demonstrable. Since the method is non-invasive it has a place in sequential evaluation of spleen size during therapy. The definitive role of both CT scanning and ultrasonography in clinical management is still under investigation.

Radiography of adjacent organs

Marked enlargement of the spleen produces displacement and distortion of adjacent organs, which may be detected by appropriate examinations. With the exception of chest radiography, such examinations are usually performed because symptoms dependent on the splenomegaly have suggested extrasplenic pathology, or because the characteristics of a detected mass have suggested an origin other than the spleen. *Chest radiography* may show the left hemidiaphragm to be raised, the left costophrenic angle to be obscured and the lower lobe of the left lung to have plate atelectases. *Intravenous pyelography* may show the left kidney to be displaced inferiorly or medially, sometimes with distortion of the calyceal pattern. *Barium meal* may show narrowing of the gastric lumen and displacement of the stomach medially, downwards and slightly forwards. *Barium enema* may show the splenic flexure displaced inferiorly or medially.

Splenic arteriography

Arteriography is principally of value in detecting the presence of focal lesions of the spleen, and in distinguishing these from splenomegaly with diffuse pathology. In blood disorders, the findings are likely to be confined to demonstrating splenic enlargement and the corresponding increase in size of the splenic artery and its branches. The method will also demonstrate splenic infarcts, and accessory spleens; splenic fibrosis may be suspected on the basis of narrowing and irregularity of the intrasplenic arteries. In Hodgkin's disease, the intrasplenic arterial pattern may be diminished and scattered focal lesions may produce an irregular appearance of focal defects in the sinus-filling phase.

Portal venography

Trans-splenic portal venography is rarely indicated in the investigation of splenomegaly secondary to haematological disorders, in which the findings are usually limited to minor changes in contrast density and elongation and tortuosity of the splenic vein. Occasionally, when portal hypertension is suspected, it may be necessary to determine whether this results from a complication of the haematological condition, such as portal-vein thrombosis, or is due to a coexisting, but unrelated condition. Prerequisites are as outlined for splenic puncture. Consideration should be given before the procedure is undertaken to the possible consequences of splenectomy in the particular case, should this be required for subsequent control of haemorrhage from the spleen.

SPLEEN SCANNING

Spleen scanning by rectilinear scanner or scintillation camera may be used:

1 for detecting displacement, enlargement or absence of the spleen;

2 for determining whether an upper abdominal mass originates in the spleen;

3 for detecting focal lesions of the spleen; and

4 for the detection of accessory spleens.

The radioisotope to be concentrated in the spleen may be used to label damaged red cells or may be in colloidal form for uptake by reticulo-endothelial cells. Each method has its advantages and ideally the particular method should be selected with regard to the specific purpose of the study [458].

Radiocolloids used for liver scanning are also suitable for examination of the spleen. For most routine clinical purposes, technetium-99m sulphur colloid provides adequate efficiency for scanning. Other available colloids are gold-198 colloid, and indium-113m colloid. The acceptable dose of gold-198 colloid limits its usefulness; the indium colloid has some advantages with respect to storage, preparation and radiation dose.

Red-cell localization in the spleen may be achieved by several methods including:

1 coating Rh(D)-positive cells with incomplete antibody [459] (this method is limited to Rh(D)-positive subjects);

2 heat treatment of cells at 49–50°C [460];

3 chemical damage with organic mercurials, such as 1-mercuri-2-hydroxypropane (MHP), which may itself carry the radioisotope [461, 462]; and

4 treatment of red cells with acid-citrate-dextrose solution [463].

It is the degree to which the red cells are damaged rather than the specific method of treatment which determines the extent of concentration of the cells in the spleen; excessive damage may lead to concentration in the liver or intravascular destruction.

Chromium-51 has commonly been used to label damaged red cells, and requires a dose of approximately 300 μCi for adults, which is in excess of the activity required for determination of red-cell lifespan. Rubi-

dium-81 labelling produces a lower radiation dose, but is of limited availability. [197]Hg-MHP and [203]Hg-MHP have been used to provide both cell damage and labelling, but the radiation dose to the kidneys is high, especially with [203]Hg. Technetium-99 pertechnate can also be used as a red-cell label [458].

The inconvenience of the methodology with labelled red cells when compared with the use of radiocolloids has limited the extension of these procedures into routine use.

SPLENIC PUNCTURE

Splenic aspiration may rarely be useful as an additional investigation in patients suspected of lymphomata, leukaemoid reactions, leukaemia, myelomatosis, primary myeloid metaplasia and Gaucher's disease [464–466]. Nucleated cells in the normal aspirate consist approximately of 60–90% lymphocytes, the remainder being mainly mature peripheral blood cells and a small number of reticulum cells. Identification of significant numbers of other cell types is made as in a marrow aspiration biopsy. The principal hazard is haemorrhage, sometimes severe enough to require prompt splenectomy. The technique requires a co-operative patient, and is usually limited to those with a firm, palpable spleen. Aspiration biopsy is usually omitted when the spleen is soft or portal hypertension is suspected. There should be no history suggestive of a haemorrhagic disorder, and the partial thromboplastin time, the prothrombin time and the tourniquet test should be normal and the platelet count above 100×10^9/l.

SPECIAL TESTS OF ABNORMAL SPLENIC ACTIVITY

The ^{51}Cr-labelled red-cell technique for the estimation of red-cell lifespan may be combined with estimates of red-cell mass, splenic pooling and the accumulation of isotope in the organ.

Red-cell mass is a useful additional estimate since the expansion of blood volume in patients with splenomegaly may lead to the haematocrit and haemoglobin estimates correlating poorly with the red-cell mass. In the presence of splenic red-cell pooling the isotope-labelled cells show delayed mixing with the total red-cell mass, and venous blood samples should be taken for estimation of the volume of expansion at six and 45 minutes from the intravenous injection of the labelled cells, or later if surface counting shows that equilibrium has not been reached. The difference between the red-cell mass estimates made from the early and late samples provides an approximate but useful measure of the volume of pooled red cells [89, 212, 242]. A plasma volume estimate by a labelled-albumin method is a useful additional estimation, since it permits calculation of the total blood volume and H_b/H_v ratio when the red-cell mass is known.

Pooling of red cells in the spleen may be detected by showing a delay in attaining a steady plateau of radioactivity in the splenic area after the injection of labelled cells, using a collimated scintillation counter with a continuous recording device [208, 209, 212].

Evidence of red-cell destruction in the spleen may be obtained by following the surface-detectable radioactivity over the organ at intervals after the injection of ^{51}Cr-labelled red cells. This requires surface counting at other sites, usually over the liver and precordium, for purposes of comparison. The method is subject to error, especially with respect to the accurate positioning of the detector for successive estimates, and adequate collimation is required for valid results. Frequently repeated counts are necessary if determination of the trend of accumulation is to be reasonably accurate.

Radioactivity detected in the splenic region arises in part from circulating red cells, both in the spleen and in neighbouring extrasplenic sites, and the fraction arising from deposited isotope varies as the activity of the red cells fall with time. Several methods of presenting the changes in activity have been proposed [467–472], but none provides a totally satisfactory quantitative estimate of the amount of isotope deposited from destroyed red cells. For example, the method of 'excess counts' [469] relates all surface activities proportionately to a standard initial precordial count of 1000; on subsequent days the 'expected count' for the spleen (or liver) is calculated in proportion to the fall in precordial count, and the difference between this and the actual corrected count constitutes the 'excess count'. An 'excess count' greater than 400 at the time when half the labelled red cells have been lost from the circulation is held to be significant of splenic red-cell destruction.

The method appears to be useful in predicting the outcome of splenectomy in a high proportion of patients with haemolytic disorders, although a significant number of exceptions occur [468, 470, 473–478]. Failure to detect red-cell destruction in the spleen does not necessarily contraindicate splenectomy, since anaemia may be improved or corrected by splenectomy in some cases without demonstrable splenic uptake of isotope [477].

^{51}Cr-labelled platelet methods have been used experimentally to study the distribution, survival and sites of destruction of platelets [107–109, 138, 314]. The experience of the individual centre appears to be important with respect to the predictive value of the method in the selection of individuals for splenectomy [479].

SPLENECTOMY

THE CONSEQUENCES OF SPLENOMEGALY

In addition to its role in the pathogenesis of haemolysis, thrombocytopenia, leucopenia, red-cell pooling, dilutional anaemia and portal hypertension, which have been discussed previously, the spleen may produce symptoms due to the local effects of enlargement. Discomfort in the left hypochondrium may vary from a dull aching pain, often with a 'dragging' component, to severe local pain, sometimes referred to the left shoulder, due to perisplenitis accompanying infarction. Marked enlargement may produce respiratory difficulty, dyspepsia, nausea and vomiting, and gross enlargement may lead to constipation and frequency of micturition.

Infarction
Splenic infarction is common, especially with marked enlargement of the spleen, and is frequently recurrent. The intrasplenic arterial pattern is essentially of end-artery type, with few interarterial connections, so that the organ is especially vulnerable to infarction following arterial occlusion. The factors predisposing to infarction remain to be critically defined, but appear to depend in part on increased sensitivity to oxygen deprivation when the mass of the spleen is increased, especially when there is extensive replacement by leukaemic cells of high metabolic rate. In addition, vascular compression may be a factor, and perfusion of the pulp may be impaired by cellular infiltration. A further factor in some instances may be extrasplenic occlusion of splenic artery radicles by enlarged lymph nodes.

Rupture
Rupture of the spleen is uncommon, but occurs more frequently with minimal trauma ('pathological' or 'spontaneous' rupture) when there is pathological enlargement. Contributing factors are the loss of protection of the thoracic cage when the spleen extends below the costal margin, and the structural weakness which results from infiltration of the stroma, invasion of the capsule, infarction and intrasplenic haemorrhage. The haematological diseases most commonly associated with the condition are infectious mononucleosis and acute and chronic leukaemias [480–493]; it has also been reported in myelomatosis [308], Gaucher's disease, polycythaemia vera [494], autoimmune haemolytic disease and congestive splenomegaly.

THE OBJECTIVES OF SPLENECTOMY
Splenectomy may be considered in haematological disorders with the following objectives.

1 For the treatment or correction of:
  (a)   haemolytic or dilutional anaemia;
  (b)   thrombocytopenia;
  (c)   leucopenia;
  (d)   persistent local discomfort;
  (e)   recurrent splenic infarction;
  (f)   splenic rupture;
  (g)   portal hypertension;
  (h)   localized splenic disease (e.g. plasmacytoma [503, 504]; splenic cysts).
2 For diagnostic purposes:
  (a)   with splenomegaly as an isolated physical finding;
  (b)   for the staging of Hodgkin's disease.
3 To improve tolerance to chemotherapy or radiation therapy.
4 To remove a major focus in a generalized disease, without expectation of cure (e.g. chronic myeloid leukaemia [505, 506]).

Diagnostic splenectomy

This is sometimes considered when splenomegaly is an isolated abnormal finding in circumstances in which the patient's condition contraindicates a further period of observation. This situation is not commonly encountered when a comprehensive evaluation is undertaken, but may occur with lymphomata, sarcoidosis, storage diseases and splenic tuberculosis. The advantages of a possible histological diagnosis need to be weighed against:
1 the possible adverse consequences of splenectomy; and
2 the possible absence of specific histological findings in the earliest stages of splenomegaly due to conditions such as lymphoma.

More frequently a histological diagnosis is made when splenectomy is undertaken for autoimmune haemolytic disease or hypersplenism which proves to be the herald state of chronic lymphocytic leukaemia, lymphoma, systemic lupus erythematosus or sarcoidosis. Nevertheless, the absence of histological findings does not preclude the later appearance of other manifestations of these diseases.

Staging of malignant disorders

Staging procedures in most cases of Hodgkin's disease require laparotomy with splenectomy, liver biopsy, bone biopsy, lymph-node biopsy and visual survey, with the objective of more precisely assessing abdominal involvement for the purposes of therapy and prognosis [495–497, 502]. Such studies have contributed significantly to the definition of the natural history of abdominal Hodgkin's disease: splenomegaly has been found in the absence of histologically identifiable lesions in the organ while, conversely, splenic

Hodgkin's disease may occur without detectable organ enlargement [495]. Likewise, involvement of the spleen appears to be an early manifestation of disease in the abdomen, and in at least one series was invariably present in patients with coeliac or para-aortic node involvement [497].

Tolerance to chemotherapy and radiotherapy

This has been stated to improve following splenectomy in Hodgkin's disease and non-Hodgkin's lymphomas, where cellular deficits in the peripheral blood may be a limiting factor for both modalities of treatment [498–501]. However, careful selection is required as these subjects are frequently not optimal patients with respect to the surgical risks, and duration of the effect of splenectomy may be no longer than several months.

THE CONSEQUENCES OF SPLENECTOMY

The reduction in immediate mortality and morbidity of splenectomy as the result of improved surgical techniques, and evidence that removal of the spleen in the otherwise healthy adult is followed by few significant sequelae has tended to diminish recognition of the hazards of the procedure in other circumstances. Since much of the information available on the effectiveness and complications of splenectomy has derived from retrospective surveys, conclusions must necessarily be tentative in many respects.

Mortality and morbidity

The overall mortality rate of splenectomy in haematological diseases in various series has been found to lie between three and 18% [511–513], with several showing a rate of approximately eight per cent [15, 308, 507–510]. The mortality appears to be significantly lower in uncomplicated cases of hereditary spherocytosis, idiopathic thrombocytopenic purpura and primary hypersplenism than with chronic leukaemias and malignant lymphomata, for which operation is likely to be considered at a time when the patient is physically impaired by extensive disease [308, 514].

The principal complications of operation include the following.

1 *Haemorrhage*, which may be immediate or delayed, and is closely related to factors such as adhesions which contribute to surgical difficulty. Avoidance is largely dependent on operative technique, but contributory factors are thrombocytopenia, coagulation defects due to associated hepatic disease, and acute fibrinolysis, for which anticipatory preparation is mandatory.

2 *Venous thrombosis*, which occurs proportionately more frequently after splenectomy than other upper

abdominal operations [515]. The two principal sites are in peripheral veins, which may be a source of pulmonary emboli, and in the tributaries of the portal vein, which may become occluded as the result of extension of thrombus from the residual segment of the splenic vein [516–518].

3 *Pulmonary complications*, including left-sided pleural effusion, left lower lobe collapse, pneumonia, pulmonary embolus and, rarely, empyema.

4 *Others*, including acute gastric distension, ileus, pancreatic trauma, septicaemia and infection of the operation site.

Infection

There is experimental evidence in laboratory animals that splenectomy increases susceptibility to infection [519, 520], and in some patients after splenectomy, abnormalities have been described in several serum components, including reduced levels of IgM [523, 553, 554], properdin [524] and tuftsin [525]. Total immunoglobulin levels, however, tend to be normal, and transferrin levels increased [539, 553]. Furthermore, in the functional hyposplenia of sickle-cell disease there is decreased clearance of $^{99}Tc^m$-sulphur colloid [526] and diminished opsonizing activity associated with a defect in the alternative complement pathway [527].

In man there is a predisposition to infection following splenectomy, the severity of which is dependent on two principal variables. These are the age of the subject and the nature of the underlying disorder for which the splenectomy is performed. In otherwise healthy adults, the additional risk of infection is present, but not high [52, 528]. However, it has long been recognized that splenectomy may reactivate malaria in previously affected persons, and that cerebral malaria is more common in these circumstances. The influence on bacterial infections has been less certain in adults, although an increase in the incidence of pneumococcal and streptococcal infection has been found following splenectomy for cryptogenic splenomegaly [381], and fulminant sepsis is more common when splenectomy is performed for the staging of lymphoma [529, 530].

Infants and children appear to be at special risk from severe bacterial infection following splenectomy. The early report of King & Shumacker [534] provoked considerable discussion, and although the association between splenectomy and infection has been denied [535–539], most reports have supported the proposition, especially for infants and where there is an associated haematological disorder or immunodeficiency [521, 522, 529, 530, 533, 540–546, 557]. The increased risk is especially related to organisms which produce polysaccharide capsules, usually *Streptococcus pneumoniae*, and infections tend to be fulminant, septicaemic or meningeal. Their frequency is especially high following splenectomy in infancy; 85% of such infections in splenectomized children occur under the age of three years. The risk is higher during the first two years following splenectomy. A comparable susceptibility is also found in hyposplenic subjects with sickle-cell disease, in whom an increased incidence of infection with *Haemophilus influenzae* has also been identified [531].

The increased susceptibility to infection gives critical importance to the question of the effectiveness of prophylactic immunization in splenectomized subjects. With respect to soluble polyvalent pneumococcal polysaccharide antigens, there appears to be an antibody response which is comparable to that of normal control subjects; furthermore, there is evidence that useful protection against overwhelming infection can be obtained [532]. Likewise, the immune response to tetanus toxoid [547] and to subcutaneously administered tularaemia vaccine [548] has been found to be normal in splenectomized subjects; the interval between splenectomy and the antigenic challenge may be important, since an early but transient depression of responsiveness following the operation has been reported [549, 550]. In this respect, a further variable is the route of administration, there being a more consistent reduction of antibody response to intravenously administered antigens [156, 551, 552].

Total immunoglobulin levels are usually normal following splenectomy [539], but mean IgM levels have been shown to be lower than normal, and transferrin levels higher, in splenectomized children [553], and in splenectomized patients with β-thalassaemia, IgM levels are lower than in non-splenectomized subjects [554].

Specific complications

Splenectomy appears to carry special hazards in certain conditions; those associated with congestive splenomegaly and Gaucher's disease have been discussed, and the possible hazard of thrombocytosis with anaemia persisting after splenectomy is considered below.

In myeloproliferative disorders, especially essential thrombocythaemia and primary myeloid metaplasia, there is the special hazard of severe thrombocytosis, with a consequent haemorrhagic disorder frequently expressed by gastro-intestinal bleeding [555, 556]. In such cases the diagnosis is often not made until after splenectomy, which may have been performed for portal hypertension or as a procedure adjuvant to gastric or oesophageal surgery, and there may be minimal evidence of the underlying condition in the peripheral blood prior to operation. Splenectomy in primary myeloid metaplasia also carries the hazards of infarction of the left hepatic lobe and extensive venous thromboses, often of bizarre distribution.

In thalassaemia major it has been reported that iron deposition in the hepatic parenchymal cells is substantially greater in patients subjected to splenectomy than in those with an intact spleen, and that this is associated with increased parenchymal damage [558].

In idiopathic thrombocytopenic purpura and autoimmune haemolytic disease it has been suggested that splenectomy may lead to the activation of latent systemic lupus erythematosus [559–561]. Later studies have failed to substantiate the relationship beyond the recognition that immunocytopenias may provide a herald state of systemic lupus erythematosus. The controversy has been reviewed by Best & Darling [562].

Splenic autotransplantation. The majority of reported instances of splenic autotransplantation, in which splenectomy is followed by the development of numerous widely distributed nodules of splenic tissue, mainly within the peritoneal cavity, have occurred when there has been preceding trauma to the spleen [563–568]. Rarely, autotransplantation may occur without prior external injury, apparently due to surgical trauma during splenectomy, and may then be the cause of relapse of the primary condition for which splenectomy is performed [569].

BLOOD AFTER SPLENECTOMY

Following splenectomy the blood shows both qualitative and quantitative changes in its cellular elements, some of which may persist indefinitely to provide continuing evidence of the absence of functioning splenic tissue. The absence of qualitative changes in the red cells, on the other hand, raises the suspicion of residual splenic tissue, such as an accessory spleen.

Red cells

The red-cell changes are principally qualitative; quantitative changes depend on the presence of underlying disease and its modification by splenectomy. Rarely, there may be post-splenectomy erythrocytosis in cases of hereditary spherocytosis [570] and primary myeloid metaplasia. The most characteristic qualitative changes are the presence of Howell–Jolly bodies, which are invariably present [331, 571, 572], and an increase in the numbers of target cells with a reduction in red-cell osmotic fragility. Specific staining also shows an increase in siderocytes and in cells containing Heinz bodies [573]. Electron microscopy may show the presence of 'autophagic vacuoles' containing haemoglobin, ferritin, and remnants of membrane and mitochondria, which may attach to the cell membrane to produce surface pits and craters [574]. Slight reticulocytosis may occur and there may be a transient normoblastosis which usually declines within a few weeks, but may reappear under the stress of haemorrhage or haemolysis. Marked normoblastosis may persist in conditions such as thalassaemia major.

The persistence of red cells with inclusion bodies after splenectomy was suggested by Crosby [90] to indicate that the normal spleen removes such cells from the circulation, or that the inclusion bodies may be removed from the cells during their passage through the spleen. Electron microscopy has confirmed the presence of both processes [294, 575, 576].

Leucocytes

Leucocytosis is commonly found within hours of the removal of the spleen and is usually maximal within the following week. This is succeeded by a gradual fall over several weeks, but in approximately one-third of patients it may persist for much longer periods. In most instances the total count is between 10 and $15 \times 10^9/l$ but rarely it may be in excess of $25 \times 10^9/l$ [572]. The initial leucocytosis is principally due to a rise in the neutrophil count, but later there is a relative or absolute lymphocytosis in approximately 60% of cases, and a relative or absolute monocytosis in approximately 30%. A slight to moderate rise in the eosinophil and basophil counts may also occur [572].

Platelets

The platelet count may show a transient depression following splenectomy [570], with a subsequent rise to a maximum between the fourth and 14th days, leading to a gradual reduction to normal levels in the next three months [52, 577–579]. Some patients show a persistent thrombocytosis which is not confined to those with myeloproliferative disorders: Hirsh & Dacie [579] found that raised platelet counts were most likely to persist when anaemia remains uncorrected by splenectomy, and cited cases of congenital non-spherocytic haemolytic anaemia, sideroblastic anaemia, haemoglobinopathies and thalassaemia. The platelet count was closely related to the severity of the anaemia. In such cases thrombotic complications are found more frequently than in non-anaemic patients, although thrombocytosis is apparently not the only causal factor.

THE DECISION FOR SPLENECTOMY

In haematological disorders removal of the spleen is seldom undertaken in the expectation of cure of the underlying disease, but principally for the correction of those secondary effects of disease which are dependent on the presence of the spleen. Ideally, the decision for splenectomy requires the assessment of the probable benefits and potential hazards of the procedure to the individual patient, but in practice the methods for predicting the outcome in the individual are limited, and reliance has principally to be placed on empirically determined results established for rather broad classes of cases. The role of splenectomy in specific disorders is discussed in appropriate sections elsewhere, but the following considerations are generally applicable.

1 Rupture of the spleen is an absolute indication for immediate splenectomy, but is an uncommon indication in haematological disorders.

2 Whenever possible the diagnosis of the underlying condition should be established prior to operation since (a) this allows the potential value of the operation to be more adequately assessed, and (b) splenectomy may be avoided in circumstances in which it is undesirable or hazardous, as with the symptomless hypersplenism of congestive splenomegaly, the increased potential for infection of the Wiskott–Aldrich syndrome and Chediak–Higashi disease and in myeloproliferative disorders with a high risk of haemorrhagic thrombocythaemia.

3 In a limited number of disorders, the advantages of splenectomy are highly predictable and the risks low: in hereditary spherocytosis the haemolytic process is usually corrected and always improved, pigmentary cholelithiasis is prevented or arrested, and the hazard of severe anaemia during a hypoplastic crisis removed. Splenectomy is therefore advisable except in rare circumstances when incidental disease precludes surgery. The haemolytic anaemia of hereditary elliptocytosis also responds in a high proportion of cases, and there is successful correction of thrombocytopenia in approximately 80% of patients with chronic idiopathic thrombocytopenic purpura. In primary hypersplenism, as at present defined, the effect of splenectomy is usually favourable and histological examination of the spleen is valuable in excluding other diagnoses.

In an intermediate group of conditions, including autoimmune haemolytic disease of 'warm-antibody' type and symptomatic secondary hypersplenism, the results of splenectomy are less easily predictable. It is in this group that isotope studies to establish the splenic destruction of red cells may improve the process of selection when haemolysis is a marked feature. Likewise, anaemia in the presence of marked splenomegaly, together with high total blood and plasma volumes in the absence of hepatic disease, suggest the presence of dilutional anaemia which may respond to splenectomy. Other factors, such as the severity of the condition, the absence or ineffectiveness of other treatment, and local symptoms related to the spleen, may also influence the decision.

In a third group of conditions, splenectomy may be justified in life-threatening circumstances, when the prognosis is otherwise uniformly poor, although its value is incompletely established. In this category are thrombotic thrombocytopenic purpura [308], the use of splenectomy to improve the response to compatible platelet transfusions in aplastic anaemia [580], and in the correction of anaemia in patients on haemodialysis [581];

4 The availability of alternative methods of treatment, such as corticosteroid therapy for autoimmune haemolysis or thrombocytopenia, also affects the decision for splenectomy and especially its timing. Even in circumstances in which the alternative therapy is not definitive, it may permit greater flexibility in choosing the time for elective splenectomy, improve the patient's fitness for operation, and allow time for the appearance of spontaneous remission. In this context, it is also relevant to consider the complications of alternative therapy: when these are potentially serious, as with long-term, high-dosage corticosteroid therapy, splenectomy may prove to be the conservative choice.

5 In childhood, susceptibility to infection presents special problems with respect to splenectomy, particularly in relation to timing. The hazard of fulminant infection is greater in conditions such as thalassaemia major, portal hypertension secondary to hepatitis and malignant histiocytosis in which resistance to infection is depressed by the underlying disorder, and much less significant in hereditary spherocytosis, idiopathic thrombocytopenic purpura, portal hypertension of extrahepatic origin and splenic trauma. In general, splenectomy should be avoided in infancy whenever possible. It is uncertain at what later age the frequency of fulminant infection declines, but the incidence is significantly higher before the age of four years than after [582] and by this age the child can complain of symptoms which may provide an early indication of the onset of infection [583]. A further relevant factor is the availability of prompt medical care in the event of infection.

THE LOSS OF SPLENIC FUNCTION

The characteristic blood changes which are found following splenectomy, especially the appearance of Howell–Jolly bodies and target cells, may also accompany other conditions in which the spleen is absent or abnormal [570].

Congenital absence of the spleen ('asplenia syndrome')
Congenital absence of the spleen is a rare defect, usually accompanied by severe congenital cardiac anomalies of cono-truncus type, partial or complete situs inversus viscerae, and accessory lobes of the lung.

The cardiac anomalies may include partial or complete ostium atrioventriculare communis, pulmonary stenosis or atresia, anomalous pulmonary venous drainage, and abnormalities of the major blood vessels [584–590], and may be sufficiently complex to be difficult to classify even at autopsy. As a consequence they are usually, but not invariably, unsuitable for surgical correction. The majority of patients fail to survive early infancy, but a small number of adults with congenital absence of the spleen have been described, and these have usually been otherwise normal, or have shown minor cardiac or gastro-intestinal anomalies [586, 591–593]. Affected infants are susceptible to infection even when there is no cardiac anomaly [594]; one adult showed recurrent episodes of the Waterhouse–Friderichsen syndrome, and most adult cases have terminated in infections, including malaria, typhoid and tuberculosis.

Hypoplasia of the spleen

Hypoplasia of the spleen is a not uncommon anomaly in Fanconi's anaemia [595].

Immaturity of the spleen

In the newborn, some Howell–Jolly bodies, nucleated red-cell precursors and siderocytes are commonly found, and 'pitted' or 'cratered' red cells, which are probably identical to vacuolated red cells [574], comprise approximately 50% of the red-cell population in the blood of the premature newborn, and about 25% of the red cells of the full-term neonate, which may be the result of functional immaturity of the spleen [596].

Atrophy of the spleen

Atrophy of the spleen occurs in idiopathic steatorrhoea, with characteristic blood changes and a reduction in the clearance rate of heat-treated red cells from the circulation [274]. In view of its association with an enteropathic disorder, it is of special interest that dermatitis herpetiformis shows a high incidence of splenic atrophy. However, the two complications do not appear to be correlated [597]. Splenic atrophy is also found in essential thrombocythaemia [598, 599]; in a series of eight cases, three showed blood changes and slow clearance of heated red cells, and failure to visualize the spleen by scintillation scanning [600]. In sickle-cell disease, splenic atrophy is common, principally as a consequence of recurrent infarction [601–604], but in this condition, evidence of depressed splenic function, as shown by the blood changes and failure to demonstrate the organ by technetium-colloid scanning, may occur while the spleen is still enlarged [605]. This can be reversed by the transfusion of normal red cells, and is probably the functional

consequence of a reduction in pulp flow due to the high viscosity of sickled cells.

REFERENCES

1 ROBB-SMITH A.H.T. (1970) Pathological lesions in surgically removed spleens. *British Journal of Hospital Medicine*, **3**, 19.
2 McCORMICK W.F. & KASHGARIAN M. (1965) The weight of the adult human spleen. *American Journal of Clinical Pathology*, **43**, 332.
3 WHITLEY J.E., MAYNARD C.D. & RHYNE A.L. (1966) A computer approach to the prediction of spleen weight from routine films. *Radiology*, **86**, 73.
4 GRAY H. (1854) *On the Structure and Use of the Spleen*. Parker, London
5 BLENDIS L.M., WILLIAMS R. & KREEL L. (1969) Radiological determination of spleen size. *Gut*, **10**, 433.
6 BOYD E. (1933) Normal variability in weight of the adult human liver and spleen, *Archives of Pathology*, **16**, 350.
7 CURTIS G.M. & MOVITZ D. (1946) The surgical significance of the secondary spleen. *Annals of Surgery*, **123**, 276.
8 OLSEN W.R. & BEAUDOIN D.E. (1966) Increased incidence of accessory spleens in haematologic disease. *Archives of Surgery*, **98**, 762.
9 ONGLEY P.A., TITUS J.L., KHOURY G.H., RAHIMTOOLA S.H., MARSHALL H.J. & EDWARDS J.E. (1965) Anomalous connections of pulmonary veins to right atrium associated with anomalous inferior vena cava, situs inversus and multiple spleens: a developmental complex. *Mayo Clinic Proceedings*, **40**, 609.
10 CRONJE R.E., HUGO L. & GRISSEL P.J.C. (1973) The association between polysplenia, asplenia and other congenital anomalies: organ isomerism. *South African Medical Journal*, **47**, 2264.
11 HALPERT B. & GYÖRKEY G. (1957) Accessory spleen in the tail of the pancreas. *Archives of Pathology*, **64**, 266.
12 HALPERT B. & GYÖRKEY G. (1959) Lesions observed in accessory spleens of 311 patients. *American Journal of Clinical Pathology*, **32**, 165.
13 GLEN J.E. (1955) Accessory spleen in the scrotum. *Journal of Urology*, **73**, 1057.
14 PUTSCHAR W.G.T. & MANNION W.C. (1956) Splenic-gonadal fusion. *American Journal of Pathology*, **32**, 15.
15 DeWEESE M.S. & COLLER G.A. (1959) Splenectomy for hematologic disorders. *Western Journal of Surgery*, **67**, 129.
16 HALPERT B. & EATON W.L. (1954) Lesions in accessory spleens. *Archives of Pathology*, **57**, 501.
17 MORRISON M., LEDERER M. & FRADKIN W.Z. (1928) Accessory spleens: their significance in essential thrombocytopenic purpura hemorrhagica. *American Journal of the Medical Sciences*, **176**, 672.
18 VAUGHAN J.M. (1937) Treatment of thrombocytopenic purpura. *British Medical Journal*, **ii**, 842.
19 THOREK P., GRADMAN R. & WELCH J. (1948) Recurrent primary thrombocytopenic purpura with accessory spleens. *Annals of Surgery*, **128**, 304.
20 ROSENTHAL N., VOGEL P., LEE S. & LIPSAY J. (1951) The role of accessory spleens in post-splenectomy recurrent

purpura hemorrhagica. *Journal of the Mount Sinai Hospital*, **17**, 1008.

21 LOEB V. JR., SEAMAN W.B. & MOORE C.V. (1952) The use of thorium dioxide sol (Thorotrast) in the roentgenologic demonstration of accessory spleens. *Blood*, **7**, 904.

22 EVANS T.S., SPINNER S., PICCOLO P., SWIRSKY M., WHITE R. & KIESEWETTER W. (1953) Recurrent hypersplenism due to accessory spleen. *Acta Haematologica*, **10**, 350.

23 MACKENZIE F.A.F., ELLIOT D.H., EASTCOTT H.H.G., HUGHES-JONES N.C., BARKHAN P. & MOLLISON P.L. (1962) Relapse in hereditary spherocytosis with proven splenunculus. *Lancet*, **i**, 1102.

24 ASPNES G.T., PEARSON H.A., SPENCER R.P. & PICKETT L.K. (1975) Recurrent idiopathic thrombocytopenic purpura with 'accessory' splenic tissue. *Pediatrics*, **55**, 131.

25 WEISS L. (1965) The structure of the normal spleen. *Seminars in Hematology*, **3**, 205.

26 WEISS L. (1973). The spleen. In: *Histology* (ed. Greep R.O. & Weiss L.), 3rd edn. p. 445. McGraw-Hill, New York.

27 LEWIS O.J. (1956) The development of the circulation in the spleen of the foetal rabbit. *Journal of Anatomy*, **90**, 569.

28 LEWIS O.J. (1957) The blood vessels of the adult mammalian spleen. *Journal of Anatomy*, **91**, 245.

29 WENNBERG E. & WEISS L. (1969) The structure of the spleen and hemolysis. *Annual Review of Medicine*, **20**, 29.

30 SCHWEIGGER-SEIDEL F. (1863) Untersuchungen über die Milz. II. Von den Arterienenden, der Pulpa und den Bahnen des Blutes. *Archiv für pathologische Anatomie und Physiologie und für klinische Medizin (Virchow)*, **27**, 460.

31 BJÖRKMAN S.E. (1947) Splenic circulation, with special reference to the function of the spleen sinus wall. *Acta Medica Scandinavica*, **191**, Suppl. 1.

32 WEISS L. (1957) Study of structure of splenic sinuses in man and in albino rat with light microscope and electron microscope. *Journal of Biophysical and Biochemical Cytology*, **3**, 599.

33 KLEMPERER P. (1938) The spleen. In: *Handbook of Haematology* (ed. Downey H.) Vol. 3, p. 1591. Hamish Hamilton, London.

34 BILLROTH T. (1861) Zur normalen und pathologischen Anatomie der menschlichen Milz. *Archiv für pathologische Anatomie und Physiologie und für klinische Medizin (Virchow)*, **20**, 409.

35 MACNEAL W.J., OTANI S. & PATTERSON M.B. (1927) The finer vascular channels of the spleen. *American Journal of Pathology*, **3**, 111.

36 KEY E.A. (1861) Zur Anatomie der Milz. *Archiv für pathologische Anatomie und Physiologie und für klinische Medizin (Virchow)*, **21**, 568.

37 MCNEE J.W. (1931) The spleen: its structure, functions and diseases. *Lancet*, **i**, 951.

38 HELLY K. (1903) Die Blutbahnen der Milz und deren funktionelle Bedeutung. *Archiv für mikroskopische Anatomie*, **61**, 245.

39 KNISELY M.H. (1936) Spleen studies. I. Microscopic observations of the circulatory system of living unstimulated mammalian spleens. *Anatomical Record*, **65**, 23.

40 SNOOK T. (1958) The histology of vascular terminations in the rabbit's spleen. *Anatomical Record*, **130**, 711.

41 WEISS L. (1962) The structure of fine splenic arterial vessels in relation to hemoconcentration and red cell destruction. *American Journal of Anatomy*, **111**, 131.

42 WEISS L. (1963) The structure of intermediate vascular pathways in the spleen of rabbits. *American Journal of Anatomy*, **113**, 51.

43 MACNEAL W.J. & PATTERSON M. (1926) The pathway of nucleated erythrocytes introduced into the splenic artery. *Proceedings of the Society for Experimental Biology and Medicine*, **23**, 420.

44 WILLIAMS R.G. (1961) Studies of the vasculature in living autografts of spleen. *Anatomical Record*, **140**, 109.

45 CHEN L.T. & WEISS L. (1972) Electron microscopy of the red pulp of the human spleen. *American Journal of Anatomy*, **134**, 425.

46 GALINDO B. & FREEMAN J.A. (1973) Fine structure of the splenic pulp. *Anatomical Record*, **147**, 25.

47 BARNHART M.I., BAECHLER C.A. & LUSHER J.M. (1976) Arteriovenous shunts in the human spleen. *American Journal of Hematology*, **1**, 105.

48 BARNHART M.I. & LUSHER J.M. (1976) The human spleen as revealed by scanning electron microscopy. *American Journal of Hematology*, **1**, 243.

49 MILLIKIN P.D. (1966) Anatomy of germinal centers in human lymphoid tissue. *Archives of Pathology*, **82**, 499.

50 MILLIKIN P.D. (1969) The nodular white pulp of the human spleen. *Archives of Pathology*, **87**, 247.

51 FLEMMING W. (1884) Studien über Regeneration der Gewebe. *Archiv für mikroskopische Anatomie und Entwicklungsmechanik*, **24**, 50.

52 EK J.I. & RAYNER S. (1950) An analytical study of splenectomised cases after traumatic rupture of healthy spleens. *Acta Medica Scandinavica*, **137**, 417.

53 ROBINETTE C.D. & FRAUMENI J.F., JR (1977) Splenectomy and subsequent mortality of veterans of the 1939–45 war. *Lancet*, **ii**, 127.

54 JORDAN H.E. (1942) Extramedullary blood production. *Physiological Reviews*, **22**, 375.

55 HARTFALL S.J. & STEWART M.J. (1933) Massive paravertebral heterotopia of bone marrow in a case of acholuric jaundice. *Journal of Pathology and Bacteriology*, **37**, 455.

56 DACIE J.V. (1943) Familial haemolytic anaemia (acholuric jaundice) with particular reference to changes in fragility produced by splenectomy. *Quarterly Journal of Medicine*, **12**, 101.

57 DACIE J.V. (1960) *The Haemolytic Anaemias: Congenital and Acquired*, Part 1, 2nd edn. Churchill, London.

58 SYMMERS D. (1948) Splenomegaly. *Archives of Pathology*, **45**, 385.

59 WILAND E.K. & SMITH E.B. (1956) The morphology of the spleen in congenital hemolytic anemia (hereditary spherocytosis). *American Journal of Clinical Pathology*, **26**, 619.

60 ERNSTRÖM U. & SANDBERG G. (1968) Migration of splenic lymphocytes. *Acta Pathologica et Microbiologica Scandinavica*, **72**, 379.

61 SANDBERG G. (1970) Release of splenic cells into the blood of guinea pigs of different ages. *Scandinavian Journal of Haematology*, **7**, 104.

62 CANNON D.C. & WISSLER R.W. (1967) Spleen cell

migration in the immune response of the rat. *Archives of Pathology*, **84**, 109.

63 FLIEDNER T.M., KESS M., CRONKITE E.P. & ROBERTSON J.S. (1964) Cell proliferation in germinal centers of the rat spleen. *Annals of the New York Academy of Sciences*, **113**, 578.

64 YOFFEY J.M., HUDSON G. & OSMOND D.G. (1965) The lymphocyte in guinea pig bone marrow. *Journal of Anatomy*, **99**, 841.

65 YOFFEY J.M. (1966) *Bone Marrow Reactions*. Edward Arnold, London.

66 OTTESEN J. (1954) On the age of human white cells in peripheral blood. *Acta Physiologica Scandinavica*, **32**, 75.

67 GOWANS J.L. & KNIGHT E.J. (1964) The route of recirculation of lymphocytes in the rat. *Proceedings of the Royal Society, Series B*, **159**, 257.

68 PARROTT D.M.V., DE SOUSA M.A.B. & EAST J. (1966) Thymus-dependent areas in the lymphoid organs in neonatally thymectomized mice. *Journal of Experimental Medicine*, **123**, 191.

69 GOLDSCHNEIDER I. & McGREGOR D.D. (1968) Migration of lymphocytes and thymocytes in the rat. I. The route of migration from blood to spleen and lymph nodes. *Journal of Experimental Medicine*, **127**, 155.

70 FORD W.L. & GOWANS J.L. (1969) The traffic of lymphocytes. *Seminars in Hematology*, **6**, 67.

71 PERRY S., IRVIN G.L. & WHANG J. (1967) Studies of lymphocyte kinetics in man. *Blood*, **29**, 22.

72 RAFF M.C. & WORTIS H.H. (1970) Thymus dependence of θ-bearing cells in the peripheral lymphoid tissues of mice. *Immunology*, **18**, 931.

73 PABST R. & TREPEL F. (1975) The predominant role of the spleen in lymphocyte recirculation. I. Homing of lymphocytes to and release from the isolated perfused pig spleen. *Cell and Tissue Kinetics*, **8**, 529.

74 PABST R. & TREPEL F. (1976) The predominant rôle of the spleen in lymphocyte recirculation. II. Pre- and postsplenectomy retransfusion studies in young pigs. *Cell and Tissue Kinetics*, **9**, 179.

75 PABST R., MUNZ D. & TREPEL F. (1977) Splenic lymphopoiesis and migration pattern of splenic lymphocytes. *Cellular Immunology*, **33**, 33.

76 WEISSMAN I.L., WARNKE R., BUTCHER E.C., ROUSE R. & LEVY R. (1978) The lymphoid system: its normal architecture and the potential for understanding the system through the study of lymphoproliferative diseases. *Human Pathology*, **9**, 25.

77 MILLER J.F.A.P. & OSOBA D. (1967) Current concepts of the immunological function of the thymus. *Physiological Reviews*, **47**, 437.

78 CAFFREY R.W., EVERETT N.B. & RIEKE W.O. (1966) Radioautographic studies of reticular and blast cells in the hemopoietic tissues of the rat. *The Anatomical Record*, **155**, 41.

79 MICKLEM H.S., FORD C.E., EVANS E.P. & GRAY J. (1966) Interrelationships of myeloid and lymphoid cells: studies with chromosome-marked cells transfused into lethally irradiated mice. *Proceedings of the Royal Society, Series B*, **165**, 78.

80 OSMOND D.G. (1969) The non-thymic origin of lymphocytes. *The Anatomical Record*, **165**, 109.

81 BARCROFT J. & BARCROFT H. (1923) Observations on the taking up of carbon monoxide by the haemoglobin in the spleen. *Journal of Physiology*, **58**, 138.

82 BARCROFT J. & STEPHENS J.G. (1927) Observations upon the size of the spleen. *Journal of Physiology*, **64**, 1.

83 BARCROFT J. & FLOREY H. (1929) The effects of exercise on the vascular conditions in the spleen and the colon. *Journal of Physiology*, **68**, 81.

84 BARCROFT J. (1932) The effect of some accidental lesions on the size of the spleen. *Journal of Physiology*, **76**, 436.

85 BARCROFT J. (1932) Alterations in the size of the denervated spleen related to pregnancy. *Journal of Physiology*, **76**, 443.

86 BARCROFT J. (1934) *Features in the Architecture of Physiological Function*. Cambridge University Press, Cambridge.

87 TURNER A.W. & HODGETTS V.E. (1959) Dynamic red cell storage function of the spleen in sheep. *Australian Journal for Experimental Biology and Medical Science*, **37**, 399.

88 GREEN H.D., OTTIS K. & KITCHEN T. (1960) Autonomic stimulation and blockade on canine splenic inflow, outflow and weight. *American Journal of Physiology*, **198**, 424.

89 MOTULSKY A.G., CASSERD F., GIBLETT E.R., BROUN G.O. & FINCH C.A. (1958) Anemia and the spleen. *New England Journal of Medicine*, **259**, 1164, 1215.

90 CROSBY W.H. (1959) Normal functions of the spleen relative to red blood cells: a review. *Blood*, **14**, 399.

91 EBERT R.V., STEAD E.A. JR. & GIBSON J.G. (1941) Response of normal subjects to acute blood loss, with special reference to the mechanism of restoration of blood volume. *Archives of Internal Medicine*, **68**, 578.

92 NYLIN G. (1947) Effect of heavy muscular work on volume of circulating red corpuscles in man. *American Journal of Physiology*, **149**, 180.

93 LUCIA S.P., AGGELER P.M., HUSSER G.D. & LEONARD M.E. (1937) Effect of epinephrine on blood count and on hematocrit value. *Proceedings of the Society for Experimental Biology and Medicine*, **36**, 582.

94 EBERT R.V. & STEAD E.A. (1941) Demonstration that in normal man no reserves of blood are mobilized by exercise, epinephrine, and hemorrhage. *American Journal of the Medical Sciences*, **201**, 655.

95 KALTREIDER N.L., MENEELY G.R. & ALLEN J.R. (1942) The effect of epinephrine on the volume of the blood. *Journal of Clinical Investigation*, **21**, 339.

96 PARSON W., MAYERSON H.S., LYONS C., PORTER B. & TRAUTMAN W.V. JR (1948) Effect of the administration of adrenalin on the circulating red cell volume. *American Journal of Physiology*, **155**, 239.

97 DORNFEST B.S., HANDLER E.S. & HANDLER E.E. (1971) Reticulocyte sequestration in spleens of normal, anaemic and leukaemic rats. *British Journal of Haematology*, **21**, 83.

98 CRUZ W.O. & ROBSCHEIT-ROBBINS F.S. (1942) Relationship between the spleen and the morphologic picture of blood regeneration. *American Journal of the Medical Sciences*, **203**, 28.

99 LORBER M. (1958) The effects of splenectomy on the red blood cells of the dog with particular emphasis on the reticulocyte response. *Blood*, **13**, 972.

100 CROSBY W.H. (1962) Hereditary non-spherocytic hemolytic anemia. *Blood*, **5**, 233.

101 BERENDES M. (1959) The proportion of reticulocytes in the erythrocytes of the spleen as compared with those of circulating blood with special reference to hemolytic states. *Blood*, **14**, 558.

102 JANDL J.H. (1960) The agglutination and sequestration of immature red cells. *Journal of Laboratory and Clinical Medicine*, **55**, 663.

103 SORBIE J. & VALBERG L.S. (1970) Splenic sequestration of stress erythrocytes in the rabbit. *American Journal of Physiology*, **218**, 647.

104 SONG S.H. & GROOM A.C. (1971) Immature and abnormal erythrocytes present in the normal healthy spleen. *Scandinavian Journal of Haematology*, **8**, 487.

105 SONG S.H. & GROOM A.C. (1972) Sequestration and possible maturation of reticulocytes in the normal spleen. *Canadian Journal of Physiology and Pharmacology*, **50**, 400.

106 SONG S.H. & GROOM A.C. (1973) Scanning electron microscope study of the splenic red pulp in relation to the sequestration of immature and abnormal red cells. *Journal of Morphology*, **144**, 439.

107 ASTER R.H. & JANDL J.H. (1964) Platelet sequestration in man. I. Methods. *Journal of Clinical Investigation*, **43**, 843.

108 ASTER R.H. (1966) Pooling of platelets in the spleen: rôle in the pathogenesis of 'hypersplenic' thrombocytopenia. *Journal of Clinical Investigation*, **45**, 645.

109 PENNY R., ROZENBERG M.C. & FIRKIN B.G. (1966) The splenic platelet pool. *Blood*, **27**, 1.

110 KUTTI J., WEINFELD A. & WESTIN J. (1972) The relationship between splenic platelet pool and spleen size. *Scandinavian Journal of Haematology*, **9**, 1.

111 LJUNGQVIST U., BERGENTZ S.E. & LEANDOUR L. (1970) Platelet adhesiveness and aggregability after acute haemorrhage in the dog. *Acta Chirurgica Scandinavica*, **137**, 1.

112 LJUNGQVIST U. & BERGENTZ S.E. (1970) The effect of experimental trauma on the platelets. *Acta Chirurgica Scandinavica*, **136**, 271.

113 LJUNGQVIST U. (1970) Platelet response to acute haemorrhage in the dog. *Acta Chirurgica Scandinavica*, **411**, Suppl. 1.

114 HIRSH J. & McBRIDE J.A. (1965) Increased platelet adhesiveness in recurrent venous thrombosis and pulmonary embolism. *British Medical Journal*, **ii**, 797.

115 HIRSH J., McBRIDE J.A. & DACIE J.V. (1966) Thromboembolism and increased platelet adhesiveness in post-splenectomy thrombocytosis. *Australasian Annals of Medicine*, **15**, 122.

116 McBRIDE J.A. & PAYLING WRIGHT H. (1968) The effect of acute anaemia on platelet adhesiveness before and after splenectomy in the rabbit. *British Journal of Haematology*, **15**, 297.

117 HAM J.M. & FURNEAUX R.W. (1969) The effect of splenectomy on blood-platelets and lipoprotein lipase activity in the dog. *British Journal of Surgery*, **56**, 527.

118 STEIMAN R.H., HENRY R.L. & MURANO G. (1969) *In-vitro* inhibition and reversal of platelet aggregation by splenic extracts. *Thrombosis et Diathesis Haemorrhagica*, **21**, 397.

119 McMILLAN R. & SCOTT J.L. (1968) Leukocyte labeling with [51]chromium. I. Technic and results in normal subjects. *Blood*, **32**, 738.

120 DUVALL C.P. & PERRY S. (1968) The use of [51]chromium in the study of leukocyte kinetics in chronic myelocytic leukemia. *Journal of Laboratory and Clinical Medicine*, **71**, 614.

121 SCOTT J.L., McMILLAN R., DAVIDSON J.G., & MARINO J.V. (1971) Leucocyte labeling with [51]chromium. II. Leukocyte kinetics in chronic myelocytic leukemia. *Blood*, **38**, 162.

122 BIERMAN H.R., BYRON R.L. & KELLY K.H. (1953) The rôle of the spleen in the leukocytosis following the intra-arterial administration of epinephrine. *Blood*, **8**, 153.

123 FIESCHI A. & SACCHETTI C. (1964) Clinical assessment of granulopoiesis. *Acta Haematologica*, **31**, 150.

124 KNISELY M.H. (1936) Spleen studies. II. Microscopic observations of the circulatory system of living traumatized spleens, and of dying spleens. *Anatomical Record*, **65**, 131.

125 BESSIS M. (1965) Cellular mechanisms for the destruction of erythrocytes. *Series Haematologica*, **2**, 59.

126 EDWARDS V.D. & SIMON G.T. (1970) Ultrastructural aspects of red cell destruction in the normal rat spleen. *Journal of Ultrastructure Research*, **33**, 187.

127 BURKE J.S. & SIMON G.T. (1970) Electron microscopy of the spleen. I. Anatomy and microcirculation. *American Journal of Pathology*, **58**, 127.

128 SIMON G.T. & BURKE J.S. (1970) Electron microscopy of the spleen. III. Erythro-leukophagocytosis. *American Journal of Pathology*, **58**, 451.

129 SINGER K. & WEISZ L. (1945) The life cycle of the erythrocyte after splenectomy and the problems of splenic hemolysis and target cell formation. *American Journal of the Medical Sciences*, **210**, 301.

130 HALL C.E., NASH J.B. & HALL O. (1957) Erythrocyte survival and blood volume in the rat as determined by labeling the red cells with Cr[51]. *American Journal of Physiology*, **190**, 327.

131 BELCHER E.H. & HARRISS E.B. (1959) Studies of red cell life span in the rat. *Journal of Physiology*, **146**, 217.

132 WALDMAN T.A., WEISSMAN S.M. & BERLIN N.I. (1960) The effect of splenectomy on erythropoiesis in the dog. *Blood*, **15**, 873.

133 TIZIANELLO A., PANNACCIULLI I., SALVIDIO E. & AJMAR F. (1961) A quantitative evaluation of the splenic and hepatic share in normal hemocatheresis. *Acta Medica Scandinavica*, **169**, 303.

134 THOMPSON J.S., GURNEY C.W., HANEL A., FORD E. & HOFSTRA D. (1961) Survival of transfused blood in rats. *American Journal of Physiology*, **200**, 327.

135 BERLIN N.I. (1964) Lifespan of the red cell. In: *The Red Blood Cell*. (ed. Bishop C. & Surgenor D.M.), p. 423. Academic Press, New York.

136 ULTMANN J.E. & GORDON C.S. (1965) Life span and sites of sequestration of normal erythrocytes in normal and splenectomized mice and rats. *Acta Haematologica*, **33**, 118.

137 HARKER L.A. (1971) The rôle of the spleen in thrombokinetics. *Journal of Laboratory and Clinical Medicine*, **77**, 247.

138 ASTER R.H. (1969) Studies of the fate of platelets in rats and man. *Blood*, **34**, 117.

139 PALMER J.G., KEMP. J., CARTWRIGHT G.E. & WINTROBE

M.M. (1951) Studies on the effect of splenectomy on the total leukocyte count in the albino rat. *Blood*, **6**, 3.

140 HJORT P.F. & PAPUTCHIS H. (1960) Platelet survival in normal, splenectomized and hypersplenic rats. *Blood*, **15**, 45.

141 LEEKSMA C.H.W. & COHEN J.A. (1956) Determination of the lifespan of human blood platelets using labeled diisopropylphosphonate. *Journal of Clinical Investigation*, **35**, 964.

142 DAMESHEK W. & ESTREN I. (1947) *The Spleen and Hypersplenism*. Grune & Stratton, New York.

143 DOAN C.A. (1949) Hypersplenism. *Bulletin of the New York Academy of Medicine*, **25**, 625.

144 CROSBY W.H. (1963) Is hypersplenism a dead issue? *Blood*, **20**, 94.

145 GOSTOMZYK J.G., ARNOLD E. & RUHENSTROTH-BAUER G. (1963) Zur Frage der Beziehung zwischen Milz und Knochenmark nach einer Ganzkörperbestrahlung. *Naturwissenschaft*, **50**, 704.

146 WETHERLEY-MEIN G., JONES N.F. & PULLAN J.M. (1961) Effects of splenectomy on red cell production in myelofibrosis. *British Medical Journal*, **i**, 84.

147 MAURICE P.A. & JEANRENAUD A. (1964) Erythropoietic depression due to splenic irradiation. *British Journal of Haematology*, **10**, 327.

148 ERNSTRÖM U. & SANDBERG G. (1970) Influence of splenectomy on thymic release of lymphocytes into the blood. *Scandinavian Journal of Haematology*, **7**, 342.

149 CROSBY W.H. & RUIZ F. (1962) Evidence of a myelo-inhibitory factor in the spleen. *Blood*, **20**, 793.

150 GOSTOMZYK J.G., FEESER C. & RUHENSTROTH-BAUER G. (1964) Stimulierung der Ausschwemmung von Granulozyten aus dem Knochenmark durch die Milz. *Klinische Wochenschrift*, **42**, 231.

151 RUHENSTROTH-BAUER G. (1965) The rôle of humoral splenic factors in the formation and release of blood cells. *Seminars in Hematology*, **2**, 229.

152 KNOSPE W.H., FRIED W., GREGORY S.A., SASSETTI R.J. & TROBAUGH F.E. JR (1970) Effect of a non-cellular spleen-derived factor on recovery of hematopoietic stem cells from irradiation. *Journal of Laboratory and Clinical Medicine*, **76**, 584.

153 BURGER M., KNYSZYNSKI A. & BERENBLUM I. (1969) Stimulation of thymic and bone marrow regeneration in irradiated mice by protein fractions of human serum and sheep spleen. *Radiation Research*, **40**, 193.

154 ASKONAS B.A. & WHITE R.G. (1956) Sites of antibody production in the guinea-pig. The relation between *in vitro* synthesis of anti-ovalbumin and γ-globulin and distribution of antibody-containing plasma cells. *British Journal of Experimental Pathology*, **37**, 61.

155 ASKONAS B.A. & HUMPHREY J.H. (1958) Formation of specific antibody and γ-globulin *in vitro*; a study of the synthetic ability of various tissues from rabbits immunized by different methods. *Biochemical Journal*, **68**, 252.

156 ROWLEY D.A. (1950) The formation of circulating antibody in the splenectomized human being following intravenous injection of heterologous erythrocytes. *Journal of Immunology*, **65**, 515.

157 FORD W.L., GOWANS J.L. & McCULLAGH P.L. (1966) The origin and function of lymphocytes. In: *The Thymus: Experimental and Clinical Studies* (ed. Wol-

stenholme G.E.W. & Porter R.), p. 58. Churchill, London.

158 FORD W.L. & GOWANS J.L. (1967) The rôle of lymphocytes in antibody formation. II. The influence of lymphocyte migration in the isolated perfused spleen. *Proceedings of the Royal Society, Series B*, **168**, 244.

159 SINGHAL S.K. & RICHTER M. (1968) Cells involved in the immune response. IV. The response of normal and immune rabbit bone marrow and lymphoid tissue lymphocytes to antigens *in vitro*. *Journal of Experimental Medicine*, **128**, 1099.

160 SINGHAL K. & RICHTER M. (1968) Cells involved in immune response. I. The response of normal rabbit bone marrow cells to antigens *in vitro*. *International Archives of Allergy and Applied Immunology*, **33**, 493.

161 RICHTER M. & ABDOU N.I. (1969) Cells involved in the immune response. VII. The demonstration, using allo-typic markers, of antibody formation by irradiation-resistant cells of irradiated rabbits injected with normal allogeneic bone marrow cells and sheep erythrocytes. *Journal of Experimental Medicine*, **129**, 1261.

162 ABDOU N.I. & RICHTER M. (1969) Cells involved in the immune response. V. The migration of antigen-reactive immunocompetent cells out of the bone marrow following antigen administration. *International Archives of Allergy and Applied Immunology*, **35**, 330.

163 MISHELL R.I. & DUTTON R.W. (1966) Immunization of normal mouse spleen cell suspensions *in vitro*. *Science*, **153**, 1004.

164 SAUNDERS G.C. & KING V.W. (1966) Antibody synthesis initiated by paired explants of spleen and thymus. *Science*, **151**, 1390.

165 TAO T.W. & UHR J.W. (1966) Primary-type antibody response *in vitro*. *Science*, **151**, 1096.

166 MARBROOK J. (1967) Primary immune response in cultures of spleen cells. *Lancet*, **ii**, 1279.

167 ROBINSON W.A., MARBROOK J. & DIENER E. (1967) Primary stimulation and measurement of antibody production to sheep red blood cells *in vitro*. *Journal of Experimental Medicine*, **126**, 347.

168 MISHELL R.I. & DUTTON R.W. (1967) Immunization of dissociated spleen cell cultures from normal mice. *Journal of Experimental Medicine*, **126**, 423.

169 GLOBERSON A. & AUERBACH R. (1965) Primary immune reactions in organ cultures. *Science*, **149**, 991.

170 BOXALL T.A., HIROSE S. & EISEMAN B. (1968) Immunological competence of the isolated perfused pig spleen. *Journal of Surgical Research*, **10**, 353.

171 ATKINS R.C., ROBINSON W.A., TRIMBLE C. & EISEMAN B. (1968) *In vitro* challenge and antibody production of the *ex vivo* perfused spleen. *Journal of Surgical Research*, **10**, 353.

172 MOORE A.R., HUMPHREY L. & EISEMAN B. (1968) The *ex vivo* perfused spleen as a source of immune lymphocytes. *Surgery, Gynecology and Obstetrics*, **126**, 1251.

173 WOOD W.B. JR, SMITH M.R., PERRY W.D. & BERRY J.W. (1951) Studies on cellular immunology of acute bacteremia: intravascular leucocytic reaction and surface phagocytosis. *Journal of Experimental Medicine*, **94**, 52.

174 BALLANTYNE B. (1968) The reticuloendothelial localization of splenic esterases. *Journal of the Reticuloendothelial Society*, **5**, 399.

175 SNODGRASS M.J. (1968) The study of some histochemi-

cal and phagocytic reactions of the sinus lining cells of the rabbit's spleen. *Anatomical Record*, **161**, 353.

176 SNODGRASS M.J. (1970) Some histochemical aspects of the sinus lining of the rabbit spleen. *Anatomical Record*, **166**, 381.

177 SNODGRASS M.J. & SNOOK T. (1971) A study of some histochemical and phagocytic reactions of the reticulo-endothelial system of the rabbit spleen. *Anatomical Record*, **170**, 243.

178 BLEYL U., KUHN W. & GRAEFF H. (1969) Reticulo-endotheliale Clearance intravasaler Fibrinmonomere in der Milz. *Thrombosis et Diathesis Haemorrhagica*, **22**, 87.

179 COBURN R.F. & KANE P.B. (1968) Maximal erythrocyte and hemoglobin catabolism. *Journal of Clinical Investigation*, **47**, 1435.

180 PALMER D.L., RIFKIND D. & BROWN D.W. (1971) ^{131}I-labeled colloidal human serum albumin in the study of reticuloendothelial system function. II. Phagocytosis and catabolism of a test colloid in normal subjects. *Journal of Infectious Diseases*, **123**, 457.

181 STUART A.E. & DAVIDSON A.E. (1964) Effects of simple lipids on antibody formation after injection of foreign red cells. *Journal of Pathology and Bacteriology*, **87**, 305.

182 COONS A.H., LEDUC E.H. & KAPLAN M.H. (1951) Localization of antigens in tissue cells. VI. The fate of injected foreign proteins in the mouse. *Journal of Experimental Medicine*, **93**, 173.

183 NOLTENIUS H. & RUHL P. (1969) Evidence of macro-phages being 19S-antibody producing cells, as shown by a modification of the plaque technic. *Experientia*, **25**, 75.

184 NOLTENIUS H. & CHAHIN M. (1969) Further evidence concerning macrophages producing 19S-antibody in mice. *Experientia*, **25**, 401.

185 WEIR D.M. (1967) The immunological consequences of cell death. *Lancet*, **ii**, 1071.

186 PRIBNOW J.F. & SILVERMAN M.S. (1967) Studies on the radiosensitive phase of the primary antibody response in rabbits. I. The rôle of the macrophage. *Journal of Immunology*, **98**, 255.

187 CROSBY W.H. (1957) Siderocytes and the spleen. *Blood*, **12**, 165.

188 CROSBY W.H. (1959) Evidence of the recycling of siderocyte iron. *Journal of Clinical Investigation*, **38**, 997.

189 CROSBY W.H. & SHEEHY T.W. (1960) Hypochromic iron-loading anaemia: studies of iron and haemoglobin metabolism by means of vigorous phlebotomy. *British Journal of Haematology*, **6**, 56.

190 NOYES W.D., BOTHWELL T.H. & FINCH C.A. (1960) The rôle of the reticuloendothelial cell in iron metabolism. *British Journal of Haematology*, **6**, 43.

191 RIZZA C.R. (1961) Effect of exercise on the level of antihaemophilic globulin in human blood. *Journal of Physiology*, **156**, 128.

192 INGRAM G.I.C. (1961) Increase in antihaemophilic globulin activity following infusion of adrenaline. *Journal of Physiology*, **156**, 217.

193 LIBRE E.P., COWAN P.H., WATKINS S.P. JR & SHULMAN N.R. (1968) Relationships between spleen, platelets and Factor VIII levels, *Blood*, **31**, 358.

194 GUNN C.G. & HAMPTON J.W. (1967) CNS influence on plasma levels of factor VIII activity. *American Journal of Physiology*, **212**, 124.

195 RIZZA C.R. & EIPE J (1971) Exercise, factor VIII and the spleen. *British Journal of Haematology*, **20**, 629.

196 MCKEE P.A., COUSSONS R.T., BUCKNER R.G., WILLIAMS G.R. & HAMPTON J.W. (1970) Effects of the spleen on canine factor VIII levels. *Journal of Laboratory and Clinical Medicine*, **75**, 391.

197 NORMAN J.C., LAMBILLIOTTE J.P., KOJIMA Y. & SISE H.S. (1967) Anti-hemophilic factor release by perfused liver and spleen. Relationship to hemophilia. *Science*, **158**, 1060.

198 WEBSTER W.P., REDDICK R.L., ROBERTS H.R. & PENICK G.D. (1967) Release of factor VIII (anti-haemophilic factor) from perfused organs and tissues. *Nature (London)*, **213**, 1146.

199 DODDS W.J. & MILLER K.D. (1968) Storage and synthesis of coagulation factors in the isolated perfused liver, kidney and spleen. *Federation Proceedings*, **27**, 373.

200 NORMAN J.C., COVELLI V.H. & SISE H.S. (1968) Transplantation of the spleen. Experimental cure of hemophilia. *Surgery*, **64**, 1.

201 WEBSTER W.P., PENICK G.D., PEACOCK E.E. & BRINKHOUS K.M. (1967) Allotransplantation of spleen in hemophilia. *North Carolina Medical Journal*, **28**, 505.

202 WEBSTER W.P., PEACOCK E.E., WAGNER J.L., PENICK G.D. & BRINKHOUS K.M. (1968) Release of factor VIII from splenic transplants in hemophilia. *Federation Proceedings*, **27**, 374.

203 WEBSTER W.P., ZUKOSKI C.F., HUTCHIN P., REDDICK R.L., MANDEL S.R. & PENICK G.D. (1971) Plasma factor VIII synthesis and control as revealed by canine organ transplantation. *American Journal of Physiology*, **220**, 1147.

204 CORNELL C.N., COOPER R.G., MUHRER M.E. & GARB S. (1972) Splenectomy and factor VIII response in bleeder swine. *American Journal of Physiology*, **222**, 1610.

205 SELAWRY H.S. & STARR J.L. (1971) Protein biosynthesis in the spleen. I. Effect of primary immunization on microsomal and ribosomal function *in vitro*. *Journal of Immunology*, **106**, 349.

206 SELAWRY H.S. & STARR J.L. (1971) Protein biosynthesis in the spleen. II. Effect of primary immunization on the mechanism of protein synthesis. *Journal of Immunology*, **106**, 358.

207 NAJJAR V.A., FIDALGO B.V. & STITT E. (1968) The physiological role of the lymphoid system. VII. The disappearance of leucokinin activity following splenectomy. *Biochemistry*, **7**, 2376.

208 HARRIS I.M., McALISTER J. & PRANKERD T.A.J. (1958) Splenomegaly and the circulating red cell. *British Journal of Haematology*, **4**, 97.

209 MOTULSKY A.G., CASSERD F. & GIBLETT E. (1956) *In vivo* measurement of splenic circulation: rapid method for demonstration of splenic red cell sequestration. *Journal of Clinical Investigation*, **35**, 725.

210 MOTULSKY A.G., GIBLETT E., CASSERD F., HOUGHTON B. & FINCH C.A. (1958) Studies on pathophysiology of splenic anemia. *Proceedings of the VIth International Congress of the International Society of Haematology, 1956*, p. 419. Grune & Stratton, New York.

211 BOWDLER A.J. (1969) Regional variations in the propor-

tion of red cells in the blood in man. *British Journal of Haematology*, **16**, 557.

212 BOWDLER A.J. (1962) Theoretical considerations concerning measurement of the splenic red cell pool. *Clinical Science*, **23**, 181.

213 PRANKERD T.A.J. (1963) The spleen and anaemia. *British Medical Journal*, **ii**, 517.

214 RICHARDS J.D.M. & TOGHILL P.J. (1967) The distribution of erythrocytes in the human spleen in health and disease. *Journal of Pathology and Bacteriology*, **93**, 653.

215 MURPHY J.R. (1962) Erythrocyte metabolism. III. The relationship of energy metabolism and serum factors to the osmotic fragility following incubation. *Journal of Laboratory and Clinical Medicine*, **60**, 32.

216 LEVESQUE M.J. & GROOM A.C. (1976) pH environment of red cells in the spleen. *American Journal of Physiology*, **231**, 1672.

217 LEVESQUE M.J. & GROOM A.C. (1978) Effects of pH and flow rate on the release of 'bound' red cells from the splenic pulp. *Canadian Journal of Physiology and Pharmacology*, **56**, 260.

218 HAM T.H. & CASTLE W.B. (1940) Studies on the destruction of red blood cells. Relation of increased hypotonic fragility and of erythrostasis to the mechanism of hemolysis in certain anemias. *Proceedings of the American Philosophical Society*, **82**, 411.

219 YOUNG L.E. (1955) Hereditary spherocytosis. *American Journal of Medicine*, **18**, 486.

220 YOUNG L.E., IZZO M.J., ALTMAN K.I. & SWISHER S.N. (1956) Studies on spontaneous *in vitro* autohemolysis in hemolytic disorders. *Blood*, **11**, 977.

221 EMERSON C.P., SHEN S.C., HAM T.H., FLEMING E.M. & CASTLE W.B. (1956) Studies on destruction of red blood cells. IX. Quantitative methods for determining osmotic and mechanical fragility of red cells in peripheral blood and splenic pulp: mechanism of increased hemolysis in hereditary spherocytosis (congenital hemolytic jaundice) as related to functions of the spleen. *Archives of Internal Medicine*, **97**, 1.

222 PRANKERD T.A.J. (1960) Studies on the pathogenesis of haemolysis in hereditary spherocytosis. *Quarterly Journal of Medicine*, **29**, 199.

223 REEVE E.B. & VEALL N. (1949) A simplified method for the determination of circulating red-cell volume with radioactive phosphorus. *Journal of Physiology*, **108**, 12.

224 BERSON S.A. & YALOW R.S. (1952) The use of K^{42} or P^{32}-labelled erythrocytes and I^{131} tagged human serum albumin in simultaneous blood volume determinations. *Journal of Clinical Investigation*, **31**, 572.

225 CHAPLIN H. JR, MOLLISON P.L. & VETTER H. (1953) The body/venous hematocrit ratio: its constancy over a wide hematocrit range. *Journal of Clinical Investigation*, **32**, 1309.

226 GRAY S.J. & FRANK H. (1953) The simultaneous determination of red cell mass and plasma volume in man with radioactive sodium chromate and chromic chloride. *Journal of Clinical Investigation*, **32**, 1000.

227 HICKS D.A., HOPPE A., TURNBULL A.L. & VEREL D. (1956) The estimation and prediction of normal blood volume. *Clinical Science*, **15**, 557.

228 BROZOVIC B., KORUBIN V., LEWIS S.M. & SZUR L. (1966) Simultaneous red cell and plasma volume deter-minations by a differential absorption method. *Journal of Laboratory and Clinical Medicine*, **68**, 142.

229 ROTHSCHILD M.A., BAUMAN A., YALOW R.S. & BERSON S.A. (1954) Effect of splenomegaly on blood volume. *Journal of Applied Physiology*, **6**, 701.

230 VEREL D. (1954) Observations on the distribution of plasma and red cells in diseases. *Clinical Science*, **13**, 51.

231 FUDENBERG H.H., BALDINI M., MAHONEY J.P. & DAMESHEK W. (1961) The body hematocrit/venous hematocrit ratio and the 'splenic reservoir'. *Blood*, **17**, 71.

232 LORÍA A., SÁNCHEZ-MEDAL L., KAUFFER N. & QUINTANER E. (1962) Relationship between body hematocrit and venous hematocrit in normal, splenomegalic and anemic states. *Journal of Laboratory and Clinical Medicine*, **60**, 396.

233 SHALDON S. & SHERLOCK S. (1962) Portal hypertension in the myeloproliferative syndrome and the reticuloses. *American Journal of Medicine*, **32**, 758.

234 OISHI N., SWISHER S.N., STORMONT S.N. & SCHWARTZ S.I. (1960) Portal hypertension in myeloid metaplasia. *Archives of Surgery*, **81**, 80.

235 ROSENBAUM D.L., MURPHY G.W. & SWISHER S.N. (1966) Hemodynamic studies of the portal circulation in myeloid metaplasia. *American Journal of Medicine*, **41**, 360.

236 GARNETT E.S., GODDARD B.A., MARKBY D. & WEBBER C.E. (1969) The spleen as an arteriovenous shunt. *Lancet*, **i**, 386.

237 BLENDIS L.M., BANKS D.C., RAMBOER, C. & WILLIAMS R. (1970) Spleen blood flow and splanchnic haemodynamics in blood dyscrasias and other splenomegalies. *Clinical Science*, **38**, 73.

238 MCFADZEAN A.J.S., TODD D. & TSANG K.C. (1958) Observations on the anemia of cryptogenetic splenomegaly. II. Expansion of the plasma volume. *Blood*, **13**, 524.

239 MCFADZEAN A.J.S. & TODD D. (1967) The blood volume in post-necrotic cirrhosis of the liver with splenomegaly. *Clinical Science*, **32**, 339.

240 BOWDLER A.J. (1963) Dilution anemia corrected by splenectomy in Gaucher's disease. *Annals of Internal Medicine*, **58**, 664.

241 BOWDLER A.J. (1967) Dilution anaemia associated with enlargement of the spleen. *Proceedings of the Royal Society of Medicine*, **60**, 44.

242 BOWDLER A.J. (1970) Blood volume changes in patients with splenomegaly. *Transfusion*, **10**, 171.

243 WEINSTEIN V.F. (1964) Haemodilution anaemia associated with simple splenic hyperplasia. *Lancet*, **ii**, 218.

244 BLENDIS L.M., RAMBOER C. & WILLIAMS R. (1970) Studies on the haemodilution anaemia of splenomegaly. *European Journal of Clinical Investigation*, **1**, 54.

245 PRYOR D.S. (1967) Splenectomy in tropical splenomegaly. *British Medical Journal*, **ii**, 825.

246 PRYOR D.S. (1967) The mechanism of anaemia in tropical splenomegaly. *Quarterly Journal of Medicine*, **34**, 337.

247 HAMILTON P.J.S., RICHMOND J., DONALDSON G.W.K., WILLIAMS R., HUTT M.S.R., & LUGUMBA V. (1967) Splenectomy in 'big spleen disease'. *British Medical Journal*, **iii**, 823.

248 HESS C.E., AYERS C.R., WEITZEL R.A., MOHLER D.N. &

SANDUSKY W.R. (1971) Dilutional anemia of splenomegaly: an indication for splenectomy. *Annals of Surgery*, **173**, 693.

249 HUMPHREY J.H. & FAHEY J.L. (1961) The metabolism of normal plasma proteins and gamma-myeloma protein in mice bearing plasma-cell tumors. *Journal of Clinical Investigation*, **40**, 1696.

250 BARTH W.F., WOCHNER R.D., WALDMANN T.A. & FAHEY J.L. (1964) Metabolism of human gamma macroglobulins. *Journal of Clinical Investigation*, **43**, 1036.

251 BIRKE G., NORBERG R., OHAGEN B. & PLANTIN L.O. (1967) Metabolism of human gamma macroglobulins. *Scandinavian Journal of Clinical and Laboratory Investigation*, **19**, 171.

252 KOPP W.L., MACKINNEY A.A. & WASSON G.W. (1969) Blood volume and hematocrit values in macroglobulinemia. *Archives of Internal Medicine*, **123**, 394.

253 HESS C., AYERS C., CARMICHAEL S. & MOHLER D. (1969) Mechanism of dilutional anemia in splenomegaly. *Clinical Research*, **17**, 329.

254 BECKER H. & SPENGLER D. (1966) Die Verdünnungsanämie. Tierexperimentelle Untersuchungen über den Einfluss des Blutvolumens auf die Erythrozytenregulation. *Acta Haematologica (Basel)*, **35**, 1.

255 BOWDLER A.J. & PRANKERD T.A.J. (1962) Anaemia in the reticuloses. *British Medical Journal*, **i**, 1169.

256 CHAPLIN H. JR, & MOLLISON P.L. (1953) Red cell lifespan in nephritis and in hepatic cirrhosis. *Clinical Science*, **12**, 351.

257 MOLLISON P.L. & HUGHES-JONES N.C. (1958) Sites of removal of incompatible red cells from the circulation. *Vox Sanguinis*, **4**, 243.

258 JANDL J.H., FILES N.H., BARNETT S.B. & MACDONALD R.A. (1965) Proliferative response of the spleen and liver to hemolysis. *Journal of Experimental Medicine*, **122**, 299.

259 HOLZBACH R.T., SHIPLEY R.A., CLARK R.E. & CHUDZIK E.B. (1964) Influence of spleen size and portal pressure on erythrocyte sequestration. *Journal of Clinical Investigation*, **43**, 1125.

260 WAGNER H.N. JR, RAZZAK M.A., GAERTNER R.A., CAINE W.P. JR, & FEAGIN O.T. (1962) Removal of erythrocytes from the circulation. *Archives of Internal Medicine*, **110**, 90.

261 HUGHES-JONES N.C., MOLLISON P.L. & VEALL N. (1957) Removal of incompatible red cells by the spleen. *British Journal of Haematology*, **3**, 125.

262 KIMBER R.J. & LANDER H. (1964) The effect of heat on human red cell morphology, fragility, and subsequent survival *in vivo*. *Journal of Laboratory and Clinical Medicine*, **64**, 922.

263 MARSH G.W., LEWIS S.M. & SZUR L. (1966) The use of ^{51}Cr-labelled heat-damaged red cells to study splenic function. I. Evaluation of method. *British Journal of Haematology*, **12**, 161.

264 RINGELHANN B. & KONOTEY-AHULU F.I.D. (1971) The removal of heat-damaged and ^{51}Cr-labelled red cells in haemoglobinopathies. *British Journal of Haematology*, **21**, 99.

265 FISCHER J. & WOLF R. (1964) Das Functionsbild der sequestratorischen Leistung des reticulohistiocytären Systems. *Helvetica Medica Acta*, **31**, 579.

266 HARRIS I.M., MCALISTER J.M. & PRANKERD T.A.J. (1957) The relationship of abnormal red cells to the normal spleen. *Clinical Science*, **16**, 223.

267 JANDL J.H. & SIMMONS R.L. (1957) Agglutination and sensitization of red cells with metallic cations: interactions between multivalent metals and red-cell membrane. *British Journal of Haematology*, **3**, 19.

268 JACOBS H.W. & JANDL J.H. (1962) Effects of sulfhydryl inhibition on red blood cells. II. Studies *in vivo*. *Journal of Clinical Investigation*, **41**, 1514.

269 SMITH C.H., SCHULMAN I., ANDO R.E. & STERN G. (1955) Studies in Mediterranean (Cooley's) anemia. I. Clinical and hematologic aspects of splenectomy, with special reference to fetal hemoglobin synthesis. *Blood*, **10**, 582.

270 LEVIN W.C., BAIRD W.D., PERRY J.E. & ZUNG W.W.K. (1957) The experimental production of splenic sequestration of erythrocytes in patients with sickle-cell trait. *Journal of Laboratory and Clinical Medicine*, **50**, 926.

271 JANDL J.H., RICHARDSON JONES A. & CASTLE W.B. (1957) The destruction of red cells by antibodies in man. I. Observations on the sequestration and lysis of red cells altered by immune mechanisms. *Journal of Clinical Investigation*, **36**, 1428.

272 MOLLISON P.L. & CUTBUSH M. (1955) The use of isotope-labelled red cells to demonstrate incompatibility *in vivo*. *Lancet*, **i**, 1290.

273 JANDL J.H. & KAPLAN M.E. (1960) The destruction of red cells by antibodies in man. III. Quantitative factors influencing the patterns of hemolysis *in vivo*. *Journal of Clinical Investigation*, **39**, 1145.

274 CROME P. & MOLLISON P.L. (1964) Splenic destruction of Rh-sensitized and of heated cells. *British Journal of Haematology*, **10**, 137.

275 MOLLISON P.L. (1962) The reticulo-endothelial system and red cell destruction. *Proceedings of the Royal Society of Medicine*, **55**, 915.

276 ROSSE W.F. (1971) Quantitative immunology of immune hemolytic anemia. II. The relationship of cell-bound antibody to hemolysis and the effect of treatment. *Journal of Clinical Investigation*, **50**, 734.

277 LACELLE R.L. (1970) Alteration of membrane deformability in hemolytic anemias. *Seminars in Hematology*, **7**, 355.

278 JANDL J.H., SIMMONS R.L. & CASTLE W.B. (1961) Red cell filtration in the pathogenesis of certain hemolytic anemias. *Blood*, **28**, 133.

279 JANDL J.H. (1966) The pathophysiology of hemolytic anemias. *American Journal of Medicine*, **41**, 657.

280 LACELLE P.L. & WEED R.I. (1969) Abnormal membrane deformability. A model for the hereditary spherocyte. *Journal of Clinical Investigation*, **48**, 48a.

281 MURPHY J.R. (1967) The influence of pH and temperature on some physical properties of normal erythrocytes and erythrocytes from patients with hereditary spherocytosis. *Journal of Laboratory and Clinical Medicine*, **69**, 758.

282 MURPHY J.R. (1968) Hemoglobin CC disease: rheological properties of erythrocytes and abnormalities in cell water. *Journal of Clinical Investigation*, **47**, 1483.

283 WEED R.I. & LACELLE P.L. (1969) ATP dependence of erythrocyte membrane deformability: relation to *in vivo* survival and blood storage. In: *Red Cell Membrane:*

Structure and Function (ed. Jamieson G.A. & Greenwalt T.J.), p. 318. J. B. Lippincott, Philadelphia.

284 DINTENFASS L. & BURNARD E. (1966) Effect of hydrogen ion concentration on *in vitro* viscosity of packed cells and blood at high haematocrits. *Medical Journal of Australia*, **1**, 1072.

285 WEED R.I. & WEISS L. (1966) The relationship of red cell fragmentation occurring within the spleen to cell destruction. *Transactions of the Association of American Physicians*, **79**, 426.

286 WEED R.I. (1968) The cell membrane in hemolytic disorders. *Plenary Session Papers. XIIth Congress of the International Society of Hematology, New York, 1968*, p. 81.

287 FESSAS P. (1963) Inclusions of hemoglobin in erythrocytes of thalassemia. *Blood*, **21**, 21.

288 RIFKIND R.A. (1966) Destruction of injured cells *in vivo*. *American Journal of Medicine*, **41**, 711.

289 SLATER L.M., MUIR W.A. & WEED R.I. (1968) Influence of splenectomy on insoluble hemoglobin inclusion bodies in β-thalassemic erythrocytes. *Blood*, **31**, 766.

290 NATHAN D.G., GABUZDA T.G., LAFORET M.T. & GARDNER F.H. (1965) Hemoglobin precipitation and erythrocyte metabolism in hemoglobin H-thalassemia. *Clinical Research*, **13**, 279.

291 NATHAN D.G. & GUNN R.B. (1966) Thalassemia: the consequences of unbalanced hemoglobin synthesis. *American Journal of Medicine*, **41**, 815.

292 WEED R.I. & REED C.F. (1966) Membrane alterations leading to red cell destruction. *American Journal of Medicine*, **41**, 681.

293 BELCHER E.H. & HUGHES JONES N.C. (1960) The mathematical analysis of ^{51}Cr deposition in organs following the injection of ^{51}Cr-labelled red cells. *Clinical Science*, **19**, 657.

294 RIFKIND R.A. (1965) Heinz body anemia. An ultrastructural study. II. Red cell sequestration and destruction. *Blood*, **26**, 433.

295 POLICARD A. & BESSIS M. (1953) Fractionnement d'hématies par les leucocytes au course de la phagocytose. *Comptes Rendus de la Société Biologique*, **147**, 982.

296 LOBUGLIO A.F., COTRAN R.S. & JANDL J.H. (1967) Red cells coated with immunoglobulin G: binding and sphering by mononuclear cells in man. *Science*, **158**, 1582.

297 VAUGHAN R.B. & BOYDEN S.V. (1964) Interactions of macrophages and erythrocytes. *Immunology*, **7**, 118.

298 ARCHER G.T. (1965) Phagocytosis by monocytes of red cells coated with Rh antibodies. *Vox Sanguinis*, **10**, 590.

299 HUBER H., POLLEY M.J., LINSCOTT W.D., FUDENBERG H.H. & MÜLLER-EBERHARD, H.J. (1968) Human monocytes: distinct receptor sites for the third component of complement and for immunoglobulin G. *Science*, **162**, 1281.

300 EVANS R.S., TAKAHASHI K., DUANE R.T., PAYNE R. & LIU C.K. (1951) Primary thrombocytopenic purpura and acquired hemolytic anemia: evidence for a common etiology. *Archives of Internal Medicine*, **87**, 48.

301 WATSON-WILLIAMS E.J., MACPHERSON A.I.S. & DAVIDSON S. (1958) The treatment of idiopathic thrombocytopenic purpura: a review of ninety-three cases. *Lancet*, **ii**, 221.

302 CARPENTER A.F., WINTROBE M.M., FULLER E.A., HAUT A. & CARTWRIGHT G.E. (1959) Treatment of idiopathic thrombocytopenic purpura. *Journal of the American Medical Association*, **171**, 1911.

303 DOAN C.A., BOURONCLE B.A. & WISEMAN B.K. (1960) Idiopathic and secondary thrombocytopenic purpura: clinical study and evaluation of 381 cases over a period of 28 years. *Annals of Internal Medicine*, **53**, 861.

304 SCHARFMAN W.B., HOSLEY H.F., HAWKINS T. & PROPP S. (1960) Idiopathic thrombocytopenic purpura. An evaluation of the patterns of response to various therapies. *Journal of the American Medical Association*, **172**, 1875.

305 MEYERS M.C. (1961) Results of treatment in 71 patients with idiopathic thrombocytopenic purpura. *American Journal of the Medical Sciences*, **242**, 295.

306 BLOCK G.E., EVANS R. & ZAJTCHUN R. (1966) Splenectomy for idiopathic thrombocytopenic purpura. *Archives of Surgery*, **92**, 484.

307 WILDE R.C., ELLIS L.D. & COOPER W.M. (1967) Splenectomy for chronic idiopathic thrombocytopenic purpura. *Archives of Surgery*, **95**, 344.

308 SCHWARTZ S.I., BERNARD R.P., ADAMS J.T. & BAUMAN A.W. (1970) Splenectomy for hematologic disorders. *Archives of Surgery*, **101**, 338.

309 LARRIEU M.J., MESHAKA G., CAEN J. & BERNARD J. (1964) Traitement du purpura thrombopénique idiopathique. *Semaine des Hôpitaux de Paris*, **40**, 403.

310 HARKER L.A. (1970) Platelet kinetics in man. In: *Formation and Destruction of Blood Cells* (ed. Greenwalt T.J. & Jamieson G.A.), Ch. 9. J. B. Lippincott, Philadelphia.

311 WRIGHT C.S., DOAN C.A., BOURONCLE B.A. & ZOLLINGER R.M. (1951) Direct splenic arterial and venous blood studies in the hypersplenic syndromes before and after epinephrine. *Blood*, **6**, 195.

312 HARRINGTON W.J., PRAGUE C.C., MINNICH V., MOORE C.V., AULVIN R.C. & DUBACH R. (1953) Immunologic mechanisms in idiopathic and neonatal thrombocytopenic purpura. *Annals of Internal Medicine*, **38**, 433.

313 COHEN P.F., GARDNER A. & BARNETT G.O. (1961) Reclassification of thrombocytopenias by the Cr-51 method for measuring platelet lifespan. *New England Journal of Medicine*, **264**, 1294, 1350.

314 NAJEAN Y., ARDAILLOU N., CAEN J., LARRIEU M.J. & BERNARD J. (1963) Survival of radiochromium-labelled platelets in thrombocytopenias. *Blood*, **22**, 718.

315 ASTER R.H. (1965) Effect of anticoagulant and ABO incompatibility on recovery of transfused human platelets. *Blood*, **26**, 732.

316 NAJEAN Y., ARDAILLOU N., DRESCH C. & BERNARD J. (1967) The platelet destruction site in thrombocytopenic purpuras. *British Journal of Haematology*, **13**, 409.

317 SOLOMON R.B. & CLATANOFF D.V. (1967) Platelet survival studies and body scanning in idiopathic thrombocytopenic purpura. *American Journal of the Medical Sciences*, **254**, 777.

318 BURGER T. & RIHMER E. (1970) Platelet life-span and sites of platelet destruction in idiopathic thrombocytopenic purpura. *Acta Medica Academiae Scientiarum Hungaricae*, **27**, 119.

319 COOPER M.R., HANSEN K.S., MAYNARD C.D., ELROD I.W. & SPURR C.L. (1972) Platelet survival and sequest-

ration patterns in thrombocytopenic disorders. *Radiology*, **102**, 89.

320 NAJEAN Y., DASSIN E. & BALITRAND N. (1977) Etude critique des méthodes de mesure du site de séquestration des plaquettes. *Journal français de Biophysique et Médicine Nucléaire*, **1**, 109.

321 LURIE A., KATZ J., LUDWIN S.K., SEFTEL H.C. & METZ J. (1969) Platelet life-span and sites of platelet sequestration in onyalai. *British Medical Journal*, **iv**, 146.

322 GREEN D., BATTIFORA H.A., SMITH R.T. & ROSSI E.C. (1971) Thrombocytopenia in Gaucher's disease. *Annals of Internal Medicine*, **74**, 727.

323 ASTER R.H. & KEENE W.R. (1969) Sites of platelet destruction in idiopathic thrombocytopenic purpura. *British Journal of Haematology*, **16**, 61.

324 ASTER R.H. & JANDL J.H. (1964) Platelet sequestration in man. II. Immunologic and clinical studies. *Journal of Clinical Investigation*, **43**, 856.

325 EVANS W.H. (1928) The blood changes after splenectomy in splenic anaemia, purpura haemorrhagica and acholuric jaundice with special reference to platelets and coagulation. *Journal of Pathology and Bacteriology*, **31**, 815.

326 WISEMAN B.K. & DOAN C.A. (1942) Primary splenic neutropenia; a newly recognized syndrome closely related to congenital hemolytic icterus and essential thrombocytopenic purpura. *Annals of Internal Medicine*, **16**, 1097.

327 DOAN C.A. & WRIGHT C.S. (1946) Primary congenital and secondary acquired splenic panhematopenia. *Blood*, **1**, 10.

328 HEINLE R.W. & HOLDEN W.D. (1949) Primary splenic panhematopenia. *Surgery, Gynecology and Obstetrics*, **89**, 79.

329 HAYHOE F.G.J. & WHITBY L. (1955) Splenic function. A study of the rationale and results of splenectomy in blood disorders. *Quarterly Journal of Medicine*, **24**, 365.

330 DACIE J.V., BRAIN M.C., HARRISON C.V., LEWIS S.M. & WORLLEDGE S.M. (1969) 'Non-tropical idiopathic splenomegaly' ('Primary hypersplenism'): a review of ten cases and their relationship to malignant lymphomas. *British Journal of Haematology*, **17**, 317.

331 SINGER K., MILLER E.B. & DAMESHEK W. (1941) Hematologic changes following splenectomy in man. *American Journal of the Medical Sciences*, **202**, 171.

332 DAMESHEK W. (1955) Hypersplenism. *Bulletin of the New York Academy of Medicine*, **31**, 113.

333 WEINREICH J., GRUSNICK D., MESSER D., OSTROWSKI R., WIEGHARDT R., BIRK K.D., KOEHLER E. & SCHLIEMANN F. (1969) Der Einfluss der Milzpassage auf Erythrozyten. *Acta Hepato-splenologica*, **17**, 297.

334 VON HAMM E. & AWNY A.S. (1948) The pathology of hypersplenism. *American Journal of Clinical Pathology*, **18**, 313.

335 RINGELHANN B., KONOTEY-AHULU F.I.D. & DODU S.R.A. (1970) The sequestration of heat damaged ^{51}Cr-tagged red cells in splenomegalies of various origins in Ghana. *Transactions of the Royal Society of Tropical Medicine and Hygiene*, **64**, 407.

336 PETTIT J.E., WILLIAMS E.D., GLASS I.H., LEWIS S.M., SZUR L. & WICKS C.J. (1971) Studies of splenic function in the myeloproliferative disorders and generalized

malignant lymphomas. *British Journal of Haematology*, **20**, 575.

337 RAMBACH W.A. & ALT H.L. (1962) A revaluation of hypersplenism: an autoimmune concept. *Medical Clinics of North America*, **46**, 3.

338 PITNEY W.R. (1968) The tropical splenomegaly syndrome. *Transactions of the Royal Society of Tropical Medicine and Hygiene*, **62**, 717.

339 THATCHER L.G., CLATANOFF D.V. & STIEHM E.R. (1968) Splenic hemangioma with thrombocytopenia and afibrinogenemia. *Journal of Pediatrics*, **73**, 345.

340 ZERVOS N., VLACHOS J., KARPATHIOS T. & MANTAS J. (1967) Giant hemangioma of the spleen with thrombocytopenia, and fibrinogen deficiency. *Acta Paediatrica Scandinavica*, **172**, Suppl. 206.

341 BLIX S. & JACOBSEN C.D. (1966) Intravascular coagulation, a possible accelerating effect of prednisone. *Acta Medica Scandinavica*, **180**, 723.

342 KWAAN H.C., McFADZEAN A.J.S. & COOK J. (1957) On plasma fibrinolytic activity in cryptogenetic splenomegaly. *Scottish Medical Journal*, **2**, 137.

343 FISHER S. (1968) Severe coagulopathy in cryptogenetic congestive splenomegaly. *Journal of the American Medical Association*, **205**, 111.

344 JANDL J.H., JACOB H.S. & DALAND G.A. (1961) Hypersplenism due to infection: a study of five cases manifesting hemolytic anemia. *New England Journal of Medicine*, **264**, 1063.

345 GEVIRZ N.R., NATHAN D.G. & BERLIN N.I. (1962) Erythrokinetic studies in primary hypersplenism with pancytopenia. *American Journal of Medicine*, **32**, 148.

346 CARTWRIGHT G.E., CHUNG H-L, & CHANG A. (1948) Studies on kala-azar. *Blood*, **3**, 249.

347 HUTT M.S.R., RICHARDSON J.S. & STAFFURTH J.S. (1951) Felty's syndrome. A report of four cases treated by splenectomy. *Quarterly Journal of Medicine*, **20**, 57.

348 DEGRUCHY G.C. & LANGLEY G.R. (1961) Felty's syndrome. *Australasian Annals of Medicine*, **10**, 292.

349 ENGELBRETH-HOLM J. (1938) A study of tuberculous splenomegaly and splenogenic controlling of the cell emission from the bone marrow. *American Journal of the Medical Sciences*, **195**, 32.

350 REINHARD E.H. & LOEB V. JR (1955) Dyssplenism secondary to chronic leukemia or malignant lymphoma. *Journal of the American Medical Association*, **158**, 629.

351 STRAWITZ J.G., SOKAL J.E., GRACE J.P. JR, MUKHPAR G. & MOORE G.E. (1961) Surgical aspects of hypersplenism in lymphoma and leukemia. *Surgery, Gynecology and Obstetrics*, **112**, 89.

352 MEDOFF A.S. & BAYRD E.D. (1955) Gaucher's disease in 29 cases: hematologic complications and effect of splenectomy. *Annals of Internal Medicine*, **40**, 481.

353 STEINBERG C.L. (1953) Splenectomy in patients having rheumatoid arthritis. *Annals of Internal Medicine*, **38**, 787.

354 STATHERS G.M., MA M.H. & BLACKBURN C.R.B. (1968) Extrahepatic portal hypertension: the clinical evaluation, investigation and results of treatment in 28 patients. *Australasian Annals of Medicine*, **17**, 12.

355 TUMEN H.J. (1970) Hypersplenism and portal hypertension. *Annals of the New York Academy of Sciences*, **170**, 332.

356 SCHULTZ J.C., DENNY W.F. & ROSS S.W. (1964)

Splenectomy in leukemia and lymphoma: report of 24 cases. *American Journal of the Medical Sciences*, **247**, 30.

357 CHILD C.G. & TURCOTTE J.G. (1964) Surgery and portal hypertension. In: *The Liver and Portal Hypertension* (ed. Child C.G.), Ch. 1. W. B. Saunders, Philadelphia.

358 GOMES M.R., SILVERSTEIN M.N. & REMINE W.H. (1967) Splenectomy for agnogenic myeloid metaplasia. *Surgery, Gynecology and Obstetrics*, **125**, 106.

359 FELTY A.R. (1924) Chronic arthritis in the adult associated with splenomegaly and leukopenia. *Bulletin of the Johns Hopkins Hospital*, **35**, 16.

360 BERTINO J. & MYERSON R.M. (1960) The role of splenectomy in sarcoidosis. *Archives of Internal Medicine*, **106**, 213.

361 GRANT G.H. & WALLACE W.D. (1954) Agammaglobulinaemia. *Lancet*, **ii**, 671.

362 PRASAD A.S. & KOZA D.W. (1954) Agammaglobulinemia. *Annals of Internal Medicine*, **41**, 629.

363 ROHN R.J., BEHNKE R.J. & BOND W.H. (1955) Acquired agammaglobulinemia with hypersplenism. *American Journal of the Medical Sciences*, **229**, 406.

364 STANDAERT L. & DEMOOR P. (1955) L'agammaglobulinémie chez l'adulte. *Acta Clinica Belgica*, **10**, 477.

365 PRASAD A.S., REINER E. & WATSON C.J. (1957) Syndrome of hypogammaglobulinemia, splenomegaly and hypersplenism. *Blood*, **12**, 926.

366 GIRSH L.S. & MYERSON R.M. (1957) Thyrotoxicosis associated with thrombocytopenia and hypersplenism. *American Journal of Clinical Pathology*, **27**, 328.

367 PITNEY W.R., PRYOR D.S. & TAIT SMITH A. (1968) Morphological observations on livers and spleens of patients with tropical splenomegaly in New Guinea. *Journal of Pathology and Bacteriology*, **95**, 417.

368 LEATHER H.M. (1961) Portal hypertension and gross splenomegaly in Uganda. *British Medical Journal*, **i**, 15.

369 HAMILTON P.J.S., HUTT M.S.R., WILKS N.E., OLWENY C., NDAWULA R.L. & MWANJE L. (1965) Idiopathic splenomegaly in Uganda. I. Pathological aspects. *East African Medical Journal*, **42**, 191.

370 WATSON-WILLIAMS E.J. & ALLEN N.C. (1968) Idiopathic tropical splenomegaly syndrome in Ibadan. *British Medical Journal*, **iv**, 793.

371 MARSDEN P.D., HUTT M.S.R., WILKS N.E., VOLLER A., BLACKMAN V., SHAH K.K., CONNOR D.H., HAMILTON P.J.S., BANWELL J.G. & LUNN H.F. (1965) An investigation of tropical splenomegaly at Mulago Hospital, Kampala, Uganda. *British Medical Journal*, **i**, 89.

372 WELLS J.V. (1967) Positive results to serological tests for rheumatoid factor in New Guinea. *Medical Journal of Australia*, **2**, 777.

373 GEBBIE D.A.M., HAMILTON P.J.S., HUTT M.S.R., MARSDEN P.D., VOLLER A. & WILKS N.E. (1964) Malarial antibodies in idiopathic splenomegaly in Uganda. *Lancet*, **ii**, 392.

374 CHARMÔT G. & VARGUES R. (1963) L'étiologie des macroglobulinémies observées en Afrique. *Semaine des Hôpitaux de Paris*, **39**, 1421.

375 WELLS J.V. (1968) Serum immunoglobulin levels in tropical splenomegaly syndrome in New Guinea. *Clinical and Experimental Immunology*, **3**, 943.

376 ZIEGLER J.L., COHEN M.H. & HUTT M.S.R. (1969) Immunological studies in tropical splenomegaly syndrome in Uganda. *British Medical Journal*, **iv**, 15.

377 MARSDEN P.D., CONNOR D.H., VOLLER A., KELLY A., SCHOFIELD F.D. & HUTT M.S.R. (1967) Splenomegaly in New Guinea. *Bulletin of the World Health Organization*, **36**, 901.

378 RICHMOND J., DONALDSON G.W.K., WILLIAMS R., HAMILTON P.J.S. & HUTT M.S.R. (1967) Haematological effects of idiopathic splenomegaly seen in Uganda. *British Journal of Haematology*, **13**, 348.

379 WATSON-WILLIAMS E.J., ALLAN N.C. & FLEMING A.F. (1967) 'Big spleen' disease. *British Medical Journal*, **iv**, 416.

380 HAMILTON P.J.S., MORROW R.H., ZIEGLER J.L., PIKE M.C., WOOD J.B., BANYIKIDDE S.K. & HUTT M.S.R. (1969) Absence of sickle trait in patients with tropical splenomegaly syndrome. *Lancet*, **ii**, 109.

381 COOK J., MCFADZEAN A.J.S. & TODD D. (1963) Splenectomy in cryptogenetic splenomegaly. *British Medical Journal*, **ii**, 337.

382 MCFADZEAN A.J.S., TODD D. & TSANG K.C. (1963) Observations on the anemia of cryptogenetic splenomegaly. I. Hemolysis. *Blood*, **13**, 513.

383 SAGOE A.S. (1970) Tropical splenomegaly syndrome: long term proguanil therapy correlated with spleen size, serum IgM, and lymphocyte transformation. *British Medical Journal*, **iii**, 378.

384 ENDE N. & CHERNISS E.I. (1958) Splenic mastocytosis. *Blood*, **13**, 631.

385 MOSCHCOWITZ E. (1948) The pathogenesis of splenomegaly in hypertension of the portal circulation; 'congestive splenomegaly', *Medicine*, **27**, 187.

386 ATKINSON M. & SHERLOCK S. (1954) Intrasplenic pressure as an index of portal venous pressure. *Lancet*, **I**, 325.

387 WILLIAMS R., CONDON R.E., WILLIAMS H.S., BLENDIS L.M. & KREEL L. (1968) Splenic blood flow in cirrhosis and portal hypertension. *Clinical Science*, **34**, 441.

388 ARMAS-CRUZ R., YAZIGI R., LOPEZ O., MONTERO E., CABELLO J. & LOBO G. (1951) Portal cirrhosis: an analysis of 208 cases with correlations of clinical, laboratory and autopsy findings. *Gastroenterology*, **17**, 321.

389 MCMICHAEL J. (1934) The pathology of hepatolienal fibrosis. *Journal of Pathology and Bacteriology*, **39**, 481.

390 JANDL J.H. (1955) The anemia of liver disease: observations on its mechanism. *Journal of Clinical Investigation*, **34**, 390.

391 PEMBERTON J. DE J. & KIERNAN P. (1945) Surgery of the spleen. *Surgical Clinics of North America*, **25**, 880.

392 MILNES WALKER R. (1962) Treatment of portal hypertension in children. *Proceedings of the Royal Society of Medicine*, **55**, 770.

393 WANTZ G.E. & PAYNE M.A. (1961) Experience with portacaval shunt for portal hypertension. *New England Journal of Medicine*, **265**, 721.

394 MORRIS P.W., PATTON T.B., BALINT J.A. & HIRSCHOWITZ B.I. (1962) Portal hypertension, congestive splenomegaly and portacaval shunt. *Gastroenterology*, **42**, 555.

395 SULLIVAN B.H. & TUMEN H.J. (1961) The effect of portacaval shunt on thrombocytopenia associated with portal hypertension. *Annals of Internal Medicine*, **55**, 598.

396 ROUSSELOT L.A., PANKE W.F., BONO R.F. & MORENO A.H. (1963) Experiences with portacaval anastomosis.

Analysis of 104 elective end-to-side shunts for the prevention of recurrent hemorrhage from esophagogastric varices. *American Journal of Medicine*, **34**, 297.

397 LIEBOWITZ H.R. (1963) Splenomegaly and hypersplenism pre- and post-portacaval shunt. *New York Journal of Medicine*, **63**, 2631.

398 PATRICK A.D. (1965) A deficiency of glucocerebrosidase in Gaucher's disease. *Biochemical Journal*, **97**, 17.

399 BRADY R.O., KANFER J.N., BRADLEY R.M. & SHAPIRO D. (1966) Demonstration of a deficiency of glucocerebroside-clearing enzyme in Gaucher's disease. *Journal of Clinical Investigation*, **45**, 1112.

400 MCCONNELL J.S., FORBES J.C. & APPERLY F.L. (1939) Notes on chemical studies of a Gaucher spleen. *American Journal of the Medical Sciences*, **197**, 90.

401 HALLIDAY M., DEUEL H.J., JR, TRAGERMAN L.J. & WARD W.E. (1940) On the isolation of a glucose-containing cerebroside from spleen in a case of Gaucher's disease. *Journal of Biological Chemistry*, **132**, 171.

402 ROSENBERG A. & CHARGAFF E. (1958) A reinvestigation of the cerebroside deposited in Gaucher's disease. *Journal of Biological Chemistry*, **233**, 1323.

403 ARANOFF B.W., RADIN N. & SUOMI W. (1962) Enzymic oxidation of cerebrosides: studies on Gaucher's disease. *Biochemica Biophysica Acta*, **57**, 194.

404 GROEN J.J. (1965) Present status of knowledge of Gaucher's disease. *Israel Journal of Medical Sciences*, **1**, 507.

405 PENNELLI N., SCARAVILLI F. & ZACCHELLO F. (1969) The morphogenesis of Gaucher cells investigated by electron microscopy. *Blood*, **34**, 331.

406 JORDAN S.W. (1964) Electron microscopy of Gaucher cells. *Experimental Molecular Pathology*, **3**, 76.

407 KATTLOVE H.E., WILLIAMS J.C., GAYNOR E., SPIVACK M., BRADLEY R.M. & BRADY R.O. (1969) Gaucher cells in chronic myelocytic leukemia: an acquired abnormality. *Blood*, **33**, 379.

408 LEE R.E. & ELLIS L.D. (1971) The storage cells of chronic myelogenous leukemia. *Laboratory Investigation*, **24**, 261.

409 LEE R.E., BALCERZAK S.P. & WESTERMAN M.P. (1967) Gaucher's disease: a morphologic study and measurements of iron metabolism. *American Journal of Medicine*, **42**, 891.

410 LORBER M. (1960) The occurrence of intracellular iron in Gaucher's disease. *Annals of Internal Medicine*, **53**, 293.

411 LORBER M. & NEMES J.L. (1970) Identification of ferritin within Gaucher cells. An electron microscopic and immunofluorescent study. *Acta Haematologica (Basel)*, **37**, 189.

412 LORBER M. (1970) Adult-type Gaucher's disease: a secondary disorder of iron metabolism. *Journal of the Mount Sinai Hospital*, **37**, 404.

413 ALBRECHT M. (1966) 'Gaucher-Zellen' bei chronisch myeloischer Leukämie. *Blut*, **13**, 169.

414 THANNHAUSER S.J. (1958) *Lipidoses: Diseases of Intracellular Lipid Metabolism*, 3rd edn. Grune & Stratton, New York.

415 PICK L. (1933) I. A classification of the diseases of lipoid metabolism and Gaucher's disease. *American Journal of the Medical Sciences*, **185**, 453.

416 MANDELBAUM H., BERGER L. & LEDERER M. (1942) Gaucher's disease. I. Case with hemolytic anemia and marked thrombopenia: improvement after removal of spleen weighing 6822 grams. *Annals of Internal Medicine*, **16**, 438.

417 FEINBERG R. & QUIGLEY G.C. (1946) Osseous Gaucher's disease with macrocytic normochromic anemia. *New England Journal of Medicine*, **234**, 527.

418 CAPPER A., EPSTEIN H. & SCHLESS R.A. (1934) Gaucher's disease: report of a case with presentation of a table differentiating the lipoid disturbances. *American Journal of the Medical Sciences*, **188**, 84.

419 DAVID F.W., GENECIN A. & SMITH E.W. (1949) Gaucher's disease with thrombocytopenia, an instance of selective hypersplenism. *Bulletin of the Johns Hopkins Hospital*, **84**, 176.

420 MATOTH Y. & FRIED K. (1965) Chronic Gaucher's disease: clinical observations on 34 patients. *Israel Journal of Medical Sciences*, **1**, 521.

421 SILVERSTEIN M.N. & KELLY P.J. (1967) Osteoarticular manifestations of Gaucher's disease. *American Journal of the Medical Sciences*, **253**, 569.

422 KAPLAN M., GRUMBACH R., FISCHGRUND A. & LUNEL J. (1953) Maladie de Gaucher chez un enfant de 6 ans; étude biologique du syndrome hémorrhagique qui l'accompagne. *Bulletins et Mémoires de la Société Médicale des Hôpitaux de Paris*, **69**, 169.

423 ABT A.F. & BLOOM W. (1928) Essential lipoid histiocytosis (type Niemann–Pick). *Journal of the American Medical Association*, **90**, 2076.

424 JOSEPHS H.W. (1936) Anaemia of infancy and early childhood. *Medicine*, **15**, 307.

425 CROCKER A.C. & FARBER S. (1958) Niemann–Pick disease: a review of eighteen patients. *Medicine*, **37**, 1.

426 LAZARUS S.S., VETHAMANY V.G., SCHNECK L. & VOLK B.W. (1967) Fine structure and histochemistry of peripheral blood cells in Niemann–Pick disease. *Laboratory Investigation*, **17**, 155.

427 LICHTENSTEIN L. (1935) Histiocytosis X: integration of eosinophilic granuloma of bone, Letterer–Siwe disease and Schüller–Christian disease as related manifestations of a single nosologic entity. *Archives of Pathology*, **61**, 84.

428 MORRISON A.N., SWILLER A.I. & MORRISON M. (1961) Asplenomegalic (cryptic) Gaucher's disease. *Archives of Internal Medicine*, **107**, 583.

429 NORMAN R.M., URICH H., TINGEY A.H. & GOODBODY R.A. (1959) Tay–Sachs' disease with visceral involvement and its relationship to Niemann–Pick's disease. *Journal of Pathology and Bacteriology*, **78**, 409.

430 DAVISON C. & JACOBSON S.A. (1936) Generalized lipidosis in a case of amaurotic family idiocy. *American Journal of Diseases of Children*, **52**, 345.

431 BAGDADE J.D., PARKER F., WAYS P.O., MORGAN T.E., LAGUNOFF D. & EIDELMAN S. (1968) Fabry's disease: a correlative clinical, morphologic and biochemical study. *Laboratory Investigation*, **18**, 681.

432 KRIVIT W., VANCE D.E., DESNICK R., WHITECAR J.P. & SWEELEY C.C. (1968) Red cell physiology in Fabry's disease. *Journal of Laboratory and Clinical Medicine*, **12**, 906.

433 FREDRICKSON D.S., ALTROCCHI P.H., AVIOLI L.V., GOODMAN D.S. & GOODMAN H.C. (1961) Tangier disease. *Annals of Internal Medicine*, **55**, 1016.

434 FREDRICKSON D.S., YOUNG O., SHIRATORI T. & BRIGGS N. (1964) The inheritance of high density lipoprotein deficiency (Tangier disease). *Journal of Clinical Investigation*, **43**, 228.

435 HOFFMAN H.N. & FREDRICKSON D.S. (1965) Tangier disease (Familial high density lipoprotein deficiency). Clinical and genetic features in two adults. *American Journal of Medicine*, **39**, 582.

436 HERBERT P.N., GOTTO A.M. & FREDRICKSON D.S., (1978) Familial lipoprotein deficiency (abetalipoproteinemia, hypobetalipoproteinemia and Tangier disease). In: *The Metabolic Basis of Inherited Disease* (ed. Stanbury J.B., Wyngaarden J.B., & Frederickson D.S.), 4th edn., Ch. 28. McGraw-Hill, New York.

437 FERRANS V.J., BUJA L.M., ROBERTS W.C. & FREDRICKSON D.S. (1971) The spleen in type I hyperlipoproteinemia. *American Journal of Pathology*, **64**, 67.

438 LAGUNOFF D., ROSS R. & BENDITT E.P. (1962) Histochemical and electron microscopic study in a case of Hurler's disease. *American Journal of Pathology*, **41**, 273.

439 REILLY W.A. (1941) The granules in the leucocytes of gargoylism. *American Journal of Diseases of Children*, **62**, 489.

440 JERMAIN L.F., ROHN R.J. & BOND W.H. (1959) Studies on the rôle of the reticuloendothelial system in Hurler's disease. *Clinical Research*, **7**, 216.

441 SAWITSKY A., ROSNER F. & CHODSKY S. (1972) The sea-blue histiocyte syndrome, a review: genetic and biochemical studies. *Seminars in Hematology*, **9**, 285.

442 SILVERSTEIN M.B. & ELLEFSON R.D. (1972) The syndrome of the sea-blue histiocyte. *Seminars in Hematology*, **9**, 299.

443 SILVERSTEIN M.N., ELLEFSON R.D. & AHERN E.J. (1970) The syndrome of the sea-blue histiocyte. *New England Journal of Medicine*, **282**, 1.

444 LAKE B.D., STEPHENS R. & NEVILLE B.G.R. (1970) Syndrome of the sea-blue histiocyte. *Lancet*, **ii**, 309.

445 GOLDE D.W., SCHNEIDER E.L., BAINTON D.F., PENTCHEV P.G., BRADY R.O., EPSTEIN C.J. & CLINE M.J. (1975) Pathogenesis of one variant of sea-blue histiocytosis. *Laboratory Investigation*, **33**, 371.

446 RYWLIN A.M., HERNANDEZ J.A., CHASTAIN D.E. & PARDO V. (1971) Ceroid histiocytosis of spleen and bone marrow in idiopathic thrombocytopenic purpura (ITP): a contribution to the understanding of the sea-blue histiocyte. *Blood*, **37**, 587.

447 RYWLIN A.M., LOPEZ-GOMEZ A., TACHMES P. & PARDO V. (1971) Ceroid histiocytosis of the spleen in hyperlipemia: relationship to the syndrome of the sea-blue histiocyte. *American Journal of Clinical Pathology*, **56**, 372.

448 TADMOR R., AGHAI E., SAROVA-PINHAS I. & BRAHAM J. (1976) Sea-blue histiocytes in a case of Takayasu arteritis. *Journal of the American Medical Association*, **235**, 2852.

449 NIXON R.K., JR (1954) The detection of splenomegaly by percussion. *New England Journal of Medicine*, **250**, 166.

450 ZELMAN S. & PICKARD C.M. (1955) Roentgen and autopsy evaluation of percussion of the liver and spleen. *Gastroenterology*, **29**, 1037.

451 RIEMENSCHNEIDER P.A. & WHALEN J.P. (1965) The relative accuracy of estimation of enlargement of the liver and spleen by radiologic and clinical methods. *American Journal of Roentgenology*, **94**, 462.

452 RÖSCH J. (1965) Roentgenologic possibilities in spleen diagnosis. *American Journal of Roentgenology*, **94**, 453.

453 RÖSCH J. (1967) *Roentgenology of the Spleen and Pancreas*. C. C. Thomas, Springfield, Illinois.

454 WYMAN A.C. (1954) Traumatic rupture of the spleen. *American Journal of Roentgenology*, **72**, 51.

455 BERGSTRAND I. & EKMAN C.A. (1957) Portal circulation in portal hypertension. *Acta Radiologica*, **47**, 1.

456 WHITLEY J.E., MAYNARD C.D. & RHYNE A.L. (1966) A computer approach to the prediction of spleen weight from routine films. *Radiology*, **86**, 73.

457 DESNICK S.J., KRIVIT W. & DESNICK R.J. (1971) Personal communication.

458 MCINTYRE P.A. & WAGNER H.N., JR (1970) Current procedures for scanning of the spleen. *Annals of Internal Medicine*, **73**, 995.

459 JOHNSON P.M., HERION J.C. & MOORING S.L. (1960) Scintillation scanning of the normal human spleen utilizing sensitized radioactive erythrocytes. *Radiology*, **74**, 99.

460 KYLE R.W., GOTSHALL E. & JOHNSON G.S. (1969) Spleen scanning with red cells simultaneously ^{51}Cr-tagged and heat-treated. *Journal of Nuclear Medicine*, **10**, 480.

461 WANG Y., WESTERMAN M.P. & HEINLE E.W. (1965) Spleen-function study with 1-mercuri-2-hydroxypropane labeled with ^{197}mercury. *Journal of the American Medical Association*, **194**, 1254.

462 WAGNER H.M., JR, WEINER I.M., MCAFEE J.G. & MARTINEZ J. (1964) 1-mercuri-2-hydroxypropane (MHP): a new radiopharmaceutical for visualization of the spleen by radioisotope scanning. *Archives of Internal Medicine*, **113**, 696.

463 MAYER K., DWYER A. & LAUGHLIN J.S. (1970) Spleen scanning using ACD-damaged red cells tagged with ^{51}Cr. *Journal of Nuclear Medicine*, **11**, 455.

464 BLOCK M.H. & JACOBSON L.O. (1950) Splenic puncture. *Journal of the American Medical Association*, **142**, 641.

465 SHAPIRO H.D. & WATSON R.J. (1953) Splenic aspirations in multiple myeloma. *Blood*, **8**, 755.

466 MOESCHLIN S. (1951) *Spleen Puncture*. Grune & Stratton, New York.

467 JANDL J.H., GREENBERG M.S., YONEMOTO R.H. & CASTLE W.B. (1956) Clinical determination of the sites of red cell sequestration in hemolytic anemias. *Journal of Clinical Investigation*, **35**, 843.

468 SCHLOESSER L.L., KORST D.R., CLATANOFF D.V. & SCHILLING R.F. (1957) Radioactivity over the spleen and liver following transfusion of chromium 51-labelled erythrocytes in hemolytic anemia. *Journal of Clinical Investigation*, **36**, 1470.

469 HUGHES-JONES N.C. & SZUR L. (1957) Determination of the sites of red-cell destruction using ^{51}Cr-labelled cells. *British Journal of Haematology*, **3**, 320.

470 MCCURDY P.R. & RATH C.E. (1958) Splenectomy in hemolytic anemia: results predicted by body scanning after injection of ^{51}Cr-tagged red cells. *New England Journal of Medicine*, **259**, 459.

471 LEWIS S.M., SZUR L. & DACIE J.V. (1960) The pattern of erythrocyte destruction in haemolytic anaemia, as

studied with radioactive chromium. *British Journal of Haematology*, **6**, 122.

472 CHRISTENSEN B.E. (1975) Quantitative determination of splenic red blood cell destruction in patients with splenomegaly. *Scandinavian Journal of Haematology*, **14**, 295.

473 VEEGER M., WOLDRING M.G., VAN ROOD J.J., EERNISSE J.G., LEEKSMA C.H.W., VERLOOP M.C. & NIEWEG H.O. (1962) The value of the determination of the site of red cell sequestration in haemolytic anaemia as a prediction test for splenectomy. *Acta Medica Scandinavica*, **171**, 507.

474 GOLDBERG A., HUTCHINSON H.E. & MACDONALD E. (1966) Radiochromium in the selection of patients with haemolytic anaemia for splenectomy. *Lancet*, **i**, 109.

475 ALLGOOD J.W. & CHAPLIN H., JR (1967) Idiopathic acquired autoimmune hemolytic anemia. *American Journal of Medicine*, **4**, 254.

476 BEN BASSAT I., SELIGSOHN U., LEIBA H., LEEF F., CHAITCHIK S. & RAMOT B. (1967) Sequestration studies with chromium-51 labeled red cells as criteria for splenectomy. *Israel Journal of Medical Sciences*, **3**, 832.

477 ALLGOOD J.W. (1967) Splenic sequestration studies in patients with autoimmune hemolytic anemia. *Clinical Research*, **15**, 130.

478 HABIBI B. & NAJEAN Y. (1971) Intérêt pratique de la cinètique érythrocytaire par marpuage au ^{51}Cr *in vitro* dans les anèmies hémolytiques autoimmunes. *Presse Médicale*, **11**, 9.

479 NAJEAN Y. & ARDAILLOU N. (1971) The sequestration site of platelets in idiopathic thrombocytopenic purpura: its correlation with the results of splenectomy. *British Journal of Haematology*, **21**, 153.

480 ARONSON W. & FOX R.A. (1940) Spontaneous rupture of the spleen: report of two unusual cases. *American Journal of Clinical Pathology*, **10**, 868.

481 YORK W.H. (1962) Spontaneous rupture of the spleen: report of a case secondary to infectious mononucleosis. *Journal of the American Medical Association*, **179**, 170.

482 FREEMAN A.R. (1962) Rupture of the spleen in infectious mononucleosis. *British Medical Journal*, **ii**, 96.

483 WOLFSON I.N., CROCE E.J. & FITE F.K. (1954) Acute leukemia with rupture of the spleen as the initial symptom. *New England Journal of Medicine*, **251**, 735.

484 FLOOD M.J. & CARPENTER R.A. (1961) Spontaneous rupture of the spleen in acute myeloid leukaemia. *British Medical Journal*, **i**, 35.

485 HYNES H.E., SILVERSTEIN M.N. & FAWCETT K.J. (1964) Spontaneous rupture of the spleen in acute leukemia: report of 2 cases. *Cancer*, **17**, 1356.

486 OLIVA L.A. & LE GRESLEY L.-E. (1969) Rupture spontanée de la rate dans la leucémie. *L'Union Medicale du Canada*, **98**, 19.

487 RAVICH R.B.M., REED C.S., STEPHENS F.O., VINCENT P.C. & GUNZ F.W. (1971) Spontaneous rupture of the spleen in acute myeloid leukaemia. *Medical Journal of Australia*, **1**, 90.

488 STEPHENS P.J.T. & HUDSON P. (1969) Spontaneous rupture of the spleen in plasma cell leukemia. *Canadian Medical Association Journal*, **100**, 31.

489 TARTAGLIA A.P., SCHARFMAN W.B. & PROPP S. (1962) Splenic rupture in leukemia. *New England Journal of Medicine*, **251**, 735.

490 STITES T.B. & ULTMANN J.E. (1966) Spontaneous rupture of the spleen in chronic lymphocytic leukemia. *Cancer*, **19**, 1587.

491 GREENFIELD M.M. & LUND H. (1944) Spontaneous rupture of the spleen in chronic myeloid leukemia. *Ohio State Medical Journal*, **40**, 950.

492 COORAY G.H. (1952) Spontaneous rupture of the leukaemic spleen. *British Medical Journal*, **i**, 693.

493 AUNG M.K., GOLDBERG M. & TOBIN M.S. (1978) Splenic rupture due to infectious mononucleosis: normal selective arteriogram and peritoneal lavage. *Journal of the American Medical Association*, **240**, 1752.

494 MACLEOD W.A.J. & LANING R.C. (1970) Spontaneous rupture of the spleen; a complication of polycythemia vera. *American Surgeon*, **36**, 569.

495 LOWENBRAUN S., RAMSEY H., SUTHERLAND J. & SERPICK A.A. (1970) Diagnostic laparotomy and splenectomy for staging Hodgkin's disease. *Annals of Internal Medicine*, **72**, 655.

496 GOLDMAN J.M. (1971) Laparotomy for staging of Hodgkin's disease. *Lancet*, **i**, 125.

497 AISENBERG A.C., GOLDMAN J.M., RAKER J.W. & WANG C.C. (1971) Spleen involvement at the onset of Hodgkin's disease. *Annals of Internal Medicine*, **74**, 544.

498 LOWENBRAUN S., RAMSEY H.E. & SERPICK A.A. (1971) Splenectomy in Hodgkin's disease for splenomegaly, cytopenias and intolerance to myelosuppressive chemotherapy. *American Journal of Medicine*, **50**, 49.

499 SALZMAN J.R. & KAPLAN H.S. (1971) Effect of prior splenectomy on hematologic tolerance during total lymphoid radiotherapy of patients with Hodgkin's disease. *Cancer*, **27**, 471.

500 ADLER S., STUTZMAN L., SOKAL J.E. & MITTELMAN A. (1975) Splenectomy for hematologic depression in lymphocytic lymphoma and leukemia. *Cancer*, **35**, 521.

501 MORRIS P.J., COOPER I.A. & MADIGAN J.P. (1975) Splenectomy for haematological cytopenias in patients with malignant lymphomas. *Lancet*, **ii**, 250.

502 JOHNSON R.E. (1971) Is staging laparotomy routinely indicated in Hodgkin's disease? *Annals of Internal Medicine*, **75**, 459.

503 STAVEM P., HJORT P.F., ELGJO K. & SOMMERSCHILD H. (1970) Solitary plasmocytoma of the spleen with marked polyclonal increase of gamma G, normalized after splenectomy. *Acta Medica Scandinavica*, **188**, 115.

504 BJØRN-HANSEN R. (1973) Primary plasmacytoma of the spleen. *American Journal of Roentgenology, Radium Therapy and Nuclear Medicine*, **117**, 81.

505 SPIERS A.S.D., BAIKIE A.G., GALTON D.A.G., RICHARDS H.G.W., WILTSHAW E., GOLDMAN J.M., CATOVSKY D., SPENCER J. & PETO R. (1975) Chronic granulocytic leukaemia: effect of elective splenectomy on the course of disease. *British Medical Journal*, **i**, 175.

506 WOLF D.J., SILVER R.T. & COLEMAN M. (1978) Splenectomy in chronic myeloid leukemia. *Annals of Internal Medicine*, **89**, 684.

507 SEDGEWICK C.E. & HUME A.H. (1960) Elective splenectomy. *Annals of Surgery*, **151**, 163.

508 DUCKETT J.W. (1963) Splenectomy in the treatment of secondary hypersplenism. *Annals of Surgery*, **157**, 737.

509 SANDUSKY W.R., LEAVELL B.S. & BENJAMIN B.I. (1964) Splenectomy: indications and results in hematologic disorders. *Annals of Surgery*, **159**, 695.

510 DEVLIN H.B., EVANS D.S. & BIRKHEAD J.S. (1970) Elective splenectomy for primary hematologic and splenic disease. *Surgery, Gynecology and Obstetrics,* **131,** 273.

511 COLLER F.A. (1955) The spleen and some of its diseases that may be treated by surgery. *Annals of the Royal College of Surgeons,* **17,** 335.

512 NORDY A. & NESET G. (1968) Splenectomy in hematologic diseases. *Acta Medica Scandinavica,* **183,** 117.

513 MAPPES G. & FISCHER J. (1969) Erfahrungen mit der Splenektomie bei Blutkrankheiten. *Deutsche Medizinische Wochenschrift,* **94,** 584.

514 MITTLEMAN A., STUTZMAN L. & GRACE J.T. (1968) Splenectomy in malignant lymphoma and leukemia. *Geriatrics,* **23,** 142.

515 BARKER N.W., NYGAARD K.K., WALTERS W. & PRIESTLEY J.T. (1940) A statistical study of postoperative venous thrombosis and pulmonary embolism. I. Incidence in various types of operations. *Proceedings of the Staff Meetings of the Mayo Clinic,* **15,** 769.

516 QUAN S. & CASTLEMAN B. (1949) Splenic vein thrombosis following transthoracic gastrectomy and incidental splenectomy. *New England Journal of Medicine,* **240,** 835.

517 BALZ J.B. & MINTON J.P. (1975) Mesenteric thrombosis following splenectomy. *Annals of Surgery,* **183,** 126.

518 MORGENSTERN L. (1977) The avoidable complications of splenectomy. *Surgery, Gynecology & Obstetrics,* **145,** 525.

519 MORRIS D.H. & BULLOCK F.D. (1919) The importance of the spleen in resistance to infection. *Annals of Surgery,* **70,** 513.

520 MARMORSTON J. (1935) The effect of splenectomy on acute *Bacterium enteritidis* infection in white mice. *Proceedings of the Society for Experimental Biology and Medicine,* **32,** 981.

521 GRUBER S., REDNER B. & KOGUT B. (1951) Congenital idiopathic thrombopenic purpura in a premature infant with splenectomy. *New York Journal of Medicine,* **51,** 649.

522 EVANS T.S., WATERS L.L. & LOWMAN R.M. (1954) Hypersplenism: indications for surgery. *Connecticut Medical Journal,* **18,** 569.

523 GAVRILIS P., ROTHENBERG S.P. & ROSCOE G. (1974) Correlation of low serum IgM levels with absence of functional splenic tissue in sickle-cell disease syndromes. *American Journal of Medicine,* **57,** 542.

524 CARLISLE H.N. & SASLAW S. (1959) Properdin levels in splenectomized persons. *Proceedings of the Society for Experimental Biology and Medicine,* **102,** 150.

525 CONSTANTOPOULOS A. & NAJJAR V.A. (1973) Tuftsin deficiency syndrome: a report of two new cases. *Acta Paediatrica Scandinavica,* **62,** 645.

526 JOHNSON R.B., JR, NEWMAN S.L. & STRUTH A.G. (1973) An abnormality of the alternate pathway of complement activation in sickle disease. *New England Journal of Medicine,* **288,** 803.

527 FALTER M.L., ROBINSON M.G., KIM O.S., GO S.C. & TAUBKIN S.P. (1973) Splenic function and infection in sickle cell anemia. *Acta Haematologica (Basel),* **50,** 154.

528 ROBINETTE C.D. & FRAUMENI J.F. (1977) Splenectomy and subsequent mortality in veterans of the 1939–45 war. *Lancet,* **ii,** 127.

529 WEITZMAN S. & AISENBERG A.C. (1977) Fulminant sepsis after the successful treatment of Hodgkin's disease. *American Journal of Medicine,* **62,** 47.

530 RAVRY M., MALDONADO N. & VELEZ-GARCIA E. (1972) Serious infection after splenectomy for the staging of Hodgkin's disease. *Annals of Internal Medicine,* **77,** 11.

531 WARD J. & SMITH A.L. (1976) Hemophilus influenzae bacteremia in children with sickle cell disease. *Journal of Pediatrics,* **88,** 261.

532 AMMAN A.J., ADDIEGO J., WARA D.W., LUBIN B., SMITH W.B. & MENTZER J. (1977) Polyvalent pneumococcal-polysaccharide immunization of patients with sickle-cell anemia and patients with splenectomy. *New England Journal of Medicine,* **297,** 897.

533 WALTER L.E. & CHAFFIN L. (1955) Splenectomized infants and children. *Annals of Surgery,* **142,** 798.

534 KING H. & SHUMACKER H.B., JR (1952) Splenic studies. I. Susceptibility to infection after splenectomy performed in infancy. *Annals of Surgery,* **136,** 239.

535 ROUSSELOT L.W. & ILLYNE C.A. (1941) Traumatic rupture of the spleen, with a consideration of early features and late sequelae in seventeen cases. *Surgical Clinics of North America,* **21,** 455.

536 MILLER E.M. & HAGEDORN A.B. (1951) Results of splenectomy: a follow-up study of 140 consecutive cases. *Annals of Surgery,* **134,** 815.

537 LASKI B. & MACMILLAN A. (1959) Incidence of infection in children after splenectomy. *Pediatrics,* **24,** 523.

538 BROBERGER O., GYULAI F. & HIRSCHFELDT J. (1960) Splenectomy in childhood. A clinical and immunological study of forty-two children splenectomized in the years 1951–1958. *Acta Paediatrica Scandinavica,* **49,** 679.

539 THURMAN W.G. (1963) Splenectomy and immunity. *American Journal of Diseases of Children,* **105,** 138.

540 GOFSTEIN R. & GELLIS S.S. (1956) Splenectomy in infancy and childhood. *American Journal of Diseases of Children,* **91,** 566.

541 SMITH C.H., ERLANDSON M., SCHULMAN I. & STERN G. (1957) Hazards of severe infections in splenectomized infants and children. *American Journal of Medicine,* **22,** 390.

542 HUNTLEY C.C. (1958) Infection following splenectomy in infants and children. *American Journal of Diseases of Children,* **95,** 477.

543 ROBINSON T.W. & STURGEON P. (1960) Post-splenectomy infection in infants and children. *Pediatrics,* **25,** 941.

544 HORAN M. & COLEBATCH J.H. (1962) Relation between splenectomy and subsequent infection. A clinical study. *Archives of Diseases in Childhood,* **37,** 398.

545 ERICKSON W.D., BURGERT E.O., JR & LYNN H.B. (1968) The hazard of infection following splenectomy in children. *American Journal of Diseases of Children,* **116,** 1.

546 WASI P. (1971) Streptococcal infection leading to cardiac and renal involvement in thalassaemia. *Lancet,* **i,** 949.

547 MYERSON R.M., STOUT R. & HAVENS W.P. (1957) The production of antibody by splenectomized persons. *American Journal of the Medical Sciences,* **234,** 297.

548 SASLAW S., BOURONCLE B.A., WALL R.L. & DOAN C.A. (1959) Studies on the antibody response in splenecto-

mized persons. *New England Journal of Medicine*, **261**, 120.

549 GOHAR M.A., EISSA A.A. & SEBAI I. (1951) Antibody response in Egyptian splenomegaly. *American Journal of Tropical Medicine*, **31**, 604.

550 ELLIS E.F. & SMITH R.T. (1966) The rôle of the spleen in immunity: with special reference to the post-splenectomy problem in infants. *Pediatrics*, **37**, 111.

551 McFADZEAN A.J.S. & TSANG K.C. (1956) Antibody formation in cryptogenetic splenomegaly. I. The response to particulate antigen injected intravenously. *Transactions of the Royal Society of Tropical Medicine and Hygiene*, **50**, 433.

552 HUANG N.N., SHENG K.T. & PILLING G.P. (1960) Antibody response to Vi antigen administered subcutaneously and intravenously following splenectomy in children. *American Journal of Diseases of Children*, **100**, 699.

553 SCHUMACHER M.J. (1970) Serum immunoglobulin and transferrin levels after childhood splenectomy. *Archives of Diseases in Childhood*, **45**, 114.

554 WASI C., WASI P. & THONGCHAROEN P. (1971) Serum-immunoglobulin levels in thalassaemia and the effects of splenectomy. *Lancet*, **ii**, 237.

555 MERSKEY C. & BUDTZ-OLSEN O.E. (1953) Splenectomy in three cases of myelophthisic anaemia. *British Medical Journal*, **ii**, 537.

556 BENSINGER G.A., LOGUE G.L. & RUNDLES R.W. (1970) Hemorrhagic thrombocythemia: control of post-splenectomy thrombocytosis with melphalan. *Blood*, **36**, 61.

557 DIAMOND L.K. (1969) Splenectomy in childhood and the hazard of overwhelming infection. *Pediatrics*, **43**, 886.

558 BERRY C.L. & MARSHALL W.C. (1967) Iron distribution in the liver of patients with thalassaemia major. *Lancet*, **i**, 1031.

559 DAMESHEK W. (1958) Systemic lupus erythematosus: a complex auto-immune disorder. *Annals of Internal Medicine*, **48**, 707.

560 DAMESHEK W. & REEVES W.H. (1956) Exacerbation of lupus erythematosus following splenectomy in 'idiopathic' thrombocytopenic purpura and autoimmune hemolytic anemia. *American Journal of Medicine*, **21**, 560.

561 RABINOWITZ Y. & DAMESHEK W. (1960) Systemic lupus erythematosus after 'idiopathic' thrombocytopenic purpura: a review. A study of systemic lupus erythematosus occurring after 78 splenectomies for 'idiopathic' thrombocytopenic purpura, with a review of pertinent literature. *Annals of Internal Medicine*, **52**, 1.

562 BEST W.R. & DARLING D.R. (1962) A critical look at the splenectomy-SLE controversy. *Medical Clinics of North America*, **46**, 19.

563 SHAW A.F.B. & SHAFI A. (1937) Traumatic transplantation of splenic tissue in man with observation of late results of splenectomy in six cases. *Journal of Pathology and Bacteriology*, **45**, 215.

564 BUCHBINDER J.M. & LIPKOFF C.J. (1939) Splenosis: multiple peritoneal splenic implants following abdominal surgery. *Surgery*, **6**, 927.

565 KRUEGER J.T. & MAST H.E. (1942) Splenic transplants following traumatic rupture of the spleen and splenectomy. *American Journal of Surgery*, **58**, 289.

566 COTLAR A.M. & CERISE E.J. (1959) Splenosis: the autotransplantation of splenic tissue following injury to the spleen. *Annals of Surgery*, **149**, 402.

567 PIROZYNSKI W.J. & ALLAN C.M. (1974) Abdominal splenosis. *Canadian Medical Association Journal*, **111**, 159.

568 GAMMILL S.L. & CRAIG H.V. (1969) Splenosis, auto-transplantation of the splenic tissue following trauma; a programmed report. *Journal of the American Medical Association*, **208**, 1387.

569 STOBIE G.H. (1947) Splenosis. *Canadian Medical Association Journal*, **56**, 374.

570 CROSBY W.H. (1963) Hyposplenism: an inquiry into normal functions of the spleen. *Annual Reviews of Medicine*, **14**, 349.

571 SCHUR H. (1908) Über eigenartige basophile Einschlüsse in den roten Blut Körperchen. *Wiener Medizinische Wochenschrift*, **58**, 441.

572 LIPSON R.L., BAYRD E.D. & WATKINS C.H. (1959) The postsplenectomy blood picture. *American Journal of Clinical Pathology*, **32**, 526.

573 SELWYN J.G. (1955) Heinz bodies in red cells after splenectomy and after phenacetin administration. *British Journal of Haematology*, **1**, 173.

574 SCHNITZER B., RUCKNAGEL D.L., SPENCER H.H. & AIKAWA M. (1971) Erythrocytes: pits and vacuoles as seen with transmission and scanning electron microscopy. *Science*, **173**, 251.

575 KOYAMA S., AOKI S. & DEGUCHI K. (1964) Electron microscopic observations of the splenic red pulp with special reference to the pitting function. *Mie Medical Journal*, **14**, 143.

576 LAWSON N.S., SCHNITZER B. & SMITH E.B. (1969) Splenic ultrastructure in drug-induced Heinz body hemolysis. *Archives of Pathology*, **87**, 491.

577 WELCH C.S. & DAMESHEK W. (1950) Splenectomy in blood dyscrasias. *New England Journal of Medicine*, **242**, 601.

578 SEDGWICK C.E. & HOME A.H. (1960) Elective splenectomy: an analysis of 220 operations. *Annals of Surgery*, **151**, 163.

579 HIRSH J. & DACIE J.V. (1966) Persistent post-splenectomy thrombocytosis and thrombo-embolism: a consequence of continuing anaemia. *British Journal of Haematology*, **12**, 44.

580 GRUMET F.C. & YANKEE R.A. (1970) Long-term platelet support of patients with aplastic anemia: effect of splenectomy and steroid therapy. *Annals of Internal Medicine*, **73**, 1.

581 HARTLEY L.C.J., INNIS M.D., MORGAN T.O. & CLUNIE G.J.A. (1971) Splenectomy for anaemia in patients on regular haemodialysis. *Lancet*, **ii**, 1343.

582 ERAKLIS A.J., KEVY S.V., DIAMOND L.K. & GROSS R.E. (1967) Hazard of overwhelming infection after splenectomy in childhood. *New England Journal of Medicine*, **276**, 1255.

583 DIAMOND L.K. (1969) Splenectomy in childhood and the hazard of overwhelming infection. *Pediatrics*, **43**, 886.

584 ADLER N.N. & VAN SLYCK E.J. (1953) Congenital absence of the spleen. *Journal of Pediatrics*, **42**, 471.

585 POLHEMUS D.W. & SCHAFER W.B. (1953) Congenital absence of the spleen; syndrome with atrioventricularis

and situs inversus; case reports and review of the literature. *Pediatrics*, **9**, 696.

586 BUSH J.A. & AINGER L.E. (1955) Congenital absence of the spleen with congenital heart disease: report of a case with ante-mortem diagnosis on the basis of hematologic morphology. *Pediatrics*, **15**, 93.

587 PUTSCHAR W.G.J. & MANION W.C. (1956) Congenital absence of the spleen and associated anomalies. *American Journal of Clinical Pathology*, **26**, 429.

588 IVEMARK B.I. (1955) Implications of agenesis of the spleen on the pathogenesis of cono-truncus anomalies in childhood. *Acta Pediatrica*, **44**, suppl. 104.

589 ROWE R.D. & MEHRIZI A. (1969) *The Neonate with Congenital Heart Disease*, p. 300. W. B. Saunders, Philadelphia.

590 SILVER W., STEIER M. & CHANDRA N. (1972) Asplenia syndrome with congenital heart disease and tetralogy of Fallot in siblings. *The American Journal of Cardiology*, **30**, 91.

591 ROSE R.G. (1918) Absence of the spleen. *British Medical Journal*, **i**, 591.

592 MCLEAN S. & CRAIG H.R. (1922) Congenital absence of the spleen. *American Journal of the Medical Sciences*, **164**, 703.

593 MYERSON R.M. & KOELLE W.A. (1956) Congenital absence of the spleen in an adult. *New England Journal of Medicine*, **254**, 1131.

594 MURPHY J.W. & MITCHELL W.A. (1957) Congenital absence of the spleen. *Pediatrics*, **20**, 253.

595 GARRIGA S. & CROSBY W.H. (1959) The incidence of leukemia in families of patients with hypoplasia of the marrow. *Blood*, **14**, 1008.

596 HOLROYDE C.P., OSKI F.A. & GARDNER F.H. (1969) The 'pocked' erythrocyte. *New England Journal of Medicine*, **281**, 516.

597 PETTIT J.E., HOFFBRAND A.V., SEAH P.O. & FRY L. (1972) Splenic atrophy in dermatitis herpetiformis. *British Medical Journal*, **ii**, 438.

598 HARDISTY R.M. & WOLFF H.H. (1955) Haemorrhagic thrombocythaemia: a clinical and laboratory study. *British Journal of Haematology*, **1**, 390.

599 GUNZ F.W. (1960) Haemorrhagic thrombocythaemia: a critical review. *Blood*, **15**, 706.

600 MARSH G.W., LEWIS S.M. & SZUR L. (1966) The use of ^{51}Cr-labelled heat-damaged red cells to study splenic function. II. Splenic atrophy in thrombocythaemia. *British Journal of Haematology*, **12**, 167.

601 DIGGS L.W. (1935) Siderofibrosis of the spleen in sickle cell anemia. *Journal of the American Medical Association*, **104**, 538.

602 WATSON R.J., LICHTMAN H.C. & SHAPIRO H.D. (1956) Splenomegaly in sickle cell anemia. *American Journal of Medicine*, **20**, 196.

603 HARRIS J.W., BREWSTER H.H., HAM T.H. & CASTLE W.B. (1956) Studies on the destruction of red blood cells. X. The biophysics and biology of sickle-cell disease. *Archives of Internal Medicine*, **97**, 145.

604 SPRAGUE C.C. & PATERSON J.C.S. (1958) The rôle of the spleen and the effect of splenectomy in sickle cell disease. *Blood*, **13**, 569.

605 PEARSON H.A., SPENCER R.P. & CORNELIUS E.A. (1969) Functional asplenia in sickle cell anemia. *New England Journal of Medicine*, **281**, 923.

606 DUNN M.A. & GOLDWEIN M.I. (1975) Hypersplenism in advanced breast cancer: report of a patient treated with splenectomy. *Cancer*, **35**, 1449.

Chapter 21
The leukaemias: pathogenesis and classification

H. E. M. KAY

Leukaemia is a neoplastic disorder of those cells whose normal purpose is to provide, by proliferation and differentiation, the mature functional cells of the blood. Of the four common varieties of leukaemia, three—acute lymphoblastic (ALL), acute myeloid (AML), and chronic granulocytic leukaemia (CGL)—are derived directly from stem cells in the bone marrow but the fourth, chronic lymphocytic leukaemia (CLL), has a less certain origin since it may originate or at least evolve in sites outside the marrow such as the spleen and lymph nodes. In the case of T-cell ALL it is open to doubt whether the origin is in the marrow with quasi-physiological spread to the thymus and blood or whether the disease starts in the thymus and later re-invades the bone marrow: probably both patterns occur. The general pattern and pathways of the normal cells and their leukaemic counterparts are indicated in Figure 21.1.

A feature that distinguishes leukaemias and some lymphomas from most 'solid' tumours is that their cell of origin is not fixed since stem cells, as well as differentiated cells, normally migrate via the bloodstream to other sites in the marrow and other haemopoietic tissues so that leukaemia nearly always presents as a widely diffused process. It is a paradox of neoplastic change that in some leukaemia-related tumours, chloromas and bone marrow lymphomas, malignant transformation seems to be accompanied by a loss of normal cell mobility.

The versatile potential of normal stem cells is reflected in the variety of different forms of leukaemia. These can be distinguished to some extent by morphological criteria, but in leukaemia, as in all neoplastic disease, the malignant clone in each and every patient is a unique species of cells characterized by one or more out of many possible deviant patterns of behaviour. The deviations from normal that accompany the malignant change often exceed the relatively trivial differences that distinguish the patterns of normal differentiation, for example neutrophil and monocyte, and may include a degree of metaplastic change, so that recognizable differentiation is not necessarily a reliable indicator of the cell of origin or of the other biochemical properties of the clone. Furthermore, leukaemic cells may respond to environmental influences, as can happen, for example, in erythroleukaemia following hypertransfusion, producing an apparent change in diagnostic category and, of course, similar changes can be part of the natural progression of the disease.

For epidemiological purposes fine distinctions have to be disregarded and the data are based on a division into the four main categories—ALL, AML, CGL and CLL. The errors inherent in this classification arise firstly from the omission of some of the chronic myeloproliferative disorders (CMD)—some will be included in CGL and others may be listed as and when they progress to AML; secondly, from the variable omission or allocation of lymphomas with leukaemic change to ALL or CLL, and thirdly, to an inevitable penumbra of borderline cases when allocation is more or less arbitrary. Finally there is plenty of sheer misdiagnosis, not least when death certificates form the basis of the data.

EPIDEMIOLOGY [1–5]

Sex and age incidence of leukaemia

The incidence of the different types of leukaemia has been the subject of extensive surveys in many countries but it remains true that variation in diagnostic accuracy and in the completeness of registration still limits the reliance which can be placed on any but large differences. For most forms of leukaemia, incidence and mortality have until recent years been almost synonymous in reality, but the methods of data collection, through cancer registries or death certificates, and the extra longevity resulting from modern treatment lead to small but important differences. Figure 21.2 shows the British incidence and mortality data three years apart (1970 and 1973) for males, and mortality alone for females. It is seen that the mortality for females is lower at all ages and, although this mainly reflects a lower incidence in women, the better survival rate for girls with ALL at present [6] must

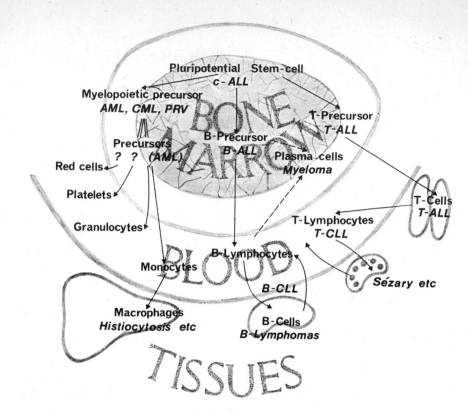

Fig. 21.1. Origins and pathways of haemopoietic cells and the neoplasms derived from them.

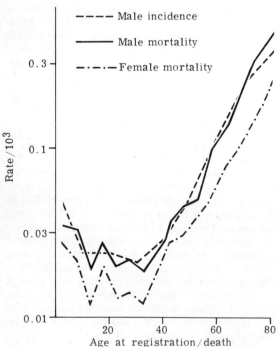

Fig. 21.2. Leukaemia incidence rates (1970) and mortality rates (1973) by age and sex.

account for some of the difference in childhood and adolescence.

When leukaemia mortality is sub-divided into the four main types of disease, four distinct patterns emerge (Fig. 21.3). Chronic lymphocytic leukaemia is the only one which has the same general trend as the majority of neoplasms, i.e. a progressive increase with age; but all the other three types have a progressive elevation above the age of fifty. It may be doubted whether in the case of ALL these are accurate observations, since typical ALL is uncommon in the elderly and various types of lymphoma or misdiagnosed poorly-differentiated AML are likely to form the majority. Similarly the peak for CML would include a higher proportion of atypical cases in the elderly so that the true line for typical (Ph[1]-positive) CGL is probably somewhat flatter. These and other data suggest that both AML and CML have two components, a peak in old age and a mid-adult plateau [7], to which may be added the third minor component of childhood AML, especially in the first year of life.

The unique age-incidence of ALL is well shown; the childhood hump comprises both the common type, with an approximately equal sex incidence and a peak age of three to four years, and the less common forms, especially T-ALL, where the peak age is slightly later and there is a more distinct male predominance, the sex ratio probably being about 3:1.

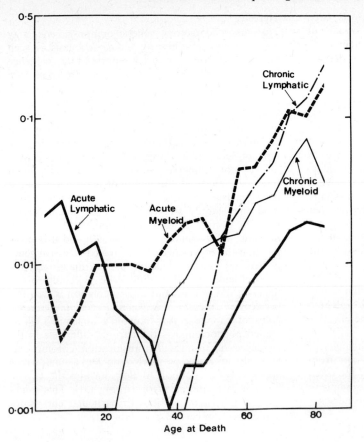

Fig. 21.3. Leukaemia: male mortality rates (1973) by cell type and age at death.

Social, racial and secular changes in incidence

Some figures of incidence related to social class have seemed to show a higher liability of classes I and II, but more recently this tendency has been eliminated and it is likely that the reported difference arose from the greater accuracy of diagnosis in the better-doctored upper social classes. No reliable evidence exists to show any correlation of incidence with class. Racial differences, however, may exist. Negroes may have a lower incidence of some forms of leukaemia and the Japanese certainly have fewer cases of CLL. Whether this is due to an environmental or hereditary factor may eventually be revealed by analysis of Japanese born in Japan and brought up there or in the U.S.A. Most of the other geographical differences must be viewed with caution and ascribed to diagnostic variation until proved to the contrary.

A similar mistrust is needed in considering evidence for secular changes in the incidence of leukaemia. The fact that the biggest increases have occurred in the oldest patients is best interpreted as a result of the greater diagnostic efforts that are now exerted in caring for the aged.

AETIOLOGICAL FACTORS

Leukaemia in other species and *in vitro* [8–21]

Before considering the aetiological factors and the pathogenetic mechanisms in human leukaemia, some mention should be made of leukaemia as it occurs in other species—both mammals and birds—and in the laboratory as well as in nature. There are some major differences: avian myeloblastosis and erythroblastosis, for example, are acute polyclonal diseases induced by variants from lymphoid leucosis virus which in nature causes a chronic monoclonal disease; and many of the leukaemias of the laboratory mouse may have no counterpart in the wild mouse, since they are the product of human manipulation and selection. Nevertheless our understanding of leukaemia as a whole largely rests on experimental studies and to some extent on epidemiology in fowls, cats, dogs and cows, etc. Some of the most important examples are listed in Table 21.1, together with examples of the cell lines which have been derived from cases of leukaemia for culture *in vitro*.

To speak of 'the cause of leukaemia' is a serious over-simplification. There are probably a number of interacting causes—necessary causes—of which one may be held to be the effective cause. Furthermore, leukaemia, as we have seen, comprises a variety of diseases and it is likely that the importance of each cause varies among the different types and at different ages. Let us suppose, for example, that a viral DNA sequence, buried in the genome and normally silent, can be activated by radiation or by another virus infection to induce a leukaemic change. Then the original virus would be a necessary cause of the leukaemia. But if it was common, if, as might be the case, almost all of us carried buried virus, it would cease to be a cause in one sense of the word, and the effective cause would be the radiation or other inductive agent. Conversely, a rare buried virus activated by common events could be held to be the effective cause.

The subject is further confused by the difficulty of distinguishing a hereditary, i.e. genetic, factor from the genetic transmission of viruses, and by the often complex interplay of circumstances, as for example in leukaemia following treatment for Hodgkin's disease or myeloma.

Heredity

That inherited factors, genetic or non-genetic, may influence susceptibility to leukaemogenesis is seen most conspicuously in a few reported high-incidence families [22, 23]. Furthermore, there are some rare hereditary diseases carrying a high risk of leukaemia—Bloom's syndrome, Fanconi's anaemia, ataxia-telangiectasia and possibly others [24–27]. In these diseases a liability to chromosome breakage is a common factor and there is some evidence that the type of leukaemia varies with the preceding syndrome, for example monocytic leukaemia with Fanconi's anaemia but lymphoblastic with ataxia-telangiectasia [28]. Even in the absence of a defined syndrome, family studies may reveal a correlation between a high rate of leukaemia and increased incidence of chromatid exchange [29] and it is possible that the prevalence of undetected recessive genes in heterozygotes plays some part in many sporadic cases of leukaemia. It is difficult to place any sort of figure in this context but one calculation is that five per cent of all cases of leukaemia occur in heterozygotes of the gene for Fanconi's anaemia [30]. A related phenomenon is the curious difference in the incidence of the 15:17 translocation chromosome anomaly in acute premyelocytic leukaemia, which appears to be common in Belgium and the U.S.A. but not in Scandinavia or Britain [31]. This might indicate inherited liabilities to particular chromosomal changes in certain populations.

Table 21.1. Examples of the characteristics of some leukaemias and leukaemic cell lines

Name	Ref.	Species	Type	Origin and Properties
L 1210	[8]	Mouse	Lymphoid	Me-cholanthrene-induced (1948). Quickest growing of all lymphomas and most widely used for drug testing, etc.
Gross AKR	[9]	,,	Thymic lymphoma	Spontaneous in AKR. Transmissible by RNA virus to other strains
Rad LV Kaplan	[10]	,,	,,	Radiation-induced RNA virus leukaemia in C57Bl
Moloney	[11]	,,	Thymic or myeloid	RNA virus leukaemia. Myeloid type in thymectomized animals.
Friend	[12]	,,	Erythroleukaemias	Polyclonal virus leukaemias; some regress spontaneously. Erythroid differentiation variable and inducible by DMSO, etc.
Mirand	[13]			
Rauscher	[14]			Variable response to erythropoietin, etc.
Sachs	[15]	,,	Myeloid cell-lines	Maturation variably dependent on MGI and/or steroids Responses related to genes on chromosomes 2 and 12
WEH1-3	[16]	,,	Myelomonocytic leukaemia	Sub-lines variably dependent on and/or productive of CSF
FeLV	[17]	Cat	Lymphoid or myeloid	Natural horizontal transmission. RNA virus also causes aplasia, immunodeficiency. ? Recombinant of rat and another virus
Marek's disease	[18]	Fowl	Lymphoma	DNA herpes virus horizontally transmitted: also causes polyneuritis
K562	[19, 20]	Man	CGL blast crisis	Some evidence of erythropoietic differentiation
HL-60	[21]	,,	Ac. promyelocytic leukaemia	Differentiation to mature granulocytes inducible by DMSO, etc.

In other hereditary conditions the important feature seems to be an immunodeficiency, although in these cases the neoplastic disorder more often resembles a lymphoma [28]. In all these examples the chain of causation is unknown, but a virus may be involved, as has been shown experimentally for lymphoma development in immunodeficient mice [32], while in the syndrome of chromosomal fragility there has been demonstrated an increased cellular susceptibility to transformation *in vitro* by SV40 virus [33], a change which in many ways resembles oncogenesis.

In the general run of cases there is no overt factor and the majority of studies (data from siblings, for example) show that inheritance can at most have some slight predisposing influence. In particular, evidence of leukaemia in monozygotic twins shows only a low rate of concordance, with an unduly high proportion of the few concordant pairs developing leukaemia in infancy [23, 34, 35]. Leukaemia is rare at this age and may be quite distinct in its aetiology from all forms with a later onset. The evidence in the case of dizygous twins is ambiguous so it is not clear whether heredity or the shared intrauterine environment is the critical factor in these cases, but conversely it would appear that in leukaemia manifest after infancy, inherited or intrauterine factors are unimportant. A weak effect may, however, be deduced from studies of immunoglobulin levels in leukaemic children, their mothers and their healthy siblings [36, 37]. As compared with controls, mothers and siblings tend to have increased IgM, mothers also having more IgG and IgA and fewer blood monocytes, while patients and siblings may have less IgA; all of which may indicate a degree of immune dysfunction predisposing to leukaemia in these families: an alternative explanation is that a virus infection in a family could cause leukaemia in one, immune dysfunction in others. Extensive analyses of the antigens at the major histocompatibility complex have not as yet shown any strong correlation with any type of leukaemia but weak associations between certain HLA groups and a good response to treatment have been claimed [38]; these await confirmation. Abnormalities of chromosome number are also associated with the leukaemia risk, as is known from the 20–30-fold increase in incidence in Down's syndrome [39]: less certainly, there may be a slightly greater incidence in disorders of other chromosomes (e.g. Klinefelter's syndrome), but these are not strictly speaking hereditary characteristics [24, 28, 40].

Radiation [2, 41, 42]

A causative role for radiation in leukaemogenesis, for which there is abundant experimental proof in the mouse and other species, has been established in man most notably through studies on patients treated for ankylosing spondylitis and other conditions and by following the survivors of atomic bombs in Japan [41, 43–45].

The form of the disease may be ALL, AML or CGL. Some cases may follow within two years of radiation exposure; there is a peak of incidence after about five years followed by a long period of lesser risk. The relationship between dose and incidence is by no means simple and depends upon variables such as age and the form of the irradiation. Children appear to be particularly susceptible, and may still be at risk from fall-out after nuclear bomb tests [46]. The form of irradiation may also determine to some extent the type of leukaemia [41]. Thus in the Japanese populations there was apparently no increase of leukaemia below a threshold of 100 rads at Nagasaki but at Hiroshima, where there was also neutron irradiation, the threshold was only 20 rads, and there were many cases of CGL compared with Nagasaki. In neither city was there any effect of low doses on fetuses *in utero* at the time of the atomic bombs. By contrast, Stewart's data on the effect of pre-natal diagnostic irradiation appear to indicate an increased incidence of acute leukaemia (and other neoplasms), with a linear relationship extending down to as little as 200 mrads [47, 48]. This surprising conclusion has been closely examined and confirmed but nowadays with reduced doses of diagnostic irradiation, the incidence of attributable leukaemia is declining. At most it only accounted for a small fraction of cases of childhood leukaemia, and similar calculations show that background radiation can at most cause one-eighth of all cases of leukaemia in the age range of 15–39 years.

Some forms of diagnostic radiation may still represent a small risk, and a few cases of leukaemia generated by therapeutic radiation may be expected. Ankylosing spondylitis is no longer so treated, and whereas the prolonged survival after radiotherapy in Hodgkin's disease and other neoplastic conditions seems to be associated with a small excess of deaths due to second neoplasms [49], leukaemia seems to be almost restricted to cases where chemotherapy has also been given. In an extensive survey of radiation treatment of carcinoma of the cervix uteri the excess of leukaemic deaths is vanishingly small [50, 51].

Acute leukaemia arising after radiophosphorus treatment for polycythaemia vera is considered in Chapter 32.

Chemical leukaemogenesis

There is probably a wide range of drugs and other chemical agents which can in some circumstances be leukaemogenic, but only in a few instances does the evidence come anywhere near proof. Benzene, which can cause chromosome damage and bone-marrow aplasia, is almost certainly a rare cause [52] and there are data hinting that other solvents and agents used in industry, e.g. petroleum refinery and rubber manufacture, may be sometimes to blame. The difficulty is to relate the degree of exposure to the excess of leukaemia incidence and to identify the agent responsible.

Rather more assurance is possible with drugs where epidemiological and experimental data can together give some notion of the probable risk [53, 54]. Both sources combine to put alkylating agents and procarbazine at the top of the list. In Hodgkin's disease [55–57] and in non-Hodgkin's lymphomas [55, 58–60] the incidence of myelomonocytic or erythroleukaemia is high in all series treated by the standard regimes which include both types of drug, whereas patients treated by radiation alone have only a slight excess of leukaemia. Myelomonocytic leukaemia is not only seen in myeloma after treatment with alkylating agents, but the two diseases also occasionally occur simultaneously [61]. This casts some doubt on the precise role of the drugs: are they perhaps revealing or precipitating disease which is already incipient in an abnormal marrow? The occurrence of leukaemia after treatment of other tumours, e.g. ovary [62], lung [63], breast [64] or melanoma [65], seems more certain to indicate a direct effect, especially, for example, in a series of 243 patients with lung carcinoma treated by busulphan in which leukaemia occurred in four, all of whom had had a period of severe marrow hypoplasia [63]. Of the other antineoplastic drugs commonly used, the long-term effects of mercaptopurine and methotrexate have been studied. These appear to be much less potent leukaemogens and mostly there is no more than suspicion, e.g. a few neoplastic conditions, including leukaemia, in a few patients treated for psoriasis by methotrexate [53]. For mercaptopurine and the related immunosuppressive azathioprine there is good evidence for an excess of lymphomas after prolonged use [66–68]. Other agents used as immunosuppressives

such as cyclophosphamide, cyclosporin A, and possibly even anti-lymphocyte globulin and corticosteroids, have similarly been suspected. The lymphomas described in these circumstances [69] have often been atypical—some, for example, appear to originate in the central nervous system—but whether the immunosuppression, as such, is the causative factor or whether, as is probably the case with the alkylating agents, there is a direct mutagenic effect, is by no means clear. Two points should be emphasized. Both radiation and anti-neoplastic drugs will not only initiate a certain number of new neoplasms in an exposed population, but they must also destroy some single cells or small clones which were destined to form neoplasms. What is observed, therefore, is always the net effect of the two opposite actions, so that any simple relation of dose to effect is hardly to be expected [40, 70].

Secondly, there are at least three distinct mechanisms whereby radiation (and other agents) may be leukaemogenic:
1 a direct mutational effect of the agent on the susceptible cell;
2 a conversion of a provirus to virus which can, as in the Rad LV system [10], induce leukaemia in other unirradiated cells; and
3 via immunosuppression;
but the idea that immunosuppression or immunodeficiency is of itself oncogenic is by no means established: in human leukaemia it is likely to be at most an infrequent and weak causative factor.

One factor, which may sometimes be of practical importance, is the relationship of the specific leukaemogenic agent to the form of leukaemia induced. The matter is not completely resolved; at present one can probably conclude that although any agent may sometimes induce any cytological type of leukaemia there is to each agent a specific pattern of probabilities. These are indicated in Table 21.2.

Viruses [71–73]
Whatever the role may be of radiation and chemical agents, in a minority of cases there is a possibility that a

Table 21.2. Relationship of leukaemogenic agents to morphological variety of leukaemia

	CML	AML	Erythroleukaemia	ALL and AUL
γ-rays } X-rays }	+	+ +	?	+
Neutrons	+ +	? +	?	? +
Benzene	? +	+ +	+	? +
Alkylating agents	?	+ (AMML)	+	?

virus can, either by itself or by interaction with other agents, including other viruses, give rise to leukaemia, and so could be directly causative in at least some, and perhaps nearly all, cases of human leukaemia.

The main strands of evidence are as follows. Practically all forms of leukaemia and lymphoma in animals which have been adequately investigated have been found to have an associated virus: these are most often C-type RNA viruses now known as retroviruses (Fig. 21.4); in a few cases a DNA virus such as a virus of the herpes group is involved (see Table 21.1). RNA viruses can be transmitted either 'horizontally' from one individual to another or 'vertically'; in the latter instance it may be conveyed as an infectious agent from the mother (a congenital infection) or may pass from either parent integrated in the genome—genetic transmission.

Several examples of horizontal transmission are known, one of the best studied being the cat, where leukaemia behaves as an infectious disease, although the majority of the infections do not result in leukaemia [71, 74]—they often, however, cause transient hypoplasia or immunodeficiency and the occasional association of such events with subsequent leukaemia in man is intriguing. Horizontal transmission implies that there is production of virus at least at the source of infection (a productive infection), but the virus is usually most prolific in cells other than leukaemic cells (e.g. the mucosa of the turbinate bones in the cat), while in the recipient the infection may be entirely non-productive. The failure to find virus in cases of leukaemia is not evidence against a viral aetiology, but the epidemiological evidence for horizontal transmission of a leukaemia virus in man is weak. If it were common one would expect minor epidemics of leukae-mia from time to time and even if the incubation period were prolonged to a few years these would often be noticed. In fact, of course, clusters of cases congregated in space and time have been recorded quite frequently, but as some clustering would be expected to occur by chance alone their significance is uncertain. The subject has provided a feast of speculative calculation for epidemiologists and the truth is still obscure but has been lucidly reviewed by Smith [75]. What one can say is that either horizontal transmission of a leukaemia virus is a rare event in man or, if it occurs commonly, then the mode of transmission is unusual or the incubation period is long, and/or that the critical event is the subsequent activation of the virus. We have seen that radiation is able to activate a latent leukaemogenic virus in the Rad LV leukaemia of mice, and chemicals such as halogenated pyrimidines, for example bromo-deoxyuridine and iododeoxyuridine, can act in the same way. A third type of interaction is where a defective virus, i.e. one which cannot form infective particles, is changed or complemented by another virus, so that complete virus particles can be formed with spread from cell to cell, or possibly the activated virus can now induce a change in the behaviour of the cell which has become doubly infected. If that were so, the occurrence of leukaemia might be related to infection by quite common viruses, e.g. those which cause common diseases such as measles, mumps or hepatitis, or viruses such as the papova viruses, at least one of which (JC) appears to be ubiquitous in man but causes no apparent disease.

Furthermore, many oncogenic viruses can infect more than one species, and where that occurs the effects differ between the species. Thus in one it may cause no known effect, in another a self-limited illness, or in another a neoplasm. A human leukaemogenic

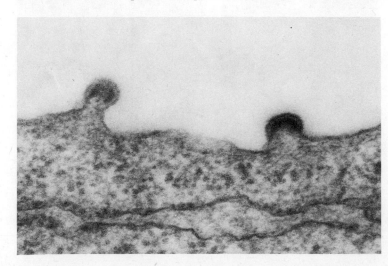

Fig. 21.4. Budding of C-type virus particles from the cell surface ($\times 135\,000$) (by kind permission of Dr M. S. C. Birbeck, Chester Beatty Research Institute).

virus could therefore be transmitted from another species in which it is not leukaemogenic.

Direct evidence for the involvement of viruses in human leukaemia is as follows.

1 Particles resembling oncornaviruses have occasionally been found in leukaemic cells (Fig. 21.5).

2 Leukaemic cells may contain cytoplasmic RNA which by hybridization techniques is found to be homologous to either a mouse leukaemia virus or certain monkey viruses—the gibbon and woolly monkey viruses.

3 Antigens found in some leukaemic cells can be shown by radioimmunoassay to resemble those of oncornaviruses.

4 Reverse transcriptase—the virus-encoded enzyme which derives a DNA copy of the virus—can be found in some leukaemic cells and is susceptible to inhibition by antibody specific to the woolly monkey and gibbon virus transcriptase.

The fact that evidence of these kinds is not consistently found in any one form of leukaemia does not diminish their significance. The leukaemic change may well be accomplished by more than one mechanism or, more probably, the signs of viral infection such as reverse transcriptase or nucleic-acid sequences may not always be retained in the leukaemic cells. This appears to be the case in feline leukaemia, since in epidemics a number of cases are recorded which are clinically identical but lack all evidence of the FeL virus [76].

In man there is also one strong but circumstantial piece of evidence for a virus: in five or six cases where leukaemia has been treated by bone-marrow transplantation, the disease has recurred in cells of donor origin [77–80]. A persistent agent which infects the donor cells is probable; alternative explanations are difficult to sustain.

Other types of virus

DNA viruses in the papovavirus, adenovirus and herpes groups have been shown to be oncogenic in some species and a lymphoma is a common type of tumour to result, for example as in Marek's disease of fowls. In man there is very strong circumstantial evidence that the Epstein–Barr (EB) virus is involved in the causation of the Burkitt lymphoma (and nasopharyngeal carcinoma) [81–83], but other factors, such as the age at which virus infection occurs, and perhaps an accompanying immune response to infection by falciparum malaria, are more critical determinants of the genesis of a lymphoma. Thus the EB virus is a necessary cause but not in a strict sense the effective cause. It should be noted that acute B-cell leukaemia, which morphologically resembles non-tropical Burkitt's lymphoma, differs in certain essential respects [84]. EB virus DNA can seldom be detected in the lymphoma cells and the clinical manifestations are distinctive. It has been shown that Hodgkin's disease follows EB virus infection more often than chance would allow, so that the virus may be one causal agent in that disease [85–86]. Other DNA viruses which are ubiquitous in human beings, for example other herpes viruses, papovaviruses and adenoviruses, must remain on the list of suspects, since many are oncogenic in other species and all have the capacity for producing life-long latent infections.

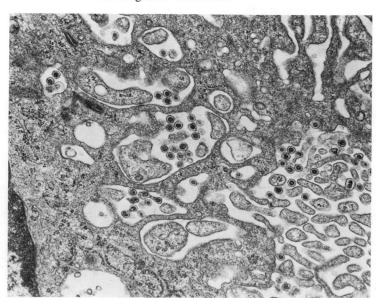

Fig. 21.5. C-type particles in HL23 V-1-infected KNRK cells (×18 600). (Reprinted from Ref. 75a, by kind permission of the authors and publishers.)

The probability with all potentially oncogenic viruses in man is that it is the circumstances which accompany the infection, e.g. acquisition around the time of birth, simultaneous events in the immune and haemopoietic systems, or the coincident infection by two defective complementary viruses, which lead by a rare chance to an alteration in one or more cells whose proliferation as a clone results in leukaemia.

In conclusion it is clear that the causes of the leukaemias are neither single nor simple. Even when some causative factors are identified it remains possible that no effective cause will be found in some cases, perhaps even in the majority. These may arise through the coincidence of rare but not essentially abnormal cellular events, of which genetic mutation is the best understood and most likely. The mutation rate at any locus has been estimated at 10^{-5} to 10^{-6} cell divisions [87] but this may be quite variable, depending on circumstances such as the properties of different DNA synthetases. The disadvantages of these 'mistakes' should not be over-emphasized. Any fatal disease resulting from them which is rare or which strikes in the post-reproductive period of life will have a negligible effect on selection and the disease will persist in the population. At the same time imperfections in the fidelity of cell reproduction, which cause genetic or epigenetic changes, may well have evolutionary advantages. Indeed the whole process of evolution would be impossible without many gross chromosomal alterations of precisely the sort which are seen in leukaemia and other neoplasms. An additional quasi-mutagenic alteration is implicit in the activity of the maverick enzyme, terminal deoxynucleotidyl transferase, which may confer both a greater range and precision of immune responses as well as perhaps an occasional liability towards harmful cell changes.

In man the incidence of most forms of leukaemia is relatively constant among different races and is so low that it can have had little selective effect in the evolution of our species. Childhood leukaemia is obviously a partial exception and, by the same argument, is most likely to have a discoverable effective cause. Similar effective causes will also, no doubt, be found to explain some cases of the other leukaemias but the possibility exists that for many other cases there is none.

CLASSIFICATION OF LEUKAEMIAS

Morphology of leukaemic cells

Many systems of classification based on morphology have been devised over the last fifty years or more,

Table 21.3. Morphology in acute myeloid leukaemias

	Romanovsky	Peroxidase or Sudan black	Non-spec. esterase NASDA	Chloro-acet. esterase F1-NASDA	PAS	Acid phosphatase	Lysozyme
Myeloblastic M1	Blasts +; few cells with granules or Auer rods	(+) rarely ++	+	+	−	−	−
Myelocytic M2	> 50% blasts + promyelocytes Auer rods common Variable mature polymorphs, often agranular or Pelger	++	++	++	Diffuse +	Diffuse +	(+)
Promyelocytic M3	Large coarse granules or Auer rods filling cytoplasm	++	++	++	+	+	−
Myelomonocytic M4	As in M2 but mono and promono >20% in BM or > 5 × 10⁹/l in blood	++	+++	+	+	+	+
Monocytic M5	Large blasts differentiating to monocytes	+	+++	−	+	−	++
Erythroleukaemia M6	As in M1, 2 or 4 with atypical erythroblasts > 30%	+	+	+	+ (often in erythroblasts)	+ (incl. erythroblasts)	+
Megakaryocytic (?M7)	As in M2 or 4 + small megakaryoblasts	+	+	+	Coarse + in megakaryocytes	+	+

Table 21.4. Proliferative patterns in chronic myeloproliferative disorders

	Granulopoiesis	Erythropoiesis	Thrombopoiesis	Blasts
CGL	↑	N or ↓	N or ↑	N
PRV	N or ↑	↑	N or ↑	N
CMML	↑(monocytes↑)	↓	↓	N
RAEB*	↓	↓	N or ↓	↑
Chronic erythroleukaemia	N or ↓	↑Dysplastic	N or ↓	(↑)
Myelofibrosis	N↑ or ↓	N or ↓	N ↓ or ↑	Late ↑

* Refractory anaemia with excess blasts.

some of great complexity, but recently more simplified systems have been gaining agreement. For example, the Franco-American-British (FAB) classification of AML [88–90] can be used with reasonable precision and consistency (Table 21.3). Most of the distinctions are possible with the aid of Romanovsky stains of blood and marrow alone, but in a minority cytochemical or antigenic analysis is needed. One important morphological distinction is the separation of hypergranular promyelocytic leukaemia (M3) from other forms of AML, since the association with intravascular coagulation and bleeding, and the prolonged remissions which are sometimes obtained, carry implications for both treatment and prognosis [91, 92]. One addition must also be made to the FAB list, a form of AML in which megakaryocytic differentiation—usually micromegakaryocytes—is a predominant feature [93]; this might conveniently be termed M7 and may be synonymous with or closely related to acute myelosclerosis [94]. One difficulty in the diagnosis of AML is to decide what is 'acute', since many, especially those with only a minor impairment of differentiation, can pursue a relatively slow course and may then be

termed 'subacute' [95–96], which, in turn, cannot be clearly demarcated from the chronic myeloproliferative disorders (CMD). Furthermore, an undoubted CMD may progress to a more acute form, and there are progressions from states considered to be 'preleukaemic' (see below) to AML. The range of tempo of disease is particularly evident where the abnormality of the erythroid series is conspicuous, i.e. in the erythroleukaemias, acute or chronic, and refractory anaemia with or without an increase of blasts in the marrow.

The CMDs can be divided into those where hyperplasia is the main abnormality (CGL, PRV and CMML) and those where dysplastic changes predominate (refractory anaemia with excess of blasts, acquired sideroblastic anaemia, chronic erythroleukaemia and myelofibrosis). The main features are listed in Table 21.4 but it should be emphasized that no system of classification can hope to embrace the many individual disease patterns that are encountered.

The FAB classification of ALL (Table 21.5) distinguishes three morphological variants: L1, where the lympholasts are relatively uniform and small; L2,

Table 21.5. Morphology in acute lymphoblastic leukaemia

	L1	L2	L3
Cell size	Small uniform	Variable	Large uniform
Nucleus	Regular shape and chromatin	Variable shape and chromatin	Oval or round. Finely and uniformly granular chromatin
Nucleoli	None or inconspicuous	Variable: may be large and conspicuous	Conspicuous
Cytoplasm	Very scarce, pale or moderate blue	Variable: often plentiful; pale or moderate blue	Moderate quantity: always deep blue
Vacuoles	Variable small	Variable small	Conspicuous, usually about 1 μm
PAS	Variable, often (c-ALL > T-ALL) single dot; sometimes multiple dots or blobs; Golgi-body positive in T-cell ALL		Negative
Acid phosphatase			Negative

where they are pleomorphic; and L3, where there is a distinctive pattern with strongly basophilic cytoplasm, multiple vacuoles and an evenly stippled chromatin pattern with a conspicuous nucleolus. This pattern is found in the rare cases of B-ALL and is of some diagnostic value. The distinction between L1 and L2, on the other hand, is largely subjective and less informative than other methods of diagnostic classification, although it may have prognostic significance. Where cell measurements have been made, a favourable prognostic group of small cell type has been demonstrated [97], though these claims have not been confirmed [98] (see Chapter 22).

A similar dispute concerns the significance of convolutions, often visible as clefts in the chromatin stained by Giemsa, but best demonstrated by electron microscopy. This is said to be a feature of T-ALL or pre-T-ALL [99] but it is not constant in that disease and is also frequent in common ALL (c-ALL), so that it is of little practical importance [100]. Leukaemic cell volumes can be measured by the Coulter counter [101] and a broad distinction can be made in this way between ALL and AML; it is also possible to determine leukaemic cell density [102] but these methods have not yet found practical application.

Cytochemistry and enzyme analysis

Diagnosis based on Romanovsky stains can often be made more precise by the use of cytochemical techniques (Tables 21.2 and 21.4), although often their contribution is merely aesthetic. It is not simply the presence or absence of a substance which can be shown by cytochemistry. In the case of acid phosphatase, for example, the location of the enzyme is critical, since in T-ALL it is concentrated in the region of the Golgi body while in AML it is found throughout the cytoplasm [103]. In many cases the main problem is that of distinguishing the population of leukaemic cells from the residual normal cells, in which event cytochemistry is no substitute for experience. The most important stains are the Sudan black and peroxidase to distinguish M1 (and M5) AML from ALL, the combined esterase stains to separate the M2, 4 and 5 types of AML and the acid phosphatase in T-ALL and AML.

One enzyme of high diagnostic value is terminal deoxynucleotidyl transferase (TdT); this is normally restricted to some thymic cells and a few cells of bone marrow—putatively lymphoid stem cells—and is found in the leukaemic cells of c-ALL and T-ALL [104, 105]. It may be demonstrated cytochemically or measured chemically and by these means the concentrations both from cell to cell and from case to case can be shown to vary by as much as a hundredfold. Other enzymes present in variable amount are adenosine deaminase (ADA) and 5-nucleotidase: the concentration of ADA is higher in ALL than in normal lymphocytes and somewhat higher in T-ALL than in c-ALL [106], whereas 5-nucleotidase is low in T-ALL and in CLL but normal in c-ALL [107].

Leukaemic cells may sometimes be characterized by a change in the concentration of the different isoenzymes in the cytoplasm as compared with normal marrow cells. This is not easily demonstrated by cytochemical methods but can be shown after extraction of the cells and chromatography. Of particular interest are the isoenzymes of hexosaminidase, since in the common form of ALL the activity of hexosaminidase I is usually increased, whereas in other forms of leukaemia and in normal cells hexosaminidases A and B account for almost all the enzymic activity [108]. Similar disproportions are seen with α-1-fucosidase [109].

Surface receptors and antigens [110–112]

Leukaemic cells exhibit at their surface antigens or receptor sites corresponding to similar configurations which characterize normal haemopoietic cells as they progress through the successive phases of maturation, although the relative concentrations in leukaemic cells may not always correspond precisely to those of a normal counterpart. In practice the most important is the common ALL antigen [113], which is present in most cases of the common type of childhood leukaemia (c-ALL) and in the lymphoblastic type of CGL blast transformation. It can be found in a few normal undifferentiated haemopoietic cells and probably signifies a primitive stage of haemopoietic ontogeny (see Chapters 2 and 3).

An antigen confined to developing and maturing T-lymphocytes serves to distinguish T-cell leukaemia from other forms of ALL and CLL and conversely an antigenic system related to the D locus of the MHC (major histocompatibility complex), also known as Ia-like (or p28, 33), can be used in diagnosis: the latter is normally present on B-lymphocytes and monocytes, and in acute leukaemia is found in B-ALL, most cases of AML and c-ALL, but only in exceptional cases of T-ALL. The reactions of appropriate antisera together with the demonstration of surface or cytoplasmic immunoglobulin, the capacity to form E-rosettes with sheep red cells and the presence of the enzymes already mentioned, permit a number of leukaemia phenotypes to be listed [114]. The common 'typical' phenotypes which account for about two-thirds of all cases are shown in Figure 21.6. The less common variants deviate in respect of one or more of the cell markers: the presence of cytoplasmic immunoglobulin in c-ALL cells demarcates a minority which may be termed pre-B [115].

A similar set of markers can be used to classify the

SURFACE & ENZYME MARKERS
IN ACUTE LEUKAEMIAS

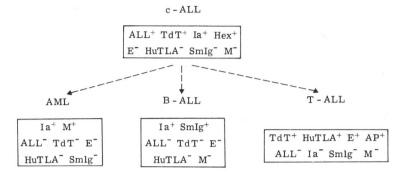

Fig. 21.6. Common phenotypes in acute leukaemia.

chronic forms of lymphocytic leukaemia and the lymphomas, the main features of which are considered in Chapters 23 and 24. Table 21.6 indicates the main markers used in classification of the leukaemias.

Leukaemia-specific antigenic changes

There have been many claims for the existence of leukaemia-specific antigens and these are undoubtedly present on the cells of virus-induced animal leukaemias. In man the position remains quite uncertain. The difficulty is to establish that the antigen is leukaemia-specific and is not a normal antigen of a haemopoietic precursor cell. Such cells may be undetectable in the marrow of adults and may be relatively scarce even in the haemopoietic tissues of the fetus during the earliest stages of ontogeny. Furthermore, a normal antigen may be present in increased concentration or in a more exposed form at the surface of a leukaemic cell and

could not therefore be called a neo-antigen. The c-ALL antigen seemed at one time to be leukaemia-specific but it is present in fetal haemopoietic stem-cells and also in a proportion of cells of regenerating marrow [116]; a similar antigen which is recognized by a monoclonal antibody has been claimed to be ALL-specific [117].

In AML the claims of immunotherapy and the apparent recognition of foreignness in leukaemic blasts by autologous lymphocytes have led to the presumption that AML leukaemia-specific antigens exist. However, the therapeutic benefit of immunotherapy is marginal at best and may rest upon non-immune mechanisms (see Chapter 22) while the significance of the stimulation of autologous lymphocytes is ambiguous since normal lymphocytes of different subsets from a single individual can be induced to recognize and react to each other in appropriate circumstances [118, 119].

Table 21.6. Immunological classification of leukaemias

		c-ALL	TdT	HUTLA	Ia	SRBC rosettes	M+	MRBC rosettes	SIgM	CIgM
AML		−	−	−	+	−	+	−	−	−
c-ALL		+	+	−	+	−	−	−	−	±
T-ALL	Early	±	+	+	−	±	−	−	−	−
	Mature	−	±	+	−	+	−	−	−	−
Sézary T-CLL		−	−	±	−	+	−	−	−	−
B-ALL		−	−	−	+	−	−	−	+	−
CLL		−	−	−	+	−	−	+	±	−
ProLL		−	−	−	+	−	−	±	++	−
Hairy Cell		−	−	−	+	−	−	±	+	−

+ Most cells positive.
± Variable or weak positivity.
++ Exceptionally strong positivity.
HUTLA Human thymic leukaemia antigen

SRBC Sheep red blood cell
MRBC Mouse red blood cell
SIgM Surface IgM
CIgM Cytoplasmic IgM

Extensive efforts to raise heterologous antisera specific to AML have on the whole failed [120] although an antibody from AML patients subjected to immunotherapy may be specific and can at least be used successfully to predict relapse [121, 122].

Losses as well as apparent gains of antigens occur in leukaemia, as in most neoplasms. These are not of great biological or clinical importance, reflecting as they do, one among many of the disorders of the phenotype. In one instance, the loss of alloantigens in CGL, the extent of the loss and the correlation with accelerated disease activity may have some clinical and possibly pathogenetic importance [123].

Cells of origin in leukaemia [110–112]

Thus, with the possible exceptions just mentioned, the phenotypes of leukaemic cells, as delineated by morphology and antigen analysis, are essentially those of normal haemopoietic cells at various stages of their maturation. In all acute leukaemias there is some degree of maturation arrest. In c-ALL the arrest takes place either in pluripotent stem cells or at an early stage of lymphoid differentiation and the block is complete, in that maturing cells of the leukaemic clone are absent. This example typifies the concept of the 'frozen phenotype' [110]; the presence of TdT or of cytoplasmic immunoglobulin in c-ALL may denote either the stage of maturation at which the phenotype has been frozen or that there is some slight degree of differentiation occurring from a more primitive type of leukaemic stem cell. T-ALLs and AML, by contrast, are mostly comprised of cells having a greater range of stages in their maturation, although the degree of differentiation varies enormously from case to case and in response to circumstances. On the whole lymphoid leukaemias and lymphomas remain restricted to the expression of either T- or B-cell characters [124] and never acquire myeloid potentials, but some cases of composite lymphomas [125] or mixed T- and B-cell leukaemias have been recorded [126]. The nature of the impediments to full maturation is unknown, nor does the analysis of phenotype fully identify the cell of origin of the leukaemia. It is tempting to assume that the most primitive cell type identified would have been the target cell of the original leukaemogenic event, but it is quite possible that the event took place at an even earlier stage of maturation. For example, a case of AML has been described with differentiation apparently restricted to granulopoiesis and monocytopoiesis [127], but the disease might not have originated in a normal cell with this restriction and could have arisen in a cell with full myeloid potential (i.e. for erythro- and thrombocytopoiesis also). Similarly in CGL, apparently a disease confined to the myeloid side of the haemopoetic range, the cells in blast crisis can carry the c-ALL phenotype so that the original target may have been a pluripotent stem cell rather than one of restricted myeloid potential [128].

In myeloma, a neoplasm of the most fully differentiated B-lineage idiotype analysis shows that a proportion of the apparently normal B lymphocytes are of the same clone, which presumably indicates a more primitive type of B-cell as the ancestor of both [129, 130]. In these instances it seems that the full potential of the cell of origin may not be expressed or else that the expression is overwhelmingly in one direction. Do leukaemic cells exhibit characteristics of more than one pathway of differentiation? There are instances where this appears to be so. For example, cells morphologically of myeloid type may contain TdT, a thymic cell character [114, 131], and leukaemic T cells may rarely also carry the Ia antigen. The latter observation may be explained by the occurrence of a small subset of normal T cells that are Ia$^+$ and are putatively activated T cells, designated T_{G1} [132] and it is possible that a similar explanation underlies the TdT + myeloid cell, i.e. there may be a small subset of normal cells with these properties; alternatively such observations may sometimes indicate distinct subclones of the original leukaemic line.

However, in other tissues metaplasia is a well-recognized phenomenon. Cells of the transitional urinary epithelium can undergo metaplastic change to squamous or mucous epithelium, so that similar 'sideways' changes in the differentiation of haemopoietic cells could be expected. Furthermore, if that can occur there is no intrinsic reason why a measure of 'de-differentiation', i.e. the re-acquisition of an abandoned potential, could not also take place. The possibility of such an event cannot be disproved, so that the key question as to the cell of origin in leukaemia remains unanswered and perhaps unanswerable (for further discussion see Ref. 133).

Chromosome changes in leukaemia [134–136]

The role of chromosome changes in oncogenesis is still uncertain. They may be causative, consequential or tenuously related epiphenomena; if all types of neoplasm are considered, these possibilities are not mutually exclusive. In human leukaemia, the changes observed have already shed some light on the pathogenesis of the disease and are becoming increasingly important in the practical classification of disease types. The limitations have been that the analyses are laborious and require considerable expertise; that, even so, well-spread metaphases may not always be procured, and that almost half of all cases show no abnormality detectable by current methods. Furthermore there are always reservations in that a sample may not be truly representative, that slowly proliferative cells are under-represented, that cells of some types may spread better for analysis than others, and that the limits of detection of a minority population are quite as poor as for orthodox morphology. Thus a population of 10^{10} cells representing one per cent of all those in marrow would often escape recognition even in an analysis of 100 cells.

A great variety of chromosome changes is seen in the myeloproliferative diseases. Some are so rarely seen that they appear to be random changes: others are observed often enough to be regarded as non-random. They can be presumed to have some pathogenetic significance but the majority are not restricted to one clinical or morphological type of disease. This creates a temporary problem in classification. Should one, for example, consider the Ph^1 anomaly as a component of variable frequency in two or three types of leukaemia (see Table 21.7) or should one categorize Ph^1-positive disease and recognize the variable manifestations of it? The former is still the conventional approach but the latter may ultimately have advantages in relation to pathogenetic analysis and therapeutic strategy.

For practical purposes the main emphasis has been on direct examination of bone-marrow cells without previous culture but sometimes examination of blood cells, both leukaemic and normal (after culture), can give valuable extra information. Most modern studies depend on banding techniques to identify each chromosome and the precise details of each deletion or translocation. However, analyses of unbanded prep-

arations can often be sufficiently accurate for most clinical purposes.

ALL [137, 138]

In a minority of patients no karyotypic abnormalities can be found and at the other extreme some seem to have no normal cells; in the majority there is a mixture of normal diploid and abnormal karyotypes but the changes appear to be non-specific. Clones can usually be detected where hyperdiploid, hypodiploid or pseudo-diploid cells form the majority but a scattering of apparently non-clonal abnormal cells is present in most cases whatever the predominant ploidy. As yet no correlation between ploidy and the phenotype of the ALL has been determined; in one series [137] pseudo-diploidy was most often associated with a high leuco-cyte count and a poor prognosis, and the rare cases with near tetraploidy seem to do badly. The most interesting association is the presence of the Ph^1 chromosome, which may be present in about 1–2% of childhood ALL, rising to 30–40% in adults [138]. Such cases also have a poor prognosis, although when treatment brings a remission the Ph^1+ve clone ceases to be detectable in the bone marrow (in contrast to CGL, in which the Ph^1-positive clone only rarely disappears when the blood count is reduced by conventional treatments).

AML [139–141]

An important division can be made into those cases

Table 21.7. Some common chromosomal changes in human leukaemias and lymphomas

Chromosome change	Conditions	Occurrence and significance
t(9q+; 22q−) (Ph¹)	CGL	>80% of typical cases
	ALL (c-ALL)	1% (childhood), 25–40% (adult)
	AML	2–3% (younger patients)
8+	CGL blast crisis	32%
	AML	5–10%
	Myelofibrosis	?
	Pre-leukaemia	?
7−	AML	5–10%
	Pre-leukaemia	
t(8q−; 21q+)	AML	c. 5% (younger patients)
		Favourable response to treatment
t(15q+; 17q−)	A. promyelocytic L.	? 50%
i(17)q	CGL blast crisis	25%
	Pre-leukaemia	
20q−	MPD esp. PRV	Usually after treatment
	Sideroblastic anaemia	Rare
14q+: often t(8q−; 14q+)	Lymphoma	Non-Hodgkin's lymphoma. Esp. Burkitt tumour
or t(11q−14q+)	B-ALL	? Specific to EB virus infection
21q−	Thrombocythaemia in MPD	? Specific to retrovirus infection
5q−	Pre-leukaemic myelodysplasia	Distinctive syndrome

where either all cells have a normal karyotype, (NN) (50% of all cases), or there is a mixture of normal and abnormal (AN) or all are abnormal, (AA). Sandberg has pointed out that prognosis is best in the first, and worst in the last of these categories. The abnormalities seen comprise a great variation of losses, gains and translocations (Figs 21.7 and 21.8). Certain anomalies are relatively common: $+8$, -7, t(8:21) and t(22:9), i.e. Ph[1]-positive. Some of these may have prognostic significance—$+8$ and t(8:21) may be relatively favourable [142] for example—but more cases must be analysed before these associations can be firmly established or before they can be used to predict the success of particular forms of treatment.

Acute promyelocytic leukaemia [143, 144]

In this disease the karyotype may either be normal or there may be a specific abnormality, t(15:17), but the frequency of these alternatives seems to vary in different countries [31]. The translocation, however, is not seen in other forms of leukaemia and thus provides useful diagnostic and prognostic information.

CGL and CMD [145, 146]

The Ph[1]-chromosome is present in over 90% of typical cases of CGL, indeed for some purposes such as a clinical trial it is held to be essential to the diagnosis, which otherwise is given as a non-specific CMD. The anomaly consists of a translocation most often between chromosomes 22 and 9, t(9:22)(q34:q11), and sometimes between chromosome 22 and others. Other anomalies such as the loss of the Y chromosome or 8-trisomy may be present in a minority of cases. The anomaly can be demonstrated in megakaryocytes and red-cell precursors, but has only once been found in the (PHA-responsive) circulating T lymphocytes or in bone-marrow fibroblasts. In a few cases where CGL has followed radiation [147, 148] or exposure to benzene [149] the anomaly has been looked for and found to be present, but these number only 21 and two

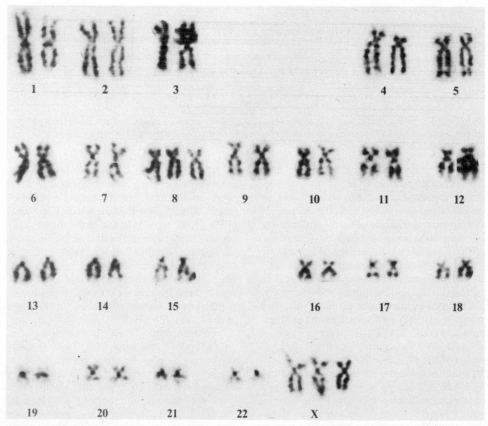

Fig. 21.7. Simple hyperdiploidy (XXX$+8$) in bone-marrow cells of a girl aged six with pancytopenia, presumed to be pre-leukaemia, but condition unchanged for two years. (Courtesy of Drs J. Steadman and J. Swansbury.)

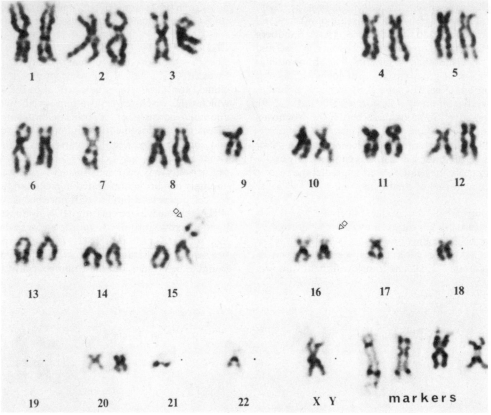

Fig. 21.8. Multiple abnormalities including four marker chromosomes in a case of pre-leukaemia progressing to erythroleukaemia. The patient, a man of 68, had received cytotoxic chemotherapy for colonic cancer 17 months earlier. (Courtesy of Drs. D. Bevan and J. Swansbury.)

cases respectively, so it is not absolutely certain that these agents cause Ph¹-positive CGL.

The Ph¹ chromosome has been widely cited as showing the clonal nature of CGL and also as evidence that the chromosomal change actually induces the alteration in cell behaviour manifest as leukaemia. Neither of these statements is proven but both are probably true. In two chromosome mosaics who developed CGL, cells were found suggesting that both types of normal cell had acquired Ph¹-positivity. However, in both cases alternative explanations, such as the acquisition by the XYPh¹-positive of an extra C chromosome to mimic XXYPh¹+, were possible or indeed preferred [148]. The aetiological role depends on the absence of the Ph¹ anomaly from normal cells and cells of other neoplasms. As we have seen it can occur in ALL and AML, also in one case of myeloma [150], but it is, at most, exceedingly rare in any normal cell *in vitro* or *in vivo*; that constitutes strong evidence that it is an essential part of one type of neoplastic conversion in haemopoietic cells.

In other types of CMD a number of miscellaneous changes have been described, mostly without specificity as to cause, classification or response to treatment. The 20q− anomaly, which is not uncommon in PRV [151], is of interest, since this usually develops during the course of the disease but is also rarely seen in acquired sideroblastic anaemia, and may represent the selection in an abnormal haemopoietic environment of an adapted clone. When CGL and other CMD are treated by cytotoxic drugs, radiation, or even by venesection, changes may occur in the populations of chromosomally marked cells. In CGL, cells with the Ph¹ chromosome usually persist and normal cells do not reappear; but rarely, especially if fairly intensive cytotoxic therapy has been given, some normal Ph¹-negative cells reappear, and occasionally prolonged remissions, with an apparently stable mixture of the two populations, can occur [145]. In other CMDs, especially PRV, such mixtures are more common both before treatment and when the blood composition is more nearly normal.

Other changes sometimes seen in CMD and preleukaemic states include monosomy-7,5q− (where refractory anaemia is associated with non-lobulating nuclei in the megakaryocytes) and i(17)q. In thrombocythaemia 21q− has been described in some cases [152] and is considered to have some specificity. Furthermore, previous infection by retroviruses in these cases was suggested by particles seen by electron microscopy and the presence of reverse transcriptase. It is possible that these are only passenger viruses but the association of a virus, a specific chromosome anomaly and a specific haematological change is, if confirmed, of some importance.

Lymphomas, myeloma and CLL [153, 154]

Of the various chromosome abnormalities described, translocation to the long arm of chromosome 14, 14q+, often t(8q−: 14q+) or t(11q−: 14q+), is the commonest. This has been found in various B-cell non-Hodgkin lymphomas including myeloma, B-ALL and the Burkitt lymphoma, and also in T-ALL [155] and T-CLL [156]. The specificity appears, therefore, to be related to lymphoid rather than myeloid tumours and there may be a close relationship to the EB virus; thus in cell hybrids, one component of which is an EB-transformed lymphoblast, the demonstration of EB DNA and of virus-determined nuclear antigen was dependent on the persistent presence of chromosome 14 [155]. In CLL [157] and hairy-cell leukaemia [158] there are relatively few observations, but trisomy, especially of chromosome 12, may be a semi-specific change.

Chromosome changes in radiation and chemically induced leukaemia

Since both radiation and cytotoxic chemicals can cause both chromosome abnormalities and leukaemia it is pertinent to ask whether the chromosome abnormalities in cases with a previous history of exposure to these cytotoxic agents are different from the general run of cases. CGL cases with a history of radiation are as likely to be Ph[1] positive as those without such a history [147, 148] although they may more often have additional abnormalities, and cases of CGL following benzene exposure have occasionally been shown to have a Ph[1] chromosome [149]. In AML, one series shows that 83% of 23 patients with a history of exposure to mutagenic or carcinogenic agents had chromosomal abnormalities (mostly −5, −7, +8 or +21) compared with only 24% of 33 without such a history, which would imply that the overall figure of 50% without abnormalities in other series is due to a chance mixture of exposed and unexposed patients [159]. The difference, however, is not a universal experience [160] and further data are needed to establish the true state of affairs. Where AML follows treatment for other neoplastic conditions chromosome changes are the rule, often with hypodiploidy, which is an uncommon finding in leukaemia *de novo* [136].

PATHOGENESIS

Differentiation and the growth of leukaemic cells in culture

The morphology and other detectable characters of leukaemic cells provide a description of the pattern of differentiation for each individual case of leukaemia which is the main basis for classification. Further detail can be added if the function or growth of the leukaemic cells can be observed *in vitro*. Where leukaemic lymphocytes and plasma cells are concerned, the demonstration of immunoglobulin in the cytoplasm, on the cell surface and actually secreted in the various phases of B-cell maturation are about as far as one can go. T-cell function is a more subtle affair but it is sometimes possible to indicate that the T cells of Sezary syndrome (and mycosis fungoides) have helper properties while in some other T-cell leukaemias (including Japanese subacute T-ALL) suppressor function may be shown [161]. The elaboration of various lymphocyte growth factors will undoubtedly enable other forms of lymphoid leukaemia and lymphoma to be grown and studied *in vitro*. The growth of normal marrow cells in culture has been described in Chapter 2 and some of these methods can be applied to leukaemic cells from the marrow and blood. In particular, the ability to culture AML cells in soft agar culture, or rarely in suspension culture, has revealed the restrictions and potentialities for differentiation. AML and CGL marrow cells in soft agar culture can exhibit a number of patterns differing from the normal, as indicated in Table 21.8 [162]. These patterns reflect

Table 21.8. Patterns of growth in seven-day agar cultures. Data from Moore [162].

Type of growth	Frequency	Remission rate in AML
No growth	AML 2%	
Macroclusters (20–40)	AML 22%	15%
Microcolonies with excess clusters	AML 13%	
Microclusters (20)	AML 54%	
Low plating efficiency (i.e. residual normal cells)	AML 4% Most ALL	75%
High plating efficiency (colony-forming cells)	AML 5% Most CGL	

both the intrinsic limitations of the colony-forming cells and their abnormal response to environmental factors; there is a variation both in the response to the colony-stimulating factor(s) (CSF) (see Chapter 2) and in the formation of CSF and lactoferrin by the cells in culture. It can also be shown that the cluster-forming cells in most instances tend to have abnormally light buoyant density (<1062) as compared with the colony-forming units of normal marrow.

In a few instances of AML from both man and mouse, continuous lines have been grown in suspension cultures, so affording a greater opportunity to explore the flexibility in differentiation that the cells retain. In a series of murine leukaemias investigated by Sachs [163], the various surface antigens and receptors have been plotted and it has been shown that, in at least one cell line, maturation which is inhibited *in vivo* can be facilitated *in vitro* by the addition of macrophage and granulocyte inducer (MGI), which is effectively one form of CSF. Perhaps more dramatically, a human line from a case of acute promyelocytic leukaemia can be induced to differentiate towards normal granulocyte formation by dimethyl sulphoxide [21], which is one of a class of compounds which can induce terminal differentiation in other circumstances (see Chapter 2). A similar induction to erythroid maturation has also been reported when sodium butyrate was added to cultures of a long-established line from a case of CGL; in that case the erythropoietic potential was already evident in the presence of glycophorin, a red-cell membrane protein, before addition of sodium butyrate [19, 20]. What significance should be attached to these abrupt changes of direction or consummations of a differentiating proclivity is uncertain, and depends upon the cell of origin of the leukaemia clone (see p. 811)

Pre-leukaemia [90, 164–166]

A number of states have been described which may be succeeded by leukaemia or lymphoma (see Table 21.9) and have given rise to the concept of pre-leukaemia, although objections to this term have suggested that the alternative of myelo-dysplastic syndromes should be preferred. Nevertheless pre-malignant conditions in other sites of the body are well recognized and the concept of pre-leukaemia is perfectly valid. All that is implied is that the degree of liability to develop overt leukaemia is greater than that for the normal individual. The fact that leukaemia does not develop during the lifetime of the affected subject is no reason to consider the term inappropriate, indeed it is the very uncertainty of the process that helps to distinguish pre-leukaemia from the earliest stages of leukaemia. A second property which may apply in some pre-leukaemic states is their reversibility. In other tissues of the

body a pre-malignant condition, such as epithelial dysplasia of the cervix uteri, may be a temporary phenomenon, with reversion to normal accompanied by a lessened liability to carcinoma formation. Most of the conditions regarded as pre-leukaemic, however, are not reversible, although it is probable that parallels will be found, for example, where there is recovery of hypoplastic states or even in the successful treatment of megaloblastic haemopoiesis which may, while it persists, predispose to leukaemia [167]. The complete remission attainable in early α-chain disease may be instanced as a reversible prelymphomatous condition [168].

Pre-leukaemia in man is characterized by either hyper-, hypo-, or dysplasia of haemopoiesis. On theoretical grounds it is valid to place CMD, including PRV and CGL, among the pre-leukaemic states, since the abnormality in the initial stages is virtually restricted to a hyperplasia. At the other extreme are hypoplastic states, some exhibiting a distinctive syndrome such as paroxysmal nocturnal haemoglobinuria (PNH) so that the probability of leukaemic change can be estimated with some accuracy [169]; others are much less well-defined, but probably all hypoplasias and acquired dysplasias have an increased tendency to advance to some sort of acute leukaemia. In general, the presence of a chromosomal abnormality increases the liability to progress to leukaemia except perhaps in myelofibrosis [170–172].

Clonal nature of leukaemia: neoplastic progression [173–175]

With the exception of some of the virus-induced leukaemias (see Table 21.1), leukaemia is a clonal disease as evidenced by chromosomal and isoenzyme analyses; that is to say, all the leukaemic cells are members of one clone, descended from a common ancestral cell in which a leukaemogenic event occurred. Within this clone further deviation can occur, giving rise to sub-clones of variant cells. The term 'neoplastic progression' implies a change in the characteristics of the neoplastic cells towards a more malignant type of disease. This may be observed as a more rapid growth rate, a loss of differentiation including a loss of antigens or enzymes peculiar to the more differentiated cells, a change from hormone-dependency to autonomy, a new ability to proliferate in metastatic sites and so forth. It is generally agreed that progression is the result of the emergence of a new 'more malignant' clone, that is to say one which outgrows and supplants the previous clone(s) of malignant cells and the term 'clonal evolution' is, therefore, sometimes preferred. This process must be distinguished from the evolution of a second neoplasm which can, of course, sometimes arise independently

Table 21.9. Neoplastic progression in leukaemia and lymphoma

Initial phase	'Progressed' disease	Incidence and circumstances of progression	Ref.
CGL	AML-like 80%	Almost constant exponential rate ($\sim 50\%$ in three years) irrespective of treatment	116 176
	ALL-like 20%	New chromosome changes usual	145
PRV	AML-like	True incidence difficult to define: ? 15% Relationship to treatment by ^{32}P and drugs obscure Multiple chromosome changes	177
Chronic myeloproliferative disorders, myelofibrosis, atypical CML, etc.	AML	Incidence not determined. Progression often gradual	164, 171
'Pre-leukaemia'			
Acquired sideroblastic leukaemia	AML	? 10–20% per annum	178
Paroxysmal nocturnal haemoglobinuria	AML	Rare	169
Aplastic anaemia	AML ALL in children	Incidence not determined. May follow directly from aplasia or after temporary recovery of normal haemopoiesis Probably frequent where aplasia is due to cytotoxic drugs Incidence not determined	
Other hypoplastic and dysplastic states	AML	Variable incidence, for example, 100% if 7−, 12% for 5q−	170–173
AML	Chloroma	Progressed non-haemopoietic clone producing tumours in bones or extra-medullary sites	179
CLL	Poorly differentiated lymphoma (Richter)	Rare	180 181
α-chain disease	B-cell lymphoma	Majority of patients progress but apparent reversion to normal with loss of α-chain over-production can occur	168, 182
Angio-immunoblastic lymphadenopathy	Immunoblastic sarcoma	? 10–20%	183–185
Sjögren's syndrome, SLE, etc.	B-cell lymphoma	Relationship obscure	186 187
Phenylhydantoin lymphadenopathy	Malignant lymphoma	Follows directly or later after resolution of lymphadenopathy	188
Myeloma	Myeloma 'escape'	Rapidly growing clone, sometimes with loss of paraprotein synthesis	189

from the same tissue of origin, either as a result of the same original oncogenic causes or as a consequence of treatment of the first neoplasm. the alternative relationships are summarized in Table 21.10.

Chromosome analysis is the main basis on which the relationship of the successive clones is deduced, and where there is, for example, a uniquely distinctive marker chromosome in both populations their common clonal origin can be accepted as proven. In the case of myeloma (and perhaps other B-cell lymphomas) the characteristic globulin idiotype provides an equally reliable clonal marker of high specificity. Where the marker is less distinctive, e.g. the Ph[1] chromosome, the clonal relationship is probable but less certain, since a change which is seen in many

individuals may also occur in more than one cell in a single individual.

Leukaemia and lymphoma in man contain a number of examples of neoplastic progression, of which the blast crisis of CGL and the evolution of some pre-leukaemic states have been studied in detail. Several examples are listed in Table 21.9, which is by no means a comprehensive list. In the simplest and all too common situation there is the emergence of a drug-resistant clone of cells after initial treatment has eliminated the majority of cells that were drug-sensitive (Table 21.10, IIIA). The rapidity of such relapses shows that very often resistant sub-clones have already been present in appreciable numbers when treatment was begun. A more natural type of progression is the

Table 21.10. Pseudo-relapse, progression and relapse in leukaemia

	Oncogenic event	Latent interval	Diagnosis and treatment	'Relapse'
I	Single leukaemic clone formed	Expansion of clone	'Successful' treatment Drug or radiation-induced second leukaemic clone	→ Second attack of leukaemia
II	Multiple unrelated leukaemic clones	Expansion of one clone	'Successful' treatment Expansion of second clone	→Second attack of leukaemia
III	Single leukaemic clone	Expansion of clone	Suppression or elimination of drug-sensitive cells	
			.... A. Emergence of drug-resistant sub-clone	→ Relapse of resistant leukaemia
			.... B. Emergence of related sub-clone	→ Relapse, e.g. blast crisis of CGL
IV	Multiple sub-clones from single leukaemic ancestor cell	Expansion of one sub-clone	'Successful' treatment Expansion of second sub-clone	→ Relapse, e.g. blast crisis

loss of differentiation seen, for example, in myelomas where the original paraprotein-producing cells are superseded by cells secreting only light chains or no protein at all. The most conspicuous example, however, is CGL blast crisis where the highly differentiated but autonomous clone of the chronic phase is succeeded by a partially differentiating AML-like clone (80%) or less commonly (20%) by an undifferentiated ALL-like stem-cell clone [116, 145, 176]. The persistence of the Ph^1 chromosome links the clones, which are assumed to be related as in IIIB or IV of Table 21.10, although if the original oncogenic cause acted specifically on chromosome 22 then the relationship of II in Table 21.10 is possible.

The difference between III and IV amounts to the time at which the second sub-clone is generated. There are data from various experimental systems which suggest that many pre-neoplastic clones are formed soon after the exposure to an oncogenic agent [190, 191]; it may be that the ancestral cells of the 'progressed' sub-clones arise at that time and remain dormant or at least proliferate more slowly during the whole of the latent period before the neoplasm is manifest. This might even be a quasi-physiological mechanism if normal haemopoiesis is maintained by a system of clonal succession [192]. On the other hand, it is highly probable that evolution of new sub-lines from the original clone can take place at any time and especially if selective pressures in the form of treatment are exerted. One unusual and rather paradoxical type of progression should be mentioned. Occasional cases have been reported where CGL [193, 194] or PRV [195] have apparently followed treatment for ALL. Such a process, which could not happen in natural circumstances, depends on the ability to treat ALL effectively and so allow a second, 'more' differentiated clone to emerge; a sequence of this sort can also be mimicked by two separate leukaemias (as in I or II of Table 21.10). Another association which may represent a form of progression is where histiocytic medullary reticulosis follows either ALL or AML [196, 197].

Progression is often accompanied by a change in the karyotype denoting the presence of the new clone(s) [145, 177, 198]. Some of these are regular associations and can be predictive, e.g. the appearance of an isochromosome 17 in CGL (i(17)q) is a reliable herald of blast crisis, but others, e.g. the appearance of a second Ph^1 chromosome, are not so closely related, and in a few cases of blast crisis there is no new abnormality. Similarly in PRV the finding of 20q− does not necessarily indicate incipient leukaemia or marrow failure, although since it increases in frequency with the duration of the disease the two events sometimes coincide.

The wide variation in the propensity of progression to leukaemia is shown in Table 21.9. On the one hand, CGL has a rather constant rate of progression to blast crisis. This is an exponential process with about 50% of all cases being affected every three years. By contrast the development of similar undifferentiated lymphomas in CLL (Richter's phenomenon) is much less common and so are most of the other conditions listed. The underlying reason for this variation is not clear but, as noted for pre-leukaemic states, the existence of chromosomal abnormalities in general and of some in particular, for example 7−, does appear to hasten the liability to progression.

Cell kinetics

Data relating to the rate of cell proliferation in acute leukaemia have been reviewed by Killmann [192] and by Mauer & Murphy [199]; and some figures are given in Table 21.11. These data are derived from diverse sources using a variety of *in vivo* and *in vitro* methods,

Table 21.11. Quantitative data in acute leukaemia

Number of blasts present at diagnosis	$\sim 10^{10}$/kg body weight
Minimum number of blasts detectable in bone marrow	$\sim 5 \times 10^8$/kg body weight
Mitotic index	$\sim 0.6\%$ $(0.3-2\%)$
[³H]thymidine labelling index (first diagnosis)	$5-10\%$ $(0.1-26.5\%)$
[³H]thymidine labelling index (relapse)	$\sim 20\%$ $(6-70\%)$
Generation time	$\sim 50-60$ hours or $15-20$ hours*
DNA-synthesis time (S)	~ 20 hours or $7-10$ hours*
Mitotic time (M)	~ 1 hour
Pre-mitotic phase (G2)	$\sim 1-3$ hours
Growth fraction (first diagnosis)	$13-35\%$
Growth fraction (relapse)	$20-100\%$
Blast-cell production rate	$\sim 10^9$/hour
Apparent doubling time	$4-10$ days

* More than one study has shown the apparent existence of two groups of cases with few intermediate values.

and must be very cautiously interpreted owing to technical uncertainties and the heterogeneity of cell populations [200–206]. The two outstanding facts are that the leukaemic blast cell, both in AML and ALL, does not proliferate at an excessive speed as compared with differentiating bone-marrow cells, and that there is a wide variation in all quanta, both from case to case and from time to time within the same case. The comparison between the situation at first diagnosis, when a great excess of blasts is present, and the situation at early relapse—diagnosed by bone-marrow aspirate before the onset of symptoms—is of particular significance. The more rapid proliferation in the latter circumstance suggests that a deceleration at higher blast-cell numbers occurs, due either to a saturation phenomenon or to a partially effective feedback. The converse effect has been seen in cases subjected to extracorporeal irradiation of the blood, where the removal of a portion of the blast population enables the remainder to resume more rapid proliferation [207].

Extrapolating backwards, on the other hand, the growth rate at relapse appears to indicate regeneration from one cell within as short a time as three months or less. This is not compatible with clinical observation of much longer remission lengths after cessation of therapy or of the latent period of radiation leukaemogenesis, so it is clear that the net growth rate at the initiation of leukaemia or of the treatment-resistant residue must also be slow.

In contrast to the variable proliferation of leukaemic blasts within the bone marrow, blast cells in the blood always show a very low rate of proliferative activity. A vexing question has been whether the majority of these cells are end-cells with no further proliferative capacity or whether they, together with the variable number of non-proliferating small blasts in the bone marrow, are resting cells capable in appropriate circumstances of re-entering further proliferative cycles within the bone marrow. There is evidence that at least some of these cells are resting cells, not end-cells; as such they become susceptible to treatment when, following reduction of cell numbers, they return to a proliferative state [201, 208–210]. This phenomenon gives some guidance to the need for continued treatment but in general the study of cell kinetics has not, despite much effort and discussion, helped in the design of more rational anti-leukaemic treatment [206, 211, 212].

In AML the maturing cells have been studied by measurement of the myelocyte-to-tissue transit time [213]. This is an aggregate estimate of the rate of maturation, release and intravascular survival and is determined by *in vivo* and *in vitro* labelling with DF³²P. It is found that whereas all labelled bone-marrow cells have matured, entered and left the blood within 17–22 days in normal subjects, in AML such cells as do complete maturation do so much more slowly (i.e. 30–40 days). Furthermore, this delay may persist even when remission has been obtained, indicating perhaps an intrinsic pre-leukaemic abnormality of the haemopoietic system.

Loss of homeostasis in leukaemia [162, 214–216]
An essential concept in leukaemia, as in all neoplastic disorders, is that there is loss of response by the neoplastic cells to homeostatic controls. The highly complex system whereby pluripotential haemopoietic stem cells normally produce an appropriate output of several different sorts of mature cells has been described in Chapter 2. The controls of the system are effected through cellular interactions both among the haemopoietic cells, and between them and the stromal cells of the marrow. These interactions are probably all mediated by diffusible substances and the major

signals from outside the marrow are also carried by hormones such as erythropoietin. Some of these mediators are readily accessible to study, especially with the aid of bone-marrow culture, but other substances such as prostaglandins whose range of action is short both in time and space are much more difficult to investigate. Our knowledge of the defects in the different forms of myeloproliferative disorder is therefore in an elementary state. Virtually nothing is known about defects in the control of thrombocyto-poiesis in leukaemia and the postulated lack of response to chalones and similar regulators has yet to be assimilated into the general framework of knowledge. Furthermore, in the leukaemic disorders there is a variable mixture of normal and leukaemic cells (see Table 21.12), the exact composition of which may be difficult to determine.

Erythropoietic abnormalities

The two myeloproliferative disorders which conspicuously affect erythropoiesis are polycythaemia rubra vera and erythroleukaemia. In the former the over-production of red cells is usually accompanied by an excess of granulocytes or platelets or both, but research has concentrated on the defect in erythropoietic control [217–219]. Thus it can be shown that the marrow in PRV contains some abnormal erythropoietic precursors at the BFU-E stage, i.e. the earliest erythropoietin-sensitive forms, which can proliferate *in vitro* without the usual requirement for erythropoietin (EPO). Elimination of all EPO, as by antibody, does depress the growth even of PRV marrow cells, but the subsequent addition of minute quantities of EPO to an anti-EPO-treated culture allows PRV erythroid colonies to grow. Thus it seems the cells are not completely autonomous but have a greatly enhanced response to small quantities of EPO. In PRV the marrow contains a mixture of cells, some of which

react normally to EPO and some of which are hypersensitive: the latter have been shown by G-6-PD isoenzyme analysis to be monoclonal and have a more rapid cell cycle [220], whereas the former are poly-clonal and thus probably represent residual normal haemopoietic cells. Similar mixtures can be demonstrated when the PRV clone carries a chromosomal abnormality [221]. The proportion of normal and abnormal cells varies, but *in vivo* when polycythaemia is present the majority of cells in division are abnormal, while after treatment to reduce the haemoglobin level, and thus to restore the production of erythropoietin, dividing normal cells become more abundant.

This provides a coherent and rational explanation of the over-production of red cells, but it remains a very incomplete account of the basis of the disease. Thus it is not clear whether there are similar hypersensitive responses of the granulopoietic and thrombocytopoie-tic precursors where these are also hyperplastic, or whether these hyperplasias have another explanation; possibly, for example, the abnormal utilization of iron might reduce the saturation of lactoferrin and thus impair its role as an inhibitor of granulocyte CSF. Nor is it known whether there is a defect in the pluripotent stem cells which induces abnormal allocation of cells to the pathways of differentiation.

In erythroleukaemia the response to EPO appears to be normal, but the capacity to make functioning red cells is impaired. As the degree of anaemia increases the largely ineffective hyperplasia of erythroid precursors is amplified, so that the marrow can contain enormous numbers of dysplastic normoblasts. If the anaemia is corrected by hypertransfusion, then the erythroid hyperplasia is almost entirely switched off and the other components of the leukaemia—blast cells and myeloid cells—predominate [222]. Again this explains no more than one part of the leukaemic abnormality. Where thrombocytopenia or granulocy-

Table 21.12. Derivation of proliferating cells in leukaemic states

| Erythro | Granulo | Megakaryo | Blasts | Lympho | | Plasma cells | Condition |
				T	B		
N	N	N	L	N	N	N	c-ALL
				(var L pre-T)	(var L pre-B)		
N	N	N	L	L	N	N	T-ALL
L (+N)	L (+N)	L (+N)	L	N	N	N	AML (1)
L	L	L	L	N	N	N	AML (2)
L	L or N	L or N		N	N	N	PRV
N	N(??L)	N		N	N(var L)	L	Myeloma

N = normal.
L = leukaemia.
( ) = sometimes or a variable proportion.

topenia is present one must assume that the response of the leukaemic cells to the analogous controls is defective while the EPO response is retained, or that there is a basic abnormality in the partitioning of differentiating progeny from the pluripotent stem cells. The converse could be assumed to exist where, as in the commoner forms of AML, there is granulopoietic hyperplasia (albeit partly ineffectual) and anaemia without the normal erythropoietic response.

Experimental erythroleukaemia, which can be induced in mice by the Friend virus [5], differs from the human disease in being polyclonal and restricted to the erythroid line. There is massive proliferation of red-cell precursors, only a few of which proceed to maturity, but maturation with haemoglobin synthesis can be induced *in vitro* by agents such as dimethyl sulphoxide [223]. The Mirand strain of the virus [6] causes a polyclonal erythropoietic hyperplasia with normal maturation and resultant polycythaemia. There may also be granulocytosis and/or thrombocytosis as in human PRV. The hyperplasia can be amplified by EPO but, unlike human PRV, removal of EPO by antibody fails to inhibit the hyperplasia.

These leukaemias, which are polyclonal and self-limited, are thought to be in the nature of artefacts, in that there has been selection in the laboratory for strains of virus which have been incorporated adjacent to portions of the regulatory DNA, the information from which is transferred in association with the viral RNA. In the experimental circumstances, there is a massive integration of such particles into the early cells of the erythropoietic line, the effect being amplified by the concurrent or immediately precedent administration of EPO. That is clearly not what happens in any type of human leukaemia but a comparable molecular change in a single pluripotent cell might be the basis for either PRV or erythroleukaemia.

Failure of granulopoietic homeostasis in leukaemia
Quantitative and qualitative variations in CSF occur in AML [162]. Leukaemic monocytes behave as their normal counterparts and so produce excessive amounts [224], to which the granulopoietic precursors are presumably unable to respond in the normal way. Where granulopoietic differentiation is present the pattern is variable and there may be only a single representative of the three species of CSF normally released by the cells in culture. Thus several patterns of abnormality involving synthesis, release and response to the different forms of CSF are possible and may be found to correlate with other variables in AML (Table 21.13). In CGL, however, the main abnormality probably resides in the lack of one of the inhibitors of granulopoiesis. The substance has now been identified as lactoferrin [225] which is a powerful inhibitor, especially in its iron-saturated form, of the formation of CSF by monocytes. Its deficiency in the polymorphs in CGL provides a mechanism whereby over-production of polymorphs fails to be prevented [226].

Another inhibitory substance termed 'leukaemia-associated inhibitory activity' (LIA) [227] has also been identified in cultures of leukaemic cells from the majority of cases of acute leukaemia. *In vitro*, the action against normal colony-forming cells is rapid and not readily reversible. It is quite distinct from lactoferrin and appears to be made by a cell of light buoyant density: it is not quite safe to assume it to be a leukaemia cell product, as it can also be derived from marrow cells in remission which are themselves resistant to its effects; thus it is possible that the resistance of the AML cells represents an adaptation to its formation in abnormal quantities. In other respects it most nearly supplies the explanation of how the leukaemic clone comes to usurp and predominate over the normal haemopoietic population. It is a key role in

Table 21.13. Abnormalities of homeostatic regulators in leukaemia

Substance	Normal source	Activity	Production	Response
Erythropoietin	Kidney (and other tissues)	Differentiation and proliferation of late erythropoiesis	Normal in all	Hypersensitive cells in polycythaemia vera; normal in erythroleukaemia
Colony-stimulating factors (CSFs)	Monocytes (and other tissues)	Required throughout granulocytopoiesis	Increased in monocytic L; qualitative restriction in some AML	Partial failure to response in some AML
Lactoferrin	Granulocytes	Inhibits CSF formation by monocytes	Defective in CGL and some AML	Possible failure of response by some leukaemic monocytes?
Leukaemia-associated inhibitory activity (LIA)	AML cells ? (light density)	Inhibits growth of normal granulopoietic cells	Increased in AML (and remission AML)	Normal cells inhibited; leukaemic and remission 'normal' cells resistant

our understanding of the pathogenesis of leukaemia although the full explanation of that process is unlikely to be so simple.

REFERENCES

1 ALDERSON M.R. (1980) The epidemiology of leukaemia. *Advances in Cancer Research*, **31**, 2.

2 DOLL R. (1972) The epidemiology of leukaemia. *Seventh Annual Guest Lecture*, Leukaemia Research Fund, London.

3 WATERHOUSE F., MURI C., CORREA P. & POWELL J. (1976) *Cancer Incidence in 5 Continents*, Vol. III. Lyon. International Agency for Research in Cancer.

4 WORLD HEALTH ORGANIZATION (1974) *World Health Statistics Report, July 1974*. World Health Organization, Geneva.

5 SEGI M., NOYE H. & SEGI R. (1977) *Age-adjusted Death Rates for Cancer for Selected Sites (A-classification) in 43 countries in 1972*. Segi Institute of Cancer Epidemiology, Nagoya, Japan.

6 WORKING PARTY ON LEUKAEMIA IN CHILDHOOD (1978) Effects of varying radiation schedule, cyclophosphamide treatment and duration of treatment in acute lymphoblastic leukaemia. (Report to the Medical Research Council). *British Medical Journal*, **ii**, 787.

7 DOLL R. (1972) Cancer following therapeutic external irradiation. *Proceedings of 10th International Cancer Congress*, Houston, 1970.

8 DURHAM L.J. & STEWART H.L. (1953) A survey of transplantable and transmissible animal tumours. *Journal of the National Cancer Institute*, **13**, 1299.

9 GROSS L. (1951) 'Spontaneous' leukaemia developing in C₃H mice following inoculation in infancy, with AK-leukaemia extracts or AK embryos. *Proceedings of the Society for Experimental Biology and Medicine*, **76**, 27.

10 KAPLAN H.S. (1964) The role of radiation in experimental leukaemogenesis. *National Cancer Institute Monograph*, **14**, 207.

11 MOLONEY J.B. (1964) The rodent leukaemias: virus-induced murine leukaemias. *Annual Review of Medicine*, **15**, 383.

12 FRIEND C. (1957) Cell-free transmission in adult Swiss mice of a disease having the character of a leukaemia. *Journal of Experimental Medicine*, **105**, 307.

13 MIRAND E.A. (1976) Autonomous erythropoiesis induced by a virus. *Seminars in Hematology*, **13**, 49.

14 RAUSCHER R.J. (1962) A virus-induced disease of mice characterized by erythrocytopoiesis and lymphoid leukaemia. *Journal of the National Cancer Institute*, **29**, 515.

15 SACHS L. (1978) Control of normal cell differentiation in leukaemic white blood cells. In: *Cell Differentiation and Neoplasia* (ed. Saunders G.F.), p. 223. Raven Press, New York.

16 METCALF D. & MOORE M.A.S. (1970) Factors modifying stem cell proliferation of myelomonocytic leukaemic cells *in vitro* and *in vivo*. *Journal of the National Cancer Institute*, **44**, 801.

17 JARRETT W.F.H. (1971) Feline leukaemia. *International Review of Experimental Pathology*, **10**, 243.

18 BRIGGS P.M. (1973) Marek's Disease. In: *The Herpes Viruses* (ed. Kaplan A.S.), p. 557. Academic Press, New York.

19 LOZZIO C.B. & LOZZIO B.B. (1973) Cytotoxicity of a factor isolated from human spleen. *Journal of the National Cancer Institute*, **50**, 535.

20 ANDERSSON L.C., NILSSON K. & GAHMBERG C.G. (1979) A human erythroleukaemia line. *International Journal of Cancer*, **23**, 143.

21 COLINS S.J., RUSCETT F.W., GALLAGHER R.E. & GALLO R.C. (1978) Terminal differentiation of human promyelocytic leukaemia cells induced by dimethyl sulfoxide and other polar compounds. *Proceedings of the National Academy of Sciences, USA*, **75**, 2258.

22 SNYDER A., LI F.P., HENDERSON E.S. & TODARO G.L. (1970) Possible inherited leukaemogenic factors in familial acute myelogenous leukaemia. *Lancet*, **i**, 586.

23 ZUELZER W.W. & COX D.E. (1969) Genetic aspects of leukemia. *Seminars in Hematology*, **6**, 228.

24 FRAUMENI J.F., MANNING M.D. & MITUS W.J. (1971) Acute childhood leukemia. Epidemiologic study by cell type 1947–65. *Journal of the National Cancer Institute*, **46**, 461.

25 LISKER R. & COBO A. (1970) Chromosome breakage in ataxia-telangiectasia. *Lancet*, **i**, 1618.

26 SCHROEDER T.M. & KURTH R. (1971) Spontaneous chromosomal breakage and high incidence of leukemia in inherited disease. *Blood*, **37**, 96.

27 FESTA R.S., MEADOWS A.T. & BOSHES R.A. (1979) Leukemia in a black child with Bloom's syndrome. *Cancer*, **44**, 1507.

28 FRAUMENI J.F. & MILLER R.W. (1967) Epidemiology of human leukemia: recent observations. *Journal of the National Cancer Institute*, **38**, 593.

29 CERVENKA J., ANDERSON R.S., NESBIT M.E. & KRIVIT W. (1977) Familial leukaemia and inherited chromosomal aberration. *International Journal of Cancer*, **19**, 783.

30 SWIFT M. (1971) Fanconi's anemia in the genetics of neoplasia. *Nature (London)*, **230**, 370.

31 TEERENHOVI L., BORSTROM G.H., MITELMAN F., BRANDT L., VUOPIO P., TIMONEN T., ALMQUIST A. & DE LA CHAPELLE A. (1978) Uneven geographical distribution of 15;17-translocation in acute promyelocytic leukaemia. *Lancet*, **ii**, 797.

32 ALLISON A.C. & TAYLOR R.B. (1967) Observations of thymectomy and carcinogenesis. *Cancer Research*, **27**, 703.

33 DOSIK H., HSU L.Y., TODARO G.J., LEE S.L., HIRSCH-HORN K., SERIRIO E.S. & ALTER A.A. (1970) Leukemia in Fanconi's anemia: cytogenetic and tumour virus susceptibility studies. *Blood*, **36**, 341.

34 ZUELZER W.W., THOMPSON R.I. & MASTRANGELO R. (1968) Evidence for a genetic factor related to leukemogenesis and congenital anomalies: chromosomal aberrations in pedigree of an infant with partial D trisomy and leukemia. *Journal of Pediatrics*, **72**, 367.

35 MILLER R.W. (1971) Deaths from childhood leukemia and solid tumours amongst twins and other sibs in the United States 1960–67. *Journal of the National Cancer Institute*, **46**, 203.

36 HANN L.H., LONDON W.T., STUNICK A.I., BLUMBERG B.S., LUSTBADER E., CARIM H.M. KAY H.E.M., EVANS A.E. & MACLENNAN I.C.M. (1975) Studies of parents of

children with acute leukemia. *Journal of the National Cancer Institute*, **54**, 1299.

37 TILL M., RAPSON N. & SMITH P.G. (1979) Family studies in acute leukaemia in childhood: a possible association with autoimmune disease. *British Journal of Cancer*, **40**, 62.

38 DE BRUYERE M., CORNU G., HEREMANS-BRACKE T., MALCHAIRE J. & SOKAL G. (1980) HLA haplotypes and long survival in childhood acute lymphoblastic leukaemia treated with transfer factor. *British Journal of Haematology*, **44**, 243.

39 STEWART A.M. (1961) Aetiology of childhood malignancies. *British Medical Journal*, **i**, 452.

40 MILLER R.W. (1967) Persons with exceptionally high risk of leukemia. *Cancer Research*, **27**, 2420.

41 MOLE R.H. (1975) Ionizing radiation as a carcinogen: practical questions and academic pursuits. *British Journal of Radiology*, **48**, 157.

42 TUBIANA M. (1978) Radioleukemogenesis in man. *Schweizerische Medizinische Wochenschrift*, **108**, 1563.

43 COURT-BROWN W.M. & DOLL R. (1957) Leukaemia and aplastic anaemia in patients irradiated for ankylosing spondylitis. *Medical Research Council Special Report Series No. 295*. HMSO, London.

44 BEEBE G.W., KATO H. & LAND C.E. (1978) Studies of the mortality of A-bomb survivors. VI. Mortality and radiation dose 1950–1974. *Radiation Research*, **75**, 138.

45 FINCH S.C. (1979) The study of atomic bomb survivors in Japan. *American Journal of Medicine*, **66**, 899.

46 LYON J.L., KLAUBER M.R., GARDNER J.W. & UDALL K.S. (1979) Childhood leukemias associated with fallout from nuclear testing. *New England Journal of Medicine*, **300**, 397.

47 STEWART A., WEBB J., GILES D. & HEWITT D. (1956) Malignant disease in childhood cancer. *Lancet*, **ii**, 447.

48 STEWART A. (1973) Factors controlling the recognition of leukaemia and childhood cancers. 1. Health physics in the healing arts. *Health Physics Society—Seventh Midyear Topical Symposium* U.S. Department of Health, Education and Welfare, Bureau of Radiological Health, Rockville, Maryland.

49 LI F.P. & STONE R. (1976) Survivors of cancer in childhood. *Annals of Internal Medicine*, **84**, 551.

50 ZIPPIN C., BAILAR J.C., KOHN H.I., LUM D. & EISENBERG H. (1971) Radiation therapy for cervical cancer: late effects on life span and on leukaemia incidence. *Cancer*, **28**, 937.

51 HUTCHINSON G.B. (1968) Leukemia in patients with cancer of the cervix uteri treated with radiation. A report covering the first 5 years of an international study. *Journal of the National Cancer Institute*, **40**, 951.

52 GOLDSTEIN B.D. (1977) Benxene haematotoxicity in humans. *Journal of Toxicology and Environmental Health*, Suppl. 2, 69.

53 SIEBER S.M. & ADAMSON R.H. (1975) Toxicity of antineoplastic agents in man: chromosomal aberrations, antifertility effects, congenital malformations and carcinogenic potential. In: *Advances in Cancer Research* (ed. Klein G. & Weinhouse S.) Vol. 22, p. 57. Academic Press, New York.

54 HARRIS C.C. (1979) A delayed complication of cancer therapy–cancer. *Journal of the National Cancer Institute*, **63**, 275.

55 ROSNER F. (1976) Acute leukemia as a delayed consequence of cancer chemotherapy. *Cancer*, **37**, 1033.

56 COLEMAN C.N., WILLIAMS C.J., FLINT A., GLATSTEIN E.J., ROSENBERG S.A. & KAPLAN H.S. (1977) Hematologic neoplasia in patients treated for Hodgkin's disease. *New England Journal of Medicine*, **297**, 1249.

57 CADMAN E.C., CAPIZZI R.L. & BERTINO J.R. (1977) Acute nonlymphocytic leukemia. A delayed complication of Hodgkin's disease therapy: analysis of 109 cases. *Cancer*, **40**, 1280.

58 COLLINS A.J., BLOOMFIELD D., PETERSON B.A. & McKENNA R.W. (1977) Acute nonlymphocytic leukemia in patients with nodular lymphoma. *Cancer*, **40**, 1748.

59 VARDIMAN J.W., GOLOMB H.M., ROWLEY J.D. & VARIAKOJIS D. (1978) Acute nonlymphocytic leukemia in malignant lymphoma. A morphologic study. *Cancer*, **42**, 229.

60 ZARRABI M.H., ROSNER F. & BENNETT J.M. (1979) Non-Hodgkin's lymphoma and acute myeloblastic leukemia. A report on 12 cases and review of the literature. *Cancer*, **44**, 1070.

61 TURSZ T., FLANDRIN G., BROUET J.C., BRIERE J. & SELIGMANN M. (1974) Simultaneous occurrence of acute myeloblastic leukaemia and multiple myeloma without previous chemotherapy. *British Medical Journal*, **ii**, 642.

62 REIMER R.R., HOOVER R., FRAUMENI J.F. & YOUNG R.C. (1977) Acute leukemia after alkylating-agent therapy of ovarian cancer. *New England Journal of Medicine*, **297**, 177.

63 STOTT H., FOX W., GIRLING D.J., STEPHENS R.J. & GALTON D.A.G. (1977) Acute leukaemia after busulphan. *British Medical Journal*, **ii**, 1513.

64 PORTUGAL M.A., FALKSON H.C., STEVENS K. & FALKSON G. (1979) Acute leukaemia as a complication of long-term treatment of advanced breast cancer. *Cancer Treatment Reports*, **63**, 177.

65 BURTON I.E., ABBOTT C.R., ROBERTS B.E. & ANTONIS A.H. (1976) Acute leukaemia after four years of melphalan treatment for melanoma. *British Medical Journal*, **ii**, 20.

66 HOOVER R. & FRAUMENI J.F. (1973) Risk of cancer in renal-transplant recipients. *Lancet*, **ii**, 55.

67 KINLEN L.J., SHEIL A.G.R., PETO J. & DOLL R. (1979) A collaborative UK-Australasian study of cancer in patients treated with immunosuppressive drugs. *British Medical Journal*, **ii**, 1461.

68 KINLEN L.J. & HOOVER R.N. (1979) Lymphomas in renal transplant recipients: a search for clustering. *British Journal of Cancer*, **40**, 798.

69 MATAS A.J., HERTEL B.F., ROSAL J., SIMMONS R.L. & NAJARIAN J.S. (1976) Post-transplant malignant lymphoma. Distinctive morphologic features related to its pathogenesis. *American Journal of Medicine*, **61**, 716.

70 GRAY L.H. (1965) In: *Cellular Radiation Biology. Eighteenth annual symposium on fundamental cancer research*, p. 7. Williams & Wilkins, Baltimore.

71 WEISS R. (1976) Transmission and expression of leukaemia viruses. *Twelfth Annual Guest Lecture for the Leukaemia Research Fund*, Leukaemia Research Fund.

72 GALLAGHER R.E. (1977) Molecular probes for components of type C viruses in human leukemia. In: *Recent*

Advances in Cancer Research (ed. Gallo R.C.) Vol. II, p. 137. C.R.C. Press, Cleveland, Ohio.

73 GALLO R.C. (1976) Current concepts of leukemia and lymphoma: The origin of the lymphomas. *Annals of Internal Medicine*, **85**, 351.

74 COTTER S.M. & ESSEX M. (1977) Animal model: feline acute lymphoblastic leukemia and aplastic anemia. *American Journal of Pathology*, **87**, 265.

75 SMITH P.G. (1978) Current assessment of 'case clustering' of lymphomas and leukemias. *Cancer*, **42**, 1026.

75a TEICH N.M., WEISS R.A., SALAHUDDIN S.Z., GALLAGHER R.E., GILLESPIE D.H. & GALLO R.C. (1975) Infective transmission and characterization of a C-type virus released by cultured human myeloid leukaemia cells. *Nature (London)*, **256**, 551.

76 FRANCIS D.P., COTTER S.M., HARDY W.D. & ESSEX M. (1979) Comparison of virus-positive and virus-negative cases of feline leukemia and lymphoma. *Cancer Research*, **39**, 3866.

77 FIALKOW P.J., THOMAS E.D., BRYANT J.I. & NEIMAN P.E. (1971) Leukaemic transformation of engrafted human marrow cells *in vivo*. *Lancet*, **i**, 251.

78 THOMAS E.D., BRYANT J.I., BUCKNER C.D., FEFER A., NEIMAN P.E., STORE R., CLIFT R.A., JOHNSON F.L. & RAMBERG R.E. (1972) Leukaemic transformation of engrafted human marrow cells *in vivo*. *Lancet*, **i**, 1310.

79 ELFENBEIN, G.J., BROGAONKAR D.S., BIAS W.B., BURNS W.H., SARAL R., SENSENBRENNER L.L., TUTSCHKA P.J., ZACZEK B.S., ZANDER A.R., EPSTEIN R.B., ROWLEY J.D. & SANTOS G.W. (1978) Cytogenetic evidence for recurrence of acute myelogenous leukemia after allogeneic bone marrow transplantation in donor hematopoietic cells. *Blood*, **52**, 627.

80 GOH K. & KLEMPERER M.R. (1977) *In vivo* leukemic transformation: cytogenetic evidence of *in vivo* leukemic transformation of engrafted marrow cells. *American Journal of Hematology*, **2**, 283.

81 KLEIN G. (1977) Medical progress: the Epstein–Barr virus and neoplasia. *New England Journal of Medicine*, **293**, 1353.

82 ROSEN F.S. (1977) Lymphoma, immunodeficiency and the Epstein–Barr virus. *New England Journal of Medicine*, **297**, 1120.

83 ZIEGLER J.L., MACGRATH I.T., GERBER P. & LEVINE P.H. (1977) Epstein–Barr virus and human malignancy. *Annals of Internal Medicine*, **86**, 323.

84 ANDERSON M., KLEIN G., ZIEGLER J.L. & HENLE W. (1976) Association of Epstein–Barr viral genomes with American Burkitt lymphoma. *Nature (London)*, **260**, 357.

85 GOTLIEB-STEMATSKY T., VONSOVER A., RAMOT B., ZAIZOV R., NORDAN U., AGHAI E., KENDE G. & MODAN M. (1975) Antibodies to Epstein–Barr virus in patients with Hodgkin's disease and leukaemia. *Cancer*, **36**, 1640.

86 MUNOZ N., DAVIDSON R.J.L., WITHOFF B., ERICSSON J.E. & DE THE G. (1978) Infectious mononucleosis and Hodgkin's disease. *International Journal of Cancer*, **22**, 10.

87 PAUL J. (1977) In: *Cell Differentiation and Neoplasia* (ed. Saunders G.F.), p. 525. Raven Press, New York.

88 MEDICAL RESEARCH COUNCIL'S WORKING PARTY ON LEUKAEMIA IN ADULTS (1975) The relation between morphology and other features of acute myeloid leukaemia, and their prognostic significance. *British Journal of Haematology*, **31**, 165.

89 BENNETT J.M. CATOVSKY D., DANIEL M.-T., FLANDRIN G., GALTON D.A.G., GRALNICK H.R. & SULTAN C. (1976) Proposals for the classification of the acute leukaemias. *British Journal of Haematology*, **33**, 451.

90 GRALNICK H.R., GALTON D.A.G., CATOVSKY D., SULTAN C. & BENNETT J.M. (1977) classification of acute leukemia. *Annals of Internal Medicine*, **87**, 740.

91 BERNARD J., WEIL M., BOIRON M., JACQUILLAT C., FLANDRIN G. & GEMON M.-F. (1973) Acute promyelocytic leukemia: results of treatment by daunorubicin. *Blood*, **41**, 489.

92 DRAPKIN R.L., GEE T.S., DOWLING M.D., ARLIN Z., MCKENZIE S., KEMPIN S. & CLARKSON B. (1978) Prophylactic heparin therapy in acute promyelocytic leukemia. *Cancer*, **41**, 2484.

93 BRETON GORIUS J., REYES F., DUHAMEL G., NAJMAN A. & GOBIN N.C. (1978) Megakaryoblastic acute leukemia. Identification by the ultrastructural demonstration of platelet peroxidase. *Blood*, **51**, 45.

94 BEARMAN R.M., PANGALIS G.A. & RAPPAPORT H. (1979) Acute ('malignant') myelosclerosis. *Cancer*, **43**, 279.

95 BLOOMFIELD C.D. & BRUNNING R.D. (1974) Prognostic implications of cytology in acute leukaemia in the adult: the case for subacute leukaemia. *Human Pathology*, **5**, 641.

96 COHEN J.R., GREGER W.P., GREENBERG P.L. & SCHRIER S.L. (1979) Subacute myeloid leukemia. A clinical review. *American Journal of Medicine*, **66**, 959.

97 PANTAZOPOULOS N. & SINKS L.F. (1974) Morphologic criteria for prognostication of acute lymphoblastic leukaemia. *British Journal of Haematology*, **27**, 25.

98 MURPHY S.B., BORELLA L., SEN L. & MADER A. (1975) Lack of correlation of lymphoblast cell size with presence of T-cell markers or with outcome in childhood acute lymphoblastic leukaemia. *British Journal of Haematology*, **31**, 95.

99 STEIN H., PETERSON N., GAEDICKE G., LENNERT K. & LANDBECK G. (1976) Lymphoblastic lymphoma of convoluted or acid phosphatase type: a tumor of T precursor cells. *International Journal of Cancer*, **17**, 292.

100 PANGALIS G.A., NATHWANI B.N., RAPPAPORT H. & ROSEN R.B. (1979) Acute lymphoblastic leukaemia. The significance of nuclear convolutions. *Cancer*, **43**, 551.

101 FACQUET-DANIS J., ZITTOUN R., BOUCHARD M., CADIOU M., BOUSSER J. & BILSKI-PASQUIER G. (1976) Cell volume measurements in acute leukaemia: method and value for diagnosis and prognosis. *Biomedicine*, **25**, 294.

102 ZIPURSKY A., BOW E., SESHADRI S. & BROWN E.J. (1976) Leukocyte density and volume in normal subjects and in patients with acute lymphoblastic leukemia. *Blood*, **48**, 361.

103 CATOVSKY D., GREAVES M.F., PAIN C., CHERCHI M., JANOSSY G. & KAY H.E.M. (1978) Acid-phosphatase reaction in acute lymphoblastic leukaemia. *Lancet*, **i**, 749.

104 MCCAFFREY R., SMOLER D. & BALTIMORE D. (1973) Terminal deoxynucleotidyl transferase in a case of

childhood acute lymphoblastic leukemia. *Proceedings of the National Academy of Sciences, USA*, **70**, 521.

105 HOFFBRAND A.V., GANESHAGURU K., JANOSSY G., GREAVES M.F., CATOVSKY D. & WOODRUFF R.K. (1977) Terminal deoxynucleotidyl-transferase levels and membrane phenotypes in diagnosis of acute leukaemia. *Lancet*, **ii**, 520.

106 SMYTH J.F., POPLACK D.G., HOLIMAN B., LEVENTHAL B.G. & YARBRO G. (1978) Correlation of adenosine deaminase activity with cell surface markers in acute lymphoblastic leukemia. *Journal of Clinical Investigation*, **62**, 710.

107 REAMAN G.H., LEVIN N., MUCHMORE A., HOLIMAN B.J. & POPLACK D.G. (1979) Diminished lymphoblast 5-nucleotidase activity in acute lymphoblastic leukemia with T-cell characteristics. *New England Journal of Medicine*, **300**, 1374.

108 ELLIS R.B., RAPSON N.T., PATRICK A.D. & GREAVES M.F. (1978) Expression of hexosaminidiase isoenzymes in childhood leukemia. *New England Journal of Medicine*, **298**, 476.

109 BESLEY G.T.N., BROADHEAD D.M., BAIN A.D. & DEAR A.E. (1978) Enzyme markers in acute lymphoblastic leukaemia. *Lancet*, **ii**, 1311.

110 GREAVES M.F. (1979) Cell surface characteristics of human leukemic cells. In: *Essays in Biochemistry* (ed. Campbell P.N. & Marshall R.D.) Vol. XV, p. 78. Academic Press, New York.

111 BROUET J.C. & SELIGMANN M. (1978) The immunological classification of acute lymphoblastic leukemias. *Cancer*, **42**, 817.

112 GREAVES M.F. (1981) *Biology of Acute Lymphoblastic Leukaemia*. Leukaemic Research Fund, London.

113 BROWN G., CAPELLARO D. & GREAVES M.F. (1975) A candidate human leukaemia antigen. *Nature (London)*, **258**, 454.

114 JANOSSY G., HOFFBRAND A.V., GREAVES M.F., GANESHAGURU K., PAIN C., BRADSTOCK K.F., PRENTICE H.G., KAY H.E.M. & LISTER T.A. (1980) Terminal transferase enzyme assay and immunological membrane markers in the diagnosis of leukaemia: a multiparameter analysis of 300 cases. *British Journal of Haematology*, **44**, 221.

115 GREAVES M.F., VERBI W., VOGLER L., COOPER M., ELLIS R., GANESHAGURU K., HOFFBRAND V., JANOSSY G. & BOLLUM F.J. (1979) Antigenic and enzymatic phenotypes of the pre-B subclass of acute lymphoblastic leukemia. *Leukemia Research*, **4**, 1.

116 GREAVES M. (1978) Cell surface structures, differentiation and malignancy in the haemopoietic system. In: *Cell–Cell Recognition*. The Society for Experimental Biology (ed. Curtis A.S.G.). Cambridge University Press, Cambridge.

117 RITZ J., PESANDO J.M., NOTIS-MCCONARTY J., LAZARUS H. & SCHLOSSMAN S.F. (1980) A monoclonal antibody to human acute lymphoblastic leukaemic antigen. *Nature (London)*, **283**, 583.

118 OPELZ G., GALE R.P. & MCCLELLAND J.D. (1977) Relationship between leukemia antigens and stimulation in mixed leukocyte culture: brief communication. *Journal of the National Cancer Institute*, **59**, 95.

119 REINSMOEN L., KERSEY J.H. & YUNIS E.J. (1978) Antigens associated with acute leukemia detected in the primed lymphocyte test. *Journal of the National Cancer Institute*, **60**, 537.

120 TUPCHONG L. & MACLENNAN I.C.M. (1978) Surface antigens in acute myeloblastic leukaemia: a study using heterologous antisera. *British Journal of Cancer*, **38**, 481.

121 BAKER M.A., FALK A. & TAUB R.N. (1978) Immunotherapy of human acute leukemia: antibody response to leukemia-associated antigens. *Blood*, **52**, 468.

122 BAKER M.A., FALK J.A., CARTER W.H., TAUB R.N. & THE TORONTO LEUKEMIA STUDY GROUP (1979) Early diagnosis of relapse in acute myeloblastic leukemia. *New England Journal of Medicine*, **301**, 1353.

123 VAN DER REIJDEN H.J., VON DEN BORNE A.E.G., VERHEUGT F.W.A., FLOOR-VAN GENT A.B., MELIEF C.J.M. & ENGELFRIET C.P. (1979) Granulocyte-specific alloantigen loss in chronic granulocytic leukaemia. *British Journal of Haematology*, **43**, 589.

124 FIALKOW P., REDDY A.L., NAJFELD V., SINGER J. & STEINMANN L. (1978) Chronic lymphocytic leukaemia: clonal origin in a committed B-lymphocyte progenitor. *Lancet*, **ii**, 444.

125 VAN DER TWELL J.G., LUKES R.J. & TAYLOR, C.R. (1979) Pathophysiology of lymphocyte transformation. A study of so-called composite lymphomas. *American Journal of Clinical Pathology*, **71**, 509.

126 HAEGERT D.G., CAWLEY J.C., KARPAS A. & GOLDSTONE A.H. (1974) Combined T and B cell acute lymphoblastic leukaemia. *British Medical Journal*, **ii**, 79.

127 FIALKOW P.J., SINGER J.W., ADAMSON J.W., BERKOW R.L., FRIEDMAN J.M., JACOBSON R.J. & MOOHR J.W. (1979) Acute nonlymphocytic leukemia. *New England Journal of Medicine*, **301**, 1.

128 JANOSSY G., WOODRUFF R.K., PAXTON A., GREAVES M.F., CAPELLARO D., KIRK B., INNES E.M., EDEN O.B., LEWIS C., CATOVSKY D. & HOFFBRAND A.V. (1978) Membrane marker and cell separation studies in Ph'-positive leukaemia. *Blood*, **51**, 861.

129 KUBAGAWA H., VOGLER L.B., CAPRA J.D., CONRAD M.E., LAWTON A.R. & COOPER M.D. (1979) Studies on the clonal origin of multiple myeloma. *Journal of Experimental Medicine*, **150**, 792.

130 VAN ACKER A., CONTE F., HULIN N. & URBAIN J. (1979) Idiotypical studies on myeloma B cells. *European Journal of Cancer*, **15**, 627.

131 SRIVASTAVA B.I.S., KHAN S.A. & HENDERSON E.S. (1976) High terminal deoxynucleotidyl transferase activity in acute myelogenous leukemia. *Cancer Research*, **36**, 3847.

132 GREAVES M.F., VERBI W., FESTENSTEIN H., PAPASTERIADIS C., JARAQUEMADA D. & HAYWARD A. (1979) 'Ia-like' antigens on human T cells. *European Journal of Immunology*, **9**, 356.

133 SAUNDERS G.F. (ed.) (1978) *Cell Differentiation and Neoplasia*. Raven Press, New York.

134 ROWLEY J.D. (1978) The cytogenetics of acute leukemia. *Clinics in Hematology*, **7**, 385.

135 ROWLEY J.D. (1978) Chromosomes in leukemia and lymphoma. *Seminars in Hematology*, **15**, 301.

136 SANDBERG A.A. (1980) *The Chromosomes in Human Cancer and Leukemia*. Elsevier/North-Holland, New York and Amsterdam.

137 SECKER-WALKER L.M., LAWLER S.D. & HARDISTY R.M.

(1978) Prognostic implications of chromosomal findings in acute lymphoblastic leukaemia at diagnosis. *British Medical Journal*, **ii**, 1529.

138 CIMINO M.C., ROWLEY J.D., KINNEALEY A., VARIAKOJIS D. & GOLOMB H.M. (1979) Banding studies of chromosomal abnormalities in patients with acute lymphocytic leukemia. *Cancer Research*, **39**, 227.

139 FIRST INTERNATIONAL WORKSHOP ON CHROMOSOMES IN LEUKAEMIA (1978) Chromosomes in acute non-lymphocytic leukaemia. *British Journal of Haematology*, **39**, 311.

140 GOLOMB H.M., VARDIMAN J.W., ROWLEY J.D., TESTA J.R. & MINTZ U. (1978) Correlation of clinical findings with quinacrine-banded chromosomes in 90 adults with acute non-lymphocytic leukemia. *New England Journal of Medicine*, **299**, 613.

141 NILSSON P.G., BRANDT L. & MITELMAN F. (1977) Prognostic implications of chromosome analysis in acute non-lymphocytic leukemia. *Leukemia Research*, **1**, 31.

142 TRUJILLO J.M., CORK A., AHEARN M.J., YOUNESS E.L. & MCCREDIE K.B. (1979) Hematologic and cytologic characterization of 8/21 translocation acute granulocytic leukemia. *Blood*, **53**, 695.

143 TESTA J.R., GOLOMB H.M., ROWLEY J.D., VARDIMAN J.W. & SWEET D.L. (1978) Hypergranular promyelocytic leukemia (APL). Cytogentic and ultrastructural specificity. *Blood*, **52**, 272.

144 VAN DEN BERGHE H., LOUWAGIE A., BROECKARET-VAN ORSHOVEN A., VERWILGHEN R., MICHAUX J.L., FERRANT A. & SOKAL G. (1979) Chromosome abnormalities in acute promyelocytic leukemia. *Cancer*, **43**, 558.

145 LAWLER S.D. (1977) The cytogenics of chronic granulocytic leukemia. *Clinics in Hematology*, **6**, 55.

146 FIRST INTERNATIONAL WORKSHOP ON CHROMOSOMES IN LEUKAEMIA (1978) Chromosomes in Ph¹-positive chronic granulocytic leukaemia. *British Journal of Haematology*, **39**, 305.

147 TOUGH I.M. (1965) Cytogenetic studies in cases of chronic myeloid leukaemia with a previous history of radiation. In: *Current Research in Leukaemia* (ed. Hayhoe F.G.J.), p. 47. Cambridge University Press, Cambridge.

148 FIALKOW P.J., GARTLER S.M. & YOSHIDA A. (1976) Clonal origin of chronic myelogenous leukemia in man. *Proceedings of the National Academy of Sciences, USA*, **58**, 1468.

149 KAY H.E.M. & LAWLER S. Unpublished data.

150 VAN DEN BERGHE H., LOUWAGLE A., BROECHAERT-VAN ORSHOVEN A., DAVID G., VERWILGHEN R., MICHAUX J.L. & SOKAL G. (1979) Philadelphia chromosome in human multiple myeloma. *Journal of the National Cancer Institute*, **63**, 11.

151 KAY H.E.M., LAWLER S.D. & MILLARD R.E. (1966) The chromosomes in polycythaemia vera. *British Journal of Haematology*, **12**, 507.

152 FUSCALDO K.E., ERLICK B.J., FUSCALDO A.A. & BRODSKY I. (1979) Correlation of a specific chromosomal marker, 21q−, and retroviral indications in patients with thrombocythemia. *Cancer Letters*, **6**, 51.

153 VAN DEN BERGHE H., PARLOIR C., DAVID G., MICHAUX J.L. & SOKAL G. (1979) A new characteristic karyotypic anomaly in lymphoproliferative disorders. *Cancer*, **44**, 188.

154 LIANG W., HOPPER J.E. & ROWLEY J.D. (1979) Karyotypic abnormalities and clinical aspects of patients with multiple myeloma and related paraproteinemic disorders. *Cancer*, **44**, 630.

155 MIVOSHI I., SUMITA M., SANO K., NISHIHARA R., MIYAMOTO K., KIMURA I. & SATO J. (1979) Marker chromosome 14q+ in adult T-cell leukemia. *New England Journal of Medicine*, **300**, 921.

156 SAXON A., STEVENS R.H. & GOLDE D.W. (1979) T-cell leukemia in ataxia telangiectasia. *New England Journal of Medicine*, **301**, 945.

157 HURLEY J.N., SHU M.F., KUNKEL H.G., CHANGANTI, R.S.K. & GERMAN J. (1980) Chromosome abnormalities of leukaemic B lymphocytes in chronic lymphocytic leukaemia. *Nature (London)*, **283**, 76.

158 GOLOMB H.M., LINDGREN V. & ROWLEY J. (1978) Chromosome abnormalities in patients with hairy cell leukaemia. *Virchow's Archiv. B: Cell Pathology*, **29**, 113.

159 MITELMAN F., BRANDT L. & NILSSON P.G. (1978) Relation among occupational exposure to potential mutagenic/carcinogenic agents. Clinical findings, and bone marrow chromosomes in acute nonlymphocytic leukemia. *Blood*, **52**, 1229.

160 LAWLER S.D., SUMMERSGILL B.M., CLINK H.McD. & MCELWAIN T.J. (1979) Chromosomes, leukaemia and occupational exposure to leukaemogenic agents. *Lancet*, **ii**, 853.

161 BRODER S., UCHIYAMA T. & WALDMANN T.A. (1979) Neoplasms of immunoregulatory cells. *American Journal of Clinical Pathology*, **70**, 724.

162 MOORE M.A.S. (1977) Regulation of leukocyte differentiation and leukemia as a disorder of differentiation. In: *Recent Advances in Cancer Research*: Vol. I. Cell biology, molecular biology and tumour virology (ed. Gallo R.C.), p. 79. CRC Press, Cleveland, Ohio.

163 SACHS L. (1979) Control of normal cell differentiation and the phenotype reversion of malignancy in myeloid leukaemia. *Nature (London)*, **274**, 535.

164 NOWELL P.C. (1977) Cytogenic clues in some confusing disorders. *American Journal of Pathology*, **89**, 459.

165 PIERRE R.B. (1974) Preleukemic states. *Seminars in Hematology*, **11**, 73.

166 DREYFUS B. (1976) Preleukemic states. Definition and classification. Refractory anemia with excess of myeloblasts in the bone marrow. *Blood Cells*, **2**, 33.

167 BLACKBURN E.K., CALLENDER S.T., DACIE J.V., DOLL R., GIRDWOOD R.H., MOLLIN D.L., SARACCI R., STAFFORD J.L., THOMPSON R.B., VARADI S. & WETHERLEY-MEIN G. (1968) Possible association between pernicious anaemia and leukaemia: a prospective study of 1,625 patients. *International Journal of Cancer*, **3**, 163.

168 SELIGMANN M. (1972) Heavy chain diseases. *Revue Européenne d'Études Cliniques et Biologiques*, **17**, 349.

169 COWALL D.E., PASQUALE D.N. & DEKKER P. (1979) Paroxysmal nocturnal hemoglobinuria terminating as erythroleukemia. *Cancer*, **43**, 1914.

170 NOWELL P., JENSEN J., GARDNER F., MURPHY S., CHAGANTI R.S.K. & GERMAN J. (1979) Chromosome studies in 'pre-leukemia'. III. Myelofibrosis. *Cancer*, **38**, 1873.

171 NOWELL P. & FINAN J. (1978) Chromosome studies in

pre-leukemic states. IV. Myeloproliferative versus cytopenic disorders. *Cancer*, **42**, 2261.

172 JUME'AN H.G. & LIBNOCH J.A. (1979) 5q— Myelodysplasia terminating in acute leukemia. *Annals of Internal Medicine*, **91**, 748.

173 McCULLOCH E.A. (1979) Abnormal myelopoietic clones in man. *Journal of the National Cancer Institute*, **63**, 883.

174 NOWELL P.C. (1978) Tumours as clonal proliferation. *Virchow's Archiv. B: Cell Pathology*, **29**, 145.

175 FIALKOW P.J. (1979) Clonal origin and stem cell evolution of human tumours. *Genetics of Human Cancer*, **3**, 439.

176 GREAVES M.F. (1979) Molecular phenotypes: a new perspective on diagnosis and classification of leukaemia. In: *Topics in Paediatrics 1: Haematology and Oncology* (ed. Morris Jones P.H.), p. 36. Pitman Medical, London.

177 LAWLER S.D., MILLARD R.E. & KAY H.E.M. (1970) Further cytogenetical investigations in polycythaemia vera. *European Journal of Cancer*, **6**, 235.

178 CHENG D.S., KUCHNER J.P. & WINTROBE M.M. (1979) Idiopathic refractory sideroblastic anemia. *Cancer*, **44**, 724.

179 REARDON G. & MOLONEY W.C. (1961) Chloroma and related myeloblastic neoplasms. *Archives of Internal Medicine*, **108**, 864.

180 LORTHOLARY P., BOIRON M., RIPAULT P., LEVY J.P., MANUS A. & BERNARD J. (1964) Leucémie lymphoïde chronique secondairement associée à une réticulopathie maligne, syndrome de Richter. *Nouvelle Revue française d'Hématologie*, **4**, 621.

181 BROUET J.C., PREUD'HOMME J.L., SELIGMANN M. & BERNARD J. (1973) Blast cells with monoclonal surface immunoglobulin in two cases of acute blast crisis supervening on chronic lymphocytic leukaemia. *British Medical Journal*, **iv**, 23.

182 RAMOT B., LEVANON M., HAHN Y., LAHAT N. & MOROZ C. (1977) The mutual clonal origin of the lymphoplasmocytic and lymphoma cell in alpha-heavy chain disease. *Clinical and Experimental Immunology*, **27**, 440.

183 FRIZZERA G., MORAN E.M. & RAPPAPORT H. (1974) Angioimmunoblastic lymphadenopathy with dysproteinaemia. *Lancet*, **i**, 1070.

184 LUKES R.J. & TINDLE B.H. (1975) Immunoblastic lymphadenopathy: a hyperimmune entity resembling Hodgkin's disease. *New England Journal of Medicine*, **59**, 803.

185 BLUMING A.Z., COHEN H.G. & SAXON A. (1979) Angioimmunoblastic lymphadenopathy with dysproteinemia. *American Journal of Medicine*, **67**, 421.

186 GREEN J.A., DAWSON A.A. & WALKER W. (1978) Systemic lupus erythematosus and lymphoma. *Lancet*, **ii**, 753.

187 ZULMAN J., JAFFE R. & TALAL N. (1978) Evidence that the malignant lymphoma of Sjögren's syndrome is a monoclonal B-cell neoplasm. *New England Journal of Medicine*, **299**, 1215.

188 ANTHONY J.J. (1970) Malignant lymphoma associated with hydantoin drugs. *Archives of Neurology*, **22**, 450.

189 HOBBS J.R. (1975) Monitoring myelomatosis. *Archives of Internal Medicine*, **135**, 125.

190 STICH H.F. (1963) Chromosomes and carcinogenesis. *Fifth Canadian Cancer Conference*, p. 99.

191 BRAND K.G. & BUOEN L.C. (1968) Polymer tumorigenesis: multiple preneoplastic clones in priority order with clonal inhibition. *Proceedings of the Society of Experimental Biology and Medicine*, **128**, 1154.

192 KILLMANN S.Å. (1968) Acute leukaemia: development, remission/relapse pattern, relationship between normal and leukaemic haemopoiesis, and the sleeper-to-feeder stem cell hypothesis. *Series Haematologica*, **1**, 103.

193 KELSEN D.P., GEE R.S. & CHAGANTI R.S.K. (1979) Philadelphia chromosome positive chronic myelogenous leukemia developing in a patient with acute lymphoblastic leukemia. *Cancer*, **43**, 1782.

194 TOSATO G., WHANG-PENG J., LEVINE A.S. & POPLACK D.G. (1978) Acute lymphoblastic leukemia followed by chronic myelocytic leukemia. *Blood*, **52**, 1033.

195 HANN H.W.L., FESTA R.S., ROSENSTOCK J.G. & CIFUENTES E. (1979) Polycythemia vera in a child with acute lymphocytic leukemia. *Cancer*, **43**, 1862.

196 GRIFFIN J.D., ELLMAN L., LONG J.C. & DVORAK A.M. (1978) Development of a histiocytic medullary reticulosis-like syndrome during the course of acute lymphocytic leukemia. *American Journal of Medicine*, **64**, 851.

197 CASTOLDI G., CRUSOVIN G.D., SCAPOLI G., GUALANDI M., SPANEDDA R. & ANZANEL D. (1977) Acute myelomonocytic leukemia terminating in histiocytic medullary reticulosis. *Cancer*, **40**, 1735.

198 TESTA J.R. (1980) Cytogenetic patterns in polycythemia vera. *Cancer Genetics and Cytogenetics*, **1**, 207.

199 MAUER A.M. & MURPHY S.B. (1979) Kinetic studies of cells in childhood leukemias. *American Journal of Clinical Pathology*, **72**, 753.

200 GAVOSTO F. (1970) The proliferative kinetics of the acute leukaemias in relation to their treatment. *Revue Européene d'Études Cliniques et Biologiques*, **15**, 1042.

201 SAUNDERS E.F. & MAUER A.M. (1969) Re-entry of nondividing leukemic cells into a proliferative phase in acute childhood leukemia. *Journal of Clinical Investigation*, **48**, 1299.

202 GAVOSTO F., PILERI A., GABUTTIE V., TAROCCO R.P., MASERA P. & PONZONE A. (1969) Unusual blast proliferation and kinetics in acute lymphoblastic leukaemia. *European Journal of Cancer*, **5**, 343.

203 SPIVAK J.L., BRUBAKER L.H. & PERRY S. (1969) Intravascular granulocyte kinetics in acute leukemia. *Blood*, **34**, 582.

204 CLARKSON B., STRIFE A., FRIED J., SAKAI Y., OTA K., OHKITA T. & MASUDA R. (1970) Studies of cellular proliferation in human leukemia. I. Behaviour of normal hematopoietic cells in three adults with acute leukemia given continuous infusion of ^{3}H-thymidine for 8 or 10 days. *Cancer*, **26**, 1.

205 SAUNDERS E.F., LAMPKIN B.C. & MAUER A.M. (1967) Variation of proliferative activity in leukemic cell populations of patients with acute leukemia. *Journal of Clinical Investigation*, **46**, 1356.

206 DE VITA V.T. (1971) Cell kinetics and the chemotherapy of cancer. *Cancer Chemotherapy Reports*, Part 3, **2**, 23.

207 CHAN B.W.B. & HAYHOE F.G.J. (1971) Changes in proliferative activity of marrow leukemic cells during and after extracorporeal irradiation of blood. *Blood*, **37**, 657.

208 STRYCKMANS P., DELALIEUX G., MANASTER J. & SOC-CUET M. (1970) The potentiality of out-of-cycle acute leukemic cells to synthesize DNA. *Blood*, **36**, 697.

209 GABUTTI V., PILERI A., TAROCCO R.P., GAVOSTO F. & COOPER E.H. (1969) Proliferative potential of out-of-cycle leukaemic cells. *Nature (London)*, **224**, 375.

210 KILLMANN S.Ä., KARLE H., ERNST P. & ANDERSEN V. (1971) Return of human leukaemic myeloblasts from blood to bone marrow. *Acta Medica Scandinavica*, **189**, 136.

211 HENDERSON E.S. (1969) Treatment of acute leukemia. *Seminars in Hematology*, **6**, 271.

212 CRONKITE E.P. (1970) Acute leukemia: is there a relationship between cell growth kinetics and response to chemotherapy? *Proceedings of the National Cancer Conference*, **6**, 113.

213 GALBRAITH P.R. & ADVINCULA E.G. (1972) Observations on the myelocyte tissue transit time (MTT) in acute leukaemia and other proliferative disorders. *British Journal of Haematology*, **22**, 453.

214 LORD B.I., MORI K.J., WRIGHT E.G. & LAJTHA L.G. (1977) Proliferation regulators in haemopoietic cell populations. *Blood Cells*, **3**, 451.

215 ADAMSON J.W. & FIALKOW P.J. (1978) The pathogenesis of the myeloproliferative syndromes. *British Journal of Haematology*, **38**, 299.

216 ADAMSON J.W. (1979) Marrow regulation by cell signals. *New England Journal of Medicine*, **300**, 378.

217 ZANJANI E.D., LUTTON J.D., HOFFMAN R. & WASSERMAN L.R. (1977) Erythroid colony formation by polycythemia vera bone marrow *in vitro*. *Journal of Clinical Investigation*, **59**, 841.

218 PRCHAL J.F., ADAMSON J.W., MURPHY S., STEINMANN L. & FIALKOW P.J. (1978) Polycythemia vera. The *in vitro* response of normal and abnormal stem cell lines to erythropoietin. *Journal of Clinical Investigation*, **61**, 1044.

219 EAVES C.J. & EVANS A.C. (1978) Eythropoietin (Ep) dose-response curves for three classes of erythroid progenitors in normal human marrow and in patients with polycythemia vera. *Blood*, **62**, 1196.

220 SINDER J.W., FIALKOW P.J., ADAMSON J.W., STEINMANN L., ERNST C., MURPHY S. & KOPECKY K.J. (1979) Increased expression of normal committed granulocytic stem cells *in vitro* after exposure of marrow to tritiated thymidine. *Journal of Clinical Investigation*, **64**, 1320.

221 LAWLER S.D., MILLARD R.E. & KAY H.E.M. (1970) Further cytogenetical investigations in polycythaemia vera. *European Journal of Cancer*, **6**, 223.

222 ADAMSON J.W. & FINCH C.A. (1970) Erythropoietin and the regulation of erythropoiesis in Di Guglielmo's syndrome. *Blood*, **36**, 590.

223 MARKS P.A., RIFKIND R.A., BANK A., TERADA M., RUEBEN R., FIBACH E., NUDEL U., SALMON J. & GAZITT Y. (1978) Induction of differentiation of murine erythroleukemia cells. In: *Cell Differentiation and Neoplasia* (ed. Saunders G.F.), p. 453. Raven Press, New York.

224 GOLDMAN J.M., TH'NG K.H., CATOVSKY D. & GALTON D.A.G. (1976) Production of colony-stimulating factor by leukemic leukocytes. *Blood*, **47**, 381.

225 BROXMEYER H.E., SMITHYMAN A. & EGER R.R. (1978) Indentification of lactoferrin as the granulocyte-derived inhibitor of colony-stimulating activity production. *Journal of Experimental Medicine*, **148**, 1052.

226 BROXMEYER H.E., BAKER F.L. & GALBRAITH P.R. (1976) *In vitro* regulation of granulopoiesis in human leukemia: application of an assay for colony-inhibiting cells. *Blood*, **47**, 389.

227 BROXMEYER H.E., GROSSBARD E., JACOBSEN N. & MOORE M.A.S. (1979) Persistance of inhibitory activity against normal bone-marrow cells during remission of acute leukemia. *New England Journal of Medicine*, **301**, 346.

Chapter 22
The acute leukaemias

J. M. CHESSELLS

NOMENCLATURE AND CLASSIFICATION

Traditionally the acute leukaemias have been classified on the basis of morphology as acute myeloid leukaemia (AML) or acute lymphoblastic leukaemia (ALL). These terms are misleading because AML is taken to comprise not only cases with myeloid differentiation, but also those with monocytic differentiation and the erythroleukaemias. Nor is there clear evidence that all cases of ALL are necessarily of lymphoid origin. This distinction has, however, been hallowed by tradition and is accepted in the Franco-American-British (FAB) classification (see Chapter 21) [1, 2].

Acute lymphoblastic leukaemias

The FAB classification of ALL is subjective and liable to observer variation, although attempts have been made to improve observer concordance by a scoring system [3]. There is no correlation between FAB subtypes and immunological class of ALL except for the association of B-ALL with L_3 morphology [4] (Fig. 22.1). It appears (see below) that the FAB subclass may have independent prognostic significance, although the factors determining FAB class L_1 or L_2 remain unclear.

The immunological classification of ALL is more widely accepted [5] and has clarified the relationship of ALL to other lymphoproliferative disorders. The distribution of immunological subtypes of ALL are outlined in Table 22.1; their clinical associations are discussed later. The lymphoblasts from the majority of cases of ALL, at least in children and young adults [6, 7], have neither T nor B characteristics but in most cases bear the c-ALL antigen [8]; the presence of intracytoplasmic immunoglobulin in some cases of c-ALL may be evidence of B-lymphoid differentiation [9]. The normal counterpart of the c-ALL cell may be a haemopoietic stem cell or cell of early B-lymphoid lineage; cells reactive with the c-ALL antigen have been found in bone marrow but not in lymphoid tissues from normal children, and in the bone marrow in a variety of non-leukaemic haematological dis-

orders [10]. Common ALL appears to have no lymphomatous counterpart: cells from patients with incontrovertible non-Hodgkin lymphoma very rarely bear the c-ALL antigen. Further indirect evidence of the derivation of c-ALL from a marrow-derived cell may be the association of the syndrome of transient marrow aplasia with c-ALL [11], and the frequency of generalized bony lesions in this, but not in other types of ALL.

In a minority of child patients, and in a larger proportion of adults with ALL, the cells, while lacking both T and B characteristics, do not possess the c-ALL antigen but are morphologically lymphoid and may show raised levels of terminal deoxynucleotidyl transferase (TdT) [12]. It is possible that these 'null'-ALL's represent a true stem-cell or undifferentiated leukaemia.

The distinction between T- or B-ALL and the related lymphoblastic or undifferentiated lymphomas occurring in children and young adults (see Chapter 24) is often imprecise and based on such arbitrary criteria as the percentage of blast cells in a bone-marrow aspirate [13]. The spectrum of T-cell lymphoid neoplasms in children and young adults embraces patients with lymphadenopathy, thymic mass and/or pleural effusion, with or without marrow infiltration, as well as patients with frank leukaemia [14]. These disorders, unlike c-ALL, have a marked male predominance, and a predilection for early CNS involvement without overt marrow infiltration. It has been suggested that T-ALL represents an advanced form of

Table 22.1. Subclasses of acute lymphoblastic leukaemia (ALL) in children ($\leqslant 15$ years) and adults (> 15 years) (From Ref. 5a, with permission)

	Children	Adults
Common-ALL	75·6%	50·5%
T-ALL	11·7%	9·7%
B-ALL	0·5%	2·0%
Null-ALL	12·1%	37·8%
Total number	701	103

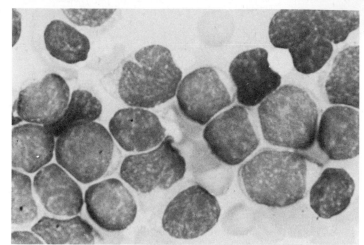

(a)

Fig. 22.1. Acute lymphoblastic leukaemia: bone-marrow appearances. (Courtesy of Prof. D. A. G. Galton; May–
Grünwald–Giemsa, ×1120.) (a) FAB
type L_1. Note the high nuclear/cytoplas-
mic ratio, the absence of conspicuous
nucleoli in most cells, the general regu-
larity of nuclear outline, and the small
size of the cells. (b) FAB type L_2. Note the
low nuclear/cytoplasmic ratio, prominent nucleoli, and large size of several
cells. The typing of L_1 and L_2 is based on a
score which records the proportions of
cells showing high or low nuclear/cyto-
plasmic ratio, inconspicuous or prominent nucleoli, irregular nuclear outline,
and of large cells. For definitions and
details see Ref. 3. The diagnosis must be
made on bone-marrow films, because the
morphology of blasts in the peripheral
blood is highly variable. N.B. Before
diagnosing undifferentiated blasts as
'lymphoblastic', myeloblastic leukaemia
without maturation (M_1) must be
excluded by Sudan-black B staining, or
by the myeloperoxidase reaction. (c) FAB
type L_3. The cells are large, with dispersed
chromatin, prominent nucleoli and
hyperbasophilic cytoplasm, often with
large vacuoles.

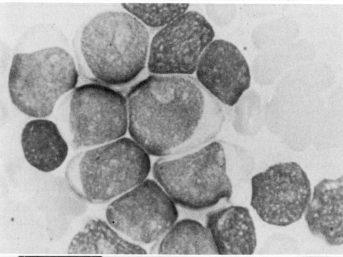

(b)

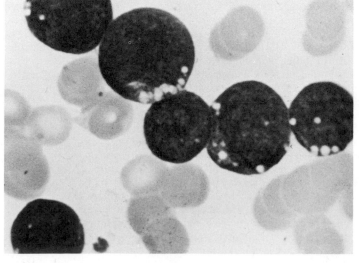

(c)

T-cell lymphoblastic lymphoma. This conclusion may be premature, as further analysis of T-cell populations may relate clinical features to T-cell sub-classes. It has been reported, for example, that lymphomatous presentation is more frequently associated with the presence on the blast cells of a suppressor cell-associated antigen, lacking in patients presenting with leukaemia [15]. Though B-ALL is rare, comprising one per cent or less of most series, marrow infiltration with B lymphoblasts is frequently seen in patients with advanced diffuse undifferentiated lymphomas, often 'Burkitt-like', and particularly of abdominal origin [14, 16].

Acute myeloid leukaemias

The FAB classification of the acute myeloid leukaemias (AML) (Fig. 22.2) is more readily reproducible and has some clinico-pathological correlations. There is an obvious overlap between AML and the subacute leukaemias [17] or dysmyelopoietic syndromes [1]. Amongst the subtypes of AML [18], M_1, M_2, M_4 and M_5 predominate. Although M_3 (hypergranular promyelocytic leukaemia) is relatively uncommon, its particular association with disseminated intravascular coagulation (DIC), sensitivity to anthracyclines and predilection for long-term remission, if the problems during induction can be overcome, render it a distinct subclass; the 15:17 chromosomal translocation, although not invariable, appears to be a specific characteristic of M_3 AML [19]. Similarly M_5 (pure monocytic leukaemia) has distinctive clinical features, notably extramedullary infiltrates, propensity for central nervous-system (CNS) involvement and relative refractoriness to conventional AML therapy [20, 21]. The pure monocytic leukaemias may represent the leukaemic counterpart of the rare true histiocytic lymphoma and of histiocytic medullary reticulosis as suggested by reports of evolution of the latter to monocytic leukaemia [22].

CLINICAL FEATURES [23–25]

Symptoms and signs

The presenting features of the acute leukaemias arise from the effects of bone-marrow failure and from the consequences of accumulation of leukaemic cells. The duration of symptoms may vary from days to months.

In children, pallor and lassitude are the commonest symptoms of anaemia and, particularly in the young child, severe anaemia (Hb < 5g/dl) may be present at diagnosis. Haemorrhagic symptoms, usually spontaneous, or excessive bruising may be of sudden or insidious onset; enlargement of cervical lymph nodes may have been noted and ascribed to an upper-respiratory-tract infection. Occasionally enlargement of mediastinal lymph nodes and/or thymus may cause symptoms of mediastinal obstruction. Bone pains or a limp are a frequent presenting symptom and lytic lesions in the spine may cause severe back pain or spinal-cord compression [26].

In adults, anaemia may cause dyspnoea, angina or oedema, and thrombocytopenia may lead to menorrhagia, melaena or even intracranial haemorrhage. Fever may be due to a complicating infection or may have no discernible cause, and lymphadenopathy to infiltration or to local sepsis. Infective lesions of the mouth and pharynx are common and patients frequently present to the dentist. Oral lesions vary from small necrotic ulcers to extensive painful necrosis and induration. The gums are frequently infected and bleed easily. True gingival hypertrophy is a characteristic feature of monocytic or myelomonocytic leukaemia; rectal and perianal sepsis are also common presenting features of this variant of AML. Generalized bone pain is less common than in childhood but symptoms may arise from localized lytic lesions, particularly in the orbit or spine.

Besides these features, examination may show enlargement of liver, spleen and, less commonly, kidneys. Skin infiltration is a feature of monocytic leukaemia and of the very rare congenital myeloid leukaemias and takes the form of multiple palpable deposits (Fig. 22.3). A search should be made for mucous-membrane haemorrhage and the fundi must be examined for evidence of haemorrhage or of leukaemic infiltration of the central nervous system.

Radiology

An X-ray of the chest should be performed in all cases of acute leukaemia; while enlargement of the hilar nodes is not infrequently seen, massive mediastinal widening or a large thymic shadow is suggestive of T-cell ALL (Fig. 22.4). Apparent infiltration of the lung fields is more likely to be due to pneumonia than to leukaemic infiltration.

Skeletal X-rays will show bony lesions in most children with ALL, including localized lytic areas, periosteal elevation and metaphyseal lucent bands (Figs 22.5 and 22.6) [27]. In the non-lymphoblastic leukaemias (AML) and in adult ALL, generalized skeletal changes are less common and lesions are usually confined to one or two sites such as the bones of the skull or the vertebral bodies. Bone pains respond rapidly to the appropriate cytotoxic chemotherapy but may tend to recur at the time of relapse.

While the characteristic skeletal lesions may suggest a diagnosis of acute leukaemia, and thus prove helpful in differential diagnosis of musculoskeletal or rheumatoid disorders, it should be emphasized that the

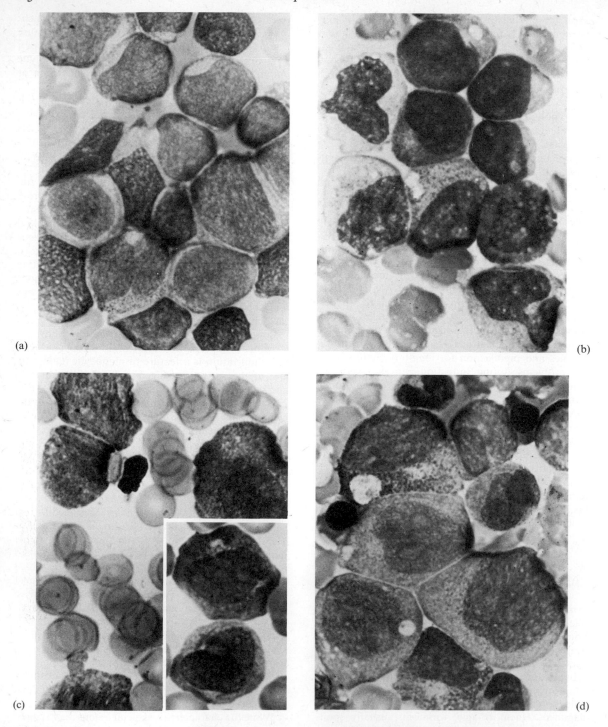

Fig. 22.2. Acute myeloid leukaemia: bone-marrow appearances. (Courtesy of Prof. D. A. G. Galton; May–Grünwald–Giemsa, ×1040.) (a) FAB type M_1 (myeloblastic without maturation). All the blast cells but one—which contains cytoplasmic azurophil granules—are undifferentiated. Most of the cells stained with Sudan black B and contained myeloperoxidase. N.B. M_1 is diagnosed even if all the blasts are undifferentiated, provided that more than three per cent of

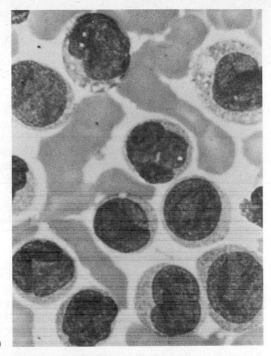

(e)

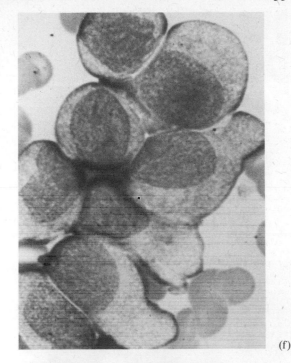

(f)

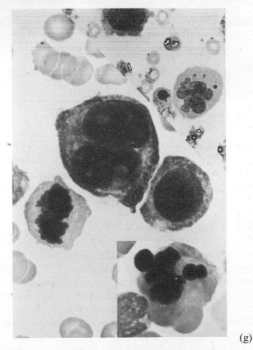

(g)

blast cells (as distinct from residual granulocytes) show positivity with Sudan black B or the myeloperoxidase reaction. The presence of azurophilic granules alone is not diagnostic of M_1: the granules may not stain with Sudan black B and may not contain myeloperoxidase. The presence of Auer rods (in a population of otherwise undifferentiated blasts, see (b)) is pathognomonic of M_1. See legend to (d) for distinction from M_4 (myelomonocytic leukaemia). (b) FAB type M_2 (myeloblastic with maturation). Note the blast cells (one with a single Auer rod), two promyelocytes, myelocytes, and a metamyelocyte. The presence of promyelocytes demarcates M_2 from M_1. (c) FAB type M_3 (hypergranular promyelocytic form). Note bizarre promyelocytes packed with coarse azurophilic granules largely obscuring the nucleus, and a 'faggot' cell packed with Auer rods. *Inset*: two 'faggot' cells; both contain multiple Auer rods, and one has a bilobed nucleus with a nucleolus in each lobe. N.B. M_3 is diagnosed on the presence of pathological promyelocytes and of faggot cells. When the majority of cells are promyelocytes of normal morphology the diagnosis is M_2. In the variant form the cells with bilobed nuclei predominate, faggot cells are scarce or absent, and granules, when present, are very small. (d) FAB type M_4 (myelomonocytic). Note monoblasts, a promonocyte (with scattered azurophilic granules), myelocytes and granulocytes. N.B. M_4 cannot be diagnosed from the bone marrow alone. The marrow may be that of M_1 or M_2, while the peripheral-blood films show mainly monocytes (see (e)). (e) FAB type M_4, peripheral blood. All but one cell, a blast, are monocytes. Similar appearances may be found in M_5. (f) FAB type M_5 (monocytic). Note the large monoblasts with abundant ground-glass (in this case basophilic) cytoplasm with amoeboid pseudopodia. In M_5 with maturation, most of the cells in the marrow are promonocytes with grey rather than basophilic cytoplasm, and azurophilic granulation, while more mature monocytes may appear in the peripheral blood. The granulocytic component in M_5 is inconspicuous or absent. (g) FAB type M_6 (erythroleukaemia). Composite of three fields. Note bizarre erythroblasts, including giant and multinucleate forms.

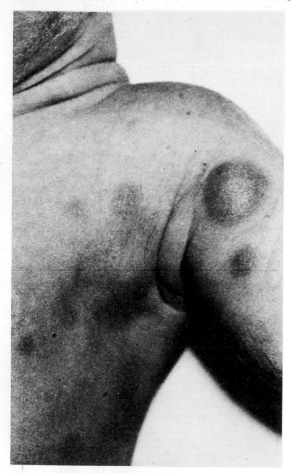

Fig. 22.3. Skin lesions in congenital AML

presence or absence of skeletal lesions *per se* is of no prognostic significance in childhood leukaemia [28]. There is therefore no need for routine skeletal X-rays and such investigations are indicated only on clinical grounds.

Biochemistry and microbiology
The only common biochemical abnormality in untreated acute leukaemia is the raised serum uric acid associated with a large leukaemic cell mass. It is essential to arrange baseline investigations of renal and hepatic function before the start of therapy but major metabolic disturbances usually occur only after the start of treatment, particularly when there is rapid cell lysis (see p. 859).

Extensive microbiological investigations may be needed in the management of suspected or actual infection (see p. 860) but it is also advisable to collect serum for storage and, in children, to measure anti-

bodies to common exanthemata, in particular measles, varicella-zoster and cytomegalovirus.

HAEMATOLOGICAL FEATURES

Anaemia is usually present at the time of diagnosis of acute leukaemia and is due to failure of red-cell production and sometimes to haemorrhage. The anaemia has no special features; reticulocytes are decreased and normoblasts are usually absent from the blood except in infancy and in erythroleukaemia (M_6). Thrombocytopenia is usual but not invariable; in patients with a raised leucocyte count at presentation and in those with hypergranular promyelocytic leukaemia (M_3) bleeding is often due to DIC [29].

The blood and bone marrow in ALL
The blood film in ALL usually shows neutropenia and monocytopenia; remaining neutrophils are normal in appearance but may show Döhle bodies. There may be a few myelocytes and metamyelocytes but the presence of large numbers of these cells is more suggestive of AML or of CML in blast crisis. Most of the nucleated cells are blasts and lymphocytes which may be difficult to distinguish from each other, particularly in L_1 ALL. Presentation with few or no blasts in the blood (previously called aleukaemic leukaemia) is not uncommon, but such patients usually have an absolute neutropenia though the platelet count may be normal.

The bone marrow is usually cellular, with blasts and lymphocytes comprising the vast majority of cells. Occasionally it is very difficult to aspirate the marrow so that needle trephine biopsy is necessary. Difficulty in aspiration may be associated with increased marrow fibrosis; this finding has no prognostic significance although fibrosis tends to decrease as remission is achieved and may recur on relapse [30, 31]. The blasts (Fig. 22.1) are usually monomorphic, about 10–15 μm in diameter, and have little cytoplasm and one or two nucleoli. Blast cells in L_1 ALL resemble small lymphocytes, but their nuclear pattern is more primitive with more prominent nucleoli. In L_2 ALL, the blasts are larger, more pleomorphic and may have more abundant cytoplasm. The distinctive features of the rare L_3 lymphoblasts of B-ALL are more easily recognized.

Cytochemistry. Blast cells in ALL are peroxidase and Sudan-black negative but frequently, particularly in L_1 ALL, show block positivity with the periodic-acid-Schiff (PAS) stain for glycogen. An acid-phosphatase stain should also be performed; polar positivity for acid phosphatase is frequently associated with T-ALL [32].

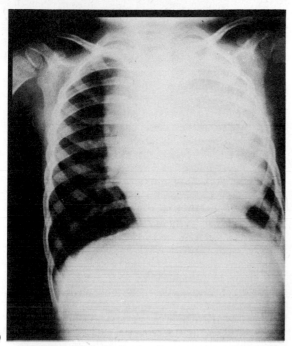
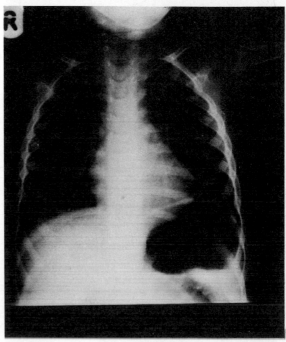

(a)

(b)

Fig. 22.4. (a) Chest X-ray showing thymic enlargement in T-ALL; (b) same case 48 hours after treatment with prednisolone and VCR.

Immunological classification. This should be performed when possible and *cytogenetic analysis* of the marrow is desirable. The Philadelphia (Ph[1]) chromosome is present in a substantial proportion of adults with ALL (possibly 20% of cases) [33, 34], but in a much smaller proportion of children—about one to two per cent [35]. A specific translocation (t8:14) has been reported in B-ALL [36], as in Burkitt's lymphoma (see Chapter 24).

The blood and bone marrow in AML

Appearances in AML show a far greater morphological diversity. Leucocytes in the blood may be increased, normal or decreased and the pattern and distribution of cells reflects the pattern of marrow activity. Usually, however, the blood contains a higher proportion of mature neutrophils and lymphocytes than the marrow and occasionally blasts predominate in the blood despite a substantial proportion of mature leucocytes in the marrow. The neutrophils frequently show morphological abnormalities such as lack of granularity or Pelger-like forms.

Marrow appearances (Fig. 22.2) depend on the degree of leukaemic differentiation and the proportion of blasts varies markedly from case to case. In the least differentiated (M₁) leukaemias there may be virtually total replacement with blast cells, whereas in the more differentiated (M₂) forms, promyelocytes and myelocytes and more mature forms are evident in varying proportions. The myeloblast is larger than the lymphoblast and has multiple nucleoli and usually more cytoplasm; the population of cells is more pleomorphic. *Auer rods*, coalescent primary granules, are pathognomic of AML but unfortunately are only prominent in a minority of cases. In hypergranular promyelocytic leukaemia (M₃) the abnormal promyelocytes contain 'faggots' of multiple coalescent granules and are very heavily granulated. Leukaemias with monocytic features comprise a spectrum from cases with myeloid predominance (myelomonocytic M₄) to pure monocytic leukaemia (M₅) in which there is almost total replacement of the marrow by leukaemic cells with only a minor granulocytic component. The blast cells are large with abundant deeply basophilic cytoplasm with or without azurophilic granules [20]. Leukaemias with a monocytic element are characterized by raised serum and urine lysozyme [37]. In erythroleukaemia (M₆) the erythroid cells constitute more than 50% of marrow cells and show bizarre morphology with giant forms, multinucleate cells and macronormoblastic change. There is usually an increase in myeloblasts and promyelocytes which

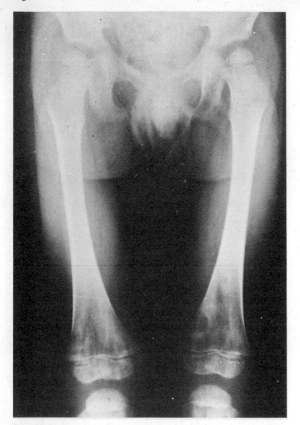

Fig. 22.5. Skeletal lesions in femora in ALL.

may predominate after recent transfusion and the illness may evolve into a predominantly myeloid leukaemia.

Cytochemical techniques. These show that blasts with a myeloid element (M_1, M_2, M_3, M_4) stain positively for peroxidase and with Sudan black. In pure monocytic leukaemia (M_5) the blast cells are negative to Sudan black but in both M_4 and M_5 non-specific esterase stains are positive and inhibited by fluoride. In erythroleukaemia (M_6) the late normoblasts often show PAS positivity.

Immunological classification of the acute myeloid leukaemias has not yet proved helpful although myeloid associated antigens have been described [38, 39]. Cases with monocytic differentiation will show receptors for the FC fragment of IgG [40]. A variety of *chromosomal abnormalities* have been described in AML and include, in addition to the (t15:17) of acute promyelocytic leukaemia, (t8:21) with loss of the sex chromosome, trisomy 8, monosomy 7 and monosomy 21 [41]. The

Ph[1] chromosome is present in about three per cent of cases of AML [33].

The diagnosis of acute leukaemia and the distinction between ALL and AML

In the great majority of cases of acute leukaemia, examination of the blood and bone marrow provides unequivocal confirmation of the diagnosis. In a minority of patients the distinction between AML and ALL is difficult to make; these cases have often been previously described as acute undifferentiated leukaemia (AUL). The use of this term has been restricted by the development of modern cytochemical techniques and methods of immunological classification; it should now be reserved for the few cases which defy classification by all these techniques. A second problem arises, particularly in AML, in assessment of the pace of evolution of the leukaemia and a distinction must be made between AML and the chronic myeloproliferative disorders.

Problems in distinguishing ALL and AML usually arise from similarity between the more pleomorphic L_2 ALL and the M_1 undifferentiated AML. The distinction between the two should be facilitated by use of the Sudan black or myeloperoxidase reaction, which is positive in AML, though occasionally problems may arise in distinguishing L_2 ALL and M_5 AML in which the Sudan black is negative. The fluoride-sensitive non-specific esterase reaction is positive in most myelomonocytic leukaemias and is very strongly positive in monocytic (M_5) leukaemias. Raised serum and urine lysozyme levels provide helpful confirmation of the monocytic element.

Immunological analysis often proves helpful in showing that blasts bear the c-ALL antigen or possess T-cell features, but the most useful investigation in the undifferentiated case is measurement of the enzyme terminal deoxynucleotidyl transferase (TdT) [42], which is raised in some otherwise unclassifiable lymphoid leukaemias [12]. The significance of raised TdT has recently been reviewed [43]: it is found in a small minority of cases of unequivocal AML [43, 44], but nevertheless it remains a useful marker. In some cases which are difficult to classify, cytogenetic investigation may show the presence of the Ph[1] chromosome: the acute leukaemias in association with the Ph[1] chromosome may show lymphoid, myeloid or mixed features [45]. In practice, careful morphological evaluation, assessment of Sudan black and non-specific esterase stains and measurement of TdT should resolve the problem. Very few cases should defy classification by all the means available, and for these cases of AUL perhaps a working rule previously used by the Medical Research Council's Working Parties on Leukaemia might apply: to treat patients under 20

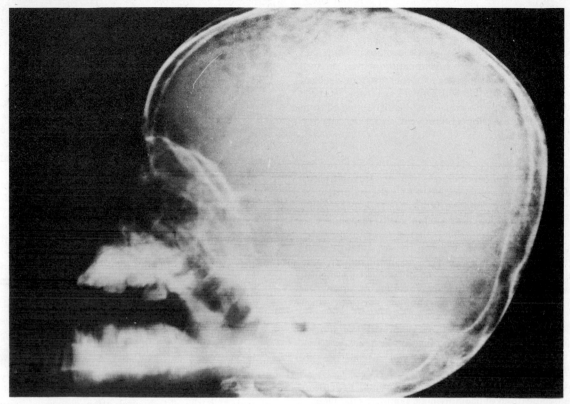

Fig. 22.6. Multiple lytic areas in the skull of a child with ALL and hypercalcaemia.

in the first instance as ALL and older patients as AML.

The second area of difficulty is in deciding whether to classify the leukaemia as 'acute'. This problem rarely arises in ALL, where widespread marrow infiltration is the rule at the time of diagnosis. In some patients with AML, however, there is a long history and the marrow may show only a moderate increase in blast cells and promyelocytes; distinction from the myelodysplastic syndromes (see p. 839) may then be a problem. If there is any doubt about the pace of evolution of the disease, a period of observation and supportive treatment is indicated. This will avoid early inappropriate therapy and is unlikely to prejudice the outcome.

DIFFERENTIAL DIAGNOSIS OF ACUTE LEUKAEMIA

Infections

Infectious mononucleosis bears a superficial resemblance to ALL, especially when it is associated with immune haemolysis or with thrombocytopenia. The pleomorphic appearance of mononuclear cells in the blood and the results of specific serological tests should distinguish it from ALL without recourse to bone-marrow aspiration in the majority of cases. Other infections, notably with cytomegalovirus, may cause a similar haematological picture.

Congenital leukaemia is extremely rare and usually myeloid; it is characterized by extensive extramedullary infiltrates including the skin. It must be distinguished from the more common congenital infections which also cause anaemia, hepatosplenomegaly and skin lesions: cytomegalovirus, toxoplasmosis, rubella and syphilis [46]. Occasionally, more exotic infections such as infantile kala-azar, causing fever, splenomegaly, neutropenia and excess of blasts in the marrow, may mimic leukaemia. In the elderly, who may present with infection and/or heart failure, diagnosis of acute leukaemia may be masked initially by the features of these complications.

Leucoerythroblastic anaemia
A leucoerythroblastic blood film with normoblasts and myelocytes in the blood may be indicative of extramedullary haemopoiesis in spleen and liver or of bone-marrow infiltration with carcinoma or other neoplasm. Bone-marrow examination will distinguish such cases from leukaemia. The increased incidence of leukaemia in children with Down's syndrome has been mentioned and leukaemia must be distinguished from the transient myeloproliferative disorder described in these infants [47].

Aplastic anaemia
There are a number of reports of bone-marrow aplasia preceding leukaemia (usually ALL); the majority were not studied by trephine biopsy and were probably cases of acute leukaemia temporarily responding to steroid therapy [48]. Nevertheless patients do occasionally present with transient marrow failure, confirmed by trephine biopsy, and then subsequently develop ALL [11]. It can be difficult to distinguish between lymphocytoid cells remaining in an aplastic marrow and leukaemic lymphoblasts, both of which may bear the common ALL antigen. The dilemma can be resolved by a period of observation and supportive therapy without recourse to cytotoxic drugs.

Idiopathic thrombocytopenic purpura (ITP)
Although to the patient and/or his parents, the acute or subacute onset of haemorrhagic symptoms in ITP may suggest leukaemia, the absence of other abnormalities on examination and the otherwise normal blood count make a distinction easy, and bone-marrow aspiration will confirm the presence of a cellular marrow with abundant megakaryocytes.

Megaloblastic anaemia
Erythroleukaemia with marked dyserythropoiesis may closely mimic megaloblastic anaemia due to deficiency of vitamin B_{12} or folic acid. It may be necessary sometimes to give these haematinics empirically in pharmacological doses pending results of determination of folate and vitamin-B_{12} levels before assuming a diagnosis of erythroleukaemia.

Juvenile rheumatoid arthritis (JRA)
Despite quite wide publicity given to the frequency of bone pain, joint pain and swelling and skeletal lesions in childhood ALL, the diagnosis of c-ALL is still too often confused with that of juvenile rheumatoid arthritis (JRA) [49]. Patients with ALL mimicking JRA may often have a near-normal blood count; true bone pain is most uncommon in JRA. Skeletal X-rays may show lytic or periosteal lesions which are quite

uncharacteristic of JRA. If there is any doubt about the diagnosis of JRA a bone-marrow examination should precede steroid therapy.

Non-Hodgkin lymphoma (NHL) and other lymphoproliferative malignancies
The problems of distinction between ALL and NHL, particularly in childhood, have been discussed above. Lymph-node biopsy in patients with ALL will show appearances indistinguishable from those of diffuse undifferentiated or lymphoblastic lymphoma. A bone-marrow examination should always precede formal surgical biopsy in children with lymph-node enlargement since it may preclude the need for further more invasive investigations. The distinction between ALL and NHL in childhood is an arbitrary one and many workers [50, 51] conventionally use a level of 25% or more lymphoblasts in the bone marrow as a cut-off point. Apparent cases of ALL in the older patient may be due to dissemination of nodular or undifferentiated lymphoma. Analysis of surface markers in such cases usually reveals their B-cell origin.

Although the lymphoblasts, particularly in L_1 ALL, may bear a superficial resemblance to the more mature lymphocytes of CLL, the pace of evolution of the disease and the age of the patient should make the distinction easy, while surface-marker analysis will confirm the B-cell lineage of the CLL cells. Similarly prolymphocytic leukaemia [52], a rare variant of CLL occurring in the elderly and often associated with very high leucocyte counts, and leukaemic reticuloendotheliosis (hairy-cell leukaemia) [53] can be distinguished by their clinical and morphological features (see Chapter 23).

Other neoplasms
Disseminated anaplastic tumours in childhood, especially neuroblastoma and Ewing's tumour, may mimic both JRA and acute leukaemia. Non-haemopoietic tumour cells are rarely seen on the blood film, which may be leucoerythroblastic. The marrow may be diffusely infiltrated with malignant cells, thus superficially resembling leukaemia, but these cells are often larger and more pleomorphic than leukaemic blast cells and under low power may be noted to occur in clumps. A suspected diagnosis of neuroblastoma may be confirmed by finding raised urine catecholamines and by demonstration of a primary tumour. Occasionally patients present with a localized bony lesion which on biopsy may be described as a 'small, round cell tumour'; an erroneous diagnosis of Ewing's sarcoma or localized bony lymphoma may be made if leukaemia is not considered and marrow sampled from a distant site.

The chronic myeloproliferative disorders

The relationship of chronic granulocytic leukaemia (CGL) to the Ph[1]-positive acute leukaemias is discussed in detail in Chapter 23. The variability of clinical expression of Ph[1]-positive leukaemia is consistent with the evidence that it is a stem-cell disorder [54]. In the chronic phase of CGL the Ph[1]-positive clone undergoes development along myeloid lines, but during the acute phase or in cases which present *de novo* with acute leukaemia, maturation may be arrested at the stage of a stem cell bearing the c-ALL antigen, thus mimicking ALL [55, 56]. Similarly, arrest during myeloid development may occur, though probably less frequently, so that Ph[1]-positive leukaemia may also mimic AML. These distinctions have practical relevance because Ph[1]-positive AML and ALL are both relatively refractory to therapy [33]. There may be no clinical clues to the true nature of these acute leukaemias but examination of the blood and marrow may show, for example, abnormalities in the myeloid series, such as degranulated polymorphs and Pelger forms, which are not seen in typical ALL.

The acute myeloid leukaemias must also be distinguished from a variety of chronic Ph[1]-negative myeloproliferative disorders. These have a variable natural history, tend to occur in older patients [57] and have been referred to as wheel-spinning or smouldering leukaemias [58]. Two broad types of syndrome have been recognized: *refractory anaemia with excess of blasts* (RAEB) and *chronic myelomonocytic leukaemia* (CMML) [1]. Both are characterized by a long history of months or years, anaemia and moderate thrombocytopenia. In both, the marrow is hypercellular with an excess of blasts and mature neutrophils may show morphological abnormalities such as agranularity or Pelger–Huet forms. In RAEB, dyserythropoietic changes are common [59] and ringed sideroblasts may be seen, so that the condition may resemble idiopathic refractory sideroblastic anaemia [60]. In CMML [61] atypical monocytes predominate in the blood while the bone marrow shows an excess of myeloblasts and promyelocytes. Serum lysozyme concentrations are increased.

In addition to the haematological abnormalities described, these dysmyelopoietic syndromes are characterized by chromosomal abnormalities, particularly of the C group, in a proportion of cases [62], and by defective maturation of myeloid cells in culture [63]. The risk of progression to acute leukaemia in patients with these myelodysplastic syndromes remains unclear; many patients succumb from infection or from intercurrent medical problems before developing acute leukaemia. Patients with all these disorders tend to develop severe and prolonged aplasia following intensive chemotherapy and every effort should therefore be made to distinguish the conditions from the acute leukaemias.

The classical myelodysplastic syndromes are very rare in the young, although RAEB is occasionally seen. In this age group and particularly in infancy, the acute myeloid leukaemias must be distinguished from juvenile CML and other less clearly defined myeloproliferative disorders. The rare juvenile (Ph[1]-negative) CML (see also Chapter 23) is characterized by splenomegaly, suppurative lymphadenopathy, a skin rash and thrombocytopenia [64]. The blood and marrow appearances are not diagnostic although monocytoid cells may predominate in the blood. The hallmark of the disease is a raised fetal haemoglobin which increases as the disease progresses and which is accompanied by other fetal red-cell characteristics such as raised i antigen and reduced carbonic anhydrase [65]. True juvenile CML is extremely refractory to cytotoxic drugs and if a suitable donor is available, the treatment of choice is bone-marrow transplantation from an HLA-identical sibling [66]. It should be distinguished from other so-called variants of juvenile CML, which may have a better prognosis, in which the progressive rise of fetal Hb is not seen. A variety of atypical cases including a familial myeloproliferative disorder have been described [67, 68].

A more clearly defined entity in the young child is a myeloproliferative syndrome characterized by hepatosplenomegaly, moderate thrombocytopenia and an excess of blasts in the marrow associated with the loss of a chromosome 7 in marrow-derived cells [69]. This monosomy 7 is a pre-leukaemic syndrome with a high risk of development of AML which is refractory to treatment [70].

PROGNOSIS AND CURABILITY

In 1967, Burchenal collected information on a worldwide series of 157 patients surviving more than five years from the time of diagnosis of acute leukaemia [71]. They comprised, of course, a tiny minority, perhaps $0.1–1.0\%$ of the total treated during the period spanning their diagnoses [72], and included relatively higher proportions of children and of patients with ALL. Till *et al.* [73], in a follow-up of 100 long-term survivors of acute leukaemia, found that patients surviving more than four years from diagnosis without relapse had a 70% chance of very long survival and that no patient died after the tenth year. More recently long-term follow-up of a group of 15 out of 229 children diagnosed in 1963/64 and surviving in remission for more than two and a half years, showed that 10 were alive and well more than 14 years from diagnosis: no relapses occurred in patients more than five years after stopping treatment [74]. It remains to be seen whether or not these findings can be extrapolated to the much larger population of patients with ALL now achieving a prolonged first remission, and to what extent clinical and haematological features at the time of diagnosis can be used as indicators of long-term prognosis. The factors determining response to induction therapy are discussed later.

Acute lymphoblastic leukaemia

Follow-up of the large series of children at St Jude Children's Hospital, who have stopped treatment after two and a half years of therapy, indicates that few patients who remain in remission four years after stopping treatment will relapse, suggesting that extrapolation from previous data is valid [75]. Occasional late relapses do occur, however, and it is not clear whether these should be regarded as failure of therapy or the induction of a new leukaemia.

There is general agreement about the prognostic significance of several clinical and haematological features in ALL; the most important of these is the height of the leucocyte count at presentation, which is inversely correlated with the duration of subsequent remission [76–78]. Other related indicators of the extent of the disease, such as the degree of organomegaly and lymph-node enlargement, show a similar correlation, although these are obviously less amenable to objective measurement. Recently recognized additional poor prognostic features include a high haemoglobin [79] and low immunoglobulins [80, 81]. Slow response to induction is associated with a higher rate of subsequent relapse [82, 83]. Children aged between two and 10 years at presentation do better than older or younger children [77, 84] and adults [85], and a particularly poor prognosis has been noted in infants under one year of age [86]. This may in part reflect a less aggressive approach to treatment. Other adverse prognostic features include the presence of a mediastinal mass [76, 87], Negro race [88] and in particular, early overt CNS disease [78]. Nevertheless, in any large group of patients survivors can be found with one or more of these features, except possibly the last.

It is possible by multivariate analysis to establish the contribution of individual factors in predicting remission duration and survival [83, 89]. In one series, six factors accounting for over 90% of total predictive value were: initial leucocyte count, nodal enlargement, age, haemoglobin, sex and platelet count [79]; of these factors, initial leucocyte count and age were the most important in influencing prognosis. In a prospective study of 724 children treated by the American Children's Cancer Study Group it was possible to define three prognostic groups using these two criteria

alone; almost 90% of the 'good-risk' group aged between three and seven years with leucocyte counts of less than $10 \times 10^9/l$ remained in complete remission four years from diagnosis, while 'poor-risk' patients, defined as having a leucocyte count of greater than $50 \times 10^9/l$ at presentation, had a median survival of only two years [90]. Except for sex, these adverse prognostic factors relate to early relapse and lose their significance in patients who remain in remission for two years or more [91, 92]. In most reported series there has been no evidence that sex materially influences prognosis, though such small differences as have been observed are usually in favour of girls. In the MRC UKALL II trial, however, boys fared significantly worse than girls, even allowing for testicular relapse [93], and George *et al.* [75] found that boys have a greater risk than girls of marrow relapse after stopping treatment. These results are now being confirmed in other series [94, 95].

It is now apparent that many of the clinical features long associated with a poor prognosis in childhood ALL, such as a high leucocyte count and mediastinal mass, are frequently associated with T-ALL [96, 97]; such patients typically respond readily to induction but tend to relapse readily [6]. Similarly, adults with T-ALL do worse than those with c-ALL [7]. It may be argued that the poor prognosis of T-ALL is merely a reflection of advanced disease, for it is certainly true that patients with localized mediastinal NHL with T-cell characteristics, if treated aggressively, do better than those with frank T-ALL [13]. B-ALL is rare and refractory to conventional anti-leukaemic therapy such as prednisolone and vincristine [4]; treatment with regimes including cyclophosphamide, as for NHL, is probably more appropriate.

While the prognostic significance of clinical features and their association with immunological subclassification of ALL have received wide acceptance, there is no universal agreement yet about the significance of morphological and cytochemical features except for the acid-phosphatase positivity of most T-ALL [32] and the B-cell characteristics of the Burkitt-like L_3 cells, which carry monoclonal surface immunoglobulin [1, 4]. The first attempt at morphological subclassification of ALL was that of Mathé *et al.* [98], but this has not been accepted by other groups. A claim that a high proportion of micro-lymphoblasts was a favourable prognostic feature [99] was not widely confirmed [100–103]. More recently, however, application of the FAB classification suggests that children with L_1 ALL may have a better prognosis than those with L_2 ALL [83, 104–106], and this distinction may also apply to adults, in whom L_1 morphology is less common [85]. In contrast to L_3 ALL, these two cytological types do not correlate with immunological subtypes of ALL, so that the potential prognostic significance of each method of classification may be independent of the other. The poorer prognosis of L_2 ALL may be related to the observation that this class of ALL is characterized by a higher proliferative activity as shown by a higher proportion of cells in S phase at diagnosis [107]. Previous investigations of cell proliferation have not supported this concept [108, 109], and the prognostic value of cytokinetic studies in ALL is at present uncertain.

It has been claimed that a high proportion of PAS-positive lymphoblasts is a favourable prognostic feature [110–112], but this association has been disputed [102]; L_1 lymphoblasts may have more PAS positivity [105] than those of L_2 ALL.

There have been attempts to correlate cytogenetic features and prognosis in ALL. A prospective study of a small number of children showed that patients with predominantly hyperdiploid blast cells at diagnosis had longer first remissions than those with predominantly pseudodiploid cells [113].

Acute myeloid leukaemias (AML)
Long-term survival is still exceptional in AML and until recently has probably been attained by fewer than five to 10% of patients [114–116]. It remains to be seen whether new, more intensive, induction and consolidation schedules or allogeneic bone-marrow transplantation will substantially increase the proportion of long-term survivors. Some recent protocols associated with a high induction rate [117, 118] have not inevitably resulted in prolonged subsequent remission. However, in a recent MRC trial more intensive induction therapy led to longer survival from the time of remission [119] and preliminary encouraging results of more intensive chemotherapy have been reported by other groups [120].

Attempts to relate clinical and haematological features at diagnosis to remission duration have produced equivocal results. There appears to be a trend for remission length to be inversely related to blast count or leucocyte count [121, 122], but this is not nearly as marked as for ALL. Similar correlations have also been noted with liver size [119], and plasma lactic dehydrogenase (LDH) and plasma fibrinogen [122].

Prospective application of the FAB classification may prove of prognostic significance; in M_3 ALL the frequency of DIC at diagnosis and subsequent propensity for long remissions in those who achieve remission have been recognized [114, 123]; by contrast, patients with M_5 AML tend to relapse readily and a have a high incidence of extramedullary leukaemia [20, 21].

Cytokinetic studies have suggested that remission duration is inversely related to the pre-treatment labelling index [121, 122] but this has been disputed by

others [109]. Cytogenetic analysis is of greater potential prognostic significance: remission rate and survival were significantly better in patients with AML and a normal marrow karyotype than in those with an abnormal karyotype, though this distinction did not hold good in myelomonocytic leukaemia [124].

TREATMENT

GENERAL PRINCIPLES
Historically, the earliest therapeutic achievement in the acute leukaemias was to obtain a remission and so to prolong survival. Although remissions were usually of short duration, a small number of patients achieving remission did survive for many years despite having received what would now be deemed inadequate treatment [71, 73]. Most such patients remained in their first remission throughout; relapse was hardly ever compatible with subsequent long-term survival. With the introduction of modern treatment a substantial proportion of patients with ALL, mainly children, and a still very small fraction of patients with AML, now experience long-term complete remission, and by extrapolation from previous experience may be considered to be cured of their disease. The aim of treatment of acute leukaemia has thus shifted from palliation to cure. It is a reflection of the present state of practice that results in ALL are usually expressed in terms of duration of the first complete remission, whereas in AML the emphasis is still on survival.

General strategy
Much of the theoretical basis for treatment of acute leukaemia is based on animal work, in particular that of Skipper *et al.* with the mouse L1210 leukaemia [125]. This clonal and homogeneous tumour can be transmitted by injection of a single cell and is characterized by rapid growth and unimpaired proliferative potential. Both leukaemic cells and normal haemopoietic stem cells co-exist in the recipient. It is possible by suitable timing of chemotherapy to reduce the leukaemic cell population to zero while sparing normal haemopoietic stem cells [125].

How relevant is this experimental model to human leukaemia? The clonal origin of AML has been confirmed by study of chromosomal markers and the G6PD locus, but the disease appears heterogeneous in that it may involve stem cells that differentiate into erythrocytes [126] or apparently be restricted to the monocyte-macrophage system [127]. The co-existence of normal and leukaemic haemopoietic cells has been questioned in AML and it has been postulated that the malignant cells may undergo continuing differentiation [128–130]. If this were the case then therapeutic strategies designed to ensure marrow repopulation with normal autologous marrow cells would be invalid. The absence of normal stem cells clearly militates against bone-marrow recovery when leukaemia supervenes on a previously existing marrow disorder such as Fanconi's anaemia and probably explains the poor response to intensive cytotoxic therapy seen in leukaemia arising in the myelodysplastic syndromes. However, the bulk of evidence derived from serial cytogenetic analysis in AML suggests that in many cases there is a residual population of normal cells [131, 132].

Chemotherapy: the use of drug combinations
The response of mouse leukaemia to chemotherapeutic agents obeys first-order kinetics: a given dose of drug destroys a given fraction of the malignant cell population and not a given number of cells [125]. As the generation time of leukaemic cells is usually longer than that of normal cells it should in theory be possible, by appropriate spacing of drugs, to reduce the leukaemic cell population to zero while sparing normal regenerating marrow. It seems intuitively likely that drugs to be maximally effective should be given in the maximum tolerated dose, although the firm evidence for this in man is scanty and is based on one trial where half-dose was inferior to full-dose therapy during remission maintenance of ALL [133].

The practice of combining different drugs is analogous to the use of two antibiotics to minimize resistant organisms: combinations are selected which inhibit different biochemical pathways and exhibit non-overlapping toxicity [134]. This has led to a system of acronyms for various drug combinations, for example, COAP (cyclophosphamide, vincristine (Oncovin), cytosine arabinoside and prednisolone). Although in theory this practice may increase cell kill and prevent the emergence of resistant cells, in practice it may result in sub-optimal dosage of individual drugs. For example, in continuing treatment of ALL in childhood, while mercaptopurine and methotrexate proved superior to methotrexate alone, the addition of cyclophosphamide or cytosine arabinoside to this combination increased toxicity without further increasing the percentage of long-term remissions [135].

Application of cell kinetics [136]. Despite the considerable amount of information available about cell proliferation in acute leukaemia at presentation and at relapse (Chapter 21), the wide variation between cases, and from time to time in the same case, makes practical application of this information difficult. There are theoretical reasons for giving non-cycle-dependent agents (e.g. anthracyclines) first to reduce tumour cell mass, followed by cycle-dependent drugs (e.g. cytosine arabinoside (ara-C)) as more neoplastic cells enter the proliferative phase when tumour burden is reduced: in practice various combinations of anthracycline and ara-C produce equivalent results in AML, irrespective of which drug is given first or whether both are given together. On the other hand, manipulation of the mitotic cycle by increasing the proliferative fraction of leukaemic cells with ara-C has resulted in a higher remission rate with 6-thioguanine and ara-C than is usually achieved with these two agents in AML [137].

Various intensive chemotherapy schedules have been developed on cell-kinetic principles [138] but as yet are of no demonstrable superiority in the treatment of any type of acute leukaemia.

Remission and relapse
Complete remission is conventionally defined as a state in which the blood count is normal, the marrow of normal cellularity with less than five per cent blast cells and there is no evidence of extramedullary disease. It has been estimated that these criteria may be compatible with the presence of as many as 10^9–10^{10} leukaemic cells in the body, a number too small to be detected by currently available techniques. Supportive evidence for this contention comes from extensive investigations of patients in apparent haematological remission [139] and from post-mortem examination of children dying in apparent remission [140]. Present techniques are also incapable of distinguishing between normal remission leucocytes and differentiated progeny of a leukaemic cell population. Leukaemic relapse is held to be due to failure of eradication of the disease, probably due to the persistence of cells which remain in the resting phase, in which they may be resistant to the chemotherapy used but retain their proliferative potential, eventually to re-enter the cell cycle [141]. An additional factor may be 're-seeding' from extramedullary tissues such as the CNS or the gonads, where anatomical barriers restrict access of drugs given systemically. Alternatively, certain instances, particularly of late relapse, may represent re-induction of a new leukaemia.

Clinical trials and record keeping
Many of the advances in treatment of acute leukaemias have been achieved by means of prospective clinical trials comparing survival or remission duration among patients allocated at random to different treatments. The principles and pitfalls of these trials and the methods of analysis of the data are clearly set out in a two-part report by Peto *et al.* [142, 143] which will be briefly summarized here, but should be read in full by all involved in the management of acute leukaemia.

The superiority of the prospective randomized trial over the use of 'historical controls' is widely accepted:

an apparent advantage for a particular new therapeutic regime may in fact reflect different referral patterns or improvements in medical supportive care. Acute leukaemia is rare and few institutions will treat enough patients to obtain an unequivocal answer to questions about management. The use of fewer and larger trials is recommended because the results of small trials are likely to be misleading: the proportion of apparently significant results from small trials that are actually due to chance is much larger than that for larger trials. The disadvantage of the multi-centre trial is of course the variability between centres, which may appear in an extreme form: in one regime AML remission rates varied between centres from 60% to nil [144]. It is perfectly possible to conduct randomized prospective trials at one large centre provided no attempt is made to ask more than one or two questions

at a time about treatment: a good example is the series of trials of different forms of prophylaxis of CNS leukaemia at St Jude Children's Research Hospital [145].

The only method of analysis of trial results that takes account of the time of follow-up is the life table (survival or remission curve); comparison of median durations is deceptive. The significance of differences between groups of patients is measured by the log-rank test from the life-table analysis, and this allows treatment differences to be analysed between subgroups and consequent retrospective stratification. One of the most serious errors is removal of patients from analysis because they deviate from the protocol; this can cause serious bias in the results.

For monitoring of individual patients' treatment the graphic recording of serial blood counts on semilog

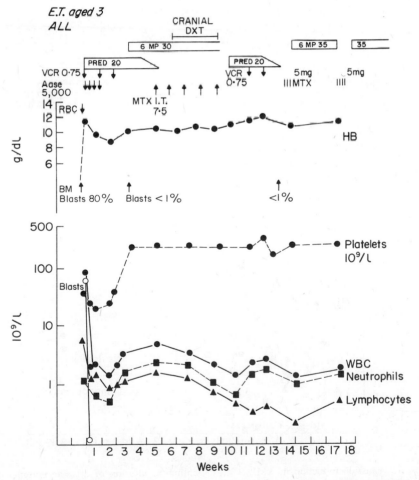

Fig. 22.7. Typical response to induction therapy in ALL. Drug doses in mg. IT = intrathecal, DXT = radiotherapy.

paper (Figs 22.7 and 22.8) is strongly recommended. It permits the early detection of trends in blood count in relation to clinical findings and treatment.

DRUGS COMMONLY USED IN THE TREATMENT OF ACUTE LEUKAEMIA [146–148]

Adrenal corticosteroids

Steroids have a specific lytic effect on normal and neoplastic lymphocytes [149] and sensitivity to steroids may be related to the presence of corticosteroid receptor proteins [150,151]. For example, non-T, non-B ALL cells have more receptors than those of T-ALL [152]. Steroids are unique among anti-leukaemic drugs in their lack of myelotoxicity.

Prednisone and prednisolone are usually chosen in preference to the other compounds because they cause less salt retention. Their undesirable metabolic side-effects preclude their use for prolonged periods; they are usually given for three to six weeks as a twice-daily dose during remission induction in ALL, and many protocols also use short pulses of prednisolone during continuing therapy. Prednisolone is mandatory during standard remission induction of ALL in combination with vincristine, with or without other drugs; even as a single agent it induced remission in 60% of children with ALL [153]. Prednisolone has some activity in AML, achieving remission in five to 15% of cases [153, 154].

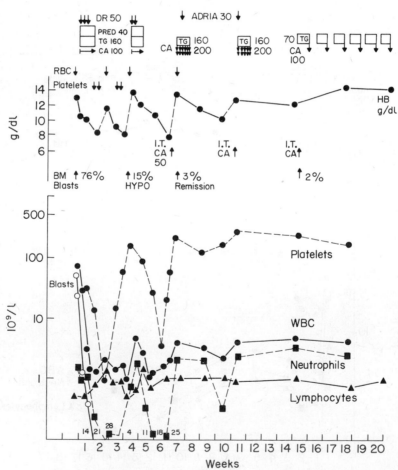

Fig. 22.8. Response to remission induction in AML. CA→ = continuous infusion of cytosine arabinoside; ↓ = 12-hourly injections.

Vinca alkaloids

The vinca alkaloids *vincristine* (VCR) and *vinblastine* are mitotic inhibitors derived from the periwinkle (*Vinca rosea*). Vincristine is the alkaloid used chiefly in treatment of acute leukaemia. The drug, poorly absorbed by mouth, is given once weekly intravenously with extreme care to avoid extravasation which causes severe tissue necrosis. It is rapidly bound to the tissues, metabolized by the liver and excreted in the bile. A new vinca alkaloid, *vindesine*, shows some evidence [155] of lack of cross-resistance and may be of value in ALL.

Vincristine binds to microtubular proteins necessary for spindle formation, thus arresting mitosis during metaphase [156]. It is important among chemotherapeutic agents because of its relative lack of myelotoxicity, which renders it especially suitable for remission induction; the combination of vincristine and prednisolone achieves remission in over 90% of children with newly diagnosed ALL [157] and about 50% of adults [158]. Vincristine is ineffective in most cases of AML but may have some activity in M₅ AML [20].

Toxicity. The vinca alkaloids cause alopecia, in common with many other cytotoxic agents, but are unusual in their neurotoxicity [159]. Loss of tendon reflexes and paraesthesiae are common during induction therapy with weekly vincristine, but more severe symptoms seldom occur if the treatment is limited to four to six injections of 1.5 mg/m² (maximum dose 2 mg). Severe constipation and/or weakness call for interruption of treatment and resumption at a reduced dose. Convulsions and coma, sometimes associated with inappropriate antidiuretic-hormone secretion, are an infrequent complication of therapy. Vincristine may cause neurological deterioration in patients with a preexisting neuropathy such as Charcot–Marie–Tooth syndrome [160].

Anthracyclines [161]

Daunorubicin and *doxorubicin* (Adriamycin) are fermentation products of the fungus *Streptomyces peucites*, var. *caessius*. Both consist of a tetracyclic ring attached to an unusual sugar, daunosamine. They differ only in that doxorubicin contains a hydroxyl radical on the carbon-14. *Rubidazone*, a new daunorubicin derivative, is active in all forms of AML but appears to be specifically effective in monocytic leukaemias (M₅) [162]. Both daunorubicin (DR) and doxorubicin (Adria) are widely used in remission induction in acute leukaemias, usually in combination with other drugs, but direct comparison of their efficacy is lacking [163]. Doxorubicin has been widely used in treatment of lymphomas and a number of non-haematological tumours; its increasing popularity in leukaemia stems from this widespread use and from its more favourable toxic/therapeutic ratio as regards the myocardium.

Both drugs are administered intravenously for one to three consecutive days and are sclerosant if extravasation occurs. They are taken up rapidly into cardiac, renal, bone-marrow and pulmonary tissue and excretion is mainly by the liver and biliary system. Drug dosage should probably be modified in the presence of hepatic dysfunction. The drugs are concentrated rapidly in cell nuclei, bind to DNA by intercalating between adjacent base pairs on the DNA strand, and inhibit both DNA and RNA synthesis. They also form free radical intermediates through catalysis of microsomal and nuclear electron-transport systems. These intermediates may cause damage and death of normal and malignant cells.

Toxicity. Both drugs cause alopecia, nausea and vomiting and stomatitis; the last symptom is more marked with doxorubicin. Both are profoundly myelotoxic, producing a nadir of leucocyte count 10–14 days after administration, and courses can therefore only be given at two- to three-weekly intervals. The most serious complication limiting their use is the cumulative cardiotoxicity. Transient ECG changes or arrhythmias may occur early in the course of treatment but the major complication is a severe cardiomyopathy causing congestive cardiac failure. The incidence of cardiomyopathy is dose-related [164] and the cumulative dose of both anthracyclines should not exceed 500 mg/m² surface area [165]. Toxicity may occur at lower dosage if there is a pre-existing cardiac abnormality, previous mediastinal irradiation [165] or concurrent cyclophosphamide therapy [166]. The mechanisms by which cardiotoxicity occurs is not clear; the pathological changes resemble those seen in other cardiomyopathies, with oedema between fibres, destruction of myocardial cells and disruption of sarcoplasm.

Routine ECG or echocardiography are not predictive of impending cardiac failure. It has recently been suggested that more sophisticated calculations such as ventricular ejection fraction or radionucleotide angiography may be more useful [167], but dose limitation remains the most practical precaution.

Purine analogues: 6-mercaptopurine (6MP) and 6-thioguanine (6TG) [168]

Both these purine analogues are readily absorbed by mouth and require activation before they become effective. 6-mercaptopurine (6MP) is activated to the ribonucleotide thioinosinic acid by the enzyme guanine-hypoxanthine phosphoribosyl transferase, and resistance to 6MP may be associated with decreased activity of this enzyme [169]. The activated product blocks DNA synthesis through inhibition of anabolic pathways of purine metabolism [170]. The catabolism of 6MP is mediated by xanthine oxidase and the dose of the drug should be reduced by 25–50% if the xanthine-oxidase inhibitor allopurinol is given simultaneously.

6-thioguanine (6TG), after conversion to ribonucleotide, is also incorporated into DNA and blocks purine biosynthesis; in combination with ara-C it is synergistic against L1210 mouse leukaemia [171]. No dose adjustment is required with allopurinol as the drug is not catabolized by xanthine oxidase; for this reason TG is preferred for remission induction in AML, while 6MP is chiefly used in the continuing treatment of ALL after remission has been induced.

Toxicity. Both drugs depress the bone marrow and some patients show marked sensitivity; nausea, vomiting and anorexia are not uncommon. Hepatotoxicity is an occasional complication [172].

Methotrexate (MTX)

Methotrexate superseded Aminopterin, the first folic-acid antagonist [173], and has been more intensively investigated than any other chemotherapeutic agent. Its pharmacology has been extensively reviewed [146, 174].

Methotrexate (MTX) binds reversibly to the enzyme dihydrofolate reductase, inhibiting the synthesis of tetrahydrofolate. This block depletes the intracellular pool of reduced folate, thus inhibiting a number of biochemical pathways including synthesis of purines and pyrimidines. In human leucocytes the reaction most sensitive to depletion is the biosynthesis of thymidylic acid, the nucleotide specific to DNA [175]. Methotrexate (MTX) is thus highly cell-cycle-specific, acting during DNA synthesis, although high doses may also arrest cells in G_1 by interfering with protein synthesis. The inhibition of DNA synthesis requires the presence of free intracellular MTX in excess of that binding to dihydrofolate reductase [176]. The intracellular concentration of MTX is increased by addition of vincristine which inhibits its transport out of the cell [177]. L-asparaginase antagonizes the cytotoxic effect of methotrexate by inhibiting protein synthesis and thus preventing cells entering S phase; however, when given at an appropriate time after MTX, asparaginase is able to limit marrow toxicity and the combination of the two drugs has been used to some advantage in ALL [178, 179].

In conventional doses (up to 30 mg/m^2) MTX is well absorbed from the gastro-intestinal tract; but its peak levels and speed of absorption are reduced by food [180]. There is some evidence that chronic MTX-induced malabsorption may ultimately affect the absorption pattern [181]. Following intravenous injec-

tion the drug disappears in a triphasic manner with half-lives of 60 minutes, four hours and 27 hours; over 90% of the drug is excreted by the kidney. The third phase of disappearance is particularly important in relation to marrow and gastro-intestinal toxicity and elevated levels will occur in the presence of renal damage. Administration of MTX in high dosage may in itself cause intrarenal precipitation of the drug, especially in an acid milieu, and impaired clearance. The toxic effect of MTX on organs such as the bowel and the marrow is more dependent on the duration of exposure to the drug rather than to the peak level [174].

Moderate doses of MTX (up to 360 mg/m^2) were used at one time as a single agent in treatment of ALL [182], and very large doses (several grams/m^2) can be given in schedules incorporating 'rescue' with folinic acid; this form of therapy is potentially lethal and suitable precautions are essential [174]. Folinic acid (5-formyltetrahydrofolic acid) is converted to tetrahydrofolate which repletes the reduced intracellular folate pool, so that the normal tissue is spared the effects of exposure to high MTX levels. An alternative approach to prevention of toxicity is thymidine rescue [183]. High-dose MTX has become fashionable in the treatment of certain solid tumours [184], but at the time of writing there seems little indication for its use in treatment in ALL.

Toxicity. Acute MTX toxicity usually produces gastro-intestinal symptoms—most often with mouth ulcers but also with peri-anal soreness, vomiting and diarrhoea. There may be skin desquamation and photosensitivity, and bone-marrow depression may occur with a nadir one to three weeks after the drug. Methotrexate pneumonitis resulting in fever, dyspnoea, cough and X-ray shadowing must be distinguished from opportunistic pulmonary infection. Uncommon side-effects include hepatic fibrosis and portal hypertension, osteoporosis and pulmonary fibrosis [185]. Prolonged intrathecal or parenteral methotrexate therapy in children irradiated to prevent or treat CNS leukaemia has resulted in MTX-radiation encephalopathy (see p. 862). The mechanism of MTX neurotoxicity is unknown but it has been shown that reduced folates are necessary for the metabolism of neurotransmitters in the CNS [186, 187].

L-asparaginase

This enzyme, extracted from bacterial cultures of *E. coli* or *Erwinia carotovorum*, hydrolyses the amino-acid L-asparaginase to L-aspartic acid and ammonia, and so impairs synthesis of protein and nucleic acids in leukaemic cells which are unable to produce intrinsic asparagine. It interferes with the synthetic phase of the cell cycle but also has some action on non-proliferating cells [188]; it may adversely affect other cells with a high rate of protein synthesis such as the liver and pancreas.

Toxicity. L-asparaginase can be given intravenously, intramuscularly or subcutaneously in the treatment of ALL [189]. It is not profoundly myelotoxic but may cause abnormal liver function, pancreatitis, hyperglycaemia and encephalopathy. The most alarming side-effect is hypersensitivity, which in the extreme case takes the form of an acute anaphylactic reaction [190]. If anaphylaxis occurs, treatment may be continued with L-asparaginase from another source [191].

Pyrimidine analogues [147]

Cytosine arabinoside (ara-C) is an analogue of deoxycytidine which causes competitive inhibition of DNA polymerase and is incorporated into DNA and RNA. It is transported readily into normal and neoplastic cells, where the factor determining its effectiveness is probably the degree of activation. The degree of sensitivity of leukaemic cells to ara-C probably relates to the relative activity of the kinase which metabolizes the drug to the active nucleotide and the deaminase which converts it to an inactive product, though attempts to correlate the clinical response to the drug with these enzyme levels have produced conflicting results.

Oral administration of the drug is ineffective because of deamination and it is usually given intravenously or subcutaneously. Following an injection the disappearance of the drug is biphasic, with an initial half-life of about 12 minutes and a slower second phase of about 116 minutes. When given intrathecally it is more slowly deaminated. With constant intravenous infusion the drug crosses into the CSF, producing levels about 40% of those in the plasma [192]. The drug is deaminated in the leucocytes, liver and kidney and 90% of an i.v. or s.c. dose is excreted within 24 hours. Since ara-C is effective in S phase and is rapidly deaminated, it should theoretically be maximally effective in courses comprising frequent (e.g. 12-hourly) pulses or a continuous infusion [193], and this seems to be the case in practice [194]. Its chief use is in treatment of AML, although it has been a component of several well-tried combination schedules for ALL.

Toxicity. Cytosine arabinoside almost invariably produces nausea and vomiting and marrow suppression with very marked megaloblastic change; less frequent side-effects are fever, rashes and arthralgia.

Azacytidine, another cytidine analogue, first used in

Czechoslovakia, is of interest because of an apparent lack of cross-resistance in patients with AML [195]. It resembles ara-C both structurally and in its requirement for activation and subsequent deamination. The cytotoxic effects of azacytidine have been ascribed to its incorporation into RNA, although it is also incorporated into DNA and inhibits protein and pyrimidine synthesis [196]. The main side-effects are nausea, vomiting and myelosuppression.

Cyclophosphamide [147]

Cyclophosphamide (CY) is one of a group of alkylating agents derived from nitrogen mustard in an attempt to obtain greater anti-tumour specificity. It is activated, not by tumour cells as originally supposed, but by microsomal enzymes in hepatocytes; the relative anti-tumour activity and toxicity of its various metabolites remain to be precisely defined. The first activation products are 4-hydroxycyclophosphamide in equilibrium with aldophosphamide; some aldophosphamide is degraded to phosphoramide mustard and acrolein, both of which are cytotoxic and may represent the active forms of the drug.

Although cyclophosphamide has been a component of several combination schedules, it is of limited value as a single agent in the treatment of ALL and of little use in AML, except in the context of bone-marrow transplantation. The drug can be given by mouth or intravenously; because it is inactive until metabolized, it is non-vesicant. Despite its activation in the liver, hepatic toxicity is rare and failure of activation has not been reported.

Toxicity. Cyclophosphamide (CY) inhibits reproduction of all rapidly dividing cells and like all alkylating agents, is more toxic to cells in division than to non-cycling cells. It causes alopecia, myelosuppression and vomiting. Long-term use has been followed by sterility in males [197]. High doses cause water intoxication [198, 199] and serious cardiac toxicity [166]. Cyclophosphamide has specific toxicity for the bladder; its active metabolite, acrolein, is excreted by the kidney in high concentration and may cause haemorrhagic cystitis [200, 201] and eventually hypertrophic changes in the bladder and even carcinoma [202]. Urothelial toxicity of CY can be reduced by ensuring an adequate urine volume.

Treatment of acute lymphoblastic leukaemia (ALL)

Although the same broad principles apply to treatment of ALL in both adults and children, including the need for measures designed to prevent overt leukaemic infiltration of the central nervous system, the relative refractoriness of adult ALL to therapy merits its separate consideration. Analysis of a large group of patients with ALL showed that the prognosis was best for children between four and 10 years of age at diagnosis followed by those aged one to three and 11–19 years [84]. In the British Medical Research Council (MRC) trials patients aged 14 or more at diagnosis are deemed 'adults' and qualify for a separate, usually more intensive, protocol, and this cut-off point has been used by others as well [203].

Acute lymphoblastic leukaemia (ALL) in children
The results of treatment of childhood ALL have substantially improved, with perhaps one-third of all children achieving long-term, disease-free survival. There is, however, still very considerable room for improvement and a clear need remains for prospective therapeutic trials. There is a bewildering variety of treatment schedules for childhood ALL and no attempt will be made to describe any of them in detail, although certain broad guide-lines for treatment will be delineated.

Remission induction and early intensification. The combination of daily oral prednisolone and weekly i.v. vincristine achieves remission in 85–95% of children with newly diagnosed ALL within three to six weeks; the two drugs are easily administered and non-myelotoxic and comparable results are therefore obtained in single-centre and multicentre trials [157, 204].

Failure to remit readily is most often seen in patients with B-ALL or null (unclassified) ALL, in Ph[1]-positive ALL and in patients with a very high leucocyte count. Slow response to remission induction is an unfavourable prognostic feature for long-term-remission duration [82, 83].

At the time of writing, the value of adding drugs to prednisolone and vincristine during induction, or of a period of 'intensification', remains uncertain. In theory, early intensive treatment may ensure maximal cell kill and thus improve the chances of subsequent long-term remission. An early report which purported to show no benefit from 'consolidation' may not have comprised the best drugs [133] and subsequent analyses have suggested that the use of a third drug in induction or a period of consolidation is associated with prolongation of remission [205]. The drug most widely used is L-asparaginase—in one study L-asparaginase given after prednisolone and vincristine gave superior results to a two-drug regimen or early asparaginase [206].

It might theoretically be best to give additional drugs at the very start of therapy; in this context neither POMP (prednisolone, VCR, 6MP and MTX) [207] nor COAP (CY, VCR, Ara-C and prednisolone) [91] have proved superior to prednisolone and vincris-tine. However, a recent study comprising an intensive multiple-agent eight-week induction with early daunorubicin and L-asparaginase, followed by further intensification for patients categorized as 'high risk', is producing some of the best results so far reported in childhood ALL, with 75% 'poor-risk' patients projected to remain in first remission at three years [208]. It must be accepted that any intensification of early treatment substantially increases the risk of infection during induction and suitable precautions should be available [204, 209].

In summary, there is sufficient evidence to warrant routine use of a third drug such as L-asparaginase during routine induction. The value of more intensive early treatment certainly deserves further critical investigation in centres with good supportive facilities. If remission induction is prolonged, or is followed by a period of intensification, it is imperative that CNS prophylaxis is started during induction with intrathecal MTX or cytosine arabinoside; this whole topic is discussed on page 857.

Continuing chemotherapy (maintenance treatment). The need for continued chemotherapy in ALL (so-called maintenance treatment) may be deduced from the fact that early short intensive regimens such as VAMP, POMP or BIKE [210] or the MRC's Concord [211], lasting from 15 to 65 weeks, were associated with a very high rate of leukaemic relapse after cessation of chemotherapy.

Continuing treatment with single drugs such as 6MP or MTX [135, 212] is less effective than treatment with at least two drugs. An almost unlimited variety of treatment schedules can be devised which vary in complexity from the time-honoured combination of daily continuous oral 6MP and weekly MTX [205, 206] to intermittent regimens incorporating multiple drug combinations, sometimes based on consideration of cytokinetic principles [213, 214]. An intermediate approach is that of the MRC UKALL I and UKALL II schedules [215] in which several drugs are given sequentially.

As most drugs are myelotoxic the addition of extra drugs in a continuous type of regime limits the dose of each individual drug; thus the addition of weekly cyclophosphamide and ara-C to daily 6MP and weekly MTX increased toxicity without improving disease-free survival [135]. Periodic re-intensification with prednisolone and vincristine does not substantially increase toxicity and is widely used, though of no proven benefit.

Drug doses are not compromised in an intermittent rotating treatment schedule, but these more complex regimens have proved to have no demonstrable therapeutic benefit over more conventional ones [213, 214].

Most treatment schedules which incorporate remission induction, CNS prophylaxis and continuing chemotherapy with two or more drugs result in a median duration of first complete remission in excess of three years, so that long-term follow-up is necessary to establish the benefit of any particular innovation. At the time of writing the best standard continuing treatment for children with ALL probably comprises 6MP and MTX with or without periodic addition of prednisolone and vincristine.

Duration of treatment. Because of the short-term and long-term complications of chemotherapy it is important to determine how soon it is safe to stop treatment without jeopardizing the patient's chances of survival. The optimum duration may of course vary with treatment schedule, but at present most centres would opt for at least two years of therapy.

In the MRC UKALL I trial, 84 weeks proved inferior to three years [216]; in UKALL II, three years of treatment proved no more effective than two [93]. Long-term follow-up of a small number of patients randomized to stop or continue at two and a half years showed that continuation was of no benefit [74]. Follow-up of a group of children randomized to stop or continue therapy at three years has shown a significantly lower relapse rate to date in boys continuing treatment for two further years but it is still too soon to determine whether relapses in these boys have merely been deferred [94]. For several years now an arbitrary decision to stop at two and a half years has been made at the St Jude Children's Research Hospital, where recent follow-up of 278 patients showed that one-fifth had relapsed after stopping therapy but that no patient surviving in remission for more than four and a half years off treatment had subsequently relapsed [75].

There thus appears at present to be no proven benefit in continuing chemotherapy beyond two to three years. Patients should have a bone-marrow examination at the time of stopping treatment and it is advisable that the CSF is also examined and that bilateral wedge biopsy of the testicles is performed in boys to detect occult testicular disease. The risk of relapse is maximal in the first year off treatment and is greater in boys than girls, a difference which is not wholly accounted for by the frequency of testicular relapse [75, 93].

Bone-marrow examination during the months following cessation of chemotherapy shows a rebound lymphocytosis with c-ALL antigen-positive cells [10], which may be interpreted by the unwary as leukaemic relapse.

Treatment after haematological relapse. So long as a patient with ALL continues in first complete remission, the aim of treatment is cure. Once a haematological relapse occurs during treatment, however, the prognosis is very poor [217, 218]. Although a second remission can be achieved with prednisolone/vincristine in over 60% of cases [219], and with added drugs such as anthracycline and asparaginase in over 90% [220], it hardly ever lasts as long as the first one: 80% of children in one series who had relapsed during treatment were dead within one year [217]. Children relapsing after the end of chemotherapy achieve a second remission more readily [217, 219], but the duration is seldom very long and few such patients become long-term survivors [221]. Further CNS prophylaxis, usually with intrathecal chemotherapy in the first instance, is essential in patients relapsing after cessation of treatment, who are at high risk of development of CNS leukaemia [221]. Central nervous system (CNS) prophylaxis with intrathecal chemotherapy should also be considered in children achieving second remission after relapsing during treatment, but in view of the poor remission duration, repeated lumbar punctures may not be justifiable in all cases.

Prolonged second remissions occasionally follow marrow relapse, usually when the initial treatment was sub-optimal [222] or after a long unmaintained remission [210]. For the majority of patients the outlook is poor and if facilities for bone-marrow transplantation are available this approach should be considered in patients with an available donor [402]. When CNS or testicular relapse accompanies haematological relapse, the prognosis is equally poor; the management of isolated CNS and testicular relapse is discussed below.

Prognostic features and treatment of ALL. The identification of certain clinical, haematological and immunological features which carry a high risk of relapse, such as age, presenting leucocyte count and mediastinal mass, has led to increasing stratification of treatment, certain groups of patients—for example those with T-ALL—being selected for special treatment. It is not yet established whether such patients will benefit from more intensive and more myelotoxic treatment; one group of 'high-risk' ALL did rather worse on intermittent intensive therapy than on conventional chemotherapy [91].

Acute lymphoblastic leukaemia (ALL) in adults [34]

Remission induction (Table 22.2). The combination of vincristine and prednisolone, so successful in children, achieves remission in only about 50% of adults. The use of additional drugs such as 6MP and MTX (POMP) or CY and cytosine arabinoside (COAP) has not markedly increased the proportion of patients achieving remission and in a recent prospective study COAP was found to be inferior to prednisolone and vincristine [91]. However, over 70% of patients achieve remission when prednisolone and vincristine are used with an anthracycline and/or L-asparaginase and it appears that at present these three or four drugs are the most suitable combination both for initial treatment of ALL [158, 223] and in treatment of relapsed patients [224]. Remission is less likely to be achieved in patients with Ph^1-positive ALL, who may comprise up to 25% of adults [33], and in the rare B-ALL [4].

There is a high risk of leukaemic infiltration of the nervous system at presentation or during remission induction in adult ALL [158], and CNS prophylaxis with intrathecal MTX should start early during induction. Intrathecal MTX alone has proved ineffective in adults with ALL, and cranial irradiation is also an essential component of therapy.

Continuing chemotherapy. There is no agreement about the best method of continuing chemotherapy in adult ALL. The intensive multiple-drug regimen from the Memorial Hospital gave a median remission duration of 25 months [228], the simpler combination of daily 6MP and weekly MTX and CY achieved 18·5 months [158]. More recently, an intermittent multiple-drug schedule has not proved superior to a simpler regime of 6MP and MTX [91, 223]. The paucity of these results emphasizes the need for further trials of treatment of ALL in which there is proper immunological subclassification and cytogenetic analysis of cases. Although remission can be achieved in the majority of cases and CNS prophylaxis appears essential, the best method of continuing treatment in adults remains undetermined.

Treatment of AML

In the majority of patients with AML the history is relatively short, the blood and marrow appearances are clearly diagnostic and prompt specific treatment is indicated. As remission in AML is only achieved (Fig. 22.8) after a period of marrow hypoplasia which may last several weeks and necessitates full supportive care, treatment should preferably only be undertaken in institutions which have facilities for such care.

In a minority of patients, intensive chemotherapy may not be appropriate. In the elderly, or those with associated medical problems, a less aggressive chemotherapeutic approach may be indicated [231]. An increasing number of patients have developed AML as a second malignancy following treatment of Hodgkin's disease, ovarian carcinoma or multiple myeloma [232–234], or following immunosuppressive therapy for non-malignant disease [235]: these patients, like those developing AML in the presence of a pre-existing marrow disorder (e.g. Fanconi's anaemia), respond very poorly to treatment.

Remission induction [236]

With the best present induction regimes this first objective of treatment can be achieved in at least 70% of patients. In the era of single-agent therapy drugs such as steroids, vincristine or 6MP induced remission in less than 25% of patients; and even with the use of combination chemotherapy such as POMP [237] rates of only about 30% were reported.

A major advance in treatment of AML came with the introduction of ara-C and the anthracyclines. When ara-C is given as a single agent by continuous i.v. or a 12-hourly injection, remission is achieved in about 30% of cases of AML [194, 238, 239], and its combination with thioguanine or with marginally active drugs

Table 22.2. Drugs for remission induction in adult ALL

Combination	Number of patients	Complete remission (%)	Reference
VCR + Prednisolone	41	46	203
	32	47	158
Prednisolone + VCR + MP + MTX (POMP)	38	61	225
COAP	21	43	226
VCR + Prednisolone + DR	33	73	227
	21	75	203
	23	78	228
VCR + Prednisolone + A′ase	149	58	223
VCR + Prednisolone + Adria + A′ase	51	71	158
TG + VCR + Dexamethasone + Pyrimethamine	17	53	229
Prednisolone + VCR + MTX	89	80	230

such as prednisolone, vincristine and cyclophospha-mide (COAP), produced modestly improved results (see Table 22.3). When daunorubicin was given alone for three consecutive days, remission was achieved in 35–50% of patients [240, 241]. The combination of one day of daunorubicin plus three to five days of cytosine, sometimes with other drugs, produced remissions in up to 50% of patients. The 'three-plus-seven' schedules introduced by Yates & Holland [242], in which three consecutive daily doses of anthracyclines are given with a seven-day infusion of ara-C, and sometimes with other drugs, appear to have raised the remission rate in AML to around 70% [243]. The present 'three-plus-seven' schedules have been chiefly explored with daunorubicin, but doxorubicin appears equally effective [244], though it is associated with a greater incidence of mucositis and gastro-intestinal toxicity. The immediate aim of treatment is to induce marrow hypoplasia rapidly, as illustrated in Figure 22.8, in the hope that normal marrow activity will recover after one or at most two courses. Prolongation of ara-C infusion from seven to 10 days [245] was not associated with undue toxicity and achieved remission after one course of drugs in the majority of patients.

The prognosis for AML resistant to anthracyclines and ara-C is very poor; a small minority of patients may respond to azacytidine [195] or VP-16-213, a podophyllin derivative [246] which has some activity in AML with a monocytic differentiation. Rubidazone appears to be an effective drug in monoblastic leukae-mia: 75% of 49 patients treated with this drug achieved complete remission [21].

Results from a number of trials are shown in Table 22.3, which demonstrates the variation in reported results with the use of broadly similar regimes; in general, reports from single centres are more en-couraging than those from multicentre trials, reflecting either the bias of small numbers or variability in supportive care and in expertise of the participants. An extreme example of such variation was seen in the MRC fourth and fifth AML trials [144].

Analysis of factors influencing the achievement of remission [144] suggested that age was the single most important factor. Presumably the young are less likely to have additional medical problems and are better able to withstand the effects of marrow hypoplasia. By contrast, remission rates in recent intensive single-centre studies have not been influenced by age [117, 118]. The early death rate is higher in patients of any age with high leucocyte counts and low platelet counts.

Table 22.3. Combination chemotherapy for induction in AML

Drugs	Trial*	Number of patients	Complete remission (%)	References
Standard therapy				
Ara-C + TG	M	66	26	144
	M	66	48	255
	S	88	56	256
	M	147	41	257
	M	162	44	241
CY + Ara-C + VCR + Prednisolone (COAP)	S	39	44	226
	M	66	48	258
DR + Ara-C	S	72	54	259
	M	71	42	144
	M	154	50	241
TG + DR + Ara-C + Prednisolone (TRAP)	M	68	34	144
	S	20	60	260
Intensive regimes (i.e. prolonged infusion or 12-hourly cytosine)				
DR + Ara-C	S	8	67	242
DR + Ara-C	M	46	70	261
DR + Ara-C + TG	S	28	79	117
TG + DR + Ara-C	S	22	85	118
Adria/DR + Ara-C	S	36	66	244
VCR + Adria + Prednisolone + Ara-C (VAPA)	S	83	70	262

* S = single centre; M = multicentre.

There have been few detailed analyses of response to treatment of the various FAB types of AML. Hypergranular promyelocytic leukaemia (M_3) is often associated with a haemorrhagic tendency due to DIC [114, 123, 247], but these patients tend to do well subsequently if they remit. Patients with erythroleukaemia (M_6) have been supposed to respond poorly to treatment, but a recent report [248] claims otherwise; it is possible that the difficulties in distinction of pure M_6 from RAEB may have previously led to inappropriate intensive therapy for some patients incorrectly diagnosed as erythroleukaemia. It has been suggested that therapeutic strategies might be improved by standard classification of the causes of failure to achieve remission. These would include: failure to induce hypocellularity of the bone marrow, hypocellularity with rapid regeneration of blasts, persistent hypocellularity with consequent death, usually from infection, and early death after an inadequate trial of therapy [249]. An analysis of early deaths in AML from one special centre with facilities for intensive support [250] revealed that 24 of 84 patients died within six weeks of starting treatment. Four patients died from bleeding, two within four days of admission; 13 of 20 patients dying from infection were in florid relapse two to six weeks after starting anti-leukaemic therapy, and their deaths were attributed to failure to control the underlying leukaemia rather than failure of supportive care.

There is some evidence that pre-treatment cytogenetic analysis may predict therapeutic response in AML: Golomb *et al.* [124] found that patients with myeloid leukaemia and a normal karyotype had a higher remission rate and survived longer than those with an abnormal karyotype; this correlation did not hold for myelomonocytic leukaemia.

Continuing treatment

The second major therapeutic objective in AML is the prevention of leukaemic recurrence; this objective is at present achieved in only a small minority of patients. The mechanism of leukaemic relapse is uncertain. The persistence of residual leukaemic cells is suggested by recurrence of cytogenetic abnormalities during relapse [251] or persistence of abnormal marrow-culture patterns during remission [252]. The whole concept of co-existence of normal and leukaemic cells has been questioned in AML and it has been suggested that during remission there is maturation and differentiation of leukaemic cells rather than their replacement by normal cell lines [129, 130].

Many treatment schedules include one or more courses of intensive (consolidation) therapy after remission is achieved and continuing treatment with the same or different drugs, perhaps at a lower dosage (so-called maintenance therapy). Although the first practice seems logical in view of the lack of absolute criteria for remission, and the second is widely accepted, there is little evidence that continued remission maintenance therapy is beneficial in AML.

Some results of treatment combinations used to maintain remission are shown in Table 22.4. It can be seen that even regimens which produce a high remission rate give disappointing long-term results, while some of the best results (e.g. Ref. 266) have been obtained with relatively simple regimens. Too many of the reports, however, involve single-arm studies with

Table 22.4. Remission duration in AML

Drugs used	No. of patients in remission	Median complete remission for patients remitting (weeks)	Reference
COAP	17	42	226
Multiple	102	26	144
Multiple (L6)	48	40	256
COAP	26	36	263
TRAP/COAP/POMP	15	66	260
TG + Ara-C	40	58	264
Nil	13	27 ⎫	265
TG + Ara-C	13	42 ⎭	
Nil (Immunotherapy)	15	35 ⎫	130
DR + Ara-C	17	35 ⎭	
TG + Ara-C	24	66	266
	22	40	117
	21	48	118
TG + Ara-C + CY + VCR	96	49	267

small numbers of patients. There is thus still a clear need for prospective controlled trials comparing the outcome in patients receiving no further therapy after induction with the results of intensive or conventional maintenance and of early allogeneic transplantation for patients who have an HLA-identical donor (see p. 854).

A further concept is late intensification therapy, given after some months of continued remission with the aim of eradicating residual leukaemic cells [253]. Encouraging results have been claimed for this form of treatment but the fact that such patients have already survived long enough to receive it must bias the results in its favour; late intensification needs to be tested by controlled trials.

Routine prophylaxis against leukaemic infiltration of the CNS, at least with irradiation, is not at present recommended in AML and has not been shown to improve survival in children or adults [117, 254] (see p. 858). The use of immunotherapy in AML is reviewed below; the present situation can be summarized by saying that immunotherapy has a marginal effect on survival after relapse but does not significantly affect overall prognosis.

Immunotherapy in the treatment of acute leukaemias [268]

There have been a number of trials of immunotherapy in the acute leukaemias. These have their theoretical basis in studies of certain animal tumours [269] in which tumour-specific antigens may be detected, and in which specific immunotherapy can prevent the development of an engrafted tumour or cause regression of established disease. In a series of experiments in mice with L1210 leukaemia, active immunotherapy with irradiated blast cells and/or BCG eradicated residual disease in some animals when the tumour load was low [270]. Thus by inference, immunotherapy in human leukaemia might be effective in prolonging remission and enabling the host's immune system to eradicate minimal residual disease. It should be emphasized, however, that despite extensive investigations in this field there is no direct evidence for the presence of tumour-specific antigens in human leukaemia and lymphoma [271]. The recent explosion of interest in the production of xenogeneic antibodies to human leukaemia cells (Chapter 21) has not resulted, to date, in detection of any antigen which is truly leukaemia-specific. All the available evidence suggests that the various antigens recognized by such antibodies are differentiation antigens present on normal cell precursors and subsequently lost during maturation.

Most attempts to use immunotherapy in man have involved non-specific stimulation with BCG or *Corynebacterium parvum* and/or 'specific' immunotherapy with irradiated allogeneic leukaemic cells, chosen because of the logistic problems in collection and processing of autologous cells. Comprehensive reviews of recent trials are available [116, 272] and only a few examples are cited here.

Acute lymphoblastic leukaemia (ALL)

The first clinical study of active immunotherapy in the acute leukaemias was that of Mathé and his colleagues [273], in which a group of children who had received two years of chemotherapy were given either no further treatment or immunotherapy with BCG by scarification, killed allogeneic leukaemic cells or both; all of the patients in the control group relapsed but some of the patients receiving immunotherapy remained in prolonged remission. Unfortunately, the control group did unusually badly while the immunotherapy group did no better than many other series of patients treated by chemotherapy alone. The original claims have never been either confirmed or disproved, but Mathé has subsequently claimed [274] that the benefits of immunotherapy are confined to certain morphological subtypes of ALL: the validity of this morphological classification is not universally recognized and it does not correlate with the recent FAB classification.

The precise conditions of Mathé's original trial have never been duplicated, but two multicentre studies [211, 275] have failed to show that patients with ALL in remission after a short course of chemotherapy are benefited by subsequent treatment with BCG; continuing chemotherapy was more effective in prolonging remissions. The long remissions now achieved in many patients with ALL using conventional chemotherapy preclude further investigation of early immunotherapy alone in treatment.

Acute myeloid leukaemia (AML)

Among the first trials of immunotherapy in AML were those of the St Bartholomew's Hospital/Royal Marsden Hospital group; the history of these trials and the pitfalls in their analysis have recently been reviewed [116]. Patients with AML who achieved remission were randomized to receive monthly chemotherapy, with or without the addition of immunotherapy in the form of BCG and irradiated allogeneic myeloblastic leukaemia cells. A preliminary analysis of the results [276] suggested that the addition of immunotherapy prolonged remission duration, but further follow-up failed to confirm this impression and suggested that the only influence of immunotherapy was on survival after relapse [277]. The combination of i.v. BCG and maintenance chemotherapy also appeared to prolong survival but not remission duration [278], and a multicentre trial also suggested that immunotherapy had this effect [279]. Reports from other centres that intradermal BCG alone prolonged remission duration in AML [280, 281] have not subsequently been confirmed [282].

It is apparent from all these reports that 'specific' or non-specific immunotherapy, while not prolonging initial remission duration, has a marginal effect on survival after relapse. It has been confirmed from several centres that patients with AML who have received immunotherapy more readily achieve a second remission; the reasons for this are not clear [283].

The role of bone-marrow transplantation in the treatment of acute leukaemia [284–286]

Thirty years ago it was observed that mice given lethal irradiation could be protected by infusion of spleen or marrow cells. Early attempts to transplant human bone marrow were made on terminally ill patients and not surprisingly, in view of the inadequate bloodproduct support available, poor understanding of the histocompatibility system and many complications, the results were extremely discouraging.

Following an era of basic research resulting in increased understanding of the HLA system, experimental transplantation in the dog and the pioneering work of the Seattle team on human bone-marrow transplantation, there has been a steady improvement in the reported results of allogeneic transplantation for acute leukaemia, although many problems remain to be solved. At the time of writing it appears that this form of treatment may offer a chance of long-term remission to certain patients with acute leukaemia. Allogeneic transplantation is based on the concept of destroying all leukaemic cells with marrow-ablative doses of chemotherapy and radiotherapy and repopulating the marrow with cells taken from a normal donor.

Selection of a donor

In marrow grafts between identical twins (syngeneic) there is no immunological barrier to transplantation. The vast majority of grafts, however, must involve allogeneic transplantation and thus carry the risk of graft rejection by the host or reaction of the donor cells against the host—graft-versus-host disease (GVHD). The major histocompatibility complex (MHC), located on chromosome 6, plays a determinant role in the degree of compatibility between donor and recipient (see Chapter 34). The complex is made up of the HLA-A, B and C loci, whose antigens are recognized by cytotoxic antisera obtained by immunization or following pregnancy, and the closely associated lymphocyte-detected HLA-D locus which governs reactivity in mixed lymphocyte cultures (MLC). Despite the large number of possible alleles at each locus, these closely linked antigens are usually inherited as a single haplotype, one from each parent. There is thus a 25% chance that any one of his siblings will be HLA-identical with the patient. Of course, HLA identity does not imply identity with other, as yet unidentified, loci, which may mediate graft rejection or GVHD. The use of random, or haplo-identical donors is an experimental concept at present, although success with an unrelated HLA-identical donor has been reported [287].

Although ABO incompatibility is not a contraindication to successful marrow grafting, patients with antibodies against the donor's red cells require plasma exchange with donor-type plasma followed by wholeblood exchange with donor-type red cells.

The harvesting of bone marrow is performed under a general or spinal anaesthetic through multiple punctures, obtaining 2–3 ml/aspirate until the desired dose of marrow, usually about 3×10^8 cells/kg body weight (a volume of 250–1000 ml), has been obtained. No untoward complications have been observed from this procedure in the largest series of procedures reported [286], although red-cell replacement may be necessary. To avoid transfusion complications it is desirable to bleed the donor some days before this procedure to facilitate auto-transfusion.

Preparation of the recipient

The aim of preparation of the recipient is to eradicate residual leukaemic cells and to prevent graft rejection. It is necessary to draw a balance between too little preparation, which carries the risk of leukaemic recurrence, and too much preparation, which may prove unacceptably toxic [288]. Thus irradiation, using totalbody irradiation (TBI) in a dose of 920 rad at 5–8 rad/minute, and cyclophosphamide (CY), 45–50 mg/kg/day for four days (as used in aplastic anaemia), were each, when used independently, accompanied by a high risk of recurrent leukaemia. The Seattle group have most frequently employed the combination of CY 60 mg/kg for two doses and irradiation 920 rad. Other, more intensive, regimens are currently under study, for example SCARI (6-thioguanine (6TG), CY, ara-C, daunorubicin and irradiation) [289], but at present it appears that the major infective complications of such regimens outweigh the decreased risk of leukaemic recurrence. Total-body irradiation (TBI) is a component of most therapeutic schedules but regimes which rely on chemotherapy alone are under investigation [290].

Subsequent treatment of the recipient

After preparation and transfusion of marrow the recipient undergoes a post-transplant period of aplasia lasting 10–20 days (Fig. 22.9) before the graft begins to function, during which time 'prophylactic' platelet support is necessary and antibiotics and granulocytes are needed if there is evidence of infection. All blood products should be irradiated to prevent transfusion of immunocompetent lymphocytes which may cause GVHD.

During the post-transplant aplasia, patients—like those with AML undergoing intensive therapy without bone-marrow transplant—are at increased risk of bacterial and fungal infection [291]. It would seem logical to attempt to reduce this risk by the use of a protective environment, special diet and oral non-absorbable antibiotics, but in practice many patients have been nursed in single rooms without these expensive measures. A recent prospective study revealed no firm evidence that patients with leukaemia undergoing allogeneic transplantation benefited from intensive isolation; the major mortality was due to interstitial pneumonitis and recurrent leukaemia [292].

It is customary to give immunosuppression after transplantation in an attempt to prevent GVHD; the drug most widely used in this context is MTX but other measures are discussed below.

Clinical results

Long-term follow-up of a group of patients with leukaemia refractory to chemotherapy who received marrow transplantation from an identical-twin donor showed that six of 16 patients were well and receiving no treatment four to six years later [293]. The first

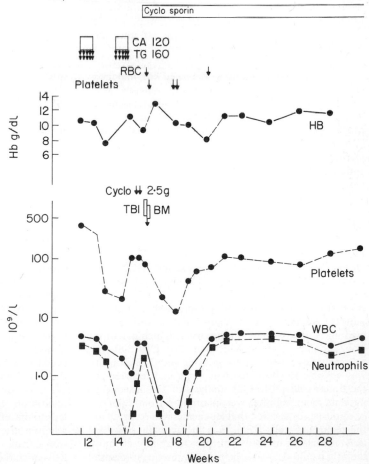

Fig. 22.9. Bone-marrow transplantation for AML in remission. Data by courtesy of Dr H. E. M. Kay. TBI = whole body irradiation, 920 rads; BM = infusion of allogeneic marrow.

encouraging report for the majority of patients, who do not have an identical twin, involved 100 patients with refractory acute leukaemia who received marrow from an HLA-identical sibling donor [294]. Patients were treated with CY and TBI; engraftment was achieved in 94, and only one of these subsequently rejected the graft; thirteen patients were alive and well one to four and a half years after transplantation and four survived with recurrent leukaemia. The major causes of death were GVHD, interstitial pneumonia, infection and recurrent leukaemia. There has been no prospective controlled trial of the benefits of transplantation in resistant leukaemia but the proportion of long-term survivors is probably sufficient evidence in itself [294, 295].

The next logical move, to offer the procedure to patients with a poor prognosis at an earlier stage in their disease, is at present under evaluation in several major centres [296–299]. At present the most clearly defined role is in AML and encouraging preliminary results have followed marrow transplantation in patients in first remission. Twelve of 19 patients so treated remained in remission and median post-graft survival was in excess of 21 months. It must be emphasized that these were a selected group of patients, several of whom had already survived in remission for some months: the need for matched comparisons, if not a controlled trial, remains. The role of transplantation in ALL is as yet unclarified, although a case can be made for its use in poor prognostic groups in first remission. Thomas *et al.* [299] reported that 50% of patients with ALL transplanted in second or subsequent remission were well and in remission at two years, an outlook substantially better than that for patients who have conventional treatment after a marrow relapse during therapy, although longer follow-up is clearly needed to confirm these results.

Problems

Despite the note of encouragement sounded by recent results, major problems remain. The chief of these are:

Recurrence of leukaemia. This is more likely to occur in patients transplanted in relapse and/or with extra-medullary disease than in those transplanted in remission, and more likely in ALL than AML [299, 300]. In two early cases prepared for grafting with TBI alone it was possible to show that leukaemia had recurred in the donor cells [301, 302]; analysis of 11 subsequent patients relapsing after transplantation from a donor of opposite sex showed that leukaemia had recurred in the recipients' cells [286]. It is theoretically possible that increased intensity of pre-transplant chemo-therapy would decrease the risk of subsequent relapse

but the possible benefits of such regimes appear at present to be outweighed by their toxicity [288].

Interstitial pneumonia. This complication occurs most frequently after marrow recovery during the second and third months after transplantation and is characterized by fever, tachypnoea, hypoxia and interstitial pulmonary infiltration. A variety of causes have been invoked for this syndrome, including cytomegalovirus [291, 303] and *Pneumocystis carinii*, but clear evidence of such agents is not present in many cases. The role of cytotoxic drugs such as MTX and of the dose and rate of administration of radiotherapy remains uncertain [286].

Graft-versus-host disease (GVHD). Despite efforts at prophylaxis with MTX, approximately 70% of patients develop some degree of GVHD. The principal organs involved are the skin, liver and gastro-intestinal tract; a system for scoring of severity has been described [285]. The disease may cause death with progressive skin lesions, jaundice and profuse diar-rhoea. Chronic GVHD chiefly involves the skin and can cause a chronic disabling syndrome resembling scleroderma.

It has been suggested that GVHD results from an attack by donor lymphocytes against non-HLA-determined histocompatibility antigens, although GVHD has been reported in recipients of marrow transplants from identical twins [304]: an association between natural killer-cell activity and GVHD has been postulated [305, 306] and imbalances of immuno-regulatory T-cell subsets have been described [307]. The drug most widely used to prevent the condition is MTX; a variety of treatments including steroids and antithymocyte globulin have been used in treatment of the established disease. Most recently cyclosporin A has shown encouraging results in treatment of GVHD [308] and is under evaluation for prevention of this complication [297]. An alternative approach is to destroy the donor lymphocytes which mediate GVHD by treating marrow *in vitro* with an anti-T serum, on the assumption that immunological reconstitution of the recipient will be achieved by maturation of stem cells or early lymphoid cells [309].

In experimental bone-marrow transplantation in the mouse, it is possible by suitable timing of immunosup-pressive therapy [310], or by prior alloimmunization of the donor [311], to obtain a graft-versus-leukaemia effect. It remains uncertain whether allogeneic trans-plantation may be associated with graft-versus-leukaemia effect in man. Two boys with ALL who relapsed after marrow engraftment went into remis-sion during subsequent GVHD without specific anti-leukaemic therapy [312]. The relation between GVHD and leukaemia was examined in 242 marrow recipients and it was tentatively concluded that the anti-leukaemic effect of GVHD was offset by the greater probability of other causes of death when this complication occurred [313]. The data appeared to show that the anti-leukaemic effect of GVHD was more marked in patients with ALL and in patients transplanted in relapse.

Autologous marrow transplantation

In view of the many complications associated with allogeneic marrow transplantation and the absence of suitable donors for the majority of patients, there has been interest in the use of cryopreserved autologous marrow. The viability of the cryopreserved stem cells has been demonstrated in the dog [314] and attempts have been made to use cryopreserved human marrow in treatment of malignancy. While this approach is logical as a means of enabling very intensive chemotherapy to be given to patients with non-haemopoietic malignancy, it seems inherently likely that stored marrow from patients with acute leukaemia, even when taken during apparently complete remission, would contain residual leukaemic cells. This approach has not so far proved successful in patients with disseminated non-Hodgkin (Burkitt-like) lymphoma [315] and although 11 of 21 patients with relapsed leukaemia treated with chemotherapy, TBI and autologous marrow were recently reported to achieve remission, the median duration of this remission was only four months [316].

Clearly if it becomes feasible to remove residual leukaemic cells *in vitro*, autologous marrow might have a place in management of acute leukaemia. Preliminary attempts to utilize this approach in c-ALL have been reported [317], but it must be remembered that removal of c-ALL antigen-positive cells may deplete stem-cell or early lymphoid populations, thus delaying or preventing marrow recovery. With increasing availability of monoclonal antibodies, this approach may become applicable in T- or B-ALL with preservation of more primitive stem cells. An alternative approach could be treatment of marrow with drugs with selective toxicity, such as 2-deoxycoformycin, a selective inhibitor of adenosine deaminase which attacks lymphoid cells and spares other haemopoietic cells [318].

EXTRAMEDULLARY LEUKAEMIA [319]

Investigations on patients in apparent clinical and haematological remission, either by multiple biopsies in life [139] or at post-mortem examination [140], have shown that despite marrow remission, there may be residual disease in many other organs. The two most important sites where disease may become clinically apparent when patients are in a state of haematological remission are the central nervous system and the testis.

THE CENTRAL NERVOUS SYSTEM (CNS)

As prolonged haematological remissions became more common, particularly in ALL, leukaemic infiltration of the CNS was noted in an increasing number of patients [320, 321]. The clinical features of CNS leukaemia in children with ALL are usually those of increased intracranial pressure—headache, vomiting, papilloedema and sixth-nerve paresis—but in adults, signs of focal CNS involvement such as cranial-nerve palsies, hemiplegia and paraplegia may also be seen [322]. Excessive appetite and weight gain are symptomatic of leukaemic infiltration of the hypothalamic region.

The diagnosis of leukaemic infiltration of the CNS should be confirmed by examination of a cytocentrifuge preparation of the cerebrospinal fluid, in which leukaemic blast cells are almost invariably seen. The distinction of leukaemic blast cells from 'reactive' mononuclear cells can be difficult; recent developments such as immunofluorescent estimation of TDT [43] may be helpful in this context. There is usually an increased cell count and the CSF glucose may be reduced. It is difficult to diagnose leukaemic infiltration of the CNS in the absence of leukaemic cells in the CSF, but computerized axial tomography may be helpful in this situation and the differential diagnosis must include the other non-leukaemic neurological complications (see p. 862).

The frequency of CNS leukaemia varies, but in the absence of specific 'prophylactic' measures it may eventually occur in over 80% of children with ALL remaining in haematological remission. The time of onset is influenced by the leucocyte count at presentation; it tends to occur earlier in patients with a high leucocyte count [323] but it is almost impossible to define a group of children free from risk of CNS infiltration. As survival improves in adult ALL, as many as 50% of patients develop symptoms of CNS involvement [34, 324] and a higher proportion have involvement at autopsy. Similarly, improved survival in AML has been associated with an increased incidence of CNS disease [325]. It seems probable that CNS involvement in AML may more frequently take the form of local deposits [326].

Pathophysiology of CNS involvement

A variety of pathological features have been described in association with leukaemic infiltration of the CNS [327]. These include infiltrations of the dura mater and nodular leukaemic lesions in the brain, but the most common finding, especially in ALL, is that of infiltration of the arachnoid mater [324, 328]. The infiltration follows a predictable anatomical pattern, the earliest evidence of which is infiltration in the walls of the superficial veins of the arachnoid mater, progressing to destruction of the arachnoid trabeculae and contamination of the CSF, dense infiltration of the superficial arachnoid and of the deep arachnoid penetrating the brain and spinal cord. Involvement of the superficial tissues causes interference with local perfusion due to compression of blood vessels and obstruction to the flow of CSF, and thus symptoms of raised intracranial pressure; while deeper infiltration may cause focal neurological signs. These observations may not be relevant to the formation of a local leukaemic mass in AML but appear to explain the insidious onset of symptoms in ALL.

It seems likely that CNS infiltration occurs at around the time of initial diagnosis of leukaemia, when there are a large number of circulating leukaemic cells [323]. This early infiltration is uninfluenced by administration of drugs to induce haematological remission, since in the conventional regimes given they do not penetrate the CNS in sufficient concentration. In the absence of measures to eradicate occult CNS leukaemia the cells proliferate, often very slowly [329], with the eventual development of overt leukaemic infiltration of the nervous system.

'Central nervous system prophylaxis'

Established leukaemic infiltration of the CNS is hard to eradicate, tends to recur and may lead to chronic disability in patients whose leukaemia is otherwise under control. It remains unclear whether or not CNS relapse is followed by increased risk of haematological relapse. An essential component of management of ALL, although not yet in regular use in AML, is treatment designed to prevent overt leukaemic infiltration of the nervous system—so-called 'CNS prophylaxis', though it presumably consists of the eradication of small numbers of leukaemic cells which have already infiltrated the CNS. Children with ALL who receive CNS prophylaxis have a higher chance of long-term survival [330, 331] than those given appropriate treatment after the clinical onset of CNS leukaemia.

In a remarkable series of prospective clinical trials from St Jude Children's Research Hospital it was shown that overt leukaemic infiltration of the CNS in children with ALL could not be prevented by prophylactic craniospinal irradiation in a dose of 1200 R, but could be prevented in the majority of children by 2400 R to the whole craniospinal axis, or by cranial irradiation at this dose with a concurrent course of five intrathecal MTX injections [332]; the latter method

was associated with less myelosuppression and serious infection and has since been preferred by the St Jude group. Confirmation of the value of CNS prophylaxis was obtained in a larger series of patients given 2400 R cranial irradiation, 1200 R to the spine and intrathecal MTX injections [331]. Comparison of this regime with full-dose (2400 R) craniospinal irradiation and with cranial irradiation alone plus intrathecal MTX showed that full-dose craniospinal irradiation was associated with a higher risk of marrow relapse, especially in patients with a high leucocyte count at presentation [93]. These studies did not explore the value of doses of cranial irradiation between 1200 and 2400 R, but it now appears that 1800 R may be adequate [403]. Attempts have been made to use repeated low doses of fractionated radiotherapy [334], but these have not received widespread acceptance.

Is cranial irradiation an essential component of 'CNS prophylaxis', or can effective prophylaxis be achieved by intrathecal MTX alone, by the lumbar or intraventricular route, or by parenteral MTX at moderate dosage? A course of six intrathecal MTX injections by lumbar puncture is inadequate for 'prophylaxis' [333]. Administration of MTX by an Ommaya intraventricular reservoir produces more reliable CSF distribution than administration by lumbar puncture [335]; it has been advocated for patients with high leucocyte counts at presentation following the observation of a high rate of CNS relapse in such patients who had received intrathecal MTX by lumbar puncture alone [336]. Another method under investigation is the use of intravenous MTX infusions at 500 mg/m^2 [337], which produce therapeutic levels in the CSF.

All patients with ALL should receive CNS prophylaxis once haematological remission is achieved; in adults and in children receiving prolonged induction, prophylaxis with intrathecal chemotherapy should start during induction. Prophylaxis should probably comprise cranial irradiation in a dose of the order of 1800–2400 R and a course of at least five intrathecal MTX injections. The only patients in whom this approach is not appropriate are very young children (certainly under one year and possibly under two), in whom it is desirable to defer cranial irradiation in view of the probable neurological and psychological sequelae [338], and to give regular intrathecal MTX alone in the first instance.

The role of CNS prophylaxis in AML is less clearly defined, although this complication does appear to be increasing in frequency [325]. Craniospinal irradiation was of no benefit in one group of children with AML [254] and cranial irradiation and intrathecal MTX did not improve remission duration or survival in adults with AML [117]. At present a reasonable compromise would seem to be the use of intrathecal cytosine arabinoside and/or MTX in patients with AML achieving remission.

Treatment of overt CNS leukaemia

A small number of patients with ALL, including a relatively high proportion of those with B-ALL, have CNS leukaemia at the time of presentation; this is a uniformly poor prognostic feature [78]. Treatment of this complication usually comprises weekly intrathecal MTX and, once complete remission is achieved, cranial irradiation and continuing intrathecal chemotherapy. For the five to 10% of patients with ALL who develop CNS relapse despite prophylaxis, treatment with weekly intrathecal MTX is usually successful in inducing a remission which may be prolonged by continuing to give MTX every four to six weeks for at least two to three years [339], though the disease is hard to eradicate. Longer CNS remissions may be obtained by the use of an Ommaya reservoir [340] or by further irradiation, which should preferably be craniospinal [341, 342], but this does carry a risk of leucoencephalopathy. Further irradiation is essential in cases with localized leukaemic deposits or hypothalamic infiltration. Intrathecal ara-C may be effective in patients resistant to MTX [343].

In summary, the management of overt CNS leukaemia depends on the anatomical site and previous therapy. In the previously unirradiated patient, craniospinal irradiation in a dose order of 2400 R is effective [330, 339]. For the patient who has received prophylactic radiotherapy, the alternatives are either regular intraventricular chemotherapy via an Ommaya reservoir or regular lumbar punctures with further irradiation at an appropriate time, bearing in mind the risk of neurological complications. The combination of radiotherapy and intraventricular chemotherapy is to be avoided. Although CNS leukaemia may be compatible with very long-term survival [339], and it remains uncertain whether it is followed by an increased risk of marrow relapse, it seems prudent to give systemic re-induction therapy at the time of CNS relapse, followed by further maintenance therapy.

TESTICULAR INFILTRATION

Leukaemic infiltration of the testicles presents as a painless swelling of one or both organs. The diagnosis is confirmed by needle or wedge biopsy; the infiltration is usually bilateral even if only one testis appears clinically involved. The incidence of leukaemic infiltration appears to vary between centres and with treatment protocols; in a recent report [344] the incidence was 13% and in a series from one hospital, 15% [319].

The reasons for the variable prevalence of testicular leukaemia are not clear but may relate to the type and intensity of systemic chemotherapy; a low incidence of testicular relapse has been reported in a schedule which included long-term doxorubicin [345] and another incorporating intensive induction and consolidation [208]. Testicular infiltration may occur during treatment in patients with a high leucocyte count at diagnosis [344, 346], but the main incidence is within one year of stopping treatment [95, 344, 346].

At the time of testicular relapse the marrow and CNS may be in apparent remission, but more extensive investigation in one small group of such patients, including lymphography and staging laparotomy, showed para-aortic lymph-node involvement in some cases, indicating that the disease was not truly localized [347].

Treatment. This consists of radiotherapy for isolated testicular relapse probably in the dose order of 2400 R [348] to both testicles, and re-introduction of systemic chemotherapy; additional CNS prophylaxis is desirable and a further course of intrathecal MTX injections seems reasonable in these circumstances. Patients treated with local radiotherapy alone usually soon develop haematological relapse. Despite the evidence cited that testicular disease is rarely localized, the prognosis for boys with 'isolated' testicular relapse, at least in the short term, is better than for those with marrow involvement at the time of relapse [349].

OTHER EXTRAMEDULLARY SITES

The CNS and the testicles are by far the commonest extramedullary sites of involvement in ALL. *Skin* infiltration is not uncommon in acute monocytic (M_5) leukaemia, either at presentation or relapse, and is a feature of the rare congenital leukaemia. *Ovarian* relapse is seldom recorded [350] and patients with ALL very occasionally relapse with lymphomatous infiltration of *lymph nodes* and a clear bone marrow. *Splenomegaly* is occasionally noted as an isolated finding during treatment of ALL; this is seldom due to leukaemic relapse but more often associated with portal fibrosis or chronic infection [351, 352]. *Ocular* involvement is usually seen in association with CNS or haematological relapse [353, 354], but leukaemic iritis and hypopyon may occasionally be the only manifestations of recurrence [355].

COMPLICATIONS OF TREATMENT

COMPLICATIONS DURING INDUCTION

Electrolyte disturbances [356]

A variety of electrolyte disturbances may occur during

the early stages of treatment of acute leukaemia. Rapid lysis of malignant cells in response to cytotoxic therapy (particularly common in patients with T- and B-cell leukaemias) can cause hyperkalaemia, hyperphosphataemia and hypermagnesaemia and consequent hypocalcaemia. These complications account for a proportion of early deaths in patients with ALL. The same electrolytic disturbances may develop as a result of acute renal failure due to uric-acid nephropathy. Hyperkalaemia should be assessed by electrocardiogram (ECG) because spurious hyperkalaemia may occur with lysis of leucocytes *in vitro* in patients with very high counts. A low serum potassium is common in AML and may be associated with renal tubular loss of potassium due to lysozyme-induced tubular damage.

The electrolyte disturbances are frequently compounded by drugs used in the treatment of acute leukaemia; for example the antibiotics gentamicin, cephalosporins and carbenicillin can all cause renal potassium loss. Other specific abnormalities include the inappropriate ADH secretion which may follow vincristine and the hypocalcaemia, hypophosphataemia and hyperphosphaturia associated with L-asparaginase therapy.

Patients with acute leukaemia, particularly those with a large cell mass and those with AML undergoing prolonged treatment with cytotoxics and antibiotics, should have regular monitoring of serum electrolytes to permit the early application of appropriate corrective measures.

Urate nephropathy [357]

The most widely recognized biochemical complication of acute leukaemia is the raised serum uric acid which may occur at presentation in patients with a large cell mass, but more often follows successful initiation of treatment. The purines liberated by lysis of leukaemic cells are converted to hypoxanthine and then to xanthine and uric acid by the enzyme xanthine oxidase. Intraluminal deposition of uric acid in the renal parenchyma can cause acute renal failure; this deposition is more likely to occur in the presence of dehydration and acidosis.

Urate nephropathy can be prevented in the majority of cases by administration of allopurinol, 300–600 mg/m^2/day in divided doses, and by ensuring adequate hydration and alkalinization of urine, particularly in patients with a large cell mass. This is effected with intravenous fluids 3000 ml/m^2 for 24 hours, with addition of NaHCO$_3$ to ensure a urine pH between 7·0 and 7·5. Allopurinol blocks the action of xanthine oxidase, preventing formation of uric acid; it does not obviate the necessity for hydration and alkalinization and large doses, particularly in dehydrated patients, may cause precipitation of xanthine crystals. Allo-purinol enhances the action of 6MP by blocking its catabolism by xanthine oxidase; the dose of 6MP should be quartered if both drugs are given together, or thioguanine may be given instead.

Hyperviscosity [358, 359]

Patients with acute leukaemia and a very high leucocyte count, like those with paraproteinaemias, may present with symptoms of the hyperviscosity syndrome: lethargy, unsteady gait, visual disturbances and coma. Early blood transfusion is contraindicated and treatment should be directed in the first instance towards reducing the leucocyte count, in selected cases by leucapheresis.

Haemorrhage

Despite improvements in supportive care, fatal intracranial haemorrhage may occur in up to 1 in 6 patients with newly diagnosed AML and in occasional patients with ALL [250]. Those with a high leucocyte count and with mucous-membrane and fundal haemorrhages are particularly at risk: thrombocytopenia may or may not be associated with evidence of disseminated intravascular coagulation (DIC). This is an almost invariable accompaniment of hypergranular promyelocytic leukaemia (M$_5$) [123], but may occur in any type of AML. The risk of haemorrhage is exacerbated by early blood transfusion in patients with a high leucocyte count.

The mainstay of management in patients at risk of bleeding, with or without DIC, is liberal use of platelet concentrates. These should be given to thrombocytopenic patients with counts of less than $20 \times 10^9/l$ or with any sign of bleeding; they should be used more liberally in patients with mucosal or fundal haemorrhages and with DIC. Debate continues about the use of prophylactic platelet transfusions, but it must be remembered in this context that there is little risk of sensitization to platelet antigens during the temporary aplasia following remission induction in AML or marrow transplantation. Platelets are usually given routinely in patients following transplantation to maintain a count of greater than $20 \times 10^9/l$, and many centres would similarly advocate prophylactic use during intensive induction schedules for AML. In the steady state, platelet transfusion twice weekly [360] should maintain adequate haemostasis; in practice the requirements are often greater because of bleeding or infection.

Bleeding in association with DIC may of course occur with high platelet counts, but here also, despite the rapid platelet consumption, the mainstay of treatment is liberal use of platelet concentrates; heparin has been advocated in this situation [123] but is less important than reduction of circulating blasts and optimal support with blood products.

Infection

Now that effective measures are available for the control of bleeding, the most frequent problem during remission induction in acute leukaemia is infection. A detailed review of the prevention and management of infection is outside the scope of this book, but a few general comments may be made.

The risk of infection during remission induction is proportional to the duration and severity of the neutropenia; serious infection is thus rarely seen in children with ALL undergoing standard remission induction with prednisolone and vincristine, but intensification of the induction regimen increases the risk of infection [209]; by contrast few patients undergoing remission induction for AML under standard ward conditions will escape a course of antibiotic therapy.

It is clearly desirable, in patients in whom marrow aplasia is anticipated, to introduce measures to try and prevent the acquisition of infection [361]. Basic precautions include provision of a single room, exclusion of visitors with infections, meticulous attention to hand washing before attending to the patient, and minimal use of in-dwelling catheters. In addition to these measures designed to prevent acquisition of infection from the environment, a variety of non-absorbable antibiotics have been given by mouth to try and prevent the patient becoming infected by his bowel flora. The combination of oral non-absorbable antibiotics and topical antiseptics [362] may be effective in reducing the acquisition of infections; unfortunately these antibiotics are nauseating, may produce diarrhoea and are frequently rejected by the patients. An attractive alternative is the use of prophylactic co-trimoxazole [361, 363], but in view of the potential hazards of drug resistance and bacterial overgrowth this alternative should await results of a proper prospective trial.

There is less agreement about the desirability of more expensive measures such as the prophylactic sterile environment; the role of such measures has been extensively reviewed [364]; although they may cause a decrease in febrile days and antibiotic usage in protected patients, they have for the most part failed to show an advantage in terms of remission induction or survival. Indeed in centres with optimum supportive care, death from infection in AML is usually associated with drug-resistant disease [250].

Infection during remission induction in a newly diagnosed patient with acute leukaemia is usually bacterial: common organisms include *Staph. aureus*, *E. coli*, *Pseudomonas aeruginosa* and *Klebsiella* spp. Although candidal infection is also seen, serious systemic fungal infection is not a common problem in the newly diagnosed patient with acute leukaemia.

In the absence of neutrophils there may be few or no signs of local infection, and fever or malaise may be the sole symptom of a septicaemia which, if untreated, may lead to death in a matter of hours. On suspicion of infection in a neutropenic patient, appropriate cultures should be taken and empirical broad-spectrum antibiotic therapy started. The initial choice of antibiotics will be dictated by local probabilities and is the subject of trials such as those organized by the EORTC; a suitable combination might be gentamicin and carbenicillin [365], but the drugs must be altered as the results of microbiological investigations become available; if there is apparent response, therapy should be continued for a minimum of five to seven days even if cultures prove negative [366]. Although it is difficult to give precise recommendations for the use of granulocyte transfusions, there is now widespread acceptance that these are of benefit in the severely neutropenic patient with Gram-negative infection [367–369]. It would seem that patients most likely to benefit are those with proven infection without likelihood of immediate marrow recovery, to whom transfusions should be given for a minimum of four days. The logistics of granulocyte transfusions are discussed in Chapter 35.

LONG-TERM COMPLICATIONS OF TREATMENT

It is perhaps a reflection of the modest success that has been achieved in the treatment of the acute leukaemias that this problem now merits consideration; regrettably the only sizeable population of long-term survivors is of children treated for ALL.

Immunosuppression

Continued treatment in ALL carries the risk of serious infection and death in remission [140]. Remission deaths are more likely in young patients [370] and those with low leucocyte counts at presentation [215]. Although treatment may cause neutropenia and transient disorders of granulocyte function have been described, for example following craniospinal irradiation [371], the risk of infection is in the main related to the degree of immunosuppression, as reflected in the lymphocyte count [372].

A variety of exotic infections have been described during continued treatment of acute leukaemia [364], but the most serious hazards are the common exanthemata, measles and varicella zoster; other childhood infections are not especially hazardous [370]. Measles may cause giant-cell pneumonia or encephalitis in the absence of a rash [373] and varicella zoster may be associated with visceral dissemination, pneumonia or encephalitis [374]. There is no effective treatment for established measles infection but acyclovir [378] shows some promise in treatment of varicella-zoster infections. Patients with no history of previous infection or immunization and no detectable immunity should receive prophylactic immune globulin as soon after exposure as possible. Live measles vaccine, like other live vaccines [375], is contraindicated during therapy, although a live varicella vaccine has been given during treatment of ALL without apparent ill effect [376, 377]. *Pneumocystis carinii* pneumonia causes cough, tachypnoea and pulmonary infiltration, often in the absence of clinical signs; it should be distinguished from other interstitial pneumonias such as those due to cytomegalovirus and measles. The incidence of *Pneumocystis* pneumonitis is related to intensity of treatment [379]; co-trimoxazole is effective both in prophylaxis of high-risk patients [380] and in treatment of established infection [381], although occasional cases are resistant to co-trimoxazole and require treatment with pentamidine isethionate.

Immunity recovers gradually after treatment is stopped and this is reflected in the rebound lymphocytosis in the bone marrow, which may be wrongly interpreted as leukaemic relapse.

Second malignancy
It is to be expected that a number of patients will eventually develop a second malignancy following successful treatment of acute leukaemia; by extrapolation from other experience, particularly in Hodgkin's disease, this may well be an AML. Acute myeloid leukaemia (AML) has been described in one child who developed a monosomy 7 during treatment of ALL [382], and other instances of AML have been recorded [90].

Neurological and psychological complications
A variety of neurological complications not directly attributable to CNS leukaemia may occur in children treated for ALL: these are more frequent and more serious in children with previous overt CNS infiltration [383]. They include viral encephalitis, transient post-irradiation somnolence [384] and arachnoiditis due to intrathecal cytotoxics [385]. Although more serious neurological complications such as a series of convulsions or a transient paraplegia can follow a single intrathecal injection, severe, sometimes fatal, progressive neurological deterioration and dementia is usually only seen in patients who have had one or more episodes of CNS leukaemia treated by cranial irradiation and long-term intrathecal MTX [386]. The neuropathological findings are those of a disseminated leuco-encephalopathy [387]. A similar syndrome has been described in patients receiving prophylactic cranial irradiation and subsequent regular intrathecal chemotherapy or parenteral MTX in doses in excess of 40 mg/m^2/week [388, 389]. These serious complications do not result from the usual treatment schedules comprising short-term intrathecal and moderate subsequent systemic MTX.

However, although children who have received conventional CNS 'prophylaxis' perform intellectually in the same range as their peers, preliminary results suggest that their performance in mathematical skills and reasoning may be below the norm [338, 390]; this is most noticeable in children treated at a young age. It is in this young group that mineralizing microangiopathy has been more frequently found [391]; and computerized axial tomography has disclosed abnormalities in some series [392] but not in others [393]. There is no apparent relationship between the extent of these findings and intellectual performance.

While these findings warrant a reappraisal of the details of CNS prophylaxis, particularly in the young child, it should be emphasized that the majority of children do function normally. It is difficult to attribute generalized psychological problems to CNS 'prophylaxis' alone in view of the many social and emotional problems faced by these children and their families [394] and the poor school attendance of many children [395].

Hormonal effects of treatment
There have been a number of reports of investigations of the hypothalamic-pituitary axis and of reproductive function in children treated for leukaemia [396, 397]. Despite biochemical evidence of growth-hormone deficiency in occasional patients, the majority of children who have completed treatment have a normal growth pattern and undergo normal pubertal progression. The effects of treatment on reproduction are not yet clear; a study of progeny of childhood-cancer survivors showed no excess of defects, but these patients received treatment which would be inadequate by modern standards [398]. There are certainly a number of girls who have given birth to normal infants following successful treatment of ALL. A study of testicular histology in boys showed a reduced fertility index compared to age-matched controls, but the findings did seem to improve with increasing time off chemotherapy [399]. Recent reports of successful fatherhood are at least encouraging [400, 401]. It is clear from all these observations that long-term follow-up is mandatory, but in the main careful observation of growth, puberty progression and school and work performance are indicated, rather than a battery of endocrinological investigations.

REFERENCES

1 BENNETT J.M., CATOVSKY D., DANIEL M.T., FLANDRIN G., GALTON D.A.G., GRALNICK H.R. & SULTAN C.

(1976) Proposals for the classification of the acute leukaemias. *British Journal of Haematology*, **33**, 451.

2 GRALNICK H.R., GALTON D.A.G., CATOVSKY D., SULTAN C. & BENNETT J.M. (1977) Classification of acute leukaemia. *Annals of Internal Medicine*, **87**, 740.

3 BENNETT J.M., CATOVSKY D., DANIEL M.T., FLANDRIN G., GALTON D.A.G., GRALNICK H.R. & SULTAN C. The French-American-British (FAB) Co-operative Group (1981) The morphological classification of acute lymphoblastic leukaemia: concordance among observers and clinical correlations. *British Journal of Haematology*, **47**, 553.

4 FLANDRIN G., BROUET J.C., DANIEL M.T. & PREUD'-HOMME J.L. (1975) Acute leukemia with Burkitt's tumor cells: a study of six cases with special reference to lymphocyte surface markers. *Blood*, **45**, 183.

5 GREAVES M.F. (1979) Molecular phenotypes: a new perspective on diagnosis and classification of leukaemias. In: *Topics in Paediatrics. I. Haematology and Oncology* (ed. Morris Jones P.H.), p. 36. Pitman Medical, Tunbridge Wells.

5a GREAVES M.F. & LISTER T.A. (1981) Prognostic importance of immunologic markers in adult acute lymphoblastic leukaemia. *New England Journal of Medicine*, **304**, 119.

6 CHESSELLS J.M., HARDISTY R.M., RAPSON N.T. & GREAVES M.F. (1977) Acute lymphoblastic leukaemia in children: classification and prognosis. *Lancet*, **ii**, 1307.

7 LISTER T.A., ROBERTS M.M., BREARLEY R.L., WOODRUFF R.K. & GREAVES M.F. (1979) Prognostic significance of cell surface phenotypes in adult acute lymphoblastic leukaemia. *Cancer Immunology and Immunotherapy*, **6**, 227.

8 GREAVES M.F., BROWN G., RAPSON N.T. & LISTER T.A. (1975) Antisera to acute lymphoblastic leukemia cells. *Clinical Immunology and Immunopathology*, **4**, 67.

9 VOGLER L.B., CRIST W.M., BOCKMAN D.E., PEARL E.R., LAWTON A.R. & COOPER M.D. (1978) Pre-B-cell leukemia. A new phenotype of childhood lymphoblastic leukemia. *New England Journal of Medicine*, **298**, 872.

10 GREAVES M.F., DELIA D., JANOSSY G., RAPSON N., CHESSELLS J., WOODS M. & PRENTICE G. (1980) Acute lymphoblastic leukaemia associated antigen. IV. Expression on non-leukaemic lymphoid cells. *Leukemia Research*, **4**, 15.

11 BREATNACH F., CHESSELLS J.M. & GREAVES M.F. (1981) The aplastic presentation of acute lymphoblastic leukaemia in childhood: a feature of common ALL. *British Journal of Haematology*, **49**, 387.

12 HOFFBRAND A.V., GANESHAGURU K., JANOSSY G., GREAVES M.F., CATOVSKY D. & WOODRUFF R.K. (1977) Terminal deoxynucleotidyl-transferase levels and membrane phenotypes in diagnosis of acute leukaemia. *Lancet*, **ii**, 520.

13 WEINSTEIN H.J. & LINK M.P. (1979) Non-Hodgkin lymphoma in childhood. *Clinics in Haematology*, **8**, 699.

14 COCCIA P.F., KERSEY J.H., KAZAMIERA J., GAJL-PECZALSKA K.J., KRIVIT W. & NESBIT M.E. (1976) Prognostic significance of surface marker analysis in childhood non-Hodgkin's lymphoproliferative malignancies. *American Journal of Hematology*, **1**, 405.

15 NADLER L.M., REINHERZ E.L., WEINSTEIN H.J., D'ORSI

C.J. & SCHLOSSMAN S.F. (1980) Heterogeneity of T-cell lymphoblastic malignancies. *Blood*, **55**, 806.

16 BRUNNING R.D., MCKENNA R.W., BLOOMFIELD C.D., COCCIA P. & GAJL-PECZALSKA K.J. (1977) Bone marrow involvement in Burkitt's lymphoma. *Cancer*, **40**, 1771.

17 COHEN J.R., GREGER W.P., GREENBERG P.L. & SCHRIER S.L. (1979) Subacute myeloid leukemia. A clinical review. *American Journal of Medicine*, **66**, 959.

18 MEDICAL RESEARCH COUNCIL'S WORKING PARTY ON LEUKAEMIA IN ADULTS (1975) The relation between morphology and other features of acute myeloid leukaemia, and their prognostic significance. *British Journal of Haematology*, **31**, 165.

19 ROWLEY J.D., GOLOMB H.M. DOUGHERTY C. (1977) C: 15/17 translocation; a consistent chromosomal change in acute promyelocytic leukaemia. *Lancet*, **i**, 549.

20 SHAW M.T. (1978) The distinctive features of acute monocytic leukemia. *American Journal of Hematology*, **4**, 97.

21 TOBELEM G., JACQUILLAT C., CHASTANG C., AUCLERC M.-F., LE CHEVALLIER T., WEIL M., DANIEL M.T., FLANDRIN G., HAROUSSEAU J.L., SCHAISON G., BOIRON M. & BERNARD J. (1980) Acute monoblastic leukemia: a clinical and biological study of 74 cases. *Blood*, **55**, 71.

22 HAROUSSEAU J.L., DEGOS L., DANIEL M.T. & FLANDRIN G. (1979) Leukemic phase of malignant histiocytosis (arguments in favour of the histiomonocytic origin of the abnormal cells). *Medical and Pediatric Oncology*, **6**, 339.

23 BOGGS D.R., WINTROBE M.M. & CARTWRIGHT G.E. (1962) The acute leukaemias. Analysis of 322 cases and review of the literature. *Medicine*, **41**, 163.

24 ROATH S., ISRAELS M.C.G. & WILKINSON J.F. (1964) The acute leukaemias: a study of 580 patients. *Quarterly Journal of Medicine*, **33**, 257.

25 LASCARI A.D. (1973) *Leukaemia in Childhood*, p. 30. C. C. Thomas, Springfield, Illinois.

26 NEWMAN A.J. & MELHORN D.K. (1973) Vertebral compression in childhood leukemia. *American Journal of Diseases of Children*, **125**, 863.

27 SIMMONS C.R., HARLE T.S. & SINGLETON E.B. (1968) The osseous manifestations of leukemia in children. *Radiological Clinics of North America*, **6**, 115.

28 AUR R.J.A., WESTBROOK H.W. & RIGGS W. (1972) Childhood acute lymphocytic leukemia. Initial radiological bone involvement and prognosis. *American Journal of Diseases of Children*, **124**, 653.

29 WEIL M., JACQUILLAT C.I., GEMON-AUCLERC M.F., CHASTANG C.L., IZRAEL V., BOIRON M. & BERNARD J. (1976) Acute granulocytic leukaemia. *Archives of Internal Medicine*, **136**, 1389.

30 HANN I.M., EVANS D.I.K., MARSDEN H.B., MORRIS JONES P. & PALMER M.K. (1978) Bone marrow fibrosis in acute lymphoblastic leukaemia of childhood. *Journal of Clinical Pathology*, **31**, 313.

31 MANOHARAN A., HORSLEY R. & PITNEY W.R. (1979) The reticulin content of bone marrow in acute leukaemia in adults. *British Journal of Haematology*, **43**, 185.

32 CATOVSKY D., CHERCHI M., GREAVES M.F., JANOSSY G., PAIN C. & KAY H.E.M. (1978) Acid phosphatase reaction in acute lymphoblastic leukaemia. *Lancet*, **i**, 749.

33 BLOOMFIELD C.D., PETERSON L.C., YUNIS J.J. & BRUN-

NING R.D. (1977) The Philadelphia chromosome (Ph¹) in adults presenting with acute leukaemia: a comparison of Ph¹+ and Ph¹− patients. *British Journal of Haematology*, **36**, 347.

34 WOODRUFF R. (1978) The management of adult acute lymphoblastic leukaemia. *Cancer Treatment Reviews*, **5**, 95.

35 CHESSELLS J.M., JANOSSY G., LAWLER S.D. & SECKER-WALKER L.M. (1979) The Ph¹ chromosome in childhood leukaemia. *British Journal of Haematology*, **41**, 25.

36 BERGER R., BERNHEIM A., BROUET J.C., DANIEL M.T. & FLANDRIN G. (1979) t(8:14) translocation in a Burkitt's type of lymphoblastic leukaemia (L₃). *British Journal of Haematology*, **43**, 87.

37 OSSERMAN E.F. & LAWLOR D.P. (1966) Serum and urinary lysozyme (muramidase) in monocytic and myelomonocytic leukemia. *Journal of Experimental Medicine*, **124**, 921.

38 ROBERTS M. & GREAVES M.F. (1978) Maturation linked expression of a myeloid cell surface antigen. *British Journal of Haematology*, **38**, 439.

39 BAKER M.A., FALK J.A., CARTER W.H., TAUB R.N. & THE TORONTO LEUKEMIA STUDY GROUP (1979) Early diagnosis of relapse in acute myeloblastic leukemia: serologic detection of leukemia-associated antigens in human marrow. *New England Journal of Medicine*, **301**, 1353.

40 KOZINER B., MCKENZIE S., STRAUS D., CLARKSON B., GOOD R.A. & SIEGAL F.P. (1977) Cell marker analysis in acute monocytic leukemias. *Blood*, **49**, 895.

41 FIRST INTERNATIONAL WORKSHOP ON CHROMOSOMES IN LEUKAEMIA (1978) Chromosomes in acute non-lymphocytic leukaemia. *British Journal of Haematology*, **39**, 311.

42 MCCAFFREY R., HARRISON T.A., PARKMAN R. & BALTIMORE D. (1975) Terminal deoxynucleotidyl-transferase activity in human leukemic cells and in normal human thymocytes. *New England Journal of Medicine*, **292**, 775.

43 BOLLUM F.J. (1979) Terminal deoxynucleotidyl transferase as a hematopoietic cell marker. *Blood*, **54**, 1203.

44 JANOSSY G., HOFFBRAND A.V., GREAVES M.F., GANESHAGURU K., PAIN C., BRADSTOCK K.F., PRENTICE H.G., KAY H.E.M. & LISTER T.A. (1980) Terminal transferase enzyme assay and immunological membrane markers in the diagnosis of leukaemia: A multiparameter analysis of 300 cases. *British Journal of Haematology*, **44**, 221.

45 ROSENTHAL S., CANNELLOS G.P., WHANG-PENG J. & GRALNICK H.R. (1977) Blast crisis of chronic granulocytic leukemia. Morphological variants and therapeutic implications. *American Journal of Medicine*, **63**, 542.

46 IVERSON T. (1966) Leukemia in infancy and childhood. *Acta Paediatrica Scandinavica*, **167** (Suppl), 9.

47 ROSNER F. & LEE S.L. (1972) Down's syndrome and acute leukemia: myeloblastic or lymphoblastic? *American Journal of Medicine*, **53**, 203.

48 MELHORN D.K., GROSS S. & NEWMAN A. (1970) Acute childhood leukemia presenting as aplastic anaemia: the response to corticosteroids. *Journal of Pediatrics*, **77**, 647.

49 SCHALLER J. (1972) Arthritis as a presenting manifestation of malignancy in children. *Journal of Pediatrics*, **81**, 793.

50 MURPHY S.B. (1978) Childhood non-Hodgkin's lymphoma. *New England Journal of Medicine*, **299**, 1446.

51 MEADOWS A.T., JENKIN R.D.T., ANDERSON J., CHILCOTE R., COCCIA P., EXELBY P., KUSHNER J., LEIKIN S., SIEGEL S., WILSON J.F. & HAMMOND D. (1980) A new therapy schedule for pediatric non-Hodgkin's lymphoma toxicity and preliminary results. *Medical and Pediatric Oncology*, **8**, 15.

52 GALTON D.A.G., GOLDMAN J.M., WILTSHAW E., CATOVSKY D., HENRY K. & GOLDENBERG G.J. (1974) Prolymphocytic leukaemia. *British Journal of Haematology*, **27**, 7.

53 CATOVSKY D., PETIT J.E., GALTON D.A.G., SPIERS A.S.D. & HARRISON C.V. (1974) Leukaemic reticuloendotheliosis (hairy cell leukaemia): a distinct clinicopathological entity. *British Journal of Haematology*, **26**, 9.

54 FIALKOW P.J. (1974) The origin and development of human tumors studied with cell markers. *New England Journal of Medicine*, **291**, 26.

55 BOGGS D.R. (1974) Haematopoietic stem cell theory in relation to possible lymphoblastic conversion of chronic myeloid leukaemia. *Blood*, **44**, 449.

56 JANOSSY G., ROBERTS M. & GREAVES M.F. (1976) Target cell in chronic myeloid leukaemia and its relationship to acute lymphoid leukaemia. *Lancet*, **ii**, 1058.

57 LINMAN J.W. & BAGBY G.C. JR (1978) The preleukemia syndrome (hematopoietic dysplasia). *Cancer*, **42**, 854.

58 KNOSPE W.H. & GREGORY S.A. (1971) Smouldering acute leukemia: clinical and cytogenetic studies in six patients. *Archives of Internal Medicine*, **127**, 910.

59 LINMAN J.W. & SAARNI M.I. (1974) The preleukemia syndrome. *Seminars in Hematology*, **ii**, 93.

60 CHENG D.S., KUSHNER J.F. & WINTROBE M.M. (1979) Idiopathic refractory sideroblastic anemia: incidence and risk factors for leukemic transformation. *Cancer*, **44**, 724.

61 MIESCHER P.A. & FARQUET J.J. (1974) Chronic myelomonocytic leukemia in adults. *Seminars in Hematology*, **ii**, 129.

62 PIERRE R.V. (1975) Cytogenetic studies in preleukemia: studies before and after transition to acute leukemia in 17 subjects. *Blood Cells*, **1**, 163.

63 KOEFFLER H.P. & GOLDE D.W. (1978) Cellular maturation in human preleukemia. *Blood*, **52**, 355.

64 HARDISTY R.M., SPEED D.E. & TILL M. (1964) Granulocytic leukaemia in childhood. *British Journal of Haematology*, **10**, 551.

65 WEATHERALL D.J., EDWARDS J.A. & DONOHUE W.T.A. (1968) Haemoglobin and red cell enzyme changes in juvenile myeloid leukaemia. *British Medical Journal*, **i**, 679.

66 SANDERS J.F., BUCKNER C.D., STEWART P. & THOMAS E.D. (1979) Successful treatment of juvenile chronic granulocytic leukemia with marrow transplantation. *Pediatrics*, **63**, 44.

67 LASCARI A.D. (1973) *Leukemia in Childhood*, p. 280. C. C. Thomas, Springfield, Illinois.

68 SMITH K.L. & JOHNSON W. (1974) Classification of chronic myelocytic leukaemia in children. *Cancer*, **34**, 670.

69 HUMBERT J.R., HATHAWAY W.E., ROBINSON A., PEAK-

MAN D.C. & GITHENS J.H. (1971) Preleukaemia in children with a missing bone marrow C chromosome and a myeloproliferative disorder. *British Journal of Haematology*, **21**, 705.

70 SIEFF C.A., CHESSELLS J.M., HARVEY B.A.M., PICK-THALL V.J. & LAWLER S.D. (1981) Monosomy 7 as a myeloproliferative disease in childhood. *British Journal of Haematology*, **49**, 235.

71 BURCHENAL J.H. (1967) Long-term survival in Burkitt's tumour and in acute leukaemia. *Cancer Research*, **27**, 2616.

72 BURCHENAL J.H. (1968) Long-term survivors in acute leukemia and Burkitt's tumor. *Cancer*, **21**, 595.

73 TILL M.M., HARDISTY R.M. & PIKE M.C. (1973) Long survivors in acute leukaemia. *Lancet*, **i**, 534.

74 NESBIT M.E., KRIVIT W., ROBISON L. & HAMMOND D. (1979) A follow-up report of long-term survivors of childhood acute lymphoblastic or undifferentiated leukemia. *Journal of Pediatrics*, **95**, 727.

75 GEORGE S.L., AUR R.J.A., MAUER A.M. & SIMONE J.V. (1979) A reappraisal of the results of stopping therapy in childhood leukemia. *New England Journal of Medicine*, **300**, 269.

76 HARDISTY R.M. & TILL M.M. (1968) Acute leukaemia 1959–64: factors affecting prognosis. *Archives of Diseases in Childhood*, **43**, 107.

77 GEORGE S.L., FERNBACH D.J., VIETTI T.J., SULLIVAN M.P., LANE D.M., HAGGARD M.E., BERRY D.H., LONS-DALE D. & KOMP D. (1973) Factors influencing survival in pediatric acute leukemia. The SWCCSG experience 1958–70. *Cancer*, **32**, 1542.

78 SIMONE J.V., VERZOSA M.S. & RUDY J.A. (1975) Initial features and prognosis in 363 children with acute lymphocytic leukemia. *Cancer*, **36**, 2099.

79 ROBISON L., SATHER H., COCCIA P.F., NESBIT M.E. & HAMMOND G.D. (1980) Assessment of the interrelationship of prognostic factors in childhood acute lymphoblastic leukemia. *American Journal of Pediatric Haematology and Oncology*, **2**, 5.

80 KHALIFA A.S., TAKE H., CEJKA J. & ZUELZER W.W. (1974) Immunoglobulins in acute leukemia in children. *Journal of Pediatrics*, **85**, 788.

81 HANN I.M., MORRIS JONES P.H., EVANS D.I.K., ADDISON G.M., PALMER M.K. & SCARFE J.H. (1980) Low IgG or IgA: a further indicator of poor prognosis in childhood acute lymphoblastic leukaemia. *British Journal of Cancer*, **41**, 317.

82 FREI E. & SALLAN S.E. (1978) Acute lymphoblastic leukemia: Treatment. *Cancer*, **42**, 828.

83 MILLER D.R., LEIKIN S., ALBO V., VITALE L., SATHER H., COCCIA P., NESBIT M., KARON M. & HAMMOND D. (1980) Use of prognostic factors in improving the design and efficiency of clinical trials in childhood leukemia: children's Cancer Study Group report. *Cancer Treatment Reports*, **64**, 381.

84 ZIPPIN C., CUTLER S.J., REEVES W.J. & LUM D. (1971) Variation in survival among patients with acute lymphocytic leukaemia. *Blood*, **37**, 59.

85 LEIMERT J.T., BURNS C.P., WILTSE C.G., ARMITAGE J.O. & CLARKE W.R. (1980) Prognostic influence of pretreatment characteristics in adults acute lymphoblastic leukemia. *Blood*, **56**, 510.

86 CARGIN A., GEORGE S. & SULLIVAN M. (1975) Unfavourable prognosis of acute leukemia in infancy. *Cancer*, **36**, 1973.

87 RAVINDRANATH Y., KAPLAN J. & ZUELZER W.W. (1975) Significance of mediastinal mass in acute lymphoblastic leukemia. *Pediatrics*, **55**, 889.

88 WALTERS T., BUSHORE M. & SIMONE J. (1972) Poor prognosis in Negro children with acute lymphocytic leukemia. *Cancer*, **29**, 210.

89 PALMER M.K., HANN I., JONES P.M. & EVANS D.I.K. (1981) A score at diagnosis for predicting length of remission in childhood acute lymphoblastic leukaemia. *British Journal of Cancer*, **42**, 841.

90 MILLER D.R. (1980) Acute lymphoblastic leukemia. *Pediatric Clinics of North America*, **27**, 269.

91 MEDICAL RESEARCH COUNCIL WORKING PARTIES ON ADULT AND CHILDHOOD LEUKAEMIA (1982) The treatment of poor-risk ALL.

92 SATHER H., COCCIA P., NESBIT M., LEVEL C. & HAMMOND D. (1981) Disappearance of the predictive value of prognostic variables in childhood acute lymphoblastic leukemia. *Cancer*, **48**, 370.

93 MEDICAL RESEARCH COUNCIL (1978a) Effects of varying radiation schedule, cyclophosphamide treatment, and duration of treatment in acute lymphoblastic leukaemia. *British Medical Journal*, **ii**, 787.

94 BAUM E., SATHER H., NACHMAN J., SEINFELD J., KRIVIT W., LEIKIN S., MILLER D., JOO P. & HAMMOND D. (1979) Relapse rates following cessation of chemotherapy during complete remission of acute lymphocytic leukemia. *Medical and Pediatric Oncology*, **7**, 25.

95 LAND V.J., BERRY D.H., HERSON J., MIALE T., RIED H., SILVA-SOSA M. & STARLING K. (1979) Long-term survival in childhood acute leukemia: 'late' relapses. *Medical and Pediatric Oncology*, **7**, 19.

96 SEN L. & BORELLA L. (1975) Clinical importance of lymphoblasts with T markers in childhood acute leukemia. *New England Journal of Medicine*, **292**, 828.

97 TSUKIMOTO I., WONG K.J. & LAMPKIN B.C. (1976) Surface markers and prognostic factors in acute lymphoblastic leukemia. *New England Journal of Medicine*, **294**, 245.

98 MATHE G., POUILLART P., STERESCU M., AMIEL J.L., SCHWARZENBERG L., SCHNEIDER R.M., HAYAT M., DE VASSAL F., JASMIN C. & LAFLEUR M. (1971) Subdivision of classical varieties of acute leukaemia. Correlation with prognosis and cure expectancy. *European Journal of Clinical and Biological Research*, **16**, 554.

99 PANTAZOPOULOS N. & SINKS L.F. (1974) Morphological criteria for prognostication of acute lymphoblastic leukaemia. *British Journal of Haematology*, **27**, 25.

100 MURPHY S.B., BORELLA L., SEN L. & MAUER A. (1975) Lack of correlation of lymphoblast cell size with presence of T-cell markers or with outcome in childhood acute lymphoblastic leukaemia. *British Journal of Haematology*, **31**, 95.

101 OSTER M.W., MARGILETH D.A., SIMON R. & LEVENTHAL B.G. (1976) Lack of prognostic value of lymphoblast size in acute lymphoblastic leukaemia. *British Journal of Haematology*, **33**, 131.

102 SHAW M.T., HUMPHREY G.B., LAWRENCE R. & FISCHER D.B. (1977) Lack of prognostic value of the periodic

acid-Schiff reaction and blast cell size in childhood acute lymphocytic leukemia. *American Journal of Hematology*, **2**, 237.

103 WAGNER V.M. & BAEHNER R.L. (1977) Lack of correlation between blast cell size and length of first remission in acute lymphocytic leukemia in childhood. *Medical and Pediatric Oncology*, **3**, 373.

104 KELETTI J., REVESZ T. & SCHULER D. (1978) Morphological diagnosis in childhood leukaemia. *British Journal of Haematology*, **40**, 501.

105 HANN I.M., EVANS D.I.K., PALMER M.K., MORRIS JONES P.H. & HOWARTH C. (1979) The prognostic significance of morphological features in childhood acute lymphoblastic leukaemia. *Clinical and Laboratory Haematology*, **1**, 215.

106 WAGNER V.M. & BAEHNER R.L. (1979) Correlation of the FAB morphologic criteria and prognosis in acute lymphocytic leukemia of childhood. *American Journal of Pediatric Hematology and Oncology*, **1**, 103.

107 SCARFE J.H., HANN I.M., EVANS D.I.K., MORRIS JONES P., PALMER M.K., LILLEYMAN J.S. & CROWTHER D. (1980) The relationship between the pre-treatment proliferative activity of bone marrow blast cells measured by flow cytometry and prognosis of acute lymphoblastic leukaemia of childhood. *British Journal of Cancer*, **41**, 764.

108 FOADI M., COOPER E.H. & HARDISTY R.M. (1968) Proliferative activity of leukaemic cells at various stages of acute leukaemia of childhood. *British Journal of Haematology*, **15**, 269.

109 MURPHY S., AUR R.J.A., SIMONE J.V., GEORGE S. & MAUER A. (1977) Pre-treatment cytokinetic studies in 94 children with acute leukemia. Relationship to other variables at diagnosis and to outcome of standard treatment. *Blood*, **49**, 683.

110 WILLOUGHBY M.L.N. & LAURIE H.C. (1968) The effect of cyclical maintenance therapy on first remission in acute leukaemia of children. *Archives of Diseases in Childhood*, **43**, 187.

111 FELDGES A.J., AUR R.J.A., VERZOSA M.S. & DANIELS S. (1975) Periodic acid-Schiff reaction, a useful index of duration of complete remission in acute childhood lymphocytic leukemia. *Acta Haematologica*, **52**, 8.

112 LILLEYMAN J.S., MILLS V., SUGDEN P.J. & BRITTON J.A. (1979) Periodic acid-Schiff reaction and prognosis in lymphoblastic leukaemia. *Journal of Clinical Pathology*, **32**, 158.

113 SECKER-WALKER L.M., LAWLER S.D. & HARDISTY R.M. (1978) Prognostic implications of chromosomal findings in acute lymphoblastic leukaemia at diagnosis. *British Medical Journal*, **ii**, 1529.

114 JACQUILLAT C., WEIL M., GEMON M.F., IZRAEL V., SCHAISON G., AUCLERC G., ABLIN A.R., GLANDRIN G., TANZER J., BUSSEL A., WEISBERGER C., DRESCH C., NAJEAN Y., GOODEMAND M., SELIGMAN M., BOIRON M. & BERNARD J. (1973) Evaluation of 216 four-year survivors of acute leukemia. *Cancer*, **32**, 286.

115 OLIFF A. & POPLACK D. (1978) Characteristics of long-term survivors in AML. *Medical and Pediatric Oncology*, **5**, 219.

116 ALEXANDER P. & POWLES R. (1978) Immunotherapy of human acute leukaemia. *Clinics in Haematology*, **7**, 275.

117 GALE R.P. & CLINE M.J. (1977) High remission-induction rate in acute myeloid leukaemia. *Lancet*, **i**, 497.

118 REES J.K.H., SANDLER R.M., CHALLENER J. & HAYHOE F.G.J. (1977) Treatment of acute myeloid leukaemia with triple cytotoxic regime: DAT. *British Journal of Cancer*, **36**, 770.

119 MEDICAL RESEARCH COUNCIL (1979) Chemotherapy of acute myeloid leukaemia in adults. *British Journal of Cancer*, **39**, 69.

120 BLOOMFIELD C.D. (1980) Treatment of adult acute nonlymphocytic leukemia—1980. *Annals of Internal Medicine*, **93**, 133.

121 CROWTHER D., BEARD M.E.J., BATEMAN C.J.T. & SEWELL R.L. (1975) Factors influencing prognosis in adults with acute myelogenous leukaemia. *British Journal of Cancer*, **32**, 456.

122 KEATING M.J., SMITH T.L., GEHAN E.A., McCREDIE K.B., BODEY G.P., SPITZER G., HERSH E., GUTTERMAN J. & FREIREICH E.J. (1980) Factors related to length of complete remission in adult acute leukemia. *Cancer*, **45**, 2017.

123 COLLINS A.J., BLOOMFIELD C.D., PETERSON B.A., McKENNA R.W. & EDSON J.R. (1978) Acute promyelocytic leukaemia: management of the coagulopathy during daunorubicin-prednisone remission induction. *Archives of Internal Medicine*, **138**, 1677.

124 GOLOMB H.M., VARDIMAN J.W., ROWLEY J.D., TESTA J.R. & MINTZ U. (1978) Correlation of clinical findings with quinacrine banded chromosomes in 90 adults with acute nonlymphocytic leukemia: an eight-year study. *New England Journal of Medicine*, **299**, 613.

125 SKIPPER H.E., SCHABEL F.M. & WILCOX W.S. (1964) Experimental evaluation of potential anticancer agents. XIII. On the criteria and kinetics associated with 'curability' of experimental leukemia. *Cancer Chemotherapy Reports*, **35**, 1.

126 BLACKSTOCK A.M. & GARSON O.M. (1974) Direct evidence for involvement of erythroid cells in acute myeloblastic leukaemia. *Lancet*, **ii**, 1178.

127 FIALKOW P.J., SINGER J.W., ADAMSON J.W., BERKOW R.L., FRIEDMAN J.M., JACOBSON R.J. & MOOHR J.W. (1979) Acute nonlymphocytic leukemia: expression in cells restricted to granulocytic and monocytic differentiation. *New England Journal of Medicine*, **301**, 1.

128 KILLMANN S.A. (1968) Acute leukemia: development, remission/relapse pattern, relationship between normal and leukemic hemopoiesis and the sleeper-to-feeder stem cell hypothesis. *Series Haematologica*, **1**, 103.

129 McCULLOCH E.A. (1979) Haemopoiesis in myeloblastic leukaemia. *Clinics in Haematology*, **8**, 501.

130 POWLES R.L., SELBY P.J., PALU G., MORGENSTERN G., McELWAIN T.J., CLINK H.M. & ALEXANDER P. (1979) The nature of remission in acute myeloblastic leukaemia. *Lancet*, **ii**, 674.

131 FITZGERALD P.H., CROSSEN P.E. & HAMER J.W. (1973) Abnormal karyotypic clones in human acute leukemia: their nature and clinical significance. *Cancer*, **31**, 1069.

132 TESTA J.R., MINTZ V., ROWLEY J.D., VARDIMAN J.W. & GOLOMB H.M. (1979) Evolution of karyotypes in acute non-lymphocytic leukemia. *Cancer Research*, **39**, 3619.

133 PINKEL D., HERNANDEZ K., BORELLA L., HOLTON C., AUR R., SAMOY G. & PRATT C. (1971) Drug dosage and

remission duration in childhood lymphocytic leukemia. *Cancer*, **27**, 247.

134 DeVita V.T., Young R.C. & Canellos G.P. (1975) Combination versus single agent chemotherapy: a review of the basis for selection of drug treatment of cancer. *Cancer*, **35**, 98.

135 Aur R.J.A., Simone J.V., Verzosa M.S., Hustu H.O., Barker L.F., Pinkel D.P., Rivera G., Dahl G.V., Wood A., Stagner S. & Mason C. (1978) Childhood acute lymphocytic leukemia: study VIII. *Cancer*, **42**, 2123.

136 Mauer A.M. (1975) Cell kinetics and practical consequences for therapy of acute leukemia. *New England Journal of Medicine*, **293**, 389.

137 Lampkin B.C., McWilliams N.B., Mauer A.M., Flessa H.C., Hake D.A. & Fisher V. (1976) Manipulation of the mitotic cycle in the treatment of acute myelogenous leukaemia. *British Journal of Haematology*, **32**, 29.

138 Arlin Z.A., Fried J. & Clarkson B.D. (1978) Therapeutic role of cell kinetics in acute leukaemia. *Clinics in Haematology*, **7**, 339.

139 Mathe G., Schwarzenberg L., Merya M., Cattan A., Scheider M., Amiel J.L., Schlumberger J.R., Poisson J. & Wajcner G. (1966) Extensive histological and cytological survey of patients with acute leukaemia in 'complete remission'. *British Medical Journal*, **i**, 640.

140 Simone J.V., Holland E. & Johnson W. (1972) Fatalities during remission of childhood leukemia. *Blood*, **39**, 759.

141 Gavosto F. (1977) Kinetic conditions preventing the eradication of human leukemia. *European Journal of Cancer*, **13**, 407.

142 Peto R., Pike M.C., Armitage P., Breslow N.E., Cox D.R., Howard S.V., Mantel N., McPherson K., Peto J. & Smith P.G. (1976) Design and analysis of randomized clinical trials requiring prolonged observation of each patient. I. Introduction and Design. *British Journal of Cancer*, **34**, 585.

143 Peto R., Pike M.C., Armitage P., Breslow N.E., Cox D.R., Howard S.V., Mantel N., McPherson K., Peto J. & Smith P.G. (1976) Design and analysis of randomized clinical trials requiring prolonged observation of each patient. II. Analysis and examples. *British Journal of Cancer*, **35**, 1.

144 Medical Research Council (1974) Treatment of acute myeloid leukaemia with daunorubicin, cytosine arabinoside, mercaptopurine, L-asparaginase, prednisone and thioguanine: results of treatment with five multiple-drug schedules. *British Journal of Haematology*, **27**, 373.

145 Simone J.V. (1974) Acute lymphocytic leukemia in childhood. *Seminars in Hematology*, **11**, 25.

146 Chabner B.A., Myers C.E., Coleman N. & Johns D.G. (1975) The clinical pharmacology of antineoplastic agents. I. *New England Journal of Medicine*, **292**, 1107.

147 Chabner B.A., Myers C.E., Coleman N. & Johns D.G. (1975) The clinical pharmacology of antineoplastic agents. II. *New England Journal of Medicine*, **292**, 1159.

148 Tattersall M.H.N. (1977) Anticancer drugs: mode of action and pharmacokinetics. In: *Recent Advances in Haematology, Vol. 2* (ed. Hoffbrand A.V., Brain M.C. & Hirsh J.), p. 325. Churchill Livingstone, Edinburgh.

149 Ernst P. & Killmann S.A. (1970) Perturbation of generation cycle of human leukemic blast cells by cytostatic therapy *in vivo*: effect of corticosteroids. *Blood*, **36**, 689.

150 Kaiser N., Milholland R.J. & Rosen F. (1974) Glucocorticoid receptors and mechanism of resistance in the cortisol-sensitive and -resistant lines of lymphosarcoma, P 1798. *Cancer Research*, **34**, 621.

151 Thompson E.B. (1979) Report on the International Union against Cancer workshop on steroid receptors in leukemia. *Cancer Treatment Reports*, **63**, 189.

152 Yarbro G.S.K., Lippmann M.E., Johnson G.E. & Leventhal B.G. (1977) Glucocorticoid receptors in subpopulations of childhood acute lymphocytic leukemia. *Cancer Research*, **37**, 2688.

153 Wolff J.A., Brubaker C.A., Murphy M.L., Pierce M.I. & Severo N. (1967) Prednisone therapy of acute childhood leukemia: prognosis and duration of response in 330 treated patients. *Journal of Pediatrics*, **70**, 626.

154 Medical Research Council (1966) Treatment of acute leukemia in adults: comparison of steroid and mercaptopurine therapy alone and in conjunction. *British Medical Journal*, **i**, 1383.

155 Bayssas M., Gouveia J., Ribaud P., Musset M., de Vassal F., Pico J.L., de Luca L., Misset J.L., Machner D., Belpomme D., Schwarzenberg L., Jasmin C., Hayat M. & Mathe G. (1979) Phase-II trial with vindesine for regression induction in patients with leukemias and hematosarcomas. *Cancer Chemotherapy and Pharmacology*, **2**, 247.

156 Bleyer W.A., Fusby S.A. & Oliverio V.T. (1975) Uptake and binding of vincristine by murine leukemia cells. *Biochemical Pharmacology*, **24**, 633.

157 Hardisty R.M., McElwain T.J. & Darby C.W. (1969) Vincristine and prednisone for the induction of remission in acute childhood leukaemia. *British Medical Journal*, **ii**, 662.

158 Lister T.A., Whitehouse J.M.A., Beard M.E.J., Brearly R.L., Wrigley P.F.M., Oliver R.T.D., Freeman J.E. & Woodruff R.K. (1978) Combination chemotherapy for acute lymphoblastic leukaemia in adults. *British Medical Journal*, **i**, 199.

159 Weiss H.D., Walker M.D. & Wiernik P.H. (1974) Neurotoxicity of commonly used antineoplastic agents. *New England Journal of Medicine*, **291**, 75.

160 Weiden P.L. & Wright S.E. (1972) Vincristine neurotoxicity. *New England Journal of Medicine*, **286**, 1369.

161 Bachur N.R. (1979) Anthracycline antibiotic pharmacology and metabolism. *Cancer Treatment Reports*, **63**, 817.

162 Jacquillat C., Weil M., Auclerc G., Izrael V., Bussel A., Boiron M. & Bernard J. (1976) Clinical study of Rubidazone (22.050 RP) A new daunorubicin derived compound in 170 patients with acute leukemias and other malignancies. *Cancer*, **37**, 653.

163 Davis H.L. & Davis T.E. (1979) Daunorubicin and adriamycin in cancer treatment: an analysis of their roles and limitations. *Cancer Treatment Reports*, **63**, 809.

164 Halazun J.F., Wagner H.R., Gaeta J.F. & Sinks L.F. (1974) Daunorubicin cardiac toxicity in children with acute lymphocytic leukemia. *Cancer*, **33**, 545.

165 Gilladoga A.C., Manuel C., Tan C.T.C., Wollner

N., Sternberg S.S. & Murphy M.L. (1976) The cardiotoxicity of Adriamycin and daunomycin in children. *Cancer*, **37**, 1070.

166 Buckner C.O., Rudolph R.H., Fefer A., Clift R.A., Epstein R.B., Funk D.D., Neiman P.E., Slichter S.J., Storb R. & Thomas E.D. (1972) High-dose cyclophosphamide therapy for malignant disease: toxicity tumour response and the effects of stored autologous marrow. *Cancer*, **29**, 357.

167 Henderson I.C. & Frei E. (1979) Adriamycin and the heart. *New England Journal of Medicine*, **300**, 310.

168 Hitchings G.H. & Elion G.B. (1954) The chemistry and biochemistry of purine analogues. *Annals of the New York Academy of Sciences*, **60**, 195.

169 Brockman R.W., Roosa R.A., Law L.W. & Stutts P. (1962) Purine ribonucleotide pyrophosphorylase activity and resistance to purine analogs in P 388 murine lymphocytic leukemia. *Journal of Cellular and Comparative Physiology*, **60**, 65.

170 Tidd D.M. & Patterson A.R.P. (1974) Distinction between inhibition of purine nucleotide synthesis and the delayed cytotoxic reaction of 6-mercaptopurine. *Cancer Research*, **34**, 733.

171 le Page G.A. & White S.C. (1973) Scheduling of arabinosyl cytosine and 6-thioguanine therapy. *Cancer Research*, **33**, 946.

172 Storey J., Schenker S., Suki W.N. & Combes B. (1968) Hepatotoxicity of mercaptopurine. *Archives of Internal Medicine*, **122**, 54.

173 Farber S., Diamond L.K., Mercer R.D., Sylvester R.F. & Wolff J.A. (1948) Temporary remissions in acute leukemia in children produced by folic acid antagonist 4-aminopteroyl-glutamic acid (aminopterin). *New England Journal of Medicine*, **238**, 787.

174 Bleyer W.A. (1977) Methotrexate: clinical pharmacology, current status and therapeutic guide lines. *Cancer Treatment Reports*, **4**, 87.

175 Hoffbrand A.V. & Tripp E. (1972) Unbalanced deoxyribonucleotide synthesis caused by methotrexate. *British Medical Journal*, **ii**, 140.

176 Goldman I.D. (1974) The mechanism of action of methotrexate. I. Interaction with a low-affinity intracellular site required for maximum inhibition of deoxyribonucleic acid synthesis in L-cell mouse fibroblasts. *Molecular Pharmacology*, **10**, 257.

177 Fyfe M.J. & Goldman I.D. (1973) Characteristics of the vincristine-induced augmentation of methotrexate uptake in Ehrlich Ascites tumor cells. *Journal of Biological Chemistry*, **218**, 5067.

178 Capizzi R., Castro O. & Aspnes G. (1974) Treatment of acute lymphocytic leukemia (ALL) with intermittent high dose methotrexate (MTX) and asparaginase (A'ase). *Proceedings of the American Association of Cancer Research*, **15**, 182.

179 Yap B.S., McCredie K.B., Benjamin R.S., Bodey G.P. & Freireich E.J. (1978) Refractory acute leukaemia in adults treated with sequential colaspase and high dose methotrexate. *British Medical Journal*, **iii**, 791.

180 Pinkerton C.R., Welshman S.G., Glasgow J.F.T. & Bridges J.M. (1980) Can food influence the absorbtion of methotrexate in children with acute lymphoblastic leukaemia? *Lancet*, **ii**, 944.

181 Craft A.W., Kay H.E.M., Lawson D.N. & Mc-
Elwain T.J. (1977) Methotrexate-induced malabsorption in children with acute lymphoblastic leukaemia. *British Medical Journal*, **ii**, 1511.

182 Djerassi I., Farber S., Abir E. & Neikirk W. (1967) Continuous infusion of methotrexate in children with acute leukemia. *Cancer*, **20**, 233.

183 Howell S.B., Herbst K., Ross G.R. & Frei E. (1980) Thymidine requirements for the rescue of patients treated with high-dose methotrexate. *Cancer Research*, **40**, 1824.

184 Frei E., Jaffe N., Tattersall M.H.N., Pitman S. & Parker L. (1975) New approaches to cancer chemotherapy with methotrexate. *New England Journal of Medicine*, **292**, 846.

185 Nesbit M., Krivit W., Heyn R. & Sharp H. (1976) Acute and chronic effects of methotrexate on hepatic, pulmonary and skeletal systems. *Cancer*, **37**, 1048.

186 Banerjee S.P. & Snyder S.H. (1973) Methyltetrahydrofolic acid mediates N− and O− methylation of biogenic amines. *Science*, **182**, 74.

187 Abelson H.T. (1978) Methotrexate and central nervous system toxicity. *Cancer Treatment Reports*, **62**, 1999.

188 Saunders E.F. (1972) The effect of L-asparaginase on the nucleic acid metabolism and cell cycle of human leukemia cells. *Blood*, **39**, 575.

189 Haskell C.M., Cannellos G.P., Leventhal B.G., Carbone P.P., Block J.B., Serpick A.A. & Selawry O.S. (1969) L-asparaginase: therapeutic and toxic effects in patients with neoplastic disease. *New England Journal of Medicine*, **281**, 1028.

190 Haskell C.M., Cannellos G.P., Leventhal B.G., Carbone P.P., Serpick A.A. & Hansen H.H. (1969) L-asparaginase toxicity. *Cancer Research*, **29**, 974.

191 King O.T., Wilbur J.R., Mumford D.M. & Sutow W.W. (1974) Therapy with *Erwinia* L-asparaginase in children with acute leukemia after anaphylaxis to *E. coli* L-asparaginase. *Cancer*, **33**, 611.

192 Ho D.H.W. & Frei E. III (1971) Clinical pharmacology of 1-β-D-arabinofuranosyl cytosine. *Clinical Pharmacology and Therapeutics*, **12**, 944.

193 Skipper H.E., Schabel F.M.J.R. & Wilcox W.S. (1967) Experimental evaluation of parenteral anticancer agents. XXI. Scheduling of arabinosylcytosine to take advantage of its S-phase specificity against leukemia cells. *Cancer Chemotherapy Reports*, **51**, 125.

194 South West Oncology Group (1974) Cytarabine for acute leukemia in adults: effects of schedule on therapeutic response. *Archives of Internal Medicine*, **133**, 251.

195 Karon M., Sieger L., Leimbrock S., Finklestein J.Z., Nesbit M.E. & Swanery J.J. (1973) 5-azacytidine: A new active agent for the treatment of acute leukemia. *Blood*, **42**, 359.

196 Li L.H., Olin E.J., Buskirk H.H. & Reineke L.M. (1970) Cytotoxicity and mode of action of 5-azacytidine on L1210 leukemia. *Cancer Research*, **30**, 2760.

197 Fairley K.F., Barrie J.V. & Johnson W. (1972) Sterility and testicular atrophy related to cyclophosphamide therapy. *Lancet*, **i**, 568.

198 Philips F.S., Sternberg S.S., Cronin A.P. & Vidal P.M. (1961) Cyclophosphamide and urinary bladder toxicity. *Cancer Research*, **21**, 1577.

199 de Fronzo R.A., Braine H., Colvin O.M. & Davis P.J. (1973) Water intoxication in man after cyclophospha-

mide therapy: time course and relation to drug activation. *Annals of Internal Medicine*, **78**, 861.

200 Cox P.J. (1979) Cyclophosphamide cystitis—identification of acrolein as the causative agent. *Biochemical Pharmacology*, **28**, 2045.

201 Brock N., Stekar J., Pohl J., Niemeyer U. & Scheffler (1979) Acrolein the causative factor of urotoxic side-effects of cyclophosphamide, fosfamide, trofosfamide and sufosfamide. *Drug Research*, **29**, 659.

202 Wall R.L. & Clausen K.P. (1975) Carcinoma of the urinary bladder in patients receiving cyclophosphamide. *New England Journal of Medicine*, **293**, 271.

203 Willenze R., Hillen H., Hartgrink-Groenveld C.A. & Haanen C. (1975) Treatment of acute lymphoblastic leukemia in adolescents and adults: a retrospective study. *Blood*, **46**, 823.

204 Johnston P.G.B., Hardisty R.M., Kay H.E.M. & Smith P.G. (1974) Myelosuppressive effect of colaspase (L-asparaginase) in initial treatment of acute lymphoblastic leukaemia. *British Medical Journal*, **iii**, 81.

205 Simone J.V. (1976) Factors that influence haematological remission duration in acute lymphocytic leukaemia. *British Journal of Haematology*, **32**, 465.

206 Jones B.F., Holland J.F., Glidewell O., Jacquillat C., Weil M., Pochedly C., Sinks L., Chevalier L., Maurer H., Koch K., Falkson G., Patterson R., Seligman B., Sartorius J., Kung F., Haurani F., Stuart M., Burgert E.O., Ruymann F., Sawitsky A., Forman E., Pluess H., Truman H. & Hakami N. (1977) Optimal use of L-asparaginase (NSC-109229) in acute lymphocytic leukemia. *Medical and Pediatric Oncology*, **3**, 387.

207 Berry D.H., Pullen J., George S., Vietti T.J., Sullivan M.P. & Fernbach D. (1975) Comparison of prednisolone, vincristine, methotrexate and 6-mercaptopurine vs vincristine and prednisone induction therapy in childhood acute leukemia. *Cancer*, **36**, 98.

208 Riehm H., Henze G., Langermann H.J., Ritter J. & Schellong G. (1981) The BFM studies 1970/76 and 1976/79 in childhood acute lymphoblastic leukaemia (ALL). In: *Modern Trends in Human Leukaemia*. Vol. IV (ed. Neth R. *et al.*). Springer-Verlag, Berlin.

209 Chessells J.M. & Leiper A.D. (1980) Infection during remission induction in childhood leukaemia. *Archives of Diseases in Childhood*, **55**, 118.

210 Leventhal B.G., Levine A.S., Graw R.G., Simon R., Freireich E.J. & Henderson E.S. (1975) Long term second remissions in acute lymphatic leukemia. *Cancer*, **35**, 1136.

211 Medical Research Council (1971) Treatment of acute lymphoblastic leukaemia. Comparison of immunotherapy (BCG), intermittent methotrexate, and no therapy after a five-month intensive cytotoxic regimen. *British Medical Journal*, **iv**, 189.

212 Lonsdale D., Gehan E.A., Fernbach D.J., Sullivan M.P., Lane D.M. & Ragab A.H. (1975) Interrupted vs continued maintenance therapy in childhood acute leukemia. *Cancer*, **36**, 341.

213 Spiers A.S.D., Roberts P.D., Marsh G.W., Parekh S.J., Franklin A.J., Galton D.A.G., Szur L.Z., Paul E.A., Husband P. & Wiltshaw E. (1975) Acute lymphoblastic leukaemia: cyclical chemotherapy with

three combinations of four drugs (COAP-POMP-CART) regimen. *British Medical Journal*, **iv**, 614.

214 Haghbin M. (1976) Chemotherapy of acute lymphoblastic leukemia in children. *American Journal of Hematology*, **1**, 201.

215 Medical Research Council (1976) Analysis of treatment in childhood leukaemia. II. Timing and the toxicity of combined 6-mercaptopurine and methotrexate maintenance therapy. *British Journal of Haematology*, **33**, 179.

216 Medical Research Council (1977) Treatment of acute lymphoblastic leukaemia: effect of variation in length of treatment on duration of remission. *British Medical Journal*, **ii**, 495.

217 Cornbleet M.A. & Chessells J.M. (1978) Bone-marrow relapse in acute lymphoblastic leukaemia in childhood. *British Medical Journal*, **ii**, 104.

218 Ekert H., Ellis W.M., Waters K.D. & Matthews R.M. (1979) Poor outlook for childhood acute lymphoblastic leukaemia with relapse. *Medical Journal of Australia*, **66**, 224.

219 Rivera G., Pratt C.B., Aur R.J.A., Verzosa M. & Hustu H.O. (1976) Recurrent childhood lymphocytic leukemia following cessation of therapy. *Cancer*, **37**, 1679.

220 Chessells J.M. & Cornbleet M. (1979) Combination chemotherapy for bone marrow relapse in childhood lymphoblastic leukaemia (ALL). *Medical and Pediatric Oncology*, **6**, 359.

221 Rivera G., Aur R.J.A., Dahl G.V., Pratt C.B., Hustu H.O., George S.L. & Mauer A.M. (1979) Second cessation of therapy in childhood lymphocytic leukemia. *Blood*, **53**, 1114.

222 Aur R.J.A., Verzosa M.S., Hustu H.O. & Simone J.V. (1972) Response to combination therapy after relapse in childhood acute lymphocytic leukemia. *Cancer*, **30**, 334.

223 Henderson E.S., Scharlau C., Cooper M.R., Haurani F.I., Silver R.T., Brunner K., Carey R.W., Falkson G., Blom J., Suny I.V.N., Levine A.S., Bank A., Cuttner J., Cornwell G.G., Henry P., Nissen N.I., Wiernik P.H., Leone L., Wohl K., Rai K., James G.W., Weinberg V., Glidewell O. & Holland J.F. (1979) Combination chemotherapy and radiotherapy for acute lymphocytic leukemia in adults. Results of CALGB protocol 7113. *Leukemia Research*, **3**, 295.

224 Woodruff R.K., Lister T.A., Paxton A.M., Whitehouse J.M.A. & Malpas J.S. (1978) Combination chemotherapy for hematological relapse in adult acute lymphoblastic leukemia (ALL). *American Journal of Hematology*, **4**, 173.

225 Rodriguez C., Hart J.S., Freireich E.J., Bodey G.P., McCredie K.B., Whitecar J.P. & Coltman C.A. (1973) POMP combination chemotherapy of adult leukemia. *Cancer*, **32**, 69.

226 Whitecar J.P., Bodey G.P., Freireich E.J., McCredie K.B. & Hart J.S. (1972) Cyclophosphamide (NSC 26271), vincristine (NSC 67574) cytosine arabinoside (NSC 63878) and prednisone (NSC 10023) (COAP). Combination chemotherapy for acute leukemia in adults. *Cancer Chemotherapy Reports*, **56**, 543.

227 Jacquillat C., Weil M., Geman M.F., Auclerc G., Loisel J.P., Delobel J., Flandrin G., Schaison G., Izrael V., Bussel A., Dresch C., Weisgerber C., Rain

D., TARZEN J., NAJEAN Y., SELIGMANN M., BOIRON M. & BERNARD J. (1973) Combination therapy in 130 patients with acute lymphoblastic leukemia (Protocol 06L A66). *Cancer Research*, **33**, 3278.

228 GEE T.S., HAGHBIN M., DOWLING M.D., CUNNINGHAM I., MIDDLEMAN M.P. & CLARKSON B.D. (1976) Acute lymphoblastic leukemia in adults and children: differences in response with similar therapeutic regimens. *Cancer*, **37**, 1256.

229 SMYTH A.C. & WIERNIK P.H. (1976) Combination chemotherapy of adult acute lymphocytic leukemia. *Clinical Pharmacology and Therapeutics*, **19**, 240.

230 OMURA G.A., MOFFITT S., VOGLER V.R. & SALTER M.M. (1980) Combination chemotherapy of adult acute lymphoblastic leukemia with randomized central nervous system prophylaxis. *Blood*, **55**, 199.

231 BURGE P.S., PRANKERD T.A.J., RICHARDS J.D.M., SARE M., THOMPSON D.S. & WRIGHT P. (1975) Quality and quantity of survival in acute myeloid leukaemia. *Lancet*, **ii**, 621.

232 CADMAN E.D., CAPIZZI R.L. & BERTINO J. (1977) Acute non lymphocytic leukemia: a delayed complication of Hodgkin's disease therapy: analysis of 109 cases. *Cancer*, **40**, 1280.

233 CHABNER B.A. (1977) Second neoplasm—a complication of cancer chemotherapy. *New England Journal of Medicine*, **297**, 213.

234 BERSAGEL D.E., BAILEY A.J., LANGLEY G.R., MACDONALD R.N., WHITE D.F. & MILLER A.B. (1979) The chemotherapy of plasma cell myeloma and the incidence of acute leukemia. *New England Journal of Medicine*, **301**, 743.

235 ROBERTS M.M. & BELL R. (1976) Acute leukaemia after immunosuppressive therapy. *Lancet*, **ii**, 768.

236 GALE R.P. (1979) Advances in the treatment of acute myelogenous leukemia. *New England Journal of Medicine*, **300**, 1189.

237 HENDERSON E.S. (1968) Treatment of acute leukemia. *Annals of Internal Mediciine*, **69**, 628.

238 ELLISON R.R., HOLLAND J.F., WEIL M., JACQUILLAT C., BOIRON M., BERNARD J., SAWITSKY A., ROSNER V., GUSSOFF B., SILVER R.T., KARANAR A., CUTTNER J., SPURR C.L., HAYES D.M., BLOM J., LEONE L.A., HAURANI F., KYLE R., HUTCHISON J.L., FORCIER R.J. & MOON J.M. (1968) Arabinosyl cytosine: a useful agent in the treatment of acute leukemia in adults. *Blood*, **32**, 507.

239 WANG J.J., SELAWRY O.S., VIETTI T.J. & BODEY G.P. (1970) Prolonged infusion of arabinosyl cytosine in childhood leukemia. *Cancer*, **25**, 1.

240 BOIRON M., JACQUILLAT C., WEIL M., TANZER J., LEVY D., SULTAN C. & BERNARD J. (1969) Daunorubicin in the treatment of acute myelocytic leukaemia. *Lancet*, **i**, 330.

241 WIERNIK P.H., GLIDEWELL O.J., HOAGLAND H.C., BRUNNER K.W., SPURR C.L., CUTTNER J., SILVER R.T., CAREY R.W., DUCA V.D., KUNG F.H. & HOLLAND J.F. (1979) A comparative trial of daunorubicin, cytosine arabinoside and thioguanine, and a combination of the three agents for the treatment of acute myelocytic leukemia. *Medical and Pediatric Oncology*, **6**, 261.

242 YATES J.W., WALLACE H.J., ELLISON R.R. & HOLLAND J.F. (1973) Cytosine arabinoside and daunorubicin

therapy in acute non-lymphocytic leukemia. *Cancer Chemotherapy Reports*, **57**, 485.

243 HOLLAND J.F., GLIDEWELL O., ELLISON R.R., CAREY R.W., SCHWARTZ J., WALLACE H.J., HOAGLAND C., WIERNIK P., RAJ K., BEKESI J.G. & CUTTNER J. (1976) Acute myelocytic leukemia. *Archives of Internal Medicine*, **136**, 1377.

244 PREISLER H.D., RUSTUM Y., HENDERSON E.S., BJORNSSON S., CREAVEN P.J., HIGBY A.J., FREEMAN A., GAILANI S. & NAEHER C. (1979) Treatment of acute non lymphocytic leukemia: use of anthracycline-cytosine arabinoside induction therapy and comparison of two maintenance regimens. *Blood*, **53**, 455.

245 PREISLER H., BJORNSSON S., HENDERSON E.S., HRYNIUK W., HIGBY D., FREEMAN A. & NAEHER C. (1979) Remission induction in acute non lymphocytic leukemia: comparison of a seven-day and ten-day infusion of cytosine arabinoside in combination with adriamycin. *Medical and Pediatric Oncology*, **7**, 269.

246 EUROPEAN ORGANIZATION FOR RESEARCH ON THE TREATMENT OF CANCER, CLINICAL SCREENING GROUP (1973) Epipodophyllotoxin VP16-213 in treatment of acute leukaemias, haematosarcomas and solid tumours. *British Medical Journal*, **iii**, 199.

247 GALTON D.A.G. & DACIE J.V. (1975) Classification of the acute leukaemias. *Blood Cells*, **1**, 17.

248 HETZEL P. & GEE T.S. (1978) A new observation in the clinical spectrum of erythroleukemia: a report of 46 cases. *American Journal of Medicine*, **64**, 765.

249 PREISLER H.D. (1978) Failure of remission induction in acute myelocytic leukemia. *Medical and Pediatric Oncology*, **4**, 275.

250 SMITH I.E., POWLES R., CLINK H.M., JAMESON B., KAY H.E.M. & MCELWAIN T.J. (1977) Early deaths in acute myelogenous leukemia. *Cancer*, **39**, 1710.

251 GUNZ F.W., BACH B.I., CROSSEN P.E., SINGH S. & VINCENT P.C. Relevance of cytogenetic status in acute leukemia in adults. *Journal of National Cancer Institute*, **50**, 55.

252 VINCENT P.C., SUTHERLAND R., BRADLEY M., LIND D. & GUNZ F.W. (1977) Marrow culture studies in adult acute leukemia at presentation and during remission. *Blood*, **49**, 903.

253 BODEY G.P., FREIREICH E.J., GEHAN E., MCCREDIE K.B., RODRIGUEZ V., GUTTERMAN J. & BURGESS M.A. (1976) Late intensification therapy for acute leukemia in remission. *Journal of the American Medical Association*, **235**, 1021.

254 DAHL G.V., SIMONE J.V., HUSTU H.O. & MASON C. (1978) Preventive central nervous system irradiation in children with acute non lymphocytic leukaemia. *Cancer*, **42**, 2187.

255 CAREY R.W., RIBAS-MUNDO M., ELLISON R.R., GLIDEWELL O., LEE S.T., CUTTNER J., LEVY R.N., SILVER R., BLOM J., HAURANI F., SPURR C.L., HARLEY J.B., KYLE R., MOON J.H., EGAN R.T. & HOLLAND J.H. (1975) Comparative study of cytosine arabinoside therapy alone and combined with thioguanine, mercaptopurine or daunorubicin in acute myelocytic leukemia. *Cancer*, **36**, 1560.

256 CLARKSON B.D., DOWLING M.D., GEE T.S., CUNNINGHAM I.B. & BURCHENAL J.H. (1975) Treatment of acute leukemia in adults. *Cancer*, **36**, 775.

257 LEWIS J.P., LINMAN J.W., MARSHALL G.J., PAJAK T.F. & BATEMAN J.F. (1977) Randomized clinical trial of cytosine arabinoside and 6-thioguanine in remission induction and consolidation of adult nonlymphocytic acute leukemia. *Cancer*, **39**, 1387.

258 BODEY G.P., COLTMAN C.A., FREIREICH E.J., BONNET J.F., GEHAN E.A., HAUT A.B., HEWLETT J.S., MCCREDIE K.B., SAIKI J.H. & WILSON H.E. (1974) Comparison between arabinosyl cytosine alone and in combination with vincristine, prednisone and cyclophosphamide. *Archives of Internal Medicine*, **133**, 260.

259 CROWTHER D., POWLES R.L., BATEMEN C.J.T., BEARD M.E.J., GAUCI C.L., WRIGLEY P.F.M., MALPAS J.S., FAIRLEY G.H. & BODLEY SCOTT R. (1973) Management of adult acute myelogenous leukaemia. *British Medical Journal*, **i**, 131.

260 SPIERS A.S.D., GOLDMAN J.M., CATOVSKY D., COSTELLO C., GALTON D.A.G. & PITCHER C.S. (1977) Prolonged remission maintenance in acute myeloid leukaemia. *British Medical Journal*, **ii**, 544.

261 GLUCKSBERG H., BUCKNER D.C., FEFER A., DE MARSH Q., COLEMAN D., DOBROW R.B., HUFF J., JOBECH C.K., HILL A.S., DITTMAN W., NEIMAN P.E., CHEEVER M.A., EINSTEIN A.B. & THOMAS E.D. (1975) Combination chemotherapy for acute non lymphoblastic leukemia in adults. *Cancer Chemotherapy Reports*, **59**, 1131.

262 WEINSTEIN H., MAYER R.J., ROSENTHAL D.S., CAMITTA B.M., CORAL F.S., NATHAN D.G. & FREI E. (1980) Treatment of acute myelogenous leukemia in children and adults. *New England Journal of Medicine*, **303**, 473.

263 BODLEY G.P., COLTMAN C.A., HEWLETT J.S. & FREIREICH E.J. (1976) Progression in the treatment of adults with acute leukemia: review of regimens containing cytarabine studied by the South West Oncology Group. *Archives of Internal Medicine*, **136**, 1383.

264 ARMITAGE J.O. & BURNS C.P. (1978) Maintenance therapy of adult acute non lymphoblastic leukaemia. *Cancer*, **41**, 497.

265 EMBURY S.H., ELIAS L., HELLER P.H., HOOD C.E., GREENPERG P.L. & SCHRIER S.L. (1977) Remission maintenance therapy in acute myelogenous leukaemia. *Western Journal of Medicine*, **126**, 267.

266 PETERSON B.A. & BLOOMFIELD C.D. (1977) Prolonged maintaned remissions of adult acute non-lymphocytic leukaemia. *Lancet*, **ii**, 158.

267 CHARD R.L., FINKLESTEIN J.Z., SONLEY M.J., NESBIT M., MCCREADIE S., WEINER J., SATHER H. & HAMMOND G.D. (1978) Increased survival in childhood acute non-lymphocytic leukemia after treatment with prednisone, cytosine arabinoside, 6-thioguanine, cyclophosphamide and oncovin (PATCO) combination chemotherapy. *Medical and Pediatric Oncology*, **4**, 263.

268 WHITTAKER J.A. (1980) Immunotherapy in the treatment of acute leukaemia. *British Journal of Haematology*, **45**, 187.

269 OLD L.J. & BOYSE E.A. (1964) Immunology of experimental tumours. *Annual Review of Medicine*, **15**, 167.

270 MATHÉ G., POUILLART P. & LAPEYRAQUE F. (1969) Active immunotherapy of LI210 leukaemia applied after the graft of tumour cells. *British Journal of Cancer*, **23**, 814.

271 LEVENTHAL B.G., MIRRO J. & KONIOR YARBRO G.S. (1978) Immune reactivity to tumor antigens in leukemia and lymphoma. *Seminars in Hematology*, **15**, 157. 157.

272 MURPHY S. & HERSH E. (1978) Immunotherapy of leukemia and lymphoma. *Seminars in Hematology*, **15**, 181.

273 MATHE G., AMIEL J.L., SCHWARZENBERG L., SCHNEIDER M., CATTAN A., SCHLUMBERGER J.R., HAYAT M. & DE VASSAL F. (1969) Active Immunotherapy for acute lymphoblastic leukaemia. *Lancet*, **i**, 697.

274 MATHE G., SCHWARZENBERG L., DE VASSAL F. & DELGARDO M. (1976) Immunotherapy for acute lymphoid leukaemia. *Lancet*, **i**, 143.

275 HEYN R.M., JOO P., KARON M., NESBIT M., SHORE N., BRESLOW N., WEINER J., REED A. & HAMMOND D. (1975) BCG in the treatment of acute lymphocytic leukemia. *Blood*, **46**, 431.

276 POWLES R.L., CROWTHER D., BATEMAN C.J.T., BEARD M.E.J., MCELWAIN T.J., RUSSELL J., LISTER T.A., WHITEHOUSE J.M.A., WRIGLEY P.F.M., PIKE M., ALEXANDER P. & HAMILTON FAIRLEY G. (1973) Immunotherapy for acute myelogenous leukaemia. *British Journal of Cancer*, **28**, 365.

277 POWLES R.L., RUSSELL J., LISTER T.A., OLIVER T., WHITEHOUSE J.M.A., MALPAS J., CHAPUIS B., CROWTHER D. & ALEXANDER P. (1977) Immunotherapy for acute myelogenous leukaemia: a controlled clinical study, two and a half years after entry of the last patient. *British Journal of Cancer*, **35**, 265.

278 WHITTAKER J.A. & SLATER A.J. (1977) The immunotherapy of acute myelogenous leukaemia using intravenous BCG. *British Journal of Haematology*, **35**, 263.

279 MEDICAL RESEARCH COUNCIL (1978) Immunotherapy of acute myeloid leukaemia. *British Journal of Cancer*, **37**, 1.

280 VOGLER W.R. & CHAN Y.K. (1974) Prolonging remission in myeloblastic leukaemia by Tice-strain bacillus. *Lancet*, **ii**, 128.

281 GUTTERMAN J.V., HERSH E.M., RODRIGUEZ V., MCCREDIE K.B., MAULIGIT G., REED R., BURGESS M.A., SMITH T., GEHAN E., BODEY G.P. & FREIREICH E.J. (1974) Chemo-immunotherapy of adult acute leukaemia. Prolongation of remission in myeloblastic leukaemia with BCG. *Lancet*, **ii**, 1405.

282 OMURA G.A., VOGLER W.R. & LYNN M.J. (1977) A controlled clinical trial of chemotherapy vs BCG immunotherapy vs no further therapy in remission maintenance of acute myelogenous leukemia (AML). *Proceedings of the American Association of Cancer Research and the American Society of Clinical Oncology*, **18**, 272.

283 GALTON D.A.G., KAY H.E.M., REIZENSTEIN P., PENCHAWSKY M., VOGLER W.R. & WHITTAKER J.A. (1977) Infection and second-remission rates in patients having immunotherapy for acute myeloid leukaemia. *Lancet*, **ii**, 973.

284 THOMAS E.D., STORB R., CLIFT R.A., FEFER A., JOHNSON F.J., NEIMAN P.E., LERNER K.G., GLUCKSBERG H. & BUCKNER C.D. (1975) Bone marrow transplantation. *New England Journal of Medicine*, **292**, 832.

285 THOMAS E.D., STORB R., CLIFT R.A., FEFER A., JOHNSON F.J., NEIMAN P.E., LERNER K.G., GLUCKSBERG H. & BUCKNER C.D. (1975) Bone marrow transplantation. *New England Journal of Medicine*, **292**, 895.

286 SANDERS J.E. & THOMAS E.D. (1978) Bone marrow

transcription for acute leukaemia. *Clinics in Haematology*, **7**, 295.

287 HANSEN J.A., CLIFT R.A., THOMAS E.D., BUCKNER C.D., STORB R. & GIBLETT E.R. (1980) Transplantation of marrow from an unrelated donor to a patient with acute leukemia. *New England Journal of Medicine*, **303**, 565.

288 THOMAS E.D., BUCKNER C.D., FEFER A., SANDERS J.E. & STORB R. (1978) Efforts to prevent recurrence of leukemia in marrow graft recipients. *Transplantation Proceedings*, **10**, 163.

289 UCLA BONE MARROW TRANSPLANTATION GROUP (1977) Bone marrow transplantation with intensive combination chemotherapy/radiation therapy (SCARI) in acute leukemia. *Annals of Internal Medicine*, **86**, 155.

290 TUTSCHKA P.J., SANTOS G.W. & ELFENBEIN G.J. (1980) Marrow transplantation in acute leukemia following busulphan and cyclophosphamide. In: *Immunobiology of Bone Marrow Transplantation* (ed. Thierfelder S., Rodt H. & Kolb H.), p. 375. Springer-Verlag, Berlin.

291 WINSTON D.J., GALE R.P., MEYER D.V., YOUNG L.S. & THE UCLA BONE MARROW TRANSPLANTATION GROUP (1979) Infectious complications of human bone marrow transplantation. *Medicine*, **58**, 1.

292 BUCKNER C.D., CLIFT R.A., SANDERS J.E., MYERS J.D., COUNTS G.W., FAREWELL V.T., THOMAS E.D. & THE SEATTLE MARROW TRANSPLANT TEAM (1978) Protective environment for marrow transplant recipients: a prospective study. *Annals of Internal Medicine*, **89**, 893.

293 FEFER A., BUCKNER C.D., THOMAS E.D., CHEEVER M.A., CLIFT R.A., GLUCKSBERG H., NEIMAN P.E. & STORB R. (1977) Cure of hematologic neoplasia with transplantation of marrow from identical twins. *New England Journal of Medicine*, **297**, 146.

294 THOMAS E.D., BUCKNER C.D., BANAJI M., CLIFT R.A., FEFER A., FLOORNOY N., GOODELL B.W., HICKMAN R.O., LERNER K.G., NEIMAN P.E., SALE G.E., SANDERS J.E., SINGER J., STEVENS M., STORB R. & WEIDEN P.L. (1977) One hundred patients with acute leukemia treated by chemotherapy, total body irradiation and allogeneic marrow transplantation. *Blood*, **49**, 511.

295 UCLA BONE MARROW TRANSPLANTATION TEAM (1977) Bone-marrow transplantation in acute leukaemia. *Lancet*, **ii**, 1197.

296 THOMAS E.D., BUCKNER C.D., CLIFT R.A., FEFER A., JOHNSON F.L., NEIMAN P.E., SALE G.E., SANDERS J.E., SINGER J.W., SCHULMAN H., STORB R. & WEIDEN P.L. (1979) Marrow transplantation for acute nonlymphoblastic leukemia in first remission. *New England Journal of Medicine*, **301**, 597.

297 POWLES R.M., MORGENSTERN G., CLINK H.M., HEDLEY D., BANDINI G., LUMLEY H., WATSON J.G., LAWSON D., SPENCE D., BARRETT A., JAMESON B., LAWLER S., KAY H.E.M. & McELWAIN T.J. (1980) The place of bone-marrow transplantation in acute myelogenous leukemia. *Lancet*, **i**, 1047.

298 BUME K.G., BEUTLER E., BROSS J., CHILLAR R.K., ELLINGTON O.B., FAHEY J.L., FARBSTEIN M.J., FORMAN S.J., SCHMIDT G.M., SCOTT E.P., SPRUCE W.E., TURNER M.A. & WOLF J.L. (1980) Bone-marrow ablation and allogeneic marrow transplantation in acute leukemia. *New England Journal of Medicine*, **302**, 1041.

299 THOMAS E.D., SANDERS J.E., FLOURNOY N., JOHNSON L., BUCKNER C.D., CLIFT R.A., FEFER A., GOODELL B.W., STORB R. & WEIDEN P.L. (1979) Marrow transplantation for patients with acute lymphoblastic leukemia in remission. *Blood*, **54**, 468.

300 HARRISON D.T., FLUORNOY N., RAMBERG R., BOYD C., ERNE K., BUCKNER D., FEFER A., SANDERS J.E., STORB R. & THOMAS E.D. (1978) Relapse following marrow transplantation for acute leukemia. *American Journal of Hematology*, **5**, 191.

301 FIALKOW P.J., THOMAS E.D., BRYANT J.I. & NEIMAN P.E. (1971) Leukaemic transformation of engrafted human marrow cells *in vivo*. *Lancet*, **i**, 251.

302 THOMAS E.D., BRYANT J.I., BUCKNER C.D., CLIFT R.A., FEFER A., JOHNSON F.L., NEIMAN P., RAMBERG R.E. & STORB R. (1972) Leukaemic transformation of engrafted human marrow cells *in vivo*. *Lancet*, **i**, 1310.

303 BESCHORNER W.E., HUTCHINS G.M., BURNS W.H., SARAL R., TUTSCHKA P.J. & SANTOS G.W. (1980) Cytomegalovirus pneumonia in bone marrow transplant recipients: miliary and diffuse patterns. *American Review of Respiratory Disease*, **122**, 107.

304 RAPPAPORT J., MIHM M., REINHERZ E., LOPRANSI R. & PARKMAN R. (1979) Acute graft-versus-host disease in recipients of bone-marrow transplants from identical twin donors. *Lancet*, **i**, 717.

305 LOPEL C., SORELL M., KIRKPATRICK D., O'REILLY R.J. & CHING C. (1979) Association between pre-transplant natural kill and graft-versus-host disease after stem cell transplantation. *Lancet*, **ii**, 1103.

306 LOPEZ C., KIRKPATRICK D., LIUNAT S. & STORB R. (1980) Natural killer cells in bone-marrow transplantation. *Lancet*, **ii**, 1025.

307 REINHERZ E.L., PARKMAN R., RAPPAPORT J., ROSEN F. & SCHLOSSMAN S.F. (1979) Aberrations of suppressor T cells in human graft-versus-host disease. *New England Journal of Medicine*, **300**, 1061.

308 POWLES R.L., BARRETT A.J., CLINK H., KAY H.E.M., SLOANE J. & McELWAIN T.J. (1978) Cyclosporin A for the treatment of graft-versus-host disease in man. *Lancet*, **ii**, 1327.

309 RODT H., NETZEL B., KOLB H.J., HAAS R., WILMS K., BENDER-GÖTZE K.C. & THIERFELDER S. (1981) Suppression of GVHD with T-lymphocyte specific antibodies: effect in animal models and application to clinical marrow transplantation in acute leukemias. In: *Modern Trends in Human Leukaemia*. Vol. IV (ed. Neth R. *et al.*). Springer-Verlag, Berlin.

310 VITALE B. & BORANIC M. (1979) Experimental bone marrow transplantation. *British Journal of Haematology*, **42**, 1.

311 BORTIN M.M., TRUITT R.L., RIMM A.A. & BACH F.H. (1979) Graft-versus-leukaemia reactivity induced by alloimmunization without augmentation of graft-versus-host reactivity. *Nature (London)*, **281**, 490.

312 ODOM L.F., AUGUST C.S., GITHENS J.H., HUMBERT J.R., MORSE H., PEAKMAN D., SHARMA B., RUSNAK S.L. & JOHNSON F.B. (1978) Remission of relapsed leukaemia during a graft-versus-host reaction. *Lancet*, **ii**, 537.

313 WEIDEN P.L., FLUORNOY N., THOMAS E.D., PRENTICE R., FEFER A., BUCKNER C.D. & STORB R. (1979) Antileukemic effect of graft-versus-host disease in human recipients of allogeneic-marrow grafts. *New England Journal of Medicine*, **300**, 1068.

314 GORIN N.C., HERZIG G., BULL M.I. & GRAW R.G. (1978) Long-term preservation of bone marrow and stem cell pool in dogs. *Blood*, **51**, 257.

315 ZIEGLER J.L., DEISSEROTH A.B., APPLEBAUM F.R. & GRAW R.G. (1977) Burkitt's lymphoma—a model for intensive chemotherapy. *Seminars in Oncology*, **4**, 317.

316 DICKE K.A., ZANDER A., SPITZER G., VERMA D.S., PETERS L., VELLEKOOP L., McCREDIE K.B. & HESTER J. (1979) Autologous bone-marrow transplantation in relapsed adult acute leukaemia. *Lancet*, **i**, 514.

317 NETZEL B., RODT H., HAAS R.J., KOLB H.J. & THIER-FELDER S. (1980) Immunological conditioning of bone marrow for autotransplantation in childhood acute lymphoblastic leukaemia. *Lancet*, **i**, 1330.

318 SMYTH J.F., CHASSIN M.M., HARRAP K.R., ADAMSON R.H. & JOHNS D.G. (1979) 2-deoxycorformycin (DCF). Phase I trial and clinical pharmacology. *Proceedings of the American Association for Cancer Research*, **20**, 47.

319 HUSTU H.O. & AUR R.J.A. (1978) Extramedullary leukemia. *Clinics in Hematology*, **7**, 313.

320 HARDISTY R.M. & NORMAN P.M. (1967) Meningeal leukaemia. *Archives of Diseases in Childhood*, **42**, 441.

321 EVANS A.E., GILBERT E.S. & ZANDSTRA R. (1970) The increasing incidence of central nervous system leukemia in children. *Cancer*, **26**, 404.

322 LAW I.P. & BLOM J. (1977) Adult acute leukemia: frequency of central nervous system involvement in long term survivors. *Cancer*, **40**, 1304.

323 WEST R.J., GRAHAM-POLE J., HARDISTY R.M. & PIKE M.C. (1972) Factors in pathogenesis of central-nervous-system leukaemia. *British Medical Journal*, **III**, 311.

324 WOLK R.W., MASSE S.R., CONKLIN R. & FREIREICH E.J. (1974) The incidence of central nervous system leukemia in adults with acute leukemia. *Cancer*, **33**, 863.

325 KAY H.E.M. (1976) Development of central nervous system leukaemia in acute myeloid leukaemia in childhood. *Archives of Diseases in Childhood*, **51**, 73.

326 PIPPARD M.J., CALLENDER S.T. & SHELDON P.W.E. (1979) Infiltration of central nervous system in adult acute myeloid leukaemia. *British Medical Journal*, **i**, 227.

327 MOORE E., THOMAS L., SHAW R. & FREIREICH E. (1960) The central nervous system in acute leukemia: a post mortem study of 117 consecutive cases. *Archives of Internal Medicine*, **105**, 451.

328 PRICE R.A. & JOHNSON W. (1973) The central nervous system in childhood leukemia. I. The arachnoid. *Cancer*, **31**, 520.

329 KUO A. H.-M., YATAGANAS X., GALICICH J.H., FRIED J. & CLARKSON B.D. (1975) Proliferative kinetics of central nervous system (CNS) leukemia. *Cancer*, **36**, 232.

330 HUSTU H.O., AUR R.J.A., VERZOSA M.S., SIMONE J.V. & PINKEL D. (1973) Prevention of central nervous system leukemia by irradiation. *Cancer*, **32**, 585.

331 MEDICAL RESEARCH COUNCIL (1973) Treatment of acute lymphoblastic leukaemia; effect of 'prophylactic' therapy against central nervous system leukaemia. *British Medical Journal*, **ii**, 381.

332 AUR R.J.A., HUSTU H.O., VERZOSA M.S., WOOD A. & SIMONE J.V. (1973) Comparison of two methods of preventing central nervous system leukaemia. *Blood*, **42**, 349.

333 NESBIT M.E., SATHER H.N., ROBISON L.L., D'ANGIO G.D., LITTMAN P., DONALDSON M. & HAMMOND G.D. (1979) Pre-symptomatic CNS treatment in childhood acute lymphoblastic leukaemia (ALL): comparison between 1800 and 2400 rads. *Proceedings of the American Society of Clinical Oncology*, **20**, 343.

334 ZUELZER W.W., RAVINDRANATH Y., LUSHER J.M., SARNAIK S. & CONSIDINE B. (1976) IMFRA (intermittent intrathecal methotrexate and fractional radiation) plus chemotherapy in childhood leukaemia. *American Journal of Hematology*, **1**, 191.

335 SHAPIRO W.R., YOUNG D.F. & MEHTA B.M. (1975) Methotrexate: distribution in cerebrospinal fluid after intravenous, ventricular and lumbar injections. *New England Journal of Medicine*, **293**, 161.

336 HAGHBIN M., TAN C., CLARKSON B., GEE T., DOWLING M., BURCHENAL J. & MURPHY M.L. (1975) Intense drug combination and Ommaya device for prophylactic chemotherapy in lymphoblastic leukemia. *Proceedings of the American Society for Cancer Research and American Society of Clinical Oncology*, **16**, 165.

337 FREEMAN A.I., WANG J.J. & SINKS L.F. (1977) High-dose methotrexate in acute lymphocytic leukemia. *Cancer Treatment Reports*, **61**, 727.

338 EISER C. & LANSDOWN R. (1977) Retrospective study of intellectual development in children treated for acute lymphoblastic leukaemia. *Archives of Diseases in Childhood*, **52**, 525.

339 GRIBBIN M.A., HARDISTY R.M. & CHESSELLS J.M. (1977) Long-term control of central nervous system leukaemia. *Archives of Diseases in Childhood*, **52**, 673.

340 BLEYER W.A. & POPLACK D.G. (1979) Intraventricular versus intralumbar methotrexate for central-nervous-system leukemia: prolonged remission with the Ommaya reservoir. *Medical and Pediatric Oncology*, **6**, 207.

341 WILLOUGHBY M.L.N. (1976) Treatment of overt meningeal leukaemia in children: results of second MRC. Meningeal leukaemia trial. *British Medical Journal*, **i**, 864.

342 WELLS R.J., WEETMAN R.M. & BAEHNER R.L. (1980) The impact of isolated central nervous system relapse following initial complete remission in childhood acute lymphocytic leukemia. *Journal of Pediatrics*, **97**, 429.

343 BAND P.R., HOLLAND J.F., BERNARD J., WEIL M., WALKER M. & RALL D. (1973) Treatment of central nervous system leukemia with intrathecal cytosine arabinoside. *Cancer*, **32**, 744.

344 MEDICAL RESEARCH COUNCIL (1978) Testicular disease in acute lymphoblastic leukaemia in childhood. *British Medical Journal*, **ii**, 334.

345 SALLAN S.E., CAMITTA B.M., CASSADY J.R., NATHAN D.G. & FREI E.I. (1978) Intermittent combination chemotherapy with adriamycin for childhood acute lymphoblastic leukemia: clinical results. *Blood*, **51**, 425.

346 NESBIT M.E., ROBISON L.L., ORTEGA J.A., SATHER H.N., DONALDSON M. & HAMMOND D. (1980) Testicular relapse in childhood acute lymphoblastic leukaemia: association with pre-treatment patient characteristics and treatment. *Cancer*, **45**, 2009.

347 BAUM E., NESBIT M. JR, TILFORD D., HEYN R. & KRIVIT W. (1979) Extent of disease in pediatric patients with acute lymphocytic leukemia experiencing an apparent

isolated testicular relapse. *Proceedings of the American Association for Cancer Research and American Society of Clinical Oncology*, **20**, 435.

348 SULLIVAN M.P., PEREZ C.A., HERSON J., SILVA-SOUSA M., LAND V., DYMENT P.G., CHAN R. & AYALA A.G. (1980) Radiotherapy (2500 Rad) for testicular leukaemia. Local control and subsequent clinical events: a South-West Oncology Group Study. *Cancer*, **46**, 508.

349 CHESSELLS J.M., NINANE J. & TIEDEMANN K. (1981) Present problems in management of childhood lymphoblastic leukaemia: experience from the Hospital for Sick Children, London. In: *Modern Trends in Leukaemia*. Vol. IV (ed. Neth R. *et al.*). Springer-Verlag, Berlin.

350 CECALUPO A.J., FRANKEL L.S. & SULLIVAN M.P. (1979) Pelvic and ovarian extramedullary leukemic relapse in young girls. *Proceedings of the American Association for Cancer Research and the American Society of Clinical Oncology*, **20**, 365.

351 MANOHARAN A., CATOVSKY D., GOLDMAN J.M., LAURIA F., LAMPERT I.A. & GALTON D.A.G. (1980) Significance of splenomegaly in childhood acute lymphoblastic leukaemia in remission. *Lancet*, **i**, 449.

352 HARDISTY R.M. & CHESSELLS J.M. (1980) Splenomegaly in childhood leukaemia. *Lancet*, **i**, 821.

353 RIDGWAY E.W., JAFFE N. & WALTON D.S. (1976) Leukemic ophthalmopathy in children. *Cancer*, **38**, 1744.

354 MURRAY K.H., PAOLINO F., GOLDMAN J.M., GALTON D.A.G. & GRINDLE C.F.J. (1977) Ocular involvement in leukemia. *Lancet*, **ii**, 829.

355 NINANE J., TAYLOR D. & DAY S. (1980) The eye as a sanctuary in acute lymphoblastic leukaemia. *Lancet*, **i**, 452.

356 O'REGAN S., CARSON S., CHESNEY R.W. & DRUMMOND K.N. (1977) Electrolyte and acid-base disturbances in the management of leukemia. *Blood*, **49**, 345.

357 JAFFE N. (1975) Metabolic and biochemical changes in leukemia. In: *Modern Problems in Paediatrics, Vol. 16. Acute Childhood Leukaemia* (ed. Pochedly C.), p. 113. Karger, Basel.

358 HARRIS A.L. (1978) Leukostasis associated with blood transfusion in acute myeloid leukaemia. *British Medical Journal*, **i**, 1169.

359 PRESTON F.E., SOKOL R.J., LILLEYMAN J.S., WINFIELD D.A. & BLACKBURN E.K. (1978) Cellular hyperviscosity as a cause of neurological symptoms in leukaemia. *British Medical Journal*, **i**, 476.

360 LISTER T.A. & YANKEE R.A. (1978) Blood component therapy. *Clinics in Haematology*, **7**, 407.

361 GURWITH M. (1978) Prevention of infection in leukaemia. *Journal of Antimicrobial Chemotherapy*, **4**, 302.

362 STORRING R.A., JAMESON B., MCELWAIN T.J., WILTSHAWE E., SPIERS A.S.D. & GAYA H. (1977) Oral non-absorbed antibiotics prevent infection in acute non-lymphoblastic leukaemia. *Lancet*, **ii**, 837.

363 ENNO A., CATOVSKY D., DARREL J., GOLDMAN J.M., HOWS J. & GALTON D.A.G. (1978) Co-trimoxazole for prevention of infection in acute leukaemia. *Lancet*, **ii**, 395.

364 LEVINE A.S., SCHIMPFF S.C., GRAW R.G. & YOUNG R.C. (1974) Hematologic malignancies and other marrow failure states: progress in the management of complicating infections. *Seminars in Hematology*, **11**, 141.

365 EORTC INTERNATIONAL ANTIMICROBIAL THERAPY PROJECT GROUP (1979) Empirical therapy in febrile granulocytopenic patients. In: *Topics in Paediatrics. I. Haematology & Oncology* (ed. Morris Jones P.H.), p. 113. Pitman Medical, Tunbridge Wells.

366 PIZZO P.A., ROBICHAUD K.J., GILL F.A., WITEBSY F.G., LEVINE A.S., DEISSEROTH A.B., GLAUBIGER D.L., MACLOWRY J.D., MAGRATH I.T., POPLACK D.G. & SIMON R.M. (1979) Duration of empiric antibiotic therapy in granulocytopenic patients with cancer. *American Journal of Medicine*, **67**, 194.

367 GRAW R.G., HERZIG G.P., PERRY S. & HENDERSON E.S. (1972) Normal granulocyte transfusion therapy; treatment of Gram-negative bacterial septicemia. *New England Journal of Medicine*, **287**, 367.

368 HERZIG R.H., HERZIG G.P., GRAW R.G., BULL M.I. & RAY K.R. (1977) Successful granulocyte transfusion therapy for Gram-negative septicemia. A prospective randomized controlled study. *New England Journal of Medicine*, **296**, 701.

369 ALAVI J.B., ROOT A.K., DJERARASSI I., EVANS A.E., CLUCKMAN S.J., MACGREGOR R.R., GUERRY D., SCHREIBER A.D., SHAW J.M., KOCH E. & COOPER R.A. (1977) A randomized clinical trial of granulocyte transfusion for infection in acute leukaemia. *New England Journal of Medicine*, **296**, 706.

370 NINANE J.N. & CHESSELLS J.M. (1981) Serious infections during continuing treatment of acute lymphoblastic leukaemia. *Archives of Diseases in Childhood*, **56**, 841.

371 BAEHNER R.L., NEIBURGER R.G., JOHNSON D.E. & MURRMAN S.M. (1973) Transient bactericidal defect of peripheral blood phagocytes from children with acute lymphoblastic leukemia receiving craniospinal irradiation. *New England Journal of Medicine*, **289**, 1209.

372 RAPSON N.T., CORNBLEET M.A., CHESSELLS J.M., BENNETT A. & HARDISTY R.M. (1980) Immunosupression and serious infections in children with acute lymphoblastic leukaemia: a comparison of three chemotherapy regimes. *British Journal of Haematology*, **45**, 41.

373 PULLAN C.R., NOBLE T.C., SCOTT D.J., WISNIEWSKI K. & GARDNER P.S. (1976) Atypical measles infections in leukemic children on immunosuppressive treatment. *British Medical Journal*, **i**, 1562.

374 FELDMAN S., HUGHES W.T. & DANIEL C.B. (1975) Varicella in children with cancer: seventy-seven cases. *Pediatrics*, **56**, 388.

375 MITUS A., HOLLOWAY A., EVANS A. & ENDERS J.F. (1962) Attenuated measles vaccine in children with acute leukaemia. *American Journal of Diseases of Children*, **103**, 413.

376 IZAWA T., IHARA T., HATTORI A., IWASA T., KAMIYA H., SAKURAI M. & TAKAHASHI M. (1977) Application of a live varicella vaccine in children with acute leukemia or other malignant diseases. *Pediatrics*, **6**, 805.

377 HA K., BABA K., IKEDA T., NISHIDA M., YABUUCHI H. & TAKAHASHI M. (1980) Application of live varicella vaccine to children with acute leukemia or other malignancies without suspension or anticancer therapy. *Pediatrics*, **65**, 346.

378 SELBY P.J., POWLES R.L., JAMESON B.J., KAY H.E.M., WATSON J.G., THORNTON R., MORGENSTERN G., CLINK

H.M., McElwain T.J., Prentice H.G., Corringham R., Ross M.G., Hoffbrand A.V. & Brigden D. (1979) Parenteral Acylovir therapy for herpesvirus infections in man. *Lancet*, ii, 1267.

379 Hughes W.T., Feldman S., Aur R.J.A., Verzosa M., Hustu H.O. & Simone J.V. (1975) Intensity of immunosuppressive therapy and the incidence of pneumocystis carinii pneumonitis. *Cancer*, **36**, 2004.

380 Hughes W.T., Kuhn S., Chaudhary S., Feldman S., Verzosa M., Aur R.J.A., Pratt C. & George S.L. (1977) Successful chemoprophylaxis for pneumocystis carinii pneumonitis. *New England Journal of Medicine*, **297**, 177.

381 Hughes W.T., Feldman S., Chaudhary S.C., Ossi M.J., Cox F. & Sanyal S.K. (1978) Comparison of pentamidine isethionate and trimethoprim-sulfamethoxazole in the treatment of pneumocystis carinii pneumonia. *Journal of Pediatrics*, **92**, 285.

382 Secker-Walker L.M. & Sandler R.M. (1978) Acute myeloid leukaemia with monosomy-7 follows acute lymphoblastic leukaemia. *British Journal of Haematology*, **38**, 359.

383 Campbell R.H.A., Marshall W.C. & Chessells J.M. (1977) Neurological complications of childhood leukaemia. *Archives of Diseases in Childhood*, **52**, 850.

384 Freeman J.E., Johnson P.G.B. & Voke J.M. (1973) Somnolence after prophylactic cranial irradiation in children with acute lymphoblastic leukaemia. *British Medical Journal*, iv, 523.

385 Geiser C.F., Bishop V., Jaffe N., Furman L., Traggis D. & Frei E. (1975) Adverse effects of intrathecal methotrexate in children with acute leukemia in remission. *Blood*, **45**, 189.

386 Kay H.E.M., Knapton P.J., O'Sullivan J.P., Wells D.G., Harris R.F., Innes E.M., Stuart J., Schwartz F.C.M. & Thompson E.N. (1972) Encephalopathy in acute leukaemia associated with methotrexate therapy. *Archives of Diseases in Childhood*, **47**, 344.

387 Rubinstein L.R., Herman M.M., Long T.F. & Wilbur J.R. (1975) Disseminated necrotizing leukoencephalopathy: a complication of treated central nervous system leukemia and lymphoma. *Cancer*, **35**, 291.

388 Price R.A. & Jamieson P.A. (1975) The central nervous system in childhood leukaemia. II. Subacute leukoencephalopathy. *Cancer*, **35**, 306.

389 McIntosh S., Klatskin E.H., O'Brien R.T., Aspnes G.T., Kammerer B.L., Snead C., Kalavsky S.M. & Pearson H.A. (1976) Chronic neurologic disturbance in childhood leukemia. *Cancer*, **37**, 853.

390 Eiser C. (1980) Effects of chronic illness on intellectual development. A comparison of normal children with those treated for childhood leukaemia and solid tumours. *Archives of Diseases in Childhood*, **55**, 766.

391 Price R.A. & Birdwell D.A. (1973) The central nervous system in childhood leukemia. III. Mineralizing microangiopathy and dystrophic calcification. *Cancer*, **42**, 717.

392 Peylan-Ramu N., Poplack D.G., Pizzo P.A., Adornato B.T. & di Chiro D. (1978) Abnormal CT scans of the brain in asymptomatic children with acute lymphoblastic leukemia after prophylactic treatment of the central nervous system with radiation and intrathecal chemotherapy. *New England Journal of Medicine*, **298**, 815.

393 Day R.E., Kingston J., Bullimore J.A., Mott M.G. & Thomson J.L.G. (1978) CAT brain scans after central nervous system prophylaxis for acute lymphoblastic leukaemia. *British Medical Journal*, ii, 1752.

394 Maguire P., Comaroff J., Ramsell P.J. & Morris Jones P.H. (1979) Psychological and social problems in families of children with leukaemia. *Topics in Paediatrics. I. Haematology and Oncology*, p. 141. Pitman Medical, Tunbridge Wells.

395 Eiser C. (1980) How leukaemia effects a child's schooling. *British Journal of Social and Clinical Psychology*, **19**, 365.

396 Siris E.S., Leventhal B.G. & Vaitukaitis J.L. (1976) Effects of childhood leukemia and chemotherapy on puberty and reproductive function in girls. *New England Journal of Medicine*, **294**, 1143.

397 Shalet S.M., Beardwell C.G., Twomey J.A., Morris Jones P.H. & Pearson D. (1977) Endocrine function following the treatment of acute leukaemia in childhood. *Journal of Pediatrics*, **90**, 920.

398 Li F.P., Fine W., Jaffe N., Holmes G.E. & Holmes F.F. (1979) Offspring of patients treated for cancer in childhood. *Journal of the National Cancer Institute*, **62**, 1193.

399 Lendon M., Hann I.M., Palmer M.K., Shalet S.M. & Morris Jones P.H. (1978) Testicular histology after combination chemotherapy in childhood for acute lymphoblastic leukaemia. *Lancet*, ii, 439.

400 Lilleyman J.S. (1979) Male fertility after successful chemotherapy for lymphoblastic leukaemia. *Lancet*, ii, 1125.

401 Matthews J.H. & Wood J.K. (1980) Male fertility during chemotherapy for acute leukemia. *New England Journal of Medicine*, **303**, 1235.

402 Johnson F.L., Thomas E.D., Clark B.S., Chard R.L., Hartmann, J.R. & Storb R. (1981) A comparison of marrow transplantation with chemotherapy for children with acute lymphoblastic leukemia in second or subsequent remission. *New England Journal of Medicine*, **305**, 846.

403 Nesbit M.E., Sather H.N., Robison L.L., Ortega J., Littman P.S., D'Angio G.J. & Hammond G.D. (1981) Presymptomatic central nervous system therapy in previously untreated childhood acute lymphoblastic leukaemia. Comparison of 1800 rad and 2400 rad. *Lancet*, i, 465.

Chapter 23
The chronic leukaemias

D. A. G. GALTON

THE CHRONIC MYELOID LEUKAEMIAS
ESPECIALLY CHRONIC GRANULOCYTIC LEUKAEMIA

The chronic myeloid leukaemias comprise five types which appear to be distinct biological entities (Table 23.1). The commonest type is the classical *Philadelphia-chromosome-positive (Ph¹ +) chronic granulocytic leukaemia (CGL)*. It is a relatively uniform condition in its clinical, haematological and cytogenetic features, and in its course, prognosis and response to treatment. Rarely, the Philadelphia chromosome is absent in otherwise typical cases, while it is present in rare cases with atypical clinical and haematological features. The majority of such cases are Ph¹ −, and the course of the disease, here designated *'atypical chronic myeloid leukaemia'*, the prognosis and response to treatment differ from those of Ph¹-positive CGL [1, 2]. *Chronic myelomonocytic leukaemia (CMML)* [3], and the even more uncommon *neutrophilic leukaemia* [4–8] are diseases of elderly subjects, while *juvenile chronic myeloid leukaemia* [9], which arises from a fetal stem cell [10], is a disease of the first few years of life. CMML has a wide spectrum of presentations, merging on the one hand with the myelodysplastic syndromes [11], as shown by the occurrence in varying degree of dyserythropoiesis and morphological abnormalities in the megakaryocytes (small mononuclear or multinuclear forms), granulocytes (hypogranularity, agranularity, presence of Pelger cells or bizarrely segmented forms), and on the other with atypical chronic myeloid leukaemia and acute myelomonocytic leukaemia [3]. Rarely the abnormalities are confined to the monocytic series [12–12b], sometimes for many years, when the condition may be diagnosed by chance, as in a patient of mine undergoing surgery for a mammary tumour, who lived without progression of the leukaemia for more than 15 years.

CGL accounts for about 15% of all cases of leukaemia, is slightly more frequent in males, and is most prevalent in young and middle-aged adults. It is rare below age five, but one case in an infant of 11 months has been reported [13]. There are no associations with social class or race, and there is no familial

incidence. Exposure to ionizing radiation is the only known aetiological factor: the incidence of CGL as well as of acute myeloid and lymphoblastic leukaemia increased one to 12 years after exposure in populations exposed to radiation received either as treatment for ankylosing spondylitis, metropathia haemorrhagica and other diseases, or from atomic bomb explosions [14–15a]. There was a higher incidence of CGL relative to other forms among the survivors of the Hiroshima explosion than among those in Nagasaki, and this is attributed to the presence of neutron radiation at Hiroshima whereas the radiation at Nagasaki was largely γ rays [16]. The leukaemogenic potential of radiation at low doses of the order encountered in background radiation is uncertain [17], and the proportion of cases of spontaneous CGL that might result from such exposure is unknown. It is likely to be very small [18].

Pathogenesis of chronic-phase CGL
CGL is a clonal myeloproliferative disorder, as shown by investigations involving cytogenetic and biochemical markers. The stem cell from which it originates appears to be a primitive haemopoietic cell of pre-lymphoid and pre-myeloid potential [19–21], which differs functionally from its normal counterpart in two respects. First, its differentiation within the myeloid compartment is unbalanced, as shown by the progressive granulocytic hyperplasia which leads to the manifestations of the chronic phase of CGL; secondly, it is at a higher risk of undergoing transformation to a malignant blast-cell clone, responsible for the events of the transformed phase of CGL which can develop at any stage in the evolution of the chronic-phase disease, or even before it has become established.

Cytogenetic evidence of monoclonality
The Philadelphia chromosome (Ph¹) [22], a chromosome 22 lacking about half of the chromosomal material of its long arm (Fig. 23.1), is found in more than 90% of all dividing cells in the bone marrow in Ph¹-positive CGL. In 90% of the positive cases only one of the two chromosomes is a Ph¹, or two of the four

Table 23.1. The chronic myeloid leukaemias

Type	Relative prevalence	Age	Cytogenetics	Remarks
Chronic granulocytic (CGL)	Common	Rare below five years	Great majority Ph^1 +	Characteristic pattern of evolution, course, response to treatment. Characteristic blood picture: essentially normal blood-cell morphology, high absolute basophil counts, low relative monocyte counts; low alkaline-phosphatase content of neutrophils. Readily controllable in chronic phase. Median duration of survival about three and a half years.
Atypical chronic myeloid	Rare	Rare below 30 years	Great majority Ph^1 −	Variable pattern of evolution, course, response to treatment. Variable blood picture; merges with acute myeloid leukaemia, CMML; basophil counts not increased, monocyte counts often increased, immature granulocytes present. Morphological abnormalities in majority. Poor response to treatment. Median duration of survival <18 months.
Chronic myelomonocytic (CMML)	Rare	Rare below 60 years	Ph^1 −	Variable pattern of evolution, course, response to treatment. High absolute neutrophil and monocyte counts (only monocytes in pure monocytic variant): immature granulocytes and monocytes absent in chronic phase. Hypogranular neutrophils, agranular polymorphs, Pelger cells common: dyserythropoiesis, ringed sideroblasts, micromegakaryocytes frequent. Splenomegaly frequent. Serum lysozyme greatly increased. Neutrophil alkaline phosphatase variable. Variable prognosis, duration of survival may exceed 10 years. Termination in blast-cell transformation. Merges with myelodysplastic syndrome and atypical CML.
Neutrophilic	Very rare	Rare below 60 years	Ph^1 −	High absolute neutrophil counts. Immature granulocytes not present. High alkaline-phosphatase content of neutrophils. Splenomegaly may be present. Terminates in blast-cell transformation.
Juvenile chronic myeloid	Very rare	Below five years	Ph^1 −	Characteristic clinical picture: splenomegaly, lymph node enlargement, rashes, septic lesions. Leucocytosis with immature granulocytes and blasts. Normoblasts in blood. Origin in fetal stem cell: high Hb F, fetal red-cell enzymes. Poor response to chemotherapy.

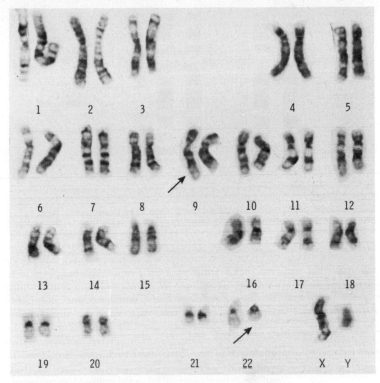

Fig. 23.1. Karyotype from a case of chronic-phase Ph¹-positive chronic granulocytic leukaemia. G-R banding technique. One member of the No. 22 pair (arrowed) lacks a portion of the long arm which has been translocated to the long arm of one member of pair No. 9 (arrowed).

in tetraploid cells, presumably megakaryocytes. The Ph¹ is present in the erythropoietic line [23, 24] and, as demonstrated in agar cultures [25–27a], in monocyte precursors and macrophages [28] as well as in granulocyte precursors, including basophil precursors [29]. The claim [30] that it is present in B-lymphocytes has been confirmed [414, 415]; it is not present in cultured marrow fibroblasts [31–32a]. Phytohaemagglutinin-stimulated peripheral blood lymphocytes do not contain the Ph¹. The Ph¹ is not present in the marrow of persons whose monozygotic twin sib has Ph¹-positive CGL [33–35], so it appears to be an acquired abnormality. In the majority of cases of CGL in constitutional mosaics, the Ph¹ is confined to one of the two cell populations characterized by their karyotypes [36], suggesting monoclonality, but the rare exceptions [37–39] are difficult to explain. However, in cases in which chromosome polymorphism is present, all the Ph¹-bearing marrow cells carry one variant, whereas the Ph¹-negative cells of other tissues contain one or other variant in equal proportions [40, 41]. The cytogenetic evidence thus supports the hypothesis of monoclonality for the Ph¹-positive cell population in CGL.

Biochemical evidence of monoclonality
In human populations which have polymorphic allo-

enzymes (A and B) for glucose-6-phosphate dehydrogenase (G6-PD), monoclonality in a cell population is shown by the presence of only one of the enzymes in all the cells, because the locus (on the X chromosome) is subject to random inactivation and in polyclonal cell populations the frequency of the two enzymes is equal. In all cases of CGL suitable for the application of this method, monoclonality has been found [42, 43]. Furthermore, the method has been used to show that in CGL, the erythrocytes, granulocytes, platelets and macrophages all arise from the same stem-cell clone [44].

The Ph¹ translocation
Rowley [45] discovered that the portion of the long arm of chromosome 22 missing in the Ph¹ was not lost to the genome as had been previously believed, but was translocated to the distal end of the long arm of one of the two chromosomes 9. The discovery was made possible by the introduction of techniques [46, 46a] for characterizing each chromosome by producing transverse banding patterns in the chromatin. The quantity of DNA lost from the Ph¹ is the same as that added to chromosome 9 [47]. The 9q+/22q− translocation (Figs 23.1, 23.2) is found in 92% of cases of CGL [48]; in the remainder, the material lost from the Ph¹ is added to one of the other chromosomes, either as a

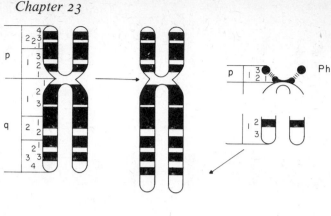

Fig. 23.2. Diagram to show the common break point in the long arm (q) of No. 22 (band q12) and the translocation to the long arm of No. 9 (q34). Note that the fate of the terminal portion of the long arm of No. 9 is uncertain. It may be reciprocally translocated to the remaining portion of the long arm of No. 22.

simple translocation or as part of a complex rearrangement involving one or more other chromosomes [48]. So far there is no evidence that the features of the disease, its evolution, response to treatment, and the duration of survival vary according to the chromosome to which the material from the Ph[1] is added [49], but the duration of follow-up is still very short. It appears to be the Ph[1] itself which is intimately associated with the pathogenesis of CGL and with the various types of blast-cell leukaemia that can arise from Ph[1]-positive stem cells.

Diagnostic features in relation to the evolution of chronic-phase CGL
Figure 23.3 is a schematic representation of the pattern of evolution in the majority of cases of classical CGL.

The early part of the chart, before the start of the time scale, is necessarily inferential. It assumes that a Ph[1]-positive clone of stem cells, once established, has a growth advantage over the normal stem cells and is able to replace them. While normal stem cells remain, the red-cell, leucocyte and platelet counts are maintained at normal levels by homeostatic mechanisms. When all the stem cells are Ph[1]-positive a defect in homeostasis results in a progressive increase in the cellularity of the bone marrow and a change in its composition. Fat spaces disappear in the red marrow and the yellow marrow becomes replaced by hypercellular red marrow. There is gross relative and absolute granulocytic hyperplasia and commonly an absolute increase in the number of megakaryocytes, a high proportion of which are often small forms of reduced

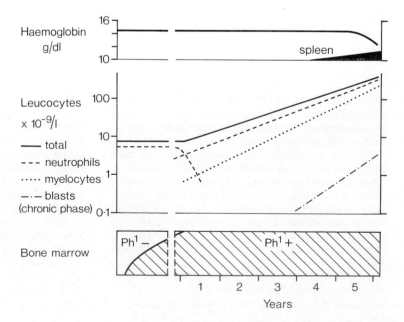

Fig. 23.3. Schematic representation of the evolution of Ph[1]-positive chronic granulocytic leukaemia, showing the temporal relationship between the replacement of the bone marrow by the Ph[1]-positive clone, the ascent of the leucocyte count, the onset of splenic enlargement and of the falling trend in the haemoglobin concentration.

ploidy [50, 51]. Quantitative estimates have shown the presence of absolute neutrophil marrow hyperplasia and increased neutrophil production [52]. The leucocyte count begins to rise exponentially, at first because of a rising neutrophil count, soon accompanied by the appearance of immature granulocytes, of which myelocytes are the most numerous [53]. The proportion of myelocytes increases as the total count increases. At an early stage absolute basophilia occurs, and sometimes eosinophilia also, but the trends in the absolute counts of these cells are variable. The relative number of monocytes declines, however, as the total leucocyte count rises [54]. The platelet counts are usually above the normal range and sometimes considerably above [53], but are not correlated with the leucocyte counts [53]. The morphology of all the cells is essentially normal, and the absolute increase in the neutrophils and myelocytes, the presence of basophils, the paucity of monocytes, and the increase in the platelets make a highly characteristic pattern. It is clear that haemopoiesis is totally disturbed, but the major derangement is in granulopoiesis, whereby the total pool of granulocyte precursor cells is progressively expanded, with an increased delivery of mature granulocytes to the circulation but little increase in the proliferation rate. The kinetics of granulopoiesis in health and in CGL are reviewed by Stryckmans *et al.* [55], Cronkite [56], and Vincent [57].

The autoregulation of granulopoiesis is extremely complex and involves subtle interactions between regulatory molecules with opposing effects [58]. It would be naive to suppose that a single defect in an integrated bioregulatory network could explain the pathogenesis of CGL, because of the high capacity for compensatory adjustment in biological systems. Nevertheless one factor in the defective homeostasis in CGL may be the reduced capacity of CGL mature granulocytes to release an inhibitor [59], believed to be iron-saturated lactoferrin [60], which decreases the production and release of granulocyte/monocyte colony-stimulating factor (CSF) by monocytes and macrophages [61]. The CGL neutrophils are, however, not always deficient in lactoferrin [62, 63], but the immunoperoxidase or immunocytochemical assays are only semiquantitative.

The exponential increase in the leucocyte count continues until the count is in the region $250 \times 10^9/l$, after which the rising trend is less regular. The rate of ascent is known only from the small number of symptomless patients whose disease is diagnosed early and who are regularly observed without treatment for one or more years. The doubling time varies from about six to more than 12 months. The spleen first becomes palpable when the leucocyte count is between 50 and $150 \times 10^9/l$, and the haemoglobin concentration begins to fall slowly thereafter in association with the increase in plasma volume and the extent of splenic red-cell pooling that accompany splenic enlargement, and eventually an absolute decrease in erythropoiesis.

This sequence of events is so characteristic of Ph[1]-positive CGL that departures from it suggest either that the condition is not Ph[1]-positive CGL or that transformation has occurred. Departures are more likely to be seen in childhood [64, 65]. Rare cases of atypical Ph[1]-positive myeloproliferative disease cannot always be interpreted as transformed CGL and are referred to below. Examples of associations unlikely to be found in uncomplicated Ph[1]-positive CGL, but commonly found in atypical (Ph[1]-negative) CML, are: anaemia in the absence of splenomegaly; massive splenomegaly with a leucocyte count below $50 \times 10^9/l$; a leucocyte count above $150 \times 10^9/l$ but no palpable enlargement of the spleen or minimal enlargement; any of the above with subnormal platelet counts; and atypical blood pictures characterized by absence of the neutrophil/myelocyte peaks in the differential count [53], morphologically abnormal neutrophils, absence of basophilia, relative and absolute monocytosis.

Unusual patterns of evolution in untreated adult CGL include the following.

1 Long periods of cyclical leucocytosis, with or without an upward trend in the peaks and troughs of the counts, and sometimes accompanied by cyclical thrombocytosis [66–69]: the cyclical oscillations persist in some cases after treatment.

2 Presentation with haemorrhagic or thrombotic symptoms resulting from thrombocythaemia in patients with normal or only moderately raised leucocyte counts and no palpable enlargement of the spleen.

3 Patients with extensive myelofibrosis who have only moderately raised leucocyte counts and usually gross enlargement of the spleen [70–73]: in these cases bone marrow cannot be aspirated and the Ph[1] can be demonstrated only in cultures of peripheral blood leucocytes, unstimulated by a mitogen. Tear-drop poikilocytes, giant platelets and megakaryocyte fragments are present in the blood films, and the neutrophil alkaline phosphatase (NAP) score may be increased. The myelofibrosis is of the 'collagen' rather than the 'reticulin' type [74].

4 Bizarre presentations such as a case [75] in which the Ph[1] with a 6p+ translocation was found in all of 40 bone-marrow metaphases: the patient had no splenic enlargement, a moderate neutrophilia, thrombocytosis, raised NAP, no circulating immature granulocytes, and a positive indirect antiglobulin reaction; the hyperplastic marrow showed granulocyte hyperplasia and increased megakaryocytes. These instances show varying degrees of departure from the common pattern of evolution of Ph[1]-positive CGL and are difficult to fit

into a general theory of the relation between the Ph[1] and granulocyte homeostasis.

Although in the majority of cases, the entire population of normal myeloid stem cells is replaced by the Ph[1]-positive clone before the rising trend in the leucocyte count begins, there are rare cases usually associated with prolonged survival [69, 76–79] in which the marrow is only partially replaced, and the proliferative advantage of the clone appears to be weak, because after treatment with busulphan, often with inadvertently produced marrow hypoplasia, prolonged remissions are associated with predominantly normal (Ph[1]-negative) stem cells, yet a minority of Ph[1]-positive cells persist [78, 80] apparently in equilibrium. The patient reported by Finney *et al.* [81] remains in remission after 17 years (McDonald G.A., personal communication). In a case of polycythaemia vera in which 10% of the bone-marrow cells were Ph[1]-positive, the Ph[1] cells disappeared following radiophosphorus treatment, none being found six years later [82]. In general, however, Ph[1]-positive clones clearly have a proliferative advantage, and a deliberate attempt to eliminate them in the hope that suppressed normal stem cells could regenerate led to only temporary restoration of the normal karyotype [83] in only seven out of 37 cases, though in five additional cases some Ph[1]-negative cells appeared transiently.

There is some evidence suggesting that the Ph[1] may be a secondary manifestation of already established leukaemia. All the marrow cells of an initially Ph[1]-negative case of otherwise typical CGL became Ph[1]-positive only after four years of observation and treatment, and remained so for three years until the patient died [84]. In another case of Ph[1]-positive CGL, the Ph[1] disappeared during the first four years of treatment, without any episode of marrow hypoplasia. Several episodes of relapse with karyotypic abnormalities ensued in the remaining one and a half years of life, but the Ph[1] never reappeared [85]. Serial chromosome examinations in a case of childhood acute lymphoblastic leukaemia showed a normal karyotype in the leukaemia cells, but some of the mitogen-stimulated normal lymphocytes had a classical Ph[1] [86]. In spite of these challenging observations, the schematic outline in Figure 23.1 for the evolution of CGL holds good for the majority of cases. It is, however, not known whether in classical CGL, when every bone-marrow cell is Ph[1]-positive, normal stem cells are present but suppressed. At least a few Ph[1]-negative cells are present in about half of all cases at presentation, but it is not known whether they are normal. At least in patients whose marrow cells are 100% Ph[1]-positive, normal cells appear to be absent rather than suppressed, because *in vitro* granulocyte/monocyte colonies from the marrow and blood of five patients

heterozygous at the G6PD locus were found to produce only one alloenzyme, whereas their normal tissues produced both [87]. It is not yet known whether Ph[1]-negative cells in the marrow of those patients who have them are monoclonal or not. It is not even certain that all the Ph[1]-negative cells are myeloid cells, because the cells in granulocyte/monocyte colonies grown from CGL blood or marrow are almost always Ph[1]-positive [26, 27], though some Ph[1]-negative colonies have been recorded [25].

The neutrophils in chronic-phase CGL

In normal subjects neutrophils circulate in the blood for only a few hours ($T_{\frac{1}{2}}$ about seven hours [88]). In CGL the $T_{\frac{1}{2}}$ is between 26 and 89 hours [89] when the leucocyte count is very high, probably because the neutrophils, which on maturation are normally retained for many hours in the marrow, are released early in CGL. Thus the age structure of circulating neutrophils in CGL differs greatly from that of normal persons, and this may account for many of the features in which CGL neutrophils differ from those in normal blood. The values that are abnormal tend to approach normal limits when the leucocyte count has been brought within the normal range by treatment. CGL neutrophils, unlike those of atypical CML, appear morphologically normal on light microscopy and in their ultrastructure [90]. Functionally, a proportion of CGL neutrophils do not adhere to glass or to nylon and are poorly phagocytic [91–93], and some of the efficient phagocytes are defective in some tests of killing capacity for ingested organisms [94], being incapable of discharging their lysosomal enzymes into the phagocytic vacuoles [95]. The proportion of defective neutrophils increases with the leucocyte count [94], and when the counts are within normal limits after treatment, the killing capacity of the neutrophils for some organisms may be normal [95a]. The decreased stickiness of CGL neutrophils may result from increased amounts of sialic acid, perhaps attached to plasma-membrane glycoproteins. The sialic acid masks the carbohydrate receptor sites responsible for adhesiveness and when removed by exposure to *Vibrio cholerae* neuraminidase the defect is partially reversed [95b]. Most of the enzymes normally present in the primary and secondary granules are present in normal amounts in CGL neutrophils [96]. A variable content of lactoferrin, a secondary granule protein, has been reported [62, 63], but more observations are needed.

Neutrophil alkaline phosphatase (NAP) is found in an organelle, the phosphasome, only recently described [97]. In CGL neutrophils the amount is greatly reduced, but sensitive assays by analytical subcellular fractionation have shown that the small amount present (13%) functions normally [96]. The NAP content, estimated cytochemically, is lower in non-phagocytic CGL neutrophils [93]. The NAP score tends to increase, though not often to normal, after the leucocyte count has been reduced to normal levels [98], and may reach normal levels for varying periods after splenectomy [99] or other operations, or during infections. The neutrophils that develop in colonies grown in agar cultures of CGL blood or marrow cells [100], in liquid cultures [101], or in diffusion chambers in mice [102], contain the enzyme, but in liquid cultures only in the presence of normal plasma [101]. Thus, in CGL, an extracellular factor seems necessary for the production of NAP: Rustin has shown that CGL neutrophils, poor in NAP, become NAP-positive when transfused into severely neutropenic recipients [103].

The neutrophils are the principal source of transcobalamin I, though the protein is released by promyelocytes and later immature granulocytes. The serum total vitamin B_{12}-binding capacity ($TB_{12}BC$) increases as the total granulocyte mass expands in CGL, and falls when it is reduced by treatment [104].

Course of CGL

CGL untreated throughout its course is no longer seen, but the duration of survival was not dissimilar from that of treated patients [105]. However, the quality of life, even in the chronic phase, must have been far worse because of the unrelieved progression of the splenic enlargement, anaemia, hypermetabolism caused by the expanding mass of myeloid tissue, the mechanical effects on the microvasculature from the increasing hyperleucocytosis, and in many cases the effects of thrombocytosis.

The chronic phase of CGL

The course of CGL is essentially biphasic. In the early or chronic phase all the manifestations are attributable to the progressive expansion of the total myeloid cell mass associated with the minor deviation, already discussed, of the homeostatic regulation of granulopoiesis, and this in turn, with the reservations mentioned, is associated with the Ph^1 defect of the stem cells. As long as the chronic phase persists, the process is controllable; all the adverse manifestations can be counteracted and their effects removed by any therapeutic measure that reduces the total granulocyte mass, the re-expansion of which begins as soon as the effects of the treatment wear off but can be prevented by maintenance treatment at suitable dosage. This is the basis of all forms of conventional treatment by chemotherapy or radiotherapy. Although patients treated in this way enjoy virtually normal health, their disease is not in 'remission' as this term is applied in the case of acute leukaemia, in which remission implies the repopulation of the bone marrow by normal myeloid tissue: in well-controlled chronic-phase CGL, normal marrow function is performed by the abnormal clone of Ph^1-positive myeloid cells which, at a total cell mass not much above the normal range, delivers almost normal numbers of erythrocytes, granulocytes, monocytes and platelets, the function of which is practically normal. The regular growth pattern of the myeloid cell mass, and the ease with which its growth can be controlled by a simple treatment, indicate a benign proliferative process, which some regard as a pre-leukaemic state [106]. The instability of the Ph^1-positive stem-cell clone, however, is shown by the almost inevitable change in the character of the disease to a frankly malignant process, variable in the speed and character of its onset, but almost always highly resistant to treatment and always ultimately lethal. The change to the malignant phase is described as 'transformation' or 'metamorphosis' [107].

Transformed CGL

Clinically, transformation manifests itself in different ways. The most dramatic, occurring in about 10% of cases, is the *fulminating blast-cell crisis* (BC), in which during apparently well-controlled symptomless chronic-phase disease, in the absence of physical signs, blast cells appear in the blood and increase exponentially with a short doubling time (four to 10 days). The bone marrow becomes rapidly replaced by blast cells, marrow failure ensues, the spleen enlarges and after a few weeks of a febrile toxic illness the patient dies. Less acute transformation, though still proving fatal within a few months, involves an increasingly disturbed blood picture, not necessarily with an increase in the blast-cell count [108] except terminally, but with an absolute and relative increase in the promyelocyte counts and a fall in the neutrophil count and in the haemoglobin concentration. This type of transformation may be preceded by a period of malaise, weight loss, and fever during which haematological evidence of transformation cannot be established, but investigation for other possible causes of the illness fails. Some patients pass through months or occasionally years of *'accelerated'* disease in which the process breaks through the smooth control hitherto maintained by treatment: they still respond to treatment, but higher doses of the drug they are receiving are needed to prevent the leucocyte count from rising, the spleen from enlarging, or the haemoglobin from falling: eventually the dose cannot be increased without reducing the platelet count below safe levels. Minor haematological changes during the otherwise stable chronic phase, especially an absolute increase in the basophil count or in the platelet count [109], may suggest early transformation. If basophilcytosis is extreme, high blood histamine levels result, and the patients may develop wheezing, urticaria, diarrhoea, pruritus, peripheral oedema and peptic ulceration [110]. The fulminating BC may be regarded as a single-step enhancement of malignancy, the other types as manifestations of multi-step progression, arising as a result of genetic instability in the Ph[1] clone with the generation of new competing clones, among which those with a proliferative advantage successively replace less hardy clones. New clones characterized by cytogenetic analysis, may arise focally during the chronic phase, in the spleen [111] and lymph nodes [112], meninges [113–115] or other extramedullary sites, or in one or more bones [116, 117], with the production of blast-cell tumours. Meningeal leukaemia in CGL/BC is most often found in lymphoid or mixed phenotype BC [65, 118, 119]. Bone pain at a single or more often at several sites is the first evidence of transformation in about three per cent of cases [117]. Scanning with bone-seeking radionuclides may reveal focal lesions even when X-rays of the painful bones fail to do so. In about one-fifth of all cases, the chronic phase is succeeded by a myelofibrotic stage [72, 74] in which the clinical picture is dominated by thrombocytosis, or more often thrombocytopenia, splenomegaly, anaemia and neutropenia, rather than by blast-cell proliferation, though in these cases also the disease may end in blast-cell crisis.

The stage in the evolution of chronic-phase CGL at which transformation occurs is discussed later.

The biology of transformed CGL

Cytogenetics. Evidence for the generation of new clones as the cause of transformation, and for competition amongst them with the ensuing survival of those with proliferative advantage, was first obtained from serial cytogenetic studies before the introduction of chromatin banding techniques [120, 121]. It is now clear that new clones in the Ph[1]-positive stem cells are usually associated with the appearance of additional chromosomal changes, sometimes detected several months before the onset of clinical evidence of transformation, in more than 75% of all chronic-phase patients. The most common changes are a second Ph[1], an extra chromosome 8, and a structural rearrangement involving chromosome 17 usually described as an isochromosome for the long arm [122]. One or other of the first two, but not the third, is found in 5–10% of chronic-phase cases, but in transformed CGL the three changes are found in various combinations, often with other chromosome changes, some of which may be treatment-related [123]. Because in more than half of the cases the modal chromosome number is unchanged, accurate karyotyping with banding is essential in the identification and characterization of additional changes [48].

Blast-cell morphology. The occurrence of blast cells of different types in transformed CGL has long been recognized and the appearance, in different cases, of blast cells with evidence of largely erythroid, granulocytic or monocytic differentiation was consistent with the concept of clonal evolution developed from cytogenetic analysis. Undifferentiated blasts, especially those resembling the 'lymphoblasts' of acute lymphoblastic leukaemia (ALL) [124], which are the only blasts in about one-fifth of all cases, were thought to belong to the myeloid stem-cell clone because they carried the Ph[1]. Classical cytochemical methods [125] can reveal the myeloid nature of some undifferentiated blasts, but those with totally negative cytochemistry require electron microscopy with cytochemistry for specific peroxidases [126] to demonstrate that they are very early megakaryoblasts [127, 128], basophil promyelocytes, or proerythroblasts. The understanding of the nature of the 'lymphoblasts' had to await the application of immunological surface-marker techniques and other methods for establishing the true phenotype of the cells [118, 129].

The phenotypes of the blast cells of transformed CGL

The possible affinity of the lymphoblast-like cells with those of ALL was suggested by their sensitivity to treatment with vincristine and prednisone, in contrast to the refractoriness of the larger granular blasts [130]. The lymphoblast-like cells from different cases are now known to exhibit the same range of phenotypes as 'common' ALL (non-T, non-B) blasts. The main characteristics examined have been:

1 the markers for haemopoietic stem cells, namely, the enzymes terminal deoxynucleotidyl transferase (TdT) [21, 131, 132], the 'common' ALL antigen (ALL[+]) [133], the p28 33 or Ia-like antigen (Ia[+]) [134];

2 the maturation markers for the lymphoid lineage, cytoplasmic IgM (Cy IgM[+]) [135] (a pre-B marker), surface membrane Ig (a B marker), sheep red-cell rosetting, human T-lymphocyte-specific antigens (T cell markers), and human fetal thymocyte-specific antigens (Thy) [136, 136a] (a thymocyte marker); and

3 a maturation marker for the myeloid lineage, the M antigen reacting with anti-myeloid serum [137].

As in common ALL, the lymphoblastic cells of transformed CGL almost always have the phenotype ALL^+, Ia^+, TdT^+, occasionally ALL^-, Ia^+, TdT^+. These cells are thought to arise in an expanded malignant clone from early pre-myeloid, pre-lymphoid stem cells that exist only in very small numbers in normal marrow [136, 138]. In most cases none of the maturation markers is present, but occasionally the cells have the pre-B lymphoid phenotype ALL^+, Ia^+, TdT^+, $Cy IgM^+$ [139]. In exceptional cases [137], the cells have reacted both with anti-ALL and with anti-myeloid serum. In equally rare cases the tests suggested some thymocyte-lineage maturation [21]: ALL^-, Ia^-, TdT^{++}, and weak reactivity with anti-*Thy* in one case, and E-rosetting (the only test performed) in another [64].

It is not possible to characterize the phenotype of the blast cells as 'lymphoid' or 'myeloid' by using a single method, for example only morphology, or only TdT or anti-ALL assays, and these terms are not synonymous with the morphologist's terms 'lymphoblastic' or 'myeloblastic'. The distribution of several markers in individual cells in a population of apparently homogeneous cells is found to vary when the same cells are labelled with several specific antisera, each antibody carrying a fluorochrome [139] which fluoresces at a particular wavelength. The majority of cases can, however, be typed as 'lymphoid' or 'myeloid' on morphology, TdT, ALL, and Ia, while a substantial minority are mixed cases with 'lymphoid' and 'myeloid' blasts coexisting. Furthermore, shifts of phenotype occur during the course of the transformed disease.

Stage of onset of transformation of Ph¹-positive ALL

Figure 23.4 illustrates schematically the temporal relationships between the onset of blast-cell and myelofibrotic transformed CGL and the evolution of chronic-phase CGL, and of Ph¹-positive leukaemia (usually ALL) in patients who never develop chronic-phase CGL. The top panel shows the onset of BC late in the course of chronic-phase CGL. However, BC, reflecting the risk of malignant change conferred by the Ph¹ on the affected stem cell, may arise at any time after its inception, as shown in the middle panel. Some patients present in BC with sufficient features of CGL to permit the diagnosis: they may have, in varying degree, splenic enlargement, neutrophilia, myelocytosis, basophilia, thrombocytosis, and a marrow containing a mixed blast-cell and granulocytic population. However, in equivocal presentations of Ph¹-positive acute myeloid leukaemia (AML) it may be difficult to find objective criteria to decide between *de-novo* AML or CGL/myeloid BC [140, 141] unless, in remission, the disease enters chronic-phase CGL. There is evidence [48] that the type and frequency of translocations other than the common 9q+/22q− of CGL may differ in *de-novo* Ph¹-positive AML from those of CGL.

Ph¹-positive ALL is now well recognized [142] as accounting for about two per cent of all cases of ALL in childhood, and about 15% in adults. The general

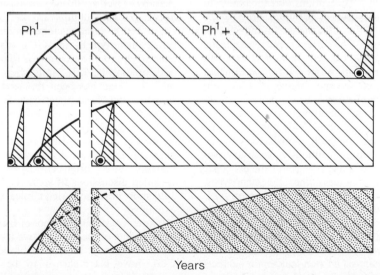

Years

Fig. 23.4. Schematic representation of the temporal relationship between the evolution of chronic-phase chronic granulocytic leukaemia (CGL) and the generation of Ph¹-positive blast-cell clones of lymphoid, myeloid, or mixed phenotype (upper and middle panels), or the development of myelofibrosis (lower panel). *Upper panel*: transformation arises during the course of established chronic-phase CGL. *Middle panel*: the event on the left illustrates Ph¹-positive acute leukaemia in a patient who does not subsequently develop chronic-phase CGL; that on the right illustrates Ph¹-positive acute leukaemia arising early in the course of chronic-phase CGL, when it may still be possible to diagnose CGL; in the case of the middle event, chronic-phase CGL develops if the patient survives. *Lower panel*: myelofibrosis may arise insidiously at any stage during the course of chronic-phase CGL (right of broken lines); presentation with myelofibrotic bone-marrow and a CGL-like peripheral blood picture is diagnosed by demonstrating Ph¹ in cultures of peripheral blood cells (left of broken lines). Light hatching: chronic-phase CGL bone marrow with 100% of metaphases Ph¹+. Dark hatching: expansion of Ph¹-positive clone of transformed blast cells arising from a single transformed cell (circle). Dotted area: myelofibrotic marrow.

relationship of this disease with CGL is shown by those cases in which chronic-phase CGL develops during remission, to be followed by one or more BC of lymphoid, myeloid, or mixed type [48, 142]. But in the majority of cases of Ph[1]-positive ALL and of the less common AML, features of chronic-phase CGL do not appear; they should therefore be called Ph[1]-positive ALL or AML and not CGL in BC. The existence of these cases raises the question of the nature of the stem cell involved in CGL and the inter-relationships of the different types of Ph[1]-positive leukaemia: this is discussed briefly below.

The lower panel in Figure 23.2 illustrates the development of myelofibrosis in CGL, either as an insidious progression in established chronic-phase CGL or as a presenting feature in which the peripheral blood values, differential count, and film appearances suggest CGL, but the marrow is densely fibrotic. The Ph[1] chromosome can be demonstrated only in cultures of blood cells unstimulated by a lymphocyte mitogen. Blast-cell crisis in any form may arise during the course of myelofibrotic transformation.

The Ph[1]-positive leukaemias: stem-cell theory
Until recently CGL was though of as *the* Ph[1]-positive disease, and the recorded exceptions were too scanty to incorporate into a comprehensive theory. We now see CGL as only one, albeit the commonest, manifestation of Ph[1]-positive disease. The current view of neoplastic change is that it can affect cell lineages at different stages in their differentiation and maturation but that once the target cell has become clonogenic, its descendants perpetuate the phenotype which represents that appropriate to the stage in development during which neoplastic conversion occurred [143]. On this basis, unusual phenotypes, formerly considered to be tumour-specific or, more cautiously, tumour-associated, are now regarded as evidence for the existence in normal fetal or adult tissues of the same phenotypes, overlooked because of their rarity. The common ALL phenotype is regarded as that of an early stage in the development of haemopoietic stem cells before differentiation to the lymphoid lineage has occurred [19], and cells of the phenotype have been demonstrated in the regenerating marrow of non-leukaemic subjects [21] as well as of leukaemic patients in remission.

If the precursor of such a cell becomes Ph[1]-positive, it appears to be altered in three respects:
1 its further proliferation is restricted, as shown by its occasional persistence for long periods at low percentage [77];
2 its capacity for differentiation and maturation is limited, for it appears only exceptionally in normal mature descendants [86, 144]; and
3 it is at risk of undergoing malignant transformation,

sometimes after many years [77]. Ph[1]-positive ALL illustrates this. To account for CGL arising either *de novo* or following Ph[1]-positive ALL after the induction of remission, we need only postulate the differentiation into the myeloid lineage of one viable clonogenic cell in the Ph[1]-positive clone precursor stem cells. This cell enters the myeloid compartment with a homeostatic defect conferred by the Ph[1], and chronic-phase CGL develops unless it is forestalled by malignant change in the parent clone. The newly established Ph[1]-positive myeloid stem-cell clone is itself at risk of undergoing malignant change and because of the homeostatic defect its proliferative potential is greater than that of the parent clone, so that myeloid-phenotype BC is more frequent than lymphoid-phenotype BC. The multiple shifts in phenotype seen in long-surviving patients in which successive relapses of lymphoid, myeloid, mixed-blast types, or of chronic-phase CGL respond to appropriate treatments [65, 145, 146] are also explained by the theory.

Deliberate attempts to eliminate the Ph[1] clone in CGL by intensive therapy have not so far succeeded in prolonging the duration of survival [83, 147, 147a] and conventional therapy does not aim at elimination. However, *de-novo* Ph[1]-positive ALL may respond to therapy as well as Ph[1]-negative common ALL, though adults are often highly resistant [148]. In responding cases the Ph[1]-positive clone may be eliminated. Lymphoid-phenotype BC in CGL tends to be responsive, at least for a time, to treatments that include vincristine and prednisone [21], and when the chronic-phase myeloid clone has been replaced by the treatment-sensitive lymphoid-phenotype BC clone, treatment with only vincristine and prednisone may occasionally lead to prolonged marrow hypoplasia, rarely followed by the regeneration of Ph[1]-negative myeloid cells [21] with the restoration for some months of a normal marrow; more often chronic-phase CGL returns. Detailed discussions of stem-cell theory [19, 48, 142, 149] show how the varied clinical phenomena may be explained.

The extent of involvement of B-lymphoid cells in the descendants of the Ph[1]-positive target cell has become clarified recently. Peripheral blood B-lymphocytes in CGL have been shown to be Ph[1]-positive by a combined cytogenetics and membrane-marker technique [414], while cultures of EBV-infected peripheral blood lymphocytes from G6PD heterozygotes with CGL showed that some colonies were monoclonal, and some of those were also Ph[1]-positive [415]. In contrast, PHA-stimulated T-lymphocytes, even in longstanding CGL cases, have always been Ph[1]-negative [150], while only one well-docmented case of Ph[1]-positive T-blast leukaemia has been reported [416]. It is not yet known why entry to the T-cell lineage is so restricted compared with that into the B-cell lineage [30, 151, 414, 415].

Features influencing the prognosis of CGL

The biological events that determine the prognosis of CGL are largely unknown. The great majority of patients die as a result of transformation, which reflects the inherent risk of the Ph^1-positive pre-myeloid/pre-lymphoid stem cell undergoing malignant change except in those patients with myelofibrotic transformation, the nature of which is totally obscure. Although the chronic phase may be regarded as an epiphenomenon in relation to the underlying threat to life of the malignant potential of the Ph^1-positive stem cell, there are features of the chronic phase that may reflect the properties of the stem-cell population and thus may have prognostic significance.

There is no doubt that the tempo of the chronic phase varies. Treatment of patients by a course of busulphan, followed by observation for a time without further treatment, shows that the duration of survival is proportional to the doubling time of the leucocyte count [152]. Although the onset of malignant transformation appears to be a random event, the magnitude of the risk varies, and is very small in the minority of patients who remain in the chronic phase for many years (e.g. 23 years in a patient treated only with busulphan (Israels L.G., personal communication)). However, the shape of survival curves [152] shows that, overall, the risk of dying increases during the course of the disease: therefore features reflecting the stage of the disease at presentation might be expected to be of prognostic significance.

The overall median duration of survival in CGL [2, 153–156] is about three and a half years from the time of diagnosis or the start of treatment [154], with about 25% of patients surviving five years and less than 10% surviving 10 years. The published series vary in the proportion of patients tested for, or known to have, Ph^1-positive CGL and this may partly explain why some presentation features were found to have prognostic significance in some series but not in others. Thus haemoglobin, total leucocyte count, platelet count, blast-cell count and spleen size were not correlated with survival in one analysis of 178 cases [157], but all had prognostic significance in another, of 798 patients [156], only 343 of whom had been tested for the presence of the Ph^1. In the series of 166 Ph^1-positive cases in the Medical Research Council's trial designed to assess the value of early elective splenectomy, features recorded at presentation that were found to have prognostic significance included performance status, spleen size, haemoglobin and total leucocyte count [157a], and the last three were significant for trend. That the magnitude of each of these

features reflects the stage of the disease, and that all three are correlated because they reflect the size of the total granulocyte mass, is evident from the evolution of the disease as recorded in untreated patients diagnosed by chance relatively early (Fig 23.1). Females lived longer than males in two series [156, 158], and the presence of Ph^1-negative as well as Ph^1-positive cells in the marrow has been associated with a good prognosis [28, 69, 76, 78, 79]. The prognostic significance of the XO karyotype in males remains controversial [159, 160].

In general, the features found to be associated with a poor prognosis [156] are those indicating more advanced disease. However, individual patients who survived for 10–20 years have had features suggesting advanced disease at presentation [161], indicating that chronic-phase disease with a slow proliferative tempo reflects a low risk of malignant transformation in the pre-myeloid/pre-lymphoid Ph^1-positive stem-cell clone. At present there is no way of identifying these patients at the time of presentation, and no evidence that different kinds of treatment might be indicated for groups of patients presumed to have good-risk or poor-risk disease.

Aspects of treatment of CGL

Chronic-phase CGL

For routine management busulphan [162, 163] is the most widely used drug, which controls the granulocytic proliferation with no inconvenience to the majority of patients [164, 165]. In a minority of cases the blood counts remain essentially normal for several years after a single course of treatment (three to five months at a daily dose of 4 mg at first, 2 mg later), but in the majority, rising counts necessitate resumption of treatment after six to 18 months. When repeated courses of treatment are administered the intervals between them become progressively shorter as the doubling time of the leucocyte count shortens [166]. Stabilization of the leucocyte count at about $10 \times 10^9/l$ by suitable adjustment (0·5–4 mg) of the daily dose administered continuously, provides smoother control and is widely used, but there is no evidence that it prolongs the duration of the chronic phase. Equally good control is possible by giving single high doses (50–100 mg) at intervals of several weeks [167–168] but there are no clear advantages. Bone-marrow hypoplasia may result from unusual sensitivity to busulphan and, on recovery, the patients may regenerate mixed Ph^1-negative and Ph^1-positive myeloid cells and experience long remissions [169, 170]: more often hypoplasia results from overdosage; on recovery the disease may revert to the chronic phase, or enter BC. Busulphan may damage the embryo or fetus, and should not be used in the early months of pregnancy [171]. The potentially lethal long-term complications of busulphan, the wasting syndrome [172] and 'busulphan lung' [173–175], are very uncommon, but to avoid them some prefer to rely on hydroxyurea (HU) to control chronic-phase CGL. Although HU provides good control, patients tend to become resistant to it. Since it is the most effective agent in the management of accelerated CGL with thrombocytopenia [176, 177], its use is probably better deferred until the onset of the accelerated phase.

Although stabilization of the leucocyte count around $10 \times 10^9/l$ does not significantly prolong the duration of the chronic phase, it is possible that stabilization at around $5 \times 10^9/l$ might. With busulphan alone, the risk of inducing marrow hypoplasia is too great to justify the attempt, but it is easily done by combining busulphan at a daily dose of 2 mg with either mercaptopurine [178] or thioguanine at a daily dose of 80 mg/m². Adjustments are made by altering the number of days in the week on which the drugs are given. This method is now being compared with standard busulphan therapy in the Medical Research Council's third trial in CGL.

Place of elective splenectomy
At the time of a retrospective analysis of 26 cases [179] in which elective splenectomy had been performed, the number of transformations was half that expected by comparison with the group of busulphan-treated patients in the Medical Research Council's first trial in CGL [154]; a controlled trial was therefore carried out but failed to show any benefit for the group allocated to elective splenectomy [157a]. There was no evidence that the quality of life of the splenectomized patients was better after the onset of transformation as shown by their transfusion requirement, proportion of the time after transformation spent in hospital, frequency and severity of infections or haemorrhagic phenomena, or proportion of the time after transformation in which the performance status was satisfactory. In other series also [180, 181] there was no evidence that elective splenectomy deferred the onset of transformation.

Transformed CGL
As described above, the chronic phase may either end abruptly with the explosive onset of fulminating BC or the fact that a change in the character of the disease has occurred may become apparent only after many months. The assessment of the efficacy of different treatments in transformed CGL is complicated by the difficulty of providing acceptable quantitative criteria for dating the onset of transformation, yet such criteria are essential if the effect of treatments on the duration

of survival after transformation are to be compared. For such trials, the definition of transformation should be restrictive so that putative new treatments are subjected to the most stringent test. The criteria [182] accepted by the Cancer and Leukaemia Group B include specifications regarding the rate of increase of the leucocyte count after the last attempt at conventional therapy, the combined blast and promyelocyte counts in the peripheral blood, and the haemoglobin or platelet-count levels. Trials concerned not with the treatment of transformed CGL, but with the possible efficacy of treatment in the chronic phase in deferring the onset of transformation, require a less restrictive definition which marks the end of the chronic phase. In the Medical Research Council's trial on the effect of elective splenectomy the date chosen was that on which treatment with busulphan was abandoned.

The treatment of transformed CGL is notoriously unsatisfactory. In the accelerated phase it is still possible to regain partial control, and HU [176, 177] has proved especially valuable in the presence of moderate thrombocytopenia when busulphan, dibromomannitol, or mercaptopurine will control the rising leucocyte count only at doses which increase the thrombocytopenia. Splenectomy helps in the presence of hypersplenism, but is contraindicated when the transformation has become frankly blastic [183]. Temporary symptomatic relief for massive splenomegaly has been obtained by the intra-arterial splenic-artery infusion of cytosine arabinoside [184].

Although the results of treatment for frank BC are very poor, in all the series reported a proportion of patients respond to some extent [165, 185]. The median survival for non-responders is two to three months, and for responders about eight months [165, 186]. On the whole, it seems likely that the capacity to respond (20–30% of patients) is inherent in the patients' disease and not due to the superiority of the treatment they receive. It appears, too, that the capacity to respond, especially to treatment combinations that include vincristine and prednisone [130, 187]—though not all trials have shown a beneficial role for these drugs [186]—is associated with the presence of the lymphoid or mixed lymphoid/myeloid phenotype [21], myeloid phenotype BC being notoriously resistant to treatment. Patients with a hypodiploid karyotype were thought to respond better, but hypodiploidy is very rare [48]. The more intensive the treatment is, the more likely it is to destroy any residual chronic-phase stem cells, or even normal stem cells that might have escaped destruction by the growth of the malignant blast-cell clone. Therefore myelotoxic treatments that produce marrow hypoplasia hardly ever induce a state of remission, and if the patient survives the hypoplasia he will shortly suffer a relapse of the BC, because treatment sufficiently intense to destroy the BC clone is likely to prove lethal. Such intensive therapy can be attempted only in conjunction with a means of restoring marrow function. The transplantation of allogeneic marrow from histocompatible sibs has been used [188], and also autografts of marrow [189] or buffy coat leucocytes [190] collected by leucapheresis and cryopreserved [191] at the time of presentation. If the treatment intended to eliminate the blast-crisis clone were successful, allografts would be expected to cure the patient, and autografts to restore chronic-phase conditions until the autografted stem-cell clone underwent transformation. Both allografts and autografts grow well in the recipients [188, 189, 191], but so far BC cells have proved to be highly resistant to intensive treatment by cyclophosphamide and whole-body irradiation, by this treatment preceded by multiple-drug chemotherapy as used for the treatment of acute myeloid leukaemia, or by chemotherapy alone.

Syngeneic grafting in chronic-phase CGL
The resistant nature of BC has led to a trial of grafting syngeneic marrow in the chronic phase in the hope that ablative therapy would be more successful in eliminating the chronic-phase Ph[1]-positive stem-cell clone [192]. Because of the high rate of complications of allogeneic grafting and the fact that some CGL patients lead essentially normal lives for many years, only identical twin donors have been used. The first graft was performed in May 1976 and, in the first five years, 11 of the 12 patients had normal bone-marrow karyotypes, and Ph[1]-positive cells had returned in only one case (Fefer A., personal communication). Although further relapses may still appear, it seems reasonable now to offer grafting to all chronic-phase patients who have healthy identical-twin sibs as donors [192a].

THE CHRONIC LYMPHOID LEUKAEMIAS

The chronic lymphoid leukaemias (CLL) are lymphoproliferative disorders characterized by the major involvement from their inception of the bone marrow and the blood, in contrast to the lymphomas in which the major involvement is in extramedullary tissues, although during the course of the disease the bone marrow, and sometimes the blood, may become secondarily involved. The characteristics of the leukaemic phase of the lymphomas are usually sufficiently different from those of the chronic lymphoid leukaemias to enable the correct diagnosis to be made. Nevertheless, the commonest chronic lymphoid leukaemia, B-cell chronic lymphocytic leukaemia (B-CLL), is closely related to its lymphoma counterpart, well-differentiated diffuse lymphocytic lym-

phoma (WDDL) [192b] or small B-cell lymphocytic lymphoma [193, 194], and intermediate forms are not uncommon. Occasionally, in a case of WDDL of several years standing, the subsequent evolution of the disease is that of classical CLL [193, 195]. The distinction between CLL and WDDL rests entirely on the pattern of evolution, with early blood and marrow involvement but minimal nodal or visceral involvement in CLL and major early nodal or visceral involvement but minimal blood and marrow involvement in WDDL. The distinction cannot yet be made on cytomorphological, ultrastructural, histological, or biochemical features or by immunological marker techniques. But it cannot be doubted that the special affinity of WDLL lymphocytes for lymphoid tissues and the high capacity of CLL lymphocytes to circulate in the blood and to infiltrate the bone marrow reflect surface-membrane differences yet to be identified.

Until recently, the lymphoproliferative diseases were characterized only by their clinical, haematological and histological features. It is now possible to characterize the tumour target cells by a spectrum of properties that defines their phenotype, and it is believed that the biological behaviour of the tumour is determined by the phenotype of its malignant cells. In each case, the tumour-cell population is thought to arise by the transformation to malignancy of a normal representative of the heterogeneous lymphoid cell population, and the transformation largely prevents the further differentiation and maturation of the cell, whose phenotype is thus perpetuated in all its descendants [143, 194]. Formal proof of monoclonality is lacking for most of the T-cell lymphomas and leukaemias though the available evidence suggests that they are monoclonal, like the B-cell lymphomas and leukaemias [196–200]. Lymphoid cells can now be characterized by a wide range of anatomical, biochemical, biophysical, immunological and functional techniques, and the great diversity of phenotypes generated by the differentiation and maturation of the lymphoid presursor cells is reflected in the diversity found in the lymphomas and leukaemias [201–203]. Indeed it is likely that 'multiparameter' characterization of tumour-cell populations will make possible the identification of subsets of normal lymphocytes hitherto unrecognized because of their rarity. The new methodology has already thrown new light on the nature of the lymphoid leukaemias, where blood cells are usually available for testing in quantity, and the results have been readily absorbed into the traditional clinical and haematological classification which has thus been clarified, refined, and expanded [204, 204a]. Clinical and cytomorphological features, formerly overlooked, are now seen to be associated with neoplasms of specific subsets of lymphocytes. Thus the association of skin lesions, splenomegaly, lymphocytosis and moderate marrow infiltration with lymphocytes suggests a chronic T-cell leukaemia, while the characteristic cerebriform nucleus of the T lymphocyte in the Sézary syndrome (Fig. 23.6d) permits the diagnosis to be made by simple inspection of a blood film that would formerly have been diagnosed as CLL. However, there is a wide range of clinical variation within the Sézary syndrome, as with all other named conditions, and it is likely that some of that variation will prove to be associated with phenotypic diversity. On the other hand, the cytomorphologically similar cells in two cases of prolymphocytic leukaemia may prove to be B cells in one case and T cells in the other [205]. Furthermore, the gross morphological changes associated with malignant progression in B-CLL, when an increasing proportion of prolymphocytoid cells [206] or the more abrupt onset of BC occurs, may involve no presently detectable change in phenotype [207, 208]. At present the full impact of the new methodology on classification, diagnosis, prognosis and management is not clear, but there can be little doubt that it will become increasingly important.

Although in a particular case the extent of variation in the malignant clone is usually limited, subclones with phenotypic shifts having a large effect can arise. Thus in B-CLL a subpopulation of cells with the capacity for immunological maturation may arise, as shown by the production of a serum paraprotein at high concentration [208, 209].

Classification of the chronic lymphoid leukaemias
Both conventional criteria and those based on immunological markers have been used in the classification given in Table 23.2. The T-cell leukaemias are almost always sufficiently distinctive in all their fea-

Table 23.2. Classification of the chronic lymphoid leukaemias

Chronic lymphocytic leukaemia (B-CLL)
Prolymphocytic leukaemia (B-PLL)
T-cell lymphocytic leukaemia
   (a) small-cell type (T-CLL)
   (b) prolymphocytic type (T-PLL)
   (c) pleomorphic-cell type
Hairy-cell leukaemia (B-HCL, T-HCL)

tures to justify their inclusion as a major group, although without marker investigations the T nature of some cases of small-cell CLL and of prolymphocytic leukaemia (PLL) may not be evident. Hairy-cell leukaemia is not easily confused with the other chronic lymphoid leukaemias, or with lymphomas, but lymphomas may present with leukaemic featues and can be misdiagnosed as CLL, PLL or T-cell lymphocytic leukaemia (T-CLL). However, as indicated above, the transition between leukaemia and lymphoma is imperceptible and intermediate forms can be allocated to one or other group only by resorting to arbitrary definitions.

LYMPHOMAS THAT MAY SIMULATE CHRONIC LYMPHOID LEUKAEMIAS
Table 23.3 lists the lymphomas that may be confused with the corresponding leukaemia when they present with lymphocytosis and bone-marrow infiltration (Fig. 23.6c and d). Conspicuous lymphocytosis is unlikely to occur unless the marrow is infiltrated [210], except in the cutaneous T-cell lymphomas. The features on which the differential diagnoses depend are considered later.

Table 23.3. Lymphomas that may simulate a chronic lymphoid leukaemia

Type of leukaemia suggested by the lymphoma	Type of lymphoma simulating leukaemia	
CLL (Fig. 23.5)	1 Small-cell lymphocytic (syn. well-differentiated diffuse lymphocytic, Rappaport) Atypical small-cell lymphocytic	
	2 Lymphoplasmacytic with paraprotein	IgM (Waldenström's macroglobulinaemia) IgA IgG
	3 Follicular (Fig. 23.11)	
PLL (Fig. 23.7)	Large-cell lymphocytic (syn. poorly differentiated diffuse lymphocytic, Rappaport)	
T-cell LL		
—small cell (Fig. 23.6)	1 Small-cell lymphocytic 2 Sézary syndrome, small cerebriform-cell type	
—pleomorphic cell (Fig. 23.10)	1 Sézary syndrome, large cerebriform-cell type (Fig. 23.12) 2 Large-cell lymphocytic	

COMMON B-CELL CHRONIC LYMPHOCYTIC LEUKAEMIA (B-CLL)

The commonest of the chronic lymphoid leukaemias is B-CLL, and national mortality figures, which include all types, therefore reflect its incidence fairly well. However, because of the long duration of subclinical CLL, the diagnosis will be made in elderly patients who die from other causes only if a blood count is performed. In western countries the rising incidence in the present century results, at least in part, from the rising frequency of routine blood counts. Even so the figures are likely to underestimate the true incidence [211]. In the west, CLL, nearly twice as common as CGL, accounts for about 25% of all deaths from leukaemia [18].

Chronic lymphocytic leukaemia is about twice as frequent in males [15a, 212], and is rare below age 40. The proportion of males appears to be declining. It is likely that many of the cases previously diagnosed below age 40 would now be recognized as cases of follicular lymphoma (FL), hairy-cell leukaemia (HCL), or T-CLL. Beyond age 40, the incidence of CLL increases from less than 10% to about 40% of all forms of leukaemia beyond age 70 [18, 213]. The incidence is low in countries with a low life expectancy, as in much of the Far East [214], but is also very low in Japan with a Western-type age structure [215]. It is higher in Japanese living in the USA, but still lower than for Europeans [216]. It now seems possible that some of the cases formerly described as CLL in Japan were cases of T-CLL. In northern Nigeria there is an excess of CLL in women of childbearing age (M:F is 1:2 below 45 years), and this had been associated with the malaria-induced depression of cell-mediated immunity [217]. The risk of familial leukaemia is higher for CLL than for any other form of leukaemia [218, 219]. An increased frequency of HLA A9 has been reported for CLL [220, 221], and also of A28, Aw30, B12, and B18 [221]. There are no clues to the aetiology of the disease. It has proved difficult to induce CLL cells to divide and, until recently, constant chromosomal abnormalities were not known in CLL; recent work, however, suggests that abnormalities of chromosome 12 may be characteristic [221a, 417].

The pathogenesis of B-CLL

There is now impressive evidence that B-CLL is a monoclonal disease [208] in which progressive accumulation of a clone of immunologically inert, long-lived B-lymphocytes occurs [222], presumably by proliferation from a single target cell. The site of origin of the target cell is not known, but its descendants retain its own pattern of immunological immaturity. They accumulate preferentially in the bone marrow and the blood, later in the lymph nodes, the spleen and

the portal tracts of the liver, frequently in that order, and they appear to recirculate as do normal lymphocytes between the blood and lymphoid tissues by way of the post-capillary venules of the lymph nodes [223] and the thoracic duct, though more slowly than normal B-lymphocytes [224, 225]. Their proliferation rate is lower than that of normal lymphocytes, but because of the greatly expanded total lymphocyte mass (TLM), the absolute daily production of lymphocytes is often increased [226, 227]. As the TLM increases, germinal centres disappear from the lymph nodes, the concentration of serum immunoglobulins falls [227a, 227b], and the capacity to produce antibodies in response to antigenic challenge declines, suggesting suppression of normal B-lymphocyte function by the CLL clone. However, autoimmune phenomena appear at some time during the course of the disease in 10–20% of all cases [152, 228–230] and in rare cases unusual allergic manifestations such as extreme hypersensitivity to insect bites [231] arise, and may be the presenting feature. Progressive lymphocytic infiltration of the bone marrow reduces the reserve capacity of the marrow and eventually exhausts it, leading to overt marrow failure. Lymphocytic infiltrates of tissues and organs other than the blood, bone marrow, lymph nodes, spleen and liver are frequently found post mortem in advanced cases, but during life they seldom cause trouble [232, 233]. Published reports of clinical disorders resulting from such infiltrates must be re-evaluated because other conditions (Tables 23.2 and 23.3) were formerly confused with CLL. Thus skin infiltrates are now especially associated with T-cell lymphoproliferative disease. There is evidence that CLL is preceded by a lymphocytopenic phase resulting from low numbers of T cells [233a].

Spontaneous remission in CLL

Unlike CGL, in which spontaneous remission (SR) has not been reported, several accounts of SR in CLL are recorded [234–240]. In the older literature, however, many of the cases, especially in younger patients, were probably examples of follicular lymphoma, in which SR occurs in about 10% of cases [241], though others appear to have been cases of genuine CLL. The remissions, which appeared to be complete or almost complete and lasted for several years, occurred spontaneously or following presumed viral infection, viral hepatitis, herpes zoster, or smallpox vaccination. In some cases the patients developed another malignant disease while their CLL was in remission. The incidence of SR appears to be less than one per cent in CLL. In one of my cases a remission lasting three months followed an attack of generalized herpes zoster.

Monoclonality of CLL

The monoclonal nature of CLL has been established by immunological methods. When the urine contains free light chains they are always monoclonal, and in a minority of patients monoclonal paraproteins are found in the serum [208]. In rare cases many of the lymphocytes contain bizarre cytoplasmic crystalline or amorphous inclusions [242–247] consisting of monoclonal Ig, usually with λ light chains [245] in crystalline and κ light chains [247] in amorphous inclusions, and sometimes without release of a paraprotein into the blood or urine. The surface-membrane immunoglobulins (SmIg) on the lymphocytes in individual cases contain a single light chain, and detailed analysis of the heavy chains has shown that they belong to the same subclass, and have the same Gm allotype on their constant regions [248], while their variable regions share the same idiotypic specificity [249–251]. Rarely, the SmIg has exhibited antibody specificity such as anti-Forssmann activity against sheep erythrocytes [252], or rheumatoid-factor activity against IgG [253], indicating identity of the variable regions of light and heavy chains.

Features of prognostic significance in CLL

It is reasonable to suppose that the steady accumulation of CLL lymphocytes and the resulting expansion of the TLM might be reflected in an orderly sequence of clinically and haematologically detectable involvement of the blood, bone marrow, lymph nodes, spleen and liver, and eventually in evidence of bone-marrow failure. If this were true, the highly variable clinical and haematological manifestations found at presentation might reflect different stages in the evolution of one disease rather than different types of disease with varying aggressiveness. Several attempts have been made to correlate the duration of survival with the incidence of various features recorded at presentation [254–256], and they have led to the formulation of staging systems of prognostic value. The best-known staging system, already widely used, is that of Rai *et al.* [254] which as originally formulated was as follows:

Stage 0:   lymphocyte count $\geqslant 15 \times 10^9$/l and lymphocytes $\geqslant 40\%$ of bone-marrow cells;
Stage I: as above with enlarged lymph nodes;
Stage II: as stage 0 or I with enlarged liver or spleen, or both;
Stage III: as stage 0, I or II, but haemoglobin concentration < 11 g/dl;
Stage IV: as stage 0, I, II or III but platelet count $< 100 \times 10^9$/l.

The prognostic value of the system is shown by the median durations of survival for staged patients in several large series. Thus in four series of 125 [254], 83 [257], 152 [258], and 167 [230] cases, the median survival for stage 0 was 150–180 months, for stage I 60–130, for stage II 47–108, for stage III 9–26, and for stage IV 19–42 months. There is thus a trend for decreasing survival with advancing stage, but with a wide overlap between I and II, and no suggestion of progression between III and IV. Phillips *et al.* [230] examined the independent prognostic significance of several features. They found significantly worse survival for lymphocyte counts $\geqslant 50 \times 10^9$/l, for enlargement of both liver and spleen, and for haemoglobin concentration < 11 g/dl. There was some association between shorter survival and enlargement of three groups of lymph nodes, bone-marrow lymphocytes $\geqslant 80\%$, and platelet counts $< 100 \times 10^9$/l. A subgroup of patients with splenic enlargement but no palpable lymph-node enlargement has been described as having a good prognosis [259]. Other features shown to be related to prognosis are the density of marrow lymphocytic infiltration in relation to the lymphocytosis, the distribution of the marrow infiltrate, the morphology of the lymphocytes, and the proportion of plasma cells in the marrow. Unfavourable features were a high ratio of marrow to blood lymphocytes, large cells, and increased marrow plasma-cell numbers [260]. The simultaneous analysis of many variables has permitted the identification of three groups of patients with widely differing prognosis [261] in two series of 86 and 169 CLL patients followed up in Paris for 120 and 42 months [261a]. The prognostic groupings are as follows.

Group A (good prognosis) Hb $\geqslant 10$ g/dl, platelet count $\geqslant 100 \times 10^9$/l, fewer than three sites of organ enlargement.

Group C (poor prognosis) Hb < 10 g/dl or platelets $< 100 \times 10^9$/l.

Group B (intermediate) Hb and platelets as group A but three or more sites of organ enlargement.

Palpable enlargement of the spleen, the liver, or of lymph nodes in the neck, axillae, or groins each count as organ enlargement at one site. This system is now being tested by several groups of workers. Like the other systems [254–256] it is simple to apply and requires no special investigations. Refinement of the definition of sites of organ enlargement by the addition of lymphography may improve the prognostic value, as it has been reported to do in the Rai [262] and Binet [263] systems.

Static and progressive CLL

None of the systems for staging or prognostic grouping allows for the clinical observation that at any stage or in any grouping some patients have almost static disease that may not progress during observation periods extending for two or more decades, whilst in other cases obvious progression occurs during observation for a year or less. Patients with static disease have almost stable lymphocyte counts that fluctuate above and below a mean level [264, 265], whereas the counts of patients with progressive disease show a persistent upward trend. In therapeutic trials it is necessary to establish for each patient whether the disease is static or progressive. In the current Medical Research Council trial, progressive disease for stages I and II is defined as a persistent downward trend in either haemoglobin or platelet count towards 10 g/dl or $100 \times 10^9/l$ respectively (when the disease enters stages III or IV) with one of the following:

1 a significant increase in physical signs;
2 a consistent upward trend of the lymphocyte count, doubling within 12 months; or
3 constitutional symptoms (sweating, malaise, weight loss).

Properties of the CLL lymphocyte

B-CLL lymphocytes

Numerous differences have been described between the blood lymphocytes from normal persons and CLL patients. However, CLL lymphocyte populations are clones of long-lived cells derived from normal precursors whose phenotypic profile might be rare in the mixture of phenotypes found in populations of normal lymphocytes. It is not known whether some or all of the 'abnormalities' of CLL lymphocytes merely reflect the properties of the normal cell of origin, or at least of populations of that cell with an abnormal age distribution, or whether they are a consequence of the malignant nature of the cell. The rare bizarre ultrastructural abnormalities [266] such as the occurrence of amorphous, fibrillary, filamentous or crystalline inclusions associated with endoplasmic reticulum appear pathological, and seem to indicate qualitative or quantitative defects in immunoglobulin synthesis or processing.

By light and electron microscopy [267], CLL lymphocytes (Fig. 23.5a) are not distinguishable from normal B lymphocytes, but in routine blood films they are more homogeneous and the marked tendency to form smudge cells is characteristic. Many attempts have been made to classify CLL into subtypes according to morphological appearances and to identify types with different prognostic significance [260, 268–271]. In different reports, however, large cells have been associated with good [269] or with bad [260, 271] prognosis, and some of the older series studied have included cases of early and late disease, untreated and

treated patients, and examples of what appear to have been B-cell prolymphocytic leukaemia (B-PLL), FL, and B-cell lymphomas. In one study, the apparent prognostic significance of morphological appearance disappeared when clinical stage was taken into account [271a]. Accurate methods for defining the size and volume distribution of cell populations are now available [270, 272], and it should be possible to assess the relation of cell size and other morphological features to prognosis in properly defined cases of untreated B-CLL. Subsets of lymphocytes in mixed populations can be fractionated by equilibrium centrifugation on linear density gradients of polysucrose-metrizoate. The CLL lymphocytes from the blood and bone marrow are homogeneous populations of high buoyant density, similar to that of normal blood B-lymphocytes; about half of the lymphocytes from CLL lymph nodes have the same density, and there is a deficiency of follicular-centre B cells of light density [273].

Immunologically, B-CLL blood cells appear to represent a restricted phase in the early maturation of B cells. They have lost the cytoplasmic IgM of the pre-B phase, and are at an early stage in synthesizing surface-membrane Ig (SmIg). The SmIg is undetectable by routine methods [274] in about 20% of cases. It is present, at low density [275, 275a], in the remainder; about 40% show SmIgM, 30% SmIgM and D, 10% IgD [204]; cases with κ chains outnumber those with λ. In a minority of cases light chains are the only detectable SmIg [276], and very rarely, crystalline light-chain inclusions but no SmIg are found [277]. As already stated, in a minority of cases subclones synthesize and export monoclonal Ig. Whether SmIg is detectable or not, B-CLL blood cells have a high capacity for forming spontaneous rosettes when, after pre-treatment with neuraminidase [278], they are incubated with mouse red cells [204, 279–282]. In 80% of cases, more than half of the cells form rosettes, in sharp contrast to B-PLL, in 80% of which less than 30% of the cells form rosettes [204]: FL, HCL, and other B-lymphoproliferative conditions are intermediate, but seldom give the high values of CLL. In individual cases of B-CLL a small proportion of the blood lymphocytes that carry other B-cell markers neither form rosettes with mouse erythrocytes, nor carry SmIg [283]. The receptor for mouse erythrocytes, confined to B cells [281], is probably expressed only during a limited period of their maturation [282].

B-cell chronic lymphocytic leukaemia lymphocytes respond poorly, in conditions of culture in which normal B cells respond well, to mitogens thought to activate normal B lymphocytes (anti-β_2-microglobulin, sepharose-bound protein A, anti-F(ab^1)$_2$ Ig serum) and the surface receptors for them cap poorly [284].

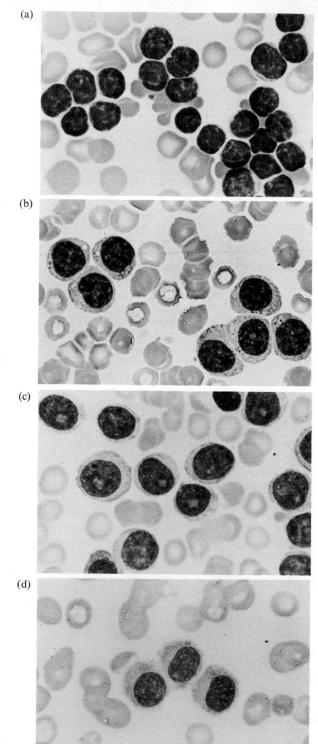

Fig. 23.5. (a) Peripheral blood; B-chronic lymphocytic leukaemia. May–Grünwald–Giemsa (×1400). Note the homogeneity of the cell population, the narrow rim of cytoplasm, the coarsely blocked chromatin; nucleolus is not visible. Smudge cells, characteristic of B-CLL, are not present in this field.–(b) Peripheral blood: T-chronic lymphocytic leukaemia. May–Grünwald–Giemsa (×1400). The nuclear structure resembles that of B-CLL, but there is more cytoplasm, which contains small numbers of azurophilic granules of varying size: the larger granules are often irregular in shape.–(c) Peripheral blood; B-prolymphocytic leukaemia. May–Grünwald–Giemsa (×1400). The cells are larger than in B-CLL, have more cytoplasm, the chromatin is condensed but the clumps are smaller than in B-CLL; note the prominent large vesicular nucleolus. This example is typical of the common type of B-PLL, with a homogeneous cell population: in a minority a variable proportion of the cell nuclei show a linear or broader indentation of varying depth. The morphology of T-PLL is indistinguishable from that of B-PLL in Romanowsky-stained films. In both forms the morphological features are seen clearly in blood films but are usually obscure in marrow smears.–(d) Peripheral blood; hairy-cell leukaemia. May–Grünwald–Giemsa (×1400). The eccentric round or ovoid nuclei have irregular small chromatin condensations with a reticular pattern. The cytoplasm, often abundant, has an ill-defined wispy border with fine projections of varying length.

From 30 seconds after exposure to the mitogens, normal but not B-CLL lymphocytes showed rapid flux of K^+ across the membrane. However, the fluidity of the plasma-membrane lipids, as determined by fluorescence polarization and fluorescent lifetime of the probe 1:6 diphenylhexatriene, is the same in normal and CLL lymphocytes [285], contrary to earlier reports [286, 287], and the content of the plasma-membrane enzymes alkaline phosphatase and alkaline phosphodiesterase I is normal in CLL cells [288], although that of L-γ-glutamyl transpeptidase, maltase, trehalase, leucine aminopeptidase, and 5′-nucleotidase is very low [289–291]. The nature of the membrane defect which blocks activation of the cell by mitogens is unknown. However, CLL lymphocytes have been found to respond normally to *Staphylococcus aureus* protein A when cultured in the presence of fetal calf serum [292]. CLL lymphocytes exposed to Sendai virus release significantly less interferon than normal lymphocytes [292a, 293]. CLL lymphocytes, and those of B-PLL [294], but not normal B-lymphocytes, are ultrasensitive to destruction when exposed to colchicine at high dilution (10^{-7} M) [295, 296], and a higher percentage of CLL than of normal cells passed through a column of polystyrene beads is retained.

The activity of several enzymes in normal blood lymphocytes has been shown to exhibit circadian rhythm. The enzymes of the blood lymphocytes in CLL retain the rhythm, but with a variable phase shift, and the pattern of activity is characteristic for each individual patient [297], yet another example of the homogeneity of CLL-lymphocyte populations.

B-CLL lymphocytes in different tissues. Lymphocytes are mobile cells programmed by their phenotypes to follow specific migration routes and to home to specific organs, sites or zones within the lymphoid system [298, 299]. It is likely that the migration and distribution patterns of the lymphocytes in lymphoproliferative diseases are determined in the same way [195, 300]. It is therefore not surprising that in CLL the distribution of subsets of the monoclone differs from one tissue to another. Thus, the great majority of peripheral-blood B-lymphocytes in CLL have the receptor for mouse erythrocytes [204, 301] whereas the proportion is lower in splenic lymphocytes, and usually much lower in lymph-node and bone-marrow lymphocytes [204, 204a]. Immunological maturation may proceed further in splenic and nodal lymphocytes than in the blood lymphocytes, as shown in cases in which SmIgG was found on the lymphocytes from the spleen and nodes but not from the blood [204, 204a].

Circulating T lymphocytes in B-CLL. The circulating T lymphocytes in B-CLL [302, 303] are believed to be normal cells and not part of the leukaemia-cell clone. However, they differ in several respects from those found in normal blood. Although their percentage decreases with advancing stage and, to some extent independently, with increasing total lymphocyte count [304], their absolute number is above the normal range in 30–80% of cases [304–306], with counts above 20×10^9/l in a few. In one report [304] no correlation with stages or with static and progressive disease was found, while in another there was a tendency for lower absolute counts in active disease and for a falling trend with time in static disease [306].

Recently, several subsets of T lymphocytes have been identified. Two of these regulate the immunological maturation of B lymphocytes by 'helper' or 'suppressor' activity [307]. It is probable that these subpopulations can be identified by the presence of surface receptors for the Fc fragment of μ chains (helper) or γ chains (suppressor). In normal blood the ratio of T_μ to T_γ cells is about 2:1. In B-CLL the ratio is almost reversed because of the disproportionate absolute increase in the number of T_γ cells [308, 309]. Differences in the functional properties of T cells in B-CLL from those of normal T cells must now be re-assessed in relation to the relative frequencies of T_μ and T_γ cells. For example the subnormal numbers of T-lymphocyte colonies that can be grown from B-CLL lymphocytes [310–313] is partly explained by the finding that T-lymphocyte colonies grow only from T_μ cells [313]. However, the response of T-cell-enriched samples of CLL lymphocytes to mitogens in different cases varies from normal [302, 303] to greatly reduced transformation [314, 315], but the variation is not accounted for by the proportions of T_γ and T_μ cells.

The absolute increase in the number of T_γ cells in B-CLL is likely to indicate a reaction against the accumulation of monoclonal B cells. It is unlikely to be a cause of the accumulation by suppressing their maturation, because the block would affect all B-cell clones equally, at least in the early stages: moreover, a suppressive mechanism could not explain the proliferative character of CLL. The increased numbers of T_γ cells may be a factor in the hypo-γ-globulinaemia of CLL, and a T-helper defect has been reported [316].

Diagnosis and differential diagnosis of B-CLL
The diagnosis is arrived at by considering each case in relation to:
1 knowledge of the evolution of B-CLL; and
2 the other chronic lymphoid leukaemias (Table 23.2) and the lymphomas (Table 23.3).

In elderly subjects under investigation for unrelated complaints B-CLL is often diagnosed by the chance isolated finding of lymphocytosis: persistent absolute

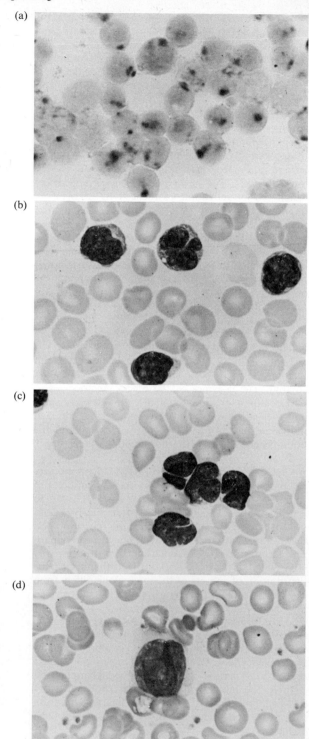

Fig. 23.6. (a) Peripheral blood; T-prolymphocytic leukaemia. Acid α-naphthyl acetate esterase reaction (×1400). Strong localized positive reaction in cytoplasm in majority of cells.–(b) Peripheral blood; pleomorphic T-cell leukaemia. May–Grünwald–Giemsa (×1400). Note heterogeneity, nuclear irregularity and multilobulation.–(c) Peripheral blood; follicular lymphoma. May–Grünwald–Giemsa (×1400). The characteristic lymphocytes ('notched-nucleus' cells, 'small cleft' cells*) are angular in outline, have scanty cytoplasm, compact chromatin, and often have one or two deep nuclear clefts which may appear to transect the nucleus.–(d) Peripheral blood; Sézary syndrome, large-cell type. May–Grünwald–Giemsa (×1400). The multiple delicate nuclear folds give the so-called cerebriform appearance which is characteristic of Sézary cells including those of the small-cell type (size of small lymphocytes).

* Small cleaved cell is a misnomer.

lymphocyte counts of $\geqslant 5 \times 10^9/l$ are suggestive, particularly when smudge cells are prominent. But for B-CLL the lymphocytes must be homogeneous small cells of normal morphology and devoid of azurophilic granules, which suggest T-CLL (Fig. 23.6b). Plasmacytoid lymphocytes suggest Waldenström's macroglobulinaemia (WM) or its IgG or IgA-secreting equivalent [316a, 316b], especially when rouleaux formation and background protein staining are present. In the absence of symptoms and signs and an otherwise normal blood count the other conditions listed are unlikely. Prolymphocytic leukaemia is only occasionally diagnosed by chance, and is recognized by the characteristic morphology of the cells [317] (Fig. 23.6a). Bone-marrow examination is necessary to confirm the diagnosis of B-CLL; infiltration with 25% or more of monomorphic small lymphocytes make the diagnosis probable but formal confirmation requires $\geqslant 40\%$. Trephine biopsy sections show either widespread but light interstitial infiltration by lymphocytes among the haemopoietic cells and between the fat cells, or fairly well circumscribed nodular collections of lymphocytes centrally placed among the haemopoietic tissue in the marrow spaces bounded by bony trabeculae. Diffuse replacement of the haemopoietic tissue is unusual in this context unless the lymphocyte counts are above $100 \times 10^9/l$. The diagnosis of B-CLL can be clinched by demonstrating the presence of receptors for mouse erythrocytes on 30% or more of the blood lymphocytes, and in 80% of cases the cells will also have SmIg at low density [204].

For patients with splenic enlargement as well as lymphocytosis, HCL must be considered as well as PLL and WM, but is unlikely in the absence of anaemia, neutropenia, thrombocytopenia, or combinations of these. The morphology of hairy cells is characteristic (Fig. 23.5d), but at lymphocyte counts of only $5 \times 10^9/l$ few may be present, and marrow examination is necessary. T-cell leukaemia must be considered also, especially if skin lesions are present and the lymphocytes have azurophilic granules.

For patients with lymph-node enlargement, PLL and HCL are unlikely; with lymphocyte counts between 5 and $10 \times 10^9/l$ the most likely alternative diagnoses are follicular lymphoma (FL) or one of the diffuse B lympomas; FL may also present with higher lymphocyte counts [318, 319]. Notched-nucleus cells (small cleft cells) [318] in the blood films are characteristic [319] but are not always present in FL, and pleomorphic lymphocytes with few or no smudge cells suggest a diffuse lymphoma rather than CLL. In bone-marrow trephine sections FL infiltrates are characteristically paratrabecular. Lymph-node biopsy serves to distinguish CLL (or small-cell diffuse lymphoma) from FL and other B-cell lymphomas including WM. The lymph-node histology of CLL is that of small-cell diffuse lymphocytic lymphoma (WDDL, Rappaport) and is usually unmistakable. There is effacement of the architecture with replacement by a monotonous infiltrate of small lymphocytes with only rare mitotic figures. There are, however, always collections of large, pale blast cells with some mitotic figures; these collections are usually inconspicuous but sometimes large enough to give a pseudofollicular appearance [193, 320] and to lead to a diagnosis of large-cell or poorly differentiated lymphoma [195].

Confusion in the diagnosis of CLL is most likely to arise:
1 in early disease before the formal requirements for both lymphocytosis and marrow infiltration are present; and
2 when there is marked enlargement of lymph nodes or of the spleen but only slightly raised or normal lymphocyte counts.

The character of the lymph-node enlargement is often helpful. In CLL they are usually soft or rubbery, discrete, mobile, and randomly distributed. Several large nodes of unequal size and consistency at one site suggest lymphoma rather than CLL, especially if they are of restricted mobility or tethered. Romanowsky-stained aspirates of lymph-node juice are helpful because of the dominance of monomorphic small lymphocytes in CLL, and of larger pleomorphic anaplastic cells in the lymphomas.

In every case of presumptive CLL, the serum immunoglobulins should be estimated, a paraprotein sought, and concentrated urine tested for free light chains. The presence of a paraprotein does not exclude the diagnosis of CLL, but the finding must be interpreted in the light of all the other features before deciding whether the case is one of CLL with a paraprotein, or lymphoplasmacytic lymphoma or other B lymphoma.

Treatment of B-CLL

The treatments now available act by destroying lymphocytes, and the benefit they confer results from the reduction in the TLM (total lymphocyte mass). None is curative, all are potentially harmful, and the disease tends to become resistant to the treatments between three and 10 years after starting. It is therefore necessary to define the extent of the benefit that can be expected from treatment before attempting to formulate aims of treatment, protocols for realizing them, and the circumstances in which treatment is likely to be helpful; the possible benefits must be balanced against the risks incurred.

Effective treatment by conventional splenic irradiation [321], alkylating-agent chemotherapy (chlorambucil or cyclophosphamide), alone or in combination with steroids [322–325], can reduce the TLM suffi-ciently to reverse most of the adverse effects resulting from its expansion. The reduction of bone-marrow infiltration will relieve bone-marrow failure and lead to an increase in the haemoglobin concentration, platelet and neutrophil counts. The reduction of splenomegaly will relieve hypersplenism. These effects can be life-saving and they relieve morbidity. The reduction of lymph-node size and of the lymphocyte count provides means of monitoring the progress of treatment. There is evidence that the reduction in the TLM affects the duration of survival, because in clinical trials, the survival of responders has been superior to that of non-responders [323, 325, 326]. All would agree that patients in bone-marrow failure (Rai stages III and IV, Binet group C) should be treated and these patients gain great symptomatic relief. There is, however, no certainty about the remainder. Most physicians would treat patients with obviously pro-gressive disease even if they have no evidence of impaired bone-marrow function, but are likely to be reluctant to treat patients with obviously static disease, though some would treat such patients if they have bulky nodal disease, very high lymphocyte counts and heavy marrow infiltration. Very few would treat early disease (stage 0, Rai), though Osgood [327] maintained that the proportion of 20-year survivors could be increased from one to 10% by treating all patients from the time of diagnosis and controlling the lymphocyte counts indefinitely. Controlled clinical trials in pro-gress are designed to discover whether treatment for the various groups of asymptomatic patients not in marrow failure prolongs survival and whether particu-lar forms of treatment are advantageous.

Methods of treatment

Radiotherapy. Radiation therapy used to be given to successive groups of enlarged lymph nodes, up to 1000 rads being delivered to each group, or the spleen was irradiated several times weekly to a total dose of 300–1000 rads [321]. After the introduction of chemo-therapy with alkylating agents, the use of radiotherapy declined; claims for whole-body irradiation [328] and for mediastinal irradiation [329] have been made but neither method has become popular. Recently, 10 exposures to splenic irradiation at weekly intervals to a total dose of 1000 rads has been introduced (Fioren-tino M., personal communication); the splenic lym-phocyte population is conceived as constantly chang-ing by recirculation [322], and the unusually long interval between exposures ensures that most of the lymphocytes killed by the previous dose will have been replaced by viable cells; thus the killing efficiency of the same dose of radiation should be greater. This method

of splenic irradiation is being tested in one arm of the Medical Research Council's current trial in CLL.

Patients with normal haemoglobin, neutrophil and platelet counts but heavily infiltrated bone marrow may have little remaining haemopoietic reserve capa-city. Unavoidable irradiation of bone marrow during the treatment of the spleen or lymph-node areas may therefore cause unacceptable falls in the neutrophil, platelet, and reticulocyte counts. Extracorporeal irra-diation of the blood (ECIB) in a coiled tube attached to an arteriovenous shunt and inserted into an irradiator permits the exposure of the blood to irradiation at very high dosage without incurring any myeloid damage. The method, though effective in lowering the lympho-cyte count [330], is unwieldy, inconvenient, and little used.

Chemotherapy. Chlorambucil and prednisone [322, 331] remain the most widely used drugs. Prednisone damages lymphocytes but is not myelosuppressive and can therefore rescue patients in bone-marrow failure, whereas the myelosuppressive chlorambucil is highly dangerous in this circumstance, but valuable once the marrow is again active following the prednisone-induced destruction of the marrow lymphocytes. Pred-nisone is indispensable as an emergency treatment for a few weeks, but is dangerous for long-term adminis-tration, especially because of its enhancement of the CLL-related immunosuppression. Chlorambucil used to be administered on a long-term basis at low daily dosage (2–6 mg), but because of the possibility that its myelosuppressive and immunosuppressive effect might be reduced, intermittent treatment at high dosage (1·0–1·5 mg/kg in 3 or 4 days every month) is becoming popular, and there is some evidence that it may be more effective [324, 325]. This method is also included in the current Medical Research Council (MRC) trial.

Treatment with prednisone and chlorambucil rarely if ever induces complete remission with disappearance of physical signs, long-lasting reduction of the lympho-cyte count below $5 \times 10^9/l$, restoration of normal blood values, of a normal bone marrow, and of immunocom-petence. Bone-marrow lymphocytes may fall below 20% but trephine sections almost always shown per-sistence of lymphocytic nodules. About 40% of patients obtain partial but worthwhile remissions. The response is often slow and optimal conditions may require treatment for one year or more. After treat-ment is discontinued the time before resumption of treatment is indicated varies from a few months to two years or more.

It is uncertain whether intensive multiple-drug ther-apy would increase the proportion of responders, of complete remissions, and of long survivors and the long-term results of a trial involving the use of vincristine, BCNU, cyclophosphamide, melphalan, and prednisone (M-2 protocol) [230] are awaited with interest. In the current MRC trial, one schedule consists of five-day courses of cyclophosphamide, vincristine and prednisone [326].

Treatment for autoimmune phenomena and hypersplenism. Overt autoimmune haemolytic anaemia (AIHA) occurs in less than one-third of the patients whose erythrocytes give a positive result in the direct antiglobulin test (DAT). Overt AIHA may be the presenting feature of CLL, or may occur at any time after diagnosis [229, 331a]. Rarely, it is precipitated by irradiation or by alkylating-agent treatment [331b, 331c]. The occurrence of AIHA does not adversely affect the prognosis; the condition usually responds dramatically to steroid therapy and once controlled may never recur. The role of alkylating agents in precipitating AIHA is difficult to establish unless the patient was known to have had a negative result of the DAT immediately before the start of treatment. In the presence of a just compensated pre-exisiting AIHA, the depression of erythropoiesis caused by treatment with an alkylating agent leads to a rapid fall in the haemoglobin concentration; the condition will respond to steroid therapy, but because of the depression of erythropoiesis the response is slow.

Like AIHA, immune thrombocytopenia may appear at any stage in the course of CLL [331d], and may be suspected when thrombocytopenia is associated with normal Hb and neutrophil count and plentiful megakaryocytes in the bone marrow. The condition may resolve spontaneously but usually requires steroid therapy and sometimes splenectomy.

Hypersplenism with erythrocyte [331e] and platelet pooling [331f] and resulting anaemia and thrombocytopenia is especially associated in CLL with spleen weights of 1 kg or more. Cautious treatment by splenic irradiation or steroid therapy followed by chlorambucil may shrink the spleen and relieve the hypersplenism. But when the spleen is very large these treatments may be only partially effective; splenectomy is indicated and is often extremely successful [332]. Patients with the 'pure' splenomegalic form of CLL [259], who have very small or no palpable lymph nodes, tend to have static disease with a good prognosis, and after splenectomy may require no treatment for several years. Splenectomy should be considered more often than it is in CLL, but caution is required when the disease is progressive because the benefits resulting from the relief of hypersplenism are likely to be short-lived. Furthermore, splenic enlargement may be due mainly to the lymphocytic infiltrate with relatively less erythrocyte and platelet pooling, while if the patient is already refractory to chemotherapy, little or nothing will have been gained by splenectomy.

Terminal CLL
The late stage of CLL is dominated by increasing resistance to treatment, the consequences of immune deficiency and of bone-marrow failure, and the development of other neoplasms. Patients with slowly progressive but treatment-resistant disease may nevertheless survive for several years even with bulky lymph-node enlargement, massive splenomegaly, high lymphocyte counts, failing bone marrow, and increasingly frequent infections which respond poorly to antibiotics. Some such patients appear to derive benefit from long-term antibiotic therapy and regular injections of γ globulin, but there is no formal proof of the efficacy of these measures. Repeated leucapheresis may help to control very high lymphocyte counts [333].

Treatment-resistant progressive CLL with a rising lymphocyte count is sometimes associated with a steady increase in the blood of the proportion of large atypical pleomorphic lymphocytes, often with prominent nucleoli. During this 'prolymphocytoid' transformation [206], the surface-marker profile of the lymphocytes does not change. A more acute type of malignant transformation, Richter's syndrome [334–340], accounts for about five per cent of deaths in CLL [331]. A subclone of treatment-resistant malignant cells bearing the same markers as the CLL clone [208] arises focally, often in para-aortic lymph nodes, to produce an invasive metastasing sarcomatous tumour of pleomorphic appearance usually with numerous multinucleate giant cells. The first clinical indication of its presence may be an unexplained pyrexia with drenching sweats, or the appearance of a paraprotein in the serum or urine. Even more uncommon is an acute blast-cell leukaemic transformation [340a] involving cells bearing the same marker profile as the CLL clone [207]. These three forms of transformation appear to reflect the risk of further malignant change in the CLL clone itself or in the stem-cell pool from which it arose, and may be analogous to the transformation of the chronic myeloid leukaemias. Acute plasma-cell leukaemia is a rare termination of CLL [341], while CLL and myelomatosis may co-exist or occur in sequence [341a–342]; phenotype characterization in future cases will show whether some of these are also examples of transformation in the CLL clone.

Acute myeloid leukaemia is another rare terminal event in CLL. Occasionally the two diagnoses are made simultaneously, the CLL being sometimes at an early stage [343–351]; when the AML is a late occurrence, the possibility that it was induced by alkylating agent [352] or radiation therapy [353] must be considered. Every clinician with long experience of CLL believes that there is a high risk of second or even multiple [354] malignant conditions. But CLL is a chronic disease of the elderly, and it is still uncertain whether the risk exceeds that expected from the number of years of exposure in the age groups affected. Most reports suggest that it does [14, 258, 331, 355–359].

PROLYMPHOCYTIC LEUKAEMIA

Prolymphocytic leukaemia (PLL) is a rare variant of CLL most often diagnosed in elderly men [317, 360]. The early subclinical stage is rarely observed, but lymphocytosis appears to be progressive, no case of static lymphocytosis having been reported; in contrast to CLL, splenic enlargement is an early feature, while clinical lymph-node enlargement may not occur at all, or is a late development. The lymphocyte counts may rise to exceed 1000×10^9/l. Unlike CLL patients, who often seek medical advice at a relatively early stage because they find enlarged lymph nodes, most PLL patients present with symptoms of anaemia: they usually have massive splenomegaly, inconspicuous or no lymph-node enlargement, and very high leucocyte counts.

Diagnosis and differential diagnosis

The diagnosis is made on the characteristic appearance of the blood films. There is a monomorphic population of round lymphoid cells, usually larger than CLL lymphocytes with more cytoplasm, a round centrally placed nucleus with a single large, central, round, vesicular nucleolus, but well-marked chromatin condensation, both peripheral and perinucleolar (Fig. 23.5b). Unlike CLL blood films, those of PLL have only rare smudge cells. In cases in which the cells are only slightly if at all larger than CLL cells, and the chromatin is as coarsely clumped as in CLL cells, the large, prominent nucleolus is nevertheless present, and there is usually more cytoplasm than in CLL cells. The differences between PLL and CLL cells are well shown by electron microscopy [361]. Cell volume measurements on the Coulter ZBI counter linked to a channelyzer confirm the large cell size and homogeneity of PLL cell populations [272].

Immunological marker studies show B-cell features in most cases, but T-PLL does occur and is cytologically indistinguishable from B-PLL. Such studies show a different pattern from that of CLL. Invariably SmIg is present, and at high density in 90% of cases. The number of SmIg antigenic sites on the PLL cell has been estimated as about 80 000, compared to about 12 000 for CLL cells [275, 275a]. In 80% of cases of PLL, less than 30% (usually < 10%) of the cells form M-rosettes [204]; a higher proportion is found in the occasional case in which the cells are close to CLL cells

but have the characteristic large nucleolus of PLL and high-density SmIg [361]. In one case of otherwise typical PLL, the cells had markers of both B and T lymphocytes. The cells, however, resembled those of CLL in their colchicine ultrasensitivity, and in their retention when passed through a column of polystyrene beads. Unlike CLL cells they were markedly radio-resistant *in vitro* [294].

The cytomorphology of PLL is so characteristic that confusion with other conditions associated with massive splenomegaly and high lymphocyte counts is unlikely to arise. The cytology of the splenomegalic form of CLL [259] is that of CLL in general. In prolymphocytoid transformation, CLL [206] shows a dimorphic lymphoid population, the residual small-cell population being mixed with larger cells, some resembling PLL cells but having the same marker profile as the accompanying small cells. Markedly heterogeneous cell populations suggest malignant lymphoma in leukaemic phase rather than B-PLL, and here the clinical and haematological features are more helpful than the marker profile.

Histological features

In one case, the histological appearance of an excised lymph node suggested an origin for the PLL cells in the mantle zone of the germinal centres [362], but lymph-node enlargement early in the disease is so unusual that this finding may not be characteristic. In other cases [363] no association of PLL infiltrates with germinal centres was apparent. In the spleen the infiltrate is, like that in CLL, primarily in the white pulp, with prominent, often bizonal, nodular infiltrates [363, 364] with diffuse infiltration of the red pulp; the only differences are the size and characteristics of the cells. In the bone marrow the location of the infiltrate, as in CLL, is intramedullary and not paratrabecular as in FL.

The nature of B-PLL

B-cell PLL is a proliferation of a B lymphocyte, immunologically more mature than the B-CLL cell, with strong affinity for the spleen, blood and bone marrow, and only weak affinity for lymph nodes. The target cell may originate in the splenic white pulp [363], but its normal counterpart is unknown.

Course, prognosis and treatment

Prolymphocytic leukaemia is almost always at a late stage when diagnosed, and its course is progressive, in contrast to the often static course of pure splenomegalic CLL. Few patients survive three years from diagnosis [363], and the outlook is perhaps similar to that of progressive stage III/IV (Rai) CLL. B-cell PLL patients usually die as a consequence of bone-marrow failure. They are, for the most part, notoriously unresponsive to conventional radiotherapy and to chemotherapy with alkylating agents. In such cases, following splenectomy, some reduction in bone-marrow infiltration and improvement in haemopoiesis has been achieved and maintained by repeated leucapheresis [365]. In two cases, good remissions have been obtained with doxorubicin [366] or with multiple-drug therapy (cyclophosphamide, doxorubicin, vincristine and prednisone) [367]. Some patients have responded to splenic irradiation; 10 exposures at weekly intervals, each of 100 rad [367a].

HAIRY-CELL LEUKAEMIA

Hairy-cell leukaemia (HCL) [368–371], formerly known as leukaemic reticulo-endotheliosis [372, 373], lymphoid myelofibrosis [374] or lymphohistiocytosis [375], is now accepted as a lymphoproliferative disease involving a unique B-lymphocyte target cell whose normal counterpart is unknown [375a, 376–377]. It affects a wider age range than CLL and PLL, being found from the third decade onwards, and males predominate. Classically the patient presents with anaemia, with recurrent infections associated with neutropenia or with bleeding or bruising resulting from thrombocytopenia. The major sign is splenomegaly; the liver is sometimes enlarged, the lymph nodes rarely, and the diagnosis is made from the examination of the blood and bone marrow. With increasing recognition of HCL, more patients are likely to be diagnosed before the spleen is palpably enlarged.

Diagnosis

The characteristic hairy cells (Fig. 23.5c) are diagnostic [369, 378]. At least a few are usually present in blood films, and with experience can be distinguished in well-spread films from other mononuclear cells mechanically distorted. The morphology is usually much better seen in films of blood than of bone marrow. Bone-marrow aspiration often either fails or yields blood only, and well-preserved hairy cells may be few. Imprints from trephine specimens are rarely satisfactory. Sections of marrow trephine samples are diagnostic in the majority of cases [370].

In well-spread blood films hairy cells (Fig. 23.5c) have round or ovoid, sometimes indented, usually eccentric nuclei about the size or slightly larger than lymphocyte nuclei, but in intact cells the cytoplasm is more abundant than that of the lymphocyte. It is grey-blue in May–Grünwald–Giemsa-stained films, has an opaque floccular, non-granular, occasionally vacuolated appearance, and its edge is variably extended into well or poorly defined wispy or hair-like projections. The nucleus has compact, variably stippled chromatin, rarely as coarsely clumped as in lymphocytes, and one or more small nucleoli are sometimes seen. The large average cell size and heterogeneity in size is well seen in histograms prepared from cell-volume channelyzer measurements [272]. Amorphous cytoplasmic purplish inclusion bodies are seen in occasional cells and are the ribosome-lamellar complexes seen in transmission electron microscopy [376, 379, 380]: they are sometimes found in other B-cell disorders also. The numerous, long, villous processes are best seen by transmission electron microscopy. A characteristic, though not quite specific [376, 381, 382] cytochemical reaction of hairy cells is that for the tartrate-resistant isoenzyme 5 of acid phosphatase [383], which accounts for 10–100% of the total enzyme activity in these cells. A negative or weak reaction or even inhibition by tartrate should not exclude the diagnosis [376]. A specific pattern of reactivity with α-naphthyl butyrate esterase, not abolished by exposure to fluoride, permits HCL to be distinguished from other haematological malignant conditions with which it might be confused [383a]. Furthermore, this reaction is usually present in a higher proportion of blood mononuclear cells than are recognizable in Romanowsky-stained films as hairy cells [383a].

When bone-marrow fragments are obtained by aspiration they appear hypercellular with little fat, and the cells look monomorphic. On the surface of the fragments numerous tissue mast cells may be seen. The trails are sparse and consist almost entirely of hairy cells, mostly damaged by the spreading. Plasma cells are usually conspicuous. The trephine sections show extensive replacement of the marrow by a highly characteristic monomorphic infiltrate in which the cells are separated from one another by faintly staining fibrillary material: the appearance is in striking contrast to the tightly packed character of most malignant infiltrates. There is diffuse and dense increase in reticulin. The extensive replacement of the marrow explains the pancytopenia. The histological appearance of hairy-cell infiltrates in the spleen, portal tracts and sinusoids of the liver, and in lymph nodes, is similar to that in the marrow [369, 381].

Hairy-cell leukaemia is not likely to be confused nowadays with any other condition, but formerly, before the characteristic clinical, haematological and histological features were recognized, it was mistaken for CLL, lymphocytic lymphoma, malignant histiocytosis, chronic monocytic leukaemia, or even acute leukaemia.

Nature of the hairy cell

Hairy cells share some features with monocytes: they adhere to glass, are weakly phagocytic [370, 376, 384, 385] and perhaps bactericidal [379, 386], and they have strong receptors for the Fc fragment of IgG [385, 386].

But they lack the major properties of monocytes [376], and are now generally accepted as monoclonal B cells. They possess SmIg with the same light chain, but unlike CLL and PLL, they often have more than one heavy-chain isotype [376, 385, 387, 387a] and very rarely they secrete an IgA or IgG [377] paraprotein. In spite of the strong Fc receptor activity, there is no doubt now that the Ig molecules are products of the cells [385, 388], which thus appear to be B cells at a later stage in immunological maturation than in CLL, though at least a proportion of hairy cells form M rosettes [388a, 389].

Like the case of PLL with cells bearing both T and B markers [294] the hairy cells in one clinically and haematologically typical case of HCL were found to have both B- and T-cell properties [390]. Other patients whose hairy cells had T-cell features have been reported [391–393].

Course, prognosis and treatment

The course of HCL is dominated by two features:
1 the progressive but sometimes very slow replacement of the haemopoietic tissue by the hairy-cell infiltrate which leads to bone-marrow failure; and
2 the progressive splenomegaly with hypersplenism.

Splenic red-cell pooling is greater in the HCL spleen than in a spleen of comparable size in other conditions [394], and when hypersplenism is gross, pancytopenia develops when there is still much functional marrow. In this circumstance splenectomy is usually beneficial and when the rate of marrow infiltration is very slow, the benefit may last for years. In a personal case, marrow function remains good 20 years after splenectomy, but occasional hairy cells are still present in blood films, while in another case [349a] the hairy-cell clone appears to have died out after 12 years. Patients who survive four years from diagnosis appear to have a good prospect for long survival [370], with 35–40% alive at 10 years [371]. However, about half of all the patients have progressive disease and die in bone-marrow failure within four years. Patients whose marrow function is severely compromised at the time of diagnosis are unlikely to benefit greatly from splenectomy [395]. A rough guide is the absolute neutrophil count, a value of $< 0.5 \times 10^9/l$ indicating a poor prognosis [370]. The post-splenectomy rise in these cases is relatively shortlived. About one-third of the patients succumb to intractable infection, and perhaps the rather constant monocytopenia [370, 371] is a factor in the unusual frequency of otherwise excessively rare infections, including atypical mycobacterial infections [396, 397] as well as tuberculosis.

Although splenectomy is beneficial in the presence of severe hypersplenism and some functioning bone marrow, it is difficult to define precise indications for the operation. It is desirable to observe progress before considering splenectomy; older patients, especially with only moderate splenomegaly, have essentially static disease and are best left untreated. The prospects for patients who do not respond to splenectomy, or who relapse after it, are poor. Steroid therapy may improve the blood values temporarily, but long-term therapy is usually both ineffective and hazardous. Alkylating-agent therapy is usually ineffective. Rarely, patients misdiagnosed as having acute leukaemia and treated by multiple-drug therapy [376, 397a] have improved, exacting supportive care being required during the phase of prolonged cytopenia, while elective doxorubicin therapy induced a temporary remission in one case after the failure of splenectomy [398].

CHRONIC T-CELL LEUKAEMIAS

Like their B-cell counterparts, the chronic T-cell leukaemias (Table 23.2) are lymphoproliferative disorders with early and predominant involvement of the blood and bone marrow. The distinction between lymphoma and leukaemia is not sharp: for example, patients with the Sézary syndrome and high lymphocyte counts were formerly diagnosed as having CLL with an associated generalized erythroderma [399], but these cases fit well in the broader group of cutaneous T-cell lymphomas (CTCL) [400]. The chronic T-cell leukaemias have been recognized only recently, but although they are now actively sought they appear to account for only about two per cent of all chronic lymphoid leukaemias. The few cases of T-PLL [205, 401–403] and T-HCL so far described do not appear to have had distinctive clinical and haematological features, though some PLL patients have palpable lymph nodes and one with T-HCL had skin lesions [392]. Morphologically T-PLL and T-HCL cells resemble their B-cell counterparts, but T-PLL cells can be distinguished by their strong acid α-naphthyl acetate esterase activity (Fig. 23.6a) [204, 403]. The small T-cell and pleomorphic T-cell leukaemias are less uncommon and are beginning to be better characterized [404].

Small T-cell leukaemia

Unlike B-CLL, small T-cell leukaemia occurs during the first two decades as well as in older subjects (Catovsky & Galton, unpublished observations), although the true age distribution is not yet known.

In some cases, discovered by chance, the only abnormal finding was a moderate T lymphocytosis increasing slowly over several years. Early enlargement of the spleen but little or no lymph node enlargement is common, and the extent of lymphocytic infiltration of the bone marrow is less in relation to the lymphocytosis than is usual in B-CLL, whereas in the

Sézary syndrome with lymphocytosis the proportion of bone-marrow lymphocytes is in the normal range. Skin infiltrations are frequent [401]. The blood lymphocytes [401] differ from those of B-CLL in their somewhat more abundant grey-blue cytoplasm which contains small numbers of azurophilic granules (Fig. 23.5b), and there are few smudge cells. The azurophilic granules vary in size, the larger ones sometimes appearing irregular in outline. Transmission electron microscopy [405] shows the larger granules to be 'parallel tubular arrays' (PTA), sometimes enclosed in a double membrane, while the smaller granules are lysosomes. Both organelles contain acid phosphatase and β-glucuronidase. So far PTA have been found only in T cells with suppressor properties from T-cell leukaemia. That small T-cell leukaemia often involves a population of T_γ cells is supported by their poor capacity for colony growth *in vitro* [204]. However, the precursor cells may be less differentiated because in one case [406] both T_γ and T_μ leukaemia cells were present. Both subsets had the same chromosome $14q+$ translocation that had been identified in 'normal' lymphocytes 11 years before during the investigation of ataxia telangiectasia.

Pleomorphic T-cell leukaemia

In recent years a rare clinicopathological entity has been described in Japan, where B-CLL is also rare. It affects adults above age 40 who were born in and around Kyushu, in contrast to T-cell leukaemias of small-cell, prolymphocytic, and blast-cell types [407–409]. There is a marked enlargement of lymph nodes, liver and spleen, but not mediastinal enlargement, and skin lesions are frequent. There is marked lymphocytosis involving highly pleomorphic, often large lymphoid cells with gross nuclear irregularities (Fig 23.6b). The cells have T-cell properties [407–413] and those tested have had suppressor activity. Although there are similarities to CTCL in some cases in respect of the cytomorphology and ultrastructure of the cells and in the histopathology of the skin lesions, the condition appears to be a distinct entity. It is possible that similar cases occur sporadically in other parts of the world [200, 204], but the precise characterization of all the chronic T-lymphoproliferative disorders is still at an early stage. The disease runs a subacute or acute course and has responded poorly to treatment with cyclophosphamide, vinca alkaloids, mercaptopurine, procarbazine and fluorouracil.

REFERENCES

1 CANELLOS G., EAGAM R.T., WHANG J. & CARBONE P.P. (1968) Clinical significance of the Philadelphia chromosome in chronic granulocyte leukaemia. *Annals of Internal Medicine*, **68**, 1166.

2 EZDINLI E.Z., SOKAL J.E., CROSSWHITE L. & SANDBERG A.A. (1970) Philadelphia chromosome-positive and -negative chronic myelocytic leukemia. *Annals of Internal Medicine*, **72**, 175.

3 GEARY C.G., CATOVSKY D., WILTSHAW E., MILNER G.R., SCHOLES M.C., VAN NOORDEN S., WARDSWORTH L.D., MULDAL S., MacIVER J.E. & GALTON D.A.G. (1975) Chronic myelomonocytic leukaemia. *British Journal of Haematology*, **30**, 289.

4 TANZER J., HAREL P., BOIRON M. & BERNARD J. (1964) Cytochemical and cytogenetic findings in a case of neutrophilic leukaemia of mature cell type. *Lancet*, **i**, 387.

5 JACKSON I.M.D. & CLARK R.M. (1965) A case of neutrophilic leukemia. *American Journal of Medical Science*, **249**, 72.

6 RUBIN H. (1966) Chronic neutrophilic leukemia. *Annals of Internal Medicine*, **65**, 93.

7 SILBERSTEIN E.B., ZELLNER D.C., SHIVAKUMAR B.N. & BURGIN L.A. (1974) Neutrophilic leukemia. *Annals of Internal Medicine*, **80**, 110.

8 SHINDO S., SAKAI C. & SHIBATA A. (1977) Neutrophilic leukemia and blastic crisis. *Annals of Internal Medicine*, **87**, 66.

9 HARDISTY R.M., SPEED D.E. & TILL M. (1964) Granulocytic leukaemia in childhood. *British Journal of Haematology*, **10**, 551.

10 WEATHERALL D.J., EDWARDS J.A. & DONAHUE W.T. (1968) Haemoglobin and red cell enzyme changes in juvenile myeloid leukaemia. *British Medical Journal*, **i**, 679.

11 BENNETT J.M., CATOVSKY, D., DANIEL M.-T., FLANDRIN G., GALTON D.A.G., GRALNICK H.R. & SULTAN C. (1976) Proposals for the classification of the acute leukaemias. *British Journal of Haematology*, **33**, 451.

12 OSGOOD E.E. (1937) Monocytic leukaemia. *Archives of Internal Medicine*, **59**, 931.

12a WATKINS C.H. & HALL B.E. (1940) Monocytic leukemia of the Naegeli and Schilling types. *American Journal of Clinical Pathology*, **10**, 387.

12b SINN C.M. & DICK F.W. (1956) Monocytic leukemia. *American Journal of Medicine*, **20**, 588.

13 SAFFHILL R., DEXTER T.M., MULDAL S., TESTA N.G., MORRIS-JONES P. & JOSEPH A. (1976) Terminal deoxynucleotidyl transferase in a case of Ph^1-positive infant chronic myelogenous leukaemia. *British Journal of Cancer*, **33**, 664.

14 FABER M. & BORUM K. (1962) Leukaemia and malignant tumour in the same patients. *British Journal of Haematology*, **8**, 313.

15 COURT BROWN W.M., DOLL R. & SMITH P. (1967) Neoplasia in patients treated with X-rays for ankylosing spondylitis or metropathia haemorrhagica. *Proceedings of the IXth International Cancer Congress. UICC Monograph Series* (ed. Harris R.J.C.), Vol. 10, p. 119. Springer-Verlag, Berlin.

15a DOLL R. (1972) The epidemiology of leukaemia. *Leukaemia Research Fund Seventh Annual Guest Lecture.* Leukaemia Research Fund, London.

16 *United Nations Report of Scientific Committee on the Effects of Atomic Radiation to the General Assembly*

(1972) 27th Session, official records. Supplement 25, A/8725.

17 MOLE R.H. (1975) Ionizing radiation as a carcinogen: practical questions and academic pursuits. *British Journal of Radiology*, **48**, 157.

18 GUNZ F.W. (1977) The epidemiology and genetics of the chronic leukaemias. In: *Clinics in Haematology: The Chronic Leukaemias* (ed. Galton D.A.G.), Vol. 6, p. 1. W. B. Saunders, London.

19 JANOSSY G., ROBERTS M. & GREAVES M.G. (1976) Target cell in chronic myeloid leukaemia and its relationship to acute lymphoid leukaemia. *Lancet*, **ii**, 1058.

20 JANOSSY G., WOODRUFF R.K., PAXTON A., GREAVES M.F., CAPELLARO D., KIRK B., INNES E.M., EDEN O.B., LEWIS C., CATOVSKY D. & HOFFBRAND A.V. (1978) Membrane marker and cell separation studies in Ph¹-positive leukemia. *Blood*, **51**, 861.

21 JANOSSY G., WOODRUFF R.K., PIPPARD M.J., PRENTICE G., HOFFBRAND A.V., PAXTON A., LISTER T.A., BUNCH C. & GREAVES M.F. (1979) Relation of 'lymphoid' phenotype and response to chemotherapy incorporating vincristine-prednisolone in the acute phase of Ph¹-positive leukaemia. *Cancer*, **43**, 426.

22 NOWELL P.C. & HUNGERFORD D.A. (1960) A minute chromosome in human chronic granulocytic leukemia. *Science*, **132**, 1197.

23 CLEIN G.P. & FLEMANS R.J. (1966) Involvement of the erythroid series in blastic crisis of chronic myeloid leukaemia. Further evidence for the presence of Philadelphia chromosome in erythroblasts. *British Journal of Haematology*, **12**, 754.

24 RASTRICK J.M., FITZGERALD P.H. & GUNZ F.W. (1974) Direct evidence for presence of Ph¹ chromosome in erythroid cells. *British Medical Journal*, **i**, 96.

25 CHERVENICK P.A., ELLIS L.D., PAN S.F. & LAWSON A.L. (1971) Human leukemic cells: *in vitro* growth of colonies containing the Philadelphia (Ph¹) chromosome. *Science*, **174**, 1134.

26 SHADDUCK R.K. & NANKIN H.R. (1971) Cellular origin of granulocytic colonies in chronic myeloid leukaemia. *Lancet*, **ii**, 1097.

27 AYE M.T., TILL J.E. & McCULLOCH E.A. (1973) Cytological studies of granulopoietic colonies from two patients with chronic myelogenous leukaemia. *Experimental Hematology*, **1**, 115.

27a MOORE, M.A.S. & METCALF D. (1973) Cytogenetic analysis of human acute and chronic myeloid leukemic cells cloned in agar culture. *International Journal of Cancer*, **11**, 143.

28 GOLDE D.W., BURGALETA C., SPARKES R.S. & CLINE, M.J. (1977) The Philadelphia chromosome in human macrophages. *Blood*, **49**, 367.

29 DENEGRI J.F., NAIMAN S.C., GILLEN J. & THOMAS J.W. (1978) *In vitro* growth of basophils containing the Philadelphia chromosome in the acute phase of chronic myelogenous leukaemia. *British Journal of Haematology*, **40**, 351.

30 BARR R.D. & WATT J. (1978) Preliminary evidence for the common origin of a lympho-myeloid complex in man. *Acta Haematologica*, **60**, 29.

31 MANIATIS A.K., AMSELS S., MITUS W.J. & COLMAN N. (1969) Chromosome pattern of bone marrow fibroblasts in patients with chronic granulocytic leukaemia. *Nature (London)*, **222**, 1278.

32 DE LA CHAPELLE A., VUOPIO P. & BERGSTRÖM H. (1973) The origin of bone marrow fibroblasts. *Blood*, **41**, 783.

32a GREENBERG B., WILSON F., WOO L. & JENKS H. (1978) Cytogenetics of fibroblastic colonies in Ph¹-positive chronic myelogenous leukaemia. *Blood*, **51**, 1039.

33 GOH K.-O. & SWISHER S.N. (1965) Identical twins and chronic myelocytic leukemia. *Archives of Internal Medicine*, **115**, 475.

34 JACOBS E.M., LUCE J.K. & CAILLEAU R. (1966) Chromosome abnormalities in human cancer. *Cancer*, **19**, 869.

35 WOODLIFF H.J., DOUGAN L. & ONESTI P. (1966) Cytogenetic studies in twins, one with chronic granulocytic leukaemia. *Nature (London)*, **211**, 533.

36 FITZGERALD P.H., PICKERING A.F. & EIBY J.A. (1971) Clonal origin of the Philadelphia chromosome and chronic myeloid leukaemia: evidence from a sex chromosome mosaic. *British Journal of Haematology*, **21**, 473.

37 COURT BROWN W.M. & TOUGH I.M. (1963) Cytogenetic studies in chronic myeloid leukemia. In: *Advances in Cancer Research* (ed. Haddow A. & Weinhouse S.), Vol. 7, p. 351. Academic Press, New York.

38 MOORE M.A.S., EKERT H., FITZGERALD M.G. & CARMICHAEL A. (1974) Further cytogenetic evolution in a sex chromosome mosaic with chronic myeloid leukemia. *Blood*, **44**, 768.

39 MOORE M.A.S. (1977) *In vitro* cultures studies in chronic granulocytic leukaemia. In: *Clinics in Haematology: The Chronic Leukaemias* (ed. Galton D.A.G.), Vol. 6, p. 97. W. B. Saunders, London.

40 GAHRTON G., LINDSTEN J. & ZECH L. (1974) Clonal origin of the Philadelphia chromosome from either the paternal or the maternal chromosome number 22. *Blood*, **43**, 837.

41 LAWLER S.D., O'MALLEY F. & LOBB D.S. (1976) Chromosome banding studies in Philadelphia chromosome positive myeloid leukaemia. *Scandinavian Journal of Haematology*, **17**, 17.

42 FIALKOW P.J., GARTLER S.M. & YOSHIDA A. (1967) Clonal origin of chronic myelocytic leukemia in man. *Proceedings of the National Academy of Sciences, USA*, **58**, 1468.

43 FIALKOW P.J. (1976) Clonal origin of human tumours. *Biochimica et Biophysica Acta Cancer Review*, **458**, 283.

44 FIALKOW P.J., JACOBSON R.J. & PAPAYÀNNOPOULOU T. (1977) Chronic myelocytic leukemia: clonal origin in a stem cell common to the granulocyte, erythrocyte, platelet and monocyte/macrophage. *American Journal of Medicine*, **63**, 125.

45 ROWLEY J.D. (1973) A new consistent abnormality in chronic myelogenous leukaemia identified by quinacrine fluorescence and Giemsa staining. *Nature (London)*, **243**, 290.

46 CASPERSSON T., ZECH L., JOHANSSON C. & MODEST E.J. (1970) Identification of human chromosomes by DNA-binding fluorescent agents. *Chromosoma*, **30**, 215.

46a CASPERSSON T., GAHRTON G., LINDSTEN J. & ZECH L. (1970) Identification of the Philadelphia chromosome as a number 22 by quinacrine mustard fluorescence analysis. *Experimental Cell Research*, **63**, 238.

47 MAYALL B.H., CARRANO A.V., MOORE D.H. & ROWLEY
J.D. (1977) Quantification by DNA-based cytophoto-
metry of the 9q+/22q− chromosomal translocation
associated with chronic myelogenous leukemia. *Cancer
Research*, 37, 3590.

48 ROWLEY J.D. (1980) Ph¹-positive leukaemia, including
chronic myelogenous leukaemia. In: *Clinics in Haematology: Cytogenetics and Haematology* (ed. Pennington
D.G.), Vol. 9, p. 155. W. B. Saunders, London.

49 SONTA S. & SANDBERG A.A. (1977) Chromosomes and
causation of human cancer and leukemia. XXIV.
Unusual and complex Ph¹ translocations and their
clinical significance. *Blood*, 50, 691.

50 FRANZEN S., STRENGER G. & ZAJICEK J. (1961) Micro-
planimetric studies on megakaryocytes in chronic
granulocytic leukaemia and polycythaemia vera. *Acta
Haematologica*, 26, 182.

51 LAGERLÖF B. & FRANZEN S. (1972) The ultrastructure of
megakaryocytes in polycythaemia vera and chronic
granulocytic leukaemia. *Acta Pathologica et Microbiologica Scandinavica Section A*, 80, 71.

52 DANCEY J.T. & VADNAIS-METZ L.H. (1978) Quantitative assessment of neutrophil marrow cellularity in
seven patients with chronic granulocytic leukaemia.
British Journal of Haematology, 39, 325.

53 SPIERS A.S.D., BAIN B.J. & TURNER J.E. (1977) The
peripheral blood in chronic granulocytic leukaemia.
Study of 50 untreated Philadelphia-positive cases. *Scandinavian Journal of Haematology*, 18, 25.

54 BAIN B.J. & WICKRAMASINGHE S.N. (1976) Relationship
between the concentration of neutrophils and monocytes in venous blood. *Acta Haematologica*, 55, 89.

55 STRYCKMANS P.A., DEBUSSCHER L. & COLLARD E.
(1977) Cell kinetics in chronic granulocytic leukaemia
(CGL). In: *Clinics in Haematology: The Chronic
Leukaemias* (ed. Galton D.A.G.), Vol. 6, p. 21. W. B.
Saunders, London.

56 CRONKITE E.G. (1979) Kinetics of granulopoiesis. In:
*Clinics in Haematology: Cellular Dynamics of Haemo-
poiesis* (ed. Lajtha L.G.), Vol. 8, p. 351. W. B. Saunders,
London.

57 VINCENT P.C. (1977) Granulocyte kinetics in health and
disease. In: *Clinics in Haematology: Radioisotopes in
Haematology* (ed. Lewis S.M.), Vol. 6, p. 695. W. B.
Saunders, London.

58 MOORE M.A.S. (1979) Humoral regulation of granulopoiesis. In: *Clinics in Haematology: Cellular Dynamics
of Haemopoiesis* (ed. Lajtha L.G.), Vol. 8, p. 287. W. B.
Saunders, London.

59 BROXMEYER H.E., MENDELSOHN N. & MOORE M.A.S.
(1977) Abnormal granulocyte feedback regulation of
colony stimulating activity-producing cells from
patients with chronic myelogenous leukaemia. *Leukemia
Research*, 1, 3.

60 BROXMEYER H.E., SMITHYMAN A., EGER R.R., MEYERS
P.A. & DE SOUSA M. (1978) Identification of lactoferrin
as the granulocyte-derived inhibitor of colony-stimulating activity production. *Journal of Experimental Medicine*, 148, 1052.

61 BROXMEYER H.E., MOORE M.A.S. & RALPH P. (1977)
Cell-free granulocyte colony inhibiting activity derived
from human PMN. *Experimental Hematology*, 5, 87.

62 MASON D.Y. (1977) Intracellular lysozyme and lactofer-

rin in myeloproliferative disorders. *Journal of Clinical
Pathology*, 30, 541.

63 RAUSCH P.G., PRYZWANSKY K.B., SPITZNAGEL J.K. &
HERION J.C. (1978) Immunocytochemical identification
of abnormal polymorphonuclear neutrophils in patients
with leukemia. *Blood Cells*, 4, 369.

64 FORMAN E.N., PADRE-MENDOZA T., SMITH P.S.,
BARKER B.E. & FARNES P. (1977) Ph¹-positive childhood
leukemias: spectrum of lymphoid-myeloid expressions.
Blood, 49, 549.

65 CHESSELLS J.M., JANOSSY G., LAWLER S.D. & SECKER
WALKER L. (1979) The Ph¹ chromosome in childhood
leukaemia. *British Journal of Haematology*, 41, 25.

66 GALTON D.A.G. (1962) Contributions of chemotherapy
to the study of leukaemia. *The Scientific Basis of
Medicine Annual Reviews*, p. 152. Athlone Press, London.

67 MORLEY A.A., BAIKIE A.G. & GALTON D.A.G. (1967)
Cyclic leucocytosis as evidence for retention of normal
homeostatic control in chronic granulocytic leukaemia.
Lancet, ii, 1320.

67a KENNEDY B.J. (1970) Cyclic leucocyte oscillations in
chronic myelogenous leukemia during hydroxyurea
therapy. *Blood*, 35, 751.

68 VODOPICK H., RUPP E.M., EDWARDS C.L., GOSWITZ
F.A. & BEAUCHAMP J.J. (1972) Spontaneous cyclic
leukocytosis and thrombocytosis in chronic granulocytic leukemia. *New England Journal of Medicine*, 286,
284.

69 GATTI R.A., ROBINSON W.A., DEINARD A.S., NESBIT M.
& McCULLOUGH J.J. (1973) Cyclic leucocytosis in
chronic myelogenous leukemia: new perspectives on
pathogenesis and therapy. *Blood*, 41, 771.

70 FORRESTER R.H. & LOURO J.M. (1966) Philadelphia
chromosome abnormality in agnogenic myeloid metaplasia. *Annals of Internal Medicine*, 64, 622.

71 KIOSSOGLOU K.A., MITUS W.J. & DAMESHEK W. (1966)
Cytogenetic studies in the chronic myeloproliferative
syndrome. *Blood*, 28, 241.

72 KRAUSS S. (1966) Chronic myelocytic leukemia with
features simulating myelofibrosis and myeloid metaplasia. *Cancer*, 19, 1321.

73 MOLONEY W.C. (1977) Natural history of chronic
granulocytic leukaemia. In: *Clinics in Haematology: The
Chronic Leukaemias* (ed. Galton D.A.G.), Vol. 6, p. 41.
W. B. Saunders, London.

74 CLOUGH V., GEARY C.G., HASHMI K., DAVSON J. &
KNOWLSON T. (1979) Myelofibrosis in chronic granulocytic leukaemia. *British Journal of Haematology*, 42,
515.

75 GRINBLAT J., MAMMON Z., LEWITUS Z. & JOSHUA H.
(1977) Chronic myelogenous leukemia with elevated
leucocyte alkaline phosphatase, positive indirect
Coombs' test, neutrophil leukocytosis, and unusual
cytogenetic findings. *Acta Haematologica*, 57, 298.

76 KENIS Y. & KOULISCHER L. (1967) Etude clinique et
cytogenetique de 21 patients atteinte de leucemie myeloide chronique. *European Journal of Cancer*, 3, 83.

77 CANELLOS G.P. & WHANG-PENG J. (1972) Philadelphia-
chromosome positive preleukaemic state. *Lancet*, ii,
1227.

78 BRANDT L., MITELMAN F., PANANI A. & LENNER H.C.
(1976) Extremely long duration of chronic myeloid

leukaemia with Ph¹-negative and Ph¹-positive bone-marrow cells. *Scandinavian Journal of Haematology*, **16**, 321.

79 SAKURAI M., HAYATA I. & SANDBERG A.A. (1976) Chromosomes and causation of human cancer and leukemia. XV. Prognostic value of chromosomal findings in Ph¹ positive chronic myelocytic leukemia. *Cancer Research*, **36**, 313.

80 GOLDE D.W., BERSCH N.L. & SPARKES A.S. (1976) Chromosomal mosaicism associated with prolonged remission in chronic myelogenous leukemia. *Cancer*, **37**, 1849.

81 FINNEY R., McDONALD G.A., BAIKIE A.G. & DOUGLAS A.S. (1972) Chronic granulocytic leukaemia with Ph¹ negative cells in bone marrow and a ten year remission after busulphan hypoplasia. *British Journal of Haematology*, **23**, 283.

82 VERHEST A. & VAN SCHOUBROECK F. (1973) Philadelphia-chromosome-positive preleukaemic state. *Lancet*, **ii**, 1386.

83 CUNNINGHAM I., GEE T., DOWLING M., CHAGANTI R., BAILEY R., HOPFAN S., BOWDEN L., TURNBULL, A., KNAPPER W. & CLARKSON B. (1979) Results of treatment of Ph+ chronic myelogenous leukemia with an intensive treatment regimen (L-5 protocol). *Blood*, **53**, 375.

84 TANZER J., FROCRAIN C. & NAJEAN Y. (1978) Rare instructive cases of chronic myelocytic leukemia (CML). *Proceedings of XVII Congress of the International Society of Hematology*, Paris. Abstract, p. 240.

85 HAGEMEIJER A., SMIT E.M.E., LÖWENBERG B. & ABELS J. (1979) Chronic myeloid leukemia with permanent disappearance of the Ph¹ chromosome and development of new clonal subpopulations. *Blood*, **53**, 1.

86 SECKER WALKER L.M. & HARDY J.D. (1976) Philadelphia chromosome in acute leukemia. *Cancer*, **38**, 1619.

87 SINGER J.W., FIALKOW P.J., STEINMANN L., NAJFELD V., STEIN S.J. & ROBINSON W.A. (1979) Chronic myelocytic leukemia (CML): failure to detect residual normal committed stem cells *in vitro*. *Blood*, **53**, 264.

88 DANCEY J.T., DEUBELBEISS K.A., HARKER L.A. & FINCH C.A. (1976) Neutrophil kinetics in man. *Journal of Clinical Investigation*, **58**, 705.

89 ATHENS J.W., RAAB S.O., HAAB O.P., BOGGS D.R., ASHENBRUCKER H., CARTWRIGHT G.E. & WINTROBE M.M. (1965) Leukokinetic studies. X. Blood granulocyte kinetics in chronic myelocytic leukemia. *Journal of Clinical Investigation*, **44**, 765.

90 ULLYOTT J.L. & BAINTON D.F. (1974) Azurophil and specific granules of blood neutrophils in chronic myelogenous leukemia: an ultrastructural and cytochemical analysis. *Blood*, **44**, 469.

91 BRANDT L. (1965) Adhesiveness to glass and phagocytic activity of neutrophilic leucocytes in myeloproliferative diseases. *Scandinavian Journal of Haematology*, **2**, 126.

92 PENNY R. & GALTON D.A.G. (1965) Studies on neutrophil function. II. Pathological aspects. *British Journal of Haematology*, **12**, 633.

93 PEDERSON B. & HAYHOE F.G.J. (1971) Relation between phagocytic activity and alkaline phosphatase content of neutrophils in chronic myeloid leukaemia. *British Journal of Haematology*, **21**, 257.

94 ODEBERG H., OLOFSSON T. & OLSSON I. (1975) Granulo-cyte function in chronic granulocytic leukaemia. I. Bactericidal and metabolic capabilities during phago-cytosis in isolated granulocytes. *British Journal of Haematology*, **29**, 427.

95 EL-MAALEM H. & FLETCHER J. (1976) Defective neutro-phil function in chronic granulocytic leukaemia. *British Journal of Haematology*, **34**, 95.

95a GOLDMAN J.M. & TH'NG K.H. (1973) Phagocytic function of leucocytes from patients wtih acute myeloid and chronic granulocytic leukaemia. *British Journal of Haematology*, **25**, 299.

95b TAUB R.N., BAKER M.A. & MADYASTHA K.R. (1980) Masking of neutrophil surface lectin-binding sites in chronic myelogenous leukemia (CML). *Blood*, **55**, 294.

96 RUSTIN G.J.S. & PETERS T.J. (1979) Studies on the subcellular organelles of neutrophils in chronic granulo-cytic leukaemia with special reference to alkaline phos-phatase. *British Journal of Haematology*, **41**, 533.

97 RUSTIN G.J.S., WILSON P.D. & PETERS T.J. (1979) Studies on the subcellular localisation of human neutro-phil alkaline phosphatase. *Journal of Cell Science*, **36**, 401.

98 XEFTERIS E., MITUS W.J., MEDNICOFF I.B. & DAMESHEK W. (1961) Leukocyte alkaline phosphatase in busul-phan-induced remissions of chronic granulocytic leu-kemia. *Blood*, **18**, 202.

99 SPIERS A.S.D., LIEW A. & BAIKIE A.G. (1975) Neutro-phil alkaline phosphatase score in chronic granulocytic leukaemia: effects of splenectomy and anti-leukaemic drugs. *Journal of Clinical Pathology*, **28**, 517.

100 HELLMANN A. & GOLDMAN J.M. (1980) Alkaline phos-phatase activity of chronic granulocytic leukaemia neutrophils in agar culture. *Scandinavian Journal of Haematology*, **24**, 237.

101 CHIYODA S. & KINUGASA K. (1978) Akaline phospha-tase activity in chronic myelogenous leukemia cells in culture. II. Suppressive effect of plasma. *Acta Haemato-logica Japonica*, **41**, 564.

102 CHIKKAPPA G., BOECKER W.R., CARSTEN A.L., CRON-KITE E.P. & OHL S. (1973) Return of leukocyte alkaline phosphatase in chronic myelocytic leukemia marrow cells cultured in a diffusion chamber system. *Journal of Clinical Investigation*, **52**, 18.

103 RUSTIN G.J.S., GOLDMAN J.M., McCARTHY D., MEES S. & PETERS T.J. (1980) An extrinsic factor controls neutrophil alkaline phosphatase synthesis in CGL. *British Journal of Haematology*, **45**, 381.

104 RACHMILEWITZ B. & RACHMILEWITZ M. (1971) Chemotherapy-induced changes in serum vitamin B_{12} binding proteins in myeloid leukemia. *Israel Journal of Medical Sciences*, **7**, 1140.

105 MINOT G.R., BUCKMAN T.E. & ISAACS R. (1924) Chronic myelogenous leukemia: age incidence, duration and benefit derived from treatment. *Journal of the American Medical Association*, **82**, 1489.

106 KILLMANN S-AA. (1972) Chronic myelogenous leuke-mia: preleukemia or leukemia? *Haematologica*, **57**, 641.

107 BAIKIE A.G. (1969) Chronic granulocytic leukaemia: metamorphosis of a conditioned neoplasm to an autonomous one. *Proceedings of the Fourth Congress of the Asian and Pacific Society of Haematology, Nagoya, Japan*, p. 197.

108 BERNARD J., SELIGMANN M. & KUICALA R. (1959) La

transformation aiguë de la leucémie myéloide chronique. *Révue française Etudes Clinique et Biologique*, **4**, 1024.

109 MASON J.E., DE VITA V.T. & CANELLOS G.P. (1974) Thrombocytosis in chronic granulocytic leukemia: incidence and clinical significance. *Blood*, **44**, 483.

110 ROSENTHAL S., SCHWARTZ J.H. & CANELLOS G.P. (1977) Basophilic chronic granulocytic leukaemia with hyperhistaminaemia. *British Journal of Haematology*, **36**, 367.

111 GOMEZ G., HOSSFELD D.K. & SOKAL J.E. (1975) Removal of abnormal clone of leukaemic cells by splenectomy. *British Medical Journal*, **i**, 421.

112 DUVALL C.P., CARBONE P.P., BELL W.R., WHANG J., TJIO J.H. & PERRY S. (1967) Chronic myelocytic leukemia with two Philadelphia chromosomes and prominent lymphadenopathy. *Blood*, **29**, 652.

113 SCHWARTZ J.H., CANELLOS G.P., YOUNG R.C. & DE VITA V.T. (1975) Meningeal leukemia in the blastic phase of chronic granulocytic leukemia. *American Journal of Medicine*, **59**, 819.

114 KWAAN H.C., PIERRE R.V. & LONG D.L. (1969) Meningeal involvement as first manifestation of acute myeloblastic transformation in chronic granulocytic leukemia. *Blood*, **23**, 348.

115 ATKINSON K.R., KAY H.E.M., LAWLER S.D., WELLS D.G. & MCELWAIN T.J. (1975) Meningeal leukemia after blastic transformation of chronic myeloid leukemia. *Cancer*, **35**, 529.

116 CRAVER L.F. & COPELAND M.M. (1935) Changes of the bone in the leukaemias. *Archives of Surgery*, **30**, 639.

117 CHABNER B.A., HASKELL C.M. & CANELLOS G.P. (1969) Destructive bone lesions in chronic granulocytic leukemia. *Medicine*, **48**, 401.

118 BEARD M.E.J., DURRANT J., CATOVSKY D., WILTSHAW E., AMESS J.L., BREARLEY R.L., KIRK B., WRIGLEY P.M.F., JANOSSY G., GREAVES M.F. & GALTON D.A.G. (1976) Blast crisis of chronic myeloid leukaemia (CML). I. Presentation simulating acute lymphoblastic leukaemia (ALL). *British Journal of Haematology*, **34**, 169.

119 WOODRUFF R.K., MALPAS J.S., WRIGLEY P.F.M., LISTER T.A., PAXTON A.M. & JANOSSY G. (1977) Meningeal leukaemia in lymphoid blast crisis of chronic myeloid leukaemia. *British Medical Journal*, **ii**, 1375.

120 PEDERSEN B. (1969) *Cytogenetic Evolution in Chronic Myelogenous Leukemia.* Munksgaard, Copenhagen.

121 DE GROUCHY J., DE NAVA C., FEINGOLD J., BILSKY-PASQUIER G. & BOUSSER J. (1968) Onze observations d'un modele precis d'évolution caryotypique au cours de la leucemie myeloïde chronique. *European Journal of Cancer*, **4**, 481.

122 FIRST INTERNATIONAL WORKSHOP ON CHROMOSOMES IN LEUKAEMIA (1978) Chromosomes in Ph¹-positive chronic granulocytic leukaemia. *British Journal of Haematology*, **39**, 305.

123 ALIMENA G., BRANDT L., DALLAPICCOLA B., MITELMAN F. & NILSSON P.G. (1979) Secondary chromosome changes in chronic myeloid leukemia. Relation to treatment. *Cancer Genetics and Cytogenetics*, **1**, 79.

124 MATHE G. & SEMAN G. (1963) *Aspects Histologiques et Cytologiques des Leucémies et Hématosarcomes*, p. 65. Librairie Maloire S.A., Paris.

125 HAMMOUDA F., QUAGLINO D. & HAYHOE F.G.J. (1964) Blastic crisis in chronic granulocytic leukaemia. Cyto-chemical, cytogenetic and autoradiographic studies in four cases. *British Medical Journal*, **i**, 1275.

126 MARIE J.P., VERNANT J.P., DREYFUS B. & BRETON-GORIUS J. (1979) Ultrastructural localization of peroxidases in 'undifferentiated' blasts during the blast crisis of chronic granulocytic leukaemia. *British Journal of Haematology*, **43**, 549.

127 BRETON-GORIUS J., REYES F., VERNANT J.P., TULLIEZ M. & DREYFUS B. (1978) Megakaryoblastic nature of cells as revealed by the presence of platelet peroxidase. A cytochemical ultrastructural study. *British Journal of Haematology*, **39**, 295.

128 BAIN B., CATOVSKY D., O'BRIEN M., SPIERS A.S.D. & RICHARDS H.G.H. (1977) Megakaryoblastic transformation of chronic granulocytic leukaemia. *Journal of Clinical Pathology*, **30**, 235.

129 JANOSSY G., GREAVES M.F., REVEZ T., LISTER T.A., ROBERTS M., DURRANT J., KIRK B., CATOVSKY D. & BEARD M.E.J. (1976) Blast crisis of chronic myeloid leukaemia (CML). II. Cell surface marker analysis of 'lymphoid' and 'myeloid' cases. *British Journal of Haematology*, **34**, 183.

130 MARMONT A.M. & DAMASIO E.E. (1973) The treatment of terminal metamorphosis of chronic granulocytic leukaemia with corticosteroids and vincristine. *Acta Haematologica*, **50**, 1.

131 MARKS S.M., BALTIMORE D. & MCCAFFREY R. (1978) Terminal transferase as a predictor of initial responsiveness to vincristine and prednisone in blastic chronic myelogenous leukemia. *The New England Journal of Medicine*, **298**, 812.

132 HOFFBRAND A.V., GANESHAGURU K., JANOSSY G., GREAVES M.F., CATOVSKY D. & WOODRUFF R.K. (1977) Terminal deoxynucleotidyl-transferase levels and membrane phenotypes in diagnosis of acute leukaemia. *Lancet*, **ii**, 520.

133 GREAVES M.F., BROWN G., RAPSON N.T. & LISTER T.A. (1975) Antisera to acute lymphoblastic leukaemia cells. *Clinical Immunology and Immunopathology*, **4**, 67.

134 JANOSSY G., GOLDSTONE A.H., CAPELLARO D., GREAVES M.F., KULENKAMPFF J., PIPPARD M. & WELSH K. (1977) Differentiation linked expression of p28, 33 (Ia-like) structures of human leukaemic cells. *British Journal of Haematology*, **37**, 391.

135 VOGLER L.B., CRIST W.M., BOCKMAN D.E., PEARL E.R., LAWTON A.R. & COOPER M.D. (1978) Pre B-cell leukaemia. A new phenotype of childhood lymphoblastic leukaemia. *New England Journal of Medicine*, **298**, 872.

136 JANOSSY G., BOLLUM F.J., BRADSTOCK K.F., MCMICHAEL A., RAPSON N. & GREAVES M. (1979) Terminal transferase positive human bone marrow cells exhibit the antigenic phenotype of common acute lymphoblastic leukaemia. *Journal of Immunology*, **123**, 1525.

136a MCMICHAEL A.J., PILCH J.R., GALFRE G., MASON D.Y., FABRE J.W. & MILSTEIN C. (1979) A human thymocyte antigen defined by a hybrid myeloma monoclonal antibody. *European Journal of Immunology*, **9**, 205.

137 ROBERTS M.M. (1979 Maturation Linked Expression of Antigens of Normal and Leukaemic Cells of the Human Haemopoietic System. Ph.D. Thesis, University of London.

138 GREAVES M.F. & JANOSSY G. (1978) Patterns of gene expression and the cellular origins of human leukaemias. *Biochemica Biophysica Acta*, **516**, 193.

139 GREAVES M.F., VERBI W., REEVES B.R., HOFFBRAND A.V., DRYSDALE H.C., JONES L., SACKER L.S. & SAMARATUNGA I. (1979) 'Pre-B' phenotypes in blast crisis of Ph[1] positive CML: evidence for a pluripotential stem cell 'target'. *Leukaemia Research*, **3**, 181.

140 WHANG-PENG J., HENDERSON E.S., KNUTSEN T., FREIREICH E.J. & GART J.J. (1970) Cytogenetic studies in acute myelocytic leukemia with special emphasis on the occurrence of Ph[1] chromosome. *Blood*, **36**, 448.

141 WAYNE A.W., SHARP J.C., JOYNER M.V., STERNDALE H. & PULFORD K.A.F. (1979) The significance of Ph[1] mosaicism: a report of six cases of chronic granulocytic leukaemia and two cases of acute myeloid leukaemia. *British Journal of Haematology*, **43**, 353.

142 CATOVSKY D. (1979) Annotation: Ph[1]-positive acute leukaemia and chronic granulocytic leukaemia: one or two diseases? *British Journal of Haematology*, **42**, 493.

143 SALMON S.E. & SELIGMANN M. (1974) B-cell neoplasia in man. *Lancet*, **ii**, 1230.

144 SECKER WALKER L.M. & HARDY J.D. (1975) Philadelphia chromosome in PHA-stimulated lymphocytes in acute leukaemia. *Lancet*, **ii**, 1301.

145 GIBBS T.J., WHEELER M.V., BELLINGHAM A.J. & WALKER S. (1977) The significance of the Philadelphia chromosome in acute lymphoblastic leukaemia. A report of two cases. *British Journal of Haematology*, **37**, 447.

146 SUMMERFIELD G.P., BELLINGHAM A.J. & WALKER S. (1979) Ph[1] positive lymphoblastic leukaemia. *British Journal of Haematology*, **42**, 161.

147 SMALLEY R.V., VOGEL J., HUGULEY C.M. & MILLER D. (1977) Chronic granulocytic leukemia: cytogenetic conversion of the bone marrow with cycle-specific chemotherapy. *Blood*, **50**, 107.

147a SHARP J.C., WAYNE A.W., CROFTS M., McARTHUR G., STERNDALE H., JOYNER M.V., KEMP J., BIRCH A.D.J., LAI S. & WILLIAMS Y. (1979) Karyotypic conversion in Ph[1]-positive chronic myeloid leukaemia with combination chemotherapy. *Lancet*, **i**, 1370.

148 BLOOMFIELD C.D., PETERSON L.C., YUNIS J.J. & BRUNNING R.D. (1977) The Philadelphia chromosome (Ph[1]) in adults presenting with acute leukaemia: a comparison of Ph[1]+ and Ph[1]− patients. *British Journal of Haematology*, **36**, 347.

149 BOGGS D.R. (1974) Hematopoietic stem cell theory in relation to possible lymphoblastic conversion of chronic myeloid leukemia. *Blood*, **44**, 449.

150 LAWLER S.D. (1977) The cytogenetics of chronic granulocytic leukaemia. In: *Clinics in Haematology: The Chronic Leukaemias* (ed. Galton D.A.G.), Vol. 6, p. 55. W. B. Saunders, London.

151 FIALKOW P.J., DENMAN A.M., JACOBSON R.J. & LOWENTHAL M.N. (1978) Chronic myelocytic leukemia: origin of some lymphocytes from leukemic stem cells. *Journal of Clinical Investigation*, **62**, 815.

152 BERGSAGEL D.E. (1967) The chronic leukemias: a review of disease manifestations and the aims of therapy. *Canadian Medical Association Journal*, **96**, 1615.

153 HAUT A., ABBOT W.S., WINTROBE H.M. & CARTWRIGHT G.E. (1961) Busulfan in the treatment of chronic myelocytic leukemia. The effect of long-term intermittent therapy. *Blood*, **17**, 1.

154 MEDICAL RESEARCH COUNCIL'S WORKING PARTY FOR THERAPEUTIC TRIALS IN LEUKAEMIA (1968) Chronic granulocytic leukaemia: comparison of radiotherapy and busulphan therapy. *British Medical Journal*, **i**, 201.

155 CONRAD F.G. (1973) Survival in chronic granulocytic leukemia. *Archives of Internal Medicine*, **131**, 684.

156 JACQUILLIAT CL., CHASTANG CL., TANZER J., BRIERE J., WEIL M., PEREIRA-NETO M., GEMON-AUCLERC M.F., SCHAISON G., DOMINGO A., BOIRON M. & BERNARD J. (1978) Prognostic factors in chronic granulocytic leukemia. A study of 798 cases. *Bolletino dell'Istituto Sieroterapico Milanese*, **57**, 237.

157 MONFARDINI S., GEE T., FRIED J. & CLARKSON B.D. (1973) Survival in chronic myelogenous leukemia; influence of treatment and extent of disease at diagnosis. *Cancer*, **31**, 492.

157a PARISH S. & CUCKLE H. (1980) Report to the Medical Research Council's Annual Review Meeting on Leukaemia Trials.

158 KARDINAL C., BATEMAN J. & WEINER J. (1976) Chronic granulocytic leukemia: review of 536 cases. *Archives of Internal Medicine*, **136**, 305.

159 LAWLER S.D., LOBB D.S. & WILTSHAW E. (1974) Philadelphia-chromosome positive bone-marrow cells showing loss of the Y in males with chronic myeloid leukaemia. *British Journal of Haematology*, **27**, 247.

160 SAKURAI M. & SANDBERG A.A. (1976) Chromosomes and causation of human cancer and leukemia. XVIII. The missing Y in acute myeloblastic leukemia and Ph[1]-positive chronic myelocytic leukemia. *Cancer*, **38**, 762.

161 WOLF D.J., SILVER R.T. & COLEMAN M. (1978) Factors associated with prolonged survival in chronic myeloid leukemia. *Cancer*, **42**, 1957.

162 HADDOW A. & TIMMIS G.M. (1953) Myleran in chronic myeloid leukaemia chemical constitution and biological action. *Lancet*, **i**, 207.

163 GALTON D.A.G. (1953) Myleran in chronic myeloid leukaemia. *Lancet*, **i**, 208.

164 GALTON D.A.G. (1969) Chemotherapy of chronic myelocytic leukemia. *Seminars in Hematology*, **6**, 323.

165 CANELLOS G.P. (1977) The treatment of chronic granulocytic leukaemia. In: *Clinics in Haematology: The Chronic Leukaemias* (ed. Galton D.A.G.), Vol. 6, p. 113. W. B. Saunders, London.

166 GALTON D.A.G. (1959) Treatment of the chronic leukaemias. *British Medical Bulletin*, **15**, 79.

167 SULLIVAN J.R., HURLEY T.H. & BOLTON J.H. (1977) Treatment of chronic myeloid leukemia with repeated single doses of busulfan. *Cancer Treatment Reports*, **61**, 43.

167a DOUGLAS I.D.C. & WILTSHAW E. (1978) Remission induction in chronic granulocytic leukaemia using intermittent high-dose busulphan. *British Journal of Haematology*, **40**, 59.

168 VICARIOT M., GOLDMAN J.M., CATOVSKY D. & GALTON D.A.G. (1979) Treatment of chronic granulocytic leukaemia with repeated single doses of busulphan. *European Journal of Cancer*, **15**, 559.

169 GALTON D.A.G. (1969) The possibility of radical

chemotherapy in chronic myelocytic leukemia. *Haematologica Latina*, **12**, 703.

170 GALTON D.A.G. (1972) Radical therapy for chronic granulocytic leukaemia. In: *Thyroid Tumours, Lymphomas, Granulocytic Leukaemia* (ed. Fiorentino M., Vangelista R. & Grigoletto E.), p. 95. Piccin Medical Books, Invicta, Padova.

171 ABRAMOVICI A., SHAKLAL M., PINKHAS J. (1978) Myeloschisis in a six weeks embryo of a leukemic woman treated by busulfan. *Teratology*, **18**, 241.

172 KYLE R.A., SCHWARTZ R.S., OLINER H.L. & DAMESHEK W. (1959) A syndrome resembling adrenal cortical insufficiency associated with long-term busulfan (Myleran) therapy. *Blood*, **18**, 497.

173 OLINER H.L., SCHWARTZ R.S., RUBIO F. & DAMESHEK W. (1961) Interstitial pulmonary fibrosis following busulfan therapy. *American Journal of Medicine*, **31**, 134.

174 HEARD B.E. & COOKE R.A. (1968) Busulphan lung. *Thorax*, **23**, 187.

175 PODOLL L.N. & WINKLER S.S. (1974) Busulfan lung. *American Journal of Roentgenology, Radium Therapy and Nuclear Medicine*, **120**, 151.

176 KENNEDY B.J. (1972) Hydroxyurea therapy in chronic myelogenous leukemia. *Cancer*, **29**, 1052.

177 SCHWARTZ J.H. & CANELLOS G.P. (1975) Hydroxyurea in the management of the hematologica complications of chronic granulocytic leukaemia. *Blood*, **46**, 11.

178 ALLAN N.C., DUVALL E. & STOCKDILL G. (1978) Combination chemotherapy for chronic granulocytic leukaemia. *Lancet*, **ii**, 523.

179 SPIERS A.S.D., BAIKIE A.G., GALTON D.A.G., RICHARDS H.G.H., WILTSHAW E., GOLDMAN J.M., CATOVSKY D., SPENCER J. & PETO R. (1975) Chronic granulocytic leukaemia: effect of elective splenectomy on the course of the disease. *British Medical Journal*, **i**, 175.

180 IHDE D.C., CANELLOS G.P., SCHWARTZ J.H. & DE VITA V.T. (1976) Splenectomy in the chronic phase of chronic granulocytic leukemia. *Annals of Internal Medicine*, **84**, 17.

181 ITALIAN COOPERATIVE STUDY GROUP ON CHRONIC MYELOID LEUKEMIA (1978) Effect of early splenectomy and cyclic acute leukemia like chemotherapy on the course of chronic myeloid leukemia. *Bolletino dell'Istitute Sieroterapico Milanese*, **57**, 360.

182 KARANAS A. & SILVER R.T. (1968) Characteristics of the terminal phase of chronic granulocytic leukemia. *Blood*, **32**, 445.

183 SPIERS A.S.D., BAIKIE A.G., GALTON D.A.G., KAUR J., CATOVSKY D., GOLDMAN J.M., WILTSHAW E., LOWENTHAL R.M. & BUSKARD N.A. (1975) Splenectomy for complications of chronic granulocytic leukaemia. *Lancet*, **ii**, 627.

184 CANELLOS G.P., SUTLIFFE S.B., DE VITA V.T. & LISTER T.A. (1979) Treatment of refractory splenomegaly in myeloproliferative disease by splenic artery infusion. *Blood*, **53**, 1014.

185 SPIERS A.S.D., GOLDMAN J.M., CATOVSKY D., COSTELLO C., BUSKARD N.A. & GALTON D.A.G. (1977) Multiple-drug chemotherapy for acute leukemia. *Cancer*, **40**, 20.

186 COLEMAN M., SILVER R.T., PAJAK T.F., CAVALLI F., RAI K.R., KOSTINAS J.E., GLIDEWELL O. & HOLLAND J.F. (1980) Combination chemotherapy for terminal phase chronic granulocytic leukemia. Cancer and Leukemia Group B studies. *Blood*, **55**, 29.

187 CANELLOS G.P., DE VITA V.T., WHANG-PENG J., CHABNER B.A., SCHEIN P.S. & YOUNG R.C. (1976) Chemotherapy of the blastic phase of chronic granulocytic leukemia: hypodiploidy and response to therapy. *Blood*, **47**, 1003.

188 DONEY K., BUCKNER C.D., SALE G.E., RAMBERG R., BOYD C. & THOMAS E.D. (1978) Treatment of chronic granulocytic leukemia by chemotherapy, total body irradiation and allogeneic marrow transplantation. *Experimental Hematology*, **6**, 738.

189 BUCKNER C.D., STEWART P., CLIFT R.A., FEFER A., NEIMAN P.E., SINGER J., STORB R. & THOMAS E.D. (1978) Treatment of blastic transformation of chronic granulocytic leukemia by chemotherapy, total body irradiation, and infusion of cryopreserved autologous marrow. *Experimental Hematology*, **6**, 96.

190 GOLDMAN J.M., CATOVSKY D., HOWS J., SPIERS A.S.D. & GALTON D.A.G. (1979) Cryopreserved peripheral blood cells functioning as autografts in patients with chronic granulocytic leukaemia in transformation. *British Medical Journal*, **1**, 1310.

191 GOLDMAN J.M., TH'NG K.H., PARK D.S., SPIERS A.S.D., LOWENTHAL R.M. & RUUTU T. (1978) Collection, cryopreservation and subsequent viability of haemopoietic stem cells intended for treatment of chronic granulocytic leukaemia in blast-cell transformation. *British Journal of Haematology*, **40**, 185.

192 FEFER A., CHEEVER M.A., THOMAS E.D., BOYD C., RAMBEEG R., GLUCKSBERG H., BUCKNER C.D. & STORB R. (1979) Disappearance of Ph¹-positive cells in four patients with chronic granulocytic leukemia after chemotherapy, irradiation and marrow transplantation from an identical twin. *New England Journal of Medicine*, **300**, 333.

192a GOLDMAN J.M., JOHNSON S.A., CATOVSKY D., AGNARSDOTTIR G., GOOLDEN A.W.G. & GALTON D.A.G. (1981) Identical twin marrow transplantation for patients with leukaemia and lymphoma. *Transplantation*, **31**, 140.

192b RAPPAPORT H. (1966) Tumors of the hematopoietic system. In *Atlas of Tumor Pathology*. Section III, Fascicle 8. Washington, D.C. Armed Forces Institute of Pathology.

193 EVANS H.L., BUTLER J.J. & YOUNESS E.L. (1978) Malignant lymphoma, small lymphocytic type. A clinicopathologic study of 84 cases with suggested criteria for intermediate lymphocytic lymphoma. *Cancer*, **41**, 1440.

194 LUKES R.J. (1979) The immunologic approach to the pathology of malignant lymphomas. *American Journal of Clinical Pathology*, **72**, Suppl. 657.

195 GALTON D.A.G., CATOVSKY D. & WILTSHAW E. (1978) Clinical spectrum of lymphoproliferative diseases. *Cancer*, **42**, 901.

196 INSEL R.A., MELEWICZ F.M., LA VIE M.F. & BALCH C.M. (1975) Morphology, surface markers and *in vitro* responses of a human leukemic T-cell. *Clinical Immunology and Immunopathology*, **4**, 382.

197 SELIGMANN M., BROUET J.-C. & PREUD'HOMME J.-L. (1977) The immunological diagnosis of human leuke-

mias and lymphomas: an overview. Immunological diagnosis of leukaemias and lymphomas. In: *Haematology and Blood Transfusion* (ed. Thierfelder S., Rodt H. & Thiel E.), Vol. 20, p. 1. Springer-Verlag, Berlin.

198 THIEL E., BAUCHINGER M., RODT H., HUHN D., THEML H. & THIERFELDER S. (1977) Evidence for monoclonal proliferation in prolymphocytic leukaemia of T-cell origin. *Blut*, **35**, 427.

199 STRYCKMANS P.A., DEBUSSCHER L., HEYDER-BRÜCKNER C., HEIMANN R., MANDELBAUM I.M. & WYBRAN J. (1978) Clonal origin of a T-cell lymphoproliferative malignancy. *Blood*, **52**, 69.

200 COLLINS R.D., WALDRON J.A. & GLICK A.D. (1979) Results of multiparameter studies of T-cell lymphoid neoplasms. *American Journal of Clinical Pathology*, **72**, 699.

201 HABESHAW J.A., MACAULEY R.A.A. & STUART A.E. (1977) Correlation of surface receptors with histological appearances in 29 cases of non-Hodgkin lymphoma. *British Journal of Cancer*, **35**, 858.

202 HABESHAW J.A., CATLEY P.F., STANSFIELD A.G. & BREARLEY R.L. (1979) Surface phenotyping, histology and the nature of non-Hodgkin lymphoma in 157 patients. *British Journal of Cancer*, **40**, 11.

203 TAYLOR C.R. (1979) Results of multiparameter studies of B-cell lymphomas. *American Journal of Clinical Pathology*, **72**, 687.

204 CATOVSKY D., PITTMAN S., O'BRIEN M., CHERCHI M., COSTELLO C., FOA R., PEARCE E., HOFFBRAND A.V., JANOSSY G., GANESHAGURU K. & GREAVES M.F. (1979) Multiparameter studies in lymphoid leukemias. *American Journal of Clinical Pathology*, **72**, Suppl. 736.

204a CHERCHI M. & CATOVSKY D. (1980) Mouse RBC rosettes in chronic lymphocytic leukaemia: different expression in blood and tissues. *Clinical and Experimental Immunology*, **39**, 411.

205 CATOVSKY D., GALETTO J., OKOS A., GALTON D.A.G., WILTSHAW E. & STATHOPOULOS G. (1973) Prolymphocytic leukaemia of B and T cell type. *Lancet*, **ii**, 233.

206 ENNO A., CATOVSKY D., O'BRIEN M., CHERCHI M., KUMARAN T.O. & GALTON D.A.G. (1979) 'Prolymphocytoid' transformation of chronic lymphocytic leukaemia. *British Journal of Haematology*, **41**, 9.

207 BROUET J.C., PREUD'HOMME J.L., SELIGMANN M. & BERNARD J. (1973) Blast cells with monoclonal surface immunoglobulin in two cases of acute blast crisis supervening on chronic lymphocytic leukaemia. *British Medical Journal*, **iv**, 23.

208 BROUET J.-C. & SELIGMANN M. (1977) Chronic lymphocytic leukaemia as an immunoproliferative disease. In: *Clinics in Haematology: The Chronic Leukaemias* (ed. Galton D.A.G.), Vol. 6, p. 169. W. B. Saunders, London.

209 ZLOTNICK A. & ROBINSON E. (1970) Chronic lymphatic leukemia associated wtih macroglobulinemia. *Israel Journal of Medical Sciences*, **6**, 365.

210 BREARLEY R.L. (1980) Relationship between Clinical and Pathological Features in Lymphoid Malignancies. M.D. Thesis, University of London.

211 KYLE R.A., NOBREGA F.T. & ELVEBACK L.R. (1968) The 30-year trend of leukemia in Olmsted County, Minnesota, 1935 through 1964. *Mayo Clinic Proceedings*, **43**, 342.

212 GAULD W.R., INNES J. & ROBSON H.N. (1953) A survey of 647 cases of leukaemia 1938–1951. *British Medical Journal*, **i**, 585.

213 DOLL R., MUIR C. & WATERHOUSE J. (1970) *Cancer Incidence in Five Continents*. Vol. 2, 388 pp. U.I.C.C. Geneva.

214 WELLS R. & LAU K.S. (1960) Incidence of leukaemia in Singapore, and rarity of chronic lymphocytic leukaemia in Chinese. *British Medical Journal*, **i**, 759.

215 WAKISAKA G., UCHINO H., YASUNAGA K., NAKAMURA T., SAKURAI M., MIYAMOTO K., YOSHINO T. & MORIGA M. (1964) Statistical investigations of leukaemia in Japan from 1956–1961. *Pathologia et Microbiologia*, **27**, 671.

216 HAENSZEL W. & KURIHARA M. (1968) Studies of Japanese migrants. I. Mortality from cancer and other diseases among Japanese in the United States. *Journal of the National Cancer Institute*, **40**, 43.

217 FLEMING A.F. (1978) Leukaemia in the Guinea Savanna of northern Nigeria. In: *Advances in Comparative Leukemia Research* (ed. Bentvelzen *et al.*), p. 53. Elsevier–North-Holland Biomedical Press, Amsterdam.

218 GUNZ F.W., GUNZ J.P., VEALE A.M.O., CHAPMAN C.J. & HOUSTON I.B. (1975) Familial leukaemia: a study of 909 families. *Scandinavian Journal of Haematology*, **15**, 117.

219 BLATTNER W.A., STROBER W., MUCHMORE A.V., BLOESE R.M., BRODER S. & FRAUMENI J.F. (1976) Familial chronic lymphocytic leukemia. *Annals of Internal Medicine*, **84**, 554.

220 JEANNET M. & MAGNIN C. (1971) HLA antigens in malignant diseases. *Transplantation Proceedings*, **3**, 1301.

221 POLLACK M.S. & DUBOIS D. (1977) Possible effects of non-HLA antibodies in common typing sera on HLA antigen frequency data in leukemia. *Cancer*, **39**, 2348.

221a GAHRTON G., ZECH L., ROBERT K.H. & BIRD A.G. (1979) Mitogenic stimulation of leukaemia cells by Epstein–Barr virus. *New England Journal of Medicine*, **301**, 438.

222 ZIMMERMAN T.S., GODWIN H.A. & PERRY S. (1968) Studies of leukocyte kinetics in chronic lymphocytic leukemia. *Blood*, **31**, 277.

223 MANASTER J., FRÜHLING J. & STRYCKMANS P. (1973) Kinetics of lymphocytes in chronic lymphocytic leukemia. I. Equilibrium between blood and a 'readily accessible pool'. *Blood*, **41**, 425.

224 FLAD G.D., HUBER C., BERMER K., MENNE H.D. & HUBER H. (1973) Impaired recirculation of B lymphocytes in chronic lymphocytic leukemia. *European Journal of Immunology*, **3**, 688.

225 BREMER K., ENGESET A. & FRÖLAND S.S. (1978) Circulation and emigration kinetics of blood lymphocytes in lymphoma patients. *Lymphology*, **11**, 231.

226 THEML H., TREPEL F., SCHICK P., KABOTH W. & BEGEMANN H. (1973) Kinetics of lymphocytes in chronic lymphocytic leukemia: studies using continuous 3H-thymidine infusion in two patients. *Blood*, **42**, 723.

227 STRYCKMANS P.A., DEBUSSCHER L. & COLLARD E. (1977) Cell kinetics in chronic lymphocytic leukaemia (CLL). In: *Clinics in Haematology: The Chronic Leukaemias* (ed. Galton D.A.G.), Vol. 6, p. 159. W. B. Saunders, London.

227a FIDDES P., PENNY R., WELLS J.V. & RCZENBERG M.C. (1972) Clinical correlations with immunoglobulin levels in chronic lymphocytic leukemia. *Australian and New Zealand Journal of Medicine*, **4**, 346.

227b FOA R., CATOVSKY D., BROZOVIC M., MARSH G.W., OOYIRILANGKUMARAN T., CHERCHI M. & GALTON D.A.G. (1979) Clinical staging and immunological findings in chronic lymphocytic leukemia. *Cancer*, **44**, 483.

228 DAMESHEK W. & GUNZ F. (1964) *Leukemia*, p. 232. Grune & Stratton, New York.

229 DACIE J.V. (1967) Secondary or symptomatic haemolytic anaemias. *The Haemolytic Anaemias. Part III.* Churchill, London.

230 PHILLIPS E.A., KEMPIN S., PASSE S., MIKE V. & CLARKSON B. (1977) Prognostic factors in chronic lymphocytic leukaemia and their implications for therapy. In: *Clinics in Haematology: The Chronic Leukaemias* (ed. Galton D.A.G.), Vol. 6, p. 203. W. B. Saunders, London.

231 WEED R.I. (1965) Exaggerated delayed hypersensitivity to mosquito bites in chronic lymphocytic leukemia. *Blood*, **26**, 257.

232 BITRAN J., GANAPATHY, R. ULTMANN J.E. & GOLOMB H.M. (1976) Malignant pleural effusion as complication of chronic lymphocytic leukaemia. *Lancet*, **ii**, 414.

233 SWEET D.L., GOLOMB H.M. & ULTMANN J.E. (1977) The clinical features of chronic lymphocytic leukaemia. In: *Clinics in Haematology: The Chronic Leukaemias* (ed. Galton D.A.G.), Vol. 6, p. 185. W.B. Saunders, London.

233a BRANDT L. & NILSSON P.G. (1980) Lymphocytopenia preceding chronic lymphocytic leukemia. *Acta Medica Scandinavica*, **208**, 13.

234 DURANT J.R. & FINKBEINER J.A. (1964) 'Spontaneous' remission in chronic lymphatic leukemia? *Cancer*, **17**, 105.

235 BOUSSER J. & ZITTOUN R. (1965) Remission spontanée prolongée d'une leucemie lymphoide chronique. *Nouvelle Révue française d'Hématologie*, **5**, 498.

236 CHERVENIK P.A., BOGGS D.R. & WINTROBE M.M. (1967) Spontaneous remission in chronic lymphocytic leukemia. *Annals of Internal Medicine*, **67**, 1239.

237 WEINTRAUB L.R. (1969) Lymphosarcoma remission associated with viral hepatitis. *Journal of the American Medical Association*, **210**, 1590.

238 HAN T. & SOKAL J.E. (1971) Spontaneous remission of leukemic lymphoproliferative disease. *Cancer*, **27**, 586.

239 WIERNIK P. (1976) Spontaneous regression of hematologic cancers. *National Cancer Institute Monograph*, **44**, 35.

240 HANSEN R.M. & LIBNOCH J.A. (1978) Remission of chronic lymphocytic leukemia after smallpox vaccination. *Archives of Internal Medicine*, **138**, 1137.

241 GATTIKER H., WILTSHAW E. & GALTON D.A.G. (1980) Spontaneous remission in malignant lymphoma. *Cancer*, **45**, 2627.

242 HUREZ D., FLANDRIN G., PREUD'HOMME J.-L. & SELIGMANN M. (1972) Unreleased monoclonal macroglobulin in chronic lymphocytic leukaemia. *Clinical and Experimental Immunology*, **10**, 223.

243 CAWLEY J.C., BARKER C.R., BRITCHFORD R.D. & SMITH J.L. (1973) Intracellular IgA immunoglobulin crystals in chronic lymphocytic leukaemia. *Clinical and Experimental Immunology*, **13**, 407.

244 CLARK C., RYDELL R.E. & KAPLAN M.E. (1973) Frequent association of IgM lymphocyte with crystalline inclusions in chronic lymphatic leukemic lymphocytes. *New England Journal of Medicine*, **289**, 113.

245 CAWLEY J.C., SMITH J., GOLDSTONE A.H., EMMINES J., HAMBLIN J. & HOUGH L. (1976) IgA and IgM cytoplasmic inclusions in a series of cases of chronic lymphocytic leukamia. *Clinical and Experimental Immunology*, **23**, 78.

246 NEIS K.M., MARSHALL J., OBERLIN M.A., HALPERN M.S. & BROWN J.C. (1976) Chronic lymphocytic leukemia with gamma chain inclusions. *American Journal of Clinical Pathology*, **65**, 948.

247 SMITH, J.L., GORDON J., NEWELL D.G. & WHISSON M. (1977) The biosynthesis and characterization of unreleased IgM in a case of CLL. *British Journal of Haematology*, **37**, 217.

248 FROLAND S.S., NATVIG J.B. & STAVEM P. (1972) Immunological characterization of lymphocytes in lymphoproliferative diseases. Restriction of classes, subclasses and Gm allotypes of membrane-bound immunoglobulins. *Scandinavian Journal of Immunology*, **1**, 351.

249 FU S.M., WINCHESTER R.J., FEIZI T., WALZER P.D. & KUNKEL H.G. (1974) Idiotypic specificity of surface immunoglobulin and the maturation of leukemic bone marrow derived lymphocytes. *Proceedings of the National Academy of Science, USA*, **71**, 4487.

250 SALSANO F., FROLAND S.S., NATVIG J.B. & MICHAELSEN T.E. (1974) Same idiotype of B lymphocyte membrane IgD and IgM. Formal evidence for monoclonality of chronic lymphocytic leukemia cells. *Scandinavian Journal of Immunology*, **3**, 841.

251 SCHROER K.R., BRILES D.E., VAN BOXEL J.A. & DAVIE J.M. (1974) Idiotypic uniformity of cell surface immunoglobulin in chronic lymphocytic leukemia. Evidence for monoclonal proliferation. *Journal of Experimental Medicine*, **140**, 1416.

252 BROUET J.C. & PRIEUR A.M. (1974) Membrane markers on chronic lymphocytic leukemia cells: a B cell leukemia with rosettes due to anti-sheep erythrocyte antibody activity of the membrane bound IgM and a T cell leukemia with surface Ig. *Clinical Immunology and Immunopathology*, **2**, 481.

253 PREUD'HOMME J.L. & SELIGMANN M. (1972) Surface-bound immunoglobulins as a cell marker in human lymphoproliferative diseases. *Blood*, **40**, 777.

254 RAI K.R., SAWITSKY A., CRONKITE E.P., CHANANA A.D., LEVY R.N. & PASTERNACK B.S. (1975) Clinical staging of chronic lymphocytic leukemia. *Blood*, **46**, 219.

255 BINET J.-L., LEPORRIER M., DIGHIERO G., CHARRON D., D'ATHIS P., VAUGIER G., MERLE BERAL H., NATALI J.C., RAPHAEL M., NIZET M.G. & FOLLEZOU J.Y. (1977) A clinical staging system for CLL: prognostic significance. *Cancer*, **40**, 855.

256 RUNDLES R.W. & MOORE J.O. (1978) Chronic lymphocytic leukemia. *Cancer*, **42**, Suppl., 941.

257 BOGGS D.R., SOFFERMAN S.A., WINTROBE M.M. & CARTWRIGHT G.E. (1966) Factors influencing the duration of survival of patients with chronic lymphocytic leukemia. *American Journal of Medicine*, **40**, 243.

258 HANSEN M.M. (1973) Chronic lymphocytic leukaemia.

Clinical studies based on 189 cases followed for a long time. *Scandinavian Journal of Haematology*, **18**, Suppl. 18.

259 DIGHIERO G., CHARRON D., DEBRE P., LE PORRIER M., VAUGIER G., FOLLEZOU J.Y., DEGOS L., JACQUILLAT C.I. & BINET J.-L. (1979) Identification of a pure splenic form of chronic lymphocytic leukaemia. *British Journal of Haematology*, **41**, 169.

260 GRAY J.L., JACOBS A. & BLOCK M. (1974) Bone marrow and peripheral blood lymphocytosis in the prognosis of chronic lymphocytic leukemia. *Cancer*, **33**, 1169.

261 BINET J.-L., AUQIER A., DIGHIERO G., CHASTANG C., PIQUET H., GOASGUEN J,. VAUGIER G., POTRON G., COLONA P., OBERLING F., THOMAS M., TCHERNIA G., JACQUILLAT C., BOIVIN P., LESTY C., DUAULT M.T., MONCONDUIT M., BELABBES S. & GREMY F. (1981) A new prognostic classification of chronic lymphocytic leukemia derived from a multivariate survival analysis. *Cancer*, **48**, 198.

261a INTERNATIONAL WORKSHOP ON CLL (1981) Chronic lymphocytic leukaemia: proposals for a revised prognostic staging system. *British Journal of Haematology*, **48**, 365.

262 MUSUMECI R., SANTORO A., CERTO A. & MONFARDINI S. (1979) Staging for chronic lymphocytic leukaemia. *Lancet*, **i**, 783.

263 BINET J.L., NIZET M.G., DIGHIERO G. & GRELLET J. (1977) La lymphographie dans la leucemie lymphoide chronique. *Nouvelle Révue française d'Hématologie*, **18**, 351.

264 GALTON D.A.G. (1963) The Natural History of Chronic Lymphocytic Leukaemia. M.D. Thesis, University of Cambridge.

265 GALTON D.A.G. (1967) Trends in the therapy of leukaemia. In: *Modern Trends in Radiotherapy* (ed. Deeley T.J. & Wood C.A.P.), p. 292. Butterworths, London.

266 STEFANI S., CHANDRA S., SCHREK R., TANAKI H. & KNOSPE W.H. (1977) Endoplasmic reticulum-associated structures in lymphocytes from patients with chronic lymphocytic leukemia. *Blood*, **50**, 125.

267 CATOVSKY D., COSTELLO C., O'BRIEN M. & CHERCHI M. (1979) Ultrastructure and cell marker studies in lymphoproliferative disorders. In: *Modern Trends in Human Leukemia III* (ed. Neth R., Gallo R.C., Hofschneider P.-H. & Mannweiler K.), p. 107. Springer-Verlag, Berlin.

268 ZACHARSKI L.R. & LINMAN J.W. (1969) Chronic lymphocytic leukemia versus chronic lymphosarcoma-cell leukemia. *American Journal of Medicine*, **47**, 75.

269 PETERSON L.C., BLOOMFIELD C.D., SUNDBERG R.D., GAJI-PECZALSKA K.J. & BRUNNING R.D. (1975) Morphology of chronic lymphocytic leukemia and its relationship to survival. *American Journal of Medicine*, **59**, 316.

270 BINET J.-L., VAUGIER G., DIGHIERO G., D'ATHIS P. & CHARRON D. (1976) Investigation of a new parameter in chronic lymphocytic leukemia: the percentage of large peripheral lymphocytes determined by the Hemalog D. *American Journal of Medicine*, **63**, 683.

271 DUBNER H.N., CROWLEY J.J. & SCHILLING R.F. (1978) Prognostic value of nucleoli and cell size in chronic lymphocytic leukemia. *American Journal of Hematology*, **4**, 337.

271a PETERSON L.C., BLOOMFIELD C.D. & BRUNNING R.D. (1980) Relationship of clinical staging and lymphocyte morphology to survival in chronic lymphocytic leukaemia. *British Journal of Haematology*, **45**, 563.

272 COSTELLO C., WARDLE J., CATOVSKY D. & LEWIS S.M. (1980) Cell volume studies in B-cell leukaemia. *British Journal of Haematology*, **45**, 209.

273 HUBER C., ZIER K., MICHLMAYR G., RODT H., NILSSON K., THEML D., LUTZ D. & BRAUNSTEINER H. (1978) A comparative study of the buoyant density distribution of normal and malignant lymphocytes. *British Journal of Haematology*, **40**, 93.

274 JAYASWAL U., ROATH S., HYDE R.D., CHISHOLM D.M. & SMITH J.L. (1977) Blood lymphocyte surface markers and clinical findings in chronic lymphoproliferative disorders. *British Journal of Haematology*, **37**, 207.

275 CHEN B.Y.-N. & HELLER P. (1978) Lymphocyte surface immunoglobulin density and immunoglobulin secretion *in vitro* in chronic lymphocytic leukemia (CLL) *Blood*, **52**, 601.

275a DIGHIERO G., BODEGA E., MAYZNER R. & BINET J.-L. (1980) Individual cell-by-cell quantitation of lymphocyte surface membrane Ig in normal and CLL lymphocytes and during ontogeny of mouse B lymphocytes by immunoperoxidase assay. *Blood*, **55**, 93.

276 CATOVSKY D., CHERCHI M., GALTON D.A.G., HOFFBRAND A.V. & GANESHAGURU K. (1978) Cell differentiation in B- and T-lymphoproliferative disorders. In: *Differentiation of Normal and Neoplastic Hematopoeitic Cells*. Cold Spring Harbor Symposium, p. 811.

277 McCANN S.R., WHELAN A. & GREALLY J. (1978) Intracellular light chain inclusions in CLL. *British Journal of Haematology*, **38**, 367.

278 BRAGANZA C.M., STATHOPOULOS G., DAVIES A.J.S., ELLIOTT E.V., KERBEL R.S., PAPAMICHAIL M. & HOLBOROW E.J. (1975) Lymphocyte:erythrocyte (L.E.) rosettes as indicators of the heterogeneity of lymphocytes in a variety of mammalian species. *Cell*, **4**, 103.

279 STATHOPOULOS G. & ELLIOTT E.V. (1974) Formation of mouse or sheep red-blood-cell rosettes by lymphocytes from normal and leukaemic individuals. *Lancet*, **i**, 600.

280 BERTOGLIO J., PEAUD P.Y., BRYON P.A., TREILLE D., FELMAN P. & DORE J.F. (1976) Prognostic value of mouse red cell rosette formation in chronic lymphocytic leukaemia. *Biomedicine (Paris)*, **25**, 277.

281 FORBES I.J. & ZELEWSKI P.D. (1976) A subpopulation of human B lymphocytes that rosette with mouse erythrocytes. *Clinical and Experimental Immunology*, **26**, 99.

282 GUPTA S., GOOD R.A. & SIEGAL F.P. (1976) Rosette formation with mouse erythroyctes. III. Studies in patients with primary immunodeficiency and lymphoproliferative disorders. *Clinical and Experimental Immunology*, **26**, 204.

283 KIROV S.M., KWANT W.O., FERNANDEZ L.A., MACSWEEN J.M. & LANGLEY G.R. (1980) Characterization of Null cells in chronic lymphocytic leukaemia with B-cell allo- and hetero-antisera. *British Journal of Haematology*, **44**, 235.

284 GODAL T., HENRIKSEN A., IVERSEN J.-G., LANDAAS T.Ø. & LINDMO T. (1978) Altered membrane-associated functions in chronic lymphocytic leukemia cells. *International Journal of Cancer*, **21**, 561.

285 JOHNSON S.M. & KRAMERS M. (1978) Membrane micro-

viscosity differences in normal and leukaemic human lymphocytes. *Biochemical and Biophysical Research Communications*, **80**, 451.

286 INBAR M. & SHINITZKY M. (1974) Cholesterol as a bioregulator in the development and inhibition of leukemia. *Proceedings of the National Academy of Sciences, USA*, **71**, 4229.

287 SHINITZKY M. & INBAR M. (1976) Microviscosity parameters and protein mobility in biological membranes. *Biochimica et Biophysica Acta*, **433**, 133.

288 KRAMERS M.T.C., CATOVSKY D. & FOA R. (1978) Cell membrane enzymes. II. Alkaline phosphatase and alkaline phosphodiesterase 1 in normal and leukaemic lymphocytes. *British Journal of Haematology*, **40**, 111.

289 KRAMERS M.T.C., CATOVSKY D., FOA R., CHERCHI M. & GALTON D.A.G. (1976) 5'nucleotidase activity in leukaemic lymphocytes. *Biomedicine*, **25**, 362.

290 LA MANTIA K., CONKLYN M., QUAGLIATA F. & SILBER R. (1977) Lymphocyte 5'-nucleotidase: absence of detectable protein in chronic lymphocytic leukemia. *Blood*, **50**, 683.

291 KRAMERS M.T.C. & CATOVSKY D. (1978) Cell membrane enzymes: L-γ-glutamyl transpeptidase, leucine aminopeptidase, maltase and trehalase in normal and leukaemic lymphocytes. *British Journal of Haematology*, **38**, 453.

292 AUTIO K., TURUNEN O., LUNDQVIST C. & SCHRÖDER J. (1978) Activation of lymphocytes in CLL by protein A from *Staphylococcus aureus*. *Clinical and Experimental Immunology*, **34**, 188.

292a LEE S.H.S., OZERE R.L. & VAN ROOYEN C.E. (1966) Interferon production by human leucocytes *in vitro*. Reduced levels in lymphatic leukemia. *Proceedings of the Society for Experimental Biology and Medicine*, **122**, 32.

293 CHISHOLM M. & CARTWRIGHT T. (1978) Interferon production in leukaemia. *British Journal of Haematology*, **40**, 43.

294 SINGH A.K., VAUGHAN-SMITH S., SAWYER B., O'CONNOR T.W.E., THOMSON A.E.R. & WETHERLEY-MEIN G. (1978) Cell studies in prolymphocytic leukaemia. *British Journal of Haematology*, **40**, 587.

295 THOMSON A.E.R., O'CONNOR T.W.E. & WETHERLEY-MEIN G. (1972) Killing and characterizing action of colchicine *in vitro* on lymphocytes of chronic lymphocytic leukaemia. *Scandinavian Journal of Haematology*, **9**, 231.

296 THOMSON A.E.R., O'CONNOR T.W.E. & WETHERLEY-MEIN G. (1974) Selective killing by cholchicine *in vitro* of lymphocytes of chronic lymphocytic leukemia. *Proceedings of Eighth Leukocyte Culture Conference, New York*. p. 665. Academic Press, New York.

297 RAMOT B., BROK-SIMONI F., CHWEIDAN E. & ASHKENAZI Y.E. (1976) Blood leucocyte enzymes. III. Diurnal rhythm of activity in isolated lymphocytes of normal subjects and chronic lymphatic leukaemia patients. *British Journal of Haematology*, **34**, 79.

298 LANCE E.M. & TAUB R.N. (1969) Segregation of lymphocyte populations through differential migration. *Nature (London)*, **221**, 841.

299 ZATZ M.M. & LANCE E.M. (1970) The distribution of chromium 51-labelled lymphoid cells in the mouse. A survey of anatomical compartments. *Cellular Immunology*, **1**, 3.

300 PILGRIM H.I. (1972) Relationship of the selective metastatic behaviour of reticular tissues to the migration patterns of their normal cells of origin. *Journal of the National Cancer Institute*, **49**, 3.

301 STATHOPOULOS G. & DAVIES A.J.S. (1976) Human lymphocytes and mouse red cells. *Lancet*, **i**, 1078.

302 WYBRAN J., CHANTLER S. & FUDENBERG H.H. (1973) Isolation of normal T cells in chronic lymphocytic leukaemia. *Lancet*, **i**, 126.

303 HAN T. & DADEY B. (1979) *In vitro* functional studies of mononuclear cells in patients with CLL. Evidence for functionally normal T lymphocytes and monocytes and abnormal B lymphocytes. *Cancer*, **43**, 109.

304 FOA R., CATOVSKY D., BROZOVIC M., MARSH G., OOYIRILANGKUMARAN T., CHERCHI M. & GALTON D.A.G. (1979) Clinical staging and immunological findings in chronic lymphocytic leukemia. *Cancer*, **44**, 483.

305 FERNANDEZ L.A., MACSWEEN J.M. & LANGLEY G.R. (1975) Separation of T lymphocytes from normal individuals and patients with B lymphocyte chronic lymphocytic leukaemia. *Immunology*, **28**, 231.

306 MELLSTEDT H., PETTERSSON D., HOLM G. (1978) Lymphocyte subpopulations in chronic lymphocytic leukemia (CLL). *Acta Medica Scandinavica*, **204**, 485.

307 MORETTA L., FERRARINI M., DURANTE M.L. & MINGARI M.C. (1975) Expression of a receptor for IgM by human T cells. *European Journal of Immunology*, **5**, 565.

308 KAY N.E., JOHNSON J.D., STANEK R. & DOUGLAS S.D. (1979) T-cell subpopulations in chronic lymphocytic leukemia: abnormalities in distribution and in *in vitro* receptor maturation. *Blood*, **54**, 540.

309 LAURIA F., FOA R. & CATOVSKY D. (1980) Increase in Tγ lymphocytes in B-cell chronic lymphocytic leukaemia. *Scandinavian Journal of Haematology*, **24**, 187.

310 DAO C., MARIE J.P., BERNADOU A. & BILSKI-PASQUIER G. (1978) T-lymphocyte colonies in the lymphoproliferative disorders. *Immunology*, **34**, 741.

311 FOA R. & CATOVSKY D. (1979) T-lymphocyte colonies in normal blood, bone marrow and lymphoproliferative disorders. *Clinical and Experimental Immunology*, **36**, 488.

312 FOA R., CATOVSKY D., LAURIA F., ZAFAR, N. & GALTON D.A.G. (1981) Reduced T-colony forming capacity by T-lymphocytes from B-chronic lymphocytic leukaemia. *British Journal of Haematology*, **46**, 623.

313 FOA R., LAURIA F. & CATOVSKY D. (1980) Evidence that T-colony formation is a property of Tμ (helper) lymphocytes. *Clinical and Experimental Immunology*, **42**, 152.

314 CHANDRA P., CHANANA A.D., CHIKKAPPA G. & CRONKITE E.P. (1977) Chronic lymphocytic leukemia: concepts and observations. *Blood Cells*, **3**, 637.

315 SCHULTZ E.F., DAVIS S. & RUBIN A.D. (1976) Further characterization of the circulating cell in chronic lymphocytic leukemia. *Blood*, **48**, 223.

316 CHIORAZZI N., FU S.M., MONTAZERI G., KUNKEL H.G., RAI K. & GEE T. (1979) T cell helper defect in patients with chronic lymphocytic leukemia. *Journal of Immunology*, **122**, 1087.

316a TURSZ T., BROUET J.-C., FLANDRIN G., DANON F.,

CLAUVEL J.-P. & SELIGMANN M. (1977) Clinical and pathological features of Waldenström's macroglobulinemia in seven patients with serum monoclonal IgG or IgA. *American Journal of Medicine*, **63**, 499.

316b LEVINE A.M., LICHTENSTEIN A., GRESIK M.V., TAYLOR C.R., FEINSTEIN D.I. & LUKES R.J. (1980) Clinical and immunologic spectrum of plasmacytoid lymphocytic lymphoma without serum monoclonal IgM. *British Journal of Haematology*, **46**, 225.

317 GALTON D.A.G., GOLDMAN J.M., WILTSHAW E., CATOVSKY D., HENRY K. & GOLDENBERG G.J. (1974) Prolymphocytic leukaemia. *British Journal of Haematology*, **27**, 7.

318 ANDAY G.J. & SCHMITZ H.L. (1952) Follicular lymphoma with transient leukemic phase. *Archives of Internal Medicine*, **89**, 621.

319 SPIRO S., GALTON D.A.G., WILTSHAW E. & LOHMANN R.C. (1975) Follicular lymphoma: a survey of 75 cases with special reference to the syndrome resembling chronic lymphocytic leukaemia. *British Journal of Cancer*, **31**, Suppl. II, 60.

320 LENNERT K., MOHRI N., STEIN H. & KAISERLING E. (1975) The histopathology of malignant lymphoma. *British Journal of Haematology*, **31**, Suppl., 193.

321 LEVITT W.M. & SCOTT R.M. (1955) Reticulosis and reticulosarcoma. In: *British Practice in Radiotherapy* (ed. Carling R., Windeyer B.W. & Smithers D.W.), p. 426. Butterworth, London.

322 GALTON D.A.G., WILTSHAW E., SZUR L. & DACIE J.M. (1961) The use of chlorambucil and steroids in the treatment of chronic lymphocytic leukaemia. *British Journal of Haematology*, **7**, 73.

323 HAN T., EZDINLI E.Z., SHIMAOKA K. & DESAI D.V. (1973) Chlorambucil versus combined chlorambucil-corticosteroid therapy in chronic lymphocytic leukemia. *Cancer*, **31**, 502.

324 KNOSPE W.H., LOEB V. & HUGULEY C.M. (1974) Bi-weekly chlorambucil treatment of chronic lymphocytic leukemia. *Cancer*, **33**, 555.

325 SAWITSKY A., RAI K.R., GLIDEWELL O., SILVER R.T. & PARTICIPATING MEMBERS OF CALGB. (1977) Comparison of daily versus intermittent chlorambucil and prednisone therapy in the treatment of patients with chronic lymphocytic leukemia. *Blood*, **50**, 1049.

326 LIEPMAN M. & VOTAW M.L. (1978) The treatment of chronic lymphocytic leukemia with COP chemotherapy. *Cancer*, **41**, 1664.

327 OSGOOD E.E. (1964) Treatment of chronic leukemias. *Journal of Nuclear Medicine*, **5**, 139.

328 JOHNSON R.E. (1977) Radiotherapy as primary treatment for chronic lymphocytic leukaemia. In: *Clinics in Haematology: The Chronic Leukaemias* (ed. Galton D.A.G.), Vol. 6, p. 237. W. B. Saunders, London.

329 RICHARDS F., SPURR C.L., FERREE C., BLAKE D.D. & RABEN M. (1978) The control of chronic lymphocytic leukemia with mediastinal irradiation. *American Journal of Medicine*, **64**, 947.

330 CRONKITE E.P. (1971) Extracorporeal irradiation of blood in the treatment of chronic lymphocytic leukemia. In: *Recent Results in Cancer Research: Current Concepts in the Management of Leukemia and Lymphoma* (ed. Ultmann J.E., Griem M.L, Kirsten W.H. & Wissler R.W.), p. 67. Springer-Verlag, Berlin.

331 WILTSHAW E. (1977) Chemotherapy in chronic lymphocytic leukaemia. In: *Clinics in Haematology: The Chronic Leukaemias* (ed. Galton D.A.G.), Vol. 6, p. 223. W. B. Saunders, London.

331a GELLER W. (1964) Chronic lymphocytic leukemia with hemolytic anemia. *Archives of Internal Medicine*, **114**, 444.

331b LEWIS F.B., SCHWARTZ R.S. & DAMESHEK W. (1966) X-irradiation and alkylating agents as possible 'trigger' mechanisms in the autoimmune complications of malignant lymphoproliferative disease. *Clinical and Experimental Immunology*, **1**, 3.

331c YONET H.M., VIGLIANO E.M. & HOROWITZ H.I. (1967) Acute hemolytic anemia associated with administration of alkylating agents: report of two cases due to cyclophosphamide and review of the literature. *American Journal of the Medical Sciences*, **254**, 71.

331d EBBE S., WITTELS B. & DAMESHEK W. (1962) Autoimmune thrombocytopenic purpura ('ITP' type) with chronic lymphocytic leukemia. *Blood*, **19**, 23.

331e CHRISTENSEN B.E. (1973) Erythrocyte pooling and sequestration in enlarged spleens. Estimations of splenic erythrocyte and plasma volume in splenomegalic patients. *Scandinavian Journal of Haematology*, **10**, 106.

331f ASTER R.H. (1966) Pooling of platelets in the spleen: rôle in the pathogenesis of 'hypersplenic' thrombocytopenia. *Journal of Clinical Investigation*, **45**, 645.

332 CHRISTENSEN B.E., HANSEN M.M. & VIDEBAEK A. (1977) Splenectomy in chronic lymphocytic leukaemia. *Scandinavian Journal of Haematology*, **18**, 279.

333 HÖCKER P., PITTERMANN E., GOBETS M. & STACKER A. (1975) Treatment of patients with chronic myeloid leukaemia and chronic lymphocytic leukaemia by leucapheresis with a continuous flow blood cell separator. In: *Leucocytes: Separation, Collection and Transfusion* (ed. Goldman J.M. & Lowenthal R.M.), p. 510. Academic Press, London.

334 RICHTER M.N. (1928) Generalized reticular cell sarcoma of lymph nodes associated with lymphatic leukemia. *American Journal of Pathology*, **3**, 285.

335 LORTHOLARY P., BOIRON M., RIPAULT P., LEVY J.P., MANUS A. & BERNARD J. (1964) Leucémie lymphoïde chronique secondairement associée à une reticulopathie maligne, syndrome de Richter. *Nouvelle Révue française d'Hématologie*, **4**, 621.

336 OBERFIELD R.A. (1966) Coexistence of chronic lymphocytic leukemia and Hodgkin's disease. *Journal of the American Medical Association*, **195**, 865.

337 TORNYOS K., MACOSSAY C.R. & GYORKEY F. (1967) Chronic lymphocytic leukemia and Hodgkin's disease in the same patient. *Cancer*, **20**, 552.

338 GIVLER R.L. (1968) Lymphocytic leukemia with coexistent localized reticulum cell sarcoma. *Cancer*, **21**, 1184.

339 ROSNER F. & GRÜNWALD H. (1975) Hodgkin's disease and acute leukemia: report of 8 cases and review of the literature. *American Journal of Medicine*, **58**, 339.

340 GOLDSTEIN J. & BADEN J. (1977) Richter's syndrome. *Southern Medical Journal*, **70**, 1381.

340a McPHEDRAN P. & HEATH C.W. (1970) Acute leukemia occurring during chronic lymphocytic leukemia. *Blood*, **35**, 7.

341 FITZGERALD P.H., RASTRICK J.M. & HAMER J.W. (1973)

Acute plasma cell leukaemia following chronic lymphatic leukaemia: transformation or two separate diseases? *British Journal of Haematology*, **25**, 171.

341a HOFFMANN K.D. & RUDDERS R.A. (1977) Multiple myeloma and chronic lymphocytic leukemia in a single individual. *Archives of Internal Medicine*, **137**, 232.

341b PEDERSEN-BJERGAARD J., PETERSEN H.D., THOMSEN M., WIIK A. & WOLFF-JENSEN J. (1978) Chronic lymphocytic leukaemia with subsequent development of multiple myeloma. *Scandinavian Journal of Haematology*, **21**, 256.

342 NARASIMHAN P., JAGATHAMBAL K., ELIZALDE A.M. & ROSNER F. (1975) Chronic lymphocytic leukemia and lymphosarcoma associated with multiple myeloma. *Archives of Internal Medicine*, **135**, 729.

343 FLANDRIN G., VARET B., DANIEL M.-T. & BERNARD J. (1970) Deux leucémies simultanées chez un même malade? Leucémie aiguë myéloblastique et leucémie lymphocytaire chronique: essai d'interpretation. *Nouvelle Révue française d'Hématologie*, **10**, 771.

344 O'NEILL B.J., McCREDIE K.B., RAIK E. & TAURO G.P. (1970) Mixed leukaemia: a report of three cases. *Medical Journal of Australia*, **ii**, 586.

345 ROBERTS P.D. & FORSTER P.M. (1973) Chronic lymphocytic leukaemia associated with acute myelomonocytic leukaemia. *British Journal of Haematology*, **25**, 203.

346 VAN HOVE W., DE BAERE H. & HAMERS J. (1974) Gelijktijdig voorkommen var acute myelocytaire en chronishe lymfocytaire leukemie. *Netherlands Tijdschrift voor Geneeskunde*, **118**, 1702.

347 HAMILTON P.J. (1976) Concomitant myeloblastic and lymphocytic leukaemia. *Lancet*, **i**, 373.

348 WARWICK R., GOLDSTONE A.H. & JANOSSY G. (1976) Chronic lymphocytic leukaemia uncovered by successful treatment of acute myeloid leukaemia. *British Medical Journal*, **iv**, 1111.

349 ADAMS P.B., CORNELL F.N., DING J.C. & COOPER I.A. (1977) Characterization of tumor cells in concomitant chronic lymphocytic leukemia and acute monocyte leukemia. *American Journal of Hematology*, **2**, 271.

350 ZARRABI M.H., GRUNWALD H.W. & ROSNER F. (1977) Chronic lymphocytic leukaemia terminating in acute leukaemia. *Archives of Internal Medicine*, **137**, 1509.

351 LAWLOR E., McCANN S.R., WHELAN A., GREALLY J. & TEMPERLEY I.J. (1979) Acute myeloid leukaemia occurring in untreated chronic lymphatic leukaemia. *British Journal of Haematology*, **43**, 369.

352 CATOVSKY D. & GALTON D.A.G. (1971) Myelomonocytic leukaemia supervening on chronic lymphocytic leukaemia. *Lancet*, **i**, 478.

353 OSGOOD E.E. (1964) Contrasting incidence of acute monocytic and granulocytic leukemia in ^{32}P-treated patients with polycythemia vera and chronic lymphatic leukemia. *Journal of Laboratory and Clinical Medicine*, **64**, 560.

354 CRYER P.E. & KISSANE J. (1975) Multiple malignancies: chronic lymphocytic leukemia, malignant melanoma, multiple myeloma and acute myelomonocytic leukemia. (Clinicopathologic Conference). *American Journal of Medicine*, **58**, 408.

355 MOERTEL C.G. & HAEDORN A.B. (1957) Leukemia or lymphoma and coexistent primary malignant lesions: a review of the literature and a study of 120 cases. *Blood*, **12**, 788.

356 BERG J.W. (1967) The incidence of multiple primary cancer. I. Development of further cancers in patients with lymphoma, leukemia, and myeloma. *Journal of the National Cancer Institute*, **38**, 5.

357 HYMAN G.A. (1969) Increased incidence of neoplasia in association with chronic lymphocytic leukemia. *Scandinavian Journal of Haematology*, **6**, 99.

358 STAVRAKY K.M., WATSON T.A., WHITE D.F. & MILES E.M. (1970) Chronic lymphocytic leukemia and subsequent cancer in the same patient. *Cancer*, **26**, 410.

359 MANUSOW D. & WEINERMAN B.H. (1975) Subsequent neoplasia in chronic lymphocytic leukemia. *American Medical Association Journal*, **232**, 267.

360 GALTON D.A.G., WILTSHAW E., BOESEN E., SPEED D.E., HOLLYHOCK V. & GOLDENBERG G.J. (1964) Prolymphocytic leukaemia. *British Empire Cancer Campaign for Research, 41st Annual Report*, p. 55. Lund Humphries, London.

361 COSTELLO C., CATOVSKY D., O'BRIEN M. & GALTON D.A.G. (1980) Prolymphocytic leukaemia. An ultrastructural study of 22 cases. *British Journal of Haematology*, **44**, 389.

362 PALLESEN G., MADSEN M. & PEDERSEN B.B. (1979) B-prolymphocytic leukaemia—a mantle zone lymphoma? *Scandinavian Journal of Haematology*, **22**, 407.

363 LAMPERT I., CATOVSKY D., MARSH G.W., CHILD J.A. & GALTON D.A.G. (1980) The histopathology of prolymphocytic leukaemia with particular reference to the spleen: a comparison with chronic lymphocytic leukaemia. *Histopathology*, **4**, 1.

364 BEARMAN R.M., PANGALIS G.A. & RAPPAPORT H. (1978) Prolymphocytic leukemia: clinical, histopathological, and cytochemical observations. *Cancer*, **42**, 2360.

365 BUSKARD N.A., CATOVSKY D., OKOS A., GOLDMAN J.M. & GALTON D.A.G. (1976) Prolymphocytic leukaemia. *Hämatologie und Bluttransfusion*, **18**, 237.

366 KÖNIG E., MEUSERS P. & BRITTINGER G. (1979) Efficacy of doxorubicin in prolymphocytic leukaemia. *British Journal of Haematology*, **42**, 487.

367 SIBBALD R. & CATOVSKY D. (1979) Complete remission in prolymphocytic leukaemia with the combination chemotherapy—CHOP. *British Journal of Haematology*, **42**, 488.

367a OSCIER D., CATOVSKY D., ERRINGTON R.D., GOOLDEN, A.W.G., ROBERTS P.D. & GALTON, D.A.G. (1981) Splenic irradiation in β-prolymphocytic leukaemia. *British Journal of Haematology* (in press).

368 PLENDERLEITH I.H. (1970) Hairy cell leukemia. *Canadian Medical Association Journal*, **102**, 1056.

369 CATOVSKY D., PETTIT J.E., GALTON D.A.G., SPIERS A.S.D. & HARRISON C.V. (1974) Leukaemic reticuloendotheliosis ('hairy' cell leukaemia): a distinct clinicopathological entity. *British Journal of Haematology*, **26**, 9.

370 GOLOMB H.M., CATOVSKY D. & GOLDE D.W. (1978) Hairy cell leukemia. *Annals of Internal Medicine*, **89**, 677.

370a GOLOMB H.M., VARDIMAN J., SWEET D.L. JR, SIMON D. & VARIAKOJIS D. (1978) Hairy cell leukaemia: evidence for the existence of a spectrum of functional characteristics. *British Journal of Haematology*, **38**, 161.

371 TURNER A. & KJELDSBERG C.R. (1978) Hairy cell leukemia: a review. *Medicine*, **57**, 477.

372 BOURONCLE B.A., WISEMAN B.K. & DOAN C.A. (1958) Leukemic reticuloendotheliosis. *Blood*, **13**, 609.

373 KATAYAMA I. & FINKEL H.E. (1974) Leukemic reticuloendotheliosis. A clinicopathologic study with a review of the literature. *American Journal of Medicine*, **57**, 115.

374 DUHAMEL G. (1971) Lymphoid myelofibrosis. *Acta Haematologica*, **45**, 89.

375 BOIRON M., FLANDRIN G., RIPAULT J., LORTHOLARY P., TEILLET F., JACQUILLAT C. & BERNARD J. (1968) Histio-lymphocytose medullaire et splenique d'apparence primitive. *Nouvelle Révue française d'Hématologie*, **8**, 179.

375a CATOVSKY D., PETTIT J.E., GALETTO J., OKOS A. & GALTON D.A.G. (1974) The B-lymphocyte nature of the hairy cell of leukaemic reticuloendotheliosis. *British Journal of Haematology*, **26**, 29.

376 CATOVSKY D. Hairy-cell leukaemia and prolymphocytic leukaemia. In: *Clinics in Haematology: The Chronic Leukaemias* (ed. Galton D.A.G.), Vol. 6, p. 245. W. B. Saunders, London.

376a BURNS G.F., CAWLEY J.C., BARKER C.R., GOLDSTONE A.H. & HAYHOE F.G.J. (1977) New evidence relating to the nature and origin of the hairy cell of leukaemic reticuloendotheliosis. *British Journal of Haematology*, **36**, 71.

377 CAWLEY J.C., BURNS G.F., BEVAN A., WORMAN C.P., SMITH J.L., GRAY L., BARKER C.R. & HAYHOE F.G.J. (1979) Typical hairy-cell leukaemia with IgGk paraproteinaemia. *British Journal of Haematology*, **43**, 215.

378 SWEET D.L., GOLOMB H.M. & ULTMANN J.E. (1977) Chronic lymphocytic leukaemia and its relationship to other lymphoproliferative disorders. In: *Clinics in Haematology: The Chronic Leukaemias* (ed. Galton D.A.G.), Vol. 6, p. 141. W. B. Saunders, London.

379 DANIEL M.-T. & FLANDRIN G. (1974) Fine structure of abnormal cells in hairy cell (tricholeukocytic) leukemia, with special reference to their *in-vitro* phagocytic capacity. *Laboratory Investigation*, **30**, 1.

380 KATAYAMA I., LI G.W. & YAM L.T. (1972) Ultrastructural characteristics of the 'hairy cells' or leukemic reticuloendotheliosis. *American Journal of Pathology*, **69**, 471.

381 BURKE J.S., BYRNE G.E. & RAPPAPORT H. (1974) Hairy cell leukemia (L-RE). I. A clinical pathologic study of 21 patients. *Cancer*, **33**, 1399.

382 SCHAEFFER H.E., HELLRIEGEL K.P., ZACH J. & FISCHER R. (1975) Zytochemischer Polymorphismus der sauren Phosphatase bei Haarzel-Leukämie. *Blut*, **31**, 365.

383 YAM L.T., LI C.Y. & FINKEL H.E. (1972) Leukemic reticuloendotheliosis. The role of tartrate-resistant acid phosphatase in diagnosis and splenectomy in treatment. *Archives of Internal Medicine*, **130**, 248.

383a HIGGY K.E., BURNS G.F. & HAYHOE F.G.J. (1978) Indentification of the hairy cells of leukaemic reticuloendotheliosis by an esterase method. *British Journal of Haematology*, **38**, 99.

384 FU S.M., WINCHESTER R.J., RAI K.R. & KUNKEL H.G. (1974) Hairy cell leukemia: proliferation of a cell with phagocytic and B-lymphocyte properties. *Scandinavian Journal of Immunology*, **3**, 847.

385 RIEBER E.P., SAAL J.G., RIETHMÜLLER G., HEYDEN H.W. & WALLER H.D. (1976) Strong expression of Fc-receptors on leukemic cells in hairy cell leukemia. *Zeitschrift für Immunitätsforschung*, **151**, 282.

386 KING G.W., HURTUBISE P.E., SAGONE A.L., LOBUGLIO A.F. & METZ E.N. (1975) Leukemic reticuloendotheliosis. A study of the origin of the malignant cell. *American Journal of Medicine*, **59**, 411.

387 JANSEN J., SCHUIT H.R.E., VAN ZWET T.L., MEIJER C.J.L.M. & HIJMANS W. (1979) Hairy-cell leukaemia: a B lymphocytic disorder. *British Journal of Haematology*, **42**, 21.

387a RIEBER E.P., HADAM M.R., LINKE R.P., SAAL J.G., RIETHMÜLLER G., VON HEYDEN H.W. & WALLER H.D. (1979) Hairy cell leukaemia: surface markers and functional capacities of the leukaemic cells analysed in eight patients. *British Journal of Haematology*, **42**, 175.

388 BURNS G.F., CAWLEY J.C., WORMAN C.P., KARPAS A., BARKER C.R., GOLDSTONE A.H. & HAYHOE F.G.J. (1978) Multiple heavy chain isotypes on the surface of the cells of hairy cell leukaemia. *Blood*, **52**, 1132.

388a CATOVSKY D., PAPAMICHAEL M., OKOS A., MILIANI E. & HOLBOROW E.J. (1975) Formation of mouse red cell rosettes by 'hairy' cells. *Biomedicine*, **23**, 81.

389 CATOVSKY D., CHERCHI M., OKOS A., HEGDE U. & GALTON D.A.G. (1976) Mouse red-cell rosettes in B-lymphoproliferative disorders. *British Journal of Haematology*, **33**, 173.

390 CAWLEY J.C., BURNS G.F., NASH T.A., HIGGY K.E., CHILD J.A. & ROBERTS B.E. (1978) Hairy-cell leukaemia with T-cell features. *Blood*, **51**, 61.

391 ADVANI S.H., TALWALKAR G.V., NADKARNI J.S., NADKARNI J.J., SIRSAT S.M. & SRINIVASAN V. (1976) Hairy-cell leukaemia. *Indian Journal of Cancer*, **13**, 283.

392 HERNANDEZ D., CRUZ C., CARNOT J., DORTICOS E. & ESPINOSA E. (1978) Hairy cell leukaemia of T-cell origin. *British Journal of Haematology*, **40**, 504.

393 SAXON A., STEVENS R.H. & GOLDE D.W. (1978) T-lymphocyte variant of hairy-cell leukemia. *Annals of Internal Medicine*, **88**, 323.

394 LEWIS S.M., CATOVSKY D., HOWS J.H. & ARDELAN B. (1977) Splenic red-cell pooling in hairy-cell leukaemia. *British Journal of Haematology*, **35**, 351.

394a SLATER N.G.P., BARKHAN P. & WILLIAMS H.J.H. (1979) Case report: Hairy cell leukaemia—apparent cure with reversal of marrow fibrosis. *Clinical and Laboratory Haematology*, **1**, 65.

395 CASTRO-MALASPINA H., NAJEAN Y. & FLANDRIN G. (1979) Erythrokinetic studies in hairy-cell leukaemia. *British Journal of Haematology*, **42**, 189.

396 WEINSTEIN R.A., GELMANN E., GOLOMB H.M. (1978) Disseminated atypical mycobacterial infection in hairy-cell leukaemia. *Lancet*, **ii**, 1052.

397 HENDRICK A.M. & HENDRICK D.J. (1979) Scotochromogen infection in hairy-cell leukaemia. *Lancet*, **i**, 109.

397a DAVIES T.E., WATERBURY L., ABELOFF M. & BURKE P.J. (1976) Leukemic reticuloendotheliosis. Report of a case with prolonged remission following intensive chemotherapy. *Archives of Internal Medicine*, **136**, 620.

398 McCARTHY D. & CATOVSKY D. (1978) Response to doxorubicin in hairy cell leukaemia. *Scandinavian Journal of Haematology*, **21**, 445.

399 EDELSON R.L., KIRKPATRICK C.H., SHEVACH E.M., SCHEIN P.S., SMITH R.W., GREEN I. & LUTZNER M.

(1974) Preferential cutaneous infiltration by neoplastic thymus-derived lymphocytes. *Annals of Internal Medicine*, **80**, 685.

400 LUTZNER M., EDELSON R., SHEIN P., GREEN I., KIRK-PATRICK C. & AHMED A. (1975) Cutaneous T-cell lymphomas: the Sézary syndrome, mycosis fungoides, and related disorders. *Annals of Internal Medicine*, **83**, 534.

401 BROUET J.-C., FLANDRIN G., SASPORTES M., PREUD'-HOMME J.-L. & SELIGMANN M. (1975) Chronic lymphocytic leukemia of T cell origin. An immunological and clinical evaulation in eleven patients. *Lancet*, **ii**, 390.

402 HUHN D., RODT H., THIEL E., GROSSE-WILDE H., FINK U., THEML H., JÄGER G., STEIDLE C. & THIERFELDER S. (1976) T-zell-leukämien des erwachsenen. *Blut*, **33**, 141.

403 WOESSNER S., LAFUENTE R., SANS-SABRAFEN J., VIVES J. & ROZMAN C. (1978) Prolymphocytic leukaemia of T-cell type: immunological, enzymatic and ultrastructural morphometric characteristics. *British Journal of Haematology*, **39**, 9.

404 HANAOKA M., SASAKI M., MATSUMOTO H., TANKAWA H., YAMABE H., TOMIMOTO K., TASAKA C., FUJIWARA H., UCHIYAMA T. & TAKATSUKI K. (1979) Adult T cell leukaemia. Histological classification and characteristics. *Acta Pathologica Japonica*, **29**, 723.

405 COSTELLO C., CATOVSKY D., O'BRIEN M., MORILLA R. & VARADI S. (1980) Chronic T-cell leukaemias. I. Morphology, cytochemistry and ultrastructure. *Leukemia Research*, **4**, 463.

406 SAXON A., STEVENS R.H. & GOLDE D.W. (1979) Helper and suppressor T-lymphocyte leukemia in ataxia telangiectasia. *New England Journal of Medicine*, **300**, 700.

407 UCHIYAMA T., YODOI J., SAGAWA K., TAKATSUKI K. & UCHINO H. (1977) Adult T-cell leukemia: clinical and hematologic features of 16 cases. *Blood*, **50**, 481.

408 TOBEN H.R. & SMITH R.G. (1977) T lymphocytes bearing complement receptors in a patient with chronic lymphocytic leukemia. *Clinical and Experimental Immunology*, **27**, 292.

409 HANAOKA M., SHIRAKAWA S., YODOI J., UCHIYAMA T. & TAKATSUKI K. (1979) Adult T cell leukemia. Histological features of the lymphoid tissues. In: *Function and Structure of the Immune System* (ed. Müller-Rucholtz W. & Müller-Hermelink H.K.), p. 613. Plenum, New York.

410 SUMIYA M., MIZOGUCHI H., KOSAKA K., MIURA Y., TAKAKU F. & YATA J.I. (1973) Chronic lymphocytic leukaemia of T cell origin? *Lancet*, **ii**, 910.

411 YODOI J., TAKATSUKI K. & MASUDA T. (1974) Two cases of T cell chronic lymphocytic leukemia in Japan. *New England Journal of Medicine*, **290**, 572.

412 UCHIYAMA T., SAGAWA K., TAKATSUKI K. & UCHINO, H. (1978) Effect of adult T-cell leukemia cells on pokeweed mitogen-induced normal B-cell differentiation. *Clinical Immunology and Immunopathology*, **10**, 24.

413 BRODER S., UCHIYAMA T. & WALDMANN T.A. (1979) Neoplasms of immunoregulatory cells. *American Journal of Clinical Pathology*, **72**, suppl., 724.

414 BERNHEIM A., BERGER R., PREUD'HOMME J.-L., LABAUME S., BUSSEL A. & BAROT-CIORBARU R. (1981) Philadelphia chromosme positive blood B lymphocytes in chronic myelocytic leukemia. *Leukemia Research*, **5**, 331.

415 FIALKOW P.J., MARTIN P.J., NAJFELD V., PENFOLD G.K., JACOBSON R.J. & HANSEN J.A. (1981) Evidence for a multistep pathogenesis of chronic myelogenous leukemia. *Blood*, **58**, 158.

416 ROOZENDAAL K.J., VAN DER REIJDEN H.J. & GERAEDTS J.P.M. (1981) Philadelphia chromosome positive acute lymphoblastic leukaemia with T-cell characteristics. *British Journal of Haematology*, **47**, 145.

417 NAJFELD V., FIALKOW P.J., KARANDE A., NILSSON K., KLEIN G. & PENFOLD G. (1981) Chromosome analysis of lymphoid cell lines derived from patients with chronic lymphocytic leukemia. *International Journal of Cancer*, **26**, 543.

Chapter 24
Malignant disorders of the lymph nodes

T. J. McELWAIN AND J. P. SLOANE

THE NORMAL LYMPH NODE

Lymph nodes (Fig. 24.1) receive lymph via afferent lymphatic vessels which drain into a subcapsular sinus extending around the full circumference of the node. From here it passes into the cortex and paracortex, and thence into the medullary sinuses which merge into larger channels and eventually discharge into the efferent lymphatic vessel.

The cortex is the outer part of the node underlying the subcapsular sinus and contains the lymphoid follicles. There is strong evidence that this is the B-cell region of the lymph node. First, isotopically labelled B cells in experimental animals specifically colonize the cortex [1]. Secondly, patients with a-γ-globulinaemia have a depleted lymph-node cortex [2], whereas in those with thymic aplasia it appears normal [3]. Thirdly, immunohistochemical studies have shown that cortical cells have complement receptors, bear surface immunoglobulin and lack the capacity to form E rosettes with sheep erythrocytes [4, 5]. Finally, hyperplasia of the cortex is associated with immune responses involving antibody production [6]. Primary follicles consist of nodular aggregates of lymphocytes, dendritic reticular cells and macrophages, and may undergo hyperplasia after exposure to antigen to form secondary follicles with germinal centres [7]. Germinal centres consist of lymphoid cells in various stages of transformation together with dendritic reticular cells and tingible-body macrophages. The *dendritic reticular cells* are large cells with long, slender cytoplasmic processes extending out between the lymphoid cells. They are best demonstrated by electron microscopy or histochemical techniques and are difficult to identify in conventional sections. Antigen can be demonstrated on the surface of the processes in immune reactions and the cells may have a role in the presentation of antigen to lymphocytes [7]. *Tingible-body macrophages* (Fig. 24.2) are also large cells with copious cytoplasm containing phagocytosed debris which appears to be derived from locally dying lymphoid cells. These macrophages do not appear to have a role in phagocytosing antigenic material [7].

The lymphoid cells exhibit a spectrum of different morphological appearances (Fig. 24.2). Some have irregular indented nuclei and are referred to as *cleaved cells* in the terminology of the Lukes–Collins classification [8] (see p. 925). These cells vary in size from slightly larger than a normal lymphocyte (*small cleaved cells*) to about the size of a histiocyte nucleus (*large cleaved cells*). Other cells have nuclei with smooth outlines and are known as small and large *non-cleaved cells*. The *small non-cleaved cells* are approximately the same size as large cleaved cells but have round nuclei with small nucleoli. *Large non-cleaved cells* have oval nuclei with a single large or two to three medium-sized nucleoli which are often applied to the nuclear membrane. *Immunoblasts* are similar to large non-cleaved cells but are generally larger, have more abundant pyroninophilic cytoplasm and usually two or three nucleoli.

In the terminology of the Kiel classification [9] (see p. 926), cleaved cells (both large and small) are referred to as *centrocytes*. The smaller cells with smooth nuclear outlines are referred to as *lymphoblasts* and the larger ones as *centroblasts* if they have several nucleoli applied to the nuclear membrane, and *immunoblasts* if they have large, centrally placed nucleoli. It is important to recognize that the term 'immunoblast' is used to describe somewhat different cells in the two different systems of nomenclature.

There is dispute about the sequence of morphological changes in transforming lymphoid cells within germinal centres. Lukes & Collins [8] believe that the lymphocyte passes through the small cleaved, large cleaved, small non-cleaved and large non-cleaved stages to become an immunoblast. Studies in experimental animals, however, have shown that large non-cleaved may precede cleaved cells in germinal-centre development [10]. A small population of immature T cells has also been identified in germinal centres [11].

The end result of germinal-centre activity is the production of plasma cells or more lymphocytes (B2 or memory cells). The paucity of plasma cells in germinal centres has been attributed to the migration of im-

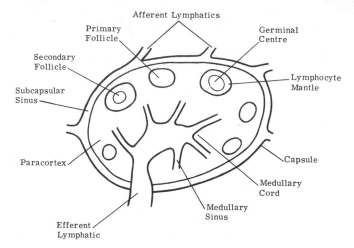

Fig. 24.1. Diagram of a normal lymph node.

munoblasts from germinal centres to the paracortex and medulla in the latter stages of transformation [8].

The *paracortex* lies in between and deep to the lymphoid follicles and is essentially the T-cell zone of the lymph node. It is hypoplastic after thymectomy in experimental animals [12] and in congenital thymic aplasia in children [3]. It contains a high proportion of cells which form E rosettes [4] and bind specific anti-T-cell antisera [5]. Isotopically labelled T cells specifically colonize this area [1], and immune reactions involving the production of sensitized T cells are associated with hyperplasia of this region of the lymph node [6]. Under such conditions lymphocytes at varying stages of transformation to immunoblasts may be

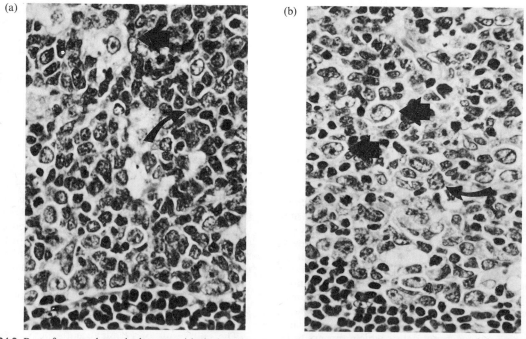

Fig. 24.2. Part of a normal germinal centre with the lymphocyte mantle at the bottom of the picture. In (a) the straight arrow indicates a tingible-body macrophage and the curved arrow a small cleaved cell (centrocyte); in (b) the curved arrow points to a large cleaved cell (centrocyte) and the straight arrows indicate two large non-cleaved cells (one a centroblast and the other an immunoblast in the Keil terminology). (H & E, × 500.)

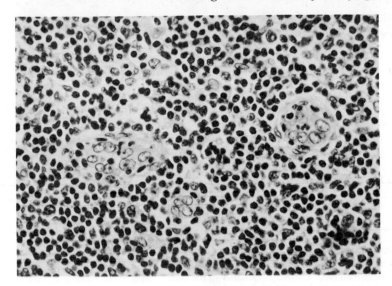

Fig. 24.3. Lymph-node paracortex showing three post-capillary venules. The one on the left shows a considerably elongated cell migrating across the endothelium. (H & E, × 400.)

observed but without the formation of cleaved cells. The paracortex also contains a number of cells which have rather convoluted nuclei and ultrastructurally exhibit numerous fine cytoplasmic processes. They are termed *interdigitating reticulum cells* by Lennert [13] and their function is unknown.

Perhaps the most conspicuous structures in the paracortex are the *post-capillary venules* (Fig. 24.3), which are lined by characteristic cuboidal or columnar endothelial cells. It is between these cells that lymphocytes pass from the blood stream into the substance of the lymph node. The traffic consists mostly of T cells but also includes some B cells and even granulocytes. The lymph-node *medulla* consists of lymphatic *sinuses*

surrounded by the *medullary cords* (Fig. 24.4). The former are lined by flattened cells and usually contain many macrophages together with a number of lymphocytes and plasma cells. These macrophages form part of the mononuclear phagocyte system and are derived from marrow stem cells [14]. They have been shown to phagocytose incoming antigen [15] and in certain reactions may fill and markedly distend the sinusoidal system (sinus histiocytosis). Macrophages may be divided into two sub-populations according to whether Langerhans-cell granules can be demonstrated ultrastructurally in the cytoplasm. These are lysosomal granules containing dense material separated from the granule membrane by a halo-like zone,

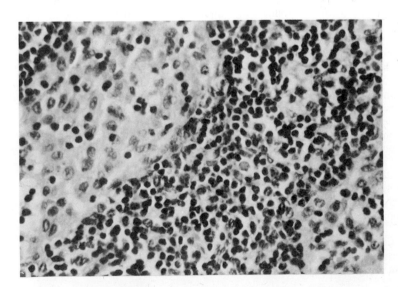

Fig. 24.4. Lymph-node medulla showing a medullary cord flanked by two medullary sinuses filled with histiocytes and a number of lymphocytes and plasma cells. (H & E, × 400.)

and cells containing them are frequently found in the skin or in lymph nodes in dermatopathic lymphadenopathy [16].

The medullary cords consist mainly of mature lymphocytes often mixed with considerable numbers of plasma cells. Reticulin fibre-forming (reticulum) cells are also scattered throughout the various regions of the lymph node, especially in the perivascular areas. Electron microscopy or enzyme histochemical techniques are usually required to demonstrate them.

TECHNIQUES EMPLOYED IN THE EXAMINATION OF LYMPH-NODE BIOPSIES

Lymph nodes should be handled with care as even minor trauma can alter histological appearances. They are best bisected as soon as possible after removal, as this aids penetration of fixative and enables the surface to be used in making touch preparations on glass slides, which may better reveal certain cytological features such as the cytoplasmic lipid inclusions in Burkitt's lymphoma. Good fixation is essential: the most usual fixative is 10% formol saline although better nuclear definition can often be obtained with formal sublimate, Zenker's or Carnoy's fixatives. Although paraffin wax is still the most commonly used embedding medium, resins such as Araldite and methyl methacrylate have recently been tried extensively. Such resin-embedded blocks allow very thin sections to be cut, in which there may be excellent resolution of cellular morphology. It is usually desirable to freeze a portion of the node as frozen sections are required for most enzyme histochemical and immunhistochemical techniques.

Conventional histological stains
The stains most widely used for the demonstration of general morphology are Giemsa and haematoxylin and eosin (H & E). Reticulin stains are useful for the demonstration of nodal architecture and its disturbances. Methyl green pyronin (MGP) is used for the demonstration of cytoplasmic RNA, which is found in high concentration in lymphoblasts, immunoblasts and, most of all, plasma cells. It is a particularly useful stain for the demonstration of plasmacytoid differentiation in malignant lymphomas. Periodic acid Schiff (PAS) is most useful for demonstrating inclusions of glycoprotein IgM in certain tumours such as the well-differentiated lymphocytic lymphomas.

Enzyme techniques
There are usually several different methods for performing the various enzyme histochemical stains

which employ different substrates and slightly different reaction conditions. Most have to be performed on frozen sections, which may be exposed to fixatives to improve enzyme localization. These variations mean that results from one laboratory are not always strictly comparable with those from another. Methodological details will not be discussed here, but references to the techniques used are given.

Non-specific esterase (α-naphthyl acetate esterase). Macrophages in sinusoids and germinal centres, as well as blood monocytes, show strong diffuse cytoplasmic staining [17, 18]. Dendritic reticular cells in germinal centres show a similar diffuse, but weaker, positivity. Mature T cells in blood and lymph nodes usually show a single intense, dot-like perinuclear zone of activity [18, 19] (Fig. 24.5), which is lost in PHA-induced transformation. A minority of thymocytes are weakly positive, suggesting that the enzyme is acquired only in the later stages of thymocyte differentiation [18].

Acid phosphatase. Many of the staining reactions are similar to those of non-specific esterase: monocytes and macrophages show strong, diffuse cytoplasmic staining and mature T cells may exhibit a single dot-like focus of activity [19]. Plasma cells, however, are positive, and dendritic reticular cells negative [17, 19]. The PHA-transformed T cells also show strong acid-phosphatase activity [20] in contrast to non-specific esterase, and fetal thymocytes are strongly positive [21].

Alkaline phosphatase. This has been identified in a population of B lymphocytes present in primary follicles of lymph nodes, and in the mantle zone of secondary follicles [22]. Endothelial cells are also strongly alkaline-phosphatase positive.

Chloroacetate esterase. This is an unusually resistant enzyme which retains its activity in conventional formalin-fixed paraffin-embedded sections [23]. It can easily be demonstrated in cells of the myeloid series and is particularly useful for distinguishing nodal infiltration by acute myeloblastic leukaemia from that of lymphoblastic lymphoma, which may often be very difficult in paraffin-embedded sections.

Terminal deoxynucleotidyl transferase. This nuclear enzyme is not detected by conventional enzyme histochemical techniques, but can be assayed in tissue extracts [24] or demonstrated immunocytochemically. It is present in cortical (but not medullary) thymocytes and in primitive bone-marrow cells, which also bear surface Ia-like antigen [25]. It thus appears to be a

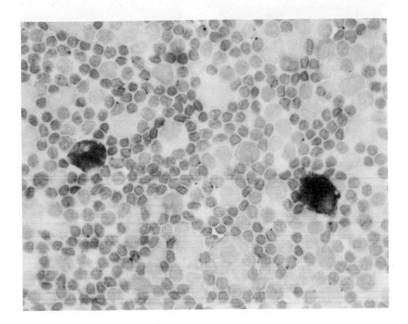

Fig. 24.5. Touch preparation of lymph node stained for non-specific esterase. Histiocytes appear as large cells with diffuse cytoplasmic staining, whereas T lymphocytes exhibit a tiny dot-like, paranuclear zone of activity. (× 490.)

marker of marrow stem cells which persists in early T cells.

Lysozyme. This enzyme may be demonstrated immunocytochemically in many cells, including histiocytes but not lymphocytes. It may thus be of value in distinguishing histiocytes from lymphoid cells [26].

Immunological tests
Lymphocyte membrane receptors are being used with increasing frequency in the investigation of malignant lymphomas. They are usually detected by the ability of cells to bind specific antisera or form rosettes with coated or uncoated red cells. They can be demonstrated in tissue sections by immunocytochemical techniques or in cell suspensions. The latter have the advantage that any adsorbed material can be removed from the cell surface by washing or even stripping with trypsin or pronase; the former, however, are easier to apply and the malignant cell population (which is often intimately mixed with reactive cells) can be identified more easily. The clinical value of these tests in the study of malignant lymphomas has yet to be firmly established, although recent work has indicated their possible value as prognostic indicators [27].

Immunoglobulin. This is bound to the surface of B lymphocytes and germinal-centre cells and is generally assumed to function as receptor for antigen. The most common class of surface immunoglobulin is IgM, followed by IgD; IgG and IgA occur less frequently [28, 29]. Only one type of light chain (κ or λ) is present in the immunoglobulin produced by any given cell, although more than one heavy chain may be identified, usually μ and δ [28].

Malignant lymphomas are usually monoclonal, and therefore express only one light-chain type in their surface immunoglobulin. Reactive lymphoid tissues, on the other hand, are polyclonal and their constituent cells exhibit surface immunoglobulin of both light-chain types (Fig. 24.6). These observations can be used in the differential diagnosis of malignant lymphoma and atypical reactive hyperplasias in lymph nodes. During the process of transformation of B lymphocytes to plasma cells, stainable surface immunoglobulin decreases and eventually becomes undetectable. This is accompanied by a corresponding rise in cytoplasmic secretory immunoglobulin [30, 31].

Complement receptors. These are usually detected by the EAC rosette method, in which cells bearing the receptor form rosettes with red cells sensitized with antibody and complement. Like surface immunoglobulin, complement receptors are present on B lymphocytes and germinal-centre cells [32], but they disappear on transformation to plasma cells. They are also detected on monocytes and histiocytes and early fetal thymocytes [21].

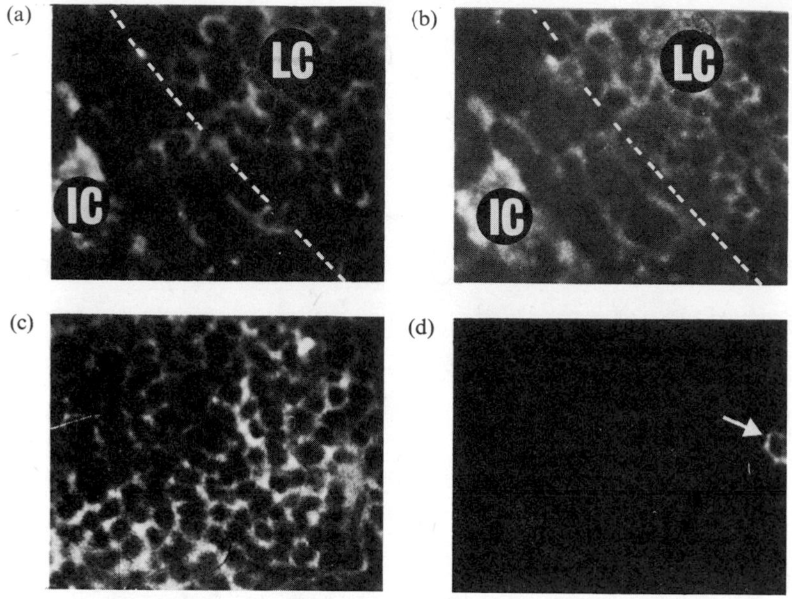

Fig. 24.6. Immunofluorescent staining of lymphoid tissue with anti-λ (a & c) and anti-κ (b & d) light chain antibodies. (a) and (b) show a germinal centre containing immune complexes (IC) surrounded by a lymphocyte mantle or corona (LC). The lymphocytes are polyclonal and exhibit surface immunoglobulin of both light-chain types. (c) and (d) show a malignant lymphoma which exhibits monoclonal staining for λ chains only, with the exception of one (probably normal) κ-positive cell. (Illustration kindly supplied by Dr G. Janossy.)

Fc receptor. This is the receptor for the Fc portion of IgG and may be detected by the ability of cells to bind immune complexes, aggregated immune complexes or aggregated immunoglobulin, or to form rosettes with red cells sensitized with IgG. It is present on B lymphocytes as well as monocytes and histiocytes.

E-rosette phenomenon. Human T lymphocytes possess on their surface membrane a receptor for a naturally occurring surface component of sheep erythrocytes. The ability of cells to form spontaneous rosettes with unsensitized sheep red blood cells is thus used as a marker of T-cell differentiation.

Ia-like (p29,34) (DR) antigen. This surface alloantigen, closely linked genetically to the HLA system, consists of two non-covalently bound glycoprotein subunits of molecular weights 29 000 and 34 000 [33]. The p29,34 complex is referred to as Ia-like in view of its chemical similarities to murine Ia antigens [34]. It is present in primitive bone-marrow cells, B lymphocytes, germinal-centre cells and a subset of T lymphocytes, although most T cells are negative. It is also present on early myeloid cells and monocytes [5, 25, 35]. Like surface immunoglobulin and complement receptor, it is lost when B lymphocytes transform into plasma cells [36].

Anti-T-cell antisera. A number of antisera have been raised to T cells [37, 38]. The human T-lymphocyte antigen (HuTLA) described by Janossy *et al.* [39] is raised in rabbits against monkey thymocytes and can be used immunocytochemically to identify thymocytes and peripheral T lymphocytes in tissue sections. Monoclonal antibodies to T cells and their subsets have recently become commercially available.

Anti-ALL antiserum. This is raised in rabbits to non-T, non-B acute lymphoblastic leukaemia cells [40]. It recognizes primitive marrow stem cells and is lost in early lymphoid differentiation (see Chapter 21).

THE NON-HODGKIN LYMPHOMAS

Classification
The classification of non-Hodgkin lymphomas is one of the most contentious issues in modern pathology. There are at least six major classifications in use at the time of writing, and one recent reviewer of the subject [41] noted that as many as 50 had been proposed in the last 50 years. The lack of any consensus of opinion among the proponents of the modern classifications renders the subject immensely complicated.

Ideally, any classification should fulfil three criteria:
1 it should be easy to apply and the subtypes should be easily recognizable, even by non-experts;
2 it should impart meaningful clinical information on how the disease is likely to behave and to what type of treatment it is likely to respond; and
3 it should not be in conflict with current scientific concepts of the nature of the disease processes.

The *Rappaport classification* (Table 24.1) is the most widely used today and is based on both the cytological appearances and growth pattern of the tumour. The system is easy to apply and has proven clinical applicability [43]. However, the classification has been shown to have some serious faults, many of which have come to light as a result of recent developments in

Table 24.1. The Rappaport classification [42]

Lymphocytic, well differentiated Lymphocytic, poorly differentiated Mixed lymphocytic and histiocytic Histiocytic Undifferentiated	Nodular or diffuse

immunology. Perhaps the most serious objection is to the use of the term 'histiocytic' to describe the large-cell lymphomas; although these cells may resemble histiocytes in tissue sections, they have now been shown to be almost exclusively of lymphoid origin. A few genuine histiocytic lymphomas do exist, but they form only a tiny proportion of the total. The histiocytic group is thus a heterogeneous one and the heterogeneity is compounded by marked morphological variations in the lymphoid types themselves. The system is inappropriate for the classification of childhood lymphoma which, histologically, often tends to be of lymphoblastic type (i.e. isomorphous with acute lymphoblastic leukaemia). Such tumours tend to be included with the poorly differentiated lymphocytic and undifferentiated lesions. The subdivision of tumours of all cell types according to growth pattern is misleading, as only certain cell types are associated with nodularity. These have been called follicular-centre-cell (FCC) lymphomas by Lukes & Collins [8]. The use of the word 'differentiation' has also been criticized as it is usually applied by pathologists to indicate the degree to which a tumour resembles its parent tissue. Poorly differentiated lymphocytes were so called because of their relative lack of resemblance to mature lymphocytes, but it is now recognized that they strongly resemble normal lymphocytes at certain stages of transformation.

Many classifications have been proposed in an attempt to overcome these inadequacies. Two in current use (Lukes & Collins [8] and Kiel [9]) are of a rather detailed and functional nature and attempt to relate the neoplastic cells to normal counterparts. As with any neoplastic-cell population, however, this can only be done to a limited extent. Some consideration will be given to these two classifications because, in spite of their obvious problems of application, they do attempt to embody modern immunological ideas and provide some conceptual understanding of the lesions. The *Lukes–Collins classification* is shown in Table 24.2. The term histiocytic is reserved for tumours of histiocytes only and the heterogeneity of the Rappaport 'histiocytic' group is further reduced by subdividing large-cell lymphomas into four further groups: the large cleaved and non-cleaved FCC lymphomas (so called because of the resemblance of the tumour cells to

Table 24.2. The Lukes–Collins classification [44]

U cell
  (undefined)

T cell
  Small lymphocyte
  Convoluted lymphocyte
  Sézary-mycosis fungoides
  Immunoblastic sarcoma
  Lennert's lymphoma

B cell
  Small lymphocyte
  Plasmacytoid lymphocyte
  Follicular-centre cell (FCC)
    small cleaved
    large cleaved
    small transformed (non-cleaved)
    large transformed (non-cleaved)
  Immunoblastic sarcoma
  Hairy-cell leukaemia

Histiocytic

the corresponding normal follicular-centre cells), and the T and B immunoblastic sarcomas (so called because of the resemblance to immunoblasts). Well-differentiated lymphocytic lymphomas are divided into T and B small-lymphocyte categories and the latter further subdivided into those with and without plasmacytoid differentiation. Tumours with lymphoblastic histology appear as the T-cell convoluted lymphocyte and B-cell small non-cleaved FCC types. Poorly differentiated lymphocytic and mixed-cell lymphomas appear as small cleaved, large cleaved and non-cleaved FCC lymphomas, depending on the relative proportions of the different cell types present. Mycosis fungoides, Lennert's lymphoma and hairy-cell leukaemia are also included. Such a classification is thus very comprehensive, overcomes many of the objections to Rappaport's classification, and attempts to impart functional as well as morphological information. However, it has also received much criticism. First, it is difficult to apply, requiring considerable expertise and very high quality sections to identify precisely all the cell types. Secondly, the classification is primarily functional (i.e. T, B, etc.), although it is based on morphological criteria. There is, thus, the implicit assertion that it is possible to determine whether neoplastic cells are T, B or histiocytic on morphological grounds alone, and this is not always the case. Thirdly, growth pattern is not taken into account, as Lukes & Collins argue that prognosis is only related to nodularity through its association with certain cell types, i.e. FCC. However, it has been claimed by others [45] that nodular FCC lymphomas of each cell type have a more favourable prognosis than their diffuse counterparts. Furthermore, growth pattern is a more objective way of categorizing lymphomas than by the rather subtle variations in cellular morphology. The convoluted lymphocyte category has been criticized as not all cases exhibit nuclear convolutions and the small non-cleaved category, which consists largely of Burkitt's lymphoma, seems to be inappropriately grouped with the FCC lymphomas. Although there is some evidence that the small non-cleaved tumours arise from germinal centres [46], they occur in a younger age group, have a poorer prognosis and do not exhibit the same mixture of cell types as the other FCC lymphomas. The undefined group contains tumours which cannot be categorized as T, B, etc. and perhaps ought to contain all those tumours which are 'null' on marker studies. This group has the same problem of heterogeneity as Rappaport's histiocytic category.

The *Kiel classification* is shown in Table 24.3. Like the Lukes–Collins classification it is comprehensive and functionally orientated but it is similarly difficult to apply for the non-expert and requires high-quality histological sections. It differs in being primarily

Table 24.3. The Kiel classification [9]

Low-grade malignancy
ML—lymphocytic (CLL, hairy-cell leukaemia and others)
ML—lymphoplasmacytoid (immunocytic)
ML—centrocytic
ML—centroblastic-centrocytic
     follicular*
     follicular* and diffuse
     diffuse*

High-grade malignancy
ML—centroblastic
ML—lymphoblastic
     Burkitt type
     convoluted-cell type
     others
ML—immunoblastic

---

* With or without sclerosis.
ML, malignant lymphoma.

descriptive and does not commit the pathologist to designate lesions as T or B cell without data from immunological studies. Growth pattern is recognized as a valuable feature and tumours of lymphoblastic histology are grouped together. Well-differentiated lymphocytic lymphomas are similarly divided into lymphocytic and lymphoplasmacytoid types but the lymphocytic type also includes hairy-cell leukaemia. Centrocytes are essentially the same as cleaved cells, both large and small, and centroblasts are a type of large non-cleaved FCC. Lymphomas are only designated as centroblastic if they can be shown to have evolved from centrocytic-centroblastic lesions and the remainder (and majority) of large-cell lymphomas are thus designated immunoblastic. The term immunoblastic is thus not used in the same sense as in the Lukes–Collins classification and the group is more heterogeneous.

The *classifications of Bennett* et al. *and Dorfman* (Tables 24.4 and 24.5) show many similarities, es-

Table 24.4. The classification of Bennett *et al.* [47]

Follicular lymphomas	
Follicle cell, predominantly small	
Follicle cell, mixed small and large	
Follicle cell, predominantly large	
Diffuse lymphomas	Grade 1
Lymphocytic, well differentiated (small round lymphocyte)	
Lymphocytic, intermediate differentiation (small follicle cell)	
Lymphocytic, poorly differentiated	
Mixed small lymphoid and undifferentiated large cell	
Undifferentiated large cell	Grade 2
Plasma cell	
True histiocyte	
Unclassified	

Plasmacytoid differentiation in lymphocytic tumours, and banded or fine sclerosis are recorded

pecially in their primary subdivision into follicular and diffuse types, thus recognizing that only lymphomas of certain cytologic subtypes have the capacity to grow in a nodular fashion. Terminology is descriptive and functional terms such as 'immunoblast' are avoided. Both classifications are relatively easy to apply. The classification of Bennett *et al.* uses the terms 'well differentiated' and 'poorly differentiated' in the same way as Rappaport, and is thus open to the same criticisms. There is also no special provision for those tumours of lymphoblastic histology.

The *WHO classification* (Table 24.6) was published

Table 24.5. The Dorfman classification [48]

Follicular lymphomas
  (Follicular or follicular and diffuse)
  Small lymphoid
  Mixed small and large lymphoid
  Large lymphoid

Diffuse lymphomas
  Small lymphocytic
  Atypical small lymphoid
  Lymphoblastic
    convoluted
      non-convoluted
  Large lymphoid
  Mixed small and large lymphoid
  Histiocytic
  Burkitt's lymphoma
  Mycosis fungoides
  Undefined

two to three years after the four which have just been discussed, and, like the last two classifications, primarily divides lesions into nodular and diffuse. It is relatively concise and easy to apply, but uses confusing terminology: lymphosarcoma is an old-fashioned term that means lymphoma to some pathologists and lymphocytic lymphoma to others; prolymphocytes are cleaved cells or centrocytes, and not the same cells as described in the prolymphocytic leukaemia by Galton *et al.* [50]; reticulosarcoma is a fibre-forming lymphoma and should not be confused with reticulum-cell sarcoma, the old, general, term for large-cell lymphomas.

No classification is entirely satisfactory and all have disadvantages and inconsistencies. Most lymphomas,

Table 24.6. The WHO classification [49]

Lymphosarcomas
  Nodular lymphosarcoma
    Prolymphocytic
    Prolymphocytic, lymphoblastic
  Diffuse lymphosarcoma
    Lymphocytic
    Lymphoplasmacytic
    Prolymphocytic
    Lymphoblastic
    Immunoblastic
    Burkitt's tumour
Mycosis fungoides
Plasmacytoma
Reticulosarcoma
Unclassified malignant lymphomas

however, appear to fall into three major categories:
1 those composed of relatively mature cells (lymphocytes, plasma cells or lymphoplasmacytoid cells);
2 those composed of lymphoblasts; and
3 the majority, which are composed of cells resembling those found in normal germinal centres.

The choice of classification is clearly a dilemma and the creation of a further one would only add to the confusion. That of Rappaport is still the most widely used but it is unacceptable in its original form. However, Rappaport has suggested alterations to his original classification [51], and recent communications from his laboratory [52] have used a modified form as shown in Table 24.7. The adoption of this modified Rappaport classification seems a useful compromise for the purpose of discussing the individual lymphoma subtypes in this chapter.

Table 24.7. Rappaport classification (modified) [52]

Nodular and/or diffuse
  Poorly differentiated lymphocytic
  Mixed
  Burkitt's
  Undifferentiated non-Burkitt's
  'Histiocytic'

Diffuse
  Well-differentiated lymphocytic
  WDL with plasmacytoid differentiation
  Intermediate lymphocytic
  Immunoblastic
  Lymphoblastic
  NHL of 'Lennert's' type
  Mycosis fungoides
  Plasmacytoma
  Unclassifiable

Composite
Malignant histiocytosis

HISTOLOGICAL SUBTYPES ACCORDING TO THE MODIFIED RAPPAPORT CLASSIFICATION

Well-differentiated lymphocytic lymphoma
This group includes lymphomas of the small lymphocytic (T and B) and plasmacytoid lymphocyte types of Lukes & Collins, and the lymphocytic and lymphoplasmacytoid (immunocytic) types of the Kiel classification. Lennert [53] also includes hairy-cell leukaemia, Sézary syndrome and mycosis fungoides under the lymphocytic heading, but these will be discussed separately. Histologically, the lymph-node architecture is replaced by a diffuse, monomorphic infiltrate of lymphoid cells (Fig. 24.7) although the capsule often remains intact. The cells are round, have a high

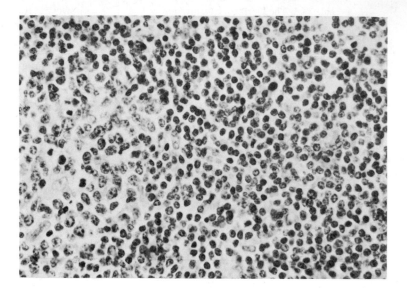

Fig. 24.7. Well-differentiated lympho-cytic lymphoma. Most of the tumour is composed of cells virtually indis-tinguishable from normal lymphocytes (right). Part of a proliferation centre is seen on the left. (H & E, × 400.)

nucleo-cytoplasmic ratio and are virtually in-distinguishable from normal lymphocytes although they may be a little larger. Interspersed among these small cells, however, is a minority population of larger, more cohesive, dividing cells, about twice the size of lymphocytes with vesicular nuclei. These cells are surrounded by others of intermediate appearance forming *pseudofollicular zones* or *proliferation centres*. Mitoses are frequently found in these areas in contrast to the remainder of the tumour.

The lymphoplasmacytoid variant exhibits essen-tially similar histological appearances except for the presence of a variable proportion of plasma cells and lymphoplasmacytoid cells which, as their name sug-gests, are intermediate in appearance between lympho-cytes and plasma cells. In most cases, the cells contain intracytoplasmic and intranuclear, PAS-positive, dias-tase-resistant, globular inclusions which are generally thought to represent retained IgM [53]. About 90% of patients with well-differentiated lymphocytic lym-phoma and associated monoclonal gammopathy exhibit this type of histology [54].

The great majority of well-differentiated lymphocy-tic lymphomas, like chronic lymphocytic leukaemias, are B-cell tumours expressing surface immunoglobu-lin, complement and Fc receptors and Ia-like antigen [55–59], although not as strongly as in normal lympho-cytes. Furthermore, their expression is variable from tumour to tumour, and as different markers are independently affected, several different phenotypes are possible [57]. A small proportion of cases may exhibit T-cell characteristics, with E-rosette formation and a high content of cytoplasmic acid phosphatase

[60]. The cells may be somewhat larger than in B-cell lesions and usually contain cytoplasmic azurophil granules.

Poorly differentiated lymphocytic lymphoma
This type is composed of cells which are larger than mature lymphocytes but smaller than histiocyte nuclei and are still recognizably lymphocytic. Most are composed of small cleaved cells or centrocytes which are morphologically similar to those observed in normal germinal centres (Fig. 24.8). It is for this reason that Lukes & Collins refer to this lesion as a FCC lymphoma. Further evidence of origin from lymphoid follicles is provided by the nodular growth pattern which is frequently observed (Fig. 24.9), and by the presence of dendritic reticulum cells in many cases [53]. Surface-marker studies also reveal similarities with normal germinal-centre cells (see below).

In addition to the small cleaved cells, these lesions contain a population of larger follicular-centre cells which vary in numbers from case to case and are found particularly within the nodules of the nodular sub-types. These cells form the so-called 'histiocytic' component of the tumours, and if they exceed about 30% of the total cell number the lesion falls into the mixed-cell category [61]. The term 'histiocyte' in this context is unfortunate, not only because it is a misnomer but because it describes a morphologically heterogeneous group of follicular-centre cells. Increase in the large-cell component is paralleled by an increase in mitotic figures and cellular proliferation rate [62].

The great majority of cases of poorly differentiated lymphocytic lymphomas are of B-cell origin, exhibit-

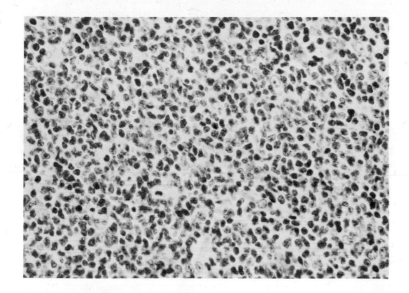

Fig. 24.8. Poorly differentiated lymphocytic lymphoma. The majority of cells are of the small cleaved type similar to those seen in normal germinal centres. (H & E, × 400.)

ing surface immunoglobulin as well as complement and Fc receptors and Ia-like antigen [56–59]. Several phenotypes are possible, as in well-differentiated lymphocytic lymphoma.

Intermediate lymphocytic lymphoma

This tumour exhibits morphological features intermediate between those of the well-differentiated and poorly differentiated types. The cells are slightly larger than normal lymphocytes, have a very high nucleocytoplasmic ratio and exhibit round-to-oval and often slightly clefted nuclei. The proliferation is usually diffuse but may exhibit a vaguely nodular pattern. Surface immunoglobulin and complement receptors have been demonstrated on the cells, and some also exhibit alkaline-phosphatase activity [63]. For this reason, it has been suggested that these lymphomas are derived from lymphocytes in the mantle zones of lymphoid follicles.

Mixed-cell lymphoma

Fortunately, the term mixed-cell lymphoma seems to

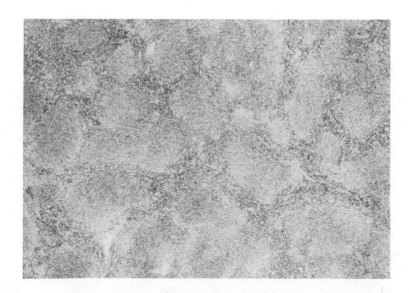

Fig. 24.9. Nodular lymphoma of the poorly differentiated lymphocytic type. (H & E, × 30.)

be replacing mixed lymphocytic and histiocytic lymphoma, as the large-cell component of these tumours is of lymphoid and not histiocytic origin. Furthermore, the large cells are generally thought to be of the same lineage as the small cells but at different stages of transformation. The histological appearances and surface-marker characteristics of most of these tumours are identical to those described for poorly differentiated lymphocytic lymphoma, although the population of large cells is higher, between about 30 and 50% [61] (Fig. 24.10). As a certain proportion of large cells is almost invariably present with the nodules of the nodular FCC lymphomas, it is not surprising that most of the tumours ascribed to the mixed-cell category exhibit a nodular growth pattern.

'Histiocytic' lymphoma

In view of the extensive modifications which have been made to Rappaport's classification, it is surprising that the term 'histiocytic' is retained to describe a group of tumours which are almost entirely lymphoid in origin. With the exclusion of the immunoblastic sarcomas, the group is less heterogeneous than it was originally, and now mainly consists of the large (cleaved and non-cleaved) FCC lymphomas. A minority of lymphomas of true histiocytic lineage which do not exhibit the characteristics of the histiocytoses also have to be included. Such tumours are very rare and are difficult to recognize in conventional sections. Indented nuclei, copious cytoplasm and phagocytosis are helpful features but enzyme histochemical and surface-marker techniques are usually required. The cells exhibit strong, diffuse, non-specific esterase and acid-phos-phatase activity and may have complement and Fc receptors. An ability to phagocytose may be demonstrated *in vitro* [63, 64].

Most of the remaining 'histiocytic' lymphomas appear to be of FCC origin and may exhibit mixtures of different FCC types. They are placed in the 'histiocytic' category when the proportion of large cells exceeds 50% [61]. There is a tendency for nodularity to be lost as the proportion of large cells increases past a certain point, and most 'histiocytic' lymphomas are thus usually diffuse in character. Not surprisingly, most of the tumours are B-cell in type [27, 59], but a small minority exhibit T-cell characteristics and some are non-T, non-B [27].

Immunoblastic sarcoma

This neoplasm is so called because the predominant cells resemble the immunoblasts found in normal lymphoid tissue. As the precise morphological definition of an immunoblast depends on the system of terminology used, and as they are difficult to distinguish from large non-cleaved cells, factors other than the histological appearances of the predominant cells should be taken into account when making the diagnosis. A mixture of cleaved cells suggests a lesion of FCC origin which should be placed in the 'histiocytic' group. Most malignant lymphomas arising in the course of lymphoproliferative disorders such as α-chain disease, angioimmunoblastic lymphadenopathy and Sjögren's syndrome are immunoblastic sarcomas [65].

Immunoblastic sarcomas may be B cell, T cell or 'null', as judged by the presence of surface immunoglo-

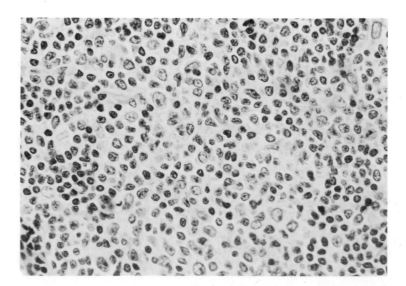

Fig. 24.10. Mixed-cell lymphoma. The lesion is composed mostly of large and small cleaved and non-cleaved cells. The large cells comprise 30–50% of the total. (H & E, ×400.)

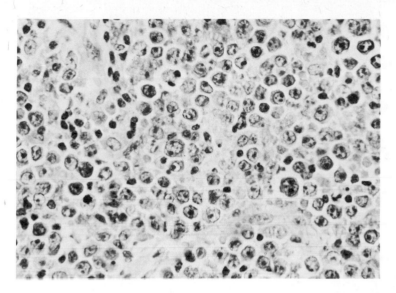

Fig. 24.11. Immunoblastic sarcoma. The larger cells resemble immunoblasts and the smaller ones exhibit plasmacytoid differentiation with eccentric nuclei. (H & E, × 400.)

bulin, complement receptors or the ability to form E rosettes [27, 58, 64, 66]. The most convincing morphological evidence of a B-cell immunoblastic sarcoma is the presence of plasmacytoid differentiation (Fig. 24.11), and the absence of this can make the diagnosis difficult. A small number of T-cell immunoblastic sarcomas have been described which may have rather characteristic histological features [66], being characterized by a diffuse pleomorphic infiltrate divided into small microscopic compartments by delicate collagenous septa. Small capillary-size blood vessels may be prominent and the neoplastic cells themselves show wide variation in size with appreciable nuclear folding and hyperlobation. A population of reactive epithelioid histiocytes may be present.

Lymphoblastic lymphoma

These tumours are composed of cells smaller than those of histiocytic lymphoma and isomorphous with those of acute lymphoblastic leukaemia (Fig. 24.12). They are divided into convoluted and non-convoluted types. The distinction between the two subtypes, however, is not clear-cut. In 1975, Barcos & Lukes [67] drew attention to a type of lymphoma characterized by a diffuse proliferation of non-cohesive blast-like cells which frequently extended outside the lymph-node capsule. The cell cytoplasm was very scanty and non-pyroninophilic, and the nucleus large and convoluted. Chromatin was finely distributed and nucleoli barely perceptible. The need for high-quality sections in the identification of these cells was stressed. Cell size varied from that of a histiocyte nucleus to that of a small lymphocyte and the proportion of large and small cells varied from case to case. Mitoses were

frequent and tended to increase with increasing proportions of large cells. Tingible-body macrophages were present in a number of cases, but were usually few, and a starry-sky pattern was only rarely observed. The tumour was found to occur predominantly in children and adolescents, who were frequently leukaemic either on presentation or later in the course of the disease. Survival was only 10 months on average. As most patients had a mediastinal (presumably thymic) mass, and as germinal centres were spared in early nodal lesions, it was suggested that the lesion might be a T-cell lymphoma possibly derived from cortical thymocytes. The T-cell nature of the lesion was later confirmed by the demonstration of E-rosette-forming ability and focal cytoplasmic acid-phosphatase activity [68]. Rather surprisingly, complement receptors have also been detected on these cells, but the simultaneous expression of receptors for complement and sheep red blood cells is a feature of immature thymocytes between 10 and 15 weeks' gestation [68]. More recent morphological studies, however, have demonstrated that nuclear convolution is not a consistent feature of this tumour and, even when present, may be confined to a minority of cells [69]. This view is supported by Lennert *et al.* [53], who found focal cytoplasmic acid-phosphatase activity to be a more reliable indicator of this type of lymphoma.

A further small subgroup of lymphoblastic lymphoma has recently been shown [57, 70] to have the same phenotype as common acute lymphoblastic leukaemia (see Chapter 21).

Burkitt's lymphoma

This tumour was first described as a commonly

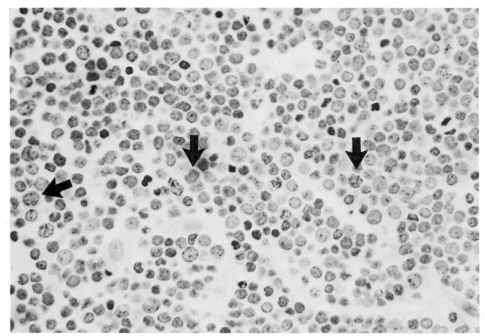

Fig. 24.12. Lymphoblastic lymphoma. There is a diffuse proliferation of uncohesive blast-like cells showing marked variation in cell size. A minority of cells show nuclear convolution (arrows). (H & E, × 500.)

occurring sarcoma of the jaw in East African children [71], and later identified as a malignant lymphoma [72]. Tumours of identical histological appearance were subsequently reported in non-African countries [73, 74], but with a much lower frequency. The tumour has now been defined as a histological and cytological entity [75] but the endemic cases occurring in Africa and Papua-New Guinea differ in certain respects from the sporadic ones in other parts of the world such as Europe and America. Although both types tend to involve extra-nodal structures, the incidence of jaw tumours is not as high in the sporadic type, in which intra-abdominal disease is more common [73, 74, 76]. Sporadic cases also exhibit a slightly later age peak [77] and a lower incidence of long-term relapses after treatment [76], though overall survival rates seem to be similar [76–78]. The relationship of the endemic and sporadic forms to the Epstein–Barr virus is clearly different, however.

Histologically, there is a proliferation of monotonous, cohesive cells resembling lymphoblasts in size and shape (Fig. 24.13). The nuclei are uniform, round, have a prominent nuclear membrane and two to five small nucleoli. The cytoplasm is scarce but strongly pyroninophilic and frequently contains small droplets of neutral lipid. Mitoses are frequent and there is an admixture of tingible-body macrophages producing the classical starry-sky appearance. The growth pattern of both Burkitt's lymphoma and the undifferentiated non-Burkitt lymphoma is almost invariably diffuse. A nodular picture usually results from multiple foci of early disease involving lymphoid follicles (see below), rather than from the intrinsic ability of the tumour to infiltrate in a nodular fashion as in the FCC lymphomas. The tumour cells are B cells bearing surface immunoglobulin (usually of the IgM class) [46, 79], and sometimes Fc and complement receptors. Histochemical stains for alkaline phosphatase, non-specific esterase and acid phosphatase are negative although acid phosphatase may be demonstrated in small quantities if very sensitive methods are used [75].

The tumour is classified by Lukes & Collins as a small non-cleaved FCC lymphoma. Although clinically and pathologically different from other FCC lymphomas, the observation that germinal centres may be selectively involved in early nodal infiltration [46] lends some support to this contention; it certainly supports the B-cell nature of the lesion.

Undifferentiated non-Burkitt lymphoma

In the past, Burkitt's lymphoma and lymphoblastic lymphoma have been termed undifferentiated [42, 69], but since the recognition of these two types as separate entities, very few lymphomas are now classified as

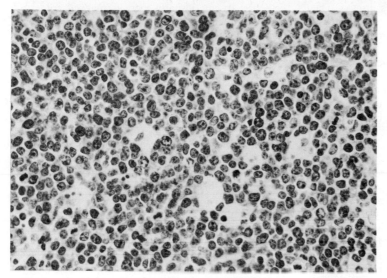

Fig. 24.13. Burkitt's lymphoma. There is a monotonous proliferation of blast-like cells interspersed with a few tingible-body macrophages. The latter have such copious cytoplasm that the nucleus is not always included in the section. (H & E, × 400.)

such, and in one recent series they comprised less than one per cent of lymphomas [61]. The tumour cells differ from those of Burkitt's lymphoma by showing considerable variation in cell size and nuclear shape [80], although mitotic figures and tingible-body macrophages may be numerous. The cell cytoplasm shows variable pyroninophilia, the nuclei are vesicular and usually contain a single prominent nucleolus. The cells may thus resemble those of many 'histiocytic' lymphomas but are distinguished by their smaller size.

Lennert's lymphoma
This was described by Lennert & Mestdagh [81] as a variant of Hodgkin's disease, but later recognized [53]

to be a type of non-Hodgkin lymphoma and termed 'lymphoepithelioid cellular lymphoma'. Subsequent authors [82–84] have referred to it as malignant lymphoma with a high content of epithelioid histiocytes, or *Lennert's lymphoma*. The lesion is characterized by a diffuse infiltrate of small and large cells which frequently breach the lymph-node capsule. The small cells often show slight nuclear irregularity, but no true clefting as in poorly differentiated lymphocytic lymphoma. The large cells may be mononuclear or multinucleate and frequently resemble Reed–Sternberg cells. The presence of numerous epithelioid histiocytes forming granulomata as well as eosinophils, neutrophils and plasma cells (Fig. 24.14) may

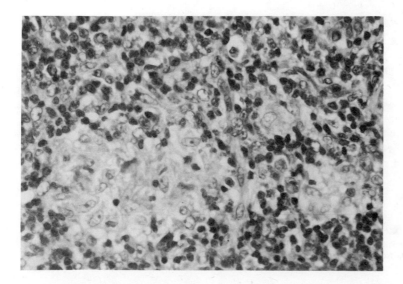

Fig. 24.14. Lennert's lymphoma. There is a small histiocyte granuloma on the left of the illustration and a smaller one to the right. The tumour shows a mixed-cell population and there are two multinucleate cells somewhat resembling Reed–Sternberg cells between the granulomata. (H & E, × 400.)

enhance the resemblance to Hodgkin's disease. The key to the distinction between the two lesions, however, rests with the identification of the small lymphoid cells in Lennert's lymphoma as an atypical and neoplastic, rather than a normal and reactive, population as in Hodgkin's disease. One study of three cases [85] showed that the neoplastic cells formed E rosettes and Lukes & Collins include this neoplasm in their T-lymphoma group; a minority of cases, however, may contain cleaved or plasmacytoid cells indicative of B-cell origin [86].

Mycosis fungoides and Sézary's syndrome

Mycosis fungoides involves the skin primarily and predominantly and evolves through three clinical and pathological stages [87]; these may overlap each other and may be present at the same time in different areas. In the first *erythematous* or *premycotic stage*, there may be only an inflammatory infiltrate in the upper dermis, making it impossible to arrive at a firm histological diagnosis. Careful examination, however, may reveal the presence of a number of neoplastic cells in some cases. In the second *plaque* or *infiltrative stage*, the picture is usually diagnostic. There is diffuse infiltration of the upper portions of the dermis and the epidermis by neoplastic cells which consist largely of small irregular lymphoid—mycosis fungoides (MF)—cells (Fig. 24.15). Histiocytes, eosinophils, plasma cells, neutrophils and fibroblasts may also be present. The polymorphism of the infiltrate may be reminiscent of Hodgkin's disease but Reed–Sternberg

cells are absent. Usually there is marked epidermal infiltration, with small intraepidermal collections of tumour cells surrounded by a clear halo known as Pautrier micro-abscesses. In the third or *tumour stage*, the picture becomes more monomorphous and more dominated by the neoplastic cells. These are more extensive masses of cutaneous tumour which may infiltrate deeply into the subcutaneous tissue, or superficially to produce ulceration. The neoplastic cells are small with a high nucleo-cytoplasmic ratio and a highly convoluted hyperchromatic nucleus. Functional studies show that they are T cells which form E rosettes [88] and react with specific anti-T-cell antisera [59]. Enzyme histochemical studies show paranuclear cytoplasmic acid-phosphatase activity [89].

Although MF primarily affects the skin, most patients also show some extracutaneous involvement, at least in the advanced stages of the disease [90]. The extracutaneous lesions have an identical histological appearance to those of the skin, and the organs most frequently involved are: lymph nodes, lung, spleen, liver, kidney, thyroid, pancreas, bone marrow and heart.

Sézary's syndrome [91] consists of chronic leukaemia and erythrodermia and is characterized by atypical cells in the skin and peripheral blood. There is a strong case for regarding Sézary's syndrome and MF as variants of the same disease process: the cells in both conditions have been shown to be T cells [88, 92], with identical morphological appearances [88]. Furthermore, the skin lesions of Sézary's syndrome may be

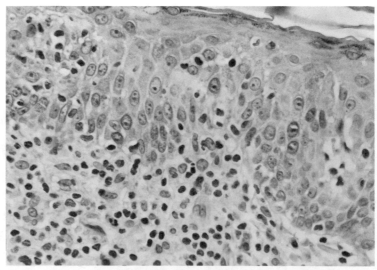

Fig. 24.15. Mycosis fungoides. The upper dermis and epidermis are infiltrated by small lymphoid cells with an irregular outline. Two rather loosely formed Pautrier micro-abscesses are seen within the epidermis on the right and left of the photograph. (H & E, ×400.)

identical to those of MF [87], and many cases of MF are found to have neoplastic cells in the blood, especially if buffy-coat samples are examined [93].

Other cutaneous lymphomas

Other lymphomas involving the skin may do so either primarily or secondarily and exhibit histological appearances identical to those arising in lymph nodes. They do not exhibit the same predilection for epidermal infiltration as MF and the tumour masses tend to occupy the lower dermis and subcutaneous tissue.

Plasmacytoma

This neoplasm is cytologically identical to multiple myeloma (Chapter 19) but limited to one osseous site. Full investigations are thus required to exclude multiple myeloma. Extra-osseous plasmacytomas may also occur, the most frequent sites being the upper respiratory tract and oral cavity [94], where they often present as polypoid tumours. Although initially localized, plasmacytomas usually progress into systemic myelomatosis after an interval of unpredictable duration.

OTHER LYMPHOMAS

Hairy-cell leukaemia
(see also Chapter 23)
There is some dispute about this lesion being regarded as a malignant lymphoma. It is not included in most classifications but does feature in that of the Kiel group, where it appears as a variety of lymphocytic lymphoma, and in that of Lukes & Collins, where it appears as a separate B-cell lymphoma. Lymph-node involvement tends to be an uncommon and late feature of the disease and the organs usually infiltrated are the bone marrow, liver and spleen [95, 96]. In histological sections, the infiltrating cells exhibit a distinctive monotonous appearance with round or oval nuclei and inconspicuous nucleoli. Mitoses are infrequent. The nuclei are similar in size to those of small lymphoid cells, but the cells of hairy-cell leukaemia are easily distinguished from the latter by their abundant clear cytoplasm (Fig. 24.16a). The characteristic cytoplasmic hairy projections which give the disease its name cannot be seen in paraffin-embedded sections by conventional light microscopy, but are readily observed in electron micrographs. Ribosomal-lamellar complexes may also be seen in the cytoplasm of the tumour cells on electron microscopy and are a useful diagnostic feature [97]. The electron microscope is thus a valuable tool in the diagnosis of this disease (Fig. 24.17).

Infiltration of the bone marrow is usually accompanied by a marked increase in reticulin fibres which makes aspiration difficult (Fig. 24.16b). The cells usually exhibit cytoplasmic acid-phosphatase activity.

Mediterranean lymphoma

This is a distinctive lymphoma which was first described in Israel [98]. Although most cases have been observed in the Middle East, not all have been confined to the Mediterranean area and examples have been recorded in other countries such as South Africa

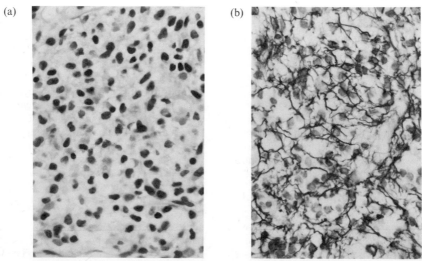

(a) (b)

Fig. 24.16. Hairy-cell leukaemia. (a) The tumour cells have small ovoid nuclei with abundant cytoplasm. (H & E, × 500.) (b) Same field as (a) stained for reticulin fibres (× 400).

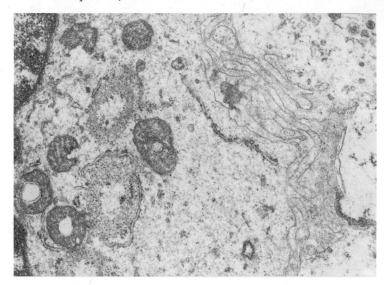

Fig. 24.17. Electron micrograph of hairy-cell leukaemia. Two ribosomal-lamellar complexes are seen on the left of the picture and interdigitating cytoplasmic 'hairy' projections are seen on the right ($\times 21\,600$).

[99] and the USA [100]. The patients tend to be younger than those with 'Western' lymphoma and usually have a history of malabsorption. The tumours tend to occur in the upper jejunum and duodenum rather than the lower ileum, which is the most frequent small-intestinal location for 'Western' lymphomas. The adjacent small intestine exhibits characteristic changes consisting of intense plasma-cell and lymphocyte infiltration associated with mucosal thickening and blunting of villi. Some patients with these histological appearances have detectable levels of α heavy chains in their serum and are then said to have α-chain disease. The lymphomas tend to have a distinctive polymorphic appearance with mixtures of large and small lymphoid cells, often exhibiting plasmacytoid differentiation. Multinucleate cells somewhat resembling Reed–Sternberg cells may also be seen [99–101].

SCLEROSIS IN MALIGNANT LYMPHOMAS

Although more usually associated with Hodgkin's disease, sclerosis may also be seen in a minority of non-Hodgkin lymphomas. There may be a nodular-sclerosing growth pattern similar to that seen in many cases of Hodgkin's disease [102], or the fibrosis may be of a more diffuse nature [103]. It is usually found in tumours of histiocytic or mixed-cell type and is probably associated with an improved prognosis.

EXTRANODAL LYMPHOMAS

Malignant lymphomas not infrequently arise from organs outside the lymphoid system. Some of these are specific histological subtypes such as MF, hairy-cell leukaemia and plasmacytoma, which involve specific organs. Most, however, exhibit appearances similar to

those seen in lymph nodes, and large-cell lymphomas are the most common. The organs most frequently involved are the gastro-intestinal tract, connective tissues, skin, thyroid, bone, testis, salivary glands, lung and breast [104].

INVOLVEMENT OF THE BONE MARROW AND BLOOD BY NON-HODGKIN LYMPHOMA

Bone-marrow infiltration by malignant lymphoma is more likely to occur in the later stages of disease, more often detected in bone-marrow biopsies than in aspirates [105], and depends on the histological type of the lymphoma. These three factors help to explain the wide variations in reported incidence of bone-marrow involvement. Lymphomas of the well, intermediate and poorly differentiated lymphocytic types often exhibit marrow infiltration and neoplastic cells are not infrequently identified in the blood [54, 106, 107]. The distinction between well-differentiated lymphocytic lymphoma and chronic lymphocytic leukaemia may thus become rather blurred, especially as the cells are identical, not only morphologically but also with respect to surface markers [55], and it could be argued that both are merely different clinical expressions of the same disease process. Stein *et al.* [106] categorized patients with lymph-node and marrow infiltration by well-differentiated lymphocytes as chronic lymphocytic leukaemia when the blood lymphocyte count exceeded $5 \times 10^9/l$.

It may sometimes be difficult to distinguish infiltrates of the lymphocytic lymphomas from normal lymphoid follicles in the marrow. The latter are small, rounded structures situated in the marrow fat, whereas the former are usually larger, irregular in outline and tend to 'hug' the bony trabeculae (Fig. 24.18). Tumours of the lymphoblastic type also exhibit a high frequency of marrow infiltration [67], and again the distinction between lymphoma and leukaemia sometimes proves difficult. Most acute lymphoblastic leukaemias are composed of cells which are non-T, non-B in type, however [108], and these account for only a small proportion of lymphoblastic lymphomas, which are usually composed of T cells [70]. Burkitt's lymphoma is also a tumour of lymphoblasts, but of B-cell type. Here bone-marrow involvement is uncommon, at least in the early stages, but, as in other lymphomas, becomes more frequent in the later stages of the disease [75, 76]. Small numbers of tumour cells are occasionally found in the blood but there is rarely any alteration of the leucocyte count.

Mixed-cell and 'histiocytic' lymphomas invade the marrow less often than those of lymphocytic type and cells are only infrequently found in the blood, usually in the terminal phases of the disease. In Lennert's lymphoma, bone-marrow infiltration usually presents as multifocal aggregates of atypical cells similar to those seen in the lymph nodes, although the epithelioid-cell component may sometimes predominate, giving the false impression of non-neoplastic granulomas [83].

'COMPOSITE' LYMPHOMAS

The term 'composite lymphoma' has been used to describe histologically different lymphomas occurring in the same patient, in the same or different tissue at the same or different times. The recognition of a lymphoma as composite clearly depends on the classification employed. For example, a lesion of mixed large cleaved follicular-centre-cell and immunoblastic sarcoma types could be described as composite using the Lukes–Collins classification, but would be described consistently as diffuse histiocytic lymphoma under the old Rappaport scheme. Composite lesions may represent two or more histogenetically different tumours arising in the same host or shifts in the degree of differentiation of transformation of the cells within the same tumour. Immunohistochemical studies on B-cell lesions have shown the latter to be the more usual explanation by demonstrating immunoglobulin of similar light- and heavy-chain types in the morphologically dissimilar areas. Immunoglobulin of similar type has even been demonstrated in cases of non-Hodgkin lymphoma combined with multiple myeloma or even Hodgkin's disease [109].

THE HISTIOCYTOSES

Neoplasia of histiocytes may take the form of monocytic or myelomonocytic leukaemia, true histiocytic lymphoma or histiocytosis. The last of these can be divided into two major groups: histiocytosis X (differentiated progressive histiocytosis) and malignant histiocytosis.

HISTIOCYTOSIS X

This is a triad of related diseases: eosinophilic granuloma, Hand–Schüller–Christian syndrome and Letterer–Siwe disease. All are characterized by the proliferation of well-differentiated, benign-appearing histiocytes which usually contain Langerhans-cell granules [16]. The justification for including all three

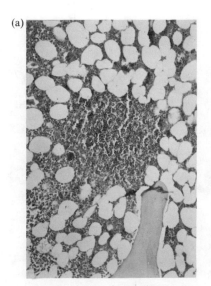
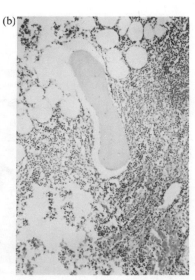

Fig. 24.18. (a) Normal lymphoid follicle in bone marrow. (b) Large irregular zone of lymphomatous marrow infiltration exhibiting a tendency to hug the bony trabecula. (H & E, × 75.)

diseases under the same general heading of histiocytosis X rests with the not infrequent identification of transitional forms which do not fit any of the types precisely. On the other hand, typical examples of the different categories differ markedly from each other in their clinical manifestations and prognosis. In the authors' experience, the main overlap is between eosinophilic granuloma and the Hand–Schüller–Christian syndrome; Letterer–Siwe disease is usually easily separated into a different category.

Eosinophilic granuloma

This is the most benign of the three and classically presents as a solitary bone lesion. It may be polyostotic, however, and involvement of skin, lymph nodes and even lungs may occur. The disease affects all age groups but is commonest in the first decade. Histologically, the lesions are composed of benign-looking histiocytes with vesicular nuclei and copious cytoplasm which may sometimes contain phagocytosed material (Fig. 24.19). Giant cells and foci of necrosis are usually present and there is a mixture of granulocytes, most of which are usually eosinophils, and lymphocytes. The lesion thus exhibits a granulomatous appearance.

Hand–Schüller–Christian syndrome

This disease is intermediate in severity between the other two, and classically presents with the clinical triad of bone lesions, exophthalmos and diabetes insipidus. The histological appearances are virtually indistinguishable from those of eosinophilic granuloma: the considerable lipid accumulation in the histiocytes which is often described usually occurs only in the later stages of the disease and may also be a feature of eosinophilic granuloma [110]. It could be argued that Hand–Schüller–Christian syndrome represents a polyostotic form of eosinophilic granuloma in which the exophthalmos and diabetes insipidus merely result from involvement of the orbital and sphenoid bones.

Letterer–Siwe disease

This is a rapidly fatal systemic disease occurring in children under three years old and involving the skin, liver, spleen, lungs and bones. Although the histiocytes are cytologically similar to those in eosinophilic granuloma and Hand–Schüller–Christian syndrome, they form diffuse, pure infiltrates unaccompanied by granulocytes, giant cells and foci of necrosis.

MALIGNANT HISTIOCYTOSIS

The term 'malignant histiocytosis' was coined by Rappaport in 1966 [111] to describe a proliferative disorder of morphologically atypical histiocytes which he and others [112, 113] regard as being synonymous with the 'histiocytic medullary reticulosis' first described by Scott & Robb-Smith [114]. The disease occurs at any age and may involve many organs including lymph nodes, bone marrow, spleen, kidney, gastro-intestinal tract and central nervous system. Abnormal cells are often found in the blood [113]. Histologically, the cells are pleomorphic: some have a 'blast-like' appearance with round nuclei with one or two nucleoli and a high nucleo-cytoplasmic ratio; others have more abundant eosinophilic cytoplasm and rather irregular nuclei. Many are much more easily recognizable as histiocytic in origin, with plenti-

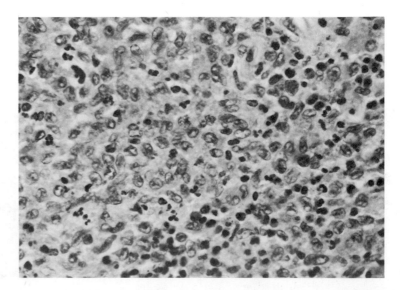

Fig. 24.19. Eosinophilic granuloma. Most of the cells are benign-looking histiocytes with vesicular nuclei and copious cytoplasm. There is a mixture of granulocytes and lymphocytes, particularly to the bottom right of the picture. (H & E, ×400.)

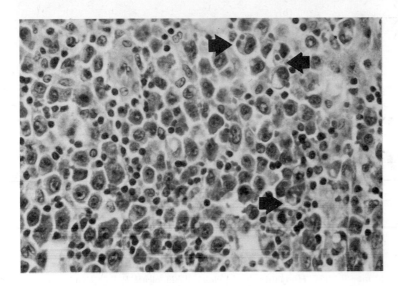

Fig. 24.20. Malignant histiocytosis. The lesion is composed of pleomorphic cells with abundant cytoplasm. A number of cells exhibit erythrophagocytosis (arrows). (H & E, × 400.)

ful non-pyroninophilic cytoplasm containing phagocytosed red cells and nuclear debris [113] (Fig. 24.20). Multinucleate giant cells and foci of necrosis are often seen.

The disease may exhibit a characteristic pattern of infiltration, being confined to the sinusoidal system of the lymph node leaving normal residual node in between. On the other hand the cells may form more cohesive masses extensively replacing the lymphoid tissue and even extending into the perinodal fat [113]. The malignant cells exhibit diffuse non-specific esterase and acid-phosphatase activity and usually contain lysozyme [113]. Malignant histiocytosis can usually be distinguished from true histiocytic lymphoma, at least until the later stages of the disease. Histiocytic lymphoma only rarely exhibits the characteristic sinusoidal pattern of infiltration and forms more cohesive cell masses. Well-differentiated histiocytes are not usually seen, and phagocytosis is rare [112]. The atypicality of the proliferating cells of malignant histiocytosis serves to distinguish them from those of histiocytosis X.

HODGKIN'S DISEASE

Unlike the non-Hodgkin lymphomas, the classification of Hodgkin's disease is fairly straightforward and generally agreed upon. It is based upon that originally proposed by Lukes & Butler [115], later modified at the Rye Conference to produce the so-called Rye classification [116]. There are four main categories:
1 lymphocyte predominance;
2 nodular sclerosis;
3 mixed cellularity; and
4 lymphocyte depletion,
based largely on the relative proportions of neoplastic and reactive cells. Hodgkin's disease is a most unusual neoplasm in that the malignant cells usually form only a minority population in the tumour mass, which is largely composed of reactive acute and chronic inflammatory cells. The abnormal cells may be mononuclear Hodgkin cells or multinucleate Reed–Sternberg cells (Fig. 24.21). Although the latter are characteristically binucleate with mirror-image nuclei, they often contain several nuclei and exhibit prominent nuclear lobation. Both the mononuclear and multinucleate forms show characteristic cytological features with a moderate amount of pyroninophilic cytoplasm and a clear nucleus surrounded by a prominent nuclear membrane and containing a very large, inclusion-like eosinophilic nucleolus. It is necessary to identify the multinucleate forms in making the diagnosis of Hodgkin's disease, as cells similar to the mononuclear variety may be seen in certain reactive conditions (see p. 944).

CLASSIFICATION

Lymphocyte predominance
The lymph-node architecture is replaced by a cellular proliferation with either a diffuse or nodular growth pattern. Although called lymphocyte predominance, histiocytes may also be prominent in about half the cases and may form giant cells or even granulomata. Hodgkin cells and Reed–Sternberg cells are rare and several low-power fields or even several sections have to be examined in order to find them. Eosinophils,

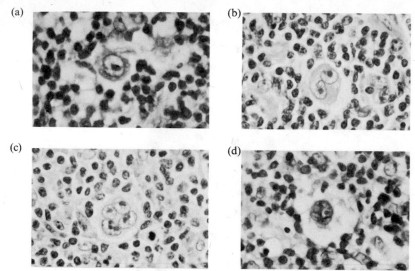

Fig. 24.21. The cells of Hodgkin's disease: (a) mononuclear Hodgkin cell; (b) classical binucleate Reed–Sternberg cell; (c) multinucleate Reed–Sternberg cell; (d) lacunar cell. (H & E, ×420.)

neutrophils and plasma cells are usually absent and there is no necrosis or fibrosis. In pure lymphocyte predominance, the appearance may thus strongly resemble well-differentiated lymphocytic lymphoma.

Nodular sclerosis
This type is characterized by capsular thickening and collagenous bands which divide the lesion into cellular nodules containing variable proportions of Reed–Sternberg cells (Fig. 24.22). The nodules may thus be lymphocyte-predominant, mixed-cellular or

lymphocyte-depleted in type, and for this reason some laboratories sub-classify nodular-sclerosing Hodgkin's disease according to the nodular content. Another feature of nodular-sclerosing Hodgkin's disease is the presence of a Reed–Sternberg-cell variant known as the lacunar cell (Fig. 24.21d). Lacunar cells have multiple lobated nuclei but small nucleoli and abundant pale, wispy cytoplasm. The cell borders are well defined and give the impression of a cell in a lacuna-like space. Nodular-sclerosing Hodgkin's disease may be difficult to recognize in its early more

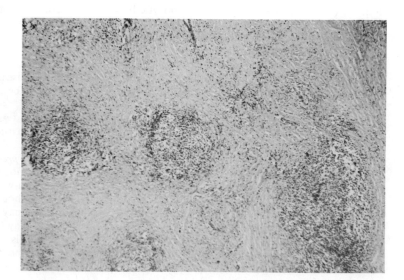

Fig. 24.22. Nodular sclerosing Hodgkin's disease. The sclerosis is very marked in this example and divides the neoplastic tissue into nodules of varying size. (H & E, ×40.)

cellular and less sclerotic phase and here the recognition of fibrous bands, capsular thickening and lacunar cells becomes important.

Mixed cellularity

This is a somewhat heterogeneous group in which the relative proportions of reactive and neoplastic cells are intermediate between the lymphocyte-predominant and lymphocyte-depleted types. In addition to Hodgkin cells, Reed–Sternberg cells, lymphocytes and histiocytes, there may also be considerable numbers of eosinophils, neutrophils and plasma cells. There is often a degree of disorderly fibrosis and foci of necrosis may be identified.

Lymphocyte depletion

Hodgkin cells and Reed–Sternberg cells predominate in this type and there is marked depletion in all reactive cell types. On occasions, the appearance may be difficult to distinguish from a large-cell non-Hodgkin lymphoma. The proliferation is often accompanied by a diffuse, disorderly fibrosis and foci of necrosis are common. In some cases, the Reed–Sternberg cells may have a highly bizarre, pleomorphic appearance.

INVOLVEMENT OF BONE MARROW AND OTHER ORGANS BY HODGKIN'S DISEASE

In Hodgkin's disease, some tissues may show infiltration by cells similar to the reactive component of the disease but without Reed–Sternberg cells or mononuclear Hodgkin cells. Thus, granulomas may be found in organs such as the liver or spleen [117], and the former may not infrequently show lymphocyte infiltration of the portal tracts, sometimes with an admixture of eosinophils. Under these circumstances, it is difficult to know whether the observed changes are simply reactive or whether the Reed–Sternberg cells have been missed through sampling error. At the Ann Arbor conference in 1971 [118], certain criteria were laid down for the diagnosis of Hodgkin's disease in staging specimens which were less stringent than those needed for diagnostic specimens. Thus if the patient already has histologically proven Hodgkin's disease, the identification of classical mononuclear Hodgkin cells is sufficient and Reed–Sternberg cells do not have to be identified.

Hodgkin's disease may involve the bone marrow: in one series [119] the incidence at presentation was 13%. Most of these patients had disease of the mixed-cellularity or lymphocyte-depleted types. Owing to its focal and cohesive nature, the detection of Hodgkin's disease in the marrow will depend on the number of sites sampled and on the techniques used; the tissue is difficult to aspirate and trephine biopsies are needed [120].

NATURE OF HODGKIN AND REED–STERNBERG CELLS

Hodgkin and Reed–Sternberg cells show aneuploidy which supports their neoplastic nature. It appears, though, that cell division is confined to the mononuclear cells and that the multinucleate forms are non-dividing [121]. The histogenesis of the cells has attracted much attention but still remains obscure. Ultrastructural studies [122, 123] have shown similarities between Reed–Sternberg cells and transformed lymphocytes, supporting their origin from lymphoid cells. Furthermore, immunocytochemical studies have shown the presence of immunoglobulin in many of the cells [124–126]. However, these same studies have shown that this immunoglobulin usually contains both κ and λ light chains. As lymphoid cells normally produce only one light-chain type, it has been suggested that the immunoglobulin is ingested, probably in the form of immune complexes. This would suggest an origin from histiocytes and, indeed, silver stains have shown that Reed–Sternberg cells may have dendritic processes which would further support a histiocytic origin. Enzyme histochemical studies, however, have failed to demonstrate significant intracellular esterase or acid-phosphatase activity [127].

AETIOLOGY AND PATHOGENESIS OF LYMPHOMAS

Little is known about the aetiology of most human malignant lymphomas, but a few important factors have been identified.

Viruses

Although viruses are known to induce malignant lymphomas readily in laboratory animals [128, 129], the only human lymphoma in which there is strong evidence of a viral aetiology is the endemic form of Burkitt's lymphoma, which is associated with the Epstein–Barr virus (EBV).

All patients with endemic Burkitt's lymphoma have antibodies to the viral capsid antigen of EBV, indicating that they have been infected by this agent. High titres of antibodies to the early antigen of the restricted type (another EBV antigen) are also observed. Furthermore, it has been shown that the presence of serum antibodies to viral capsid antigen precedes the development of lymphoma [130]. Although EBV particles have not been identified in freshly taken samples of Burkitt's lymphoma, the tumour cells exhibit an

EBV-determined membrane antigen [131], and virus particles do appear after the cells are grown in culture [132].

Even if EBV does play a causative role in endemic Burkitt's lymphoma, other factors also seem to be necessary, as the virus has world-wide distribution while the lymphoma is confined to certain areas. Burkitt [133] suggested that malaria may be an important cofactor, as this disease is hyperendemic in East Africa and Papua-New Guinea where the lymphoma occurs. Furthermore, the incidence of the tumour is reduced in areas where malaria has been eradicated, and subjects with sickle-cell trait (which confers partial protection against malaria) have a reduced incidence of tumour. However, even the combination of EBV and malaria does not seem to explain the predisposition totally, and genetic factors may also be involved.

Only a small minority of patients with non-endemic Burkitt's lymphoma show the same close association with EBV as in the endemic form [134].

Pre-existing immune disorders
It has been estimated that the risk of malignancy in patients with primary immunodeficiency syndromes such as infantile X-linked a-γ-globulinaemia, severe combined immunodeficiency, Wiskott–Aldrich syndrome, common variable immunodeficiency and ataxia telangiectasia is about 10 000 times that of an age-matched population. Most of these malignancies are lymphoid in origin [135]. Further evidence of a relationship between immunodeficiency and lymphoma is the increased incidence observed in patients who have undergone organ transplantation [136]. These lymphomas are unusual in that they are generally of the immunoblastic sarcoma type [137], and have a tendency to involve extranodal structures, particularly the central nervous system. However, the risk appears to be related not only to the immunosuppression necessary, but also to the presence of the organ transplant itself, possibly by providing chronic antigenic stimulation, which has been shown to be important in producing lymphomas in animals [138, 139].

Pre-existing 'autoimmune diseases' such as Mikulicz disease (Sjögren's syndrome), rheumatoid arthritis and systemic lupus erythematosus [140–144] may be associated with the development of lymphomas, usually of the immunoblastic sarcoma type [65].

Drugs and irradiation
Lymphomas have been reported following the administration of cancer chemotherapy and irradiation [145]. The hydantoin drugs have also been associated with malignant lymphomas as well as with the atypical reactive proliferations [146].

CONDITIONS COMMONLY MISTAKEN FOR MALIGNANT LYMPHOMA AND HODGKIN'S DISEASE

Although it is usually easy for the experienced pathologist to distinguish between reactive proliferation and malignant lymphoma, this is not always the case. Problems may arise because the normal responses of the three major compartments of the lymph node (follicular hyperplasia, paracortical hyperplasia, sinus histiocytosis) are merely exaggerated. Reactive follicular hyperplasia is usually the most troublesome, as there may be considerable nodal enlargement and architectural distortion mimicking nodular lymphoma. No single criterion can be used to distinguish between the two and the diagnosis rests upon the consideration of many factors. In follicular hyperplasia, the architecture is distorted rather than effaced and the follicles tend to be located predominantly in the cortex, rather than throughout the node. Variation in size and shape of follicles is more prominent in reactive nodes and there is usually a sharp cut-off between the germinal centre and the lymphocyte mantle which itself is composed of small, mature lymphocytes. The germinal centres differ from the centres of neoplastic nodules by showing greater variation in cell type, and tingible-body macrophages are usually prominent. Infiltration of the capsule and perinodal fat may occur in reactive conditions but is more usually associated with malignant lymphoma, especially if extensive.

There is also a small number of well-defined entities which exhibit atypical features and may be confused with lymphoma. The more common of these are briefly discussed.

Angio-immunoblastic lymphadenopathy
This entity has only recently been recognized [143, 147]. It usually occurs in elderly patients who present with generalized lymphadenopathy, hepatosplenomegaly and a polyclonal increase in serum γ globulin. There may be an antiglobulin-positive haemolytic anaemia. Histologically, the nodal architecture is diffusely obliterated by tissue composed of immunoblasts showing extensive plasma-cell differentiation, mixed with lymphocytes, eosinophils and histiocytes (Fig. 24.23). The polymorphism may give rise to confusion with Hodgkin's disease but true Reed–Sternberg cells are absent. The polymorphism, together with the proliferation of small blood vessels and the presence of extensive PAS-positive intercellular sludgy material, also helps to distinguish the lesion from immunoblastic sarcoma. Terminally, the lymph nodes usually show cellular depletion and fibrosis; lymphoma has supervened in a number of cases [143].

(a)

(b)

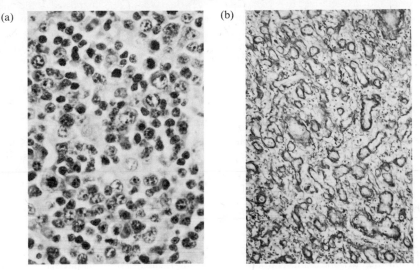

Fig. 24.23. Angio-immunoblastic lymphadenopathy. (a) The tissue is composed largely of immunoblasts and plasma cells in various stages of differentiation. (H & E, × 500.) (b) Reticulin stain showing extensive proliferation of small blood vessels (× 100).

Sinus histiocytosis with lymphadenopathy [148]

This condition usually involves the cervical lymph nodes and most commonly occurs in young Negroes who have lymphadenopathy, fever, leucocytosis and hyper-γ-globulinaemia. Histologically, the nodes show marked sinusoidal dilatation by histiocytes and plasma cells. The histiocytes have clear and sometimes foamy cytoplasm which may contain phagocytosed lymphocytes or other cells (Fig. 24.24). They may be somewhat atypical in appearance and are often multinucleated. The appearance may thus be confused

with malignant histiocytosis, but the cells show more atypicality in the latter and usually exhibit prominent erythrophagocytosis, rather than the less obvious ingestion of lymphocytes. Although the disease may follow a protracted clinical course, there is usually spontaneous and total recovery.

Angiofollicular lymph-node hyperplasia (Castleman's disease)

Although originally described in mediastinal lymph nodes [149], this disease may occur in many other sites.

(a)

(b)

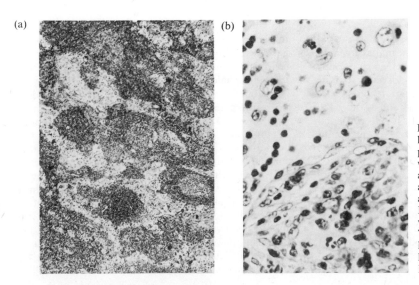

Fig. 24.24. Sinus histiocytosis with lymphadenopathy. (a) This low-power view shows sinusoids distended with histiocytes. Structural features are preserved in this field but in other areas there was greater distension with architectural loss. (H & E, × 50.) (b) High-power view of a sinus (above) with adjacent medullary cord (below). The sinus contains somewhat atypical histiocytes containing phagocytosed lymphocytes and granulocytes. (H & E, × 420.)

It is usually localized and characterized by hyperplasia of lymphoid follicles which contain prominent capillary-sized blood vessels exhibiting endothelial hyperplasia. These vessels may undergo hyalinization, forming structures reminiscent of the Hassall corpuscles of the thymus.

Lymphadenopathy associated with Hodgkin-like cells
In infectious mononucleosis, lymph-node hyperplasia may manifest as follicular hyperplasia, or as a more diffuse proliferation of lymphocytes and immunoblasts, which may infiltrate the perinodal connective tissue and cause considerable architectural distortion [150]. The immunoblasts may resemble mononuclear Hodgkin cells, so that the overall picture may be reminiscent of Hodgkin's disease. Similar appearances may be seen in postvaccinial lymphadenitis [151] and in patients receiving hydantoin drugs [152]. In the latter, eosinophils and neutrophils may form a conspicuous part of the infiltrate. In none of these conditions, however, can true Reed–Sternberg cells be found, emphasizing the need for the identification of these cells in making the diagnosis of Hodgkin's disease.

Anaplastic carcinoma
Problems may be encountered in distinguishing large-cell lymphomas from large-cell anaplastic carcinomas and, less commonly, lymphocytic lymphomas from small-cell anaplastic (oat-cell) carcinomas. Electron microscopy [153] and immunocytochemical methods may be of great value in this context [59, 154].

CLINICAL FEATURES AND MANAGEMENT OF MALIGNANT LYMPHOMAS

Hodgkin's disease
Major advances have been made in the management of Hodgkin's disease in the past 20 years, so that today the majority of patients can look forward to long remissions and probable cure. The new techniques of management are not without risk of short- and long-term complications and this is of particular importance in growing children and young adults. Fundamental to good management is accurate staging (see p. 945).

CLINICAL FEATURES
Hodgkin's disease is more common in males than females and the age incidence is bimodal, with a peak at the age of 25 and a smaller one in late middle age. The disease is very rare in childhood, with boys greatly outnumbering girls, and with a relatively high frequency of lymphocyte-predominant and mixed-cellu-

larity types. The increased male incidence is most marked in the youngest age group (three to six years), where in one series [155] boys outnumbered girls by nine to one. After puberty girls become affected more commonly, their commonest histological subtype being nodular sclerosis. By adulthood, nodular sclerosis is the commonest histological type in Europeans, although in Indians and Africans it is much rarer: this is reflected in a relative absence of mediastinal involvement in these races, involvement of this site being a hallmark of nodular sclerosis.

In most cases, the first manifestation of Hodgkin's disease is painless enlargement of lymph nodes, usually in the neck, less commonly in the axillae and inguinal regions. Chest X-ray may show mediastinal nodal enlargement, which characteristically affects the para-tracheal lymph nodes with or without concomitant involvement of the hilar nodes. It is unusual for hilar lymphadenopathy to occur without paratracheal node enlargement, and this pattern raises the possibility of tuberculosis or sarcoidosis. Lung involvement usually occurs in association with mediastinal disease, the commonest pattern being direct spread of tumour from the mediastinum into the lung parenchyma. Less common patterns of lung involvement, in order of frequency, are large lung nodules, small (miliary) nodules and coarse and fine reticular shadowing. Pleural effusions may occur: these may contain malignant cells, but in the presence of large mediastinal masses, tumour-cell-free chylous effusions may arise as a result of obstruction to lymphatic pathways by the tumour.

Palpable abdominal masses may occasionally occur, with or without enlargement of the liver and spleen. Bones, when involved, show a mixed lytic/sclerotic radiological pattern; extradural deposits can compress the spinal cord. In advanced disease, almost any organ in the body may be involved, including the skin, gastro-intestinal tract and kidneys. It is rare for the central nervous system to be involved directly, but leucoencephalopathy and peripheral neuropathy are occasionally reported. Classically, the tumour does not cause pain, but alcohol intolerance, with pain in sites involved by tumour, is well known though uncommon.

In addition to these local features, systemic symptoms including fever, malaise, weight loss and pruritus may occur. Pruritus, usually generalized and severe enough to cause intense scratching, is sometimes reported by adults, almost never by children. By itself this symptom has no prognostic significance, but it is usually associated with other symptoms which do. Sweating, particularly at night and severe enough to soak the bedclothes, is a characteristic symptom.

Anaemia occurs in Hodgkin's disease and may be

due to autoimmune haemolysis, hypersplenism, ineffective erythropoiesis, bone-marrow infiltration or an expanded plasma volume. It is generally a feature of advanced disease. A raised ESR is a common, but by no means universal finding. Before treatment the leucocyte count may be normal or slightly reduced by lymphopenia. The 'classical' findings of neutrophil leucocytosis and absolute eosinophilia are nowadays quite rare and are features of aggressive, widespread disease. In the late stages of the disease, thrombocytopenia may occur due to marrow infiltration or treatment with radiotherapy and cytotoxic drugs. At this point it is important to stress that today patients with Hodgkin's disease are being diagnosed increasingly early. Most present with none of these features other than painless lymphadenopathy, with or without night sweats and weight loss.

Infections are not uncommon in Hodgkin's disease, partly owing to impairment of cellular immunity and partly due to the immunosuppressive and myelosuppressive effects of treatment. Herpes zoster (see p. 954) is a frequent complication in treated patients, but uncommon in newly presenting ones. Tuberculosis, although historically commonly associated with Hodgkin's disease, has become rare as its incidence has declined in developed countries, but should still be thought of in Hodgkin's patients from countries in which it is still a problem. Rare opportunistic infections such as cryptococcosis and torulosis should be remembered in debilitated febrile patients, whose fever should not be assumed to be due to Hodgkin's disease. Nowadays, it is uncommon for patients to *present* with severe infections, which are mostly related to treatment.

Diagnosis
Clearly, most patients presenting with lymphadenopathy do not have a lymphoma. However, painless, rubbery, non-tender lymph nodes, not obviously associated with infection and not regressing after antibiotic therapy, should alert the clinician to this possibility. At this stage, other diagnoses such as tuberculosis, toxoplasmosis and sarcoidosis need to be considered, but once simple diagnostic tests have been done it is better not to delay but to proceed directly to biopsy, which is the only way of making the diagnosis. Usually a lymph node is taken but occasionally a liver or bone-marrow biopsy may be done. In the unusual situation where the mediastinal nodes are enlarged in the absence of peripheral lymphadenopathy, a mediastinoscopy or limited thoracotomy may be needed. Once the diagnosis has been made the patient must be fully staged.

STAGING
The purpose of staging in Hodgkin's disease is to gather enough information to permit the choice of the appropriate treatment. Procedures which do not assist in this process may be of academic interest and are sometimes justified in this setting, but they are inappropriate in a routine context. The investigations commonly done in patients with Hodgkin's disease are shown in Table 24.8 and further discussed below.

Table 24.8. Investigations in Hodgkin's disease

1 Review histology, subtype
2 Full blood count, ESR, liver-function tests, urea, uric acid, electrolytes, protein studies
3 Chest X-ray, tomography if indicated
4 Bipedal lymphography and CT scanning
5 Radionuclide scanning
6 Bone-marrow biopsy
7 Laparotomy with splenectomy, liver and node biopsies and bone biopsy

Histological review. This is mandatory and has already been discussed.

Full blood count and ESR, blood chemistry. It is important that this includes a platelet count and a differential white-cell count. The ESR is not specific but is a useful way of monitoring the progress of treatment. A raised serum alkaline-phosphatase level may indicate bone or liver involvement and can be used to monitor treatment [156]. Two or more abnormal liver function tests are regarded as indicative of liver involvement in patients whose staging does not include liver biopsy. Hyperuricaemia is an indication for allopurinol treatment before chemotherapy is given. Protein studies are largely of academic interest. Hypercalcaemia occurs very rarely in the presence of bone disease.

Radiological investigations. These include chest X-rays, bipedal lymphography and excretion urography. A standard postero-anterior and lateral *chest X-ray* will often give enough information about the mediastinum and lungs if these are obviously affected. Whole-lung tomography may reveal undetected involvement in 10–20% of cases [157]. Indications for tomography are equivocal plain films, bulky mediastinal disease and unusual chest-wall shape which may obscure parenchymal lesions.

Lymphography with oily contrast media is essential in all patients with Hodgkin's disease unless there is a specific contraindication. These include orthopnoea, which is aggravated by the pulmonary oil embolism that occurs to some extent in every case, active thrombophlebitis which may increase the danger of pulmonary embolism, right-to-left intracardiac shunts, which introduce the risk of systemic oil embolism, and therapeutic irradiation of the lungs, which paralyses the pulmonary capillaries and permits systemic oil embolism with the risk of cerebral damage. Youth is not a contraindication in experienced hands, although smaller doses of contrast medium must be used to avoid the risk of excessive pulmonary embolism [158]. In young children, a light general anaesthetic is necessary. Bipedal lymphography permits the inguinal, iliac and para-aortic lymph nodes to be visualized. The contrast medium then passes up the thoracic duct to the root of the neck. Nodes may be opacified in the mediastinum and root of the neck; opacification of mediastinal nodes is uncommon and suggestive of their involvement by tumour. Large masses of tumour in the abdomen may not fill with contrast medium at all, but their presence may be inferred from the displacement of the normal lymphatic architecture or ureters, as seen on the excretion urogram, which should be done 24 hours after the lymphogram and must be regarded as an essential part of the investigation [158].

Retroperitoneal lymph-node involvement occurs in about 40% of patients with Hodgkin's disease. The accuracy of lymphography in most series is 75–85%. Lymphographically involved nodes show a foamy or reticular pattern and are frequently enlarged. Filling defects may be present; a less common pattern is for nodes to look more dense than normal. The accuracy of lymphography is increased by taking follow-up films, since affected nodes enlarge if not treated and shrink on treatment, whereas unaffected nodes usually remain static. Sometimes, unaffected nodes shrink on treatment, but they do so symmetrically, whereas affected nodes shrink more than their normal counterparts. The oily contrast medium remains in the lymph nodes for two years or longer in adults, usually less in children, so that follow-up films can easily be taken.

Bipedal lymphography does not fill the coeliac axis, splenic hilar, porta hepatis or mesenteric lymph nodes and these should be sampled if a staging laparotomy is done. 'Refill' lymphograms can be done up to three times in selected patients. It is wise to keep previously involved lymph nodes filled with contrast medium for at least two years after treatment has been completed.

Computerized axial tomographic (CT) scanning can be used to complement lymphography. It does not replace lymphography but may be useful for looking at those nodal sites which are not opacified by lymphography [159]. If the lymphogram is positive it is likely that other abdominal sites are involved.

Isotopic scanning. Scanning of the *liver* and *spleen* seldom does more than provide information about the size of the organs, and is no longer warranted as a standard procedure. Occasionally, filling defects due to the presence of lymphoma may be seen but these still require confirmation by histology.

It is uncommon for *bone* to be involved at presentation in Hodgkin's disease in the absence of a raised serum calcium or alkaline phosphatase, or without bone pain. In these circumstances bone scanning may be useful to identify sites of involvement.

Gallium-67 citrate has been used as a 'tumour-seeking' isotope and will detect Hodgkin's disease in about 70% of cases. It is probably most useful in the mediastinum, where it can distinguish between fibrosis (scan-negative) and tumour (scan-positive). However, not only is there a 30% false-negative rate in patients with obvious tumour, but the isotope is taken up by inflammatory non-malignant lesions to give a significant false-positive rate. Small (less than 2 cm diameter) lesions are not visualized by this technique and it is of little value in the abdomen, where the excretion of isotope into the bowel produces a high background of radiation which may obscure lesions detectable by other means. For all these reasons gallium scanning has found little favour as a routine investigation. The position of isotope scanning has recently been well reviewed [160].

Trephine biopsy of the bone marrow. This, preferably from more than one site, is useful in patients with clinical evidence of advanced disease. In patients with limited disease it is very seldom positive. At presentation only five per cent of all patients have involvement of the bone marrow but, in patients with Stage IIIB or IV disease, lymphocyte-depletion histology or an unexplained elevation of the serum alkaline phosphatase, marrow involvement has been reported in 10–13% [119, 161]. Its detection may save the patient from a laparotomy and is an absolute indication for treatment with chemotherapy. It is important to stress that a *trephine* biopsy is necessary: aspiration biopsy is not worth doing on its own.

Staging laparotomy

Laparotomy with splenectomy, node sampling, liver biopsy and bone biopsy was introduced by the Stanford group over a decade ago [162] and has become a routine in many centres. The basis for it was the observation that patients with disease above the diaphragm tended to relapse first in the para-aortic lymph nodes after treatment with involved field radiation, and it was argued that if occult abdominal disease could be detected at presentation it could be eradicated if appropriate treatment was given. Many series now confirm the truth of this [163–166]. What has been learned from laparotomy can be summarized as follows.

1 About one-third of patients with disease apparently confined above the diaphragm have occult abdominal disease.

2 The commonest site of occult abdominal involvement is the spleen.

3 Small spleens may be involved and the pattern of involvement is frequently focal, with small nodules which may be only a few millimetres in diameter. These may only be detected by careful cutting of the spleen into thin slices. The likelihood of splenic involvement increases with spleen size and is almost invariable in spleens weighing more than 400 g.

4 Liver involvement in Hodgkin's disease is virtually always accompanied by splenic involvement, but the reverse is not the case. Wedge biopsies of the liver are superior to needle biopsies in the detection of diseases.

5 In most patients, laparotomy results in an increase in disease stage (up-staging) but in about 10%, apparently involved nodes (on lymphogram) will be found not to contain disease and this may result in the patient finishing up in an earlier stage than was previously suspected (down-staging).

6 Lymphography is an accurate way of assessing abdominal nodal status in most patients.

7 In experienced hands laparotomy is a safe procedure with a low mortality (less than one per cent) and morbidity.

8 Splenectomy in children and adolescents increases the risk of overwhelming, sometimes fatal, bacterial sepsis [167]. This usually, but not always, is caused by *Streptococcus pneumoniae* or *Haemophilus influenzae*, and can be prevented in most cases by administering prophylactic oral penicillin post-operatively until the age of 20 years. However, it is felt by some to be a contraindication to diagnostic laparotomy in children.

9 Despite more than a decade of diagnostic laparotomies there is no clear evidence that pathological staging improves the overall survival of patients with Hodgkin's disease. Patients with early-stage disease appear to do better when pathologically staged, but this is due to the elimination by laparotomy of patients with more advanced disease than would be apparent from non-invasive staging. This group of patients, if pathologically staged, can be given more appropriate therapy from the outset, and this will frequently be chemotherapy. If they had not been pathologically staged they would have been treated with radiotherapy, subsequently relapsed and then been given effective chemotherapy. Thus, in terms of final outcome, the results are much the same whether laparotomy is done or not. The attraction of staging laparotomy is that it spares some patients from inappropriate treatment which carries its own morbidity.

Hodgkin's disease is staged by the Ann Arbor system [168] which is shown in Table 24.9. In this staging system the suffix 'E' is used to denote involvement of an extranodal site, either where the disease is confined to that site or where there has been direct extension from an adjacent affected lymph node. The implication is that this extranodal disease is still localized and can be treated with radiotherapy. As soon as there is widespread extranodal disease which cannot be treated with radiotherapy the disease becomes Stage IV. The 'E' concept was introduced by Musshoff [169], who found that localized extranodal spread did not alter the prognosis provided the disease could be included in a radiation field, but these findings have been challenged by Levi & Wiernik [170] and opinion is now moving to the position of regarding

Table 24.9. Ann Arbor staging of Hodgkin's disease

Stage I
Involvement of a single lymph-node region (I) or of a single extralymphatic site (I$_E$)

Stage II
Involvement of two or more lymph-node regions on the same side of the diaphragm (II), which may also include the spleen (II$_S$), localized extralymphatic involvement (II$_E$), or both (II$_{SE}$) if confined to the same side of the diaphragm

Stage III
Involvement of lymph-node regions on both sides of the diaphragm (III), which may also include the spleen (III$_S$), localized extralymphatic involvement (III$_E$) or both (III$_{SE}$)

Stage IV
Diffuse or disseminated involvement of extralymphatic sites (e.g. lung, liver, bone, bone marrow, skin)

Systemic symptoms
Unexplained weight loss (more than 10% of body weight in six months before diagnosis), fever, sweating: if absent = 'A'; if present = 'B'

---

all extranodal disease as carrying a bad prognosis and representing an indication for treatment with chemotherapy.

In the Ann Arbor system, patients are assigned both a clinical stage (CS) and a pathological stage (PS). Clinical staging stops short of laparotomy, pathological staging includes laparotomy findings. Thus an asymptomatic patient with disease in the neck and mediastinum, normal blood chemistry and lymphogram and negative scans who was found at laparotomy to have liver, spleen and abdominal node involvement would be staged CSIIA PSIVA$_{H+,S+,N+}$. In this system the suffixes are as follows: H, liver; S, spleen; N, nodes; M, marrow; and O, bone. The system allows more accurate comparisons of treatment results to be made between different centres and also allows the influence of laparotomy on the outcome of treatment to be more readily assessed. However, as Lewis & De Vita have pointed out [171], the source of greatest difficulty in understanding the role of staging laparotomy in Hodgkin's disease has come from failure to separate its use as a research tool from its role in the management of the individual patient. They have eloquently made the point that for many patients with Hodgkin's disease laparotomy makes no difference to their choice of treatment or to its outcome. In other words, the majority of patients with clinically limited disease are curable with radiotherapy and those with more extensive disease probably with chemotherapy. Patients who relapse following 'curative' radiotherapy are increasingly effectively retreated with combination chemotherapy and will go on to become long survivors. In this context, it is perhaps unfortunate that diagnostic laparotomy was introduced before the spectacular results of modern chemotherapy became apparent, at a time when radiotherapy was still the only form of treatment that offered a real prospect of cure. Today, the need for laparotomy in the individual patient with apparently early disease must be assessed in terms of what is already known about the likelihood of his having more advanced disease, requiring treatment with chemotherapy or combined-modality therapy. Paradoxically the accuracy of assessment of these odds has been increased by information from staging laparotomies performed on series of patients in the past. What is now required is the development of treatment which increases remission rates and which is even better than available forms of treatment in salvaging patients who relapse following a period of disease control.

TREATMENT

Hodgkin's disease can be treated with radiotherapy, chemotherapy or both treatments combined. Choice of treatment depends first on stage of disease, but also on the age of the patient, the histological subtype, the volume (as distinct from the distribution) of the disease, and upon an assessment of prognosis based on past experience with either form of treatment used alone.

There is no doubt that the most effective treatment for localized Hodgkin's disease is radiotherapy. As long ago as 1958 Peters & Middlemiss [172] showed that the prognosis in Stages I and IIA was considerably improved if, in addition to irradiating the involved areas, the adjacent lymph-node regions were also treated. Subsequently Easson & Russell [173] and Kaplan [174] have extended this further, and wide-field high-dose supervoltage techniques are now the accepted form of treatment. Localized disease above the diaphragm is treated by the 'mantle' technique which involves irradiating both sides of the neck, both axillae, the mediastinum and possibly the upper para-aortic areas, while disease below the diaphragm is treated by an inverted Y field which includes the para-aortic, pelvic and inguinal regions. Kaplan [174] has shown that with Stage I and II disease, 80% of the patients are alive at five years, none have subsequently relapsed and many may well be cured.

Just as the correct treatment for localized disease is radiotherapy, the treatment for generalized disease (Stage IV and probably Stage IIIB) is chemotherapy. It is now 100 years since chemotherapy was first used for the treatment of Hodgkin's disease by Billroth [175], who used arsenic. There was no advance until the end of the Second World War, when nitrogen mustard was introduced by Gilman & Philips [176] and Wilkinson & Fletcher [177]. Following this, many agents with different actions were introduced and today there are three major groups of cytotoxic drugs known to be effective in this disease: the alkylating agents such as mustine hydrochloride, chlorambucil and cyclophosphamide; the vinca alkaloids—vincristine and vinblastine; and a methylhydrazine derivative—procarbazine. These drugs, when used singly, will produce complete remission of the disease in about 25% of patients, and partial remission in a further 50% [178]. When two agents are used there is a significant increase in the percentage of complete remissions, as shown by Lacher & Durant [179], who used a combination of vincristine and chlorambucil. However, the most dramatic improvement in the prognosis of generalized Hodgkin's disease occurred when de Vita, Carbone and their colleagues introduced quadruple chemotherapy, using nitrogen mustard (mustine hydrochloride), vincristine, procarbazine and prednisone (MOPP). Their results in patients who had not received any treatment in the past (i.e. patients presenting with disseminated disease) showed a complete remission rate of 80%, and a further 10% obtained a partial regression of the disease [180].

These two events, the introduction of extended-field radiotherapy and MOPP chemotherapy, ushered in the era of radical treatment for Hodgkin's disease, and with it the prospect of cure for most of its victims. The two methods of treatment will now be considered in more detail.

Radiotherapy

Modern treatment of Hodgkin's disease with radiotherapy requires the use of megavoltage equipment, either linear accelerators producing high-energy X-rays or ^{60}Co equipment producing γ rays. These permit the radiotherapist to treat large volumes of tissue so that multiple lymph-node groups may be treated in a single field, either the 'mantle' field in which all the major lymph-node regions above the diaphragm are treated, or the 'inverted Y' field in which subdiaphragmatic lymphoid regions including para-aortic, splenic pedicle, iliac, inguinal and femoral lymph nodes are irradiated. Lead blocks are inserted in the field to shield the larynx, humeral epiphyses, lungs, spinal cord, kidneys, pelvic bone marrow and gonads.

High-energy radiation is skin-sparing, as the maximum dose is delivered at least 1 cm deep to the skin surface. Skin erythema and desquamation are therefore not a dose-limiting problem. An opposed-field technique should be used, since it provides a more homogeneous dose distribution and reduces the amount of radiation received by normal tissues. The tumoricidal dose of radiation lies between 3500 and 4000 rads at a dose rate of 1000 rads/week [181]. In general, bulky disease requires larger doses of irradiation for eradication than does small-volume disease. Definition of 'bulk' is necessarily arbitrary, but nodes of greater than 5 cm in diameter are usually taken as bulky. To assess the bulk of mediastinal nodes the ratio between the width of the mediastinum and the thoracic-cage diameter at the same level (the M/T ratio) is calculated. An M/T ratio of more than 1:3 is taken as evidence of bulky mediastinal disease. Details of radiation technique are outside the scope of this chapter, but the subject has recently been reviewed by Hoppe [182].

Chemotherapy

The drugs effective against Hodgkin's disease are listed in Table 24.10. It can now be stated firmly that these should never be used singly, except for palliation in end-stage disease, since to do so prejudices both quality and quantity of survival. MOPP [180] (Table 24.11) has become the standard against which all other combinations are judged. With this regimen, or with vinblastine substituted for vincristine (MVPP) [183] (Table 24.12), complete remission rates of 70–80% can

Table 24.10. Drugs effective against Hodgkin's disease

Alkylating agents	mustine hydrochloride
	cyclophosphamide
	chlorambucil
Vinca alkaloids	vincristine
	vinblastine
Corticosteroids	prednisone
	prednisolone
Antibiotics	bleomycin
	doxorubicin
	(adriamycin)
Procarbazine	
Epipodophyllotoxins	VM 26
	VP 16-213
Dimethyltriazenoimidazole carboxamide (DTIC)	

Table 24.11. MOPP*

Mustine hydrochloride	6 mg/m^2 i.v. on days 1 and 8
Vincristine (Oncovin)	1·4 mg/m^2 i.v. on days 1 and 8
Procarbazine	100 mg/m^2 orally on days 1–14 inclusive
Prednisone†	40 mg/m^2 orally on days 1–14 inclusive

* Six courses are given with two-week intervals between courses.
† Prednisone originally given in courses 1 and 4 only but now usually given with each course.

be achieved in patients presenting with untreated advanced disease or following relapse from primary treatment with radiotherapy. It has recently been shown that oral chlorambucil can be substituted for mustine to give ChlVPP [184] (Table 24.13), which produces equivalent remission rates to MOPP and MVPP but spares patients the nausea and vomiting associated with mustine. It is not known yet whether ChlVPP will produce survivals as long as those achieved with MOPP or MVPP; these combinations

Table 24.12. MVPP*

Mustine hydrochloride	6 mg/m^2 i.v. on days 1 and 8
Vinblastine	6 mg/m^2 i.v. on days 1 and 8
Procarbazine	100 mg/m^2 orally on days 1–14 inclusive
Prednisolone†	40 mg orally on days 1–14 inclusive

* Six to 10 courses given with four-week intervals between courses.
† 40 mg never exceeded but may be reduced for children.

Table 24.13. ChlVPP*

Chlorambucil†	6 mg/m² orally on days 1–14 inclusive
Vinblastine	6 mg/m² i.v. on days 1 and 8
Procarbazine	100 mg/m² orally on days 1–14 inclusive
Prednisolone‡	40 mg orally on days 1–14 inclusive

* Six to 10 courses given with two-week intervals between courses.
† A maximum daily dose of 10 mg is not exceeded.
‡ 40 mg never exceeded, but may be reduced for children.

both produce a high proportion of long survivors and it can be expected that approximately 60% of patients achieving complete remission will be alive and free of disease at five years. The tendency to relapse is highest in the first two years from the discontinuation of treatment, after which relapses are uncommon. This has raised the question whether relapsing patients are really patients who never truly achieved complete remission and has prompted studies of intensive restaging, including 'second-look' laparotomy on cessation of chemotherapy. The results of these studies are not yet available.

The value of maintenance chemotherapy following six or more courses of combination chemotherapy has been studied in two controlled trials. Young *et al.* [185], in a trial in which patients in remission after six courses of MOPP were randomized to no further treatment, maintenance with MOPP or maintenance with BCNU, showed no influence of maintenance treatment on survival or disease-free survival, but an increased complication rate, mainly due to infection in maintained patients. Frei *et al.* [186], in a trial in which MOPP-treated patients were randomized to MOPP maintenance or no maintenance, showed that although the maintained patients had a higher relapse-free rate than the unmaintained ones at two years and five years of follow-up, there was no difference in survival between the groups. This was because unmaintained relapsing patients could be effectively retreated with further MOPP, a fact noted by other workers including de Vita [187].

The value of steroids in first-line combinations for Hodgkin's disease is controversial. The British National Lymphoma Investigation study [188], which compared MOPP with MOPr (MOPP without prednisone) showed a complete remission rate of 80% for MOPP compared with 44% for MOPr, but no difference in survival between the groups. The Stanford group [189], in a retrospective study, found that complete remission rates and six-year survivals were identical (MOPP 90% and 64% respectively, MOPr 93% and 60%). At present it would seem wise to include steroids in first-line combinations.

In summary, therefore, first-line combinations of alkylating agent, vinca alkaloid, steroid and procarbazine produce high remission rates and probable cures in advanced disease. There is little evidence that continuing treatment beyond six to 10 courses is of any benefit, although clearly it is prudent to give several courses of treatment after complete remission has been obtained. This has varied from two to five in different series. Many patients who relapse following a period of disease-free remission will remit again when treated with the same combination, which should probably contain a corticosteroid.

The factors which prejudice response to chemotherapy have been reviewed by Coltman [190]. These include age (patients over 40 years fare less well than younger patients), performance status, weight loss and Stage IV disease, particularly IVB. Many clinicians also feel that lymphocyte-depleted and 'bulky' disease patients do badly, although this requires formal confirmation. In contrast, several studies have shown that prior radiotherapy is associated with particularly high remission rates and survival. This is probably because a large proportion of previously irradiated patients relapse with small-volume disease in comparatively few sites, and this is easily eradicated by chemotherapy.

Alternative chemotherapy in Hodgkin's disease. Many alternative drug combinations have been devised to treat Hodgkin's disease and these have been fully reviewed by Coltman [190]. They are conveniently thought of as:
1 those in which alternative drugs have been substituted for those in MOPP;
2 those in which drugs have been added to MOPP; and
3 those which are essentially completely different from MOPP and have been designed in an attempt to treat MOPP-resistant disease.

Examples of the first category are MVPP and ChlVPP. Other examples are C-MOPP in which cyclophosphamide substitutes for mustine, BOPP in which BCNU substitutes for mustine and BCVPP in which BCNU and cyclophosphamide substitute for mustine and vinblastine substitutes for vincristine. These combinations show no advantage over MOPP in terms of remission rate, although toxicity may be different.

In the second category are MOPPLDB, in which low-dose bleomycin is added to MOPP, and a similar combination MOPPHDB, which employs high-dose bleomycin. There is no good evidence that these show any advantage over MOPP either.

In the third category are B-DOPA: bleomycin, DTIC, vincristine, prednisone and adriamycin; PAVe: phenylalamine mustard, procarbazine and vinblastine;

and SCAB: streptozoticin, CCNU, adriamycin and bleomycin. The most widely studied of these combinations is ABVD (Table 24.14): adriamycin, bleomycin, vinblastine and DTIC. This was developed in Milan [191] and a complete remission rate of 62% was observed in advanced disease. More important, an apparent lack of cross-resistance with MOPP was seen,

Table 24.14. ABVD

Adriamycin	25 mg/m^2 i.v. on days 1 and 14
Bleomycin	25 mg/m^2 i.v. on days 1 and 14
Vinblastine	6 mg/m^2 i.v. on days 1 and 14
DTIC	150 mg/m^2 i.v. on days 1, 2, 3, 4 and 5

with a 70% disease-free rate at three years in patients achieving complete remission. This has not been the experience of other groups [192–194], who have all noted much lower complete-remission rates (seven per cent, 29% and zero per cent respectively) with marked evidence of cross-resistance with MOPP, and few patients surviving beyond 18 months. Thus, at present, it must be concluded that patients in whom complete remission is not obtained with first-line chemotherapy are unlikely to be long survivors, and there is still an urgent need for chemotherapy that will both increase the complete-remission rate in advanced disease and effectively salvage patients who fail first-line treatment. A recent report from Bonadonna *et al.* [195], in which six cycles of MOPP alternating with six cycles of ABVD was compared with 12 cycles of MOPP in two randomized groups of patients with Stage IV disease, gives some grounds for hope, although further follow-up is needed. In the MOPP/ABVD group there was a 55% remission rate with 100% survival of remitters at two years, whereas in the MOPP alone group, although 53% complete-remission rate was observed, only 65% of these patients were in remission at two years.

The choice of treatment for Hodgkin's disease
Conventionally, patients with pathological Stages IA, IB, IIA, IIB and IIIA disease are treated with radiotherapy and those with IIIB, IVA and IVB disease are given chemotherapy. There is controversy over the extent of the radiotherapy field in patients with above-diaphragm Stage I and II disease, some radiotherapists preferring to treat with a mantle field alone, others opting for a mantle plus para-aortic node extension, and others for a mantle plus full inverted Y field ('total nodal' irradiation). The use of the total nodal field results in a five-year relapse-free survival of about 70% in Stages IA and IIA with a survival rate of 85%, the difference between the two representing

effective salvage of relapsing patients with combination chemotherapy. There is little difference in the results if the pelvic lymph nodes are not irradiated, since although the relapse rate is slightly higher this is reclaimed by chemotherapy. Most radiotherapists therefore prefer to use an 'Anchor' or 'Spade' field in which only the para-aortic nodes are irradiated following mantle radiotherapy. In patients with pathological Stage IB or IIB disease, total nodal radiotherapy produces results equivalent to those obtained in Stages IA and IIA. However, in many patients with *clinical* Stage IB or IIB disease, occult abdominal disease will be detected at laparotomy, moving them into Stages IIIB or IV. Therefore if a patient in this category is not pathologically staged many therapists will give chemotherapy as first-line treatment. Other factors may strongly influence the tendency to relapse in patients with Stage II disease. These are the presence of more than three nodal areas involved above the diaphragm, lymphocyte-depleted histology and large-volume (M/T ratio less than 1:3) mediastinal adenopathy. In the group with more than three nodal areas involved above the diaphragm, we [196] have observed a cure rate with radiotherapy alone of less than 20%, and in those patients with bulky mediastinal disease we [197] and others [198] have seen a similar failure of radiotherapy to control disease, with patients relapsing both in the mediastinum, at the edge of the radiotherapy field, and outside the irradiated volume. For these reasons it has become increasingly fashionable to treat this group of patients with chemotherapy to remission, followed by mantle radiotherapy. Since adopting this policy 12 out of our own series of 16 patients with bulky mediastinal disease are alive and disease-free with a median follow-up time of 24 months [196].

In patients with pathological Stage IIIA disease, total nodal radiation produces a disease-free rate at five years of about 65% in patients whose disease is confined to lymph nodes. If the spleen is extensively involved there is evidence [182] that more than half the patients will relapse following radiotherapy alone and it is probably better to treat these patients with chemotherapy, although this has not been the subject of a controlled trial.

In some respects the management of Stages IIIB and IV Hodgkin's disease is easier, or at any rate, less controversial. If six to 10 courses of MOPP or MVPP are given, approximately 75% of patients will remit and more than half of these patients will be disease-free at five years. The problems of non-remitting or relapsing patients have already been discussed—only about 20% will be cured by further therapy. Those who are most likely to benefit from treatment on relapse are those whose relapse is in a few nodal sites only. These can sometimes be controlled by further chemotherapy or by radiotherapy and here it is appropriate to restage the patient intensively, including laparotomy in selected cases. If the relapse is truly local, radiotherapy can then be given appropriately as though the patient was a new case presenting with localized disease.

In an attempt to lower the relapse rate in chemotherapy-treated patients, the influence of 'adjuvant' radiotherapy given to sites of major pre-treatment involvement has been studied by a number of groups (reviewed by Coltman [190]). Although there is only one controlled study [198] which did not show a difference in disease-free survival when total nodal radiotherapy was added to MOPP, other studies do suggest that 'bulk' irradiation may reduce the relapse rate in patients with large-volume nodal disease. Further studies are needed to identify those patients likely to benefit from this approach, but it seems likely that the target for radiotherapy should be previously involved lymph nodes, which have been shown in one series [199] to be the site of relapse in most cases.

The use of chemotherapy as an adjuvant to radio-therapy in patients with Stage I, II and III disease has been most fully studied by the Stanford group [198]. A group of 244 patients was treated with radiotherapy alone or radiotherapy followed by six cycles of MOPP. Although the use of adjuvant chemotherapy significantly improved the duration of freedom from relapse it did not significantly prolong survival, since most patients relapsing after radiotherapy alone could be reclaimed by chemotherapy given at the time of relapse. There was also a suggestion that those patients relapsing after elective radiotherapy and chemo-therapy had shorter survival following their second remission than those who had received radiotherapy alone as their first treatment, and that this was due to shorter second remissions in the combined-treatment group. Clearly the routine use of adjuvant chemo-therapy after radiotherapy cannot be recommended, since a large proportion of patients who have already been cured by radiotherapy will be unnecessarily overtreated by toxic chemotherapy. The use of chemo-therapy before radiotherapy in selected patients at high risk of nodal relapse is a more attractive proposi-tion and has already been discussed.

HODGKIN'S DISEASE IN CHILDREN

Childhood Hodgkin's disease is similar to the disease in adults except that males greatly outnumber females and nodular sclerosis is a relatively unusual histologi-cal finding. Symptoms are similar, although severe night sweats are not so common as in adults. What is different is the growing child himself and investiga-tions and treatment need to be designed to interfere as little as possible with his physical and emotional development.

Since overall five-year survival rates now approach 90% in several series [200], great care must be taken before orthodox treatment is modified. However it is now clear that there are two main areas where there is beginning to be agreement about the need for approaches that differ from those in adults. These are the use of laparotomy for staging and extended-field irradiation for treatment.

Staging laparotomy in children reveals about the same proportion of occult disease as it does in adults [200], but the hazards, particularly of splenectomy, are greater. It has been found [167] that about 10% of splenectomized children experience overwhelming post-splenectomy infection, the chief organisms being the pneumococcus, meningococcus and *H. influenzae*. In Chilcoate's series [167] half these infections were fatal. Patients remain at risk up to the age of 20 years. Any child undergoing this operation needs to take prophylactic penicillin until early adulthood and there are inevitably problems with compliance in some patients. In patients who are allergic to penicillin, erythromycin or cotrimoxazole can be substituted. Prophylaxis with polyvalent pneumococcal vaccines is currently being studied but results are not yet avail-able. With this major problem in mind, there is an increasing feeling that patients, particularly young children under the age of 10 years, should not be subjected to laparotomy, particularly since there is little evidence that pathologically staged patients sur-vive longer than those staged clinically. In addition, since the purpose of laparotomy is, in one sense, to define radiocurability, it becomes superfluous if for other reasons a decision has already been taken not to use radiotherapy as primary treatment for apparently early-stage disease. This topic has been reviewed by Jenkin & Berry [200] and McElwain & Smith [201]. In essence, it has been found that extended-field radio-therapy using the mantle, inverted Y and total nodal techniques interferes with spinal bone growth, and young children so treated are at risk of becoming short adults [202]. In addition, hypothyroidism may develop in children who have received irradiation to the neck [203]. If irradiation with involved fields only is substi-tuted, there is a high relapse rate, although patients can often be reclaimed with subsequent combination chemotherapy. Thus, there is an increasing tendency to treat children with chemotherapy as primary treat-ment irrespective of stage, either reserving radio-therapy for bulky local sites, or reducing the dose of radiotherapy if extended-field treatment needs to be given. Such combined-modality treatment produces excellent results but its long-term morbidity may still be considerable (see below), since chemotherapy is not

without complications, including sterility in males and an increased risk of second tumours. There is no easy solution to these problems, but it would be fair to say that increasing numbers of centres would recommend:
1 clinical staging, without laparotomy;
2 radiotherapy only for non-bulky Stage I and II disease; and
3 chemotherapy for all other stages, with or without adjuvant radiotherapy for sites of previously bulky disease, and as 'reclaim' treatment for irradiated patients who subsequently relapse.

Further trials to settle these issues are in progress.

COMPLICATIONS OF TREATMENT

Radiotherapy

Radiation pneumonitis and fibrosis. These occur to some extent in all patients treated with mantle radiotherapy and typically appear one to three months after completing treatment. Usually, the only symptom is mild dry cough and some shortness of breath on exertion, though retrosternal pain and severe dyspnoea may sometimes develop. Active pneumonitis occurs in the upper mediastinum and upper-lung zones and is later replaced by streaky shadowing as fibrosis and scarring develop. The condition is nearly always self-limiting and patients recover without noticeable disability, although lung-function studies have shown that there is about a 10% reduction in vital capacity [204]. In severe cases, high-dose steroid treatment may give relief in the acute phase. Prednisolone, 20–30 mg daily, is usually sufficient and this may be required for several weeks before being slowly tapered and discontinued.

If the whole lung is irradiated severe pneumonitis may develop. This has been reviewed by Thar & Million [205].

Radiation-induced hypothyroidism. This occurs in patients whose neck has been irradiated in the mantle field. Clinical hypothyroidism is rare (about three per cent) but chemical hypothyroidism is more common. Many patients have normal thyroxine (T_4) levels with elevated TSH levels ('compensated hypothyroidism') [206]: this requires no treatment, but these patients should be carefully watched for evidence of later clinical hypothyroidism, which will require standard replacement therapy.

Radiation pericarditis. This is very rare in patients who receive doses of less than 4500 rads to the mediastinum. In patients receiving higher doses, acute pericarditis with fever, dyspnoea, pericardial friction rub and abnormal chest X-ray and ECG may develop,

usually about one year after treatment; in a few cases, this may be followed by constrictive pericarditis, necessitating pericardectomy. Acute radiation-induced pericarditis should be treated with steroids in addition to routine treatment with digoxin and diuretics.

Radiation hepatitis. This may appear four to six weeks after whole-liver irradiation. It is characterized by liver pain, increase in abdominal girth, ascites and fever. All the liver enzymes may be elevated. It is dose-related and seldom seen at doses below 3000 rads [207]. It may be fatal, but usually recovers, and can be managed with bed rest, diet and appropriate diuretics such as spironolactone. Steroids are given, but their benefit is uncertain.

Radiation myelitis. This may develop if long segments of spinal cord are irradiated. With the radiation doses used for Hodgkin's disease it is very rare [205].

Testicular damage from radiation. This can be minimized by effective shielding [205]. The testis receives about 100 rads, which results in temporary aspermia. Ovarian failure results from irradiation in the 'inverted Y' field, and to prevent this the ovaries can be transposed to the mid-line and sutured to the uterus in patients staged by laparotomy [208].

Chemotherapy

The side-effects of the drugs used to treat Hodgkin's disease are numerous and are listed in Table 24.15. They have been reviewed by Gams [209].

Successful avoidance of major side-effects results from careful attention to protocols and skill on the part of the chemotherapist. In general, young patients are far more drug-tolerant than older ones and in patients over the age of 50 years dosage modifications often need to be made. Two major drug-related side-effects are infertility and the development of second tumours in long survivors.

Infertility. In males treated with MOPP, C-MOPP, MVPP and ChlVPP infertility is inevitable and was first reported by de Vita [210] for MOPP. Aspermia develops rapidly and is probably permanent for most patients, although recovery in some has been reported some years after cessation of therapy. In our own experience, this applies to children as well—none of five children treated for Hodgkin's disease has developed spermatogenesis after puberty. For this reason sperm-banking should be offered to men who want a family before they begin a programme of chemotherapy, so that their wives may be artificially inseminated later.

Table 24.15. Side-effects of cytotoxic drugs used to treat Hodgkin's disease

---

Nausea and vomiting
  (a) Severe
     Nitrogen mustard, BCNU, CCNU
  (b) Mild to moderate
     Adriamycin, bleomycin, vinblastine, procarbazine, DTIC, VP 16-213, cyclophosphamide

Fever
  Bleomycin, DTIC

Peripheral neuropathy
  Vincristine, vinblastine

Cardiotoxicity
  Adriamycin

Alopecia
  Adriamycin, cyclophosphamide, vincristine (mild), VP 16-213

Pulmonary toxicity
  Bleomycin, alkylating agents (rarely), BCNU (rare, hypersensitivity)

Myelosuppression
  Nearly all except vincristine and prednisone or prednisolone.
  Severe with BCNU, CCNU, cyclophosphamide, adriamycin at high doses

---

In women, combination chemotherapy may produce oligomenorrhoea or amenorrhoea in premenopausal patients. In some of these the amenorrhoea remains permanent after stopping treatment and there is biochemical evidence of ovarian failure, often associated with menopausal symptoms such as hot flushes. The nearer the patient is to her natural menopause, the more likely this is to happen, and it can lead to severe psychosexual problems. In young women, hormone-replacement therapy should always be offered and psychiatric help may be needed.

Second malignant tumours. These are increasingly being reported in long-term survivors treated with chemotherapy. The subject is fully reviewed by Getaz [211]. The tumours usually occur some few years after cessation of treatment, and in some series the highest frequency has occurred in patients treated with both chemotherapy and radiotherapy. The proportion of long survivors developing second tumours has varied from about two per cent to about five per cent and seems to be increasing with time. About half of the second tumours are acute myeloid leukaemia, mostly the myelomonocytic or monocytic variety. These are nearly always refractory to treatment. There has also been an unexplained increase in the incidence of Kaposi's sarcoma. Common tumours such as skin cancers, carcinoma of the bronchus and colonic cancer make up most of the rest and there is an apparent tendency for skin tumours to occur on the edge of radiation-treatment fields. Carcinoma may arise in the thyroid if it has been irradiated.

The aetiology of these second tumours is probably multifactorial, representing an interplay between drug/radiation-induced carcinogenesis and immunological deficiencies in the patient which may relate both to the lymphoma itself and its treatment. Although the risk of second tumours is not a reason to stop the aggressive treatment of what was a previously incurable disease, it is sufficiently worrying to stimulate the careful examination of current treatment programmes in the hope that programmes that are associated with the development of fewer tumours can be developed.

Herpes zoster
A high incidence of herpes zoster is seen in patients with Hodgkin's disease [212–214] and this seems to have risen as treatment has become more intensive. Between one-quarter and one-third of patients now develop shingles or disseminated infection while receiving treatment or, more commonly, some time after treatment has been given. Children and adults are both affected, about equally. Some workers have suggested that splenectomy increases the incidence of zoster [212]; others, such as Reboul *et al.* [214], have found an association with the intensity of treatment, observing a rising incidence when patients are grouped respectively into those receiving limited-field radiotherapy, extensive-field radiotherapy or extensive-field radiotherapy plus chemotherapy. Stage also correlates with incidence, which rises with the extent of the Hodgkin's disease. In most people's experience the

development of zoster does not correlate with the prognosis for the patient's Hodgkin's disease.

Herpes zoster in Hodgkin patients can be severe, though it is rarely fatal. Dissemination is common, occurring to some extent in about one-third of patients. In most cases, the disease will run its course and the lesions will heal without treatment. Attempts to treat with cytosine arabinoside and adenine arabinoside have produced equivocal results and it is not certain whether these drugs are of any real benefit. Recently, an experimental antiviral agent, acyclovir (acycloguanosine), has shown promise and is the subject of clinical trial [215].

Non-Hodgkin lymphomas

There are many clinical similarities between the non-Hodgkin lymphomas and Hodgkin's disease. The clinical presentation can be much the same, the diagnosis is made by biopsy, usually of an enlarged lymph node or site of extranodal involvement such as gut or bone marrow, and the principles of treatment are the same: radiotherapy for localized, and chemotherapy for generalized disease. There are, however, many differences as well.

Non-Hodgkin lymphomas are far more common than Hodgkin's disease in the middle-aged and elderly, although young adults and children can be affected; they are frequently seen to involve multiple nodal sites at presentation and extranodal sites are often involved, notably the bone marrow, gut and, more rarely, the nervous system. Thus a wide variety of clinical presentations are possible and there is a high probability that patients will be found to have widely disseminated disease. This dissemination appears to be more disorderly and less predictable than in Hodgkin's disease, with the bone marrow frequently representing the 'final common pathway' for this group of diseases. Put another way, few patients with non-Hodgkin lymphomas have Stage I or II disease, many have Stage III or IV disease. Stage II disease is less curable with radiotherapy. This means that chemotherapy is the major method of treatment for most patients, with radiotherapy reserved for local problems, although there is currently an interest in the use of low-dose radiotherapy given to the whole body to control widely disseminated disease.

Although non-Hodgkin lymphomas as a class are less curable than Hodgkin's disease, this observation must be set against the fact that many, particularly the nodular ones, can pursue a very indolent course and are compatible with long survival for the patient, even though treatment does nothing more than palliate his disease.

Finally, faced with the diversity of pathological classifications, some descriptive, some functional and some a mixture of both, it is little wonder that clinicians involved in treating these tumours sometimes experience feelings of confusion and despair which are not dispelled by their frequent failure to obtain long remissions or good quality of life for their patients. Under these circumstances, it is perhaps wisest to look for clinical associations or 'syndromes', which are sufficiently commonly associated with particular histological types of disease to aid in deciding on the most appropriate available treatment. Attempts at staging, largely based upon concepts derived from experience with Hodgkin's disease, have helped, although it is likely that staging systems will change as the biology of this heterogeneous group of tumours is increasingly revealed.

STAGING

No completely standard plan of staging can be adopted for the non-Hodgkin lymphomas as in Hodgkin's disease. For the time being the Ann Arbor system [168] (Table 24.9) is still employed. Clinical assessment must include a full clinical examination, including an assessment of the lymphoid tissue in Waldeyer's ring which is best done by a laryngologist. In patients with suspected lymphomas of the small bowel, a barium meal and follow-through may reveal mucosal abnormalities, oedema, intrinsic or extrinsic narrowing of the bowel, or displacement of the bowel by mesenteric lymph-node masses. *Lymphography* may show the typical changes of lymphomatous involvement, but it is not uncommon for the opacified axial lymph nodes to be normal in the presence of gross mesenteric nodal disease. Here *CAT scanning* may reveal disease and in general this investigation is far more helpful for investigating abdominal non-Hodgkin lymphomas than for Hodgkin's disease.

Patients in whom there are symptoms or signs of meningeal involvement by tumour—headache, vomiting, photophobia and papilloedema—should have a *lumbar puncture* and the CSF cytology examined, preferably using the cytocentrifuge technique to concentrate the malignant cells on the slide, since it is their nature, not their number, which is important. As with leukaemia, papilloedema is *not* a contraindication to lumbar puncture. Patients with proven bone-marrow involvement are more likely to have central-nervous-system involvement and should have a lumbar puncture even in the absence of neurological symptoms or signs. Clinical features of extradural spinal-cord compression should be investigated by myelography.

The thorough investigation of the *bone marrow* is of enormous importance in patients with non-Hodgkin lymphoma, since it is so frequently involved. About half the patients with lymphocytic histology will be found to have marrow involvement [105–107, 216], but it is much rarer in patients with diffuse histiocytic pathology (less than 10%). Each subtype of disease tends to have an identifiable pattern of bone-marrow involvement, patients with nodular poorly differentiated lymphocytic lymphomas having a paratrabecular location of the tumour, while the diffuse variant shows a more diffuse than focal pattern. Patients with histiocytic lymphomas tend to have malignant cells diffusely distributed throughout the marrow, sometimes with associated fibrosis. Although in diffuse histiocytic lymphoma this pattern is uncommon, it is associated with central-nervous-system involvement [217] and it is important to detect it.

Because focal marrow involvement is common, aspiration biopsy is insufficient for diagnosis of involvement. Trephine biopsies should be done, preferably from more than one site. A single trephine biopsy has about a five times greater chance of revealing disease than an aspirate, and the yield increases by a further 10% if two trephines are done.

The *liver* can be investigated by percutaneous or laparoscopic biopsy. By this method about 30% of patients with lymphographically Stage III disease, or Stage IV disease by other criteria, will be found to have liver involvement. For most patients, this will not affect management since they will already have a stage of disease which would be treated with chemotherapy. For this reason liver biopsy is not an essential staging procedure except in patients who, by all other criteria, have Stage I disease. For the same reason, laparotomy is of very little value in non-Hodgkin lymphoma and in our view it is not justified.

The systematic clinical staging of patients, followed by chest X-ray, lymphography and scanning, marrow biopsy and lumbar puncture, places most patients in Stages III and IV. The few that remain with Stage I and II nodal disease (Stage II is rare) are properly treated with local radiotherapy and the majority will not relapse. Those that do so will require chemotherapy, the nature of which is determined by an assessment of the responsiveness of the disease type and its behaviour if left untreated. In a series of 133 patients with Stage I and II lymphoma, treated with local radiotherapy at the Royal Marsden Hospital, approximately 60% were alive and disease-free at four years. This is likely, in part, to reflect the longer natural history of nodular lymphomas since there was a clear survival advantage for this group when compared with those with diffuse histology.

THE CHOICE OF TREATMENT FOR NON-HODGKIN LYMPHOMAS

As stated previously, patients with Stages I and II disease can be treated with local radiotherapy, but those with Stages III and IV need chemotherapy.

There is no evidence that radiotherapy is more effective if the extended fields routinely employed to treat Hodgkin's disease are used, since localized disease is more likely to have spread to extranodal sites, particularly bone marrow, and not to so-called 'contiguous' lymph nodes. The main problem, therefore, is the choice of chemotherapy for advanced disease, and this depends largely on the histological grade of lymphoma, but also upon the age and fitness of the patient and whether the presence of disease in a particular anatomical site dictates a special treatment strategy. Five sites—the gastro-intestinal tract, the central nervous system, the bone marrow, the testis and the head and neck—require special consideration before choices based upon histology and age are considered. Two others—anterior mediastinal convoluted-cell lymphoma of T cells (so-called Sternberg's sarcoma), and mycosis fungoides—will be considered later.

Gastro-intestinal tract lymphomas

Bowel lymphomas may complicate advanced disseminated disease or occur as a primary phenomenon. Primary lymphoma of the gastro-intestinal (GI) tract may arise in a normal bowel or complicate coeliac disease [218]. In adults in this country, GI lymphomas tend to occur in the stomach and proximal small bowel, whereas in children they are commonly ileal. In elderly adults, GI lymphomas may be nodular and are usually associated with widespread dissemination to mesenteric lymph nodes, though they are usually confined to the abdomen. In younger adults and children they are either diffuse histiocytic or diffuse poorly differentiated lymphocytic and may disseminate widely, particularly in children. Their treatment is unsatisfactory. If they are confined to a single segment of bowel and can be resected surgically, there is a small chance of cure. In most patients, complete surgical excision is impossible, although local excision is usually necessary to bypass obstruction. Treatment with chemotherapy should then be given: this gives reasonable palliation but seldom cures. The value of abdominal radiation, either as an adjunct to chemotherapy or on its own, is uncertain. Many patients are too old and unfit for such an aggressive approach and palliative chemotherapy is all that is possible. In children, aggressive multi-agent chemotherapy should follow surgery where possible. There is early evidence that an increasing proportion of children may be cured by this means [220].

Central-nervous-system lymphomas

Extradural spinal-cord compression is commonly seen in patients with diffuse histiocytic and poorly differentiated lymphocytic diffuse lymphomas. It is a medical emergency which in the face of advancing signs of cord compression should be managed with decompressive laminectomy followed by radiotherapy. Myelography should be done as a routine, but is not a substitute for careful clinical examination, since several segments of cord may be involved with 'skip' areas between, and radiological screening may only reveal the lowest site of involvement. If this is suspected the whole spinal cord should be irradiated and not just the site of major involvement. Since the tumour is extradural, it is accessible to chemotherapy, which should also be given when the neurological disability has been relieved. Failure to act quickly may result in permanent neurological disability.

Meningeal involvement commonly accompanies bone-marrow involvement with diffuse lymphocytic or histiocytic lymphomas. It is treated like meningeal involvement in acute leukaemia (see Chapter 22) with intrathecal chemotherapy and whole neuraxis radiation.

Bone-marrow lymphomas

In elderly patients with indolent nodular lymphomas, bone-marrow involvement may be sparse and have little effect on outcome; in patients with diffuse lymphocytic poorly differentiated and diffuse histiocytic lymphomas it indicates a poor prognosis. Lister *et al.* [219], using an aggressive multidrug regimen combined with central-nervous-system radiation and intrathecal chemotherapy, followed by 'antileukaemic' maintenance treatment with 6-mercaptopurine and methotrexate, had no patients alive at two years, compared with 75% of patients without bone-marrow involvement. In the face of these results it is difficult to see where to go next. A few younger patients with bone-marrow involvement might be suitable for a bone-marrow allograft from an HLA-matched sibling donor following treatment with total-body irradiation. For the majority of adults, however, the outlook will remain dismal. For children the outlook may be a little better if they are treated with intensive antileukaemic-type treatment from the outset [220].

Testicular lymphomas

Testicular lymphomas are usually found in elderly men. They are always of diffuse histology, either histiocytic or poorly differentiated lymphocytic. Those staged as I or II can sometimes be cured by orchidectomy and radiotherapy to the pelvic and para-aortic nodes [221]. Progressive involvement of the lymphoid tissue in Waldeyer's ring or adjacent structures in the nasopharynx or oropharynx occurs in about one-quarter. Systemic chemotherapy should follow radiotherapy. In patients presenting with widespread disease outside the testicle, chemotherapy should be used

as primary treatment. A few of these Stage III and IV patients survive for five years or longer.

Head and neck lymphomas

Lymphomas may present with involvement of Waldeyer's ring, usually in association with cervical node involvement. Some are truly localized to these sites, but others may be associated with nodal involvement in other sites, or with gut or testicular involvement [221, 222]. In those patients with localized disease, cure with radical radiotherapy may be achieved; these probably represent about 25% of the whole group.

CHOICE OF TREATMENT BASED UPON HISTOLOGY

'Favourable' histology

This includes diffuse lymphocytic well-differentiated, nodular lymphocytic well- and poorly differentiated, nodular mixed lymphocytic and histiocytic. These diseases represent about half of all non-Hodgkin lymphomas. About 70% are nodular lymphocytic poorly differentiated (NLPD), 25% nodular mixed (NM) and most of the rest diffuse lymphocytic well-differentiated (DLWD). Nodular lymphocytic well-differentiated (NLWD) are very rare. The patients are usually in late middle age or old age and present with a history of non-tender bulky lymphadenopathy in many sites, waxing and waning with time and often present for many years. Systemic symptoms are usually absent and the patients may not present until the nodes are large enough to be a nuisance, or systemic symptoms develop. They may occasionally present with the symptoms of bone-marrow failure and be found to be anaemic. Massive mesenteric node involvement may result in a lumpy feel to the abdomen—the so-called 'sack-of-potatoes' sign. Many patients require no treatment for years, particularly those with NLPD and DLWD. Those with NM usually require treatment within a year of presentation, but in all patients who are asymptomatic it is sensible to observe them for a period before deciding to give any treatment.

Although there is evidence that patients who achieve complete remission live longer than those who do not (for review, see Ref. 223), it remains uncertain whether these patients would have fared just as well if no treatment had been given, their ability to respond to chemotherapy being a feature of disease diagnosed earlier than in those patients in whom remission does not occur. There is little evidence at present that aggressive treatment with combination chemotherapy is superior to that with single agents. For example, the Stanford group [224] compared a combination of cyclophosphamide, vincristine and prednisone (CVP) with split-course CVP plus total lymphoid irradiation (CVP-TLI) and with daily cyclophosphamide or chlorambucil (SA) in patients with Stage IV NLPD, NML and DLWD. The SA group responded more slowly than the other two groups but the final response rates were not significantly different, and there was no survival difference between the groups: at last analysis [223] the median relapse-free survival was 50 months in all groups with an actuarial survival of 70% at seven years; histological subtype had made no difference to survival. These conclusions have been endorsed by Lister *et al.* [225], but the NCI group have recently suggested [223] that nodular mixed lymphomas may be an exception to the finding that multiple-drug chemotherapy is no more effective than single agents. Using either C-MOPP, CVP or BACOP (Table 24.16), they achieved a complete remission rate of 77% in a group of patients with NM: 79% of these patients remained disease-free at over 90 months, compared with median remission durations of 16 months for NLPD and 23 months for DLWD, though there was no difference in survival between the groups at the time of reporting. It would nevertheless seem prudent to offer combination chemotherapy to younger patients with NM in the hope that their survival may ultimately be shown to be prolonged.

In another study [226], low-dose total-body irradiation (TBI: 10 rads/day to a total dose of 150–300 rads) was compared with CVP in patients with nodular and diffuse poorly differentiated lymphomas. There was no significant difference between CVP and TBI in either group although, as expected, the patients with nodular disease survived longer (80% at five years) than those with diffuse disease (approximately 30% at five years).

In summary, patients with 'favourable' lymphomas can be treated gently when treatment is needed. A possible exception may be young patients with NM. A satisfactory regimen is chlorambucil, 5–10 mg daily, reducing the dose or suspending treatment if there is evidence of bone-marrow toxicity. There seems to be no advantage for low-dose TBI over this approach, although there is a need to test the performance of TBI in patients who have first achieved a chemotherapy-induced remission. The purpose of such a study would be to attempt to achieve cure or at least very long survival. It should not be forgotten that although many elderly patients can comfortably co-exist with their disease and die of old age, the 'favourable' lymphomas are the cause of death in a significant number of patients who would have lived longer without them.

Table 24.16. Drug combinations for lymphomas of unfavourable histology

Regimen	Dosage schedule	Reference
CVP		
Cyclophosphamide	400 mg/m^2 p.o. daily for 5 days	233
Vincristine	1·4 mg/m^2 i.v. day 1	
Prednisone	100 mg/m^2 p.o. daily for 5 days	
Repeat every 3 weeks as tolerated		
C-MOPP		
Cyclophosphamide	650 mg/m^2 i.v. days 1 and 8	228
Vincristine	1·4 mg/m^2 i.v. days 1 and 8	
Procarbazine	100 mg/m^2 p.o. daily for 14 days	
Prednisone	40 mg/m^2 p.o. daily for 14 days	
Repeat monthly		
BACOP		
Bleomycin	5 mg/m^2 i.v. days 15 and 21	232
Doxorubicin (adriamycin)	25 mg/m^2 i.v. days 1 and 8	
Cyclophosphamide	650 mg/m^2 i.v. days 1 and 8	
Vincristine	1·4 mg/m^2 i.v. days 1 and 8	
Prednisone	60 mg/m^2 p.o. days 15 and 29	
Repeat monthly		
CHOP		
Cyclophosphamide	750 mg/m^2 i.v. day 1	229
Doxorubicin	50 mg/m^2 i.v. day 1	
Vincristine	1·4 mg/m^2 i.v. day 1	
Prednisone	100 mg/m^2 p.o. days 1, 2, 3, 4 and 5	
Repeat every 3 weeks		

'Unfavourable' histology

This includes diffuse lymphocytic poorly differentiated (DLPD), diffuse mixed (DM), diffuse histiocytic (DH) and Lennert's lymphoma. In comparison with the lymphomas of favourable histology, these have a more acute onset, progress rapidly if untreated, frequently present with widespread disease and are often associated with systemic symptoms. These symptoms are usually the same as those associated with Hodgkin's disease—fever, weight loss, sweating and pruritus. Dyspnoea may be associated with lung or pleural infiltration, bone pain may be due to multiple bone deposits or marrow infiltration, and hypochondrial pain may result from rapid enlargement of the liver or spleen. Central-nervous-system involvement may manifest with features of meningeal disease or spinal-cord compression and gut involvement may produce abdominal pain, ascites or the symptoms of obstruction. Some patients present with symptoms of bone-marrow failure due to lymphomatous infiltration. Backache or hydronephrosis due to massively enlarged retroperitoneal lymph nodes may be a feature, as may biliary obstruction from enlarged nodes in the porta hepatis. Superior vena caval obstruction sometimes occurs, most commonly with DH. In general, DH has a greater tendency to involve extranodal sites other than bone marrow, whereas DLPD more commonly involves lymph nodes and bone marrow and at times can produce a frankly leukaemic picture.

Unless treated, these lymphomas are rapidly fatal and unless truly localized, when treatment with radiotherapy may be appropriate, they should be treated with intensive combination chemotherapy (Table 24.16). In contrast to the nodular lymphomas, intensive treatment that produces complete remission of disease is clearly associated with an improvement in the quality and quantity of survival. Indeed, in the DH group, evidence is accumulating that a high proportion of patients who achieve complete remission become long-term disease-free survivors and may be cured [227]. In DH, reported complete-remission rates range from 41% for C-MOPP [228] to 68% for CHOP [229], which contains adriamycin. Other studies have also shown an advantage for adriamycin-containing combinations [230, 231] and it now seems proper to recommend their use in patients with DH and to treat the patients with the utmost vigour in an attempt to secure complete remission.

Of particular interest in this setting is a report [234] in which CHOP chemotherapy was given to a group of 22 DH patients with *early*-stage disease (Stages I and II): 14 patients received chemotherapy alone and eight also received local radiotherapy. All patients achieved complete remission and 21 remained disease-free, with a median relapse-free survival from completion of chemotherapy of over 23 months. Several other groups have reported impressive relapse-free survival rates in early disease using combinations of chemotherapy and radiotherapy, to the point where the need for radiotherapy is being questioned. This is now the subject of controlled clinical trials.

In contrast to patients with DH, those with DLPD show no evidence of potential cure with the currently tested combinations. Here the complete-remission rates are lower than with DH and there is a constant tendency for patients to relapse: half have relapsed within about 15 months and few survive beyond two years [233]. In this setting, it is less reasonable to give aggressive treatment, at least to old people, but young patients should be treated vigorously with combination chemotherapy, since a handful may become long survivors.

STERNBERG'S SARCOMA

This term describes a syndrome in which an anterior mediastinal lymphomatous mass is associated with bone-marrow infiltration and leukaemia. The histological features are those of the lymphoblastic lymphoma. It is best regarded as a variant of T-cell acute leukaemia and should be treated as such (see Chapter 22). About three-quarters of patients present with a massive anterior mediastinal shadow, often with a left-sided pleural effusion, associated with frank leukaemia, frequently with very high leukaemic-cell counts in the peripheral blood. However, it is very important to realize that while about one-quarter of patients may present with the thymic mass but without evidence of overt bone-marrow involvement, this *always* develops, usually within a few weeks or months. The disease should therefore always be treated as acute lymphoblastic leukaemia from the outset. Local treatment with radiotherapy to the mediastinum is of uncertain value, despite the fact that the disease is exquisitely radiosensitive and the mass will usually have vanished after a few hundred rads have been given, behaviour which led to misplaced optimism on the part of physicians in the past, which rapidly disappeared when the patient developed frank leukaemia.

The typical patient with Sternberg's sarcoma is an adolescent boy. Girls are infrequently affected and the disease is uncommon in young children, being more a condition of adolescence and early adulthood. The syndrome probably accounts for about half the patients with T-cell leukaemia, the other half presenting without clinical evidence of lymphomatous involvement of the thymus.

MYCOSIS FUNGOIDES

Clinical features

Mycosis fungoides (MF) is a chronic lymphoma which arises in the skin. In its later stages, nodal and other systemic involvement may occur. It evolves through three stages—the first a *premycotic* stage consisting of lesions similar to eczema or psoriasis. The lesions are sometimes itchy and may be very sparsely distributed throughout the skin. This phase can persist for many years before giving way to the *infiltrative* or *plaque* stage. Here the lesions become infiltrated with the characteristic tumour cells, and these plaques increase in both size and number. During the plaque stage, the skin may become generally erythematous to produce the so called 'homme rouge', or invasion of the blood with typical convoluted T-cell-derived tumour cells may occur—the so-called *Sézary syndrome*, which is best thought of as a variant of MF with a leukaemic phase. At this point the skin becomes intensely itchy.

Further progression of the skin lesions with deeper infiltration leads to the nodular or *tumour* phase. At this point infiltration of lymph nodes and viscera with tumour cells frequently occurs, producing signs or symptoms of pulmonary infiltration, hepatomegaly and lymphadenopathy. Few patients survive longer than two years from the onset of the tumour phase, but the time from the onset of the first premycotic lesion to death in MF can be very long—as much as 15 years—and the interval from the very first onset of symptoms to biopsy confirmation of the disease varies widely and can last eight years or more in some cases. Thus patients can co-exist with the disease for long periods although they progressively deteriorate, and this makes any assessment of the influence of treatment difficult. The subject is fully reviewed by Broder & Bunn [235].

Treatment

Four types of treatment can bring about useful palliation at different stages of the disease: topical application of nitrogen mustard [236], photochemotherapy with psoralens and ultraviolet light (PUVA), electron-beam therapy and systemic chemotherapy.

Topical nitrogen mustard. This is useful in the infiltrative stage and consists of the application of 10 mg of nitrogen mustard dissolved in 50 mg of water to the whole skin surface daily. In responding patients this can be continued for six to 12 months and the frequency of treatment then reduced.

Photochemotherapy. Treatment with psoralen and ultraviolet light A [235] gives good long-term palliation in patients with non-tumorous lesions.

Electron-beam therapy. This has been used by many groups, notably those at Stanford [237]. It produces a high remission rate and about 20% of patients remain relapse-free at three years. It is expensive and technically rather difficult but is a useful option in those centres possessing radiotherapy equipment which can produce electron beams capable of treating large fields.

Chemotherapy. Chemotherapy with those agents that have been widely employed to treat other lymphomas can be employed in MF, and can be combined with electron-beam therapy and PUVA in patients with advanced disease. It does not cure but can palliate patients with advanced disease for several years. For further details the reader is again referred to the excellent review by Broder & Bunn [235].

REFERENCES

1 HOWARD J.C., HUNT S.V. & GOWANS J.L. (1972) Identification of marrow-derived small lymphocytes in the lymphoid tissue and thoracic duct lymph of normal rats. *Journal of Experimental Medicine*, **135**, 200.

2 GOOD R.A. (1955) Failure of plasma cell formation in the bone marrow and lymph nodes of patients with agammaglobulinemia. *Journal of Laboratory and Clinical Medicine*, **46**, 167.

3 CLEVELAND W.W., FOGEL B.J., BROWN W.T. & KAY H.E.M. (1968) Foetal thymic transplant in a case of DiGeorge's syndrome. *Lancet*, **ii**, 1211.

4 SILVEIRA N.P.A., MENDES N.F. & TOLNAI M.E.A. (1972) Tissue localization of two populations of human lymphocytes distinguished by membrane receptors. *Journal of Immunology*, **108**, 1456.

5 SEYMOUR G.J., GREAVES M.F. & JANOSSY G. (1980) Identification of cells expressing T and P.28,33 (Ia-like) antigens in sections of human lymphoid tissue. *Clinical and Experimental Immunology*, **39**, 66.

6 OORT J. & TURK J.L. (1965) A histological and autoradiographic study of lymph nodes during the development of contact sensitivity in the guinea-pig. *British Journal of Experimental Pathology*, **46**, 147.

7 NOSSAL G.J.V., ABBOT A., MITCHELL J. & LUMMUS Z. (1968) Ultrastructural features of antigen capture in primary and secondary lymphoid follicles. *Journal of Experimental Medicine*, **127**, 277.

8 LUKES R.J. & COLLINS R.D. (1975) New approaches to the classification of the lymphomata. *British Journal of Cancer*, **31** (Suppl. II), 1.

9 GERARD-MARCHANT R., HAMLIN I., LENNERT K., RILKE F., STANSFELD A.G. & VAN UNNIK J.A.M. (1974) Classification of non-Hodgkin's lymphomas. *Lancet*, **ii**, 406.

10 LENNERT K. (1978) *Malignant Lymphomas other than Hodgkin's Disease*, p. 38. Springer-Verlag, New York.

11 LAMELIN J.P., THOMASSET N., ANDRE C., BROCHIER J. & REVILLARD J.P. (1978) Studies of human T and B lymphocytes with heterologous antisera. III. Immuno-

fluorescent studies on tonsil sections. *Immunology*, **35**, 463.

12 DAVIES A.J.S., CARTER R.L., LEUCHARS E., WALLIS V. & KELLER P.C. (1969) The morphology of immune reactions in normal, thymectomized and reconstituted mice. *Immunology*, **16**, 57.

13 LENNERT K. (1978) *Malignant Lymphomas other than Hodgkin's Disease*, p. 65. Springer-Verlag, New York.

14 VAN FURTH R., LANGEVOORT H.L. & SCHABERG A. (1975) Mononuclear phagocytes in human pathology— proposal for an approach to improved classification. In: *Mononuclear Phagocytes in Immunity, Infection and Pathology* (ed. Van Furth R.), p. 1. Blackwell Scientific Publications, Oxford.

15 NOSSAL G.J.V., ABBOT A. & MITCHELL J. (1967) Electron microscopic radioautographic studies of antigen capture in lymph node medulla. *Journal of Experimental Medicine*, **127**, 263.

16 GLICK A.D., BENNETT B. & COLLINS R.D. (1980) Neoplasms of the mononuclear phagocyte system: criteria for diagnosis. *Investigative and Cell Pathology*, **3**, 259.

17 LENNERT K. (1978) *Malignant Lymphomas other than Hodgkin's Disease*, p. 48. Springer-Verlag, New York.

18 KULENKAMPFF J., JANOSSY G. & GREAVES M.F. (1977) Acid esterase in human lymphoid cells and leukaemic blasts: a marker for T lymphocytes. *British Journal of Haematology*, **36**, 231.

19 SEYMOUR G.J., DOCKRELL H.M. & GREENSPAN J.S. (1978) Enzyme differentiation of lymphocyte subpopulations in sections of human lymph nodes, tonsils and periodontal disease. *Clinical and Experimental Immunology*, **32**, 169.

20 BIBERFELD P. (1971) Morphogenesis in blood lymphocytes stimulated with phytohaemagglutinin (PHA). *Acta Pathologica et Microbiologica Scandinavica*, **223** (Suppl.), 29.

21 STEIN H. & MÜLLER-HERMELINK H.K. (1977) Simultaneous presence of receptors for complement and sheep red blood cells on human fetal thymocytes. *British Journal of Haematology*, **36**, 225.

22 NANBA K., JAFFE E.S., BRAYLAN R.C., SOBAN E.J. & BERARD C.W. (1977) Alkaline phosphatase-positive malignant lymphoma. *American Journal of Clinical Pathology*, **68**, 535.

23 LEDER L.D. (1964) Über die selektive fermentcytochemische Darstellung von neutrophilen myeloischen Zellen und Gewebsmastzellen im Paraffinschnitt. *Klinische Wochenschrift*, **42**, 553.

24 MCCAFFREY R., HARRISON T.A., PARKMAN R. & BALTIMORE D. (1975) Terminal deoxynucleotidyl transferase activity in human leukemic cells and in normal human thymocytes. *New England Journal of Medicine*, **292**, 775.

25 BRADSTOCK K.F., JANOSSY G., PIZZOLO G., HOFFBRAND A.V., MCMICHAEL A., PILCH J.R., MILSTEIN C., BEVERLEY P. & BOLLUM F.J. (1980) Subpopulations of normal and leukemic human thymocytes: an analysis using monoclonal antibodies. *Journal of the National Cancer Institute*, **65**, 33.

26 MASON D.Y. & TAYLOR C.R. (1975) The distribution of muramidase (lysozyme) in human tissues. *Journal of Clinical Pathology*, **28**, 124.

27 BLOOMFIELD C.D., GAJL-PECZALSKA K.J., FRIZZERA G.,

KERSEY J.H. & GOLDMAN A.I. (1979) Clinical utility of lymphocyte surface markers combined with the Lukes–Collins histologic classification in adult lymphoma. *New England Journal of Medicine*, **301**, 512.

28 EHLENBERGER A.G., MCWILLIAMS M., PHILLIPS-QUAGLIATA J.M., LAMM M.E. & NUSSENZWEIG V. (1976) Immunoglobulin-bearing and complement-receptor lymphocytes constitute the same population in human peripheral blood. *Journal of Clinical Investigation*, **57**, 53.

29 BROUET J.C., LABAUME S. & SELIGMANN M. (1975) Evaluation of T and B lymphocyte membrane markers in human non-Hodgkin malignant lymphomata. *British Journal of Cancer*, **31** (Suppl. II), 121.

30 TAYLOR C.R. (1979) *Hodgkin's Disease and the Lymphomas*, p. 8. Eden Press, Montreal.

31 ANDERSSON J., BUXBAUM J., CITRONBAUM R., DOUGLAS S., FORNI L., MELCHERS F., PERNIS B. & STOTT D. (1974) IgM-producing tumours in the BALB/c mouse. *Journal of Experimental Medicine*, **140**, 742.

32 JAFFE E.S., SHEVACH E.M., FRANK M.M., BERARD C.W. & GREEN I. (1974) Nodular lymphoma—evidence for origin from follicular B lymphocytes. *New England Journal of Medicine*, **290**, 813.

33 SPRINGER T.A., KOUFMAN J.F., TERNHORST C. & STROMINGER J.L. (1977) Purification and structural characterisation of human HLA-linked B-cell antigens. *Nature (London)*, **268**, 213.

34 ALLISON J.P., WALKER L.E., RUSSELL W.A., PELLEGRINO M.A., FERRONE S., REISFELD R.A., FRELINGER J.A. & SILVER J. (1978) Murine Ia and human DR antigens: homology of amino-terminal sequences. *Proceedings of the National Academy of Sciences, USA*, **75**, 3953.

35 GREAVES M.F., VERBI W., FESTENSTEIN H., PAPSTERIADIS C., JARAQUEMADA D. & HAYWOOD A. (1979) 'Ia-like' antigens on human T cells. *European Journal of Immunology*, **9**, 356.

36 BURNS G.F., WORMAN C.P., ROBERTS B.E., RAPER C.G.L., BARKER C.R. & CAWLEY J.C. (1979) Terminal B cell development as seen in different human myelomas and related disorders. *Clinical and Experimental Immunology*, **35**, 180.

37 BROCHIER J., ABOU-HAMED Y.A., GUEHO J.P. & REVILLARD J.P. (1976) Study of human T and B lymphocytes with heterologous antisera. *Immunology*, **31**, 749.

38 GREAVES M.F. & JANOSSY G. (1976) Antisera to human T lymphocytes. In: *In-vitro Methods in Cell-mediated and Tumour Immunity* (ed. Bloom B.R. & David J.R.). Academic Press, London.

39 JANOSSY G., GREAVES M.F. & SUTHERLAND R. (1977) Comparative analysis of membrane phenotypes in acute lymphoid leukaemia and in lymphoid blast crisis of chronic myeloid leukaemia. *Leukaemia Research*, **1**, 289.

40 GREAVES M.F. & BROWN G. (1975) Antisera to acute lymphoblastic leukemia cells. *Clinical Immunology and Immunopathology*, **4**, 67.

41 TAYLOR C.R. (1978) Classification of lymphoma. *Archives of Pathology and Laboratory Medicine*, **102**, 549.

42 RAPPAPORT H. (1966) Atlas of tumour pathology, section III. Fascicle 8. *Tumours of the Haemopoietic*

System, p. 97. Armed Forces Institute of Pathology, Washington DC.

43 JONES S.E., FUKS Z., BULL M., KADIN M.E., DORFMAN R.F., KAPLAN H.S., ROSENBERG S.A. & KIM H. (1973) Non-Hodgkin's lymphomas. IV. Clinicopathologic correlation in 405 cases. *Cancer*, **43**, 806.

44 LUKES R.J. & COLLINS R.D. (1977) Lukes–Collins classification and its significance. *Cancer Treatment Reports*, **61**, 971.

45 BUTLER J.J., STRYKER J.A. & SHULLENBERGER C.C. (1974) A clinicopathological study of stages I and II non-Hodgkin's lymphomata using the Lukes–Collins classification. *British Journal of Cancer*, **31** (Suppl. II), 208.

46 MANN R.B., JAFFE E.S., BRAYLAN R.C., NANBA K., FRANK M.M., ZIEGLER J.L. & BERARD C.W. (1976) Non-endemic Burkitt's lymphoma—a B-cell tumour related to germinal centers. *New England Journal of Medicine*, **295**, 685.

47 BENNETT M.H., FARRER-BROWN A., HENRY K. & JELLIFFE A.M. (1974) Classifications of non-Hodgkin's lymphomas. *Lancet*, **ii**, 405.

48 DORFMANN R.F. (1977) Pathology of the non-Hodgkin's lymphomas: new classifications. *Cancer Treatment Reports*, **61**, 945.

49 MATHE G., RAPPAPORT H., O'CONOR G.T. & TORLONI H. (1976) *International Histological Classification of Tumours*. XIV. Histological and cytological typing of neoplastic diseases of haematopoietic and lymphoid tissues. World Health Organisation, Geneva.

50 GALTON D.A.G., GOLDMAN J.M., WILTSHAW E., CATOVSKY D., HENRY K. & GOLDENBERG G.J. (1974) Prolymphocytic leukaemia. *British Journal of Haematology*, **27**, 7.

51 BERARD C.W. (1977) Round table discussion of histopathologic classification. *Cancer Treatment Reports*, **61**, 1037.

52 NATHWANI B.N. (1979) A critical analysis of the classifications of non-Hodgkin's lymphomas. *Cancer*, **44**, 347.

53 LENNERT K., MOHRI N., STEIN H. & KAISERLING E. (1975) The histopathology of malignant lymphoma. *British Journal of Haematology*, **31**, 193.

54 PANGALIS G.A., NATHWANI B.N. & RAPPAPORT H. (1977) Malignant lymphoma, well-differentiated lymphocytic. *Cancer*, **39**, 999.

55 BRAYLAN R.C., JAFFE E.S., BURBACH J.W., FRANK M.M., JOHNSON R.E. & BERARD C.W. (1976) Similarities of surface characteristics of neoplastic well-differentiated lymphocytes from solid tissues and from peripheral blood. *Cancer Research*, **36**, 1619.

56 PINKUS G.S. & SAID J.W. (1979) Characterization of non-Hodgkin's lymphomas using multiple cell markers. *American Journal of Pathology*, **94**, 349.

57 HABESHAW J.A., CATLEY P.F., STANSFELD A.G. & BREARLEY R.L. (1979) Surface phenotyping, histology and the nature of non-Hodgkin lymphoma in 157 patients. *British Journal of Cancer*, **40**, 11.

58 LUKES R.J., TAYLOR C.R., PARKER J.W., LINCOLN T.L., PATTENGALE P.K. & TINDLE B.H. (1978) A morphologic and immunologic surface marker study of 299 cases of non-Hodgkin lymphomas and related leukemias. *American Journal of Pathology*, **90**, 461.

59 PIZZOLO G., SLOANE J.P., BEVERLEY P., THOMAS J.A., BRADSTOCK K.F. & JANOSSY G. (1980) Differential diagnosis of malignant lymphoma and non-lymphoid tumours using monoclonal anti-leucocyte antibody. *Cancer*, **46**, 2640.

60 BROUET J.C., FLANDRIN G., SASPORTES M., PREUD'-HOMME J.L. & SELIGMANN M. (1975) Chronic lymphocytic leukaemia of T-cell origin. *Lancet*, **ii**, 890.

61 NATHWANI B.N., KIM H., RAPPAPORT H., SOLOMON J. & FOX M. (1978) Non-Hodgkin's lymphomas: a clinicopathologic study comparing two classifications. *Cancer*, **41**, 303.

62 SILVESTRINI R., PIAZZA R., RICCARDI A. & RILKE F. (1977) Correlation of cell kinetic findings with morphology of non-Hodgkin's malignant lymphomas. *Journal of National Cancer Institute*, **58**, 499.

63 JAFFE E.S., BRAYLAN R.C., NANBA K., FRANK M.M. & BERARD C.W. (1977) Functional markers: a new perspective on malignant lymphomas. *Cancer Treatment Reports*, **61**, 953.

64 FRIZZERA G., GAJL-PECZALSKA K.J., BLOOMFIELD C.D. & KERSEY J.H. (1979) Predictability of immunologic phenotype of malignant lymphomas by conventional morphology. *Cancer*, **43**, 1216.

65 LUKES R.J. & COLLINS R.D. (1974) Immunologic characterization of human malignant lymphomas. *Cancer*, **34**, 1488.

66 WALDRON J.A., LEECH J.H., GLICK A.D., FLEXNER J.M. & COLLINS R.D. (1977) Malignant lymphoma of peripheral T-lymphocyte origin. *Cancer*, **40**, 1604.

67 BARCOS M.P. & LUKES R.J. (1975) Malignant lymphoma of convoluted lymphocytes: a new entity of possible T-cell type. In: *Conflicts in Childhood Cancer: An Evaluation of Current Management, Vol. 4* (ed. Sinks L.F. & Godden J.O.), p. 147. Alan Liss Inc., New York.

68 STEIN H., PETERSEN N., GAEDICKE G., LENNERT K. & LANDBECK G. (1976) Lymphoblastic lymphoma of convoluted or acid phosphatase type—a tumour of T precursor cells. *International Journal of Cancer*, **17**, 292.

69 NATHWANI B.N., KIM H. & RAPPAPORT H. (1976) Malignant lymphoma, lymphoblastic. *Cancer*, **38**, 964.

70 BERNARD A., BOUMSELL L., BAYLE C., RICHARD Y., COPPIN H., PENIT C., ROUGET P., MICHAEU C., CLAUSSE B., GERARD-MARCHANT R., DAUSSET J. & LEMERLE J. (1979) Subsets of malignant lymphomas in children related to the cell phenotype. *Blood*, **54**, 1058.

71 BURKITT D. (1958) A sarcoma involving the jaws in African children. *British Journal of Surgery*, **46**, 218.

72 O'CONOR G.T. & DAVIES J.N.P. (1960) Malignant tumours in African children. *Journal of Pediatrics*, **56**, 526.

73 O'CONOR G.T., RAPPAPORT H. & SMITH E.B. (1965) Childhood lymphoma resembling 'Burkitt tumor' in the United States. *Cancer*, **18**, 411.

74 DORFMAN R.F. (1965) Childhood lymphosarcoma in St Louis, Missouri, clinically and histologically resembling Burkitt's tumor. *Cancer*, **18**, 418.

75 BERARD C., O'CONOR G.T., THOMAS I.B. & TORLONI H. (1969) Histopathological definition of Burkitt's tumour. *Bulletin of the World Health Organisation*, **40**, 601.

76 ARSENEAU J.C., CANELLOS G.P., BANKS P.M., BERARD C.W., GRALNICK H.R. & DE VITA V.T. (1975) American

Burkitt's lymphoma: a clinicopathologic study of 30 cases. *American Journal of Medicine*, **58**, 314.

77 LEVINE P.H., CHO B.R., CONNELLY R.R., BERARD C.W., O'CONOR G.T., DORFMAN R.F., EASTON J.M. & DE VITA V.T. (1975) The American Burkitt lymphoma registry: a progress report. *Annals of Internal Medicine*, **83**, 31.

78 NKRUMAH F.K. & PERKINS I.V. (1973) Burkitt's lymphoma in Ghana: clinical features and response to chemotherapy. *International Journal of Cancer*, **11**, 19.

79 FLANDRIN G., BROUET J.C., DANIEL M.T. & PREUD'-HOMME J.L. (1975) Acute leukemia with Burkitt's tumor cells: a study of six cases with special reference to lymphocyte surface markers. *Blood*, **45**, 183.

80 BERARD C.W. & DORFMAN R.F. (1974) Histopathology of malignant lymphomas. *Clinics in Haematology*, **3**, 39.

81 LENNERT K. & MESTDAGH J. (1968) Lymphogranulomatosen mit konstant hohem Epitheloidzellgehalt. *Virchows Archiv Abteilung Pathologische Anatomie*, **344**, 1.

82 BURKE J.S. & BUTLER J.J. (1976) Malignant lymphoma with a high content of epithelioid histiocytes (Lennert's lymphoma). *American Journal of Clinical Pathology*, **66**, 1.

83 KIM H., JACOBS C., WARNKE R.A. & DORFMAN R.F. (1978) Malignant lymphoma with a high content of epithelioid histiocytes. *Cancer*, **41**, 620.

84 HAYES D. & ROBERTSON J.H. (1979) Malignant lymphoma with a high content of epithelioid histiocytes. *Journal of Clinical Pathology*, **32**, 675.

85 TINDLE B.H. & LONG J.C. (1977) Case records of the Massachusetts General Hospital. *New England Journal of Medicine*, **297**, 206.

86 KIM H., NATHWANI B.N. & RAPPAPORT H. (1980) 'So called Lennert's lymphoma'. Is it a clinico-pathological entity? *Cancer*, **45**, 1379.

87 LEVER W.F. (1975) *Histopathology of the Skin*. 5th edn., p. 696. J. P. Lippincott Co., Philadelphia.

88 ROBINOWITZ B.N., NOGUCHI S. & ROENIGK H.H. JR (1976) Tumor cell characterization in mycosis fungoides. *Cancer*, **37**, 1747.

89 SCHWARZE E.W. (1975) T-cell origin of acid-phosphatase-positive lymphoblasts. *Lancet*, **ii**, 1264.

90 RAPPAPORT H. & THOMAS L.B. (1974) Mycosis fungoides: the pathology of extracutaneous involvement. *Cancer*, **34**, 1198.

91 SEZARY A. & BOUVRAIN Y. (1938) Erythrodermie avec présence de cellules monstrueuses dans le derme et le sang circulant. *Société de Dermatologie et de Syphiligraphie*, **45**, 254.

92 BROUET J.C., FLANDRIN G. & SELIGMANN M. (1973) Indications of the thymus-derived nature of the proliferating cells in six patients with Sézary's syndrome. *New England Journal of Medicine*, **289**, 341.

93 LUTZNER M.A., HOBBS J.W. & HORVATH P. (1971) Ultrastructure of abnormal cells in Sézary syndrome, mycosis fungoides and para-psoriasis en plaque. *Archives of Dermatology*, **103**, 375.

94 CARSON C.P., ACKERMAN L.V. & MALTBY J.D. (1955) Plasma cell myeloma: a clinical pathologic and roentgenologic review of 90 cases. *American Journal of Clinical Pathology*, **25**, 819.

95 CATOVSKY D., PETTIT J.E., GALTON D.A.G., SPIERS A.S.D. & HARRISON C.V. (1974) Leukaemic reticuloendotheliosis ('hairy' cell leukaemia): a distinct clinico-pathological entity. *British Journal of Haematology*, **26**, 9.

96 BURKE J.S., BYRNE G.E. & RAPPAPORT H. (1974) Hairy cell leukemia (Leukemic reticuloendotheliosis). *Cancer*, **33**, 1399.

97 BURKE J.S., MACKAY B. & RAPPAPORT H. (1976) Hairy cell leukemia (leukemic reticuloendotheliosis: ultrastructure of the spleen. *Cancer*, **37**, 2267.

98 RAMOT B., SHAHIN N. & BUBIS J.J. (1965) Malabsorption syndrome in lymphoma of small intestine. *Israel Journal of Medical Science*, **1**, 221.

99 LEWIN K.J., KAHN L.B. & NOVIS B.H. (1976) Primary intestinal lymphoma of 'Western' and 'Mediterranean' type, alpha chain disease and massive plasma cell infiltration. *Cancer*, **38**, 2511.

100 LEWIN K.J., RANCHOD M. & DORFMAN R.F. (1978) Lymphomas of the gastrointestinal tract: a study of 117 cases presenting with gastrointestinal disease. *Cancer*, **42**, 693.

101 AL-SALEEM T. & ZARDAWI I.M. (1979) Primary lymphomas of the small intestine in Iraq: a pathological study of 145 cases. *Histopathology*, **3**, 89.

102 BENNETT M.H. & MILLETT Y.L. (1969) Nodular sclerotic lymphosarcoma, a possible new clinico-pathological entity. *Clinical Radiology*, **20**, 339.

103 ROSAS-URIBE A. & RAPPAPORT H. (1972) Malignant lymphoma, histiocytic type with sclerosis (sclerosing reticulum cell sarcoma). *Cancer*, **29**, 946.

104 FREEMAN C., BERG J.W. & CUTLER S.J. (1972) Occurrence and prognosis of extranodal lymphomas. *Cancer*, **29**, 252.

105 JONES S.E., ROSENBERG S.A. & KAPLAN H.S. (1972) Non-Hodgkin's lymphomas. I. Bone marrow involvement. *Cancer*, **29**, 954.

106 STEIN R.S., ULTMANN J.E., BYRNE G.E., MORAN E.M., GOLOMB H.M. & OETZEL N. (1976) Bone marrow involvement in non-Hodgkin's lymphoma. *Cancer*, **37**, 629.

107 DICK F., BLOOMFIELD C.D. & BRUNNING R.D. (1974) Incidence, cytology, and histopathology of non-Hodgkin's lymphomas in the bone marrow. *Cancer*, **33**, 1382.

108 BELPOMME D., MATHE G. & DAVIES A.J.S. (1977) Clinical significance and prognostic value of the T-B immunological classification of human primary acute lymphoid leukaemias. *Lancet*, **ii**, 555.

109 VAN DEN TWEEL J.G., LUKES R.J. & TAYLOR C.R. (1979) Pathophysiology of lymphocyte transformation: a study of so-called composite lymphomas. *American Journal of Clinical Pathology*, **71**, 509.

110 LICHTENSTEIN L. (1953) Histiocytosis X. Integration of eosinophilic granuloma of bone, 'Letterer–Siwe disease' and 'Schüller–Christian disease' as related manifestations of a single nosologic entity. *Archives of Pathology*, **56**, 84.

111 RAPPAPORT H. (1966) Atlas of tumor pathology, section III. Fascicle 8. *Tumours of the Haematopoietic System*, p. 49. Armed Forces Institute of Pathology, Washington DC.

112 WARNKE R.A., KIM H. & DORFMAN R.F. (1975) Malignant histiocytosis (histiocytic medullary reticulosis). *Cancer*, **35**, 215.

113 LAMPERT I.A., CATOVSKY D. & BERGIER N. (1978)

Malignant histiocytosis: a clinico-pathological study of 12 cases. *British Journal of Haematology*, **40**, 65.

114 SCOTT R.B. & ROBB-SMITH A.H.T. (1939) Histiocytic medullary reticulosis. *Lancet*, **ii**, 194.

115 LUKES R.J. & BUTLER J.J. (1966) The pathology and nomenclature of Hodgkin's disease. *Cancer Research*, **26**, 1063.

116 LUKES R.J. (1966) Report of the Nomenclature Committee. *Cancer Research*, **26**, 1311.

117 KADIN M.E., DONALDSON S.S. & DORFMAN R.F. (1970) Isolated granulomas in Hodgkin's disease. *New England Journal of Medicine*, **28**, 859.

118 RAPPAPORT H., BERARD C.W., BUTLER J.J., DORFMAN R.F., LUKES R.J. & THOMAS L.B. (1971) Report of the committee on histopathological criteria contribution to staging of Hodgkin's Disease. *Cancer Research*, **31**, 1864.

119 WEISS R.B., BRUNNING R.D. & KENNEDY B.J. (1975) Hodgkin's disease in the bone marrow. *Cancer*, **36**, 2077.

120 WEBB D.I., UBOGY G. & SILVER R.T. (1970) Importance of bone-marrow biopsy in the clinical staging of Hodgkin's disease. *Cancer*, **26**, 313.

121 PECKHAM M.J. & COOPER E.H. (1969) Proliferation characteristics of the various classes of cells in Hodgkin's disease. *Cancer*, **24**, 135.

122 DORFMAN R.F., RICE D.F., MITCHELL A.D., KEMPSON R.L. & LEVINE A. (1973) Ultrastructural studies of Hodgkin's disease. *National Cancer Institute Monograph*, **36**, 221.

123 GLICK A.D., LEECH J.H., FLEXNER J.M. & COLLINS R.D. (1978) Ultrastructural study of Reed–Sternberg cells. *American Journal of Pathology*, **85**, 195.

124 CURRAN R.C. & JONES E.L. (1978) Hodgkin's disease: an immunohistochemical and histological study. *Journal of Pathology*, **125**, 39.

125 CURRAN R.C. & JONES E.L. (1978) Immunoglobulin in Reed–Sternberg and Hodgkin cells. *Journal of Pathology*, **126**, 35.

126 TAYLOR C.R. (1974) The nature of Reed–Sternberg cells and other malignant 'reticulum' cells. *Lancet*, **ii**, 802.

127 STUART A.E., WILLIAMS A.R.W. & HABESHAW J.A. (1977) Rosetting and other reactions of the Reed–Sternberg cell. *Journal of Pathology*, **122**, 81.

128 PATTER M., SKLAR M.D. & ROWE W.P. (1973) Rapid viral induction of plasmacytosis in pristane-primed BALB/c mice. *Science*, **182**, 592.

129 OLDING L.B., JENSEN F.C. & OLDSTONE M.B.A. (1975) Pathogenesis of cytomegalovirus infection. Activation of virus from bone marrow-derived lymphocytes by *in-vitro* allogeneic reaction. *Journal of Experimental Medicine*, **141**, 561.

130 EPSTEIN M.A. & ACHONG B.G. (1979) The relationship of the virus to Burkitt's lymphoma. In: *The Epstein–Barr Virus* (eds. Epstein M.A. & Achong B.G.), p. 322. Springer-Verlag, Berlin.

131 KLEIN G., CLIFFORD P., KLEIN E. & STJERNSWARD J. (1966) Search for tumour specific immune reactions in Burkitt lymphoma patients by the membrane immunofluorescence reaction. *Proceedings of the National Academy of Sciences, USA*, **55**, 1628.

132 EPSTEIN M.A., ACHONG B.G. & BARR Y.M. (1964) Virus particles in cultured lymphoblasts from Burkitt's lymphoma. *Lancet*, **i**, 702.

133 BURKITT D.P. (1969) Etiology of Burkitt's lymphoma—an alternative hypothesis to a vectored virus. *Journal of the National Cancer Institute*, **42**, 19.

134 ZIEGLER J.L., ANDERSSON M., KLEIN G. & HENLE W. (1976) Detection of Epstein–Barr virus DNA in American Burkitt's lymphoma. *International Journal of Cancer*, **17**, 701.

135 GATTI R.A. & GOOD R.A. (1971) Occurrence of malignancy in immunodeficiency disease. *Cancer*, **28**, 89.

136 PENN I. (1975) The incidence of malignancies in transplant patients. *Transplant Proceedings*, **7**, 323.

137 MATAS A.J., HERTEL B.F., ROSAI J., SIMMONS R.L. & NAJARIAN J.S. (1976) Post-transplant malignant lymphoma: distinctive morphological features related to its pathogenesis. *American Journal of Medicine*, **61**, 716.

138 WALFORD R.L. (1966) Increased incidence of lymphoma after injections of mice with cells differing at weak histocompatibility loci. *Science*, **152**, 78.

139 ARMSTRONG M.Y.K., GLEICHMANN E., GLEICHMANN H., BELDOTTI D., SCHWARTZ J.A. & SCHWARTZ R.S. (1970) Chronic allogeneic disease: development of lymphomas. *Journal of Experimental Medicine*, **132**, 417.

140 AZZOPARDI J.G. & EVANS D.J. (1971) Malignant lymphoma of parotid associated with Mikulicz disease (benign lymphoepithelial lesion). *Journal of Clinical Pathology*, **24**, 744.

141 TALAL N. & BUNIM J.J. (1964) The development of malignant lymphoma in the course of Sjögren's syndrome. *American Journal of Medicine*, **36**, 529.

142 GREEN J.A., DAWSON A.A. & WALKER W. (1978) Systemic lupus erythematosus and lymphoma. *Lancet*, **ii**, 753.

143 LUKES R.J. & TINDLE B.H. (1975) Immunoblastic lymphadenopathy: a hyperimmune entity resembling Hodgkin's disease. *New England Journal of Medicine*, **292**, 1.

144 RAPPAPORT H., RAMOT B., HULU N. & PARK J.K. (1972) The pathology of so-called Mediterranean abdominal lymphoma with malabsorption. *Cancer*, **29**, 1502.

145 KRIKORIAN J.G., BURKE J.S., ROSENBERG S.A. & KAPLAN H.S. (1979) Occurrence of non-Hodgkin's lymphoma after therapy for Hodgkin's disease. *New England Journal of Medicine*, **300**, 452.

146 HYMAN G.A. & SOMMERS S.C. (1966) The development of Hodgkin's disease and lymphoma during anticonvulsant therapy. *Blood*, **28**, 416.

147 FRIZZERA G., MORAN E.M. & RAPPAPORT H. (1974) Angio-immunoblastic lymphadenopathy with dysproteinaemia. *Lancet*, **ii**, 1070.

148 ROSAI J. & DORFMAN R.F. (1972) Sinus histiocytosis with massive lymphadenopathy: a pseudolymphomatous benign disorder. *Cancer*, **30**, 1174.

149 CASTLEMAN B., IVERSON L. & MENENDEZ V.P. (1956) Localised mediastinal lymph node hyperplasia resembling thymoma. *Cancer*, **9**, 822.

150 SALVADOR A.H., HARRISON E.G. & KYLE R.A. (1971) Lymphadenopathy due to infectious mononucleosis: its confusion with malignant lymphoma. *Cancer*, **27**, 1029.

151 HARTSOCK R.J. (1968) Postvaccinial lymphadenitis:

hyperplasia of lymphoid tissue that simulates malignant lymphomas. *Cancer*, **21**, 632.

152 SALTZSTEIN S.I. & ACKERMAN L.V. (1950) Lymphadenopathy induced by anticonvulsant drugs and mimicking clinically and pathologically malignant lymphomas. *Cancer*, **12**, 164.

153 ROSAI J. & RODRIGUEZ H.A. (1968) Application of electron microscopy to the differential diagnosis of tumors. *American Journal of Clinical Pathology*, **50**, 555.

154 SLOANE J.P. & ORMEROD M.G. (1981) Distribution of epithelial membrane antigen in normal and neoplastic tissues and its value in diagnostic tumour pathology. *Cancer*, **47**, 1786.

155 SMITH I.E., PECKHAM M.J., McELWAIN T.J., GAZET J.-C. & AUSTIN D.E. (1977) Hodgkin's disease in children. *British Journal of Cancer*, **36**, 120.

156 FRIEDMAN M.A. & ROSENBERG S.A. (1974) Diagnostic and therapeutic aspects of marrow positive (Stage IV) Hodgkin's disease. *Blood*, **44**, 928.

157 CASTELLINO R.A., FILLY R. & BLANK N. (1976) Routine full lung tomography in the initial staging and treatment planning of patients with Hodgkin's disease and non-Hodgkin's lymphoma. *Cancer*, **38**, 1130.

158 MACDONALD J.S. (1973) Diagnostic radiology in Hodgkin's disease. *British Journal of Hospital Medicine*, **9**, 443.

159 REDMAN H.C., GLATSTEIN E., CASTELLINO R.A. & FEDERAL W.A. (1977) Computed tomography as an adjunct in the staging of Hodgkin's disease and non-Hodgkin's lymphomas. *Radiology*, **124**, 381.

160 JONES S.E. & SALMON S.E. (1976) The role of radionuclides in clinical oncology. *Seminars in Nuclear Medicine*, **6**, 331.

161 ROSENBERG S.A. (1971) Hodgkin's disease of the bone marrow. *Clinical Research*, **31**, 1733.

162 ROSENBERG S.A. (1971) A critique of the value of laparotomy and splenectomy in the evaluation of patients with Hodgkin's disease. *Cancer Research*, **31**, 1737.

163 CANNON W.B. & NELSEN T.D. (1976) Staging of Hodgkin's disease: a surgical perspective. *American Journal of Surgery*, **132**, 224.

164 HELLMAN S. (1974) Current studies in Hodgkin's disease. What laparotomy has wrought. *New England Journal of Medicine*, **290**, 894.

165 EDITORIAL (1978) Staging laparotomy for Hodgkin's disease—reassessment. *Lancet*, **ii**, 875.

166 PECKHAM M.J., FORD H.T., McELWAIN T.J., HARMER C.L., ATKINSON K. & AUSTIN D.E. (1975) The results of radiotherapy for Hodgkin's disease. *British Journal of Cancer*, **32**, 391.

167 CHILCOATE R.R., BAEHNER R.L., HAMMOND D. & THE INVESTIGATORS AND SPECIAL STUDIES COMMITTEE OF THE CHILDREN'S CANCER STUDY GROUP (1976) Septicemia and meningitis in children splenectomised for Hodgkin's disease. *New England Journal of Medicine*, **295**, 798.

168 CARBONE P.P., KAPLAN H.S., MUSSHOFF K., SMITHERS D.W. & TUBIANA M. (1971) Report of the committee on Hodgkin's disease staging classification. *Cancer Research*, **31**, 1860.

169 MUSSHOFF K. (1971) Prognostic and therapeutic implications of staging in extranodal Hodgkin's disease. *Cancer Research*, **31**, 1814.

170 LEVI J.A. & WIERNIK P.H. (1977) Limited extranodal Hodgkin's disease: unfavourable prognosis and therapeutic implications. *American Journal of Medicine*, **63**, 365.

171 LEWIS B.J. & DE VITA V.T. (1978) Combination therapy of the lymphomas. *Seminars in Hematology*, **15**, 431.

172 PETERS M.V. & MIDDLEMISS K.C.H. (1958) A study of Hodgkin's disease treated by irradiation. *American Journal of Roentgenology, Radium Therapy and Nuclear Medicine*, **79**, 114.

173 EASSON E.L. & RUSSELL M.H. (1963) The cure of Hodgkin's disease. *British Medical Journal*, **i**, 1704.

174 KAPLAN H.S. (1966) Role of intensive radiotherapy in the management of Hodgkin's disease. *Cancer*, **19**, 356.

175 BILLROTH T. (1871) Chirurgische Reminiscanzen aus dem Sommersemester 1871. V. Multiple Lymphome. Erfolgreiche Behandlung mit Arsenik. *Wiener Medizinische Wochenschrift*, **44**, 1065.

176 GILMAN A. & PHILLIPS F.S. (1946) Biological actions and therapeutic implications of the data re chloroethyl amines and sulphides. *Science*, **103**, 409.

177 WILKINSON J.F. & FLETCHER F. (1947) Effect of B-chloroethylamine hydrochlorides in leukaemia. *Lancet*, **ii**, 540.

178 CARBONE P.P. (1967) Hodgkin's disease. *Annals of Internal Medicine*, **67**, 424.

179 LACHER M.J. & DURANT J.R. (1965) Combined vinblastine and chlorambucil therapy of Hodgkin's disease. *Annals of Internal Medicine*, **62**, 468.

180 DE VITA V.T., SERPICK A.A. & CARBONE P.P. (1970) Combination chemotherapy in the treatment of advanced Hodgkin's disease. *Annals of Internal Medicine*, **73**, 881.

181 KAPLAN H.S. (1966) Evidence for a tumoricidal dose level in the radiotherapy of Hodgkin's disease. *Cancer Research*, **26**, 1221.

182 HOPPE R.T. (1980) Radiation therapy in the treatment of Hodgkin's disease. *Seminars in Oncology*, **7**, 144.

183 SUTCLIFFE S.B., WRIGLEY P.F.M., PETO J., LISTER T.A., STANSFELD A.G., WHITEHOUSE J.M.A., CROWTHER D. & MALPAS J.S. (1978) MVPP chemotherapy regimen for advanced Hodgkin's disease. *British Medical Journal*, **i**, 679.

184 KAYE S.B., JUTTNER C.A., SMITH I.E., BARRETT A., AUSTIN D.E., PECKHAM M.J. & McELWAIN T.J. (1979) Three years' experience with ChlVPP (a combination of drugs of low toxicity) for the treatment of Hodgkin's disease. *British Journal of Cancer*, **39**, 168.

185 YOUNG R.C., CANELLOS G.P., CHABNER B.A., SCHEIN P.S. & DE VITA V.T. (1973) Maintenance chemotherapy for advanced Hodgkin's disease in remission. *Lancet*, **i**, 1339.

186 FREI E., LUCE J.K. & GAMBLE J.F. (1973) Combination chemotherapy in advanced Hodgkin's disease. Introduction and maintenance of remission. *Annals of Internal Medicine*, **79**, 376.

187 DE VITA V.T., CANELLOS G.P. & MOXLEY J.H. (1972) A decade of combination chemotherapy in advanced Hodgkin's disease. *Cancer*, **30**, 1495.

188 BRITISH NATIONAL LYMPHOMA INVESTIGATION (1975) Value of prednisone in combination chemotherapy of

Stage IV Hodgkin's disease. *British Medical Journal*, **iii**, 413.

189 JACOBS C., PORTLOCK C.S. & ROSENBERG S.A. (1976) Prednisone in MOPP chemotherapy for Hodgkin's disease. *British Medical Journal*, **ii**, 1469.

190 COLTMAN C.A. (1980) Chemotherapy of advanced Hodgkin's disease. *Seminars in Oncology*, **7**, 155.

191 SANTORO A. & BONADONNA G. (1979) Prolonged disease-free survival in MOPP resistant Hodgkin's disease after treatment with ABVD. *Cancer Chemotherapy and Pharmacology*, **2**, 101.

192 SUTCLIFFE S.B., WRIGLEY P.F.M., STANSFELD A.G. & MALPAS J.S. (1979) Adriamycin, bleomycin, vinblastine and imidazole carboxamide (ABVD) therapy for advanced Hodgkin's disease resistant to MVPP. *Cancer Chemotherapy and Pharmacology*, **2**, 209.

193 CASE D.C., YOUNG C.W. & LEE B.J. (1977) Combination chemotherapy of MOPP-resistant Hodgkin's disease with ABDV. *Cancer*, **39**, 1382.

194 CLAMON G.H. & CORDER M.P. (1978) ABVP treatment of MOPP—failures with Hodgkin's disease. *Cancer Treatment Reports*, **63**, 363.

195 BONADONNA G., FOSSATI V. & DE LENA M. (1978) MOPP vs MOPP plus ABVD in Stage IV Hodgkin's disease. *Proceedings of the American Association for Cancer Research*, **19**, 363.

196 VELENTJAS E., BARRETT A., MCELWAIN T.J. & PECKHAM M.J. (1980) Mediastinal involvement in early-stage Hodgkin's disease. *European Journal of Cancer*, **16**, 1065.

197 MAUCH P., GOODMAN R. & HELLMAN S. (1978) The significance of mediastinal involvement in early stage Hodgkin's disease. *Cancer*, **42**, 1039.

198 ROSENBERG S.A., KAPLAN H.S., GLATSTEIN E.J. & PORTLOCK C.S. (1978) Combined modality therapy of Hodgkin's disease. A report on the Stanford trials. *Cancer*, **42**, 991.

199 YOUNG R.C., CANELLOS G.P., CHABNER B.A., HUBBARD S.M. & DE VITA V.T. (1978) Patterns of relapse in advanced Hodgkin's disease treated with combination chemotherapy. *Cancer*, **42**, 1001.

200 JENKIN R.D.T. & BERRY M.P. (1980) Hodgkin's disease in children. *Seminars in Oncology*, **7**, 202.

201 MCELWAIN T.J. & SMITH I.E. (1979) Hodgkin's disease: present concepts and advances in management. In: *Topics in Paediatrics. 1. Haematology and Oncology* (ed. Morris Jones P.), p. 84. Pitman Medical, London.

202 PROBERT J.C. & PARKER B.R. (1975) The effects of radiation therapy on bone growth. *Radiology*, **114**, 115.

203 SHALET S.M., ROSENSTOCK J.D., BEARDWELL C.G., PEARSON D. & MORRIS JONES P.H. (1977) Thyroid dysfunction following external irradiation to the neck for Hodgkin's disease in children. *Clinical Radiology*, **28**, 511.

204 HOST H. & VALE J.R. (1973) Lung function after mantle field irradiation in Hodgkin's disease. *Cancer*, **31**, 328.

205 THAR T.L. & MILLION R.R. (1980) Complications of radiation treatment in Hodgkin's disease. *Seminars in Oncology*, **7**, 174.

206 GLATSTEIN E., MCHARDY-YOUNG S. & BRAST N. (1971) Alterations in serum thyrotropin (TSH) and thyroid function following radiotherapy in patients with malig-nant lymphoma. *Journal of Clinical Endocrinology and Metabolism*, **32**, 833.

207 INGOLD J.A., REED G.B. & KAPLAN H.S. (1965) Radiation hepatitis. *American Journal of Roentgenology*, **93**, 200.

208 RAY G.R., TRUEBLOOD H.W., ENWRIGHT L.P., KAPLAN H.S. & NELSEN T.S. (1970) Oophoropexy: a means of preserving ovarian function following pelvic megavoltage radiotherapy for Hodgkin's disease. *Radiology*, **96**, 175.

209 GAMS R.A. (1980) Complications of chemotherapy in the treatment of Hodgkin's disease. *Seminars in Oncology*, **7**, 184.

210 SHERINS R.J. & DE VITA V.T. (1973) Effect of drug treatment for lymphoma on male reproductive capacity. *Annals of Internal Medicine*, **79**, 216.

211 GETAZ E.P. (1979) Second malignant neoplasms in Hodgkin's disease. *Cancer Chemotherapy and Pharmacology*, **2**, 143.

212 GOFFINET D.R., GLATSTEIN E. & MERIGAN T.C. (1972) Herpes zoster—varicella infections and lymphoma. *Annals of Internal Medicine*, **76**, 235.

213 SCHIMPFF S., SERPICK A., STOLER B., RUMACK B., MELLIN H., JOSEPH J.M. & BLOCK J. (1972) Varicella zoster infection in patients with cancer. *Annals of Internal Medicine*, **76**, 241.

214 REBOUL F., DONALDSON S. & KAPLAN H.S. (1978) Herpes zoster and varicella infections in children with Hodgkin's disease. *Cancer*, **41**, 95.

215 SELBY P.J., POWLES R.L., JAMESON B., KAY H.E.M., WATSON J.G., THORNTON R., MORGENSTERN G., CLINK H.M., MCELWAIN T.J., PRENTICE H.G., CORRINGHAM R., ROSS M.G., HOFFBRAND A.V. & BRIGDEN D. (1979) Parenteral acyclovir therapy for Herpes virus infections in man. *Lancet*, **ii**, 1267.

216 CHABNER B.A., JOHNSON R.E., YOUNG R.C., CANELLOS G.P., HUBBARD S.P., JOHNSON S.K. & DE VITA V.T. (1976) Sequential non-surgical and surgical staging of non-Hodgkin's lymphoma. *Annals of Internal Medicine*, **85**, 149.

217 BUNN P.A., SCHEIN P.S., BANKS P.M. & DE VITA V.T. (1976) Central nervous system complications in patients with diffuse histiocytic and undifferentiated lymphoma: leukaemia revisited. *Blood*, **47**, 3.

218 GOUGH K.R., READ A.E. & NAISH J.M. (1962) Intestinal reticulosis as a complication of idiopathic steatorrhoea. *Gut*, **3**, 232.

219 LISTER T.A., CULLEN M.H., BREARLEY R., BEARD M.E.J., STANSFELD A.G., WHITEHOUSE J.M.A., WRIGLEY P.F.M., FORD J.M., MALPAS J.S. & CROWTHER D. (1978) Combination chemotherapy for advanced non-Hodgkin's lymphoma of unfavourable histology. *Cancer Chemotherapy and Pharmacology*, **1**, 107.

220 WOOLNER N., BURCHENAL J.H., LIEBERMAN P.H., EXELBY P., D'ANGIO G. & MURPHY M.L. (1976) Non-Hodgkin lymphoma in children. A comparative study of two modalities of therapy. *Cancer*, **37**, 123.

221 DUNCAN P.R., CHECA F., GOWING N.F.C., MCELWAIN T.J. & PECKHAM M.J. (1980) Extranodal non-Hodgkin's lymphoma presenting in the testicle. *Cancer*, **45**, 1578.

222 BANFI A., BONADONNA G., RICCI S.B., MILANI F., MOLINARI R., MONFARDINI S. & ZUCALI R. (1972)

Malignant lymphomas of Waldeyer's ring. Natural history and survival after radiotherapy. *British Medical Journal*, **iii**, 140.

223 PORTLOCK C.S. (1980) Management of indolent lymphomas. *Seminars in Oncology*, **7**, 292.

224 PORTLOCK C.S., ROSENBERG S.A., GLATSTEIN E. & KAPLAN H.S. (1976) Treatment of advanced non-Hodgkin lymphomas with favourable histologies: preliminary results of a prospective trial. *Blood*, **47**, 747.

225 LISTER T.A., CULLEN M.H., BEARD M.E.J., BREARLEY R.L., WHITEHOUSE J.M.A., WRIGLEY P.F.M., STANSFELD A.G., SUTCLIFFE S.B.J., MALPAS J.S. & CROWTHER D. (1978) Comparison of combined and single agent chemotherapy in non-Hodgkin lymphoma of favourable histological type. *British Medical Journal*, **i**, 533.

226 JOHNSON R.E., CANELLOS G.P., YOUNG R.C., CHABNER B.A. & DE VITA V.T. (1978) Chemotherapy (CVP) versus radiotherapy (TBI) for Stage III–IV poorly differentiated lymphocytic lymphoma. *Cancer Treatment Reports*, **62**, 321.

227 ANDERSON T., BENDER R.A., FISHER R.I., DE VITA V.T., CHABNER B.A., BERARD C.W., NORTON L. & YOUNG R.C. (1977) Combination chemotherapy of non-Hodgkin lymphomas: results of long-term follow up. *Cancer Treatment Reports*, **61**, 1057.

228 DE VITA V.T., CANELLOS G.P., CHABNER B., SCHEIN P., HUBBARD S. & YOUNG R.C. (1975) Advanced diffuse histiocytic lymphoma, a potentially curable disease. *Lancet*, **i**, 248.

229 McKELVEY E.M., GOTTLIEB J.A., WILSON H.E., HAUT A., TALLEY R.W., STEPHENS R., LANE, M., GAMBLE J.F., JONES S.E., GROZEA P.N., GUTTERMAN J., COLTMAN C. & MOON T.E. (1976) Hydroxydaunomycin (adriamy- cin) combination chemotherapy in malignant lymphoma. *Cancer*, **38**, 1484.

230 CABANILLAS F., RODRIGUEZ V. & FREIREICH E.J. (1978) Improvement in complete response rate, duration of response and survival with adriamycin combination chemotherapy for non-Hodgkin lymphomas. A prognostic factor comparison of two regimens. *Medical and Pediatric Oncology*, **4**, 321.

231 JONES S.E., GROZEA P.N. & METZ E.N. (1979) Superiority of adriamycin-containing combination chemotherapy in the treatment of diffuse lymphoma. *Cancer*, **43**, 417.

232 SCHEIN P.S., DE VITA V.T., HUBBARD S., CHABNER B.A., CANELLOS G.P., BERARD C. & YOUNG R.C. (1976) BACOP combination chemotherapy in the treatment of advanced diffuse histiocytic lymphoma. *Annals of Internal Medicine*, **85**, 417.

233 SCHEIN P.S., CHABNER B.A., CANELLOS G.P., YOUNG R.C., BERARD C. & DE VITA V. (1974) Potential for prolonged disease-free survival following combination chemotherapy of non-Hodgkin's lymphoma. *Blood*, **43**, 181.

234 MILLER T.P. & JONES S.E. (1979) Chemotherapy of localised histiocytic lymphoma. *Lancet*, **i**, 358.

235 BRODER S. & BUNN P.A. (1980) Cutaneous T-cell lymphomas. *Seminars in Oncology*, **7**, 310.

236 VONDERHEID E.C., VAN SCOTT E.J., WALLNER P.E. & JOHNSON W.C. (1979) A ten year experience with topical mechlorethamine for mycosis fungoides. *Cancer Treatment Reports*, **63**, 681.

237 HOPPE R.T., COX R.S., FUKS Z., PRICE N.M., BAGSHAW M.A. & FARBER E.M. (1979) Electron beam therapy in the treatment of mycosis fungoides—the Stanford experience. *Cancer Treatment Reports*, **63**, 691.

SECTION 4
THE HAEMOSTATIC MECHANISM
AND ITS DISORDERS

Chapter 25
Platelet production and turnover: thrombocytopenia and thrombocytosis

C. N. CHESTERMAN AND D. G. PENINGTON

PLATELET PRODUCTION AND TURNOVER

The cellular basis of platelet production

Comprehension of platelet production involves an understanding of megakaryocytes. These are unusual polyploid cells which follow a pattern of cellular proliferation and endomitosis which is unique in mammalian biology. They are derived from a hierarchy of stem cells, as yet poorly understood, but the immediate precursor of the megakaryoblast is now identified as a diploid cell of lymphoid morphology [1, 2]. These cells undergo cell division and then enter the complex endomitotic proliferative pattern or 'ploidy ladder' which, when DNA synthesis is complete [3], gives rise to the differentiating basophil and granular megakaryocytes of the three major ploidy classes (Fig. 25.1). Once fully mature, the granular megakaryocyte assumes an amoeboid form and penetrates the sinusoidal endothelium of the bone marrow either to release fragments or itself to pass into the sinusoid, and be carried with the venous bloodstream to the lungs. The final step of platelet production is the further break-up of these cytoplasmic fragments to produce discoid platelets and here, again, much remains to be learned. The regulation of platelet production is now partially understood, particularly in so far as it applies to the morphologically recognizable megakaryocyte compartment in the bone marrow, but there remain many uncertainties concerning the stem cells from which megakaryocytes are derived and also the final stages of megakaryocyte and platelet development.

Multipotent stem cells

Till & McCulloch [4], using the technique of infusion of marrow cells into lethally irradiated recipients, established that colonies formed in the spleen could either contain cells of all three major haemopoietic lines or be comprised of a single cell line, which might be megakaryocytic. The multipotent stem cells which give rise to such colonies are not normally in cell cycle, and Ebbe & Stohlman [5] have shown that stimulation of production of platelets by the induction of acute thrombocytopenia has little effect on these cells. The reserve for increased platelet production is normally met by stem cells of a more differentiated nature than those which give rise to splenic colonies. From recent studies [6] it appears likely that only the penultimate step in the sequence from the multipotent stem cell to the immediate diploid precursor of the megakaryoblast is involved in the regulatory adjustments in megakaryocyte proliferation induced by acute thrombocytopenia or an excess of circulating platelets; it is likely that earlier stem cells are only activated once this immediate precursor compartment is depleted. There is now increasing evidence to suggest that between the multipotent stem cell and the committed stem cell, which may be cultured in semi-solid supporting media, there is a hierarchy of stem cells of differing degrees of differentiation and repopulating potential [7, 8].

In human disease, the importance of this group of stem cells is coming to be understood in relation to chronic granulocytic leukaemia (CGL) [9] and polycythaemia vera [10]. Clearly, analysis of diseases such as essential thrombocythaemia and paroxysmal nocturnal haemoglobinuria in terms of basic lesions affecting stem cells of this class is likely to assume increasing importance as techniques are developed to study the more primitive human stem cells under *in-vitro* conditions.

Committed megakaryocytic stem cells

The immediate precursor stem cell of the megakaryocytic series may be grown in tissue culture using a soft agar supporting medium [11–14]. A plasma clot system has also been used for the growth of both murine [15, 16] and human [17] megakaryocytic colonies. Methyl cellulose has also proved to be a successful supporting medium for human colonies and Fauser & Messner [18] have recently reported the growth of colonies from human marrow which contain each of the major cell lines (including megakaryocytes); presumably these represent a more primitive stem cell than that grown from murine marrow in agar. The cells from which colonies are grown are lymphoid in appearance [2] and have reproducible characteristics on both velocity

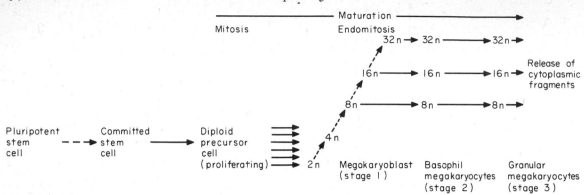

Fig. 25.1. Megakaryocyte maturation and ploidy changes. Note that the committed stem-cell pool is self-replicating and only intermittently requires replenishment from a pluripotent stem-cell pool, which is not normally in cell cycle. The diploid precursor cell undergoes frequent mitoses as maturation commences, but as endomitosis develops the cell climbs the 'ploidy ladder'. Most cells reach 16n before endomitosis ceases but some cease endomitosis at either 8n or 32n. With stimulation of platelet production a brief surge of endomitosis to 64n occurs and with suppression of platelet production following transfusion of platelets, more cells mature in the 4n class.

sedimentation [14] and density separation [19], by which means they may be concentrated from the general marrow population.

The immediate stem cell of the megakaryocyte series has been shown to be suppressed by cycle-specific inhibitors *in vivo* [5, 20, 21] and *in vitro* [22] but these studies suggest that in the resting state a proportion of these stem cells are not in cell cycle but may be recruited to divide when there is a stimulus to increased platelet production [22]. Recent studies of the stem cells cultured *in vitro* [14] support the view that only a proportion of these cells are in cell cycle, as shown by the effects of high-dose tritiated thymidine *in vivo* and hydroxyurea *in vitro*, although under culture conditions used by other investigators the great majority of these stem cells appear to be in cycle [16, 22].

The characteristics of megakaryocytic colonies grown *in vitro* vary somewhat with the technique. In the agar-culture system, however, a number of investigators have reported two distinct colony types. Metcalf [11] referred to these as 'mixed' and 'pure', the former being so described because of the presence of substantial numbers of smaller cells; these findings have been confirmed by others [13, 14]. Recent studies which have included the analysis of ploidy and cytochemical characteristics of cells from individual colonies point to both being purely megakaryocytic in type but one representing, almost certainly, a more primitive stem-cell type than the other [23]. The more mature colony type shows the same pattern with respect to ploidy as appears in megakaryocytes of the bone marrow so that a single diploid stem cell must give rise to progeny with the full range of polyploid

content of DNA as seen *in vivo*, rather than the high ploidy classes being derived from polyploid precursor cells as had previously been proposed [24].

Megakaryocytes in the marrow
The earliest megakaryocytic cell which may be identified in rodents is a cell the size of a lymphocyte which stains positively for the enzyme acetyl-cholinesterase. This cell may also be identified immunologically as having antigens on its surface identical with at least some of those in the circulating platelet [1, 25]. These cells are most probably capable of true cell division [23] before endomitosis commences and the cells ascend the 'ploidy ladder' (Fig. 25.1) by successive steps of chromosomal replication without cell division.

From the time a cell is morphologically recognizable as a megakaryoblast, generally beyond the tetraploid stage of endoreduplication, it is committed to maturation without further cell division [3, 24]. This initial stage of polyploid development, the megakaryoblast, is termed Stage 1; as the cell matures, intense basophilia becomes apparent and the basophil megakaryocyte is termed Stage 2; Stage 3 is the granular megakaryocyte in which the basophilia has decreased to the extent that the azurophil cytoplasmic granules can be seen on normal light microscopy with Romanowsky staining.

Stage-1 cells or *megakaryoblasts* (Fig. 25.2(a)) are cells of variable size and ploidy which, when identified with normal staining of a marrow smear, are principally cells of the 4n, 8n and 16n ploidy classes. Probably only very small numbers of 32n cells are normally found at this stage of maturation [26, 27]. Megakaryoblasts undergo rapid DNA synthesis [3, 27,

(a)

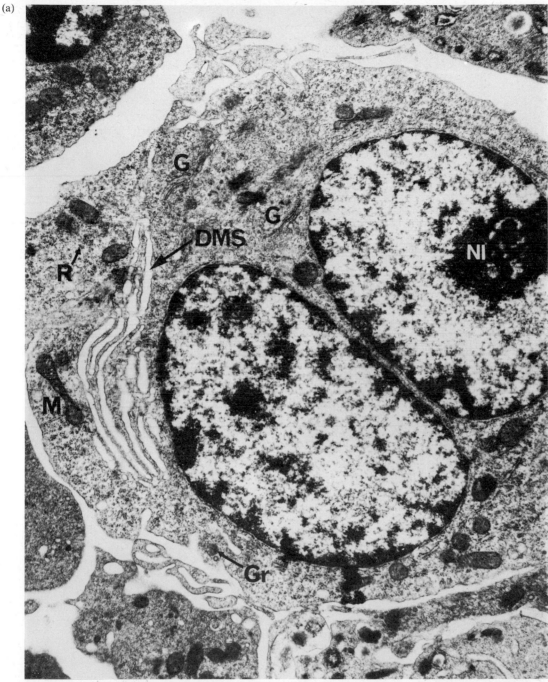

Fig. 25.2. Electronmicrographic appearances of maturing megakaryocytes. (a) Megakaryoblast (Stage 1). Note demarcation membrane system (DMS), Golgi apparatus (G), ribosomes (R), large mitochondria (M) and a small number of specific granules (Gr). Nucleolus (Nl) is prominent in the nucleus ($\times 15\,120$).

(b)

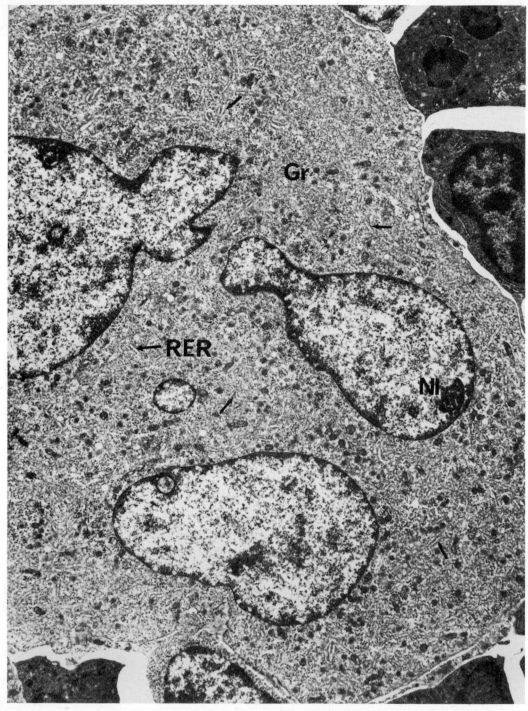

Fig. 25.2. *(cont.)* (b) Basophil megakaryocyte (stage 2). The cell is much larger. Demarcation membrane system (→) is spread throughout the cell as are polyribosomes. Rough endoplasmic reticulum (RER) is prominent. Nuclear lobes are dispersed and nucleoli (Nl) are prominent and active (× 8100).

(c)

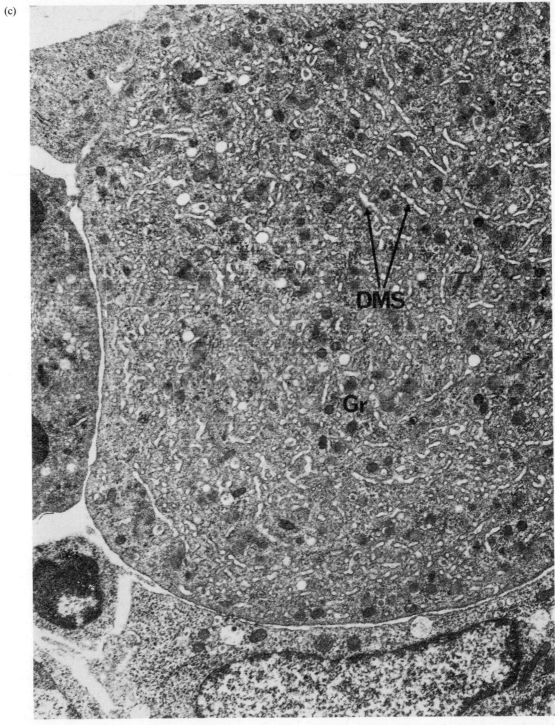

Fig. 25.2 *(cont.)* (c) Granular megakaryocyte (Stage 3). Note numerous granules (Gr) and empty demarcation membrane system (DMS) (× 12 150).

28] and their size varies with their ploidy. All show a high nuclear to cytoplasmic ratio and although the nucleus is often large, it is generally only partially segmented [3]. On electron microscopy, the cytoplasm shows some of the characteristic dense-core granules present in more mature megakaryocytes and platelets [3, 29] and at this stage the surface membrane is invaginated and arborizes with rapidly progressive folding and proliferation within the cytoplasm of the cell [30].

Stage 2 or *basophil megakaryocytes* (Fig. 25.2(b)) are characterized by intense development of nucleoli and associated RNA synthesis. Polyribosomes spread throughout the cytoplasm of the cell and many segments of rough endoplasmic reticulum are seen with features suggestive of active protein synthesis; many sets of Golgi apparatus are apparent with associated vesicles. The demarcation membrane system continues to arborize throughout the cell and granule synthesis proceeds apace, most probably arising in the vicinity of the Golgi apparatus. Specialized dense-core segments become evident and may play some role in the synthesis of the membrane system [29–31]. The cells reach their full ploidy level during this stage of cytoplasmic maturation and only the most immature cells of this stage show evidence of DNA synthesis [3, 24, 29]. It would appear that once a certain level of cytoplasmic maturation has been reached, further DNA synthesis is inhibited [3] but the nature of the signal suppressing synthesis of DNA is unknown. The principal ploidy class in this stage is 16n, representing approximately two-thirds of the cells with near to one-sixth in both the 8n and 32n classes [26, 27].

Stage 3 or *granular megakaryocytes* (Fig 25.2(c)) represent the majority of recognizable megakaryocytes in the bone marrow. Protein synthesis continues at this stage, but with increasing production of granules and membranes and increasing size of the cell [32], polyribosomes become steadily less prominent. The demarcation membrane system is in communication with the external environment of the cell through pores in its surface [31]. It is uncertain, however, whether the proliferation of membrane system within the cell is by direct extension of folding sheets [30] or by a process involving both fusion and fission [33]. As the cell matures it adopts an amoeboid form with projections apparently seeking out marrow sinusoids [34]. These projections owe their rigidity to long microtubular structures which follow the long axis of the pseudopodia and push their way through the substance of endothelial cells lining the marrow sinusoids to project into the bloodstream [35, 36] (Fig. 25.3). The adventitial cell supporting the marrow sinusoid may play some role in regulating access of megakaryocyte pseudopodia to the sinusoid but relatively little is known concerning this aspect of regulation of platelet production [37].

Fragmentation of megakaryocytes

The pseudopodia which penetrate the marrow–sinusoid barrier differ from platelets in that they contain microtubules either randomly orientated as seen in megakaryocyte cytoplasm, or running with the long axis of the more attenuated pseudopodia [32, 34]. Presumably these give rigidity to the protruding cytoplasm. The same feature is seen in the circumscribed fragments which are observed within the sinusoid after the break-up of the pseudopodium [32, 38] (Fig. 25.3) and distinguishes these fragments from true platelets with their discoid form and marginal microtubular bundles. Whole megakaryocytes may sometimes be observed in transit to the sinusoid [39] and may be recovered from central venous blood [40, 41] and the lung [42].

It has been postulated that a very significant proportion of the platelets produced in the body can be accounted for by shedding of cytoplasm of pulmonary megakaryocytes [41]. Both whole megakaryocytes and cytoplasmic fragments released into marrow sinusoids would be carried to the pulmonary capillary bed and be subjected there to the gentle massaging which must occur in the course of respiration [43]. If further fragmentation occurs and particles of an appropriate size are formed, these presumably acquire a discoid shape with marginal microtubules and submarginal dense-tubular system [44] as they move within the circulation. Whether these large fragments, if they pass through the capillary bed, represent some of the megathrombocytes seen in states of increased platelet production [45, 46] remains unknown.

Significance of ploidy in megakaryocytes

Two alternative theories have been proposed to account for the striking pattern of endomitosis and maturation of megakaryocytes in three major ploidy classes (Fig. 25.1):

1 Harker [47, 48] has proposed that the variable pathway of maturation provides a means whereby the body modulates the volume of megakaryocyte cytoplasm available for release as platelets. As the body responds to acute thrombocytopenia, the size [49] and ploidy [27, 47, 50] of megakaryocytes increases within 48 hours. The very large 32n cells become the most common form of maturing megakaryocyte and certainly this shift in ploidy appears to be a critical element in the response of the marrow to the sudden stress of thrombocytopenia. However, with sustained depletion of platelets, the number of megakaryocytes differentiating from the stem-cell compartment increases [47, 50, 51] so that an increase in number of

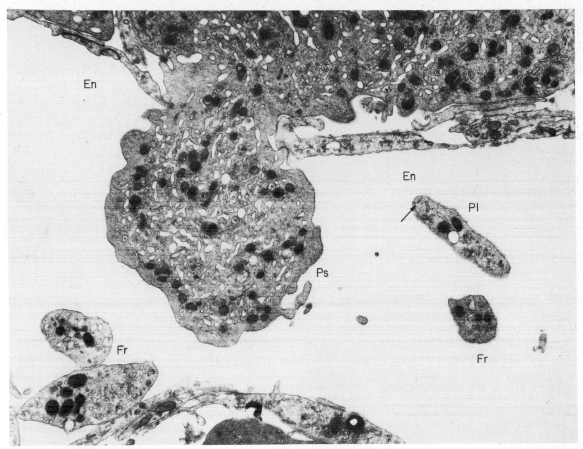

Fig. 25.3. Cytoplasmic shedding from megakaryocyte in a marrow sinusoid. A pseudopodium (Ps) is seen penetrating through the endothelial lining of the sinusoid (En). Three other cytoplasmic fragments are seen within the sinusoid (Fr) and also a normal platelet (Pl). The platelet has a normal discoid form and shows a marginal microtubular bundle (arrowed) which maintains the discoid form (× 6300). (Reproduced with permission from *British Journal of Haematology* [32].)

cells differentiating provides the major source of increased production of platelets, and the shift to the high ploidy class becomes very much less prominent. Biologically, therefore, the 32n cell line can be seen only as a relatively temporary source of increased megakaryocyte cytoplasm, perhaps of importance in the production of large or 'stress' platelets seen in this situation [27, 52] (see p. 978).

2 The alternative view is based on ultrastructural observations by Penington and others of the cytoplasm of cells of each ploidy class [32]. The cells of the 8n class show a greater concentration of granules and mitochondria in their cytoplasm than the more numerous 16n cells and presumably give rise to platelets with similar characteristics. The cells of the 32n class have a greater content of internalized membrane system (demarcation membrane system) and a lesser concentration of granules and mitochondria. From studies on megakaryocytes in disease, Paulus [53] has proposed that cells with less membrane system give rise to larger platelets, and those with more membrane, small platelets. If this is correct, the low ploidy megakaryocytes would give large platelets and the higher ploidy cells smaller platelets, a postulate which is consistent with findings in morphometric analysis of platelets in the peripheral circulation following separation by buoyant density [32].

Biologically, each cell division is associated with a major stimulus to plasma-membrane synthesis in order to provide membrane for the two daughter cells. Endomitosis in megakaryocytes may be viewed as a form of specialized differentiation in which this drive to membrane synthesis is diverted to synthesis of an internalized membrane which has all the characteristics of plasma membrane and is indeed in communication with the external environment of the cell [31].

The higher the ploidy, the larger the amount of membrane produced [32]. This provides not only more surface membrane for the platelet progeny, facilitating the production of smaller platelets, but would be expected to result in platelets with a higher content of surface-connected canalicular system from the higher ploidy cells. This is borne out by morphometric studies [32]. The surface membrane plays a very important role in the platelet in a number of ways and functional differences between populations of platelets derived from different ploidy classes of megakaryocytes remain to be clarified.

Heterogeneity of circulating platelets
Platelets in the circulation are known to vary greatly in size [53], in buoyant density [32, 54–56], in biochemical characteristics [54, 57], in morphology [32, 58] and in certain characteristics which have been shown to be related to age [59]. The extent to which these various features can be presumed to be interrelated remains a matter of debate, but the observations that the most dense platelets have a greater mean size than the lightest platelets, and that they are metabolically more active in several respects and show a slightly more rapid labelling pattern with a cohort label such as [75Se]selenomethionine than the lightest platelets, have led to the postulate by Karpatkin and his colleagues [54, 55] that all of these features of heterogeneity may be ascribed primarily to the effects of platelet ageing.

Further evidence has been presented in support of this view [56, 57, 60] and includes studies of platelets produced during recovery from acute thrombocytopenia (Fig. 25.4). These are larger than normal [27, 57] and are metabolically more active in some respects [57, 61]. They do not, however, show increased buoyant density [57, 61] and many are larger than any found in the normal circulation [27]. Platelet size in patients with ITP shows a log-normal distribution, suggesting production of both large and small platelets simultaneously [53]. The megathrombocytes characteristic of increased platelet turnover [45, 46] should be regarded as 'stress' platelets with their own particular properties [52].

Hirsh *et al.* [59] have clearly shown variation in properties of platelets during ageing, identified by the use of cohort labelling. Young platelets are more reactive to collagen but not to ADP either *in vivo* or *in vitro*. The cohort-labelling pattern of density-separated platelets using [75Se]selenomethionine is compatible with a small diminution in platelet density with age [62] but suggests that the greater contribution to heterogeneity with respect to buoyant density of platelets under physiological conditions is conferred on platelets by the megakaryocytes from which they

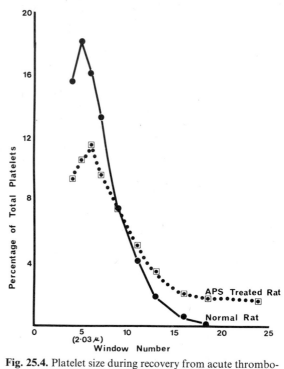

Fig. 25.4. Platelet size during recovery from acute thrombocytopenia. Distribution of platelets according to window number on a Coulter size plotter, comparing animals 48 hours after injection of an anti-platelet serum with a normal animal.

are derived [32]. Ageing may be associated with diminution in size and under pathological conditions, when platelet degranulation occurs *in vivo*, a significant increase in the proportion of light platelets would be expected [63]: this phenomenon may prove to be of great importance in clinical disorders such as disseminated intravascular coagulation.

Regulation of platelet production
The circulating platelet count is maintained at a very constant number, the normal range in man being $150–400 \times 10^9/l$, and any disturbance such as depletion or infusion of platelets is rapidly followed by compensatory changes in platelet production [47, 50, 64, 65].

Mediation of the signal to increase platelet production in acute thrombocytopenia is by means of a humoral factor, termed *thrombopoietin*. This factor has not yet been isolated and characterized, but the evidence for its physiological role is sufficiently clear to justify the use of a term which equates it in many respects to the erythroid-regulating hormone, erythro-poietin [65–67].

Thrombopoietin

Assay of this factor continues to present many diffi-culties [68]. In most studies, evidence of stimulation of platelet production in recipient animals is based on an increase in incorporation of a cohort label, [^{75}Se]selenomethionine [69–71] or [^{35}S]sulphate [72], into newly produced platelets. Although in some studies an increase in platelet count has been regularly observed [73], in most the platelet count is unaltered in the recipient, suggesting the production of larger platelets or platelets richer in protein, as occurs with 'stress' thrombopoiesis (see p. 978). In some studies the sensitivity of the assay system is enhanced by inducing a temporary suppression of platelet production in the recipient animals [70, 71, 74].

Thrombopoietin appears to be a relatively small protein which may be precipitated, like erythropoietin, between 60 and 80% saturation with ammonium sulphate and may be chromatographed on DEAE cellulose and Sephadex G100 [68, 75]. It is believed by some to be derived from the kidneys like erythro-poietin [76], and McDonald has demonstrated a similar factor produced by an embryonic cell line derived from the kidney [77]. However, bilateral nephrectomy does not impair the recovery from acute thrombocytopenia [64, 73] and does not result in sustained thrombocyto-penia in man. Siemensma *et al.* [78] have shown that sub-total hepatectomy results in immediate slowing of platelet production in rats, which recovers as the liver regenerates. Whether this phenomenon, which has also been observed in man, is related to production of thrombopoietin or to some metabolic consequence of sub-total hepatectomy has not yet been resolved.

Other stimulators of platelet production

Odell [79] showed that a variety of non-specific insults stimulate platelet production in animals. The same phenomenon may be seen in the variety of factors which give rise to non-specific thrombocytosis in man [80]. Evidence has been presented from animal studies that the platelets produced in response to 'non-specific' stimuli do not show the increase in size characteristic of 'stress' thrombopoiesis induced by acute thrombocytopenia [81]. It is likely, therefore, that at least one major mechanism of stimulation of platelet production exists outside the thrombopoietin system.

Relationship between thrombopoiesis and erythropoiesis

Independence of erythrocyte and platelet production has been demonstrated in many studies [64, 82]. However, haemolysis appears capable of stimulating platelet production both in animals [83] and in man

[84], and this may be by a mechanism other than that involving thrombopoietin. The likely existence of a second mechanism to account for 'non-specific throm-bocytosis' and contamination of some preparations of erythropoietin with thrombopoietin [82] may well account for certain observations which suggest a common humoral regulator for the two cell lines [85].

Sustained iron deficiency is associated with defective megakaryocyte maturation [86] and its correction with a brisk rise in platelet numbers. This phenomenon may account for the occasional observation of very high platelet counts in association with clinical iron defi-ciency [87].

Response of megakaryocytes to thrombocytopenia

The first recognizable change in the bone marrow following the induction of severe thrombocytopenia is in the number of small cells, presumably diploid, which in rodents carry the enzymic marker of the megakaryo-cyte series, acetyl-cholinesterase [1, 25]. A striking increase in these cells is observed at four hours after administration of platelet antiserum, but with a large dose of antiserum the change may appear as soon as one hour. Within 16 hours after antiserum, an increase in ploidy first becomes apparent in megakaryoblasts [27] so that the increase in synthesis of DNA must have commenced some nine hours earlier.

The increase in ploidy of maturing megakaryocytes which follows acute thrombocytopenia is striking [27, 50] (Fig. 25.5). The cells are larger [47, 49, 50] and follow a more accelerated course of maturation [51]. Platelets are released from cells which show persisting basophilia [27, 52] and an increase in content of glycogen [52]. Many of the platelets released early after the induction of acute thrombocytopenia are larger than any seen in the normal circulation [27] (Fig. 25.4) and their special properties of size, protein and carbohydrate metabolic characteristics [57, 88] should be regarded as features of 'stress' thrombopoiesis rather than as properties of normal, young platelets. As previously noted, the buoyant density of these platelets is no greater than that of average normal platelets [57], but from human studies they may well be more reactive than normal [89].

Platelet survival time

The survival of circulating platelets is probably a function both of intrinsic changes due to ageing and of extrinsic influences, in particular interaction with the blood vessel wall. Normal endothelium constitutes a non-reactive surface by virtue of surface components and charge. Endothelial cells also synthesize and release prostacyclin (PGI$_2$), a powerful inhibitor of platelet adhesion and aggregation [90, 91]. However, while pathological changes in the vessel wall may result

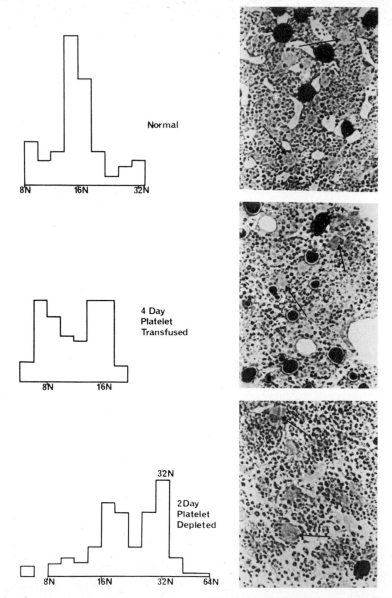

Fig. 25.5. Changes in megakaryocytes (arrowed on right) and their ploidy in rats. Above is the normal ploidy distribution; middle shows the effects of transfusion of platelets to suppress thrombopoiesis; shown below is the effect of stimulation of platelet production by the administration of a platelet antiserum. (Reproduced with permission from Ref. 52.)

in a dramatic shortening of platelet lifespan, under normal circumstances senescence is probably the major influence responsible for the disappearance of platelets from the circulation. Intrinsic platelet changes associated with ageing have been described (p. 978). While there is disagreement over the interpretation of platelet heterogeneity it is likely that metabolic changes are associated with ageing. For example, it has been postulated that there is progressive increase in lipid peroxidation products. This latter may reflect increasing susceptibility to oxidative stress and the toxic effect of lipid peroxides on enzyme systems and sulphydryl groups [92]. A progressive loss of surface glycoprotein with subsequent reduction in functional capability has also been attributed to senescence [93, 94]. That surface glycoproteins are important for platelet viability is suggested by their shortened survival in the circulation following *in-vitro* treatment by neuraminidase [95] or oxidation by sodium periodate [96].

Platelet-survival techniques

Measurement of platelet survival *in vivo* has been used for elucidation of physiological and pathological mechanisms, and to study the effects of both *in-vitro* and *in-vivo* treatment of platelets. Numerous methods have been used and these can be conveniently divided into non-isotopic and isotopic.

Non-isotopic methods. These have not gained widespread support. Direct counting to evaluate the disappearance of transfused platelets has been used in thrombocytopenic patients [96a]. This has obvious limitations in being inappropriate in individuals with normal platelet counts and comparatively inaccurate. Two methods utilizing the dramatic effect of acetylation of platelet cyclo-oxygenase by aspirin have been described recently. The first method [97] is based on the assay of malondialdehyde (MDA), a by-product of prostaglandin synthesis, which is completely inhibited by an adequate single dose of aspirin. The lifespan is calculated from the reappearance of platelet MDA over a period of days following such a dose. A particular methodological problem lies in the difficulty of measuring small amounts of MDA reliably, and a more recent technique using radioimmunoassay of thromboxane B_2, the stable end-product of thromboxane synthesis by platelets, is likely to prove more accurate [98]. Both, however, rely on the assumptions that platelet cyclo-oxygenase is completely inhibited by the single dose of aspirin, that megakaryocytes, and thus platelets newly formed following the dose, are unaffected, and that platelets treated by aspirin remain in the circulation unaltered with respect to lifespan.

Isotopic labelling of platelets for survival measurement has been used in two ways, namely cohort labelling and random labelling. *Cohort techniques* utilize the uptake of radio-labelled precursor substances with the subsequent appearance of labelled platelets followed by their disappearance as they are removed from the circulation; ^{32}P [99], [^{32}P]diisopropyl fluorophosphate (DF^{32}P) [100], ^{35}S and [^{75}Se]selenomethionine [101, 102] have been used as such precursors. While theoretically attractive, their routine use has been precluded for a number of reasons. Because of a comparatively protracted availability of the precursors there is concurrent appearance of labelled platelets during the disappearance phase; added to this there may be some re-utilization of isotope which confuses the analysis of disappearance time further. Finally, comparatively large doses of long-lived isotope are required to produce adequate isotope counts in the isolated platelets.

Random labelling of platelets has proved technically superior to cohort methods. Three comparatively specific agents have been used in the past to randomly label platelets. These are [^{32}P]orthophosphate, DFP labelled with ^{32}P, and [^{3}H] or [^{14}C]serotonin. Of these, DFP has had the most use but all three suffer from unacceptable elution of isotope from platelets in the circulation as well as subsequent reutilization [103–106].

Most information regarding platelet survival has been accumulated from studies using ^{51}Cr-labelling of platelets [107]. The technique has been modified over a number of years, particularly with regard to anticoagulant mixture, the use of plastic bags and changes in manipulation of the labelled platelets. A summary of the method has been published by the panel on diagnostic applications of radio-isotopes in haematology [108]. Despite improvements in methodology, ^{51}Cr-labelling still involves *in-vitro* handling of platelets. Furthermore the comparatively low efficiency of labelling means that a substantial volume of blood is required and a platelet count of less than 50×10^9/l precludes using autologous platelets. Elution of label and re-utilization are probably minor problems but there is evidence that the labelling procedure can produce significant dysfunction which may alter platelet survival [109].

^{111}Indium-labelling is a recent addition to the methodology of platelet survival. ^{111}In-hydroxyquinoline complex, which is lipid-soluble, has been shown to label dog, rabbit and human platelets with high efficiency, apparently without affecting *in-vitro* function or *in-vivo* survival [110–112]. The method has considerable theoretical advantages over previous techniques. ^{111}In has a relatively short half-life (2·8 days) and emits γ photons which are detectable by γ-camera imaging, so making it theoretically possible to record the *in-vivo* distribution of labelled platelets and their accumulation at thrombogenic foci. Because of efficient labelling (27–67%) only comparatively small numbers of platelets are required [111] which is a distinct advantage over chromium. The technique is still in the developmental phase and there are differences in methodology [112, 113].

Analysis of platelet-survival curves

^{51}Cr-labelled platelet disappearance in normal subjects is usually regarded as being linear [114–116], suggesting an age-related removal (Fig. 25.6, Table 25.1). In

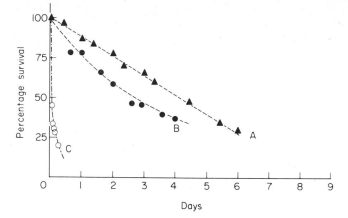

Fig. 25.6. Platelet survival curves obtained from disappearance of ^{51}Cr-labelled platelets from the circulation; (a) normal disappearance is approximately linear; (b) shortened platelet survival is associated with an exponential disappearance curve in the presence of severe vasculitis; (c) grossly reduced platelet lifespan in a patient with ITP.

conditions where disappearance is more rapid the curves may approach an exponential, suggesting random platelet removal [114–116]. In other situations the disappearance curve clearly lies somewhere between the two, and a number of attempts have been made to express the data in a satisfactory mathematical fashion. Three methods have found favour [108], but all are prone to artefact as one or two inaccurate data points can produce marked changes in the final calculated survival time. In addition there is no consensus as to whether the initial slope of the disappearance curve is the most important or whether analyses should take cognisance of samples counted over a period of days.

An adaptation of the Mills–Dornhorst equation is based on a maximum lifespan and a decay parameter. This model provides a curve which lies between the extremes of linear and exponential disappearance [108, 117]. A second method employs regression analysis of data by least squares computer fitting to a sum of γ functions [118–120]. This method of analysis, known also as the 'multiple hit', provides an estimation of the shape of the disappearance curve. A further method of analysing platelet-survival data which requires less sophisticated computation is the weighted mean, being

the mean survival time calculated from both linear and exponential estimates based on the experimental data. Finally the platelet count divided by platelet survival has been used to derive platelet turnover [116] which, with correction for splenic pooling and in the steady state, is a measure of platelet production.

The splenic pool of platelets

Following the injection of ^{51}Cr-labelled platelets, approximately one-third disappears from the circulation and is thought to remain in the splenic pool, which exchanges with the general circulation. Support for this concept is derived from studies with asplenic subjects in which the recovery of labelled platelets from the circulation is almost 100%. Further, in patients with significant splenomegaly there is an increase in splenic pooling so that as little as 10% of an injected dose of radio-labelled platelets may be found in the circulation [48, 121].

Interpretation of platelet-survival measurement

A reduced circulating lifespan of platelets may reflect intrinsic platelet defects or mechanisms external to the platelets themselves. *In-vitro* changes have been studied extensively in relation to techniques of platelet

Table 25.1. Normal laboratory values for platelets

		Ref.
Volume (*median*)	5·4 (4·0–6·4) fl (in ACD)	53
(*mode*)	3·7 (2·8–4·6) fl (in ACD)	53
	8·14 (6·48–10·2) fl (in EDTA)	148
Number in whole blood	150–400 × 10⁹/l	136, 137
Lifespan	8–12 days	48, 97, 112–116, 121
Turnover	35 000 ± 4300/µl/day	48

labelling (see above) and in the assessment of various storage conditions for platelet transfusion. It is of interest that treatment with enzymes such as neuraminidase causes significant shortening of platelet survival [95] but that thrombin-induced platelet degranulation, at least in the rabbit, does not affect the survival of such platelets when reinjected into the circulation [122].

Platelet-survival measurement has been invaluable in the investigation of mechanisms underlying thrombocytopenic diseases (see appropriate disease categories below). In some cases of thrombocytopenia it may be an informative clinical investigation when other less sophisticated procedures fail to yield a definite diagnosis.

More controversial are the results of platelet-survival data in vascular diseases, in which subtle shortening of lifespan may imply involvement in such disorders [123, 124]. A relation between the plasma concentration of proteins released from the platelets and platelet survival [125], and prolongation of abnormally short survival times by drugs which interfere with platelet function [123, 124], suggests that platelet consumption in vascular disease may be related to surface-mediated reactions to a diseased vessel wall.

THROMBOCYTOPENIA

Thrombocytopenia, the term for a reduced number of blood platelets, is defined as a blood-platelet count of less than $150 \times 10^9/l$, although normal haemostasis is maintained with $50–60 \times 10^9/l$, one-third the lower limit of normal. A platelet count greater than $30 \times 10^9/l$ is adequate to control minor bleeding and serious haemorrhage is exceptional with platelet counts above $20 \times 10^9/l$ [126, 127]. Below this level spontaneous haemorrhage is potentially dangerous. Departures from this general rule are met in situations where the functional capacity of the platelets is altered by disease or treatment. The haemostatic defect in disorders in which the proportion of young or 'stress' platelets in the circulation is high (e.g. in ITP) is often not as severe as in patients with thrombocytopenia due to reduced platelet production by the bone marrow [89, 128]. Thrombocytopenia secondary to splenic pooling is usually not associated with severe haemorrhage as the platelet pool is interchangeable. The converse applies in patients with combined thrombocytopenia and functional defects, in particular acute leukaemia and hereditary thrombocytopenias, following the ingestion of drugs likely to affect platelet function and when plasma factors interfere with platelet function—for example in uraemia [129], dysproteinaemias [130] and von Willebrand's disease. Associated fibrinolysis with plasma-factor abnormalities, classically with disseminated intravascular coagulation (DIC), is also likely to produce haemorrhage greater than that expected from the degree of thrombocytopenia.

Clinical effects

The clinical picture of thrombocytopenia is dominated by skin and mucous-membrane bleeding. *Purpura*, ranging from small petechial spots to large ecchymoses, is commonly concentrated on the lower extremities and at areas where pressure from tight clothing results in minor trauma. Petechiae may appear anywhere on the skin, however, and buccal purpura and haemorrhagic bullae are common, the latter seen especially when thrombocytopenia develops rapidly. *Bruising* with minimal trauma, *mucous-membrane bleeding* (e.g. epistaxis, bleeding from the gums) and also *menorrhagia* are common manifestations of platelet disorders. Internal haemorrhage, including renal, gastro-intestinal and intracerebral haemorrhage, is a significant danger with severe thrombocytopenia. Excessive bleeding following trauma, especially operative or tooth extraction, may be a presenting manifestation and tends to be immediately apparent, in contrast to coagulation defects which characteristically show normal primary haemostasis with subsequent breakdown and oozing.

The tourniquet test (Hess test) [131] is a useful clinical manoeuvre to detect a significant tendency to skin bleeding. A sphygmomanometer cuff inflated to 100 mg of mercury is maintained around the upper arm for a period of five minutes. Following removal of the cuff the appearance of more than 20 petechial spots within a circle of 3 cm diameter is indicative of a capillary or platelet disorder, usually thrombocytopenia.

Differentiation of purpura due to vascular defects and platelet dysfunction may be necessary but should be straightforward with comparatively simple laboratory investigations. Paradoxically thrombocytosis due to myeloproliferative disorders may result in haemorrhagic manifestations probably based on more than one abnormal mechanism; these conditions are fully described in Chapters 26 and 32.

Laboratory assessment of thrombocytopenia

A detailed description of techniques is outside the scope of this book, but the principles involved in laboratory investigation are outlined. Normal values for laboratory tests are shown in Table 25.1. A platelet count and examination of the peripheral-blood film are the basis of the investigation of suspected platelet disorders. A skin bleeding time is of particular value if haemorrhage is excessive for the degree of thrombocytopenia. If a significant divergence exists then platelet function studies may be indicated (Chapter 26). The underlying cause of thrombocytopenia is usually ascertained by means of a bone-marrow aspiration and trephine and by employing other more specialized tests (see below). Thrombocytopenia due to coagulation disturbances may occur and an investigation of the coagulation profile, particularly in the case of suspected DIC, may be indicated. Nutritional deficiencies are similarly investigated by appropriate assays.

Skin bleeding time. This test permits a more precise assessment of platelet disorders than does the tourniquet test. The time taken for a small skin puncture or laceration to stop bleeding is measured under standard conditions. The ear-lobe puncture technique described by Duke [132] is comparatively insensitive; the Ivy method modified by the application of a standard template [133] is the most commonly performed. The skin bleeding time has a reasonably close relationship to the platelet count in uncomplicated thrombocytopenias [128] due to reduced platelet production (Fig. 25.7), so that a disparity between these two requires investigation.

Blood platelet count. Platelet counts are commonly performed by automated systems, either electronic particle counters [134] or enumeration based on light scattering of platelets in suspension [135]. Both methods give good correlations with the visual techniques, which are described by Dacie & Lewis [136] and Brecher & Cronkite [137]. Errors in platelet counting are not uncommon [136]: in particular, the ease with which poor technique may result in the formation of a small clot makes it essential for a low platelet count to be confirmed on a second blood sample and by examination of a blood smear. Minor

degrees of *in-vitro* platelet aggregation may result in a falsely low platelet count, while other cellular fragments may be counted as platelets, resulting in an erroneously high platelet count: target cells, red-cell inclusions, sickle cells, fragmented red cells and white-cell components are potential sources of error.

Examination of blood film. With the platelet count, examination of a blood smear made from either anticoagulated blood or a finger-prick specimen is essential for assessment of platelet disorders. A standard technique is important; platelets may form aggregates in both thin and thick areas of the film. In anticoagulated blood such aggregates are less common than with direct finger-prick. With normal platelet counts, several platelets should be seen in each oil immersion field, analyses suggesting that one platelet/field is equivalent to about $20 \times 10^9/l$ [138, 139]. An assessment of platelet size and morphology may be of value in thrombocytopenic states, in particular giant platelets in Bernard–Soulier syndrome (Chapter 26) and in myeloproliferative disorders (Chapter 32), and both large and small platelets in immune thrombocytopenia (p. 988). Morphological abnormalities of the red cells and white cells may lead to an immediate diagnosis of the cause of thrombocytopenia.

Bone-marrow aspiration and trephine. Morphology of the bone marrow and, in particular, examination of megakaryocytes, remains the most useful diagnostic investigation in patients with thrombocytopenia. In disorders associated with decreased platelet production, marrow examination is frequently diagnostic (e.g. in leukaemias, marrow infiltrations, aplasia and nutritional deficiencies). In isolated thrombocytopenia, marrow examination is equally important.

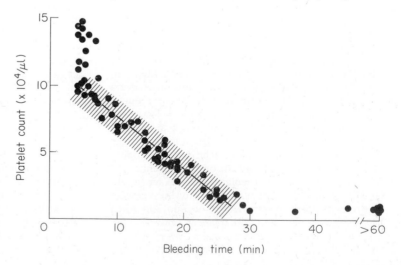

Fig. 25.7. The inverse relation of skin bleeding time to circulating platelet count in patients with thrombocytopenia due to impaired platelet production when the number of platelets is between $10 \times 10^9/l$ and $100 \times 10^9/l$. 95% confidence limits are indicated by the shaded area. (Reprinted, by permission, from *New England Journal of Medicine* [128].)

Most commonly normal or increased numbers of megakaryocytes are seen and this implies peripheral destruction of platelets. Sometimes specific megakaryocyte abnormalities such as hypoplasia or morphological changes associated with dyshaemopoiesis may be seen. Specific marrow changes are instanced in their appropriate sections.

In-vitro *coagulation tests related to platelets*. Several *in-vitro* aspects of coagulation become abnormal in the presence of thrombocytopenia. *Clot retraction* is largely dependent on normal numbers of functioning platelets. Inspection of a clot formed from 1 ml of blood at 37°C allows a qualitative assessment of retraction and red-cell 'fall-out'; quantification of the process has been described [140]. The *whole-blood coagulation time* is normal except in severe thrombocytopenia, when it may be prolonged. The *thromboplastin generation test* [141], *prothrombin consumption test* [142] and *platelet-factor-3 availability* [143] also depend on normal platelet numbers, but are not routinely used as diagnostic techniques for thrombocytopenia. The *thromboelastogram* pattern reflects thrombocytopenia by showing lack of retraction of the formed clot. Radioimmunoassays of the *platelet-specific proteins* β-thromboglobulin (βTG) and platelet factor 4 (PF4) in the plasma may be of value in differentiating causes of thrombocytopenia [144, 145].

Other specific platelet studies. Platelet-survival techniques (see p. 981) and platelet antibody tests, both drug-associated (see p. 999) and autoimmune (see p. 986), are of value in specific cases where the routine tests leave the diagnosis in reasonable doubt. Assessment of platelet function is discussed in Chapter 26.

Aetiology of thrombocytopenia

Causes of thrombocytopenia are numerous and varied (Table 25.2). The majority are secondary to an underlying process and are frequently associated with other haematological derangements involving either cellular components or coagulation mechanisms. Isolated thrombocytopenia is less common and these cases require more careful evaluation to exclude an infection, drug or other toxin as the cause.

In broad terms thrombocytopenia is associated with:

1 reduced platelet production;
2 increased destruction or utilization of platelets in the circulation; and
3 pooling (sequestration) of platelets in the spleen.

Normal physiological variations in platelet count do occur and these may be cyclical, the periodicity being 21–35 days [146]. In addition, a small drop in platelet

Table 25.2. Causes of thrombocytopenia

Impaired production (Table 25.6)
  Marrow aplasia (acquired)
  Metabolic (megaloblastosis, drugs)
  Megakaryocyte abnormalities (congenital, acquired)
  Infiltration of marrow (leukaemia, lymphoma)

Increased utilization or destruction
  (a) Immune platelet destruction (Table 25.3)
     Primary (idiopathic)
     Secondary
     Drug-induced (Table 25.5)
  (b) Intravascular coagulation
     Disseminated (malignancy, sepsis, obstetric accidents)
     Local (massive thromboembolism, giant haemangioma)
  (c) Intravascular platelet utilization, deposition or loss
     Thrombotic thrombocytopenic purpura
     Haemolytic-uraemic syndrome
     Viraemia
     Drugs (ristocetin, heparin)
     Extracorporeal circulations
     Haemorrhage
     Thrombocytapheresis

Distribution abnormalities
  Splenic pooling in splenomegaly
  Dilution by massive blood transfusion

count sometimes occurs in women at the time of menstruation [146, 147].

Racial differences in normal platelet count have also been described. For example, Mediterranean migrants in Australia have been reported to have lower platelet counts and higher mean platelet volumes than their northern European counterparts [148]. Such considerations are important in the assessment of minor deviations from the 'normal'.

Pseudothrombocytopenia. Technical artefacts may account for apparent thrombocytopenia (see p. 984). In addition platelet agglutination or platelet 'satellitism' occasionally occurs. The latter phenomenon, in which platelets are grouped around neutrophils in the blood smear, is likely to be due to a plasma factor acting in the presence of EDTA [149, 150].

Immune thrombocytopenic purpura

Immune thrombocytopenias constitute a substantial proportion of all cases of thrombocytopenia. The term does not denote a single disorder, but includes several entities (Table 25.3), the common aetiological factor being immune destruction of platelets. In addition to primary acquired (autoimmune) thrombocytopenia, underlying aetiologies such as lymphoproliferative disorders, systemic lupus erythematosus, viral infec-

Table 25.3. Immune thrombocytopenias

Primary (idiopathic)
    Acute
    Intermittent
    Chronic
Secondary
    Systemic lupus erythematosus
    Chronic lymphocytic leukaemia
    Lymphoma
    Hodgkin's disease
    Hashimoto's thyroiditis
    Hyperthyroidism
Drug-induced (Table 25.5)
Neonatal thrombocytopenia due to maternal antibody
    Passive—maternal autoantibody
    Active—maternal isoantibody (anti Pl^{Al}, Pl^{E2})
Post-transfusion purpura

tion or drugs may be present. There is a haemorrhagic tendency associated with a low platelet count, normal or increased numbers of megakaryocytes in the bone marrow and, in most cases, a short platelet survival and antibodies directed against platelets can be demonstrated.

IDIOPATHIC THROMBOCYTOPENIC PURPURA (ITP)
(Autoimmune thrombocytopenia; primary or essential thrombocytopenia)
Originally described by Werlhof in 1735 [151] as 'morbus haemorrhagicus maculosis', this disorder embraces thrombocytopenia in which, by process of exclusion, no underlying disorder or drug cause can be detected. In many cases there may well be an inciting agent prior to the development of thrombocytopenic purpura. The syndrome can be clearly differentiated into acute, intermittent and chronic. While there are a number of common features there are several differences, particularly in relation to incidence, the course of the condition and the prognosis.

Aetiology and pathogenesis
That excessive destruction of platelets by the spleen was the basic abnormality in ITP was first suggested by Kaznelson [152]. The concept of an underlying immune mechanism was mooted by Evans *et al.* when they reported the association of thrombocytopenia and autoimmune haemolytic anaemia [153] and by Epstein *et al.* [154] in a study of thrombocytopenia in children born to mothers with ITP.

Harrington *et al.* [155] reported a 'thrombocytopenic factor' in eight out of 10 patients with ITP which produced thrombocytopenia in normal individuals transfused with their blood or plasma. Further obser-

vations on 35 ITP patients [156] indicated that platelet agglutinins were present *in vitro* in about 65%. Harrington *et al.* concluded that the 'thrombocytopenic factor' was probably an anti-platelet antibody. Shulman *et al.* [157] isolated the factor and found that it was present in the IgG fraction of plasma and could be absorbed by normal platelets. The antibody in adults appears to be exclusively in the IgG_3 subclass [158].

Since the original observations suggesting a humoral anti-platelet antibody, numerous attempts have been made to devise more specific and more sensitive methods for the demonstration of these antibodies. Conventional serological methods including precipitation, haemagglutination, and platelet lysis [159–161], platelet agglutination [162] and antihuman globulin techniques [163] have all been tried, but on the whole the degree of reproducibility of these tests was disappointing: the percentage of positive tests in ITP patients ranged from zero to 90%. More recent techniques for autoantibodies in serum of patients with ITP appear more successful. These include, for example, the PF3 availability test [164, 165]; ^{51}Cr release from labelled platelets of patients with paroxysmal nocturnal haemoglobinuria (PNH) by ITP sera (based on the hypersusceptibility to complement-dependent lysis of platelets of patients with this disorder) [166, 167], or from enzyme-treated platelets [167]; and ^{14}C-labelled serotonin release from platelets by immuno-injury. In general, approximately 60% of patients with ITP have serum anti-platelet antibodies detectable by these techniques.

In the past decade, several techniques have suggested that in almost all cases of immune thrombocytopenia there is an increased amount of immunoglobulin on the platelet surface. The first direct measurement of platelet-bound antibody was based on competitive binding between the ^{125}I-labelled Fab fragment of IgG and its respective antibody [168]. Other techniques have been developed by Rosse and others [169–172]. They appear to provide a clinically useful quantitative assessment of antibody levels on platelets as an increment over that observed on normal, washed platelets. There are significant discrepancies between reports with respect to the amount of immunoglobulin on both normal and ITP platelets: normal platelets have been reported to carry 65–311 $ng/10^9$ platelets [168] by one group and up to 400 $\mu g/10^9$ platelets by another [169]. Using a radio-labelled antiglobulin test it has been estimated that there are approximately 5×10^3 anti-IgG combining sites per normal platelet [172]. In ITP and other immune thrombocytopenias the quantities of platelet-bound IgG are increased up to 10 times normal and the quantities appear to correlate well with severity of disease and resistance to various forms of treatment (p. 990). Platelet-bound immunoglobulin has also been demonstrated by immunofluorescence [173] and using immunoperoxidase techniques [174, 175].

One-half to two-thirds of patients with ITP have demonstrable platelet-bound complement (C3) [172, 176]. Despite other differences between adults and children with ITP, the incidence of platelet-bound immunoglobulin and complement appears to be similar in the two groups.

Platelet survival determined by isotope-disappearance techniques is grossly decreased in patients with ITP [177, 178] and scintillation scanning has demonstrated various patterns of sequestration of the destroyed platelets. Splenic, hepatic, and combinations of sequestration site have been reported, the more severe and more resistant to therapy usually being associated with hepatic sequestration and the less severe and more amenable to treatment showing splenic sequestration (p. 991).

The role of the spleen as a major site of destruction in ITP is strengthened by the finding of increased histiocytes with lipid and platelet remnants in spleens removed at operation [179]. *In-vitro* splenic anti-platelet-antibody formation has been reported [180] and splenic IgG-synthesis rates greatly increased [181]. Cellular immunity has been postulated by some authors: lymphocytes were stimulated by platelets incubated with serum in 25 of 26 patients with ITP reported in one study [182] and six out of seven in another [183]. Lymphocytes from ITP patients have been reported to show a significantly reduced response to phytohaemagglutinin compared to normal persons [184]. Finally the possibility that circulating immune complexes may result in platelet consumption in at least some immune thrombocytopenias cannot be excluded. This is more likely in acute forms of ITP and in the uncommon post-transfusion thrombocytopenia (p. 995).

Prevalence and incidence

The overall prevalence rate of thrombocytopenia has been reported from hospital diagnosis in Sweden as 4·5 male and 7·5 female patients per 100 000 inhabitants per year. Of these approximately half were categorized as 'essential thrombocytopenia' [185]. In another well-documented study ITP was found to account for 0·18% of 132 235 hospital admissions analysed over a 10-year period [186]. ITP or 'essential thrombocytopenia' makes up a more moderate proportion of patients with thrombocytopenia in other series: 73 out of 500 [187] and 65 out of 827 [188].

Age and sex distribution

Overall, females predominate in a ratio of approximately two to one [186]. When analysed in age groups a striking difference emerges, as the sex incidence is approximately equal in the first decade of life while females in their third and fourth decades are affected somewhere between three and four times more commonly than males. This difference becomes less marked over the age of 60 [186, 189, 190] (Fig. 25.8).

The differences in sex incidence are further resolved when separated into acute and chronic forms. Acute ITP most commonly affects children between the ages of two and six with a peak incidence at three years [191]; it most commonly develops during spring, coinciding with the seasonal increase in viral infections, and the sexes are affected with equal frequency. Chronic ITP is comparatively rare in children, usually

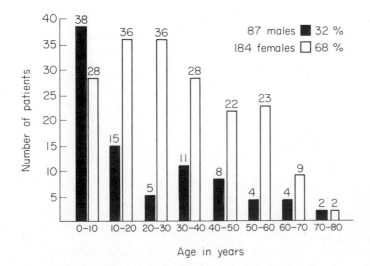

Fig. 25.8. Age and sex distribution in 271 patients with idiopathic thrombocytopenic purpura. (Reprinted, by permission, from *Annals of Internal Medicine* [186].)

affecting young and middle-aged adults, and females predominate with a sex ratio of three or four to one [186, 189, 190].

There is apparently a low incidence of immune thrombocytopenia in Negroes [191, 192]; and while it is possible that bruises and petechae might more easily pass unnoticed in dark-skinned individuals, this is probably not the full explanation [193].

Clinical features

Acute ITP. This is usually an acute and transient illness which most frequently occurs following a viral infection in the preceding few days to three weeks [191, 193, 194]. Occasionally it may follow vaccination [195, 196]. Characteristically the onset of skin purpura is sudden, often with haemorrhagic bullae in mucous membranes. Bleeding is usually confined to these sites. In 25% of children, epistaxis occurs, and in five per cent, haematuria. The extent of the purpura is variable and in only three to four per cent is there massive purpura including retinal haemorrhages [191, 193]. Despite such a major bleeding tendency no cases of intracranial haemorrhage were found in 350 children consecutively diagnosed as acute ITP [193]. Gastro-intestinal haemorrhage is uncommon and haemorrhage into parenchymal organs, muscles or joints is rare enough to suggest a coagulation disturbance rather than a platelet disorder when it arises. Acute ITP in the adult is more likely to be associated with gastro-intestinal bleeding, haematuria, epistaxis and central-nervous bleeding [197]. Lymphadenopathy may be present and a minor degree of splenomegaly occurs in up to 10% of children [193].

Chronic ITP. In chronic ITP there is usually no antecedent history, but purpura, a tendency to bruise, or some form of local bleeding may be manifest for some time before presentation, the onset being insidious in many instances. Menorrhagia and metrorrhagia are common and in fact may be the only manifestations. As with acute ITP, gastro-intestinal haemorrhage, haematuria and intracerebral bleeds are comparatively uncommon. Retinal haemorrhage may indicate the risk of an intracerebral bleed which is usually subarachnoid. A palpable spleen is rare and significant splenomegaly excludes the diagnosis of ITP.

Intermittent ITP. In a small group of patients the disease follows a pattern of alternating remissions and exacerbations. Acute episodes lasting for some weeks are followed by prolonged periods with normal platelet count and no evidence of bleeding. In most cases such remissions probably represent a compensated state with increased platelet turnover [46, 198–200] but in others both platelet count and platelet survival are normal [198].

Laboratory investigation

The blood picture is characteristic. Thrombocytopenia is the essential feature and is usually more severe in acute cases, the platelet count being less than $10 \times 10^9/l$ and occasionally zero. In chronic ITP the count tends to be in the range $20–80 \times 10^9/l$ in the majority of cases [197, 201]. On the blood smear both large (megathrombocytes) and small platelets (microthrombocytes) are characteristically present [46, 199, 202]. Megathrombocytes, which may measure up to 10 μm in diameter, represent accelerated thrombopoiesis; whether they have the true discoid platelet form or whether some may be megakaryocyte cytoplasmic fragments is as yet uncertain, but the fact that in most patients showing these large forms the bleeding time is less prolonged than might be anticipated from the platelet count [128], would favour the view that these megathrombocytes are functionally highly active.

Haemoglobin, red-cell count, white-cell count and morphology are usually normal although some variations have been observed. In chronic ITP with increased blood loss there is the possibility of iron deficiency developing. In a small percentage of cases evidence for immune red-cell destruction with a positive direct antiglobulin test is present (Evans' syndrome [153]). Ultrastructural studies indicate that minor degrees of red-cell fragmentation are probably quite common [203].

The white cells may show minor aberrations in acute ITP with mild eosinophilia or lymphocytosis [191] and neutropenia is found in a small proportion of cases otherwise characterized as ITP.

Bone-marrow changes are minor: normal or increased numbers of megakaryocytes are the rule, with an increased proportion of immature forms, some with lower than normal ploidy, scanty cytoplasm, few granules and prominent basophilia. The 'platelet-releasing megakaryocyte', the mature, amoeboid form, is not seen in smears of patients with ITP but as this form is not easily detected in all normal marrow smears, its absence is not of great significance from the diagnostic viewpoint.

Coagulation tests in which platelets play a part (clot retraction, prothrombin consumption test, thromboplastin generation and thromboelastogram) are abnormal.

Platelet survival. Studies of platelet survival in ITP

patients indicate that the lifespan is shortened in almost all cases. The shortest survival curves are commonly seen in acute ITP and there appears to be a good relationship between platelet count and platelet survival in most. Various estimates of platelet production suggest that it is increased from three to eight times normal [48, 177, 178, 204]; this occurs with mean platelet survival shortened to less than 10% of normal. It is stated that platelet production is inappropriately depressed in some cases of ITP [197] and this has been attributed to immune disruption of megakaryocytopoiesis [205].

Platelet antibodies have been demonstrated in the serum of approximately two-thirds of patients with ITP by a variety of methods (p. 986). Significantly increased amounts of immunoglobulin bound to platelets have been demonstrated by a number of laboratories [168–175] (p. 986). In a substantial proportion, components of complement have been detected either with Ig or alone [172, 176]. Increase in platelet-bound Ig has been reported in other situations, notably in hyper-γ-globulinaemic states [206] and in association with sepsis [207].

A number of other laboratory features have been described in ITP which are not routinely required for diagnosis. Platelet function tests, when the numbers are adequate for investigation, may show reduced adhesion to glass, poor clot retraction, impaired platelet factor-3 availability and aggregation [208]. These abnormalities have been described in patients with chronic and intermittent ITP in which the platelet count and bleeding time have returned to normal. Both increased [209] and decreased [208] antiheparin activity of platelets have been described in ITP. The antiheparin activity in plasma [210] and platelet factor 4 [144] and β-thromboglobulin [145] content of plasma by radioimmunoassay are reduced.

Diagnosis

The diagnosis of ITP usually remains one of exclusion. The development of cutaneous and mucous-membrane bleeding in an otherwise well individual without significant splenomegaly is clinically most suggestive. In the case of children a preceding viral illness is additional suggestive evidence. A positive tourniquet test and increased skin bleeding time, and the presence of isolated thrombocytopenia with normal or increased numbers of megakaryocytes in an otherwise normal marrow, further strengthen the diagnosis. Marrow aspiration is necessary to exclude an underlying marrow disorder or impaired thrombopoiesis.

Other causes of peripheral platelet destruction or pooling need to be considered. Intravascular coagulation (Chapter 29) may be suspected in the appropriate clinical setting and should be excluded by coagulation studies, in particular those relating to abnormalities of fibrinogen metabolism. Splenic pooling is unlikely to be responsible for thrombocytopenia unless the spleen is significantly enlarged and, except in children or in the presence of some other complicating disorder, splenic enlargement is very unusual in ITP. Hereditary thrombocytopenias should be considered and associated features, age of onset and family history elicited (p. 1008). Pseudothrombocytopenia produced by an *in-vitro* phenomenon must be excluded (p. 985).

The demonstration of abnormal platelet kinetics, namely a low recovery rate, short survival, and sequestration in spleen or liver [211] is further strong evidence for ITP. The demonstration of increased immunoglobulin on the platelet surface or a circulating anti-platelet antibody is of value. Caution should be exercised in the interpretation of increased platelet-bound immunoglobulin.

An underlying cause must be sought. Of first importance is to exclude the intake of one of the large number of drugs which may be responsible for thrombocytopenia. Although techniques to detect drug-dependent antibodies may be of value, a close history and, if possible, the suspension of all likely medications should be undertaken. An acute onset following recent drug ingestion is suggestive but by no means always present. Systemic lupus erythematosus and other autoimmune disorders such as Hashimoto thyroiditis [212], hyperthyroidism [213], lymphoma [214, 215] and chronic lymphocytic leukaemia (CLL) [215, 216] need to be considered. The presence of appropriate clinical features is likely to lead to the diagnosis in most instances but lupus erythematosus in particular may present with thrombocytopenia alone, other manifestations only developing at a later date. For this reason antinuclear factor, DNA antibody or LE cells should be sought on diagnosis of ITP.

Course and prognosis

As indicated above, the course of the acute and chronic ITP syndromes differ significantly. The acute disease is usually self-limiting, lasting from a few days to a few weeks and rarely exceeding six months [191, 193]. In less than 10% of children a chronic course is reported [191, 217]. The mortality rate in children with acute ITP is probably less than one per cent [191, 193, 197].

The course of chronic ITP is protracted, lasting from months to years. Characteristically there are fluctuations in severity both in platelet count and in bleeding manifestations. Exacerbations may be associated with viral infections, other intercurrent illness, drug ingestion or changes in nutrition. In general the prognosis is good, even in patients who show a poor therapeutic response and remain thrombocytopenic. An overall mortality rate of 4·4% has been reported [218] although in older patients this may be significantly higher [197]. In a small number of cases manifestations of systemic lupus erythematosus or an underlying lymphoma may supervene at a later date.

Treatment

It is wise to admit to hospital all patients presenting with symptomatic thrombocytopenia. General measures which are appropriate in ITP, be it acute or chronic, include bed rest, avoidance of trauma and the prohibition of drugs which might affect platelet function, in particular aspirin, other nonsteroidal antiflammatory agents and alcohol. The treatment of intercurrent problems (e.g. fever and infection which are likely to exacerbate thrombocytopenia and platelet dysfunction) should be undertaken [219].

Specific therapy aimed at either reducing the production of immunoglobulin or interfering with its detrimental effect on the platelet consists of immunosuppression either with corticosteroid or cytotoxic drugs, or splenectomy.

ACTH and cortisone. These were introduced into the treatment of ITP in 1950 [220]. Corticosteroids have subsequently become the mainstay of initial therapy.

An apparently non-specific, beneficial effect on capillary integrity is somewhat controversial [193, 219]. Animal experiments suggest that thrombocytopenia is associated with the development of endothelial cell 'thin spots' and diminished vessel-wall thickness. Treatment with prednisone corrects these abnormalities in the absence of a rise in the platelet count [221]. Other animal experiments provide evidence that steroids in high dose reduce endothelial prostacyclin production, resulting in the maintenance of vasoconstriction and hence haemostasis [222]. There is a clinical impression that steroids enhance capillary resistance [220, 223]. Counter-arguments are that a lessening of the bleeding tendency prior to a significant rise in the platelet count may be part of a natural history, for example in childhood purpura [193], and may reflect an absolute increase in the number of platelets, supporting the needs of the endothelium and haemostasis before enough change has occurred to be apparent in the platelet count. Further possible beneficial effects may be via the inhibition of binding of antiplatelet antibody, with correction of qualitative platelet defects, or by inhibition of splenic sequestration of younger more haemostatically effective platelets [224].

Aside from their possible effect on endothelial integrity, corticosteroids act in one or more of three ways and these are almost certainly through effects on the immune system; corticosteroids have no effect on platelet survival or platelet count in normal individuals [225]. Reduction of surface-bound and serum antibody is usually achieved by the administration of corticosteroids [169, 170, 172, 226] over a period of days to weeks (Fig. 25.9). There may, however, be remission in the thrombocytopenia before a normal level of platelet-associated IgG [172] is achieved or without the disappearance of anti-platelet antibody [169]. Antibody binding to the cell-surface antigen may be impaired [172] in a manner similar to that observed with erythrocyte antibody [169]. Similarly there may be impairment of the ability of reticuloendothelial cells to remove opsonized platelets from the circulation [226, 227].

Complete remissions are achieved in 15–60% of patients treated with corticosteroids, the response taking several days or weeks to become apparent [186, 219, 228]. Sustained remissions following discontinuance of therapy are much less common [186, 219, 229]. Lack of response to corticosteroids is usually related to comparatively large quantities of immunoglobulin on the platelet surface [170, 230].

An initial dosage of 1–1·5 mg/kg/day of prednisolone or equivalent is used, continuing for a period of two to three weeks [219]. Higher doses may be required to obtain a therapeutic effect. Full dosage should not be continued beyond three or four weeks because of the dangers of adverse steroid effects. With a complete remission (platelet count greater than $250 \times 10^9/l$) the dosage of steroids may be reduced over a period of two to three weeks to the minimum dose necessary to control the condition. If the platelet count does not reach $50 \times 10^9/l$ in the initial two to three weeks it is unlikely that substantial or sustained remission will occur and in adults splenectomy should be performed [219]. With a partial remission of greater degree, a period of expectant therapy or maintenance at a lower dose is advised before consideration is given to splenectomy. The choice of the appropriate alternative is a matter for individual judgment but prolonged treatment with corticosteroids carries hazards, particularly in older patients. There is no necessity to maintain the platelet count at greater than $50–100 \times 10^9/l$ and an even lower count is acceptable if there are no haemorrhagic manifestations

Splenectomy. This has been used for the treatment of ITP since 1916 [152]. Under normal circumstances splenectomy has no effect on platelet survival [225, 231] despite the consequent rise in platelet count. In the presence of anti-platelet immunoglobulin, platelets are removed by reticuloendothelial macrophages in the spleen and elsewhere. The spleen is also responsible for production of autoantibody and levels of both platelet-

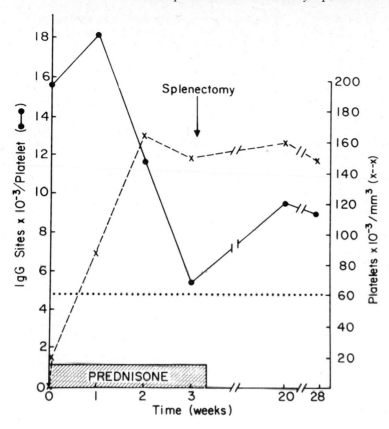

Fig. 25.9. Platelet-associated IgG shown in relation to the platelet count and treatment with prednisolone and splenectomy in a patient with ITP. (Reprinted, by permission, from *New England Journal of Medicine* [172].)

bound and circulating anti-platelet immunoglobulin are usually reduced by splenectomy [169, 170, 172] (Fig. 25.9).

The overall response rate to splenectomy varies from 70 to 90% [186, 229, 232–234], but up to 10% of patients will subsequently relapse. The indications for splenectomy are failure of, or contraindications to, continuing corticosteroid therapy. In patients requiring more than a low dosage of corticosteroid to control the purpura it is probably not reasonable to wait longer than six to eight weeks before proceeding to splenectomy, though some would advocate waiting as long as six months [234]. In cases of life-threatening bleeding, immediate splenectomy is indicated. In children, particularly younger children, splenectomy should be delayed for at least six months (p. 992).

Following splenectomy, the risk of severe infection (especially pneumococcal) and the development of disseminated intravascular coagulation with Waterhouse–Friedrichsen syndrome is particularly significant in children [235, 236]. This risk is by no means abolished by age [237] although it is clearly lessened. Splenectomy should be avoided in children under the age of two and should preferably wait until at least

four or five years of age to minimize the risk of infection [193]. Prophylactic oral penicillin should be given for at least two years postsplenectomy [193], even in older children [224], and polyvalent pneumococcal vaccines should probably be administered to all postsplenectomy patients [238].

In reaching a decision with respect to splenectomy, the pointers towards a favourable response should be taken into account. Good response to corticosteroid therapy (e.g. prenisolone 1 mg/kg) has been reported to indicate 100% success in subsequent splenectomy [239]. Less severe disease bodes well for a good response: this is often reflected by splenic rather than hepatic sequestration, as shown by ^{51}Cr-labelled platelet-uptake studies [233], and may be predictable even more precisely by the quantity of platelet-bound immunoglobulin [169, 170]. The other major prognostic feature is comparative youth: Harrington [239] observed an 88% response to splenectomy below the age of 45, as compared to 59% response above that age. As might be expected there is some correlation between splenic sequestration and age [233]. A non-immune aetiology for ITP may also be a good prognostic feature for splenectomy [219]. Splenectomy should not be withheld from a patient on the basis of the above criteria alone, however, as they are by no means exclusive, and other forms of therapy are also less likely to be effective in the more severe case or the older patient.

The development of an accessory spleen, which may occur in the area of the splenic pedicle or in more distant sites, has been described within weeks or months following splenectomy, resulting in a curtailment of remission [266]. This is an uncommon occurrence and should be easily excluded by the presence of Howell–Jolly bodies and other red-cell changes. Otherwise appropriate radionuclide scanning may be used to outline such splenic tissue.

Immunosuppression. Of the 20–25% of patients who fail to respond to splenectomy and corticosteroids or in those in whom splenectomy is contraindicated, immunosuppression with cytotoxic agents may produce a remission in perhaps one-half. Azathioprine, cyclophosphamide and vinca alkaloids have proved to be the most useful. Early experience was gained with mercaptopurine and azathioprine [218, 240], corticosteroids usually being administered concurrently. Unfortunately the response to this treatment is comparatively slow, usually taking two to three months for a rise in platelet count, and persistent treatment is necessary for one to two years. Cyclophosphamide may be more active in the dosages used but is more toxic; the response rate reported has varied from 25 to 68% [219, 241, 242]. Dosages of 50–200 mg/day maintained for at least 10 days after remission (ordinarily no longer than two months) resulted in complete remissions in more than half of a group of 22 patients [242], and partial remissions in three of this group. Cyclophosphamide has also been administered successfully in a single large dose (300–600 mg/m² i.v. or orally every two to three weeks) [243].

Finally, the vinca alkaloids, vincristine and vinblastine, have been advocated for refractory thrombocytopenia [244–249]. These drugs are not only potent immunosuppressants but induce thrombocytosis in animals [250, 251] and in man [250, 252] (p. 1014). The response rate to vincristine is approximately 50% in terms of complete remission without maintenance therapy; others require continued use of vinca alkaloids to achieve control of the disease and about 25% fail to respond at all. More recently it has been reported that patients non-responsive to vincristine or vinblastine given by conventional means may respond to 'vinblastine-loaded platelets' [249]. This technique consists of *in-vitro* incubation of the patient's own platelets with a high concentration of vinblastine and their subsequent reinfusion. It is believed that in such a way selective delivery of vinblastine into the macrophage may lead to its dysfunction and alleviation of platelet destruction.

Each of the immunosuppressive agents carries its own side-effects but, in general, alopecia, gastrointestinal side-effects and possible teratogenic and mutagenic effects make them unsuitable for use in children and, ideally, they should be avoided in women of child-bearing age. These and other considerations also make splenectomy a preferable form of management where possible. Particular side-effects of these drugs are discussed in Chapter 22.

Platelet transfusion. This has only a small part in the management of ITP, as transfused platelets rarely improve bleeding or result in a rise in the circulating platelet count [217]: the more severe the thrombocytopenia the more rapidly are transfused platelets removed from the circulation. It is used by some in association with corticosteroid and emergency splenectomy in severe life-threatening haemorrhage [193, 217]. Platelet transfusion both before and during splenectomy for ITP has been both recommended [197] and denigrated [219]. In the authors' view it has little role in such situations.

Plasma infusions. These have been reported to result in a rise in platelet numbers in some individuals with ITP. This phenomenon has been described in particular in children, both with acute and chronic ITP, the rise in count occurring within 72 hours and reaching a peak after four to five days [253–255]. The mechanism of this action is uncertain and at least in some cases it is likely that the treatment coincided with spontaneous cure at the time the plasma was given.

Plasma exchange. This has been reported to be effective in two cases of ITP [256]. This approach may be rational if immune complexes are responsible for *in-vivo* platelet destruction: this is more likely to be the case in the acute forms of ITP and those associated with systemic lupus erythematosus, drug allergy, infectious diseases and anaphylactic reations.

Management of ITP in specific circumstances

Childhood. While the therapeutic measures outlined in the preceding sections are used in the management of children with ITP, the overall philosophy of management differs because of the self-limiting, transient nature of the disease in childhood. In general, avoidance of trauma until bleeding manifestations subside or the platelet count begins to rise is all that is required

[193]. For practical purposes intracranial haemorrhage is the only significant risk and appears to be extremely rare in childhood [193, 194, 197]. This comment applies to infants and young children; in teenagers the disease is more likely to follow the adult pattern.

Corticosteroids have been advocated by some on the basis of improvement in capillary function and interference with phagocytosis at least of lightly sensitized platelets as discussed above. There is clearly a wide spectrum of opinion regarding their use, as experienced clinicians have regarded corticosteroids as unnecessary in children under the age of 12 [193], while some recommend the use of prednisolone during the initial acute phase in selected children. The criteria for selection of such cases vary [217, 257, 258], but reasonable indications for steroids are a history of recent head injury, severe haemorrhagic manifestations or a platelet count less than $5 \times 10^9/l$ [258]. A recent prospective, randomized study [259] suggests that corticosteroids used early in the disease result in a greatly accelerated remission of thrombocytopenia. It should be borne in mind that a transient drop in platelet count frequently occurs when steroid dosages are reduced [191, 193, 217, 258].

In the small number of children with chronic ITP the approach to management should be similar to that for adults with due regard to the problems of postsplenectomy sepsis in infants and to the mutagenic effects of immunosuppressive drugs which assume greater importance in the younger patient. A decision to perform an elective splenectomy should be delayed for at least six months [193].

Pregnancy. This poses a real problem in ITP with regard to management of the mother, the fetus and neonate. Maternal mortality may be as high as 10% [260, 261] and the fetal mortality between 15 and 25% [260, 262]. As most women with ITP give birth to thrombocytopenic infants [262] (see p. 994) the greatest threat to the infant is intracranial haemorrhage due to trauma during delivery. In the first trimester, corticosteroids and immunosuppressants should be avoided and splenectomy carried out, although this may precipitate abortion [219, 263]. Corticosteroids may be used later in pregnancy but if thrombocytopenia is not easily controlled splenectomy should be performed [219, 263]. When the infant is viable a combined splenectomy and Caesarian section may be appropriate [219, 264, 265]. If severe thrombocytopenia is present in the mother or if she has had previous infants with significant neonatal thrombocytopenia, delivery should in any case be accomplished by Caesarian section; otherwise delivery should be as atraumatic as possible.

SECONDARY FORMS OF IMMUNE THROMBOCYTOPENIC PURPURA

Thrombocytopenia associated with systemic lupus erythematosus (SLE)

Thrombocytopenia is common in SLE, being manifest in more than one-third of one series of 200 patients [267]. Of this group 32% had platelet counts between 100 and $150 \times 10^9/l$ and five per cent less than $100 \times 10^9/l$. In a further analysis of SLE, platelet counts of less than $100 \times 10^9/l$ were found in 19% [268]. Patients diagnosed as suffering from ITP occasionally develop manifestations of SLE subsequently [186, 269]: thus in one large series, five of 243 patients with thrombocytopenic purpura were diagnosed as having SLE, three of these patients developing the disease over a 10-year period. Despite the inference [270] that splenectomy might accelerate the development of SLE, the sporadic association and the weak temporal relationship make this notion unlikely [186, 269].

The anti-platelet antibody associated with SLE differs in some respects from the ITP antibody. It occurs in all four subgroups of IgG rather than just IgG_3 [230]. In addition the anti-platelet antibody binds serum complement to the platelet membrane [176, 230] and requires the presence of complement for antibody-induced platelet damage. There is some physico-chemical evidence to suggest that the lupus anti-platelet factor may be an immune complex [230].

Some patients with SLE have circulating antibodies to platelets without thrombocytopenia [176, 271] and a small number may have platelet dysfunction and easy bruising [272].

Thrombocytopenia associated with lymphoproliferative disorders and Hodgkin's disease

Thrombocytopenia is a common complication of lymphoproliferative diseases, particularly later in the course of CLL. It may develop as a result of marrow infiltration, hypersplenism, chemotherapy or occasionally as an immune thrombocytopenic purpura [215, 216]. Of 36 patients with CLL, 11 had elevated membrane-bound IgG and in each of these the platelet count was decreased [215]. There was no consistent relationship between the disease activity and the degree of thrombocytopenia or platelet-bound IgG. In eight of the 11 patients there was a favourable platelet response to corticosteroids, cytotoxic agents and/or splenectomy. In this series, thrombocytopenia did not indicate a poor prognosis as suggested by others [273]. A small number of patients with Hodgkin's disease [214, 215, 274] and non-Hodgkin lymphoma [215] have been described with thrombocytopenia and elevated membrane-bound IgG.

The diagnosis of immune thrombocytopenia in

these conditions may be suggested by the same criteria as in ITP. A bone-marrow trephine is more likely to allow a quantitative assessment of megakaryocytes in the presence of infiltration. The effect of cytotoxic agents may confuse the diagnosis and it is in these situations that measurements of platelet survival and platelet-bound immunoglobulin are likely to be of diagnostic value. Drugs as a cause of immune thrombocytopenia should not be forgotten [275].

The treatment of thrombocytopenia in these conditions is dependent on a clear diagnosis and may include manipulation of chemotherapy and platelet transfusion (p. 1010) as an interim measure. In cases of immune thrombocytopenia associated with lymphoproliferative disorders, splenectomy may be required [215, 274].

Neonatal thrombocytopenia

The chief causes of neonatal thrombocytopenia are listed in Table 25.4. Several of these are considered elsewhere, in relation to their pathogenesis, the present section being concerned primarily with immune thrombocytopenias. In practice, crops of petechiae are often seen over the presenting part of normal infants at birth, as a result of venous compression during delivery, but more generalized purpura, or other signs of haemorrhage, call for a platelet count. Apart from

Table 25.4. Neonatal thrombocytopenia

Intrauterine infections
    Rubella, cytomegalovirus, herpes
    Toxoplasmosis
    Syphilis

Platelet antibodies
    Maternal ITP and SLE (autoantibody)
    Fetomaternal incompatibility
      (isoantibody)
    Drug-induced

Disseminated intravascular coagulation
    Maternal pre-eclampsia
    Hypothermia, asphyxia, shock, sepsis
    Rhesus isoimmunization

Congenital megakaryocytic hypoplasia
    TAR syndrome
    Maternal drug ingestion

Hereditary thrombocytopenias
    Wiskott–Aldrich syndrome
    Others

Giant haemangioma

Congenital and neonatal leukaemia and histiocytosis

Metabolic disorders: hyperglycinaemia, methylmalonic
    acidaemia, etc.

Post-exchange transfusion

---

the immune causes, intrauterine infections and DIC are the most important: in each case, the haemorrhagic signs are usually associated with other clinical features, while infants with immune thrombocytopenia are commonly otherwise healthy.

Passive immune thrombocytopenia. Since neonatal thrombocytopenia associated with maternal ITP was initially recognized in the early 1950s [154, 156], it has been clear that maternal anti-platelet antibodies can cross the placenta. Thrombocytopenia is present in approximately three-quarters of infants born to mothers with ITP [219, 262], the incidence varying from 34 to 90% [262, 264, 265, 276]. Consistent with the observation that platelet antibody may persist in patients successfully treated by splenectomy, infants born to such women may be affected. In general, however, the severity of thrombocytopenia in the infant is related to the maternal platelet count [265]. The clinical manifestations are most marked at, or shortly after, birth and are related to delivery. They may vary from a mild petechial rash to major internal haemorrhage and umbilical-cord bleeding. The course of the disease is between two and three months [276]. Improperly managed, the mortality may be of the order of 15–25% [260, 262]. Death is almost always due to intracranial haemorrhage following birth trauma.

The diagnosis is clear in the setting of maternal ITP or SLE, with the presence of marked thrombocytopenia (platelet count 10×10^9/l or less) and the absence of signs of other causes. With extensive haemorrhage, absorption of bilirubin may produce jaundice after 12–24 hours [193]. Differential diagnosis includes the various other conditions in Table 25.4. The condition is self-limiting and usually requires no active therapy unless there is evidence of a severe haemorrhagic state, intracranial haemorrhage or other potentially serious bleeding. It is unlikely that steroids will effect the course, unless perhaps by inhibiting the sequestration of antibody-coated platelets, and splenectomy is contraindicated because of the risk of later fulminating infection. Other measures such as exchange transfusion, to lower the antibody titre, and platelet transfusion, may occasionally be of value. The platelet count usually begins to rise spontaneously during the second or third week, but may not reach normal values until six to eight weeks after birth.

Not all mothers with ITP produce thrombocytopenic infants, and the antenatal detection of circulating anti-platelet antibodies is not an entirely reliable guide. Particular care should obviously be taken in delivering such women, and in those who have borne a thrombocytopenic infant previously, Caesarean section should be considered as a means of avoiding birth trauma.

Active immune neonatal thrombocytopenia. About 20% of immune neonatal thrombocytopenia falls into this category. Long-standing maternal antibodies directed against the platelet-specific or histocompatibility (HLA) antigens of fetal platelets may be acquired transplacentally with consequent thrombocytopenia in the fetus. Neonatal alloimmune thrombocytopenia is most often due to antibodies to the Pl^{A1} antigen on platelets, less commonly to Pl^{E2} [280] or other antigens. Since 97% of the population are Pl^{A1}-positive, immunization is rare. Histocompatibility immunization probably occurs more commonly, but seldom results in severe thrombocytopenia. In the event of a severe haemorrhagic state requiring active treatment, transfusion with platelet concentrates from the mother in ABO-compatible plasma is an effective source of 'compatible' platelets [281], and removal of antibodies by exchange transfusion may also be advisable. Most cases require no treatment, however, and the platelet count returns to normal within a month or so.

Intrauterine infections. Thrombocytopenia occurs in 40–80% of cases of the congenital rubella syndrome [277, 278], the incidence varying from one epidemic to another, in about half of congenital CMV infections [279], and occasionally in congenital toxoplasmosis and syphilis. Both defective platelet production and increased turnover may play a part in the pathogenesis, the latter resulting either from DIC or from the effect of virus or immune complexes on the platelets themselves. Purpura is maximal on the first day of life and usually disappears during the first weeks, though hepatosplenomegaly commonly persists.

DIC in the newborn [279a]. This condition is further considered in Chapter 29, but is mentioned here in order to contrast its clinical presentation with that of other causes of neonatal thrombocytopenia. It is seen in association with various complications of pregnancy and delivery, including premature separation of the placenta, haemolytic disease, birth asphyxia and haemorrhagic shock. Prematurity and sepsis are amongst other predisposing factors, as are the respiratory-distress syndrome and necrotizing enterocolitis. In contrast to those with immune thrombocytopenia, these infants present as acute emergencies in which hypoxia, hypothermia and shock are usually more urgent problems than the bleeding disorder itself. Prompt attention to resuscitation and to the treatment of the underlying condition take precedence over management of the DIC itself.

Post-transfusion purpura

This rare condition occurs almost exclusively in multiparous women and is transient, lasting up to six weeks.

Approximately seven days after the transfusion of blood or platelets, acute and severe thrombocytopenia develops. In most cases post-transfusion purpura is a result of an antibody response to the Pl^{A1} antigen in those who lack it [280]. The mechanism whereby the patient's own platelets are destroyed by an alloantibody directed against donor platelets has been perplexing. There is evidence that complement activation is instrumental in the lysis of the patient's platelets [280, 282]. The condition may be treated effectively by repeated plasmapheresis [283] if intervention becomes necessary. Transfusion with Pl^{A1}-negative platelets was ineffective in the one reported case of its use [284].

Drug-induced thrombocytopenia

Drugs may induce thrombocytopenia as part of the process of bone-marrow aplasia. In many cases these are predictable responses, as in cytotoxic therapy. Some drugs may also cause selective thrombocytopenia, and these are not predictable. While there is some overlap between those drugs capable of causing sporadic marrow aplasia and selective thrombocytopenia, this chapter deals primarily with the latter group; the former is considered in Chapter 31.

Drugs as a cause of thrombocytopenia are important numerically from two points of view: two recent analyses suggest that thrombocytopenia and granulocytopenia are the commonest types of blood dyscrasia due to drugs [285, 286]; and an analysis of 359 cases of thrombocytopenia reported from Sweden [287] suggested that 13% of cases were possibly, and five per cent probably, due to drugs. This association was particularly common in older age groups. The capricious nature of reporting of drug reactions means that the overall incidence is probably understated and prevalence rates are highly inaccurate; the reaction rates for particular drugs are likely to be even more misleading. A comprehensive list of drugs reported to result in thrombocytopenia is shown in Table 25.5. The table is compiled from a number of sources [286–289] as well as more recent case reports, and includes a number of drugs for which the evidence implicating the cause of thrombocytopenia is slim. Heparin (three to 30%), gold preparations (one per cent), thiazide diuretics and cinchona alkaloids appear to produce thrombocytopenia most commonly.

Pathogenesis

Drug-induced thrombocytopenia may be due to peripheral destruction of platelets or to decreased production of platelets in the bone marrow. Peripheral destruction of circulating platelets is most commonly due to an immune mechanism but occasionally platelet activation and *in-vivo* aggregation may be caused directly by a drug [290] or in association with an

Table 25.5. Drugs reported to cause thrombocytopenia

Category and name	Numbers reported		Probable mechanism	References
	(Ref. 286)	(Ref. 289)		
Cinchona alkaloids				295, 305, 362–364, 368, 369, 376, 377
quinidine	52	185+	Immune	
quinine		90+		
Anti-inflammatory and analgesic				
gold	17	250	Immune	325, 375
phenylbutazone	48	124	Impaired production	
oxyphenbutazone	47	47	Impaired production (? immune)	326, 327, 371
indomethacin	40	12		
acetylsalicylic acid	12	48	Immune	342
paracetamol (acetaminophen)		20	Immune (? to metabolite)	298
ibuprofen		4		
fenoprofen				328
penicillamine		60+		
Diuretics				
chlorothiazide		42	Immune: impaired production	288, 365, 370
hydrochlorothiazide		2	Immune	302
frusemide	20	30		286
chlorthalidone		36		
clopamide				
acetazolamide		2	Immune	286
spironolactone		3	Immune	342
ethacrynic acid		6		
Antibiotics				
sulphonamides		34	Immune	167, 330, 331
sulphamethoxazole-trimethoprim	73	160+	Immune: impaired production	322, 335
trimethoprim		25		
chloramphenicol	19	125+		332, 333
ampicillin	11	17		334
penicillin		15	? Immune, TTP	319, 320
methicillin		1		337
cephalothin		7	Immune	336
ristocetin		11	Platelet aggregation	290, 306
streptomycin		20		
tetracycline		11		
novobiocin		4	Immune	338
lincomycin		4		
Anti-tuberculous				
para-amino-salicylic acid		14	Immune (? to metabolite)	299
rifampicin	18	53	Immune	301
pyrazinamide				
isoniazid		30		
Hypoglycaemic				
chlorpropamide	11	43		339–341
tolbutamide		17		
carbutamide				

Table 25.5 (*continued*)

Category and name	Numbers reported		Probable mechanism	References
	(Ref. 286)	(Ref. 289)		
Antidepressants and tranquilizers				
desipramine		3	Immune	300
imipramine		11		
amitriptyline		10		
doxepin		1		343
meprobamate		8		
thioridazine		11		
diazepam		6+	Immune	167
ethchlorvynol		2	Immune	347
Antiepileptic				
diphenylhydantoin		22	Immune (TTP)	167, 318
sodium valproate			Immune	303, 348
carbamazepine		12	? Immune	349
Miscellaneous				
amodiaquine		2		367
antazoline		3		
apronal (Sedormid)			Immune	291–294, 297
arsenicals (organic)		55+		
barbiturates		16		
chloroquine		24		350
hydroxychloroquine		6		
diazoxide		4		351
digitoxin		5	Immune	352
ethanol		230+	Impaired production	323, 324
heparin		15		307–314
levodopa		2		353
methyldopa		25	Immune	354, 355
oestrogens		5	Impaired production	
oral contraceptives		8		321
phenindione		10		357
procainamide		5	Impaired production (immune)	342, 356, 358
propranolol		10		
pyrimethamine		90+		359
stibophen		6	Immune	360
thioguanine			Immune: impaired production	342
xylocaine				361

Non-referenced entries are from reviews of drug-induced blood dyscrasias [286, 289].

Italicized entries are comparatively poorly documented causes of thrombocytopenia.

Assumption of an immune mechanism may be premature in some cases but is based on either the rapid production of thrombocytopenia on rechallenge with the drug, the presence of *in-vitro* evidence for the presence of an antibody which is active in the presence of drug, or the demonstration of normal megakaryocytes in bone marrow.

ill-defined endothelial-cell-platelet interaction resulting in a thrombotic thrombocytopenic purpura syndrome. These mechanisms will be discussed below.

Immunological mechanism. The classical theory to explain immune drug reactions was developed by Ackroyd [291–294], originally with respect to apronal (Sedormid) thrombocytopenia. Sera of patients with 'Sedormid purpura' were found to contain an anti-platelet factor which agglutinated the patient's own platelets in the presence of the drug; furthermore, addition of apronal inhibited clot retraction in sensitive patients. In the presence of the drug and complement, the patient's plasma caused platelet lysis and the anti-platelet activity was found in the γ-globulin fraction. These findings suggested that the anti-platelet factor was an antibody. In view of the fact that the anti-platelet antibody activity required the presence of drug, Ackroyd postulated that the antigen was a hapten formed by a drug–platelet complex. In support of this mechanism, recent studies have shown a requirement for both drug and platelets to induce *in-vitro* lymphocyte transformation and synthesis of specific IgG in patients sensitive to quinine or quinidine [295]. A plasma component is also required for lymphocyte transformation in this system.

The second hypothesis to explain drug-induced platelet destruction invoked the formation of soluble immune complexes as the anti-platelet factor. Early investigations [296, 297] showed that antigen–antibody complexes were capable of absorption to rabbit platelets resulting in agglutination, destruction and resultant thrombocytopenia. Shulman [296] suggested that the hapten was a complex of drug and plasma protein which resulted in the stimulation of antibody production. The resulting antigen–antibody complex was not specifically absorbed on the platelets, but resulted in their destruction as 'innocent bystanders'.

Both mechanisms require the formation of a drug–macromolecule complex to stimulate antibody formation. In a few isolated cases strong evidence has been presented for drug metabolites being the active component of the immunogenic complex. These include cases of thrombocytopenia related to ingestion of phenacetin [298] and para-amino-salicylic acid (PAS) [299]. While clinically it has been the rule that there is no cross-reactivity between quinine- and quinidine-induced purpura and some *in-vitro* studies would support this observation, more sensitive tests suggest that some degree of cross-reactivity exists in almost all cases [295].

The antibody involved in drug-induced thrombocytopenia has usually been IgG [293, 300] but has been present in both IgG and IgM [301], IgG and IgA [298] and in IgM alone [302, 303]. The antibody titre rises rapidly to a peak about a week after ingestion [304] and falls off slowly over a period of months [304, 305]. Increased immunoglobulin may be detected on the platelet during an episode of thrombocytopenia [303].

Other mechanisms of peripheral platelet destruction. There is strong evidence that direct platelet aggregation is sometimes a cause of peripheral platelet destruction and thrombocytopenia. A classical example is that of ristocetin, the thrombocytopenia which it causes being dose-dependent and predictable [290]. The knowledge gained from studying *in-vitro* aggregation induced by ristocetin, which requires von Willebrand factor for this activity [306], makes this mechanism highly likely.

A more complex situation exists with respect to heparin-induced thrombocytopenia. It is not clear whether heparin itself or contaminants in the preparations are responsible, nor whether preparations from different sources (intestinal mucosa or lung) may cause different types of reaction. Normal numbers of megakaryocytes in the marrow suggest that the reduced platelet count is due to increased platelet consumption [307, 308]. A direct immunological mechanism for this consumption is supported by the results of *in-vitro* testing for heparin-dependent anti-platelet antibody in some patients [307–312]. Furthermore the onset of thrombocytopenia has usually been towards the end of the first treatment week or later, unless there has been previous exposure. Contrary evidence has been presented to suggest that platelet consumption during heparin therapy is due to disseminated intravascular coagulation [313, 314]. This concept is supported by reports of myocardial infarction [307], priapism [315], pulmonary emboli [316] and peripheral vascular complications [317], with and without the development of thrombocytopenia, during heparin treatment. An immune-mediated mechanism and tendency to intravascular platelet aggregation are probably not mutually exclusive.

Thrombotic thrombocytopenic purpura has occasionally been reported following or during drug administration. Such a syndrome has been described with serum sickness due to diphenylhydantoin [318] and in patients receiving penicillin [319, 320], and the haemolytic-uraemic syndrome (HUS) has been associated with oral contraceptive drugs [321].

Thrombocytopenia due to drug interference with platelet production. Drugs which regularly cause thrombocytopenia as part of generalized bone-marrow depression, and those which produce generalized marrow aplasia and pancytopenia by idiosyncratic mechanisms, are discussed in Chapter 31. While there is some overlap with these categories, a number of drugs result in selective thrombocytopenia due to interference with platelet production in the bone marrow, while in some instances thrombocytopenia is associated with neutropenia or anaemia but not total marrow aplasia. The mechanisms involved are for the most part poorly understood: thrombocytopenia associated with the use of trimethoprim and co-trimoxazole is usually due to interference with folate metabolism, but an immune mechanism may occasionally be involved [322]. The thrombocytopenia induced by ethanol may represent a defect in thrombopoiesis due to a metabolic disturbance. In this situation there are normal numbers of megakaryocytes with increased ploidy (as assessed by lobe counting) in response to the thrombocytopenia, but defective platelet production [323, 324]. With other drugs in this category the bone marrow has sometimes shown reduced megakaryocyte numbers and this has been taken as evidence for the drug-induced damage.

Clinical manifestations

The clinical expression of drug-induced thrombocytopenia was well described in 1865 [362]. The features of *immune drug thrombocytopenias* are most fully documented with quinidine and quinine. The purpura may appear at any time whilst the patient is taking the drug and this applies both to continuous or intermittent medication. Not infrequently the onset follows a small dose when there has been prior exposure some time before. It is unusual for purpura to occur after less than a week of initial exposure although it has been described after as little as five days [363]. When the thrombocytopenia develops in a sensitized individual it may appear only a few hours after ingestion of the drug. Purpura frequently develops rapidly and may be very severe, with haemorrhagic bullae in the buccal mucosa and fulminating bleeding. Constitutional symptoms, when they occur, may coincide with bleeding or may precede it by some hours. They vary considerably in severity, and may include warmth, flushing, chills, headache, fever, weakness, nausea, vomiting, abdominal pains and joint pains [364]. In other respects the manifestations are those of acute ITP (p. 988).

The thrombocytopenia produced as a result of *suppression of platelet production* may be of less dramatic onset, may produce a less severe thrombocytopenia and takes longer, perhaps two to three weeks, for the platelet count to recover. Ethanol [323, 324], oral diuretics (in particular chlorothiazide, hydrochlorothiazide and frusemide [365]), co-trimoxazole [366] and oral antidiabetic drugs [339–341] may all produce thrombocytopenia by interfering with platelet production and in many cases the thrombocytopenia may be so mild as to escape detection [365].

Diagnosis

In many cases the diagnosis is straightforward, with a clear association between the onset of purpura and the recent initiation of treatment with a drug well recognized to cause the disorder. In others, however, particularly when thrombocytopenia develops in a patient taking a number of drugs or one who has been treated with a potentially offending drug for some time, the precise association may be more difficult to establish. A careful history is required, with specific questioning about potential drugs and the possibility of self-administration of proprietary medicines, including cold cures, tonics and purgatives, which may contain quinine in association with other ingredients. Tonic water and bitter soft drinks may also contain quinine and may be responsible for so-called 'cocktail purpura' [286].

ITP may present a clinical and haematological picture which is identical, the only ingredient missing being a drug history. However, other possible external agents must also be considered, including benzene, insecticides, solvents, turpentine and other immunological causative agents such as vaccines.

Clinical investigation

Thrombocytopenia, often of considerable severity, is the predominant feature and counts below $10 \times 10^9/l$ are usual in cases due to immune mechanisms [287]. The blood picture otherwise resembles ITP although concomitant leucopenia, agranulocytosis [367, 368] or haemolytic anaemia [369] occasionally occurs. Bone-marrow examination reveals a picture identical with that in ITP. In cases in which no immune mechanism has been demonstrated, reduced numbers of megakaryocytes in the marrow have sometimes been reported [370, 371].

In-vitro tests for drug-induced antibodies. A number of methods have been developed for the detection of drug-dependent antibodies. They range from comparatively crude and insensitive tests to sophisticated techniques unlikely to be available in routine laboratories. Technical difficulties [286] include poor solubility of many drugs in appropriate buffer solutions, the presence of contaminating solvents or other vehicles for the drug and variation in reaction with differing concentrations of drug.

The earliest and the least sensitive tests are those involving clot retraction-inhibition [291] and platelet agglutination [372] in the presence of drug and serum. Evidence for platelet activation or damage by patient's serum or an immunoglobulin fraction in the presence of drug has been used for the detection of antibodies. Such techniques include platelet factor 3 (PF3) release [164, 165, 342, 373] release of ^{14}C-labelled serotonin

[374] or ^{51}Cr from pre-labelled platelets [166, 167] and also platelet aggregation induced by the drug [304]. Recently, increased lymphocyte blastogenesis and IgG synthesis in the presence of platelets and drug have been used to record the association of thrombocytopenia with gold [375] and the cinchona alkaloids [295]. Quantification of Ig or complement bound to the platelet membrane (p. 986) may prove of value in the investigation of drug purpura [376].

In routine diagnostic testing, the PF3 release [373, 374] and platelet aggregometry [304] tests combine reasonable simplicity and sensitivity and are of value in the management of this condition.

Course and prognosis

The course of drug-induced thrombocytopenia depends on the underlying mechanism. In the case of immune mechanisms [286, 364], recovery to normal platelet count is the rule within one to two weeks of stopping the drug. The major exception to this rule is with gold salts, where poor excretion results in a protracted course in many cases. Recovery of thrombocytopenia associated with toxic effects on the megakaryocyte varies according to the agent but tends to be slower. For example, thrombocytopenia due to diuretics may take two to three weeks to recover. Mortality due to selective thrombocytopenia induced by drugs is probably less than five per cent [285, 286], although mortality rates based on cases reported to drug safety committees have been reported as high as 20% [286].

Treatment

General measures with respect to the treatment of any form of thrombocytopenia apply to drug-induced cases. The rationale for the use of corticosteroids in their 'capillary-function' enhancement has been discussed on page 990 and applies equally to drug-induced thrombocytopenia. Because of the transient nature of this disorder such treatment is unlikely to be unduly prolonged and it is probably advisable to administer corticosteroids in cases with significant bleeding and low platelet counts. Prednisolone has been advocated [286] in a dosage of 1 mg/kg until clinical bleeding has ceased, with subsequent reduction over seven to 10 days.

If the platelet count remains low and the bleeding diathesis is severe despite withdrawal of the drug responsible for thrombocytopenia, platelet transfusion may have a place: both control of bleeding and a rise in the platelet count have been reported in a few cases (e.g. in association with quinidine [377] and heparin [378]). Platelet transfusion is likely to be of more value in drug-induced thrombocytopenia due to bone-marrow toxicity in which there is normal platelet survival and a more protracted recovery.

Clearly the most important aspect of treatment is the recognition and immediate withdrawal of the responsible drug. Identification is not always easy and it may be that a number of drugs are potentially causative, in which case all should be suspended if possible. Adequate explanation and warning are essential as recurrent attacks are not infrequently due to misunderstanding on the part of the patient and his medical advisers. A warning card with the appropriate information is a useful precaution [286].

Thrombocytopenia induced by other agents

Chemical and industrial agents. A number of these have been reported to cause thrombocytopenia. Benzene is implicated in a comparatively large number of cases, but this is usually associated with other marrow abnormalities and is a manifestation of aplastic anaemia. Selective thrombocytopenia has been described following exposure to the combination spray of dichlorvos and dieldrin [379] and toluene [380], and after ingestion of turpentine [381]. Poorly documented cases have been reported with other solvents, insecticides and inorganic arsenicals [289].

Anti-lymphocyte and anti-thymocyte globulin. These frequently result in thrombocytopenia and occasionally in thrombotic complications [382]. Such reactions are due to antibodies against HLA antigens common to both lymphocytes and platelets. *In-vitro* platelet aggregation is induced by anti-lymphocyte globulin and appears to be a specific reaction due to such antibodies; it is probably responsible for the *in-vivo* observations [383]. Thrombocytopenia caused by administration of anti-lymphocyte globulin is usually brief and self-limiting.

Vaccination. This occasionally results in thrombocytopenia. The commonest association appears to be with live attenuated measles vaccines. Thrombocytopenia following measles vaccine is more common in children under four years of age and the onset is usually within seven days of vaccination, with recovery over the following two to three weeks. Some patients have had decreased [384] and others increased [385, 386] numbers of megakaryocytes in the bone marrow. Rubella [195], typhoid and paratyphoid, and rarely smallpox vaccination [387] have also been implicated. As with other forms of acute thrombocytopenia the natural history is usually one of complete recovery within weeks of onset. The management of this condition is essentially that of acute ITP with bed rest, and the possible options of corticosteroid therapy and platelet transfusion.

Thrombocytopenia due to intravascular coagulation syndromes

Thrombocytopenia is a common accompaniment of a wide variety of conditions in which intravascular coagulation or intravascular platelet deposition is an integral part of the overall reaction to insult. Thrombocytopenia develops when the consumption of platelets in the circulation exceeds the replacement potential; in most instances the marrow production of platelets is probably increased to meet this demand, though in some instances associated bone-marrow toxicity may reduce the response. In the spectrum of conditions included in this section it is possible to make an artificial distinction between platelet involvement and activation of the coagulation system. In many instances of intravascular coagulation, platelets may be involved secondarily following thrombin generation, though they are not a necessary component for the development or indeed the progression of intravascular coagulation (see Chapter 29). In certain well-defined conditions, particularly thrombotic thrombocytopenic purpura (TTP) and the haemolytic-uraemic syndrome (HUS), platelet thrombus formation and platelet–endothelial cell interaction appear to be the most important aspects of involvement of haemostatic components and intravascular coagulation, when it occurs, is of only minor degree.

Disseminated intravascular coagulation (DIC)

Disorders associated with DIC are discussed more fully in Chapter 29. In general the degree of thrombocytopenia mirrors the severity of the intravascular coagulation process. In acute DIC, such as that associated with obstetric accidents of abruptio placentae and amniotic-fluid embolism, almost complete defibrination is associated with gross thrombocytopenia [388]. The platelet count, in common with coagulation factors, returns to normal within a few days following correction of the underlying abnormality; in obstetric cases this usually implies evacuation of the uterus.

In the coagulation disturbance associated with disseminated malignancy or generalized sepsis, thrombocytopenia is one of the commonest laboratory manifestations [389–391]. In most cases it is of moderate degree and parallels the coagulation defect. Platelet counts of the order of $30–100 \times 10^9/l$ are the rule, although gross thrombocytopenia sometimes occurs. The bleeding tendency is usually more severe than the thrombocytopenia alone would be expected to produce, owing to the coagulation disturbance and secondary fibrinolysis. Effective treatment of the un-derlying condition and the correction of metabolic and fluid abnormalities frequently result in improvement of coagulation defects. There is evidence [389, 390] that heparin therapy may sometimes hasten the improvement. An improvement in the platelet count commonly follows coagulation improvement by some three to four days [389] or even weeks [390]. Bone-marrow depression due to infection, drugs or metabolic changes may be instrumental in this delay. In malignant disease bone-marrow infiltration may be a major component in the production of thrombocytopenia, while in DIC complicating liver disease, hypersplenism may be an additional factor contributing to a delayed or reduced platelet response.

Viral infections

Thrombocytopenia of mild degree is probably a common occurrence during the course of viral illnesses [193]. It has been reported following vaccination, for example with attenuated live measles vaccine [384–386], and as an incidental finding in children with viral illnesses [191]. Significant thrombocytopenia has been described during the course of infectious mononucleosis [392], rubella [393] and influenza [394] in particular. The mechanism may be through damage to circulating platelets [394, 395] with consequent reduction in platelet lifespan, or to an effect on megakaryocytes [395] with impairment of platelet production [385, 396].

Giant haemangiomata (Kasabach–Merritt syndrome)

Thrombocytopenia in association with giant haemangioma was described in 1940 by Kasabach & Merritt [397]. Originally reported in infants [397–399], the condition has also been observed in adults [391]. Thrombocytopenia has also been seen in association with venous haemangioma and with the Klippel–Trenaunay syndrome [391, 399a]. The pathogenesis of the thrombocytopenia in these conditions is related to the continuous deposition of coagulation factors and platelets in the multiple vascular channels. In haemangio-endothelioma of the mouse [400] and in man a microangiopathic haemolytic anaemia has been described with shortened red-cell survival. Associated coagulation abnormalities include reduced plasma concentrations of factors I, II, V and VIII [398, 399] and reduced fibrinogen survival [391].

The syndrome may present with spontaneous purpura and bruising or as massive haemorrhage following trauma or surgery. Exacerbation of acute DIC may supervene on an otherwise chronic condition. The haemangiomata are ordinarily subcutaneous but may be elsewhere [391] (e.g. liver [400] or spleen [401]). They may subside spontaneously in infants but in adults they tend to remain static or enlarge in size [399].

Coagulation abnormalities may be corrected by systemic heparin [399], and this has been used successfully prior to surgery. Vascular tumours have been treated by X-irradiation or surgical removal.

Thrombotic thrombocytopenic purpura (TTP)
This is a rare disorder characterized by thrombocytopenia, microangiopathic haemolytic anaemia, fluctuating neurological abnormalities and renal impairment. The disease was first described in 1925 by Moschowitz [402], who interpreted the pathological lesions as thrombi in terminal arterioles and capillaries with 'fibroblasts' surrounding them. While there is still argument concerning the nature of the lesion and underlying aetiological factors, recent progress in treatment appears to have improved the outcome from that of an almost universally fatal disease. The condition is also described in Chapter 12.

Incidence. The disease may occur at any age but is particularly common among females in the second and third decades [403]. Although a rare disorder, over 340 cases had been reported by 1976 [404]. The disease appears sporadically but has been reported in siblings [405] and in marital partners [406]. It has been described in association with a wide variety of external agents, including influenza vaccination [407], combined triple antigen and TAB vaccination [408], as a possible sequel of infection with *M. pneumoniae* [404] and with drugs, in particular penicillin and diphenylhydantoin (p. 998). A similar syndrome has been described in association with systemic lupus erythematosus [409], meningococcal infection [410] and malignancy [411], and with other systemic disorders such as rheumatoid arthritis, polyarthritis and Sjögren's syndrome [412].

Pathology and pathogenesis. The underlying lesion consists of thrombotic vascular occlusions in arterioles and capillaries, particularly in the brain and kidneys, though other tissues may be involved including the heart, adrenals and spleen. Other vessels are occluded by hyaline material associated with local endothelial proliferation; similar hyaline material is also present in the subendothelium. A further feature of the vascular lesion is dilatation and cylindrical aneurysm formation at arteriolar-capillary junctions [413]. The hyaline material appears to be composed of fibrin and platelets [414, 415], but complement and immunoglobulins have also been demonstrated in the lesions [416, 417]. Plasminogen activator activity has been found to be absent in vessels affected by the TTP lesion and normal in those blood vessels not affected [416]. The morphological changes in the affected segments of blood vessel and the reduction in endothelial-cell function with respect to plasminogen activator might suggest interference in other endothelial-cell functions, in particular reduced production of prostacyclin (PGI_2). Such an hypothesis has been suggested by reports of patients lacking plasma prostacyclin-like activity during relapse [418]. The situation has been further clouded by the description of a platelet-aggregating factor in the plasma of some [419] but not all patients [420] with TTP. The platelet-aggregating factor could be reduced by incubation with normal plasma at 37°C, and clinical responses were obtained by plasma infusions in these patients [419]. It has thus been suggested that in some cases of TTP there is a deficiency of a plasma component which inhibits a platelet-aggregating factor, or which stimulates prostacyclin production in the vessel wall. The nature of such plasma components is unknown.

While the endothelial-cell proliferation and subendothelial changes have been interpreted to indicate that the primary event is vascular damage, with secondary platelet adhesion and aggregation, primary intravascular platelet agglutination is possible. The underlying cause of the lesion, be it endothelial or platelet, is still obscure and although the occasional case is associated with 'immune' disorders and immunoglobulin and complement have been discerned in the lesions, changes in serum complement and evidence for immune complexes in the circulation are lacking [421]. Despite the gross thrombocytopenia and evidence for markedly shortened platelet survival in TTP [116], changes in other coagulation components are usually mild [415, 422, 423] and fibrinogen consumption is not usually significantly increased [116]. Other manifestations of the disorder can be explained by the thrombocytopenia and small-vessel occlusion, which are responsible for widespread haemorrhage and organ dysfunction. The microangiopathic anaemia results from red-cell fragmentation due to mechanical trauma consequent on fibrin deposition, leading to premature removal from the circulation [424].

Clinical manifestations. The onset of TTP may be acute and rapidly progressive, or a prodromal period with headache, malaise and weight loss may extend over weeks or months [425]. The commonest symptoms are thrombocytopenia with purpura, bruising and other bleeding manifestations such as gastro-intestinal haemorrhage or menorrhagia. Fever is usually a feature. Neurological symptoms and signs may vary from minor episodes of confusion to the effects of focal lesions, including pareses, paraesthesiae, convulsions or coma. Though the neurological symptoms tend to fluctuate in severity, a proportion of deficits are permanent. Abdominal pain is often present; it may be mild and colicky but is occasionally severe, often with radiation to the back, so that pancreatitis or other 'acute abdomen' may be diagnosed. Symptoms of anaemia are frequently present early in the disease. Renal involvement may be suggested by haematuria or oliguria.

Clinical signs apart from purpura include conjunctival pallor and mild icterus. The spleen is commonly palpable and sometimes tender. There may be other areas of abdominal tenderness and, in severe cases, rigidity and muscular guarding. Tachycardia is present and a wide pulse pressure and systolic bruits over the heart may be evidence of anaemia. Signs of left-ventricular failure with pulmonary oedema may also be found [426].

Laboratory manifestations. Severe thrombocytopenia, microangiopathic haemolytic anaemia and renal impairment are the hallmarks of this condition. The haemoglobin is usually reduced to 6–8 g/dl and haematocrit to 20–30%. The platelet count is almost invariably below $20 \times 10^9/l$ and usually less than $10 \times 10^9/l$. There is frequently a leucocytosis of $15-25 \times 10^9/l$. The blood film shows grossly reduced platelet numbers and marked fragmentation of the red cells with schistocytes and burr cells. The red-cell fragments may result in erroneously high platelet counts when electronic particle counters are employed [404]. Polychromasia and sometimes nucleated red cells are present. The reticulocyte count is raised, often to five to 30%. A neutrophil leucocytosis and toxic granulation are often present. Bone-marrow aspiration reveals an active marrow with evidence of increased production of all cell lines.

Coagulation studies are often mildly abnormal but it is rare to find evidence of marked intravascular coagulation [422, 423]. The usual abnormalities are a mild increase in serum fibrin degradation products (FDP) and some evidence of activation of the coagulation system, with positive paracoagulation tests or shortening of the partial thromboplastin time. The platelet-survival time may be grossly shortened but fibrinogen survival has been found normal [116].

Serum biochemistry affords evidence of intravascular haemolysis and renal impairment. The bilirubin may be two to three times the normal value, and raised plasma haemoglobin, positive tests for methaemalbumin, increase in lactic dehydrogenase and absent haptoglobins are the rule. The blood urea and serum creatinine and sometimes the serum uric acid are raised, the degree of renal dysfunction varying considerably from case to case. The severity of the renal lesion is also indicated by the presence of proteinuria, which may be of the order of several grams per 24

hours. Casts and red cells in the urine are further evidence of renal involvement.

Tests for evidence of immune involvement, including the antiglobulin test, antinuclear factor, LE cells, complement levels and immune complex assays, are routinely unhelpful. Occasionally the antiglobulin test has been reported positive [404, 425], with weak reaction to components of complement [404].

Radiological changes with diffuse alveolar infiltrates and pulmonary dysfunction with arterial hypoxaemia and reduced compliance have recently been reported as a common finding [426]. Tissue biopsy, while not universally positive, may reveal the characteristic occluding hyaline microthrombi. Bone marrow [427], lymph node [428], gingiva [429], skin and kidney [425] have been the usual biopsy sites.

Diagnosis. The clinical features of anaemia, purpura, fever and fluctuating neurological symptoms and signs are highly suggestive of TTP. Icterus and splenomegaly are frequently present and strengthen the clinical diagnosis. The major laboratory findings of microangiopathic changes on the blood film with evidence of severe haemolysis and thrombocytopenia in addition to the characteristic urinary changes and renal impairment are the major pointers to the diagnosis of TTP. Demonstration of the TTP vascular lesion by skin biopsy or gingival biopsy is of value in making a definitive diagnosis.

A fine line divides the classification of TTP from HUS in the adult. The presence of neurological manifestations, more severe thrombocytopenia and haemorrhagic manifestations are more in keeping with the diagnosis of TTP, while the predominance of renal failure and hypertension is more in keeping with the clinical diagnosis of HUS. In particular, a syndrome developing post partum or in women taking oral contraceptives (p. 1005) tends to fit the description of HUS.

Other neurological disorders may be diagnosed mistakenly, in particular vascular accidents and cerebral tumour. Abdominal symptoms may be initially diagnosed as pancreatitis, cholecystitis, appendicitis and other acute surgical emergencies and laparotomy has been mistakenly performed in TTP. The presence of fever and other manifestations of TTP should alert the clinician to this possibility.

Difficulty may arise in differentiating TTP from DIC, but the comparatively normal coagulation results in the face of severe thrombocytopenia and purpura make the diagnosis of DIC unlikely. Similarly, thrombocytopenia due to other causes, in particular ITP, may be confused with TTP, though the clinical features, the presence of microangiopathic haemolysis and renal impairment should serve to exclude them.

Course and prognosis. Of 116 cases of TTP reviewed in 1959 [425], all but four died, 98 succumbing to a rapid febrile illness within weeks. In a few cases the illness, though fatal, lasted over three months and the longest survival was 16 years. The immediate outlook has been improved by the introduction of a number of both empirical and semi-specific means of treatment, but recurrence, often fatal, is unfortunately still common. Death may be due to intracerebral haemorrhage, renal failure, cardiac failure or respiratory insufficiency.

Treatment. The treatment of TTP has passed through a number of fashions, some based on empiricism, some on hypotheses of causation, while others were suggested by chance observation. The comparatively unsatisfactory nature of many of the treatments proposed is indicated by the rapidity with which fashions have swung from one to another. Problems in assessing the value of any given therapy relate to the rarity of the condition, its heterogeneous nature, the tendency to recur and the vagaries of medical reporting. In many instances where one form of therapy was claimed effective, other treatments had been given previously or were being administered concurrently.

Anti-coagulation with heparin was one of the earliest forms of treatment used and has subsequently been used in combination with other therapy. As recent evidence suggests a comparatively minor coagulation component in this disorder, heparin has largely been replaced by anti-platelet agents. In the intervening period, treatment with massive doses of corticosteroids with or without splenectomy has had a vogue. A combination of steroids and splenectomy was reported to result in comparatively long-term remissions in 39 cases reviewed in 1976 [404]. In some of these cases other agents were used, namely heparin, dextran and combinations of anti-platelet agents. Anti-platelet therapy was used first in 1970 [430]: dextran [423], aspirin and dipyridamole [430, 431] and sulphinpyrazone [432] have all been used and the timing of response has favoured a beneficial effect.

Exchange transfusion [433], plasma exchange [403] and intensive plasmapheresis [434, 435] have been reported to result in dramatic improvement of both clinical and laboratory abnormalities in TTP. In the small series of patients reported, remission rates were from 60% [403] to 80% [435]. It was originally assumed that these procedures removed immune complexes. Recently, however [419, 436], three patients with TTP have been treated with simple infusions of normal plasma with abrupt reversal of the disease process, suggesting the correction of a deficiency. Fresh frozen and outdated plasma and plasma from which cryoprecipitate had been removed were successful in the treatment of at least one of these cases. This treatment is not universally successful [420]. Plasmapheresis has been repeated at intervals of 12–24 hours initially and subsequently every two to three days. Plasma infusion has been given daily at doses of between three and 10 donor units and in successful cases has resulted in remission over a period of several days, but with a continuing requirement, often for some weeks [419].

Controlled trials of treatment in this uncommon but serious disorder are unlikely ever to be feasible. Combined treatment with high-dose corticosteroid, anti-platelet therapy such as sulphinpyrazone, aspirin or dipyridamole and immediate plasma exchange would seem to be the most appropriate management. Following a useful response, withdrawal of one or more forms of therapy may then be cautiously undertaken. In the face of lack of response with the above treatment, splenectomy should be carried out. A continued follow-up is essential, as recurrence following complete remission is common even months or years later.

Haemolytic-uraemic syndrome (HUS)

In 1955 Gasser *et al.* [437] described an illness in five children characterized by acute renal failure, thrombocytopenia and haemolytic anaemia. The disorder has many features akin to TTP, particularly in adults, but in children HUS presents such a characteristic picture that it is classified as a separate entity. Because of the involvement of both red cells and platelets, it is described below as well as in Chapter 12.

Incidence. In childhood the age of onset is generally before the age of four, though hardly ever before three months; the sexes are equally affected [438]. The disease tends to occur either sporadically or in microepidemics, with a peak incidence in late summer. In certain areas, notably Argentina and South Africa, it seems to be endemic. The disease is uncommon in adults and may be associated with a number of unrelated disorders (see below). In many instances the distinction between HUS and TTP may be conjectural. Familial occurrence of HUS has been reported [439, 440]: sibs may be affected together or at different times, the latter event being associated with a worse prognosis.

Aetiological factors. A number of aetiological factors associated with its development suggest that HUS is a broad syndrome manifested by a final common pathology. The disorder commonly follows an infectious process, usually with a prodrome of vomiting and diarrhoea. Both viral infections such as Coxsackie, influenza, ECHO, mumps and myxovirus [441–443] and bacterial infections particularly with Shigella [444], but also with *Salmonella typhi, E. coli* and bacteroides [445, 446], have been implicated. Such associations are strengthened by reports of epidemics. Vaccination against poliomyelitis, smallpox or measles may also be a precipitating factor. Numerous cases have occurred following a normal pregnancy [447, 448] and in association with the use of oral contraceptives. Further sporadic cases have been reported following renal transplantation and in association with SLE and malignancy.

Pathogenesis. The primary injury in HUS involves the endothelial cells of glomerular capillaries with the production of a distinctive glomerulitis [449]. In common with TTP, however, an initial platelet activation cannot be totally excluded. The frequent association of HUS with infection and the documented relation with circulating endotoxin [444] support the notion that a bacterial product produces the endothelial damage [256, 261]. The clinical associations are supported by the similarity of the endotoxin-mediated, experimental Shwartzman reaction to HUS [450].

In the absence of an infective cause, immunological factors have been implicated, as in the case of TTP. Similar deposits of IgM, complement components and occasional IgG have been observed in the lesions obtained by renal biopsy [451, 452] and hypocomplementaemia has been reported [452, 453]. The association of HUS with pregnancy and oral contraceptives is difficult to explain on this basis and suggests a platelet or coagulation-initiated disorder with secondary endothelial damage.

It has been suggested [453a] that the intravascular deposition of platelets results from a defect of prostacyclin (PGI$_2$) production by the vessel wall, and that this in turn is due to deficiency of a plasma factor which stimulates PGI$_2$ synthesis. The demonstration of such a deficiency in a patient with HUS and two of her children [453b, 453c] provides a possible explanation of familial predisposition to the disease.

The renal failure of HUS is related to small-vessel occlusion and glomerular subendothelial deposits. If the latter predominate, recovery is faster and more complete than when small arterioles are involved. Thrombocytopenia is due to reduced platelet survival [454] but while adhesion of platelets to glomerular basement membrane may occur, ^{51}Cr-labelled platelets appear to be sequestered in liver and spleen [454] rather than the kidney. Anaemia is presumably due to mechanical fragmentation of red cells by roughened and narrowed small vessels.

Clinical manifestations. The onset in children is sudden, usually following a mild non-specific gastroenteritis or less commonly an upper-respiratory-tract infection. After seven to 10 days the acute illness develops, with malaise, pallor, clinical bleeding (usually skin purpura) and oliguria [438, 455, 456]. Occasionally neurological abnormalities occur. In adults the disease may be complicated by an associated condition (e.g. malignancy or SLE). In HUS developing post partum or in association with oral contraceptive use, the disease may either be acute and sudden or develop insidiously over a period of a few weeks.

The major signs on physical examination include lethargy, conjunctival pallor, tachycardia and a hyperdynamic circulation. Purpura occurs in 30–40% of patients and hypertension is commonly present, with signs of circulatory overloading with oedema, or less commonly dehydration [321, 438, 455, 456]. Fever may be present and hypertensive encephalopathy may develop. Oliguria is almost universal and anuria may occur in up to one-third of cases [321, 455, 456].

Laboratory findings. Anaemia (Hb 4–10 g/dl) and a reticulocytosis of two to 20% are commonly found. The platelet count is almost invariably below 100×10^9/l but usually not as grossly reduced as in TTP. Fibrinogen degradation products (FDP) are raised, but there is seldom evidence of significant consumption of clotting factors: fibrinogen and factors V and VIII are more often raised than reduced. The leucocyte count is commonly raised and there may be a leukaemoid picture. There is red-cell fragmentation with schistocytes and burr cells, and as in TTP, red-cell fragments may produce falsely high platelet counts when electronic particle counters are used. Serum biochemistry reveals evidence of haemolysis and severe renal failure, with markedly raised blood urea and serum creatinine. Proteinuria, haematuria and urinary casts are present.

Course and prognosis. The course of the disease is variable, but the prognosis appears to be worse in adults than in children. In children, older age and an insidious onset, without antecedent diarrhoea, are adverse features. A good correlation has been reported between the severity of renal changes and the ultimate prognosis [457]. In general, prolonged anuria or oliguria and persistent hypertension are suggestive of poor prognosis. Recovery usually begins within two to three weeks but renal function may continue to improve for up to 18 months. In patients whose renal function remains impaired, hypertension and cardiac failure may supervene, and this group has a comparatively poor prognosis. Before the modern management of acute renal failure the mortality was as high as 40%, but it has now fallen to five to 10% [456]. In a few patients, recurrent episodes of the syndrome have occurred over periods of three months to 20 years [458].

Treatment. A major component of the management of HUS is careful fluid and electrolyte balance, control of blood pressure and correction of metabolic problems, particularly acidosis. In more severely affected children peritoneal dialysis may be employed; haemodialysis is more commonly used in adults. The use of anticoagulants [459] is controversial. Steroids [460], fibrinolytic therapy [461, 462] and anti-platelet agents [463, 464] have been advocated, but the results of these forms of therapy are equally difficult to assess. More recently, plasma exchange, or even simple plasma infusions, have been claimed to produce remissions, perhaps by stimulating PGI_2 production. If transfusion is undertaken, great care must be taken to avoid circulatory overloading: it is best to establish dialysis first.

Thrombocytopenia in association with splenomegaly
The splenic platelet pool is discussed on page 982 and in Chapter 20. Splenomegaly of any degree results in enlargement of the pool and is frequently associated with thrombocytopenia. It is unusual, however, for splenomegaly alone to account for thrombocytopenia severe enough to cause major haemorrhagic problems. Common causes of thrombocytopenia due to hypersplenism include liver disease, myeloproliferative disorders, malignant lymphoma, chronic leukaemias, chronic malaria and kala-azar, thalassaemia major and Gaucher's disease.

Liver disease
Thrombocytopenia is probably the commonest platelet abnormality in liver disease, platelet counts of $70–100 \times 10^9/l$ being usual in hepatic cirrhosis. Abnormal platelet function (see Chapter 26) may also contribute to haemostatic failure, as may coagulation disorders (see Chapter 29). While splenomegaly due to portal hypertension is the commonest cause of thrombocytopenia in such patients, chronic DIC with intermittent exacerbations may complicate the course of cirrhosis, leading to further reduction of the platelet count to potentially dangerous levels. The direct toxic effect of ethanol on the bone marrow is a further cause of thrombocytopenia in alcoholic patients, whose platelet counts often rise after admission to hospital as a result of withdrawal of alcohol.

Mild thrombocytopenia has been described in Wilson's disease [465], sometimes in association with defects of platelet aggregation *in vitro*.

Malignant lymphomas
Thrombocytopenia in these diseases may have numerous causes, including bone-marrow involvement, cytotoxic chemotherapy and immune mechanisms (p. 993) as well as hypersplenism. In the presence of widespread disease or sepsis, DIC may also contribute to the haemostatic defects. Differentiation of the contributions of these various factors may be a complex problem, requiring assessment of bone marrow, full coagulation studies, a search for anti-platelet antibodies (p. 986) and possibly platelet-survival studies with surface scanning for hepatic and splenic sequestration.

Chronic myeloid leukaemia (CML) and myeloproliferative disorders
Thrombocytopenia in these disorders is multifactorial. When the spleen becomes significantly enlarged, hypersplenism may assume a prominent role. Splenectomy has been advocated in the routine management of CML, partly as prophylaxis against cytopenia later in the disease [466], but the dangers of thrombocytosis and other postsplenectomy morbidity have prevented its general adoption.

Other diseases
Thrombocytopenia may result from hypersplenism in various other diseases characterized by splenomegaly (see Chapter 20), and splenectomy may be indicated for this complication. Thrombocytopenia is also described as an early sign of vinyl-chloride disease [467], in which it is suggested that besides splenomegaly there are structural changes in red-pulp cords, affecting the splenic microcirculation and causing increased pooling and destruction of platelets. Similar qualitative changes in splenic tissue may be responsible for variable degrees of splenic pooling in other disorders.

Thrombocytopenia due to dilution or loss of platelets

Transfusion-induced thrombocytopenia
Blood transfusion may cause thrombocytopenia. The rare immune-mediated post-transfusion thrombocytopenia is described on page 995. Thrombocytopenia may also develop *during* blood transfusion, usually in the face of massive replacement of 50% or more of the patient's blood volume. Coagulation deficiencies in general are common and can be at least partly attributed directly to dilution. The loss of platelets and clotting factors is often greater than can be accounted for by simple dilution [468], however, and may also be related to consumption at the site of haemorrhage; gross thrombocytopenia occasionally results. Red-cell breakdown products and activated clotting factors in stored blood may also induce a degree of DIC

responsible for further consumption. Impairment of platelet function has also been described in association with massive transfusion [469, 470].

In practice, dilutional thrombocytopenia is a usual accompaniment of massive transfusion, but the platelet count seldom falls below $50 \times 10^9/l$, which is usually adequate for haemostasis. When severe thrombocytopenia (less than $50 \times 10^9/l$) results from massive blood transfusion, fresh platelet concentrates are probably indicated.

Extracorporeal circulations

Passage of blood through extracorporeal circulations results in platelet adherence to foreign surfaces and activation of coagulation unless specific measures are taken to prevent this. Specific surface-reactive groups, surface charge and texture, in addition to absorbed plasma protein [471–473], all influence the behaviour of platelets and coagulation proteins, and further effects are due to blood pooling and gas-fluid interfaces in oxygenators. The haemostatic changes induced are complex and include those due to anti-coagulation, DIC, excessive fibrinolysis, dilutional effects of transfusion, hypocalcaemia and platelet abnormalities. The contribution of these various factors may vary from case to case, but the platelet abnormality includes functional defects [474, 475] as well as thrombocytopenia. These are probably related to thromboxane production [476] and granule content release [144, 476]. The infusion of prostacyclin (PGI$_2$) has already met with some success in preventing the development of thrombocytopenia associated with extracorporeal circulations [477, 478]. By further reducing the problems associated with platelet activation and thrombocytopenia, its use opens the way to the possibility of long-term cardiopulmonary bypass in the treatment of respiratory failure.

During *cardiopulmonary bypass* the degree of thrombocytopenia is variable: in earlier reported series, platelet counts fell to 33% of their pre-operative value [479] or even lower, but with technical improvements the degree of thrombocytopenia is comparatively mild [480, 481]. Thrombocytopenia develops within the first few minutes of bypass and this is followed by a slower progressive fall after an hour, the platelet count dropping by as much as 50% of the initial value [482, 483]. The platelet count tends to fall by a further 10% after heparin neutralization by protamine sulphate, and there may be a subsequent reduction over two to three days post-operatively [484], with increase to preoperative levels by the sixth to eighth days. Frequently there is a 'rebound' thrombocytosis maximal between the ninth and 13th days. Although thrombocytopenia is usual, excessive bleeding is uncommon unless it is associated with coagulation defects.

Management. In the comparatively small proportion of patients who develop a significant haemorrhagic diathesis, particularly following lengthy bypass, transfusion of platelet concentrates following neutralization of heparin is appropriate. Coagulation abnormalities should also be investigated and corrected.

Thrombocytopenia associated with thrombocytapheresis

Following leucapheresis and thrombocytapheresis by either continuous or discontinuous flow cell separation, a transient reduction in platelet count and coagulation factors may occur [485, 486]. With daily consecutive thrombocytapheresis, platelet production is stimulated and significant thrombocytopenia does not occur [324, 486].

Thrombocytopenia due to impaired platelet production

Thrombocytopenia is common in disorders affecting the bone marrow (Table 25.6). The major features are fully covered in other chapters but certain selected aspects with respect to thrombocytopenia and its diagnosis are considered below.

Aplastic anaemia (see Chapter 31)

Thrombocytopenia may be the major component in cases of aplastic anaemia, and occasionally predates the development of anaemia and agranulocytosis by some weeks [487]. In such cases the bone marrow may temporarily present the appearance of megakaryocytic aplasia alone; pure megakaryocytic aplasia is otherwise a very rare condition, which may be acquired as a manifestation of immune disorders [488, 489] or inherited in the syndrome of thrombocytopenia with absent radii (TAR) (p. 1009).

A haemorrhagic tendency is the most frequent presenting symptom of aplastic anaemia, and thrombocytopenia is almost always found at diagnosis [490]. It may be comparatively mild, with a platelet count of $20–80 \times 10^9/l$, or very severe, in which case it is a common cause of death: in a series of 101 cases of drug-induced aplastic anaemia [487], haemorrhage was responsible for 22 deaths though neither the initial nor the lowest platelet count in the course of the disease correlated with a fatal outcome in the group as a whole. Others have found the platelet count to be of prognostic value [490]. During the recovery of aplastic anaemia, thrombocytopenia is usually the last element to show improvement and a low platelet count is the commonest abnormality to persist [487], sometimes for years.

Table 25.6. Thrombocytopenia due to impaired platelet production

Aplastic anaemia
    Idiopathic
    Drug-induced
    Ionizing radiation
Megakaryocytic aplasia
    Idiopathic
    Associated with immune disorders (SLE, red-cell aplasia)
    Congenital (with absent radii)
Paroxysmal nocturnal haemoglobinuria
Megaloblastic anaemia
    Vitamin-B_{12} deficiency
    Folate deficiency
    Folate antagonists
Refractory anaemia
    Dyserythropoiesis (pre-leukaemia)
Marrow infiltration
    Carcinoma
    Lymphoma
    Myeloma
    Leukaemia
    Myelofibrosis
Infections
    Virus
    Dengue
Drugs
    Ethanol
    Thiazides
Hereditary thrombocytopenias
    Wiskott–Aldrich syndrome
    May–Hegglin anomaly
    (Thrombocytopenia with absent radii)

Paroxysmal noctural haemoglobinuria (PNH)
(see Chapter 12)
The platelet count in PNH is normal or reduced and in patients with marrow hypoplasia may be very low: Dacie [491] has commented that thrombocytopenia may dominate the clinical picture. In Dacie's series, 35 out of 43 patients had a platelet count of less than $150 \times 10^9/l$, 17 less than $50 \times 10^9/l$ and nine less than $20 \times 10^9/l$ at some time during clinical observation. It is not certain whether impaired platelet production is wholly responsible for the thrombocytopenia [492]; the thrombotic tendency in many patients with PNH, coupled with the demonstration of 'hypersensitivity' of platelets in one such a patient [493], suggest that in some instances intravascular coagulation may be a contributory factor.

Thrombocytopenia in acute leukaemias
Before the introduction of improved chemotherapy and sophisticated support with platelet transfusions,

haemorrhage accounted for approximately two-thirds of deaths in acute leukaemia [494]. While improved treatment has reduced this overall figure, haemorrhage remains a significant problem during remission induction and was the direct cause of 17% of early deaths in a recent series of patients [495]. The major sites of bleeding in a series of 222 cases of fatal haemorrhage [496] were pulmonary (33%), intracranial (27%) and gastro-intestinal (25·5%). Non-fatal bleeding is commonly into the skin, mucous membranes and retina [497].

The haemorrhagic defect in acute leukaemia is complex and contributing factors are DIC, fibrinolysis and leucostasis as well as thrombocytopenia. In addition to reduced numbers of platelets, abnormal *in-vitro* platelet function has been reported [498], as evidenced by prolonged bleeding time in the presence of a normal platelet count [499]. Morphological abnormalities are well recognized [500]. The underlying natural history may be complicated by platelet functional defects in association with chemotherapy and antibiotic usage (see Chapters 22 and 26). The management of thrombocytopenia in acute leukaemias rests very much on the use of both prophylactic and therapeutic platelet transfusion (p. 1010).

Thrombocytopenia and platelet abnormalities may develop as the major manifestation of the pre-leukaemic syndromes or indolent leukaemias [501, 502]. The diagnosis and classification of such conditions is outlined in detail in Chapter 22.

Thrombocytopenia in chronic leukaemias
During the course of chronic granulocytic leukaemia there is a tendency for a progressive drop in platelet count [503]. This is a function of leukaemic proliferation, toxic effects of therapy and also hypersplenism; early splenectomy may reduce this tendency (see p. 1006). The rapid onset of thrombocytopenia may herald the onset of blast crisis or 'transformation'. This is associated with a decrease in the number of megakaryocytes in the marrow and the appearance of more immature megakaryoblasts and promegakaryocytes. A haemorrhagic tendency in chronic granulocytic leukaemia (CGL) may also relate to dysfunction of platelets [504] (see Chapter 26) and occasionally to coagulation and fibrinolytic abnormalities. The thrombocytopenia of chronic lymphocytic leukaemia is discussed on page 993.

Hereditary thrombocytopenia
Thrombocytopenia forms part of certain well-recognized though uncommon hereditary syndromes, and also occasionally occurs as an isolated hereditary abnormality. In the latter case especially, it may be difficult to distinguish on clinical grounds from chronic

ITP; this distinction is obviously important in relation to both treatment and prognosis.

Bernard–Soulier syndrome

This disorder is discussed fully in Chapter 26. Though some degree of thrombocytopenia is usually present, the predominating feature is the functional platelet abnormality.

Wiskott–Aldrich syndrome

This is a sex-linked recessive disorder characterized by recurrent infections, eczema and thrombocytopenia. The susceptibility to infection is due to a complex disorder of both cellular and humoral immune mechanisms, which is discussed in Chapter 18. The haemorrhagic effects are usually seen first: purpura and rectal haemorrhage often occur in the neonatal period. Eczema commonly appears in infancy, but infections may not become a serious problem until later. Thrombocytopenia in a male infant should therefore always raise the suspicion of the Wiskott–Aldrich syndrome, and prompt a search for clinical and laboratory evidence of immunodeficiency. The condition is usually fatal during childhood, chiefly as a result of infection, though deaths from intracranial or gastro-intestinal haemorrhage also occur. There is also an increased incidence of lymphoreticular malignancy [505].

The thrombocytopenia has been ascribed to both ineffective platelet production [506] and shortened platelet survival [507, 508] and the platelets are distinguished by their small mean size [506, 507]. Electronic particle sizing is required to demonstrate the reduction in size of platelets, a blood smear being inadequate for this purpose. Defective function, including reduced aggregation *in vitro* and storage-pool deficiency [508, 509], may contribute to the haemorrhagic tendency. The bone marrow usually contains normal or increased numbers of megakaryocytes, and does not distinguish the condition clearly from others, such as ITP, in which thrombocytopenia is due chiefly to diminished platelet survival.

Management. For boys with compatible sibling donors, tissue-matched bone-marrow transplantation would seem to be the treatment of choice: it has been effective in correcting the immune deficiency in one case [510] and the thrombocytopenia as well in others [511, 512]. Moderately encouraging results have been claimed for treatment with transfer factor, including not only improvement in the eczema and diminution in infections, but a reduction in bleeding symptoms [513, 514]. Thymus transplantation plus transfer factor was ineffective in two cases, however [515]. Despite the obviously increased post-operative risk of sepsis [516],

splenectomy has proved a useful means of correcting the thrombocytopenia: in a recent series of 16 patients [517] the platelet count rose above $100 \times 10^9/l$ after the operation in every case, and serious infections could be successfully prevented by means of prophylactic antibiotics for periods up to 16 years. The platelet size also reverted to normal after splenectomy, suggesting that the small size of Wiskott–Aldrich platelets is due to a splenic effect rather than a defect of production. Platelet survival and function were also found to be normal after splenectomy [517].

May–Hegglin anomaly

The May–Hegglin anomaly is a rare autosomal-dominant trait, less than 30 families having been reported [500], characterized by giant platelets [518] in association with basophilic inclusions not unlike Döhle bodies in the granulocytes [519]. The platelet count may be normal, mildly reduced or fluctuating, but is seldom so low as to cause serious bleeding. Platelet ultrastructure appears to be comparatively normal despite the greatly increased size (up to 20 μm in length) [509], but an increase in the number of giant granules has been reported [520]. Platelet function studies have usually been normal, although defective pseudopod formation and lack of platelet spreading have been observed [509]. Platelet survival is probably within normal limits [521]. The clinical presentation is frequently as an incidental finding on blood examination, though occasional patients have a significant bleeding tendency [522, 523].

Thrombocytopenia with absent radii (TAR)

This is an autosomal-recessive disorder. The underlying haematological abnormality is an absence or decrease in the number of bone-marrow megakaryocytes, the other cell series being unaffected. In some cases the megakaryocytes appear immature [524]. Thrombocytopenia is a constant finding, though variable in degree [524]. Early reports suggested normal platelet survival and function, but storage-pool deficiency has been observed in some cases [525, 526]. All patients have the typical bilateral absence of the radii and about one-third also have congenital cardiac defects [524]; various other skeletal abnormalities have also been observed.

Typical thrombocytopenic bleeding usually starts in the first weeks of life, and almost all patients have clinical bleeding before the age of four months [524]. The bleeding tendency is severe from the onset: almost half of a series of 40 patients died in infancy, often of intracranial haemorrhage [524]. After the first year of life, however, the clinical severity tends to ameliorate, and the platelet count to rise somewhat. Platelet transfusions are effective interim measures but unfortunately splenectomy and corticosteroids are of no therapeutic benefit [516].

Hereditary thrombocytopenia resembling ITP

This condition may be transmitted as an autosomal-dominant [527] or rarely as an autosomal-recessive trait [507]. The defect appears to be intrinsic to the patient's platelets, as megakaryocytes are present in normal or increased numbers in the bone marrow [527]; platelet survival has been reported as short in some cases [516] and normal in others [527]. In patients with shortened platelet survival the lifespan of infused normal platelets is not reduced [507]. Differentiation from ITP is sometimes difficult but is of practical importance. An early onset (in the first year of life) and a family history are clinical indications, while a negative anti-platelet antibody test in serum and more specifically normal platelet-bound Ig (p. 986) are aids in excluding ITP. The survival of labelled normal platelets will be found to be normal [507], in sharp contrast to ITP. *In-vitro* platelet function studies have been reported normal in many cases [516], but abnormal aggregation observed in others [507, 528]. Corticosteroids are not indicated, but splenectomy may result in partial correction of thrombocytopenia [516] and platelet transfusion is effective in the treatment of emergency bleeding.

Hereditary hypogranular thrombocytopenia

This disorder, one of extreme rarity, appears to be transmitted as an autosomal dominant. Families have been reported from a number of countries [529–531] with thrombocytopenia of moderate degree associated with reduced numbers of granules. Ultrastructural defects [529, 531] were associated with abnormal aggregation with collagen and ADP but a normal response to thrombin and ristocetin [531]. The condition, which results in a haemorrhagic tendency of variable severity, is probably the same as that described as the 'gray platelet syndrome' (Chapter 26, p. 1050).

Epstein's syndrome

This is an autosomal-dominant trait in which thrombocytopenia and macrothrombocytosis are combined with Alport's syndrome of hereditary nephritis and deafness [532, 533] (Chapter 26, p. 1050).

Platelet transfusion

In general, the severity of haemorrhagic symptoms, like the bleeding time, correlates fairly closely with the platelet count in the circulating blood. In some cases, however, platelet functional defects or associated coagulation changes alter this relationship and the platelet count is no longer a reliable guide to the haemostatic defect. Such factors must be taken into account when considering platelet transfusion in the management of thrombocytopenia.

Practical aspects of management

The available methods for preparing platelet-rich plasma and platelet concentrates are fully reviewed in Chapter 35. The source of platelet concentrates is frequently dictated by availability from local blood banks. In general, when repeated transfusion is unlikely to be necessary, as in thrombocytopenia associated with massive transfusion, cardiac bypass, DIC and other emergencies, platelet concentrates are derived from random blood donations. A similar approach may be used in the case of patients likely to be thrombocytopenic only transiently during the treatment of acute leukaemia.

The alternative is single-donor transfusions from an appropriate donor, frequently a relative, from whom the platelets are obtained by thrombocytapheresis [485, 486]. A refractory state due to antibody formation to random donor platelets or those of non-HLA-compatible siblings develops over a period of 10 days to three months [534, 535]. While the refractory state relates chiefly to the HLA system, other platelet antigens are clearly important, since isoimmunization may occur against platelets apparently fully compatible with respect to antigens of the HLA A and B series [535]. The development of a refractory state is evidenced by a failure to increase the circulating platelet count or lower the bleeding time by platelet transfusion, though this may be related to other factors (Table 25.7). Tests for assessing the suitability of

Table 25.7. Factors resulting in a poor response to platelet transfusion

Collection and storage
    Storage methods (anticoagulant, volume, pH, etc.)
    Temperature
    Duration of storage

Immune destruction
    Iso-antibodies (maternal, multiple transfusion)
    Auto-antibody (ITP, drug)

Intravascular utilization
    Disseminated intravascular coagulation
    Thrombotic thrombocytopenic purpura
    Massive haemorrhage

Splenic pooling

Infection

Fever

Induction of functional defect
    Uraemia, dysproteinaemia
    Drug

prospective donors include platelet aggregometry [535] and serotonin release [536], using the patient's serum and the prospective donor's citrated platelet-rich plasma; if patients become refractory a further search can be made among siblings for compatible donors. Centralized identification of potentially compatible, unrelated donors is desirable but costly.

A further sophistication, at present available only in a few units, is the storage at −120°C of autologous platelets collected during remission phases of acute leukaemia, for subsequent reinfusion [537]. This technique clearly circumvents some of the problems of recurrent platelet transfusion.

Administration

In the presence of active bleeding, 6 u/m² should be given [538]; with minor bleeding and for prophylaxis 3–4 u/m² is adequate. At about 10^{11} platelets/unit of platelet concentrate this implies the transfusion of approximately $4–8 \times 10^{11}$ platelets. Shortening of the bleeding time would be an ideal method of assessing response [538], but platelet counts one and 24 hours after transfusion provide a good indication: an increment at one hour of $10–20 \times 10^9/l/m^2$ is expected for each unit of platelet concentrate, and ideally 85–90% of this increment should remain after 24 hours [538]. An immediate increment of less than $8 \times 10^9/l/u/m^2$ or less than $5 \times 10^9/l/u/m^2$ after 24 hours has been suggested as an arbitrary limit to indicate failure [538]. Common reasons for a poor response are excessive utilization due to the presence of DIC, fever or infection, inadequate platelet preparation, splenic pooling or the development of isoimmune antibodies. A poor clinical result with continuing haemorrhage may suggest one of the above, but complicating factors such as associated coagulation disorders or the administration of drugs likely to affect platelet function may also be operative.

Adverse effects and precautions

As with other blood components, patients may develop chills and fever, particularly following multiple transfusions. This presumably indicates a reaction to contaminating granulocytes. With stored concentrates, however, bacterial contamination should be considered [539], particularly if storage is above 4°C. A further major disadvantage of random-donor platelet transfusion is the increased risk of hepatitis due to exposure to a comparatively large number of donors. Platelet transfusion in patients with DIC or TTP may result in a worsening of the coagulation disturbance, and concomitant treatment of the underlying coagulation disturbance should therefore be given.

The development of a refractory state, particularly in aplastic anaemia but also in acute leukaemia, is

discussed above and necessary precautions outlined. Besides resulting in chills and fever and a disappointing rise in the platelet count, incompatible platelet transfusions may produce granulocytopenia [540]; the mechanism of this is unclear. In the face of impaired marrow reserve such granulocytopenia may persist for days and be seriously detrimental.

ABO and Rh incompatibility have not been regarded as particularly important in platelet transfusion therapy, though a mildly reduced *in-vivo* recovery may result. While platelets from Rh-positive donors may stimulate antibody formation in Rh-negative recipients, this is usually of no great import [541]. Immunization may be prevented by the prophylactic administration of anti-D γ globulin.

Indications

Indications for platelet transfusion are shown in Table 25.8. Patients with active thrombocytopenic bleeding, particularly when it is due to inadequate platelet production, are clearly likely to benefit. Platelet transfusion has also proved invaluable as prophylactic support during transient periods of thrombocytopenia, the prime examples being during remission induction in acute leukaemia, following cytotoxic therapy for other tumours, and during bone-marrow

Table 25.8. Indications for platelet transfusion

---

1 Definite indications

Treatment of bleeding episodes in:
  Acute leukaemia
  Aplastic anaemia
  Drug-induced thrombocytopenia due to marrow suppression
  Platelet functional disorders (e.g. thrombasthenia)
  Hereditary thrombocytopenias
  Thrombocytopenia due to:
    massive transfusion
    extracorporeal circulation
  Iso-immune neonatal thrombocytopenia

Prophylaxis
  During cytotoxic therapy for:
    acute leukaemia
    other malignancy
  Surgical procedures in patients with:
    thrombocytopenia
    platelet functional defects

2 Possible indications

Treatment
  Severe haemorrhage in:
    ITP and drug-induced immune thrombocytopenia
    intravascular coagulation

Prophylaxis
  Splenectomy for ITP

---

engraftment; or in the presence of thrombocytopenia or platelet functional defects where surgery is contemplated. Some particular indications for platelet transfusion are further considered below.

Acute leukaemia. Bleeding complications are relatively uncommon in children with acute lymphoblastic leukaemia, as remission induction is rapid and associated with only transient thrombocytopenia [542], but in adults with acute myeloid leukaemia, thrombocytopenia is usually more severe and prolonged. Since the introduction of platelet transfusion the mortality associated with haemorrhage has been reduced from approaching 65% [494, 496] to less than 25% [495, 538]. Repeated regular platelet transfusion has been shown in comparative studies to reduce the incidence of serious haemorrhage [543]. As the time to remission is usually within eight to 10 weeks, the risk of introducing a refractory state is not excessive. Prophylactic transfusions of platelets may be given three times weekly during remission induction [538] when the platelet count is below $20 \times 10^9/l$ [485], and may even be required on a daily basis in the presence of infection, fever or DIC.

Aplastic anaemia. A different approach is required in the case of patients with aplastic anaemia, who are at risk over a long period of time. If regular transfusions are administered they will become immunized and develop resistance to the transfused platelets some time between 10 days and three months. It may be possible to avoid this refractory state by the use of related donors compatible for the A and B systems of HLA antigens, though this places a considerable burden on the donor, who may also be the only suitable donor for marrow transplantation. Prior transfusion from a prospective marrow donor may jeopardize subsequent marrow transplantation [544], and family members should not be used as platelet donors for patients awaiting transplants. The problems of platelet compatibility are discussed further in Chapter 34.

Hereditary thrombocytopenia. In hereditary thrombocytopenias, haemorrhagic episodes should be treated by platelet transfusion. As with aplastic anaemia, such transfusion should be kept to a minimum to avoid immunization and a refractory state. The same applies to hereditary disorders of platelet function, such as thrombasthenia and the Bernard–Soulier syndrome.

Cardiac-bypass surgery and massive blood replacement. In both these situations the platelet count may be as low as $20 \times 10^9/l$. In cardiac surgery, platelet dysfunction may compound the haemorrhagic tendency and

transfusion of six to eight units of platelet concentrate may prove of considerable benefit [485].

Thrombocytopenia due to accelerated platelet destruction. Arguments for employing platelet transfusion in ITP and DIC are complex. In ITP, the lower the platelet count the more rapid the destruction of transfused platelets and hence the less likely are they to be of value, though some have advocated their use in life-threatening conditions and during splenectomy. On the other hand, platelet transfusion is of benefit in isoimmune neonatal thrombocytopenia (p. 995), since the maternal platelets lack the specific antigen and may be used suspended in ABO-compatible plasma. Platelet transfusion may also be of value in drug-induced thrombocytopenia [377, 378], especially cases when impairment of thrombopoiesis is operative.

Platelet transfusion may be used in DIC associated with severe thrombocytopenia, but theoretical considerations would suggest that simultaneous transfusion of fresh frozen plasma (FFP) or coagulation-factor concentrates should be used, together with attempts to interfere with the coagulation process by treatment of the underlying disorder and with heparin: the survival of transfused platelets is likely to be brief in the face of continuing intravascular coagulation.

THROMBOCYTOSIS

Causes and mechanisms
The finding of a platelet count consistently greater than $450 \times 10^9/l$ should evoke a search for underlying causes. These are listed in Table 25.9; in broad terms, they fall into two groups. The first group are termed thrombocythaemias and are characterized by an autonomous increase in platelet production associated with abnormal stem-cell proliferation, as in polycythaemia vera, chronic granulocytic anaemia [10] and other myeloproliferative disorders (Chapter 32). In the second there is either a stimulus to platelet production (reactive thrombocytosis) or altered distribution, as occurs following splenectomy (see below). Difficulties in diagnosis may arise when thrombocythaemia associated with a myeloproliferative disorder is complicated by haemorrhage, tissue damage, infection or a second neoplastic process, in which case extremely high platelet numbers are found. It is also important to note that thrombocythaemia may be exaggerated by splenectomy.

Little is known of the mechanisms involved in some forms of thrombocytosis. Rebound following acute haemorrhage or thrombocytopenia may be presumed to be mediated via the thrombopoietin mechanism (p. 978), but the reactive thrombocytosis associated with

Table 25.9. Common causes of a raised platelet count

Autonomous thrombocytosis (thrombocythaemia)
    Essential thrombocythaemia
    Polycythaemia vera
    Myelofibrosis
    Chronic granulocytic leukaemia

Reactive thrombocytosis
    Neoplastic disease
        Carcinoma
        Hodgkin's disease
        Non-Hodgkin lymphoma
    Chronic inflammatory disorders
        Rheumatoid arthritis
        Polyarteritis nodosa
        Wegener's granulomatosis
        Crohn's disease
        Ulcerative colitis
    Tissue necrosis
        Post-operative thrombocytosis
        Post-infarction syndromes
    Haemolytic anaemia
    Rebound thrombocytosis
        Post-haemorrhage or cardiac bypass
        Post-acute thrombocytopenia
    Drug-induced
        Vincristine and vinblastine

Distributional thrombocytosis
    Splenectomy
    Adrenaline administration

tissue damage is unaccompanied by the usual increase in platelet size [81] or increase in megakaryocyte ploidy [78] and must be presumed to be mediated by an independent mechanism. This is likely to be the same as is responsible for non-specific stimulation of platelet production in experimental animals [79]. Whether the thrombocytosis associated with malignancy, chronic inflammatory disorders and haemolysis are all mediated in the same manner remains unknown.

Diagnosis
Differentiation between reactive thrombocytosis and thrombocythaemia may be made simple in the individual case by the presence of undoubted features of myeloproliferative disease affecting cell lines other than the platelets (see Chapter 32). Sometimes, however, the platelets may be the only abnormal cell line, or the diagnosis may be obscured by the possibility that the enlargement of spleen or liver is due to a neoplastic or inflammatory process, which itself is the cause of a reactive thrombocytosis. In this situation, both clinical and laboratory evidence should be sought for any of the possible underlying causes. Tests of platelet function should be performed, as defects of aggregation in response to adrenaline, ADP or col-

lagen, or of PF3 availability, are common in thrombocythaemia of the myeloproliferative type [545–548] but rare in reactive thrombocytosis [545–547], providing aspirin medication can be excluded.

Notes on particular causes of thrombocytosis

Carcinoma. This is an important cause of thrombocytosis. In a survey of causes of reactive thrombocytosis Levin & Conley [549] reported 35 cases in association with carcinoma, the tumours being in stomach, colon, lung, breast and ovary. In lung cancer requiring chemotherapy, the platelet count is seldom greater than $1000 \times 10^9/l$, though more extreme thrombocytosis may occur [550], remitting after effective treatment of the primary lesion [549, 550]. Thrombocytosis is a common accompaniment of Hodgkin's disease and other lymphomas [549], especially when the patient suffers systemic symptoms such as fever, night sweats and weight loss.

Inflammatory diseases. Various types of inflammatory diseases, particularly those associated with vasculitis, may raise the platelet count to levels greater than $1000 \times 10^9/l$ [545, 549]. Rheumatoid arthritis and the other collagen diseases are important in this context, and chronic inflammation of the bowel, including Crohn's disease, ulcerative colitis [551] and coeliac disease [552], may have a similar effect. Other features of chronic inflammation, such as a high sedimentation rate, are usually apparent.

Post-operative thrombocytosis. A mild degree of this is common, reaching a peak eight to 12 days after surgery [553]. Similar thrombocytosis is seen following soft tissue injuries, fractures and parturition [553–555]. In a carefully documented study, Mustard [556] showed that post-operative thrombocytosis did not necessarily follow an initial thrombocytopenia. The mechanism is likely to be similar to that which applies in inflammatory or neoplastic disease, since the increase in platelet count is not associated with an increase in platelet size, either in human subjects [557] or animals [81].

Splenectomy. This presents a complex picture: superimposed on post-operative reactive thrombocytosis is the effect of removal of the splenic platelet pool [121]. When platelet production is already increased, as in ITP [189], or abnormal, as in myeloproliferative disorders [558], the post-operative rise may be more rapid than usual and more extreme. When haemolytic anaemia or some other disease process persists, such as in patients with congenital haemolytic anaemia, the thrombocytosis may remain at a high level for many years [84], but otherwise it usually subsides within three to eight weeks to a level about 30% above normal.

Haemolysis. This is associated with increased platelet production, both in the experimental animals [83] and in man [84]. The mechanism involved remains uncertain (p. 979).

Iron deficiency. This has been reported to be associated with both low [559] and high [560] platelet counts. Iron therapy is commonly followed by an increase in low platelet counts [559] and by a fall of high ones [560, 561]. In the experimental animal, iron deficiency is regularly associated with disturbance of megakaryocyte maturation together with high platelet counts [562] but the mechanisms involved remain obscure [87].

Rebound thrombocytosis, comparable to that in the experimental animal (p. 979) is seen following massive haemorrhage [563]. It may also be seen following correction of megaloblastosis [564] and recovery from thrombocytopenia due to agents such as cytotoxic drugs [565] or alcohol [566, 567].

Vincristine-induced thrombocytosis appears to differ in mechanism from that which follows the action of other cytotoxic drugs. Thrombocytosis develops without preceding thrombocytopenia [252, 568]. Vincristine almost certainly stimulates platelet production by more than one mechanism. In rats, vincristine in high dosage induces megakaryocytopenia by a direct toxic action on maturing megakaryocytes; this appears to be followed by differentiation of cells from the stem-cell pool with subsequent accelerated maturation [569, 570]. This action appears to be similar to that recently observed following 5-fluorouracil administration [7, 8]. The second mechanism is stimulation of platelet production through an effect of vincristine, even in relatively low dosage, on circulating platelets: platelets exposed to vincristine are altered in such a way that they do not participate in the normal regulatory process governing platelet production [571]. Vincristine [572] and vinblastine [573] have both been reported to stimulate release of thrombopoietin, and the enhanced rate of production of platelets which follows administration of the drug is almost certainly mediated in part by stimulation of this normal regulatory process. In immune thrombocytopenia yet a further mechanism operates in that vinca alkaloids almost certainly interfere with removal of sensitized platelets by phagocytic cells [249]. However, as platelet lifespan under normal steady-state conditions is unaffected by vincristine [571], this mechanism does not contribute to the thrombocytosis which follows the administration of the drug in other conditions.

Management of thrombocytosis

Raised platelet counts may be reduced by thrombocytapheresis [574] or by the use of myelosuppressive therapy. However, in contrast to the high incidence of thrombotic and haemorrhagic complications which occur in thrombocythaemia (see Chapter 32), these are relatively uncommon in reactive thrombocytosis, even if prolonged [575–577].

In a study of 318 patients undergoing splenectomy for a variety of reasons, Boxer *et al.* [575] observed significant thrombocytosis in 75%. Amongst these the incidence of clinically recognized thromboembolic complications was 3·8%, not significantly greater than in those without thrombocytosis. Hirsh & Dacie [84] noted that some of their cases had maintained high platelet counts over some 20 years without thromboembolic episodes, although thromboembolism had occurred in others. Clearly in the post-operative period after splenectomy, as with other abdominal surgery, there is a risk of thromboembolism, and prophylaxis with heparin [578], or with drugs inhibiting platelet aggregation [579], should be considered in its own right. Treatment with myelosuppressive drugs or thrombocytapheresis is not warranted in post-splenectomy thrombocytosis other than that associated with myeloproliferative disorders. In other forms of reactive thrombocytosis the risk of thromboembolism is small compared with that in thrombocythaemia [546, 576, 577], and long-term therapy with anticoagulants or other anti-thrombotic agents is not recommended.

REFERENCES

1 JACKSON C.W. (1973) Cholinesterase as a possible marker for early cells of the megakaryocytic series. *Blood*, **42**, 413.
2 TRANUM-JENSEN J. & BEHNKE O. (1977) Electron microscopical identification of the committed precursor cell of the megakaryocyte compartment of rat bone marrow. *Cell Biology International Reports*, **1**, 445.
3 PAULUS J.-M. (1970) DNA metabolism and development of organelles in guinea-pig megakaryocytes: a combined ultrastructural, autoradiographic and cytophotometric study. *Blood*, **35**, 298.
4 TILL J.E. & McCULLOCH E.A. (1961) A direct measurement of the radiation sensitivity of normal mouse bone marrow cells. *Radiation Research*, **14**, 213.
5 EBBE S. & STOHLMAN F. JR (1970) Stimulation of thrombocytopoiesis in irradiated mice. *Blood*, **35**, 783.
6 GOLDBERG J., PHALEN E., HOWARD D., EBBE S. & STOHLMAN F. JR (1977) Thrombocytotic suppression of megakaryocyte production from stem cells. *Blood*, **49**, 59.
7 HODGSON G.S. & BRADLEY T.R. (1979) Properties of haematopoietic stem cells surviving 5-fluorouracil treatment: evidence for a pre-CFU-S cell? *Nature (London)*, **281**, 381.

8 JONES B.C., RADLEY J.M., BRADLEY T.R. & HODGSON G.S. (1980) Enhanced megakaryocyte repopulation ability of stem cells surviving 5-fluorouracil treatment. *Experimental Hematology*, **8**, 61.

9 WHANG-PENG J., FREI E. III, TJIO J.H., CARBONE P.P. & BRECHER G. (1963) The distribution of the Philadelphia chromosome in patients with chronic myelogenous leukemia. *Blood*, **22**, 664.

10 ADAMSON J.W., FIALKOW P.J., MURPHY S. PRCHAL J.F. & STEINMANN L. (1976) Polycythemia vera: stem-cell and probable clonal origin of the disease. *New England Journal of Medicine*, **295**, 913.

11 METCALF D., MACDONALD H.R., ODARTCHENKO N. & SORDAT B. (1975) Growth of mouse megakaryocyte *in vitro*. *Proceedings of the National Academy of Sciences, USA*, **72**, 1744.

12 NAKEFF A. & DANIELS-MCQUEEN S. (1976) *In-vitro* colony assay for a new class of megakaryocyte precursor: colony-forming unit megakaryocyte (CFU-M). *Proceedings of the Society for Experimental Biology and Medicine*, **151**, 758.

13 WILLIAMS N., JACKSON H., SHERIDAN A.P.C., MURPHY M.J. JR, ELSTE A. & MOORE M.A.S. (1978) Regulation of megakaryopoiesis in long-term murine bone marrow cultures. *Blood*, **51**, 245.

14 BURSTEIN S.A., ADAMSON J.W., THORNING D. & HARKER L.A. (1979) Characteristics of murine megakaryocytic colonies *in vitro*. *Blood*, **54**, 169.

15 MCLEOD D.L.M., SHREEVE M.M. & AXELRAD A.A. (1976) Induction of megakaryocyte colonies with platelet formation *in vitro*. *Nature (London)*, **261**, 492.

16 MIZOGUCHI H., KUBOTA K., MIURA Y. & TAKAKU F. (1979) An improved plasma culture system for the production of megakaryocyte colonies *in vitro*. *Experimental Hematology*, **7**, 345.

17 VAINCHENKER W., GUICHARD J. & BRETON-GORIUS J. (1979) Growth of human megakaryocyte colonies in culture from fetal, neonatal and adult peripheral blood cells. Ultrastructural analysis. *Blood Cells*, **5**, 25.

18 FAUSER A.A. & MESSNER H.A. (1979) Identification of megakaryocytes, macrophages and eosinophils in colonies of human bone marrow containing neutrophilic granulocytes and erythroblasts. *Blood*, **53**, 1023.

19 NAKEFF A. & FLOEH D.P. (1976) Separation of megakaryocytes from mouse bone marrow by density gradient centrifugation. *Blood*, **48**, 133.

20 EBBE S., HOWARD D., PHALEN E. & STOHLMAN F. JR (1975) Effects of vincristine on normal and stimulated megakaryocytopoiesis in the rat. *British Journal of Haematology*, **29**, 593.

21 EBBE S. & PHALEN E. (1979) Does autoregulation of megakaryocytopoiesis occur? *Blood Cells*, **5**, 123.

22 WILLIAMS N. & JACKSON H. (1978) Regulation of the proliferation of murine megakaryocyte progenitor cells by cell cycle. *Blood*, **52**, 163.

23 LEVIN J., LEVIN F.C., PENINGTON D.G. & METCALF D. (1981) Measurement of ploidy distribution in megakaryocyte colonies obtained from cultures: With studies of the effects of thrombocytopenia. *Blood* (in press).

24 EBBE S. & STOHLMAN F. JR (1965) Megakaryocytopoiesis in the rat. *Blood*, **26**, 20.

25 JACKSON C.W. (1974) Some characteristics of rat megakaryocyte precursors identified using cholinester-ase as a marker. In: *Platelets: Production, Function, Transfusion and Storage* (ed. Baldini M.G. & Ebbe S.), p. 33. Grune & Stratton, New York.

26 ODELL T.T. JR & JACKSON C.W. (1968) Polyploidy and maturation of rat megakaryocytes. *Blood*, **32**, 102.

27 ODELL T.T., MURPHY J.R. & JACKSON C.W. (1976) Stimulation of megakarocytopoiesis by acute thrombocytopenia in rats. *Blood*, **48**, 765.

28 FEINENDEGEN L.E., ODARTCHENKO N., COTTIER H. & BOND V.P. (1962) Kinetics of megakaryocyte proliferation. *Proceedings of the Society for Experimental Biology and Medicine*, **111**, 177.

29 MACPHERSON G.G. (1971) Development of megakaryocytes in bone marrow of the rat: an analysis by electron microscopy and high resolution autoradiography. *Proceedings of the Royal Society of London, Series B*, **177**, 265.

30 MACPHERSON G.G. (1972) Origin and development of the demarcation system in megakaryocytes of rat bone marrow. *Journal of Ultrastructure Research*, **40**, 167.

31 BEHNKE O. (1968) An electron microscope study of the megakaryocyte of the rat bone marrow. I. The development of the demarcation membrane system and the platelet surface coat. *Journal of Ultrastructure Research*, **24**, 412.

32 PENINGTON D.G., STREATFIELD K. & ROXBURGH A.E. (1976) Megakaryocytes and the heterogeneity of circulating platelets. *British Journal of Haematology*, **34**, 639.

33 TAVASSOLI M. (1979) Fusion-fission reorganization of membrane: a developing membrane model for thrombocytogenesis in megakaryocytes. *Blood Cells*, **5**, 89.

34 BEHNKE O. (1969) An electron microscope study of the megakaryocyte of the rat bone marrow. II. Some aspects of platelet release and microtubules. *Journal of Ultrastructure Research*, **26**, 110.

35 BECKER R.P. & DE BRUYN P.P.H. (1976) The transmural passage of blood cells into myeloid sinusoids and the entry of platelets into the sinusoidal circulation: a scanning electron microscopic investigation. *American Journal of Anatomy*, **145**, 183.

36 LICHTMAN M.A., CHAMBERLAIN J.K., SIMON W. & SANTILLO P.A. (1978) Parasinusoidal location of megakaryocytes in marrow: A determinant of platelet release. *American Journal of Hematology*, **4**, 303.

37 TAVASSOLI M. (1979) The marrow-blood barrier. *British Journal of Haematology*, **41**, 297.

38 PENINGTON D.G. (1979) The cellular biology of megakaryocytes. *Blood Cells*, **5**, 5.

39 PENINGTON D.G., STREATFIELD K. & WESTE S.M. (1974) Megakaryocyte ploidy and ultrastructure in stimulated thrombopoiesis. In: *Platelets: Production, Function, Transfusion and Storage* (ed. Baldini M.G. & Ebbe S.), p. 115. Grune & Stratton, New York.

40 MELAMED M.R., CLIFTON E.E., MERCER C. & KOSS L.G. (1966) The megakaryocyte blood count. *American Journal of the Medical Sciences*, **252**, 301.

41 KAUFMAN R.M., AIRO R., POLLACK S., CROSBY W.H. & DOBERNECK R. (1965) Origin of pulmonary megakaryocytes. *Blood*, **25**, 767.

42 TINGAARD PEDERSEN N. (1974) The pulmonary vessels as a filter for circulating megakaryocytes in rats. *Scandinavian Journal of Haematology*, **13**, 225.

43 CROSBY W.H. (1977) Delivery of megakaryocytes by the

marrow—the derivation of platelets. In: *Topics in Hematology* (ed. Seno S., Takaku F. & Irino S.), p. 416. Excerpta Medica, Amsterdam.

44 BEHNKE O. (1970) The morphology of blood platelet membrane systems. *Series Haematologica*, 3 (Suppl. 4), 3.

45 WEINTRAUB A.H. & KARPATKIN S. (1974) Heterogeneity of rabbit platelets. II. Use of the megathrombocyte to demonstrate a thrombopoietic stimulus. *Journal of Laboratory and Clinical Medicine*, 83, 896.

46 GARG S.K., AMOROSI E.L. & KARPATKIN S. (1971) Use of the megathrombocyte as an index of megakaryocyte number. *New England Journal of Medicine*, 284, 11.

47 HARKER L.A. (1968) Kinetics of thrombopoiesis. *Journal of Clinical Investigation*, 47, 458.

48 HARKER L.A. & FINCH C.A. (1969) Thrombokinetics in man. *Journal of Clinical Investigation*, 48, 963.

49 EBBE S., STOHLMAN F. JR, OVERCASH J., DONOVAN J. & HOWARD D. (1968) Megakaryocyte size in thrombocytopenic rats. *Blood*, 32, 787.

50 PENINGTON D.G. & OLSON T.E. (1970) Megakaryocytes in states of altered platelet production: Cell numbers, size and DNA content. *British Journal of Haematology*, 18, 447.

51 ODELL T.T. JR, JACKSON C.W., FRIDAY T.J. & CHARSHA D.E. (1969) Effects of thrombocytopenia on megakaryocytopoiesis. *British Journal of Haematology*, 17, 91.

52 PENINGTON D.G. & STREATFIELD K. (1975) Heterogeneity of megakaryocytes and platelets. *Series Haematologica*, 8, 22.

53 PAULUS J.-M. (1975) Platelet size in man. *Blood*, 46, 321.

54 KARPATKIN S. (1969) Heterogeneity of human platelets. I. Metabolic and kinetic evidence suggestive of young adult platelets. *Journal of Clinical Investigation*, 48, 1073.

55 CHARMATZ A. & KARPATKIN S. (1974) Heterogeneity of rabbit platelets. I. Employment of an albumin density gradient for separation of a young platelet population identified with Se[75] selenomethionine. *Thrombosis et Diathesis Haemorrhagica*, 31, 485.

56 BUSCH C. & OLSON P.S. (1973) Density distribution of ^{51}Cr-labelled platelets within the circulating dog platelet population. *Thrombosis Research*, 3, 1.

57 GINSBURG A.D. & ASTER R.H. (1972) Changes associated with platelet ageing. *Thrombosis et Diathesis Haemorrhagica*, 27, 407.

58 CORASH L., TAN H. & GRALNICK H.R. (1977) Heterogeneity of human whole blood platelet subpopulations. I. Relationship between buoyant density, cell volume and ultrastructure. *Blood*, 49, 71.

59 HIRSH J., GLYNN M.F. & MUSTARD J.F. (1968) The effect of platelet age on platelet adherence to collagen. *Journal of Clinical Investigation*, 47, 466.

60 CORASH L., SHAFER B. & PERLOW M. (1978) Heterogeneity of whole human blood platelet subpopulations. II. Use of a subhuman primate model to analyse the relationship between density and platelet age. *Blood*, 52, 726.

61 MINTER F.M. & INGRAM M.L. (1971) Platelet volume: density relationships in normal and acutely bled dogs. *British Journal of Haematology*, 20, 55.

62 PENINGTON D.G., LEE N.Y.L., ROXBURGH A.E. &

63 CIESLAR P., GREENBERG J.P., RAND M.L., PACKHAM M.A., KINLOUGH-RATHBONE R.L. & MUSTARD J.F. (1979) Separation of thrombin-treated platelets from normal platelets by density-gradient centrifugation. *Blood*, 53, 867.

64 DE GABRIELE G. & PENINGTON D.G. (1967) Physiology of the regulation of platelet production. *British Journal of Haematology*, 13, 202.

65 HARKER L.A. (1970) Regulation of thrombopoiesis. *American Journal of Physiology*, 218, 1376.

66 ABILDGAARD C.F. & SIMONE J.V. (1967) Thrombopoiesis. *Seminars in Hematology*, 4, 424.

67 LEVIN J. (1970) Humoral control of thrombopoiesis. In: *Formation and Destruction of Blood Cells* (ed. Greenwalt T.J. & Jamieson G.A.), p. 143. Lippincott, Philadelphia.

68 LEVIN J. & EVATT B.L. (1979) Humoral control of thrombopoiesis. *Blood Cells*, 5, 105.

69 EVATT B.L. & LEVIN J. (1969) Measurement of thrombopoiesis in rabbits using [75]selenomethionine. *Journal of Clinical Investigation*, 48, 1615.

70 SHREINER D.P. & LEVIN J. (1970) Detection of thrombopoietic activity in plasma by stimulation of suppressed thrombopoiesis. *Journal of Clinical Investigation*, 49, 1709.

71 PENINGTON D.G. (1970) Isotope bioassay for thrombopoietin. *British Medical Journal*, i, 606.

72 COOPER G.W., COOPER B. & CHANG C.-Y. (1970) Demonstration of a circulating factor regulating blood platelet production using ^{35}S-sulfate in rats and mice. *Proceedings of the Society for Experimental Biology and Medicine*, 134, 1123.

73 KRIZSA F. (1971) Study on the development of post-haemorrhagic thrombocytosis in rats. *Acta Haematologica*, 46, 228.

74 McDONALD T.P. (1973) Bioassay for thrombopoietin utilizing mice in rebound thrombocytosis. *Proceedings of the Society for Experimental Biology and Medicine*, 144, 1006.

75 McDONALD T.P. (1975) Assay of thrombopoietin utilizing human sera and urine fractions. *Biochemical Medicine*, 13, 101.

76 McDONALD T.P. (1976) Role of the kidneys in thrombopoietin production. *Experimental Hematology*, 4, 27.

77 McDONALD T.P., CLIFT R., LANGE R.D., NOLAN C., TRIBBY I.I.E. & BARLOW G.H. (1975) Thrombopoietin production by human embryonic kidney cells in culture. *Journal of Laboratory and Clinical Medicine*, 85, 59.

78 SIEMENSMA N.P., BATHAL P.S. & PENINGTON D.G. (1975) The effect of massive liver resection on platelet kinetics in the rat. *Journal of Laboratory and Clinical Medicine*, 86, 817.

79 ODELL T.T. JR, McDONALD T.P. & HOWSDEN F.L. (1964) Native and foreign stimulators of platelet production. *Journal of Laboratory and Clinical Medicine*, 64, 418.

80 LEVIN J. & CONLEY C.L. (1964) Thrombocytosis associated with malignant disease. *Archives of Internal Medicine*, 114, 497.

81 KRAYTMAN M. (1973) Platelet size in thrombocyto-

penias and thrombocytosis of various origin. *Blood*, **41**, 587.

82 EVATT B.L., SPIVAK J.L. & LEVIN J. (1976) Relationships between thrombopoiesis and erythropoiesis with studies of the effects of preparations of thrombopoietin and erythropoietin. *Blood*, **48**, 547.

83 FREEDMAN M.L. & KARPATKIN S. (1975) Heterogeneity of rabbit platelets. IV. Thrombocytosis with absolute megathrombocytosis in phenylhydrazine-induced hemolytic anemia in rabbits. *Thrombosis et Diathesis Haemorrhagica*, **33**, 335.

84 HIRSH J. & DACIE J.V. (1966) Persistent post-splenectomy thrombocytosis and thromboembolism: a consequence of continuing anaemia. *British Journal of Haematology*, **12**, 44.

85 JACKSON C.W., SIMONE J.V. & EDWARDS C.C. (1974) The relationship of anemia and thrombocytosis. *Journal of Laboratory and Clinical Medicine*, **84**, 357.

86 CHOI S.I., SIMONE J.V. & JACKSON C.W. (1974) Megakaryocytopoiesis in experimental iron deficiency anemia. *Blood*, **43**, 111.

87 KARPATKIN S., GARG S.K. & FREEDMAN M.L. (1974) Role of iron as a regulator of thrombopoiesis. *American Journal of Medicine*, **57**, 521.

88 STEINER M. & BALDINI M. (1969) Protein synthesis in aging blood platelets. *Blood*, **33**, 628.

89 JOHNSON C.A., ABILGAARD C.F. & SCHULMAN I. (1971) Functional studies of young versus old platelets in a patient with chronic thrombocytopenia. *Blood*, **37**, 163.

90 MONCADA S., GRYGLEWSKI R., BUNTING S. & VANE J.R. (1976) An enzyme isolated from arteries transforms prostaglandin endoperoxides to an unstable substance that inhibits platelet aggregation. *Nature (London)*, **263**, 663.

91 MONCADA S., HIGGS E.A. & VANE J.R. (1977) Human arterial and venous tissues generate prostacyclin (prostaglandin X), a potent inhibitor of platelet aggregation. *Lancet*, **i**, 18.

92 KARPATKIN S. (1972) Human platelet senescence. *Annual Review of Medicine*, **23**, 101.

93 NURDEN A.T. & CAEN J.P. (1976) Role of surface glycoproteins in human platelet function. *Thrombosis and Haemostasis*, **35**, 139.

94 GEORGE J.N. & LEWIS P.C. (1977) Membrane glycoprotein loss from circulating platelets: inhibition by dipyridamole and aspirin. *Thrombosis and Haemostasis*, **38**, 111.

95 GREENBERG J., PACKHAM M.A., CAZENAVE J.P., REIMERS H.-J. & MUSTARD J.F. (1975) Effects on platelet function of removal of platelet sialic acid by neuramidinase. *Laboratory Investigation*, **32**, 476.

96 CAZENAVE J.P., REIMERS H.J., KINLOUGH-RATHBONE R.L., PACKHAM M.A. & MUSTARD J.F. (1976) Effects of sodium periodate on platelet function. *Laboratory Investigation*, **34**, 471.

96a HIRSCH E.O. & GARDNER F.H. (1952) The transfusion of human blood platelets. *Journal of Laboratory and Clinical Medicine*, **39**, 556.

97 STUART M.J., MURPHY S. & OSKI F.A. (1975) A simple non-radioisotope technic for the determination of platelet life-span. *New England Journal of Medicine*, **292**, 1310.

98 GREAVES M., ROCHE R. & CASTALDI P.A. (1981) Assessment of the recovery of platelet cyclooxygenase from aspirin effect using a radioimmunoassay for thromboxane B_2. *Clinical and Experimental Pharmacology and Physiology*. (In press).

99 MUELLER J.F. (1953) Pathologic physiology of mammalian blood platelets utilising P^{32} tagged rabbit platelets. *Proceedings of the Society of Experimental Biology and Medicine*, **83**, 557.

100 LEEKSMA C.H.W. & COHEN J.A. (1956) Determination of the life-span of human blood platelets using diisopropyl fluorofosphonate. *Journal of Clinical Investigation*, **35**, 964.

101 ODELL T.T. JR & ANDERSON B. (1959) Production and life-span of platelets. In: *The Kinetics of Cellular Proliferation* (ed. Stohlman F. jr.), p. 278. Grune & Stratton, New York.

102 BRODSKY I., ROSS E.M., PETKOV G. & KAHN S.B. (1972) Platelet and fibrinogen kinetics with (^{75}Se)-selenomethionine in patients with myeloproliferative disorders. *British Journal of Haematology*, **22**, 179.

103 GROSSMAN C.N., KOHN R. & KOCH R. (1963) Possible errors in the use of P^{32} orthophosphate for the estimation of platelet lifespan. *Blood*, **22**, 9.

104 GINSBURG A.D. & ASTER R.H. (1969) Kinetic studies with Cr^{51}-labelled platelet cohorts in rats. *Journal of Laboratory and Clinical Medicine*, **74**, 138.

105 DEUBELBEISS K.A., DANCEY J.T., HARKER L.A. & FINCH C.A. (1975) Neutrophil kinetics in the dog. *Journal of Clinical Investigation*, **55**, 833.

106 HANSON S. & HARKER L.A. (1977) Simultaneous Cr^{51} and ^{14}C-serotonin platelet survival measurements. *Thrombosis and Haemostasis*, **38**, 140.

107 AAS K. & GARDNER F. (1958) Survival of blood platelets labelled with chromium. *Journal of Clinical Investigation*, **37**, 1257.

108 PANEL ON DIAGNOSTIC APPLICATIONS OF RADIOISOTOPES IN HEMATOLOGY (1977) Recommended methods for radioisotope platelet survival studies. *Blood*, **50**, 1137.

109 KATTLOVE H.E. & SPAET T.H. (1970) The effect of chromium on platelet function *in vitro*. *Blood*, **35**, 659.

110 THAKUR M.L., WELCH M.J., JOIST J.H. & COLEMAN R.E. (1976) Indium-111 labelled platelets: Studies on preparation and evaluation of *in-vitro* and *in-vivo* functions. *Thrombosis Research*, **9**, 345.

111 SCHEFFEL U., McINTYRE P.A., EVATT E., DVORNICKY J.A., NATARAJAN T.K., BOLLING D.R. & MURPHY E.A. (1977) Evaluation of Indium-111 as a new high photon yield gamma-emitting 'physiological' platelet label. *Johns Hopkins Medical Journal*, **140**, 285.

112 HEATON W.A., DAVIS H.H., WELCH M.J., MATHIAS C.J., JOIST J.H., SHERMAN L.A. & SIEGEL B.A. (1979) Indium-111: A new radionuclide label for studying human platelet kinetics. *British Journal of Haematology*, **42**, 613.

113 SCHEFFEL U., TSAN M.-F. & McINTYRE P.A. (1979) Labelling of human platelets with (^{111}In) 8-hydroxyquinoline. *Journal of Nuclear Medicine*, **20**, 524.

114 O'NEILL B. & FIRKIN B.G. (1964) Platelet survival studies in coagulation disorders, thrombocythemia and conditions associated with atherosclerosis. *Journal of Laboratory and Clinical Medicine*, **64**, 188.

115 ABRAHAMSEN A.F. (1968) Platelet survival studies in man—with special reference to thrombosis and athero-

sclerosis. *Scandinavian Journal of Haematology*, **3** (Suppl.), 7.

116 HARKER L.A. & SLICHTER S.J. (1972) Platelet and fibrinogen consumption in man. *New England Journal of Medicine*, **287**, 999.

117 PAULUS J.-M. (1971) Measuring mean life span, mean age and variance of longevity in platelets. In: *Platelet Kinetics* (ed. Paulus J.-M.), p. 60. North Holland, Amsterdam.

118 MURPHY E.A. & FRANCIS M.E. (1971) Estimation of blood platelet survival. II. The multiple hit model. *Thrombosis et Diathesis Haemorrhagica*, **25**, 53.

119 MURPHY E.A. (1971) The estimation of blood platelet survival. III. The robustness of the basic models. *Thrombosis et Diathesis Haemorrhagica*, **26**, 431.

120 MURPHY E.A., FRANCIS M.E. & MUSTARD J.F. (1972) The estimation of blood platelet survival. IV. Characteristics of the residual errors from regression. *Thrombosis et Diathesis Haemorrhagica*, **28**, 447.

121 ASTER R.J. (1966) Pooling of platelets in the spleen: Role in the pathogenesis of 'hypersplenic' thrombocytopenia. *Journal of Clinical Investigation*, **45**, 645.

122 REIMERS H.J., KINLOUGH-RATHBONE R.L., CAZENAVE J.P., SENYI A.F., HIRSH J., PACKHAM M.A. & MUSTARD J.F. (1976) *In-vitro* and *in-vivo* functions of thrombin-treated platelets. *Thrombosis and Haemostasis*, **35**, 151.

123 RITCHIE J.L. & HARKER L. (1977) Platelet and fibrinogen survival in coronary atherosclerosis: response to medical and surgical therapy. *American Journal of Cardiology*, **39**, 595.

124 STEELE P., CARROLL J., OVERFIELD D. & GENTON E. (1977) Effect of sulphinpyrazone on platelet survival time in patients with transient cerebral ischaemic attacks. *Stroke*, **8**, 396.

125 DOYLE D.J., CHESTERMAN C.N., CADE J.F., McGREADY J.R., RENNIE G.C. & MORGAN F.J. (1980) Plasma concentration of platelet-specific proteins correlated with platelet survival. *Blood*, **55**, 82.

126 CASH J.D. (1972) Platelet transfusion therapy. *Clinics in Haematology*, **1**, 395.

127 MURPHY S. (1976) Platelet transfusion. *Progress in Hemostasis and Thrombosis*, **3**, 289.

128 HARKER L.A. & SLICHTER S.J. (1972) The bleeding time as a screening test for evaluation of platelet function. *New England Journal of Medicine*, **287**, 155.

129 STEWART J.H. & CASTALDI P.A. (1967) Uraemic bleeding: reversible platelet defect corrected by dialysis. *Quarterly Journal of Medicine*, **36**, 409.

130 LACKNER H. (1973) Hemostatic abnormalities associated with dysproteinemias. *Seminars in Hematology*, **10**, 125.

131 STAVEM P. (1965) The tourniquet test and the influence of age or haemorrhagic disorders on the distribution and size of petechiae. *Scandinavian Journal of Clinical and Laboratory Investigation*, **17**, 607.

132 DUKE W.W. (1912) The pathogenesis of purpura haemorrhagica with especial reference to the part played by blood platelets. *Archives of Internal Medicine*, **10**, 445.

133 MIELKE C.H., KANESHIRO I.A., MAHER J.M., WEINER J.M. & RAPAPORT S.H. (1969) The standardised normal Ivy bleeding time and its prolongation by aspirin. *Blood*, **34**, 204.

134 BULL B.S., SCHNEIDERMAN M.A. & BRECHER G. (1965)

Platelet counts with the Coulter counter. *American Journal of Clinical Pathology*, **44**, 678.

135 ROWAN R.M., ALLAN W. & PRESCOTT R.J. (1972) Evaluation of an automatic platelet counting system utilizing whole blood. *Journal of Clinical Pathology*, **25**, 218.

136 DACIE J.V. & LEWIS S.M. (1975) *Practical Haematology*, 5th edn. Churchill Livingstone, Edinburgh, London and New York.

137 BRECHER G. & CRONKITE E.P. (1950) Morphology and enumeration of human blood platelets. *Journal of Applied Physiology*, **3**, 365.

138 ABBEY A.P. & BELLIVEAU R.R. (1978) Enumeration of platelets. *American Journal of Clinical Pathology*, **69**, 55.

139 NOSANCHUK J.S., CHANG J. & BENNETT J.M. (1978) The analytic basis for the use of platelet estimates from peripheral blood smears. *American Journal of Clinical Pathology*, **69**, 383.

140 MACFARLANE R.G. (1939) A simple method for measuring clot-retraction. *Lancet*, **i**, 1199.

141 BIGGS R. & DOUGLAS A.S. (1953) The thromboplastin generation test. *Journal of Clinical Pathology*, **6**, 23.

142 BIGGS R. (1976) *Human Blood Coagulation, Haemostasis and Thrombosis*, p. 673. Blackwell Scientific Publications, Oxford.

143 HARDISTY R.M. & HUTTON R.A. (1966) Platelet aggregation and the availability of platelet factor 3. *British Journal of Haematology*, **12**, 664.

144 CHESTERMAN C.N., McGREADY J.R., DOYLE D.J. & MORGAN F.J. (1978) Plasma levels of platelet factor 4 measured by radioimmunoassay. *British Journal of Haematology*, **40**, 489.

145 HAN P., TURPIE A.G.G. & GENTON E. (1979) Plasma β-thromboglobulin: differentiation between intravascular and extravascular platelet destruction. *Blood*, **54**, 1192.

146 MORLEY A. (1969) A platelet cycle in normal individuals. *Australasian Annals of Medicine*, **18**, 127.

147 YGGE J. (1969) Variation in the individual subject of some parameters in blood coagulation and fibrinolysis. A longitudinal study in young healthy women. *Scandinavian Journal of Haematology*, **6**, 343.

148 VON BEHRENS W.E. (1975) Mediterranean macrothrombocytopenia. *Blood*, **46**, 199.

149 ANSFORD A.J., FINDLAY A.B. & BRUSHE J.M. (1975) Cold platelet agglutinins. *Lancet*, **ii**, 417.

150 SHREINER D.P. & BELL W.R. (1973) Pseudothrombocytopenia: Manifestation of a new type of platelet agglutinin. *Blood*, **42**, 541.

151 WERLHOF P.G. (1735) *Disquisitio medica et philologica de variolis et anthracibus*. Hannover. Kap. 315, note 65.

152 KAZNELSON P. (1916) Verschwinden der hämorrhagischen Diathese bei einem Falle von 'essentieller Thrombopenie' (Frank) nach Milzexstirpation. *Wiener Klinische Wochenschrift*, **29**, 1451.

153 EVANS R.S., TAKAHASHI K., DUANE R.T., PAYNE R. & LIU C.K. (1951) Primary thrombocytopenic purpura and acquired hemolytic anaemia. Evidence for a common etiology. *Archives of Internal Medicine*, **87**, 48.

154 EPSTEIN R.D., LOZNER E.L., COFFEY T.S. & DAVIDSON C.S. (1950) Congenital thrombocytopenic purpura. Purpura haemorrhagica in pregnancy and in the newborn. *American Journal of Medicine*, **9**, 44.

155 HARRINGTON W.J., MINNICH V., HOLLINGWORTH J.W. & MOORE C.V. (1951) Demonstration of a thrombocytopenic factor in the blood of patients with thrombocytopenic purpura. *Journal of Laboratory and Clinical Medicine*, **38**, 1.

156 HARRINGTON W.J., SPRAGUE C.C., MOORE C.V., AULVIN B.S. & DUBACH R. (1953) Immunologic mechanisms in idiopathic and neonatal thrombocytopenic purpura. *Annals of Internal Medicine*, **38**, 433.

157 SHULMAN N.R., MARDER V.J. & WEINRACH R.S. (1965) Similarities between known antiplatelet antibodies and the factor responsible for thrombocytopenia in idiopathic purpura. *Annals of New York Academy of Sciences*, **124**, 499.

158 KARPATKIN S., SCHUR P.M., STRICK N. & SISKIND G.W. (1973) Heavy chain subclass of human antiplatelet antibodies. *Clinical Immunology and Immunopathology*, **2**, 1.

159 CORN M. & UPSHAW J.D. (1962) Evaluation of platelet antibodies in idiopathic thrombocytopenic purpura. *Archives of Internal Medicine*, **109**, 157.

160 KISSMEYER-NIELSEN F. & JENSEN K.G. (1969) Immunology of platelets. *Progress in Clinical Pathology*, **2**, 141.

161 DAUSSET J. & COLOMBANI J. (1964) Reactions immunologiques au cours du purpura thrombopenique idiopathique. *Semaine des Hôpitaux de Paris*, **40**, 387.

162 SVEJGAARD A. (1969) Iso-antigenic system of human blood platelets. A survey. *Series Haematologica*, **2**, 3.

163 COOMBS R.R.A., MARKS J. & BEDFORD D. (1956) Specific mixed agglutination: mixed erythrocyte platelet antiglobulin reaction for the detection of platelet antibodies. *British Journal of Haematology*, **2**, 84.

164 HOROWITZ H.I., RAPPAPORT H.I., YOUNG R.C. & FUJIMOTO M.M. (1965) Change in platelet factor 3 as a means of demonstrating immune reactions involving platelets: Its use as a test for quinidine-induced thrombocytopenia. *Transfusion*, **5**, 336.

165 KARPATKIN S. & SISKIND G.W. (1969) *In-vitro* detection of platelet antibody in patients with idiopathic thrombocytopenic purpura and systemic lupus erythematosus. *Blood*, **33**, 795.

166 ASTER R.H. & ENRIGHT S.E. (1969) A platelet and granulocyte membrane defect in paroxysmal nocturnal hemoglobinuria: Usefulness for the detection of platelet antibodies. *Journal of Clinical Investigation*, **48**, 1199.

167 CIMO P.L., PISCIOTTA A.V., DESAI R.G., PINO J.L. & ASTER R.H. (1977) Detection of drug-dependent antibodies by the Cr^{51} platelet lysis test: documentation of immune thrombocytopenia induced by diphenylhydantoin, diazepam and sulfisolazone. *American Journal of Hematology*, **2**, 65.

168 MCMILLAN R., SMITH R.S., LONGMIRE R.L., YELENOSKY R., REID R.T. & CRADDOCK C.G. (1971) Immunoglobulins associated with human platelets. *Blood*, **37**, 316.

169 DIXON R.H., ROSSE W.F. & EBBERT L. (1975) Quantitative determination of antibody in idiopathic thrombocytopenic purpura. *New England Journal of Medicine*, **292**, 230.

170 HEGDE U.M., GORDON-SMITH E.C. & WORLLEDGE S. (1977) Platelet antibodies in thrombocytopenic patients. *British Journal of Haematology*, **35**, 113.

171 KELTON J.G., NEAME P.B., BISHOP J., ALY M., GAULDIE J. & HIRSH J. (1979) The direct assay for platelet-associated IgG (PAIgG): Lack of association between antibody level and platelet size. *Blood*, **53**, 73.

172 CINES D.B. & SCHREIBER A.D. (1979) Immune thrombocytopenia. Use of a Coombs' antiglobulin test to detect IgG and C3 on platelets. *New England Journal of Medicine*, **300**, 106.

173 VAN BOXTEL C.J., OOSTERHOF F. & ENGELFRIET C.P. (1975) Immunofluorescence microphotometry for the detection of platelet antibodies. III. Demonstration of autoantibodies against platelets. *Scandinavian Journal of Immunology*, **4**, 657.

174 TATE D.Y., SORENSON R.L., GERRARD J.M., WHITE J.G. & KRIVIT W. (1977) An immuno-enzyme histochemical technique for the detection of platelet antibodies from the serum of patients with idiopathic (autoimmune) thrombocytopenic purpura (ITP). *British Journal of Haematology*, **37**, 265.

175 LEPORRIER M., DIGHIERO G., AUZEMERY M. & BINET J.L. (1979) Detection and quantification of platelet-bound antibodies with immunoperoxidase. *British Journal of Haematology*, **42**, 605.

176 HAUCH T.W. & ROSSE W.F. (1977) Platelet-bound complement (C3) in immune thrombocytopenia. *Blood*, **50**, 1129.

177 BRANEHÖG I. & WEINFIELD A. (1974) Platelet survival and platelet production in idiopathic thrombocytopenic purpura (ITP) before and during treatment with corticosteroids. *Scandinavian Journal of Haematology*, **12**, 69.

178 ASTER R.H. & KEENE W.R. (1969) Sites of platelet destruction in idiopathic thrombocytopenic purpura. *British Journal of Haematology*, **16**, 61.

179 FIRKIN B.G., WRIGHT R., MILLER S. & STOKES E. (1969) Splenic macrophages in thrombocytopenia. *Blood*, **33**, 240.

180 MCMILLAN R., LONGMIRE R.L., YELENOSKI R., SMITH R.S. & CRADDOCK C.G. (1972) Immunoglobulin synthesis *in vitro* by splenic tissue in idiopathic thrombocytopenic purpura. *New England Journal of Medicine*, **286**, 681.

181 LIGHTSEY A.L., KOENIG H.M., MCMILLAN R. & STONE J.R. (1979) Platelet-associated immunoglobulin G in childhood idiopathic thrombocytopenic purpura. *Journal of Pediatrics*, **94**, 201.

182 HANDIN R.I., PIESSENS W.F. & MOLONEY W.C. (1973) Stimulation of nonimmunised lymphocytes by platelet-antibody complexes in idiopathic thrombocytopenic purpura. *New England Journal of Medicine*, **289**, 714.

183 CLANCY R. (1972) Cellular immunity to autologous platelets and serum-blocking factors in idiopathic thrombocytopenic purpura. *Lancet*, **i**, 6.

184 WALDSCHMIDT R. & MUELLER-ECKHARDT C. (1979) Stimulation of lymphocytes by platelet-antibody complexes and their role in the pathogenesis of idiopathic thrombocytopenia. *Blut*, **39**, 53.

185 BOTTIGER L.E. & WESTERHOLM B. (1972) Thrombocytopenia. I. Incidence and aetiology. *Acta Medica Scandinavica*, **191**, 535.

186 DOAN C.A., BOURONCLE B.A. & WISEMAN B.K. (1960) Idiopathic and secondary thrombocytopenic purpura: clinical study and evaluation of 381 cases over a period of 28 years. *Annals of Internal Medicine*, **53**, 861.

187 KING H.E. & COOPER T. (1962) Thrombocytopenia: A clinical analysis of 500 cases. *Postgraduate Medicine*, **31**, 532.

188 WURZEL H.A. (1961) Incidence of various coagulation defects and their association with different diseases. *American Journal of the Medical Sciences*, **241**, 625.

189 CHARLESWORTH D. & TORRANCE H.B. (1968) Splenectomy in idiopathic thrombocytopenic purpura. *British Journal of Surgery*, **55**, 437.

190 LOZNER E.L. (1954) The thrombocytopenic purpuras. *Bulletin of the New York Academy of Medicine*, **30**, 184.

191 LUSHER J.M. & ZUELZER W.W. (1966) Idiopathic thrombocytopenic purpura in childhood. *Journal of Pediatrics*, **68**, 971.

192 BRECKENRIDGE R.T., MOORE R.D. & RATNOFF O.D. (1967) A study of thrombocytopenia—new histologic criteria for the differentiation of idiopathic thrombocytopenia and thrombocytopenia associated with disseminated lupus erythematosus. *Blood*, **30**, 39.

193 LUSHER J.M. & IYER R. (1977) Idiopathic thrombocytopenic purpura in children. *Seminars in Thrombosis and Hemostasis*, **3**, 175.

194 CHOI S.I. & MCCLURE P.D. (1967) Idiopathic thrombocytopenic purpura in childhood. *Canadian Medical Association Journal*, **97**, 562.

195 SHARA O.M. (1973) Thrombocytopenia following measles-mumps-rubella vaccination in a one year old infant. *Clinical Pediatrics* (Philadelphia), **12**, 315.

196 DAMESHEK W. (1960) Controversy in idiopathic thrombocytopenic purpura. *Journal of the American Medical Association*, **173**, 1025.

197 BALDINI M.G. (1972) Idiopathic thrombocytopenic purpura and the ITP syndrome. *Medical Clinics of North America*, **56**, 47.

198 DAMESHEK W., EBBE S., GREENBERG L. & BALDINI M. (1963) Recurrent acute idiopathic thrombocytopenic purpura. *New England Journal of Medicine*, **269**, 647.

199 GARG S.K., AMOROSI E.L. & KARPATKIN S. (1972) The increased percentage of megathrombocytes in various clinical disorders. *Annals of Internal Medicine*, **77**, 361.

200 KARPATKIN S., GARG S.K. & SISKIND G.W. (1971) Autoimmune thrombocytopenic purpura and the compensated thrombocytolytic state. *American Journal of Medicine*, **51**, 1.

201 MUELLER-ECKHARDT C. (1977) Idiopathic thrombocytopenic purpura (ITP): Clinical and immunologic considerations. *Seminars in Thrombosis and Hemostasis*, **3**, 125.

202 KHAN I., ZUCKER-FRANKLIN D. & KARPATKIN S. (1975) Microthrombocytosis and platelet fragmentation associated with idiopathic/autoimmune thrombocytopenic purpura. *British Journal of Haematology*, **31**, 449.

203 ZUCKER-FRANKLIN D. & KARPATKIN S. (1977) Red-cell and platelet fragmentation in idiopathic autoimmune thrombocytopenic purpura. *New England Journal of Medicine*, **297**, 517.

204 HARKER L.A. (1970) Thrombokinetics in idiopathic thrombocytopenic purpura. *British Journal of Haematology*, **19**, 95.

205 ROLOVIC Z., BALDINI M. & DAMESHEK W. (1970) Megakaryocytopoiesis in experimentally induced immune thrombocytopenia. *Blood*, **35**, 173.

206 MCGRATH K.M., STUART J.J. & RICHARDS F. II (1979) Correlation between serum IgG, platelet membrane IgG, and platelet function in hypergammaglobulinaemic states. *British Journal of Haematology*, **42**, 585.

207 KELTON J.G., NEAME P.B., GAULDIE J. & HIRSH J. (1979) Elevated platelet-associated IgG in the thrombocytopenia of septicemia. *New England Journal of Medicine*, **300**, 760.

208 CLANCY R., JENKINS E. & FIRKIN B. (1972) Qualitative platelet abnormalities in idiopathic thrombocytopenic purpura. *New England Journal of Medicine*, **286**, 622.

209 SOKAL G. (1965) Approaches de la pathogenie de la maladie de Werlhof. *Revue Belgique Pathologie*, **31**, 186.

210 CONLEY C.L., HARTMANN R.C. & LALLEY J.S. (1948) Relationship of heparin activity to platelet concentration. *Proceedings of the Society for Experimental Biology and Medicine*, **69**, 284.

211 ASTER R.H. (1966) Observations on survival time, sites of sequestration, and production rate of platelets in idiopathic thrombocytopenic purpura. *Blood*, **28**, 1014.

212 CRABTREE G.R., LEE J.C. & CORNWELL G.G. (1975) Autoimmune thrombocytopenic purpura and Hashimoto's thyroiditis. *Annals of Internal Medicine*, **83**, 371.

213 CATTAN D., CAEN J., FERNANDEZ Y., IZARD J., LECLERE H., TANGUY A. & LEMENAGER J. (1970) Purpura thrombopénique chronique, hyperthyroidie pre-tibial et LATS. *Presse Médicale*, **78**, 1535.

214 JONES A. (1973) Autoimmune disorders and malignant lymphoma. *Cancer*, **31**, 1092.

215 KADEN B.R., ROSSE W.F. & HAUCH T.W. (1979) Immune thrombocytopenia in lymphoproliferative diseases. *Blood*, **53**, 545.

216 EBBE S., WITTELS D. & DAMESHEK W. (1962) Autoimmune thrombocytopenic purpura ('ITP' type) with chronic lymphocytic leukaemia. *Blood*, **19**, 23.

217 MCCLURE P.D. (1975) Idiopathic thrombocytopenic purpura in children: diagnosis and management. *Pediatrics*, **55**, 68.

218 BOURONCLE B.A. & DOAN C.A. (1966) Refractory idiopathic thrombocytopenic purpura treated with imuran. *New England Journal of Medicine*, **275**, 630.

219 AHN Y.S. & HARRINGTON W.J. (1977) Treatment of idiopathic thrombocytopenic purpura (ITP). *Annual Review of Medicine*, **28**, 299.

220 ROBSON H.N. & DUTHIE J.J.R. (1950) Capillary resistance and adrenocortical activity. *British Medical Journal*, **ii**, 971.

221 KITCHENS C.S. (1977) Amelioration of endothelial abnormalities by prednisone in experimental thrombocytopenia in the rabbit. *Journal of Clinical Investigation*, **60**, 1129.

222 BLAJCHMAN M.A., SENYI A.F., HIRSH J., SURYA Y. & BUCHANAN M. (1979) Shortening of the bleeding time in rabbits by hydrocortisone caused by inhibition of prostacyclin generation by the vessel wall. *Journal of Clinical Investigation*, **63**, 1026.

223 SHULMAN I. (1964) Diagnosis and treatment: management of idiopathic thrombocytopenic purpura. *Pediatrics*, **33**, 979.

224 KARPATKIN S. (1978) Autoimmune thrombocytopenic purpura. In: *Immunological Diseases* (ed. Samter M.) 3rd edn, p. 1228. Little, Brown, Boston.

225 SHULMAN N.R., MARDER V.J. & WEINRACH R.S. (1965) Similarities between known antiplatelet antibodies and

the factor responsible for thrombocytopenia in idiopathic purpura. Physiologic, serologic and isotopic studies. *Annals of the New York Academy of Sciences*, **124**, 499.

226 RHINEHART J.J., BALCERZAK S.P., SAGONE A.L. & LOBUGLIO A.F. (1974) The effects of corticosteroids on human monocyte function. *Journal of Clinical Investigation*, **54**, 1337.

227 SCHREIBER A.D., PARSONS J., MCDERMOTT P. & COOPER R.A. (1975) The effect of corticosteroids on the human monocyte IgG and complement receptors. *Journal of Clinical Investigation*, **56**, 1189.

228 THOMPSON R.L., MOORE R.A., HESS C.E., WHEBY M.S. & LEAVELL B.S. (1972) Idiopathic thrombocytopenic purpura. Long-term results of treatment and prognostic significance of response to corticosteroids. *Archives of Internal Medicine*, **130**, 730.

229 MEYERS M.C. (1961) Results of treatment in 71 patients with idiopathic thrombocytopenic purpura. *American Journal of the Medical Sciences*, **242**, 295.

230 DIXON R.H. & ROSSE W.F. (1975) Platelet antibody in autoimmune thrombocytopenia. *British Journal of Haematology*, **31**, 129.

231 COHEN P., GARDNER R.H. & BARNETT G.O. (1961) Classification of the thrombocytopenias by the Cr51-labelling method for measuring platelet lifespan. *New England Journal of Medicine*, **264**, 1294.

232 WILDE R.C., ELLIS L.D. & COOPER W.M. (1967) Splenectomy for chronic idiopathic thrombocytopenic purpura. *Archives of Surgery*, **95**, 344.

233 NAJEAN Y., ARDAILLOU N., DRESCH C. & BERNARD J. (1967) The platelet destruction site in thrombocytopenic purpuras. *British Journal of Haematology*, **13**, 409.

234 MACPHERSON A.I.S. & RICHMOND J. (1975) Planned splenectomy in treatment of idiopathic thrombocytopenic purpura. *British Medical Journal*, **1**, 64.

235 ERAKLIS A.J., KEVY S.V., DIAMOND L.K. & GROSS R.E. (1967) Hazard of overwhelming infection after splenectomy in childhood. *New England Journal of Medicine*, **276**, 1225.

236 ERICKSON W.D., BURGERT E.O. & LYNN H.B. (1968) The hazard of infection following splenectomy in children. *American Journal of Diseases of Children*, **116**, 1.

237 WHITAKER A.N. (1969) Infection and the spleen: association between hyposplenism, pneumococcal sepsis and disseminated intravascular coagulation. *Medical Journal of Australia*, **1**, 1213.

238 SULLIVAN J.L., SHIFFMAN G., MISER J., OCHS H.D., HAMMERSCHLAG M.R., VICHINSKY E. & WEDGWOOD R.J. (1978) Immune response after splenectomy. *Lancet*, **i**, 178.

239 HARRINGTON W.J. & ARIMURA G. (1961) Immune reactions of platelets. In: *Blood Platelets* (ed. Johnson S.A., Monto R.W., Rebuck J.W. & Horn R.J.), p. 659. Little, Brown, Boston.

240 SUSSMAN L.M. (1967) Azathioprine in refractory idiopathic thrombocytopenic purpura. *Journal of the American Medical Association*, **202**, 259.

241 FINCH S.C., CASTRO O., COOPER M., COVEY W., ERICHSON R. & MCPHEDRAN P. (1974) Immunosuppressive therapy of chronic idiopathic thrombocytopenic purpura. *American Journal of Medicine*, **56**, 4.

242 VERLIN M., LAROS R.K. & PENNER J. (1976) Treatment of refractory thrombocytopenic purpura with cyclophosphamide. *American Journal of Hematology*, **1**, 97.

243 WEINERMAN B., MAXWELL I. & HRYNIUK W. (1974) Intermittent cyclophosphamide treatment of autoimmune thrombocytopenia. *Canadian Medical Association Journal*, **111**, 1100.

244 SULTAN Y., DELABEL J., JEANNEAU C. & CAEN J.P. (1971) Effect of periwinkle alkaloids in idiopathic thrombocytopenic purpura. *Lancet*, **i**, 496.

245 AHN Y.S., HARRINGTON W.J., SEELMAN R.C. & EYTEL C.S. (1974) Vincristine therapy of idiopathic and secondary thrombocytopenias. *New England Journal of Medicine*, **291**, 376.

246 VAN ZYL-SMIT R. & JACOBS P. (1974) The use of vincristine in refractory autoimmune thrombocytopenic purpura. *South African Medical Journal*, **48**, 2039.

247 BURTON I.E., ROBERTS B.E., CHILD J.A., MONTGOMERY D.A. & RAPER C.G.L. (1976) Responses to vincristine in refractory idiopathic thrombocytopenic purpura. *British Medical Journal*, **ii**, 918.

248 RIES C.A. (1976) Vincristine for treatment of refractory autoimmune thrombocytopenia. *New England Journal of Medicine*, **295**, 1136.

249 AHN Y.S., BYRNES J.J., HARRINGTON W.J., CAYER M.L., SMITH D.S., BRUNSKILL D.E. & PALL L.M. (1978) The treatment of idiopathic thrombocytopenia with vinblastine-loaded platelets. *New England Journal of Medicine*, **298**, 1101.

250 ROBERTSON J.H. & MCCARTHY G.M. (1969) Periwinkle alkaloids and the platelet count. *Lancet*, **ii**, 353.

251 ROBERTSON J.H., CROZIER E.H. & WOODEND B.E. (1970) The effect of vincristine on the platelet count in rats. *British Journal of Haematology*, **19**, 331.

252 CARBONE P.P., BONO V., FREI E. & BRINDLEY C.O. (1963) Clinical studies with vincristine. *Blood*, **21**, 640.

253 SCHULMAN I. & CURRIMBHOY Z. (1960) Platelet stimulating properties of human plasma with observations on the role of the spleen and the pathogenesis in treatment of ITP. *American Journal of Diseases of Children*, **100**, 747.

254 SCHULMAN I., ABILDGAARD C.F., CORNET J., SIMONE J.V. & CURRIMBHOY Z. (1965) Studies on thrombopoiesis. II. Assay of human plasma thrombopoietic activity. *Journal of Pediatrics*, **66**, 604.

255 REIQUAM C.W. & PROSPER J.C. (1966) Fresh plasma transfusions in the treatment of acute thrombocytopenic purpura. *Journal of Pediatrics*, **68**, 880.

256 BRANDA R.F., MOLDOW C.F., MCCULLOUGH J.J. & JACOB H.S. (1975) Plasma exchange in the treatment of immune disease. *Transfusion*, **15**, 570.

257 MCELFRESH A.E. (1975) Idiopathic thrombocytopenic purpura—to treat or not to treat? *Journal of Pediatrics*, **87**, 160.

258 SIMONS S.M., MAIN C.A., YAISH H.M. & RUTZKY J. (1975) Idiopathic thrombocytopenic purpura in children. *Journal of Pediatrics*, **87**, 16.

259 MCWILLIAMS N.B. & MAURER H.M. (1977) Controlled clinical trial of prednisone in childhood ITP. *Pediatric Research*, **11**, 476.

260 ROBSON H.N. & DAVIDSON L.S. (1950) Purpura in pregnancy with special reference to idiopathic thrombocytopenic purpura. *Lancet*, **ii**, 164.

261 HEYS R.F. (1966) Childbearing and idiopathic thrombocytopenic purpura. *Journal of Obstetrics and Gynaecology of the British Commonwealth*, **73**, 205.

262 PETERSON O.H. JR & LARSON P. (1954) Thrombocytopenic purpura in pregnancy. *Obstetrics and Gynecology*, **4**, 454.

263 LAROS R.K. & SWEET R.L. (1975) Management of idiopathic thrombocytopenic purpura during pregnancy. *American Journal of Obstetrics and Gynecology*, **122**, 182.

264 JONES W.R., STOREY B., NORTON G. & NEISCHE F.W. JR (1974) Pregnancy complicated by acute idiopathic thrombocytopenic purpura. *Journal of Obstetrics and Gynaecology of the British Commonwealth*, **81**, 330.

265 TERRITO M., FINKLESTEIN J., OH W., HOBEL C. & KATTLOVE H. (1973) Management of autoimmune thrombocytopenia in pregnancy and in the neonate. *Obstetrics and Gynecology*, **41**, 579.

266 THOREK P., GRABMAN R. & WELCH J.S. (1948) Recurrent primary thrombocytopenic purpura with accessory spleen. *Annals of Surgery*, **128**, 304.

267 TAN E.M. & ROTHFIELD N.F. (1978) Systemic lupus erythematosus. In: *Immunological Diseases* (ed. Samter M.) 3rd edn, p. 1038. Little, Brown, Boston.

268 ESTES D. & CHRISTIAN C.L. (1971) The natural history of systemic lupus erythematosus by prospective analysis. *Medicine* (Baltimore), **50**, 85.

269 BEST W.R. & DARLING D.R. (1962) A critical look at the splenectomy-SLE controversy. *Medical Clinics of North America*, **46**, 19.

270 RABINOWITZ Y. & DAMESHEK W. (1960) Systemic lupus erythematosus after 'idiopathic' thrombocytopenic purpura: a review. A study of systemic lupus erythematosus occurring after 78 splenectomies for 'idiopathic' thrombocytopenic purpura, with a review of the pertinent literature. *Annals of Internal Medicine*, **52**, 1.

271 KARPATKIN S., STRICK N., KARPATKIN M.B. & SISKIND G.W. (1972) Cumulative experience in the detection of antiplatelet antibody in 234 patients with idiopathic thrombocytopenic purpura, systemic lupus erythematosus and other clinical disorders. *American Journal of Medicine*, **52**, 776.

272 KARPATKIN S. & LACKNER H.L. (1975) Association of antiplatelet antibody with functional platelet disorders. *American Journal of Medicine*, **59**, 599.

273 RAI K.R., SAWITSKY A. & CRONKITE E.P. (1975) Clinical staging of chronic lymphocytic leukaemia. *Blood*, **46**, 219.

274 HASSIDIM K., McMILLAN R., CONJALKA M.S. & MORRISON J. (1979) Immune thrombocytopenic purpura in Hodgkin's disease. *American Journal of Hematology*, **6**, 149.

275 SHALEV O. & BREZIS M. (1977) Methyldopa-induced thrombocytopenia in chronic lymphocytic leukemia. *New England Journal of Medicine*, **297**, 1471.

276 ANTHONY B. & KRIVIT W. (1962) Neonatal thrombocytopenic purpura. *Pediatrics*, **30**, 776.

277 REISS J.S. & PRYLES C.V. (1966) Thrombocytopenia in congenital rubella. *New England Journal of Medicine*, **275**, 264.

278 RAUSEN A.K., RICHTER P., TALLAL L. & COOPER L.Z. (1967) Hematologic effects of intrauterine rubella. *Journal of the American Medical Association*, **199**, 75.

279 BIRNBAUM G., LYNCH J.I., MARGILETH A.M., LONERGAN W.M. & SEVER J.L. (1969) Cytomegalovirus infection in newborn infants. *Journal of Pediatrics*, **75**, 789.

279a HATHAWAY W.E. & BONNAR J. (1978) *Perinatal Coagulation*, p. 132. Grune & Stratton, New York.

280 SHULMAN N.R., MARDER V.J., HILLER M.C. & COLLIER E.M. (1964) Platelet and leukocyte isoantigens and their antibodies: serologic, physiologic and clinical studies. *Progress in Hematology*, **4**, 222.

281 ADNER M.M., FISCH G.R., STAROBIN S.G. & ASTER R.H. (1969) Use of 'compatible' platelet transfusions in treatment of congenital isoimmune thrombocytopenic purpura. *New England Journal of Medicine*, **280**, 244.

282 CINES D.B. & SCHREIBER A.D. (1979) Effect of anti Pl^{A1} antibody on human platelets. I. The role of complement. *Blood*, **53**, 567.

283 ABRAMSON N., EISENBERG P.D. & ASTER R.H. (1974) Post-transfusion purpura: immunologic aspects and therapy. *New England Journal of Medicine*, **291**, 1163.

284 GERSTNER J.B., SMITH M.J., DAVIS K.D., CIMO P.L. & ASTER R.H. (1979) Post-transfusion purpura: therapeutic failure of Pl^{A1}-negative platelet transfusion. *American Journal of Hematology*, **6**, 71.

285 BOTTIGER L.E. & WESTERHOLM B. (1973) Drug-induced blood dyscrasias in Sweden. *British Medical Journal*, **iii**, 339.

286 DEGRUCHY G.C. (1975) *Drug-induced Blood Disorders*, p. 7. Blackwell Scientific Publications, Oxford.

287 BOTTIGER L.E. & WESTERHOLM B. (1972) Thrombocytopenia. I. Incidence and aetiology. *Acta Medica Scadinavica*, **191**, 535.

288 BOTTIGER L.E. & WESTERHOLM B. (1972) Thrombocytopenia. II. Drug-induced thrombocytopenia. *Acta Medical Scandinavica*, **191**, 541.

289 SWANSON M. & COOKE R. (1977) *Drugs, Chemicals and Blood Dyscrasias*. Drug Intelligence Publications, Illinois.

290 GANGAROSA E.J., JOHNSON T.R. & RAMOS H.S. (1960) Ristocetin-induced thrombocytopenia. *Archives of Internal Medicine*, **105**, 83.

291 ACKROYD J.F. (1949) The pathogenesis of thrombocytopenic purpura due to hypersensitivity to sedormid. *Clinical Science*, **7**, 249.

292 ACKROYD J.F. (1954) The role of sedormid in the immunological reaction that results in platelet lysis in sedormid purpura. *Clinical Science*, **13**, 409.

293 ACKROYD J.F. (1958) Thrombocytopenic purpura due to drug hypersensitivity. In: *Sensitivity Reactions to Drugs* (ed. Rosenheim M.L. & Moulton R.), p. 28. Blackwell Scientific Publications, Oxford.

294 ACKROYD J.F. & ROOK A.J. (1968) Allergic drug reactions. In: *Clinical Aspects of Immunology* (ed. Gell P.G.H. & Coombs R.R.A.) 2nd edn, p. 693. Blackwell Scientific Publications, Oxford.

295 HOSSEINZADEH P.K., FIRKIN B.G. & PFUELLER S.L. (1980) Study of the factors that cause specific transformation in cultures of lymphocytes from patients with quinine and quinidine-induced immune thrombocytopenia. *Journal of Clinical Investigation*, **66**, 638.

296 SHULMAN N.R. (1964) A mechanism of cell destruction in individuals sensitised to foreign antigens and its implications in autoimmunity. *Annals of Internal Medicine*, **60**, 506.

297 MIESCHER P. & MIESCHER A. (1952) Die Sedormid anaphylaxie. *Schweitzer Medizinische Wochenschrift*, **82**, 1279.

298 EISNER P.V. & SHAHIDI N.T. (1972) Immune thrombocytopenia due to a drug metabolite. *New England Journal of Medicine*, **287**, 376.

299 EISNER P.V. & KASPER K. (1972) Immune thrombocytopenia due to a metabolite of para-amino-salicylic acid. *American Journal of Medicine*, **53**, 793.

300 RACHMILEWITZ E.A., DAWSON R.B. JR & RACHMILEWITZ B. (1968) Serum antibodies against desipramine as a possible cause for thrombocytopenia. *Blood*, **32**, 524.

301 BLAJCHMAN M.A., LOWRY R.C., PETTIT J. & STRADLING P. (1970) Rifampicin-induced immune thrombocytopenia. *British Medical Journal*, **iii**, 24.

302 EISNER E.V. & CROWELL E.B. (1971) Hydrochlorothiazide-dependent thrombocytopenia due to IgM antibody. *Journal of the American Medical Association*, **215**, 480.

303 SANDLER R.M., EMBERSON C., ROBERTS G.E., VOAK D., DARNBOROUGH J. & HEELEY A.F. (1978) IgM platelet autoantibody due to sodium valproate. *British Medical Journal*, **ii**, 1683.

304 DEYKIN D. & HELLERSTEIN L.J. (1972) The assessment of drug-dependent and isoimmune antiplatelet antibodies by the use of platelet aggregometry. *Journal of Clinical Investigation*, **51**, 3142.

305 HELMLY R.B., BERGIN J.J. & SHULMAN N.R. (1967) Quinine-induced purpura: observation on antibody titres. *Archives of Internal Medicine*, **120**, 59.

306 HOWARD M.A. & FIRKIN B.G. (1971) Ristocetin—a new tool in the investigation of platelet aggregation. *Thrombosis et Diathesis Haemorrhagica*, **26**, 362.

307 RHODES G.R., DIXON R.H. & SILVER D. (1973) Heparin-induced thrombocytopenia with thrombotic and haemorrhagic manifestations. *Surgery, Gynecology and Obstetrics*, **136**, 409.

308 BABCOCK R.B., DUMPER C.W. & SCHARFMAN W.D. (1976) Heparin-induced immune thrombocytopenia. *New England Journal of Medicine*, **295**, 237.

309 GREEN D., HARRIS K., REYNOLDS N., ROBERTS M. & PATTERSON R. (1978) Heparin immune thrombocytopenia: evidence for a heparin-platelet complex as antigenic determinant. *Journal of Laboratory and Clinical Medicine*, **91**, 167.

310 TROWBRIDGE A.A., CARAVEO J., GREEN J.B., AMARAL B. & STONE M.J. (1978) Heparin-related immune thrombocytopenia. *American Journal of Medicine*, **65**, 277.

311 FRANTANTONI J.C., POLLET R. & GRALNICK H.R. (1975) Heparin-induced thrombocytopenia: confirmation of diagnosis with *in-vitro* methods. *Blood*, **45**, 395.

312 GALLUS A.S., GOODALL K.T., BESWICK W. & CHESTERMAN C.N. (1980) Heparin-associated thrombocytopenia: case report and prospective study. *Australian and New Zealand Journal of Medicine*, **10**, 25.

313 KLEIN H.G. & BELL W.R. (1974) Disseminated intravascular coagulation during heparin therapy. *Annals of Internal Medicine*, **80**, 477.

314 BELL W.R., TOMASULO P.A., ALVING B.M. & DUFFY T.P. (1976) Thrombocytopenia occurring during the administration of heparin. A prospective study of 52 patients. *Annals of Internal Medicine*, **85**, 155.

315 DUGGAN M.L. & MORGAN C. JR (1970) Heparin: a cause of priapism. *Southern Medical Journal*, **63**, 1131.

316 NELSON J.C., LERNER R.G., GOLDSTEIN R. & CAGIN M.A. (1978) Heparin-induced thrombocytopenia. *Archives of Internal Medicine*, **138**, 548.

317 TOWNE J.B., BERNHARD V.M., HUSSEY C., GARANCIS J.C. (1979) White clot syndrome. Peripheral vascular complications of heparin therapy. *Archives of Surgery*, **114**, 372.

318 ZIDAR B.L., MENDELOW H., WINKELSTEIN A. & SHADDUCK R.K. (1975) Diphenylhydantoin-induced serum sickness with fibrin-platelet thrombi in a lymph node microvasculature. *American Journal of Medicine*, **58**, 704.

319 WALLACE D.C. (1951) Diffuse disseminated platelet thrombosis (thrombotic thrombocytopenic purpura) with a report of two cases. *Medical Journal of Australia*, **2**, 9.

320 PARKER J.C. & BARRETT D.A. (1971) Microangiopathic haemolysis and thrombocytopenia related to penicillin drugs. *Archives of Internal Medicine*, **127**, 474.

321 BROWN C.B., CLARKSON A.R., ROBSON J.S., CAMERON J.S., THOMSON D. & OGG C.S. (1973) Haemolytic uraemic syndrome in women taking oral contraceptives. *Lancet*, **i**, 1479.

322 CLAAS F.H.J., VAN DER MEER J.W.M. & LANGERAK J. (1979) Immunological effect of co-trimoxazole on platelets. *British Medical Journal*, **ii**, 898.

323 SULLIVAN L.W. & HERBERT V. (1964) Suppression of haematopoiesis by ethanol. *Journal of Clinical Investigation*, **43**, 2048.

324 SULLIVAN L.W., ADAMS W.H. & YONG K.L. (1977) Induction of thrombocytopenia by thrombophoresis in man: patterns of recovery in normal subjects during ethanol ingestion and abstinence. *Blood*, **49**, 197.

325 DEREN B., MASI R., WEKSLER M. & NACHMAN R.L. (1974) Gold-associated thrombocytopenia. *Archives of Internal Medicine*, **134**, 1012.

326 ARMSTRONG F.B. & SCHERBEL A.L. (1961) Review of toxicity of oxyphenbutazone. *Journal of the American Medical Association*, **175**, 614.

327 HANDLEY A.J. (1971) Thrombocytopenia and LE cells after oxyphenbutazone. *Lancet*, **i**, 245.

328 SIMPSON R.E., GOLDSTEIN V.J., HJELTE G.S. & EVANS E.R. (1978) Acute thrombocytopenia associated with phenoprofen. *New England Journal of Medicine*, **298**, 629.

329 KARPATKIN S. (1971) Drug-induced thrombocytopenia. *American Journal of the Medical Sciences*, **262**, 68.

330 JANOVSKY R.C. (1960) Fatal thrombocytopenic purpura after administration of sulfamethoxypyridazine. *Journal of the American Medical Association*, **172**, 155.

331 SCHWARTZ M.J. & NORTON W.S. II. (1958) Thrombocytopenia and leukopenia associated with the use of sulfamethoxypyridazine. *Journal of the American Medical Association*, **167**, 457.

332 FRIEDMAN A. (1954) An evaluation of chloramphenicol therapy in typhoid fever in children. *Pediatrics*, **14**, 28.

333 BOUTTON E.M. (1955) Thrombocytopenic purpura during chloramphenicol therapy. *British Medical Journal*, **ii**, 106.

334 BROOKS A.P. (1974) Thrombocytopenia during treatment with ampicillin. *Lancet*, **ii**, 723.

335 GLECKMAN R.A. (1975) Trimethoprimsulfamethoxazole vs ampicillin in chronic urinary tract infection. *Journal of the American Medical Association*, **233**, 427.

336 GRALNICK H.R., McGINNES M. & HALTERMAN R. (1972) Thrombocytopenia with sodium cephalothin therapy. *Annals of Internal Medicine*, **77**, 401.

337 SCHIFFER C.A., WEINSTEIN H.J. & WIERNIK P.H. (1976) Methicillin-associated thrombocytopenia. *Annals of Internal Medicine*, **85**, 338.

338 DAY H.J., CONRAD F.G. & MOORE J.E. (1958) Immunothrombocytopenia induced by novobiocin. *American Journal of the Medical Sciences*, **236**, 475.

339 GRACE W.J. (1959) Thrombocytopenia in a patient taking chlorpropamide. *New England Journal of Medicine*, **260**, 711.

340 FITZPATRICK W.J. (1963) Thrombocytopenia occurring during chlorpropamide therapy. *Diabetes*, **12**, 457.

341 MORLEY A. & HIRSH J. (1964) A case of thrombocytopenia associated with chlorpropamide therapy. *Medical Journal of Australia*, **2**, 988.

342 KARPATKIN M., SISKIND G.W. & KARPATKIN S. (1977) The platelet factor 3 immuno injury technique re-evaluated. Development of a rapid test for antiplatelet antibody detection in various clinical disorders, including immunologic drug-induced and neonatal thrombocytopenias. *Journal of Laboratory and Clinical Medicine*, **89**, 400.

343 NIXON D. (1972) Thrombocytopenia following doxepin treatment. *Journal of the American Medical Association*, **220**, 418.

344 KARPATKIN S., STRICK N., KARPATKIN M.B. & SISKIND G.W. (1972) Cumulative experience in the detection of anti-platelet antibody in 234 patients with idiopathic thrombocytopenic purpura, systemic lupus erythematosus and other clinical disorders. *American Journal of Medicine*, **52**, 776.

345 SILBERSTEIN P. (1972) Melleril and thrombocytopenia. *Australian Paediatric Journal*, **8**, 219.

346 TURNER O.A., FISHER C.J. & BERNSTEIN L.L. (1966) Intrathecal sodium diatrizoate. *Neurology*, **16**, 230.

347 JACOBSON E.S. (1972) Fatal immune thrombocytopenia induced by ethchlorvynol. *Annals of Internal Medicine*, **77**, 73.

348 RAWORTH R.E. & BIRCHALL G. (1978) Sodium valproate and platelet-count. *Lancet*, **i**, 671.

349 PEARCE J. & RON M.A. (1968) Thrombocytopenia after carbamazepine. *Lancet*, **ii**, 223.

350 NIEWIG H.O., BOUMA H.G., DeVRIES K. & JANSZ A. (1963) Haematological side effects of some anti-rheumatic drugs. *Annals of Rheumatic Diseases*, **22**, 440.

351 WALES J.K. & WOLFF F. (1967) Haematological side effects of diazoxide. *Lancet*, **i**, 53.

352 YOUNG R.C., NACHMAN R.L. & HOROWITZ H.I. (1966) Thrombocytopenia due to digitoxin. *American Journal of Medicine*, **41**, 605.

353 WANAMAKER W.M., WANAMAKER S.J., CELESIA G.G. & KOELLER J.A. (1976) Thrombocytopenia associated with long-term levodopa therapy. *Journal of the American Medical Association*, **235**, 2217.

354 BENRAAD A.H. & SCHOENAKER A.M. (1965) Thrombocytopenia after use of methyldopa. *Lancet*, **ii**, 292.

355 MANOHITHARAJAH S.M., JENKINS W.J., ROBERTS P.D. & CLARKE R.C. (1971) Methyldopa and associated thrombocytopenia. *British Medical Journal*, **i**, 494.

356 ROTHMAN I.K. & AMOROSI E.L. (1979) Procainamide-induced agranulocytosis and thrombocytopenia. *Archives of Internal Medicine*, **139**, 246.

357 MOHAMED S.T. (1965) Sensitivity reaction to phenindione with urticaria, hepatitis and pancytopenia. *British Medical Journal*, **ii**, 1475.

358 STOFFER R.P. (1966) Adverse drug reaction. Thrombocytopenic purpura due to pronestyl. *Journal of Kansas Medical Society*, **67**, 20.

359 KAUFMAN H.E. & GEISLER P.H. (1960) The hematologic toxicity of pyrimethamine (daraprim) in man. *Archives of Ophthalmology*, **64**, 170.

360 RIVERA J.B., RODRIGUEZ H.F. & PEREZ-SANTIAGO E. (1956) Thrombocytopenic purpura due to fuadin (stibophen). *American Journal of Tropical Medicine and Hygiene*, **5**, 863.

361 STEFANINI M. & HOFFMAN M.N. (1978) Studies on platelets. XXVIII. Acute thrombocytopenic purpura due to lidocaine (xylocaine)-mediated antibody. Report of a case. *American Journal of the Medical Sciences*, **275**, 365.

362 VIPAN W.H. (1865) Quinine as a cause of purpura. *Lancet*, **ii**, 37.

363 COLLINS D.C. (1950) Atypical secondary or symptomatic thrombocytopenic purpura developing with the use of quinidine sulphate. *Circulation*, **2**, 438.

364 BOLTON F.G. & DAMESHEK W. (1956) Thrombocytopenic purpura due to quinidine. I. Clinical studies. *Blood*, **11**, 527.

365 KUTTI J. & WEINFELD A. (1968) The frequency of thrombocytopenia in patients with heart disease treated with oral diuretics. *Acta Medica Scandinavica*, **183**, 245.

366 FLEMING A.F., WARRELL D.A. & DICKMEISS H. (1974) Co-trimoxazole and the blood. *Lancet*, **ii**, 284.

367 LIND D.E., LEVI J.A. & VINCENT P.C. (1973) Amodiaquine-induced agranulocytosis: toxic effect of amodiaquine in bone marrow cultures *in vitro*. *British Medical Journal*, **i**, 458.

368 KISSMEYER-NIELSEN F. (1956) Thrombocytopenic purpura following quinine medication. *Acta Medica Scandinavica*, **154**, 289.

369 ZEIGLER Z., SHADDUCK R.K., WINKELSTEIN A. & STROUPE T.K. (1979) Immune hemolytic anemia and thrombocytopenia secondary to quinidine: *in-vitro* studies of quinidine-dependent red cell and platelet antibodies. *Blood*, **53**, 396.

370 RODRIQUEZ S.U., LEIKIN S.L. & HILLER M.C. (1964) Neonatal thrombocytopenia associated with antepartum administration of thiazide drugs. *New England Journal of Medicine*, **270**, 881.

371 GREENBAUM D. & WENLEY W.G. (1963) Blood dyscrasia with oxyphenbutazone. *British Medical Journal*, **ii**, 385.

372 ACKROYD J.F. (1964) The diagnosis of disorders of the blood due to drug hypersensitivity caused by an immune mechanism. In: *Immunological Methods* (ed. Ackroyd J.F.), p. 453. Blackwell Scientific Publications, Oxford.

373 HARDISTY R.M. & HUTTON R.A. (1965) The kaolin clotting time of platelet-rich plasma. A test of platelet factor-3 availability. *British Journal of Haematology*, **11**, 258.

374 HIRSCHMAN R.J. & SHULMAN N.R. (1973) The use of

platelet serotonin release as a sensitive method for detecting anti-platelet antibodies and the plasma anti-platelet factor in patients with idiopathic thrombocytopenic purpura. *British Journal of Haematology*, **24**, 793.

375 LEVIN H.A., McMILLAN R., TAVASSOLI N., LONGMIRE R.L., YELENOSKY R. & SACKS P.V. (1975) Thrombocytopenia associated with gold therapy. Observations on the mechanism of platelet destruction. *American Journal of Medicine*, **59**, 274.

376 KEKOMAKI R., RAJAMOKI A. & MYLLYLÄ G. (1980) Detection of quinidine-specific antibodies with platelet ^{125}J-labelled staphylococcal protein A test. *Vox Sanguinis*, **38**, 12.

377 MOSS R.A. & CASTRO O. (1973) Platelet transfusion for quinidine-induced thrombocytopenia. *New England Journal of Medicine*, **288**, 522.

378 HOAK J.C. & KOEPKE J.A. (1976) Platelet transfusion. *Clinics in Haematology*, **5**, 69.

379 KULIS J.C. (1965) Chemically induced, selective thrombocytopenic purpura. *Archives of Internal Medicine*, **116**, 559.

380 JENNINGS G.H. & GOWER N.D. (1963) Thrombocytopenic purpura in toluene di-isocyanate workers. *Lancet*, **i**, 406.

381 WHALBERG P. & NYMAN D. (1969) Turpentine and thrombocytopenic purpura. *Lancet*, **ii**, 215.

382 HENRICSSON A., HEDNER U. & BERGENTZ S.-E. (1978) The effect of ALG on coagulation and fibrinolysis. *Thrombosis Research*, **12**, 1099.

383 ROSENBERG J.C., LEKAS M., LYSZ K. & MORRELL R. (1975) Effect of antithymocyte globulin and other immune reactants on human platelets. *Surgery*, **77**, 520.

384 OSKI F.A. & NAIMAN J.L. (1966) The effect of live measles vaccine on the platelet count. *New England Journal of Medicine*, **275**, 352.

385 BACHAND A.J., RUBENSTEIN J. & MORRISON A.N. (1967) Thrombocytopenic purpura following live measles vaccine. *American Journal of Diseases of Children*, **113**, 283.

386 ALTER H.J., SCANLON R.T. & SCHECHTER G.R. (1968) Thrombocytopenic purpura following vaccination with attenuated measles virus. *American Journal of Diseases of Children*, **115**, 111.

387 LANE J.M., RUBEN F.L., NEFF J.M. & MILLAR J.D. (1969) Complications of smallpox vaccination 1968. National Surveillance in the United States. *New England Journal of Medicine*, **281**, 1204.

388 BONNAR J. (1973) Blood coagulation and fibrinolysis in obstetrics. *Clinics in Haematology*, **2**, 213.

389 CORRIGAN J.J. JR & JORDAN C.M. (1970) Heparin therapy in septicemia with disseminated intravascular coagulation. Effect on mortality and on correction of hemostatic defects. *New England Journal of Medicine*, **283**, 778.

390 MINNA J.D., ROBBOY S.J. & COLMAN R.W. (1974) *Disseminated Intravascular Coagulation in Man.* C. C. Thomas. Springfield, Illinois, USA.

391 AL-MONDHIRY H. (1975) Disseminated intravascular coagulation. Experience in a major cancer center. *Thrombosis et Diathesis Haemorrhagica*, **34**, 181.

392 FERNBACH D. & STARLING K.A. (1972) Infectious mononucleosis. *Pediatric Clinics of North America*, **19**, 957.

393 BAYER W.L., SHERMAN F.E., MICHAELS R.H., SZETO I.L.F. & LEWIS J.H. (1965) Purpura in congenital and acquired rubella. *New England Journal of Medicine*, **273**, 1362.

394 TERADA H., BALDINI M., EBBE S. & MEDOFF M. (1966) Interaction of influenza virus with blood platelets. *Blood*, **28**, 213.

395 TURPIE A.G.G., CHERNESKY M.A., LARKE R.P.B., PACKHAM M.A. & MUSTARD J.F. (1973) Effect of Newcastle disease virus on human or rabbit platelets. Aggregation and loss of constituents. *Laboratory Investigation*, **28**, 575.

396 ESPINOZA C. & KUHN C. (1974) Viral infection of megakaryocytes in varicella with purpura. *American Journal of Clinical Pathology*, **61**, 203.

397 KASABACH H.H. & MERRITT K.K. (1940) Capillary hemangioma with extensive purpura. *American Journal of Diseases of Children*, **59**, 1063.

398 WACKSMAN S.J., FLESSA H.C., GLUECK H.I. & WILL J.J. (1966) Coagulation defects in giant cavernous hemangioma: A case study in infancy. *American Journal of Diseases of Children*, **111**, 71.

399 HAGERMAN L.J., CZAPEK E.E., DONNELLAN W.L. & SCHWARTZ A.D. (1975) Giant hemangioma with consumption coagulopathy. *Journal of Pediatrics*, **87**, 766.

399a KUFFER F.R., STARZYNSKI T.E., GIROLAMI A., MURPHY L. & GRABSTALD H. (1968) Klippel–Trenaunay syndrome, visceral angiomatosis and thrombocytopenia. *Journal of Paediatric Surgery*, **3**, 65.

400 MARTINEZ J., SHAPIRO S.S., HOLBURN R.R. & ARABASI R.A. (1973) Hypofibrinogenemia associated with hemangioma of the liver. *American Journal of Clinical Pathology*, **60**, 192.

401 SHANBERGE J.N., TANAKA K. & GRUHL M.C. (1971) Chronic consumption coagulopathy due to hemangiomatous transformation of the spleen. *American Journal of Clinical Pathology*, **56**, 723.

402 MOSCHOWITZ E. (1925) An acute febrile pleiochromic anaemia with hyaline thrombosis of the terminal arterioles and capillaries. An undescribed disease. *Archives of Internal Medicine*, **36**, 89.

403 BUKOWSKI R.M., HEWLETT J.S., HARRIS J.W., HOFFMAN G.C., BATTLE J.D., SILBERBLATT E. & YANG I.-Y. (1976) Exchange transfusions in the treatment of thrombotic thrombocytopenic purpura. *Seminars in Hematology*, **13**, 219.

404 REYNOLDS B.M., JACKSON J.M., BRINE J.S. & VIVIAN A.B. (1976) Thrombotic thrombocytopenic purpura—remission following splenectomy. *American Journal of Medicine*, **61**, 439.

405 WALLACE D.C., LOVRIC A., CLUBB J.S. & CARSELDINE D.B. (1975) Thrombotic thrombocytopenic purpura in four siblings. *American Journal of Medicine*, **58**, 724.

406 WATSON C.G. & COOPER W.M. (1971) Thrombotic thrombocytopenic purpura. Concomitant occurrence in husband and wife. *Journal of the American Medical Association*, **215**, 1821.

407 BROWN R.C., BELCHER T.E., FRENCH E.A. & TOGHILL P.J. (1973) Thrombotic thrombocytopenic purpura after influenza vaccination. *British Medical Journal*, **ii**, 303.

408 FRICK E.G. & HITZIG W.H. (1960) Simultaneous thrombotic thrombocytopenic purpura and agammaglobulinaemia. *Lancet*, **ii**, 1401.

409 AMOROSI E.L. & ULTMANN J.E. (1966) Thrombotic thrombocytopenic purpura: report of 16 cases and a review of the literature. *Medicine* (Baltimore), **45,** 139.

410 USSBAUM M. & DAMESHEK W. (1957) Transient hemolytic and thrombocytopenic episode (acute transient thrombohemolytic thrombocytopenic purpura), with probable meningococcemia. *New England Journal of Medicine,* **256,** 448.

411 REAGAN T.J. & OKAZAKI H. (1974) The thrombotic syndrome associated with carcinoma. *Archives of Neurology,* **31,** 390.

412 KWAAN H.C. (1979) Pathogenesis of thrombotic thrombocytopenic purpura. *Seminars in Thrombosis and Hemostasis,* **5,** 184.

413 ORBISON J.L. (1952) Morphology of thrombotic thrombocytopenic purpura with demonstration of aneurysms. *American Journal of Pathology,* **28,** 129.

414 CRAIG J.M. & GITLIN D. (1957) The nature of the hyaline thrombi in thrombotic thrombocytopenic purpura. *American Journal of Pathology,* **33,** 251.

415 NEAME P.B., LECHAGO J., LING E.T. & KOVAL A. (1973) Thrombotic thrombocytopenic purpura: A report of a case with disseminated intravascular platelet aggregation. *Blood,* **42,** 805.

416 KWAAN H.C., GALLO G., POTTER E.V., CUTTING H. & STANZLER R. (1968) The nature of the vascular lesion in thrombotic thrombocytopenic purpura. *Annals of Internal Medicine,* **68,** 1169.

417 MANT M.J., CAUCHI M.N. & MEDLEY G. (1972) Thrombotic thrombocytopenic purpura: report of a case with possible immune etiology. *Blood,* **40,** 416.

418 REMUZZI G., MISIANA R., MECCA G., DE GAETANO G. & DONATI M.B. (1978) Thrombotic thrombocytopenic purpura—a deficiency of plasma factors regulating platelet-vessel-wall interaction. *New England Journal of Medicine,* **299,** 311.

419 LIAN E.C.-Y., HARKNESS D.R., BYRNES J.J., WALLACH H. & NUNEZ R. (1979) Presence of a platelet aggregating factor in the plasma of patients with thrombotic thrombocytopenic purpura (TTP) and its inhibition by normal plasma. *Blood,* **53,** 333.

420 ANSELL J.E., SLEPCHUK J.I. JR & PECHET L. (1979) Letter. *Blood,* **54,** 959.

421 NEAME P.B. & HIRSH J. (1978) Circulating immune complexes in thrombotic thrombocytopenic purpura (TTP). *Blood,* **51,** 559.

422 LERNER R.G., RAPAPORT S.I. & MELTZER J. (1967) Thrombotic thrombocytopenic purpura—serial clotting studies, relation to the generalised Shwartzman reaction and remission after adrenal steroid and dextran therapy. *Annals of Internal Medicine,* **66,** 1180.

423 JAFFE E.A., NACHMAN R.L. & MERSKEY C. (1973) Thrombotic thrombocytopenic purpura—coagulation parameters in twelve patients. *Blood,* **42,** 499.

424 BRAIN M.C., DACIE J.V. & HOURIHANE D.O. (1962) Microangiopathic haemolytic anaemia. The possible role of vascular lesions in pathogenesis. *British Journal of Haematology,* **8,** 358.

425 CAHALANE S.F. & HORN R.C. (1959) Thrombotic thrombocytopenic purpura of long duration. *American Journal of Medicine,* **27,** 333.

426 BONE R.C., HENRY J.E., PETTERSON J. & AMARE M. (1978) Respiratory dysfunction in thrombotic thrombo-cytopenic purpura. *American Journal of Medicine,* **65,** 262.

427 BLECHER T.E. & RAPER A.B. (1967) Early diagnosis of thrombotic microangiopathy by paraffin sections of aspirated bone marrow. *Archives of Disease in Childhood,* **42,** 158.

428 ALCORN M.O. JR & FADELL E.J. (1961) A note on the antemortem histologic diagnosis of thrombotic thrombocytopenic purpura. *American Journal of Clinical Pathology,* **35,** 546.

429 GOODMAN A., RAMOS R., PETRELLI M., HIRSCH S.A., BUKOWSKI R. & HARRIS J.W. (1978) Gingival biopsy in thrombotic thrombocytopenic purpura. *Annals of Internal Medicine,* **89,** 501.

430 JOBIN F. & DE LARGE J.M. (1970) Aspirin and prednisolone in microangiopathic haemolytic anaemia. *Lancet,* **ii,** 208.

431 ZACHARSKI L.R., WALWORTH C. & MCINTYRE O.R. (1971) Antiplatelet therapy for thrombotic thrombocytopenic purpura. *New England Journal of Medicine,* **285,** 408.

432 AMOROSI E.L. & KARPATKIN S. (1977) Antiplatelet treatment of thrombotic thrombocytopenic purpura. *Annals of Internal Medicine,* **86,** 102.

433 RUBENSTEIN M.A., KEGAN E.M., MACGILVRAY M.H., RUBEN M. & SACKS H. (1959) Unusual remission in a case of thrombotic thrombocytopenic purpura syndrome following fresh blood exchange and transfusion. *Annals of Internal Medicine,* **51,** 1419.

434 BUKOWSKI R.M., KING J.W. & HEWLETT J.S. (1977) Plasmapheresis in the treatment of thrombotic thrombocytopenic purpura. *Blood,* **50,** 413.

435 RYAN P.F.J., COOPER I.A. & FIRKIN B.G. (1979) Plasmapheresis in the treatment of thrombotic thrombocytopenic purpura: A report of five cases. *Medical Journal of Australia,* **1,** 69.

436 BYRNES J.J. & KHURANA M. (1977) Treatment of thrombotic thrombocytopenic purpura with plasma. *New England Journal of Medicine,* **297,** 1386.

437 GASSER C., GAUTIER E., STECK A., SIEBENMANN R.E. & OCHSLIN R. (1955) Hämolytisch-urämische syndrome: Bilaterale Nierenrindennekrosen bei akuten erworbenen hämolytischen Anämien. *Schweizer Medizinische Wochenschrift,* **85,** 905.

438 LIEBERMAN E. (1972) Hemolytic-uremic syndrome. *Journal of Pediatrics,* **80,** 1.

439 KAPLAN B.S., CHESNEY R.W. & DRUMMOND K.N. (1975) Hemolytic uremic syndrome in families. *New England Journal of Medicine,* **292,** 1090.

440 FARR M.J., ROBERTS S., MORLEY A.R., DEWAR T.J., ROBERTS B.F. & ULDALL P.R. (1975) The haemolytic-uraemic syndrome—a family study. *Quarterly Journal of Medicine,* **44,** 161.

441 GLASGOW L.A. & BALDUZZI P. (1965) Isolation of Coxsackie virus group A type 4 from a patient with hemolytic uremic syndrome. *New England Journal of Medicine,* **273,** 754.

442 DAVIDSON A.M., THOMSON D. & ROBSON J.S. (1973) Intravascular coagulation complicating influenza A2 infection. *British Medical Journal,* **i,** 654.

443 AUSTIN T.W. & RAY C.G. (1973) Coxsackie virus group B infections and haemolytic-uraemic syndrome. *Journal of Infectious Diseases,* **127,** 698.

444 KOSTER F., LEVIN J., WALKER L., TUNG K.S.K., GILMAN R.H., RAHAMAN M.M., MAJID M.A., ISLAM S. & WILLIAMS R.C. JR (1978) Hemolytic-uremic syndrome after shigellosis. Relation to endotoxemia and circulating immune complexes. *New England Journal of Medicine,* **298,** 927.

445 MCKAY D.B. & WAHLE G.H. JR (1955) Epidemic gastroenteritis due to Escherichia coli O111B4. *Archives of Pathology,* **60,** 679.

446 RAPAPORT S.E., TATTER D., COEUR-BARROW N. & HJORT, P.F. (1964) Pseudomonas septicemia with intravascular clotting leading to the generalised Shwartzman reaction. *New England Journal of Medicine,* **271,** 80.

447 ROBSON J.S., MARTIN A.M., RUCKLEY D.A. & MAC-DONALD M.K. (1968) Irreversible post-partum renal failure. *Quarterly Journal of Medicine,* **37,** 423.

448 CLARKSON A.R., MEADOW R. & LAWRENCE J.R. (1969) Post-partum renal failure? The generalised Shwartzman reaction. *Australasian Annals of Medicine,* **18,** 209.

449 LIEBERMAN E., HEUSER E., DONNELL G.N., LANDING D.H. & HAMMOND G.C. (1966) Hemolytic-uremic syndrome: clinical and pathological considerations. *New England Journal of Medicine,* **275,** 227.

450 HAMMOND D. & LIEBERMAN E. (1970) The hemolytic uremic syndrome: renal cortical thrombotic microangiopathy. *Archives of Internal Medicine,* **126,** 816.

451 MCCOY R.C., ABRAMOWSKY C.R. & KRUEGER R. (1974) The hemolytic-uremic syndrome with positive immunofluorescent studies. *Journal of Pediatrics,* **85,** 170.

452 BARRE P., KAPLAN B.S., DE CHADAREVIAN J.P. & DRUMMOND K.N. (1977) Hemolytic-uremic syndrome with hypocomplementemia serum C3 NeF, and glomerular deposits of C3. *Archives of Pathology and Laboratory Medicine,* **101,** 357.

453 KIM Y., MILLER K. & MICHAEL A.F. (1977) Breakdown products of C3 and Factor B in hemolytic-uremic syndrome. *Journal of Laboratory and Clinical Medicine,* **89,** 845.

453a REMUZZI G., MISIANI R., MARCHESI D., LIVIO M., MECCA G., DE GAETANO G. & DONATI M.B. (1978) Hypothesis: haemolytic-uraemic syndrome: deficiency of plasma factor(s) regulating prostacyclin activity? *Lancet,* **ii,** 871.

453b REMUZZI G., MARCHESI R., MISIANI R., MECCA G., DE GAETANO G. & DONATI M.B. (1979) Familial deficiency of a plasma factor stimulating vascular prostacyclin activity. *Thrombosis Research,* **16,** 517.

453c REMUZZI G., MECCA G., LIVIO M., DE GAETANO G., DONATI M.B., PEARSON J.D. & GORDON J.L. (1980) Prostacyclin generation by cultured endothelial cells in haemolytic uraemic syndrome. *Lancet,* **i,** 656.

454 KATZ J., LURIE A., KAPLAN B.S., KRAWITZ S. & METZ J. (1971) Coagulation findings in the hemolytic-uremic syndrome of infancy: similarity to hyperacute renal allograft rejection. *Journal of Pediatrics,* **78,** 426.

455 GIANANTONIO C.A., VITACCO M., MENDELAHARZU J., MENDELAHARZU F. & RUTTY A. (1962) Acute renal failure in infancy and childhood. Clinical course and treatment in 41 patients. *Journal of Pediatrics,* **61,** 660.

456 TUNE B.M., LEAVITT T.J. & GRIBBLE T.J. (1973) Hemolytic-uremic syndrome in California: A review of twenty-eight non-heparinised cases with long-term follow up. *Journal of Pediatrics,* **82,** 304.

457 GOLDSTEIN M.H., CHURG J., STRAUSS L. & GRIBETZ D. (1979) Hemolytic-uremic syndrome. *Nephron,* **23,** 263.

458 KAPLAN B.S. (1977) Hemolytic uremic syndrome with recurrent episodes: an important subset. *Clinical Nephrology,* **8,** 495.

459 VITACCO M., AVALOS J.S. & GIANANTONIO C.A. (1973) Heparin therapy in the hemolytic-uremic syndrome. *Journal of Pediatrics,* **83,** 271.

460 PIEL C.F. & PHIBBS R.H. (1966) Hemolytic-uremic syndrome. *Pediatric Clinics of North America,* **13,** 295.

461 MONNENS L.A.H. (1973) Localized intravascular coagulation. *Postgraduate Medical Journal,* **49** (Suppl. 5), 102.

462 POWELL H.R. & EKERT H. (1974) Streptokinase and anti-thrombotic therapy in the hemolytic-uremic syndrome. *Journal of Pediatrics,* **84,** 345.

463 ARENSON G.B. & AUGUST C.S. (1975) Preliminary report. Treatment of the hemolytic-uremic syndrome with aspirin and dipyridamole. *Journal of Pediatrics,* **86,** 957.

464 THORSEN C.A., ROSSI E.C., GREEN D. & CARONE F.A. (1979) The treatment of the hemolytic-uremic syndrome with inhibitors of platelet function. *American Journal of Medicine,* **66,** 711.

465 OWEN C.A. JR, GOLDSTEIN N.P. & BOWIE E.J.W. (1976) Platelet function and coagulation in patients with Wilson's disease. *Archives of Internal Medicine,* **136,** 148.

466 SPIERS A.S.D., BAIKIE A.G., GALTON D.A.G., RICHARDS H.G.H., WILTSHAW E., GOLDMAN J.M., CATOVSKY D., SPENCER J. & PETO R. (1975) Chronic granulocytic leukaemia: effect of elective splenectomy on the course of disease. *British Medical Journal,* **i,** 175.

467 HEUSERMANN U. & STUTTS H.J. (1977) Aetiology of the thrombocytopenia in vinyl chloride disease. *Blut,* **35,** 317.

468 COLLINS J.A. (1976) Massive blood transfusion. *Clinics in Haematology,* **5,** 201.

469 MCNAMARA J.J., BURRAN E.L., STREMPLE J.F. & MOLOT M.D. (1972) Coagulopathy after major combat injury: Occurrence, management and pathophysiology. *Annals of Surgery,* **176,** 243.

470 LIM R.C., OLCOTT C., ROBINSON A. & BLAISDELL F.W. (1973) Platelet response and coagulation changes following massive blood replacement. *Journal of Trauma,* **13,** 577.

471 MASON R.G., MOHAMMAD S.F., CHUANG H.Y.K. & RICHARDSON P.D. (1976) The adhesion of platelets to subendothelial, collagen and artificial surfaces. *Seminars in Thrombosis and Hemostasis,* **3,** 98.

472 DUTTON R.C., BAIER R.E., DEDRICK R.L. & BOWMAN R.L. (1968) Initial thrombus formation on foreign surfaces. *Transactions of the American Society of Artificial Internal Organs,* **14,** 57.

473 SCARBOROUGH D.E., MASON R.G., DALLDORF F.G. & BRINKHOUS K.M. (1969) Morphologic manifestations of blood–solid interfacial reactions. *Laboratory Investigation,* **20,** 164.

474 BICK R.L., SCHMALHORST W.R. & ARBEGAST M.R. (1976) Alterations of haemostasis associated with cardiopulmonary bypass. *Thrombosis Research,* **8,** 285.

475 STASS S., BISHOP C., FOSBERG R., HARTLEY M. & CRAMER A. (1976) Platelets as affected by cardiopul-

monary bypass. *Transactions of the American Society of Clinical Pathology*, Dallas, p. 35.

476 ADDONIZIO V.P., SMITH J.B., GUIOD L.R., STRAUSS J.F., COLMAN R.W. & EDMUNDS L.H. (1979) Thromboxane synthesis and platelet protein release during simulated extracorporeal circulation. *Blood*, **54**, 371.

477 LONGMORE D.B., BENNETT G., GUEIRRA D., SMITH M., BUNTING S., MONCADA S., REED P., READ N.G. & VANE J.R. (1979) Prostacyclin: a solution to some problems of extracorporeal circulation. Experiments in greyhounds. *Lancet*, **i**, 1002.

478 GIMSON A.E.S., LANGLEY P.G., HUGHES R.D., CANALESE J., MELLON P.J., WILLIAMS R., WOODS H.F. & WESTON M.J. (1980) Prostacyclin to prevent platelet activation during charcoal haemoperfusion in fulminant hepatic failure. *Lancet*, **i**, 173.

479 PORTER J.N. & SILVER D. (1968) Alterations in fibrinolysis and coagulation associated with cardiopulmonary bypass. *Journal of Thoracic and Cardiovascular Surgery*, **56**, 869.

480 BICK R.L. (1976) Alterations of hemostasis associated with cardiopulmonary bypass: pathophysiology, prevention, diagnosis and management. *Seminars in Thrombosis and Hemostasis*, **3**, 59.

481 MULLER N., POPOV-CENIC S., BUTTNER W., KLADETSKY R.G. & EGLI H. (1975) Studies of fibrinolytic and coagulation factors during open-heart surgery. II. Postoperative bleeding tendencies and changes in the coagulation system. *Thrombosis Research*, **7**, 589.

482 KEVY S.V., GLICKMAN R.M., BERNHARD W.F., DIAMOND L. & GROSS R. (1966) The pathogenesis and control of the hemorrhagic defect in open-heart surgery. *Journal of Surgery, Gynecology and Obstetrics*, **123**, 313.

483 SIGNORI E.E., PENNER J.A. & KAHN D.R. (1969) Coagulation defects and bleeding in open heart surgery. *Annals of Thoracic Surgery*, **8**, 521.

484 MCKENZIE F.N., DHALL D.P., ARFORS K.-E., NORDLUND S. & MATHESON N.A. (1969) Blood platelet behaviour during and after open heart surgery. *British Medical Journal*, **ii**, 795.

485 URBANIAK S.J. & CASH J.D. (1977) Blood replacement therapy. *British Medical Bulletin*, **33**, 273.

486 KISKER C.T., STRAUSS R.G., KOEPKE J.A., MAGUIRE L.D. & THOMPSON J.S. (1979) The effects of combined platelet and leukapheresis on the blood coagulation system. *Transfusion*, **19**, 173.

487 WILLIAMS D.M., LYNCH R.E. & CARTWRIGHT G.E. (1973) Drug-induced aplastic anemia. *Seminars in Hematology*, **10**, 195.

488 GRINER P.L. & HOYER L.W. (1970) Amegakaryocytic thrombocytopenia in systemic lupus erythematosus. *Archives of Internal Medicine*, **125**, 328.

489 FOX R.M. & FIRKIN F.C. (1978) Sequential pure red cell and megakaryocyte aplasia associated with chronic liver disease and ulcerative colitis. *American Journal of Hematology*, **4**, 79.

490 LEWIS S.M. (1965) Course and prognosis in aplastic anaemia. *British Medical Journal*, **i**, 1027.

491 DACIE J.V. (1967) *The Haemolytic Anaemias: Congenital and Acquired, Part IV*, 2nd edn, p. 1128. Churchill Livingstone, London.

492 GARDNER F.H. & MURPHY S. (1972) Granulocyte and platelet functions in proxysmal nocturnal haemoglobinuria. *Series Haematologica*, **5**, 78.

493 STEINBERG D., CARVALHO A.C., CHESNEY C. & COLMAN R.W. (1975) Platelet hypersensitivity and intravascular coagulation in paroxysmal nocturnal hemoglobinuria. *American Journal of Medicine*, **59**, 845.

494 HAN T., STUTZMAN L., COUHEN E. & KIM U. (1966) Effect of platelet transfusion on haemorrhage in patients with acute leukaemia. *Cancer*, **19**, 1937.

495 SMITH I.E., POWLES R., CLINK H.M., JAMESON B., KAY H.E.M. & MCELWAIN T.J. (1977) Early deaths in acute myelogenous leukemia. *Cancer*, **39**, 1710.

496 HERSH E.M., BODEY G.P., NIES B.A. & FREIREICH E.J. (1965) Causes of death in acute leukemia. A 10 year study of 414 patients from 1954–1963. *Journal of the American Medical Association*, **193**, 105.

497 HOLT J.M. & GORDON-SMITH E.G. (1969) Retinal abnormalities in diseases of the blood. *British Journal of Ophthalmology*, **53**, 145.

498 COWAN D.M. & HAUT M.J. (1972) Platelet function in acute leukemia. *Journal of Laboratory and Clinical Medicine*, **79**, 893.

499 ROSNER F., DOBBS J.V., RITZ D.M. & LEE S.L. (1970) Disturbances of hemostasis in acute myeloblastic leukemia. *Acta Haematologica* (Basle), **43**, 65.

500 COWAN D.H., GRAHAM R.C. & BAUNACH D. (1975) The platelet defect in leukemia. Platelet ultrastructure, adenine nucleotide metabolism, and the release reaction. *Journal of Clinical Investigation*, **56**, 188.

501 LINMAN J.W. & BAGBY G.C. (1976) The preleukaemic syndrome: clinical and laboratory features, natural course, and management. *Blood Cells*, **2**, 11.

502 MALDONADO J.E. (1975) Giant platelet granules in refractory anaemia (preleukaemia) and myelomonocytic leukaemia: a cell marker? *Blood Cells*, **1**, 129.

503 LISIEWICZ J. (1978) Mechanisms of hemorrhage in leukemias. *Seminars in Thrombosis and Hemostasis*, **4**, 241.

504 CARDAMONE J.M., EDSON R., MCARTHUR J.R. & JACOB H.S. (1972) Abnormalities in platelet function in the myeloproliferative disorders. *Journal of the American Medical Association*, **221**, 270.

505 TEN BENSEL R.W., STADLAN E.M. & KRIVIT W. (1966) The development of malignancy in the course of the Aldrich syndrome. *Journal of Pediatrics*, **68**, 761.

506 OCHS H.D., SLICHTER S.J., HARKER L.A., VAN BOHRENS W.E., CLARK R.A. & WEDGWOOD R.J. (1980) The Wiskott–Aldrich syndrome: studies of lymphocytes, granulocytes and platelets. *Blood*, **55**, 243.

507 MURPHY S., OSKI F.A. & NAIMAN J.L. (1972) Platelet size and kinetics in hereditary and acquired thrombocytopenia. *New England Journal of Medicine*, **286**, 499.

508 GRÖTTUM K.A., HOVIG T., HOLMSEN H., ABRAHAMSEN A.F., JEREMIC M. & SEIP M. (1969) Wiskott–Aldrich syndrome: qualitative defects and short platelet survival. *British Journal of Haematology*, **17**, 373.

509 LUSHER J.M. & BARNHART M.I. (1977) Congenital disorders affecting platelets. *Seminars in Thrombosis and Hemostasis*, **4**, 123.

510 BACH F.H., ALBERTINI R.J., JOO P., ANDERSON J.T. & BORTIN M.M. (1968) Bone marrow transplantation in a patient with Wiskott–Aldrich Syndrome. *Lancet*, **i**, 1364.

511 MEUWISSEN H.J., KIESERMAN M.A., TAFT E.G., POL-
LARA B. & PICKERING J. (1978) Marrow transplantation
in Wiskott–Aldrich syndrome: T-cell engraftment with
cyclophosphamide, complete engraftment with total
body irradiation. (Abstract.) *Pediatric Research*, **12**,
482.

512 PARKMAN R., RAPPEPORT J., GEHA R., BELLI J., CAS-
SADY R., LEVEY R., NATHAN D.G. & ROSEN F.S. (1978)
Complete correction of the Wiskott–Aldrich syndrome
by allogeneic bone-marrow transplantation. *New England Journal of Medicine*, **298**, 921.

513 LAWTON A.R. & COOPER M.D. (1977) Immune defi-
ciency diseases. In: *Harrison's Principles of Internal
Medicine* (ed. Thorn G.W., Adams R.D., Brunwald E.,
Isselbacher K.J. & Petersdorf R.G.), p. 402. McGraw-
Hill, New York.

514 SPITLER L.E. (1979) Transfer factor therapy in the
Wiskott–Aldrich syndrome. Results of long term follow-up in 32 patients. *American Journal of Medicine*, **67**,
59.

515 PAHWA S. (1976) Review of thymus transplants. In:
*International Co-operative Group for Bone Marrow
Transplantation in Man*. Third Workshop. Tarytown,
New York.

516 MURPHY S. (1972) Hereditary thrombocytopenia.
Clinics in Haematology, **1**, 359.

517 LUM L.G., TUBERGEN D.G., CORASH L. & BLAESE R.M.
(1980) Splenectomy in the management of the thrombocytopenia of the Wiskott–Aldrich syndrome. *New England Journal of Medicine*, **302**, 892.

518 BUCHANAN J.G., PEARCE L. & WETHERLEY-MEIN G.
(1964) The May–Hegglin anomaly: a family report and
chromosome study. *British Journal of Haematology*, **10**,
508.

519 CAWLEY J.C. & HAYHOE F.G.J. (1972) The inclusions of
the May–Hegglin anomaly and Dohle bodies of infection: an ultrastructural comparison. *British Journal of
Haematology*, **22**, 491.

520 WHITE J.G. & GERRARD J.M. (1976) Ultrastructural
features of abnormal blood platelets. *American Journal
of Pathology*, **83**, 590.

521 GODWIN H.A. & GINSBERG A.D. (1971) May–Hegglin
anomaly: ? defect in megakaryocyte fragmentation.
*Fourteenth Annual Meeting of the American Society of
Hematology*, San Francisco. Abstract 279.

522 NAJEAN Y. (1966) Le syndrome de Hegglin. *Presse
Médicale*, **74**, 1649.

523 WOODFIELD D.G. (1974) The May–Hegglin anomaly.
An account of a New Zealand family. In: *Platelets* (ed.
Ulutin O.N.), Excerpta Medica Amsterdam Interna-
tional Congress Series, **357**, 221.

524 HALL J.G., LEVIN J., KUHN J.P., OTTENHEIMER E.J., VAN
BERKUM K.A.P. & MCKUSICK V. (1969) Thrombocytopenia with absent radius. *Medicine* (Baltimore), **48**,
411.

525 SULTAN Y., SCROBOHACI M.L., RENDU F. & CAEN J.P.
(1972) Abnormal platelet function, population and
survival time in a boy with congenital absent radii and
thrombocytopenia. *Lancet*, **ii**, 653.

526 ZAHAVI J., GALE R. & SACKS Z. (1977) Storage pool
disease of platelets in an infant with thrombocytopenic
absent radii syndrome simulating Fanconi anaemia.
Thrombosis and Haemostasis, **38**, 283.

527 SEIP M. (1963) Hereditary hypoplastic thrombocytopenia. *Acta Paediatrica Scandinavica*, **52**, 370.

528 SHETH N.K. & PRANKERD T.A.J. (1968) Inherited
thrombocytopenia with thrombasthenia. *Journal of
Clinical Pathology*, **21**, 154.

529 LIBANSKA J., FALCÃO L., GAUTIER A., AMMON J., SPAHR
A., VAINER H. & CAEN J. (1975) Thrombocytopénie
thrombocytopathique hypogranulaire héréditaire. *Nouvelle Revue française d'Hématologie*, **15**, 182.

530 KURSTJENS R., BOLT C., VOSSEN M. & HAANEN C. (1968)
Familial thrombopathic thrombocytopenia. *British
Journal of Haematology*, **15**, 305.

531 ARDLIE N.G., COUPLAND W.W. & SCHOEFL G.I. (1976)
Hereditary thrombocytopathy: a familial bleeding dis-
order due to impaired platelet coagulant activity.
Australian and New Zealand Journal of Medicine, **6**, 37.

532 EPSTEIN C.J., SAHUD M.A., PIEL C.F., GOODMAN J.R.,
BERNFIELD M.R., KUSHNER J.H. & ABLIN A.R. (1972)
Hereditary macrothrombocytopathia, nephritis and
deafness. *American Journal of Medicine*, **52**, 299.

533 BERNHEIM J., DE CHAVANNE M., BRYON P.A., LAGARDE
M., COLON S., POZET N. & TRAGER J. (1976) Thrombocytopenia, macrothrombocytopathia, nephritis and
deafness. *American Journal of Medicine*, **61**, 145.

534 YANKEE R.A., GRUMET F.C. & ROGENTINE G.N. (1969)
Platelet transfusion therapy. The selection of compatible platelet donors for refractory patients by lymphocyte HL-A typing. *New England Journal of Medicine*,
281, 1208.

535 WU K.K., HOAK J.C., THOMPSON J.S. & KOEPKE J.A.
(1975) Use of platelet aggregometry in the selection of
compatible platelet donors. *New England Journal of
Medicine*, **292**, 130.

536 GOCKERMAN J.P., BOWMAN R.P. & CONRAD M.E.
(1975) Detection of platelet isoantibodies by '³H' serotonin platelet release and its clinical application to the
problem of platelet matching. *Journal of Clinical Investigation*, **55**, 75.

537 SHIFFER C.A., AISNER J. & WIERNIK P.H. (1978) Frozen
autologous platelet transfusion for patients with leukemia. *New England Journal of Medicine*, **299**, 7.

538 MURPHY S. (1976) Platelet transfusion. *Progress in
Hemostasis and Thrombosis*, **3**, 289.

539 CUNNINGHAM M. & CASH J.D. (1973) Bacterial contamination of platelet concentrates stored at 20°C.
Journal of Clinical Pathology, **26**, 401.

540 HERZIG R.H., POPLACK D.G. & YANKEE R.A. (1974)
Prolonged granulocytopenia from incompatible platelet
transfusions. *New England Journal of Medicine*, **290**,
1220.

541 GOLDFINGER D. & MCGINNISS M.H. (1971) Rh-incompatible platelet transfusions—risks and consequences of
sensitising immunosuppressed patients. *New England
Journal of Medicine*, **284**, 942.

542 SIMONE J.V. (1971) Use of fresh blood components
during intensive combination therapy of childhood
leukemia. *Cancer*, **28**, 562.

543 HIGBY D.J., COHEN E., HOLLAND J.F. & SINKS L. (1974)
The prophylactic treatment of thrombocytopenic leu-
kemia patients with platelets: a double blind study.
Transfusion, **14**, 440.

544 THOMAS E.D., STORB R., CLIFT R.A., FEFER A., JOHN-
SON F.L., NEIMAN P.E., LERNER K.G., GLUCKSBERG H.

& BUCKNER C.D. (1975) Bone marrow transplantation. *New England Journal of Medicine*, **292**, 832.

545 GINSBURG A.D. (1975) Platelet function in patients with high counts. *Annals of Internal Medicine*, **82**, 506.

546 McCLURE P.D., INGRAM G.I.C., STACEY R.S., GLASS U.H. & MATCHETT M.D. (1966) Platelet function test in thrombocythaemia and thrombocytosis. *British Journal of Haematology*, **12**, 478.

547 ZUCKER S. & MIELKE C.H. (1972) Classification of thrombocytosis based on platelet function tests: correlations with hemorrhagic and thrombotic complications. *Journal of Laboratory and Clinical Medicine*, **80**, 385.

548 NEEMEH J.A., BOWIE E.J.W., THOMPSON J.H., DIDISHEIM P. & OWEN C.A. (1972) Quantitation of platelet aggregation in myeloproliferative disorders. *American Journal of Clinical Pathology*, **57**, 336.

549 LEVIN J. & CONLEY C.L. (1964) Thrombocytosis associated with malignant disease. *Archives of Internal Medicine*, **114**, 497.

550 SPIGEL S.C. & MOONEY L.R. (1977) Extreme thrombocytosis associated with malignancy. *Cancer*, **39**, 339.

551 MOROWITZ D.A., ALLEN L.W. & KIRSNER J.B. (1968) Thrombocytosis in chronic inflammatory bowel disease. *Annals of Internal Medicine*, **68**, 1013.

552 NELSON E.W., ERTAN A., BROOKS F.P. & CERDA J.J. (1976) Thrombocytosis in patients with celiac sprue. *Gastroenterology*, **70**, 1042.

553 DAWBARN R.Y., EARLAM F. & HOWEL EVANS W. (1928) The relation of the blood platelets to thrombosis after operation and parturition. *Journal of Pathology and Bacteriology*, **31**, 833.

554 FORBES-GALLOWAY J. (1931) The blood platelet after fracture. *Lancet*, **i**, 1032.

555 INNES D. & SEVITT S. (1964) Coagulation and fibrinolysis in injured patients. *Journal of Clinical Pathology*, **17**, 1.

556 MUSTARD J.F. (1957) Changes in platelet levels of nontransfused patients following surgical operation. *Acta Haematologica*, **17**, 257.

557 ENTICKNAP J.B., LANSLEY T.S. & DAVIS T. (1970) Reduction in platelet size with increase in circulating numbers in the post-operative period and a comparison of the glass bead and rotating bulb method for detecting changes in function. *Journal of Clinical Pathology*, **23**, 140.

558 BENSINGER T.A., LOGUE G.L. & RUNDLES R.W. (1970) Hemorrhagic thrombocythemia: control of postsplenectomy thrombocytosis with melphalan. *Blood*, **36**, 61.

559 DINCOL K. & AKSOY M. (1969) On the platelet levels in chronic iron deficiency anemia. *Acta Haematologica*, **41**, 135.

560 SCHLOESSER L.L., KIPP M.A. & WENZEL F.J. (1965) Thrombocytosis in iron deficiency anemia. *Journal of Laboratory and Clinical Medicine*, **66**, 107.

561 GROSS M.A., KEEFER V. & NEWMAN A.J. (1964) The platelets in iron deficiency anemia. I. The response to oral iron and parenteral iron. *Journal of Pediatrics*, **34**, 315.

562 CHOI S.I., SIMONE J.V. & JACKSON C.W. (1974) Mega-

karyocytopoiesis in experimental iron deficiency anemia. *Blood*, **43**, 111.

563 DESFORGES J.F., BIGELOW F.S. & CHALMERS T.C. (1954) The effects of massive gastrointestinal hemorrhage on hemostasis. *Journal of Laboratory and Clinical Medicine*, **43**, 501.

564 OGSTON D. & DAWSON A.A. (1969) Thrombocytosis following thrombocytopenia in man. *Postgraduate Medical Journal*, **45**, 754.

565 OGSTON D., DAWSON A.A. & PHILIP J.F. (1968) Methotrexate and the platelet count. *British Journal of Cancer*, **22**, 244.

566 COWAN D.H. & HINES J.D. (1971) Thrombocytopenia of severe alcoholism. *Annals of Internal Medicine*, **74**, 37.

567 HASELAGER E.N. & VREEKEN J. (1977) Rebound thrombocytosis after alcohol abuse: a possible factor in the pathogenesis of thromboembolic disease. *Lancet*, **i**, 774.

568 ROBERTS J.H. & McCARTHY G.M. (1969) Periwinkle alkaloids and the platelet count. *Lancet*, **i**, 353.

569 CHOI S.I., SIMONE J.V. & EDWARDS C.C. (1974) Effects of vincristine on platelet production. In: *Platelets: Production, Function, Transfusion and Storage* (ed. Baldini M. & Ebbe S.), p. 51. Grune & Stratton, New York.

570 EBBE S., HOWARD D., PHALEN E. & STOHLMAN F. (1975) Effects of vincristine on normal and stimulated megakaryocytopoiesis in the rat. *British Journal of Haematology*, **29**, 593.

571 JACKSON C.W. & EDWARDS C.C. (1977) Evidence that stimulation of megakaryocytopoiesis by low dose vincristine results from an effect on platelets. *British Journal of Haematology*, **36**, 97.

572 RAK K. (1972) Effect of vincristine on platelet production in mice. *British Journal of Haematology*, **22**, 617.

573 KLENER P., MARCIPAL O., DONNER L. & KORNALIK F. (1977) Serum thrombopoietic activity following administration of vinblastine. *Scandinavian Journal of Haematology*, **19**, 287.

574 COLMAN W., SIEBERG C.A. & PUGH R.P. (1966) Thrombocytopheresis: a rapid and effective approach to symptomatic thrombocytosis. *Journal of Laboratory and Clinical Medicine*, **68**, 389.

575 BOXER M.A., BRAUN J. & ELLMAN L. (1978) Thromboembolic risk of postsplenectomy thrombocytosis. *Archives of Surgery*, **113**, 808.

576 WU K.K. (1978) Platelet hyperaggregability and thrombosis in patients with thrombocythemia. *Annals of Internal Medicine*, **88**, 7.

577 WALSH P.N., MURPHY S. & BARRY W.E. (1977) The role of platelets in the pathogenesis of thrombosis and hemorrhage in patients with thrombocytosis. *Thrombosis and haemostasis*, **38**, 1085.

578 INTERNATIONAL MULTICENTRE TRIAL (1975) Prevention of fatal postoperative pulmonary embolism by low doses of heparin. *Lancet*, **ii**, 45.

579 MUSTARD J.F. & PACKHAM M.A. (1975) The role of blood platelets in atherosclerosis and complications of atherosclerosis. *Thrombosis et Diathesis Haemorrhagica*, **33**, 444.

Chapter 26
Platelets, blood vessels and haemostasis: disorders of platelet and vascular function

R. M. HARDISTY

The term haemostasis is usually taken to apply to the arrest of haemorrhage from damaged blood vessels, but may usefully be extended to include the prevention of leakage of red cells from small vessels which are apparently uninjured. Both mechanisms involve interaction between platelets and components of the vessel wall, and both are considered here. Pathological extension of similar platelet–vessel-wall interactions within the lumen of the vessel leads to thrombosis, which is the subject of Chapter 30. The haemodynamic effects of vascular injury include the pressure changes resulting from the accumulation of blood in the tissues and the central and peripheral control of blood flow; while these obviously contribute to the haemostatic mechanism, their detailed consideration is outside the scope of this book.

BLOOD VESSELS AND HAEMOSTASIS

The endothelial cell
So long as the endothelial lining of the vasculature remains intact, haemorrhage does not occur, and the haemostatic mechanism is not brought into play. Such a bald statement implies that apparently spontaneous haemorrhage, as in various purpuric states, or that following venous obstruction, reflects some degree of damage to endothelial cells, or at least the appearance of gaps between them, with the exposure of underlying structures. These gaps may be due either to desquamation of endothelial cells, or retraction of their margins.

The endothelial cell was formerly thought to be inert with respect to platelets and blood coagulation factors, but its role in haemostasis is now recognized to be an active one. The chief functions of vascular endothelial cells related to haemostasis are listed in Table 26.1. The property of removing various substances from plasma which are potential platelet-aggregating agents has been observed in the pulmonary microcirculation [1–3], and might be specific to endothelial cells in this site; serotonin, however, has also been shown to be taken up by bovine aortic endothelial cells in culture [4], and the angiotensin-converting enzyme has been demonstrated in vascular endothelium from many different organs [5]. The synthesis of the various active principles listed has been demonstrated in cultured endothelial cells from human umbilical vessels and/or large vessels of other species [6–11]. Endothelial cells are the chief site of synthesis of PGI_2, factor-VIII-related antigen and von Willebrand factor, and plasminogen activator (see Chapters 27 and 28), but a relatively minor source of tissue thromboplastin, which comes predominantly from the deeper layers of the vessel wall [8] (see also Chapter 27).

Prostaglandin I_2.
In 1976, Moncada et al. [12] showed that microsomes from rabbit or pig aortas transformed the prostaglandin (PG) endoperoxides PGG_2 and PGH_2 into an unstable substance which was a potent inhibitor of human platelet aggregation as well as a vasodilator. This substance, first designated PGX, and subsequently prostacyclin [13], is now known as PGI_2. It is formed by human arterial and venous tissues [14], the intima being a more potent source than the media or adventitia [15], and is synthesized by cultured endothelial cells, but not by aortic smooth muscle cells [6,

Table 26.1. Haemostatic functions of vascular endothelial cells

Synthesis of:
  prostaglandin I_2
  factor-VIII-related antigen, von Willebrand factor
  tissue thromboplastin
  plasminogen activator
  basement membrane collagen, elastin
  fibronectin
  mucopolysaccharides

Removal from plasma of platelet-aggregating agents:
  5-hydroxytryptamine (5HT)
  adenine nucleotides
  prostaglandin $F_{1\alpha}$
  bradykinin
  angiotensin I
  (converted to angiotensin II)

16]. The pathway of formation from arachidonic acid is shown in Figure 26.1. Comparison with Figure 26.7 (p. 1040) shows that both endothelial cells and platelets form PGG_2 and PGH_2 by a similar mechanism, and that the pathways then diverge, endothelial cells converting the endoperoxides to the aggregation inhibitor PGI_2, while platelets form the aggregating agent thromboxane A_2. Thus both pathways are blocked by cyclo-oxygenase inhibitors such as acetylsalicylic acid (aspirin) and indomethacin. While the effect of aspirin on platelet cyclo-oxygenase is irreversible, however, that on the endothelial-cell enzyme is less profound [17] and relatively short-lived [18]. These observations are of potential importance in relation to the clinical use of aspirin as an anti-thrombotic agent (see Chapter 30).

Since vessel-wall preparations were found to produce PGI_2 more readily from the endoperoxides PGG_2 and PGH_2 than from arachidonate, it was proposed that the chief natural substrate for PGI_2 formation *in vivo* was endoperoxides released from platelets in contact with the vessel wall [19]. This would provide a mechanism by which the formation or extension of a platelet aggregate would be prevented by contact with intact endothelium. The weight of evidence, however, is against this hypothesis: cultured endothelial cells and fibroblasts have been shown to produce PGI_2 on incubation with arachidonate, and endothelial cells synthesize PGI_2 from endogenous arachidonate in response to stimulation by thrombin, trypsin or the calcium ionophore A23187 [6, 20, 21], and have no need of exogenous endoperoxides; PGI_2 is also formed from both exogenous and endogenous arachidonate, but not from PGH_2, by the isolated perfused rabbit heart [22]. Basal PGI_2 production by intact vascular endothelium may perhaps be sufficient to prevent platelet aggregation in uninjured vessels, while increased production in response to mechanical injury, thrombin or other stimuli provides a control mechanism for the limitation of haemostatic plugs and thrombi. PGI_2 has also been found to inhibit the adhesion of platelets to subendothelium, but at much higher concentrations than are required for the inhibiton of aggregation [23, 24].

PGI_2 has a half-life of less than five minutes at neutral pH, being rapidly metabolized to its stable derivative, 6-keto-$PGF_{1\alpha}$ (Fig. 26.1). Its inhibitory effect on platelet aggregation is mediated by the stimulation of platelet adenyl cyclase. Two classes of binding sites for PGI_2 on platelets have been identified, of which the higher affinity site appears to be the specific receptor through which it exerts its effect [25].

Effect of corticosteroids on endothelial cells
It has been recognized clinically for many years that

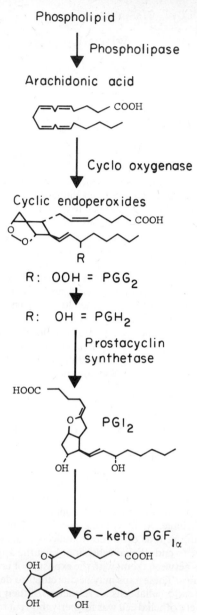

Fig. 26.1. Synthesis of PGI_2 (prostacyclin) by vascular tissues.

the spontaneous purpuric haemorrhage which characterizes thrombocytopenia can often be at least partially controlled by corticosteroid therapy, even in the absence of a rise of platelet count. It has been suggested that this is due to a trophic effect of the steroids on endothelial cell growth: thinning and fenestration of vascular endothelial cells in thrombocytopenic rabbits was prevented by prednisone [26], and glucocorticoids enhanced the confluency of endothelial cell mono-layers in culture [27]. Another likely explanation of the effect of corticosteroids in shortening the bleeding time in thrombocytopenia is that they inhibit PGI_2 synthesis in the vessel wall through their inhibitory effect on phospholipase A_2, and so allow vasoconstriction to be maintained [28].

Adherence of platelets to endothelial cells

Although platelets do not adhere to intact endothelial cells in culture, they do so in response to thrombin, though less avidly than to smooth muscle cells or fibroblasts [29]. Thrombin-induced platelet adherence is enhanced when PGI_2 production is blocked by pre-treatment of the endothelial cells with aspirin [30].

Synthesis of connective tissue elements

The subendothelium, on which the endothelial cells rest, is composed of basement membrane, microfibrils, fibrillar collagen, elastin and mucopolysaccharides [31]. At least two types of collagen are present—type III, which is also found in the deeper layers of the vessel wall, and type IV, which is specific for basement membranes. Both of these are synthesized by vascular endothelial cells [10, 32], as are microfibrillar materials, elastin [10] and mucopolysaccharides [33]. Fibronectin, the protein responsible for the attachment of cells to collagen, is also synthesized by endothelial cells [11], as well as by smooth muscle cells.

Adhesion of platelets to vascular connective tissue

A lesion of continuity of the endothelial lining of a blood vessel leads, within a second or two, to the adhesion of platelets to the exposed connective tissues in the vessel wall [34]. Depending on the nature and extent of the lesion, these may be the subendothelium itself or structures in the deeper layers of the vessel. The scale on which platelets adhere, and the degree to which they subsequently undergo the release reaction and aggregate, will depend on the conditions of blood flow and also on the nature of the connective tissue to which they are exposed.

Subendothelium

When the endothelium is removed from an artery, as by stripping with a balloon catheter, and the vessel perfused with blood *in vivo* or *in vitro*, platelets adhere to the exposed subendothelium, and this adhesion leads to aggregation of further platelets on top of the adherent monolayer [35, 36]. Of the various constituents of the subendothelium (see above), fibrillar collagen is the most active in inducing platelet adhesion, the amorphous basement membrane being much less so [37]; microfibrils evidently contribute to platelet

adhesion, though they do not cause aggregation [38], and elastin is essentially inert. There is some evidence to suggest that collagenous and non-collagenous components of the basement membrane may interact to potentiate the adhesion and aggregation reactions [39].

Collagen

When a vessel is transected, so that blood comes into contact with the media and adventitia, it is to the collagen in these deeper layers that the platelets especially adhere [40]. Of the various kinds of collagen found in vessel walls, type I is present chiefly in the outer layers of larger arteries, type IV is confined to basement membranes and type III is present in the subendothelium as well as the media and adventitia. All these types are capable of inducing adhesion but type IV is much less active in inducing platelet release and aggregation than types I and III, perhaps because of its higher carbohydrate content and lower fibrillo-genesis [41, 42]; this may be one reason why mural thrombi, originating from platelets adherent to basement membrane, tend to propagate less rapidly than haemostatic plugs formed after deeper vascular injury.

The chemical and structural requirements for the adhesion of platelets to collagen, and for their subsequent release reaction and aggregation, are not clearly understood. On the one hand, the adhesive and aggregating properties of collagen have been related to elements of its primary structure, such as the ε-amino groups of lysine [43] or specific short amino-acid sequences [44, 45]; on the other hand, much evidence has been presented that these properties depend largely on its quaternary structure, or degree of polymerization and fibril formation [46–49], though the native fibrillary structure itself is evidently not essential [50]. The factor-XII-activating property of collagen (see Chapter 27) appears to be quite distinct from its effect on platelets, being associated with free carboxyl groups of glutamic and aspartic acids [51].

THE PLATELETS

Ultrastructure and function

A century has elapsed since Hayem [52] and Bizzozero [53], using light microscopy, recognized that platelets played an essential part in the formation of haemostatic plugs and thrombi. The electron microscope has contributed significantly to the great increase in knowledge of these mechanisms during the last 30 years or so, by revealing the ultrastructural basis of many aspects of platelet function. The following account may be supplemented by reference to the profusely illustrated reviews of Hovig [54], White [55] and White & Gerrard [56].

Platelets which have been rapidly fixed in their resting, intact state have a round or oval discoid shape with a smooth surface and few, if any, cytoplasmic protrusions or pseudopodia. Athough non-nucleated, they contain many intracellular structures in common with most other cell types. The chief features revealed by electron microscopy are illustrated in Figures 26.2–26.5.

The plasma membrane

The platelet surface, including that of the surface-connected canalicular system, which consists of invaginations of the surface membrane into the cytoplasm, is formed by a trilamellar unit membrane about 7–9 nm thick, of which the lipid bilayer is partially or completely penetrated by glycoprotein molecules. The carbohydrate part of these glycoproteins projects from the outer surface of the membrane to form an exterior coat or glycocalyx, some 15–20 nm thick, which can be revealed as a fuzzy layer on electron microscopy by the use of ruthenium red or other appropriate stains. This exterior coat is the site of adsorption of various plasma proteins, including particularly fibrinogen and factor VIII, and clearly plays an essential part in the interaction of the platelet with components of the vessel wall and other foreign surfaces (*adhesion*) and with platelets (*aggregation*). It also carries various group-specific and other antigenic sites.

Analysis of platelet membrane glycoproteins by surface labelling and SDS-polyacrylamide gel electrophoresis has revealed three major components, with apparent molecular weights of the order of 155 000, 120 000 and 95 000 daltons, and these were originally designated glycoproteins I, II and III respectively [57, 58]. The use of various refinements of technique has subsequently led to improved resolution of minor components and so to some terminological confusion; a provisional classification is set out in Table 26.2, which also indicates some properties and functions of

these glycoproteins. From the observed deficiency of glycoprotein I in the Bernard–Soulier syndrome (p. 1047), and glycoproteins IIb and IIIa in thrombasthenia (p. 1048), it may be inferred that these two membrane components are involved in adhesion to subendothelium and aggregation respectively (see p. 1038), while the identification of glycoprotein IIIa with α-actinin [67] suggests a role in the platelet contraction-secretion reaction and in clot retraction.

The platelet membrane also carries receptor sites and transducing mechanisms for a range of aggregating agents and inhibitors of aggregation which do not themselves enter the cell. Amongst the various enzyme activities associated with the membrane, those most evidently concerned with haemostatic functions include the adenylate cyclase system [69] and phospholipases (see below).

Contractile elements

Just under the cell membrane, in the equatorial plane, runs a circumferential band of *microtubules*, which serves a skeletal function in maintaining the normal platelet shape [70]. The microtubules disappear in the cold (when the platelets lose their disc shape) and reappear on warming (when they regain it) [71]. During aggregation they contract towards the centre of the cell, where they surround the centrally displaced organelles, and they are also prominent within the giant pseudopodia formed in response to higher concentrations of aggregating agents.

The *microfilaments* are widely distributed throughout the platelet cytoplasm, and are the morphological expression of the platelet contractile protein [72, 73]. They are difficult to visualize in thin sections of intact platelets, but become clearly visible in the activated state, particularly in the pseudopodia.

Since the original description by Bettex-Galland & Lüscher [74] of an actomyosin-like protein in platelets, which they later [75] named thrombosthenin, it has

Table 26.2. Platelet membrane glycoproteins

	Components	Properties	Refs
I	Is (glycocalicin)	Thrombin receptor	59, 60
	Ib	Sialic-acid-rich	
		Defective in Bernard–Soulier syndrome	61
		Drug-dependent antibody receptor	62
II	IIa		
	IIb		
III	IIIa (III)	Defective in thrombasthenia	63, 64
		Pl^A (Zw) antigenic site	65, 66
		α-actinin	67
	IIIb (IV)		
V	V	Thrombin receptor	68

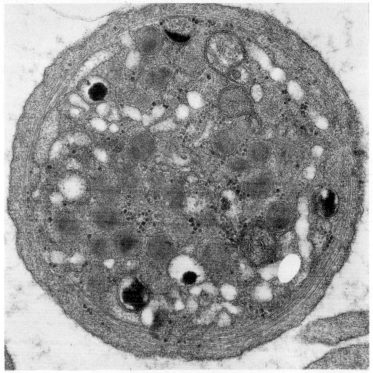

Fig. 26.2. Electron micrograph of a platelet, sectioned in the equatorial plane.

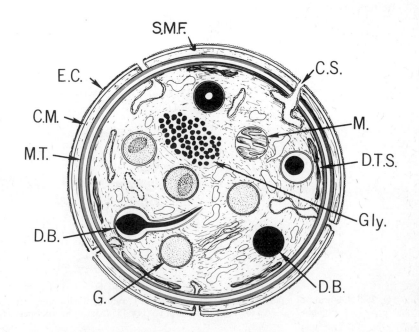

Fig. 26.3. Diagram of a platelet in equatorial section. EC, external coat; CM, cell membrane; SMF, submembranous microfilaments; MT, microtubules; DTS, dense tubular system; CS, surface-connected system; G, α granule; DB, dense body; M, mitochondrion; Gly, glycogen granules.

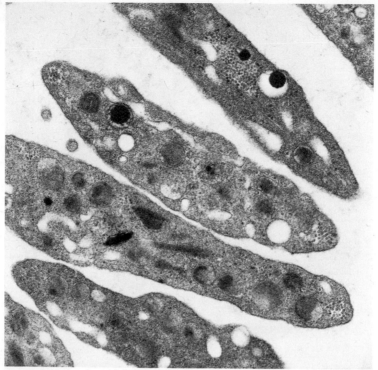

Fig. 26.4. Electron micrograph of platelets sectioned transversely to the equatorial plane.

become clear that platelets contain a complete system of muscle proteins, including tropomyosin, troponin and α-actinin [76–78], in addition to actin and myosin. Actin comprises about 10% of the total platelet protein, and myosin about one per cent [79]. Platelet actin is very similar to muscle actin, but platelet myosin differs from muscle myosin in various ways, including its filament size and the mechanism of its interaction with actin. The platelet contractile system is involved in the change of shape of the platelets in response to

stimulation, in platelet contraction and secretion, and in clot retraction. Further details of its structure and function are given in the recent reviews by Adelstein & Pollard [79] and Cohen [80].

Platelet organelles
Platelets contain collections of glycogen particles throughout the cytoplasm, and in a minority of sections a Golgi apparatus is seen. Besides these, a series of highly specialized structures is present, includ-

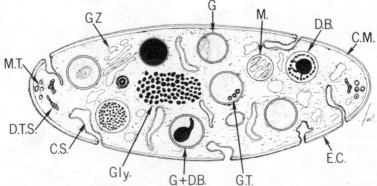

Fig. 26.5. Diagram of a platelet in transverse section. GT, tubules within an α granule; GZ, Golgi zone; other symbols as in Figure 26.3. Figures 26.2–26.5 are reproduced from White [55, 55a, b] by kind permission of the author and publishers.

ing deeply osmiophilic *dense bodies*, other secretory granules known as α *granules*, lysosomes, peroxisomes, mitochondria and the *dense tubular system*. The *surface-connected canalicular system*, considered above as an extension of the plasma membrane, appears as a series of spaces lined by a unit membrane, with a glycocalyx on its inner surface.

Dense bodies. A small number of the granules in human platelets fixed with glutaraldehyde and osmic acid are very electron-dense, probably because of their relatively high calcium content. They are lined by a unit membrane, within which the dense material sometimes fails to fill the whole space, producing a 'bull's-eye' appearance (Figs 26.2 and 26.5). These dense bodies, which are slightly smaller than α granules, are the storage site (Table 26.3) for 5-hydroxytryptamine (serotonin) [81], the non-metabolic pool of adenine nucleotides [82], adrenaline [83] and calcium [84], all of which are secreted from them during the platelet release reaction (see p. 1041).

Table 26.3. Platelet granules and their contents

Dense bodies	ATP, ADP (storage pool)
	5-hydroxytryptamine
	Adrenaline
	Ca^{2+}
α granules	Platelet factor 4 (PF4)
	Low affinity PF4,
	β thromboglobulin
	Fibrinogen
	Growth factor(s)
	Fibronectin
	Factor V
	Factor VIII-related antigen,
	von Willebrand factor
	Permeability factor
Lysosomes	Acid hydrolases
Peroxisomes	Catalase

Alpha granules. This term was originally applied to the moderately electron-dense granules, bounded by unit membranes, found evenly distributed throughout the cytoplasm of the intact platelet. In recent years, the use of cell fractionation and cytochemical techniques has shown that these structures are functionally heterogeneous. They include *lysosomes*, containing acid hydrolases [85, 86], *peroxisomes* containing catalase [87], and a third population, which may itself be heterogeneous, consisting of secretory organelles which are the site of storage and release of a series of platelet-specific and other proteins [88–92]. If the term α granule continues to be used, it is to this last category that it should now be applied. The contents of these granules, which are secreted from them during the platelet-release reaction (p. 1041), are listed in Table 26.3. It is not known whether a given α granule can store many different proteins, or whether individual granules exhibit different storage specificities.

Mitochondria. Platelet mitochondria are few in number and simple in structure, with few cristae. They make an important contribution, through oxidative phosphorylation, to the metabolic pool of ATP within the platelet, which provides the energy for aggregation, secretion, clot retraction and other functions.

Dense tubular system. This highly specialized membrane system, seen as an irregular series of channels lying just under the band of microtubules, appears to be the analogue of the sarcoplasmic reticulum of muscle—the source and repository of the calcium ions required for the contractile activities of the platelet. Gerrard *et al.* [93, 94] have produced evidence that the dense tubular system is the site of synthesis of prostaglandin endoperoxides and thromboxane A_2, and have proposed that the function of the latter is to transport calcium from the dense tubular system to the cytoplasm.

Haemostatic functions of platelets
The platelets play a central role in the sequence of events which follows injury to a blood vessel, by virtue of their properties of adhering to structures in the vessel wall, of aggregating together to form the main mass of the haemostatic plug, and of contributing both to vasoconstriction and to blood coagulation. But besides this, the platelets are essential for the maintenance of the integrity of the walls of small vessels which are not the site of obvious injury—hence the spontaneous purpura which characterizes severe thrombocytopenia. This function probably depends largely on the ability of the platelets to plug small gaps in the vascular endothelium [38, 95], where the subendothelium has become exposed by the shedding of endothelial cells, by retraction of their margins or by vasodilatation. Like haemostatic plug formation, it depends on the adhesive property of the platelets. Thrombocytopenia in rabbits has also been found to cause thinning, fenestration and increased permeability of the endothelial cells themselves [96], and platelets have been shown to stimulate the replication of endothelial cells in culture [97, 98]; there may thus be various means whereby they maintain vascular integrity.

The formation of a haemostatic plug begins within seconds of injury to a vessel with the adherence of platelets to subendothelial structures, and involves a closely interwoven sequence of reactions. These include the synthesis within the platelets of prostaglandin endoperoxides and thromboxane A_2, contraction of platelet actomyosin and the secretion from the storage organelles of various active principles (the platelet release reaction), platelet aggregation, activation of the blood coagulation mechanism by vessel-wall constituents and also by the platelets themselves, fibrin formation between and around the aggregated platelets, and finally retraction of the fibrin clot. The interrelationships between the various components of this sequence are complex and imperfectly understood; any attempt to dissect them one from another in print must be as fraught with difficulty, and as prone to oversimplification, as the interpretation of *in-vitro* experiments in terms of physiological function. The following brief account is intended chiefly as a basis for the understanding of clinical disorders of platelet function; those requiring more detailed information are advised to consult recent reviews and conference proceedings [e.g. 99, 100].

Platelet adhesion

The properties of connective tissues related to the platelet adhesion reaction have been briefly considered above (p. 1033). The requirements of the platelets themselves for adhesion to connective tissues are still unresolved. Jamieson *et al.* [101] proposed that a glucosyl transferase on the outer side of the platelet membrane might interact with galactosyl residues on collagen, but subsequent findings make this hypothesis unlikely [46, 102, 103]. Evidence has been presented that platelets have fibronectin on their cell surface, and that this is a receptor for collagen [104]. From the defects of adhesion to subendothelium observed in the Bernard–Soulier syndrome (p. 1047) and von Willebrand's disease (p. 1125), it may be inferred that platelet membrane glycoprotein I and the plasma factor VIII molecule are also involved in this platelet–vessel-wall interaction. Plasma factor VIII has been shown to bind both to normal platelets in the presence of ristocetin [105, 106], and to human arterial subendothelium [107], and it may be that it acts as the glue which binds platelets and subendothelial structures together.

Platelet adhesion to connective tissue, unlike aggregation, appears to be an irreversible process [36]. Unlike adhesion to glass and other inorganic surfaces, it does not require the presence of fibrinogen or divalent cations. In the presence of calcium ions, however, platelets will also adhere to polymerizing fibrin [108], and in certain circumstances this may form an adhesive surface *in vivo*.

Platelet shape change and aggregation

Adenosine diphosphate (ADP). The adhesion of rela-tively few platelets to connective tissue is rapidly followed by the aggregation of larger numbers arriving at the site, with the formation of a platelet plug. Since the pioneer observations of Hellem [109] and Gaarder *et al.* [110], the function of ADP as a platelet-aggregating agent has become well established [111] and there is little doubt that it plays an essential role as one of the chief physiological mediators of platelet aggregation *in vivo*. Adenosine diphosphate is derived from damaged red cells and connective tissue at the site of injury, but its chief source for platelet aggregation is probably the platelets themselves: several times as much ADP is released from platelets by collagen as is necessary for the induction of aggregation, and ADP aggregation itself promotes further nucleotide release, leading to an extension of the process [112].

The initial step in the action of ADP on platelets involves its binding to specific receptors on the outside of the platelet membrane. The nature and number of these, and the mechanisms by which the stimulus is transmitted from the receptor sites to elicit the aggregation response, have been the subject of extensive investigation and debate. For a review of this complex field, the reader is referred to Refs 113 and 114.

The first directly observable effect of ADP on platelets, as of most other aggregating agents, is the change in shape from smooth discs to 'spiny spheres', with the formation of many small pseudopodia ('filo-podia'); this produces a transient decrease in light transmission in the aggregometer, accompanied by a decrease in amplitude of the oscillations (Fig. 26.6). It occurs within two to three seconds, and results in an increase of platelet surface area and of exposed sialic-acid residues [115, 116]. Unlike aggregation, it does not require extracellular cations, but it does appear to be associated with intracellular calcium shifts and is inhibited by cyclic AMP [117, 118].

The details of the mechanism of the platelet–platelet interaction in response to the stimulus of ADP are still unresolved. The process of aggregation requires the presence of extracellular divalent cations, calcium being more active than magnesium, and of fibrinogen at a concentration of not less than about $0 \cdot 2 \, \text{g/l}$ [119]. It has been shown [120–123] that ADP induces, in the presence of divalent cations, a receptor for fibrinogen on the platelet membrane. Since fibrinogen does not bind to thrombasthenic platelets [120, 122, 123], which are deficient in membrane glycoproteins IIb and IIIa [63, 64], it may be that this glycoprotein complex carries the fibrinogen receptor, and that it becomes exposed on the outer surface of the platelet in the course of the initial shape change.

The measurement of platelet aggregation *in vitro*, whether in platelet-rich plasma (PRP) or in suspensions of isolated platelets, has proved a most valuable

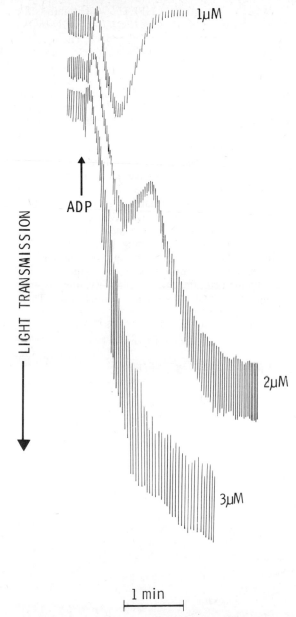

Fig. 26.6. Platelet shape change and aggregation in response to ADP: 1 μM, first phase only; 2 μM, biphasic; 4 μM, maximal aggregation. The initial decrease in light transmission represents the shape change.

research procedure for studying the effect and mode of action of various aggregating agents and inhibitors, but is of limited value in clinical investigation, owing to the large number of variables, many of them difficult or impossible to control, which may affect the response of an individual sample of PRP. Certain broad patterns

of response may be recognized in the aggregometer tracing, however, depending on the presence or absence of an increase in light transmission due to the primary aggregating effect of the inducer, or of a second wave associated with the release from the platelets themselves of thromboxane A_2, ADP and other products of secretion. Typical aggregometer tracings of the effect of various concentrations of ADP on normal citrated PRP are shown in Figure 26.6. The second wave is dependent on low concentrations of ionized calcium, such as are present in citrated plasma; it is not seen in heparinized PRP [124].

Other aggregating agents. A number of compounds besides ADP cause platelet aggregation *in vitro*. Some of these, such as collagen, do not cause aggregation directly, but only through the release of ADP and thromboxane A_2 (see below), but the following (most of which also stimulate the release reaction) seem to have a direct primary aggregating effect:

Thrombin
Adrenaline, noradrenaline
5-hydroxytryptamine
Cyclic endoperoxides (prostaglandins G_2
    and H_2) and thromboxane A_2
'Platelet-activating factor' (PAF-acether)
Vasopressin

All of these compounds except adrenaline and noradrenaline [125] cause a shape change, and all of them, like ADP, require the presence of extracellular calcium ions for aggregation. Thrombin aggregates platelets at concentrations below those required to clot fibrinogen and will do so, unlike ADP, in the absence of fibrinogen in the medium [119], probably because it also causes the secretion of fibrinogen from the platelets themselves. Low concentrations of adrenaline and of thrombin also potentiate the aggregating activity of ADP [126, 127]. The aggregating activity of the cyclic endoperoxides and thromboxane A_2 can be demonstrated indirectly by the aggregation of platelets by their precursor, arachidonic acid (see p. 1040); failure of arachidonic acid to aggregate platelets which respond to ADP or thrombin indicates a defect or inhibition of the prostaglandin–thromboxane pathway, of which the most likely cause is inhibition of cyclo-oxygenase by aspirin or other similar drugs (see p. 1055).

The 'platelet-activating factor' (PAF), a phospholipid released from basophils and macrophages in response to antigenic challenge [128], is a potent inducer of platelet aggregation and secretion [129]. It has recently been found to be released from the platelets themselves by a calcium-dependent mechanism independent of ADP release and thromboxane synthesis [130], and its structure has been determined [130a, b], leading to its designation as PAF-acether. As an aggregating agent, it is about four orders of magnitude more potent than ADP, and it may well prove to play an important part in normal haemostasis.

Vasopressin is about 40 times as active as ADP in aggregating platelets in heparinized PRP, but almost inactive in citrated PRP; it appears to require bound, as well as extracellular, calcium ions for its effect [131].

Prostaglandin and thromboxane synthesis

Contact of platelets with collagen fibres, or the action upon them of various other aggregating agents (see above), including thrombin, ADP and adrenaline, results in the release of arachidonic acid from platelet phospholipids, particularly phosphatidylcholine and phosphatidylinositol, and so triggers the synthesis within the platelet of prostaglandins, cyclic endoperoxides and thromboxane A_2 [132–136]. The pathways of conversion of arachidonic acid by the platelet are illustrated in Figure 26.7. The lipoxygenase pathway

leads to the formation of HPETE, which inhibits the conversion of prostaglandin (PG)G_2 to PGI_2 by the vessel wall [137] (see p. 1031) and HETE, which is chemotactic for neutrophils [138]. Cyclo-oxygenase (endoperoxide synthetase) converts arachidonic acid to the cyclic endoperoxides, PGG_2 and PGH_2, from which the potent platelet-aggregating and vasoconstrictor agent, thromboxane (TX)A_2, is formed by the action of the enzyme thromboxane synthetase. Thromboxane A_2 is very unstable, with a half-life of only about 30 seconds in water (but several minutes in plasma [139]), and is rapidly hydrolyzed to the stable TXB_2. The major alternative pathway for PGH_2 metabolism is degradation to malonyl dialdehyde (MDA) and the hydroxy fatty acid HHT, and small amounts are also converted to PGE_2, PGF_2 and PGD_2; the first two of these have little effect on platelets, but the last is an inhibitor of aggregation [140], and may have a regulatory role in the haemostatic mechanism.

The initiating event in this sequence, the release of arachidonic acid, depends on the activation of phospholipases A_2 and C by an aggregating agent. These

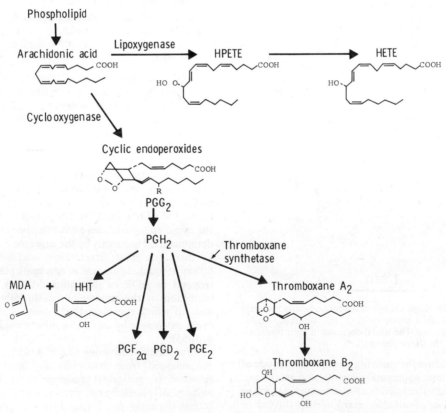

Fig. 26.7. Pathways of arachidonic-acid metabolism in human platelets. HPETE, 12-hydroperoxy-eicosatetranoic acid; HETE, 12-hydroxy-eicosatetraenoic acid; MDA, malonyl dialdehyde; HHT, 12-hydroxy-hepatadecatrienoic acid.

enzymes require calcium for their activity, and it seems likely that the effect of the various aggregating agents, acting on their several receptors on the plasma membrane, is mediated through the liberation of calcium from intracellular storage sites, so as to make it available to the phospholipases. This process, which is energy-dependent, requiring metabolic ATP [141], is inhibited by cyclic AMP [142], which stimulates the uptake of calcium ions from the cytoplasm into membranes [143], and by local anaesthetics, which block the transport of calcium ions across membranes. Thromboxane formation can also be blocked by inhibitors of enzymes in the pathway from arachidonic acid (see Fig. 26.7). The chief of these are aspirin, indomethacin and other non-steroidal anti-inflammatory agents, which inhibit cyclo-oxygenase [144, 145].

The dense tubular system may be the chief site of endoperoxide and thromboxane synthesis; it has been proposed that TXA$_2$ acts as an ionophore, transporting calcium from the membrane of the dense tubular system, where the enzymes of the pathway are situated, into the cytoplasm, where it is made available for the contractile mechanism of the cell [91, 92]. This would provide a mechanism for the stimulation of the release reaction by TXA$_2$, and another point at which cyclic AMP may inhibit platelet activation by removing calcium ions from the cytoplasm. The interdependence of the endoperoxide and cyclic AMP systems is further underlined by the fact that the endoperoxides and TXA$_2$ themselves inhibit adenylate cyclase [146]. Thromboxane A$_2$. moreover, is itself released from the cell, and causes direct platelet aggregation independently of the secretion of ADP and other granule contents [147].

The activation of phospholipase C also leads to the production of diglycerides and phosphatidic acids from phosphatidylinositol in the platelet membrane [148]. Since phosphatidic acid behaves as an ionophore [149], this may well provide another pathway for calcium-mediated intracellular reactions.

The platelet release reaction

The adhesion of platelets to collagen, or the action upon them of thrombin and various other agents (Table 26.4), results in the secretion of the contents of various specific storage organelles (see p. 1036). The term 'release reaction' was originally coined by Grette [150] to describe the specific effect of thrombin on platelets, but has now come to be applied more generally to this active secretory process of the platelet, however induced. The process has many points of similarity with that of other secretory cells, including dependence on metabolic ATP as an energy source, the involvement of contractile proteins, regulation by intracellular calcium ions and cyclic nucleotides, and

Table 26. 4. Inducers of the platelet release reaction

Collagen	Bovine factor VIII
Thrombin	Ristocetin
Plasmin	Antigen–antibody complexes
Trypsin	γ-globulin-coated sufaces
Calcium ionophores	Endotoxin
Polymerizing fibrin	Zymosan
ADP	Particulate fatty acids
Adrenaline	Viruses, bacteria
Arachidonic acid	Snake venoms

finally exocytosis by fusion of granule membranes with the plasma membrane of the cell—in the case of the platelet, the membrane of the surface-connected canalicular system. The release reaction has been the subject of several recent reviews [151–153].

The substances released include the contents of the dense bodies, α granules, and, in response to more powerful stimuli, lysosomes (Table 26.3, p. 1037). Some of these contents are discussed below.

Adenine nucleotides. Platelets contain two separate pools of adenine nucleotides [82, 112]: a 'metabolic pool', consisting mainly of ATP, which is rapidly labelled on incubating platelets with radioactive adenine or adenosine and which takes part in energy-requiring metabolic activities, and a 'storage pool' containing more ADP than ATP, which is only slowly labelled and is not metabolized within the platelet. It is the storage pool which is contained within the dense bodies and secreted from them during the release reaction. Typical normal values for nucleotides in the two pools are shown in Table 26.5.

Table 26.5. Platelet nucleotides (nmoles/10^8 platelets)

	Metabolic pool	Storage pool	Total
ATP	3·7	2·8	6·5
ADP	0·6	3·6	4·2
AMP	0·1	0·4	0·5
Total	4·4	6·8	11·2
ATP/ADP ratio	6·2	0·8	1·5

5-hydroxytryptamine (5HT, serotonin) and adrenaline. Serotonin is secreted by the argentaffin cells of the intestine and transported in the circulation by the platelets, which normally contain almost all the 5HT in the blood. Platelets takes up 5HT at 37°C against a concentration gradient by an active transport mechanism [154, 155] and store it in an intact form. Although platelets also contain monoamine oxidase activity, the great majority of the 5HT which they take up is evidently inaccessible to it: the 5HT is stored in the dense bodies from which it is secreted during the release reaction.

Platelets also take up adrenaline at 37°C, though much more slowly than 5HT [83], and store most of it intact in the dense bodies. Nearly half the adrenaline, and a much smaller proportion of 5HT, is also taken up by another process which does not involve the storage organelles. The amines taken up in this way are metabolized within the platelet, and are not available for release. Reserpine blocks the uptake of both amines into storage organelles, but does not affect the second uptake mechanism: it therefore depletes the platelets of both amines, but increases the concentration of their metabolites [83, 156].

Platelet factor 4 and β thromboglobulin. Platelet factor 4 (PF4) is the name given to the heparin-neutralizing activity of platelets. It has also been claimed to neutralize the inhibitory effects of fibrin-degradation products on thrombin and on platelet aggregation [157], but this has been disputed, and its biological function remains unclear. It is composed of four identical polypeptide subunits, each containing 70 amino acids [158], and is released from the platelets as a complex with a proteoglycan carrier [159, 160]. Another protein with antiheparin activity has been isolated from platelets and designated low-affinity PF4 [161]; this material now appears to be almost identical with β thromboglobulin (βTG) [162], which differs from it only in lacking the four N-terminal amino acids [163]. It has been suggested that βTG is a proteolytic breakdown product of LA-PF4, formed after its secretion from the α granules.

Both PF4 and βTG (or its precursor) have been shown to be secreted from the α granules during the release reaction [90]; highly sensitive radioimmunoassays have been developed for both proteins, and are currently being used for the detection of spontaneous release of platelet contents *in vivo* in a variety of clinical states. Like that of PF4, the biological function of βTG remains uncertain; it has recently been shown to inhibit the formation of PGI_2 by arterial endothelial cells [164], and may thus contribute to the propagation of platelet plugs and thrombi.

Amongst other proteins secreted from the platelets are the platelet-derived growth factor(s) for arterial smooth muscle, fibroblasts and other cells [165–167], a permeability-enhancing factor [168], fibrinogen [169], fibronectin [90a], activated factor V [170] and factor-VIII-related antigen [171]. Fibrinogen [88], the growth factor [90] and fibronectin [90a] have been localized to

the α granules, which also seem to be the most likely storage site for the other releasable proteins.

Release inducers. The release reaction can be induced by many different stimuli (Table 26.4), including contact with foreign surfaces or particles, or with other platelets, immune reactions at the platelet surface, various enzymes and divalent cation ionophores. The most important physiological stimuli are collagen fibrils, thrombin, ADP, and perhaps also adrenaline and 5HT—the last three because of the positive feedback mechanism which they provide on release from the dense bodies themselves. Many of the others may contribute to abnormal platelet aggregation *in vivo* in various disease states.

Mechanism. The release reaction is presumed to be brought about by contraction of the actomyosin filaments within the cytoplasm, causing centralization of the secretory granules, which come into contact with the membrane of the surface-connected canalicular system, through which their contents are discharged by exocytosis [151] (Fig. 26.8). The contractile mechanism involves the phosphorylation of cytoplasmic proteins [172], including the light chain of myosin [173], and the polymerization of actin. It is accompanied by disassembly of the circumferential band of microtubules, which later reassemble so as to form a skeletal structure for the pseudopodia. These changes all require the presence of calcium [174], which is liberated from intracellular storage sites, both through the endoperoxide–thromboxane pathway (see above), and by an independent mechanism; thrombin and collagen liberate calcium by both these mechanisms, but ADP and adrenaline, which are weaker inducers of release, only by the first. Extracellular calcium is essential for aggregation and thus for the release which is secondary to it, but is not required for release by thrombin or collagen [175]. Secretion of the contents of dense bodies and α granules occurs in parallel in response to ADP, adrenaline or low concentrations of collagen or thrombin [90], but lysosomal secretion requires higher concentrations of collagen or thrombin and is not induced by ADP or adrenaline [112].

Inhibitors of release. The release reaction can be partly or completely inhibited, depending on the potency and mode of action of the inducer, by reagents which interfere with any of the contributory mechanisms: endoperoxide and thromboxane synthesis, permeability of intracellular membranes to calcium ions, or contraction of microfibrils. The process is also inhibited by agents which increase the cyclic AMP concentration within the platelet, and thus remove available calcium ions from the cytoplasm. The chief representatives of these various classes of inhibitors are listed in Table 26.6.

Interrelations of aggregation, thromboxane synthesis and release

It was formerly believed that aggregation in response to collagen and thrombin, the agents most likely to be primarily involved in initiating platelet plug formation *in vivo*, depended on the release of ADP from the storage granules; following the discovery of TXA_2, the simplest explanation of its role in platelet activation was that it was required for the release of ADP by thrombin, collagen and other agents. Although these agents do indeed cause both thromboxane synthesis and the release of ADP, and TXA_2 does induce the release reaction, this simple causal relationship is not a sufficient explanation of many subsequent observations. Thus ATP, which inhibits ADP aggregation competitively, does not inhibit aggregation by adrenaline, thrombin, vasopressin or 5HT [176]. Thromboxane A_2, which is itself released from the platelets by aggregating agents, causes platelet aggregation independently of the release reaction [147], while thrombin, like the calcium ionophore, A23187, promotes platelet aggregation even in the presence of inhibitors of both ADP and thromboxane synthesis [177], and must therefore also act through a third mechanism. It has been suggested that this may be mediated by the release of the 'platelet-activating factor' [130] (see p. 1039). ADP and adrenaline themselves cause release, but this appears to be dependent on aggregation, and to be mediated through the endoperoxide pathway [178]. The time course of aggregation and nucleotide release gives no reason for believing that the former is solely dependent on the latter, even when collagen is the inducing agent [178]. It therefore seems that aggregation, thromboxane synthesis and secretion from dense bodies exert a synergistic effect rather than having a direct linear causal relationship with a single end result. All of them are energy-dependent processes, involving the breakdown of metabolic ATP, and all can be inhibited by blocking both glycolysis and oxidative phosphorylation, on which mechanisms the platelet depends roughly equally for its ATP production [179]. Progressively more energy is required for the initial shape change of platelets, aggregation, thromboxane synthesis, secretion from dense bodies and α granules, and the release of lysosomal enzymes. Aggregation is the only one of these functions which requires the presence of extracellular divalent cations, but all the rest are dependent on the intracellular mobilization of calcium, and it seems likely that this is the essential mechanism by which the stimulus of the binding of an aggregating agent to its receptor on the platelet membrane is coupled to each of these responses [180]. Figure 26.8 represents an attempt to portray some of these interrelations in a simple diagrammatic form.

Platelets and blood coagulation

Platelets are essentially inert with respect to blood coagulation in their normal circulating state, but during adhesion, release and aggregation they contribute to the coagulation mechanism at several points, with the result that thrombin and fibrin are rapidly formed in close association with the surface of the aggregating platelets.

Contact phase activation. Walsh [181] found that factor XII was activated by platelets which had undergone a shape change, but not necessarily aggregation, in response to ADP, but this finding has recently been disputed [182]. The activation of factor XII, which has also been demonstrated with collagen-treated platelets, appears to require the presence of kallikrein and to be enhanced by high-molecular-weight (HMW) kininogen [183]; factor-XII activation by collagen-

Table 26.6. Inhibitors of the release reaction

Cyclo-oxygenase inhibitors
Aspirin, indomethacin

Membrane stabilizers
Chlorpromazine
Propranolol
Local anaesthetics (tetracaine, dibucaine, etc.)

Inhibitors of contractile elements
Cytochalasin B
Colchicine
Vinca alkaloids

Components which increase cyclic AMP
Prostaglandins E_1, D_2, I_2
Phosphodiesterase inhibitors (dipyridamole, theophylline, etc.)

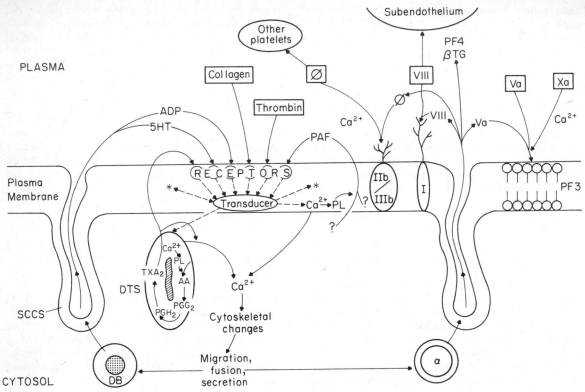

Fig. 26.8. Interrelations of some platelet functions. SCCS, surface-connecting canalicular system; DTS, dense tubular system; DB, dense body; α, α granule; PL, phospholipases; AA, arachidonic acid; PAF, platelet-activating factor; φ, fibrinogen; PF3, platelet factor 3; PF4, platelet factor 4; βTG, β thromboglobulin; I, IIb/IIIa, glycoproteins; *, alteration of membrane structure, leading to exposure of fibrinogen receptor sites and procoagulant phospholipids (PF3). Agents extrinsic to the platelet are shown in square boxes.

treated platelets is abolished by indomethacin, suggesting that the release of TXA_2 or ADP is necessary for the reaction [183]. Collagen- or ADP-treated platelets also activate factor XI; this reaction, which also requires kallikrein, is enhanced by factor XII and HMW kininogen, but will occur in the absence of factor XII [184, 185]. This alternative pathway for factor-XI activation thus provides a possible explanation for the absence of haemostatic failure in most patients with factor-XII deficiency. Platelets not only bind factor XI from the plasma, but contain endogenous factor-XI-like activity in their plasma membranes, which is itself capable of activation by collagen in the absence of plasma factor XI [186, 187]; this may explain why some patients with factor-XI deficiency (but with factor-XI-like activity in their platelet membranes) have only minor bleeding symptoms.

Activation of factor X. The activation of factor X by factors IXa and VIII is enhanced by their adsorption to

a phospholipid surface in the presence of calcium. Such a surface is provided by the platelet membrane, to which factors VIII and IX are loosely adsorbed. Walsh & Biggs [188] have proposed that factor XIa on the platelet membrane (see above) where it is protected from its natural inhibitor in the plasma, activates adsorbed factor IX *in situ*, with subsequent factor-X activation. The platelet membrane requirements for this sequence of reactions appear to be distinct from platelet factor 3 (PF3) [189], though like the latter, they involve the availability of membrane phospholipids. Although endogenous platelet factor-VIII-related antigen is secreted from the granules in the course of the release reaction [171], and bound to the platelet membrane, there is no evidence that it is associated with procoagulant activity, and therefore no reason to suppose that it contributes to factor-X activation.

Conversion of prothrombin. Platelet factor 3 is the name given to that procoagulant activity of the platelets which becomes available on the platelet membrane during aggregation and release, providing a phospholipid surface at which factors Xa and V react to convert prothrombin to thrombin [190]. The surface of the intact circulating platelet is inactive in this respect, and the availability of PF3 has been ascribed to a reorientation of specific phospholipids in the platelet membrane bilayer [191], phosphatidylserine and phosphatidylethanolamine, which are mostly in the inner layer in the resting state, becoming exposed in the outer layer during activation of the platelet. Such an effect might be due to a 'flip-flop' mechanism in the plasma membrane, or to fusion of granule membranes, known to be rich in PF3 activity [192], with those of the cell surface.

Platelets are capable of adsorbing factor V to their surface—the activity described as platelet factor 1 is attributable to adsorbed factor V [193]—and also contain factor V which is released by collagen, probably in an activated form [170, 194]. The release reaction exposes factor-Xa binding sites on the platelet surface, and the binding of factor Xa to these sites requires the presence of factor-V activity and of calcium ions [195]. A synthesis of these observations suggests that aggregation and release make active phospholipid sites available on the outside of the platelet membrane, to which the factor Va released from the platelet binds; this bound factor Va forms the receptor site for factor Xa in the presence of calcium ions, and binding of Xa is rapidly followed by thrombin formation on the platelet surface.

Fibrin formation. Platelet fibrinogen forms about 10–15% of the total protein of the cell, and consists partly of plasma fibrinogen adsorbed to the surface, and partly of intracellular fibrinogen [196, 197]. The latter is chiefly located in the α granules, from which it is secreted during the release reaction [88, 90]. This intracellular platelet fibrinogen, which is probably synthesized in the megakaryocytes and perhaps to some extent within the platelets themselves, differs from plasma fibrinogen in its structural and functional characteristics [198]; this may be attributable to its partial degradation by proteases within the platelet [199, 200]. Its specific function in haemostasis is uncertain, but fibrinogen on the platelet surface, whether derived from the plasma or from the platelets themselves after release, is essential for aggregation by ADP as well as for consolidation of the platelet plug through fibrin formation.

Platelets also contain factor XIII, but this differs from plasma factor XIII in being composed of an *a*-chain dimer, while the plasma factor consists of two *a* and two *b* chains [201]. Unlike fibrinogen, of which the platelets contain only about 0·03% of that in whole blood, factor XIII is approximately equally distributed between plasma and platelets [202]. Platelet factor XIII is found in the cytosol and not in the granules, and is not released from the platelets by thrombin or collagen [202, 203]. Its function in the haemostatic mechanism is unknown, but it may render platelet fibrinogen less susceptible to fibrinolysis [204], and it may perhaps be a source of the *a* chain of plasma factor XIII. It is evidently synthesized in megakaryocytes [205].

Two other platelet constitutents whose biological function is unknown, but which may play a role in thrombin–fibrinogen interaction, are PF2 and PF4. Platelet factor 2 accelerates the conversion of fibrinogen by thrombin, and is said also to aggregate platelets and to neutralize antithrombin III [206]. Platelet factor 4 may neutralize not only heparin, but also the inhibitory effects of fibrinogen-degradation products on thrombin and on platelet aggregation [157], and its haemostatic role may therefore be more closely related to aggregation than to blood coagulation. Low-affinity PF4 may be more important as the precursor of β thromboglobulin (see p. 1042) than for its antiheparin activity.

Platelets also exhibit antithrombin activity; it has been suggested that this is mediated mainly by thrombin binding to the platelet membrane and partly by adsorption of thrombin on to released platelet fibrinogen [207, 208].

Platelets and fibrinolysis. Platelets appear to have a role in both the activation and inhibition of fibrinolysis. They contain plasminogen [209], and have both adsorbed and intrinsic antiplasmin activity amounting to about one per cent of that of whole plasma [210]. The intrinsic antiplasmin of pig platelets is released by collagen and thrombin, probably from the dense bodies [211]. Plasminogen activator is present, if at all, in only trace amounts in platelets [212], but its release from vascular endothelium is probably mediated by 5HT and other amines secreted by them. An inhibitor of plasminogen activation has also been isolated from platelets [212]. The net biological effect of all these platelet activities cannot be assessed, but it seems reasonable to suppose that the secretion of inhibitors of fibrinolysis may contribute to consolidation of the fibrin clot formed in the immediate vicinity of the platelet plug.

Clot retraction

Platelets have long been known to be essential for clot retraction, which has been used as a test of platelet function for many years. *In vitro*, the phenomenon is most strikingly observed in PRP, in which the clot may retract to as little as one-tenth of its original volume; in whole blood, the process is limited by mechanical interference by the red cells. Since fibrin forms a relatively minor part of haemostatic plugs *in vivo*, clot retraction seems unlikely to play an important part in haemostasis, though it can easily be imagined to contribute to the compactness of a haemostatic plug, and to recanalization of a vessel obstructed by clot.

Clot retraction depends on contraction of the actomyosin microfibrils, particularly within the platelet pseudopodia, where they are seen to have a predominantly longitudinal orientation following activation *in vitro* by an aggregating agent [72]. The microfibrils are attached to α-actinin on the inner surface of the plasma membrane, while fibrin is formed from fibrinogen molecules attached to the outer surface—perhaps also to glycoprotein IIIa, with which α-actinin has been identified [67]. Extracellular calcium ions are required for clot retraction, which occurs only following aggregation. Like the other platelet functions discussed above it is energy-dependent, and can be abolished by inhibiting both glycolysis and oxidative phosphorylation.

Other functions of platelets

While the chief function of the platelets is to confine the circulating blood within the vasculature, they also contribute to inflammatory and immune reactions, including transplant rejection, and to wound healing, and are capable of engulfment of viruses, bacteria and other particles. Their role in the pathogenesis of thrombosis and atherosclerosis is discussed in Chapter 30.

Inflammation. Platelets accumulate at sites of tissue damage and release constituents which increase vascular permeability and are chemotactic for granulocytes. These include a cationic protein released from the α granules [168] which has both these effects, the latter being mediated through the fifth component of complement [213]; and two products of arachidonic-acid metabolism: PGE_2, which increases vascular permeability [214], and HETE, which is chemotactic for leucocytes [138]. The release of 5HT from the platelet dense bodies will also influence vascular permeability, as may the liberation of elastase and collagenase from the platelets [215, 216].

Engulfment of particles. Platelets can ingest very small particles and can also engulf larger particles by aggregating around them. Engulfment of bacteria by platelets is not followed by bacterial killing [217], and may therefore be deleterious to the host. Aggregation around carbon particles leads to their clearance from the circulation by the reticulo-endothelial system [218].

Immune reactions. Human platelets aggregate and undergo the release reaction in response to preformed immune complexes, aggregated IgG and zymosan particles, and contribute to their removal from the circulation. These reactions lead to transient thrombocytopenia, and are probably concerned in the pathogenesis of acute thrombocytopenia in various clinical circumstances (see Chapter 25). The vascular occlusion and injury associated with transplant rejection is largely attributable to platelet aggregation and release in response to immune complex formation, and can be partially overcome by treatment with inhibitors of these platelet responses [219]. Further details of the role of platelets in immune reactions are given in Refs 220 and 221.

Wound healing. During the release reaction, platelets secrete from their α granules a basic protein which stimulates the growth of arterial smooth muscle [165] and skin fibroblasts [166]. This platelet-derived growth factor, which may play an important part in the pathogenesis of atherosclerosis (see Chapter 30), perhaps also contributes to the proliferation of fibroblasts during wound healing. Serotonin released from the platelets may also contribute, since it has been shown to stimulate the secretion of collagen by fibroblasts [222].

DISORDERS OF PLATELET FUNCTION

Bleeding disorders may result from abnormalities of platelet function affecting any one or more of the steps involved in the formation of a haemostatic plug—adhesion to subendothelial connective tissue, endoperoxide and thromboxane synthesis, contraction, secretion, aggregation, the contribution of platelets to blood coagulation, and clot retraction. As in the field of blood coagulation, genetic defects of platelet function are more specific in their effects than acquired disorders, and their investigation has taught us much about normal platelet function.

Inherited disorders of platelet function

As shown in Table 26.7, these may be classified into abnormalities of the plasma membrane and those affecting intracellular structures and mechanisms. The former group includes defects of adhesion, aggregation and blood coagulation mechanisms, while the latter group all result in defects of secretion. Defects of adhesion may also be due to hereditary disorders of the connective tissue with which the platelets normally react, as in the Ehlers–Danlos syndrome (see p. 1061), or of the factor-VIII complex (von Willebrand's disease, Chapter 28), and aggregation will be defective in afibrinogenaemia [223] (Chapter 28), but this section is confined to defects of the platelets themselves.

Table 26.7. Inherited disorders of platelet function

Membrane abnormalities
  Bernard–Soulier syndrome
  Thrombasthenia
  Platelet factor-3 deficiency

Intracellular abnormalities
  Storage-pool (dense body) deficiency
    Hermansky–Pudlak syndrome
    Wiskott–Aldrich syndrome
    Chediak–Higashi syndrome
    Thrombocytopenia with absent radii
    Idiopathic storage-pool disease
  α-granule deficiency
    Gray platelet syndrome
  Combined deficiency of dense bodies and α granules
  Defects of thromboxane synthesis
    Cyclo-oxygenase deficiency
    Thromboxane synthetase deficiency
    Defective response to thromboxane

Miscellaneous
  Epstein's syndrome
  May–Hegglin anomaly

MEMBRANE ABNORMALITIES

Bernard–Soulier syndrome

This condition, first described in 1948 [224], is a rare autosomal-recessive trait of which the typical features are a long bleeding time, a normal or variably reduced platelet count, defective prothrombin consumption and unusually large platelets, commonly showing a wide variation in size and appearance on a stained film. The haemorrhagic symptoms consist of numerous superficial bruises and ecchymoses, often apparently spontaneous, mucosal bleeding and excessive and prolonged haemorrhage following trauma; like the prolongation of the bleeding time, their severity is characteristically disproportionate to the degree of thrombocytopenia. Symptoms are usually observed during the first months or years of life, and several deaths have occurred from haemorrhage during childhood. The clinical severity of the disease varies from one patient to another, but is not well correlated with the results of laboratory investigations.

Pathogenesis. Platelets of patients with the Bernard–Soulier syndrome adhere normally to collagen *in vitro*, and aggregate and release normally in response to ADP or collagen, but fail to agglutinate in the presence of bovine factor VIII [225] or of human factor VIII and ristocetin [226]. They are defective in their capacity to adhere to the subendothelium of rabbit aorta, but not in their ability to form microthrombi by aggregation at sites where platelets do adhere [227]. The defect of adhesion presumably explains the long bleeding time and the haemostatic failure; like the defect of ristocetin-induced agglutination, it appears to be due to a specific deficiency of the sialic-acid-rich glycoprotein I complex in the platelet membrane [228]. This glycoprotein is evidently essential for the interaction of platelets with the plasma factor-VIII-von Willebrand factor, which is required for both these reactions [228, 229] and may perhaps be the site of a factor-VIII receptor. The defective prothrombin consumption, first recognized by Bernard & Soulier [224], is due to impaired coagulant activity of the platelets and has been shown to be associated with a failure to bind and activate plasma factor XI [230]; this may be another effect of the glycoprotein deficiency, as may the short platelet survival which is the probable cause of the thrombocytopenia. The receptor for quinine- and quinidine-dependent antibodies, which is absent from Bernard–Soulier platelets, is evidently also situated on the glycoprotein complex [62].

Diagnosis. The clinical features of the Bernard–Soulier syndrome are no different from those of von Willebrand's disease, thrombasthenia or other inherited platelet disorders, and the diagnosis rests on the results of laboratory tests. The combination of a long bleeding time and giant platelets suggests the diagnosis, particularly if there is evidence of autosomal-recessive inheritance, such as consanguinity; confirmation comes from the finding of defective ristocetin agglutination of the patient's platelets, not corrected by normal plasma (Fig. 26.9). Other diagnostic features are shown in Table 26.8, page 1051.

Management. Bleeding from superficial cuts can usually be adequately controlled by local measures, but platelet transfusions are the only means available for treating serious bleeding episodes or for controlling surgical haemorrhage. Splenectomy has been performed in a few cases, and has sometimes resulted in a moderate increase of platelet count and partial amelioration of the bleeding tendency; it is a hazardous undertaking, however, and cannot be expected to be effective. Corticosteroids are contraindicated. Serious menorrhagia may require use of anovulatory drugs.

A patient with the Bernard–Soulier syndrome who had received muliple platelet transfusions developed an IgG antibody which agglutinated normal platelets carrying a wide range of group-specific antigens, but not the patient's own platelets or those of other patients with the Bernard–Soulier syndrome [231]. The antibody inhibited both ristocetin agglutination and adhesion to subendothelium of normal platelets, and was probably directed against the glycoprotein lacking from the patient's own platelets [232]. This represents a potential hazard of replacement therapy in this condition.

Thrombasthenia (Glanzmann's disease)

This is an autosomal-recessive trait resulting in a lifelong bleeding tendency, usually of moderate severity, the typical symptoms being multiple superficial bruises, epistaxis and menorrhagia, and prolonged haemorrhage from superficial cuts. The platelets are normal in number and size, but the bleeding time is greatly prolonged and clot retraction is defective, as noted by Glanzmann in his original description [233]. The essential diagnostic feature is the complete failure of the platelets to aggregate in response to ADP. Although the defect is absolute, the clinical severity can vary widely from one patient to another, and not infrequently seems to diminish somewhat during adult life.

Pathogenesis. Thrombasthenic platelets adhere normally to collagen fibres *in vitro* and undergo the release reaction normally in response to collagen or thrombin [234], but they completely fail to aggregate in response to either of these reagents or to ADP, adrenaline or 5HT [234–236]. In contrast to Bernard–Soulier platelets, they are agglutinated by bovine factor VIII [236] and by ristocetin [237], and adhere normally to subendothelium, though they fail to form microthrombi by aggregating on top of the adherent monolayer [238]. Though ADP and thrombin fail to aggregate them, they bind normally to the membrane [239, 240] and cause a normal shape change [234]. This initial reaction is not accompanied, however, as in the case of normal platelets, by the induction of a fibrinogen receptor on the platelet membrane [120, 122, 123]. The platelets of most, but not all, thrombasthenic patients are deficient in fibrinogen [236], and a deficiency of platelet factor-VIII-related antigen has also been observed [241]. The defect of clot retraction is more profound in those cases with a deficiency of platelet fibrinogen than in those without, but the aggregation defect is absolute in both groups.

Thrombasthenic platelets are deficient in two closely associated membrane glycoproteins, IIb and IIIa [63, 64], and it may be that these carry the fibrinogen receptor inducible by ADP on normal platelets. Since α-actinin, which is deficient in thrombasthenic platelets, has been identified with glycoprotein III [67], this specific glycoprotein deficiency, by depriving the platelet of points of attachment for fibrinogen on the outer surface of the membrane and actin on the inner surface, may well account for the defects of both aggregation and clot retraction. Glycoprotein IIIa also carries the Pl^A (Zw) platelet alloantigens, which are partially or wholly deleted in thrombasthenia [242]. An IgG antibody developing in the plasma of a thrombasthenic patient after platelet transfusion, induced a thrombasthenia-like state in normal platelets [243, 244], and appeared to be directed against the glycoprotein IIb/IIIa complex from normal platelet membranes [245].

Although thrombasthenic platelets neither aggregate nor promote clot retraction (both of which require extracellular cations), they appear to be capable of fulfilling all the functions for which intracellular calcium ions are necessary. Thus they synthesize prostaglandin endoperoxides and thromboxanes, and undergo contraction and secretion of dense-body constituents, in response to thrombin or the ionophore A23187 [234, 246], though not in response to ADP [247], which can evidently only produce these effects when aggregation occurs [178]. The failure to make PF3 available [235] is a constant feature, which is presumably secondary to the aggregation defect [190]. Defects of activation of factors XII and XI by thrombasthenic platelets have also been observed, and appear to be more closely correlated with clinical severity [248].

Diagnosis. The condition is indistinguishable on clinical grounds from other hereditary platelet disorders, and the diagnosis depends on the demonstration of the characteristic aggregation defect (Table 26.8, Fig. 26.9). Complete failure of aggregation in response to any concentration of ADP is virtually pathognomic of thrombasthenia.

Detection of heterozygotes. There is preliminary evidence that heterozygotes, though they have neither abnormal bleeding nor a demonstrable aggregation defect, may have reduced amounts of glycoprotein IIb/IIIa in their platelet membranes, detectable either biochemically [249] or immunologically [250].

Management. Corticosteroids and splenectomy are contraindicated. Bleeding episodes require local haemostatic measures and platelet transfusion, but the potential risk of development of platelet antibodies [243] must be borne in mind. Suppression of ovulation may be required for serious menorrhagia.

Platelet factor-3 deficiency

A failure of ADP or kaolin to make PF3 available is a constant feature of thrombasthenia, in which the platelets do not aggregate in response to these stimuli, and a partial defect of PF3 availability is frequently seen in many other conditions which result in minor defects of platelet aggregation and release [251, 252], presumably as a secondary effect of these. Weiss *et al.* [253] have recently reported the case of a young woman whose long-standing bleeding disorder appeared to be due to a primary defect of PF3, unassociated with any abnormality of platelet aggregation or secretion. The bleeding time was consistently normal, but prothrombin consumption was defective and PF3 availability was not restored to normal by lysing the platelets, as in aggregation defects. The underlying defect appeared to consist of a deficiency of factor-V binding sites on the platelet membrane, resulting in impaired binding of factor Xa in addition [254]. Platelet transfusion was effective in securing surgical haemostasis. The aetiology of the condition remains unexplained; bleeding symptoms were first noticed during the second decade of life, and there was no evidence of a platelet abnormality in the patient's parents, or of a bleeding tendency amongst her other relatives.

INTRACELLULAR DEFECTS

In 1967, Hardisty & Hutton [251] described a series of patients with mild haemorrhagic tendencies associated with a variety of clinical conditions, whose platelets failed to aggregate in response to collagen, and gave only first-phase aggregation with ADP or adrenaline, without the second wave usually associated with the release reaction. Similar defects of platelet aggregation have since been described in a wide variety of conditions, both hereditary and acquired, and the association of this pattern of aggregation response with defects of the release reaction has been abundantly confirmed [255–257]. Hereditary disorders of the release reaction fall into two groups (Table 26.7): 'storage-pool deficiency', in which the failure of release is due to a lack of the dense bodies in which the releasable pool of adenine nucleotides and 5HT are normally stored; and defects of induction of the release mechanism, including defects of thromboxane synthesis from arachidonic acid or of response to thromboxane. A third type of hereditary intracellular defect, which may coexist with dense-body deficiency, or occur separately from it, is deficiency of the α granules. All of these give rise to mild bleeding disorders which seldom require any special therapeutic measures except in the case of surgery or serious accidental trauma, when platelet transfusions may be indicated.

Storage-pool deficiency

Pathogenesis and diagnosis. Besides the characteristic pattern of aggregation described above and in Table 26.8, and shown in Figure 26.9, the chief diagnostic features of this condition are those of a deficiency of dense-body constituents from the patient's platelets. Thus the 5HT content of the platelets will be low, and their saturation capacity for [^{14}C]5HT and ability to release it in reponse to thrombin will be defective

[257–259]; ATP will be somewhat reduced, and ADP much more so, giving a total nucleotide distribution within the platelets equivalent to that of the metabolic pool alone of normal platelets (see Table 26.5), with an abnormally high ATP/ADP ratio [256–258], and incubation with labelled adenine will lead to an abnormally high specific activity of ADP within the platelets, since there is no unlabelled storage pool to dilute the rapidly labelled metabolic pool [260]. Electron microscopy will reveal the paucity of dense bodies [261, 262], and platelet calcium content will also be found to be reduced [263].

In at least some cases of storage-pool deficiency, ADP, adrenaline and collagen also fail to induce thromboxane formation, apparently because of a failure to activate phospholipase [264]. The conversion of arachidonic acid to endoperoxides and thromboxane is normal, however [264, 265], and aggregation in response to sodium arachidonate is therefore a useful test for distinguishing storage-pool deficiency from disorders of this pathway (see Table 26.8).

Clinical associations. Storage-pool deficiency occurs in a variety of hereditary bleeding disorders with distinguishing clinical features and also as an isolated hereditary defect, when it has been termed *storage-pool disease* [260]. This latter group is itself heterogeneous, since some patients have been found to have an associated deficiency of α granules [266]. In three families studied [255, 265, 267] an autosomal-dominant pattern of heredity has been observed. Amongst other syndromes of which storage-pool deficiency forms a part, the *Hermansky–Pudlak syndrome* is the best studied with regard to the platelet defect [258, 261, 268]. This is an autosomal-recessive trait characterized by the triad of oculocutaneous albinism, a lifelong bleeding tendency and the presence of pigmented macrophages in the bone marrow [269]. The albinism is of the tyrosinase-positive variety, and the ceroid-like pigment is found throughout the reticulo-endothelial system [270], including macrophages in the lung and intestine; this may lead to pulmonary fibrosis and inflammatory bowel disease [271]. The platelet count is normal, and the bleeding tendency and long bleeding time are attributable to the defect of platelet function. Heterozygotes are clinically unaffected, but in one family they have been found to have low levels of platelet 5HT [271a].

Storage-pool deficiency has also been observed in the Wiskott–Aldrich syndrome [272], the Chediak–Higashi syndrome [273, 274], and the syndrome of thrombocytopenia with absent radii [275]. In all of these, however (see Chapter 25), the main cause of bleeding symptoms is the thrombocytopenia. Shapiro *et al.* [276], on the other hand, found that carriers of the

Wiskott–Aldrich syndrome had a defect of oxidative phosphorylation in their platelets, so that the second wave of aggregation in response to adrenaline was abolished by inhibition of glycolysis alone. This was thought to provide a method for carrier detection, and also suggested that the release defect observed in Wiskott–Aldrich patients might be due to a metabolic abnormality rather than a storage-pool deficiency. Subsequent investigations, however, have failed to substantiate these findings.

Defect of induction of the release reaction
In these disorders the releasable nucleotides and 5HT are normally present, but the mechanism for their release is defective. Since this situation is most commonly produced by the ingestion of aspirin, the naturally-occurring condition has been referred to as 'aspirin-like defect' [256, 257]. Although the actual mechanism involved has not been elucidated in most such cases, a few have been shown to have a deficiency of platelet *cyclo-oxygenase* [277–279], the enzyme in the cyclic endoperoxide pathway which is inhibited by aspirin, and one a deficiency of *thromboxane synthetase* [279a]. The pattern of aggregation responses to ADP and collagen in these patients resembles that of storage-pool deficiency, but their platelets also fail to aggregate, or to synthesize thromboxanes, in response to sodium arachidonate. The chief difficulty in diagnosis is to exclude aspirin ingestion as the cause of the platelet abnormality. One patient with cyclo-oxygenase deficiency was found to have a defect of PGI_2 synthesis in venous tissue as well as of thromboxanes by platelets [279]: the net clinical effect was a mild bleeding tendency without thrombotic problems. In several cases a similar aggregation pattern has been shown to be due to a failure of the platelets to respond to thromboxane, though they synthesize it normally [412, 413].

This group of defects of release induction may well prove to be still more heterogeneous, particularly since some of them appear to be enhanced by aspirin [280], suggesting a mechanism independent of thromboxane synthesis. Many such patients have bleeding times within the normal range, but becoming unusually prolonged after taking aspirin [280].

Gray platelet syndrome: hereditary hypogranular thrombocytopenia
An autosomal-dominant bleeding disorder, characterized by ecchymoses and mucosal haemorrhages, a long bleeding time, mild thrombocytopenia and a greatly reduced number of platelet granules, has been reported in Dutch and Swiss families [280a, 280b], and given the name of 'hereditary hypogranular thrombocytopenia'. Raccuglia [281] described a boy with an evidently similar condition, whose thrombocytopenia responded partially to corticosteroids and splenectomy, and called it the 'gray platelet syndrome', from the appearance of the platelets on electron microscopy. Further investigations on this and subsequent investigation of another similar patient have shown that their platelets are larger than normal and have a specific deficiency of α granules, with normal numbers of dense bodies and other organelles [282]. The condition is extremely rare, and usually causes only relatively minor haemorrhagic symptoms.

MISCELLANEOUS HEREDITARY DISORDERS

Epstein's syndrome [283] consists of the association of thrombocytopenia and giant platelets with Alport's syndrome of hereditary nephritis and nerve deafness. The details of the functional defect of the platelets have not been fully worked out; there appears to be a defect of aggregation and release [283, 284] though this has been disputed [285]. Heredity is autosomal dominant.

Defects of platelet function have also been described in *Down's syndrome* [286], and in various hereditary connective-tissue disorders [287, 288]. None of these are associated with major bleeding tendencies: haemorrhage in the latter group, when it occurs, is more likely to be due to the abnormality of the connective tissue itself (see p. 1061).

Seven members of a family, in which a mild bleeding disorder appeared to be inherited as an autosomal-dominant trait, have been found to have a defect of platelet aggregation by arachidonate, but normal responses to ADP, adrenaline and collagen [289]. These observations are difficult to reconcile with current views on the interrelations of platelet functions, and require further investigation.

DIAGNOSIS OF HEREDITARY DISORDERS
From the clinical point of view, the diagnosis of a hereditary disorder of platelet function is suggested by a lifelong history of multiple superficial bruises, perhaps associated with apparently spontaneous haemorrhages into the skin or from mucous membranes. The nature of the haemorrhagic lesions themselves does not distinguish one platelet disorder from another, but clues to a more specific diagnosis may come from the genetic pattern or from associated clinical features characteristic of particular syndromes (Table 26.8). The characteristic laboratory pointers to a defect of platelet function are a long bleeding time and a normal (or possibly moderately reduced) platelet count: this combination indicates the need for platelet function tests, as may a strongly suggestive clinical history even in the absence of a prolonged bleeding time. Assays of the various activities of the factor-VIII

Table 26.8. Diagnosis of inherited disorders of platelet function

Disorder	Platelet count	Platelet size	Aggregation			Ristocetin agglutination		Heredity	Associated features
			ADP	Collagen	Arachidonic acid	Platelets	Plasma		
Bernard–Soulier syndrome	↓ (or N)	↑	N	N	N	↓	N	AR	
von Willebrand's disease*	N	N	N	N	N	N	↓	Variable*	Factor-VIII defects
Thrombasthenia	N	N	Nil	Nil	Nil	N	N	AR	Clot retraction ↓
Storage-pool disease	N	N or ↓	↓	↓	N	↓	N	AD	
Hermansky–Pudlak syndrome	N	N	↓	↓	N	↓	N	AR	Albinism, pigmented macrophages
Wiskott–Aldrich syndrome	↓	↓	↓	↓	N	↓	N	X-borne	Recurrent infections, eczema
Disorders of thromboxane synthesis	N	N	↓	↓	↓	↓	N	?	
Gray platelet syndrome	↓ or N	N or ↑	N	N	N	↓	N	?	

N, normal; 1, first phase only; AR, autosomal recessive; AD, autosomal dominant.
* See Chapter 28.

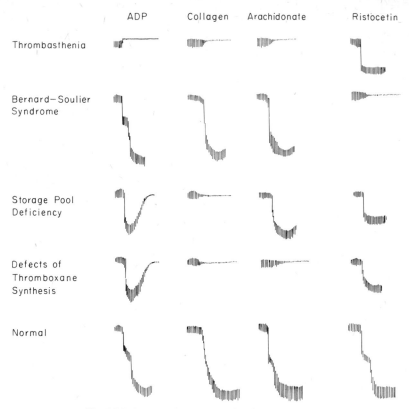

Fig. 26.9. Aggregation patterns in platelet disorders.

complex will be required for the diagnosis or exclusion of von Willebrand's disease (see Chapter 28), and tests of aggregation by ADP, collagen, arachidonic acid and ristocetin will serve to identify most of the recognized platelet abnormalities: typical aggregation patterns are shown in Figure 26.9. Other confirmatory investigations in particular circumstances may include measurement of platelet size by means of an electronic particle sizer (see Table 26.8), electron microscopy, content and secretion of dense-body and α-granule constituents, platelet coagulant activities, clot retraction, endoperoxide and thromboxane synthesis and surface membrane glycoproteins. In practice, these special investigations are seldom necessary for routine diagnostic purposes, though they may help to identify and explain new and unusual disorders.

Acquired disorders of platelet function
Platelet function may be disturbed in a wide range of diseases, and by the action of several different classes of drugs. The platelet abnormalities in many of the conditions listed in Table 26.9 are less well defined than in the hereditary platelet disorders, and even the degree

to which they contribute to the bleeding tendency may be in doubt, since other defects of the haemostatic mechanism not infrequently coexist.

Uraemia
The bleeding tendency associated with uraemia is probably largely due to defective platelet function,

Table 26.9. Causes of acquired platelet dysfunction

Uraemia
Myeloproliferative disorders
Acute leukaemias and pre-leukaemic states
Dysproteinaemias
Chronic hypoglycaemia
Liver disease
Valvular and congenital heart disease
Severe burns
Scurvy
Drugs*

---

* See Table 26.10.

though coagulation defects and thrombocytopenia may contribute in some cases. The bleeding time is frequently prolonged, and amongst other abnormalities that have been demonstrated are reduced platelet retention in glass-bead columns and defective PF3 availability and clot retraction [290–293]. Aggregation findings have been inconsistent, and have included defects of primary ADP-induced aggregation, patterns suggesting defects of release, and normal results [290, 291, 294–296]. It is therefore perhaps not surprising that there is equal lack of agreement about the pathogenesis of the defects. They can be corrected by haemodialysis or peritoneal dialysis, which also corrects the bleeding tendency [297], suggesting that they are due to the inhibitory effect of retained metabolites in the plasma. Urea [298, 299], the urea metabolite guanidino-succinic acid [295] and phenolic acids [300] have all been proposed as the agents responsible, and Rabiner [301] has concluded that both classes of compound contribute to the platelet abnormality, each by a different mechanism. More recently, uraemic bleeding has been found to be associated with reduced prostaglandin-endoperoxide production and adenylate-cyclase activity in platelets [302], and with increased PGI_2 production by vessel walls [303]: the resulting imbalance between PGI_2 and thromboxane-A_2 production may be largely responsible for the defect of aggregation. Raised plasma levels of low-affinity PF4 [304] and β thromboglobulin [305] have also been observed in patients with chronic renal failure; both increase further after haemodialysis, owing to mechanical damage to the platelets.

Myeloproliferative disorders

Patients with these disorders (see Chapter 32) may suffer from a severe bleeding tendency, with a prolonged bleeding time, in the presence of a normal or even a greatly raised platelet count. Ecchymoses, epistaxis and gastro-intestinal haemorrhage are the commonest symptoms. Thrombosis of peripheral arteries is another frequent complication, particularly in patients with thrombocythaemia, and may coexist with haemorrhagic symptoms.

Many different abnormalities of platelet function have been described in these patients, and none of them can be regarded as especially characteristic of any single disease entity: similar defects have been observed in patients with essential thrombocythaemia, polycythaemia vera, myelofibrosis and chronic granulocytic leukaemia. The results of platelet function tests have sometimes [306, 307], but by no means always [308–310], been found to correlate with clinical evidence of bleeding and/or thrombosis. Secondary thrombocytosis, in contrast to essential thrombocythaemia, does not usually result in either a bleeding

tendency or a demonstrable defect of platelet function [306, 308, 311, 312].

Amongst the abnormalities which have been described are defects of platelet coagulant activity, retention in glass-bead columns, and aggregation. The patterns of aggregation observed have included defects both of the first and the second wave in response to various aggregating agents, but the commonest abnormality is a failure of response to adrenaline or noradrenaline [308, 310, 313, 314], which may be due to a deficiency of α-adrenergic receptors on the membrane of these platelets [315]. Defects of the release reaction in response to other inducing agents, particularly collagen, are also frequently seen, however, and may have a multiple pathogenesis, including defects of endoperoxide and thromboxane synthesis in some patients [307, 316] and storage-pool deficiency in others [317, 318]. Changes in the distribution of membrane glycoproteins have also been reported in myeloproliferative disorders [319], but are of doubtful relevance to the haemostatic mechanism. In contrast to the aggregation defects discussed above, evidence of hyperaggregability has been obtained in a number of patients, and has been found to correlate well with the incidence of arterial thrombotic episodes [320]. A possible explanation for such hyperaggregability is provided by the resistance of platelets from patients with various myeloproliferative disorders to the aggregation inhibitor prostaglandin D_2 [321], which has been shown to be due to the loss of specific membrane receptors [322].

Platelet function usually returns towards normal in response to myelosuppressive therapy, though this is not always the case; even venesection has had this effect in polycythaemia vera [309]. Thrombotic complications may respond to anti-platelet drugs such as aspirin and dipyridamole [320, 323]. Treatment of these disorders is considered in detail in Chapter 32.

Acute leukaemias and pre-leukaemic states. The usual cause of bleeding in the acute leukaemias is thrombocytopenia, but defects of platelet function may sometimes play a role during the overt disease, as well as in various pre-leukaemic states. Defects in PF3 availability, aggregation and release have all been observed [324–326]; storage-pool deficiency and a metabolic defect may both contribute to the failure of release [327].

Dysproteinaemias

Amongst the many haemostatic abnormalities observed in this group of diseases, including also disorders of coagulation and fibrinolysis, defects of platelet function and hyperviscosity seem to be the most closely correlated with clinical bleeding [328,

329]. The bleeding time is often prolonged, and laboratory findings include defects of platelet retention in glass-bead columns, PF3 availability, aggregation and adhesion to connective tissues [328–331]. These defects are due to the inhibitory effect of the paraprotein, which probably acts by coating the platelet and collagen surfaces; they can be corrected by plasmapheresis. Further details are given in Chapter 19.

Chronic hypoglycaemia

A mild haemorrhagic tendency, characterized by superficial bruising, epistaxis and prolonged bleeding after trauma, and by a long bleeding time, forms part of the syndrome resulting from *glycogen-storage disease type I (glucose-6-phosphatase deficiency)*. Similar bleeding symptoms result from *fructose-1, 6-diphosphatase deficiency*. In both these disorders, there is a defect of platelet aggregation and nucleotide release in response to ADP, collagen or adrenaline [332–334]; this platelet abnormality is not a direct result of the underlying hereditary metabolic defect, but is evidently due to a defect of platelet nucleotide synthesis secondary to the chronic hypoglycaemia [334], which itself results from the hereditary enzyme defect in the liver cells. Continuous intravenous administration of glucose produces a gradual correction of the haemostatic defect by restoring the capacity of the platelets to synthesize sufficient ATP to perform their haemostatic functions.

Liver disease

Coagulation disorders are the chief cause of haemostatic failure in liver disease (see Chapter 29), but thrombocytopenia and disorders of platelet function may also occur, including defective aggregation in response to ADP and thrombin [335, 336]. It has been suggested [335] that the aggregation defect is largely attributable to the presence of fibrinogen degradation products (FDP) in the circulation, which are well known to impair this function *in vitro* [337, 338], but it is doubtful whether sufficiently high concentrations of FDP are reached *in vivo* to produce this effect [339].

Other conditions

Acquired storage-pool deficiency has been described in patients with severe valvular heart disease, in whom the defect was intensified by cardiopulmonary bypass surgery [340]; in severely burnt patients [341]; and in one patient with autoimmune disease characterized by nephritis, polyarthralgia, chondritis and antiplatelet antibodies [342], and another with a post-operative deep-vein thrombosis and pulmonary embolism who also had evidence of disseminated intravascular coagulation [343]. It is to be presumed that all these clinical circumstances led to intravascular platelet damage, with partial release of their dense-body contents. Less well-defined defects of platelet function have been observed in a variety of other conditions, including scurvy [344], pernicious anaemia [345], congenital heart disease [346] and infectious mononucleosis [347].

Bartter's syndrome [348] is an uncommon metabolic disorder associated with hyerplasia of the renal juxtaglomerular apparatus and characterized by hypokalaemic alkalosis, hyper-reninaemia, aldosteronism, increased excretion of urinary prostaglandins and normal blood pressure. Defective platelet aggregation has been reported [349] and appears to be due to a plasma factor; it is improved by indomethacin. It seems likely that the aggregation defect results from over-production of prostacyclin [350] or a more stable related substance [351].

Drug-induced defects of platelet function

Various classes of drugs are known to interfere with platelet function: some of them are used as potential anti-thrombotic agents on account of their anti-platelet effects (see Chapter 30), while others may cause bleeding symptoms as a side-effect of their use for other purposes; acetylsalicylic acid (aspirin) falls into both these groups. Others again, while known to inhibit various aspects of platelet function *in vitro*, do not significantly impair haemostasis at pharmacological dosage; amongst these are tricyclic anti-depressants, anti-histamines, phenothiazines and both general and local anaesthetics. Several excellent reviews of the effects of drugs on platelet function are available [352–354]; the present account is confined to those (Table 26.10) whose clinical use may cause bleeding as a side-effect. It is essential, before performing platelet function tests in the course of investigating a possible bleeding tendency, to ensure that the patient has not taken any drugs which may have interfered with platelet function during the preceding seven to 10 days.

Table 26.10. Drugs which may cause bleeding through interference with platelet function

Acetylsalicylic acid
Other non-steroidal anti-inflammatory agents
    Indomethacin
    Sulphinpyrazone
    Phenylbutazone
Dextrans
Heparin
Penicillins, cephalosporins

Acetylsalicylic acid. Aspirin has long been known to prolong the bleeding time, and to provoke bleeding in some patients; its use is contraindicated in patients with known bleeding disorders. It has been shown to impair platelet aggregation by inhibiting the release reaction [355–358], and this effect is now known to be due to its inhibition of the enzyme cyclo-oxygenase, leading to a failure of endoperoxide and thromboxane synthesis by the platelets [144, 145] (and incidentally also to a failure of synthesis of I_2 by the vascular endothelium). Aspirin inhibits cyclo-oxygenase irreversibly by acetylation [359], and the effect of a single pharmacological dose (300–600 mg) can be detected for up to a week or more—throughout the lifespan of the platelets exposed to it. Other non-steroidal anti-inflammatory drugs, including indomethacin, sulphinpyrazone and phenylbutazone, have a similar but less prolonged effect. Some of these (but not aspirin itself) have also been claimed to inhibit platelet adhesion to subendothelial structures [354].

Dextrans. These have been shown to prolong the bleeding time [360] and to inhibit PF3 availability, retention in glass-bead columns and collagen-induced aggregation [361–363]. These effects are dose-related and are more pronounced with HMW dextrans [362, 363]; they reach a maximum four to eight hours after the end of an infusion, implying that they are not due to simple absorption of dextran to the platelet surface, since this occurs rapidly. It has been suggested that dextran may act by causing reversible platelet aggregation, with subsequent refractoriness to further aggregating stimuli [364].

Penicillins and cephalosporins. McClure *et al.* [365] observed purpuric bleeding in patients receiving carbenicillin in high dosage, and found that the drug prolonged the bleeding time and impaired ADP-induced platelet aggregation. Several other penicillins have been found to have a similar effect, including penicillin G and ampicillin, and to a lesser extent, ticarcillin and methicillin [366, 367]; cephalosporins have also been incriminated [368]. Adhesion to collagen-coated surfaces and subendothelium, shape change, aggregation, release, PF3 availability and clot retraction have all been shown to be inhibited by high concentrations of pencillin G and cephalothin *in vitro* [369], and it has been suggested that all these antibiotics act by coating the platelet surface [366, 369]. They produce bleeding symptoms only when given in very high dosage, particularly to patients in renal failure, whose platelet function may already be defective and in whom clearance of the drug is impaired.

DISORDERS OF VASCULAR FUNCTION

The non-thrombocytopenic purpuras

In a wide variety of conditions, both hereditary and acquired, a tendency to bleed from small vessels seems to result from an abnormality of the vessels themselves, or of their supporting structures, in the absence of any demonstrable defect of the platelets or coagulation mechanism. In some of these disorders, the bleeding is related to focal vascular abnormalities, as in hereditary haemorrhagic telangiectasia, or to local inflammation or pressure (e.g. exanthemata, cough purpura), while in others, such as the Schönlein–Henoch syndrome, it may be more generalized. Vascular lesions of various sorts may also contribute to the pathogenesis of abnormal bleeding, together with disorders of the platelets and/or coagulation mechanism, as in the purpuras due to some drugs and snake venoms, and in association with scurvy and giant haemangiomata.

Besides these examples, Table 26.11 lists a miscellany of disorders of which the haemorrhagic component seems to have a predominantly vascular origin. In the absence of reliable clinical tests of vascular function, this assumption often rests largely on the failure to demonstrate defects of the other components of the haemostatic mechanism. In practice, the diagnosis of this group of disorders depends very largely on clinical features rather than laboratory tests. Some of them are considered in more detail below, and some in other chapters; others again are mentioned only briefly, on account of their differential diagnostic significance.

MECHANICAL PURPURAS

Local purpura may occur as a result of an acute or chronic increase in intravascular pressure, particularly in small venules, in a wide variety of clinical contexts, in subjects with no generalized bleeding tendency. For example, purpura is commonly seen over the presenting part in newborn infants as a result of compression of small vessels during the birth process, and prolonged coughing or vomiting may lead to purpura of the face and neck, or even subconjunctival haemorrhage.

Orthostatic purpura. This may develop over the lower legs of elderly people after prolonged standing, particularly in association with varicose veins; atrophy of supporting structures, as in senile purpura of the upper limbs (p. 1058), may be a contributory factor as well as the increased hydrostatic pressure. This condition may result in a permanent dusky discoloration of the skin due to deposition of haemosiderin.

Table 26.11. Bleeding disorders due mainly to vascular abnormalities

---

Mechanical
    Cough purpura
    Neonatal (compression) purpura
    Orthostatic purpura
    Pigmented dermatoses

Allergic
    Schönlein–Henoch syndrome
    Drug purpuras

Atrophic
    Senile purpura
    Steroid purpura
    Cushing's syndrome
    Scurvy

Inflammatory, toxic (Chs 25 and 29)
    Exanthemata
    Bacterial and rickettsial infections
    Purpura fulminans
    Snake venoms

Hereditary disorders of blood vessels and connective tissues
    Hereditary haemorrhagic telangiectasia
    Ehlers–Danlos syndrome
    Pseudoxanthoma elasticum
    Osteogenesis imperfecta
    Marfan's syndrome
    Fabry's disease (Ch. 33)

Paraproteinaemias, amyloidosis (Ch. 19)

Proliferative vascular disorders
    Kaposi's sarcoma
    Haemangiomata (Ch. 25)

Miscellaneous
    Purpura simplex
    Factitious purpura
    Autoerythrocyte sensitization, DNA sensitivity

Pigmented dermatoses. These are a group of chronic skin diseases affecting mainly dependent areas and characterized by capillary proliferation with inflammation and rupture of skin vessels, leading, as in other cases of chronic orthostatic purpura, to extravasation of red cells and deposition of haemosiderin. The group includes annular telangiectatic purpura (Majocchi's disease), the pigmentary dermatoses of Schamberg, and the pigmented purpuric lichenoid dermatitis of Gougerot and Blum, in which purpuric papules are scattered among larger purpuric lesions. The three are probably not distinct entities [370]; their importance to the haematologist consists only in the need to distinguish them from other causes of chronic purpura of the lower limbs, including paraproteinaemias and amyloidosis.

ALLERGIC PURPURAS
The terms *allergic* or *anaphylactoid purpura* are com-
monly used to refer to a group of non-thrombocytopenic purpuras characterized by aseptic inflammation of the vessels of the skin and other tissues, in association with other allergic features, such as urticaria and oedema. The syndrome may occur acutely and transiently following the ingestion of certain drugs or foods in sensitive individuals, or may form part of a more chronic and widespread autoimmune disorder. The association of the skin lesions with joint pains and/or gastro-intestinal symptoms leads to the diagnosis of the Schönlein–Henoch syndrome.

Schönlein–Henoch syndrome
In 1837, under the name 'peliosis rheumatica', Schönlein [371] described the syndrome of a red macular and purpuric rash with acute joint symptoms. Many years later, his former student, Henoch [372], reported four cases of a similar condition in children associated with colic and bloody diarrhoea, and in 1895 he was the first to draw attention to the important association of renal disease with the syndrome [373]. Osler [374] pointed out the similarities of the condition to serum sickness, attributed it to an anaphylactic response to foreign antigens and coined the term 'anaphylactoid purpura'.

Pathogenesis. Since Osler's original suggestion, the Schönlein–Henoch syndrome has been regarded as a manifestation of a disordered immune response to a variety of antigens. Of these, β-haemolytic streptococci were probably once the most important, but more recent observations suggest that this is no longer the case [375–377]; many different antigenic stimuli (see below) may evidently precipitate the disease. The characteristic lesion is an aseptic vasculitis, demonstrable in skin and renal biopsy material [376], and present also in affected areas of the bowel and other organs. The renal lesions are those of focal glomerulonephritis, with fibrinoid deposition and mesangial proliferation [378]. Deposits of IgA, and occasionally IgG and complement components (C3 and C4) can be demonstrated by immunofluorescence in vessels of both clinically affected and unaffected skin and in the mesangium of the glomeruli [379]. Levinsky & Barratt [380] found raised levels of IgA immune complexes in the serum of most children with the syndrome, irrespective of the presence of nephritis, but IgG immune complexes only in those in whom nephritis developed. They suggest that IgA complexes are probably not the direct cause of vascular damage, but may interfere with the clearance of IgG complexes, which bind complement and are thus toxic to the renal vessels.

Clinical features. The Schönlein–Henoch syndrome is an acute condition, chiefly of children, in which a characteristic exanthem is associated with various combinations of the following: localized subcutaneous oedema, painful periarticular swellings, gastro-intestinal symptoms and haematuria. The skin lesions are an invariable feature, and other types of lesion each occur in about half to two-thirds of affected children, though somewhat less frequently in adults, in which the course tends to be rather more benign and chronic. The incidence is rather higher in the spring and autumn than at other times of the year, and boys seem to be somewhat more commonly affected than girls, though there is no evidence of an unequal sex incidence in adults. The peak age incidence is between about three and seven years.

The onset usually follows about one to three weeks after an acute upper respiratory or other infection, various organisms having been implicated; less commonly, it appears to have been precipitated by the ingestion of certain foods [381] or drugs [382] and cases have also been reported following smallpox vaccination, insect bites or exposure to cold. There remains a proportion of cases—perhaps one in three—in which no precipitating cause can be identified.

The skin, joint and gastro-intestinal symptoms occur as the presenting feature with roughly equal frequency in children, and are commonly accompanied by moderate fever. The exanthem (Fig. 26.10) has been described in great detail by Gairdner [383]: it is fairly symmetrical, usually urticarial at the onset, later turning to a red maculopapular rash, which may become confluent before fading to a brown colour; ecchymoses are a patchy and inconstant feature, and are seldom extensive. The rash typically occurs in successive crops, chiefly on the buttocks and the extensor surfaces of the lower legs and arms; the face is often involved but the trunk seldom.

The knees and ankles are the joints most frequently affected, and after them the elbows, wrists and finger joints. The periarticular swelling is accompanied by moderate pain and tenderness, but the joint rarely becomes hot, red or acutely tender. Intra-articular effusions seldom occur, and although the joint manifestations tend to recur during the course of the disease, eventual resolution is complete, leaving no residual deformity. Acute colicky abdominal pain is the commonest symptom of intestinal involvement, and may present a difficult diagnostic problem when it antedates the rash. It is frequently recurrent, and often accompanied by melaena. In young children, evidence of intestinal bleeding not infrequently occurs in the absence of colic. Vomiting is fairly common, and haematemesis sometimes occurs. Occasionally, massive intestinal haemorrhage or intussusception may endanger life, and call for rapid treatment; when intussusception occurs after the age of two years, the Schönlein–Henoch syndrome is a likely diagnosis.

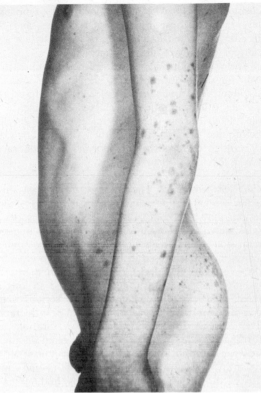

Fig. 26.10. Typical rash of Schönlein–Henoch syndrome. Reproduced from Ref. 411, by kind permission of the authors and publishers.

Localized subcutaneous oedema is common, particularly of the dorsum of the hands and feet, and less frequently of the scalp and periorbital region. Oedema of the face and scalp is a particularly common and distressing feature under the age of three, while involvement of the joints, gastro-intestinal tract and kidneys is more common in older children. In adults, the purpura usually occurs alone or in erythematous macules; raised skin lesions are not seen, but skin necrosis may occur. Joint and gastro-intestinal symptoms are seen somewhat less commonly than in children, being present in about half the patients [382].

Severe epistaxes and various neurological complications are occasionally seen [384], but much the most serious manifestation of the syndrome is renal involvement, which may lead to acute or chronic renal failure.

Diagnosis. This depends essentially on the clinical features. Laboratory tests may be of value in monitoring the course of the disease, but do not contribute to the diagnosis. There is usually a mild neutrophil leucocytosis and a raised ESR, and there may also be eosinophilia. The platelet count is normal, or moderately raised in response to haemorrhage, and the bleeding time and capillary resistance tests are also normal, as is the coagulation mechanism.

The skin lesions are usually sufficiently characteristic for diagnostic purposes, though they must be distinguished from the rash of rheumatic fever and various other exanthemata. Diagnostic difficulty is most likely to arise when systemic symptoms develop before the rash. In adults, the syndrome may be difficult to distinguish from polyarteritis nodosa or systemic lupus erythematosus.

Course and prognosis. The condition usually lasts up to a few weeks, during which successive crops of skin lesions may be accompanied by repeated episodes of intestinal or joint symptoms, before a spontaneous remission occurs. In about half the cases, one or more symptoms recur subsequently from time to time, but these recurrences seldom continue for more than a few months. The ultimate prognosis is good so long as renal involvement does not persist; serious acute complications such as gastro-intestinal or intracranial haemorrhage, intussusception and perforation, are fortunately rare. The mortality from renal disease is between one and five per cent, and the course of the renal involvement can be predicted with some confidence from the urinary and renal biopsy findings in the early stages of the disease [384]: early acute nephritis, marked proteinuria and haematuria at onset, and diffuse glomerular changes on renal biopsy are all adverse prognostic features, carrying an increased risk of chronic renal disease.

Treatment. The variability and relapsing nature of the syndrome makes the assessment of therapy very difficult, and no well-controlled trials have been carried out. Corticosteroids have been advocated for the relief of joint and abdominal symptoms, but have little, if any, effect on the skin lesions [385]; nor is there any good evidence that they influence the course of the renal disease [378]. Immunosuppressive therapy with azathioprine or cyclophosphamide has been used for chronic renal disease, but its value remains unproven. In summary, mild cases require nothing but symptomatic treatment, and active measures are needed only for the major complications when they occur. If food or drugs are suspected as the precipitating cause, they should obviously be eliminated.

Non-thrombocytopenic purpura due to drugs
Skin purpura, without thrombocytopenia, has been observed from time to time following the administration of a wide variety of drugs. No drugs produce it as a regular effect, and it may be assumed that it represents an idiosyncrasy of the particular patient. Among the drugs which have been associated with this form of purpura are penicillin, sulphonamides, salicylates, barbiturates and other hypnotics, meprobamate, iodides, quinine and many others. It is noteworthy that some drugs in this group have also been thought to provoke thrombocytopenic purpura on occasion, either by an immune mechanism or as a result of bone-marrow depression; these various effects may possibly be brought about by similar immune mechanisms with different sites of action. Non-thrombocytopenic purpura is the least serious form, and calls for no treatment but withdrawal of the offending drug.

ATROPHIC DISORDERS OF CONNECTIVE TISSUES

Senile purpura
The clinical and histological features of this condition have been well described by Tattersall & Seville [386]. It occurs with increasing frequency in both sexes from the seventh decade of life onwards, and is almost always confined to the extensor surface of the forearms (Fig. 26.11) and backs of the hands and neck; in a few patients, lesions may be found on the face in relation to spectacle frames. The ecchymotic lesions are quite distinctive, being 1–4 cm in diameter, irregular in shape with clear-cut margins, dark purple in colour, fading to brown, and of variable duration. The skin in the affected areas is always thin, inelastic and pigmented. Fresh lesions can be produced by applying blunt pressure to the skin in the affected areas, but purpura cannot be produced in this way in other sites, or in other elderly subjects. The results of the bleeding time and capillary resistance tests are within normal limits. The lesions appear to result from extravasation of blood in response to minor trauma, from vessels which are inadequately supported, owing to the extreme degree of senile degeneration of the surrounding skin and subcutaneous tissues. The vessels in such atrophic skin are easily ruptured by slight shearing strains, and blood spreads more widely and is absorbed more slowly than in the skin of younger subjects [387].

Steroid purpura
The purpura which sometimes develops in middle-aged patients who have received adrenal corticosteroids for long periods may occur on the lower legs as well as the backs of the forearms, but is closely similar in other respects to senile purpura, and probably has a similar pathogenesis [388]. The same type of purpura is sometimes seen in Cushing's syndrome, and also, in association with osteoporosis, in middle-aged subjects with long-standing rheumatoid disease, whether or not they have been treated with steroids [389]. In whatever circumstances it occurs, this easily recognized type of

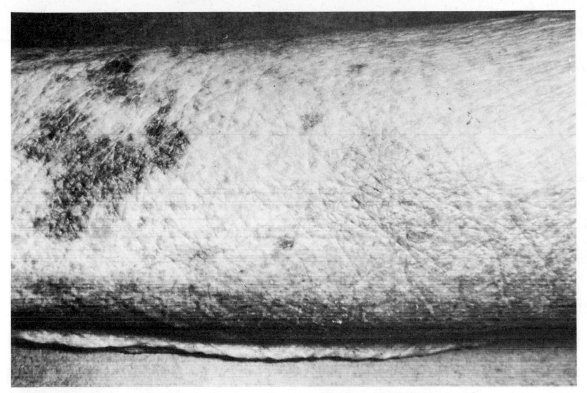

Fig. 26.11. Senile purpura. (Courtesy of Professor M. W. Greaves.)

purpura is a benign condition and requires no treatment.

Scurvy
In infants, acute limb pain from subperiosteal haemorrhage is the usual presenting feature, though widespread mucosal haemorrhage may also occur. In adults, the clinical onset is more insidious, with irritability and anorexia, accompanied usually by haemorrhage into the gums, often leading to infection. Skin petechiae are typically perifollicular in distribution, and more widespread ecchymoses may occur, sometimes accompanied by deep haematomata and haemarthroses. The bleeding is attributed to a defect of synthesis of collagen and intercellular cement substance in and around vessel walls, but a defect of platelet function may also play a part [344]. The condition responds rapidly to oral ascorbic acid.

PURPURA ASSOCIATED WITH INFECTIONS

Purpura and internal haemorrhage may complicate many different acute infections, and may be attributable to a variety of causes, including disseminated intravascular coagulation (Chapter 29) and thrombo-

cytopenia due to other mechanisms (Chapter 25). Besides these, direct vascular injury may be responsible for non-thrombocytopenic purpura in bacterial, viral or rickettsial infections: the purpuric element in the rash of severe scarlet fever or measles affords a good example. The role of infections in the pathogenesis of Schönlein–Henoch syndrome is discussed on page 1056.

HEREDITARY DISORDERS OF BLOOD VESSELS AND CONNECTIVE TISSUES

Hereditary haemorrhagic telangiectasia
This is an autosomal-dominant trait, first well defined by Rendu [390], Osler [391] and Weber [392], by whose names it is commonly known.

Pathology [393, 394]. The typical vascular lesions consist of thinning of the wall, dilatation and tortuosity of veins, leading to cavernous angiomatous formations. These are scattered widely thoughout all organ systems, and range in size from pinpoint up to some 3 mm. Arteriovenous fistulae commonly occur in the lungs, and less commonly in the brain and other organs.

Clinical features. Although hereditary, the condition does not usually present clinically until late childhood or early adult life, as the vascular lesions develop. The symptoms are those of haemorrhage, which occurs only from the lesions, and of the resulting anaemia. Epistaxis is much the commonest symptom, but the patient may also bleed from telangiectases in the gut, genitourinary tract, bronchial mucosa or skin (Fig. 26.12). Surgical and accidental wounds do not result in excessive bleeding, unless a telangiectatic lesion is injured. The severity of the condition is likely to increase with age, as more lesions develop and enlarge. Pulmonary arteriovenous fistulae (often multiple) are also detected more frequently in older patients: of 91 patients with telangiectasia in a large family studied by Hodgson *et al.* [395], 14 (17%) also had pulmonary arteriovenous fistulae. Conversely, up to 60% of patients with pulmonary arteriovenous fistulae are found to have hereditary haemorrhagic telangiectasia [396]: diagnosis of either condition should prompt a search for the other.

Diagnosis. The diagnosis rests on the family history and the detection of telangiectases. These must be distinguished from purpuric spots, which do not blanch on pressure, and from spider naevi. They may not be present in the skin, particularly in the younger patient, but should be sought in the nasal and buccal mucosa. The bleeding time and other tests of the haemostatic mechanism give normal results. The diagnosis should always be considered in patients with unexplained recurrent epistaxis or gastro-intestinal haemorrhage; in the latter case, angiography may reveal the vascular lesions [397].

Treatment. This consists of local measures for the arrest of haemorrhage, and correction of the anaemia with iron, or by transfusion in the event of major acute blood loss. Pressure may be applied to bleeding lesions in the nasal mucosa by attaching a lubricated finger-stall to a catheter, passing it up the nostril and inflating it. Cautery may be temporarily effective, but its repeated use should be avoided. Oestrogen therapy has

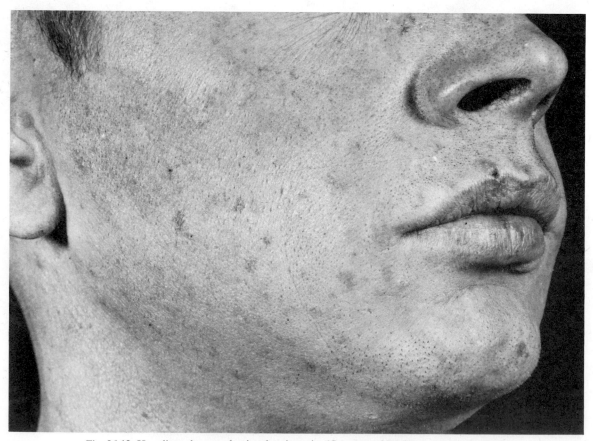

Fig. 26.12. Hereditary haemorrhagic telangiectasia. (Courtesy of Professor M. W. Greaves.)

been recommended for the control of epistaxis [398, 399], but at the cost of many side-effects, from the discomfort caused by squamous metaplasia of the nasal mucosa to feminization and carcinogenicity. Surgery may be required for gastro-intestinal lesions or pulmonary arteriovenous fistulae.

Connective-tissue disorders

A tendency to bleed on slight or no provocation is a characteristic feature of several hereditary disorders of connective tissues, and is presumably due either to a mechanical failure of blood vessels or their supporting tissues, or a defect of platelet–vessel-wall interaction resulting from the collagen abnormality. In the *Ehlers– Danlos syndrome*, hyperextensibility of the joints and hyperelasticity and friability of the skin are associated with easy bruising and haematoma formation, and sometimes with more serious bleeding complications. The condition is now known to be heterogeneous, and six types are recognized [400]. The bleeding tendency is most severe in type IV, in which there is a deficiency of type-III collagen [401]. Skin collagen from patients with the Ehlers–Danlos syndrome has been shown to be defective in its ability to aggregate normal platelets [402, 403], and this would seem to be the most likely explanation for the bleeding tendency.

Bleeding complications are the chief medical problem in *pseudoxanthoma elasticum*: gastro-intestinal haemorrhage may even occur in childhood, and it and intracranial haemorrhage are the commonest causes of death; genitourinary, retinal and skin bleeding and haemarthroses also occur. Easy bruising and epistaxes are also seen in *osteogenesis imperfecta* and *Marfan's syndrome*, but serious bleeding is seldom a problem in these conditions.

PROLIFERATIVE VASCULAR DISORDERS

Kaposi's haemorrhagic sarcoma

This is a multifocal disorder of blood vessels, particularly of the lower limbs, but sometimes also affecting the lungs, gastro-intestinal tract, lymph nodes and other organs. Its chief incidence is in middle-aged and elderly men, though women and children may also be affected; it is particularly common in central Africa. It is generally held to be of reticulo-endothelial origin, and not infrequently coexists with other lymphoproliferative disorders. Bleeding occurs from the skin lesions, which tend to assume a reddish-brown colour from the extravasation of blood and deposition of haemosiderin. Haemorrhage from visceral lesions may necessitate surgery.

Giant haemangiomata

Although these proliferative vascular lesions may be

associated with a bleeding disorder, they are seldom the site of bleeding themselves, but rather of a chronic thrombotic process. This leads secondarily to the consumption of platelets and clotting factors and so to a generalized haemorrhage state, the Kasabach– Merritt syndrome. This is considered in Chapter 25 (p. 1001).

OTHER NON-THROMBOCYTOPENIC PURPURAS

Purpura simplex (simple easy bruising)

Many otherwise healthy girls and young women complain of frequent spontaneous bruising of the legs, sometimes associated with ecchymoses, but without other bleeding symptoms. The tendency to bruise easily may be lifelong or may be confined to adolescence and early adult life; it often appears to have a familial incidence [404]. The lesions are painless and non-tender, and are usually a cause for complaint on cosmetic grounds alone: this may well account for the apparent predilection for the female sex. Tests of the haemostatic mechanism give normal results, except perhaps for the capillary resistance test, and no treatment is required other than reassurance. The chief importance of the condition lies in the necessity of distinguishing it from more serious conditions, particularly thrombocytopenia and the hereditary bleeding states. With the development of new tests of platelet function, it seems likely that a proportion of patients who would previously have been placed in this category actually suffer from minor defects of platelet secretion and/or aggregation [405], whether hereditary in origin or induced by aspirin or other drugs [280].

Factitious purpura

Self-inflicted purpuric lesions may sometimes present a difficult diagnostic problem, whether they are an isolated physical manifestation of a psychological disorder or a component of Munchausen's syndrome. The unusual distribution of lesions and the presence of other evidence of psychological disturbance are most likely to suggest the diagnosis, and tests of the haemostatic mechanism will, of course, give normal results.

Auto-erythrocyte sensitization and DNA sensitivity

Gardner & Diamond [406] described four women, between the ages of 19 and 60, who showed an abnormal response to bruising, characterized by the development of painful ecchymoses with local oedema. They presented evidence that these women had become sensitized against their own red cells, and named the condition 'auto-erythrocyte sensitization'. Many similar cases have subsequently been described, virtually all in adult women.

The onset usually follows an injury or operation.

The typical lesions occur mainly on the limbs, usually but not necessarily at the site of the trauma. The patient's attention is often first drawn to the site by local irritation and pain, and this is shortly followed by the appearance of an itchy urticarial and erythematous nodule, which develops in the course of the next few hours into an extensive painful ecchymosis, usually with a tender nodular centre. The lesion gradually disappears during the next week or two, to be succeeded at intervals by other similar lesions, either at the site of minor trauma or arising spontaneously. Headache, nausea and vomiting are common, and abdominal pain, melaena and haematuria may also occur from time to time, so that the clinical condition may come to resemble the Schönlein–Henoch syndrome. Cerebral vascular accidents have also occurred. Once started, the condition runs a protracted course, successive crops of lesions appearing over the years, but there may be a tendency for the lesions to become gradually less severe and less frequent. These patients often have profound emotional disturbances, and tend to be of a hysterical and masochistic nature, with signs of suppressed hostility, usually towards men; the condition must be regarded as a psychosomatic disorder [407, 408]. Although some of the lesions may be self-inflicted, it has often been possible to exclude this.

The platelet count, bleeding time and tests of blood coagulation all give normal results, but the diagnosis may be confirmed by the reaction of the patient to the intradermal injection of her own blood. If 0·1 ml or less of whole venous blood, washed red cells or red-cell stroma is injected intradermally, a spreading, painful, indurated ecchymosis develops over the course of 24 hours or so, in sharp contrast to the small local bleb produced in the skin of a normal subject.

The natural fluctuations in the course of the condition make it difficult to evaluate the effect of treatment. Splenectomy, corticosteroids and desensitization with the patient's red cells have all been tried without success, and the last method may result only in the production of typical lesions at injection sites. Even if steroid therapy affords temporary symptomatic relief, its long-term continuation should be avoided. Psychotherapy may be of value [408].

DNA sensitivity [409]. This is a similar but less common syndrome, also confined to women, in which the lesions can be provoked by the intradermal injection of lysed autologous leucocytes or heterologous DNA, but not by red cells. The clinical features differ from those of auto-erythrocyte sensitization in that a history of trauma is often lacking, and that the lesions are usually confined to the limbs: skin tests may be positive on the limbs and negative on the trunk, and reciprocal skin grafting has shown that it is the recipient rather than the donor site which determines sensitivity [410]. A reaction is not provoked by RNA, and incubation of DNA or leucocytes with deoxyribonuclease or chloroquine abolishes their effect. Treatment with chloroquine (250 mg q.d.s. for one week) produces a rapid clinical response; maintenance therapy at lower dosage is necessary for the prevention of relapses.

REFERENCES

1 STRUM J.M. & JUNOD A.F. (1972) Radioautographic demonstration of 5-hydroxytryptamine-^{3}H uptake by pulmonary endothelial cells. *Journal of Cell Biology*, **54**, 456.

2 SMITH U. & RYAN J.W. (1972) Pulmonary endothelial cells and the metabolism of adenine nucleotides, kinins and angiotensin I. *Advances in Experimental Medicine and Biology*, **4**, 267.

3 RYAN J.W., NIEMEYER R.S. & RYAN U. (1975) Metabolism of prostaglandin $F_{1\alpha}$ in the pulmonary circulation. *Prostaglandins*, **10**, 101.

4 SHEPPARD D., BATBOUTA J.C., ROBBLEE L.S., CARSON M.P. & BELAMARICH F.A. (1975) Serotonin transport by cultured bovine aortic endothelium. *Circulation Research*, **36**, 799.

5 CALDWELL P.R.B., SEEGAL B.C., HSU K.C., DAS M. & SOFFER R.L. (1976) Angiotensin-converting enzyme: vascular endothelial localization. *Science*, **191**, 1050.

6 WEKSLER B.B., MARCUS A.J. & JAFFE E.A. (1977) Synthesis of prostaglandin I_2 (prostacyclin) by cultured human and bovine endothelial cells. *Proceedings of the National Academy of Sciences, USA*, **74**, 3922.

7 JAFFE E.A., HOYER L.W. & NACHMAN R.L. (1974) Synthesis of von Willebrand factor by cultured human endothelial cells. *Proceedings of the National Academy of Sciences, USA*, **71**, 1906.

8 MAYNARD J.R., DRYER B.E., STEMERMAN M.B. & PITLICK F.A. (1977) Tissue-factor coagulant activity of cultured human endothelial and smooth muscle cells and fibroblasts. *Blood*, **50**, 387.

9 LOSKUTOFF D.J. & EDGINGTON T.S. (1977) Synthesis of a fibrinolytic activator and inhibitor by endothelial cells. *Proceedings of the National Academy of Sciences, USA*, **74**, 3903.

10 JAFFE E.A., MINICK C.R., ADELMAN B., BECKER C.G. & NACHMAN R. (1976) Synthesis of basement membrane collagen by cultured human endothelial cells. *Journal of Experimental Medicine*, **144**, 209.

11 JAFFE E.A. & MOSHER D.F. (1978) Synthesis of fibronectin by cultured human endothelial cells. *Annals of the New York Academy of Sciences*, **312**, 122.

12 MONCADA S., GRYGLEWSKI R., BUNTING S. & VANE J.R. (1976) An enzyme isolated from arteries transforms prostaglandin endoperoxides to an unstable substance that inhibits platelet aggregation. *Nature (London)*, **263**, 663.

13 JOHNSON R.A., MORTON D.R., KINNER J.H., GORMAN R.R., McGUIRE J.C., SUN F.F., WHITTAKER N., BUNTING S., SALMON J., MONCADA S. & VANE J.R. (1976) The chemical structure of prostaglandin X (prostacyclin). *Prostaglandins*, **12**, 915.

14 MONCADA S., HIGGS E.A. & VANE J.R. (1977) Human arterial and venous tissues generate prostacyclin (prostaglandin X), a potent inhibitor of platelet aggregation. *Lancet*, **i**, 18.

15 MONCADA S., HERMAN A.G., HIGGS E.A. & VANE J.R. (1977) Differential formation of prostacyclin (PGX or PGI_2) by layers of the arterial wall. An explanation for the anti-thrombotic properties of vascular endothelium. *Thrombosis Research*, **11**, 323.

16 MacINTYRE D.E., PEARSON J.D. & GORDON J.L. (1978) Localisation and stimulation of prostacyclin production in vascular cells. *Nature (London)*, **271**, 549.

17 BURCH J.W., BAENZIGER N.L., STANFORD N. & MAJERUS P.W. (1978) Sensitivity of fatty acid cyclooxygenase from human aorta to acetylation by aspirin. *Proceedings of the National Academy of Sciences, USA*, **75**, 5181.

18 JAFFE E.A. & WEKSLER B.B. (1979) Recovery of endothelial cell prostacyclin production after inhibition by low doses of aspirin. *Journal of Clinical Investigation*, **63**, 532.

19 MONCADA S. & VANE J.R. (1978) Unstable metabolites of arachidonic acid and their role in haemostasis and thrombosis. *British Medical Bulletin*, **34**, 129.

20 BAENZIGER N.L., DILLENDER M.J. & MAJERUS P.W. (1977) Cultured human skin fibroblasts and arterial cells produce a labile platelet-inhibitory prostaglandin. *Biochemical and Biophysical Research Communications*, **78**, 294.

21 WEKSLER B.B., LEY C.W. & JAFFE E.A. (1978) Stimulation of endothelial cell prostacyclin (PGI_2) production by thrombin, trypsin, and the ionophore A23187. *Journal of Clinical Investigation*, **62**, 923.

22 NEEDLEMAN P., BRONSON S.D., WYCHE A., SIVAKOFF M. & NICOLAOU K.C. (1978) Cardiac and renal prostaglandin I_2. Biosynthesis and biological effects in isolated perfused rabbit tissues. *Journal of Clinical Investigation*, **61**, 839.

23 HIGGS E.A., MONCADA S., VANE J.R., CAEN J.P., MICHEL H. & TOBELEM G. (1978) Effect of prostacyclin (PGI_2) on platelet adhesion to rabbit arterial subendothelium. *Prostaglandins*, **16**, 17.

24 WEISS H.J. & TURITTO V.T. (1979) Prostacyclin (prostaglandin I_2, PGI_2) inhibits platelet adhesion and thrombus formation on subendothelium. *Blood*, **53**, 244.

25 SIEGL A.M., SMITH J.B., SILVER M.J., NICOLAOU K.C. & AHERN D. (1979) Selective binding site for [3H] prostacyclin on platelets. *Journal of Clinical Investigation*, **63**, 215.

26 KITCHENS C.S. (1977) Amelioration of endothelial abnormalities by prednisone in experimental thrombocytopenia in the rabbit. *Journal of Clinical Investigation*, **60**, 1129.

27 MACA R.D., FRY G.L. & HOAK J.C. (1978) The effects of glucocorticoids on cultured human endothelial cells. *British Journal of Haematology*, **38**, 501.

28 BLAJCHMAN M.A., SENYI A.F., HIRSH J., SURYA Y., BUCHANAN M. & MUSTARD J.F. (1979) Shortening of the bleeding time in rabbits by hydrocortisone caused by inhibition of prostacyclin generation by the vessel wall. *Journal of Clinical Investigation*, **63**, 1026.

29 CZERVIONKE R.L., HOAK J.C. & FRY G.L. (1978) Effect of aspirin on thrombin-induced adherence of platelets to cultured cells from the blood vessel wall. *Journal of Clinical Investigation*, **62**, 847.

30 CZERVIONKE R.L., SMITH J.B., FRY G.L., HOAK J.C. & HAYCRAFT D.L. (1979) Inhibition of prostacyclin by treatment of endothelium with aspirin. *Journal of Clinical Investigation*, **63**, 1089.

31 STEMERMAN M.B. (1975) Vascular intimal components: precursors of thrombosis. *Progress in Hemostasis and Thrombosis*, **2**, 1.

32 HOWARD B.V., MACARALE E.J., GUNSON D. & KEFALIDES N.A. (1976) Characterization of the collagen synthesis by endothelial cells in culture. *Proceedings of the National Academy of Sciences, USA*, **73**, 2361.

33 BUONASSISI V. (1973) Sulfated mucopolysaccharide synthesis and secretion in endothelial cell cultures. *Experimental Cell Research*, **76**, 363.

34 HUGUES J. (1962) Accolement des plaquettes aux structures conjonctives périvasculaires. *Thrombosis et Diathesis Haemorrhagica*, **8**, 241.

35 BAUMGARTNER H.R. & MUGGLI R. (1976) Adhesion and aggregation: morphological demonstration and quantitation *in vivo* and *in vitro*. In: *Platelets in Biology and Pathology* (ed. Gordon J.L.), p. 23. North-Holland, Amsterdam.

36 BAUMGARTNER H.R., MUGGLI R., TSCHOPP T.B. & TURITTO V.T. (1976) Platelet adhesion, release and aggregation in flowing blood: effects of surface properties and platelet function. *Thrombosis and Haemostasis*, **35**, 124.

37 BAUMGARTNER H.R. & HAUDENSCHILD C. (1972) Adhesion of platelets to subendothelium. *Annals of the New York Academy of Sciences*, **201**, 22.

38 STEMERMAN M.B., BAUMGARTNER H.R. & SPAET T.H. (1971) The subendothelial microfibril and platelet adhesion. *Laboratory Investigation*, **24**, 179.

39 FREYTAG J.W., DALRYMPLE P.N., MAGUIRE M.H., STRICKLAND D.K., CARRAWAY K.L. & HUDSON B.G. (1978) Glomerular basement membrane: studies on its structure and interaction with platelets. *Journal of Biological Chemistry*, **253**, 9069.

40 HUGUES J. & LAPIERE C.M. (1964) Nouvelles recherches sur l'acolement des plaquettes aux fibres de collagène. *Thrombosis et Diathesis Haemorrhagica*, **11**, 327.

41 MICHAELI D. & ORLOFF K.G. (1976) Molecular considerations of platelet adhesion. *Progress in Hemostasis and Thrombosis*, **3**, 29.

42 BARNES M.J. & MacINTYRE D.E. (1979) Collagen-induced platelet aggregation. The activity of basement membrane collagens relative to other collagen types. *Frontiers in Matrix Biology*, **7**, 246.

43 WILNER G.D., NOSSEL H.L. & LEROY E.C. (1968) Aggregation of platelets by collagen. *Journal of Clinical Investigation*, **47**, 2616.

44 KANG A.H., BEACHEY E.H. & KATZMAN R.L. (1974) Interaction of an active glycopeptide from chick skin collagen (α1-CB5) with human platelets. *Journal of Biological Chemistry*, **249**, 1054.

45 FAUVEL F., LEGRAND Y.J., KÜHN K., BENTZ H., FIETZEK P.P. & CAEN J.P. (1979) Platelet adhesion to type III collagen: involvement of a sequence of nine aminoacids from α_1 (III) CB4 peptide. *Thrombosis Research*, **16**, 269.

46 MUGGLI R. & BAUMGARTNER H.R. (1973) Collagen-induced platelet aggregation: requirement for tropocollagen multimers. *Thrombosis Research*, **3**, 715.

47 JAFFE R.M. & DEYKIN D. (1974) Evidence for structural requirement for the aggregation of platelets by collagen. *Journal of Clinical Investigation*, **53**, 875.

48 BRASS L.F. & BENSUSAN H.B. (1974) The role of collagen quaternary structure in platelet-collagen interaction. *Journal of Clinical Investigation*, **54**, 1480.

49 KRONIK P. & JIMINEZ S. (1975) Collagen structure and binding to platelets. *Federation Proceedings*, **34**, 855.

50 MUGGLI R. (1978) Collagen-induced platelet aggregation: native collagen quaternary structure is not an essential structural requirement. *Thrombosis Research*, **13**, 829.

51 WILNER G.D., NOSSEL H.L. & LEROY E.C. (1968) Activation of Hageman factor by collagen. *Journal of Clinical Investigation*, **47**, 2608.

52 HAYEM G. (1882) Pathologie experimentale — sur le méchanism de l'arret des hémorrhagies. *Comptes Rendus Hebdomadaires des Séances de l'Académie des Sciences, Paris*, **95**, 18.

53 BIZZOZERO J. (1882) Ueber einen neuen Formbestandtheil des Blutes und dessen Rolle bei der Thrombose und der Blutgerinnung. *Archiv für Pathologische Anatomie und Physiologie und für klinische Medicin*, **90**, 261.

54 HOVIG T. (1968) The ultrastructure of blood platelets in normal and abnormal states. *Series Haematologica*, **1**, 3.

55 WHITE J.G. (1971) Platelet morphology. In: *The Circulating Platelet* (ed. Johnson S.A.), p. 45. Academic Press, New York.

55a WHITE J.G. (1971) Platelet microtubules and microfilaments: effects of cytochalasin B on structure and function. In: *Platelet Aggregation* (ed. Caen J.), p. 15. Masson et Cie, Paris.

55b WHITE J.G. (1968) The origin of dense bodies in the surface coat of negatively stained platelets. *Scandinavian Journal of Haematology*, **5**, 241.

56 WHITE J.G. & GERRARD J.M. (1976) Ultrastructural features of abnormal blood platelets. *American Journal of Pathology*, **823**, 590.

57 NACHMAN R.L. & FERRIS B. (1972) Studies on the proteins of human platelet membranes. *Journal of Biological Chemistry*, **247**, 4468.

58 PHILLIPS D.R. (1972) Effect of trypsin on the exposed polypeptides and glycoproteins in the human platelet membrane. *Biochemistry*, **11**, 4582.

59 OKUMURA T. & JAMIESON G.A. (1976) Platelet glycocalycin. I. Orientation of glycoproteins of the human platelet surface glycoproteins in platelet function. *Nature (London)*, **255**, 720.

60 GANGULY P. & GOULD N.L. (1979) Thrombin receptors of human platelets: thrombin binding and antithrombin properties of glycoprotein I. *British Journal of Haematology*, **42**, 137.

61 NURDEN A.T. & CAEN J.P. (1975) Specific roles for platelet surface glycoproteins in platelet function. *Nature (London)*, **255**, 720.

62 KUNICKI T.J., JOHNSON M.M. & ASTER R.H. (1978) Absence of the platelet receptor for drug-dependent antibodies in the Bernard–Soulier syndrome. *Journal of Clinical Investigation*, **62**, 716.

63 NURDEN A.T. & CAEN J.P. (1974) An abnormal platelet glycoprotein pattern in three cases of Glanzmann's thrombasthenia. *British Journal of Haematology*, **28**, 253.

64 PHILLIPS D.R. & AGIN P.P. (1977) Platelet membrane defects in Glanzmann's thrombasthenia. Evidence for decreased amounts of two major glycoproteins. *Journal of Clinical Investigation*, **60**, 535.

65 KUNICKI T.J. & ASTER R.H. (1979) Isolation and immunologic characterization of the human platelet alloantigen Pl^Al. *Molecular Immunology*, **16**, 353.

66 van LEEUWEN E.F., ZONNEFELD G.T.E., von RIESZ L.E., JENKINS C.S.P., van MOURIK J.A. & von DEM BORNE A.E.G.K. (1979) Absence of the complete platelet-specific alloantigens Zw (Pl^A) on the platelets in Glanzmann's thrombasthenia and the effect of anti-Zw^a antibody on platelet function. *Thrombosis and Haemostasis*, **42**, 422.

67 GERRARD J.M., SCHOLLMEYER J.V., PHILLIPS D.R. & WHITE J.G. (1979) α-actinin deficiency in thrombasthenia: possible identity of α-actinin and glycoprotein III. *American Journal of Pathology*, **94**, 509.

68 PHILLIPS D.R. & AGIN P.P. (1977) Platelet plasma membrane glycoproteins. Identification of a proteolytic substrate for thrombin. *Biochemical and Biophysical Research Communications*, **75**, 940.

69 MILLS D.C.B. (1977) Platelet aggregation and the adenylate cyclase system. In: *Platelets and Thrombosis* (ed. Mills D.C.B. & Pareti F.I.), p. 63. Academic Press, London.

70 BEHNKE O. (1965) Further studies on microtubules. A marginal bundle in human and rat thrombocytes. *Journal of Ultrastructure Research*, **13**, 469.

71 WHITE J.G. & KRIVIT W. (1967) An ultrastructural basis for the shape changes induced in platelets by chilling. *Blood*, **30**, 625.

72 ZUCKER-FRANKLIN D. (1969) Microfibrils of blood platelets: their relationship to microtubules and the contractile protein. *Journal of Clinical Investigation*, **48**, 165.

73 BEHNKE O., KRISTENSEN B.I. & NIELSEN L.E. (1971) Electron microscopical observations of actinoid and myosinoid filaments in blood platelets. *Journal of Ultrastructure Research*, **37**, 351.

74 BETTEX-GALLAND M. & LÜSCHER E.F. (1959) Extraction of an actomyosin-like protein from human platelets. *Nature (London)*, **184**, 276.

75 BETTEX-GALLAND M. & LÜSCHER E.F. (1961) Thrombosthenin—a contractile protein from thrombocytes. Its extraction from human blood platelets and some of its properties. *Biochimica et Biophysica Acta*, **49**, 536.

76 COHEN I. & COHEN C. (1972) A tropomyosin-like protein from human platelets. *Journal of Molecular Biology*, **68**, 383.

77 MUSZBEK L., KUZNICKI J., SZABO T. & DRABIKOWSKI W. (1977) Troponin C-like protein of blood platelets. *FEBS Letters*, **80**, 308.

78 PUSZKIN E.G., SPAET T.H., MAIMON J. & PUSZKIN S. (1977) Platelet α-actinin: effect on actin properties. *Circulation*, **56**, 285a.

79 ADELSTEIN R.S. & POLLARD T.D. (1978) Platelet contractile proteins. *Progress in Hemostasis and Thrombosis*, **4**, 37.

80 COHEN I. (1979) The contractile system of blood

platelets and its function. *Methods and Achievements in Experimental Pathology*, **9**, 40.

81 DA PRADA M., PLETSCHER A., TRANZER J.P. & KNUCHEL H. (1967) Subcellular localization of 5-hydroxytryptamine and histamine in blood platelets. *Nature (London)*, **216**, 1315.

82 HOLMSEN H., DAY H.J. & STORM E. (1969) Adenine nucleotide metabolism of blood platelets. VI. Subcellular localization of nucleotide pools with different functions in the platelet release reaction. *Biochimica et Biophysica Acta*, **186**, 254.

83 BORN G.V.R. & SMITH J.B. (1970) Uptake, metabolism and release of [^{3}H]-adrenaline by human platelets. *British Journal of Pharmacology*, **39**, 765.

84 SKAER R.J., PETERS P.D. & EMMINES J.P. (1974) The localization of calcium and phosphorus in human platelets. *Journal of Cell Science*, **15**, 679.

85 SIEGEL A. & LÜSCHER E.F. (1967) Non-identity of the α-granules of human blood platelets with typical lysosomes. *Nature (London)*, **215**, 745.

86 BENTFIELD M.E. & BAINTON D.F. (1975) Cytochemical localization of lysosomal enzymes in rat megakaryocytes and platelets. *Journal of Clinical Investigation*, **56**, 1635.

87 BRETON-GORIUS J. & GUICHARD J. (1975) Two different types of granules in megakaryocytes and platelets as revealed by the diaminobenzidine method. *Journal de Microscopie et de Biologie Cellulaire*, **23**, 197.

88 BROEKMAN M.J., HANDIN R.I. & COHEN P. (1975) Distribution of fibrinogen, and platelet factors 4 and XIII in subcellular fractions of human platelets. *British Journal of Haematology*, **31**, 51.

89 DA PRADA M., JAKABOVA M., LÜSCHER E.F., PLETSCHER A. & RICHARDS J.G. (1976) Subcellular localization of the heparin-neutralizing factor in blood platelets. *Journal of Physiology*, **257**, 495.

90 KAPLAN K.L., BROEKMAN M.J., CHERNOFF A., LESZNIK G.R. & DRILLINGS M. (1979) Platelet α-granule proteins: studies on release and subcellular localization. *Blood*, **53**, 604.

91 ZUCKER M.B., BROEKMAN M.J. & KAPLAN K.L. (1979) Factor VIII-related antigen in human blood platelets. Localization and release by thrombin and collagen. *Journal of Laboratory and Clinical Medicine*, **94**, 675.

92 ZUCKER M.B., MOSESSON M.W., BROEKMAN M.J. & KAPLAN K.L. (1979) Release of platelet fibronectin (cold-insoluble globulin) from alpha granules induced by thrombin or collagen: lack of requirement for plasma fibronectin in ADP-induced platelet aggregation. *Blood*, **54**, 8.

93 GERRARD J.M., WHITE J.G., RAO G.H.R. & TOWNSEND D. (1976) Localization of platelet prostaglandin production in the platelet dense tubular system. *American Journal of Pathology*, **83**, 283.

94 GERRARD J.M., WHITE J.G. & PETERSON D.A. (1978) The platelet dense tubular system: its relationship to prostaglandin synthesis and calcium flux. *Thrombosis and Haemostasis*, **40**, 224.

95 TRANZER J.P. & BAUMGARTNER H.R. (1967) Filling gaps in the vascular endothelium with blood platelets. *Nature (London)*, **216**, 1126.

96 KITCHENS C.S. & WEISS L. (1975) Ultrastructural changes of endothelium associated with thrombocytopenia. *Blood*, **46**, 567.

97 SABA S.R. & MASON R.G. (1975) Effects of platelets and certain platelet components on growth of cultured human endothelial cells. *Thrombosis Research*, **7**, 807.

98 MACA R.D., FRY G.L., HOAK J.C. & LOH P.T. (1977) The effects of intact platelets on cultured human endothelial cells. *Thrombosis Research*, **11**, 715.

99 GORDON J.L. (1976) *Platelets in Biology and Pathology*. North-Holland, Amsterdam.

100 SIXMA J.J. (1981) Role of blood vessel, platelet and coagulation interactions in haemostasis. In: *Haemostasis and Thrombosis* (ed. Bloom A.L. & Thomas D.P.), p. 252. Churchill-Livingstone, Edinburgh.

101 JAMIESON G.A., URBAN C.L. & BARBER A.J. (1971) Enzymatic basis for platelet:collagen adhesion as the primary step in haemostasis. *Nature (New Biology)*, **234**, 5.

102 PUETT D., WASSERMAN B.K., FORD J.D. & CUNNINGHAM L.W. (1973) Collagen-mediated platelet aggregation: effects of collagen modification involving the protein and carbohydrate moieties. *Journal of Clinical Investigation*, **52**, 2495.

103 MENASHI S., HARWOOD R. & GRANT M.E. (1976) Native collagen is not a substrate for the collagen glucosyltransferase of platelets. *Nature (London)*, **264**, 670.

104 BENSUSAN H.B., KOH T.L., HENRY K.G., MURRAY B.A. & CULP L.A. (1978) Evidence that fibronectin is the collagen receptor on platelet membranes. *Proceedings of the National Academy of Sciences, USA*, **75**, 5864.

105 ZUCKER M.B., KIM S.J., MCPHERSON J. & GRANT R.A. (1977) Binding of factor VIII to platelets in the presence of ristocetin. *British Journal of Haematology*, **35**, 535.

106 KAO K.J., PIZZO S.V. & MCKEE P.A. (1979) Demonstration and characterization of specific binding sites for factor VIII/von Willebrand factor on human platelets. *Journal of Clinical Investigation*, **63**, 656.

107 SAKARIASSEN K.S., BOLHUIS P.A. & SIXMA J.J. (1979) Human blood platelet adhesion to artery subendothelium is mediated by factor VIII–von Willebrand factor bound to the subendothelium. *Nature (London)*, **279**, 636.

108 NIEWIAROWSKI S., REGOECZI C., STEWART G.J., SENYI A.F. & MUSTARD J.F. (1972) Platelet interaction with polymerizing fibrin. *Journal of Clinical Investigation*, **51**, 685.

109 HELLEM A.J. (1960) The adhesiveness of human blood platelets *in vitro*. *Scandinavian Journal of Clinical Investigation*, **12** (Suppl.), 51.

110 GAARDER A., JONSEN J., LALAND S., HELLEM P.A. & OWREN P.A. (1961) Adenosine diphosphate in red cells as a factor in the adhesiveness of human blood platelets. *Nature (London)*, **192**, 531.

111 BORN G.V.R. & CROSS M.J. (1963) The aggregation of blood platelets. *Journal of Physiology*, **168**, 178.

112 MILLS D.C.B., ROBB I.A. & ROBERTS G.C.K. (1968) The release of nucleotides, 5-hydroxytryptamine and enzymes from human blood platelets during aggregation. *Journal of Physiology*, **195**, 715.

113 MILLS D.C.B. & MACFARLANE D.E. (1976) Platelet receptors. In: *Platelets in Biology and Pathology* (ed. Gordon J.L.), p. 159. North-Holland, Amsterdam.

114 MILLS D.C.B. (1981) The basic biochemistry of the

platelet. In: *Haemostasis and Thrombosis* (ed. Bloom A.L. & Thomas D.P.), p. 50. Churchill-Livingstone, Edinburgh.

115 BORN G.V.R. (1970) Observations on the change in shape of blood platelets brought about by adenosine diphosphate. *Journal of Physiology*, **209**, 487.

116 MOTAMED M., MICHAL F. & BORN G.V.R. (1976) Increase in sialic acids removable by neuraminidase during the shape change of platelets. *Biochemical Journal*, **158**, 655.

117 LE BRETON G.C., DINERSTEIN R.J., ROTH L.J. & FEINBERG H. (1976) Direct evidence for intracellular divalent cation redistribution associated with platelet shape change. *Biochemical and Biophysical Research Communications*, **71**, 362.

118 NACHMIAS V.T., SULLENDER J. & ASCH A. (1977) Shape and cytoplasmic filaments in control and lidocaine-treated human platelets. *Blood*, **50**, 39.

119 MCLEAN J.R., MAXWELL R.E. & HERTLER D. (1964) Fibrinogen and adenosine diphosphate-induced aggregation of platelets. *Nature (London)*, **202**, 605.

120 BENNETT J.S. & VILAIRE G. (1979) Exposure of platelet fibrinogen receptors by ADP and epinephrine. *Journal of Clinical Investigation*, **64**, 1393.

121 MARGUERIE G.A., PLOW E.F. & EDGINGTON T.S. (1979) Human platelets possess an inducible and saturable receptor specific for fibrinogen. *Journal of Biological Chemistry*, **254**, 5357.

122 MUSTARD J.F., KINLOUGH-RATHBONE R.L., PACKHAM M.A., PERRY D.W., HARFENIST E.J. & PAI K.R.M. (1979) Comparison of fibrinogen association with normal and thrombasthenic platelets on exposure to ADP or chymotrypsin. *Blood*, **54**, 987.

123 PEERSCHKE E.I., GRANT R.A. & ZUCKER M.B. (1979) Relationship between aggregation and binding of ^{125}I fibrinogen and ^{45}calcium to human platelets. *Thrombosis and Haemostasis*, **42**, 358.

124 MUSTARD J.F., PERRY D.W., KINLOUGH-RATHBONE R.L. & PACKHAM M.A. (1975) Factors responsible for ADP-induced release reaction of human platelets. *American Journal of Physiology*, **228**, 1757.

125 O'BRIEN J.R. (1965) Effects of adenosine diphosphate and adrenaline on mean platelet shape. *Nature (London)*, **207**, 306.

126 MILLS D.C.B. & ROBERTS G.C.K. (1967) Effects of adrenaline on human blood platelets. *Journal of Physiology*, **193**, 443.

127 NIEWIAROWSKI S. & THOMAS D.P. (1966) Platelet aggregation by ADP and thrombin. *Nature (London)*, **212**, 1544.

128 BENVENISTE J. (1974) Platelet-activating factor, a new mediator of anaphylaxis and immune complex deposition from rabbit and human basophils. *Nature (London)*, **249**, 581.

129 BENVENISTE J., LE COUEDIC J.P. & KAMOUN P. (1975) Aggregation of human platelets by platelet-activating factor. *Lancet*, **i**, 344.

130 CHIGNARD M., LE COUEDIC J.P., TENCE M., VARGAFTIG B.B. & BENVENISTE J. (1979) The role of platelet-activating factor in platelet aggregation. *Nature (London)*, **279**, 799.

130a BENVENISTE J., TENCE M., VARÈNE P., BIDAULT J., BOULLET C. & POLONSKY J. (1979) Immunologie, semi-synthèse et structure proposée du facteur activant les plaquettes (PAF): PAF-acether, un alkyl ether analogue de la lysophosphatidyl-choline. *Compte Rendu de l'Académie des Sciences*, **289**, 1037.

130b DEMOPOULOS C.A., PINCKARD R.N. & HANAHAN D.J. (1979) Platelet-activating factor. Evidence for 1-0-alkyl-2-acetyl-sn-glyceryl-3-phosphorylcholine as the activating component. (A new class of rapid chemical mediators.) *Journal of Biological Chemistry*, **254**, 9355.

131 HASLAM R.J. & ROSSON G.M. (1972) Aggregation of human blood platelets by vasopressin. *American Journal of Physiology*, **223**, 958.

132 SMITH J.B. & WILLIS A.L. (1970) Formation and release of prostaglandins in response to thrombin. *British Journal of Pharmacology*, **40**, 545P.

133 SMITH J.B., INGERMAN C.M., KOCSIS J.J. & SILVER M.J. (1974) Formation of an intermediate in prostaglandin biosynthesis and its association with the platelet release reaction. *Journal of Clinical Investigation*, **53**, 1468.

134 HAMBERG M., SVENSSON J. & SAMUELSSON B. (1975) Thromboxanes: a new group of biologically active compounds derived from prostaglandin endoperoxides. *Proceedings of the National Academy of Sciences, USA*, **72**, 2994.

135 BILLS T.K., SMITH J.B. & SILVER M.J. (1976) Metabolism of [^{14}C] arachidonic acid by human platelets. *Biochimica et Biophysica Acta*, **424**, 303.

136 BILLS T.K., SMITH J.B. & SILVER M.J. (1977) Selective release of arachidonic acid from the phospholipids of human platelets in response to thrombin. *Journal of Clinical Investigation*, **60**, 1.

137 MONCADA S., GRYGLEWSKI R.J., BUNTING S. & VANE J.R. (1976) A lipid peroxide inhibits the enzyme in blood vessel microsomes that generates from prostaglandin endoperoxides the substance (prostaglandin X) which prevents platelet aggregation. *Prostaglandins*, **12**, 715.

138 TURNER S.R., TAINER J.A. & LYNN W.S. (1975) Biogenesis of chemotactic molecules by the arachidonate lipoxygenase systems of platelets. *Nature (London)*, **257**, 680.

139 SMITH J.B., INGERMAN C. & SILVER M.J. (1976) Persistence of thromboxane A_2-like material and platelet release-inducing activity in plasma. *Journal of Clinical Investigation*, **58**, 119.

140 SMITH J.B., SILVER M.J., INGERMAN S.M. & KOCSIS J.J. (1974) Prostaglandin D_2 inhibits the aggregation of human platelets. *Thrombosis Research*, **5**, 291.

141 RITTENHOUSE-SIMMONS S. & DEYKIN D. (1977) The mobilization of arachidonic acid in platelets exposed to thrombin or ionophore A23187. Effects of adenosine triphosphate deprivation. *Journal of Clinical Investigation*, **60**, 495.

142 MINKES M., STANFORD N., CHI M.M.-Y., ROTH G.J., RAZ A., NEEDLEMAN P. & MAJERUS P.W. (1972) Cyclic adenosine 3'5'-monophosphate inhibits the availability of arachidonate to prostaglandin synthetase in human platelet suspensions. *Journal of Clinical Investigation*, **59**, 449.

143 KÄSER-GLANZMANN R., JAKABOVA M., GEORGE J.N. & LÜSCHER E.F. (1977) Stimulation of calcium uptake in platelet membrane vesicles by adenosine 3'5'-cyclic

monophosphate and protein kinase. *Biochimica et Biophysica Acta*, **466**, 429.

144 VANE J.R. (1971) Inhibition of prostaglandin synthesis as a mechanism of action for aspirin-like drugs. *Nature (New Biology)*, **231**, 232.

145 SMITH J.B. & WILLIS A.L. (1971) Aspirin selectively inhibits prostaglandin production in human platelets. *Nature (New Biology)*, **231**, 235.

146 SALZMAN E.W. (1977) Interrelation of prostaglandin endoperoxide (prostaglandin G_2) and cyclic 3′,5′-adenosine monophosphate in human blood platelets. *Biochimica et Biophysica Acta*, **499**, 48.

147 CHARO I.F., FEINMAN R.D., DETWILER T.C., SMITH J.B., INGERMAN C.H. & SILVER M.J. (1977) Prostaglandin endoperoxides and thromboxane A_2 can induce platelet aggregation in the absence of secretion. *Nature (London)*, **269**, 66.

148 MAUCO G., CHAP H., SIMON M.-F. & DOUSTE-BLAZY L. (1978) Phosphatidic and lysophosphatidic acid production in phospholipase C- and thrombin-treated platelets. Possible involvement of a platelet lipase. *Biochimie* **60**, 653.

149 GERRARD J.M., BUTLER A.M., PETERSON S.A. & WHITE J.G. (1978) Phosphatidic acid releases calcium from a platelet membrane fraction *in vitro*. *Prostaglandins and Medicine*, **1**, 387.

150 GRETTE K. (1962) Studies on the mechanism of thrombin-catalyzed hemostatic reactions in blood platelets. *Acta Physiologica Scandinavica*, **56** (Suppl.), 195.

151 WHITE J.G. (1974) Electron microscopic studies of platelet secretion. *Progress in Hemostasis and Thrombosis*, **2**, 49.

152 HOLMSEN H. (1975) Biochemistry of the platelet release reaction. *Ciba Foundation Symposium*, **35**, 175.

153 MACINTYRE D.E. (1976) The platelet release reaction: association with adhesion and aggregation, and comparison with secretory responses in other cells. In: *Platelets in Biology and Pathology* (ed. Gordon J.L.), p. 61. North-Holland, Amsterdam.

154 HARDISTY R.M. & STACEY R.S. (1955) 5-hydroxytryptamine in normal human platelets. *Journal of Physiology*, **130**, 711.

155 BORN G.V.R. & GILLSON R.E. (1959) Studies on the uptake of 5-hydroxytryptamine by blood platelets. *Journal of Physiology*, **146**, 472.

156 PLETSCHER A. (1968) Metabolism, transfer and storage of 5-hydroxytryptamine in blood platelets. *British Journal of Pharmacology and Chemotherapy*, **32**, 1.

157 NIEWIAROWSKI S., LIPINSKI B., FARBISZEWSKI R. & POPLAWSKI A. (1968) The release of platelet factor 4 during platelet aggregation and the possible significance of this reaction in haemostasis. *Experientia*, **24**, 343.

158 MORGAN F.J., BEGG G.S. & CHESTERMAN C.N. (1979) Complete covalent structure of human platelet factor 4. *Thrombosis and Haemostasis*, **42**, 1652.

159 KÄSER-GLANZMANN R., JAKABOVA M. & LÜSCHER E.F. (1972) Isolation and some properties of the heparin neutralizing factor (PF4) released from human blood platelets. *Experientia*, **28**, 1221.

160 MOORE S., PEPPER D.S. & CASH J.D. (1975) Platelet anti-heparin activity: the isolation and characterization of platelet factor 4 released from thrombin-aggregated washed human platelets and its dissociation into subunits and the isolation of membrane-bound anti-heparin activity. *Biochimica et Biophysica Acta*, **379**, 370.

161 RUCINSKI B., NIEWIAROWSKI S. & BUDZYNSKI A.Z. (1977) Separation of two antiheparin proteins secreted by human platelets. *Federation Proceedings*, **36**, 4278.

162 MOORE S., PEPPER D.S. & CASH J.D. (1975) The isolation and characterization of a platelet-specific beta-globulin (beta-thromboglobulin) and the detection of anti-urokinase and antiplasmin released from thrombin-aggregated washed human platelets. *Biochimica et Biophysica Acta*, **379**, 360.

163 HOLT J.C. & NIEWIAROWSKI S. (1979) On the relationship between low affinity PF4 and β-thromboglobulin. *Thrombosis and Haemostasis*, **42**, 271.

164 HOPE W., MARTIN T.J., CHESTERMAN C.N. & MORGAN F.J. (1979) Human β-thromboglobulin inhibits PGI_2 production and binds to a specific site in bovine aortic endothelial cells. *Nature (London)*, **282**, 210.

165 ROSS R., GLOMSET J., KARIYA B. & HARKER L. (1974) A platelet-dependent serum factor stimulates the proliferation of arterial smooth muscle cells *in vitro*. *Proceedings of the National Academy of Sciences, USA*, **71**, 1207.

166 RUTHERFORD R.B. & ROSS R. (1976) Platelet factors stimulate fibroblasts and smooth muscle cells quiescent in plasma serum to proliferate. *Journal of Cell Biology*, **69**, 196.

167 WITTE C.D., KAPLAN K.L., NOSSEL H.L., LAGES B.A., WEISS H.J. & GOODMAN D. (1978) Studies of the release from human platelets of the growth factor for cultured human arterial smooth muscle cells. *Circulation Research*, **42**, 402.

168 NACHMAN R.L., WEKSLER B. & FERRIS B. (1972) Characterization of human platelet vascular permeability-enhancing activity. *Journal of Clinical Investigation*, **51**, 549.

169 KEENAN J.P. & SOLUM N.O. (1972) Quantitative studies on the release of platelet fibrinogen by thrombin. *British Journal of Haematology*, **23**, 461.

170 ØSTERUD B., RAPAPORT S.I. & LAVINE K.K. (1977) Factor V activity of platelets: evidence for an activated factor V molecule and for a platelet activator. *Blood*, **49**, 819.

171 KOUTTS J., WALSH P.N., PLOW E.F., FENTON J.W., BOUMA B.N. & ZIMMERMAN T.S. (1978) Active release of human platelet factor VIII-related antigen by adenosine diphosphate, collagen, and thrombin. *Journal of Clinical Investigation*, **62**, 1255.

172 HASLAM R.J. & LYNHAM J.A. (1976) Increased phosphorylation of specific blood platelet proteins in association with the release reaction. *Biochemical Society Transactions*, **4**, 694.

173 DANIEL J.L., HOLMSEN H. & ADELSTEIN R.S. (1977) Thrombin-stimulated myosin phosphorylation in intact platelets and its possible involvement in secretion. *Thrombosis and Haemostasis*, **38**, 984.

174 CHARO I.F., FEINMAN R.D. & DETWILER T.C. (1976) Inhibition of platelet secretion by an antagonist of intracellular calcium. *Biochemical and Biophysical Research Communications*, **72**, 1462.

175 FEINMAN R.D. & DETWILER T.C. (1975) Absence of a requirement for extracellular calcium for secretion from platelets. *Thrombosis Research*, **7**, 677.

176 MACFARLANE D.E. & MILLS D.C.B. (1975) The effects of ATP on platelets: evidence against the central role of released ADP in primary aggregation. *Blood*, **46**, 309.

177 PACKHAM M.A., GUCCIONE M.A., GREENBERG J.P., KINLOUGH-RATHBONE R.L. & MUSTARD J.F. (1977) Release of ^{14}C-serotonin during initial platelet changes induced by thrombin, collagen or A23187. *Blood*, **50**, 915.

178 CHARO I.F., FEINMAN R.D. & DETWILER T.C. (1977) Interrelations of platelet aggregation and secretion. *Journal of Clinical Investigation*, **60**, 866.

179 HOLMSEN H. (1977) Platelet energy metabolism in relation to function. In: *Platelets and Thrombosis* (ed. Mills D.C.B. & Pareti F.I.), p. 45. Academic Press, London.

180 MASSINI P. (1977) The role of calcium in the stimulation of platelets. In: *Platelets and Thrombosis* (ed. Mills D.C.B. & Pareti F.I.), p. 33. Academic Press, London.

181 WALSH P.N. (1972) The role of platelets in the contact phase of blood coagulation. *British Journal of Haematology*, **22**, 237.

182 VICIC W.J., RATNOFF O.D., SAITO H. & GOLDSMITH G.H. (1979) Platelets and surface-mediated clotting activity. *British Journal of Haematology*, **43**, 91.

183 WALSH P.N. & GRIFFIN J.H. (1979) Human platelets promote the proteolytic activation of factor XII. *Thrombosis and Haemostasis*, **42**, 36.

184 WALSH P.N. (1972) The effects of collagen and kaolin on the intrinsic coagulant activity of platelets. Evidence for an alternative pathway in intrinsic coagulation not requiring factor XII. *British Journal of Haematology*, **22**, 393.

185 WALSH P.N. & GRIFFIN J.H. (1979) Platelet-dependent proteolytic activation of factor XI. *Thrombosis and Haemostasis*, **42**, 236.

186 CONNELLAN J.M., CASTALDI P.A. & MUNTZ R.H. (1977) The role of factor XI in the coagulant activity of platelets. *Haemostasis*, **6**, 41.

187 LIPSCOMB M.S. & WALSH P.N. (1979) Human platelets and factor XI. Localization in platelet membranes of factor XI-like activity and its functional distinction from plasma factor XI. *Journal of Clinical Investigation*, **63**, 1006.

188 WALSH P.N. & BIGGS R. (1972) The role of platelets in intrinsic factor-Xa formation. *British Journal of Haematology*, **22**, 743.

189 WALSH P.N. (1978) Different requirements for intrinsic factor-Xa forming activity and platelet factor 3 activity and their relationship to platelet aggregation and secretion. *British Journal of Haematology*, **40**, 311.

190 HARDISTY R.M. & HUTTON R.A. (1966) Platelet aggregation and the availability of platelet factor 3. *British Journal of Haematology*, **12**, 764.

191 ZWAAL R.F.A., COMFURIUS P. & VAN DEENAN L.L.M. (1977) Membrane asymmetry and blood coagulation. *Nature (London)*, **268**, 358.

192 BROECKMAN M.J., HANDIN R.I., DERKSEN A. & COHEN P. (1976) Distribution of phospholipids, fatty acids and platelet factor 3 activity among subcellular fractions of human platelets. *Blood*, **47**, 963.

193 HJORT P.F., RAPAPORT S.I. & OWREN P.A. (1955) Evidence that platelet accelerator (platelet factor I) is adsorbed plasma proaccelerin. *Blood*, **10**, 1139.

194 BREEDERVELD K., GIDDINGS J.C., TEN CATE J.W. & BLOOM A.L. (1975) The localization of factor V within normal human platelets and the demonstration of a platelet-factor V antigen in congenital factor V deficiency. *British Journal of Haematology*, **29**, 405.

195 MILETICH J.P., JACKSON C.M. & MAJERUS P.W. (1978) Properties of the factor Xa binding site on human platelets. *Journal of Biological Chemistry*, **253**, 6908.

196 CASTALDI P.A. & CAEN J. (1965) Platelet fibrinogen. *Journal of Clinical Pathology*, **18**, 579.

197 NACHMAN R.L., MARCUS A.J. & ZUCKER-FRANKLIN D. (1967) Immunologic studies of proteins associated with subcellular fractions of normal human platelets. *Journal of Laboratory and Clinical Medicine*, **69**, 651.

198 JAMES H.L., GANGULY P. & JACKSON C.W. (1977) Characterization and origin of fibrinogen in blood platelets. *Thrombosis and Haemostasis*, **38**, 939.

199 DOOLITTLE R.F., TAKAGI T. & COTTRELL B.A. (1974) Platelet and plasma fibrinogens are identical gene products. *Science*, **185**, 368.

200 PLOW E.F. & EDGINGTON T.S. (1975) Unique immunochemical features and intracellular stability of platelet fibrinogen. *Thrombosis Research*, **7**, 729.

201 SCHWARTZ M.L., PIZZO S.V., HILL R.L. & McKEE P.A. (1973) Human factor XIII from plasma and platelets: molecular weights, subunit structures, proteolytic activation, and cross-linking of fibrinogen and fibrin. *Journal of Biological Chemistry*, **248**, 1395.

202 LOPACIUK S., LOVETTE K.M., McDONAGH J., CHUANG H.Y.K. & McDONAGH R.P. (1976) Subcellular distribution of fibrinogen and factor XIII in human blood platelets. *Thrombosis Research*, **8**, 453.

203 JOIST J.H. & NIEWIAROWSKI S. (1973) Retention of platelet fibrin stabilizing factor during the platelet release reaction. *Thrombosis et Diathesis Haemorrhagica*, **29**, 679.

204 McDONAGH J., KIESSELBACH T.H. & WAGNER R.H. (1969) Factor XIII and antiplasmin activity in human platelets. *American Journal of Physiology*, **216**, 508.

205 KIESSELBACH T.H. & WAGNER R.H. (1972) Demonstration of factor XIII in human megakaryocytes by a fluorescent antibody technique. *Annals of the New York Academy of Sciences*, **202**, 318.

206 NIEWIAROWSKI S., FARBISZEWSKI R. & POPLAWSKI A. (1967) In: *Biochemistry of Blood Platelets* (ed. Kowalski E. & Niewarowski S.), p. 35. Academic Press, London.

207 DETWILER T.C. & FEINMAN R.D. (1973) Kinetics of the thrombin-induced release of calcium (II) by platelets. *Biochemistry*, **12**, 282.

208 WATANABE K., CHAO F.C. & TULLIS J.L. (1977) Platelet antithrombins: role of thrombin binding and the release of platelet fibrinogen. *British Journal of Haematology*, **35**, 123.

209 NACHMAN R.L. (1965) Immunologic studies of platelet protein. *Blood*, **25**, 703.

210 EKERT H., FRIEDLANDER I. & HARDISTY R.M. (1970) The role of platelets in fibrinolysis. Studies on the plasminogen activator and anti-plasmin activity of platelets. *British Journal of Haematology*, **18**, 575.

211 JOIST J.H., NIEWIAROWSKI S., NATH N. & MUSTARD J.F. (1976) Platelet antiplasmin: its extrusion during the release reaction, subcellular localization, characteriza-

tion, and relationship to antiheparin in pig platelets. *Journal of Laboratory and Clinical Medicine*, **87**, 659.

212 MURRAY J., CRAWFORD G.P.M., OGSTON D. & DOUGLAS A.S. (1974) Studies on an inhibitor of plasminogen activators in human platelets. *British Journal of Haematology*, **26**, 661.

213 WEKSLER B.B. & COUPAL C.E. (1973) Platelet-dependent generation of chemotactic activity in serum. *Journal of Experimental Medicine*, **137**, 1419.

214 SILVER M.J., SMITH J.B. & INGERMAN C. (1974) Blood platelets and the inflammatory process. *Agents and Actions*, **4**, 233.

215 ROBERT B., SZIGETTI M., ROBERT L., LEGRAND Y., PIGNAUD G. & CAEN J. (1970) Release of elastolytic activity from blood platelets. *Nature (London)*, **227**, 1248.

216 CHESNEY C.M., HARPER E. & COLMAN R.W. (1974) Human platelet collagenase. *Journal of Clinical Investigation*, **53**, 1647.

217 CLAWSON C.C. & WHITE J.G. (1971) Platelet interaction with bacteria. I. Reaction phases and effects of inhibitors. *American Journal of Pathology*, **65**, 367. II. Fate of the bacteria. *American Journal of Pathology*, **65**, 381.

218 VAN AKEN W.G. & VREEKEN J. (1969) Accumulation of macro-molecular particles in the reticuloendothelial system (RES) mediated by platelet aggregation and disaggregation. *Thrombosis et Diathesis Haemorrhagica*, **22**, 496.

219 MOWBRAY J.F. (1975) The role of platelets in rejection of organ transplants. In: *Platelets, Drugs and Thrombosis* (ed. Hirsh J. *et al.*), p. 200. Karger, Basel.

220 PFUELLER S.L. & LÜSCHER E.F. (1972) The effects of immune complexes on blood platelets and their relationship to complement activation. *Immunochemistry*, **9**, 1151.

221 BROWN D.L. (1976) Platelets in immunological reactions. In: *Platelets in Biology and Pathology* (ed. Gordon J.L.), p. 313. North-Holland, Amsterdam.

222 AALTO M. & KULONEN E. (1972) Effects of serotonin, indomethacin and other anti-rheumatic drugs on the synthesis of collagen and other proteins in granulation tissue slices. *Biochemical Pharmacology*, **21**, 2835.

223 INCEMAN S., CAEN J. & BERNARD J. (1966) Aggregation, adhesion and viscous metamorphosis of platelets in congenital fibrinogen deficiencies. *Journal of Laboratory and Clinical Medicine*, **68**, 21.

224 BERNARD J. & SOULIER J.P. (1948) Sur une nouvelle variété de dystrophie thrombocytaire hémorrhagipare congenitale. *Semaine des Hôpitaux, Paris*, **24**, 3217.

225 BITHELL T.C., PAREKH S.J. & STRONG R.R. (1972) Platelet function in the Bernard–Soulier syndrome. *Annals of the New York Academy of Sciences*, **201**, 145.

226 HOWARD M.A., HUTTON R.A. & HARDISTY R.M. (1973) Hereditary giant platelet syndrome: a disorder of a new aspect of platelet function. *British Medical Journal*, **ii**, 586.

227 WEISS H.J., TSCHOPP T.B., BAUMGARTNER H.R., SUSSMAN I.I., JOHNSON M.M. & EGAN J.J. (1974) Decreased adhesion of giant (Bernard–Soulier) platelets to subendothelium. Further implications on the role of the von Willebrand factor in hemostasis. *American Journal of Medicine*, **57**, 920.

228 CAEN J.P., NURDEN A.T., JEANNEAU C., MICHEL H.,

TOBELEM G., LEVY-TOLEDANO S., SULTAN Y., VALENSI F. & BERNARD J. (1976) Bernard–Soulier syndrome—a new platelet glycoprotein abnormality. Its relationship with platelet adhesion to subendothelium and with the factor VIII von Willebrand protein. *Journal of Laboratory and Clinical Medicine*, **87**, 586.

229 NACHMAN R.L., JAFFE E.A. & WEKSLER B.B. (1977) Immunoinhibition of ristocetin-induced platelet aggregation. *Journal of Clinical Investigation*, **59**, 143.

230 WALSH P.N., MILLS D.C.B., PARETI F.I., STEWART G.I., MACFARLANE D.E., JOHNSON M.M. & EGAN J.J. (1975) Hereditary giant platelet syndrome: absence of collagen-induced coagulant activity and deficiency of factor XI binding to platelets. *British Journal of Haematology*, **29**, 639.

231 TOBELEM G., LEVY-TOLEDANO S., BREDOUX R., MICHEL H., NURDEN A. & CAEN J.P. (1976) New approach to determination of specific functions of platelet membrane sites. *Nature (London)*, **263**, 427.

232 DEGOS L., TOBELEM G., LETHIELLEUX P., LEVY-TOLEDANO S., CAEN J. & COLOMBANI J. A molecular defect in platelets from patients with Bernard–Soulier syndrome. *Blood*, **50**, 899.

233 GLANZMANN E. (1918) Hereditäre hämorrhagische thrombasthenie. Ein Beitrag zur Pathologie der Blutplättchen. *Jahrbuch der Kinderheilkunde*, **88**, 1.

234 ZUCKER M.B., PERT J.H. & HILGARTNER M.W. (1966) Platelet function in a patient with thrombasthenia. *Blood*, **28**, 524.

235 HARDISTY R.M., DORMANDY K.M. & HUTTON R.A. (1964) Thrombasthenia: studies on three cases. *British Journal of Haematology*, **10**, 371.

236 CAEN J.P., CASTALDI P.A., LECLERC J.C., INCEMAN S., LARRIEU M.J., PROBST M. & BERNARD J. (1966) Congenital bleeding disorders with long bleeding time and normal platelet count. I. Glanzmann's thrombasthenia. *American Journal of Medicine*, **41**, 4.

237 HOWARD M.A. & FIRKIN B.G. (1971) Ristocetin: a new tool in the investigation of platelet aggregation. *Thrombosis et Diathesis Haemorrhagica*, **26**, 362.

238 TSCHOPP T.B., WEISS H.J. & BAUMGARTNER H.R. (1975) Interaction of thrombasthenic platelets with subendothelium: normal adhesion, absent aggregation. *Experientia*, **31**, 113.

239 LEGRAND C. & CAEN J.P. (1976) Binding of ^{14}C-ADP by thrombasthenic platelet membranes. *Haemostasis*, **5**, 231.

240 WHITE G.C., WORKMAN E.F. & LUNDBLAD R.L. (1978) Thrombin binding to thrombasthenic platelets. *Journal of Laboratory and Clinical Medicine*, **91**, 76.

241 HOWARD M.A., MONTGOMERY D.C. & HARDISTY R.M. (1974) Factor-VIII-related antigen in platelets. *Thrombosis Research*, **4**, 617.

242 KUNICKI T.J. & ASTER R.H. (1978) Deletion of the platelet-specific alloantigen Pl^{A1} from platelets in Glanzmann's thrombasthenia. *Journal of Clinical Investigation*, **61**, 1225.

243 CAEN J.P., MICHEL H., TOBELEM G., BODEVIN E. & LEVY-TOLEDANO S. (1977) Adhesion and aggregation of human platelets to rabbit subendothelium. A new approach for investigation: specific antibodies. *Experientia*, **33**, 91.

244 LEVY-TOLEDANO S., TOBELEM G., LEGRAND C., BRE-

DOUX R., DEGOS L., NURDEN A. & CAEN J.P. (1978) An acquired IgG antibody occurring in a thrombasthenic patient: its effect on human platelet function. *Blood*, **51**, 1065.

245 HAGEN I., NURDEN A.T., BJERRUM O.J., SOLUM N.O. & CAEN J.P. (1980) Immunochemical evidence for protein abnormalities in platelets from patients with Glanzmann's thrombasthenia and the Bernard–Soulier syndrome. *Journal of Clinical Investigation*, **65**, 722.

246 LEVY-TOLEDANO S., MACLOUF J., RENDU F., RIGAUD M. & CAEN J.P. (1979) Ionophore A 23187 and thrombasthenic platelets: a model for dissociating serotonin release and thromboxane formation from true aggregation. *Thrombosis Research*, **16**, 453.

247 MALMSTEN C., KINDAHL H., SAMUELSSON B., LEVY-TOLEDANO S., TOBELEM G. & CAEN J.P. (1977) Thromboxane synthesis and the platelet release reaction in Bernard–Soulier syndrome, thrombasthenia Glanzmann and Hermansky–Pudlak syndrome. *British Journal of Haematology*, **35**, 511.

248 WALSH P.N. (1972) Platelet coagulant activities in thrombasthenia. *British Journal of Haematology*, **23**, 553.

249 PHILLIPS D. (1978) In: *Platelet Function Testing* (ed. Day H.J., Holmsen H. & Zucker M.B.) DHEW publication no. (NIH) 78–1087, p. 240.

250 DEGOS L., DAUTIGNY A., BROUET J.C., COLOMBANI M., ARDAILLOU N., CAEN J.P. & COLOMBANI J. (1975) A molecular defect in thrombasthenic platelets. *Journal of Clinical Investigation*, **56**, 236.

251 HARDISTY R.M. & HUTTON R.A. (1967) Bleeding tendency associated with 'new' abnormality of platelet behaviour. *Lancet*, **i**, 983.

252 WEISS H.J. (1967) Platelet aggregation, adhesion and adenosine diphosphate release in thrombopathia (platelet factor 3 deficiency): a comparison with Glanzmann's thrombasthenia and von Willebrand's disease. *American Journal of Medicine*, **43**, 570.

253 WEISS H.J., VICIC W.J., LAGES B.A. & ROGERS J. (1979) Isolated deficiency of platelet procoagulant activity. *American Journal of Medicine*, **67**, 206.

254 MILETICH J.P., KANE W.H., HOFMANN S.L., STANFORD N. & MAJERUS P.W. (1979). Deficiency of factor Xa-factor Va binding sites on the platelets of a patient with a bleeding disorder. *Blood*, **54**, 1015.

255 WEISS H.J., CHERVENICK P.A., ZALUSKY R. & FACTOR A. (1969) A familial defect in platelet function associated with impaired release of adenosine diphosphate. *New England Journal of Medicine*, **281**, 1264.

256 WEISS H.J. & ROGERS J. (1972) Thrombocytopathia due to abnormalities in platelet release reaction—studies on six unrelated patients. *Blood*, **39**, 187.

257 PARETI F.I., DAY H.J. & MILLS D.C.B. (1974) Nucleotide and serotonin metabolism in platelets with defective secondary aggregation. *Blood*, **44**, 789.

258 HARDISTY R.M., MILLS D.C.B. & KETSA-ARD K. (1972) The platelet defect associated with albinism. *British Journal of Haematology*, **23**, 679.

259 WEISS H.J., TSCHOPP T., BRAND H. & ROGERS J. (1974) Studies of platelet 5-hydroxytryptamine (serotonin) in patients with storage-pool disease and albinism. *Journal of Clinical Investigation*, **54**, 421.

260 HOLMSEN H. & WEISS H.J. (1972) Further evidence for a deficient storage pool of adenine nucleotides in platelets from some patients with thrombocytopathia—'storage pool disease'. *Blood*, **39**, 197.

261 WHITE J.G., EDSON J.R., DESNICK S.J. & WITKOP C.J. (1971) Studies of platelets in a variant of the Hermansky–Pudlak syndrome. *American Journal of Pathology*, **63**, 319.

262 WEISS H.J. & AMES R.P. (1973) Ultrastructural findings in storage pool disease and aspirin-like defects of platelets. *American Journal of Pathology*, **71**, 447.

263 LAGES B., SCRUTTON M.C., HOLMSEN H., DAY H.J. & WEISS H.J. (1975) Metal ion content of gel-filtered platelets from patients with storage pool disease. *Blood*, **46**, 119.

264 MINKES M.S., JOIST J.H. & NEEDLEMAN P. (1979) Arachidonic acid-induced platelet aggregation independent of ADP-release in a patient with a bleeding disorder due to platelet storage pool disease. *Thrombosis Research*, **15**, 169.

265 INGERMAN C.M., SMITH J.B., SHAPIRO S., SEDAR A. & SILVER M.J. (1978) Hereditary abnormality of platelet aggregation attributable to nucleotide storage pool deficiency. *Blood*, **52**, 332.

266 WEISS H.J., WITTE L.D., KAPLAN K.L., LAGES B.A., CHERNOFF A., NOSSEL H.L., GOODMAN D.S. & BAUMGARTNER H.R. (1979) Heterogeneity in storage pool deficiency: studies on granule-bound substances in 18 patients including variants deficient in α-granules, platelet factor 4, β-thromboglobulin, and platelet-derived growth factor. *Blood*, **54**, 1296.

267 MAURER H.M., STILL W.J.S., CAUL J., VALDES O.S. & LAUPUS W.E. (1971) Familial bleeding tendency associated with microcytic platelets and impaired release of platelet adenosine diphosphate. *Journal of Pediatrics*, **78**, 86.

268 MAURER H.M., WOLFF J.A., BUCKINGHAM A.R. & SPIELVOGEL A.R. (1972) 'Impotent' platelets in albinos with prolonged bleeding times. *Blood*, **39**, 490.

269 HERMANSKY F. & PUDLAK P. (1959) Albinism associated with hemorrhagic diathesis and unusual pigmented reticular cells in the bone marrow: report of two cases with histochemical studies. *Blood*, **14**, 162.

270 WITKOP C.J., WHITE J.G. & KING R.A. (1974) Oculocutaneous albinism. In: *Heritable Disorders of Amino Acid Metabolism* (ed. Nyhan W.L.), p. 177. Wiley, New York.

271 GARAY S.M., GARDELLA J.E., FAZZINI E.P. & GOLDRING R.M. (1979) Hermansky–Pudlak syndrome: pulmonary manifestations of a ceroid storage disorder. *American Journal of Medicine*, **66**, 737.

271a GERRITSEN S.M., AKKERMAN J.W.N., NIJMEIJER B., SIXMA J.J., WITKOP C.J. & WHITE J. (1977) The Hermansky–Pudlak syndrome: evidence for a lowered 5-hydroxytryptamine content in platelets of heterozygotes. *Scandinavian Journal of Haematology*, **18**, 249.

272 GRÖTTUM K.A., HOVIG T., HOLMSEN H., ABRAHAMSEN A.F., JEREMIC M. & SEIP M. (1969) Wiskott–Aldrich syndrome: qualitative platelet defects and short platelet survival. *British Journal of Haematology*, **17**, 373.

273 BUCHANAN G.R. & HANDIN R.I. (1976) Platelet function in the Chediak–Higashi syndrome. *Blood*, **47**, 941.

274 BOXER G.J., HOLMSEN H., ROBKIN L., BANG N.U., BOXER L.A. & BAEHNER R.L. (1977) Abnormal platelet

function in Chediak–Higashi syndrome. *British Journal of Haematology*, **35**, 521.

275 DAY H.J. & HOLMSEN H. (1972) Platelet adenine nucleotide 'storage pool deficiency' in thrombocytopenic absent radii syndrome. *Journal of the American Medical Association*, **221**, 1053.

276 SHAPIRO R.S., GERRARD J.M., PERRY G.S. III, WHITE J.G., KRIVIT W. & KERSEY J.H. (1978) Wiskott–Aldrich syndrome: detection of the carrier state by metabolic stress of platelets. *Lancet*, **i**, 121.

277 MALMSTEN C., HAMBERG M., SVENSSON J. & SAMUELSSON B. (1975) Physiological role of an endoperoxide in human platelets: hemostatic defect due to platelet cyclo-oxygenase deficiency. *Proceedings of the National Academy of Sciences, USA*, **72**, 1446.

278 LAGARDE M., BRYON P.A., VARGAFTIG B.B. & DECHAVANNE M. (1978) Impairment of platelet thromboxane A$_2$ generation and of the platelet release reaction in two patients with congenital deficiency of platelet cyclo-oxygenase. *British Journal of Haematology*, **38**, 251.

279 PARETI F.I., MANNUCCI P.M., D'ANGELO A., SMITH J.B., SAUTERIN L. & GALLI G. (1980) Congenital deficiency of thromboxane and prostacyclin. *Lancet*, **i**, 898.

279a DEFREYN G., MACHIN S.J., CARRERAS L.O., VERGERA DAUDON M., CHAMONE D.A.F. & VERMYLEN J. (1981) Familial bleeding tendency with partial platelet thromboxane synthetase deficiency: reorientation of cyclic endoperoxide metabolism. *British Journal of Haematology*, **49**, 29.

280 CZAPEK E.E., DEYKIN D., SALZMAN E., LIAN E.C., HELLERSTEIN L.J. & ROSOFF C.B. (1978) Intermediate syndrome of platelet dysfunction. *Blood*, **52**, 103.

280a KURSTJENS R., BOLT C., VOSSEN M. & HAANEN C. (1968) Familial thrombopathic thrombocytopenia. *British Journal of Haematology*, **15**, 305.

280b LIBANSKA J., FALCÃO L., GAUTIER A., AMMON J., SPAHR A., VAINER H. & CAEN J. (1975). Thrombocytopénie thrombocytopathique hypogranulaire héréditaire. *Nouvelle Revue française d'Hématologie*, **15**, 165.

281 RACCUGLIA G. (1971) Gray platelet syndrome. A variety of qualitative platelet disorder. *American Journal of Medicine*, **51**, 818.

282 WHITE J.G. (1979) Ultrastructural studies of the gray platelet syndrome. *American Journal of Pathology*, **95**, 445.

283 EPSTEIN C.J., SAHUD M.A., PIEL C.F., GOODMAN J.R., BERNFIELD M.R., KUSHNER J.H. & ABLIN A.R. (1972) Hereditary macrothrombocytopathia, nephritis and deafness. *American Journal of Medicine*, **52**, 299.

284 BERNHEIM J., DECHAVANNE M., BRYON P.A., LAGARDE E.M., COLON S., POZET N. & TRAEGER J. (1976) Thrombocytopenia, macrothrombocytopathia, nephritis and deafness. *American Journal of Medicine*, **61**, 145.

285 ECKSTEIN J.D., FILIP D.J. & WATTS J.C (1975) Hereditary thrombocytopenia, deafness and renal disease. *Annals of Internal Medicine*, **82**, 639.

286 BOULLIN D.J. & O'BRIEN R.A. (1971) Abnormalities of 5-hydroxytryptamine uptake and binding by blood platelets from children with Down's syndrome. *Journal of Physiology*, **212**, 287.

287 ESTES J.W. (1968) Platelet size and function in the heritable disorders of connective tissue. *Annals of Internal Medicine*, **68**, 1237.

288 HATHAWAY W.E., SOLOMONS C.C. & OTT J.E. (1972) Platelet function and pyrophosphates in osteogenesis imperfecta. *Blood*, **39**, 500.

289 NYMAN D., ERIKSSON A.W., LEHMANN W. & BLOMBÄCK M. (1979) Inherited defective platelet aggregation with arachidonate as the main expression of a defective metabolism of arachidonic acid. *Thrombosis Research*, **14**, 739.

290 CASTALDI P.A., ROZENBERG M.C. & STEWART J.H. (1966) The bleeding disorder of uraemia. *Lancet*, **ii**, 66.

291 SALZMAN E.W. & NERI L.J. (1966) Adhesiveness of blood platelets in uremia. *Thrombosis et Diathesis Haemorrhagica*, **15**, 84.

292 HOROWITZ H.I., COHEN B.D., MARTINEZ P. & PAPAYOANOU M.F. (1967) Defective ADP-induced platelet factor 3 activation in uremia. *Blood*, **30**, 331.

293 RABINER S.F. & HRODEK O. (1968) Platelet factor 3 in normal subjects and patients with renal failure. *Journal of Clinical Investigation*, **47**, 901.

294 HUTTON R.A. & O'SHEA M.J. (1968) Haemostatic mechanism in uraemia. *Journal of Clinical Pathology*, **21**, 406.

295 HOROWITZ H.I., STEIN I.M., COHEN B.D. & WHITE J.G. (1970) Further studies on the platelet inhibitory effect of guanidinosuccinic acid: its role in uremic bleeding. *American Journal of Medicine*, **49**, 336.

296 BALLARD H.S. & MARCUS A.J. (1972) Primary and secondary platelet aggregation in uraemia. *Scandinavian Journal of Haematology*, **9**, 198.

297 STEWART J.H. & CASTALDI P.A. (1967) Uraemic bleeding: a reversible platelet defect corrected by dialysis. *Quarterly Journal of Medicine*, **36**, 409.

298 EKNOYAN G., WACKSMAN S.J., GLUECK H.I. & WILL J.J. (1969) Platelet function in renal failure. *New England Journal of Medicine*, **280**, 677.

299 DAVIS J.W., McFIELD J.R., PHILLIPS P.L. & GRAHAM B.A. (1972) Effects of exogenous urea, creatinine, and guanidinosuccinic acid on human platelet aggregation *in vitro*. *Blood*, **39**, 388.

300 RABINER S.F. & MOLINAS F. (1970) The role of phenol and phenolic acids on the thrombocytopathy and defective platelet aggregation of patients with renal failure. *American Journal of Medicine*, **49**, 346.

301 RABINER S.F. (1972) Uremic bleeding. *Progress in Hemostasis and Thrombosis*, **1**, 233.

302 MATTHIAS F.F. & PALINSKI W. (1977) Prostaglandinendoperoxides and cyclic 3'-5'-AMP in platelets of patients with uremia. *Thrombosis and Haemostasis*, **38**, 34.

303 REMUZZI G., MARCHESI D., LIVIO M., CAVENAGHI A.E., MECCA G., DONATI M.B. & DE GAETANO G. (1978) Altered platelet and vascular prostaglandin generation in patients with renal failure and prolonged bleeding times. *Thrombosis Research*, **13**, 1007.

304 NIEWIAROWSKI S., GUZZO J., RAO A.K., BERMAN I. & JAMES P. (1979) Increased levels of low affinity platelet factor 4 in plasma and urine of patients with chronic renal failure. *Thrombosis and Haemostasis*, **42**, 416.

305 GREEN D., SANTHANAM S., KRUMLOVSKY F.A. & DEL GRECO F. (1979) β-thromboglobulin in patients with

chronic renal failure: effect of hemodialysis. *Thrombosis and Haemostasis*, **42**, 416.

306 ZUCKER S. & MIELKE C.H. (1972) Classification of thrombocytosis based on platelet function tests. Correlation with hemorrhagic and thrombotic complications. *Journal of Laboratory and Clinical Medicine*, **80**, 385.

307 KEENAN J.P., WHARTON J., SHEPHERD A.J.N. & BELLINGHAM A.J. (1977) Defective lipid peroxidation in myeloproliferative disorders: possible defect of prostaglandin synthesis. *British Journal of Haematology*, **35**, 275.

308 SPAET T.H., LEJNIEKS I., GAYNOR E. & GOLDSTEIN M.L. (1969) Defective platelets in essential thrombocythaemia. *Archives of Internal Medicine*, **124**, 135.

309 BERGER S., ALEDORT L.M., GILBERT H.S., HANSON J.P. & WASSERMAN L.R. (1973) Abnormalities of platelet function in patients with polycythemia vera. *Cancer Research*, **33**, 2683.

310 ADAMS T., SCHULTZ L. & GOLDBERG L. (1974) Platelet function abnormalities in the myeloproliferative disorders. *Scandinavian Journal of Haematology*, **13**, 215.

311 McCLURE P.D., INGRAM G.I.C., STACEY R.S., GLASS U.H. & MATCHETT M.O. (1966) Platelet function tests in thrombocythaemia and thrombocytosis. *British Journal of Haematology*, **12**, 478.

312 GINSBURG A.D. (1975) Platelet function in patients with high platelet counts. *Annals of Internal Medicine*, **82**, 506.

313 CARDAMONE J.M., EDSON J.R., McARTHUR J.R. & JACOB H.S. (1972) Abnormalities of platelet function in the myeloproliferative disorders. *Journal of the American Medical Association*, **221**, 270.

314 NEEMEH J.A., BOWIE E.J.W., THOMPSON J.H., DIDISHEIM P. & OWEN C.A. (1972) Quantitation of platelet aggregation in myeloproliferative disorders. *American Journal of Clinical Pathology*, **57**, 336.

315 KAYWIN P., McDONOUGH M., INSEL P.A. & SHATTIL S.J. (1978) Platelet function in essential thrombocythaemia. Decreased epinephrine responsiveness associated with deficiency of platelet α-adrenergic receptors. *New England Journal of Medicine*, **299**, 505.

316 RUSSELL N.H., KEENAN J.P. & BELLINGHAM A.J. (1979) Thrombocytopathy in preleukaemia: association with a defect of thromboxane A_2 activity. *British Journal of Haematology*, **41**, 417.

317 GERRARD J.M., STODDARD S.F., SHAPIRO R.S., COCCIA P.F., RAMSAY N.K.C., NESBIT M.E., RAO G.H.R., KRIVIT W. & WHITE J.G. (1978) Platelet storage pool deficiency and prostaglandin synthesis in chronic granulocytic leukaemia. *British Journal of Haematology*, **40**, 597.

318 NISHIMURA J., OKAMOTO S. & IBAYASHI H. (1979) Abnormalities of platelet adenine nucleotides in patients with myeloproliferative disorders. *Thrombosis and Haemostasis*, **41**, 787.

319 BOLIN R.B., OKUMURA T. & JAMIESON G.A. (1977) Changes in distribution of platelet membrane glycoproteins in patients with myeloproliferative disorders. *American Journal of Hematology*, **3**, 63.

320 WU K.K. (1978) Platelet hyperaggregability and thrombosis in patients with thrombocythemia. *Annals of Internal Medicine*, **88**, 7.

321 COOPER B., SCHAFER A.I., PUCHALSKY D. & HANDIN R.I. (1978) Platelet resistance to prostaglandin D_2 in patients with myeloproliferative disorders. *Blood*, **52**, 618.

322 COOPER B. & AHERN D. (1979) Characterization of the platelet prostaglandin D_2 receptor—loss of prostaglandin D_2 receptors in platelets of patients with myeloproliferative disorders. *Journal of Clinical Investigation*, **64**, 586.

323 BIERME R., BONEU B., GUIRAUD B. & PRIS J. (1972) Aspirin and recurrent painful toes and fingers in thrombocythaemia. *Lancet*, **i**, 432.

324 FRIEDMAN I.A., SCHWARTZ S.O. & LEITHOLD S.L. (1964) Platelet function defects with bleeding: early manifestations of acute leukemia. *Archives of Internal Medicine*, **113**, 177.

325 COWAN D.H. & HAUT M.J. (1972) Platelet function in acute leukemia. *Journal of Laboratory and Clinical Medicine*, **79**, 893.

326 SULTAN Y. & CAEN J.P. (1972) Platelet dysfunction in preleukemic states and in various types of leukemia. *Annals of the New York Academy of Sciences*, **201**, 300.

327 COWAN D.H., GRAHAM R.C. & BAUNACH D. (1975) The platelet defect in leukemia, platelet ultrastructure, adenine nucleotide metabolism, and the release reaction. *Journal of Clinical Investigation*, **56**, 188.

328 PERKINS H.A., McKENZIE M.R. & FUDENBERG H.H. (1970) Hemostatic defects in dysproteinemias. *Blood*, **35**, 695.

329 LACKNER H. (1973) Hemostatic abnormalities associated with dysproteinemias. *Seminars in Hematology*, **10**, 125.

330 VIGLIANO E.M. & HOROWITZ H.I. (1967) Bleeding syndrome in a patient with IgA myeloma: interaction of protein and connective tissue. *Blood*, **29**, 823.

331 PENNY R., CASTALDI P.A. & WHITSED H.M. (1971) Inflammation and haemostasis in paraproteinaemias. *British Journal of Haematology*, **20**, 35.

332 CZAPEK, E.E., DEYKIN D. & SALZMAN E.W. (1973) Platelet dysfunction in glycogen storage disease type I. *Blood*, **41**, 235.

333 CORBY D.G., PUTNAM C.W. & GREENE H.L. (1974) Impaired platelet function in glucose-6-phosphatase deficiency. *Journal of Pediatrics*, **85**, 71.

334 HUTTON R.A., MacNab A.J. & RIVERS R.P.A. (1976) Defect of platelet function associated with chronic hypoglycaemia. *Archives of Disease in Childhood*, **51**, 49.

335 THOMAS D.P., REAM V.J. & STUART R.K. (1967) Platelet aggregation in patients with Laennec's cirrhosis of the liver. *New England Journal of Medicine*, **276**, 1344.

336 BALLARD H.S. & MARCUS A.J. (1976) Platelet aggregation in portal cirrhosis. *Archives of Internal Medicine*, **136**, 316.

337 JERUSHALMY Z. & ZUCKER M.B. (1966) Some effects of fibrinogen degradation products (FDP) on blood platelets. *Thrombosis et Diathesis Haemorrhagica*, **15**, 413.

338 STACHURSKA J., LATALLO Z. & KOPEĆ M. (1970) Inhibition of platelet aggregation by dialysable fibrinogen degradation products (FDP). *Thrombosis et Diathesis Haemorrhagica*, **23**, 91.

339 SOLUM N.O., RIGOLLOT C., BUDZYŃSKI A.Z. & MARDER V.J. (1973) A quantitative evaluation of the inhibition of platelet aggregation by low molecular weight degradation products of fibrinogen. *British Journal of Haematology*, **24**, 419.

340 BEURLING-HARBURY C. & GALVAN C.A. (1978) Acquired decrease in platelet secretory ADP associated with increased postoperative bleeding in post-cardio-pulmonary bypass patients and in patients with severe valvular heart disease. *Blood*, **52**, 13.

341 HOURDILLÉ P., BERNARD P., BELLOC F., PRADET A., SANCHEZ R. & BOISSEAU M.R. (1981) Platelet abnormalities in thermal injury. *Haemostasis*, **10**, 141.

342 ZAHAVI J. & MARDER V.J. (1974) Acquired 'storage pool disease' of platelets associated with circulating anti-platelet antibodies. *American Journal of Medicine*, **56**, 883.

343 PARETI F.I., CAPITANIO A. & MANNUCCI P.M. (1976) Acquired storage pool disease in platelets during disseminated intravascular coagulation. *Blood*, **48**, 511.

344 WILSON P.A., McNICOL G.P. & DOUGLAS A.S. (1967) Platelet abnormality in human scurvy. *Lancet*, **i**, 975.

345 LEVINE P.H. (1973) A qualitative platelet defect in severe vitamin B_{12} deficiency: response, hyperresponse and thrombosis after vitamin B_{12} therapy. *Annals of Internal Medicine*, **78**, 533.

346 MAURER H.M., McCUE C.M., CAUL J. & STILL W.J.S. (1972) Impairment in platelet aggregation in congenital heart disease. *Blood*, **40**, 207.

347 CLANCY R., JENKINS E. & FIRKIN B. (1971) Platelet defect of infectious mononucleosis. *British Medical Journal* **iv**, 646.

348 BARTTER F.C., GILL J.R. JR, FROLICH J.C. *et al.* (1976) Prostaglandins are overproduced by the kidneys and mediate hyperreninaemia in Bartter's syndrome. *Transactions of the Association of American Physicians*, **89**, 77.

349 GULLNER H.-G., CERLETTI C., BARTTER F.C., SMITH J.B. & GILL J.R. JR (1979) Prostacyclin overproduction in Bartter's syndrome. *Lancet*, **ii**, 767.

320 STOFF J.S., STEMERMAN M., STEER M., SALZMAN E. & BROWN R.S. (1978) A unique defect in platelet aggregation in Bartter's syndrome: improvement by indomethacin. *Clinical Research*, **26**, 508A.

351 STOFF J.S, MacINTYRE D.E., BROWN R.S. & SALZMAN E.W. (1979) Prostacyclin overproduction in Bartter's syndrome. *Lancet*, **ii**, 1196.

352 DE GAETANO G., DONATI M.B. & GARATTINI S. (1975) Drugs affecting platelet function tests: their effects on haemostasis and surgical bleeding. *Thrombosis et Diathesis Haemorrhagica*, **34**, 285.

353 WEISS H.J. (1976) Antiplatelet drugs: a new pharmacologic approach to the prevention of thrombosis. *American Heart Journal*, **92**, 86.

354 PACKHAM M.A. & MUSTARD J.F. (1977) Clinical pharmacology of platelets. *Blood*, **50**, 555.

355 WEISS H.J. & ALEDORT L.M. (1967) Impaired platelet-connective tissue reaction in man after aspirin ingestion. *Lancet*, **ii**, 495.

356 O'BRIEN J.R. (1968) Effects of salicylates on human platelets. *Lancet*, **i**, 779.

357 ZUCKER M.B. & PETERSON J. (1968) Inhibition of adenosine diphosphate-induced secondary aggregation and other platelet functions by acetylsalicylic acid ingestion. *Proceedings of the Society for Experimental Biology and Medicine*, **127**, 547.

358 EVANS G., PACKHAM M.A., NISHIZAWA E.E., MUSTARD J.F. & MURPHY E.A. (1968) The effect of acetylsalicylic acid on platelet function. *Journal of Experimental Medicine*, **128**, 877.

359 ROTH G.J., STANFORD N. & MAJERUS P.W. (1975) Acetylation of prostaglandin synthetase by aspirin. *Proceedings of the National Academy of Sciences, USA*, **72**, 3073.

360 LANGDELL R.D., ADELSON E.A., FURTH F.W. & CROSBY W.H. (1958) Dextran and prolonged bleeding time; results of a 60 gram, 1 liter infusion given to one hundred sixty three normal human subjects. *Journal of the American Medical Association*, **166**, 346.

361 EWALD R.A., EICHELBERGER J.W., YOUNG A.A., WEISS H.J. & CROSBY W.H. (1965) The effect of dextran on platelet factor 3 activity: *in-vitro* and *in-vivo* studies. *Transfusion*, **5**, 109.

362 BYGDEMAN S. & ELIASSON R. (1967) Effect of dextrans on platelet adhesiveness and aggregation. *Scandinavian Journal of Clinical and Laboratory Investigation*, **20**, 17.

363 WEISS H.J. (1967) The effect of clinical dextran on platelet aggregation, adhesion, and ADP release in man: *in-vivo* and *in-vitro* studies. *Journal of Laboratory and Clinical Medicine*, **69**, 37.

364 EVANS R.J. & GORDON J.L. (1974) Mechanisms of the antithrombotic action of dextran. *New England Journal of Medicine*, **290**, 748.

365 McCLURE P., CASSERLY J., MONSIER CH. & CROZIER D. (1970) Carbenicillin-induced bleeding disorder. *Lancet*, **ii**, 1307.

366 BROWN C.H. III, NATELSON E.A., BRADSHAW M.W., ALFREY C.P. & WILLIAMS T.W. JR (1975) Study of the effects of ticarcillin on blood coagulation and platelet function. *Antimicrobial Agents and Chemotherapy*, **7**, 652.

367 BROWN C.H. III, BRADSHAW M.W., NATELSON E.A., ALFREY C.P. & WILLIAMS T.W. (1976) Defective platelet function following the administration of penicillin compounds. *Blood*, **47**, 949.

368 NATELSON E.A., BROWN C.H. III, BRADSHAW M.W., ALFREY C.P. & WILLIAMS T.W. JR (1976) Influence of cephalosporin antibiotics on blood coagulation and platelet function. *Antimicrobial Agents and Chemotherapy*, **9**, 91.

369 CAZENAVE J.P., GUCCIONE M.A., PACKHAM M.A. & MUSTARD J.F. (1977) Effects of cephalothin and penicillin G on platelet function *in vitro*. *British Journal of Haematology*, **35**, 135.

370 GOTTLIEB A.J. (1977) Non allergic purpura. In: *Hematology* (ed. Williams W.J., Beutler E., Erslev A.J. & Rundles R.W.) 2nd edn., p. 1385. McGraw-Hill, New York.

371 SCHÖNLEIN J.L. (1837) *Allgemeine und specielle Pathologie und Therapie,* 3rd edn., Vol. II, p. 48. Freyburg.

372 HENOCH E. (1874) Uber eine eigenthümliche Form von Purpura. *Berliner klinische Wochenschrift*, **11**, 641.

373 HENOCH E. (1895) Neunter Abschnitt. III. Die Hämorrhagische Diathese—Purpura. In: *Vorlesungen über Kinderkrankheiten*, p. 847. Hirschwald, Berlin.

374 OSLER W. (1914) The visceral lesions of purpura and allied conditions. *British Medical Journal*, **i**, 517.

375 BYWATERS E.G.L., ISDALE I. & KEMPTON J.J. (1957) Schönlein–Henoch purpura. Evidence for a group A β-haemolytic streptococcal aetiology. *Quarterly Journal of Medicine*, NS **26**, 161.

376 VERNIER R.L., WORTHEN H.G., PETERSON R.D., COLLE E. & GOOD R.A. (1961) Anaphylactoid purpura. I.

Pathology of the skin and kidney and frequency of streptococcal infection. *Pediatrics*, **27**, 181.

377 AYOUB E.M. & HOYER J. (1969) Anaphylactoid purpura: streptococcal antibody titres and β_{1c}-globulin levels. *Journal of Pediatrics*, **75**, 193.

378 MEADOW S.R., GLASGOW E.F., WHITE R.H.R., MONCRIEFF M.W., CAMERON J.S. & OGG C.S. (1972) Schönlein–Henoch nephritis. *Quarterly Journal of Medicine*, NS **41**, 241.

379 BAART DE LA FAILLE-KUYPER E.H., KATER L., KOOIKER C.J. & DORHOUT MEES E.J. (1973) IgA-deposits in cutaneous blood-vessel walls and mesangium in Henoch–Schönlein syndrome. *Lancet*, i, 892.

380 LEVINSKY R.J. & BARRATT T.M. (1979) IgA immune complexes in Henloch–Schönlein purpura. *Lancet*, ii, 1100.

381 ACKROYD J.F. (1953) Allergic purpura, including purpura due to foods, drugs and infections. *American Journal of Medicine*, **14**, 605.

382 CREAM J.J., GUMPEL J.M. & PEACHEY R.D.G. (1970). Schönlein–Henoch purpura in the adult. *Quarterly Journal of Medicine*, NS **39**, 461.

383 GAIRDNER D. (1948) The Schönlein–Henoch syndrome (anaphylactoid purpura). *Quarterly Journal of Medicine*, NS **17**, 95.

384 MEADOW R. (1978) Schönlein–Henoch syndrome. In: *Pediatric Kidney Disease* (ed. Edelmann C.J., jr), p. 788. Little Brown, Boston.

385 ALLEN D.M., DIAMOND L.K. & HOWELL A. (1960) Anaphylactoid purpura in children (Schönlein–Henoch syndrome). Review with a follow-up of the renal complications. *American Journal of Diseases of Children*, **99**, 833.

386 TATTERSALL R.N. & SEVILLE R. (1950) Senile purpura. *Quarterly Journal of Medicine*, NS **19**, 151.

387 SHUSTER S. & SCARBOROUGH H. (1961) Senile purpura. *Quarterly Journal of Medicine*, NS **30**, 33.

388 SCARBOROUGH H. & SHUSTER S. (1960) Corticosteroid purpura. *Lancet*, i, 93.

389 McCONKEY B., FRASER G.M. & BLIGH A.S. (1962) Osteoporosis and purpura in rheumatoid disease: prevalence and relation to treatment with corticosteroids. *Quarterly Journal of Medicine*, NS **31**, 419.

390 RENDU H.J.L. (1896) Epistaxis repétés chez un sujet porteur de petits angiomes cutanés et muqueux. *Gazette des Hôpitaux, Paris*, **69**, 1322.

391 OSLER W. (1901) On a family form of recurring epistaxis, associated with multiple telangiectases of the skin and mucous membranes. *Bulletin of the Johns Hopkins Hospital*, **12**, 333.

392 WEBER F.P. (1907) Multiple hereditary developmental angiomata (telangiectases) of the skin and mucous membranes associated with recurring haemorrhages. *Lancet*, ii, 160.

393 BIRD R.M. & JAQUES W.E. (1959) Vascular lesion of hereditary hemorrhagic telangiectasia. *New England Journal of Medicine*, **260**, 597.

394 HASHIMOTO K. & PRITZKER M.S. (1972) Hereditary hemorrhagic telangiectasia: an electron microscopic study. *Oral Surgery*, **34**, 752.

395 HODGSON C.H., BURCHELL H.B., GOOD C.A. & CLAGGETT O.T. (1959) Hereditary hemorrhagic 'telangiectasia' and pulmonary arteriovenous fistula. Survey of a large family. *New England Journal of Medicine*, **261**, 625.

396 DINES D.E., ARMS R.A., BERNATZ P.E. & GOMES M.R. (1974) Pulmonary arteriovenous fistulas. *Mayo Clinic Proceedings*, **49**, 460.

397 CAMPBELL E.W. JR, JEWSON D. & GILBERT E. (1970) Angiographic identification of enteric lesions. Guide to therapy in hereditary hemorrhagic telangiectasis. *Archives of Internal Medicine*, **125**, 705.

398 KOCH H.J., ESCHER G.C. & LEWIS J.S. (1952) Hormonal management of hereditary hemorrhagic telangiectasia. *Journal of the American Medical Association*, **149**, 1376.

399 HARRISON D.F.N. (1964) Familial haemorrhagic telangiectasia: 20 cases treated with systemic oestrogen. *Quarterly Journal of Medicine*, NS **33**, 25.

400 McKUSICK V.A. (1972) *Heritable Disorders of Connective Tissue*, 4th edn. Mosby, St. Louis.

401 POPE F.M., MARTIN G.R., LICHTENSTEIN J.R., PENTINEN R., GERSON E., ROWE D.W. & McKUSICK V.A. (1975) Patients with Ehlers–Danlos syndrome type IV lack type III collagen. *Proceedings of the National Academy of Sciences, USA*, **72**, 1314.

402 KARACA M., CRONBERG L. & NILSSON I.M. (1972) Abnormal platelet-collagen reaction in Ehlers–Danlos syndrome. *Scandinavian Journal of Haematology*, **9**, 465.

403 HARDISTY R.M. (1975) Hereditary disorders of platelet function. In: *Platelets, Recent Advances in Basic Research and Clinical Aspects. Excerpta Medica International Congress Series*, **357**, 201.

404 DAVIS E. (1941) Hereditary familial purpura simplex. Review of 27 families. *Lancet*, i, 145.

405 LACKNER H. & KARPATKIN S. (1975) On the 'easy bruising' syndrome with normal platelet count. A study of 75 patients. *Annals of Internal Medicine*, **83**, 190.

406 GARDNER F.H. & DIAMOND L.K. (1955) Autoerythrocyte sensitization. A form of purpura producing painful bruising following autosensitization to red blood cells in certain women. *Blood*, **10**, 675.

407 ÅGLE D.P. & RATNOFF O.D. (1962) Purpura as a psychosomatic entity. A psychiatric study of autoerythrocyte sensitization. *Archives of Internal Medicine*, **109**, 685.

408 RATNOFF O.D. & AGLE D.P. (1968) Psychogenic purpura: a re-evaluation of the syndrome of autoerythrocyte sensitization. *Medicine*, **47**, 475.

409 CHANDLER D. & NALBANDIAN R.M. (1966) DNA autosensitivity. *American Journal of Medical Sciences*, **251**, 145.

410 LITTLE A.S. & BELL H.E. (1964) Painful subcutaneous hemorrhages of the extremities with unusual reaction to injected deoxyribonucleic acid. *Annals of Internal Medicine*, **60**, 886.

411 BARRATT T.M. & DRUMMOND K.N. (1981) The vasculitis syndromes: Henoch–Schönlein syndrome or anaphylactoid purpura. In: *Practice of Pediatrics* (ed. Wedgwood R.V.). Harper & Row, Hagerstown.

412 LAGES B., MALMSTEN C., WEISS H.J. & SAMUELSSON B. (1981) Impaired platelet response to thromboxane-A_2 and defective calcium mobilization in a patient with a bleeding disorder. *Blood*, **57**, 545.

413 WU K.K., LE BRETON G.C., TAI H.H. & CHEN Y.C. (1981) Abnormal platelet response to thromboxane A_2. *Journal of Clinical Investigation*, **67**, 1801.

Chapter 27
Physiology and biochemistry of blood coagulation and fibrinolysis

C. D. FORBES AND C. R. M. PRENTICE

Blood coagulation and fibrinolysis represent only two of the complex interlinked triggered-enzyme systems in blood plasma. It is considered that both represent basic examples of haemostasis: blood coagulation protecting the body from loss of blood volume by sealing the defect in the vessel wall, and fibrinolysis removing excess fibrin from the endothelial-cell lining of vessels which might obstruct blood flow.

Blood coagulation factors play a key role in haemostasis. Damage to the vessel wall results in simultaneous activation of platelets (Chapter 26) and the coagulation mechanism. Platelet aggregation may be sufficient to occlude the damaged vessel temporarily but the platelet thrombus needs fibrin to be generated by an intact coagulation mechanism for stability. In addition the enzyme thrombin is a powerful platelet-aggregating agent and enhances the effects of adenosine diphosphate and serotonin.

The importance of integrity of the coagulation system is illustrated clinically by the sequence of events when a patient with a coagulation defect, such as haemophilia, has a surgical procedure. Because of the normality of his platelet function, immediate bleeding is often not excessive. However, oozing starts within a few hours as vasoconstriction passes off and the platelet thrombus, unstabilized by fibrin generation, is swept away.

Fibrinolysis represents that part of the healing process associated with removal of fibrin clot. The production of the active enzyme plasmin from its inert precursor plasminogen may result from a series of reactions including, for example, the activation of factor XII, or from activators in the tissues, white or red cells or in the plasma itself. The end result is digestion of fibrin and its removal as degradation products.

The importance of studying such factors in blood coagulation and fibrinolysis, and their relationship with each other and with the other triggered-enzyme systems in plasma is the possibility that an imbalance enhances the chance of haemorrhage or thrombosis. It is also possible that atheroma may be produced by a similar imbalance.

Blood coagulation

The cascade (waterfall) concept of blood coagulation was formulated in 1964 [1, 2] to encompass all the known clotting factors which had been revealed by the study of patients with genetically determined haemorrhagic defects. Since then, additional factors have been found and the current scheme for the cascade is shown in Figure 27.1. It is postulated that most of the clotting factors circulate as inert pro-enzymes (zymogens) which are converted to an active form, which in turn activates the following zymogen. It is the recommendation of the International Committee on Blood Clotting Factors that these factors be given Roman numerals and the activated form be indicated by the addition of the suffix (a) (see Table 27.1).

BLOOD COAGULATION FACTORS

The contact factors

Development of knowledge
In early research into blood coagulation William Hewson suggested that solidification of 'the coagulable lymph' was initiated by exposure to air [3], a view which was extended in 1819 by Thackrah [4], who postulated a 'vital influence' in the vessel wall which prevented clotting. This was confirmed experimentally by Brücke in 1857 [5], using turtle blood which clotted rapidly in a glazed basin but remained fluid if kept in an isolated heart. In 1863, Joseph Lister [6] confirmed the importance of the type of surface in contact with blood by allowing blood to clot in India rubber and glass tubes. He then extended these observations *in vivo* and was able to show that in the intact circulation exposure to a foreign surface initiated a 'contact' mechanism and rapidly led to clotting on the foreign surface.

Further elucidation of the contact mechanism of blood coagulation resulted from the work of Margolis [7], Shafrir & de Vries [8] and Waaler [9]. They showed that initiation of coagulation was due to a particular plasmatic factor or factors. This was confirmed by the

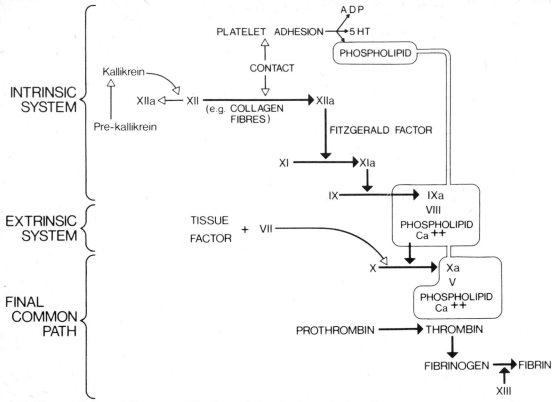

Fig. 27.1. The cascade (waterfall) concept of blood coagulation showing activation of inert plasma precursors to active enzymes with negative feedback and accelerator properties

Table 27.1. Clotting factors in blood

Factor*	Synonyms
XII	Hageman factor (HF)
Pre-kallikrein	Fletcher factor
High MW kininogen	Fitzgerald, Flaujeac, Williams factor
XI	Plasma thromboplastin antecedent (PTA), antihaemophilic factor C
X	Stuart–Prower factor
IX	Christmas factor, plasma thromboplastin component (PTC), antihaemophilic factor B, autoprothrombin II
VIII	Antihaemophilic factor (AHF), antihaemophilic globulin (AHG)
VII	Proconvertin, stable factor, serum prothrombin conversion accelerator (SPCA)
V	Proaccelerin, labile factor, plasma ac-globulin
II	Prothrombin
I	Fibrinogen
XIII	Fibrin-stabilizing factor (FSF), fibrinase

* The numbers III, IV and VI are no longer used.

discovery by Ratnoff & Colopy [10] of a patient (John Hageman) whose blood did not clot in a glass tube. They showed that this patient's plasma was deficient in a factor localized to the intrinsic pathway, which they named the Hageman factor, and which is now known as factor XII. Several hundred such patients have been described. It is now appreciated that at least three other factors are involved in the contact phase of blood coagulation and these include plasma thromboplastin antecedent (PTA, factor XI), Fletcher factor (pre-kallikrein) and Fitzgerald factor (high-molecular-weight kininogen).

Factor XII
Deficiency of factor XII is a rare abnormality which surprisingly is not usually associated with any tendency to excess bleeding, despite the key role the factor has in *in-vitro* coagulation. Deficiency of factor XII is usually inherited as an autosomal-recessive characteristic [11]. The site of synthesis is unknown, but its level is reduced in liver disease and shows remarkable variations in various races. In Caucasians its concentration in plasma is about 29–40 μg/ml. Infusion experiments suggest a half time in plasma of between two and three days.

Factor XII may be purified by a variety of means but the initial step is usually to adsorb it from the plasma on to one of the diatomaceous earths; this is followed by further adsorption and elution on cation-exchange resins. By such simple means preparations of 5000-fold purity may be obtained and surprisingly little of the factor is activated [12].

Human factor XII is a single-chain polypeptide which migrates in the β-globulin band. The sedimentation constant of purified factor XII has been variously estimated between 4·5S and 5·5S with the iso-electric point between 5·8 and 7·5 [13]. The molecular weight measured by a variety of techniques is about 80 000 [14, 15]. A diagrammatic representation of the molecule is shown in Figure 27.3 (p. 1084). Patients with the defect may be discovered when their blood fails to clot in a glass tube or if they are related to a known patient. Specific assay of factor XII requires the use of a known deficient substrate in a one-stage assay. These deficient substrates are now readily available from a variety of commercial sources. Factor XII can also be assayed using a variety of synthetic substrates.

Factor XI
Factor XI is a protein lacking in a small number of patients with a mild autosomal recessive bleeding tendency [16, 17]. The site of synthesis is unknown but its level is reduced in patients with chronic liver disease. The concentration in human plasma is 4 μg/ml. Infusion experiments suggest a half time in plasma of

two to three days. Purification of both factors XI and XIa depends on their adsorption on to diatomaceous earths (such as Celite 512) and elution, followed by passage through an ion-exchange resin. By such means it may be separated from pre-kallikrein and HF cofactor [17]. Human factor XI has an apparent molecular weight of about 160 000, a sedimentation constant of 6·9–7·5S and an iso-electric point of 8·0–8·2. It migrates in plasma as a γ globulin [17, 18]. After reduction and acetylation, single-chain subcomponents of MW 80 000 are found, suggesting that the structure consists of two identical polypeptide chains with similar properties, joined by disulphide bridges [19] (see Fig. 27.4, p. 1084).

The diagnosis is suggested by prolongation of the activated partial thromboplastin time (APTT) with normality of the other screening tests. Assay of the plasma factor level is dependent on the use of substrate plasma deficient in factor XI. These are now readily available commercially. If naturally occurring deficient substrates are not available, adequate materials can be prepared by adsorption of normal plasma with a diatomaceous earth (celite) or from factor-XI deficient cows [20, 21].

Fletcher and Fitzgerald factors
The discovery of these factors has resulted from the investigation of extremely rare coagulation abnormalities in patients with defects in the initial, surface-mediated reactions of blood clotting. Hathaway *et al.* [22] have described a coagulation abnormality in a family resulting from a consanguineous union. In affected members, the partial thromboplastin time was abnormally long (with a normal prothrombin time) and prolonged exposure to surface activating agents corrected this defect [23]. The deficient protein, *Fletcher factor*, is identical to plasma pre-kallikrein [19]. It may also be called factor-XII-dependent plasminogen proactivator. The protein has a single-chain structure of MW 85 000 and migrates in the γ-globulin band. In human plasma the concentration is about 50 μg/ml. Artificial Fletcher-deficient plasma may be prepared by adding antiserum against plasma pre-kallikrein to normal plasma [24]. Fletcher-factor-deficient plasma is defective not only in clotting ability, but also in tests for the generation of fibrinolytic and esterolytic activity, chemotaxis and permeability factors. Assay of this factor should be carried out using deficient plasma from patients who have an identical defect with the index case. As there may be more than one pre-kallikrein [25], caution should be exercised in the use of substrate plasmas prepared artificially by the use of pre-kallikrein antisera.

Deficiency of yet another contact factor (*Fitzgerald factor*) (high MW kininogen) was described by Waldman & Abraham [26] in an asymptomatic patient who was found to have prolongation of the APTT, which, unlike Fletcher-factor deficiency, was not corrected by prolonged incubation with kaolin. Since the original case, several patients have been described with rather different deficiencies but the common factor is probably an abnormality in the level of high-MW kininogen. These have been variously called Flaujeac, Williams or contact-activation cofactor. These patients are asymptomatic and the defect is transmitted by an autosomal recessive gene. Assay is dependent on reference to the plasma of the index case. High-MW kininogen is a single-chain protein of MW 110 000 and migrates in the α-band. In human plasma its concentration is 70–90 μg/ml.

Factor IX

Factor IX is a vitamin-K-dependent glycoprotein containing carboxyglutamic-acid residues necessary for the binding of calcium. Factor IX is the factor deficient in patients with Christmas disease [27, 28]. In normal plasma the concentration is about 3 μg/ml [29] and infusion experiments suggest a half life of 18–24 hours in plasma.

Purification, using plasma as the starting material, involves adsorption of factors II, VII, IX and X with barium sulphate, then elution, followed by DEAE-cellulose column chromatography. Partially pure factor IX may also be made by gel filtration, isoelectric focusing and preparative polyacrylamide gel electrophoresis. A valuable additional step is affinity chromatography on a heparin-agarose column. This results in approximately 2500-fold purification. In the presence of calcium ions factor IX may be separated from factors II and VII [30, 31]. Such purification procedures suggest a molecular weight of about 55 000 for human factor IX. It is a single-chain glycoprotein containing hexose, hexosamine, and sialic acid with an amino-terminal glycine (see Fig. 27.5, p. 1085). Vitamin K is necessary for synthesis of the molecule, and its absence, due either to malabsorption of vitamin K or anticoagulant therapy, results in the appearance of a circulating competitive inhibitor—'protein induced by vitamin K absence/antagonism' (PIVKA) [32]. This protein, which is functionally inert, may be detected immunologically [33]. Such PIVKAs also exist for factors II, VII and X and they may interfere with the coagulation process by competitive inhibition.

Factor VIII

Factor VIII is the protein which is deficient in its activity in patients with classical haemophilia (haemophilia A). Numerous purification procedures have been described. The starting material for most of these is a cryoglobulin precipitate of plasma which is then chromatographed on large-pore agarose gels [34, 35]. By such means purification up to 10 000-fold may be achieved and the material is homogeneous by ultracentrifugation and zone electrophoresis. Sedimentation analysis of this material reveals a symmetrical peak with a sedimentation coefficient of 27S and reduction with mercaptoethanol or dithiothreitol and SDS-polyacrylamide gel electrophoresis results in one component of MW 270 000.

In addition to its activity in the coagulation cascade, factor VIII is necessary for agglutination of human platelets by the antibiotic ristocetin, for platelet adhesion to subendothelium and correction of the prolonged bleeding time in patients with von Willebrand's disease. Separation of the procoagulant activity (FVIIIC) from the platelet-aggregating activity (FVIII:vWF) can be achieved with high ionic strength solutes or in the presence of calcium ions (0·25 M) [36–38]. This reversible dissociation produces a low-molecular-weight fragment (approximately 120 000) which retains procoagulant activity, and a fragment with von Willebrand activity which has a molecular weight of over one million. This large molecule is composed of identical chains of molecular weight 210 000 [39]. Recombination of the small fragment with the large carrier molecule occurs in the absence of calcium ions. It is not clear whether in native plasma the two molecules are in combination or exist separately. In classical haemophilia the evidence is that the factor-VIII molecule is defective at the site of coagulant activity [40] but the factor-VIII-related antigen (FVIIIR:Ag) is identical to normal [35, 41].

Factor VIII is probably synthesized in the vascular endothelium and antigenic material has been demonstrated in endothelial cells and platelets [42, 43]. The plasma level is of the order of 10 μg/ml but little is known of the physiological mechanisms which maintain this. There is a four-fold range in the normal population (0·5–2·0 u/ml) and in an individual the level may be elevated by exercise, stress and age, in pregnancy and by the use of oral contraceptives. The half life in the circulation is about eight to 10 hours. There is a statistically higher level of factor VIII in people with blood group A than blood group O [44] and it has been suggested that elevation of factor VIII may be associated with an increased risk of thrombosis [45, 46].

Laboratory diagnosis of factor-VIII and factor-IX deficiency

Laboratory diagnosis is usually straightforward in the severely affected patient. The APTT is prolonged, and the prothrombin time, thrombin time, and bleeding time are normal. Specific assays of factors VIII and IX establish the diagnosis and baseline factor level (and hence the type of plasma concentrate required for replacement therapy). In very mild cases the APTT can be normal; occasionally these patients may bleed severely after major surgery or trauma, and if there is reasonable suspicion from the history that mild haemophilia is possible then specific assays of factors VIII and IX should be performed in spite of a normal APTT in the 'coagulation screen'. The differentiation of mild haemophilia A from mild von Willebrand's disease requires determination of factor-VIII-related antigen, bleeding time and platelet function studies (see Chapter 28).

Assays of factor-VIII and factor-IX activity

The activity of factor VIII and factor IX is usually assayed using modifications of the APTT (one-stage assay) or of the thromboplastin generation test (two-stage assay). Only the principles of the assays will be considered here; suitable methods are described by Austen & Rhymes [47] and Denson [48] and computer programming of the assays is possible [49].

One-stage assays. Serial dilutions of pooled normal and test plasmas are added to substrate plasma from a severe haemophiliac with a factor-VIII (or IX) level less than 0·5 u/dl. It is important to ensure that the chosen substrate does not contain an inhibitor. Kaolin, platelet substitute and calcium are added to each mixture and the APTT performed. The results are plotted on double logarithmic graph paper and parallel straight line calibration curves are obtained. As all factors other than factor VIII (or IX) are present in excess, the clotting times are assumed to be proportional to the concentration of the deficient factor. The clotting times obtained with the test plasma are converted to factor VIII (or IX) activity by comparison with the normal calibration curve.

One-stage assays are widely used despite many disadvantages, because they are rapid and simple to perform. Supplies of substrate plasma from severely affected patients may be difficult to obtain as they are now frequently treated, and patients with severe haemophilia B are few. The development of assays using artificially depleted plasma may help to solve this problem [50]. Standards of normality also present difficulty. Laboratory standards (deep-frozen or freeze-dried large-pool normal plasma, or factor concentrates) may now be compared with International factor VIII Standard Preparations [51]. Activated clotting factors may cause falsely high assays; conversely, inhibitors can result in falsely low assays. The method becomes progressively less reliable at low concentrations of factors, but this is not of major importance for diagnosis or management. Random errors and variations in reagents, equipment, environment and technique combine to give poor reproducibility both within and between laboratories [51]. The large range of error should be considered when clinical decisions are based on these assays.

Two-stage assays. These assays are more complex than the one-stage methods, but the results are more reliable both between and within laboratories [51]. The method is based on the thromboplastin generation test [52]. For factor-VIII assay, dilutions of the test plasma and normal plasma are incubated with normal serum, factor V, phospholipid and calcium to generate activated factor X, which is measured by adding normal substrate plasma and calcium and recording the clotting time. The results are plotted on double logarithmic paper, parallel straight lines obtained, and factor VIII activity derived. Two-stage factor-IX assay requires testing of test and normal sera, incubated with haemophilia B sera, adsorbed plasma, phospholipid and calcium. Generation of thromboplastin is measured by sub-sampling into normal substrate plasma when the plateau of prothrombin activator is achieved.

Ristocetin-induced platelet agglutination

Ristocetin, an antibiotic rendered obsolete because of its side-effect of thrombocytopenia, induces platelet agglutination in normal platelet-rich plasma but not in that of patients with von Willebrand's disease [53]. The aggregation response to other commonly used agents (ADP, collagen, thrombin, adrenaline) is normal. The defect is due to deficiency of a plasma factor related to factor VIII—von Willebrand factor (FVIIIR:WF)—and is corrected *in vitro* by the addition of normal or haemophilic platelet-poor plasma, or factor VIII, and *in vivo* by transfusion of plasma or factor VIII. Some patients who appear to have von Willebrand's disease have normal agglutination with ristocetin, and the defect is not specific for von Willebrand's disease [54]. Nevertheless, ristocetin-induced agglutination is a useful screening test for von Willebrand's disease and is easier to perform than platelet retention in glass bead columns.

Von Willebrand factor assay (FVIIIR:WF)

Following screening of the patient's platelet-rich plasma with ristocetin a variety of semi-quantitative methods may now be used for measurement of this activity [55, 56]. Formaldehyde-fixed platelets are also suitable for use in assay of von Willebrand factor and these may be stored for some weeks.

Factor-VIII-related antigen (FVIIIR:Ag)

The preparation of specific precipitating rabbit antibodies to semi-purified human factor VIII [40] allowed the demonstration that patients with von Willebrand's disease had reduced levels of factor-VIII-related antigen, whereas patients with haemophilia A had normal or raised levels. Quantitative estimation of FVIIIR : Ag is usually performed by the immunoelectrophoresis technique of Laurell [57] or by immunoradiometric methods [57a, 57b].

Factor-VIII coagulant activity (FVIIIC)

Procoagulant activity is reduced in most patients with von Willebrand's disease, often to only a moderate degree (5–50% of normal). Patients with levels under five per cent of normal usually have severe clinical symptoms; levels of under one per cent are rare, in contrast to severe haemophilia A. Rises in factor-VIII activity (and antigen) occur following exercise, pregnancy, oral-contraceptive consumption and transfusion and these effects may complicate the diagnosis of mildly affected patients.

Tissue Factor

It has been known for many years that certain tissue extracts activate and accelerate the clotting of plasma. Tissue factor has been identified as a cell membrane component in a variety of cells and has been found in the brain, lung, kidney, liver and large vessels [58]. Attempts have been made to purify it and it seems to be a lipoprotein complex with a molecular weight between 220 000 and 300 000. The apoprotein has been partially characterized and that from human brain has a molecular weight of 52 000. The lipid-protein complex is required for coagulant activity and although it also has peptidase activity this does not appear to be associated with its procoagulant activity.

Factor VII

Factor VII is a single-chain glycoprotein of MW 45 000. It is produced by the liver and requires the presence of vitamin K for synthesis. The liver pathway may be inhibited by oral anti-coagulants and this results in an immunologically identical but inert protein (PIVKA) (see p. 1078). The half life of infused factor VII is between four and six hours.

The assay depends on the availability of specific deficient substrates from a human source but such patients are extremely rare. Attempts have also been made to use dog plasma congenitally deficient in factor VII.

Factor X

Factor X was originally discovered as a result of giving patients dicoumarol [59] and later a series of cases of congenital factor-X deficiency were described, characterized by a minor bleeding tendency [60].

Factor X is present in human plasma in a concentra-

tion of about 10 mg/l; it is a glycoprotein with a molecular weight of about 52 000 containing 10% carbohydrate in a heavy chain (MW 35 000) which contains the active centre and is joined to a light chain (MW 17 000) by disulphide bonds [61] (see Fig. 27.6, p. 1086). It contains γ-carboxyglutamic-acid residues necessary for calcium binding.

Factor X may be purified by chromatography on DEAE cellulose, then on DEAE-Sephadex and finally by gel filtration. This produces two components, X_1 and X_2, which behave as distinct species on repeated chromatography but which are in all other respects identical. In clotting assays X_2 has a higher specific activity. The more acidic behaviour of X_2 on chromatography is due to the presence of an extra six γ-carboxyglutamic-acid residues in its light chain. The primary structures of the heavy and light chains are documented, and it is of interest that the N-terminal portion of the light chain shows close sequence homology with the equivalent chain of factors IX, VII and II, suggesting a common ancestral gene.

Factor X is produced in the liver and requires vitamin K for its synthesis. Oral anti-coagulants inhibit this synthesis and result in formation of a functionally inert protein. Infusion experiments suggest a half life *in vivo* of about two to three days. Little is known about the physiological control of factor-X synthesis.

Factor V

The existence of factor V was postulated when it was appreciated that partially purified prothrombin required an additional factor to convert it rapidly to thrombin [62]. It was then observed that the clotting time of stored plasma lengthened progressively, suggesting the presence of a labile factor [63]. A patient with a congenital deficiency of such a factor was then described [64]. Congenital factor-V deficiency (see Chapter 28) is a rare disorder which is associated with a minor to moderate bleeding tendency: something over 50 cases have been recorded [65]. There is evidence that factor V is synthesized in the liver and when transfused into man it has a half life of about 24 hours.

Because of its labile nature, purification of human factor V has proved difficult and much of the information on its structure comes from studies of bovine material. Purification procedures start from barium-sulphate-adsorbed plasma and the protein is then adsorbed onto triethyl-amino-ethyl (TEAE) cellulose. The final step is adsorption and elution from phosphorylated cellulose [66]. There is dispute over the molecular weight of the protein and estimates range from 70 000 to 350 000. It is probable that the basic active unit is of the order of 60 000–70 000 and the functional protein exists as a multiple of this with calcium ions maintaining the integrity of the polymer [67].

The function of factor V is to accelerate the conversion of prothrombin to thrombin in the presence of factor Xa, the evidence being that it has no other activity. However, thrombin splits the molecule —probably the heavy chain. This results in a 10-fold increase in activity and a fall in molecular weight with production of two chains of MW 115 000 and 73 000 [68]. Assay of factor V (labile factor) depends on the availability of congenitally deficient plasma or the use of oxalated plasma exhausted of factor-V activity by prolonged incubation at 37°C.

Prothrombin

Prothrombin is the inactive plasma precursor of thrombin; it is a single chain glycoprotein of MW 70 000 and is produced, like factors VII, IX, and X, in the liver [69, 70]. The plasma concentration is about 100 mg/l and infused material has a half life in plasma of three to five days. Synthesis is dependent on vitamin K and may be inhibited by oral anti-coagulants. In the purification procedures, advantage is taken of its metal-binding properties to adsorb it to barium sulphate or calcium phosphate, which gives a 100-fold purification in the first step. Passage through DEAE cellulose separates factor X, and rechromatography on DEAE and ammonium sulphate fractionation produces a protein suitable for analysis.

Assay of prothrombin. Prothrombin may be measured functionally by the rate of thrombin generation or the total amount of thrombin formed or by an immunochemical assay. In functional assays there may be significant differences between the one-stage and two-stage methods. The one-stage assay measures the initial velocity of thrombin generation, and the two-stage assay the amount of thrombin formed. Discrepancies occur when an abnormal prothrombin is activated slowly. In the original one-stage assay [71], prothrombin was measured in association with other factors; the assay has been improved by use of purified preparations, but it remains tedious and time-consuming. Using tiger snake venom, however, which acts like activated factor X, only factor V, phospholipid and fibrinogen are necessary [72]. A still easier, more rapid, method is the use of the coagulant venom of the Taipan snake (*Oxyuranus scutellatus*). This venom converts prothrombin directly to thrombin without the need for other clotting factors and forms the basis of a specific one-stage assay [75].

In the two-stage prothrombin time assay of Warner *et al.* [73] as modified by Biggs & Douglas [52], and that of Ware & Seegers [74], brain extract and calcium are added to preparations of factors V, VII, X and prothrombin, and the thrombin generated is added to a standard solution of fibrinogen. By using dilutions of prothrombin and the minimum clotting times of the fibrinogen a hyperbolic curve is obtained. This can be converted to a straight line by plotting concentration of prothrombin as a reciprocal. The number of thrombin units present can be found by reference to a standard dilution curve of purified thrombin.

A variety of abnormal prothrombins have now been described in patients with reduced biological prothrombin activity but normal levels of immunoreactive material [76]. In these patients, activation of prothrombin was abnormally slow and abnormal products of splitting were found in the serum. Several molecular variants have subsequently been found by immunological means [77] (see also Chapter 28).

Fibrinogen

Fibrinogen is a glycoprotein synthesized in the liver parenchymal cells. It is the inert circulating precursor of fibrin and as such it plays a key role in haemostasis.

Fibrinogen is a β globulin with a molecular weight of approximately 340 000, of which three per cent is carbohydrate. The molecule is a dimer, each half consisting of three dissimilar polypeptide chains (Aα, Bβ, γ) with respective molecular weights of approximately 63 000, 56 000 and 47 000, joined by disulphide bridges [78, 79]. These chains are linked by disulphide bonds near the N-terminal end of the α and γ chains (Fig. 27.2).

The normal plasma concentration is 1·5–4 g/l. However, multiple forms of fibrinogen are present in normal plasma; they differ in solubility, association with cold insoluble globulin, molecular weight, mobility on electrophoresis and chromatography, and in the oligosaccharide and phosphate residues which are bound to the protein chains. These differences in the molecule may be due to alteration by plasmin or by thrombin [79].

In addition to its function in coagulation, fibrinogen, because of its molecular size and shape, has important effects on red-cell aggregation and is the most important protein determinant of plasma viscosity, and therefore plays a part in determining blood flow [80, 81]. There is also some evidence which links fibrinogen as a risk association in atherosclerosis. It is essential for the aggregation of platelets by ADP (see Chapter 26), has a role in the inflammatory response in defence mechanisms against invasion by bacteria and by malignant cells, and is of importance in providing a scaffold for fibroblastic growth in wound healing.

Assay of fibrinogen

Many methods for the assay of plasma fibrinogen have been described, based on clotting by thrombin,

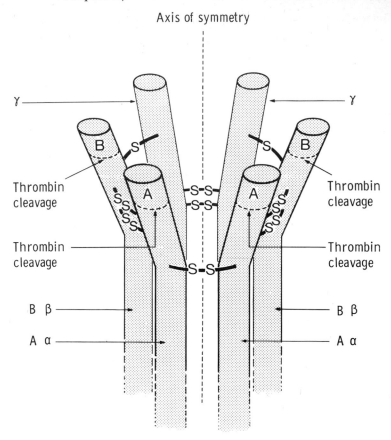

Axis of symmetry

Fig. 27.2. Diagrammatic representation of the N-terminal end of the fibrinogen molecule.

physicochemical transformation and precipitation by heat, salt, or immunological detection.

Clotting methods. Methods employing clotting of fibrinogen are most widely used, as thrombin-clottable protein is more likely to be of physiological importance than that detected by other methods. These include the following:
1 *Turbidimetric method* [82]. The degree of plasma turbidity after clotting with thrombin is proportional to the fibrinogen concentration. This test is rapid and simple, and can also be used in screening for defibrination.
2 *Thrombin-time method* [83]. The thrombin clotting time is inversely proportional to the fibrinogen concentration. It may be determined automatically on the diluted test plasma, and the fibrinogen concentration read from a standard curve prepared from known fibrinogen standards. The test is rapid and simple.
3 *Clot collection methods.* Many methods of clot collection and estimation have been described: they are accurate but time-consuming. Tyrosine release

methods are widely used [84]. The most accurate method for research purposes is that of Nilsson & Olow [85].

Physicochemical methods.
1 *Heat precipitation methods.* Incubation of plasma at 56°C for a few minutes causes heat denaturation and precipitation of fibrinogen. A rapid, simple method, which uses standard microhaematocrit tubes and centrifuge, has been described [86]. After heating, the tubes are recentrifuged and the depth of precipitated fibrinogen read using a microscope with Vernier scale and eye piece grid. The results correlate well with clotting techniques.

2 *Salt-denaturation methods.* Sodium sulphite has the most specific action on fibrinogen, splitting its disulphide bonds; an accurate method using this agent has been described by Rampling & Gaffney [87].

Immunological methods. These methods detect fibrinogen-related antigen (FR antigen), which persists in

FDP as well as intact fibrinogen. They are thus less reliable for plasma fibrinogen estimation than the methods described above, but are in routine use for estimation of FDP in serum. Immunological assays may, however, be of use in the detection of dysfibrinogenaemias, in which normal immunological levels contrast with low fibrinogen clotting assays and prolonged thrombin clotting times.

Factor XIII

In the final stage of blood coagulation fibrin becomes insoluble as a result of the cross-linking of fibrin monomer by the action of a transpeptidating enzyme (FXIII) first described by Lorand & Jacobsen [88]. This enzyme is responsible for the strengthening of fibrin-to-fibrin bonds by inter-glutamyl-ε-lysine bridges. Plasma factor XIII is composed of two *a* chains (MW 75 000) and two *b* chains (MW 88 000); the whole molecule has an $a_2 b_2$ structure with a molecular weight of 320 000 [89]. Factor XIII circulates as an inactive percursor in plasma, and is activated to XIIIa by the action of thrombin in the presence of ionic calcium. Its half life in the circulation is of the order of 12 days.

Deficiency of factor XIII is a rare disorder which may be associated with a moderate or severe bleeding disorder, characterized by delayed onset of haemorrhage after trauma. It is considered in detail in Chapter 28. The screening test for factor-XIII deficiency (solubility in 5 M urea) is rather insensitive because as little as one per cent of factor-XIII activity will result in insolubility of fibrin. Accurate determination of enzyme levels is now possible using simple rate assays. These include the incorporation of labelled primary amines such as putrescine or fluorescent dansylcadaverine [90]. Immunoassay of factor XIII antigen may be of value in addition to activity studies. It is reported that heterozygotes for factor-XIII deficiency have normal levels of factor XIII antigen and homozygotes about half normal amounts of antigen which is still in marked excess compared to activity [91].

ACTIVATION OF BLOOD COAGULATION FACTORS

This complex mechanism is best described in five phases:
1 The contact phase of blood coagulation.
2 Formation of factor IXa.
3 Formation of factor Xa.
4 Formation of thrombin.
5 Formation of fibrin and its stabilization.

THE CONTACT PHASE

Activation of factor XII

Activation of factor XII may occur after exposure to a wide variety of foreign surfaces such as glass, kaolin, bentonite, diatomaceous earths, dacron, nylon, and homocystine. Of more interest is the wide range of physiological substances which may also cause activation; these include collagen, sebum, basement membrane, uric-acid crystals, endotoxins and the soaps of saturated fatty acids.

The mechanism of activation seems to be related to the negative surface charge of the material and inhibition of activation follows exposure of the surface to a positively charged agent such as protamine sulphate, hexadimethrine bromide or cytochrome *c* [92]. It has been suggested that activation of factor XII results from conformational changes in the molecule following its adsorption on to rigidly spaced, negatively charged sites [93]. Additional support for this comes from studies suggesting that the molecular weight is unaltered by activation [94, 95]. In addition, phenylglyoxal hydrate, which reacts with the positively charged guanide groups of arginine residues, inhibits activation of factor XII by kaolin, suggesting that at least one action of negatively charged surfaces is on these sites [96]. The surface binding sites are situated on the heavy (amino terminal) chain (Fig. 27.3). It is probable that activation is associated with unfolding of the molecule which in the process exposes functional sites.

The end result of such activation is the development of active sites with esterase and proteolytic activity, as shown by the ability to hydrolyse a series of synthetic esters (e.g. acetylglycyl lysine methyl ester, and N-benzoylphenyl-alanyl-valyl-arginine-p-nitroanalide). These active sites are on the light (carboxy terminal) chain. In addition activated factor XII initiates the clotting, fibrinolytic and kallikrein-kinin systems and enhances vascular permeability and chemotaxis. In the coagulation cascade, activated factor XII acts on factor XI. It is also possible to split factor XII into two fragments with trypsin or plasma kallikrein to give fragments of MW 52 000 and 28 000, the latter being associated with functional activity.

Surface activation of factor XII is associated with a positive feedback mechanism in which HMW-kininogen (Fitzgerald factor) enhances the activation of pre-kallikrein (Fletcher factor) to kallikrein. This in turn activates more factor XII. Further degradation of factor XIIa occurs with production of fragments, one of which, fragment E (MW 28 000), retains esterolytic activity.

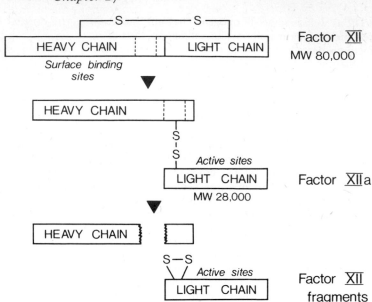

Fig. 27.3. Structure and activation of factor XII, showing light and heavy chains, sites of cleavage and production of fragments.

Activation of factor XI

The activation of factor XI by factor XIIa (Fig. 27.4) does not require the presence of ionized calcium and the process consists of cleavage of internal peptide bonds in the two chains, resulting in two subunits (heavy chains) with a molecular weight of 50 000 each and two subunits (light chains) with a molecular weight of 33 000 each. The active site is located on the light chains. Trypsin, but not plasmin, kallikrein or thrombin, will also activate factor XI in a similar fashion [97], and platelets, treated with collagen or kaolin, may also activate factor XI in the absence of factor XII [98]. Factor XII requires the presence of

HMW kininogen (Fitzgerald factor) to activate purified factor XI [99]. Activated factor XI is a hydrolytic enzyme which converts factor IX to its activated form and may also act on N-benzoyl-L-phenylalanyl-valyl-arginyl-p-nitroanilide and arginine and lysine esters [19]. Activated factor XI is inhibited by a variety of agents including di-isopropylfluorophosphonate (DFP), phenylmethyl sulphonylfluoride (PMSF), heparin, apyrase and the plasma inhibitor C1 inactivator and α_1-anti-trypsin [100, 101].

Contact reactions and platelet function

It has been known for many years that the clotting time

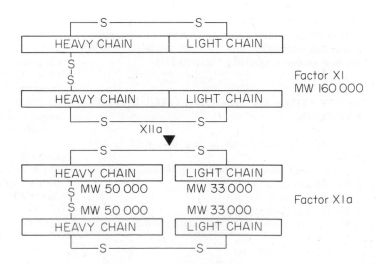

Fig. 27.4. Structure of factor XI and the molecular changes induced by activation by factor XIIa.

of platelet-rich plasma from patients with factor-XII deficiency is accelerated by any contact procedure [102]. This is probably due to the presence of factor XI adsorbed to the platelet membrane [103]. In normal platelet-rich plasma, factor XII may also be present on the platelet membrane in small amounts but this can be readily removed by washing [104].

Walsh [105] has demonstrated that addition of adenosine diphosphate (ADP) to platelets releases a clot-promoting agent into the plasma, but only if factor XII is present. Also, addition of collagen to platelets generated activity attributable to activated factor XI [98]. A variety of platelet function tests in patients with factor-XII and -XI deficiency have given different results, and while it seems clear that platelets may produce a clot-promoting contact product the exact mechanism is unclear.

FORMATION OF FACTOR IXa

Factor IX is activated by factor XIa in the presence of calcium ions in a reaction which occurs in two steps. In the first (slow reaction) an arginine–alanine bond is cleaved, giving rise to a two-chain intermediate held together by a disulphide bond. This intermediate, which is inert, is then cleaved in a second step at an arginine–valine bond to give rise to activated factor IX and a polypeptide residue (fast reaction). Activated factor IX consists of a heavy chain (MW 38 800) and light chain (MW 16 000) held together by disulphide bonds. The light chain originates from the amino-terminal end of the molecule and contains the γ-carboxyglutamic acid residues, necessary for binding calcium, and the heavy chain contains the active site which functions as a serine esterase. A schematic representation of this reaction is shown in Figure 27.5. In addition there is some evidence that factor IX may be activated by factor Xa and by kallikrein [106], and a protease in Russell's viper venom may also cleave the molecule at the arginine–valine bond.

FORMATION OF FACTOR Xa

The intrinsic pathway—slow factor-Xa generation
This step involves the participation of factor VIII, activated factor IX, phospholipid and ionic calcium. These factors form a complex which converts factor X to Xa [107]. It is probable that the phospholipid micelles for this reaction are produced by platelets, and both factors VIII and IXa require to be adsorbed onto the micelle surface for the reaction to occur. There is also evidence of a feedback mechanism in that the reaction may be accelerated by alteration of the physical structure of the factor-VIII molecule by thrombin [108], which may be due to conformational changes in the molecule rather than cleavage [109]. Factor VIII acts as a regulatory protein enhancing the rate of factor-X activation, its role being similar to that of factor V in the activation of prothrombin.

The extrinsic pathway—rapid factor-Xa generation
The extrinsic pathway of factor-Xa generation involves the participation of tissue factor, factor VII and calcium ions. These components form a complex during which factor VII is activated and in turn activates factor X.

Factor VII is activated by tissue factor, by exposure of plasma to cold and by prolonged contact with glass, celite or kaolin. Other factors which modify its function are factor Xa, thrombin, factor XII(a), kallikrein, factor IXa, and plasmin [94, 110–112].

Factor VII exists in plasma as a single-chain glycoprotein and in this form has weak proteolytic activity. When activated by thrombin or factor Xa this activity may be increased several hundred-fold and results in

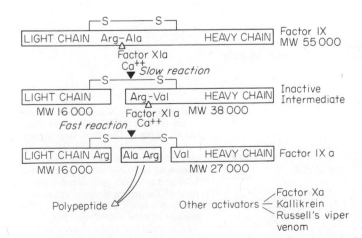

Fig. 27.5. Factor IX: structure and activation by factor XIa in the presence of ionic calcium. The initial slow reaction produces an inert intermediate. In the second, fast reaction factor XIa cleaves the heavy chain at an arginine–valine bond to release a polypeptide, leaving the activated factor which functions as a serine esterase.

the formation of a two-polypeptide chain. On further incubation, activity disappears due to continued proteolysis.

The role of tissue factor appears to be that of a cofactor similar to the role of factor VIII, factor V and HMW kininogen [113].

Factor-X activation

Factor X may be activated either by a complex formed by factor VIII, activated factor IX, phospholipid and ionized calcium or by tissue factor and factor VII, or *in vitro* by Russell's viper venom or trypsin. During activation (Fig. 27.6) there is a cleavage of a single specific arginyl–isoleucine bond in the heavy chain of factor X, with release of one or more polypeptide fragments. This gives rise to the formation of a glycoprotein of molecular weight 45 300 (α Xa) and a peptide chain of MW 10 000 which is split from the amino-terminal end of the heavy chain. The result is the formation of the active enzyme.

A further degradation may occur either in α Xa or in the zymogen as a result of cleavage of a peptide of molecular weight 2700 from the carboxy terminal portion of the heavy chain. For this second degradation, thrombin is necessary and the product is β Xa. The activity of activated factor X does not depend on this reaction.

FORMATION OF THROMBIN

The enzyme thrombin (MW 38 000) is formed by activation of the inert precursor prothrombin (factor

II) by a complex formed by factor Xa, factor V and phospholipid in the presence of ionic calcium. The phospholipid is derived mainly from platelets and is in micellar form. The exact mode of action of factor V is unknown but it appears to be bound onto the surface of phospholipid in association with prothrombin fragment 2, and the calcium ions bind to prothrombin fragment 1 by virtue of its γ-carboxyglutamic acid content.

Activation of prothrombin

The sequence of events during activation, which is complex, has been described by Magnusson *et al.* [114]. It is probable that activation occurs in several steps (Fig. 27.7) and the reaction is further complicated by digestion of the molecule by nascent thrombin. It is probable that more than one pathway of thrombin production exists *in vivo*.

In the factor-Xa-mediated pathway, prothrombin is cleaved to give two products: prethrombin 2 (intermediate II) and fragment 1:2 (Fig. 27.7D). Prethrombin 2 is then cleaved at an arginine–isoleucine bond to give thrombin. This is the pathway when pure systems are used and the reaction takes place in the presence of a thrombin inhibitor. If thrombin is *not* inhibited at the time of formation, it acts on the prothrombin molecule itself and cleaves off fragment 1 to give prethrombin 1 (intermediate I) (Fig. 27.7B), which is then slowly converted to thrombin by the factor-Xa complex. Thrombin also acts on fragment 1:2 (Fig. 27.7D) to give fragment 1 and this competitively inhibits pro-

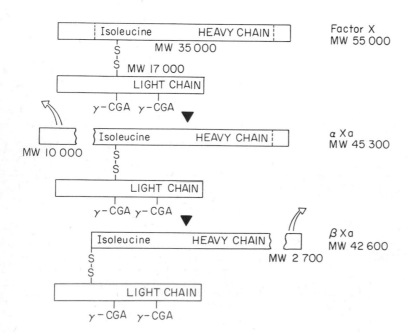

Fig. 27.6. Factor X consists of a heavy chain (MW 35 000) and a light chain (MW 17 000). The first step in activation is cleavage of a specific arginyl–isoleucine bond in the heavy chain with release of one or more polypeptides of MW about 10 000. Additional degradation of the active enzyme (αXa) may occur as a result of cleavage of a polypeptide of MW 2700 from the carboxy terminal portion of the heavy chain.

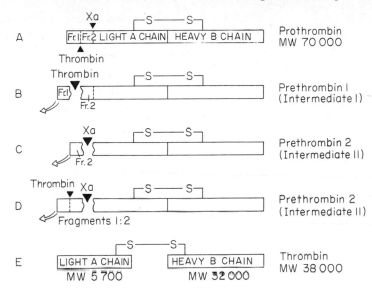

Fig. 27.7. Prothrombin conversion to thrombin and the intermediates produced (for details see text).

thrombin conversion [115]. Since the calcium-binding sites of prothrombin are in fragment 1:2 and fragment 1, the removal of fragment 1 by thrombin generation prevents the factor-Xa complex from binding properly and results in slow generation of further thrombin. Factor V competes with fragment 1 for a common binding site on the prothrombin molecule and reduces this inhibitory action, thus accelerating the reaction. Phospholipid also increases the reaction rate by about 10-fold, perhaps by binding the reactants to the lipid surface and so raising the local concentration of the molecules or by inducing conformational changes in the protein.

The product of prothrombin activation is the two-chain (A and B) serine protease thrombin, with a molecular weight of approximately 38 000. The larger B chain has sequence homology with other serine proteases, particularly those from the pancreas. The short A chain restricts the specificity of the enzyme. Thrombin has numerous activities in coagulation: it converts fibrinogen to fibrin, activates factor XIII, digests fragment 1:2 of prothrombin, alters the structure of factors V and VIII, induces platelet aggregation

and release. It also digests a variety of synthetic substrates *in vitro*.

CONVERSION OF FIBRINOGEN TO FIBRIN

The conversion of fibrinogen to fibrin involves proteolysis, polymerization and stabilization (Fig. 27.8). The enzyme thrombin cleaves the fibrinogen molecule at arginyl–glycine bonds in the amino terminal end of the Aα chains [116, 117]. This leads to conformational change with end-to-end associations of the intermediate fibrin monomer molecules. In addition the B-peptide is now exposed to thrombin and is cleaved from the Bβ chain. The two acidic fibrinopeptides A and B are released, A being released first, and B after a lag phase.

During release of these peptides the molecules polymerize with side-to-side association. These polymers have a molecular weight of 5 million and a length of 4000 Å (this is fibrin$_S$—the 'S' denoting solubility to 5 M urea). Fibrin polymer is then acted on by factor XIIIa with the formation of ε-(γ-glutamyl) lysine isopeptide bonds to form γ–γ dimers, followed

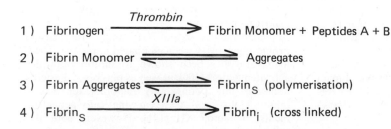

Fig. 27.8. Fibrinogen–fibrin transformation. The subscript 'S' represents solubility in 5 M urea and the subscript 'i' represents insolubility in urea.

by linkage across α chains [118]. This fibrin is designated fibrin$_i$, indicating insolubility in 5 M urea.

Some fibrin monomer may complex with fibrinogen and with high-molecular-weight FDP to form soluble fibrin–fibrinogen complexes of high molecular weight [119, 120]. This may be one of the pathways of fibrinogen catabolism but in excess they reflect evidence of intravascular thrombin generation [121].

Activation of factor XIII
Activation of factor XIII may occur with either thrombin or activated factor X, the latter reaction requiring calcium ions. It takes place in two steps: in the first step a peptide chain of MW 4000 is split from the amino terminal end of the A chains, producing an inert intermediate, and in the second, this dissociates into an active dimer of modified *a* chains and an inactive dimer of *b* chains. This activated factor XIII (factor XIIIa, fibrinoligase) catalyses the formation of ε-(γ-glutamyl)-lysine isopeptide bonds between γ chains to form γ–γ dimers and between α chains to form an α-polymer [122].

PHYSIOLOGICAL INHIBITORS OF BLOOD COAGULATION

It is probable that every activated coagulation factor in the cascade has one or more inhibitors which regulate the rate of generation of the active product or determine its rate of destruction. The purpose of these would seem to be limitation of activation of coagulation and protection against inadvertent deposition of fibrin in the vascular tree.

ANTITHROMBIN III (AT III)
The presence of an inhibitor of thrombin has been postulated since Morawitz showed a gradual decline in coagulant activity of clotted blood [123]. It was initially suggested that this might be due either to some specific antithrombin or to adsorption of thrombin to fibrinogen. It was soon appreciated that when heparinized plasma was used, acceleration of this inhibitory effect occurred, and it was though to be due to the presence of a heparin cofactor in plasma [124]. Deficiency of antithrombin activity and low heparin cofactor activity in plasma were associated with a genetic predisposition to thrombosis by Egeberg [125] and the antithrombin associated with heparin cofactor activity was later purified [126].

AT III is the most important of at least six different antithrombins, three of which ($α_1$-antitrypsin, $α_2$-macroglobulin and AT III) play a physiological role. It is estimated that 75% of antithrombin activity is due to AT III.

AT III has now been purified about 500 times relative to plasma and its structure and functions have been characterized. It is an $α_2$-globulin with a molecular weight of about 65 000 and is present in plasma at a concentration of about 0·2 g/l [127, 128]. AT III reacts with thrombin to produce a complex in which both components are inactivated. The rate of the reaction depends on the concentrations of thrombin and AT III, and there is some evidence that the mechanism of antithrombin activity is made more efficient by activation of the system during the early stages of coagulation. Thrombin and AT III react in a 1:1 stoichiometric ratio to form a complex with a molecular weight varying between 90 000 and 250 000 [129].

AT III also has inhibitory actions on factor Xa [130], but this is largely protected when associated with platelets, factor V–phospholipid complex or phospholipid. Neutralization of factor Xa generated in plasma is rapid and complete within 15 minutes [131]. This is analogous to the situation with thrombin and suggests that the inhibitory system is primed by the earlier stages of the cascade.

There is also evidence that AT III plays a part in neutralization of factors IXa [132, 133], XIa [134], XIIa [135] and plasmin: the rate of inactivation of all these factors is accelerated by the addition of heparin.

AT III is synthesized by the liver, and in cirrhosis and chronic hepatitis the level falls to about 60% of normal [136]. Similar levels are also found in the nephrotic syndrome. There is a tendency for the levels to fall with age, and in women taking the combination contraceptive pill [137]. Acute-onset disseminated intravascular coagulation results in lower levels, as does deep venous thrombosis. In hereditary AT-III deficiency, lower levels are associated with an increased tendency to thrombosis in veins and rarely in arteries [125, 138]. Turnover studies have shown a half life of 2·8 days in the normal population [128].

AT III may be assayed in terms of its ability to neutralize thrombin or factor Xa, either in the presence or absence of heparin. Synthetic substrates may also be used and immunoassay has a place, although the results must be interpreted with caution because of the possible presence of abnormally functioning molecules with immunological identity [139].

INHIBITORS OF THE CONTACT PHASE OF COAGULATION
Activated factors XI and XII rapidly lose their clot-promoting activity when incubated in plasma. The C1 inactivator has been shown to inhibit both these activated factors [100], as well as plasmin, C1 esterase, kallikrein and permeability factors [140]. The C1 inhibitor also acts on the enzymatically active fragments of factor XII [141]. However, both these

activated factors have additional, as yet uncharacterized, inhibitors [142, 143], and activated factor XI is also inhibited by AT III, an effect augmented by heparin. Little is known about tissue inhibitors of surface activation, but in animal experiments the isolated, perfused liver of the rat and rabbit destroy activated contact factors [144].

ROUTINE SCREENING TESTS FOR ABNORMALITIES OF BLOOD COAGULATION

A variety of tests are used and numerous laboratory manuals are available with technical details [45, 48, 145, 146]. Unfortunately there is no single test which will screen for all types of coagulation defect. It is necessary to select a panel of proven tests which can be used to demonstrate normality of different parts of the coagulation system. Many such screening tests have been hallowed by time but are of little practical value because of their non-specific nature and insensitivity. Examples of these are the Hess test, whole-blood clotting time, thromboplastin generation test, and prothrombin consumption index. The tests which we believe to be of value are the bleeding time, activated partial thromboplastin time (APTT), one-stage prothrombin time, thrombin clotting time and factor-XIII clot solubility test.

It is usual to perform the one-stage prothrombin time (OSPT) as a measure of integrity of the extrinsic pathway and the activated partial thromboplastin time (APTT) as a measure of the intrinsic pathway. Both tests have a final common pathway and the inference from the finding of normality in either test is that this final common path is intact. In addition, routine screening for a factor-XIII defect, using the urea solubility test, and a thrombin clotting time for a fibrinogen defect are required. Abnormality of a particular section of the cascade may then be defined. Immunoassay for the defective factor is also recommended, so that variants of these disorders can be recognized.

Bleeding time
The bleeding time is prolonged in patients with thrombocytopenia, platelet function defects and some vascular defects. Its main use in the investigation of congenital bleeding disorders is in the diagnosis of von Willebrand's disease.

The original method was described by Duke [147]. A small cut is made in an ear lobe and the blood touched onto a filter paper every 30 seconds. By this method the normal bleeding time is less than three minutes, but the depth and length of the cut are not standardized.

The Ivy method [148] is a modification in which the forearm is used. A sphygmomanometer cuff is placed on the upper arm and the pressure raised to 40 mm Hg. Using a stylet set with a guard at 3 mm, a cut is made in the pronator surface of the forearm skin, avoiding any obvious superficial veins, and the bleeding time recorded [149]. The upper normal limit is four minutes using the average of three cuts. In an attempt to increase accuracy a variety of modifications have been made to these methods and the authors currently favour that of Mielke *et al.* [150]. In this test a template is laid on the skin of the forearm and a cut 3 mm deep and 9 mm long is made in triplicate. Bleeding time is recorded as above.

A simple method has also been used by Ratnoff (personal communication, 1968). This requires no sphygmomanometer. The patient sits with the arm and hand dependent over a bucket and a cut, 3 mm deep, is made in the pulp of the index finger with a No. 11 Bard-Parker scalpel blade. The time taken for bleeding to stop is recorded and this is less than ten minutes in all normals. If an abnormal bleeding time is found it is easy to ensure haemostasis by pressure to the digit.

Activated partial thromboplastin time (APTT); kaolin cephalin clotting time (KCCT)
This test is recommended for screening the intrinsic coagulation system. Although relatively sensitive, the APTT can be normal in patients with factor-VIII levels greater than 10% of normal, and cannot therefore be relied upon to diagnose 'mild' cases of haemophilia or von Willebrand's disease, who may nevertheless experience serious bleeding after major surgery or trauma.

Platelet-poor plasma is incubated with kaolin (to standardize contact activation) and cephalin (substitute for platelet lipid) prior to recalcification. The normal range is usually 40–60 seconds. Abnormal samples exceed the control clotting time by seven seconds or more. The APTT is prolonged in patients with deficiencies of clotting factors XII, XI, IX, VIII, X, V, prothrombin or fibrinogen. It is normal in factor-VII deficiency. If in the test sample there is a normal one-stage prothrombin time and thrombin time, haemophilia A or B is the most likely diagnosis and specific assays of factor-VIII and factor-IX activity should be performed. Further tests for von Willebrand's disease, factor-VIII inhibitors, factor XI or factor XII may be indicated if the diagnosis is still uncertain.

One-stage prothrombin time (OSPT)
This test bypasses that part of the intrinsic coagulation cascade above factor X and the clotting of the plasma sample is dependent on the concentration of factors

VII, X, V, prothrombin and fibrinogen. Equal volumes of test plasma and brain extract are recalcified and the clotting time recorded. The normal range obtained varies from laboratory to laboratory and depends on the reagents used. However, in any one laboratory the day-to-day variation is very small (usually only plus or minus one second). Prolongation of the test-sample clotting time more than two seconds beyond the control suggests a defect of one of the above factors providing that no heparin has been given to the patient. A prolonged OSPT in combination with a normal thrombin time suggests a deficiency of factors X, V or prothrombin (APTT also prolonged) or factor VII (APTT normal), and specific assays of these factors are then indicated. Russell's viper venom directly activates factor X, and is therefore useful as an indirect screening test in the detection of deficiency of factor VII, i.e. a patient with a prolonged OSPT but a normal Russell's viper venom time.

Thrombin clotting time (TCT) [151]

Thrombin is added to plasma in a concentration adjusted to clot normal plasma in approximately 15 seconds. Abnormal samples exceed the control clotting time by three seconds or more. The thrombin time is prolonged in patients with fibrinogen defects whether quantitative or qualitative (dysfibrinogenaemia), but is also prolonged when the thrombin–fibrinogen reaction is inhibited by heparin, paraproteins, or high levels of fibrinogen–fibrin degradation products.

THE FIBRINOLYTIC ENZYME SYSTEM

Fibrinolysis and thrombolysis are the processes by which fibrin, in the form of either a clot or a thrombus, is enzymatically degraded into soluble fibrin degradation products (FDP). The dominant mechanism is the plasminogen–plasmin system; in this, the inactive protein precursor (plasminogen) is activated to the enzyme plasmin by an activator, the reaction being controlled by the presence of inhibitors. Such activators may be of tissue, plasma or synthetic origin and this step may be inhibited by a variety of physiological or therapeutic inhibitors (Fig. 27.9). It is known that alternative mechanisms of fibrinolysis exist, but these seem to be of minor importance [152].

The fibrinolytic process probably functions as a major homeostatic mechanism in the maintenance of patency in the vascular tree by controlling deposition of fibrin. The physiological control of the system remains controversial, however, and the importance of deficiencies of part or all of the system in the production of vascular occlusion is not yet clear. Activation of

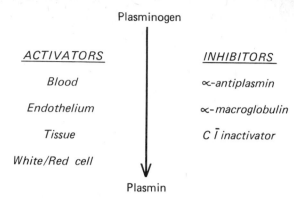

Fig. 27.9. Activation of plasminogen to plasmin is possible under the control of a variety of activators and the reaction may be inhibited by a series of naturally occurring inhibitors.

fibrinolysis for therapeutic purposes is possible and in selected situations is of proven value [153].

A variety of theories have been proposed to explain the selective digestion of fibrin intravascularly: plasminogen may be bound selectively to fibrin [154]; plasmin may be dissociated from anti-plasmin in contact with fibrin [155]; plasminogen activator may be bound to fibrin [156].

The four components of plasminogen–plasmin system are plasminogen, plasmin, plasminogen activator and inhibitors.

PLASMINOGEN

Human plasminogen is a single-chain β globulin of approximate MW 90 000 and is found in Cohn plasma Fraction III-3. It is present in normal adult plasma in a concentration of 200 ng/ml and in the infant at a lower level, and is present in all body fluids. It is precipitated in the euglobulin fraction of plasma at pH 5·3 with plasmin, activator and fibrinogen and this forms the starting material in many purification processes. Because of the high affinity of plasminogen for fibrin, pure preparations are difficult to make using Cohn Fraction III as a starting material. Two forms of the molecule have been prepared and their biochemical and physiological activities intensively studied. They differ in the composition of their amino terminals: native human plasminogen has glutamic acid in the N-terminal position (glu-plasminogen) [157], and the other main form has lysine (lys-plasminogen) [158] (Fig. 27.10). The biological importance of this biochemical difference is controversial. Both types occur in multiple but electrophoretically distinct forms [159]. The MW values of glu- and lys-plasminogen have been estimated variously as being of the order of 97 000 and 84 000 [160] and 85 000 and 82 000 respectively [161]. It seems likely that the lys-form results from limited

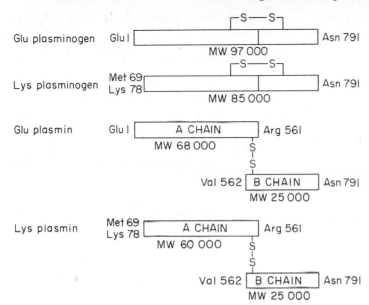

Fig. 27.10. At least two main forms of plasminogen and plasmin exist in native human plasma. They differ in composition of the amino terminals. Glu-plasminogen (MW about 97 000) has glutamic acid in the N-terminal position and lys-plasminogen has lysine in the N-terminal position. Cleavage of an arginine–valine bond in the A-chain by an activator releases a polypeptide to produce plasmin.

proteolysis of the glu-form by plasmin formed during the purification procedure [159, 160, 167]. Lys-plasminogen is more readily adsorbed to fibrin and more readily activated than glu-plasminogen [162], and for these reasons may be of greater potential value in thrombolysis [163]. Estimation of levels of plasminogen by enzymic and immunological methods correlate poorly, probably owing to the presence of inhibitors [164–166]: the functional assay gives lower values.

PLASMIN

Plasmin is a proteolytic enzyme formed from its inactive precursor plasminogen by any of a variety of activators. The action of plasmin is not restricted to fibrin: it splits peptide bonds in practically all protein substrates and a wide variety of esters of arginine and lysine. Such synthetic esters form the basis for assays of activity. It is not normally detected in human plasma as it is rapidly neutralized by inhibitors. The molecule consists of two amino-acid chains of different sizes connected by a disulphide bond (Fig. 27.10). These two chains result from splitting of an arginine–valine bond during activation to produce a heavy (A) chain (MW approximately 68 000) and a light (B) chain (MW approximately 25 000). The A chain contains the N-terminal end and the B chain contains the C-terminal end and the active serine centre.

The mechanism of activation of human plasminogen is complex and varies with the activator used; tissue activator seems to differ from urokinase and streptokinase. Streptokinase itself has no protease activity but in suitable concentrations it forms equimolar complexes with plasminogen and plasmin, with the development of an active enzyme site. The complex of plasminogen–streptokinase then functions as an activator with resultant degradation of the streptokinase molecule itself [167–169]. Urokinase has a direct proteolytic action on plasminogen, cleaving the arginine–valine bond and producing a conformational change which exposes an active centre.

The activity of plasmin is usually measured in caseinolytic units, one unit being defined as that quantity of plasmin which liberates 450 μg trichloracetic-acid-soluble tyrosine from a four per cent solution at pH 7·4 and 35°C within one hour [170]. One millilitre of average normal human plasma produces an amount of plasmin equivalent to three to four caseinolytic units, which is equivalent to approximately 200 ng/l plasma [171].

PLASMINOGEN ACTIVATORS

Activators of plasminogen occur in most body tissues and fluids, including plasma, and may be synthesized by certain bacteria.

Tissue activators

Plasminogen activator is found in body tissues in varying concentrations [172]. It may be present in two forms: labile, which is extractable by saline, and stable, which is extractable by potassium thiocyanate [173, 174]. By use of a histochemical technique [175] it has been shown that most activators are associated with the endothelial layer of vessels, especially small veins, and the fibrinolytic activity is a reflection of tissue vascularity [176]. A modification of this method may be used for the quantitative assay of activator [177]. Activator has also been found in epithelial cells, synovium, mesothelium, red cells, white cells and platelets, uterus, ovaries, lungs, thyroid and prostate [152, 178, 179]. It is of interest that a variety of tumours may produce plasminogen activator, which may interfere with local haemostasis [180] but may also be implicated in the metastasis of malignant cells [181].

A variety of activators from human and animal tissues have been highly purified and characterized. They vary greatly in molecular weight, electrophoretic mobility and amino-acid content. They activate plasminogen by cleaving arginyl–valine bonds in the C-terminal part of the plasminogen molecule and are inhibited by a wide range of proteinase inhibitors.

Urinary activator

Fibrinolytic activity has been known to be present in urine for almost a century, and crude concentrates of human urine have been used in the laboratory and in patients with a variety of thrombotic disorders [182]. Such preparations of urinary activator (*urokinase*) contain at least two components with molecular weights of approximately 31 000 and 55 000. They are partially identical, as shown by cross-reactivity with specific antisera, and it is though that the higher MW material is degraded during purification. Activator produced by renal cell cultures has been shown to have corresponding properties and immunological identity [183, 184]. Such urokinase activates plasminogen by first-order kinetics, probably by splitting lysine or arginine bonds. Urokinase is a serine protease and is irreversibly inhibited by DFP. In addition to activating plasminogen it can hydrolyse casein and a variety of amino-acid esters, including lysine ethyl ester, N-α-acetyl-glycyl-L-lysine methyl ester and p-toluenesulphonyl-L-arginine methyl ester. These reactions form the basis of assays of activity. In addition urokinase seems to possess a special affinity for fibrin thrombus.

Activators from other body fluids

Epithelial cells of other tubular systems commonly produce activators to dissolve fibrin which may be potentially produced in their lumens. Plasminogen activators are found in human milk, seminal fluid, cerebrospinal fluid, saliva, tears and bile.

Bacterial activators

Although many bacteria produce plasminogen activators, the only one of therapeutic importance is that produced by β-haemolytic streptococci, *streptokinase* (SK). This is an α_2-globulin with MW 46 000. For therapeutic purposes it may be produced relatively free of other streptococcal proteins, but it remains antigenic and administration may be associated with allergic and immune reactions. Streptokinase does not possess any enzymatic activity. The mechanism of activation of plasminogen by SK is complex and probably involves the formation of intermediates. Equimolar complexes of plasminogen–SK form, and an active centre develops immediately in plasminogen [185]. The plasminogen–SK complex is then converted into plasmin–SK complex with concomitant structural modification and fragmentation of SK [186, 187]. There are major interspecies differences in this activation mechanism and human plasminogen–SK complex may be used as an activator of non-SK-sensitive zymogens [188]. In a human equimolar complex there is a single DFP-sensitive residue which is probably the active site serine of the plasmin moiety [189, 190]. Several different fragments of SK have been isolated from the complex and one of MW 36 000 has activator activity [191].

Vascular endothelial activator

Small quantities of plasminogen activator may be detected in normal plasma but this level may be elevated by venous occlusion, exercise, stress, infusion of catecholamines, nicotinic acid and vasopressin analogues [192–194]. Plasminogen activator may be identified using a histological technique [175] and has been localized to the endothelial layer of both arteries and veins, although the vein wall is several times richer as a source than the artery. Attempts have been made to purify this material from the vascular tree of the human cadaver and the material so produced [195] was found to have a MW of 65 000. Other workers have shown activators to be present with molecular weight values ranging from 15 000 to 120 000 [196], probably representing polymerized forms of a basic unit of MW 15 000.

As an index of the fibrinolytic potential of vascular endothelium, release of vascular activator into blood can be assayed using standardized stimuli such as exercise, adrenaline or venous occlusion [197]. Such data must be interpreted with caution in the investigation of patients with arterial diseases as the major source is venous endothelium.

Factor-XII-dependent activator

An additional source of 'physiological' activator is found in plasma which has been activated with kaolin or glass, and this is lacking in plasma from patients deficient in factor XII [198, 199]. Formation of this plasminogen activator is complex and involves a Hageman-factor cofactor [200], Fletcher factor [201] and a factor deficient in Fitzgerald trait [99, 202]. In addition it has been suggested that plasma kallikrein

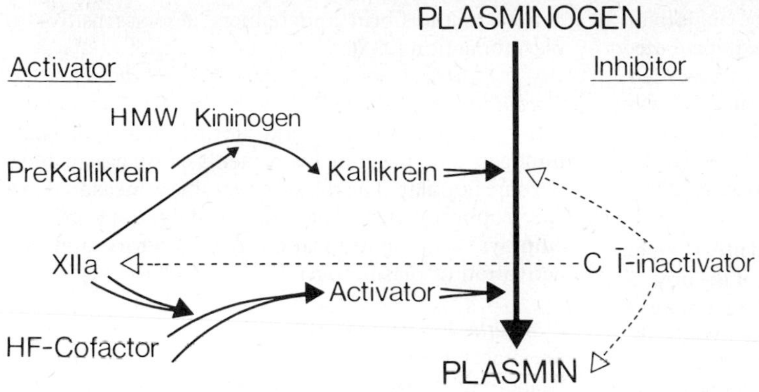

PLASMINOGEN

Fig. 27.11. Intrinsic activation of plasminogen mediated by factor XIIa.

directly activates plasminogen and is the sole intermediary in factor-XII-dependent fibrinolytic activity [203, 204] (Fig. 27.11). Furthermore, Kapland & Austen [205] have shown that plasmin-induced factor-XII fragments are capable of inducing fibrinolytic activity.

Yet another activator may be precipitated from plasma by dextran sulphate and this system does not require factor XII [206]. The physiological and pathological significance of these plasma activators of plasminogen is unknown.

White- and red-cell plasminogen activators
Human granulocytes contain an activator of plasminogen [207, 208]. This has not been isolated and characterized in man and its place in haemostasis is obscure. Human erythrocytes also contain an activator, which is present in the stroma-free haemolysate [178]; it appears to have different characteristics from urokinase and other tissue activators.

INHIBITORS OF PLASMIN
At least six inhibitors of plasmin exist in plasma [209–213]. These are α_2 macroglobulin, α_1-antitrypsin, antithrombin-III–heparin complex, C1 inactivator, α_2-antiplasmin and inter-α-trypsin inhibitor. Most react with plasmin to form inactive complexes [214]. It is probable that under physiological conditions α_2-macroglobulin and α_2-antiplasmin are the two main inhibitors.

Platelets, white cells and a variety of other tissues contain inhibitors of plasmin, but their function and importance is not clear. Placenta also contains an inhibitor [215] and this may be of importance in implantation of the ovum [216].

Inhibitors of plasminogen activation
A variety of poorly defined inhibitors of plasminogen activation have been described in plasma [217, 218]. At least three have been partially characterized; they have

no antiplasmin activity. They range in MW from 20 000 to 75 000 and inhibit vascular and tissue activators as well as urokinase [209, 219–222].

TESTS OF FIBRINOLYSIS

Plasminogen activators
Plasminogen activators are usually measured by their ability to lyse fibrin in the presence of plasminogen. All these tests are rather non-specific and may be influenced by the quality of the reagents used and the presence of inhibitors. In measuring baseline levels of plasminogen activator it should be remembered that variation occurs as a result of ingestion of lipid, after exercise, stress, emotion and following prolonged venous occlusion. In addition, activators are labile and the samples should be handled at 4°C. The screening tests of value are the dilute whole-blood clot lysis time, euglobulin clot lysis time, fibrin plate assay, and the fibrinolytic response to venous occlusion. Activator may also be measured by the release of radioactivity from ^{131}I-fibrinogen-labelled clots, by use of chromogenic substrates, and in tissue slices covered with fibrin. For a recent review see Ref. 223.

Dilute whole-blood clot lysis time. Blood is diluted in buffer and clotted with thrombin, incubated at 37°C and the lysis time recorded. The lysis time is shorter than that of undiluted blood, owing to reduction of fibrinolytic inhibitor activity relative to activator activity. The test has been used to measure physiological variations in fibrinolysis, and for estimation of fibrinolysis in patients treated with antifibrinolytic drugs. The original method used phosphate buffer, but acetate buffer has been advocated, as the lysis time is shorter and the endpoint clearer [224, 225].

Euglobulin clot lysis time. Dilution and acidification of plasma precipitates euglobulins, which include most of the plasma fibrinogen and plasminogen, as well as plasminogen activators and plasmin. The euglobulin precipitate is resuspended in buffer, clotted, incubated at 37°C, and lysis of the euglobulin clot recorded. Removal of fibrinolytic inhibitors shortens the lysis time compared to whole or diluted blood (or plasma). However, most of the antiplasmin, C1 inactivator, may co-precipitate and hence affect the results [226].

Fibrin plate assay [227]. Plasminogen activators can be assayed by measuring the mean diameter of the area of lysis around a euglobulin fraction placed on a plate of fibrin. A standard preparation of fibrin avoids the variation in clot lysis time assays due to variable fibrinogen and plasminogen content of the test samples. Plasminogen-free fibrin plates can be prepared by heating and used to assay lysis due to plasmin. There is a linear correlation between the diameter of the lysis area on fibrin plates and the logarithm of the euglobulin clot lysis time [228].

Fibrinolytic response to venous occlusion and other stimuli. Venous occlusion is a relatively simple and repeatable stimulus of activator release. A 20-minute occlusion test is used. Blood is sampled after the period of occlusion and plasminogen activator measured on fibrin plates. Other workers have used a five-minute occlusion period, which is less painful than the 20-minute one: using this method, impaired response has been demonstrated in some patients with coronary artery disease [229].

Exercise and adrenaline tests have been described which are reproducible and correlate well with each other, and which have been used to investigate groups of patients prone to vascular disease [230, 231]. However, such tests cannot be used in all subjects.

Assay of plasminogen and plasmin
Levels of plasminogen and plasmin may be assayed functionally by recording lysis of fibrin or other proteins (such as casein), synthetic esters, or synthetic chromogenic substrates. In functional assays, plasminogen must be activated by SK or urokinase, and inhibitors neutralized by dilution, acidification or precipitation. Plasminogen may also be measured immunologically.

Functional assays give lower values than immunological assays—probably due in part to inhibitor action. Assays using synthetic chromogenic substrates are simple to perform, and correlate well with immunological and caseinolytic methods [232].

Fibrin substrates. The methods described are based on clot lysis times [233, 234]. Plasminogen can be destroyed by heating the fibrin plates, but the heat partly denatures the fibrin and renders it less sensitive to plasmin action [235].

Casein substrates. Owing to the difficulties of separation of plasminogen and fibrin, assays of plasminogen and plasmin by proteolysis of casein have become popular. The released tyrosine is measured in a spectrophotometer. The most widely used method employs acid neutralization of inhibitors and SK activation of plasminogen [154, 170, 236, 237].

Synthetic ester substrates. Plasmin lyses esters of arginine, e.g. tosyl arginine methyl ester (TAME), and lysine, e.g. acetyl lysine methyl ester (ALME), and esterolytic assays have been described [238].

Chromogenic substrate. The tripeptide H-D-valyl-L-leucyl-lysine-p-nitroanilide (S-2251, Kabi) is relatively sensitive to the action of plasmin and SK-activated plasminogen, and much less sensitive to other proteases (thrombin, trypsin, kallikrein). These enzymes release p-nitroaniline from the colourless substrate.

Immunological assays. Monospecific antisera are available and allow immunological assay of plasminogen and plasmin. Methods described include modifications of the Laurell immunoelectrophoresis technique, radioimmunoassay and radioimmunodiffusion [164, 239–241]. Agar plates containing plasminogen antiserum for plasminogen assay are available commercially.

DEGRADATION OF FIBRINOGEN/FIBRIN BY PLASMIN

Fibrinogen interaction with plasmin (Fig. 27.12)
The first stage of degradation involves the symmetrical splitting of a peptide of MW 40 000 from both carboxyl ends of the Aα chains of fibrinogen, leaving a high-MW fragment X (MW 260 000), which consists of the Aα-chain remnants disulphide-bonded to intact Bβ- and γ-chains [242, 243]. This high MW fragment may still clot under the action of thrombin. In the next step a peptide of MW 6000 is split from the N-terminal ends of the Bβ chains [244], then all three chains are cleaved on one side of the partially degraded dimer to release fragment D (MW 94 000), leaving fragment Y (MW 150 000) [79, 245, 246]. Fragment Y is then rapidly cleaved to produce a second fragment D and a third fragment, E (MW 50 000). Fragment E is a dimer made up of the N-terminal sections of the three chains of fibrinogen [247]. Fragments Y, D and E do not clot on addition of thrombin, but inhibit the conversion of fibrinogen to fibrin by thrombin. The larger of these fragments have a greater effect on inhibition of clotting, purified Y being most active; it has been

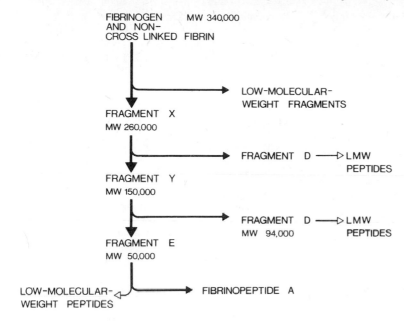

Fig. 27.12. Production of FDPs from fibrinogen and non-cross-linked fibrin by plasmin.

shown that they inhibit the enzymatic as well as the polymerization phase of clotting [248, 249].

Non-cross-linked fibrin and plasmin degradation
The fragments released are electrophoretically similar to those generated during plasmin-fibrinogen degradation [250, 251]. However, fragment E differs in that fibrinopeptide A is lacking, though this seems to produce only minor immunological differences [252].

Cross-linked fibrin and plasmin degradation
Degradation of cross-linked fibrin proceeds at a slower rate, as the cross-linking of chains confers resistance to the initial steps of plasmin digestion [253]. Unique fragments called D dimer and E are formed. The D-dimer fragments contain the cross-linked γ-chain remnants of the original fibrin [251, 254]. It has been suggested that detection of D dimer may provide a means of monitoring thrombolytic treatment [253]. The MW of the D dimer is between 63 000 and 80 000 and there is evidence of D-dimer and fragment-E complexing.

Biological functions of FDP
As well as inhibiting polymerization of fibrin and the action of thrombin, FDP have the following actions.
1 *Effects on platelet function.* FDP inhibit platelet aggregation, adhesion and the release reaction, the high-MW products being more active than low-MW products [255–257]. Their action is probably due to adsorption of fragments onto the platelet membrane

[258] and is found whether the production of fragments is due to SK, defibrase or ancrod [255, 259, 260].
2 *Effects on heart and blood vessels.* These are due to low-MW peptides which potentiate the effects of bradykinin, angiotensin, adrenaline and serotonin [261, 262]. Low-MW fragments also increase the permeability of skin capillaries [263].

ASSAYS OF FIBRINOGEN/FIBRIN DEGRADATION PRODUCTS
Degradation products of fibrinogen and fibrin can be measured by virtue of their biological activities or by immunological means.

Biological activity

Thrombin clotting time [264]. The thrombin time is prolonged by low fibrinogen levels, heparin, dysfibrinogenaemia or dysproteinaemia. Although nonspecific, it is a useful rapid screening test in suspected defibrination [265]. In patients treated with heparin the thrombin time cannot be used as a measure of fibrinogen and FDP. An alternative is to use the snake venom reptilase (batroxobin) which is not affected by heparin [145].

Staphylococcal clumping test [266]. Fibrinogen and FDP agglutinate certain strains of staphylococci. Equal volumes of staphylococcal suspension and serial dilutions of test serum are mixed and clumping is observed. The test is sensitive to fragments X and Y but not to D and E: results correlate with the tanned red-cell method [267]. The reaction depends on the presence of a clumping factor in the bacterial wall. This peptide seems to be distinct from staphylococcal coagulase.

Immunological methods

These methods are based on detection of fibrinogen/fibrin-related antigen (FR antigen), which is present in intact fibrinogen and persists in FDP, or new antigenic sites (neo-antigens) which are exposed in later fragments (D and E) by the action of plasmin or thrombin [152, 268]. Methods detecting FR antigen use antisera raised against human fibrinogen and are performed on serum. Blood is collected into tubes containing an excess of thrombin (to ensure total fibrinogen conversion) and inhibitors of fibrinolysis (EACA). Early, thrombin-clottable FDP (fragment X) are also removed from the serum, while other FDP complex with the fibrin clot, or are non-specifically retained within the meshwork of the clot [269].

Direct latex agglutination tests. Latex particles can be coated with fibrinogen antiserum and tested for agglutination against dilutions of test serum [270]. The tests are rapid, but relatively insensitive to FDP compared to fibrinogen, and measure only fragments X and Y [267]. Coating of the latex particles with a mixture of antibodies to fragments D and E increases sensitivity to these later FDP.

Tanned red-cell haemagglutination inhibition immunoassay (TRCHII) [271]. This assay is sensitive and is widely used for measurement of FDP. Serial dilutions of the test serum are incubated with fibrinogen antiserum: the antibodies are consumed in proportion to the amount of FR antigen. Tanned group-O red cells, coated with fibrinogen, are then added, and agglutination of the cells follows further incubation. Dilutions of a fibrinogen standard are tested in parallel, and the results expressed as equivalents of micrograms of fibrinogen per ml. Less than 5–10 μg/ml are found in normal serum. The test is more sensitive to fragments X and Y than D, and is insensitive to E: levels of 3 μg/ml are detectable [267].

Indirect latex agglutination tests [272]. Latex particles coated with fibrinogen may be substituted for the tanned red cells. The sensitivity of the test is similar to the TRCHII and the results correlate well.

Immunoelectrophoresis. The Laurell technique has been adapted to measure FR antigen and fragments D and E [169, 273]. The sensitivity is similar to the TRCHII, particularly if D and E antisera are used.

Radioimmunoassays. These assays are highly sensitive and specific. Specific assays of fragments D and E have been developed, and differentiation of fibrinogen-derived FDP and fibrin-derived FDP is possible [268, 274, 275], as is measurement of fibrinopeptide A.

REFERENCES

1 DAVIE E.W. & RATNOFF O.D. (1964) Waterfall sequence for intrinsic blood clotting. *Science*, **145**, 1310.
2 MACFARLANE R.G. (1964) An enzyme cascade in the blood clotting mechanism and its function as a biochemical amplifier. *Nature (London)*, **202**, 498.
3 GULLIVER G. (1846) *The Works of William Hewson, F.R.S.* p. 40. The Sydenham Society, London.
4 THACKRAH C.T. (1819) *An Inquiry into the Nature and Properties of the Blood, as Existent in Health and Disease.* Cox, London.
5 BRÜCKE V.E. (1857) Ueber die Ursache der Gerinnung des Blutes. *Archiv für Pathologische Anatomie und Physiologie und für Klinische Medicin*, **12**, 81.
6 LISTER J. (1863) On the coagulation of blood. *Proceedings of the Royal Society*, **12**, 580.
7 MARGOLIS J. (1957) Glass surface and blood coagulation. *Nature (London)*, **178**, 805.
8 SHAFRIR E. & DE VRIES A. (1956) Studies on clot-promoting activity of glass. *Journal of Clinical Investigation*, **35**, 1183.
9 WAALER B.A. (1959) Contact activation in the intrinsic blood clotting system: studies on a plasma product formed on contact with glass and similar surfaces. *Scandinavian Journal of Clinical and Laboratory Investigation*, Suppl. **11**, 1.
10 RATNOFF O.D. & COLOPY J.E. (1955) Familial hemorrhagic trait associated with deficiency of clot-promoting fraction of plasma. *Journal of Clinical Investigation*, **34**, 602.
11 RATNOFF O.D. & MARGOLIUS A. JR (1955) Hageman trait: an asymptomatic disorder of blood coagulation. *Transactions of the Association of American Physicians (Philadelphia)*, **68**, 149.
12 RATNOFF O.D. & DAVIE E.W. (1962) The activation of Christmas Factor (factor IX) by activated plasma thromboplastin antecedent (activated factor XI). *Biochemistry (Washington)*, **1**, 677.
13 SPRAGG J.A., KAPLAN A.P. & AUSTEN K.F. (1973) The use of iso-electric focusing to study components of the human kinin-forming system. *Annals of the New York Academy of Sciences*, **209**, 372.
14 SCHOENMAKERS J.C.G., MATZE R., HAANEN C. & ZILLIKEN F. (1965) Hageman factor, a novel sialoglycoprotein with esterase activity. *Biochimica et Biophysica Acta*, **101**, 166.
15 REVAK S.D., COCHRANE C.G., JOHNSTON A.R. & HUGLI T.E. (1974) Structural changes accompanying enzymatic activation of human Hageman factor. *Journal of Clinical Investigation*, **54**, 619.
16 ROSENTHAL R.L., DRESKIN O.H. & ROSENTHAL N. (1953) New hemophilia-like disease caused by deficiency of third plasma thromboplastin factor. *Proceed-*

ings of the Society for Experimental Biology and Medicine, **82**, 171.

17 FORBES C.D. & RATNOFF O.D. (1972) Studies on plasma thromboplastin antecedent (factor XI), PTA deficiency and inhibition of PTA by plasma, pharmacologic inhibitors and specific antiserum. *Journal of Laboratory and Clinical Medicine*, **79**, 113.

18 SCHIFFMAN S. & LEE P. (1974) Preparation, characterisation and activation of a highly purified factor XI: evidence that a hitherto unrecognised plasma activity participates in the interaction of factors XI and XII. *British Journal of Haematology*, **27**, 101.

19 WUEPPER K.D. (1972) Biochemistry and biology of components of the plasma kinin-forming system. In: *Inflammation, Mechanisms and Control* (ed. Lepow I.W. & Ward P.A.), p. 93. Academic Press, New York.

20 NOSSEL H.L. (1964) *The Contact Phase of Blood Coagulation*. Blackwell Scientific Publications, Oxford.

21 KOCIBA G.J., RATNOFF O.D., LOEB W.F., WALL R.L. & HEIDER L.E. (1969) Bovine plasma thromboplastin antecedent (Factor XI) deficiency. *Journal of Laboratory and Clinical Medicine*, **74**, 37.

22 HATHAWAY W.E., BELHASEN L.P. & HATHAWAY H.S. (1965) Evidence for a new plasma thromboplastin factor. Case report coagulation studies and physicochemical properties. *Blood*, **26**, 521.

23 HATHAWAY W.E. & ALSEVER J. (1970) The relationship of Fletcher factor to factors XI and XII. *British Journal of Haematology*, **18**, 161.

24 SAITO H. & RATNOFF O.D. (1974) Inhibition of normal clotting and Fletcher factor activity by rabbit antikallikrein antiserum, *Nature (London)*, **248**, 597.

25 DONALDSON V.A., GLUECK H.I. & FLEMING T. (1972) Brief recordings: Rheumatoid arthritis in a patient with Hageman trait. *New England Journal of Medicine*, **286**, 528.

26 WALDMAN R. & ABRAHAM J.B. (1974) Fitzgerald factor, a heretofore unrecognised coagulation factor. *Blood*, **44**, 934.

27 BIGGS R., DOUGLAS A.S., MACFARLANE R.G., DACIE J.V., PITNEY W.R., MERSKEY C. & O'BRIEN J.R. (1952) Christmas disease: a condition previously mistaken for haemophilia. *British Medical Journal*, **ii**, 1378.

28 AGGELER P.M., WHITE S., GLENDENNING M.B., PAGE E.W., LEAKE T.B. & BATES G. (1952) Plasma thromboplastin component (PTC) deficiency; a new disease resembling haemophilia. *Proceedings of the Society for Experimental Biology and Medicine*, **79**, 692.

29 FUJIKAWA K., THOMPSON A.R., LEGAZ M.E., MEYER R.G. & DAVIE E.W. (1973) Isolation and characterisation of bovine factor IX. *Biochemistry*, **12**, 4938.

30 GENTRY P.W. & ALEXANDER B. (1973) Specific coagulation factor adsorption to insoluble heparin. *Biochemistry and Biophysics* **50**, 500.

31 OSTERUD B. & FLENGSRUD R. (1975) Purification and some characteristics of the coagulation factor IX from human plasma. *Biochemical Journal*, **145**, 469.

32 HEMKER H.C., VELTKAMP J.J., HENSEN A. & LOELIGER E.A. (1963) Nature of prothrombin biosynthesis: preprothrombinaemia in vitamin-K deficiency. *Nature (London)*, **200**, 589.

33 REEKERS P.P.M., LINDHOAT M.J., KOP-KLAASSEN B.H.M. & HEMKER H.C. (1973) Demonstration of three anomalous plasma proteins induced by a vitamin K antagonist. *Biochimica et Biophysica Acta*, **317**, 559.

34 KASS L., RATNOFF O.D. & LEON M.A. (1969) Studies on the purification of antihemophilic factor (factor VIII). Separation of partially purified antihemophilic factor by gel filtration of plasma. *Journal of Clinical Investigation*, **48**, 351.

35 BENNETT B., FORMAN W.B. & RATNOFF O.D. (1973) Studies on the nature of antihemophilic factor (factor VIII). Further evidence relating the AHF-like antigens in normal and hemophilic plasmas. *Journal of Clinical Investigation*, **52**, 2191.

36 RICK M.E. & HOYER L.W. (1973) Immunologic studies of anti-hemophilic factor (AHF, Factor VIII). V. Immunologic properties of AHF subunits produced by salt dissociation. *Blood*, **42**, 737.

37 WAGNER R.H., COOPER H.A. & OWEN W.G. (1973) Dissociation of antihaemophilic factor and separation of a small active fragment. *Thrombosis et Diathesis Haemorrhagica*, **54**, 185.

38 AUSTEN D. (1974) Factor VIII of small molecular weight and its origin, *British Journal of Haematology*, **27**, 89.

39 LEGAZ M.E., SCHMER G., COUNTS R.B. & DAVIE E.W. (1973) Isolation and characterisation of human factor VIII (antihaemophilic factor). *Journal of Biological Chemistry*, **248**, 3946.

40 ZIMMERMAN T.S., RATNOFF O.D. & POWELL, A.E. (1971) Immunologic differentiation of classic hemophilia (factor VIII deficiency) and von Willebrand's disease. *Journal of Clinical Investigation*, **50**, 244.

41 HOYER L.W. & BRECKENRIDGE R.I. (1970) Immunologic studies of antihemophilic factor. II; properties of CRM. *Blood*, **35**, 809.

42 BLOOM A.L., GIDDINGS J.C. & WILKS C.J. (1973) Factor VIII on the vascular intima: possible importance in haemostasis and thrombosis. *Nature (New Biology)*, **241**, 217.

43 HOWARD M.A., MONTGOMERY D.C. & HARDISTY R.M. (1974) Factor VIII-related antigen in platelets. *Thrombosis Research*, **4**, 617.

44 PRESTON A.E. & BARR A. (1964) The plasma concentration of Factor VIII in the normal population. II. The effects of age, sex, and blood group. *British Journal of Haematology*, **10**, 238.

45 DAVIES J.A. & MCNICOL G.P. (1978) Blood coagulation and thrombosis. *British Medical Bulletin*, **34**, 113.

46 MEADE T.W. & NORTH W.R.S. (1977) Population-based distributions of haemostatic variables. *British Medical Bulletin*, **33**, 283.

47 AUSTEN D.E.G. & RHYMES I.L. (1975) *A Laboratory Manual of Blood Coagulation*. Blackwell Scientific Publications, Oxford.

48 DENSON K.W.E. (1976) Techniques. In: *Human Blood Coagulation, Haemostasis and Thrombosis*, 2nd edition (ed. Biggs, R.), p. 602. Blackwell Scientific Publications, Oxford.

49 WILLIAMS K.N., DAVIDSON J.M.F. & INGRAM G.I.C. (1975) A computer program for the analysis of parallel-line bioassays of clotting factors. *British Journal of Haematology*, **31**, 13.

50 CHANTARANGKUL V., INGRAM G.I.C. & DARBY S. (1977) An artificial haemophilic plasma for one-stage factor VIII assay. *Thrombosis and Haemostasis*, **38**, 344.

51 BANGHAM D.R., BIGGS R., BROZOVIC M., DENSON K.W.E. & SKEGG J.L. (1971) A biological standard for measurement of blood coagulation factor VIII activity. *Bulletin of the World Health Organisation*, **45**, 337.

52 BIGGS R. & DOUGLAS A.S. (1953) The thromboplastin generation test. *Journal of Clinical Pathology*, **6**, 23.

53 HOWARD M.A. & FIRKIN B.G. (1971) Ristocetin; a new tool in the investigation of platelet aggregation. *Thrombosis et Diathesis Haemorrhagica*, **26**, 362.

54 WEISS H.J. (1975) Abnormalities of factor VIII and platelet aggregation—use of ristocetin in diagnosing von Willebrand's syndrome. *Blood*, **45**, 403.

55 MEYER D., JENKINS C.S.P., DREYFUS M. & LARRIEU M. (1973) Experimental model for von Willebrand's disease. *Nature (London)*, **234**, 293.

56 BRINKHOUS K.M., GRAHAM J.B. & COOPER H.A. (1975) Assay of von Willebrand factor in von Willebrand's disease and haemophilia—use of a macroscopic platelet aggregation test. *Thrombosis Research*, **6**, 267.

57 ZIMMERMAN T.S., HOYER L.W., DICKSON L. & EDGINGTON T.S. (1975) Determination of the von Willebrand's disease antigen (Factor VIII-related antigen) in plasma by quantitative immunoelectrophoresis. *Journal of Laboratory and Clinical Medicine*, **86**, 152.

57a HOYER L.W. (1972) Immunologic studies of antihemophilic factor (AHF, factor VIII). IV. Radio-immunoassay of AHF antigen. *Journal of Laboratory and Clinical Medicine*, **80**, 822.

57b PEAKE I.R. & BLOOM A.L. (1977) The use of an immunoradiometric assay for factor VIII-related antigen in the study of atypical von Willebrand's disease. *Thrombosis Research*, **10**, 27.

58 ASTRUP T. (1965) Assay and content of tissue thromboplastin in different organs. *Thrombosis et Diathesis Haemorrhagica*, **14**, 401.

59 DUCKERT F., FLUCKIGER P., MATTER M. & KOLLER F. (1955) Clotting factor X. Physiologic and physicochemical properties. *Proceedings of the Society of Experimental Biology and Medicine*, **90**, 17.

60 TELFER T.P., DENSON K.W.E. & WRIGHT D.R. (1956) A 'new' coagulation defect. *British Journal of Haematology*, **2**, 308.

61 FUJIKAWA K., LEGAZ M.E. & DAVIE E.W. (1972) Bovine factors X_1 and X_2 (Stuart Factor). Isolation and characterisation. *Biochemistry*, **11**, 4882.

62 NOLF P. (1908) Préparation et propriétés coagulantes de la thrombozyme. *Archives of Internal Physiology*, **6**, 1.

63 QUICK A.J. (1943) On the constitution of prothrombin. *American Journal of Physiology*, **140**, 212.

64 OWREN P.A. (1947) The coagulation of blood. Investigation of a new clotting factor. *Acta Medica Scandinavia*, Suppl. **1**, 194.

65 MALLIGER E.J. & DUCKERT F. (1971) Major surgery in a subject with factor V deficiency. Cholecystectomy in a parahaemophilic woman and a review of the literature. *Thrombosis et Diathesis Haemorrhagica*, **25**, 438.

66 ESNOUF M.P., JOBIN F. & PEDEN J.C. (1963) The isolation of factor V from bovine plasma. *Biochemical Journal*, **89**, 44.

67 DAY W.C. & BARTON P.G. (1972) Studies on the stability of bovine plasma factor V. *Biochimica et Biophysica Acta*, **261**, 457.

68 PAPAHADJOPOULOS D. & HANAHAN D.J. (1964) Observations on the interaction of phospholipids and certain clotting factors in prothrombin activator formation. *Biochimica et Biophysica Acta*, **90**, 436.

69 SEEGERS W.H., McCLAUGHRY R.I. & FAHEY J.L. (1950) Some properties of purified prothrombin and its activation with sodium citrate. *Blood*, **5**, 421.

70 SEEGERS W.H., HASSOUNA H.I., HEWETT-EMMETT D., WALZ D.A. & ANDARY T.J. (1975) Prothrombin and thrombin: selected aspects of thrombin formation, properties, inhibition, and immunology. *Seminars in Thrombosis and Hemostasis*, **1**, 211.

71 QUICK A.J. (1935) Prothrombin in hemophilia and in obstructive jaundice. *Journal of Biological Chemistry*, **109**, 73.

72 JOBIN F. & ESNOUF M.P. (1966) Coagulant activity of tiger snake (*Notechis scutatus scutatus*) venom. *Nature (London)*, **211**, 873.

73 WARNER E.D., BRINKHOUS K.M. & SMITH H.P. (1936) A quantitative study on blood clotting. Prothrombin fluctuations under experimental conditions. *American Journal of Physiology*, **114**, 667.

74 WARE A.G. & SEEGERS W.H. (1949) Two stage procedure for the quantitative determination of prothrombin concentration. *American Journal of Clinical Pathology*, **19**, 471.

75 DENSON K.W.E., BARRETT R. & BIGGS R. (1971) The specific assay of prothrombin using the Taipan snake venom. *British Journal of Haematology*, **21**, 219.

76 SHAPIRO S.S., MARTINEZ J. & HOLBURN R.R. (1969) Congenital dysprothrombinaemia: an inherited structural disorder of human prothrombin. *Journal of Clinical Investigation*, **48**, 2251.

77 GIROLAMI A. (1975) Prothrombin Padua. In: *Prothrombin and Related Coagulation Factors* (ed. Hemker H.C. & Veltkamp J.J.), p. 213. Boerhave Series, No. 10, Leiden University Press.

78 McKEE P.A., MATTOCK P. & HILL R.L. (1970) Subunit structure of human fibrinogen, soluble fibrin and cross-linked insoluble fibrin. *Proceedings of the National Academy of Sciences, U.S.A.*, **66**, 738.

79 GAFFNEY P.J. (1977) Structure of fibrinogen and FDP. *British Medical Bulletin*, **33**, 245.

80 DINTENFASS L. (1971) *Blood Microrheology—Viscosity Factors in Blood Flow, Ischaemia and Thrombosis*. p. 267. Butterworth, London.

81 LOWE G.D.O., DRUMMOND M.M., FORBES C.D. & BARBENEL J.C. (1980) Occlusive arterial disease and blood rheology. In: *Clinical Aspects of Blood Viscosity and Cell Deformability* (ed. Lowe G.D.O., Barbenel J.C. & Forbes C.D.), p. 219. Springer-Verlag, New York.

82 ELLIS B.C. & STRANSKY A. (1961) A quick and accurate method for the determination of fibrinogen in plasma. *Journal of Laboratory and Clinical Medicine*, **58**, 477.

83 CLAUSS A. (1957) Gerinnungsphysiologische Schnellmethode zur Bestimmung des Fibrinogens. *Acta Haematologica*, **17**, 237.

84 RATNOFF O.D. & MENZIE C. (1951) A new method for the determination of fibrinogen in small samples of plasma. *Journal of Laboratory and Clinical Medicine*, **37**, 316.

85 NILSSON I.M. & OLOW B. (1962) Determination of fibrinogen and fibrinogenolytic activity. *Thrombosis et Diathesis Haemorrhagica*, **8**, 297.

86 MILLAR H.R., SIMPSON J.G. & STALKER A.L. (1971) An evaluation of the heat precipitation method for plasma fibrinogen estimation. *Journal of Clinical Pathology*, **24**, 827.

87 RAMPLING M.W. & GAFFNEY P.J. (1976) The sulphite precipitation method for fibrinogen measurement. Its use on small samples in the presence of fibrinogen degradation products. *Clinica Chimica Acta*, **67**, 43.

88 LORAND L. & JACOBSEN A. (1958) Studies on the polymerization of fibrin; the role of the globulin:fibrin stabilising factor. *Journal of Biological Chemistry*, **230**, 421.

89 SCHWARTZ M.L., PIZZO S.V., HILL R.L. & McKEE P.A. (1973) Human factor XIII from plasma and platelets. Molecular weights, subunit structures, proteolytic activation, and cross-linking of fibrinogen and fibrin. *Journal of Biological Chemistry*, **248**, 1395.

90 LORAND L., LOCKRIDGE O.M., CAMPBELL L.K., MYHRMAN R. & BRUNE-LORAND J. (1971) Transamidating enzymes. II. A continuous fluorescent method suited for automating measurements of factor XIII in plasma. *Annals of Biochemistry*, **44**, 221.

91 DUCKERT F. (1972) Documentation of plasma factor XIII deficiency in man. *Annals of the New York Academy of Sciences*, **202**, 190.

92 NOSSEL H.L., RUBIN H., DRILLINGS M. & HSIEH R. (1968) Inhibition of Hageman factor activation. *Journal of Clinical Investigation*, **47**, 1172.

93 GRIFFIN J.H. (1978) The role of surface in the surface-dependent activation of Hageman factor (Factor XII). *Proceedings of National Academy of Sciences, USA*, **75**, 1998.

94 COCHRANE C.G., REVAK S.D. & WUEPPER K.D. (1973) Activation of Hageman factor in solid and fluid phases. A critical role of kallikrein. *Journal of Experimental Medicine*, **138**, 1564.

95 McMILLAN C.R., SAITO H., RATNOFF O.D. & WALTON A.G. (1974) The secondary structure of human Hageman factor (factor XII). *Journal of Clinical Investigation*, **54**, 1312.

96 RATNOFF O.D. & SAITO H. (1975) Inhibition of Hageman factor, plasma thromboplastin antecedent, thrombin and other clotting factors by phenyl-glyoxalhydrate. *Proceedings of the Society for Experimental Biology and Medicine*, **148**, 177.

97 SAITO H., RATNOFF O.D., MARSHALL J.S. & PENSKY J. (1973) Partial purification of plasma thromboplastin antecedent (factor XI) and its activation by trypsin. *Journal of Clinical Investigation*, **52**, 850.

98 WALSH P.N. (1972) The effects of collagen and kaolin on intrinsic coagulation activity of platelets: Evidence for an alternate pathway in intrinsic coagulation not requiring factor XII. *British Journal of Haematology*, **22**, 393.

99 SAITO H., RATNOFF O.D., WALDMANN R. & ABRAHAM J.P. (1975) Fitzgerald trait. Deficiency of a hitherto unrecognised agent, Fitzgerald factor, participating in surface-mediated reactions of clotting, fibrinolysis, generation of kinins and the property of diluted plasma enhancing vascular permeability (PF/dil). *Journal of Clinical Investigation*, **55**, 1082.

100 FORBES C.D., PENSKY J. & RATNOFF O.D. (1970) Inhibition of activated Hageman factor and activated plasma thromboplastin antecedent by purified C1 inactivator. *Journal of Laboratory and Clinical Medicine*, **76**, 80.

101 HECK L.W. & KAPLAN A.P. (1974) Substrates of human Hageman factor. 1. Isolation and characterisation of PTA (factor XI) and its inhibition by α_1-antitrypsin. *Journal of Experimental Medicine*, **140**, 1615.

102 RATNOFF O.D. & ROSENBLUM J.H. (1959) Role of Hageman factor in the initiation of clotting by glass: evidence that glass frees Hageman factor from inhibitors. *American Journal of Medicine*, **25**, 160.

103 HOROWITZ H.I. & FUJIMOTO M.M. (1965) Association of factors XI and XII with blood platelets. *Proceedings of the Society for Experimental Biology and Medicine*, **119**, 487.

104 IATRIDIS P.G. & FERGUSON J.H. (1965) The plasmatic atmosphere of blood platelets. Evidence that only fibrinogen AcG and activated Hageman factor are present on the surface of platelets. *Thrombosis et Diathesis Haemorrhagica*, **13**, 114.

105 WALSH P.N. (1972) The role of platelets in the contact phase of blood coagulation. *British Journal of Haematology*, **22**, 237.

106 KALOUSEK F., KONINGSBERG W. & NEMERSON Y. (1975) Activation of factor IX by activated factor X: A link between the extrinsic and intrinsic coagulation systems. *Federation of European Biochemical Societies: Letters (Amsterdam)*, **50**, 382.

107 HEMKER K.C. & KAHN M.J.P. (1967) Reaction sequence of blood coagulation. *Nature (London)*, **215**, 1201.

108 RAPAPORT S.I., SCHIFFMAN S., PATCH M.J. & AMES S.B. (1963) The importance of activation of antihaemophilic globulin and proaccelerin by traces of thrombin in the generation of intrinsic prothrombinase activity. *Blood*, **21**, 221.

109 DAVIE E.W. & FUJIKAWA K. (1975) Basic mechanisms in blood coagulation. *Annual Revues of Biochemistry*, **44**, 799.

110 ALEXANDER B. & LANDWEHR G. (1949) Evolution of prothrombin conversion accelerator in stored human plasma and prothrombin fractions. *American Journal of Physiology*, **159**, 322.

111 COLMAN R.W., MATTLER L. & SHERRY S. (1969) Studies on the pre-kallikrein (kallikreinogen)—kallikrein enzyme system of human plasma. II. Evidence relating the kaolin-activated arginine esterase to plasma kallikrein. *Journal of Clinical Investigation*, **48**, 23.

112 ØSTERUD B., BERRE A., OTNAESS A.-B., BJORKILD E. & PRYDZ H. (1972) Activation of the coagulation factor VII by tissue thromboplasin and calcium. *Biochemistry*, **ii**, 2853.

113 REZVAN H. & HOWELL R.M. (1977) Protein-magnetic-resonance studies of the interaction of thromboplastin apoprotein with lipids. *Biochemical Society Transcripts*, **5**, 1549.

114 MAGNUSSON S., PETERSEN T.E., SETTRUP-JENSON L. & CLAEYS H. (1975) Complete primary structure of pro-thrombin; isolation structure and reactivity of ten carboxylated glutamic acid residues and regulation of pro-thrombin activation by thrombin. In: *Proteases and Biological Control* (ed. Reich E., Rifkind D.B. & Shaw E.), p. 123. Cold Harbor Conferences on Cell Proliferation, Vol. II. Cold Spring Harbor Laboratory, New York.

115 PROWSE C.V., MATTOCK P., ESNOUF M.P. & RUSSELL A.M. (1976) A variant of prothrombin induced in cattle by prolonged administration of warfarin. *Biochimica et Biophysica Acta*, **434**, 265,

116 LORAND L. (1952) Fibrino-peptide. *Biochemical Journal*, **52**, 200.

117 BLOMBACK B. & YAMASHINA I. (1958) On the N-terminal amino acids in fibrinogen and fibrin. *Arkiv För Kemi*, **12**, 299.

118 LORAND L. (1972) Fibrinoligase: the fibrin-stabilizing factor system of blood plasma. *Annals of the New York Academy of Sciences*, **202**, 6.

119 SHAINOFF J.R. & PAGE I.H. (1960) Cofibrin and fibrin intermediates as indicators of thrombin activity *in vivo*. *Circulation Research*, **8**, 1013.

120 MCKILLOP C., EDGAR W., FORBES C.D. & PRENTICE C.R.M. (1975) *In vivo* production of soluble complexes containing fibrinogen–fibrin related antigen during ancrod therapy. *Thrombosis Research*, **7**, 361.

121 BANG N.U. & CHANG M.L. (1974) Soluble fibrin complexes. *Seminars in Thrombosis and Hemostasis*, **1**, 91.

122 LORAND L. (1975) Controls in the clotting of fibrinogen. In: *Proteases and Biological Control* (ed. Reich E., Rifkind D.B. & Shaw E.), p. 79. Cold Spring Harbor Conferences on Cell Proliferation, Vol. II. Cold Spring Harbor Laboratory, New York.

123 MORAWITZ P. (1905) Die Chemie der Blutgerinnung. *Ergebnis der Physiol*, **4**, 307.

124 CLARK A.J. (1938) The normal anti-thrombin of the blood and its relation to heparin. *American Journal of Physiology*, **123**, 712.

125 EGEBERG O. (1965) Inherited antithrombin deficiency causing thrombophilia. *Thrombosis et Diathesis Haemorrhagica*, **13**, 516.

126 ABILDGAARD U. (1968) Highly purified anti-thrombin III with heparin cofactor activity prepared by disc electrophoresis. *Scandinavian Journal of Clinical and Laboratory Investigation*, **21**, 89.

127 ABILDGAARD U. (1967) Purification of two progressive antithrombins of human plasma. *Scandinavian Journal of Clinical and Laboratory Investigation*, **19**, 190.

128 COLLEN D., SCHETZ J., DE COCK F., HOLMER E. & VERSTRAETE M. (1977) Metabolism of antithrombin III (Heparin cofactor) in man: effects of venous thrombosis and of heparin administration. *European Journal of Clinical Investigation*, **7**, 27.

129 ROSENBERG R.D. & DAMUS P.S. (1973) The purification and mechanism of action of human antithrombin-heparin cofactor. *Journal of Biological Chemistry*, **248**, 6490.

130 SEEGERS W.H., COLE E.R. & HARMISON C.R. (1964) Neutralisation of autoprothrombin C with antithrombin. *Canadian Journal of Biochemistry*, **42**, 359.

131 ØDEGÅRD O.R., LIE M. & ABILDGAARD U. (1975) Heparin co-factor activity measured by an amidolytic method. *Thrombosis Research*, **6**, 287.

132 ROSENBERG J.S., MCKENNA P. & ROSENBERG R.D. (1975) Inhibition of human factor Xa by human antithrombin-heparin cofactor. *Journal of Biological Chemistry*, **250**, 8883.

133 ØSTERUD B., MILLER-ANDERSSON M., ABILDGAARD U. & PRYDZ H. (1976) The effect of antithrombin III on the activity of the coagulation factors VII, IX, and X. *Thrombosis and Haemostasis*, **35**, 295.

134 DAMUS P.S., HICKS M. & ROSENBERG R.D. (1973) Anticoagulant action of heparin. *Nature (London)*, **246**, 355.

135 STEAD N., KAPLAN A.P. & ROSENBERG R.D. (1976) Inhibition of activated factor XII by antithrombin-heparin cofactor. *Journal of Biological Chemistry*, **251**, 6481.

136 ØDEGÅRD O.R., LIE M. & ABILDGAARD U. (1976) Antifactor Xa activity measured with amidolytic methods. *Haemostasis*, **5**, 265.

137 FAGERHOL M.K. & ABILDGAARD U. (1970) Immunological studies on human antithrombin III. Influence of age, sex and use of oral contraceptives on serum concentration. *Scandinavian Journal of Haematology*, **7**, 10.

138 VAN DER MEER J., STOEPMAN-VAN DALEN E.A. & JANSEN J.M.S. (1973) Antithrombin III in a Dutch family. *Journal of Clinical Pathology*, **26**, 532.

139 SAS G., BLASKO G., BANHEGYI D., JAKO J. & PALOS L.A. (1974) Abnormal antithrombin III (Antithrombin III Budapest) as a cause of familial thrombophilia. *Thrombosis et Diathesis Haemorrhagica*, **32**, 105.

140 RATNOFF O.D., PENSKY J., OGSTON D. & NAFF G.B. (1969) The inhibition of plasmin, plasma kallikrein, permeability factor and the C1r subcomponent of the first component by serum C1 esterase inhibitor. *Journal of Experimental Medicine*, **129**, 315.

141 SCHREIBER A.D., KAPLAN A.P. & AUSTEN K.E. (1973) Inhibition of C1 INH of Hageman factor fragment activation of coagulation, fibrinolysis and kinin generation. *Journal of Clinical Investigation*, **52**, 1402.

142 RATNOFF O.D. & ROSENBLUM J.H. (1957) The role of Hageman factor on the initiation of clotting by glass. *Journal of Laboratory and Clinical Medicine*, **50**, 941.

143 NOSSEL H. & NIEMETZ J. (1965) A normal inhibitor of the blood coagulation contact reaction product. *Blood*, **25**, 712.

144 DEYKIN D. (1966) The role of liver in serum-induced hypercoagulability. *Journal of Clinical Investigation*, **45**, 256.

145 GIDDINGS J.C. (1980) The investigation of hereditary coagulation disorders. In: *Blood Coagulation and Haemostasis: A Practical Guide* (ed. Thomson J.M.), p. 48. Churchill-Livingstone, London.

146 OWEN C.A., BOWIE E.J.W. & THOMPSON J.H. (1975) *The Diagnosis of Bleeding Disorders*. p. 155. Little, Brown & Co., Boston.

147 DUKE W.W. (1910) The relation of blood platelets to haemorrhagic disease. *Journal of the American Medical Association*, **55**, 1185.

148 IVY A.C., NELSON D. & BUCHER G. (1941) Standardization of certain factors in cutaneous 'venostasis' bleeding time technique. *Journal of Laboratory and Clinical Medicine*, **26**, 1812.

149 BORCHGREVINK C.F. & WAALER B.A. (1958) The secondary bleeding time. A new method for the differentiation of haemorrhagic diseases. *Acta Medica Scandinavica*, **162**, 361.

150 MIELKE C.H. JR, KANESHIRO M.M., MAHER I.A., WEINER J.M. & RAPPAPORT S.I. (1969) The standardised normal Ivy bleeding time and its prolongation by aspirin. *Blood*, **34**, 204.

151 FLETCHER A.P., ALKJAERSIG N. & SHERRY S. (1959) The

maintenance of a sustained thrombolytic state in man. I. Induction and effect. *Journal of Clinical Investigation*, **38**, 1096.

152 PLOW E.F. & EDGINGTON T.S. (1973) An alternative pathway for fibrinolysis. I. The cleavage of fibrinogen by leucocyte proteases at physiological pH. *Journal of Clinical Investigation*, **56**, 30.

153 FORBES C.D., LOWE G.D.O. & PRENTICE C.R.M. (1978) Thrombolytic therapy—indications, advantages and disadvantages. *Angiology*, **29**, 783.

154 ALKJAERSIG N., FLETCHER A.P. & SHERRY S. (1959) The mechanism of clot dissolution by plasmin. *Journal of Clinical Investigation*, **38**, 1086.

155 AMBRUS C.M. & MARKUS G. (1960) Plasmin–antiplasmin complex as a reservoir of fibrinolytic enzyme. *American Journal of Physiology*, **199**, 491.

156 CHESTERMAN C.N., ALLINGTON M.J. & SHARP A.A. (1972) Relationship of plasminogen activator to fibrin. *Nature (New Biology)*, **238**, 15.

157 WALLEN P. & WIMAN B. (1970) Characterisation of human plasminogen. I. On the relationship between different molecular forms of plasminogen demonstrated in plasma and found in purified preparations. *Biochimica et Biophysica Acta*, **221**, 20.

158 ROBBINS K.C., SUMMARIA L., HSIEH B. & SHAH R.J. (1967) The peptide chains of human plasmin. Mechanisms of activation of human plasminogen to plasmin. *Journal of Biological Chemistry*, **242**, 2333.

159 COLLEN D. & DE MAEYER L. (1975) Molecular biology of human plasminogen. I. Physio-chemical properties and microheterogeneity. *Thrombosis et Diathesis Haemorrhagica*, **34**, 396.

160 COLLEN D., ONG E.B. & JOHNSTON A.J. (1975) Human plasminogen; *in-vitro* and *in-vivo* evidence for the biological integrity of NH_2-terminal glutamic acid plasminogen. *Thrombosis Research*, **7**, 515.

161 ROBBINS K.C., SUMMARIA L. & BARLOW G.H. (1975) Activation of plasminogen. In: *Proteases and Biological Control* (ed. Reich E., Rifkind D.B. & Shaw E.), p. 305. Cold Spring Harbor Conferences on Cell Proliferation, Vol. II. Cold Spring Harbor Laboratory, New York.

162 THORSEN S. (1975) Differences in the binding of native plasminogen and plasminogen modified by proteolytic degradation. *Biochimica et Biophysica Acta*, **393**, 55.

163 KAKKAR V.V. (1978) Advances in thrombolytic therapy. In: *Fibrinolysis: Current Fundamental and Clinical Concepts* (ed. Gaffney P.J. & Balkuv-Ulutin S.), p. 191. Academic Press, London.

164 RABINER S.F., GOLDFINE I.D., HART A., SUMMARIA L. & ROBBINS K.C. (1969) Radio-immunoassay of human plasminogen and plasmin. *Journal of Laboratory and Clinical Medicine*, **74**, 265.

165 MANNUCCI P.M., STABILINI R., BRAGOTTI R., MARASINI B. & AGOSTORI A. (1971) Enzymatic and immunochemical determination of plasminogen and plasmin in different physiological and pathological states. *Journal of Clinical Pathology*, **24**, 228.

166 NANNINGA L.B. (1975) Molar concentrations of fibrinolytic components, especially free fibrinolysis *in vivo*. *Thrombosis et Diathesis Haemorrhagica*, **33**, 244.

167 MARKUS G., EVES J.L. & HOBIKA G.H. (1976) Activator activities of the transient forms of the human plasminogen–streptokinase complex during its proteolytic conversion to the stable activator complex. *Journal of Biological Chemistry*, **251**, 6495.

168 SUMMARIA L. & ROBBINS K.C. (1976) Isolation of a human plasmin-derived, functionally active, light (B) chain capable of forming with streptokinase and equimolar light (B) chain streptokinase complex with plasminogen activator activity. *Journal of Biological Chemistry*, **251**, 5810.

169 LANDMAN H. (1978) Biochemistry of the factors of the fibrinolytic system. In: *Fibrinolytics and Antifibrinolytics* (ed. Markwardt F.), p. 3. Springer-Verlag, Berlin.

170 REMMERT L.F. & COHEN P. (1949) Partial purification and properties of a proteolytic enzyme of human serum. *Journal of Biological Chemistry*, **181**, 431.

171 COLLEN D. & VERSTRAETE M. (1975) Molecular biology of human plasminogen. II. Metabolism in physiological and some pathological conditions in man. *Thrombosis et Diathesis Haemorrhagica*, **34**, 403.

172 ALBRECHTSEN O.K. (1957) The fibrinolytic activity of human tissues. *British Journal of Haematology*, **3**, 284.

173 ASTRUP T. (1966) Tissue activators of plasminogen. *Federation Proceedings*, **25**, 42.

174 ASTRUP T. (1978) Fibrinolysis: an overview. In: *Progress in Chemical Fibrinolysis and Thrombolysis* (ed. Davidson J.F.), Vol. 3, p. 1. Raven Press, New York.

175 TODD A.S. (1959) The histological localisation of fibrinolytic activator. *Journal of Pathology and Bacteriology*, **78**, 281.

176 TODD A.S. (1964) Localisation of fibrinolytic activity in tissues. *British Medical Bulletin*, **20**, 210.

177 NILSSON I.M. & PANDOLFI M. (1970) Fibrinolytic activity of the vascular wall. *Thrombosis et Diathesis Haemorrhagica*, Suppl. **40**, 231.

178 SEMAR M., SKOZA L. & JOHNSON A.J. (1969) Partial purification and properties of a plasminogen activator from human erythrocytes. *Journal of Clinical Investigation*, **48**, 1777.

179 EKERT H., FRIEDLANDER I. & HARDISTY R.M. (1970) The rôle of platelets in fibrinolysis. Studies on the plasminogen activator and antiplasmin activity of platelets. *British Journal of Haematology*, **18**, 575.

180 DAVIDSON J.F., McNICOL G.P., FRANK G.L., ANDERSON T.J. & DOUGLAS A.S. (1969) Plasminogen-activator-producing tumour. *British Medical Journal*, **i**, 88.

181 CHRISTMAN J.K., ACS G., SILAGI S. & SILVERSTEIN S.C. (1975) Plasminogen activator: biochemical characterisation and correlation with tumorigenicity. In: *Proteases and Biological Control* (ed. Reich E., Rifkind D.B. & Shaw E.), Vol. II, p. 827. Cold Spring Harbor Conferences on Cell Proliferation. Cold Spring Harbor Laboratory, New York.

182 SOBEL G.W., MOHLER S.R., JONES N.W., DOWDY A.B.C. & GUEST M.M. (1952) Urokinase: an activator of plasma profibrinolysis extracted from urine. *American Journal of Physiology*, **171**, 768.

183 BERNIK M.B. & KWAAN H.C. (1969) Plasminogen activator activity in cultures from human tissues. An immunological and histochemical study. *Journal of Clinical Investigation*, **48**, 1740.

184 BARLOW G.H., RUETER A. & TRIBBY I. (1975) Production of plasminogen activator by tissue culture technique. In: *Proteases and Biological Control* (ed. Reich E., Rifkind D.B. & Shaw E.), Vol. II. p. 325. Cold

Spring Harbor Conferences on Cell Proliferation. Cold Spring Harbor Laboratory, New York.

185 McCLINTOCK D.K. & BELL P.H. (1971) The mechanism of activation of human plasminogen by streptokinase. *Biochemical and Biophysical Research Communications*, **43**, 694.

186 SUMMARIA L., ROBBINS K.C. & BARLOW G.H. (1971) Dissociation of the equimolar human plasmin–streptokinase complex. Partial characterisation of the isolated plasmin and streptokinase moieties. *Journal of Biological Chemistry*, **246**, 2136.

187 SUMMARIA L., ARZADON L., BERNABE P. & ROBBINS K.C. (1974) The interaction of streptokinase with human, cat, dog, and rabbit plasminogen. The fragmentation of streptokinase in the equimolar plasminogen–streptokinase complexes. *Journal of Biological Chemistry*, **249**, 4760.

188 WULF R.J. & MERTZ E.T. (1969) Plasminogen. VIII. Species specificity of streptokinase. *Canadian Journal of Biochemistry*, **47**, 927.

189 SUMMARIA L., LING C.-M., GROSKOPF W.R. & ROBBINS K.C. (1968) The active site of bovine plasminogen activator. Interaction of streptokinase with human plasminogen and plasmin. *Journal of Biological Chemistry*, **243**, 144.

190 BUCK F.F., HUMMEL B.C. & DE RENZO E.C. (1968) Interaction of streptokinase and human plasminogen. V. Studies of the nature and mechanism of formation of the enzymatic site of the activator complex. *Journal of Biological Chemistry*, **243**, 3648.

191 BROCKWAY W.J. & CASTELLINE F.J. (1974) A characterisation of native streptokinase and altered streptokinase isolated from a human plasminogen activator complex. *Biochemistry*, **13**, 1063.

192 ÅBERG M. & NILSSON I.M. (1975) Fibrinolytic response to venous occlusion and vasopressin in health and thrombotic disease. In: *Progress in Clinical Fibrinolysis and Thrombolysis* (ed. Davidson J.F., Sanara H.M. & Desnoyers P.C.), Vol. I, p. 121. Raven Press, New York.

193 CASH J.D. (1975) Short term enhancement of plasminogen activator *in vivo* by drugs. *Thrombosis et Diathesis Haemorrhagica*, **34**, 648.

194 BRITTON B.J., WOOD W.G., SMITH M., HAWKEY C. & IRVING M.H. (1976) The effect of β-adrenergic blockade upon exercise-induced changes in blood coagulation and fibrinolysis. *Thrombosis and Haemostasis*, **35**, 396.

195 AOKI N. & VON KAULLA K.N. (1971) Human serum plasminogen anti-activator: distinction from antiplasmin. *American Journal of Physiology*, **220**, 1137.

196 AUERSWALD W., BINDER B. & DOLESCHEL W. (1971) Angiokinase-molecular weight of proteins representing a perivascular plasminogen activator. *Thrombosis et Diathesis Haemorrhagica*, **26**, 411.

197 CASH J.D. & ALLAN A.G.F. (1967) The fibrinolytic response to moderate exercise and intravenous adrenaline in the same subjects. *British Journal of Haematology*, **13**, 376.

198 NIEWIAROWSKI S. & PROU-WARTELLE O. (1959) Rôle du facteur contact (Facteur Hageman) dans la fibrinolyse. *Thrombosis et Diathesis Haemorrhagica*, **3**, 593.

199 IATRIDIS S.G. & FERGUSON J.H. (1961) Effect of surface and Hageman factor on the endogenous or spontaneous

activation of the fibrinolytic system. *Thrombosis et Diathesis Haemorrhagica*, **6**, 411.

200 OGSTON D., OGSTON C.M., RATNOFF O.D. & FORBES C.D. (1969) Studies of a complex mechanism for the activation of plasminogen by kaolin and by chloroform: the participation of Hageman factor and additional co-factors. *Journal of Clinical Investigation*, **48**, 1786.

201 SAITO H., RATNOFF O.D. & DONALDSON V.H. (1974) Defective activation of clotting, fibrinolytic and permeability enhancing systems in human Fletcher trait plasma. *Circulation Research*, **34**, 641.

202 DONALDSON V.H., GLUECK V.I. & MILLER M.A. (1975) Kininogen deficiency and defective surface activation of blood coagulation and fibrinolysis in a kindred with Fitzgerald trait. *Abstract Vth Congress International Society Thrombosis and Haemostasis*, Paris.

203 COLEMAN R.W. (1969) Activation of plasminogen by human plasma kallikrein. *Biochemical and Biophysical Research Communications*, **35**, 273.

204 LAAKE K. & VENNEROD A.U. (1974) Studies on the separation of pre-kallikrein plasminogen proactivator and factor XI in human plasma. *Thrombosis Research*, **4**, 285.

205 KAPLAN A.P. & AUSTEN K.F. (1972) The fibrinolytic pathway of human plasma. Isolation and characterisation of the plasminogen proactivator. *Journal of Experimental Medicine*, **136**, 1378.

206 ASTRUP T. & ROSA A.T. (1974) A plasminogen proactivator–activator system in human blood effective in absence of Hageman factor. *Thrombosis Research*, **4**, 609.

207 GANS H. (1964) Fibrinolytic properties of proteases derived from human, dog and rabbit leukocytes. *Thrombosis et Diathesis Haemorrhagica*, **10**, 379.

208 GOLDSTEIN I.M., WUNSCHMAN B., ASTRUP T. & HENDERSON E.S. (1971) Effects of bacterial endotoxin on the fibrinolytic activity of normal human leukocytes. *Blood*, **37**, 447.

209 MARKWARDT F. (1978) Naturally occurring inhibitors of fibrinolysis. In: *Fibrinolytics and Antifibrinolytics* (ed. Markwardt F.), p. 487. Springer-Verlag, Berlin.

210 SCHWICK H.G., HEIMBURGER N. & HAUPT H. (1967) Antiproteinasen des Humanserums. *Zeitschrift für die Gesamte innere Medizin und ihre Grenzgebiete (Leipzig)*, **21**, 193.

211 CRAWFORD G.P.M., OGSTON D. & DOUGLAS A.S. (1976) The contribution of plasma protease inhibitors to antiplasmin activity in man. *Clinical Science and Molecular Medicine*, **51**, 215.

212 MOROI M. & AOKI N. (1976) Isolation and characterisation of an α_2-plasmin inhibitor from human plasma. A novel proteinase inhibitor, which inhibits activator-induced clot lysis. *Journal of Biological Chemistry*, **251**, 5956.

213 COLLEN D. (1976) Identification and some properties of a new fast-reacting plasmin inhibitor in human plasma. *European Journal of Biochemistry*, **69**, 209.

214 HEIMBURGER N. (1975) Proteinase inhibitors of human plasma—their properties and control function. In: *Proteases and Biological Control*. (ed. Reich E., Rifkind D.B. & Shaw E.), Vol. II, p. 367. Cold Spring Harbor Conferences on Cell Proliferation. Cold Spring Harbor Laboratories, New York.

215 FORNASARI P.H., PANDOLFI M. & ASTEDT B. (1976) On the proteolytic inhibitory effect of human fetal and neoplastic tissues. *Thrombosis Research*, **8**, 829.

216 LIEDHOLM P. (1975) On fibrinolysis in reproduction. *Acta Obstetricia et Gynecologica Scandinavica.* Suppl. **4**, 1.

217 MCNICOL G.P., GALE S.G. & DOUGLAS A.S. (1963) *In-vitro* and *in-vivo* studies of a preparation of uro-kinase. *British Medical Journal*, **i**, 909.

218 LAURITSEN O.S. (1968) Urokinase inhibitor in human plasma. *Scandinavian Journal of Clinical and Laboratory Investigation*, **22**, 314.

219 HEDNER U. (1973) Studies on an inhibitor of plas-minogen activation in human serum. *Thrombosis et Diathesis Haemorrhagica*, **30**, 414.

220 BENNETT N.B. (1967) A method for the quantitative assay of inhibitor of plasminogen activation in human serum. *Thrombosis et Diathesis Haemorrhagica*, **17**, 12.

221 AOKI N. & MOROI M. (1974) Distinction of serum in-hibitor of activator-induced clot lysis from α_1-antitryp-sin. *Proceedings of the Society for Experimental Biology and Medicine*, **146**, 567.

222 BEATTIE A., OGSTON D., BENNETT B. & DOUGLAS A.S. (1976) Inhibitors of plasminogen activation in human blood. *British Journal of Haematology*, **32**, 135.

223 LOWE G.D.O. & PRENTICE C.R.M. (1980) The labora-tory investigation of fibrinolysis. In: *Blood Coagulation and Haemostasis—A Practical Guide*, (ed. Thomson J.), p. 222. Churchill-Livingstone, London.

224 FEARNLEY G.R., BALMFORTH G. & FEARNLEY E. (1957) Evidence of a diurnal fibrinolytic rhythm; with a simple method of measuring natural fibrinolysis. *Clinical Science*, **16**, 645.

225 CHOHAN I.S., VERMYLEN J., SINGH I., BALAKRISHNAN K. & VERSTRAETE M. (1975) Sodium acetate buffer—a diluent of choice in the clot lysis time technique. *Thrombosis et Diathesis Haemorrhagica*, **33**, 226.

226 KLUFT C. & BRAKMAN P. (1975) Effect of flufenamate on euglobulin fibrinolysis: involvement of C1-inactiva-tor. In: *Progress in Chemical Fibrinolysis and Thrombo-lysis* (ed. Davidson J.F., Samama M.M. & Desnoyers P.C.), Vol. I, p. 375. Raven Press, New York.

227 ASTRUP T. & MULLERTZ S. (1952) The fibrin plate method for estimating fibrinolytic activity. *Archives of Biochemistry and Biophysics*, **40**, 346.

228 HAVERKATE F. & BRAKMAN P. (1975) Fibrin plate assay. In: *Progress in Chemical Fibrinolysis and Thrombolysis* (ed. Davidson J.F., Samama M.M. & Desnoyers P.C.), Vol. I, p. 151. Raven Press, New York.

229 WALKER I.D., DAVIDSON J.F., HUTTON I. & LAWRIE T.D.V. (1977) Disordered 'fibrinolytic potential' in coronary heart disease. *Thrombosis Research*, **10**, 509.

230 CASH J.D. & WOODFIELD D.G. (1967) Fibrinolytic re-sponse to moderate exhaustive and prolonged exercise in normal subjects. *Nature (London)*, **215**, 628.

231 CASH J.D. & MCGILL R.C. (1969) Fibrinolytic response to moderate exercise in young male diabetics and non-diabetics. *Journal of Clinical Pathology*, **22**, 32.

232 SORIA J., SORIA C. & SAMAMA M.M. (1978) A plas-minogen assay using a chromogenic synthetic substrate: results from clinical work and from studies of thrombo-lysis. In: *Progress in Chemical Fibrinolysis and Thrombo-lysis* (ed. Davidson J.F., Rowan R.M., Samama M.M.

& Desnoyers P.C.), Vol. III, p. 337. Raven Press, New York.

233 BERG W., KORSAN-BENGSTEN K. & YGGE J. (1966) Determination of plasminogen in human plasma by the lysis time method. *Thrombosis et Diathesis Haemor-rhagica*, **21**, 1.

234 BRAKMAN P. & TRAAS D.W. (1976) Assay of plas-minogen in blood on fibrin plates. In: *Progress in Chemi-cal Fibrinolysis and Thrombolysis* (ed. Davidson J.F., Samama M.M. & Desnoyers P.C.), Vol. II, p. 79, Raven Press, New York.

235 LASSEN M. (1952) Heat denaturation of plasminogen in the fibrin plate method. *Acta Physiologica Scandinavica*, **27**, 371.

236 DERECHIN M. (1962) Hydrolysis of some casein frac-tions with plasmin. *Biochemistry*, **82**, 42.

237 ROBERTS P.S. (1960) The esterase activities of human plasmin during purification and subsequent activation by streptokinase or glycerol. *Journal of Biological Chemistry*, **235**, 2262.

238 SHERRY S., ALKJAERSIG N. & FLETCHER A.P. (1966) Activity of plasmin and streptokinase-activator on substituted arginine and lysine esters. *Thrombosis et Diathesis Haemorrhagica*, **16**, 18.

239 GANROT P.O. & NILEHN J.E. (1968) Immunochemical determination of human plasminogen. *Clinica Chimica Acta*, **22**, 335.

240 NUSSENZWEIG V., SELIGMAN M. & GRABER P. (1961) Les produits de dégradation du fibrinogène par la plasmine. II. Étude immunologique: mise en évidence d'anticorps antifibrinogène notif possédant des spécificités différ-entes. *Annales de l'Institut Pasteur*, **100**, 490.

241 STORIKO K. (1968) Normal values for 23 different human plasma proteins determined by single radial immunodiffusion. *Blut*, **16**, 200.

242 GAFFNEY P.J. & DOBOS P. (1971) A structural aspect of human fibrinogen suggested by its plasmin degradation. *Federation of European Biochemical Societies Letters*, **15**, 13.

243 MARDER V.J. & BUDZYNSKI A.Z. 1975) Data for defin-ing fibrinogen and its plasmic degradation products. *Thrombosis et Diathesis Haemorrhagica*, **33**, 199.

244 MOSESSON M.W., FINLAYSON J.S. & GALANAKIS D.K. (1973) The essential covalent structure of human fibrinogen evinced by analysis of derivatives formed during plasmic hydrolysis. *Journal of Biological Chemistry*, **249**, 7913.

245 FURLAN M., KEMP G. & BECK E.A. (1975) Plasmic degradation of human fibrinogen. III. Molecular model of the plasmin-resistant disulphide knot in monomeric fragment D. *Biochimica et Biophysica Acta*, **400**, 95.

246 MARDER V.J., SCHULMAN N.R. & CARROLL W.R. (1969) High molecular weight derivatives of human fibrinogen produced by plasmin. 1. Physiochemical and immuno-logical characterisation. *Journal of Biological Chemis-try*, **244**, 2111.

247 KOWALSKA-LOTH B., GARDLUND B., EGBERG N. & BLOMBÄCK B. (1973) Plasmic degradation products of human fibrinogen. 1. Chemical and immunological reactions between fragment E and N-DSK. *Thrombosis Research*, **2**, 423.

248 LATALLO Z.S., BUDZYNSKI A.Z., LIPINSKI B. & KOW-ALSKI E. (1964) Inhibition of thrombin and of fibrin

polymerisation. Two activities derived from plasmin-digested fibrinogen. *Nature (London)*, **203**, 1184.

249 LIPINSKY B., WEGRZYNOWICZ Z., BUDZYNSKI A., KOPEC M., LATALLO Z.S. & KOWALSKI E. (1967) Soluble un-clottable complexes formed in the presence of fibrinogen degradation products (FDPs) during the fibrinogen-fibrin conversion and their potential significance in pathology. *Thrombosis et Diathesis Haemorrhagica*, **17**, 65.

250 DUDEK G.A., KLOCZEWIAK M., BUDZYNSKI A.Z., LATALLO Z.S. & KOPEC M. (1970) Characterisation and comparison of macromolecular end products of fibrinogen and fibrin proteolysis by plasmin. *Biochimica et Biophysica Acta*, **214**, 44.

251 PIZZO S.V., SCHWARTZ M.L., HILL R.L. & MCKEE P.A. (1973) The effect of plasmin on the subunit structure of human fibrin. *Journal of Biological Chemistry*, **248**, 4574.

252 SLADE C.L., PIZZO S.V., TAYLOR L.M. JR, STEINMAN H.M. & MCKEE P.A. (1976) Characterisation of fragment E from fibrinogen and cross-linked fibrin. *Journal of Biological Chemistry*, **251**, 1591.

253 GAFFNEY P.J. & BRASHER M. (1973) Subunit structure of the plasmin-induced degradation products of cross linked fibrin. *Biochimica et Biophysica Acta*, **295**, 308.

254 KOPEC M., TEISSEYRE E., DUDEK-WEJCIECHOWSKA G., KLOCZEWIAK M., PANKIEWICZ A. & LATALLO Z.S. (1973) Studies on the 'Double D' fragment from stabilised bovine fibrin. *Thrombosis Research*, **2**, 283.

255 KOWALSKI E., KOPEC M. & WEGRZYNOWICZ Z. (1964) Influence of fibrinogen degradation products (FDP) on platelet aggregation, adhesiveness, and viscous meta-morphosis. *Thrombosis et Diathesis Haemorrhagica*, **10**, 406.

256 JERUSHALMY Z. & ZUCKER M.B. (1966) Some effects of fibrinogen degradation products (FDP) on blood plate-lets. *Thrombosis et Diathesis Haemorrhagica*, **15**, 413.

257 STACHURSKA J., LATALLO Z.S. & KOPEC M. (1970) Inhi-bition of platelet aggregation by dialysable fibrinogen degradation products (FDP). *Thrombosis et Diathesis Haemorrhagica*, **23**, 91.

258 KOPEC M., BUDZYNSKI A.Z., STACHURSKA J., WEGR-ZYNOWICZ Z. & KOWALSKI E. (1966) Studies on the mechanism of interference by fibrinogen degradation products (DFP) with the platelet function. Rôle of fibrinogen in the platelet atmosphere. *Thrombosis et Diathesis Haemorrhagica*, **15**, 476.

259 OLSSON P.I. & JOHNSSON H. (1972) Interference of acetyl salicylic acid, heparin and fibrinogen degradation pro-ducts in haemostasis of Reptilase-defibrinated dogs. *Thrombosis Research*, **1**, 135.

260 PRENTICE C.R.M., TURPIE A.G.G., HASSANEIN A.A. & MCNICOL G.P. (1969) Changes in platelet behaviour during Arvin therapy. *Lancet*, **i**, 644.

261 BULUK K. & MALOFIEJEW M. (1969) The pharmacologi-cal properties of fibrinogen degradation products. *British Journal of Pharmacology*, **35**, 79.

262 TAKAKI A., VAMAGUCHI T. & OHSATO K. (1974) Kinin-like activities of the synthetic low molecular weight fragment of fibrinogen degradation products. *Thrombosis et Diathesis Haemorrhagica*, **32**, 350.

263 MALOFIEJEW M. (1971) The biological and pharmacolo-gical properties of some fibrinogen degradation pro-ducts. *Scandinavian Journal of Haematology*, Suppl. **13**, 303.

264 KOWALSKI E., BUDZYNSKI A.Z., KOPEC M., LATALLO Z.S., LIPINSKI B. & WEGRZYNOWICZ Z. (1965) Circulat-ing fibrinogen degradation products (FDP) in dog blood after intravenous thrombin infusion. *Thrombosis et Diathesis Haemorrhagica*, **13**, 12.

265 LATALLO Z.S., WEGRZYNOWICZ Z., BUDZYNSKI A.Z. & KOPEC M. (1971) Effect of protamine sulphate on the solubility of fibrinogen, its derivatives and other plasma proteins. *Scandinavian Journal of Haematology*, Suppl. **13**, 151.

266 ALLINGTON M.J. (1967) Fibrinogen and fibrin degrada-tion products and the clumping of staphylococci by serum. *British Journal of Haematology*, **13**, 550.

267 MARDER V.J., MATCHETT M.O. & SHERRY S. (1971) Detection of serum fibrinogen and fibrin degradation products. Comparison of six technics using purified products and application in clinical studies. *American Journal of Medicine*, **51**, 71.

268 MARDER V.J. (1968) Immunologic structure of fibrinogen and its plasmin degradation products: theoretical and clinical considerations. In: *Fibrinogen* (ed. Laki K.). Marcel Dekker, New York.

269 NILEHN J.E. (1967) Separation and estimation of 'split products' of fibrinogen and fibrin in human serum. *Thrombosis et Diathesis Haemorrhagica*, **18**, 487.

270 MELLIGER E.J. (1970) Detection of fibrinogen degrada-tion products by use of antibody-coated latex particles. *Thrombosis et Diathesis Haemorrhagica*, **23**, 211.

271 MERSKEY C., LALEZARI P. & JOHNSON A.J. (1969) A rapid, simple, sensitive method for measuring fibrinoly-tic split products in human serum. *Proceedings of the Society for Experimental Biology and Medicine*, **131**, 871.

272 ALLINGTON M.J. (1971) Detection of fibrin(ogen) degra-dation products by a latex clumping method. *Scandina-vian Journal of Haematology*, Suppl. **13**, 115.

273 HEDNER U. (1976) Immunochemical methods for deter-mination of fibrin/fibrinogen degradation products. In: *Progress in Chemical Fibrinolysis and Thrombolysis* (ed. Davidson J.F., Samama M.M. & Desnoyers P.C.), Vol. II, p. 107. Raven Press, New York.

274 GORDON Y.V., MARTIN M.J., MCNEILE A.T. & CHARD T. (1973) Specific and sensitive determination of fibrinogen degradation products by radioimmunoassay. *Lancet*, **ii**, 1168.

275 CHEN J.P. & SHURLEY H.M. (1975) A simple, efficient production of neoantigenic antisera against fibrinolytic degradation products: radio-immunoassay of fragment E. *Thrombosis Research*, **7**, 425.

Chapter 28
Hereditary disorders of blood coagulation

A. L. BLOOM

Nearly all the hereditary disorders of blood coagulation are due to deficiency or abnormality of single clotting factors, but in a few instances defects of two or more factors have been described. The importance of this relatively uncommon group of disorders is out of proportion to their numerical incidence; not only have they provided unique information concerning the physiology of haemostasis but their clinical management has imposed immense burdens on national blood transfusion services and other resources. In this chapter the pathogenesis, diagnosis and management of individual disorders will be reviewed systematically.

INCIDENCE

Classical haemophilia (A) is the least uncommon in this group of disorders and occurs in all ethnic groups. Its incidence in developed countries such as the UK is about 5:100 000 [1] but there is probably a smaller number of less severely affected patients who are not yet diagnosed but who may bleed excessively after trauma. The incidence of haemophilia B (Christmas disease) is usually quoted as about one-fifth that of haemophilia A except in certain defined localities where, perhaps due to the presence of a very large family, it is a little more common. An example is the famous Tenna family of Switzerland [2]. The incidence of von Willebrand's disease is much more difficult to determine because of its variable nature. The overall incidence of heterozygous von Willebrand's disease in the author's centre is about one-half that of haemophilia A, but the incidence of homozygous patients who suffer frequent haemarthroses and other haemophilic lesions is very much less—only about one per million of the population. Inherited deficiencies and defects of other coagulation factors severe enough to cause a significant tendency to bleed are very uncommon, and together contribute only a few per cent of the total. Factor-XI deficiency is largely confined to Ashkenazi Jews [3].

NOMENCLATURE

The Roman numerical nomenclature of coagulation factors was established in 1962 by international convention [4] although some workers still prefer to retain descriptive or trivial names. The term 'haemophilia' is sometimes used in a general sense referring to all inherited coagulation defects, or more often and specifically to deficiencies of factor VIII ('classical haemophilia', haemophilia A), factor IX (haemophilia B) or factor XI (haemophilia C). In this chapter the terms 'haemophilia A' will be used for sex-linked factor-VIII deficiency and 'haemophilia B' for factor-IX deficiency (Christmas disease). Other deficiencies will be referred to by their Roman number or by the trivial or descriptive name of the relevant factor as seems appropriate by common usage.

It has become conventional to refer to molecular variants of individual clotting factors by the town or location in which the abnormality was first described, for example fibrinogen 'Detroit', prothrombin 'Barcelona', factor-X 'Friuli', etc. Graham et al. [5] tried to establish a more rational nomenclature but their recommendations have not been widely adopted.

Additional to the problem of general nomenclature is the specific problem of the nomenclature of factor VIII. The physiological aspects of this factor have been reviewed by Bloom [8, 9] and are described in Chapter 27. The symbols used in this chapter to describe factor-VIII-related activities are shown in Table 28.1.

HAEMOPHILIA A

Historical background
A familial bleeding disorder of males was recognized as early as the second century in the Talmud [11]. The subsequent growth of knowledge concerning haemophilia has been the subject of several reviews [12–16]. Apparently the first case of haemophilia was recorded in the modern medical literature in 1793 [17] but a more detailed account was presented by Otto [18] and the first major study was that of Bulloch & Fildes [19].

Table 28.1. Nomenclature of factor VIII

Name	Symbol	Activity
Factor-VIII-related von Willebrand factor	VIIIR:WF	Required for platelet adhesion in primary haemostasis
Factor-VIII-related ristocetin cofactor of human plasma	RiCoF	Required for mediating ristocetin-induced platelet aggregation
Factor-VIII-related antigen	VIIIR:Ag	The antigenic determinants of the molecule which exhibits VIIIR:WF (and presumably RiCoF) activity
Procoagulant factor VIII	VIIIC	Antihaemophilic-factor activity— the procoagulant activity deficient in haemophilia A
Factor-VIII-clotting antigen [10]	VIIICAg	The antigenic determinants associated with VIIIC activity

The name 'haemophilia' was introduced in 1823 and the sex-linked nature of the disease was suspected as long ago as 1813 [13]. This was more firmly established after the work of Bulloch & Fildes and confirmed in haemophilic dogs by selective mating, including the breeding of 'true' bleeder females [20]. It is likely, however, that most cases of 'female haemophilia' in fact represent patients with von Willebrand's disease or heterozygotes for haemophilia A with inactivation of most of the normal X chromosomes in the cells which synthesize VIIIC.

The slow clotting of haemophilic blood was documented by Wright [21] but Sahli (cited by Brinkhous [13]) noted the accelerated clotting *in vitro* with tissue extract and the normal fibrinogen levels. Soon afterwards Weil [22] and Addis [23] demonstrated the corrective effect of normal blood and plasma *in vitro*. Unfortunately Addis attributed the corrective effect of a plasma fraction to the presence of prothrombin and hence concluded that haemophilia was due to a prothrombin defect. Because prothrombin was found to be normal in haemophilia Addis' findings were forgotten or ignored for 25 years. Patek & Taylor [24] then showed that a fraction derived from normal plasma accelerated the clotting of haemophilic blood and this was subsequently referred to as antihaemophilic globulin (AHG) or antihaemophilic factor (AHF). Brinkhous [25] demonstrated that prothrombin conversion to thrombin was impaired in haemophilic blood unless normal blood 'thromboplastin' was added and later both he [26] and Quick [27] concluded that AHG reacted with platelets to generate thromboplastin. These observations were extended into clinical practice by the establishment of the prothrombin consumption index [28] and the thromboplastin generation test [29] as standard clinical tests. Thus by

1952, haemophilia was defined as a sex-linked haemorrhagic disease characterized by defective prothrombin consumption and deficiency of AHG. The International Committee on Blood Clotting Factors later assigned the Roman numeral VIII to AHF [4], by which symbol it is now generally known (*vide supra*).

In 1947 Pavlovsky [30] showed that mixing blood of certain haemophilic patients *in vitro* with that of most others resulted in mutual correction of the clotting defects. Later Aggeler *et al.* [31] studied one such patient who had no affected family members and Biggs *et al.* [32], in studies on several patients, showed that the inheritance pattern was similar to that of classical haemophilia. The defect in these patients was shown to be due to lack of a clotting factor with characteristics different from that of AHG in that it was present in normal serum and was adsorbed by inorganic adsorbents. The factor was termed plasma thromboplastin component (PTC) by Aggeler *et al.* and Christmas factor by Biggs *et al.* after the name of the propositus of their series. Later, Christmas factor was allocated the Roman numeral IX by international convention. It is interesting to speculate that the 'haemophilia' which affected European royalty may in fact have been Christmas disease and not 'classical' haemophilia, but there is now no definite way of determining this.

Pathogenesis

The corrective effect of normal blood in haemophiliacs is consistent with deficiency in the patient's blood of a normal component. Even so, various workers have considered that the basic defect in haemophilia is the presence of an abnormal inhibitor [33, 34] but these concepts seem to have arisen from misinterpretation or laboratory artefacts [35, 36]. In any case, the great majority of uncomplicated haemophiliacs respond quantitatively to treatment as though the disorder were simply due to a deficiency of VIIIC. These proposed 'inhibitors' have always been distinguished from the antibodies to VIIIC which develop in the blood of a small proportion of haemophiliacs and others and which make these patients resistant to treatment with factor VIII. It is thus generally accepted that haemophilia is due to a deficiency of normal VIIIC activity.

The biochemical nature of normal factor VIII is described in Chapter 27 and briefly alluded to below. Haemophilia may be expected to result from failure to synthesize VIIIC, reduced synthesis of VIIIC, or synthesis of an abnormal variant of the protein carrying VIIIC activity (Fig. 28.1). The concept of abnormal coagulation-factor variants was introduced by Fantl *et al.* [37] who noted that the plasma of a patient with haemophilia B neutralized an inhibitor of Factor IX. Similar evidence for inherited variants of VIIIC has been derived from studies with acquired inhibitors. These develop in some haemophilic patients after treatment and are thought to be alloantibodies; autoantibodies with similar specificity sometimes develop in non-haemophilic patients. Using antibody neutralization tests with coagulation techniques, cross-reacting material (CRM) was found in about

10% of haemophilic patients [38–40]. The term 'haemophilia A+' was given by Denson *et al.* [38] to this type and it was concluded that such patients synthesize abnormal variants of VIIIC. Later studies in antibody excess suggested the presence of CRM in an even greater number of patients [41]. Peake *et al.* [10, 42] have recently described an immunoradiometric assay for factor-VIII clotting antigen (VIIICAg) using alloantibodies, but CRM was found in only one of 30 haemophilic kindreds tested. Although there are technical reasons for these discrepancies the nature of possible molecular variants of VIIIC in haemophilia awaits further characterization. It should be noted that xenogeneic antisera to factor VIII such as those raised in rabbits react primarily with VIIIR:Ag. This is deficient or abnormal in von Willebrand's disease and is synthesized under autosomal control (see below). Thus the presence in haemophilic plasma of material giving precipitin reactions with rabbit antisera does not necessarily indicate the presence of abnormal VIIIC. In fact, levels of VIIIR:Ag are normal or even raised in haemophilia [43]. Whilst available evidence indicates that VIIIR:Ag is synthesized in vascular endothelial cells [44, 45], there is no evidence that VIIIC is synthesized at this site [9]. It is possible that VIIIR:Ag circulates to another site, possibly in the liver [46], where it is joined to, or activated to acquire, VIIIC activity by an X-linked system. The basic

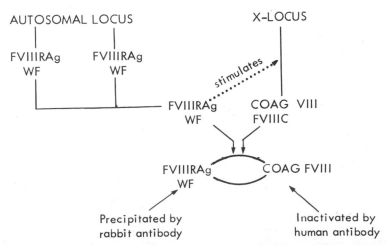

Fig. 28.1. Diagrammatic representation of the inheritance and relationship of factor-VIII-related antigen (VIIIR:Ag) and procoagulant factor VIII (VIIIC). Haemophilia is due to deficiency or abnormality of VIIIC. von Willebrand's disease is due primarily to deficiency or abnormality of VIIIR:Ag with secondary deficiency of VIIIC. The dotted arrow indicates the possibility that VIIIR:Ag stimulates the synthesis or release of VIIIC or is altered to acquire this activity (e.g. the secondary transfusion response in von Willebrand's disease). (Modified from Bloom [404].)

pathogenetic defect in haemophilia at the cellular level thus remains to be determined.

A condition indistinguishable from human haemophilia A also occurs in dogs [47], horses [48] and cats [49].

Clinical features

The clinical features of haemophilia A and haemophilia B are indistinguishable from each other and apart from the mode of inheritance, those of several other inherited coagulation deficiencies are very similar. The features of haemophilia A will therefore be described in detail. Important differences or additional features exhibited by patients with other disorders will be described in the appropriate sections of the chapter.

Haemophilia is an episodic disorder in which abnormally prolonged or repeated bleeding occurs at one or a few sites at a time, characteristically producing a haematoma, haemathrosis or other form of deep tissue bleeding; excessive external blood loss may occur but it is very much less common. Primary haemostasis at capillary level is normal so that petechiae and purpura do not occur and, except for haematuria, excessive mucous-membrane bleeding is not a usual feature. Secondary haemostasis is impaired so that bleeding occurs from larger vessels—hence the tendency to form deep tissue haematomata following trauma. Bleeding is particularly likely to occur when the effect of the initial vasoconstrictive axon reflex wanes—hence the tendency to delayed intra-operative or post-operative bleeding.

The severity of the disease usually parallels the degree of deficiency of VIIIC. This varies from family to family but is usually constant within kindreds, possibly because the same abnormality is inherited at molecular level. In addition the underlying defect is almost always constant throughout life in individual patients, though a remarkable variant called Heckathorn's disease has been described [50], in which levels of VIIIC fluctuate from time to time.

Levels of VIIIC in normal individuals expressed in terms of average normal plasma (100 u/dl) range from 50–200 u/dl [51]. One unit of VIIIC is defined as that present in one millilitre of fresh normal plasma as standardized internationally and it should be noted that local standards may be influenced by ethnic characteristics; thus VIIIC levels are high in the black African population [52]. It is convenient to express VIIIC activity in u/dl; the numerical value is then similar to the older expressions of activity as a percentage of average normal. Haemophiliacs do not suffer from excessive bleeding unless plasma levels are below 30 u/dl. Definition of individuals with levels between 30 and 50 u/dl as 'haemophiliacs' is therefore one of semantics. Patients (and hence families) are usually classified as 'severe', 'moderate' and 'mild' [53]. Severely affected patients usually have VIIIC levels of 0–1 u/dl. Such patients may suffer frequent and apparently 'spontaneous' haemarthroses etc., although probably bleeding is triggered by trauma which is not noticed. Moderately affected patients have VIIIC levels of 2–5 u/dl: they suffer from occasional haemarthroses or deep tissue haematomata, usually after noticeable trauma. Sometimes chronic arthropathy develops in one particular joint, which then becomes a 'target' joint for frequent episodes of bleeding, so that the patient may appear to be more severely affected than would be suggested by his basal VIIIC level. Occasionally patients with 2–5 u/dl of VIIIC activity *in vitro* behave clinically in a manner more appropriate to those with lower levels. In these patients it is possible that the VIIIC measured *in vitro* is not effective *in vivo*. Conversely, occasional patients with 0–1 u/dl VIIIC activity seldom bleed; this is particularly true of well-built, muscular individuals of phlegmatic temperament. Mildly affected patients have over 5 u/dl VIIIC activity and bleed excessively only after significant trauma such as dental or general surgery. Although most patients fall roughly into the above clinical categories there is a considerable degree of overlap so that the disease represents a continuous spectrum of severity.

Factor-VIIIC levels are reduced in haemophilic infants even at birth, but they rarely present with bleeding in the neonatal period. Occasionally progressively enlarging cephalhaematoma, intramuscular haematoma from vitamin-K injection or excessive bleeding after circumcision are observed. Bleeding from small accidental lacerations of the frenulum or from the gum or tongue as the primary dentition erupts are common and quite difficult to manage. Lumpy subcutaneous haematomata develop as the child grows older and begins to crawl, and haemarthroses make their appearance as the toddler walks. In severely affected patients the most commonly presenting and important lesions are haemarthroses, haematomata at various sites (sometimes with neurological signs from nerve compression), haematuria and, later, gastro-intestinal bleeding. Intracranial bleeding, although serious, is relatively uncommon. Less severely affected patients may not present until they participate in the more vigorous activities of later childhood or until they undergo dental extractions or other forms of surgical trauma. Mildly affected adults may first present with bleeding due to other pathological lesions such as peptic ulcer. Patients sometimes experience 'good' and 'bad' periods during which the incidence of episodes of bleeding vary; the 'bad' patches are sometimes related to emotional disturbances at home, work or school, such as examinations, etc.

Haemarthroses

Haemarthroses are the characteristic and most important haemophilic lesions. Almost any joint may be
involved but those which bear weight or are relatively
unstable, such as the knee, ankle, elbow, hip, shoulder
and wrist, are affected most frequently, whilst some,
such as the temporo-mandibular joint, are rarely
affected. Initially blood may be reabsorbed, leaving no
obvious residual effect, but repeated intra-articular
bleeding leads to gross joint changes [54]. The synovial
membrane becomes thickened and coloured with
haemosiderin; villi develop and extend into the articular space. It has been suggested that the iron stimulates
secretion of proteinases by the synovium, with resultant progression of the arthropathy even in the absence
of further bleeding [55].

Later the cartilage becomes irregular, loose fragments may detach and it is completely lost in the
weight-bearing areas with consequent narrowing of
the joint space. Cystic changes occur in the bones
underlying the articular surfaces, possibly from
haemorrhage in the bone or adjacent subperiosteal
area. Osteoporosis is common as a result of hyper-
aemia and decreased use. Eventually damage to the
stabilizing structures of the joint results in varying
degrees of disorganization and sometimes fibrous
ankylosis, but bony ankylosis is uncommon [56, 57].
These pathological changes refer to the natural progression of the untreated disease and will be modified
by treatment. Radiological changes occur in almost
all joints which have been subjected to even a few
episodes of bleeding and reflect the pathological
lesions described above. In the knee there is enlargement of the intercondylar fossa and the patella sometimes appears to have a squared-off distal edge—
although this is not characteristic only of haemophilia
(Fig. 28.2). At the elbow there may be overgrowth of
the head of the radius and in the ankle the articular top
of the talus may be flattened. In the hip the radiological
appearances may superficially resemble those of Legg–
Perthes disease although there are significant differences. These changes are comprehensively reviewed by
Schreiber [57] and Jaffe [58]. Clinically, bleeding into a
joint is heralded by the onset of discomfort which
usually develops rapidly to more or less severe pain,
especially in the case of elbows and knees but also in
other joints. There is often, but not invariably, a
history of trauma; in mild cases the degree of trauma
needed is correspondingly greater. If untreated, the
joint becomes swollen, hot and tense with restricted
movement. Sometimes even when there is clearly a
joint effusion present, the extra-articular tissues are
also involved, and bruising may develop around the
joint, possibly as a result of the initial trauma.
Eventually the signs and symptoms subside but if

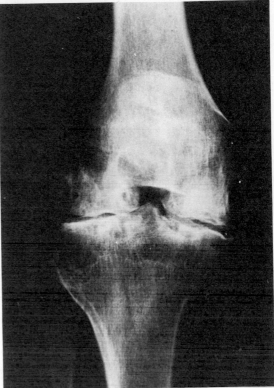

Fig. 28.2. Radiographic appearances of a haemophilic knee
showing loss of joint space, erosion of articular surfaces and
adjacent small cystic areas with enlargement of the intercondylar fossa (from *Haemostasis and Thrombosis*, ed. A. L.
Bloom & D. P. Thomas, Churchill-Livingstone, 1981).

treatment has not been quickly or effectively administered chronic arthropathy is likely to develop. Sometimes, particularly in the knee, the joint cavity appears
to become distensible, with thickening of the periarticular tissues, and sometimes a small chronic residual effusion. The knee may then become the site of
repeated painless haemarthroses which are particularly difficult to manage. Eventually there may
be flexion, genu valgum with external rotation and
posterior subluxation of the tibia producing a characteristic haemophilic gait. Limitation of both flexion
and extension of the elbows is also quite common.
Except when antibodies to VIIIC develop (see p. 1120),
the development and progression of these joint
changes should be more or less retarded by effective
treatment, atlhough it is becoming apparent that
complete prevention will be very difficult to achieve.

Haematomata

Superficial bruising and lumpy subcutaneous haematomata are the rule in severe haemophilia but rarely
need treatment unless very extensive. On the other

hand, haematomata in muscles are extremely important. They present as a painful swelling following trauma of greater or lesser severity. In the limbs—e.g. the calf, thigh or forearm—they may, if not effectively treated, lead to considerable oedema and necrosis; if the haematoma is large there may be shock and anaemia, and jaundice of the prehepatic type may develop. At first there may be no superficial discoloration but this may appear later as the blood tracks to the surface. Necrosis of the overlying skin may occur if the haematoma 'points'. Ischaemic damage may occur distally leading to Volkmann's contracture or other similar lesions. Bleeding into the calf muscles may predispose to subsequent haemarthroses of the ankle and shortening of the tendo achilles. Compression of peripheral nerves may lead to neuropathies with pain, paraesthesiae and sensory loss as well as motor impairment and muscular atrophy. The femoral and ulnar nerves are most frequently involved.

Haematomata in two sites deserve special consideration:

Iliopsoas haematoma. This occurs within the iliopsoas sheath just above the inguinal ligament or more superiorly. There is frequently a characteristic clinical history of mild trauma—coughing, for example, or a bumpy automobile journey—followed by abdominal pain leading to spasm of the iliopsoas muscle, flexion of the hip and involvement of the femoral nerve or plexus leading to sensory loss over the patella or more extensively, as well as weakness of the quadriceps muscle which rapidly wastes. A mass may be palpable in the iliac fossa and pressure on it may exacerbate the neurological symptoms. In the acute phase the flexion of the hip and neurological changes are important differential points from acute appendicitis when the lesion is situated in the right iliac fossa. The lesion may be visualized radiologically as bulging of the psoas shadow or displacement of the ureter on intravenous pyelography, but it can be followed conveniently during therapy by ultrasonic scan or computer-assisted tomography.

Sublingual haematoma. This occurs usually as a result of intra-oral trauma and presents as a blue submucous mass which may displace the tongue and extend into the neck causing respiratory obstruction. Sublingual or peritonsillar haematoma in a haemophiliac is a real medical emergency calling for high-level antihaemophilic therapy.

Blood cysts and pseudotumours
If haematomata are inadequately treated for any reason cystic collections of blood may develop [59]. Once established, untreated haemophilic cysts develop thick fibrous walls and contain thick liver-like inspissated clot. They tend to enlarge from repeated bleeding, with infiltration of fascial planes, erosion of adjacent structures and eventually rupture and infection. Complete surgical excision is then usually needed to prevent death, although regression may occur after prolonged antihaemophilic treatment. Pseudotumour or cysts may occur at any site—e.g. the heel (Fig. 28.3) or the temporal bone [60]—but are commonest in the pelvis and thigh where they may lead to pathological fracture [61].

Renal-tract abnormalities
Microscopic haematuria is often detectable in patients with severe haemophilia. Gross haematuria is also common but probably occurs less frequently in patients who often receive antihaemophilic therapy. Blood loss may be prolonged but is usually small and transfusion is seldom required. Persistent gross haematuria should be treated by specific antihaemophilic therapy in spite of the risk of inducing clot colic, but antifibrinolytic therapy is definitely contraindicated because of the risk of inducing ureteric obstruction. In the last decade there have been several reports of obstructive uropathies in haemophilia [62–66] as well as lesions resembling papillary necrosis [64]. A recent study [67], however, suggests that renal function is well preserved and the condition does not appear to be related to analgesic abuse. There are probably multiple causes for the renal-tract abnormalities related to intrarenal or periureteric bleeding, but these are not always apparent.

Neurological and intracranial bleeding
Compression neuropathies from intramuscular or other localized sites of bleeding are relatively common and may lead to both sensory and motor loss with loss of deep tendon reflexes and muscular wasting. Although such neurological lesions are often reversible, recovery may be incomplete with permanent sequelae. Intracranial bleeding was at one time thought to be relatively common but its frequency has diminished, possibly as a result of prompt antihaemophilic therapy for head injuries. Nevertheless, intracranial bleeding is still the commonest cause of death in haemophilia [1] and in spite of prolonged intensive treatment 47% of patients in one recent series had neurological sequelae [68]. The presence of hypertension may predispose to intracranial bleeding [69]. It is important to treat all significant head injuries with antihaemophilic therapy, and to differentiate intracranial bleeding from other neurological conditions such as meningitis, if necessary by lumbar puncture under cover of appropriate high-level treatment. Non-invasive diagnostic techniques such as computer-

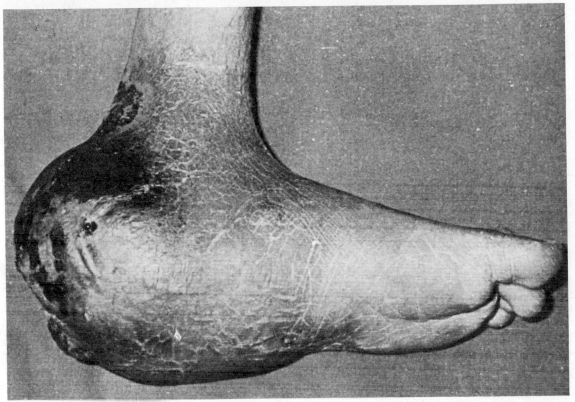

Fig. 28.3. Haemophilic cyst of the heel which involved the talus and calcaneum. The cyst was surgically excised.

assisted tomography are invaluable. Haemorrhage into the spinal canal is uncommon but can lead to paraplegia.

Other sites of bleeding
Epistaxes are common in haemophilia but are rarely the presenting symptom. Gastro-intestinal bleeding is also common but is sometimes associated with the presence of an organic lesion such as peptic ulcer, particularly in mildly or moderately affected patients. Bleeding of this type occurring for the first time in later life should be investigated as in a normal person, and endoscopy may be needed.

Bleeding after injury
For a given injury haemophilic bleeding is not more rapid than normal, but continues for longer, either continuously or intermittently. Superficial skin wounds or pin pricks do not usually bleed abnormally because haemostasis depends upon platelet and vascular integrity which is normal. Full thickness skin cuts may stop bleeding in the usual time but bleeding may recur later as vasodilatation occurs, with small move-

ments of the wound or as ligatures loosen; a local haematoma will interrupt healing and if effective treatment is not applied bleeding may then continue intermittently for several weeks. Crushing injuries with spreading haematomata are particularly likely to give trouble.

Dental extractions. These provide a sensitive index of the haemostatic defect, but exfoliation of primary dentition is not usually accompanied by excessive bleeding. Extraction of secondary dentition, if untreated, may be followed by prolonged intermittent bleeding lasting several days or weeks. Mild haemophiliacs often present in this way but prolonged bleeding may not follow every extraction.

Surgical operations. These are commonly followed by extensive bruising, prolonged bleeding, haematoma formation, wound disruption and infection unless effective treatment is applied (see below). Sometimes in relatively bloodless operations where the muscle layers are separated carefully and sutured in layers the wounds may heal relatively normally, but this cannot be relied on even in mildly affected patients. Indeed it is in the latter type of person for whom adequate treatment has not been given that the most disastrous results are sometimes seen.

The above account of physical haemophilic lesions refers in the main to untreated patients. Moderately affected patients are, of course, much less incapacitated, whilst mildly affected patients may lead a virtually normal life. The natural history of severe haemophilia used to be one of progressive incapacity leading to early death, often in the third decade. The use of intensive and early antihaemophilic therapy as described below has completely altered the prognosis but has not entirely prevented progressive arthropathies and has led to the appearance of other complications. The prognosis of treated haemophilia will be described later.

Other effects of the disease
Haemophilia affects every member of an affected person's immediate family. The mother usually has feelings of guilt because she has transmitted the disease to her son. Unaffected siblings may be relatively neglected, and may suffer psychological disturbance as well as their affected brother. For the affected boy, repeated episodes of painful bleeding interrupt school and work, and disorganize social life. Educational progress may be slowed and employment difficult to find and keep. Some haemophiliacs come to be dependent on the Social Services and are unable or unwilling to find employment; such lack of self-sufficiency may lead to problems as their parents grow old. Others react aggressively to their disorder by running unnecessary risks at sport or work [70], but some show great courage and develop self-reliant mature personalities. Recent progress in home therapy has considerably modified the psychological climate for many haemophilic families.

Diagnosis
The full clinical picture of severe haemophilia will readily suggest the diagnosis. Mild haemophilia should be considered in any male presenting with prolonged post-traumatic bleeding; it is important to make the diagnosis before surgery or dental extractions so that appropriate treatment can be initiated beforehand.

History
It is convenient first to enquire about the various manifestations of apparently spontaneous or post-traumatic bleeding site by site. A history of lumpy subcutaneous bruises, muscle haematomata or joint swelling is particularly relevant; petechiae and purpura are never seen in the uncomplicated haemophilias.

Enquiry should be made concerning a history and frequency of haematuria. The effect of surgical intervention and dental extractions should be documented for each episode, taking care not to forget circumcision and tonsillectomy, which are not considered as operations by some patients. Even slight bleeding persisting for over 24 hours after dental extractions, particularly if recurrent, should be investigated, but occasionally mildly affected patients can escape excessive bleeding after extractions. On the other hand, tonsillectomy presents a particularly severe haemostatic challenge and a history of uneventful surgery of this type makes haemophilia very unlikely. It should be noted that except in the rare, possibly homozygous, severe form of disease, haemarthroses are uncommon in von Willebrand's disease (p. 1125), whereas mucous-membrane bleeding frequently occurs. Details of the family history should be systematically recorded, including complete sex distribution as well as the presence or absence of a history of bleeding, and a family tree should be drawn.

Clinical examination
This should include an assessment of the joints and of any residual neuro-muscular disability—although of course in many patients with mild haemophilia and in young severely affected haemophiliacs there may be no abnormal physical signs.

Laboratory investigation
The platelet count and primary bleeding time are characteristically normal in haemophilia. The prothrombin time is also normal because the extrinsic system (*in vitro*) is intact. The whole-blood clotting time may be prolonged in some severely affected patients but is often within the normal range and usually so in those who are mildly affected. The prothrombin consumption index is more often abnormal but is also a poor screening test for haemophilia. Characteristically an abnormality may be demonstrated by tests of the intrinsic pathway, e.g. Hicks–Pitney thromboplastin screening test (TST) and the activated partial thromboplastin time (e.g. kaolin cephalin clotting time—KCCT). In patients with normal prothrombin time and abnormal KCCT or TST the level of VIIIC (or, if normal, of factor IX) should be determined and the presence of an inhibitor excluded by mixing tests with normal plasma. If facilities for assays are not available, correction tests with alumina-adsorbed normal plasma and aged normal serum may be performed. Alumina removes the vitamin-K-dependent factors (II, VII, IX and X) but not most of factors V and VIIIC; factors V and VIIIC are inactivated during clotting but serum contains significant amounts of factors VII, IX and X. Theoreti-

cally, normal alumina plasma corrects the KCCT in haemophilia A and normal serum corrects the KCCT in haemophilia B. Unfortunately, unless carefully prepared, normal serum often contains activated intermediaries (e.g. factor Xa) which may correct the KCCT in both types of haemophilia. Similar diagnostic conclusions can be reached by applying the full thromboplastin generation test, but this is rarely required. The diagnosis should also be confirmed by noting lack of mutual correction in mixtures of patient's plasma with that of a known haemophiliac of appropriate type. The tests based on the TST are usually abnormal in patients with VIIIC levels below 20–25 u/dl. If these tests are normal but the patient has a convincing history of a tendency to bleed, specific assays should be performed, because significant post-surgical bleeding can occur even in very mildly affected patients. In infants, the initial diagnosis may have to be provisional because of sampling problems. In this case the diagnosis must be confirmed on a good venous sample obtained from a superficial vein when the child is older. Except in an emergency requiring treatment, no attempts should be made to obtain blood from jugular, femoral or other deep veins, because of the real risk of causing a serious haematoma at a time when intravenous access for therapy is difficult. Levels of VIIIR:Ag measured with xenogeneic antisera are normal or even raised in haemophilia [43], as are ristocetin-induced platelet aggregation in platelet-rich plasma (PRP) and the level of ristocetin cofactor activity [71], but these tests should be performed to exclude the possibility of von Willebrand's disease [72].

Assays of VIIIC have recently come under renewed scrutiny. There are two main types: one-stage assays based on the KCCT and two-stage assays based on the TST. The two-stage assays are usually more precise [73] but they do not necessarily give identical results to one-stage assays, particularly when comparing plasma and factor-VIII concentrates [74]. Standardization of the VIIIC assay has been considerably improved by the introduction of biological standards [75]. Recently an immunoradiometric assay for the factor-VIII clotting antigen (VIIICAg) has been described and levels are reduced in most haemophilic kindreds [42].

The laboratory diagnosis of haemophilia is described in detail in several recent monographs [76–79].

Inheritance

In haemophilia A the failure to synthesize or release VIIIC normally is due to a mutation on the X chromosome at a locus closely linked to those for a glucose-6-phosphate dehydrogenase (G6PD) variant, for deutan colour blindness [80, 81] and possibly X-linked hereditary persistence of fetal haemoglobin [82], but not to that for the Xg^z blood group and haemophilia B [83]. Affected males are hemizygous for the mutant allele which they carry on their single X chromosome. Heterozygous females carry the allele on one X-chromosome and although true homozygosity is possible, its calculated frequency is only about $3:10^9$ [84]. The possible causes of lifelong factor-VIII deficiency in women have been discussed in detail by Barrow & Graham [84]: they include the diagnosis of von Willebrand's disease and extreme lyonization (see below), as well as abnormalities of the X chromosome.

Detection of carriers

Carrier detection is important in genetic counselling and may enable individual heterozygotes to consider several eugenic options including family planning, fetal sexing and, more recently, prenatal diagnosis of haemophilia. Information which may be of value in carrier detection may be derived from:
1 genetic data;
2 linkage studies; and
3 haematological studies.

Genetic data. Haemophilias A and B are inherited as X-linked characteristics. Thus, all the sons of a haemophiliac will be normal and all his daughters will be carriers. At each pregnancy the sons of an obligate carrier will each have a 0·5 chance of being an affected hemizygote and the daughters will each have a 0·5 chance of being a heterozygous carrier. In about 30–40% of cases of haemophilia there is no preceding family history [15]. This may be due to passage of the carrier state through several generations of females without affected male relatives, or to a mutation, the rate of which has been estimated at $1·3–4·2 \times 10^{-5}$ [86]. Obligate carriers are thus:
1 a woman whose father is a haemophiliac;
2 a woman who has had more than one haemophilic son at separate births; and
3 a woman with a haemophilic son and well-documented evidence of a haemophilic relative on her side of the family.

It is essential that the diagnosis is supported by reliable coagulation factor assays in the affected male relative, not only to differentiate between factor-VIII and factor-IX deficiency, but also to determine the severity of the disorder in that particular family and to exclude the possibility that the condition is some other haemostatic defect (e.g. of platelets). Such disorders are often loosely described as 'haemophilia' by patients, relatives or even their medical advisors.

Possible carriers include:
1 women with a haemophilic relative on the maternal side, but who have not yet given birth to an affected son; and

2 women who have given birth to a haemophilic son but who have no other family history of haemophilia.

It should be noted that the *a priori* probability that a female member of a haemophilic family is a carrier may be modified by the presence of affected or normal individuals within the kindred and quantitated by the application of Bayes' theorem [87].

Linkage studies. These are possible in some families with haemophilia A because the genetic locus for VIIIC is closely linked to that for G6PD [80]. This linkage has been used for carrier detection in a Negro family by electrophoretic determination of G6PD variants [88].

Haematological studies. In normal individuals the level of VIIIC is usually within the range 50–200 u/dl with a mean value of about 100 u/dl. As described in Chapter 26 and briefly discussed above, VIIIC is biologically, and possibly biochemically, related to VIIIR:Ag so that they are quantitatively related to each other in normal individuals. In male haemophiliacs, whereas levels of X-chromosomally controlled VIIIC are reduced, those of autosomally controlled VIIIR:Ag are not. Consistent with these facts, levels of VIIIC in carriers of haemophilia follow the general principles of Lyon's hypothesis [89]. Average values of VIIIC are about 50 u/dl [90] but they vary depending upon the frequency of inactivation of the maternally or paternally derived X chromosomes in the somatic cells which synthesize VIIIC. Thus levels of VIIIC may be reduced in some carriers of haemophilia, and this fact alone is of some value in carrier detection [90]. Indeed in some cases, as would be expected, the reduction of VIIIC may be such that the carrier suffers from clinically excessive bleeding resembling, to a greater or lesser degree, that seen in males with haemophilia. However, as in the case of hemizygous males, levels of VIIIR:Ag are normal in carriers. The ratio of VIIIC to VIIIR:Ag is therefore reduced in most carriers of haemophilia A and this ratio can also be incorporated into statistical assessments much more effectively than consideration of VIIIC levels alone [91, 92]. These data have been applied to carrier detection using regression analysis, but can be more effectively applied together with pedigree data by other forms of statistical discrimination to derive a final probability ratio. The reader is referred to a Bulletin of the World Health Organisation [93] and to Graham [94]. It should be noted, however, that just as a certain proportion of carriers have reduced VIIIC levels as described above, so a small proportion, variously estimated as up to 16%, will be indistinguishable from normal. It is therefore always unwise to assure a possible carrier that she is, in fact, normal.

Prenatal diagnosis

The object of carrier detection is to assist in genetic counselling and to try to give a statistical probability to individual women that they may or may not be carriers. Further counselling includes advice on genetic risks, family planning and the possibility of amniocentesis, fetal sexing and termination of male pregnancies. The possibility of prenatal diagnosis of haemophilia would allow a carrier to have a normal son and reduce the number of elective pregnancy terminations. Until recently the technological barriers to fetal blood sampling for VIIIC assay seemed to present insurmountable obstacles to prenatal diagnosis. Improvements in fetoscopic sampling techniques [95] as well as the development of an appropriate coagulation assay [96] and an immunoradiometric assay for VIIIC antigen which is less susceptible to coagulation artefacts [10, 97] have made successful prenatal diagnosis of haemophilia possible [96, 98], although the methods still remain to be fully validated [99].

In addition to direct fetal blood sampling, prenatal diagnosis—like carrier detection—has been successfully attempted by linkage studies on variants of G6PD, in this case in cultured amniotic fetal cells from a black woman [100]. As originally suggested by McCurdy [88], this method may also be applicable in other ethnic groups.

Management

There is no permanent cure for haemophilia nor, except in certain special circumstances, is continuous prophylaxis feasible in a way analogous to that used in diabetes. Patients and their families must therefore try to adapt to the limitations imposed by their disability. Although the emphasis of management in developed countries has shifted from hospital to home, many old problems remain and some serious new ones have emerged. Nevertheless the mainstay of modern management is the provision and effective use of blood-coagulation-factor concentrates.

TREATMENT OF BLEEDING EPISODES

Sources and administration of factor VIII

Transfusion of whole blood is an efficient method of administration of factor VIII only when massive acute blood loss requires the rapid transfusion of large volumes and when fresh blood is available, because factor VIII is only present in the plasma and it deteriorates on storage. In practice, external blood loss is not usually a major problem in haemophilia and in any case it is generally far more effective and convenient to administer factor-VIII concentrate rapidly (see below) to correct haemostasis, and stored whole blood or plasma protein solutions according to general haemodynamic requirements.

If fresh or fresh-frozen plasma (FFP) alone is given, the dose of factor VIII in a single administration is limited by the volume of plasma the circulation can receive without overloading, say 15–20 ml/kg for an average, otherwise healthy, man over a period of one hour. The concentration of VIIIC in FFP is less than that normally circulating because of dilution with anticoagulant, lability during venesection and separation, and loss during freezing and thawing; the average is about 60 u/dl [101]. Simple calculation will indicate that it is not usually possible to raise the plasma level of VIIIC by more than 15–20 u/dl by infusing a single dose of FFP. Concentrates of factor VIII allow the dose to be given in a small volume over a short period of time without risk of overloading the circulation; they are obligatory for safe management of major surgery and serious bleeding.

Cryoprecipitate. If plasma is snap-frozen and allowed to thaw in the cold, i.e. between +4°C and +8°C, then VIIIC activity remains in suspension with other cryoproteins (e.g. fibrinogen) and can be separated by centrifugation. Pool & Shannon [102] described a simple process for producing cryoprecipitate from single donors in a closed-bag system. The bags are stored at −30°C and when needed the contents are thawed at 37°C, pooled and administered by intravenous infusion or injection. The specific activity of VIIIC in cryoprecipitate is purified about seven to 20 times [103] but there is considerable variation in individual packs [104] so that it is essential to use pooled doses, if necessary discarding the unused balance in the case of infants. In one study an average donor pack of cryoprecipitate contained about 85 units [104] but this figure falls to about 70 u/pack with mass production. Cryoprecipitate must therefore be assessed locally and doses calculated accordingly, but there is no reason why it cannot be used even for major surgery without overloading the patient's circulation.

Freeze-dried concentrates. An ether-precipitated fraction [105] or Cohn fraction 1–0 [106] was used for some years but required relatively large volumes of solvent. Small-volume freeze-dried concentrates have recently been developed, usually using cryo-ethanol precipitation (intermediate purity) with about 30 times purification, or high-potency cryo-polyethylene glycol-glycine precipitation with 100–400 times purification. The high-potency concentrates have the advantage of very rapid solubility and low protein content. The advantages and disadvantages of concentrates are shown in Table 28.2.

Animal concentrates. Both porcine and bovine factor VIII have been concentrated for therapeutic use. Recent commercial preparations of porcine factor VIII are soluble but cause thrombocytopenia because of the presence of 'platelet-aggregating factor' (PAF) [107]—a part of the factor-VIII complex analogous to human von Willebrand factor. In addition, resistance to treatment develops after about a week to 10 days, presumably as a result of antibody formation, but it has not been established if these are directed mainly against VIIIR:Ag or VIIIC. Very recently porcine VIIIC has been separated from PAF for therapeutic use in resistant patients (see p. 1120).

Calculation of the dose. Following infusion of FFP the maximum rise of VIIIC expected is about 2 u/dl/unit infused/kg body weight [101]. Recovery of modern

Table 28.2. The advantages and disadvantages of freeze-dried factor-VIII concentrate and cryoprecipitate

	Cryoprecipitate	Freeze-dried
Advantages	1 made locally 2 small plasma pool 3 relatively cheap 4 gives adequate factor-VIII levels 5 may reduce bleeding time in vWd	1 standardized product, pre-assayed 2 consistent low volume, easily made up 3 stored at 4°C 4 relatively long shelf-life 5 low protein content 6 low incidence of reactions 7 can be administered in large amounts (e.g. to antibody patients)
Disadvantages	1 unstandardized 2 awkward to make up 3 less suitable for home treatment 4 may cause reactions 5 needs storage at −30°C	1 cost 2 risk of hepatitis even if HBsAg excluded 3 iso-agglutinins and haemolysis 4 theoretical risk of denaturation of factor VIII 5 not effective in correcting bleeding time in vWd

concentrates in the patient's circulation is usually about 75–80% [108]. Bloom & Emmanuel [104] calculated that, on average, one pack of cryoprecipitate (85 u VIIIC) would raise the VIIIC level 2·5 u/dl in a 70 kg man, and this is still a good working rule applicable also to other concentrates. Doses can be scaled down or up from this proportionally. It should be appreciated that it is only necessary to calculate the dose approximately because there are large individual variations in recovery. Complicated formulae are therefore not necessary.

Fate of factor VIII. The concentration of VIII activity falls exponentially after infusion with a half-life of about 12 hours [109], but this may increase slightly with continued infusion, perhaps because high-molecular-weight (HMW) forms of FVIIIR:Ag (which 'carry' VIIIC activity) are removed rapidly from the circulation, to the reticulo-endothelial system, which may become saturated [110].

Methods of administration. Factor-VIII concentrate and FFP have to be given intravenously; FFP is given by drip infusion but freeze-dried concentrates and small doses of cryoprecipitate can be given by slow intravenous injection. When treatment is needed over prolonged periods it is economical to administer treatment by continuous infusion but this often leads to local thrombophlebitis, so that in practice concentrates are usually administered in divided doses once daily, every 12 hours or more frequently according to the lesion under treatment. It is important to conserve veins and cut-down should be avoided unless absolutely essential. Plastic cannulae inserted into the superior vena cava can be of value during surgery and construction of an arterio-venous fistula may facilitate access to superficial veins in the arms when frequent injections are needed. The recent claim by Hemker *et al.* [111] that oral administration of factor VIII packaged in liposomes resulted in prolonged elevation of plasma factor-VIII levels, if confirmed, could revolutionize the treatment of haemophilia as well as open many fascinating lines of study regarding the molecular structure of factor VIII.

MANAGEMENT OF DIFFERENT TYPES OF BLEEDING
The principles of intravenous therapy described above are applied in various clinical situations. It is useful to distinguish between episodes of bleeding arising apparently spontaneously or after minor injury and those following more severe injury, or after dental or general surgery.

Unless he has an anti-factor-VIII antibody, a haemophiliac should be given factor VIII as soon as it is reasonably suspected that he is bleeding. Sufficient evidence will be available from the patient's symptoms and his own assessment alone for treatment to be given immediately he presents. Any further medical observation or detailed physical examination should be deferred until after the patient has been treated. This policy is deliberately at variance with established practice in other clinical fields, but it must be realized that in haemophilia to delay treatment reduces its effectiveness, and that physical examination of an untreated patient may aggravate bleeding. It must be accepted that in a lifelong disorder the opinion of parents and patients that a bleed has commenced is usually correct and it is almost always an error of judgement to ignore the symptoms and await the development of signs. Indeed, this tenet forms a main rationale for home therapy.

Closed or 'spontaneous' bleeding

Musculo-skeletal lesions. As soon as it is reasonably certain that bleeding has occurred a suitable factor-VIII preparation is administered intravenously. The levels to be aimed for in treating various haemarthroses, haematomata and other lesions are outlined in Table 28.3. If a haemarthrosis is very tense or painful, aspiration of the joint may be of value, but in practice it is rarely needed. It has been recommended that factor-VIII concentrate should not be given until aspiration is concluded, in order to avoid clotting the blood in the joint. It is sometimes useful to prepare a light removable polystyrene splint, particularly for haemarthroses of ankle, knee and elbow. These can be worn for a few days after the event and especially at night, because bleeding sometimes recurs at that time, presumably as a result of involuntary movements.

No attempt should be made to aspirate or drain a haematoma unless there is a real risk of ischaemia, when formal decompression under full operative cover should be undertaken (see p. 1118). Patients with ilio-psoas haematomata will usually need admission to hospital, rest in bed and quite intensive factor-VIII therapy during the acute phase. Subsequent ambulation and physiotherapy in bed or in the pool may need additional cover. The resolution of the lesion can often be conveniently monitored by ultrasonic scan. Haematomata in the neck and sublingual haematomata are potentially very dangerous and require high-level factor-VIII therapy, but they usually then resolve rapidly.

Epistaxis. In haemophilia this is not very common but can be troublesome. If it does not respond to simple local measures a modest dose of factor VIII should be given. If the bleeding is recurrent, especially if from one nostril and not associated with coryza, cauterization of

Table 28.3. Guide to factor-VIII therapy in severe haemophilia (70 kg man)

| Lesion | Hospital treatment* | | Immediate home treatment* | |
	Dose (u)	Level (u/dl)	Dose (u)	Level (u/dl)
Early haemarthrosis of non-weight-bearing joints; early muscle haematoma	500–750 One dose usually sufficient	15–25	250	10
Haemarthrosis of knee, ankle, elbow	1000 Repeated next day if needed	30	500	15
Severe haemarthrosis, iliopsoas haematoma, etc.	1500 Repeated daily or more frequently as needed	50	Patient contacts centre for advice and transfer	
Dental extractions	1500 + antifibrinolytic therapy	> 50	Not applicable	
Minor surgery and injuries requiring sutures	1500 Repeated once or twice daily until healed	50	Not applicable	
Major surgery; head injuries and severe injury	3000 Repeated to maintain level > 40 u/dl until healed	100	1500 For significant head injury and contact centre for transfer	50

* Hospital treatment presupposes some delay, hence higher dosages.

Little's area may be needed as in normal people. This should be done by an experienced operator under cover of factor VIII. An antifibrinolytic agent may also be given.

Gastro-intestinal bleeding. This is relatively uncommon in haemophilia and often complicates an organic lesion. In the case of haematemesis, factor-VIII therapy should be administered and endoscopy performed to try to visualize the bleeding point. Especially in milder haemophiliacs, barium and other studies should be performed as with a haemostatically normal person, although the vigour with which the studies are pursued requires experienced clinical judgement.

Haematuria may occur in severe haemophilia without a demonstrable local lesion; a few haemophiliacs have numerous attacks whereas others remain relatively free of the symptom. Microscopic or 'chemical' haematuria is, however, often present on casual examination. The incidence of overt haematuria seems to be decreasing, possibly as a result of more frequent use of factor-VIII concentrates and home therapy. Mild haematuria may subside with rest alone but if it is severe or prolonged, several doses of factor VIII should be given in order to raise the VIIIC to peak levels of 50 u/dl. If too little is given, clot colic or obstruction may be precipitated without arresting the bleeding. Antifibrinolytic agents may induce obstructive uropathy [112, 113] and are contraindicated, especially as minor degrees of obstructive uropathy and other renal-tract lesions are, in any case, common in haemophilia (see above). Investigation of haematuria in a known haemophiliac requires careful judgement, but as with gastro-intestinal bleeding, it must be remembered that sufferers may also develop non-haemophilic lesions. Tight abdominal binders for intravenous pyelography should be used only with care, and invasive or endoscopic examinations require antihaemophilic cover.

Orthopaedic management. Many haemophiliacs who have suffered repeated bleeds into joints develop chronic arthropathies or contractures. Repeated painless haemarthroses into a chronically distended knee joint due to synovial hypertrophy are particularly difficult to manage. Synovectomy has been advocated for these [114] but the results of operation are still controversial [115, 116]; the role of synoviorthesis or chemical synovectomy, e.g. with radioactive gold [117], also remains to be established. Other orthopaedic manoeuvres may be needed to correct deformities: for flexion deformity of the knee, Stein & Dickson [118] recommended the use of the reversed dynamic sling and we have found this procedure useful, especially in children, even in the presence of antibody to factor VIII. Lengthening of the tendo achilles and other surgical procedures may also be required. Physiotherapy, especially in the pool, is an indispensible adjunct to muscular recovery, not only after operation, but during ambulation, from any serious neuromuscular or locomotor lesion. The orthopaedic aspects of haemophilia have been fully described in several reviews [118–122].

Bleeding after injury
Contrary to popular belief, external blood loss is not a conspicuous symptom in haemophilia except after serious injury. Minor injuries and cuts rarely cause trouble, but if intermittent bleeding does not respond to local pressure, application of topical thrombin or Russell's viper venom can be tried, although they are rarely very effective; a small dose of factor VIII is sometimes needed and for minor external bleeding can be supplemented with an antifibrinolytic agent. Small lacerations in the mouth can be troublesome in infants and if an excrescence of granulation tissue and a clot develops this should be removed manually with a piece of gauze after administration of factor VIII and necessary sedation. Suturing should be covered by factor VIII and treatment continued until healing is complete and the sutures removed. For superficial lacerations a single daily dose aiming for post-infusion levels of 50 u/dl will suffice. More extensive injuries should be treated as for surgery (see below).

Management of surgery. All forms of major surgery can be performed safely in haemophiliacs provided no antibody to factor VIII is present and provided certain rules are followed. Hepatitis antigen, liver function and general coagulation status, including prothrombin time, should be checked before operation. It should be emphasized that if adequate laboratory facilities for monitoring therapy and medical, nursing and physiotherapy staff specifically experienced in haemophilia management are not available, then surgery should not be attempted, even on patients with mild haemophilia, except in dire emergency: a procedure which may be dealt with routinely at a large haemophilia centre can monopolize the attention of the staff of a whole ward for several days or weeks if attempted at an inappropriate location.

It is impossible to guarantee adequate haemostasis, even in mild haemophilia, by the use of surgical technique alone—although good technique is obviously desirable. Blood vessels constrict when injured but bleeding may occur when they relax during the post-operative period if factor-VIII levels are inadequate. Ligated vessels are end-vessels: antihaemophilic factor administered only after ligation does not enter the vessel to reinforce the haemostatic plug. Ligatures loosen after operation and the ineffective plug may then be pushed out of the vessel, even if systemic levels of VIIIC are then adequate. Arterial bleeding may then recommence and disrupt the wound. It is therefore absolutely vital that adequate factor-VIII therapy is administered *before* the operation is commenced, and maintained throughout the operative and post-operative period until healing is complete. If levels are allowed to fall below 40 u/dl then movements of the wound may cause rebleeding, wound disruption, haematoma formation, infection and disaster. The surgeon should ensure meticulous surgical haemostasis, but excessive use of diathermy should be avoided. Drains may delay healing and are not necessary on account of haemophilia alone, if adequate treatment with factor VIII is available. Surgery should not be rushed; a major case such as excision of a large cyst should be scheduled as the only one on the list. Nursing procedures, use of bed pans, etc., should be delayed until after one of the daily doses of factor VIII; house-staff must therefore be instructed to administer one early in the day and not to relax the rules at weekends. Sutures should be left in for a few days longer than is customary in non-haemophilic patients. Healing is sometimes a little slow and secondary haemorrhage may occur at about 10 days, even with adequate VIII levels. Ambulation and mobilization may require additional factor-VIII cover.

Dental surgery in haemophilia. Haemophiliacs should have a dental examination every six months and receive appropriate instruction in dental hygiene. Fluoridation of water or use of appropriate medication is desirable. Local anaesthesia by gentle infiltration, particularly in the upper jaw, does not usually require factor-VIII therapy. More circumspection is required for procedures in the lower jaw because of the risk of sublingual haematoma, and factor-VIII therapy is certainly needed for submandibular block. Factor-VIII antibody should be excluded before undertaking any dental procedure which entails risk of bleeding or haematoma formation.

Dental extractions can be undertaken safely following administration of factor VIII sufficient to raise levels of VIIIC to over 50 u/dl in combination with antifibrinolytic and antibiotic therapy [123]. Additional doses of factor VIII are then only needed if bleeding occurs. The provision of dental splints is not usually necessary: indeed, if not well fitting, they may actually cause bleeding as the gum shrinks.

There are many other individual considerations in planning both surgical procedure and antihaemophilic cover for different operations, for details of which larger texts should be consulted [124–127].

Ancillary methods of treatment

Local therapy with topical thrombin and snake venom have been mentioned above but are not very effective. Corticosteroids have been advocated for the prevention of haemarthroses and in the control of haematuria, but the evidence that they are effective is not convincing [128–130].

Antifibrinolytic drugs. These have a definite part to play in dental extractions (see above) and in the treatment of mucous-membrane bleeding, particularly in the mouth. They may therefore reduce the amount of factor-VIII concentrate needed. Epsilon-amino-caproic acid (EACA) (0·1 g/kg) may be given intravenously for the first dose if the patient is to be anaesthetized and can subsequently be given orally in similar doses six-hourly. The drug sometimes causes gastro-intestinal upset and tranexamic acid (cyclokapron) (0·015 g/kg) may be used instead. Antifibrinolytic therapy is of doubtful value in other forms of surgery and has the theoretical drawback that it may delay resolution of clot should a haematoma form. Similar reservations apply to its use in haemarthroses and although this objection may not in fact be valid there is, equally, no convincing evidence of its efficacy in the treatment or prevention of these lesions.

Deamino-d-arginine vasopressin. Following observation during neurohypophyseal stimulation, Mannucci et al. [131, 132] found that a non-vasoactive analogue of vasopressin, deamino-d-arginine vasopressin (DDAVP), raised the levels of VIIIC (and VIIIR:Ag) in patients with mild haemophilia and von Willebrand's disease sufficiently to perform minor surgery or dental extractions. The effect of the drug wears off after a day or two and it is not effective in severe disease. Additionally, DDAVP also stimulates release of plasminogen activator and concomitant treatment with tranexamic acid is desirable [133]. This combination may have a limited role in haemophilia therapy especially as it may prevent exposure to hepatitis viruses in a susceptible group of patients (see below).

Relief of pain. The relief of pain is an important aspect of haemophilia management. Probably the most effective analgesic is specific antihaemophilic therapy with factor-VIII concentrate, but in the acute phase of an episode of bleeding more rapidly effective relief may be needed. Chronic arthropathies are painful even in the absence of active bleeding. Drugs which inhibit platelet function such as aspirin and other anti-rheumatic drugs are clearly contraindicated, since they may induce bleeding. Paracetamol may be too mild to be effective except in children. Thus drug dependence may become a problem and, especially in large cities, even drug addiction. Nevertheless, it is cruel and counterproductive to withhold potent analgesics in the presence of obvious severe pain, particularly during acute episodes of bleeding. Appropriate drugs and combinations have been reviewed by Jones [134] and include promazine, 25 mg, for intermittent acute pain and dihydrocodeine (DF118), pentazocine and dextropropoxyphene for chronic pain. As concluded by Jones, relief of pain in specific joints may eventually require surgical intervention such as arthrodesis, whilst early and effective treatment with factor-VIII concentrate is the best method of prophylaxis.

COMPLICATIONS OF TREATMENT WITH FACTOR-VIII CONCENTRATE

General complications

Pulmonary oedema due to overloading of the circulation is rarely seen now that FFP has given way to concentrates. Nevertheless, large infusions should be covered by a diuretic and care taken in patients with already compromised haemodynamic equilibrium. Allergic reactions are relatively common with repeated plasma or cryoprecipitate infusions but less so with purified concentrates: they include headache, urticaria, etc., and may be relieved by an antihistamine, e.g. chlorpheniramine (piriton), 4–10 mg by mouth or intravenously. Antihistamine drugs may stabilize platelet membranes [135] and may theoretically compromise haemostasis in haemophilia; they should probably not be used routinely but experience suggests that this is not a major problem. For severe anaphylactoid-type reactions intravenous hydrocortisone (50–100 mg) may be needed. In a small number of patients severe pulmonary reactions may occur, with oedema unrelated to fluid overload [136, 137], and may be fatal unless energetically treated. Haemolytic anaemia has always been a potential complication of antihaemophilic therapy: unless group-specific plasma, cryoprecipitate or concentrates are used there is a risk of inducing haemolysis in the recipient owing to the presence of anti-A or anti-B isoagglutinins, especially when large amounts of concentrates are administered [138, 139]. At one time it was thought that the high fibrinogen levels achieved, particularly after the use of the older concentrates, might also contribute to haemolysis by causing red-cell sludging. Selected batches of commercial concentrates are obtainable which the manufacturers claim to have low isoagglutinin titres, but these are not needed routinely.

The two most important complications of treatment are the development of antibodies to factor VIII and various forms of hepatitis.

Antibodies to factor VIII

These develop in a small proportion of treated haemophiliacs, variously estimated at between five and 14% [1, 140, 141] of large populations, and render the patients more or less resistant to specific treatment. They usually arise in severely affected patients but occasionally in those who are only mildly affected [142]. They presumably develop because of antigenic differences between the patient's factor VIII (if any) and that of one or more donors. The antibodies are IgG immunoglobulins with restricted heterogeneity, often $\gamma G_4 k$, although in other patients oligoclonal types may coexist. They usually react specifically with the VIIIC activity and antigens of the factor-VIII molecular complex. Patients can be divided into 'high responders', who exhibit brisk anamnestic responses following infusion of factor VIII, and 'poor responders' (in an immunological sense), who have little anamnestic response; the latter group often have low antibody titres. The strength of the antibodies has been assessed by various methods, utilizing different relative concentrations of antigen and antibody and incubation times [143, 144]; a method popular in the USA (Bethesda units) was described by Kasper *et al.* [145]. The reactions of some antibodies follow second-order kinetics, whilst those of others are more complex and it is doubtful if it is possible to make other than an approximate estimate of their relative strength. One thing which is clear, however, is that one unit of antibody, assessed by whatever method, does not necessarily neutralize the activity of one unit of VIIIC *in vivo*. In general one 'old Oxford' unit [143] is approximately equivalent to two Bethesda units and to three to four 'new Oxford' [144] units, but this relationship is not always valid.

Development of antibodies to VIIIC represents the most serious complication of haemophilia therapy. Management of bleeding in these patients has been reviewed by Blatt *et al.* [146] and Bloom [147].

Immunosuppression with steroids, azathioprine or cyclophosphamide has given disappointing results, unlike the situation in non-haemophilic patients with auto-antibodies to VIIIC [148]. In haemophilia, immunosuppression has most chance of success if given during the actual immunizing course—when this is detected [149].

Plasmapheresis can be used to reduce the antibody concentration during a bleeding episode or, using saline replacement, to prepare a patient for elective surgery [150].

Activated clotting factors. Some batches of factor-IX-prothrombin concentrates used for the treatment of haemophilia B have been observed to be thrombogenic, in spite of manufacturers' precautions to exclude this effect. It is thought that such concentrates contain 'activated' clotting intermediates and Kurczynski & Penner [151] claimed that such 'accidentally' activated preparations were effective in securing haemostasis in haemophilia-A patients with antibodies to VIIIC. Presumably they 'bypassed' the activity of normal VIIIC in the coagulation sequence at the site of haemostasis without inducing generalized intravascular coagulation. Later, purposely activated concentrates were prepared to contain this factor-VIII-bypassing activity, such as Feiba (Immuno, Vienna) and Autoplex (Travenol, USA), but the nature of the active ingredient (if any) is obscure. Numerous reports on the effectiveness of these materials have yielded conflicting results [146, 147, 152] and neither is it known if non-activated 'cold' factor-IX-prothrombin concentrates have any therapeutic benefit in these patients. It is certain that none of them are as effective as are factor-VIII concentrates in haemophilic patients without antibodies. In addition these factor-IX concentrates may produce an anamnestic rise of the VIII antibodies, presumably because they are contaminated with factor VIII [153]. There are few reports that they cause unpleasant side-effects, but controlled clinical trials and further assessment of this material is necessary before they can be recommended confidently for clinical use.

Factor-VIII concentrates. In theory, factor-VIII concentrates should not be effective in patients with antibodies to VIIIC and until recently they were though to be contraindicated, in order to avoid inducing an anamnestic response. Lately this view has been revised [154], and it is illogical to allow patients to become incapacitated for this reason. With low-titre antibodies it may be possible to obtain a haemostatic level of VIIIC, but even if this is not achieved bleeding may stop. It is the author's practice to administer a dose of factor-VIII concentrate approximately equivalent to the patient's plasma volume, repeated if necessary. Results of this regime have seemed to be at least as good as the admittedly equally subjective results of using activated concentrates. There is at present no confirmation of the induction of permanent immune tolerance claimed for the prolonged use of massive and repeated doses of factor VIII [155].

Occasionally the antibody does not cross-react with porcine factor VIII *in vitro*. This material may then be useful for a short period, but it tends to cause thrombocytopenia; a recent new preparation may not produce this effect.

Hepatitis

Hepatitis is one of the commonest complications of haemophilia treatment. It is usually due to hepatitis-B virus but the importance of non-A, non-B viruses has recently been appreciated. Other virus diseases in which hepatitis forms part of the clinical picture may complicate transfusions with fresh blood or plasma but cytomegalovirus and the Epstein–Barr virus do not usually survive the freezing and fractionation processes used in the preparation of concentrates.

In the early days of transfusion therapy using FFP, the risks of individual haemophiliacs developing hepatitis were relatively small. Application of a sensitive radioimmunoassay test for HBsAg indicates its presence in about 1:1000 of the volunteer blood-donor population [156], but it is probably more common in paid donors. The use of plasma from large pools will thus increase the risk of transmitting hepatitis B even if donors are individually tested. Presumably this increased rate of transmission is even greater in the case of non-A, non-B hepatitis, for which there are no routine laboratory tests. The importance of commercial concentrates of factors VIII and IX as a source of hepatitis B has been emphasized by the studies of Hoofnagle *et al.* [157], and later studies have stressed the importance of short-incubation non-A, non-B hepatitis [158, 159], of which there may be two types [160]. The importance of hepatitis-A virus in transfusion-induced hepatitis is uncertain [159]. A disturbing feature of recent studies has been not just the modest incidence of overt jaundice—about four per cent of haemophilic patients in the UK [1]—but the high incidence of abnormal liver function tests [161–163], and especially of histopathological changes on liver biopsy. The latter have included changes consistent with chronic active hepatitis, chronic persistent hepatitis and even cirrhosis [162–164]. Although it is likely that the presence of antibodies to HBsAg in patients' plasma can protect against hepatitis B, with intensive treatment the hepatocytes can remain infected [164]. In addition it is likely that non-A, non-B hepatitis can also lead to chronic liver disease. The role of immune complexes in the pathogenesis of hepatitis remains to be determined [165], as does the significance of the high incidence of splenomegaly recently reported in haemophiliacs [166].

The long-term prognosis of chronic hepatitis in haemophiliacs is not known. The histopathological and clinical indications for steroid therapy are controversial and the case for routine liver biopsy in patients with abnormal liver function tests is therefore debatable. The operation is risky and is probably best confined to centres with special expertise in dealing with both haemophilia and liver disorders.

Acute hepatitis tends to be more severe in the very young and the elderly. Use of commercial concentrates should be avoided if possible in mildly affected patients, especially of these age groups, because such individuals may also lack immunity. Recourse should be made to cryoprecipitate from 'safe' donors and, if possible, to use of DDAVP for minor episodes (see above).

GENERAL MANAGEMENT OF THE HAEMOPHILIAC

In addition to specific therapy already described, it is important that the haemophiliac and his family receive general support and advice. Episodes of bleeding often come in cycles. These may be precipitated by psychological causes (e.g. an examination at school) and may be aggravated if a particular episode is mismanaged. The introduction of home therapy and the development of specialized haemophilia centres have done much to improve general management and minimize untoward psychological and physical effects.

Home therapy

Until recently, specific treatment was usually administered in hospital. This necessitated frequent absences from school or work and, because of the distances involved, sometimes led to delay in treatment. The development of home therapy has overcome some of these problems. Patients or their parents are taught to administer intravenous treatment at home or at work [125, 134, 166, 167], usually using freeze-dried concentrates, which are more convenient to handle than cryoprecipitate. This therapy has proved to be remarkably successful [168] even in young children. Of course, not all patients are suitable for training because of lack of intelligence or other constraints, and individual training programmes are required. Patients on home treatment become less dependent on the hospital and the dose of factor VIII needed for the usual bleed may possibly be reduced, for example to 250 units [169, 170]. Nevertheless, it is important not to take this reduction too far in case residual arthropathies occur and higher doses of factor VIII may be needed to control the majority of bleeds [171, 172].

Prophylactic therapy. Permanent regular prophylactic therapy on a daily basis is probably neither practical nor even desirable for most patients, both on account of expense and because of the risks of known and unknown (e.g. immunological) complications. Nevertheless, daily or less frequent prophylaxis has a definite role in some circumstances. Thus, when a patient is receiving a great deal of therapy on an 'on-demand' basis, morbidity and the amount of treatment may actually be reduced by regular infusions. Prophylaxis can also be used on a temporary basis to allow individual arthropathies to resolve or to tide patients over periods of social need or psychological tension (e.g. examinations, holidays, etc.). It is important that patients on home or prophylactic therapy are seen by the physician at regular intervals for clinical and laboratory assessment. This should include liver and renal function tests, hepatitis antigen screening and exclusion of factor-VIII antibody.

Organization of haemophilia therapy
Haemophilia is an uncommon disorder requiring specialized haematological care. It is important to realize that there is more to haemophilia management than the mere administration of factor VIII. In addition, the advent of home therapy has to a certain extent placed increased responsibility on the haemophiliac and his family. It is essential, therefore, that patients and family members are able to obtain expert advice at all times. In the UK, management of haemophilia is organized around Haemophilia Centres. The functions of centres are to provide:
1 a laboratory service for diagnosis, treatment and genetic studies;
2 a 24-hour clinical service;
3 an advisory service in preventive medicine and dentistry, education, employment, genetic counselling, social medicine, and to General Practitioners; and
4 maintenance of records.

In addition, centres which deal with many patients and are thus appropriately staffed may act as reference centres and advise on difficult problems, undertake specialized or general surgery and co-ordinate special services such as those necessary for carrier detection and prenatal diagnosis.

It is important that the haemophilic child is brought up in an atmosphere of confidence and encouraged to lead an active life. Whilst contact sports should be avoided, every effort must be made to encourage muscular development, by swimming and gymnastics, etc. In this way the joints are stabilized and haemarthroses prevented.

The haemophilia team [134] includes a haematologist (or a physician or paediatrician experienced in haemophilia), orthopaedic surgeon, dental surgeon, nurses, scientific staff, physiotherapists, a social worker cognizant of the problems of haemophilia, and

secretarial staff. The services of other specialists (e.g. an educational psychologist) may be needed at certain times and in some centres, notably in the USA, multidisciplinary case conferences are a regular feature of haemophilia care.

Education and employment are particularly important for patients with severe haemophilia, who will need to live relatively sedentary lives. In general it is best if children can attend their normal local schools but in some instances (e.g. in the presence of antibody to factor VIII, permanent disability or social problems at home) attendance at a special school may be required; home tuition may be needed at times.

The educational programme should be specifically directed to appropriate occupations and local authority and other agencies consulted at an early stage. With advances in treatment, employers can be reassured adequately and their fears regarding emergency bleeding or absenteeism allayed. The Haemophilia Centre staff must therefore develop appropriate links with health and local administrative authorities, ambulance services, employment agencies and social and voluntary services. Severe haemophilia poses problems to the whole family; an unaffected sibling may resent the attention given to the less fortunate brother, whilst parents may experience feelings of guilt as well as more obvious difficulties such as enforced absences from work. Contact with others with similar experiences through associations such as the Haemophilia Society may help to resolve some of these difficulties and give direction and purpose to an otherwise burdensome life. These aspects of haemophilia have been the subject of several reviews [125, 134, 173].

HAEMOPHILIA B (CHRISTMAS DISEASE)

Pathogenesis
Haemophilia B is due to a deficiency of factor IX. This is a vitamin-K-dependent factor synthesized in the liver which, as far as is known, is not associated with any activity other than its role in blood coagulation. It is activated by factor XIa and in its activated form (IXa) interacts with thrombin-activated VIIIC, phospholipid and calcium as a serine protease in the activation of factor X (see Chapter 27). Factor IX has close biochemical homologies with the other vitamin-K-dependent factors II, VII and X, but whereas abnormalities of these are inherited as autosomal traits, haemophilia B is a sex-linked disease. This does not negate a close similarity between the synthetic mechanisms of these factors, but may merely mean that abnormalities of hypothetical X-chromosome loci concerned with II, VII and X synthesis or at an

autosomal locus concerned with factor-IX synthesis are excessively rare.

The concept of abnormal coagulation-factor variants originated with the observation of inhibitor-neutralizing material in one patient with haemophilia B [37]. This concept was extended by observation of an abnormal reaction to ox-brain 'thromboplastin' in the plasma of some patients—so-called haemophilia B_M (the subscript refers to the surname of the propositus) [174, 175]. The syndrome appears to be due to the presence of a factor-IX variant which acts as a competitive inhibitor in the extrinsic system with bovine thromboplastin. Abnormal variants of factor IX were later detected immunologically using both allogeneic [176] and xenogeneic antibodies [177], but there is not necessarily a correlation between the immunological status and the reaction with ox brain. Various methods for measuring factor-IX antigen (IXAg) have been developed, including electro-immunoassay [178], radioimmunoassay [179] and immunoradiometric assay [180]. By the use of either allogeneic [181] or xenogeneic antisera [182, 183] haemophilia-B patients have been described without cross-reacting material (CRM−, B−), with normal levels of IXAg (CRM+, B+), and with reduced levels of both activity and antigen, usually, but not always, with the antigen in excess (CRM-reduced; CRM^R, B^R) (Table 28.4). From the point of view of carrier detection in particular, it is important to note that in about 33–50% of patients the antigen level is significantly higher than the coagulant activity (IXC) [184] and that about 50% of patients are B−. The latter definition, however, depends on the sensitivity of the immunoassay, radioimmunoassays being more sensitive than the electroimmunoassay [185]. These basic immunological and coagulant patterns are usually [185] but not always [183] consistent within kindreds.

In addition to this simple classification, more or less distinct variants of factor IX have been described according to other criteria. With factor IX Leyden [186], levels of IXC increase with age so that patients become progressively less severely affected. With factor IX Alabama [187, 188] there was defective interaction of IXC with phospholipid, demonstrated when the latter was diluted in determining the partial thromboplastin time. With factor IX Chapel Hill [189] there was an abnormality of activation by factor XIa (Table 28.4). Bertina & Veltkamp [190] pointed out that functional abnormalities can be sought at three levels:
1 proteolytic activation of factor-IX zymogen by factor XIa;
2 high-affinity binding of Ca^{2+} ions—presumably necessary for efficient binding to phospholipid and requiring the normally reactive carboxyglutamic acid

residues at the amino-terminal end of the molecule; and
3 the esterolytic (serine protease) centre actually responsible for IXC activity.

On the basis of these and other biochemical studies, several characteristics of apparent factor-IX variants have been distinguished [191, 194, 195]. It was observed that one of the variants [190, 191] resembled PIVKA IX and that haemophilia B_M is not a homogeneous disorder. In addition to the above abnormalities, minor deficiencies of factor VII have been reported in some patients [192] and in one patient with combined deficiency of factors II, VII, IX and X there was evidence of a deficiency of the γ-carboxylation mechanism for prothrombin and, it was presumed, for the other factors [193]. In due course, variants of haemophilia B− may also be reported, because IXC is not completely absent in some B− patients [183, 187].

Diagnosis

The clinical and family history in haemophilia B are identical to those in haemophilia A, including the wide variation in severity. For purposes of clinical management, even at a sophisticated level, knowledge of the 'variant' status of individual patients as described above is not necessary, although it may conceivably be of value in the future. Haemophilia B can therefore be diagnosed adequately using relatively simple methods. The platelet count, primary bleeding time and prothrombin time (except with ox brain as noted above) are normal. Tests of intrinsic coagulation are abnormal: the partial thromboplastin time is prolonged and is corrected by alumina eluate but not by alumina-adsorbed plasma [196]; in the thromboplastin generation test the patient's serum is defective whereas the alumina-adsorbed plasma reacts normally. Factor IX can be measured in plasma by a one-stage assay based on the partial thromboplastin time or by a two-stage method based on the thromboplastin generation test, but the two methods sometimes give widely divergent results. It has been reported that in comparison with haemophilia A, low levels of factor IX may be found in patients with relatively mild bleeding symptoms; this may be because some assay methods underestimate factor IX [197, p. 239] or because haemostasis really requires a lower proportion of the average normal level of factor IX than of factor VIII. This problem has still not been resolved.

As with factor VIII in haemophilia A, factor-IX levels are usually constant throughout life, except in patients with haemophilia B Leyden described above.

Detection of carriers
As with factor VIII in haemophilia A, the average level of IXC in heterozygotes for haemophilia B is about

Table 28.4. Factor-IX variants: general classification (after Parekh *et al.* [182] and Kasper *et al.* [183])

Factor-IX variants	B−		B+	B$_M$	B^R			FIX Leyden [186]	FIX Alabama [187, 188]	FIX Chapel Hill [189]
	B−(a)	B−(b)†			B^R(a)	B^R(b)	B^R(c)‡			
IXC	severe	mild	severe (or moderate)	severe	mild	severe	mild	severe becoming mild	'moderate'	5 u/dl
IXAg	undetected*	undetected	normal	normal or raised	reduced but >IXC	reduced but >IXC	reduced ≡IXC	reduced ≡IXC	N	N
Bovine thromboplastin time	N	N	N	greatly prolonged	N	N (or slightly prolonged)	N	N	N	N
Approximate incidence	50%	10%†	10%	5–7%	—	20–30%	—	...	...	...

* Small amounts (2–6 u/dl) detected by Thompson *et al.* [185] in similar patients.
† Kasper *et al.* only.
‡ Parekh *et al.* only.

one-half that in the normal population [183, 198–201]. Allowing for observational errors, however, only about one-quarter of all heterozygotes have IXC levels so low that they may be identified with confidence by the coagulation assay [198, 199]. In some of these, the IXC levels may be low enough to suggest the homozygous state [202] but similar levels may also occur in undoubted heterozygotes [203]. Kasper *et al.* [183] describe a formula, including family as well as IXC data, for obtaining an estimate of probability that a potential carrier is a true carrier.

The development of immunoassays for IXAg has provided additional data for carrier detection but the situation is not straightforward. About 50% of patients with haemophilia B are CRM− (B−) and hence, in addition to IXC activity, levels of IXAg may also be more or less reduced in carriers of this type depending upon inactivation (or not) of the abnormal X-chromosome. For this reason measurement of IXAg was considered to offer only limited predictive improvement, mainly in B+ kindreds [183, 184]. Recently, however, Graham *et al.* [204] have concluded that the most effective way of classifying haemophilia-B− carriers is by univariate discrimination based only on IXAg assay; for B+ carriers bivariate linear discrimination using both IXC and IXAg assays gave the most acceptable results. Orstavik *et al.* [205] have also found that estimation of IXAg levels is of discriminant value for carrier detection in both B− and B+ kindreds. In addition the presence of the B_M defect, or electrophoretic or other abnormalities of factor IX, may be of considerable help in carrier detection in B+ kindreds [191], depending upon the extent of inactivation of the normal X chromosome.

Treatment

The principles of treatment in haemophilia B are the same as for haemophilia A (pp. 1114–22).

Sources and administration of factor IX

Factor IX may be given as whole plasma. Although it is more stable than VIIIC, plasma stored at 4°C is not suitable, and fresh plasma or FFP must be used for optimal effect. The half-life of factor IXC after infusion is rather longer than that of VIIIC—about 18–24 hours—but this advantage is more than offset by the fact that *in-vivo* recovery is much lower [126]. The reason for this is not certain, but in practice it means that it is not usually possible to obtain an adequate post-infusion level of factor IX using plasma, even taking into account the possibility that the haemostatic levels needed may be slightly lower than those of factor VIIIC in haemophilia A. Concentrates containing

higher specific activity of factor IX are therefore needed for the treatment of most lesions. Freeze-dried concentrates containing factors II, VII, IX and X, as well as three-factor concentrates which lack factor VII (e.g. Oxford DE or Edinburgh DEFIX) are available, and their production is described in some detail by Bidwell *et al.* [103]. Their factor-IX activity is assessed against an international standard and it is important to realize that one unit of activity may not therefore be strictly equivalent to the activity present in 1 ml of fresh normal plasma. Dosage schemes are inevitably empirical but the post-infusion levels which should be aimed for are similar to those of factor VIIIC needed in haemophilia A. Because of the low *in-vivo* recovery it may be estimated that 100 u of factor IXC infused into a 70 kg man will result in a rise of about 1–1·5 u/dl (*cf.* p. 1116). The frequency of injections or infusions needed may be a little less than in haemophilia A because of the relatively longer half-life of factor IX, although a recent report indicates a very rapid initial component of the decay curve [206].

It seems that in the past some batches of certain factor-IX concentrates may have contained activated clotting factors or intermediates and thromboembolic complications were recorded following their use in haemophilia B, notably after surgery [207]. Although the nature of the agent responsible and the ideal test to exclude its presence are uncertain, improved manufacturing controls have reduced this risk. Indeed, with some concentrates, notably those produced in the UK, there has never been significant evidence of similar complications. Nevertheless, circumspection is advisable when considering concurrent use of antifibrinolytic agents and factor-IX concentrates.

Because of the longer *in-vivo* half-life of factor IX, prophylactic therapy with concentrate is easier and possibly more effective in haemophilia B than in haemophilia A. In other respects the principles of treatment and complications are similar in the two conditions. In particular there is strong evidence that factor-IX concentrates may contain hepatitis viruses [208], and antibodies to factor IX develop, though only in a very small proportion, perhaps one to two per cent, of treated patients [126, 209].

VON WILLEBRAND'S DISEASE

History and pathogenesis

A familial bleeding disorder affecting both sexes was described by von Willebrand among the inhabitants of the Åland Islands in the mouth of the Gulf of Bothnia [210]. Patients presented with excessive mucous-membrane bleeding and prolonged bleeding times. At first, platelet [211] and later capillary [212] defects were suspected, but a relationship to factor VIII was indicated by the observations of reduced levels of this factor in similar patients [213], and later confirmed in affected Åland islanders [214, 215]. It was noted that following infusion of plasma, factor-VIII concentrates or even haemophilic plasma there was a well recognized, but inconsistent, secondary rise of VIIIC activity above that originally attained.

In addition to these basic original findings further abnormalities have been detected in this disorder. There are reduced levels of factor-VIII-related antigen (VIIIR:Ag) detected by Laurell electroimmunoassay [43] or immunoradiometric assay [216, 217], using precipitating xenogeneic antisera to factor-VIII-rich plasma fractions. With relevance to primary haemostasis and possibly to the bleeding time, there are deficiencies of certain platelet-related activities, notably platelet retention in glass-bead columns [218], platelet adhesion to exposed subendothelial connective tissue [219] and of a plasma factor needed for platelet aggregation or agglutination by the antibiotic ristocetin [220]. It should be noted that defective ristocetin aggregation also occurs in the Bernard–Soulier giant platelet syndrome, but in this it is due to a platelet and not a plasma defect (see p. 1047). Porcine and bovine plasma aggregate human platelets without ristocetin [107]; this activity is also thought to be related to factor VIII [221] and is, for instance, deficient in porcine von Willebrand's disease (vWd) [222].

The biochemical nature of the molecules which normally exhibit these activities has been extensively investigated and is described in Chapter 27. Recent evidence from large-pore agarose and polyacrylamide gel electrophoresis reviewed by Sixma et al. [223] suggests that VIIIR:Ag/WF exists as a series of homologous oligomers and that those of the highest molecular weight—up to 20×10^6 daltons—show the greatest platelet-related activities. Factor VIIIR:Ag/WF is synthesized under autosomal control and is linked, possibly by non-covalent bonds, to a molecule or antigen which exhibits VIIIC activity and which is under X-chromosomal control. In the genetic context (Fig. 28.1) vWd in its usual heterozygous state would be expected to be associated with reduced levels of VIIIR:Ag/WF or with the presence of abnormal VIIIR:Ag/WF with secondary reduction of factor VIIIC activity.

Studies of the biochemical lesion in vWd have indicated several abnormalities of VIIIR:Ag in some patients. These include increased electrophoretic mobility [224, 225], reduced carbohydrate content [226], defective precipitation with concanavalin A [227], abnormal dose-response curves in the immuno-radiometric assay for VIIIR:Ag and a lack of the electrophoretically slow-moving higher-molecular-weight oligomers [223]. These features have led to suggestions [228] that vWd may be due to:

1 reduced synthesis or release of the whole range of oligomers of VIIIR:Ag;

2 selective reduction of synthesis or release of the higher oligomers of VIIIR:Ag (e.g. a post-translational defect due to a deficiency of a polymerase or a glycosyl transferase); and

3 a true amino-acid sequence defect of the subunit of VIIIR:Ag with resultant failure to polymerize.

Graham [229] has recently resurrected the regulatory-gene hypothesis to explain the pathogenesis of vWd. However, available evidence seems to suggest that in most patients the polymers of VIIIR:Ag are abnormal in structure or distribution and not merely quantitatively reduced. If a regulatory-gene mutation is involved, it is most likely to be so in the relatively uncommon type-4 disease described below.

In normal individuals there is strong evidence that VIIIR:Ag/WF (but not necessarily VIIIC) is localized to and synthesized by vascular endothelial cells [44, 230]. von Willebrand's disease may therefore represent a primary endothelial-cell defect [231]. Other endothelial-cell defects such as reduced production of plasminogen activator have also been reported in vWd [133], as well as morphological vascular disorders such as angiodysplasia [232] and telangiectasia [233], recalling Blackburn's earlier suggestion of a capillary defect in this disease [212].

In addition to endothelial cells, VIIIR:Ag is also present in normal platelets [230]. It is located in the membrane [234] and in granules [235] from which it may be released during aggregation [236, 237]. The antigen seems to be synthesized in megakaryocytes [238] and there is evidence for the presence of two different platelet pools [239]. Tschopp et al. [219] have shown that the defective adhesion of platelets in vWd blood to exposed subendothelium can be corrected by a source of VIIIR:Ag/WF. The defective subendothelial platelet adhesion and ristocetin-induced platelet aggregation in the Bernard–Soulier syndrome (see p. 1047) involves an abnormality of the platelet membrane glycoprotein-I complex [240]. It appears that there is normally an interaction between a subendothelial component—possibly collagen [241]—the higher oligomers of VIIIR:Ag/WF and platelet membrane glycoprotein I, and that this interaction is defective in vWd. VIIIR:Ag may be absent from the platelets in severe vWd [242] and abnormalities of the electrophoretic characteristics of platelet VIIIR:Ag have been described in other types of the disease [243], but the role of platelet VIIIR:Ag in normal haemostasis and in the pathogenesis of vWd is uncertain.

Genetic and clinical features

Genetic features

Much controversy has centred on the descriptions of different types of vWd (Table 28.5). It is often described as being inherited as an autosomal dominant characteristic. In its usual heterozygous form mucous-membrane bleeding is common, haemarthroses are rare and factor-VIII-related activities are concordantly (type 1, Table 28.5) or disproportionately (type 2, Table 28.5) reduced. Often the electrophoretic pattern, most easily demonstrated on two-dimensional crossed immunoelectrophoresis, suggests a lack of slower moving forms of VIIIR:Ag. Although in general these types of the disease are relatively mild compared to severe haemophilia, bleeding can be troublesome and dangerous, particularly after trauma, from the gastro-intestinal tract and from menorrhagia.

In addition to this 'usual' type of the disease there is a much less common, very severe, autosomal 'recessive' type (type 3, Table 28.5), in which haemophilic-type lesions such as haemarthroses occur, in addition to purpura and the more usual type of bleeding. The parents are usually symptomless but may be consanguineous and have slightly reduced levels of VIIIR:Ag. In this type of patient all factor-VIII-related activities are very low and VIIIR:Ag may be undetectable except, in some cases, by a very sensitive method [244].

In patients with a fourth type of vWd (Table 28.5) the bleeding time is usually normal although levels of VIIIR:Ag, VIIIC and RiCoF are concordantly reduced. This syndrome, originally referred to as 'autosomal haemophilia', is now recognized to be a form of vWd [72] and it has been suggested that in this type of the disease there is reduced synthesis of normal VIIIR:Ag/WF [245]. Although the classification into autosomal dominant and recessive patterns is an acceptable generalization, exceptions may occur and patients who exhibit features of each type of inheritance may be present within individual kindreds [246, 247]. This is possibly due to interaction between maternally and paternally derived polymers of VIIIR:Ag or the synthetic mechanisms which control these, so that a range of different oligomers is present in different family members [247].

In addition to these relatively well-characterized patients, vWd has been described in association with a variety of other defects including haemorrhagic telangiectasia [233] and angiodysplasia [232], as well as with platelet defects of various types [248–251] and with abnormal fibrinogen [252] or Factor XII [509] (e.g. vWd San Diego [254]). It is not known if these combinations represent distinct disease entities or are coincidental.

Clinical features

In its usual heterozygous form vWd often presents in early childhood, usually with mucous-membrane

Table 28.5. Types of von Willebrand's disease*†

Type	BT	Concentration of:			Comments
		VIIIC	VIIIR:Ag	RiCoF	
1	prolonged	moderately reduced ≡VIIIR:Ag	moderately reduced (Laurell assay)	usually very reduced	possibly two subtypes: 1 ? normal VIIIR:Ag quality 2 abnormal antigen or polymerization: (i) increased EM (ii) IRMA dose-response curve not similar to normal
2	prolonged	normal	normal (Laurell assay)	usually very reduced	abnormal antigen or polymerization: 1 increased electrophoretic mobility 2 abnormal IRMA dose-response curve 3 ? abnormal carbohydrate
3	prolonged	0–1 u/dl	<0·01 u/dl	very reduced	parents 'silent' but VIIIR:Ag < VIIIC 'recessive' von Willebrand's disease
4	normal	reduced	reduced	reduced	VIIIC ≡ VIIIR:Ag ≡ RiCoF ? antigen quality normal (so-called 'autosomal haemophilia')

* Note: possibility of double (compound) heterozygotes.
† VIIIR:Ag, factor-VIII-related antigen; VIIIC, procoagulant factor VIII; RiCoF, ristocetin cofactor; BT, bleeding time; EM, electrophoretic mobility; IRMA, immunoradiometric assay.

bleeding such as epistaxis and melaena. Excessive bruising is common and bleeding may be excessive after dental extractions and surgery, but post-partum bleeding is relatively rare. This may be due to the fact that levels of factor-VIII-related activities rise during pregnancy [253], although the bleeding time may remain prolonged. Menorrhagia, on the other hand, is common and may be the most troublesome symptom. The symptoms are often quite variable in different family members and even in the same patient at different times. Some affected members, detected during family studies, are symptomless.

On the other hand, patients with homozygous vWd are severely affected: haemarthroses, retroperitoneal bleeding and other haemophilia-like lesions may occur, in addition to mucous-membrane bleeding and even purpura.

Diagnosis

In most cases in which vWd is suspected the diagnosis can be made on the basis of the clinical picture, autosomal inheritance and relatively simple laboratory tests. The bleeding time is prolonged, especially if measured by the sensitive template modification of the Ivy technique [255], and the VIIIC concentration is moderately reduced. The secondary rise of VIIIC which occurs after treatment with a source of factor VIII (possibly due to VIIIR:Ag) is inconsistent and usually only of confirmatory value in diagnosis. The level of VIIIR:Ag is usually reduced when measured by the Laurell electroimmunoassay; in some patients (type 2, Table 28.5), however, it is relatively normal, but its electrophoretic mobility may be increased [224, 225] or there may be a lack of slow-moving forms [223]. Platelet ristocetin agglutination in PRP is impaired, but is corrected *in vitro* by addition of a small proportion of a factor-VIII-rich plasma fraction such as cryoprecipitate—a test which distinguishes the abnormality from that seen in the Bernard–Soulier syndrome. Measurement of plasma ristocetin cofactor activity (e.g. on fixed platelets [256]) is more sensitive and usually gives very low results, but it should be noted that this test is technically demanding and tends to be imprecise. However, reduced levels of ristocetin cofactor activity probably represent most closely the abnormality of biological function of the higher oligomers of VIIIR:Ag/WF which may be present in vWd. In the majority of clinically significant cases the diagnosis can be established using the above tests. In a small number, additional studies (e.g. using an immunoradiometric assay of VIIIR:Ag) may be of value [217, 257]. Platelet retention may be impaired when native or heparinized, but not citrated, blood is passed through glass-bead filters, but this test is imprecise.

It is apparent that the diagnostic criteria for vWd usually include some indication of an abnormality of the molecule which exhibits VIIIR:Ag/WF (ristocetin cofactor) activity. In addition, it must be shown that other tests of platelet reactivity (e.g. aggregation with ADP, collagen and thrombin) are all normal. All abnormalities may not be present in all patients—particularly those who are mildly affected (see also Table 28.5). Family studies (e.g. of electrophoretic mobility of VIIIR:Ag) may be helpful and such studies, combined with clinical data in discriminant function analyses, have detected transmitting heterozygotes even when all individual tests were within the normal range [258]. Clearly, therefore, definitive diagnosis is occasionally difficult. It is sometimes better not to label a borderline patient as definitely affected unless this information is clinically relevant, in order not to prejudice employment or insurance prospects.

Treatment

The principles underlying the treatment of vWd do not differ from those of haemophilia, for example, with regard to general management, education, provision of social services and the delivery of health care, but there are several differences in detail.

Replacement therapy

Following infusion of plasma there is not only an immediate rise of VIIIC activity but the level may continue to rise above that expected from the amount infused, so that peak levels may be reached at about 12–24 hours. Activity declines thereafter with much the same rapidity as in haemophilia A. After infusion of material containing the highest-molecular-weight polymers of factor VIII such as cryoprecipitate, there may also be short-lived correction of the bleeding time, ristocetin cofactor activity and levels of VIIIR:Ag. The bleeding time effect is not so marked after infusion of high-potency concentrates of factor VIII [259–261], possibly because the VIIIR:Ag in such preparations is less highly polymerized [262, 263]. It seems that the higher-molecular-weight polymers of VIIIR:Ag/WF bind preferentially to subendothelium and to platelets [264, 265]. Even so, correction of the bleeding time is difficult to achieve in vWd for more than a few hours, even with cryoprecipitate, possibly because VIIIR:Ag/WF is not taken up by platelets and endothelial cells [242, 266] and is cleared rapidly from the circulation [110, 267, 268]. Nevertheless, cryoprecipitate is usually the treatment of choice for bleeding in this disorder.

Deamino-d-arginine vasopressin

As in mild haemophilia (p. 1119), this drug may be effective in raising the levels of factor-VIII-related activities in vWd and may also correct the bleeding time, although its effect is variable [131, 269]. It is given slowly by intravenous injection in doses of 0·3 μg/kg, and tranexamic acid should also be given to prevent increased fibrinolysis [133]. Injections of DDAVP may be repeated at six- to 12-hourly intervals, but it may lose its effect after a day or two. In more concentrated solution it can be administered by intranasal instillation (e.g. 1 μg/kg in 0·2 ml [270]). This method was of value when given for menorrhagia in one woman with vWd (one or two doses on the third day of the period (personal observation)). Repeated administration of DDAVP may theoretically cause water retention, but this is not usually a problem when used as above.

Specific problems in vWd

Menorrhagia may be troublesome and require hormonal or other forms of gynaecological management. Antifibrinolytic therapy and DDAVP may be of value. Hysterectomy may be needed in intractable cases. Gastro-intestinal bleeding may also present problems and a local cause is not always found: treatment is with cryoprecipitate, antifibrinolytic agents or DDAVP as described above. Replacement therapy for major surgery follows similar principles to those in haemophilia. Factor-VIII levels are usually easy to maintain but correction of the bleeding time is difficult, even with the most effective agents such as cryoprecipitate or fraction 1–0 [261]. However, correction of VIIIC levels is more important for securing surgical haemostasis.

Antibody to VIIIR:Ag may develop in some severely affected, apparently homozygous patients [271, 272]. The antibody may be precipitating or non-precipitating and inhibits ristocetin cofactor activity. It may be possible to maintain VIIIC levels in such patients by means of high-purity concentrate more easily than by using cryoprecipitate, possibly because the inhibitor reacts preferentially with the higher oligomers of VIIIR:Ag which are present in cryoprecipitate [273], but it is not possible to correct the bleeding time in this way.

Acquired von Willebrand's syndrome

A syndrome closely resembling the inherited disease has been reported in patients who previously did not suffer from a haemostatic defect and in whom there was no family history of such a disorder [274]. The syndrome has usually been reported in association with autoimmune or lymphoproliferative disease, including SLE [275] and monoclonal gammopathy [276]. The patients developed reduced levels of VIIIC and VIIR:Ag [277] and an IgG antibody with inhibitory activity against ristocetin cofactor was demonstrated in one case [278]. A further parallel with the inherited

disorder was drawn by the observation by Joist *et al.* [279] of abnormal electrophoretic mobility of VIIIR:Ag in a patient with acquired vWd complicating lymphocytic lymphoma, and angiodysplastic lesions have also been reported [280, 281]. Acquired von Willebrand's syndrome is usually thought to be associated with an autoimmune reaction to VIIIR:Ag/WF, but the interrelationship with the vascular lesions remains to be explained adequately.

FIBRINOGEN (FACTOR I) DEFICIENCIES

In general disorders of fibrinogen synthesis can be divided into:
1 deficient synthesis—afibrinogenaemia, hypofibrinogenaemia; and
2 defective synthesis—dysfibrinogenaemia.

It is not known if the basic lesion in patients who exhibit deficient synthesis is related to gene deletions analogous to those of thalassaemia or to the synthesis of a very unstable fibrinogen chain. Examples of deficient synthesis confined to one chain have not yet been described.

In some cases of defective fibrinogen synthesis there is a point mutation causing substitution of a specific amino acid (see fibrinogen Detroit below) and a corresponding allotypic disorder; in others the abnormality may be due to a post-translational defect.

From the practical point of view, in afibrinogenaemia there is absence (or virtual absence) of circulating fibrinogen, whereas in hypofibrinogenaemia there are reduced levels of apparently normal fibrinogen. In dysfibrinogenaemia circulating fibrinogen exhibits abnormal characteristics; it is present in normal or reduced amounts, but quantification may depend critically on the method used. This group of disorders has been the subject of several reviews [282–287].

Afibrinogenaemia and hypofibrinogenaemia

Afibrinogenaemia

Absence of fibrinogen from the plasma was first described by Rabe & Solomon [288] and part of the report was translated from the German by Beck [287]. Since then over 100 patients have been recorded [282, 284]. The condition also occurs in dogs [289] and goats [290]. Consanguinity is often present in the parents and the disease probably represents a homozygous genotype of an autosomally inherited trait. Bleeding frequently starts in the first year of life, sometimes from the umbilical cord. Haematomata, gastro-intestinal and mucous-membrane bleeding are common. Haemarthroses occur in about 20% of cases but joint sequelae are less common than in severe haemophilia.

Menorrhagia is sometimes a problem. Cerebral hae-morrhage has been noted as a cause of death.

Laboratory investigations. These reveal abnormalities of all tests which depend upon the formation of fibrin, including prothrombin time, thrombin clotting time, reptilase time, etc., but tests which do not, such as the thromboplastin generation test, are normal. The abnormal test results can be corrected by addition of normal plasma or fibrinogen solution. All coagulation assays are normal except for that of fibrinogen, which is absent when measured by conventional clotting, chemical or immunological methods, although trace amounts may be detected by very sensitive techniques. There is no evidence of increased fibrinolysis or disseminated intravascular coagulation and survival of transfused human fibrinogen is normal except, rarely, when antibodies to fibrinogen have developed after transfusion therapy [291]. Mild thrombocytopenia has been observed in about 25% of cases [284] but the platelet count is rarely below $100 \times 10^9/1$. The bleeding time may be prolonged even when the platelet count is normal: this may be associated with reduction of the normal intraplatelet pool of fibrinogen and with abnormalities of platelet retention in glass-bead columns and impaired aggregation with ADP, collagen, adrenaline and thrombin [292–296]. These platelet abnormalities can be corrected by addition of fibrinogen: it appears that low concentrations (of the order of 0·4 g/l) are necessary for normal platelet function. It is important to exclude acquired disorders of fibrinogen and disseminated intravascular coagulation. The presence of anti-coagulants such as heparin can be excluded by the greatly prolonged reptilase time. It is also necessary to confirm the virtual absence of fibrinogen by immuno-logical tests.

Treatment. This is relatively easy because fibrinogen has a long half-life. Levels above 1 g/l are needed in order to secure haemostasis. Manufacture of fibrinogen concentrate has been discontinued in the USA on account of the risk of hepatitis, but alternative sources of fibrinogen are available in the form of cryoprecipitate or the older Cohn fraction 1–0 factor-VIII concentrate. As a rough guide, cryoprecipitate from one donor contains, on average, about 200 mg of fibrinogen and 2–4 g is needed to achieve haemostatic levels in an adult patient.

Antibodies to fibrinogen have been reported after replacement therapy and may reduce the survival rate of infused material [291]. Paradoxically, thrombo-embolic episodes may also follow treatment [297, 298], possibly due to an immunological reaction with the vessel wall. A more likely explanation, which may also

apply in dysfibrinogenaemia, is based on the fact that thrombin is adsorbed to normal fibrin from which it is released during fibrinolysis [299]. In this way fibrinogen itself may act as an anticoagulant [287] and this activity may be lacking if its concentration is reduced (e.g. in treated afibrinogenaemia) or if it is abnormal as in dysfibrinogenaemia [300].

Hypofibrinogenaemia
The parents of patients with afibrinogenaemia often show reduced levels of apparently normal fibrinogen, consistent with the heterozygous state. It is likely that hypofibrinogenaemia is in fact the heterozygous form of afibrinogenaemia. As pointed out by Flute [284], the condition is 'recessive' by clinical expression but 'dominant' on laboratory testing; thus, as in the case of vWd, the terms 'dominant' and 'recessive' are best avoided [5]. Some patients, originally thought to be suffering from hypofibrinogenaemia of the above type [301] were shown later to have a form of dysfibrino-genaemia [302]. This condition is sometimes given the awkward title 'hypo-dysfibrinogenaemia' and will be described below. It is thus important to assess fibrinogen levels by both physicochemical and immunological methods in order to establish a diag-nosis of hypofibrinogenaemia.

Inherited dysfibrinogenaemia
The first report of a molecular abnormality of fibrinogen is usually attributed to Imperato & Dettori [303], although family studies failed to confirm that the condition studied was inherited and both Fanconi [304] and Ingram [305] had previously made similar suggestions on the basis of clinical studies. The first well-documented report of abnormal fibrinogen as an inherited disorder—dysfibrinogenaemia—was that of Ménaché [306]. Beck [307] established the convention of naming 'new' abnormal fibrinogens after the town of discovery (e.g. fibrinogen 'Baltimore'). Thus the variant of Imperto & Dettori later became known as fibrinogen Parma and that of Ménaché as fibrinogen Paris I. Although over 50 kindreds with dysfibrino-genaemia have now been designated, comparative investigations are incomplete so that the exact number of distinct variants is uncertain.

Mode of inheritance
The condition is usually inherited as an autosomal trait. Homozygous genotype has been postulated in the propositus of fibrinogen Metz [308] and possibly in fibrinogen Detroit [309]. In some families presumed heterozygotes are asymptomatic, but biochemical co-agulation abnormalities may be detected, particularly when there are polymerization defects. In some patients the heterozygous state has been suggested by

the separation of normal and abnormal fibrinogens, using, for example, reptilase polymerization [310], immunoelectrophoresis [309, 311], cellulose chromatography [312] and ethanol fractionation [313]. The coagulation and clinical abnormalities tend to be similar within families but variation of both has been described, as in fibrinogen Bethesda I and III [313, 314] and fibrinogen New York [315]. In one family with fibrinogen St. Louis, a gene for factor-VIII deficiency was also segregating [316] and in another family dysfibrinogenaemia was associated with von Willebrand's syndrome [252].

Pathogenesis and biochemical abnormalities

Dysfibrinogenaemia appears to be due to a qualitative defect of the fibrinogen molecule and is usually assumed, often without proof, to be the result of inheritance of a mutant form of the protein. In at least seven variants, Vancouver [301, 302], Leuven [317], Bethesda II [318], Philadelphia [319], Bethesda III [313], New York [315] and Valencia [320], circulating fibrinogen concentrations were reduced. In some cases (Bethesda II and III, Philadelphia) this was due, at

least in part, to increased catabolism, while in others there may have been reduced synthesis.

It is customary to classify the disorders into
1 those affecting fibrinopeptide release;
2 those affecting fibrin polymerization; and, with less certainty,
3 those involving abnormalities of cross-linking or digestion by plasmin.

Dysfibrinogenaemia with impaired fibrinopeptide release

This has been described in at least 14 kindreds (Table 28.6), but in some of these it is associated with defective polymerization which may, in fact, be the major defect. Most of these patients exhibit prolonged thrombin time and discrepant values when fibrinogen is investigated by coagulation assay (low) and by chemical or immunological methods (normal or elevated). Measurement of fibrinopeptide release has indicated that this is abnormal with respect to that of peptide A or B or both, as indicated in Table 28.6. Presumed heterozygotes for fibrinogen Detroit, Metz and Giessen I showed no release of fibrinopeptides and no

Table 28.6. Dysfibrinogenaemia with disordered fibrinopeptide release (modified from Flute [284] and updated)

Type	Defective release of fibrinopeptide	Fibrin polymerization	Immuno-electrophoresis	Thrombin time inhibition by fibrinogen	Clinical	Molecular data or comments	Reference
Detroit	B only	Slow	Anodal	+	Bleeding	Aα (Arg^{19}→serine)	309
Seattle	B only	Fast	Normal	...	None		325
Baltimore	A	Slow	Anodal	0	Bleeding: thrombosis	Defective α polymers	338
Cleveland II	A	Slow	Normal	+	Bleeding	Defect in N=DSK†	339
Giessen I	A	Slow	Normal	+	Bleeding	Decreased sensitivity to plasmin	340
Metz	A	Slow	Cathodal	+	Bleeding abortions	Aα chain abnormal	321
Freiburg	A	Slow	Normal	+	Bleeding possible	—	341
Manchester	A	Slow	Normal	0	Not stated	—	342
Copenhagen	A	Slow	Normal	...	Thrombosis	Normal plasminogen binding	343
Bethesda I	A+B	Normal	Anodal	+	Bleeding		314
Bethesda II	A+B (slight)	Slow*	Anodal	0	None	Increased catabolism	318
New York	A+B	Slow	Anodal	+	Thrombosis	Low fibrinogen	315
St. Louis	A+B (slight)	Slow*	Normal	+	None	...	316
New Orleans	A+B (A slower)	Normal	Anodal	+	Bleeding	...	324

* Major defect.
† N=DSK, N-terminal disulphide knot.

clot with thrombin. Disordered release of fibrinopeptides may lead to impaired polymerization of fibrin monomers as well as altered kinetics of cross-linking. It is thus necessary to measure fibrinopeptide release in order to characterize the condition. Various other biochemical defects have been described in different fibrinogens, including abnormal elution on DEAE chromatography, carbohydrate and electron-microscopic analysis; these have been reviewed by Flute [284] and Gralnick [285]. Several fibrinogens have been shown to migrate abnormally on immunoelectrophoresis (Table 28.6), but the migration of individual reduced chains on SDS polyacrylamide gels has usually been found to be normal. Nevertheless, an abnormality of the Aα chain was demonstrated in fibrinogen Metz [321], and the Aα chain of fibrinogen Baltimore also appears to be abnormal. It is not known if the abnormalities observed represent unbalanced over-production of minor normal populations of Aα chains.

Fibrinogen Detroit remains the only abnormal fibrinogen in which the exact nature of the molecular defect has been elucidated [322]: examination of the tryptic digest of the Aα chain from the N-terminal disulphide knot (N-DSK) showed that the arginine at position 19 had been replaced by a serine residue. Release of fibrinopeptide A by thrombin was normal, but release of fibrinopeptide B was unexpectedly impaired, possibly as a result of steric hindrance [323]. The only fibrinogen other than Detroit to show impaired release of fibrinopeptide B alone is fibrinogen Seattle [325], but the two fibrinogens seem to be different from each other.

Hereditary dysfibrinogenaemia with delayed fibrin polymerization

At least 34 named fibrinogen variants with delayed fibrin polymerization have been described. According to Flute [284], fibrinopeptide release was normal in at least 20 of these variants (Table 28.7). As with the other abnormal fibrinogens, various additional defects have been described, such as abnormal migration of plasma or purified fibrinogen on immunoelectrophoresis; these are summarized in Table 28.7. Fibrinogens Philadelphia and Bethesda III have certain similarities by virtue of reduced levels in patients and increased fractional catabolic rate, but differences were noted in the correcting effect of thrombin and other reactions. The proposita with fibrinogen Bethesda III and her sister had bleeding only during pregnancy, sometimes associated with spontaneous abortion. Plasma became incoagulable with thrombin during pregnancy, although the amount of fibrinogen present was constant when measured by immunoassay. This suggests an alteration of the ratio of abnormal to normal

fibrinogen. In fibrinogens Valencia and Bethesda III the euglobulin lysis times were below the normal range—probably related to deficient α-polymer formation.

Other abnormal fibrinogens

The thrombin clotting time of fibrinogen Oslo [6] was shorter than normal and that of fibrinogen Tokyo [326] was reported as being normal. Fibrinogen Oslo was described in a family in which affected members showed a high incidence of venous thromboembolism. Fibrinogen Tokyo was associated with defective cross-linking and an abnormal fragment D on plasmin digestion. Fibrinogen Oklahoma [327] was also associated with defective cross-linking and showed an abnormality of the tryptic digest. Both fibrinogens Tokyo and Oklahoma were associated with a moderate bleeding tendency but it is uncertain if the abnormalities of cross-linking and proteolysis indicate the presence of an abnormal fibrinogen. In the case of fibrinogen Parma [303], tested family members were not affected and although this is often quoted as the index case for dysfibrinogenaemia, the real nature of the defect is uncertain.

Fetal fibrinogen

The prolonged thrombin clotting time of newborn plasma was recognized by Biggs [328] and later confirmed by Roberts *et al.* [329] and others. It has been suggested that this phenomenon is due to the persistence in the blood of fetal fibrinogens analogous to the fetal haemoglobins. Fetal fibrinogen is supposed to differ from that of adults in several respects, including monomer aggregation, pH dependence and biochemical reactions [330–334]. It has been suggested that fibrinogen Paris I [330] may represent hereditary persistence of fetal fibrinogen, but otherwise there is no evidence that this protein is of any clinical significance.

Clinical features

Excessive bleeding does not occur in all patients with dysfibrinogenaemia. It was prominent in the apparently homozygous patient with fibrinogen Detroit and in patients with several other variants as indicated in the tables. It is more commonly observed in patients with defective fibrinopeptide release than in those in whom the major defect is one of fibrin polymerization. When it occurs, bleeding is usually of the mucous-membrane type with epistaxes, menorrhagia and excessive bleeding after surgery or trauma. Bleeding from the umbilical cord may occur in affected neonates. The tendency to bleed may vary between individual members of the same family who show identical laboratory defects, and is more likely to

Table 28.7. Dysfibrinogenaemia with delayed polymerization of fibrin monomers (modified from Flute [284] and updated)

	Immuno-electrophoresis	Thrombin-time inhibition by fibrinogen	Clinical associations	Comments	Reference
(i) Fibrinopeptide release normal					
Amsterdam	Cathodal	+	None	α_2 globulin needed for polymer defect	346
Cleveland I	Cathodal	+	Wound dehiscence		311
Buenos Aires	Anodal	?	Bleeding: wound dehiscence		347
Caracas	Anodal	+	Bleeding: wound dehiscence	Defective α polymers	348
Nancy	Anodal	+	None		349
Paris I	Anodal	+	Wound dehiscence	Abnormal γ chain: no γ–γ dimers	7
Alba/Geneva	Normal	0	Abortions		350
Leuven	Normal	+	None		317
Manila	Normal	+	None		351
Marburg	Normal	+	Bleeding: thrombosis		352
Montreal I	Normal	0	Wound dehiscence	Increased mobility of Aα chain	353
Paris II	Normal	+	Thrombosis		354
Paris III	Normal	+	Thrombosis		355
Philadelphia	Normal	+	Bleeding	Low fibrinogen, cf. Bethesda III	319
Troyes	Normal	0	None		308
Weisbaden	Normal	+	Bleeding: thrombosis		356
Zurich I	Normal	+	None		310
Zurich II	Normal	+	None		357
Bethesda III	Normal	+	Bleeding	Low fibrinogen	313
London	Normal	+	Coronary artery disease		344
Logrono	Abnormal	0	?		358
(ii) Fibrinopeptide release not reported					
Boulogne	?	?	None		359
Clermond-Ferrand	?	?	None		359
Giessen II	?	?	Bleeding	Low fibrinogen	360
Hanover	?	+	Bleeding		361
Iowa City	Normal	0	None		362
Los Angeles	Abnormal	+	None		363
Montreal II	?	0	Bleeding		364
Parma	?	0	Bleeding	Low fibrinogen	303
Vancouver	Anodal	0	Abortions		302
Valencia	?	0	Bleeding	Low fibrinogen	320
Vienna	Normal	0	Bleeding		365
Homberg	?	?	None		345
Nagoya	?	?	None	3 abnormal γ chains	366

be absent in those families detected by routine, pre-operative screening, for example.

A significant number of patients have shown a tendency to thrombosis. Others, particularly in the group with defective fibrin polymerization (e.g. Paris I and Cleveland I), have shown a tendency to wound dehiscence, whilst haemorrhagic and spontaneous abortions have been reported in women with fibrinogens Bethesda III, Vancouver, Metz and Alba/Geneva. It has been suggested that the tendency to thrombosis may be linked to the fact that normal fibrinogen acts as an antithrombin, thrombin being absorbed to fibrin. The interaction could be defective in some disfibrinogenaemic states with consequent predisposition to thrombosis [300]. In any case anti-coagulant therapy seems to be of value in such patients. It is remarkable that the symptoms in some patients resemble those which occur in factor-XIII deficiency and it may be that this is associated with defective cross-linking of the abnormal fibrinogen (e.g. of fibrinogen Paris I) so that it has defective tensile strength or increased susceptibility to proteolysis.

Diagnosis

In almost all of the patients with abnormal fibrinogen the thrombin clotting time is prolonged; some exceptions (e.g. fibrinogen Oslo) have been noted above. The reptilase time (Bothrops' venom time) is also prolonged: reptilase releases only fibrinopeptide A and the reptilase time is not prolonged in heparin therapy—an important point of differential diagnosis. The thrombin clotting time is often more or less corrected by calcium. Other tests which depend on conversion of fibrinogen may also be prolonged but the partial thromboplastin time is not usually as abnormal as the one-stage prothrombin time. Fibrinogen concentrations determined by coagulation or thrombin-clotting-time techniques are often reduced, whereas those depending upon immunological or chemical precipitation are usually normal or even raised. Exceptions with reduced fibrinogen levels as measured by any method (e.g. Bethesda III, Philadelphia, Vancouver, Leuven, Bethesda II, Valencia and New York) have been described. The discrepancy noted with the other fibrinogens is presumably the result of defective polymerization of the abnormal monomers with each other or with any normal monomers which may be present. As a result 'serum' may contain unpolymerized fibrin which will give false positive tests for 'fibrin-degradation products'. The latter may be excluded by immunoelectrophoretic studies. Determination of immunoelectrophoretic mobility of plasma fibrinogen may also be of value in detecting abnormal variants by comparison with normal plasma fibrinogen and may thus help to characterize the disorder. These abnormalities are more often detected with plasma than with purified fibrinogen, possibly because the purification processes preferentially select a normal component. Studies of the survival of labelled fibrinogen may indicate increased catabolism of the abnormal fibrinogen (Bethesda III, Philadelphia) or normal intravascular survival (Bethesda I and II), but these studies are not usually essential for diagnosis. In a significant number of patients lysis of plasma clots, and in particular euglobulin lysis times, have been accelerated. This seems to be a result of the abnormal fibrin and does not necessarily indicate increased activation of the fibrinolytic system. Levels of other coagulation factors, including factor XIII, have usually been normal except for the coincidental defect of factor VIII (e.g. with fibrinogen St. Louis). Additional defects may be demonstrated using sophisticated techniques such as SDS polyacrylamide gel electrophoresis of reduced chains, but these are not necessary for clinical diagnosis.

It is important to differentiate inherited dysfibrinogenaemia from acquired disorders. Thus acquired dysfibrinogenaemia has been reported in association with hepatocellular carcinoma [335, 336] and relatively frequently in other liver disease [337]. The presence of inhibitors of fibrin polymerization such as fibrindegradation products can be excluded by the clinical context, the family history and possibly by immunoelectrophoretic studies. The presence of heparin is usually easy to exclude by performing the reptilase clotting time and the presence of paraproteins (e.g. in myeloma) which may interfere with fibrin polymerization can be excluded by appropriate immunoassays.

Treatment

Many patients with dysfibrinogenaemia are symptomless and do not require treatment even for surgery. Those who present with thrombosis may require anti-coagulant therapy, while those with excessive bleeding may respond to treatment with fibrinogen. As in the case of afibrinogenaemia discussed above, cryoprecipitate or factor-VIII concentrates may be needed to provide a source of fibrinogen. In general, however, the bleeding diathesis is not severe and even in patients who present with thrombosis, the prognosis for life is good.

FACTOR-XIII DEFICIENCY

The existence of fibrin-stabilizing factor (factor XIII) in normal plasma was suspected by Robbins [367] long before the first deficient patient was described [368]; in most other coagulation disorders the patients preceded characterization of the defect. Although factor-XIII deficiency is uncommon, over 100 patients have been described [369] and recent genetic, biochemical and immunological studies have revealed considerable heterogeneity both of the molecule and of its disorders. The condition has been the subject of several reviews [370–372].

Pathogenesis

Plasma factor XIII is a zymogen, which after activation by thrombin [373] forms a transamidase. This, in the presence of Ca^{2+}, catalyses the formation of γ-glutamyl-ε-lysine crosslinks between fibrin monomers. Factor XIII consists of two A subunits joined as a dimer and two B subunits, i.e. A_2B_2. These have also been referred to as A (activity) and S (support) subunits [374]. Most of the transamidase activity is associated with the A subunits but the B subunits may play a role in regulating the rate of calcium-dependent activation of the zymogen. Factor XIII is present in platelets and placenta, but in the form of the active A subunit only. Deficiency of factor XIII renders clots 'unstable'. This means that they are soluble in 5 M urea or 1% monochloroacetic acid, lack elasticity and are more susceptible than normal to digestion by plasmin.

There is a high incidence of consanguinity in affected families [375]. Ratnoff & Steinberg [376] suggested a sex-linked component to the inheritance pattern but recent evidence supports the conclusion that it is an autosomal trait. In apparently homozygous individuals, factor XIII is virtually absent when measured biochemically [377–379]; earlier studies by Duckert [382] showed less severe deficiencies because the antiserum used was not specific for subunit A. In most heterozygous individuals transamidase activity and subunit A are reduced to intermediate levels; in several families the level of subunit S was also reduced but the specificity of the antiserum used was in doubt. Recent biochemical studies by Board [383, 384] have clarified the position regarding the inheritance of A and B subunits. A subunit has two alleles, giving rise to three electrophoretically distinguishable phenotypes; B subunit has three alleles with six possible electrophoretic phenotypes. These studies [380] have confirmed that the structural loci for the A and B subunits lie on autosomal chromosomes and indicated that in one family the deficiency resulted from the inheritance of a null allele at the A subunit locus. The cases reported by Barbui *et al.* [381] may represent similar defects, but the existence of patients with non-functional forms of factor XIII was suggested by the studies of Forman *et al.* [385]. Further details of the molecular and genetic heterogeneity of factor XIII and its disorders remain to be determined.

Clinical picture
Severe factor-XIII deficiency, in homozygous individuals for example, often presents with excessive bleeding from the umbilical stump during the first few days of life, and continues throughout life with bruising, haematoma formation and post-traumatic bleeding. Haemarthroses sometimes occur [375, 386–389]. Although bleeding may occur immediately after trauma, it is characteristically delayed for several hours or days. Healing is also delayed, possibly because the clot is unstable and susceptible to fibrinolysis and does not support the proper growth of fibroblasts [390]. There is a relatively high incidence of intracranial bleeding and spontaneous abortion occurs in females [388, 391, 392]; sterility may occur in affected males [85].

Diagnosis
Characteristically all the tests of coagulation based on the formation of fibrin are normal, as are the bleeding time, platelet count and platelet function tests. Plasma clots are soluble in 5 M urea or 1% monochloroacetic acid and this test is convenient for screening for a severe defect, though it may not detect heterozygous subjects. The diagnosis can be confirmed by specific biochemical or immunological assays (see above) and these are needed to detect carriers.

The disorder must be differentiated from other inherited haemostatic defects and especially from dysfibrinogenaemia and afibrinogenaemia, in which there may be similar symptoms of wound dehiscence and haemorrhagic abortion and in which there may also be defective fibrin cross-linking and increased clot solubility in 5 M urea. The recently described syndrome of α_2-antiplasmin deficiency (see p. 1143) must also be excluded. Acquired deficiencies of factor XIII may occur in liver disease and disseminated intravascular coagulation and inhibitors to factor XIII may develop, particularly in association with anti-tuberculous therapy. These and other acquired deficiencies of factor XIII have been reviewed by Losowsky & Miloszewski [372].

Treatment
The treatment of an episode of bleeding is easy; only one to five per cent of normal factor-XIII activity is necessary to maintain haemostasis [393]; it is well preserved in plasma *in vitro* and the half-life *in vivo* is about 12 days [394]. Development of antibodies to factor XIII was suggested in one case [377] but has not proved to be a problem in the inherited disorder [372]. A concentrate of placental factor XIII has been on clinical trial [372, 395] and is said to be useful in patients who suffer plasma reactions, but availability on a long-term basis is in doubt. Prophylactic treatment with FFP, 500 ml every five to six weeks, seems to produce satisfactory results and allows patients, including children, to lead a normal life.

DEFICIENCIES OF PROTHROMBIN, FACTOR X AND FACTOR VII

These deficiencies will be considered in the same section; pathogenesis and diagnosis of each will be described separately and clinical presentation and treatment together.

Prothrombin deficiency
Prothrombin deficiency probably represents one of the rarest hereditary coagulation defects: by 1978 Owen *et*

al. [396] were able to describe only 24 affected pedigrees. Of these, 11 seemed to represent true deficiency of prothrombin (hypoprothrombinaemia), while seven involved the inheritance of abnormal molecular variants of prothrombin (dysprothrombinaemia). Since then Gill *et al.* [397] and Montgomery *et al.* [398] have described further kindreds with hypoprothrombinaemia and the apparent molecular variants prothrombin Molise [399], prothrombin Madrid [400] and prothrombin Metz [401] have been described.

Pathogenesis

True prothrombin deficiency is assumed when reduced levels of the protein are detected by both functional and immunological methods. In functional methods the ability of prothrombin to yield thrombin is measured in a two-stage system with brain extract or in one-stage systems based on prothrombin-deficient substrate plasma. Other techniques involve the use of prothrombin-converting snake venoms including the taipan, *Echis carinatus*, the tiger snake (*Notechis scutatis scutatis*) and *Dispholidus typus*, or the use of staphylocoagulase which combines with prothrombin to produce a thrombin-like activity [411]. The nature of these reactions is summarized and referenced by Bezeaud *et al.* [400]. Immunological assay methods involve the use of precipitating antisera in the Mancini radial immunodiffusion, Laurell electroimmunoassay or similar methods. Antisera can also be used to demonstrate other abnormal biochemical characteristics of prothrombin variants (e.g. on standard Scheidegger or two-dimensional immunoelectrophoresis); these methods have been summarized and referenced by Girolami *et al.* [399]. Biochemical abnormalities involving the calcium- and phospholipid-binding region containing γ-carboxyglutamic-acid residues have been sought using inorganic adsorbents and electrophoresis. Calcium-related abnormalities have been detected in prothrombin San Juan [402] and prothrombin Brussels [403], but the nature of the molecular abnormalities has not been established.

In severe hypoprothrombinaemia, levels of prothrombin measured by functional assay have parallelled those measured by immunoassay [396], but many families have been poorly characterized. The patient reported by Gill *et al.* [397] appears to be a homozygote (or compound heterozygote) with heterozygous parents. Occasionally there is a co-existing mild deficiency of factor VII (see p. 1140). The characteristics of the earlier reported dysprothrombinaemias have been reviewed by Bloom [404], and are summarized together with those of the few additional reported cases, in Table 28.8.

Diagnosis

The characteristic features on laboratory examination are prolonged one-stage prothrombin times not corrected by adsorbed normal plasma, aged serum or Russell's viper venom. The partial thromboplastin time (KCCT) may also be prolonged, but levels of fibrinogen and of factors V, VII and X are usually normal, although slightly reduced levels of factor VII have occasionally been reported [396]. Prothrombin measured by one- or two-stage methods using tissue extract is virtually always reduced, but levels using other activators may be variable in patients with dysprothrombinaemia (see Table 28.8). Immunological assay is characteristically reduced in hypoprothrombinaemia and normal in dysprothrombinaemia. Other immunological and biochemical features of dysprothrombinaemia have been described above. The condition must be differentiated from acquired disorders including vitamin-K-deficient states (which may be difficult in the newborn) and 'lupus-like' anti-coagulants.

Factor-X deficiency

Pathogenesis

Factor-X deficiency was originally described in the Prower [412] and Stuart [413] kinships. The abnormality in these and similar patients was characterized by a prolonged prothrombin time using either brain extract or Russell's viper venom and by deficiency of factor Xa in intrinsic coagulation, as indicated by the KCCT and the thromboplastin generation test. In several earlier studies no antigen attributable to factor X was detected by antibody neutralization [414] or by immunoelectrophoresis [415], but subsequent immunological and other coagulation methods have revealed a variety of abnormalities related to factor X [416, 417]. It seems that even the index patients, Miss Prower and Mr Stuart, have themselves inherited different variants.

Denson *et al.* [416] investigated six patients with a factor-X defect and claimed to distinguish at least five different forms using tests of factor-X activation in the intrinsic system (KCCT), the extrinsic system (prothrombin time) and the Russell's viper venom test in combination with xenogeneic antibody neutralization and double immunodiffusion tests. Girolami *et al.* [417] described a remarkable group of patients in the Friuli valley in northern Italy: 11 homozygous patients (one was not from Friuli) and about 60 heterozygotes were studied subsequently [418, 419]. The main features of factor X Friuli are that it is activated slowly or not at all in the presence of tissue extract or phospholipid, but reacts normally in the presence of Russell's viper venom and phospholipid. Trypsin and the

Table 28.8. Dysprothrombinaemias

Anomaly	Reference	Inheritance	Prothrombin level assayed by†						Immunoelectrophoresis		Bleeding	Comments
			Coag.	Staph.	E. car.	Taipan	Tiger	Immuno.	Plasma	Serum		
Cardeza	405	heterozygous	R*	?	?	?	?	N*	normal	normal and abnormal	No	Associated with Ehlers–Danlos syndrome
Barcelona	406, 407	homo- and heterozygous	R	N	almost N	?	?	N	increased anodal	?	Yes	Absence of one Xa cleavage site
San Juan	402, 409	compound heterozygous	R	N	N	?	?	N	normal and abnormal (anodal)	anodal band	Yes	Decreased Ca^{2+} binding
Padua	399, 408	heterozygous	R	N	N‡	R	R	N	normal	normal and abnormal bands	Yes	
Brussels	403	homo- and heterozygous	R	R or N	R	?	?	N	normal	second line in presence of Ca^{2+}	Yes	Slow activation. Two stage assays higher than one stage
Molise	399	? compound heterozygous	R	R	R	R	R	R§	normal	slightly less anodal	Yes	
Quick	396, 410	? homozygous compound heterozygous	R	?	R	R	?	R§	?	?	Yes	Normal Ca^{2+} binding. Abnormal cleavage. Xa activates amidolytic activity but not clotting
Metz	401		?	?	?	?	?	?	?	?	?	
Madrid	400	homo- and heterozygous	R	?	N	R	?	N	almost normal	?	Yes	Slow conversion to thrombin. Binds tightly to DEAE Sephadex

* R = reduced, N = normal.
† Coag: conventional coagulation assay; Staph : staphylocoagulase; *E. car.*, Taipan, Tiger: snake venoms; Immuno: immunoassay.
‡ See Girolami *et al.* [399].
§ 'Hypo-dysprothrombinaemia'.

venoms of *Bothrops atrox* or *Vipera aspis* activated it to an intermediate degree. Immunologically factor X Friuli was indistinguishable from normal factor X; it had normal electrophoretic mobility different from that of PIVKA-X and did not exert an inhibitory effect in blood coagulation. The importance of the above studies is the implication that many families with factor-X deficiency may have inherited abnormal variants: there are relatively clear-cut differences between the Stuart, Prower and Friuli defects (Table 28.9), and other less well characterized patients with atypical immunological reactions to factor-X antisera have been described by Denson *et al.* [416]. In addition to these possible variants, two kindreds with factor-X deficiency were described by Porter *et al.* [420]; in one there was no apparent excess of factor-X antigen, but in the other there was disproportionate reduction of the activity-to-antigen ratio. Factor X Vorarlberg was described by Lechner *et al.* [421] in two apparently unrelated families from the same region of Austria: in these families also there was evidence of inheritance of a reduced amount of a functionally abnormal molecule. Recently Fair *et al.* [422] have studied plasma samples from eight unrelated patients: only modest differences in factor-X activities (Russell's viper venom, extrinsic and intrinsic activation) were observed and with one possible exception, levels of factor X measured by radioimmunoassay paralleled procoagulant activity. Thus, while Denson, his co-workers and most others have concluded that there is genetic heterogeneity, Fair and co-workers consider that there is genetic homogeneity between the inherited factor-X-deficient states. Direct comparisons are difficult because the patients, antisera and methods have been different and this dilemma remains to be resolved.

Diagnosis
The prothrombin time is prolonged but the Russell's viper venom-cephalin time may be normal (e.g. in factor-X-Friuli defect as described above). The latter test is thus not a good screening procedure for factor-X deficiency. The abnormalities are corrected by normal plasma and aged serum but not by alumina-adsorbed plasma. The partial thromboplastin time is prolonged and there is a serum abnormality in the thromboplastin generation test. The possibility of this deficiency should be considered in any patient with an otherwise unexplained slight prolongation of the partial thromboplastin time (KCCT), because in one patient tests of the intrinsic system were more abnormal than those of the extrinsic system [416]. Inherited factor-X deficiency must be distinguished from the acquired disorder, specifically in vitamin-K-deficient states and especially from the isolated deficiency of factor X which may accompany amyloidosis.

Factor-VII deficiency

Pathogenesis and inheritance
The first patient with inherited deficiency of factor VII was described in 1957 by Alexander *et al.* [423]; by 1964 some 40 cases had been added in which the factor-VII level was below 10% [424]. Factor VII (proconvertin) participates in the extrinsic coagulation system during the activation of factor X in the presence of tissue factor, phospholipid and calcium. Its activity can be increased by factors Xa, XIIa, fragments of factor XII and by storage at 0–4°C, apparently due to the action of kallikrein. It may also play a part in the activation of factor IX [425]. The activities of all these pathways must be borne in mind when considering the pathophysiology of factor-VII deficiency.

There is little information concerning the nature of the biochemical defect in factor-VII deficiency. Immunological studies have been hampered by the lack of a precipitating antiserum which can be used in immunoelectrophoretic techniques, and recourse has been made to imprecise antibody (inhibitor) neutralization tests. Using this technique, cross-reacting material has been detected in a varying number of affected kindreds [426–429]. Using a carefully standardized inhibitor neutralization assay, Mazzuconi *et al.* [430] detected normal levels of factor-VII antigen in one patient out of seven kindreds studied; in this family the ratio of VIIC to VIIAg was useful in detecting symptomless heterozygotes. Girolami and colleagues [431–433] have recently demonstrated a number of apparent variants of factor VII in defined areas of

Table 28.9. Factor-X deficiency: main types (after Girolami *et al.* [419])

Type	Factor-X level (tissue extract)	Factor-X level (Russell's viper venom— cephalin)	Factor-X antigen (immunologically reactive)
Prower	Low	Low	Present
Stuart	Very low	Very low	Absent
Friuli	Low	Normal	Present

Table 28.10. Factor-VII deficiency states

Report	Number of pedigrees studied	VIIC level in relation to type of tissue extract used in assay	VII C:VIIAg*	Comments
Goodnight et al. [426]	4	Only human reported	C≡Ag and C<Ag	Hereditary VII deficiency
Denson et al. [427]	5	Source of tissue not stated	C≡Ag and C<Ag	VII deficiency+Dubin–Johnson syndrome Antigen inhibitory in ox-brain coagulation system
Levanon et al. [428]	1	Only rabbit reported	C≡Ag	
Briet et al. [429]	9 patients	Only rabbit reported	C≡Ag in 8 & C < Ag in 1	
	2	Human≡ox?	C≡Ag and C<Ag	
Mazzuconi et al. [430]	1	Only human reported	C<Ag	C:Ag ratio reduced in carriers
	6	Only human reported	C≡Ag	
Girolami et al. [431]	2	Simian or rabbit or human<ox† (porcine not reported)	C<Ag‡	VII Verona (? double heterozygous)
Girolami et al. [432]	1	Rabbit<human<porcine <ox or simian	C (rabbit brain) < Ag‡	VII Padua (? homozygous)
Girolami et al. [433]	1	Ox or porcine<rabbit or simian or human	C (ox brain) < Ag‡	VII Padua 2 (? double heterozygous)

* VIIAg by antibody neutralization.
† Data in Girolami et al. [433].
‡ VIIAg measured by inhibitor neutralization test using rabbit tissue extract.

northern Italy by testing the reaction of plasma in the factor-VII assay with tissue extracts from different species, in conjunction with immunoassay by an antibody neutralization technique: the findings in these and other families are summarized in Table 28.10. In kindreds with factor VII Verona and Padua 2, double heterozygosity for dysproconvertinaemia and hypoproconvertinaemia was suspected on the basis of family studies. Factor-VII deficiency has been reported in association with congenital hyperbilirubinaemia, Gilbert's disease [434] and Dubin–Johnson syndrome [428], but the conditions may segregate separately [435] and are not necessarily genetically related.

Diagnosis

Factor-VII deficiency prolongs the one-stage prothrombin time with tissue extract but not with Russell's viper venom [436], and tests of intrinsic coagulation pathways are normal. In doubtful cases, it may be profitable to test the effect of tissue extract from different species [431–433]. Assays for factor VII are based on a one-stage system using factor-VII-deficient plasma substrate. This is difficult to obtain from patients, but factor-VII deficiency also occurs in dogs [437, 438] and an assay based on canine plasma has been devised [439].

Clinical picture and treatment of prothrombin and factors-X and -VII deficiency

All these syndromes are inherited as autosomal characteristics. The clinical pictures of prothrombin and factor-X deficiency are similar. Homozygous patients sometimes have consanguineous parents. They, and those with compound heterozygous genotype, have a more or less severe haemorrhagic syndrome with excessive bruising, mucous-membrane and gastro-intestinal bleeding, menorrhagia and occasional muscle haematomata and haemarthroses. Heterozygous patients are symptomless or have only a mild tendency to bleed. Most patients with homozygous factor-VII deficiency have a lifelong bleeding tendency [424, 440], but coincident thromboembolic complications have been reported [432, 441, 442]. Intracranial bleeding in the neonate is a particular dangerous lesion [443]. The severity varies widely between individuals and bleeding symptoms may be delayed until adolescence or the menarche; other patients may remain almost symptomless throughout life. It is not known if this variation is due to the presence of variant forms of factor VII but the tendency to bleed is not necessarily related to factor-VII levels; possibly the latter may depend upon the source of substrate plasma and tissue extract used for the assays (Table 28.10).

The treatment of these deficiencies is by infusion of FFP or specific concentrates. The exact levels needed to maintain normal haemostasis are not known with certainty, but are presumably similar to those for other coagulation defects, i.e. 15–20 u/dl for minor episodes and over 30–40 u/dl for major surgery. These levels are comparatively easy to obtain in prothrombin and factor-X deficiency because of the relatively long half-lives of these factors *in vivo*—up to 90 hours in the case of prothrombin and up to 30 hours, with a biphasic decay curve, in the case of factor X [103, 420]. Fresh-frozen plasma can be administered for minor bleeds, and concentrates (e.g. of factors II, IX and X) for more severe lesions or to cover surgery.

The varying symptomatology recorded in patients with severe deficiency of factor VII makes it difficult to assess the intensity of treatment needed and this is compounded by the very short half-life of factor VII after infusion—about two to six hours [444, 445]—but it would be unwise not to treat affected patients if the occasion arises, as has been suggested [446]. Because the half-life of infused factor VII is so short, use of FFP may be limited by problems of fluid overload. Factor VII is present in some, but not all, preparations of 'factor-IX-prothrombin' concentrates and a specific concentrate of factor VII is available [103]. The subject has been reviewed by Zimmerman *et al.* [440].

Combined deficiencies of the vitamin-K-dependent factors

Factors II, VII, IX and X are all synthesized in the liver and depend upon the activity of vitamin K for the post-translational carboxylation of γ-glutamyl residues. There is evidence of biochemical homologies between these factors. Although the mode of inheritance of factor-IX deficiency (X-linked) differs from that of deficiencies of the other three factors (autosomal), it is not surprising that inherited combined deficiencies have been reported. What is not always clear is whether these represent true combined deficiencies, or merely apparent deficiencies due to aberrant or atypical reactions of one or other of the factors in *in-vitro* tests. Combined deficiency of factors VII and IX was originally reported by Bell & Alton [447] and reports of the combination have been reviewed by Hall *et al.* [448]. Girolami *et al.* [192] reported further examples. Factor-VII deficiency has also been reported in patients with prothrombin deficiency [396]. Combined deficiency of factors VII and X was reported in a large kindred in association with carotid-body tumour [449]. Combined congenital deficiency of factors II, VII, IX and X was recently reported in two patients: investigation suggested that some prothrombin molecules lacked γ-carboxy-glutamic-acid residues, as if there was a defect of the γ-carboxylation mechanism or of vitamin-K transport [193, 450]. An apparently similar deficiency was previously described by Newcomb *et al.* [451].

FACTOR-V DEFICIENCY

Pathogenesis and inheritance

'Parahaemophilia' was first described by Owren [452] as a haemorrhagic disease due to a deficiency of a clotting factor other than the four recognized at the time. The deficiency was thus defined as that of factor V, which was soon identified with the 'labile factor' already described by Quick [453]. It is an uncommon disorder: Seeler [454] reviewed the syndrome and defined 58 recorded cases. The inheritance pattern is autosomal and consanguinity has often been observed [455]. Symptomatic patients are usually homozygous, but the disease is sometimes manifested mildly in heterozygotes, in whom factor-V concentrations may be below the normal range. In others, apparently heterozygous on genetic grounds, factor-V levels have been recorded as being normal [454]. It is not clear if these findings are a function of the assay techniques used or of the nature of the factor-V molecule, because little is known of its chemical structure.

Immunological studies of factor V have been hampered by the fact that all antisera so far raised have been non-precipitating (*cf.* antibodies to factors VIIIC and VII). So far no antibody-neutralizing material has been detected in the plasma of the few patients studied [456–458], though paradoxically antibody-neutralizing material was detected in the platelets of one patient [459].

Clinical features and diagnosis

Symptoms, if they occur, consist mainly of bruising, epistaxis, and haemorrhage, bleeding after minor lacerations and dental extractions, and menorrhagia. Muscle haematomata and haemarthroses occur but are uncommon. Intracranial bleeding has been recorded as a cause of death. An association with congenital anomalies has often been reported, including renal, cardiovascular and skeletal abnormalities [454].

The bleeding time is prolonged in about one-third of recorded cases, possibly owing to an abnormality of platelet factor V. The prothrombin time and activated or non-activated partial thromboplastin times are prolonged, and are corrected by adsorbed normal plasma but not by aged serum or Russell's viper venom. In the thromboplastin generation test, incubation mixtures containing adsorbed patient's plasma are abnormal. Hougie [460] points out that normal platelets must not be used in diagnostic tests for

factor-V deficiency, as they contain this factor. Assays for factor V depend upon the use of artificially depleted substrate (e.g. aged oxalated plasma [79]).

Treatment

There is no concentrate of factor V available for therapeutic use and because it is relatively labile *in vitro*, specific treatment consists of the transfusion of FFP: factor V is not concentrated in cryoprecipitate. The minimum haemostatic level is not known with certainty but is probably in the order of 20 u/dl for post-operative care [461, 462]. The recovery of factor V in the circulation is approximately 50% of the expected level and the half-life is about 15–24 hours, so that frequent plasma infusions may be needed.

Combined deficiency of factors V and VIII

The combination of factor-V and -VIII deficiency occurs more frequently than can be accounted for by chance and in affected families the deficiencies are usually transmitted together [468]. Data from reported kindred have been reviewed by several authors [463–467]. The condition is clinically similar to isolated deficiency of factor V and follows an autosomal pattern of inheritance. Immunological tests have revealed normal levels of VIIIR:Ag [43, 467, 469, 470] and also cross-reacting material to human antibodies (VIIICAg and VCAg) in significant amounts [470]. Ristocetin cofactor was normal in one case [465].

Giddings *et al.* [470] and Graham [229] discuss the possible pathogenesis of the combined defect. Factors VC and VIIIC have much in common; both act with phospholipid as co-enzymes in the coagulation sequence, are activated by thrombin, and have similar stability and adsorption characteristics. It is thus possible that they will prove to have biochemical homologies and that the abnormalities are derived either from structural defects of a common precursor or by a common failure at a step in post-translational modification. Recently a defect of an inhibitor of activated protein C has been suggested [470a]: protein C is a vitamin-K-dependent factor which on activation destroys the activity of factors V and VIII.

CONTACT-FACTOR DEFICIENCIES

The interaction of factors XI and XII, prekallikrein (Fletcher factor) and high-molecular-weight kininogen in homeostatic mechanisms including the blood coagulation, fibrinolytic and complement systems are described elsewhere (Chapter 27). Deficiencies of each of these factors and, possibly, of less well-characterized ones which interact with them have been described; all are inherited as autosomal traits.

Factor-XI (plasma thromboplastin antecedent, PTA) deficiency

This was first described by Rosenthal *et al.* [471] and occurs mainly in Jews [472, 473], specifically of Ashkenazi descent from families emigrating from eastern Europe [3]; it is rare in Jews of other origins (e.g. Oriental and Sephardic) and in other population groups. The disease is inherited as an autosomal trait and thus occurs in homozygous and heterozygous forms. Basic levels of factor XI in homozygous individuals vary between kindreds (*cf.* haemophilia A and B); levels in heterozygotes tend to be higher but are variable. Normal levels have been recorded in some carriers, whilst in other kindreds transmission from heterozygotes of similar severity ('dominant' inheritance) occasionally occurs [3]. Seligsohn [3] recorded a low incidence of admitted consanguinity, suggesting a high mutation rate for the abnormal gene. Immunological studies in factor-XI deficiency are few, mainly because available antisera are non-precipitating. No excess of antigen over activity has been detected in over 20 patients studied [474–476].

Clinical picture, diagnosis and treatment

The haemorrhagic tendency is usually mild, even in patients with homozygous disease, and is not necessarily related to the level of factor-XI coagulant or antigen [475]. Excessive bruising may be associated and coincident with menorrhagia, and is much more common in women than in men. Other symptoms include epistaxis, post-operative and post-extraction bleeding; haemarthroses and intramuscular bleeding are rare.

The bleeding time is usually normal. The prothrombin time is normal but the activated and non-activated partial thromboplastin times are prolonged. In the thromboplastin generation test there is an abnormality when both adsorbed plasma and serum are tested together. The lack of contact activation can be detected by the glass contact activation [477] and celite eluate tests [478], or more specifically localized using the celite-6 test [478] or assay of factor XI [479]. Since tests of contact activation factors may be influenced by freezing and thawing, initial assessment should be performed on fresh plasma.

Treatment for factor-XI deficiency is not usually required, and no concentrate is available. Specific treatment for bleeding or to cover surgery consists of the administration of FFP: this is effective because the half-life of factor XI *in vivo* is long—in the region of 60 hours [103]. Modest doses of plasma are all that are needed for minor procedures but it was necessary to maintain factor-XI levels at over 30 u/dl for two weeks to cover major prostatic surgery [480].

Factor XII, prekallikrein and kininogen deficiencies

FACTOR-XII DEFICIENCY

Factor-XII deficiency was first discovered by Ratnoff & Colopy [481] in a patient called Hageman during the course of routine pre-operative assessment. In spite of a prolonged clotting time, the patient had no haemorrhagic symptoms; in fact he and several other similarly affected persons died from thromboembolic disease or myocardial infarction [482]. The deficiency is usually fully expressed only in homozygous individuals, though in some kindreds vertical transmission through heterozygotes ('dominant' inheritance) has been reported [483]. Abnormal variants have been detected by immunological methods [484] but the biochemical defects could not be characterized. Most patients with factor-XII deficiency (Hageman trait) are asymptomatic, but rarely there may be a mild bleeding tendency [485]: an association with subarachnoid haemorrhage was reported in one case [486]. Factor XII is more fully reviewed by Ratnoff [485] and elsewhere in this book (Chapter 27).

FLETCHER-FACTOR DEFICIENCY

This was described by Hathaway *et al.* [487] in asymptomatic offspring of a consanguineous marriage. The defect is fully manifested in homozygous individuals [488]. Affected persons have a prolonged kaolin-cephalin clotting time which shortens on prolonged exposure to glass or kaolin [487, 489]. Fletcher factor has been identified by Wuepper [490] as prekallikrein, but some unexpected reactions have been observed in experiments using rabbit plasma and eluates from diatomaceous earths, suggesting that plasma may contain more than one prekallikrein [485].

FITZGERALD-FACTOR DEFICIENCY

This condition was described by Waldmann & Abraham [491] and studied in more detail by Saito *et al.* [492]. The subject was a 71-year-old asymptomatic man who was unexpectedly found to have a prolonged activated partial thromboplastin time. All recognized coagulation factors were normal but Fletcher factor (prekallikrein) was present at only about 10–15% of normal concentration. Prolonged incubation with kaolin did not shorten the partial thromboplastin time. Subjects with similar defects were independently reported and named after the affected kindreds: Flaujeac-factor deficiency [493], Williams factor [494] and Reid trait [495]. These plasmas are not mutually corrective and subsequent studies have indicated that they are deficient in components of the kininogen system. Fitzgerald-factor-deficient plasma lacks high-molecular-weight kininogen, and defective kinin production is not corrected by addition of purified kallikrein. The Reid trait appears to be similar, but in both the Williams and Flaujeac traits there is a deficiency of both high- and low-molecular-weight kininogens. Factor XII, prekallikrein and kininogen are necessary for the generation of contact-activated fibrinolytic activity and the vascular permeability factor (PF/dil) and for stimulating the migration of leucocytes in inflammatory reactions (see Chapter 16). None of these functions are abnormal in Fletcher-factor-deficient individuals but an atypical inflammatory response was reported in the Fitzgerald trait [496]. Most people with prekallikrein and kininogen deficiencies are symptomless and do not have tendencies to abnormal bleeding, thrombosis or infections, suggesting that alternative homeostatic mechanisms exist *in vivo* (see Chapter 27).

The coagulation findings in deficiencies of factor XII and in Fletcher, Fitzgerald and related traits are very similar. The activated partial thromboplastin time (KCCT) is prolonged—most severely in factor-XII deficiency; the prothrombin and bleeding times are normal. In Fletcher-factor deficiency the KCCT may be shortened by prolonging the incubation with kaolin for 10–20 minutes. Definitive coagulation studies depend upon cross-correction with known defective plasmas, but a chromogenic assay has been described for plasma prekallikrein [497] and immunological assays for kallikrein [498] and kininogen [494]. The role of these in clinical diagnosis remains to be established, but they may be of value in characterizing the abnormality in patients with otherwise unexplained prolongation of the KCCT.

One other possible member of this group of disorders was described by Hougie *et al.* [499] in subjects with a mild bleeding diathesis; the trait was called the Passovoy defect. In affected individuals the KCCT was shortened by prolonged incubation with kaolin, but the defect seemed to be distinct from Fletcher-factor deficiency and remains to be more fully characterized. Treatment is not necessary for subjects with the Hageman, Fletcher, Fitzgerald and related traits, but plasma transfusion was needed post-operatively in some patients with the Passovoy trait.

COMBINED AND UNUSUAL DEFECTS

Combined deficiencies of factors V and VIII and of the vitamin-K-dependent factors have already been discussed above. In addition a number of uncommon or isolated kindreds or patients with other combined deficiencies have been described. These include deficiencies of factors VII and VIII [500], VIII and IX [501], VIII and IX with a platelet defect [502] and VIII

and XI [503]. Some of these reports may represent coincidental inheritance of otherwise distinct defects fortuitously present in the same individual. In older reports it is sometimes difficult to evaluate the techniques used in the light of current knowledge and in any event most of the deficiencies reported were relatively mild.

A number of relatively uncharacterized coagulation defects have also been described. The Dynia defect [504] seemed to involve an abnormality in the interaction between factor IXa and factor VIII during the activation of factor X. An atypical inherited disorder in which the only definite laboratory abnormality was a severe defect of prothrombin conversion was described by Robinson *et al.* [505], and three further families have recently been described by Parry *et al.* [506]. The defect was inherited as an autosomal characteristic and was sometimes associated with a mild bleeding tendency, mainly after trauma or childbirth. Assays of all coagulation factors were normal and in one kindred the abnormality seemed to involve the presence of a factor which interfered with the interaction of plasma with platelet phospholipid. This condition remains to be characterized, but indicates the importance of performing a prothrombin consumption test in otherwise unexplained haemorrhagic diseases. An abnormality of a platelet receptor for factors V and activated X was reported in a similar case (see Chapter 26, p. 1048).

One further inherited haemostatic abnormality deserves mention. A severe haemorrhagic defect resembling haemophilia has been reported in one patient in association with complete deficiency of α_2-antiplasmin [507, 508] and called 'Miyasato's disease'. Intermediate levels were noted in the consanguineous parents and other apparently heterozygous family members. The euglobulin lysis time was moderately accelerated and excessive bleeding responded to treatment with tranexamic acid.

HEREDITARY COAGULATION DISORDERS WITH THROMBOTIC TENDENCY

A tendency to thromboembolic episodes may occur in certain forms of dysfibrinogenaemia and during treatment of afibrinogenaemia (see p. 1130), as well as possibly in factor-XII deficiency. In addition there is the uncommon but well-documented syndrome of inherited deficiency of antithrombin-III activity.

Inherited antithrombin-III deficiency
Antithrombin III (ATIII) is a single-chain glycoprotein of molecular weight approximately 65 000. It is the

main physiological inhibitor of thrombin and factor Xa but it also has some effect on factors IXa, XIa and XIIa.

Inherited quantitative deficiency of ATIII was first described by Egeberg [510] and since then there have been over 20 reports of similar families. In most kindreds, ATIII has been reduced when measured by coagulation, amidolytic or immunological methods. In one family [511] ATIII activity was reduced in functional assays but its level measured by immunological methods was normal, suggesting the presence of a molecule of similar immunological specificity to normal ATIII but lacking function. This condition has been called ATIII Budapest.

Antithrombin-III deficiency is inherited as an autosomal dominant characteristic. Levels in affected heterozygous individuals are usually about 50–60% of those in normal relatives [512, 513]. It thus seems that a thrombotic tendency may be associated with quite modest reduction of ATIII. Clinically, patients present with recurrent venous thromboembolic manifestations such as pulmonary embolism, deep-vein thrombosis, mesenteric-vein thrombosis and priapism; arterial lesions occur but are rare. The onset of symptoms is usually delayed until after puberty and in females may be associated with pregnancy. In other patients thromboembolic episodes may complicate trauma or surgery or coincide with ingestion of oral contraceptive agents. The latter may reduce ATIII levels even in normal subjects.

Antithrombin-III deficiency should thus be suspected in any patient with recurrent thromboses, especially in young individuals and those with a positive family history. The diagnosis is confirmed by functional or amidolytic assay. Immunological assay is best reserved for detection of molecular variants. It should be remembered that ATIII levels may be reduced by heparin therapy even in hitherto normal individuals so that diagnosis may be difficult at this time. The methods for measuring ATIII are reviewed by Conard [514].

The optimum treatment for ATIII deficiency has not been fully established. On theoretical grounds the use of heparin during an acute thrombotic episode could be questioned not only because heparin acts through ATIII as cofactor but also because it may cause a further reduction of the ATIII level. Nevertheless, heparin treatment has been recommended [515]. It is possible that the optimum regime may combine heparin with a recently described concentrate of human ATIII [516]. Coumarin therapy may result in elevation of plasma ATIII, although not to normal levels, and this type of treatment may be useful for long-term and prophylactic therapy. Subcutaneous heparin has also been reported to prevent recurrent thrombosis [515]. The role of long-term treatment with human ATIII concentrate remains to be assessed.

REFERENCES

1 BIGGS R. (1977) Haemophilia treatment in the United Kingdom from 1969 to 1974. *British Journal of Haematology*, **35**, 487.

2 DUCKERT F. & KOLLER F. (1975) The old Swiss haemophilia families of Tenna and Wald. In: *Handbook of Hemophilia* (ed. Brinkhous K.M. & Hemker H.C.), p. 21. Excerpta Medica, Amsterdam.

3 SELIGSOHN U. (1978) High gene frequency of factor IX (PTA) deficiency in Ashkenazi Jews. *Blood*, **51**, 1223.

4 WRIGHT I.S. (1962) The nomenclature of blood clotting factors. *Thrombosis et Diathesis Haemorrhagica*, **7**, 381.

5 GRAHAM J.B., BARRETT D.A., BLOMBÄCK B., CANN H.M., HARDISTY R.M., LARRIEU M.J. & RENWICK J.H. (1973) Reports from the International Committee of Haemostasis and Thrombosis. A genetic nomenclature for human blood coagulation. *Thrombosis et Diathesis Haemorrhagica*, **30**, 2.

6 EGEBERG O. (1976) Inherited fibrinogen abnormality causing thrombophilia. *Thrombosis et Diathesis Haemorrhagica*, **17**, 176.

7 BUDZYNSKI A.Z., MARDER V.J., MÉNACHÉ D. & GUILLIN M.-C. (1974) Defect in the gamma polypeptide chain of a congenital abnormal fibrinogen. *Nature (London)*, **252**, 66 (letter).

8 BLOOM A.L. (1977) The physiology of Factor VIII. In: *Recent Advances in Blood Coagulation* (ed. Poller L.) 2nd edn, p. 141. Churchill-Livingstone, Edinburgh.

9 BLOOM A.L. (1979) The biosynthesis of factor VIII. *Clinics in Haematology*, **8**, 53.

10 PEAKE I.R. & BLOOM A.L. (1978) Immunoradiometric assay of procoagulant factor VIII antigen in plasma and serum and the reduction in haemophilia. Preliminary studies on adult and fetal blood. *Lancet*, **i**, 473.

11 ROSNER F. (1969) Hemophilia in the Talmud and Rabbinic writings. *Annals of Internal Medicine*, **70**, 833.

12 QUICK A.J. (1942) *The Hemorrhagic Diseases and Physiology of Hemostasis*, p. 192. C. C. Thomas, Springfield, Illinois.

13 BRINKHOUS K.M. (1975) A short history of hemophilia with some comments on the word 'hemophilia'. In: *Handbook of Hemophilia* (ed. Brinkhous K.M. & Hemker H.C.), p. 3. Excerpta Medica, Amsterdam.

14 KERR C.B. (1965) Genetics of human blood coagulation. *Journal of Medical Genetics*, **2**, 154.

15 OWEN C.A., BOWIE E.J.W., DIDISHEIM P. & THOMPSON J.M. (1969) *The Diagnosis of Bleeding Disorders*, p. 23. Churchill, London.

16 RATNOFF O.D. (1977) Blood clotting mechanisms: an overview. In: *Haemostasis: Biochemistry, Physiology and Pathology* (ed Ogston D. & Bennett B.), p. 1. J. Wiley & Sons, London.

17 HYNES H.E., OWEN C.A., JR, BOWIE E.J.W. & THOMSON J.R., JR (1969) Development of the present concept of hemophilia. *Mayo Clinical Proceedings*, **44**, 193.

18 OTTO J.C. (1803) An account of an haemorrhagic disposition existing in certain families. *Medical Repository*, **6**, 1.

19 BULLOCH W. & FILDES P. (1911) Haemophilia: treasury of human inheritance, parts V and VI. *Eugenic Laboratory Memoirs XII*, Dulan & Co., London.

20 BRINKHOUS K.M., GRAHAM J.B., PENICK G.D. & LANGDELL R.D. (1951) Studies on canine hemophilia. In: *Blood Clotting and Allied Problems. Transactions of the Fourth Conference* (ed. Flynn J.E.), p. 51. Josiah Macy Jr Foundation, New York.

21 WRIGHT A.E. (1893) On a method of determining the condition of blood coagulability for clinical and experimental purposes, and on the effect of calcium salts in haemophilia and actual or threatened haemorrhage. *British Medical Journal*, ii, 223.

22 WEIL P.E. (1906) Étude de sang chez les hémophiles. *Bulletins et Mémoires de la Société Medicale des Hôpitaux de Paris*, 23, 1001.

23 ADDIS T. (1911) The pathogenesis of hereditary haemophilia. *Journal of Pathology and Bacteriology*, 15, 427.

24 PATEK A.J. & TAYLOR F.H.C. (1937) Hemophilia II. Some properties of a substance obtained from normal human plasma effective in accelerating the coagulation of hemophilic blood. *Journal of Clinical Investigation*, 16, 113.

25 BRINKHOUS K.M. (1939) A study of the clotting defect in hemophilia. The delayed formation of thrombin. *American Journal of Medical Sciences*, 198, 509.

26 BRINKHOUS K.M. (1947) Clotting defect in hemophilia: deficiency in a plasma factor required for platelet utilisation. *Proceedings of the Society for Experimental Biology and Medicine*, 66, 117.

27 QUICK A.J. (1947) Studies on the enigma of the hemostatic dysfunction in hemophilia. *American Journal of Medical Sciences*, 214, 272.

28 MERSKEY C. (1950) The laboratory diagnosis of haemophilia. *Journal of Clinical Pathology*, 3, 301.

29 BIGGS R. & DOUGLAS A.S. (1953) The thromboplastin generation test. *Journal of Clinical Pathology*, 6, 23.

30 PAVLOVSKY A. (1974) Contribution to the pathogenesis of hemophilia. *Blood*, 2, 185.

31 AGGELER P.M., WHITE S.G., GLENDENNING M.B., PAGE E.W., LEAKE T.B. & BATES G. (1952) Plasma thromboplastin component (PTC) deficiency: A new disease resembling hemophilia. *Proceedings of the Society for Experimental Biology and Medicine*, 79, 692.

32 BIGGS R., DOUGLAS A.S., MACFARLANE R.G., DACIE J.V., PITNEY W.R., MERSKEY C. & O'BRIEN J.R. (1952) Christmas disease: A condition previously mistaken for haemophilia. *British Medical Journal*, ii, 1378.

33 TOCANTINS L.M., CARROL R.T. & HOLBURN R.H. (1951) The clot accelerating effect of dilution on blood and plasma: Relation to the mechanism of coagulation of normal and hemophilic blood. *Blood*, 6, 720.

34 NOUR-ELDIN F. & WILKINSON J.F. (1958) *In-vivo* study on the relation between Bridge anticoagulant and antihaemophilic globulin. *British Journal of Haematology*, 4, 292.

35 GRAHAM J.B. & BARROW E.M. (1957) The pathogenesis of hemophilia. An experimental analysis of the anticephalin hypothesis in hemophilic dogs. *Journal of Experimental Medicine*, 106, 273.

36 INGRAM G.I.C., TANNER E.I. & MATCHETT M.O. (1959) Experiments on the 'Bridge effect'. *British Journal of Haematology*, 5, 307.

37 FANTL P., SAWERS R.J. & MARR A.G. (1956) Investigation of a haemorrhagic disease due to betaprothromboplastin deficiency complicated by a specific inhibitor of thromboplastin formation. *Australasian Annals of Medicine*, 5, 163.

38 DENSON K.W.E., BIGGS R., HADDON M.E., BORRETT R. & COBB K. (1969) Two types of haemophilia (A+ and A−). A study of forty-eight cases. *British Journal of Haematology*, 17, 163.

39 HOYER L.W. & BRECKENRIDGE R.T. (1968) Immunologic studies of antihemophilic factor (AHF, factor VIII): cross-reacting material in a genetic variant of hemophilia A. *Blood*, 32, 962.

40 FEINSTEIN D., CHONG M.N.Y., KASPER C.K. & RAPAPORT S.I. (1969) Hemophilia A: polymorphism detectable by a factor VIII antibody. *Science*, 163, 1071.

41 BIGGS R. (1974) The absorption of human factor-VIII neutralising antibody for factor VIII. *British Journal of Haematology*, 26, 259.

42 PEAKE I.R., BLOOM A.L., GIDDINGS J.C. & LUDLAM C.A. (1979) An immunoradiometric assay for procoagulant factor VIII antigen: Results in haemophilia, von Willebrand's disease and fetal plasma and serum. *British Journal of Haematology*, 42, 269.

43 ZIMMERMAN T.S., RATNOFF O.D. & POWELL A.E. (1971) Immunologic differentiation of classic hemophilia (factor VIII deficiency) and von Willebrand's disease. With observations on combined deficiencies of antihemophilic factor and proaccelerin (factor V) and on an acquired circulating anticoagulant against antihemophilic factor. *Journal of Clinical Investigation*, 50, 244.

44 JAFFE E.A., HOYER L.W. & NACHMAN R.S. (1973) Synthesis of antihemophilic factor antigen by cultured human endothelial cells. *Journal of Clinical Investigation*, 52, 2757.

45 SHEARN S.A.M., PEAKE I.R., GIDDINGS J.C., HUMPHRYS J. & BLOOM A.L. (1971) The characterisation and synthesis of antigens related to factor VIII in vascular endothelium. *Thrombosis Research*, 11, 43.

46 OWEN C.A., JR, BOWIE E.J.W. & FASS D.N. (1979) Generation of factor-VIII coagulant activity by isolated, perfused neonatal pig livers and adult rat livers. *British Journal of Haematology*, 43, 307.

47 GRAHAM J.B., BRINKHOUS K.M. & DODDS W.J. (1975) Canine and equine hemophilia. In: *Handbook of Hemophilia* (ed. Brinkhous K.M. & Hemker H.C.), p. 119. Excerpta Medica, Amsterdam.

48 ARCHER R.K. (1961) True haemophilia (haemophilia A) in a thoroughbred foal. *Veterinary Record*, 73, 338.

49 COTTER S.M., BRENNER R.M. & DODDS W.J. (1978) Hemophilia A in three unrelated cats. *Journal of the American Veterinary Association*, 172, 166.

50 RATNOFF O.D. & LEWIS J.H. (1975) Heckathorn's disease: variable functional deficiency of antihemophilic factor (factor VIII). *Blood*, 46, 161.

51 DENSON K.W.E. & BIGGS R. (1976) Laboratory diagnosis, tests of clotting function and their standardisation. In: *Human Blood Coagulation, Haemostasis and Thrombosis* (ed. Biggs R.), 2nd edn, p. 510. Blackwell Scientific Publications, Oxford.

52 ESSIEN E.M. & AYENI O. (1978) Factor VIII coagulant activity in an African population in relation to a

recognised standard. *British Journal of Haematology*, **39**, 225.

53 RIZZA C.R. (1976) The clinical features of clotting factor deficiencies. In: *Human Blood Coagulation, Haemostasis and Thrombosis* (ed. Biggs R.), 2nd edn, p. 231. Blackwell Scientific Publications, Oxford.

54 HOEDEMAEKER P.H.J. & WAGENVOORT C.A. (1975) Pathological changes in joints of patients suffering from hemophilia. In: *Handbook of Hemophilia* (ed. Brinkhous K.M. & Hemker H.C.), p. 301. Excerpta Medica, Amsterdam.

55 MAINARDI C.L., LEVINE P.H., WERB Z. & HARRIS E.D., JR (1978) Proliferative synovitis in hemophilia: biochemical and morphologic observations. *Arthritis and Rheumatism*, **21**, 137.

56 AHLBERG A. (1965) Haemophilia in Sweden. VIII. Incidence, treatment and prophylaxis of orthropathy and other musculo-skeletal manifestations of haemophilia A and B. *Acta Orthopaedica Scandinavica*, **77** (Suppl.), 5.

57 SCHREIBER R.R. (1975) Musculo-skeletal system—radiologic findings. In: *Handbook of Hemophilia* (ed. Brinkhous K.M. & Hemker H.C.), p. 333. Excerpta Medica, Amsterdam.

58 JAFFE H.L. (1972) *Metabolic, Degenerative and Inflammatory Diseases of Bones and Joints*, p. 728, Lea & Febiger, Philadelphia.

59 VALDERRAMA J.A.F. & MATTHEWS J.M. (1965) The haemophilic pseudotumour or haemophilic subperiosteal haematoma. *Journal of Bone and Joint Surgery*, **47B**, 256.

60 KILBY D., BLOOM A.L. & RICHARDS S.H. (1972) Haemophilic pseudotumour of the temporal bone. A case successfully treated by a closed mastoidectomy technique. *Journal of Laryngology and Otology*, **86**, 657.

61 BLOOM A.L., ENOCH B.A. & RICHARDS H.J. (1968) Major surgery in haemophilia. Prolonged substitution therapy for surgical treatment of haemophilic cyst and pathological fracture of the femur. *British Journal of Surgery*, **55**, 109.

62 PRENTICE C.R.M., LINDSAY R.M., BARR R.D., FORBES C.D., KENNEDY A.C., McNICOL G.P. & DOUGLAS A.S. (1971) Renal complications in haemophilia and Christmas disease. *Quarterly Journal of Medicine* (NS), **40**, 47.

63 WRIGHT F.W., MATTHEWS J.M. & BROCK L.G. (1971) Complications of haemophilic disorders affecting the renal tract. *Radiology*, **98**, 571.

64 BECK P. & EVANS K.T. (1972) Renal abnormalities in patients with haemophilia and Christmas disease. *Clinical Radiology*, **23**, 349.

65 DALINKA M.K., LALLY J.F., RANCIER L.F. & MATA J. (1975) Nephromegaly in haemophilia. *Radiology*, **115**, 337.

66 DHOLAKIA A.M. & HOWARTH F.H. (1979) The urinary tract in haemophilia. *Clinical Radiology*, **30**, 533.

67 ROBERTS G.M., EVANS K.T., BLOOM A.L. & AL-GAILANI F. (1982) Renal papillary necrosis in haemophilia and Christmas disease. *Clinical Radiology* (in press).

68 EYSTER M.E., GILL F.M., BLATT P.M., HILGARTNER M.W., BALLARD J.C. & KINNEY T.R. (1978) Central nervous system bleeding in hemophiliacs, *Blood*, **51**, 1179.

69 LEVINE P.H., McVERRY B.A., SEGELMAN A.E., CRANFORD C.M. & ZIMBLER S. (1976) Comprehensive health care clinic for hemophiliacs. *Archives of Internal Medicine*, **136**, 792.

70 MATTSSON A. & GROSS S. (1966) Social and behavioural studies on hemophilic children and their families. *Journal of Pediatrics*, **68**, 952.

71 MEYER D. (1977) Von Willebrand's disease. In: *Recent Advances in Blood Coagulation* (ed. Poller L.), 2nd edn, p. 183. Churchill-Livingstone, Edinburgh.

72 VELTKAMP J.J. & VAN TILBURG N.H. (1974) Autosomal haemophilia—a variant of von Willebrand's disease. *British Journal of Haematology*, **26**, 141.

73 KIRKWOOD T.B.L., RIZZA C.R., SNAPE T.J., RHYMES I.L. & AUSTEN D.E.G. (1977) Identification of sources of inter-laboratory variation in factor VIII assay. *British Journal of Haematology*, **37**, 559.

74 KIRKWOOD T.B.L. & BARROWCLIFFE T.W. (1978) Discrepancy between one-stage and two-stage assay of factor VIII:C. *British Journal of Haematology*, **40**, 333.

75 BANGHAM D.R., BIGGS R., BROZOVIC M., DENSON K.W.E. & SKEGG J.L. (1971) A biological standard for measurement of blood coagulation factor VIII activity. *Bulletin of the World Health Organisation*, **45**, 331.

76 AUSTEN D.E.G. & RHYMES I.L. (1975) *A Laboratory Manual of Blood Coagulation*. Blackwell Scientific Publications, Oxford.

77 DENSON K.W.E. (1976) Appendices 1 and 2. In: *Human Blood Coagulation, Haemostasis and Thrombosis* (ed. Biggs R.), 2nd edn, p. 655. Blackwell Scientific Publications, Oxford.

78 GIDDINGS J.C. (1980) Hereditary coagulation disorders: laboratory techniques. In: *A Practical Guide to Blood Coagulation and Haemostasis* (ed. Thomson J.M.), 2nd edn, p. 117. Churchill-Livingstone, Edinburgh.

79 GIDDINGS J.C. (1980) The investigation of hereditary coagulation disorders. In: *A Practical Guide to Blood Coagulation and Haemostasis* (ed. Thomson J.M.), 2nd edn, p. 48. Churchill-Livingstone, Edinburgh.

80 BOYERS S.H. & GRAHAM J.B. (1965) Linkage between the X-chromosome loci for glucose-6-phosphate dehydrogenase electrophoretic variation and hemophilia A. *American Journal of Human Genetics*, **17**, 320.

81 WHITTAKER D.L., COPELAND D.L. & GRAHAM J.B. (1962) Linkage of color blindness to hemophilias A and B. *American Journal of Human Genetics*, **14**, 149.

82 MIYOSHI K., SASAKI N. SHIRAKAMI A., INOUE H., SHIGEKIO T., HERADA H., KAWACHI S., KANETO Y., NIKO S., ONICHI H. & KAWAI H. (1978) Hereditary persistence of fetal hemoglobin and Xg blood group in hemophilia and von Willebrand's disease. *Japanese Journal of Human Genetics*, **23**, 268.

83 DAVIES S.H., CAVIN J., GOLDSMITH K.L.G., GRAHAM J.B., HAMPER J., HARDISTY R.M., HARRIS J.B., HOLMAN C.A., INGRAM G.I.C., JONES T.G., McAFEE L.A., McKUSICK V.A., O'BRIEN J.R., RACE R.R., SANGER R. & TIPPETT P. (1963) The linkage relations of hemophilia A and hemophilia B (Christmas disease) to the Xg blood group system. *American Journal of Human Genetics*, **15**, 481.

84 BARROW E.M. & GRAHAM J.B. (1974) Blood coagulation factor VIII (antihemophilic factor): with comments

on von Willebrand's disease and Christmas disease. *Physiological Reviews*, **54**, 23.

85 KITCHENS C.S. & NEWCOMB T.F. (1979) Factor XIII. *Medicine*, **58**, 413.

86 BARRAI I., CANN H.M., CAVALLI-SFORZA L.L. & DE NICOLA P. (1968) The effect of prenatal age on rates of mutation for hemophilia and evidence for differing mutation rates for hemophilia A and B. *American Journal of Human Genetics*, **20**, 175.

87 BARRAI I. & CANN H.M. (1972) Inherited blood clotting disorders: Report of a WHO Scientific Group. *World Health Organisation Technical Report Series No. 504*, 47.

88 McCURDY P.R. (1971) Use of genetic linkage for the detection of female carriers of hemophilia. *New England Journal of Medicine*, **285**, 218.

89 LYON M. (1962) Sex chromatin and gene action in the mammalian X-chromosome. *American Journal of Human Genetics*, **14**, 135.

90 KERR C.B., PRESTON A.E., BARR A. & BIGGS R. (1965) Inheritance of factor VIII. In: *Genetics and the Interaction of Blood Clotting Factors* (ed Hunter R.B., Wright I.S., Koller F. & Streuli F.), p. 173. Schattauer-Verlag, Stuttgart.

91 BENNETT E. & HUEHNS E.R. (1970) Immunological differentiation of three types of haemophilia and identification of some female carriers. *Lancet*, **ii**, 956.

92 ZIMMERMAN T.S., RATNOFF O.D. & LITTELL A.S. (1971) Detection of carriers of classic hemophilia using an immunological assay for antihemophilic factor (Factor VIII). *Journal of Clinical Investigation*, **50**, 255.

93 AKHMETELI M.A., ALEDORT L.M., ALEXANIANTS S., BULANOV A.G., ELSTON R.C., GINTER E.K., GOUSSEV A., GRAHAM J.B., HERMANS J., LARRIEU M.J., LOTHE F., McLAREN A.D., MANUCCI P.M., PRENTICE C.R.M. & VELTKAMP J.J. (1977) Methods for the detection of haemophilia carriers: a memorandum. *Bulletin of the World Health Organisation*, **55**, 675.

94 GRAHAM J.B. (1979) Genotype assignment (carrier detection) in the hemophilias. *Clinics in Hematology*, **8**, 115.

95 RODECK C.H. & CAMPBELL S. (1979) Umbilical cord insertion as a source of pure fetal blood for prenatal diagnosis. *Lancet*, **i**, 1244.

96 MIBASHAN R.S., RODECK C.H., THUMPSON J.K., EDWARDS R.J., SINGER J.D., WHITE J.M. & CAMPBELL S. (1979) Plasma assay of fetal factors VIIIC and IX for prenatal diagnosis of haemophilia. *Lancet*, **i**, 1309.

97 LAZARCHICK J. & HOYER L.W. (1978) Immunoradiometric measurement of the factor VIII procoagulant antigen. *Journal of Clinical Investigation*, **62**, 1048.

98 FIRSHEIN S.I., HOYER L.W., LAZARCHICK J., FORGET B.E., HOBBINS J.C., CLYNE L.P., PITLICK F.A., MUIR W.A., MERKATZ I.R. & MAHONEY M.J. (1979) Prenatal diagnosis of classical hemophilia. *New England Journal of Medicine*, **300**, 937.

99 BLOOM A.L. & PEAKE I.R. (1980) Prenatal diagnosis of haemophilia. In: *Fetoscopy* (ed. Rocker I. & Laurence M.) Elsevier, Amsterdam (in press).

100 EDGELL C.J.S., KIRKMAN H.N., CLEMONS E., BUCHANAN P.D. & MILLER C.H. (1978) Prenatal diagnosis by linkage: Hemophilia A and polymorphic glucose-6-phosphate dehydrogenase. *American Journal of Human Genetics*, **30**, 80.

101 BIGGS R. & MATTHEWS J.M. (1966) The plasma concentration of factor VIII in the treatment of haemophilia. In: *The Treatment of Haemophilia and Other Coagulation Disorders* (ed. Biggs R. & Macfarlane R.G.), p. 107. Blackwell Scientific Publications, Oxford.

102 POOL J.G. & SHANNON A.E. (1965) Production of high potency concentrate of antihemophilic globulin in a closed bag system. *New England Journal of Medicine*, **273**, 1443.

103 BIDWELL E., DIKE G.W.R. & SNAPE T.J. (1976) Therapeutic materials. In: *Human Blood Coagulation, Haemostasis and Thrombosis* (ed. Biggs R.), 2nd edn, p. 249. Blackwell Scientific Publications, Oxford.

104 BLOOM A.L. & EMMANUEL J.H. (1968) Use of cryoprecipitate antihaemophilic factor for the treatment of haemophilia. *Quarterly Journal of Medicine*, **37**, 291.

105 KEKWICK R.A. & WOLF P. (1957) A concentrate of human antihaemophilic factor: its use in six cases of haemophilia. *Lancet*, **i**, 647.

106 BLOMBÄCK M. (1958) Purification of antihaemophilic globulin. I. Some studies on the stability of the antihaemophilic globulin activity in fraction 1–0 and a method for its partial separation from fibrinogen. *Arkiv for Kemi*, **12**, 387.

107 FORBES C.D. & PRENTICE C.R.M. (1973) Aggregation of human platelets by purified porcine and bovine antihaemophilic factor. *Nature (New Biology)*, **241**, 149.

108 BIGGS R. (1978) The amount of blood required annually to make concentrates to treat patients with haemophilia A and B. In: *Treatment of Haemophilia A and B and von Willebrand's disease* (ed. Biggs R.), p. 89. Blackwell Scientific Publications, Oxford.

109 BIGGS R. & DENSON K.W.E. (1963) The fate of prothrombin and factors VIII, IX and X transfused to patients deficient in these factors. *British Journal of Haematology*, **9**, 532.

110 OVER J., SIXMA J.J., DOUCET-DE-BRUINE M.H.M., TRIESCHNIGG A.M.C., VLOOSWIJK R.A.A., BISSER-VISSER N.H. & BOUMA B.N. (1978) Survival of ^{125}iodine-labelled factor VIII in normals and patients with classic hemophilia. Observations on the heterogeneity of human factor VIII. *Journal of Clinical Investigation*, **62**, 223.

111 HEMKER H.C., HERMENS W.TH., MULLER A.D. & ZWAAL R.F.A. (1980) Oral treatment of haemophilia A by gastrointestinal absorption of factor VIII entrapped in liposomes. *Lancet*, **i**, 70.

112 LINDARGH G. & ANDERSSON L. (1966) Clot retention in the kidneys as a probable cause of anaemia during treatment of haematoma with epsilon-aminocaproic acid. *Acta Medica Scandinavica*, **180**, 469.

113 VAN ITTERBEEK H., VERMYLEN J. & VERSTRAETE M. (1968) High obstruction of urine flow as a complication of the treatment with fibrinolysis inhibitors of haematuria in haemophiliacs. *Acta Haematologica*, **39**, 237.

114 STORTI E., TRALDI A., TOSATTI E., & DAVOLI P.G. (1969) Synovectomy, a new approach to haemophilic arthropathy. *Acta Haematologica*, **41**, 193.

115 ARNOLD W.D. & HILGARTNER M.W. (1977) Hemophilic arthropathy: current concepts and management. *Journal of Bone and Joint Surgery*, **59A**, 287.

116 SNEPPEN O., BECK H. & HOLSTEEN V. (1978) Synovectomy as a prophylactic measure in recurrent haemophilic haemarthroses. *Acta Paediatrica Scandinavica*, **67**, 491.

117 AHLBERG A. (1975) Synoviorthesis in haemophilia with special reference to the use of radioactive gold. In: *Handbook of Hemophilia* (ed. Brinkhous K.M. & Hemker H.C.), p. 727. Excerpta Medica, Amsterdam.

118 STEIN H. & DICKSON R.A. (1975) Reversed dynamic slings for knee-flexion contractures in the hemophiliac. *Journal of Bone and Joint Surgery*, **57A**, 282.

119 DUTHIE R.B., MATTHEWS J.M., RIZZA C.R., STEEL W.M. & WOODS C.G. (1972) *The Management of Musculo-Skeletal Problems in the Haemophiliac*. Blackwell Scientific Publications, Oxford.

120 BOONE D.C. (1976) Common musculo-skeletal problems and their management. In: *Comprehensive Management of Hemophilia* (ed. Boone D.C.), p. 52. F. A. Davis, Philadelphia.

121 RHODES J.M. & MARTINSON A.M. (1976) Surgical management of musculo-skeletal problems. In: *Comprehensive Management of Hemophilia* (ed. Boone D.C.), p. 86. F. A. Davis, Philadelphia.

122 KINGMA J.M. (1975) Orthopaedic treatment in Haemophilia. In: *Handbook of Hemophilia* (ed. Brinkhous K.M. & Hemker H.C.), p. 715. Excerpta Medica, Amsterdam.

123 WALSH P.N., RIZZA C.R., MATTHEWS J.M., EIPE J., KERNOFF P.B.A., COLES M.D., BLOOM A.L., KAUFMAN B.M., BECK P., HANAN C.M. & BIGGS R. (1971) Epsilon-aminocaproic acid therapy for dental extractions in haemophilia and Christmas disease: a double-blind controlled trial. *British Journal of Haematology*, **20**, 463.

124 BIGGS R. (ed.) (1976) *Human Blood Coagulation, Haemostasis and Thrombosis*, 2nd edn. Blackwell Scientific Publications, Oxford.

125 BOONE D.C. (ed.) (1976) *Comprehensive Management of Hemophilia*. F. A. Davis, Philadelphia.

126 BIGGS R. (ed.) (1978) *The Treatment of Haemophilia A and B and von Willebrand's Disease*. Blackwell Scientific Publications, Oxford.

127 BRINKHOUS, K.M. & HEMKER H.C. (ed.) (1975) *Handbook of Hemophilia*. Excerpta Medica, Amsterdam.

128 SINGHER L.J. (1975) Renal and urological complications of hemophilia. In: *Handbook of Hemophilia* (ed. Brinkhous K.M. & Hemker H.C.), p. 377. Excerpta Medica, Amsterdam.

129 BENNETT A.E. & INGRAM G.I.C. (1967) A controlled trial of long-term steroid treatment in haemophilia. *Lancet*, **i**, 967.

130 RIZZA C.R., KERNOFF P.B.A., MATTHEWS J.M., McLENNAN C.R. & RAINSFORD S.G. (1977) A comparison of coagulation factor replacement with and without prednisolone in the treatment of haematuria in haemophilia and Christmas disease. *Thrombosis and Haemostasis*, **37**, 86.

131 MANNUCCI P.M., RUGGERI Z.M., PARETI F.I. & CAPITANIO A. (1977) 1-deamino-8-D-arginine vasopressin: a new pharmacological approach to the management of haemophilia and von Willebrand's disease. *Lancet*, **i**, 869.

132 MANNUCCI P.M., RUGGERI Z.M., PARETI F.I. & CAPITANIO A. (1977) DDAVP in haemophilia. *Lancet*, **ii**, 1171.

133 LUDLAM C.A., PEAKE I.R., ALLEN N., DAVIES B.L., FURLONG R.A. & BLOOM A.L. (1980) Factor VIII and fibrinolytic response to deamino-8-D-arginine vasopressin in normal subjects and dissociate response in some patients with haemophilia and von Willebrand's disease. *British Journal of Haematology*, **45**, 499.

134 JONES P. (1977) Developments and problems in the management of hemophilia. *Seminars in Hematology*, **14**, 375.

135 MILLS D.C.B. & ROBERTS G.C.K. (1967) Membrane active drugs and the aggregation of human blood platelets. *Nature (London)*, **213**, 35.

136 KERNOFF P.B.A., DURRANT I.J., RIZZA C.R. & WRIGHT F.W. (1972) Severe allergic pulmonary oedema after plasma transfusion. *British Journal of Haematology*, **23**, 777.

137 REESE E.P., JR, McCULLOUGH J.J. & CRADDOCK P.R. (1975) An adverse pulmonary reaction to cryoprecipitate in a hemophiliac. *Transfusion*, **15**, 583.

138 SEELER R.A. (1972) Hemolysis due to anti-A and anti-B in factor VIII preparations. *Archives of Internal Medicine*, **130**, 101.

139 TAMAGNINI G.P., DORMANDY K.M., ELLIS D. & MAYCOCK W.D'A. (1975) Factor VIII concentrate in haemophilia. *Lancet*, **ii**, 188.

140 BRINKHOUS K.M., ROBERTS H.R. & WEISS A.E. (1972) Prevalence of inhibitors in hemophilia A and B. *Thrombosis et Diathesis Haemorrhagica*, **51** (Suppl.), 315.

141 SHAPIRO S.S. (1979) Antibodies to blood coagulation factors. *Clinics in Hematology*, **8**, 207.

142 BECK P., GIDDINGS J.C., & BLOOM A.L. (1969) Inhibitor of factor VIII in mild haemophilia. *British Journal of Haematology*, **17**, 283.

143 BIGGS R. & BIDWELL E. (1959) A method for the study of antihaemophilic globulin inhibitors with reference to six cases. *British Journal of Haematology*, **5**, 379.

144 RIZZA C.R. & BIGGS R. (1973) The treatment of patients who have factor VIII antibodies. *British Journal of Haematology*, **24**, 65.

145 KASPER C.K., ALEDORT L.M., COUNTS R.B., EDSON J.R., FRATANTONI J., GREEN D., HAMPTON S.W., HILGARTNER M.W., LAZERSON J., LEVINE P.H., McMILLAN C.W., POOL J.G., SHAPIRO S.S., SHULMAN N.R. & VAN EYS J. (1975) A more uniform measurement of factor VIII inhibitors. *Thrombosis et Diathesis Haemorrhagica*, **34**, 869.

146 BLATT P.M., WHITE G.C. II, McMILLAN C.W. & ROBERTS H.R. (1977) Treatment of anti-factor VIII antibodies. *Thrombosis and Haemostasis*, **38**, 514.

147 BLOOM A.L. (1978) Clotting factor concentrates for resistant haemophilia. *British Journal of Haematology*, **40**, 21.

148 GREEN D. (1971) Suppression of an antibody to factor VIII by a combination of factor VIII and cyclophosphamide. *Blood*, **37**, 381.

149 DORMANDY K.M. & SULTAN Y. (1975) The suppression of factor VIII antibodies in haemophilia. *Pathologie et Biologie*, **23** (Suppl.), 17.

150 COBCROFT R., TAMAGNINI G. & DORMANDY K.M. (1971) Serial plasmapheresis in a haemophiliac with

antibodies to FVIII. *Journal of Clinical Pathology*, **30**, 763.

151 KURCZYNSKI E. & PENNER J.A. (1974) Activated pro-thrombin concentrate for patients with factor VIII inhibitors. *New England Journal of Medicine*, **291**, 164.

152 PARRY D.H. & BLOOM A.L. (1978) Failure of factor VIII inhibitor bypassing activity (Feiba) to secure haemo-stasis in haemophilic patients with antibodies. *Journal of Clinical Pathology*, **31**, 1102.

153 ONDER O. & HOYER L.W. (1979) Factor VIII coagulant antigen in factor IX complex concentrates. *Thrombosis Research*, **15**, 569.

154 RIZZA C.R. (1977) Clinical management of haemophi-lia. *British Medical Bulletin*, **33**, 225.

155 BRACKMANN H.H. & GORMSEN J. (1977) Massive factor-VIII infusion in a haemophiliac with factor-VIII inhibi-tor, high responder. *Lancet*, **ii**, 933.

156 BURRELL C.J., BLACK S.H. & RAMSEY D.M. (1978) Antibody to hepatitis B surface antigen in haemophi-liacs on long-term therapy with Scottish factor VIII. *Journal of Clinical Pathology*, **31**, 309.

157 HOOFNAGLE J.H., GERETY R.J., THIEL J. (1976) The prevalence of hepatitis B surface antigen in commer-cially prepared plasma products. *Journal of Laboratory and Clinical Medicine*, **88**, 102.

158 HRUBY M.A. & SCHAUF V. (1978) Transfusion-related short-incubation hepatitis in hemophilic patients. *Jour-nal of the American Medical Association*, **240**, 1355.

159 CRASKE J., KIRK P., COHEN B. & VANDERVELDE E.M. (1978) Commercial factor VIII associated hepatitis, 1974–75, in the United Kingdom: a retrospective study. *Journal of Hygiene* (Cambridge), **80**, 327.

160 CRASKE J., SPOONER R.J.D. & VANDERVELDE E.M. (1978) Evidence for existence of at least two types of Factor-VIII-associated non-B transfusion hepatitis. *Lancet*, **ii**, 1051.

161 HASIBA U.W., SPERO J.A. & LEWIS J.H. (1977) Chronic liver dysfunction in multi-transfused hemophiliacs. *Transfusion*, **17**, 490.

162 MANNUCCI P.M., RONCHI G., ROTA L. & COLOMBO M. (1978) A clinico-pathological study of liver disease in haemophiliacs. *Journal of Clinical Pathology*, **31**, 779.

163 PRESTON F.E., TRIGER D.R., UNDERWOOD J.C.E., BARDHAN G., MITCHELL V.E., STEWART R.M. & BLACKBURN E.K. (1978) Percutaneous liver biopsy and chronic liver disease in haemophiliacs. *Lancet*, **ii**, 592.

164 SPERO J.A., LEWIS J.H., VAN THIEL D.H., HASIBA U. & RABIN B.S. (1978) Asymptomatic structural liver dis-ease in hemophilia. *New England Journal of Medicine*, **298**, 1373.

165 MCVERRY B.A., VOKE J., MOHAMMED I., DORMANDY K.M. & HOLBOROW E.J. (1977) Immune complexes and abnormal liver function in haemophilia. *Journal of Clinical Pathology*, **30**, 1142.

166 LEVINE P.H. & BRITTEN A.F.H. (1973) Supervised patient management in hemophilia. A study of 45 patients with hemophilia A and B. *Annals of Internal Medicine*, **78**, 195.

167 LEVINE P.H. (1974) Efficacy of self-therapy in hemophi-lia. *New England Journal of Medicine*, **291**, 1381.

168 INGRAM G.I.C., DYKES S.R., CREESE A.L., MELLOR P., SWAN A.V., KAUFERT J., RIZZA C.R., SPOONER R.J.D. & BIGGS R. (1979) Home treatment of haemophilia:

clinical, social and economic advantages. *Clinical and Laboratory Haematology*, **1**, 13.

169 STIRLING M.L. & PRESCOTT R.J. (1979) Minimum effective dose of intermediate factor VIII concentrate in haemophiliacs on home therapy. *Lancet*, **i**, 813.

170 HARRIS R.I. & STUART J. (1979) Low-dose factor VIII in adults with haemophilic arthropathy. *Lancet*, **i**, 93.

171 JONES P., FEARNS M., FORBES C. & STUART J. (1978) Haemophilia A home therapy in the United Kingdom. *British Medical Journal*, **i**, 1447.

172 ALLAIN J.P., (1979) Dose requirement for replacement therapy in hemophilia A. *Thrombosis and Haemostasis*, **42**, 825.

173 KATZ A.H. (1970) *Hemophilia—A Study in Hope and Reality*. C. C. Thomas, Springfield, Illinois.

174 KIDD P., DENSON K.W.E. & BIGGS R. (1963) The thrombotest and Christmas disease. *Lancet*, **ii**, 522.

175 HOUGIE C. & TWOMEY J.J. (1967) Haemophilia B_M: a new type of factor IX deficiency. *Lancet*, **i**, 698.

176 ROBERTS H.R., GRIZZLE J.E., MCLESTER W.D. & PENICK G.D. (1968) Genetic variants of hemophilia B: detection by means of a specific inhibitor. *Journal of Clinical Investigation*, **47**, 360.

177 DENSON K.W.E., BIGGS R. & MANNUCCI P.M. (1968) An investigation of three patients with Christmas disease due to an abnormal type of factor IX. *Journal of Clinical Pathology*, **12**, 160.

178 ØRSTAVIK K.H., ØSTERUD B., PRYDZ H. & BERG K. (1975) Electroimmunoassay of factor IX in hemophilia B. *Thrombosis Research*, **7**, 373.

179 THOMPSON A.R. (1977) Factor IX antigen by radioim-munoassay: abnormal factor IX protein in patients on warfarin therapy and with hemophilia B. *Journal of Clinical Investigation*, **59**, 900.

180 YANG H.C. (1978) Immunologic studies of factor IX (Christmas factor). II. Immunoradiometric assay of factor IX antigen. *British Journal of Haematology*, **39**, 215.

181 NEAL W.R., TAYLOR D.T., JR, CEDERBAUM A.L. & ROBERTS H.R. (1973) Detection of genetic variants of hemophilia B with an immunosorbent technique. *Bri-tish Journal of Haematology*, **25**, 63.

182 PAREKH V.R., MANNUCCI P.M. & RUGGERI Z.M. (1978) Immunological heterogeneity of haemophilia B: a mul-ticulture study of 98 kindreds. *British Journal of Haema-tology*, **40**, 643.

183 KASPER C.K., ØSTERUD B., MINAMI J.Y., SHONICK W. & RAPAPORT S.I. (1977) Hemophilia B: characterization of genetic variants and detection of carriers. *Blood*, **50**, 351.

184 PECHET L., TIARKS C.Y., STEVENS J., SUDHINDRA R.R. & LIPWORTH L. (1978) Relationship of factor IX antigen and coagulant in hemophilia B patients and carriers. *Thrombosis and Haemostasis*, **40**, 465.

185 THOMPSON A.R. (1977) Factor IX antigen by radioim-munoassay in heterozygotes for hemophilia B. *Throm-bosis Research*, **11**, 193.

186 VELTKAMP J.J., MEILOF J., REMMELTS H.G., VAN DER VLERK D. & LOELIGER E.A. (1970). Another genetic variant of haemophilia B: haemophilia B Leyden. *Scandinavian Journal of Haematology*, **7**, 82.

187 CHUNG K.S., GOLDSMITH J.C. & ROBERTS H.R. (1978) Isolation and characterization of factor IX Chapel Hill.

Comparison to normal human factor IX. *Bibliotheca Haematologica*, **44**, 68.

188 ROBERTS H.R., CHUNG K.S. & GOLDSMITH J.C. (1977) Mutant forms of factor IX. *Thrombosis and Haemostasis*, **38**, 338.

189 CHUNG K.S., MADAR D.A., GOLDSMITH J.C., KINGDON H.S. & ROBERTS H.R. (1978) Purification and characterization of an abnormal factor IX (Christmas factor) molecule. Factor IX Chapel Hill. *Journal of Clinical Investigation*, **62**, 1078.

190 BERTINA R.M. & VELTKAMP J.J. (1978) The abnormal factor IX of hemophilia B⁺ variants. *Thrombosis and Haemostasis*, **40**, 335.

191 BERTINA R.M. & VELTKAMP J.J. (1979) A genetic variant of factor IX with decreased capacity for Ca^{2+} binding. *British Journal of Haematology*, **42**, 623.

192 GIROLAMI A., STICCHI A., BURUL A., DAL B.O. & ZANON R. (1977) An immunological investigation of hemophilia B with tentative classification of the disease into five variants. *Vox Sanguinis*, **32**, 230.

193 CHUNG K.S., BESEAUD A., GOLDSMITH J.C., McMILLAN C.W., MÉNACHÉ, D. & ROBERTS H.R. (1979) Congenital deficiency of blood clotting factors II, VII, IX and X. *Blood*, **53**, 776.

194 ØSTERUD B., LEVINE K., KASPER C.K. & RAPAPORT S. (1977) Isolation and properties of the abnormal factor IX molecule in hemophilia B_M. *Thrombosis and Haemostasis*, **38**, 51.

195 ØSTERUD B., KASPER C.K. & PRODANOS C. (1979) Factor IX variants of hemophilia B. The effect of activated factor XI and the reaction product of factor VII and tissue factor on the abnormal factor IX molecules. *Thrombosis Research*, **15**, 235.

196 KNIGHTS S.F. & INGRAM G.I.C. (1967) Partial thromboplastin time with kaolin: diagnosis of haemophilia and Christmas disease without natural reference plasma. *Journal of Clinical Pathology*, **20**, 616.

197 BIGGS R. & MACFARLANE R.G. (1966) *Treatment of Haemophilia and Other Coagulation Disorders*. Blackwell Scientific Publications, Oxford.

198 BARROW E.M., BULLOCK W.R. & GRAHAM J.B. (1960) A study of the carrier state for plasma thromboplastin component (PTC, Christmas factor) deficiency, utilising a new assay procedure. *Journal of Laboratory and Clinical Medicine*, **55**, 936.

199 SIMPSON N.E. & BIGGS R. (1962) The inheritance of Christmas factor. *British Journal of Haematology*, **8**, 191.

200 FROTA-PESSOA O., GOMES E.L. & CALICCHIO T.R. (1963) Christmas factor: dosage compensation and the production of blood coagulation factor IX. *Science*, **139**, 348.

201 WALL R.L., McCONNEL J., MOORE D., MacPHERSON C.R. & MARSON A. (1967) Christmas disease, color-blindness and blood group Xgᵃ. *American Journal of Medicine*, **43**, 214.

202 HASHMI K.Z., MacIVER J.E. & DELAMORE I.W. (1978) Christmas disease in a female. *Lancet*, **ii**, 965.

203 HOLMBERG L., NILSSON I.M., HENRIKSSON P. & ØRSTAVIK K.H. (1978) Homozygous expression of haemophilia B in a heterozygote. *Acta Medica Scandinavica*, **204**, 231.

204 GRAHAM J.B., FLYER P., ELSTON R.C. & KASPER C.K. (1979) Statistical study of genotype assignment (carrier detection) in hemophilia B. *Thrombosis Research*, **15**, 69.

205 ØRSTAVIK K.H., VELTKAMP J.J., BERTINA R.M. & HERMANS J. (1979) Detection of carriers of haemophilia B. *British Journal of Haematology*, **42**, 293.

206 ZAUBER N.P. & LEVIN J. (1977) Factor IX levels in patients with hemophilia B (Christmas disease) following transfusion with concentrates of factor IX or fresh frozen plasma (FFP). *Medicine*, **56**, 213.

207 KASPER C.K. (1973) Postoperative thrombosis in hemophilia B (letter). *New England Journal of Medicine*, **289**, 160.

208 WYKE R.J., TSIQUAYE K.N., THORNTON A., WHITE Y., PORTMANN B., DAS P.K., ZUCKERMAN A.J. & WILLIAMS R. (1979) Transmission of non-A-non-B hepatitis to chimpanzees by factor-IX concentrates after fatal complications in patients with chronic liver disease. *Lancet*, **i**, 520.

209 ROBERTS H.R., GROSS G.P., WEBSTER W.P., DEJANOV I.I. & PENICK G.D. (1966) Acquired inhibitors of plasma factor IX: a study of their induction, properties and neutralization. *American Journal of the Medical Sciences*, **251**, 43.

210 VON WILLEBRAND E.A. (1926) Hereditäre pseudo-hemofili. *Finska Läkaresällskapits Handlingar*, **67**, 7.

211 VON WILLEBRAND E.A. & JURGENS R. (1933) Über ein neues vererbbares blutungsübel: die constitutionelle thrombopathy. *Deutsches Archiv für Klinische Medizin*, **175**, 453.

212 BLACKBURN E.K. (1961) Primary capillary haemorrhage (including von Willebrand's disease). *British Journal of Haematology*, **7**, 239.

213 ALEXANDER B. & GOLDSTEIN R. (1953) Dual hemostatic defect in pseudohemophilia. *Journal of Clinical Investigation*, **32**, 551.

214 JÜRGENS R., LEHMANN W., WEGELIUS O., ERIKSSON A.W. & HIEPLER E. (1957) Mitteilung über den Mangel an antihämophilen Globulin (Factor VIII) bei der Aaländischen Thrombopathie (v. Willebrand-Jurgens). *Thrombosis et Diathesis Haemorrhagica*, **1**, 257.

215 NILSSON I.M., BLOMBÄCK, M. & VON FRANCKEN I. (1957) On an inherited autosomal hemorrhagic diathesis with antihemophilic globulin (AHG) deficiency and prolonged bleeding time. *Acta Medica Scandinavica*, **159**, 35.

216 HOYER L.W. (1972) Immunologic studies of antihemophilic factor (AHF, factor VIII). IV. Radioimmunoassay of AHF antigen. *Journal of Laboratory and Clinical Medicine*, **80**, 822.

217 PEAKE I.R. & BLOOM A.L. (1977) The use of an immunoradiometric assay for factor VIII-related antigen in the study of atypical von Willebrand's disease. *Thrombosis Research*, **10**, 27.

218 SALZMAN E.W. (1963) Measurement of platelet adhesiveness. A simple *in vitro* technique demonstrating an abnormality in von Willebrand's disease. *Journal of Laboratory and Clinical Medicine*, **62**, 724.

219 TSCHOPP T.P., WEISS H.J. & BAUMGARTNER H.R. (1974) Decreased adhesion of platelets to subendothelium in von Willebrand's disease. *Journal of Laboratory and Clinical Medicine*, **83**, 296.

220 HOWARD M.A. & FIRKIN B.G. (1971) Ristocetin—a

new tool in the investigation of platelet aggregation. *Thrombosis et Diathesis Haemorrhagica*, **26**, 362.

221 DONATI M.B., DE GAETANO G. & VERMYLEN J. (1973) Evidence that bovine factor VIII, not bovine fibrinogen, aggregates human platelets. *Thrombosis Research*, **2**, 97.

222 DE GAETANO G., DONATI M.B. & VERMYLEN J. (1974) Evidence that human platelet aggregating activity in porcine plasma is a property of von Willebrand factor. *Thrombosis et Diathesis Haemorrhagica*, **32**, 549.

223 SIXMA J.J., OVER J., BOUMA B.M., BLOOM A.L. & PEAKE I.R. (1978) Predominance of normal low molecular weight forms of factor VIII in 'variant' von Willebrand's disease. *Thrombosis Research*, **12**, 929.

224 KERNOFF P.B.A., GRUSON R. & RIZZA C.R. (1974) A variant of factor VIII related antigen. *British Journal of Haematology*, **26**, 435.

225 PEAKE I.R., BLOOM A.L. & GIDDINGS J.C. (1974) Inherited variants of factor VIII-related protein in von Willebrand's disease. *New England Journal of Medicine*, **291**, 113.

226 GRALNICK H.R., COLLER B.S. & SULTAN Y. (1975) Studies of the human factor VIII/von Willebrand factor protein. III. Qualitative defects in von Willebrand's disease. *Journal of Clinical Investigation*, **56**, 814.

227 PEAKE I.R. & BLOOM A.L. (1977) Abnormal factor VIII-related antigen (FVIIIRAg) in von Willebrand's disease (vWd): decreased precipitation by concanavalin A. *Thrombosis and Haemostasis*, **37**, 361.

228 BLOOM A.L. (1980) The von Willebrand syndrome. *Seminars in Hematology*, **17**, 215.

229 GRAHAM J.B. (1980) Hypothesis: The genetic control of factor VIII. *Lancet*, **i**, 340.

230 BLOOM A.L., GIDDINGS J.C. & WILKS C.J. (1973) Factor VIII on the vascular intima: possible importance in haemostasis and thrombosis. *Nature (New Biology)*, **241**, 217.

231 CAEN J.P. & SULTAN Y. (1965) von Willebrand's disease as an endothelial-cell abnormality. *Lancet*, **ii**, 1129.

232 RAMSAY P.M., BUIST T.A.S., MACLEOD D.A.D. & HEADING R.C. (1976) Persistent gastrointestinal bleeding due to angiodysplasia of the gut in von Willebrand's disease. *Lancet*, **ii**, 275.

233 AHR D.J., PICKLES F.R., HOYER L.W., O'LEARY D.S. & CONRAD M.E. (1977) von Willebrand's disease and hemorrhagic telangiectasia. Association of two complex disorders of hemostasis resulting in life-threatening hemorrhage. *American Journal of Medicine*, **62**, 452.

234 HOWARD M.A., MONTGOMERY D.C. & HARDISTY R.M. (1974) Factor VIII-related antigen in platelets. *Thrombosis Research*, **4**, 617.

235 SLOT J.W., BOUMA B.N., MONTGOMERY R. & ZIMMERMAN T.S. (1978) Platelet factor VIII-related antigen: immunofluorescent localization. *Thrombosis Research*, **13**, 871.

236 SULTAN Y., MAISONNEUVE P. & ANGLES-CANO E. (1979) Release of VIIIR:Ag and VIIIR:WF during thrombin and collagen-induced aggregation. *Thrombosis Research*, **15**, 415.

237 KOUTTS J., WALSH P.N., PLOW E.F., FENTON J.W., BOUMA B.N. & ZIMMERMAN T.S. (1978) Active release of human platelet factor VIII related antigen by adenosine diphosphate, collagen and thrombin. *Journal of Clinical Investigation*, **62**, 1255.

238 NACHMAN R., LEVINE R. & JAFFE E.A. (1977) Synthesis of factor VIII antigen by cultured guinea pig megakaryocytes. *Journal of Clinical Investigation*, **60**, 914.

239 MEUCCI P., PEAKE I.R. & BLOOM A.L. (1978) Factor-VIII-related activities in normal, haemophilic and von Willebrand's disease platelet fractions. *Thrombosis and Haemostasis*, **40**, 288.

240 NURDEN A.T. & CAEN J.P. (1978) Membrane glycoproteins and human platelet function. *British Journal of Haematology*, **38**, 155.

241 LEGRAND Y.J., RODRIGUEZ-ZEBALLOS A., KARTALIS G., FAUVEL F. & CAEN J.P. (1978) Adsorption of factor VIII antigen-activity complex by collagen. *Thrombosis Research*, **13**, 909.

242 GREEN D. & POTTER E.V. (1976) Platelet-bound ristocetin aggregating factor in normal subjects and patients with von Willebrand's disease. *Journal of Laboratory and Clinical Medicine*, **87**, 976.

243 SULTAN Y., BOUMA B.N., DE GRAAF S., SIMEON J., CAEN J.P. & SIXMA J.J. (1977) Factor-VIII-related antigen in platelets of patients with von Willebrand's disease. *Thrombosis Research*, **11**, 23.

244 ZIMMERMAN T.S., ABILDGAARD C.F. & MEYER D. (1979) The factor VIII abnormality in severe von Willebrand's disease. *New England Journal of Medicine*, **301**, 1307.

245 BLOOM A.L., PEAKE I.R. & GIDDINGS J.C. (1974) Factor-VIII-related antigen or von Willebrand factor? *Lancet*, **i**, 576.

246 MILLER C.H., GRAHAM J.B., GOLDIN L.R. & ELSTON R.C. (1979) Genetics of classic von Willebrand's disease. I. Phenotypic variation within families. *Blood*, **54**, 117.

247 BLOOM A.L. & PEAKE I.R. (1979) Apparent 'dominant' and 'recessive' inheritance of von Willebrand's disease within the same kindreds. Possible biochemical mechanisms. *Thrombosis Research*, **25**, 505.

248 VALENTE A., VOLPE E., GANDINI M. & BUONANNO G. (1972) von Willebrand's disease: platelet nucleotide alterations in a case with marked platelet adhesiveness and aggregation defects. *Acta Haematologica*, **47**, 182.

249 SULTAN Y., BERNAL-HOYOS E.J., LEVY-TOLEDANO S., JEANNEAU C. & CAEN J.P. (1974) Dominant inherited familial factor VIII deficiency (von Willebrand's disease) associated with thrombocytopathic thrombocytopenia (biologic and genetic implications). *Pathologie et Biologie*, **22**, 27.

250 DOWLING S.V., MUNTZ R.M., D'SOUZA S. & EKERT H. (1976) Platelet release abnormality associated with a variant of von Willebrand's disease. *Blood*, **47**, 265.

251 RIVARD G.E., DEVIAULT M.B., BRAULT N., D'ARAGON L. & RAYMOND R. (1977) von Willebrand's disease associated with thrombocytopenia and a fast migrating factor VIII related antigen. *Thrombosis Research*, **11**, 507.

252 OWEN C.A., BOWIE E.J.W., FASS D.N., PEREZ R.A., COLE T.L. & STEWART M. (1979) Hypofibrinogenemia—dysfibrinogenaemia and von Willebrand's disease in the same family. *Mayo Clinic Proceedings*, **54**, 375.

253 VAN ROYEN E.A. & TEN CATE J.W. (1973) Antigen/biological activity ratio for factor VIII in late pregnancy. *Lancet*, **ii**, 449.

254 CRAMER A.D., MELARAGNO A.J., PHIFER S.J. & HOUGIE

C. (1976) von Willebrand's disease San Diego; a new variant. *Lancet*, **ii**, 12.

255 MIELKE C.H., JR, KANESHIRO M.M., MAHER I.A., WEINER J.M. & RAPAPORT S.I. (1969) The standardised normal Ivy bleeding time and its prolongation by aspirin. *Blood*, **34**, 204.

256 MACFARLANE D.E., STIBBE K., KIRBY E.P., ZUCKER M.B., GRANT R.A. & MCPHERSON J. (1975) A method for assaying von Willebrand factor (ristocetin co-factor). *Thrombosis et Diathesis Haemorrhagica*, **34**, 306.

257 RUGGERI Z.M., MANNUCCI P.M., JEFFCOATE S.L. & INGRAM G.I.C. (1976) Immunoradiometric assay of factor-VIII-related antigen with observations in 32 patients with von Willebrand's disease. *British Journal of Haematology*, **33**, 221.

258 MILLER C.H., GRAHAM J.B., GOLDIN L.R. & ELSTON R.C. (1979) Genetics of classic von Willebrand's disease. II. Optimal assignment of the heterozygous genotype (diagnosis) by discriminant analysis. *Blood*, **54**, 137.

259 BLATT P.M., BRINKHOUS K.M., CULP H.R., KRAUSS J.S. & ROBERTS H.R. (1976) Antihemophilic factor concentrate therapy in von Willebrand's disease. Dissociation of bleeding time and ristocetin co-factor activities. *Journal of the American Medical Association*, **236**, 2770.

260 GREEN D. & POTTER E.V. (1976) Failure of AHF concentrate to control bleeding in von Willebrand's disease. *American Journal of Medicine*, **60**, 357.

261 NILSSON I.M. & HEDNER U. (1978) Characteristics of various factor VIII concentrates used in treatment of haemophilia A. *British Journal of Haematology*, **37**, 543.

262 EKERT H. & CHAVIN S.I. (1977) Changes in electrophoretic mobility of human factor-VIII-related antigen: evidence for a subunit structure. *British Journal of Haematology*, **36**, 271.

263 WEINSTEIN M. & DEYKIN D. (1979) Comparison of factor-VIII-related von Willebrand factor proteins prepared from human cryoprecipitate and factor VIII concentrate. *Blood*, **53**, 1095.

264 DOUCET-DE-BRUINE M.H.M., SIXMA J.J., OVER J. & BISSER-VISSER N.H. (1978) Heterogeneity of human factor VIII. II. Characterisation of forms of factor VIII binding to platelets in the presence of ristocetin. *Journal of Laboratory and Clinical Medicine*, **92**, 96.

265 BOLHUIS P.A., SAKARIASSEN K.S. & SIXMA J.J. (1979) Platelet adhesion by subendothelium-bound factor VIII-vWF: kinetics and molecular weight dependence. *Thrombosis and Haemostasis*, **42**, 270.

266 MANNUCCI P.M., PARETI F.I., HOLMBERG L., NILSSON I.M. & RUGGERI Z.M. (1976) Studies on the prolonged bleeding time in von Willebrand's disease. *Journal of Laboratory and Clinical Medicine*, **88**, 662.

267 BENNETT B. & RATNOFF O.D. (1972) Studies on the response of patients with classic hemophilia to transfusion with concentrates of antihemophilic factor. A difference in the half-life of antihemophilic factor as measured by procoagulant and immunologic techniques. *Journal of Clinical Investigation*, **51**, 2593.

268 BLOOM A.L., PEAKE I.R. & GIDDINGS J.C. (1973) The presence and reactions of high and lower molecular weight procoagulant factor VIII in the plasma of patients with von Willebrand's disease after treatment:

significance for a structural hypothesis for factor VIII. *Thrombosis Research*, **3**, 389.

269 THEISS W. & SCHMIDT G. (1978) DDAVP in von Willebrand's disease: repeated administration and the behaviour of the bleeding time. *Thrombosis Research*, **13**, 1119.

270 KOBAYASHI I. (1979) Treatment of hemophilia A and von Willebrand's disease patients with an intranasal dripping of DDAVP. *Thrombosis Research*, **16**, 775.

271 MANNUCCI P.M., MEYER D., RUGGERI Z.M., KOUTTS J., CIAVERALLA N. & LAVERGNE I.M. (1976) Precipitating antibodies in von Willebrand's disease. *Nature (London)*, **262**, 141.

272 STRATTON R.D., WAGNER R.H., WEBSTER W.P. & BRINKHOUS K.M. (1975) Antibody nature of circulating inhibitor of plasma von Willebrand factor. *Proceedings of the National Academy of Sciences, USA*, **72**, 4167.

273 BLOOM A.L., PEAKE I.R., FURLONG R.A. & DAVIES B.L. (1979) High potency factor VIII concentrate: more effective than cryoprecipitate in a patient with von Willebrand's disease and inhibitor. *Thrombosis Research*, **16**, 847.

274 INGRAM G.I.C., KINGSTON P.J., LESLIE J. & BOWIE E.J.W. (1971) Four cases of acquired von Willebrand's syndrome. *British Journal of Haematology*, **21**, 189.

275 SIMONE J.V., CORNET J.A. & ABILDGAARD C.F. (1968) Acquired von Willebrand's syndrome in systemic lupus erythematosus. *Blood*, **31**, 806.

276 MANT M.J., HIRSH J., GAULDIE J., BIENSTOCK J., PINEO G.F. & LUKE K.H. (1973) von Willebrand's syndrome presenting as an acquired bleeding disorder in association with a monoclonal gammopathy. *Blood*, **42**, 429.

277 INGRAM G.I.C., PRENTICE C.R.M., FORBES C.D. & LESLIE J. (1973) Low factor-VIII-like antigen in acquired von Willebrand's syndrome and response to treatment. *British Journal of Haematology*, **25**, 137.

278 HANDIN R.I., MARTIN V. & MOLONEY W.C. (1976) Antibody-induced von Willebrand's disease: a newly defined inhibitor syndrome. *Blood*, **48**, 393.

279 JOIST J.H., COWAN J.F. & ZIMMERMAN T.S. (1978) Acquired von Willebrand's disease. Evidence for a quantitative and qualitative factor VIII disorder. *New England Journal of Medicine*, **298**, 988.

280 ROSBOROUGH T.K. & SWAIM W.R. (1978) Acquired von Willebrand's disease, platelet release defect and angiodysplasia. *American Journal of Medicine*, **65**, 96.

281 WAUTIER J.L., CAEN J.P. & RYMER R. (1976) Angiodysplasia in acquired von Willebrand's disease. *Lancet*, **ii**, 973.

282 MAMMEN E.F. (1974) Congenital abnormalities of the fibrinogen molecule. *Seminars in Thrombosis and Hemostasis*, **1**, 184.

283 RATNOFF O.D. & FORMAN W.B. (1976) Criteria for the differentiation of dysfibrinogenemic states. *Seminars in Hematology*, **13**, 141.

284 FLUTE P.T. (1977) Disorders of plasma fibrinogen synthesis. *British Medical Bulletin*, **33**, 253.

285 GRALNICK H.R. (1977) Congenital disorders of fibrinogen. In: *Hematology* (ed. Williams W.J., Beutler E., Erslev A.R. & Rundles R.W.), 2nd edn, p. 1423. McGraw-Hill, New York.

286 MORSE E.E. (1978) The fibrinogenopathies. *Annals of Clinical and Laboratory Science*, **8**, 234.

287 BECK E.A. (1979) Congenital abnormalities of fibrinogen. *Clinics in Hematology*, **8**, 169.

288 RABE F. & SALOMON E. (1920) Ueber Faserstoffmangel im Blut bein einem Falle von Hämophilie. *Deutsches Archiv für Klinische Medizin*, **132**, 240.

289 KAMMERMANN B., GMUR J. & STÜNZI H. (1971) Afibrinogenämie beim Hund. *Zentralblatt für Veterinärmedizin*, **18**, 192.

290 BREVINK H.J., HART H.C. & VAN ARKEL C. (1972) Congenital afibrinogenemia in goats. *Zentralblatt für Veterinärmedizin*, **19**, 661.

291 DE VRIES A., ROZENBERG T., KOCHWA S. & BOSS J.H. (1961) Precipitating antifibrinogen antibody appearing after fibrinogen infusions in a patient with congenital afibrinogenemia. *American Journal of Medicine*, **30**, 486.

292 GUGLER E. & LÜSCHER E.F. (1965) Platelet function in congenital afibrinogenemia. *Thrombosis et Diathesis Haemorrhagica*, **14**, 361.

293 NACHMAN R.L. & MARCUS A.J. (1968) Immunological studies of proteins associated with subcellular fractions of thrombasthenic and afibrinogenaemic platelets. *British Journal of Haematology*, **15**, 181.

294 WEISS H. & ROGERS J. (1971) Fibrinogen and platelets in the primary arrest of bleeding; studies in two patients with afibrinogenemia. *New England Journal of Medicine*, **285**, 369.

295 MCCLEAN J.R., MAXWELL R.E. & HERTLER D. (1964) Fibrinogen and adenosine diphosphate-induced aggregation of platelets. *Nature (London)*, **202**, 605.

296 BANG N.U., HEIDENREICH R.O. & MATSUDA M. (1970) Plasma protein requirement for human platelet aggregation. *Thrombosis et Diathesis Haemorrhagica*, **42** (Suppl.), 37.

297 INGRAM G.I.C., MCBRIEN D.J. & SPENCER H. (1966) Fatal pulmonary embolus in congenital fibrinopenia: report of two cases. *Acta Haematologica* (Basel), **35**, 56.

298 EBRING R., ANDRASSY K., EGLI H. & MEYER-LINDENBERG J. (1971) Diagnostische und therapeutische Probleme bei congenitaler Afibrinogenämie. *Blut*, **22**, 175.

299 BLOOM A.L. (1962) The release of thrombin from fibrin by fibrinolysin. *British Journal of Haematology*, **8**, 129.

300 LIU C.Y., NOSSEL H.L. & KAPLAN K.L. (1979) The binding of thrombin by fibrin. *Journal of Biological Chemistry*, **254**, 10421.

301 HASSELBACK R., MARION R.B. & THOMAS J.W. (1963) Congenital hypofibrinogenemia in five members of a family. *Canadian Medical Association Journal*, **88**, 19.

302 JACKSON D.P. & BECK E.A. (1970) Inherited abnormal fibrinogen. In: *Hemophilia and New Hemorrhagic States* (ed. Brinkhous K.M.), p. 225. University of North Carolina Press, Chapel Hill.

303 DI IMPERATO C. & DETTORI A.G. (1958) Ipofibrinogenemia congenita con fibrinoastenia. *Helvetica Paediatrica Acta*, **13**, 380.

304 FANCONI G. (1941) 'Fibrinasthenia' als Ursache einer schweren hämorrhagischen Diathese bei lues congenita. *Schweizerische Medizinische Wochenschrift*, **71**, 255.

305 INGRAM G.I.C. (1955) Variations in the reaction between thrombin and fibrinogen and their effects on the prothrombin time. *Journal of Clinical Pathology*, **8**, 318.

306 MÉNACHÉ D. (1964) Constitutional and familial abnormal fibrinogen. *Thrombosis et Diathesis Haemorrhagica*, **13**, 173.

307 BECK E.A. (1964) Abnormal fibrinogen (fibrinogen 'Baltimore') as a cause of a familial hemorrhagic disorder. *Blood*, **24**, 853.

308 SORIA J., SORIA C., SAMAMA M., POIROT E. & KLING C. (1972) Fibrinogen Troyes-fibrinogen Metz, two new cases of congenital dysfibrinogenemia. *Thrombosis et Diathesis Haemorrhagica*, **27**, 619.

309 MAMMEN E.F., PRASAD A.S., BARNHART M.I. & AU C.C. (1969) Congenital dysfibrinogenemia: fibrinogen Detroit. *Journal of Clinical Investigation*, **48**, 235.

310 VON FELTEN A., FRICK P.G. & STRAUB P.W. (1969) Studies on fibrin monomer aggregation in congenital dysfibrinogenaemia (fibrinogen Zurich). *British Journal of Haematology*, **16**, 253.

311 FORMAN W.B., RATNOFF O.D. & BOYER M.H. (1968) An inherited qualitative abnormality in plasma fibrinogen: fibrinogen Cleveland. *Journal of Laboratory and Clinical Medicine*, **72**, 455.

312 MOSESSON M.W. & BECK E.A. (1969) Chromatographic, ultracentrifugal, and related studies on fibrinogen 'Baltimore'. *Journal of Clinical Investigation*, **48**, 1656.

313 GRALNICK H.R., COLLER B.S., FRATANTONI J.C. & MARTINEZ J. (1979) Fibrinogen Bethesda III: a hypodysfibrinogenemia. *Blood*, **53**, 28.

314 GRALNICK H.R., GIVELBER H.M., SHAINOFF J.R. & FINLAYSON J.S. (1971) Fibrinogen 'Bethesda': a congenital dysfibrinogenemia with delayed fibrinopeptide release. *Journal of Clinical Investigation*, **50**, 1819.

315 AL-MONDHIRY H.A.B., BILEZIKIAN S.B. & NOSSEL H.L. (1975) Fibrinogen New York, an abnormal fibrinogen associated with thromboembolism. *Blood*, **45**, 607.

316 SHERMAN L.A., GASTON L.W., KAPLAN M.E. & SPIVAK A.R. (1972) Fibrinogen St. Louis: a new inherited fibrinogen variant, coincidentally associated with hemophilia. *Journal of Clinical Investigation*, **51**, 590.

317 VERHAEGHE R., VERSTRAETE M., VERMYLEN J. & VERMYLEN C. (1974) Fibrinogen Leuven, another genetic variant. *British Journal of Haematology*, **26**, 421.

318 GRALNICK H.R., GIVELBER H.M. & FINLAYSON J.S. (1973) A new congenital abnormality of human fibrinogen, fibrinogen Bethesda II. *Thrombosis et Diathesis Haemorrhagica*, **29**, 562.

319 MARTINEZ J., HOLBURN R.R., SHAPIRO S.S. & ERSLEV A.J. (1974) Fibrinogen Philadelphia: a hereditary hypofibrinogenemia characterised by fibrinogen hypercatabolism. *Journal of Clinical Investigation*, **53**, 600.

320 AZNAR J., FERNANDEZ-PAVÓN A., REGANÓN E., VILA V. & ARELLNA F. (1974) Fibrinogen Valencia: a new case of congenital dysfibrinogenemia. *Thrombosis et Diathesis Haemorrhagica*, **32**, 564.

321 SORIA J., SORIA C. & BOULARD C. (1972) Anomalie de structure du fibrinogène 'Metz' localisée sur la chaine (A) de la molecule. *Biochemie*, **54**, 415.

322 BLOMBÄCK M., BLOMBÄCK B., MAMMEN E. & PRASAD A.S. (1968) Fibrinogen 'Detroit', a molecular defect in the N-terminal disulphide knot of human fibrinogen. *Nature (London)*, **218**, 134.

323 KUDRYK B., BLOMBÄCK B. & BLOMBÄCK M. (1976) Fibrinogen Detroit—an abnormal fibrinogen with non-

functional NH$_2$-terminal polymerization domain. *Thrombosis Research*, **9**, 25.

324 CHAVIN S.I., ABE ANDES W., BELTRAN G. & STUCKEY W.J. (1980) Fibrinogen New Orleans: hereditary dysfibrinogenemia with an A(α) chain abnormality (personal communication).

325 BRANSON H.E., THEODOR I., BAUMGARTNER R., SCHMER G. & PIRKLE H. (1979) Fibrinogen Seattle: a heritable disfibrinogen with an isolated impairment in fibrinopeptide B release. *Thrombosis and Haemostasis*, **42**, 138.

326 SAMORI T., YATABE M., UKITA M., FUJIMAKI M., FUKUTAKE K. (1975) A new type of congenital dysfibrinogenemia (fibrinogen Tokyo) with defective stabilization of fibrin monomers. *Thrombosis et Diathesis Haemorrhagica*, **34**, 329.

327 HAMPTON J.W. (1968) Qualitative fibrinogen defect associated with abnormal fibrin stabilization. *Journal of Laboratory and Clinical Medicine*, **72**, 882.

328 BIGGS R. (1951) *Prothrombin Deficiency*, p. 52. Blackwell Scientific Publications, Oxford.

329 ROBERTS J.T., GRAY O.P. & BLOOM A.L. (1966) An abormality of the thrombin-fibrinogen reaction in the newborn. *Acta Paediatrica Scandinavica*, **55**, 148.

330 GUILLIN M.-C. & MÉNACHÉ D. (1973) Fetal fibrinogen and fibrinogen Paris. I. Comparative fibrin monomer aggregation studies. *Thrombosis Research*, **31**, 117.

331 TEGER-NILSSON A.-M. & EKELUND H. (1974) Fibrinogen to fibrin transformation in umbilical cord blood and purified normal fibrinogen. *Thrombosis Research*, **5**, 601.

332 WITT I., MÜLLER H. & KÜNZER W. (1969) Evidence for the existence of fetal fibrinogen. *Thrombosis et Diathesis Haemorrhagica*, **22**, 101.

333 WITT I. & MÜLLER H. (1970) Phosphorus and hexose content of human foetal fibrinogen. *Biochimica Biophysica Acta*, **221**, 402.

334 WITT I. & TESCH R. (1979) Molecular characterization of human foetal fibrinogen. *Thrombosis and Haemostasis*, **42**, 79.

335 VON FELTEN A., STRAUB P.W. & FRICK P.G. (1969) Dysfibrinogenemia in a patient with primary hepatoma. *New England Journal of Medicine*, **280**, 495.

336 GRALNICK H., ABRAMS E. & KROLIKOWSKI J. (1975) Acquired dysfibrinogenaemia in hepatocellular carcinoma. *Clinical Research*, **23**, 338A.

337 LANE, D.A., SCULLY M.F., THOMAS D.P., KAKKAR V.V., WOOLF I.L. & WILLIAMS R. (1977) Acquired dysfibrinogenaemia in acute and chronic liver disease. *British Journal of Haematology*, **35**, 301.

338 BECK E.A., CHARACHE P. & JACKSON D.P. (1965) A new inherited coagaulation disorder caused by an abnormal fibrinogen ('fibrinogen Baltimore'). *Nature (London)*, **208**, 143.

339 CRUM E.D., SHAINOFF J.R., GRAHAM R.C. & RATNOFF O.D. (1974) Fibrinogen Cleveland II, an abnormal fibrinogen with defective release of fibrinopeptide A. *Journal of Clinical Investigation*, **53**, 1308.

340 KRAUSE W.H., HEENE D.L. & LASCH H.G. (1973) Congenital dysfibrinogenemia (fibrinogen Giessen). *Thrombosis et Diathesis Haemorrhagica*, **29**, 547.

341 BÖTTCHER D., HASLER K., KÖTGEN E. & MARUATH J. (1979) Hereditary hypodysfibrinogenemia with defective release of fibrinogenopeptide A (fibrinogen Freiburg). *Thrombosis and Haemostasis*, **42**, 78.

342 LANE D.A., VAN ROSS M., KAKKAR V.V., DHIR K., HOLT L.P.J. & MACIVER J.E. (1979) An abnormal fibrinogen with delayed fibrinopeptide A release. *Thrombosis and Haemostasis*, **42**, 77.

343 HANSEN M.S. & CLEMMENSEN I. (1979) An abnormal fibrinogen (Copenhagen) associated with severe thromboembolic disease, but with normal adsorption of plasminogen. *Thrombosis and Haemostasis*, **42**, 137.

344 LANE D.A., CUDDIGAN B., VAN ROSS M. & KAKKAR V.V. (1980) Dysfibrinogenaemia characterized by abnormal fibrin monomer polymerization and normal fibrinopeptide A release. *British Journal of Haematology*, **44**, 483.

345 DUMITRESCU E., TAUBERT W., NIEWHAUS K. & WENZEL E. (1979) Observations on a new variant of hereditary dysfibrinogenaemia ('Homburg'?) with delayed fibrin polymerization and without clinical abnormality. *Thrombosis and Haemostasis*, **42**, 139.

346 JANSSEN C.L. & VREEKEN J. (1971) Fibrinogen Amsterdam, another hereditary abnormality of fibrinogen. *British Journal of Haematology*, **20**, 287.

347 BURASCHI J.A., SACK E.S., QUIROGA E. & HEWDLER H. (1975) A new fibrinogen anomaly: fibrinogen Buenos Aires. *Thrombosis et Diathesis Haemorrhagica*, **34**, 570.

348 DE BOSCH N.B., AROCHA-PIÑANGO C.L., SORIA J., SORIA C., RODRIGUEZ A. & RODRIGUEZ S. (1977) An abnormal fibrinogen in a Venezuelan family. *Thrombosis Research*, **10**, 253.

349 STREIFF F., ALEXANDRE P., VIGNERON C., SORIA J., SORIA C. & MESTER L. (1971) Un nouveau cas d'anomalie constitutionelle et familiale de fibrinogène sans diathèse hémorrhagique. *Thrombosis et Diathesis Hamorrhagica*, **26**, 565.

350 ACQUERCIF M., SORIA J., SORIA C., RITSCHARD J., SAMAMA M. & BOUVIER C. (1973) A new family with dysfibrinogenemia, fibrinogen Alba/Geneva. *Abstracts Fourth International Congress on Thrombosis and Haemostasis*, **1**, 38.

351 WOHL R.C. & BRADLEY T.B. (1974) Impaired monomer aggregation in congenital dysfibrinogenemia. *Blood*, **44**, 935.

352 FUCHS G., EBRING R. & HAVERMANN K. (1977) Fibrinogen Marburg, a new genetic variant of fibrinogen. *Blut*, **34**, 107.

353 LACOMBE M., SORIA J., SORIA C., D'ANGELA G., LAVALLÉE R. & BONNY Y. (1973) Fibrinogen Montreal—a new case of congenital dysfibrinogenemia with defective aggregation of monomers. *Thrombosis et Diathesis Haemorrhagica*, **29**, 536.

354 SAMAMA M., SORIA J., SORIA C. & BOUSSER J. (1969) Dysfibrinogénémie congentiale et familiale sans tendance hémorrhagique. *Nouvelle Revue française d'Hématologie*, **9**, 817.

355 SORIA J. & SORIA C. (1974) Dysfibrinogénémie familiale avec anomalie de l'aggregation des monomères; le fibrinogène Paris III. *Pathologie et Biologie*, **22** (Suppl.), 72.

356 WINKELMANN G. (1973) Kongenitale dysfibrinogenämie — Bericht über eine neue familie (Fibrinogen Wiesbaden). *Thrombosis et Diathesis Haemorrhagica*, **55**, 345.

357 FUNK C. & STRAUB P.W. (1970) Hereditary abnormality

of fibrin monomer aggregation (fibrinogen Zurich II). *European Journal of Clinical Investigation*, **1**, 131.

358 FERNANDEZ J., LASIERRA J., NARVAIZA M.J., VILADES E., PALACIOS E. & ROCHA Y.E. (1979) Fibrinogen Logroño. A new fibrinogen molecular variant. *Thrombosis and Haemostasis*, **42**, 138.

359 SAMAMA M., SORIA J. & SORIA C. (1977) Congenital and acquired dysfibrinogenaemia. In: *Recent Advances in Blood Coagulation* (ed. Poller L.), 2nd edn, p. 313. Churchill-Livingstone, Edinburgh.

360 KRAUSE W.H., HUTH K., HEENE D.L. & LASCH H.G. (1975) Hypodysfibrinogenämie: fibrinogen Giessen II. *Klinische Wochenschrift*, **53**, 781.

361 BARTHELS M. & SANDROSS G. (1977) 'Fibrinogen Hannover', ein Weiteres atypisches Fibrinogen. *Blut*, **34**, 99.

362 JACOBSEN C.D. & HOAK J.C. (1973) Fibrinogen Iowa city: an abnormal fibrinogen with no clinical symptoms. *Thrombosis Research*, **2**, 261.

363 ZIETZ B.H. & SCOTT J.L. (1970) An inherited defect in fibrinogen polymerization: fibrinogen Los Angeles. *Clinical Research*, **18**, 179.

364 d'ANGELO C., LACOMBE M., LEMAY J. LAVALLÉE R., BONNY Y. & BOILEAU J. (1975) Fibrinogen Montreal II. *Thrombosis et Diathesis Haemorrhagica*, **34**, 570.

365 THALER E. Quoted by Samama *et al.* [359].

366 TAKAMATSU J., OGATA K., KAMIYA T. & KOIE K. (1979) A novel dysfibrinogenemia with abnormal γ-chain (fibrinogen Nagoya). *Thrombosis and Haemostasis*, **42**, 78.

367 ROBBINS K.C. (1944) A study on the conversion of fibrinogen to fibrin. *American Journal of Physiology*, **142**, 581.

368 DUCKERT F., JUNG E. & SCHMERLING D.H. (1960) Hitherto undescribed congenital haemorrhagic diathesis probably due to fibrin-stabilising factor deficiency. *Thrombosis et Diathesis Haemorrhagica*, **5**, 179.

369 GIROLAMI A., BURUL A., FABRIS F., CAPPELLATO G. & BETTERLE C. (1978) Studies on factor XIII antigen in congenital factor XIII deficiency. A tentative classification of the disease into two groups. *Folia Haematologica*, **105**, 131.

370 DUCKERT F. & BECK E.A. (1968) Clinical disorder due to the deficiency of factor XIII (fibrin stabilising factor, fibrinase). *Seminars in Hematology*, **5**, 83.

371 WILLIAMS W.J. (1977) Congenital deficiency of factor XIII (fibrin-stabilising factor). In; *Hematology* (ed. Williams W.J., Beutler E., Erslev A.J. & Rundles R.W.), 2nd edn, p. 1431. McGraw-Hill, New York.

372 LOSOWSKY M.S. & MILOSZEWSKI K.J.A. (1977) Factor XIII. *British Journal of Haematology*, **37**, 1.

373 LORAND L. & KONISHI K. (1964) Activation of the fibrin-stabilising factor of plasma by thrombin. *Archives of Biochemistry and Biophysics*, **105**, 58.

374 ISRAELS E.D., PARASKEVAS F. & ISRAELS G.L. (1973) Immunological studies of coagulation factor XIII. *Journal of Clinical Investigation*, **52**, 2398.

375 BRITTEN A.F.H. (1967) Congenital deficiency of factor XIII (fibrin-stabilising factor): report of a case and review of the literature. *American Journal of Medicine*, **43**, 751.

376 RATNOFF O.D. & STEINBERG A.G. (1972) Fibrin cross-linking and heredity. *Annals of the New York Academy of Sciences*, **202**, 186.

377 LORAND L., URAYAMA T., DE KIEWIET J.W.C. & NOSSEL H.L. (1969) Diagnostic and genetic studies on fibrin-stabilising factor with a new assay based on amine incorporation. *Journal of Clinical Investigation*, **48**, 1054.

378 DVILANSKY A., BRITTEN A.F.H. & LOEWY A.G. (1970) Factor XIII assay by an isotope method. I. Factor XIII (transamidase) in plasma, serum, leucocytes, erythrocytes and platelets and evaluation of screening tests of clot solubility. *British Journal of Haematology*, **18**, 399.

379 SCHMER G. (1973) A solid-phase radioassay for factor-XIII activity (fibrin stabilising activity) in human plasma. *British Journal of Haematology*, **24**, 735.

380 BOARD P.G., COGGAN M. & HAMER J.W. (1980) An electrophoretic and quantitative analysis of coagulation factor XIII in normal and deficient subjects. *British Journal of Haematology*, **45**, 633.

381 BARBUI T., RODEGHEIRO F., DINI E., MARIANI G., PAPA M.L., DE BIASI R., CORDERO MURICCO R. & MONTERO UMANA C. (1978) Subunits A and S inheritance in four families with congenital factor XIII deficiency. *British Journal of Haematology*, **38**, 267.

382 DUCKERT F. (1972) Documentation of the plasma factor XIII deficiency in man. *Annals of the New York Acadamy of Sciences*, **202**, 190.

383 BOARD P.G. (1979) Genetic polymorphism of the A subunit of human coagulation factor XIII. *American Journal of Human Genetics*, **31**, 116.

384 BOARD P.G. (1980) Genetic polymorphism of the B sununit of human coagulation factor XIII. *American Journal of Human Genetics*, **32**, 348.

385 FORMAN W.B., BYER R., HADADY H., KRILL C. & LUBIN A. (1977) Congenital fibrin-stabilising factor deficiency: evidence for dys-FSF. *Blood*, **50** (Suppl.), 266.

386 AMRIS C.J. & RANEH L. (1965) A case of fibrin stabilising factor (FSF) deficiency. *Thrombosis et Diathesis Haemorrhagica*, **14**, 332.

387 GREENBERG L.H., SCHIFFMAN S. & WONG Y.S.S. (1969) Factor XIII deficiency: treatment with monthly plasma infusions. *Journal of the American Medical Association*, **209**, 264.

388 IKKALA E., MYLLYLÄ G. & NEVANLINNA H.R. (1964) Transfusion therapy in factor XIII (FSF) deficiency. *Scandinavian Journal of Haematology*, **1**, 308.

389 BARRY A. & DELAGE J.M. (1965) Congenital deficiency of fibrin stabilising factor. *New England Journal of Medicine*, **272**, 943.

390 BECK E., DUCKERT F. & ERNST M. (1961) The influence of fibrin stabilising factor on the growth of fibroblasts *in vitro* and wound healing. *Thrombosis et Diathesis Haemorrhagica*, **6**, 485.

391 FISHER S., RICKOVER M. & NADY S. (1966) Factor 13 deficiency with severe hemorrhagic diathesis. *Blood*, **28**, 34.

392 GIROLAMI A., BURUL A. & STICCHI A. (1977) Congenital deficiency of factor XIII with normal subunit S and lack of subunit A: report of a new family. *Acta Haematologica*, **58**, 17.

393 WALLS W.D. & LOSOWSKY M.S. (1968) Congenital deficiency of fibrin-stabilising factor. *Coagulation*, **1**, 111.

394 MILOSZEWSKI K. & LOSOWSKY M.S. (1970) The half-life

of factor XIII *in vivo. British Journal of Haematology,* **19**, 685.

395 TROBISCH H. & EGBRING R. (1972) Substitution mit einem neuen Faktor-XIII-konzentrat bei kongenitalem Faktor-XIII-Mangel. *Deutsches Medizinische Wochenschrift,* **97**, 499.

396 OWEN C.A., HENRIKSEN R.A., McDUFFIE F.C. & MANN K.G. (1978) Prothrombin Quick: A newly identified dysprothrombinaemia. *Mayo Clinic Proceedings,* **53**, 29.

397 GILL F.M., SHAPIRO S.S. & SCHWARTZ E. (1978) Severe congenital hypoprothrombinaemia. *Journal of Pediatrics,* **93**, 264.

398 MONTGOMERY R.R., OTSAKU A. & HATHAWAY W.E. (1978) Hypoprothrombinaemia: Case report. *Blood,* **51**, 299.

399 GIROLAMI A., COCCHERI S., PALARETI G., POGGI I., BURUL A. & CAPPELLATO G. (1978) Prothrombin Molise: a 'new' congenital dysprothrombinemia, double heterozygosis with an abnormal prothrombin and 'true' prothrombin deficiency. *Blood,* **52**, 115.

400 BEZEAUD A., GUILLIN M.-C., OLMEDA F., QUINTANA M. & GOMEZ M. (1979) Prothrombin Madrid: a new familial abnormality of prothrombin. *Thrombosis Research,* **16**, 47.

401 RABIET M.-J., ELION J., LABIE D. & JOSSO F. (1979) Prothrombin Metz: purification and characterization of a variant of human prothrombin. *Thrombosis and Haemostasis,* **42**, 57.

402 SHAPIRO S.S. (1975) Prothrombin San Juan: A new complex dysprothrombinemia. In: *Prothrombin and Related Coagulation Factors* (ed. Hemker H.C. & Veltkamp J.J.), p. 205. Leiden University Press, Leiden.

403 KAHN M.J.P. & GOVAERTS A. (1974) Prothrombin Brussels, a new congenital defective protein. *Thrombosis Research,* **5**, 141.

404 BLOOM A.L. (1977) Immunological detection of blood coagulation factors in haemorrhagic disorders. In: *Recent Advances in Haematology* (ed. Hoffbrand A.V., Brain M.C. & Hirsh J.), p. 387. Churchill-Livingstone, Edinburgh.

405 SHAPIRO S.S., MARTINEZ J. & HOLBURN R.H. (1969) Congenital dysprothrombinemia: an inherited structural disorder of human prothrombin. *Journal of Clinical Investigation,* **48**, 2251.

406 JOSSO F., MONASTERIO DE SANCHEZ J., LAVERGNE J.M., MÉNACHÉ D. & SOULIER J.P. (1971) Congenital abnormality of the prothrombin molecule (factor II) in four siblings: prothrombin Barcelona. *Blood,* **38**, 9.

407 RABIET M.-J., ELION J., BENAROUS R., LABIE D. & JOSSO F. (1979) Activation of prothrombin Barcelona: evidence for active high molecular-weight intermediates. *Biochimica et Biophysica Acta,* **584**, 66.

408 GIROLAMI A., BAREGGI G., BRUNETTI A. & STICCI A. (1974) Prothrombin Padua: a 'new' congenital dysprothrombinemia. *Journal of Laboratory and Clinical Medicine,* **84**, 654.

409 SHAPIRO S.S., MALDONADO M., FRADERA J. & McCORD S. (1974) Prothrombin San Juan: a complex new dysprothrombinemia. *Journal of Clinical Investigation,* **53**, 73.

410 QUICK A.J., PISCIOTTA A.V. & HUSSEY C.V. (1955) Congenital hypoprothrombinemic states. *Archives of Internal Medicine,* **95**, 2.

411 BAS B.M. & MULLER A.D. (1975) Staphylocoagulase. In: *Prothrombin and Related Coagulation Factors* (ed. Hemker H.C. & Veltkamp J.J.), p. 99. Leiden University Press, Leiden.

412 TELFER T.P., DENSON K.W. & WRIGHT D.R. (1956) A 'new' coagulation defect. *British Journal of Haematology,* **2**, 308.

413 HOUGIE C., BARROW E.M. & GRAHAM J.B. (1957) Stuart clotting defect. I. Segregation of an hereditary hemorrhagic state from a heterogeneous group heretofore called 'stable factor' (SPCA, proconvertin, factor VII) deficiency. *Journal of Clinical Investigation,* **36**, 485.

414 RATNOFF O.D. (1972) The molecular basis of hereditary clotting disorders. *Progress in Hemostasis and Thrombosis,* **1**, 39.

415 PRYDZ H. & GLADHAUG A. (1971) Factor X. Immunological studies. *Thrombosis et Diathesis Haemorrhagica,* **25**, 157.

416 DENSON K.W.E., LURIE A., DE CATALDO F. & MANNUCCI P.M. (1970) The factor X defects: recognition of abnormal forms of factor X. *British Journal of Haematology,* **18**, 317.

417 GIROLAMI A., MOLARO G., LAZZARIN M., SCARPA R. & BRUNETTI A. (1970) A 'new' congenital haemorrhagic condition due to the presence of an abnormal factor X (factor X Friuli): a study of a large kindred. *British Journal of Haematology,* **19**, 179.

418 GIROLAMI A. (1975) Factor X Friuli. In: *Prothrombin and Related Coagulation Factors* (ed. Hemker H.C. & Veltkamp J.J.), p. 230. Leiden University Press, Leiden.

419 GIROLAMI A., BAREGGI G. & BORSATO N. (1975) Factor X Friuli: an immunological study in plasma and serum using several methods. *Blut,* **30**, 203.

420 PORTER N.R., MALIA R.G., COOPER P.C. & PRESTON F.E. (1979) The heterogeneity of congenital factor X deficiency. A study of two unrelated patients. *Thrombosis and Haemostasis,* **42**, 58.

421 LECHNER K., MÄHR G., MARGARITELLER P. & DEUTSCH E. (1979) Factor X Vorarlberg, a new variant of hereditary factor X deficiency. *Thrombosis and Haemostasis,* **42**, 58.

422 FAIR D.S., PLOW E.F. & EDGINGTON T.S. (1979) Combined functional and immunochemical analysis of normal and abnormal human factor X. *Journal of Clinical Investigation,* **64**, 884.

423 ALEXANDER B., GOLDSTEIN R., LANDWEHR G. & COOK C.D. (1951) Congenital SPCA deficiency: a new hitherto unrecognised defect with hemorrhage rectified by serum and serum fractions. *Journal of Clinical Investigation,* **30**, 596.

424 MARDER V.J. & SHULMAN N.R. (1964) Clinical aspects of congenital factor VII deficiency. *American Journal of Medicine,* **37**, 182.

425 ØSTERUD B. & RAPAPORT S.I. (1977) Activation of factor IX by the reaction product of tissue factor and factor VII: additional pathway for initiating blood coagulation. *Proceedings of the National Academy of Sciences, USA,* **74**, 5260.

426 GOODNIGHT S.H., JR, FEINSTEIN D.I., ØSTERUD B. & RAPAPORT S.I. (1971) Factor VII antibody-neutralising material in hereditary and acquired factor VII deficiency. *Blood,* **38**, 1.

427 DENSON K.W.E., CONARD J. & SAMAMA M. (1972) Genetic variants of factor VII. *Lancet*, **ii**, 1234.

428 LEVANON M., RIMON S., SHANI M., RAMOT B. & GOLDBERG E. (1972) Active and inactive factor VII in Dubin–Johnson syndrome with factor VII deficiency, hereditary factor VII deficiency and on coumadin administration. *British Journal of Haematology*, **23**, 669.

429 BRIËT E., LOELIGER E.A., VAN TILBURG N.H. & VELT-KAMP J.J. (1976) Molecular variants of factor VII. *Thrombosis and Haemostasis*, **52**, 289.

430 MAZZUCCONI M.G., MANDELLI F., MARIANI G., BRIËT E. & VELTKAMP J.J. (1977) A CRM-positive variant of factor VII deficiency and the detection of heterozygotes with the assay of factor-like antigen. *British Journal of Haematology*, **36**, 127.

431 GIROLAMI A., FALEZZA G., PATRASSI G., STENICO M. & VETTORE L. (1977) Factor VII Verona coagulation disorder: double heterozygosis with an abnormal factor VII and heterozygous factor VII deficiency. *Blood*, **50**, 603.

432 GIROLAMI A., FABRIS F., DAL B.O., ZANON R., GHIOTTO G. & BURUL A. (1978) Factor VII Padua: a congenital coagulation disorder due to an abnormal factor VII with a peculiar activation pattern. *Journal of Laboratory and Clinical Medicine*, **91**, 387.

433 GIROLAMI A., CATTAROZZI G., DAL B.O., ZANON R., CELLA G. & TOFFANIN F. (1979) Factor VII Padua$_2$: another factor VII abnormality with defective ox brain thromboplastin activation and a complex hereditary pattern. *Blood*, **54**, 46.

434 SELIGSOHN U., SHANI M. & RAMOT B. (1970) Gilbert syndrome and factor VII deficiency. *Lancet*, **i**, 1398.

435 SELIGSOHN U., SHANI M., RAMOT B., ADAM A. & SHEBA C. (1970) Dubin–Johnson syndrome in Israel. II. Association with factor VII deficiency. *Quarterly Journal of Medicine* N.S. **39**, 569.

436 DISCHE F.E. (1958) Blood-clotting substances with 'factor VII' activity: a comparison of some congenital and acquired deficiencies. *British Journal of Haematology*, **4**, 201.

437 MUSTARD J.F., SECORD D., HOEKSEMA T.D., DOWNIE H.G. & ROWSELL H.C. (1962) Canine factor VII deficiency. *British Journal of Haematology*, **8**, 43.

438 GARNER R., HERMOSO-PEREZ C. & CONNING D.M. (1967) Factor VII deficiency in beagle dog plasma and its use in the assay of human factor VII. *Nature (London)*, **216**, 1130.

439 GARNER R. & CONNING D.M. (1970) The assay of human factor VII by means of modified factor VII deficient dog plasma. *British Journal of Haematology*, **18**, 57.

440 ZIMMERMAN R., EHLERS G., EHLERS W., VON VOSS H., GÖBEL U. & WAHN U. (1979) Congenital factor VII deficiency: a report of four new cases. *Blut*, **38**, 119.

441 GODAL C., MADSEN K. & NISSEN-MEYER R. (1962) Thromboembolism in patients with total proconvertin (factor VII) deficiency. *Acta Medica Scandinavica*, **171**, 325.

442 GERSHWIN M.E. & GUDE J.K. (1973) Deep vein thrombosis and pulmonary embolism in congenital factor VII deficiency. *New England Journal of Medicine*, **288**, 141.

443 MATTHAY K.H., KOERPER M.A. & ABLIN A.R. (1979) Intracranial hemorrhage in congenital factor VII deficiency. *Journal of Pediatrics*, **94**, 413.

444 HOAG M.S., AGGELER P.M. & FOWELL A.H. (1960) Disappearance rate of concentrated proconvertin extracts in congenital and acquired hypoproconvertinemia. *Journal of Clinical Investigation*, **39**, 554.

445 STRAUSS H.S. (1965) Surgery in patients with congenital factor VII deficiency (congenital hypoproconvertinemia). Experience with one case and review of the literature. *Blood*, **25**, 325.

446 YORKE A.Y. & MANT M.J. (1977) Factor VII deficiency and surgery. Is preoperative replacement therapy necessary? *Journal of the American Medical Association*, **238**, 424.

447 BELL W.N. & ALTON H.G. (1955) Christmas disease associated with factor VII deficiency. Case report with family survey. *British Medicial Journal*, **i**, 330.

448 HALL C.A., LONDON A.R., MOYNIHAN A.C. & DODDS W.J. (1975) Hereditary factor VII and IX deficiencies in a large kindred. *British Journal of Haematology*, **29**, 319.

449 KROLL A.J., ALEXANDER B., COCHIOS F. & PECHET L. (1964) Hereditary deficiencies of clotting factors VII and X associated with carotid-body tumours. *New England Journal of Medicine*, **270**, 6.

450 JOHNSON C.A., CHUNG K.S., McGRATH K.M., BEAN P.E. & ROBERTS H.R. (1980) Characterization of variant prothrombin in a patient congenitally deficient in factors II, VII, IX and X. *British Journal of Haematology*, **44**, 461.

451 NEWCOMB T., MATTER M., CONROY L., DeMARSH Q.B. & FINCH C.A. (1956) Congenital hemorrhagic diathesis of the prothrombin complex. *American Journal of Medicine*, **20**, 798.

452 OWREN P.A. (1947) Parahaemophilia, haemorrhagic diathesis due to absence of a previously known clotting factor. *Lancet*, **i**, 446.

453 QUICK A.J. (1943) On the constitution of prothrombin. *American Journal of Physiology*, **140**, 212.

454 SEELER R.A. (1972) Parahemophilia. Factor V deficiency. *Medical Clinics of North America*, **56**, 119.

455 MITTERSTEILER G. & MULLER W., (1978) Congenital factor V deficiency. A family study. *Scandinavian Journal of Haematology*, **21**, 9.

456 FEINSTEIN D.I., RAPAPORT S.I., McGEHEE W.G. & PATCH M.J. (1970) Factor V anticoagulants: clinical, biochemical and immunological observations. *Journal of Clinical Investigation*, **49**, 1578.

457 FRANTANTONI J.W., HILGARTNER M. & NACHMAN R.L. (1972) Nature of the defect in congenital factor V deficiency: study in a patient with acquired circulating anticoagulant. *Blood*, **39**, 751.

458 GIDDINGS J.C., SHEARN S.A.M. & BLOOM A.L. (1975) the immunological localization of factor V in human tissue. *British Journal of Haematology*, **29**, 57.

459 BREEDERVELD K., GIDDINGS J.C., TEN CATE J.W. & BLOOM A.L. (1975) The localization of factor V within normal human platelets and the demonstration of a platelet-factor V antigen in congenital factor V deficiency. *British Journal of Haematology*, **29**, 405.

460 HOUGIE C. (1977) Hemophilia and related conditions—congenital deficiencies of prothrombin (factor II), factor V, and factors VII to XII. In: *Hematology* (ed.

Williams W.J., Beutler E., Erslev A.J. & Rundles R.W.), 2nd edn, p. 1404. McGraw-Hill, New York.

461 MELLIGER E.J. & DUCKERT F. (1971) Major surgery in a subject with factor V deficiency. *Thrombosis et Diathesis Haemorrhagica*, **33**, 645.

462 RUSH B. & ELLIS H. (1965) Treatment of patients with factor V deficiency. *Thrombosis et Diathesis Haemorrhagica*, **14**, 74.

463 SMIT SIBINGA C.T., GÖKEMEYER J.D.M., TEN CATE L.P. & BOS-VAN ZWOL F. (1972) Combined deficiency of factors V and VIII: report of a family and genetic analysis. *British Journal of Haematology*, **23**, 467.

464 GIROLAMI A., BRUNETTI A. & DE MARCO L. (1974) Congenital combined factor V and factor VIII deficiency in a male born from a brother–sister incest. *Blut*, **28**, 33.

465 CIMO P.L., MOAKE J.L., GONZALEZ M.F., NATELSON E.A. & FOX K.R. (1977) Inherited combined deficiency of factor V and factor VIII: report of a case with normal factor VIII antigen and ristocetin-induced platelet aggregation. *American Journal of Hematology*, **2**, 385.

466 GOBBI F., ASCARI E. & BARBIERI U. (1967) Congenital combined deficiency of factor VIII (anti-haemophiliac globulin) and factor V (pro-accelerin) in two siblings. *Thrombosis et Diathesis Haemorrhagica*, **17**, 194.

467 GIROLAMI A. & BAREGGI G. (1974) Normal factor VIII antigen level in combined congenital deficiency of factor V and factor VIII. *Acta Haematologica*, **51**, 362.

468 SELIGSOHN U. & RAMOT B. (1969) Combined factor V and factor VIII deficiency: report of four cases. *British Journal of Haematology*, **16**, 475.

469 GIROLAMI A., GASTALDI G., PATRASSI G. & GALLETTI A. (1976) Combined congenital deficiency of factor V and factor VIII. Report of a further case with some considerations on the hereditary transmission of the disorder. *Acta Haematologica*, **55**, 234.

470 GIDDINGS J., SELIGSOHN U. & BLOOM A.L. (1977) Immunological studies in combined factor V and factor VIII deficiency. *British Journal of Haematology*, **37**, 257.

470a MARLAR R.A. & GRIFFIN J.H. (1980) Deficiency of protein C-inhibitor in combined factor V/VIII deficiency disease. *Journal of Clinical Investigation*, **66**, 1186.

471 ROSENTHAL R.L., DRESKIN O.H. & ROSENTHAL M. (1953) New hemophilia-like disease caused by deficiency of a third plasma thromboplastin factor. *Proceedings of the Society for Experimental Biology and Medicine*, **82**, 171.

472 RAPAPORT S.I., PROCTOR R.R., PATCH M.J. & YETTRA M. (1961) The mode of inheritance of PTA deficiency: evidence for the existence of major PTA deficiency and minor PTA deficiency. *Blood*, **18**, 149.

473 LEIBA H., RAMOT B. & MANY A. (1965) Heredity and coagulation studies in ten families with factor XI (plasma thromboplastin antecedent) deficiency. *British Journal of Haematology*, **11**, 654.

474 FORBES C.D. & RATNOFF O.D. (1972) Studies on plasma thromboplastin antecedent (factor XI, PTA) deficiency and inhibition of PTA by plasma: pharmacologic inhibitors and specific antiserum. *Journal of Laboratory and Clinical Medicine*, **79**, 113.

475 RIMON A., SCHIFFMAN S., FEINSTEIN D.I. & RAPAPORT S.I. (1976) Factor IX activity and factor XI antigen in homozygous and heterozygous factor XI deficiency. *Blood*, **48**, 165.

476 SAITO H. & GOLDSMITH G.H. (1977) Plasma thromboplastin antecedent (PTA, factor XI); a specific and sensitive radioimmunoassay. *Blood*, **50**, 377.

477 MARGOLIS J. (1957) Initiation of blood coagulation by glass and related surfaces. *Journal of Physiology*, **137**, 95.

478 NOSSEL H.L. (1964) *The Contact Phase of Blood Coagulation*. Blackwell Scientific Publications, Oxford.

479 GIDDINGS J.C. (1971) Preparation and use of a new artificial system for factor XI assay. *Medical Laboratory Technology*, **28**, 284.

480 SIDA A., SELIGSOHN U., JONAS P. & MANY M. (1978) Factor XI deficiency: detection and management during urological surgery. *Journal of Urology*, **119**, 528.

481 RATNOFF O.D. & COLOPY J.H. (1975) A familial hemorrhagic trait associated with a deficiency of clot-promoting fraction of plasma. *Journal of Clinical Investigation*, **34**, 601.

482 RATNOFF O.D., BUSSE R.J. & SHEON R.P. (1968) The demise of John Hageman. *New England Journal of Medicine*, **279**, 760.

483 BENNETT B., RATNOFF O.D., HOLT J.B. & ROBERTS H.R. (1972) Hageman trait (factor XII deficiency): a probable second genotype inherited as an autosomal dominant characteristic. *Blood*, **40**, 412.

484 SAITO H., SCOTT J.C., MOVAT H.Z. & SCIALLA S.J. (1979) Molecular heterogeneity of Hageman trait (factor XII deficiency): evidence that two of 49 subjects are cross-reacting material positive (CRM+). *Journal of Laboratory and Clinical Medicine*, **94**, 256.

485 RATNOFF O.D. (1977) The surface-mediated initiation of blood coagulation and related phenomena. In: *Haemostasis: Biochemistry, Physiology and Pathology* (ed. Ogston D. & Bennett B.), p. 25. John Wiley & Sons, London.

486 KOVALAINEN S., MYLLYLÄ V.V., TOLONEN U. & HOKKANEN E. (1979) Recurrent subarachnoid haemorrhages in patients with Hageman factor deficiency. *Lancet*, **i**, 1035.

487 HATHAWAY W.E., BELHASEN L.P. & HATHAWAY H.S. (1965) Evidence for a new plasma thromboplastin factor. I. Case report, coagulation studies and physicochemical properties. *Blood*, **26**, 521.

488 ABILDGAARD C.F. & HARRISON J. (1974) Fletcher factor deficiency: family study and detection. *Blood*, **43**, 641.

489 HATHAWAY W.E. & ALSEVER J. (1970) The relationship of 'Fletcher factor' to factors XI and XII. *British Journal of Haematology*, **18**, 161.

490 WUEPPER K.D. (1973) Prekallikrein deficiency in man. *Journal of Experimental Medicine*, **138**, 1345.

491 WALDEMANN R. & ABRAHAM J.B. (1974) Fitzgerald factor: a heretofore unrecognised coagulation factor. *Blood*, **44**, 934.

492 SAITO H., RATNOFF O.D., WALDEMANN R. & ABRAHAM J.P. (1975) Fitzgerald trait. Deficiency of a hitherto unrecognised agent—Fitzgerald factor, participating in surface-mediated reactions of clotting, fibrinolysis, generation of kinins, and the property of diluted plasma enhancing vascular permeability. *Journal of Clinical Investigation*, **55**, 1082.

493 LACOMBE M., VARET B. & LEVY J. (1975) A hitherto

undescribed plasma factor acting at the contact phase of blood coagulation (Flaujeac factor): case report and coagulation studies. *Blood*, **46**, 761.

494 COLMAN R.W., BAGDASARIAN A., TALAMO R.C., SCOTT C.F., SEAVEY M., GUIMARAES J.A., PIERCE J.V., KAPLAN A.P. & WEINSTEIN L. (1975) Williams trait: human kininogen deficiency with diminished levels of plasminogen proactivator and prekallikrein associated with abnormalities of the Hageman factor-dependent pathways. *Journal of Clinical Investigation*, **56**, 1650.

495 LUTCHER C.L. (1967) Reid trait: a new expression of high molecular weight kininogen deficiency. *Clinical Research*, **24**, 440.

496 WALDMAN R., ABRAHAM J.P., REBUCK J.W., CALDWELL J., SAITO H. & RATNOFF O.D. (1975) Fitzgerald factor: A hitherto unrecognised coagulation factor. *Lancet*, **i**, 949.

497 KLUFT C., TRUMPI-KALSHOVEN M.M. & JIE A.F.H. (1979) Crucial conditions for the determination of prekallikrein levels in plasma with chromogenic substrates. In: *Chromogenic Peptide Substrates, Chemistry and Clinical Usage* (ed. Scully M.F. & Kakkar V.V.), p. 84. Churchill-Livingstone, Edinburgh.

498 HAIMBURGER N. & KARGES H.E. (1978) The immunological diagnosis of coagulation defects. *Medical Laboratory*, **5**, 1.

499 HOUGIE C., McPHERSON R.A. & ARONSON L. (1975) Passovoy factor: hitherto unrecognised factor necessary for haemostasis. *Lancet*, **ii**, 290.

500 CONSTANDOULAKIS M. (1958) Familial haemophilia and factor VII deficiency. *Journal of Clinical Pathology*, **11**, 412.

501 VERSTRAETE M. & VANDENBROUCKE J. (1955) Combined antihaemophilic globulin and Christmas factor deficiency in haemophilia. *British Medical Journal*, **ii**, 1533.

502 INGRAM G.I.C. (1956) Observations in a case of multiple haemostatic defect. *British Journal of Haematology*, **2**, 180.

503 LIAN C.-Y.E., DEYKIN D. & HARKNESS D.R. (1976) Combined deficiencies of factor VIII (AHF) and factor XI (PTA). *American Journal of Hematology*, **1**, 319.

504 PECHET L., COCHIOS F. & DEYKIN D. (1967) Further studies on the 'Dynia' clotting abnormality. *Thrombosis et Diathesis Haemorrhagica*, **17**, 365.

505 ROBINSON A.J., AGGELER P.M., McNICOL G.P. & DOUGLAS A.S. (1967) An atypical genetic haemorrhagic disease with increased concentration of a natural inhibitor of prothrombin consumption. *British Journal of Haematology*, **13**, 510.

506 PARRY D.H., GIDDINGS J.C. & BLOOM A.L. (1980) Familial haemostatic defect associated with reduced prothrombin consumption. *British Journal of Haematology*, **44**, 323.

507 KOIE K., KAMIYA T., OGATA K. & TAKAMATSU J. (1978) α_2-plasmin-inhibitor deficiency (Miyasato's disease). *Lancet*, **ii**, 1334.

508 AOKI N., SAITO H., KAMIYA T., KOIE K., SAKATA Y. & KOBAKURA M. (1979) Congenital deficiency of α_2-plasmin inhibitor associated with severe hemorrhagic tendency. *Journal of Clinical Investigation*, **63**, 877.

509 BUCHANAN G.R., GREEN D.M. & HANDIN R.I. (1977) Combined von Willebrand's disease and Hageman factor deficiency. *Journal of Pediatrics*, **90**, 779.

510 EGEBERG O. (1965) Inherited antithrombin deficiency causing thrombophilia. *Thrombosis et Diathesis Haemorrhagica*, **13**, 516.

511 SAS G., BLASKO G., BANHEGYI D., JAKO J. & PALOS L.A. (1974) Abnormal antithrombin III (antithrombin III 'Budapest') as a cause of familial thrombophilia. *Thrombosis et Diathesis Haemorrhagica*, **32**, 105.

512 ØDEGÅRD O.R. & ABILDGAARD U. (1977) Antifactor Xa activity in thrombophilia: studies in a family with ATIII deficiency. *Scandinavian Journal of Haematology*, **18**, 86.

513 MACKIE M., BENNETT B., OGSTON D. & DOUGLAS A.S. (1978) Familial thrombosis: inherited deficiency of antithrombin III. *British Medical Journal*, **1**, 136.

514 CONARD J. (1980) Inhibitors of blood coagulation. In: *Blood Coagulation and Haemostasis. A Practical Guide* (ed. Thomson J.M.), 2nd edn, p. 200. Churchill-Livingstone, Edinburgh.

515 VON KAULLA E. & VON KAULLA K.N. (1972) Deficiency of antithrombin III activity associated with hereditary thrombosis tendency. *Journal of Medicine* (Basel), **3**, 349.

516 THALER E., NIESSNER H., KLEINBERGER G. & GABNER A. (1979) Antithrombin III replacement therapy in patients with congenital and acquired antithrombin III deficiency. *Thrombosis and Haemostasis*, **42**, 327.

Chapter 29
Acquired disorders of blood coagulation

P. T. FLUTE

Disorders of blood coagulation may appear in previously normal individuals who develop a failure of coagulation-factor synthesis, abnormal loss of coagulation factors, or unusual inhibitors. Acquired defects in synthesis, which may be quantitative or qualitative, usually involve several coagulation factors; they are associated with alterations in vitamin-K metabolism, with anticoagulant therapy, or with liver disease. Abnormal loss of coagulation factors by internal consumption in the process of coagulation, or loss to the exterior by bleeding, often with thrombocytopenia, or via the urine, also gives multiple deficiencies. Unusual inhibitors, often immunoglobulins, account for most acquired changes of a single coagulation factor.

DISORDERS OF VITAMIN-K METABOLISM

Vitamin K (Koagulations vitamin) prevents bleeding in chicks fed on fat-free diets [1]. Its activity is associated with a series of napthoquinone derivatives found in structures responsible for active photosynthesis; green vegetables of the diet are the main source [2], possibly supplemented by bacterial synthesis in the intestine [3]. Naturally occurring vitamin K_1 (phylloquinone) is fat-soluble. The large amount of vitamin K in the stool is mainly menaquinone (vitamin K_2), synthesized by Gram-positive intestinal bacteria, but also a constituent of the diet [4]. The water-soluble synthetic analogues of the vitamin are slower and less successful than vitamin K_1 in correcting deficiencies [5].

Vitamin K provides for calcium-binding prosthetic groups in the amino-terminal regions of certain proteins, including coagulation factors II, VII, IX and X. Under the influence of the vitamin an extra carboxyl group is introduced into specific glutamic-acid residues to give γ-carboxyglutamic acid [6]. Inactive precursors of the coagulation factors in the plasma were recognized by Hemker in patients treated with the oral anticoagulants which antagonize the action of vitamin

K. He called them 'Protein induced by vitamin-K absence or antagonists (PIVKA)' [7–9]. These inactive precursors represent the protein factors complete except for their γ-carboxyglutamic-acid residues, the last stage of their assembly. Deficiency or antagonism of vitamin K is clinically manifest as an unusual bleeding tendency. The clinical significance of other vitamin-K-dependent proteins [10, 11], found in plasma, in bone, in dentine, in kidney and in other organs, remains to be assessed. Protein C, one of these vitamin-K-dependent proteins found in plasma, is of particular interest; it is activated by thrombin to a protease which inhibits coagulation by degrading Factor V [12].

Clinically significant lack or antagonism of vitamin K occurs in neonates as haemorrhagic disease of the newborn, and in adults due to malabsorption, after ingestion of oral anticoagulants, or in liver disease. A long prothrombin time is sometimes a feature of renal failure, when it responds to vitamin-K administration; it may be due to associated liver disease, poor diet, or malabsorption due to uraemic enteritis.

Haemorrhagic disease of the newborn
In this disease persistent rather than violent bleeding occurs before the age of five or six days in an otherwise well-seeming child. It may come from the umbilical cord or be seen as melaena, haematuria, cephalhaematoma or bleeding at the sites of birth injury. This bleeding can be controlled by the administration of vitamin K [13] and the disease is therefore linked with a deficiency of the vitamin in the neonate. In the normal neonate the plasma concentration of coagulation factors is such that the one-stage prothrombin and partial thromboplastin times are prolonged when referred to a control of normal adult plasma, the actual result depending on the particular reagents employed. Diagnosis of haemorrhagic disease of the newborn depends on finding prothrombin and partial thromboplastin times which are unusually prolonged, while the thrombin time, plasma fibrinogen and platelet count will be within the usual adult range for the laboratory. The newborn infant should have normal

adult levels of plasma fibrinogen, factor V and factor VIII pro-coagulant activity (VIIIC) and a normal platelet count [14, 15]. Plasma concentration of factor VIII-related antigen (VIIIR:Ag) should also be normal, although the protein from half of a series of neonates studied was found to show abnormal electrophoretic mobility [16]. Mildly reduced plasma levels are found for factors XI, XII [17], and XIII [18] and for antithrombin III [19, 20]. Further details are given in Chapter 3, pp. 88–91. The vitamin-K-dependent factors show [21] more definite, though still very variable, reductions, from 25–70% of adult values, with even lower values in premature infants. In all neonates the levels may drop further during the first week of life. This further fall is prevented by the administration of vitamin K [22], but whatever the dose of the vitamin, adult values for the vitamin-K-dependent coagulation factors are not achieved in the plasma for weeks or even months, suggesting an immaturity of the synthetic mechanism in the liver [23]. Intake of vitamin K is low during the first few days of life [24]; human breast milk contains little and the gut has not yet been colonized by bacteria, although the evidence for a significant contribution from this source remains doubtful [25]. Drugs which the mother has taken may exaggerate the effects of the vitamin lack; the oral anticoagulants cross the placenta [26] and anticonvulsant therapy, particularly with diphenylhydantoinate, exaggerates the problem [27].

Premature infants should be given not more than 1 mg of vitamin K_1 intramuscularly on the first day of life, repeated every eight hours if there is any sign of bleeding. The dose is low, and water-soluble analogues of vitamin K are avoided in order to reduce the risk of haemolytic anaemia with consequent bilirubinaemia and kernicterus [15]. In babies who are bleeding the response to vitamin K is often slow and cannot be expected in less than 12 hours, so that severe defects require the transfusion of fresh-frozen plasma [22, 28].

Neonatal bleeding may also be due to birth injury, disseminated intravascular coagulation or thrombocytopenia from other causes [22, 24, 29]. Melaena may be a manifestation of congenital intestinal malformations or swallowed maternal blood; the latter will not resist alkali denaturation and the infant is not anaemic. Inherited congenital coagulation-factor deficiencies, especially deficiency of factor XIII, may occasionally cause bleeding from the umbilical cord. Vaginal bleeding on the seventh or eight day may signify withdrawal of maternal hormones.

Malabsorption states
Vitamin-K deficiency in later infancy [30] or after should raise the suspicion of intestinal malabsorption.

Poor diet and sterilization of the intestine have to coincide for either to produce clinically significant deficiency [31]. Any cause of steatorrhoea may produce deficiency of vitamin K, as may high intestinal fistulae and extensive resections or bypassing of the small intestine. The most severe changes are seen in obstructive jaundice, where the lack of bile salts in the intestine so reduces absorption that severe coagulation abnormalities may occur within a few weeks of the onset. In gluten-induced enteropathy, sprue, cystic fibrosis and ulcerative lesions of the gut, deficiency is seldom severe, but may be accentuated by oral administration of broad-spectrum antibiotics.

Oral anticoagulants
The investigation of spoiled sweet clover disease in cattle which led to the discovery of the anticoagulant action of the substituted 4-hydroxycoumarins such as warfarin has been reviewed by Link [32]. These and the indanediones, such as phenindione [33], act as antagonists of vitamin K. As well as their use in therapeutics the drugs may be encountered in suicide attempts and chronic surreptitious self-administration is a recognized problem, particularly in hospital workers. The syndrome is recognized by deficiencies confined to the vitamin-K-dependent factors, the absence of any other cause, and the presence of the inhibitory effect in laboratory tests of the precursor proteins, PIVKA [34]. It may be confirmed by chemical demonstration of the drug in the plasma. Even surreptitious self-administration of heparin has been encountered [35].

Control of anticoagulant therapy
Oral anticoagulant therapy is usually monitored by the one-stage prothrombin time [36], the Thrombotest [37] or the Prothrombin and Proconvertin (P & P) test [38]. The reagents used vary in sensitivity to changes of factors II, VII and X and are relatively insensitive to changes in factor IX. Standardization of the tests, and of the reporting of the results, is therefore most important [39, 40]. Standard and reference preparations of various brain thromboplastins are now available [41, 42]; these may be compared with reagents by the prothrombin ratio method [36]. The maximum fall in concentration in the early stages of anticoagulant treatment is of factors VII and X [43]; after a change in dose a new steady-state plasma concentration is reached for factor VII within 20 hours, but for factor II this takes eight days [44, 45].

The large number of drug interactions which are possible [44], the fact that one drug may have more than one type of interaction, and the individual variability of response, account for the need for stringent laboratory control whenever any drug is added to, or subtracted from, the treatment regime. Patients should be specifically warned against self-medication. No use of the oral antibiotics or chemotherapeutic agents is free from the risk of potentiating the anticoagulant in at least some individuals. However, cardiac glycosides, chlordiazepoxide, diazepam, paracetamol, dextropropoxyphene, pethidine, and nitrazepam interact with warfarin very rarely, if at all.

Increased sensitivity to oral anticoagulants. Once stabilization has been achieved the anticoagulant response may still change for one or more of four reasons [46]: increased catabolism of coagulation factors, increased sensitivity of liver drug-receptors, decreased availability of vitamin K, or increased availability of 'free' drug.

The *rate of loss of coagulation factors* is known to be increased by fever and hyperthyroidism and an increased loss is probably a part of the complex changes in plasma proteins which follow injury [47]. Apparent *increase in sensitivity of the drug receptors* is part of any interference with liver function; congestive cardiac failure is a frequent cause in this group of patients. Many drugs may also reduce liver function (e.g. cinchophen, phenothiazines) and some appear to reduce coagulation-factor synthesis (e.g. salicylates). The effect of alcohol varies between individuals but clinical experience suggests that an excessive intake increases sensitivity to coumarins. The *availability of vitamin K* is reduced by a poor diet, by gastro-intestinal hurry, or by interference with vitamin-K absorption, as by liquid paraffin. There is probably little absorption of the vitamin K produced by gut bacteria; the administration of oral antibiotics may, however, potentiate the anticoagulant effect by other means, for example, inhibition of coumarin metabolism by chloramphenicol and tetracycline. An *increase in the 'free' drug* available to the liver may be caused first by an increase in dose, prescribed or taken in error, secondly by displacement from protein binding, or thirdly by decreased drug metabolism [44]. Many drugs, particularly those acidic in nature, including phenylbutazone and clofibrate, compete with the coumarins for binding to serum albumin. Only the 'free' drug has pharmacological activity or is available for metabolism, so that drugs which displace warfarin from its plasma protein-binding sites increase the anticoagulant effect of a given dose, and yet the plasma concentration of drug falls as its metabolism increases. The enzymes reponsible for drug metabolism may be the site of primary change. They are inhibited, and the anticoagulant effect potentiated, by drugs such as allopurinol, nortryptiline, chloramphenicol, or tetracycline. It seems likely that many drugs that are metabolized by the same hepatic enzyme system will inhibit coumarin metabolism competitively. Other drugs, considered below, stimulate the activity of the hepatic microsomal enzyme systems by a process of 'enzyme induction', which includes synthesis of increased amounts of enzyme protein [48]. It is when these drugs are withdrawn that a slow increase in sensitivity to the coumarins occurs as the enzymes decay and the rate of drug metabolism gradually falls over a period of several weeks.

Decreased sensitivity to oral anticoagulants. The dose of drug may be forgotten, inadequate, or not absorbed, for example if cholestyramine, which forms insoluble complexes with warfarin, has been given. However, acquired decrease in responsiveness is usually due to an increase in the availability of vitamin K or to increased drug metabolism [49]. An increase in dietary vitamin-K absorption is sometimes seen in food faddists who eat large quantities of green vegetables. Over 20 drugs, including many barbiturates, glutethimide, meprobamate, phenylbutazone, and griseofulvin, have been shown to cause induction of hepatic microsomal enzymes, leading to increased metabolism of warfarin and decreased anticoagulant effect. There is considerable individual variability in the rate of response and a new steady state may not be reached for several weeks [50].

If the anticoagulant effect needs to be reversed, a decrease of dose begins to take effect within 24–36 hours. For serious bleeding, vitamin K_1 is given, not more than 5 mg if anticoagulants are to be continued, for then resistance to treatment may last for one or two weeks. Vitamin K has a delayed effect, up to 24 hours, while liver synthesis increases [51]. For life-endangering bleeding, transfusion of plasma or of factor concentrates [52] provides immediate replacement of the necessary coagulation factors. Treatment with ε-aminocaproic acid may control minor external bleeding (e.g. menorrhagia or epistaxis), and allow continued anticoagulation within the therapeutic range. Recommendations for the therapeutic range have been reviewed [53].

LIVER DISEASE

In liver disease, derangements of coagulation may involve quantitative or qualitative changes in hepatic synthesis of coagulation enzyme precursors, of fibrinolytic enzyme precursors, or of the inhibitors of either [54–56]. There may also be disorders of clearance of the active enzymes and their products from the blood, a normal property of the reticulo-endothelial cells of the liver and elsewhere [57, 58]. While defective hepatic synthesis accounts for the major changes in coagulation in liver disease, an increased catabolism of coagulation factors is also demonstrable in many patients, thus exaggerating deficiencies of the various plasma components.

Simple screening tests of blood coagulation—prothrombin time, kaolin partial thromboplastin time, and thrombin time—are often abnormal in liver disease. They are therefore sensitive tests of liver function, even in the absence of an obvious bleeding diathesis, but are of less value in determining prognosis. It is most important that subtle interrelationships of vessel and platelet function and more obvious anatomical changes in vessels, such as those associated with portal hypertension, are taken into account in addition to changes in coagulation and fibrinolysis when considering the reasons for bleeding in hepatic disorders [59, 60].

HEPATIC SYNTHESIS

The liver is thought to synthesize fibrinogen [61], the zymogen factors II, VII, IX, X, XI, XII, XIII, the cofactor factor V [62–64] and the inhibitors of both coagulation and fibrinolysis, including antithrombin III and α_2-antiplasmin [65, 66]. The liver may also be a site of plasminogen synthesis [62]. Synthesis of any constituent may be quantitatively deficient or qualitatively abnormal. Acquired derangements are characteristically multiple.

Biosynthetic studies of liver slices and suspensions of hepatocytes confirm that the hepatocyte is the main and probably the only source of *plasma fibrinogen* [67]. Fibrinogen synthesized by platelets does not appear to contribute to plasma levels. Fibrinogen is one of the acute-phase reactants whose concentration increases dramatically in response to inflammation anywhere in the body. In liver disease the output of fibrinogen is maintained until a very late stage; low plasma levels of this protein are found in terminal hepatic coma [54]. Many patients with liver disease have abnormal molecules of fibrinogen in their plasma which cause a delay in fibrin monomer polymerization, that is to say show evidence of dysfibrinogenaemia [68, 69]. This is easily recognizable from the prolonged clotting time of plasma with thrombin and also with extracts of the venoms of the snakes *Bothrops jararaca* or *Agkistrodon rhodostoma*. Unlike the thrombin time, the clotting times with these venoms are not affected by heparin. Other causes of a long thrombin time such as a plasma-fibrinogen level of less than 1 g/l, very high levels of fibrin(ogen) degradation products of fibrinolysis (FDP), or the nonspecific inhibitory effects of paraproteins, must be excluded. While a defect of fibrinogen synthesis is postulated, damage to the preformed molecule by mechanical stress or proteolytic attack in the circulation has yet to be eliminated. The original observations of such abnormal fibrinogens were made by Fanconi in 1941 in a child with congenital syphilis, jaundice, and hepatomegaly, but dysfibrinogenaemia has since been found in many cases of hepatic coma, uncompensated cirrhosis, and primary hepatic carcinoma [70]. Detailed analysis of a number of cases gave normal electrophoretic patterns for the isolated fibrinogen, its constituent chains, and its plasmin degradation products, but fibrin monomers prepared from the fibrinogen showed delayed polymerization [71]. The change has been compared with the unusual production of α-fetoprotein in liver disease, but no clearly recognizable fetal fibrinogen [72] has yet been isolated, and the defects are clearly heterogeneous.

The liver is the main source of the *vitamin-K-dependent coagulation factors* [73]: multiple deficiencies of these factors are common in all forms of liver disease [74]. The earliest changes and the greatest reductions usually affect factor VII, with its short half-life of six hours [75]. Immunological methods give values corresponding to the functional assays if overall synthesis is reduced by hepatocellular disease; in contrast, levels of inactive protein are in excess of demonstrable biological activity if vitamin K is deficient.

Perfusion of isolated rat liver suggests that *factor V* is synthesized by hepatocytes [76]. Since this is independent of vitamin K, the demonstration of a low factor V helps to differentiate between a vitamin-K-responsive disorder and reduced synthesis owing to hepatocyte loss. High plasma levels of factor V have been reported in obstructive jaundice [77].

Although *factor VIII* has been obtained from perfused livers and rises have sometimes followed transplantation of livers between normal and haemophilic dogs [78], there is little to suggest that the hepatocyte is involved in the synthesis of factor-VIII procoagulant activity (VIIIC) or of factor-VIII-related antigen (VIIIR:Ag) [79]. Many physiological and pathological stimuli cause a parallel increase in VIIIC and VIIIR:Ag, which may perhaps be considered as 'acute-phase reactants'. During normal pregnancy a sustained increase of both VIIIC and VIIIR:Ag suggests an increased rate of synthesis [80]. In states of intravascular coagulation, however, VIIIC may be consumed at a faster rate than normal, and since VIIIR:Ag is detectable in equal amounts in serum and in plasma, a reduction in VIIIC relative to VIIIR:Ag may result [81]. Such a finding is common in hepatocellular disease.

The synthesis of the '*contact factors*' (factors XI and XII, prekallikrein and high-molecular-weight kininogen) is thought to occur in the liver, since hepatocellular necrosis is associated with decreased plasma levels [74, 82]. There is, however, no conclusive evidence. Similarly, *plasminogen* levels are decreased in hepatocellular disease, but liver perfusion studies have failed to provide positive support for its synthesis [83]. Plasma *factor-XIII* levels have sometimes been reported as low in hepatocellular disease [74, 84].

The *protease inhibitors* of plasma are probably synthesized by the hepatocyte, but perhaps not exclusively [85]. Reduced plasma concentration of antithrombin III is characteristic of hepatocellular disease [86, 87]: values are normal or increased in patients with cholestasis. The plasma concentration of the main inhibitor of fibrinolysis, α_2-antiplasmin, follows a similar pattern of changes [66].

INCREASED CATABOLISM

Normally, approximately 20% of the circulating fibrinogen is lost each day, and this fractional catabolic rate is remarkably constant and independent of the plasma concentration of fibrinogen [88]. The fractional loss of fibrinogen is increased in many types of liver disease, particularly in fulminant hepatic failure [89] and cirrhosis [90] but also in severe acute viral hepatitis and chronic active hepatitis [91]. The increased catabolism is usually counterbalanced by increased synthesis, giving normal or even increased plasma fibrinogen concentrations [92]. Turnover studies of labelled prothrombin and labelled plasminogen in patients with cirrhosis showed that increased fractional catabolic rate and decreased synthetic rate of these proteins accounted for their low plasma levels [93]. The increase in the fractional catabolic rate for fibrinogen that occurs in liver disease suggests that an unusual route of loss is involved. The association of increased prothrombin and plasminogen turnover and of many other changes suggests that this route may, at least in part, be via accelerated intravascular coagulation [94]. This is supported by finding microthrombi in the organs at autopsy in some series [95], though they were infrequent in others [96]; by excessive deposition of isotopically labelled fibrinogen in the organs of animals subjected to experimental hepatic necrosis [97–99]; by discrepancy between VIIIC and VIIIR:Ag levels typical of intravascular coagulation [100–102]; by an associated thrombocytopenia; by increase of circulating FDP; and by circulating soluble fibrin complexes [103, 104]. Heparin has no effect on the rate of fibrinogen loss in normal subjects but slows the rate of loss in liver disease, which is further evidence to support the role of intravascular coagulation [105]. Stimuli to coagulation would be expected to arise from necrotic hepatocytes or from defective clearance of intestinal endotoxin. Defective hepatic clearance of activated enzymes, soluble fibrin, and FDP could accentuate the tendency. Also to be considered as possible routes of increased loss, by no means excluded as important in liver disease, are bleeding, loss into extravascular compartments (e.g. ascites, areas of liver necrosis), intravascular proteolysis by enzymes other than thrombin (e.g. plasmin) and accelerated removal by the reticulo-endothelial system (possibly the normal route) [99].

FIBRINOLYSIS

The blood of many patients with cirrhosis has increased plasminogen activator and decreased plasminogen concentration [106, 107], possibly owing to impaired clearance of activator by the liver [108] and perhaps accentuated by defective hepatic synthesis of plasminogen and of α_2-antiplasmin. In fulminant hepatic failure [103] and after hepatic transplantation [109], plasma plasminogen is often low, with normal or decreased plasminogen activator and a mild increase in FDP. However, none of the latter group of changes is greater than similar changes frequently found in response to mild physiological stimuli (such as pregnancy), and their clinical significance is uncertain.

COAGULATION PATTERNS IN LIVER DISEASE

Despite considerable overlap, patterns characteristic of three main types of hepatic disorder can be identified: those of portal hypertension, cholestasis, or hepatocellular disease (Table 29.1).

Patients with *portal hypertension* tend to have extensive new collateral blood vessels of varying distribution which pose a severe haemostatic hazard, especially to the surgeon, because of the unusual anatomy. There may be defective clearance of plasminogen activator from the blood, resulting in short lysis times of blood clots. Thrombocytopenia often complicates portal hypertension [59].

Patients with *cholestasis* ultimately develop a deficiency of blood-clotting factors limited to those that are vitamin-K-dependent, since the absorption of this fat-soluble vitamin is impaired. Prothrombin time is prolonged (deficiency of factors II, VII and X), partial thromboplastin time becomes prolonged (deficiency of factors II, IX and X), and immunological determination of these factors gives higher values than do the corresponding procoagulant assays. Specific assays show normal or high factor-V concentration. There is often an acute-phase reaction with increased plasma fibrinogen, VIIIR:Ag, a corresponding increase of VIIIC, and little evidence of increased catabolism. Inhibitor assays are normal. High plasma levels of any of the coagulation factors may be found in the early stages and of the non-vitamin-K-dependent proteins at any stage.

With *acute or chronic hepatocellular disease*, the

Table 29.1. Blood tests in liver disease: patterns of abnormality*

Test	Portal hypertension	Bile flow obstruction	Hepato-cellular dysfunction
Prothrombin time		long	long
Partial thromboplastin time		long	long
Thrombin time			long
Bleeding time	long		normal or long
Platelet count	low		normal or low
FII, VII, IX, X functional assay		low	low
immunological assay		normal	low
FVIIIC	normal	normal	high or low
FVIIIR:Ag	or	or	high
FV	high	high	low
Fibrinogen		high	high→low
Ethanol gel			positive
FDP			raised
Plasminogen activator	normal or high		normal or low
Plasminogen	normal or low		low
Antithrombin III			low
α_2-antiplasmin			low

* Gaps signify that the test is usually normal.

predominant finding is deficient or defective hepatic synthesis producing a pattern of changes maximal in fulminant hepatic failure. There are multiple deficiencies of all factors and inhibitors synthesized by the hepatocytes and it is in this group that the changes thought to be associated with intravascular coagulation have been described. Platelets may be reduced and show defective function [110, 111]. Plasminogen activator is usually decreased in the blood, plasminogen levels are low and serum FDP slightly increased, a non-specific pattern of changes common to many disorders. Inhibitors of coagulation and fibrinolysis are decreased. Prothrombin time and partial thromboplastin time are prolonged by the coagulation-factor deficiencies, and unusual inhibitors have been postulated but never clearly identified. Plasma thrombin and 'reptilase' times are prolonged if abnormal fibrinogen molecules are formed.

MANAGEMENT AND PROGNOSIS

Frequently repeated simple screening tests, such as platelet count, prothrombin time, partial thromboplastin time, and thrombin time, give all the information needed for practical management and are among the most sensitive of laboratory tests of liver function. Many authors, however, have noted the dissociation between the results of these tests and the incidence of clinical bleeding [54, 112]. The presence or absence of bleeding depends both on the efficiency of the haemostatic systems and the level of challenge to which they are subjected. Even the severe multiple defects of

fulminant hepatic failure may cause no bleeding unless vessels are damaged (e.g. by ill-advised needle puncture, or by gastric ulceration). One study of 105 deaths among 132 consecutive admissions for fulminant hepatic failure showed major bleeding, usually from the gastro-intestinal tract, as the cause of death in 28 patients [113]. The incidence of bleeding was not related to the coagulation screening tests, the presence of renal failure, or the cause of the hepatic failure, but to the presence of oesophageal or gastric erosions. Administration of histamine antagonists in sufficient amounts to maintain intragastric pH above 5 proved effective in reducing the incidence of these erosions and of fatal gastro-intestinal bleeding in hepatic coma [114].

In determining overall prognosis in terms of survival in liver disease the coagulation-factor levels are of little importance compared with the presence or absence of significant bleeding [115]. Once bleeding has occurred, however, the prognosis is better in patients with normal rather than with abnormal results of coagulation tests [116].

The prothrombin time has proved of some value in predicting the outcome for patients suffering from an overdose of paracetamol [103]. There is a characteristic latent interval of three to four days between ingestion of the drug and maximum abnormalities in results of coagulation tests. Hepatic coma developed only in those patients in whom the ratio of patient's to normal result in the prothrombin time was greater than 2·2 before the fourth day. However, the level of serum bilirubin was of greater predictive value for the outcome than the prothrombin time.

Patients with coagulation-factor deficiencies who are not bleeding and who do not face an identifiable challenge to haemostasis need no special treatment for their deficiencies. This includes the majority of patients with uncompensated chronic liver disease. *Vitamin K_1* should be given when the clinical circumstances and laboratory tests indicate the need, and it is usually given routinely to patients with fulminant hepatic failure. Prophylaxis against bleeding in these patients should be directed to the protection of blood vessels, including the use of *histamine antagonists* to abolish gastric acidity.

Replacement of missing coagulation factors by transfusion is neither easy to accomplish nor free from hazard [56, 112, 113], but should be attempted in those who are bleeding or in those who face a definite haemostatic challenge (including biopsy). *Fresh-frozen plasma* supplies all the coagulation factors and may also be used after the cryoprecipitate fraction (rich in fibrinogen and factor VIII) has been removed. Large volumes are needed because of the accelerated loss of coagulation factors, and the prothrombin time is difficult to correct completely. The short biological survival of factor VII makes frequent administration necessary. Yet 300 ml of plasma every six hours approaches the limits of tolerance for continuous administration to patients in hepatic coma and carries with it the risk of overloading the circulation or causing electrolyte imbalance; there is no convincing evidence of prophylactic benefit. Fresh-frozen plasma is the mainstay of treatment in any patient actually bleeding, when larger amounts may be given rapidly. *Concentrates* of the vitamin-K-dependent coagulation factors are available but their place in therapeutics remains undecided [117]. They carry the risk of transmitting hepatitis; some, but not all, lack factor VII. The factors concerned may be partially in their active form and thus precipitate intravascular microthrombosis. This risk is greatest in patients with fulminant hepatic failure already predisposed to intravascular coagulation. Thus in a trial [118] of one such concentrate in fulminant hepatic failure, clinical evidence of intravascular coagulation appeared in two patients and laboratory evidence progressed in others, even those given simultaneous heparin. The magnitude of this risk is uncertain, however, and further controlled trials in different types of liver disease are in progress.

Similar arguments suggest that in the presence of severe hepatocellular necrosis the use of *inhibitors of fibrinolysis*, 6-aminohexanoic acid (ε-aminocaproic acid: EACA), tranexamic acid, or Trasylol may predispose to microthrombi [97]. The value of these inhibi-

tors may be in other forms of liver disease where the risk of associated intravascular coagulation seems less, particularly where portal hypertension is not accompanied by major hepatocellular disease [119].

Heparin has been used by several groups in an attempt to reduce the loss of coagulation factors. The only controlled trial in man showed no benefit [120]. The use of EACA increased the incidence of microthrombi in animals with experimental galactosamine-induced hepatitis, while heparin prevented their formation, but heparin did not prolong the survival time of the animals nor reduce liver cell damage [98].

Platelet transfusions are being used with increasing frequency in the treatment of bleeding in liver disease associated with thrombocytopenia, giving emphasis, if such were needed, to the importance of considering all aspects of haemostasis. Undoubtedly the most important seems to be the condition of the blood vessels themselves; challenges to haemostasis should be scrupulously avoided.

DISSEMINATED INTRAVASCULAR COAGULATION

An important cause of increased loss of coagulation factors, which affects platelets as well, is disseminated intravascular coagulation. Almost any human disease may provide a stimulus to coagulation, which is often necessary for haemostasis or tissue repair but potentially harmful if it occurs within blood vessels. In the most severe examples of disease, massive coagulation may consume many coagulation factors and platelets faster than they can be produced. The consequent drop in plasma concentration was first recognized for fibrinogen, which may disappear from the plasma: virtually incoagulable blood with bleeding and shock result and were designated the '*defibrination (defibrinogenation) syndrome*' [121]. When the defects of so many other coagulation factors and of platelets were recognized in the severe stages, the alternative name was proposed of '*consumption coagulopathy*' [122]. Others have emphasized the harmful effects of multiple thrombi in small vessels and the generalized nature of the process which they have called '*disseminated (diffuse) intravascular coagulation*' [123] or '*intravascular coagulation with fibrinolysis*' [124]. The initials 'DIC' have come into popular use to cover this group of heterogeneous disorders, of which acute, subacute and chronic examples have been recognized [125].

Increased losses of coagulation factors may also be due to other causes. Loss due to haemorrhage is often exaggerated by massive transfusion of stored blood. Rarely, stimulation of fibrinolysis may release sufficient plasmin to overwhelm the antiplasmins and allow this enzyme to digest fibrinogen and other coagulation factors. This is a feature of thrombolytic therapy with streptokinase or urokinase; idiopathic spontaneous hyperfibrinolysis of similar degree is almost unknown [126]. Possible additional causes of loss, which are not yet known to play a significant part in any clinical syndrome, are transfer of coagulation factors from the intravascular to the extravascular pool, loss via the urine in the nephrotic syndrome [127], hyperactivity of the reticulo-endothelial system, or an acceleration of the normal, as yet undefined, route of metabolism for coagulation factors which appears to be independent of activation of blood coagulation or fibrinolytic enzyme systems.

PATHOGENESIS OF INTRAVASCULAR COAGULATION

The stimulus
Both coagulation and fibrinolysis may respond to the same original stimulus, whether this be the entry of foreign material into the blood or contact between normal blood constituents and the foreign surfaces provided by damaged tissue. The agent which actually initiates coagulation has been called the 'trigger' [128, 129]. Much further research is needed before the precise trigger can be defined for each group of disorders; often multiple triggers can be postulated. The action of the trigger may be direct, if the agent is one which will cause coagulation *in vitro*—thromboplastins from inflamed, necrotic, or neoplastic cells, for example, or the toxins of venomous animals—or indirect where a mediator is needed. Such indirect triggers would include bacterial endotoxin, immune complexes, particulate agents and lipid. These may stimulate the intrinsic coagulation mechanisms, perhaps by a direct effect upon factor XII [130], stimulate platelet aggregation and release phenomena [131]; or damage cell membranes with release of direct triggers from the leucocytes, red cells or vascular endothelium [132–134]. In addition the stimulus may come from blood perfusing vessels in which the endothelium has been damaged by physical agents, or by ischaemia and acidosis in hypovolaemic shock [123].

The compensation
Opposed to the stimulus are a number of exceptionally potent mechanisms. The blood contains, in considerable excess, powerful specific and non-specific natural inhibitors of the active coagulation and fibrinolytic enzymes, antithrombin III and α_2-antiplasmin factors being of greatest biological importance. Blood flow will carry activated factors away from the site of stimulus to those places where cells of the reticulo-endothelial system can remove them from the blood

[57, 58, 135, 136]. Stimulation of coagulation may produce fibrin monomer and stimulation of fibrinolysis may produce fibrin/fibrinogen degradation products (FDP); these end-products of the coagulation and fibrinolytic systems may form soluble complexes with each other and be held in solution in the plasma [137] to be cleared by the reticulo-endothelial system.

The result
Thus the final intravascular effect of a stimulus to blood coagulation may fall short of fibrin formation, be limited to the formation of soluble fibrin-monomer complexes with fibrinogen or FDP, proceed to transient fibrin deposits which are rapidly dissolved by fibrinolysis, lead to persistent thrombosis, especially of small vessels, with resultant tissue necrosis, or cause bleeding due to massive consumption of coagulation factors and platelets. What happens will depend on the quantity, quality, portal of entry, and persistence of the stimulus, balanced against the efficiency of the plasma inhibitors and fibrinolytic enzymes, the activity of reticulo-endothelial cells and, in particular, the amount of regional blood flow. The effects are mediated by the enzyme thrombin, which in addition to its action on various coagulation factors causes aggregation, release, and therefore loss, of platelets.

A particular example of intravascular coagulation which illustrates many important points is given by the experimental *Shwartzman phenomenon*. A symptom complex of shock, widespread haemorrhages, and bilateral renal cortical necrosis characteristically follows two spaced intravenous injections of bacterial endotoxin into experimental animals. The first 'preparatory' injection is without clinical effect, while the second 'provocative' injection, spaced 6–72 hours after the first, produces the syndrome. Endotoxin is the trigger for intravascular coagulation; at the time of the second injection the animal is particularly vulnerable because the already extended compensating mechanisms are easily overwhelmed. The syndrome also follows continued infusion of the preparatory agent for 8–14 hours [138], or single injections after reticulo-endothelial blockage [139], or inhibition of fibrinolysis [140] or treatment with cortisone [141], or, in some species at least, during pregnancy [142]. The effects may be prevented by prior treatment with heparin [143, 144] or by stimulation of fibrinolysis [145]. Leucocytes must also be present for the fully developed reaction. Blood flow is also important: unilateral sympathectomy prevents fibrin deposition in the glomeruli on the denervated side [146]. A similar protective effect has been reported after the administration of α-adrenergic blockers and vasoactive amines, such as bradykinin and serotonin [147]. Although it would be dangerous to assume identical effects in human disease, the principles concerned are well illustrated by this experimental parallel.

CLINICAL MANIFESTATIONS OF INTRAVASCULAR COAGULATION

When so many factors are involved it is perhaps not surprising that laboratory tests are a poor guide to clinical effects. Bleeding is unlikely if plasma fibrinogen concentration is within the normal range and may not occur even when fibrinogen is virtually absent from the blood unless there is a local lesion of blood vessels. Surgical wounds, needle punctures, the atonic uterus after childbirth, and benign or malignant ulcers may then bleed profusely.

Fibrin, together with platelets, may be deposited anywhere in the vascular system. Deposits may be 'localized', when confined to a major artery or vein, or 'disseminated' throughout the microcirculation of one or many organs. Disseminated lesions are formed in capillaries and their draining venules, a process of 'microthrombosis'. This may cause shock if it affects the lungs, local necrotic lesions in other organs, and haemolytic anaemia. Since all of the possible clinical effects may be due to many other causes, which may in their turn precipitate thrombosis, the true aetiological role of intravascular fibrin is often obscure. Many of the possibilities have been reviewed [123, 125, 148–153] and are shown in Table 29.2.

A particular form of intravascular haemolysis, characterized by irregularly distorted and fragmented red cells (schistocytes), has been called '*microangiopathic haemolytic anaemia*' [154]. Some examples are due to intravascular coagulation [155]: typical red-cell changes have been produced *in vitro* by passage of blood through a fibrin mesh [156], similar mechanical changes to red cells can arise in other ways, however, such as from malfunction of cardiac-valve prostheses

[157] and perhaps following disseminated platelet aggregation [158].

LABORATORY MANIFESTATIONS OF INTRAVASCULAR COAGULATION

Histology

Intravascular fibrin deposition may be apparent but this is not invariable since active fibrinolysis may remove the deposits, and since incompletely polymerized fibrin is notoriously difficult to demonstrate by conventional staining methods. 'Haematoxylinophil bodies' in capillaries may represent an early stage of the process [159]. They are believed to be extruded nuclei of endothelial cells damaged by, or responding to, fibrin on their surface. Immunofluorescence microscopy of frozen sections [160] demonstrates fibrin directly, but the antigen may have been derived from the fibrinogen of plasma or of the platelets, and sometimes represents a non-specific association of fibrinogen with deposits of immunoglobulins. Organs with a high incidence of microthrombosis are the kidney, adrenal, lung and testes [149, 161]. Extravascular precipitates, which form a hyaline membrane in the lung alveoli in the respiratory-distress syndrome of the neonate or the 'shock lung' of the adult, may include fibrin as judged by transverse striations on electron-microscopy and by immunofluorescence with specific antibodies [160]. These hyaline membranes also include other plasma proteins, including plasminogen and immunoglobulins, and miscellaneous cellular debris including DNA. They are often associated histologically with intravascular microthrombi; the problem centres on whether these thrombi are the cause of the membrane, since this has therapeutic implications. The fact that laboratory changes of DIC may not be found even in those with undoubted

Table 29.2. Examples of the selective clinical syndromes of DIC

| Organ | Grade of change | |
	Moderate	Severe
Blood	Microangiopathic haemolytic anaemia	Haemostatic failure
Lungs	Reduced P_{O_2} with cyanosis	Acute cor pulmonale
Kidneys	Oliguria	Renal cortical necrosis
Brain	Confusion	Coma
Skin	Purpura	Gangrene
Heart	Arrhythmia	Arrest
Gut	Melaena	Pseudomembranous colitis
Endocrines	Temporary dysfunction	Haemorrhagic infarction (e.g. Waterhouse–Friderichsen syndrome, Sheehan's syndrome)

histological pulmonary hyaline membranes, suggests that these lesions are more often the cause of the coagulation changes, via the anoxia and acidosis they provoke, than their consequence [22].

The haemostatic mechanism
(Table 29.3)

Tests of blood coagulation. Massive consumption of platelets and coagulation factors may remove so much fibrinogen that the blood cannot clot, and then simple observation of the process of clotting is enough to raise suspicion of the diagnosis. Clots may be absent altogether or collapse rapidly into almost invisible fragments. One-stage tests of coagulation—prothrombin, partial thromboplastin (kaolin-cephalin) and thrombin times—are prolonged. Repeating each test on a mixture of equal parts of patient's and control plasma gives substantially shorter results, indicating a deficiency of coagulation factors, but this correction may not be as complete as one might expect, owing to the presence of FDP. Detailed analysis, which it must be emphasized is not required for diagnosis, shows that many coagulation factors are reduced in concentration, especially factors II, V, VII, X and XIII, but all the coagulation factors may be involved. Factor VIIIR:Ag concentration is raised in the blood, some-

times greatly, while the increase in VIIIC is less; this leads to abnormal ratios of VIIIC to VIIIR:Ag [81]. Only in the more severe states is the absolute plasma concentration of VIIIC below normal levels [153]. Another early sign of DIC is a fall in antithrombin-III concentration [87, 162, 163]. It is noteworthy that falls in the concentration of zymogens such as factors VII and X, which are not consumed by *in-vitro* clotting in glass, do occur during intravascular coagulation, presumably because of accelerated clearance of enzyme–inhibitor complexes [125].

A low plasma fibrinogen assumes special significance, as this seldom occurs unexpectedly in other disorders. Inherited defects of synthesis of fibrinogen are rare and will be apparent from the history; in liver disease, fibrinogen synthesis is maintained in all but the most severe cases of acute hepatic necrosis. The significance of the results of the fibrinogen estimation will depend on the method employed. Precipitation methods using heat or ammonium sulphate and immunological methods will include all the circulating complexes of fibrinogen and its derivatives, many of which play no part in effective haemostasis and may even be inhibitory. It is important, therefore, to use a method which demonstrates the amount of fibrinogen which can be formed as a recognizable clot after the addition of thrombin to the patient's plasma. Thrombin added to

Table 29.3. Blood changes of DIC

| Test | Grade of DIC | | |
	Severe (i.e. haemostatic failure)	Moderate (microthrombosis a possibility; often no clinical effect)	Mild
Defining			
Platelet count	$<75 \times 10^9/1$	low or normal	normal or high
Plasma fibrinogen	<1 g/l	normal or high	normal or high
Thrombin time 25 u/ml	incoagulable	normal or long	normal
2·5 u/ml	incoagulable	long	long
FDP	high	high	high
Ethanol-gel test	usually +	usually +	+ or −
Supporting			
Bleeding time	very long	long or normal	normal
Clotting time			
Prothrombin time	often incoagulable	long or normal	normal or short
Partial thromboplastin time			
FVIIIR:Ag	high	high	high
FVIIIC	low	low, normal or high	normal or high
FII, V, VII, IX, X, XI, XII	low	low, normal or high	normal
Antithrombin III	very low	low	low or normal
Plasminogen activator	low, normal or high	low, normal or high	often low
Plasminogen	low	low or normal	low, normal or high
α_2-antiplasmin	low	low or normal	low or normal
Fragmented red cells	+ or −	+ or −	+ or −

serial-doubling dilutions of normal plasma in physio-logical saline will usually give a recognizable clot to a titre of 128 or 256 [164]. Alternatively, a measured volume of plasma can be treated with thrombin and the result determined by measuring the time to clot formation [165], or by the fibrin which has formed being removed, dried, and weighed [166], estimated chemically [167], or determined from the change in opacity of the solution [168, 169]. A clottable fibrinogen of less than 1 g/l of plasma usually confirms the diagnosis of acute 'defibrination'. However, plasma fibrinogen is typically raised in pregnancy, after operation or injury, and in those with inflamma-tory disorders; the amount of fibrinogen found has to be compared with that expected for the patient. In subacute or chronic DIC, increased synthesis of fibrinogen may more than compensate for the exces-sive loss, so that a normal or even high plasma fibrinogen concentration is possible. Even so, it remains an important measurement, since bleeding is unlikely if the plasma fibrinogen is normal. In the less severe states the one-stage prothrombin time and partial thromboplastin time may be normal or even shorter than normal and one-stage assays of VIIIC may give exceptionally high results. Factor VIIIR:Ag is also increased, and plasma levels may be even higher than those of factor VIIIC [81].

Platelets. A fall in the blood platelet count is often the first sign of intravascular coagulation and the count tends to remain low for several days after an acute episode. Platelet-survival studies show their rapid removal from the circulation [170]. In the less severe or chronic forms, increased production of platelets may give normal or even increased counts.

Activation of fibrinolysis. Stimulation of fibrinolysis may become evident in the blood in four different ways:
1 by an increase in circulating plasminogen activator;
2 by an increase in the products of lysis of fibrin or fibrinogen (FDP);
3 by a fall in plasminogen concentration, due to increased consumption following absorption to fibrin and local activation to plasmin [171]; and
4 by a fall in plasma concentration of α_2-antiplasmin [66].

An increase of plasminogen activator in the blood is unusual in DIC, but may be encountered as a transient phenomenon. If the patient's own blood is used to provide the substrate for a test such as the whole blood-clot or euglobulin clot-lysis time [172], the result may be artificially short if fibrinogen is deficient, or artificially prolonged if plasminogen is deficient. A true measure of circulating activator can be obtained by using a substrate of known fibrinogen and plas-minogen content, such as the fibrin plate [173, 174] or a radioactive clot-lysis method [175]. These tests need not be included in emergency studies: the first treat-ment should assume intravascular coagulation as the cause of an unexpectedly low level of plasma fibrinogen.

A prolonged thrombin time indicates either a very low or abnormal plasma fibrinogen or an unusual antithrombin effect, such as that produced by FDP. Care should be taken to exclude the presence of heparin, given in therapeutic doses or contaminating the catheter through which the blood sample is collected, for this will produce the same effect. Where there is doubt the clotting time of citrated plasma with ancrod or reptilase may help to differentiate the cause, since these are unaffected by heparin but prolonged by FDP [176]. The FDP may also be recognizable by immunological methods [177] or staphylococcal clumping tests in the supernatant serum left after the removal of the clot [178]. Very sensitive radio-immunoassays are available [179] and identification of individual FDP may come to be of clinical importance [180]. There is no evidence to suggest that FDP in the circulating blood ever reach the urine [66]: urinary FDP usually represent the degradation of fibrinogen or fibrin from within the urinary tract.

A fall in α_2-antiplasmin may represent decreased synthesis or increased consumption, only the latter indicating an activation of fibrinolysis. The two may be differentiated by turnover studies [181] or perhaps by the immunochemical measurement of the plasmin–antiplasmin complex [182]. Molecular interactions between plasminogen activator, plasminogen and fibrin, direct and confine the action of plasmin to fibrin, where it is protected from the otherwise inevi-table and virtually instantaneous inactivation of α_2-antiplasmin [66]. However, plasma concentration of plasminogen (1·5 μM) exceeds that of α_2-antiplasmin (1 μM), and once the neutralizing power of the latter is saturated the slower inhibitory action against plasmin of α_2-macroglobulin allows time for the enzyme to cause fibrinogenolysis and digestion of other coagula-tion factors. It is not yet known how often this happens in human disease, but it seems to be uncommon. It has been demonstrated directly only in thrombolytic ther-apy with high loading doses of streptokinase. It is not known how many of the earlier reports of primary fibrinolysis in liver disease [183], neoplasia [184] and surgical operations [185] really represent the secondary fibrinolysis of DIC in these conditions. Plasminogen activator has a poor efficiency in the absence of fibrin, when even high plasma concentrations of activator, such as those released by exercise or adrenaline, will not lead to significant plasmin formation. However, with the appearance of fibrin the activator can readily react with fibrin-bound plasminogen, hence the 'secondary' fibrinolysis of DIC which appears to be the most likely explanation. Here activator levels are variable, but fibrin degradation products are produced and these may have significant antihaemostatic effects interfering with platelet function, thrombin activation and fibrin polymerization [137]. Once α_2-antiplasmin had been neutralized, fibrinogen degradation products could further contribute to the bleeding diathesis by similar actions.

Soluble fibrin-monomer complexes. Thrombin liberates fibrinopeptides from fibrinogen, leaving the remainder of the molecule as fibrin monomer. This can polymerize spontaneously to form the insoluble three-dimensional network of a fibrin gel. However, fibrin monomer may also form soluble complexes, either with fibrinogen or with FDP [186]. The finding of soluble fibrin-monomer complexes (SFMC) in plasma strongly suggests intravascular thrombin formation. The SFMC can be precipitated from solution by cooling to 4°C when another plasma protein (fibronectin) is present [187], by diluting with water, by ethanol, or by certain basic materials including protamine sulphate [188]. These have been used as the basis of tests of clinical importance [189, 190]. It is easy to produce false positive results by poor venepuncture.

Fibrinogen turnover. Analysis of the kinetic behaviour of ^{125}I-labelled fibrinogen has made important contributions to the study of intravascular coagulation [88, 170]. Normal catabolism of fibrinogen molecules occurs randomly at a relatively constant rate without regard to the age of the individual molecules; the mass of fibrinogen catabolized each day appears to be a constant fraction, around 20%, of the total amount in the circulation [88]. An increase in the fractional catabolic rate suggests an unusual method of breakdown (e.g. coagulation or fibrinolysis [191]). This change has been demonstrated in primary and secondary polycythaemia and in cirrhosis of the liver [90], in acute hepatic necrosis [89], after burns and major tissue injury [192], after surgical operations [193], and in several conditions causing microangiopathic haemolysis including metastatic neoplasm, abruptio placentae, malignant hypertension and pre-eclamptic toxaemia [194]; all these are conditions in which potent stimulation of coagulation could be expected. In many the rate of loss of fibrinogen can be reduced by heparin, which supports the suggestion that the loss is due to intravascular coagulation. Accelerated turnover of platelets and prothrombin has also been demonstrated in some cases [170].

CLINICAL ASSOCIATIONS OF INTRAVASCULAR COAGULATION

The very concept of disease implies that there has been some form of tissue damage; this can always act as a stimulus to coagulation. Thus a comprehensive list of potential clinical associations with intravascular coagulation might include all known diseases. While it is easy to demonstrate the blood changes of coagulation in many patients, it is comparatively rare to find the severe changes of 'defibrination' with levels of fibrinogen low enough to be associated with bleeding. How often the less severe changes are associated with morbidity due to microthrombosis is uncertain; but even this phenomenon seems to be distinctly uncommon. Some special examples will be considered.

Obstetrics

During normal pregnancy the increased concentration of some coagulation factors, including fibrinogen and factor VIIIC, and a progressive increase of serum FDP, suggests general activation of coagulation [195]. The blood changes are maximal in the uterine veins during labour [196]. Massive intravascular coagulation may reduce the fibrinogen concentration to very low values in many complications of pregnancy. Hypothetical triggers include the entry of tissue fragments, amniotic fluid, activated coagulation factors, incompatible red cells, or bacterial products into the maternal circulation [197]. In abruptio placentae a 'pathway of auto-extraction' [121] has been described whereby products of cell necrosis in the placenta and activated coagulants derived from the retroplacental haematoma may be the trigger. The most florid acute haemostatic failure, combined with widespread microthrombosis of the pulmonary vasculature, is produced by amniotic-fluid embolism [195]. Bleeding and thrombosis are frequent complications of septic abortions. Subacute states, often clinically latent, accompany a retained dead fetus and have been reported with hydatidiform mole or degenerating leiomyoma [198]. The renal lesions of eclampsia deserve special mention; intrarenal fibrin deposits have been frequently demonstrated [199–201] and the blood changes suggestive of intravascular coagulation found in normal pregnancy are accentuated [202, 203].

Coagulant stimuli are not limited to the mother; intravascular coagulation is also a risk to the fetus and the neonate. Stillbirth, or delivery with widespread haemorrhage and thrombosis, are possible results [204, 205]. The condition has been described in infants of mothers suffering from toxaemia or abruptio placentae, in one of twins where the other had died *in utero*, in generalized virus infections, and as a complication of rhesus isoimmunization [206, 207]; predisposing factors in the infant include prematurity, birth asphyxia, hypoglycaemia, and hypothermia [22].

Surgery and trauma

Any surgical operation or injury will tend to increase the consumption of platelets and of coagulation factors. Accelerated losses are inevitable, due to bleeding and the necessity to form haemostatic plugs in damaged vessels, and increased capillary permeability at sites of tissue damage may also increase the transfer from the intravascular to the extravascular pool; in addition there are the effects of intravascular coagulation [208, 209]. Loss is enhanced by major operations, particularly those on the lung, prostate, or neoplastic tissues, by the foreign surfaces provided by external cardiopulmonary-bypass machines [185], or by hypovolaemia and metabolic acidosis. Intravascular haemolysis, resulting from mechanical damage or from transfusions of stored cells, may contribute. Cardiac arrest causes a particularly severe depletion of coagulation factors [210]. Intravascular coagulation has been studied after burns [192], in the crush syndrome [211], in heat stroke [212], and after head injury [213].

Blood stored for longer than 24 hours is deficient in factor V, VIIIC, and viable platelets. A single transfusion of stored blood equal to the total blood volume of the patient is likely to cause impaired haemostasis during surgery unless a proportion of fresh blood is given [214].

Infections

Overwhelming general infection of any type may produce the acute syndrome [215, 216]; cases of septicaemia due to clostridia [217] or meningococci [218] have been reported in detail. In the latter, haemorrhagic infarction of the adrenal may cause the Waterhouse–Friderichsen syndrome. Less acute changes are found in malaria [219]. Thrombocytopenia may occur without evidence of coagulation, particularly in viral infections [220, 221].

Neoplasm

Subacute intravascular coagulation is a characteristic of many disseminated neoplasms, including carcinoma of the prostate, breast, lung, gastro-intestinal tract, cervix and pancreas [222–225]. Intravascular coagulation is common in acute promyelocytic leukaemia [226], but may also occur in other types of leukaemia and lymphoma [227, 228].

Intravascular haemolysis

Intravascular haemolysis liberates coagulant materials into the blood [229]. Animal experiments suggest that relatively large volumes of blood, of the order of 100 ml in the dog, need to be suddenly destroyed before detectable coagulation is produced [230]. The coagulation is increased if reticulo-endothelial activity is depressed [231]. Examples of coagulation have been described after transfusion of ABO-incompatible blood [232], in malaria [233, 234], and in G6PD deficiency [235]. Intravascular coagulation may contribute to the thrombotic crises of sickle-cell disease [236, 237].

Renal disease

Intrarenal fibrin may be a manifestation of intravascular coagulation due to any of the known causes. In other patients fibrin has been found only in the kidney, where it may have been produced by local damage. Evidence of intraglomerular fibrin is found in acute ischaemic renal failure [238], post-partum renal failure [239], proliferative glomerulonephritis [240], and the haemolytic-uraemic syndrome of childhood or adults [158, 241, 242].

The haemolytic-uraemic syndrome of renal failure and haemolytic anaemia with distorted and fragmented red cells (microangiopathic haemolysis) may occur without obvious precipitating cause, especially in childhood. Microangiopathy and renal lesions are also associated with auto-allergic disease, malignant hypertension, septicaemia, and disseminated neoplasm [242]. The blood changes of intravascular coagulation may be found, but not always [243].

Thrombotic thrombocytopenic purpura. This is a particular syndrome described by Moschowitz in 1925 [244], characterized by the sudden onset of fever, thrombocytopenic purpura, microangiopathic haemolytic anaemia, fluctuating neurological signs and renal failure. The disease may occur at any age, in either sex, and if untreated usually runs a rapidly fatal course. At autopsy, occluding hyaline microthrombi are found in the terminal arterioles and capillaries of many organs [245, 246] with heavy involvement of heart, kidneys, adrenals and brain; none show any associated inflammatory change. There may be aneurysmal dilatation of the arteriolocapillary junction [247, 248]. The blood changes of DIC are absent or minimal in many of these patients and it has been suggested that the lesions represent disseminated intravascular platelet aggregation [170, 243]. This aggregation may perhaps be in response to primary vessel damage [158, 248] or due to the absence of a normal, as yet unidentified, platelet aggregation inhibitor to be found in plasma [249], including outdated plasma, but not in plasma protein concentrates available for transfusion. Although none of the lesions are specific the presence of hyaline microthrombi with no surrounding inflammatory change or vascular necrosis, may help to differentiate thrombotic thrombocytopenic purpura from the other associations of microangiopathic haemolytic anaemia and the haemolytic-uraemic syndrome. Biopsies to show the lesions may be taken from bone marrow, kidney, lymph node or skin; the last is preferred, the thrombi being found in dermal capillaries in relation to petechial lesions [243]. Successful treatment of this otherwise fatal disease by splenectomy together with corticosteroids and antiplatelet agents has been reported [250]; more recently, intensive plasma transfusion has been advocated [249]. Heparin and thrombolytic therapy appear to play no part in the treatment of this syndrome. The condition is considered more fully in Chapters 12 and 25.

Allergic reactions

Intravascular thrombi are characteristic of the Arthus reaction and generalized changes may be associated with anaphylactic shock [251]. Intravascular coagulation is associated with the rejection of renal transplants [252] and liver transplants [109].

Purpura fulminans, which may have an allergic basis, is a rare but severe complication which follows acute infections, particularly with β-haemolytic streptococci or varicella virus [253]. Extensive purpuric and echymotic lesions develop some weeks after the infection, enlarge, and undergo necrosis due to thrombotic occlusion of small vessels [254, 255]. Purpura after infection may also be due to the Schönlein–Henoch syndrome or post-infective thrombocytopenia; neither shows the necrosis of purpura fulminans.

Local vascular lesions

Bleeding, with thrombocytopenia and low plasma fibrinogen, has frequently been observed in association with a giant haemangioma due to deposition of platelets and fibrin within it [256] (see Chapter 25, p. 1001). A similar syndrome may be associated with large aortic aneurysms or vascular tumours.

Venomous animals

The complex toxins produced by venomous animals frequently produce intravascular coagulation and fibrinolysis. The effects of the snake venoms have been reviewed [257]. Bleeding with low plasma fibrinogen has been reported after contact with caterpillars of the Saturnidae family found in restricted areas of Venezuela [258].

Patients bitten by the Malayan pit viper, *Agkistrodon rhodostoma*, have a very low plasma fibrinogen concentration for many days afterwards; bleeding is unusual [259]. The venom contains an enzyme now purified and available as ancrod (Arvin), which splits fibrinopeptide A but not fibrinopeptide B from fibrinogen, without activating other blood-coagulation factors and without any direct effect on platelets [260, 261]. The fibrinogen is rendered insoluble so that microclots form, but these are rapidly removed from the circulation by reticulo-endothelial cells and the patient appears 'defibrinated'. Plasminogen activator is not increased in the blood, but there is a considerable fall in the plasminogen suggesting local activation of fibrinolysis by absorption of plasminogen to fibrin. There is no evidence that ancrod actively increases fibrinolysis in pre-existing thrombi [262].

In experimental animals, large doses of ancrod, given rapidly, cause death with multiple thrombi in the lungs. Much larger doses, given slowly, do not overwhelm the clearance mechanisms and the margin of clinical safety appears high [263]. Laboratory control is by a simple clot-observation test or the measurement of clottable plasma fibrinogen. If bleeding occurs an antivenom is available and may be supplemented by transfusion of fibrinogen concentrates. Ancrod may be given intravenously or by the subcutaneous route, but the latter has been associated with resistance to long-term therapy due to the formation of neutralizing antibodies [264].

MANAGEMENT OF INTRAVASCULAR COAGULATION

General principles

Removal of the cause is always necessary, though often impossible. The need for other active treatment must be assessed in relation to the nature and expected duration of the coagulation stimulus, the type and site of any bleeding, and whether or not the haemostatic mechanism must withstand the challenge of trauma or merely prevent spontaneous bleeding. The minimum laboratory tests needed are the plasma fibrinogen, the thrombin clotting time, the PCV and an estimate of the platelet count. Deficiencies need not be treated automatically 'because they are there'; a period of observation and assessment with attempts to alleviate the stimulus is often worthwhile if the patient is not bleeding.

Transfusion

Prompt, complete, and therefore carefully monitored blood volume replacement is essential in the acute bleeding states. The nature of the transfusion fluid is less important than the completeness of the volume replacement, but as soon as possible, fresh materials should be obtained, blood or fresh-frozen plasma as appropriate. Massive transfusion with stored materials deficient in platelets, factors V and VIII may exaggerate the deficiencies. Plasma protein fraction BP contains only insignificant quantities of any of the coagulation factors; fresh-frozen plasma supplies all the major clotting factors. A fibrinogen concentrate or fresh platelet concentrates may be shown to be needed by repeated measurements of blood fibrinogen and platelet levels in the individual patient. These general measures take precedence over all other considerations. The concept that the transfusion of clottable materials may 'feed the fire', allowing further microthrombosis, has never been established and can for practical purposes be discounted [151].

Heparin therapy
Heparin may decrease intravascular coagulation but will also decrease extravascular coagulation, which is needed for haemostasis; thus the indications for its use in these disorders have yet to be established. The control of intravascular coagulation in experimental animals requires heparin in large doses, and these often have to be given before the trigger to coagulation, in order to achieve real protection [144]. There is no single clinical condition in which the adminstration of heparin is generally agreed to be of benefit, but many in which it has been advocated. Heparin has been used in obstetric cases with abruptio placentae [197], and the hyperacute syndrome of pulmonary vascular obstruction in amniotic-fluid embolism is often considered an indication [198, 265]. Several reports suggest the effectiveness of anticoagulants in purpura fulminans [151, 253] and during the acute phase of septicaemia [217, 266]. Rhesus monkeys infected with yellow fever have been given heparin, which reversed the coagulation effects but did not prolong the life of the animals [267]; similar results were obtained in another animal model, fowl plague in chickens [268]. Heparin combined with antimalarials gave a more rapid control of infection with drug-resistant strains of *Plasmodium falciparum* than antimalarial drugs used alone [233]. Transfusion reactions have been treated with anticoagulants [232]. Heparin has also been used to control bleeding in acute hepatic necrosis, but a controlled trial showed no clinical benefit [120]. The improved prognosis in the haemolytic-uraemic syndrome of childhood has coincided with the use of heparin in some centres, and with a better understanding of the methods of treatment of renal failure, so that either may be the responsible factor [269, 270]. Most animal venoms are unaffected by heparin, which is therefore contraindicated in their management [271].

Two groups of patients must be separately considered, the fundamental division between them depending on whether their vascular system is damaged or intact. First, in defibrinated patients with already damaged major vessels, and therefore with acute bleeding, the use of heparin has never gained general acceptance, though it has not been the subject of a formal trial. Careful attention to the general

principles already enunciated should be used alone first, and heparin reserved for those in whom other measures have failed. There is one possible exception, amniotic-fluid embolism. Prompt intravenous injection of heparin, in full anticoagulant doses, is logical as soon as the clinical diagnosis is suspected, in order to reduce the obstructive effects of the pulmonary thrombi [195]. Secondly, when the vascular system is largely intact but consumption by intravascular coagulation has reduced fibrinogen and platelets below haemostatic levels and the patient has a haemostatic challenge to face, heparin has a real place. The consumption can be reduced by the intravenous infusion of heparin, beginning at 1000 units hourly for an adult and continued for 24–48 hours. In some cases the dose may need to be increased temporarily in order to achieve a definite prolongation of the patients' partial thromboplastin or thrombin time. This and similar regimes have often been reported as returning fibrinogen and platelets to normal levels in patients with disseminated neoplasia, including myeloma, retained dead fetus, or vascular malformations such as aneurysms or giant haemangiomas. The syndrome in these patients may be suspected because of purpura and a minor bleeding tendency in a patient with one of the underlying disorders. Its presence is easily confirmed by blood tests which reveal the low level of fibrinogen and platelets. Treatment with heparin should certainly precede any surgical or needle-biopsy procedure in these patients; the need for anticoagulants in those for whom no such procedure is contemplated will depend on the possibility of treating the underlying cause. Thus when a dead fetus is retained *in utero*, only one-third of the patients have a low plasma fibrinogen and spontaneous delivery by the natural route is usually possible without bleeding. However, heparin is indicated if blood levels are low and Caesarian section or episiotomy is contemplated [195]. In susceptible neoplasms, heparin may reduce the effects of consumption and prevent major bleeding during the course of cytotoxic therapy. It has often been combined with infusions of platelets and cytotoxic drugs in the initial management of acute promyelocytic leukaemia.

One very great problem remains. There are many disease processes where DIC changes are marked not so much by consumption with imperilled haemostasis as by the possibility of damage to organs by microthrombosis. Changes in the blood are easy to demonstrate, but the importance of fibrin in the pathogenesis of the lesions and the benefits conferred by heparin are much less easy to assess. In general, opinion has veered away from the use of heparin in such disorders, including eclampsia, traumatic or septicaemic shock, and renal failure.

Other treatments

Although there are good theoretical reasons for using fibrinolytic therapy in DIC there are also obvious hazards, since further damage to haemostatic function may imperil already damaged organs. The role of antiplatelet drugs, the infusion of antithrombin III without heparin [162], and the use of low-dose heparin have yet to be adequately explored. Inhibitors of fibrinolysis have no definite role and may well be dangerous [162, 272].

UNUSUAL INHIBITORS OF COAGULATION

No abnormal bleeding has been ascribed to acquired disorders of the normal inhibitors of blood coagulation. Pathological endogenous inhibitors may develop and reveal their presence by giving abnormal coagulation test results for the patient, and for normal plasma to which plasma from the patient has been added [273]. These unusual inhibitors may be immunoglobulins active against a specific clotting factor, often factor VIII [274], or abnormal proteins which block one or more stages of the coagulation mechanism. There is no modern evidence to support earlier reports of endogenous heparin in human disease.

Antibodies specific for a single factor in the coagulation mechanism may develop in those with congenital coagulation-factor deficiencies, usually following repeated transfusion of the missing factor, or in otherwise normal individuals with or without a previous history of blood transfusion. Sometimes there is no associated abnormality in the latter group, but more frequently the antibodies appear up to some months after childbirth, in the elderly, or in association with a variety of chronic disorders of auto-allergic type. The latter include rheumatoid arthritis, rheumatic heart disease, systemic lupus erythematosus, pemphigus, dermatitis herpetiformis, penicillin hypersensitivity and regional enteritis.

ANTIBODIES TO FACTOR VIII

In the UK [275], Sweden, USA and France [276] 5–10% of patients with haemophilia A develop antibodies to factor-VIII procoagulant activity (VIIIC). With one possible exception [277], inhibitors in haemophilic patients have appeared only after transfusion with factor VIII, but there is no indication that the chance of developing an antibody is related to the frequency of exposure to this antigen [278]. Most inhibitors occur in patients with the severe form of the disease, more than 97% being in patients with VIIIC less than 2 u/dl before the antibody developed [276]. Half the antibodies had appeared by the age of 10

years, another 20% by the age of 20 years, but the remainder came later in life. In non-haemophilic subjects the incidence rises with age.

The antibodies inactivate VIIIC in a time-consuming reaction following second-order or complex kinetics and are non-precipitating [278, 279]. The interaction is to some extent species-specific, many antibodies of human origin having little effect against bovine or porcine factor VIII [280]. In most cases the antibody has restricted specificity for VIIIC, but a very few have been reported to interfere with ristocetin-induced platelet aggregation [281, 282]. A different type of precipitating antibody to other activities of factor VIII has been reported in patients with von Willebrand's disease [283], or in previously normal subjects producing an acquired von Willebrand's syndrome. The latter may be asssociated with lupus erythematosus [284], lymphosarcoma [285], pesticide injection [286] or without apparent underlying disease [287]. These antibodies do not usually inhibit VIIIC unless they do so by co-precipitation rather than specific combination [288].

The majority of the antibodies to VIIIC are of the IgG class [288, 289]. Exceptionally they have been reported as exclusively IgM [290], IgA in a patient with myeloma [291], or IgM with IgG [292]. In haemophiliacs detailed studies show very high, but not exclusive, occurrence of a single light-chain type, usually kappa. Heavy-chain typing also shows a restricted heterogeneity with an unusually high incidence of the less common subtypes [293]. Greater variability is found in non-haemophilic individuals in both respects. It has been suggested that there may be a linkage between the major histocompability locus and a gene controlling the immune response to factor VIII, but no correlation has been found with a specific HLA type [294].

The appearance of an antibody often has no obvious clinical effect, the frequency and severity of bleeding usually being unchanged. However, a few patients with initially mild haemophilia exposed to unusually intensive therapy with factor VIII have developed an antibody which has converted their disease into the severe form. In these patients withdrawal of factor-VIII therapy has usually been followed by disappearance of the antibody and subsequent smaller exposures to factor VIII have not caused it to reappear [276].

The antibodies can be detected by incubating test plasma at 37°C with a source of VIIIC and performing serial coagulation tests to measure any loss of activity with time. The slow nature of the inactivation makes incubation necessary for two to four hours. Various units of inhibitor activity have been suggested from Oxford [295] or Bethesda [296].

In haemophiliacs receiving transfusions of factor

VIII, occasional checks for the presence of an antibody are advisable; they are obligatory before any major predictable challenge to haemostasis. Antibody producers have been described as two types known as 'weak' or 'strong' responders [297]. The former, some 25% of those affected, seldom develop over three Bethesda units of inhibitor per ml of plasma even after repeated exposure to factor VIII by transfusion. The strong responder reacts to such exposure by a rise in inhibitor, often beginning within four days, to reach a maximum after about 14–21 days, thereafter declining slowly over many months or not at all. In some well-substantiated patients, haemophilic and non-haemophilic, with or without factor-VIII treatment, antibodies have disappeared spontaneously [278].

In the management of a bleeding episode in a patient with an inhibitor, much depends on knowledge of the level of antibody, whether the patient is known to be a 'weak' or 'strong' responder, and the nature of the challenge to haemostasis. The options have been reviewed [298] and include human [297] or animal [298] factor-VIII concentrates, perhaps by continuous infusion [299], factor-IX concentrates either activated [300] or non-activated [301, 302], immunosuppression [303–305], platelet concentrates [306] and either exchange transfusion [278] or plasmapheresis [307, 308] (see also Chapter 28, p. 1120). The normal routine of home therapy and even prophylactic therapy with factor VIII is now accepted practice for the 'weak' responder, but must be avoided in the 'strong' responder. Some factor-IX concentrates have contained enough material to stimulate an anamnestic rise in anti-factor-VIIIC antibodies [309] in these patients.

ANTIBODIES TO OTHER COAGULATION FACTORS

Immunoglobulin inhibitors against other coagulation factors, the great majority of the immunoglobulins being of the IgG class, are being reported frequently both from transfused patients having a genetic coagulation-factor deficiency, and from previously normal individuals, who often give no history of blood transfusion before the inhibitor is recognized.

Factor IX

Antibodies to factor IX are found in one per cent of patients with Christmas disease in the UK [275], and up to three per cent elsewhere [276]. The severely affected patient is more likely to develop an antibody than the mildly affected; in both cases the inhibitor follows transfusion with factor IX. Antigen–antibody interaction is faster than with anti-factor-VIIIC antibodies. Examples have been reported in non-Christmas disease patients [274, 310–312].

Factor V

Antibodies to factor V have been reported in normal persons [276, 313–315], often those treated with aminoglycosides or other antibiotics, and in one patient with congenital deficiency of factor V. The inhibitor may disappear within a few months, but meanwhile the bleeding tendency may be severe.

Contact factors

Reported antibodies to factor XI [316, 317] and factor XII [318] tended to persist, and were associated with only a mild bleeding tendency. In all but one of the reported instances (a patient with congenital factor-XI deficiency) the patients were female and suffering from systemic lupus erythematosus.

Factor XIII

Antibodies have been described [319, 320] specific either for factor XIII, the active enzyme factor XIIIa, or the specific receptor site for XIIIa on the α or γ chains of the fibrin monomer [321]. Such antibodies have been associated with serious bleeding tendencies; many of the patients had systemic lupus erythematosus or had been treated with isoniazid.

Fibrinogen

At least one patient with congenital afibrinogenaemia has developed precipitating antibodies to fibrinogen after transfusion [322]. Antibodies to fibrinogen have also been reported in a patient with recurrent thrombophlebitis [323], and in one patient with a mild bleeding tendency where the IgG antibody delayed fibrinopeptide-A release [324].

LUPUS-LIKE ANTICOAGULANT

Bleeding in systemic lupus erythematosus may be associated with thrombocytopenia, liver failure, renal failure, or the production of antibodies to specific coagulation factors, including factors V, VIII, XI, XII or XIII [274, 284, 325]. Patients with this disease may also develop immunoglobulin inhibitors, either IgG or IgM [326], which are not directed against a particular factor but which appear to inhibit the coagulant action of phospholipid [327–329]. First described in patients with systemic lupus erythematosus [330] and therefore dubbed the 'lupus anticoagulant', these non-specific inhibitors are now known to occur in other autoimmune disorders [331], sometimes with a familial predisposition [332], following infections [333], after long-term therapy with chlorpromazine [334] or procainamide [335], and even in patients without demonstrable underlying disease who are found to have abnormal results in routine screening tests for haemostasis [336]. Hence the proposal to call the phenomenon that of the 'lupus-like anticoagulant'. In most cases the demonstration of the anticoagulant is of no clinical significance. In many patients there has been no bleeding tendency, even with the haemostatic challenge of major surgery. However, the presence of the inhibitor has been associated with a predisposition to thrombosis [333, 337] and sometimes with a mild bleeding tendency [336].

Characteristically the presence of the lupus-like anticoagulant prolongs the partial thromboplastin time with or without kaolin, and a mixture of equal parts of normal and control plasma also has an abnormal partial thromboplastin time; this may be even longer than that of the patient alone [336]. The inhibition in the mixture is immediate and clotting factors are not inactivated progressively. The pro-thrombin time may be normal or—with higher titres of inhibitor—prolonged. It then shows similar inhibitory properties for normal plasma. One-stage assays for factors VIII, IX, XI, or XII often given abnormal results for one or more of these factors with non-parallel dose-response curves, the effect of the inhibitor being less at the higher plasma dilutions.

Most lupus-like anticoagulants disappear spontaneously within a few months or as any underlying disease responds to treatment. They are of greater academic interest than clinical significance.

PARAPROTEINS

Patients with high plasma levels of monoclonal immunoglobulin due to myeloma or macroglobulinaemia may show multiple abnormalities of haemostasis. Bleeding is usually associated with the 'hyperviscosity syndrome' [338], disturbed platelet function [339–341], or antibody specific for factor VIII [342, 343]. Independently of these processes, however, the monoclonal protein may block one or more phases of blood coagulation [344] to give prolonged prothrombin, partial thromboplastin or thrombin-clotting times. The inhibition most often affects the thrombin–fibrinogen reaction [340, 345] and resembles the effects of an inhibitor described as antithrombin V in a man with rheumatoid arthritis and hyper-γ-globulinaemia [346]. Bleeding in any of these states can sometimes be relieved by plasmapheresis or by specific chemotherapy [347].

ACQUIRED DEFICIENCY OF COAGULATION FACTORS OF UNCERTAIN CAUSE

Plasma factor X as low as 1–20% of normal, with other coagulation factors normal, has been recorded in a number of patients with amyloidosis [348, 349]. Recovery of transfused factor X is poor but no inhibitory effect on normal plasma can be demonstrated *in vitro*. It has been suggested that the abnormal amyloid material itself is the neutralizing factor [350]. An element of DIC may also contribute [351]. Acquired deficiency of factor X has occurred as a transient phenomenon, in the absence of associated disease, after exposure to methyl bromide used as a fungicide, and in a patient with renal and adrenal neoplasm [352]. Isolated, apparently acquired, deficiencies of factor VII [353] and prothrombin [354] not associated with detectable anticoagulants have also been reported.

Acquired deficiency of factor IX has been associated with Gaucher's disease [355] and the nephrotic syndrome [127, 356]. Although patients with Gaucher's disease frequently have a mild bleeding disorder due to thrombocytopenia, a deficiency of factor IX was found in seven of 10 patients studied, with values as low as 1 u/dl. Low levels of factor VIII were found in three of these patients, low factor VII and X in one patient each, and low factor V in two patients. It was suggested that the accumulated cerebroside may have acted as an anticoagulant; the possibility of intravascular coagulation was also discussed [355]. Deficiency of factor IX in the nephrotic syndrome was related to excessive loss in the urine [356]. Asparaginase used in therapy is known to decrease the synthesis of fibrinogen [357].

Acquired, often transient, apparent deficiencies of factor XIII which return to normal as the associated condition recovers have been reported in many conditions, including pregnancy and after major surgery [358, 359]. It has been suggested that a fall in plasma factor XIII may be a non-specific finding of disease, proportional to its severity, but the wide variation in results for different methods of measurement, even in the same patient, makes interpretation difficult. The virtual absence of cross-linking activity which would be needed to cause or exacerbate bleeding is seldom found except in the few patients in whom acquired neutralizing antibodies to factor XIII have been demonstrated. Many of these antibodies appear in patients treated with isoniazid, which in other patients receiving long-term therapy has been considered responsible for the production of non-antibody inhibitors of uncertain nature, but also associated with serious bleeding [360, 361].

REFERENCES

1 DAM H. & SCHONHEYDER F. (1934) A deficiency disease in chicks resembling scurvy. *Biochemical Journal*, **28**, 1355.

2 SHEARER M.J., ALLAN V., HAROON Y. & BARKHAN P. (1980) Nutritional aspects of vitamin K in the human. In: *Vitamin K Metabolism and Vitamin-K-dependent Proteins* (ed. Suttie J.W.), p. 317. University Park Press, Baltimore.

3 SHEARER M.J., McBURNEY A., BRECKENRIDGE A.M. &

BARKHAN P. (1977) Effect of warfarin on the metabolism of phylloquinone (vitamin K_1): dose response relationships in man. *Clinical Science and Molecular Medicine*, **52**, 621.

4 UDALL J.A. (1965) Human sources and absorption of vitamin K in relation to anticoagulation stability. *Journal of the American Medical Association*, **194**, 127.

5 FINKEL M.J. (1961) Vitamin K_1 and the vitamin K analogues. *Clinical Pharmacology and Therapeutics*, **2**, 794.

6 FERNLUND P., STENFLO J., ROEPSTORFF R. & THOMSEN J. (1975) Vitamin K and the biosynthesis of prothrombin. V. γ-carboxyglutamic acids, the vitamin K-dependent structures in prothrombin. *Journal of Biological Chemistry*, **250**, 6125.

7 HEMKER H.C., VELTKAMP J.J., HENSEN A. & LOELIGER E.A. (1963) Nature of prothrombin biosynthesis: prethrombinaemia in vitamin K deficiency. *Nature (London)*, **200**, 589.

8 HEMKER H.C. & LOELIGER E.A. (1968) Kinetic aspects of the interaction of blood clotting enzymes. III. Demonstration of the presence of an inhibitor of prothrombin conversion in vitamin K deficiency. *Thrombosis et Diathesis Haemorrhagica*, **19**, 346.

9 GANROT P.O. & NILÉHN J.E. (1968) Plasma prothrombin during treatment with Dicumarol. II. Demonstration of an abnormal prothrombin fraction. *Scandinavian Journal of Clinical and Laboratory Investigation*, **22**, 23.

10 GALLOP P.M., LIAN J.B. & HAUSCHKA P.V. (1980) Carboxylated calcium-binding proteins and vitamin K. *New England Journal of Medicine*, **302**, 1460.

11 PRYDZ H. (1977) Vitamin K-dependent clotting factors. *Seminars in Thrombosis and Hemostasis*, **4**, 1.

12 KISIEL W. (1979) Human plasma protein C: isolation, characterization and mechanism of activation by α-thrombin. *Journal of Clinical Investigation*, **64**, 761.

13 LUCEY J.F. & DOLAN R.G. (1958) Injections of a vitamin K compound in mothers and hyperbilirubinemia in the newborn. *Pediatrics*, **22**, 605.

14 CADE J.F., HIRSH J. & MARTIN M. (1969) Placental barrier to coagulation factors: its relevance to the coagulation defect at birth and to haemorrhage in the newborn. *British Medical Journal*, **ii**, 281.

15 BUCHANAN G.R. (1978) Neonatal coagulation: normal physiology and pathophysiology. *Clinics in Hematology*, **7**, 85.

16 FUKUI H., TAKASE T., IKARI H., MURAKAMI, Y., ŌKUBO Y. & NAKAMURA K. (1979) Factor-VIII procoagulant activity, factor-VIII-related antigen and von Willebrand factor in newborn cord blood. *British Journal of Haematology*, **42**, 637.

17 HATHAWAY W.E. (1975) The bleeding newborn. *Seminars in Hematology*, **12**, 175.

18 HENRIKSSON P., HEDNER U., NILSSON I.M., BOEHM J., ROBERTSON B. & LORAND L. (1974) Fibrin stabilizing factor (factor XIII) in the fetus and the newborn infant. *Pediatric Research*, **8**, 789.

19 NEUMANN L.L., HATHAWAY W.E., CLARKE S. & BORDEN C. (1974) Antithrombin III levels in term and preterm newborn infants. *Clinical Research*, **22**, 226A.

20 HATHAWAY W.E., NEUMANN L.L., BORDEN C.A. & JACOBSON L.J. (1978) Immunologic studies of antithrombin III heparin cofactor in the newborn. *Thrombosis and Haemostasis*, **39**, 624.

21 FOLEY M.E., CLAYTON J.K. & McNICOL G.P. (1977) Haemostatic mechanisms in maternal, umbilical vein, and umbilical artery blood at the time of delivery. *British Journal of Obstetrics and Gynaecology*, **84**, 81.

22 CHESSELLS J.M. & HARDISTY R.M. (1974) Bleeding problems in the newborn infant. In: *Progress in Hemostasis and Thrombosis* (ed. Spaet T.H.), Vol. II, p. 333. Grune & Stratton, New York.

23 SCHETTINI F., DE MATTIA D., MAUTONE A. & ALTOMARE M. (1976) Post natal development of factor II (preprothrombin and prothrombin) in man. *Biology of the Neonate*, **29**, 82.

24 ABALLI A.J. (1974) Hemorrhagic disease of the newborn. *Pediatric Annals*, **3**, 35.

25 KEENAN W.J., JEWETT T. & GLUECK H.I. (1971) Role of feeding and vitamin K in hypoprothrombinemia of the newborn. *American Journal of Diseases of Children*, **121**, 271.

26 HIRSH J., CADE J.F. & O'SULLIVAN E.F. (1970) Clinical experience with anticoagulant therapy during pregnancy. *British Medical Journal*, **i**, 270.

27 BLEYER W.A. & SKINNER A.L. (1976) Fatal neonatal hemorrhage after maternal anticonvulsant therapy. *Journal of the American Medical Association*, **235**, 626.

28 SUTHERLAND J.M., GLUECK H.I. & GLESER G. (1967) Hemorrhagic disease of the newborn. *American Journal of Diseases of Children*, **113**, 524.

29 UTTLEY W.S., ALLAN A.G.E. & CASH J.D. (1969) Fibrin/fibrinogen degradation products in sera of normal infants and children. *Archives of Disease in Childhood*, **44**, 761.

30 LUKENS J.N. (1972) Vitamin K and the older infant. *American Journal of Diseases of Children*, **124**, 639.

31 KLIPPEL A.P. & PITSINGER B. (1968) Hypoprothrombinemia secondary to antibiotic therapy and manifested by massive gastro-intestinal haemorrhage. *Archives of Surgery*, **96**, 266.

32 LINK K.P. (1959) The discovery of Dicumarol and its sequels. *Circulation*, **19**, 97.

33 KABAT H., STOHLMAN E.F. & SMITH M.T. (1944) Hypoprothrombinemia induced by administration of indandione derivatives. *Journal of Pharmacology and Experimental Therapeutics*, **80**, 160.

34 O'REILLY R.A. & AGGELER P.M. (1976) Covert anticoagulant ingestion: study of 25 patients and review of world literature. *Medicine*, **55**, 389.

35 MARTIN C.M., ENGSTROM P.F. & BARRETT O. JR (1970) Surreptitious self-administration of heparin. *Journal of the American Medical Association*, **212**, 475.

36 POLLER L. (1969) Progress in laboratory control of anticoagulant therapy. In: *Recent Advances in Blood Coagulation* (ed. Poller L.), p. 137. Churchill, London.

37 OWREN P.A. (1963) Control of anticoagulant therapy. The use of new tests. *Archives of Internal Medicine*, **111**, 248.

38 OWREN P.A. & AAS K. (1951) The control of dicumarol therapy and the quantitative determination of prothrombin and proconvertin. *Scandinavian Journal of Clinical and Laboratory Investigation*, **3**, 201.

39 BROZOVIĆ M. (1978) Oral anticoagulants in clinical practice. *Seminars in Hematology*, **15**, 27.

40 ICTH/ICSH (1979) Prothrombin time standardization: Report of the expert panel on oral anticoagulant control. *Thrombosis and Haemostasis*, **42**, 1073.

41 DENSON K.W.E. (1971) International and national standardization of control of anticoagulant therapy in patients receiving coumarin and indanedione drugs using calibrated thromboplastin preparations. *Journal of Clinical Pathology*, **24**, 460.

42 ALDERSON M.R., POLLER L. & THOMSON J.M. (1970) Validity of the British system for anticoagulant control using the national reagent. *Journal of Clinical Pathology*, **23**, 281.

43 LOELIGER E.A., VAN DER ESCH B., MATTERN M.J. & DEN BRABANDER A.S. (1963) Behaviour of factors II, VII, IX and X during long-term treatment with coumarin. *Thrombosis et Diathesis Haemorrhagica*, **9**, 74.

44 KOCH-WESER J. & SELLERS E.M. (1971) Drug interactions with coumarin anticoagulants. *New England Journal of Medicine*, **285**, 487 and 547.

45 O'REILLY R.A. (1976) Vitamin K and the oral anticoagulant drugs. *Annual Review of Medicine*, **27**, 245.

46 KELTON J.G. & HIRSH J. (1980) Bleeding associated with antithrombotic therapy. *Seminars in Hematology*, **17**, 259.

47 MINCHIN CLARKE H.G., FREEMAN T. & PRYSE-PHILLIPS W. (1971) Serum protein changes after injury. *Clinical Science*, **40**, 337.

48 BRECKENRIDGE A. & ORME M. (1971) Clinical implications of enzyme induction. *Annals of the New York Academy of Sciences*, **179**, 421.

49 LEWIS R.J., SPIVACK M. & SPAET T. (1967) Warfarin resistance. *American Journal of Medicine*, **42**, 620.

50 VESELL E.S. & PAGE J.G. (1969) Genetic control of the phenobarbital-induced shortening of plasma antipyrine half-lives in man. *Journal of Clinical Investigation*, **48**, 2202.

51 O'REILLY R.A. & AGGELER P.M. (1970) Determinants of the response to oral anticoagulant drugs in man. *Pharmacology Reviews*, **22**, 35.

52 TABERNER D.A., THOMSON J.M. & POLLER L. (1976) Comparison of prothrombin complex concentrate and vitamin K_1 in oral anticoagulant reversal. *British Medical Journal*, **ii**, 83.

53 LOELIGER E.A. (1979) The optimal therapeutic range in oral anticoagulation. History and proposal. *Thrombosis and Haemostasis*, **42**, 1141.

54 RATNOFF O.D. (1963) Hemostatic mechanisms in liver disease. *Medical Clinical of North America*, **47**, 721.

55 WALLS W.D. & LOSOWSKY M.S. (1971) The haemostatic defect of liver disease. *Current Clinical Concepts*, **60**, 108.

56 ROBERTS H.R. & CEDERBAUM A.I. (1972) The liver and blood coagulation: physiology and pathology. *Gastroenterology*, **63**, 297.

57 SPAET T.H., HOROWITZ H.I., ZUCKER-FRANKLIN D., CINTRON J. & BIEZENSKI J.J. (1961) Reticulo-endothelial clearance of blood thromboplastins by rats. *Blood*, **17**, 196.

58 DEYKIN D., COCHIOS F., DECAMP G. & LOPEZ A. (1968) Hepatic removal of activated factor X by the perfused rabbit liver. *American Journal of Physiology*, **214**, 414.

59 ASTER R.H. (1972) Annotation: platelet sequestration studies in man. *British Journal of Haematology*, **22**, 259.

60 FLUTE P.T. (1971) Haemostasis in fulminant hepatic failure. *British Medical Journal*, **i**, 215.

61 BOUMA H. III., KWAN S.W. & FULLER G.M. (1975) Radioimmunological identification of polysomes synthesizing fibrinogen polypeptide chains. *Biochemistry*, **14**, 4787.

62 WORKMAN E.F.J. & LUNDBLAD R.L. (1977) The role of the liver in biosynthesis of the non-vitamin-K-dependent clotting factors. *Seminars in Thrombosis and Hemostasis*, **4**, 15.

63 OLSON J.P., MILLER L.L. & TROUP S.B. (1966) Synthesis of clotting factors by the isolated perfused rat liver. *Journal of Clinical Investigation*, **45**, 690.

64 JEEJEEBHOY K.N., HO J., GREENBERG G.R., PHILLIPS M.J., BRUCE-ROBERTSON A. & SODTKE V. (1975) Albumin, fibrinogen and transferrin synthesis in isolated rat hepatocyte suspensions: a model for the study of plasma protein synthesis. *Biochemical Journal*, **146**, 141.

65 DUCKERT F. (1973) Behaviour of antithrombin III in liver disease. *Scandinavian Journal of Gastroenterology*, **8** (Suppl. 19), 109.

66 COLLEN D. (1980) On the regulation and control of fibrinolysis. *Thrombosis and Haemostasis*, **43**, 77.

67 REEVE E.B. & FRANKS J.J. (1974) Fibrinogen synthesis, distribution and degradation. *Seminars in Thrombosis and Hemostasis*, **1**, 129.

68 FLUTE P.T. (1977) Disorders of plasma fibrinogen synthesis. *British Medical Bulletin*, **33**, 253.

69 PALASCAK J.E. & MARTINEZ J. (1977) Dysfibrinogenemia associated with liver disease. *Journal of Clinical Investigation*, **60**, 89.

70 SORIA J., SORIA C., SAMAMA M., COUPIER J., GIRARD M.L., BOUSSER J. & BILSKI-PASQUIER G. (1970) Dysfibrinogénémies acquises dans les atteintes hépatiques sévères. *Coagulation*, **3**, 37.

71 LANE D.A., SCULLY M.F., THOMAS D.P., KAKKAR V.V., WOOLF I.L. & WILLIAMS R. (1977) Acquired dysfibrinogenaemia in acute and chronic liver disease. *British Journal of Haematology*, **35**, 301.

72 GUILLIN M.-C. & MENACHÉ D. (1973) Fetal fibrinogen and fibrinogen Paris I. Comparative fibrin monomers aggregation studies. *Thrombosis Research*, **3**, 117.

73 SUTTIE J.W. & JACKSON C.M. (1977) Prothrombin structure, activation, and biosynthesis. *Physiological Reviews*, **57**, 1.

74 LECHNER K., NIESSNER H. & THALER E. (1977) Coagulation abnormalities in liver disease. *Seminars in Thrombosis and Hemostasis*, **4**, 40.

75 GREEN G., POLLER L., THOMSON J.M. & DYMOCK I.W. (1976) Factor VII as a marker of hepatocellular synthetic function in liver disease. *Journal of Clinical Pathology*, **29**, 971.

76 GIDDINGS J.C., SHAW E., TUDDENHAM E.G.D. & BLOOM A.L. (1975) The synthesis of factor V in tissue culture and isolated organ perfusion. *Thrombosis et Diathesis Haemorrhagica*, **34**, 321.

77 CEDERBLAD G., KORSAN-BENGTSEN K. & OLSSON R. (1976) Observations of increased levels of blood coagulation factors and other plasma proteins in cholestatic liver disease. *Scandinavian Journal of Gastroenterology*, **11**, 391.

78 SHAW E., GIDDINGS J.C., PEAKE I.R. & BLOOM A.L. (1979) Synthesis of procoagulant factor VIII, factor

VIII related antigen and other coagulation factors by the isolated perfused rat liver. *British Journal of Haematology*, **41**, 585.

79 BLOOM A.L., PEAKE I.R., GIDDINGS J.C., SHEARN S.A.M. & & TUDDENHAM E.G.D. (1976) Endothelial cells and factor-VIII-related protein. *Lancet*, **i**, 46.

80 BENNETT B. & RATNOFF O.D. (1972) Changes in anti hemophilic factor (AHF, factor VIII) procoagulant activity and AHF-like antigen in normal pregnancy, and following exercise and pneumoencephalography. *Journal of Laboratory and Clinical Medicine*, **80**, 256.

81 DENSON K.W.E. (1977) The ratio of factor-VIII-related antigen and factor VIII biological activity as an index of hypercoagulability and intravascular clotting. *Thrombosis Research*, **10**, 107.

82 RAPAPORT S.I. (1961) Plasma thromboplastin antecedent levels in patients receiving coumarin anticoagulants and in patients with Laennec's cirrhosis. *Proceedings of the Society for Experimental Biology and Medicine (New York)*, **108**, 115.

83 MATTII R., AMBRUS J.L., SOKAL J.E. & MINK I. (1964) Production of members of the blood coagulation and fibrinolysin systems by the isolated perfused liver. *Proceedings of the Society for Experimental Biology and Medicine (New York)*, **116**, 69.

84 WALLS W.D. & LOSOWSKY M.S. (1969) Plasma fibrin stabilising factor (FSF) activity in normal subjects and patients with chronic liver disease. *Thrombosis et Diathesis Haemorrhagica*, **21**, 134.

85 CHAN V. & CHAN T.K. (1979) Antithrombin III in fresh and cultured human endothelial cells: a natural anticoagulant from the vascular endothelium. *Thrombosis Research*, **15**, 209.

86 HARPEL P.C. & ROSENBERG R.D. (1976) α_2-Macroglobulin and antithrombin-heparin cofactor: modulators of hemostatic and inflammatory reactions. In: *Progress in Haemostasis and Thrombosis* (ed. Spaet T.H.), Vol. III, p. 145. Grune and Stratton, New York.

87 CHAN V., CHAN T.K., WONG V., TSO S.C. & TODD D. (1979) The determination of antithrombin III by radioimmunoassay and its clinical application. *British Journal of Haematology*, **41**, 563.

88 McFARLANE A.S., TODD D. & CROMWELL S. (1964) Fibrinogen catabolism in humans. *Clinical Science*, **26**, 415.

89 RAKE M.O., FLUTE P.T., PANNELL G. & WILLIAMS R. (1970) Intravascular coagulation in acute hepatic necrosis. *Lancet*, **i**, 533.

90 TYTGAT G.N., COLLEN D. & VERSTRAETE M. (1971) Metabolism of fibrinogen in cirrhosis of the liver. *Journal of Clinical Investigation*, **50**, 1690.

91 CLARK R.D., GAZZARD B.G., LEWIS M.L., FLUTE P.T. & WILLIAMS R. (1975) Fibrinogen metabolism in acute hepatitis and active chronic hepatitis. *British Journal of Haematology*, **30**, 95.

92 VERSTRAETE M., VERMYLEN J. & COLLEN D. (1974) Intravascular coagulation in liver disease. *Annual Review of Medicine*, **25**, 447.

93 COLLEN D. & VERSTRAETE M. (1975) Molecular biology of human plasminogen. II. Metabolism in physiological and some pathological conditions in man. *Thrombosis et Diathesis Haemorrhagica*, **34**, 403.

94 BLOOM A.L. (1975) Intravascular coagulation and the liver. *British Journal of Haematology*, **30**, 1.

95 HILLENBRAND P., PARBHOO S.P., JEDRYCHOWSKI A. & SHERLOCK S. (1974) Significance of intravascular coagulation and fibrinolysis in acute hepatic failure. *Gut*, **15**, 83.

96 OKA K. & TANAKA K. (1979) Intravascular coagulation in autopsy cases with liver diseases. *Thrombosis and Haemostasis*, **42**, 564.

97 RAKE M.O., FLUTE P.T., PANNELL G., SHILKIN K.B. & WILLIAMS R. (1973) Experimental hepatic necrosis: Studies on coagulation abnormalities, plasma clearance, and organ distribution of ^{125}I-labelled fibrinogen. *Gut*, **14**, 574.

98 MÜLLER-BERGHAUS G., REUTER C. & BLEYL U. (1976) Experimental galactosamine-induced hepatitis. *American Journal of Pathology*, **82**, 393.

99 STRAUB P.W. (1977) Diffuse intravascular coagulation in liver disease. *Seminars in Thrombosis and Hemostasis*, **4**, 29.

100 MEILI E.O. & STRAUB P.W. (1970) Elevation of factor VIII in acute fatal liver necrosis. *Thrombosis et Diathesis Haemorrhagica*, **24**, 161.

101 GAZZARD B.G., CLARK R., FLUTE P.T. & WILLIAMS R. (1975) Factor VIII levels during the course of acute hepatitis in a haemophiliac. *Journal of Clinical Pathology*, **28**, 972.

102 BAELE G., MATTHUS E., & BARBIER F. (1977) Antihaemophilic factor A activity, FVIII-related antigen and von Willebrand factor in hepatic cirrhosis. *Acta Haematologica*, **57**, 290.

103 CLARK R., RAKE M.O., FLUTE P.T. & WILLIAMS R. (1973) Coagulation abnormalities in acute liver failure: pathogenetic and therapeutic implications. *Scandinavian Journal of Gastroenterology*, **8** (suppl. 19), 63.

104 GUREVITCH V. & HUTCHINSON E. (1971) Detection of intravascular coagulation by a serial dilution protamine sulphate test. *Annals of Internal Medicine*, **75**, 895.

105 COLEMAN M., FINLAYSON N., BETTIGOLE R.E., SADULA D., COHN M. & PASMANTIER M. (1975) Fibrinogen survival in cirrhosis: improvement by 'low-dose' heparin. *Annals of Internal Medicine*, **83**, 79.

106 DAS P.C. & CASH J.D. (1969) Fibrinolysis at rest and after exercise in hepatic cirrhosis. *British Journal of Haematology*, **17**, 431.

107 MOWAT N.A.G., BRUNT P.W. & OGSTON D. (1974) The fibrinolytic enzyme system in acute and chronic liver injury. *Acta Haematologica*, **52**, 289.

108 FLETCHER A.P., BIEDERMAN O., MOORE D., ALKJAERSIG N. & SHERRY S. (1964) Abnormal plasminogen-plasmin system activity (fibrinolysis) in patients with hepatic cirrhosis: its cause and consequences. *Journal of Clinical Investigation*, **43**, 681.

109 FLUTE P.T., RAKE M.O., WILLIAMS R., SEAMAN M.J. & CALNE R.Y. (1969) Liver transplantation in man. IV. Haemorrhage and thrombosis. *British Medical Journal*, **iii**, 20.

110 THOMAS D.P., REAM V.J. & STUART R.K. (1967) Platelet aggregation in patients with Laennec's cirrhosis of the liver. *New England Journal of Medicine*, **276**, 1344.

111 RUBIN M.H., WESTON M.J., BULLOCK G., ROBERTS J., LANGLEY P.G., WHITE Y.S. & WILLIAMS R. (1977) Abnormal platelet function and ultrastructure in ful-

minant hepatic failure. *Quarterly Journal of Medicine*, **44**, 339.

112 SPECTOR I. & CORN M. (1967) Laboratory tests of hemostasis. The relation to hemorrhage in liver disease. *Archives of Internal Medicine*, **119**, 577.

113 GAZZARD B., PORTMANN B., MURRAY-LYON I.M. & WILLIAMS R. (1975) Causes of death in fulminant hepatic failure and relationship to quantitative histological assessment of parenchymal damage. *Quarterly Journal of Medicine*, **44**, 615.

114 MACDOUGALL B.R.D., BAILEY R.J. & WILLIAMS R. (1977) H₂-receptor antagonists and antacids in the prevention of acute gastrointestinal haemorrhage in fulminant hepatic failure. Two controlled trials. *Lancet*, **i**, 617.

115 BILAND L., DUCKERT F., PRISENDER S. & NYMAN D. (1978) Quantitative estimation of coagulation factors in liver disease. The diagnostic and prognostic value of factor XIII, factor V and plasminogen. *Thrombosis and Haemostasis*, **39**, 646.

116 DYMOCK I.W., TUCKER J.S., WOOLF I.L., POLLER L. & THOMPSON J.M. (1975) Coagulation studies as a prognostic index in acute liver failure. *British Journal of Haematology*, **29**, 385.

117 BICK R.L. (1975) Prothrombin complex concentrates and chronic liver disease. *Thrombosis et Diathesis Haemorrhagica*, **34**, 873.

118 GAZZARD B.G., LEWIS M.L., ASH G., RIZZA C.R., BIDWELL E. & WILLIAMS R. (1974) Coagulation factor concentrate in the treatment of the haemorrhagic diathesis of fulminant hepatic failure. *Gut*, **15**, 993.

119 GROSSI C.E., ROUSSELOT L.M. & PANKE W.F. (1964) Control of fibrinolysis during portacaval shunts. *Journal of the American Medical Association*, **187**, 1005.

120 GAZZARD B.G., CLARK R., BORIRAKCHANYAVAT V. & WILLIAMS R. (1974) A controlled trial of heparin therapy in the coagulation defect of paracetamol-induced hepatic necrosis. *Gut*, **15**, 89.

121 SCHNEIDER C.L. (1959) Etiology of fibrinopenia: fibrination, defibrination. *Annals of the New York Academy of Sciences*, **75**, 634.

122 RODRIGUEZ-ERDMANN F. (1965) Bleeding due to increased intravascular blood coagulation; hemorrhagic syndromes caused by consumption of blood-clotting factors (consumption coagulopathies). *New England Journal of Medicine*, **273**, 1370.

123 McKAY D.G. (1965) *Disseminated Intravascular Coagulation: an Intermediary Mechanism of Disease*. Hoeber Harper, New York.

124 OWEN C.A. JR & BOWIE E.J.W. (1977) Chronic intravascular coagulation and fibrinolysis (ICF) syndromes (DIC). *Seminars in Thrombosis and Hemostasis*, **3**, 268.

125 MERSKEY C., JOHNSON A.J., KLEINER G.J. & WOHL H. (1967) The defibrination syndrome: clinical features and laboratory diagnosis. *British Journal of Haematology*, **13**, 528.

126 MERSKEY C. (1968) Diagnosis and treatment of intravascular coagulation. *British Journal of Haematology*, **15**, 523.

127 NATELSON E.A., LYNCH E.C., HETTIG R.A. & ALFREY C.P. (1970) Acquired factor IX deficiency in the nephrotic syndrome. *Annals of Internal Medicine*, **73**, 373.

128 MÜLLER-BERGHAUS G. (1969) Pathophysiology of disseminated intravascular coagulation. *Thrombosis et Diathesis Haemorrhagica*, **36** (Suppl.), 45.

129 CASH J.D. (1977) Disseminated intravascular coagulation. In: *Recent Advances in Blood Coagulation 2* (ed. Poller L.), p. 293. Churchill-Livingstone, Edinburgh.

130 McKAY D.G., MÜLLER-BERGHAUS G. & CRUSE V. (1969) Activation of Hageman factor by ellagic and the generalized Shwartzman reaction. *American Journal of Pathology*, **54**, 393.

131 EVENSEN S.A. & JEREMIC M. (1970) Platelets and the triggering mechanism of intravascular coagulation. *British Journal of Haematology*, **19**, 33.

132 McGRATH J.M. & STEWART G.J. (1969) The effects of endotoxin on vascular endothelium. *Journal of Experimental Medicine*, **129**, 833.

133 GARG S.K. & NIEMETZ J. (1973) Tissue factor activity of normal and leukemic cells. *Blood*, **42**, 729.

134 RIVERS R.P.A., HATHAWAY W.E. & WESTON W.L. (1975) The endotoxin-induced coagulant activity of human monocytes. *British Journal of Haematology*, **30**, 311.

135 GANS H. & LOWMAN J.T. (1967) The uptake of fibrin and fibrinogen degradation products by the isolated perfused rat liver. *Blood*, **29**, 526.

136 WESSLER S., YIN E.T., GASTON L.W. & NICOL I. (1967) A distinction between the role of precursor and activated forms of clotting factors in the genesis of stasis thrombi. *Thrombosis et Diathesis Haemorrhagica*, **18**, 12.

137 KOWALSKI E. (1968) Fibrinogen derivatives and their biologic activities. *Seminars in Hematology*, **5**, 45.

138 BELLER F.K. & GRAEFF H. (1967) Deposition of glomerular fibrin in the rabbit after infusion with endotoxin. *Nature (London)*, **215**, 295.

139 BEESON P.B. (1947) Effect of reticulo-endothelial blockage on immunity to the Shwartzman phenomenon. *Proceedings of the Society for Experimental Biology and Medicine*, **64**, 146.

140 MARGARETTEN W. & McKAY D.G. (1963) Production of the generalized Shwartzman reaction (GSR) in rats by intravenous infusion of thrombin. *Federation Proceedings*, **22**, 251.

141 THOMAS L. & GOOD R.A. (1952) The effect of cortisone on the Shwartzman reaction; the production of lesions resembling the dermal and generalised Shwartzman reactions by a single injection of bacterial toxin in cortisone-treated rabbits. *Journal of Experimental Medicine*, **95**, 409.

142 McKAY D.G., WONG T. & GALTON M. (1960) Effect of pregnancy on the disseminated thrombosis caused by bacterial endotoxin. *Federation Proceedings*, **19**, 246.

143 CLUFF L.E. & BERTHRONG M. (1953) The inhibition of the local Shwartzman reaction by heparin. *Bulletin of the Johns Hopkins Hospital*, **92**, 353.

144 CORRIGAN J.J. JR (1970) Effect of anticoagulating and non-anticoagulating concentrations of heparin on the generalized Shwartzman reaction. *Thrombosis et Diathesis Haemorrhagica*, **24**, 136.

145 KLIMAN A. & McKAY D.G. (1958) The prevention of the generalised Shwartzman reaction by fibrinolytic activity. *Archives of Pathology*, **66**, 715.

146 PALMERIO C., MING S.C., FRANK E. & FINE J. (1962) The role of the sympathetic nervous system in the gener-

alised Shwartzman reaction. *Journal of Experimental Medicine*, **115**, 609.

147 MÜLLER-BERGHAUS G. & McKAY D.G. (1967) Prevention of the generalised Shwartzman reaction in pregnant rats by α-adrenergic blocking agents. *Laboratory Investigation*, **17**, 276.

148 HARDAWAY R.M. (1970) The significance of coagulative and thrombotic changes after haemorrhage and injury. *Journal of Clinical Pathology*, **23**, Suppl. (Royal College of Pathologists) **4**, 110.

149 MINNA J.D., ROBBOY S.J. & COLMAN R.W. (1974) *Disseminated Intravascular Coagulation in Man.* C. C. Thomas, Springfield, Illinois.

150 AL-MONDHIRY H. (1975) Disseminated intravascular coagulation: experience in a major cancer center. *Thrombosis et Diathesis Haemorrhagica*, **34**, 181.

151 SHARP A.A. (1977) Diagnosis and management of disseminated intravascular coagulation. *British Medical Bulletin*, **33**, 265.

152 SIEGAL T., SELIGSOHN U., AGHAI E. & MODAN M. (1978) Clinical and laboratory aspects of disseminated intravascular coagulation (DIC): a study of 118 cases. *Thrombosis and Haemostasis*, **39**, 122.

153 SPERO J.A., LEWIS J.H. & HASIBA U. (1980) Disseminated intravascular coagulation: findings in 346 patients. *Thrombosis and Haemostasis*, **43**, 28.

154 BRAIN M.C., DACIE J.V. & HOURIHANE D.O'B. (1962) Microangiopathic haemolytic anaemia: the possible role of vascular lesions in pathogenesis. *British Journal of Haematology*, **8**, 358.

155 BRAIN M.C. & HOURIHANE D.O'B. (1967) Microangiopathic haemolytic anaemia: the occurrence of haemolysis in experimentally produced vascular disease. *British Journal of Haematology*, **13**, 135.

156 BULL B.S., RUBENBERG M.L., DACIE J.V. & BRAIN M.C. (1968) Microangiopathic haemolytic anaemia. Mechanisms of red cell fragmentation: *in-vitro* studies. *British Journal of Haematology*, **14**, 643.

157 MARSH G.W. & LEWIS S.M. (1969) Cardiac hemolytic anemia. *Seminars in Hematology*, **6**, 133.

158 KWAAN H.C. (1979) The pathogenesis of thrombotic thrombocytopenic purpura. *Seminars in Thrombosis and Hemostasis*, **5**, 184.

159 SIMPSON J.G. & STALKER A.L. (1973) The concept of disseminated intravascular coagulation. *Clinics in Hematology*, **2**, 189.

160 BLEYL U. (1977) Morphologic diagnosis of disseminated intravascular coagulation: histologic, histochemical and electronmicroscopic studies. *Seminars in Thrombosis and Hemostasis*, **3**, 247.

161 REGOECZI E. & BRAIN M.C. (1969) Organ distribution of fibrin in disseminated intravascular coagulation. *British Journal of Haematology*, **17**, 73.

162 SCHIPPER H.G., JENKINS C.S.P., KAHLE L.H. & TEN CATE J.W. (1978) Antithrombin-III transfusion in disseminated intravascular coagulation. *Lancet*, **i**, 854.

163 DAMUS P.S. & WALLACE G.A. (1975) Immunologic measurement of antithrombin III—heparin cofactor and α2-macroglobulin in disseminated intravascular coagulation and hepatic failure coagulopathy. *Thrombosis Research*, **6**, 27.

164 SHARP A.A., HOWIE B., BIGGS R. & METHUEN D.T. (1958) Defibrination syndrome in pregnancy. Value of various diagnostic tests. *Lancet*, **ii**, 1309.

165 CLAUSS A. (1957) Gerinnungsphysiologische Schnellmethode zur Bestimmung des Fibrinogens. *Acta Haematologica*, **17**, 237.

166 INGRAM G.I.C. (1961) A suggested schedule for the rapid investigation of acute haemostatic failure. *Journal of Clinical Pathology*, **14**, 356.

167 RATNOFF O.D. & MENZIE A.B. (1951) A new method for the determination of fibrinogen in small samples of plasma. *Journal of Laboratory and Clinical Medicine*, **37**, 316.

168 ELLIS B.C. & STRANSKY A. (1961) A quick and accurate method for the determination of fibrinogen in plasma. *Journal of Laboratory and Clinical Medicine*, **58**, 477.

169 BURMESTER H.B.C., AULTON K. & HORSFIELD G.I. (1970) Evaluation of a rapid method for the determination of plasma fibrinogen. *Journal of Clinical Pathology*, **23**, 43.

170 HARKER L.A. & SLICHTER S.J. (1972) Platelet and fibrinogen consumption in man. *New England Journal of Medicine*, **287**, 999.

171 FLUTE P.T. (1964) Assessment of fibrinolytic activity in the blood. *British Medical Bulletin*, **20**, 195.

172 CHAKRABARTI R., BIELAWIEC M., EVANS J.F. & FEARNLEY G.R. (1968) Methodological study and a recommended technique for determining the euglobulin lysis time. *Journal of Clinical Pathology*, **21**, 698.

173 BRAKMAN P., ALBRECHTSEN O.K. & ASTRUP T. (1966) A comparative study of coagulation and fibrinolysis in blood from normal men and women. *British Journal of Haematology*, **12**, 74.

174 BISHOP R., EKERT H., GILCHRIST G., SHANBROM E. & FEKETE L. (1970) The preparation and evaluation of a standardized fibrin plate for the assessment of fibrinolytic activity. *Thrombosis et Diathesis Haemorrhagica*, **23**, 202.

175 HICKMAN J.A. & GORDON-SMITH I.C. (1972) Timed fibrin digestion: a simplified technique for the measurement of the fibrinolytic activity of the blood. *Journal of Clinical Pathology*, **25**, 191.

176 FUNK C., GMÜR J., HEROLD R. & STRAUB P.W. (1971) Reptilase-R—a new reagent in blood coagulation. *British Journal of Haematology*, **21**, 43.

177 ELLMAN L., CARVALHO A. & COLMAN R.W. (1973) The thrombo-wellcotest as a screening test for disseminated intravascular coagulation. *New England Journal of Medicine*, **288**, 633.

178 THOMAS D.P., NIEWIAROWSKI S., MYERS A.R., BLOCH K.J. & COLMAN R.W. (1970) A comparative study of four methods for detecting fibrinogen degradation products (FDP) in patients with various diseases. *New England Journal of Medicine*, **283**, 663.

179 GORDON Y.B., MARTIN M.J., LANDON T. & CHARD T. (1975) The development of radioimmunoassays for fibrinogen degradation products: fragments D and E. *British Journal of Haematology*, **29**, 109.

180 MARDER V.J. & BUDZYNSKI A.Z. (1974) Degradation products of fibrinogen and crosslinked fibrin; projected clinical applications. *Thrombosis et Diathesis Haemorrhagica*, **32**, 49.

181 COLLEN D. & WIMAN B. (1979) Turnover of antiplas-

min, the fast-acting plasmin inhibitor of plasma. *Blood*, **53**, 313.

182 COLLEN D., DECOCK F., CAMBIASCO C.L. & MASSON P. (1977) A latex agglutination test for rapid quantitative estimation of the plasmin-antiplasmin complex in human plasma. *European Journal of Clinical Investigation*, **7**, 21.

183 KWAAN H.C. (1972) Disorders of fibrinolysis. *Medical Clinics of North America*, **56**, 163.

184 RATNOFF O.D. (1952) Studies on a proteolytic enzyme in human plasma. VII. A fatal hemorrhagic state associated with excessive plasma proteolytic activity in a patient undergoing surgery for carcinoma of the head of the pancreas. *Journal of Clinical Investigation*, **31**, 521.

185 BICK R.L. (1976) Alterations of hemostasis associated with cardiopulmonary bypass: pathophysiology, prevention, diagnosis and management. *Seminars in Thrombosis and Hemostasis*, **3**, 59.

186 LIPINSKI B., WEGRZYNOWICZ Z., BUDZYNSKI A.Z., KOPÉC M., LATALLO Z.S. & KOWALSKI E. (1967) Soluble unclottable complexes formed in the presence of fibrinogen degradation products (FDP) during the fibrinogen-fibrin conversion and their potential significance in pathology. *Thrombosis et Diathesis Haemorrhagica*, **17**, 65.

187 MOSESSON M.W. & AMRANI D.L. (1980) The structure and biologic activities of plasma fibronectin. *Blood*, **56**, 145.

188 LIPINSKI B. & WOROWSKI K. (1968) Detection of soluble fibrin monomer complexes in blood by means of protamine sulphate test. *Thrombosis et Diathesis Haemorrhagica*, **20**, 44.

189 BREEN F.A. JR & TULLIS J.L. (1968) Ethanol gelation: a rapid screening test for intravascular coagulation. *Annals of Internal Medicine*, **69**, 1197.

190 NIEWIAROWSKI S. & GUREVICH V. (1971) Laboratory identification of intravascular coagulation. The serial dilution protamine sulphate test for the detection of fibrin monomer and fibrin degradation products. *Journal of Laboratory and Clinical Medicine*, **77**, 665.

191 REGOECZI E. (1971) Iodine-labelled fibrinogen: a review. *British Journal of Haematology*, **20**, 649.

192 DAVIES J.W.L., RICKETTS C.R. & BULL J.P. (1966) Studies of plasma protein metabolism. III. Fibrinogen in burned patients. *Clinical Science*, **30**, 305.

193 HICKMAN J.A. (1971) A study of the metabolism of fibrinogen after surgical operations. *Clinical Science*, **41**, 141.

194 BAKER L.R.I., RUBENBERG M.L., DACIE J.V. & BRAIN M.C. (1968) Fibrinogen catabolism in microangiopathic haemolytic anaemia. *British Journal of Haematology*, **14**, 617.

195 BONNAR J. (1973) Blood coagulation and fibrinolysis in obstetrics. *Clinics in Hematology*, **2**, 213.

196 BONNAR J., PRENTICE C.R.M., MCNICOL G.P. & DOUGLAS A.S. (1970) Haemostatic mechanism in the uterine circulation during placental separation. *British Medical Journal*, **ii**, 564.

197 VERSTRAETE M. & VERMYLEN J. (1968) Acute and chronic 'defibrination' in obstetrical practice. *Thrombosis et Diathesis Haemorrhagica*, **20**, 444.

198 BONNAR J. (1977) Acute and chronic coagulation problems in pregnancy. In: *Recent Advances in Blood Coagulation 2* (ed. Poller L.), p. 363. Churchill-Livingstone, Edinburgh.

199 PIRANI C.L., POLLAK V.E., LANNIGAN R. & FOLLI G. (1963) The renal glomerular lesions of pre-eclampsia: electron microscopic studies. *American Journal of Obstetrics and Gynecology*, **87**, 1047.

200 MORRIS R.H., VASSALI P., BELLER F.K. & McCLUSKEY R.T. (1964) Immunofluorescent studies of renal biopsies in the diagnosis of toxemia of pregnancy. *Obstetrics and Gynecology*, **24**, 32.

201 McKAY D.G., MERRILL S.J., WEINER A.E., HERTIG A.T. & REID D.E. (1953) The pathologic anatomy of eclampsia, bilateral renal cortical necrosis, pituitary necrosis, and other fatal complications of pregnancy, and its possible relationship to the generalised Shwartzman phenomenon. *American Journal of Obstetrics and Gynecology*, **66**, 507.

202 HENDERSON A.H., PUGSLEY D.J. & THOMAS D.P. (1970) Fibrin degradation products in pre-eclamptic toxaemia and eclampsia. *British Medical Journal*, **iii**, 545.

203 PRESTON F.E., MALIA R.G., TIPTON R.H. & SMITH A.J. (1972) Intravascular coagulation and pre-eclamptic toxaemia. *Lancet*, **i**, 34.

204 ROBERTS J.T., DAVIES A.J. & BLOOM A.L. (1966) Coagulation studies in massive pulmonary haemorrhage of the newborn. *Journal of Clinical Pathology*, **19**, 334.

205 BOYD J.F. (1969) Disseminated fibrin thromboembolism among neonates dying more than 48 hours after birth. *Journal of Clinical Pathology*, **22**, 663.

206 HEY E. & JONES P. (1979) Coagulation failure in babies with rhesus isoimmunization. *British Journal of Haematology*, **42**, 441.

207 HATHAWAY W.E., MULL M.M. & PECHET G.S. (1969) Disseminated intravascular coagulation in the newborn. *Pediatrics*, **43**, 233.

208 SHARP A.A. & EGGLETON M.J. (1963) Haematology and the extracorporeal circulation. *Journal of Clinical Pathology*, **16**, 551.

209 FLUTE P.T. (1970) Coagulation and fibrinolysis after injury. *Journal of Clinical Pathology*, **23**, Suppl. 4 (Royal College of Pathologists), 102.

210 MEHTA B., BRIGGS D.K., SOMMERS S.C. & KARPATKIN M. (1972) Disseminated intravascular coagulation following cardiac arrest: a study of 15 patients. *American Journal of Medical Science*, **264**, 353.

211 McKAY D.G. & HARDAWAY R.M. (1959) Alterations in the hemostatic mechanism in the experimental crush syndrome. *Laboratory Investigation*, **8**, 979.

212 WEBER M.B. & BLAKELY J.A. (1969) The haemorrhagic diathesis of heat stroke. A consumption coagulopathy successfully treated with heparin. *Lancet*, **i**, 1190.

213 GOODNIGHT S.H., KENOYER G., RAPAPORT S.I., PATCH M.J., LEE J.A. & KURZE T. (1974) Defibrination after brain-tissue destruction: a serious complication of head injury. *New England Journal of Medicine*, **290**, 1043.

214 INGRAM G.I.C. (1965) The bleeding complications of blood transfusion. *Transfusion*, **5**, 1.

215 McKAY D.G. & MARGARETTEN W. (1967) Disseminated intravascular coagulation in virus diseases. *Archives of Internal Medicine*, **120**, 129.

216 CORRIGAN J.J., JR, JORDAN C.M. & BENNETT B.B. (1973) Disseminated intravascular coagulation in septic shock:

Report of three cases not treated with heparin. *American Journal of Diseases of Children*, **126**, 629.

217 RUBENBERG M.L., BAKER L.R.I., MCBRIDE J.A., SEVITT L.H. & BRAIN M.C. (1967) Intravascular coagulation in a case of Clostridium perfringens septicaemia: treatment by exchange transfusion and heparin. *British Medical Journal*, **iv**, 271.

218 GÉRARD P., MORIAU M., BACHY A., MALVAUX P. & DEMEYER R. (1973) Meningococcal purpura: report of 19 patients treated with heparin. *Journal of Pediatrics*, **82**, 780.

219 REID H.A. (1975) Adjuvant treatment of severe falciparum malaria, intravascular coagulation, and heparin. *Lancet*, **i**, 167.

220 RICHARDSON S.G.N., MATTHEWS K.B., CRUICKSHANK J.K., GEDDES A.M. & STUART J. (1979) Coagulation activation and hyperviscosity in infection. *British Journal of Haematology*, **42**, 469.

221 NEAME P.B., KELTON J.G., WALKER I.R., STEWART I.O., NOSSEL H.L. & HIRSH J. (1980) Thrombocytopenia in septicemia: the role of disseminated intravascular coagulation. *Blood*, **56**, 88.

222 TAGNON H.J., WHITMORE W.F. JR & SHULMAN N.R. (1952) Fibrinolysis in metastatic cancer of the prostate. *Cancer (Philadelphia)*, **5**, 9.

223 MCKAY D.G., MANSELL H. & HERTIG A.T. (1953) Carcinoma of the body of the pancreas with fibrin thrombosis and fibrinogenopenia. *Cancer (Philadelphia)*, **6**, 862.

224 MCKAY D.G. & WAHLE G.H. JR (1955) Disseminated thrombosis in colon cancer. *Cancer (Philadelphia)*, **8**, 970.

225 MCKAY D.G., HASSETT A. & FENNELL R.H. JR (1955) Renal capillary thrombosis in a post-partum patient with squamous cell carcinoma of the cervix. *Obstetrics and Gynecology*, **5**, 341.

226 ROSENTHAL R.L. (1963) Acute promyelocytic leukemia associated with hypofibrinogenemia. *Blood*, **21**, 495.

227 PITNEY W.R. (1971) Disseminated intravascular coagulation. *Seminars in Hematology*, **8**, 65.

228 RODEGHIERO F., BARBUI T., BATTISTA R., CHISESI T., RIGONI G. & DINI E. (1980) Molecular subunits and transamidase activity of factor XIII during disseminated intravascular coagulation in acute leukaemia. *Thrombosis and Haemostasis*, **43**, 6.

229 QUICK A.J. (1960) Influence of erythrocytes on the coagulation of blood. *American Journal of the Medical Sciences*, **239**, 51.

230 HARDAWAY R.M., MCKAY D.G., WAHLE G.H. JR, TARTOCK D.E. & EDELSTEIN R. (1956) Pathologic study of intravascular coagulation following incompatible blood transfusion in dogs. I. Intravenous injection of incompatible blood. *American Journal of Surgery*, **91**, 24.

231 RABINER S.F. & FRIEDMAN L.H. (1968) The role of intravascular haemolysis and the reticuloendothelial system in the production of a hypercoagulable state. *British Journal of Haematology*, **14**, 105.

232 ROCK R.C., BOVE J.R. & NEMERSON Y. (1969) Heparin treatment of intravascular coagulation accompanying haemolytic transfusion reactions. *Transfusion*, **9**, 57.

233 DENNIS L.H., EICHELBERGER J.W., INMAN M.M. & CONRAD M.E. (1967) Depletion of coagulation factors in drug-resistant Plasmodium falciparum malaria. *Blood*, **29**, 713.

234 REID H.A. & NKRUMAH F.K. (1972) Fibrin-degradation products in cerebral malaria. *Lancet*, **i**, 218.

235 CASPER J. & SHULMAN J. (1956) Bilateral cortical necrosis of the kidneys in an infant with favism. *American Journal of Clinical Pathology*, **26**, 42.

236 MAHMOOD A., MACKINTOSH D.M. & SHAPER A.G. (1967) Fibrinolytic activity in the clinical crisis of sickle-cell anaemia. *British Medical Journal*, **iii**, 653.

237 RICHARDSON S.G.N., MATTHEWS K.B., STUART J., GEDDES A.M. & WILCOX R.M. (1979) Serial changes in coagulation and viscosity during sickle cell crisis. *British Journal of Haematology*, **41**, 95.

238 CLARKSON A.R., MACDONALD M.K., FUSTER V., CASH J.D. & ROBSON J.S. (1970) Glomerular coagulation in acute ischaemic renal failure. *Quarterly Journal of Medicine*, **39**, 585.

239 ROBSON J.S., MARTIN A.M., RUCKLEY V.A. & MACDONALD M.K. (1968) Irreversible post-partum renal failure. A new syndrome. *Quarterly Journal of Medicine*, **37**, 423.

240 CLARKSON A.R., MACDONALD M.K., PETRIE J.J.B., CASH J.D. & ROBSON J.S. (1971) Serum and urinary fibrin/fibrinogen degradation products in glomerulonephritis. *British Medical Journal*, **iii**, 447.

241 CLARKSON A.R., LAWRENCE J.R., MEADOWS R. & SEYMOUR A.E. (1970) The haemolytic uraemic syndrome in adults. *Quarterly Journal of Medicine*, **39**, 227.

242 BRAIN M.C. (1969) The hemolytic-uremic syndrome. *Seminars in Hematology*, **6**, 162.

243 NALBANDIAN R.M., HENRY R.L. & BICK R.L. (1979) Thrombotic thrombocytopenic purpura: an extended editorial. *Seminars in Thrombosis and Hemostasis*, **5**, 216.

244 MOSCHOWITZ E. (1925) An acute febrile pleiochromic anaemia with hyaline thrombosis of the terminal arterioles and capillaries. An undescribed disease. *Archives of Internal Medicine*, **36**, 89.

245 SYMMERS W.ST.C. (1952) Thrombotic microangiopathic haemolytic anaemia (thrombotic microangiopathy). *British Medical Journal*, **ii**, 897.

246 AMOROSI E.L. & ULTMANN J.E. (1966) Thrombotic thrombocytopenic purpura: report of 16 cases and review of the literature. *Medicine (Baltimore)*, **45**, 139.

247 ORBISON J.L. (1952) Morphology of thrombotic thrombocytopenic purpura with demonstration of aneurysms. *American Journal of Pathology*, **28**, 129.

248 GORE I. (1950) Disseminated arteriolar and capillary platelet thrombosis: a morphological study of its histogenesis. *American Journal of Pathology*, **26**, 155.

249 BYRNES J.J. & LIAN E.C.Y. (1979) Recent therapeutic advances in thrombotic thrombocytopenic purpura. *Seminars in Thrombosis and Hemostasis*, **5**, 199.

250 CUTTNER J. (1980) Thrombotic thrombocytopenic purpura: a ten-year experience. *Blood*, **56**, 302.

251 BLOMBÄCK M., JOHANSSON S.-A. & SJÖBERG H.-E. (1967) Coagulation factors and defibrinogen syndrome in anaphylaxis. *Acta Physiologica Scandinavica*, **69**, 313.

252 CLARKSON A.R., MORTON J.B. & CASH J.D. (1970) Urinary fibrin/fibrinogen degradation products after renal homotransplantation. *Lancet*, **ii**, 1220.

253 HJORT P.F., RAPAPORT S.I. & JORGENSEN L. (1964)

Purpura fulminans. Report of a case successfully treated with heparin and hydrocortisone. Review of 50 cases from the literature. *Scandinavian Journal of Haematology*, **1**, 169.

254 ANTLEY R.M. & MCMILLAN C.W. (1967) Sequential coagulation studies in purpura fulminans. *New England Journal of Medicine*, **276**, 1287.

255 DUDGEON D.L., GILCHRIST G.S. & WOOLLEY M.M. (1971) Purpura fulminans *Archives of Surgery*, **103**, 351.

256 KASABACH H.H. & MERRITT K.K. (1940) Capillary hemangioma with extensive purpura. *American Journal of Diseases of Children*, **59**, 1063.

257 DE VRIES A. & COHEN I. (1969) Haemorrhagic and blood coagulation disturbing action of snake venoms. In: *Recent Advances in Blood Coagulation* (ed. Poller L.), p. 277. Churchill, London.

258 AROCHA-PINANGO C.L. & LAYRISSE M. (1969) Fibrinolysis produced by contact with a caterpillar. *Lancet*, i, 810.

259 REID H.A. & CHAN H.E. (1968) The paradox in therapeutic defibrination. *Lancet*, i, 485.

260 EWART M.R., HATTON M., BASFORD J.M. & DODGSON K.S. (1969) The proteolytic action of Arvin on human fibrinogen. *Biochemical Journal*, **115**, 17.

261 BELL W.R., BOLTON G. & PITNEY W.R. The effect of Arvin on blood coagulation factors. *British Journal of Haematology*, **15**, 589.

262 KAKKAR V.V., FLANC C., HOWE C.T., O'SHEA M. & FLUTE P.T. (1969) Treatment of deep vein thrombosis. A trial of heparin, streptokinase, and Arvin. *British Medical Journal*, i, 806.

263 SHARP A.A., WARREN B.A., PAXTON A.M. & ALLINGTON M.J. (1968) Anticoagulant therapy with a purified fraction of Malayan pit viper venom. *Lancet*, i, 493.

264 PITNEY W.R., BRAY C., HOLT P.J.L. & BOLTON G. (1969) Acquired resistance to treatment with Arvin. *Lancet*, i, 79.

265 HOWIE P.W., PRENTICE C.R.M. & FORBES C.D. (1975) Failure of heparin therapy to affect the clinical courses of severe pre-eclampsia. *British Journal of Obstetrics and Gynaecology*, **82**, 711.

266 CORRIGAN J.J., RAY W.L. & MAY N. (1968) Changes in the blood coagulation system associated with septicemia. *New England Journal of Medicine*, **279**, 851.

267 DENNIS L.H., REISBERG B.E., CROSBIE J., GROZIER D. & CONRAD M.E. (1969) The original haemorrhagic fever: yellow fever. *British Journal of Haematology*, **17**, 455.

268 GAGEL C.H., LINDER M., MÜLLER-BERGHAUS G. & LASCH H.G. (1970) Virus infection and blood coagulation. *Thrombosis et Diathesis Haemorrhagica*, **23**, 1.

269 KATZ J., LURIE A. & KAPLAN B. (1969) Haemolyticuraemic syndrome and heparin therapy. *Lancet*, ii, 700.

270 MONCRIEFF M.W. & GLASGOW E.F. (1970) Haemolyticuraemic syndrome treated with heparin. *British Medical Journal*, iii, 188.

271 WARRELL D.A. POPE H.M. & PRENTICE C.R.M. (1976) Disseminated intravascular coagulation caused by the Carpet Viper (*Echis carinatus*): trial of heparin. *British Journal of Haematology*, **33**, 335.

272 RATNOFF O.D. (1969) Epsilon-aminocaproic acid: a dangerous weapon. *New England Journal of Medicine*, **280**, 1124.

273 MARGOLIUS A. JR, JACKSON D.P. & RATNOFF O.D. (1961) Circulating anticoagulants. A study of 40 cases and a review of the literature. *Medicine*, **40**, 145.

274 SHAPIRO S.S. & HULTIN M. (1975) Acquired inhibitors to the blood coagulation factors. *Seminars in Thrombosis and Hemostasis*, **1**, 336.

275 BIGGS R. (1974) Jaundice and antibodies directed against factor VIII and IX in patients treated for haemophilia or Christmas disease in the United Kingdom. *British Journal of Haematology*, **26**, 313.

276 SHAPIRO S.S. (1979) Antibodies to blood coagulation factors. *Clinics in Hematology*, **8**, 207.

277 HARMON M.C., ZIPURSKY A. & LAHEY M.E. (1957) A study of hemophilia. *America Journal of Diseases in Children*, **93**, 375.

278 BIGGS R., AUSTEN D.E.G., DENSON K.W.E., RIZZA C.R. & BORRETT R. (1972) The mode of action of antibodies which destroy factor VIII. I. Antibodies which have second-order concentration graphs. *British Journal of Haematology*, **23**, 125.

279 BIGGS R., AUSTEN D.E.G., DENSON K.W.E., BORRETT R. & RIZZA C.R. (1972) The mode of action of antibodies which destroy factor VIII. II. Antibodies which give complex concentration graphs. *British Journal of Haematology*, **23**, 137.

280 BLOOM A.L., DAVIES A.J. & REES J.K. (1966) A clinical and laboratory study of a patient with an unusual factor VIII inhibitor. *Thrombosis et Diathesis Haemorrhagica*, **15**, 12.

281 KOUTTS J., MEYER D., RICKARD K., STOTT L. & FIRKIN B.G. (1975) Heterogeneity in biological activity of human factor VIII antibodies. *British Journal of Haematology*, **29**, 99.

282 MAZURIER C., KACEM M., PARQUET-GERNEZ A. & GOUDEMAND M. (1977) Action of insolubilized homologous anti-factor VIII antibodies on factor-VIII related antigen. *Thrombosis Research*, **10**, 661.

283 MANNUCCI P.M., MEYER D., RUGGERI Z.M., KOUTTS J., CIAVARELLA N. & LAVERGNE J.-M. (1976) Precipitating antibodies in von Willebrand's disease. *Nature (London)*, **262**, 141.

284 INGRAM G.I.C., KINGSTON P.J., LESLIE J. & BOWIE E.J.W. (1971) Four cases of acquired von Willebrand's syndrome. *British Journal of Haematology*, **21**, 189.

285 HANDIN R.I., MARTIN V. & MOLONEY W.C. (1976) Antibody-induced von Willebrand's disease. A newly defined inhibitor syndrome. *Blood*, **48**, 393.

286 VELTKAMP J.J., STEVENS P., PLAS M.V.D. & LOELIGER E.A. (1970) Production site of bleeding factor. Acquired morbus von Willebrand. *Thrombosis et Diathesis Haemorrhagica*, **23**, 412.

287 GOUAULT-HEILMANN M., DUMONT M.D., INTRATOR L., CHENAL C. & LEJONC J.L. (1979) Acquired von Willebrand's syndrome with IgM inhibitor against von Willebrand's factor. *Journal of Clinical Pathology*, **32**, 1030.

288 SHAPIRO S.S. (1967) The immunologic character of acquired inhibitors of antihemophilic globulin (FVIII) and the kinetics of their interaction with factor VIII. *Journal of Clinical Investigation*, **46**, 147.

289 FEINSTEIN D.I., RAPAPORT S.I. & CHONG M.N.Y. (1969) Immunologic characterization of 12 factor VIII inhibitors. *Blood*, **34**, 85.

290 CASTALDI P.A. & PENNY R. (1970) A macroglobulin

with inhibitory activity against coagulation factor VIII. *Blood*, **35**, 370.

291 GLUECK H.I. & HONG R. (1965) A circulating anti-coagulant in γ₁A multiple myeloma: its modification by penicillin. *Journal of Clinical Investigation*, **44**, 1866.

292 LUSHER J.M., SHUSTER J., EVANS R.K. & POULIK M.D. (1968) Antibody nature of an AHG (factor VIII) inhibitor. *Journal of Pediatrics*, **72**, 325.

293 ROBBOY S.J., LEWIS E.J., SCHUR P.H. & COLMAN R.W. (1970) Circulating anticoagulants to factor VIII. *American Journal of Medicine*, **49**, 742.

294 FROMMEL D. & ALLAIN J.-P. (1977) Genetic predisposition to develop factor VIII antibody in classic haemophilia. *Clinical Immunology and Immunopathology*, **8**, 34.

295 RIZZA C.R. & BIGGS R. (1973) The treatment of patients who have factor-VIII antibodies. *British Journal of Haematology*, **24**, 65.

296 KASPER C.K., ALEDORT L.M., COUNTS R.B., EDSON J.R., FRATANTONI J., GREEN D., HAMPTON J.W., HILGARTNER M.W., LAZERSON J., LEVINE P.M., McMILLAN C.W., POOL J.G., SHAPIRO S.S., SHULMAN N.R. & van EYS J. (1975) A more uniform measurement of factor VIII inhibitors. *Thrombosis et Diathesis Haemorrhagica*, **34**, 869.

297 ALLAIN J.-P. & FROMMEL D. (1976) Antibodies for factor VIII. V. Patterns of immune response to factor VIII in haemophilia A. *Blood*, **47**, 973.

298 BLOOM A.L. (1978) Clotting factor concentrates for resistant haemophilia. *British Journal of Haematology*, **40**, 21.

299 BLATT P.M., WHITE G.C.II, McMILLAN C.W. & ROBERTS H.R. (1977) Treatment of anti-factor VIII antibodies. *Thrombosis and Haemostasis*, **38**, 514.

300 BUCHANAN G.R. & KEVY S.V. (1978) Use of prothrombin complex concentrates in hemophiliacs with inhibitors: clinical and laboratory studies. *Pediatrics*, **62**, 767.

301 KELLY P. & PENNER J.A. (1976) Management of anti-hemophilic factor inhibitors: management with prothrombin complex concentrates. *Journal of the American Medical Association*, **236**, 2061.

302 LUSHER J.M., SHAPIRO S.S., PALASCAK J.E., RAO A.V., LEVINE P.H., BLATT P.M. & THE HEMOPHILIA STUDY GROUP (1980) Efficacy of prothrombin-complex concentrates in hemophiliacs with antibodies to factor VIII: a multicenter therapeutic trial. *New England Journal of Medicine*, **303**, 421.

303 SHERMAN L.A., GOLDSTEIN M.A. & SISE H.S. (1969) Circulating anticoagulant (anti factor VIII) treated with immunosuppressive drugs. *Thrombosis et Diathesis Haemorrhagica*, **21**, 249.

304 HULTIN M.B., SHAPIRO S.S., BOWMAN H.S., GILL F.M., ANDREWS A.T., MARTINEZ J., EYSTER M.E. & SHERWOOD W.C. (1976) Immunosuppressive therapy of factor VIII inhibitors. *Blood*, **48**, 95.

305 NILSSON I.M. & HEDNER U. (1976) Immunosuppressive treatment in haemophiliacs with inhibitors to factor VIII and factor IX. *Scandinanvian Journal of Haematology*, **16**, 369.

306 BLOOM A.L. & HUTTON R.D. (1975) Fresh platelet transfusions in haemophiliac patients with factor-VIII antibody. *Lancet*, **ii**, 369.

307 COBCROFT R., TAMAGNINI G. & DORMANDY K.M. (1977) Serial plasmapheresis in a haemophiliac with antibodies to factor VIII. *Journal of Clinical Pathology*, **30**, 763.

308 KELLER A.J., CHIRNSIDE A. & URBANIAK S.J. (1979) Coagulation abnormalities produced by plasma exchange on the cell separator with special reference to fibrinogen and platelet levels. *British Journal of Haematology*, **42**, 593.

309 KASPER C.K. & FEINSTEIN D.I. (1976) Rising factor VIII inhibitor titres after Konyne factor IX complex. *New England Journal of Medicine*, **295**, 505.

310 HARDISTY R.M. (1962) A naturally occurring inhibitor of Christmas factor (factor IX). *Thrombosis et Diathesis Haemorrhagica*, **8**, 67.

311 GEORGE J.N., MILLER G.M. & BRECKENRIDGE R.T. (1971) Studies on Christmas disease: investigation and treatment of a familial acquired inhibitor of Factor IX. *British Journal of Haematology*, **21**, 333.

312 FRICK P.G. (1953) Hemophilia-like disease following pregnancy with transplacental transfer of an acquired circulating anticoagulant. *Blood*, **8**, 598.

313 FEINSTEIN D.I., RAPAPORT S.I., McGEHEE W.G. & PATCH M.J. (1967) Biochemical and immunological properties of an acquired inhibitor of factor V. *Blood*, **30**, 863.

314 LANE T.A., SHAPIRO S.S. & BURKA E.R. (1978) Factor V antibody and disseminated intravascular coagulation. *Annals of Internal Medicine*, **89**, 182.

315 FEINSTEIN D.I. (1978) Acquired inhibitors of factor V. *Thrombosis and Haemostasis*, **39**, 663.

316 JOSEPHSON A.M. & LISKER R. (1958) Demonstration of a circulating anticoagulant in plasma thromboplastin antecedent deficiency. *Journal of Clinical Investigation*, **37**, 148.

317 LEONE G., ACCORRA F. & BONI P. (1977) Circulating anticoagulant against factor XI and thrombocytopenia with platelet aggregation inhibition in systemic lupus erythematosus. *Acta Haematologica*, **58**, 240.

318 GANDOLFO G.M., AFELTRA A., AMOROSO A., BIANCOLELLA F. & FERRI G.M. (1977) Circulating anticoagulant against factor XII and platelet antibodies in systemic lupus erythematosus. *Acta Haematologica*, **57**, 135.

319 GRAHAM J.E., YOUNT W.J. & ROBERTS H.R. (1973) Immunochemical characterization of a human antibody to factor XIII. *Blood*, **41**, 661.

320 MILNER G.R., HOLT P.J.L., BOTTOMLEY J. & MacIVER J.E. (1977) Practolol therapy associated with a systemic lupus erythematosus-like syndrome and an inhibitor to factor XIII. *Journal of Clinical Pathology*, **30**, 770.

321 ROSENBERG R.D., COLMAN R.W. & LORAND L. (1974) A new haemorrhagic disorder with defective fibrin stabilisation and cryofibrinogenaemia. *British Journal of Haematology*, **26**, 269.

322 de VRIES A., ROSENBERG T., KOCHWA S. & BOSS J.H. (1961) Precipitating antifibrinogen antibody appearing after fibrinogen infusions in a patient with congenital afibrinogenemia. *American Journal of Medicine*, **30**, 486.

323 MAMMEN E.F., SCHMIDT K.P. & BARNHART M.I. (1967) Thrombophlebitis migrans associated with circulating antibodies against fibrinogen. *Thrombosis et Diathesis Haemorrhagica*, **18**, 605.

324 MARCINIAK E. & GREENWOOD M.F. (1979) Acquired

coagulation inhibitor delaying fibrinopeptide release. *Blood*, **53**, 81.

325 REGAN M.G., LACKNER H. & KARPATKIN S. (1974) Platelet function and coagulation profile in lupus erythematosus. *Annals of Internal Medicine*, **81**, 462.

326 LECHNER K. (1974) Acquired inhibitors in non-haemophilic patients. *Haemostasis*, **3**, 65.

327 HOUGIE C. (1964) Naturally occurring species specific inhibitor of human prothrombin in lupus erythematosus. *Proceedings of the Society for Experimental Biology and Medicine*, **116**, 359.

328 YIN E.T. & GASTON K.W. (1965) Purification and kinetic studies on a circulating anticoagulant in a suspected case of lupus erythematosus. *Thrombosis et Diathesis Haemorrhagica*, **14**, 88.

329 FEINSTEIN D.I. & RAPAPORT S.I. (1972) Acquired inhibitors of blood coagulation. *Progress in Thrombosis and Hemostasis*, **1**, 75.

330 CONLEY C.L. & HARTMANN R.C. (1952) A hemorrhagic disorder caused by circulating anticoagulant in patients with disseminated lupus erythematosus. *Journal of Clinical Investigation*, **31**, 621.

331 SCHLEIDER M.A., NACHMAN R.L., JAFFE E.A., & COLEMAN M. (1976) A clinical study of the lupus anticoagulant. *Blood*, **48**, 499.

332 EXNER T., BARBER S., KRONENBERG H. & RICKARD K.A. (1980) Familial association of the lupus anticoagulant. *British Journal of Haematology*, **45**, 89.

333 MUEH J.R., HERBST K.D. & RAPAPORT S.I. (1980) Thrombosis in patients with the lupus anticoagulant. *Annals of Internal Medicine*, **92**, 156.

334 ZARRABI M.H., ZUCKER S., MILLER F., DERMAN R.M., ROMANO G.S., HARTNETT J.A. & VARMA A.O. (1979) Immunologic and coagulation disorders in chlorpromazine treated patients. *Annals of Internal Medicine*, **91**, 194.

335 BELL W.R., BOSS G.R. & WOLFSON J.S. (1977) Circulating anticoagulant in the procainamide-induced lupus syndrome. *Archives of Internal Medicine*, **137**, 147.

336 MANNUCCI P.M., CANCIANI M.T., MARI D. & MEUCCI P. (1979) The varied sensitivity of partial thromboplastin and prothrombin time reagents in the demonstration of the lupus-like anticoagulant. *Scandinavian Journal of Haematology*, **22**, 423.

337 BOWIE E.J.W., THOMPSON J.H., PASCUZZI C.A. & OWEN C.A. JR (1963) Thrombosis in systemic lupus erythematosus despite circulating anticoagulants. *Journal of Laboratory and Clinical Medicine*, **62**, 416.

338 FAHEY J.L. (1963) Serum protein disorders causing clinical symptoms in malignant neoplastic disease. *Journal of Chronic Disease*, **16**, 703.

339 PACHTER M.R., JOHNSON S.A. & BASINSKI D.H. (1959) The effect of macroglobulins and their dissociation units on release of platelet factor 3. *Thrombosis et Diathesis Haemorrhagica*, **3**, 501.

340 LACKNER H., HUNT V., ZUCKER M.B. & PEARSON J. (1970) Abnormal fibrin ultrastructure polymerization and clot retraction in multiple myeloma. *British Journal of Haematology*, **18**, 625.

341 LACKNER H. (1973) Hemostatic abnormalities associated with dysproteinemias. *Seminars in Hematology*, **10**, 125.

342 PENNY R., CASTALDI P.A. & WHITSED H.M. (1971) Inflammation and haemostasis in paraproteinaemias. *British Journal of Haematology*, **20**, 35.

343 BRODY J.I., HAIDAR M.E. & ROSSMAN R.E. (1979) A hemorrhagic syndrome in Waldenström's macroglobulinemia secondary to immunoabsorption of factor VIII. *New England Journal of Medicine*, **300**, 408.

344 COOPER M.R., COHEN H.J., HUNTLEY C.C., WAITE B.M., SPEES L. & SPURR C.L. (1974) A monoclonal IgM with antibody-like specificity for phospholipids in a patient with lymphoma. *Blood*, **43**, 493.

345 COLEMAN M., VIGLIANO E.M., WEKSLER M.E. & NACHMAN R.L. (1972) Inhibition of fibrin monomer polymerization by lambda myeloma globulins. *Blood*, **39**, 210.

346 LOELIGER E.A. & HERS J.F. PH. (1957) Chronic antithrombinaemia (antithrombin V) with haemorrhagic diathesis in a case of rheumatoid arthritis with hypergammaglobulinaemia. *Thrombosis et Diathesis Haemorrhagica*, **1**, 499.

347 PERKINS H.A., MACKENZIE M.R. & FUDENBERG H.H. (1970) Hemostatic defects in dysproteinemias. *Blood*, **35**, 695.

348 GALBRAITH P.A., SHARMA N., PARKER W.L. & KILGOUR J.M. (1974) Acquired factor X deficiency: altered plasma antithrombin activity and association with amyloidosis. *Journal of the American Medical Association*, **230**, 1658.

349 KORSAN-BENGSTEN K., HJORT P.F. & YGGE J. (1962) Acquired factor X deficiency in a patient with amyloidosis. *Thrombosis et Diathesis Haemorrhagica*, **7**, 558.

350 FURIE B., GREENE E. & FURIE B.C. (1977) Syndrome of acquired factor X deficiency and systemic amyloidosis: in vivo studies of the metabolic fate of factor X. *New England Journal of Medicine*, **297**, 81.

351 GREIPP P.R., KYLE R.A. & BOWIE E.J.W. (1979) Factor X deficiency in primary amyloidosis. Resolution after splenectomy. *New England Journal of Medicine*, **301**, 1050.

352 BAYER W.L., CURIEL D., SZETO I.L.F. & LEWIS J.H. (1969) Acquired factor X deficiency in a negro boy. *Pediatrics*, **44**, 1007.

353 PINKHAS J., COHEN I., KRUGLAK J. & DE VRIES A. (1972) Hobby-induced factor VII deficiency. *Haemostasis*, **1**, 52.

354 KARPATKIN S., INGRAM G.I.C. & GRAHAM J.B. (1962) Severe isolated prothrombin deficiency: an acquired state with complete recovery. *Thrombosis et Diathesis Haemorrhagica*, **8**, 221.

355 BOKIAN B.F. & SAWITSKY A. (1976) Factor IX deficiency in Gaucher's disease. *Archives of Internal Medicine*, **136**, 489.

356 THOMSON C., FORBES C.D., PRENTICE C.R.M. & KENNEDY A.C. (1974) Changes in blood coagulation and fibrinolysis in the nephrotic syndrome. *Quarterly Journal of Medicine*, **43**, 399.

357 BETTIGOLE R.E., HIMELSTREIN E.S., OETTGEN H.F. & CLIFFORD G.O. (1969) Hypofibrinogenemia due to L-asparaginase: studies using ^{131}I-fibrinogen. *Clinical Research*, **17**, 399.

358 KITCHENS C.S. & NEWCOMB T.F. (1979) Factor XIII. *Medicine*, **58**, 413.

359 LORAND L., LOSOWSKY M.S. & MILOSZEWSKI K.J.M. (1980) Human factor XIII: fibrin-stabilizing factor. In:

Progress in Hemostasis and Thrombosis, Vol. V (ed. Spaet T.H.), p. 245. Grune & Stratton, New York.

360 LORAND L., JACOBSEN A. & BRUNER-LORAND J. (1968) A pathological inhibitor of fibrin cross-linking. *Journal of Clinical Investigation*, **47**, 268.

361 OTIS P.T., FEINSTEIN D.I., RAPAPORT S.I. & PATCH M.J. (1974) An acquired inhibitor of fibrin stabilization associated with isoniazid therapy: clinical and biochemical observations. *Blood*, **44**, 771.

Chapter 30
Thrombosis and anti-thrombotic therapy

J. A. DAVIES AND G. P. McNICOL

Epidemiology of thrombotic disorders

All physicians and many laymen know that in the developed countries thrombo-occlusive vascular disease kills more young people than any other single cause. In the UK in 1976 deaths in those under 55 years of age amounted to 11 717 from ischaemic heart disease, 2973 from cerebral vascular disease and 193 from pulmonary embolism [1]. In patients with diabetes mellitus, who are more at risk of vascular disorders than the general population, half of deaths from all causes may be from vascular disease of some kind [2]. Thrombotic disease in its widest sense presents easily the largest and most serious challenge to the health of the developed communities of the world and the concept of the risk factor has evolved from epidemiological studies designed to identify those characteristics which mark a population for this affliction. It is recognized that cigarette smoking, raised plasma cholesterol and plasma lipids, raised blood glucose, increased blood pressure and the presence of a number of other lesser factors all increase the risk of developing coronary heart disease [3] though risk factors for other forms of arterial disease are less clearly delineated. However, in coronary heart disease the presence of the identified factors accounts for only about 50% of the risk indicating that other, as yet unrecognized, factors are important. Risk of developing venous thromboembolic disease is also linked firmly to certain precipitating circumstances: surgical operations, development of malignant disease, or heart failure; use of oral contraceptives, obesity and the presence of superficial varicose veins. These factors should be partly amenable to preventive measures. Clearly cigarette smoking, obesity and the use of oral contraceptives are, theoretically at least, open to control, though factors such as plasma cholesterol concentration or necessity for an operation would be much harder to influence. Although there is evidence in some countries of a falling mortality from coronary heart disease [4, 5] which some have interpreted as reflecting the success of exhortatory programmes in primary prevention, it is likely that any significant impact from such measures lies some way in the future. In the short-term and in the real world, the development and use of anti-thrombotic drugs remains the most promising mode of intervention.

Thrombosis as a disorder of haemostasis

There is little evidence to support the view that any of the known risk factors in arterial thrombo-occlusive disease operates through disturbance of the haemostatic mechanism. In venous thrombosis, however, some abnormalities of coagulation function have been recognized and are discussed later. Yet in both instances, the symptomatic event is usually related to occlusion of the vessel, undeniably the consequence of solidification of some normally fluid elements of the blood. The visible contribution of blood constituents to a thrombotic event has proved a compulsive stimulus of efforts to find links between the haemostatic mechanism and thrombogenesis. Surprisingly, relatively few of these efforts have examined mechanisms and most have involved trials of treatment. During the last 50 years, millions of patients have been treated with anticoagulants with the intention of inhibiting thrombus deposition on both the venous and arterial sides of the circulation. Studies of haemostatic function in arterial disease have so far yielded little encouragement for this approach, yet a strong emotional urge persists to consider thrombosis as a disorder of the blood. This chapter examines some of the evidence which links thrombosis, blood clotting and haemostatic disorder, and the validity of current therapeutic use of anti-thrombotic drugs.

MECHANISMS OF THROMBOSIS

Vascular components

It is traditional to consider that thrombosis involves the vessel wall, the blood itself and the characteristics of flow and to invoke Virchow to justify doing so. Study of the relationship in life between blood and the intact circulation is obviously extremely difficult, and this has bedevilled attempts to obtain firm evidence that deranged vascular structure or function contribute to clinical thrombosis.

Vasoactive substances

Tissue trauma, by exposing the blood to various extravascular structures, and by the release of active substances, may have a significant role. In general, accumulated metabolic products and material released from damaged cells (e.g. lactate, potassium, hydrogen ion, adenosine) work towards relaxation of vascular tone, restoration of flow to anoxic areas being paramount. There are a number of vasoactive substances which attract particular interest because of their presence in platelets (prostaglandins, serotonin and adenosine diphosphate (ADP)). Interaction between platelets and the vessel wall to generate a pro-thrombotic environment seems a particularly plausible mechanism. There is ample experimental evidence to indicate that ADP can promote vasoconstriction and platelet microthrombus formation in arterioles [6]. Serotonin, released during the platelet release reaction, also promotes further platelet aggregation and is a potent constrictor of peripheral vessels when released into the arterial circulation [7]. Prostaglandins have a complex role, some acting as vasodilators, others as vasoconstrictors, and the response varying according to species and target organ [8]. Thromboxane A_2, an unstable intermediate of platelet prostaglandin biosynthesis, is especially notable as a possible thrombogenic agent, being both a powerful platelet-aggregating agent and also a potent vasoconstrictor [9, 10].

Atherogenesis

The blood vessel wall has a number of characteristics, whose significance remains to be fully explained, which may contribute to the thrombotic process. Recently, endothelial cells have been found to generate two of the three recognized properties of the factor-VIII molecule (Chapter 28). The evidence is now conclusive that endothelial cells synthesize the von Willebrand factor and also the moiety recognized by antisera to factor VIII raised in rabbits, although the coagulant property which is absent in haemophilia is not produced. The physiological purpose of this site of synthesis is unknown, as at the moment factor VIII has no defined vascular function. However, there is increasing circumstantial evidence to suggest that the von Willebrand factor may be involved in platelet–vessel-wall interactions: in the absence of von Willebrand factor, platelet adhesion to subendothelium is reduced [11] and in subjects with von Willebrand's disease, platelet plug formation at sites of injury is defective [12]. The observation that pigs with von Willebrand's disease appear to be resistant to the development of atherosclerosis [13, 14] is particularly intriguing in its implication that platelet adhesion to the vessel wall mediated by von Willebrand factor may play a part in atherogenesis. Further evidence of a vascular role in the development of atheroma comes from the finding that the smooth muscle cells proliferating in the fibro-muscular lesions are monoclonal in origin [15], a property conventionally associated with tumour cells. That the cells originate through mutation rather than selection is born out by the observation that different regions of the plaque tend to have similar clonal characteristics [16]. Atheromatous plaques may therefore, in some sense, be analogous to benign tumours, smooth muscle cells continuing to proliferate spontaneously following an initiating stimulus at a time of vascular injury.

Inhibitor systems

Loss of physiological defence mechanisms in the vessel wall may contribute to thrombosis. At least two inhibitor systems are known which protect the intima from platelet-aggregate formation. Vascular cells show strong ADPase activity [17] which would tend to disperse platelet aggregates. However a much more important defence mechanism is provided by prostaglandin I_2 (PGI$_2$; prostacyclin) a prostaglandin synthesized in the vessel wall [18] (see also Chapter 26). PGI$_2$ is a vasodilator [10] and powerfully inhibits both platelet aggregation [10] and platelet adhesion to subendothelium [19]. In the light of current knowledge this is the most active of the agents which confer on the vascular endothelium a uniquely non-thrombogenic surface. Small fibrin thrombi initiated on the vessel wall are probably normally cleared by fibrinolytic mechanisms. It has been shown that fibrinolytic activator is produced by endothelial cells and released continuously into the bloodstream [20]. There is also evidence that in patients with venous thrombosis, fibrinolytic activity of the vessel walls is impaired, even at sites not actively involved in the thrombotic process [21]. Failure of these normally protective functions of the vessel wall may promote thrombosis.

Response to injury

Some indication of a possible role of the vessel wall in thrombogenesis comes from observation of the effects of injury. Endothelial cells may be damaged during intercurrent illness by circulating substances such as thrombin, bacterial endotoxin, and neuraminidase, all of which have been shown experimentally to injure endothelial cells and promote platelet and fibrin deposition [22]. Homocystine, the amino acid present to excess in the hereditary disorder homocystinuria, in which recurrent thrombosis is a feature, has been shown to promote atherosclerosis-like lesions and thrombosis in primates as a result of primary damage to the endothelium [23]. In patients with clinical thrombosis it is hard to be certain whether vascular damage has preceded or followed the thrombotic process. However, some confirmation for the hypothesis comes from the observation of endothelial damage in the arteries and veins of women dying from pulmonary embolism thought to have been induced by administration of oestrogen-containing contraceptive pills [24]. On the arterial side of the circulation Mitchell & Schwartz [25] have noted extensive vessel-wall disease in arteries at sites of thrombosis, although they note the relationship may not be causal. Damage to the intima has also been observed in the coronary arteries of healthy young men who were the victims of violent death [26].

Haemodynamic factors

The potential importance of haemodynamic factors in thrombogenesis has been convincingly illustrated by experiments using branching extracorporeal shunts. In experiments in which branched plastic tubes were inserted between carotid artery and jugular vein in pigs, Mustard *et al.* [27] showed that platelet microthrombi formed downsteam of flow dividers on the walls of the tube. Platelets were deposited preferentially at these sites of turbulent flow and did not attach elsewhere on the tube surface. There is a notable similarity between the distribution of thrombi in this model and the siting of human thrombo-atherosclerotic deposits. Much subsequent laboratory experiment has confirmed the close relationship between haemodynamic characteristics and thrombus formation, at least in relation to platelet deposition. The factors which seem to be critically important are shear rate and the presence of red cells. In various types of experiment, platelet deposition and platelet microthrombus formation have been shown to increase linearly with increasing shear rate [6, 28, 29]. Experiments using glass models of branched and curved arteries have shown that platelet microthrombus formation occurs selectively where turbulence and vortex formation can lead to stagnation point flow [30]. Thrombosis may also be promoted by the effect of shear stress in sensitizing blood platelets [31].

Experiments on platelet thrombus formation have also emphasized the importance of red cells. Red cells provide a major force contributing to the movement of platelets from the axial stream towards the vessel wall [32, 33]. The presence of red cells increases diffusion of platelets to the vessel surface and increases platelet-surface collision energy [34]. This phenomenon increases the rate of platelet microthrombus formation at the vessel surface [35, 36].

It is difficult to obtain evidence which relates experimental observations directly to human disease. There is better evidence for the relevance of factors which by reducing blood flow may contribute to thrombogenesis as a result of stasis in the vessel lumen. Patients with diabetic vascular disease [37, 38] and severe peripheral vascular disease [39] have increased blood viscosity compared to normal subjects. Thrombotic episodes in patients with polycythaemia are more frequent in those patients with a high haematocrit [40], an effect probably mediated by stasis since small changes in haematocrit lead to proportionately much larger changes in blood flow [41]. It seems all the more likely that reduction in flow may contribute to thrombosis, since it has been shown experimentally that following contact activation, thrombi form only in static blood [42]. Stasis may particularly encourage thrombosis on the venous side of the circulation. Pathological studies indicate that deep venous thrombi form preferentially at sites where ligaments or tendons may compress the vein, or valve cusps interrupt laminar flow [43].

It is unlikely that the evidence for a haemodynamic component in the origin of thrombosis will be other than circumstantial, until better methods become available for studying flow in the intact circulation. It is a reasonable inference that turbulence contributes to thrombosis in the arterial circulation, while stasis may be a more potent factor in the genesis of venous thrombi.

Platelet component

There is a substantial body of evidence that blood platelets are involved in the development of thrombosis, particularly in the arterial circulation [44–48]. The evidence is the result of experimental observation and rational hypothesis, rather that the inevitable conclusion of clinical investigation. However, drugs which inhibit platelet function have been tested and are being used in patients with the rationale that inhibition of platelet activity should decrease thromboembolic events [49–51]. Data which infer that platelets are intimately involved in thrombogenesis are extensive, though platelets may well be mediators rather than initiators of the process.

Platelet adhesion

Platelets do not adhere to normal endothelial cells [52], though they can be induced to adhere at the junctional complex between cells by minimal external forces [53, 54]. If the endothelium is removed experimentally, it has been shown that platelets adhere avidly to the exposed subendothelium, using both *in-vitro* models [55] and the intact animal [56, 57]. Following attachment of the initial platelet monolayer, there is accretion of further platelets, a process probably controlled mainly through the release of ADP [58, 59]. However, potent intermediates of platelet prostaglandin metabolism, particularly thromboxane A_2, probably strongly augment the reaction by inducing further platelet aggregation and vasoconstriction [10]. Under some circumstances this process can give rise to a platelet microthrombus, from which platelet emboli break off [6]. Alternatively white cells and fibrin may add to the platelet mass, building up a stabilized, mature thrombus [48].

Aggregate formation

Platelets stick to each other following exposure to a variety of stimuli in the phenomenon known as aggregation, without prior attachment to a surface. This process is easily studied because of the difference produced in the light-transmitting properties of the platelet suspension [60]. Partly as a result, investigations of platelet function have been disproportionately centred on the process of aggregation. Whether platelet aggregates can be present in the intact circulation is not known, although there are observations to suggest that they occur [61] and that such aggregates are found more frequently in patients with thromboembolic disorders [62]. The question cannot be resolved using current technology because it is impossible to be certain that the aggregates have not formed at the point where the circulation was breached for blood sampling. Aggregates may form as a result of platelet exposure to physiological compounds such as thrombin, serotonin, ADP, adrenaline and noradrenaline, all of which occur in the normal circulation, even if only in trace amounts. During intercurrent disease, platelets are also exposed to bacterial endotoxin, viruses, and antigen–antibody complexes, which have been shown experimentally to induce platelet aggregation [45].

Interaction with the vessel wall

Adhesion or aggregation leading to secretion of platelet contents in the immediate vicinity of the blood vessel wall may produce vascular effects. Platelets can release acid hydrolases [63] and also a cationic protein capable of altering vascular permeability [64]. Such substances have potentially destructive effects on the intima which may augment minor localized thrombotic activity. It is likely that platelets also contribute to atherogenesis, by provision of a cell mitogen which stimulates smooth muscle cell proliferation [65]. Further evidence to support this hypothesis comes from observations that platelet material can be demonstrated in histological sections from human plaques [66] and that induction of thrombocytopenia can protect against experimental atherosclerosis in animals [67].

Platelet coagulant activity

Interaction of platelets with blood coagulation mechanisms may provide an additional pathway by which trivial vascular insult results in thrombosis. Platelets can initiate activity in the intrinsic pathway of coagulation [68]. In addition, following certain stimuli they make membrane phospholipid available to accelerate a number of reactions in the clotting sequence [69]. Heparin-neutralizing activity, designated platelet factor 4 [70], and antiplasmin are also extruded by platelets [71]. Platelets have receptors for factor Xa on their surface which, following the release reaction, bind factor Xa and accelerate the local rate of thrombin formation about 1000-fold [72]. This combination of pro-thrombotic properties makes the platelet micro-environment an ideal nidus for initiation of thrombosis [73].

Coagulation component

On superficial consideration, it seems inevitable that disturbance of the blood-coagulation mechanism should be a prime element in thrombogenesis. Full waiting-rooms at anticoagulant clinics attest to persisting faith in this view. Yet there is accumulating evidence, outlined earlier, that other factors play a crucial role. Definition of the part played by coagulant proteins in thrombosis is hampered by the fragility of haemostatic equilibrium; however delicately blood may be removed from the circulation, it clots. Increasing application of biochemical skills is helping to resolve the mechanism of coagulation (Chapter 27). But the problem of studying blood without in some way inhibiting clotting persists and renders it much more difficult to ascertain how the uninhibited system might function *in vivo* in relation to thrombogenesis.

Activation of the intrinsic system

Thrombus forms in static blood exposed to activators of factor XII [42]. Flow normally helps to prevent this by dispersal of the stimulus and mobilization of plasma inhibitors. Most recognized activators of factor XII are charged particles [74] which rarely occur in the circulation. However, this may be part of the mechanism for the intravascular thrombosis which follows amniotic fluid or fat embolism [75]. Contact activation may also result from exposure of the blood to free fatty acids [76] and collagen [77], bacterial endotoxin [78], proteolytic enzymes [79], isoimmune IgG [80] and homocystine [76]. It is plausible to consider that the circulation might be exposed to such compounds during illness or following trauma, leading to thrombus formation in regions of stagnant flow. It is less certain that exposure of blood to de-endothelialized areas of blood vessel in the live animal might trigger intrinsic activation. Purified preparations of factor XII and factor XI do not generate coagulant activity when exposed to kaolin [81] and it seems probable that contact activation of factor XII has a limited role both in haemostasis and in thrombosis because alternative pathways adequately compensate for deficiency of factor XII. Hageman-factor deficiency is usually asymptomatic [74] and John Hageman died of pulmonary embolism. It is likely that most of those stimuli which might induce activation of factor XII *in vivo* also stimulate blood platelets and possibly generate intrinsic coagulation activity through the inherent pro-coagulant function of platelets [73].

Activation of the extrinsic system
Involvement of the coagulation mechanism in thrombosis might more feasibly arise via the extrinsic pathway. Factor VII circulates in plasma with an active serine residue and can bind di-isopropyl fluorophosphate [82]. Addition of tissue factor causes correspondingly rapid generation of factor Xa which autocatalyzes the reaction by conversion of native factor VII to a more potent, two-chain form [83]. Tissue factor, present in the plasma membrane of endothelial cells and also atheromatous plaques [84, 85], is likely to be released into the circulation not only by trauma but by superficial damage to the endothelium. Additionally, factor VII may be activated by factors IXa and XIIa, plasmin and kallikrein [86] which may prime the system for rapid generation of factor Xa after trivial vascular insult.

Evidence of thrombin generation
A logical case can be made out along these lines to indicate pathways by which the coagulation system might be involved in the earliest stages of thrombogenesis. Experimental evidence that this is so is much harder to find. Recent technical advances have deployed sensitive assays for demonstration of thrombin activity in the circulation (e.g. assay of fibrinopeptide A [87]; radioimmunoassay of thrombin [88]; immunoassay of neo-antigenic sites on antithrombin III formed after complexing with thrombin [89]). However, the precision and sensitivity of these tests is irrelevant to the central dilemma, which is whether thrombin generation is causal or consequential. It is not surprising that forming thrombus generates thrombin; it is much more difficult to demonstrate that hyperactivity of mechanisms for thrombin generation is concerned in the pathogenesis of thrombosis.

Deficiency of coagulation factors
Case reports from patients with congenital deficiency of clotting factors in relation to thrombosis have disproportionate impact because of their apparently paradoxical nature. There are reports of venous thrombosis occurring in patients with deficiency of factor VII [90] and, as already noted, factor XII [91]; venous thrombosis has not been reported in patients with deficiency of factors VIII and IX [92] though there may be a number of reasons for this. Further inconclusive evidence comes from observations on the clinical effectiveness of anti-coagulant drugs, discussed in more detail later in this chapter. Both heparin and warfarin have a marked effect on blood clotting, sufficient to induce a bleeding tendency, which can be profound in overdosage. Yet even used prophylactically they are relatively ineffective in the prevention of thrombosis. The reasons for their clinical inadequacy are complex, but argue further against a central role for coagulation disturbance in the pathogenesis of thrombosis.

The pre-thrombotic state
Study of the pre-thrombotic state partially circumvents the frustrations associated with the successful prophecy of the onset of thrombosis [93, 94]. There are certain difficulties in this approach, not least in deciding which changes in haemostatic function indicate hypercoagulability. Reduction in the concentration of coagulation factors may reflect active consumption of coagulant protein, as occurs in severe intravascular coagulation [95]. However, low levels may arise due to failure of synthesis, e.g. in liver failure [96], a condition in which alterations in coagulant protein concentration are easily misinterpreted. Only a minute proportion of zymogen need be activated for fibrin generation to ensue [97], and it therefore seems likely that in most instances of hypercoagulability the fraction of coagulant protein consumed will be too small for reliable measurement. The thrombogenic potential of increase in the concentration of coagulation factors is equally open to argument. Fibrinogen, factors V and VIII and fibrin-degradation products may behave as acute-phase reactants and rise non-specifically in disease [98]. Nor, since there is substantial excess of coagulant protein above the level required for normal function, is there any particular reason why the system should become self-generating because of greater availability of substrate.

In spite of these difficulties, there are a number of conditions which provide sound circumstantial evidence for the concept of a pre-thrombotic state. *Oestrogen administration* provides one of the most convincing examples. There is incontrovertible documentation of an increased risk of thrombotic disease in patients given oestrogen; and good evidence that synthetic oestrogens raise levels of coagulation factors [99]. The conclusion that the relationship is causal is almost irresistible. However, there are studies which indicate that oestrogen administration increases the risk of other vascular mishaps [100], suggesting that oestrogens may have deleterious effects on the vessel wall as well.

Patients with *malignant disease* are well-recognized to be at greater risk of suffering various forms of thrombotic disease than patients without malignancy. Disseminated intravascular coagulation occurs more commonly in these patients [101], who are also at risk of developing non-bacterial thrombotic endocarditis [102]. Post-operative venous thrombosis has been shown to be three times more common in surgical patients with cancer than in a group with non-malignant disease [102a]. The basis of the pro-thrombotic status of these patients is ill-understood and probably complex [102b]. However, animal experiments have indicated that tumour material can activate platelets [102c], and mucus extracted from human adenocarcinoma has been shown to activate factor X and produce intravascular coagulation following infusion into rabbits [102a].

Patients with *diabetes mellitus* are generally accepted to be at greater risk of thrombo-occlusive vascular disease than the general population, and provide a further example of a group at risk of thrombosis in whom certain tests of haemostatic function are abnormal. The situation is far from straightforward however, since damage to vascular structures is a feature of the disease and an undoubted major contributory factor. None the less diabetics, particularly those with vascular complications, have hyper-reactive platelets which can be demonstrated in a number of different laboratory tests of platelet function [102d]. Such patients are also prone to abnormalities of plasma lipid composition, and *hyperlipidaemia*, besides being a risk factor for atheromatous disease, additionally affects haemostatic function in apparently adverse ways. Feeding fat to normal volunteers has been shown to shorten the Russell-viper-venom time [102e]. Patients with hyperlipoproteinaemia have shorter bleeding times than control subjects and their platelets exhibit enhanced sensitivity to agonists in a range of platelet function tests [102f].

Indecision over the precise interpretation of raised concentrations of plasma coagulant proteins or altered platelet function in patients with disease is likely to persist until results of prospective studies are available [102g]. Preliminary data from this one study are at least compatible with the concept that raised levels of clotting factors and lowered blood fibrinolytic capacity may promote overt thrombotic disease [102h].

DISORDERED HAEMOSTASIS IN THROMBOEMBOLIC DISEASE

As tests of haemostatic function are increasingly applied in the study of thrombotic disease (see Ref. 94), it is clear that the tests are frequently abnormal in patients with established thrombosis. This is not particularly surprising in view of the haemostatic stimulus likely to be provided by fresh thrombi. It is much harder to be certain of the significance of such tests in relation to pathogenesis, for reasons earlier outlined. Evidence for disordered haemostasis in established cases of thrombosis is therefore likely to reflect mainly the secondary consequences of thrombus deposition.

Venous thrombosis
Venous thrombi more closely resemble clots which form in blood freshly drawn into glass, than do thrombi from the arterial circulation. Their physical appearance may not be entirely misleading. Although the resemblance initially encouraged greater effort into the investigation of haemostatic function in venous disease, the results increasingly indicate that disordered coagulation may have a significant role.

Oestrogen
It has long been known that pregnancy and the puerperium are times of increased risk of venous thrombosis. Venous thromboembolic disease is one of the most frequent causes of maternal death in the UK [103]. There are undoubtedly a number of major changes in circulatory function during pregnancy, which may contribute to this process. More significantly there are changes in haemostatic function which can be broadly interpreted to indicate a lower threshold for coagulation and a reduction in fibrinolytic activity. They seem a sound adaptive manoeuvre, in view of the challenge to the haemostatic system which childbirth represents. There is a rise in plasma concentration of factors VII, VIII and X [104, 105] and concentrations of fibrinogen and plasminogen also rise [106]. There is reduction in factor-XIII activity [107] and plasminogen-activator activity in plasma falls [106]. That there is an increased thrombotic risk conferred by these changes is supported by observations that soluble fibrin monomer complexes are present in the maternal circulation [108] and that fibrin is laid down in arterioles of the placenta [109]. This stage of apparent hypercoagulability persists during labour and into the puerperium [103].

Administration of oral contraceptives provides an apparently analogous situation. Increased risk of venous thrombosis in women taking oestrogen-containing oral contraceptives is well established [110].

There have been a large number of studies of coagulation function in women taking oestrogen and there is a general consensus that tests of haemostatic function are altered in the direction of greater pro-coagulant activity [99]. Although not all the numerous studies have been in agreement, there have been demonstrated increases in plasma concentrations of fibrinogen [111], factors VII [112], VIII [113], XI [114] and X [112]. Levels of antithrombin III are reduced in women taking oestrogen compared to controls [115] and there may be an increase in fibrinolytic activity [99] suggestive of an increased propensity for fibrin formation.

Predictive studies
There have been a number of studies of coagulation function in patients with established deep venous thrombosis though under these circumstances any changes may only be indicators of disease activity. Three months after acute deep venous thrombosis proved by venography, only a minority of patients were found to have increased levels of fibrinogen and factor-VIII coagulant activity [116]. More notably, a study in 73 patients prior to surgery showed shortened partial thromboplastin times and higher levels of antiplasmin in those patients who subsequently developed positive ^{125}I-labelled fibrinogen leg scans [117]. In a similar prospective study, shortened partial thromboplastin time, increased haematocrit, and increased platelet adhesiveness were found to distinguish between 29 patients with established DVT and appropriate controls, with 90% precision [118]. In a larger study of 126 gynaecological patients, designed to develop a predictive formula, it was found that increased plasma concentrations of fibrinogen, factor-VIII coagulant activity, and fibrin(ogen)-related antigen (FR antigen) with reduced euglobulin lysis activity, measured in blood samples taken the day before surgery, all proved highly discriminant in distinguishing those patients who subsequently developed post-operative DVT from those who did not [119]. A combination of two of the laboratory tests (euglobulin lysis time and FR antigen) and three items of clinical information (age, percentage overweight for height and presence of varicose veins) when incorporated in a predictive index was more discriminatory than either clinical factors or laboratory data considered independently [119]. Almost identical findings were reported when this study was repeated elsewhere [120].

Increased platelet reactivity has also been demonstrated in patients developing post-operative DVT. It was found that patients who developed DVT after surgery had a significant rise in platelet pro-coagulant activities, which remained normal in patients who did not [121]. Findings of apparently spontaneous platelet aggregates in the plasma of patients with recurrent DVT has also been taken to indicate that platelets are more reactive in these patients [122]. For reasons discussed earlier, it is by no means axiomatic that these findings indicate a causal role for disordered haemostatic function in venous thrombosis. However, the results, particularly of those studies carried out prospectively, indicate that disordered haemostatic function may at the least act synergistically with other factors in the development of venous thrombi.

Pulmonary embolism
There is relatively little information relating changes in laboratory measurements of coagulation function to occurrence of pulmonary embolism. Amongst other reasons, this is because of the relative rarity of the condition, the difficulty of timing its onset, and frequently the greater urgency for prompt treatment which limits investigation. An interesting experimental study in animals has indicated that there is accretion and dissolution of fibrin on the surface of emboli in the pulmonary tree [123], suggesting that haemostatic changes may be provoked by the embolic material rather than being concerned in its origin. Following symptomatic pulmonary embolism, there is usually a substantial increase in fibrin(ogen)-related antigen in the serum [124]. Fibrin(ogen) fragments can be demonstrated in the circulation [125] and free fibrinopeptide A is released at high concentration [126].

Coronary heart disease
Heroic struggles, over a period of more than 20 years, to establish a benefit from anti-coagulant therapy in the secondary prevention of myocardial infarction, yielded discouraging results [127]. Reasons for this outcome might include inadequate trial design, small numbers of patients and inappropriate dosage schedules of the drugs. However, in view of the pronounced effects of coumarin anticoagulants upon the haemostatic mechanism it may indicate that coagulation mechanisms are not centrally involved in pathogenesis of the disease.

Acute myocardial infarction
It is difficult to draw any conclusion about the role of the haemostatic system in the development of coronary heart disease from the results of studies performed on patients following acute myocardial infarction. The rate of fibrinopeptide-A generation is increased (indicating accelerated thrombin generation) in the plasma of some patients after various thrombotic episodes [128] and it is likely that abnormal laboratory tests of coagulation and platelet function in patients following acute myocardial infarction are a non-specific consequence of the disease. Reported abnormalities include

increased levels of heparin-neutralizing activity in plasma and less anti-thrombin activity than controls [129] and a fall in fibrinolytic activity in the days following the infarction [130]. Patients in the recovery phase have increased concentrations of soluble fibrin monomer complexes in their plasma [131] although levels of fibrin-related antigen in serum are rarely increased [132]. The concentration of plasma fibrinogen is raised, and platelets are more adhesive to glass beads [133]. Sharma & Seth [133], in contrast to Rawles *et al.* [130], found a rise in fibrinolytic activity. Platelets may also be more reactive in the plasma of such patients [134] and tend to form spontaneous aggregates more readily than in plasma from controls [135].

Myocardial infarction is commoner in women who use oral contraceptives than in those who do not [136], though it is not known whether this is in any way related to the effect of such drugs on the haemostatic mechanism [99].

Prospective studies

The prospect of better information on the relationship between coagulation function and coronary heart disease is encouraged by the development of long-term prospective studies [137]. Measurement of a panel of laboratory tests of coagulation function in a large cohort of normal individuals is related to their subsequent history of the disease [102g]. Very preliminary information indicated that at least two of the measurements, plasma fibrinogen concentration and fibrinolytic activity, have a general epidemiological pattern which suggests that they may be implicated in the pathogenesis of ischaemic heart disease [102h]. This does not necessarily indicate that the relationship is directly one of cause and effect.

Cerebrovascular disease

There is an increased risk of cerebrovascular disease in women taking oestrogen-containing oral contraceptives [100], as there is of other forms of thrombotic disorder. The relationship of these observations to any alteration in haemostatic function is presumptive. Observations in stroke patients are few and changes may merely reflect constitutional disturbance. Warlow *et al.* [138] found little change in haemostatic function of patients with recent stroke, other than elevated levels of fibrinogen (an acute-phase reactive protein). Finding of increased soluble-fibrin monomer complexes in plasma of stroke patients [139] has greater significance as an indicator of intravascular fibrin formation, but probably no greater relevance in regard to pathogenesis. Interestingly, normolipaemic patients with episodes of transient cerebral ischaemia have been found to have increased platelet pro-coagulant

activity compared to controls [140]. In this study, slight shortening of partial thromboplastin time was noted and an increased tendency for platelet aggregation. Others have reported similarly increased sensitivity of platelets to aggregating agents [141]. These findings are supported by the observation of spontaneous aggregate formation in the blood of patients with transient cerebral ischaemia [62].

Peripheral vascular disease

There has been little work on haemostatic disorder in this group of conditions. Patients have been found to have greater heparin-neutralizing capacity of their plasma compared to controls [129]. As in other forms of arterial thrombo-occlusive disease, spontaneous platelet aggregates may form in blood taken from a majority of patients with peripheral vascular insufficiency [135].

Disseminated intravascular coagulation (see Chapter 29)

Disseminated intravascular coagulation (DIC) is a syndrome complex. Clinical states range from acute bleeding episodes threatening life, to unsuspected fibrin deposition in small vessels leading to failure of organs such as the kidney. Clinical heterogeneity thwarts precise classification and definition of diagnostic criteria [75]. Two major problems in pathogenesis remain unresolved. The first is why clinically important DIC should develop relatively infrequently when presumed triggering factors are quite commonly present. The second is the recognition of those factors which determine whether the disease presents primarily as a bleeding or thrombotic disorder.

Clinical evaluation indicates that bleeding is the commonest manifestation and nearly 10 times more frequent than overt thrombosis [142]. Conversely, autopsy studies show that thrombosis is present in 90% of patients who die [143]. These data may only be apparently discordant since activation of fibrinolysis occurs in parallel with intravascular coagulation, though simultaneous occurrence of haemorrhage and thrombosis is unlikely [75]. More plausible is that bleeding and fibrin deposition occur at different phases of the illness, or that patients that come to autopsy are a distinct sub-group.

Disseminated intravascular coagulation is one of the thrombotic disorders in which disturbance of haemostasis is most clearly demonstrable. In most patients there is a fall in platelet count and fibrinogen concentration with prolongation of thrombin, kaolin-cephalin and occasionally prothrombin times [142]. Less frequently, changes which may indicate consumption of other coagulation protein become apparent, with reduction in levels of factors V, VIII, X and XIII [144].

High levels of fibrin(ogen)-breakdown products can usually be found in serum [132] and thrombin activity in plasma can be shown by increased incorporation of glycine methyl ester (^{14}C) into ethanol-precipitated plasma [145] and by high levels of free fibrinopeptide A [126].

Ways in which DIC might develop have been recently reviewed [75, 146] and depend principally on trigger mechanisms [147]. In massive DIC associated with extensive tissue damage, it is probable that released tissue thromboplastin causes inappropriate activation of coagulation and fibrinolysis. The chain of causality with other recognized triggering factors is more speculative. Sepsis is a frequent predisposing cause of DIC [148] and may provoke DIC through platelet aggregation induced by bacteria [149] or antigen–antibody complexes [150]; and by effects of endotoxaemia leading to endothelial damage [22] and activation of factor XII [78]. Plausible though such mechanisms seem, none is firmly established, and experimental evidence introduces some discrepancies. Endotoxin does not cause DIC in animals following a single injection unless there is prior blockade of the reticulo-endothelial system [75]. White blood cells are also necessary for development of DIC in animal models.

While there are many areas of ignorance in knowledge of pathogenesis in DIC, it seems a plausible thesis that in most cases, inappropriate activation of the coagulation system is a major contributor.

THE BASIS OF ANTI-THROMBOTIC THERAPY

Avoidance of recognized risk factors

Venous thrombosis
Surgical operations are the major recognized determinant of venous thromboembolic disease, and can rarely be avoided. Attention has centred on offsetting this particular risk by other methods. Of the lesser risk factors, oestrogen in general, and the contraceptive pill in particular, should be prescribed in the knowledge of their thrombogenic potential [99]. Obesity and the presence of varicose veins have also been shown to predispose to post-operative venous thrombosis [119]. While avoidance of exogenous oestrogen clearly removes this iatrogenic risk, there is no direct evidence that weight reduction and treatment of varicose veins are beneficial. However, it would seem sensible to encourage the obese to slim before elective operations. The association with venous stasis is harder to quantify, but it may be beneficial to discourage long periods of immobility in patients at risk of venous thrombosis.

Arterial thrombosis
In contrast, the relative failure of therapeutics in the field of arterial thromboembolism, and the huge investment in identification of risk factors [151, 152] have encouraged the concept of primary prevention through avoidance of recognized injurious agents. Regrettably, application has not yielded the hoped-for results. Abstaining from smoking cigarettes has been shown to lower the risk of subsequent coronary heart disease [3] and reduction of high blood pressure to reduce the incidence of stroke [153]. Although measures designed to reduce the risk of CHD associated with high plasma cholesterol, obesity, lack of exercise, and personality traits have not been proved to be effective, many physicians would regard it as reasonable to eliminate risk factors where this is possible. Equally, aggressive control of blood glucose concentration in diabetic patients has not clearly been shown to reduce the risks from vascular disease and thrombosis, though there is some experimental encouragement for this approach. The potential complexities involved in primary prevention are well illustrated by the outcome of the very large and extended primary intervention study with clofibrate [154]. This meticulously planned and carefully conducted investigation showed that clofibrate reduced plasma cholesterol in treated individuals by about nine per cent, reduced their risk of developing ischaemic heart disease, but did not reduce overall mortality and may even have increased it. Manipulation of plasma cholesterol levels may not be the obvious panacea it appears on first consideration.

Smoking and diet
Women over the age of 35 years who use oral contraceptives and particularly those who smoke cigarettes as well have a substantially increased risk of developing arterial thrombosis compared to women who avoid both [155]. It seems rational to advise women in this age group not to take oral contraceptives, particularly if they smoke.

In the light of available knowledge, stopping the habit of cigarette smoking would seem to be the most powerful preventive measure of those which could realistically be implemented. Advocacy of dietary change in patients with established disease and even more so in the healthy population, should be cautious. It seems entirely rational to advise individuals in developed countries to eat less in general and less fat in particular. Pressure to substitute one form of fat for another may be premature, until we know more about the long-term effects on human lipid metabolism [156, 157]. Encouragement to eat more vegetable fibre is most unlikely to do harm and may have some benefit [158].

Heparin

Chemistry and biological activity

Heparin is a highly negatively charged organic acid with an extended chain structure and molecular weight varying from 3000 to 37 500. It is a mucopolysaccharide (glucosaminoglycan) composed of repeated sequences of glucosamine, which is heavily sulphated, and linked in alternating fashion to glucuronic or iduronic acid [159]. The molecule defies precise chemical description because of a heterogeneity which depends partly on its source and also almost certainly on its inherent chemical structure. One group of workers, for example, have claimed to identify more than 20 different sub-unit chains from the molecule separated on the basis of electrical charge [160], although this finding has been disputed [161].

Heparin is located mainly in mast cells, but increasingly many extracellular locations are being reported. Heparin-containing mast cells are found mainly in the gut, lungs and vessel wall but there are marked species differences, with human tissues containing little analysable heparin [162]. Physiological function is unknown, but circumstantial evidence suggests that it may be concerned in mast-cell function; that it may contribute to the biological non-thrombogenicity of vascular endothelium; and that it may play a role in fat absorption and metabolism [162].

For therapeutic purposes, heparin is prepared principally from bovine lung and pig intestinal mucosa. Heterogeneity of the material has proved a considerable problem in clinical use. There is no precise chemical assay and the biological assays yield different potency for the same material, depending on the test system employed [160]. Standardization of commercial heparins and comparison in potency of different preparations has been a major problem as a result [163, 164]. Control of heparin administered intravenously in therapy remains an unresolved problem. Use of the whole-blood clotting time is traditional [165] but use of a wider range of coagulation tests indicates that heparin affects different parts of the coagulation system with variable potency [164].

Mode of action

The fundamental mechanism of action of heparin is still in dispute [166]. It was recognized shortly after its initial isolation that a cofactor in plasma was required for anticoagulant effect [167]. More recently, work from a number of different centres has shown the cofactor to be a plasma protein, antithrombin III [166]. The most attractive and unifying concept of heparin activity has been that it exerts its effect by binding to antithrombin III and altering the configuration of the molecule so that subsequent binding to, and inactiva-

tion of, the serine protease coagulant proteins of plasma is vastly accelerated [168, 169]. Blockade of the active serine residues of thrombin and activated factors IX, X and XI inhibits their enzymic action in the coagulation sequence and, as might be predicted, has a profound anticoagulant effect. However, it is probable that the action of heparin is more complex than this. There is evidence that heparin activity against activated factor X is distinct from its antithrombin activity [170]. There is also evidence that heparin may bind directly to thrombin [171]. In the low dosage administered subcutaneously and used in prophylaxis rather than treatment of thrombosis, there is little doubt that heparin acts by accelerating the inactivation of activated factor X by antithrombin III [172]. This action can be shown at very low concentrations of heparin [173]. It is known that small amounts of activated factor X are capable of producing much larger amounts of thrombin [174], a low-dose heparin regime thus functioning very effectively to prevent this amplification effect. Heparin also has an effect on blood platelets [175] and prolongs the bleeding time in man [176]. While the anti-thrombotic effect of heparin is probably due almost entirely to its anticoagulant properties there may be a variable component related to antiplatelet activity.

Coumarins

Drugs of the coumarin group were developed as a result of studies into the active ingredient in spoiled sweet clover, which caused a bleeding disorder in cattle. The investigations culminated in the isolation of 3,3′-methylene bis (4-hydroxycoumarin) [177] from which a number of substituted derivates were produced. Sodium warfarin has been the most successful of these compounds because of the convenience and greater safety conferred by its particular pharmacodynamics [178]. Substituted indandiones (e.g. phenindione) were also deployed as oral anticoagulants but are obsolete because of the frequency with which they cause sensitivity reactions [179].

The development of oral anticoagulants and investigation of the action of vitamin K had a synergistic effect upon each other [178] and it was quickly appreciated that coumarins acted as antagonists of vitamin K in the haemostatic mechanism. A precursor protein for prothrombin was found in the plasma of anticoagulated patients in 1963 [180]. This was shown to be antigenically similar to prothrombin, though lacking biological activity [181] because of defective calcium-binding properties. Inability to bind calcium renders the precursor protein physiologically inert, because calcium is required to anchor prothrombin to a phospholipid surface during prothrombin–thrombin conversion [182]. The vitamin-K-dependent step was shown to involve modification of amino-acid structures in the calcium-binding region of the precursor molecule [183]. In the presence of vitamin K, glutamic-acid residues are carboxylated to form γ-carboxyglutamic acid, a newly discovered, natural amino acid [184]. This post-ribosomal step in the synthesis of vitamin-K-dependent clotting factors probably takes place in microsomes, the carboxylase activity being present in a washed microsomal preparation [185]. In spite of the intensive efforts which have been invested in characterization of the effect of coumarins, the precise method by which they antagonize the action of vitamin K in this carboxylation reaction is unknown [186]. However, it is clear that administration of coumarin drugs results in modification of the molecular structure of factors VII, IX and X in addition to prothrombin. As a result, utilization of calcium and phospholipid as catalysts of activation is grossly impaired. Although immunologically closely related proteins which are functionally inert circulate, the plasma of individuals treated with coumarins behaves as though it were deficient in factors II, VII, X and, to a lesser extent, IX. These immunologically similar precursors have shorter half-lives than the active proteins and were initially designated by the acronym PIVKA, for protein induced by vitamin-K absence [186a]. The defect in function is reflected in marked prolongation of the prothrombin time (factors II, VII and X) or thrombotest (also sensitive to deficiency of factor IX). Current thinking about vitamin-K antagonism by anticoagulants and its effect on blood coagulation has been reviewed by Jackson & Suttie [186b].

Fibrinolytic drugs

A drug able to dissolve thrombus in the circulation carries an almost magical aura. Regrettably in practice it has been difficult to demonstrate that fibrinolytic drugs are of real therapeutic utility, except in a few restricted circumstances. Two agents, streptokinase and urokinase, have been used extensively (for review see Ref. 187), others on only an experimental basis.

Streptokinase

Action of streptokinase. Streptokinase (perhaps largely on grounds of cost) has been more widely used in Europe. It is a protein usually purified from type-C streptococci (for review see Ref. 188). In a series of impressive experiments which might now be considered unethical, Johnson & McCarty showed the material would lyse experimental thrombi induced in forearm veins of human volunteers [189]. Precisely how it does this is still unclear. Streptokinase has no intrinsic enzymic activity and in plasma forms a complex with plasminogen [190]. The interaction

provokes a conformational change in the single-chain plasminogen molecule which invests the complex with plasminogen-activator activity [191]. Plasmin, a disulphide-linked two-chain molecule, is formed from residual, non-complexed plasminogen. The reaction involves proteolytic cleavage of an arginyl–valine bond [192], and may be autocatalytic. Plasmin can release a small peptide from plasminogen, converting it from a molecule with N-terminal glutamic acid (glu-plasminogen) into a form with N-terminal lysine (lys-plasminogen) [193]. Under certain conditions this partial degradation can greatly accelerate the rate of activation to plasmin [194].

At the start of streptokinase infusion, plasminogen is used up in this process and the plasma concentration of plasminogen falls rapidly. During this initial burst of activity, free plasmin may appear in the circulation, but thereafter plasmin generation is rate-limited by plasminogen synthesis.

A large proportion of formed plasmin is bound almost instantaneously to α_2 antiplasmin and circulates as an inactive complex [195]. Plasmin binds to other inhibitors in plasma only after available sites on antiplasmin have been saturated. Plasmin can form a complex with α_2 macroglobulin which retains slight fibrinolytic activity [196].

Mechanism of thrombolysis. Ingenious hypotheses have been advanced over the years to explain how fibrinolysis occurs in the absence of free plasmin in the circulation. There have been three principal explanations of this apparent paradox (for review see Refs 197 and 198). In outline, the Sherry hypothesis proposed that plasmin was formed locally in the immediate vicinity of its substrate fibrin, from plasminogen which had been incorporated in the thrombus during its development [199]. Ambrus & Markus suggested that plasmin dissociated from an inhibitor complex in the neighbourhood of the thrombus, because fibrin had greater affinity than antiplasmin for plasmin [200]. Chesterman *et al.* proposed that activators selectively bound to fibrin activated plasminogen which diffused into the thrombus from the plasma [201].

There has recently been a major advance in understanding the way in which fibrin can be preferentially degraded by plasmin [195]. Briefly, activators and plasminogen (particularly lys-plasminogen) have a high affinity for lysine residues in fibrin and bind strongly to fibrin polymerizing in the circulation. Binding to fibrin greatly accelerates the rate of plasminogen activation by physiological activators and also prevents inactivation of plasmin by plasma inhibitors, since the lysine-binding sites on plasmin are inaccessibly complexed with the fibrin [195].

Administration of streptokinase. It is still not clear that activation of plasminogen by streptokinase proceeds by the same mechanism as activation by physiological activators. The potential complexities give rise to certain difficulties in the clinical use of streptokinase. A loading dose of very variable size is required to neutralize antibody almost always present in plasma from earlier streptococcal infection [202]. Reduction in the rate of streptokinase infusion, by allowing plasminogen levels to rise, may produce unexpected hyperplasminaemia. And the non-linearity of the dose-response relationship, with variability between subjects, makes guesswork of the dosage schedule [203]. Variations on the basic theme have been introduced to try and offset these disadvantages. Pulsed doses may be both more effective and safer [197] and more consistent fibrinolytic activity may be attainable by simultaneous administration of plasminogen [204].

Urokinase

In contrast, therapy with urokinase is more straightforward, though also much more expensive. Urokinase is the active ingredient responsible for the long-recognized fibrinolytic activity of human urine (for brief review see Refs 203 and 205). It is synthesized by kidney cells and can be demonstrated in fetal kidney-cell culture [206]. It is a proteolytic enzyme which directly activates plasminogen to plasmin. Dosage calculated on body weight therefore produces a reasonably predictable response. Sensitivity reactions are highly unlikely to occur because it is a protein of human origin.

A number of other fibrinolytic agents has been tried but there is nothing specifically to encourage their therapeutic application [198]. Drugs which, when given orally, enhance fibrinolysis over a period of weeks or months have also been studied. These probably act by enhancing the production of vascular fibrinolytic activator. The diguanide phenformin and the anabolic steroid ethyloestranol, which are active individually and synergistically [207], were the first described. There are others [198] but there is no convincing evidence from clinical trials that these agents have worthwhile anti-thrombotic activity.

Ancrod

Reid was intrigued by the observation that patients bitten by the Malayan pit-viper (*Agkistrodon rhodostoma*) had incoagulable blood yet rarely suffered from serious haemorrhage [208]. He thought the active principal in the venom might be therapeutically useful and went on to demonstrate that it produced defibrination [209]. Esnouf & Tunnah [210] isolated and characterized the defibrinating enzyme which became the therapeutic agent ancrod (Arvin).

Mechanism of action. The mechanism of action of ancrod has been fairly recently reviewed [211]. It has a thrombin-like action, reacting directly with fibrinogen to release fibrinopeptide A [212]. Unlike thrombin, it does not release the B peptide. The fibrin so formed is rapidly cleared from the circulation, probably mainly by the reticulo-endothelial system and partly by secondary fibrinolysis. The reluctance of fibrin produced by ancrod to polymerize and form clot may be an inherent property of the molecule, or because it forms a polymer more susceptible to lysis [213]. Absence of intravascular clot formation may also relate to lack of activation of factor XIII and failure of the normal cross-linking mechanism [214].

The action of ancrod appears to be confined to fibrinogen and it does not affect other coagulant proteins [210]. It also seems fairly certain that it has no direct effect on fibrinolytic systems [215], although there is increased secondary fibrinolysis due to intravascular fibrin formation. Ancrod does have some additional proteolytic action on fibrinogen, partially degrading the α chain of the molecule [216]. This may provide an additional explanation for the apparently increased susceptibility to lysis of ancrod-formed clots under certain conditions [215, 216]. The anti-thrombotic benefit of ancrod is probably largely confined to its anticoagulant effect. Experimental studies in animals have hinted at the possibility that it may have additional properties which could alter the nature of the thrombus [217]. It is conceivable that ancrod might have minimal advantages over more conventional anticoagulants because of concomitant reduction in plasma viscosity [218] or because of secondary activation of fibrinolysis.

Anti-platelet drugs

Most drugs with clinically applicable anti-platelet activity are non-steroidal anti-inflammatory agents. Interest in this group has been continuous since the mid-1960s when it was appreciated that they inhibited platelet aggregation and the release reaction [45].

Aspirin

Aspirin has been the most intensively studied of these agents. In 1971 it was proposed that it might act by inhibition of prostaglandin synthesis [219]. This made little sense at the time in relation to platelet function, since none of the known prostaglandin products of platelets was pro-aggregatory. Later, it was shown that a metabolic product of arachidonic acid induced platelet aggregation [220] and that this was an unstable prostaglandin precursor, PGH_2 [221]. A further intermediate with more potent pro-aggregatory properties was discovered in thromboxane A_2 [222]. These powerful, short-lived intermediates of prostaglandin biosynthesis modulate the platelet release reaction evoked by certain concentrations of thrombin and collagen, although there are pathways for aggregation and release which are independent of prostaglandin activity. Aspirin inhibits the prostaglandin-dependent mechanism by irreversible acetylation of the enzyme cyclo-oxygenase [223]. This enzyme catalyses the formation of the endoperoxides PGG_2 and PGH_2 from arachidonate. While exposure to aspirin inhibits prostaglandin production for the lifespan of the treated platelet, aggregation and release can still occur in response to sufficient concentrations of collagen and thrombin via prostaglandin-independent pathways. The permanent nature of the inactivation produced by aspirin explains the clinical observation that aspirin affected platelets for the lifetime of the cell [224]. This apparently straightforward mechanism for an anti-thrombotic action of aspirin has been complicated by the discovery of prostacyclin [18].

Effect on prostacyclin. Prostacyclin (PGI_2) is synthesized in the vessel wall, and is dependent on cyclo-oxygenase for processing of precursor arachidonate. It is a highly potent inhibitor of platelet aggregation [10] and, at higher concentration, also inhibits platelet adhesion to vascular subendothelium [19, 225]. The suggestion has been made that PGI_2 supplies the principal defensive mechanism of the vessel wall against deposition of platelet microthrombi [10]. Not surprisingly, realization that aspirin also inhibits vascular cyclo-oxygenase and hence prostacyclin production has led to a reappraisal of the clinical role of aspirin as an anti-thrombotic agent [10]. There is some evidence from experimental thrombosis in animals to suggest that, at very high doses, aspirin treatment may actually promote thrombus formation [226], an effect ascribed to inhibition of vascular PGI_2 production. It is, however, likely that the action of drugs which inhibit prostacyclin synthesis will not affect the platelet and the vessel wall equally *in vivo*. Endothelial cells, unlike platelets, can rapidly resynthesize cyclo-oxygenase [227] and are likely to be exposed to lower drug concentrations than the platelet circulating in plasma.

Anti-thrombotic activity. While the intracellular site of action of aspirin has been localized, the precise way in which the inhibition of prostaglandin synthesis limits platelet incorporation into thrombi is still debatable. In the platelet, prostaglandins may act by modulating changes in levels of cyclic AMP [10] and ionized calcium. There is good evidence from models of experimental thrombosis that aspirin can inhibit platelet microthrombus formation [228–230]. It is unclear whether this effect is mediated by inhibition of platelet adhesion to the vessel wall [231] or solely by interfer-

ence with subsequent interplatelet reactions [232]. Experiments using human volunteers have shown that administration of aspirin by mouth results in suppression of platelet-aggregatory activity in plasma [233, 234]. It has also been found to prolong bleeding time in the majority of studies [235].

The other non-steroidal anti-inflammatory drugs, like aspirin, inhibit prostaglandin synthesis by reversible or irreversible inhibition of cyclo-oxygenase [236]. They similarly inhibit *in-vitro* tests of platelet function [237] and platelet vessel-wall reactions [238] and can be shown experimentally to have anti-thrombotic effects [239, 240].

Sulphinpyrazone
Of these compounds only sulphinpyrazone has achieved any particular currency as an anti-thrombotic drug. Sulphinpyrazone has attracted particular interest because it was shown early on to prolong platelet survival time in man [241]. In this respect, which may be an important indicator of anti-thrombotic potential [242], sulphinpyrazone differs from aspirin in prolonging survival in patients with thrombotic disorders [243] while aspirin does not [244, 245]. It may also be relevant to possible differences between these two drugs as anti-thrombotic agents that sulphinpyrazone is a competitive rather than irreversible inhibitor of cyclo-oxygenase [236].

Dipyridamole
Pyrimido-pyrimidines (of which dipyridamole is the archetype) form the other major group of compounds which have been used clinically as anti-platelet drugs in man. Dipyridamole was found to inhibit platelet white-body formation in the rabbit [246] and has since been shown to inhibit platelet aggregation *in vitro* [247, 248]. It probably acts by raising the level of intraplatelet cyclic AMP due to inhibition of phosphodiesterase [249]. Dipyridamole may act synergistically with prostacyclin to raise cyclic AMP levels [250]. Experimentally, dipyridamole used alone has been shown to inhibit platelet adhesion to collagen [36] and thrombus formation in rabbits [251]. However, it may be more effective in combination with aspirin [252, 253]. Other pyrimido-pyrimidine compounds have more powerful anti-platelet function *in vitro* [254] though they have not been used therapeutically to any extent.

Ticlopidine
This agent does not affect platelets when added to blood in a test tube. Following oral administration to normal volunteers and after a lag of 12–24 hours, bleeding time has been found to be prolonged and platelet aggregation in blood samples inhibited [255]. Ticlopidine has also been shown to inhibit thrombus

formation induced by lactic acidosis in rats [256]. The mode of action of the drug is not clear, but recent evidence indicates that it activates basal and PGE_1-stimulated adenyl cyclase activity in platelets leading to increased levels of cyclic AMP [257]. Although it has been used for some time on the continent, there is as yet insufficiently firm evidence available to encourage its use in anti-thrombotic therapy.

Dextran, dihydroergotamine and calf stimulation

Dextran

Dextran has been used for a number of years as an anti-thrombotic agent, although its action on blood is obscure [45]. It has little effect on platelet function *in vitro*, but appears to reduce platelet adhesiveness in blood taken a few hours after dextran infusion [258] and alters the characteristics of thrombi produced in treated blood [259]. It also prolongs the bleeding time [258]. Whether these experimental observations are related to its postulated therapeutic benefit is unknown. It is possible that dextran has wider effects on the haemostatic mechanism. The molecular size of the polymer may determine whether dextran interferes non-specifically with coagulation reactions. Its physico-chemical characteristics would also be compatible with an action dependent on surface coating, a dextran film coming between vascular intima and the blood. It has been shown experimentally to inhibit thrombosis in the microvasculature [260].

Dihydroergotamine

Dihydroergotamine has been used as an adjunct to low-dose heparin prophylaxis, with the aim of reducing venous stasis by pharmacological means [261]. Experiments in human volunteers showed that administration of dihydroergotamine constricted the capacitance vessels of the venous circulation [262], thereby increasing the velocity of venous blood flow in the legs. When used in combination with low-dose heparin, it was found that velocity of calf-muscle blood flow was significantly increased for several hours after subcutaneous injection [263].

Calf stimulation

Avoidance of venous stasis has also been attempted by use of mechanical and electrical devices to stimulate the pumping action of the calf muscles [264, 265]. Mechanical dorsiflexion of the foot has also been shown to increase both venous flow and pulsatility of the blood column in the femoral vein by several orders of magnitude [266]. Intermittent compression of the leg, produced by inflation of a plastic legging, more effectively increases pulsatility of flow, which may be the critical characteristic of the flow pattern in relation to venous thrombosis [264]. Electrical stimulation of the calf muscles to produce sporadic contraction during operation may achieve the same purpose [267].

EFFICACY OF ANTI-THROMBOTIC AGENTS

Clinical trial design

Evaluation of anticoagulant drugs served as an important proving ground in the development of the design of clinical trials. The necessity for effective trials was underlined by the painful experience of evaluating anticoagulant drugs in myocardial infarction [268]. Accurate evaluation of anti-thrombotic drugs is vital for the very reasons which make a trial laborious to organize: difficulty of diagnosis, heterogeneity of the cases, imprecision of the end points to be measured, number of unforeseen variables affecting the outcome, emotional attitudes to the disease, and methods of treatment by both patients and physicians. The size of the health problem posed by thrombosis accentuates the need for sensitive and reliable assays of therapeutic efficiency. Inability to prove the value of a drug which reduced the death rate from a rare congenital disorder by 10% is a shortcoming the community might decide to accept; the same reduction in the death rate from many thrombotic diseases would represent a major therapeutic success. Good clinical trials of anti-thrombotic drugs are therefore an essential prerequisite of therapy, both for the selection of agents whose effectiveness is too small to be apparent to individual judgement, and the rejection of treatments adopted because of unreasonable emotional prejudice.

The principles of clinical trial design have been admirably and succinctly described recently [269–271]. Amongst a number of points crucial to proper analysis of the result, emphasis is placed on: estimation of the necessary number of patients required to have a reasonable prospect of achieving a result; importance of the time taken for therapy to fail in relation to entry; advantage of comparing only two treatment groups; absolute necessity for strict randomization; inclusion of all patients entered into the final analysis, with care over withdrawals; and circumspection over preliminary analysis of data [270]. This importance of basically effective design has been stressed by a number of others [272, 273].

A dispiriting sidelight on the ultimate outcome of trials of anti-thrombotic drugs is cast by the history of anticoagulant administration to patients with fractured femur. In one of the seminal controlled trials, it was shown that prophylactic administration of phenindione to patients with hip fractures substantially reduced the incidence of deep venous thrombosis and pulmonary embolism [274]. Other trials have subsequently confirmed this finding, yet few orthopaedic surgeons give anticoagulants to their patients and most are firmly against doing so [275]. While it is rarely stated as an aim of the clinical trial, one additional design specification should perhaps indicate ways of propagating the result and ensuring its acceptability.

Venous thrombosis

Venous thrombosis is a common complication of serious illness and an occasional complication of minor ailments and trivial disability. The incidence ranges from about 15% of patients undergoing routine gynaecological surgery [276] to nearly 70% of elderly patients with hip fracture [277]. Amongst the problems which confront those dealing with the disease, two have principally determined the pattern of management. The first is the inaccuracy and unreliability of clinical diagnosis, which is correct in only about half the suspected cases [278]. The second is the disappointing results obtained from the treatment of established thrombosis. These two factors mainly account for the enthusiasm with which clinicians have pursued prevention as the best point of therapeutic intervention.

Established venous thrombosis

Prevention of embolism. Treatment of established deep venous thrombosis is intended to prevent pulmonary embolism and to minimize residual damage to the deep venous system of the leg with consequent development of the post-phlebitic syndrome. Treatment instituted with heparin and continued with an oral anticoagulant is probably reasonably effective in prevention of pulmonary embolism but the voluminous evidence is far from conclusive [279]. Anticoagulant treatment became accepted on the basis of enthusiastic reports of the value of heparin [280] which pre-dated modern techniques of evaluation. Later studies as a result have not included an untreated control group, but have shown that heparin treatment reduces the incidence of pulmonary embolism to between one and two per cent of patients with venous thrombosis, compared to the 20–40% incidence quoted in earlier studies [281]. Most practising clinicians therefore accept that anticoagulation should be instituted in patients with established thrombosis to prevent embolism, whatever qualms they may have about the scientifically inadequate evidence on which such practice is based [282].

Having accepted that anticoagulation is probably effective, a number of unresolved lesser issues remain with regard to duration of heparin therapy, dosage and method of administration. The argument deployed to justify prolongation of heparin administration is that it is a more effective anticoagulant than warfarin. The evidence for this is tenuous, depending on a single series of experiments with artificial thrombi in animals [283] and indirect clinical observation [284]. In routine clinical practice there is likely to be minimal effective difference and on grounds of cost, safety and saving of time to patients and hospitals, heparin should be used for 48–72 hours to cover the period of warfarin induction. Continuous infusion of 1000–1200 units hourly, monitored by the activated partial thromboplastin time, provides a satisfactory regime which results in fewer bleeding problems than when heparin is given by injection or without laboratory control [285].

The time at which warfarin is started owes more to personal inclination than any objective factor. The aim should be to establish a prothrombin time of about two and a half times the normal value. At higher levels of anticoagulation, bleeding is likely to be frequent [286] while at lower levels, pulmonary embolism during treatment is much more likely to occur [287]. Treatment should probably be continued for a minimum of six weeks, the period for which available evidence suggests minor emboli may continue [288]. After three months' anticoagulation, there seems to be little advantage from prolonging therapy [289].

Post-phlebitic syndrome. For most patients with significant venous thrombosis, there is persisting disability. Deep veins in which thrombus has formed may recanalize after a fashion, but the valve mechanism is destroyed [290] and the pressures transmitted through the system lead to superficial venous distension, oedema and eventually a risk of venous ulceration (the post-phlebitic syndrome). Conventional anticoagulants probably do nothing to prevent this and studies comparing heparin, ancrod and streptokinase have shown that significant clearance of thrombi can be achieved only with thrombolytic treatment [291–293].

In the management of the individual patient with suspected deep venous thrombosis, sequential decisions have therefore to be made. Initially the diagnosis should be substantiated by venography when available. Next, the risk: benefit equation for the use of fibrinolytic agents has to be evaluated considering suitability of the clot for lysis, likelihood of severe post-phlebitic symptoms, age of the patient and importance, usually to her, of the cosmetic consequences of a swollen leg. Finally the anticoagulant policy must be considered using similar information; there is little point in anticoagulating a patient in whom venous thrombosis is one aspect of an advanced malignant process, or of prescribing warfarin to an out-patient incapable of rational self-administration.

In severe venous thrombosis with total obstruction to venous return and incipient venous gangrene there is a temptation to press for surgery, motivated by a desire at least to clear the blockage. Surgery probably has a very limited place in the management of venous thrombosis, with a third of patients re-thrombosing the occluded segment and more than half having serious residual symptoms [294]. It may serve to gain time in that very small number of patients in whom tissue necrosis might occur without temporary restoration of partial venous flow.

Prophylaxis in venous thrombosis

For reasons touched on earlier, much of the effort to improve management in venous thrombosis has centred on efficient prevention [295]. This relies on the availability of cheap, safe and effective agents and the ability to identify patients particularly at risk of sustaining a venous thrombosis. The selection of patients for prophylaxis has usually been determined simply by their classification in a category known to be at high risk, e.g. following surgical operation or while confined to bed with heart failure. Using multivariate discriminant analysis it may be possible to narrow the selection further by making a few clinical and laboratory measurements and applying them in a simple formula [119, 120]. Preliminary evidence already indicates that this approach can satisfactorily limit expensive prophylactic measures to those in need [296].

Existing forms of prophylaxis comprise the pharmacological [295] and the mechanical [297]. Controversy has arisen over how these should be judged, whether by effect on overall mortality, incidence of fatal or non-fatal pulmonary emboli, or reduction in ^{125}I-labelled fibrinogen leg-scans [298]. While none has been shown to reduce overall mortality, this is equally true of almost all the treatments currently prescribed for most illness. However, and more pertinently, few have been shown to limit the incidence of pulmonary emboli.

Post-operative pulmonary embolism. In one of only two large-scale studies so far carried out, low-dose calcium heparin was compared against no treatment in the prevention of post-operative venous thrombosis. The results were interpreted to indicate that fatal pulmonary emboli were reduced [299], though not all the participants were in agreement [300] and some doubt remains about the validity of the conclusion [298]. In spite of reservations about interpretation of the International Multicentre Trial taken in isolation, support for the effectiveness of low-dose heparin comes from a smaller study in which it was found that fewer fatal pulmonary emboli occurred in treated patients [301]. Administration of dextran is the only alternative form of prophylaxis which has been shown to prevent death

from pulmonary embolism [302, 303]. Although there has been some disagreement about the conclusions of the earlier of these two trials [302], the finding of the recent large-scale study [303] firmly establishes the value of prophylaxis with dextran 70 against post-operative pulmonary embolism.

Post-operative venous thrombosis. A very large number of studies has shown that low-dose heparin significantly inhibits the development of positive ^{125}I-labelled fibrinogen leg-scans both in post-surgical patients and those with disabling medical problems known to predispose to venous thrombosis [296]. While few would dispute this finding, enthusiasm for low-dose heparin as the solution to the problem is tempered by appreciation of some shortcomings of the ^{125}I-labelled fibrinogen scan as an index of risk from pulmonary embolism. There is some doubt as to whether the dangerous proximal thrombi are necessarily preceded by small clots in calf veins [294]; proximal venous thrombi may certainly occur without positive ^{125}I-labelled fibrinogen scanning [304]; and low-dose heparin, while suppressing the small calf-vein lesions picked up by isotope scan, may have no effect on large ileo-femoral thrombi [305].

Hip surgery. These theoretically derived reservations about the invariable efficacy of low-dose heparin prophylaxis are substantiated by reports of trials carried out in patients following hip-joint surgery. The operative technique—inflicting torsion damage to the femoral vein and occluding venous flow—is particularly liable to promote formation of the large, potentially fatal, proximal thrombi [306]. In these circumstances, low-dose heparin was found to be ineffective in one study [307] and less effective than aspirin, dextran or oral anticoagulants in another [308]. Recently, it has been shown that the poor results obtained using low-dose heparin alone can be substantially improved by combination with dihydroergotamine [261].

The value of aspirin shown in the earlier study [308] was subsequently confirmed by the same group, although the effect was restricted to men [304]. This curious sex difference lends credibility to the findings since the same sex difference emerged for the beneficial effect of aspirin in transient cerebral ischaemia [51]. Hip surgery also provided the testing ground for the original trials of anti-thrombotic prophylaxis, in which oral anticoagulation was shown to prevent DVT and fatal pulmonary embolism in patients with fractured neck of femur [274], a finding since fully confirmed [277]. An original approach, worth further evaluation in orthopaedic patients, is to use the defibrinating enzyme ancrod, which has been shown to reduce the incidence of major DVT in patients with fractured neck of femur [309].

Sometimes, pragmatic decisions to use a drug in clinical practice may be necessary before full evidence is available to satisfy strict scientific criteria. We believe that this situation pertains in the prophylaxis of venous thrombosis. For routine prophylaxis of patients at risk from immobility, reversible medical conditions and post-operatively, low-dose heparin is the most satisfactory agent on current evidence. In a high-risk situation, full oral anticoagulation is more effective although unwanted bleeding is also enhanced [310].

Pulmonary embolism

The pressures which have led to the application of maximal investigative effort in venous thrombosis towards successful prevention have applied with even greater force to pulmonary embolism; and obviously success with the first largely precludes the second. Effective prophylaxis against venous thrombosis should prevent most cases of pulmonary embolism although sporadic, unpredictable cases are bound to occur [311].

Management of acute life-threatening emboli

Treatment of established embolism is directed to preventing death from circulatory failure, reducing residual disability due to damage to the pulmonary circulation and preventing recurrence. In the majority of patients who survive the first two hours, death from circulatory obstruction is not an issue. Where the patient seems at risk of imminent death, three treatment options exist:
1 surgical embolectomy;
2 thrombolytic therapy with streptokinase or urokinase; and
3 infusion of heparin.
Most patients with potentially fatal acute massive pulmonary embolism will not survive long enough for treatment to be instituted [312] so that these measures are only applicable to a very small minority. Embolectomy using cardiac bypass is probably the treatment of choice in patients with persistently low blood pressure, urine output and arterial oxygen pressure [313, 314]. There is lack of total agreement about the value of embolectomy [315] and there is certainly a wide variation in reported mortality rates [316]. However, there do seem to be some patients who survive long enough for implementation of full medical resuscitative measures, despite which they appear to be deteriorating progressively [313]. If the surgical resources are available, it is difficult not to proceed to embolectomy in such cases; in these circumstances, survival rates as high as 75% have been reported [314].

The value of thrombolytic therapy is hard to assess. There is good evidence from angiography and catheter studies that treatment with urokinase or streptokinase reduces right-heart outflow obstruction and often causes partial dissolution of the embolus [313, 317–319]. Since outflow-tract obstruction is the cause of death in most patients it seems logical that accelerated relief of the obstruction should improve survival. However, this is only an assumption and likely to remain unproven. The other alternative is to proceed with anticoagulation without recourse to surgery or fibrinolytic therapy. There is some experimental evidence from animals to suggest that heparin in large doses may suppress platelet-mediated respiratory distress associated with platelet adhesion to the emboli [320], and high-dose heparin has been claimed to improve survival in man by this mechanism [321]. Heparin has the additional virtue of being the only treatment for which there is evidence of improvement in survival when compared to untreated controls [322]. There are some disquieting features about this celebrated study: for example, diagnostic criteria were inadequate by today's standards, and the high mortality rate in the control patients was 25%. However, it has to be accepted that while the study might be technically inadequate by present standards, heparin was shown to reduce mortality on the only occasion when the drug was compared directly with a non-treatment regime. On this basis it is both rational and usual to give heparin if embolectomy and fibrinolytic therapy are considered unsuitable.

Initial management of the patient with suspected massive pulmonary embolism should include confirmation of the diagnosis, with pulmonary angiography where available, and supportive measures designed to maintain cardiac filling pressure so far as that is possible [314]. External cardiac massage may have some value in breaking up large embolic masses and distributing them to the lung periphery [323].

Reduction in disability

In lesser degrees of pulmonary embolism, death is most unlikely to occur from the primary event. Standard anticoagulation with heparin and warfarin is instituted largely with the aim of preventing detachment of further emboli.

There is little available evidence on which to base a rational approach to prevention of residual damage to the pulmonary vasculature. Early experimental studies in dogs suggested that untreated pulmonary emboli lysed spontaneously *in situ* [324]. This appeared to be true also in man, on the basis of serial angiographic studies in patients treated with heparin [325]. However, the weight of later evidence indicates overwhelmingly that pulmonary emboli do not spontaneously dissolve completely although they contract and become endothelialized [313, 326–328]. In the largest study with long-term follow-up, some patients had residual filling defects on lung scan as long as one year after the initial event [319]. Fibrinolytic therapy does not seem to have much effect on long-term sequelae. Patients treated with streptokinase may still have filling defects on angiography and slight elevation of right-heart pressures six months after the embolus [313]. The large urokinase and urokinase-streptokinase trials conducted for the National Institutes of Health also failed to demonstrate any long-term advantage for fibrinolytic agents compared to heparin in minimizing perfusion defects in the pulmonary tree [319, 329]. Successful embolectomy should theoretically fully restore normal flow, though there are no adequate long-term follow-up studies to prove this.

Prevention of recurrence

The final essential of successful management is that recurrent emboli should be prevented. The trials of preventive treatment in venous thrombosis indicate that adequate anticoagulation does at least partially achieve this. It may also provide a more logical explanation of the successful outcome of the study of Barritt & Jordan [322] that anticoagulation reduced mortality by prevention of subsequent emboli rather than by attenuating the haemodynamic consequences of the first. Surgery has provided a more aggressive approach to this problem and has been used particularly in the USA. In the preliminary assessment, bilateral venography of the lower limb is essential. Large thrombi whose free end lies distal to the junction of the profunda femoris vein may be successfully incarcerated by ligation of the superficial femoral vein just below the profunda orifice [294]. Interruptive procedures on the more proximal veins and particularly on the inferior vena cava are probably scarcely ever indicated. The evidence for and against caval surgery has recently been meticulously and rationally analysed [279]. It can be summarized for practical purposes by pointing out that such procedures frequently result in venous obstructive symptoms and signs; that recurrent embolism is by no means uncommon and may originate from new thrombi laid down at the site of caval interruption; and that adequate anticoagulation is probably at least as effective, and certainly less traumatic to the patient.

A rational approach to patients with pulmonary embolism requires first that those with shock should receive immediate treatment to prevent death from the consequences of acute right-heart obstruction. Often availability of cardiological facilities determines whether embolectomy, fibrinolytic therapy or heparin infusion is preferred, although angiography followed by thrombolytic therapy with cardiac bypass on stand-by is probably the most logical. Patients not at imminent risk of death should receive standard heparin therapy. After the acute phase patients should be maintained on anticoagulants for three months to minimize the risk of recurrence. Detailed radiology of the veins is only justifiable where surgery to reduce recurrent embolism is contemplated.

Coronary heart-disease

'Coronary thrombosis' was a satisfying term, evocative of an underlying process and implying an understanding of pathogenesis. It would certainly seem reasonable on semantic grounds to treat coronary thrombosis with anticoagulants or anti-thrombotic drugs. And yet it is not certain that acute myocardial infarction resulting from coronary heart disease is always due to thrombosis [330, 331]. Thrombi are readily demonstrable post mortem in the coronary arteries of patients who have died from acute myocardial infarction [332]. In spite of some evidence to the contrary [333] it is likely that in most cases the infarct was precipitated by the thrombotic occlusion of the vessel lumen [332]. However, in patients dying suddenly and those with subendocardial infarction, other mechanisms involving platelet aggregates or vascular spasm may be important [330].

Anticoagulants

Anti-thrombotic treatment of myocardial infarction was started with anticoagulants well before the controversy over whether coronary thrombi were causal or consequential had been joined. The therapeutic intention was to reduce the death rate following myocardial infarction largely by preventing the thromboembolic sequelae from which about 25% of the patients died [334, 335]. In the 1950s and early 1960s it seemed clear that the benefit of anticoagulant therapy in acute myocardial infarction had been established. Later it became apparent that most of the early drug trials had been inadequate in design and potentially heavily biased [268]. While the advocates of anticoagulant therapy [336] continue the argument with their critics [337] it is likely that we have attained our ultimate insight into this particular therapeutic dilemma. Further trials will not be undertaken and the problem is one of interpretation. By the usual scientific criteria the case for anticoagulation has not been proven [338]. If there were some benefit observed in the early trials it seems entirely plausible that this was achieved by reduction in thromboembolic complications [339]. These are now a rare cause of death following myocardial infarction and more suitable forms of prophylaxis are available.

In the longer term, anticoagulants may be of

marginal benefit. This equally difficult topic has been reviewed in some detail [127, 340]. The conclusion, drawn from a number of trials, would be that anticoagulation may result in a marginal improvement in survival rate, any effect being most applicable to young males and those with a history of previous ischaemia. It is extremely doubtful whether in practical terms the limited gain justifies the difficulties for both the health-care team and the patient.

Anti-platelet agents

Work in the field was much stimulated by the report of the Boston Drug Surveillance Programme [341] that regular aspirin takers had only about 20% of the risk of non-aspirin takers of leaving hospital with a discharge diagnosis of myocardial infarction. The possibility that aspirin might be beneficial was reinforced by the report of the Coronary Drug Project Research Group [49], in which in 1629 patients admitted to the trial, in some cases many years after myocardial infarction, there appeared to be a benefit from regular aspirin use (1 g/day), although conventional levels of statistical significance were not achieved.

Two trials have been carried out by the Medical Research Council. In the first [342] there was a 24% reduction in mortality in a 12-month period in men taking 300 mg of aspirin daily as compared with control patients; this difference was not significant. The findings were reinforced by the second Medical Research Council study [343], in which there was a 17% reduction in the incidence of death in the year of follow-up in patients of both sexes taking 300 mg of aspirin three times a day; the five per cent significance level once again was not achieved.

The results of an important negative study were reported by the Aspirin Myocardial Infarction Research Study Group [344]. In this study, there was random allocation to either aspirin (1 g/day) or placebo for three years. The end-points determined before the beginning of the trial included total mortality, coronary incidence (that is the combination of coronary deaths plus proved non-fatal myocardial infarction and fatal or non-fatal stroke). Entry was eight weeks to five years after myocardial infarction and analysis was by life tables and final outcome. As regards the three primary end-points, the results for aspirin and placebo were almost identical. However, a positive outcome emerged for both aspirin and an aspirin–dipyridamole combination in the report of the Persantin Aspirin Reinfarction Study Research Group [345]. In this study there were three treatment groups: one group received 75 mg dipyridamole (Persantin) and 324 mg aspirin three times a day; the second group received aspirin and placebo, and a third group placebo only. The primary end-points were total mortality, coronary deaths and coronary incidence. There was a trend in favour of aspirin and dipyridamole, and of aspirin as compared with placebo, but statistical significance was not achieved. Life-table analysis, however, showed that dipyridamole and aspirin were significantly better than placebo at four, eight, 12, 16, 20 and 24 months, and aspirin was significantly better than placebo at eight and 24 months. Subgroup analysis showed that the effect on the three primary end-points was much more marked in those who entered the study within six months of myocardial infarction.

The effects of sulphinpyrazone (Anturane) in the secondary prevention of myocardial infarction were investigated by the Anturane Reinfarction Trial Research Group [346]. In this trial patients were allocated at random to sulphinpyrazone, 200 mg four times daily, or to placebo, for 12–24 months. Entry to the trial was 25–35 days after myocardial infarction. Before the trial began it was decided to restrict the analysis to so-called eligible patients and analysable events. In other words, the designers of the study decided to restrict analysis to patients suffering from their disease, dying their kind of deaths, while under the influence of their drug. It was decided that four per cent of patients were 'non-eligible' and three per cent of deaths were regarded as 'non-analysable'. Deaths from all causes, and cardiac deaths, were reduced at up to 24 months, although conventional levels of significance were not achieved. If the results are analysed on an 'intention-to-treat' basis, including all patients and all deaths, the difference between the placebo and treatment groups was trivial (nine per cent deaths in the sulphinpyrazone-treated patients and 11% deaths in the placebo patients). There was, however, a marked and significant reduction in sudden deaths which took place almost entirely during the first six months of treatment. It is of course by no means clear that a reduction in sudden deaths is due to an effect on platelets or the vessel wall, and other mechanisms, such as an anti-arrythmic effect, may be involved. The design of the trial has been the subject of some criticism [346a] and, in addition, at the time of writing (September 1980) an unfortunate difficulty has arisen with the interpretation of the data. It is reported [346b] that in the USA the Food and Drug Administration had reservations concerning the classification of deaths and was of the opinion that although there was suggestive evidence that sulphinpyrazone may be effective in preventing sudden death, the study did not provide the quality of scientific evidence required by American law to approve the drug for use after myocardial infarction. The data are being re-examined by the Food and Drug Administration and the Trial Policy Committee.

Platelet-inhibitor drugs in the secondary prevention of myocardial infarction: the present position. At present no confident statement can be made about the place of agents which inhibit platelet function, or platelet–vessel-wall interaction, in the secondary prevention of myocardial infarction. In several trials, aspirin has appeared to be beneficial, although one major study has been negative. It has recently been suggested [346c] that trials involving aspirin can be legitimately grouped together. If the pooled data from six trials are analysed, aspirin appears to be significantly effective in reducing cardiovascular mortality after myocardial infarction. Despite all the efforts which have been made up to the present the practising physician cannot yet be given firm guidelines. Each individual clinician must make up his own mind on the basis of existing evidence, but it would be unwise to drift into premature acceptance of the value of anti-platelet intervention after myocardial infarction until more information is available. Further large-scale, well-designed, randomized prospective clinical trials are needed.

Thrombolytic therapy
Thrombolytic therapy has also been used in acute myocardial infarction on the basis that dissolution of thrombus would improve tissue oxygenation and limit infarct size. Several trials have been published, but the four which had been conducted on patients admitted to a coronary care unit up to 1976 had agreed in finding no significant effect on morbidity or mortality from thrombolytic treatment [347]. Recently a collaborative European group have reported beneficial effects from streptokinase administered to patients within 12 hours of the onset of symptoms [348]. There are a number of factors in this study urging caution in appraisal of the result, most notably the observation that the improvement in survival of the treated group did not become apparent until three weeks after treatment.

Cerebrovascular disease
In thrombotic cerebrovascular disease the assessment of medication poses a problem which in some ways is more difficult than that in coronary heart disease, because there is much less diagnostic precision. In other ways the problem is less acute in social terms because it afflicts an older population in whom imminent death from some cause is a high probability. However, even from the most materialistic viewpoint, there would be considerable benefit to individual patients and the community from reduction in morbidity from stroke, though it would be over-optimistic to hope for a large effect on survival.

Anticoagulants
The greatest difficulty in stroke patients is to distinguish those with vascular occlusion from those with haemorrhage. Computerized tomography has probably had little real impact, although in theory it should enable diagnostic precision to be increased. Perhaps partly because of the diagnostic difficulties, attempts to treat acute stroke with oral anticoagulants have been unsuccessful [338]. A small trial of urokinase was even less successful, being abandoned because of haemorrhage in the treated group [349]. In the very restricted group of patients considered to have evolving stroke (a term not easily defined) there is a more general consensus that anticoagulation may abort the attack, although the evidence is far from convincing [350]. It seems hard to imagine that anti-thrombotic drugs could have any effect other than to limit secondary brain damage by reducing vascular occlusion with propagated clot. If this small effect is achieved, it is obscured by the scarcely surprising complication of haemorrhage into ischaemic or necrotic brain tissue.

Anti-platelet agents
Use of anti-thrombotic agents has more to commend it theoretically in prevention of stroke in high-risk patients, such as those who have had a transient ischaemic attack (TIA), an embolic episode, or who are likely to have a cerebral embolus, as for example in mitral stenosis with atrial fibrillation. It has been customary to anticoagulate these latter patients and most clinicians would do so, though the body of scientific evidence to support such action is rather thin [338].

In the case of transient cerebral ischaemic attacks the accent has shifted recently to the use of anti-platelet agents. This approach has considerable logic in view of the evidence from pathological studies that most patients have vestiges of platelet-fibrin emboli in the cerebral circulation, and many have ulcerating carotid plaques from which such emboli might feasibly originate. Two large studies have supported the value of aspirin 1200 mg daily in prevention of stroke and death in patients with TIA. In one from the USA, 88 patients treated with aspirin were significantly more likely to be alive without having suffered stroke or further emboli or TIA than 90 controls [351]. In a larger Canadian study, also looking at sulphinpyrazone, aspirin was found to reduce the risk of stroke or death by 30% compared to placebo, though only in men [51]. Sulphinpyrazone had a smaller, statistically insignificant effect, the trial data also being compatible with a synergistic action of the two drugs. It would seem reasonable on currently available evidence to treat males having TIA with aspirin and females with sulphinpyrazone. Surgery (endarterectomy of the carotid artery) may well be a suitable treatment in selected cases with a clearly defined atherosclerotic source of emboli.

Peripheral vascular disease

Occlusion of arteries to the lower limb is usually a late, acute phase in a chronic process, during which atherosclerosis has narrowed and partially obstructed the major vessels. The outcome may depend more on the state of the collateral vessels than on the form of therapeutic intervention. In most instances where survival of the limb is in doubt, or ischaemic symptoms very severe, reconstructive surgery is the only treatment worth consideration.

Anticoagulants

No large study on the effect of oral anticoagulants has been attempted. In a small trial with numbers adequate to detect only a very large effect, no benefit was observed from anticoagulation [352]. While this does not exclude the possibility of improvement in flow resulting from anticoagulation, the negative outcome conforms to the general view that anticoagulation in peripheral vascular disease is not useful [338]. Ancrod has been used in a small group of patients in whom peripheral blood flow and clinical symptoms appeared to improve with treatment [218]. The basis of this effect was thought to be reduction in blood viscosity produced by depletion of fibrinogen by ancrod.

Thrombolytic therapy

Thrombolytic therapy with streptokinase has been used in a number of studies [353]. In patients with recent thromboembolic occlusion of a limb, streptokinase infusion may avert amputation [354] though surgical management is certainly preferable in all but the least fit patients [355]. In chronic arterial insufficiency, streptokinase infusion has been of little value [356]. Except in those few patients unfit for surgery, with acute, localized thrombi, thrombolytic therapy is probably of little benefit in peripheral vascular disease.

Anti-platelet agents

There is little evidence of the possible value of anti-platelet drugs. Encouraging preliminary results have been reported following intra-arterial infusion of prostacyclin [357] which resulted in clinical improvement in a small number of patients. In loosely analogous circumstances, the combination of aspirin and dipyridamole was found to have no effect on preservation of the patency of coronary artery grafts [358]. Aspirin alone did not prevent thrombosis following catheterization of the brachial artery [359]. Peripheral arterial disease is the result of advanced atheroma affecting the vascular wall and it seems

unlikely, in view of the time-scale over which atherosclerosis develops, that anti-thrombotic drugs administered to symptomatic individuals could make much difference to the underlying disease process. Limitation of secondary thrombosis may have relatively little effect, even were the ideal anti-thrombotic drug available.

Disseminated intravascular coagulation (DIC) (see Chapter 29)

Indecision in the management of the DIC syndrome is the inevitable consequence of conflict between theoretical considerations of pathogenesis and clinical manifestations of bleeding. Even if haemorrhage is the result of consumption of coagulation material, it is a bold decision to put the patient's life at more immediate risk by administering anticoagulants.

This therapeutic dilemma has been concisely annotated by Sharp [75]. The first essential of therapy is to treat vigorously the underlying cause. This is frequently sepsis and treatment involves the rational choice of antibiotic and maintenance of plasma volume with appropriate fluids. When the problem is acute, as in obstetric accident, more urgent attention may need to be given to securing haemostasis. In these circumstances, administration of fresh-frozen plasma to restore clotting proteins or fresh whole blood if blood loss is severe, may be life-saving without other therapy. If the patient continues to deteriorate consideration may need to be given to treatment with heparin [75].

An ingenious approach has recently been suggested [360]: antithrombin III, activated *in vitro* with small amounts of heparin, is given in place of heparin itself. This may avoid increasing the risk of haemorrhage, while subserving the same role of inhibiting activated coagulation proteins; in addition it enhances plasma concentrations of antithrombin III which may be depleted in patients with DIC.

Some of the problems associated with heparin treatment have been considered by Merskey [361]. The essence of the difficulty is to decide in the short term whether symptoms and results of laboratory investigations are due to continuing intravascular thrombosis with secondary fibrinolysis, in which case anticoagulation may abort the episode by inhibiting further fibrin formation; or alternatively whether there is intense activation of fibrinolysis with minimal continuing fibrin deposition, for which anticoagulation may be disastrous. In general it seems unwise to administer anticoagulants to patients with acute DIC, in whom bleeding is known to be the most prominent symptom. In addition, the rather simple logic which underpins the case for heparin therapy has been increasingly undermined by our more detailed knowledge of the complex interaction which ensues when haematological systems are activated in shock states [146]. In the more chronic states associated with renal and hepatic disease and malignancy, heparin therapy may be more logical (as well as safer) although results in the haemolytic-uraemic syndrome of childhood [362] and hepatic disease [363] have not been clear cut. In view of the difficulty of mounting adequate clinical trials in DIC, it is improbable that more reliable evidence of therapeutic benefit will be forthcoming soon [75].

Claims of benefit have also been made for thrombolytic and anti-platelet drugs in the DIC syndromes. In view of the fundamental ignorance of pathogenesis in most instances, the reasoning behind use of these drugs is speculative, although on an empirical basis, anti-platelet drugs should have less potential to do harm.

POSSIBLE FUTURE DEVELOPMENTS

Looking back at the history of the development of pharmaceutical agents does not encourage confidence in looking forward to predict areas for future therapeutic advance. Most successful drugs have been the outcome of serendipity, not the brain children of scientists and planners. Drugs with a useful clinical function which have been discovered as the result of a directed pharmacological search, such as the beta-blockers and histamine (H$_2$) receptor antagonists, are rarities. The likeliest future development in the field of thrombosis is that something totally unexpected will turn up. However, we cannot rely on this Micawber-like philosophy; and while hoping for a novel compound to select itself, we may reasonably expect limited, if useful, advance in some of the following fields.

Improved diagnosis and prediction

Much of the difficulty alluded to in earlier sections in the choice of therapeutic agents stems from present inability to identify those patients who may benefit from the large numbers of others who will not. Greater precision in diagnosis of thrombosis may be as important to the future success of an anti-thrombotic agent as the inherent properties of the drug. We might make more sense of anti-thrombotic treatment for acute myocardial infarction if we knew which patients had suffered coronary arterial occlusion, which spasm, and which hypoxia-induced dysrhythmia. Similarly, anti-thrombotic drugs are unlikely to be restored to favour in treatment of stroke until it is easier to be sure that there is not a haemorrhagic infarct present.

It is in the field of prediction that the largest potential for improved direction of therapy lies. It is highly probable that by the time clinical consequences of thrombotic disease appear, treatment can merely be palliative. Prevention, even mediated pharmacologically, makes more sense. In patients undergoing gynaecological surgery, it has already been shown that patients at risk of post-operative venous thrombosis can be reliably identified [119, 120]. Restriction of preventive measures to high-risk patients will reduce costs and side-effects; and, equally important, it will allow new preventive measures to be tested more thoroughly and quickly by restricting the trial group to those at risk. In the wider field of thrombotic disease similar identification of a high-risk group may be possible. Coronary heart disease has been a field in which this approach has been practised for some time: smoking cigarettes increases the risk of developing the disease, while stopping smoking reduces it [3]. It may be possible similarly to isolate thrombotic factors and to show that they predispose to development of manifestations of disease. Preliminary data from such studies are encouraging [102h, 364]. If there is an identifiable subgroup of the population with an apparent thrombotic tendency, which increases the risk of acute myocardial infarction or sudden death, it seems rational that it is this group to whom present and future anti-thrombotic agents will have most to offer.

Cheap urokinase

The occasional astounding effectiveness of thrombolysis achieved with streptokinase, usually in recent massive deep venous thrombosis, makes a powerful impression on the witnesses. Unfortunately total clearance of a large thrombus is a relatively rare event. The reasons why streptokinase frequently fails are often not known and likely to be complex. One of the disadvantages of streptokinase as a thrombolytic agent is the complexity of its biochemical activity *in vivo* and in this respect urokinase has distinct advantages. However, urokinase suffers from the equally compelling disadvantage of very high cost: average doses for systemic fibrinolytic effect in a 70 kg man would exceed £100 per hour at October 1979 prices.

Were urokinase very much cheaper, there is a definite possibility that fibrinolytic therapy for acute thrombotic vascular obstruction might become both much more effective and much safer. The prospect of this is perhaps not too remote. Urokinase until very recently has been concentrated and purified from vast volumes of male human urine, both collection and purification being expensive. Urokinase (Abbokinase®) produced by human fetal kidney cells in culture [206] is now commercially available in this country and while very costly at present may become cheaper, particularly as its use becomes more widespread.

Oral heparin

Heparin is not absorbed from the gastro-intestinal tract and the need for parenteral administration limits therapeutic utility. Although the complexity of the molecule and the ease with which the anticoagulant property can be lost [159] discourages optimism, it may be possible to produce a heparin which has anti-thrombotic potential and can be given by mouth. An oral preparation might be particularly useful in pregnancy because of its short duration of action and because it does not have the teratogenic effect of oral anticoagulants [365]. A semi-synthetic heparin analogue which has greater activity than the parent compound against factor Xa for a standard anticoagulant effect [366] has already been prepared.

Effective oral fibrinolytic agents

Fibrinolytic activity measured in the vein wall [367] and as plasma euglobulin lysis activity [119] may be reduced in patients developing venous thrombosis; and lytic activity in the blood is reduced in men at higher risk of developing overt coronary heart disease [102h]. The hypothesis that decreased fibrinolytic activity might predispose to thrombosis is as convincing as many others and may justify evaluation of long-term prophylaxis with agents which significantly enhance fibrinolysis. A number of fibrinolytic agents are available and have been discussed earlier. Of these, several are active when given by mouth, including the combination of phenformin with ethyloestranol or stanozolol [207], the combination having greater activity than either compound used alone [368]. A diguanide and anabolic steroid together have been used clinically in treatment of vasculitis, Raynaud's phenomenon and recurrent venous thrombosis but no large preventive study has been mounted. If a more potent single agent were developed which resulted in sustained increase in endogenous fibrinolytic activity, it would have considerable promise as a prophylactic agent when administered to high-risk patients.

Inhibition of von Willebrand factor

Lack of the von Willebrand factor (see Chapter 28) partly accounts for the bleeding tendency of von Willebrand's disease. The way in which the von Willebrand factor functions is not known but there is evidence that it is required for normal platelet adhesion to damaged vessel surfaces [369]. A possible link between this property and thrombotic disease is provided by the observation that strains of pigs with von Willebrand's disease are resistant to experimental atherosclerosis [13, 14]. It may be that von Willebrand factor is required for adherence of platelets to vessel surfaces, lack of the factor resulting in protection against platelet-mediated thrombo-atherosclerosis.

These observations require to be considerably extended before any useful therapeutic advance could result. One obvious problem would rest with the bleeding tendency likely to be induced by a drug which inhibited von Willebrand factor. However, the experimental findings indicate that this may be a further point at which the haemostatic mechanism could be manipulated to produce an anti-thrombotic effect.

Inhibition of thromboxane A_2

Thromboxane A_2 is an unstable intermediate of platelet prostaglandin synthesis and a potent platelet-aggregating agent and vasoconstrictor [8, 10]. It is probably a crucial agent in the recruitment of platelets into the haemostatic plug, or platelet microthrombus, forming at sites of vessel injury [330]. Drugs such as aspirin, which inhibit platelet function by inhibition of cyclo-oxygenase, have the potential disadvantage previously discussed, that they also inhibit prostacyclin production in the vessel wall. If thromboxane A_2 is the principal pro-aggregatory compound released from platelets in addition to ADP, then a drug which inhibits thromboxane synthesis or antagonizes the action of thromboxane A_2 may have powerful anti-thrombotic effects. Inhibitors of thromboxane synthetase [370, 371] and thromboxane antagonists [372] have been described. None is yet available for clinical evaluation though this is an immediate prospect.

PGI_2 analogues

It has been proposed that PGI_2 provides the principal defence of the vascular intima against interaction with sensitized blood platelets [10]. PGI_2 may also function as a hormone, circulating in the bloodstream to depress the formation of platelet aggregates [373]. Experimentally in sensitive assay systems it has not proved possible to detect adequate levels of PGI_2 to achieve this latter role [374] but PGI_2, whatever its physiological function, is undoubtedly a very powerful inhibitor both of platelet adhesion to damaged surfaces and of platelet aggregation [19].

In itself PGI_2 is not suitable for general clinical use because of its vasodilator action, which produces hypotension in man [375], and its short half-life. These properties may not restrict its use in special circumstances. For example, it has been found to be an acceptable substitute for heparin in experimental extracorporeal circulations, with the additional advantage that because of its short half-life it does not affect haemostatic function in the main circulation [376]. The possible benefit of PGI_2 infusion in peripheral arterial disease has been noted earlier. Unfortunately the disadvantages are unlikely to be overcome for use systemically as an anti-thrombotic agent. However, a PGI_2 analogue may be found which will retain platelet inhibitory activity, but have greater stability and trivial adverse side-effects. Such a substance is likely to prove elusive.

Conclusion

Thrombotic disease is heterogeneous. Post-operative thrombosis of the superficial femoral vein probably shares little of the pathogenesis of occlusive disease in an adjacent atherosclerotic femoral artery. Much of what we think we know about thrombogenesis is rational supposition rather than established fact and new observations (along the lines of the recent discovery of prostacyclin) may radically alter current concepts. We can advance reasoned explanations as to how thrombi occur but we do not know which factors start the process. Nor do we know whether thrombosis is a failure of endogenous mechanisms or an inevitable response to unidentified insults from the environment. The uncertainties in our assessment of what causes thrombosis inevitably limit the ability to design anti-thrombotic drugs. Some available compounds are quite effective in certain circumstances and considerable advances have been made recently in pharmacological prevention of venous thrombotic disease. Similar success in the field of thrombo-atherosclerosis probably depends on a more precise definition and identification of the thrombotic component in a multifactorial disease.

REFERENCES

1 OFFICE OF POPULATION CENSUSES & SURVEYS (1978) *Mortality Statistics 1976 (Cause)*. HMSO, London.

2 BELL E.T. (1952) A postmortem study of vascular disease in diabetics. *Archives of Pathology*, **53**, 444.

3 JOINT WORKING PARTY OF THE ROYAL COLLEGE OF PHYSICIANS AND THE BRITISH CARDIAC SOCIETY (1976) Prevention of coronary heart disease. *Journal of the Royal College of Physicians*, **10**, 1.

4 WALKER W.J. (1977) Changing United States life-style and declining vascular mortality: cause or coincidence. *New England Journal of Medicine*, **297**, 163.

5 FLOREY C. DU V., MELIA R.J.W. & DARBY S.C. (1978) Changing mortality from ischaemic heart disease in Great Britain 1968–76. *British Medical Journal*, **i**, 635.

6 BEGENT N.A. & BORN G.V.R. (1970) Growth rate *in vivo* of platelet thrombi produced by iontophoresis of ADP as a function of mean blood flow velocity. *Nature (London)*, **227**, 926.

7 RODDIE I.C., SHEPHERD J.T. & WHELAN R.F. (1955) The action of 5-hydroxytryptamine on the blood vessels of the human hand and forearm. *British Journal of Pharmacology*, **10**, 445.

8 MARCUS A.J. (1978) The role of lipids in platelet function: with particular reference to the arachidonic acid pathway. *Journal of Lipid Research*, **19**, 793.

9 NEEDLEMAN P., MINKES, M. & RAZ, A. (1976) Throm-boxanes: selective biosynthesis and distinct biological properties. *Science*, **193**, 163.

10 MONCADA S. & VANE J.R. (1978) Unstable metabolites of arachidonic acid and their role in haemostasis and thrombosis. *British Medical Bulletin*, **34**, 129.

11 WEISS H.J., BAUMGARTNER H.R., TSCHOPP T.B., TURITTO V.T. & COHEN D. (1978) Correction by factor VIII of the impaired platelet adhesion to subendothelium in von Willebrand's disease. *Blood*, **51**, 267.

12 JORGENSEN L. & BORCHGREVINK C.F. (1964) The haemostatic mechanism in patients with haemorrhagic diseases. *Acta Pathologica et Microbiologica Scandinavica*, **60**, 55.

13 FUSTER V. & BOWIE E.J.W. (1978) The von Willebrand pig as a model for atherosclerosis research. *Thrombosis and Haemostasis*, **39**, 322.

14 FUSTER V., BOWIE E.J.W., JOSA A., KAYE M.P. & FASS D.N. (1979) Atherosclerosis in normal and von Willebrand pigs: cross aortic transplantation studies. *Thrombosis and Haemostasis*, **42** (Suppl), 1. 425.

15 BENDITT E.P. & BENDITT J.M. (1973) Evidence for a monoclonal origin of human atherosclerotic plaques. *Proceedings of the National Academy of Sciences, USA*, **70**, 1753.

16 PEARSON T.A., DILLMAN B.A., SOLEZ K. & HEPTINSTALL R.H. (1978) Clonal characteristics in layers of human atherosclerotic plaques. *American Journal of Pathology*, **93**, 93.

17 LIEBERMAN G.E., LEWIS G.P. & PETERS T.J. (1977) A membrane-bound enzyme in rabbit aorta capable of inhibiting adenosine-diphosphate-induced platelet aggregation. *Lancet*, **ii**, 330.

18 MONCADA S., HIGGS E.A. & VANE J.R. (1977) Human arterial and venous tissues generate prostacyclin (prostaglandin X) a potent inhibitor of platelet aggregation. *Lancet*, **i**, 18.

19 CAZENAVE J.-P., DEJANA E., KINLOUGH-RATHBONE R.L., RICHARDSON M., PACKHAM M.A. & MUSTARD J.F. (1979) Prostaglandins I$_2$ and E$_1$ reduce rabbit and human platelet adherence without inhibiting serotonin release from adherent platelets. *Thrombosis Research*, **15**, 273.

20 PANDOLFI M., NILSSON I.M., ROBERTSON B. & ISACSON S. (1967) Fibrinolytic activity of human veins. *Lancet*, **ii**, 127.

21 PANDOLFI M., ISACSON S. & NILSSON I.M. (1969) Low fibrinolytic activity in the walls of veins in patients with thrombosis. *Acta Medica Scandinavica*, **186**, 1.

22 BARNHART M.I. & CHEN S. (1978) Vessel wall models for studying interaction capabilities with blood platelets. *Seminars in Thrombosis and Haemostasis*, **5**, 112.

23 HARKER L.A., ROSS R., SLICHTER S.J. & SCOTT C.R. (1976) Homocystine-induced arteriosclerosis. The role of endothelial cell injury and platelet response in its genesis. *Journal of Clinical Investigation*, **58**, 731.

24 IREY N.S., MANION W.C. & TAYLOR H.B. (1970) Vascular lesions in women taking oral contraceptives. *Archives of Pathology*, **89**, 1.

25 MITCHELL J.R.A. & SCHWARTZ C.J. (1965) *Arterial Disease*, p. 191. Blackwell Scientific Publications, Oxford.

26 ENOS W.F., BEYER J.C. & HOLMES R.H. (1955) Pathogenesis of coronary disease in American soldiers killed

in Korea. *Journal of the American Medical Assocation*, **158**, 912.

27 MUSTARD J.F., MURPHY E.A., ROWSELL H.C. & DOW-NIE H.G. (1962) Factors influencing thrombus formation *in vivo*. *American Journal of Medicine*, **33**, 621.

28 FRIEDMAN L.I., LIEM H., GRABOWSKI E.F., LEONARD E.F. & MCCORD C.W. (1970) Inconsequentiality of surface properties for initial platelet adhesion. *Transactions of the American Society for Artificial Internal Organs*, **16**, 63.

29 TURITTO V.T., MUGGLI R. & BAUMGARTNER H.R. (1977) Physical factors influencing platelet deposition on subendothelium: importance of blood shear rate. *Annals of the New York Academy of Sciences*, **283**, 284.

30 BALDAUF W., WURZINGER L.J. & KINDER J. (1978) The role of stagnation point flow in the formation of platelet thrombi on glass surfaces in tubes with various geometry. *Pathology Research and Practice*, **163**, 9.

31 BROWN C.H., LEVERETT L.B., LEWIS C.W., ALFREY C.P. & HELLUMS J.D. (1975) Morphological, biochemical and functional changes in human platelets subjected to shear stress. *Journal of Laboratory and Clinical Medicine*, **86**, 462.

32 GRABOWSKI E.F., FRIEDMAN L.I. & LEONARD E.F. (1972) Effects of shear rate on the diffusion and adhesion of blood platelets to a foreign surface. *Industrial & Engineering Chemical Fundamentals*, **11**, 224.

33 GOLDSMITH H.L. (1972) The flow of model particles and blood cells and its relation to thrombogenesis. In: *Progress in Hemostasis and Thrombosis* (ed. Spaet T.H.) **1**, 97. Grune & Stratton, New York.

34 BRASH J.L., BROPHY J.M. & FEUERSTEIN I.A. (1976) Adhesion of platelets to artificial surfaces: effect of red cells. *Journal of Biomedical Materials Research*, **10**, 429.

35 TURITTO V.T. & BAUMGARTNER H.R. (1975) Platelet interaction with subendothelium in a perfusion system: physical role of red blood cells. *Microvascular Research*, **9**, 335.

36 CAZENAVE J.-P., PACKHAM M.A., DAVIES J.A., KIN-LOUGH-RATHBONE R.L. & MUSTARD J.F. (1978) Studies of platelet adherence to collagen and the subendothelium. In: *Platelet Function Testing* (ed. Day H.J., Holmsen H. & Zucker M.B.), p. 181. DHEW Publication No. (NIH) 78–1087.

37 MCMILLAN D.E. (1976) Plasma protein changes, blood viscosity and diabetic microangiopathy. *Diabetes*, **25** (Suppl. 2), 858.

38 BARNES A.J., LOCKE P., SCUDDER P.R., DORMANDY T.L., DORMANDY J.A. & SLACK J. (1977) Is hyperviscosity a treatable component of diabetic microcirculatory disease? *Lancet*, **ii**, 789.

39 DORMANDY J.A., HOARE E., KHATTAB A.H., ARROWS-MITH D.E. & DORMANDY T.L. (1973) Prognostic significance of rheological and biochemical findings in patients with intermittent clandication. *British Medical Journal*, **iv**, 581.

40 PEARSON T.C. & WETHERLEY-MEIN G. (1978) Vascular occlusive episodes and venous haematocrit in primary proliferative polycythaemia. *Lancet*, **ii**, 1219.

41 THOMAS D.J., DU BOULAY G.H., MARSHALL J., PEARSON T.C., ROSS RUSSELL R.W., SYMON L., WETHERLEY-MEIN G. & ZILKHA E. (1977) Effect of haematocrit on cerebral blood flow in man. *Lancet*, **ii**, 941.

42 BOTTI R.E. & RATNOFF O.D. (1964) Studies on the pathogenesis of thrombosis: an experimental hypercoagulable state induced by intravenous injection of ellagic acid. *Journal of Laboratory and Clinical Medicine*, **64**, 385.

43 SEVITT S. & GALLAGHER N. (1961) Venous thrombosis and pulmonary embolism. A clinico-pathological study in injured and burned patients. *British Journal of Surgery*, **48**, 475.

44 MUSTARD J.F., KINLOUGH-RATHBONE R.L. & PACKHAM M.A. (1974) Recent status of research in the pathogenesis of thrombosis. *Thrombosis et Diathesis Haemorrhagica*, **59** (Suppl.), 157.

45 MUSTARD J.F. & PACKHAM M.A. (1975) Platelets, thrombosis and drugs. *Drugs*, **9**, 19.

46 PATON R.C. & DOUGLAS A.S. (1976) Mechanisms of thrombotic disease. In: *Pathobiology Annual* (ed. Ioachim H.L.), p. 59. Appleton-Century-Crofts, New York.

47 WHITE A.M. & HEPTINSTALL S. (1978) Contribution of platelets to thrombus formation. *British Medical Bulletin*, **34**, 123.

48 MUSTARD J.F., PACKHAM M.A. & KINLOUGH-RATH-BONE R.L. (1978) Platelets and thrombosis in the development of atherosclerosis and its complications. *Advances in Experimental Medicine and Biology*, **102**, 7.

49 CORONARY DRUG PROJECT RESEARCH GROUP (1976) Aspirin in coronary heart disease. *Journal of Chronic Diseases*, **29**, 625.

50 ANTURANE REINFARCTION TRIAL RESEARCH GROUP (1978) Sulfinpyrazone in the prevention of cardiac death after myocardial infarction. *New England Journal of Medicine*, **298**, 289.

51 CANADIAN COOPERATIVE STROKE STUDY GROUP (1978) A randomised trial of aspirin and sulfinpyrazone in threatened stroke. *New England Journal of Medicine*, **299**, 53.

52 STEMERMAN M.B. (1974) Vascular intimal components: precursors of thrombosis. In: *Progress in Haemostasis and Thrombosis* (ed. Spaet T.H.) **2**, 1. Grune & Stratton, New York.

53 TRANZER J.P. & BAUMGARTNER H.R. (1967) Filling gaps in the vascular endothelium with blood platelets. *Nature (London)*, **216**, 1126.

54 ASHFORD T.P. & FREIMAN D.G. (1968) Platelet aggregation at sites of minimal endothelial injury. *American Journal of Pathology*, **53**, 599.

55 BAUMGARTNER H.R. (1974) Morphometric quantitation of adherence of platelets to an artificial surface and components of connective tissue. *Thrombosis et Diathesis Haemorrhagica*, **60** (Suppl.), 39.

56 TS'AO C.H. (1970) Graded endothelial injury of the rabbit aorta. *Archives of Pathology*, **90**, 222.

57 HAUDENSCHILD G. & STUDER A. (1971) Early interactions between blood cells and severely damaged rabbit aorta. *European Journal of Clinical Investigation*, **2**, 1.

58 CAZENAVE J.-P., PACKHAM M.A., GUCCIONE M.A. & MUSTARD J.F. (1975) Inhibition of platelet adherence to damaged surface of rabbit aorta. *Journal of Laboratory and Clinical Medicine*, **86**, 551.

59 TSCHOPP T.B. & BAUMGARTNER H.R. (1976) Enzymatic removal of ADP from plasma: unaltered platelet adhesion but reduced aggregation on subendothelium and collagen fibrils. *Thrombosis and Haemostasis*, **35**, 334.

60 BORN G.V.R. (1962) Aggregation of blood platelets by adenosine diphosphate and its reversal. *Nature (London)*, **194**, 927.

61 WU K.K. & HOAK J.C. (1974) A new method for the quantitative detection of platelet aggregates in patients with arterial insufficiency. *Lancet*, **ii**, 924.

62 DOUGHERTY J.H., LEVY D.E. & WEKSLER B.B. (1977) Platelet activation in acute cerebral ischaemia. *Lancet*, **i**, 821.

63 DAY H.J. & HOLMSEN H. (1971) Concepts of the blood platelet release reaction. *Series Haematologica*, **4**, 3.

64 NACHMAN R.L., WEKSLER B.B. & FERRIS B. (1972) Characterization of human platelet vascular permeability-enhancing activity. *Journal of Clinical Investigation*, **51**, 549.

65 ROSS R., GLOMSET J.A. & HARKER L.A. (1977) Response to injury and atherogenesis. *American Journal of Pathology*, **86**, 675.

66 WOOLF N. (1978) Thrombosis and atherosclerosis. *British Medical Bulletin*, **34**, 137.

67 MOORE S., FRIEDMAN R.J., SINGHAL D.P., GAULDIE J., BLAJCHMAN M.A. & ROBERTS R.S. (1976) Inhibition of injury-induced thromboatherosclerotic lesions by anti-platelet serum in rabbits. *Thrombosis and Haemostasis*, **35**, 70.

68 WALSH P.N. (1972) The role of platelets in the contact phase of blood coagulation. *British Journal of Haematology*, **22**, 237.

69 HARDISTY R.M. & HUTTON R.A. (1966) Platelet aggregation and the availability of platelet factor 3. *British Journal of Haematology*, **12**, 764.

70 NATH N., NIEWIAROWSKI S. & JOIST J.H. (1973) Platelet factor 4-anti-heparin protein releasable from platelets, purification and properties. *Journal of Laboratory and Clinical Medicine*, **82**, 754.

71 JOIST J.H., NIEWIAROWSKI S., NATH N. & MUSTARD J.F. (1976) Platelet antiplasmin: its extrusion during the release reaction, subcellular localization, characterization and relationship to antiheparin in pig platelets. *Journal of Laboratory and Clinical Medicine*, **87**, 659.

72 MILETICH J.P., JACKSON C.M. & MAJERUS P.W. (1977) Interaction of coagulation factor Xa with human platelets. *Proceedings of the National Academy of Sciences, USA*, **74**, 4033.

73 WALSH P.N. (1974) Platelet coagulant activities and hemostasis: a hypothesis. *Blood*, **43**, 597.

74 RATNOFF O.D. (1977) The surface-mediated initiation of blood coagulation and related phenomena. In: *Haemostasis: Biochemistry, Physiology and Pathology* (ed. Ogston D. & Bennett B.), p. 25. John Wiley & Sons, London.

75 SHARP A.A. (1977) Diagnosis and management of disseminated intravascular coagulation. *British Medical Bulletin*, **33**, 265.

76 NOSSEL H.L. (1976) The contact system. In: *Human Blood Coagulation, Haemostasis and Thrombosis* (ed. Biggs R.), p. 81. Blackwell Scientific Publications, Oxford.

77 WILNER G.D., NOSSEL H.L. & LEROY E.C. (1968) Activation of Hageman factor by collagen. *Journal of Clinical Investigation*, **47**, 2608.

78 MORRISON D.C. & COCHRANE C.G. (1974) Direct evidence for Hageman factor (factor XII) activation by

bacterial lipopolysaccharides (endotoxins). *Journal of Experimental Medicine*, **140**, 797.

79 KAPLAN A.P. & AUSTEN K.F. (1971) A prealbumin activator of prekallikrein. II. Derivation of activators of prekallikrein from active Hageman factor by digestion with plasmin. *Journal of Experimental Medicine*, **133**, 696.

80 LOPAS H., BIRNDORF N.I., BELL C.E., ROBBOY S.J. & COLMAN R.W. (1973) Immune hemolytic transfusion reactions in monkeys: activation of the kallikrein system. *American Journal of Physiology*, **225**, 372.

81 SCHIFFMAN S. & LEE P. (1974) Preparation, characterization and activation of a highly purified factor XI: evidence that a hitherto unrecognized plasma activity participates in the interaction of factors XI and XII. *British Journal of Haematology*, **27**, 101.

82 ESNOUF M.P. (1977) Biochemistry of blood coagulation. *British Medical Bulletin*, **33**, 213.

83 RADCLIFFE R.D. & NEMERSON Y. (1975) Activation and control of factor VII by activated factor X and thrombin. Isolation and characterization of a single chain form of factor VII. *Journal of Biological Chemistry*, **250**, 388.

84 ZELDIS S.M., NEMERSON Y., PITLICK F.A. & LENTZ T.L. (1972) Tissue factor (thromboplastin): localisation to plasma membranes by peroxidase-conjugated antibodies. *Science*, **175**, 766.

85 NEMERSON Y. & PITLICK F.A. (1972) The tissue factor pathway of blood coagulation. In: *Progress in Hemostasis and Thrombosis* (ed. Spaet T.H.) **1**, 1. Grune & Stratton, New York.

86 LAAKE K. & ÖSTERUD B. (1974) Activation of purified plasma factor VII by human plasmin, plasma kallikrein and activated components of the human intrinsic blood coagulation system. *Thrombosis Research*, **5**, 729.

87 NOSSEL H.L., YUDELMAN I., CANFIELD R.E., BUTLER V.P., SPANONDIS K., WILNER G.D. & QURESHI G.D. (1974) Measurement of fibrinopeptide A in human blood. *Journal of Clinical Investigation*, **54**, 43.

88 SHUMAN M.A. & MAJERUS P.W. (1976) The measurement of thrombin in clotting blood by radioimmunoassay. *Journal of Clinical Investigation*, **58**, 1249.

89 COLLEN D. & DE COCK F. (1975) A tanned red cell haemagglutination inhibition immunoassay (TRCHII) for the quantitative estimation of thrombin-antithrombin III and plasmin-alpha 1-antiplasmin complexes in human plasma. *Thrombosis Research*, **7**, 235.

90 GODAL H.C., MADSEN K. & NISSEN-MEYER R. (1962) Thrombo-embolism in patients with total proconvertin (factor VII) deficiency. A report on two cases. *Acta Medica Scandinavica*, **171**, 325.

91 RATNOFF O.D., BUSSE R.J. & SHEON R.P. (1968) The demise of John Hageman. *New England Journal of Medicine*, **279**, 760.

92 RAWLES J.M., OGSTON D. & DOUGLAS A.S. (1973) Hemostatic factors in the diagnosis of thrombosis. *Clinics in Hematology*, **2**, 79.

93 HIRSH J. (1977) Hypercoagulability. *Seminars in Hematology*, **14**, 409.

94 DAVIES J.A. & McNICOL G.P. (1981) Detection of a pre-thrombotic state. In: *Haemostasis and Thrombosis* (ed. Bloom A.L. & Thomas D.P.), p. 593. Churchill Livingstone, Edinburgh.

95 DENSON K.W.E. (1977) The ratio of factor VIII-related antigen and factor VIII biological activity as an index of hypercoagulability and intravascular clotting. *Thrombosis Research*, **10**, 107.

96 BLOOM A.L. (1975) Annotation. Intravascular coagulation and the liver. *British Journal of Haematology*, **30**, 1.

97 WESSLER S. & YIN E.T. (1968) Experimental hypercoagulable state induced by factor X: comparison of the non-activated and activated forms. *Journal of Laboratory and Clinical Medicine*, **72**, 256.

98 ISACSON S. & NILSSON I.M. (1972) Coagulation and fibrinolysis in acute cholecystitis. *Acta Chirurgica Scandinavica*, **138**, 179.

99 POLLER L. (1978) Oral contraceptives, blood clotting and thrombosis. *British Medical Bulletin*, **34**, 151.

100 BERAL V. (1977) Mortality among oral contraceptive users. Royal College of General Practitioners Oral Contraceptive Study. *Lancet*, **ii**, 727.

101 PECK S.D. & REIQUAM C.W. (1973) Disseminated intravascular coagulation in cancer patients: supportive evidence. *Cancer*, **31**, 1114.

102 KIM H.S., SUZUKI M., LIE J.T. & TITUS J.L. (1977) Non-bacterial thrombotic endocarditis (NBTE) and disseminated intravascular coagulation (DIC). *Archives of Pathology and Laboratory Medicine*, **101**, 65.

102a PINEO G.G., BRAIN M.C., GALLUS A.S., HIRSH J., HATTON M.W.C. & REGOECZI E. (1974) Tumours, mucous production and hypercoagulability. *Annals of the New York Academy of Sciences*, **230**, 262.

102b WARREN B.A. (1978) Platelet-tumour cell interactions. Morphological studies. In: *Platelets: a Multidisciplinary Approach* (ed. de Gaetano G. & Garattini S.), p. 427. Raven Press, New York.

102c GASIC G.J., GASIC T.B. & JIMENEZ S.A. (1977) Platelet aggregating material in mouse tumour cells. Removal and regeneration. *Laboratory Investigation*, **36**, 413.

102d COLWELL J.A., HALUSHKA P.V., SARJI K.E. & SAGEL J. (1978) Platelet function and diabetes mellitus. *Medical Clinics of North America*, **62**, 753.

102e FERGUSON J.C., MACKAY N. & MCNICOL G.P. (1970) Effect of feeding fat on fibrinolysis, Stypven time and platelet aggregation in Africans, Asians and Europeans. *Journal of Clinical Pathology*, **23**, 580.

102f JOIST J.H., KENDALL BAKER R. & SCHONFIELD G. (1979) Increased *in-vivo* and *in-vitro* platelet function in type II and type IV hyperlipoproteinaemia. *Thrombosis Research*, **15**, 95.

102g MEADE T.W. & NORTH W.R.S. (1977) Population based distributions of haemostatic variables. *British Medical Bulletin*, **33**, 283.

102h MEADE T.W., CHAKRABARTI R., HAINES A.P., NORTH W.R.S. & STIRLING Y. (1979) Characteristics affecting fibrinolytic activity and plasma fibrinogen concentration. *British Medical Journal*, **i**, 153.

103 BONNAR J. (1977) Acute and chronic coagulation problems in pregnancy. In: *Recent Advances in Blood Coagulation* (ed. Poller L.), p. 363. Churchill Livingstone, Edinburgh.

104 TALBERT L.M. & LANGDELL R.D. (1964) Normal values of certain factors in the blood clotting mechanism in pregnancy. *American Journal of Obstetrics and Gynecology*, **90**, 44.

105 NILSSON I.M. & KULLANDER S. (1967) Coagulation and fibrinolytic studies during pregnancy. *Acta Obstetrica et Gynecologica Scandinavica*, **46**, 273.

106 BONNAR J., MCNICOL G.P. & DOUGLAS A.S. (1969) Fibrinolytic enzyme system and pregnancy. *British Medical Journal*, **iii**, 387.

107 COOPLAND A., ALKJAERSIG N. & FLETCHER A.P. (1969) Reduction in plasma factor XIII (fibrin stabilising factor) concentration during pregnancy. *Journal of Laboratory and Clinical Medicine*, **73**, 144.

108 MCKILLOP C., HOWIE P.W., FORBES C.D. & PRENTICE C.R.M. (1976) Soluble fibrinogen/fibrin complexes in pre-eclampsia. *Lancet*, **i**, 56.

109 SHEPPARD B.L. & BONNAR J. (1974) The ultrastructure of the arterial supply of the human placenta in early and late pregnancy. *Journal of Obstetrics and Gynaecology of the British Commonwealth*, **81**, 497.

110 VESSEY M.P. & DOLL R. (1969) Investigation of relation between use of oral contraceptives and thromboembolic disease. A further report. *British Medical Journal*, **ii**, 651.

111 AMBRUS J.L., NISWANDER K.R., COUREY N.G., WAMSTEKER E.F. & MINK I.B. (1969) Progestational agents and blood coagulation. *American Journal of Obstetrics and Gynecology*, **103**, 994.

112 POLLER L. & THOMSON J.M. (1966) Clotting factors during oral contraception: further report. *British Medical Journal*, **ii**, 23.

113 MINK I.B., COUREY N.G., NISWANDER K.R., MOORE R.H., WILLIE M.A. & AMBRUS J.L. (1974) Progestational agents and blood coagulation. V. Changes induced by sequential oral contraceptive therapy. *American Journal of Obstetrics and Gynecology*, **119**, 401.

114 DAVIES T., FIELDHOUSE G. & MCNICOL G.P. (1976) The effects of therapy with oestriol succinate and ethinyloestradiol on the haemostatic mechanism in postmenopausal women. *Thrombosis and Haemostasis*, **35**, 403.

115 HOWIE P.W., MALLINSON A.C., PRENTICE C.R.M., HORNE C.H.W. & MCNICOL G.P. (1970) Effect of combined oestrogen-progestogen oral contraceptives, oestrogen and progestogen on antiplasmin and antithrombin activity. *Lancet*, **ii**, 1329.

116 ISACSON S. & NILSSON I.M. (1972) Coagulation and platelet adhesiveness in recurrent 'idiopathic' venous thrombosis. *Acta Chirurgica Scandinavica*, **138**, 263.

117 GALLUS A.S., HIRSH J. & GENT M. (1973) Relevance of preoperative and postoperative blood tests to postoperative leg-vein thrombosis. *Lancet*, **ii**, 805.

118 HUME M. & CHAN Y.K. (1967) Examination of the blood in the presence of venous thrombosis. *Journal of the American Medical Association*, **200**, 747.

119 CLAYTON J.K., ANDERSON J.A. & MCNICOL G.P. (1976) Preoperative prediction of postoperative deep vein thrombosis. *British Medical Journal*, **ii**, 910.

120 RAKOCZI I., CHAMONE D., COLLEN D. & VERSTRAETE M. (1978) Prediction of postoperative leg-vein thrombosis in gynaecological patients. *Lancet*, **i**, 509.

121 WALSH P.N., ROGERS P.H., MARDER V.J., GAGNATELLI G., ESCOVITZ E.S. & SHERRY S. (1976) The relationship of platelet coagulant activities to venous thrombosis following hip surgery. *British Journal of Haematology*, **32**, 421.

122 WU K.K., BARNES R.W. & HOAK J.C. (1975) Role of

platelets in recurrent deep vein thrombosis. *Thrombosis et Diathesis Haemorrhagica*, **34**, 357.

123 CADE J., HIRSH J. & REGOECZI E. (1975) Mechanism for elevated fibrin/fibrinogen degradation products in acute experimental pulmonary embolism. *Blood*, **45**, 563.

124 RUCKLEY C.V., DAS P.C., LEITCH A.G., DONALDSON A.A., COPLAND W.A., REDPATH A.T., SCOTT P. & CASH J.D. (1970) Serum fibrin/fibrinogen degradation products associated with postoperative pulmonary embolus and venous thrombosis. *British Medical Journal*, **iv**, 395.

125 COOKE E.D., GORDON Y.B., BOWCOCK S.A., SOLA C.M., PILCHER M.F., CHARD T., IBBOTSON R.M. & AINSWORTH M.E. (1975) Serum fibrin(ogen) degradation products in diagnosis of deep-vein thrombosis and pulmonary embolism after hip surgery. *Lancet*, **ii**, 51.

126 NOSSEL H.L. (1976) Radioimmunoassay of fibrinopeptides in relation to intravascular coagulation and thrombosis. *New England Journal of Medicine*, **295**, 428.

127 INTERNATIONAL ANTICOAGULANT REVIEW GROUP (1970) Collaborative analysis of long-term anticoagulant administration after acute myocardial infarction. *Lancet*, **i**, 203.

128 NOSSEL H.L., TI M., KAPLAN K.L., SPANONDIS K., SOLAND T. & BUTLER V.P. (1976) The generation of fibrinopeptide A in clinical blood samples: evidence for thrombin activity. *Journal of Clinical Investigation*, **58**, 1136.

129 O'BRIEN J.R., ETHERINGTON M.D., JAMIESON S., LAWFORD P., LINCOLN S.V. & ALKJAERSIG N.J. (1975) Blood changes in atherosclerosis and long after myocardial infarction and venous thrombosis. *Thrombosis et Diathesis Haemorrhagica*, **34**, 483.

130 RAWLES J.M., WARLOW C. & OGSTON D. (1975) Fibrinolytic capacity of arm and leg veins after femoral shaft fracture and acute myocardial infarction. *British Medical Journal*, **ii**, 61.

131 FLETCHER A.P. & ALKJAERSIG N. (1977) The use and monitoring of antithrombotic drug therapy. The need for a new approach. *Thrombosis and Haemostasis*, **38**, 881.

132 NILSSON I.M. (1974) *Haemorrhagic and Thrombotic Diseases*, p. 133. John Wiley & Sons, New York.

133 SHARMA S.C. & SETH H.M. (1978) Platelet adhesiveness, plasma fibrinogen and fibrinolytic activity in acute myocardial infarction. *British Heart Journal*, **40**, 526.

134 SZCZEKLIK A., GRYGLEWSKI R.J., MUSIAL J., GRODZINSKA L., SERWONSKA M. & MARCINKIEWICZ E. (1978) Thromboxane generation and platelet aggregation in survivals of myocardial infarction. *Thrombosis and Haemostasis*, **40**, 66.

135 WU K.K. & HOAK J.C. (1976) Spontaneous platelet aggregation in arterial insufficiency: mechanisms and implications. *Thrombosis and Haemostasis*, **35**, 702.

136 MANN J.I., VESSEY M.P., THOROGOOD M. & DOLL R. (1975) Myocardial infarction in young women with special reference to oral contraceptive practice. *British Medical Journal*, **ii**, 241.

137 MEADE T.W. (1973) The epidemiology of thrombosis. *Thrombosis et Diathesis Haemorrhagica*, **54** (Suppl.), 317.

138 WARLOW C.P., RENNIE J.A.N., OGSTON D. & DOUGLAS A.S. (1976) Platelet adhesiveness and fibrinolysis after recent cerebrovascular accidents and their relationship with subsequent deep venous thrombosis of the legs. *Thrombosis and Haemostasis*, **36**, 127.

139 FLETCHER A.P., ALKJAERSIG N., DAVIES A., LEWIS M., BROOKS J., HARDIN W., LANDAU W. & RAICHLE M.E. (1976) Blood coagulation and plasma fibrinolytic enzyme system pathophysiology in stroke. *Stroke*, **7**, 337.

140 WALSH P.N., PARETI F.I. & CORBETT J.J. (1976) Platelet coagulant activities and serum lipids in transient cerebral ischaemia. *New England Journal of Medicine*, **295**, 854.

141 ANDERSON L.A. & GORMSEN J. (1976) Platelet aggregation and fibrinolytic activity in transient cerebral ischaemia. *Acta Neurologica Scandinavica*, **55**, 76.

142 SIEGAL T., SELIGSOHN U., AGHAI E. & MODAN M. (1978) Clinical and laboratory aspects of disseminated intravascular coagulation (DIC): a study of 118 cases. *Thrombosis and Haemostasis*, **39**, 122.

143 MINNA J.D., ROBBOY S.J. & COLMAN R.W. (1974) *Disseminated Intravascular Coagulation in Man*. C. C. Thomas, Springfield, Illinois.

144 MERSKEY C., JOHNSON A.J., KLEINER G.J. & WOHL H. (1967) The defibrination syndrome: clinical features and laboratory diagnosis. *British Journal of Haematology*, **13**, 528.

145 KISKER C.T. & RUSH R. (1971) Detection of intravascular coagulation. *Journal of Clinical Investigation*, **50**, 2235.

146 PRESTON F.E. (1979) Haematological problems associated with shock. *British Journal of Hospital Medicine*, **21**, 232.

147 MÜLLER-BERGHAUS G. (1969) Pathophysiology of disseminated intravascular coagulation. *Thrombosis et Diathesis Haemorrhagica*, **36** (Suppl.), 45.

148 AL-MONDHIRY H. (1975) Disseminated intravascular coagulation. Experience in a major cancer center. *Thrombosis et Diathesis Haemorrhagica*, **34**, 181.

149 CLAWSON C.C. & WHITE J.G. (1971) Platelet interaction with bacteria. I. Reaction phases and effects of inhibitors. *American Journal of Pathology*, **65**, 367.

150 EVENSEN S.A. & ELGJO R.F. (1972) Antibody-induced platelet injury: its potency as a trigger of intravascular clotting. *Scandinavian Journal of Haematology*, **9**, 61.

151 KANNEL W.B., CASTELLI W.P. & MCNAMARA P.M. (1967) The coronary profile: 12 year follow-up in the Framingham study. *Journal of Occupational Medicine*, **9**, 611.

152 KEYS A. (1970) Coronary heart disease in seven countries. *Circulation*, **41** (Suppl. 1), 1.

153 VETERANS ADMINISTRATION CO-OPERATIVE STUDY GROUP (1970) Effects of treatment on morbidity in hypertension. *Journal of the American Medical Association*, **213**, 1152.

154 COMMITTEE OF PRINCIPAL INVESTIGATORS (1978) A co-operative trial in the primary prevention of ischaemic heart disease using clofibrate. *British Heart Journal*, **40**, 1069.

155 VESSEY M.P., MCPHERSON K. & JOHNSON B. (1977) Mortality among women participating in the Oxford Family Planning Association Contraceptive Study. *Lancet*, **ii**, 731.

156 MANN G.V. (1977) Diet-heart: end of an era. *New England Journal of Medicine*, **297**, 644.

157 TRUSWELL A.S. (1978) Diet and plasma lipids—a reappraisal. *American Journal of Clinical Nutrition*, **31**, 977.

158 MORRIS J.N., MARR J.W. & CLAYTON D.G. (1977) Diet and heart—a postscript. *British Medical Journal*, **ii**, 1307.

159 LINDAHL U., HÖÖK M., BÄCKSTRÖM G., JACOBSSON I., REISENFELD J., MALMSTRÖM A., RODEN L. & FEINGOLD D.S. (1977) Structure and synthesis of heparin-like polysaccharides. *Federation Proceedings*, **36**, 19.

160 JACQUES L.B. & MCDUFFIE N.M. (1978) The chemical and anticoagulant nature of heparin. *Seminars in Thrombosis and Haemostasis*, **4**, 277.

161 RIGHETTI P.G. & GIANAZZA E. (1978) Isoelectric focusing of heparin. Evidence for complexing with carrier ampholytes. *Biochemica Biophysica Acta*, **532**, 137.

162 JACQUES L.B. (1978) Endogenous heparin. *Seminars in Thrombosis and Haemostasis*, **4**, 326.

163 LANE D.A., MACGREGOR I.R., MICHALSKI R. & KAKKAR V.V. (1978) Anticoagulant activities of four unfractionated and fractionated heparins. *Thrombosis Research*, **12**, 257.

164 BARROWCLIFFE T.W., JOHNSON E.A., EGGLETON C.A. & THOMAS D.P. (1978) Anticoagulant activities of lung and mucous heparins. *Thrombosis Research*, **12**, 27.

165 MACKIE M.J. & DOUGLAS A.S. (1976) Anticoagulants. *British Journal of Hospital Medicine*, **16**, 118.

166 BARROWCLIFFE T.W., JOHNSON E.A. & THOMAS D.P. (1978) Antithrombin III and heparin. *British Medical Bulletin*, **34**, 143.

167 HOWELL W.H. (1925) The purification of heparin and its presence in blood. *American Journal of Physiology*, **71**, 553.

168 ROSENBERG R.D. (1975) Actions and interactions of antithrombin and heparin. *New England Journal of Medicine*, **292**, 146.

169 ROSENBERG R.D. (1977) Biologic actions of heparin. *Seminars in Hematology*, **14**, 427.

170 BIGGS R., DENSON K.W.E., AKMAN N., BORRETT R. & HADDEN M. (1970) Antithrombin III, antifactor Xa and heparin. *British Journal of Haematology*, **19**, 283.

171 SMITH G.F. (1977) The heparin-thrombin complex in the mechanism of thrombin inactivation by heparin. *Biochemical and Biophysical Research Communications*, **77**, 111.

172 YIN E.T., WESSLER S. & STOLL P.J. (1971) Biological properties of the naturally occuring plasma inhibitor to activated factor X. *Journal of Biological Chemistry*, **246**, 3703.

173 DENSON K.W.E. & BONNAR J. (1973) The measurement of heparin. A method based on the potentiation of anti-factor Xa. *Thrombosis et Diathesis Haemorrhagica*, **30**, 471.

174 WESSLER S. & YIN E.T. (1974) On the antithrombotic action of heparin. *Thrombosis et Diathesis Haemorrhagica*, **32**, 71.

175 ZUCKER M.B. (1977) Biological aspects of heparin action. Heparin and platelet function. *Federation Proceedings*, **36**, 47.

176 HEIDEN D., MIELKE C.H. & RODVIEN R. (1977) Impairment by heparin of primary haemostasis and platelet (^{14}C) 5-hydroxytryptamine release. *British Journal of Haematology*, **36**, 427.

177 STAHMANN M.A., HUEBNER C.F. & LINK K.P. (1941) Studies on the haemorrhagic sweet clover disease. V. Identification and synthesis of the haemorrhagic agent. *Journal of Biological Chemistry*, **138**, 513.

178 O'REILLY R.A. (1976) Vitamin K and the oral anticoagulant drugs. *Annual Review of Medicine*, **27**, 245.

179 PERKINS J. (1962) Phenindione sensitivity. *Lancet*, **i**, 127.

180 HEMKER H.C., VELTKAMP J.J., HENSEN A. & LOELIGER E.A. (1963) Nature of prothrombin biosynthesis: pre-prothrombinaemia in vitamin K deficiency. *Nature (London)*, **200**, 589.

181 GANROT P.O. & NILEHN J.E. (1968) Plasma prothrombin during treatment with Dicumarol. II. Demonstration of an abnormal prothrombin fraction. *Journal of Clinical and Laboratory Investigation*, **22**, 23.

182 GITEL S.N., OWEN W.G., ESMON G.T. & JACKSON C.M. (1973) A polypeptide region of bovine prothrombin specific for binding to phospholipids. *Proceedings of the National Academy of Sciences, USA*, **70**, 1344.

183 NELSESTUEN G.L. & SUTTIE J.W. (1973) The mode of action of vitamin K. Isolation of a peptide containing the vitamin K-dependent portion of prothrombin. *Proceedings of the National Academy of Sciences, USA*, **70**, 3366.

184 STENFLO J., FERNLUND P., EGAN W. & ROEPSTORFF P. (1974) Vitamin K-dependent modifications of glutamic acid residues in prothrombin. *Proceedings of the National Academy of Sciences, USA*, **71**, 2730.

185 SADOWSKI J.A., ESMON C.T. & SUTTIE J.W. (1976) Vitamin K-dependent carboxylase. Requirements of the rat liver microsomal enzyme system. *Journal of Biological Chemistry*, **251**, 2770.

186 SUTTIE J.W. (1977) Oral anticoagulant therapy: the biosynthetic basis. *Seminars in Hematology*, **14**, 365.

186a BROZOVIC M. (1976) Oral anticoagulants, vitamin K and prothrombin complex factors. *British Journal of Haematology*, **32**, 9.

186b JACKSON C.W. & SUTTIE J.W. (1977) Recent developments in understanding the mechanism of vitamin K and vitamin K-antagonist drug action and the consequences of vitamin K action in blood coagulation. *Progress in Hematology*, **10**, 333.

187 KAKKAR V.V. & SCULLY M.F. (1978) Thrombolytic therapy. *British Medical Bulletin*, **34**, 191.

188 BROGDEN R.N., SPEIGHT T.M. & AVERY G.S. (1973) Streptokinase: a review of its clinical pharmacology, mechanism of action and therapeutic uses. *Drugs*, **5**, 357.

189 JOHNSON A.J. & MCCARTY W.R. (1959) The lysis of artifically induced intravascular clots in man by intravenous infusions of streptokinase. *Journal of Clinical Investigation*, **38**, 1627.

190 BROCKWAY W.J. & CASTELLINO F.J. (1974) A characterization of native streptokinase and altered streptokinase isolated from a human plasminogen activator complex. *Biochemistry*, **13**, 2063.

191 REDDY K.N.N. & MARCUS G. (1972) Mechanism of activation of human plasminogen by streptokinase. Presence of active center in streptokinase-plasminogen complex. *Journal of Biological Chemistry*, **247**, 1683.

192 SUMMARIA L., HSIEH B. & ROBBINS K.C. (1967) The

specific mechanism of activation of human plasminogen to plasmin. *Journal of Biological Chemistry*, **242**, 4279.

193 CLAEYS H., MOLLA A. & VERSTRAETE M. (1973) Conversion of NH₂-terminal glutamic acid to NH₂-terminal lysine human plasminogen by plasmin. *Thrombosis Research*, **3**, 515.

194 WALLEN P. (1978) Chemistry of plasminogen and plasminogen activation. In: *Progress in Chemical Fibrinolysis and Thrombolysis* (ed. Davidson J.F., Rowan R.M., Samama M.M. & Desnoyers P.C.), p. 167. Raven Press, New York.

195 WIMAN B. & COLLEN D. (1978) Molecular mechanism of physiological fibrinolysis. *Nature* (London), **272**, 549.

196 HARPEL P.C. & MOSESSON M.W. (1973) Degradation of human fibrinogen by plasma α₂-macroglobulin enzyme complexes. *Journal of Clinical Investigation*, **52**, 2175.

197 FLUTE P.T. (1976) Thrombolytic therapy. *British Journal of Hospital Medicine*, **16**, 135.

198 KERNOFF P.B.A. & McNICOL G.P. (1977) Normal and abnormal fibrinolysis. *British Medical Bulletin*, **33**, 239.

199 ALKJAERSIG N., FLETCHER A.P. & SHERRY S. (1959) The mechanism of clot dissolution by plasmin. *Journal of Clinical Investigation*, **38**, 1086.

200 AMBRUS C.M. & MARKUS G. (1960) Plasmin-antiplasmin complex as a reservoir of fibrinolytic enzyme. *American Journal of Physiology*, **199**, 491.

201 CHESTERMAN C.N., ALLINGTON M.J. & SHARP A.A. (1972) Relationship of plasminogen activator to fibrin. *Nature (New Biology)*, **238**, 15.

202 VERSTRAETE M., VERMYLEN J., AMERY A. & VERMYLEN C. (1966) Thrombolytic therapy with streptokinase using a standard dosage scheme. *British Medical Journal*, **i**, 454.

203 McNICOL G.P. & DAVIES J.A. (1972) Fibrinolytic enzyme system. *Clinics in Hematology*, **2**, 23.

204 KAKKAR V.V., SAGAR S. & LEWIS M. (1975) Treatment of deep-vein thrombosis with intermittent streptokinase and plasminogen infusion. *Lancet*, **ii**, 674.

205 McNICOL G.P. & DOUGLAS A.S. (1976) Thrombolytic therapy and fibrinolytic inhibitors. In: *Human Blood Coagulation, Haemostasis and Thrombosis* (ed. Biggs R.), p. 436. Blackwell Scientific Publications, Oxford.

206 BERNIK M.B. & KWAAN H.C. (1969) Plasminogen activator activity in cultures from human tissues. An immunological and histochemical study. *Journal of Clinical Investigation*, **48**, 1740.

207 CHAKRABARTI R., EVANS J.F. & FEARNLEY G.R. (1970) Effects on platelet stickiness and fibrinolysis of phenformin combined with ethyloestranol or stanozolol. *Lancet*, **i**, 591.

208 REID H.A., THEAN P.C., CHAN K.E. & BAHAROM A.R. (1963) Clinical effects of bites by Malayan viper (Ancistrodon rhodostoma). *Lancet*, **i**, 617.

209 REID H.A., CHAN K.E. & THEAN P.C. (1963) Prolonged coagulation defect (defibrination syndrome) in Malayan viper bite. *Lancet*, **i**, 621.

210 ESNOUF M.P. & TUNNAH G.W. (1967) The isolation and properties of the thrombin-like activity from Ancistrodon rhodostoma venom. *British Journal of Haematology*, **13**, 581.

211 TURPIE A.G.G., McNICOL G.P. & DOUGLAS A.S. (1976) Ancrod (Arvin) a new anticoagulant. In: *Human Blood Coagulation, Haemostasis and Thrombosis* (ed. Biggs R.), p. 476. Blackwell Scientific Publications, Oxford.

212 EWART M.P., HATTON M., BASFORD J.M. & DODGSON K.S. (1970) The proteolytic action of arvin on human fibrinogen. *Biochemical Journal*, **118**, 603.

213 SHARP A.A., WARREN B.A., PAXTON A.M. & ALLINGTON M.J. (1968) Anticoagulant therapy with a purified fraction of Malayan pit viper venom. *Lancet*, **i**, 493.

214 BARLOW G.H., HOLLEMAN W.H. & LORAND L. (1970) The action of arvin on fibrin stabilizing factor (factor XIII). *Research Communications in Chemical Pathology and Pharmacology*, **1**, 1.

215 TURPIE A.G.G., PRENTICE C.R.M., McNICOL G.P. & DOUGLAS A.S. (1970) *In-vitro* studies with ancrod (Arvin). *British Journal of Haematology*, **20**, 217.

216 PIZZO S.V., SCHWARTZ M.L., HILL R.L. & McKEE P.A. (1972) Mechanism of ancrod anticoagulation. A direct proteolytic effect on fibrin. *Journal of Clinical Investigation*, **51**, 2841.

217 OLSEN E.G.J. & PITNEY W.R. (1969) The effect of arvin on experimental pulmonary embolism. *British Journal of Haematology*, **17**, 425.

218 DORMANDY J.A., GOYLE K.B. & REID H.L. (1977) Treatment of severe intermittent claudication by controlled defibrination. *Lancet*, **i**, 625.

219 SMITH J.B. & WILLIS A.L. (1971) Aspirin selectively inhibits prostaglandin production in human platelets. *Nature (New Biology)*, **231**, 235.

220 WILLIS A.L. & KUHN D.C. (1973) A new potential mediator of arterial thrombosis whose biosynthesis is inhibited by aspirin. *Prostaglandins*, **4**, 127.

221 HAMBERG M. & SAMUELSSON B. (1973) Detection and isolation of an endoperoxide intermediate in prostaglandin biosynthesis. *Proceedings of the National Academy of Sciences, USA*, **70**, 899.

222 HAMBERG M., SVENSSON J. & SAMUELSSON B. (1975) Thromboxanes: A new group of biologically active compounds derived from prostaglandin endoperoxides. *Proceedings of the National Academy of Sciences, USA*, **72**, 2994.

223 ROTH G.J. & MAJERUS P.W. (1975) The mechanism of the effect of aspirin on human platelets. I. Acetylation of a particulate fraction protein. *Journal of Clinical Investigation*, **56**, 624.

224 HIRSH J., STREET D., CADE J.F. & AMY H. (1973) Relation between bleeding time and platelet connective tissue reaction after aspirin. *Blood*, **41**, 369.

225 WEISS H.J. & TURITTO V.T. (1979) Prostacyclin (prostaglandin I₂, PGI₂) inhibits platelet adhesion and thrombus formation on subendothelium. *Blood*, **53**, 244.

226 KELTON J.G., HIRSH J., CARTER C.J. & BUCHANAN M.R. (1978) Thrombogenic effect of high-dose aspirin in rabbits. *Journal of Clinical Investigation*, **62**, 892.

227 JAFFE E.A. & WEKSLER B.B. (1979) Recovery of endothelial cell prostacyclin production after inhibition by low doses of aspirin. *Journal of Clinical Investigation*, **63**, 532.

228 KRICHEFF I.I., ZUCKER M.B., TSCHOPP T.B. & KOLODJIEZ A. (1973) Inhibition of thrombosis on vascular catheters in cats. *Radiology*, **106**, 49.

229 JUSTICE C., PAPAVANGELOU E. & EDWARDS W.S. (1974)

Prevention of thrombosis with agents which reduce platelet adhesiveness. *American Surgeon*, **40**, 186.

230 FOLTS J.D., CROWELL E.B. & ROWE G.G. (1976) Platelet aggregation in partially obstructed vessels and its elimination with aspirin. *Circulation*, **54**, 365.

231 DAVIES J.A., ESSIEN E., CAZENAVE J.-P, KINLOUGH-RATHBONE R.L., GENT M. & MUSTARD J.F. (1979) The influence of red blood cells on the effects of aspirin or sulphinpyrazone on platelet adherence to damaged rabbit aorta. *British Journal of Haematology*, **42**, 283.

232 BAUMGARTNER H.R., MUGGLI R., TSCHOPP T.B. & TURITTO V.T. (1976) Platelet adhesion, release and aggregation in flowing blood: effects of surface properties and platelet function. *Thrombosis and Haemostasis*, **35**, 124.

233 HORNSTRA G. & TEN HOOR F. (1975) The filtragometer: a new device for measuring platelet aggregation in venous blood of man. *Thrombosis et Diathesis Haemorrhagica*, **34**, 531.

234 FLEISCHMAN A.I., BIERENBAUM M.L. & STIER A. (1976) The effect of aspirin on *in-vivo* platelet function in humans. *Thrombosis Research*, **8**, 797.

235 DE GAETANO D., DONATI M.B. & GARATTINI S. (1975) Drugs affecting platelet function tests. Their effect on haemostasis and surgical bleeding. *Thrombosis et Diathesis Haemorrhagica*, **34**, 285.

236 ALI M. & MCDONALD J.W.D. (1978) Reversible and irreversible inhibition of platelet cyclo-oxygenase and serotonin release by nonsteroidal anti-inflammatory drugs. *Thrombosis Research*, **13**, 1057.

237 DAVIES T., LEDERER D.A., SPENCER A.A. & MCNICOL G.P. (1974) The effect of flurbiprofen [2-(2-fluro-4-biphenyl) propionic acid] on platelet function and blood coagulation. *Thrombosis Research*, **5**, 667.

238 PACKHAM M.A., CAZENAVE J.-P., KINLOUGH-RATHBONE R.L. & MUSTARD J.F. (1978) Drug effects on platelet adherence to collagen and damaged vessel walls. *Advances in Experimental Medicine and Biology*, **109**, 253.

239 BOURGAIN R.H. (1978) The effect of indomethacin and ASA on *in-vivo* induced white platelet arterial thrombus formation. *Thrombosis Research*, **12**, 1079.

240 KAEGI A., PINEO G.F., SHIMUZU A., TRIVEDI H., HIRSH J. & GENT M. (1975) The role of sulphinpyrazone in the prevention of arterio-venous shunt thrombosis. *Circulation*, **52**, 497.

241 SMYTHE H.A., ORGYZLO M.A., MURPHY E.A. & MUSTARD J.F. (1965) The effect of sulphinpyrazone (Anturan) on platelet economy and blood coagulation in man. *Canadian Medical Association Journal*, **92**, 818.

242 WEILY H.S., STEELE P.P., DAVIES H., PAPPAS G. & GENTON E. (1974) Platelet survival time in patients with substitute heart valves. *New England of Medicine*, **290**, 534.

243 STEELE P.P., WEILY H.S. & GENTON E. (1973) Platelet survival and adhesiveness in recurrent venous thrombosis. *New England Journal of Medicine*, **288**, 1148.

244 HARKER L.A. & SLICHTER S.J. (1970) Studies of platelet and fibrinogen kinetics in patients with prosthetic heart valves. *New England Journal of Medicine*, **283**, 1302.

245 ABRAHAMSEN A.F., EIKA C., GODAL H.C. & LORENTSEN E. (1974) Effect of acetylsalicylic acid and dipyridamole on platelet survival and aggregation in patients with

246 EMMONS P.R., HARRISON M.J.G., HONOUR A.J. & MITCHELL J.R.A. (1965) Effect of a pyrimido-pyrimidine derivative on thrombus formation in the rabbit. *Nature (London)*, **208**, 255.

247 ZUCKER M.B. & PETERSON J. (1970) Effect of acetylsalicylic acid, other non-steroidal anti-inflammatory agents, and dipyridamole on human blood platelets. *Journal of Laboratory and Clinical Medicine*, **76**, 66.

248 RAJAH S.M., CROW M.J., PENNY A.F., AHMAD R. & WATSON D.A. (1977) The effect of dipyridamole on platelet function: correlation with blood levels in man. *British Journal of Clinical Pharmacology*, **4**, 129.

249 MILLS D.C.B. & SMITH J.B. (1971) The influence on platelet aggregation of drugs that affect the accumulation of adenosine $3':5'$ cyclic monophosphate in platelets. *Biochemical Journal*, **121**, 185.

250 MONCADA S. & KORBUT R. (1978) Dipyridamole and other phosphodiesterase inhibitors act as antithrombotic agents by potentiating endogenous prostacyclin. *Lancet*, **I**, 1286.

251 GUREWICH V. & LIPINSKI B. (1976) Evaluation of antithrombotic properties of suloctidil in comparison with aspirin and dipyridamole. *Thrombosis Research*, **9**, 101.

252 HONOUR A.J., HOCKADAY T.D.R. & MANN J.I. (1977) The synergistic effect of aspirin and dipyridamole upon platelet thrombi in living blood vessels. *British Journal of Experimental Pathology*, **58**, 268.

253 OBLATH R.W., BUCKLEY F.O., GREEN R.M., SCHWARTZ S.I. & DE WEESE J.A. (1978) Prevention of platelet aggregation and adherence to prosthetic vascular grafts by aspirin and dipyridamole. *Surgery*, **84**, 37.

254 HASSANEIN A.A., TURPIE A.G.G., MCNICOL G.P. & DOUGLAS A.S. (1970) Effect of RA233 on platelet function *in vitro*. *British Medical Journal*, **ii**, 83.

255 DAVID J.-L., MONFORT F. & RASKINET R. (1979) Compared effects of three dose-levels of ticlopidine on platelet function in normal subjects. *Thrombosis Research*, **14**, 35.

256 TOMIKAWA M., ASHIDA A., KAKIHATA K. & ABIKO Y. (1978) Anti-thrombotic action of ticlopidine, a new platelet aggregation inhibitor. *Thrombosis Research*, **12**, 1157.

257 ASHIDA S.-I. & ABIKO Y. (1979) Mode of action of ticlopidine in inhibition of platelet aggregation in the rat. *Thrombosis and Haemostasis*, **41**, 436.

258 WEISS H.J. (1967) The effect of clinical dextran on platelet aggregation, adhesion and ADP release in man. *Journal of Laboratory and Clinical Medicine*, **69**, 37.

259 ÅBERG M. & RAUSING A. (1978) The effect of dextran 70 on the structure of *ex-vivo* thrombi. *Thrombosis Research*, **12**, 1113.

260 ARFORS K.-E., HINT H.C., DHALL D.P. & MATHESON N.A. (1968) Counteraction of platelet activity at sites of laser-induced endothelial trauma. *British Medical Journal*, **iv**, 430.

261 KAKKAR V.V., STAMATAKIS J.D., BENTLEY P.G., LAWRENCE D., DE HAAS H.A. & WARD V.P. (1979) Prophylaxis for postoperative deep-vein thrombosis. *Journal of the American Medical Association*, **241**, 39.

262 MELLANDER S. & NORDENFELT I. (1970) Comparative

effects of dihydroergotamine and noradrenaline on resistance, exchange and capacitance functions in the peripheral circulation. *Clinical Science*, **39**, 183.

263 SAGAR S., NAIRN D., STAMATAKIS J.D., MAFFEI F.H., HIGGINS A.F., THOMAS D.P. & KAKKAR V.V. (1976) Efficacy of low-dose heparin in prevention of extensive deep-vein thrombosis in patients undergoing total hip replacement. *Lancet*, **i**, 1151.

264 SABRI S., ROBERTS V.C. & COTTON L.T. (1971) Prevention of early post-operative deep vein thrombosis by intermittent compression of the leg during surgery. *British Medical Journal*, **iv**, 394.

265 ROBERTS V.C. (1977) Passive stimulation of venous flow as a prophylactic against deep vein thrombosis. *Triangle*, **16**, 35.

266 ROBERTS V.C., SABRI S., PIETRONI M.C., GUREWICH V. & COTTON L.T. (1971) Passive flexion and femoral vein flow: a study using a motorized foot mover. *British Medical Journal*, **iii**, 78.

267 BROWSE N.L. & NEGUS D. (1970) Prevention of postoperative leg vein thrombosis by electrical muscle stimulation. An evaluation with ^{125}I-labelled fibrinogen. *British Medical Journal*, **iii**, 615.

268 GIFFORD R.H. & FEINSTEIN A.R. (1969) Critique of studies of anticoagulant therapy for myocardial infarction. *New England Journal of Medicine*, **280**, 351.

269 PETO R. (1978) Clinical trial methodology. *Biomedicine Special Issue*, **28**, 24.

270 PETO R., PIKE M.C., ARMITAGE P., BRESLOW N.E., COX D.R., HOWARD S.V., MANTEL N., MCPHERSON K., PETO J. & SMITH P.G. (1976) Design and analysis of randomized clinical trials requiring prolonged observation of each patient. I. Introduction and design. *British Journal of Cancer*, **34**, 585.

271 PETO R., PIKE M.C., ARMITAGE P., BRESLOW N.E., COX D.R., HOWARD S.V., MANTEL N., MCPHERSON K., PETO J. & SMITH P.G. (1977) Design and analysis of randomized clinical trials requiring prolonged observation of each patient. II. Analysis and examples. *British Journal of Cancer*, **35**, 1.

272 BYAR D.P., SIMON R.M., FRIEDEWALD W.T., SCHLESSELMAN J.J., DEMETS D.L., ELLENBERG J.H., GAIL M.H. & WARE J.H. (1976) Randomized clinical trials: perspectives on some new ideas. *New England Journal of Medicine*, **295**, 74.

273 HARKER L.A., HIRSH J., GENT M. & GENTON E. (1975) Critical evaluation of platelet-inhibiting drugs in thrombotic disease. In: *Progress in Hematology* (ed. Brown E.B.), p. 229. Grune & Stratton, New York.

274 SEVITT S. & GALLAGHER N.G. (1959) Prevention of venous thrombosis and pulmonary embolism in injured patients. *Lancet*, **ii**, 981.

275 MORRIS G.K. & MITCHELL J.R.A. (1976) Prevention and diagnosis of venous thrombosis in patients with hip fractures. A survey of current practice. *Lancet*, **ii**, 867.

276 BONNAR J. & WALSH J. (1972) Prevention of thrombosis after pelvic surgery by British dextran 70. *Lancet*, **i**, 614.

277 MORRIS G.K. & MITCHELL J.R.A. (1976) Warfarin sodium in prevention of deep venous thrombosis and pulmonary embolism in patients with fractured neck of femur. *Lancet*, **ii**, 869.

278 BROWSE N. (1978) Diagnosis of deep-vein thrombosis. *British Medical Bulletin*, **34**, 163.

279 GALLUS A.S. & HIRSH J. (1976) Treatment of venous thromboembolic disease. *Seminars in Thrombosis and Haemostasis*, **2**, 291.

280 MORRIS G.K. & MITCHELL J.R.A. (1978) Clinical management of venous thromboembolism. *British Medical Bulletin*, **34**, 169.

281 ZILLIACUS H. (1946) On the specific treatment of thrombosis and pulmonary embolism with anticoagulants with particular reference to the post-thrombotic sequelae. *Acta Medica Scandinavica*, **171** (Suppl.), 13.

282 MCNICOL G.P. (1974) Conventional uses of heparin. *Thrombosis et Diathesis Haemorrhagica*, **33**, 97.

283 WESSLER S., MORRIS L.E. & MORAN C.J. (1955) Studies in intravascular coagulation. IV. The effect of heparin and dicoumarol on serum-induced venous thrombosis. *Circulation*, **12**, 553.

284 COON W.W. & WILLIS P.W. (1972) Thromboembolic complications during anticoagulant therapy. *Archives of Surgery*, **105**, 209.

285 SALZMAN E.W., DEYKIN D., SHAPIRO R.M. & ROSENBERG R. (1975) Management of heparin therapy. *New England Journal of Medicine*, **292**, 1046.

286 COON W.W. & WILLIS P.W. (1974) Hemorrhagic complications of anticoagulant therapy. *Archives of Internal Medicine*, **133**, 386.

287 COON W.W. & WILLIS P.W. (1969) Assessment of anticoagulant treatment of venous thromboembolism. *Annals of Surgery*, **170**, 559.

288 WALKER R.H.S., JACKSON J.A. & GOODWIN J. (1970) Resolution of pulmonary embolism. *British Medical Journal*, **iv**, 135.

289 COON W.W. & WILLIS P.W. (1973) Recurrence of venous thromboembolism. *Surgery*, **73**, 823.

290 KAKKAR V.V., HOWE C.T., LAWS J.W. & FLANC C. (1969) Late results of treatment of DVT. *British Medical Journal*, **i**, 810.

291 KAKKAR V.V., FLANC C., HOWE C.T., O'SHEA M. & FLUTE P.T. (1969) Treatment of deep venous thrombosis. A trial of heparin, streptokinase and Arvin. *British Medical Journal*, **i**, 806.

292 DAVIES J.A., MERRICK M.V., SHARP A.A. & HOLT J.M. (1972) Controlled trial of ancrod and heparin in treatment of deep vein thrombosis of lower limb. *Lancet*, **i**, 113.

293 TIBBUTT D.A., WILLIAMS E.W., WALKER N.W., CHESTERMAN C.N., HOLT J.M. & SHARP A.A. (1974) Controlled trial of ancrod and streptokinase in the treatment of deep vein thrombosis of lower limb. *British Journal of Haematology*, **27**, 407.

294 MAVOR G.E. & GALLOWAY J.M.D. (1969) Ileofemoral venous thrombosis: pathological considerations and surgical management. *British Journal of Surgery*, **56**, 45.

295 GALLUS A.S. & HIRSH J. (1976) Prevention of venous thromboembolism. *Seminars in Thrombosis and Haemostasis*, **2**, 232.

296 CRANDON A.J., PEEL K.R. & MCNICOL G.P. (1979) Post-operative deep vein thrombosis: prophylaxis in high risk patients. *British Journal of Haematology*, **43**, 494.

297 COTTON L.T. & ROBERTS V.C. (1977) The prevention of deep vein thrombosis with particular reference to mechanical methods of prevention. *Surgery*, **81**, 228.

298 MITCHELL J.R.A. (1979) Can we really prevent post-

operative pulmonary emboli? *British Medical Journal*, **i**, 1523.

299 INTERNATIONAL MULTICENTRE TRIAL (1975) Prevention of fatal postoperative pulmonary embolism by low doses of heparin. *Lancet*, **ii**, 45.

300 GRUBER V.F., DUCKERT F., FRIDRICH R., TORHORST J. & REM J. (1977) Prevention of postoperative thromboembolism by Dextran 40, low doses of heparin or xantinol nicotinate. *Lancet*, **i**, 207.

301 KIIL J., KIIL J., AXELSEN F. & ANDERSEN D. (1978) Prophylaxis against postoperative pulmonary embolism and deep vein thrombosis by low-dose heparin. *Lancet*, **i**, 1115.

302 KLINE A., HUGHES L.E., CAMPBELL H., WILLIAMS A., ZLOSNICK J. & LEACH K.G. (1975) Dextran 70 in prophylaxis of thromboembolic disease after surgery: a clinically orientated randomized double-blind trial. *British Medical Journal*, **ii**, 109.

303 BROKOP T., EKLÖF B., ERIKSSON I., GOLDIE I., GRAN L., GRUBER U.F., HOHL M., JONSSON T., KRISTERSSON S., LJUNGSTRÖM K.G., LUND T., MAARTMAN MOE H., SALDEEN T., SVENSJÖ E., THOMSON D., TORHORST J., TRIPPESTAD A. & ULSTEIN M. (1979) Prevention of fatal postoperative pulmonary embolism by Dextran 70 or low doses of heparin. An international multicentre trial. *Thrombosis and Haemostasis*, **42**, 248.

304 HARRIS W.H., SALZMAN E.W., ATHANASOULIS C.A., WALTMAN A.C. & DE SANCTIS R.W. (1977) Aspirin prophylaxis of venous thromboembolism after total hip replacement. *New England Journal of Medicine*, **297**, 1246.

305 GROOTE SCHUUR HOSPITAL THROMBOEMBOLUS STUDY GROUP (1979) Failure of low-dose heparin to prevent significant thromboembolic complications in high-risk surgical patients: interim report of a prospective trial. *British Medical Journal*, **i**, 1447.

306 STAMATAKIS J.D., KAKKAR V.V., SAGAR S., LAWRENCE D., NAIRN D. & BENTLEY P.G. (1977) Femoral vein thrombosis and total hip replacement. *British Medical Journal*, **ii**, 223.

307 HAMPSON W.G.J., HARRIS F.C., LUCAS H.K., ROBERTS P.H., McCALL I.W., JACKSON P.C., POWELL N.L. & STADDON G.E. (1974) Failure of low-dose heparin to prevent deep vein thrombosis after hip replacement arthroplasty. *Lancet*, **ii**, 795.

308 HARRIS W.H., SALZMAN E.W., ATHANASOULIS C., WALTMAN A.C., BAUM S. & DE SANCTIS R. (1974) Comparison of warfarin, low-molecular-weight dextran, aspirin and subcutaneous heparin in prevention of venous thromboembolism following total hip replacement. *Journal of Bone and Joint Surgery*, **56A**, 1552.

309 LOWE G.D.O., CAMPBELL A.F., MEEK D.R., FORBES C.D. & PRENTICE C.R.M. (1978) Subcutaneous ancrod in prevention of deep-vein thrombosis after operation for fractured neck of femur. *Lancet*, **ii**, 698.

310 HULL R., DELMORE T., GENTON E., HIRSH J., GENT M., SACKETT D., McLOUGHLIN D. & ARMSTRONG P. (1979) Warfarin sodium versus low-dose heparin in the long-term treatment of venous thrombosis. *New England Journal of Medicine*, **301**, 855.

311 BRECKENRIDGE R.T. & RATNOFF O.D. (1964) Pulmonary embolism and unexpected death in supposedly normal persons. *New England Journal of Medicine*, **270**, 298.

312 COON W.W. & COLLER F.A. (1959) Clinico-pathological correlation in thromboembolism. *Surgery, Gynecology and Obstetrics*, **109**, 259.

313 TIBBUTT D.A., DAVIES J.A., ANDERSON J.A., FLETCHER E.W.L., HAMILL J., HOLT J.M., LEA THOMAS M., LEE G. DE J., MILLER G.A.H., SHARP A.A. & SUTTON G.C. (1974) Comparison by controlled clinical trial of streptokinase and heparin in treatment of life-threatening pulmonary embolism. *British Medical Journal*, **i**, 343.

314 MILLER G.A.H. (1977) The management of acute pulmonary embolism. *British Journal of Hospital Medicine*, **18**, 26.

315 ALPERT J.S., SMITH R.E., OCKENE I.S., ASKENAZI J., DEXTER L. & DALEN J.E. (1975) Treatment of massive pulmonary embolism: the role of pulmonary embolectomy. *American Heart Journal*, **89**, 413.

316 CROSS F.S. & MOWLEM A. (1967) A survey of the current status of pulmonary embolectomy for massive pulmonary embolism. *Circulation*, **35** (Suppl. 1), 86.

317 HIRSH J., McDONALD I.G. & HALE G.S. (1970) Streptokinase in the treatment of major pulmonary embolism—experience with 25 patients. *Australasian Annals of Medicine*, **19** (Suppl. 1), 54.

318 MILLER G.A.H., SUTTON G.C., KERR I.H., GIBSON R.V. & HONEY M. (1971) Comparison of streptokinase and heparin in treatment of isolated acute massive pulmonary embolism. *British Medical Journal*, **ii**, 681.

319 UROKINASE-STREPTOKINASE EMBOLISM TRIAL (1974) Phase 2 results. A cooperative study. *Journal of the American Medical Association*, **229**, 1606.

320 THOMAS D.P., GUREWICH V. & STUART R.K. (1968) Epinephrine potentiation of platelet aggregation: its effect on death from experimental pulmonary emboli. *Journal of Laboratory and Clinical Medicine*, **71**, 955.

321 CRANE C., HARTSUCK J., BIRTCH A., COUCH N.P., ZOLLINGER R., MATLOFF J., DALEN J. & DEXTER L. (1969) The management of major pulmonary embolism. *Surgery, Gynecology and Obstetrics*, **128**, 27.

322 BARRITT D.W. & JORDAN S.C. (1960) Anticoagulant drugs in the treatment of pulmonary embolism. A controlled trial. *Lancet*, **i**, 1309.

323 HEIMBECKER R.O., KEON W.J. & RICHARDS K.U. (1973) Massive pulmonary embolism. A new look at surgical management. *Archives of Surgery*, **107**, 740.

324 ALLISON P.R., DUNNILL M.S. & MARSHALL R. (1960) Pulmonary embolism. *Thorax*, **15**, 273.

325 FRED H.L., AXELRAD M.A., LEWIS J.M. & ALEXANDER J.K. (1966) Rapid resolution of pulmonary thromboemboli in man. *Journal of the American Medical Association*, **196**, 1137.

326 TOW D.E. & WAGNER H.N. (1967) Recovery of pulmonary arterial blood flow in patients with pulmonary embolism. *New England Journal of Medicine*, **276**, 1053.

327 DALEN J.E., BANAS J.S., BROOKS H.L., EVANS G.E., PARASKOS J.A. & DEXTER L. (1969) Resolution rate of acute pulmonary embolism in man. *New England Journal of Medicine*, **280**, 1194.

328 McDONALD I.G., HIRSH J. & HALE G.S. (1971) Early rate of resolution of major pulmonary embolism. *British Heart Journal*, **33**, 432.

329 UROKINASE PULMONARY EMBOLISM TRIAL (1970) Phase

l results. A cooperative study. *Journal of the American Medical Association*, **214**, 2163.

330 MUSTARD J.F. (1976) Function of blood platelets and their role in thrombosis. *Transactions of the American Clinical and Climatological Association*, **87**, 104.

331 SHORT D. (1977) The great circulatory paradox. *Lancet*, **i**, 1244.

332 FRIEDMAN M. (1975) The pathogenesis of coronary plaques, thromboses and haemorrhages: an evaluative review. *Circulation*, **51/52** (Suppl. 3), 34.

333 ROBERTS W.C. & FERRANS V.J. (1976) The role of thrombosis in the aetiology of atherosclerosis (a positive one) and in precipitating fatal ischaemic heart disease (a negative one). *Seminars in Thrombosis and Haemostasis*, **2**, 123.

334 WRIGHT I.S., MARPLE C.D. & BECK D.F. (1948) Report of the committee for the evaluation of anticoagulants in the treatment of coronary thrombosis with myocardial infarction. *American Heart Journal*, **36**, 801.

335 TULLOCH J.A. & GILCHRIST A.R. (1950) Anticoagulants in treatment of coronary thrombosis. *British Medical Journal*, **ii**, 965.

336 CHALMERS T.C., MATTA R.J., SMITH H. & KUNZLER A.-M. (1977) Evidence favoring the use of anticoagulants in the hospital phase of acute myocardial infarction. *New England Journal of Medicine*, **297**, 1091.

337 GOLDMAN L. & FEINSTEIN A.R. (1979) Anticoagulants and myocardial infarction. The problems of pooling, drowning and floating. *Annals of Internal Medicine*, **90**, 92.

338 MACKIE M.J. & DOUGLAS A.S. (1978) Oral anticoagulants in arterial disease. *British Medical Bulletin*, **34**, 177.

339 SELZER A. (1978) Use of anticoagulant agents in acute myocardial infarction: Statistics or clinical judgement? *American Journal of Cardiology*, **41**, 1315.

340 DOUGLAS A.S. & MCNICOL G.P. (1976) Anticoagulant therapy. In: *Human Blood Coagulation, Haemostasis and Thrombosis* (ed. Biggs R.), p. 557. Blackwell Scientific Publications, Oxford.

341 JICK S. & MIETTINEN O.S. (1976) Regular aspirin use and myocardial infarction. *British Medical Journal*, **i**, 1057.

342 ELWOOD P.C., COCHRANE A.C., BURR M.L., SWEETNAM P.M., WILLIAMS G., WELSBY E., HUGHES J.S. & RENTON R. (1974) A randomised controlled trial of acetyl salicylic acid in the secondary prevention of mortality from myocardial infarction. *Lancet*, **i**, 436.

343 ELWOOD P.C. & SWEETNAM P.M. (1979) Aspirin and secondary mortality after myocardial infarction. *Lancet*, **ii**, 1313.

344 ASPIRIN MYOCARDIAL INFARCTION STUDY RESEARCH GROUP (1980) A randomised controlled trial of aspirin in persons recovered from myocardial infarction. *Journal of the American Medical Association*, **243**, 661.

345 PERSANTINE-ASPIRIN REINFARCTION STUDY RESEARCH GROUP (1980) Persantine and aspirin in coronary heart disease. *Circulation*, **62**, 449.

346 ANTURANE REINFARCTION TRIAL RESEARCH GROUP (1980) Sulfinpyrazone in the prevention of sudden death after myocardial infarction. *New England Journal of Medicine*, **302**, 250.

346a MITCHELL J.R.A. (1980) Secondary prevention of myocardial infarction. *British Medical Journal*, **280**, 1128.

346b SCIENCE (1980) FDA says no to Anturane. *Science*, **208**, 1130.

346c LEADING ARTICLE (1980) Aspirin after myocardial infarction. *Lancet*, **i**, 1172.

347 ABER C.P., BASS N.M., BERRY C.L., CARSON P.H.M., DOBBS R.J., FOX K.M., HAMBLIN J.J., HAYDU S.P., HOWITT G., MACIVER J.E., PORTAL R.W., RAFTERY E.B., ROUSELL R.H. & STOCK J.P.P. (1976) Streptokinase in acute myocardial infarction: a controlled multicentre study in the United Kingdom. *British Medical Journal*, **ii**, 1100.

348 EUROPEAN COOPERATIVE STUDY GROUP FOR STREPTOKINASE TREATMENT IN ACUTE MYOCARDIAL INFARCTION (1979) Streptokinase in acute myocardial infarction. *New England Journal of Medicine*, **301**, 797.

349 FLETCHER A.P., ALKJAERSIG N., LEWIS M., TULEVSKI V., DAVIES A., BROOKS J.E., HARDIN W.B., LANDAU W.M. & RAICHLE M.E. (1976) A pilot study of urokinase therapy in cerebral infarction. *Stroke*, **7**, 135.

350 MILLIKAN C.H. (1971) Reassessment of anticoagulation therapy in various types of occlusive cerebrovascular disease. *Stroke*, **2**, 201.

351 FIELDS W.S., LEMAK N.A., FRANKOWSKI R.F. & HARDY R.J. (1977) Controlled trial of aspirin in cerebral ischaemia. *Stroke*, **8**, 301.

352 RICHARDS R.L. & BERG T.B. (1967) Long-term anticoagulant therapy in atherosclerotic peripheral arterial disease. *Vascular Diseases*, **4**, 27.

353 FRATANTONI J.C., NESS P. & SIMON T.L. (1975) Thrombolytic therapy. *New England Journal of Medicine*, **293**, 1073.

354 AMERY A., DELOOF W., VERMYLEN J. & VERSTRAETE M. (1970) Outcome of recent thromboembolic occlusions of limb arteries treated with streptokinase. *British Medical Journal*, **iv**, 639.

355 PERSSON A.V., THOMSON J.E. & PATMAN R.D. (1973) Streptokinase as an adjunct to arterial surgery. *Archives of Surgery*, **107**, 779.

356 VERSTRAETE M., VERMYLEN J. & DONATI M.B. (1971) The effect of streptokinase infusion on chronic arterial occlusions and stenoses. *Annals of Internal Medicine*, **74**, 377.

357 SZCZEKLIK A., NIZANKOWSKI R., SKAWINSKI S., SZCZEKLIK J., GLUSZKO P. & GRYGLEWSKI R.J. (1979) Successful therapy of advanced arteriosclerosis obliterans with prostacyclin. *Lancet*, **i**, 1111.

358 PANTELY G.A., GOODNIGHT S.H., RAHIMTOOLA S.H., HARLAN B.J., DEMOTS H., CALVIN L. & RÖSCH J. (1979) Failure of antiplatelet and anticoagulant therapy to improve patency of grafts after coronary-artery bypass. *New England Journal of Medicine*, **301**, 962.

359 HYNES K.M., GAU G.T., RUTHERFORD B.D., KAZMIER F.J. & FRYE R.L. (1973) Effect of aspirin on brachial artery occlusion following brachial arteriotomy for coronary arteriography. *Circulation*, **47**, 554.

360 SCHIPPER H.G., JENKINS C.S.P., KAHLE L.H. & TEN CATE J.W. (1978) Antithrombin-III transfusion in disseminated intravascular coagulation. *Lancet*, **i**, 854.

361 MERSKEY C. (1976) Defibrination syndrome. In *Human Blood Coagulation, Haemostasis and Thrombosis* (ed.

Biggs R.), p. 492. Blackwell Scientific Publications, Oxford.

362 VITACCO M., SANCHEZ AVALOS J. & GIANANTONIO C.A. (1973) Heparin therapy in the hemolytic-uremic syndrome. *Journal of Pediatrics*, **83**, 271.

363 GAZZARD B.G., CLARK R., BORIRAKCHANYAVAT V. & WILLIAMS R. (1974) A controlled trial of heparin therapy in the coagulation defect of paracetamol-induced hepatic necrosis. *Gut*, **15**, 89.

364 FULLER J.H., KEEN H., JARRETT R.J., OMER T., MEADE T.W., CHAKRABARTI R., NORTH W.R.S. & STIRLING Y. (1979) Haemostatic variables associated with diabetes and its complications. *British Medical Journal*, **ii**, 964.

365 TEJANI N. (1973) Anticoagulant therapy with cardiac valve prosthesis during pregnancy. *Obstetrics and Gynecology*, **42**, 785.

366 THOMAS D.P., LANE D.A., MICHALSKI R., JOHNSON E.A. & KAKKAR V.V. (1977) A heparin analogue with specific action on antithrombin III. *Lancet*, **i**, 120.

367 PANDOLFI M., ISACSON S. & NILSSON I.M. (1969) Low fibrinolytic activity in the walls of veins in patients with thrombosis. *Acta Medica Scandinavica*, **186**, 1.

368 DAVIDSON J.F. (1977) Recent advances in fibrinolysis. In: *Recent Advances in Blood Coagulation* (ed. Poller L.), p. 91. Churchill Livingstone, Edinburgh.

369 BAUMGARTNER H.R., TSCHOPP T.B. & WEISS H.J. (1978) Defective adhesion of platelets to subendothelium in von Willebrand's disease and Bernard–Soulier syndrome. *Thrombosis and Haemostasis*, **39**, 782.

370 GRYGLEWSKI R.J., ZMUDA A., KORBUT R., KRECIOCH E. & BIERON K. (1977) Selective inhibition of thromboxane A_2 biosynthesis in blood platelets. *Nature (London)*, **267**, 627.

371 ALLAN G. & EAKINS K.E. (1978) Burimamide is a selective inhibitor of thromboxane—A_2 biosynthesis in human platelet microsomes. *Prostaglandins*, **15**, 659.

372 FITZPATRICK F.A., BUNDY G.L., GORMAN R.R. & HONOHAN T. (1978) 9,11-Epoxyiminoprosta-5, 13-dienoic acid is a thromboxane A_2 antagonist in human platelets. *Nature (London)*, **275**, 764.

373 MONCADA A., KORBUT R., BUNTING S. & VANE J.R. (1978) Prostacyclin is a circulating hormone. *Nature (London)*, **273**, 767.

374 HASLAM R.J. (1979) Roles of cyclic nucleotides in the inhibition of platelet function by physiological and pharmacological agents. *Thrombosis and Haemostasis*, **42**, 86.

375 FITZGERALD G.A., FRIEDMAN L.A., LEWIS P.J., MYAMORI I. & O'GRADY J. (1979) A double-blind placebo controlled cross-over study of prostacyclin in man. *Clinical Science*, **57**, 6P.

376 WOODS H.F., ASH G., WESTON M.J., BUNTING S., MONCADA S. & VANE J.R. (1978) Prostacyclin can replace heparin in haemodialysis in dogs. *Lancet*, **ii**, 1075.

SECTION 5
DISORDERS AFFECTING
ALL THE
FORMED ELEMENTS OF
THE BLOOD

Chapter 31
Aplastic and dysplastic anaemias

S. M. LEWIS AND E. C. GORDON-SMITH

Bone-marrow failure may occur as a result of either *failure of cell production* ('aplastic anaemia') or *abnormal cell production with failure of maturation* ('dysplastic anaemia'). In reality, there is often considerable overlap between the two, as the same bone-marrow injury may induce either effect whilst a marrow recovering from aplasia might become dysplastic during the recovery phase. Any or all of the cell lines may be affected. Depending on which, there will be anaemia, thrombocytopenia and/or leucopenia with neutropenia. When there is reduction in all the formed elements in the peripheral blood (i.e. pancytopenia) the disorder should be termed aplastic anaemia; when there is anaemia but without involvement of leucocytes and platelets, the term red-cell aplasia is more appropriate. The equivalent terms to describe qualitative abnormalities are dyshaemopoiesis and dyserythropoiesis respectively. Abnormalities which give rise exclusively to neutropenia or thrombocytopenia are described in Chapters 15 and 25.

In addition to the various causes of aplastic and dysplastic anaemia which are described in this chapter, anaemia or pancytopenia may result from hypersplenism. In this condition the bone marrow is of normal or increased cellularity; the spleen is enlarged to a significant extent (see Chapter 20).

The main causes of reduced bone-marrow activity are listed in Table 31.1. The other cell lines may be variably affected but anaemia is a constant feature. As a rule, many of these causes are readily identifiable by the presence in peripheral blood of abnormal or primitive cells or a leuco-erythroblastic reaction, by characteristic bone-marrow appearances, by clinical features, by haematological course, and by response to specific therapy. In some cases diagnosis may be assisted by means of special investigations, including ferrokinetic studies with radioactive iron, erythropoietin assay and various microbiological assays.

APLASTIC ANAEMIAS

The concept of aplastic anaemias appears to have been introduced by Paul Erlich who, in 1886, reported the case of a 21-year-old girl who presented with haemorrhage associated with anaemia, thrombocytopenia, leucopenia and a bone marrow devoid of all cells. He drew attention to the absence of red-cell regeneration and recognized that the primary defect was one of decreased blood-cell production [1].

Within 50 years, 150 cases had been reported and a diagnostic picture was established of a uniformly acute and rapidly fatal disease of adolescents and young adults, associated with a rapidly developing anaemia without regeneration, and a bone marrow which had undergone complete fatty degeneration [2]. Subsequently, variations from this uniform picture were noted with an increasing frequency, and it is now apparent that 'aplastic anaemia' comprises a number of different conditions with varying aetiology, course and prognosis [3–10]. Various classifications have been suggested; Table 31.2 shows variants which can be distinguished by clinical and haematological criteria. This classification is based on whether only erythropoiesis is involved (red-cell aplasia) or whether other cells are affected also. Although the latter group is referred to as 'pancytopenias' there may not necessarily be a total pancytopenia. In many cases, there may be a normal leucocyte and neutrophil count, at least at some stage of a fluctuating course. However, thrombocytopenia (less than 100×10^9/l) is always present and this feature is essential for making a diagnosis. It is not clear whether the occurrence of pancytopenia rather than red-cell aplasia, in response to a causative agent, is a reflection of the intensity of the toxic action, or the level of its effect (i.e. whether at stem cell or later). In general, the variants of the pancytopenias have their parallel in the red-cell aplasias, but some causes will affect only the red cells, e.g. the immune-type of red-cell aplasia, and the types associated with renal failure; conversely, irradiation and certain chemicals, drugs and other toxic substances are more likely to cause pancytopenia with thrombocytopenia rather than anaemia as the most serious aspect.

Pathogenesis of aplastic anaemia

An understanding of the pathogenesis of aplastic

Table 31.1. Causes of reduction in normal marrow activity*

Haemopoietic cell defects
Aplastic anaemia
Red-cell aplasia

Deficiency or defect of erythropoietic factor(s)
Renal insufficiency diseases (e.g. glomerulitis, pyelonephritis, congenital polycystic kidneys: especially with uraemia)
Endocrine hypofunction
    Thyroid
    Pituitary
'Refractory anaemia' (? smouldering leukaemia)

Nutritional deficiencies
Vitamin-B_{12} and folate deficiencies
Iron deficiency
Pyridoxine deficiency
Protein deficiency (especially kwashiorkor)

Bone-marrow infiltration or replacement
Myelofibrosis
Osteomyelosclerosis
Osteopetrosis
Leukaemias and malignant lymphomas
Multiple myelomatosis
Metastatic carcinoma of bone-marrow
Histiocytosis X (Letterer–Siwe disease, Hand–Schuller–Christian disease)
Primary xanthomatoses (Gaucher's disease, Niemann–Pick disease)
Miliary tuberculosis

*This aetiological classification is a rough guide only, as there may be a variable degree of marrow depression in some of the conditions listed; also there may be concomitant quantitative and qualitative disorders of haemopoiesis. In some cases, e.g. vitamin-B_{12} or folate deficiency, the overall marrow activity may be increased with a marked degree of ineffective erythropoiesis.

Table 31.2. Variants of aplastic anaemia

Pancytopenias
Inevitable
    Radiation
    Cytotoxic drugs
    Benzene (Benzol)*
Idiosyncratic (chronic acquired)
    Drugs—chemicals
    Viral infection (especially hepatitis)
    Idiopathic
Acute transient (? immune)
    Viral infections (especially infectious mononucleosis)
    Drugs (e.g. amidopyrine)
    Systemic immune disorders (e.g. SLE)
Familial (Fanconi)
Aplastic–PNH syndrome

Red-cell aplasia
Idiosyncratic (chronic acquired)
    Drugs—chemicals
    Idiopathic
Immune
    Infections
    Thymoma
Familial (Diamond–Blackfan)
Renal
Acute transient
    Riboflavin deficiency
    Haemolytic anaemia

*Distinguish from *benzine*, a petroleum distillate which may contain a variable amount of benzene. Benzol is an alternative for benzene.

anaemia is still largely speculative, but the past few years have witnessed a major upsurge of experimental work especially bone-marrow culture with assay of stem cells and committed progenitor cells [11–14]. In culture assays of granulocyte progenitor cells, a marked reduction in both CFU-C colonies and clusters (see Chapter 2) has been demonstrated in bone marrow and blood from patients with aplastic anaemia [12–15]. These studies, together with observations on the effects of marrow transplants, immunosuppressive therapy and other forms of treatment, provide evidence on the nature of the disorder, albeit still largely circumstantial [16]. The most likely cause of aplastic anaemia is damage by drug or toxin to the haemopoietic stem cell which may then become defective in absolute number, or in its ability for self renewal or its ability to differentiate into committed stem cells in response to normal stimuli [6, 11, 12, 17]. There are

three ways in which toxins may damage the haemopoietic stem cell, namely:
1 dose-dependent effect,
2 idiosyncratic effect, and
3 immunological effect.

Some chemotherapeutic agents, e.g. cytotoxic and antimetabolite drugs such as busulphan, melphalan, nitrogen mustards and 6-mercaptopurine, will invariably cause marrow depression with direct dose-dependent and predictable effect; when the drug is stopped the marrow recovers and the red blood cells, leucocytes and platelets usually return rapidly to normal levels. Other compounds only cause aplastic anaemia occasionally when administered in the usual therapeutic dose. Thus, for example, it has been estimated that one in 60 000 patients risk developing aplastic anaemia as a result of chloramphenicol [18] and a similar extent of risk exists with the pyrazoles (butazones): about one in 90 000 persons receiving organic arsenicals develops a variable degree of bone-marrow depression [19] and one in 35 000 for quinacrine [20].

Drugs containing the benzene ring, especially when

it has a closely attached amino (NH_2) group, are particularly liable to affect the haemopoietic cell, but it is not easy to identify all drugs with harmful potential. Thus, for example, 'Stoddard solvent' was developed as a ('safe') non-benzene petroleum distillate but exposure to this, too, has resulted in aplastic anaemia [21].

There are a number of ways in which haemopoietic cell depression may occur [22, 23]. Some drugs and toxins are known to affect nucleic-acid and protein synthesis, although the site of action varies. Thus, for example, actinomycin inhibits DNA-dependent RNA synthesis whereas streptomycin inhibits protein synthesis by binding irreversibly to ribosomes while allowing continued RNA and DNA synthesis. Chloramphenicol inhibits protein synthesis in mitochondria. Benzene and a number of other chemicals have been shown to inhibit DNA synthesis in erythroid cells at the stage of the basophilic normoblast, and in the myeloid line at the stage of the myelocyte.

There is no method available to detect the susceptible subject and the cause of individual susceptibility is not clear. For example, in the case of chloramphenicol, inhibition of protein synthesis is demonstrable *in vitro* only with high concentrations of the drug, in excess of 250 mg/ml [24], whereas in patients a usual oral dose of 4 g results in a blood content of 40–60 mg/ml, a level which thus appears to be well below that which is apparently necessary for marrow inhibition. One possibility is that a patient may have a biochemical defect of marrow cells, perhaps genetically determined, which may lead to metabolic inhibition at a drug concentration which is relatively harmless to normal cells. The possibility of a genetically determined factor is supported by the occurrence of aplastic anaemia in identical twins exposed to similar (low) doses of chloramphenicol [25]. However, in contrast to most genetically determined blood disorders there is no clear evidence of any racial or ethnic variations in susceptibility [26]. An alternative possibility is that the sensitive subject may have a defect in a detoxification or excretion mechanism, so that a higher concentration of the toxic substance accumulates for a given dose. There is some evidence that there is an impaired clearance of administered chloramphenicol in patients who have manifested signs of erythropoietic depression, for example, in patients with liver or renal disease in whom chloramphenicol is less readily conjugated or excreted, so that six to eight hours after administration of the drug, plasma concentration of the free drug is higher than in other patients receiving similar doses for various conditions [27, 28]. It should be noted, however, that even when there has been no major bone-marrow injury chloramphenicol is likely to produce a (reversible) suppression of erythropoiesis; early evidence of this may be detected by ferrokinetic studies as reduced ^{59}Fe utilization, increased levels of serum iron and increased saturation of transferrin antedate perceptible changes in blood and bone marrow [28–31].

The haemopoietic stem cell can be injured by immune mechanisms involving both humoral antibodies and cell-mediated cytotoxicity. Antibodies have been demonstrated to erythroblasts in pure red-cell aplasia [32, 33] to CFU-C and myeloid precursors [34] in granulocytopenia and to CFU-E in aplastic anaemia [34]. Antibodies have also been identified which act by inhibiting erythropoietin [33, 35], and possibly other humoral factors [36]. There is also some preliminary evidence to suggest that inhibition may be due to the effects on stem cells of suppressor (T) lymphocytes which are found in some cases of aplastic anaemia [37–38]. The likelihood of an immunological mechanism being involved is supported by the fact that a number of drugs which are known or suspected to cause aplastic anaemia, such as diphenylhydantoin, gold salts and sulphonamides, may also cause immune thrombocytopenia or agranulocytosis [39] and sometimes autoimmune haemolytic anaemia.

Yet another factor which has been incriminated is the micro-environment within the bone marrow. This includes the matrix of endothelial (epithelioid) cells, fat cells and macrophages, and the sinusoidal microcirculation. An intact matrix is necessary for maintaining CFU-S proliferation and differentiation [11], and an intact microvasculature for adequate oxygenation and for transport of nutritional factors, erythropoietin and other humoral factors. Damage to the micro-environment by X-irradiation [40] and by mechanical means [41] has been shown to induce marrow failure in experimental animal models.

Incidence of drugs and toxins as a cause of aplastic anaemia

Information on adverse haematological effects of drugs is based on published case reports, reviews and on the Registry of Blood Dyscrasias of the Council on Drugs of the American Medical Association [23, 26]. The Registry was established in 1953, but was abandoned in 1964. By that time 782 cases of drug-induced aplastic anaemias had been reported. Undoubtedly this figure represents only a fraction of the cases which actually occurred during this period, but it served a valuable purpose as a source of raw data and as a means of providing early warnings regarding potentially toxic drugs. In Britain a similar service, but concerned with all drug reactions, is provided by the Department of Health Committee on Safety of Drugs which was established in 1964 [42]. Drugs in common use in Britain which had been incriminated as probable causes of aplastic anaemia were reviewed in 1968 [43].

Similar information is also provided in a world-wide survey of the side-effects of drugs [44] which is now published annually.

Some chemical substances which seem especially likely to cause marrow depression are shown in Table 31.3. They include therapeutic drugs and also chemicals used in industry or in the home, and some which are likely to be occupational causes of aplastic anaemia. Frequently only one of the marrow elements is affected, most often the white-cell precursors leading to neutropenia, or there may only be thrombocytopenia. If the drug is stopped immediately after the onset of the neutropenia or thrombocytopenia, anaemia may not develop, and recovery may take place. With some drugs, e.g. chlorpromazine, the toxic effect is selectively on the leucocytes, whilst other drugs selectively affect platelets. In some cases, pure red-cell aplasia may occur with a substance which, at other times, is associated with pancytopenia [45]. Some drugs and chemicals cause marrow depression regularly while others cause it only rarely.

In addition to the substances shown in Table 31.3 there is a large list of suspect drugs and chemicals, but it is frequently impossible to be sure whether a drug taken by a patient prior to the onset of the disease should be incriminated, especially in these days of therapeutic overabundance when few people are not subjected to a drug at some time and where 'innocent' drugs may be potentially toxic to the susceptible subject, and even aspirin has been shown to be a cause of marrow depression [46]. There appears to be a progressively increasing incidence of aplastic anaemia [47]. Definite association with a drug or chemical has been noted in about one-third of all patients in whom aplastic anaemia is the established diagnosis [3]. The course and outcome are identical in the idiopathic

Table 31.3. Drugs and chemicals which may cause aplastic anaemia

	Definite association	Possible association
Antibiotics	Chloramphenicol*	Thiamphenicol
	Sulphonamides	Streptomycin
		Penicillin
		Methicillin
		Tetracycline
		Nitrofurantion
		Para-aminosalicylic acid
		Isoniazid
Anti-inflammatory agents	Phenylbutazone*	Indomethacin
	Oxyphenbutazone*	Penicillamine
	Amidopyrine*	Colchicine
	Gold salts	
Anti-epileptic drugs	Phenytoin	
	Methoin	
	Troxidone	
Oral hypoglycaemic agents	Tolbutamide	
	Chlorpropamide	
Drugs used for parasite infections	Mepacrine	Amodiaquine
	Organic arsenicals	Pyrimethamine
Antithyroid drugs	Potassium perchlorate	Carbimazole
		Thiouracil
Antihistamines		Chlorpheniramine
		Tripelennamine
Psychoactive drugs		Penothiazines
		Chlordiazepoxide
		Meprobamate
Diuretics		Acetazolamide
		Chlorthiazide
		Hydroflumethiazide
Others		Quinidine bisulphate
		Gamma benzene hexachloride
		Naphthalene

*These drugs have a strong association with aplastic anaemia and are often used when there is no specific clinical indication.

cases and those in whom a cause is established (see below); the difference seems to be failure to identify the causal agent rather than the absence of one, and undoubtedly the majority of cases may be caused by drugs or chemicals.

Benzene effect on haemopoiesis

Benzene (C_6H_6) is an aromatic hydrocarbon which is obtained as a by-product in the manufacture of coke and in the refinement of petroleum. It is used as a solvent for rubber resins, plastics, fats and alkaloids and is used extensively in a wide range of industries from aeroplane manufacture to dry-cleaning, as well as in the house as a cleaning agent and paint remover. Substances related to benzene which also have myelotoxic potential include trinitrotoluene, hydrocarbon-containing glues and kerosene. Since it is volatile, benzene is readily absorbed, usually by inhalation in badly ventilated rooms; it is an important cause of haemopoietic damage [48, 49], leading to depression of one or more cell lines with resultant cytopenia.

Benzene inhibits DNA synthesis and cell division, probably in the committed compartments. In the erythroid series this is at the stage of the basophilic normoblast, and in the myeloid series at the myelocyte. There is some controversy as to which is the most susceptible cell line. Anaemia is said to be the commonest abnormality, but in an extensive study [48] carried out in 217 apparently healthy workers exposed to benzene for periods of between three months and 17 years, 9·7% had leucopenia alone, 4·6% had leucopenia and thrombocytopenia, and 2·7% had pancytopenia. Thrombocytopenia occurred in 9·2% of the group but thrombocytopenia alone in only four individuals. Anaemia was common and 38% had haemoglobin levels below 12 g/dl, although in at least some subjects the anaemia was due to apparently unrelated iron deficiency. Undoubtedly, however, anaemia is a frequent finding in chronic benzene poisoning, increasing in severity in proportion to the extent of exposure [49].

Pancytopenia occurs in the most severe form of benzene poisoning. Although very serious, this is by no means necessarily fatal and spontaneous remission may occur quite suddenly. Other manifestations of toxicity which have been observed are transient neutrophil leucocytosis, eosinophilia or basophilia, whilst immature cells may appear in the circulating blood, and there may be a leuco-erythroblastic anaemia. Lymphocytosis is an occasional occurrence whereas lymphopenia is frequent. There are also manifestations of qualitative abnormalities of haemopoiesis, including pseudo-Pelger–Huet anomaly [48] and, in the marrow, features of dyserythropoiesis with hyperplasia rather than aplasia. In some cases the bone marrow contains areas of fibrosis, and excessive reticulin is demonstrable. When pancytopenia occurs the course is, in general, similar to that of aplastic anaemia, with a mortality that is similar or slightly lower [50]. There appears, however, to be a much higher incidence of leukaemia, which has been reported to occur in 15–20% of patients [50]. This is consistent with the frequent occurrence of chromosomal damage [51, 52].

Infection

Bacterial or viral infections may cause pancytopenia, either during or following the infection. Marrow failure is extremely rare in bacterial infection although it has been reported in association with miliary tuberculosis [53] and brucellosis [54]. Many viruses, particularly those containing RNA, are likely to be a potential cause of marrow damage, and pancytopenia, with temporary bone-marrow hypoplasia, has been noted in rubella, influenza caused by myxoviruses, parainfluenza, mumps and infectious mononucleosis [54a]. There appears to be a special association with infectious hepatitis. Since the first report in 1955 [55], more than 200 cases have been reported [6, 56, 57], including some familial cases [58]. The incidence has been estimated as one and two cases per 1000 cases of hepatitis [59]. The prognosis varies but, in general, it is a serious condition, with a high mortality rate—in one series this was 88% and the mean survival was only 10 weeks after onset of marrow failure [60].

The reason for this course is unclear. There might be a direct effect of the virus on the bone-marrow stem cell or microenvironment, perhaps due to an individual patient's susceptibility to the virus, which is not ordinarily myelotoxic, or the concomitant liver insufficiency may prevent some detoxification mechanism. It has also been suggested that the bone-marrow failure may be explained on the basis of an autoimmune mechanism consequent on the virus infection [54a, 61].

Radiation

Radiation effects are dose-dependent. Some cells are killed directly; others are affected by the production of mitotic abnormalities so that the progeny are short-lived or can divide only a few times before dying out; or there may be undue prolongation of the resting phase with interruption in the cell cycle [62, 63]. Erythroblasts which are killed directly and promptly become pyknotic and are rapidly removed from the marrow, so that within 24 hours after exposure, nuclear debris is no longer evident in the marrow. Erythroblasts which survive the initial exposure continue to mature and to divide, producing mitotically abnormal cells as described above; the abnormalities include chromosomal and internuclear bridges, nuclear fragmentation, binucleated and multinucleated cells, and giant cells.

The blood reticulocyte count remains constant for about 24 hours and then falls to a level which reflects the extent of suppression of erythropoiesis. Anaemia develops later because of the long lifespan of erythrocytes, as the mature cells tend not to be susceptible to radiation injury. Lymphocytes are very susceptible. Within a few hours after exposure, disintegration of the nuclei of the lymphocytes occurs, followed by the break-up of the cells and their removal by phagocytosis, with marked lymphopenia by the third day. The differentiated cell lines of granulocytopoiesis and megakaryocytopoiesis continue to mature and divide in a relatively uninterrupted fashion. Thus the most immature cells disappear from circulating blood at a rate which depends on their lifespan; neutropenia will occur by the sixth day, thrombocytopenia on the seventh to eighth day. Transient neutrophil leucocytosis precedes the neutropenia. Eosinophils may be affected in parallel to the neutrophils but there may be a persistent and striking eosinophilia.

Types of radiation. The effect of radiation depends on the type of rays, their dose, and the variable sensitivity of different tissues. As α and β rays have little penetration, external irradiation with these rays has no effect on haemopoietic tissue, which is well beyond their reach. However, they can be damaging when ingested or given parenterally. Gamma rays, X-rays and neutrons penetrate easily and are all likely to cause an aplastic anaemia. Radiation effects occur at the site of irradiation but leucopenia and thrombocytopenia may be caused by intense localized X-irradiation even though the bone marrow is not in the path of the rays. In practice, although various forms of irradiation cause some degree of marrow depression, and acute radiation injury can cause severe haemopoietic damage, the clinical picture of chronic aplastic anaemia is a rare occurrence. It has been reported amongst radiologists, and others exposed to unshielded radiation over a long period of time [64, 65] and also amongst patients with ankylosing spondylitis treated by radiation [66, 67]. There have been a few reports of aplastic anaemia as an early effect of intense radiation, e.g. amongst atomic bomb survivors [68] and immediately after radiation accidents [63, 69], but it also appears to occur as a delayed complication of exposure [70]. As has been indicated above, the most sensitive haemopoietic cells are lymphocytes and erythroblasts, followed in decreasing order of sensitivity by myeloblasts, monocytes and megakaryocytes, while the most resistant cells are the reticulum cells. The sinusoidal endothelial cells are also resistant (see below).

Recovery from irradiation depends on the extent of initial marrow damage and whether the microvasculature has been affected. It is correlated with the fraction of stem cells that survive. Only 0·1% of cells survive 700 rad, and five per cent of stem cells survive after a dose of 300 rad [62, 71]. With lower doses recovery is increasingly likely. These doses do not affect the endothelial cells of the sinusoids, and haemopoietic recovery begins within a few weeks of exposure. At doses of 2000 rad or more the sinusoidal cells are damaged and haemopoietic cells will only regenerate when the microenvironment recovers sufficiently after about six months; with doses of 4000–6000 rad the sinusoidal cells are irreversibly damaged and aplasia is permanent [40]. In the recovery phase the peripheral-blood findings are determined by the rate of regeneration of the various precursor cells. Lymphocytes begin to increase in the peripheral blood very soon after lymphopoiesis is restored. The neutrophils and platelets return to normal soon thereafter. A sustained reticulocytosis occurs at about 30 days after bone-marrow regeneration becomes established. The pattern of haematological recovery from a relatively low dose of irradiation is illustrated in Figure 31.1 which is of a patient with polycythaemia vera whose bone-marrow activity was seriously depressed as a result of an injection of ^{32}P [72].

Chronic acquired aplastic anaemia

From a clinical standpoint, chronic acquired aplastic anaemia is the most important condition involving depressed haemopoiesis. It requires careful and arduous management of the patient, in some cases for many years. It is difficult to judge the relative incidence, as transient marrow failure, especially when caused by an identifiable disease, is less likely to be investigated from the haematological point of view than the primary types which are usually referred to haematological centres. Doubtless, it is the commonest form of aplastic anaemia and it is this condition which is usually implied when a diagnosis of 'aplastic anaemia' is made. An incidence of 0·91–2·39 per thousand hospital admissions has been reported from one leading haematological centre in Paris [73]. Several extensive reviews of a relatively large number of patients from several centres [3–5, 15, 73, 74] give further indication that the frequency of chronic acquired aplastic anaemia is far from insignificant.

There are no apparent differences in haematological and clinical course or in prognosis between the idiopathic cases and the drug or toxin-induced cases [75]. Accordingly they will be dealt with together in the following section.

Age and sex

The disease occurs at all ages; children of two years and old people of 80 years have been reported as having

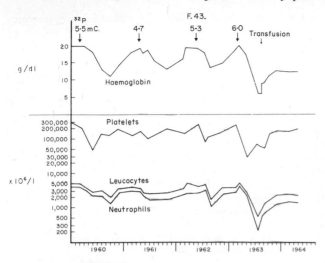

Fig. 31.1. Haematological effects of ^{32}P in a 43-year-old woman with polycythaemia vera. Transient pancytopenia followed a dose of 6 mCi; with recovery, the platelet count returned to normal levels at about the same time as the leucocytes and red cells.

chronic acquired anaemia and there is no significant preponderance of any age group. Some reports have indicated that there is a slightly greater incidence amongst females than males in a proportion of approximately 1·2:1 [47, 75], but in other series the ratio was reversed [76].

Clinical features

Patients present with signs and symptoms that relate to the severity of the anaemia, thrombocytopenia, or neutropenia. If thrombocytopenia is sufficiently severe, there will be a bleeding tendency, either as ecchymosis and purpura or as retinal haemorrhages and bleeding into organs, especially cerebral haemorrhage. It is difficult to say at what level of thrombocytopenia bleeding may occur. At any given platelet count, one patient may bleed while another will not. In general, bleeding is common when the platelet count is less than 20×10^9/l and rare when it is more than 50×10^9/l. However, the tendency to bleed will be greater, at any level of platelet count, when there is concomitant infection, and even when the platelet count is 50×10^9/l bleeding may occur when infection is present [4]. In early stages of aplastic anaemia, infection does not seem to be a serious problem, although many have minor infections such as skin pustules, thrombophlebitis, bronchitis, and upper-respiratory-tract infections. Infections may become more serious later in the course of the illness; however, the availability of antibiotics makes this relatively easier to control than bleeding, and death occurs more frequently as the result of haemorrhage. There is not, as a rule, any significant splenomegaly, hepatomegaly or lymph-node enlargement.

Blood count

By definition there is anaemia; its severity varies, and may be obscured by blood transfusion. There may not necessarily be a pancytopenia, and in many cases, during the fluctuating course, the patient may at some stage have a normal leucocyte and neutrophil count. However, thrombocytopenia (less than 100×10^9/l is always present and this feature is essential for making the diagnosis. The degree of thrombocytopenia varies. At its worst a platelet count of less than 1×10^9/l may be found; in most cases the platelets range between 10 and 80×10^9/l.

Lymphopenia also occurs in many cases at some stages in the course of the disease, and a lymphocyte count of $0.5-1 \times 10^9$/l is not an unusual finding. There is an absolute and relative decrease of B-cell and a relative increase of T-cell fractions [7]. It is of interest to note that the low lymphocyte count is seen predominantly in patients with subnormal immunoglobulin levels [77].

There is usually a reticulocytopenia but it is not present throughout the illness, and the diagnosis may be confused by the presence of a normal reticulocyte count and even a relative reticulocytosis when expressed as a percentage of the red cells. This suggests that the marrow may not be uniformly affected, or perhaps that in some cases there may be premature release of reticulocytes from the marrow. Expressing the reticulocyte count in absolute numbers provides a more reliable index. Extramedullary haemopoiesis is not a feature of aplastic anaemia.

The blood films shows anisocytosis with macrocytosis and a variable degree of poikilocytosis and other abnormalities of erythrocyte morphology. In Romanowsky-stained films the neutrophils often show morphological abnormalities in the form of coarse red granules in the cytoplasm, and they have an extremely high content of alkaline phosphatase [78].

Bone marrow

As a rule, aspirated material contains a few hypocellular fragments and few cells in the trails of the fragments. However, bone-marrow cellularity may vary, and normal, or even hypercellular, marrow may be obtained from any one site. The presence of a focus of hypercellular marrow adjacent to an aplastic area may result in a misleading sample from a single aspiration (Fig. 31.2). If there is a discrepancy between peripheral blood and marrow a further marrow aspiration should be carried out from another site, and, if necessary, a trephine biopsy of the iliac crest, in order to obtain a more reliable representative specimen. When sufficient material is aspirated to enable cell morphology to be studied, erythroblasts will often show evidence of dyserythropoiesis, including cytoplasmic vacuolation, nuclear lobulation, fragmentation, karyorrhexis, and other abnormalities of nu-

clear shape and structure. Abnormal sideroblasts may be seen.

Ferrokinetics

An injected dose of ^{59}Fe is cleared slowly from the plasma. The normal half-life ($T_\frac{1}{2}$) is 90–160 minutes; in aplastic anaemia, $T_\frac{1}{2}$ may be three to four hours or even longer. By surface-counting only a small amount of radioactivity reappears in the circulation; most is retained as stored iron, mainly in the liver (Fig. 31.3). In the most serious cases, less than five per cent of the radioactive iron is utilized for red-cell production; in other cases there is, as a rule, 10–20% utilization although this may be misleading if there is any significant degree of ineffective erythropoiesis or haemolysis. Similarly, plasma iron turnover may be misleading because of the amount of iron taken up by non-erythroid tissue [79].

Radio-iron studies are usually performed with ^{59}Fe. A cyclotron-produced isotope ^{52}Fe which is available in some centres is the best radiochemical for measuring the relative contributions of erythropoiesis and iron storage by means of quantitative scanning; a characteristic scan is obtained in aplastic anaemia (Fig. 31.3). Some workers have used, instead, indium-111 as this is also bound to plasma transferrin; however, this complex does not behave quite like iron-transferrin and misleading results may be obtained [80].

Erythrocyte survival studies

There is frequently an increased rate of erythrocyte destruction with a mean cell life in the order of 20–40 days and $T_\frac{1}{2}{}^{51}$Cr of 10–15 days. In about one-third of the cases, the spleen is the site of red-cell destruction [78]. In some cases, haemolysis is compounded with haemorrhage; gastro-intestinal bleeding can be estimated by measurement of radioactivity in stools after administration of ^{51}Cr.

Clinical course

In recent years, advances in treatment and improved general support measures (p. 1241) have undoubtedly influenced the course and prognosis in many cases. It may, however, be difficult to assess the effectiveness of treatment in any individual cases because of great variability in the natural course of the disease; it is thus important to distinguish the various ways in which the disease may progress and to try to establish criteria for prognosis.

In some patients the disease is explosive, with rapid deterioration and death within a few weeks. In others it may be long continued, with remissions, relapses and the occasional complete recovery, but recovery usually takes place very slowly, and the platelet count may become normal only after months or even years (Fig.

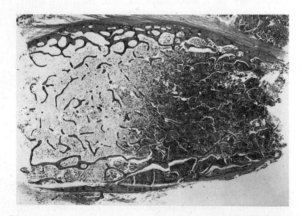

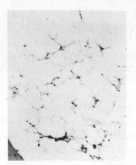
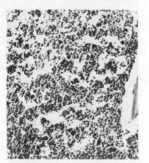

Fig. 31.2. Section of sternum obtained at autopsy from a patient with chronic acquired aplastic anaemia. Note adjacent areas of hypocellularity and hypercellularity, shown below at higher magnification.

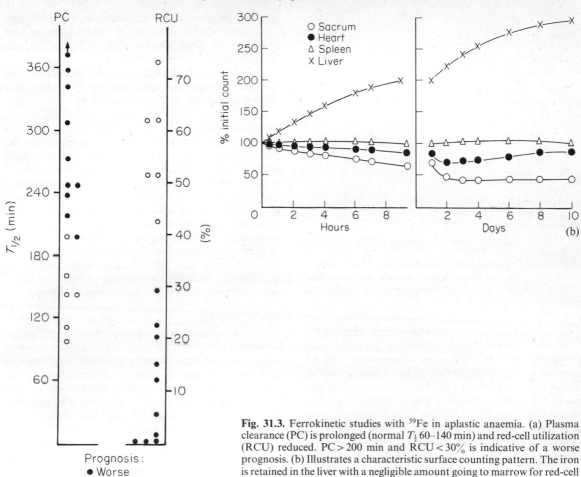

Fig. 31.3. Ferrokinetic studies with ^{59}Fe in aplastic anaemia. (a) Plasma clearance (PC) is prolonged (normal $T_{\frac{1}{2}}$ 60–140 min) and red-cell utilization (RCU) reduced. PC > 200 min and RCU < 30% is indicative of a worse prognosis. (b) Illustrates a characteristic surface counting pattern. The iron is retained in the liver with a negligible amount going to marrow for red-cell production. There is no evidence of extramedullary erythropoiesis.

31.4) [75, 81]. This slow recovery of the platelets is in contrast to the situation when marrow has been damaged by irradiation or by cytotoxic drugs. A partial remission may be followed by relapse and subsequent death (Fig. 31.5).

The serious nature of aplastic anaemia is indicated by the fact that 10–15% of the patients are likely to die within three months (if untreated) and half the patients within 15 months of onset (Fig. 31.6). The outlook is equally poor whether or not there has been an identifiable cause. Patients who live beyond 18 months have a relatively good chance of survival, and the longer a patient survives, the better his chance of an ultimate recovery or even cure.

It is impossible to be sure of the ultimate prognosis when the patient is first seen. A number of factors have been suggested as prognostic indicators to enable an assessment to be made of the extent of bone-marrow injury and thus the likelihood of eventual recovery,

and also to provide an indication of the clinical severity, and thus the risk of death [73, 75, 82–86]. Patients with severe anaemia in whom the platelet count is less than $20 \times 10^9/l$, and the neutrophils less than $0 \cdot 1 \times 10^9/l$ seem to have the worst prognosis. On the whole neutropenia appears to be less serious than thrombocytopenia and the patients are more likely to die as a result of haemorrhage than from infection. A partial remission cannot be taken as an indication of an improving prognosis as this may be followed by a relapse and subsequent death (see Fig 31.5). It seems likely that the platelet count is the most reliable criterion as to whether or not the marrow has recovered. Once the platelet count has become normal it seems unlikely that there will be another relapse. The reticulocyte count appears to be a good discriminant factor when expressed as an absolute number; a count of less than $10 \times 10^9/l$ indicates a high-risk patient. However, a low reticulocyte count may be a falsely

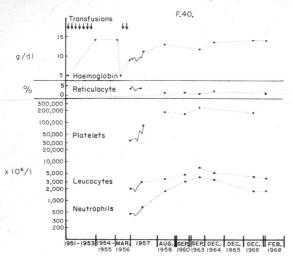

Fig. 31.4. Haematological course in a 40-year-old woman with chronic acquired (idiopathic) aplastic anaemia, illustrating slow recovery. The platelet count became normal only after several years.

the same prognostic significance as severe neutropenia.

In early studies of acquired aplastic anaemia of children, the fetal haemoglobin concentration was thought to have prognostic value, with better survival prospects when the Hb F level was 400 mg/dl or higher [89], but this has not been confirmed in subsequent studies in children [88] or in adults [90].

Prognostic index

Lynch *et al.* [85] proposed an index based on scoring the various haematological parameters described above, together with the sex of the patient and clinical manifestations of bleeding, etc., in order to distinguish the patients who are likely to die within four to six months of onset of their illness. This index has been criticized as being no more useful than a clinical impression in predicting the patient's final outcome [83]. However, there is no doubt that a reliable method for predicting the risk of early death would be particularly valuable for selecting patients for bone-marrow transplant or alternate forms of therapy.

Ferrokinetic studies

From the observations on bone-marrow cellularity described above it is obvious that random marrow sampling is of little value in assessing total marrow function. For this, ferrokinetic studies are more informative. It has been suggested that normal, or near normal, plasma clearance of radio-iron is an indicator of a better prognosis [73] and also that red-cell utilization gives a reasonably good prediction of prognosis [91]. A more recent study failed to show any significant relationship between marrow cellularity, reticulocyte count and red-cell utilization [92], but confirmed the value of ferrokinetic studies for providing

pessimistic index in patients with acute infection [87].

Bone-marrow cellularity does not correlate with prognosis, and in even severe cases there may be normal or hypercellular foci of haemopoetic cells at one site of aspiration [75, 86]. An increase in the relative number of lymphocytes is associated with a worse prognosis [83, 85, 86, 88]. It is of interest to note that there is no correlation between blood lymphocyte count and marrow lymphoid cell content but there is a close direct relationship between the blood neutrophil count and marrow myeloid cell content [86], so that a low content of myeloid cells in the marrow will have

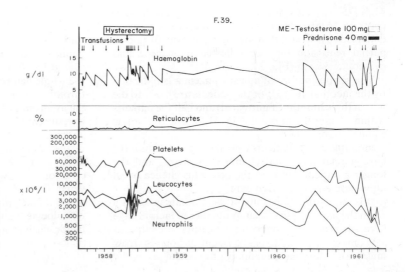

Fig. 31.5. Haematological course in a 39-year-old woman with chronic acquired aplastic anaemia, showing a partial remission which, however, was followed by relapse and death.

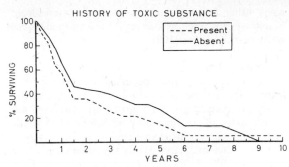

Fig. 31.6. Survival rate in chronic acquired aplastic anaemia. Prognosis is not materially different between cases where there has been an identifiable aetiological factor and idiopathic cases.

prognostic information, in that a plasma clearance $T_{\frac{1}{2}}$ of less than 200 minutes and red-cell utilization above 35% generally identifies the patients with a better outlook.

With recovery from aplastic anaemia the patient may develop paroxysmal nocturnal haemoglobinuria (PNH) or, less frequently, leukaemia (see p. 1252); obviously, these complications will alter the course and prognosis.

Aplastic anaemia following hepatitis
This occurs especially in younger persons, the age distribution being that of infectious hepatitis. In general, the aplastic anaemia has its clinical onset within 10 weeks after the hepatitis. The hepatitis is, as a rule, mild but the aplastic anaemia is especially severe with poor prognosis [57, 60]. It has been said that hepatitis A is more likely to cause aplastic anaemia than hepatitis B [93] but this has not yet been confirmed by serological studies. In one patient, hepatitis A was identified [94]; this was a six-year-old

child with severe aplastic anaemia who eventually had a spontaneous remission.

Aplastic anaemia in pregnancy
Aplastic anaemia has been reported as a transient event during the course of pregnancy, possibly related in some way to the pregnancy [95, 96]. In other cases, where chronic acquired aplastic anaemia has been present as an underlying disease and pregnancy has occurred, it has been generally considered that the pregnancy exacerbates the marrow depression and results in a rapid deterioration [95, 97], or at least carries the same serious prognosis as aplastic anaemia due to drugs or unknown causes [98]. Most authors have suggested that in these situations pregnancy should be rapidly terminated. However, pregnancy is not necessarily harmful in aplastic anaemia, and recovery from a chronic aplastic anaemia may even occur after a spontaneous abortion [99] or a normal delivery [100]. Recovery from aplastic anaemia after pregnancy is illustrated in Figure 31.7 which relates to a 24-year-old woman who had chloramphenicol-induced aplastic anaemia of two years' duration when she became pregnant. The thrombocytopenia worsened to some extent during pregnancy but delivery was followed by a significant increase in platelet count. A second pregnancy resulted in a similar pattern and subsequent complete remission. Both babies were normal and have thrived since their birth, as has their mother. The reason for the unusual haematological course is not clear. In experimental studies the pituitary hormone, prolactin, and the plasma of pregnant and lactating mice have been shown to have a stimulatory effect of erythropoiesis [101, 102] and it is possible in the case described here that remission could have been brought about by lactogenic and other hormones of late pregnancy and the puerperium.

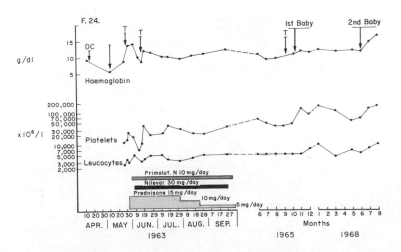

Fig. 31.7. Haematological course in a 24-year-old woman with chloramphenicol-induced aplastic anaemia who became pregnant. Improvement occurred after each of two normal deliveries.

Aplastic anaemia at puberty

It is not clear whether aplastic anaemia occurring in young people at, or about, the time of puberty has a unique cause. Clinically, the picture is one of chronic acquired aplastic anaemia. There is no familial incidence and no constitutional manifestation other than pancytopenia. However, it certainly seems to be more amenable to treatment than the chronic acquired aplastic anaemia of adults, and spontaneous remission may occur after puberty [100]. A similar remission at puberty has been noted in Fanconi's anaemia [103, 104]. It should be remembered that other cases occur at this age without such puberty remission and with the same course and prognosis as at any other age.

Gold-induced aplastic anaemia

Gold salts are a recognized cause of thrombocytopenia and neutropenia as well as aplastic anaemia [105] but there is an unusual course in that treatment with dimercaprol (BAL) results in rapid recovery with an early return of platelets to normal (Fig. 31.8). The bone marrow is one of the principal organs of the body in which administered gold accumulates, as it is taken up predominantly by reticulo-endothelial cells [106] and response to BAL suggests that the gold exerts a direct dose-dependent action on haemopoietic precursor cells when it has accumulated in a sufficiently high concentration to exert its toxic effect. However, as there is no consistent marrow depression in every case, an idiosyncratic reaction to gold cannot be excluded [105, 107].

Other metals, notably arsenical compounds, have also been identified as the cause of marrow depression; there is a direct effect on DNA synthesis or possibly some other facet of protein synthesis in erythroid precursor cells, and this also results in a marked degree of dyserythropoiesis [108].

Transient aplasias

Marrow depression may occur as a transient event during the course of various chronic haemolytic anaemias. As a rule only erythropoiesis is affected but occasionally all cell lines may be depressed. Aplastic crisis has been reported in hereditary spherocytosis, sicke-cell anaemia, and in autoimmune haemolytic anaemias [109, 110]. Although these incidents have been referred to as transient, they may be serious and indeed be responsible for the death of the patient.

The incidence of aplastic crises probably varies in the different diseases; they are far less common, for example, in hereditary spherocytosis than in sickle-cell disease and there is no report of the occurrence of either pancytopenia or erythroid aplasia in thalassaemia major [110]. PNH is frequently accompanied by a degree of marrow depression (see Chapter 12); however, acute aplasia during the course of 'haemolytic' PNH is uncommon [110–112].

The aetiology of aplastic crises in haemolytic disorders is not well understood. There have been reports of their occurrence when the patient has become infected, and an acute viral infection seems to be a particular hazard in patients who are suffering from a haemolytic disorder [110]. Marrow failure should be suspected whenever the anaemia of a congenital haemolytic disease suddenly becomes more severe, but in acquired haemolytic disease variation in severity of the anaemia may reflect either marrow failure or fluctuation in the haemolytic process. As any disorder

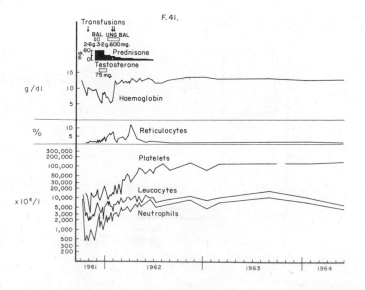

Fig. 31.8. Haematological course in a 41-year-old woman with rheumatoid arthritis in whom aplastic anaemia followed administration of gold. There was a rapid complete remission following treatment with BAL (dimercaprol).

with shortened red-cell survival and compensatory marrow hyperplasia is likely to lead to folate deficiency [113], the possibility must always be considered that the advent of an increasing anaemia or pancytopenia might be due to this factor rather than to marrow hypoplasia. Characteristic megaloblastic changes in the marrow and/or peripheral blood, and folate assay, will be helpful in reaching a diagnosis.

Treatment of aplastic anaemia

The treatment of aplastic anaemia depends to some extent on the type and severity. Relatively mild cases with a moderate degree of anaemia, neutropenia and thrombocytopenia can be kept under surveillance without active treatment. Severe cases should be looked after in a centre where there is considerable experience and expertise in the management of bone-marrow failure.

Identification and removal of cause

The difficulty in deciding whether a drug or other toxic agent has actually been responsible for the bone-marrow depression has been referred to above. Unfortunately, in the majority of cases removal of the cause or presumed cause does not seem to influence the ultimate prognosis which depends on the extent of the initial damage to the bone marrow. Usually it is not possible to identify susceptible subjects in advance and great care must be taken in using drugs that are known to be especially liable to cause aplastic anaemia. Although it is important on medico-legal grounds to perform regular blood counts in patients on such drugs, it should be remembered that aplastic episodes may be of very rapid onset and it is much more important to warn the patient to report immediately with any unusual symptoms such as bleeding, a sore throat or simply if they feel 'off colour'. Cytotoxic drugs affect the bone marrow of all subjects and administration of such drugs must be carefully controlled by regular blood counts, especially platelet counts. It should be remembered that drugs like busulphan show a significant 'hangover' effect, i.e. the blood count may fall for several weeks after stopping them, and therefore it is most important that patients should be taken off such agents while the count is still higher than that which is desired at the end point of chemotherapy.

If aplastic anaemia follows the administration of gold or arsenical compounds the patient can be treated with dimercaprol (BAL), 800 mg/day intramuscularly in divided doses for two to three days, then reducing to 100–200 mg/day over the next few days; the problems of intramuscular injections in severely thrombocytopaenic patients must be remembered.

Alleviation of anaemia

Blood transfusion requirements for anaemia will vary from patient to patient; in some patients a state of equilibrium will become established at a reasonably satisfactory haemoglobin level, whereas others may require blood transfusion at intervals over a period of months or even years. There is no point in attempting to maintain the haemoglobin at a normal level if the patient is free of distress and can undertake an acceptable amount of activity at a lower level. It is undesirable to overtransfuse and the risks of transfusion such as serum hepatitis, transfusion reaction and iron loading must always be borne in mind. It should be added that there is some controversy about the ideal haemoglobin level to maintain in patients with aplastic anaemia. On the one hand it is suggested that a relatively low haemoglobin level between 6 and 9 g/dl will produce maximum erythropoietic drive, and hence accelerate recovery. On the other hand it is possible that the haemoglobin level should be kept higher because there is a reciprocal relationship between granulopoiesis and erythropoiesis. Since there is no real evidence that the level of haemoglobin influences recovery, common sense dictates that as few transfusions as possible should be given. In patients who require an intravenous line for treatment of acute infective episodes a cannula should be inserted into the peripheral veins and changed every 24 hours; metal and teflon cannulae are less irritant to blood vessels than polystyrene. In seriously ill patients it is useful to set up a central venous line. A catheter introduced into the subclavian vein, under platelet cover and aseptic conditions, is most convenient. It should be remembered that lines of this type are a potent source of infection and they should not be left in longer than one to two weeks. They are of particular value when irritant antibiotic solutions are used.

Packed red cells are suitable for most patients, but in those who develop transfusion reactions white-cell-poor or washed blood should be used. Blood which has been stored by freezing has certain advantages; it is less viscous than conventional blood, the absence of lymphocytes and other white cells means that reactions are rare, and there is some evidence that there is less risk of developing antibodies to platelets. Furthermore, virus infections are less likely to be transmitted by frozen blood.

Control of haemorrhage

Bleeding due to thrombocytopenia is a major problem in the management of bone-marrow failure. Because of the danger that repeated platelet infusions will provoke the production of platelet antibodies, most workers now believe that there is only a limited place for prophylactic platelet infusions and that this type of therapy should be reserved for serious bleeding episodes. Although the particular level of circulating platelets at which bleeding occurs varies between patients, in general it is common when the platelet count is less than $20 \times 10^9/l$ and rare when it is more than $50 \times 10^9/l$. It is unusual for a massive and life-threatening bleed to occur without some kind of previous warning and particular regard should be taken of mucous-membrane bleeding, haematuria, rapidly progressive skin purpura, unexplained headache, gastro-intestinal bleeding and retinal haemorrhages. The latter seem to be more common in patients who are also anaemic, and a combination of severe thrombocytopenia and anaemia requires urgent treatment as severe retinal bleeding may lead to permanent blindness. It should be remembered that thrombocytopenia and associated bleeding may be exacerbated by intercurrent infection. Menstrual blood loss may be difficult to control and it is reasonable to suppress menstruation completely using oestrogens and norethisterone. Once bleeding is established any few remaining platelets will be consumed and a vicious circle ensues which must be broken by platelet infusion.

Initially, platelet concentrates from six donors should be given. The latter should yield approximately $3–4 \times 10^{11}$ platelets and this should raise the platelet count by $25–35 \times 10^9/l$. However, in many of these patients, platelet consumption is increased and the rise may be only 25–50% of this figure or even less. If the bleeding is not stopped by one infusion of six units a similar dose should be repeated immediately. If the presence of platelet antibodies is suspected, it is useful to measure the increment in circulating platelet counts at five, 15 and 60 minutes after the transfusion of platelets; if antibody is present no rise is seen in the circulating count. It is probably wise to give platelets even in the absence of bleeding to any patient with aplastic anaemia who has a severe intercurrent infection and whose platelet count at presentation is less than $50 \times 10^9/l$. In the patient who has retinal haemorrhages and is anaemic as well as thrombocytopenic it is essential to correct the anaemia rapidly with packed cells at the same time as giving platelet infusions.

Prolonged use of platelet transfusion eventually results in resistance to the infused platelets with the development of allo-antibodies against specific platelet antigens. This phenomenon usually becomes manifest six to eight weeks after starting therapy. To avoid sensitization of the patient, HLA-matched platelets should be used when feasible; alternatively, the use of a leucocyte-free platelet preparation may delay anti-platelet antibody formation [114]. When an antibody does develop, and if it has HLA-specificity, it may be possible to improve the effectiveness of platelet transfusions by using HLA-compatible platelets [115] but when antibody is directed against other platelet antigens it is much more difficult to find compatible donors and the outlook is poor if platelets are required to control bleeding in long continued disease.

Control of infection

Infection is a major cause of death in bone-marrow failure when neutropenia is severe; it may develop at great speed and be caused by organisms which are not usually pathogenic in man. It is important to consider the prevention of infection as well as the management of established cases.

To avoid exogenous infection the patient should be in a protected environment with barrier nursing and out of contact with other patients during any period of hospital admission. Patients who have chronic aplastic anaemia should spend as much time out of hospital as possible. During periods of severe bone-marrow failure, a scrupulous oral toilet regime should be set up on a four-hourly basis which should include regular antiseptic mouth washes, and anti-fungal lozenges. This is combined with regular use of antiseptic and antibiotic skin creams. The motions should be kept soft and on no account should rectal examinations be carried out. There is some evidence that decontamination of the gastro-intestinal tract is worth carrying out. Broad-spectrum antibiotics which are not absorbed are usually employed, a suitable combination being framycetin sulphate 500 mg six hourly, colistin sulphate $1·5 \times 10^6$ units six hourly and nystatin $0·5 \times 10^6$ units six hourly (FRACON), although nystatin syrup is unpleasant to take and may be nauseating; amphotericin syrup is more suitable but more expensive. The anti-fungal agent (nystatin or amphotericin) is usually given for 48 hours before the antibacterial drugs in order to eradicate yeasts, since the absence of bacteria may encourage fungal overgrowth. If possible the low absorbable antibiotics are used in association with low-bacterial-content food. During the period of severe marrow failure scrupulous care must be taken of drip sites and all intravenous lines must be changed at regular intervals.

The development of a serious infection with organisms such as *Pseudomonas aeruginosa*, *Proteus* and *Klebsiella* may be extremely rapid and there may be few prodromal symptoms; some patients simply feel 'peculiar' or generally unwell and although there may be a rising fever some overwhelming infections are not associated with a temperature change. The infection may develop at such a speed that there may be only a history of a matter of hours between the initial onset and irreversible Gram-negative shock. Hence there is no time to wait for bacteriological reports and in any patient in whom infection is suspected a blood culture should be taken and antibiotic therapy started immediately. For general use, a combination of gentamycin and carbenicillin is recommended at the following dose: gentamicin: loading dose 2 mg/kg maintenance dose 4–5 mg/kg/24 hours in three divided doses depending on peak and trough plasma levels; carbenicillin: 5 g four hourly intravenously. These antibiotics should not be mixed together and it should be remembered that the carbenicillin introduces a heavy sodium load and that any patient on this antibiotic regime will lose large amounts of potassium and hence potassium supplements should always be added. This combination will deal with the majority of organisms encountered in patients with bone-marrow failure apart from some anaerobes such as *Bacteroides*. Since many patients respond dramatically to this regime it is always difficult to know when to stop treatment, but a useful rule is to maintain antibiotics for at least five days after the fever has settled and, after stopping therapy, to watch the patient carefully for 24–48 hours before they leave hospital.

Failure of response to treatment suggests the presence of an unusual organism or a viral or fungal agent. With increasing availability of cell separators, granulocyte transfusions have become used more often although there is no case for their prophylactic administration. If the fever persists for more than 24–48 hours after stopping antibiotics, or if there is localized spreading cellulitis, a granulocyte infusion should be used if available. To be effective, granulocytes have to be given on at least four successive days; donors should be ABO-compatible and ideally HLA-compatible. Granulocyte transfusion therapy is considered in greater detail in Chapter 35.

It is impossible to deal with all the possible organisms that may be encountered in patients with bone-marrow failure in this short account. Where there is severe perineal infection and the patient's general condition does not improve on the regime outlined above, organisms of the *Bacteroides* class should be considered. Antibiotics like clindamycin have now been largely abandoned for the treatment of this organism because of the high incidence of colitis, and metronidazole is the drug of choice at a dose of 500 mg intravenously eight hourly. Systemic fungus infections with organisms such as *Candida albicans* can be treated with amphotericin B alone or in combination with 5-fluorocytosine but the combination is extremely toxic. Miconazole has a wide anti-fungal spectrum and can be used in a dose of 600 mg three times a day intravenously diluted in 300–500 ml of saline or dextrose over 30 minutes. This drug should not be used in combination with amphotericin B. In patients with disseminated herpes zoster infections the use of immune sera or anti-viral agents such as adenine arabino-side should be tried. Infections with *Pneumocystis carcnii* should be treated with high-dose cotrimoxazole (20 mg trimethoprim/100 mg sulphamethoxazole/kg in divided doses/24 hours for 10–14 days).

In addition to instituting immediate antibiotic regimes patients with septicaemic shock require urgent general management, ideally in an intensive care unit. It is essential to insert a central venous pressure line and to monitor the venous pressure continuously. Such patients are frequently collapsed, hypotensive and show clear evidence of poor perfusion. Renal failure is a common complication. Apart from treatment with antibiotics as outlined above it is essential to maintain volume with saline or plasma. In many centres it is customary to use intravenous hydrocortisone at a dose of 100–500 mg four to six hourly although there is no real evidence that this is beneficial. Occasionally, disseminated intravascular coagulation may occur and this should be treated as outlined in Chapter 29. It may be necessary to tide these patients through a period of renal shutdown and subsequent tubular necrosis with appropriate haemodialysis regimes.

Home treatment of patients with aplastic anaemia and bone-marrow failure

It is most important that patients with chronic aplastic anaemia should be kept out of hospital as much as possible.

It is believed that patients at home are relatively safe from antibiotic-resistant pathogens as compared with those in a hospital environment. Gut decontamination is usually stopped before discharge. The safest way of stopping decontamination and recolonizing the gastro-intestinal tract is still uncertain. Some centres use *Lactobacillus* at the time of withdrawal of antibiotics, while others recommend the use of stored encapsulated faecal material so that the patients are recolonized with their original flora. They should continue with their oral toilet at home and pay scrupulous attention to personal hygiene. They should be given a facility for direct access to a centre with experience of managing bone-marrow failure and they should report any unusual symptoms or the development of septic or purpuric lesions. They are advised to avoid crowds or similar sources of infection.

Patients with severe thrombocytopenia require very careful outpatient surveillance. It is sometimes possible to keep these patients at home by giving prophylactic platelet infusions as an outpatient. The number of infusions and time intervals vary very much from case to case, but many patients with platelet counts of less than $10 \times 10^9/l$ can be maintained at home on twice-weekly platelet infusions. The problems associated with repeated platelet transfusions have been discussed above.

The treatment of bone-marrow failure has been dealt with here in outline only; the detailed management is described in two recent reviews [116, 117].

Haemopoietic stimulus

Androgens and anabolic steroids (androstanes) influence erythropoiesis in normally functioning bone marrow. Their use in the treatment of aplastic anaemia was stimulated by Shahidi & Diamond's observations [118] of the beneficial effect of testosterone in the treatment of childhood aplastic anaemia. Since then a search has gone on for an anabolic agent which has fewer side effects than testosterone. Preparations that have been used include methyltestosterone, testosterone propionate, testosterone enanthate, fluoxymesterone, oxymetholone, methandienone and nandrolone phenylpropionate (Fig. 31.9).

There is a great diversity of opinion with regard to the effectiveness of the various preparations, their relative hepatotoxicity and virilizing side-effects, optimal dose and duration of treatment. Because of the problems associated with injections in patients with thrombocytopenia, oral preparations are preferable. Early reports of the use of oxymetholone were encouraging [4, 119, 120], although the high doses which were necessary to be effective (e.g. in the order of 2·5 mg/kg/day) were likely to produce troublesome side-effects including jaundice and fluid retention [121]. More recent studies have given conflicting results [116, 122–126]. One prospective multicentre trial showed no advantages for androgen therapy [122]; however, in another extensive multicentre trial of 352 patients with severe aplastic anaemia it appeared to influence favourably the long-term prognosis of patients who did not succumb within the first three months [124].

Remission with stabilization of the haemoglobin may occur after two to three months of treatment with oxymetholone or methandienone in a dose of 2–3 mg/kg/day. There may be an accompanying neutrophil increase but this may be delayed for several months. Platelets are least responsive and it seems to be worthwhile to continue treatment for 20 months in patients who have begun to show signs of partial remission in the hope of inducing a full remission [124]. Indeed, regardless of the persistence of thrombocytopenia, the bleeding tendency seems to decrease strikingly in the responding patient [119]. Examples of the response to androgens are illustrated in Figures 31.10–31.12. After remission, therapy is not, as a rule, required in chronic acquired aplastic anaemia.

All androgenic steroids have side-effects which include virilization, deepening of the voice, body

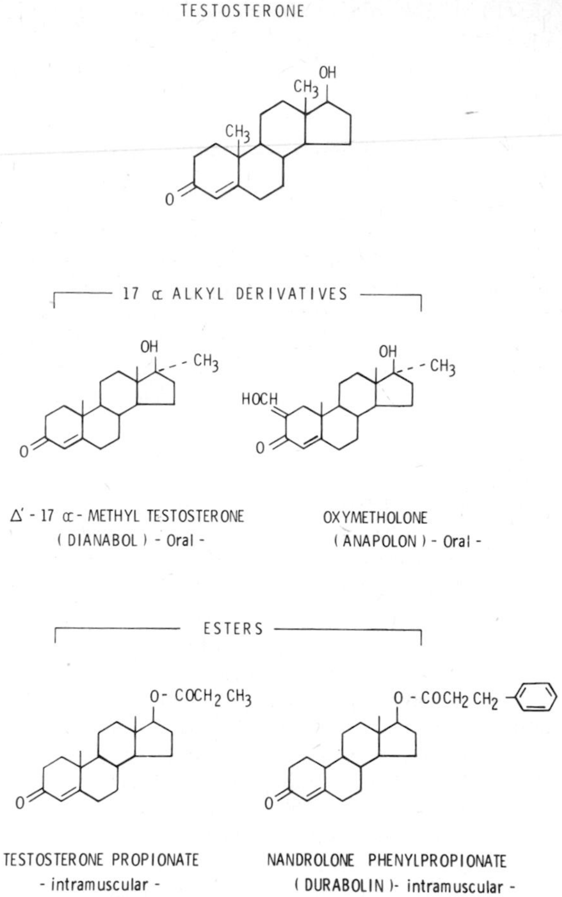

Fig. 31.9. Formulae of testosterone and related steroids (androstanes) used for treatment of aplastic anaemia.

hirsutism and alopecia, severe acne, amenorrhoea, prostatic hypertrophy, salt retention with oedema, hypercholesterolaemia and hypertriglyceridaemia. The 17-α substituted androgens also cause liver toxicity with cholestatic jaundice. These effects are reversible when the drug is withdrawn or used in a lower dose. Other pathological effects in the liver are hepatocellular carcinoma [126] and peliosis hepatitis [127]. There have been occasional reports of acute leukaemia occurring in patients with aplastic anaemia receiving androgens [128]. It is debatable whether the androgens should be incriminated, since leukaemia is known to occur as a natural event in the course of aplastic anaemia (see below), and there is no clear evidence that patients on high-dose androgens are more likely to develop leukaemia than any other aplastic anaemia patient.

Corticosteroids

There is no convincing evidence that corticosteroids

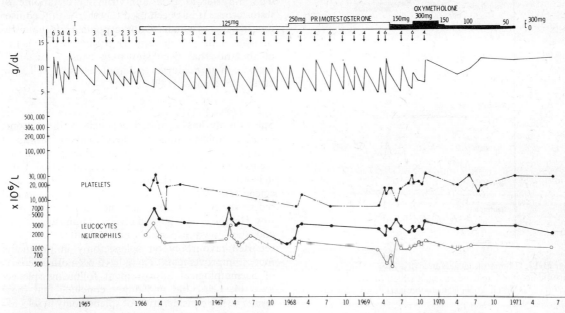

Fig. 31.10. Response to oxymetholone therapy in a 31-year-old man with chronic acquired aplastic anaemia. Previously he had required blood transfusions at approximately two-monthly intervals; since onset of remission this need has ceased. Thrombocytopenia persisted for several years before he recovered completely.

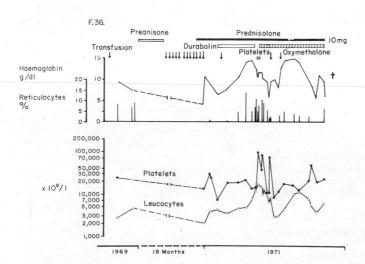

Fig. 31.11. Haematological course in a 36-year-old woman with chronic acquired aplastic anaemia, showing response to androgen therapy. There appeared to be a partial remission with durabolin, but this was followed by relapse. A second partial remission occurred with oxymetholone, but neither was this sustained, and the patient died of haemorrhage.

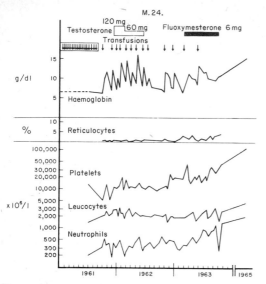

Fig. 31.12. Haematological course in a 24-year-old man with chronic acquired aplastic anaemia which followed administration of Miracil D for schistosomiasis. This illustrates a slow recovery.

have any beneficial effect either alone or as an adjunct to androgens. Moreover, they may be dangerous if given in high doses because they increase the risk of infections, especially in patients with marked granulocytopenia. Low-dose corticosteroids probably do no harm and may reduce skin-bleeding complications.

Aetiocholanolone

This 5-β steroid is a non-virilizing metabolite of testosterone. It has been used together with prednisolone in patients who have not responded adequately to previous androgen therapy. In preliminary trials this combination has been shown to cause a sustained increase in granulocytes and in platelets, as well as an erythroid response [129].

Splenectomy

Splenectomy has a limited beneficial value in some cases. In aplastic anaemia there is almost always a haemolytic element and in a third of cases the spleen seems to be the site of red-cell sequestration [78]. Thus, it is not unreasonable to expect that in these cases splenectomy will lessen transfusion requirements and reduce the erythropoietic demands made on the marrow. Heaton *et al.* [130] in a review of published results and their own experience, and Scott *et al.* [131] reported favourably on splenectomy in producing modest improvements. There have been other reports of haematological improvement following splenectomy [4, 131a] and one might conclude that these results justify consideration of splenectomy in selected patients. There is, however, no evidence that splenectomy improves the ultimate prognosis, and indeed the operative hazards may outweigh the advantages.

Bone-marrow transplantation

After an uncertain start [132, 133], better understanding of human histocompatibility typing, greater use of immunosuppressive drugs and improved methods for

Table 31.4. Example of regimens used for bone-marrow transplantation in aplastic anaemia

Day	Conventional	If patient sensitized by prior exposure to family transfusions
−7		ALG*
−6		Procarbazine 12·5 mg/kg
−5	Cyclophosphamide 50 mg/kg	+ ALG*
−4	Cyclophosphamide 50 mg/kg	+ Procarbazine 12·5 mg/kg
−3	Cyclophosphamide 50 mg/kg	+ ALG*
−2	Cyclophosphamide 50 mg/kg	+ Procarbazine 12·5 mg/kg
−1	—	—
0	Bone-marrow infusion	
+1	Methotrexate 10 mg/m^2	
+3	Methotrexate 10 mg/m^2	
+6	Methotrexate 10 mg/m^2	
+11	Methotrexate 10 mg/m^2	
Weekly to 102 days	Methotrexate 10 mg/m^2	

*ALG = Antilymphocyte globulin—dosage depends on source and manufacture.

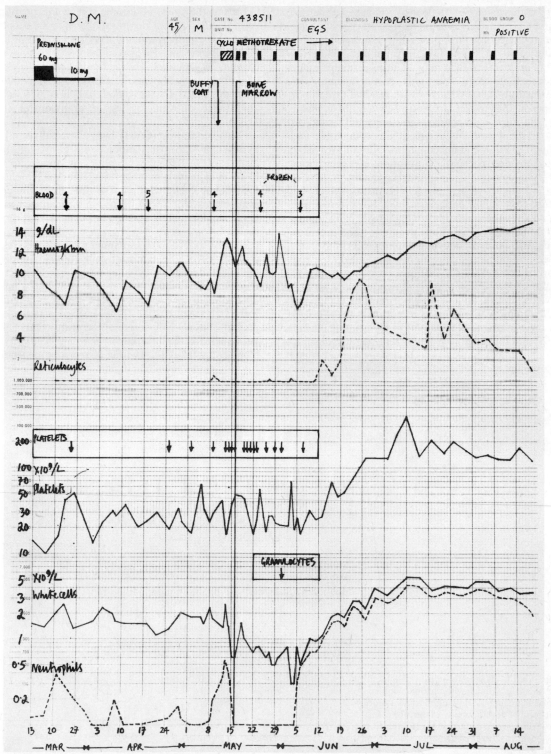

Fig. 31.13. Actual record of haematological course in a 45-year-old man with chronic acquired aplastic anaemia who has shown a satisfactory response to bone-marrow transplantation.

the management of patients with immune defence mechanisms have led to increasing attempts at bone-marrow grafting, with promising results with success rates of 40–50% [134–139]. Infusion of bone marrow from an identical twin may result in permanent cure, although in some cases only partial haemopoietic reconstitution has occurred with residual thrombocy-topenia [134]. When an identical twin is not available, an allogeneic bone-marrow graft may still be success-ful if the donor and recipient are compatible with regard to HLA and mixed lymphocyte culture (MLC) and provided that special precautions are taken by way of immunosuppression to protect against graft rejec-tion and graft-versus-host (GVH) disease which may result from minor antigen systems. For precondition-ing, various combinations of high doses of cyclophos-phamide, total lymph-node irradiation and procarba-zine with antilymphocyte globulin (ALG) have been used and immunosuppression is continued, as a rule, with methotrexate for 100 days after the transplan-tation. A typical protocol is illustrated in Table 31.4. Cyclosporin A, an anti-T-cell drug, [140] is currently undergoing evaluation for prevention of GVH disease in bone-marrow transplantation for acute leukaemia [141] and for the prevention of rejection in transplan-tation for aplastic anaemia [142].

During the preconditioning and in the post-graft period, at least until the granulocyte count becomes normal, the patient is confined to an isolation tent. Supportive measures are taken to avoid infections and bleeding as described above. Evidence for successful engraftment usually appears between 15 and 30 days after the graft. In the blood, the first sign is the appearance of reticulocytes or granulocytes (Fig. 31.13).

Graft-versus-host (GVH) disease is usually heralded by fever or skin rash, jaundice and gastro-intestinal disturbances. Reactive lymphocytes appear in the blood in increasing numbers and a marked lymphocy-tosis is an ominous sign. No treatment presently available is particularly effective in the management of GVH disease; ALG and cyclosporin A may prove useful in some cases [141–143]. Virus infections are a particular hazard in transplanted patients, more espe-cially if GVH disease is present. Interstitial pneu-monitis induced by cytomegalic virus is especially common and disseminated spread of herpex-simplex infection is a special danger. The course in a patient with GVH disease is illustrated in Figure 31.14.

Graft rejection, or failure of the graft to take, must be assumed if no increase in marrow cellularity or blood count takes place within 30 days; a transient rise

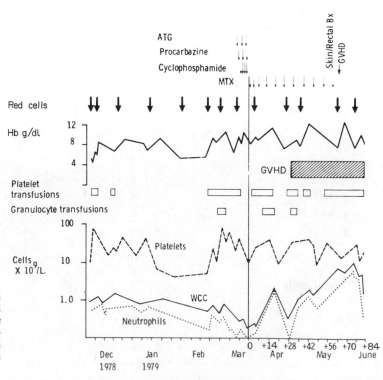

Fig. 31.14. Haematological course in 22-year-old woman with chronic acquired aplastic anaemia, showing marrow failure following development of graft-versus-host disease after marrow transplantation (indicated as day 0). The patient died from bacterial infection.

in granulocyte counts is indication of a temporary transplant with subsequent rejection. Failure of engraftment is a particular feature of aplastic anaemia, about 30% of the transplantations failing for this reason. Apart from cyclosporin A [142], total body irradiation [144] and total nodal irradiation [145] have been used in conditioning. If transplantation is to be undertaken, it should be performed without delay, to reduce the risk of complications and also to restrict the patient's blood or platelet transfusions, as these are likely to cause presensitization which makes the task of finding a compatible donor increasingly difficult. Thus, HLA typing of the patient and the family should be performed when the patient is first seen. Mixed-lymphocyte culture studies are performed if transplantation seems to be feasible and the patient should be referred to a specialized marrow-transplant unit with facilities for intensive medical and nursing care.

Marrow transplantation is an important development in the treatment of aplastic anaemia but the hopes of the patient and family must not be raised too high; its application is at present generally limited to patients with HLA-, MLC-compatible siblings and even in this selected group only about 60% of the patients appear likely to have a favourable response. When a graft fails, a decision to regraft requires serious consideration; the results of second grafting have not been very encouraging [146], clinical management is even more difficult and the prospect puts great strain on the patient, relatives and nursing staff.

Antilymphocyte globulin (ALG)
Antilymphocyte globulin has been used for pre-graft conditioning with encouraging results [147–149], including some cases where the patients received mismatched marrows [150]. Similarly good responses have been found in patients receiving ALG alone without subsequent bone-marrow infusion [148, 151, 151a] (Fig. 31.15). However, ALG results in anaphylactic reactions, thrombocytopenia, vomiting and haemorrhage; serum sickness occurs in about one-third to-half of the patients, appearing 10 days after treatment. Thus its use should be carefully monitored and reactions controlled by intravenous corticosteroids and analgesics.

Haematological complications of aplastic anaemia
Aplastic anaemia may be followed by paroxysmal nocturnal haemoglobinuria (PNH), less commonly by leukaemia. In the evolution of aplastic anaemia and of these complications the significance of the occurrence of dyserythropoiesis must also be considered.

Paroxysmal nocturnal haemoglobinuria (PNH)
A remarkable relationship exists between aplastic anaemia and PNH (see also Chapter 12), and a relatively large number of cases have been reported [111, 152–159] and reviewed [111, 112, 159, 160]. Occasionally the course of PNH may be complicated by transient marrow failure. More frequently, PNH is accompanied by a degree of marrow depression as evidenced by slight to moderate thrombocytopenia and reticulocytosis that is lower than expected for the degree of marrow depression. In other cases a patient may present with aplastic anaemia and only later will PNH become manifest. About 15% of patients presenting with chronic aplastic anaemia develop PNH or PNH-like defect during the course of their disease. In some of these cases PNH remains a laboratory phenomenon without significant effect on the course of the patient's illness; in others PNH becomes the serious clinical problem, while sometimes it is impossible to say whether the disease was primarily PNH or aplastic anaemia, and the unfortunate patient may suffer from the worst aspects of both diseases.

In some of the cases the initial aplastic anaemia phase has appeared to be drug-induced: chloramphenicol has been incriminated as the possible toxic agent in several cases [155, 156] and also other antibiotics, resorcin, benzene, sedatives, tranquillizers, insecticides and weed killers [161]; PNH has also followed Fanconi's congenital aplastic anaemia [162]. It is now generally thought that PNH develops as a somatic mutation affecting the haemopoietic stem cell and leading eventually to the marrow becoming occupied, to a greater or lesser extent, by a clone of erythroid progenitors which give rise to defective haemopoietic cells. The somatic mutation may be particularly likely to occur in aplastic anaemia in which early or abortive attempts at regenerative haemopoiesis were occurring. An alternative explanation is that the aetiological factors which lead to aplastic anaemia may also cause PNH; however, in the majority of cases no identifiable cause can be established for the aplastic anaemia, and PNH has followed the familial type as well. It seems more likely that the link is the occurrence of marrow hypoplasia with its associated dyshaemopoiesis.

Neutrophil alkaline phosphatase provides useful information on the transformation of aplastic anaemia to PNH. The alkaline phosphatase score is very high in aplastic anaemia, and markedly reduced, or zero, in typical severe cases of PNH [163]. When PNH supervenes on aplastic anaemia the previously high score falls (Fig. 31.16).

In conclusion, it should be emphasized that in all cases of aplastic anaemia, diagnostic tests for PNH (*in-vitro* lysis tests, haemosiderinuria, neutrophil alkaline phosphatase, red-cell acetylcholinesterase) should be carried out at regular intervals.

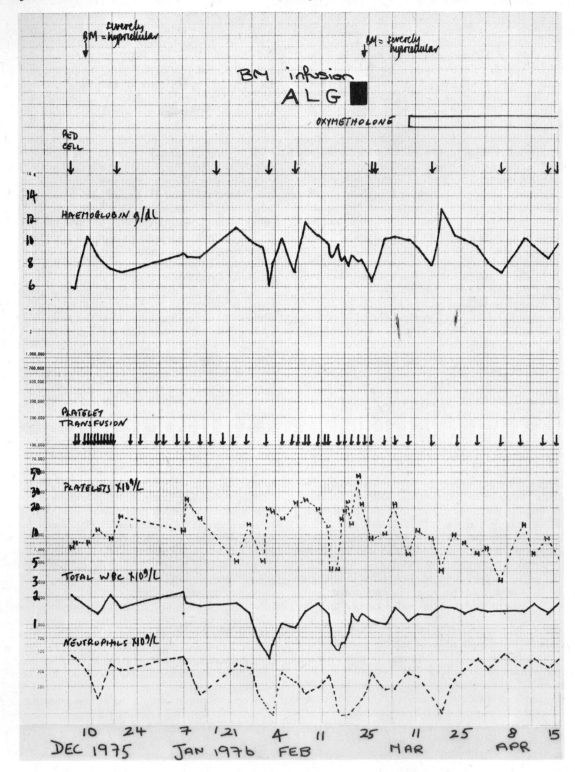

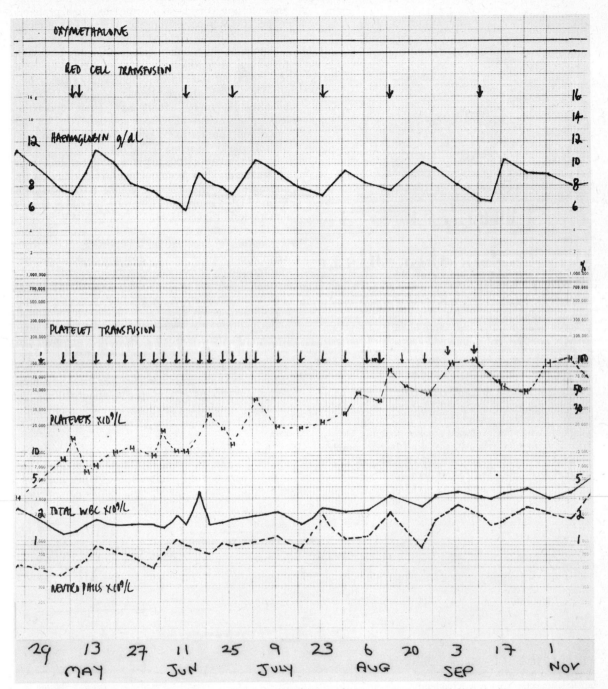

Fig. 31.15. Actual record of haematological course in patient with chronic acquired aplastic anaemia, showing response to anti-lymphocyte globulin.

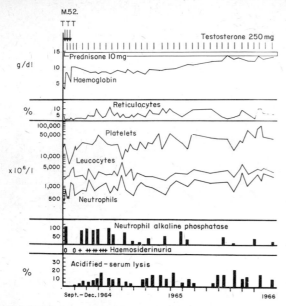

Fig. 31.16. Occurrence of paroxysmal nocturnal haemoglobinuria (PNH) in a 52-year-old man with chronic acquired aplastic anaemia. Onset of PNH was detected by a positive acidified-serum lysis test, reduction in score of neutrophil alkaline phosphatase and the appearance of haemosiderin in the urine.

Leukaemia

A transformation of aplastic anaemia into acute leukaemia was first reported by Frank in a case of idiopathic aplastic anaemia [164]. The patient was 13 years old when he developed aplastic anaemia. He was treated with blood transfusion and had a complete remission after about two and a half years, with a rise in platelets from the initial level of $25 \times 10^9/l$ to

$120 \times 10^9/l$. One year after remission he again became anaemic, and a diagnosis of acute leukaemia, probably monocytic, was made from the appearances of blood and bone marrow. He died a few months later.

Subsequently, further cases of acute leukaemia following idiopathic aplastic anaemia have been reported [100] and especially following benzene toxicity [165, 166], phenylbutazone [167] and chloramphenicol [168, 169]. There have been reports of leukaemia in cases of red-cell aplasia [170, 171] and leukaemia appears to be especially common in congenital aplastic anaemia [172–175].

In some reports [100, 121, 176, 177] the occurrence of leukaemia has been related to treatment with androgens. A characteristic course is illustrated in Figure 31.17. Leukaemia following red-cell aplasia is illustrated in Figure 31.18.

The association of aplastic anaemia and leukaemia is a matter for speculation. It is possible that a toxic agent which causes aplastic anaemia could also cause chromosomal injury that subsequently leads to leukaemia. There are certainly some similarities between the chromosome abnormalities in Fanconi's anaemia and in leukaemia [170] and similar chromosomal abnormalities have been recorded following irradiation and benzene poisoning [166], both of which can lead to either marrow aplasia or leukaemia. In chronic acquired aplastic anaemia, there are not, as a rule, any chromosomal abnormalities [180] but there have been occasional reports of non-specific abnormalities, including trisomy-21, chromosomal breaks and gaps, chromatid exchanges and extra chromosomes [178, 179].

There are various possible mechanisms of leukaemogenesis in aplastic anemia [181]. It may be analogous to the occurrence of PNH (see above) with a leukaemic

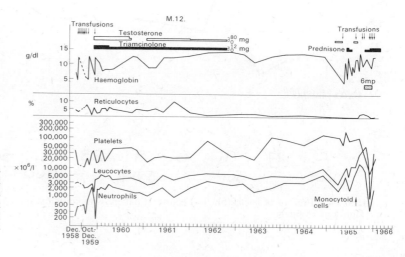

Fig. 31.17. Haematological course in a 12-year-old boy with chronic acquired aplastic anaemia. There was a remission following testosterone and steroids, but the patient subsequently developed acute leukaemia to which he succumbed.

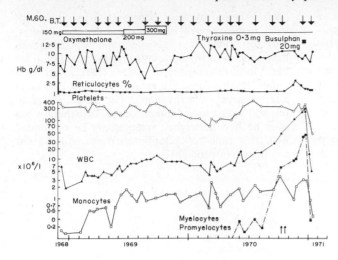

Fig. 31.18. Haematological course in a 60-year-old man with red-cell aplasia, treated with oxymetholone and transfusions. After two years there was transformation to chronic granulocytic leukaemia. During the course of his illness he developed myxoedema, apparently primary, for which he was given thyroxine.

clone developing; it is interesting to note that in a few patients both PNH and leukaemia have occurred sequentially [182, 183].

Dyserythropoiesis

The extent of dyserythropoiesis (see p. 1257) in aplastic anaemia may be obscured by the paucity of bone-marrow material available for cytological examination, but in almost all cases dyserythropoiesis occurs to a greater or lesser extent [86, 184], affecting five to 95% of the erythroid cells seen in a smear. The morphological features of dyserythropoiesis may be seen in cells at all stages of maturation. In some cases it occurs as a transient phenomenon [185]; in other cases it persists when the marrow recovers from the aplasia.

Red-cell aplasia

As a rule, haemopoietic depression involves all cell lines. Pure red-cell aplasia without involvement of platelets and leucocytes is uncommon but not rare and there have been several extensive reviews [10, 186–188]. There is a chronic idiopathic type, drug or toxin-induced types, and a transient acute type. This last form may be associated with infection or with a haemolytic condition.

The diagnosis of red-cell aplasia is made from peripheral-blood and bone-marrow findings. Anaemia is chronic and usually severe. There is a reticulocytopenia, leucocytes and platelets are normal, and there is a normal leucocyte response to infections. The bone marrow is cellular but there is a virtual absence of nucleated erythroid cells; the myeloid cells show normal maturation and morphology.

In addition to the conditions in which red-cell aplasia has its counterpart in aplastic anaemias, there are other conditions in which only erythropoiesis is affected. Erythropoietic failure leading to red-cell aplasia may be an important factor in the anaemia of renal insufficiency, either because of reduced erythropoietin production by the kidneys or because of inhibition of erythropoiesis by uraemia. In other cases defective tryptophan metabolism may be involved in the genesis of the erythroblastic hypoplasia and this may be associated with riboflavine deficiency [189, 190]. Transient erythroblastopenia, without obvious cause, has been reported in infants and children, with spontaneous recovery after about three months [191].

Red-cell anaemia and thymoma

An association of red-cell aplasia with thymoma was recognized in 1928 [192]. It occurs in about five per cent of cases [188], and about half the cases of red-cell aplasia appear to be associated with thymic tumour [186, 193, 194]. Occasionally it has also been associated with myasthenia gravis, systemic lupus erythematosus, autoimmune haemolytic anaemia and other immune processes [188].

The significance of the association of red-cell aplasia with thymic tumours and the question of whether red-cell aplasia is an autoimmune disease have been the subject of much debate and speculation [186]. Red-cell aplasia may occur without a thymoma; it may persist after thymectomy and, conversely, spindle-cell tumours and other thymic abnormalities may occur without the development of red-cell aplasia. Thus, it is possible that the tumour of the thymus may have nothing directly to do with red-cell aplasia, but that an alteration in the function of the thymus might be the end result of some abnormality which simultaneously results in development of tumour and red-cell hypoplasia [186]. There is, however, convincing evidence that erythroblastic hypoplasia may be associated with or be due to abnormal immunological mechanisms: an antibody against erythroblast nuclei has been demonstrated [32, 195, 196] and an anti-erythropoietic inhibitor of erythropoiesis has been described [33, 195, 197–199]. Hypogammaglobulinaemia and other immunological anomalies have been reported [200–204].

Treatment of red-cell aplasia

In aplastic anaemia with pancytopenia the most serious effects are due to neutropenia and thrombocytopenia. Accordingly, red-cell aplasia is, as a rule, relatively less severe, although the outlook is hardly satisfactory for a patient with red-cell aplasia who requires regular blood transfusions for survival. The general principles of management are similar to those for aplastic anaemia. Androgens are sometimes effective and patients who do have a remission do not appear to require subsequent maintenance therapy. (Fig. 31.19).

Where there is an antibody directed against the marrow erythroblasts, and/or plasma inhibitor of erythroid function, good response has been obtained by immunosuppressive therapy [35, 194, 205, 206] cyclophosphamide (150 mg daily) or azathioprine (100 mg daily) together with prednisone (20–40 mg daily) have been found to be effective in inducing remission; after remission it may be necessary to continue the drugs at a lower dose which should be titrated in each individual case. Antilymphocyte globulin has also been used in combination with immunosuppressants [35, 205]. Splenectomy seems to have a beneficial effect in some cases, although remission, if it occurs at all, will occur only gradually [188]. Splenectomy should be considered if immunosuppressive therapy fails; conversely, immunosuppressive therapy should be tried again after an apparently unsuccessful splenectomy

[194]. When a thymoma is present, it requires treatment. While removal of the tumour does not invariably result in remission, it is said that only patients who have undergone thymectomy or thymic irradiation are likely to have complete remissions [187]. In one case report, however, red-cell aplasia appeared two years after removal of a thymoma. The patient failed to respond to a course of immunosuppressive therapy but after he had undergone splenectomy he responded well, this time to cyclophosphamide, with almost complete remission [207].

FAMILIAL APLASTIC ANAEMIA

Two forms of familial haemopoietic hypoplasia occur: one results in a pancytopenia, and has been referred to as *familial constitutional panmyelocytopathy, constitutional aplastic anaemia, congenital pancytopenia* and by the eponym *Fanconi's anaemia* [208]; the other affects erythroid cells alone, and has been referred to as *erythrogenesis imperfecta, chronic congenital aregenerative anaemia, congenital (erythroid) hypoplastic anaemia,* and also by the eponym *Diamond–Blackfan anaemia* [209]. These are both rare diseases.

Fanconi's anaemia

The criteria for diagnosing Fanconi's anaemia are as follows [209, 210]:
(1) pancytopenia;
(2) hyperpigmentation;
(3) malformations, especially of the skeleton;
(4) small stature from birth;
(5) hypogonadism;
(6) familial occurrence.

The skeletal malformations include aplasia or

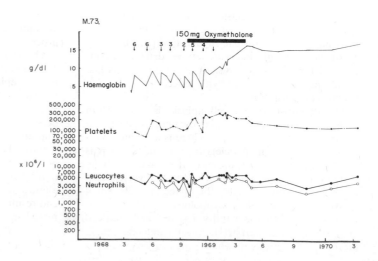

Fig. 31.19. Haematological course in a 73-year-old man with an essentially pure red-cell aplasia, showing good response to oxymetholone therapy.

hypoplasia of thumb, radius, carpal bones, and poly-
dactyl; other abnormalities include microcephaly and
mental retardation, deafness, strabismus and renal
malformation, especially ectopy and hypoplasia.

With regard to familial occurrence, while more than
one member may be affected, this is not invariable and
the diagnosis may be made if the other manifestations
are present even in the absence of a familial incidence.
Conversely, in some instances the constitutional anomalies may be present without anaemia in one sibling,
and anaemia without other manifestations in another
sibling. It is, of course, important to exclude the
possibility that siblings who develop aplastic anaemia
at the same time have not been exposed to the same
toxic substance. In Fanconi's anaemia, while the
malformations will be present at birth the severe
manifestations of anaemia and thrombocytopenia
occur later: on average at seven and a half years for
boys and eight and a half years for girls. This does of
course vary, and anaemia may occur even in the
newborn or only after the age of 20 [210], but the age of
onset tends to be the same within a family [211].
Environmental factors such as malnutrition or infections, especially viral, may precipitate the onset.

Bone-marrow findings are variable; at first the
marrow may even be hyperactive, but eventually it
becomes hypoplastic. There is an increased number of
plasma cells, reticulum cells and lymphocytes, and
even tissue mast cells may appear [211, 212].

In the majority of cases cytogenetic abnormalities
are demonstrable. These are mainly chromatid-type
abnormalities in the form of endoreduplication, chromatid exchange, or gaps and breaks, whereas chromo-
some-type aberrations appear to be rare [212–220].
Thus it seems less likely that chromosome breakage is
the primary cause of the disease than that some factor,
as yet unknown, which is lethal to haemopoietic cells,
results in chromatid damage as a secondary effect
[214]. Fibroblasts and lymphocytes as well as all types
of bone-marrow cells may be affected [216, 217].

Cytogenetic abnormalities occur in Fanconi's anaemia even in the absence of other manifestations. The
rare occurrence of leukaemia in acquired aplastic
anaemias has been referred to earlier (see p. 1252).
Leukaemia appears to occur relatively more commonly in Fanconi's anaemia [165, 173] and there also
seems to be a predisposition to the development of
solid tumours [217, 218]. There are some similarities
between the cytogenetic abnormalities in Fanconi's
anaemia and those found in leukaemia; it is of interest
to note that similar abnormalities have also been
recorded in irradiation and in benzene intoxication,
both of which can induce either marrow aplasia or
leukaemia. It is possible that the cytogenetic abnormalities are a manifestation of somatic alterations that

may lead to the production of some cells with selective
growth advantage (resulting in leukaemia) and to
others with growth defect (resulting in aplasia); PNH
has also been reported in Fanconi's anaemia [162].

Fetal haemoglobin is raised in both familial and
acquired aplastic anaemia [219] and it does not
distinguish one type from the other.

Dyskeratosis congenita is a rare condition which
appears to have some relationship with Fanconi's
anaemia [212, 220]; it is also associated with bone-marrow failure, hypogenitalism, mental retardation, skin
pigmentation and poor growth. However, there are
features which are characteristic of dyskeratosis and
which do not occur in Fanconi's anaemia. These are
telangiectatic erythrema, lachrymal-duct atresia, alopecia and abnormal sweating, and leukoplakia of
mucosal surfaces; furthermore, the chromosome pattern in dyskeratosis is normal.

Diamond–Blackfan anaemia

Some 200 cases have been recorded in the literature
[221]. The essential defect is that of red-cell production. Skeletal anomalies have been described but in
contrast to Fanconi's anaemia renal abnormalities do
not occur and there are no chromosomal changes. The
condition becomes manifest soon after birth and in
most cases it is recognized in the first six months of life.
Hepatomegaly may occur but splenomegaly is unusual. A familial incidence has been noted in some
cases.

The anaemia is normocytic and normochromic and
may be severe, while reticulocytes are usually less than
one per cent. Leucocyte and platelet counts are
normal. In the bone marrow there is a remarkable
absence of erythroid precursors but all other elements
are normal. The course is progressive and blood
transfusions may be necessary to sustain life. An
intensive transfusion regime may lead to siderosis and
the risk of serum hepatitis, with severe liver damage;
these can be considered as complications of the disease.
They lead to the growth retardation, failure of sexual
maturation and portal hypertension which has been
associated with the disease. Spontaneous remissions
do occur (see below), although the remissions have
sometimes been only temporary.

The cause of Diamond–Blackfan anaemia is not
known. Culture studies have suggested that there is a
quantitative or qualitative deficiency of BFU-E which
gives rise to erythropoietin-unresponsive CFU-E, and
in turn to proerythroblasts with poor erythropoietic
response [222, 223]. There is no evidence for an
immune mechanism and normal T-cell function has
been demonstrated [224]. The familial incidence and
early age of onset suggest that the abnormality is
genetically determined. In some cases an abnormality

(a)

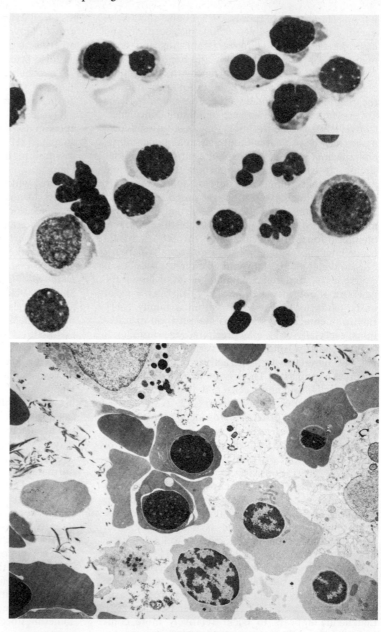

Fig. 31.20 (a). Characteristic features of dyserythropoiesis by light microscopy. For description see text.

of tryptophan metabolism has been described [225], but subsequent investigations have given variable results [226].

Treatment of familial aplastic anaemias

Fanconi's anaemia. General management is similar to that for acquired aplastic anaemia (p. 1241). Some cases respond well to androgens, although they rarely produce permanent cure, and the high doses which are necessary to induce remission result in unpleasant side-effects such as virilization with its associated physical and emotional problems in young male children, deepening of the voice and hirsutism in girls, and embarrassing sexual activity in both boys and girls. Bone-marrow transplantation is described on page 1246. As some patients will undergo spontaneous remission and others will respond well to conservative

(b)

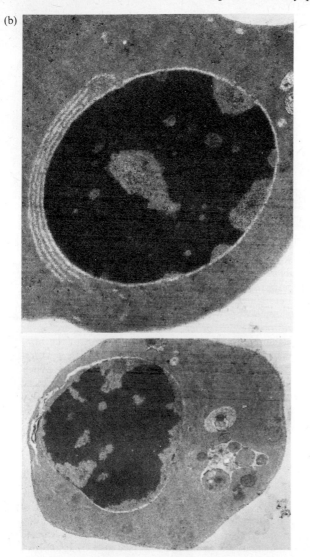

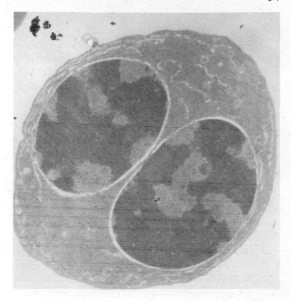

Fig. 31.20 (b). Characteristic features of dyserythropoiesis by transmission electron microscopy. For description see text.

treatment, the problem is to decide whether to undertake this arduous and hazardous procedure in the individual case.

Diamond–Blackfan anaemia. Most patients respond to corticosteroids; treatment is commenced in a dose of 2 mg/kg daily in divided doses. After remission (usually within a few weeks) the dose is reduced to a maintenance level which varies from case to case; it may be necessary to continue treatment with an adjusted dose for months or years. Androgens in low dosage may counteract the growth depression associated with corticosteroid treatment. Patients who fail to respond to corticosteroids may require long-term treatment

with regular transfusions; these patients may be considered for bone-marrow transplantation, but it must be remembered that spontaneous remission occurs in a quarter of all cases, sometimes only after many years [221, 226, 227].

DYSERYTHROPOIESIS

By contrast to *aplasia* or *hypoplasia* which describe a quantitative defect of the bone marrow, the term *dyshaemopoiesis* or *dyserythropoiesis,* when erythropoiesis alone is affected, describes the situation where there is a qualitative abnormality of the bone marrow (*dysplasia*) resulting in inefficient haemopoiesis with extramedullary death of at least some cells which have failed to mature (see Chapter 4).

Dyserythropoiesis may occur in a wide range of diseases which primarily affect synthesis of the nucleus or the cytoplasm. In some cases the cause of the defect is easily identified, e.g. deficiencies of vitamin B_{12} or folate, iron deficiency or iron-utilization defects including thalassaemia and primary sideroblastic anaemias (see Chapters 9 and 13). In other cases, the cause of dyserythropoiesis is more obscure: it occurs in aplastic anaemia, myelosclerosis, infections and in a group of congenital disorders [161, 228, 229]. In dyshaemopoiesis the bone marrow is, as a rule, of normal or increased cellularity. There is, however, an overlap between decreased and defective erythropoiesis. As mentioned above, dyserythropoiesis is frequently a feature in aplastic anaemia and indeed hypoplasia alone is the exception rather than the rule. It is necessary to distinguish the (rare) cases where dyserythropoiesis is of primary importance from cases in which aplastic (aregenerative) anaemia is the essential disorder, and dyserythropoiesis is a secondary event.

Morphological abnormalities characteristic of dyserythropoiesis include binuclearity and multinuclearity of the normoblasts, internuclear bridging, asynchrony between nuclear and cytoplasmic maturation and premature nuclear extrusion, nuclear budding, fragmentation and degeneration (karyorrhexis) and various abnormalities of mitosis. There is persistence of intercellular cytoplasmic connections and abnormalities of the cytoplasm itself, such as vacuolation, basophilic stippling and the presence of an excessive amount of siderotic granules. The extent to which these abnormalities are apparent in a bone marrow and the relative preponderance of one or other type of abnormality varies considerably between cases.

Electron microscopy reveals other structural abnormalities [184, 230, 231]. Anomalies of nuclear division include incomplete separation of nuclei which range from slight indentations, to deep clefts in the nuclear substance, to chromatin bridges between two nuclei, or the nuclei might be completely divided but the cells remain joined by cytoplasmic junctions, with a persistent spindle bridge containing microtubules.

In the cytoplasm, siderotic material is prominent both free-lying and in mitochondria, whilst the mitochondria themselves are swollen with disintegrating internal structure, and loss of normal configuration. Microtubules similar in size to those of the spindle bridge are found within the cytoplasm and there is persistence of endoplasmic reticulum and stacks of annulated lamellae occur adjacent to the nucleus. The nuclear membrane itself is abnormal and loses its integrity so that one sees mitchondria and cytoplasmic vesicles in the nuclear area and, conversely, oozing of nuclear material into the cytoplasm. The nuclear pores are widened and contain disintegrating structures. There are ribosomal anomalies: some cells have few or no ribosomes, other ribosomes may not have characteristic distribution in the cytoplasm, but may instead be found in arrays attached to the nuclear membrane. Large autophagic vacuoles are present in the cytoplasm. Some characteristic features are shown in Figure 31.20 (a) and (b).

Other indications of dyserythropoiesis [229]

In the secondary dyserythropoietic anaemias there will be clinical and haematological features of the primary disease. There are, in addition, certain non-specific clinical and haematological manifestations of dyserythropoiesis *per se*. There is anaemia and usually some degree of haemolysis. The reticulocyte count is usually increased, but as a rule, the reticulocyte response is relatively low for the degree of anaemia. Ferrokinetic studies show an accelerated clearance of plasma iron with a decreased erythrocyte incorporation in the order of 25–50%, and there is an accumulation and retention of the iron in the bone marrow. A useful parameter of ineffective erythropoiesis is the serum bilirubin. An unconjugated hyperbilirubinaemia is observed in many dyserythropoietic conditions and this is evidence of increased haemoglobin catabolism. More specialized investigations include the use of an appropriate isotope to demonstrate the appearance of an early bilirubin peak after administration of labelled haem precursors, and the demonstration of high carbon-monoxide production which, in the absence of peripheral-blood haemolysis, is a pointer to ineffective erythropoiesis. Intramedullary destruction of cytoplasm results in the liberation of various enzymes, notably lactic dehydrogenase and aldolases, and destruction of nuclear material leads to an increased level of uric acid (see also Chapter 4).

Serology [232]

Another feature of dyserythropoiesis is that the erythrocytes adsorb an increased amount of antibody on their membranes, demonstrated *in vitro* by increased agglutination and by a positive cold-antibody (anti-I) lysis test. The cold-antibody lysis test is also positive in PNH (see Chapter 12), but in contrast to PNH, in the dyserythropoietic anaemias there is no increased sensitivity to complement, although of course complement is necessary for lysis to occur.

A positive cold-antibody lysis test is most frequently observed in aplastic anaemia, leukaemia, erythraemic myelosis, myelosclerosis, and megaloblastic anaemias. The reason for this phenomenon is not known. At least one aspect of the defect is the presence of enhanced I- and i-antigen activity, and the antigenic modifications have features characteristic of neonatal cells [232]. This may be due to disturbed synthesis of membrane protein consequent to disturbed nucleic-acid metabolism, or it may reflect membrane immaturity caused by an abnormally short marrow transit time, or by the re-activation of fetal erythropoiesis. There are also alterations in red-cell enzymes, notably a deficiency in pyruvate kinase and increased activities of hexokinase, G6PD and 6PGD [233].

Congenital dyserythropoietic anaemia

This is a fairly well-defined clinical and haematological syndrome of a congenital disorder of variable severity with recessive inheritance. It may simulate a thalassaemic-like condition or a hereditary haemolytic anaemia. There is hyperbilirubinaemia of the unconjugated type. However, the reticulocyte count is low and there is no evidence for a major degree of haemolysis. Ferrokinetic studies demonstrate ineffective erythropoiesis. The peripheral-blood and bone-marrow picture distinguish this condition from thalassaemia. Peripheral-blood film shows anisocytosis, poikilocytosis and irregularly crenated and contracted cells. The marrow shows one of three patterns [234].

Type I: Megaloblastoid changes, macrocytosis, internuclear chromatin bridges, but binuclearity not prominent; pro-erythroblasts and basophilic erythroblasts especially affected.

Type II: Binuclearity especially of late erythroblasts, multinuclearity, pluripolar mitoses, karyorrhexis.

Type III: Multinuclearity with up to 12 nuclei, gigantoblasts and macrocytosis. There is an overlap between Types I and II and each type includes variants which differ in some of their features.

CDA Type I [235, 236]

This is less common than CDA Type II (see below). It has an autosomal recessive inheritance; no method is available to identify heterozygous subjects. The clinical manifestations include a variable degree of jaundice, hepatomegaly and splenomegaly. General symptoms are usually slight or absent and a number of patients are only diagnosed by chance, e.g. when a blood count is performed as a screening procedure in pregnancy. However, some patients are diagnosed because of the symptoms of anaemia, and in others iron overload occurs, even in patients who have neither been transfused nor treated with iron; this may lead to secondary haemochromatosis and cirrhosis. Haematologically, CDA Type I differs from Type II by its bone-marrow morphological appearances and a negative acidified serum lysis test (see below).

CDA Type II [237–241]

Type II is the most common type of the CDAs. It is transmitted as an autosomal recessive disease; the geographical distribution of the recorded cases suggests a particularly high frequency in north-west Europe, in Italy and in northern Africa. As with Type I the clinical manifestations include a variable degree of jaundice, hepatomegaly and splenomegaly, iron overload with cirrhosis and diabetes, and a few patients have been mentally retarded. The serum iron levels and transferrin saturation rate are increased.

CDA II has an acronym: 'HEMPAS'—hereditary erythroblast multinuclearity with positive acidified serum [238]. This is because of a unique feature: the red cells are haemolysed by some acidified normal sera, but unlike PNH, where lysis in the acidified serum test is due to marked sensitivity to complement, in HEMPAS there is a specific antigen on the erythrocytes and only sera which contain an IgM anti-HEMPAS antibody in sufficient amount (about 30% of normal people) will induce lysis of HEMPAS cells [232]. HEMPAS is readily distinguished from PNH because lysis does not occur when the patient's own serum is used and also because lysis occurs with only about one-third of normal sera. Another point of difference is that lysis may be enhanced if the cell/serum mixture is chilled before it is incubated at 37°C. Furthermore, sucrose lysis is negative.

Aberrant types [242–247]

There have been a number of reports of cases where the morphological features are uncharacteristic and/or the serological behaviour is unexpected. It is convenient to classify the cases into Types I and II on the basis of the acidified serum lysis test, irrespective of any other features.

CDA Type III [248–251]

Type III is the rarest form, which was the first to be described in 1951. It is notable for the multinuclearity and gigantoblasts in the bone marrow. Indeed, the erythroblasts are especially remarkable for being present with up to 12 nuclei in a cell. Morphologically the condition is more likely to be confused with erythroleukaemia than with the other types of CDA, but the clinical picture is of a mild anaemia with good prognosis, and there is no granulocytopenia or thrombocytopenia. In the few cases studied the red cells have been strongly haemolysed by both anti-I and anti-i sera but acidified serum lysis test has been negative.

The pathogenesis of the CDAs has not yet been established. The abnormality appears to be in the committed erythroid stem cell [252, 253]. HEMPAS red cells are deficient in neuraminic acid [254, 255] and have an aberrant expression of membrane antigens

(232]. There is evidence for repressed induction of DNA synthesis [256], and ultrastructural studies suggest that the disturbance in protein synthesis may stem from a defect in the nuclear membrane [230, 231, 257]. It is of interest to note that apparently identical defects can be induced by some toxic agents, infections, and even in normal bone marrow under artificial culture conditions [231, 257].

REFRACTORY ANAEMIAS

There are two types of chronic refractory cytopenia in which defects of the myeloid stem cell is the prominent feature. They are sometimes referred to collectively as 'myelodysplastic syndromes'. Individually, they are termed:
1 refractory anaemia with excess of blasts (RAEB) or refractory anaemia with excess myeloblastosis (RAEM), and
2 refractory anaemia with proliferative dysplasia.

Refractory anaemia with excess of myeloblasts [258, 259]

This occurs in men and women over the age of 50 who present with symptoms of chronic anaemia without palpable lymph nodes or enlarged spleen or liver. There is pancytopenia with qualitative abnormalities of all cell lines—poikilocytosis, agranular polymorphs with Pelger-like anomaly and giant platelets. The bone marrow is of normal or increased cellularity. The erythroid cells show the full range of dyserythropoietic features, but the most outstanding feature is the presence of up to 30–35% of morphologically abnormal myeloblasts and promyelocytes: the latter cells have blast-like nuclei without chromatin condensation, sometimes large azurophilic granules and sometimes deficient granulation. Megakaryocytes are present but may also be morphologically abnormal with small, round nuclei, scanty basophilic cytoplasm, and surrounded by a few giant platelets.

This condition is related to dyserythropoiesis not only by the morphological features, but also by the demonstration of membrane antigenic and enzyme anomalies—there may be decrease in blood group antigens, especially A, B and H, and an increase in I [260]; pyruvate kinase is decreased and other enzymes are increased [233].

It is not clear whether this is in fact pre-leukaemia (or 'smouldering leukaemia'). It may certainly remain stable with an unchanging bone marrow for years, although a proportion of cases undoubtedly terminate in acute leukaemia [261, 262]. Bone-marrow culture may be of value in distinguishing non-leukaemia RAEB from pre-leukaemia or at least for monitoring the progress of the dysplastic condition. Change in the growth pattern or a modification of cluster to colony ratio is said to precede, often for many months, the evolution towards leukaemic proliferation [263–265]. By means of CFU-C assay and co-culture with normal marrow, three growth patterns have been observed in refractory anaemias [226]:
1 low colony formation, not suppressed by normal marrow;
2 low colony formation with suppression by normal marrow;
3 normal colony formation without suppression.
These findings suggest that there are three different pathogenetic mechanisms, namely:
1 an intrinsic defect in the stem cell;
2 suppressor-cell action against the stem cell; and
3 an abnormality in the micro-environment rather than a direct cellular defect.

There has been some debate as to whether patients with RAEB should receive chemotherapy as for acute leukaemia or be considered as having a form of aplastic anaemia and be treated with androgens [261, 267]; in view of the fact that many cases do not progress to leukaemia, cytotoxic agents should be withheld at least until there is clear evidence of evolution to leukaemia in the individual patient. The CFU-C assay and co-culture studies [266] may be helpful in deciding in an individual patient whether treatment should be directed towards stem-cell replacement, stimulation of erythropoiesis or immuno-suppression.

Proliferative dysplasia [268]

This condition occurs in elderly patients, equally in men and women. There is a pancytopenia and reticulocytopenia. The bone marrow has normal cellularity with the morphological features of dyserythropoiesis, and with no increase in the proportion of myeloblasts to promyelocytes, whilst megakaryocytes are present in normal numbers. There is no difficulty in aspirating marrow but when bone-biopsy material is examined there is seen to be an increased amount of reticulin although no obvious fibrosis. The first impression is of a myeloproliferative disorder, but there is no leuco-erythroblastic anaemia, the spleen is not enlarged, ferrokinetic studies show an aplastic pattern with marked reduction in red-cell iron incorporation and no extramedullary erythropoiesis. This seems most likely to be a variant of aplastic anaemia with especially marked dyserythropoiesis. Management should be along lines similar to that for aplastic anaemia.

REFERENCES

1 ERLICH P. (1886) Uber einen Fall von Anämie mit Bemerkungen über regenerative Veränderungen des Kockenmarks. *Charité-Annalen*, **13**, 300.

2 CAREY J.B. & TAYLOR J.H. (1931) Primary aplastic anaemia: discussion and report of two cases. *Annals of Internal Medicine*, **5**, 471.

3 LEWIS S.M. (1971) Aplastic anaemia. *British Journal of Hospital Medicine*, **6**, 593.

4 VINCENT P.C. & DE GRUCHY G.C. (1967) Complications and treatment of acquired aplastic anaemia. *British Journal of Haematology*, **13**, 977.

5 WILLIAMS D.M., LYNCH R.E. & CARTWRIGHT G.E. (1978) Prognostic factors in aplastic anemia. *Clinics in Hematology*, **7**, 467.

6 ALTER B.P., POTTER N.U. & LI F.P. (1978) Classification and etiology of the aplastic anemias. *Clinics in Hematology*, **7**, 431.

7 MORLEY A, HOLMES K. & FORBES I. (1974) Depletion of B lymphocytes in chronic hypoplastic marrow failure (aplastic anaemia). *Australian and New Zealand Journal of Medicine*, **4**, 538.

8 O'GORMAN-HUGHES D.W. (1966) The varied pattern of aplastic anaemia in childhood. *Australian Paediatric Journal*, **2**, 228.

8a O'GORMAN-HUGHES D.W. (1973) Aplastic anaemia in childhood: a reappraisal. II. Idiopathic and acquired aplastic anaemia. *Medical Journal of Australia*, **2**, 361.

9 GEARY C.G. (1979) Red-cell aplasia. In: *Aplastic Anaemia* (ed. Geary C.G.), p.195. Baillière Tindall, London.

10 KRANTZ S.B. (1976) Diagnosis and treatment of pure red-cell aplasia. *Medical Clinics of North America*, **60**, 945.

11 GEARY C.G. & TESTA N.G. (1979) Pathophysiology of marrow hypoplasia. In: *Aplastic Anaemia* (ed. Geary C.G.), p. 1. Baillière Tindall, London.

12 KERN P., HEIMPEL H., HEIT W. & KUBANEK B. (1977) Granulocyte progenitor cells in aplastic anaemia. *British Journal of Haematology*, **35**, 613.

13 MORIYAMA Y., SATO M & KINOSHITA Y. (1979) Studies on hematopoietic stem cells. XI. Lack of erythroid burst-forming units (BFU-E) in patients with aplastic anemia. *American Journal of Hematology*, **6**, 11.

14 SINGER J.W. & BROWN J.E. (1978) *In vitro* marrow culture techniques in aplastic anemia and related disorders. *Clinics in Hematology*, **7**, 487.

15 BARRETT A.J., FAILLE A., BALITRAND N., KETELS F. & NAJEAN Y. (1979) Bone-marrow culture in aplastic anaemia. *Journal of Clinical Pathology*, **32**, 660.

16 FITCHEN J.H. & CLINE M.J. (1978) Recent developments in understanding the pathogenesis of aplastic anemia. *American Journal of Hematology*, **5**, 365.

17 HEIMPEL H. & KUBANEK B. (1975) Pathophysiology of aplastic anaemia. *British Journal of Haematology*, **31** (Suppl.), 57

18 SMICK K.M., CONDIT P.K., PROCTOR R.L. & SUTCHER V. (1964) Fatal aplastic anemia. *Journal of Chronic Diseases*, **17**, 899.

19 MAILE J.B. (1977) *Laboratory Medicine—Hematology*, 5th edn, p. 799. C. V. Mosby, St. Louis.

20 CUSTER R.P. (1946) Aplastic anemia in soldiers treated with atabrine (Quinacrine). *American Journal of Medical Science*, **212**, 211.

21 PRAGER D. & PETERS C. (1970) Development of aplastic anemia and the exposure to Stoddard solvent. *Blood*, **35**, 286.

22 GOLDBERG I.H. (1965) Mode of action of antibiotics. II. Drugs affecting nucleic acid and protein synthesis. *American Journal of Medicine*, **39**, 722.

23 BITHELL T.C. & WINTROBE M.M. (1967) Drug-induced aplastic anemia. *Seminars in Hematology*, **4**, 194.

24 YUNIS A.A. & HARRINGTON W.J. (1960) Patterns of inhibition by chloramphenicol of nucleic acid synthesis in human bone marrow and leukemic cells. *Journal of Laboratory and Clinical Medicine*, **56**, 831.

25 NAGAO T. & MAUER A.M. (1969) Concordance for drug-induced aplastic anemia in identical twins. *New England Journal of Medicine*, **281**, 7.

26 BEST W. (1967) Chloramphenicol-associated blood dyscrasias. *Journal of American Medical Association*, **201**, 363.

27 McCURDY P.R. (1963) Plasma concentration of chloramphenicol and bone-marrow suppression. *Blood*, **21**, 363.

28 SUHRLAND L.G. & WIESBERGER A.S. (1963) Chloramphenicol toxicity in liver and renal disease. *Archives of Internal Medicine*, **112**, 747.

29 RUBIN D., WEISBERGER A.S., BOTTI R.E. & STORAASLI J.P. (1958) Changes in iron metabolism in early chloramphenicol toxicity. *Journal of Clinical Investigation*, **37**, 1286.

30 SCOTT J.L., FINEGOLD S.M., BELKIN G.A. & LAWRENCE J.S. (1965) A controlled double blind study of the hematologic toxicity of chloramphenicol. *New England Journal of Medicine*, **272**, 1137.

31 RUBIN D., WEISBERGER A.S. & CLARK D.R. (1960) Early detection of drug-induced erythropoietic depression. *Journal of Laboratory and Clinical Medicine*, **56**, 453.

32 KRANTZ S.B. & KAO V. (1969) Studies on red-cell aplasia. II. Report of a second patient with an antibody to erythroblast nuclei and a remission after immunosuppressive therapy. *Blood*, **34**, 1.

33 PESCHLE C. & CONDORELLI M. (1976) Physiopathology of pure red-cell aplasia, type I and II. In: *Leukaemia and Aplastic Anaemia* (ed. Metcalf D., Condorelli M. & Peschle C.), p. 51. Il Pasiero Scientifico, Rome.

34 CLINE M.J. & GOLDE D.W. (1978) Immune suppression of hematopoiesis. *American Journal of Medicine*, **64**, 301.

35 MARMONT A., PESCHLE C., SANGUINETI M. & CONDORELLI M. (1975) Pure red-cell aplasia (PRCA): response of three patients to cyclophosphamide and/or antilymphocytic globulin (ALG) and demonstration of two types of serum IgG inhibitors to erythropoiesis. *Blood*, **45**, 247.

36 GORDON M.Y. (1978) Circulating inhibitors of granulopoiesis in patients with aplastic anaemia. *British Journal of Haematology*, **39**, 491.

37 KAGAN W.A., ASCENSAO J.A., PAHWA R.N., HANSEN J.A., GOLDSTEIN G., VALERA E.B., ICEFY G.S., MOORE M.A.S. & GOOD R.A. (1976) Aplastic anemia: presence in human bone marrow of cells that suppress myelopoiesis. *Proceedings of National Academy of Sciences, USA*, **73**, 2890.

38 GOOD R.A. (1977) Aplastic anemia—suppressor lymphocytes and hematopoiesis. *New England Journal of Medicine*, **296**, 41.

39 PETZ L.D. & FUDENBERG H.H. (1975) Immunologic mechanisms in drug-induced cytopenias. *Progress in Hematology*, **9**, 185.

40 KNOSPE W.H. & CROSBY W.H. (1971) Aplastic anaemia: a disorder of the bone-marrow sinusoidal microcirculation rather than stem-cell failure? *Lancet*, **i**, 20.

41 PATT H.M. & MOLONY M.A. (1975) Bone-marrow regeneration after local injury: a review. *Experimental Hematology*, **3**, 135.

42 COMMITTEE ON SAFETY OF DRUGS (1965) *Annual Report for 1964*. H.M. Stationery Office, London.

43 DAVIES D.M. (ed.) (1968) Drugs and anaemia. In: *Adverse Drug Reaction Bulletin* No. 8, p. 16. Newcastle Regional Hospital Board, Newcastle upon Tyne.

44 DUKES M.N.G. (ed.) (1975) *Meyler's Side Effects of Drugs*, Vol. VIII and *Side Effects of Drugs Annual*, Vol. 1, 1977, Vol. 2, 1978. Excerpta Medica, Amsterdam, Oxford.

45 KRANTZ S.B. & ZAENTZ S.D. (1977) Pure red-cell aplasia. In: *A Year of Hematology* (ed. Silber R., Gordon A.S. & LoBue J.) p.153. Plenum Press, London.

46 WIJNJA J., SNUDER J.A.M. & NIEWEG H.O. (1966) Acetylsalicyclic acid as a cause of pancytopenia from bone-marrow damage. *Lancet*, **ii**, 768.

47 DONSKI S. & BUCHER U. (1968) Increase of the number of pancytopenias between 1954 and 1964. *Helvetica Medica Acta*, **34**, 337.

48 AKSOY M., DINCOL, K., AKGUN T., ERDEM S. & DINCOL G. (1971) Haematological effects of chronic benzene poisoning in 217 workers. *British Journal of Industrial Medicine*, **28**, 296.

49 BROWNING E. (1965) *Toxicity and Metabolism of Industrial Solvents*, p. 3. Elsevier, Amsterdam.

50 AKSOY M. & ERDEM S. (1978) Follow-up study on the mortality and the development of leukemia in 44 pancytopenic patients with chronic exposure to benzene. *Blood*, **52**, 285.

51 RONDANELLI E.G., GORINI P., PECORARI D., TROTTA N. & COLOMBI R. (1961) Effets du benzène sur la mitose érythroblastique. Investigations à la microcinématographie en contrate de phase. *Acta Haematologica*, **26**, 281.

52 SPECK B. (1975) Toxische Knochenmarkinsuffinzienz. *Haematologie und Bluttransfusion*, **16**, 235.

53 COOPER W. (1959) Pancytopenia associated with disseminated tuberculosis. *Annals of Internal Medicine*, **50**, 1497.

54 LYNCH E.C., MCKECHNIE J.C. & ALFREY C.P. (1968) Brucellosis with pancytopenia. *Annals of Internal Medicine*, **69**, 319.

54a SHADDUCK R.K., WINKELSTEIN A., ZEIGLER Z., LICHTER J., GOLDSTEIN M., MICHAELS M. & RABIN B. (1979) Aplastic anemia following infectious mononucleosis: possible immune etiology. *Experimental Hematology*, **7**, 264.

55 LORENZ E. & QUAISER K. (1955) Panmyelopathie nach Hepatitis epidemica. *Weiner Medizinische Wockenschrift*, **105**, 19.

56 CAMITTA B.M., NATHA D.G., FORMAN E.N., PARKMAN A., RAPPEPORT J.M. & ORELLANA T.D. (1974) Posthepatitis severe aplastic anemia—an indication for early bone-marrow transplantation. *Blood*, **43**, 473.

57 HAGLER L., PASTORE R.A., BERGIN J.J. & WRENSCH M.R. (1975) Aplastic anaemia following viral hepatitis: report of two fatal cases and literature review. *Medicine*, **54**, 139.

58 SEARS D.A., GEORGE J.N. & GOLD M.S. (1975) Transient red blood cell aplasia in association with viral hepatitis. Occurrence four years apart in siblings. *Archives of Internal Medicine*, **135**, 1585.

59 BÖTTIGER L.E. & WESTERHOLM B. (1972) Aplastic anaemia. III. Aplastic anaemia and infectious hepatitis. *Acta Medica Scandinavica*, **192**, 323.

60 AJLOUNI K. & DOEBLIN T.D. (1974) The syndrome of hepatitis and aplastic anaemia. *British Journal of Haematology*, **27**, 345.

61 DELLER J.J., CIRKSENA W.J. & MARCURELLI J. (1962) Fatal pancytopenia associated with viral hepatitis. *New England Journal of Medicine*, **266**, 297.

62 CRONKITE E.P. (1967) Radiation-induced aplastic anemia. *Seminars in Hematology*, **4**, 273.

63 FLIEDNER T.M., ANDREWS G.A., CRONKITE E.P. & BOND V.P. (1964) Early and late cytologic effects of whole body irradiation on human marrow. *Blood*, **23**, 471.

64 COURT BROWN W.M. & DOLL R. (1965) Leukaemia and aplastic anaemia in patients irradiated for ankylosing spondylitis. *Medical Research Council Special Report Series* (London), **295**, 1.

65 LEWIS E.B. (1963) Leukemia, multiple myeloma and aplastic anemia in American radiologists. *Science*, **142**, 1492.

66 SHADDUCK, R.K., WINKSELSTE A., ZEIGLER Z., LICHTER J., GOLDSTEIN M., MICHAELS M. & RABIN B. (1979) Aplastic anemia following infectious mononucleosis: possible immune etiology. *Experimental Hematology*, **7**, 264.

67 COURT BROWN W.M. & DOLL R. (1965) Mortality from cancer and other causes after radiotherapy for ankylosing spondylitis. *British Medical Journal*, **ii**, 1327.

68 WARREN S. & BOWERS J. (1950) The acute radiation syndrome in man. *Annals of Internal Medicine*, **32**, 207.

69 JAMMET H., MATHÉ G., PENDIC B., DUPLAN J.F., MAUPIN B., LANTARJET R., KALIE D., SCHWARZENBERG L., DJUKIC Z. & VIGNE J. (1959) Étude de six cas d'irradiation totale aiguë accidentale. *Revue française d'Études Cliniques et Biologiques*, **4**, 210.

70 KIRSCHBAUM J.D., MATSUO T., SATO K., ICHIMARU M., TSUCHIMOTO T. & ISCHIMARU T. (1971) A study of aplastic anemia in an autopsy series with special reference to atomic bomb survivors in Hiroshima and Nagasaki. *Blood*, **38**, 17.

71 MCCULLOCH E.A. & TILL E.A. (1962) The sensitivity of cells from normal mouse bone marrow to γ radiation *in vitro* and *in vivo*. *Radiation Research*, **16**, 822.

72 SZUR L. & LEWIS S.M. (1966) The haematological complications of polycythaemia vera and treatment with radioactive phosphorus. *British Journal of Radiology*, **39**, 122.

73 BERNARD J. & NAJEAN Y. (1965) Evolution and prognosis of the idiopathic pancytopenias. *Series Haematologica*, **5**, 1.

74 MOHLER D.N. & LEAVELL B.S. (1958) Aplastic anemia: an analysis of 50 cases. *Annals of Internal Medicine*, **49**, 326.

75 LEWIS S.M. (1965) Course and prognosis in aplastic anaemia. *British Medical Journal*, **i**, 1027.

76 WHANG K.S. (1978) Aplastic anemia in Korea: a clinical study of 309 cases. In: *Aplastic Anemia*. Japanese

Medical Research Foundation, Publ. no. 4, p. 225. University of Tokyo Press.

77 HUHN D., FATEH-MOGHADAM A., DEMMLER K., KRONSEDER A., ERHART H. (1975) Hämatologische und immunologische Befunde bei Knochenmarkplasia. *Klinische Wochenschrift*, **53**, 7.

78 LEWIS S.M. (1962) Red-cell abnormalities and haemolysis in aplastic anaemia. *British Journal of Haematology*, **8**, 322.

79 HAURANI F.I. & MARCOLINA M.J. (1971) Expression of plasma iron turnover in aplastic anemia. *American Journal of Clinical Pathology*, **55**, 659.

80 CHIPPING P., KLONIZAKIS I. & LEWIS S.M. (1980) Indium chloride scanning: a comparison with iron as a tracer for erythropoiesis. *Clinical and Laboratory Haematology*, **2**, 255.

81 BJORKMAN S.E. (1962) Case of aplastic anaemia caused by chlormaphenicol with recovery after 22 months. *Acta Haematologica*, **27**, 124.

82 HELLRIEGEL K.-P., ZÜGER M. & GROSS R. (1977) Prognosis in acquired aplastic anemia. An approach in the selection of patients for allogeneic bone-marrow transplantation. *Blut*, **34**, 11.

83 TE VELDE J. & HAAK H.L. (1977) Aplastic anaemia. Histological investigation of methacrylate embedded bone-marrow biopsy specimens; correlation with survival after conventional treatment in 15 adult patients. *British Journal of Haematology*, **35**, 61.

84 LOHRMANN H.-P., KERN P., NIETHAMMER D. & HEIMPEL H. (1976) Indentification of high-risk patients with aplastic anaemia in selection for allogeneic bone-marrow transplantation. *Lancet*, **ii**, 647.

85 LYNCH R.E., WILLIAMS D.M., READING T.C. & CARTWRIGHT G.E. (1975) The prognosis in aplastic anemia. *Blood*, **45**, 517.

86 FRISCH B. & LEWIS S.M. (1974) The bone marrow in aplastic anaemia: diagnostic and prognostic features. *Journal of Clinical Pathology*, **27**, 231.

87 GRAY C.G. (1976) Selection for bone-marrow transplantation. *Lancet*, **ii**, 810.

88 LI F.P., ALTER B.P. & NATHAN D.G. (1972) The mortality of acquired aplastic anemia in children. *Blood*, **40**, 153.

89 BLOOM G.E. & DIAMOND L.K. (1968) Prognostic value of fetal hemoglobin levels in acquired aplastic anemia. *New England Journal of Medicine*, **278**, 304.

90 AKSOY M. & ERDEM S. (1973) Letter. *Blood*, **41**, 742.

91 NAJEAN Y., BERNARD J., WAINBERGER M., DRESCH C., BOIRON M. & SELIGMANN M. (1965) Évolution et prognostic des paucytopenies idiopathiques. Étude de 116 observations. *Nouvelle Revue française d'Hématologie*, **5**, 639.

92 MCCARTHY D.M., OSCIER D.G. & LEWIS S.M. (1980) Ferrokinetic studies and prognosis in aplastic anaemia. *Acta Haematologica*, **64**, 297.

93 VIALA J.J., BRYON P.A., CARDEL J.C., REVEL L. & CROIZAT P. (1970) Discussions du role des hepatitis virales dans le declenchment des insuffisances médullaires chroniques. *Lyon Médicine*, **223**, 1019.

94 SMITH D., GRIBBLE T.J., YEAGER A.S., GREENBERG H.B., PURCELL R.H., ROBINSON W. & SCHWARTZ H.C. (1978) Spontaneous resolution of severe aplastic anemia associated with viral hepatitis A in a six year old child. *American Journal of Hematology*, **5**, 247.

95 ROVINSKY J.J. (1959) Primary refractory anaemia complicating pregnancy and delivery: review. *Obstetrical and Gynaecological Survey*, **14**, 149.

96 FLEMING A.F. (1973) Hypoplastic anemia in pregnancy. *Clinics in Hematology*, **2**, 477.

97 TAYLOR J.J., STUDD J.W.W. & GREEN J.D. (1968) Primary refractory anaemia and pregnancy. *Journal of Obstetrics and Gynaecology of the British Commonwealth*, **75**, 963.

98 KNISPEL J.W., LYNCH V.A. & VIELE B.D. (1976) Aplastic anemia in pregnancy: a case report, review of the literature and a re-evaluation of management. *Obstetrical and Gynaecological Survey*, **31**, 523.

99 HILDEN M., LETH A. & HILDEN T. (1968) Aplastic anaemia in pregnancy remitting after abortion. *British Medical Journal*, **iii**, 166.

100 LEWIS S.M. (1969) Aplastic anaemia: problems of diagnosis and of treatment. *Journal of the Royal College of Physicians of London*, **3**, 253.

101 JEPSON J.H. & LOWENSTEIN L. (1964) Effects of prolactin on erythropoiesis in the mouse. *Blood*, **24**, 726.

102 JEPSON J.H. & LOWENSTEIN L. (1966) Erythropoiesis during pregnancy and lactation in the mouse. II. Role of erythropoietin. *Proceedings of the Society for Experimental Biology and Medicine*, **121**, 1077.

103 MCDONALD R. & MIBASHAN R.S. (1968) Prolonged remission in Fanconi-type anemia. *Helvetica Paediatrica Acta*, **23**, 565.

104 ZAIZOV R., MATOTH Y. & MAMON Z. (1978) Long-term observations in children with Fanconi's anaemia. In: *Aplastic anaemia*, p. 2. Japanese Medical Research Foundation Publication No. 4. University of Tokyo Press.

105 DENMAN A.M., HUBER H., WOOD P.H.N. & SCOTT J.T. (1965) Reticulocyte count in patients with rheumatoid arthritis, with observations on the effect of gold therapy on bone-marrow function. *Annals of the Rheumatic Diseases*, **24**, 278.

106 GOTTLIEB N.L., SMITH P.M. & SMITH E.M. (1972) Tissue gold concentration in a rheumatoid arthritic receiving chrysotherapy. *Arthritis and Rheumatism*, **15**, 16.

107 BALDWIN J.L. & STORB R. (1977) Bone-marrow transplantation in patients with gold-induced marrow aplasia. *Arthritis and Rheumatism*, **20**, 1043.

108 FEUSSNER J.R., SHELBOURNE J.D., BREDEHOEFT S. & COHEN H.J. (1979) Arsenic-induced bone-marrow toxicity: ultrastructural and electron probe analysis. *Blood*, **53**, 820.

109 DACIE J.V. (1960) *The Haemolytic Anaemias: Congential and Acquired. Part I: The Congenital Anaemias*, 2nd edn, pp. 110, 176, 263. Churchill Livingstone, London.

110 BAUMAN A.W. & SWICHER S.N. (1967) Hyporegenerative processes in hemolytic anemia. *Seminars in Hematology*, **4**, 265.

111 DACIE J.V. & LEWIS S.M. (1961) Paroxysmal nocturnal haemoglobinuria: variation in clinical severity and association with bone-marrow hypoplasia. *British Journal of Haematology*, **7**, 442.

112 SIRCHIA G. & LEWIS S.M. (1975) Paroxysmal nocturnal hemoglobinuria. *Clinics in Hematology*, **4**, 199.

113 Chanarin I. (1979) The Megaloblastic Anaemias, 2nd edn, p. 527. Blackwell Scientific Publications, Oxford.

114 Eernisse J.G. & Brand A. (1977) Postponement (or prevention?) of immunization against HLA-antigens by blood and platelet transfusions. British Journal of Haematology, 35, 674.

115 Mittal K.K., Ruder E.A. & Green D. (1976) Matching of histocompatibility (HL-A) antigens for platelet transfusion. Blood, 47, 31.

116 Gordon Smith E.C. (1979) Treatment of aplastic anaemia. I. Conservative management. In: Aplastic Anaemia (ed. Geary C.G.), p. 108. Baillière Tindall, London.

117 Clift R.A. & Buckner C.D. (1978) Supportive measures for patients with aplastic anemia. Clinics in Hematology, 7, 623.

118 Shahidi N.T. & Diamond L.K. (1959) Testosterone-induced remission in aplastic anemia. American Journal of Diseases of Children, 98, 293.

119 Sanchez-Medal L., Gomez-Leal A., Duarte L. & Guadalupe R.M. (1969) Anabolic androgens in the treatment of acquired aplastic anemia. Blood, 34, 283.

120 Daiber A., Herve L., Con J. & Donoso A. (1970) Treatment of aplastic anemia with nandrolone decanoate. Blood, 36, 748.

121 Gordon Smith E.C. & Lewis S.M. (1972) Treatment of aplastic anaemia and allied disorders with oxymetholone. Symposium on Steriods in Modern Medicine, p. 9. Excerpta Medica, Amsterdam.

122 Camitta B.M. & Thomas E.D. (1978) Severe aplastic anemia: a prospective study of the effect of androgens or transplantation on hematological recovery and survival. Clinics in Hematology, 7, 587.

123 van Hengstum M., Steenbergen J. & Yoffey J.M. (1979) Clinical course in 28 unselected patients with aplastic anaemia treated with anabolic steroids. British Journal of Haematology, 41, 323.

124 Najean Y., Pecking A. & le Danvic M. (1979) Androgen therapy of aplastic anaemia—a prospective study of 352 cases. Scandinavian Journal of Haematology, 22, 343.

125 Hirota Y. & Hibino S. (1978) Effect of andostanes on aplastic anaemia in Japan. In: Aplastic Anaemia, p. 377. Japanese Medical Research Foundation, Publication No. 4. University of Tokyo Press.

126 Johnson, F.L., Feagler J.R., Lerner K.G. Majerus P.W., Siegel M., Harmann R.R. & Thomas E.D. (1973) Association of androgenic-anabolic steroid therapy with development of hepatocellular carcinoma. Lancet, ii, 1274.

127 Bagheri S.A. & Boyer J.L. (1974) Peliosis hepatitis associated with androgenic-anabolic steroid therapy. A severe form of hepatic injury. Annals of Internal Medicine, 81, 610.

128 Delamore I.W. & Geary C.G. (1971) Aplastic anaemia, acute myeloblastic leukaemia and oxymetholone. British Medical Journal, ii, 743.

129 Besa E.C., Dale D.C., Wolff S.M. & Gardner F.H. (1977) Aetiocholanolone and prednisolone therapy in patients with severe bone-marrow failure. Lancet, i, 728.

130 Heaton L.D., Crosby W.H. & Cohen A. (1957) Splenectomy in the treatment of hypoplasia of the bone marrow. Annals of Surgery, 146, 637.

131 Scott J.L., Cartwright G.E. & Wintrobe M.M. (1959) Acquired aplastic anemia: an analysis of 39 cases and review of the pertinent literature. Medicine (Baltimore), 38, 119.

131a Koch J.L. (1967) Aplastic anemia and splenectomy. Archives of Internal Medicine, 119, 305.

132 McFarland W., Granville N., Schwartz R., Oliver H., Misra D.K. & Dameshek W. (1961) Therapy of hypoplastic anemia with bone-marrow transplantation. Archives of Internal Medicine, 108, 91.

133 Bortin M.M. (1970) A compendium of reported human bone-marrow transplants. Transplantation, 9, 571.

134 Gordon Smith E.C. (1979) Treatment of aplastic anaemia. II. Bone-marrow transplantation and the use of antilymphocyte globulin. In: Aplastic Anaemia (ed. Geary C.G.), p. 131. Baillière Tindall, London.

135 Camitta B.M., Thomas E.D., Nathan D.G., Gale R.P., Kopecky K.J., Rappaport J.M., Santos G., Gordon Smith E.C. & Storb R. (1979) A prospective study of androgens and bone-marrow transplantation for treatment of severe aplastic anemia. Blood, 53, 504.

136 UCLA Bone Marrow Transplant Team (1976) Bone-marrow transplantation in severe aplastic anaemia. Lancet, ii, 921.

137 Storb R. & Thomas E.D. (1978) Marrow transplantation for treatment of aplastic anemia. Clinics in Hematology, 7, 597.

138 Storb R., Thomas E.D., Buckner C.D., Clift R.A., Fefer A., Fernando L.P., Giblett E.R., Johnson F.L. & Neilman P.E. (1976) Allogeneic marrow grafting for treatment of aplastic anemia: a follow-up on long-term survivors. Blood, 48, 485.

139 Storb R., Thomas E.D., Weiden P.L., Buckner C.D., Clift R.A., Fefer A., Fernando L.P., Giblett E.R., Goodell, B.W., Johnson F.L., Lerner K.G., Neiman P.E. & Sanders J.E. (1976) Aplastic anemia treated by allogeneic bone-marrow transplantation: a report on 49 new cases from Seattle. Blood, 48, 817.

140 Borel J.F., Feever C., Gubler H.L. & Stahelin H. (1976) Biological effects of cyclosporin A: a new antilymphocyte agent. Agents and Actions, 6, 468.

141 Powles R.L., Clink H.M., Spence D., Morgenstern G., Watson J.G., Selby P.J., Woods, M., Baretta A., Jameson B., Sloane J., Lawler S.D., Kay H.E.M., Lawson, D., McElwain T.J. & Alexander P. (1980) Cyclosporin A to prevent graft-versus-host disease in man after allogeneic bone-marrow transplantation. Lancet, i, 327.

142 Hows, J., Harris R., Palmer S.J. & Gordon Smith E.C. (1981) Immunosuppression with Cyclosporin A in allogeneic bone-marrow transplantation for severe aplastic anaemia—preliminary studies, British Journal of Haematology, 48, 227

143 Storb B., Gluckman E., Thomas E.D., Buckner C.D., Clift R.A., Fefer A., Glucksberg H., Graham T.C., Johnson F.L., Lerner K.G., Neiman P.E. & Ochs H. (1974) Treatment of established human graft-versus-host disease by antithymocyte globulin. Blood, 44, 57.

144 Gluckman E., Devergie A., Dutreix A., Dutreix J., Boirin M. & Bernard J. (1979) Total body irradiation in bone-marrow transplantation: Hôpital Saint Louis results. Pathologie et Biologie (Paris), 27, 349.

145 Ramsay N.K.C., Trewan K., Nesbit M.E., Krivit W.,

COCCIA P.F., LEVITT S.H., WOODS W.G. & KERSEY J.H. (1980) Total lymphoid irradiation and cyclophosphamide as preparation for bone-marrow transplantation in severe aplastic anemia. *Blood*, **55**, 344.

146 WRIGHT S.E., THOMAS E.D., BUCKNER C.D., CLIFT R.A., FESSER A., NEIMAN P.E. & STORB R. (1976) Experience with second marrow transplants. *Experimental Haematology*, **4**, 221.

147 MATHE G., AMIEL J.L., SCHWARZENBERG L., CHOAY J., TROLARD P., SCHNEIDER M., HAYAT M., SCHLUMBERGER J.R., JASMIN C. (1970) A bone-marrow graft in man after conditioning by antilymphocyte serum. *British Medical Journal*, **II**, 131.

148 SPECK B., GLUCKMAN E., HAAK L. & VAN ROOD J.J. (1977) Treatment of aplastic anaemia by antilymphocyte globulin with and without allogeneic bone-marrow infusions. *Lancet*, **ii**, 1145.

149 SPECK B., GLUCKMAN E., HAAK H.L. & VAN ROOD J.J. (1978) Treatment of aplastic anemia with or without marrow infusion. *Clinics in Hematology*, **7**, 611.

150 MATHE G. & SCHWARZENBERG L. (1976) Treatment of bone-marrow aplasia by mismatched bone-marrow transplantation after conditioning with antilymphocyte globulin—long-term results. *Transplant Proceedings*, **8**, 595.

151 AMARE M., ABDOU N.L., ROBINSON M.G. & ABDOU N.I. (1978) Aplastic anemia associated with bone-marrow suppressor T-cell hyperactivity: successful treatment with antithymocyte globulin. *American Journal of Hematology*, **5**, 25.

151a PEDERSON-BJERGAARD J., ERNST J. & NISSEN N.I. (1978) Severe aplastic anaemia with complete autologous marrow reconstitution following treatment with antithymocyte globulin—report of a case and review of the literature. *Scandinavian Journal of Haematology*, **21**, 14.

152 LEWIS S.M. & DACIE J.V. (1967) The aplastic anaemia-paroxysmal nocturnal haemoglobinuria syndrome. *British Journal of Haematology*, **13**, 236.

153 LETMAN H. (1952) Possible paroxysmal nocturnal hemoglobinuria with pronounced pancytopenia, reticulocytopenia, and without hemoglobinuria simulating aplastic anemia. *Blood*, **7**, 842.

154 SCHUBOTHE H. (1958) Bone-marrow aplasia and paroxysmal nocturnal haemoglobinura following administration of resorcin and metracresol. In: *Sensitivity to Drugs: a Symposium*, p. 101. Blackwell Scientific Publications, Oxford.

155 ROSS J.D. & ROSENBAUM E. (1964) Paroxysmal nocturnal hemoglobinuria presenting as aplastic anemia in a child. Case report with evidence of deficient leukocyte acetylcholinesterase activity. *American Journal of Medicine*, **37**, 130.

156 QUAGLIANA J.M., CARTWRIGHT G.E. & WINTROBE M.M. (1964) Paroxysmal nocturnal hemoglobinura following drug-induced aplastic anemia. *Annals of Internal Medicine*, **61**, 1045.

157 DAMESHEK W. (1967) Riddle: what do aplastic anemia, paroxysmal nocturnal hemoglobinuria (PNH) and 'hypoplastic' leukemia have in common? *Blood*, **30**, 251.

158 BEAL R.W., KRONENBERG H. & FIRKIN B.G. (1964) The syndrome of paroxysmal nocturnal hemoglobinuria. *American Journal of Medicine*, **37**, 899.

159 GARDNER F.H. & BLUM S.F. (1967) Aplastic anemia in paroxysmal nocturnal hemoglobinuria. Mechanisms and therapy. *Seminars in Hematology*, **4**, 250.

160 HARTMAN R.C. & ARNOLD A.B. (1977) Paroxysmal nocturnal hemoglobinuria (PNH) as a clonal disorder. *Annual Review of Medicine*, **28**, 187.

161 LEWIS S.M. (1979) Dyserythropoiesis in aplastic anaemia. In: *Aplastic Anaemia* (ed. Geary C.G.), p. 82. Baillière Tindall, London.

162 DACIE J.V. & GILPIN A., (1944) Refractory anemia (Fanconi type): its incidence in three members of one family, with in one case a relationship to chronic haemolytic anaemia with nocturnal haemoglobinuria (Marchiafava-Micheli disease or 'nocturnal haemoglobinuria'). *Archives of Disease in Childhood*, **19**, 155.

163 LEWIS S.M. & DACIE J.V. (1965) Neutrophil (leucocyte) alkaline phosphatase in paroxysmal nocturnal haemoglobinuria. *British Journal of Haematology*, **11**, 549.

164 FRANK E. (1951) A case of aleucia hemorrhagica (idiopathic aplastic anaemia) apparently healed by repeated blood transfusions, which after three years of complete recovery turned into acute leukaemia. *Istanbul Contributions to Clinical Science*, **1**, 461.

165 DE GOWIN R.L. (1963) Benzene exposure and aplastic anemia following by leukemia 15 years later. *Journal of the American Medical Association*, **185**, 748.

166 ROZMAN C., WOESSNER S. & SAEZ-SERRANIA J. (1968) Acute erythromyelosis after benzene poisoning. *Acta Haematologica*, **40**, 234.

167 DOUGAN L. & WOODLIFF H.J. (1965) Acute leukaemia association with phenylbutazone treatment. A review of the literature and report of a further case. *Medical Journal of Australia*, **1**, 217.

168 BRAUER M.J. & DAMESHEK W. (1967) Hypoplastic anemia and myeloblastic leukemia following chloramphenicol therapy. Report of three cases. *New England Journal of Medicine*, **277**, 1003.

169 COHEN T. & CREGER W.P. (1967) Acute myeloid leukemia following seven years of aplastic anemia induced by chloramphenicol. *American Journal of Medicine*, **43**, 762.

170 SOUTTER L. & EMERSON C.P. (1960) Elective thymectomy in the treatment of aregenerative anemia associated with monocytic leukemia. *American Journal of Medicine*, **28**, 609.

171 SCHMID J.R., KIELEY J.M., PEASE G.L. & HARGRAVES M.M. (1963) Acquired pure red-cell agenesis. Report on 16 cases and review of the literature. *Acta Haematologica*, **30**, 255.

172 DOSIK H., HSU L.Y., TODARO G.J., LEE S.L., HISCHHORN K., SELIRIO E.S. & ALTER A.A. (1970) Leukemia in Fanconi's anemia: cytogenetic and tumour virus susceptibility studies. *Blood*, **36**, 341.

173 GARRIGA S. & CROSBY W.H. (1959) The incidence of leukemia in families of patients with hypoplasia of the marrow. *Blood*, **14**, 1008.

174 PRINDULL G., JENTSCH E. & HANSMANN I. (1979) Fanconi's anemia developing erythroleukaemia. *Scandinavian Journal of Haematology*, **23**, 59.

175 WASSER J.S., YOLKEN R., MILLER D.R. & DIAMOND L. (1978) Congenital hypoplastic anemia (Diamond–Blackfan syndrome) terminating in acute myelogenous leukemia. *Blood*, **51**, 991.

176 DELAMORE I.W. & GEARY C.G. (1971) Aplastic anae-

mia, acute myeloblastic leukaemia and oxymetholone. *British Medical Journal*, ii, 743.

177 GARDNER F.H. (1978) Androgen therapy for aplastic anemia. *Clinics in Hematology*, 7, 571.

178 HAAK H.L., HARTGRINK-GROENVELD C.A., EERNISSE J.G., SPECK B. & VAN ROOD J.J. (1977) Acquired aplastic anaemia in adults. I. A retrospective analysis of 40 cases: single factors influencing the prognosis. *Acta Haematologica*, 58, 257.

179 ERDOGAN G., AKSOY M. & DINCOL K. (1967) A case of idiopathic aplastic anaemia associated with trisomy-21 and partial endoreduplication. *Acta Haematologica*, 37, 137.

180 COBO A., LISKER R., SOLEDAD CORDOVA M. & PIZZUTO J. (1970) Cytogenetic findings in acquired aplastic anemia. *Acta Haematologica*, 44, 32.

181 MILNER G.R. & GEARY C.G. (1979) The aplastic-leukaemic syndrome. In: *Aplastic Anaemia* (ed. Geary C.G.), p. 230. Baillière Tindall, London.

182 SEAMAN A.J. (1969) Sequels to chloramphenicol aplastic anemia: acute leukemia and paroxysmal nocturnal hemoglobinuria. *Northwest Medicine*, 69, 831.

183 WASI P., KRUETRACHUE M. & NA-NAKORN S. (1970) Aplastic anemia-paroxysmal nocturnal hemoglobinuria syndrome—acute leukemia in the same patient. The first record of such an occurrence. *Journal of the Medical Association of Thailand*, 53, 656.

184 FRISCH B., LEWIS S.M. & SHERMAN D. (1975) The ultrastructure of dyserythropoiesis in aplastic anaemia. *British Journal of Haematology*, 29, 545.

185 MARMONT A.M. (1978) Congenital hypoplastic anaemia refractory to corticosteroids but responding to cyclophosphamide and antilymphocytic globulin. Report of a case having responded with a transitory wave of dyserythropoiesis. *Acta Haematologica*, 60, 90.

186 DAMESHEK W., BROWN S.M. & RUBIN A.D. (1967) 'Pure' red-cell anemias (erythroblastic hypoplasia) and thymoma. *Seminars in Hematology*, 4, 222.

187 HIRST E. & ROBERTSON T.I. (1967) The syndrome of thymoma and erythroblastopenic anemia. *Medicine* (Baltimore), 46, 225.

188 GEARY C.G. (1979) Red-cell aplasia. In: *Aplastic Anaemia* (ed. Geary C.G.), p. 195. Baillière Tindall, London.

189 FOY H., KONDI A. & MACDOUGALL L. (1961) Pure red-cell aplasia in marasmus and kwashiorkor treated with riboflavine. *British Medical Journal*, i, 937.

190 KANE M. & ALFREY C.P. (1965) The anemia of human riboflavin deficiency. *Blood*, 25, 432.

191 WRANNE L. (1970) Transient erythroblastopenia in infancy and childhood. *Scandinavian Journal of Haematology*, 7, 76.

192 MATRAS A. & PRIESEL A. (1928) Über einige Gewachse des Thymus. *Beiträge zur Pathologischen Anatomie*, 80, 270.

193 HAVARD C.W.H. (1965) Thymic tumours and refractory anaemia. *Series Haematologica*, 5, 18.

194 ROLAND A.S. (1964) The syndrome of benign thymoma and primary aregenerative anemia: an analysis of 43 cases. *American Journal of Medical Science*, 247, 719.

195 KRANTZ S.B. & KAO V. (1967) Studies on red-cell aplasia. I. Demonstration of a plasma inhibitor to heme synthesis and an antibody to erythroblast nuclei. *Proceedings of the National Academy of Sciences, USA*, 58, 493.

196 BJORKHOLM M., HOLM G., MELLSTEDT H., CARBERGER G. & NISELL J. (1976) Membrane bound IgG on erythroblasts in pure red-cell aplasia following thymectomy. A case report. *Scandinavian Journal of Haematology*, 17, 341.

197 SCHOOLEY J.C. & GARCIA J.F. (1962) Immunochemical studies of human urinary erythropoietin. *Proceedings of the Society for Experimental Biology and Medicine*, 109, 325.

198 JEPSON J.H. & LOWENSTEIN L. (1966) Inhibition of erythropoiesis by a factor present in the plasma of patients with erythroblastopenia. *Blood*, 27, 425.

199 PESCHLE C., MARMONT A.M., MARONE G., GENOVESE A., SASSO G.F. & CONDORELLI M. (1975) The cellular basis for the defect in haemopoiesis in flexed-tailed mice. III. Restriction of the defect to erythropoietic progenitors capable of transient colony formation *in vivo*. *British Journal of Haematology*, 30, 411.

200 KORN D., GELDERMAN A., CAGE G., NATHANSON D. & STRAUSS A.J.L. (1967) Immune deficiencies, aplastic anemia and abnormalities of lymphoid tissue in thymoma. *New England Journal of Medicine*, 276, 1333.

201 ROGERS B.H.G., MANALIGOD R.J. & BLAZEK W.V. (1968) Thymoma associated with pancytopenia and hypogammaglobulinaemia. Report of a case and review of the literature. *American Journal of Medicine*, 44, 154.

202 ROBINS-BROWNE R.M., GREEN R., KATZ J. & BECKER D. (1977) Thymoma, pure red-cell aplasia, pernicious anaemia and candidiasis: a defect in immunohomeostasis. *British Journal of Haematology*, 36, 5.

203 WOLF J.K. (1962) Primary acquired agammaglobulinaemia with a family history of collagen and hematologic disorders. *New England Journal of Medicine*, 266, 473.

204 LINSK J.A. & MURRAY C.K. (1961) Erythrocyte aplasia and hypogammaglobulinaemia. Response to steroids in a young adult. *Annals of Internal Medicine*, 55, 831.

205 ZAENTZ S.D., KRANTZ S.B. & BROWN E.B. (1976) Studies on pure red-cell aplasia. VIII. Maintenance therapy with immunosuppressive drugs. *British Journal of Haematology*, 32, 47.

206 BOTTIGER L.E. & RAUSING A. (1972) Pure red-cell anemia: immunosuppressive treatment. *Annals of Internal Medicine*, 76, 593.

207 SAFDAR S.H., KRANTZ & BROWN E.B. (1970) Successful immunosuppressive treatment of erythroid aplasia appearing after thymectomy. *British Journal of Haematology*, 19, 435.

208 FANCONI G. (1927) Familiare infantile periziosaartige Anämie (pernisiöses Blutbild und Konstitution). *Jahrbuch für Kinderheilkunde*, 117, 257.

209 DIAMOND L.K. & BLACKFAN K.E. (1938) Hypoplastic anemia. *American Journal of Diseases of Children*, 56, 464.

210 ROHR K. (1949) Familial panmyelophthisis. *Blood*, 4, 130.

211 FANCONI G. (1967) Familial constitutional panmyelocytopathy, Fanconi's anemia (FA). I. Clinical aspects *Seminars in Hematology*, 4, 233.

212 BEARD M.E.J. (1976) Fanconi anaemia. In: *Congenital Disorders of Erythropoiesis*. Ciba Foundation Symposium 37NS, p. 103. Elsevier, Amsterdam.

213 BLOOM G.E., WARNER S., GÉRALD P.S. & DIAMOND

L.K. (1966) Chromosome abnormalities in constitutional aplastic anemia. *New England Journal of Medicine*, **274,** 8.

214 SCHMID W. (1967) Familial constitutional panmyelocytopathy. Fanconi's anemia (FA). II. A discussion of the cytogenic findings in Fanconi's anemia. *Seminars in Hematology*, **4,** 241.

215 POLANI P.E. (1976) Cytogenetics of Fanconi anaemia and related chromosome disorders. In: *Congenital disorders of Erythropoiesis*. Ciba Foundation Symposium 37NS, p. 261. Elsevier, Amsterdam.

216 SWIFT M.R. & HIRSCHORN K. (1966) Fanconi's anemia. Inherited susceptibility to chromosome breakage in various tissues. *Annals of Internal Medicine*, **65,** 496.

217 SWIFT M. (1976) Fanconi anaemia: cellular abnormalities and clinical predisposition to malignant disease. In: *Congenital Disorders of Erythropoiesis*, Ciba foundation Symposium 37NS, p. 115. Elsevier, Amsterdam.

218 SWIFT M., ZIMMERMAN D. & McDONOUGH E.R. (1971) Squamous cell carcinomas in Fanconi's anemia. *Journal of the American Medical Association*, **216,** 325.

219 SHAHIDI N.T., GERALD P.S. & DIAMOND L.K. (1962) Alkali-resistant hemoglobin in aplastic anemia of both acquired and congenital types. *New England Journal of Medicine*, **266,** 117.

220 STEIER W., VAN WOOLEN G.A. & SELMANOWITZ V.J. (1972) Dyskeratosis congenita: relationship to Fanconi's anemia. *Blood*, **39,** 510.

221 HARDISTY R.M. (1976) Diamond–Blackfan anaemia. In: *Congenital Disorders of Erythropoiesis*. Ciba Foundation Symposium 37NS, p. 89. Elsevier, Amsterdam.

222 NATHAN D.G., CLARKE B.J., HILLMAN D.G., ALTER B.P. & HOUSMAN D.E. (1978) Erythroid precursors in congenital hypoplastic (Diamond–Blackfan) anemia. *Journal of Clinical Investigation*, **61,** 489.

223 SAUNDERS E.F. & FREEDMAN M.H. (1978) Constitutional aplastic anaemia: defective haemopoietic stem cell growth *in vitro*. *British Journal of Haematology*, **40,** 277.

224 NATHAN D.G., HILLMAN D.G., CHESS L., ALTER B.P., CLARKE B.J., BEARD J. & HOUSMAN D.E. (1978) Normal erythropoietic helper T cells in congenital hypoplastic (Diamond–Blackfan) anemia. *New England Journal of Medicine*, **298,** 1049.

225 ALTMAN K.I. & MILLER G. (1953) A disturbance of tryptophan metabolism in congenital hypoplastic anaemia. *Nature (London)*, **172,** 868.

226 DIAMOND L.K., WANG W.C. & ALTER B.P. (1976) Congenital hypolastic anemia. *Advances in Pediatrics*, **22,** 349.

227 DIAMOND L.K., ALLEN D.M. & MAGILL F.B. (1961) Congenital (erythroid) hypoplastic anemia. *American Journal of Diseases of Children*, **102,** 403.

228 LEWIS S.M. & VERWILGHEN R.L. (1972) Annotation: dyserythropoiesis and dyserythropoietic anaemias. *British Journal of Haematology*, **23, 1.**

229 LEWIS S.M. & VERWILGHEN R.L. (1977) Dyserythropoiesis: definition, diagnosis and assessment. In: *Dyserythropoiesis* (ed. Lewis S.M. & Verwilghen R.L.), p. 3. Academic Press, London.

230 FRISCH B. & BROECKAERT-VAN ORSHOVEN A. (1977) Ultrastructure of normal and abnormal erythropoiesis. In: *Dyserythropoiesis* (ed. Lewis S.M. & Verwilghen R.L.), p. 271. Academic Press, London.

231 LEWIS S.M. & FRISCH B. (1976) Congenital dyserythropoiesis anaemias: electron microscopy. In: *Congenital Disorders of Erythropoiesis*. Ciba Foundation Symposium 37 NS, p. 171. Elsevier, Amsterdam.

232 WORLLEDGE S.M. (1977) Red-cell antigens in dyserythropoiesis. In: *Dyserythropoiesis* (ed. Lewis S.M. & Verwilghen R.L.), p. 191. Academic Press, London.

233 BOIVIN P. (1977) Red blood cell enzyme abnormalities in dyserythropoietic anaemias. In: *Dyserythropoiesis* (ed. Lewis S.M. & Verwilghen R.L.), p. 221. Academic Press, London.

234 HEIMPEL H. & WENDT F. (1966) Congenital dyserythropoietic anaemia with karyorrhexis and multinuclearity of erythroblasts. *Helvetica Medica Acta*, **34,** 103.

235 HEIMPEL H. (1977) Congenital dyserythropoietic anemias. Type I. In: *Dyserythropoieisis* (ed. Lewis S.M. & Verwilghen R.L.), p. 55. Academic Press, London.

236 LEWIS S.M., NELSON D.A. & PITCHER C.S. (1972) Clinical and ultrastructural aspects of Congenital dyserythropoietic anaemia Type I. *British Journal of Haematology*, **23,** 113.

237 VERWILGHEN R.L., LEWIS S.M., DACIE J.V., CROOKSTON J.H. & CROOKSTON M.C. (1973) HEMPAS: Congenital dyserythropoietic anaemia (type II). *Quarterly Journal of Medicine*, **42,** 257.

238 CROOKSTON J.H., CROOKSTON M.C., BURNIE K.L., FRANCOMBE W.H., DACIE J.V., DAVIS J.A. & LEWIS S.M. (1969) Hereditary erythroblastic multinuclearity associated with a positive acidified-serum test: a type of congenital dyserythropoietic anaemia. *British Journal of Haematology*, **17,** 11.

239 PUNT K., BORST-EILERS E. & NIJESSEN J.G. (1977) Congenital dyserythropoietic anaemia Type II (HEMPAS). In: *Dyserythropoiesis* (ed. Lewis S.M. & Verwilghen R.L.), p. 71. Academic Press, London.

240 VERWILGHEN R.L. (1976) Congenital dyserythropoietic anaemia type II (HEMPAS). In: *Congenital Disorders of Erythropoiesis*. Ciba Foundation Symposium 37NS, p. 151. Elsevier, Amsterdam.

241 RICCI P., BACCARANI M., BIAGINI G., PREDA P., TOMASINI I., ZUCCHELLI P. & TURA S. (1979) Congenital dyserythropoietic anemia Type II: serological and morphological family study. *Nouvelle Revue française d'Hematologie*, **21,** 197.

242 SEIP M., SKREDE S., BJERVE K.S., HOVIC T. & GAARDER P.I. (1975) Congenital dyserythropoietic anaemia with features of both type I and II. *Scandinavian Journal of Haematology*, **15,** 272.

243 DAVID G. (1977) The contribution of cytogenetics in the classification of acquired idiopathic dysmyelopoiesis. In *Dyserythropoiesis* (ed. Lewis S.M. & Verwilghen R.L.), p. 183. Academic Press, London.

244 LOWENTHAL R.M., MARSDEN K.A., DEWAR C.L. & THOMPSON G.R. (1980) Congenital dyserythropoietic anaemia with severe gout, rare Kell phenotype and erythrocyte, granulocyte and platelet membrane reduplication: a new variant of CDA type II. *British Journal of Haematology*, **44,** 211.

245 SANSONE G. (1978) A new type of congenital dyserythropoietic anaemia. *British Journal of Haematology*, **39,** 537.

246 WEATHERALL D.J., CLEGG J.B., KNOX-MACAULEY H.H.M., BUNCH C., HOPKINS R. & TEMPERLEY I.J. (1973) A genetically determined disorder with features both of thalassaemia and congenital dyserythropoietic anaemia. *British Journal of Haematology*, **24**, 681.

247 SCHUPPLER J., CORNU P., KREY G., GUDAT F. & SPECK B. (1976) Congenital dyserythropoietic anaemia with ultrastructural features of Type I and Type II. *Blut*, **31**, 271.

248 WOLFF J.A. & VON HOFE F.H. (1951) Familial erythroid multinuclearity. *Blood*, **6**, 1274.

249 GOUDSMITH R. (1977) Congenital dyserythropoietic anaemia, Type III. In: *Dyserythropoiesis* (ed. Lewis S.M. & Verwilghen R.L.), p. 83. Academic Press, London.

250 BJÖRKSTEN B., HOLMGREN G., ROOS G. & STENLING R. (1978) Congenital dyserythropoietic anaemia type III: an electron microscope study. *British Journal of Haematology*, **38**, 37.

251 WICKRAMASINGHE S.N. & GOUDSMITH R. (1979) Some aspects of the biology of multinucleate and giant mononucleate erythroblasts in a patient with CDA, type III. *British Journal of Haematology*, **41**, 485.

252 TEBBI K. & GROSS S. (1978) Absence of morphological abnormalities in marrow erythrocyte colonies (CFU-E) from a patient with HEMPAS-II. *Journal of Laboratory and Clinical Medicine*, **91**, 797.

253 VAINCHENKER W., GUICHARD J. & BRETON-GORIUS J. (1979) Morphological abnormalities in cultured erythroid colonies (CFU-E) from the blood of two patients with HEMPAS. *British Journal of Haematology*, **42**, 363.

254 JACOBS H.S. (1977) Erythroid cell membrane abnormalities in HEMPAS. In: *Dyserythropoiesis* (ed. Lewis S.M. & Verwilghen R.L.), p. 209. Academic Press, London.

255 GERMAN J.P., DUROCHER J.R. & CONRAD M.E. (1975) The abnormal surface characteristics of the red blood cell membranes in congenital dyserythropoietic anaemia type II (HEMPAS). *British Journal of Haematology*, **30**, 383.

256 QUEISSER W., SPIERTZ E., JOSTE E. & HEIMPEL H. (1971) Proliferation disturbances of erythroblasts in dyserythropoietic anemia types I and II. *Acta Haematologica*, **45**, 65.

257 FRISCH B. (1977) Ultrastructural aspects of pathogenetic mechanisms in dyserythropoiesis. In: *Dyserythropoiesis* (ed. Lewis S.M. & Verwilghen R.L.), p. 339. Academic Press, London.

258 DREYFUS B., ROCHANT H. & SULTAN C. (1969) Anémies réfractaires: enzymopathies acquises de cellules souches hematopoiétiques. *Nouvelle Revue française d'Hématologie*, **9**, 65.

259 DUHAMEL G., MURATORE R. & BYRON P. (1976) Anémies réfractaire avec myéloblastose partielle. Analyse d'un protocol, portant sur 77 cas. II. Résultats de l'examen des biopsies médullaire. *Nouvelle Revue française d'Hématologie*, **16**, 81.

260 DREYFUS B., SULTAN C., ROCHANT H., SALMON C.H., MANNONI P., CARTRON J.P., BOIVIN P. & GALAND C. (1969) Anomalies of blood group antigens and erythrocyte enzymes in two types of chronic refractory anaemia. *British Journal of Haematology*, **16**, 303.

261 NAJEAN Y., PECKING A. & BROQUET M. (1976) Anémies réfractaires avec myéloblastose partielle. Analyse d'un protocol, groupant 79 cas. I. Caractères cliniques et evolution sous androgénothérapies. *Nouvelle Revue française d'Hématologie*, **16**, 67.

262 RICCI P., BACCARANI M., ZACCARIA A., SANTUCCI M.A. & TURA S. (1968) Clinical contribution to the knowledge of hemopoietic dysplasias: long-term follow-up of 13 patients with refractory anaemia. *Acta Haematologica*, **60**, 10.

263 SULTAN C., IMBERT M., RICARD M.F. & MARQUET M. (1977) Myelodysplastic syndromes. In: *Dyserythropoiesis* (ed. Lewis S.M. & Verwilghen R.L.), p. 171. Academic Press, London.

264 MILNER G.R., TESTA N.G., GEARY C.G., DEXTER T.M., MULDAL S., MACIVER J.E. & LAJTHA L.G. (1977) Bone-marrow culture studies in refractory cytopenia and 'smouldering leukaemia'. *British Journal of Haematology*, **35**, 251.

265 FAILLE A., DRESCH C., POIRIER O., BALITRANS & NAJEAN Y. (1978) Prognostic value of *in vitro* bone marrow culture in refractory anaemias with excess of myeloblasts. *Scandinavian Journal of Haematology*, **20**, 280.

266 KAGAN W.A., FIALK M.A., COLEMAN M., ASCENSO J.L., VALERA E. & GOOD R.A. (1980) Studies on the pathogenesis of refractory anemia. *American Journal of Medicine*, **68**, 381.

267 NAJEAN Y. & PECKING A. (1977) Refractory anaemia with excess of myeloblasts in the bone marrow: a clinical trial of androgens in 90 patients. *British Journal of Haematology*, **37**, 25.

268 GORDON SMITH E.C. (1972) Bone-marrow failure: diagnosis and treatment. *British Journal of Haematology*, **23** (Suppl.), 167.

Chapter 32
The myeloproliferative disorders

G. WETHERLEY-MEIN AND T. C. PEARSON

The term 'myeloproliferative disorder' requires some definition. Originally it was coined to crystallize the concept that such conditions as the lymphomas, the leukaemias, primary polycythaemia and myelofibrosis were all related disease processes [1]. The basis of this idea was that such disorders had a common histogenesis from a cell system with a wide anatomical distribution, which retained the capacity for multipotential differentiation of the primitive mesenchymal cell, and that they were expressions of abnormal proliferation of this population [2–8]. This comprehensive and unifying concept was of considerable value in that it simplified an increasingly confused nomenclature, explained observed transitions from one condition to another, made it unnecessary to be surprised by atypical anatomical and morphological presentations [9] and had, as an additional attraction, a ring of truth about it. The concept still has some value and merit providing it is clearly recognized that this is a histogenetic classification which does not imply common aetiology [10]. However, although the term is still perfectly reasonably used in its original comprehensive sense, the lymphomas, and particularly the leukaemias, have become more clearly defined by their various cytogenetic, histochemical, biochemical, immunological, cultural and clinical characteristics. There is, therefore, an increasing tendency to define the myeloproliferative disorders as primary polycythaemia, myelofibrosis, thrombocythaemia and a miscellaneous group of evidently proliferative conditions which are sufficiently atypical to defy more precise classification. It is in this more restricted sense that the myeloproliferative disorders are considered here.

THE POLYCYTHAEMIAS

Although the main objective here is to consider primary proliferative polycythaemia ('polycythaemia rubra vera'), a number of conditions have in common the finding of an abnormally high packed cell volume. These disorders fall into two main groups, the true polycythaemias and the apparent polycythaemias. In the true polycythaemias there is an absolute increase in the red-cell mass above normal; included in this group are primary proliferative polycythaemia, the secondary polycythaemias and a number of conditions classified as 'idiopathic erythrocytosis' (p. 1278). In the apparent polycythaemias the red-cell mass is in the normal range and the raised packed cell volume is due either to an abnormal reduction in plasma volume or to the combination of a high normal red-cell mass and a low normal plasma volume. The interpretation of red-cell mass and plasma volume data in the differential diagnosis of these groups is considered later (p. 1288).

On this basis the general classification of the polycythaemias suggested in Table 32.1 emphasizes that there are several forms of true polycythaemia and implies that, in spite of common usage, the term polycythaemia vera should not be used to describe the primary form of polycythaemia which is generally regarded as one of the myeloproliferative disorders.

The role of erythropoietin, in the various forms of polycythaemia, is discussed in more detail elsewhere (pp. 1275, 1282, 1283) but as indicated in Tables 32.1 and 32.3, there are, in terms of erythropoietin, two major groupings. In primary proliferative polycythaemia, plasma erythropoietin levels are normal or reduced and the increase in red-cell mass is independent of erythropoietin. In the secondary true polycythaemias the increase is, in the majority of instances, determined by an increased production of erythropoietin which may be due either to activation of the normal physiological mechanism or to inappropriate synthesis of the hormone.

THE TRUE POLYCYTHAEMIAS

Primary proliferative polycythaemia

Pathogenesis
The aetiology of the myeloproliferative disorders as a group, in terms of their nature and causation, is considered elsewhere (p. 1305). There has been recent

Table 32.1. General classification of the polycythaemias

The polycythaemias	
True polycythaemias	*Apparent polycythaemias*
Primary proliferative*	Relative*
Secondary	Overt fluid loss
Hypoxic†	Idiopathic
Inappropriate	High normal red-cell mass‡
erythropoietin induced	Physiological variant‡
Hypertransfusion*	
Idiopathic erythrocytosis‡	

* Not erythropoietin-mediated.
† Erythropoietin-mediated—activated physiological mechanism.
‡ Role of erythropoietin uncertain—probably heterogeneous groups.

clarification of the nature of primary polycythaemia. It has long been thought, on the basis of clinical, haematological and chromosome findings (p. 1274), that this condition, often loosely called polycythaemia rubra vera, is a primary proliferative process comparable to such conditions as chronic myeloid leukaemia. Only now has acceptable support for this assumption emerged. Elegant studies on G6PD variants in females with primary polycythaemia have indicated that there is a mutant red-cell clone present [11–13]. These views have been confirmed by marrow culture studies which have demonstrated that in primary polycythaemia there are two populations of erythroid progenitors. Essentially, one population behaves normally in that it is erythropoietin-dependent, whereas the second population has colony-forming capacity even in the absence of erythropoietin. This second population is therefore likely to represent an autonomous mutant clone [14–16]. Quite separate studies on the distribution of Hb F in primary polycythaemia also support this concept [17, 18]. This condition can now, therefore, be justifiably called primary proliferative polycythaemia (PPP).

Presentation

There are two main groups. In the first the patient complains of symptoms which are the result of the disease itself and, in the second, the incidental finding of, for example, plethora, a high packed cell volume or splenomegaly during the investigation of an unrelated disease process, indicates that the patient may also have an apparently symptomless polycythaemia. Occasional cases are reported in the third and fourth decades, but the average age of onset is between 40 and 60 years [8, 19–21] and most cases are diagnosed in the fifth decade [20]. Polycythaemia in the young is uncommon in the absence of cardiac or pulmonary cyanotic disease. Neonatal polycythaemia, defined as a packed cell volume of 0·70 or more during the first month of life, is usually explicable in terms of maternal–fetal or twin-to-twin transfusion [22, 23], and is obviously secondary. In childhood occasional, sometimes familial, cases described as primary erythrocytosis or benign familial polycythaemia have been reported [24–26]. Although the condition is well authenticated there is, in spite of the occasional finding of splenomegaly and chromosomal abnormalities, little to suggest that it is comparable to the primary polycythaemia of adults. These uncommon forms of sometimes familial polycythaemia, which also present in adult life, need further definition in terms of haemoglobinopathy, erythropoietin measurement, chromosome analysis and marrow culture studies. Some aspects of this probably heterogeneous group are discussed elsewhere (pp. 1282 and 1283).

The range of presenting symptoms directly determined by PPP is indicated in Table 32.2. The frequency of these and other symptoms has been reported by a number of authors [19–21, 27]. There are wide differences in the reported frequency of symptoms in these reports and this is probably due to variations in interpretation of the relevance of particular symptoms. It is nevertheless clear that all reports emphasize the overriding importance of vascular lesions.

Vascular lesions

Major vascular lesions. In PPP these are the most serious complications. Occlusive cerebral lesions may produce effects ranging from transient ischaemic attacks to irreversible stroke and death [28]. Episodes of arterial occlusion, of deep vein thrombosis and of

Table 32.2. Symptoms at presentation in primary proliferative polycythaemia

Symptom	Approximate incidence	Possible mechanisms
Headache Dizziness Cerebro-vascular lesions Peripheral vascular lesions Visual defect Myocardial infarction Other occlusive vascular lesions	+ + + +	Viscosity Platelet defect
Pruritus	+ +	? Histamine effect
Bleeding	+	Platelet defect
Gout	+	Abnormal urate production
Splenic pain	+	Enlargement Infarct
Dyspepsia and peptic ulcer	+	? Coincidental ? Histamine effect
Incidental diagnosis	+ +	—

superficial thrombophlebitis are also common and arterial and venous episodes occur with equal frequency [29]. Less commonly, visceral thrombosis involving, for example, mesenteric vessels occurs and, particularly in patients with splenomegaly, splenic vein thrombosis may lead to portal hypertension with bleeding from oesophageal varices [30]. Less serious, but probably more frequent in communities where diagnosis is early, is the complaint of fullness in the head, dizziness, headache and true migraine. Loss of concentration and intellectual impairment are not uncommon, but are often only recognized retrospectively by the patient after treatment has produced improvement. Psychometric studies before and after venesection have provided objective evidence of this improvement [31].

Peripheral vascular symptoms—commonly of an erythromelalgic type with reddening of feet and burning sensations particularly when warmed—occur without evidence of arterial insufficiency and may be associated with small local ischaemic lesions, usually in the toes [29, 32]. In patients, particularly the elderly, with existing arterial insufficiency, polycythaemia may enhance the ischaemic effects. When there is an association of polycythaemia and thrombocythaemia, the latter may itself be more responsible for vascular and haemostatic abnormalities than the former [33]. The role of platelets and other factors in the pathogenesis of vascular lesions is discussed elsewhere (pp. 1285 and 1286).

Other vascular lesions. There are often changes in the retina, with tortuous distended retinal veins [34] and

even papilloedema [28], and occasionally venous thrombosis with severe visual loss may occur. Quantitative studies indicate that the retinal vascular dilatation is due primarily to increase in blood viscosity rather than to increase in blood volume [34]. Radiological increase in pulmonary vascular shadowing is not uncommon but symptoms are probably not produced by polycythaemia unless there is local thrombosis or embolism. Hypertension, when it occurs, is generally regarded as incidental. Increased liability to myocardial infarction is to be expected in a disease process in which one of the main causes of morbidity is vascular occlusion [35, 36]. However, the incidence of stroke as compared to myocardial infarction appears to be considerably greater in PPP than in the normal population [21, 29]; the mechanism is not established. It may reflect difference in age incidences of uncomplicated myocardial infarction, polycythaemia and stroke or may be related to some physiological difference in the characteristics of cerebral and coronary blood flow.

Abnormal bleeding. This is an important, but relatively uncommon, presenting symptom which is more usually post-traumatic than spontaneous. It can usually be attributed to the defective function of thrombocythaemic platelets (p. 1291) but coagulation abnormalities have also been reported (p. 1273).

Pathogenesis of vascular lesions. It is likely that there are multiple factors, including blood viscosity, blood flow and platelet abnormalities, which contribute to the development of the vascular lesions. This is discussed elsewhere (p. 1285).

Skin changes

Those associated with peripheral vascular lesions are common but a number of other dermatological lesions have been observed in polycythaemia. Probably the most common is itching; a considerable proportion of patients complain of this, and in a number it is the major presenting symptom. Characteristically, it is intermittent, induced or enhanced by warmth, and has a distribution affecting limbs and back. The pathogenesis is not established and although it may improve when the polycythaemia is treated, it usually persists or recurs in spite of a maintained normal packed cell volume. High leucocyte and blood histamine levels have been reported in PPP and there is a good correlation between histamine level and basophil count [37]; it has been suggested that there is also a good correlation between these and the incidence of pruritus [38, 39]. However, increased histamine levels have also been found in patients with chronic myeloid and acute leukaemia [40, 41], in which pruritus does not seem to occur. Other studies, although confirming that there are increases in basophils and in histamine turnover in PPP, do not support the view that there is a direct causative relationship between histamine and pruritus [41, 42]. The pathogenesis of pruritus in PPP is, therefore, not yet clearly understood.

Increased urate production

This produces symptoms in about 10% of patients during the course of the disease [8, 27] and is more common in PPP than in chronic myeloid leukaemia, the acute leukaemias or the secondary polycythaemias. Most commonly the symptoms are those of acute gout, although occasionally gouty tophi, sometimes numerous and widespread, is the only manifestation. In a few patients dysuria or renal colic due to passage of urate crystals or calculi may prompt extensive urinary-tract investigations if the possibility of polycythaemia is not considered.

Peptic ulceration

This is traditionally considered to have a higher incidence in PPP than in the normal population and although dyspepsia may occasionally be the presenting symptom it is more commonly an incidental complaint [8, 20, 43]. It has been suggested that like pruritus this can also be related to increased histamine production [38, 39]. A more recent analysis, however, suggests that the incidence of peptic ulcer in PPP may be no greater than in a comparable non-polycythaemic population [101].

Clinical findings

Plethora. This is the most obvious clinical finding in all forms of polycythaemia, with conjunctival injection and reddening of hands and feet but not usually of covered skin surfaces. It may be absent, certainly its presence is not diagnostic, and it is more likely to be due to the vasodilation associated with increased blood volume than to mere increase in haemoglobin level.

Splenomegaly. This is the most useful and significant clinical finding in PPP but in a number of patients who have, or develop, unequivocal PPP the spleen may be impalpable on presentation and in a few may remain so throughout the course of the disease. The disease in some of these patients without splenomegaly, particularly if it is associated with normal leucocyte and platelet counts, may be so benign that it is considered by some observers to be a separate entity—'benign polycythaemia' [44] or 'benign erythrocytosis' [45]. The nature of this group of patients is considered in greater detail under the heading of 'idiopathic erythrocytosis' (p. 1278). In about 60% of patients, however, modest or considerable splenomegaly is present when they are first seen [20, 27, 46] and slowly increases, usually over a period of years, so that in the later phases of the disease the symptoms and effects of splenomegaly may be dominant. It is in patients with progressive splenomegaly that transition to myelofibrosis most frequently occurs [46].

Other clinical findings are those which might be expected in association with the various, mainly vascular, clinical presentations which have already been considered.

Laboratory findings

Haemoglobin level, PCV and red-cell count. By definition all forms of polycythaemia should be, and normally are, characterized by abnormal elevation of these values in venous or capillary samples. The PCV is, however, an unreliable index of the degree of true polycythaemia for there is not a proportional rise in PCV as the red-cell mass increases above normal [47, 48] and polycythaemic patients occasionally present with a normal or reduced PCV either because there is gross splenomegaly, with raised plasma volume and splenic red-cell pooling, or because of recent haemorrhage or iron deficiency. Except in some patients who are iron-deficient, usually as the result of treatment by repeated venesection, red-cell morphology, absolute red-cell values and corrected reticulocyte count are normal. The recent evidence (pp. 1270 and 1305) that in PPP there is, in the peripheral circulation, a heterogeneous population of cells derived from the original normal cell line and from an abnormal proliferative red-cell line is not reflected by any abnormalities of red-cell morphology. Several intrinsic red-cell metabolic abnormalities, usually in relation to red-cell enzymes, have been observed [49–52]. At present the majority of these findings make no cohesive contribution to the understanding of any fundamental abnormality of red-cell metabolism in PPP. Some studies on red-cell phosphofructokinase (PFK) and aldolase are of interest. First, the evidence that PFK is a mutant enzyme fits with the concept of a mutant red-cell clone in PPP and secondly, changes in PFK and aldolase appear to occur when there is transition of PPP to acute leukaemia [53, 54]. Further studies in this area are necessary.

Actual red-cell mass. This is increased, since this a true polycythaemia. Indications and methods for measuring it and the relationship between red-cell mass and splenomegaly are considered later (pp. 1288, 1289 and Table 32.4).

Leucocyte count. This is characteristically raised in PPP. Although a number of patients have normal counts the majority have a modest granulocytosis ($12–30 \times 10^9$/l). The predominant cells are segmented neutrophils, in which the lysozyme content is normal [55], with small numbers of immature granulocytes. This finding is often taken to indicate that there is co-existent polycythaemia and chronic granulocytic leukaemia, and the association in the occasional patient of raised packed cell volume, considerable splenomegaly and exceptionally high leucocyte count ($>40 \times 10^9$/l) encourages this view. However, the resemblance is superficial, and does no more than reinforce the concept that red cells, granulocytes and platelets have some commonality of stem-cell origin. In PPP the leucocyte alkaline phosphatase (LAP) score is sometimes normal (e.g. 16–90), particularly in the early stages of the disease, but in the majority of patients it is raised (e.g. 100–350), while in chronic granulocytic leukaemia (CGL) the LAP is invariably below normal (e.g. 0–5), except when there is incidental acute infection or transition to acute leukaemia or myelofibrosis (pp. 1275 and 1276). Again, the chromosome findings distinguish the two conditions: in classical CGL the Philadelphia (Ph^1) chromosome is invariably present, while in PPP it has never been found, except in one patient [56] who probably had a true CGL with the transient elevation of packed cell volume which occasionally occurs during the course of the disease, and in three ^{32}P-treated patients with polycythaemia in whom a Ph^1-like chromosome was found in phytohaemagglutinin-stimulated peripheral-blood cultures [57]. This distinction between the granulocytosis of PPP and CGL is of considerable practical importance, for in CGL the granulocyte proliferation is invariably progressive and is associated with anaemia and clinical deterioration, and treatment is mandatory. In contrast, reduction of the granulocytosis of PPP is not a primary objective of treatment except, perhaps, in patients in whom it is associated with unacceptably high urate production or pruritus. The granulocytosis of PPP is also distinct from that found in the so-called Ph^1-negative CGL (see Chapter 23). Although the chromosome and LAP findings in this condition may resemble those in PPP, it is characterized by anaemia, often thrombocytopenia and a poor prognosis with progressive clinical and haematological deterioration which is not modified by busulphan therapy [58, 59].

Platelet count. In PPP this may often be normal but is characteristically raised ($400–2000 \times 10^9$/l) and associated with abnormalities of morphology and function. The morphological abnormalities consist of variation in size and shape of platelets with, most characteristically, the presence of large and bizarre forms. These abnormalities, which may be associated with haemorrhage or microvascular lesions, are identical with those which may also be found in myelofibrosis and thrombocythaemia. They emphasize the close association between these conditions and are considered in greater detail later (pp. 1286 and 1291).

Coagulation studies
In PPP these have included observations on fibrinogen, fibrinolytic activity, factors V, VII, VIII, X and XII. These results have shown multiple, usually minor and sometimes contradictory anomalies [60–64]. These defects, some of which may also be found in hypoxic polycythaemia [65], may contribute to the high incidence of spontaneous and post-traumatic bleeding but there has been no observed correlation between the coagulation abnormalities and either occlusive vascular lesions or abnormal bleeding.

In PPP the major factor in the causation of haemorrhagic complications is almost certainly the defective platelet function (p. 1291). The pathogenesis of occlusive vascular lesions is discussed elsewhere (p. 1285).

Bone marrow
The findings, particularly in histological preparations, tend to correlate well with the peripheral-blood findings in the individual patient. In the untreated patient, films from aspirates are sometimes misleadingly normal [66] but are usually cellular and easily withdrawn;

in patients without associated granulocytosis or thrombocythaemia, there is normoblastic hyperplasia, the cellularity correlating well with the packed cell volume [67]. In some untreated patients, and in all those treated predominantly by repeated venesection, the normoblasts may have the ragged cytoplasm of iron deficiency and there may be no free stainable iron or sideroblasts seen. In patients with raised peripheral-granulocyte counts, the proportion of morphologi-cally normal marrow granulocyte precursors is in-creased; similarly, thrombocythaemia is associated with an often striking increase in megakaryocytes, which show a wide range of nuclear morphology. In all patients who are effectively treated by chemotherapy or ^{32}P, the marrow changes become less defined and apart from evidence of iron deficiency the aspirate may appear normal [67]. Transition to myelofibrosis, acute leukaemia or treatment-induced acellular marrow failure produces alterations in the characteristics of the aspirate which are described later. Histological sec-tions of marrow obtained by trephine biopsy, which have a more consistent abnormality than aspirates, show reduction of fat spaces and the increased cellular-ity and cell-type distribution already described. In addition there is the increased density of reticulin fibrils, with the retention of normal pattern, which is found in many hypercellular marrows [68]. Some increase in coarse reticulin fibrils is often found but this does not necessarily presage transition to myelofi-brosis [69]. These histological findings have been confirmed in a comprehensive review in which a quantitative analysis of the observed abnormalities was made [70].

Chromosome abnormalities

There is now a considerable number of observations on marrow chromosomes in PPP. There is, particularly in irradiated patients, a significant increase in certain anomalies such as partial F deletion, C-group anom-alies and the emergence of aneuploid lines, and these findings have considerable interest in terms of the aetiology and evolution of the disease [71–74]. How-ever, in many patients with unequivocal primary polycythaemia, particularly if they have not been treated with chemotherapy or irradiation [75, 76] no chromosome abnormality is found, and in those with anomalies there is not sufficient consistency, either within patients or between patients, for this investiga-tion to have, as yet, the diagnostic or prognostic value which it has in CGL [76–78]. The matter has been well reviewed by Lawler [79].

Metabolic abnormalities

These have been observed in PPP. Clinically the most important of them is increased uric-acid production.

At some stage in the disease 70% of patients show increased plasma urate levels [80] and increased urinary urate excretion. This reflects an increased nucleic-acid synthesis and breakdown with metabolic pathways which are different from those in primary gout [81]. Since the plasma level is a function of both urate production and excretion it is not, by itself, a reliable index of the activity of the polycythaemic process but considerable increase may occur in the early stages of treatment and in patients who develop high granulocyte counts. Some patients, particularly those with progressive splenomegaly and increasing granulocytosis, develop considerable elevation of basal metabolic rate [27]. This finding, often associated with raised creatine values, is similar to that observed in many patients with proliferative disorders such as CGL [82, 83].

Iron metabolism

The changes are those which might be anticipated where there is increased red-cell production, often with some associated iron deficiency. Reduced serum iron with raised iron-binding capacity is almost invariably found in venesected patients and is surprisingly com-mon even before treatment. ^{59}Fe studies show in-creased plasma clearance rates and increased plasma and red-cell iron turnover [84]; ^{59}Fe utilization is usually above normal and there is nothing, certainly in the early phases of the disease, to suggest ineffective erythropoiesis. The ^{59}Fe surface pattern, based on changes of radioactivity in blood, sacrum, spleen and liver, is essentially normal, and it is only when there is increasing splenomegaly with transition to myelofi-brosis that it shows evidence of extramedullary splenic erythropoiesis and this is confirmed by quantitative ^{52}Fe scanning [85]. Regional scanning shows extension of erythropoiesis to the distal long bones with patterns of distribution varying according to the stage of the disease [86, 87].

^{51}Cr studies

These show a normal red-cell lifespan [84], indicating that the increased red-cell mass is a function of increased production rather than excessive accumu-lation, and this is supported, not only by the ^{59}Fe data, but by studies of haem synthesis [88] and of erythro-blast DNA synthesis [89]. As the disease progresses there may be shortening of red-cell and platelet life-span; while it has been suggested that this may be due to the evolution of clones which retain increased capacity for proliferation but produce cells which have decreased capacity for survival [84], in patients with splenomegaly it is more readily explained by the haemolytic effect which any enlarged spleen may have on normal red cells (see Chapter 20).

Vitamin B₁₂ and folic acid

Pernicious anaemia has been reported in established PPP [90] and although, conversely, a few patients with unequivocal pernicious anaemia have developed PPP following treatment, the association of these two conditions is almost certainly fortuitous [91]; serum vitamin-B_{12} levels in PPP are either normal or show the abnormal elevation often found in other myeloproliferative disorders. This is the result of abnormal and high plasma B_{12}-binding capacity [92, 93]; since there is evidence that B_{12}-binding protein is produced by intact granulocytes it has been suggested [94], although there are reservations [95], that it could be a useful measure of the total granulocyte mass in myeloproliferative disorders. A study of transcobalamins I, II and III in primary polycythaemia showed that changes, particularly in transcobalamin III, appeared to be associated with changes in the disease process, response to treatment and, possibly, with transition to an acute leukaemic phase [96]. As in many other proliferative conditions, such as the leukaemias, laboratory investigation may establish that there is folate deficiency, but in PPP this is only occasionally of practical significance.

Erythropoietin

The diagnostic value of erythropoietin assay in the polycythaemias is considered later (p. 1289). In PPP, assays of plasma and urinary erythropoietin activity show that it is either decreased or normal, and there is additional evidence that the erythropoietin mechanism itself is intrinsically normal [97]. Clinical and experimental evidence, including study of erythropoietic colony-forming units (CFU-E), indicates that both normal and PPP stem cells are responsive to erythropoietin stimulation. However, CFU-E are developed by normal marrow only in the presence of erythropoietin while CFU-E may be derived from PPP marrow in the absence of erythropoietin [14–16, 389]. The significance of these findings in terms of aetiology and treatment is considered elsewhere (pp. 1269 and 1277).

Diagnosis of primary proliferative polycythaemia

The course and treatment of the various types of polycythaemia is so different that no patient should be regarded as having PPP unless the diagnosis is unequivocally established. In many patients, with or without symptoms, the association of an unequivocally high packed cell volume with splenomegaly, granulocytosis, a high platelet count and characteristic marrow findings virtually establishes the diagnosis of PPP. In the individual patient the demonstration of various combinations of these and other abnormalities, such as raised red-cell mass, a high serum B_{12} level and high leucocyte-alkaline-phosphatase score, has been regarded as requisite for the diagnosis [98], particularly in relation to therapeutic trials [99]. Even with these findings the diagnosis should not be accepted without further investigations which exclude other forms of polycythaemia. In many patients, however, the findings are less clear cut: in some, the combination of abnormal leucocyte and platelet counts with considerable splenomegaly and a normal or even reduced packed cell volume, may be more suggestive of chronic granulocytic leukaemia, myelofibrosis or one of the many alternative causes of splenomegaly; more commonly, the isolated finding of only a raised packed cell volume establishes that the patient has some form of polycythaemia and further investigations, which differentiate the various types of polycythaemia, are necessary. The differential diagnosis of the polycythaemias is discussed later (p. 1288).

Course and prognosis

The rate of rise of the packed cell volume following simple venesection indicates that, in most patients, PPP is a relatively slow proliferative process which has probably been present for several years before the diagnosis is made. In the untreated or inadequately treated patient there is a considerable morbidity, predominantly from vascular occlusive lesions, with, in one untreated series, a mortality of about 50% within 18 months of diagnosis [21]. With effective treatment there is a very considerable reduction in mortality from vascular causes in the early years of the disease and the median survival improves to 10–14 years from diagnosis. However, even in reported series of apparently effectively treated patients with this improved median survival, cerebral and myocardial vascular lesions appear to be the cause of death in 30–60% of cases [35, 36, 46, 100]. It is not clear whether this is the natural sequel of extension of life into a susceptible age group or whether polycythaemia is a factor. The pathogenesis and prevention of these vascular complications is discussed elsewhere (p. 1278).

With effective treatment, two main patterns of disease emerge. The first is that of a simple polycythaemia, often without splenomegaly, granulocytosis or thrombocythaemia, which over many years may require no more than intermittent treatment to maintain the packed cell volume at an acceptable level. These patients with increased red-cell mass alone appear to correspond to the group defined by Modan [45, 102] as 'benign erythrocytosis', but it now seems likely that it is heterogeneous. The majority of such patients develop some combination of splenomegaly, thrombocythaemia, granulocytosis and elevation of leucocyte alkaline phosphatase which justifies their reclassification as PPP [103]. In others no such changes occur over periods of nine or 10 years and their nature is obscure. It is for this reason that 'idiopathic erythrocytosis' seems an appropriate initial diagnosis in these patients (p. 1278).

The second pattern is characterized by ultimate transformation to myelofibrosis—an intermediate and sometimes prolonged state has been described as 'transitional myeloproliferative disorder' [104]—to acute leukaemia and very rarely to erythroleukaemia [105], and the subsequent course is that of these conditions. The incidence of these complications is greater in patients presenting with splenomegaly or leucocytosis and in those who are treated with ^{32}P, but these two factors seem to operate independently of each other [106]. The transition to myelofibrosis, which occurs in 10–20% of patients [1, 106, 107], is usually gradual, and generally associated with progressive splenomegaly, anaemia and thrombocytopenia; the leucocyte count may be low, normal or high, with increase in circulating granulocyte precursors. At this stage the findings may suggest that transition to classical chronic granulocytic leukaemia has occurred, but the high leucocyte alkaline phosphatase, absence of the Ph[1] chromosome and indifferent response to busulphan or splenic irradiation establish that this is a

different condition, while the diagnosis of myelofibrosis is established by marrow aspiration ('dry tap') and biopsy. Transition to acute leukaemia is usually more abrupt, with rapidly progressive anaemia and thrombocytopenia and increasing numbers of blast cells in peripheral blood and marrow. Morphologically these are primitive white cells, and PPP only rarely transforms to erythroleukaemia. Previous treatment with ^{32}P undoubtedly increases the incidence of acute leukaemic transition [100, 106, 108]. This transition does, however, occur in non-irradiated patients [109]. While this suggests that acute leukaemia can also develop as part of the natural history of PPP, this question is not easily resolved since many non-irradiated patients are treated with alkylating agents [78] which may themselves be capable of inducing the mutation* which is presumably the mechanism of transition (Fig. 32.1). There is no clear association between previous therapy and the development of myelofibrosis [46] however, and this is most probably part of the natural history of primary polycythaemia. Chromosome studies show that some patients with primary polycythaemia develop abnormal cell lines and there is some evidence that this may be related to subsequent development of acute leukaemia or myelofibrosis [79]. Earlier recognition of transition to

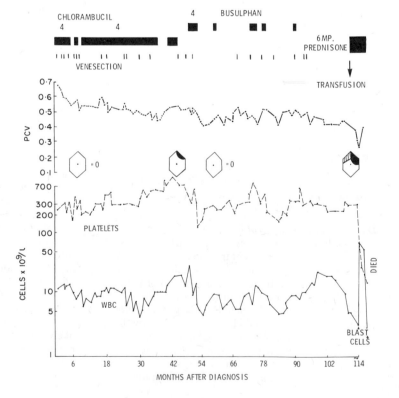

Fig. 32.1. Non-irradiated primary polycythaemia with transition to acute leukaemia. A woman of 48 presented with itching, no splenomegaly, high venous haematocrit and increased red-cell mass, normal platelet count and granulocytosis. Maintained in well state, apart from itching, for 10 years with venesection and intermittent chemotherapy. Sudden transition to blast-cell leukaemia with rapid death.

* In the recent Polycythaemia Study Group trial the incidence of acute leukaemia in patients treated with chlorambucil was 2·3 times that of the ^{32}P treated group and 13 times that in the group treated by venesection alone (390). It is possible that other alkylating agents (Fig 32.1) may have a similar leukaemogenic effect in polycythaemia but, as yet, proof is lacking.

myelofibrosis can be achieved by serial marrow biopsy or by radioactive iron scanning [87] but this information has, at present, little practical application in management.

Treatment

The primary objectives of treatment are to reduce the packed cell volume (PCV), to maintain it at an optimal level and to control any associated thrombocythaemia.

Evidence that there is continuing risk of vascular lesions even when the PCV is only modestly raised (p. 1285) indicates that the PCV which should be achieved and maintained by treatment is lower than is generally accepted and retrospective studies [110] suggest a value of 0·45 or less. The pathogenesis of vascular lesions in the polycythaemias is considered elsewhere (p. 1285).

Control of packed cell volume and thrombocythaemia. It is generally agreed that to produce immediate symptomatic relief and to remove the risk of thrombotic lesions, reduction of the red-cell mass is initially best achieved by venesection, of the order of 400 ml at three to five day intervals, until the PCV comes within the desired range. Disagreement as to how it should subsequently be maintained at this level centres around the use of radioactive phosphorus (^{32}P). Administration of ^{32}P in a single intravenous dose of approximately 5 mCi is effective, convenient, and controls thrombocythaemia, granulocytosis and red-cell mass; methods for calculating optimal dose are established [111, 112]. It produces its effect rather slowly, which is irrelevant if the patient is venesected, but the effect is prolonged and most patients only require repeat administration at intervals of nine to 18 months. For these reasons many centres regard ^{32}P as the treatment of choice and Osgood, who made an analysis of available data, considered that ^{32}P-treated patients have an increased survival of approximately four years as compared with those treated by other methods [112]. The main argument against its use is that there is about a 10-fold higher incidence of transition to acute leukaemia in ^{32}P-treated patients (p. 1276) and that equally satisfactory results, and equal survival, can be obtained by repeated venesection alone, when increased PCV is the only problem, or by a combination of venesection and chemotherapy when there is associated granulopoiesis or thrombocythaemia [48, 113, 114]. While there is reputable support for both views, there has been no adequately controlled trial to establish which is correct, though such a trial is now under way [99]. Such a reasonable divergence of views indicates that both regimes may have a place in the treatment of the condition—at least until the results of an objective study are available—and that selection should be determined by the clinical, haemato-logical and general situation of each individual patient. It is on this basis that the following approach is suggested.

In all patients, following the initial period of venesection, a rising PCV should be returned to the low normal range (< 0.45) by repeated single venesections rather than by ^{32}P. Since this is often a slow proliferative process, many patients will, after the initial treatment, only require a clinical and haematological check every six to eight weeks, with single 400 ml venesection about two to four times a year, and will be spared the risk of developing the acute leukaemia which, in a proportion of patients receiving ^{32}P and chemotherapy, is induced within two to five years of its administration. This is particularly relevant to the so called 'idiopathic erythrocytosis' group (p. 1278). The concept that venesection will stimulate erythropoiesis in primary polycythaemia is fallacious, since the physiological erythropoietin mechanism only operates in these patients when they become anaemic or hypoxic [97]. In primary polycythaemia venesection itself will diminish red-cell production, mainly by inducing iron deficiency but also, possibly, by reducing the level of some erythropoietic stimulating substance which may be an independent product of the increased red-cell mass itself [115]. The iron deficiency, which almost invariably follows the venesection regime, is usually asymptomatic, confirming the observations of Wood & Elwood [116] that symptoms due to iron deficiency are not inevitable until the haemoglobin falls to around 8 g/dl. Although there is now evidence suggesting that iron deficiency could adversely affect such functions as cerebral metabolism and the immune response [117] there is, as yet, no evidence that this has clinical relevance. It should be emphasized that patients treated by venesection alone require closer supervision than those treated by ^{32}P. If such supervision is impracticable, recurrent rise of the PCV to unacceptable levels is likely. This may explain some of the less satisfactory results in venesected groups of patients [118] and, unless adequate continuous control of PCV can be obtained by venesection, the patient is probably unsuitable for this regime.

In patients in whom rate of relapse or symptoms of iron deficiency make control of red-cell mass by venesection alone unacceptable, chemotherapy will often control red-cell production by itself, decrease the need for venesection and, in some patients, reduce spleen size. In the presence of thrombocythaemia the platelet count must also be reduced to the normal range and, for this, chemotherapy such as busulphan, 2–6 mg daily, is effective. The role of high-dose intermittent chemotherapy is being examined in current trials [119]. In patients without thrombocythaemia, busulphan may induce an unacceptable thrombocytopenia, but various other drugs have been used [119–122]. The results suggest that there may be advantages in the selection of a particular drug to meet a specific clinical or haematological situation. Gilbert [114], for example, compared the effects of cyclophosphamide, chlorambucil and busulphan and found that, while all were useful, chlorambucil was the most effective in reducing splenomegaly while cyclophosphamide produced the least thrombocytopenia.

In a small group of patients the venesection-chemotherapy regime is ineffective, either because it does not control the process effectively, or because the very careful supervision it requires is impracticable. There is then a clear-cut indication for the use of ^{32}P, particularly in patients in the seventh and eighth decades, in whom death from unrelated causes is likely to precede transition to acute leukaemia. While the aetiology of the disease was uncertain, there was a natural reluctance to use blood from venesected polycythaemics for routine transfusion. Hyman & Carlsen [123] found no short- or long-term adverse effects in 300 patients transfused with polycythaemic blood over a 15-year period. Therefore, in spite of the recent evidence suggesting that PPP is due to the existence of a mutant clone, there is a case for using this source in selected recipients with, for example, acellular marrow failure or leukaemia.

Acute gout. This obviously requires immediate and appropriate management, but in the early phases of chemotherapy or treatment with ^{32}P, urate production may increase, and this should be prophylactically controlled by allopurinol (*c.* 400 mg daily) particularly to obviate the risk of renal complications. In the later stages of effectively treated polycythaemia, urate production usually decreases and no specific treatment is necessary. Plasma urate levels should, however, be measured throughout the course of the disease and if raised levels persist it is sensible to control them with allopurinol.

Itching. This may occasionally decrease as counts revert to normal with chemotherapy or ^{32}P, but itching is normally persistent and unresponsive to conventional antihistamine therapy. The marginal and transient value of topical applications is outweighed by their inconvenience, and the management of intolerable itching is extremely difficult. Studies by Gilbert & Krauss [38, 39] on blood histamine levels prompted trials of drugs which either antagonize the effects of histamine on receptor sites (cyproheptadine) or inhibit the synthesis of histamine. They considered that both approaches could be effective in controlling itching but found that both produced side-effects, which were serious with the synthesis inhibitor. The concept is

interesting and the trials of cyproheptadine suggested that this drug might be of value. Cholestyramine, sometimes useful in the pruritus of obstructive jaundice, has also been reported as useful in the treatment of polycythaemic itching [124]. However, limited personal experience suggests that neither cyproheptadine or cholestyramine are very effective. There is similar uncertainty about the value of the histamine H_2 antagonist cimetidine. Some authors have reported dramatic relief with the administration of 300 mg four times daily [125] while others have found no consistent benefit [126]. In patients with distressing pruritus, trial use of these drugs is worthwhile but if this is ineffective nocturnal sedatives, mild analgesics and avoidance of individual precipitating factors, such as undue warmth or hot baths, may be helpful.

Peripheral vascular symptoms. Symptoms and signs which are the result of transient or reversible vascular lesions, particularly in the microvasculature—such as erythromelalgia—often show a dramatic improvement when the PCV and platelet count become normal. Surgery—amputation or sympathectomy—should, if possible, be avoided until the haematological abnormalities have been corrected, since this may result in recovery without operation. Failure to respond after effective haematological treatment suggests some unrelated cause or irreversible situation which should then be treated in its own right.

Surgery in PPP. Patients with PPP requiring surgical operations for unrelated conditions are particularly susceptible to post-operative bleeding and thrombosis [60]. Surgery should, if possible, be avoided in PPP until the haematological abnormalities have been corrected for two to three months since the untreated or recently treated patient is particularly vulnerable to these complications.

Transition to acute leukaemia or myelofibrosis. The treatment appropriate to these conditions is discussed elsewhere (Chapter 22 and p. 1301).

Idiopathic erythrocytosis

Definition
The term idiopathic erythrocytosis has been used (pp. 1269 and 1276) to define patients with abnormal elevation of PCV and red-cell mass who do not, at the time of presentation, have any of the other characteristics which enable them to be classified as primary proliferative polycythaemia (PPP) or as some form of secondary polycythaemia. It is generally accepted that for classification as PPP (p. 1269) a patient should have

not only a raised red-cell mass, but also splenomegaly or some combination of abnormalities which includes at least two of the following: granulocytosis, thrombocytosis, and a raised leucocyte alkaline phosphatase. In current therapeutic trials, raised serum B_{12} level or raised B_{12}-binding capacity are regarded as additional diagnostic features [99]. While there may be some variations in the criteria regarded as necessary for the diagnosis of PPP there would be general agreement that, in patients with a raised red-cell mass, the absence of these associated abnormalities would make the diagnosis of PPP unacceptable. If, in such patients, there is no evidence of hypoxia, inappropriate erythropoietin production or other recognizable cause of secondary polycythaemia, they emerge as examples of unexplained, but unequivocal, increase in red-cell mass alone. Such cases, which are common and probably

present with greater frequency than classical primary polycythaemia, in some ways correspond to the group described by Modan [45] as 'benign erythrocytosis' because it was considered that they remained unchanged over time. However, there are now reasons for considering the term 'benign' as inappropriate. Long-term follow-up of a group of patients presenting with only an increased red-cell mass has shown that a considerable proportion will, often after several years, develop some combination of splenomegaly or leucocytosis, thrombocythaemia and leucocyte alkaline-phosphatase change which permits their reclassification as PPP [103]. The findings in such a study are shown in Figure 32.2. Although the initial progress of the condition in such patients may be slow and unaggressive, the transition to PPP which occurs indicates that they are not 'benign'. In addition it will

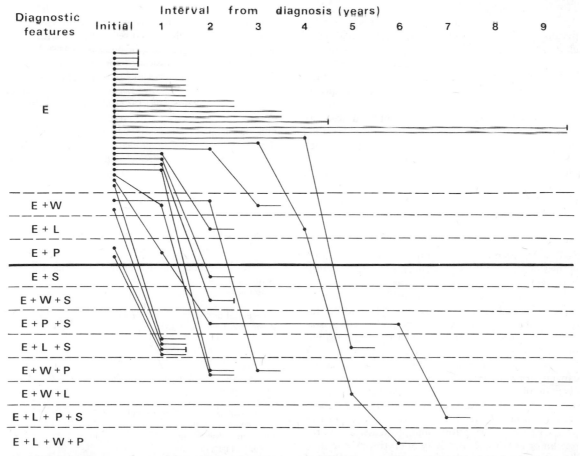

Fig. 32.2. Haematological and clinical features developing in the period after initial diagnosis in patients with idiopathic erythrocytosis. Each line represents one patient. A vertical bar at the end of a line denotes the death of the patient. (E = definite polycythaemia; L = raised LAP score; W = neutrophilia; P = thrombocytosis; S = splenomegaly.) Patients crossing the central horizontal line developed features enabling them to be reclassified as primary proliferative polycythaemia.

be seen in Figure 32.2 that a proportion of patients presenting with erythrocytosis do not, even after many years, undergo this transition to PPP. The pathogenesis of the polycythaemia in these patients is, at present, not known. It therefore seems sensible to recognize that this group of polycythaemia patients, who are not distinguishable from each other on presentation, may eventually be shown to be heterogeneous. For these reasons the most useful and least misleading initial diagnosis in these patients would appear to be 'idiopathic erythrocytosis'.

Presentation

As with other forms of polycythaemia, these patients may present with an occlusive vascular lesion, symptoms related to hyperviscosity or following the incidental finding of an elevated PCV.

Course and management

As already indicated, many of these patients eventually develop features of PPP while others remain unchanged for many years. In the idiopathic erythrocytosis and PPP phases the behaviour of the condition will depend largely on the level of the PCV with a general correlation between PCV level and incidence of vascular occlusive lesions [101, 103]. It is for this reason that the condition requires continued observation and control of PCV (p. 1277). If overt PPP develops, the subsequent course and treatment is that described for this condition (p. 1275). However, for idiopathic erythrocytosis there is a good argument for treatment by venesection alone, thus avoiding the unnecessary risks associated with exposure to ^{32}P or chemotherapy [102, 103].

Pathogenesis

Since a considerable proportion of patients presenting with idiopathic erythrocytosis eventually develop PPP it is likely that their erythrocytosis is due from the onset, like PPP itself, to autonomous proliferation of a mutant red-cell clone. In those patients who do not develop characteristics of PPP the pathogenesis is at present obscure but a number of theoretical possibilities exist. First it is possible that it could be the result of primary proliferation of a stem-cell line which has no capacity for differentiation in the direction of granulocytes or platelets. Secondly, it could be a secondary proliferation of red-cells conditioned by, and dependent on, some as yet unrecognized primary factor: primary production of abnormal or excessive erythropoietin or abnormal sensitivity of erythropoietic stem cells to normal erythropoietin are some of the more obvious possibilities. Some examples of such abnormalities have recently been described [127–130, 387]. Definition of this group of patients is likely to be

clarified by longer observation, by increased application of stem-cell kinetic study techniques and by development of more sensitive and practicable methods of erythropoietin assay.

THE SECONDARY TRUE POLYCYTHAEMIAS

By definition, the secondary polycythaemias are a group of conditions in which an increased red-cell mass can be shown to be the sequel of some other disease process. The classification of the polycythaemias, which is confused, is discussed elsewhere (p. 1270, Table 32.1) but this secondary group must be distinguished from a separate, heterogeneous group of patients in which a raised packed cell volume is due either to an unequivocal and abnormal reduction in plasma volume (the relative polycythaemias), or to a combination of high normal red-cell mass with a low normal plasma volume. In the present context detailed description and discussion of the secondary polycythaemic group is unnecessary but the conditions in it need to be clearly defined because, in a number of patients, the diagnosis of PPP or idiopathic erythrocytosis can be assumed only when secondary polycythaemia has been excluded. A general classification of the secondary polycythaemias is given in Table 32.3. Some aspects of this group, which are due to the effect of increased production of erythropoietin on an essentially normal marrow, should be considered here.

Table 32.3. The secondary true polycythaemias

Hypoxic (activation of normal erythropoietin mechanism)
Altitude
Pulmonary
Cardiac
Congenital methaemoglobinaemia
Abnormal haemoglobins
Smoking
Red-cell metabolic defects
Cobalt

Inappropriate erythropoietin-induced
Renal lesions
Hepatoma
Cerebellar haemangioblastoma
Uterine fibromyoma
Phaeochromocytoma
Bronchial carcinoma
Hormonal
Unexplained high erythropoietin activity

Hypertransfusion

The hypoxic polycythaemias

Altitude, pulmonary and cardiac polycythaemias and the polycythaemias associated with certain abnormal haemoglobins, congenital methaemoglobinaemia and some red-cell metabolic defects are all predictable responses to a hypoxic situation which activates the physiological erythropoietin mechanism. The possibility that smoking may have a similar effect is discussed later (p. 1282).

Altitude polycythaemia. The changes in PCV which occur at altitude are complex and vary according to rate of ascent, altitude reached and duration of stay. Initially there appears to be a fall in PCV due, possibly, to a retention of fluid or to a shift from the extravascular to the intravascular compartment. This is followed by a diuresis which returns the PCV to normal or even produces a relative polycythaemia [19, 131, 132]. These effects, which may occur during the first 14 days of ascent, are followed in most individuals who remain at altitude by the more gradual development of a true hypoxic-induced polycythaemia [133, 134]. An alternative form of apparent adaptation, probably genetically determined, has been reported in Sherpas who appear, skilfully, to avoid the hazards of polycythaemia by maintaining a normal PCV but shift their O_2 dissociation curve to the left [135, 136]. This is in contrast to the changes in indigenous high-altitude Peruvians who shift their O_2 dissociation curve to the right and develop a true polycythaemia, which may be associated with pulmonary hypertension and chronic mountain sickness (Monge's disease) [137]. The polycythaemias of altitude, like other forms, produce an increased risk of permanent or transient occlusive vascular episodes in high-altitude expeditions but, in contrast, there is some evidence that long-term dwellers at high altitude may have a normal or even decreased risk of such episodes, particularly of myocardial infarction [138].

Pulmonary and cardiac polycythaemia. In these hypoxic situations there is, in the majority of patients with chronic disease, a predictable relationship between the reduced arterial Po_2 and the raised PCV [139, 140], and the symptoms and signs are those of the primary disease and of the associated polycythaemia. In practice, a number of anomalous situations occur. In a number of patients with clinically obvious hypoxic pulmonary disease, with classically abnormal arterial gas tensions, the PCV is normal; although there is an increase in plasma erythropoietin in many but not all of such patients [97] there is no increase in red-cell mass. There is at present no agreed explanation for this, but there have been a number of suggestions, the most reasonable of which is that erythropoiesis is inhibited by associated chronic inflammatory lung disease [141–145]. Conversely, other patients with equally obvious hypoxic pulmonary disease present with plethora, high PCV and true increase in red-cell mass but have normal arterial-gas tensions. The mechanism of this is not established, but it is possible that these patients develop polycythaemia as a result of the intermittent hypoxia which is known to occur in patients with pulmonary dysfunction during sleep [146]. During exercise and with exacerbations of pulmonary infection a similar mechanism may operate. In patients without lung disease hypoxic polycythaemia may be due to defects in ventilation as found in the Pickwickian syndrome [147], sleep apnoea syndromes [148] and neurological abnormalities affecting respiration. The most obvious neurological lesion is poliomyelitis, but more rarely central-nervous-system lesions may have a similar effect and it has, paradoxically, been described as a complication of primary polycythaemia [149]. Finally, in all forms of hypoxic polycythaemia it is difficult to imagine that the exceptionally high PCV levels (>0.75) which are occasionally observed, particularly in pulmonary and congenital cardiac hypoxic conditions, represent optimal compensation in view of the high viscosity associated with such levels, and there is some evidence that clinical improvement may follow cautious reduction of excessive PCV in such patients by venesection [150, 151]. This is particularly relevant to the pre-operative preparation of patients with congenital cardiac lesions who may, in addition, have a thrombocytopenia of unknown cause [65, 152, 153].

Congenital methaemoglobinaemia. This is a rare condition in which deficiency or abnormality of methaemoglobin reductase (diaphorase) in the red cells results in intracellular accumulation of methaemoglobin; the metabolic aspects are fully considered elsewhere (Chapters 7 and 8). Between patients the amount of methaemoglobin varies between 20% and 50% of the total cell pigment but within patients the level remains fairly constant and the symptoms and clinical findings correlate reasonably well with the amount present. In the untreated patient, lifelong cyanosis, which may be very pronounced, is the most striking characteristic and while the majority of patients are asymptomatic and lead an active existence with normal life expectancy, the more severely affected may have symptoms of hypoxia and it is in this group that a raised PCV will establish a diagnosis of polycythaemia. No data on red-cell mass and plasma volume are available in this condition and other clinical and laboratory findings are essentially negative: there is no splenomegaly, no clubbing and the leucocyte and platelet counts are normal. The diagnosis rests on the laboratory identification of methaemoglobinaemia and on the demonstration that it is due to methaemoglobin reductase deficiency. This is obviously an uncommon cause of polycythaemia but it is a possibility which should be borne in mind in the inexplicably cyanotic patient since treatment with oral reducing agents, such as ascorbic acid 300–500 mg daily, is specific and effective, clearing not only the symptoms but also the cyanosis.

Abnormal haemoglobins and polycythaemia. In recent years it has been increasingly recognized that certain congenital abnormalities of haemoglobin structure are associated with defects of oxygen transport with resultant tissue hypoxia, increased erythropoietin production and consequent polycythaemia. The nature of these abnormalities is fully discussed elsewhere (Chapter 8) but in essence there are two main groups: in the first [154, 155] the abnormal haemoglobin (Hb Chesapeake was the first of the variants so far described) has an increased oxygen affinity resulting in tissue hypoxia but, in contrast to other abnormal haemoglobins such as Köln and Zürich (Chapter 8), no haemolysis; the second group comprises the Hb M variants which result in excessive formation of methaemoglobin (p. 1281) and may, like methaemoglobin reductase deficiency, cause polycythaemia.

These patients, when polycythaemic, may present because of the incidental finding of a high PCV or with symptoms related to it. There is no splenomegaly; red-cell morphology, leucocyte and platelet counts are normal and erythropoietin levels are raised. Ultimately the diagnosis depends on identification of the abnormal haemoglobin and, if necessary, confirmation of its role in inducing the polycythaemia by demonstration that the O_2 dissociation curve is shifted to the left (Chapter 8). In the individual patient a family history of polycythaemia gives an immediate indication of the possible diagnosis. There is no specific treatment and there is rarely sufficient increase in red-cell mass to produce viscosity symptoms or occlusive vascular lesions. Recent studies in families with polycythaemia due to high-oxygen-affinity haemoglobin variants have shown that, unlike most polycythaemic individuals, they have abnormally high cardiac outputs and cerebral blood flows [156]. This finding reinforces the view that this group may be less at risk of cerebral occlusive vascular lesions and therefore not in need of therapy to reduce the packed cell volume.

Smoking. It has been established that very heavy smokers tend to have higher than normal PCV values and that, in individuals, abstention from smoking is followed by a fall in PCV [157]. Particularly in habitual smokers this is due to an increase in red-cell mass but there may also be a reduction in plasma volume especially when rapid change in PCV level is associated with abrupt change in smoking habit [157, 158]. The mechanism of the acute plasma volume change is unknown. The increase in red-cell mass has been attributed either to a left shift of the oxygen dissociation curve in the presence of carbonmonoxyhaemoglobin or to hypoxia secondary to nocturnal pulmonary ventilation defects [159]. The relation between smoking and polycythaemia needs further examination but since the reported studies suggest that heavy smoking may raise the PCV to a level of 0·55 it is possible that it may, in this way, contribute to the development of occlusive vascular lesions in smokers.

Red-cell metabolic defects and hypoxia. High PCV values have been found in families in association with increased red-cell ATP [160] and with reduced 2,3-DPG levels [161]. In one report the reduced 2,3-DPG level was attributed to 2,3-DPG mutase deficiency [162] but the primary defect in these situations is not generally established although it presumably results in a shift of the oxygen dissociation curve to the left with consequent tissue hypoxia.

Cobalt. Administration of cobalt salts, such as cobaltous chloride, produces an increase in red-cell mass, haemoglobin and PCV [163]. This is due to increased erythropoietin production [164] which follows cobalt-induced tissue or renal hypoxia. It has been used therapeutically but the obvious side-effects outweigh any advantage produced by the rise in haemoglobin.

True polycythaemia due to inappropriate erythropoietin activity
There is a well-recognized but relatively uncommon group of disorders which are sometimes associated with excessive erythropoietin production and resultant true polycythaemia. This form of polycythaemia has been observed with a variety of renal lesions, which are considered in more detail later, and with cerebellar haemangioblastoma [165], phaeochromocytoma [166], uterine fibromyoma [167, 168], hamartoma of the liver [169], hepatoma [170], Bartter's syndrome [171] and, possibly, bronchial carcinoma [172, 173]. These patients may present with symptoms and signs related to the primary lesion but the majority probably present simply as a polycythaemia (see also Chapter 33). The haematological findings, which are similar in all members of this group, are those of an uncomplicated increase in red-cell production with raised PCV, normoblastic hyperplasia in marrow and normal leucocyte and platelet counts. The leucocyte alkaline phosphatase is normal and splenomegaly is not found, except perhaps as an incidental result of pre-existing portal hypertension in patients with portal fibrosis

who have developed a hepatoma. A further and characteristic feature of this group is that removal of the primary lesions, when this is practicable, is followed by rapid reversion of plasma erythropoietin and red-cell mass to normal levels and it is for this reason that, although most of these are rare conditions, their presence should be positively excluded in all cases of polycythaemia in which the cause is not obvious.

Renal polycythaemia. This, the most commonly reported member of the inappropriate erythropoeitin group, has been found in association with renal parenchymal cysts [174, 175], polycystic kidneys [176], hydronephrosis [177] and, more frequently, with renal carcinoma [173, 178–180]. One survey has shown a 2·6% incidence of polycythaemia in patients with renal carcinoma, and a 4·4% incidence of renal carcinoma in patients with an initial diagnosis of polycythaemia [178]. Transient elevation of packed cell volume up to 0·65 has been observed following renal transplantation and it appears that this is a true, erythropoietin-mediated polycythaemia [181]. This change has practical significance in renal transplantation since five out of six patients in one series developed serious thromboembolic lesions during the polycythaemic phase [182]. Other renal lesions, such as 'chronic glomerular nephritis' have occasionally been found to be associated with an increase in the red-cell mass [183].

Hepatoma. Polycythaemia due to this must be extremely uncommon in the United Kingdom, where hepatoma itself is a rare disease. The incidence of polycythaemia in primary hepatoma in Hong Kong, where hepatocellular carcinoma is common and has been well investigated, is about 12% [170]. In Africa, where there is also a high incidence of liver carcinoma, it seems that this type of polycythaemia occurs very rarely, possibly because of the high incidence of anaemia caused by coincident but unrelated disease [184]. In a patient with known liver disease, such as portal fibrosis, the development of polycythaemia strongly suggests either primary malignant change in the liver [185] or, less probably, a hypoxic polycythaemia due to the reduced oxygen saturation which may be the result of porto-pulmonary anastomoses [186].

Hormonal polycythaemia. Polycythaemia may develop in Cushing's disease and after administration of androgens. The pathogenesis is not clear but the available evidence suggests that there may be a hormonal potentiation of erythropoietin activity [187–191].

Unexplained increase in erythropoietin activity. There are a number of reports of polycythaemia in families or individuals where obvious causes, such as abnormal haemoglobins, have been excluded. Studies on these patients, which include erythropoietin assay and CFU-E activity, have suggested a variety of mechanisms. These include, first, primary excessive production of erythropoietin [127, 129, 130] and, secondly, a situation where there is no measurable erythropoietin but the primary defect is considered to be an expanded, erythropoietin responsive, erythropoietic precursor pool [128, 192].

Pathogenesis. The mechanism by which these apparently quite unrelated lesions induce excess erythropoietin production is not completely understood. The known physiological involvement of the kidney in erythropoietin production (Chapter 4) suggests that tumours of the kidney might themselves produce abnormal amounts and that anatomical distortion of renal tissue by cysts, hydronephrosis or vascular lesions might produce increased, possibly hypoxic, stimulation of the normal erythropoietin mechanism. Primary renal tumours and renal cysts have been found to contain excess erythropoietin [175, 179] and polycythaemia has been found in experimental nephritis [193] and, with increased erythropoietin production, in hypertrophy of the juxta-glomerular apparatus in man [194], but it is of interest that in the case of complete hydronephrosis reported by Jones *et al.* [177], where red-cell mass and erythropoietin reverted to normal after total nephrectomy, virtually no renal tissue could be found in the specimen. Similarly, although in some of the polycythaemias of hepatoma, cerebellar haemangioblastoma and myoma, excess erythropoietin has been found in plasma, urine and tumour [165, 168, 179, 195, 196], in others there are inconsistencies [170, 179, 195], the most obvious anomaly being absence of erythropoietin activity in causative lesions where polycythaemia is associated with observed increase in circulating erythropoietin. Some of these discrepancies may be the result of assay difficulty but they indicate that the production of erythropoietin under physiological and pathological conditions is a complex and not exclusively renal function. This is discussed in greater detail elsewhere (see Chapter 4) but in the present context of polycythaemia the common endpoint is an inappropriate stimulus of erythropoiesis by abnormal and excessive erythropoietin production.

Hypertransfusion
The commonest and most obvious cause of polycythaemia in this category is simple miscalculation of the amount of blood required by a patient receiving direct therapeutic transfusion, exchange transfusion or some

form of plasmapheresis. Less commonly neonatal polycythaemia occurs and is due to twin-to-twin or materno-fetal transfusion *in utero* [22, 23].

THE APPARENT POLYCYTHAEMIAS

The term 'apparent polycythaemia' is used here to define the group of conditions in which a raised PCV is not associated with a raised red-cell mass. Understanding of the polycythaemias has suffered from a confusion of nomenclature. It has been generally recognized that patients presenting with an unacceptably raised PCV fall into two main groups. The first comprises those with a true increase in red-cell mass which is due either to a primary proliferation of abnormal erythropoietic stem cells or to the response of a normal erythropoietic stem cell population to an exogenous stimulus, such as appropriate or inappropriate erythropoietin production. These, which already have been considered in detail (pp. 1280–1283), are recognized as true polycythaemias of primary or secondary types.

The major confusion has arisen in the definition of the second group, in which a raised PCV is not associated with an unequivocal rise in the red-cell mass. The nature of this group has not been clarified by the use of such terms as stress polycythaemia, pseudo-polycythaemia, relative polycythaemia and Gaisböck's disease. It is for this reason that the term 'apparent polycythaemia' is suggested to describe those patients with a raised PCV which is not due to a raised red-cell mass. Recognition of apparent polycythaemia and its sub-groups is dependent on measurement and interpretation of red-cell mass and plasma volume data in the individual patient and this is discussed elsewhere (p. 1288). On the basis of such interpretation (p. 1289) the apparent polycythaemias can perhaps be usefully subdivided into three main groups (Table 32.1). The first comprises the relative polycythaemias, in which there is an unequivocal abnormal reduction in plasma volume. The second is defined as the high normal red-cell mass group, where there is no notable alteration in plasma volume but in which the red-cell mass, though within defined normal limits, is at the upper end of the normal range. The third group consists of patients who do not fall into either the relative or the high normal red-cell mass categories in that they have a plasma volume which, though normal, is at the lower end of the range, and a red-cell mass which is again normal but towards the upper end of the range. Alone, either of these variations would be acceptable as a physiologically normal value but in combination they produce a significant elevation of PCV.

The relative polycythaemias

Conditions such as severe burns and excessive gastro-intestinal fluid loss, which produce a raised PCV by reducing the plasma volume (Table 32.1) do not require any detailed examination in the present context. Although in these situations the increased blood viscosity may contribute adversely to the clinical situation, the dominant problem is appropriate fluid replacement and management of the primary condition. Serial measurement of PCV may merely be one of the parameters by which the effectiveness of the appropriate therapy is measured.

There remains a group of relative polycythaemias, with undoubted depletion of plasma volume, which cannot be explained in terms of obvious overt fluid loss. The patients commonly present because of the incidental finding of raised PCV or with some characteristic symptom referable to it. They do not have any features of primary polycythaemia such as splenomegaly, leucocytosis and thrombocythaemia and can only be distinguished from other forms of polycythaemia by measurement of red-cell mass and plasma volume. A variety of mechanisms have been considered as causative. They include stress [197], abnormality of the aldosterone mechanism [198], disturbances of nocturnal ADH secretion [199], smoking [158], alcohol [200], diuretics [201, 202] and abnormalities of venous tone [203]. There is very limited evidence to support any of these hypotheses and, since the causative mechanism of this form of relative polycythaemia therefore remains uncertain, it seems more appropriate at the present juncture to regard it as idiopathic. Although, for excellent historical reasons, Gaisböck's name has been associated with this disorder, it is not now possible to be certain that the patients he described [204], many of whom died of occlusive vascular lesions, were relative polycythaemics since techniques essential for distinguishing this condition from true polycythaemia were not at that time available.

The long-term course of idiopathic relative polycythaemias is uncertain because the condition is uncommon and adequate follow-up studies have not been reported. In the short-term, however, there is satisfactory evidence [205, 206] that these patients are susceptible to occlusive vascular lesions. This is not surprising in view of the recent observations that these patients, like other patients with elevated PCVs, have an abnormal reduction in cerebral blood flow [207].

There is still uncertainty about the treatment of these patients. Some authors, who considered that there was an unexpectedly high incidence of associated risk factors, such as hypertension, in this group felt that the appropriate treatment was the control of these factors rather than of the haematological abnormality.

However, in view of the unequivocal risk of occlusive vascular lesions and those symptoms which could be associated with an elevated PCV, it seems sensible that attempts should also be made to modify the raised PCV. Venesection therapy would at first sight appear to be illogical and some authors have suggested therapy with fludrocortisone, a salt-retaining steroid, in order to retain fluid and expand the plasma volume [205]. While there is no reported evidence which establishes any particular regime, limited experience suggests that fludrocortisone is ineffective [208] and that a venesection regime, which produced plasma volume expansion without hypovolaemic effect, has been useful in maintaining an acceptable PCV and modifying symptoms [209].

The high normal red-cell mass and physiological variant groups

There is no general agreement on the upper normal PCV level. Measurement of red-cell mass and plasma volume in subjects with a PCV in the conventional upper normal range shows that some have one of the types of unequivocal true or relative polycythaemia already described. Others with PCV values above the accepted normal limit have red-cell mass and plasma volume values which are normal and it is suggested that these patients should be classified as belonging to either the 'high-normal red-cell mass' group or the 'physiological variant' group. The recognition that an individual patient is undoubtedly polycythaemic, undoubtedly normal, or in the high-normal red-cell mass (HNRCM) or physiological variant categories will depend on the definitions of the normal values for red-cell mass and plasma volume which are accepted, and this is considered elsewhere (p. 1288).

The pathogenesis and course of the processes in these patients are not yet established, but it is likely that they are a heterogeneous group which, for example, will certainly contain some patients who will eventually develop true or relative polycythaemia. As a group they cannot, for several reasons, be ignored. First, because despite the often modest elevation of PCV found, they may, even if asymptomatic, be at unnecessary risk of occlusive vascular episodes. Secondly because, particularly in the HNRCM group, there may be some treatable primary cause. Possible primary causes such as renal lesions, hypoxic disorders and abnormal haemoglobins, should therefore be sought in these patients. Finally, because these patients may, as mentioned, progress to some form of true or relative polycythaemia they require long-term observation.

Management, in patients without obvious associated causative disease, is determined by the need to control the PCV and reduce the risk of occlusive vascular lesions (p. 1286). This is a matter for judgement in the individual patient. It is, for example, reasonable that, in patients either aged over 50 with probable degenerative vascular disease or in the hypertensive range, an initial PCV of > 0.50 should be maintained by venesection at or below the 0.45 level. Conversely, in a fit young man or a patient with known hypoxic lung disease, there is a strong argument for observation rather than immediate treatment when the PCV is 0.50 or below. It is particularly important that none of these patients should be formally diagnosed as polycythaemic since this may cause the patient unnecessary anxiety and may lead to unjustifiable difficulties with life insurance. It is more sensible to explain the situation to the patient and then, as indicated, to regard, and use, him or her as a blood donor.

Pathogenesis of vascular occlusive lesions in the polycythaemias

The high frequency of vascular occlusive lesions in untreated PPP, idiopathic erythrocytosis and apparent polycythaemia has been noted. These lesions occur in the larger arteries and veins as well as in the microvasculature. This widespread distribution and the complexity of the interacting factors leading to vascular occlusive events make it unlikely that any single factor or abnormality acts alone. A number of the factors which must be considered are the PCV level, platelet numbers and function, and the role of associated diseases such as hypertension and degenerative vascular conditions.

PCV and occlusive vascular lesions

In PPP the incidence of occlusive vascular lesions (OVL) in the follow-up period has been shown to be related to the PCV level [110]. This is illustrated in Figure 32.3 which shows not only the expected high incidence of OVL at high PCV levels but an increasing risk as the PCV rises from the low normal (0.40–0.45) to high normal (0.45–0.50). A smaller but similar study has shown a higher incidence of OVL in idiopathic erythrocytosis when the PCV was maintained above rather than below 0.50 [101]. The association of raised PCV or haemoglobin level with an increased incidence of OVL has been further emphasized by autopsy studies which showed increased cerebral infarction in high-normal as opposed to low-normal PCV groups [210] and in the Framingham study where a high-normal haemoglobin appeared to be a factor in determining the incidence of stroke [211]. There is, therefore, no doubt that an elevated PCV level is a major factor in producing vascular occlusive events in these conditions.

The mechanism by which it does this is less clear. Increased whole blood viscosity has long been sug-

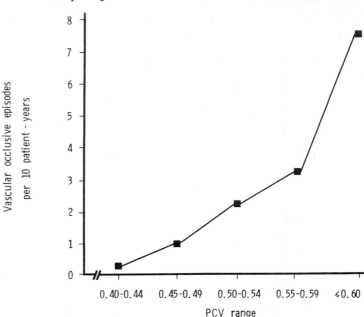

Fig. 32.3. Relationship of PCV and incidence of vascular occlusive episodes in primary proliferative polycythaemia.

gested as a major factor particularly in patients who, usually with age, have developed vessel-wall changes. PCV is the single most important factor determining whole blood viscosity and this has been confirmed in samples from patients with primary polycythaemia [212].

Since blood is a non-Newtonian fluid the relationship between PCV and viscosity is complex and is considerably dependent on variations in shear rate. In the present context shear rate may be taken to correspond to flow rate. This is illustrated in Figure 32.4 which demonstrates that at lower shear rates, as found in the venous circulation, a given change in PCV will produce much greater changes in whole blood-viscosity than at the higher shear rates in the arterial circulation. Though there has been doubt about the *in-vivo* relevance of very low shear rates [213] recent views indicate that, particularly when there are local vascular abnormalities, there may be very low shear rate effects producing extreme increases in viscosity and even cessation of flow [214]. While, therefore, there are obvious local variations in the effects of PCV and viscosity, it is now well established that there is an inverse relationship between PCV and blood flow, certainly in the cerebral circulation [207, 215, 216] and in limb circulation [217]. In primary and relative polycythaemias the abnormally low flows found in the cerebral circulation with high PCV levels revert to normal when the haematocrit is reduced by venesection [207, 215]. These relationships, which are particularly relevant to the high increase of cerebral vascular

occlusion in these forms of polycythaemia are illustrated in Figure 32.5. It is tempting, in view of this evidence, to assume that, because of the undoubted relationship between PCV level and the incidence of occlusive vascular lesions, the mechanism by which these lesions are induced is the direct result of increase in viscosity with consequent slowing of blood flow. This assumption is not completely justified, for although decreased blood flow has been related to an increased incidence of thrombus formation [218, 219], there is convincing evidence that, while an increase in viscosity may diminish cerebral blood flow [220], the major factor producing this change in polycythaemia is increased oxygen delivery to the brain [156]. Thus, although PCV, viscosity, flow and vascular occlusive lesions are probably linked in the mechanism of thrombosis, other factors such as changes in axial flow [221], red-cell aggregation and platelet distribution, which may all be modified by PCV increase [222, 223], could be contributory.

The role of platelets

Microvascular lesions are seen in patients with PPP who have an associated thrombocythaemia, and are comparable to the lesions found in primary thrombocythaemia without polycythaemia. Their pathogenesis is discussed elsewhere (p. 1291). These lesions, which are distinct from the larger vessel occlusions which occur in the polycythaemias, do not occur in idiopathic erythrocytosis [103]. Conversely, large vessel occlusion is uncommon in pure thrombocythaemia [224].

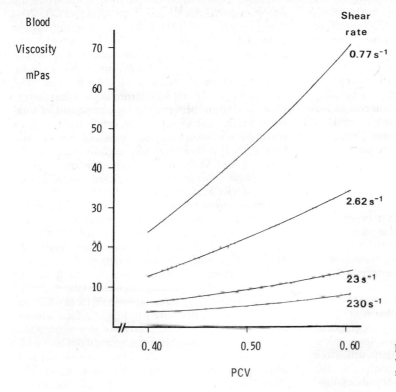

Fig. 32.4. Relationship between PCV and whole blood viscosity at different shear rates.

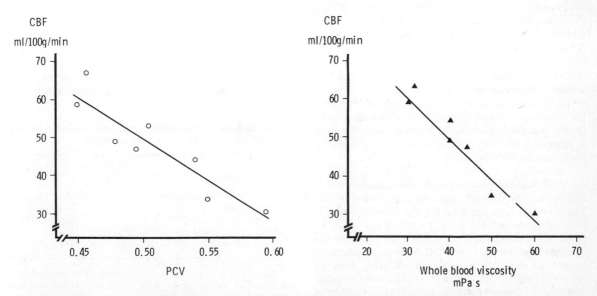

Fig. 32.5. Effect on whole blood viscosity and cerebral blood flow (CBF) of reduction of PCV in a patient with primary proliferative polycythaemia. (Shear rate -0.67 s^{-1}; 37°C.)

The possibility that platelets are involved in the pathogenesis of larger vessel occlusions is a separate and less clear-cut matter. While some observers have reported a significant correlation between platelet count and incidence of OVL [33] others have not [21, 110, 225]. Similarly, there is at present such a conflict of evidence on the incidence and nature of abnormalities of platelet function in polycythaemia, particularly when it is of primary type, that no certain conclusion can be drawn concerning the possible role of platelets in the causation of larger vessel occlusion [226–231]. Again, although a variety of coagulation abnormalities have been reported in primary polycythaemia [60–62, 64] their significance is uncertain.

Other factors
Arterial disease and hypertension both occur with increasing frequency in the age groups in which most forms of polycythaemia are commonest and it is highly probable that the association of polycythaemia with either or with both of these conditions increases the risk of vascular lesions.

The differential diagnosis of the polycythaemias
From the preceding description of the various types of polycythaemia, it will be evident that the clinical findings and simple haematological data will often indicate the correct differential diagnosis. In the patient with associated splenomegaly, thrombocythaemia and granulocytosis the diagnosis of PPP is virtually established; conversely, the combination of high PCV, impalpable spleen and otherwise normal peripheral-blood findings in patients with gross pulmonary or cardiac cyanotic disease will justify the diagnosis of secondary hypoxic polycythaemia. Similarly, only relative polycythaemia is likely to be considered in a patient with severe burns or cholera.

Often, however, the differential diagnosis of a raised PCV cannot be made without more elaborate investigation, and even when the diagnosis appears obvious it is desirable, if time and facilities are available, to confirm it by such means.

Red-cell mass and plasma volume measurement in the diagnosis of the true and apparent polycythaemias
The essential data required for the diagnosis of true polycythaemia are the patient's actual red-cell mass (ARCM) and expected normal red-cell mass. In the true polycythaemias the ARCM will significantly exceed the expected normal red-cell mass, while in apparent polycythaemia it will not. However, identification of the various forms of apparent polycythaemia (relative, HNRCM, and the 'physiological variant': Table 32.1 and pp. 1284–1285) requires simultaneous measurement of red-cell mass and plasma volume.

Actual red-cell mass can be directly measured by simple and well-established ^{51}Cr techniques [232–234] (see Chapter 1, p. 38). Although the result can be expressed as ml/kg of body weight and compared with a normal range, this is unsatisfactory and should perhaps now be abandoned in favour of a more precise and equally simple method of interpretation. The disadvantage of the ml/kg interpretation is that there is poor correlation between the fat component of total body weight and red-cell mass, while there is good correlation between lean body mass and red-cell mass [234, 236]. It is therefore more useful to measure the patient's ARCM by the ^{51}Cr technique and compare this with his or her own mean predicted normal red-cell mass (MNRCM). The individual's MNRCM can be determined by one of two methods. In the first, the lean body mass may be directly determined by measurement of urea space [236], antipyrine space [235] or total body water [237]; given the lean body mass, the MNRCM, to which it bears a direct relationship, can be derived from established normal data. In the second more practicable and convenient method the bias of fat weight is removed by using tables [238] from which the MNRCM can be derived by using the subject's height and weight; the practical validity of this technique is confirmed by the good correlation between lean body mass and height and weight [239]. Examples of such observations are given in Table 32.4, which also illustrates the unreliability of the PCV as a measure of red-cell mass in polycythaemia with splenomegaly.

The percentage increase of the ARCM above the MNRCM which is great enough to establish a diagnosis of definite polycythaemia has received attention. Examination of the confidence limits of the MNRCM based on the blood-volume prediction (BV) of Nadler [238] shows that males with ARCM 25% above and females with ARCM 30% above their MNRCM

Table 32.4. Actual red-cell mass and mean predicted normal red-cell mass (MNRCM) in polycythaemia

Measurement	Results	
	Case 1*	Case 2†
Packed cell volume (PCV)	0·55	0·44
Mean predicted normal red-cell mass (ml)	2173	1354
Actual red-cell mass (^{51}Cr) (ml)	3149	2274

* In Case 1, with no splenomegaly, there is an unequivocal increase in red-cell mass (45% above MNRCM) and the patient has true polycythaemia.
† In Case 2, with gross splenomegaly, the undoubted polycythaemia (actual red-cell mass 68% above MNRCM) is concealed by the hypersplenic effect and the PCV is normal.

should in practice be diagnosed as having true poly-cythaemia [240].

These predictions and interpretations, based on height and weight, are closely similar to those based on surface area [241] and the confidence limits are similar to those given by other authors [242].

The use of measured and predicted red-cell mass and plasma volume values in establishing the diagnosis in the relative polycythaemia, HNRCM and physiologi-cal variant groups (p. 1283) is less easily defined. Some arbitrary criteria can be suggested. Relative polycy-thaemia may be defined by the association of normal measured red-cell mass and a measured plasma volume which is greater than 12·5% below the indi-vidual's mean predicted normal plasma volume (MNPV). For this purpose it is reasonable to assume that $MNPV = BV - MNRCM$ where BV is the indi-vidual's predicted normal blood volume as derived from the Nadler height and weight tables [238]. The HNRCM group can be defined by an ARCM which is only 12·5–25% above the individual patient's MNRCM. For females the comparable range is 15–30%. Finally, the 'physiological variant' group may be defined when similar variations in measured red-cell mass and plasma volume are less extreme but summate to produce the raised PCV.

Differential diagnosis of the true polycythaemias
Distinction between PPP and the erythropoietin-mediated polycythaemias by assay of plasma or uri-nary erythropoietin is a logical approach which would be of great practical value if such assays were easily performed. Unfortunately, no simple *in-vitro* assay method has yet been developed and the complexity of biological assay techniques makes their routine use impracticable. In a very small number of patients reference of samples to a special centre may be necessary but fortunately, in the majority, a convinc-ing differential diagnosis can be established by simpler methods.

Renal polycythaemia. This must always be positively excluded in all patients in whom the cause of polycy-thaemia is not clearly established. Intravenous and retrograde pyelography will establish or exclude most causative renal lesions but in doubtful cases renal arteriography or renography may be necessary. The presence of a renal lesion does not establish a renal aetiology, for radiological renal abnormalities have been observed in a number of patients with unequivo-cal primary polycythaemia [243] and ultimate proof may depend on the haematological responses to removal of an observed renal lesion. The association of definite renal-induced polycythaemia and thrombocy-tosis in some patients with renal carcinoma has been

reported [224] and this re-emphasizes the importance of a routine renal investigation in all cases of polycy-thaemia. The much less common erythropoietin-producing lesions—cerebellar haemangioma, primary hepatoma, etc.—must, in cases of persistently obscure aetiology, be considered and excluded by appropriate investigation.

The hypoxic polycythaemias. The hypoxic polycythae-mias in which the diagnosis is not clinically obvious can be defined by measurement of arterial Po_2 and Po_2, by the recognition of methaemoglobinaemia (see Chapter 7) or by the demonstration of a high oxygen-affinity haemoglobin by measurement of oxygen affinity (see Chapter 8). The finding of normal blood gases at rest in patients with pulmonary disease does not exclude hypoxia as a cause of the polycythaemia, and in such patients pulmonary function tests and blood gas measurement, either after exercise or at night, might be of value. Conversely, the finding of a low arterial Po_2 in a patient with polycythaemia may be coincidental and not causative [149].

Primary proliferative polycythaemia. This cannot be diagnosed in the absence of some combination of splenomegaly, granulocytosis or thrombocythaemia (p. 1270). The recognition of splenomegaly is virtually diagnostic. At present, spleen scanning with radio-active isotopes has limited general application, but it may become useful in demonstrating enlargement of a clinically impalpable spleen [245, 246]. A persistently raised leucocyte alkaline phosphatase makes the diag-nosis probable and the finding of relevant chromo-some abnormalities by direct marrow techniques (p. 1274) would suggest, but not establish, the diagnosis. While histological examination of marrow biopsy material may help to distinguish primary polycythae-mia from other types in terms of granulocyte/erythro-cyte ratio, number of megakaryocytes and absence of stainable iron [247], there will still remain a group, defined elsewhere as idiopathic erythrocytosis (p. 1278), in whom the firm diagnosis of PPP can only be made when, over an observation period, the patient develops splenomegaly, granulocytosis or thrombo-cythaemia.

Some of the observations which are of value in the differential diagnosis of the more common polycythae-mias are summarized in Table 32.5.

THROMBOCYTHAEMIA

Thrombocythaemia, alternatively known as essential, primary or haemorrhagic thrombocythaemia, is char-

Table 32.5. Some typical diagnostic findings in the more common polycythaemias

Type of polycythaemia	Splenomegaly	Granulocytosis	Thrombocythaemia	Raised L.A.P.	Raised red-cell mass	Reduced plasma volume	Abnormal blood gases	Abnormal I.V.P.	Raised erythropoietin
Primary proliferative	+	+	+	+	+	0	0	0	0
Hypoxic	0	0	0	0	+	0	+	0	+
Renal	0	0	0	0	+	0	0	+	+
Other erythropoietin-producing lesions	0	0	0	0	+	0	0	0	+
Relative polycythaemia	0	0	0	0	0	+	0	0	0

acterized by an increase in the number of circulating platelets, many of which are abnormal in morphology and function. It is occasionally called megakaryocytic myelosis, usually in the rare patient in whom the most striking abnormality is excessive proliferation of megakaryocyte-like cells not only in the marrow, but also in extramedullary sites. Recently, a process with many of the clinical and haematological features of an acute blast-cell leukaemia has been described in which the 'blast' cells have been identified as primitive circulating megakaryocytes [248] (see p. 1303). Thrombocythaemia is distinct from thrombocytosis, where there is an increased number of circulating platelets of normal morphology and function; the justification for regarding it as a myeloproliferative disorder is that, although it may present as an isolated platelet abnormality, it is frequently associated with PPP and myelofibrosis and closely resembles, but is not identical with, the platelet proliferation found in many patients with classical Ph[1]-positive chronic granulocyic leukaemia. In addition, a proportion of patients initially presenting with pure-line thrombocythaemia eventually show transition to myelofibrosis (pp. 1293 and 1294) or develop the type of granulocytosis found in PPP (p. 1273). The view that this is a primary proliferative disorder is reinforced by studies of platelet kinetics and of megakaryocyte morphology and enzyme characteristics [249, 250].

Presentation
A number of patients are asymptomatic when the diagnosis is established by the incidental finding of a raised platelet count with abnormal forms present. In some of these patients, the only clinical finding may be modest, unexpected splenomegaly, which is found in about 60% of patients at first presentation. Symptoms relating to the disease fall into two main groups: abnormal, spontaneous or post-traumatic, bleeding and symptoms of microvascular occlusive lesions. In this section, the various aspects of uncomplicated thrombocythaemia are described but comparable platelet changes may be associated with PPP, myelofibrosis or chronic granulocytic leukaemia.

The haemorrhagic group
These patients may present, following accidental trauma or surgery, with the formation of a massive haematoma or severe open-wound bleeding. In some patients there may be little more than a complaint of minor spontaneous or post-traumatic bruising. Purpura does not occur in this condition but in some severe cases the patient may develop very large extravasating haematomas, often subcutaneous but sometimes, for example, retroperitoneal. Bleeding occasionally occurs from the gut, sometimes from oesophageal varices due to splenic vein thrombosis [251]. The precise mechanism of the bleeding is not established but primary defects of coagulation are very rare and it is undoubtedly related to interaction of some of the abnormalities of platelet function observed in this condition. These include defective platelet thromboplastic activity, decreased platelet adhesiveness, reduced uptake of 5-hydroxytryptamine, defects of aggregation, enzyme abnormalities, notably of lactate dehydrogenase, and platelet membrane changes [226, 250, 252–258]. Abnormality of *in-vivo* platelet function is probably also related to the number of platelets, since there is evidence that the effectiveness of thrombocythaemic platelets *in vitro* decreases as the concentration increases [252, 254, 259]: this may partly account for the clinical response to any therapy which reduces the platelet count.

The microvascular occlusive syndromes
These are not uncommon in thrombocythaemic patients and are not usually associated with large vessel occlusion or simultaneous spontaneous thrombocythaemic bleeding [224]. The basic condition is often unrecognized unless a routine platelet count is done or the possibility of thrombocythaemia is considered. The initial symptoms may be erythromelalgic, there may be livedo reticularis of the feet [260], the patient may complain of chilblains, or the findings may suggest arterial insufficiency, with gangrene or ulceration of extremities, particularly the toes [224, 260, 261]. Occasionally, disseminated small-vessel symptoms may suggest a diagnosis of polyarteritis or diffuse vasculitis [224]. Neurological disorders may sometimes

be explicable in terms of intra-cranial haemorrhage but in other patients the pattern, often of transient ischaemic episodes, is more suggestive of reversible microvascular lesions [262, 263]. The pathogenesis of these occlusive syndromes is not unequivocally established, but since they are often intermittent and are often rapidly improved by administration of drugs which inhibit platelet aggregation (p. 1294) or eventually cured by reducing the platelet count, it seems possible that the primary abnormality is platelet sludging in small vessels and, certainly, migrating emboli have been observed in the retinal arteries of thrombocythaemic patients in whom transient visual disturbance was cleared by chemotherapeutic reduction of the high platelet count [264].

This view receives some support from *in-vitro* studies of platelet function. In thrombocythaemia and primary polycythaemia, the platelets although characteristically showing diminished *in-vitro* response to aggregating agents such as ADP and serotonin may, in some patients, show increased, aspirin-reversible, spontaneous aggregation [258, 261, 263] and a diminished inhibition of the normal aggregation produced by prostaglandin D_2 [231]. Quite separate observations indicate abnormalities of platelet and plasma β-thromboglobulin levels in thrombocythaemia and primary polycythaemia, which are again aspirin-reversible [229].

The paradoxical association of abnormal bleeding and microvascular occlusion in thrombocythaemia is probably attributable to the multiple abnormalities of platelet function separately affecting haemostasis and the microvascular circulation. A more precise correlation of clinical findings and platelet function tests will be necessary before the mechanisms are properly understood.

Laboratory findings

In pure thrombocythaemia the outstanding abnormality is the high platelet count which ranges from $500-2500 \times 10^9/l$. Platelet morphology is usually strikingly abnormal although occasionally, particularly when the count is relatively low, the proportion of abnormal forms may be unremarkable. Some of the platelets are large, with diameters around 7 μm, others may have gross abnormalities of shape, granular material may comprise the bulk of the cell or may be nearly absent and, particularly when the count is high, syncytial fragments may appear in the peripheral-blood film. Electron microscopy has shown ultrastructural abnormalities but the functional significance of these is not established [265]. Except in patients who have had a recent bleed, have developed iron deficiency, or have associated polycythaemia, myelofibrosis or chronic granulocytic leukaemia, the haemoglobin level and the red-cell morphology are normal. As in primary polycythaemia the leucocyte count may be normal or there may be a modest granulocytosis, of the order of $12-20 \times 10^9/l$, with some left shift and occasional metamyelocytes and myelocytes; the leucocyte alkaline-phosphatase score is usually raised. The bone marrow is easily aspirated, cellular and, in pure thrombocythaemia, normal apart from increased numbers of platelets and megakaryocytes. Histologically, the marrow usually shows some increased cellularity, decrease in fat spaces, increase in reticulin of normal pattern and increase in morphologically abnormal megakaryocytes [249] which, in some patients, may be so striking that the term 'megakaryocytic myelosis' has been used. Direct marrow chromosome studies have shown occasional random abnormalities but no specific markers: the Ph[1] chromosome has not yet been found [266]. Investigation of haemostatic mechanisms shows that the bleeding time, particularly after aspirin [266], may be prolonged and that there may be marginal deficiencies of factors II, V and VII. The multiple abnormalities of platelet function tests, which have already been described above are the most obvious laboratory indices of haemostatic defect.

Diagnosis

This presents few problems in the patient with haemorrhagic symptoms, modest splenomegaly, a high count of morphologically abnormal platelets, granulocytosis, raised leucocyte alkaline phosphatase and compatible marrow findings. The diagnosis may be overlooked in patients with occlusive vascular lesions and it is important that it should be considered and excluded in such patients before they are subjected to operation, such as sympathectomy, as this may not only be ineffective but may be associated with excessive haemorrhage.

Since thrombocythaemia may be associated with PPP, myelofibrosis or chronic granulocyte leukaemia, these possibilities must be considered when a high count of abnormal platelets is found. If the distinction is not obvious, the presence of the Ph[1] chromosome will establish the diagnosis of chronic granulocytic leukaemia, while marrow aspiration and biopsy will demonstrate myelofibrosis. An associated PPP process, masked by a recent acute bleed or by iron deficiency due to chronic thrombocythaemic bleeding, may only become apparent after these have been treated (Fig. 32.6).

Outside the myeloproliferative group, pure thrombocythaemia must be differentiated from other bleeding disorders and from thrombocytosis. The platelet findings, the history, the absence of purpura and negative laboratory evidence of major congenital or

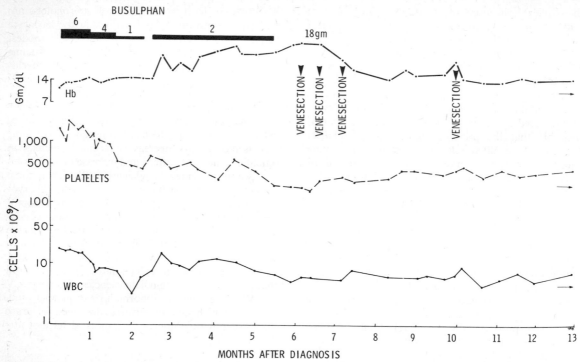

Fig. 32.6. Polycythaemia and thrombocythaemia presenting with anaemia. A woman of 60 presented with a very large spontaneous haematoma, anaemia and typical thrombocythaemic platelet count and morphology. Primary polycythaemia, concealed by the bleed, emerged after satisfactory control of thrombocythaemia by busulphan. Well controlled by occasional busulphan for six years after diagnosis, then lost to follow-up.

acquired coagulation defects will exclude other bleeding disorders. Some of the causes of thrombocytosis are given in Table 32.6. The reason for the thrombocytosis will usually be obvious but two situations need comment. First, in patients previously splenectomized or having a non-functioning spleen, platelets of abnormal morphology may be identical to those found in primary thrombocythaemia. Splenic atrophy has been reported in several cases where the thrombocythaemia [278] is probably the consequence, rather than the cause, of splenic non-function. The history and other evidence of splenic non-function—Howell–Jolly bodies, Heinz bodies and siderocytes—differentiate it

from primary thrombocythaemia. Secondly, since in some patients with thrombocythaemia there is only minimal abnormality of platelet morphology, serial platelet counts over a period of weeks may be the only way of distinguishing the patient who has bled because of thrombocythaemia from the patient with transient thrombocytosis due to recent unrelated haemorrhage (Fig. 32.7). Studies of platelet function, including the bleeding time, may be of practical value in identifying those patients with high platelet counts who are at particular risk of bleeding or thrombosis [226, 257] and differentiating thrombocythaemia from thrombocytosis. From the practical point of view, the most useful

Table 32.6. Some causes of thrombocytosis

Common	Uncommon
Post-haemorrhagic [267]	Infection
Post-operative [268]	Citrovorum factor [273]
Malignant disease [267, 269, 270]	Vinblastine [274] and vincristine [275]
Splenectomized patients [271]	Chronic inflammatory bowel disease [276, 277]
Non-functioning spleen	
Exercise [272]	

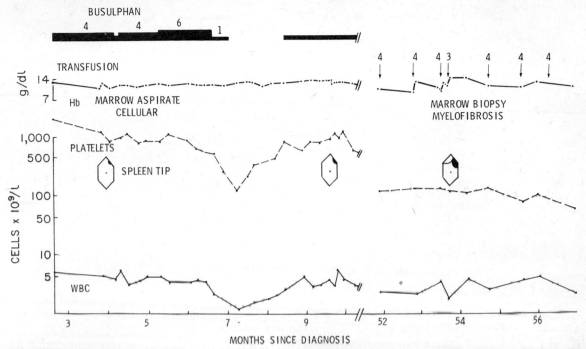

Fig. 32.7. Haemorrhage with high platelet count. A man of 53 presented with a large gastro-intestinal bleed, a raised count of mainly normal-appearing platelets and no splenomegaly. Maintained high platelet count and development of splenomegaly established the diagnosis of thrombocythaemia rather than post-haemorrhagic thrombocytosis. Transition to myelofibrosis 52 months after diagnosis.

tests at present available appear to be the bleeding time, the aspirin bleeding time, platelet adhesiveness and platelet aggregation in response to serotonin [226].

Course and prognosis

Like primary polycythaemia, thrombocythaemia is generally a slow proliferative process. The frequency with which it is found incidentally in the asymptomatic patient, the relatively slow increase in platelet count in the untreated patient and the equally slow relapse after initial treatment, support this view. Platelet kinetic studies confirm that there is increased platelet production and that platelet lifespan is either normal or, occasionally, reduced [249, 279]. Although the haemorrhagic or occlusive vascular lesions already described may produce considerable morbidity in the untreated patient, the prognosis is good and many treated patients lead normal lives 10–15 years after initial diagnosis.

In a number of patients—the proportion is not established—there is eventual transition to myelofibrosis (Fig. 32.7), and the development of increasing splenomegaly, thrombocytopenia not produced by excessive therapy, or anaemia should suggest this

possibility. Transition to acute leukaemia rarely, if ever, occurs [224].

Treatment

The central aim of treatment is to reduce the platelet count to around $250–400 \times 10^9/l$ for, at these levels, although a proportion of morphologically abnormal platelets remain, haemorrhagic and occlusive vascular lesions disappear, and there is some revision of platelet function towards normal [226, 257]. ^{32}P [280], melphalan [251] and uracil mustard [281] have been used but busulphan (2–6 mg daily by mouth) is probably the treatment of choice [282]. The response is more gradual than in, for example, chronic granulocytic leukaemia, reinforcing the view that this is a slow proliferative process, and it may require four to eight weeks of carefully monitored treatment before the platelet count is within the acceptable range. Once this is achieved, relapse, as might be expected, is slow and only intermittent treatment is required. The asymptomatic patient should be treated in the same way since, untreated, there is persistent risk of severe post-traumatic bleeding (Fig. 32.8).

Active thrombocythaemic bleeding cannot, of course, be immediately managed by chemotherapy

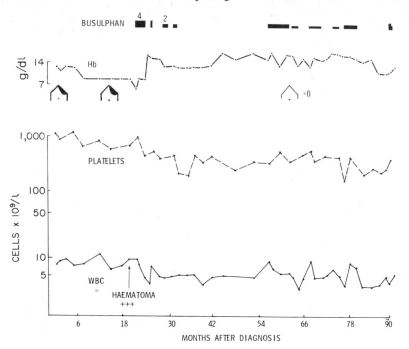

Fig. 32.8. Asymptomatic, untreated thrombocythaemia with severe post-traumatic haematoma. Incidentally diagnosed, this man of 42 should have been treated. A large psoas haematoma, following a fall, could have been prevented. Well 216 months after diagnosis on, intermittent busulphan.

because of its lag effect and in the acute situation, or when a thrombocythaemic patient requires incidental surgery, corticosteroids often have an immediate, though unexplained, haemostatic effect and short-term high dosage (prednisone 20 mg t.d.s.) is indicated. Replacement of blood lost may of course be required and there is some evidence that massive platelet transfusion may control acute thrombocythaemic bleeding [283].

In some patients with microvascular occlusive lesions and severe pain, anti-platelet drugs, particularly aspirin in small doses (300 mg daily) with or without dipyridamole (150 mg daily) may produce dramatic relief and there may also be simultaneous regression of the ischaemic lesions [224, 261, 263, 284]. This form of therapy must be used cautiously because of the special risk of inducing thrombocythaemic bleeding. In patients with very high platelet counts and severe microvascular occlusive lesions, particularly of the central nervous system, platelet pheresis, using intermittent or continous flow cell separation, has been used with dramatically good immediate response [263, 285].

The management of associated primary polycythaemia and myelofibrosis is discussed elsewhere (pp. 1277 and 1301).

MYELOFIBROSIS

The term myelofibrosis is used here to describe the process which most commonly presents with gross splenomegaly, moderate to severe anaemia, a very variable peripheral-blood picture and a marrow which, though it is extremely difficult to aspirate ('dry tap'), is found on biopsy to be cellular and to contain an excess of reticulin fibrils with a varying admixture of megakaryocytes, 'reticulum-type' cells and other hae-mopoietic precursor cells. 'Myelofibrosis' is not an entirely satisfactory descriptive term since the process is not confined to the marrow and collagen formation is not an outstanding finding. Other terms used—my-eloid metaplasia, agnogenic myeloid metaplasia, my-elosclerosis, osteomyelosclerosis—are equally unsatis-factory: metaplasia implies that the formation of extramedullary haemopoietic tissue which occurs, is secondary to some primary marrow change, and this is almost certainly not the case; myelosclerosis and osteomyelosclerosis suggest that the connective tissue changes found in the marrow are reactive rather than primary, which is debatable (p. 1296), and that increased bone formation is a constant feature, which it is not. However, providing their meaning is under-stood, all these terms have the validity of common usage and, in the present context, 'myelofibrosis' is used because it is familiar and not because it has exclusive merit.

The close relationship between myelofibrosis, thrombocythaemia and PPP suggests a common aetiology and this is discussed later (p. 1305). Increase in marrow connective tissue, often with obvious collagen formation, is found in a number of other conditions, notably when the marrow is the site of metastatic carcinoma or is involved in a generalized tuberculous process [286]. In the case of carcinoma, the 'myelofibrosis' is obviously reactive rather than primary and this may also be the mechanism in some cases of tuberculosis. Such types of secondary marrow fibrosis are aetiologically unrelated to the primary form considered here. It should, however, be recognized that local or generalized tuberculosis may develop in patients with primary myelofibrosis and that the finding of tuberculous lesions in a myelofibrotic marrow does not establish that the marrow changes are reactive [287]. In the majority of patients the findings suggest that an incidental tuberculous infection has developed in the course of a primary myelofibrosis. The pathogenesis of the 'fibrosis' in primary myelofibrosis is considered later (p. 1296).

Presentation

Myelofibrosis may develop during the course of PPP, pure thombocythaemia or, less commonly, Ph^1+ chronic granulocytic leukaemia [288–290]. Rather more frequently, there is no previous history of any of these conditions, although the first two are difficult to exclude, since they may be asymptomatic for long periods. For example, in two large series of cases of myelofibrosis [8, 107] the proportions of patients with antecedent polycythaemia were 58% and 10% respectively; in a third series intermediate figures were obtained [291]. Myelofibrosis is most commonly diagnosed in the fifth to eighth decades, with a peak incidence in the 50–70 age group and an even sex distribution [107, 291, 292]. It has, however, been reported in childhood [293] and although occasional cases resemble the adult type, many seem to be examples of acute leukaemia with increased marrow reticulin formation. Like primary polycythaemia and thrombocythaemia, myelofibrosis is a clinically slow proliferative process which in most patients has probably been present for several years before diagnosis. For this reason there are two main types of presentation: in the first, the incidental finding of splenomegaly, anaemia or an atypical blood picture leads to the diagnosis in a patient being investigated for unrelated symptoms; in the second group, symptoms may be simply related to the anatomical effects of gross splenomegaly with complaints of abdominal swelling, postprandial discomfort, reflux oesophagitis, unilateral or bilateral ankle oedema or, less commonly, acute abdominal pain due to local splenic infarction. Many patients are remarkably unaware of enormous splenomegaly and complain of a variety of symptoms—fatigue, weight loss, heat intolerance—which can be explained in terms of anaemia or hypermetabolism. Gout, related to high urate production, is not uncommon, but unless there is associated thrombocythaemia, peripheral vascular lesions, except for pruritus, do not occur.

Myelofibrosis is a common cause of splenic vein thrombosis which may produce typical portal hypertension. Portal hypertension may also be due to extramedullary portal-tract proliferation or increased portal-tract blood flow [294, 295]. All these patients may, therefore, present with ascites or acute bleeding from oesophageal varices. In addition, patients may present with or develop spontaneous or post-traumatic bleeding, most commonly involving skin or gastrointestinal tract [291, 292]. This is, most probably, due to abnormalities of platelet function (p. 1291).

Clinical findings

Although in occasional patients with unequivocal myelofibrosis the spleen is not palpable [7, 107, 296] splenomegaly is the most consistent clinical finding; the spleen may extend into the pelvis and virtually fill the abdomen. A splenic rub is often present after splenic infarction. The haematological effects of such splenomegaly are considered fully later (p. 1298). Other findings vary considerably. The patient may be active and well or feeble and emaciated, while signs of anaemia may be absent or very obvious. Cardiac failure is not uncommon and anaemia, hypervolaemia, hypermetabolism [82, 83] and the sometimes considerable splenic arterio-venous shunt [297–299] may make varying contributions to its cause. Hepatomegaly is common and ascites, which if present is usually slight, may occasionally be gross and recurrent. Although lymph-node histology is often abnormal, palpable enlargement of nodes is very uncommon [289, 291]. Pulmonary signs do not occur but radiological changes—usually an evenly distributed increase in fine linear marking—are occasionally seen and are, probably correctly, interpreted as extramedullary involvement of the lungs in the proliferative process. Similarly, although there is only occasional clinical evidence of bone involvement [292, 300] radiological bone change is common. Periosteal new bone formation, with severe bone pain [301] and osteolytic lesions, sometimes with hypercalcaemia, occur but are rare [300] and the appearances are usually those of increased bone density. Some of the descriptive

terms—'sandwich' or 'rugger-jersey' effect at verte-
bral-body end plates, 'jail-bar' effect of densely sclerotic ribs on chest X-ray—clearly reflect some of the
characteristic findings. These have been analysed by
Pettigrew & Ward [302] in a report of 23 patients in
whom the clinical, histological and radiological findings were compared. They found osteosclerosis in 40%
of patients, usually symmetrical and mostly involving
the axial skeleton and proximal ends of humerus and
femur, although other sites, such as the cranium, were
occasionally affected. There was good correlation of
histology and radiology, marrow osteosclerosis and
fibrosis being proportionately associated with radiological appearances varying from increased trabecula-
tion to extreme density, while X-ray findings were
normal or osteoporotic in patients with predominantly
cellular marrows. There was no apparent correlation
between age, sex, duration of disease, survival or
spleen size. Since these X-ray changes are not found in
the leukaemias they may, in doubtful cases, be of
diagnostic value.

Laboratory findings

Bone marrow. Just as splenomegaly is the most consistent clinical abnormality, so the bone-marrow abnormalities are the most characteristic laboratory findings. The initial haematological findings, which are
considered later, indicate the need for marrow
examination and the extreme difficulty experienced in
aspirating even a small volume of marrow, the 'dry
tap', strongly supports any clinical evidence that the
patient may have myelofibrosis. If any aspirate is
obtained it is either completely acellular or hypocellular, and may contain scattered normoblasts and
granulocyte precursors, disrupted nuclear material
(smudge cells) and occasional primitive cells. The 'dry
tap' is not diagnostic of myelofibrosis since, for
example, it may occur for technical reasons, in secondary marrow carcinoma, in the sternum following
irradiation for carcinoma of the breast, and in some of
the atypical myeloproliferative disorders which are
considered later (p. 1301). It is an indication for
bone-marrow biopsy. In most patients biopsy material
can be obtained from the anterior or posterior iliac
crest using local anaesthesia and a small trephine of the
Gardner or Jamshidi type. If this is unsatisfactory a
larger iliac-crest sample, using a larger trephine, can be
taken, preferably under general anaesthesia. Rib
biopsy, which gives the most satisfactory preparations,
[303] carries some risk and is rarely necessary. Proper
fixation of the sample, using for example Bouin's fluid
rather than formalin, with careful decalcification, is
essential [304] and even more satisfactory histology
can be produced by embedding in, for example,

methacrylate rather than paraffin [305]. Haematoxylin
and eosin-stained sections show considerable morphological variation, not only between patients with
similar clinical and haematological findings but also
within the individual patient [7, 289, 306]. Most
commonly, the pattern is pleomorphic with areas of
dense, eosinophilic, hypocellular connective tissue
adjacent to more cellular areas containing varying
admixtures of red-cell and granulocyte precursors,
immature spindled 'reticulum cells' and often a considerable excess of multinucleate, megakaryocyte-like
cells. In some patients there may be no obvious excess
of connective tissue elements and the marrow is
predominantly hypercellular, while in others there is
virtually complete replacement by amorphous, hypocellular, fibrotic-looking tissue (Fig. 32.9). In spite of
the morphological appearance, special staining usually
shows minimal collagen formation, but whether the
marrow is cellular or apparently fibrotic, the normal
reticulin pattern is always lost and there is a striking
increase in coarse reticulin fibrils which tend to be
arranged in parallel interlacing bundles (Fig. 32.9 (d)).
It has been pointed out that this reticulin pattern is
neither invariably present nor exclusively found in
myelofibrosis [67, 290] but while this is probably true,
it still remains a most consistent and useful histological
marker in this condition. Quantitative study of the
amount of fibrillary tissue showed that, although there
was some correlation with the amount of granulocytic
proliferation, there was no correlation of fibrillary
content with any other haematological or clinical
feature [307]. In some patients there is considerable
increase in bone trabeculae and this correlates with the
radiological abnormalities which may be found (see
above).

Histogenesis of myelofibrosis. It has long been considered that the clinical and haematological features
and the pleomorphic histology of myelofibrosis were
expressions of mutant proliferation of a primitive
mesenchymal-type cell which had the capacity to
differentiate between red cells, granulocytes, platelets
and 'fibroblast'-like cells. Recent studies of chromosome characteristics and G6PD variants have supported the view that red-cell, granulocyte and megakaryocyte abnormalities are due to abnormal proliferation of a pluripotential stem cell in bone marrow,
spleen and other extramedullary sites. These studies
have, however, shown that simultaneously isolated
'fibroblastic' colonies are normal in terms of chromosomes and variant enzymes. It has therefore been
suggested, with varying degrees of conviction, that the
'fibrotic', reticulin fibre component of myelofibrosis is
a reactive and not a primary proliferative process
[308–314]. The evidence is persuasive though not yet

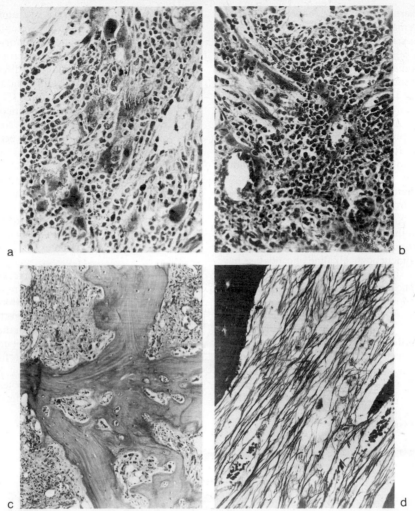

Fig. 32.9. (a), (b) and (c): marrow biopsies illustrating variations in histological pattern (see text). All haematoxylin and eosin. (a) and (b) × 200; (c) × 70; (d) marrow biopsy in myelofibrosis showing characteristic reticulin pattern, reticulin × 200.

conclusive, but is of interest in the context of separate observations suggesting that immune complexes in phagocytic cells are a particular feature of myelofibrosis [315].

Peripheral-blood findings
These are very variable and in patients with clinical findings suggestive of myelofibrosis, this lack of specificity is, paradoxically, almost diagnostic. Anaemia may be negligible, moderate or very severe. Partial or complete red-cell production failure, sometimes with reversible folate deficiency [316] and haemolysis, probably due to factors extrinsic to the red cell, make varying contributions to its causation [317–319] but in patients with severe anaemia the effects of gross

splenomegaly may be the dominant factor (p. 1298). Autoimmune haemolysis is extremely uncommon, but occasional patients do develop paroxysmal nocturnal haemoglobinuria with positive Ham's and sucrose lysis tests and low red-cell acetylcholinesterase levels [320, 321]. It has been suggested, however, that in patients with splenomegaly the main mechanism of haemolysis may be an induced metabolic abnormality of the red cells following prolonged exposure to abnormal conditions in the slow-flow splenic compartment (see Chapter 20).

The red cells show anisocytosis and poikilocytosis and 'tear-drop' cells which, though not exclusive to myelofibrosis, are often present in large numbers. The mechanism of production of these tear-drop cells is not established. There are occasional reports in myelofibrosis of abnormalities of red-cell antigens [323], or red-cell metabolism [324] and of erythroblast RNA synthesis [325], but little to establish whether these are intrinsic to the disease or merely secondary changes. The leucocyte count may be normal, reduced or raised to $20–40 \times 10^9/l$. There is granulocyte preponderance with mainly mature neutrophils, occasional band cells, metamyelocytes, neutrophil myelocytes and nucleated red cells. The presence of blast cells, which may constitute five to 10% of the leucocyte population, does not necessarily indicate a poor prognosis or impending transition to an acute phase [296]. The leucocyte alkaline-phosphatase score is almost invariably raised and transition from low to high levels in chronic granulocytic leukaemia may indicate that myelofibrosis is developing [288] (Fig. 32.10). Normal or low values are occasionally found, but there is no evidence that variations in leucocyte alkaline phosphatase have any prognostic significance in established cases of myelofibrosis. The neutrophil lysozyme activity, raised in infectious granulocytosis, is normal in both myelofibrosis and primary polycythaemia [55]. The platelet count is, again, extremely variable both between patients and within individual patients during the course of the disease. The count may be normal, low or raised, but in all situations varying proportions of morphologically and functionally abnormal platelets are present (p. 1291). It is almost certain that the

abnormal spontaneous or post-traumatic bruising or bleeding which may occur in myelofibrosis (p. 1295) is secondary to these functional abnormalities.

Chromosome data in myelofibrosis are limited by the difficulty of obtaining good direct marrow preparations. A number of clonal anomalies have been reported; these include trisomy C1–3 translocation [308, 310–312, 326]. They are inconsistent and no specific marker abnormality has so far been found [327, 328]. Except in myelofibrosis occurring by transition from chronic granulocytic leukaemia, no convincing Ph[1] chromosome has been found and the sharp distinction between the granulocytosis of CGL and of myelofibrosis is reinforced by the observation that while an abnormal form of mitochondrial DNA was observed in CGL it did not occur in myelofibrosis [329] and that the characteristics of stem cells in myelofibrosis and CGL are different [311, 330].

Haematological effects of splenomegaly
These effects are for the most part non-specific and are found in many unrelated conditions which have nothing in common except considerable splenomegaly (see Chapter 20). The way in which the enlarged spleen causes anaemia is complex. First, it can be involved in the shortening of red-cell lifespan, for this will often return to normal after splenectomy. Secondly, it may inhibit effective marrow erythropoiesis, although the evidence for this—derived partly from animal studies

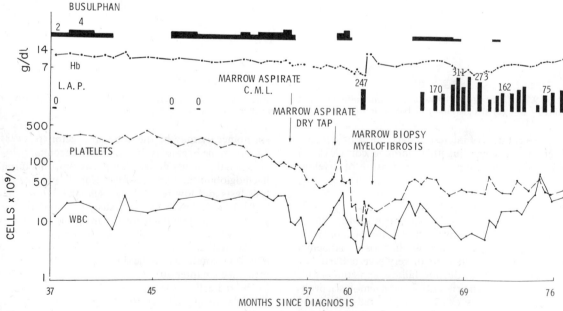

Fig. 32.10. Transition of classical Ph[1]-positive CGL to myelofibrosis. Illustrates the peripheral-blood changes associated with transition: note the change from low to high leucocyte alkaline phosphatase values.

[331, 332] and partly from limited pre- and post-splenectomy studies in man [333, 334]—needs extension. Thirdly, its most important effect is to produce an 'apparent' anaemia which is partly due to increase in plasma volume and partly to pooling of a variable fraction of the red-cell mass in the spleen [335, 336]. This mechanism, which has, for example, been well studied in idiopathic splenomegaly in Uganda [337] and in a variety of splenomegalic disease processes [338–341] can also be shown to operate in most myelofibrotic patients with large spleens [319]. There is also evidence, in myelofibrosis with splenomegaly, that platelets are often normal or increased in number and have a normal lifespan, and that the peripheral thrombocytopenia is largely due to splenic pooling which is dependent on spleen size [279, 342–344]. The hypersplenic anaemic mechanism can be demonstrated by comparing the actual red-cell mass (ARCM), measured by a ^{51}Cr technique, with the patient's mean predicted normal red-cell mass (MNRCM)—determined by calculation or measurement (p. 1288). With these data the expected red-cell mass for the patient's observed PCV can be calculated using the formula:

$$\frac{\text{Expected red-cell mass}}{\text{for observed PCV}} = \text{MNRCM} \times \frac{\text{Observed PCV}}{\text{Mean normal PCV}}$$

When, in the absence of hypersplenic effect, there is true anaemia, the measured red-cell mass will equal or closely approximate to the expected red-cell mass for the observed PCV. In contrast when there is 'apparent' anaemia due to splenomegaly the measured red-cell mass will be considerably in excess of that which would be expected from the patient's observed PCV. An example of such observations in a patient with myelofibrosis, anaemia and splenomegaly is given in Table

32.7. This splenic effect is abolished by splenectomy, and the relevance of this to treatment is discussed later. In addition, the relative contributions of splenic red-cell pooling and increased plasma volume to the

Table 32.7. 'Apparent' anaemia in myelofibrosis

Measurement*	Result
Packed cell volume (PCV)	0·30
Expected normal red-cell mass (mean) (ml)	1827
Expected red-cell mass for PCV of 0·30 (mean) (ml)	1275
Actual red-cell mass (^{51}Cr) (ml)	2227

* Observations in a woman of 46 with unequivocal myelofibrosis and gross splenomegaly which demonstrates that her measured red-cell mass was not only greater than might be expected for her low PCV (+1034 ml), but that it also exceeded her expected mean normal value (+400 ml). This 'apparent' anaemia was corrected by splenectomy.

anaemia can, if desired, be distinguished by simultaneous measurement of red-cell mass and plasma volume.

Some laboratory findings have lent support to the view that, in myelofibrosis, extramedullary erythropoiesis, particularly in the spleen, makes a useful contribution to red-cell production, but this is probably incorrect. For instance, ^{59}Fe tracer studies [345, 346] show a characteristic surface-counting pattern with apparently absent uptake of iron by the marrow and a splenic curve showing uptake and release of iron comparable to that produced by a normal marrow (Fig. 32.11). This finding, which is quite distinct from that usually found in chronic granulocytic leukaemia [346, 388], certainly confirms that splenic erythro-

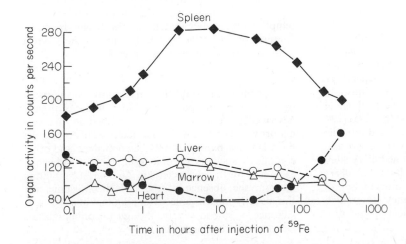

Fig. 32.11. ^{59}Fe surface pattern characteristic of myelofibrosis. Peak activity in spleen and marrow is synchronous but geometry of counting gives disproportionate significance to erythropoietic activity of spleen compared to marrow.

poiesis occurs in myelofibrosis and is virtually diagnostic of the condition, but even in the presence of normal ^{59}Fe utilization, it does not justify the assumption that the spleen is commonly an effective site of red-cell production. The geometry of counting exaggerates splenic radioactivity and underestimates the marrow erythropoiesis which may be diffused through an enlarged marrow mass. This is confirmed by the observation that splenectomy may appear to increase red-cell production [333] and by quantitative [52]Fe studies of splenic erythropoiesis which showed very wide variations between patients [85]. [59]Fe utilization, plasma and red-cell iron turnover give variable results from patient to patient and indicate that marrow red-cell production may be normal or that there may be partial or complete erythropoietic failure. Electron-microscopic and erythrokinetic studies in myelofibrosis support the view that splenic erythropoiesis is ineffective [319, 347]. From the practical point of view, ^{59}Fe and ^{51}Cr studies may be of value in predicting the outcome of splenectomy [319, 348] although [52]Fe studies, which require cyclotron facilities and are therefore less generally practicable, may give more precise prediction [85]. The quantification of splenic erythropoiesis is discussed in greater detail in Chapter 1.

Histological findings

The marrow histology has already been described (p. 1296). In spleen, lymph nodes and liver a similar pleomorphic accumulation of granulocyte precursors, red-cell precursors, 'reticulum' cells and, most characteristically, multinucleate megakaryocyte-like cells occurs. There may be evidence of recent or old splenic infarction. The abnormal cells are generally evenly distributed through the spleen in which, although the germinal centres disappear, there may still be a considerable residual lymphocyte population. In lymph nodes, the normal architecture is usually retained and the abnormal cells are found mainly in the sinusoids. In the liver there may be only an occasional intra-sinusoidal megakaryocyte-like cell in an otherwise normal liver but, particularly after splenectomy, there may be extensive portal-tract and sinusoidal pleomorphic proliferation with liver-cell damage, hepatomegaly and portal hypertension (p. 1295) [294, 295]. In all these sites there may be increased reticulin formation, but the pattern is seldom as distinctive as it is in the marrow. Though other extramedullary sites, such as the cranial dura [349] and the kidney [350] are rarely involved, the occurrence and morphology of such lesions reinforces the view that they are predictable manifestations of a potentially widespread proliferative process.

Metabolic and immunological abnormalities

In myelofibrosis the metabolic changes are similar to those already described in PPP (p. 1274): raised plasma urate levels are common, and plasma vitamin-B_{12} levels, as in many myeloproliferative disorders, may be very high due to abnormal B_{12} binding in the plasma (p. 1275). Some patients have an increased basal metabolic rate which may be as high as $+60\%$ [83]. The mechanism of this change, which is also found in the chronic leukaemias [82], is not established, although it is certainly not thyroid-mediated. It is usually without apparent clinical effect, but may be associated with considerable weight loss and heat intolerance. All these patients with hypermetabolism have raised serum creatine levels, and this change, which may be observed in the absence of a raised basal metabolic rate, is comparable to that found in such unrelated conditions as pregnancy, childhood and epithelial neoplasia, where the common factor may be the release of creatine from young cell populations which are known to have a high creatine content [83, 351]. Abnormal paraproteins have occasionally been found in patients diagnosed as having myelofibrosis [352, 353]; this is an unexpected finding in a disease in which, histogenetically, there is no primary involvement of the lymphocyte/plasma cell system.

Although the majority of studies have indicated that immunological status is normal in myelofibrosis, some observers, reporting abnormalities of immunoglobulins, mitogen response of lymphocytes and delayed hypersensitivity, have suggested that these changes are either secondary to the primary disease process and its treatment, or that there is a primary involvement of lymphocytes in myeloproliferative disorders [354, 355]. Other workers have described a high incidence of immune complexes in phagocytic cells in myelofibrosis but not in primary polycythaemia, chronic granulocytic leukaemia or normal controls [315]. The available evidence does not justify any hypothesis but it is tempting to speculate that, if the 'fibroblastic-reticulin' component is reactive (p. 1296), it may be the product of an abnormal immune response.

Diagnosis

The diagnosis of established myelofibrosis, suggested by the clinical and peripheral-blood findings already described, is unequivocally established in the vast majority of patients by the characteristic histology of a bone-marrow biopsy. It may be confirmed, and other conditions such as chronic granulocytic leukaemia excluded, by the characteristic ^{59}Fe surface-counting pattern, the absence of the Ph[1] chromosome and the usually raised leucocyte alkaline phosphatase. Absence of splenomegaly, though uncommon, does not preclude the diagnosis.

Transition to myelofibrosis. In established PPP, thrombocythaemia or chronic granulocytic leukaemia this should be suspected if there is an unexplained fall in haemoglobin, leucocyte count or platelet count, particularly if this is associated with increasing splenomegaly. In PPP and thrombocythaemia, the leucocyte alkaline phosphatase will probably already be high, but in chronic granulocytic leukaemia the change from an abnormally low to an abnormally high figure, which occurs in the more common blast-cell transformation, also occurs in transition to myelofibrosis (Fig. 32.10). In all these transitions, which may be abrupt or prolonged [104, 290], the diagnosis is established by marrow histology.

Atypical myeloproliferative disorders. These, which comprise acute myelofibrosis and a heterogeneous group of similar conditions, are discussed later (p. 1303). In practice these conditions are usually easily distinguished from classical myelofibrosis by obvious differences in clinical behaviour and laboratory findings. The main difficulties they present are in the achievement of a precise diagnosis and a logical regime of treatment.

Reactive marrow fibrosis. This is usually due to secondary carcinoma, irradiation or tuberculosis and can generally be distinguished from myelofibrosis by the history, absence of splenomegaly or the finding of a primary carcinoma, commonly of breast or prostate (see Chapter 33). Tuberculosis is often generalized and produces more fever and malaise than primary myelofibrosis. The blood findings in all may be of the leuco-erythroblastic type and not readily distinguishable. Marrow biopsy may be diagnostic if there is typical tuberculous histology or if islands of obvious carcinoma cells are found. True collagen formation is more common in reactive fibrosis and the differential diagnosis is rarely difficult but in occasional patients repeated marrow biopsy, continued observation or therapeutic trial with anti-tuberculous drugs may be necessary (see also Chapter 33, p. 1328).

Course and prognosis

Like PPP and thrombocythaemia, myelofibrosis is a relatively slow proliferative process. Nearly all patients present with well-established disease and the time of initial onset is difficult to determine. From the time of first diagnosis, the average reported survival ranges from about three to six years [107, 291, 319] but the scatter is wide and a steady-state situation, with modest anaemia, splenomegaly and well-being, may persist for as long as 10 years; in one survey approximately 30% of deaths were due to apparently unrelated disease [356]. On average, however, slow clinical and haematological deterioration occurs within two to three years of diagnosis, usually with increasing splenomegaly and gradual fall in haemoglobin and platelet count; transfusion becomes necessary with an increasing requirement and a progressively diminishing response (Fig. 32.12). These changes may in part be due to progressive haemopoietic failure and haemolysis, but as discussed earlier (p. 1298), the dominant mechanism is usually non-specific 'hypersplenism'. The same mechanism may produce leucopenia, but in some patients there may be a well-differentiated granulocytosis. Untreated, or if treatment is ineffective, the characteristic picture of an increasingly emaciated patient harbouring a massive spleen develops, and death results from unmanageable anaemia and cardiac failure. The course following effective treatment is considered below. Transition to an acute blast-cell process occasionally occurs [291, 357, 358] and, rarely, patients may develop a generalized, or sometimes focal, anaplastic process.

Treatment

Myelofibrosis, like chronic lymphatic leukaemia (Chapter 23), is one of the few proliferative blood disorders in which diagnosis may be an indication for observation rather than immediate treatment. In, for example, the elderly patient who is well and has few symptoms, the haematological state and spleen size may remain unchanged for several years and chemotherapy or splenic irradiation may induce unacceptable thrombocytopenia before there is any useful modification of splenomegaly or anaemia. In all patients folate deficiency should be considered and, if found, treated [316]. Until more specific therapy is available there is therefore an argument against treatment of these steady-state patients unless they have a high granulocyte count, high urate production or thrombocythaemia, when administration of chemotherapy, such as busulphan (2–4 mg daily) and allopurinol (400 mg daily), is indicated. There is no general agreement on this conservative management of the relatively asymptomatic phase of myelofibrosis, and reputable observers have reported satisfactory modification of anaemia and splenomegaly following treatment with busulphan, testosterone or oxymetholone [107, 189, 359]. The finding of immune complexes in myelofibrosis (p. 1297) has led to the suggestion that immuno-suppressive therapy, using chlorambucil and prednisone, is logical. Beneficial effects are reported [315] but further study is required. Only a minority of patients respond to conventional chemotherapy and a number may experience the adverse side-effects of these drugs without benefit. However, in the younger asymptomatic patient or in the older patient in whom symptoms of anaemia or splenomegaly are not severe

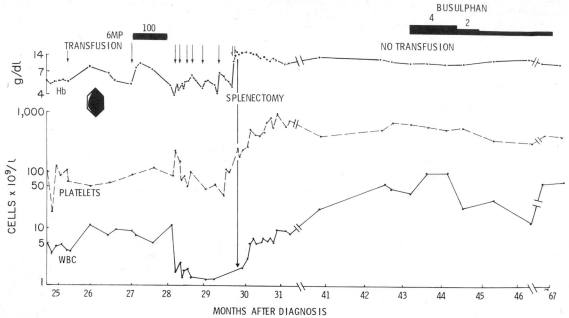

Fig. 32.12. Splenectomy in myelofibrosis. A woman of 42 with gross splenomegaly developed an unmanageable anaemia and was extremely ill 26 months after initial diagnosis. Well for 48 months following splenectomy with haemoglobin maintained without transfusion.

enough to justify splenectomy, there is a good case for therapy, busulphan or chlorambucil in low continuous or high intermittent dosage being the drugs of choice. Careful supervision is essential since patients with myelofibrosis are haematologically more sensitive to alkylating agents than those with chronic granulocytic leukaemia, and readily develop thrombocytopenia. High-dosage splenic irradiation is contraindicated, not only because it is ineffective and may produce thrombocytopenia, but also because it may produce adhesions between the spleen and adjacent peritoneal surfaces which may prejudice the ease and success of later splenectomy. Anecdotal but as yet inadequately documented experience suggests that in patients with symptomatic splenomegaly, in whom chemotherapy is ineffective or splenectomy impracticable, low-dose splenic irradiation, of the order of 3 × 100 rad at three to six-week intervals, may produce a worthwhile response.

Splenectomy. The place of splenectomy in the treatment of myelofibrosis is still disputed. The main arguments advanced against it are that the spleen is a site of effective, compensatory erythropoiesis and that the operation has a high morbidity and mortality which outweigh any advantage it may confer. However, the contribution of the spleen to red-cell production, which has already been discussed (p. 1300), is

generally negligible when compared with the apparent anaemia produced by gross splenic enlargement (p. 1298). Splenectomy can be a formidable procedure in elderly patients with very large spleens, severe anaemia and cardiac failure, but the concept of unacceptable hazard is largely based on experience of the operation before platelet transfusion and intensive-care techniques were available [360, 361]. In patients in whom there is an indication for splenectomy it is now possible, with careful pre- and post-operative care and a surgeon experienced in the operation, to remove massive spleens without inevitable complications. Nevertheless, even with adequate resources there may, in the occasional patient, be intractable post-operative thrombocythaemic bleeding and there should be some reservations about splenectomy in patients with gross morphological and functional platelet abnormality or, particularly, a prolonged pre-operative bleeding time. Operation in such patients should not be considered unless resources for providing massive platelet transfusions are available [283]. The dramatically beneficial effect of successful operation (Fig. 32.12) is mainly due to ablation of the 'hypersplenic' effect: the PCV may be returned to near normality without change in the red-cell mass. Splenectomy may also modify a haemolytic component [317] and may possibly be followed by increased red-cell production. The operation is also effective in the occasional patient with left-sided portal hypertension due to splenic vein thrombosis and in patients with frequent recurrent, painful splenic infarction.

In the individual patient the main indication for splenectomy is the association of considerable splenomegaly with a falling haemoglobin and increasing thrombocytopenia, leucopenia and transfusion requirement. An inadequate immediate post-transfusion rise in haemoglobin is not usually due to haemolysis of the transfused cells but to their dilution in an increased plasma volume and splenic pool, and this further supports the view that splenectomy may be effective. If measurement of actual red-cell mass, predicted normal red-cell mass and plasma volume confirm that 'hypersplenism' is the predominant mechanism of anaemia there is, given proper facilities for pre- and post-operative care, a clear case for splenectomy, particularly if chemotherapy has proved ineffective. There is at present limited evidence to support prophylactic splenectomy on diagnosis [362] but in the well, steady-state patient it is probably inadvisable. Following splenectomy the immediate complications may be bleeding due to abnormal platelet function or perisplenic adhesions, cardiac failure from operative over-transfusion of a hypervolaemic patient and the gradual development of subphrenic infection. In the later post-operative phases, thrombocythaemia and granulocytosis may require suppressive chemotherapy with, for example, busulphan; and in some patients there is slow intra-hepatic proliferation of abnormal cells with gross hepatomegaly and eventual liver failure. Similar extramedullary proliferation has occurred in other sites [349] following splenectomy; whether these changes are the direct sequel of splenectomy or merely reflect longer survival is unresolved. In a review of the data on over 300 published reports of splenectomy in myelofibrosis the median post-operative survival was found to be only 13 months [361] but the operation can, in selected patients, control an unmanageable anaemia and offer an extension of worthwhile lifespan of up to four or five years (Fig. 32.12).

OTHER MYELOPROLIFERATIVE DISORDERS

The characteristics which PPP, thrombocythaemia and classical myelofibrosis have in common make it possible to regard them as a closely related group of disorders, each having defined and recognizable features. However, most physicians and haematologists have observed occasional patients with less definable conditions which, either from the onset or during the course of their disease, have shown clinical and haematological abnormalities indicating a primary proliferative disorder of bone marrow. The heterogeneity of these conditions has made, and still makes, it difficult to define and classify individual cases. A number of attempts have been made and, although the situation is still confused, several main groupings, based either on clinical and haematological findings, on cytogenetic studies or on colony-forming characteristics, emerge. First, there are patients in whom a phase of haematological abnormality precedes an unequivocal transition to a recognizable, often demonstrably clonal, proliferation which is very commonly some form of acute leukaemia. This group includes pre-leukaemia [363, 364] (see p. 1260), certain 'dyserythropoietic' anaemias [365] (see p. 1260), 'aregenerative anaemia with hypercellular marrow' [366] (see p. 1260), the 'aplasia-leukaemia syndrome' [367] (see p. 1252), and possibly some patients with idiopathic primary acquired sideroblastic anaemia [368] (see p. 536). The second group consists of patients in whom there is, from the outset, strong or certain haematological evidence of a definitive proliferative process. This group includes the syndrome of 'refractory anaemia with excess myeloblasts' [369, 370] (see p. 1260), acute myelofibrosis and a variety of 'atypical myeloproliferative' disorders. With the exception of acute myelofibrosis and the 'atypical myeloproliferative' disorders, all these conditions are, as indicated, considered in more detail elsewhere in the book.

Acute myelofibrosis

This is a relatively uncommon disorder which itself probably comprises a heterogeneous group of conditions which have in common a proliferation of poorly differentiated cells in the marrow, usually with an excess of reticulin formation and a resultant difficulty in aspirating marrow—'dry tap'. Following the original description of 'acute myelofibrosis' in 1963 [371] some observers have suggested that the primitive cells are of megakaryocytic origin and that acute myelofibrosis is, in fact, an acute megakaryoblastic leukaemia [248, 372]. In the cases reported this view is well-supported by cytochemical and electron-microscopical findings but the concept that 'acute myelofibrosis' and 'acute megakaryoblastic leukaemia' are identical disorders has been challenged [373]. Until there is further evidence it is probably reasonable to take the view that acute myelofibrosis is a recognizable syndrome and that in some, but by no means all, patients it is certainly an expression of a poorly differentiated megakaryocyte proliferation.

Presentation and clinical findings
Although the condition has been reported in children, the onset, which is generally acute, occurs most commonly after the age of 40. It usually appears *de*

novo and is not reported as a sequel of chronic classical myelofibrosis [374]. In occasional cases, described as acute myelofibrosis, developing in the course of such conditions as Hodgkin's disease and non-Hodgkin lymphoma, the transition was associated with clonal chromosome changes and attributed to previous chemotherapy or radiotherapy [375, 376]. The patient with the acute myelofibrotic syndrome is usually ill, anaemic and febrile, and may have purpura or active bleeding; the spleen may be impalpable or slightly enlarged.

Laboratory findings

There is, characteristically, pancytopenia with a leuco-erythroblastic picture and occasional primitive cells. The marrow aspirate, obtained with difficulty, is of small volume ('dry tap') containing few cells which comprise a non-specific admixture of normal precursors, 'smudge' cells and primitive cells. Marrow biopsy is cellular with a dominance of immature cells and an increase in reticulin fibres but with little of the amorphous pseudo-collagen formation found in classical chronic myelofibrosis.

Marker chromosomes have been found in this condition [310, 377, 378], but although the findings indicate that this is a clonal proliferative process in the individual patient, there is no consistent abnormality between patients. The finding of an abnormal marker chromosome in the blast cells, but not in marrow fibroblasts, has led, as in classical myelofibrosis, to the view, which requires confirmation, that this condition is primarily a leukaemic-type process with reactive rather than proliferative connective tissue change in the marrow [308].

Course and treatment

This is usually short, with death from anaemia, bleeding or infection within six to nine months. There is as yet no evidence that the process is modified by any specific treatment, although transient improvement may obviously be produced by red-cell and platelet transfusion and appropriate antibiotic therapy. However, the rarity of the condition limits the value of any views on prognosis and treatment and it would seem reasonable to treat patients with obviously aggressive disease as for acute leukaemia, initially using, with caution, some modest combined therapy regime such as vincristine, 6-mercaptopurine and prednisone. With less aggressive disease more conservative treatment, as for acellular marrow failure, using androgenic steroids, corticosteroids and blood transfusion may be preferable.

Atypical myeloproliferative disorders

The main feature of this group of disorders is that it is indefinable. It does not include the more clear-cut group of disorders which have been previously mentioned. Most physicians and haematologists have observed occasional patients with some of the hallmarks of the well-recognized myeloproliferative disorders, but in whom other features of the disease precluded definite diagnosis [7, 9, 379]. The variation between patients is an example of the versatility of proliferating primitive mesenchymal cells and these

Table 32.8. Examples of atypical myeloproliferative disorders*

Case	Age, sex	Presentation and clinical findings	Blood and marrow findings	Course
1	60 F	Incidental finding of gross splenomegaly	Compatible with acute leukaemia. Hb 11·0 g/dl, WBC 60×10^9/l. (90% blasts) Platelets 90×10^9/l. Marrow hypercellular, easily aspirated: 90% blasts	Steady-state and well without treatment for six years, then splenectomy for 'hypersplenism'. Subsequent survival for four years. Autopsy = acute leukaemia
2	53 M	Anaemia; Nodes and spleen impalpable	Pancytopenia. Very hypocellular marrow aspirate and biopsy, both containing islands of unequivocal blasts	As 'aplastic' anaemia. Well with transfusion for 15 months. Died suddenly with pneumonia.
3	60 M	Anaemia; Nodes and spleen impalpable	Pancytopenia. 'Dry-tap' marrow aspirate. Cellular marrow biopsy with occasional groups of blast cells in otherwise normal marrow. No sideroblasts	Rapid deterioration with refractory anaemia, thrombocytopenia and death within six months without further marrow change

* Only those features which demonstrate the spectrum of atypicality in this group are given.

conditions are really only atypical because they are uncommon. Some examples of such conditions are given in Table 32.8, and the 18 patients described by Pegrum & Risdon [380] also illustrate the difficulties of classification and prognosis in these syndromes.

The majority of such patients have a poor prognosis and have proved to be refractory to any specific therapy. Other patients (Case 1, Table 32.8) may maintain a well steady-state, particularly if they are spared the complications of aggressive therapy. Management is difficult but it is probably advisable to determine the natural rate of progress in individual patients by an initial phase of observation, using only blood transfusion and other supportive measures as necessary. Evident deterioration provides a case for empirical therapy, perhaps using oxymetholone for patients who behave as acellular marrow failure, or combination chemotherapy for those with a more obviously cellular proliferative process.

The heterogeneity of these conditions emphasizes the need for a re-assessment of all the myeloproliferative disorders by the most recently developed cytogenetic, cytochemical and cell-culture techniques.

AETIOLOGY OF THE MYELOPROLIFERATIVE DISORDERS

The aetiology of the secondary true polycythaemias (p. 1280) is obviously that of the primary disease, and that of the apparent polycythaemias has already been briefly considered elsewhere (pp. 1284–1285). The aetiology of primary polycythaemia, thrombocythaemia and myelofibrosis, in terms of nature and causative factors, is considered here.

Nature

It is now reasonably well established that classical primary polycythaemia is a proliferative disorder in which there is an identifiable mutant red-cell line (p. 1269). It is for this reason that it is suggested that the term 'primary *proliferative* polycythaemia' now defines this condition more precisely than such terms as 'polycythaemia rubra vera'.

The development of classical PPP in a high proportion of patients initially only diagnosable as 'idiopathic erythrocytosis' (p. 1278) suggests that the nature of the disease in patients showing this change is similar. The nature of the disorder in patients with idiopathic erythrocytosis who do not develop PPP, or do not have one of the abnormalities of erythropoietin production which are more appropriately classified with the secondary polycythaemias, is not yet known.

As in primary polycythaemia, cytogenetic and cell-culture studies support the view that myelofibrosis is a mutant, clonal proliferation involving a stem cell which has the capacity for differentiation to red cells, granulocytes and platelets (pp. 1296–1297). The considerable morphological abnormality of the 'fibrotic' connective tissue component of myelofibrosis seen in some patients has suggested that it was also an expression of the primary proliferative process. There is now, however, evidence (p. 1297) which suggests that in at least some instances this component may be reactive to the primary proliferation rather than part of it.

The nature of thrombocythaemia is, at present, less clearly established, but it is generally felt that, like PPP, it is due to the emergence of an autonomous, mutant cell line. The existing evidence for this is persuasive. The clinical and haematological findings, for example, indicate a close relationship between PPP, thrombocythaemia and myelofibrosis in that all, at some stage, may show simultaneous proliferation of red cells, granulocytes and 'reticulum-type' cells, and there may be transition from one member of the group to another.

Causative factors

Genetic. Racially there is some evidence that amongst Jews the incidence of PPP is higher in those of Eastern European origin than in other Jews [381]. The occasional familial incidence of polycythaemia indicates a genetic factor but further studies of such disorders, particularly to exclude such conditions as haemoglobinopathies, are necessary before it can be accepted that there is a hereditary type of PPP.

Age and sex. PPP, thrombocythaemia and myelofibrosis are predominantly diseases of the elderly and most series show that in all these conditions there is only a slight male predominance. By contrast, in the 'benign erythrocytosis' type of primary polycythaemia as defined by Modan [45] the male/female ratio was 5·5:1. A similar sex ratio has been reported in the comparable group of patients described as 'idiopathic erythrocytosis' in this chapter (p. 1278).

Radiation. The role of radiation in inducing these conditions in man has only really been explored in atomic bomb survivors in Japan [382–384]: there appeared to be a genuinely increased incidence of primary myelofibrosis with two peaks, at three to five years and 10 years after exposure, incidence being related to distance from the epicentre; there was no observed increase in primary polycythaemia, which apparently has a low incidence in the Japanese, nor in thrombocythaemia, but the number of subjects studied was considered too small to provide meaningful data. *Chemical agents.* Benzene has long been recognized as a cause of abnormal marrow reactions and of acellular marrow failure. In one study of the role of benzene in blood disorders, two out of 13 patients with myelofibrosis had a history of benzene exposure [385]. A similar history of considerable exposure was noticed in two patients who developed atypical myeloproliferative disorders [386]. It is increasingly clear that second malignancies may be induced by anti-tumour chemotherapy. There is, as yet, little evidence of this mechanism in the myeloproliferative disorders but acute myelofibrosis has been described following chemotherapy and radiotherapy [376].

In summary, it is now virtually established that primary polycythaemia, thrombocythaemia and myelofibrosis are abnormal clonal proliferations of closely related stem cells. A more satisfactory and meaningful classification of the other myeloproliferative disorders is likely to be achieved by application of recently developed cytogenetic, cell-culture and immunological techniques.

REFERENCES

1 DAMESHEK W. (1951) Some speculations on the myeloproliferative syndromes. *Blood*, **6**, 372.

2 WETHERLEY-MEIN G. (1951) Malignant lymphoma. *St. Thomas's Reports*, **7**, Second Series, 5.

3 CUSTER R.P. & BERNHARD W.G. (1948) The inter-relationship of Hodgkin's disease and other lymphatic tumors. *American Journal of Medical Sciences*, **216**, 625.

4 PULLINGER B.D. (1932) Histology and histogenesis. In: *Rose Research on Lymphadenoma*. John Wright & Son, Bristol.

5 ROSS J.M. (1933) The pathology of the reticular tissue illustrated by two cases of reticulosis with splenomegaly and a case of lymphadenoma. *Journal of Pathology and Bacteriology*, **37**, 311.

6 WETHERLEY-MEIN G., SMITH P., GEAKE M.R. & ANDERSON H.J. (1952) Follicular lymphoma. *Quarterly Journal of Medicine*, **21**, 327.

7 HUTT M.S.R., PINNIGER J.L. & WETHERLEY-MEIN G. (1953) The myeloproliferative disorders with special reference to myelofibrosis. *Blood*, **8**, 295.

8 WASSERMAN L.R. (1954) Polycythemia vera—its course and treatment: relation to myeloid metaplasia and leukemia. *Bulletin of the New York Academy of Medicine*, **30**, 343.

9 WETHERLEY-MEIN G. (1960) The myeloproliferative syndromes. In: *Lectures on Haematology* (ed. Hayhoe F.G.J.), p. 126. Cambridge University Press, Cambridge.

10 GILBERT H.S. (1970) A reappraisal of the myeloproliferative disease concept. *Mount Sinai Journal of Medicine, NY*, **37**, 426.

11 ADAMSON J.W., FIALKOW P.J., MURPHY S., PRCHAL J.F. & STEINMANN L. (1976) Polycythemia vera: stem-cell and probable clonal origin of the disease. *New England Journal of Medicine*, **295**, 913.

12 PRCHAL J.F., ADAMSON J.W., STEINMANN L. & FIALKOW P.J. (1978) Human erythroid colony formation *in vitro*: evidence for clonal origin. *Journal of Cellular Physiology*, **89**, 489.

13 PRCHAL J.F., ADAMSON J.W., MURPHY S., STEINMANN L. & FIALKOW P.J. (1978) Polycythemia vera. The *in vitro* response of normal and abnormal stem-cell lines to erythropoietin. *Journal of Clinical Investigation*, **61**, 1044.

14 GOLDE D.W. & CLINE M.J.(1975) Erythropoietin responsiveness in polycythaemia vera. *British Journal of Haematology*, **29**, 567.

15 GOLDE D.W., BERSCH N. & CLINE M.J. (1977) Polycythemia vera: hormonal modulation of erythropoiesis *in vitro*. *Blood*, **49**, 399.

16 ZANJANI E.D., LUTTON J.D., HOFFMAN R. & WASSERMAN L.R. (1977) Erythroid colony formation by polycythemia vera bone marrow *in vitro*. *Journal of Clinical Investigation*, **59**, 841.

17 PAPAYANNOPOULOU T., BUCKLEY J., NAKAMOTO B., KURACHI S., NUTE P.E. & STAMATOYANNOPOULOS G. (1979) Hb F production in endogenous colonies of polycythemia vera. *Blood*, **53**, 446.

18 HOFFMAN R., PAPAYANNOPOULOU T., LANDAW S., WASSERMAN L.R., de MARSH Q.B., CHEN P. & STAMATOYANNOPOULOS G. (1979) Fetal hemoblogin in polycythemia vera: cellular distribution in 50 unselected patients. *Blood*, **53**, 1148.

19 LAWRENCE J.H. (1955) *Polycythemia: Physiology, Diagnosis and Treatment Based on 303 Cases.* Grune & Stratton, New York.

20 PERKINS J., ISRAELS M.C.G. & WILKINSON J.F. (1964) Polycythaemia vera: clinical studies on a series of 127 patients managed without radiation therapy. *Quarterly Journal of Medicine*, **33**, 499.

21 CHIEVITZ E. & THIEDE T. (1962) Complications and causes of death in polycythaemia vera. *Acta Medica Scandinavica*, **172**, 513.

22 OSKI F.A. & NAIMAN J.L. (1966) Hematologic problems in the newborn. Vol. IV in the series *Major Problems in Clinical Pediatrics*. W. B. Saunders, Philadelphia and London.

23 DUNN P.M. (1970) Neonatal polycythaemia. *Archives of Diseases in Childhood*, **45**, 273.

24 AUERBACK M.L., WOLFF J.A. & METTIER S.R. (1958) Benign familial polycythemia in childhood. Report of two cases. *Pediatrics*, **21**, 54.

25 ABILDGAARD C.F., CORNET J.A. & SCHULMAN I. (1964) Primary erythrocytosis. *Journal of Pediatrics*, **63**, 1072.

26 SCHARFMAN W.B., AMAROSE A.P. & PROPP S. (1969) Primary erythrocytosis of childhood. *Journal of the American Medical Association*, **210**, 2274.

27 CALABRESI P. & MEYER O.O. (1959) Polycythemia vera. I. Clinical and laboratory manifestations. *Annals of Internal Medicine*, **50**, 1182.

28 SILVERSTEIN A., GILBERT H. & WASSERMAN L.R. (1962) Neurological complications of polycythemia. *Annals of Internal Medicine*, **57**, 909.

29 BARABAS A.P., OFFEN D.N. & MEINHARD E.A. (1973)

The arterial complications of polycythaemia vera. *British Journal of Surgery*, **60**, 183.

30 ALFORD F.P., MYERS K.A. & SYME J. (1968) Portal hypertension and bleeding varices due to thrombosis in the portal venous system complicating polycythaemia vera. *Medical Journal of Australia*, **2**, 64.

31 WILLISON J.R., THOMAS D.J., DU BOULAY G.H., MARSHALL J., PAUL E.A., PEARSON T.C., ROSS RUSSELL R.W., SYMON L. & WETHERLEY-MEIN G. (1980) The effect of high haematocrit on alertness. *Lancet*, **i**, 846.

32 EDWARDS E.A. & COOLEY M.H. (1970) Peripheral vascular symptoms as the initial manifestation of polycythemia vera. *Journal of the American Medical Association*, **214**, 1463.

33 DAWSON A.A. & OGSTON D. (1970) The influence of the platelet count on the incidence of thrombotic and haemorrhagic complications in polycythaemia vera. *Postgraduate Medical Journal*, **46**, 76.

34 HUME R. & BEGG I.S. (1969) The relationship of blood volume and blood viscosity to retinal vessel size and circulation time in polycythaemia. In: *The Ocular Circulation In Health and Disease* (William Mackenzie Centenary Symposium), p. 158. Kimpton, London.

35 HALNAN K.E. & RUSSELL M.H. (1965) Comparison of survival and causes of death in patients managed with and without radiotherapy. *Lancet*, **ii**, 760.

36 WATKINS P.J., HAMILTON FAIRLEY G. & BODLEY SCOTT R. (1967) Treatment of polycythaemia vera. *British Medical Journal*, **ii**, 664.

37 BRANDT L., CEDERQUEST E., RORSMAN H. & TRYDING N. (1964) Blood histamine and basophil leucocytes in polycythaemia. *Acta Medica Scandinavica*, **176**, 745.

38 GILBERT H.S., WARNER R.R.P. & WASSERMAN L.R. (1966) A study of histamine in myeloproliferative disease. *Blood*, **28**, 795.

39 GILBERT H.S. & KRAUSS S. (1970) The relation of histamine metabolism to the clinical picture and pathophysiology of myeloproliferative disorders. In: *Myeloproliferative Disorders of Animals and Man*, p. 429. United States Atomic Energy Commission, Division of Technical Information Extension, Oak Ridge, Tennessee.

40 SUZUKI S., ISHIDA F., KONO T. & MURANAKA M. (1971) Histamine contents of blood plasma and cells in patients with myelogenous leukemia. *Cancer*, **28**, 384.

41 WESTIN J., GRANERUS G., WEINFELD A. & WETTERQUIST H. (1975) Histamine metabolism in polycythaemia vera. *Scandinavian Journal of Haematology*, **15**, 45.

42 GHOSH M.L., HUDSON G. & BLACKBURN E.F. (1975) Skin window studies in polycythaemia rubra vera. *British Journal of Haematology*, **29**, 461.

43 MODAN B. (1965) Polycythemia—a review of epidemiological and clinical aspects. *Journal of Chronic Diseases*, **18**, 605.

44 RUSSELL R.P. & CONLEY C.L. (1964) Benign polycythemia: Gaisböck's syndrome. *Archives of Internal Medicine*, **114**, 734.

45 MODAN B. & MODAN M. (1968) Benign erythrocytosis. *British Journal of Haematology*, **14**, 375.

46 CAMPBELL A., GODLEE J.N., EMERY E.W. & PRANKERD T.A. (1970) Diagnosis and treatment of primary polycythaemia. *Lancet*, **i**, 1074.

47 HUBER H., LEWIS S.M. & SZUR L. (1964) Influence of anaemia, polycythaemia and splenomegaly on the relationship between venous haematocrit and red-cell volume. *British Journal of Haematology*, **10**, 567.

48 BRODSKY I., KAHN S.B. & BRADY L.W. (1968) Polycythaemia vera: differential diagnosis by ferrokinetic studies and treatment with Busulphan (Myleran). *British Journal of Haematology*, **14**, 351.

49 BARTOS H.R. & DESFORGES J.F. (1967) Brief report: erythrocyte enzymes in polycythemia vera. *Blood*, **29**, 916.

50 BOIVIN P., GALAND C. & AUDOLLENT M. (1970) Erythroenzymopathies acquises. I. Anomalies quantitatives observées dans 100 cas d'hémopathies diverses. *Pathologie Biologie* (Paris), **18**, 175.

51 ZITTOUN R., BERNADOU A., LECLERC M., POUILLART P., SORIA J., COSSON G., VAGNER D., BILSKI-PASQUIER G. & BOUSSER J. (1970) Recherche de différentes anomalies erythrocytaires dans les leucémies. *Revue française d'Études Cliniques et Biologiques*, **15**, 215.

52 FUNAKOSHI S. & DEUTSCH H.F. (1971) Human carbonic anhydrases. V. Levels in erythrocytes in various states. *Journal of Laboratory and Clinical Medicine*, **77**, 39.

53 ZATONSKI W., KWIATKOWSKA J., BARANOWSKI T. & TAWLAS N. (1971) Investigations on the activity of glycolytic erythrocytic enzymes in polycythemia vera. *Polish Medical Journal*, **X**, 819.

54 KWIATKOWSKA J., ZATONSKI W. & BARANOWSKI T. (1972) Erythrocyte phosphofructokinase alterations in polycythaemia vera. *Clinica Chimica Acta*, **40**, 101.

55 HANSEM N.E. & ANDERSON V. (1973) Lysozyme activity in human neutrophilic granulocytes. *British Journal of Haematology*, **24**, 613.

56 KEMP N.H., STAFFORD J.L. & TANNER R. (1961) Cytogenetic studies in polycythaemia vera. *Proceedings of the 8th Congress of the European Society of Haematology, Vienna*. Vol. I, p. 92. Karger, Basel.

57 MODAN B., PADEH B., KALLNER H., AKSTEIN E., MEYTES D., CZERNIAK P., RAMOT B., PINKHAS J. & MODAN M. (1970) Chromosomal aberrations in polycythemia vera. *Blood*, **35**, 28.

58 HARDISTY R.M., SPEED D.E. & TILL M. (1964) Granulocytic leukaemia in childhood. *British Journal of Haematology*, **10**, 551.

59 EZDINLI E.Z., SOKAL J.E., CROSSWHITE L. & SANDBERG A.A. (1970) Philadelphia chromosome-positive and -negative chronic myelocytic leukemia. *Annals of Internal Medicine*, **72**, 175.

60 WASSERMAN L.R. & GILBERT H.S. (1964) Surgical bleeding in polycythemia vera. *Annals of the New York Academy of Sciences*, **115**, 122.

61 NAGY G., ASZODI L., HATVANI I. & ANTAL L. (1968) Blood coagulation in polycythaemia vera. *Acta Medica Academie Scientiarum Hungaricae*, **25**, 157.

62 TYTGAT G.N., COLLEN D. & VERMYLEN J. (1972) Metabolism and distribution of fibrinogen. II. Fibrinogen turnover in polycythaemia, thrombocytosis, haemophilia A, congenital afibrinogenaemia and during streptokinase therapy. *British Journal of Haematology*, **22**, 701.

63 STATHAKIS N.E., PAPAYANNIS A.G., ARAPAKIS G. & GARDIKAS C. (1974) Haemostatic defects in polycythaemia vera. *Blut*, **29**, 77.

64 CARVALHO A. & ELLMAN L. (1976) Activation of the coagulation system in polycythemia vera. *Blood,* **47,** 669.

65 KOMP D.M. & SPARROW A.W. (1970) Polycythaemia in cyanotic heart disease—a study of altered coagulation. *Journal of Pediatrics,* **76,** 231.

66 WASSERMAN L.R., LAWRENCE J.H., BERLIN N.I., DOBSON R.L. & ESTREN S. (1952) The bone marrow picture in polycythemia vera before and after treatment with radioactive phosphorus. *Acta Medica Scandinavica,* **143,** 442.

67 ROBERTS B.E., MILES D.W. & WOODS C.G. (1969) Polycythaemia vera and myelosclerosis: a bone study. *British Journal of Haematology,* **16,** 75.

68 BURSTON J. & PINNINGER J.L. (1963) The reticulin content of bone marrow in haematological disorders. *British Journal of Haematology,* **9,** 172.

69 DUHAMEL G., NAJMAN A. & ANDRE R. (1970) L'histologie de la moelle osseuse dans la maladie de Vaquez et la problème de la myelosclérose. *Nouvelle Revue française d'Hématologie,* **10,** 209.

70 ELLIS J.T., SILVER R.T., COLEMAN M. & GELLER S.A. (1975) The bone marrow in polycythemia vera. *Seminars in Hematology,* **12,** 433.

71 KAY H.E.M., LAWLER S.D. & MILLARD R.E. (1966) The chromosomes in polycythaemia vera. *British Journal of Haematology,* **12,** 507.

72 MILLARD R.E., LAWLER S.D., KAY H.E.M. & CAMERON C.B. (1968) Further observations on patients with a chromosomal abnormality associated with polycythaemia vera. *British Journal of Haematology,* **14,** 363.

73 KAY H.E.M., LAWLER, S.D. & MILLARD R.E. (1969) Chromosomes in polycythaemia vera. *British Journal of Haematology,* **17,** 305.

74 LAWLER S.D., MILLARD R.E. & KAY H.E.M. (1970) Further cytogenetical investigations in polycythaemia vera. *European Journal of Cancer,* **6,** 223.

75 GRIMES E. & WETHERLEY-MEIN G. (1971) Serial chromosome studies in un-irradiated primary polycythaemia. (Unpublished observations.)

76 WESTIN J., WAHLSTROM J. & SWOLIN B. (1976) Chromosome studies in untreated polycythaemia vera. *Scandinavian Journal of Haematology,* **17,** 183.

77 WESTIN J. (1976) Chromosome abnormalities after chlorambucil therapy of polycythaemia vera. *Scandinavian Journal of Haematology,* **17,** 197.

78 WEINFELD A., WESTIN J., RIDELL B. & SWOLIN B. (1977) A clinical, cytogenetic and morphologic study in eight patients treated with alkylating agents. *Scandinavian Journal of Haematology,* **19,** 255.

79 LAWLER S.D. (1980) Cytogenetic studies in Philadelphia chromosome-negative myeloproliferative disorders, particularly polycythemia rubra vera. *Clinics in Hematology,* **9,** 159.

80 WASSERMAN L.R. (1968) The treatment of polycythemia. A panel discussion. *Blood,* **32,** 483.

81 YU T.F., WEISSMANN B., SHARNEY L., KUPFER S. & GUTMAN A.B. (1956) On the biosynthesis of uric acid from glycine-N^{15} in primary and secondary polycythemia. *American Journal of Medicine,* **21,** 901.

82 GRIFFITHS W.J., WETHERLEY-MEIN G. & COTTAM D.G. (1958) Metabolic studies in leukemia with special reference to the BMR and serum creatine. *Proceedings of the International Society of Hematology.* Grune & Stratton, New York.

83 GRIFFITHS W.J. & WETHERLEY-MEIN G. (1971) Metabolic studies in leukaemia and allied disorders with special reference to the BMR and serum creatine. (Unpublished observations.)

84 POLLYCOVE M., WINCHELL H.S. & LAWRENCE J.H. (1966) Classification and evolution of patterns of erythropoiesis in polycythemia vera as studied by iron kinetics. *Blood,* **28,** 807.

85 PETTIT J.E., LEWIS S.M., WILLIAMS E.D., GRAFTON C.A., BOWRING C.S. & GLASS H.I. (1976) Quantitative studies of splenic erythropoiesis in polycythaemia vera and myelofibrosis. *British Journal of Haematology,* **34,** 465.

86 ALFREY C.P., JR., LYNCH E.C. & HETTIG R.A. (1969) Studies of iron kinetics using a linear scanner. I. Distribution of sites of uptake of plasma iron in hematological disorders. *Journal of Laboratory and Clinical Medicine,* **73,** 405.

87 VAN DYKE D., LAWRENCE J.H. & ANGER H.O. (1970) Whole body marrow distribution studies in polycythemia vera. In: *Myeloproliferative Disorders of Animals and Man,* p. 721. United States Atomic Energy Commission, Division of Technical Information Extension, Oak Ridge, Tennessee.

88 LONDON I.M., SHEMIN D., WEST R. & RITTENBERG D. (1949) Heme synthesis and red blood cell dynamics in normal humans and in subjects with polycythemia vera, sickle-cell anemia and pernicious anemia. *Journal of Biological Chemistry,* **179,** 463.

89 JAROSHEVSKY A.J., PLOTKIN V.J. & SHEKTER C.J. (1968) DNA synthesis by erythroblasts in normal man and in some disorders of erythropoiesis. *Acta Haematologica* (Basel), **40,** 315.

90 SAGE R.E. (1969) Polycythemia rubra vera with pernicious anemia. Some observations on vitamin B_{12} metabolism. *Blood,* **34,** 14.

91 ENGLAND J.M., CHANARIN I., PETTY J. & SZUR L. (1968) Pernicious anaemia and polycythaemia rubra vera. *British Journal of Haematology,* **15,** 473.

92 HERBERT V. (1968) Diagnostic and prognostic values of measurement of serum vitamin B_{12}-binding proteins. *Blood,* **32,** 305.

93 HALL C.A. (1969) Transport of vitamin B_{12} in man. *British Journal of Haematology,* **16,** 429.

94 CHIKKAPPA G., CORCINO J., GREENBERG M.L. & HERBERT V. (1971) Correlation between various blood white cell pools and the serum B_{12}-binding capacities. *Blood,* **37,** 142.

95 GULLBERG R. & RIEZENSTEIN P. (1975) Granulocyte release of vitamin B_{12}-binders *in vivo* and *in vitro* in leukaemia and non-neoplastic leucocytosis. *Scandinavian Journal of Haematology,* **15,** 377.

96 RACHMILEWITZ B., MANNY N. & RACHMILEWITZ M. (1977) The transcobalamins in polycythaemia vera. *Scandinavian Journal of Haematology,* **19,** 453.

97 ADAMSON J.W. (1968) The erythropoietin/hematocrit relationship in normal and polycythemic man: implications of marrow regulation. *Blood,* **32,** 597.

98 BERLIN N.I. (1975) Diagnosis and classification of the polycythemias. *Seminars in Hematology,* **12,** 339.

99 WASSERMAN L.R. (1971) The management of polycy-

themia vera. *British Journal of Haematology*, **21**, 371.

100 HARMAN J.B. & LEDLIE E.M. (1967) Survival of poly-cythaemia vera patients treated with radioactive phosphorus. *British Medical Journal*, **ii**, 146.

101 PEARSON T.C. (1977) Clinical and Laboratory Studies in the Polycythaemias. M.D.Thesis, London University.

102 MODAN B. & MODAN M. (1970) Treatment of primary polycythaemia. *Lancet*, **ii**, 525.

103 PEARSON T.C. & WETHERLEY-MEIN G. (1979) The course and complications of idiopathic erythrocytosis. *Clinical and Laboratory Haematology*, **1**, 189.

104 PETTIT J.E., LEWIS S.M. & NICHOLAS A.W. (1979) Transitional myeloproliferative disorder. *British Journal of Haematology*, **43**, 167.

105 SCOTT R.B., ELLISON R.R. & LEY A.B. (1964) A clinical study of twenty cases of erythroleukemia (di Guglielmo's syndrome). *American Journal of Medicine*, **37**, 162.

106 TUBIANA M., FLAMANT R., ATTIE E. & HAYAT M. (1968) A study of hematological complications occurring in patients with polycythemia vera treated with ^{32}P (based on a series of 296 patients). *Blood*, **32**, 536.

107 BOURONCLE B.A. & DOAN C.A. (1962) Myelofibrosis. Clinical, hematologic and pathologic study of 110 patients. *American Journal of the Medical Sciences*, **243**, 697.

108 MODAN B. & LILIENFIELD A.M. (1965) Polycythemia vera and leukemia—the role of radiation treatment: a study of 1222 patients. *Medicine*, **44**, 305.

109 LANDAW S.A. (1976) Acute leukemia in polycythemia vera. *Seminars in Hematology*, **13**, 33.

110 PEARSON T.C. & WETHERLEY-MEIN G. (1978) Vascular occlusive episodes and venous haematocrit in primary proliferative polycythaemia. *Lancet*, **ii**, 1219.

111 HUME R., COWELL M.A.C. & GOLDBERG A. (1966) Prediction of the dose of radioactive phosphorus in the treatment of polycythaemia vera. *Clinical Radiology*, **17**, 295.

112 OSGOOD E.E. (1968) The case for ^{32}P in treatment of polycythemia vera. *Blood*, **32**, 492.

113 DAMESHEK W. (1968) The case for phlebotomy in polycythemia vera. *Blood*, **32**, 488.

114 GILBERT H.S. (1968) Problems relating to control of polycythemia vera: the use of alkylating agents. *Blood*, **32**, 500.

115 PAYNE R.W. (1960) Erythropoietin in Human Blood. M.D.Thesis, University of Cambridge.

116 WOOD M.M. & ELWOOD P.C. (1966) Symptoms of iron deficiency anaemia: a community survey. *British Journal of Social and Preventive Medicine*, **20**, 117.

117 DALLMAN P.R., BEUTLER E. & FINCH C.A. (1978) Effects of iron deficiency exclusive of anaemia. *British Journal of Haematology*, **40**, 179.

118 VIDEBAEK A. (1950) Polycythaemia vera. Course and prognosis. *Acta Medica Scandinavica*, **138**, 179.

119 WASSERMAN L.R. (1976) The treatment of polycythemia vera. *Seminars in Hematology*, **13**, 57.

120 LOGUE G.L., GUTTERMAN J.U., McGINN T.G., LASZLO J. & RUNDLES R.W. (1970) Melphalan therapy of polycythemia vera. *Blood*, **36**, 70.

121 LASZLO J. (1968) Effective treatment of polycythemia vera with phenylalanine mustard. *Blood*, **32**, 506.

122 DECONTI R.C. & CALABRESI P. (1970) Treatment of polycythemia vera with azauridine and azaribine. *Annals of Internal Medicine*, **73**, 575.

123 HYMAN G.A. & CARLSEN E. (1970) Polycythemic donors—are they useful and safe? *Transfusion*, **10**, 10.

124 CHANARIN I. & SZUR L. (1975) Relief of intractable pruritus in polycythaemia rubra vera with cholestyramine. *British Journal of Haematology*, **29**, 669.

125 EASTON P. & GALBRAITH P.R. (1978) Cimetidine treatment of pruritus in polycythemia vera. *New England Journal of Medicine*, **299**, 1134.

126 SCOTT G.L. & HORTON R.J. (1979) Pruritus, cimetidine and polycythemia. *New England Journal of Medicine*, **300**, 434.

127 YONEMITSU H., YAMAGUCHI K., SHIGETA H., OKUDA K. & TAKAKU F. (1973) Two cases of familial erythrocytosis with increased erythropoietin activity in plasma and urine. *Blood*, **42**, 793.

128 GREENBERG B.R. & GOLDE D.W. (1975) Studies in erythropoiesis in familial erythrocytoses. *Blood*, **46**, 1025.

129 DAINIAK N., HOFFMAN R., LEBOWITZ A.I., SOLOMON L., MAFFEI L. & RITCHEY K. (1979) Erythropoietin-dependent primary pure erythrocytosis. *Blood*, **53**, 1076.

130 DAVIES S.A., GOOLDEN A.W.G., LEWIS S.M. & ZAAFRAN A. (1979) Autonomous erythropoietin induced erythrocytosis. *Scandinavian Journal of Haematology*, **22**, 105.

131 SINGH I., KHANNA P.K., SRIVASTAVA M.C., LAL M., ROY S.B. & SUBRAMANYAM C.S.V. (1969) Acute mountain sickness. *New England Journal of Medicine*, **280**, 175.

132 HOWELL A. & COVE D.H. (1979) The diuresis and related changes during a trek to high altitude. *Postgraduate Medical Journal*, **55**, 471.

133 MERINO C.F. (1950) Studies on blood formation and destruction in the polycythemia of high altitudes. *Blood*, **5**, 1.

134 SANCHEZ C., MERINO C. & FIGALLO M. (1970) Simultaneous measurement of plasma volume and cell mass in polycythemia of high altitude. *Journal of Applied Physiology*, **28**, 775.

135 ADAMS W.H. & STRANG L.J. (1975) Hemoglobin levels in persons of Tibetan ancestry living at high altitude. *Proceedings of the Society for Experimental Biology and Medicine*, **149**, 1036.

136 MORPURGO G., ARESE P., BOSIA A., PESCARMONA G.P., LUZZANA M., MODIANO G. & RANJIT S.K. (1976) Sherpas living permanently at high altitude: a new pattern of adaptation. *Proceedings of the National Academy of Sciences, USA*, **76**, 747.

137 HEATH D. (1977) Hypoxia and the pulmonary circulation. *Journal of Clinical Pathology*, Suppl. 30 (Royal College of Pathology) **11**, 21.

138 EDITORIAL (1980) Cardiovascular mortality and altitude. *British Medical Journal*, **i**, 5.

139 HUME R. & GOLDBERG A. (1964) Actual and predicted normal red cell and plasma volumes in primary and secondary polycythaemia. *Clinical Science*, **26**, 499.

140 BALCERZAK S.P. & BROMBERG P.A. (1975) Secondary polycythemia. *Seminars in Hematology*, **12**, 353.

141 HAMMARSTEN J.F., WHITCOMB W.H., JOHNSON P.C. & LOWELL J.R. (1958) The hematologic adaptation of patients with hypoxia due to pulmonary emphysema.

American Revue of Tuberculosis and Pulmonary Diseases, **78**, 391.

142 TURA S., POLLYCOVE M. & GELPI A.P. (1962) Erythrocyte and iron-kinetics in patients with chronic pulmonary emphysema. *Journal of Nuclear Medicine*, **3**, 110.

143 VANIER T., DULFANO M.J., WU C. & DESFORGES J.F. (1963) Emphysema, hypoxia and the polycythemic response. *New England Journal of Medicine*, **269**, 169.

144 FREEDMAN B.J. & PENNINGTON D.G. (1963) Erythrocytosis in emphysema. *British Journal of Haematology*, **9**, 425.

145 GALLO R.C., FRAIMOW W., CATHCART R.T. & ERSLEV J. (1964) Erythropoietic response in chronic pulmonary disease. *Archives of Internal Medicine*, **113**, 559.

146 WARD H.P., BIGELOW D.B. & PETTY T.L. (1968) Postural hypoxemia and erythrocytosis. *American Journal of Medicine*, **45**, 880.

147 BURWELL C.S., ROBIN E.D., WHALEY R.D. & BICKELMANN A.G. (1956) Extreme obesity associated with alveolar hypertension—a Pickwickian syndrome. *American Journal of Medicine*, **21**, 811.

148 LUGARESI E., COCCAGNA G. & MANTOVANI M. (1978) *Hypersomnia with Periodic Apneas*. S. P. Medical & Scientific Books, New York and London.

149 NEIL J.F., REYNOLDS C.F., SPIKER D.G. & KUPFER D.J. (1980) Polycythaemia vera and sleep apnoea. *British Medical Journal*, **i**, 19.

150 PENGELLY C.D.R. (1969) Reduction of excessive haematocrit levels in patients with polycythaemia due to hypoxic lung disease by phenylhydrazine hydrochloride and pyrimethamine. *Postgraduate Medical Journal*, **45**, 583.

151 HARRISON B.D.W., DAVIES J., MADGWICK R.G. & EVANS M. (1973) The effects of therapeutic decrease in packed cell volume on the responses to exercise of patients with polycythaemia secondary to lung disease. *Clinical Science and Molecular Medicine*, **45**, 833.

152 JOHNSON C.A., ABILDGAARD C.F. & SCHULMAN I. (1968) Absence of coagulation abnormalities in children with cyanotic congenital heart-disease. *Lancet*, **ii**, 660.

153 EKERT H., GILCHRIST G.S., STANTON R. & HAMMOND D. (1970) Hemostasis in cyanotic congenital heart disease. *Journal of Pediatrics*, **76**, 221.

154 ADAMSON J.W. (1975) Familial polycythemia. *Seminars in Hematology*, **12**, 383.

155 STEPHENS A.D. (1977) Polycythaemia and high affinity haemoglobins. *British Journal of Haematology*, **36**, 153.

156 WADE J.P.H., DU BOULAY G.H., MARSHALL J., PEARSON T.C., ROSS RUSSELL R.W., SHIRLEY J.A., SYMON L., WETHERLEY-MEIN G. & ZILKHA E. (1980) Cerebral blood flow, haematocrit and viscosity in subjects with a high oxygen affinity haemoglobin variant. *Acta Neurologica Scandinavica*, **61**, 210.

157 EISEN M.E. & HAMMOND E.C. (1956) The effect of smoking on packed cell volume, red blood cell counts, haemoglobin and platelet counts. *Canadian Medical Association Journal*, **75**, 520.

158 SMITH J.R. & LANDAW S.A. (1978) Smokers' polycythemia. *New England Journal of Medicine*, **298**, 6.

159 GOLDSTEIN R. (1978) Smokers' polycythemia. *New England Journal of Medicine*, **298**, 972.

160 ZÜRCHER C., LOOS J.A. & PRINS H.K. (1965) Hereditary high ATP content of human erythrocytes. *Folia Haematologica Liepzig*, **84**, 366.

161 CARTIER P., LABIE D., LEROUX J.P., NAJMAN A. & DEMAUGRE F. (1972) Deficit familial en diphosphoglycérate-mutase: étude hématologique et biochimique. *Nouvelle Revue française d'Hématologie*, **12**, 269.

162 LABIE D., LEROUX J.P. & NAJMAN A. (1970) Familial diphosphoglycerate-mutase deficiency. Influence on the oxygen affinity curves of hemoglobin. *Federation of European Medical Societies Letters*, **9**, 37.

163 BERK L., BURCHENAL J.H. & CASTLE W.B. (1949) Erythropoietic effect of cobalt in patients with or without anemia. *New England Journal of Medicine*, **240**, 754.

164 GOLDWASSER E., JACOBSON L.O., FRIED W. & PLZAK L.F. (1958) Studies on erythropoiesis. V. The effect of cobalt on the production of erythropoietin. *Blood*, **13**, 55.

165 WALDMANN T.A., LEVIN E.H. & BALDWIN M. (1961) The association of polycythemia with a cerebellar hemangioblastoma: the production of an erythropoiesis stimulating factor by the tumor. *American Journal of Medicine*, **31**, 318.

166 WALDMANN T.A. & BRADLEY J.E. (1961) Polycythaemia secondary to a pheochromocytoma with production of an erythropoiesis stimulating factor by the tumour. *Proceedings of the Society for Experimental Biology and Medicine*, **108**, 425.

167 PAYNE P., WOODS H.F. & WRIGLEY P.F. (1969) Uterine fibromyomata and secondary polycythaemia. *Journal of Obstetrics and Gynaecology of the British Commonwealth*, **76**, 845.

168 WRIGLEY P.F.M., MALPAS J.S., TURNBULL A.L., JENKINS G.C. & McART A. (1971) Secondary polycythaemia due to a uterine fibromyoma producing erythropoietin. *British Journal of Haematology*, **21**, 551.

169 JOSEPHS B.N., ROBBINS G. & LEVINE A. (1962) Polycythemia secondary to hamartoma of the liver. *Journal of the American Medical Association*, **179**, 867.

170 KAN Y.W., McFADZEAN A.J.S., TODD D. & TSO S.C. (1961) Further observations on polycythemia in hepatocellular carcinoma. *Blood*, **18**, 592.

171 ERKELENS D.W. & STATIUS VAN EPPS L.W. (1973) Bartter's syndrome and erythrocytosis. *American Journal of Medicine*, **55**, 711.

172 VIDEBAEK A. (1950) Polycythaemia vera. Co-existing with malignant tumours (particularly hypernephroma). *Acta Medica Scandinavica*, **138**, 239.

173 DONATI R.M., McCARTHY J.M., LANGE R.D. & GALLAGHER N.I. (1963) Erythrocythemia and neoplastic tumors. *Annals of Internal Medicine*, **58**, 47.

174 LUKE R.G., KENNEDY A.C., BARR STIRLING W. & McDONALD G.A. (1965) Renal artery stenosis, hypertension and polycythaemia. *British Medical Journal*, **i**, 164.

175 ROSSE W.F., WALDMAN T.A. & COHEN P. (1963) Renal cysts, erythropoietin and polycythemia. *American Journal of Medicine*, **34**, 76.

176 ANDERSON E.T. & WALKER B.R. (1969) Polycystic kidney disease, polycythemia, and azotemia. *Journal of the American Medical Association*, **208**, 2472.

177 JONES N.F., PAYNE R.W., HYDE R.D. & PRICE T.M.L. (1960) Renal polycythaemia. *Lancet*, **i**, 299.

178 DAMON A., HOLUB D.A., MELICOW M.M. & USON A.C. (1958) Polycythemia and renal carcinoma. *American Journal of Medicine*, **25**, 182.

179 MURPHY G.P., KENNY G.M. & MIRAND E.A. (1970) Erythropoietin levels in patients with renal tumors or cysts. *Cancer*, **26**, 191.

180 SPERBER M.A. (1969) Malignant renal lesions and erythrocytosis. *British Medical Journal*, i, 51.

181 WU K.K., GIBSON T.P., FREEMAN R.M., BONNEY W.W., FRIED W. & DEGOWIN R.L. (1973) Erythrocytosis after renal transplantation. *Archives of Internal Medicine*, **132**, 898.

182 SWALES J.D. & EVANS D.B. (1969) Erythraemia in renal transplantation. *British Medical Journal*, ii, 80.

183 HOPPIN E.C., DEPNER T., YAMUCHI H. & HOPPER J. (1976) Erythrocytosis associated with diffuse parenchymal lesions of the kidney. *British Journal of Haematology*, **32**, 557.

184 SANKALÉ M., BAO O., SOW A.M. & MEROUEH F. (1969) Les syndromes paranéoplasiques au cours du cancer primitif du foie. *Semaine des Hôpitaux de Paris*, **45**, 279.

185 BROWNSTEIN M.H. & BALLARD H.S. (1966) Hepatoma associated with erythrocytosis: report of eleven new cases. *American Journal of Medicine*, **40**, 204.

186 CALABRESI P. & ABELMANN W.H. (1957) Porto-caval and porto-pulmonary anastomases in Laennec's cirrhosis and in heart failure. *Journal of Clinical Investigation*, **36**, 1257.

187 PLOTZ C.M., KNOWLTON A.I. & RAGAN C. (1952) The natural history of Cushing's syndrome. *American Journal of Medicine*, **11**, 597.

188 NAETS J.P. & WITTEK M. (1968) The mechanism of action of androgens on erythropoiesis. *Annals of the New York Academy of Sciences*, **149**, 366.

189 GARDNER F.H., NATHAN D.G., PIOMELLI S. & CUMMINS J.F. (1968) Further studies on the erythropoietic effects of androgens. *Journal of Laboratory and Clinical Medicine*, **65**, 775.

190 GARDNER F.H., NATHAN D.G., PIOMELLI S. & CUMMINS J.F. (1968) The erythrocythaemic effects of androgen. *British Journal of Haematology*, **14**, 611.

191 SHAHIDI N.T. (1973) Androgens and erythropoiesis. *New England Journal of Medicine*, **289**, 72.

192 WHITCOMB W.H., PESCHLE C., MOORE M., NITSCHKE R. & ADAMSON J.W. (1980) Congenital erythrocytosis: a new form associated with an erythropoietin-dependent mechanism. *British Journal of Haematology*, **44**, 17.

193 DAVIES S.W. (1968) Erythraemia in experimental nephritis. *British Journal of Haematology*, **15**, 237.

194 JEPSON J. & McGARRY E.E. (1968) Polycythemia and increased erythropoietin production in a patient with hypertrophy of the juxta-glomerular apparatus. *Blood*, **32**, 370.

195 NAKAO K., KIMURA K., MIURA Y. & TAKAKU F. (1966) Erythrocytosis associated with carcinoma of the liver (with erythropoietin assay of tumor extract). *American Journal of the Medical Sciences*, **251**, 161.

196 OSSIAS A.L., ZANJANI E.D., ZALUSKY R., SOLOMON E. & WASSERMAN L.R. (1973) Case report: studies on the mechanism of erythrocytosis associated with a uterine fibromyoma. *British Journal of Haematology*, **25**, 179.

197 LAWRENCE J.H. & BERLIN N.I. (1952) Relative polycythemia—the polycythemia of stress. *Yale Journal of Biology and Medicine*, **24**, 498.

198 PRANKERD T.A.J. (1966) Polycythaemia: diagnosis and variants. *Proceedings of the Royal Society of Medicine*, **59**, 1089.

199 EL-YOUSEF M.K. & BAKEWELL W.E. (1972) The Gaisböck syndrome. *Journal of the American Medical Association*, **220**, 864.

200 SMITH J.F.B. & LUCIE N.P. (1973) Alcohol—a cause of stress erythrocytosis? *Lancet*, i, 637.

201 DAVIES S.W., GLYNNE-JONES E. & LEWIS E.P. (1974) Red face and reduced plasma volume. *Journal of Clinical Pathology*, **27**, 109.

202 LETH A. (1970) Changes in plasma and extracellular fluid volumes in patients with essential hypertension during long-term treatment with hydrochlorothiazide. *Circulation*, **XLII**, 479.

203 VELASQUEZ M.T., SCHECHTER G.P., McFARLAND W. & COHN J.N. (1974) Relative polycythaemia: a state of high venous tone. *Clinical Research*, **22**, 409A.

204 GAISBÖCK F. (1905) Die Bedeutung der Blutdruckmessung für die artzliche Praxis. *Deutsche Archive für Klinische Medizin*, **83**, 363.

205 BURGE P.S., JOHNSON W.S. & PRANKERD T.A.J. (1975) Morbidity and mortality in pseudopolycythaemia. *Lancet*, i, 1266.

206 WEINREB N.J. & SHIH C.F. (1975) Spurious polycythemia. *Seminars in Hematology*, **12**, 397.

207 HUMPHREY P.R.D., DU BOULAY G.H., MARSHALL, J., PEARSON T.C., ROSS RUSSELL R.W., SYMON L., WETHERLEY-MEIN G. & ZILKHA E. (1979) Cerebral blood-flow and viscosity in relative polycythaemia. *Lancet*, ii, 873.

208 HUMPHREY P.R.D., MICHAEL J. & PEARSON T.C. (1980) Management of relative polycythaemia: studies of cerebral blood flow and viscosity. *British Journal of Haematology*, **46**, 427.

209 HUMPHREY P.R.D., MICHAEL J. & PEARSON T.C. (1980) Red-cell mass and plasma volume before and after venesection in relative polycythaemia. *British Journal of Haematology*, **46**, 435.

210 TOHGI H., YAMANOUCHI H., MURAKAMI M. & KAMEYAMA M. (1978) Importance of the hematocrit as a risk factor in cerebral infarction. *Stroke*, **9**, 369.

211 KANNEL W.B., GORDON T., WOLF P.A. & McNAMARA P. (1972) Hemoglobin and the risk of cerebral infarction: The Framingham Study. *Stroke*, **3**, 409.

212 PEARSON T.C., RING C.P. & WETHERLEY-MEIN G. (1980) Plasma and whole blood viscosity in treated primary polycythaemia. *Clinical and Laboratory Haematology*, **2**, 73.

213 WEAVER J.P.A., EVANS A. & WALDER D.N. (1969) The effect of increased fibrinogen content on the viscosity of the blood. *Clinical Science*, **36**, 1.

214 SCHMID-SCHÖNBEIN H. (1977) Rheological properties of the blood under normal and pathological conditions. In: *Brain and Heart Infarct* (ed. Zülch K.J., Kaufmann W., Hossmann K.-A. & Hossmann V.), p. 96. Springer-Verlag, Berlin.

215 THOMAS D.J., DU BOULAY G.H., MARSHALL J., PEARSON T.C., ROSS RUSSELL R.W., SYMON L., WETHERLEY-MEIN G. & ZILKHA E. (1977) Cerebral blood-flow in polycythaemia. *Lancet*, ii, 161.

216 THOMAS D.J., DU BOULAY G.H., MARSHALL J., PEARSON T.C., ROSS RUSSELL R.W., SYMON L., WETHERLEY-MEIN G. & ZILKHA E. (1977) Effect of haematocrit on cerebral blood-flow in man. *Lancet*, **ii**, 941.

217 YATES C.J.P., BERENT A., ANDREWS V. & DORMANDY J.A. (1979) Increase in leg blood-flow by normovolaemic haemodilution in intermittent claudication. *Lancet*, **ii**, 166.

218 McLACHLIN A.D., McLACHLIN J.A., JORY T.A. & RAWLING E.G. (1960) Venous stasis in the lower extremities. *Annals of Surgery*, **152**, 678.

219 CLARK C. & COTTON L.T. (1968) Blood-flow in deep veins of leg: recording technique and evaluation of methods to increase flow during operation. *British Journal of Surgery*, **55**, 211.

220 HUMPHREY P.R.D., DU BOULAY G.H., MARSHALL J., PEARSON T.C., ROSS RUSSELL R.W., SLATER N.G.P., SYMON L., WETHERLEY-MEIN G. & ZILKHA E. (1980) Viscosity, cerebral blood flow and haematocrit in patients with paraproteinaemia. *Acta Neurologica Scandinavica*, **61**, 201.

221 BUGLIARELLO G., KAPUR C. & HSIAO G. (1965) The profile viscosity and other characteristics of blood flow in a non-uniform shear field. *Proceedings of the 4th International Congress on Rheology. Interscience, New York*, **4**, 351.

222 PALMER A.A. (1967) Platelet and leucocyte skimming. 4th European Conference on Microcirculation, Cambridge 1966, *Bibliotheca Anatomica*, **9**, 300. Karger, Basel and New York.

223 DINTENFASS L. (1971) *Blood Microrheology—Viscosity Factors in Blood Flow, Ischaemia and Thrombosis*. Butterworth, London.

224 SINGH A.K. & WETHERLEY-MEIN G. (1977) Microvascular occlusive lesions in primary thrombocythaemia. *British Journal of Haematology*, **36**, 553.

225 SZUR L., LEWIS S.M. & GOOLDEN A.W.G. (1959) Polycythaemia vera and its treatment with radioactive phosphorus. *Quarterly Journal of Medicine*, **28**, 397.

226 ADAMS T., SCHUTZ L. & GOLDBERG L. (1974) Platelet function abnormalities in the myeloproliferative disorders. *Scandinavian Journal of Haematology*, **13**, 215.

227 BERGER S., ALEDORT L.M., GILBERT H.S., HANSON, J.P. & WASSERMAN L.R. (1973) Abnormalities of platelet function in patients with polycythemia vera. *Cancer Research*, **33**, 2683.

228 BOUGHTON B.J., CORBETT W.E.N. & GINSBURG A.D. (1977) Myeloproliferative disorders: a paradox of *in vivo* and *in vitro* platelet function. *Journal of Clinical Pathology*, **30**, 228.

229 BOUGHTON B.J., ALLINGTON M.J. & KING A. (1978) Platelets and plasma β-thromboglobulin in myeloproliferative syndromes and secondary thrombocytosis. *British Journal of Haematology*, **40**, 125

230 KWAAN H.C. & SUWANWELA N. (1971) Inhibitors of fibrinolysis in platelets in polycythaemia vera and thrombocytosis. *British Journal of Haematology*, **21**, 313.

231 COOPER B., SCHAFER A.I., PUCHALSKY D. & HANDIN R.I. (1978) Platelet resistance to prostaglandin D_2 in patients with myeloproliferative disorders. *Blood*, **52**, 618.

232 MOLLISON P.L. (1979) *Blood Transfusion in Clinical Medicine*, 6th edn. Blackwell Scientific Publications, Oxford.

233 DACIE J.V. & LEWIS S.M. (1975) *Practical Haematology*, 5th edn. J. & A. Churchill, London.

234 CARTWRIGHT G.E. (1968) *Diagnostic Laboratory Haematology*, 4th edn. Grune & Stratton, New York.

235 MULDOWNEY F.P. (1957) The relationship of total red cell mass to lean body mass in man. *Clinical Science*, **16**, 163.

236 HYDE R.D. & JONES N.F. (1962) Red cell volume and total body water. *British Journal of Haematology*, **8**, 283.

237 RETZLAFF J.A., NEWLON TAUXE W., HIELY J.M. & STROEBEL C.F. (1969) Erythrocyte volume, plasma volume, and lean body mass in adult men and women. *Blood*, **33**, 649.

238 NADLER S.B., HIDLAGO J.U. & BLOCH T. (1962) Prediction of blood volume in normal human adults. *Surgery*, **51**, 224.

239 HUME R. (1966) Prediction of lean body mass from height and weight. *Journal of Clinical Pathology*, **19**, 389.

240 PEARSON T.C., GLASS U.H. & WETHERLEY-MEIN G. (1978) Interpretation of measured red cell mass in the diagnosis of polycythaemia. *Scandinavian Journal of Haematology*, **21**, 153.

241 HURLEY P.J. (1975) Red cell and plasma volumes in normal adults. *Journal of Nuclear Medicine*, **16**, 46.

242 NAJEAN Y. & CACCHIONE R. (1977) Blood volume in health and disease. *Clinics in Hematology*, **6**, 543.

243 BRANDT P.W.T., STEINER R.E., DACIE J.V. & SZUR L. (1963) Incidence of renal lesions in polycythaemia. *British Medical Journal*, **ii**, 468.

244 MODAN B. (1971) *The Polycythemic Disorders*, p. 55. C. C. Thomas, Springfield, Illinois.

245 McREADY V.R. & AHUJA S. (1969) Spleen scanning. *Proceedings of the Royal Society of Medicine*, **62**, 794.

246 BATEMAN S., LEWIS S.M., NICHOLAS A. & ZAAFFRAN A. (1978) Splenic red cell pool in differential diagnosis of polycythaemia. *XVII Congress of the International Society of Hematology—XV Congress of the International Society of Blood Transfusion* (Abstracts) **I**, 338.

247 BLOCK M. & BETHARD W. (1952) Bone marrow studies in polycythemia. *Journal of Clinical Investigation*, **31**, 618.

248 DEN OTTOLANDER G.J., TE VELDE J., BREDEROO, P., GERAEDTS J.P.M., SLEE P.H.T., WILLEMZE R., ZWAAN F.E., HAAK H.L., MULLER H.P. & BIEGER R. (1979) Megakaryoblastic leukaemia (acute myelofibrosis): a report of three cases. *British Journal of Haematology*, **42**, 9.

249 BRANEHÖG I., RIDELL B., SWOLIN B. & WEINFELD A. (1975) Megakaryocyte quantifications in relation to thrombokinetics in primary thrombocythaemia and allied disorders. *Scandinavian Journal of Haematology*, **15**, 321.

250 KASS L. (1973) Enzymatic abnormalities in megakaryocytes. *Acta Haematologica*, **49**, 193.

251 BENSINGER T.A., LOGUE G.L. & RUNDLES R.W. (1970) Hemorrhagic thrombocythemia: control of postsplenectomy thrombocytosis with melphalan. *Blood*, **36**, 61.

252 GLASS U.H. (1961) Platelet function tests in thrombo-

cythaemia. *Journal of Medical and Laboratory Technology*, **18**, 82.

253 McClure P.D., Ingram G.I.C., Stacey R.S., Glass U.H. & Matchett M.O. (1966) Platelet function tests in thrombocythaemia and thrombocytosis. *British Journal of Haematology*, **12**, 478.

254 Spaet T.H., Gaynor E. & Goldstein M.L. (1969) Defective platelets in essential thrombocythemia. *Archives of Internal Medicine*, **124**, 135.

255 Knudsen F.U. & Gormsen J. (1968) Lactate dehydrogenase isoenzymes in thrombocytes in various diseases. *Scandinavian Journal of Haematology*, **5**, 361.

256 Knudsen F.U. & Gormsen J. (1970) Subbands of lactate dehydrogenase isoenzymes in human thrombocytes. *Scandinavian Journal of Haematology*, **7**, 100.

257 Zucker S. & Mielke C.H. (1972) Classification of thrombocytosis based on platelet function tests: correlation with hemorrhagic and thrombotic complications. *Journal of Laboratory and Clinical Medicine*, **80**, 385.

258 Cortelazzo S., Barbui T., Viero P., Bassan R., Dini E. & Ferro Milone F. (1979) Platelet malonyldialdehyde and spontaneous aggregation during ischaemic attacks of patients with polycythaemia vera. *Thrombosis and Haemostasis* (Stuttgart), **42**, 1344.

259 Glass U.H. (1960) *Platelet Function Tests in Thrombocythaemia*. Thesis accepted for Fellowship of the Institute of Medical Laboratory Technology, London.

260 Champion R.H. & Rook A. (1963) Idiopathic thrombocythemia. *Archives of Dermatology*, **87**, 302.

261 Preston F.E., Emmanuel I.G., Winfield D.A. & Malia R.G. (1974) Essential thrombocythaemia and peripheral gangrene. *British Medical Journal*, **iii**, 548.

262 Singer G. (1969) Migrating emboli of retinal arteries in thrombocythaemia. *British Journal of Ophthalmology*, **53**, 279.

263 Preston F.E., Martin J.F., Stewart R.M. & Davies-Jones G.A.B. (1979) Thrombocytosis, circulating platelet aggregates, and neurological dysfunction. *British Medical Journal*, **ii**, 1561.

264 Korenman G. (1969) Neurologic syndromes associated with primary thrombocythemia. *Journal of the Mount Sinai Hospital, N.Y.*, **36**, 317.

265 Simar L.J. & Hughes J. (1969) Ultra-structure des plaquettes dans deux cas de thrombocythémie. *Acta Haematologica* (Basel), **41**, 33.

266 Grimes E. & Wetherley-Mein G. (1971) Marrow chromosome findings in 16 cases of thrombocythaemia. (Unpublished observations.)

267 Silvis E.S., Turkbas N., Swaim W.R. & Doscherholman A. (1969) Thrombocytosis. A clinical evaluation of 322 patients. *Minnesota Medicine*, **52**, 1603.

268 Breslow A., Kaufman R.M. & Lawsky A.R. (1968) The effect of surgery on the concentration of circulating megakaryocytes and platelets. *Blood*, **32**, 393.

269 Silvis S.E., Turkbas N. & Doscherholmen A. (1970) Thrombocytosis in patients with lung cancer. *Journal of the American Medical Association*, **211**, 1852.

270 Levin J. & Conley C.L. (1964) Thrombocytosis associated with malignant disease. *Archives of Internal Medicine*, **114**, 497.

271 Hirsh J. & Dacie J.V. (1966) Persistent post-splenectomy thrombocytosis and thrombo-embolism: a conse-quence of continuing anaemia. *British Journal of Haematology*, **12**, 44.

272 Dawson A.A. & Ogston D. (1969) Exercise-induced thrombocytosis. *Acta Haematologica*, **42**, 241.

273 Eastham R.D. & Morgan E.H. (1969) Thombocytosis induced by citrovorum factor. *Lancet*, **ii**, 1258.

274 Hwang Y.F., Hamilton H.E. & Sheets R.F. (1969) Vinblastine-induced thrombocytosis. *Lancet*, **ii**, 1075.

275 Jackson C.W. & Edwards C.C. (1977) Evidence that stimulation of megakaryocytopoiesis by low dose vincristine results from an effect on platelets. *British Journal of Haematology*, **36**, 97.

276 Morowitz D.A., Allen L.W. & Kirsner J.B. (1968) Thrombocytosis in chronic inflammatory bowel disease. *Annals of Internal Medicine*, **68**, 1013.

277 Jansen E., Hartling O. & Nielsen B. (1970) Colitis ulcerosa og trombocytose. *Ugeskrift für Laeger*, **132**, 2079.

278 Hardisty R.M. & Wolff H.H. (1955) Haemorrhagic thrombocythaemia: a clinical and laboratory study. *British Journal of Haematology*, **1**, 390.

279 Harker L.A. & Finch C.A. (1969) Thrombokinetics in man. *Journal of Clinical Investigation*, **48**, 963.

280 Fountain J.R. (1958) Haemorrhagic thrombocythaemia. Report of two cases treated with radioactive phosphorus. *British Medical Journal*, **ii**, 126.

281 Robertson J.H. (1970) Uracil mustard in the treatment of thombocythemia. *Blood*, **35**, 288.

282 Edgcumbe J.O.P. & Wetherley-Mein G. (1960) Haemorrhagic thrombocythaemia treated with myleran (busulphan). *Proceedings of the VII Congress of the European Society of Haematology, London, 1959*, Part II, p. 324. Karger, Basel.

283 Toolis F. & Paton L. (1979) Massive platelet transfusion after splenectomy in a case of myelofibrosis. *Scandinavian Journal of Haematology*, **23**, 317.

284 Hansen M.S., Christensen B.E. & Jønsson V. (1979) The effect of acetyl salicylic acid and dipyridamole on thromboembolic complications in splenectomized patients with myelofibrosis. *Scandinavian Journal of Haematology*, **23**, 177.

285 Taft E.G., Babcock R.B., Scharfman W.B. & Tartaglia A.P. (1977) Plateletpheresis in the management of thrombocytosis. *Blood*, **50**, 927.

286 Crail H.W., Alt H.L. & Nadler W.H. (1948) Myelofibrosis associated with tuberculosis. A report of four cases. *Blood*, **3**, 1426.

287 Samuelsson S-M., Killander A., Werner I. & Stenkvist B. (1966) Myelofibrosis associated with tuberculous lymphadenitis. *Acta Medica Scandinavica*, Suppl. 445, p. 326.

288 Gralnick H.R., Harbor J. & Vogel C. (1971) Myelofibrosis in chronic granulocytic leukemia. *Blood*, **37**, 152.

289 Buyssens N. & Bourgeois N.H. (1977) Chronic myelocytic leukemia versus idiopathic myelofibrosis. A diagnostic problem in bone marrow biopsies. *Cancer*, **40**, 1548.

290 Clough, V., Geary C.G., Hashmi K., Davson J. & Knowlson T. (1979) Myelofibrosis in chronic granulocytic leukaemia. *British Journal of Haematology*, **42**, 515.

291 Rosenthal D.S. & Moloney W.C. (1969) Myeloid

metaplasia: a study of 98 cases. *Postgraduate Medicine*, **45**, 136.

292 LEONARD B.J., ISRAËLS M.C.G. & WILKINSON J.F. (1957) Myelosclerosis. *Quarterly Journal of Medicine*, **36**, 131.

293 TOBIN M.S., TAN C. & ARGANO S.A.P. (1969) Myelofibrosis in pediatric age group. *New York State Journal of Medicine*, **69**, 1080.

294 LIGUMSKI M., POLLIACK A. & BENBASSAT J. (1978) Nature and incidence of liver involvement in agnogenic myeloid metaplasia. *Scandinavian Journal of Haematology*, **21**, 81.

295 COLKER J.L., BAKER W.G., JR. & KOLODNY M. (1968) Agnogenic myeloid metaplasia with portal hypertension. *Gastrointestinal Endoscopy*, **15**, 70.

296 CHENG D.S. (1979) Idiopathic myelofibrosis without splenomegaly. *Cancer*, **43**, 1761.

297 GARNETT E.S., GODDARD B.A., MARKBY D. & WEBBER C.E. (1969) The spleen as an arteriovenous shunt. *Lancet*, **i**, 386.

298 BOWDLER A.J. (1969) The spleen as an arteriovenous shunt. *Lancet*, **i**, 841.

299 BLENDIS L.M., BANKS D.C., RAMBOER C. & WILLIAMS R. (1970) Spleen blood flow and splanchnic haemodynamics in blood dyscrasia and other splenomegalies. *Clinical Science*, **38**, 73.

300 LICHT A., MANY N. & RACHMILEWITZ E.A. (1973) Myelofibrosis, osteolytic bone lesions and hypercalcemia in chronic myeloid leukemia. *Acta Haematologica* (Basel), **49**, 182.

301 MASON B.A., KRESSEL B.R., CASHDOLLAR M.R., BERNATH A.M. & SCHECHTER G.P. (1979) Periostitis associated with myelofibrosis. *Cancer*, **43**, 1568.

302 PETTIGREW J.D. & WARD H.P. (1969) Correlation of radiologic, histologic and clinical findings in agnogenic myeloid metaplasia. *Radiology*, **93**, 541.

303 HUTT M.S.R., SMITH P., CLARK A.E. & PINNIGER J.L. (1952) The value of rib biopsy in the study of marrow disorders. *Journal of Clinical Pathology*, **5**, 246.

304 THE ASSOCIATION OF CLINICAL PATHOLOGISTS (1960) *The Preparation of Bone for Diagnostic Histology.* Broadsheet No. 29 (New Series).

305 ZAMBERNAND J., BLOCK M., VATTER A. & TRENNER L. (1969) An adaptation of methacrylate embedding for routine histopathological use. *Blood*, **33**, 444.

306 NELSON B. & KNISELEY R.M. (1970) Marrow fibrosis in myeloproliferative disorders. In: *Myeloproliferative Disorders of Animals and Man*, p. 533. United States Atomic Energy Commission, Division of Technical Information Extension, Oak Ridge, Tennessee.

307 BENTLEY S.A. & HERMAN C.J. (1979) Bone marrow fibre production in myelofibrosis: a quantitative study. *British Journal of Haematology*, **42**, 51.

308 VAN SLYCK E.J., WEISS L. & DULLY M. (1970) Chromosomal evidence for the secondary role of fibroblastic proliferation in acute myelofibrosis. *Blood*, **36**, 729.

309 GREENBERG B.R., WILSON F.D., WOO L. & JENKS H.M. (1978) Cytogenetics of fibroblastic colonies in Ph[1]-positive chronic myelogenous leukemia. *Blood*, **51**, 1039.

310 NOWELL P.C. & FINAN J.B. (1978) Cytogenetics of acute and chronic myelofibrosis. *Virchows Archive, Part B, Cell Pathology*, **29**, 45.

311 JACOBSON R.J., SALO A. & FIALKOW P.J. (1978) Agnogenic myeloid metaplasia: a clonal proliferation of hematopoietic stem cells with secondary myelofibrosis. *Blood*, **51**, 189.

312 ADAMSON J.W. & FIALKOW P.J. (1978) Annotation: The pathogenesis of the myeloproliferative syndromes. *British Journal of Haematology*, **38**, 299.

313 MANIATIS A.K., AMSEL S., MITUS W.J. & COLEMAN N. (1969) Chromosome pattern of bone marrow fibroblasts in patients with chronic granulocytic leukaemia. *Nature (London)*, **222**, 1278.

314 DE LA CHAPELLE A., VUOPIO P. & BORGSTRÖM G.H. (1973) The origin of bone marrow fibroblasts. *Blood*, **41**, 783.

315 LEWIS C.M. & PEGRUM G.D. (1978) Immune complexes in myelofibrosis: a possible guide to management. *British Journal of Haematology*, **39**, 233.

316 HOFFBRAND A.V., CHANARIN I., KREMENCHUZKY S., SZUR L., WATERS A.H. & MOLLIN D.L. (1968) Megaloblastic anaemia in myelosclerosis. *Quarterly Journal of Medicine*, **147**, 493.

317 WETHERLEY-MEIN G. (1960) Anaemia in leukaemia and allied disorders. *Proceedings of the VII Congress of the European Society of Haematology, London, 1959.* Part II, p. 231. Karger, Basel.

318 SZUR L. & SMITH M.D. (1961) Red-cell production and destruction in myelosclerosis. *British Journal of Haematology*, **7**, 147.

319 NAJEAN Y., CACCHIONE R., CASTRO-MALASPINA H. & DRESCH C. (1978) Erythrokinetic studies in myelofibrosis: their significance for prognosis. *British Journal of Haematology*, **40**, 205.

320 HANSEN N.E. & KILLMAN S.-AA. (1970) Paroxysmal nocturnal hemoglobinuria in myelofibrosis. *Blood*, **36**, 428.

321 KUO C-Y., VAN VOOLEN G.A. & MORRISON A. (1972) Primary and secondary myelofibrosis: its relationship to 'PNH-like defect'. *Blood*, **40**, 875.

322 JANDL J.H. & ASTER R.H. (1967) Increased splenic pooling and the pathogenesis of hypersplenism. *American Journal of the Medical Sciences*, **253**, 383.

323 MANNONI P., BRACQ C., YVART J. & SALMON C. (1970) Anomalie du functionnement du locus Rh au cours d'une myélofibrose. *Nouvelle Revue française d'Hématologie*, **10**, 381.

324 GOSWITZ F. (1966) Erythrocyte reduced glutathione, glucose-6-phosphate dehydrogenase, and 6-phosphogluconic dehydrogenase in patients with myelofibrosis. *Journal of Laboratory and Clinical Medicine*, **67**, 615.

325 TORELLI U.L., VACCARI G.L. & MAURI C. (1970) Characteristics of the RNA synthesized *in vitro* by human erythroblasts. *Acta Haematologica* (Basel), **43**, 1.

326 KIOSSOGLOU K.A., MITUS W.J. & DAMESHEK W. (1966) Cytogenetic studies in chronic myeloproliferative syndrome. *Blood*, **28**, 241.

327 KIOSSOGLOU K.A., MITUS W.J. & DAMESHEK W. (1965) Chromosomal aberrations in acute leukemia. *Blood*, **26**, 610.

328 BAIKIE A.G., TOUGH I. & WETHERLEY-MEIN G. Peripheral blood chromosomes in myelofibrosis. (Unpublished observations.)

329 CLAYTON D.A. & VINOGRAD J. (1969) Complex mito-

chondrial DNA in leukemic and normal human myeloid cells. *Proceedings of the National Academy of Sciences (USA)*, **62**, 1077.

330 CHERVENICK P.A. (1973) Increase in circulating stem cells in patients with myelofibrosis. *Blood*, **41**, 67.

331 PALMER J.G., EICHWALD E.J., CARTWRIGHT G.E. & WINTROBE M.M. (1953) The experimental production of splenomegaly, anemia and leukopenia in albino rats. *Blood*, **8**, 72.

332 PÉREZ-TAMAYO R., MORA J. & MONFORT I. (1960) Humoral factor(s) in experimental hypersplenism. *Blood*, **16**, 1145.

333 WETHERLEY-MEIN G., JONES N.F. & PULLAN J.M. (1961) Effects of splenectomy on red-cell production in myelofibrosis. *British Medical Journal*, **i**, 84.

334 TUBIANA M., PARMENTIER C., LACOUR J. & MATHÉ G. (1966) Résultats d'explorations isotopiques pratiquées avant et après splenectomie. *Revue française d'Études Cliniques et Biologiques*, **11**, 790.

335 BOWDLER A.J. (1969) Regional variations in the proportion of red cells in the blood in man. *British Journal of Haematology*, **16**, 557.

336 DONALDSON G.W.K., McARTHUR M., MacPHERSON A.I.S. & RICHMOND J. (1970) Blood volume changes in splenomegaly. *British Journal of Haematology*, **18**, 45.

337 RICHMOND J., DONALDSON G.W.K., WILLIAMS R., HAMILTON P. & HUTT M.S.R. (1967) Haematological effects of the idiopathic splenomegaly seen in Uganda. *British Journal of Haematology*, **13**, 348.

338 BLENDIS L.M., CLARKE M.M. & WILLIAMS R. (1969) Effect of splenectomy on the haemodilutional anaemia of splenomegaly. *Lancet*, **i**, 795.

339 PRYOR D.S. (1967) The mechanism of anaemia in tropical splenomegaly. *Quarterly Journal of Medicine*, **36**, 337.

340 BOWDLER A.J. (1963) Dilution anemia corrected by splenectomy in Gaucher's disease. *Annals of Internal Medicine*, **58**, 664.

341 WEINSTEIN V.F. (1964) Haemodilution anaemia associated with simple splenic hyperplasia. *Lancet*, **ii**, 218.

342 PENNY R., ROZENBERG M.C. & FIRKIN B.G. (1966) The splenic platelet pool. *Blood*, **27**, 1.

343 HARKER L.A. (1970) Platelet production. *New England Journal of Medicine*, **282**, 492.

344 BRANEHOG I., WEINFELD A. & ROOS B. (1973) The exchangeable splenic platelet pool studied with epinephrine infusion in idiopathic thrombocytopenic purpura and in patients with splenomegaly. *British Journal of Haematology*, **25**, 239.

345 WETHERLEY-MEIN G., HUTT M.S.R., LANGMEAD W.A. & HILL M.J. (1956) Radioactive iron studies in routine haematological practice. *British Medical Journal*, **ii**, 1445.

346 HUTT M.S.R., JONES N.F. & WETHERLEY-MEIN G. (1960) Radioactive iron studies in myelofibrosis and chronic myeloid leukaemia. *Proceedings of the VII Congress of the European Society of Haematology, London, 1959*, Part II, p. 581. Karger, Basel.

347 TAVASSOLI T. & WEISS L. (1973) An electron microscopic study of spleen in myelofibrosis with myeloid metaplasia. *Blood*, **42**, 267.

348 MILNER G.R., GEARY C.G., WADSWORTH D.L. & DOSS A. (1973) Erythrokinetic studies as a guide to the value of splenectomy in primary myeloid metaplasia. *British Journal of Haematology*, **23**, 467.

349 POLLIACK A. & ROSENMANN E. (1969) Extramedullary hematopoietic tumors of the cranial dura mata. *Acta Haematologica* (Basel), **41**, 43.

350 WETHERLEY-MEIN G. Renal involvement in myelofibrosis. (Unpublished observations.)

351 GRIFFITHS W.J. & FITZPATRICK M. (1967) The effect of age on the creatine in red cells. *British Journal of Haematology*, **13**, 175.

352 RITZMANN S.E., STOUFFLET E.J., HOUSTON E.W. & LEVIN W.C. (1966) Coexistent chronic myelocytic leukemia, monoclonal gammopathy and multiple chromosomal abnormalities. *American Journal of Medicine*, **41**, 981.

353 HOBBS J.R. (1969) Paraproteins. *Proceedings of the Royal Society of Medicine*, **62**, 773.

354 DIBELLA N.J. & BROWN G.L. (1978) Immunologic dysfunction in the myeloproliferative disorders. *Cancer*, **42**, 149.

355 SELROOS O., SKRIFVARS B. & WASASTJERNA C. (1973) Immunological deficiency in myelofibrosis. *Scandinavian Journal of Haematology*, **11**, 307.

356 SILVERSTEIN M.N. & LINMAN J.W. (1969) Causes of death in agnogenic myeloid metaplasia. *Mayo Clinic Proceedings*, **44**, 36.

357 EMBERGER J.M., WAGNER A. & IZARN P. (1969) La terminaison en leucémie aigue de l'osteomyelofibrose avec metaplasie myeloide hepato-splenique. *Nouvelle Revue française d'Hématologie*, **9**, 375.

358 BENTLEY S.A., MURRAY K.H., LEWIS S.M. & ROBERTS P.D. (1977) Erythroid hypoplasia in myelofibrosis: a feature associated with blastic transformation. *British Journal of Haematology*, **36**, 41.

359 McCREDIE K.B. (1969) Oxymetholone in refractory anaemia. *British Journal of Haematology*, **17**, 265.

360 HUTT M.S.R., PINNIGER J.L. & WETHERLEY-MEIN G. (1958) Splenectomy in myelofibrosis. *Proceedings of the International Society of Hematology*. Grune & Stratton, New York.

361 BENBASSAT J., PENCHAS S. & LIGUMSKI M. (1979) Splenectomy in patients with agnogenic myeloid metaplasia: an analysis of 321 published cases. *British Journal of Haematology*, **42**, 207.

362 MULDER H., STEENBERGEN J. & HAANEN C. (1977) Clinical course and survival after elective splenectomy in 19 patients with primary myelofibrosis. *British Journal of Haematology*, **35**, 419.

363 LINMAN J.W. & BAGBY G.C., JR. (1978) The preleukemic syndrome (hemopoietic dysplasia). *Cancer*, **42**, 854.

364 ALTER B.P., POTTER N.U. & LI F.P. (1978) Classification and aetiology of the aplastic anaemias. *Clinics in Haematology*, **7**, 431.

365 LEWIS S.M. (1979) Dyserythropoiesis in aplastic anaemia. In: *Aplastic Anaemia* (ed. Geary C.G.), p. 82. Baillière Tindall, London.

366 HAST R. & REIZENSTEIN P. (1977) Studies on human preleukaemia. I. Erythroblast and iron kinetics in aregenerative anaemia with hypercellular bone marrow. *Scandinavian Journal of Haematology*, **19**, 347.

367 MILNER G.R. & GEARY C.G. (1979) The aplasia-leukaemia syndrome. In: *Aplastic Anaemia* (ed. Geary C.G.), p. 230. Baillière Tindall, London.

368 DAMESHEK W. (1969) The Di Guglielmo Syndrome revisited. *Blood*, **34**, 567.

369 DREYFUS B. (1976) Preleukemic states. I. Definition and classification. II. Refractory anemia with an excess of myeloblasts in the bone marrow (smouldering acute leukemia). *Blood Cells*, **7**, 33.

370 FAILLE A., DRESCH C., POIRIER O., BALITRAND N. & NAJEAN Y. (1978) Prognostic value of *in vitro* bone marrow culture in refractory anaemia with excess of myeloblasts. *Scandinavian Journal of Haematology*, **20**, 280.

371 LEWIS S.M. & SZUR L. (1963) Malignant myelosclerosis. *British Medical Journal*, **ii**, 472.

372 BRETON GORIUS J.B., DANIEL M.T., FLANDRIN G. & DENOEL G.K. (1973) Fine structure and peroxidase activity of circulating micromegakaryoblasts and platelets in a case of acute myelofibrosis. *British Journal of Haematology*, **25**, 331.

373 MANOHARAN A. & ISLAM A. (1979) Acute megakaryoblastic leukaemia or acute myelofibrosis? *British Journal of Haematology*, **42**, 157.

374 ROJER R.A., MULDER N.H. & NIEWEG H.O. (1978) 'Classic' and 'acute' myelofibrosis. A retrospective study. *Acta Haematologica* (Basel), **60**, 108.

375 WHANG-PENG J., KNUTSEN T., O'DONNELL J.F. & BRERETON H.D. (1979) Acute non-lymphocytic leukemia and acute myeloproliferative syndrome following radiation therapy for non-Hodgkin's lymphoma and chronic lymphocytic leukemia. Cytogenetic studies. *Cancer*, **44**, 1592.

376 ALI N.A. & JANES W.O. (1979) Malignant myelosclerosis (acute myelofibrosis). Report of two cases following cytotoxic chemotherapy. *Cancer*, **43**, 1211.

377 MITUS W.J., COLEMAN N. & KIOSSOGLOU K.A. (1969) Abnormal (marker) chromosomes in two patients with acute myelofibrosis. *Archives of Internal Medicine*, **123**, 192.

378 NOWELL P., JENSEN J., GARDNER F., MURPHY S., CHANGANTI R.S.K. & GERMAN J. (1976) Chromosome studies in 'Preleukemia'. III. Myelofibrosis. *Cancer*, **38**, 1873.

379 HAYHOE F.G.J. (1957) Diagnostic and nosological problems at the borderline of leukemia. In: *The Leukemias: Etiology, Pathophysiology and Treatment* (ed.

Rebuck J.W., Bethell F.H. & Monto R.W.). Academic Press, New York.

380 PEGRUM G.D. & RISDON R.A. (1970) The haematological and histological findings in 18 patients with clinical features resembling those of myelofibrosis. *British Journal of Haematology*, **18**, 475.

381 MODAN B., KALLNER H., ZEMER D. & YORAN C. (1971) A note on the increased risk of polycythemia vera in Jews. *Blood*, **37**, 172.

382 ANDERSON R.E., YAMAMOTO T., YAMADA A. & WILL D.W. (1964) Autopsy study of leukaemia in Hiroshima. *Archives of Pathology*, **78**, 618.

383 ANDERSON R.E., HOSHINO T. & YAMAMOTO T. (1964) Myelofibrosis with myeloid metaplasia in survivors of the atomic bomb in Hiroshima. *Annals of Internal Medicine*, **60**, 1.

384 ANDERSON R.E. & YAMAMOTO T. (1970) Myeloproliferative disorders in atomic bomb survivors. In: *Myeloproliferative Disorders of Animals and Man*. United States Atomic Energy Commission, Division of Technical Information Extension, Oak Ridge, Tennessee.

385 GIRARD R. & REVOL L. (1970) La frequence d'une exposition benzenique au cours des hemopathies graves. *Nouvelle Revue française d'Hématologie*, **10**, 477.

386 VAN DEN BERGHE H., LOUWAGIE A., BROECKAERT-VAN ORSHOVEN A., DAVID G. & VERWILGHEN R. (1979) Chromosome analysis in two unusual malignant blood disorders presumably induced by benzene. *Blood*, **53**, 558.

387 ADAMSON J.W., STAMATOYANNOPOULOS G., KONTRAS S., LASCARI A. & DETTER J. (1973) Recessive familial erythrocytosis: aspects of marrow regulation in two families. *Blood*, **41**, 641.

388 WETHERLEY-MEIN G., EPSTEIN I.S., FOSTER W.D. & GRIMES A.J. (1958) Mechanisms of anaemia in leukaemia. *British Journal of Haematology*, **4**, 281.

389 ZANJANI E.D. (1976) Hematopoietic factors in polycythemia vera. *Seminars in Hematology*, **13**, 1.

390 BERK P.D., GOLDBERG J.D., SILVERSTEIN N., WEINFELD A., DONOVAN P.B., ELLIS J.T., LANDAW S.A., LAZLO J., NAJEAN Y., PISCIOTTA A.V. & WASSERMAN L.R. (1981) Increased incidence of acute leukemia in polycythemia vera associated with chlorambucil therapy. *New England Journal of Medicine*, **304**, 441.

SECTION 6
THE BLOOD IN SYSTEMIC DISEASE

Chapter 33
The haematological manifestations of systemic disease

C. BUNCH AND D. J. WEATHERALL

THE HAEMATOLOGICAL MANIFESTATIONS OF SYSTEMIC DISEASE

One of the greatest fascinations and occasional frustrations of haematology is that it encroaches on practically all branches of medicine. Indeed, there can be few diseases which do not produce some alteration in the blood. In this chapter some of the general systemic diseases which produce well-defined haematological changes are reviewed. Many of these topics have been discussed in detail elsewhere in this book but are briefly discussed here in order to present a relatively complete picture of the blood changes in this important group of conditions.

THE ANAEMIA OF CHRONIC DISORDERS

A refractory anaemia accompanies a wide variety of conditions such as infection, malignancy, rheumatoid arthritis, collagen-vascular disease and similar disorders. The haematological and ferrokinetic characteristics which accompany these diverse conditions have so much in common as to suggest a common pathophysiology [1–3], and this is reflected in the now widely used term 'anaemia of chronic disorders'. In their classical review, however, Cartwright & Lee [3] pointed out that this term should not be taken to describe all possible mechanisms of anaemia in chronic disease, and have suggested the cumbersome though more descriptive *sideropenic anemia with reticuloendothelial siderosis.*

The condition is characterized by a mild normochromic normocytic anaemia; on occasions the red-cell indices may be slightly hypochromic and microcytic, though usually not so strikingly as in iron-deficiency anaemia of similar degree. The haemoglobin falls progressively over the first month or two of illness, levelling out between 8 and 12 g/dl. Within these limits the degree of anaemia reflects the activity of the underlying condition as judged by the presence of fever, inflammation or a raised erythrocyte sedimentation rate. The anaemia may on occasion be found in association with a localized neoplasm, and does not necessarily indicate spread of the disease. On the other hand, a haemoglobin level of much less than 8 g/dl should suggest the presence of some other complication.

The diagnosis of this condition can be made by serum iron and total iron binding capacity (TIBC) estimations together with an examination of the distribution of iron in the bone marrow. The main diagnostic criteria are summarized in Table 33.1. The characteristic findings are a reduced serum iron level and iron-binding capacity so that the percentage saturation of the TIBC is relatively normal. There are usually normal or increased amounts of storage iron in the marrow but a marked decrease in the number of red-cell precursors which contain iron granules. In other words, there is adequate iron in the marrow stores but it does not appear to be transported normally to the erythroblasts. Additional findings are in increased concentration of plasma copper and red-cell protoporphyrin.

Pathophysiology
Various factors contribute to the development of this anaemia. There is a moderate shortening of the red-cell lifespan, which cross-transfusion experiments have shown to be due to an extracorpuscular defect. The cause of this is unknown, but it has been suggested that there is an increase in reticuloendothelial activity as part of the general defence mechanism, which results in premature destruction of circulating erythrocytes. The degree of haemolysis is slight and well within the capacity of normal marrow to compensate, indicating that the marrow response is impaired. It has been suggested that the anaemia might be an adaptive response to reduced tissue oxygen demand, but many of the underlying conditions are associated with increased metabolic activity such as fever and weight loss. Furthermore, 2,3-DPG levels and P_{50} estimations indicate that oxygen transport is in fact increased appropriate to the degree of anaemia (Chapter 4) [4]. Erythropoietin production in response to the anaemia

Table 33.1. Laboratory findings in the anaemia of chronic disorders (from Cartwright & Lee [3])

Determination	Normal subjects	Chronic disease
Plasma iron (μg/dl)	100 (70–150)	30 (10–70)
Total iron-binding capacity (μg/dl)	350 (300–400)	200 (100–300)
Transferrin saturation (%)	30 (25–50)	15 (10–25)
Sideroblasts (%)	40 (30–50)	10 (5–20)
Reticulo-endothelial iron	2+ (1 to 2+)	3+ (2 to 6+)
Plasma copper (μg/dl)	114 (81–147)	191 (118–267)
Free erythrocyte protoporphyrin (μg/dl)	36 (14–79)	180 (36–634)

has been extensively studied with conflicting results [4–11] though serum and urinary erythropoietin or ESF levels are generally less than would be expected for the degree of anaemia. The variability may in part reflect difficulties associated with the assay of erythropoietin. Indirect support for a degree of erythropoietin lack comes from observations that administration of cobalt, which increases erythropoietin production, improves the anaemia to some extent. Zucker and colleagues [10, 11] have suggested that the marrow response to erythropoietin is normal in the anaemia of infection or inflammation, but is reduced in the anaemia of malignancy, particularly when there is marrow involvement. However, these results are questionable as their patients had a variety of different malignancies and some had received radiotherapy or cytotoxic drugs before study.

There is much evidence to suggest that a major factor in the pathogenesis of the anaemia of chronic disorders is a 'block' in the movement of iron from reticulo-endothelial stores to the developing erythroblasts. The condition is characterized by a reduced serum iron, transferrin and transferrin saturation with a demonstrable increase in marrow storage iron and a decrease in iron staining of developing erythroblasts. In addition, serum ferritin levels are elevated unless there is concomitant iron deficiency [12–14]. The erythroblasts have an intact haem synthetic pathway [15] and produce increased amounts of protoporphyrin, as in iron deficiency. Ferrokinetic studies show an increased plasma iron turnover and utilization of transferrin-bound iron [16] but a decreased utilization of iron from damaged erythrocytes [17] in keeping with the concept of a 'block' in iron release. The serum iron level falls rapidly following the onset of inflammation [1, 18], and the levels found in this condition would themselves tend to limit the erythropoietic response of the marrow [19]. The fall in serum iron is preceeded by an increase in ferritin synthesis by the liver and spleen [20] which parallels the production of the 'acute-phase' reactants such as haptoglobins, and there is also a marked increase in the synthesis of ferritin from iron released by heat-damaged erythrocytes [21, 22]. It is thus clear that iron metabolism is severely disturbed in inflammatory disorders, with a shift of iron into ferritin and away from the developing erythroid cells.

In summary, there appear to be at least three different mechanisms contributing to this anaemia—a moderately shortened red-cell lifespan, impaired erythropoietin response, and a block in the flow of iron from reticulo-endothelial cells to developing erythroblasts. However, the clinical importance of the anaemia of chronic disorders is that it be recognized as such. Although it occurs in a wide variety of conditions, it presents a broadly uniform picture, and the relative importance of these pathogenetic mechanisms is not known. Indeed it may vary between patients or depend on the nature of the underlying illness. In conditions such as cancer and rheumatoid arthritis, where blood loss may complicate the picture, iron deficiency may coincide with anaemia of chronic disorders. This can be difficult to sort out, but examination of marrow iron stores and estimation of serum ferritin may be useful [12–14]. A suboptimal response to iron may be expected in this situation unless the underlying condition can be corrected, and this may be one way in which the anaemia of chronic disorders first comes to light.

Treatment

The anaemia only improves after treatment of the underlying disorder. It can be partly corrected in man and in experimental animals by the administration of cobalt or erythropoietin. Unfortunately, the former causes unacceptable side-effects whilst the latter is not yet available in sufficient quantities for clinical use.

MALIGNANT DISEASE

There are few malignant disorders which are not associated with changes in the blood at some time during their course; indeed, haematological complications may be the presenting features of the illness. Some of the protean haematological abnormalities associated with carcinoma and the reticuloses are summarized in Table 33.2. Many of these features have been reviewed elsewhere in this book but are briefly summarized here as it is important that the haematologist be aware of the blood changes in malignant disease, and recognizes that they may mimic practically any primary haematological disorder. The blood changes in the leukaemias and lymphomas are considered in detail elsewhere (Chapters 22–24).

By far the commonest haematological finding in malignancy is the anaemia of chronic disorders described above. It may occur in the presence of localized or widespread disease and is frequently associated with an elevated erythrocyte sedimentation rate. This type of anaemia is found in association with practically every type of carcinoma and reticulosis; as one would expect it is refractory to haematinics, but it may respond to successful removal or treatment of the tumour. The various pathogenetic factors contributing to the development of this anaemia have already been discussed.

The anaemia of many patients with carcinoma, particularly of the gastro-intestinal tract, may be complicated by chronic blood loss and superimposed iron deficiency. The development of an iron-deficiency anaemia in middle to later life without overt nutritional cause should always suggest the possibility of an occult neoplasm of the caecum or ascending colon. One should be equally suspicious when an apparently straightforward iron-deficiency anaemia fails to respond completely to iron therapy because of the presence of an underlying malignancy. In occasional patients with splenomegaly or very large tumour

Table 33.2. Principal haematological changes in malignant disorders

Haematological changes	Type (or site) of malignancy
Erythrocytes	
Anaemia of chronic disorders	All forms
Iron deficiency	Gastro-intestinal; cervix, uterus
Leucoerythroblastic anaemia	Stomach, breast, thyroid, prostate, bronchus, kidney
Microangiopathic haemolytic anaemia	Mucin-secreting tumours; stomach
Secondary myelosclerosis	As for leucoerythroblastic; also reticuloses
Selective red-cell aplasia	Thymus, lymphoma, bronchus
Immune haemolytic anaemia	Ovary; lymphoma
Megaloblastic anaemia	Myeloma; rarely others
Sideroblastic anaemia	All forms; myeloproliferative disorders
Polycythaemia	Kidney, liver, posterior fossa, uterus
Leucocytes	
Leucocytosis	All forms
Leukaemoid reactions	As for leucoerythroblastic anaemia
Eosinophilia	Miscellaneous carcinoma and reticuloses
Monocytosis	All forms
Basophilia	Myeloproliferative disease; mastocytosis
Lymphopenia	Carcinoma, reticulosis
Platelets	
Thrombocytosis	Gastro-intestinal with bleeding; bronchus and others without bleeding
Thrombocytopenia	As for the microangiopathies
Acquired thrombocytopathy	Macroglobulinaemia; other paraproteinaemias
Coagulation	
Disseminated intravascular coagulation	Prostate, many others
Primary activation of fibrinolysis	Prostate
Thrombophlebitis	All forms
Miscellaneous	
Abnormal proteins—cryofibrinogens	Prostate, others
Fetal proteins	α-feto protein—liver and others
	Carcino-embryonic antigen (CEA)—gastro-intestinal neoplasms
	Fetal haemoglobin—leukaemia, other tumours
Circulating tumour cells	All forms
Effects of cytotoxic drugs	All forms

masses the anaemia may also be complicated by haemodilution.

Disseminated malignancy

Disseminated malignancy may produce a number of striking haematological pictures in addition to the more straightforward anaemias described above. The commonest abnormalities are leucoerythroblastic or leukaemoid blood pictures, and the spectrum of microangiopathic haemolytic anaemia and disseminated intravascular coagulation.

A leucoerythroblastic picture is characterized by the appearance in the blood of immature myeloid cells together with some nucleated red cells and usually a reticulocytosis. Anaemia is usual but not invariable. The red cells show a moderate degree of anisocytosis and poikilocytosis, and there may be some tear-drop forms. The total leucocyte and platelet counts are variable; occasionally the leucocyte count may be greatly increased, producing a 'leukaemoid' picture. Distinction from chronic myeloid leukaemia can be made by the finding of a raised leucocyte alkaline phosphatase and the absence of the Philadelphia

chromosome. A leucoerythroblastic picture is generally considered to be pathognomonic of marrow infiltration, but this is not always the case, and other mechanisms may be responsible [23]. Disseminated tuberculosis was once the commonest cause of a leucoerythroblastic picture, and this fact is reflected in the North American term *myelophthisic anemia*, though nowadays such infiltrations are usually malignant [23]. The carcinomas which most commonly metastasize to the marrow are those of prostate, breast and stomach, although almost any type of cancer may be responsible. The picture may sometimes be difficult to distinguish from a primary myeloproliferative disorder such as myelofibrosis or chronic myeloid leukaemia, particularly if the primary tumour is occult. Splenomegaly is sometimes seen in association with disseminated carcinoma, but it is only rarely marked [24] and gross splenomegaly should suggest a myeloproliferative disorder. Localized bone pain, radiological lytic areas and hypercalcaemia are all suggestive of malignancy. The diagnosis of metastasizing carcinoma can often be made by marrow examination, but carcinomatosis can produce a surprising degree of

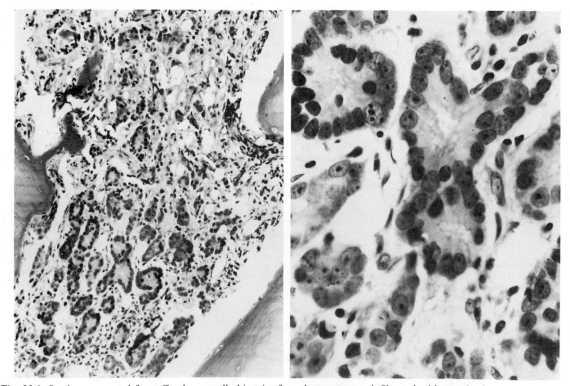

Fig. 33.1. Sections prepared from Gardner-needle biopsies from bone marrow infiltrated with neoplastic cells; the primary tumour was in the prostate (H. & E. Stain): (a) ×230; (b) ×920. (Prepared by Dr George MacDonald.)

fibrosis, and the success rate is variable [25] (Fig. 33.1). There is no doubt that a marrow trephine biopsy produces a higher yield than routine marrow aspiration smears, but the choice of site is often important. Prior localization by palpation for tender areas of the skeleton is helpful, and multiple biopsies may be necessary. Recent advances in radioisotope imaging techniques have made the bone-marrow scan a most useful tool in this difficult diagnostic area. An example of the use of technetium-99m sulphur colloid for this purpose is illustrated in Figure 33.2.

The association between disseminated carcinoma and microangiopathic haemolytic anaemia is well established [26–30], and this is probably the commonest form of frank haemolysis in patients with malignancy. In most cases the tumour is a mucin-secreting adenocarcinoma, usually of stomach, although there have been a few well-documented reports of this type of anaemia in association with disseminated mucin-secreting tumours of the ovary, lung and breast [29]. The clinical picture is typically that of a microangiopathic process as described in Chapter 29. Examination of the peripheral blood reveals striking anisocytosis and poikilocytosis together with red-cell fragmentation (schizocytes) and a reticulocytosis. Indeed it is likely that the poikilocytosis that has been frequently noted in association with cancer [31] is the result of a microangiopathic process. In some cases the haemolytic anaemia is found together with haemorrhagic phenomena characteristic of disseminated intravascular coagulation. There is a variable degree of thrombocytopenia with an increase in the rate of fibrinogen turnover and elevated levels of fibrin-degradation products (FDPs).

It has been suggested that this complication develops secondarily to intravascular coagulation brought about by thromboplastins liberated from the mucin-secreting cells which have gained access to the circulation [29, 32]. Additional erythrocyte damage may be caused by contact between circulating red cells and tumour emboli within small vessels [33], particularly within the lung where vascular changes have been noted in relation to tumour emboli [30].

Other forms of anaemia associated with malignancy

Autoimmune haemolytic anaemia. Immune haemolytic anaemia, either of the 'warm' or 'cold' antibody type, is not infrequently found in association with the reticuloses and chronic lymphatic leukaemia; these conditions have been fully described in Chapters 23 and 24. Immune haemolysis occurs rarely in other forms of malignancy; the classical association is with tumours of the ovary [34], but there have been reports of autoimmune haemolysis occurring in a wide variety

of tumours including lung, stomach, breast, kidney, cervix, colon and testis [35]. Most of the patients have been elderly, and many have presented with symptoms of anaemia. In most instances the antibody has not been characterized, but anti-Kell, anti-E and anti-c have each been reported. In one recent report four patients with different non-haematological malignancies were reported with haemolytic anaemia due to cold agglutinins of anti-I specificity [36]. In some patients, removal of the tumour has been associated with cessation of haemolysis, improvement in the anaemia and reversion of the Coombs' test. The pathogenesis of autoimmune haemolysis complicating these tumours is not fully understood. In one report of haemolysis associated with an ovarian teratoma, antibody was found within the cyst fluid in concentrations ten times that of the serum, and it was suggested that the tumour itself (which contained lymphoid tissue) was responsible for the antibody production [37]. Alternative mechanisms have been suggested in other instances. For example, the tumour may produce substances which alter the red cell surface to render it antigenic, or it may induce the production of antibodies which cross-react with the red cells [38].

Selective red-cell aplasia. The association of selective red-cell aplasia with tumours of the thymus [39] has been fully described in Chapter 31. In addition there have been rare reports of red-cell aplasia occurring with other neoplasms including carcinoma of the bronchus [40] and the reticuloses [39].

Megaloblastic anaemia. The relationship between malignant disorders and vitamin B_{12} and folic-acid metabolism has been described in Chapter 6 and reviewed by Chanarin in his monograph on megaloblastic anaemia [41]. There have been many reports of megaloblastic anaemia in patients with malignancy, in most cases due to folate deficiency [42, 43]. The factors which lead to folate deficiency in these patients are complex and include such mechanisms as reduced intake, malabsorption and increased utilization by the tumour mass. Myelomatosis is particularly associated with an increased folic-acid turnover [42, 44]. There have been conflicting reports of the overall incidence of folic-acid deficiency in patients with malignancy and although serum folate levels are often reduced, red-cell levels are usually normal. In one series, whole blood folate levels were reduced in 22% of patients with disseminated disease but in only 2·5% of patients with localized disease [43].

The relationship between vitamin-B_{12} deficiency and gastric carcinoma is discussed in Chapter 6. High serum vitamin-B_{12} levels are occasionally seen in patients with hepatic metastases.

Sideroblastic anaemia. The sideroblastic anaemias have been reviewed in Chapter 5. There is a well-established relationship between sideroblastic anaemia and carcinoma [45]; thus Mollin & Hoffbrand studied 62 patients with secondary sideroblastic anaemia and found underlying malignancy in 10 [45]. Clearly any patient presenting with sideroblastic anaemia should be carefully screened for an associated malignancy. The relationship between sideroblastic anaemia and the myeloproliferative disorders and leukaemia is discussed in Chapter 13.

Polycythaemia

The polycythaemias secondary to malignant disease have been reviewed in Chapter 32. Very occasionally in clinical practice a patient with polycythaemia is encountered in whom there is an underlying neoplasm [46]. This association has been found in patients with a hypernephroma [47], Wilms' tumour [48], solitary cysts of the kidney [49] and polycystic kidney disease. It has also been found in patients with hepatomas [50],

hamartomas of the liver [51], myxomas, uterine fibroids [52], vascular tumours of the cerebellum [53] and carcinoma of the lung [54]. In some cases increased amounts of erythropoietin have been found, either in the plasma and urine or in the tumour or cyst. This type of secondary polycythaemia must be clearly differentiated from that due to hypoxia and the other causes of secondary polycythaemia as outlined in Chapter 32. It should be pointed out that in clinical practice polycythaemia secondary to neoplasia is extremely uncommon and that this rare group makes up less than one per cent of all secondary polycythaemias.

Abnormalities of the platelets and blood coagulation

Quantitative abnormalities of the platelets are not uncommon in patients with malignant disorders. While a thrombocytosis may often be associated with chronic gastro-intestinal blood loss secondary to carcinoma, there is good evidence that malignancy—even in the absence of blood loss—may result in a high

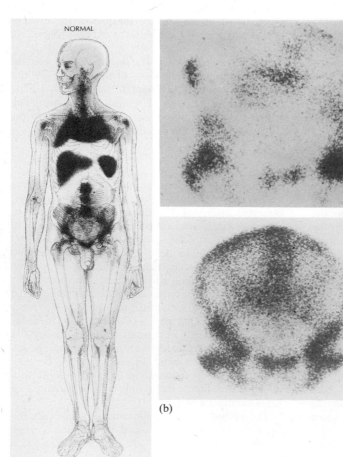

(a)

(b)

Fig. 33.2. The demonstration of tumour deposits in the bone marrow and liver by scanning with radioactive colloids (^{99m}Tc-S-colloid). (a) Normal distribution of RES marrow activity in the axial bones and proximal parts of the humeri and femora. (b) (top) Normal pelvis; (bottom) a pelvis of a patient with Hodgkin's disease. (c) On following page.

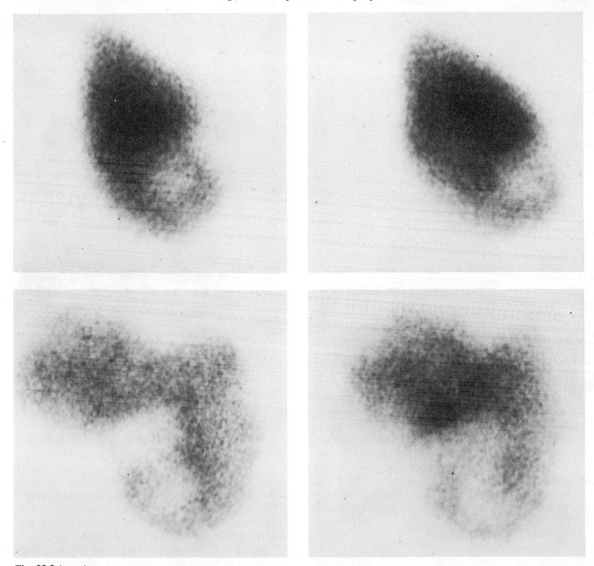

Fig. 33.2 (*cont.*)
(c) Views of the liver scan showing multiple metastatic lesions: (upper left) anterior; (upper right) anterior oblique; (lower left) posterior; (lower right) posterior oblique. (By courtesy of Dr P. McIntyre and editors of *Hospital Practice* and *Johns Hopkins Medical Journal*.)

platelet count [55–57]. Thus an elevated platelet count was found in 60% of 153 patients with bronchial carcinoma [56] and similar findings have been noted in association with other tumours. In fact the finding of an increased number of platelets on a peripheral blood film, or a raised platelet count, may be the first indication of an underlying neoplasm. In one platelet kinetic study, platelet lifespan was slightly reduced but platelet turnover was increased two- to fourfold suggesting that the thrombocytosis is due to an increased production of platelets [57]. Thombocyto-

penia is a less frequent finding in patients with carcinoma except as part of the disseminated intravascular coagulation syndrome or secondary myelosclerosis. Acquired functional thrombocytopathies have been observed in those malignancies in which paraproteins are produced, particularly myelomatosis and macroglobulinaemia.

Generalized haemostatic failure is a very well recognized complication of malignant disease (Fig. 33.3). Although particularly associated with disseminated carcinoma of the prostate it has been well documented

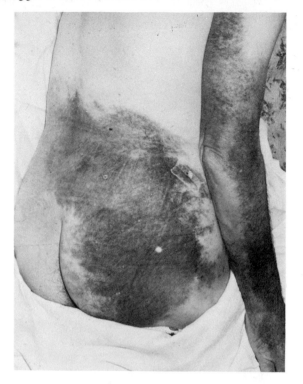

Fig. 33.3. Disseminated intravascular coagulation in association with disseminated carcinoma of the prostate. The patient started to bleed extensively from the iliac-crest marrow biopsy site and from venesection sites. The bleeding was controlled with replacement therapy and heparin and the condition gradually improved with the use of massive doses of oestrogens. The patient was symptom-free and well six months later. Marrow biopsy showed widespread tumour metastasis.

in patients with tumours of the gastro-intestinal tract and lung. It may result from disseminated intravascular coagulation or primary activation of fibrinolysis. The clinical and laboratory findings in these disorders are fully described in Chapter 29. A migrating thrombophlebitis is also a well-recognized accompaniment of carcinoma and may precede the presentation of the primary tumour by several months. It is possible that this is associated with chronic intravascular coagulation.

Leucocyte abnormalities
A variety of changes in the total or differential leucocyte counts may occur in association with carcinoma or other malignant tumours. While the leukaemoid reactions described earlier in the chapter are rare, a persistent neutrophil leucocytosis is not uncommon. The mechanism is unknown, but it is tempting to think that at least in some instances the tumour might produce substances which stimulate granulopoiesis. Human lung tissue is known to elaborate colony-stimulating activity (Chapter 2), and in one recent report tumour cells from a patient with a poorly differentiated squamous cell carcinoma of the lung who had developed a mild neutrophilia were transplanted into nude mice. Growth of the tumour was associated with the development of neutrophilia in the

recipient mice, and the tumour cells were shown to produce human granulopoietic colony-stimulating activity [58].

A monocytosis is also a well-documented finding in patients with carcinoma. Thus in a group of 100 such patients, 62% had an absolute monocyte count of more than 5×10^9/l and 21% more than 10×10^9/l; this was a highly significant increase over a well-matched control series [59]. Monocytosis also occurs in association with Hodgkin's disease and the myeloproliferative disorders. While an absolute eosinophilia is also a well-recognized feature in some cases of Hodgkin's disease, it is found less commonly with carcinoma. However, well-documented cases of eosinophilia in association with ovarian neoplasms and disseminated malignancies of other types, particularly involving the pancreas, stomach and breast, have been reported [60]. More recently, eosinophilia has been recognized as a complication of carcinoma of the lung. In one report of extreme eosinophilia associated with an anaplastic large cell carcinoma of the lung, the tumour itself was found to be infiltrated with eosinophils and a substance was isolated from the tumour which was indistinguishable from the eosinophilic chemotactic factor of anaphylaxis (Chapter 15) [61]. Further reports of the association between eosinophilia and bronchogenic carcinoma have since followed [62, 63].

Basophilia is a well-recognized feature of the myeloproliferative diseases and Hodgkin's disease, but does not usually occur in association with carcinoma. The changes in the total lymphocyte count which occur in Hodgkin's disease and the reticulosis are summarized in Chapter 24. There is no consistent alteration in lymphocyte count in association with carcinoma although lymphopenia may occur in patients with disseminated tumours, or as a result of treatment [64].

BACTERIAL INFECTION

Acute and chronic bacterial infections can produce a variety of blood changes which can mimic practically any primary haematological disorder; indeed there are few infections which do not occasionally alter the blood picture. In the account which follows only those disorders which produce well-defined haematological changes will be considered.

Acute bacterial infection

The most consistent haematological changes in bacterial infection are alterations in the relative or absolute numbers of the leucocytes, anaemia, and the haemorrhagic phenomena which result from thrombocytopenia and disseminated intravascular coagulation.

The leucocyte changes in response to infection were considered in detail in Chapter 15. Most acute bacterial infections are associated with a neutrophil leucocytosis: this is particularly common in staphylococcal, streptococcal, pneumococcal, gonococcal and meningococcal infections and also in some bacillary infections (e.g. those with *E. coli*, *Pseudomonas* spp., *C. diphtheriae* and *P. tularenis*). During the course of such infections total leucocyte count usually climbs into the $10-25 \times 10^9/l$ range, although occasionally higher counts are seen—particularly with pneumococcal pneumonia or with local abscess formation. The leucocytosis is invariably associated with the appearance of increased numbers of band neutrophils and even metamyelocytes or myelocytes in the peripheral blood—the so-called 'shift-to-the-left'. This may be seen in the absence of overt neutrophilia and can be a sensitive indicator of infection [65] particularly in the neonatal period [66] or in patients with sickle-cell anaemia [67]. Neutrophil cytoplasmic changes are commonly seen in severe infections. *Toxic granulation* is the term given to the presence of deeply basophilic cytoplasmic granules though these are not specific to bacterial infection. In some instances toxic granulation may be accompanied by the presence of Döhle bodies (Chapter 16) or cytoplasmic vacuolation.

Occasionally the leucocytosis of acute bacterial infection may be extreme, reaching the levels found in chronic granulocytic leukaemia. These leukaemoid reactions are easily distinguished from the latter by the presence of a raised leucocyte alkaline phosphatase and the absence of the Philadelphia chromosome.

Patients are sometimes encountered who are severely ill with acute bacterial infections in whom the neutrophil response seems inadequate or who may be frankly neutropenic. Some will prove to have an underlying haematological disorder or a debilitating condition such as alcoholism [68], but a proportion of patients who recover from their infection show no such underlying abnormality subsequently. This situation can be very worrying for the clinician who will take little solace from the fact that the mechanism of this type of neutropenia is poorly understood. Marrow examination usually reveals a paucity of mature granulocytes even in the absence of an underlying disorder. This picture is sometimes erroneously described as a maturation arrest, but it is more likely due to exhaustion of the marrow-reserve granulocyte pool by the demands of infection. A shift from the circulating to marginating compartments, as occurs following endotoxin administration could be another factor contributing to this picture. It is rarely possible to measure neutrophil kinetics directly, but the appearance of local accumulations of pus should indicate that neutrophil production is probably adequate. One group of patients which commonly shows a neutropenic response to acute bacterial infection are newborn infants, especially when premature. Marrow neutrophil reserves are low at birth, and neonatal infections thus prove especially hazardous and require careful management [66].

Other leucocyte changes in acute infection are less spectacular and of doubtful significance. Eosinophilia is extremely uncommon—indeed eosinophils are typically absent from the peripheral blood of patients with acute bacterial infection, although an eosinophilia has been observed in patients with scarlet fever [69]. Monocytosis is also unusual although it has been reported in typhoid fever and may sometimes occur in brucellosis and subacute bacterial endocarditis [69]. In the latter disorder, particularly when caused by *Streptococcus viridans*, the total leucocyte count may be normal, subnormal or increased. Occasionally monocytosis may be associated with the presence of undifferentiated reticulo-endothelial cells in the blood which show erythrophagocytosis, and which may also engulf neutrophils or lymphocytes. These cells are found more frequently in blood obtained from the ear lobe than from a finger prick [70]. A similar phenomenon has been noted in patients with bacterial endocarditis, even in the absence of a positive blood culture [71].

Some degree of anaemia is found almost invariably in patients with bacterial infections of any duration. This is frequently a normochromic normocytic anaemia of the type seen in chronic disorders and described above. Haemolytic anaemia has been reported in a wide variety of bacterial infections [72] including those due to streptococci, staphylococci, pneumococci, *H. influenzae* and *S. typhi*. It is likely that this complication is associated with disseminated intravascular coagulation (see below and Chapter 29). *Cl. welchii* produces an α-toxin which acts as a lecithinase and causes fulminating intravascular haemolysis. Infection occurs most commonly post partum or after a septic abortion [72]. The clinical picture is one of septic shock with marked intravascular haemolysis, haemoglobinuria and disseminated intravascular coagulation [73]. A severe haemolytic anaemia also occurs with *Bartonella bacilliformis* infection (Oroya fever). This is described in Chapter 12.

Clinically the most striking haematological abnormality in acute bacterial infection is undoubtedly the haemorrhagic diathesis which frequently accompanies overwhelming sepsis [74]. This is seen more commonly in infections with Gram-negative organisms, possibly because of endotoxin release, but it may occur in the course of virtually any severe infection. The clinical features are extremely variable, and range from the development of a few scattered petechiae to major haemostatic failure with widespread tissue damage from the dual effects of intravascular coagulation and consumption of coagulation factors. Such patients may develop respiratory failure (shock lung), altered consciousness, hypotension, anuria and circulatory collapse. In some patients microangiopathic haemolysis may be prominent. Prior to the appreciation of the role of disseminated intravascular coagulation (DIC), particular associations between haemostatic failure and bacterial infection were recognized. The most striking of these are the *Waterhouse–Friderischen syndrome* in which meningococcal septicaemia is associated with widespread skin and internal haemorrhage, and *purpura fulminans*—characterized by the development of severe peripheral haemorrhagic lesions which rapidly become gangrenous. The latter is classically associated with streptococcal sepsis, but both conditions can occur in infections with a wide variety of organisms, and are generally thought to be non-specific manifestations of DIC.

The laboratory findings in DIC are fully discussed in Chapter 29, but briefly include evidence of consumption of coagulation factors (particularly V and VIII), fibrinogen, thrombocytopenia, elevation of circulating levels of fibrin split products and enhanced fibrinolysis. In addition, the blood film may show evidence of microangiopathic red-cell damage.

More recently it has become appreciated that thrombocytopenia may complicate acute bacterial infection without evidence for DIC [75, 76]. This has been especially noted in Gram-negative infections, and appears to be due to platelet injury rather than to reduced production or splenic sequestration. In one study it appeared that antigen–antibody complexes might be responsible for the platelet damage [75]. Immune complexes have also been found in a high proportion of patients with the haemolytic-uraemic syndrome complicating shigella dysentery [77]. The role of immune complexes in the pathogenesis of this complication was not clear, however, and many of the patients also had detectable circulating endotoxin which itself may have been responsible.

Chronic bacterial infection

Most chronic bacterial infections are associated with some degree of anaemia and usually with an elevated erythrocyte sedimentation rate. The haematological picture is that of the anaemia of chronic disorders described earlier in this chapter. Indeed the presence of this type of blood picture in the absence of any obvious cause such as rheumatoid arthritis or malignancy should suggest the presence of a hidden focus of chronic infection. By far the commonest site is the urinary tract; chronic pyelonephritis is a frequent case of low-grade anaemia, particularly in females. A similar blood picture, often associated with a monocytosis or lymphocytosis, is a well-recognized part of the syndrome of chronic brucellosis. However, the chronic bacterial infection which produces the most striking and variable haematological picture is tuberculosis.

Tuberculosis. The haematological findings in patients with tuberculosis are extremely variable (Table 33.3); indeed there is considerable doubt as to whether many of the reported findings in this disorder are due to the disease itself, or due to tuberculous infection occurring in patients with underlying blood dyscrasias.

The haematological findings in patients with active pulmonary tuberculosis are fairly characteristic. There is usually a normochromic normocytic anaemia with all the characteristics of the anaemia of chronic disorders. This is usually associated with a raised erythrocyte sedimentation rate which, together with the degree of anaemia, bears a fairly good relationship to the activity of the disease. After therapy the anaemia usually improves and persistent severe anaemia in patients on anti-tuberculous drug therapy should raise the possibility of a secondary sideroblastic anaemia due to one of the drugs, particularly INAH. This association has been fully reviewed in Chapter 13.

Other forms of anaemia in patients with active pulmonary tuberculosis are unusual. Megaloblastic anaemia is not common but may be associated with a malabsorption syndrome secondary to abdominal tuberculosis. Chanarin [41] has reviewed the literature

Table 33.3. Haematological changes in tuberculosis

Type of tuberculosis or therapy	Haematological changes
(1) Pulmonary	Anaemia of chronic disorders; iron-deficiency anaemia; anaemia due to therapy; high ESR
(2) Ileo-caecal	Anaemia of chronic disorders; megaloblastic anaemia due to vitamin-B_{12} or folate deficiency; high ESR
(3) Cryptic miliary (aregenerative)	Leukaemoid reaction Myelosclerosis Pancytopenia Polycythaemia Anaemia of chronic disorders
(4) Antituberculous drugs 　PAS or streptomycin allergy 　INAH, Cycloserine 　Rifampicin	Fever, lymphadenopathy, eosinophilia Sideroblastic anaemia Thrombocytopenic purpura

on serum vitamin-B_{12} and folate levels in patients with tuberculosis. There seems to be a genuine increase in the prevalence of low serum folate levels and although this finding has been related in part to the use of drugs such as INAH and cycloserine, its basis it not absolutely clear. It may simply result from the poor physical condition of the patients and hence a deficient dietary intake. Certainly, a florid megaloblastic anaemia due to folate deficiency is most unusual except in cases with associated abdominal tuberculosis.

A variety of haematological disorders have been described as part of the clinical picture of disseminated tuberculosis, particularly of the cryptic miliary type. These clinical pictures include leukaemoid reactions with a blood picture very similar to acute or chronic myeloid leukaemia [78, 79], pancytopenia [80, 81], myelofibrosis [82] and polycythaemia [82]. Furthermore, a postmortem study [83] revealed a high incidence of myelosclerotic marrows associated with infection with atypical mycobacteria. Similarly Gordon-Smith & Holt [84] described four patients, two with myelosclerosis and two with aplastic anaemia, who had evidence of infection with atypical mycobacteria of Runyon groups 1 and 3. The diagnosis was made in these cases by liver biopsy but none of the patients responded to anti-tuberculous drugs.

The main problem in assessing all these reports is whether the patients had tuberculous infections or infections due to atypical mycobacteria superimposed on an underlying blood disease, or whether disseminated tuberculosis can occasionally produce a clinical picture fairly similar to leukaemia or myelosclerosis. In an attempt to answer this question, Glasser *et al.* [85] studied 40 patients with miliary tuberculosis and a further 24 with tuberculosis and significant haematological abnormalities. They concluded that anaemia, monocytosis, leucopenia and leucocytosis could all be secondary to infection as these abnormali-

ties disappeared with treatment of the tuberculosis. On the other hand patients with pancytopenia or leukaemoid blood pictures did not respond to anti-tuberculous therapy alone and may have had an underlying blood dyscrasia.

The relationship between disseminated cryptic tuberculosis and blood disease has been extensively reviewed by Proudfoot [86]. In an analysis of over 27 000 reports of autopsies on patients of all ages the incidence of tuberculosis was 6·5%, and 5·6% in patients with leukaemia [87]. These findings suggest that the association between these two diseases is not significant, and this conclusion has been confirmed by others [88]. However, if these studies are subjected to more detailed analysis it appears that disseminated tuberculosis is slightly commoner in patients with blood disorders and indeed the incidence in patients with chronic granulocytic leukaemia is twice that in the normal population [88]. If the distinction is made between reactive and areactive tuberculosis the association becomes stronger. For example, Oswald [89] found only four cases of blood disorders out of 120 individuals with reactive disease, compared with six out of eight with areactive tuberculosis.

It is quite clear therefore that if a patient presents with a bizarre form of aplastic anaemia, leukaemoid reaction, myelosclerosis or a condition resembling chronic granulocytic or monocytic leukaemia, the possibility of tuberculosis should always be borne in mind, remembering that the infection may simply have modified an underlying haematological disorder. This is particularly important in the aged, where cryptic disseminated tuberculosis may be extremely difficult to diagnose. Similarly, if the clinical course of a patient with a primary blood disorder suddenly deteriorates for no apparent reason, infection of this type should be considered. If disseminated tuberculosis is suspected, probably the most useful investigations are liver and marrow biopsies. In addition to histological examination it may be very useful to culture the marrow for tuberculosis. The use of large marrow aspirates (up to 15 ml) have been recommended for this purpose [86, 90]. If these investigations do not help, and if the clinical picture deteriorates without any obvious haematological cause, a therapeutic trial of isoniazid and para-aminosalicyclic acid is certainly indicated. Unfortunately, there are no really well-documented cases of patients with these bizarre haematological manifestations of tuberculosis who have reverted to complete normality after anti-tuberculous treatment; this observation is probably the strongest evidence to suggest that in most of these cases the tuberculous infection is superimposed on a pre-existing blood disorder.

SPIROCHAETAL INFECTIONS

Secondary syphilis is often associated with a leucocytosis and lymphocytosis. There is also an eosinophilia and a mild normochromic anaemia in some cases. The relationship between paroxysmal cold haemoglobinuria and syphilis is described in Chapter 11.

Most leptospiral illnesses are associated with marked changes in the blood [91]. There is usually a polymorphonuclear leucocytosis and leukaemoid reactions have been recorded. Leptospiral haemolysins are active *in vivo*, and in acute infections there may be marked intravascular haemolysis. In addition, reduction in the platelet count has been recorded, possibly with a microangiopathic basis in some cases. The marked bleeding tendency of these disorders has a complex basis including thrombocytopenia and acute renal and hepatic failure.

VIRUS INFECTIONS

There is increasing interest in the relationship between virus infections and the blood. The possible relationships between virus infection and leukaemia, malignant lymphoma, the haemolytic-uraemic syndrome, aplastic anaemia, haemolytic anaemia and other conditions are reviewed elsewhere in this book. The account which follows emphasizes those viral infections which cause specific haematological syndromes.

Viral infections of the respiratory tract
A wide variety of viruses can affect the upper and, less commonly, lower respiratory tract. These include the rhinoviruses, adenoviruses, influenza and para-influenza viruses. There are no specific haematological abnormalities associated with these infections. Early in the course of the illness there is usually a mild leucopenia with a relative lymphocytosis and this is followed by a slight neutrophil leucocytosis. In primary influenzal pneumonia, neutrophilia may be marked and does not necessarily indicate secondary bacterial infection.

Rubella
The haematological manifestations of acquired rubella have been well documented by Morse [92] and McKay & Margaretten [93]. During the acute phase there is a leucocytosis with atypical lymphocytes ranging from two to 21%. Anaemia is uncommon unless associated with blood loss due to thrombocytopenia. The most important complication is the rare occurrence of thrombocytopenic purpura. The majority of Morse's patients were children and the median interval between the onset of the rubelliform rash and the appearance of purpura was four days. The illness was usually self-limiting but in several cases the thrombocytopenia was extreme and in one instance it was fatal. Platelet survival studies indicated an extremely shortened lifespan. As in idiopathic thrombocytopenic purpura the bleeding appeared to be controlled by corticosteroids, though splenectomy was performed in one case.

Congenital rubella infection is much more commonly complicated by haematological abnormalities, particularly haemorrhagic phenomena [94–96]. The commonest abnormality is thrombocytopenia; this is maximal on the first day of life and generally recovers within four to six weeks [97], though rarely it may be more persistent [98]. The cause is not known; its transient nature suggests the involvement of a transplacental factor, but maternal platelet counts are unaffected. Marrow examination occasionally shows megakaryocytic hypoplasia [99], and phagocytosis of blood cells has been described [100]. McKay & Margaretten [93] have reviewed the histological findings in infants dying with the haemorrhagic complications of congenital rubella and have presented a good case for an underlying disseminated intravascular coagulation. A mild haemolytic anaemia has been reported in 15–30% of cases, with exaggeration of the post-natal fall in haemoglobin level (Chapter 3). Once again the cause is not known: the blood film shows an appropriate reticulocytosis with marked poikilocytosis including fragmented and burr cells. The Coombs' test is negative and osmotic fragility and red-cell enzymes are normal [100]. There is an associated hepatosplenomegaly in about half the affected infants.

Morbilli
Haematological complications of measles infection are extremely uncommon. In the acute phase the leucocyte count is variable and there may be a leucocytosis or a leucopenia with occasional atypical lymphocytes.

Anaemia is uncommon, but there have been isolated reports of paroxysmal cold haemoglobinuria (Chapter 11) following measles infection [72, 101] and, in one instance, measles immunization [102]. This anaemia has differed from that classically associated with syphilis in being acute and transient.

Whilst purpuric staining of the measles rash is quite common in mild infections, marked haemorrhagic phenomena in measles are extremely rare [93, 103]. Thrombocytopenic purpura may occur: it typically appears after the true rash has faded or even as late as 14 days after the acute illness. In an extensive review of the literature, McKay & Margaretten were able to find only 26 cases reported between 1890 and 1956. The complication occurred mainly in young children and was fatal in 23%. Once again, disseminated intravascular coagulation has been implicated as the cause of these severe haemorrhagic manifestations [93].

Varicella

The haematological complications of varicella are similar to those of the other exanthemata although haemorrhagic phenomena are probably slightly commoner. In the acute phase the leucocyte count is variable, and atypical lymphocytes are often present. Anaemia is uncommon. Thrombocytopenia may occur either during the acute phase or during convalescence. It may be explosive in onset with generalized skin and mucous-membrane bleeding, and several cases of adrenal haemorrhage have been reported [93]. McKay & Margaretten have described five clinical syndromes of haemorrhagic complications in chickenpox: febrile purpura; post-infectious purpura; anaphylactoid purpura; malignant chickenpox with purpura; and purpura fulminans.

About two per cent of patients with chickenpox show minor haemorrhages including bleeding into vesicles and scattered petechiae. The platelet count is usually decreased in such cases. Severe thrombocytopenia may occur after the rash has faded and bleeding may persist for four or five weeks. The platelet count may reach extremely low levels but usually returns spontaneously to normal. A typical anaphylactoid reaction resembling Henoch–Schönlein purpura can also occur. In the syndrome of malignant chickenpox with purpura, bleeding appears at the same time as the measles rash, which is usually confluent; there is a marked systemic upset including convulsions and coma. Bleeding may be generalized and thrombocytopenia is usually profound. This complication develops mainly in immunosuppressed patients such as those with leukaemia or lymphoma.

INFECTIOUS MONONUCLEOSIS (GLANDULAR FEVER)
Infectious mononucleosis is an acute viral illness caused by the Epstein–Barr (EB) virus. The disease principally affects adolescents and young adults and is characterized by fever, sore throat, lymphadenopathy and the appearance in the peripheral blood of abnormal lymphocytes. The early history of the disorder has been well reviewed by Carter & Penman [104]; more recently, principally through the work of Henle et al. [105], the relationship with the EB virus has become firmly established, and of particular interest at the present time is the possible relationship of the disease and the EB virus with malignant disorders.

Aetiology [105]
For many years after the clinical syndrome of glandular fever had been firmly established, its cause was completely unknown. Indeed its infectious nature was in some doubt as numerous attempts to isolate a causative agent had failed completely, and attempts to transmit the disease to humans using a variety of pathological materials met with little success. In 1964 Epstein et al. [106] identified herpes-like virus particles by electron microscopy in cultured tumour cells from African children with Burkitt's lymphoma, and in 1966 the Henles detected antibodies to the viral capsid antigen (VCA) of the new virus in sera from normal healthy adults and children as well as from patients with Burkitt's lymphoma [107]. In 1968 the same workers reported a serendipitous observation in one of their technicians who had contracted clinical infectious mononucleosis [108]: before infection her serum contained no antibodies to the EB virus, but these appeared with the onset of her illness. This and subsequent epidemiological evidence have established beyond doubt that infectious mononucleosis is caused by the EB virus [105], and the compelling evidence for this as outlined by the Henles is summarized in Table 33.4.

The discovery that infectious mononucleosis is caused by an agent which has a strong association with a malignant lymphoma has led to much speculation that the virus might be oncogenic and that infectious mononucleosis might be a pre-malignant condition. A more recently recognized association is that between the EB virus and nasopharyngeal carcinoma. These issues are not fully resolved at the present time, and it is beyond the scope of this chapter to discuss them in depth, but the interested reader is referred to excellent reviews by Klein [109] and Henle et al. [105].

Pathogenesis and pathology [110, 105]
Transmission of infectious mononucleosis is principally via saliva; the communicability is low, and close or intimate contact—as might occur by kissing or perhaps sharing a drinking vessel—is probably required [111]. The cells initially infected may be the

Table 33.4. Summary of the evidence that the Epstein–Barr virus (EBV) causes infectious mononucleosis (IM)

Serological	Other
(1) Classical, heterophil antibody-positive IM only develops in EBV-negative persons	(1) Lymphocytes from patients with IM will readily establish *in-vitro* cultures whilst lymphocytes from EBV-antibody-negative persons do not
(2) The titre of EBV antibody rises following typical IM infection; IgM transiently and IgG permanently	(2) Normal lymphocytes transform *in vitro* after exposure to EBV-containing lymphocytes
	(3) EBV can be isolated from throat washings from patients who have or have had IM
	(4) IM can be transmitted by transfusion of blood containing EBV-positive lymphocytes

epithelial cells of the mouth and pharynx but the infection soon spreads to the B-lymphocytes in the lymphoid tissues of Waldeyer's ring and subsequently to lymphoid tissue elsewhere. Infection of B-lymphocytes with the EB virus has a number of consequences. The majority of cells do not produce new virus particles but are transformed into a state of active proliferation, and copies of the viral genome and virally induced antigens can be detected in the progeny of these cells. Further transmission of the virus is ensured by a smaller proportion of cells in which the viral genome can be activated to produce new virus particles. Infectious mononucleosis may thus be viewed as a polyclonal lymphoproliferative disorder affecting B-cells. One consequence of this B-cell activation is the production of a wide variety of immunoglobulins, including the heterophil antibody. In addition to this indiscriminate activity, the presence of viral antigens also induces the specific synthesis of appropriate antibodies. The next stage of the illness is characterized by an aggressive T-cell response to the presence of virally altered infected B-cells. The 'abnormal' lymphocytes characteristic of this condition are in fact proliferating T-cells. This situation has been likened to a type of graft-versus-host disease [112], and it is possible that much of the damage to organs such as the liver is a consequence of this aggressive T-cell activity.

Following this humoral and cell-mediated immune response, the virally infected cells are largely but not completely eliminated. Latent infection is characteristic of the herpes viruses including the EB virus, and shedding of the virus can be detected in the saliva for a considerable time following infection. Furthermore, a small proportion of B-cells from previously infected persons will grow spontaneously in tissue culture, contain the EB virus genome, and are capable of producing new virus particles. Cells from individuals who have not previously been infected do not show these characteristics.

The pathological changes in infectious mononucleosis are confined mainly to the lymphoid organs. The lymph nodes show follicular hyperplasia and in some cases there is such marked reticulo-endothelial hyperplasia as to resemble a lymphoma, though invasion of the capsule does not occur. There are widespread perivascular aggregates of normal and abnormal lymphocytes throughout the body, while in the nervous system perivascular cuffing and disruption of myelin occurs. Granulomatous lesions have been reported on marrow biopsies but are not specific to this disorder.

Clinical features
Infectious mononucleosis affects mainly young adults, and 85% or more of well-documented cases have occurred between the ages of 15 and 30 years [113]. Epidemiological and serological studies suggest that in low socio-economic groups infection is common in infancy and early childhood, when it is usually subclinical or very mild. Infection in the elderly is rare and may run an atypical course [114].

The incubation period is uncertain but is probably between 33 and 49 days. There may then follow two or three days of prodomal symptoms including fatigue, malaise, chills, sweating, headache, anorexia, nausea and a distaste for cigarette smoking, though the onset of the illness is usually abrupt with the development of the most constant symptom of infectious mononucleosis: a sore throat. This is frequently associated with lymphadenopathy; the cervical glands are most consistently affected and are often slightly tender and usually noticed by the patient. In addition to these symptoms about 10% of patients develop fleeting skin rashes which usually last for about 24–48 hours, though administration of ampicillin in the early stages of the illness is associated with a much more striking rash in over 70% of instances [115]. Mild jaundice has been noted in up to five per cent of cases.

On examination the patient is usually pyrexial with

peaks between 38 and 39·5°C. There is usually a moderate bradycardia and the throat is red and injected, with slight oedema of the pharynx, uvula, soft palate and peritonsillar region. About half the patients have some degree of pharyngeal exudate while in other cases there may be more severe membranous ulceration. About one-third develop small purpuric lesions over the soft palate. There is usually anterior and posterior cervical or more generalized lymphadenopathy: the nodes are small, discrete and often slightly tender. In over half of the cases the spleen is enlarged; it is usually soft and non-tender and is not usually felt much more than 5 cm below the costal margin. Hepatomegaly occurs in 10–20% of cases and may be associated with clinical jaundice. Other useful physical signs include periorbital oedema, and skin rashes which are usually maculopapular and distributed over the trunk and proximal parts of the limbs. In the majority of cases the disease is a short self-limiting disorder which lasts from five to 10 days. Usually all manifestations have disappeared by the end of the third week. However, as in other virus disorders, a considerable period of lethargy and depression may follow and this is usually more severe in patients who have had an acute illness.

Laboratory findings

The total leucocyte count is usually normal or slightly elevated in the first week of the illness but a mild leucocytosis in the range $10-15 \times 10^9/l$ occurs in some patients throughout the entire clinical course. In some cases there is an initial leucopenia, but during the second week there is usually a moderate leucocytosis with maximum values in the third week. The total leucocyte count rarely exceeds $20 \times 10^9/l$ but a few leukaemoid reactions have been reported with counts in the $30-80 \times 10^9/l$ range. The pathognomonic finding in this disorder is the presence of large numbers of atypical lymphocytes (Fig. 33.4), which by the end of the first week usually constitute more than 60% of the total circulating leucocytes. The atypical lymphocytes are large cells but vary considerably in size and have

irregular outlines, showing a tendency to 'flow' round adjacent erythrocytes in blood smears. The nucleus is large and often eccentric with coarse chromatin and occasional nucleoli. The abundant cytoplasm is basophilic and may contain vacuoles and a few eosinophilic granules. Attempts by Downey, and later by Wood & Frenkel [116], to classify different morphological characteristics of these cells were once fashionable, but are of little clinical help and are no longer used.

Many patients show a slight neutropenia with a shift to the left, and about five per cent of patients show a mild eosinophilia which often occurs as late as four to five months after the onset of the clinical symptoms. The leucocyte alkaline phosphatase level falls during the acute phase. Except in cases where there is associated haemolysis, the red-cell morphology is normal, but 50% of cases have a slight thrombocytopenia. The marrow findings are non-specific with a shift to the left in the myeloid series and a slight increase in mature lymphocytes. On histological section of the marrow about 50% of cases show scattered epithelioid-cell granulomata [117].

Diagnosis

The diagnosis of the disorder is confirmed by the presence of a typical heterophil antibody. Heterophil antibodies react with antigens found in a variety of animal species which could not, of course, have been the immunizing antigens. These antigens are immunologically related to the so-called Forssmann antigens which are glycolipids found in the red cells and tissues of many species as well as certain bacteria and plants. In the original test devised by Paul & Bunnell, heterophil antibodies were demonstrated by simple titration of sheep-cell agglutinins but this technique was subsequently modified in order to distinguish between agglutinins formed in patients with infectious mononucleosis and the Forssman-type antibodies found in normal serum and in other conditions such as leukaemia and serum sickness. Tissues rich in Forssman antigen, such as guinea-pig kidney, absorb these antibodies but not the heterophil antibodies of infec-

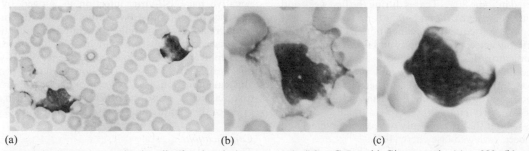

(a) (b) (c)

Fig. 33.4. Infectious mononucleosis cells (for description, see text); (May–Grünwald–Giemsa stain (a) ×920, (b) ×2300, (c) ×2300). (By courtesy of Dr George MacDonald.)

tious mononucleosis. The latter are, however, absorbed by ox cells. Thus in the modified Paul–Bunnell–Davidsohn test the two types of sheep-cell agglutinin are distinguished by titrating them before and after absorption with guinea-pig kidney and ox cells. When adequately performed this test is specific for infectious mononucleosis and false-positive results are extremely uncommon [118].

Heterophil antibody is detected in over 80% of patients with infectious mononucleosis; titres rise during the first two or three weeks but there is little relationship between the titre and the severity of the disease. The antibody is an IgM; its level gradually declines and by 12 weeks after the onset of the illness it is no longer detectable. A rapid spot test has been developed based on the principle that horse erythrocytes are more sensitive than sheep erythrocytes, and are therefore useful for demonstrating the low titres of antibodies that are found early in the disease. Furthermore, fine suspensions of guinea-pig kidney or beef-erythrocyte stromata absorb antibodies instantly and give clear-cut differentiation between infectious mononucleosis and other sera. Thus, in the spot test, serum is mixed thoroughly with guinea-pig kidney on one spot and with beef-erythrocyte stromata on another and washed, preserved horse erythrocytes are added immediately to each spot. In contrast to the Paul–Bunnell test, the spot test remains positive for up to 18 months in 75% of individuals. It is a reliable test though false positives are occasionally encountered, particularly with cytomegalovirus infections (see below). False negative are rare, but may occur if plasma is used instead of serum. For more extensive discussion of the serological testing for infectious mononucleosis the reader is referred to several reviews [118–120].

Tests for the heterophil antibody were developed before the EB virus has been discovered and remain the cornerstone of serological diagnosis. Various antibodies are produced to the EB virus or to its products during the course of infection. The most useful clinically are IgM and later IgG antibodies to the viral capsid antigen (VCA). These antibodies can be detected in some 80% of cases during the first week and virtually all cases by the end of the third week. The IgM antibodies subsequently decline, more or less in parallel with the heterophil antibody and its presence is thus an indicator of recent infection. In contrast, IgG antibody persists indefinitely and probably confers life-long immunity against further attacks. Other antibodies produced to the EB virus include those to the EBV early antigen (EA) and nuclear antigen (EBNA), but these are mainly of research interest and have been reviewed elsewhere [105].

The production of heterophil antibody is but one example of the effects of polyclonal B-cell expansion by the EB-virus infection. A wide variety of other non-specific antibodies may be found including rheumatoid factor, antinuclear factor, increased levels of cryoglobulins and antibodies against certain strains of proteus, streptococci, salmonella and brucella.

Other laboratory findings include evidence of abnormal liver function (elevated transaminases and alkaline phosphatase) in the vast majority of patients, with, less commonly, a slight elevation in bilirubin.

The differential diagnosis of infectious mononucleosis and the problem of the seronegative form

It has been suggested that infectious mononucleosis should only be diagnosed in the presence of posterior cervical lymphadenopathy, heterophil antibodies and a differential white-cell count of which 20% or more are atypical lymphocytes [113]. To this should now be added the presence of a raised titre of antibody to EB virus. Where the onset of the illness is associated with marked inflammatory changes in the pharynx the condition may be confused with a streptococcal throat infection or even diphtheria. Practically all the common virus infections of childhood may present with a sore throat, lymphadenopathy and a rash, although the further development of the illness usually makes the distinction from infectious mononucleosis relatively easy. It should be remembered that these conditions may all be associated with atypical lymphocytes in the peripheral blood. The condition can also be confused with Hodgkin's disease and the other reticuloses. When in doubt it is most important *not* to do an immediate lymph-node biopsy but to wait for two or three weeks and see if the affected group of nodes is settling spontaneously. A lymph-node biopsy performed in the acute phase of any viral illness may produce an equivocal histological picture and necessitate the patient being followed up for years, with much unnecessary anxiety.

The problem of seronegative mononucleosis has been well reviewed by Penman [121]. A significant proportion of patients with the clinical features of infectious mononucleosis who are heterophil antibody negative have EB-virus infection as judged by the presence of IgM anti-EBV antibody. This situation is found relatively commonly with childhood infections. One occasionally observes patients who have neither a heterophil antibody response nor evidence of EB-virus infection. Many of these can be shown to have cytomegalovirus infection (see below) or, less commonly, toxoplasmosis. These and other conditions which may produce this picture are summarized in Table 33.5.

Complications

The complications of infectious mononucleosis have been the subject of several excellent reviews [104, 113,

Table 33.5. Some causes of 'sero-negative' IM-like disorders (modified from Ref. 121)

Disorder	Features
Toxoplasmosis	Less pharyngitis than IM, lymphadenopathy marked, myocarditis commoner. More prolonged than IM
Cytomegalovirus infection	Less pharyngitis and lymphadenopathy than IM This includes the post-perfusion and post-transfusion syndromes
Drug reactions	Sulphones, PAS, phenylbutazone, hydantoinates Rashes common, pharyngitis less marked
Listeriosis	May have sheep-cell agglutinins. Rare cause of IM picture
Rickettsial infection (*R. sennetsa*)	Described in Japan; not seen in Europe or USA
IM treated with steroids	Steroid therapy may reduce agglutinin titre
Other viruses	Likely that other viruses may cause IM-like illness In some cases there is increased titre to EB virus in absence of heterophil antibody Other virus infections include those due to adenoviruses, rubella and hepatitis virus

122] and they will only be broadly outlined here. They are all uncommon; exact incidence figures are extremely difficult to obtain because in many cases critical diagnostic criteria for infectious mononucleosis have not been obtained.

There are a variety of neurological complications which may occur occasionally in patients with infectious mononucleosis. These include encephalitis, meningoencephalitis, meningitis, a Guillain–Barré-like syndrome and peripheral neuritis. In one large series of neurological complications the overall mortality rate was approximately eight per cent, while another 12% had serious residual neurological damage [113]. However, the finding that approximately 25% of patients with infectious mononucleosis have abnormalities of the cerebrospinal fluid, and 30% have abnormal electroencephalograms indicates that subclinical neurological involvement may be very common. The neurological complications can occur at any time during the illness although most commonly in the second or third week. A disorder resembling Bell's palsy may also occur.

A slight to moderate thrombocytopenia occurs in about 50% of patients during the first four weeks of the illness. This rarely causes bleeding and up to 1969 there were only 35 well-documented reports of excessive bleeding due to thrombocytopenia [123]. The distribution and pattern of bleeding is similar to that found in other forms of thrombocytopenic purpura. Once established it usually lasts between two weeks and two months. The mechanism of thrombocytopenia is not clear; it is possible that the virus infection can induce the production of platelet antibodies [124] or reduce the platelet count by a direct interaction between virus and circulating platelets. A few cases have been reported in which other abnormalities of the coagulation mechanism have occurred, and a patient with the haemolytic-uraemic syndrome has been described

[125a], though there appear to have been no systematic studies of the possible occurrence of disseminated intravascular coagulation in this disorder.

Acquired haemolytic anaemia is another rare but well-documented complication of infectious mononucleosis and has been the subject of several extensive reviews [122]. The haemolytic anaemia usually develops about two weeks after the onset of symptoms and is associated with weakness, fever, anaemia and jaundice and, in a few cases, haemoglobinuria. The peripheral blood picture shows findings typical of an immune haemolytic process. There is now good evidence that the majority of these cases result from the increased production of anti-i antibody during the course of the illness. The anti-i titre rises in at least 50% of patients with infectious mononucleosis and it has been suggested that the presence or absence of haemolysis is related to the magnitude of this rise; the few patients who develop a sufficient titre develop haemolysis *in vivo*. It seems likely that the anti-i antibody combines with red cells and complement in the small vessels of the skin at temperatures of about 28–32°C. Presumably some of the cells are then lysed intravascularly while others, coated by sublytic amounts of complement, are sequestered in the spleen, liver and bone marrow. There is a positive direct antiglobulin test of the complement or non-IgG type. Thus the immunological abnormalities bear a close resemblance to those of individuals with primary atypical pneumonia except that in the latter the antibody is usually anti-I (Chapter 11). In a few cases the patients may have been more susceptible to anti-i antibody by having increased amounts of antigen on their red cells in association with such disorders as hereditary spherocytosis and thalassaemia.

As with the other virus infections occasional cases of aplastic anaemia have been recorded, with several fatalities [122] (see also Chapter 31, p. 1233). Paroxysmal nocturnal haemoglobinuria has also been described [125b]. There have also been reports of severe neutropenia, which in some instances may have an immune basis [125c].

Hepatitis of varying severity occurs in most cases of infectious mononucleosis. Transient jaundice occurs in about eight to 10% of cases; this is usually short-lived and is without morbidity or mortality [113]. Rupture of the spleen is now a well-recognized complication. There have been about 50 well-documented instances of this complication which usually occurs during the second or third week of the illness in cases where the spleen is unusually large [113]. The clinical picture is characterized by a sudden onset of pain in the left upper quadrant followed by the symptoms and signs of profound shock.

Other rare complications of the disorder include respiratory obstruction due to massive oedema of the pharynx and peritonsillar region, and pulmonary involvement with radiological appearances similar to primary atypical pneumonia. There have been one or two reports of the occurrence of unilateral pleural effusion. Although transient abnormalities of the electrocardiogram are not uncommon, significant cardiac abnormalities are very rare. Similarly, while slight albuminuria or a slight increase in the number of red cells in the urine is not uncommon, nephritis is not observed in this disorder.

The main causes of death in infectious mononucleosis have been assessed by Finch [113] as follows: rupture of the spleen 25%, neurological complications 25%, infectious or toxic complications 25%, with a wide variety of complications making up the remaining 25%.

Treatment

In most cases no treatment is required except for mild analgesia or sedation. Secondary infections of the pharynx may require appropriate antibiotics, but ampicillin must be avoided [115]. Corticosteroid therapy is not indicated in the uncomplicated case, and should be reserved for life-threatening complications (see above). Its effect on the immune response to the EB-virus-infected B cells will at best be unpredictable. Haemolytic anaemia usually requires little treatment except for keeping the patient warm; corticosteroid therapy is not usually effective.

CYTOMEGALOVIRUS INFECTION [126]

The cytomegalovirus (CMV) is a herpes virus which gets its name from the striking cytopathic effect that it produces in tissue culture, characterized by the development of large intranuclear inclusions. The virus itself was first recognized in relation to congenital infection, but it is now known to have world-wide distribution. Serological studies have demonstrated that the majority of people will at some stage in their life develop antibodies to the virus, yet overt disease is distinctly uncommon. The virus has been isolated from a variety of body secretions including saliva, urine, milk, cervical secretions, semen, faeces and from circulating leucocytes. Its communicability is very low, and transmission depends on close or intimate physical contact, though it may occasionally be transmitted by blood transfusion.

Clinical disease due to CMV infection is of three main types:
1 congenital infection;
2 a disorder resembling infectious mononucleosis; and
3 disseminated CMV infection in the immunosuppressed.

Infection of the fetus with CMV is probably quite common, some 0·5–1·5% of newborns being virus positive [95], but the majority of these are asymptomatic. Symptomatic infections [94, 95, 126] are characterized by hepato-splenomegaly, jaundice, purpura, microcephaly, pneumonia and chorioretinitis. There is often a moderate degree of anaemia with morphological changes of the red cells and the appearance of many normoblasts in the peripheral blood. In addition there may be a reticulocytosis of 10–30%. The anaemia may persist for many weeks. Often there is an associated thrombocytopenia and bone-marrow examination reveals a marked reduction in the number of megakaryocytes. The diagnosis can be confirmed by finding cells with intranuclear or cytoplasmic inclusions in the spinal fluid or urine. The inclusion bodies are about 9 μm in diameter and stain reddish-violet with haematoxylin and eosin. The best method of confirming the diagnosis is the direct isolation of CMV from the urine.

There is good evidence that a clinical disorder indistinguishable from infectious mononucleosis may be associated with a rising titre of antibody against CMV [126, 127]. The route of transmission is probably the same as for infectious mononucleosis. In such patients the infection tends to last for two to five weeks but as compared with infectious mononucleosis, pharyngeal involvement is not a prominent feature and the lymphadenopathy is much less marked. the haematological changes are very similar to those of infectious mononucleosis. Complications of the disorder include inner-ear damage, arthritis, pneumonia, polyneuritis, myocarditis and a significant rise in cold-agglutinin titres. Abnormal liver-function tests are common and although clinical hepatitis is unusual, several cases with severe liver damage have been reported. The condition can be diagnosed by the finding of a rising titre against CMV or by isolation of the virus from the throat during the acute part of the illness.

There are well-documented cases of an infectious

mononucleosis-like disorder occurring after transfusion with fresh blood or after perfusion for open-heart surgery [127]. The syndrome usually occurs one to three months after the blood transfusion and is self-limiting, resolving within a few weeks. The illness is characterized by a moderate rise in temperature with transient hepatomegaly and splenomegaly. A slight lymphadenopathy has been noted in occasional cases as have transient maculopapular rashes. There is a lymphocytosis with atypical lymphocytes indistinguishable from those of true infectious mononucleosis. As in the latter disorder, occasional leukaemoid reactions have occurred although usually the leucocyte count does not exceed $15 \times 10^9/l$. During the acute part of the illness some degree of anaemia is not uncommon; the mechanism has not been worked out adequately. In some cases it is associated with a high titre of cold agglutinins or a positive Coombs' test but this is by no means always so. As in infectious mononucleosis, other immunological abnormalities occur during the acute phase including the appearance of rheumatoid factor, cryoglobulins and antinuclear antibodies. These post-transfusion and perfusion syndromes can be avoided by the use of blood which is 48 hours or more old (Chapter 35).

With increasing use of immunosuppression in the treatment of malignant disease and in transplantation, disseminated infections with the cytomegalovirus have become a major problem [128]. Infection may occur by reactivation of latent infection or by introduction of fresh virus by transfusion or in the transplanted organ itself. The clinical picture is varied and ranges from a mild febrile illness to a rapidly fatal condition often with hepatic or pulmonary failure. There are no specific haematological manifestations in this situation and the blood picture is often complicated by the underlying condition. Any of the blood changes seen in other CMV infections may occur.

INFECTIOUS HEPATITIS

There are two main forms of this disease [129]. Hepatitis-A is synonymous with infectious, short-incubation or hepatitis-associated-antigen (HAA) negative hepatitis. Hepatitis-B covers the various forms of serum hepatitis, also called long-incubation or HAA-positive hepatitis. HAA (previously the Australian antigen) is found in a high proportion of patients with the clinical diagnosis of serum hepatitis and occurs with a high frequency in a variety of groups including institutionalized patients with Down's syndrome, leukaemics, haemophiliacs and thalassaemics who have had many transfusions with blood or blood products. It is detected by a variety of serological and immunological techniques (see Chapter 35).

Serious haematological complications of infectious hepatitis are rare. There is often an alteration in the total or differential leucocyte count early on in the illness, with a moderate degree of leucopenia or relative lymphocytosis as the commonest abnormalities. The leucocyte alkaline phosphatase level is reduced. Occasionally there is an overt haemolytic anaemia and there is substantial evidence that a severe aplastic anaemia may sometimes follow the disorder.

The extensive literature on haemolytic anaemia and infectious hepatitis has been reviewed by Dacie [72]. A whole variety of haemolytic syndromes have been reported. Some are associated with a positive Coombs' test while in others both direct and indirect antiglobulin tests are negative. Occasionally high titres of cold agglutinins have been observed. Some shortening of the ^{51}Cr red-cell survival has been noted in over 50% of patients in the acute phase of hepatitis. In addition there are now several well-documented cases of acute intravascular haemolysis occurring in patients with infectious hepatitis who were also glucose-6-phosphate dehydrogenase (G6PD) deficient.

There are now a considerable number of reports of aplastic anaemia occurring in patients with infectious hepatitis [130]. The majority of patients have been young, with half of the reported cases occurring between the ages of 10 and 20, and males have been affected twice as frequently as females. This age and sex distribution parallels that of the underlying hepatitis rather than that of idiopathic aplastic anaemia, suggesting that this is not purely a chance association. The onset of aplastic anaemia has been within nine weeks of the onset of hepatitis in the majority of cases. The condition is associated with a mortality of nearly 90%, and those patients who have survived have taken between three and 20 months from the onset of symptoms to full recovery.

ACUTE INFECTIOUS LYMPHOCYTOSIS

This is a short, self-limiting illness which occurs predominantly in young people. Outbreaks have occurred throughout the American continent, Europe and Africa. A causative organism has not yet been isolated although there is some evidence that infections with various enteroviruses, and at least one virus resembling those of the Coxsackie A subgroup, may occasionally be involved.

There are no specific clinical features. Many patients are asymptomatic but occasionally there is fever, signs of an upper-respiratory-tract infection and a morbilliform rash with some enlargement of the superficial nodes.

There is a striking leucocytosis which is largely the result of an increase in the number of small lymphocytes. Total white-cell counts in the $40–50 \times 10^9/l$ range are not infrequent while levels of up to $100 \times 10^9/l$ have been reported. The lymphocytosis usually lasts from three to five weeks and there may occasionally be an associated eosinophilia. The condition can easily be distinguished from infectious mononucleosis because of the absence of systemic symptoms, the magnitude of the leucocyte count, and the lack of atypical mononuclear cells and heterophil antibody. No treatment is required.

THE VIRAL HAEMORRHAGIC FEVERS

Apart from the uncommon haemorrhagic complications of the exanthemata and infectious mononucleosis mentioned earlier in the chapter, there are a large number of viral illnesses in which haemorrhagic phenomena predominate. This group, known collectively as the viral haemorrhagic fevers, have now been encountered in many parts of the world and increasing numbers of viruses are being isolated and named as the causative organisms [93, 131]. The conditions may be transmitted by many blood-sucking arthropods or may be acquired through close contact with infected animals or their excreta.

Viruses which multiply in arthropods are classified as arboviruses. There are several groups of arboviruses which can produce haemorrhagic disorders. One family, the togaviruses, which includes mosquito-borne arboviruses, was originally isolated in Africa from patients with dengue-like disorders but it has been found more recently in individuals with severe haemorrhagic fevers in both Thailand and India. Other types of haemorrhagic fever in South-east Asia have been shown to follow infections with the dengue virus group. Another group of the arboviruses, the flaviviruses, are responsible for yellow fever which occurs commonly in a haemorrhagic form. Other disorders which are transmitted by the arboviruses include Bukovinian haemorrhagic fever and Kyasanur forest disease in India. The Argentinian and Bolivian forms of haemorrhagic fever are different in that they are acquired from infected rodents and are due to a group of viruses now classed as the arenaviruses. This name is derived from the appearance of sandy granules seen in virus particles under the electron microscope. Several other arenaviruses have been isolated from patients with severe haemorrhagic fevers in Latin and Central America and similar disorders have now been reported from West Africa. Finally there is the syndrome of haemorrhagic fever with renal involvement, or haemorrhagic nephroso-nephritis, which is endemic in parts of Korea, Hungary, Czechoslovakia and the Soviet Union. This disorder is clearly associated with infected rodents and voles and is probably a zoonotic, rather than an arbovirus, infection.

The clinical features of these haemorrhagic fevers are extremely variable. Thus they range from mild dengue-like infections characterized by severe headache, pyrexia and generalized myalgia associated with scarlatiniform rash, leucopenia and thrombocytopenia, to the severe haemorrhagic fever so well described in the first Thai epidemic of 1954 [93]. This disorder is characterized by severe cough, dyspnoea and cyanosis. The marked bleeding tendency, which is seen in all cases, is characterized by purpura with severe bleeding at injection sites and from the gastrointestinal tract and other mucous membranes. The mortality in the original outbreak was 38% in infants under one year and 19% for all age groups. The coagulation findings in these patients were well reviewed by McKay & Margaretten [93]. There was gross thrombocytopenia in the severe cases with prolongation of the prothrombin time, reduced levels of factors VII and X and abnormalities of the thromboplastin-generation test. These findings, together with autopsy evidence of generalized fibrin deposition, provide strong evidence of disseminated intravascular coagulation. Similar abnormalities of coagulation have been reported in individuals with Bolivian and Argentine haemorrhagic fever and Kyasanur forest disease. In some cases the autopsy findings have been rather similar to those of purpura fulminans.

The use of heparin in the treatment of these disorders is reviewed by McKay & Margaretten [93] who describe this form of therapy in patients with Philippine haemorrhagic fever. They treated 20 patients with heparin and maintained a control group without anticoagulant therapy. There was a very impressive difference between the groups in that the duration of the haemorrhagic phenomena was shorter in the treated group.

PARASITIC DISEASES

One-third of the world's population has some form of parasitic infestation and many of these disorders produce haematological changes [132]. A full description of all these conditions is beyond the scope of this book and only those which show major haematological alterations will be mentioned. A classified account of some of the main haematological changes which occur with parasitic disease is given in Table 33.6.

PROTOZOAL DISEASE

Toxoplasmosis [133, 134]

Toxoplasma gondii infection can produce a variety of haematological manifestations, which may accompany

Table 33.6. Blood findings in nematode infections in man (from Ref. 132)

Disease	Organism	Reservoir	Transmission	Haematology	Diagnosis
Amoebiasis	*E. histolytica*	Man	Faeces	Anaemia Leucocytosis Eosinophilia	Trophozoites or cysts in stool CF*, HT*
Giardiasis	*Giardia lamblia*	Man	Faeces	Anaemia. Mild eosinophilia	Steatorrhoea. Cysts or trophozoites in faeces
Toxoplasmosis	*T. gondii*	Mammals Birds	Meat Ticks Faeces Placental	Anaemia Lymphocytosis Atypical mononuclear cells. Mild eosinophilia	Dye test Serology Organism in RE cells
Malaria	*Plasmodium falciparum vivax malariae ovale*	Man	Mosquito	Haemolytic anaemia Leucopenia Thrombocytopenia Monocytosis Eosinophilia DIC Changes in immune globulins Hypersplenism	Parasites in red blood cells Specific antibodies
Kala-azar	*Leishmania donovani*	Man Dog Cat Rodent	Sandfly	Splenomegaly Anaemia Thrombocytopenia Leucopenia Monocytosis Hyperglobulinaemia	L–D bodies in marrow, spleen, liver, lymph nodes. Culture *in vivo*. CF
Oriental sore	*Leishmania tropica*	Rodent Dog	Sandfly	Monocytosis	Biopsy or culture from lesion
Mucocutaneous Leishmaniasis	*Leishmania braziliensis*	Rodent	Sandfly	Monocytosis	As above
African trypanosomiasis	*T. gambiense* and *rhodesiense*	Man Cattle	Tsetse fly	Adenopathy Anaemia Leucopenia Lymphocytosis Monocytosis	Trypanosomes in lymph, blood or CSF. Animal inoculation
Chagas' disease	*T. cruzi*	Man Animals	Bug Faeces	Adenopathy Leucocytosis Lymphocytosis Hypergammaglobulinaemia	Blood film Animal, inoculation CF
Trichuriasis	*Trichuris trichiuria*	Man	Faeces	Anaemia Eosinophilia	Eggs in faeces
Enterobiasis	*Eterobius vermicularis*	Man	Faeces	Eosinophilia	Worms around anus. Eggs in faeces
Ascariasis	*Ascaris lumbricoides*	Man	Faeces	Eosinophilia	Eggs in faeces
Hookworm disease	*Necator americanus Ancylostoma duodenale*	Man	Faeces	Iron-deficiency anaemia Eosinophilia Hypoproteinaemia	Eggs in faeces

Table 33.6. (*cont.*)

Disease	Organism	Reservoir	Transmission	Haematology	Diagnosis
Stronglyoidiasis	*Strongyloides stercoralis*	Man Dog	Faeces Autoinfection	Anaemia Leucocytosis Eosinophilia	Larvae in faeces
Filariasis	*Wuchereria bancrofti Brugia malayi*	Man	Mosquito	Adenopathy Leucocytosis Eosinophilia	Microfilariae in blood or lymph
Onchocercosis	*Onchocerca volvulus*	Man	Flies (Simuliidae)	Eosinophilia	Microfilariae in skin or eye
Loiasis	*Loa loa*	Man	Mango fly (*Chrysops*)	Eosinophilia	Microfilariae in blood. Skin test
Trichinosis	*Trichinella spiralis*	Swine Wild mammals	Uncooked meat	Eosinophilia Leucocytosis	Parasite in blood. Larvae in muscle. Skin test CF*, PT*
Creeping eruption	*Ancylostoma braziliensis*	Dog Cat	Faeces	Eosinophilia Leucocytosis	Biopsy
Visceral larva migrans	*Toxocara canis* and *cati*	Dog Cat	Faeces	Hepatomegaly Leucocytosis Eosinophilia Hyperglobulinaemia Changes in anti-A and/or anti-B titre	Biopsy

CF = complement fixation; HT = haemagglutination test; PT = precipitin test.

both the congenital and acquired forms of the disorder.

Congenital toxoplasmosis. This can produce a condition resembling erythroblastosis fetalis. The clinical picture is of a pale hydropic infant with marked hepatosplenomegaly who may be stillborn or who may live for only a few minutes. There is usually anaemia, thrombocytopenia and a leucocytosis; an eosinophilia has been noted in approximately 20% of infants with the generalized form of the disease. In less severe cases the disease can manifest itself during the first week of life with the appearance of fever, jaundice, lymphadenopathy, hepatosplenomegaly, a diffuse maculopapular rash and ocular or neurological symptoms. The picture is very similar to that seen in congenital cytomegalovirus infection.

Toxoplasmosis acquired in later life. This may produce a clinical disorder resembling infectious mononucleosis and characterized by fever, malaise, generalized lymphadenopathy and hepatosplenomegaly. There is usually a lymphocytosis with atypical mononuclear cells or a monocytosis, and the liver function tests are frequently abnormal. A myocarditis may occur. There is good evidence from epidemiological surveys that subclinical infections are extremely common, although immunosuppressed patients are particularly prone to severe infection [135]. Autopsy in such cases reveals generalized organ involvement, with toxoplasma cysts in the heart, brain, pancreas and kidney and the presence of free toxoplasma in the myocardium.

Toxoplasmosis can be diagnosed by a variety of laboratory investigations. The dye test (Sabin–Feldman) is fairly specific. Whilst 20–40% of normal adults give a positive dye test at titres between 1/8 and 1/128, higher titres are suggestive of recent infection, and for a definitive diagnosis a rising titre should be sought with serial samples. Complement fixation and haemagglutination tests have also been used but are less useful than the original dye test.

Since most adult cases remit spontaneously, no treatment is required for the mononucleosis-like form of the disease. In the congenital form treatment will not reverse existing damage but is probably worthwhile in the hope of averting further progression. Active treatment with pyrimethamine, sulphadiazine and folinic acid is indicated for immunosuppressed patients and for patients with ocular involvement.

Malaria

Malarial infection causes a variety of haematological abnormalities. It is beyond the scope of this chapter to cover the clinical aspects of malaria, and to augment the brief description of the haematological changes which follows the reader is referred to standard texts on tropical medicine and to more extensive haematological reviews elsewhere [132, 136].

The species of plasmodia which produce malaria in humans are *Plasmodium falciparum, vivax, malariae* and *ovale*. These parasites are transmitted either by a bite from an anopheline mosquito or from the injection of malarious blood during a blood transfusion or intravenous injection. It is most important to identify the species of malarial parasite since the clinical disorders due to infection with the various types are quite different. Furthermore, there has been an emergence of treatment-resistant strains over the last few

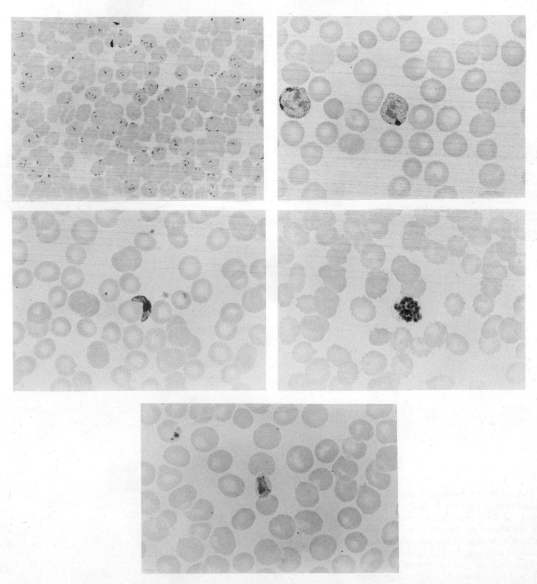

Fig. 33.5. Peripheral blood films showing different forms of malarial parasites (May–Grünwald–Giemsa stain): (a) *P. falciparum*, rings (× 2000); (b) *P. falciparum*, gametocyte (× 400); (c) *P. vivax*, amoeboid trophozoites (× 400); (d) *P. vivax*, schizont (× 400); (e) *P. malariae*, band form (× 400). (By courtesy of Professor H. M. Gilles.)

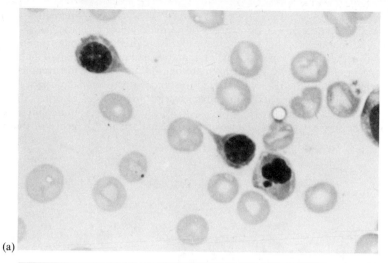

(a)

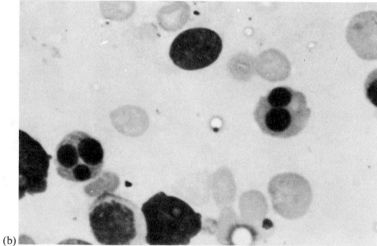

(b)

Fig. 33.6. Dyserythropoietic features in the bone marrow of patients with *P. falciparum* malaria. (a) Two intermediate normoblasts which are joined together with a long inter-cytoplasmic bridge. Also an intermediate normoblast showing nuclear fragmentation. (b) Multinuclearity of erythroblasts. (c) A group of erythroblasts of varying degrees of maturation. Three erythroblasts showing incomplete and irregular amitotic nuclear division.

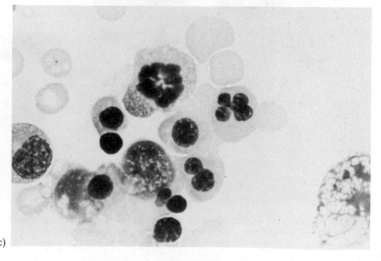

(c)

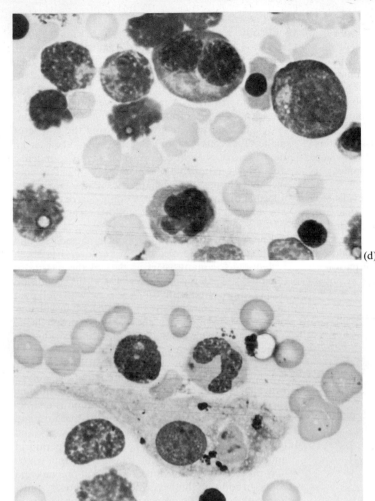

(d)

(e)

Fig. 33.6. (*cont.*) (d) One binucleate erythroblast and erythroblast with irregular nuclear division. (e) Erythrophagocytosis by a bone-marrow macrophage in a case of acute malaria. The macrophage shown has phagocytosed two erythrocytes which appear to be parasitized. In addition, there is malaria pigment in the cytoplasm of the macrophage. (By courtesy of Dr S. Abdulla and the editors of *British Journal of Haematology* [140].)

years so that many *P. falciparum* are now chloroquine-resistant. Primaquine therapy is required for the treatment of the exoerythrocytic forms of *P. vivax*, *ovale* and *malariae* but not for the treatment of *P. falciparum* which has no secondary exoerythrocytic stage. The morphological appearances of the different forms of parasite are illustrated in Figure 33.5. The characteristics which distinguish *P. falciparum* from the others include the presence of only ring forms in circulating erythrocytes and the absence of mature trophozoites or schizonts; the presence of more than one parasite in an erythrocyte; the double chromatin dots in the ring forms; and the presence of crescent-shaped gametocytes.

From a biological standpoint it is useful to consider not only the effects of the parasite on the host erythrocyte but also the effects of the host cell on the parasite. The widespread endemicity of malaria has ensured that genetic alterations in the red cell which adversely affect this relationship have become equally prominent. This topic has been extensively reviewed recently [137]; the most important genetic red-cell alterations which may provide some protection from malaria are the presence of HbS (see Chapter 8), G6PD deficiency (see Chapter 7), and the absence of the Duffy blood group antigen which confers resistance against *P. vivax*. The presence of HbF has been shown to impair the growth of, but not invasion by, *P. falciparum* [138, 139]; this may be one explanation for the relative resistance to malarial infection in early infancy, and for the high gene frequencies of thalassaemia and related conditions in which HbF levels are elevated, in areas where malaria is endemic.

A degree of anaemia is an almost inevitable consequence of malarial infection, but its pathophysiology is complex and has relatively little in common with the anaemia of other infections so far discussed. At first sight the very nature of malaria—with invasion and rupture of red cells—suggests a possible mechanism, but this is not sufficient explanation as the proportion of parasitized cells observed bears little relation to the severity of anaemia. Because of its high morbidity and mortality, falciparum malaria has received the most attention, and much of the following discussion refers particularly to this form of malaria. Factors which may to a variable extent influence the development of anaemia are listed in Table 33.7.

Notwithstanding that anaemia may be prevalent in endemic malarial areas for other reasons, the pattern of anaemia in malaria depends to some extent on the pattern of infection. With acute falciparum infection and high levels of parasitaemia, anaemia is mild on presentation but worsens transiently as the parasites are successfully eradicated [140]. This is followed by a

Table 33.7. Factors contributing to anaemia in malaria

Increased red-cell destruction—haemolysis
Direct or indirect damage by parasites
? Immune mechanisms
Hypersplenism
Drugs—blackwater fever

Decreased production
Hyperplastic marrow
  Ineffective erythropoiesis
  Megaloblastic anaemia: folate deficiency [421]
Hypoplastic marrow [422]

---

gradual recovery over the next few weeks. Patients with 'chronic' malarial infection and a low level of parasitaemia may be severely anaemic at presentation, with an inappropriately low reticulocyte count. Paradoxically, the marrow in such patients is hyperplastic but shows a gross degree of ineffective erythropoiesis (Fig. 33.6). Successful treatment of the malaria is followed by a reticulocytosis and an improvement in the anaemia.

An explanation for this diverse pathophysiology is hard to find. It has been suggested that in acute attacks the principal mechanism is haemolysis, partly as a result of direct or indirect damage by parasites and partly by an autoimmune mechanism [140, 141]. The direct antiglobulin test is commonly positive in falciparum infections when tested with a broad spectrum reagent, though less commonly with an anti-IgG reagent. The nature of any antigen(s) involved is not

yet known and the role of immune haemolysis must presently remain speculative [142]. From animal studies it has been suggested that the spleen can remove parasites from the red cell, which can then return to the circulation as spherocytes with a shortened lifespan [143, 144]. This phenomenon has not been demonstrated in man, however, and spherocytosis is not a typical feature of the malarial blood film.

Splenic enlargement is usual during the course of malarial infection, and has even been taken as an indication of the prevalence of malaria in endemic areas. The relationship of malaria to 'tropical' splenomegaly is discussed in Chapter 20. Patients with the anaemia of malaria often have some degree of thrombocytopenia and leucopenia, and hypersplenism may partly explain this in some cases.

Episodes of marked intravascular haemolysis and haemoglobinuria, termed blackwater fever, have been recognized for many years as part of the picture of falciparum malaria (Chapter 12). This condition occurs more frequently in patients with relapsed malaria on quinine therapy, and there is often a history of irregular or inadequate therapeutic or prophylactic anti-malarial drug administration. Although there is some evidence that this phenomenon results from the effect of quinine rather than malaria, this is certainly not always the case because fulminating haemolysis with haemoglobinuria may occur before quinine therapy has been instituted. The condition is characterized by a sudden rise in temperature with rigors, and this is associated with a variable degree of shock and the passage of dark urine. There follows a period of anuria or a marked reduction in urinary output which may proceed to the full clinical picture of uraemia and coma. In addition there is evidence of hepatic dysfunction with tender hepatomegaly. The major causes of death in this syndrome are anaemia, renal failure and acute cardiac failure.

It has been suggested that some patients who die with fulminating falciparum malaria have disseminated intravascular coagulation (DIC). Widespread thrombi with surrounding haemorrhage is commonly found at autopsy, and multiple coagulation abnormalities have been described including thrombocytopenia, shortened lifespan of labelled platelets and fibrinogen, diminished levels of factors V, VII, VIII and X, diminished fibrinogen, prolonged euglobulin-lysis times and increased levels of fibrin-degradation products (FDP) [145–148]. Unfortunately, the true incidence and importance of DIC is far from clear and there is lack of agreement between several of the published series [149]. Thrombocytopenia has been explained on the basis of increased splenic pooling with a decreased platelet lifespan [150], which has been ascribed to an immune mechanism [145]. It seems likely that many of the thrombotic lesions described are secondary to local vascular damage rather than to a generalized coagulation abnormality.

The leucocyte changes in malaria are variable [148]. In most forms of malaria a leucopenia is usual, and in falciparum malaria a neutropenia and monocytosis have been described [136]. In one study, six patients with acute vivax malaria had a total leucocyte count of $3 \cdot 0 \pm 0 \cdot 37 \times 10^9/l$ (± 1 s.d.) with $1 \cdot 65 \pm 0 \cdot 63 \times 10^9/l$ neutrophils. There was a marked shift to the left and neutrophil kinetic studies showed a normal or increased total blood neutrophil pool and an increased half-disappearance time. There was a marked shift from the circulating to marginating pools, and a decrease in marrow neutrophil reserve [151]. The circulating eosinophils may be decreased for 24–36 hours before a paroxysm while convalescence may be associated with a moderate eosinophilia.

Giardiasis

Infestation with *Giardia lamblia* may be associated with watery diarrhoea and steatorrhoea. The only haematological change which is associated with this infestation is a very mild eosinophilia. There is an increased incidence of infestation with this parasite in patients with dysgammaglobulinaemia type 1 (see Chapter 19).

Amoebiasis

Infestation with *Entamoeba histolytica* is often associated with anaemia, leucocytosis and an elevated blood sedimentation rate, but eosinophilia is rare. The anaemia is principally that of chronic disorders, but may be complicated by gastro-intestinal blood loss. In patients with amoebic liver abscess the leucocytosis may be extreme.

Leishmaniasis [132, 136, 152]

Visceral leishmaniasis or kala-azar is caused by infection with *Leishmania donovani* and is transmitted by the bite of infected sandflies. It occurs in two forms: the Mediterranean form, which is also endemic in China and South America and occurs predominantly in young children, and the Indian form, which occurs mainly in adolescents and young adults. The condition is characterized by bouts of irregular fever associated with malaise, weight loss and increasing hepatosplenomegaly, lymphadenopathy, and pancytopenia. Thus the condition can mimic a variety of primary haematological disorders. Early in the course of the disease there may be a marked neutropenia with a relative or absolute lymphocytosis and occasionally a monocytosis. The marrow becomes grossly infiltrated with parasitized macrophages (Fig. 33.7) and the spleen may become massively enlarged due to a similar process. The disorder should be suspected by the finding of very high globulin levels with a positive Sia (water) or formol gel test; a positive diagnosis can be made by the finding of typical Leishman–Donovan bodies in the marrow or spleen (Fig. 33.7), a positive skin test (Montenegro) or by a complement fixation test.

The traditional view that the anaemia of kala-azar is caused by a 'crowding-out' of the marrow by parasit-

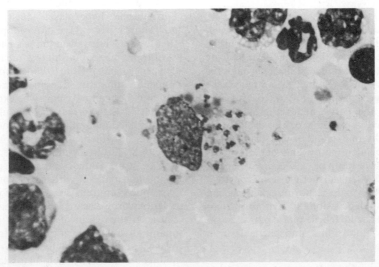

Fig. 33.7. A bone-marrow aspiration showing a *Leishmania* macrophage (LD body) (May–Grünwald–Giemsa stain ×400). (By courtesy of Professor H. M. Gilles.)

ized reticulo-endothelial cells is no longer tenable [152, 153]. Erythrokinetic and ferrokinetic studies show a rapid iron clearance but reduced incorporation of iron into erythrocytes, and a markedly shortened red-cell survival with peripheral sequestration, principally by the spleen [154]. Thus the anaemia is complex, and there is evidence for haemolysis as well as reduced or ineffective erythropoiesis. Complement has been found on the red-cell membrane, and it has been suggested that immune mechanisms may play a part in the shortened red-cell survival [153]. Neutropenia and thrombocytopenia are most likely a manifestation of hypersplenism [155]. Multiple haemostatic abnormalities have been described [156] but in spite of this, serious bleeding is uncommon.

African trypanosomiasis

African trypanosomiasis is a protozoal disease caused by the haemoflagellates *Trypanosoma rhodiense* and *Trypanosoma gambiense*, which are transmitted by the tsetse fly, *Glossina*. Infection with *T. rhodiense* is usually more fulminating than with *T. gambiense*. During the initial part of the illness there may be fever, headache, transient oedema of the hands and feet and enlargement of the posterior cervical lymph nodes. The spleen is often enlarged at this stage. Although the total leucocyte count remains normal there is often relative or absolute monocytosis. Parasites may be observed in the peripheral blood, and the preparation of fixed buffy-coat smears increases the likelihood of their identification. In the later stages of the disease, with central nervous system involvement, there is a moderate increase in serum IgM.

American trypanosomiasis (Chagas' disease)

This condition is caused by infection with *Trypanosoma cruzi* which is transmitted via the faeces of biting reduviid bugs of the family Triatominae. The parasite gains entry through the abraided skin or through the mucous membrane. It may also be transmitted via the placenta as a congenital infection, or by infected mother's milk. In the early stages there is often unilateral conjunctivitis, oedema of the eyelids and swelling of the lachrymal glands, while later there is generalized lymphadenopathy and hepatosplenomegaly with evidence of brain or cardiac involvement. The haematological changes include a leucocytosis and absolute lymphocytosis, a normocytic anaemia with a high ESR, and occasionally hypoprothrombinaemia. During the acute febrile phase parasites can be demonstrated in blood films, and particularly in thick buffy-coat smears.

HELMINTHIC DISEASES—NEMATODES

The most characteristic haematological change in the helminthic infections is a eosinophilia. Although this is most marked in those infestations associated with a systemic phase such as ascariasis and ankylostomiasis, it may also be found in those localized to the gastro-intestinal tract. It should be remembered that the diagnosis of helminthic infestation in patients with eosinophilia may not become obvious for weeks or months until the adult worms have produced progeny. Such cases thus require careful long-term observation with frequent examination of stool or tissue specimens.

Hookworm disease [132, 136]

Infection with *Ankylostoma duodenale* is common in temperate climates including southern Europe, the Middle East, North Africa and China, whilst *Necator americanus* infestation is widespread throughout the tropics. Both worms are found in South-east Asia, India, Africa and South America. The larvae typically enter through the skin of bare feet following contact with infected soil, or occasionally by inhalation.

Following penetration by the parasite a local patch of dermatitis with regional lymphadenopathy may develop. During the systemic phase when the larvae invade the lungs there may be a severe bronchitis with eosinophils in the sputum. After about six weeks the eggs appear in the stools, indicating that the larvae have migrated from the lung through the tracheobronchial tree into the intestine and have matured into adult worms. During this phase there is a leucocytosis with a variable degree of eosinophilia; total leucocyte counts as high as 50×10^9/l with 50% eosinophils have been reported. The eosinophilia usually persists for about one year after the infection. The marrow shows normoblastic hyperplasia whilst the myeloid series may show a percentage of eosinophils out of proportion to that observed in the peripheral blood.

Chronic infestation almost invariably causes iron-deficiency anaemia due to consumption by the worms. Hypoalbuminaemia due to gastro-intestinal loss is common but can only partly be explained by a loss of protein to the worms. Each adult worm consumes between 0·02 ml and 0·2 ml of blood daily [132, 157]; the rate at which anaemia and hypoalbuminaemia develop will thus depend upon the total worm load as well as the nutritional status of the patient. In addition to anaemia, patients with heavy worm loads may suffer dyspeptic symptoms suggestive of peptic ulceration.

Hookworm disease is diagnosed by the finding of characteristic ova in the faeces. It is useful to make a quantitative estimate of the worm load by counting the ova in 2 g of faeces: each female worm is represented by about 50 ova. It is also helpful to examine the stools for the worms themselves after treatment. The anaemia responds completely to oral iron therapy but will relapse if iron is withdrawn without the patient first being dewormed [157].

Trichinosis [132]

Infestation with *Trichinella spiralis* follows the eating of raw pork. About one week later there is severe muscle pain, facial oedema, dyspnoea and difficulty in swallowing. At this stage there is a marked leucocytosis with an eosinophilia and the larvae may be found in the peripheral blood. During the acute phase, bruising and thromboembolic phenomena are common and coagulation studies may show increased fibrinolysis.

Visceral larva migrans [132]

This disorder is due to the ingestion of the eggs of *Toxocara canis* from soil contaminated with dog or cat faeces. It is thus a disease of young children who keep pets. The condition is characterized by hepatomegaly, bizarre forms of pneumonia and neurological and ophthalmological disturbances. Haematological changes are common and include mild anaemia and a leucocytosis with a marked eosinophilia [158].

Some patients show marked elevation in heterophil antibody titre (p. 1333). The antibody is completely adsorbed by guinea-pig kidney but only partially by beef erythrocytes, suggesting that it is a Forssman-type antibody. There may also be a marked increase in the titre of anti-A and anti-B blood group antibodies. This is most striking in patients of blood group O, who may have anti-A and anti-B titres of over 1/100 000.

Other nematode infections

Other nematode infections including filariasis, onchocerciasis and loiasis may be associated with a marked eosinophilia. Filariasis is also associated with a thrombotic tendency.

HELMINTHIC INFECTIONS—TREMATODES

Schistosomiasis [132]

These disorders result from the presence of the ova of the schistomasomes *S. mansoni* and *S. japonicum* in the venules of the intestine and of *S. haematobium* in the bladder and pelvic vessels. The developing worms cause local injury to the blood vessels with petechial haemorrhages and, subsequently, inflammatory changes in the liver, lungs and central nervous system. During the incubation period there may be asthma, urticaria, diarrhoea and hepatomegaly accompanied by a striking leucocytosis and eosinophilia. Once the schistosomes mature and lay eggs, bleeding may occur from the bladder or gut and there may be fever and abdominal pain with leucocytosis, eosinophilia and an elevated blood sedimentation rate.

The chronic phase of mansoni and japonicum infection is characterized by the development of periportal fibrosis in the liver, with portal hypertension, splenomegaly and the attendant problems of hypersplenism. The picture may be further complicated by gastro-intestinal bleeding. This phase of the disease responds well to splenectomy, though some kind of porto-systemic shunt procedure is usually also required.

Other trematode infestations including clonorchiasis, fascioliasis and paragonamiasis may all be associated with eosinophilia, leucocytosis and anaemia. Antibody to the P_1 blood group antigen has been found in grossly elevated titres in the blood of most patients with acute fascioliasis [159].

HELMINTHIC INFECTIONS—CESTODES

There are many tapeworms which can produce cestodiasis in man. The commonest are *Taenia saginata* (beef tapeworm), *Taenia solium* (pork tapeworm), *Diphyllobothrium latum* (fish tapeworm) and *Dipylidium canium* (dog tapeworm). Most of these infections are asymptomatic but a mild eosinophilia may be found. Infections due to *D. latum* have been considered in Chapter 6, page 217. The clinical picture is that of a macrocytic anaemia due to vitamin-B_{12} deficiency.

Infections due to the larvae of *Echinococcus granulosus* result in hydatid disease with the production of large unilocular cysts in the liver and lungs. There is sometimes an associated eosinophilia, and in patients with multiple hepatic cysts there may be coagulation abnormalties, presumably related to abnormal liver function. Hydatid cyst fluid is rich in P_1 blood group substance, and moderate titres of anti-P_1 antibody have been noted in about 50% of patients with hydatid disease [159].

RHEUMATOID ARTHRITIS AND THE COLLAGEN VASCULAR DISORDERS

There are a variety of haematological changes which may accompany rheumatoid arthritis and the collagen vascular disorders. These conditions are now all recognized to be multisystem disorders and it is not surprising that there are many ways in which they can affect the blood. The principal blood changes in these conditions are listed in Table 33.8 and are discussed briefly in this section.

RHEUMATOID ARTHRITIS

Anaemia

Some degree of anaemia is extremely common in patients with active rheumatoid arthritis and this is

Table 33.8. Principal blood changes in rheumatoid arthritis and collagen disease

---

Rheumatoid arthritis
Anaemia
   Anaemia of chronic disorders. Iron deficiency; blood loss due to salicylates. Folic-acid deficiency.
   Hypersplenism in Felty's syndrome. Marrow depression due to gold or phenylbutazone
Leucopenia
   Felty's syndrome. Gold or phenylbutazone
Thrombocytopenia
   Felty's syndrome. Gold or phenylbutazone
Leukocytosis
   Septic arthritis. Steroid therapy

Systemic lupus erythematosus
Anaemia
   Anaemia of chronic disorders. Immune haemolytic anaemia. Hypoplastic anaemia. Blood loss due to thrombocytopenia.
   Anaemia of renal failure. Marrow depression due to immuno-suppressive therapy
Thrombocytopenia
   Picture similar to idiopathic thrombocytopenic purpura. May be complicated by marrow hypoplasia due to disease or
   therapy
Neutropenia or lymphopenia
Splenic atrophy
   Typical blood changes of hyposplenism
LE-cell phenomena
Circulating anticoagulant

Polyarteritis nodosa
Anaemia
   Anaemia of chronic disorders. Blood loss. Renal failure
Leucocytosis, eosinophilia

Temporal arteritis and polymyalgia rheumatica
Anaemia
   Anaemia of chronic disorders. High ESR

---

probably the commonest systemic manifestation of this disease. The anaemia is usually that of chronic disorders and has been described in detail above; the features that are particularly relevant to rheumatoid arthritis have been well reviewed by Bennett [160]. This anaemia is occasionally complicated by genuine iron deficiency, which may result from a variety of causes including poor diet and chronic intestinal blood loss due to the effects of treatment—particularly the ingestion of salicylates and phenylbutazone. A potentially major source of inapparent blood loss has been described by Bennett using ^{59}Fe-labelled transferrin [161]. He has shown that significant bleeding occurs into actively inflamed joints and has estimated that if only two knee joints were affected the annual blood loss could amount to 2500 ml. Although this iron is not lost from the body, the red cells are degraded within the synovial membrane and the iron is deposited in the synovium as haemosiderin. It is not known how much if any of this sequestered iron is available for erythropoiesis. The diagnosis of iron deficiency complicating rheumatoid arthritis may not be straightforward: the serum iron and iron-binding capacity levels may be difficult to interpret because of co-existing inflammation, but examination of the marrow iron stores and estimation of serum ferritin may be useful [12, 13].

Macrocytic anaemia is uncommon in patients with rheumatoid arthritis, and when present is usually due to folic-acid deficiency. Several reports suggesting an increased incidence of pernicious anaemia in patients with rheumatoid arthritis have been reviewed by Chanarin [41]. In many of the cases the diagnosis was not proven, and in one large series with matched controls there was no increase in the incidence of pernicious anaemia or of parietal-cell antibodies [162]. Folic-acid deficiency is found occasionally and may result from poor diet or increased requirements due to chronic gastro-intestinal blood loss [163]. Low serum or red-cell folate values are often found in the absence of frank macrocytic anaemia [164, 165].

Management. In general, the severity of anaemia follows the degree of activity of the arthritis and tends to improve as the condition comes under control with anti-inflammatory drugs. It is important to rule out the presence of a complicating factor such as genuine iron or folic-acid deficiency, the side-effects of the various anti-inflammatory agents which the patient may be receiving, and hypersplenism due to Felty's syndrome. Iron deficiency, if present, should be treated with oral iron but the response may be tempered by the presence of active inflammation. Parenteral iron therapy has been advocated and it has been suggested that some improvement in the anaemia of rheumatoid arthritis may be expected even in the absence of genuine iron deficiency [166]. It must be remembered, however, that patients with chronic disorders have increased iron stores, and the regular administration of parenteral iron will ultimately result in severe iron loading with consequent tissue damage. In the authors' opinion this form of therapy is rarely justified.

Leucocytes and platelets

In uncomplicated rheumatoid arthritis the leucocyte count may be normal, slightly elevated or slightly depressed, though when the disease is particularly active there is frequently a mild neutrophil leucocytosis [167]. A more marked leucocytosis may occur as a response to steroid therapy or may indicate a super-added infection such as a septic arthritis. The neutrophil alkaline phosphatase tends to be slightly reduced during the active phase of the disease. There have been a number of reports of impaired neutrophil function *in vitro* [160], though it is not clear if this is responsible for an increased tendency to infection. Circulating immune complexes have been demonstrated in over half the sera of patients with rheumatoid arthritis [168], and are associated with defective neutrophil chemotaxis.

The platelet count is elevated in 12–52% of patients with rheumatoid arthritis [169–171]. The degree of thrombocytosis parallels the level of disease activity and the presence of extra-articular manifestations such as cutaneous vasculitis, and correlates inversely with the level of haemoglobin. The cause of the thrombocytosis is unexplained; although patients taking anti-inflammatory medication may have increased gastrointestinal blood loss, this did not explain the thrombocytosis in the reported series [169, 170]. In one case report thrombocytosis was associated with fatal arterial thromboembolism [171]. Thrombocytopenia occurs much less commonly and is usually associated with significant splenomegaly.

FELTY'S SYNDROME

In 1924, Felty described five patients with active rheumatoid arthritis, splenomegaly, leucopenia, skin pigmentation and weight loss, and felt that the triad of chronic arthritis, leucopenia and splenomegaly might constitute a distinct clinical disorder [172]. The term *Felty's syndrome* was first used in 1932 by Hanrahan & Miller who described the effects of splenectomy in a patient with this triad of symptoms [173]. Although the syndrome has now become firmly established in the medical literature, it has attracted an interest out of proportion to its incidence [174], and present evidence suggests that it should be considered as one aspect of the spectrum of rheumatoid disease with extra-articular manifestations rather than as a separate entity. Indeed some degree of lymphoid hypertrophy and splenomegaly is found in many patients [175], though relatively few have specific symptoms due to this complication.

Clinical findings [174, 176]

Felty's syndrome is a complication of long-standing seropositive rheumatoid arthritis. The arthritis is usually severe with rheumatoid nodules and considerable ankylosis and deformity. The spleen is palpably enlarged but does not usually weigh more than 1000 g after removal [177]; the histological changes are non-specific with large germinal centres and increased mononuclear infiltration. Hepatomegaly is found in some cases with slight alterations in liver-function tests; it is associated with a diffuse lymphocytosis infiltration of both the sinusoids and portal tracts.

Several complications may arise in patients with Felty's syndrome. These include splenic rupture or abscess formation, and an increased incidence of infections, presumably due to the associated neutrophil defect. Particularly common are recurrent pneumonia, cellulitis and septic arthritis superimposed on the underlying rheumatoid condition.

Haematological changes

Anaemia is found in nearly 90% of patients with Felty's syndrome [174]; in addition to the anaemia of chronic disorders characteristic of rheumatoid arthritis, there is frequently a marked shortening of the red-cell survival with evidence of splenic sequestration [178]. There is usually a marked leucopenia with absolute neutrophil counts of less than 0.6×10^9/l and often an associated lymphopenia. There is no direct relationship between the leucocyte count and the incidence of infections or the size of the spleen, and many patients with this disorder seem to remain well for years despite profound neutropenia. The serological changes are those of seropositive rheumatoid arthritis; thus rheumatoid factor is always present in high titres, anti-nuclear factor can be found in two-thirds of cases [174], and there is often an associated hypocomplimentaemia.

The cause of the neutropenia in Felty's syndrome is complex, and a number of different though not mutually exclusive mechanisms have been proposed [174]. These include reduced production, immune destruction, and sequestration by the enlarged spleen.

The marrow shows a non-specific picture with myeloid hyperplasia and often a paucity of mature neutrophils, the so-called 'shift-to-the-left' [176, 179]. Neutrophil production is reduced in some patients as judged by the performance of neutrophil progenitors *in vitro*, reductions in serum and urinary levels of CSF and a reduced response to etiocholanolone. Of particular interest is a recent report that peripheral blood, marrow and spleen cells from patients with Felty's syndrome suppressed normal marrow cells in a CFU-C assay [180]. The cells responsible were thought to be predominantly T-cells but monocytes also had suppressor activity. Neutrophil kinetics have been studied in 17 patients with Felty's syndrome by Vincent *et al.* [181]; the blood neutrophil half-life was normal but the proportion of marginating neutrophils was sufficiently increased to explain the neutropenia entirely in all but five patients, in whom production appeared suboptimal. It was not possible in this study to determine if the spleen was the major site of margination, though this seems likely.

There has been considerable interest in a possible role for antineutrophil antibodies; in one study, transfusion of blood from patients with Felty's syndrome into normal individuals produced a transient leucopenia [182], and in another series, granulocyte-specific antinuclear factor was present in all patients [183]. Using an indirect anti-human-globulin consumption test for leucocytes, Rosenthal *et al.* [184] found IgG leucocyte antibodies in 13 out of 15 patients; this could not be explained by previous pregnancy or transfusion, and the antibody appeared to be genuinely leucocyte-specific. Similarly, Logue has demonstrated that neutrophils from patients with Felty's syndrome have markedly increased amounts of surface IgG and that this was corrected by splenectomy [185]. This evidence suggests that the role of the spleen in the neutropenia Felty's syndrome could be as a producer of antibody as well as a site of sequestration.

Management

Therapy with corticosteroids in safe therapeutic doses and other anti-inflammatory agents has little effect on the leucocyte count in Felty's syndrome. After splenectomy there is sometimes a dramatic rise in the neutrophil and total leucocyte counts, but this is not always associated with an decreased incidence of infection [176, 177, 179, 186]. Thus in a study of six patients who underwent splenectomy with recurrent infection as the main indication, three died of infection within six months and two continued with recurrent infections [179]. In another report 12 patients in a series of 34 underwent splenectomy; there was a significant increase in neutrophil, lymphocyte, total leucocyte and platelet counts in the group as a whole,

but although recurrent infections has been noted prior to splenectomy in eight patients, these persisted after splenectomy in four [176]. Thus at the present time no clear-cut recommendation can be made for splenectomy in this disorder, though it may be beneficial in some patients who have recurrent life-threatening infections (Fig. 33.8).

HAEMATOLOGICAL CHANGES SECONDARY TO DRUG THERAPY IN RHEUMATOID ARTHRITIS AND RELATED DISORDERS

The drugs commonly used in the management of rheumatoid arthritis have a wide range of side-effects and many of them can affect the blood. Salicylates may produce chronic blood loss while drugs containing phenacetin can produce methaemoglobinaemia and Heinz-body haemolytic anaemia. Corticosteroids produce a neutrophil leucocytosis and may exacerbate peptic ulcers and produce chronic bleeding. Gold may produce a pancytopenia or selective reduction in the platelet or granulocyte counts. Patients with gold dermatitis may develop a marked eosinophilia and this may precede the skin reaction and is a useful early-warning sign of the development of this serious complication. Phenylbutazone occasionally causes a pancytopenia which may be severe and irreversible. Increased chromosome breaks are found in the marrow cells of patients on phenylbutazone [187], but although there have been reports of the development of leukaemia in patients who were taking this drug, a causal relationship is far from proven. Oxyphenbutazone and penicillamine have also caused aplastic anaemia.

SYSTEMIC LUPUS ERYTHEMATOSUS

Systemic lupus erythematosis (SLE) is a multisystem disorder of unknown aetiology, which is characterized by major alterations in the immune system with manifestations in a wide variety of organ systems. It is beyond the scope of this chapter to review the immunological aspects of this disorder, for which the reader is referred elsewhere [188]. The haematological manifestations have been well annotated in a recent review by Budman & Steinberg [189].

Anaemia

The commonest haematological abnormality in SLE is an anaemia which affects practically all patients at some stage of their illness [190, 191]. This is usually the anaemia of chronic disorders and is generally mild. More severe anaemia may be due to blood loss from analgesic or anti-inflammatory medication, from renal impairment, and in particular from haemolysis. Acquired autoimmune haemolytic anaemia may be the sole presenting feature of SLE and may antedate the

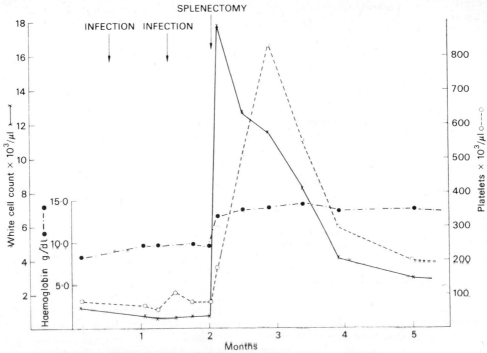

Fig. 33.8. The clinical course after splenectomy in a patient with Felty's syndrome. The patient maintained a satisfactory leucocyte count for five years after the operation.

appearance of other typical features by a number of years. More commonly, however, this anaemia is present from the onset with other symptoms suggestive of SLE. The incidence of this complication varies in reported series but occurs overall in approximately five per cent of all cases. The Coombs' test is almost invariably positive with anti-complement reagents, and is positive with anti-IgG reagents more often during periods of acute haemolysis than in quiescent phases, though the incidence of positive reactions is greater when very sensitive techniques are used. A pure IgG reaction without complement probably never occurs in SLE. The antibodies involved are of the 'warm' type and are usually IgG, though occasionally IgM and rarely IgA antibodies are found. They are usually complement-fixing and show no blood group specificity, in contrast to antibodies found in idiopathic autoimmune haemolytic anaemias.

Occasionally other forms of anaemia are encountered in patients with SLE. Repeated blood loss secondary to thrombocytopenia may lead to the picture of iron deficiency and the anaemia may also be exacerbated by superimposed renal failure. In patients with splenomegaly there may be the added complication of hypersplenism. The marrow in SLE is usually hyperplastic with a 'shift-to-the-left' in the myeloid series. Occasionally a relatively hypocellular marrow picture is found, and this is probably due to involvement of the small vessels of the marrow by the disease process. A severe hypoplastic anaemia has been reported in very acute forms of SLE [192, 193], and there is an association with splenic atrophy.

Leucocytes
The most consistent leucocyte abnormality in SLE is a leucopenia, which is found in up to half of the patients at some time during the illness [190, 191]. The leucopenia is often due to a reduction in both the neutrophils and lymphocytes, though neutropenia is usually the most striking feature. A number of factors which could be responsible for these changes have been reviewed by Budman & Steinberg [189] and are summarized in Table 33.9. Abnormalities of neutrophil function have also been reported, but these have largely been explained by humoral abnormalities rather than defects in the phagocytes themselves. A leucocytosis may occur in SLE during intercurrent infection, acute haemolytic episodes, or with corticosteroid therapy. A mild eosinophilia has been noted occasionally, particularly when there is extensive skin involvement [190].

Table 33.9. Factors contributing to the development of leucopenia in SLE (after Ref. 189)

Neutropenia

Peripheral destruction
  ? immune mechanisms
  hypersplenism

Reduced production
  central destruction
  inadequate marrow response
  drug-induced (e.g. phenylbutazone, azathioprine)

Lymphopenia

Non-immune mechanisms
  drug-induced
  ? environmental or genetic loss

Immune mechanisms
  IgM complement-dependent antilymphocyte antibody
  IgG non-complement-dependent antilymphocyte antibody
  non-lymphocyte-specific antibody cross-reacting with lymphocytes
  ? non-cytotoxic antilymphocyte antibodies

Platelets

A mild thrombocytopenia with platelet counts of less than $100 \times 10^9/l$ has been reported in between eight and 26% of cases [190, 194], although the overall incidence of this complication may be much higher. The thrombocytopenia of SLE has much in common with idiopathic thrombocytopenic purpura (ITP). It is associated with increased numbers of megakaryocytes in the bone marrow, an increase in the number of large platelets (megathrombocytes) in the peripheral blood, and a markedly decreased platelet survival [195]. However, there is some evidence to suggest that platelet destruction in SLE may be mediated by immune complexes rather than by anti-platelet antibody, as is thought to be the case in ITP [189, 196].

Thrombocytopenia may occur many years before the onset of clinical SLE, or the two conditions may present together. The frequency with which SLE develops after ITP has been much disputed: Dameshek *et al.* [197] recorded eight cases of SLE in a series of 51 patients with ITP but Carpenter *et al.* [198] found no cases after a long follow-up of 41 individuals similarly affected. Doan *et al.* [199] found an incidence of two per cent of patients with SLE in a series of 381 patients with ITP. There is no evidence that splenectomy tends to precipitate SLE in patients with the clinical picture of ITP. The clinical and haematological changes in thrombocytopenic purpura and the management of the condition is dealt with in detail in Chapter 25.

Purpura in SLE may result from causes other than thrombocytopenia. There is occasionally an element of vascular purpura, particularly in patients receiving corticosteroids. Similarly, where renal failure occurs there may be an increased bleeding tendency. Bleeding may also occur due to the deficiency to the vitamin-K-dependent clotting factors in patients where there is associated liver damage. A characteristic coagulation inhibitor has been described in SLE and can be detected by routine coagulation tests in five to 10% of patients with this disorder. The inhibitor is an immunoglobulin which interferes with the interaction between the factor-V–factor-Xa–phospholipid–calcium complex, possibly by inhibition of phospholipid. This anticoagulant is not specific for SLE [200] and, even though it may be present in high titres, it is rarely a cause of serious bleeding. Indeed, recent reports have highlighted an increased tendency to venous thrombosis in the presence of this inhibitor [201].

The LE-cell phenomenon [188, 194, 202]

In 1948 Hargreaves *et al.* described the appearances of two types of abnormal cell in the bone marrow of patients with systemic lupus erythematosis. Both of these, the 'LE cell' and the 'Tart cell' result from the phagocytosis of cellular material. The LE-cell phenomenon depends on the presence of an antinuclear antibody which appears to combine directly with nuclear protein, and it is probably only leucocytes which have been slightly damaged and lost their membrane integrity that are capable of showing this phenomenon. After the entrance of the antibody the nucleus swells and loses its chromatin structure and finally becomes a fairly homogeneous mass which then ruptures through the nuclear membrane. The nuclear

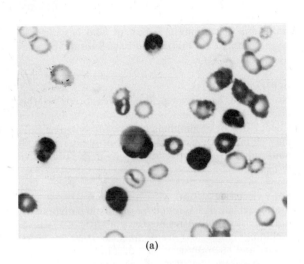

(a)

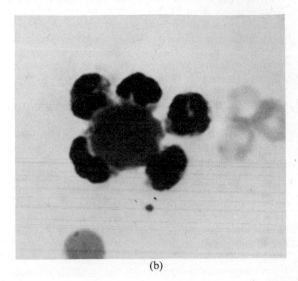

(b)

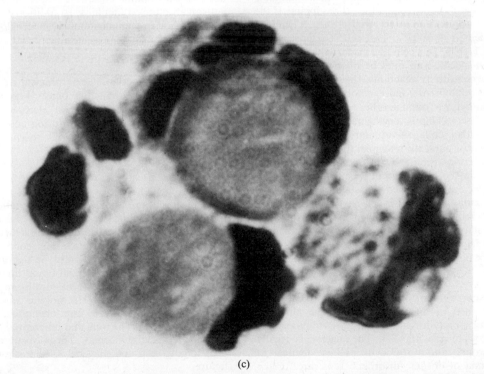

(c)

Fig. 33.9. LE cells: (a) LE cell (×920); (b) Rosette formation (×920); (c) LE cell (×2875). (By courtesy of Dr George MacDonald.)

material so discharged, or free 'LE body', varies in size from about a third of the size of a red-blood cell to about three or four times that size. It tends to attract neutrophils and monocytes which cluster around it to form a rosette, and ultimately the material is engulfed by one or more of the phagocytes so producing a typical LE cell (Fig. 33.9). This contains a large, round, bluish homogeneous body while the darker-stained nucleus of the phagocyte is squashed against the periphery of the cell. Thus in buffy-coat samples prepared after suitable incubation of the blood of patients with SLE, several abnormalities may be observed: these include increased rouleux formation, extracellular material, rosettes, LE cells and occasional erythrophagocytosis. The LE cell is essentially an *in-vitro* phenomenon, though large numbers of LE cells may be seen in direct smears from serous effusions, and the characteristic haematoxylin bodies found in the tissues represent the *in-vivo* counterpart of the LE body.

It is important to distinguish the so-called pseudo-LE cell and Tart cell from true LE cells. Pseudo-LE cells are polymorphonuclear leucocytes or monocytes that have engulfed a nuclear mass which maintains some nuclear structure and which is basophilic. If the engulfed nucleus is an intact, well-preserved lymphocyte nucleus it is called a Tart cell. The presence of pseudo-LE cells, Tart cells and erythrophagocytosis is quite non-specific and may be observed in patients with hypersensitivity reactions, rheumatoid arthritis, infections, malignancy and haemolytic anaemia.

LE cells may be found in other conditions including chronic discoid lupus erythematosus, rheumatoid arthritis, other collagen-vascular disorders, chronic active hepatitis, aplastic anaemia, the lymphomas and in drug reactions. Similarly, the finding of haematoxylin bodies in the tissues is not specific for SLE since they have been observed in such conditions as Hodgkin's disease. The LE-cell test has largely been superceded by the more convenient tests for antinuclear factor in the serum [188], but the test should still be performed in difficult cases as it may occasionally be positive in the absence of antinuclear factor [203].

ANKYLOSING SPONDYLITIS

The incidence of anaemia in the active phase of ankylosing spondylitis is variable; it was found in 25% of one series of patients [204]. The anaemia is usually normochromic and normocytic and is identical to the anaemia of chronic disorders. It is rare for the haemoglobin to fall much below 10 g/dl [205]. The leucocyte and platelet counts are usually normal, but the ESR is usually elevated in the active phase of the disease.

If radiotherapy has been given to the lumbosacral region, the marrow in that area may remain hypoplastic for many years and extensive chromosomal abnormalities are readily demonstrable. The risk of leukaemia developing in a patient who has received such treatment is 10 times that of the normal population [206].

DERMATOMYOSITIS

No specific haematological features occur in this disease. Mild anaemia is noted occasionally and a leucocytosis or eosinophilia may be present. The ESR may be markedly elevated; values of greater than 60 mm/hour are indicative of severe and progressive disease [207].

POLYARTERITIS NODOSA

The anaemia which is found frequently in patients with polyarteritis nodosa results from a variety of causes including blood loss from mucosal surfaces, renal failure and haemolysis as part of a microangiopathy.

A moderate elevation of the white-cell count is typical of polyarteritis nodosa. The increase is usually due to a neutrophilia but this is frequently associated with an absolute eosinophilia. In addition to a generalized increase in gammaglobulins, macroglobulins or cryoglobulins may be present in increased amounts.

REITER'S DISEASE

There are no specific haematological features of Reiter's disease. In the active phase there may be a normochromic anaemia and an elevated ESR. A neutrophil leucocytosis occurs during acute attacks, and the total leucocyte count may reach as high as $30 \times 10^9/l$ [208].

PROGRESSIVE SYSTEMIC SCLEROSIS (SCLERODERMA)

Anaemia occurs in about one-third of patients with progressive systemic sclerosis. Although this is usually the anaemia of chronic disorders, iron deficiency due to bleeding from telangiectases may complicate the picture [209]. Anaemia may also be aggravated by renal failure. In cases with small bowel involvement, malabsorption of folic acid or vitamin B_{12} may lead to a megaloblastic anaemia. Haemolytic anaemia has also been reported as a rare accompaniment of scleroderma [210]. The total and differential leucocyte counts are usually normal. Thrombocytopenia is occasionally seen and may be associated with renal failure.

POLYMYALGIA RHEUMATICA AND GIANT-CELL ARTERITIS [211]

It is not uncommon for patients with polymyalgia

rheumatica, or a variant of this disorder, to present to the haematologist. These patients usually complain of severe stiffness in the region of the neck, shoulders, buttocks and thighs of fairly sudden onset. This is associated with marked constitutional symptoms and signs, with weight loss, fatigue, anorexia, sweating and nocturnal fever. In some cases the clinical features of temporal arteritis may also be present, with severe pain in the scalp and visual disturbance sometimes progressing to blindness.

The haematological changes in this disorder are usually marked, and include the anaemia of chronic disorders and a marked elevation of the ESR, often to over 100 mm/hour. The leucocyte count is usually normal although there may occasionally be a mild eosinophilia. The marrow shows no specific changes. Rheumatoid factor is usually absent and there is a general increase in α_2 and γ globin. The levels of muscle enzymes are normal.

The major problem for the clinician is to distinguish this disorder from primary haematological conditions such as myeloma, and from the haematological complications of disseminated malignancy. Whilst the former can usually be excluded quite simply by blood, marrow and urine examination, occult malignancy can be very difficult to exclude. A trial of corticosteroids is often useful: relatively small doses of prednisolone (5–10 mg/day) typically produce dramatic and complete resolution of the symptoms of polymyalgia rheumatica, but will have little if any effect on the symptoms of the anaemia of disseminated malignancy. Temporal arteritis, however, demands more active management as visual loss is common and usually severe. A temporal artery biopsy should be performed and treatment commenced with high doses of prednisolone (60–80 mg/day).

In clinical practice it is not uncommon to encounter elderly patients who have a mild normochromic normocytic anaemia associated with a very high ESR. Full investigations fail to reveal a cause for the anaemia and the condition responds dramatically to corticosteroid treatment. It seems very likely that this is a variant of polymyalgia rheumatica.

RENAL DISEASE

A wide variety of blood changes are associated with the various conditions that affect the kidney (Table 33.10). The most important haematological abnormality is anaemia, which develops rapidly after renal shutdown, and which has a complex aetiology as discussed below. Renal tumours, cysts and hydronephrosis may all be associated with polycythaemia [212] and a variable haemorrhagic tendency is commonly seen in renal failure. Several systemic disorders affect both the

Table 33.10. Haematological changes in renal disease

Acute renal shutdown
  Anaemia
  Erythroid hypoplasia
Chronic renal failure
  Anaemia
  Bleeding diathesis
Chronic pyelonephritis
  Anaemia of chronic disorders
Renal tumours
  Anaemia
  Leuco-erythroblastic anaemia
  Polycythaemia
Renal cysts
  Polycythaemia
Vascular disease (Acute nephritis, malignant hypertension, haemolytic-uraemic syndrome, eclampsia, acute tubular or cortical necrosis, allograft rejection etc.)
  Microangiopathic haemolytic anaemia
Post-renal transplantation
  Thrombocytosis
  Polycythaemia
  Leucocytosis
  Thrombotic tendency
Effects of dialysis
  Anaemia
  Folic-acid deficiency
  Iron deficiency

blood and the kidney: these include the microangiopathies which accompany malignant hypertension, preeclampsia, disseminated malignancy, the haemolytic uraemic syndrome, disseminated intravascular coagulation and the collagen vascular disorders. Finally, primary blood disorders may affect the kidney, the most notable being sickle-cell disease [213] and myeloma [214]. The majority of these conditions have been described in detail elsewhere in this book; in the section which follows the blood changes characteristic of chronic renal failure are briefly reviewed.

THE ANAEMIA OF CHRONIC RENAL FAILURE (CRF)
Some degree of anaemia is invariable in patients with chronic renal failure (CRF) [215, 216]. In the early stages, anaemia may be mild though it usually becomes more severe with progression of the disease. In most instances its severity is roughly proportional to the degree of uraemia, though patients with an underlying microangiopathy may be more severely anaemic, whilst patients with polycystic disease are often less anaemic than other patients with similar renal impairment [217].

Haematological changes
In milder cases the anaemia is normochromic and

normocytic with only mild changes in red-cell morphology, typically occasional burr cells or other distorted forms. In severe renal failure with blood urea values of over 25 mmol/l, the blood film usually shows a considerable degree of poikilocytosis with irregularly contracted cells including burr, triangular, helmet and other bizarre forms [218–220]. Burr cells can be produced by incubation of normal erythrocytes with uraemic serum and result from an alteration of membrane lipids, though the nature of the factor responsible has not been determined [221]. Continued blood loss during dialysis or due to gastro-intestinal haemorrhage may lead to the changes of iron deficiency. The absolute reticulocyte count may be normal, subnormal or moderately increased [222]. Leucocyte and platelet morphology is usually normal though neutrophil hypersegmentation has been reported. In some cases this is related to associated folate deficiency but in others the abnormality persists after treatment with folic acid and the mechanism is unknown.

In some patients, progressive renal failure is associated with a microangiopathic haemolytic anaemia [223] (see Chapter 12). In such cases there is marked erythrocyte fragmentation together with a reticulocytosis, evidence of both intravascular haemolysis and coagulation, and a variable haemorrhagic tendency with thrombocytopenia. This haematological picture may occur in primary renal disease such as acute nephritis, in the haemolytic-uraemic syndrome, or as part of a more generalized vascular disorder such as toxaemia of pregnancy or thrombotic thrombocytopenic purpura.

The most striking feature of the marrow in CRF is its apparent normality in the face of moderate or severe anaemia. Whilst there may be mild erythroid hyperplasia [224, 225], it is not of a degree that is commensurate with the severity of the anaemia. Erythroid hypoplasia has been observed in acute renal failure.

The mechanism of the anaemia of renal failure

The aetiology of the anaemia of renal failure is complex and results from the interaction of several factors, including haemolysis, a reduced erythropoietic response and a variable degree of haemodilution. Many studies have confirmed that the red-cell lifespan is shortened in the majority of cases, even in the absence of microangiopathic haemolysis [222, 223, 225, 226], and that the reduction in lifespan correlates with the degree of impaired renal function rather than the type of renal damage. Cross-transfusion experiments have shown that the shortened survival is due to an extracorpuscular defect. A number of metabolic defects can be demonstrated in the erythrocytes [225–227]; these are reversible and are caused by factors in the uraemic serum. Autohaemolysis of both uraemic and normal erythrocytes is increased in uraemic serum, and there is a reduction in Na^+, K^+-ATPase activity with a resulting loss of potassium and increase in intracellular sodium content. A variety of other metabolic changes have been noted, including impairment of glycoclysis, glutathione metabolism and the pentose pathway. Although some of these abnormalities can be related to acidosis or to the concentration of guanidine or related substances, no single factor can be identified as a major cause.

The effect of a shortened red-cell lifespan is aggravated in many patients by blood loss, either by bleeding or during haemodialysis. Gastro-intestinal haemorrhage is particularly common and is often due to gastric erosions or peptic ulceration, though a haemostatic defect may also be present (see Chapter 29). It is clear, however, that these factors alone are insufficient to account fully for the anaemia of CRF, and that the haemopoietic response must also be impaired. This has been confirmed by ferrokinetic studies; the rate of clearance of iron from the plasma is reduced and plasma iron turnover is less than normal [222, 224, 225]. Utilization of iron for erythropoiesis is reduced and an increased proportion is deviated to the iron stores. The marrow transit time is not increased as it is in other forms of anaemia and 'skip' reticulocytes are not seen in the peripheral blood [228].

The cause of the subnormal marrow response in CRF has not been fully elucidated. As the kidney plays a major role in erythropoietin production, measurements of erythropoietin levels have received considerable attention in patients with renal disease. The majority of studies have shown that plasma erythropoietin activity is inappororiately low for the degree of anaemia, but with present bioassay techniques it is difficult to demonstrate significant erythropoietin activity in normal plasma and it is therefore not absolutely certain whether subnormal secretion of the hormone plays a major role in the pathogenesis of renal anaemia. Erythropoietin is elaborated in response to tissue hypoxia, and patients with CRF have reduced intracellular pH and increased erythrocyte 2,3-DPG (see Chapter 3). Both of these factors enhance oxygen delivery relative to the degree of anaemia, and may partly explain why erythropoietin levels are inappropriately low. *In-vitro* studies have shown an inhibitory effect of uraemic serum on the incorporation of ^{59}Fe into erythroblasts. In one study this effect was shown to be independent of the presence of urea, creatinine and guanidosuccinic acid.

In summary, the anaemia of CRF is characterized by an inadequate erythropoietic response to a reduced red-cell lifespan and to increased blood loss. Production of erythropoietin is impaired, presumably due to underlying renal damage, but erythropoiesis may be further depressed by ill-defined circulating substances present in uraemia.

The haematological effects of dialysis

The haematological response to dialysis follows two main patterns [215, 229]. In patients dialysed for the first time there is often temporary improvement in erythropoiesis which is not associated with an elevation in plasma erythropoietin activity. This observation suggests the temporary removal of metabolites inhibitory to red-cell production [230]. In patients who have been on long-term maintenance haemodialysis treatment (MHDT), however, there is frequently a chronic anaemia which often becomes stable at a haemoglobin concentration similar to that seen in anephric patients. A number of factors may complicate the anaemia in patients on MHDT [231]. A major problem is blood loss, not just from dialysis itself but also from blood sampling, and leakage from shunt or fistula sites. This loss may lead to iron deficiency, which may be further aggravated by direct loss of iron at dialysis. Paradoxically, recognition of this fact has lead to a number of patients becoming iron loaded from indiscriminate parenteral iron therapy.

Iron metabolism in MHDT patients has recently been studied by Gokal *et al.* [415] who report a high incidence of iron loading in patients receiving regular parenteral iron therapy. Mechanisms regulating iron absorption were intact in these patients, and there would thus seem to be little justification for routine parenteral iron replacement during haemodialysis. Genuine iron deficiency can be diagnosed from the red-cell indices and oral iron therapy is both appropriate and effective. Interestingly, iron-loaded patients have been found to have a slight macrocytosis which reverts on cessation of iron therapy [232]. This macrocytosis is not related to B_{12} or folate levels, nor to the reticulocyte count, and appears to be directly induced by iron overload.

In addition to the factors contributing to the shortened red-cell survival in CRF [223], patients on MHDT may develop haemolysis related to a variety of physico-chemical factors in the dialysis fluid. These include excessive heat, copper, cholamines, nitrates, formaldehyde and mechanical causes, and have been reviewed by Whitehead [231].

A transient granulocytopenia has been observed in patients dialysed with cellophane-membrane apparatus. This has been found within two hours of commencement of dialysis in all patients studied, and is associated with complement-mediated pulmonary sequestration of leucocytes [233a]. In the majority of instances there have been no untoward consequences, but patients with pre-existing cardiac or respiratory disease may develop acute breathlessness and hypoxia.

Renal transplantation [215, 233b]

The effects of transplantation on erythropoiesis are striking: following kidney grafting there is a significant increase in erythropoiesis which is accompanied by increased production of erythropoietin, a marked reticulocytosis, and often a normoblastaemia. In a small proportion of cases frank polycythaemia develops which may persist for several months. Thromboembolic complications are common unless the polycythaemia is controlled by phlebotomy. This complication has been seen as early as two months and as late as 20 months after renal grafting.

Leucocyte changes following transplantation are variable. A neutrophil leucocytosis may result from corticosteroid administration or intercurrent infection, whilst azathioprine administration or hyperacute rejection may be associated with leucopenia. Platelet counts are generally normal but may be reduced. Impaired platelet production may result from cytotoxic drugs whilst pathological deposition of platelets and fibrin in the grafted kidney occurs during rejection crises.

The management of the anaemia of CRF

Probably no treatment is required for most patients with mild or moderate degrees of anaemia associated with stable renal failure. However, it is important to ensure that there is no complicating iron or folic-acid deficiency. Similarly, many patients on chronic dialysis may manage quite well with relatively low haemoglobin levels, but it is important to ensure that blood loss is kept to a minimum. On the whole, blood transfusion should be avoided in patients with CRF or in those who are on regular dialysis. Transfusion depresses the patient's endogenous erythropoiesis and there is a danger of producing transfusion siderosis. The role of blood transfusion in the preparation of recipients for renal transplantation remains controversial. Whilst several studies suggest a beneficial effect of transfusion on graft survival [234], the mechanism is not clear. Furthermore, there is a significant risk of hepatitis in these patients, and frequent exposure to leucocyte antigens may make tissue typing for subsequent renal transplantation extremely difficult.

A variety of substances have been used in the hope of stimulating erythropoiesis in this disorder. These have included androgens and cobalt, but there is no real evidence that any of them have proved of any value. A logical approach might be the administration of erythropoietin, but unfortunately sufficient quantities are not yet available for therapeutic use. The management of microangiopathic haemolysis is considered in detail in Chapter 12.

Haemostasis in renal failure

The abnormalities of platelet function and coagulation

which are found in renal failure are considered in Chapters 26 and 29.

THE GASTRO-INTESTINAL TRACT

There are numerous ways in which primary disease of the gastro-intestinal tract and liver may present to the haematologist, and many aspects of this subject have been dealt with in detail in other parts of this book. In the section which follows, the gastro-intestinal and liver disorders which are of particular haematological importance are summarized briefly.

GASTRO-INTESTINAL BLOOD LOSS

The results of increased blood loss from the GI tract on iron balance and the subsequent development of iron-deficiency anaemia have been fully reviewed in Chapter 5. It is quite clear that blood loss in excess of 20 ml/day will result ultimately in iron-deficiency anaemia, the time taken depending on the body stores of iron at the time when the bleeding started. Apart from nutritional iron deficiency, this group of conditions represent the most important group of iron-deficiency anaemias encountered in clinical practice. Although in many cases the diagnosis is obvious from the history and a few simple investigations, patients are occasionally encountered in whom the elucidation of the site of bleeding may be extremely difficult.

Aetiology

Blood loss may occur throughout the alimentary tract. There are few causes of chronic blood loss from the oro- or naso-pharynx but it should be remembered that repeated epistaxes in old people are not infrequently associated with the development of chronic iron-deficiency anaemia. The common oesophageal causes of bleeding are hiatus hernia, oesophageal varices and, occasionally, carcinoma of the oesophagus. Bleeding from the stomach most commonly results from peptic ulceration, superficial erosive gastritis following the use of drugs such as salicylates, or from gastric carcinoma. Gastro-intestinal bleeding as a late complication of gastric surgery is uncommon and should suggest the presence of a stomal ulcer, although occasionally inflammation at the site of anastamosis is the only demonstrable abnormality. Peptic ulceration is the commonest cause of bleeding from the duodenum; duodenal tumours are rare but carcinomas of the ampulla of Vater may bleed, and the finding of obstructive jaundice and iron-deficiency anaemia should suggest this diagnosis. Bleeding may also result from other lesions in the biliary tract [235]. Bleeding due to primary disease of the small bowel is uncommon; it may occur occasionally with small bowel neoplasms, such as lymphomas or leiomyo-

mata, or from polyps as part of the Peutz–Jeghers syndrome. The bleeding which occurs with inflammatory diseases of the small bowel is considered in the next section. Recurrent iron-deficiency anaemia due to gastro-intestinal bleeding in children should always suggest the diagnosis of a Meckel's diverticulum. The major causes of bleeding from the large bowel and rectum include haemorrhoids, carcinoma, diverticular disease, polyps and ulcerative colitis. It is particularly important to remember that the right-sided colonic neoplasms cause obstructive symptoms very late and chronic iron deficiency is one of the most frequent presenting symptoms. Although recurrent haemorrhage may occur from colonic diverticular disease, this should not be diagnosed without a careful search for other causes of gastro-intestinal bleeding. The parasitic causes of intestinal blood loss were reviewed earlier in this chapter.

Recurrent gastro-intestinal bleeding may also occur in a variety of systemic disorders. It is extremely common in patients with chronic renal failure and may occasionally be the presenting symptom. It is also a frequent complication of severe thrombocytopenia, though the skin manifestations usually make this diagnosis obvious, and it may also be the presenting feature in other haemorrhagic disorders; this is particularly the case in von Willebrand's disease where recurrent gastro-intestinal haemorrhage may be the major clinical problem (see Chapter 28). Similarly abnormal platelet function, either in the acquired disorders such as the myeloproliferative states and the paraproteinaemias, or in the congenital thrombocytopathies, may be associated with recurrent gastro-testinal bleeding. It may also be an important feature of some of the collagen vascular disorders, particularly polyarteritis nodosa and SLE (see pp. 1350–1354). Finally it may be the presenting feature in several of the inherited disorders of connective tissue [236]. It is particularly well documented in patients with pseudoxanthoma elasticum, but it has also been reported in Ehlers–Danlos syndrome. It also forms an important part of the clinical picture of hereditary telangiectasia (Osler–Rendu–Weber syndrome) (see p. 1373).

Diagnosis

An approach to the differential diagnosis of gastro-intestinal bleeding is outlined in Table 33.11. It is important to take an accurate family history, and to enquire about visits abroad and for symptoms suggestive of hiatus hernia, peptic ulceration, carcinoma of the stomach or a change in bowel habit due to a neoplasm of the large bowel. It is also important to ask specifically for any history of fresh bleeding on passing of the motions. A very careful drug history should be elicited as many patients consider household remedies

Table 33.11. Some causes of gastro-intestinal blood loss

Local causes within the gastro-intestinal tract
Oesophagus
  Hiatus hernia, varices, Mallory–Weiss syndrome, carcinoma
Stomach
  Gastric ulcer, erosion, salicylates and other drugs, carcinoma, simple tumours, reticuloses
Duodenum
  Duodenal ulcer, simple tumour
Biliary tract
  Calculi, tumours, heterotopic gastric mucosa
Small bowel
  Simple tumours (including Peutz–Jeghers syndrome), Meckel's diverticulum, regional ileitis
Large bowel and rectum
  Colitis, polyps, carcinoma, haemorrhoids, diverticular disease, angiodysplasia
Parasites
  Hookworm, schistosomiasis

General systemic disease
Haemostatic and coagulation disorders
  Congenital bleeding disorders including the thrombocytopathies, von Willebrand's disease and specific factor deficiencies.
  Acquired disorders including thrombocytopathies, particularly myeloproliferative disease; uraemia and paraproteinaemias;
  thrombocytopenic purpura (primary and secondary); defibrination syndromes; acquired factor deficiencies, particularly in
  liver disease; Henoch–Schönlein purpura
Connective tissue disorders
  Pseudoxanthoma elasticum, Ehlers–Danlos syndrome, Marfan syndrome
Vascular anomalies
  Hereditary telangiectasia, blue-rubber bleb naevus disease, Fabry's disease
Vasculitis and arteriosclerosis
  Periarteritis, SLE, cersoid aneurysm, Goodpasture's syndrome

such as aspirin to be hardly worthy of mention, and are indeed often unaware just how many such remedies contain salicylates! Clinical examination must include a careful search for telangiectases in the mouth, round the lips and over the skin of the face. It is important to examine the skin carefully for purpura and to assess its texture and elasticity—to rule out an inherited disorder of connective tissue such as pseudoxanthoma elasticum. This should be followed by careful palpation of the abdomen for tenderness indicative of peptic ulceration, hepatosplenomegaly or masses in either iliac fossae. Stigmata of liver failure such as jaundice, spider naevi, gynaecomastia, large parotids, pink palms, testicular atrophy, white nails or finger clubbing should be sought. Rectal examination should be carried out in every case, and an occult-blood test performed on a fingerstall sample. Finally, examination should include proctoscopic examination for internal haemorrhoids.

Once an iron-deficiency anaemia has been established on haematological grounds, the most important step is the unequivocal demonstration of gastro-intestinal bleeding. In most cases a simple faecal occult-blood test will suffice, but in cases of obscure iron-deficiency anaemia where negative or equivocal occult-blood results are being obtained, it is well worthwhile measuring the actual rate of blood loss with ^{51}Cr-labelled red cells. Where facilities are avail-

able it is much more convenient to use a whole-body counter for this purpose. Stools should also be examined for worms and ova by a concentration method. Once gastro-intestinal blood loss has been demonstrated, the most important investigation is an adequate radiological examination of the gastro-intestinal tract. This should include a barium swallow, a barium meal including examination of the lower oesophagus and an adequate barium enema. Unless there is good reason from the history to suggest an upper gastro-intestinal lesion, a barium enema should be performed first. This should be of the double-contrast type, and adequate preparation is critical; it should be combined with proctoscopy and sigmoidoscopy in order not to miss lesions in the rectum or recto-sigmoid junction. Where a small-bowel lesion is suspected, a small-bowel meal should be carried out by intubation. If this does not outline the lesion itself it may show some dilated segments proximal to it. It may be necessary to combine these examinations with endoscopy and biopsy.

In most cases the investigations outlined above will be adequate to demonstrate the site of bleeding; should they fail it is important to exclude the various systemic causes. Investigations will therefore include assessment of renal function, full haematological studies, examination of the plasma proteins and screening tests for liver function and the collagen vascular disorders. It is not uncommon to meet a patient in whom all these investigations have proved negative but in whom there is still a continuous or intermittent gastro-intestinal blood loss. In such cases selective mesenteric angiography may be helpful. Small vascular lesions (Fig. 33.10) or occasionally tumours may be demonstrated by this technique. If the patient is actually bleeding, angiography may also show leakage of contrast at the site of bleeding. A variety of other tests designed to indicate the level of bleeding have been reported but none of them seems to be regularly useful.

Should all else fail, laparotomy may be considered, though the success of this operation performed 'blind' varies considerably between series and it is certainly not something to be embarked on without really exhaustive study by every other available technique.

DISEASE OF THE SMALL AND LARGE BOWEL

Inflammatory bowel disease

Anaemia is a common accompaniment of inflammatory bowel disease; it is observed frequently in patients with regional enteritis (Crohn's disease), ileocaecal tuberculosis, ulcerative colitis and other forms of proctocolitis. This anaemia has a complex aetiology: in many cases it takes the form of the anaemia of chronic disorders, often complicated by intermittent blood loss or dietary iron deficiency. In some cases of extensive regional enteritis there may be an added factor of malabsorption [41, 237]. In one series, anaemia was present in 79% of males and 54% of females [238]. Marrow biopsies were performed on two-thirds of the patients and 39% of these were megaloblastic. Eleven patients in the megaloblastic group were folate-

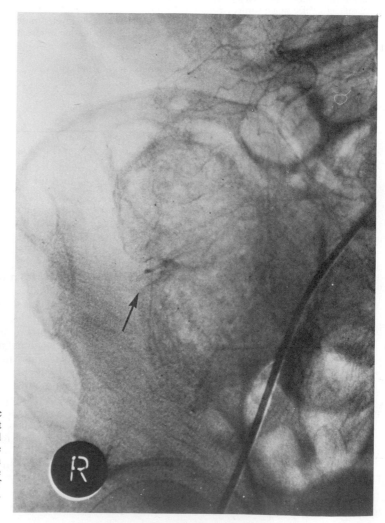

Fig. 33.10. Selective superior mesenteric angiography in a patient with recurrent gastro-intestinal blood loss: (a) arterial phase; (b) (page 1361), venous phase. The arrow points to an angio-dysplastic lesion in the lateral border of the caecum. In the venous phase (b) characteristic dilatation of a vein draining the lesion is seen. (By courtesy of Dr E. W. L. Fletcher.)

deficient, six B_{12}-deficient, and one patient had both deficiencies. This study underlined the importance of the anaemia of chronic disorders in this condition, and that the response to treatment of folate or B_{12} deficiency may be suboptimal until the inflammatory process has been suppressed. While blood loss may occur occasionally in patients with regional enteritis, continuous bleeding suggests either extensive colonic involvement or that the patient has ulcerative colitis. Anaemia in ulcerative colitis is usually secondary to blood loss [239]. Macrocytic anaemia is unusual, but there have been occasional reports of autoimmune haemolytic anaemia [72, 239]. In several cases the antibody has shown Rhesus specificity.

The anaemia of inflammatory bowel disease may be aggravated by the drugs which are used in its management. Thus patients who are receiving salazopyrine for colitis occasionally develop an acute haemolytic anaemia associated with Heinz-body formation (see also Chapter 12, p. 524). This may precipitate a megaloblastic anaemia in patients with depleted folic-acid stores, due to increased utilization resulting from the shortened red-cell survival. Marrow depression may also occur in patients receiving immunosuppressive treatment for colitis or regional enteritis. Ileocaecal tuberculosis [240] may be associated with any of the bizarre manifestations of tuberculosis described earlier in this chapter and the anaemia may be complicated by the side-effects of anti-tuberculous drug therapy. Patients receiving corticosteroid therapy for ulcerative colitis may lose blood from the stomach, so adding to their iron deficit.

In most of the inflammatory diseases of the bowel there is a neutrophil leucocytosis. There is often an

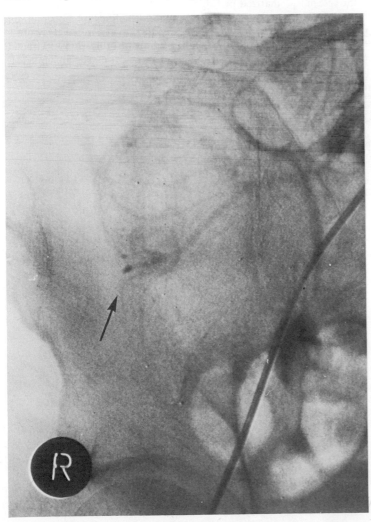

Fig. 33.10. (b)

increased number of mast cells in the wall of the large bowel in ulcerative colitis, and the blood basophil count is sometimes raised during the acute phase, returning to normal during remission. Occasionally there may be a marked eosinophilia during the active phase of ulcerative colitis [241]. Similarly, eosinophilic (allergic) gastro-enteritis is associated with a marked eosinophilia together with infiltrative lesions in the stomach and, more rarely, the large bowel.

Whipple's disease may produce a clinical picture and blood changes which can mimic several primary haematological disorders. The typical clinical triad of diarrhoea, arthropathy and enlarged lymph nodes is usually associated with a mild normochromic normocytic anaemia, a raised erythrocyte sedimentation rate and a neutrophil leucocytosis. There may be an associated lymphopenia or eosinophilia. In cases with less typical presentation, particularly where the spleen is enlarged, the condition may closely mimic a primary reticulosis. Malabsorption of vitamin B_{12} or folic acid may be occasionally encountered in this disorder [41]. The diagnosis is confirmed by lymph-node or intestinal biopsy which show macrophages containing PAS-staining material. Under the electron microscope, bacilliform bodies are visible close to the macrophages [242].

Structural disease of the stomach, small and large bowel
By far the most important haematological manifestations of the anatomical abnormalities of the stomach and small bowel and of the malabsorption syndromes are iron deficiency, due to impaired iron absorption, and megaloblastic anaemia secondary to either vitamin-B_{12} or folic-acid deficiency. These subjects have been dealt with in detail in Chapter 6 and will only be summarized briefly here. The relationships between gastric surgery and vitamin-B_{12} and iron metabolism are discussed in Chapters 5 and 6 respectively. An approach to the diagnosis of malabsorption is summarized in Table 33.12.

Several anatomical abnormalities of the small gut have in common the production of a relatively profuse bacterial flora with subsequent utilization of vitamin B_{12} with the production of megaloblastic anaemia [41,

Table 33.12. Investigation of malabsorption

A. Demonstration of malabsorption
Stool examination
  Macroscopic, microscopic (ova, cysts and parasites)
  3-day fat excretion or full fat balance
Haematological data
  Routine blood and marrow examination
  Serum iron, serum vitamin B_{12}, serum or red-cell folate
  Vitamin-B_{12} absorption
  Prothrombin time
Biochemical data
  Serum protein, calcium, phosphorus, magnesium and alkaline phosphatase
  Protein electrophoretic pattern
  Immunoglobulin assay
  Xylose tolerance test
  Glucose tolerance
  Labelled-albumin excretion
  Lipoprotein fractionation
Radiological examination
  Skeletal survey
  Splenic function with heat-treated red cells

B. Cause of malabsorption
Biopsy
  Jejunal mucosal biopsy, node biopsy, liver biopsy
Radiological examination
  Barium meal and follow through or small bowel enema
  Chest X-ray, lymphangiography
Biochemical data
  Pancreatic function tests. Gastric function tests. Liver function tests. Thyroid function tests
Haematological data
  Vitamin-B_{12} absorption before and after broad-spectrum antibiotic
Therapeutic trial
  Gluten-free diet

243] (see also Chapter 6, p. 216). These conditions include surgically produced blind loops, anastomotic strictures, diverticulae, fistulae between various sections of the bowel, malfunctioning gastro-enterostomy, interference of gut motility in conditions such as scleroderma, Whipple's disease or after vagotomy, and extensive gut resection. In the latter case, malabsorption may be due to removal of part of the absorbing area for either B_{12} or folic acid. The megaloblastic anaemia found in these patients is nearly always due to vitamin-B_{12} deficiency and there is a marked reduction in the degree of B_{12} absorption. Provided that the terminal ileum is intact, this can be corrected by the administration of a broad-spectrum antibiotic such as tetracyline but not by intrinsic factor.

In the malabsorption syndromes, anaemia may be due to iron, folate or B_{12} deficiency, or to a combination of these. This group of disorders includes childhood and adult coeliac disease, tropical sprue, and other rare causes of malabsorption such as chronic pancreatitis, Zollinger–Ellison syndrome, reticulosis, parasitic infestations, and vascular disease. Iron deficiency is particularly common [244], and is occasionally the only detectable abnormality in patients presenting with coeliac disease. In one series of 31 patients with this disorder, 21 had serum iron values of less than 10μm/l at presentation, and radioactive iron absorption studies using a double isotope (^{55}Fe and ^{59}Fe) technique showed reduced iron absorption which improved on a gluten-free diet. Megaloblastic anaemia in the malabsorption syndrome has been fully reviewed in Chapter 6. In the large majority of patients it is due to folic-acid deficiency secondary to folate malabsorption [41, 243, 244], but there is also a defect in B_{12} absorption in between one-third and one-half of patients with idiopathic steatorrhoea [41].

The malabsorption syndromes and related disorders may present to the haematologist in other ways. There is now a clear-cut relationship between the presence of intestinal malabsorption and splenic atrophy [245] (see Chapter 20). Indeed, if surgical removal of the spleen is excluded, the finding of the changes of splenic atrophy on a routine blood film should strongly suggest the presence of intestinal malabsorption.

In some patients with steatorrhoea there may be a marked deficiency of prothrombin due to a defective absorption of vitamin K. The resulting bleeding diathesis may occasionally be the presenting feature, and severe hypoprothrombinaemia in the absence of obvious liver disease should suggest the possibility of an underlying malabsorption syndrome. Although subnormal levels of α tocopherol have been found in the serum of patients with a variety of intestinal malabsorption syndromes [246], it has been difficult to relate any anaemia found in those patients to a basic deficiency of vitamin E. Thus, although there have been abnormal peroxide-haemolysis tests the results of red-cell-survival studies have been equivocal; both normal and shortened half-lives have been described in different series. The whole relationship between vitamin-E deficiency and anaemia in man is uncertain and requires further investigation, particularly in patients with extensive disease of the small bowel.

Enterogenous cyanosis
This term was formerly applied to patients who were thought to develop methaemoglobinaemia and sulphaemoglobinaemia due to the absorption of nitrites and sulphides from the gut as the result of abnormal bowel function [247]. In addition to a slate-blue appearance, the patients had abdominal pain, dyspnoea, syncope and collapse. Some of them had indicanuria and were anaemic. It is likely that many of these symptoms resulted from drug ingestion. A woman has been described with long-standing methaemoglobinaemia, sulphaemoglobinaemia and Heinz-body haemolytic anaemia together with an unusual aromatic amine in the urine [248]. Following neomycin therapy there was a dramatic fall in methaemoglobin levels. Furthermore it has been shown that Heinz-body anaemia in experimental rats fed phenacetin occurs only if the rats have an intestinal blind loop. The production of a blind loop alone does not produce anaemia of this type [249]. These results raise again the question of whether products of bacteria in the bowel can cause methaemoglobin production, or in some way sensitize red cells to the action of oxidant or other drugs.

LIVER DISEASE

A variety of haematological changes are associated with liver disease (Table 33.13). The blood changes in acute viral hepatitis have been described earlier in this chapter. The changes which accompany chronic liver disease are complex, and in many cases the picture is complicated by the presence of portal hypertension or alcoholism. There is frequently an increase in plasma volume with anaemia, thrombocytopenia and leucopenia suggestive of hypersplenism, and gastrointestinal blood loss may result from peptic ulceration or varices. The picture may be further complicated by folic-acid deficiency, particularly in alcoholics. Primary liver tumours may occasionally cause polycythaemia, while patients with metastatic liver deposits may show a leukaemoid reaction in their peripheral blood. Finally, many forms of liver failure

Table 33.13 Haematological changes in liver disease

---

(1) *Virus hepatitis*
   Haemolytic anaemia. Hypoplastic anaemia
(2) *Chronic active hepatitis*
   Immune haemolytic anaemia. LE cells in blood. Hyperglobulinaemia
(3) *Chronic liver failure*
   Chronic anaemia is often complicated by:
      (a) blood loss and iron deficiency
      (b) alcohol; direct effect on marrow
      (c) folate deficiency
      (d) portal hypertension and hypersplenism
      (e) acute haemolytic episodes (e.g. Zieve's syndrome, spur-cell syndrome)
   Thrombocytopenia. Leucopenia.
   Haemorrhagic diathesis due to:
      (a) deficiency of vitamin-K-dependent factors
      (b) portal hypertension
      (c) increase fibrinolysis
      (d) thrombocytopenia
(4) *Portal hypertension*
   Anaemia, leucopenia, thrombocytopenia, bleeding from varices
(5) *Obstructive jaundice*
   Mild anaemia. Target-cell formation
(6) *Tumours*
   Polycythaemia. Leukamoid reactions. α-feto-protein production
(7) *Liver transplantation*
   Haemorrhagic and hypercoagulable states

---

are associated with chronic thrombocytopenia and a marked haemorrhagic tendency due to deficiency of the vitamin-K-dependent clotting factors (see Chapter 29).

THE ANAEMIA OF LIVER DISEASE

Haematological findings
Mild to moderate anaemia is common in patients with chronic liver disease. In uncomplicated cases the haemoglobin level rarely falls below 10 g/dl, and the red cells are normochromic and normocytic or slightly macrocytic, with MCV values ranging from 100 to 115 fl. The cells are not so well filled and show less variation in shape and size than the macrocytes of megaloblastic anaemia, and have been described as 'thin' macrocytes [250, 251]. Target cells and a variable degree of polychromasia associated with a slight macrocytosis are usually found. The degree of macrocytosis and target-cell formation correlates reasonably well with the degree of liver failure.

The marrow tends to be hypercellular in all forms of liver failure and shows erythroid hyperplasia with macronormoblastic changes [252, 253]. The red-cell precursors are large and show abnormalities of nuclear chromatin with some premature haemoglobinization of the cytoplasm, though maturation is not as abnormal as in megaloblastic anaemia. There are no marked abnormalities of leucocyte maturation and megakaryocytes are present.

Variable changes in the red-cell osmotic fragility are found in liver disease. Quite often the bulk of the fragility curve lies within the normal limits but there is a small proportion at the top which is in the range of increased resistance due to the presence of underfilled cells. This shift may be magnified after sterile incubation of the red cells for 24 hours. The plasma volume is increased in some patients and there is usually a reduced red-cell mass [254, 255].

Pathogenesis of the anaemia liver failure
Although the anaemia tends to be macrocytic, there is no evidence in the majority of cases that it results from a genuine deficiency of either vitamin B_{12} or folic acid, and the administration of these haematinics is usually ineffective. Several studies have shown a reduced red-cell lifespan, and there is thus an increased production of unconjugated bilirubin and excretion of faecal and urinary urobilinogen [256–258]. Both intra- and extracorpuscular defects have been demonstrated [257, 258]. There is no evidence for an immune haemolytic process in the majority of patients with liver disease, and the nature of the defects is unknown.

Although there is an increased rate of red-cell destruction this is of limited magnitude and well within the capacity of a normal marrow to compensate fully.

This does not occur, however, and there appears to be a relatively inadequate bone-marrow response in all forms of liver failure [259, 260]. Furthermore, the anaemia in many cases is aggravated by an increase in plasma volume.

Factors complicating the anaemia of liver disease
In clinical practice it is not uncommon to encounter patients with severe anaemia and liver disease. This usually indicates that the mild anaemia of liver failure has been exacerbated by such factors as acute or chronic blood loss, folic-acid deficiency, infection, obstructive jaundice, iron overload, the effects of alcoholism or acute haemolytic episodes of uncertain aetiology.

Vitamin B-12 and folate metabolism in hepatic disease. Although megaloblastic anaemia secondary to folate deficiency is common in patients with liver disease, most of them are chronic alcoholics with a history of inadequate diet, and there is little evidence that liver disease itself has an adverse effect on folate metabolism [41].

In several large series, low serum folate levels have been found in about 50% of patients with liver disease; in each series a high proportion of the patients were alcoholics [261, 262]. Almost all patients who showed megaloblastic anaemia had low serum folate values but these are also observed in patients with normoblastic haemopoiesis. In patients with non-alcoholic cirrhosis the rate of plasma clearance of folate is normal [41]. There is frequently an elevated excretion of formiminoglutamic acid in patients with chronic alcoholism and cirrhosis [263]. In addition high levels of urocanic acid are found in the urine after histidine loading [264]. It is not clear whether these findings are a reflection of liver disease or folate deficiency; probably both factors play a part. The absorption of folate is normal [265].

The serum vitamin-B_{12} level is either normal or elevated in liver disease, whether or not there is a marked degree of anaemia [266, 267]. Vitamin-B_{12} absorption is normal but there is diminished hepatic uptake [268]. The high levels may result from release of vitamin B_{12} into the serum following liver damage [41]. There is no evidence that the anaemia of liver disease is in any way related to vitamin-B_{12} deficiency.

Iron deficiency and iron metabolism. Iron-deficiency anaemia is commonly superimposed on the anaemia of liver disease [254]. This results from a variety of causes, including chronic intestinal blood loss from peptic ulceration or from oesophageal or gastric varices, and a poor diet.

Where there is no superadded iron deficiency the serum iron level may be normal or slightly elevated and the iron-binding capacity of the serum is usually reduced. Studies of iron absorption in 76 patients with liver disease, 29 of whom had undergone a portocaval shunt one to 11 years previously, demonstrated that although none was iron deficient, iron absorption was increased in 50% of the group who had undergone surgery and 38% of those who had not. Siderosis was present in about 50% of both groups [269]. The degree of iron overload is seldom severe enough to cause confusion with idiopathic haemochromatosis, and in several large series has only been found in a very small proportion of patients [270, 271].

Haemolytic anaemia. Although there is a definite haemolytic component to the uncomplicated anaemia of chronic liver failure, this is usually mild. There are, however, a variety of situations in which the degree of haemolysis may suddenly increase. This may occur as an acute episode in association with abnormalities of the serum lipids: Zieve described a syndrome consisting of jaundice, hyperlipidaemia, hypercholesterolaemia, and haemolytic anaemia which follows an excessive alcohol intake in people with alcoholic fatty livers or cirrhosis [272]. This is often accompanied by general malaise, anorexia and vomiting, low-grade fever, and pain in the upper abdomen or lower chest, which may be so troublesome as to lead to laparotomy. In this condition, cholesterol levels of up to 1000 mg/dl may occur, but these fall when the alcohol intake is reduced [273], and there is rapid improvement in the condition when the intake of alcohol ceases. Analysis of red-cell lipids during the acute stage of Zieve's syndrome reveals that the total lipid, cholesterol and phospholipid fractions are increased [274]; these changes are accompanied by a decrease in red-cell osmotic fragility. In addition, the degree of shortening of red-cell survival can be correlated with the magnitude of the increase in red-cell lipids.

The observation that increased serum lipid levels could provoke a haemolytic anaemia was first made by Okey & Greaves [275], who fed one per cent cholesterol to guinea-pigs. After five weeks the animals became severely anaemic and at seven to 10 weeks the spleen had enlarged until it was 10 times normal size. The red cells were observed to be larger than normal and resistant to osmotic lysis. Similar changes have been reported when cholesterol has been fed to rabbits [276].

Other forms of overt haemolytic anaemia may occur in liver disease. In virus hepatitis an acute haemolytic episode may occur and if G6PD deficiency is also present the degree of haemolysis is out of proportion to the severity of liver disease but correlates with the degree of enzyme deficiency [277]. An acquired haemolytic anaemia with positive Coombs' test may occur occasionally in chronic active hepatitis [72]. Another form of haemolytic anaemia in liver disease, usually alcoholic cirrhosis, has been observed in which there are marked red-cell abnormalities with burr- and spur-shaped forms predominating. Indeed the blood picture may resemble that of a β-lipoproteinaemia with many acanthocytes [278]. There is a marked increase in membrane cholesterol and the rigid cells are sequestered in the spleen.

Obstructive jaundice. In pure jaundice with normal liver function the red cells have normal or near-normal lifespan [279] and normal metabolic function, but are enlarged with target forms and increased osmotic resistance. The latter is acquired by normal cells transfused into such patients. Normally cholesterol is in rapid flux between the red-cell membrane and plasma. When bile salts accumulate in the blood the equilibrium is displaced and cholesterol accumulates in the red-cell membrane [280–282]. This results from an inhibition of cholesterol esterification and shift in the serum/red-cell cholesterol partition under the action of bile salts. The surface area of the cells is increased by the accumulation of cholesterol although the cell contents and metabolism are unaltered. This results in a 'thin' macrocyte with target-cell formation an in an increased osmotic resistance. The content of phospholipid remains normal. It seems likely that the red cell associated with the accumulation of cholesterol alone is stable, whereas that associated with accumulation of cholesterol and other metabolites (e.g. lithocolic acid [283]) may be subject to increased destruction, as occurs in Zieve's syndrome.

The effect of alcohol [284, 285]. As already mentioned the haematological changes of liver disease are frequently complicated by the direct or indirect results of alcohol on the haemopoietic system. Many alcoholics have poor diets resulting in iron or folic-acid deficiency and alcohol may cause impairment of folic-acid absorption. In addition it has several direct effects on normal red-cell production.

The evolution of the anaemia of alcoholism seems to go through three main stages [286]:
1 a 'dietetic' phase in which the serum and red-cell folate levels fall in the absence of anaemia;
2 megaloblastic conversion occurs, probably as a result of the direct effect of alcohol on the marrow. This is associated with marked vacuolization of the red- and white-cell precursors [287];
3 the marrow may become sideroblastic, again due to direct effect of alcohol [288].

These morphological changes may occur within a week of very heavy alcohol intake. After withdrawal of alcohol they are rapidly reversible, further evidence that they are not due to folate deficiency but follow the direct toxic effect of alcohol on the red-cell precursors. The improvement in marrow morphology is associated with a reticulocytosis.

Thus in alcoholic cirrhosis a variety of complicated blood and marrow pictures may be superimposed on the basic anaemia of chronic liver disease. These are only sorted out after withdrawal of alcohol, adequate replacement therapy and repeated blood and marrow studies. It should be emphasized that it is well worth waiting for a week to 10 days after withdrawal of alcohol and following the reticulocyte count, before administering haematinics to patients with severe anemia and liver disease.

CHANGES IN THE LEUCOCYTES AND PLATELETS IN LIVER DISEASE

Changes in the leucocyte count in viral hepatitis have been considered on page 1337. In chronic liver disease leucopenia is common with total leucocyte counts ranging between 1.5 and $3.0 \times 10^9/l$. The leucopenia is mainly due to a neutropenia which in some cases may be extreme [289]. The exact cause has not been determined; in many cases there is a clear element of hypersplenism with associated portal hypertension and splenomegaly, but the degree of neutropenia is not always related to the size of the spleen and chronic liver failure may have other effects of leucocyte kinetics. In patients with multiple hepatic metastases there is frequently a marked neutrophil leucocytosis with occasionally a leukaemoid picture. Similar changes may occur with infections of the liver, particularly an amoebic abscess.

Thrombocytopenia is found frequently with chronic liver disease. The platelet count is usually in the $60–120 \times 10^9/l$ range but may be much lower. The mechanism is not understood; although frequently associated with splenomegaly and portal hypertension [290], it is often more profound than one would expect from the size of the spleen. In some cases consumption of platelets due to gastro-intestinal bleeding, or reduced production due to folate deficiency, or the effects of alcohol on thrombopoiesis, may add to the degree of thrombocytopenia.

Although the neutropenia and thrombocytopenia may be corrected by splenectomy in patients with portal hypertension, the operation carries a high mortality and should only be embarked upon if there are life-threatening infections or thrombocytopenic bleeding. Furthermore, the bleeding which occurs in these patients is due to several factors and can rarely be ascribed to thrombocytopenia alone. Surgery to relieve portal hypertension has no effect on the neutropenia and thrombocytopenia unless the spleen is also removed [291].

HAEMORRHAGIC DIATHESIS IN LIVER DISEASE

The bleeding of chronic liver disease has an extremely complex aetiology [292]. This includes the mechanical effects of portal hypertension combined with a series of defects in haemostasis and coagulation. In addition to thrombocytopenia there is evidence of abnormal platelet function [293]. There is a deficiency of the vitamin-K-dependent clotting factors, prothrombin and factors VII, IX and X and also of factor V. There is sometimes evidence of increased fibrinolysis, disseminated intravascular coagulation, or of a 'hypercoagulable state' with elevated levels of factor VIII. In addition to these abnormalities there are frequently problems of coagulation which result from massive replacement therapy in patients with acute bleeding from varices [294]. These coagulation problems are fully reviewed in Chapter 29.

CONGENITAL HYPERBILIRUBINAEMIA

There are several syndromes characterized by chronic jaundice which are probably due to genetically determined abnormalities of liver function [295]. These conditions fall into two groups: the first comprises congenital familial non-haemolytic jaundice (Crigler–Najjar syndrome) and constitutional hepatic dysfunction (Gilbert's syndrome); the second group includes the Dubin–Johnson syndrome which probably involves the hepatic excretory functions.

The Crigler–Najjar syndrome is a rare inherited disorder characterized by high concentrations of unconjugated bilirubin in the plasma and often irreversible brain damage. This condition does not usually present to the haematologist. However, patients with milder hyperbilirubinaemia (Gilbert's syndrome) are frequently referred as possible cases of chronic haemolytic anaemia. It seems likely that Gilbert's syndrome represents a group of mild metabolic abnormalities of bilirubin metabolism. In most affected individuals there is no haemolytic component but a few have been reported in which there is a very slight shortening of the red-cell survival. However, in these cases there must have been an associated defect in bilirubin metabolism.

Gilbert's syndrome can be diagnosed if there are no haematological abnormalities or evidence of haemolysis as judged by an increased reticulocyte count, decreased haptoglobin level or shortened red-cell survival. In addition, standard liver-function tests, BSP excretion and liver histology must be normal. It is helpful to study close relatives because in some instances several family members are affected. It should be remembered that the jaundice of Gilbert's syndrome shows a marked degree of fluctuation and many affected patients have non-specifc symptoms such as tiredness and malaise, and it may be quite difficult to rule out a low-grade haemolytic process without red-cell survival studies. No treatment is required.

It is possible to determine the rate of bilirubin clearance and turnover using labelled unconjugated bilirubin: in patients with Gilbert's syndrome there is an abnormal plasma disappearance pattern while in patients with haemolysis the disappearance curves are normal but there is increased bilirubin turnover. Using this technique it is possible to diagnose a third disorder in this group, i.e. patients in whom there is both the Gilbert defect and associated low-grade haemolysis. It has been suggested that this combination represents the chance association of two relatively common disorders [296].

DISEASES OF THE PANCREAS

There seems to be a genuine association between pancreatic insufficiency in early childhood, unrelated to fibrocystic disease, and chronic neutropenia [297]. Affected children have symptoms suggestive of pancreatic malabsorption together with neutropenia and repeated infections, and in a few cases there has been a moderate degree of thrombocytopenia. The bone marrow is hypocellular. The pancreatic function seems to improve as the children develop. There is no explanation for this interesting association.

Chronic pancreatitis may be accompanied by a malabsorption syndrome. Although there have been reports of increased iron absorption in this condition this appears to be related to iron-store depletion rather than to a deficiency of pancreatic secretion. It is of little clinical importance [298].

ENDOCRINE DISEASE

DISEASES OF THE THYROID

Patients with thyroid disorders commonly show blood changes of a fascinating and complex nature. The relationship between the thyroid and haemopoiesis has been recognized for many years, and recently there have been considerable advances in our understanding of the actions of thyroid hormones on erythropoiesis at the cellular level. Furthermore, as the autoimmune nature of much thyroid pathology has become apparent, associations with immune disorders affecting the blood are being increasingly recognized. Finally, one is occasionally reminded that the drugs used for the treatment of hyperthyroidism may have calamitous consequences for marrow function.

Effects of thyroid hormones on the red cell and erythropoiesis

The major physiological effect of the thyroid hormones is to increase metabolic activity and thus tissue oxygen requirements, so one might expect to find evidence of adaptation to altered oxygen demands in patients with thyroid disorders. Oxygen delivery to the tissues is governed by cardiac output, the red-cell mass and by the oxygen affinity of haemoglobin (Chapter 8), and predictable alterations in these parameters have been described in patients with hypo- or hyperthyroidism.

There have been few studies of the red-cell mass and plasma volume in thyroid disease [299–302], and only one in which isotope methods were used [302]. These studies indicate that on average the red-cell mass is increased in uncomplicated hyperthyroidism, and decreased in hypothyroidism and that concomitant changes in plasma volume may mask or reduce the expected alterations in haemoglobin and haematocrit. Unfortunately, changes in the red-cell mass in hyperthyroid states are difficult to assess as these patients have generally lost weight prior to diagnosis and red-cell-mass estimations are usually expressed in relation to body weight or lean body mass. A further complication is the fact that weight loss in thyrotoxicosis is largely from tissues which, in the basal state, consume relatively small amounts of oxygen and it it thus not at all clear that the red-cell mass actually expands during the development of thyrotoxicosis. Further studies would obviously be of interest.

Whether real or apparent, changes in the red-cell mass are reflected in alterations in the rate of erythropoiesis as assessed by morphological examination of the marrow [303] and by ferrokinetic studies in both man [302, 304] and animals [305–309]. The traditional view has been that these changes in erythropoiesis are appropriate, reflecting the body's altered requirements for oxygen, and that they are mediated indirectly via modulation of erythropoietin secretion [310]. A number of reports have indicated that erythropoietin levels are decreased in hypothyroidism and increased in hyperthyroidism [302, 305, 307, 308]. However, erythropoietin assays are notoriously difficult to interpret, particularly at low or normal levels, and recent evidence suggests that the effect of thyroid hormones on erythropoiesis is independent of their effect on metabolic rate [306]. Furthermore, *in-vitro* studies of erythropoiesis have shown that thyroid hormones directly stimulate erythroid colony growth, but only in the presence of erythropoietin [311]. This facilitatory effect has much in common with that produced by catecholamines and can be blocked by specific β_2-adrenergic antagonists. A close relationship between thyroid hormone action and adrenergic receptors has been shown for other tissues [312]; indeed most of the peripheral effects of excess thyroxine may be effectively controlled by β blockers such as pro-

pranolol. Responsiveness to β_2-adrenergic agonists is lost in marrow cells from hypothyroid dogs but is restored to normal after pre-incubation of the cells with L-thyroxine, suggesting that thyroid hormones actively modulate the number and type of adrenergic receptors on the target-cell surface [313].

Appropriate changes in erythrocyte oxygen affinity have been described in both hypo- and hyperthyroid states [314, 315], but are not found consistently, and measurements of erythrocyte 2,3-DPG levels in patients with thyroid disease and in normal cells incubated *in vitro* with thyroid hormones have shown conflicting results [316] suggesting that other adaptive mechanisms are more important in the regulation of oxygen transport in thyroid disorders. Levels of other red-cell enzymes are altered in thyroid disease: G6PD activity is increased in thyrotoxicosis [317] and the activity of many other enzymes is reduced in hypothyroidism [318]. Furthermore, on treatment of hypothyrodism, enzyme activities are increased despite whether or not they had previously been depressed. It has been suggested that this reflects differences in mean age of the cell populations studied, the thyroid-induced increase in erythropoiesis producing a younger average population [318]. In contrast to other red-cell enzymes, the levels of carbonic anhydrase show an inverse correlation with plasma thyroxine. Other clinical conditions also produce alterations in carbonic-anhydrase levels, and the subject has been extensively reviewed by Tashian [319], although the mechanism of these changes is not understood.

Hypothyroidism

Anaemia may occur in all forms of hypothyroidism including the various forms of cretinism and juvenile and adult myxoedema [301, 320]. In one series [320], anaemia was present at diagnosis in 39 of 172 women and 14 of 30 men, although the mean overall haemoglobin level was 12·9 g/dl. There is a tendency for the blood picture to be macrocytic, and in this series the average MCV was 90 fl (s.d. 9·1 fl). Macrocytosis appears to be a particular feature of hypothyroidism as, although the average MCV was higher in those patients who had low B_{12} levels, and lower with those who had reduced serum iron, it was still 90 fl in patients with normal B_{12}, folate and iron levels. In some patients the erythrocytes include small numbers of irregularly crenated cells which disappear after therapy [321]. There is an improvement in anaemia and a return of the MCV to normal with hormone replacement.

The anaemia of hypothyroidism appears to be due principally to reduced erythropoiesis as discussed above. This is reflected in a reduction in marrow-erythroid activity [322, 323]. The picture may be complicated by concomitant iron deficiency [324], which may be due to a variety of factors including a poor intake due to anorexia, increased menstrual loss, and a high incidence of histamine-fast achlorhydria [301]. The incidence of pernicious anaemia is increased in patients with thyroid disease. There are histological similarities between the atrophic stomach and the thyroid gland in chronic thyroiditis, and there is a marked increase in the frequency of focal thyroiditis in patients coming to autopsy [325]. Furthermore, patients with pernicious anaemia have a high incidence of gastric parietal-cell antibodies but over half also have antibodies against the thyroid [326]. There is also a high incidence of gastric parietal-cell antibodies in patients with primary myxoedema and Graves' disease, and a high incidence of gastric and thyroid antibodies can be found in their relatives [327, 328]. The whole topic of autoimmunity and thyroid disease has been reviewed elsewhere [329]. Megaloblastic anaemia due to folate deficiency has also been seen in association with hypothyroidism [330].

Hyperthyroidism

Although there is evidence for increased erythropoiesis in hyperthyroid states (see above), and in some instances the red-cell mass may be increased, polycythaemia is not a feature of this condition, and the majority of patients have a normal haemoglobin level [331]. Indeed, some patients become anaemic and in one series of 239 patients the haemoglobin was less than 12·0 g/dl in 37 of 207 women and less than 13·0 g/dl in nine of 32 men [331]. Some but not all of these patients were iron deficient. Why some patients with hyperthyroidism should become anaemic in the face of increased erythropoiesis is not clear. To some extent it may be due to an increase in plasma volume, and in one study a reduced red-cell lifespan was found [332], though this has not been confirmed by others [302, 333]. In some patients, particularly with severe or prolonged hyperthyroidism, reduced iron utilization has been noted, with improvement after therapy [333]. An interesting recent observation is that patients with hyperthyroidism have, on average, a lower MCV than normal even in the absence of demonstrable iron deficiency [331]. There was a rise in MCV on treatment in 95% of patients, suggesting that a reduction in red-cell volume—even within the normal range—is an inevitable consequence of the hyperthyroid state. The relationship between thyroid disease and the stomach has been discussed above. True megaloblastic anaemia is uncommon in patients with thyrotoxicosis, though the incidence of pernicious anaemia is increased in patients who have been treated for this condition [41].

Leucocyte changes in hyperthyroidism.
Patients with thyrotoxicosis often have a moderate degree of leuco-penia with a relative or absolute neutropenia [334]. Lymphocyte counts are generally normal and no changes have been found in lymphocyte subpopulations. Splenomegaly and lymphadenopathy are occasionally observed. It should be remembered that leucopenia is a frequent side-effect of the antithyroid drugs including the thioureas, carbimazole and potassium chlorate, and that fatal agranulocytosis has occurred. Autoimmune neutropenia has been reported [335].

Platelets and coagulation in thyroid disease
Abnormalities of coagulation have been observed in patients with thyroid disease; in general these are mild [336], though clinical bleeding has been observed in patients with myxoedema coma [337]. Factor-VIII levels are elevated in hyperthyroidism and reduced in hypothyroidism [338], but return to normal with treatment. There have been several reports of the association of immune thrombocytopenic purpura with hyperthyroidism [339–341]. It seems likely that this is yet another example of the association of two autoimmune diseases.

PITUITARY DISEASE
Normochromic normocytic anaemia is very frequently observed in patients with reduced function of the anterior lobe of the pituitary. This is most frequently due to post-partum necrosis as part of Sheehan's syndrome. The anaemia may be the presenting feature. On clinical examination, apart from anaemia there are signs of hypopituitarism including pallor in excess of that expected with mild anaemia, loss of body hair and depigmentation of the areolae with atrophy of the breasts and genital organs. The anaemia responds well to replacement therapy with thyroid, testosterone and corticosteroids and appears to have the same metabolic basis as the anaemia of hypothyroidism [342].

There is some evidence that growth hormone plays a role in erythropoiesis, possibly via the release of renal erythropoietic factor. This may be of importance in the management of pituitary dwarfs [343]. Crude extracts of human pituitary gland have been shown to have an erythropoietic effect on normal and polycythaemic mice [344].

ADRENAL DISEASE
There is frequently a mild normochromic normocytic anaemia in patients with chronic adrenal failure (Addison's disease). This is associated with leucopenia, an increase in the eosinophil count and a relative lymphocytosis. The lymphocytes are often large. these changes are all corrected with adequate replacement therapy.

There is good evidence of an association between idiopathic adrenal insufficiency and pernicious anaemia. There have been many case reports of this association and, in some of these, organ-specific antibodies against both tissues were found. Thus in one series of patients with adrenal insufficiency, adrenal antibodies were found in 18 out of 35 individuals and of these, eight had parietal-cell antibodies and 11 had thyroid antibodies [345]. In a further study [346] associated disease or antibodies against other organs were found in 75 out of 118 patients with adrenal insufficiency. Of these, seven had pernicious anaemia, six of them being less than 17 years old. Half of the patients had adrenal antibodies and 12% parietal-cell antibodies.

Cushing's disease may be associated with a mild polycythaemia, though the basis for this is not known. In addition there is a neutrophil leucocytosis with a lymphopenia and eosinopenia.

PARATHYROID DISEASE

There are no particular haematological changes in hypoparathyroidism, though there seems to be a genuine association with pernicious anaemia. The nature of this association has been clarified by the demonstration of organ-specific antibodies against these tissues [345]. Thus a high incidence of parietal-cell and thyroid antibody has been found in children with pernicious anaemia and hypoparathyroidism.

Anaemia may occur in primary hyperparathyroidism [347]. Causes include renal failure, the anaemia of chronic disorders and gastro-intestinal blood loss.

ENDOCRINE OBESITY

There is a well-recognized association between marked obesity and polycythaemia [348]. This condition has been named the Pickwickian syndrome and the polycythaemia appears to be corrected by weight reduction. These patients have hypoxia but the mechanism is complex. In some instances there may be mechanical impairment of ventilation, reflex abnormalities, sleep apnoea or combinations of these factors [349–351].

CARDIORESPIRATORY DISEASE

CARDIAC DISEASE

Congenital heart disease

Cyanosis and polycythaemia are found regularly in children with congenital heart disease associated with right-to-left shunt [352]. In severe cases the arterial oxygen saturation may be as low as 50% and red-cell counts in excess of $10^{13}/l$ have been reported. Some degree of right shift in the oxygen dissociation curve is observed, probably due to an increased production of 2,3-diphophoglycerate [353]. Although there is a rela-

tively high incidence of thrombotic episodes in such children [354], a definite bleeding tendency is found in a proportion [355]. In one large series the most frequently encountered abnormalities were thrombocytopenia (52%), impaired clot retraction (59%), low fibrinogen levels (78%) and the formation of soft friable clots [356]. In another study, reduced levels of one or more coagulation factors, typically factor V and platelets, were found [357]. Improvement was noted after venesection or heparinization, suggesting an element of intravascular consumption. Venesection should be performed with great care as there have been several reports of death immediately following phlebotomy [356]. A significant improvement in systemic blood flow, peripheral resistance and systemic oxygen transport can be achieved if the red-cell mass is reduced acutely without lowering the total blood volume, by replacement of blood withdrawn with plasma or 5% albumin [358].

There is a specific association between congenital absence of the spleen and severe congenital heart disease of the cono-truncus type associated with situs inversus viscerae. Thus the finding of red-cell changes characterized by burr cells, target cells and the presence of Howell–Jolly bodies in a newborn infant with cyanosis and respiratory distress is pathognomonic of this type of cardiac abnormality [359].

Valvular disease of the heart

Patients with severe valvular disease may develop low-grade haemolysis [360–362]. This occurs particularly with severe aortic-valve disease, but has also been noted in mitral disease, It seems likely that red-cell damage is the result of abnormally turbulent blood flow through the affected valve. There is frequently a low-grade anaemia with a reticulosis and absent haptoglobins, and in one series of 21 patients, red-cell survival times ranged between 14 and 21 days [360].

Haemolytic anaemia after cardiac surgery may be produced either as part of the post-perfusion syndrome or due to abnormal turbulence following valve replacement [362] (see Chapter 12). The haemorrhagic complications of cardiac bypass are considered in Chapter 29, whilst the haematological manifestations of bacterial endocarditis and the post-perfusion syndrome are dealt with earlier in this chapter (see pp. 1327 and 1336).

Cardiac tumours [363]

In addition to the more usual presentation with fainting attacks and transient cardiac murmurs, atrial myxoma may occasionally present for the first time to the haematologist because of the severity of the associated blood changes. Some degree of normochromic normocytic anaemia is common, and this is associated with a high ESR, rouleaux formation in the blood smear, and elevated immunoglobulin levels. In addition there may be a persistent leucocytosis. These haematological changes may be confused with a variety of primary disorders of the blood including macroglobulinaemia and myelomatosis. However, the hypergammaglobulinaemia of this disorder is of the diffuse variety and monoclonal proteins are not seen.

Hypereosinophilic syndrome [364]

Whilst marked eosinophilia may occur in a variety of pathological situations such as allergy, parasitic infestation, neoplasia and collagen-vascular diseases, it has become increasingly clear that there is a distinct clinical syndrome characterized by marked eosinophilia with widespread tissue infiltration and organ dysfunction, but without demonstrable cause. Earlier reports have stressed the association between eosinophilia, splenomegaly and cardiac disease [365, 366], though more recently it has become clear that the condition may be more generalized, and the term 'hypereosinophilic syndrome' seems appropriate [364].

The disorder predominantly affects middle-aged males. The patient usually presents with fever, fatigue and weight loss, with or without other features such as abdominal or chest pain, dyspnoea, diarrhoea and night sweats. Examination may reveal splenomegaly, hepatomegaly, cardiomegaly with or without overt failure or murmurs, or a pruritic rash. A recent review has stressed a high incidence of neurological complications [364], which may be due either to central thrombotic or embolic phenomena or to peripheral nerve infiltration. The striking haematological findings is a marked eosinophilia of both blood and marrow. The absolute eosinophil count is usually in the range $5–50 \times 10^9/l$, but may be higher; anaemia, if present, is mild and the platelet count is usually normal. Pathologically, there is widespread tissue infiltration with eosinophils. In the heart there may be mural thrombosis, endomyocardial fibrosis and valvular damage (Löffler's fibroplastic parietal endocarditis [365]). It is not clear if the tissue damage is due to the presence of eosinophils, or whether the infiltration occurs in response to tissue damage by an unknown agent. In this respect it is of interest that similar cardiac lesions have been observed in patients with eosinophilia due to filariasis [367] and drug reactions [368].

The underlying cause of this disorder is not known. The magnitude of the leucocyte count suggests a leukaemic process, although blast-cell proliferation is rare, even in the terminal stages. Chromosome abnormalities were sought in one series of 14 patients [364]: in one patient the Ph^1 chromosome was detected in all cells examined, whilst in another it was found on one occasion in one per cent of cells. Aneuploidy was detected in five patients, two of whom showed a C-group deletion. In many patients it is extremely difficult to make a convincing diagnosis of leukaemia, and it is likely that this syndrome represents a heterogeneous group of conditions. Whatever the cause, patients have significant morbidity and a mortality of about 75% at three years. Recent reports suggest that aggressive therapy with corticosteroids, hydroxyurea and supportive measures may significantly improve the outlook [369].

PULMONARY DISEASE

There are a variety of haematological manifestations which occur with pulmonary disease although in the majority of cases the clinical presentation is nearly always due to the effects of the chest disorder rather than its haematological complications. The haematological changes which occur with pulmonary tuberculosis or malignant disease have been described earlier in this chapter. There remain, however, a few chest diseases which regularly produce haematological changes which have not been considered elsewhere in this book.

Purpura due to coughing

Mechanical purpura due to vascular damage resulting from an increase in the intraluminal pressure occurs after severe bouts of coughing. 'Cough purpura' is particularly common in young children and occurs most commonly in association with pertussis infection, but may occur with any childhood upper-respiratory infection. The condition is characterized by showers of petechia occurring particularly around the eyelids and upper half of the face. This may be associated with conjunctival haemorrhages and, less commonly, ecchymotic lesions over the face.

Pneumonia

Most bacterial pneumonias are associated with a neutrophil leucocytosis. This is usually in the range $10–25 \times 10^9/l$, but may be more marked in *Strep. pneumoniae* infection. Haemophilus and klebsiella pneumonias are less consistently associated with neutrophilia, though there is usually some left shift even with normal leucocyte counts. Gram-negative pneumonias are most commonly seen in patients with some degree of marrow failure but are otherwise associated with a leucocytosis. In viral pneumonias the leucocyte count is not usually strikingly elevated.

In mycoplasma pneumonia [370, 371], the leucocyte count is usually normal, though in some cases there is a leucocytosis and, rarely, a leucopenia. Cold agglu-

Chapter 33

tinins can be detected in increased amounts towards the end of the first week in up to 76% of cases [374], but are not especially diagnostic, particularly if present in titres of 1:40 or less. The cold agglutinins are polyclonal IgM antibodies to the red-cell I antigen (see Chapters 11 and 34). Although a positive Coombs' test has been described in 83% and a reticulocytosis in 64% of cases [373], overt haemolysis is rare [371]. A fatal case complicated by disseminated intravascular coagulation has been reported [372].

In pneumonia caused by *Legionella pneumophila* (Legionnaires' disease [375]), a neutrophil leucocytosis is common, and there may be an absolute lymphopenia [376]. Thrombocytopenia has been described [372], and a case of Legionnaires' disease with concomitant mycoplasma pneumonia complicated by disseminated intravascular coagulation has been reported [423].

Chronic bronchitis and emphysema

Patients with chronic obstructive-airways disease fall into two main groups [377]. Type A, the so-called 'pink puffers', tend to have severe dyspnoea with hyperinflation of the lungs, but normal blood gas tensions and no evidence of right-heart failure or clubbing. Type B, the 'blue bloaters', have less limitation of exercise tolerance and tend to be oedematous, plethoric and cyanosed. They have a variable degree of arterial desaturation and in the more severe cases this leads to a secondary polycythaemia, though the degree of polycythaemia does not correlate well with the level of erythropoietin production [378]. A better correlation exists between the degree of hypoxia and the red-cell mass [379, 380], and oxygen administration is followed by a significant fall in the latter [380].

The reasons for the poor correlation between the degree of hypoxia and red-cell production in chronic pulmonary hypoxia, as compared with other diseases, is not clear. It may result from such complicating factors as cardiac failure, chronic pulmonary infection and iron deficiency. Certainly, the anaemia of chronic disorders may be superimposed on chronic pulmonary infection. An additional factor may be the decreased oxygen affinity which results from increased levels of 2,3-diphosphoglycerate which are found in the red cells of some patients with chronic hypoxic lung disease [353]. This would lead to increased delivery of oxygen to the tissues and a decreased erythropoietin response. Recent evidence suggests that 'blue bloaters' have a reduced ventilatory response to hypoxia, and that this could have a genetic basis [351].

It should be remembered that some patients with chronic bronchitis, particularly 'blue boaters', may give a minimal history of respiratory distress and be referred as possible cases of primary polycythaemia. It is most important to include an arterial P_{O_2} estimation as part of the routine study of polycythaemic patients. With very high haematocrits the increased blood viscosity may increase the cardiac load and it has been suggested that careful venesection may help patients with severe hypoxaemia and polycythaemia [381]. This is still a controversial topic, however, and the reader may feel happier to follow the advice of Castle and Jandl that in 'achieving the best balance between increased cardiac work and decreased tissue hypoxia, the wisdom of the body probably exceeds that of the physician' [382].

Pulmonary eosinophilia [383–385]

This term refers to a group of disorders which have in common a raised eosinophil count in the peripheral blood in association with pulmonary infiltrates on the chest X-ray. The exact nature of many of the disorders which make up this syndrome is uncertain. In the simplest form there may be a brief period of respiratory distress in association with eosinophilia and transient pulmonary infiltrates. This condition is sometimes called Löffler's syndrome. At the other end of the spectrum there is a severe illness associated with repeated pulmonary infiltrates and eosinophilia which may culminate with many of the features of polyarteritis nodosa.

Löffler described a condition characterized by fleeting pulmonary infiltrates in association with a raised blood eosinophil count. This condition probably represents a heterogeneous group of disorders and in many cases there is associated parasitic infection. Many parasitic disorders have caused this type of syndrome, including ascariasis, ankylostomiasis, trichiuriasis, taeniasis and fascioliasis. However, the condition can occur in the absence of demonstrable parasitic infection. A similar clinical disorder has been well documented as part of a hypersensitivity reaction to certain drugs. The commonest is para-aminosalicylic acid but a similar reaction has been observed in patients receiving penicillin, sulphonamides and nitrofurantoin. There are often associated features of drug hypersensitivity such as fever, rashes and muscle pain. In addition, a similar clinical picture is associated with the syndrome of so-called allergic alveolitis, including farmers' lung, bird-fancier's lung and a variety of other occupational disorders complicated by allergic reactions to inhaled allergens [386].

Another disorder characterized by marked eosinophilia with pulmonary infiltrates goes under the general descriptive term 'tropical eosinophilia'. This disorder is characterized by fever, dry cough and asthmatic symptoms. The chest X-ray shows diffuse pulmonary mottling and eosinophil counts as high as $100 \times 10^9/l$ have been observed. There is considerable evidence that this disorder is due to occult filarial infection. The disorder responds well to diethylcarba-mazine in doses of 6 mg/kg body weight three times daily for five days.

Another cause of pulmonary eosinophilia is hyper-sensitivity to fungi, particularly *Aspergillus fumigatus*. The clinical manifestations include recurrent asthmatic attacks associated with a variable eosinophilia and pulmonary mottling; the latter has been described as both infiltrative and atelectatic. Affected patients frequently cough up brown plugs of sputum which contain eosinophils, mycelia and mucus.

Finally a pulmonary-eosinophilia syndrome may complicate polyarteritis nodosa. The haematological changes in this disorder were described earlier in this chapter but in this particular syndrome the patients frequently present with asthmatic attacks associated with pulmonary infiltration and very high eosinophil counts.

Idiopathic pulmonary haemosiderosis and Goodpasture's syndrome

Idiopathic pulmonary haemosiderosis most commonly affects children and young adults although it may occur at any age. It is a disorder characterized by episodes of haemorrhage into the pulmonary alveolae due to capillary rupture. The patients complain of attacks of cough, haemoptysis, shortness of breath and the symptoms and signs of anaemia. The anaemia of this disorder is predominantly hypochromic and microcytic with some elements of the anaemia of chronic disorders. In haematological practice it is a rare cause of refractory iron-deficiency anaemia but the clinical history, the finding of macrophages laden with iron in the sputum and the characteristic changes on the chest X-ray usually make the diagnosis relatively easy [387].

A condition very similar to idiopathic pulmonary haemosiderosis, but associated with an acute glomerulonephritis, is known as Goodpasture's syndrome [388]. Again there may be a striking iron-deficiency anaemia with a considerable loss of iron through the alimentary canal due to swallowing of iron-laden macrophages in the sputum. In Goodpasture's syndrome there is frequently a superadded anaemia due to progressive renal failure.

Wegener's granulomatosis [389, 390]

This condition is probably a form of collagen-vascular disorder, but because of its protean haemorrhagic manifestations, involving particularly the upper respiratory tract and lungs, it may occasionally present to the haematologist. The characteristic features are giant-cell granulomata in the naso-pharynx and antra with similar lesions in the lungs, and an associated glomerulonephritis. In addition there may be a general-ized focal necrotizing vasculitis affecting veins as well as arteries. Presenting symptoms are those of an intractable ulcerative rhinitis and sinusitis with severe episodes of nose-bleeding associated with nasal obstruction and a continuous sanguinous discharge. Pulmonary lesions result in haemoptysis and marked dyspnoea. There is usually a progressive nephritis. This condition usually presents to the haematologist as a bleeding disorder due to the striking haemorrhagic changes in the upper respiratory tract. Furthermore there are often vascular haemorrhages in the skin and nail beds which may mimic a primary bleeding disorder. The peripheral blood findings include a normochromic normocytic anaemia which is often complicated by an anaemia of renal failure. The ESR is usually raised and there is a neutrophil leucocytosis but not usually an eosinophilia. The platelet count is normal.

SKIN DISEASE

Although minor haematological abnormalities may occur with a large number of dermatological disorders there are a few in which important blood changes are regularly found. The vascular purpuras are considered in detail in Chapter 26. Many widespread dermatoses are associated with the anaemia of chronic disorders which has been discussed earlier.

DERMATOLOGICAL DISORDERS ASSOCIATED WITH BLOOD LOSS

In any refractory hypochromic anaemia, particularly in young persons, a full dermatological examination must always be performed. There are a variety of primary dermatological conditions which are associated with lesions in the gastro-intestinal tract and hence with gastro-intestinal bleeding. Some of these have already been mentioned earlier in this chapter, and also in Chapter 26.

Hereditary telangiectasia or the Osler–Rendu–Weber syndrome [391–393] is transmitted as a simple dominant trait. Pathologically the lesions are characterized by a defect in vessel walls leading to visible dilation of capillaries and arterioles and occasionally to the development of arteriovenous aneurysms. The skin lesions appear as either violaceous haemangiomas or spiders. Involvement of both skin and mucous membranes is the rule and occasionally there may be aneurysms in the lungs, liver, spleen or central nervous system [393, 395]. Although these lesions may be found in childhood, they increase with advancing years and bleeding is only observed commonly in adult life. The blood picture is that of a simple iron-deficiency anaemia. The commonest forms of bleeding are epistaxis and gastro-intestinal loss. Abnormal platelet function has been observed in a high proportion of these patients [396]. Affected persons can often be maintained on regular iron therapy combined with simple measures such as nasal packs.

Other dermatological disorders which may be associated with intestinal blood loss include the Peutz–Jeghers syndrome [397], Degos' disease and the blue-rubber bleb naevus syndrome. A full description of these dermatological disorders is beyond the scope of this book and the reader is referred to an excellent review of the subject by Wheeler [398].

MEGALOBLASTIC ANAEMIA AND THE SKIN

The whole relationship between dermatological disorders and megaloblastic anaemia is extremely complex and much of the work in this field is still rather controversial. This subject is discussed in Chapter 6 and has been the subject of an extensive review [399] and will only be summarized briefly here.

There are a variety of skin rashes which occur in patients with genuine coeliac disease or tropical sprue. An incidence as high as 10–20% has been reported. The rashes are rather non-specific, are usually eczematous or psoriasiform and are often associated with abnormalities of skin pigmentation. It should be remembered that reticulosis may be superimposed on coeliac disease and skin involvement may be the first indication of this complication.

The relationship between specific skin disorders and megaloblastic anaemia is much more controversial. There is no doubt that a proportion of patients with various dermatoses show evidence of folate depletion, at least as judged by increased urinary excretion of formimino-glutamic acid (FIGLU). Thus Shuster et al. noticed increased FIGLU levels in the urine of 19 out of 30 patients and reduced serum folate levels in 21 out of 28 patients with erythroderma, psoriasis or extensive eczema [400]. In addition, of 13 patients with dermatitis herpetiformis, 11 had low serum folate levels and five had low red-cell folate levels [401]. Although megaloblastic anaemia is not found frequently in association with disorders of the skin, some of the patients in these series did have megaloblastic changes. Earlier reports suggested that a significant proportion of patients with severe skin disease have abnormalities of small intestinal function and structure [402]. It was suggested that the skin disorder is the primary cause of these changes and the intestinal malabsorption is secondary; hence the term 'dermatogenic enteropathy' has been coined [403]. In a recent review Marks & Shuster [399] have stated that there is now general agreement that a completely flat small bowel mucosa, similar to that found in coeliac disease, is never found in dermatogenic enteropathy. The basis for intestinal malabsorption in dermatological disorders remains unclear.

The relationship between dermatitis herpetiformis (DH) and malabsorption of the coeliac type seems to be a rather special case. Several series have shown a high incidence of the small bowel changes of coeliac disease in patients with DH. Thus in Marks & Shuster's series approximately 25% of patients with DH had an intestinal biopsy abnormality [399]. Furthermore, there seems to be a high incidence of splenic hypoplasia in patients with DH (see Chapter 6). Apart from the results of malabsorption and hyposplenism, a variety of other haematological changes occur in DH including eosinophilia, the occasional presence of thromboplastin inhibitors, and the results of drug therapy including the Heinz-body anaemia which follows the administration of dapsone.

Finally, it must be remembered that some systemic disorders which present frequently with dermatological manifestations may be associated with small-bowel disease and malabsorption. Such conditions include the collagen-vascular disorders, particularly disseminated lupus erythematosus and polyarteritis nodosa.

SKIN DISORDERS WITH ALTERATIONS IN THE WHITE CELLS [398]

A variety of mild alterations in the white-cell count occur in association with widespread dermatological disease. Eosinophilia is a common accompaniment of atopic eczema, drug reactions, certain pre-reticuloses, infestations, Behcet's syndrome and polyarteritis. The lymphocyte count varies in the cutaneous reticuloses. In some cases there is a lymphocytosis while in cutaneous Hodgkin's disease and in dermatomyositis there is often a lymphopenia. A slight elevation in the neutrophil count is observed in many skin diseases; high levels may be associated with polyarteritis nodosa and particularly with the acute neutrophilic dermatosis of Sweet [404].

SKIN DISORDERS PARTICULARLY ASSOCIATED WITH HAEMATOLOGICAL CHANGES

The various components of the systemic mast-cell syndrome produce regular haematological changes [405, 406]. This syndrome is divided into urticaria pigmentosa of childhood and systemic mastocytosis which occurs in adult life. Changes in the bone marrow and peripheral blood in association with urticaria pigmentosa have only been reported occasionally. Affected children show repeated eruptions of macular lesions, with nodular and plaque-like forms, over the neck, face, scalp, extremities and oral mucosa. This is associated with flushing, itching and hypotension.

There may be lymphadenopathy, splenomegaly and increased numbers of mast cells in the bone marrow.

Systemic mastocytosis is a disease of adult life. The clinical manifestations resemble those of a lymphoma or leukaemia and the disease should probably be classified as a reticulo-endotheliosis. The skin and mucous-membrane manifestations are rather similar to those of childhood urticaria pigmentosa; however, the macules tend to become confluent with persistent telangiectasia. Furthermore, there is extensive involvement of the mouth, nose and rectal mucosa and progressive cutaneous changes characterized by a chronic lichenified dermatitis and generalized infiltration of the skin with a 'scotch-grain' appearance. As in the childhood form of the disease adults have flushing attacks and shock-like episodes. The skin changes are associated with generalized lymphadenopathy, splenomegaly and hepatomegaly and the bone marrow contains an abnormal accumulation of mast cells. In addition there may be anaemia, leucopenia, thrombocytopenia and leukaemoid features. These include a monocytosis, lymphocytosis or eosinophilia.

Liver function is impaired and there may be a bleeding tendency from a combination of thrombocytopenia and prothrombin deficiency. Occasionally mast cells 'spill' into the peripheral blood in large numbers with the picture of 'mast-cell leukaemia'. There is no treatment which seems to alter the natural course of this fatal illness.

Another skin disorder which presents sometimes to the haematologist is *angiokeratoma corporis diffusum universale* (Fabry's disease) [407, 408]. This is an inherited disorder of glycolipid metabolism characterized by telangiectatic skin lesions, hypohidrosis, corneal opacities, fever and cardiovascular and central nervous system disturbances. It is inherited as an X-linked incompletely recessive factor. The basic defect in this disorder is absence of the enzyme trihexosyl ceramide galactosyl hydrolase which can be demonstrated in cultured skin fibroblasts. The lesions which may bring these patients to the haematologist are the telangiectatic spots which vary in size from a pin-pont to several millimetres. They are bright red to blue-black and have a slight covering scale (Fig. 33.11).

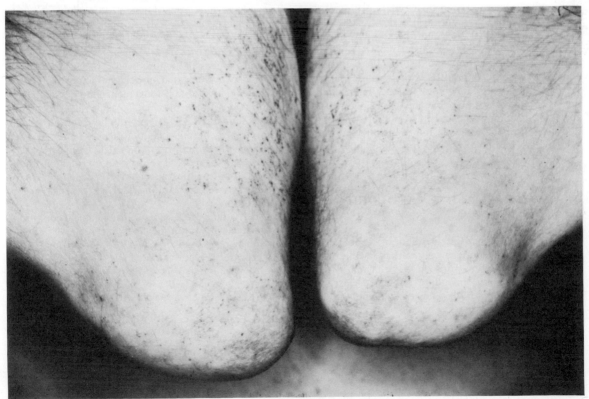

Fig. 33.11. The elbows of a patient with Fabry's disease. The purpuric lesions and atrophy and pigmentation of the skin are shown.

They tend to occur in clusters around the umbilicus, scrotum, penis, buttocks, thighs and elbows and also on the oral mucosa. These lesions have to be distinguished from other forms of purpuric spots including the vascular and thrombocytopenic purpuras and hereditary telangiectasia. The distinction is usually easy because there is decreased sweating, scantiness of hair, paraesthesia of the hands and feet and obvious evidence of a multisystem disorder including renal failure, vascular disease and eye changes. The condition can be diagnosed with certainty by the finding of 'Maltese-cross' material in the urine on polaroscopy or by direct enzyme assay of skin fibroblasts (see p. 1375). Furthermore, 'mulberry cells' containing glycolipid may be found in the urinary sediment. With progression of the disease there is progressive renal failure. The blood changes include a mild normochromic normocytic anaemia, raised ESR and a neutrophil leucocytosis. The anaemia of renal failure may be an additional complication.

There are a variety of other rare dermatoses which may present to the haematologist because of their tendency to be associated with purpuric lesions [409]. These conditions occur particularly in the dependent areas and are characterized by capillary proliferation with inflammation and rupture of skin vessels. Skin pigmentation results from the liberation of haemosiderin by the chronic extravasation of blood cells. The characteristic finding in these disorders is pigmented purpuric lichenoid dermatitis with purpuric papules scattered among large purpuric lesions. These conditions have a variety of names including pigmentary dermatosis of Shamberg, purpura annularis telangiectoides (Majocchi's disease) and pigmented purpuric lichenoid dermatitis of Gougerot & Blum [409].

OTHER GENERALIZED SYSTEMIC DISORDERS WITH HAEMATOLOGICAL CHANGES

There are a few inherited disorders of carbohydrate metabolism which produce well-marked haematological changes and thus may present to the haematologist. The storage diseases, inlcuding Tangier disease, are considered in Chapter 20, and the remaining conditions in this group are listed briefly below.

Acanthocytosis with a-beta-lipoproteinaemia [410]
This condition is inherited in an autosomal recessive fashion. The fully expressed clinical picture consists of fat malabsorption, ataxic neuropathy, retinitis pigmentosa and acanthocytosis. The red cells resemble crenated spheres with spiny excrescences (Fig. 33.12). They are best seen in wet preparations and since the

cells do not form rouleaux there is a low sedimentation rate. The red-cell osmotic fragility is normal and there is an increased mechanical fragility. Some affected individuals have been anaemic and this seems to result from several mechanisms including folic-acid deficiency and, in a few cases, a definite haemolytic process. The bone marrow is usually normal and the red-cell precursors do not show acanthocytosis.

The changes in the red-cell membrane lipids in this condition have been reviewed in Chapters 10 and 12. In summary, the cells contain less phosphatidylcholine and more sphingomyelin, but the same amount of phospholipids as normal cells. The basic molecular defect is not known, but probably resides in the lipoprotein apoproteins. There is a total deficiency of low-density lipoproteins in this condition.

Hypo-beta-lipoproteinaemia [411]
This is an autosomal recessive condition characterized by a low-density lipoprotein level of about 10% of normal. Acanthocytes are not present in the blood, but poikilocytosis was noted on the blood films of some family members in the first reported kindred study; some of these persons had clear-cut evidence of haemolysis but in subsequent families the blood picture has been essentially normal.

Acanthocytosis with normal lipoproteins [412]
Several families have now been reported in which a chronic neurological disorder characterized by tics, grimacing, involuntary movements and dementia was associated with the presence of many acanthocytes in the blood (Fig. 33.12). A full description of this disorder, including haematological and red-cell enzyme studies has been reported elsewhere [412]. Apart from the red-cell deformities no other haematological abnormalities were noted except for a slight increase in red-cell autohaemolysis after 48 hours' incubation.

Clearly there are a series of neurological conditions associated with acanthocytosis and it is very easy to miss this group of disorders if wet preparations of the erythrocytes are not examined in all cases of bizarre neurological illness.

Familial lecithin-cholesterol-acyltransferase deficiency [413]
This condition is characterized by anaemia, corneal infiltrates, proteinuria and progressive renal failure. There is a reduced level of cholesterol and cholesterol esters and increased unesterified cholesterol and lecithin in the blood. The red-cell membrane changes have been reviewed briefly in Chapter 7. The peripheral blood film shows many target cells and increased amounts of cholesterol and lecithin in the membrane.

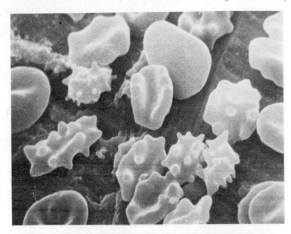

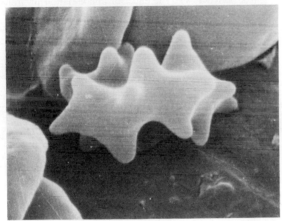

Fig. 33.12. Scanning electron microscope photographs of the cells of a patient with acanthocytosis, normal lipoproteins and a degenerative disease of the nervous system associated with dementia and involuntary movement. (From Ref. 412 and by courtesy of Dr J. A. Salisbury and Dr J. A. Clarke.)

These patients have a shortened red-cell survival and the anaemia is usually complicated by progressive renal failure.

The mucopolysaccharidoses
The bleeding tendency which occurs in this group of inherited disorders of connective tissue has been mentioned earlier in this chapter (p. 1359).

Hurler's syndrome (gargoylism) [414]. This syndrome is characterized by dwarfism, grotesque facies, protuberance of the abdomen and mental retardation. Inclusion bodies occur in both the polymorphonuclear leucocytes and in the lymphocytes. These appear as large dark granules on Giemsa's stain, but are seen better by metachromatic staining with toluidine blue.

These bodies are also found in the bone marrow in large histiocytes and lymphocytes. They are also observed in skin exudates after trauma.

PREGNANCY

Although pregnancy can hardly be considered as a systemic disease, it is appropriate to consider at this point some of the haematological changes that may occur during its course.

There is an increased drive to erythropoiesis from early pregnancy, mediated through increased production of erythropoietin and possibly other hormones, and this is reflected in an absolute rise in the red-cell mass of—on average—300 ml [416]. In spite of this, some degree of anaemia is commonly manifest by the end of the second trimester, but this is generally due to haemodilution as there is a concomitant rise in plasma volume averaging 1000 ml. This has given rise to the concept of a 'physiological anaemia of pregnancy', though it should be remembered that true anaemia is common and haemoglobin values of less than 10 g/dl in the second and third trimester are probably abnormal and should be investigated further.

The relationship between pregnancy and iron and folate metabolism, and the anaemias which occur from lack of these substances, are considered in Chapter 9 and 10 respectively. Iron deficiency is by far the commonest cause of anaemia in pregnancy, although folate deficiency is still often seen when prophylactic folic acid has not been taken. Furthermore, iron deficiency is not always easy to diagnose in pregnancy. The red-cell appearances and indices are relatively insensitive and there is usually a reduced serum iron value and increased total iron-binding capacity as part of the normal response to pregnancy. Serum iron values of less than 60 μg/100 ml are significant, however. Iron stores may be assessed by marrow examination or by estimation of serum ferritin [417], and one of these investigations should always be carried out if the haemoglobin level does not rise after iron therapy, and there is no other obvious cause for the anaemia. It should be remembered that pyelonephritis is a fairly frequent complication of pregnancy, and may be complicated by the anaemia of chronic disorders.

Hypoplastic anaemia occurs occasionally in pregnancy (Chapter 31). In many instances it is precipitated by infection or renal disease, less commonly by drugs. Idiopathic aplastic anaemia is rare: Fleming has reviewed 41 cases from the literature: 28 patients died but in 11 of the 13 survivors spontaneous remission occurred at or shortly after the time of delivery [418].

A mild leucocytosis is common during pregnancy

[419]; the neutrophils are larger than normal with pronounced granulation. The alkaline phosphatase score is increased but myeloperoxidase activity is decreased [420]. This is reflected in a mild impairment of the ability to kill phagocytosed *Candida*. These changes do not appear to be of clinical significance.

REFERENCES

1 CARTWRIGHT G.E. & WINTROBE M.M. (1952) The anemia of infection. XVII. A review. *Advances in Internal Medicine*, **5**, 165.

2 CARTWRIGHT G.E. (1966) The anemia of chronic disorders. *Seminars in Hematology* **3**, 351.

3 CARTWRIGHT G.E. & LEE G.R. (1971) The anaemia of chronic disorders. *British Journal of Haematology* **21**, 147.

4 DOUGLAS S.W. & ADAMSON J.W. (1975) The anemia of chronic disorders: studies of marrow regulation and iron absorption. *Blood*, **45**, 55.

5 WARD H.P., GRODON B. & PICKETT J.C. (1969) Serum levels of erythropoietin in rheumatoid arthritis. *Journal of Laboratory and Clinical Medicine*, **74**, 93.

6 WARD H.P., KURNICK J.E. & PISARCZYK M.J. (1971) Serum levels of erythropoietin in anemias associated with chronic infection, malignancy and primary hematopoietic disease. *Journal of Clinical Investigation*, **50**, 332.

7 WALLNER S.F., KURNICK J.E., VAUTRIN R.M., WHITE M.J., CHAPMAN R.G. & WARD H.P. (1977) Levels of erythropoietin in patients with the anaemias of chronic disease and liver failure. *American Journal of Hematology*, **3**, 37.

8 ALEXANIAN R. (1972) Erythropoietin excretion in hemolytic anemia and in the hypoferremia of chronic disease. *Blood*, **40**, 946.

9 KURNICK J.E., WARD H.P. & PICKETT J.C. (1972) Mechanism of the anemia of chronic disorders. Correlation of haematocrit value with albumin, vitamin B_{12}, transferrin and iron stores. *Archives of Internal Medicine*, **130**, 323.

10 ZUCKER S., FRIEDMAN S. & LYSIK R.M. (1974) Bone marrow erythropoiesis in the anemia of infection, inflammation and malignancy. *Journal of Clinical Investigation*, **53**, 1132.

11 ZUCKER S., LYSIK R.M. & FRIEDMAN S. (1976) Diminished bone marrow responsiveness to erythropoietin in myelopthisic anemia. *Cancer*, **37**, 1308.

12 LIPSHITZ D.A., COOK J.D. & FINCH C.A. (1974) A clinical evaluation of serum ferritin. *New England Journal of Medicine*, **290**, 1213.

13 WALSH J.R. & FREDRICKSON M. (1977) Serum ferritin, free erythrocyte protoporphyrin and urinary iron excretion in patients with iron disorders. *American Journal of the Medical Sciences*, **273**, 293.

14 BIRGEGARD G., HALLGREN R., KILLANDER A., STROMBERG A., VENGE P. & WIDE L. (1978) Serum ferritin during infection. A longitudinal study. *Scandinavian Journal of Haematology*, **21**, 333.

15 CAMPBELL B.C., RENNIE N., THOMPSON G.G., MOORE M.R. & GOLDBERG A. (1978) Haem biosynthesis in rheumatoid disease. *British Journal of Haematology*, **240**, 563.

16 FINCH C.A., DEUBELBEISS K., COOK J.D., ESCHBACH J.W., HARKER L.A., FUNK D.D., MARSAGLIA G., HILLMAN R.S., SLICHTER S., ADAMSON J.W., GANZONI A. & GIBLETT E.R. (1979) Ferrokinetics in man. *Medicine (Baltimore)*, **49**, 17.

17 FREIREICH E.J., MILLER A., EMERSON C.P. & ROSS J.F. (1957) The effect of inflammation on the utilization of erythrocyte and transferrin bound radioiron for red cell production. *Blood*, **12**, 972.

18 ELIN R.J., WOLFF S.M. & FINCH C.A. (1977) Effect of induced fever on serum iron and ferritin concentrations in man. *Blood*, **49**, 147.

19 HILLMAN R.S. & HENDERSON P.A. (1969) Control of marrow production by the level of iron supply. *Journal of Clinical Investigation*, **48**, 454.

20 HERSHKO C., COOK J.D. & FINCH C.A. (1974) Storage iron kinetics. VI. The effect of inflammation on iron exchange in the rat. *British Journal of Haematology*, **28**, 67.

21 TORRANCE J.D., CHARLTON R.W., SIMON M.O., LYNCH S.R. & BOTHWELL T.H. (1978) The mechanism of endotoxin-induced hypoferraemia. *Scandinavian Journal of Haematology*, **21**, 403.

22 FILLET G., COOK J.D. & FINCH C.A. (1974) Storage iron kinetics. VII. A biologic model for reticuloendothelial iron transport. *Journal of Clinical Investigation*, **53**, 1527.

23 WEICK J.K., HAGEDORN A.B. & LINMAN J.W. (1974) Leukoerythroblastosis: diagnosis and prognostic significance. *Mayo Clinic Proceedings*, **49**, 111.

24 KIELEY J.M. & SILVERSTEIN M.N. (1969) Metastatic carcinoma simulating agnogenic myeloid metaplasia and myelofibrosis. *Cancer*, **24**, 1041.

25 CONTRERAS E., ELLIS L.D. & LEE R.E. (1972) Value of the bone marrow biopsy in the diagnosis of metastatic carcinoma. *Cancer*, **29**, 778.

26 BROOK J. & KONWALER B.E. (1965) Thrombotic thrombocytopenic purpura in association with metastatic gastric carcinoma and a possible autoimmune disorder. *California Medicine*, **102**, 222.

27 DUMONT J., BIORON M., LEDUC C., FRESSINAUD L. & BERNARD J. (1965) Association d'une anemie hemolytique et d'un purpura thrombopenique a un cancer de l'estomac. *Presse Medicale*, **73**, 877.

28 LYNCH E.C., BAKKEN C.L., CASEY T.H. & ALFREY C.P. JR (1967) Microangiopathic hemolytic anemia in carcinoma of the stomach. *Gastroenterology*, **52**, 88.

29 BRAIN M.C., AZZOPARDI J.G., BAKER L.R.I., PINEO G.F., ROBERTS P.D. & DACIE J.V. (1970) Microangiopathic haemolytic anaemia and mucin-forming adenocarcinoma. *British Journal of Haematology*, **18**, 183.

30 ANTMAN K.H., SKARIN A.T., MAYER R.J., HARGREAVES H.K. & CANELLOS G.P. (1979) Microangiopathic haemolytic anaemia and cancer: A review. *Medicine (Baltimore)*, **58**, 377.

31 FORSHAW J. & HARWOOD L. (1966) Poikilocytosis associated with carcinoma. *Archives of Internal Medicine*, **117**, 203.

32 PINEO C.F., REGOECZI E., HATTON M.W.C. & BRAIN M.C. (1973) Activation of coagulation by extracts of mucus. A possible pathway of intravascular coagulation

accompanying adenocarcinoma. *Journal of Laboratory and Clinical Medicine*, **82**, 255.

33 HILGARD P. & GORDON-SMITH E. (1974) Microangiopathic haemolytic anaemia and experimental tumour-cell embolism. *British Journal of Haematology*, **26**, 651.

34 JONES E. & TILLMAN C.A. (1945) A case of hemolytic anemia relieved by removal of an ovarian tumour. *Journal of the American Medical Association*, **128**, 225.

35 SPIRA M.A. & LYNCH E.C. (1980) Autoimmune hemolytic anemia and carcinoma: an unusual association. *American Journal of Medicine*, **67**, 753.

36 WORTMAN J., ROSSE W. & LOGUE G. (1979) Cold agglutinin autoimmune hemolytic anaemia in non-hematologic malignancies. *American Journal of Hematology*, **6**, 275.

37 DE BRUYERE M., SOKAL G., DEVOITILLE J.M., FAUCHET-DUTRIEUX M.C. & DE SPA V. (1971) Autoimmune haemolytic anaemia and ovarian tumours. *British Journal of Haematology*, **20**, 83.

38 GORDON P.A., BAYLIS P.H. & BIRD G.W.G. (1976) Tumour-induced haemolytic anaemia. *British Medical Journal*, **i**, 1569.

39 DAMESHEK W., BROWN S.M. & RUBIN A.D. (1967) 'Pure' red cell anemia (erythroblastic hypoplasia) and thymoma. *Seminars in Hematology*, **4**, 222.

40 ENTWISTLE C.C., FENTEM P.H. & JACOBS A. (1964) Red cell aplasia with carcinoma of the bronchus. *British Medical Journal*, **ii**, 1504.

41 CHANARIN I. (1979) *The Megaloblastic Anaemias*, 2nd edn. Blackwell Scientific Publications, Oxford.

42 HOFFBRAND A.V., HOBBS J.R., KREMENCHUZKY S. & MOLLIN D.L. (1967) Incidence and pathogenesis of megaloblastic erythropoiesis in multiple myeloma. *Journal of Clinical Pathology*, **20**, 699.

43 MAGNUS E.M. (1967) Folate activity in serum and red cells of patient with cancer. *Cancer Research*, **27**, 490.

44 FORSHAW J. (1963) Megaloblastic erythropoiesis in multiple myeloma. *British Medical Journal*, **ii**, 101.

45 MOLLIN D.L. & HOFFBRAND A.V. (1968) Sideroblastic anaemia. In: *Recent Advances in Clinical Pathology, Series V* (ed. Dyke S.C.), p. 273. Churchill, London.

46 DONATI R.M., McCARTHY J.M., LANGE R.D. & GALLAGHER N.I. (1963) Erythrocythemia and neoplastic tumours. *Annals of Internal Medicine*, **58**, 47.

47 ROSENBACK L.M. & XEFTERIS E.D. (1961) Erythrocytosis associated with carcinoma of the kidney. *Journal of the American Medical Association*, **176**, 136.

48 SHALET M.F., HOLDER T.M. & WALTERS T.R. (1967) Erythropoietin-producing Wilms' tumor. *Journal of Pediatrics*, **70**, 615.

49 VERTEL R.M., MORSE B.S. & PRINCE J.E. (1967) Remission of erythrocytosis after damage of a solitary renal cyst. *Archives of Internal Medicine*, **120**, 54.

50 BROWNSTEIN M.H. & BALLARD H.S. (1966) Hepatoma associated with erythrocytosis. *American Journal of Medicine*, **40**, 204.

51 JOSEPHS B.N., ROBBINS G. & LEVINE A. (1962) Polycythemia secondary to hamartoma of the liver. *Journal of the American Medical Association*, **179**, 867.

52 HERTKO E.J. (1963) Polycythemia (erythrocytosis) associated with uterine fibroids and apparent surgical cure. *American Journal of Medicine*, **34**, 288.

53 BOIVIN P. (1965) Polycythemia and cerebellar hemangioma. *Presse Medicale*, **73**, 2799.

54 SHAH P.C., PATEL A.R., DIMARIA F., RABA J. & VOHRA R.M. (1979) Polycythaemia in lung cancer. *Clinical and Laboratory Haematology*, **1**, 329.

55 LEVIN J. & CONLEY C.L. (1964) Thrombocytosis associated with malignant disease. *Archives of Internal Medicine*, **114**, 497.

56 SILVIS S.E., TURBAS N. & DOSCHERHOLMEN A. (1970) Thrombocytosis in patients with lung cancer. *Journal of the American Medical Association*, **211**, 1852.

57 TRANUM B.L. & HAUT A. (1974) Thrombocytosis: platelet kinetics and neoplasia. *Journal of Laboratory and Clinical Medicine*, **84**, 615.

58 ASANO S., URABE A., OKABE T., SATO N., KONDO Y., UEYAMA Y., CHIBA S., OSHAWA N. & KOSAKA K. (1977) Demonstration of granulopoietic factor(s) in the plasma of nude mice transplanted with a human lung cancer and in the tumor tissue. *Blood*, **49**, 845.

59 BARRETT O'N. (1970) Monocytosis in malignant disease. *Annals of Internal Medicine*, **73**, 991.

60 ISAACSON N.H. & RAPAPORT P. (1946) Eosinophilia in malignant tumors. *Annals of Internal Medicine*, **25**, 893.

61 WASSERMAN S.I., GOETZL E.J., ELLMAN L. & AUSTEN K.F. (1974) Tumor associated eosinophilotactic factor. *New England Journal of Medicine*, **290**, 420.

62 DELLON A.L., HUME R.B. & CHRETIEN P.B. (1974) Eosinophilia in bronchogenic carcinoma. *New England Journal of Medicine*, **291**, 207.

63 HEALY T.M. (1974) Eosinophilia in bronchogenic carcinoma. *New England Journal of Medicine*, **291**, 794.

64 CROWTHER D. & BATEMAN C.J.T. (1972) Malignant disease. *Clinics in Hematology*, **1**, 447.

65 MARSH J.C., BOGGS D.R., CARTWRIGHT G.E. & WINTROBE M.M. (1967) Neutrophil kinetics in acute infection. *Journal of Clinical Investigation*, **46**, 1943.

66 ZIPURSKY A. & JABER H.M. (1978) The hematology of bacterial infection in newborn infants. *Clinics in Hematology*, **7**, 175.

67 SEELER R.A., METZGER W. & MUFSON M.A. (1972) *Diplococcus pneumoniae* infection in children with sickle cell anemia. *American Journal of Diseases of Children*, **123**, 8.

68 EMERSON W.A., ZIEVE P.D. & KREVANS J.R. (1970) Hematologic changes in septicemia. *Johns Hopkins Medical Journal*, **126**, 69.

69 WINTROBE M.W. (1974) *Clinical Hematology*, 7th edn. Lea and Febiger, Philadelphia.

70 BEESON P.B. (1975) Infective endocarditis (bacterial endocarditis, prosthetic valve endocarditis). In: *Textbook of Medicine*, 14th edn (ed. Beeson P.B. & McDermott W.), p. 308. W.B. Saunders, Philadelphia.

71 HILL R.W. & BAYRD E.D. (1960) Phagocytic reticuloendothelial cells in subacute bacterial endocarditis with negative cultures. *Annals of Internal Medicine*, **52**, 310.

72 DACIE J.V. (1967) *Secondary or Symptomatic Haemolytic Anaemias. III. The haemolytic anaemias*, 2nd edn. Churchill, London.

73 RUBENBERG M.L., BAKER L.R.I., McBRIDE J.A., SEVITT L.H. & BRAIN M.C. (1967) Intravascular coagulation in a case of *Clostridum perfringens* septicaemia; treatment by exchange transfusion and heparin. *British Medical Journal*, **iv**, 271.

74 YOSHIKAWA T., TANAKA K.R. & GUZE L.B. (1971) Infection and disseminated intravascular coagulation. *Medicine (Baltimore)*, **50**, 237.

75 KELTON J.G., NEAME P.B., GAULDIE J. & HIRSH J. (1979) Elevated platelet-associated IgG in the thrombocytopenia of septicemia. *New England Journal of Medicine*, **300**, 760.

76 ROWE M.I., MARCHILDON M.B., ARANGO A., MALININ T. & GANS A. (1978) The mechanisms of thrombocytopenia in experimental Gram-negative septicaemia. *Surgery*, **84**, 87.

77 KOSTER F., LEVIN J., WALKER L., TUNG K.S.K., GILMAN R.H., RAHAMAN M.M., MAJID M.A., ISLAM S. & WILLIAMS R.C. JR (1978) Hemolytic uremic syndrome after shigellosis. Relation to endotoxemia and circulating immune complexes. *New England Journal of Medicine*, **298**, 927.

78 TWOMEY J.J. & LEAVELL B.S. (1965) Leukemoid reactions to tuberculosis. *Archives of Internal Medicine*, **116**, 21.

79 SKARBERG K.O., LANGERLOF B. & REIZENSTEIN P. (1967) Leukaemia, leukaemoid reaction and tuberculosis. *Acta Medica Scandinavica*, **182**, 427.

80 BALL K., JOULES H. & PAGEL W. (1951) Acute tuberculous septicaemia with leucopenia. *British Medical Journal*, **ii**, 869.

81 MEDD W.E. & HAYHOE F.G.J. (1955) Tuberculous miliary necrosis with pancytopenia. *Quarterly Journal of Medicine (New Series)*, **24**, 351.

82 ANDRE J., SCHWARTZ R. & DAEMSHEK W. (1961) Tuberculosis and myelosclerosis with myeloid metaplasia; report of three cases. *Journal of the American Medical Association*, **178**, 1169.

83 ZAMORANO J. JR & TOMPSETT R. (1968) Disseminated atypical mycobacterial infection and pancytopenia. *Archives of Internal Medicine*, **121**, 424.

84 GORDON-SMITH E. & HOLT J.M. (1967) Areactive generalised tuberculosis as a diagnostic problem in clinical haematology. *Quarterly Journal of Medicine (New Series)*, **36**, 602.

85 GLASSER R.M., WALKER R.I. & HERION J.C. (1970) The significance of hematologic abnormalities in patients with tuberculosis. *Archives of Internal Medicine*, **125**, 691.

86 PROUDFOOT A.T. (1971) Cryptic disseminated tuberculosis. *British Journal of Hospital Medicine*, **5**, 773.

87 LOWTHER C.P. (1959) Leukemia and tuberculosis. *Annals of Internal Medicine*, **51**, 52.

88 MORROW L.B. & ANDERSON R.E. (1965) Active tuberculosis in leukemia. *Archives of Pathology*, **79**, 484.

89 OSWALD N.C. (1963) Acute tuberculosis and granulocytic disorders. *British Medical Journal*, **ii**, 1489.

90 SCHLEICHER E.M. (1966) Demonstration of tuberculosis in the human bone marrow. *Minnesota Medicine*, **49**, 221.

91 ALSON J.M. & BROOM J.C. (1958) *Leptospirosis in Man and Animals*. Livingstone, Edinburgh.

92 MORSE E.E., ZINKHAM W.H. & JACKSON D.P. (1966) Thrombocytopenic purpura following rubella infection in children and adults. *Archives of Internal Medicine*, **117**, 573.

93 McKAY D.G. & MARGARETTEN W. (1967) Disseminated intravascular coagulation in virus diseases. *Archives of Internal Medicine*, **120**, 129.

94 OSKI F.A. & NAIMAN J.L. (1966) *Hematologic Problems in the Newborn*. W.B. Saunders, Philadelphia.

95 HANSHAW J.B. & DUDGEON J.A. (1978) *Viral Diseases of the Fetus and Newborn*. W.B. Saunders, Philadelphia.

96 LUKENS J.N. (1978) Neonatal hematological abnormalities associated with maternal disease. *Clinics in Hematology*, **7**, 155.

97 PAYNE M.C. & GLUCK L. (1965) Rubella syndrome and thrombocytopenic purpura in newborn infants: clinical and virologic observations. *New England Journal of Medicine*, **273**, 474.

98 RIESS J.S. & PRYLES C.V. (1966) Thrombocytopenia in congenital rubella. *New England Journal of Medicine*, **275**, 264.

99 PLOTKIN S.A., OSKI F.A., HARTNETT E.M., HERVADA A.R., FRIEDMAN S. & GOWING J. (1965) Some recently recognized manifestations of the rubella syndrome. *Journal of Pediatrics*, **67**, 182.

100 ZINKHAM W.H., MEDEARIS D.N. & OSBORN J.E. (1967) Blood and bone marrow findings in congenital rubella. *Journal of Pediatrics*, **71**, 512.

101 O'NEILL B.J. & MARSHALL W.C. (1967) Paroxysmal cold haemoglobinuria and measles. *Archives of Disease in Childhood*, **42**, 183.

102 BUNCH C., SCHWARTZ F.C.M. & BIRD G.W.G. (1972) Paroxysmal cold haemoglobinuria following measles immunization. *Archives of Disease in Childhood*, **47**, 299.

103 CHRISTIE A.B. (1969) *Infectious Disease: Epidemiology and Clinical Practice*. Livingstone, Edinburgh.

104 CARTER R.L. & PENMAN H.G. (1969) *Infectious Mononucleosis*. Blackwell Scientific Publications, Oxford.

105 HENLE W., HENLE G. & LENNETTE E.T. (1979) The Epstein–Barr virus. *Scientific American*, **241**, 40.

106 EPSTEIN M.A., ACHONG B.C. & BARR Y.M. (1964) Virus particles in cultured lymphoblasts from Burkitt's lymphoma. *Lancet*, **i**, 702.

107 HENLE G. & HENLE W. (1966) Immunofluorescence in cells derived from Burkitt's lymphoma. *Journal of Bacteriology*, **91**, 1248.

108 HENLE G., HENLE W. & DIEHL V. (1968) Relation of Burkitt's tumor associated herpes-type virus to infectious mononucleosis. *Proceedings of the National Academy of Sciences, USA*, **59**, 94.

109 KLEIN G. (1975) The Epstein–Barr virus and neoplasia. *New England Journal of Medicine*, **293**, 1353.

110 EPSTEIN M.A. & ACHONG B.G. (1977) Pathogenesis of infectious mononucleosis. *Lancet*, **ii**, 1270.

111 NIEDERMAN J.C., MILLER G., PEARSON H.A., PAGANO J.S. & DOWALIBY J.M. (1976) Infectious mononucleosis. Epstein–Barr-virus shedding in saliva and the oropharynx. *New England Journal of Medicine*, **294**, 1355.

112 PURTILO D.T. (1980) Epstein–Barr-virus-induced oncogenesis in immune-deficient individuals. *Lancet*, **i**, 300.

113 FINCH S.C. (1969) Clinical symptoms and signs of infectious mononucleosis. In *Infectious Mononucleosis* (ed. Carter R.L. & Penman H.G.), p. 19. Blackwell Scientific Publications, Oxford.

114 McKENDRICK M.W., GEDDES A.M. & EDWARDS J.M.B. (1979) Atypical infectious mononucleosis in the elderly. *British Medical Journal*, **iv**, 970.

115 SPECK W.I. (1971) High frequency of ampicillin rashes

in infectious mononucleosis. Clinical implications and case report. *Clinical Pediatrics*, **10**, 59.

116 WOOD T.A. & FRENKEL E.P. (1967) The atypical lymphocyte. *American Journal of Medicine*, **42**, 923.

117 FINCH S.C. (1969) Laboratory findings in infectious mononucleosis. In: *Infectious Mononucleosis* (ed. Carter R.L. & Penman H.G.), p. 42. Blackwell Scientific Publications, Oxford.

118 DAVIDSOHN I. & LEE C.L. (1969) The clinical serology of infectious mononucleosis. In: *Infectious Mononucleosis* (ed. Carter R.L. & Penman H.G.), p. 177. Blackwell Scientific Publications, Oxford.

119 STITES D.P. & LEIKOLA J. (1971) Infectious mononucleosis. *Seminars in Hematology*, **8**, 243.

120 HOAGLAND R.J. (1967) *Infectious Mononucleosis*. Grune & Stratton, New York.

121 PENMAN H.G. (1969) The problem of seronegative infectious mononucleosis. *Infectious Mononucleosis* (ed. Carter R.L. & Penman H.G.), p. 201. Blackwell Scientific Publications, Oxford.

122 WORLLEDGE S.M. & DACIE J.V. (1969) Haemolytic and other anaemias in infectious mononucleosis. In: *Infectious Mononucleosis* (ed. Carter R.L. & Penman H.G.), p. 82. Blackwell Scientific Publications, Oxford.

123 SHARP A.A. (1969) Platelets, bleeding and haemostasis in infectious mononucleosis. In: *Infectious Mononucleosis* (ed. Carter R.L. & Penman H.G.), p. 99. Blackwell Scientific Publications, Oxford.

124 ELLMAN L., CARVALHO A., JACOBSON B.M. & COLMAN R.W. (1973) Platelet autoantibody in a case of infectious mononucleosis presenting as thrombocytopenic purpura. *American Journal of Medicine*, **55**, 723.

125a SHASHATY G.G. & ATAMER M.A. (1974) Hemolytic uremic syndrome associated with infectious mononucleosis. *American Journal of Diseases of Children*, **127**, 720.

125b VOGEL S.J. & REINHARD E.H. (1979) Paroxysmal nocturnal haemoglobinaemia associated with infectious mononucleosis. *Blood*, **54**, 351.

125c KOZINER B., HADLER N., PARRILLO J. & ELLMAN L. (1973) Agranulocytosis following infectious mononucleosis. *Journal of the American Medical Association*, **225**, 1235.

126 WELLER T.H. (1971) The cytomegaloviruses; ubiquitous agents with protean clinical manifestations. *New England Journal of Medicine*, **285**, 267.

127 KANTOR G.L. & GOLDBERG L.S. (1971) Cytomegalovirus-induced postperfusion syndrome. *Seminars in Hematology*, **8**, 261.

128 BETTS R.F. & HANSHAW J.B. (1977) Cytomegalovirus (CMV) in the compromised host(s). *Annual Review of Medicine*, **28**, 103.

129 SHERLOCK S. (1975) *Disease of the Liver and Biliary System*, 5th edn, p. 305. Blackwell Scientific Publications, Oxford.

130 AJLOUNI K. & DOEBLIN T.D. (1974) The syndrome of hepatitis and aplastic anaemia. *British Journal of Haematology*, **27**, 345.

131 EDITORIAL (1971) Viral haemorrhagic fevers. *Lancet*, **ii**, 858.

132 CONRAD M.E. (1971) Hematologic manifestations of parasitic infections. *Seminars in Hematology*, **8**, 267.

133 FELDMAN H.A. (1968) Toxoplasmosis. *New England Journal of Medicine*, **279**, 1370.

134 FELDMAN H.A. (1968) Toxoplasmosis. *New England Journal of Medicine*, **279**, 1431.

135 RUSKIN J. & REMINGTON J.S. (1976) Toxoplasmosis in the compromised host. *Annals of Internal Medicine*, **84**, 193.

136 MAEGRAITH B.G. (1980) *Clinical Tropical Disease*, 7th edn. Blackwell Scientific Publications, Oxford.

137 LUZATTO L. (1979) Genetics of red cells and susceptibility to malaria. *Blood*, **54**, 961.

138 PASVOL G., WEATHERALL, D.J., WILSON R.J.M., SMITH D.H. & GILLES H.M. (1976) Fetal haemoglobin and malaria. *Lancet*, **i**, 1269.

139 WILSON R.J.M., PASVOL G. & WEATHERALL D.J. (1977) Invasion and growth of *Plasmodium falciparum* in different types of human erythrocyte. *Bulletin of the World Health Organisation*, **55**, 179.

140 ABDULLA S., WEATHERALL D.J., WICKRAMASINGHE S.N. & HUGHES M. (1980) The anaemia of *Plasmodium falciparum* malaria. *British Journal of Haematology*, **46**, 171.

141 FACER C.A., BRAY R.S. & BROWN J. (1978) Direct Coombs' antiglobulin reaction in Gambian children with *Plasmodium falciparum* malaria. I. Incidence and class specificity. *Clinical and Experimental Immunology*, **35**, 119.

142 FACER C.A. (1980) Direct Coombs' antiglobulin reactions in Gambian children with *Plasmodium falciparum* malaria. II. Specificity of erythrocyte-bound IgG. *Clinical and Experimental Immunology*, **39**, 279.

143 CONRAD M.E. & DENNIS L.H. (1968) Splenic function in experimental malaria. *American Journal of Tropical Medicine and Hygiene*, **17**, 170.

144 SCHNITZER B., SODEMAN T.M., MEAD M.L. & CONTALOS P.G. (1973) An ultrastructural study of the red pulp of the spleen in malaria. *Blood*, **41**, 207.

145 BEALE P.J., CORMACK J.D. & OLDREY T.B.H. (1972) Thrombocytopenia in malaria with immunoglobulin (IgM) changes. *British Medical Journal*, **i**, 345.

146 REID H.A. & NKRUMAH F.K. (1972) Fibrin degradation products in cerebral malaria. *Lancet*, **i**, 218.

147 JAROONVESAMA N. (1972) Intravascular coagulation in falciparum malaria. *Lancet*, **i**, 221.

148 ESAN G.J.F. (1975) Hematological aspects of malaria. *Clinics in Hematology*, **4**, 247.

149 VREEKEN J. & CREMER-GOOTE T.L.M. (1978) Haemostatic defect in non-immune patients with falciparum malaria: no evidence of diffuse intravascular coagulation. *British Medical Journal*, **ii**, 533.

150 SKUDOWITZ R.B., KATZ J., LURIE A., LEVIN J. & METZ J. (1973) Mechanisms of thrombocytopenia in malignant tertian malaria. *British Medical Journal*, **ii**, 515.

151 DALE D.C. & WOLFF S.M. (1973) Studies of the neutropenia of acute malaria. *Blood*, **41**, 197.

152 CARTWRIGHT G.E., CHUNG H.-L. & CHANG A. (1948) Studies on the pancytopenia of kala azar. *Blood*, **3**, 249.

153 WOODRUFF A.W., TOPLEY E., KNIGHT R. & DOWNIE C.G.B. (1972) The anaemia of kala-azar. *British Journal of Haematology*, **22**, 219.

154 MUSMECI S., ROMEO M. & D'AGATA A. (1974) Red cell survival and iron kinetics in kala-azar. *Journal of Tropical Medicine and Hygiene*, **77**, 106.

155 MUSMECI S., D'AGATA A., SCHILIRO G. & FISHER A. (1976) Studies on the neutropenia in kala-azar: results in

two patients. *Transactions of the Royal Society of Tropical Medicine and Hygiene*, **70**, 500.

156 BASU A.K., CHATTERJEA J.B., GUPTA P.C.S. & MUKHERJEE A.M. (1970) Hemostasis in kala azar. *Transactions of the Royal Society of Tropical Medicine and Hygiene*, **64**, 581.

157 GILLES H.M., WATSON WILLIAMS E.J. & BALL P.A. (1964) Hookworm infection and anaemia. An epidemiological, clinical and laboratory study. *Quarterly Journal of Medicine (New Series)*, **33**, 1.

158 ZINKHAM W.H. (1968) Visceral larva migrans due to *Toxocara* as a cause of eosinophilia. *Johns Hopkins Medical Journal*, **123**, 41.

159 BEN-ISMAIL R., ROUGER P., CARME B., GENTILINI M. & SALMON C. (1980) Comparative automated assay of anti-P_1 antibodies in acute hepatic distomiasis (fascioliasis) and in hydatidosis. *Vox Sanguinis*, **38**, 165.

160 BENNETT R.M. (1977) Haematological changes in rheumatoid disease. *Clinics in Rheumatic Diseases*, **3**, 433.

161 BENNETT R.M., WILLIAMS E.D., LEWIS S.M. & HOLT P.J.L. (1973) Synovial iron deposition in rheumatoid arthritis. *Arthritis and Rheumatism*, **16**, 298.

162 CARTER M.E., ARDEMAN S., WINOCOUR V., PERRY J. & CHANARIN I. (1968) Rheumatoid arthritis and pernicious anaemia. *Annals of Rheumatic Diseases*, **27**, 454.

163 GOUCH K.R., McCARTHY C., READ A.E., MOLLIN D.L. & WATERS A.H. (1964) Folic acid deficiency in rheumatoid arthritis. *British Medical Journal*, **i**, 212.

164 MARKKANEN T. & KAJANDER A. (1966) Folic acid activity of serum in rheumatoid arthritis. *Rheumatism*, **22**, 71.

165 OMER A. & MOWAT A.G. (1968) Nature of anaemia in rheumatoid arthritis. IX. Folate metabolism in patients with rheumatoid arthritis. *Annals of Rheumatic Diseases*, **27**, 414.

166 MOWAT A.G. (1972) Connective tissue diseases. *Clinics in Hematology*, **1**, 573.

167 SHORT C.L., BAUER W. & REYNOLDS W.E. (1957) *Rheumatoid Arthritis*. Harvard University Press, Cambridge, Massachusetts.

168 ROBERTS-THOMSON P.J., HAZLEMAN B.L., BARNETT I.G., MacLENNAN I.C.M. & MOWAT A.G. (1976) Factors relating to circulating immune complexes in rheumatoid arthritis. *Annals of Rheumatic Diseases*, **35**, 314.

169 SELROOS O. (1972) Thrombocytosis in rheumatoid arthritis. *Scandinavian Journal of Rheumatology*, **1**, 136.

170 HUTCHMAN R.M., DAVIS D. & JAYSON M.I. (1976) Thrombocytosis in rheumatoid arthritis. *Annals of Rheumatic Diseases*, **35**, 138.

171 EHRENFELD M., PENCHAS S. & ELIAKIM M. (1977) Thrombocytosis in rheumatoid arthritis. Recurrent arterial thromboembolism and death. *Annals of Rheumatic Diseases*, **36**, 579.

172 FELTY A.R. (1924) Chronic arthritis in the adult associated with splenomegaly and leukopenia. A report of five cases of an unusual clinical syndrome. *Johns Hopkins Hospital Bulletin*, **35**, 16.

173 HANRAHAN E.M. JR & MILLER S.R. (1932) Effects of splenectomy in Felty's syndrome. *Journal of the American Medical Association*, **99**, 1247.

174 SPIVAK J.L. (1977) Felty's syndrome: an analytical review. *Johns Hopkins Medical Journal*, **141**, 156.

175 MOTULSKY A.G., WEINBERG S., SAPHIR O. & ROSENBERG E. (1952) Lymph nodes in rheumatoid arthritis. *Archives of Internal Medicine*, **90**, 660.

176 SIENKNECHT C.W., VROWITZ M.B., PRUZANSKI W. & STEIN H.B. (1977) Felty's syndrome. Clinical and serological analysis of 34 cases. *Annals of Rheumatic Diseases*, **36**, 500.

177 LOUIE J.S. & PEARSON C.M. (1971) Felty's syndrome. *Seminars in Hematology*, **8**, 216.

178 HUME R., DAGG J.H., FRASER T.N. & GOLDBERG A. (1964) Anaemia of Felty's syndrome. *Annals of Rheumatic Diseases*, **23**, 267.

179 RUDERMAN M., MILLER L.M. & PINALS R.S. (1968) Clinical and serologic observations on 27 patients with Felty's syndrome. *Arthritis and Rheumatism*, **11**, 377.

180 ABDOU N.I., NAPOMBEJARA C., BALENTINE L. & ABDOU N.L. (1978) Suppressor cell-mediated neutropenia in Felty's syndrome. *Journal of Clinical Investigation*, **61**, 738.

181 VINCENT P.C., LEVI J.A. & MacQUEEN A. (1974) The mechanism of neutropenia in Felty's syndrome. *British Journal of Haematology*, **27**, 463.

182 CALABRESI P., EDWARDS E.A. & SCHILLING R.F. (1959) Fluorescent antiglobulin studies in leukopenia and related disorders. *Journal of Clinical Investigation*, **38**, 2091.

183 FABER V. & ELLING P. (1966) Leucocyte specific antinuclear factors in patients with Felty's syndrome, rheumatoid arthritis, systemic lupus erythematosus and other diseases. *Acta Medica Scandinavica*, **179**, 257.

184 ROSENTHAL F.D., BEELEY J.M., GELSTHORPE K. & DOUGHTY R.W. (1974) White-cell antibodies and the aetiology of Felty's syndrome. *Quarterly Journal of Medicine (New Series)*, **170**, 187.

185 LOGUE G. (1976) Felty's syndrome: granulocyte-bound immunoglobulin G and splenectomy. *Annals of Internal Medicine*, **85**, 437.

186 HOLLINGSWORTH J.W. (1968) *Local and Systemic Complications of Rheumatoid Arthritis*, p. 99. W.B. Saunders, Philadelphia.

187 STEVENSON A.C., BEDFORD J., HILL A.G.S. & HILL H.F.H. (1971) Chromosomal studies in patients taking phenylbutazone. *Annals of Rheumatic Diseases*, **30**, 487.

188 HUGHES G.R.V. & LACHMANN P.J. (1975) Systemic lupus erythematosus. In: *Clinical Aspects of Immunology*, 3rd edn (ed. Gell P.G.H., Coombs R.R.A. & Lachmann P.J.), p. 1117. Blackwell Scientific Publications, Oxford.

189 BUDMAN D.R. & STEINBERG A.D. (1977) Hematologic aspects of systemic lupus erythematosus. Current concepts. *Annals of Internal Medicine*, **86**, 220.

190 HARVEY A.M., SHULMAN L.E., TUMULTY P.A., CONLEY C.L. & SCHOENRACH E.H. (1954) Systemic lupus erythematosus. Review of the literature and clinical analysis of 138 cases. *Medicine (Baltimore)*, **33**, 291.

191 DUBOIS E.L. & TUFANELLI D.L. (1964) Clinical manifestations of systemic lupus erythematosus. Computer analysis of 520 cases. *Journal of the American Medical Association*, **190**, 104.

192 FLOOD F.T. & LIMARZI L.R. (1950) Bone marrow studies in lupus erythematosus before and after ACTH and cortisone therapy. *Journal of Laboratory and Clinical Medicine*, **36**, 823.

mononucleosis-like disorder occurring after transfusion with fresh blood or after perfusion for open-heart surgery [127]. The syndrome usually occurs one to three months after the blood transfusion and is self-limiting, resolving within a few weeks. The illness is characterized by a moderate rise in temperature with transient hepatomegaly and splenomegaly. A slight lymphadenopathy has been noted in occasional cases as have transient maculopapular rashes. There is a lymphocytosis with atypical lymphocytes indistinguishable from those of true infectious mononucleosis. As in the latter disorder, occasional leukaemoid reactions have occurred although usually the leucocyte count does not exceed $15 \times 10^9/l$. During the acute part of the illness some degree of anaemia is not uncommon; the mechanism has not been worked out adequately. In some cases it is associated with a high titre of cold agglutinins or a positive Coombs' test but this is by no means always so. As in infectious mononucleosis, other immunological abnormalities occur during the acute phase including the appearance of rheumatoid factor, cryoglobulins and antinuclear antibodies. These post-transfusion and perfusion syndromes can be avoided by the use of blood which is 48 hours or more old (Chapter 35).

With increasing use of immunosuppression in the treatment of malignant disease and in transplantation, disseminated infections with the cytomegalovirus have become a major problem [128]. Infection may occur by reactivation of latent infection or by introduction of fresh virus by transfusion or in the transplanted organ itself. The clinical picture is varied and ranges from a mild febrile illness to a rapidly fatal condition often with hepatic or pulmonary failure. There are no specific haematological manifestations in this situation and the blood picture is often complicated by the underlying condition. Any of the blood changes seen in other CMV infections may occur.

INFECTIOUS HEPATITIS

There are two main forms of this disease [129]. Hepatitis-A is synonymous with infectious, short-incubation or hepatitis-associated-antigen (HAA) negative hepatitis. Hepatitis-B covers the various forms of serum hepatitis, also called long-incubation or HAA-positive hepatitis. HAA (previously the Australian antigen) is found in a high proportion of patients with the clinical diagnosis of serum hepatitis and occurs with a high frequency in a variety of groups including institutionalized patients with Down's syndrome, leukaemics, haemophiliacs and thalassaemics who have had many transfusions with blood or blood products. It is detected by a variety of serological and immunological techniques (see Chapter 35).

Serious haematological complications of infectious hepatitis are rare. There is often an alteration in the total or differential leucocyte count early on in the illness, with a moderate degree of leucopenia or relative lymphocytosis as the commonest abnormalities. The leucocyte alkaline phosphatase level is reduced. Occasionally there is an overt haemolytic anaemia and there is substantial evidence that a severe aplastic anaemia may sometimes follow the disorder.

The extensive literature on haemolytic anaemia and infectious hepatitis has been reviewed by Dacie [72]. A whole variety of haemolytic syndromes have been reported. Some are associated with a positive Coombs' test while in others both direct and indirect antiglobulin tests are negative. Occasionally high titres of cold agglutinins have been observed. Some shortening of the ^{51}Cr red-cell survival has been noted in over 50% of patients in the acute phase of hepatitis. In addition there are now several well-documented cases of acute intravascular haemolysis occurring in patients with infectious hepatitis who were also glucose-6-phosphate dehydrogenase (G6PD) deficient.

There are now a considerable number of reports of aplastic anaemia occurring in patients with infectious hepatitis [130]. The majority of patients have been young, with half of the reported cases occurring between the ages of 10 and 20, and males have been affected twice as frequently as females. This age and sex distribution parallels that of the underlying hepatitis rather than that of idiopathic aplastic anaemia, suggesting that this is not purely a chance association. The onset of aplastic anaemia has been within nine weeks of the onset of hepatitis in the majority of cases. The condition is associated with a mortality of nearly 90%, and those patients who have survived have taken between three and 20 months from the onset of symptoms to full recovery.

ACUTE INFECTIOUS LYMPHOCYTOSIS

This is a short, self-limiting illness which occurs predominantly in young people. Outbreaks have occurred throughout the American continent, Europe and Africa. A causative organism has not yet been isolated although there is some evidence that infections with various enteroviruses, and at least one virus resembling those of the Coxsackie A subgroup, may occasionally be involved.

There are no specific clinical features. Many patients are asymptomatic but occasionally there is fever, signs of an upper-respiratory-tract infection and a morbilliform rash with some enlargement of the superficial nodes.

There is a striking leucocytosis which is largely the result of an increase in the number of small lymphocytes. Total white-cell counts in the $40–50 \times 10^9/l$ range are not infrequent while levels of up to $100 \times 10^9/l$ have been reported. The lymphocytosis usually lasts from three to five weeks and there may occasionally be an associated eosinophilia. The condition can easily be distinguished from infectious mononucleosis because of the absence of systemic symptoms, the magnitude of the leucocyte count, and the lack of atypical mononuclear cells and heterophil antibody. No treatment is required.

THE VIRAL HAEMORRHAGIC FEVERS

Apart from the uncommon haemorrhagic complications of the exanthemata and infectious mononucleosis mentioned earlier in the chapter, there are a large number of viral illnesses in which haemorrhagic phenomena predominate. This group, known collectively as the viral haemorrhagic fevers, have now been encountered in many parts of the world and increasing numbers of viruses are being isolated and named as the causative organisms [93, 131]. The conditions may be transmitted by many blood-sucking arthropods or may be acquired through close contact with infected animals or their excreta.

Viruses which multiply in arthropods are classified as arboviruses. There are several groups of arboviruses which can produce haemorrhagic disorders. One family, the togaviruses, which includes mosquito-borne arboviruses, was originally isolated in Africa from patients with dengue-like disorders but it has been found more recently in individuals with severe haemorrhagic fevers in both Thailand and India. Other types of haemorrhagic fever in South-east Asia have been shown to follow infections with the dengue virus group. Another group of the arboviruses, the flaviviruses, are responsible for yellow fever which occurs commonly in a haemorrhagic form. Other disorders which are transmitted by the arboviruses include Bukovinian haemorrhagic fever and Kyasanur forest disease in India. The Argentinian and Bolivian forms of haemorrhagic fever are different in that they are acquired from infected rodents and are due to a group of viruses now classed as the arenaviruses. This name is derived from the appearance of sandy granules seen in virus particles under the electron microscope. Several other arenaviruses have been isolated from patients with severe haemorrhagic fevers in Latin and Central America and similar disorders have now been reported from West Africa. Finally there is the syndrome of haemorrhagic fever with renal involvement, or haemorrhagic nephroso-nephritis, which is endemic in parts of Korea, Hungary, Czechoslovakia and the Soviet Union. This disorder is clearly associated with infected rodents and voles and is probably a zoonotic, rather than an arbovirus, infection.

The clinical features of these haemorrhagic fevers are extremely variable. Thus they range from mild dengue-like infections characterized by severe headache, pyrexia and generalized myalgia associated with scarlatiniform rash, leucopenia and thrombocytopenia, to the severe haemorrhagic fever so well described in the first Thai epidemic of 1954 [93]. This disorder is characterized by severe cough, dyspnoea and cyanosis. The marked bleeding tendency, which is seen in all cases, is characterized by purpura with severe bleeding at injection sites and from the gastrointestinal tract and other mucous membranes. The mortality in the original outbreak was 38% in infants under one year and 19% for all age groups. The coagulation findings in these patients were well reviewed by McKay & Margaretten [93]. There was gross thrombocytopenia in the severe cases with prolongation of the prothrombin time, reduced levels of factors VII and X and abnormalities of the thromboplastin-generation test. These findings, together with autopsy evidence of generalized fibrin deposition, provide strong evidence of disseminated intravascular coagulation. Similar abnormalities of coagulation have been reported in individuals with Bolivian and Argentine haemorrhagic fever and Kyasanur forest disease. In some cases the autopsy findings have been rather similar to those of purpura fulminans.

The use of heparin in the treatment of these disorders is reviewed by McKay & Margaretten [93] who describe this form of therapy in patients with Philippine haemorrhagic fever. They treated 20 patients with heparin and maintained a control group without anticoagulant therapy. There was a very impressive difference between the groups in that the duration of the haemorrhagic phenomena was shorter in the treated group.

PARASITIC DISEASES

One-third of the world's population has some form of parasitic infestation and many of these disorders produce haematological changes [132]. A full description of all these conditions is beyond the scope of this book and only those which show major haematological alterations will be mentioned. A classified account of some of the main haematological changes which occur with parasitic disease is given in Table 33.6.

PROTOZOAL DISEASE

Toxoplasmosis [133, 134]

Toxoplasma gondii infection can produce a variety of haematological manifestations, which may accompany

193 HEINIVAARA O. & EISALO A. (1961) Anaemia due to systemic lupus erythematosus. *Annales Medicine Internae Fenniae*, **50**, 73.

194 DUBOIS E.L. (1966) *Lupus Erythematosus*. McGraw-Hill, New York.

195 KARPATKIN S., GARG S.K. & SISKIND G.W. (1971) Auto-immune thrombocytopenic purpura and the compensated thrombocytic state. *American Journal of Medicine*, **51**, 1.

196 DIXON R.H. & ROSSE W.F. (1975) Platelet antibody in autoimmune thrombocytopenia. *British Journal of Haematology*, **31**, 129.

197 DAMESHEK W., RUBIO F. JR, MAHONEY J.P., REEVES W.H. & BURGIN L.A. (1958) Treatment of idiopathic thrombocytopenic purpura (ITP) with prednisone. *Endocrinology*, **166**, 1805.

198 CARPENTER A.F., WINTOBE M.M., FULLER E.A., HAUT A. & CARTWRIGHT G.E. (1959) Treatment of idiopathic thrombocytopenic purpura. *Journal of the American Medical Association*, **171**, 1911.

199 DOAN C.A., BOURONCLE B.A. & WISEMAN B.K. (1960) Idiopathic and secondary thrombocytopenic purpura: clinical study and evaluation of 381 cases over a period of 28 years. *Annals of Internal Medicine*, **53**, 861.

200 SCHLEIDER M.A., NACHMAN R.L., JAFFE E.A. & COLEMAN M. (1976) A clinical study of the lupus anticoagulant. *Blood*, **48**, 499.

201 WILLIAMS H., LAURENT R. & GIBSON T. (1980) The lupus coagulation inhibitor and venous thrombosis: a report of four cases. *Clinical and Laboratory Haematology*, **2**, 139.

202 HARGREAVES M.M., RICHMOND H. & MORTON R. (1948) Presentation of two bone marrow elements: the 'Tart' cell and the 'LE' cell. *Mayo Clinic Proceedings*, **23**, 25.

203 KOLLER S.R., JOHNSTON C.L., MONCURE C.W. & WALLER M.V. (1976) Lupus erythematosus cell preparation—antinuclear factor incongruity. A review of diagnostic tests for systemic lupus erythematosus. *American Journal of Clinical Pathology*, **66**, 495.

204 ROSEN P.S. & GRAHAM D.C. (1962) Ankylosing (Strumpell–Marie) spondylitis. (A clinical review of 128 cases.) *Archives of Interamerican Rheumatology*, **5**, 158.

205 POLLEY H.F. & SLOCUMB C.H. (1947) Rheumatoid spondylitis, a study of 1035 cases. *Annals of Rheumatic Diseases*, **6**, 95.

206 COURT-BROWN W.M. & DOLL R. (1957) Leukaemia and aplastic anaemia in patients irradiated for ankylosing spondylitis. *Special Report Series; Medical Research Council (London), No. 295*. HMSO, London.

207 DIESSNER G.R., HOWARD F.M. JR, WINKELMAN R.K., LAMBERT E.H. & MULDER D.W. (1966) Laboratory tests in polymyositis. *Archives of Internal Medicine*, **117**, 757.

208 HALL W.H. & FINEGOLD S. (1953) A study of 23 cases of Reiter's syndrome. *Annals of Internal Medicine*, **38**, 533.

209 HOLT J.M. & WRIGHT R. (1967) Anaemia due to blood loss from the telangiectases of scleroderma. *British Medical Journal*, **iii**, 537.

210 FUDENBERG H. & WINTROBE M.M. (1955) Scleroderma with symptomatic hemolytic anemia: a case report. *Annals of Internal Medicine*, **43**, 201.

211 DIXON A.ST.J., BEARDWELL A.K., WANKA J. & WONG Y.T. (1966) Polymyalgia rheumatica and temporal arteritis. *Annals of Rheumatic Diseases*, **25**, 203.

212 JEPSON J.H. (1979) Secondary erythrocytosis and the kidney. In: *Hematologic Problems in Renal Disease* (ed. Jepson J.H.). Addison-Wesley, Menlo-Park, California.

213 BESA E.C. & JEPSON J.H. (1979) Sickle cell anemia and the kidney. In: *Hematologic Problems in Renal Disease* (ed. Jepson J.H.). Addison-Wesley, Menlo-Park, California.

214 CHANG F.-F., BARTUSKA D. & JEPSON J.H. (1979) Renal manifestation of dysproteinemias. In: *Hematologic Problems in Renal Disease* (ed. Jepson J.H.). Addison-Wesley, Menlo-Park, California.

215 PENINGTON D.G. & KINCAID-SMITH P. (1971) Anaemia in renal failure. *British Medical Bulletin*, **27**, 218.

216 ANAGNOSTOU A. & FRIED W. (1979) Anemia of renal disease. In: *Hematologic Problems in Renal Disease* (ed. Jepson J.H.). Addison-Wesley, Menlo-Park, California.

217 FRIEND D., HOSKINS R.G. & KIRKIN M.W. (1961) Relative erythrocytemia (polycythemia) and polycystic disease with uremia. Report of a case with comments on frequency of occurrence. *New England Journal of Medicine*, **264**, 17.

218 AHERNE W.A. (1957) The 'burr' red cell and azotaemia. *Journal of Clinical Pathology*, **10**, 252.

219 LOCK S.P. & DORMANDY K.M. (1961) Red-cell fragmentation syndrome: a condition of multiple aetiology. *Lancet*, **i**, 1020.

220 BRAIN M.C., DACIE J.V. & HOURIHANE D.O'B. (1962) Microangiopathic haemolytic anaemia: the possible role of vascular lesions in pathogenesis. *British Journal of Haematology*, **8**, 358.

221 COOPER R.A. (1970) The pathogenesis of burr cells in uremia. *Journal of Clinical Investigation*, **49**, 229.

222 SHAW A.B. (1967) Haemolysis in chronic renal failure. *British Medical Journal*, **ii**, 213.

223 BRAIN M.C. (1979) Hemolysis in renal disease. In: *Hematologic Problems in Renal Disease* (ed. Jepson J.H.). Addison-Wesley, Menlo-Park, California.

224 JOSKE R.A., McALISTER J.M. & PRANKERD T.A.J. (1956) Isotope investigations of red cell production and destruction in chronic renal disease. *Clinical Science*, **15**, 511.

225 DESFORGES J.F. & DAWSON J.P. (1958) The anemia of renal failure. *Archives of Internal Medicine*, **101**, 326.

226 SHAW A.B. & SCHOLES M.C. (1967) Reticulocytes in renal failure. *Lancet*, **i**, 799.

227 GIOVANNETTI S., BALESTRI P.L. & CIONI L. (1965) Spontaneous *in-vitro* autohaemolysis of blood from chronic uraemic patients. *Clinical Science*, **29**, 407.

228 ADAMSON J.W., ESCHBACH J. & FINCH C.A. (1968) The kidney and erythropoiesis. *American Journal of Medicine*, **44**, 725.

229 KURTIDES E.S., RAMBACH W.A., ALT H.L. & DEL GRECO F. (1964) Effect of hemodialysis on erythrokinetics in anemia of uremia. *Journal of Laboratory and Clinical Medicine*, **63**, 469.

230 MANN D.L., DONATI R.M. & GALLAGHER N.I. (1965) Erythropoietin assay and ferrokinetic measurements in anemic uremic patients. *Journal of the American Medical Association*, **194**, 1321.

231 WHITEHEAD V.M. (1979) Regular dialysis treatment and the hematologic systems. In: *Hematologic Problems in*

Renal Disease (ed. Jepson J.H.). Addison-Wesley, Menlo-Park, California.

232 GOKAL R., WEATHERALL D.J. & BUNCH C. (1979) Iron-induced increase in red cell size in haemodialysis patients. *Quarterly Journal of Medicine (New Series)*, **48**, 393.

233a CRADDOCK P.R., FEHR J., BRIGHAM K.L., KRONENBERG R.S. & JACOB H.S. (1977) Complement and leukocyte-mediated pulmonary dysfunction in hemodialysis. *New England Journal of Medicine*, **296**, 769.

233b JEPSON J.H. (1979) Hematologic complications of renal homotransplantation. In: *Hematologic Problems in Renal Disease* (ed. Jepson J.H.). Addison-Wesley, Menlo-Park, California.

234 KISSMEYER-NIELSEN F. (1979) Matching for HL-A. In: *Kidney Transplantation. Principles and Practice* (ed. Morris P.J.). Academic Press, London.

235 ARNESON L.A., VINES D.H., MILLER R.E. & DEUTSCH D.L. (1965) Ulceration of the common bile duct as a cause of hemobilia. *Gastroenterology*, **48**, 648.

236 MCKUSICK V.A. (1960) *Heritable Disorders of Connective Tissue*, 2nd edn. Mosby, St Louis.

237 HOFFBRAND A.V., STEWART J.S., BOOTH C.C. & MOLLIN D.L. (1968) Folate deficiency in Crohn's disease: incidence, pathogenesis, and treatment. *British Medical Journal*, **ii**, 71.

238 DYER N.H., CHILD J.A., MOLLIN D.L. & DAWSON A.M. (1972) Anaemia in Crohn's Disease. *Quarterly Journal of Medicine (New Series)*, **41**, 419.

239 ORMEROD T.P. (1967) Observations on the incidence and cause of anaemia in ulcerative colitis. *Gut*, **8**, 107.

240 ANSCOMBE A.R., KEDDIE N.C. & SCHOFIELD P.F. (1967) Caecal tuberculosis. *Gut*, **8**, 337.

241 WRIGHT R. & TRUELOVE S.C. (1966) Circulating and tissue eosinophils in ulcerative colitis. *American Journal of Digestive Diseases*, **11**, 831.

242 DOBBINS W.D. (1968) Electron microscopy of intestinal fat absorption under normal conditions in malabsorptive states. In: *Progress in Gastroenterology* (ed. Glass G.B.J.), p. 473. Grune & Stratton, New York.

243 HALSTED J.A., LEWIS P.M. & GASSTER M. (1956) Absorption of radioactive vitamin B_{12} in the syndrome of megaloblastic anemia associated with intestinal stricture of anastomosis. *American Journal of Medicine*, **20**, 42.

244 COOKE W.T. (1968) Adult celiac disease. In: *Progress in Gastroenterology* (ed. Glass G.B.J.), p. 299. Grune & Stratton, New York.

245 MARTIN J.B. & BELL H.E. (1965) The association of splenic atrophy and intestinal malabsorption: report of a case and review of the literature. *Canadian Medical Association Journal*, **92**, 875.

246 SILBER R. & GOLDSTEIN B.D. (1970) Vitamin E and the hematopoietic system. *Seminars in Hematology*, **7**, 40.

247 FINCH C.A. (1948) Methemoglobinemia and sulfhemoglobinemia. *New England Journal of Medicine*, **239**, 470.

248 ROSSI E.C., BRYAN G.T., SCHILLING R.F. & CLATANOFF D.V. (1966) Remission of chronic methemoglobinemia following neomycin therapy. *American Journal of Medicine*, **40**, 440.

249 NEALE G., CANELLOS G.P., PATTERSON M.J.L., EVANS

D.J. & BRAIN M.C. (1967) Effects of phenacetin on rats with small intestinal blind loops. *Gut*, **8**, 636.

250 BINGHAM J. (1959) Macrocytosis of hepatic disease. I. Thin macrocytosis. *Blood*, **14**, 694.

251 BINGHAM J. (1960) The macrocytosis of hepatic disease. II. Thick macrocytosis. *Blood*, **15**, 244.

252 BERMAN L., AXELROD A.R., HORAN T.M., JACOBSON S.D., SHARP E.A. & VON DER HEIDE E.C. (1949) Blood and bone marrow in patients with cirrhosis and other disorders of liver. *Blood*, **4**, 511.

253 NUNNALLY R.M. & LEVINE I. (1961) Macronormoblastic hyperplasia of the bone marrow in hepatic cirrhosis. *American Journal of Medicine*, **30**, 972.

254 KIMBER C., DELLER D.J., IBBOTSON R.N. & LANDER H. (1965) The mechanism of anaemia in chronic liver disease. *Quarterly Journal of Medicine (New Series)*, **34**, 33.

255 LIEBERMAN F.L. & REYNOLDS T.B. (1967) Plasma volume in cirrhosis of the liver. Its relation to portal hypertension ascites, and renal failure. *Journal of Clinical Investigation*, **46**, 1297.

256 ADLUNG J., UTHGENANNT H. & WEINREICH J. (1969) Studies on the anemia in liver cirrhosis both on the basis of nuclear medicine and hematological methods. *Zeitschrift für Gastroenterologie*, **7**, 157.

257 PITCHER C.S. & WILLIAMS R. (1963) Reduced red cell survival in jaundice and its relation to abnormal glutathione metabolism. *Clinical Science*, **24**, 239.

258 KATZ R., VELASCO M., GUZMAN C. & ALESSANDRI H. (1964) Red cell survival estimated by radioactive chromium in hepatobiliary disease. *Gastroenterology*, **46**, 399.

259 GIBLETT E.R., COLEMAN D.H., PIRZIO-BIROLI G., DONOHUE D.M., MOTULSKY A.G. & FINCH C.A. (1956) Erythrokinetics: quantitative measurements of red cell production and destruction in normal subjects and patients with anemia. *Blood*, **11**, 291.

260 HALL C.A. (1960) Erythrocyte dynamics in liver disease. *American Journal of Medicine*, **28**, 541.

261 LEEVY C.M., BAKER H., TEN HOVE W.W., FRANK O. & CHORNICK G.R. (1965) B-complex vitamins in liver disease of the alcoholic. *American Journal of Clinical Nutrition*, **16**, 339.

262 BAKER H., FRANK O., ZIFFER H., GOLDFARB S., LEEVY C.M. & SOBOTKA H. (1964) Effect of hepatic disease on liver B-complex vitamin titers. *American Journal of Clinical Nutrition*, **14**, 1.

263 KNOWLES J.P., SHALDON S. & FLEMING A. (1963) Folic acid metabolism in liver disease. *Clinical Science*, **24**, 39.

264 MERRITT A.D., RUCKNAGEL D.L., SILVERMAN M. & GARDINER R.C. (1962) Urinary urocanic acid in man: the identification of urocanic acid and the comparative excretions of urocanic acid and N-formiminoglutamic acid after oral histidine in patients with liver disease. *Journal of Clinical Investigation*, **41**, 1472.

265 KLIPSTEIN F.A. & LINDENBAUM J. (1965) Folate deficiency in chronic liver disease. *Blood*, **25**, 443.

266 HERBERT V. (1965) Hematopoietic factors in liver disease. In: *Progress in Liver Diseases* (ed. Popper H. & Schaffner F.), p. 57. Grune & Stratton, New York.

267 RETIEF F.P., VANDENPLAS L. & VISSER H. (1969) Vitamin B_{12} binding proteins in liver disease. *British Journal of Haematology*, **16**, 231.

268 GLASS G.B.J. (1959) Deposition and storage of vitamin B$_{12}$ in the normal and diseased liver. *Gastroenterology*, **36**, 180.

269 WILLIAMS R., WILLIAMS H.S., SCHEUER P.J., PITCHER C.S., LOISAAN E. & SHERLOCK S. (1967) Iron absorption and siderosis in chronic liver disease. *Quarterly Journal of Medicine (New Series)*, **36**, 151.

270 ZIMMERMANN H.J., CHOMET B., KULESH M.H. & McWHORTER C.A. (1961) Hepatic hemosiderin deposits. *Archives of Internal Medicine*, **107**, 494.

271 SCHEUER P.J., WILLIAMS R. & MUIR A.R. (1962) Hepatic pathology in relatives of patients with haemochromatosis. *Journal of Pathology and Bacteriology*, **84**, 53.

272 ZIEVE L. (1958) Jaundice, hyperlipemia, and hemolytic anemia: a heretofore unrecognized syndrome associated with alcoholic fatty liver and cirrhosis. *Annals of Internal Medicine*, **48**, 471.

273 KESSEL L. (1962) Acute transient hyperlipemia due to hepatopancreatic damage in chronic alcoholics (Zieve's syndrome). *American Journal of Medicine*, **32**, 747.

274 WESTERMAN M.P., BALCERZAK S.P. & HEINLE E.W. JR (1968) Red cell lipids in Zieve's syndrome: their relation to hemolysis and to red cell osmotic fragility. *Journal of Laboratory and Clinical Medicine*, **72**, 663.

275 OKEY R. & GREAVES V.D. (1939) Anemia caused by feeding cholesterol to guinea pigs. *Journal of Biological Chemistry*, **129**, 111.

276 SILVER M.M., McMILLAN G.C. & SILVER M.D. (1964) Haemolytic anaemia in cholesterol fed rabbits. *British Journal of Haematology*, **10**, 271.

277 CLEARFIELD H.R., BRODY J.I. & TUMEN H.J. (1969) Acute viral hepatitis, glucose-6-phosphate dehydrogenase deficiency and hemolytic anemia. *Archives of Internal Medicine*, **123**, 689.

278 SMITH J.A., LONERGAN E.T. & STERLING K. (1964) Spur-cell anemia: hemolytic anemia with red cells resembling acanthocytes in alcoholic cirrhosis. *New England Journal of Medicine*, **271**, 396.

279 POWELL L.W., DUNNICLIFF M.A. & BILLING B.H. (1968) Red cell survival in experimental cholestatic jaundice. *British Journal of Haematology*, **15**, 429.

280 COOPER R.A. & JANDL J.H. (1966) Mechanism of 'target cell' formation in jaundice. *Clinical Research*, **14**, 314.

281 COOPER R.A. & JANDL J.H. (1969) The selective and conjoint loss of red cell lipids. *Journal of Clinical Investigation*, **48**, 906.

282 JANDL J.H. & COOPER R.A. (1969) Red cell cholesterol content: a manifestation of the serum affinity for free cholesterol. *Clinical Research*, **17**, 462.

283 COOPER R.A., ADMIRAND W.H., GARCIA F. & TREY C. (1969) The role of lithocholic acid in the pathogenesis of spur red cells and hemolytic anemia. *Journal of Clinical Investigation*, **48**, 18a.

284 CHANARIN I. (1979) Alcohol and the blood. *British Journal of Haematology*, **42**, 333.

285 COLMAN N. & HERBERT V. (1980) Hematological complications of alcoholism: overview. *Seminars in Hematology*, **17**, 164.

286 EICHNER E.R. & HILLMANN R.S. (1971) The evolution of anemia in alcoholic patients. *American Journal of Medicine*, **50**, 218.

287 McCURDY P.R., PIERCE L.E. & RATH C.E. (1962) Abnormal bone marrow morphology in acute alcoholism. *New England Journal of Medicine*, **266**, 505.

288 HINES J.D. (1969) Reversible megaloblastic and sideroblastic marrow abnormalities in alcoholic patients. *British Journal of Haematology*, **16**, 87.

289 SHERLOCK S. (1968) *Diseases of the Liver and Biliary System*, 5th edn, p. 57. Blackwell Scientific Publications, Oxford.

290 ASTER R.H. (1966) Pooling of platelets in the spleen: role in the pathogenesis of 'hypersplenic' thrombocytopenia. *Journal of Clinical Investigation*, **45**, 645.

291 MACPHERSON A.I.S. & INNES J. (1953) Peripheral blood picture after operation for portal hypertension. *Lancet*, **i**, 1120.

292 RATNOFF O.D. (1963) Hemostatic mechanisms in liver disease. *Medical Clinics of North America*, **47**, 721.

293 THOMAS D.P., REAM V.J. & STUART R.K. (1967) Platelet aggregation in patients with Laennec's cirrhosis of the liver. *New England Journal of Medicine*, **276**, 1344.

294 KREVANS J.R. & JACKSON D.P. (1955) Hemorrhagic disorder following massive whole blood transfusion. *Journal of the American Medical Association*, **159**, 171.

295 SCHMID R. & McDONAGH A.F. (1978) Hyperbilirubinemia. In: *The Metabolic Basis of Inherited Disease*, 4th edn (ed. Stanbury J.B., Wyngaarden J.B. & Fredrickson D.S.), p. 1221. McGraw-Hill, New York.

296 BERK P.D. & BLASCHKE T.F. (1972) Detection of Gilbert's syndrome in patients with hemolysis. *Annals of Internal Medicine*, **77**, 527.

297 BURKE V., COLEBATCH J.H., ANDERSON C.M. & SIMONS M.J. (1967) Association of pancreatic insufficiency and chronic neutropenia in childhood. *Archives of Disease in Childhood*, **42**, 147.

298 BOTHWELL T.H. & CHARLTON R.W. (1971) Absorption of iron. *Annual Review of Medicine*, **21**, 145.

299 GIBSON J.G. & HARRIS A.W. (1939) Clinical studies of the blood volume. V. Hyperthyroidism and myxedema. *Journal of Clinical Investigation*, **18**, 59.

300 MULDOWNEY F.P., CROOKS J. & WAYNE E.J. (1957) The total red cell mass in thyrotoxicosis and myxoedema. *Clinical Science*, **16**, 309.

301 TUDHOPE G.R. & WILSON G.M. (1960) Anaemia in hypothyroidism. *Quarterly Journal of Medicine (New Series)*, **29**, 513.

302 DAS K.G., MUKHERJEE M., SARKAR T.K., DASH R.J. & RASTOGI G.K. (1975) Erythropoiesis and erythropoietin in hypo- and hyperthryroidism. *Journal of Clinical Endocrinology and Metabolism*, **40**, 211.

303 AXELROD A.R. (1951) The bone marrow in hyperthyroidism and hypothyroidism. *Blood*, **6**, 436.

304 KIELY J.M., PURNELL D.C. & OWEN C.A. (1967) Erythrokinetics in myxedema. *Annals of Internal Medicine*, **67**, 533.

305 DINATO R.M., FLETCHER J.W., WARNICKE M.A. & GALLAGHER N.I. (1973) Erythropoiesis in hypothyroidism. *Proceedings of the Society for Experimental Biology and Medicine*, **144**, 78.

306 HOLLANDER C.S., THOMPSON R.H., BARRETT P.V.D. & BERLIN N.I. (1967) Repair of the anemia and hyperlipidemia of the hypothyroid dog. *Endocrinology*, **81**, 1007.

307 NAKAO K., MAEKAWA T., SHIRAKURA T. & YAGINUMA M. (1965) Anaemia due to hypothyroidism. *Israel Journal of Medical Science*, **1**, 742.

308 PESCHLE C., ZANJANI E.D., GIDARI A.S., McLAURIN W.D. & GORDON A.S. (1971) Mechanism of thyroxine action on erythropoiesis. *Endocrinology*, **89**, 609.

309 SHALET M., COE D. & REISSMAN K.R. (1966) Mechanism of erythropoietic action of thyroid hormone. *Proceedings of the Society for Experimental Biology and Medicine*, **123**, 443.

310 FISHER J.W. & GROSS D.M. (1977) Hormonal influences on erythropoiesis: anterior pituitary, adrenocortical, thyroid, growth and other hormones. In: *Kidney Hormones. II. Erythropoietin* (ed. Fisher J.W.), p. 415. Academic Press, New York.

311 ADAMSON J.W., POPOVIC W.J. & BROWN J.E. (1978) Modulation of *in-vitro* erythropoiesis: normal interactions and erythroid colony growth. In: *Differentiation of Normal and Neoplastic Hematopoietic Cells, Book A* (ed Clarkson B., Marks P.A. & Till J.E.), p. 235. Cold Spring Harbor.

312 WILLIAMS L.T., LEFKOWITZ R.J., WATANABE D.R., HATHAWAY D.R. & BESCH H.R. JR (1977) Thyroid hormone regulation of beta-adrenergic receptor number. *Journal of Biological Chemistry*, **252**, 779.

313 POPOVIC W.J., BROWN J.E. & ADAMSON J.W. (1979) Modulation of *in-vitro* erythropoiesis. Studies with euthyroid and hypothyroid dogs. *Journal of Clinical Investigation*, **64**, 56.

314 GAHLENBECK H. & BARTELS H. (1968) Veränderung der Sauerstoffbindungskurven des Blutes bei Hyperthyreosen und nach Gabe von Trijodothyronin bei Gesunden und bei Ratten. *Klinische Wochenschrift*, **46**, 547.

315 GROSZ H.J. & FARMER B.B. (1969) Reduction-oxidation potential of blood determined by oxygen releasing factor in thyroid disorders. *Nature (London)*, **222**, 875.

316 ZAROULIS C.G., KOURIDES I.A. & VALERI C.R. (1978) Red cell 2,3-diphosphoglycerate and oxygen affinity of hemoglobin in patients with thyroid disorders. *Blood*, **52**, 181.

317 PEARSON H.A. & DRUYAN R. (1961) Erythrocyte glucose-6-phosphate dehydrogenase activity related to thyroid activity. *Journal of Laboratory and Clinical Medicine*, **57**, 343.

318 BUTENANDT O. (1972) Erythrocytic enzyme activities in hypothyroid children. *Acta Haematologica*, **47**, 335.

319 TASHIAN E.D. & CARTER N.D. (1976) Biochemical genetics of carbonic anhydrase. *Advances in Human Genetics*, **7**, 1.

320 HORTON L., COBURN R.J., ENGLAND J.M. & HIMSWORTH R.L. (1976) The haematology of hypothyroidism. *Quarterly Journal of Medicine (New Series)*, **45**, 101.

321 WARDROP C. & HUTCHINSON H.E. (1969) Red-cell shape in hypothyroidism. *Lancet*, **i**, 1243.

322 BOMFORD R. (1938) Anaemia in myxoedema: role of the thyroid gland in erythropoiesis. *Quarterly Journal of Medicine (New Series)*, **7**, 495.

323 CAPLAN R.H., DAVIS K., BENGSTON B. & SMITH M.J. (1975) Serum folate and vitamin B_{12} levels in hypothroid and hyperthyroid patients. *Archives of Internal Medicine*, **135**, 701.

324 LARSSON S.D. (1957) Anemia and iron metabolism in hypothyroidism. *Acta Medica Scandinavica*, **157**, 349.

325 WILLIAMS E.D. & DONIACH I. (1962) The post-mortem incidence of focal thyroiditis. *Journal of Pathology and Bacteriology*, **83**, 255.

326 DONIACH D. & ROITT I.M. (1964) An evaluation of gastric and thyroid auto-immunity in relation to hematologic disorders. *Seminars in Hematology*, **1**, 313.

327 DONIACH D., ROITT I.M. & TAYLOR K.B. (1965) Autoimmunity in pernicious anemia and thyroiditis: a family study. *Annals of the New York Academy of Sciences*, **124**, 605.

328 EVANS A.W.H., WOODROW J.C., McDOUGALL C.D.M., CHEW A.R. & EVANS R.W. (1967) Antibodies in the families of thyrotoxic patients. *Lancet*, **i**, 637.

329 VOLPE R. (1977) The role of autoimmunity in hypoendocrine and hyperendocrine function. With special emphasis on autoimmune thyroid disease. *Annals of Internal Medicine*, **87**, 86.

330 HINES J.D., HALSTED C.H., GRIGGS R.C. & HARRIS J.W. (1968) Megaloblastic anemia secondary to folate deficiency associated with hypothyroidism. *Annals of Internal Medicine*, **68**, 792.

331 NIGHTINGALE S., VITEK P.J. & HIMSWORTH R.L. (1978) The haematology of hyperthyroidism. *Quarterly Journal of Medicine (New Series)*, **47**, 35.

332 McCLELLAN J.E., DONEGAN C., THORUP O.A. & LEAVER B.S. (1979) Survival time of the erythrocyte in myxedema and hypothyroidism. *Journal of Laboratory and Clinical Medicine*, **81**, 91.

333 RIVLIN R.S. & WAGNER H.N. JR (1969) Anemia in hyperthyroidism. *Annals of Internal Medicine*, **70**, 507.

334 IRVINE W.J., WU F.C.W., URBANIAK S.T. & TOOLIS F. (1977) Peripheral blood leucocytes in thyrotoxicosis (Graves' disease). *Clinical and Experimental Immunology*, **27**, 216.

335 LIGHTSEY A.L., CHAPMAN R.M., McMILLAN R., MUSCHEVIC J., YEZEWOSKY R. & LONGMIRE R.L. (1977) Immune neutropenia. *Annals of Internal Medicine*, **86**, 60.

336 BECHGAARD P. (1946) Tendency to haemorrhage in thyrotoxicosis. *Acta Medica Scandinavica*, **124**, 79.

337 ORR F.R. (1962) Haemorrhage in myxoedema coma. *Lancet*, **ii**, 1012.

338 TUDHOPE G.R. (1972) Endocrine diseases. *Clinics in Hematology*, **1**, 475.

339 EVANS H. & PERRY K.M.A. (1943) Thrombocytopenic purpura. *Lancet*, **ii**, 410.

340 MARSHALL J.S., WEISBERGER A.S., LEVY R.P. & BRECKENBRIDGE R.T. (1967) Coexistent idiopathic thrombocytopenic purpura and hyperthyroidism. *Annals of Internal Medicine*, **67**, 411.

341 LAMBERG B.-A., KIVIKANGAS V., PLEKONEN R. & VUOPIO P. (1971) Thrombocytopenia and decreased lifespan of thrombocytes in hyperthyroidism. *Annals of Clinical Research*, **3**, 98.

342 RODRIGUEZ J.M. & SHAHIDI N.T. (1971) Erythrocyte 2,3-diphosphoglycerate in adaptive red-cell volume deficiency. *New England Journal of Medicine*, **285**, 479.

343 JEPSON J.H. & McGARRY E.E. (1968) Effect of growth hormone and other hormones on erythropoiesis and erythropoietin excretion of pituitary dwarfs. *Annals of Internal Medicine*, **68**, 1169.

344 LINDEMANN R., TRYGSTAD O. & HALVORSEN S. (1969) Pituitary control of erythropoiesis. *Scandinavian Journal of Haematology*, **6**, 77.

345 GOUDIE R.B., ANDERSON J.R., GRAY K.K. & WHYTE W.G. (1966) Autoantibodies in Addison's disease. *Lancet*, **i**, 1173.

346 BLIZZARD R.M., CHEE D. & DAVIS W. (1967) The incidence of adrenal and other antibodies in the sera of patients with idiopathic adrenal insufficiency (Addison's disease). *Clinical and Experimental Immunology*, **2**, 19.

347 FALKO J.M., GUY J.T., SMITH R.E. & MAZZAFERRI E.L. (1976) Primary hyperparathyroidism and anemia. *Archives of Internal Medicine*, **136**, 887.

348 AUCHINCLOSS J.H. JR, COOK E. & RENZETTI A.D. (1955) Clinical and physiological aspects of a case of obesity, polycythemia and alveolar hypoventilation. *Journal of Clinical Investigation*, **34**, 1537.

349 LOURENCO R.V. (1969) Diaphragm activity in obesity. *Journal of Clinical Investigation*, **48**, 1609.

350 WARD H.P., BIGELOW D.B. & PETTY T.L. (1968) Postural hypoxemia and erythrocytosis. *American Journal of Medicine*, **45**, 880.

351 FLENLEY D.C. (1978) Clinical hypoxia; causes, consequences, and correction. *Lancet*, **i**, 542.

352 STROEBEL C.G. & FOWLER W.S. (1956) Secondary polycythemia. *Medical Clinics of North America*, **40**, 1061.

353 OSKI F.A., GOTTLIEB A.J., DELIVORIA-PAPADOPOULOS M. & MILLER W.W. (1969) Red cell 2,3-diphosphoglycerate levels in subjects with chronic hypoxemia. *New England Journal of Medicine*, **280**, 1165.

354 PARSONS C.G., ASTLEY R., BURROWS F.G.O. & SINGH S.P. (1971) Transposition of great arteries. A study of 65 infants followed for 1 to 4 years after balloon septostomy. *British Heart Journal*, **33**, 725.

355 HARTMANN R.C. (1952) Hemorrhagic disorder occurring in patients with cyanotic congenital heart disease. *Bulletin of the Johns Hopkins Hospital*, **91**, 49.

356 JACKSON D.P. (1964) Hemorrhagic diathesis in patients with cyanotic congenital heart disease: preoperative management. *Annals of the New York Academy of Sciences*, **115**, 235.

357 IHENACHO H.N.C., BREEZE G.R., FLETCHER D.J. & STUART J. (1973) Consumption coagulopathy in congenital heart-disease. *Lancet*, **i**, 231.

358 ROSENTHAL A., NATHAN D.G., MARTY A.T., BUTTON L.N., MIETTINEN O.S. & NADAS A.S. (1970) Acute hemodynamic effects of red cell volume reduction in polycythemia of cyanotic congenital heart disease. *Circulation*, **42**, 297.

359 BUSH J.A. & AINGER L.E. (1955) Congenital absence of the spleen with congenital heart disease; report of a case with ante-mortem diagnosis on the basis of hematologic morphology. *Pediatrics*, **15**, 93.

360 BRODEUR M.T.J., SUTHERLAND D.W., KOLER R.D., STARR A., KIMSEY J.A. & GRISWOLD H.E. (1965) Red blood cell survival in patients with aortic valvular disease and ball valve prostheses. *Circulation*, **32**, 570.

361 GROSSE-BROCKHOFF F. & GEHRMANN G. (1967) Mechanical hemolysis in patients with valvular heart disease and valve prosthesis. *American Heart Journal*, **74**, 137.

362 GOODWIN J.F. (1963) Diagnosis of left atrial myxoma. *Lancet*, **i**, 464.

363 MARSH G.W. & LEWIS S.M. (1969) Cardiac hemolytic anemia. *Seminars in Hematology*, **6**, 133.

364 CHUSHID M.J., DALE D.C., WEST B.C. & WOLFF S.M. (1975) The hypereosinophilic syndrome: analysis of fourteen cases with review of the literature. *Medicine (Baltimore)*, **54**, 1.

365 LOEFFLER W. (1936) Endocarditis parietalis Fibroplastica mit Bluteosinophilie. *Schweizerische Medizinische Wochenschrift*, **66**, 817.

366 SHEPHERD A.J.N., WALSH C.H., ARCHER R.K. & WETHERLEY-MEIN G. (1971) Eosinophilia, splenomegaly and cardiac disease. *British Journal of Haematology*, **20**, 233.

367 STERNON J., PARMENTIERI R. & KENIS J. (1962) Filariose et endocarditi fibroplastique. *Annales de la Societe Belge de Medecina Tropicale*, **3**, 351.

368 EDGE J.R. (1946) Myocardial fibrosis following arsenical therapy. *Lancet*, **ii**, 676.

369 PARRILLO J.E., FAUCI A.S. & WOLFF S.M. (1977) The hypereosinophilic syndrome: dramatic response to therapeutic intervention. *Transactions of the Association of American Physicians*, **90**, 135.

370 MURRAY H.W., MASUR H., SENTERFIT L.B. & ROBERTS R.B. (1975) The protean manifestations of *Mycoplasma pneumoniae* infection in adults. *American Journal of Medicine*, **58**, 229.

371 LEVINE D.P. & LERNER A.M. (1978) The clinical spectrum of *Mycoplasma pneumoniae* infections. *Medical Clinics of North America*, **62**, 961.

372 GASPER T.M., FARNDON P.A. & DAVIES R. (1978) Thrombocytopenia associated with Legionnaires' disease. *British Medical Journal*, **ii**, 1611.

373 JACOBSON L.B., LONGSTRETH G.F. & EDGINGTON T.S. (1973) Clinical and immunologic features of transient cold agglutinin hemolytic anemia. *American Journal of Medicine*, **54**, 514.

374 FEIZI T. (1967) Cold agglutinins, the direct Coombs' test and serum immunoglobulins in *Mycoplasma pneumoniae* infection. *Annals of the New York Academy of Sciences*, **143**, 801.

375 SANFORD J.P. (1979) Legionnaires' disease—the first thousand days. *New England Journal of Medicine*, **300**, 654.

376 MILLER A.C. (1979) Early clinical differentiation between Legionnaires' disease and other sporadic pneumonias. *Annals of Internal Medicine*, **90**, 526.

377 BURROWS B., FLETCHER C.M., HEARD B.E., JONES N.L. & WOOTLIFF J.S. (1966) The emphysematous and bronchial types of chronic airways obstruction. *Lancet*, **i**, 830.

378 GALLO R.C., FRAIMOW W., CATHCART T. & ERSLEV A.J. (1964) Erythropoietic response in chronic pulmonary disease. *Archives of Internal Medicine*, **113**, 559.

379 HUME R. (1968) Blood volume changes in chronic bronchitis and emphysema. *British Journal of Haematology*, **15**, 131.

380 CHAMBERLAIN D.A. & MILLARD F.J.C. (1963) The treatment of polycythaemia secondary to hypoxic lung disease by continuous oxygen administration. *Quarterly Journal of Medicine (New series)*, **32**, 341.

381 AUCHINCLOSS J.H. JR & DUGGAN J.J. (1957) Effects of venesection on pulmonary and cardiac function in patients with chronic pulmonary emphysema and

secondary polycythemia. *American Journal of Medicine*, **22,** 74.

382 CASTLE W.B. & JANDL J.H. (1966) Blood viscosity and blood volume; opposing influences upon oxygen transport in polycythemia. *Seminars in Hematology*, **3,** 193.

383 CROFTON J.W., LIVINGSTON J.L., OSWALD N.C. & ROBERTS A.T.M. (1952) Pulmonary eosinophilia. *Thorax*, **7,** 1.

384 HARDY W.R. & ANDERSON R.E. (1968) The hypereosinophilic syndromes. *Annals of Internal Medicine*, **68,** 1220.

385 LIEBOW A.A. & CARRINGTON C.B. (1969) The eosinophilic pneumonias. *Medicine (Baltimore)*, **48,** 251.

386 STRETTON T.B. & LEE H.Y. (1972) Respiratory diseases. *Clinics in Hematology*, **1,** 645.

387 SOERGEL K.H. & SOMMERS S.C. (1962) Idiopathic pulmonary hemosiderosis and related syndromes. *American Journal of Medicine*, **32,** 499.

388 PROSKEY A.J., WEATHERBEE L., EASTERLING R.E., GREENE J.A. JR & WELLER J.M. (1970) Goodpasture's syndrome: A report of five cases and review of the literature. *American Journal of Medicine*, **48,** 162.

389 FAHEY J.L., LEONARD E., CHURG J. & GODMAN G.C. (1954) Wegener's granulomatosis. *American Journal of Medicine*, **17,** 168.

390 FAUCI A.S. & WOLFF S.M. (1973) Wegener's granulomatosis: studies in 18 patients and a review of the literature. *Medicine (Baltimore)*, **52,** 535.

391 OSLER W. (1901) On a family form of recurring epistaxis, associated with multiple telangiectases of the skin and mucous membranes. *Bulletin of the Johns Hopkins Hospital*, **12,** 333.

392 RENDU H.J.L. (1896) Epistaxis repetes chez un sujet porteur de petits angiomes cutanes et muqueux. *Gazette des Hôpitaux Civils et Militaires*, **69,** 1322.

393 WEBER F.P. (1907) Multiple hereditary developmental angiomata (telangiectases) of the skin and mucous membranes associated with recurring haemorrhages. *Lancet*, **ii,** 160.

394 HODGSON C.H., BURCHELL H.B., GOOD C.A. & CLAGETT O.T. (1959) Hereditary hemorrhagic telangiectasia and pulmonary arterio-venous fistula. *New England Journal of Medicine*, **261,** 625.

395 CHANDLER D. (1965) Pulmonary and cerebral arteriovenous fistula with Osler's disease. *Archives of Internal Medicine*, **116,** 277.

396 MUCKLE T.J. (1964) Low *in-vivo* adhesive platelet count in hereditary haemorrhagic telangiectasia. *Lancet*, **ii,** 880.

397 DORMANDY T.L. (1957) Gastrointestinal polyposis with mucocutaneous pigmentation (Peutz–Jeghers syndrome). *New England Journal of Medicine*, **256,** 1093, 1141, 1186.

398 WHEELER C.E. (1975) Certain cutaneous diseases with significant systemic manifestations. In: *Textbook of Medicine*, 14th edn (ed. Beeson P.B. and McDermott W.). W.B. Saunders, Philadelphia.

399 MARKS J. & SHUSTER S. (1972) Dermatological disorders. *Clinics in Hematology*, **1,** 533.

400 SHUSTER S., MARKS J. & CHANARIN I. (1967) Folic acid deficiency in patients with skin disease. *British Journal of Dermatology*, **79,** 398.

401 FRY L., KEIR P., McMINN R.M.H., COWAN J.D. & HOFFBRAND A.V. (1967) Small intestinal structure and function and haematological changes in dermatitis herpetiformis. *Lancet*, **ii,** 729.

402 SHUSTER S., WATSON A.J. & MARKS J. (1967) Small intestine in psoriasis. *British Medical Journal*, **iii,** 458.

403 SHUSTER S. & MARKS J. (1965) Dermatogenic enteropathy: a new cause of steatorrhoea. *Lancet*, **i,** 1367.

404 EVANS S. & EVANS C.C. (1971) Acute febrile neutrophilic dermatosis—two cases. *Dermatologica*, **143,** 152.

405 SAGHER F. & EVEM-PAZ Z. (1967) *Mastocytosis and the Mast Cell.* Year Book Publishers, Chicago.

406 ULTMANN J.E., MUTTER R.D., TANNENBAUM M. & WARNER R.R.P. (1964) Clinical, cytologic, and biochemical studies in systemic mast cell disease. *Annals of Internal Medicine*, **61,** 326.

407 WISE D., WALLACE H.J. & JELLINEK E.H. (1962) Angiokeratoma corporis diffusum. A clinical study of eight affected families. *Quarterly Journal of Medicine (New Series)*, **31,** 177.

408 VON GEMMINGEN G., KIERLAND R.R. & OPITZ J.M. (1965) Angiokeratoma corporis diffusum (Fabry's disease). *Archives of Dermatology*, **91,** 206.

409 GOTTLIEB A.J. (1977) Disorders of hemostasis—non-thrombocytopenic purpuras. In: *Hematology*, 2nd edn (ed. Williams W.J., Beutler E., Erslev A.J. & Rundles R.W.), p. 1385. McGraw-Hill, New York.

410 HERBERT P.N., GOTTO A.M. & FREDRICKSON D.S. (1978) Familial lipoprotein deficiency (abetalipoproteinemia, hypobetalipoproteinemia, and Tangier Disease). In: *The Metabolic Basis of Inherited Disease*, 4th edn (ed. Stanbury J.B., Wyngaarden J.B. & Fredrickson D.S.), p. 544. McGraw-Hill, New York.

411 VAN BUCHEM F.S.P., POL G., DE GIER J., BOTTCHER C.J.F. & PRIES C. (1966) Congenital β-lipoprotein deficiency. *American Journal of Medicine*, **40,** 794.

412 CRITCHLEY E.M.R., NICHOLSON J.Y., BETTS J.J. & WEATHERALL D.J. (1970) Acanthocytosis, normolipoproteinaemia and multiple tics. *Postgraduate Medical Journal*, **46,** 698.

413 GJONE E., GLOMSET J.A. & KAARE N.K. (1978) Familial lecithin: cholesterol acyl transferase deficiency. In: *The Metabolic Basis of Inherited Disease*, 4th edn (ed. Stanbury J.B., Wyngaarden J.B. & Fredrickson D.S.), p. 589. McGraw-Hill, New York.

414 McKUSICK V.A., NEUFELD E.F. & KELLY T.E. (1978) The mucopolysaccharide storage diseases. In: *The Metabolic Basis of Inherited Disease*, 4th edn, (ed. Stanbury J.B., Wyngaarden J.B. & Fredrickson D.S.), p. 1282. McGraw-Hill, New York.

415 GOKAL R., MILLARD P.R., WEATHERALL D.J., CALLENDER S.T.E., LEDINGHAM J.G.G. & OLIVER D.O. (1979) Iron metabolism in haemodialysis patients. *Quarterly Journal of Medicine (New Series)*, **48,** 369.

416 LANGE R.D. & DYNESIUS R. (1973) Blood volume changes during normal pregnancy. *Clinics in Hematology*, **2,** 433.

417 PUOLAKKA J. (1980) Serum ferritin as a measure of iron stores during pregnancy. *Acta Obstetrica et Gynecologica Scandinavica*, Suppl. 95.

418 FLEMING A.F. (1973) Hypoplastic anemia in pregnancy. *Clinics in Hematology*, **2,** 477.

419 MITCHELL G.W., McRIPLEY R.J., SELVARAJ R.J. & SBARRA A.J. (1966) The role of the phagocyte in

host-parasite interactions. IV. The phagocytic activity of leucocytes in pregnancy and its relationship to urinary tract infections. *American Journal of Obstetrics and Gynecology*, **96**, 687.

420 EL-MAALLEM H. & FLETCHER J. (1980) Impaired neutrophil function and myeloperoxidase deficiency in pregnancy. *British Journal of Haematology*, **44**, 375.

421 STRICKLAND G.T. & KOSTINAS J.E. (1970) Folic acid deficiency complicating malaria. *American Journal of Tropical Medicine and Hygiene*, **19**, 910.

422 SRICHAIKUL T., SIRIASAWAKUL T., POSHYACHINDA M. & POSHYACHINDA V. (1973) Ferrokinetics in patients with malaria: normoblasts and iron incorporation *in vitro. American Journal of Clinical Pathology*, **60**, 166.

423 OLDENBURGER D., CARSON, J.P., DUNDLACH, W.J., GHALY, F.I. & WRIGHT, W.H. (1979) Legionnaires' disease. Association with *Mycoplasma* pneumonia and disseminated intravascular coagulation. *Journal of the American Medical Association*, **241**, 1269.

SECTION 7
BLOOD GROUPS
AND TRANSFUSION

Chapter 34
The blood groups

G. W. G. BIRD AND G. H. TOVEY

Blood groups are important not only in haematology but also in anthropology, biochemistry, clinical medicine and surgery, forensic science, genetics, oncology and immunology.

There are at least 14 major blood-group systems in man and several minor systems. Some of the systems, particularly ABO and Rhesus, are of great importance in blood transfusion and clinical medicine.

GENERAL PRINCIPLES

Blood-group serology is fundamentally a study of antigens, antibodies and antigen–antibody reactions. Some knowledge of the principles of immunology is therefore necessary for a clear understanding of blood groups. The account which follows is specifically related to blood-group serology; many other aspects of the subject are considered in greater detail in Chapters 17 and 19.

Antigens and antibodies

An antigen is a substance which can stimulate the production of an antibody, a serum globulin, with which it reacts in a specific manner. The term immunoglobulin is used to denote all globulins which act as antibodies. There are five classes of immunoglobulin distinguished by their electrophoretic, physicochemical and chemical properties. They are IgG, IgM, IgA, IgD and IgE. At present only IgG, IgM and IgA are relevant to blood-group serology. The immunoglobulin molecule (Fig. 34.1) is composed of four polypeptide chains, two heavy chains characteristic of each class, and two light chains common to all classes. The heavy chains are named γ, μ, α, δ and ε in IgG, IgM, IgA, IgD and IgE respectively. The light chains are κ and λ. Each immunoglobulin molecule has either κ or λ chains but not both. The heavy and light chains are connected by disulphide bonds.

The IgG molecule occurs as a monomer. IgA may also occur as a monomer but is most frequently found as a dimer or trimer; the IgM molecule is a pentamer. IgM antibody therefore has 10 combining sites, IgG

only two. Important differences between IgG and IgM antibodies are shown in Table 34.1. IgA antibodies usually accompany IgG or IgM antibodies of the same specificity.

Immunization

The injection of a foreign antigen into the animal body sets off a series of complex events which lead to production of antibodies. If the antigen is obtained from another species the response is known as heteroimmunization; if it is from the same species it is termed alloimmunization. According to Ehrlich's principle of *horror autotoxicus* an animal does not produce antibodies to its own antigens. There are, however, exceptions to this principle; erythrocyte autoantibodies are described in Chapter 11.

If the injected animal has never been previously exposed to the antigen, a primary response occurs in which the peak of antibody production is attained in 10–30 days. Subsequent exposure to antigen produces a secondary or anamnestic response in which antibody is produced more rapidly (a few hours to 10 days); the secondary antibody is stronger and more avid than the primary antibody.

Antigen–antibody interaction

The manifestations of antigen–antibody interaction are dependent on various factors which include the conditions of the reaction, the nature and size of antigen and antibody, and whether the antigen is particulate or in solution. Erythrocytes are, of course, particulate antigens so that union with antibodies is manifested by agglutination (or clumping) of erythrocytes or by haemolysis in the presence of Complement.

Agglutination

Agglutination of erythrocytes takes place in two stages: antibody first combines rapidly with antigen and then the agglutination of red cells occurs. Visible agglutinates will not form if the distance between individual cells is greater than the length of the adherent antibody.

Erythrocytes have a negative electrical charge,

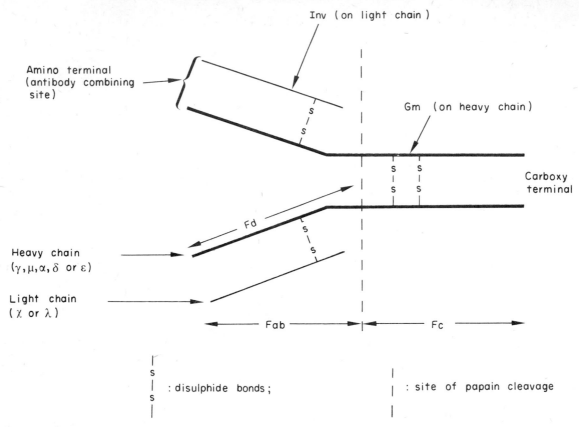

Fig. 34.1. Diagrammatic representation of an immunoglobulin molecule (monomer).

largely derived from N-acetylneuraminic (sialic) acid, a constituent of the cell membrane. The charge is equal in all normal erythrocytes. Since like charges repel, erythrocytes are normally separated from one another. When red cells are suspended in physiological saline the Na$^+$ and Cl$^-$ ions form an electrical double layer around each cell. The positively charged Na$^+$ ions are attracted by the negative charge of the cells and form the inner layer of the ionic 'cloud'; the negatively charged Cl$^-$ ions form the outer layer. This serves to decrease the force of repulsion between erythrocytes

and allows them to approach each other more closely. The electrical potential that develops between the cells' negative charge and the ionic 'cloud' is known as the ζ potential, a force which must be overcome if agglutination is to take place. The ζ potential is usually sufficient to maintain a space of about 100 nm between erythrocytes. IgM antibody is long enough to agglutinate erythrocytes suspended in physiological saline, whereas IgG antibody is shorter and cannot bridge the gap between red cells in a saline medium, so that other methods are required to demonstrate IgG antibody.

Table 34.1. A comparison of IgG and IgM antibodies

	IgG	IgM
Optimal reaction temperature	37°C	4°C
Molecular weight (approx.)	150 000	900 000
Sedimentation constant (Svedberg units)	7 S	19 S
Placental transfer	Yes	No
Serological type	'Incomplete'	Saline

Reduction of ζ potential is not the only factor involved. Vicinal water may be an important factor. Tightly bound water molecules may contribute to the maintenance of cell separation and their displacement may be conducive to cell agglutination.

Haemolysis

Some human blood-group antibodies haemolyse the corresponding red cells in the presence of Complement (C'), a group of components of fresh serum, most of which are β globulins. Complement activation begins with its interaction with the antigen–antibody complex. Complement may fix to the antigen–antibody complex or the erythrocyte surface in close proximity to the complex. The latter is the more likely possibility because it is known that antibody can be eluted from the cell surface, leaving C' adherent to it. A single IgM molecule can establish a C'-fixing site on the cell surface. A single IgG molecule cannot establish a C'-fixing site: two molecules are required. Since IgG molecules are normally distributed singly over the erythrocyte surface, IgM antibodies are more efficient in causing haemolysis than IgG. Reactions which involve C' do not necessarily cause haemolysis; the detection of some C'-fixing antibodies therefore requires demonstration of C' or its components on the red-cell surface. Some C' components have blood-group activity (p. 1417).

Antibody notation

We use the undermentioned system [1], as applied to antibodies against hypothetical antigens X and Y.

Mixtures of separable antibodies:	anti-X + anti-Y
Cross-reacting antibody:	anti-X + Y

Antibody which acts only when X and Y are both present on the erythrocyte surface: anti-XY

ABO BLOOD GROUPS

Antigens

The ABO blood groups, which are fundamental to successful blood transfusion, were discovered by Landsteiner [2, 3] at the beginning of this century. The four common groups of this system, AB, A, B and O, are determined by the presence or absence of two erythrocyte antigens (agglutinogens) A and B (Table 34.2). The rare O_h group is described on page 1397.

Antibodies

The corresponding antibodies (agglutinins), anti-A (α) and anti-B (β), are present in serum in accordance with the simple 'law' that an antigen and its corresponding antibody are never present together in the blood of the same person (Table 34.2). The interactions of the antigens and antibodies of the ABO blood-group system are shown in Table 34.2.

Inheritance of the ABO blood groups

The ABO blood groups are inherited [4] in accordance with Mendelian principles [5] by means of three allelic genes *A*, *B* and *O*. The *A* and *B* genes are co-dominant; the *O* gene is thought to be an amorph, a gene which has no demonstrable product. The genotypes and phenotypes of the ABO system are shown in Table 34.3.

A blood-group character cannot appear in a child unless it is present in one or other of its parents. If a person is homozygous for a blood-group gene, the

Table 34.2. ABO blood-group interactions

Group	Serum Antibodies normally present	Red cells Phenotype: Genotype: Genotype*:	AB AB HH or Hh	A AA or AO HH or Hh	B BB or BO HH or Hh	O OO HH or Hh	O_h hh
AB	—		—	—	—	—	—
A	anti-B		+	—	+	—	—
B	anti-A		+	+	—	—	—
O	anti-A anti-B		+	+	+	—	—
O_h	anti-A anti-B anti-H		+	+	+	+	—

* The Hh genes are independent of the ABO genes.

Table 34.3. Inheritance of the ABO blood groups

Gene from one parent	Gene from other parent	Genotype	Phenotype (serologically demonstrable blood group)
A	B	AB	AB
A	A	AA	A
A	O	AO	A
B	B	BB	B
B	O	BO	B
O	O	OO	O

character determined by that gene must appear in all his children. These are the principles of blood-grouping tests in paternity disputes.

The primary products of blood-group genes are enzymes (p. 1404) which build blood-group-active structures by the sequential addition of component molecules.

Cis *AB*

A few families have been described in which A and B have been inherited together, usually as A_2B [6]. An example of *cis* A_1B has also been described [7, 8]. In *cis* AB the B antigen is weaker than normal and anti-B is usually present in the serum. The *cis* arrangement with A(AB/O) is thought to weaken the effect of the B gene in comparison with the normal *trans* disposition (A/B). *Cis* AB could result from recombination within a complex locus or from a rare allele which produces an antigen with the properties of both A and B. *Cis* AB does not detract from the value of ABO blood groups in paternity tests; the weak B and the presence of anti-B in the serum should draw attention to the true situation in most examples. The serum *A*-gene-specified glycosyltransferase levels (p. 1407) are slightly, and *B*-gene transferase very much lower than normal [9]. *Cis* AB could be also be due to the fact that *B*-gene-specified glycosyltransferase can also produce some A-antigen [10]. This would not, however, be a typical *cis* AB.

Development of ABO antigens

The A and B antigens can be detected on the red cells of five-week-old embryos, but are nevertheless not fully developed at birth. Their strength increases up to about the age of 20 years and then remains constant.

Origin of ABO antibodies

Agglutinins derived from the mother by placental transfer are demonstrable in about 50% of newborn babies. Maternal antibody completely disappears in about six months, by which time the baby has developed agglutinins characteristic of its own group. The titre rises to about the age of puberty and then gradually falls towards old age.

Anti-A and anti-B are generally held to be naturally occurring antibodies, of which they have the typical characteristics: ability to agglutinate erythrocytes suspended in physiological saline solution and to act more strongly at lower temperatures than at body temperature. Some authorities, however, believe that they are really hetero-agglutinins produced as an immune response to ubiquitous bacterial antigens which have a chemical structure similar to A or B. This hypothesis is supported by the observations of Springer *et al.* [11] on germ-free chicks, which never develop antibodies, whereas ordinary chicks develop antibodies within 30 days of hatching. On the other hand, when germ-free chicks are fed *E. coli* O_{86}, which contains a B-like antigen, anti-B agglutinins quickly develop.

Cross-reacting antibodies in group-O sera

Group-O sera may contain, besides specific anti-A and anti-B, cross-reacting (anti-A + B) antibodies. Cross-reacting antibody has been extensively studied and three hypotheses have been offered in explanation:
1 Wiener [12], reviving an old idea conceived by Moss [13], claimed that cross-reacting agglutinins are anti-C and react with a blood factor C, common to A and B.
2 Dodd [14] and Bird [15] thought that cross-reacting antibodies had separate combining sites for A and B.
3 Owen [16] was the first to suggest that cross-reacting antibody was directed towards a chemical structure shared by A and B.

The subject has been reviewed and discussed by Dodd *et al.* [17] and by Race & Sanger [6]. The problem has not been completely solved; however, in view of the chemical similarity between A and B, the third hypothesis is probably the best.

Bird [18] focused attention on asymmetric varieties of cross-reacting antibody, which were further studied by Richardson-Jones *et al.* [19]. It seems that there exists a wide spectrum of cross-reacting antibodies, some better adapted to A and others to B depending, as suggested by Dodd *et al.* [17], on the chemical nature of the inciting antigen.

Immune anti-A and anti-B
Whereas naturally occurring anti-A and anti-B are IgM antibodies, immune anti-A and anti-B may be either IgG or IgM. Naturally occurring IgM anti-A does not readily cause haemolysis of human A or react with pig A (A^p) cells [20, 21]. Immune IgM anti-A readily haemolyses A cells and agglutinates A^p cells. Some sera, usually from group-O persons, contain IgG anti-A and anti-B. These antibodies readily haemolyse not only the corresponding cells but also A^p cells and may cause haemolytic disease of the newborn. Anti-A and anti-B may occur partly as IgA. IgA antibodies, unlike IgM and IgG, do not bind Complement. All anti-A and anti-B antibodies agglutinate the corresponding red cells in saline. IgG anti-A or anti-B in dilutions which no longer agglutinate red cells will, however, sensitize them to an anti-IgG serum.

To predict or diagnose ABO haemolytic disease it may be useful to estimate the amount of IgG anti-A or anti-B in the serum. Witebsky [22] added enough blood-group substance to inhibit IgM anti-A (agglutination in saline) and then titrated the serum against A_1 cells suspended in AB serum. Although this method demonstrates IgG antibody, it does not estimate it accurately. A modification described by Polley *et al.* [23] is more useful: in this method enough human A substance is added to just fail to inhibit IgG anti-A and the serum is then tested by the indirect antiglobulin method, using a specific anti-IgG serum.

Antigen-site density
Knowledge of the density of antigen sites on the erythrocyte surface is fundamental to a clear understanding of antigen–antibody interactions.

Each A_1 erythrocyte has about a million A-antigen sites; each B red cell has about 700 000 B-antigen sites [24]. Subgroup distinctions (p. 1398) are probably mainly dependent on differences in antigen-site density.

Secretors and non-secretors
The antigens of the ABO system are not confined to erythrocytes; they are also present in leucocytes (p. 1422), platelets (p. 1423) and tissue cells. Blood-group-active substances are also present in soluble form in most of the body fluids of the majority of persons. Those persons whose body fluids contain blood-group-active substances are known as secretors. The saliva of secretors contains appreciable amounts of blood-group substance; pseudo-mucinous ovarian cyst fluid contains high concentrations of blood-group-active material.

Capacity to secrete blood-group substances is inherited independently of the ABO blood groups as a simple Mendelian character [25]. The genes concerned are *Se* (dominant) and *se* (an amorph); persons of the genotypes *SeSe* and *Sese* are secretors; those of the genotypes *sese* are non-secretors. About 78% of British people are secretors.

The H character
Almost all human erythrocytes contain H substance in the descending quantitative order: O, A_2, A_2B, B, A_1, A_1B. H is inherited independently of the ABO groups and the Secretor character. The genes involved are *H* and *h*; *H* is dominant, *h* is very rare and is an amorph. The genotypes *HH* and *Hh* are H-positive, the genotype *hh* is H-negative. The red cells of H-negative persons (group O_h or 'Bombay' blood group) are not agglutinated by anti-A, anti-B or anti-H; their serum contains anti-A, anti-B and anti-H (Table 34.2), so that if they require transfusion, only O_h blood can be given.

H is believed to be the substrate on which the *A* and *B* genes act to form the A and B characters (p. 1407). Group-O cells are therefore richly endowed with H; in A_1B cells most of the substrate is used up so that there is relatively little H. Even if O_h persons have *A* or *B* genes, the genes are not expressed because of absence of substrate.

Whereas in erythrocytes H is expressed in the presence of an *H* gene, the presence of H in body fluids is controlled by the *Se* gene. H substance is therefore present in secretor but not in non-secretor saliva.

Anti-H
Anti-H agglutinates red cells in the following descending order of strength: O, A_2, A_2B, B, A_1, A_1B. It is inhibited by secretor but not by non-secretor saliva. Human anti-H is regularly present in the serum of O_h persons; it sometimes occurs as a weak cold agglutinin in A_1 and A_1B, and rarely in B sera. In O_h sera, anti-H is about as strong as anti-A and anti-B. Since most erythrocytes contain H, separation of anti-H from anti-A and anti-B in O_h serum by absorption with A_1B cells reduces its titre. Neutralization of anti-A and anti-B by pure A and B group-specific substances effectively isolates anti-H. Anti-H can be produced by injecting *Shigella shigae* into goats or other animals. This is a time-consuming procedure and gives rise to a strong anti-H antibody which needs high dilution before it can effectively classify the erythrocytes of the various ABO groups and subgroups or distinguish secretor from non-secretor saliva. Eel (*Anguilla*

anguilla) serum may contain a naturally occurring anti-H. The most convenient sources of anti-H, however, are the seeds of various plants (p. 1417), such as the common gorse, *Ulex europaeus*. *Ulex* anti-H is particularly useful for making the secretor/non-secretor distinction [26].

A_h *and* B_h

The symbols A_h and B_h have been given to persons whose red cells have little or no H with varying amounts of A or B. A number of H-deficient bloods associated with varying strengths of A, B and H on red cells and in saliva have been described [27, 28].

The subgroups of A

A_1 *and* A_2

When some B sera are absorbed with certain A erythrocytes (A_2) until they no longer agglutinate such erythrocytes, they are still capable of agglutinating most other A (A_1) cells. A_1 and A_2 are variants of the agglutinogen A; there are therefore two subgroups of A, A_1 and A_2, and two of AB, A_1B and A_2B. As a general rule the antigen A_2 is less sensitive to agglutination than A_1, particularly in A_2B cells, so that A_2 is likely to be mistaken for O and A_2B for B.

The existence of variants of the antigen A does not invalidate the Bernstein theory of inheritance of the ABO groups. The theory can be extended to include an A_2 gene, recessive to A_1. Further extension can accommodate the weaker subgroups described below.

Besides anti-A (α), human sera may contain the 'extra' agglutinins anti-A_1 (α_1) and anti-H (α_2), their distribution being as shown in Table 34.4. Anti-A_1 and anti-H usually act only at low temperatures. Anti-A agglutinates A_1, A_1B, A_2 and A_2B cells; anti-A_1 agglutinates A_1 and A_1B but not A_2 or A_2B cells. The anti-H agglutinin is much weaker than the anti-H regularly found in the sera of O_h persons and usually reacts with only O, A_2 and A_2B cells.

Table 34.4. Antibodies of the ABO system

	Normal	Additional agglutinins sometimes present
A_1B	—	anti-H
A_2B	—	anti-A_1
A_1	anti-B	anti-H
A_2	anti-B	anti-A_1
B	anti-A	anti-H
O	anti-A	—
	anti-B	—
O_h	anti-A	—
	anti-B	—
	anti-H	—

Group-B (or O) sera regularly contain both anti-A and anti-A_1 in varying amounts and proportions. Some B sera may have good titres of anti-A and anti-A_1 and would then agglutinate A_2 cells appreciably; others may have low titres of anti-A with adequate titres of anti-A_1 and act poorly on A_2 cells. Group-B sera intended for blood grouping must be titrated against both A_1 and A_2 cells and issued only if A_2 cells are strongly agglutinated.

Whether the difference between A_1 and A_2 is qualitative or quantitative has been debated for many years. It now seems that the difference is primarily qualitative, but is also quantitative; the qualitative difference is determined by the fact that the biosynthesis of A_1 and A_2 involves different gene-specified glycosyltransferases which are believed by Kisailus & Kabat [29] to synthesize different chemical structures, and the quantitative difference depends on the number of antigen sites, each A_2 red cell having about a quarter as many antigen sites (about 250 000) as A_1 cells [24].

Many methods of distinguishing A_1 from A_2 red cells have been described. A quick and sharp distinction is made by the agglutinin from *Dolichos biflorus* seeds (p. 1418). *D. biflorus* seed extract forms a heavy precipitate with A_1 and a weaker precipitate with A_2 secretor saliva, indicating a quantitative difference. Similar concentrations of purified blood-group-specific substance prepared from ovarian cyst fluids from A_1 and A_2 persons give a reaction of identity in Ouchterlony tests when they are allowed to diffuse against the *Dolichos* precipitin [30]. This observation supports the view that A_1 and A_2 are qualitatively identical.

Clinical importance. Anti-A_1 in the serum of A_2 or A_2B persons can cause haemolytic transfusion reactions.

A_3

An even weaker form of A is A_3. A_3 cells are very weakly agglutinated by B or O sera, giving, under the microscope, a typical mixed-field appearance of very small agglutinates against a background of unagglutinated cells. Anti-A_1 is very seldom present in A_3 sera. A_3 persons secrete both A and H.

A_x

The A_x variant (also known as A_4, A_o, A_z, etc.) is peculiar in that the red cells are not agglutinated (rarely weakly agglutinated) by B serum, but are strongly agglutinated by many O sera. O serum must therefore be used in addition to A and B sera in routine blood grouping. Although A_x cells are not agglutinated by the anti-A of B serum, they absorb the antibody, which can be eluted from the cells. Anti-A_1 or anti-A may be present in the serum [31]. A_x persons secrete H but little or no A.

Table 34.5. Comparison of A_1, A_2, A_3, and A_x subgroups

	B serum	O serum	Additional agglutinins which may be present in serum
A_1	$+++$	$+++$	anti-H
A_2	$+$ (some B sera$-$)	$+++$	anti-A_1
A_3	w (mixed-field)	w (mixed-field)	anti-A_1
A_x	$-$	$+++$ (most O sera)	anti-A_1 or anti-A

In some families the inheritance of A_x appears straightforward; in others there are indications of the action of suppressor genes [6, pp. 16–17]. As measured by B serum, A_x is a weaker form of A than A_3: as measured by O serum it is not. The properties of A_1, A_2, A_3 and A_x are compared in Table 34.5.

Yokoyama & Plocinik [32] found evidence of a specific anti-A_x antibody in O sera. As far as we know this evidence has not been corroborated.

A_{end}
A_{end} cells are not agglutinated by naturally occurring anti-A but may be agglutinated by immune anti-A (by the centrifugation technique), and give a weak mixed-field reaction with O serum [33, 34].

A_m and A_y
These variants of A are very rare. A_m red cells are not agglutinated by B or O sera but do absorb anti-A. The saliva of A_m secretors contains A and H. This phenotype is inherited as an allele at the ABO locus [35]. The properties of A_y are virtually identical with those of A_m; details are given by Cartron *et al.* [35]. A_m and A_y can be distinguished by serum gene-specified glycosyltransferase assays. In A_m, *A*-gene-specified glycosyltransferase levels are 30–50% of the average values for A_1 or A_2 persons respectively, whereas no *A*-gene-specified glycosyltransferase is demonstrable in A_y [35].

It is thought that the A_y phenotype represents homozygosity for a very rare gene *y*, whose very common allele *Y* is necessary for the development of A in red cells [36].

A_{el}
This variant is the weakest form of A [37]. The red cells are not agglutinated by the anti-A of B or O sera and the saliva of secretors contains H but no A. The only evidence that the red cells are indeed group A is provided by the demonstration that they absorb anti-A which can be subsequently eluted. The essential differences between A_x, A_m, A_{end} and A_{el} are shown in Table 34.6.

Other forms of weak A
Several weak A variants, some named and others as yet unchristened, have been described. We doubt if any useful purpose is served by making minor distinctions at this level. For example, A_g [38] is not a true variant of A but an acquired weakening of the A antigen associated with leukaemia. (For A_{mos} and B_{mos} see p. 1424.)

Reciprocity with H
Whereas A is progressively weaker as one descends from A_1 to A_{el}, the strength of H increases. Anti-H reagents may therefore be used in subgrouping; for example *Ulex europaeus* anti-H agglutinates A_2 cells more strongly than A_1 and may be used in parallel with

Table 34.6. Comparison of A_x, A_{end}, A_m and A_{el} subgroups

	B serum (anti-A)	O serum (anti-A + B)	α_1 in serum	Secretion	Eluate from red cells after exposure to anti-A
A_x	$-$	$+++$	Usually $+$	H only	anti-A
A_{end}	$-$*	w (mixed-field)		H only	anti-A
A_m	$-$	$-$	$-$	A and H	anti-A
A_{el}	$-$	$-$	$-$	H only	anti-A

* Agglutinated by immune anti-A.

the agglutinin from *Dolichos biflorus* in making the A_1/A_2 distinction.

A_{int}

Landsteiner & Levine [39] classified bloods which were agglutinated both by anti-A_1 and anti-H as A-intermediate (A_{int}). This variant is correctly placed between A_1 and A_2 if reactions with anti-A and anti-A_1 are considered. If A_{int} is intermediate between A_1 and A_2 it would be expected to have more H than A_1 and less H than A_2. A_{int} cells, however, may have as much or even more H than A_2 [6].

A_{int} cells react much more weakly than A_1 with the *Dolichos biflorus* agglutinin and are agglutinated by seed anti-H reagents which are so diluted as to just fail to agglutinate A_1 cells.

Subgroups of B

B variants are rarer than A variants. Weak forms of B may be inherited or acquired. An inherited variant, B_2, corresponding in strength to A_2, has been described by Jacobowicz *et al.* [40]. Inherited weak B, besides B_2, *cis* AB (p. 1396) and B_h (p. 1398) have been divided by Race & Sanger [6] into three categories (Table 34.7) depending on the presence or absence of anti-B in the serum and B in saliva. Notation for B variants is not in line with that for A variants; furthermore, the same notation, for example B_x, has been used for examples belonging to different Race & Sanger categories.

Table 34.7. Subgroups of B; weak Bs other than B_2*, *cis* AB, B_h or acquired B

Race & Sanger category	Anti-B in serum	Saliva	Notation allocated to some examples
1	+	H, B	B_v
2	–	H, B	B_w
	(or very weak cold anti-B)		B_x
			B_m
3	–	H, but little or no B	B_3
			B_x

* B_2 is a stronger form of weak B than any of those included in the table.

The variant B_v is thought by Boorman & Zeitlin [41] to lack part of the normal B antigen so that the serum contains an antibody specific for the missing part, which agglutinates all normal B cells.

Salmon and his associates [42, 43] have applied fine quantitative techniques to the study of weak B antigens. Antigen strength is expressed as the percentage of cells agglutinated by selected anti-B sera at a definitive dilution and temperature. Weak B cells ranging from B_0 to B_{80} (normal B_{100}) were described.

Although weak B cells are agglutinated very weakly or not at all, they absorb anti-B and yield potent eluates. Such eluates may agglutinate weak B cells which are not agglutinated by the serum used to prepare the eluate.

The B antigen may be weakened in leukaemia [44].

Kogure & Iseki [45] have described a family in which a weak B, B_m (category 2 of Race & Sanger), was clearly shown to have a genetic basis corresponding to that of A_m. They suggest that B_m occurs in persons homozygous for a recessive gene z allelic to a dominant gene Z responsible for the development of B in red cells.

Salmon & Cartron believe that the notation for the weak forms of B should correspond to that for the weak forms of A, for example B_3, B_x, B_m, B_{el}. They have therefore re-classified various forms of weak B previously reported in the literature [46].

Acquired or 'pseudo' B

Cameron *et al.* [47] described seven A_1 persons whose red cells had acquired a B-like antigen. Most of the patients had cancer and were over 60 years old; two examples of acquired B in 'normal' individuals have been reported [48]. A and H, but not B, were present in the saliva of secretors. All seven sera contained normal anti-B.

The red cells were agglutinated by some anti-B sera. The reactions were weaker than those of normal B cells; many unagglutinated cells were observed.

It is attractive to suppose that the acquisition of B is due to the coating of red cells by B-like substance given up by *E. coli* O_{86} [49]. However, since bacterial products adhere to A_1 and O cells alike, this does not explain why *in vivo* only A_1 cells acquire B. A more likely possibility, suggested by Gerbal *et al.* [50], is that N-acetylgalactosamine, the structural determinant of A, is converted by a bacterial deacetylase to galactosamine which cross-reacts with galactose, the structural determinant of B.

LEWIS GROUPS

The Lewis blood-group system is unusual in man because the antigens are not an integral part of the red-cell membrane but are acquired by absorption from the plasma [51].

Body fluids

The Lewis system is primarily a system of the body fluids [52]. The Lewis antigen (or blood-group-active substance) is inherited independently of the ABO antigens and capacity to secrete ABH substances, from a pair of allelic genes, *L* and *l*. *L* is dominant; *l* is an amorph. Persons of the genotype *LL* and *Ll* have Lewis substance in their body fluids (Lewis secretors); those of the genotype *ll* have none (non-secretors of Lewis). The unqualified terms secretor and non-secretor refer to the presence or absence of ABH substance in body fluids.

The *L* gene acts on a precursor substance present in body fluids and converts it to Lewis substance by adding certain chemical groupings (p. 1409). The *H* gene acts on the same substrate so that the two genes interact in their phenotypic expression. Since H is only found in body fluids in the presence of an *Se* gene, the Lewis system can only be understood clearly if Lewis, H and Secretor phenotypes are considered together [53] (Table 34.8). The product of the *L* gene is Le^a. Le^b was originally believed to be the product of a gene *Le^b* allelic to the gene for Le^a. It is now thought that Le^b is the product of interaction of the *L* and *H* genes.

Erythrocytes

The relationship of the Lewis and H phenotypes of erythrocytes to the Lewis, H and secretor phenotypes of the body fluids is shown in Table 34.8. The numbers in the first vertical column of this table serve only as a guide and their use does not constitute an attempt to create a notation. In genotype combinations 2, 3 and 4, the Lewis gene has unrestricted access to the substrate, so that a relatively large amount of Le^a is formed and then taken up by the red cells. In combination 1, the interaction of the *L* and *H* genes results in the production of much Le^b and relatively little Le^a, so that there is insufficient Le^a for coating the red cells.

Cord cells are Le(a−b−). From soon after birth to about the age of 18 months the red cells of children of genotype combination 1 (Table 34.8) are Le(a+b+) after which they become Le(a−b+). For as yet unexplained reasons Le^a and Le^b are weakened during pregnancy.

Lewis antibodies

Anti-Le^a and anti-Le^b are naturally occurring antibodies, usually IgM, rarely IgG. They bind Complement and act best at 16°C. Many anti-Le^a and a few anti-Le^b antibodies haemolyse red cells at 37°C. The antibodies act on red cells in saline; their action is enhanced by proteolytic enzymes. They can be demonstrated by indirect Coombs' tests; C′ must be added if the serum under test is not sufficiently fresh. The agglutinates formed by anti-Le^a and anti-Le^b have a characteristic appearance. Agglutination by some Lewis antibodies is prone to reversal ('disagglutination') if the agglutinated cells are spread out on a slide [54]. Indeed Lewis antibodies sometimes act very well on slides or tiles. For strong antibodies, red cells in saline are adequate for slide tests; weaker sera should be inactivated and tested against papainized cells.

There are two kinds of anti-Le^b: anti-Le^{bH} and anti-Le^{bL}. Anti-Le^{bH} reacts with Le(b+) cells in the descending order of strength—O, A$_2$, B, A$_1$, and is inhibited by all ABH secretor salivas. The specificity of anti-Le^{bL} is not influenced by the ABO status of red cells: it is inhibited only by the salivas of those who secrete both ABH and Lewis substances.

Kornstad [55] suggests anti-Le^{bH} may be divided into two categories: anti-H(Le^b), found in the serum of an A$_1$Le(a+b−) person, which shows strong cross-reaction with H, and anti-Le^b(H), found in Le(a−b−) persons, which shows appreciably less cross-reactivity.

Bird [56] studied the cross-reaction of H and Le^b and

Table 34.8. Lewis, H and secretor genotypes and phenotypes, modified from Giblett [84]

	Genotypes			Phenotypes						Approximate frequency
	Lewis	Hh	ABH Secretor	Body fluids			Erythrocytes			
				ABH	Le^a	Le^b	H	Le^a	Le^b	
1		*HH* or *Hh*	*SeSe* or *Sese*	+	+	+	+	−	+	74%
2			*sese*	−	+	−	+	+	−	23%
3	*LL* or *Ll*	*hh*	*SeSe* or *Sese*	−	+	−	−	+	−	Extremely rare
4			*sese*	−	+	−	−	+	−	Extremely rare
5		*HH* or *Hh*	*SeSe* or *Sese*	+	−	−	+	−	−	3%
6			*sese*	−	−	−	+	−	−	Rare: 6 per 1000
7	*ll*	*hh*	*SeSe* or *Sese*	−	−	−	−	−	−	Extremely rare
8			*sese*	−	−	−	−	−	−	Extremely rare

indeed suggested that Le^b could be considered a part of H, so that H could be visualized as just H or a broader H, HH$_1$, or HLe^b. Anti-H would agglutinate both H and HH$_1$ and anti-Le^b (or anti-H$_1$) HH$_1$ only. This idea is compatible with the chemical structure of H and Le^b (p. 1406).

Anti-Le^x, an antibody once believed to be a separable or inseparable mixture of anti-Le^a and anti-Le^b, is now thought to define a specific receptor Le^x [57]. Le^x is closely related to Le^a and has no connection with secretor/non-secretor status or with Le^b; it is well developed in cord cells.

An unusual antibody, anti-A$_1$Le^b, found in the serum of a 'blood-group chimaera', has been described by Crookston *et al.* [58].

Clinical importance of Lewis antibodies

Lewis antibodies rarely cause haemolytic transfusion reactions, because they are neutralized by Lewis substance in the donor's plasma. In a few days the transfused red cells take up Lewis substance from the recipient's plasma and thus acquire the Lewis phenotype of the recipient. Nevertheless, a few moderately severe haemolytic transfusion reactions have occurred.

When Le(a$-$b$-$) persons, whose sera contains anti-Le^a and anti-Le^b, require to be transfused with many bottles of blood, as in heart-bypass operations, it might be difficult to obtain sufficient compatible blood. An ingenious solution to this problem has been offered by Mollison [59], who neutralized the antibodies by first transfusing Le(a$+$) and Le(b$+$) plasma and later Le(a$-$b$-$) and Le(a$-$b$+$) blood. There was no reaction, despite the reappearance of anti-Le^a and anti-Le^b within two days.

Anti-Le^c and anti-Le^d

Anti-Le^c reacts with the red cells of Le(a$-$b$-$) non-secretors of ABH, i.e. with those of persons of the genotype *ll sese* and *ll hh*: the saliva of such individuals inhibits the antibody [60].

Anti-Le^d reacts with the red cells of Le(a$-$b$-$) secretors [61], i.e. persons of the genotype *ll*, *HH* or *Hh*, *SeSe* or *Sese*.

The notations Le^c and Le^d are unfortunate because their characters are not products of the *L* or *l* genes and are therefore not part of the Lewis system.

Anti-A$_1$Le^b and anti-BLe^b

Anti-A$_1$Le^b, first described by Seaman *et al.* [62], is an interesting antibody. It is inhibited only by saliva from A$_1$,Le(b$+$) persons. The A$_1$Le^b glycosphingolipid is present in the plasma of persons who have *L*, *H*, *Se* and *A^1* genes. Anti-A$_1$Le^b is a useful reagent in the study of blood group chimaeras [58, 63, 64]. To the best of our knowledge anti-BLe^b has only so far been demonstrated in lymphocytotoxicity tests.

Magard

The antibody 'Magard' has been known but little understood for many years [65]. It reacts only with the red cells of A,Le(a$-$b$-$) secretors of ABH. It is now thought to have the specificity anti-A$_1$Le^d [66].

THE P SYSTEM

For many years the P blood-group system consisted of P-positives (strong or weak) and P-negatives, distinguished by an antibody, anti-P. The recognition of the antigen Tj^a [67] and its relationship with the P system [68] showed the system to be complex.

The original notations for the P and Tj^a groups had to be modified. The phenotype P$+$ became P$_1$, P$-$ became P$_2$ and Tj(a$-$) became p. It was proposed that genes *P$_1$*, *P$_2$* and *p* controlled the P$_1$, P$_2$ and p characters respectively. Anti-P was renamed anti-P$_1$, and anti-Tj^a became anti-P or anti-P$+$P$_1$.

The discovery of the P^k groups [69] provided further evidence of intricacy. The antibody anti-Tj^a was shown to be anti-P$+$P^k.

The autoantibody in paroxysmal cold haemoglobinuria (Donath–Landsteiner antibody) usually if not invariably has the specificity anti-P. It reacts with P$_1$ and P$_2$ but not P^k or p cells. Anti-P$+$P^k is both haemolytic and haemagglutinating, whereas the Donath–Landsteiner antibody is only haemolytic.

The present position of the P phenotypes and their reactions with the antibodies of this system is shown in Table 34.9. Further complexity was introduced by the discovery of the Luke antibody [70]. This antibody reacts with the red cells of most, but not all, P$_1$ and P$_2$ persons and fails to react with P^k or p cells. Although obviously related to the P system, the Luke character

Table 34.9. P blood-group interactions

Red cell phenotype	Antibodies		
	anti-P$_1$*	anti-P†	anti-P$+$P^k‡
P$_1$	$+$	$+$	$+$
P$_2$	$-$	$+$	$+$
P^k	$+$	$-$	$+$
P$^k_2$	$-$	$-$	$+$
P	$-$	$-$	$-$

* Formerly anti-P.
† Donath–Landsteiner antibody.
‡ Formerly anti-Tj^a.

segregates independently of the genes of the P-system antigens. Luke also has a mysterious association with ABO: weak and negative reactions are more common with P_2 than with P_1 cells and with A_1 and A_1B than with O, A_2, A_2B or B.

Clinical aspects

Strong anti-P_1 is associated with hydatid disease and hydatid cyst fluid has been found to be a valuable source of P_1 substance. Round worms and the liver fluke also contain P_1 substance, so that strong anti-P_1 may be present in the serum of those who harbour these parasites [71]. The association of the P system with paroxysmal cold haemoglobinuria is mentioned above.

In Western Australia a transient anti-Tj^a antibody, which is agglutinating but not haemolytic, was found in women who were threatening to abort for the second time [72]. Its significance is far from clear.

THE Ii SYSTEM

The I blood-group system has so far defied clear genetic analysis. The system fundamentally consists of two antigens, I and i, and two antibodies, anti-I and anti-i. Cord cells are rich in i and poor in I. The strength of I increases and that of i decreases until the age of 18 months, when the I antigen reaches adult strength. It has been suggested [73] that a regulator gene Z is responsible for the switch from I to i; there is as yet no firm proof of its existence. The switchover is retarded when there is 'marrow stress', as in thalassaemia, hypoplastic anaemia, or leukaemia. Certain rare adults (I −ve) have little or no I.

Anti-I is usually seen as a cold autoagglutinin in the serum of normal persons or, in much greater strength, after pneumonia due to *Mycoplasma* or after certain viral infections. The antibody is sometimes strong enough to produce an autoimmune haemolytic anaemia (Chapter 11). Anti-I is almost invariably IgM; IgG anti-I occurs very rarely. Anti-I may also occur as an allo-antibody in the serum of I-negative adults. Anti-i frequently occurs as a cold autoantibody in lymphomata and in infectious mononucleosis, and may occur in both IgM and IgG classes.

Anti-I binds Complement. At temperatures above 30°C anti-I is eluted from the erythrocyte surface leaving C′ adherent to it. Red cells sensitized by anti-I will therefore give a positive Coombs test if the antiglobulin serum contains not only anti-IgG and anti-IgM but also anti-C′ antibodies (the so-called 'broad-spectrum' antiglobulin serum).

There is clearly a serological association between the ABO and Ii systems. Some antibodies react as if they were anti-HI, anti-A_1I or anti-BI. Anti-HI, for example, reacts only when H and I are present on the red-cell surface; it does not react with HI or O_hI cells. This has given rise to the assumption that the antibody reacts with a joint product of the *H* and *I* genes, despite the fact that there is no clear evidence of the existence of *I* and *i* genes.

Rosse & Lauf [74] extracted the I antigen from adult and cord cells and found little or no difference in the strength of the extracted antigen; furthermore, it reacted as well at 37°C as at 0°C. They suggested that the 'placement' of the antigen in the membrane largely determines its reactivity with antibody; at 37°C the antigen may be 'hidden' whereas at 0°C it may be available to combine with antibody.

There are at least four categories of I antigens: I^D, I^F, I^S and I^T, which can be distinguished by means of a panel of I-adult, i-adult and cord cells and by other properties (Table 34.10).

There is much heterogeneity not only in the Ii status of erythrocytes but also among various anti-I anti-

Table 34.10. Classification of I antigens

Notation	Definition	Reactions with red cells			Effect of enzymes
		I adult	i adult	cord	
I^D	Developed: the I antigen of adults	+++	−	− or w	Enhanced*†
I^F	Fetal I	+++	+++	+++	Unaffected†
I^S	Present in secretors: inhibited by saliva, milk	+++	−	− or w	Enhanced*
I^T	Transition: present during the change from i to I	++	w	+++	Enhanced*

* Proteolytic enzymes.
† Neuraminidase.

Table 34.11. Glycosphingolipids of red cells (globoside series)

Activity	Structure*	Chemical name
	Galβ1-4Glc Cer	Lactosylceramide
P^k	Galα1-4Galβ1-4Glc Cer	Trihexosylceramide
P	GalNAcβ1-3Galα1-4Galβ1-4Glc Cer	Globoside

* For explanation of abbreviations see Table 34.17. The Forssman (Fs) antigen of the tissue cells of some human subjects is a globoside derivative and has the structure: GalNAcαa1-3GalNAcβ1-3Galα1-4Galβ1-4Glc Cer.

bodies. Anti-I is inhibited by sheep hydatid cyst fluid and by substances derived from milk. Dzierzkowa-Borodej *et al.* [75] studied a true anti-I antibody which was unusual in being highly susceptible to inhibition by saliva. They showed that the saliva of I-negative adults and newborn infants contained high concentrations of I substance. This accords with the observations of Rosse & Lauf [74], whose experiments indicate that adult and cord cells actually have about the same amount of I. Some antibodies are perfectly straightforward anti-I, others show a spectrum of activity as if they were detecting parts of an I mosaic, and others again react as if they were anti-HI, anti-Hi, anti-A$_1$I, and anti-BI, or even anti-P$_1$I or anti-Le^{b}I.

BIOSYNTHESIS OF ABH, LEWIS, Ii AND P BLOOD-GROUP-SYSTEM ANTIGENS AND THE CHEMICAL BASIS OF THEIR SPECIFICITIES

The ABH, Lewis, Ii and P blood-group antigens of red cells and plasma are glycolipids; ABH antigens of red cells also occur as glycoproteins, but the carbohydrate part of the ABH glycolipid or glycoprotein which constitutes their reactive sites is exactly the same. It is convenient to consider the chemistry of these antigens in a single section of this chapter because these antigens share a common substrate.

The primary products of genes which determine carbohydrate blood-group antigens are enzymes known as transferases. The blood-group gene-specified transferase adds the characteristic end-sugar to a preformed substrate assembled by the sequential action of other transferases.

The ABH, Lewis, and Ii blood-group-specific substances of various human body fluids, such as saliva, are glycoproteins. Whereas the structure of the distal part of their carbohydrate structure is the same as the corresponding red-cell glycolipid, there is a difference between the glycolipid and glycoprotein chains in as much as the glycolipid is a single chain and the glycoprotein consists of two chains, 1 and 2, of almost identical structure. The carbohydrate chain of the blood-group-specific glycolipids is bound to ceramide (N-acylsphingosine). The blood-group-specific glycolipids are therefore glycosphingolipids. The chemistry and biosynthesis of the various blood-group glycosphingolipids are described below.

Chemistry of antigens of the P system

It is convenient first to consider antigens of the P system because the genes for these antigens act early in the biosynthetic pathway. It seemed at first that the various P antigens all belonged to one system. It is now clear, however, that the biosynthetic pathway of P$_1$ is not the same as that of P^k and P: the P and P^k structures belong to the globoside series of glycosphingolipids (Table 34.11), whereas P$_1$ belongs to the paraglboside series (Table 34.12).

Table 34.12. Glycosphingolipids of red cells (paragloboside series)

Activity	Structure*	Chemical name
?Tk	GlcNAcβ1-3Galβ1-4Glc Cer	Lacto-N-triosylceramide
XIV	Galβ1-4GlcNAcβ1-3Galβ1-4Glc Cer	Lacto-N-neotetraosylceramide (paragloboside)
P$_1$	Galα1-4Galβ1-4GlcNAcβ1-3Galβ1-4Glc Cer	
?	NeuNAcα2-3Galβ1-4GlcNAcβ1-3Galβ1-4Glc Cer	Sialosylparagloboside

* For explanation of abbreviations see Table 34.17.

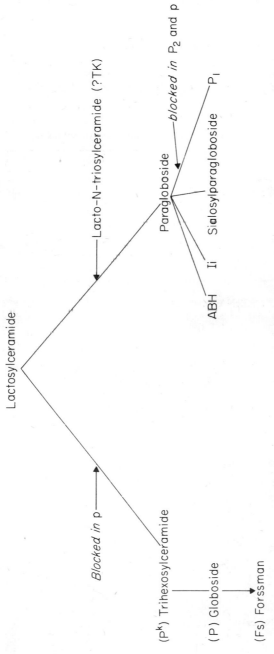

Fig. 34.2. Summary of biosynthetic pathways in the formation of glycosphingolipid antigens of the ABH, P and Ii systems.

In the globoside series (Fig. 34.2) the precursor lactosylceramide is converted by an, as yet, not understood genetic mechanism to P^k, and P^k is converted by a *P* gene to P (globoside).

Events relevant to the paragloboside series are more complex (Fig. 34.2) and need to be further discussed. It should be remembered that whereas paragloboside (lacto-N-neotetraose) is an intermediate stage in the biosynthesis of glycosphingolipid antigens of cells and plasma, lacto-N-tetraose (Table 34.13) represents the corresponding intermediate stage in the biosynthesis of the glycoprotein blood-group-active substances of body fluids.

Schwarting *et al.* [76] propose that the biosynthesis of antigens of the P system proceeds as shown in Figure 34.2. In P_2 cells the conversion of paragloboside to P_1 is blocked, and in p cells there is also a block in the conversion of lactosylceramide to P^k. The block is presumably due to absence or malfunction of the appropriate transferases. Paragloboside is also con-

Table 34.13. Structure of the ABH and Lewis antigens (glycosphingolipids) of plasma

Activity	Structure*	Chemical name
Precursor	Galβ1-3GlcNAcβ1-3Galβ1-4Glc Cer	Lacto-N-tetraose

H

$$\text{Gal}\beta\text{1-3GlcNAc}\beta\text{1-3Gal}\beta\text{1-4Glc Cer}$$
$$|\ (\alpha\text{1-2})$$
$$\text{Fuc}$$

Le^a

$$\text{Gal}\beta\text{1-3GlcNAc}\beta\text{1-4Glc Cer}$$
$$|\ (\alpha\text{1-4})$$
$$\text{Fuc}$$

Le^b

$$\text{Gal}\beta\text{1-3GlcNAc}\beta\text{1-3Gal}\beta\text{1-4Glc Cer}$$
$$(\alpha\text{1-2})\ |\quad |\ (\alpha\text{1-4})$$
$$\text{Fuc}\quad\text{Fuc}$$

A

$$\text{GalNAc}\alpha\text{1-3Gal}\beta\text{1-3GlcNAc}\beta\text{1-3Gal}\beta\text{1-4Glc Cer}$$
$$|\ (\alpha\text{1-2})$$
$$\text{Fuc}$$

B

$$\text{Gal}\alpha\text{1-3Gal}\beta\text{1-3GlcNAc}\beta\text{1-3Gal}\beta\text{1-4Glc Cer}$$
$$|\ \alpha(\text{1-2})$$
$$\text{Fuc}$$

ALe^b

$$\text{GalNAc}\alpha\text{1-3GalGlcNAc}\beta\text{1-3Gal}\beta\text{1-4Glc Cer}$$
$$(\alpha\text{1-2})|\ |\ \alpha(\text{1-4})$$
$$\text{Fuc}\quad\text{Fuc}$$

* For explanation of abbreviations see Table 34.17.

Table 34.14. Structure of the ABH antigens (glycosphingolipids) of red cells

Activity	Structure*	Chemical name
	Galβ1-4GlcNAcβ1-4Galβ1-4Glc Cer	Lacto-N-neotetraosylceramide (Paragloboside)
H	Galβ1-4GlcNAcβ1-3Galβ1-3Glc Cer	
	|(α1-2)	
	Fuc	
A	GalNAcα1-3Galβ1-4GlcNAcβ1-3Galβ1-4Glc Cer	
	|(α1-2)	
	Fuc	
B	Galα1-3Galβ1-4GlcNAcβ1-3Galβ1-4Glc Cer	
	|(α1-2)	
	Fuc	

* For explanation of abbreviations see Table 34.17.

verted to sialosylparagloboside (Fig. 34.2). The relationship of sialosylparagloboside to antigens of the P system is obscure. It is perhaps present in increased quantity in p cells or it may just be that it is more readily accessible to the rare antibodies which act preferentially on p cells.

Chemistry of the ABH antigens of red blood cells
Paragloboside is not only the substrate of P_1 but also of H, which is the precursor of A and B. The P_1 gene codes for an αD-galactosaminyltransferase which adds galactose in an α(1–4) position to the terminal galactose of paragloboside, whereas, in the formation of the H-glycosphingolipid, the primary product of the *H* gene, an α-fucosyltransferase adds fucose in an α(1–2)-linked position (Table 34.14).

The primary product of an *A* gene, an N-acetyl-galactosaminyltransferase, adds N-acetyl-D-galactos-amine to H in an α(1–3)-linked position to form A, and the primary product of a *B* gene, a galactosyltransferase, adds galactose to H in an α(1–3)-linked position to form B (Table 34.14).

Chemistry of Ii antigens
The study of I and i is difficult because of heterogeneity of anti-I antibodies. At present it seems probable that a straight-chain glycosphingolipid, lacto-N-norhexaosyl ceramide (Table 34.15), i.e. paragloboside to which is added a terminal β(1–4)-linked galactose residue, probably represents the i-structure and that glycosphingolipid with a branched carbohydrate chain, lacto-N-iso-octosyl ceramide (Table 34.15), also formed from paragloboside, represents the I-structure. Further details are given by Feizi *et al.* [77].

It should be noted at this stage that the cryptantigen

Table 34.15. Probable structure of the I and i antigens (glycosphingolipids)

Activity	Structure*	Chemical name
	Galβ1-4GlcNAcβ1-3Galβ1-4Glc Cer	Lacto-N-neotetraosylceramide (paragloboside)
I	Galβ1-4GlcNAc(β1-6)⟍ Galβ1-4GlcNAc(β1-3)⟋Galβ1-4GlcNAcβ1-3Galβ1-4Glc Cer	Lacto-N-iso-octaosylceramide
i	†Galβ1-4GlcNAcβ1-3Galβ1-4GlcNAcβ1-3Galβ1-4Glc Cer	Lacto-N-norhexaosylceramide

* For explanation of abbreviations see Table 34.17.
† There may be repeating Galβ1-4GlcNAcβ1-3 sequences.

Table 34.16. ABH and Lewis antigens (glycoproteins) in saliva and other secretions

Chain	Activity	Structure*
1		Galβ1-3GlcNAc............αGalNAc Ser or Thr
2	XIV	Galβ1-4GlcNAc............αGalNAc Ser or Thr

1	H	Galβ1-3GlcNAc............αGalNAc Ser or Thr
		   |(α1-2)
		   Fuc

2	H	Galβ1-4GlcNAc............αGalNAc Ser or Thr
		   |(α1-2)
		   Fuc

1	A	GalNAcα1-3Galβ1-3GlcNAc...αGalNAc Ser or Thr
		   |(α1-2)
		   Fuc

2	A	GalNAcα1-3Galβ1-4GlcNAc...αGalNAc Ser or Thr
		   |(α1-2)
		   Fuc

1	B	Galα1-3Galβ1-3GlcNAc....αGalNAc Ser or Thr
		   |(α1-2)
		   Fuc

2	B	Galα1-3Galβ1-4GlcNAc.....αGalNAc Ser or Thr
		   |(α1-2)
		   Fuc

1	Le^a	Galβ1-3GlcNAc.........αGalNAc Ser or Thr
		   |α1-4
		   L Fuc

2		Galβ1-4GlcNAc............ αGalNAc Ser or Thr

1	Le^b	Galβ1-3GlcNAc............αGalNAc Ser or Thr
		  |(α1-2) |α1-4
		  L Fuc L Fuc

2	H	Galβ1-4GlcNAc............αGalNAc Ser or Thr
		   |(α1-2)
		   L Fuc

* For explanation of abbreviations see Table 34.17.

Tk (p. 1418) is probably the paragloboside precursor, lacto-N-triosylceramide (Table 34.12).

ABH and Lewis antigens in secretions and plasma

The ABH and Lewis antigens of secretions and plasma are determined by the interaction of four sets of genes: *Hh*, *Sese*, *ABO* and *Ll*. H substance is found only when both the *Se* and *H* genes are present. *Se* is a regulator gene. As in the case of the *H*, *A* and *B* genes, the primary product of an *L* gene is a glycosyltransferase. The ABH and Lewis antigens of secretions consist of two glycoprotein chains, 1 and 2 (Table 34.16). The carbohydrate part is linked to a serine or threonine residue of the protein backbone through N-acetyl-D-galactosamine. The structure of chains 1 and 2 is as follows:

1 Gal 1–3GlcNAc ....αGalNAc-serine (or threonine)
2 Gal 1–4GlcNAc ....αGalNAc-serine (or threonine)

The *H*, *A* and *B*-transferases act on the precursor chains in the same way as they do on the precursor chain of the red-cell antigens, *which is a Type-2 chain only*. The transferases act on both glycoprotein chains, converting them first to H substance and then to A or B substances or both.

The A_1 and A_2 transferases are different enzymes: the optimal pH for the A_1 transferase is 6 and for the A_2 transferase is 8. According to Kisailus & Kabat [29] there are structural differences between A_1 and A_2

Table 34.17. Explanation of abbreviations in Tables

Cer	Ceramide (N-acylsphingosine)
Glc	Glucose
Gal	Galactose
Fuc	Fucose
GlcNAc	N-acetyl-D-glucosamine
GalNAc	N-acetyl-D-galactosamine
NeuNAc	N-acetylneuraminic (sialic) acid
Ser	Serine
Thr	Threonine
XIV	Pneumococcus Type XIV polysaccharide

glycoproteins in that A_1 specificity is determined by Type-1 chains, and A_2 specificity by Type-2 chains: we doubt that this is true.

The *L*-gene specified glycosyltransferases can only act on a Type-1 chain. *Lewis antigens are therefore present only in body fluids, for example saliva, and are not an intrinsic part of the red-cell membrane.* They are adsorbed by red cells from the plasma, where they occur as glycosphingolipids. The *L* gene codes for the antigen Le^a. The Le^b antigen is an interaction product of the *H* (and *Se*) and *L* genes. If *A* or *B* genes are

present the glycosphingolipids ALe^b or BLe^b may also be formed (Table 34.13). Table 34.13 shows the structure of Le^a and Le^b glycosphingolipids.

Further details of the biochemistry and biosynthesis of the ABH, Lewis, P and Ii systems are given in an excellent review by Watkins [78].

RHESUS BLOOD GROUPS

Rh and LW

In 1940 Landsteiner & Wiener [79] reported that they had injected Rhesus-monkey red cells into rabbits and guinea-pigs and produced an antibody which, after absorption, agglutinated the red cells of about 85% of white Americans. The antibody was called anti-Rh and the antigen it detected, Rh. In the previous year Levine & Stetson [80] had reported the finding of an unnamed antibody in the serum of a previously untransfused group-O woman who had had a reaction after being transfused with the blood of her group-O husband. The patient subsequently gave birth to a macerated fetus. Levine & Stetson suggested that she had produced an antibody to a fetal erythrocyte antigen inherited from her husband.

The human and animal antibodies appeared to be identical and the name anti-Rh was therefore accepted for the human antibody. It was later found [81, 82] that the two antibodies were not quite the same, for the following reasons:

1 although the animal antibody does not agglutinate Rh-negative cells it combines with them and can be recovered by elution;

2 the animal antibody can distinguish Rh-positive and Rh-negative red cells of adult but not cord bloods; and

3 antibodies of exactly the same specificity can be produced in guinea-pigs in response to injections of either Rh-positive or Rh-negative cells.

By the time these discoveries were made, the name anti-Rh for the human antibody had become widely established; the animal antibody was therefore renamed anti-LW [83] in honour of Landsteiner & Wiener.

The relationship of Rh and LW may be simply illustrated (Fig. 34.3) on the lines suggested by Giblett [84].

Clinical importance

After Levine & Stetson's discovery, many anti-Rh antibodies were found in the serum of both males and females, and the clinical importance of the Rh blood groups became established. Rhesus isoimmunization may occur in an Rh-negative person transfused with Rh-positive blood or in an Rh-negative mother bear-

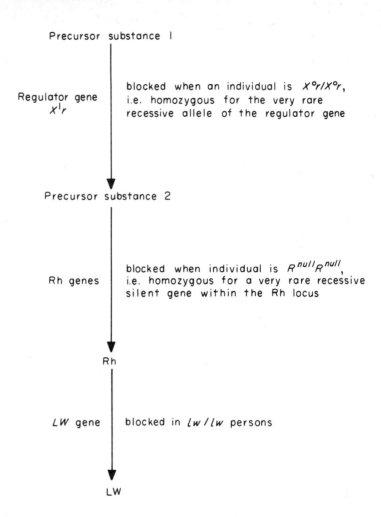

Fig. 34.3. Genetic pathways in the synthesis of Rh and LW antigens: modified from Giblett [84].

Table 34.18. The Wiener and Fisher–Race notations for Rhesus blood groups

	Wiener			Fisher–Race			Frequency in England [6]
	Allele	Antigen	Factors	Gene complex	Antigen	Shorthand notation	
$Rh_0(D)$ positive	R^1	Rh_1	Rh_0, rh′, hr″	*CDe*	CDe	R_1	0·40356
	R^2	Rh_2	Rh_0, hr′, rh″	*cDE*	cDE	R_2	0·16701
	R^0	Rh_0	Rh_0, rh′, hr″	*cDe*	cDe	R_0	0·01855
	R^z	Rh_z	Rh_0, rh′, rh″	*CDE*	CDE	R_z	0·00082
$Rh_0(D)$ negative	r	rh	hr′, hr″	*cde*	ce	r	0·38205
	r′	rh′	rh′, hr″	*Cde*	Ce	r′	0·00489
	r″	rh″	hr′, rh″	*cdE*	cE	r″	0·00295
	r^y	rh^y	rh′, rh″	*CdE*	CE	r_y	Very rare

ing an Rh-positive child. Since fetal red cells usually enter the maternal circulation at or near delivery, the first Rh-positive baby of a Rh-negative mother is usually normal. Subsequent Rh-positive babies, however, are likely to be affected with haemolytic disease as the result of passage of re-stimulated maternal antibody through the placenta.

ABO incompatibility between mother and fetus, as in the case of a group-O mother with a group-A fetus, tends to protect against isoimmunization, probably because the incompatible fetal cells are destroyed in the maternal circulation before they can act as a stimulus to antibody formation.

Extended Rhesus system

Besides the original Rh antigen, which permits a simple subdivision into Rh-positive and Rh-negative, there are other antigens in the Rhesus system. Before describing these antigens it is necessary to comment on Rhesus blood-group notation. At present three notations are used—Wiener, Fisher–Race and Rosenfield; the Wiener notation has priority.

The Wiener and Fisher–Race notations (Table 34.18) are based on different genetic concepts.

Wiener holds that a gene at a single locus on each chromosome controls the entire system, and that there are multiple alleles of this gene. Each gene produces an agglutinogen which consists of various factors which can be identified by specific antibodies. For example,

the gene R^I determines the agglutinogen Rh, which consists of three factors, Rh_o, hr′ and hr″. The Fisher–Race theory postulates three closely linked loci, each of which has two alternative genes. Each gene, with one exception, produces an antigen which is given the same notation as the gene. The gene pairs are C, c; D, d; E, e; the genes give rise to the antigens C, c, D, E and e. The d gene is thought to have no product.

Rosenfield et al. [85] have adopted a numerical notation, first proposed by Murray [86]. This notation has no genetic basis; it is entirely a phenotype notation based on serological reactions, for example Rh: 1, 2, −3, 4, −5 indicates that red cells are positive with anti-Rh_1, anti-Rh_2 and anti-Rh_4 and negative with anti-Rh_3 and anti-Rh_5. This corresponds to the phenotype Rh_1 of Wiener and the CcDee phenotype or the CDe/cde genotype of the CDE notation. The numerical notation gives a clear indication of which antisera were used and has the additional merit of easy application to the storage and retrieval of computer data. The three notations for Rhesus antigens are shown in Table 34.19.

Since the Fisher–Race notation is adequate for general clinical use we shall use it hereafter. In this notation the human anti-Rh of Levine & Stetson is anti-D. Each of the other antigens, C, c, E and e has its corresponding antibody so that the fundamental importance of the Rhesus system may be restated as follows. If an individual lacks any of the Rhesus

Table 34.19. Notations for Rhesus antigens

Rosenfield	Rh–Hr	CDE and miscellaneous notations	Rosenfield	Rh–Hr	CDE and miscellaneous notations
Rh 1	Rh_o	D	21		C^G
2	rh′	C	22		CE
3	rh″	E	23		D^{Wiel}
4	hr′	c	24		E^t
5	hr″	e	25		LW
6	hr	ce	26		Deal (C-like)
7	rh_1	Ce	27		cE
8	rh^{w1}	C^w	28	hr^H	
9	rh^x	C^x	29		Total Fh
10	hr^v	V, ce^s	30		$D^{Cor}Go^a$
11	rh^{w2}	E^w	31	hr^B	
12	rh^G	G	32		Troll
13	Rh^A		33		Har
14	Rh^B		34	Hr^B	Baaso
15	Rh^C		35		1114
16	Rh^D		36		Be^a
17	Hr_o		37		Evans
18	Hr		38		Duclos
19	hr^s		39		C-like
20		VS, e^s	40		Tar

antigens, for example c, and is transfused with red blood cells which carry that antigen, he is likely to produce the corresponding antibody, anti-c: or, if a pregnant woman who lacks any of the antigens, for example, c, has a fetus that has the antigen, she may develop the corresponding antibody, anti-c, so that a subsequent c-positive child may develop haemolytic disease.

According to the Fisher–Race theory the three loci for the Rh genes never separate, so that the genes are transmitted as a gene complex. The three pairs of genes give rise to the eight gene complexes shown in Table 34.18, which also shows the corresponding 'shorthand' notations used to simplify written or verbal communication. Combination of the eight units gives rise to 36 genotypes, for example CDe/cDE. Without anti-d, genotyping requires a family study. If a single individual is phenotyped, his probable genotype is guessed from the frequency of the chromosomes in the population (Table 34.18).

D is the strongest Rhesus antigen and anti-D is therefore the antibody most commonly produced. Anti-C by itself is comparatively rare; it occurs more commonly with anti-D. Of the other antibodies anti-c and anti-E are found much more often than anti-e.

Rhesus antigens and Rhesus-antigen variants

Rare forms of C and E
C^w, C^u and C^x are antigens derived from genes allelic to C and c and E^w, E^u and E^T are antigens derived from genes allelic to E and e.

D^u
D^u is a weak form of D. It is of practical importance in that D^u cells are agglutinated by some anti-D sera but not by others: 'high-grade' D^u cells are agglutinated by many anti-D sera, and 'low-grade' D^u is demonstrable either by a positive indirect antiglobulin test with incomplete (IgG) anti-D or by fixation-elution techniques.

Some examples of D^u represent an inherited weakness of the D antigen; this type of D^u is regularly transmitted from one generation to the next. Other D^us are the result of a 'position effect' in which a *Cde* gene complex depresses a normal D in the 'opposite' gene complex, for example *Cde/CDe*. This type of D^u is not regularly transmitted from one generation to the next: if the *CDe* complex accompanies a gene complex other than *Cde* this D antigen is fully expressed. D^u blood is D-positive. Many clinicians, however, regard D^u persons to be D-positive as blood donors but to be D-negative as transfusion recipients or expectant mothers, because of reports that D^u persons may very rarely form anti-D antibodies in response to exposure to the D-antigen. It is very doubtful, however, if this

actually happens. It is much more likely that all the persons who make anti-D are either D variants or D^u variants (see below).

D variant
The D-antigen is a mosaic of several parts. The red cells of an individual may lack one of the parts, so that after exposure to red cells with normal D antigens, he may make antibody to the missing part. Since normal D-positive cells contain this part the antibody would appear to be anti-D.

D^u variant
When essentially the same situation occurs in a D^u person, he is classified as a D^u variant.

Anti-D in the serum of a D-positive person
If anti-D is found in the serum of a truly D-positive person it is suggestive evidence that the person is a D variant. Two other possibilities need to be excluded. The anti-D may in fact be an autoantibody which appears to be D-specific, or it may really be the closely similar alloantibody or autoantibody anti-LW.

The subject of depressed Rhesus phenotypes is reviewed by Tippett [87].

Compound antigens
There are four antigens in the Rhesus system which may be visualized as the joint products of the theoretically inseparable *CDE* genes. They are *ce* (formerly f). *Ce* (rh₁), *CE* and *cE*. There are four corresponding antibodies, anti-ce, anti-Ce, anti-CE and anti-cE. The antibodies react only if the antigen determinants are in the same gene complex: anti-ce, for example, reacts with CDe/cde but not CDe/cDE.

The Rhesus antigen G
Allen & Tippett studied a sample of red cells which reacted with anti-C+D sera but not with specific anti-C or anti-D [6]. They explained their observations by suggesting that the red cells contained an antigen G which occurs with C or D and that the anti-C+D sera were really anti-D+G or anti-C+D+G.

Six of the eight *CDE* gene complexes give rise to G; the exceptions are cde and cdE. The discovery of G provided a solution to two previously unexplained serological puzzles. The first was how previously untransfused pregnant cde/cde women with C-negative husbands apparently made anti-C+D, and the second was how cde/cde mothers with Cde/cde fetuses made anti-C+D. The explanation, of course, is that anti-D+G was the antibody in the first example and anti-C+G in the second.

Rhesus antigens in Negroes

The Rhesus antigens of Negroes present special problems which space does not permit us to discuss; a detailed account is given by Race & Sanger [6].

Suppression

Rare bloods which lack representation of one or more of the three pairs of allelic genes have been discovered; for example $cD/cD-$, $-D-/-D-$ and Rh_{null} or $---/---$. It would readily be understood that if a $-D-/-D-$ person is immunized against the bloods of normal persons he may develop anti-C, anti-c, anti-E and anti-e or more complex antibodies, so that only other $-D-/-D-$ bloods would be compatible. Similarly, Rh_{null} persons could make anti-C, anti-c, anti-D, anti-E and anti-e or more complex antibodies. The Rh_{null} state may be associated with changes in other blood-group antigens, such as those of the MNSsUu system, and with a chronic mild haemolytic anaemia [88].

It will be seen from Figure 34.3 that the Rh_{null} condition could arise either when a person is homozygous for a rare recessive gene X^0r, allelic to a common regulator gene X^1r, or when there is homozygosity for a rare silent or amorphic gene R_{null} within the Rh locus. The regulator type can be recognized when a parent or child has Rhesus antigens. In the amorphic type of Rh_{null}, family studies may show, for example, an apparently homozygous CDe/CDe parent with an apparently homozygous cDE/cDE child; the true genotypes are $CDe/---$ and $---/cDE$ respectively.

Rh_{mod} is similar to Rh_{null}: the Rhesus antigens are present but depressed. Other depressed Rhesus antigens are described by Tippett [87].

Rhesus antigen sites

The number of D-antigen sites on the red cells has been calculated to range from 9900 in CDe/cde to 333 000 in cDE/cDE [20].

Rhesus antibodies

Rhesus antibodies occur as complete (IgM) or, much more commonly, as incomplete (IgG) antibodies. Incomplete antibodies combine with antigen sites on the erythrocyte surface but are too small to cause agglutination unless the normal state of inter-erythrocytic repulsion is reduced by lowering their negative charge. This can be done by treating the red cells with certain proteolytic enzymes, e.g. trypsin, ficin or bromelin. Proteolytic enzymes also serve to reduce steric hindrance and promote coalescence of antigen sites. Incomplete antibody can also be demonstrated by suspending the red cells in 20–30% bovine albumin. Albumin acts by raising the dielectric constant of the erythrocyte medium [89].

Another very effective method of demonstrating incomplete antibody is by the antiglobulin (Coombs) test [90]. This test demonstrates incomplete antibody adherent to the red-cell surface. The test is carried out by washing the red cells to reduce contamination by plasma to negligible proportions, resuspending the cells in 'saline' to make a 20% suspension, and adding anti-human-globulin serum usually prepared in rabbits or goats. The antiglobulin antibodies bridge the gap between incomplete blood-group antibody bound to the erythrocytes and cause the cells to agglutinate. The direct antiglobulin test also detects erythrocytes sensitized *in vivo* and is invaluable in the diagnosis of haemolytic disease of the newborn and autoimmune haemolytic anaemia.

The indirect test is used to detect incomplete antibodies. Here the red cells are first exposed to antibody in the appropriate way and the same procedure as for the direct test is then adopted.

Chemistry and biosynthesis of Rhesus antigens

Relatively little is known about the chemistry of Rhesus antigens. They are probably proteins, structurally linked to membrane lipid [91]. The biosynthetic pathway in their formation is unknown.

Prevention of Rhesus Isoimmunization

Since ABO incompatibility between mother and fetus (e.g. group-O mother, group-A fetus) protects against Rhesus isoimmunization, probably because fetal red cells are destroyed by maternal antibody before they can stimulate antibody formation, it was thought that anti-D antibody, administered as soon as possible after delivery, and certainly within 72 hours, could prevent Rhesus haemolytic disease [92]. This proved to be true. It is unlikely that rapid removal of fetal cells from the maternal circulation is the sole protective mechanism; it could be that blocking of antigen sites on the erythrocyte surface prevents their attachment to antibody-forming cells.

In Britain all D-negative women, regardless of parity or ABO groups, who give birth to a D-positive child are given 100 μg of anti-D immunoglobulin intramuscularly; all D-negative women who have had therapeutic abortions and who are not sterilized simultaneously are given 50 μg. D-negative women whose pregnancy is terminated after the 20th week and whose fetus is D-positive should receive 100 μg. The blood of all D-negative women giving birth to D-positive fetuses after the 20th week is screened for fetal cells by the Kleihauer method. The size of the bleed is calculated by comparison with a prepared standard representing a transplacental haemorrhage of 5 ml. If a larger bleed occurs the dose of the anti-D is increased proportionately (see below). Failure to prevent isoimmunization is almost invariably due to previous sensitization, either in a previous pregnancy or earlier in the one which has just ended.

In massive transplacental haemorrhage or in transfusion of D-positive blood to an unimmunized woman of child-bearing age, 25 μg anti-D immunoglobulin per ml of red cells transfused should be given intramuscularly.

Since primary isoimmunization occurs during pregnancy it would seem logical to give anti-Rh immunoglobulin antenatally to all Rhesus-negative mothers. Fears that this may adversely affect the fetus are probably groundless because relatively little of the injected dose would actually cross the placenta. Trials in Canada and elsewhere have shown this practice to be safe and effective. Whether the increased workload and cost involved in such a scheme is justified in terms of the marginal improvement observed in success rates needs to be carefully considered: the subject is discussed by Tovey [93].

OTHER BLOOD GROUP SYSTEMS

The MN system

This system consists fundamentally of the antigens M, N, S, s and U and their corresponding antibodies. The antigens M and N are derived from allelic genes M and N; the antigens S and s are controlled by allelic genes S and s. The loci for the M and N and the S and s genes are situated so close together that it seems that the inheritance of the MNSs antigens is controlled by the gene complexes MS, Ms, NS, Ns. Nevertheless, there are striking differences between M and N on the one hand and S and s on the other. For example, M and N are poor antigens in man, so that immune anti-M and anti-N are rare; S and s, however, are potent antigens so that immune anti-S and anti-s are more common, and they give rise to transfusion reactions or haemolytic disease of the newborn. Recently, antibodies similar, but not completely identical to anti-N have been reported in the case of patients on renal dialysis when formaldehyde-sterilized dialysers are used [94].

The antigen U is derived from a very frequent gene U allelic to a silent gene u. Most U-negatives are S- and s-negative; rare bloods have been described which are S- and s-negative and U-positive.

The complexity of the MN system is increased by the existence of many antigen variants, such as M_1. M^c, M^g, M^k, M^z, M^v, M^r, N_2, and of 'satellite' antigens, for example Hu, He, Mi^a, Vw, Mur and Hil. M and N variants have been studied in great depth by Metaxas *et al.* [95] (for information on 'satellite' antigens see Ref. 6).

The MN system is potentially the most useful of all blood-group systems in paternity investigations.

Chemistry and biosynthesis

The antigens of the MN system are glycoproteins. The carbohydrate part of the glycoprotein is attached to a serine or threonine residue of the protein component and is believed to have the structure shown in Table 34.20. The chief structural determinant of M and N is N-acetyl-neuraminic acid (NeuNAc), also known as sialic acid.

There are two different concepts of the chemical basis of MN specificity. The prevailing view [96–99] is that there is no difference whatever in the carbohydrate structure of M and N and that the serological differences between them are dependent on conformational differences in the outward 'display' of the carbohydrate chains, secondary to differences in the aminoacid sequence of the protein chains. It has been shown that serine is the NH_2 terminus for M, and leucine for N. Furthermore the fifth amino acid from the NH_2 terminus is glycine for M and glutamic acid for N. In this concept M and N genes control the differences in amino-acid sequence. The other view [100] is that the carbohydrate structures of M and N are different, and that M and N genes determine glycosyltransferases

Table 34.20. Carbohydrate structure of M and N

	Structure*	Remarks
Ser . . . . (or Thr)	αGalNAcβGalNeuNAc	M or N
Ser . . . . (or Thr)	αGalNAcβGalNeuNAc	N
Ser . . . . (or Thr)	αGalNAcβGalNeuNAcNeuNAc	M

* For meaning of the abbreviations see Table 34.17.

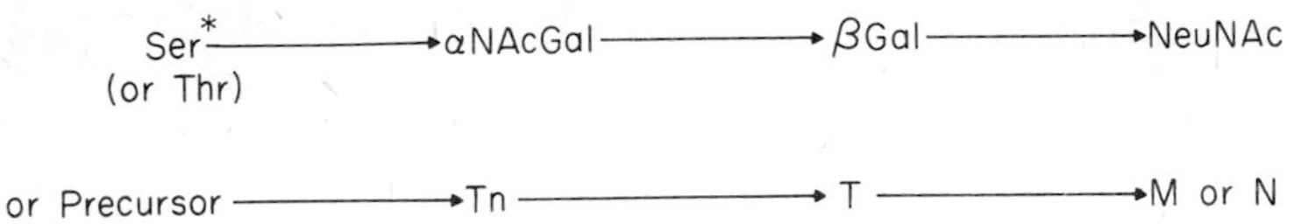

$$\begin{array}{ccccc}
\text{Ser}^* & \longrightarrow \alpha\text{NAcGal} & \longrightarrow \beta\text{Gal} & \longrightarrow \text{NeuNAc} \\
\text{(or Thr)} & & & \\
\end{array}$$

$$\text{or Precursor} \longrightarrow \text{Tn} \longrightarrow \text{T} \longrightarrow \text{M or N}$$

Fig. 34.4. MN biosynthetic pathway.

responsible for the synthesis of the different carbohydrate chains. In this concept N is the precursor of M. Both schools of thought are agreed that Tn and T (p. 1418) are intermediate stages in the biosynthesis of M and N. The MN biosynthetic pathway is shown in Figure 34.4.

The MN antigens are carried on the major sialoglycoprotein (PAS-1, Glycophorin A). The Ss antigens are not carried on this glycoprotein but on another membrane glycoprotein (PAS-3, Glycophorin B) [99]: they are probably part of the polypeptide component of the glycoprotein.

The Lutheran blood groups

The antigens of this system are Lu^a and Lu^b, derived from Lu^a and Lu^b genes. The phenotypes are:

Lu(a+b−)	rare
Lu(a+b+)	about 8% of English people
Lu(a−b+)	about 92% of English people
Lu(a−b−)	very rare

The antibodies are anti-Lu^a, anti-Lu^b and anti-$Lu^a + Lu^b$.

Family studies show that there are two kinds of Lu(a−b−), dominant and recessive.

The system is of little clinical importance. However, it has provided two 'firsts' in blood-group genetics—the first example of autosomal linkage in man when it was shown that the Lutheran and ABH secretor genes were carried on the same chromosome, and the first example of a 'minus-minus' phenotype, Lu(a−b−), which occurs as a dominant character. There are other Lutheran antigens and para-antigens each detected by the corresponding rare antibody [6].

The Kell system

The main antigens of this system are K and k, which are controlled by allelic K and k genes. Genotype frequencies in England are KK: 0·0021; Kk: 0·0872; kk: 0·9197.

Other antigens in this system are Kp^a, Kp^b and Js^a and Js^b, each controlled by a pair of allelic genes.

The antibodies of this system are anti-K, anti-k, anti-Kp^a, anti-Kp^b, anti-Js^a, and anti-K^u. The antibodies of the Kell system are best demonstrated by the antiglobulin method. Anti-K^u is found in immunized persons of the very rare phenotype K^o, i.e. in the serum of persons who are K-k-Kp(a−b−)Js(a−b−); this antibody agglutinates all bloods except K^o.

The Kell system is clinically important because Kell antibodies give rise to haemolytic transfusion reactions and to haemolytic disease of the newborn. There are other Kell antigens and para-antigens, each detected by the corresponding rare antibody [6]. Since anti-K is not infrequently associated with haemolytic transfusion reactions, blood transfused in an emergency without crossmatching should be K-negative.

Kell groups and chronic granulomatous disease

Giblett *et al.* [101] drew attention to an association between rare Kell groups and some patients with chronic granulomatous disease (CGD), an inherited X-linked defect in neutrophil function, in which there is a high susceptibility to infection, even by low-grade pathogens (see Chapter 16). A potential transfusion hazard arises from the capacity of CGD patients to make Kell-system antibodies which react with the red cells of almost everyone else. Indeed Giblett *et al.* [101] advise that transfusion should be avoided for as long as possible and that CGD should be suspected in any child with recurrent infection for whom it is difficult to find compatible blood.

Both normal erythrocytes and normal leucocytes carry the K_x antigen, a substrate for the formation of normal Kell antigens. The rare erythrocyte Kell group variant associated with CGD is the McLeod phenotype. Most, but not all, persons of this phenotype have CGD. To identify this phenotype and distinguish it from another rare Kell variant, K_o, an antibody, anti-K_x, is required. This antibody does not agglutinate McLeod cells, which lack K_x, but agglutinates K_o cells, which are very rich in K_x.

There are two types of CGD: in Type I the red-cell Kell antigens, including K_x, are normal; in Type II the red cells are of the McLeod phenotype. In both types the leucocytes lack K_x.

McLeod erythrocytes are morphologically abnormal: anisocytosis and acanthocytosis are seen in blood films. McLeod himself, who does not have CGD and is apparently healthy, has an enlarged spleen, reticulocytosis and a reduced haptoglobin level, indicative of a compensated haemolytic anaemia.

Further details, along with a discussion of the mode of inheritance of CGD, are given by Marsh *et al.* [102].

The Duffy system

The Duffy blood-group system fundamentally involves two antigens, Fy^a and Fy^b (derived from allelic genes *Fy^a* and *Fy^b*), and the two antibodies anti-Fy^a and anti-Fy^b. About two-thirds of the English population are Fy(a+), and belong either to the phenotype Fy(a+b−) or Fy(a+b+). About two-thirds of Negroes have the phenotype Fy(a−b−), which is almost unknown in Caucasians.

Duffy antibodies may cause haemolytic transfusion reactions or haemolytic disease of the newborn. They are usually demonstrated only by the indirect antiglobulin technique; their reactions are delicate and the tests require special care. The Fy^a and Fy^b antigens are destroyed by some proteolytic enzymes.

The existence of a gene *Fy*, allelic to *Fy^a* and *Fy^b*, which has no product, is postulated to explain the Negro phenotype Fy(a−b−). Fy(a−b−) is very rare in Whites. The genotypes Fy^{a}Fy and Fy^{b}Fy have however been demonstrated. There are thought to be two other genes in Whites, *Fy*, which, as in Negroes, produces no antigen, and *Fy^x* which produces an antigen Fy^x. Fy^x reacts only with certain anti-Fy^b sera; the cells take up antibody, which on elution is shown to be anti-Fy^b. An antibody, anti-Fy3, has been described by Albrey *et al.* [103]. This antibody reacts with all red cells except Fy(a−b−). Absorption failed to reveal separate anti-Fy^a and anti-Fy^b antibodies; the antibody must therefore be regarded as anti-Fy^a + Fy^b. Oddly enough, treatment of red cells with papain enhances the reactions of anti-Fy3; Albrey *et al.* think the antibody is specific for the precursor substance for Fy^a and Fy^b. Fy4 is an antigen detected by anti-Fy4, an antibody which reacts with all Fy(a−b−) cells and with the majority of Negro Fy(a+b−) and Fy(a−b+) cells [104]. Fy5 is an antigen detected by anti-Fy5, an antibody which was found to react with all red cells which have either Fy^a or Fy^b and with Fy(a−b−) cells of a White person, but not Negro Fy(a−b−) or with Rh$_{null}$ cells [105].

Duffy blood groups and malaria
There is an incompletely understood relationship between Duffy groups and malaria [106]. Fy(a−b−) persons appear to be resistant to *Plasmodium vivax* malaria: the parasites are unable to enter Fy(a−b−) cells. This would account for the evolution of a high incidence of Fy(a−b−) in West Africa, and the resistance of its people to *Plasmodium vivax* malaria.

The Kidd system
This system consists of the antigens Jk^a and Jk^b and the corresponding antibodies. The antigens are determined by *Jk^a* and *Jk^b* genes. The phenotypes are Jk(a+b−), Jk(a−b+), Jk(a+b+) and the rare Jk(a−b−). About 76% of persons are Jk(a+).

Because of difficulty in obtaining monospecific anti-Jk^b it is difficult to give a precise figure for Jk(b+). Anti-Jk^a + Jk^b antibodies have been demonstrated in a few Jk(a−b−) persons after transfusion. Kidd antibodies are sometimes difficult to demonstrate and may require antiglobulin tests on enzyme-treated cells. All Kidd antibodies bind Complement and the best results are obtained with fresh serum and an antiglobulin serum which contains anti-Complement antibody. The proteolytic enzyme trypsin is widely recommended for this purpose; we prefer papain. Kidd antibodies may cause immediate or delayed haemolytic transfusion reactions or haemolytic disease of the newborn.

Diego blood groups
The genes *Di^a* and *Di^b* give rise to the antigens Di^a and Di^b. Di^a is almost entirely confined to Mongoloid races. The phenotypes are Di(a+b−), Di(a−b+) and Di(a+b+).

Yt blood groups
This system consists of a very common antigen Yt^a and a very rare one Yt^b. The antigens are under the control of *Yt^a* and *Yt^b* genes. The phenotypes of this system are Yt(a+b−), Yt(a−b+) and Yt(a+b+). The antibodies are anti-Yt^a and anti-Yt^b. Because of the high incidence of Yt^a it is difficult to find compatible blood for any Yt(a−) patient who has made anti-Yt^a.

The Xg^a system
The discovery of Xg^a and the demonstration that the relevant gene was carried on the X chromosome [107] was without doubt the most exciting event in blood-group genetics. Males have only one gene for this system, instead of two as in all other systems. Xg(a+) males pass Xg^a to their daughters but not to their sons. About 65% of males and 88% of females in Britain are Xg(a+).

Anti-Xg^a was first found in a man who had had many transfusions. Studies of Xg^a have been useful in determining the origin of X chromosomes in cases of aneuploidy (e.g. Turner's syndrome), and in the mapping of the X chromosome.

The Dombrock system
The demonstration of the Dombrock (Do^a) antigen is possible with certain antiglobulin sera. About 64% of northern Europeans are Do(a+). So far only a few examples of anti-Do^a have been found, all in transfused patients and usually in combination with other antibodies such as anti-Fy^a and anti-E.

Auberger blood group
The antibody anti-Au^a, defining the only known antigen, Au^a, of this system was produced in response

to transfusion. Tests carried out in Paris and London show that 80–85% of Caucasians are Au(a +).

The Colton system

There are two antigens in this system, Co^a (very common) and Co^b (comparatively rare) determined by *Co^a* and *Co^b* genes respectively. There are three antibodies, anti-Co^a, anti-Co^b and anti-Co^{a}Co^b. Anti-Co^{a}Co^b was made by a person whose red cells are Co(a − b −). The antibodies are best demonstrated by antiglobulin tests on papain-treated red cells [6].

The Sd^a blood group

Sd^a is an unusual blood-group character. Even red cells which react 'strongly' with anti-Sd^a give a weak mixed-field reaction, so that both good antisera and some expertise are required to distinguish weak positives from negatives. About 91% of English people are Sd(a +).

Sd^a substance is present, independently of ABH and Lewis substances, in saliva and other secretions; the highest concentrations are found in urine.

Recently some evidence has been obtained in support of a relationship between Sd^a and the red-cell character Cad (p. 1420).

The Scianna system

There are two antigens in the Scianna system: the common Sc1 (formerly Sm) and the rare Sc2 (formerly Bu^a). There are very rare persons whose red cells lack both antigens. The antibodies of this system are anti-Sc1 and anti-Sc2 [6].

'Indefinite' blood groups

A number of blood-group antigens have proved difficult to understand genetically or serologically. Among these is Bg^a, which probably includes the Bennett, Goodspeed, Sturgeon or Donna antigens and the antigens Ho and Ot. There is evidence to show that Bg^a and the leucocyte antigen HLA-B7 may be identical and that anti-Bg^a may be regarded as a leucocyte antibody. Further details are given on page 1422.

The antigen Cs^a also fits into this category, as do the Chido and Rodgers blood-group antigens. Chido and Rodgers blood-groups have recently acquired scientific importance.

Chido, Rodgers and C4

The genes which determine Chido and Rodgers blood groups are carried on chromosome 6; i.e. they are linked to the genes for HLA, Bf, C2 and C4. O'Neill *et al.* [108] have shown that Chido and Rodgers blood groups are distinct antigenic components of the fourth component, C4, of human Complement; the electrophoretic pattern of C4 is dependent on the Chido and Rodgers phenotype. These antigens, detectable on red cells, are more easily demonstrated in plasma. Most persons are both Chido (Ch^a)- and Rodgers (Rg^a)-positive. On electrophoresis their plasma forms four slow-moving and four fast-moving bands. Chido-negative plasma shows only the four fast-moving and Rodgers-negative plasma only the four slow-moving bands. Persons who are both Chido and Rodgers negative are C4-deficient. Chido and Rodgers determinants are probably located on the C4d fragment of C4 [109].

'Private' or very infrequent antigens

The best known antigen of this class is Wr^a. Some antigens are so rare that they have been found only in a single individual or in a single family. A complete list of very infrequent antigens is given in Ref. 6, page 431. Some private antigens have been found to belong to established blood-group systems. For example, the infrequent antigen Go^a has been accommodated in the Rhesus system (Table 34.19).

'Public' or very frequent antigens

Besides H, U, Tj^a, Yt^a, I and other frequent antigens which are part of well-established blood-group systems, there are other common antigens which demand attention. These antigens include Ve^a (Vel), Ge, Lan, Co^a, Gy^a, At^a amd En^a, each detected by its corresponding antibody. If a person negative for any of these very frequent antigens produces the corresponding antibody it will obviously be extremely difficult to obtain compatible blood; the first search must be made among the patient's siblings.

AGGLUTININS FROM SEEDS

The seeds of many plants, chiefly legumes, contain proteins which agglutinate red cells. Most seed agglutinins react unspecifically; some are blood-group-specific [110, 111]. The various specificities which have so far been found are anti-A$_1$, anti-(A + B), anti-B, anti-H, anti-M, anti-N, anti-(A + N) anti-T, anti-Tk, anti-Tn and anti-Cad. Seed agglutinins are widely referred to as lectins; the term, originally proposed by Boyd [112], is derived from the latin word *legere* which means to choose or to pick out. Seed agglutinins have proved to be useful in blood grouping and in blood-group research.

The most widely used seed agglutinins are those derived from *Dolichos biflorus* and *Ulex europaeus*. *Dolichos biflorus* seeds contain an anti-A agglutinin which reacts so much more strongly on A_1 or A_1B than on A_2 or A_2B cells that it is virtually A_1 specific. In fact, mere dilution of *Dolichos* seed extract provides a reagent which distinguishes A_1 and A_1B cells from those of the weaker subgroups of A and AB in a few seconds. Useful anti-A agglutinins are obtained from many varieties of Lima bean. Extracts of the tree fungus *Fomes (Polyporus) fomentarius* contain a fairly good anti-B.

Ulex europaeus seeds contain anti-H; *Ulex* extract is very useful in the classification of secretors and non-secretors, particularly in group-O persons (p. 1397). Other good sources of anti-H are the seeds of *Lotus tetragonolobus*, *Laburnum alpinum* and *Cytisus sessilifolius*.

Vicia graminea seeds are a useful source of anti-N. Peanuts (*Arachis hypogaea*) contain strong anti-T [113]. *Salvia sclarea* contains a useful anti-Tn [114], and *Leonurus cardiaca* an anti-Cad lectin [115].

Seed agglutinins are easily inhibited by monosaccharide components of blood-group-active structures. In fact, some of the earliest indications of the chemical basis of human blood-group specificity were obtained from studies of the inhibition of seed agglutinins by simple sugars.

Seed agglutinins have proved useful in the elucidation of polyagglutination (see below).

AGGLUTININS FROM INVERTEBRATE ANIMALS

Many invertebrate animals contain agglutinins for human red cells [116]. The albumin glands [116] or, better still, the eggs [117] of certain snails, e.g. *Helix hortensis*, *Helix pomatia*, *Helix aspersa*, *Otala lactea*, *Euhadra periomphala* and others, contain very strong anti-A agglutinins. Some snail anti-A reagents withstand very high dilution and are therefore economical in automated blood grouping. These agglutinins were named protectins [118] because it is thought that they serve to protect snail eggs during their exposure to open air. They are now classified as lectins.

POLYAGGLUTINATION

Polyagglutination is the agglutination, irrespective of blood group, by a variable number of sera, of altered, defective or otherwise abnormal erythrocytes. It there-fore gives rise to blood-grouping problems. The subject has been reviewed by Bird [119, 120].

Polyagglutination may occur in the following circumstances:

1 *Due to adsorption by erythrocytes of extraneous antigens.* In this form of polyagglutination bacteria or bacterial antigen is adsorbed on to the surface of the red cells, which are then agglutinated by sera which contain specific anti-bacterial antibody.

2 *Due to structural peculiarities of the erythrocyte membrane.* (i) Enzyme alteration of the erythrocyte membrane with exposure of cryptantigens T, Tk. (ii) Specific transferase deficiency, for example Tn. (iii) Rare inherited erythrocyte receptors, for example Cad and those present on HEMPAS red cells.

The various red cells are polyagglutinable because the corresponding antibodies are present in most adult human sera.

T transformation

This is the commonest form of red-cell polyagglutinability. It is due to the action of bacterial or viral neuraminidase on the erythrocyte surface. The enzyme splits off sialic acid and exposes the T receptor. It is usually seen as an *in-vitro* state when blood specimens are contaminated after collection; *in-vivo* T transformation is not uncommon and is usually a transient condition. T-transformed red cells are strongly agglutinated by the peanut (*Arachis hypogaea*) lectin. T is an intermediate stage in MN biosynthesis (Fig. 34.4).

Tk polyagglutination

For 47 years T polyagglutination was the only known polyagglutination caused by exposure of a cryptantigen by a microbial enzyme. In 1972 Bird & Wingham [121] described a second form of this type of polyagglutination, which they named Tk. Although Tk cells were agglutinated by peanut extract, there were clear differences between Tk and T (Table 34.21). Tk cells have normal levels of sialic acid and are agglutinated by sera from which anti-T has been removed by absorption. Treatment of the red cells with papain enhances agglutination by the peanut lectin. Inglis *et al.* [121a, 121b] studied a patient whose red cells were both T- and Tk-polyagglutinable. Tk can co-exist with T or with other forms of red-cell polyagglutinability.

Bacteriological studies suggested the involvement of *Bacteroides fragilis*. Shortly afterwards Bird *et al.* [122] examined the blood of a patient with *Bacteroides fragilis* septicaemia and found the red cells to be Tk-polyagglutinable. The involvement of *Bacteroides fragilis* in the pathogenesis of Tk was therefore supported. Inglis later studied a patient with *Bacteroides fragilis* septicaemia whose red cells were not Tk-polyagglutinable. This was shown to be due to the

Table 34.21. Some reactions of polyagglutinable erythrocytes

	Erythrocytes				
Reagent	T	Tk	Th	Tn	Cad
Dolichos biflorus	−	−	−	+	+
Arachis hypogaea (peanut)	+	+ or −	+	−	−
Glycine soja (soya bean)	+	−	−	+	+
BS II	−	+	−	−	−
Salvia sclarea	−	−	−	+	−
Leonurus cardiaca	−	−	−	−	+
Polybrene	−	+	+	−	+
Effect of papain on erythrocyte receptor	Nil	Enhanced		Destroyed	Enhanced

presence of a powerful inhibitor in the patient's plasma. Further studies of Tk by Inglis *et al.* [121b] suggested that exposure of Tk was the result of an enzyme present in certain strains of *Bacteroides fragilis*. A very important advance was the demonstration that *Bandeiraea simplicifolia* II (BS II) lectin studied by Judd *et al.* [123] had the specificity anti-Tk. BS II is therefore a very useful lectin in the elucidation of erythrocyte polyagglutination (Table 34.21).

Many examples of Tk have now been studied and it is becoming increasingly evident that Tk cells often show gross depression of H, A, B, I and i receptors.

It was many years after the discovery of T transformation that neuraminidase was incriminated as the enzyme which was responsible. However, the difficult search for the enzyme responsible for Tk may not last so long and indeed may already be over. Doinel *et al.* [124] have found that an endo-β-galactosidase isolated from *Escherichia freundii* can expose Tk receptors on red cells and cause extreme depression of H, I and i. Presumably some strains of *Bacteroides fragilis* contain the same, or a similar, enzyme. We have also found that certain *Clostridia* and *Pneumococci* expose Tk receptors on red cells.

It seems very likely that Tk is situated deep in the biosynthetic pathway common to the ABH and Ii and P$_1$ antigens. Studies of the endo-β-galactosidase from *Escherichia freundii* show that the enzyme splits deeply situated Galβ1-4GlcNAc linkages and these observations support the view of Judd *et al.* [123] that N-acetyl-glucosamine is the immunodominant sugar in Tk specificity. The chemical structure of Tk is probably lacto-N-triosylceramide GlcNAcβ1-3Galβ1-4Glu-Cer (p. 1404).

Various examples of Tk cover a wide serological spectrum. In some examples red cells are not agglutinated by the peanut lectin but are agglutinated by BS II, which is a better detector of Tk. In some examples,

pre-treatment of the red cells by proteolytic enzymes is necessary for the demonstration of Tk.

Th polyagglutination

Th polyagglutination, probably also of microbial origin, was first described in 1978 [125]. Th polyagglutinable red cells are also agglutinated by the peanut lectin but are distinguished from T and Tk as shown in Table 34.21.

VA polyagglutination

Two examples have been reported of an odd form of polyagglutination named VA [126–128], one co-existent with Tk [128]. VA is associated with depressed H receptors, and may represent one end of the Tk spectrum. On the other hand, there are serological distinctions between Tk and VA, and VA has some properties not yet known to be associated with Tk. VA may well be due to a bacterial α fucosidase; one cannot say much more about it until other examples are found and studies of the action of various α fucosidases on red cells are performed.

Tn polyagglutination

Tn polyagglutination is also acquired. It has been found in persons previously known to have had normal erythrocytes; once it appears it persists for years. Tn polyagglutination usually gives a mixed-field appearance, which depends on the fact that there are virtually two erythrocyte populations, one of which is deficient in sialic acid. The condition may be associated with haemolytic anaemia, leucopenia and thrombocytopenia [129]. Three examples of Tn polyagglutination in association with acute myelomonocytic leukaemia have been reported [130–132]. In one patient Tn polyagglutination preceded the development of leukaemia [131]; Tn may therefore be a pre-leukaemic state, and all persons with Tn-polyagglutinable red cells should have regular haematological checks. Tn is a precursor of T and is an intermediate stage in MN biosynthesis (p. 1415).

Cad polyagglutination

This is a rare inherited form of polyagglutination described by Cazal *et al.* [133]. New interest in Cad has been aroused by the observation [134] that Cad red cells are very strongly agglutinated by anti-Sd^a. This suggests that Cad may be a very strong Sd^a, so strong that Cad red cells are polyagglutinable. This would mean that most sera contain anti-Sd^a which is too weak to be detected by testing with ordinary Sd(a+) cells. The fact that 91% of the population is Sd(a+) does not necessarily contradict this view, because the co-existence of antigen and weak specific antibody, inactive at body temperature, is not unknown in blood-group serology. An alternative explanation is that strong Sd^a antigen is an associated change in Cad erythrocytes. N-acetyl-D-galactosamine is the chief determinant of Cad specificity.

Seed agglutinins and polyagglutinable erythrocytes

The classification of polyagglutinable erythrocytes once required time-consuming absorption tests to establish identity with known examples. Seed agglutinins are now used for the rapid identification of polyagglutinable red cells (Table 34.21).

Effect of polybrene on polyagglutinable erythrocytes

The highly positively charged substance polybrene is a very strong aggregator of normal erythrocytes. It acts by neutralizing their negative charge and forming ionic bonds with them. Erythrocytes which are appreciably deficient in sialic acid are not aggregated by polybrene. Polybrene therefore fails to aggregate T-transformed cells, or Tn cells, but strongly aggregates Cad cells.

Effect of papain

Papain has little or no effect on T, destroys Tn, impairs or destroys Th, and enhances Tk and Cad. The correct ABO blood group of Tn cells can be determined by testing papainized cells.

Elucidation of polyagglutination

The various forms of polyagglutination can quickly be distinguished (Table 34.21) by the reactions obtained with seed agglutinins and polybrene and by tests done before and after treatment of red cells with papain.

Clinico-pathological aspects of red-cell polyagglutinability

Red-cell polyagglutinability due to microbial enzymes may occur both as an *in-vitro* condition (contaminated blood samples) or as an *in-vivo* state. The *in-vivo* condition may be due to enzymes derived from bacteria or viruses actually present in the bloodstream, or which enter the bloodstream from infected sites in other parts of the body. There must be enough enzyme first to neutralize enzyme inhibitors normally present in plasma. The condition is usually transient but may persist for months, especially in bowel disorders in children (e.g. congenital megacolon [135], neonatal necrotizing enterocolitis [136]). T-, Tk- or Th-polyagglutination, or combinations of two or of all of them, are usually demonstrated.

Some examples of the haemolytic-uraemic syndrome may be due to T transformation of red cells, platelets and kidney cells giving rise to anaemia, thrombocytopenia and renal dysfunction [137].

T and Tn receptors are exposed on the cells of patients with breast and other cancers [138, 139].

Red-cell polyagglutinability may present problems in blood transfusion. Apart from delays due to blood-grouping difficulties, haemolytic transfusion reactions may result from the transfusion of whole blood, because adult plasma normally contains antibodies for polyagglutinable red cells. The potential hazard is avoided by transfusion of washed cells.

BLOOD GROUPS AND LINKAGE

Besides the Lutheran-Secretor linkage mentioned above, other linkages have been established (Table 34.22). The subject is discussed by Race & Sanger [6] and by Giblett [84].

BLOOD GROUPS AND DISEASE

Apart from various associations of blood groups and disease mentioned in the preceding pages, such as the weakening of blood-group antigens in leukaemia, the relationship of anti-P to paroxysmal cold haemoglobinuria, and of the Ii system to various clinical disorders, there are other associations between blood groups and disease. Autoagglutinins showing specificities other than anti-P, anti-I and anti-i may cause autoimmune haemolytic anaemia: the specificity of autoagglutinins is fully treated in Chapter 11.

Whether persons of a particular blood group are more liable to develop a particular disease has been investigated for many years. It seems that group-A persons are more likely than those of groups B or O to develop carcinoma of the stomach or pernicious anaemia, and that non-secretors of group O are more likely to develop duodenal ulcer.

According to Mourant *et al.* [140], group-A persons are more liable to thromboembolic disease. This

Table 34.22. Red-cell blood groups and linkage

Blood-group system	Chromosome number	Condition or marker
ABO	9	Nail–patella syndrome Adenylate kinase
MNSs	4	Sclerotylosis
Rhesus Duffy } Scianna	1	Elliptocytosis 6-phosphogluconate dehydrogenase (PGD) Phosphoglucomutase (PGM_1) A form of congenital cataract
Chido } Rodgers	* 6	HLA Bf C2 C8 PGM_3 Glyoxylase (GLO) Superoxide dismutase (SOD_2)
Xg	X	X-borne ichthyosis Ocular albinism Retinoschisis

* Components of C4.

applies to women taking oral contraceptives, pregnant and puerperal women, and patients with coronary thrombosis. Mourant *et al.* suggest that this association, and the increased liability to haemorrhage in group-O persons with duodenal ulcer, is related to the curious fact, well known to producers of cryoprecipitate, that group-A persons tend to have higher levels of antihaemophilic globulin than others.

Because erythrocytes and microbes have chemically similar antigens, Pettenkofer and his associates [141] suggested that the distribution of blood groups in various populations, discussed in the next section, might be an example of natural selection brought about by epidemic diseases. From the probably erroneous assumption that smallpox virus contains an A-like substance, they concluded that B or O persons whose sera normally contain anti-A antibodies would tend to have milder smallpox than A or AB persons.

The relations of HLA types to various diseases are mentioned below.

POPULATION GENETICS

The incidence of blood-group antigens varies from one race to another. Understandably, most anthropological blood-group surveys have involved the ABO system. The distribution of ABO groups in some populations is shown in Table 34.23. It is seen from the Table that European gypsies have a blood-group distribution similar to that of Asiatic Indians, from whom they are thought to have originated.

Various theories have been offered to explain the racial differences in blood-group distribution. According to one theory there were originally three human races of groups A, B and O respectively, and the modern distribution was the result of migration and intermarriage. Another theory is that the blood groups arose by mutation from one group, probably O; the fact that many isolated South American tribes are exclusively group O (Table 34.23) supports this view. The A gene is thought to have arisen in Europe and the B gene in Asia. The third theory is a reversal of the second: it is postulated that the original group was AB and that A and B, and eventually O, arose from 'loss' mutation. The possible role of epidemics in population genetics is mentioned in the previous section.

Negroid and Mongoloid races have a very high

Table 34.23. Distribution of ABO blood groups in various populations

	O	A	B	AB
United Kingdom	47	42	8	3
European Gypsies	31	27	35	7
Asiatic Indians	33	24	34	9
Japanese	30	39	22	9
Maoris (Polynesians)	40	56	3	1
Some South American tribes	100	0	0	0

incidence of Rh-positives, and the Basques an un-usually high incidence of Rh-negatives (30%). Extensive data on blood-group distribution are given by Boyd [142], Mourant *et al,* [143] and Kopeć [144].

LEUCOCYTE ANTIGENS

In 1952 Dausset & Nenna [145] detected, in the serum of multi-transfused recipients, antibodies which agglutinated human leucocytes. The alloantigens most readily detected on leucocytes are those of the HLA (human leucocyte antigen) system. Monospecific antisera for their determination are generally obtained from pregnant women, the antibody having been stimulated by an HLA alloantigen of the fetus. Although HLA typing was at first determined by an agglutination test, this has largely been replaced by a cytotoxic micro-technique based on dye exclusion [146]. This technique depends on the fact that some dyes, such as trypan blue and eosin, cannot pass through intact cell membranes, but will enter cells, e.g. lymphocytes, when the membrane has been damaged by Complement-fixing antibodies in the presence of Complement. In this procedure, therefore, a suspension of the lymphocytes to be tissue-typed, prepared by flotation, is incubated with micro-volumes of the appropriate test sera in the presence of Complement; trypan blue or eosin is then added. Staining of the cells indicates a positive antigen–antibody interaction. Lymphocytes are used because they give greater reproducibility, and cytotoxic antibodies are more readily found than are leucoagglutinins. HLA antigens are not confined to leucocytes but are present on most tissue cells and, using the red-cell reagent anti-Bg^a, Morton *et al.* [147] have found a correlation between the blood group Bg^a and the HLA-B7 antigen. Subsequent work by the same group [148] has shown that Bg^b is correlated with B17 and Bg^c with A28. Following an attack of infectious mononucleosis the red cells of HLA-B7 patients may show an enhanced reactivity with anti-Bg^a [149]. HLA antigens identified on leucocytes have also been detected on platelets using a micro-Complement-fixing technique [150].

The cluster of linked genes controlling the HLA alloantibodies is located on the autosomal chromosome 6. These antigens recognized by humoral antibodies are determined by the *A, B* and *C* loci and referred to as SD (serum-defined). Other HLA antigens are determined by products of the *D* locus and are recognized by their ability to stimulate T lymphocytes to divide in mixed-lymphocyte culture. These are referred to as LD or lymphocyte-defined antigens. Serological techniques may be used to identify determinants in B lymphocytes which are closely associated,

if not identical with HLA-D determinants, and are known as DR (D-related) alloantigens [151]. B cells are isolated from human lymphocyte suspensions by adding an equal volume of a one per cent suspension of neuraminidase-treated sheep red cells and layering on to Ficoll-Triosil. After centrifugation the rosetted T cells sediment to the bottom of the tube whilst the B lymphocytes remain at the interface; the sheep red cells are removed by hypotonic lysis. The isolated B cells may then be typed by a modified microcytotoxicity technique using pregnancy sera from which antibodies to HLA antigens carried on T lymphocytes have been removed by platelet absorption.

Nomenclature for the HLA antigens is regularly updated at International Histocompatibility Workshops: specificities agreed following the seventh Workshop in 1980 [172] are listed in Table 34.24. The prefix 'w' signifies a provisional specificity.

Analysis of the survival times of skin allografts and the results of renal allografts suggest that the HLA system is the only genetic system besides ABO which has a major influence on human transplantations. On current evidence a successful outcome when a kidney graft is performed between unrelated individuals is most likely to obtain when both donor and recipient are identically matched for HLA-A, -B and -DR antigens [152]. The significance of HLA-C antigen matching has not yet been adequately investigated. Oriol *et al.* [153] claim that when there is HLA non-identity, an Le^a-negative recipient is less likely to reject an Le^a-negative kidney than one from an Le^a-positive donor; this has not yet been confirmed by other workers, however. The clinical importance of HLA-typing in blood transfusion is discussed in Chapter 35. HLA-typing has a considerable potential in medico-legal work, such as problems of disputed paternity, and it has been established that susceptibility of individuals to various diseases is related to their HLA types. Ankylosing spondylitis, for example, is found almost exclusively in persons who are HLA-B27 positive [154], and in a number of diseases in which there are abnormalities of immune response such as coeliac disease, dermatitis herpetiformis, myasthenia gravis, chronic active hepatitis and juvenile diabetes there are significant associations with HLA antigens B8 and DR3. Associations between HLA antigens and disease have been reviewed by Bodmer [155].

Although most HLA antibodies in the blood of pregnant women are IgG in type, they have no adverse effect upon the fetus [156]. Moulinier *et al.* [157] claim that the degree of fetal haemolytic disease is more severe when the mother is doubly sensitized, i.e. to HLA as well as Rh antigens, but this was not confirmed by Tovey *et al.* [158] or Ahrons [156].

Table 34.24. HLA antigen specificities

HLA-A	HLA-B		HLA-C	HLA-D	HLA-DR
A1	B5	Bw46	Cw1	Dw1	DR1
A2	B7	Bw47	Cw2	Dw2	DR2
A3	B8	Bw48	Cw3	Dw3	DR3
A9	B12	Bw49(w21)	Cw4	Dw4	DR4
A10	B13	Bw50(w21)	Cw5	Dw5	DR5
A11	B14	Bw51(5)	Cw6	Dw6	DRw6
Aw19	B15	Bw52(5)	Cw7	Dw7	DR7
Aw23(9)	Bw16	Bw53	Cw8	Dw8	DRw8
Aw24(9)	B17	Bw54(w22)		Dw9	DRw9
A25(10)	B18	Bw55(w22)		Dw10	DRw10
A26(10)	Bw21	Bw56(w22)		Dw11	
A28	Bw22	Bw57(17)		Dw12	
A29	B27	Bw58(17)			
Aw30	Bw35	Bw59			
Aw31	B37	Bw60(40)			
Aw32	Bw38(w16)	Bw61(40)			
Aw33	Bw39(w16)	Bw62(15)			
Aw34	B40	Bw63(15)			
Aw36	Bw41				
Aw43	Bw42				
	Bw44(12)	Bw4			
	Bw45(12)	Bw6			

Koskimies *et al.* [159] report a case of neonatal hyperbilirubinaemia in which anti-HLA B7 was present in high titre in the mother's blood. Since B7 was present in the baby's erythrocytes as the red-cell antigen Bg^a, they suggest that in this instance the fetal haemolytic disease was caused by maternal anti-HLA antibodies.

Neutrophil-specific antigens

Verheught and his colleagues [160] have developed an immunofluorescence test for the detection of granulocyte-specific antibodies and confirm that granulocyte antigens play a major role in causing febrile reactions during blood transfusion (see Chapter 35). Neutrophil-specific antibodies are also associated with alloimmune neonatal neutropenia [161] and autoimmune neutropenia [162, 163], and when present either in donor or recipient plasma may cause pulmonary infiltration by granulocytes. A number of alleles have been described and are given the specificities NA_1, NA_2, NB_1, NC_1, etc. [164].

PLATELET GROUPS

Some human platelet antigens are exclusive to platelets, others are shared with other blood cells. The antigens A and B are common to erythrocytes, leucocytes and platelets, and most if not all HLA antigens are present in platelets.

Antigen systems peculiar to platelets are Pl^A or Zw, Ko and Pl^E. The first platelet antigen to be described was named DUZO; it is not known if DUZO is identical with or related to any antigen of the Pl^A, Ko or Pl^E systems (Table 34.25).

The Pl^A system consists of two antigens Pl^{A1}(Zw^a) and Pl^{A2}(Zw^b) and their corresponding antibodies. In the Ko system, there are two antigens, Ko^a and Ko^b, and two specific antibodies. A rare but serious haemorrhagic complication following transfusion may occur when the recipient's plasma contains anti-Pl^{A1} (Chapter 25, p. 995), and platelet-specific antibodies are also responsible for alloimmune neonatal thrombocytopenia (Chapter 25, p. 994).

Antibodies to platelets are difficult to detect. At present it seems that immunofluorescence microphotometry tests on paraformaldehyde-fixed platelets [165] are best.

SERUM GROUPS

The chief serum- (or plasma-) group systems are immunoglobulins (Gm and Km), haptoglobins, transferrins, Gc, and β-lipoprotein (Ag). An excellent account is given by Giblett [84]. Gm and Ag antibodies may cause transfusion reactions (see Chapter 35).

Table 34.25. Platelet antigens and gene frequencies

System	Antigen	Country	Number tested	% positive	Gene frequency
Pl^A	Pl^{A1}	The Netherlands	287	97·6	0·845
	Pl^{A2}	The Netherlands	597	26·8	0·144
Ko	Ko^a	North America	1696	14·3	0·074
	Ko^b	North America	1980	99·4	0·920
Pl^E	Pl^{E1}	North America	1025	? all	
	Pl^{E2}	North America	200	5	0·025
DUZO	DUZO	France	82	22	

MOSAICS AND CHIMAERAS

Mosaics and chimaeras are of wide scientific interest. A mosaic is an individual with two cell populations of a single zygote lineage, whereas a chimaera is an individual with cells of two zygote lineages.

Mosaics

Blood-group mosaicism is usually acquired as the result of somatic mutation and may be associated with myeloproliferative disorders. An example of blood-group mosaicism in a patient with acute erythroleukaemia has been described by Bird *et al.* [166]. The patient had two red-cell populations, one group B, and the other apparently group O, because the red cells did not react with anti-B. It was shown, however, that the apparent O cells carried weak B antigens, because they were found to adsorb anti-B antibodies.

Other forms of blood-group mosaicism are inherited. One is known as inherited mosaicism within the ABO blood-group system and the terms A$_{mos}$ or B$_{mos}$ are used to indicate whether the A or B antigens are involved. In some families the proportion of A or B to O cells is exactly the same in each affected member. The literature has been reviewed, and an example of a B$_{mos}$ family has been described, by Bird *et al.* [167]. In this family, affected members had significantly reduced levels of serum B-gene-specified glycosyltransferase, which suggests that B$_{mos}$ is a form of weak B. B$_{mos}$ cells, however, can be distinguished from conventional forms of weak B as shown in Table 34.26.

Chimaeras

Blood-group chimaerism is a rare condition with interesting scientific implications; this subject has been reviewed by Race & Sanger [6].

There are two types of chimaerism:
1 twin (haemopoietic) chimaerism; and
2 dispermic (whole-body) chimaerism.

Twin chimaeras

Twin chimaerism is thought to be due to placental vascular anastomoses in dizygotic twins. Blood-cell precursors from one twin lodge in the bone marrow of the other and continue to function in a state of immunological tolerance. Since the grafted cells are genetically programmed to produce blood cells with surface characters (e.g. blood groups) which differ in certain respects to those of the host cells, two blood-cell populations are demonstrable in chimaeric twins. Rushton (personal communication) suggests that the vascular anatomoses may occur in the yolk sac, the earliest site of haemopoiesis. Twin chimaerism usually presents by mixed-field haemagglutination reactions

Table 34.26. Differences between A$_{mos}$ or B$_{mos}$ and inherited weak forms of A and B

	Inherited weak A or B	A$_{mos}$ or B$_{mos}$
Anti-A + B	Stronger than anti-A or anti-B	Not stronger than anti-A or anti-B
Treatment of red cells with proteolytic enzymes	Increases proportion of agglutinable cells	Does not increase proportion of agglutinable cells
Adsorption of anti-A or anti-B	Yes	No

or violations of 'Landsteiner's Law', such as an apparent group-O person who lacks either anti-A or anti-B; other causes of these phenomena must be excluded. The diagnosis of twin chimaerism is easy when both twins are alive and are available for study; when the subject is unaware that he or she is a twin the diagnosis is less obvious. If chimaerism is confined to haemopoietic cells it is almost certain, in the absence of a living twin, that there indeed had been a twin, who failed to thrive or was aborted.

Dispermic chimaeras

Dispermic chimaerism is thought to be due to the fertilization of an egg by two sperms which entered it simultaneously. What happens after that is not known. However, the result is an individual who is 'two persons in one body' or a 'self-contained twin'. The chimaerism affects all body cells, apparently at random: haemopoietic cells may not be involved. The subject may have, for example, one blue and one brown eye, or skin patches of different colours. If the cells of the genital organs are involved there are genital abnormalities. Dispermic chimaeras usually present as genital abnormalities, but may also present in the same way as twin chimaeras.

Examples of chimaerism

A brief description of three chimaeras studied by one of us (GWGB) is presented below.

Twin (haemopoietic) chimaerism: subject unaware of being a twin. The observation of mixed fields in routine antenatal ABO and Rhesus blood-group tests led to the demonstration of chimaerism. There were two red-cell populations: one population (93%) was group O, *MN*, cde/cde, Fy(a−), and the other (7%) was group A_1, *NN*, CDe/cde, Fy(a+). Lymphocyte karyotyping showed that 96% of cells were of the normal male karyotype, 46XY, and four per cent were of the normal female karyotype 46XX. The patient is a normal female. No evidence of chimaerism was found in other tissues. The patient was a secretor of A and H substances; her true blood group is therefore A. This means that her truly begotten red cells constitute the minor red-cell population and that the major population is no doubt derived from a twin. Confirmation that her true blood groups are those of the minority red-cell population was obtained from the following observations:

1 the levels of ABH blood-group gene-specified glycosyltransferases were those expected of an A_1 person;
2 since she inherited *A_1, L, H* and *Se* genes she had the hybrid glycosphingolipid A_1Le^b in her plasma; this substance coated her red cells, which were agglutinable by the rare antibody anti-A_1Le^b; and

3 she had a baby who was Fy(a+): since her husband is Fy(a−) her baby must have inherited this character from her. Thus the blood-forming cells of her long-dead twin survive in her bone marrow, producing the cells they have been programmed to form. We now know that the dead twin was a male, and we know his blood groups. Details are given by Battey *et al.* [168] and Bird *et al.* [63].

Dispermic (whole body) chimaerism. A normal healthy blood donor was found on routine blood grouping to be group B. His serum, however, lacked anti-A. Further investigation [169] showed that his red cells carried a very weak A antigen, A_{el}, which could not be demonstrated by agglutination, but only by the fact that anti-A could be adsorbed on to and eluted from his red cells. He is a non-secretor of ABH. His serum contains A_1 blood-group gene-specified glycosyltransferase at the lower limit of normal, whereas his serum B-gene-specified transferase is at a much lower level than normal. His true blood group is therefore A_1B, and there is clearly a discrepancy between his red-cell phenotype and serum transferases. A family study showed that his wife is group A_2, his first son A_2 and his second son B. Since his first son has inherited neither an A_1 nor a B gene from his father he would have been held, in normal circumstances, to be illegitimate. However, further studies showed that 60% of the donor's skin fibroblasts were female. The donor is therefore a dispermic chimaera with two cell lines, one of the genotype A_1A_1 or A_1O, and the other *BO*. There is therefore no reason whatever to assume his first son is illegitimate. The majority of the donor's skin cells are group A_1 and female, and the minority group B and male. His sex organs are obviously male. His red-cell transferase levels are in accordance with his red-cell phenotype. Serum transferases are not derived from the bone marrow and do not act on red cells in the bloodstream; if they did we would never be able to find mixtures of red cells of different ABO groups in chimaeras. They are responsible only for the synthesis of blood-group substances in body fluids or secretions. Red-cell antigens are synthesized solely from transferases derived from the bone marrow.

A most remarkable example of a very unusual dispermic chimaera has been investigated in Vienna by Mayr *et al.* [170]. A group-A_2B woman was apparently excluded as the mother of a newborn group-O child. Further investigation of the mother and father, the newborn child and three older children, showed that the mother was excluded from the parentage of all four children. Baby exchange at birth or 'wilful substitution' were considered to be very highly improbable. The mother was not a twin, and showed no evidence of more than one cell line in various tissues. The authors propose that the mother has two populations of genetically different cells, one present in her blood and the other in her gonads.

Twin (haemopoietic) chimaerism: both twins available for study. The propositus is a healthy blood donor. A mixed-field reaction was observed during examination of the filter paper 'read-out' of a Technicon™ 15-channel blood-grouping machine. This observation was confirmed by manual tests. The two red-cell populations were separated: one population (80%) was group O, *ss*, Jk(b−), and the other (20%) group B, *Ss*, Jk(b+). The propositus is a secretor of B and H substances: his true ABO group is therefore B. This was confirmed by transferase studies. His lymphocytes are 81% female, 46XX, and 19% male, 46XY. His twin sister was also studied, with similar findings. She secretes H but not B substance, and her true ABO blood group is therefore O. Details of this study are presented elsewhere [171].

REFERENCES

1 BIRD G.W.G. (1969) Blood group antibody notation. *Vox Sanguinis*, **17**, 468.

2 LANDSTEINER K. (1900) Zur kenntnis der antifermentativen, lytischen und agglutinierenden Wirkungen des Butserums und der Lymphe. *Zentralblatt für Bakteriologie*, **27**, 357.

3 LANDSTEINER K. (1901) Über Agglutinationserscheinungen normalen menschlichen Blutes. *Wiener Klinische Wochenschrift*, **14**, 1132.

4 VON DUNGERN E. & HIRSZFELD L. (1910) Über Vererbung gruppen-spezifischer Strukturen des Blutes. *Zeitschrift für Immunitätsforschung*, **6**, 284.

5 BERNSTEIN F. (1924) Ergebnisse einer biostatischen zussamenfassenden Betrachtung über die erblichen Blutstructuren des Menschen. *Klinische Wochenschrift*, **3**, 1495.

6 RACE R.R. & SANGER R. (1975) *Blood Groups in Man*, 6th edn. Blackwell Scientific Publications, Oxford.

7 REVIRON J., JACQUET A., DELARUE F., LIBERGE F., SALMON D. & SALMON CH. (1967) Interaction allélique des gènes de groupes sanguines ABO. Résultats préliminaires avec l'anti-B d'un sujet 'cis A₁B' et étude quantitative avec l'anti-B d'un sujet A₁O. *Nouvelle Revue française d'Hématologie*, **7**, 425.

8 REVIRON J., JACQUET A. & SALMON CH. (1968) Un exemple de chromosome 'cis A₁B'. Étude immunologique et genetique du phénotype induit. *Nouvelle Revue française d'Hématologie*, **8**, 323.

9 SABO B.H., BUSH M., GERMAN J., CARNE L.R., YATES A.D. & WATKINS W.M. (1978) The *cis* AB phenotype in three generations of one family—serological, enzymic and cytogenetic studies. *Journal of Immunogenetics*, **5**, 87.

10 YATES A.D. & WATKINS W.M. (1980) Biosynthesis of A antigenic determinants on group O erythrocytes mediated by the blood group B gene specified transferase (Abstract No. 1125). *Joint Meeting of the 18th Congress of the International Society of Hematology and 16th Congress of the International Society of Blood Transfusion*, Montreal, p. 214.

11 SPRINGER G.F., HORTON R.E. & FORBES M. (1959) Origin of anti-human blood group B antigens in white leghorn chicks. *Journal of Experimental Medicine*, **110**, 221.

12 WIENER A.S. (1953) The blood factor C of the A–B–O system, with special reference to the rare blood group C. *Annals of Eugenics*, **18**, 1.

13 MOSS W.L. (1910) Studies on isoagglutinins and isohemolysins. *Bulletin of the Johns Hopkins Hospital*, **21**, 63.

14 DODD B.E. (1952) Linked anti-A and anti-B antibodies from group O sera. *British Journal of Experimental Pathology*, **33**, 1.

15 BIRD G.W.G. (1953) Observations on haemagglutinin 'linkage' in relation to isoagglutinins and autoagglutinins. *British Journal of Experimental Pathology*, **34**, 131.

16 OWEN R.D. (1954) Heterogeneity of antibodies to the human blood groups in normal and immune sera. *Journal of Immunology*, **73**, 29.

17 DODD B.E., LINCOLN P.J. & BOORMAN K.E. (1967) The cross-reacting antibodies of group O sera: Immunological studies and possible explanation of the observed facts. *Immunology*, **12**, 39.

18 BIRD G.W.G. (1954) The hypothetical factor C of the ABO system of blood groups. *Vox Sanguinis* (Old Series), **4**, 66.

19 RICHARDSON JONES A. & KANEB L. (1960) Some properties of cross-reacting antibody of the ABO group system. *Blood*, **15**, 395.

20 MOLLISON P.L. (1967) *Blood Transfusion in Clinical Medicine*, 4th edn., p. 249. Blackwell Scientific Publications, Oxford.

21 TOVEY G.H. (1964) Serological prediction of haemolytic disease in the newborn In: *Recent Advances in Clinical Pathology*, Series IV (ed. Dyke S.C.), p. 209. Churchill, London.

22 WITEBSKI E. (1948) Interrelationship between the Rh system and the ABO system. *Blood*, **3** (Suppl. 2), 66.

23 POLLEY M.J., MOLLISON P.L., ROSE J. & WALKER W. (1965) A simple serological test for antibodies causing ABO-haemolytic disease of the newborn. *Lancet*, **i**, 291.

24 ECONOMIDU J. (1966) A study of the reactions between certain human blood group antigens and their respective antibodies with special reference to the ABO system. Ph.D. Thesis, University of London.

25 SCHIFF F. & SASAKI H. (1932) Der Ausscheidungstypus, ein auf serologischen Wege nachweisbares mendelndes Merkmal. *Klinische Wochenschrift*, **11**, 1426.

26 BOYD W.C. & SHAPLEIGH E. (1954) Separation of individuals of any blood group into secretors and non-secretors by use of a plant agglutinin (lectin). *Blood*, **9**, 1195.

27 FAWCETT K.J., ECKSTEIN E.G., INNELLA F. & YOKOYAMA M. (1970) Four examples of B_m^h blood in one family. *Vox Sanguinis*, **19**, 457.

28 HRUBIŠKO M., LALUHA J., MERGANCOVÁ O. & ZAKOVICOVÁ S. (1970) New variants in the ABOH blood group

system due to interaction of recessive genes controlling the formation of H antigen in erythrocytes: the 'Bombay'-like phenotypes O_{Hm}, $O_{Hm}B$ and $O_{Hm}AB$. *Vox Sanguinis*, **19**, 113.

29 KISAILUS E.C. & KABAT E.A. (1978) Immunochemical studies on blood groups. LXVI. Competitive binding assays of A_1 and A_2 blood group substances with insolubilized anti-A serum and insolubilized A agglutinin from *Dolichos biflorus*. *Journal of Experimental Medicine*, **147**, 830.

30 BIRD G.W.G. (1959) Agar gel studies of blood group specific substances and precipitins of plant origin. I. The precipitins of *Dolichos biflorus*. *Vox Sanguinis*, **4**, 307.

31 BIRD G.W.G., ROBERTS K.D. & WINGHAM J. (1975) Change of blood group from A_2 to A_x in a child with congenital abnormalities. *Journal of Clinical Pathology*, **28**, 962.

32 YOKOYAMA M. & PLOCINIK B. (1965) Serologic and immuno-chemical characterization of A_x blood. *Vox Sanguinis*, **10**, 149.

33 STURGEON P., MOORE B.P.L. & WIENER W. (1964) Notations for two weak A variants: A_{end} and A_{el}. *Vox Sanguinis*, **9**, 214.

34 WEINER W., SANGER R. & RACE R.R. (1959) A weak form of the blood group antigen A. An inherited character. *Proceedings of the 7th Congress of the International Society of Blood Transfusion, Rome, 1958.* p. 720. Karger, Basel.

35 CARTRON J.P., GERBAL A., BADET J., ROPARS C. & SALMON C. (1975) Assay of α-N-acetylgalactosaminyltransferases in human sera. Further evidence for several types of A_m individuals. *Vox Sanguinis*, **28**, 347.

36 WEINER W., LEWIS H.B.M., MOORES P., SANGER R. & RACE R.R. (1957) A gene Y, modifying the blood group antigen A. *Vox Sanguinis*, **2**, 25.

37 MOORE B.P.L., NEWSTEAD P.H. & JOHNSON J. (1961) A weak example of the blood group antigen A. *Vox Sanguinis*, **6**, 151.

38 VON LOGHEM J.J., DORFMEIER H. & VAN DER HART M. (1957) Two A antigens with abnormal serological properties. *Vox Sanguinis*, **2**, 16.

39 LANDSTEINER K. & LEVINE P. (1930) Differentiation of a type of human blood by means of normal animal serum. *Journal of Immunology*, **18**, 87.

40 JAKOBOWICZ R., SIMMONS R.T. & WHITTINGHAM S. (1961) A subgroup of group B blood. *Vox Sanguinis*, **6**, 706.

41 BOORMAN K.E. & ZEITLIN R.A. (1964) B_v—a subgroup of B which lacks part of the normal human B antigen. *Vox Sanguinis*, **9**, 278.

42 SALMON CH. & REVIRON J. (1964) Trois phénotypes 'B faible': B_{80}, B_{60}, B_0 définis par leur agglutinabilité, comparée à celle du phénotype normal. *Nouvelle Revue française d'Hématologie*, **4**, 655.

43 SALMON CH., SALMON D. & REVIRON J. (1964) Données quantitative et thermodynamiques comparées, concernant les antigènes B_{100}, B_{80}, B_{60}, et B_0. Applications à l'étude de l'agglutination. *Nouvelle Revue française d'Hématologie*, **4**, 739.

44 VAN DER HART M., VAN DER VEER M. & VAN LOGHEM J.J. (1962) Change of blood group B in a case of leukaemia. *Vox Sanguinis*, **7**, 449.

45 KOGURE T. & ISEKI S. (1970) A family of B_m, due to a modifying gene. *Proceedings of the Japan Academy*, **46**, 728.

46 SALMON CH. & CARTRON J.P. (1977) ABO phenotypes. In: *Handbook Series in Clinical Laboratory Science. Section D. Blood Banking* (ed. Greenwalt T.J. & Steane E.A.), p. 71. CRC Press, Cleveland, Ohio.

47 CAMERON C., GRAHAM F., DUNSFORD I., SICKLES G., MACPHERSON C.R., CAHAN A., SANGER R. & RACE R.R. (1959) Acquisition of a B-like antigen by red blood cells. *British Medical Journal*, **ii**, 29.

48 LANSET S. & ROPARTZ C. (1971) A second example of acquired B-like antigen in a healthy person. *Vox Sanguinis*, **20**, 82.

49 SPRINGER G.F. & ANSELL N.J. (1960) Acquisition of blood-group B-like bacterial antigens by human A and O erythrocytes. *Federation Proceedings*, **19**, 70.

50 GERBAL A., LIBERGE G., LOPEZ M. & SALMON CH. (1970) Un antigène B acquis chez un sujet de phénotype erythrocytaire A_h^m. *Revue française de Transfusion*, **13**, 61.

51 SNEATH J.S. & SNEATH P.H.A. (1955) Transformation of the Lewis groups of human red cells. *Nature (London)*, **176**, 172.

52 GRUBB R. (1951) Observations on the human group system Lewis. *Acta Pathologica et Microbiologica Scandinavica*, **28**, 61.

53 CEPPELLINI R. (1955) On the genetics of secretor and Lewis characters: a family study. *Proceedings of the 5th Congress of the International Society of Blood Transfusion, Paris, 1954*, p. 207.

54 STRATTON F. (1958) Lewis antibodies—with a note on their preservation. *Proceedings of the 6th Congress of the International Society of Blood Transfusion, Boston, Mass., 1956. Bibliotheca Haematologica, Fasc.* 7, p. 7. Karger, Basel.

55 KORNSTAD L. (1969) Anti-Le^b in the serum of $Le(a+b-)$ and $Le(a-b-)$ persons: adsorption studies with erythrocytes of different ABO and Lewis phenotypes. *Vox Sanguinis*, **16**, 124.

56 BIRD G.W.G. (1958) Erythrocyte agglutinins from plants. Ph.D. Thesis, University of London.

57 STURGEON P. & ARCILLA M.B. (1970) Studies on the secretion of blood group substances. I. Observations on the red cell phenotype $Le(a+b+x+)$. *Vox Sanguinis*, **18**, 301.

58 CROOKSTON M.C., TILLEY C.A. & CROOKSTON J.H. (1970) Human blood group chimaera with seeming breakdown of immunological tolerance. *Lancet*, **ii**, 1110.

59 MOLLISON P.L. (1979) *Blood Transfusion in Clinical Medicine*, 6th edn., p. 535. Blackwell Scientific Publications, Oxford.

60 GUNSON H.H. & LATHAM V. (1972) An agglutinin in human serum reacting with cells from $Le(a-b-)$ non-secretor individuals. *Vox Sanguinis*, **22**, 344.

61 POTAPOV M.I. (1970) Detection of the antigen of the Lewis system characteristic of the erythrocytes of the secretory group $Le(a-b-)$. *Problems of Hematology and Blood Transfusion*, **15**, 45.

62 SEAMAN M.J., CHALMERS D.G. & FRANKS D. (1968) Siedler: an antibody which reacts with $A_1 Le(a-b+)$ red cells. *Vox Sanguinis*, **15**, 25.

63 BIRD G.W.G., BATTEY D.A., GREENWELL P., MORTIMER C.W., WATKINS W.M. & WINGHAM J. (1976) Further

observations of the Birmingham chimaera. *Journal of Medical Genetics*, **13**, 70.

64 SZYMANSKI I.O., TILLEY C.A., CROOKSTON M.C., GREENWALT T.J. & MOORE S. (1977) A further example of human blood group chimaerism. *Journal of Medical Genetics*, **14**, 279.

65 ANDERSEN J. (1958) Modifying influence of the secretor gene on the development of the ABH substance. *Vox Sanguinis*, **3**, 251.

66 HIRSCH H.F., GRAHAM H.A. & DAVIES D.M. (1975) The relationship of the Le^c and Le^d antigens to the Lewis, Secretor and ABO systems (Abstract). *Program, 28th Annual Meeting of the American Association of Blood Banks, Chicago*, p. 109.

67 LEVINE P., BOBBITT O.B., WALLER R.K. & KUMICHAEL A. (1951) Isoimmunization by a new blood factor in tumor cells. *Proceedings of the Society of Experimental Biology, New York*, **77**, 403.

68 SANGER R. (1955) An association between the P and Jay systems of blood groups. *Nature (London)*, **176**, 1163.

69 MATSON G.A., SWANSON J., NOADES J., SANGER R. & RACE R.R. (1959) A 'new' antigen and antibody belonging to the P blood group system. *American Journal of Human Genetics*, **9**, 274.

70 TIPPETT P., SANGER R., RACE R.R., SWANSON J. & BUSCH S. (1965) An agglutinin associated with the P and ABO blood group system. *Vox Sanguinis*, **10**, 269.

71 BEVAN B., HAMMOND W. & CLARKE R.L. (1970) Anti-P₁ associated with liver-fluke infection. *Vox Sanguinis*, **18**, 188.

72 VOS G.H. (1966) The serology of anti-Tj^a-like haemolysins observed in the serum of threatened aborters in Western Australia. *Acta Haematologica*, **35**, 272.

73 FEIZI T., KABAT E.A., VICARI G., ANDERSON B. & MARSH W.L. (1971) Immunochemical studies on blood groups XLVII. The I antigen complex—Precursors in the A, B, H, Le^a and Le^b blood group system—Haemagglutination–inhibition studies. *Journal of Experimental Medicine*, **133**, 39.

74 ROSSE W.F. & LAUF P.K. (1970) Reaction of cold agglutinins with I antigen solubilized from human red cells. *Blood*, **36**, 777.

75 DZIERZKOWA-BORODEJ W., SEYFRIED H., NICHOLS M., REID M. & MARSH W.L. (1970) The recognition of water-soluble I blood group substance. *Vox Sanguinis*, **18**, 222.

76 SCHWARTING G.A., MARCUS D.M. & METAXAS M. (1977) Identification of sialosylparagloboside as the erythrocyte receptor for an 'anti-p' antibody. *Vox Sanguinis*, **32**, 257.

77 FEIZI T., CHILDS R.A., WATANABE K. & HAKOMORI S.I. (1979) Three types of blood group I specificity among monoclonal anti-I autoantibodies revealed by analogues of a branched erythrocyte glycolipid. *Journal of Experimental Medicine*, **149**, 975.

78 WATKINS W.M. (1980) Biochemistry and genetics of the ABO, Lewis and I systems. In: *Advances in Human Genetics*. Vol 10 (ed. Harris H. & Hirschorn K.), p. 1. Plenum Publishing Corporation, New York.

79 LANDSTEINER K. & WIENER A.S. (1940) An agglutinable factor in human blood recognized by immune sera for Rhesus blood. *Proceedings of the Society of Experimental Biology, New York*, **43**, 223.

80 LEVINE P. & STETSON R.E. (1939) An unusual case of intragroup agglutination. *Journal of the American Medical Association*, **113**, 126.

81 FISK R.T. & FOORD A.G. (1942) Observations on the Rh agglutination of human blood. *American Journal of Clinical Pathology*, **12**, 545.

82 MURRAY J. & CLARKE E.C. (1952) Production of anti-Rh in guinea-pigs from human erythrocytes. *Nature (London)*, **169**, 886.

83 LEVINE P. (1968) Rh and LW bloodfactors. *International Convention on Immunology, Buffalo, New York*, p. 140. Karger, Basel.

84 GIBLETT E.R. (1969) *Genetic Markers in Human Blood*. Blackwell Scientific Publications, Oxford.

85 ROSENFIELD R.E., ALLEN F.H., SWISHER S.N. & KOCHWA S. (1962) A review of Rh serology and presentation of a new terminology. *Transfusion*, **2**, 287.

86 MURRAY J. (1944) A nomenclature of subgroups of the Rh factor. *Nature (London)*, **154**, 701.

87 TIPPETT P. (1978) Depressed Rh phenotypes. *Revue française de Transfusion et d'Immuno-hématologie*, **21**, 135.

88 STURGEON P. (1970) Hematological observations on the anaemia associated with blood type Rh_null. *Blood*, **36**, 310.

89 POLLACK W. & RECKEL R.P. (1970) The ζ potential and haemagglutination with Rh antibodies. A physiochemical explanation. *International Archives of Allergy and Applied Immunology*, **38**, 482.

90 COOMBS R.R.A., MOURANT A.E. & RACE R.R. (1945) Detection of weak and 'incomplete' Rh agglutinins: a new test. *Lancet*, **ii**, 15.

91 GREEN F.A. (1968) Phospholipid requirements of Rh antigenic activity. *Journal of Biological Chemistry*, **243**, 5519.

92 WOODROW J.C. (1970) Rh immunization and its prevention. *Series Haematologica, Vol. III, No. 3*. Munksgaard, Copenhagen.

93 TOVEY G.H. (1980) Should anti-D immunoglobulin be given antenatally? *Lancet*, **ii**, 466.

94 FASSBINDER W., SEIDL S. & KOCH K.M. (1978) The role of formaldehyde in the formation of haemodialysis-associated anti-N-like antibodies. *Vox Sanguinis*, **35**, 41.

95 METAXAS M., METAXAS-BÜHLER M. & IKIN E.W. (1968) Complexities of the MN locus. *Vox Sanguinis*, **15**, 102.

96 DAHR R., UHLENBRUCK G. & BIRD G.W.G. (1975) Influence of free amino and carboxyl groups on the specificity of plant anti-N. *Vox Sanguinis*, **28**, 389.

97 LISOWSKA E. & DUK M. (1975) Effect of modification of amino groups of human erythrocytes on M, N and N_Vg specificities. *Vox Sanguinis*, **28**, 392.

98 WALKER M.E., RUBINSTEIN P. & ALLEN F.H. JR (1977) Biochemical genetics of MN. *Vox Sanguinis*, **32**, 111.

99 ANSTEE D.J., BARKER D.M., JUDSON P.A. & TANNER M.J.A. (1977) Inherited sialoglycoprotein deficiencies in human erythrocytes of the type En(a−). *British Journal of Haematology*, **35**, 309.

100 DESAI P.R. & SPRINGER G.F. (1980) Sialylation of Thomsen-Friedenreich (T) and blood type NM antigens by transferases in human sera measured by [¹⁴C] NAN uptake. *Journal of Immunogenetics*, **7**, 149.

101 GIBLETT E.R., KLEBANOFF S.J., PINCUS S.H., SWANSON J., PARK B.H. & McCULLOUGH J. (1971) Kell pheno-

types in chronic granulomatous disease: A potential transfusion hazard. *Lancet*, **i**, 1235.

102 MARSH W.L., ØYEN R., NICHOLS M.E. & ALLEN F.H. JR (1975) Chronic granulomatous disease and the Kell groups. *British Journal of Haematology*, **29**, 247.

103 ALBREY J.A., VINCENT E.E.R., HUTCHINSON J., MARSH W.L., ALLEN F.H., GAVIN J. & SANGER R. (1971) A new antibody, anti-Fy3, in the Duffy blood group system. *Vox Sanguinis*, **20**, 29.

104 BEHZAD O., LEE C.L., GAVIN J. & MARSH W.L. (1973) A new anti-erythrocyte antibody in the Duffy system: anti-Fy4. *Vox Sanguinis*, **24**, 337.

105 COLLEDGE K.I., PEZZULICH M. & MARSH W.L. (1973) Anti-Fy5, an antibody disclosing a probable association between the Rhesus and Duffy blood group genes. *Vox Sanguinis*, **24**, 193.

106 MILLER L.H., MASON S.J., CLYDE D.F. & McGINNISS M.H. (1976) The resistance factor to *Plasmodium vivax* in blacks. The Duffy blood-group genotype, FyFy. *New England Journal of Medicine*, **295**, 302.

107 MANN J.D., CAHAN A., GELB A.G., FISHER N., HAMPER J., TIPPETT P., SANGER R. & RACE R.R. (1962) A sex-linked blood group. *Lancet*, **i**, 8.

108 O'NEILL G.J., YANG S.Y., TEGOLI J., BERGER R, & DUPONT B. (1978) Chido and Rodgers blood groups are distinct antigenic components of human complement C4. *Nature (London)*, **273**, 668.

109 TILLEY C.A., ROMANS D.G. & CROOKSTON M.C. (1978) Localisation of Chido and Rodgers determinants to the C4d fragment of human C4. *Nature (London)*, **276**, 713.

110 BIRD G.W.G. (1959) Haemagglutinins in seeds. *British Medical Bulletin*, **15**, 165.

111 BIRD G.W.G. (1963) The contribution to blood group knowledge of substances obtained from higher plants. *Proceedings of the 1st Asian Congress of Blood Transfusion, Hakone, Japan*, p. 24.

112 BOYD W.C. & SHAPLEIGH E. (1954) Antigenic relations of blood group antigens as suggested by tests with lectins. *Journal of Immunology*, **73**, 226.

113 BIRD G.W.G. (1964) Anti-T in peanuts. *Vox Sanguinis*, **9**, 748.

114 BIRD G.W.G. & WINGHAM J. (1973) Seed agglutinin for the rapid identification of Tn polyagglutination. *Lancet*, **i**, 677.

115 BIRD G.W.G. & WINGHAM J. (1979) Anti-Cad lectin from the seeds of *Leonurus cardiaca*. *Clinical and Laboratory Haematology*, **1**, 57.

116 PROKOP O., UHLENBRUCK G. & KÖHLER W. (1968) A new source of antibody-like substances having anti-blood group specificity. *Vox Sanguinis*, **14**, 321.

117 LOCKYER J.W. & CANN G. (1966) *Agglutinins from the Hedgerow*. Paper read at the National Blood Transfusion Service Scientific and Technical Conference, Birmingham.

118 PROKOP O. & UHLENBRUCK G. (1969) *Human Blood and Serum Groups* (Translated by Raven J.L.), p. 67. Maclaren, London.

119 BIRD G.W.G. (1971) Erythrocyte polyagglutination. *Nouvelle Revue française d'Hématologie*, **11**, 57.

120 BIRD G.W.G. (1978) Significant advances in lectins and polyagglutinable red cells. *Plenary Session. Main lectures, XVII Congress of the International Society of Blood Transfusion*, p. 87. Librairie Arnette, Paris.

121 BIRD G.W.G. & WINGHAM J. (1972) Tk: a new form of red cell polyagglutination. *British Journal of Haematology*, **23**, 759.

121a INGLIS G., BIRD G.W.G., MITCHELL A.A.B., MILNE G.R. & WINGHAM J. (1975) Erythrocyte polyagglutination showing properties of both T and Tk, probably induced by *Bacteroides fragilis* infection. *Vox Sanguinis*, **28**, 314.

121b INGLIS G., BIRD G.W.G., MITCHELL A.A.B. & WINGHAM J. (1978) Tk: polyagglutination associated with reduced A and H activity. *Vox Sanguinis*, **35**, 370.

122 BIRD G.W.G., WINGHAM J., INGLIS G. & MITCHELL A.A.B. (1975) Tk polyagglutination in *Bacteroides fragilis* septicaemia. *Lancet*, **i**, 286.

123 JUDD W.J., BECK M.L., HICKLIN B.L., SHANKAR IYER P.N. & GOLDSTEIN I.J. (1977) BS II lectin: a second hemagglutinin isolated from *Bandeiraea simplicifolia* seed with affinity for type III polyagglutinable cells. *Vox Sanguinis*, **33**, 246.

124 DOINEL C., ANDREU G., CARTRON J.P., SALMON C. & FUKUDA M.N. (1980) Tk polyagglutination produced *in vitro* by an endo-beta-galactosidase. *Vox Sanguinis*, **38**, 94.

125 BIRD G.W.G., WINGHAM J., BECK M.L., PIERCE S.R., OATES G.D. & POLLOCK A. (1978) Th, a 'new' form of erythrocyte polyagglutination. *Lancet*, **i**, 1215.

126 GRANINGER W., RAMEIS H., FISCHER K., POSCHMANN A., BIRD G.W.G., WINGHAM J. & NEUMANN E. (1977) 'VA' a new type of erythrocyte polyagglutination characterized by depressed H receptors and associated with hemolytic anemia. I. Serological and hematological observations. *Vox Sanguinis*, **32**, 195.

127 GRANINGER W., POSCHMANN A., FISCHER K., SCHEDL-GIOVANNONI I., HÖRANDER H. & KLAUSHOFER K. (1977) 'VA' a new type of erythrocyte polyagglutination characterized by depressed H receptors and associated with hemolytic anemia. II. Observations by immunofluorescence electron microscopy, cell electrophoresis and biochemistry. *Vox Sanguinis*, **32**, 201.

128 BECK M.L., MYERS M.A., MOULDS J., PIERCE S.R., HARDMAN J., WINGHAM J. & BIRD G.W.G. (1978) Coexistent Tk and VA polyagglutinability. *Transfusion*, **18**, 680.

129 BIRD G.W.G., SHINTON N.K. & WINGHAM J. (1971) Persistent mixed-field polyagglutination. *British Journal of Haematology*, **21**, 443.

130 BIRD G.W.G., WINGHAM J., PIPPARD M.J., HOULT J.G. & MELIKIAN V. (1976) Erythrocyte membrane modification in malignant diseases of myeloid and lymphoreticular tissues. I. Tn-polyagglutination in acute myelocytic leukaemia. *British Journal of Haematology*, **33**, 289.

131 NESS P.M., GARRATTY G., MOREL P.A. & PERKINS H.A. (1979) Tn-polyagglutination preceding acute leukemia. *Blood*, **54**, 30.

132 BALDWIN M.L., BARRASSO C. & RIDOLFI R.L. (1979) Tn-polyagglutinability associated with acute myelomonocytic leukemia. *American Journal of Clinical Pathology*, **72**, 1024.

133 CAZAL P., MONIS M., CAUBEL J. & BRIVES J. (1968) Polyagglutinabilité héréditaire dominante: antigène privé (Cad) correspondant à un anticorps public et à une lectine de Dolichos biflorus. *Revue française de Transfusion*, **11**, 209.

134 SANGER R., GAVIN J., TIPPETT P., TEESDALE P. & ELDON K. (1971) Plant agglutinins for another human blood group. *Lancet,* **i,** 1130.

135 OBEID D., BIRD G.W.G. & WINGHAM J. (1977) Prolonged erythrocyte T-polyagglutination in two children with bowel disorders. *Journal of Clinical Pathology,* **30,** 953.

136 SEGER R., JOLLER P., BIRD G.W.G., WINGHAM J., KENNY A., RAPP A., GARZONI D., HITZIG W.H. & DUC G. (1980) Necrotising enterocolitis and neuraminidase-producing bacteria. *Helvetica Paediatrica Acta,* **35,** 121.

137 KLEIN P.J., BULLA M., NEWMAN R.A., MÜLLER P., UHLENBRUCK G., SHAEFER H.E., KRUGER G. & FISHER R. (1977) Thomson-Friedenreich antigen in haemolytic–uraemic syndrome. *Lancet,* **ii,** 1024.

138 SPRINGER G.F., DESAI P.R., YANG H.J. & MURTHY M.S. (1977) Carcinoma-associated blood group MN precursor antigens against which all humans possess antibodies. *Clinical Immunology and Immunopathology,* **7,** 426.

139 ANGLIN J.H. JR, LERNER M.P. & NORDQUIST R.E. (1977) Blood group-like activity released by human mammary carcinoma cells in culture. *Nature (London),* **269,** 254.

140 MOURANT A.E., KOPÉC A.C. & DOMANIEWSKA-SOBCZAK K. (1971) Blood groups and blood-clotting. *Lancet,* **i,** 223.

141 PETTENKOFER H.J. (1962) New aspects on the mechanism of the present blood group distribution in the world. *Proceedings of the 8th Congress of the International Society of Blood Transfusion, Tokyo, 1960,* p. 154. Karger, Basel.

142 BOYD W.C. (1939) Blood Groups. *Tabulae Biologicae,* **17,** 113.

143 MOURANT A.E., KOPEĆ A.C. & DOMANIEWSKA-SOBCZAK K. (1976) *The Distribution of the Human Blood Groups and Other Biochemical Polymorphisms,* 2nd edn. Oxford University Press, Oxford.

144 KOPEĆ A.C. (1970) *The Distribution of the Blood Groups in the United Kingdom.* Oxford University Press, London.

145 DAUSSET J. & NENNA A. (1952) Présence d'une leuco-agglutinine dans le serum d'un cas d'agranulocytose chronique. *Comptes Rendues des Séances, Société Biologie et de les Filiales,* **146,** 1539.

146 TERASAKI P.I. & McCLELLAND J.D. (1964) Microdroplet assay of human serum cytotoxins. *Nature (London),* **206,** 998.

147 MORTON J.A., PICKLES M.M. & SUTTON O. (1969) The correlation of the Bg^a blood group with the HL-A7 leucocyte group: demonstration of antigenic sites on red cells and leucocytes. *Vox Sanguinis,* **17,** 536.

148 MORTON J.A., PICKLES M.M., SUTTON L. & SKOV F. (1971) Identification of further antigens as red cells and lymphocytes. Association of Bg^b with W17(Te57) and Bg^a with W28(Da 15, Ba*). *Vox Sanguinis,* **21,** 141.

149 MORTON J.A., PICKLES M.M. & DALEY J.H. (1977) Increase in strength of red cell Bg^a antigen following infectious mononucleosis. *Vox Sanguinis,* **32,** 26.

150 SVEJGAARD A., KISSMEYER-NIELSEN F. & THORSBY E. (1970) HL-A typing of platelets. In: *Histocompatibility Testing* (ed. Terasaki P.I.), p. 153. Munksgaard, Copenhagen.

151 VAN ROOD J.J., VAN LEEUWEN A., TERMIJTELEN A. &

KEUNING J.J. (1976) B-cell antibodies. Ia-like determinants, and their relationship to MLC-determinants in man. *Transplantation Reviews,* **30,** 122.

152 TING A. & MORRIS P.J. (1978) Matching for B-cell antigens of the HLA-DR genes in cadaver renal transplantation. *Lancet,* **i,** 575.

153 ORIOL R., CARTRON J., YVART J., BEDROSSIAN J., DUBOUST A., BARIETY J., GLUCKMAN J.C. & GAGNADOUX M.F. (1978) The Lewis system: new histocompatibility antigens in renal transplantation. *Lancet,* **i,** 574.

154 DAUSSET J. & SVEJGAARD A. (1977) *HLA and disease.* Munksgaard, Copenhagen.

155 BODMER W.F. (1980) The HLA system and disease. *Journal of the Royal College of Physicians of London,* **14,** 43.

156 AHRONS S. (1971) HL-A antibodies: influence on the human foetus. *Tissue Antigens,* **1,** 121.

157 MOULINIER J., MERLE M.C., MESNIER F. & SERVANTIER X. (1971) Les anticorps anti-tissulaires de la femme immunisée anti-Rh. *Proceedings of the 12th Congress of the International Society of Blood Transfusion, Moscow, 1969,* p. 860. Karger, Basel.

158 TOVEY G.H., DARKE C. & FRASER I.D. (1970) Significance of HL-A cytotoxic antibodies in Rh haemolytic disease. *Lancet,* **i,** 1234.

159 KOSKIMIES S., PIRKOLA A. & JULIN M. (1980) Maternal lymphocytotoxic antibodies as possible cause of neonatal hyperbilirubinaemia. *Lancet,* **i,** 879.

160 VERHEUGT F.W.A., VON DEM BORNE A.E.G. KR., DECARY F. & ENGELFRIET C.P. (1977) The detection of granulocyte alloantibodies with an indirect immunofluorescent test. *British Journal of Haematology,* **36,** 533.

161 VERHEUGT F.W.A., VAN NOORD-BOKHORST J.C., VON DEM BORNE A.E.G. KR. & ENGELFRIET C.P. (1979) A family with allo-immune neonatal neutropenia: group-specific pathogenicity of maternal antibodies. *Vox Sanguinis,* **36,** 1.

162 VERHEUGT F.W.A., VON DEM BORNE A.E.G. KR., VAN NOORD-BOKHORST J.C., NIJENHUIS L.E. & ENGELFRIET C.P. (1976) Autoimmune granulocytopenia: the detection of granulocyte antibodies with the immunofluorescence test. *British Journal of Haematology,* **39,** 339.

163 VALBONESI M., CAMPELLI A., MORAZZI M.G., COTTAFAVA F. & JANNUZZI C. (1979) Autoimmune neutropenia due to anti-NA1 antibodies. *Vox Sanguinis,* **36,** 9.

164 LALEZARI P. & RADEL E. (1974) Neutrophil specific antigens: immunology and clinical significance. *Seminars in Hematology,* **11,** 281.

165 VON DEM BORNE A.E.G. KR., VERHEUGT F.W.A., OOSTERHOF F., VON REISZ E., BRUTEL DE LA RIVIERE E. & ENGELFRIET C.P. (1978) A simple immunofluorescence test for the detection of platelet antibodies. *British Journal of Haematology,* **39,** 195.

166 BIRD G.W.G., WINGHAM J., CHESTER G.H., KIDD P. & PAYNE R.W. (1976) Erythrocyte membrane modification of malignant disease of myeloid and lymphoreticular tissues. II. Erythrocyte mosaicism in acute erythroleukaemia. *British Journal of Haematology,* **33,** 295.

167 BIRD G.W.G., WINGHAM J., WATKINS W.M., GREENWELL P. & CAMERON A.H. (1978) Inherited 'mosaicism' within the ABO blood group system. *Journal of Immunogenetics,* **5,** 215.

168 BATTEY D.A., BIRD G.W.G., McDERMOTT A., MORTIMER

C.W., MUTCHINIK O.M. & WINGHAM J. (1974) Another human chimaera. *Journal of Medical Genetics*, **11**, 283.

169 WATKINS W.M., YATES A.D., GREENWELL P., BIRD G.W.G., GIBSON M., ROY T.C.F., WINGHAM J. & LOEB W. (1978) Human chimaera first suspected from analysis of blood group gene-specified glycosyltransferases. (Abstract). *XVII Congress of the International Society of Haematology. XV Congress of the International Society of Blood Transfusion. Abstracts*, Vol. I, p. 443.

170 MAYR W.R., PAUSCH V. & SCHNEDL W. (1979) Human chimaera detected only by investigation of her progeny. *Nature (London)*, **277**, 210.

171 BIRD G.W.G., GIBSON M., WINGHAM J., MACKINTOSH P., WATKINS W. & GREENWELL P. (1980) Another example of haemopoietic chimaerism in dizygotic twins. *British Journal of Haematology*, **46,** 439.

172 TERASAKI P.I. (ed.) (1980) *Histocompatibility Testing 1980*. UCLA Tissue Typing Laboratory.

Chapter 35
Blood transfusion and the use of blood products

G. H. TOVEY AND G. W. G. BIRD

Blood transfusion is a form of replacement therapy. Whole blood collected into a suitable anticoagulant preservative may be prescribed and will, of course, provide red cells for the correction of anaemia and, for example, if freshly drawn, platelets and factor VIII for the treatment of a haemorrhagic diathesis. Since, however, many of the separate components of blood can be isolated and are available for transfusion, they should preferably be prescribed individually whenever this is appropriate. Moreover, to transfuse these in the form of whole blood represents a waste of those components for which the patient has no specific need.

Transfusion of blood, a blood component or a blood product almost inevitably introduces an extra risk for the recipient additional to that of the technical procedure itself. In assessing the need for transfusion the clinician must be aware of these hazards and must weigh them against the expected benefits. He must also be aware of some of the problems of availability of the biological fluids he is prescribing.

PROBLEMS AND COMPLICATIONS OF TRANSFUSION

The complications of transfusion may occur as acute reactions during or shortly after the transfusion, or the effects may be delayed, as is the case with disease transmission or sensitization to antigens present in the blood or blood constituents (Table 35.1).

Febrile reactions
A rise in temperature to 37·5 or 38°C is not uncommon during or following transfusion and, if unaccompanied by chills or symptoms such as pain in the back or urticaria, is probably due to the presence of pyrogens in the anticoagulant fluid or apparatus and is of little consequence or significance. The severity of the reaction may be lessened by keeping the patient warm during transfusion, slowing the drip rate to the minimum for at least 30 minutes and giving a simple antipyretic such as aspirin.

When the reaction is more severe, and particularly if the patient has received previous transfusions or has been pregnant, it should be remembered that pyrexia may be the first sign of sensitization to antigens on red cells, white cells, platelets or plasma proteins, and tests should be made for alloimmunization.

Haemolytic transfusion reactions
An acute haemolytic transfusion reaction is most often due to the combination *in vivo* of an antibody with red cells possessing the corresponding antigen. In the most severe cases the antibody is anti-A, anti-B, anti-D, anti-c, anti-C, anti-E, or anti-Kell in the recipient's plasma reacting with the corresponding antigen on the red cells of the blood transfused. The reverse situation, in which an antibody in the donor plasma reacts with an antigen on the recipient's red cells, may also cause haemolysis, but the reaction then is generally less severe. The risk of a reaction from either of these causes is minimized by:
1 exercising care when grouping the patient and the donor;
2 selecting donor blood that is of the same ABO and Rh(D) group as the recipient;
3 testing both the donor and the recipient blood for irregular blood-group antibodies; and
4 performing a direct matching test before every blood transfusion (p. 1446).
The techniques employed in the antibody and matching tests must be capable of detecting immune antibodies, which may be present in the plasma of patients who have been pregnant or have received a previous blood transfusion, as well as the so-called naturally occurring antibodies, anti-A and anti-B, which are present in almost all recipients. Despite every care being taken in carrying out these tests, a severe or fatal haemolytic reaction may occur if blood intended for another patient is inadvertently transfused. As the final step, therefore, before each unit of blood is transfused a procedure must be included to check that the blood for transfusion is that prepared for the recipient.

In addition to interaction of antigen and antibody,

Table 35.1. Complications of transfusion

Immediate	Delayed
Febrile reactions	Transmission of disease:
Haemolytic reactions	(i) viral hepatitis
Allergic reactions	(ii) syphilis
Reactions to plasma proteins	(iii) cytomegalovirus infection
Reactions to leucocyte antigens	(iv) malaria
Reactions to platelet antigens	(v) brucellosis
Bacteraemic shock	(vi) other infections
Citrate toxicity	Post-transfusion purpura
Air embolism	Haemosiderosis
Circulatory overload	Haemolytic disease of the newborn
	Rejection of a transplant

haemolysis of the donor red cells may result from other causes. Storage in a poorly controlled refrigerator so that the blood becomes frozen; prolongation of storage beyond three to four weeks; warming the blood at a temperature above 40°C prior to transfusion; or exposure to dextrose solutions (p. 1446) may all cause the red cells to become excessively fragile, so that their transfusion is followed either by extensive haemolysis or by a critically reduced red-cell survival.

In its most acute form a haemolytic reaction occurs shortly after the start of a transfusion. The commonest signs and symptoms are a feeling of heat along the vein into which the blood is being transfused, flushing of the face, a rigor accompanied by pain in the lumbar region and constricting pain in the chest. The last may be due partly to blocking of pulmonary vessels by agglutinates, but also to vasoconstriction following release of histamine. The symptoms may be abolished by anaesthesia and the only signs which may then draw attention to the incompatible transfusion are a sudden hypotension and/or abnormal bleeding. Disseminated intravascular coagulation is one of the most dangerous complications and is probably initiated by the liberation of thromboplastins from the damaged red cells (Chapter 29, p. 1173). When the red-cell destruction is predominantly intravascular, e.g. in ABO incompatibility, the haemoglobin released binds with the plasma haptoglobin. Each 100 ml of plasma combines with about 100 mg of haemoglobin and the resultant complex is not excreted by the kidneys but is cleared by the reticulo-endothelial system. A massive haemolysis will saturate the haptoglobin binding mechanism so that free haemoglobin then appears in the plasma. When this reaches about 25 mg/100 ml, haemoglobin will be excreted in the urine. Haemoglobinaemia is followed by the combination of haem with albumin, and methaemalbumin may be detectable in the plasma from about five to 24 hours after an acute haemolytic episode. The breakdown of haemoglobin is also fol-

lowed by bilirubinaemia with a maximum blood level at about three to six hours.

Renal failure does not always follow gross intravascular haemolysis, but it is more likely to occur after incompatible blood transfusion than after the transfusion of fragile red cells. Yuile *et al.* [1] suggest that acute renal failure accompanies haemoglobinuria only when there is some degree of previous or concomitant renal damage, such as that occasioned by the oligaemic anoxia of unreplaced blood loss or severe dehydration. It follows, therefore, that as soon as a haemolytic reaction is suspected, the causative transfusion should be stopped, but any oligaemia must be corrected where necessary by the further transfusion of a 'safe' fluid such as plasma protein solution (p. 1443). An attempt should be made to provoke a diuresis by intravenous injection of frusemide, 60–80 mg, and administration of fluid by mouth or intravenously. Should there not be a resultant diuresis, treatment then becomes a matter of expert fluid and electrolyte management and, in severe cases, haemodialysis. Mannitol must be avoided as it may produce hypervolaemia and pulmonary oedema [2]. If the patient is seen sufficiently early, and particularly when 500 ml or more of incompatible blood has been transfused, prompt exchange transfusion with compatible blood stored less than four days may be of benefit.

Sometimes, and especially when the antibody is initially undetectable or is in very low titre, transfusion of incompatible red cells may provoke no immediate reaction but provides a secondary antigenic stimulus. The recipient then becomes jaundiced and may even have transient haemoglobinuria five to seven days after an apparently successful transfusion [3]. This will be accompanied by a fall in haemoglobin to the pre-transfusion level. In 69% of a series of cases reviewed by Howard [4] the delayed reactions occurred in women who had been pregnant. In some cases no overt reaction is observed but the donor red cells fail to show the expected survival and their disappearance is followed by the appearance of detectable blood-group antibodies in the patient's plasma.

Sensitization to red-cell antigens

From an analysis of 671 patients who developed blood-group antibodies following transfusion, Giblett [5] has determined that after the D antigen, Kell, E and c are those most likely to cause alloimmunization when transfused to patients whose red cells lack these factors. Anti-Kell, anti-E and anti-c may each cause haemolytic disease of the newborn (Chapter 11, p. 485) and since haemolytic disease from these antibodies is not as yet prevented by the prophylactic injection of the appropriate immunoglobulin, blood transfusion should be avoided whenever possible to female patients who may subsequently bear children, in case they become sensitized to any of these antigens. When such patients must be transfused and are known to be Rh-positive, Tovey [6] recommends that c-negative, Kell-negative blood is given in emergency, as well as to any female patient already known to be c-negative.

Should an Rh(D)-negative female accidentally receive a transfusion of Rh(D)-positive blood, it is advised that anti-D immunoglobulin in a dose of 25 μg/ml of red cells should be injected in an attempt to prevent primary immunization.

Transmission of disease

Blood collected from apparently healthy donors may contain viruses, bacteria or protozoa and induce the corresponding disease in the recipient when transfused.

Viral hepatitis. The transmission of viral hepatitis is the most serious complication of the transfusion of blood and blood products. A Medical Research Council Survey conducted in Britain in 1974 [7] before the introduction of total screening of donations for the hepatitis-B antigen, indicated a morbidity of 27 cases per 10 000 units of blood transfused and would mean approximately 4000 cases of post-transfusion hepatitis per annum in the UK using untested donations. An important step towards the eventual elimination of this complication was taken when in a search for new alloantigens using an immunodiffusion technique, Blumberg and his colleagues [8] discovered an unknown antigen in the serum of an Australian aborigine and later [9] found it to occur in 20–30% of patients with hepatitis, leukaemia or mongolism. This so-called Australia or Au antigen was subsequently demonstrated by Prince [10] in the blood of patients in the prodromal and acute phases of serum hepatitis, but not of infectious hepatitis. Prince, therefore, called it the SH (serum hepatitis) antigen but it is now generally

referred to as HBsAg, i.e. hepatitis-B surface antigen. HBsAg is thought not to be the infectious agent itself but probably a particle of the protein coat of the hepatitis-B virus which by its presence serves as an indicator of virus activity. Electron microscopy of serum containing HBsAg reveals particles of diameter 42 nm, so called Dane particles, made up of a core consisting of double-stranded DNA and DNA polymerase surrounded by a coat of surface antigen. These particles are considered to be the hepatitis-B virus (HBV); the core carries an independent antigen known as HBcAg. Some sera containing HBsAg also contain a soluble antigen HBeAg. The presence of HBeAg appears to be related to the infectivity of the serum [11]. Antibodies to core antigen (anti-HBc) are a sensitive indicator of persistent viral replication. Minute amounts of infected blood introduced parenterally may transmit HBV; the minimum dose by subcutaneous or intravenous injection is of the order of 4×10^{-5} ml [12]. All blood and blood components for transfusion should therefore be tested for HBsAg. Development of a test for anti-HBc in donations may also help to prevent the transmission of hepatitis type B. Blood containing anti-HBs is acceptable for transfusion, as are donations from persons with a history of jaundice, provided the attack occurred more than 12 months ago and HBsAg is not detected in the serum by reversed passive haemagglutination or a test of equal sensitivity [13]. Detection of anti-HBe in the serum of a donor previously found to be a carrier of HBV mostly correlates with a low risk of infectivity [14].

The virus remains viable in whole blood or any of its components such as red-cell concentrates, plasma, platelet concentrates and cryoprecipitates which have been prepared by simple physical means. It is killed by heating at 60°C for 10 hours. This cannot be applied to whole blood or plasma because of denaturation of globulins and damage to the red cells, but preparations from which the globulin has been separated, such as concentrated albumin and plasma protein solution, can be heated at 60°C and are then non-infective. Human γ globulin, including anti-D immunoglobulin used in the prevention of haemolytic disease of the newborn (p. 1413), prepared by either an alcohol or ether-fractionation technique, carries little or no risk of transmitting hepatitis, but the transfusion of concentrated fibrinogen is followed by a case incidence similar to that of whole blood or plasma. The transfusion of red cells which have been stored at -196°C in liquid nitrogen rarely, if ever, causes hepatitis [15]; Alter *et al.* [16], however, have transmitted HBV to chimpanzees by such transfusions.

The incubation period of post-transfusion hepatitis is generally between 50 and 160 days with a peak incidence at 60–90 days. The clinical disease may be so mild as to cause only transient liver dysfunction, or so severe as to cause fatal hepatic necrosis. The more severe forms occur mostly in persons above the age of 40 and the overall mortality of 12% is considerably greater than that of infectious hepatitis. The reported case incidence of post-transfusion hepatitis varies from country to country. It is further dependent upon the extent to which donations are tested for HBsAg, the sensitivity of the technique used, and whether both icteric and non-icteric cases are included. In a survey carried out in the UK, mainly before testing was introduced, and which included both icteric and non-icteric cases, the incidence was one per cent [7]. Of 768 patients transfused, five developed icteric viral hepatitis and four of these five (of which two were fatal) were due to HBV. By contrast, in a more recent survey in the USA [17], post-transfusion hepatitis was reported in 10·2% of 2204 patients and in approximately 80% of these the illness was non-icteric.

Although transmission of HBV infection by transfusion has been greatly reduced by testing donations for HBsAg, Hoofnagle *et al.* [18] claim that in the USA as many as 90% of cases of post-transfusion hepatitis are now due to other viruses, currently known as non-A, non-B, for which no suitable screening tests are as yet available. In Britain the proportion of cases due to these viruses is almost certainly not as high; few have been reported following transfusion of blood from UK donors, but of 72 haemophilic patients undergoing surgery at the Oxford Haemophilia Centre from 1977 to 1979 who were treated with imported factor VIII concentrates from commercial sources, five (seven per cent) contracted non-A, non-B hepatitis [19]. Whilst most cases of non-A, non-B post-transfusion hepatitis are mild, some fatal infections have been reported. In a recent study Seef & Hoofnagle [17] found that in 10% of cases associated with whole-blood transfusions the patient went on to develop a chronic active hepatitis confirmed by liver biopsy.

Attempts to sterilize whole blood or plasma by irradiation with ultra-violet light, by the addition of chemicals or, in the case of liquid plasma, by storage at room temperature have proved ineffective; so also has the attempted protection of the recipient by repeated injections of γ globulin [20]. A report of the World Health Organization [21] suggests that until improved techniques are available, the routine testing of donor blood for HBsAg will reduce the case incidence of post-transfusion hepatitis by not more than 25%. *It is clear therefore that the best single step available to reduce this potentially serious hazard is avoidance of unnecessary transfusions.*

Syphilis. This is a hazard only to patients receiving fresh blood or a component which has been prepared from blood which has been stored at 4°C for fewer than four days. The treponeme does not survive storage at this temperature for 96 hours or in plasma kept at −20°C for 48 hours [22]; blood which has been stored for even 24 hours is safer than fresh blood. Routine syphilis testing of the donor blood is not a complete safeguard, since about one-third of persons with primary syphilis are serologically negative.

Cytomegalovirus infection (see also Chapters 18 and 33). Although serological evidence of primary infection has been reported following transfusion of stored blood [7], clinical disease is limited to those transfused with fresh whole blood or components. Perham *et al.* [23] estimate that 12% of donors are potentially infective, but generally the causative virus does not survive cooling to a temperature of 4°C for 48 hours. The case incidence is highest amongst patients who receive several units of fresh blood as, for example, during open-heart surgery (the so-called post-perfusion syndrome) and in the replacement therapy of thrombocytopenia, and takes the form of a febrile, influenza-like illness with splenomegaly, occurring three to five weeks after the transfusion. At this time abnormal mononuclear cells resembling those of infectious mononucleosis may be demonstrable in the patient's blood, and cytomegalovirus (CMV) and/or the corresponding antibodies in the plasma and urine. Patients whose immunological function is impaired by disease or by immunosuppressive treatment are particularly prone to CMV infection; so are the fetus and the newborn child. Except in these the disease is rarely of itself fatal, but may be sufficiently severe to jeopardize recovery in an otherwise seriously ill patient. Dijkmans *et al.* [24] report successful treatment of a fulminating CMV infection by passive immunization with hyperimmune CMV plasma.

Malaria. All known species of malaria parasites may survive for at least 14 days in blood stored at 4°C. Examining blood films from potential donors as a routine is not practicable and Hutton & Shute [25] have reported a fatal case in which examination for several hours resulted in finding only two parasites.

Precautions to be taken to prevent accidental transmission by transfusion differ for services in endemic and non-endemic areas. In non-endemic areas, donors should have a negative history for malaria exposure within the past three months and may donate blood if they have remained asymptomatic for three years following recovery from an attack of malaria. In a high-risk area, donors should be given a single dose of 600 mg (base) chloroquine phosphate six hours before their blood donation [26].

While the case incidence is not high, the disease is an

unpleasant and potentially grave complication for a patient who is already seriously ill or injured.

Brucellosis. Undulant fever occurring 13 weeks after transfusion has been reported by Wood [27], who gives reference also to two other cases.

Other diseases. There is a risk of the recipient developing a virus encephalitis if transfused with blood donated during the phase of viraemia following a recent vaccinia or poliomyelitis vaccination. In South America the trypanosomes of Chagas' disease have sometimes been transmitted by transfusion [28], and Kostman & Bengtsson [29] have reported two cases of Leishmaniasis which occurred in newborn babies in Sweden after transfusion of blood from a donor recently returned from a holiday in Spain.

Allergic reactions

Although severe allergic reactions such as laryngeal oedema or bronchial spasm during or following transfusion are rare, the development of urticaria is common and complicates about one per cent of transfusions [30]. Mostly it occurs in patients who are already sensitized to an allergen present in such foods as milk, eggs or chocolate, and who receive the atopen in the blood transfused. Less commonly the recipient may be transfused with plasma containing 'reaginic' IgE antibodies to an allergen, for example, in chocolate, so that following the transfusion they quite unwittingly ingest the corresponding atopen and thus experience an attack of urticaria.

Allergic reactions are minimized when donors who give a history of severe allergy are rejected, when washed red cells are transfused and by giving an antihistamine (e.g. chlorprophenpyridamine maleate 10 mg) before transfusion to those recipients with a history of previous allergic manifestations [31]. Antihistamines, or any other drugs, should be given by mouth or by injection and not added to the blood to be transfused, since the latter procedure may result in damage to the blood components or, in some cases, to inactivation of the drug [32] (see also p. 1440).

If an allergic reaction develops, 25 or 50 mg of diphenhydramine hydrochloride ('Benadryl') should be given intravenously. If symptoms are severe the transfusion must be discontinued and adrenaline should be given with or without a corticosteroid such as prednisolone.

Reactions to transfused proteins

The presence of antibodies reacting with antigens carried by human γ globulin was first demonstrated in the serum of patients with rheumatoid arthritis [33]

and has since been found not infrequently after transfusion and after pregnancy. The first antigenic determinants so described were named Gm and the antibodies anti-Gm, and it was shown by Harboe *et al.* [34] that the anti-γ-globulin factors are all γM and react with Fc fragments of the γG molecule. Light chains of immunoglobulins also carry specific determinants classified as Km and interact with corresponding antibodies anti-Km. Other antibodies (anti-Ag^a) to a lipoprotein (Ag^a) have been identified by Allison & Blumberg [35]. Serum antibodies do not usually cause a reaction during transfusion unless they are present in high titre. Fudenberg *et al.* [36], Fischer [37], and Prentice *et al.* [38], however, have all reported cases in which Gm(1) plasma transfused to patients with anti-Gm(1) at titres of 128–512 caused severe febrile reactions with collapse and hypotension. No reaction followed the transfusion of Gm(1)-negative plasma.

Anti-IgA is present in low titre in the serum of about two per cent of persons, but Vyas *et al.* [39] have found potent anti-IgA in the serum of patients suffering from conditions such as ataxia telangiectasia and dys-γ-globulinaemia, in which there is a low level or total absence of IgA (aIgA). Anti-IgA of this type will interact with all IgA globulins, by contrast with a second group of multi-transfused patients who have normal levels of IgA and who develop anti-IgA of a more limited specificity. It would seem that this latter group has produced anti-IgA to an antigenic determinant of IgA which they do not themselves possess. When transfused with plasma containing incompatible IgA, the patient with high titre anti-IgA may react alarmingly with a severe erythema and anaphylaxis.

It is clearly not practicable to attempt to determine the serum groups of all patients requiring multiple transfusions. This should be done, however, in the small number who develop reactions, and plasma compatible with the causative antibody found. Transfusion should be avoided whenever possible and, when appropriate, well-washed red cells or the patient's own stored blood should be transfused. One in approximately 500 apparently healthy persons lacks IgA and a small number of blood banks are in the process of building up a donor panel of such aIgA subjects [40]. In a difficult situation one of these banks should be contacted via a national reference centre.

Reactions to leucocyte antigens

Using a lymphocytotoxic technique, antibodies which react with donor leucocytes can be found in about one in three women who have been pregnant [41] and in a similar proportion of patients who have had three blood transfusions [42]. Perkins [43] has found weak anti-leucocyte antibodies in almost 50% of patients between one and two months after large transfusions given during cardiac surgery.

Transfusion of incompatible leucocytes to patients with antibodies causes a characteristic reaction of fever, headache and vomiting. Leucocyte-poor red cells may be prepared by dextran sedimentation for the transfusion of such patients [44]. Reconstituted frozen red cells also have few leucocytes and usually result in a reaction-free transfusion.

One of the important side-effects of the development of leucocyte antibodies is inherent in the relationship of the HLA antigens to histocompatibility (p. 1422). Patel & Terasaki [45] reported that 80% of patients undergoing kidney transplant had a prompt rejection when cytotoxic incompatibility had been detected at a crossmatch between the recipient's serum and the donor's lymphocytes; this contrasted with only four per cent acute rejections when the leucocyte crossmatch was negative. Because of the risk of stimulating lymphocytotoxic antibodies it was therefore recommended that blood transfusion to patients who may have to undergo a transplant should be avoided. More recent surveys [46–48] have indicated, however, that, providing the crossmatch is negative, transfusion before transplantation may have a beneficial effect upon the survival of the grafted kidney and the previous recommendation has now therefore been reversed. The number of units of blood to be transfused, and whether these should be given as whole blood or as washed or reconstituted frozen red cells, is still, however, unresolved. By contrast, blood transfusion, particularly from family donors, seriously prejudices the success of a subsequent bone-marrow graft (p. 1450).

Identification of HLA antigens specific for B-lymphocytes, so-called DR antigens, established that hyperacute rejection of a transplanted kidney is most likely to occur when the crossmatch shows T-cell incompatibility. Lymphocytotoxic B-cell antibodies may be 'cold' or 'warm' reacting. Those found to be incompatible at 37°C are deleterious to the graft. Cold B-cell antibodies, on the other hand, not only do not harm the transplanted kidney but may have an enhancing effect on graft survival [49, 50].

Reactions to platelet antigens
In patients who receive repeated transfusions, platelet survival may become progressively shorter. In most cases this is accompanied by the appearance of platelet alloantibodies in the serum, but in others no antibodies can be detected [51]. Platelets carry A and B antigens, and Aster [52] found that when ABO incompatible platelets were transfused, an average of only 19% were present in the circulation at the end of the transfusion compared with 67% when the platelets were ABO

compatible. The subsequent survival of the incompatible platelets was also shorter. Platelets also carry HLA antigens and Grumet & Yankee [53] reported that, whilst seven patients with aplastic anaemia had all become refractory within about eight weeks to platelets transfused from random donors and non-HLA-matched family donors, platelets from HLA-identical siblings were tolerated twice weekly for 77 weeks without adverse reactions and with excellent clinical responses.

Because of the complexity of the HLA system the probability of finding sufficient HLA-compatible donors from outside a patient's own family is remote and would demand a very large panel of fully typed donors, any one of whom would have to be willing to undergo plateletpheresis twice weekly during the entire course of the patient's illness. Yankee *et al.* [54] found that the transfusion of platelets from a 'nearly identical' related donor was tolerated no better than those from random donors. It would be necessary, therefore, to type for every known HLA antigen and it is questionable whether HLA typing on this scale is a justifiable use of the limited supplies of the rarer HLA typing sera. It would seem reasonable, therefore, to attempt to find HLA-identical platelets only for those patients who have a number of siblings willing to undergo repeated plateletpheresis and from amongst whom, it is hoped, at least one HLA-identical donor will be found, and also for those who have already developed platelet alloantibodies [55].

Post-transfusion purpura
This is a rare complication in which severe purpura with acute thrombocytopenia occurs four to eight days after blood transfusion [56]. In all reported cases except one the patient has been female and, again in all cases but one, an alloantibody specific for the platelet alloantigen Pl^{A1} has been identified in the patient's serum [57]; the patient's own platelets were Pl^{A1}-negative. It is suggested that when such patients are transfused with Pl^{A1}-positive platelets, the alloantibodies not only destroy the transfused platelets but at the height of the immune response cross-react with the recipient's own platelets and produce a profound thrombocytopenia [58]. Treatment consists of transfusion of platelets from a Pl^{A1}-negative donor, blood replacement, administration of corticosteroids, and removal of antibody by exchange transfusion or plasmapheresis. In two of 15 reported cases the outcome was fatal; both patients were elderly and the thrombocytopenia occurred within seven days of major surgery [59].

Transfusion of heavily contaminated blood
Although a small number of units of blood are

contaminated with bacteria at the time of collection, these are usually killed during storage. Exceptionally, some cryophilic organisms such as pseudomonad and coli-aerogene groups may grow slowly at 4°C, or more rapidly if the blood is allowed to warm up intermittently to temperatures above 10°C. Heavily contaminated blood is not always haemolysed; Braude *et al.* [60] found that 25% of bacteria grown in blood at 4°C produced no haemolysis. The longer the infected blood has been stored before transfusion, the greater will be the degree of contamination and the greater the effects upon the recipient.

Generally within a few minutes of the start of the transfusion there will be a profound collapse accompanied by a rigor, vomiting, acute abdominal pain and diarrhoea. The patient may become hyperpyrexial and death may ensue within 12–24 hours. The risk of this grave hazard is increased if strict refrigeration at 4°C is not maintained during the storage life of the blood; or if containers are entered, for example, to obtain a sample for crossmatching or to prepare red-cell concentrates, when bacteria may be introduced. Even though the blood is stored at 4°C after the puncture, the British Pharmacopoeia recommends that a time limit of 12 hours should not be exceeded before its subsequent transfusion.

Because all connecting tubes can be made as an integral part of the system and plasma can be separated in a 'closed system' for the preparation of components, it was expected that a change to plastic containers for blood would eliminate the hazard of bacterial infection. Unfortunately this has not proved as absolute a safeguard as was expected, principally because of the development of 'pin-hole' leaks in the plastics [61]. With improvements in the manufacture of plastics it is to be expected that this risk will eventually be overcome.

Citrate toxicity

Serious toxic effects may occur if the plasma level of citrate rises during transfusion to 1 g/l. Because of the normal metabolism of citrate in the liver and excretion via the kidneys, dangerous levels are unlikely unless the circulation to these organs is impaired or there is liver damage. Hypothermia may inhibit citrate metabolism and babies undergoing exchange transfusion with citrated blood are also at risk. Citrate toxicity usually causes hypotension with cardiac dysrhythmia. In the case of massive transfusion in which more than two litres of citrated blood are being transfused in 20 minutes, prophylactic therapy may be given by injecting 10% calcium gluconate solutions, 10 ml for every litre of citrated blood. Injection of 1 ml of the same preparation after each 100 ml of blood is recommended by most authorities for babies undergoing

exchange transfusion. Solutions containing calcium must not be injected into the lumen of the giving set since they may clot the donor blood. Injection should be made into another vein or, during exchange transfusion, be preceded and followed by the injection of 1–2 ml of heparin-saline. Calcium overdose may result in cardiac arrest: Wolf *et al.* [62] report the death of a child who was transfused with 1250 ml of citrated blood in 20 hours following cardiac surgery and was given 2 ml of 10% calcium chloride with each 50 ml of blood.

Transfusion haemosiderosis (see also Chapters 5 and 9). Each unit (500 ml) of blood contains as much iron as is normally lost from the body in about 250 days. Following repeated transfusions to patients who are not losing blood—e.g. in patients with refractory anaemia—iron deposits are likely to be found in almost all the cells of the body. The serum iron concentration is greatly increased and the iron-binding capacity of the serum is fully saturated. Widespread tissue damage is associated with steadily increasing iron stores and the liver damage of iron overload may be further exacerbated by the consequences of post-transfusion hepatitis. Treatment with desferrioxamine (Chapter 5, p. 183) may reduce the iron overload, but this end is achieved more easily if the transfusions are kept to as few as possible and blood that is less than seven days old is used for such patients.

Technical and procedural hazards

These are conditioned more by the skill, experience and care of the transfusionist and those looking after the patient than are most of the complications already detailed. They include air embolism, circulatory overload, thrombophlebitis and septicaemia from the giving set.

Air embolism. The accidental introduction of more than 40 ml of air into the circulation may be followed by alarming signs, and in a patient already dangerously ill, even 10 ml may be fatal [63]. The patient suddenly becomes cyanosed, there is circulatory collapse; a millwheel murmur can be heard over the precordium and there is syncope from cerebral ischaemia. Treatment consists in putting the patient on his left side in a head-low position [64].

The risk of air embolism is greatest when air pressure is applied to secure the rapid transfusion of blood from a glass bottle. The hazard is minimal in the case of collapsible plastic containers, since blood can be rapidly transfused from them by the application of external pressure, but air embolism may occur even with this system when the giving set is changed during transfusion. Yackel [65] advises that if the set must be changed before the bag is emptied, the defective set should be occluded and left in place, the replacement set being inserted into the second port by the usual procedure.

Circulatory overload. Transfusion of patients with already increased plasma volumes may lead to pulmonary oedema. The severely anaemic patient is especially at risk. Only red-cell concentrates should be transfused to avoid overload from unwanted plasma. It is wise to limit the initial transfusion to 250 ml at a drip rate of 10–15 minutes. The patient should be kept warm and propped up in a sitting position to reduce right-auricular pressure. Except when there is potassium depletion a rapidly acting diuretic such as ethacrynic acid (50 mg intravenously) may be given just before the transfusion. Harrison *et al.* [66] have found this to be as valuable in reducing cardiac overload as the more elaborate procedure of exchange transfusion. Some severely anaemic patients may be dangerously deficient in potassium, however, particularly if they have already been treated by diuretics and/or there is polyuria or diarrhoea. Such cases are more safely treated by exchange transfusion with frequent monitoring of the serum potassium and electrocardiograph [67].

If, despite these precautions, signs of overload develop, such as a dry cough and tightness in the chest with moist râles, the transfusion should be stopped and, unless there is a rapid relief of symptoms, venesection of 500 ml carried out.

Circulatory overload may also occur when products such as triple-strength plasma or cryoprecipitate with a high protein and sodium content are given to non-oligaemic patients. The volume of tissue fluid attracted into the circulation by the hypertonic solution may be more than the patient can tolerate.

Particulate emboli from stored blood. Microaggregates of leucocytes and platelets form within 24 hours and may be numerous and up to 200 μm in diameter after eight to 10 days' storage of blood at 4–6°C [68]. In standard administration sets, the nylon filter has a pore size of 170 μm. Special filters have been designed, therefore, to hold back particles down to a size of 20–40 μm. Hypoxia may develop in patients receiving massive transfusions of stored blood and it has been suggested that pulmonary microembolism from transfused aggregates is a possible cause. Although some studies of battle casualties have appeared to support this view [69], an experimental study of exsanguinated baboons, resuscitated with large volumes of blood containing aggregates similar to those found in stored human blood, resulted in no detectable changes in lung function and no rise in pulmonary arterial pressure [70]. In an International Forum reported in *Vox Sanguinis*, Bredenberg [71] concluded that although particulate emboli from stored blood may contribute to pulmonary failure following massive transfusion, their role was probably minor. Other opinions vary widely as to the necessity for using special microfilters when transfusing large volumes of stored blood: Solis & Walker [72] consider they should probably be used whenever more than 2·5 l of blood are administered rapidly.

Pulmonary embolism from severed catheter. Many instances have been reported of the loss of the distal end of a plastic catheter into a vein [73]. In some the lost catheter has been recovered from the right auricle; in others the patient has died from pulmonary embolism. This hazard is most likely to occur when attempting to withdraw a catheter through a needle and is best avoided by using the type of catheter which fits over the outside of the inserting needle.

Addition of drugs to transfusion fluids. Laboratory studies have shown that the addition to the transfusion fluid of some preparations suitable for intravenous use may have an inhibiting effect upon the drug, alternatively the drug may have toxic effects upon the red cells. When ethacrynic acid is added, for example, there may be damage to the red-cell membrane with efflux of potassium and influx of sodium [74]. Despite the convenience, therefore, medicaments should never be added to the blood in the container but should be given intravenously via a different vein or injected through the special device incorporated in the giving set close to the intravenous needle.

Thrombophlebitis. The most effective prophylactic measure is to change the site of infusion every eight hours. Addition of heparin to the fluid infused is ineffective [75].

Septicaemia from the giving set. Bacteria may be introduced at the time of setting up a transfusion, or may be present in minimal and non-dangerous numbers in the blood transfused. They may then multiply within the filter if the same giving set is used during treatment spread over several days [76]. This potentially dangerous complication is prevented by changing the giving set twice daily.

Necrotizing enterocolitis after exchange transfusion. Perforation of the bowel after neonatal exchange transfusion has been reported by Corkery *et al.* [77] and Orme & Eades [78]. There is no clear reason for the association, and it may occur in babies not subjected to transfusion or infusion via an umbilical catheter.

Refusal to feed, abdominal distension and vomiting are characteristic features. Passage of blood per rectum is an early sign of colonic perforation. Emergency surgery, peritoneal lavage and broad-spectrum antibiotics are indicated.

Problems of availability

The difficulty of finding blood for patients who have developed alloantibodies which react with the majority of donor bloods is generally well understood. Not so well appreciated, however, is that supplies of Rh(D)-negative blood are only one-sixth those of Rh-positive, so that rarely are large amounts of Rh-negative blood available. In Britain approximately six per cent of donors are O Rh-negative and only 1·5% are B Rh-negative. A large blood centre collecting 2000 donations per week can therefore expect an intake of only 120 units of O and 30 units of B Rh-negative blood and this may have to suffice for 10 or 20 hospital blood banks. Care must therefore be taken to group as many recipients as possible in advance of transfusion so as to avoid an emergency situation in which group O Rh-negative blood is needlessly transfused to a patient subsequently found to be Rh-positive. In many circumstances transfusion of plasma protein solution or a plasma volume expander may suffice, or at least buy time whilst emergency ABO and Rh-typing are being performed.

INDICATIONS FOR TRANSFUSION OF BLOOD AND BLOOD COMPONENTS

As already stated, only when the clinician is fully aware of the complications which may arise, and when he has an appreciation of some of the problems of supply, is he really in a position critically to assess the need of his patient for transfusion. The overall risk of a transfusion causing the death of the patient is similar to that of an 'interval' appendicectomy and the decision to transfuse should only be taken after a full appraisal of the clinical situation.

In the majority of cases transfusions are given to correct:
1 a blood volume deficit;
2 deficient oxygen transport;
3 a bleeding disorder; or
4 susceptibility to infection.

The modern approach to transfusion must be to give the patient only those components required to achieve the necessary therapeutic end. Not only does this make blood components available for other patients' needs (e.g. factor VIII for the treatment of haemophilia or platelets for those with thrombocytopenia) but eliminates to a considerable extent sources of reaction and sensitization. In addition, most of the components are preserved better when separated from whole blood and stored under conditions appropriate to the particular component.

Whole blood

The essential value of whole blood is that it increases both intravascular fluid volume and oxygen carrying capacity, and only if these require simultaneous augmentation should its transfusion be considered. In general, this situation arises when there has been a recent acute blood loss of more than 20–25% of the total blood volume. Nevertheless, in many instances in which the haemorrhage is only moderate, resuscitation may be accomplished satisfactorily by the rapid initial transfusion of 500–1000 ml of physiological saline or Ringer lactate solution, followed by 500–1000 ml of concentrated red cells. Transfusion of whole blood is then required only if blood volume has not been adequately restored or there is continued or renewed haemorrhage. This practice became established through extensive experience with battle casualties in Vietnam [79] and, by its adoption, many hospitals have found it possible to transfuse 60–70% of blood donated as red-cell concentrates and thus to facilitate a policy of component therapy. It is axiomatic, however, that when the decision is taken to treat haemorrhage by transfusion of red-cell concentrates, plasma protein solution or albumin is not used as a supplement, since this will not only defeat the basic philosophy underlying this plan of therapy but detract significantly from its cost effectiveness.

Freshly drawn blood should be avoided whenever possible because of the hazard of cytomegalovirus infection and syphilis (p. 1436), but is necessary when platelet replacement is required and platelet concentrates are not available, or for the exchange transfusion treatment of hepatic coma [80]. In the treatment of severe blood loss, when the volume transfused approaches or exceeds a total blood volume replacement, the patient may become deficient in platelets because of platelet consumption and loss resulting from the haemorrhage and its replacement with stored blood. This may cause a general oozing, mild purpura and sometimes haematuria, and will respond rapidly to the transfusion of two or three units of fresh blood.

Blood used for the exchange transfusion of the newly born, or in open-heart surgery, should not be more than five days stored, otherwise there may be adverse effects from hyperkalaemia. Fresh blood is not required during either of these procedures unless the patient shows bleeding from thrombocytopenia.

Red-cell concentrates

Anaemic patients who require transfusion are in no

way benefited by the protein and other components of the plasma portion of whole blood. The additional fluid may cause circulatory overload as well as the unnecessary hazard of sensitizing the recipient to plasma components (p. 1437). Transfusion should therefore be with red-cell concentrates, which may be regarded as a by-product of the preparation of plasma components, and are generally available.

The red cells from a single blood donation will raise the haemoglobin in an adult recipient by about 1 g/dl and the total number of units required to restore the haemoglobin to a safe level may therefore be conveniently calculated. The precautions to be taken in a severely anaemic patient are given on page 1440. In general, because of the increase in blood viscosity when red-cell concentrates are transfused, it is unwise to attempt to raise the haemoglobin by more than 4 g/dl during a period of 24 hours. When exceptionally this is necessary, exchange transfusion is to be preferred.

If the container is not entered when the red-cell concentrate is prepared, for example when a plastic container with a transfer pack is used, the expiry date remains the same as that of the original whole blood. If the container is entered, there is a risk of bacterial contamination and the red cells should be transfused only within the next 12 hours.

Frozen red cells. Red cells undergo irreversible damage during freezing from the excessive concentration of solutes within the red-cell envelope. This may be prevented either by very rapid freezing or by adding a preparation such as glycerol which will minimize the degree of intracellular solute hyperconcentration. In the method developed by Krijnen *et al.* [81] concentrated red cells from ACD or CPD blood are suspended in 20% w/v glycerol and are then frozen in liquid nitrogen at $-196°C$ in about 2·5 minutes. They may be stored for several years in the frozen state and when required for transfusion are thawed at $40°C$ and then washed in 17·5% sorbitol and 0·9% NaCl. The 24-hour ^{51}Cr survival of such cells is greater than 90%.

The indications for the transfusion of frozen red cells are the same as those of red-cell concentrates, but they have the additional advantage that, probably because of the washing, they are more or less free of leucocytes and carry a lesser risk of transmitting hepatitis. An individual's own red cells may be stored pending subsequent transfusion. This is of special value when the risk of sensitization to white-cell antigens must be avoided (p. 1438) or when the recipient has a rare blood group or has developed alloantibodies reacting with most donor bloods.

Small-pool plasma

This is prepared in Britain by pooling plasma separated from 10 donations, which is then freeze-dried. The content of anti-A and anti-B is artificially lowered by including in the pool some A and B plasma to allow for the inhibition of high-titre anti-A and anti-B by the A and B substances (p. 1397). Plasma may therefore be transfused to a patient of any group and is useful as a volume expander after blood loss when whole blood or red-cell concentrates are not available, and as a replacement fluid in cases of burns, or skin or intestinal disease in which protein-containing fluid is lost from the body. One unit is reconstituted by the addition of 400 ml of sterile pyrogen-free water and must be transfused within 12 hours of reconstitution. Since small-pool plasma is prepared from 10 donations one might expect a greater incidence of hepatitis following its transfusion than after whole blood or a red-cell concentrate. In practice there is no significant difference. Freeze-dried plasma can be stored, protected from direct sunlight, for up to 10 years provided the temperature is kept below $25°C$.

Fresh-frozen plasma (FFP)

Acid-citrate-dextrose (ACD) or citrate-phosphate-dextrose (CPD) plasma separated from the red cells within 18 hours of donation, frozen rapidly and stored at $-30°C$, has a coagulation factor content which will remain at near normal levels for up to 12 months. If kept at $-20°C$ it should not be stored for more than six months. For use, FFP should be thawed rapidly at $37°C$ (with continuous agitation) and transfused within 30 minutes to avoid rapid post-thaw deterioration of coagulation factors. Fresh-frozen plasma can also be prepared in a freeze-dried form: stored in the dark at $-25°C$ it is satisfactory for use for up to eight years. It is of particular value in the management of inherited deficiencies of factors V, VII, X, XI and XIII [82]. Fresh-frozen plasma is also indicated for control of haemorrhage in patients with multiple haemostatic defects from underlying liver disease (p. 1167). In a severe case of liver disease as much as 20 ml/kg body weight may be required within six hours and, because of the risk of overloading, some authorities prefer to use a factor-IX concentrate [83]. Some preparations of the latter may induce a massive thrombosis, however, and should be resorted to only when transfusion of FFP is contraindicated or has failed. Fresh-frozen plasma is recommended by some clinicians for transfusion as a 'non-specific haemostatic agent' to patients requiring massive blood replacement. Unless the patient has received oral anticoagulants prior to transfusion or has significant liver disease, FFP is rarely required and transfusion of platelet concentrates is more likely to be indicated.

Plasma protein solution

This is the solution remaining after the preparation of components such as cryoprecipitate, fibrinogen and immunoglobulins. The protein content of about 5 g/dl is mostly albumin and the solution is heated at 60°C for 10 hours to destroy the causative viruses of hepatitis and cytomegalovirus disease. Plasma protein solution is a valuable volume expander in a case of haemorrhage when whole blood or red-cell concentrates are not available, and for replacement therapy in protein-losing states such as burns and exfoliative dermatitis. Since it contains no fibrinogen or other coagulation factors it is not suitable for the treatment of coagulation defects.

Albumin

Infusions of albumin are indicated in three main circumstances:
1 to restore plasma volume;
2 to increase the intravascular binding of bilirubin in babies with haemolytic disease of the newborn; and
3 as replacement therapy in chronic hypoalbuminaemia.

Human albumin may be provided as a solution or as a freeze-dried powder to be reconstituted with sterile water immediately prior to transfusion. The preparation contains a low proportion of salts and an albumin content of 15–25% w/v of protein. The product is sometimes termed 'salt-poor' concentrated albumin. During preparation it is heated at 60°C for 10 hours to inactivate any hepatitis viruses which may be present.

In a case of nephrosis or cirrhosis, Davison [84] advises that infusions of albumin are given only when the patient fails to lose weight after treatment with 500 mg of frusemide plus 200 mg of spironolactone for five days when on a sodium intake restricted to 0·5 g/day. If under these conditions the urinary sodium excretion is less than 100 mEq/24 hours, 50 g albumin should be infused in 350 ml of water three times per week. In Davison's experience albumin infusions alone are not as effective as when they are given in combination with diuretics.

Fibrinogen

The fibrinogen component of plasma is available for transfusion as a freeze-dried concentrate containing 4 g of fibrinogen, which is reconstituted with 200 ml of sterile water to make a two per cent solution. The concentrate is prepared from large pools of plasma ranging from 500–5000 donations and despite the routine testing of all donations and the final product for HBsAg, its transfusion carries a significant risk of transmitting hepatitis. The potential hazard of non-A, non-B hepatitis (p. 1436) must be borne in mind, particularly when transfusing fibrinogen from commercial sources [18]. Cryoprecipitate (see below) contains 0·1–0·3 g of fibrinogen per pack and when available is a safer alternative.

Fibrinogen replacement therapy is not generally required in a haemorrhagic state unless the level of fibrinogen is below 1 g/l. Under these circumstances the patient should be given an initial transfusion of cryoprecipitate from 10–12 packs or, if these are not available, one to two units of concentrated fibrinogen. Triple-strength plasma, prepared by reconstituting three units of freeze-dried plasma in 400 ml of water, is another useful alternative.

Factor-VIII concentrates (see also Chapter 28)

Plasma separated from ACD or CPD blood within 18 hours of donation is an excellent source of factor VIII (AHF) for the control of haemorrhage in haemophilia or von Willebrand's disease. Since AHF is stable only when freeze-dried or frozen at temperatures below −25°C, the sooner the plasma is separated and deep frozen, the greater is the potency of the final preparation. The amount of AHF in the plasma of different donors varies considerably and in a few is outside the usual range of 50–150% [85]. This matters little when an adult patient is treated with a concentrate prepared from the plasma of several donors, but may be important when cryoprecipitate prepared from only one or two units of plasma is used to treat a haemophilic child. In such a case the donors selected should be known to have a factor-VIII level of at least 100%.

Table 35.2 lists the AHF content of the preparations generally available for replacement therapy. Pool & Shannon [86] discovered that when FFP thaws between 4° and 8°C a white gelatinous precipitate remains which contains most of the factor VIII as a cryoprecipitate. After removal of the supernatant this material can be stored frozen (preferably at −40°C), to be thawed at 37°C when required for transfusion. On average one unit of cryoprecipitate per 7 kg of body weight is needed to raise the circulating level of AHF to 25%. Recent technical developments, by which the supernatant is removed continuously as the FFP thaws, enhance the factor-VIII content of the cryoprecipitate [87]. Cryoprecipitate is effective only if given intravenously and it should be noted that the preparation contains no factor IX. In the emergency treatment of a suspected case of haemophilia, FFP, which contains factors VIII and IX, is the treatment of choice until laboratory tests have established that the patient is deficient only in factor VIII, when cryoprecipitate or factor-VIII concentrate is to be preferred.

Table 35.2. Concentration of factor VIII in plasma and available concentrates

Factor-VIII preparation	Volume containing 100 units	Times concentrated
Fresh plasma	100 ml	1
Fresh-frozen plasma	120 ml	1
Cryoprecipitate	20–30 ml	3–5
Freeze-dried concentrate		
Type 1	16–22 ml	4·5–6
Type 2	8–10 ml	10–12

Cryoprecipitate also contains the von Willebrand factor.

The more concentrated freeze-dried preparations of human AHF currently prepared in Britain have a potency equivalent in the one case to about 600 ml of fresh plasma, and in the other to about 1200 ml (Table 35.2). The latter should be reserved for grave situations, such as major surgery complicating haemophilia, since only limited supplies are available. A highly purified concentrate has been developed by the American National Red Cross, using polyethylene glycol, and is assessed as being purified about 150-fold. Similar material is also available commercially. Because freeze-dried AHF can be stored at ordinary refrigerator temperature and, after reconstitution, administered by a syringe, it is the ideal product for home treatment of haemophilia. When in short supply, however, freeze-dried cryoprecipitate is a suitable alternative.

Apart from cryoprecipitate, concentrates factor VIII are prepared from multiple donor pools. Consequently they are more likely to transmit hepatitis than is cryoprecipitate. There is increasing evidence that most haemophilic adults are now, as the result of repeated treatments, immune to infection with HBsAg [18]. Few in Britain appear to have an immunity to non-A, non-B viruses, however, and this must be borne in mind before resorting to commercial sources of factor VIII, all of which are prepared from plasma collected from non-British donors [19]. This will be of even greater clinical significance if subsequent studies confirm a greater likelihood of chronic active hepatitis following a non-A, non-B infection (p. 1436).

Factor-IX concentrates

Factor IX is relatively stable at 4°C, so that plasma prepared from blood stored up to seven days may be used for replacement therapy in Christmas disease. Fresh-frozen plasma is an alternative and convenient source. There is a rapid loss of factor IX from the circulation following transfusion, probably due to rapid diffusion into a large extravascular pool [88], and

concentrates of this material are therefore required for treating haemorrhage of any severity. Because of the difficulty of preparation, they are, however, available only in limited amounts.

Most of the products currently available have a factor-IX content of between 25 and 30 units/ml and also contain factors II, VII and X. The concentrate is freeze-dried and prepared from a plasma pool of up to 5000 donations [82]. Stability at 4°C is for up to two years and when reconstituted with sterile pyrogen-free water, 10 ml contains 200–300 units of factors II, VII, IX and X. The hazard of transmitting hepatitis viruses must be regarded as similar to that of concentrates of fibrinogen or factor VIII.

Thrombogenicity is also recognized as a serious potential hazard, particularly in patients with liver disease (Chapter 29). Urbaniak & Cash [83] consider that thrombogenicity may be enhanced when factor-IX concentrates are left at room temperature after reconstitution. Injection should therefore be completed within 15 minutes of reconstitution.

Certain 'activated' factor-IX concentrates, particularly those which when tested *in vitro* are thought to have a thrombogenic potential, have been claimed to be of value in the control of bleeding in severe haemophilia A complicated by the development of factor-VIII inhibitors (see also Chapters 28 and 29).

Platelets

The indications for platelet transfusions are outlined in Chapters 22, 25, 29 and 31. Dangerous bleeding is rarely seen if the platelet count is above $20\,000/mm^3$. Platelets deteriorate rapidly in stored blood, about 50% loss of function occurring within 24 hours. Platelet replacement therapy may be by means of fresh whole blood drawn into ACD or CPD anticoagulant, platelet-rich plasma (PRP) or platelet concentrates (PC).

Transfusion of fresh whole blood to arrest thrombocytopenic haemorrhage is of doubtful efficacy and should be employed only when there is no alternative. A single donation contains about 1×10^{11} platelets and, since three to four times this number are required in the average adult to raise the platelet count by $25-35 \times 10^9/l$, transfusion of sufficient whole blood is likely to result in circulatory overload unless the recipient is oligaemic from blood loss or transfusion is practised as a 'mini exchange' [89].

Slichter & Harker [90] have described a method of preparing PRP and PC which yields more than 85% of platelets from a unit of citrated blood. Blood is collected into ACD or CPD in a plastic bag and centrifuged at 100 g for nine minutes. The supernatant PRP is expressed into an integral satellite pack, which may then be sealed and detached ready for transfusion or centrifuged at 3000 g for 20 minutes and left for 90 minutes to allow the platelets to disaggregate spontaneously. When required for immediate transfusion the platelet pellet is resuspended in 20 ml of residual plasma by gentle manipulation. For storage as a PC, 70 ml of plasma should be left in the satellite pack. All procedures must be carried out at room temperature (c. 22°C), and constant gentle mixing by resting the pack on a mechanical stage is essential during storage. Under these conditions platelet concentrates may be stored at 22°C for up to 72 hours. If stored at 4°C the platelets achieve only an immediate but short-lived haemostatic effect. Platelets from CPD blood have a slightly better viability after storage than those from ACD blood [91]. Attempts to preserve platelets for long periods in the frozen state in dimethyl sulphoxide or glycerol have as yet proved only partially successful [92].

The risks of transmitting hepatitis and of alloimmunization are lessened when all platelets transfused to a recipient are collected from a single donor; this can be accomplished by so-called plateletpheresis, using either an intermittent-flow or a continuous-flow cell separator (p. 1446). It is important that the donor should not have taken aspirin within the previous 72 hours. Disaggregated platelets will pass satisfactorily through a blood administration set filter; some 10–35% may be removed, however, when a filter designed to remove microaggregates is used [93].

Many published studies evaluate the response to platelet replacement in terms of the rise in platelet count per square metre of body surface area, the latter being determined from a nomogram. Whilst such accuracy is admittedly desirable for any serious evaluation, there are so many variables that assessing the anticipated increase in platelet level as $10 \times 10^9/l$/unit transfused is generally satisfactory for clinical use; an adjustment upwards related to body weight being made in paediatric cases. Although platelets may circulate for up to 12 days following transfusion, it is often necessary to transfuse patients with severe thrombocytopenia at four- or five-day intervals and

sometimes more frequently. The decision to transfuse is generally better based on the clinical situation, e.g. recurrence of purpura, than on the platelet count.

ABO-compatible platelets survive better in the recipient than do ABO-incompatible (p. 1438), and since PRP or PC always contains some red cells it is advisable to give Rh-negative platelets to Rh-negative recipients. When this is not possible, sensitization to the D antigen may be prevented by administration of anti-D immunoglobulin (p. 1413). Platelet concentrates are also contaminated by leucocytes and the pyrexial reactions which sometimes occur with PC are often due to antibodies reacting with leucocytes rather than platelets. Patients receiving repeated platelet transfusions may develop a refractory state in which further transfusions from random donors become progressively less effective. Post-transfusion platelet survival has been reported to decrease as the number of HLA incompatibilities increased [94]. In such cases a search should be made for HLA-compatible donors (see p. 1438) and, using plateletpheresis, it may be possible to provide clinically effective platelets from a single donor, who should ideally be a sibling of the patient. In others alloimmunization may have resulted from platelet-specific rather than HLA antigens, and in these donor platelets may be found by selecting those which are not aggregated by the recipient's serum [95] or are compatible in a direct platelet fluorescence matching test [96]. Despite care in matching and donor selection, however, some patients continue to respond poorly, suggesting that factors other than alloimmunization may play an important role in determining the haemostatic response to platelet transfusion therapy [97].

Transfusion of leucocytes

Control of infection by granulocyte transfusions may increase the survival of patients with neutropenia, particularly when there is septicaemia failing to respond to antibiotic therapy. Higby [98] advises that granulocyte transfusions should begin within 48 hours of the onset of the infection and that at least $1·5 \times 10^{10}$ should be transfused daily for a minimum of four days. Leucocytes harvested from as many as 40 units of normal blood are required to raise the peripheral-blood granulocyte level by $1 \times 10^9/l$ in a recipient of 1 m^2 body surface area [99]. Patients with chronic myelocytic leukaemia and very high leucocyte counts are therefore sometimes preferentially used as donors; because of the delay in the rise of the leucocyte count following treatment with myleran those treated with hydroxyurea are more likely to be suitable as donors.

The introduction of cell separators is particularly valuable for the preparation of leucocyte concentrates and they may also be used for plateletpheresis. Several different models and systems are now available, but a cell separator consists essentially of a sealed sterile bowl into which blood from the donor is fed continuously or intermittently through a closed circuit for centrifugation. There is then an upward flow of blood in the bowl with the separation of red cells in the outer portion, plasma in the central area and the leucocytes in the form of a buffy-coat layer at the plasma red-cell interface. Three collecting ports permit the continuous collection from each of these layers and the separated components are removed at a rate controlled by individual peristaltic pumps. The red cells and the platelet-rich plasma may then be recombined and returned to the donor as buffy-coat-poor blood, or the platelet-rich plasma and the buffy coat may be directed separately into plastic bags containing ACD for the preparation of leucocyte and platelet concentrates and the platelet-poor plasma and red cells returned to the donor. The procedure is known as continuous-flow centrifugation and yields about four or five times as many leucocytes or platelets per hour as would a conventional plasmapheresis. Two methods may be used, separately or in combination, to increase the yield of granulocytes. Administration of corticosteroids to the donor (dexamethasone 6–12 mg) will cause a shift of cells from the marginated to the circulating granulocyte pool [100], or a rouleaux-forming agent such as hydroxyethyl starch (HES) may be added to the input line of the cell separator to effect an improved separation between red cells and white cells. Hydroxyethyl starch has been used extensively and is devoid of serious side-effects in the donor other than an occasional pyrogenic reaction or a mild urticaria. With the addition of HES a total of $7-10 \times 10^9$ granulocytes can be harvested from 4–10 l of blood in two to four hours; this can be increased three- or fourfold when dexamethasone is also given to the donor.

Filtration leucapheresis, in which venous blood is passed through a nylon filter, to which the granulocytes adhere before the blood is returned via another vein, has been developed as a simpler and less costly procedure for collecting leucocytes. The granulocytes are eluted from the filter using ACD-plasma-saline. There is evidence, however, that granulocytes obtained in this way are less effective therapeutically than those collected by cell separation [101].

Using HLA-identical donors minimizes the risk of sensitization to leucocyte antigens and a direct matching test between the donor granulocytes and the recipient's serum should be carried out before transfusion. Verheugt *et al.* [102] recommend an immuno-fluorescence technique using Fab fragments of anti-human immunoglobulins so as to avoid non-specific binding to the leucocyte Fc receptors. When leucocytes are transfused to recipients in whom the immune mechanism is suppressed, the transfused lymphocytes may survive in the patient's circulation and initiate a graft-versus-host reaction. This may be prevented by irradiating the blood prior to transfusion (p. 1450).

TECHNIQUE OF TRANSFUSION

Practical considerations

Most transfusions are given via a peripheral vein; exceptionally, in catastrophic haemorrhage, blood may be transfused intra-arterially [103] and, in children when the intravenous route is difficult or it is necessary to conserve the peripheral veins, into the peritoneal cavity [104]. This last route is used also for intrauterine transfusion of the fetus [105]. A vein in the forearm is to be preferred to one in the antecubital fossa or in the leg; there is then less restriction of movement and any subsequent thrombophlebitis is less incapacitating. If it is necessary to start the transfusion with an electrolyte solution, one containing five or 10% dextrose is to be avoided. Red cells coming into contact with the dextrose may suffer osmotic damage, lose potassium rapidly and show an impaired post-transfusion survival [106]. Those still present on the filter of a giving set which is then used for a dextrose infusion may haemolyse and, in the case of a small child, cause a subsequent haemoglobinuria [107].

Whenever possible, blood of the same ABO and Rh(D) group as the patient should be selected. Subgroups of A and AB are unimportant unless the recipient has anti-A or anti-H active at a temperature of 20°C in the serum. In emergency, group-O, Kell-negative blood may be transfused, but if the recipient is not group O the donor plasma must be free of high-titre anti-A/anti-B agglutinins and haemolysins. Donor blood for Rh(D)-negative recipients should be Rh-negative and Kell-negative. Serum from both the donor and the recipient should be tested routinely for irregular antibodies and the red cells of the donor and the serum of the recipient should be tested directly together at 20 and 37°C under conditions designed to detect incompatibility from any IgM or IgG antibodies in the patient's serum. A detailed procedure using saline, albumin, indirect antiglobulin and Liss techniques has been drawn up by Tovey & Jenkins [108].

Special care must be taken at the bedside to identify:
1 the patient;
2 the blood sample at the time it is collected; and
3 the blood or blood component before every transfusion.

Most fatal accidents from incompatible transfusion are due to a lack of care in identification. Accurate records must be kept of the batch numbers of all blood and blood products transfused to make possible donor identification in the event of a post-transfusion reaction.

Laboratory investigation of a reaction to transfusion

So that they are available to investigate a suspected transfusion reaction, all pilot tubes and patient samples used for cross matching, together with remnants of the blood transfused, should be kept at 4°C for two days after every transfusion. As soon as possible after the reaction, samples of the recipient's blood should be collected, one into heparin and the other clotted, to be examined for free haemoglobin or bile pigments. Any urine passed during or after the transfusion should be tested for haemoglobin and urobilinogen. The immediate examination of the residue of the donor blood should include tests for free haemoglobin and inspection of a hanging drop preparation and a stained film for bacteria. A serious haemolytic reaction or one due to infected fluid will usually be detected by these investigations. Less urgent tests will include a check grouping (ABO and Rh) of all samples, a direct antiglobulin test of the post-transfusion sample to test for red-cell sensitization, a repeat of the direct matching tests, a search for immune antibodies in the recipient's serum and, where appropriate, investigation for white cell, platelet and anti-serum protein antibodies. Details of the procedures to be employed have been given by Tovey & Gillespie [109].

Storage of blood

Blood products which have been freeze-dried, such as plasma, fibrinogen and albumin, may be stored at normal room temperature, 18–28°C, for several years, but must not be exposed to sunlight since ultra-violet light denatures plasma proteins. The adequacy of red-cell storage at other than sub-zero temperatures is dependent upon the active metabolism of glucose. Therefore not only must the anticoagulant-preservative solution used provide glucose in adequate amounts, but the conditions of storage must be such as to facilitate its conversion to adenosine triphosphate (ATP). There is a good correlation between the ATP content of stored red cells and their post-transfusion survival [110]. Dextrose consumption in red cells at 4°C is at least 30 times slower than it is at 37°C [111]. Glycolysis is therefore retarded when blood is stored between 2 and 6°C and at this temperature the likelihood of bacterial growth is minimized.

The most generally used anticoagulant-preservative solutions are acid-citrate-dextrose (ACD) and citrate-phosphate-dextrose (CPD) solutions. The ACD solution used in Britain has the following composition:

Disodium citrate (monohydric)	2·5 g
Dextrose (anhydrous)	3·0 g
Water	120 ml

to which is added 420 ml of donor blood. In the USA the formula for ACD (solution NIHA) contains the same amount of disodium citrate (as a mixture of trisodium citrate and citric acid) but has only half as much dextrose (1·5 g) and 67·5 ml of water: 450 ml of blood is collected into this solution.

The formula for CPD solution is:

Trisodium citrate (dihydrate)	26·30 g
Citric acid (monohydrate)	3·27 g
Sodium dihydrogen phosphate (monohydrate)	2·22 g
Dextrose	25·50 g
Water to	1 litre

63 ml of this solution are mixed with 450 ml whole blood.

Among the advantages claimed for CPD preservative is that blood collected into this solution has an initial pH of 7·2, by contrast with ACD blood in which the pH is 7·0, and that the higher pH minimizes the initial damage to the red-cell membrane known as the 'lesion of collection' [112]. In consequence, blood collected into CPD maintains its ATP level better and may be stored for seven days longer than that collected into ACD. Further advantages claimed are a decreased incidence of transfusion-induced acidosis and proportionately less risk of citrate toxicity in massive transfusion, and that CPD blood may be better able to release oxygen to tissues immediately after transfusion [113]. Valtis & Kennedy [114] reported that the oxygen dissociation curve of red cells stored in ACD is 'shifted to the left' and it has been established that the affinity of haemoglobin for oxygen varies inversely with the red cell concentration of 2,3-diphosphoglycerate (2,3-DPG). Red cells stored in CPD for seven days contain twice as much 2,3-DPG as those stored in ACD. In theory, therefore, transfusion of CPD-stored blood should be of greater benefit to the patient requiring a massive transfusion. As yet, however, no convincing evidence has been produced to show that a decrease in 2,3-DPG content of stored red cells, and hence the possible impairment in the release of oxygen to the tissues, has any adverse clinical effect upon the recipient.

The addition of either adenosine or adenine to the preservative leads to an increased concentration of ATP and to an enhanced post-transfusion survival of the stored cells. In the amount that might be given in a massive transfusion, adenosine would be toxic, but this is not the case with adenine. A CPD-adenine solution, in which whole blood or red cells are stored for up to 35 days, is now used routinely in blood banks in Sweden [115].

During storage of blood at 4°C there is a slow but constant loss of potassium from the red cells into the plasma in exchange for sodium ions and by 21 days the concentration of potassium in the plasma may have risen to 20–30 mEq/l. This level may be dangerous during the transfusion of a patient with severe kidney disease and only relatively fresh blood or packed cells should be transfused in such cases. The plasma ammonia level also rises during storage from an initial level of 1 mg/l to about 9 mg/l by three weeks. This is only likely to be a hazard in severe liver disease and in such patients blood stored less than seven days is indicated. (Storage of red cells at $-196°C$ has been described on p. 1442.)

Use of plasma expanders

Human blood and blood products are costly fluids, both in actual monetary terms and in personal inconvenience to the donor. When volume replacement only is required, as in a case of moderate blood loss, this may be achieved more cheaply and with less risk of serious complication by use of plasma-volume expanders. Amongst the fluids available are dextrans, artificial colloids as hydroxethyl starch and modified gelatin derivatives. There is a growing appreciation, however, that simple salt solutions have a place in the treatment of moderate blood loss (p. 1441) and do not introduce some of the side-effects common to the artificial colloid plasma-volume expanders.

Dextrans are polysaccharides produced by the action of *Leuconostoc mesenteroides* on media containing sucrose. Dextrans (MW 50 000 or less) are rapidly excreted by the kidney but solutions with molecules slightly above this figure, e.g. Macrodex (70 000) or dextran 110 (110 000), are excreted at such a rate that after 24 hours approximately 40% of the infused amount has appeared in the urine. Since the dextran remaining in the circulation has a molecular size similar to that of plasma albumin it exerts osmotic effects and will satisfactorily restore and maintain plasma volume. Clinical evaluation [116] has confirmed dextran to be a safe and effective plasma-volume expander in a dose of up to 15 ml/kg body weight. Dextran solutions are contraindicated in patients with coagulation defects or thrombocytopenia, and although the more recent preparations are unlikely to cause rouleaux formation it is advisable to collect a blood sample before infusion to forestall any possible subsequent interference in crossmatching. Toxic reactions to dextrans are few but there have been occasional reports of urticaria and, exceptionally, anaphylaxis [117]. Vickers and his colleagues [118] detected no significant difference in the clinical response between two groups of patients undergoing routine surgery, in one of which the patients were infused with up to 1000 ml of dextran and in the other stored blood, for the replacement of operative blood loss. Low MW dextrans were at one time claimed to have special rheological properties but are no longer advised because of reported renal complications [119].

Hydroxyethyl starch (HES) (MW about 400 000) is supplied as a six per cent solution in saline. It persists longer in the blood than dextran—within seven days about 80% is excreted in the urine [120]. Solanke *et al.* [121] investigated in human volunteers the plasma-volume expansion given by 500 ml of HES and found it to be about twice that following infusion of a similar volume of plasma, dextran-70, or a commercial gelatin derivative (Haemacel). Few adverse clinical effects have been reported following its infusion (see below).

The gelatins are produced by hydrolysis of animal collagen, are non-toxic and completely metabolized in the body. Preparations of a molecular size large enough to be well retained in the circulation have the disadvantage, however, that they do not remain fluid at low temperatures. In those that remain fluid at ambient temperatures only about 30% of molecules remain intravascular; the remainder are excreted in the urine [122]. Probably because of this and in contrast to dextrans and HES, no evidence has been found of abnormal bleeding, even in patients receiving 4 l or more of a modified fluid gelatin within a period of 24 hours [123].

An occasional severe anaphylactic reaction, with an incidence comparable to that following penicillin, has been reported following transfusion of each of these three fluids. Ring & Messmer [124] give the following incidence: dextran, 1 in 6000 units transfused; hydroxyethyl starch, 1 in 16 000; and gelatin, 1 in 2500. Using a different fluid gelatin prepared in Switzerland, Lundsgaard-Hansen [123] found an incidence, however, of only 1/20 000 units transfused. The reported incidence of anaphylaxis from plasma protein solution is 1/50 000 [124].

In a study of 25 patients receiving blood transfusions because of sickle-cell thalassaemia, Kontopoulou-Griva (personal communication) found that seven of 14 patients (50%) who had been given infusions of dextran-40 (Rheomacrodex) in addition to blood had developed alloantibodies, mostly anti-E, anti-c and anti-Kell. None of the remaining 11 patients had been given dextran as well as blood and only two (18%) of these were immunized. The number of units of blood transfused to both groups was similar and Kontopoulou-Griva suggests that infusion of dextran may have an enhancing effect upon the formation of alloantibodies.

Red-cell substitutes

Both stroma-free haemoglobin (SFH) and synthetic perfluorocarbons will transport oxygen and carbon dioxide and are under investigation as substitutes for whole blood for transfusion. The presence of even traces of stroma and cell-membrane lipids in a haemoglobin solution will give rise on transfusion to disseminated intravascular coagulation and kidney damage [125]. Stroma-free haemoglobin has proved difficult to prepare, it carries the risk of transmitting hepatitis and other viruses and during storage, even at 4°C, is prone to undesirable methaemoglobin formation [126]. Extensive clinical trials of SFH have been carried out, particularly in Poland, and have demonstrated that whilst oxygen transport is satisfactory and current preparations are generally well tolerated, the solution is excreted rapidly with a massive haemoglobinuria [127].

Perfluorocarbons can be prepared as an oxygen-carrying emulsion with the properties of a colloid plasma expander, but tend to produce lesions in the lungs and interact with platelets and coagulation factors [128]. Perfluorotributylamine and perfluorodecaline are the most stable preparations currently under investigation, but much further work is necessary before it will be known whether either fulfils the requirements of an artificial blood substitute [129].

Selection and care of blood donors

The aim of donor selection is to exclude any whose blood may transmit disease or whose own health may suffer as the result of donation. Age limits are universally accepted as minimum 18 years and maximum 60–65 years; it is advisable to limit first time donors to those below the age of 60. The donor is usually the best judge of whether he is in normal health and truthful answers to simple questions concerning his medical history form the main part of the medical examination. Completion of a questionnaire to include a list of transmissible diseases, which should form part of the donor's permanent record, is advisable; the record should also include the blood pressure and haemoglobin levels. Female donors with less than 12·5 g or males with less than 13·1 g Hb/dl should not be bled. Hazardous occupations or hobbies, such as gliding, power flying, motor racing, climbing, driving heavy vehicles or operating hazardous machinery, should be regarded as contraindications, unless they can be deferred for 24 hours after donation. Donors who have undergone major surgery, have suffered severe trauma, received a transfusion of blood or blood products, been tattooed or subject to acupuncture, should be deferred for a period of at least six months. Women should not normally be bled during or for 12 months after pregnancy.

Any chronic illness or infection is generally a reason for disqualification, as well as a history of syphilis, cancer or significant cardiovascular disease. Prospective donors who suffer from allergy should not donate at a time when they are subject to a clinical attack. Persons with a history of jaundice or hepatitis, or in whose blood anti-HBsAg is present, may be accepted as donors provided they have not suffered the attack within the previous 12 months and have not been in house contact with hepatitis within the previous six months. A sensitive test for HBsAg (RIA or RPH) must be performed each time a donor is bled, as well as an accepted test for syphilis. Persons found positive to either test should be permanently excluded from the donor panel. Measures to minimize the risk of transmitting malaria are outlined on page 1436.

The above recommendations must be regarded only as guidelines and more detailed accounts should be consulted [130]. Other measures to be taken to minimize transmission of disease depend partly upon what infections are endemic to the geographic area in which the prospective donor normally resides. More stringent codes of practice are required for plasmapheresis donors and for those being bled by cell separator [131]. Plasmapheresis should not normally exceed 600 ml on each occasion with a maximum of 15 l/year. The interval between plasmaphereses should not in general be less than two weeks. All members of the staff of a cell separator team must be especially trained in the procedure; such training to include instruction in the selection and care of donors, all aspects of the operation of cell separators, the associated hazards and the action to be taken in the event of harm occurring to the donor. There are some who consider that a continuous-flow cell separator should be used only where a cardiac-arrest team is available to deal with a collapse of the donor during donation. Care must be exercised to ensure that unrelated, specially motivated donors are not placed in a position where it is difficult for them to withdraw from giving further donations.

BONE-MARROW TRANSPLANTATION

Before 1970 nearly all attempts at marrow transplantation failed [132]. A number of factors contributed to these discouraging results: the importance of HLA matching was not clearly recognized; immunosuppressive regimes were inadequate for conditioning the recipient to accept genetically different marrow; intensive treatment of infections and haemorrhagic complications was not fully developed, nor had methods to prevent or treat graft-versus-host disease (GVHD) been fully developed at the clinical level.

Important progress was made when it was found that acquired aplastic anaemia in man will usually respond to the intravenous infusion of syngeneic marrow from a monozygous twin without preceding imunosuppressive therapy [133]. On the basis of subsequent studies in rodents and dogs and combined results from various marrow-transplant centres, Storb & Thomas [134] advise that, in the absence of a monozygous twin, donors of marrow for transplantation should be limited so far as is possible to siblings compatible with the recipient for antigens of the HLA-A, B and D (or DRW) series. Only a few successful transplants from well-matched unrelated donors have so far been reported. Donor and recipient lymphocytes must be mutually non-stimulatory in the mixed-lymphocyte culture (MLC). There is some evidence that antigens on the X and Y chromosomes are associated with GVHD, and that GVHD is less likely when donor and recipient are of the same sex [134]. Successful engraftment of ABO-incompatible marrow has been reported following massive plasmapheresis of the recipient to lower the titre of the incompatible anti-A/anti-B [135].

It is mandatory that the immune defence system of the patient be suppressed for the allogeneic marrow graft to be accepted. This is generally accomplished by intravenous injection of cyclophosphamide and/or total body irradiation. Some groups also use anti-lymphocyte serum [136]. The place of anti-thymocyte serum in conditioning patients for marrow grafting has still to be determined.

The immediate post-grafting period is characterized by a complete loss of haemopoietic function, with a grave hazard of haemorrhage and infection. Frequent transfusions of platelet concentrates should be given to maintain the level of platelets above 20 000/mm^3. Transfusion of granulocytes to control infection is discussed on pages 1445–6. All blood and blood products transfused should be irradiated *in vitro* with 1500 rads to inactivate immunologically competent cells and thus to minimize the risk of GVHD. In patients receiving an allogeneic marrow graft for the treatment of aplastic anaemia, Storb & Thomas [134] administer methotrexate intermittently for approximately 100 days post-grafting as a further measure to induce immunological tolerance and prevent GVHD.

The fate of a subsequent marrow transplant may be seriously jeopardized by preceding blood transfusion (p. 1438). Blood or blood products must not, therefore, be transfused prior to transplantation unless indicated by urgent medical necessity. Transfusions from family members must particularly be avoided. There is evidence that graft rejection may result when minor histocompatibility antigens are present in both the blood donor and the marrow graft donor; this is less likely to be the case when transfusion donor and graft donor are unrelated.

The current position of bone-marrow transplantation in the treatment of acute leukaemia and aplastic anaemia is reviewed in Chapters 22 and 31. Powles and his colleagues [137] advise transplantation as an alternative treatment to chemo-immunotherapy for patients with acute myelogenous leukaemia who have an HLA-identical sibling. Substantially fewer of their transplanted patients (four out of 22) than chemo-immunotherapy patients (19 out of 28) relapsed and 14 (64%) transplanted patients remain alive, well and disease-free.

REFERENCES

1 YUILE C.L., VAN ZANDT T.F., ERVIN D.M. & YOUNG L.E. (1949) Haemolytic reactions produced in dogs by transfusion of incompatible dog blood and plasma. *Blood*, **4**, 1232.

2 GOLDFINGER D. (1974) Acute haemolytic transfusion reactions—a fresh look at pathogenesis and considerations regarding therapy. *Transfusion*, **17**, 85.

3 JOSEPH J.I., AWER E., LAULICHT M. & SCUDDER J. (1964) Delayed haemolytic transfusion reaction due to appearance of multiple antibodies following transfusions of apparently compatible blood. *Transfusion*, **4**, 367.

4 HOWARD P.L. (1973) Delayed haemolytic transfusion reactions. *Annals of Clinical and Laboratory Science*, **3**, 13.

5 GIBLETT E.R. (1961) A critique of the theoretical hazard of inter- vs intra-racial transfusion. *Transfusion*, **1**, 233.

6 TOVEY G.H. (1974) Preventing the incompatible blood transfusion. *Haematologia*, **8**, 389.

7 MEDICAL RESEARCH COUNCIL (1974) Post-transfusion hepatitis in a London hospital: results of a two-year prospective study, *Journal of Hygiene*, **73**, 173.

8 BLUMBERG B.S., ALTER H.J. & VISNIC S. (1965) A 'new' antigen in leukaemia sera. *Journal of the American Medical Association*, **191**, 541.

9 BLUMBERG B.S., GERSTLEY B.J.S., HUNGERFORD D.A., LONDON W.T. & SUTNICK A.I. (1967) A serum antigen (Australia antigen) in Down's Syndrome, leukaemia and hepatitis. *Annals of Internal Medicine*, **66**, 924.

10 PRINCE A.M. (1968) Relation of Australia and SH antigens. *Lancet*, **ii**, 462.

11 TONG M.J., STEVENSON D. & GORDON I. (1977) Correlation of e antigen, DNA polymerase activity, and Dane particles in chronic benign and chronic active type B hepatitis infections. *Journal of Infectious Diseases*, **135**, 980.

12 DRAKE M.E., HAMPIL B., PENNELL R.B., SPIZIZEN J., HENLE W. & STOKES J. (1952) Effect of nitrogen mustard on virus of serum hepatitis in whole blood. *Proceedings of the Society for Experimental Biology, New York*, **80**, 310.

13 REPORT OF NATIONAL HEALTH SERVICE ADVISORY GROUP (1975) *Second Report of the Advisory Group on Testing for the Presence of Hepatitis B Surface Antigen*

and its Antibody. Her Majesty's Stationery Office, London.

14 MAGNIUS L., LINDHOLM A, LUNDIN P. & IWARSON S. (1975) Clinical significance in long-term carriers of hepatitis B surface antigen. *Journal of the American Medical Association*, **231**, 356.

15 HUGGINS C.E., RUSSELL P.S., WYNN H.S., FULLER T.C. & BECK C.H. (1972) Frozen blood in transplant patients: hepatitis and HL-A isosensitization. *Transplantation Abstracts, Fourth International Congress of the Transplantation Society*, p. 144. Grune & Stratton, New York.

16 ALTER H.J., TABOR E., MERYMAN H.T., HOOFNAGLE J.H., KAHN R.A., HOLLAND P.V., GERETY R.J. & BARKER L.F. (1978) Transmission of hepatitis B virus infection by transfusion of frozen-deglycerolized red blood cells. *New England Journal of Medicine*, **298**, 637.

17 SEEF L.B. & HOOFNAGLE, J. (1977) Leader. *Annals of Internal Medicine*, **86**, 818.

18 HOOFNAGLE J.H., GERETY R.J., TABOR E., FEINSTONE S.M., BARKER L.F. & PURCELL R.H. (1977) Transmission of non-A, non-B hepatitis. *Annals of Internal Medicine*, **87**, 14.

19 CRASKE J. (1979) Factor VIII and factor IX associated transfusion hepatitis in the UK. *Report to Department of Health and Social Security*, London.

20 GRADY G. & BENNET A.J.E. (1970) Prevention of post-transfusion hepatitis by gammaglobulin: a co-operative study. *Journal of the American Medical Association*, **214**, 140.

21 WORLD HEALTH MEMORANDUM (1970) *Bulletin of the World Health Organization*, **42**, 957.

22 RAVITCH M.M. & CHAMBERS J.W. (1942) Spirochaetal survival in frozen plasma. *Bulletin of the Johns Hopkins Hospital*, **71**, 299.

23 PERHAM T.G.M., CAUL E.O., CONWAY P.J. & MOTT M.G. (1971) Cytomegalovirus in blood donors. *British Journal of Haematology*, **20**, 307.

24 DIJKMANS B.A.C., VERSKEEG J., KAUFFMAN R.H., VAN DEN BROEK P.J., EERNISSE J.G., VAN ZUNKEN J.J., BAKKER W., KALFF M.W. & VAN HOOF J.P. (1979) Treatment of cytomegalovirus pneumonitis with hyper-immune plasma. *Lancet*, **i**, 820.

25 HUTTON E.L. & SHUTE P.G. (1939) The risk of transmitting malaria by blood transfusion. *Journal of Tropical Medicine and Hygiene*, **42**, 309.

26 WORLD HEALTH ORGANIZATION REPORT (1955) Chemotherapy of malaria. *World Health Organization Monograph Series*, No. 27.

27 WOOD E.E. (1955) Brucellosis as a hazard of blood transfusion. *British Medical Journal*, **i**, 27.

28 VILASECA J.A., CERISOLA J.A., OLARTE J.A. & SOTHNER A. (1966) The use of crystal violet in the prevention of the transmission of Chagas-Mazza disease (South American Trypansomiasis). *Vox Sanguinis*, **11**, 711.

29 KOSTMANN R. & BENGTSSON E. (1964) Leishmaniasis transmitted by replacement transfusions. *Proceedings of the 10th Congress of the International Society of Blood Transfusion, Stockholm*.

30 DEGOWIN E.L., HARDIN R.C. & ALSEVER J.B. (1949) *Blood Transfusion*. W. B. Saunders, London.

31 SIMON S.W. & ECKMAN W.G. (1954) Use of chlor-

trimeton in the prevention of blood transfusion reactions. *Annals of Allergy*, **12**, 182.

32 DRUG AND THERAPEUTICS BULLETIN (1970) Mixing drugs with intravenous infusions, **8**, 53. Consumers' Association, London.

33 Grubb R. (1956) The existence of human serum groups. *Acta Pathologica et Microbiologica Scandinavica*, **39**, 195.

34 HARBOE M., RAU B. & AHO K. (1965) Properties of various anti-globulin factors in human sera. *Journal of Experimental Medicine*, **121**, 503.

35 ALLISON A.C. & BLUMBERG B.S. (1961) An isoprecipitation reaction distinguishing human serum protein types. *Lancet*, **i**, 634.

36 FUDENBERG H.H., STIEHM E.R., FRANKLIN E.C., MELTZER M. & FRANGIONE B. (1964) Antigenicity of hereditary human gamma-globulin (Gm) factors. *Cold Spring Harbor Symposia on Quantitative Biology*, **29**, 463.

37 FISCHER K. (1964) Immunhämatologische und Klinische Befund bei einem Transfusionszwischenfall infolge Gm(a)-Antikörperbildung. *Proceedings of 10th Congress, International Society of Blood Transfusion, Stockholm*, p. 434.

38 PRENTICE C.R.M., IZATT M.M., ADAMS J.F., McNICOL G.P. & DOUGLAS A.S. (1971) Amyloidosis associated with the nephrotic syndrome and transfusion reactions in a haemophiliac. *British Journal of Haematology*, **21**, 305.

39 VYAS G.N., PERKINS H.A. & FUDENBERG H.H. (1968) Anaphylactoid transfusion reactions associated with anti-IgA. *Lancet*, **ii**, 312.

40 HOLT P.D.J., TANDY N.P. & ANSTEE D.J. (1977) Screening of blood donors for IgA deficiency. A study of the donor population of the South West of England. *Journal of Clinical Pathology*, **30**, 1007.

41 TOVEY G.H. & DARKE C.C. (1970) Prevention of leucocyte-antibody formation. *Lancet*, **i**, 1396.

42 ENGELFRIET C.P. & VAN LOGHEM J.J. (1961) Studies on leucocyte iso- and auto-antibodies. *British Journal of Haematology*, **7**, 223.

43 PERKINS H.A. (1968) Isoantibodies following open heart surgery. *Proceedings of 11th Congress, International Society of Blood Transfusion, Sydney, 1966*, p. 831.

44 CHAPLIN H. JR, BRITTINGHAM T.E. & CASSELL M. (1959) Methods for preparation of suspensions of buffy-coat-poor red blood cells for transfusion. *American Journal of Clinical Pathology*, **31**, 373.

45 PATEL R. & TERASAKI P.I. (1969) Significance of the positive cross-match test in kidney transplantation. *New England Journal of Medicine*, **280**, 735.

46 OPELZ G. & TERASAKI P.I. (1974) Poor kidney transplant survival in recipients with frozen-blood transfusions or no transfusions. *Lancet*, **ii**, 696.

47 MURRAY S., DEWAR P.J., ULDALL P.R., WILKINSON R., KERR D.N.S., TAYLOR R.M.R. & SWINNEY J. (1974) Some important factors in cadaver-donor kidney transplantation. *Tissue Antigens*, **4**, 548.

48 VAN HOOFF J.P., KALFF M.W., VAN POELGEEST A.E., PERSIJN G.G. & VAN ROOD J.J. (1976) Blood transfusions and kidney transplantation. *Transplantation*, **22**, 306.

49 TING A. & MORRIS P.J. (1978) Matching for B-cell

antigens of the HLA-DR genes in cadaver renal transplantation. *Lancet*, **i**, 575.

50 MARTINS-DA SILVA B., VASSALLI C. & JEANNET M. (1978) Matching renal grafts. *Lancet*, **i**, 1047.

51 ASTER R.H. & BECKER G.A. (1972) Platelet preservation. In: *Progress in Transplantation and Transfusion.* Proceedings of Plenary Session, AABB & ISBT Congress. Published by the American Association of Blood Banks.

52 ASTER R.H. (1965) Effect of anticoagulant and ABO incompatibility on recovery of transfused human platelets. *Blood*, **26**, 732.

53 GRUMET F.C. & YANKEE R.A. (1970) Long-term platelet support of patients with aplastic anaemia. *Annals of Internal Medicine*, **73**, 1.

54 YANKEE R.A., GRUMET F.C. & ROGENTINE G.N. (1969) Platelet transfusion therapy. *New England Journal of Medicine*, **280**, 1208.

55 TOVEY G.H. (1972) Platelet groups and transfusion: International Forum. *Vox Sanguinis*, **22**, 283.

56 SHULMAN N.R., ASTER R.H., LEITNER A. & HILLER M.C. (1961) Immuno-reactions involving platelets. *Journal of Clinical Investigation*, **40**, 1587.

57 ZEIGLER Z.R., MURPHY S. & GARDNER F.H. (1975) Post-transfusion purpura: a heterogeneous syndrome. *Blood*, **45**, 529.

58 MORRISON F.S. & MOLLISON P.L. (1966) Post-transfusion purpura. *New England Journal of Medicine*, **275**, 243.

59 GERSTNER J.B., SMITH M.J., DAVIS K.D., CINO P.L. & ASTER R.H. (1979) Post-transfusion purpura: therapeutic failure of Pl^{A1}-negative platelet transfusion. *American Journal of Hematology*, **6**, 71.

60 BRAUDE A.I., CAREY F.J. & SIEMIENSKI J. (1955) Studies of bacterial transfusion reactions from refrigerated blood: the properties of cold-growing bacteria. *Journal of Clinical Investigation*, **34**, 311.

61 TOVEY G.H. (1969) *Trends in Clinical Pathology*, p. 289. Eyre & Spottiswoode, London.

62 WOLF P.L., MCCARTHY L.J. & HAFLEIGH B. (1970) Extreme hypercalcaemia following blood transfusion combined with intravenous calcium. *Vox Sanguinis*, **19**, 544.

63 SIMPSON K. (1942) Air accidents during transfusion. *Lancet*, **i**, 697.

64 RUESCH M., MIYATAKE S. & BALLINGER C.M. (1960) Continuing hazard of air embolism during pressure transfusions. *Journal of the American Medical Association*, **172**, 1476.

65 YACKEL A.E. (1968) Lethal air embolism from plastic blood storage container. *Journal of the American Medical Association*, **204**, 267.

66 HARRISON K.A., AJABOR L.N. & LAWSON J.B. (1971) Ethacrynic acid and packed-blood-cell transfusion in treatment of severe anaemia in pregnancy. *Lancet*, **i**, 11.

67 LAWSON D.H., MURRAY R.M. & PARKIN J.L.W. (1972) Early mortality in the megaloblastic anaemias. *Quarterly Journal of Medicine*, **41**, 1.

68 SWANK R.L. (1961) Alteration of blood on storage: measurement of adhesiveness of 'aging' platelets and leucocytes and their removal by filtration. *New England Journal of Medicine*, **265**, 728.

69 REUL G.J., BEALL A.C. & GREENBERG S.D. (1974) Protection of the pulmonary microvasculature by fine screen blood filtration. *Chest*, **66**, 4.

70 TOBEY R.E., KOPRIVA C.J., HOMER L.D., SOLIS R.T., DICKSON L.G. & HERMAN C.M. (1974) Pulmonary gas exchange following hemorrhagic shock and massive transfusion in the baboon. *Annals of Surgery*, **179**, 316.

71 BREDENBERG C.E. (1977) Does a relationship exist between massive blood transfusions and the adult respiratory distress syndrome? *Vox Sanguinis*, **32**, 311.

72 SOLIS R.T. & WALKER B.D. (1977) In: International Forum, *Vox Sanguinis*, **32**, 319.

73 BENNETT P.J. (1963) The use of intravenous plastic catheters. *British Medical Journal*, **ii**, 1252.

74 LIEBERMAN J. & KANESHIRO W. (1971) Ethacrynic acid with packed red cells. *Lancet*, **i**, 911.

75 MCNAIR T.J. & DUDLEY H.A.F. (1959) The local complications of intravenous therapy, *Lancet*, **ii**, 365.

76 MICHAELS L. & REUBENER B. (1953) Growth of bacteria in intravenous infusion. *Lancet*, **i**, 772.

77 CORKERY J.J., DUBOWITZ V., LISTER J. & MOOSA A. (1968) Colonic perforation after exchange transfusion. *British Medical Journal*, **iv**, 345.

78 ORME R.L.E. & EADES S.M. (1968) Perforation of the bowel in the newborn as a complication of exchange transfusion. *British Medical Journal*, **iv**, 349.

79 COLLINS J.A. (1972) Fluid replacement in trauma. In: *Practice of Surgery: Current Review* (ed. Ballinger E.J. & Drapanes T.L.). Mosby, St. Louis.

80 BERGER R.L., LIVERSAGE R.M., CHALMERS T.C., GRAHAM J.H., MCGOLDRICK D.M. & STOHLMAN F. (1966) Exchange transfusion in the treatment of fulminating hepatitis. *New England Journal of Medicine*, **274**, 497.

81 KRIJNEN H.W., DE WIT J.J., KUIVENHOVEN A.C.J., LOOS J.A. & PRINS H.K. (1964) Glycerol-treated human red cells frozen with liquid nitrogen. *Vox Sanguinis*, **9**, 559.

82 RIZZA C.R. (1976) Coagulation factor therapy. *Clinics in Hematology*, **5**, 113.

83 URBANIAK S.J. & CASH J.D. (1977) Blood replacement therapy. *British Medical Bulletin*, **33**, 273.

84 DAVISON A.M. (1972) *Clinical Uses of Albumin.* Joint Symposium, Blood and Blood Products. *Proceedings RSE* Suppl. **71B**.

85 PRESTON A.E. (1967) The factor VIII activity in fresh and stored plasma. *British Journal of Haematology*, **13**, 42.

86 POOL J.G. & SHANNON A.E. (1965) Production of high potency concentrates of antihemophilic globulin in a closed bag system. *New England Journal of Medicine*, **273**, 1443.

87 PROWSE C.V. & MCGILL A. (1979) Evaluation of 'Mason' (continuous-thaw-syphon) method of cryoprecipitate production. *Vox Sanguinis*, **37**, 235.

88 BIGGS R. & DENSON K.W.E. (1963) The fate of prothrombin and factors VIII, IX and X transfused to patients deficient in these factors. *British Journal of Haematology*, **9**, 532.

89 SHAW A.E. (1971) Platelet transfusion. *British Medical Journal*, **i**, 404.

90 SLICHTER S.J. & HARKER L.A. (1976) Preparation and storage of platelet concentrates. *British Journal of Haematology*, **34**, 395.

91 SLICHTER S.J. & HARKER L.A. (1976) Storage variables

influencing platelet viability and function. *British Journal of Haematology*, **34**, 403.

92 SCHIFFER C.A., AISNER J. & WIERNIK P.H. (1978) Platelet transfusion therapy for patients with leukaemia. In: *The Blood Platelet in Transfusion Therapy* (ed. Greenwalt T.J. & Jamieson G.A.), p. 267. Alan R. Liss Inc., New York.

93 DUNBAR R.W., PRICE K.A. & CANNARELLA C.F. (1974) Microaggregate blood filters: effects on filtration time, plasma haemoglobin, and fresh blood platelet counts. *Anaesthesia & Analgesia*, **53**, 577.

94 MITTAL K.M., RUDER E.A. & GREEN D. (1976) Matching of histocompatibility (HLA) antigens for platelet transfusion *Blood*, **47**, 31.

95 WU K.K., THOMPSON J.S., KOEPKE J.A., HOAK J.C. & FLINK R. (1976) Heterogeneity of antibody response to human platelet transfusion. *Journal of Clinical Investigation*, **58**, 432.

96 BRAND A., VAN LEEUWEN A., EERNISSE J.G. & VAN ROOD J.J. (1978) Platelet transfusion therapy. Optimal donor selection with a combination of lymphocytotoxicity and platelet fluorescence tests. *Blood*, **51**, 781.

97 TOSATO G., APPLEBAUM F.R. & DEISSEROTH A.B. (1978) HLA matched platelet transfusion therapy of severe aplastic anaemia. *Blood*, **52**, 846.

98 HIGBY D.J. (1977) Controlled prospective studies of granulocyte transfusion therapy. *Experimental Hematology*, **5** (Suppl. 1), 57.

99 BUCKNER D., GRAW R.J. JR, EISEL R.J., HENDERSON E.S. & PERRY S. (1969) Leukapheresis by continuous flow centrifugation in patients with chronic myelocytic leukemia. *Blood*, **33**, 353.

100 MISHLER J.M. (1977) The effects of corticosteroids on moblisation and function of neutrophils. *Experimental Hematology*, **5** (Suppl. 1), 15.

101 ROY A.J., YANKEE R.A., BRIVKALNS A. & FITCH M. (1975) Viability of granulocytes obtained by filtration leukopheresis. *Transfusion (Philadelphia)*, **2**, 342.

102 VERHEUGT F.W.A., VON DEM BORNE A.E.G.K., DECARY F. & ENGELFRIET C.P. (1977) The detection of granulocytic alloantibodies with an indirect immunofluorescence test. *British Journal of Haematology*, **36**, 533.

103 LENNON G.G. & TOVEY G.H. (1956) Massive blood transfusion for traumatic post-partum haemorrhage. *British Medical Journal*, **i**, 547.

104 SCOPES J.W. (1963) Intraperitoneal transfusion of blood in newborn babies. *Lancet*, **i**, 1027.

105 HOLT F.M., BOYD I.E., DEWHURST C.J., MURRAY J., NAYLOR C.H. & SMITHAM J.H. (1973) Intrauterine transfusion: 101 consecutive cases treated at Queen Charlotte's Maternity Hospital. *British Medical Journal*, **iii**, 39.

106 JONES J.H., KILPATRICK G.S. & FRANKS E.H. (1962) Red cell aggregation in dextrose solutions. *Journal of Clinical Pathology*, **15**, 161.

107 NOBLE T.C. & ABBOTT J. (1959) Haemolysis of stored blood mixed with isotonic dextrose-containing solutions in transfusion apparatus. *British Medical Journal*, **ii**, 865.

108 TOVEY G.H. & JENKINS W.J. (1981) Compatibility tests for blood transfusion. *Association of Clinical Pathologists Broadsheet*, No. 57. Swan Press, London.

109 TOVEY G.H. & GILLESPIE W.A. (1966) The investigation of transfusion reactions. *Association of Clinical Pathologists Broadsheet*, No. 54, Swan Press, London.

110 RAPAPORT S. (1947) Dimensional, osmotic and chemical changes of erythrocytes in stored blood. *Journal of Clinical Investigation*, **26**, 591.

111 HUGHES-JONES N.C., MOLLISON P.L. & ROBINSON M.A. (1957) Factors affecting the viability of erythrocytes stored in the frozen state. *Proceedings of the Royal Society, Series B*, **147**, 476.

112 GIBSON J.G., REES S.B., MCMANUS T.J. & SCHEITLIN W.A. (1957) A citrate-phosphate-dextrose solution for the preservation of human blood. *American Journal of Clinical Pathology*, **28**, 569.

113 KEVY S.V., GIBSON J.G. & BUTTON L. (1965) A clinical evaluation of the use of citrate-phosphate-dextrose solution in children. *Transfusion*, **5**, 427.

114 VALTIS D.J. & KENNEDY A.C. (1954) Defective gas-transport function of stored red blood cells. *Lancet*, **i**, 119.

115 KREUGER A., ACKERBLOM O. & HOGMAN C.F. (1975) A clinical evaluation of citrate-phosphate-dextrose-adenine blood. *Vox Sanguinis*, **29**, 81,

116 DERRICK J.R. & MASON GUEST M. (1971) *Dextrans: Current Concepts of Basic Actions and Clinical Applications*. C. C. Thomas, Springfield, Illinois.

117 HEISTO H. & LUND I. (1953) Studies on allergic reactions following administration of dextran. *Journal of the Oslo City Hospitals*, **3**, 159.

118 VICKERS M.D., HEATH M.L. & DUNLAP D. (1969) A comparison of Macrodex and stored blood as replacement for blood loss during planned surgery. *British Journal of Anaesthesia*, **41**, 667.

119 RUSH B.F. (1974) Volume replacement: when, what and how much? In: *Treatment of Shock: Principles and Practice* (ed. Schumer W. & Nyhus L.M.). Lea & Febiger, Philadelphia.

120 MISHLER J.M. (1975) Hydroxyethyl starch as an adjunct to leucocyte separation by centrifugal means: a review of safety and efficacy. *Transfusion (Philadelphia)* **15**, 449.

121 SOLANKE T.F., KHWAJA M.S. & MODOJEMU E.I. (1971) Plasma volume studies with four different plasma volume expanders. *Journal of Surgical Research*, **11**, 140.

122 RUDOWSKI W. & KOSTRZEWSKA E. (1976) Aspects of treatment: blood substitutes. *Annals of the Royal College of Surgeons of England*, **58**, 115.

123 LUNDSGAARD-HANSEN P. & TSCHIRREN B. (1978) Modified fluid gelatin as a plasma substitute. In: *Blood Substitutes and Plasma Expanders* (Greenwalt T.J. & Jamieson G.A.), p. 227. Alan R. Liss Inc., New York.

124 RING J. & MESSMER K. (1977) Incidence and severity of anaphylactoid reactions to colloid volume substitutes. *Lancet*, **i**, 446.

125 RABINER S.F., O'BRIEN K., PESKIN G.W. & FREDMAN L.H. (1970) Further studies with a stroma-free haemoglobin solution. *Annals of Surgery*, **171**, 615.

126 KRAMLOVA M., PRISTOUPIL T.I., ULRYCH S. & HRKAL Z. (1976) Stroma-free haemoglobin solution for infusion: changes during storage. *Haematologia*, **10**, 365.

127 RUDOWSKI W.J. (1980) Evaluation of modern plasma expanders and blood substitutes. *British Journal of Hospital Medicines* **23**, 389.

128 SLOVITER H.A. (1975) Perfluoro compounds as artificial erythrocytes. *Federation Proceedings*, **34,** 184.

129 CLARK L.C. (1978) Perfluorodecalin as a red cell substitute. In: *Blood Substitutes and Plasma Expanders* (ed. Jamieson G.A. & Greenwalt T.J.), p. 57. Liss, New York.

130 SECOND REPORT OF THE ADVISORY GROUP ON TESTING FOR THE PRESENCE OF HEPATITIS B SURFACE ANTIGEN AND ITS ANTIBODY (1975) Her Majesty's Stationery Office, London.

131 MOLLISON P.L. (1979) *Blood Transfusion in Clinical Medicine* (6th edn), p. 9. Blackwell Scientific Publications, Oxford.

132 BORTIN M.M. (1970) A compendium of reported human bone marrow transplants. *Transplantation*, **9,** 571.

133 ROBINS M.M. & NOYES W.D. (1961) Aplastic anaemia treated with bone-marrow infusion from identical twins. *New England Journal of Medicine*, **265,** 974.

134 STORB R. & THOMAS E.D. (1978) Marrow transplantation for treatment of aplastic anemia. *Clinics in Hematology*, **7,** 597.

135 GALE R.P., FEIG S., HO W., FALK P., RIPPEE C. & SPARKES R. (1977) ABO blood group system and bone marrow transplantation. *Blood*, **50,** 185.

136 SPECK B., CORNU P., NISSEN C., GROFF P. & JEANNET M. (1977) On the immune pathogenesis of aplastic anemia. *Experimental Hematology*, **5** (Suppl. 2), 2.

137 POWLES R.L., CLINK H.M., BANDINI G. *et al.* (1980) The place of bone-marrow transplantation in acute myelogenous leukaemia. *Lancet*, **i,** 1047.

SECTION 8
THE INVESTIGATION OF
THE PATIENT WITH
A HAEMATOLOGICAL
DISORDER

Chapter 36
The investigation of the patient with a haematological disorder

S. T. E. CALLENDER AND M. J. PIPPARD

In each of the previous sections the major groups of haematological disorders have been described as separate entities. In this final chapter we shall attempt to summarize some of this information and present it in the context of the clinician faced with the investigation of a patient who may have a haematological disorder.

As in other branches of clinical medicine, the problem is approached by history-taking and physical examination followed by some basic laboratory screening tests. At this stage a differential diagnosis can be established and then a more detailed analysis of the condition can be carried out as set out in previous sections of this book.

HISTORY-TAKING AND CLINICAL EXAMINATION

History

A careful history is often the key to the further investigation and treatment of a patient with a haematological disorder.

If the presenting symptoms suggest anaemia (see Chapter 4, p. 134) the commonest causes are anaemia of chronic disorders and iron deficiency. In the case of the former, attention should be directed towards obtaining a history of the underlying disease, e.g. renal disease, chronic infection, neoplasm, and in the elderly the polymyalgia/arteritis syndromes.

In relation to suspected iron deficiency, questions should be directed towards the diet and possible sources of blood loss, particularly menstrual periods, peptic ulcer, piles and aspirin ingestion. It is quite inadequate to ask a woman whether she considers her menstrual loss to be normal or heavy. If she uses only internal tampons, she probably does not have menorrhagia. On the other hand, the use of more than one packet of one of the more absorbent brands of external pads (e.g. Dr White's) suggests a heavy loss, as does the need for her to stay at home for one or more days of the period, or to get up at night to change the pad. It is often overlooked that a blood donor loses 200–250 mg of iron at each blood donation, and this, in a frequent, regular donor, may lead to a negative iron balance. Previous surgery, particularly involving the stomach, is often significant, especially when the indication for operation has been repeated haemorrhage. Many patients of this kind go to surgery with depleted iron stores and following the operation are unable to replenish them. Operations which might have given rise to a blind loop should also be noted as vitamin-B_{12} deficiency can occur in these circumstances.

If a patient is reputed to be refractory to iron treatment, the first step should be to establish the type of iron given. Some preparations, especially those of slow-release type, may be quite inadequate, as a simple change to a well-absorbed preparation such as ferrous sulphate or ferrous fumarate will readily demonstrate. Secondly, it is important to know whether the iron prescribed has been taken. If a rectal examination shows a normal-coloured stool it almost certainly has not.

There may be no obvious symptoms of malabsorption but direct questioning about episodes of loose stools which are pale, bulky and difficult to flush may suggest such a diagnosis, as may evidence that the patient is smaller in stature than other members of the family or has had a delayed puberty.

Many haematological disorders are hereditary and a detailed family history is essential. This is particularly so in the case of haemolytic anaemias and many haemorrhagic disorders (see later). Even in conditions such as pernicious anaemia, a personal or family history of thyroid disease, rheumatoid arthritis, diabetes, carcinoma of the stomach or early greying may point to the diagnosis.

A careful drug history should always be taken, including special enquiry into any tablets which the patient may have used but not regarded as significant, e.g. one of the many aspirin preparations which can be bought over the counter. Phenylbutazone, chloramphenicol, sulphonamides, penicillin, thiazide diuretics, methyl-dopa and, more recently, cimetidine, are some of the most commonly prescribed drugs in the UK which may be implicated in blood disorders. The use of quinine or quinidine may give rise to acute purpura, and it should be remembered that quinine is a component of tonic water and of some compound aspirin preparations such as Anadin.

Symptoms referable to the mouth are common in many haematological disorders and should always be asked about. A sore, burning tongue may accompany iron deficiency or vitamin-B_{12} deficiency. Mouth ulceration is more a feature of folate deficiency and conditions associated with severe neutropenia—e.g. acute leukaemia—or it may be the result of a viral infection such as infectious mononucleosis.

Dysphagia related to the post-cricoid region may be indicative of a past or present iron deficiency.

If the general appearance suggests a diagnosis of polycythaemia, special enquiry should be made about pruritus since this symptom, particularly after a hot bath, is a useful distinguishing feature between primary and secondary polycythaemia. Pruritus may also suggest a diagnosis of lymphoma in a patient with lymph-node enlargement.

A history of bone pain is important in the diagnosis of infiltrative disorders of the bone marrow. Very severe pain may suggest bone infarction such as is associated with sickle-cell disease and some cases of leukaemia.

Patients who present with a history of rapid onset of signs of spinal-cord compression, or with cranial-nerve lesions, may be suspected of having leukaemic, lymphomatous or myeloma deposits. In the case of the latter, vertebral collapse may produce similar symptoms. A history of gross central-nervous-system disease associated with vitamin-B_{12} deficiency is rare nowadays, but minor symptoms of paraesthesiae may be elicited on enquiry and will help to distinguish between vitamin-B_{12} and folate deficiency.

History-taking is of particular importance in patients who present with a suspected haemorrhagic disorder. It is essential to obtain a clear picture regarding the extent and severity of the haemorrhagic tendency. For example, many women claim that they bruise easily and indeed have small, unexplained bruises from time to time. The size and site of bruising is of particular importance and it is essential to determine whether there is any *unusual* bruising. It should be remembered that purpura over the face is not at all uncommon in otherwise normal children who have bouts of coughing associated with upper respiratory infections. In any patient who presents with purpura a careful drug history should be taken. A patient with purpura who is likely to have serious bleeding may often give a history of mucous-membrane blood loss, blood blisters in the mouth, headaches, or neck stiffness. The history in patients with the painful bruising syndrome can be almost diagnostic with the typical story of subcutaneous tingling and the later appearance of a bruise, usually on an extremity.

Where genetic disorders of haemostasis are suspected the history may also be extremely helpful (see p. 1478). There may be a family history and the pattern of bleeding may aid the distinction between vascular or platelet defects and deficiency of clotting factors. It is important to ask for history of bleeding at circumcision, during dental extraction, following any other operative procedure, or of spontaneous bleeding into joints or muscles. A patient who has undergone any major operative procedure or extensive dental extraction without significant blood loss is unlikely to have a serious hereditary disorder of haemostasis.

Physical examination
Every patient who presents with a haematological disorder should have a full clinical examination, but there are some features which may be particularly helpful in making a diagnosis. Of particular interest are the skin, eyes, mouth, hands, lymph nodes, spleen and skeletal structure.

Skin. The combination of pallor and a lemon-yellow tinge to the skin suggests the mild haemolysis of pernicious anaemia, while marked icterus may point to a more severe haemolytic anaemia. A biscuity pallor, especially if associated with bruising or pruritus, may indicate renal failure. Vitiligo is found in association with various organ-specific autoimmune diseases but particularly pernicious anaemia. Increased pigmentation may be the result of haemosiderosis or haemochromatosis if it is not racial in origin. Liver disease is sometimes accompanied by quite marked pigmentation and a search should be made for other evidence of disordered liver function such as spider naevi or signs of portal hypertension (e.g. splenomegaly).

Skin infiltration may occur in the leukaemias or lymphoma, being particularly common in monocytic leukaemias and chronic lymphocytic leukaemia (CLL). The rythroderma of Sézary syndrome (see Chapter 23, p. 902) is virtually diagnostic.

In a patient presenting with a haemorrhagic problem many clues can be obtained by careful examination of the skin. The Schönlein–Henoch type of non-thrombocytopenic purpura has a typical distribution over the buttocks and the backs of the arms and legs. The vascular purpura of amyloidosis has a periorbital distribution, while that of scurvy is found in the perifollicular regions. Patients with thrombocytopenia, from whatever cause, may have both bruises and petechiae more widely distributed; pressure areas are particularly likely to be involved. Disseminated intravascular coagulation (DIC) should be suspected if there is widespread purpura and bleeding from vene-puncture sites in a very sick patient, with a tendency for the purpuric areas to become necrotic. The DIC of purpura fulminans presents a striking picture, with large areas of ecchymoses which are remarkable in their symmetrical distribution. Areas of purpura with necrosis may also occur in cryoglobulinaemia.

Unexplained bleeding, particularly from the gastro-intestinal tract, may occur in some of the rarer genetic disorders which may be suggested by the presence of telangiectases, especially on the face, palms of the hands and soles of the feet, or the appearance of paper-thin scars, hyperextensibility of the joints, and increased elasticity of the skin. Pseudoxanthoma elas-ticum (PXE) produces a characteristic 'plucked-chicken' appearance of the skin, particularly in the axillary folds and in the neck area.

Eyes. A unilateral proptosis or a squint may suggest orbital infiltration or cranial-nerve involvement, par-ticularly with a leukaemic deposit. The conjunctivae may show mild icterus which has not been apparent in the skin, or there may be conjunctival haemorrhages in association with purpura elsewhere. Pingueculae in the conjunctivae in association with splenomegaly make a diagnosis of Gaucher's disease likely. Periorbital oedema is characteristic of infectious mononucleosis.

The fundi should always be examined, particularly in patients with thrombocytopenia from any cause. Haemorrhages are most likely to be found if there is anaemia as well as a platelet deficiency. The fundi should also be examined to detect papilloedema, especially in leukaemia, since this may indicate meningeal involvement.

The appearance of the fundal vessels may be informative (e.g. in sickle-cell disease and related disorders there may be tortuous vessels, microaneur-ysms or proliferative lesions). In patients with macro-globulinaemia the veins may become tortuous, and segmentation of the blood may be seen in the vessels. In patients with excessively high white counts, the blood flowing through the vessels may appear creamy. In PXE, typical angioid streaks may be seen in the retina.

The mouth. The lips, tongue, throat and buccal mucosa are frequently involved in haematological disorders. The lips should be examined carefully, especially in patients with iron deficiency, for evidence of telangiec-tases, naevi, 'blue-rubber blebs', or the pigmented lesions of the Peutz–Jeghers syndrome.

In both iron deficiency and pernicious anaemia there may be atrophy of the papillae of the tongue but there is seldom frank ulceration. The latter is more likely to occur in association with folate deficiency, drug-induced agranulocytosis, and acute leukaemia. Ul-ceration may extend to the gums, palate and throat. There is often complicating monilial infection.

In infectious mononucleosis, the throat may be red and oedematous or may show more severe ulceration; purpuric lesions are sometimes seen on the soft palate. These findings, together with some lymphadenopathy, skin rash and occasionally orbital oedema or mild jaundice, should make one suspect the diagnosis.

If the patient is not edentulous, changes in the gums may be diagnostic. Striking hypertrophy of the gums may occur in acute monocytic leukaemia, often in association with skin infiltrates and perianal lesions, and a somewhat similar hypertrophy may be seen in patients on phenytoin therapy. Vitamin-C deficiency is indicated by haemorrhagic spongy gums, and lead poisoning by a characteristic blue line along the gums. Edentulous patients may well show fissuring and soreness of the corners of the mouth in the presence of iron deficiency. It is an uncommon finding in patients who have their own teeth.

The hands. Rheumatoid arthritis may be associated with three kinds of haematological disorder. First, the anaemia of chronic disorders, secondly, iron deficiency as the result of the medication the patient is taking and, thirdly, Felty's syndrome. Raynaud's phenomenon in the absence of arterial disease may suggest the presence of a cryoglobulin or cold agglutinins. Koilonychia is indicative of iron deficiency, and clubbing of the nails, in the absence of any significant lung or heart disease, suggests the presence of coeliac or Crohn's disease.

Lymph nodes (see p. 1477). Lymph nodes should be examined systematically, and the distribution, texture and mobility of enlarged nodes noted. The size of nodes should be recorded, preferably by actual measurement rather than reference to peas, walnuts, eggs, etc. A diagram of the distribution is useful for future reference.

Spleen. Splenomegaly should be looked for in any haematological case. In patients with gross spleno-megaly the outline may be seen on simple inspection of the abdomen. With less obvious degrees of spleno-megaly the patient should be examined first when lying supine and with the arms at the sides. The left hand should be placed behind the lower ribs to bring the spleen forward and the right hand should be used to palpate the abdomen while the patient relaxes and takes deep breaths. If the spleen cannot be felt in this position it may be useful to ask the patient to lie on the right side with the legs flexed and the left arm hanging over the side of the bed. It may be difficult in some cases to distinguish, on clinical examination alone, between splenomegaly, renal tumours, tumours of the stomach or retroperitoneal masses, particularly where such a mass displaces the spleen downwards. The size of a palpable spleen should be recorded by the measurement made at right angles to the costal margin. The measurement should be made in centimetres and not recorded as finger-breadths. Massive splenomegaly will suggest a diagnosis of myelofibrosis, chronic granulocytic leukaemia (CGL), some forms of lymphatic leukaemia, or infiltrative disorders such as Gaucher's disease. A splenic rub indicates that there is an infarction involving a serous surface.

Skeletal abnormalities. A small stature may indicate long-standing anaemia dating from childhood; it can occur in iron deficiency with or without an associated malabsorption syndrome. Other chronic anaemias such as the thalassaemias may also retard growth. In this latter case there may also be gross skeletal changes associated with the expansion of the bone marrow. Congenital hypoplastic anaemias such as Fanconi's anaemia are often accompanied by skeletal abnormalities. Other skeletal changes which may be important in diagnosis are bony tenderness, which is found particularly in leukaemia and myeloma and sometimes in other neoplastic infiltrations, or pathological fractures which are found particularly in myeloma. Myelomatous deposits in the skull can sometimes be felt as raised indurated areas under the scalp.

THE FURTHER EVALUATION OF HAEMATOLOGICAL DISORDERS

Having suspected a haematological disorder from the history and physical examination, the next step is to carry out a series of laboratory screening tests, in particular an examination of the stained blood film combined with a full blood count, preferably using an automated counting system. In the sections which follow, an approach to the differential diagnosis of the major haematological disorders, described in detail in earlier sections of this book, will be considered.

ANAEMIA

Investigation of an anaemic patient involves:
1 assessment of the significance of the haemoglobin concentration;
2 preliminary classification based on red-cell morphology and indices; and
3 a determination of the cause.

The haemoglobin concentration

Anaemia is defined on the basis of normal population studies as a haemoglobin concentration below 13·0 g/dl (adult males) or 11·5 g/dl (adult females) (see Chapter 1, p. 30). In children, the lower limits increase from 11·0 g/dl at one year to adult levels by age 15 [1]. Though very few people have levels lower than these, they remain arbitrary for a particular individual. For example, a significant overlap in haemoglobin concentration exists between normal and mildly iron-deficient subjects [2, 3]. In addition, the haemoglobin concentration is one link in the chain of oxygen transport from lungs to tissues which is modified by environment or in disease. Altitude [4] and cardiac or respiratory disease must be taken into account in deciding whether an apparently normal haemoglobin concentration is suboptimal in terms of the particular demands for oxygen transport. Further problems occasionally arise with disturbances in the distribution of body fluids. A relative, dilutional anaemia with no reduction in red-cell mass may be seen as part of the normal physiology of pregnancy [5], with massive splenomegaly, or with plasma protein abnormalities such as macroglobulinaemia. In contrast, dehydration is associated with a fall in plasma volume and an increase in haematocrit. The delayed expansion of plasma volume after acute bleeding [6] means that changes in haemoglobin concentration initially underestimate the degree of blood-loss anaemia.

These problems present little difficulty with marked anaemia, but they may obscure the presence of mild anaemia and thus prevent recognition of serious underlying disease. In practice, clinical assessment combined, where possible, with a comparison with previous haemoglobin levels is often helpful in deciding whether the current level is abnormal for a particular patient.

Type of anaemia

Basic investigations of an anaemia include determination of red-cell 'absolute' indices, examination of the peripheral-blood smear, and a reticulocyte count. The first two investigations allow a classification on the basis of red-cell morphology, particularly cell size and haemoglobin content [7]. The reticulocyte count is a measure of the bone marrow's response to anaemia. It allows a further tentative division of anaemias into those due primarily to impaired red-cell production (with an inappropriately low reticulocyte count) and those due to red-cell loss such as haemolysis (where the reticulocyte count usually shows an increase consonant with the stress of the anaemia).

Red-cell indices

Most laboratories now use particle counters such as

the Coulter S [8] to provide an automated print-out of haemoglobin concentration, red-cell count, packed cell volume (PCV), total nucleated cell count, and the red-cell 'absolute' indices—the mean cell volume (MCV), the mean cell haemoglobin (MCH), and the mean cell haemoglobin concentration (MCHC). The MCV is calculated from the mean height of the pulses generated during the erythrocyte count, and the MCH from the haemoglobin concentration and the erythrocyte count (see Chapter 1, p. 33). These values are therefore much more reliable than in the past when they depended on manual red-cell counts. They allow an initial classification of an anaemia on the basis of the MCV as normocytic (MCV 76–96 fl), macrocytic (MCV > 96 fl) or microcytic (MCV < 76 fl).

Blood film

Whenever the haemoglobin concentration is low, or any of the red-cell indices abnormal, a stained blood film should be examined. (In laboratories where an automated print-out is not available, determination of the haemoglobin concentration and examination of the blood film constitute a minimum screen for the presence of red-cell abnormalities.) The two examinations are complementary. A uniform change in cell size or haemoglobin content may be difficult to detect on the blood film but will be reflected in the red-cell indices, whereas a small population of abnormal cells is more obvious on the blood film. Furthermore, leucocyte abnormalities (e.g. the hypersegmented neutrophils of megaloblastic erythropoiesis), and changes in platelet numbers or morphology, may indicate a more generalized disorder of haemopoiesis (or cell loss), rather than an isolated anaemia. Changes in red-cell morphology are often important additional clues to the disordered physiology underlying an anaemia.

Red-cell morphology
(see also Chapter 1, p. 45)

Abnormal red-cell production. This is accompanied by the non-specific changes of anisocytosis and poikilocytosis. Their severity is generally proportional to the degree of anaemia, but they may be visible before there has been any great change in haemoglobin concentration. The nuclear maturation defects of megaloblastic haemopoiesis are accompanied by an increase in erythrocyte size without change in intracellular haemoglobin concentration. However the increase is rarely uniform: associated poikilocytosis and cell fragmentation usually reflect damage to abnormal cells as they are released into marrow sinusoids, as part of the pathophysiology of ineffective erythropoiesis.

Microcytosis, hypochromia and poikilocytosis suggest defects in cytoplasmic maturation and haemoglobin synthesis, such as those found in iron deficiency and the thalassaemias. These maturation defects may initially affect only a small proportion of cells. Thus the presence of occasional true macrocytes or microcytes should lead to a consideration of the appropriate group of maturation abnormalities.

The presence of nucleated red blood cells in the peripheral blood suggests a disturbance of release of red cells from the marrow, though there may also be small numbers after splenectomy. They are seen with intense erythropoietin stimulation in almost any severe anaemia, but otherwise suggest marrow damage such as that caused by infiltration with tumour metastases, leukaemia, or myelofibrosis. With marrow damage, early myeloid cells are also likely to be present, to give the peripheral-blood picture of a leuco-erythroblastic anaemia. Tear-drop poikilocytes are particularly characteristic of myelofibrosis.

Changes related to red-cell injury. Red-cell fragmentation, with the formation of schistocytes, occurs in microangiopathic haemolytic anaemias, in association with cardiac valve replacement, and is produced by heat damage after severe burns. As already discussed, red-cell fragmentation may also result from ineffective erythropoiesis, but in these circumstances the reticulocyte count (see below) is likely to be low, in contrast to the increase usual with haemolysis. Irregularly contracted cells are characteristic of drug-induced haemolysis and are also seen in unstable haemoglobinopathies (e.g. Hb Köln) (see Chapter 8). Spherocytes indicate red-cell membrane abnormalities such as those resulting from immune damage or due to the genetic abnormality of hereditary spherocytosis. Acanthocytes and burr cells are also indicative of red-cell membrane damage. The former are found after splenectomy, in a-β-lipoproteinaemia, and in chronic liver diseases. Burr cells may also be seen in association with liver disease as well as in uraemia.

Characteristic changes in red-cell morphology may provide a direct clue to the specific aetiology of several haemolytic anaemias. Target cells are prominent in the thalassaemias, sickle-cell disease and Hb C disease though they may also be found with liver disease, severe iron deficiency, and following splenectomy. Irreversibly sickled cells are characteristic of homozygous sickle-cell disease. In hereditary elliptocytosis, 50–90% of red cells are oval compared with less than 15% in normals, though some increase in elliptocytes is also seen in iron deficiency, thalassaemia, myelosclerosis and megaloblastic anaemias. Stomatocytes are commonly seen in normal blood films, but larger numbers may indicate a rare haemolytic anaemia associated with increased red-cell sodium permeability [9].

Changes due to splenectomy. These include prominent Howell–Jolly bodies (nuclear remnants) which may be particularly numerous in the face of a continuing haemolytic disorder. Siderotic granules (Pappenheimer bodies), target cells, and occasional nucleated red cells are also a feature of a post-splenectomy blood film. In the absence of splenectomy, these changes may indicate splenic atrophy as is common, for example, in sickle-cell disease. They may be the first clue to malabsorption as the cause of an iron or folate deficiency anaemia, for coeliac disease is associated with splenic hypofunction.

Compensatory increase in erythropoiesis. This is suggested by the presence of polychromatic macrocytes on the peripheral-blood film, though like nucleated red blood cells these may also be seen with marrow infiltration [10]. Basophilic stippling is occasionally found in normal films as a variant of the diffuse basophilia of reticulocytes. Where stippling is prominent and coarse-grained, the possibility of thalassaemia or lead poisoning should be considered. The further assessment of the marrow response to anaemia is discussed in the next section.

Reticulocyte count

An increase in effective marrow erythroid activity in response to the stimulus of anaemia results in the delivery of younger red cells to the peripheral blood. However, the significance of the reticulocyte count as a measure of the functional capacity of the marrow is dependent on the degree of anaemia. This determines the number of adult red cells, of which the reticulocytes are expressed as a percentage, and is also related to the reticulocyte maturation time in the circulation [11] (see also Chapter 4, p. 126). The first factor may be eliminated by adjusting the reticulocyte percentage to a normal PCV or haemoglobin concentration:

Adjusted reticulocyte % =

$$\text{observed reticulocyte \%} \times \frac{\text{observed PCV}}{45}$$

The second factor is due to the premature release of bone-marrow reticulocytes into the blood under the stimulus of increased levels of erythropoietin [12]. This stimulus is found in all anaemias except those due directly to failure of erythropoietin production such as may accompany renal disease. The stimulated or 'shift' reticulocytes can be recognized as polychromatic macrocytes on the peripheral-blood smear and have an MCV approximately 25% greater than adult cells. The 'shift' cells have a maturation time of two to three days in the circulation compared with one day for normal reticulocytes. Their accumulation therefore results in a falsely high estimate of marrow production unless a second correction is made to the reticulocyte count for the extended maturation time. Though the alteration in reticulocyte lifespan is proportional to the degree of anaemia [12], an approximate correction for the presence of 'shift' cells is to divide the adjusted reticulocyte count by two, representing an increase in overall maturation time to two days [11]. Alternatively, the twice-corrected reticulocyte count (reticulocyte production index) (see Chapter 4, p. 126), can be obtained directly from a nomogram based on the PCV [13] or by using correction factors derived from this nomogram (Table 36.1). A normal marrow can increase reticulocyte production from an index of one at PCV 45% to two at 35%, and more than three at 25% or less [14]. Lower values suggest impaired red-cell production while values greater than three are characteristic of haemolytic anaemias. It should be remembered, however, that these estimates are only semi-quantitative. Several days are required for the marrow to mount a full reticulocyte response to sudden anaemia; changes in P_{50} of the blood may mean that the PCV does not always reflect the extent of erythropoietin drive and stimulus to 'shift'; splenectomy, by removing a site of reticulocyte maturation, may also lead to an apparent increase in the production index. Despite these limitations the index provides a useful basis for the initial classification of anaemia.

Table 36.1. Factors for double correction of reticulocyte count to a reticulocyte production index

PCV %	Multiplication factor
45	1·00
35	0·50
25	0·25
20	0·20
15	0·15
10	0·10

Initial classification of the anaemia

The initial studies, together with the clinical setting, may be sufficient to reach a firm diagnosis. A microcytic hypochromic anaemia in a young woman with menorrhagia, a previously normal haemoglobin concentration and no other blood changes requires no further haematological investigation. Other anaemias may be more tentatively categorized as shown in Figure 36.1.

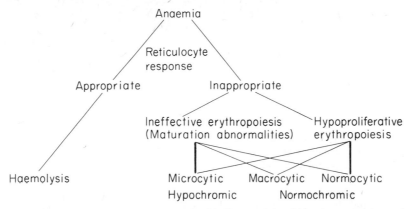

Fig. 36.1. Preliminary classifications of anaemia based on red-cell indices, peripheral-blood examination and reticulocyte count. Note that the categories define the predominant abnormality but are not mutually exclusive. Separation of ineffective from hypoproliferative erythropoiesis may require bone-marrow examination.

A haemolytic anaemia is likely if the reticulocyte response is appropriate. However, delay in mounting a response to red-cell loss and relative failure of response due to exhaustion of iron or folate may mislead, as may a reticulocyte response to prior haematinic therapy, or withdrawal of a toxin such as alcohol. As already indicated, specific red-cell changes may allow a firm diagnosis in several haemolytic disorders, but others may require considerable further study. A bone-marrow examination is not usually helpful in these conditions.

The morphological classification of the anaemias due primarily to inadequate red-cell production has the advantage of emphasizing the maturation defects associated with treatable haematinic deficiencies, though these are certainly not the only cause of changes in cell size. The separation of maturation defects accompanied by ineffective erythropoiesis from hypoproliferative anaemias may be possible on the basis of changes in red-cell morphology, but a bone-marrow examination is often required.

Bone-marrow examination
This may indicate qualitative and quantitative disturbances of erythropoiesis, associated abnormalities of other haemopoietic cell lines, infiltration by haematological or other malignancy, as well as the state of iron stores. Disturbances of marrow architecture due to infiltration and decreased overall marrow cellularity are best appreciated with histological sections of marrow particles or, particularly where marrow aspiration fails, of a marrow trephine biopsy. In the absence of marrow infiltration, and where the circulating granulocytes are normal, the erythroid precursor : myeloid cell (E:M) ratio in the marrow gives a measure of the size of the erythron (see Chapter 4). The normal

ratio is approximately one to three, but may vary widely [1]. However, with even mild anaemias the ratio should increase to at least one to one within three to five days of the onset of the anaemia. A lesser response suggests a hypoproliferative anaemia due to impaired erythropoietin production, a limited iron supply or intrinsic marrow disease. The ratio is increased with both maturation abnormalities and haemolytic anaemias. However, the ineffective nature of erythropoiesis in the former (e.g. in megaloblastic anaemias, sideroblastic disorders and a heterogeneous group of pre-leukaemic conditions with hypercellular bone marrows) is shown by a low circulating reticulocyte count.

Ferrokinetic studies
Discussed in Chapter 5 and recently reviewed in detail [15, 16], ferrokinetic studies using a radioisotope of iron to label transferrin can give quantitative measures of red-cell production that have greatly increased understanding of its physiology and pathophysiology. They have provided a yardstick with which to compare more standard morphological investigations of blood and bone marrow. For example the reticulocyte index, despite its semi-quantitative nature as a measure of effective red-cell production, shows a close correlation with ferrokinetic measurements in both normal subjects and patients with a variety of anaemias [17]. As a result the added precision of ferrokinetic measurements is seldom required for the delineation of individual clinical problems.

The cause of the anaemia
Appropriate further investigations that may be necessary to determine the specific cause of the anaemia will be considered under the four main categories shown in

Figure 36.1 (i.e. microcytic/hypochromic, macrocytic, normocytic and haemolytic anaemias).

Microcytic hypochromic anaemias

The main causes of microcytic, hypochromic anaemias are shown in Table 36.2. All are associated with maturation abnormalities, but limitation of erythroid proliferation by the supply of iron may be the most prominent characteristic of iron-deficient erythropoiesis [14]. An increased reticulocyte count is exceptional and indicates additional factors such as response to haematinic therapy or a major haemolytic component to the anaemia. The latter may be seen, for example, in the thalassaemias and in lead poisoning, or in paroxysmal nocturnal haemoglobinuria where chronic urinary iron loss may give rise to iron deficiency.

The most frequent causes of hypochromic anaemia are iron deficiency and chronic inflammatory disease. The anaemia of chronic diseases is most often normocytic and normochromic, but the reticulo-endothelial trapping of iron [18] can give rise to mild hypochromia. Though the clinical situation and peripheral-blood changes in florid anaemias may make the diagnosis clear without further investigation, separation of this group of anaemias is often dependent on an assessment of body-iron status.

Table 36.2. Microcytic/hypochromic anaemia

---

1 Iron-deficient erythropoiesis
Negative iron balance—blood loss
                                malabsorption
                                nutritional deficiency
                                haemosiderinuria (e.g. PNH)
Increased iron need—pregnancy
                                adolescence
Impaired iron utilization—anaemia of chronic disorders
2 Non-sideropenic hypochromic anaemias
Impaired globin synthesis—thalassaemia disorders
Abnormal haem synthesis—sideroblastic anaemias
                                lead poisoning

Assessment of iron status
(see also Chapter 5).
Iron supply for erythropoiesis is most easily determined by measurement of the serum iron and percentage saturation of the total iron-binding capacity (TIBC). A percentage saturation of less than 16 is unable to support normal haemoglobin synthesis [14, 19]. It should be noted that blood for serum iron determinations is best taken early in the day when values are at the upper limits of the daily range in normal individuals. The serum iron responds within

hours to events such as bleeding or infection, and evidence of impaired iron supply is therefore not always associated with anaemia. A red-cell protoporphyrin level of more than 1 mg/l of red blood cells is a more direct measurement of the imbalance between erythron iron requirements and iron supply [20]. It is also stable over longer periods than the serum iron. Changes in the red-cell indices occur late—after several months—in the development of iron-deficient erythropoiesis. Of these, the MCH is most sensitive in identifying impaired haemoglobin synthesis since it combines the effects of a reduced MCV and MCHC. A marked reduction in MCHC (to less than 30 g/dl) has been shown by automated cell counting to be a late result of iron deficiency, and by the time it is present there is nearly always marked hypochromia on the blood film. Reticulo-endothelial iron stores may be directly estimated in a bone-marrow aspirate [21]. Haemosiderin appears as golden-brown refractile granules in unstained smears, and its nature may be confirmed by staining for iron with potassium ferrocyanide (Prussian Blue). An indirect estimate, more convenient for the patient, is obtained by a serum ferritin assay [22, 23], now becoming more widely available as a laboratory test. A subnormal ferritin concentration correlates well with reduced bone-marrow iron (see Chapter 5, p. 169). However, inflammation, liver disease and increased red-cell turnover can elevate the serum ferritin to a degree disproportionate to the iron stores [23]. Interpretation of normal or increased levels is therefore uncertain in these situations and bone-marrow examination may still be necessary.

Fortunately, in many instances changes in the serum iron and TIBC can be used to differentiate anaemias due to reduced iron supply from the alternative causes of hypochromic anaemias.

Iron-deficient erythropoiesis
A severe microcytic and hypochromic anaemia associated with reduced serum iron and percentage saturation of the TIBC presents little diagnostic problem. Difficulties are greatest with mild anaemias where the red-cell indices may still be in the low normal range. In this situation observers may disagree about the presence or absence of the peripheral-blood abnormalities of iron deficiency [24], and separation of this from other normocytic, hypoproliferative anaemias may be the central problem. The differences in the measurements of iron status between the anaemias of iron deficiency and chronic inflammation are summarized in Table 36.3. Also included are the features of the relative iron deficiency that may accompany recent bleeding, where the rate of mobilization of iron stores limits erythroid proliferation. The clinical picture,

Table 36.3. Iron-deficient erythropoiesis

	Iron deficiency	Inflammation	Recent bleeding
Degree of anaemia	Any severity	Rarely < 10 g/dl	Any severity
Red-cell morphology	Normal or microcytic/ hypochromic	Normal or mild hypochromia	Normal
Reticulocyte index	1	1–2	1–3
Serum iron (normal 10–30 μmol/l)	< 10	< 10	10–20
Serum TIBC (normal 45–70 μmol/l)	> 65	< 50	55–70
Percentage saturation of TIBC (normal 20–60)	Usually < 16	Usually > 16	16–30
Serum ferritin (normal 20–200 μg/l)	Low	Normal or high	Normal or reduced
Bone-marrow iron	Absent	Normal or increased	Normal or reduced

together with the characteristic changes in TIBC (increased in iron deficiency and decreased with inflammation), may be sufficient to identify the likely cause of reduced iron supply. Where doubt remains, a serum ferritin estimation and/or bone-marrow examination may be crucial in distinguishing the absent iron stores of iron deficiency from the block in reticuloendothelial iron release, and accumulation of iron in the anaemia of chronic diseases. A bone-marrow examination is rarely indicated for any other reason where iron deficiency is suspected. The morphological changes are subtle, erythropoiesis being characterized by small erythroblasts with reduced cytoplasm, and only moderate erythroid hyperplasia.

Where iron-deficiency anaemia is established, a search for the underlying cause of negative iron balance is always necessary. In the adult male this is usually haemorrhage, but malabsorption and haemosiderin loss (e.g. in paroxysmal nocturnal haemoglobinuria) may also be considered. In the absence of obvious external bleeding, gastro-intestinal blood loss is likely and may be confirmed by tests for faecal occult blood. However, even if negative, radiological examination of the gut is indicated, looking particularly for evidence of peptic ulceration and neoplasia. The same guidelines apply to post-menopausal women. The decision as to whether gastro-intestinal investigations are necessary in pre-menopausal women has to be based on assessment of diet and menstrual losses (unreliable unless directly measured) and whether faecal occult blood is found. In infants, particularly the premature, iron deficiency is usually dietary in origin.

Non-sideropenic hypochromic anaemias
A hypochromic anaemia in the presence of a normal iron supply (as judged by the serum iron and percentage saturation of the TIBC) should raise the possibility of a defect in either globin chain or haem synthesis.

Thalassaemia syndromes (see also Chapter 9). The presence of the more severe thalassaemia syndromes (e.g. homozygous β thalassaemia, Hb H disease) is usually suggested by the clinical picture (race, family history, age of onset, splenomegaly and skeletal changes) and blood findings of marked poikilocytosis, hypochromia, target cells, nucleated red cells and basophilic stippling. The diagnosis may be confirmed by staining the blood with methyl violet for α-chain inclusion bodies, or cresyl violet for Hb H inclusions; cellulose acetate or starch-gel electrophoresis to identify the major haemoglobin components (and any abnormal haemoglobins) and quantify Hb A$_2$; and determination of Hb F by alkali denaturation.

The blood findings in the minor thalassaemia syndromes, heterozygous β and α thalassaemia, may sometimes be confused with those of iron deficiency. The main points of distinction are shown in Table 36.4.

Table 36.4. Distinction between thalassaemia minor and iron deficiency

	Iron deficiency	Thalassaemia minor
Anaemia	Variable severity	Rarely < 10 g/dl
Red-cell count	< 5 × 10^{12}/l	> 5 × 10^{12}/l
Basophilic stippling	Absent	Present
Serum iron	Reduced	Normal
Serum TIBC	Increased	Normal
Hb A$_2$	< 4%	> 4%
Family history	Absent	Present

The red-cell changes are typically out of proportion to the mild or absent anaemia, the red-cell count is frequently raised, and there is usually a marked reduction in MCV and MCH. Diagnosis in β thalassaemia trait may be confirmed by finding elevated levels of Hb A_2 [25], a rise in Hb F being much less constant. There is no such change in α thalassaemia trait and confirmation is therefore much more dependent on family studies. Where iron deficiency and β thalassaemia minor co-exist there may be a reduction in Hb A_2 levels and the diagnosis can be made with certainty only after treatment of the iron deficiency [26].

Defects in haem synthesis (see Chapter 13). The finding of a dual population of hypochromic and normochromic cells in the blood, combined with a normal or increased serum iron and transferrin saturation, may suggest the diagnosis of a sideroblastic anaemia. This can be confirmed by bone-marrow examination, the usual findings being of erythroid hyperplasia with ringed sideroblasts on the iron stain. In some patients, particularly men with a sex-linked sideroblastic anaemia, the hypochromic microcytic cells may form a single population, though with a large variation. An increase in MCV is common in secondary forms of the disorder [27], where the underlying disease gives a clue to diagnosis. Of particular note are the changes associated with excessive alcohol ingestion, where megaloblastic changes associated with abnormalities in folate metabolism may be followed by the development of ringed sideroblasts in the marrow [28]. Lead poisoning may be suspected, particularly in young children. However, sideroblastic changes are not an invariable accompaniment, and marked basophilic stippling of red cells [29] may lead to a suspicion that can be confirmed by measuring blood or urine lead levels.

Confusion may occasionally arise between inherited sideroblastic anaemias and the thalassaemia disorders, both of which are iron-loading anaemias associated with hypochromia and ineffective erythropoiesis. Although an increase in marrow sideroblasts is typical in the thalassaemias, the majority are not ring forms and haemoglobin electrophoresis studies clearly distinguish the two types of anaemia.

Macrocytic anaemias
The Coulter S has greatly aided the early recognition of macrocytic anaemias, for changes in MCV may occur before the development of anaemia or the typical red-cell and granulocyte changes of megaloblastic erythropoiesis. Macrocytosis is not necessarily due to megaloblastic red-cell production (Table 36.5), but the greater the increase in MCV the more likely this is

[30–32]. Very occasionally a normal MCV may be associated with a megaloblastic marrow (e.g. where there is coincidental iron deficiency resulting in a dimorphic anaemia, in thalassaemia with associated folate deficiency, or after cytotoxic drug therapy). In these instances, however, the white-cell changes of hypersegmentation and granulocytopenia are often present to suggest megaloblastic haemopoiesis. In most cases a bone-marrow examination is performed to confirm the megaloblastic state or to exclude other haematological diseases associated with normoblastic macrocytosis.

Investigation of megaloblastic anaemias centres on assay of vitamin-B_{12} and folate levels followed by identification of the cause of the vitamin deficiency. There is nothing specific about the initial haematological findings to distinguish between folate and vitamin-B_{12} deficiency. A defect in spinal-cord posterior column or peripheral-nerve function makes lack of vitamin-B_{12} the likely cause, though neuropsychiatric disorders accompanying folate deficiency are receiving increasing attention [33], and some malabsorption syndromes may result in both folate deficiency and neurological disease. Underlying diseases in which one deficiency is more likely than the other are shown in Table 36.5. However, the interrelationships of folate and vitamin-B_{12} metabolism mean that regardless of the clinical suspicion, assays of both vitamins should wherever possible be performed simultaneously.

Serum vitamin B_{12}. This can be measured by microbiological- or radio-assay (see Chapter 6, p. 220). The radioassay has the advantage of speed and of being uninfluenced by concurrent antibiotic therapy, but in the past assay artefacts may occasionally have given falsely high serum levels in patients with unquestionable vitamin-B_{12} deficiency [34]. Very exceptionally a high serum vitamin-B_{12}-binding capacity in chronic granulocytic leukaemia may also give a normal level with untreated pernicious anaemia [35]. Low serum vitamin-B_{12} levels in the presence of normal stores may occur in pregnancy, in some haematological malignancies such as multiple myeloma and aplastic anaemia (where macrocytosis may further confuse the issue), in severe iron deficiency and, most important from a diagnostic point of view, in primary folate deficiency. However, with only the rarest exceptions already discussed, and in the absence of premature vitamin-B_{12} therapy, a normal serum vitamin-B_{12} level excludes its deficiency and indicates lack of folate as the cause of a megaloblastic anaemia.

Serum and red-cell folate levels. These are usually measured by microbiological assay, though a reliable

Table 36.5. Macrocytic anaemias

Megaloblastic erythropoiesis
   Vitamin-B_{12} deficiency
      Intrinsic-factor deficiency—pernicious anaemia, post-gastrectomy
      Malabsorption—regional ileitis, stagnant-loop syndrome, tropical sprue, drugs (e.g. neomycin, colchicine)
      Nutritional deficiency—rarely in vegans
      Fish tapeworm (Finland)
      Congenital malabsorption of B_{12} (Chapter 6)
   Folate deficiency
      Nutritional deficiency
      Malabsorption—coeliac disease, tropical sprue
      Increased requirements—pregnancy, haemolytic anaemias
                            myeloproliferative disorders, malignancy
     Associated with alcoholism
     Anticonvulsant drugs
     Congenital malabsorption of folate (Chapter 6)
   Not due to B_{12} or folate deficiency
      Drugs interfering with folate metabolism—folic-acid antagonists (e.g. methotrexate, trimethoprim), alcohol
      Drugs interfering with B_{12} metabolism—nitrous-oxide anaesthesia
      Other antimetabolites—cytosine arabinoside, 6-mercaptopurine, etc.
      Some cases of erythroleukaemia, other myeloid leukaemias, sideroblastic anaemias
      Congenital dyserythropoietic anaemias
      Congenital metabolic defects—of B_{12} or folate and others (e.g. orotic aciduria)

Normoblastic erythropoiesis
   Macrocytosis associated with systemic disease
      Liver disease
      Alcoholism
      Myxoedema and hypopituitarism
   Macrocytosis associated with marrow disease
      Leukaemia
      Aplastic anaemia
      Marrow infiltration—myelofibrosis, multiple myeloma, disseminated carcinoma
      Sideroblastic anaemias
   Physiological macrocytosis
      Haemolytic anaemia
      Post-haemorrhagic anaemia

---

radioassay is now available for serum folate measurements (see Chapter 6, p. 234). The serum folate responds quickly to changes in diet with illness, and when reduced suggests a negative folate balance. However, many hospital patients are found to have equivocal or low serum folate levels, in spite of adequate tissue folate levels. Stores are estimated more accurately by red-cell folate assay. Even this may mislead, however, for a relatively sudden increase in folate requirements (e.g. in pregnancy) takes time to be reflected in the mature red cells which have a comparatively long lifespan. The higher folate content of younger red cells may also give normal values in folate-deficient megaloblastic anaemias complicating chronic haemolytic states [36]. An additional complication is that low red-cell folate levels are common in vitamin-B_{12} deficiency [36, 37]. In these circumstances the serum folate is normal or elevated, as the defect appears to be one of impaired red-cell uptake of folate [38].

Despite the interrelationship of vitamin-B_{12} and folate metabolism the deficiency at fault can nearly always be clearly identified by these assays (Table 36.6).

Vitamin-B_{12} deficiency megaloblastic anaemias (see Chapter 6).

Pernicious anaemia (PA). This may be suspected on clinical grounds with a positive family history, and an association with vitiligo, thyroid disease, Addison's disease and hypoparathyroidism, as well as idiopathic thrombocytopenic purpura and autoimmune haemolytic anaemias. Confirmation depends upon the demonstration of pentagastrin-fast achlorhydria (pH remains greater than 4·0–5·0) and a gross reduction of

Table 36.6. Separation of megaloblastic anaemias using B_{12} and folate assays

	Serum		
	B_{12}	Folate	Red-cell folate
Normal range [1]	160–925 μg/l	3–20 μg/l	160–640 μg/l
B_{12} deficiency	Low	Normal or high	Often low
Folate deficiency	Normal (rarely low)	Low	Low
B_{12} + folate deficiency	Low	Low	Low

intrinsic factor secretion. The latter can be indirectly demonstrated by measurement of radiolabelled vitamin-B_{12} absorption, repeating the test with exogenous intrinsic factor if the vitamin B_{12} alone is poorly absorbed. The tests of absorption use urinary excretion (Schilling test) [39], plasma radioactivity at eight hours (less reliable) [40], or whole-body counting [41] to monitor absorption. They can be performed after treatment with vitamin B_{12} and indeed this may have the advantage that any gastro-intestinal mucosal abnormalities due to the vitamin-B_{12} deficiency will then have been reversed.

Intrinsic-factor antibodies are found in the serum of over 50% of patients with PA; their association with a megaloblastic anaemia is virtually diagnostic. Parietal-cell antibodies, though more frequently present, are less specific. Additional studies that may be necessary include radiology of the stomach (where history or examination suggests the possibility of carcinoma), and assessment of thyroid function.

Other causes of vitamin-B_{12} deficiency (Table 36.5). These are usually clear from the clinical features and do not require specific tests of absorption. However, where these are carried out for suspected PA and show no correction of vitamin-B_{12} malabsorption by intrinsic factor, an unsuspected small-bowel abnormality (e.g. Crohn's disease or diverticuli) is likely and requires appropriate X-ray studies. Megaloblastic anaemia due to nutritional deficiency is rare, in spite of the low serum vitamin-B_{12} levels that are frequent in people eating a deficient diet (mainly vegans). Confirmation of the diagnosis depends on the response to low doses (2–5 μg) of vitamin-B_{12} daily by mouth.

Folate-deficiency megaloblastic anaemias
The cause may be clear from the history (particularly of the diet). Occasionally folate deficiency may be the sole indicator of coeliac disease though other features including steatorrhoea are more often present. Diagnosis in the malabsorption syndromes requires small bowel radiology and jejunal biopsy.

Megaloblastic anaemia not due to vitamin-B_{12} or folate deficiency
The megaloblastic changes due to therapeutic, cytotoxic agents have an obvious cause. Those due to alcohol (reducing tissue availability of folate) or to nitrous-oxide anaesthesia (blocking cobalamin metabolism) may be less obvious.

The rare congenital dyserythropoietic anaemias occasionally escape detection until adult life (see Chapter 31, p. 1259). They are characterized by erythroid hyperplasia and multinuclearity of erythroblasts. Type 1 is megaloblastic; type 2 (HEMPAS) is normoblastic with a red-cell membrane abnormality giving rise to a positive acidified serum test (though, unlike paroxysmal nocturnal haemoglobinuria, with only a proportion of normal sera and not with the patient's own acidified serum); type 3 is characterized by gigantoblasts.

The erythroleukaemias show erythroid hyperplasia with bizarre nucleated red-cell precursors which are often megaloblastic in appearance. Vitamin-B_{12} and folate levels are normal. An associated increase in myeloblasts, the presence of ringed sideroblasts, and PAS-positive staining of the nucleated red cells, may all be diagnostically helpful.

Normoblastic macrocytosis
This occurs in haemolytic and some dyserythropoietic anaemias and is discussed in the next section.

Normocytic anaemias
Normocytic, normochromic anaemias (Table 36.7) form a large proportion of those seen in clinical practice. Many are associated with the systemic disorders discussed in Chapter 33. Their severity is usually related to that of the underlying disease. Others are due to marrow failure (whether related to intrinsic marrow disease, toxic agents, or infiltration), or to reduced erythropoietin production. The anaemia of renal failure is largely due to the latter, and the mild anaemias of the endocrinopathies and protein malnutrition [42] may result in part from reduced tissue oxygen requirements and a consequent decrease in

Table 36.7. Normocytic anaemias

Hypoproliferative	
Mild iron deficiency	
Chronic disorders	Infection
	Disseminated malignancy
	Collagen disorders
	Liver diseases
Marrow failure	Aplastic anaemia
	Pure red-cell aplasia
	Infiltration by haematological or other malignancies
Reduced erythropoietin production	Renal failure
	Reduced need for O_2-carrying capacity
	—endocrine disorders (hypothyroidism, hypopituitarism, Addison's disease)
	—haemoglobinopathy with decreased O_2 affinity
	—protein malnutrition
Acute blood loss	
Haemolytic anaemias (see separate section)	

erythropoietin production. There may be characteristic peripheral-blood findings with some disorders (e.g. target cells in liver disease, burr cells or fragmented cells in renal disease. eosinophilia in polyarteritis and giant-cell arteritis), and an increase in white-cell count is frequent. A raised ESR (out of proportion to the mild degree of anaemia) is common in many of the anaemias of chronic disorders. Where appropriate, investigation for underlying infection, liver, renal and endocrine function, or for a collagenosis (e.g. rheumatoid factor, antinuclear factor and LE cells) may be necessary. Further haematological investigation is indicated when there is a suspicion of intrinsic or infiltrative marrow disease, or of a haematinic deficiency accompanying the underlying disorder.

Apart from the haemolytic disorders, which are commonly normocytic or mildly macrocytic and are considered separately, the normocytic anaemias are predominantly hypoproliferative and are characterized by an inappropriately low reticulocyte count without evidence of maturation abnormalities. Marked anisocytosis and poikilocytosis are rare in the anaemias of chronic disorders, aplastic anaemia or pure red-cell aplasia. However, these features may be more marked, and sometimes accompanied by mild macrocytosis, when the marrow architecture is disturbed due to infiltration by leukaemia, lymphoma, multiple myeloma or myelofibrosis. In many of these conditions a pancytopenia or a leucoerythroblastic blood picture indicates the need for bone-marrow examination, though early red and white cells may also be seen in the blood in severe acute infections. Where infiltration is suspected areas of bone tenderness may

be most appropriately aspirated for bone marrow. A dry tap may necessitate a trephine biopsy, a bloody tap can sometimes be redeemed by making histological sections of the clot, and marrow-particle sections should be obtained where possible. Tumour cells from disseminated carcinoma may be identified [43], and silver staining of a trephine biopsy will demonstrate myelofibrosis. A bone-marrow examination may also be necessary where the degree of anaemia is out of proportion to the severity of the underlying disorder, or where no such disorder is apparent. An isolated deficiency of red-cell precursors indicates a pure red-cell aplasia. Chest radiography for a possible thymoma [44] may then be necessary unless the red-cell aplasia is clearly related to an aplastic crisis (e.g. after intercurrent infection in a chronic haemolytic anaemia).

As discussed under hypochromic anaemias, the initial development of iron deficiency may be marked by a mild normocytic, normochromic anaemia. The features which distinguish the hypoproliferative anaemias of mild iron deficiency from those of chronic disorders have been summarized in Table 36.3. This table also shows the features of the normochromic anaemia associated with the recent onset of bleeding, where erythropoiesis is limited by the rate of mobilization of iron stores that have not yet been completely exhausted. Investigation of a normocytic anaemia with no obvious cause should therefore include assessment of iron status, examination of stools for occult blood, and radiology of the gut if appropriate. The anaemia of renal failure may also be complicated by iron deficiency related to blood loss, often due to impaired platelet function and slow gastro-intestinal oozing of blood. Haemodialysis is a further source of blood loss [45, 46] and folate deficiency may also develop. However, potentially toxic iron overload has recently been noted after parenteral-iron replacement therapy has been given to patients on long-term dialysis [47]. Separation of contributory factors in anaemia associated with renal failure may thus depend on measurements of iron stores, including serum ferritin and bone-marrow examination for iron. In addition, where hypersegmented neutrophils are seen in the peripheral blood, determination of serum and red-cell folate and bone-marrow examination may be necessary to exclude a megaloblastic element in the anaemia. The anaemia of hypothyroidism is normocytic [48], and if there is a macrocytosis, associated pernicious anaemia should be suspected.

Haemolytic anaemias

Anaemia in the presence of reticulocytes (reticulocyte index greater than three) suggests a haemolytic process. Unrecognized haematinic therapy of a deficiency anaemia and the erythroid response to blood loss may occasionally be confused with haemolysis, and stool examination may be necessary to investigate the latter possibility. Diagnosis involves confirmation of red-cell damage and increased destruction (Table 36.8), followed by elucidation of the specific cause (Table 36.9). A combination of the clinical setting and blood findings often indicates the likely diagnosis or most profitable line of investigation. Despite the wide range of investigation available in this group of disorders, the

Table 36.8. Haemolytic anaemias—initial assessment

1 Clinical features—history and examination (see text)
2 Complete blood count
3 Assessment of red-cell production
      Reticulocyte count and production index
      Bone-marrow examination if associated haematological
        abnormality is suspected (e.g. folate deficiency,
        marrow infiltration or aplastic crisis)
4 Examination of blood film for evidence of red-cell
      damage and specific red-cell shape abnormalities (e.g.
      sickle cells) (see p. 1461)
5 Confirmation of increased red-cell destruction
      Urine for urobilinogen, haemoglobin, haemosiderin
      Serum unconjugated bilirubin level
      Plasma haptoglobin level
      In selected patients: plasma haemoglobin and
                        methaemalbumin levels.
                  ^{51}Cr-labelled red-cell
                      survival studies (with
                      surface counting)

aetiology may remain obscure in a small number of patients [49].

Clinical features

The history and clinical examination can provide information both as to the likelihood of haemolysis and its cause. The patient's ethnic origin and family history (e.g. of anaemia, jaundice, and splenectomy) may suggest a congenital haemolytic anaemia. For example, the thalassaemia disorders and glucose-6-phosphate dehydrogenase (G6PD) deficiency affect predominantly Mediterranean, Asian and African peoples, and sickle-cell disease those of African origin. The pattern of inheritance may be helpful, whether present in successive generations as an autosomal dominant trait such as hereditary spherocytosis, or sex-linked as with G6PD deficiency. Associated illness, particularly systemic lupus erythematosus (SLE), chronic lymphocytic leukaemia and lymphomas, infectious mononucleosis, and the convalescent phase of *Mycoplasma pneumoniae* pneumonia suggests the possibility of an immune haemolytic anaemia. Cold agglutinins may result in Raynaud's phenomenon. Drug exposure may give rise to haemolysis whether due to an immune mechanism (e.g. methyldopa), or to oxidant stress, particularly in patients with G6PD deficiency or an unstable haemoglobinopathy. Many infections are associated with a shortened red-cell lifespan, but in patients with a haemoglobinopathy or enzyme defect they may precipitate frank haemolysis. A setting of previous cardiac-valve surgery, or one of the variety of disorders that can give rise to a microangiopathic haemolytic anaemia, may suggest a red-cell fragmentation haemolysis.

Acute abdominal, back or limb pains, associated with dark urine, suggest a severe intravascular haemolysis with haemoglobinuria, as may occur with an incompatible blood transfusion, thermal burn or the α toxin of a *Clostridium welchii* septicaemia. Where these symptoms arise after travel to endemic areas, malaria should be suspected. Abdominal and limb pains may also occur with sickle-cell crises.

A more chronic history of haemoglobinuria may be obtained with paroxysmal nocturnal haemoglobinuria (PNH), march haemoglobinuria, paroxysmal cold haemoglobinuria and cold-agglutinin haemolysis, where a relationship to sleep, exertion or cold respectively may be obtained.

The cardinal signs of haemolysis—pallor, jaundice and splenomegaly—may be absent. Marked splenomegaly with the bone changes of marrow expansion suggests a congenital haemolytic anaemia such as one of the thalassaemia disorders. A large spleen in lymphoma, myelosclerosis, chronic granulocytic or lymphocytic leukaemia, malaria and kala-azar may

Table 36.9. Haemolytic anaemias—further investigations

1 Where an acquired defect is suspected
  (a) Due to an immune reaction
      Direct antiglobulin (Coombs) tests with broad-spectrum, anti-Ig, and anti-complement sera
      Titration of IgM cold agglutinins
      Donath–Landsteiner test for IgG cold lytic antibody in paroxysmal cold haemoglobinuria
      Tests for underlying disease (e.g. LE cell preparation, antinuclear-factor measurement, Mycoplasma
          antibody titre, Wasserman and VDRL tests)
  (b) Due to drugs and chemicals
      Heinz-body preparation for denatured haemoglobin
      Screening test for G6PD deficiency
      Identification of methaemoglobin and sulphaemoglobin
      Tests for drug-dependent antibodies using red cells preincubated with the appropriate drug
  (c) Due to mechanical fragmentation
      Identification of underlying disease (e.g. cardiac valve replacement, microangiopathic haemolytic
          anaemias)
  (d) Due to hypersplenism
      ^{51}Cr red-cell mass and sequestration studies in selected patients
  (e) Associated with haemoglobinuria, hypoplastic anaemia or any obscure haemolytic anaemia
      Sucrose lysis screening test
      Acidified-serum (Ham's) test (for enhanced complement lysis in paroxysmal nocturnal haemoglo
          binuria)
2 Where a congenital haemolytic anaemia is suspected
  (a) General screen for defects in membrane and metabolic function (including hereditary spherocytosis)
      Osmotic fragility test, with and without incubation at 37°C for 24 hours
      Autohaemolysis test, with and without the addition of glucose
  (b) Identification of haemoglobinopathies (including the thalassaemias, Hb S and C disease, and unstable
      haemoglobins)
      Haemoglobin electrophoresis (cellulose acetate, starch gel, etc.)
      Estimation of Hb A_2 and F
      Sickling tests
      Screening tests for unstable haemoglobins
        Heinz-body preparation
        Heat instability test
        Isopropanol precipitation test
  (c) Identification of metabolic deficiency (including the inherited red-cell enzyme defects)
      G6PD and PK screening tests and assays
      Other red-cell enzyme assays as indicated
  (d) Family studies
      If congenital haemolysis confirmed

itself be associated with hypersplenism and shortened red-cell survival. Mild enlargement of the spleen is common in hereditary spherocytosis and pyruvate kinase (PK) deficiency, less common in immune haemolytic anaemias and PNH, and rare in G6PD deficiency and sickle-cell anaemia after the early years of life. Cyanosis may raise the question of an unstable haemoglobin with low oxygen affinity [50].

Blood film
The blood film may provide evidence of red-cell injury and often gives the specific cause of the haemolysis (see p. 1461). In addition to the morphological changes already discussed, erythrophagocytosis by monocytes is occasionally seen in immune haemolytic anaemias, and cold agglutinins may be suspected from the presence of agglutination on the blood film.

Confirmation and assessment of the severity of increased red-cell destruction
There are no good direct measures of increased red-cell destruction. Many of the indicators are non-specific, being common to conditions of ineffective erythropoiesis, or in some cases a result of liver disease or gallstones (see Chapter 4, p. 129).

Measures of bile-pigment turnover. These are insensitive and non-specific for haemolysis. A plasma bilirubin of less than 7 µmol/l makes significant haemolysis unlikely, and though an increase of unconjugated bilirubin to 25–50 µmol/l may be present with haemolysis, this is not always the case. Increased levels of urobilinogen in the urine are characteristic, but non-specific for haemolytic anaemias. The demonstration of increased faecal urobilinogen [51] has obvious disadvantages in addition to the doubts that it accurately reflects red-cell turnover [52], and is now of historical interest only (see Chapter 4, p. 129).

Plasma red-cell enzyme (SGOT and LDH) levels. These are increased in haemolytic disorders, but also with ineffective erythropoiesis and after other tissue damage, particularly of heart, liver and muscle.

Haemoglobinuria. This indicates severe intravascular haemolysis and occurs at the time of an acute haemolytic attack. Increased plasma haemoglobin levels (greater than 0·03 g/dl) in blood samples drawn with care to avoid haemolysis, and the detection of methaemalbumin in plasma (Schumm's test) have a similar significance.

Haemosiderinuria. This, detected by staining the urinary sediment from a random, or preferably early morning, urine specimen for iron, indicates chronic intravascular haemolysis.

Depletion of plasma haptoglobins. This occurs with both intravascular and extravascular haemolysis [53]. However, low levels are also found in hepatocellular disease due to impaired synthesis, and higher than expected levels may be seen in inflammatory disorders [54] where haptoglobins behave as acute-phase proteins.

Red-cell survival studies
(see Chapter 4, p. 114)

Where doubts remain as to the contribution of a significant haemolytic element to an anaemia, ^{51}Cr-labelled, red-cell survival studies [1, 55] offer a sensitive measure of red-cell lifespan, as well as giving the opportunity for surface counting over liver and spleen to determine major sites of sequestration. In addition, a comparison of the survival of the patient's and donor cells may allow extracellular and intracellular mechanisms of cell destruction to be distinguished where this remains in doubt. These time-consuming ^{51}Cr studies are seldom necessary, however; the severity of haemolysis can be deduced indirectly from the reticulocyte production index combined with the degree of anaemia, and though splenic sequestration studies frequently correlate with the results of subsequent splenectomy, patients may show benefit despite a poor splenic uptake of ^{51}Cr [56].

Tests to determine the cause of haemolysis

The initial assessment usually indicates whether the haemolysis is of acute onset or chronic in nature, whether there is significant intravascular haemolysis, and whether the disorder is likely to be inherited or acquired. Further studies are directed to identification of specific defects intrinsic to the red cell (intracorpuscular defects which, with the exception of PNH, are inherited disorders), or to defining an acquired extracorpuscular defect. The main lines of investigation are shown in Table 36.9. More detailed analysis of the abnormalities found in the different disorders may be found in Chapters 7–12 and the methodology in Ref. 1.

The immune haemolytic anaemias are in most cases identified by a positive direct antiglobulin test. A negative test does not completely exclude the diagnosis, however, because the amount of immunoglobulin coating of the red cells has to be substantially increased before the antiglobulin test becomes positive [56]. Furthermore, the presence of a positive direct antiglobulin test is not synonymous with haemolysis, and other mechanisms for the anaemia should be considered if the reticulocyte count is not substantially raised (index greater than three). By the use of specific antisera, and specificity testing of antibodies both in serum and after elution from the red cells, the presence of immunglobulin, with or without complement, may be demonstrated on the red cells, and the autoantibody more precisely characterized. The significance of the various types of antibodies is summarized in Chapter 11.

Sudden, severe intravascular haemolysis in a previously healthy patient may be due to autoimmune haemolysis, infection (particularly clostridial) or to toxic drugs or chemicals. These are especially likely to be implicated in cases of previously unsuspected G6PD deficiency, when oxidative drugs such as aspirin, phenacetin, nitrofurantoin, sulphonamides and probenecid may precipitate a Heinz-body anaemia. More chronic intravascular haemolysis with haemosiderinuria should lead to consideration of fragmentation haemolysis and PNH.

The various tests of osmotic fragility and autohaemolysis are non-specific screening investigations for disorders of membrane function and intracellular metabolism (see Chapter 7, p. 280). In hereditary spherocytosis, which may be suspected from the red-cell appearances, family history and negative antiglobulin test, there is a variable increase in osmotic fragility which becomes more marked after incubation at 37°C for 24 hours. By contrast, in autoimmune haemolytic anaemias there is often a population of relatively more resistant cells in addition to the fragile spherocytes. In the autohaemolysis test the amount of lysis after 48 hours' sterile incubation is measured with and without added glucose [60] (see Chapter 7, p. 280). In many, but not all, patients with inherited membrane defects (hereditary spherocytosis and elliptocytosis), the increase in autohaemolysis, compared with normal blood, is significantly reduced by the addition of glucose (type-I autohaemolysis). In contrast, metabolic enzyme deficiencies resulting in a non-spherocytic haemolytic anaemia (e.g. PK deficiency) show no correction with glucose (type-II autohaemolysis). Increased autohaemolysis due to congenital, unstable haemoglobinopathies may also show a partial correction with glucose; in addition Heinz bodies and methaemoglobin are likely to be detected at the end of the incubation period [50]. Further investigation of the non-spherocytic congenital haemolytic anaemias is considered under the headings of haemoglobinopathies and metabolic deficiencies in Table 36.9, and in Chapters 7 and 8. Investigation of the thalassaemia disorders has been briefly considered under microcytic, hypochromic anaemias and is discussed in detail in Chapter 9.

POLYCYTHAEMIA

As with the definitions of anaemia, the upper limits for normal haemoglobin (or PCV) levels are based on population data and are arbitrary for any particular individual. Haemoglobin levels greater than 18 g/dl in males and 16·5 g/dl in females are above the 95% range [1]. Absolute, or true, polycythaemia implies an increase in red-cell mass and is usually present if the haemoglobin is greater than 20 g/dl (PCV > 60%) in men, or 18·5 g/dl (PCV > 55%) in women [61]. Lesser increases are not invariably accompanied by an increased red-cell mass, and may result from plasma-volume disturbances in relative or spurious [62] polycythaemia. The clinical setting may help in determining the likelihood of an absolute polycythaemia in a particular patient, whether there is an obvious cause such as chronic hypoxia, and whether further investigation is warranted.

Clinical setting

Hypoxia is the commonest cause of true polycythaemia. Cyanosis and clinically obvious cardiac or respiratory disease may indicate secondary polycythaemia which does not require further haematological investigation. A history of smoking may be important in patients with mild increases in PCV, and suggests the need to measure carboxyhaemoglobin levels in the blood [63]. Diuretic therapy or a history of nausea and vomiting point to a relative polycythaemia with reduced plasma volume. A florid case of polycythaemia rubra vera should lead to appropriate confirmatory investigations: itching, especially after warm baths, splenomegaly, and microvascular disease of fingers and toes are all highly suggestive of the disease and are not a feature of the secondary polycythaemias.

Determination of red-cell mass and plasma volume
(see Chapter 1, p. 38)

Measurement of red-cell mass using ^{51}Cr-labelled red cells, and plasma volume using radioiodinated albumin, permits the separation of relative and true polycythaemias, though mild elevations in red-cell mass may be as difficult to interpret as mild increases in haemoglobin concentration. Direct measurements are probably not essential where the haemoglobin levels are grossly elevated and there are additional findings pointing to a specific cause for a true polycythaemia.

Blood examination in polycythaemia rubra vera

Neutrophilia (> 12×10^9/l) in the absence of infection, and/or thrombocytosis (> 400×10^9/l) in addition to a true polycythaemia, are highly suggestive of polycythaemia rubra vera. An increase in basophils or eosinophils is also supporting evidence for this diagnosis. The red-cell indices and film commonly show a degree of hypochromia and microcytosis, and serum iron measurements may demonstrate a reduced level consistent with a relative impairment of iron supply.

Further investigation for polycythaemia rubra vera

In the absence of palpable splenomegaly a spleen scan can be helpful in recording splenic enlargement. A raised leucocyte-alkaline-phosphatase score (> 100) is also a feature of the disease. A bone-marrow examination typically shows a non-specific increase in all cellular elements, and does not add greatly to the information from the peripheral blood. Where thrombocytosis is present, an increase in size as well as number of megakaryocytes may be helpful in identifying the autonomous, rather than reactive, nature of the thrombopoiesis.

Further investigations for secondary polycythaemias

In the absence of clear evidence for a myeloproliferative disorder further studies are needed. Hypoxia may be demonstrated by a reduced arterial oxygen tension and saturation, and lead to a search for underlying cardiopulmonary disease. A mild elevation in PCV may be related to increased amounts of carboxyhaemoglobin in the blood due to smoking.

Tissue hypoxia and polycythaemia may result from an abnormal haemoglobin with a high affinity for oxygen. This should be suspected with a positive family history, and particularly when the patient is young and otherwise healthy. Confirmation requires determination of the position of the haemoglobin oxygen dissociation curve and the P_{50}, which is shifted to the left. More simply, a greater-than-expected oxygen saturation may be seen at the particular oxygen tension of a venous blood sample [64]. An inherited polycythaemia due to inappropriate erythropoietin

Table 36.10. Diagnosis in polycythaemia

Relative polycythaemia: Dehydration
                       Diuretics
                       Idiopathic
Absolute polycythaemia:
    (a) Primary (independent of erythropoietin)
         Polycythaemia rubra vera
    (b) Secondary (erythropoietin dependent)
         Tissue hypoxia: Smoking (carboxyhaemoglobinaemia)
                        Pulmonary disease
                        Cyanotic cardiac disease
                        Alveolar hypoventilation
                        Abnormal haemoglobin with high O_2 affinity
                        High altitude
         Inappropriate increase in erythropoietin production:
             Renal artery stenosis, masses (cysts, hydronephrosis), transplantation
             Neoplasia (hypernephroma, hepatoma, cerebellar angioma, carcinoma of lung, uterine fibroids)
             Familial erythropoietinaemia

---

production has also been described, diagnosis being dependent on the demonstration of a marked increase in erythropoietin with no underlying cause and an inappropriate response to venesection [65].

Inappropriate erythropoietin production may result from a number of renal diseases (Table 36.10) and the investigation of an isolated erythrocytosis requires intravenous pyelography and the further investigation of any abnormality detected. Various neoplasms have also been associated with polycythaemia, though the commonest are renal in origin [66].

Despite full assessment there are certain patients in whom the diagnosis will remain unclear. Some may develop frank polycythaemia rubra vera at a later date. Serum erythropoietin levels, which offer the hope of separating autonomous marrow production in polycythaemia rubra vera (depressed levels) from the secondary polycythaemias (elevated levels), are not yet generally available for the assessment of these difficult problems.

LEUCOCYTE DISORDERS

Neutrophilia

By far the commonest causes of a neutrophil leucocytosis are bacterial infections and tissue injury. The history and clinical examination will usually suggest a cause for the neutrophilia, but if not, investigation should be directed towards finding occult infection. particularly in the chest, renal and biliary tracts, or identifying tumours, especially those associated with much tissue destruction. Perinephric, subphrenic and liver abscesses may be particularly difficult to identify,

although the newer radiological techniques of ultrasound and scanning are helpful.

The usual degree of leucocytosis in infection is $12–30 \times 10^9/l$ but sometimes, and particularly in young children, the white count may reach $50 \times 10^9/l$ or higher and a few early myeloid cells may be present in the peripheral blood. This type of leukaemoid reaction to infection has to be distinguished from a primary haematological disorder. In young children this is not usually a problem, since juvenile CGL is rare and the accompanying clinical features of rashes, purpura, lymphadenopathy and splenomegaly should suggest the diagnosis. If there is any doubt, other features of this rare condition should be looked for, such as the high haemoglobin F, low haemoglobin A_2 and decreased red-cell carbonic anhydrase (see Chapter 23).

In older subjects with leukaemoid reactions, the distinction again has to be made between primary and secondary disorders. The greatest confusion will arise between the leucoerythroblastic picture of primary myelofibrosis and the very similar picture produced by disseminated tuberculosis or metastatic carcinoma. In all three there may be hepatosplenomegaly, anaemia and thrombocytopenia, although splenomegaly is a more dominant feature of primary myelofibrosis. If there is no obvious site of a primary neoplasm nor any evidence of tuberculosis (such as miliary lesions in the lung), a bone-marrow examination with a trephine biopsy is one of the most useful diagnostic tests. The smears may be acellular in all three conditions, but in tuberculosis acid-fast bacilli are occasionally found, and in disseminated neoplasia carcinoma cells may be recognized. The histological preparation is, however, more likely to give a definitive diagnosis. Liver biopsy is helpful if tuberculosis is suspected, since it often reveals miliary lesions. Bone X-rays and bone scans may show diagnostic appearances in myelosclerosis or may indicate metastatic deposits in the case of carcinoma.

Chronic granulocytic leukaemia in its more florid state seldom presents any diagnostic difficulty. The combination of a very high leucocyte count with the presence of early myeloid cells and often a basophilia, together with hepatosplenomegaly, make the diagnosis obvious; but at an earlier stage, or when a leucocytosis is discovered during the investigation of another complaint, there may be only a moderate increase in white cells and little, if any, splenomegaly. If the disease is suspected the leucocyte alkaline phosphatase should be measured, as it is characteristically reduced in CGL, and the bone marrow should be examined both morphologically and for the presence of the Philadelphia chromosome, although the absence of the latter does not entirely exclude the diagnosis.

Neutropenia

Patients who present with neutropenia (neutrophils less than $1 \cdot 5 \times 10^9/l$) may have few complaints apart from a history of an increased tendency to bacterial infection, and the low count may be an incidental finding. Severe agranulocytosis (less than $0 \cdot 5 \times 10^9/l$) is usually symptomatic, producing mouth and throat ulceration and often being accompanied by septicaemia.

From the diagnostic point of view the history may be the most helpful investigation. It may indicate whether the neutropenia is of recent onset or is long-standing and, if the latter, whether it is congenital, familial or cyclical in nature. Apart from giving a name to the condition and perhaps providing genetic counselling, little can be done about the congenital or familial conditions apart from early recognition of intercurrent infections and the use of appropriate antibiotics. The acquired conditions deserve more detailed investigation.

Any association with other diseases should be noted; for example, rheumatoid arthritis will suggest that the neutropenia may be due to Felty's syndrome, or a history of liver disease or any other condition which may give rise to splenomegaly will suggest a cause for the neutropenia. The medication received for other conditions is also important, since neutropenia may be drug-induced. Besides drugs prescribed by doctors, attention should be paid to any self-medication or exposure to chemicals in the home or in industry.

Apart from drugs, the commonest causes of acute neutropenia are viral infections. Associated symptoms and signs may point towards such a diagnosis, as may the morphology of the reactive lymphocytes in the blood, and appropriate viral tests should be instituted.

Some bacterial infections, such as typhoid and brucellosis, are also associated with neutropenia and in a patient with pyrexia of unknown origin the low neutrophil count may suggest such a diagnosis. It is important to realize that overwhelming septicaemia, particularly with Gram-negative organisms or staphylococci, may present with neutropenia rather than a leucocytosis. This is a serious sign in any febrile, seriously ill patient, calling for the immediate use of wide-spectrum antibiotics as soon as blood cultures have been taken.

Neutropenia is a frequent feature of systemic lupus erythematosus and if there is any other clinical evidence to suggest such a diagnosis, tests for SLE should be made.

Neutropenia and severe agranulocytosis may occasionally be the presenting feature of folate deficiency in coeliac disease. There may not be any history suggestive of bowel disturbance and only on specific investigation into the biopsy appearances of the small bowel is the underlying disease revealed. Vitamin-B_{12} deficiency also produces a neutropenia but this is overshadowed by the other changes and is not in itself symptomatic.

Occasionally other primary haematological diseases present as a neutropenia; for example it may be an early feature of aplastic anaemia or acute leukaemia. A bone-marrow examination will usually clarify the diagnosis. If the marrow is hypocellular there is a possibility of paroxysmal nocturnal haemoglobinuria being associated with the condition and tests for PNH should be done on the blood.

Eosinophilia

Eosinophilia is characteristic of conditions associated with an immune response. Investigation therefore should be directed towards finding the agent which has triggered such a response. The ethnic background may make a parasitic infection the most likely cause, and the faeces should be examined carefully for evidence of hookworm, roundworm and tapeworm. Toxocara may be suggested, particularly if there is a history of respiratory symptoms and contact with dogs or cats with roundworm. In patients coming from sheep-farming areas, echinococcal infection should be considered.

Ingestion of undercooked pork or sausages, in association with a febrile illness and swelling of the eyelids, will suggest *Trichinella* infection, and consumption of watercress grown in an area where there may be infected snails will make one look for evidence of liver fluke. If ova are not found in the stools, liver biopsy may be necessary for diagnosis.

In the absence of any evidence of parasitic infestation, the possibility of a drug reaction should be considered, particularly after the use of para-amino-salicylic acid, penicillin or a sulphonamide derivative.

Eosinophilia may be a sign of underlying neoplastic disease, particularly when the liver is involved with necrotic tumour. Although often considered to be a classical finding in Hodgkin's disease, eosinophilia is in fact rare in this condition.

Symptoms of peripheral neuropathy and collagen-vascular disease may suggest a diagnosis of polyarteritis nodosa, and a variety of other symptoms, including endocarditis, are manifestations of the eosinophilic syndrome.

In many patients the precise cause of the eosinophilic reaction may never become apparent, but apart from the obvious search for parasitic infestation, biopsy of lymph nodes, liver or muscle may be indicated.

Basophilia

An increase in the basophil count is frequently found in the myeloproliferative disorders, especially CGL, and it tends to persist even when the blood count is otherwise well controlled by treatment. In the absence of other classical signs of CGL, bone-marrow chromosome studies may confirm the diagnosis. The rare condition of systemic mastocytosis is accompanied by a basophilia. Clinical examination will reveal hepatosplenomegaly, skeletal changes, and the characteristic skin lesions of urticaria pigmentosa: the diagnosis can be confirmed by skin biopsy.

Lymphocytosis

The significance of a lymphocytosis must be assessed in relation to the age of the patient as it is a normal finding in young children. An increase in the lymphocytes may be either reactive to an infection or neoplastic. The morphological characteristics of the cells in the blood film, together with the clinical picture, will often distinguish between these groups. There may, however, be some difficulty in certain cases in distinguishing between viral infections such as glandular fever, cytomegalovirus (CMV) and toxoplasma infection,

and a non-Hodgkin lymphoma. If a Paul–Bunnell test and virological tests for these specific infections are inconclusive, a bone-marrow aspiration and lymph-node biopsy will be needed.

Immature lymphoid cells in the blood may be difficult to distinguish from myeloblasts and enzyme stains and immunological cell markers may be needed to make the differentiation (see Chapters 21 and 22). The neoplastic nature of more mature cells may be indicated by their monoclonal production of immunoglobulins and by evidence of immune paresis. Most of those lymphoproliferative disorders which result in a peripheral lymphocytosis are B-cell disorders. From the point of view of the prognosis, B-cell chronic lymphocytic leukaemia should be distinguished from the rarer T-cell type, which carries a worse prognosis.

PANCYTOPENIA

The investigation of isolated deficiencies of one of the cellular elements of the blood is discussed in the appropriate sections of this chapter. Combined deficiencies of blood cells may present with the classical features of anaemia, infection and bleeding, although symptoms referable to a single cell line may be found on examination to be accompanied by a pancytopenia. As with the isolated defects, the deficiency may be due to impaired production or increased destruction of mature blood cells. General disorders associated with hypersplenism (e.g. Felty's syndrome) or with an autoimmune disorder (e.g. SLE) may suggest the presence of increased destruction. A bone-marrow examination is central to the separation of these disorders (Fig. 36.2). In patients with aplasia or marrow infiltration it may be difficult to obtain a particulate aspirate even on repeated attempts, and a trephine biopsy may be necessary. The finding of increased marrow cellularity may be a normal response to increased destruction of blood cells, may result from a maturation defect such as occurs in the

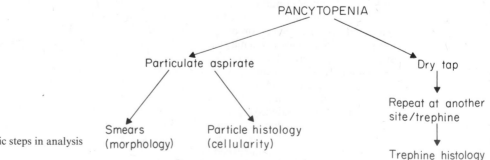

Fig. 36.2. Diagnostic steps in analysis of pancytopenia.

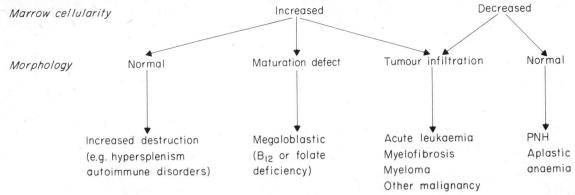

Fig. 36.3. Further analysis of pancytopenia based on bone-marrow findings.

megaloblastic marrow, or may be due to tumour infiltration (Fig, 36.3). In an ill-understood group of disorders pancytopenia is found in association with a hypercellular marrow showing a variety of maturation abnormalities: these may persist unchanged for long periods, or may progress to a more frankly leukaemic picture. Decreased cellularity may be seen with myelofibrosis, where special stains will demonstrate an increase in reticulin, and also in aplastic anaemias, including the hypoplastic anaemia associated with PNH. A normal or increased marrow cellularity may occasionally be found in patients with a hypoplastic anaemia where, by chance, the biopsy is taken from an isolated cellular island. This finding may be suspected as atypical of the entire marrow if blood examination provides no evidence of increased haemopoiesis (e.g. no increase in reticulocytes). Such a discrepancy should lead to sampling of marrow at a different site, and a bone-marrow scan may be helpful in confirming reduced marrow uptake or an abnormal distribution of the marrow uptake. Where atypical cells are seen in the blood, as in acute leukaemia, occasional cases of myeloma and in patients with myelofibrosis, the marrow may provide confirmation of the malignant infiltration. Where a haematological or other malignancy is suspected, areas of bony tenderness may prove a particularly profitable site from which to take the marrow biopsy.

ENLARGED LYMPH NODES

Lymphadenopathy may be reactive or neoplastic. Some guidance as to the cause may be obtained from a careful history and examination, but it is often necessary to proceed to biopsy of the node to be sure of the diagnosis.

The age of the patient is important, for example children are likely to have an infective cause or to have leukaemia; young adults may have viral infections, especially glandular fever, or they may have leukaemia or Hodgkin's disease, whereas older patients are more likely to have a neoplastic cause, either carcinoma, non-Hodgkin lymphoma or Hodgkin's disease.

Racial origin is also important, as in recent immigrants, particularly from India and Pakistan, tuberculous adenitis needs serious consideration.

A history of erythema nodosum, arthralgia or iridocyclitis would suggest the diagnosis of sarcoidosis.

With cervical lymphadenopathy, a recent history of sore throat or any suggestion of a viral infection should be noted. With inguinal or axillary adenopathy, enquiries should be made about injuries or infections of the foot or hand or any recent exposure to cat scratches. Posterior cervical lymphadenopathy in childhood suggests infestation of the hair and scalp.

The length of history should be assessed, though an asymptomatic lymph node is often found by chance. On the other hand, some patients present with lymph nodes which have varied in size over a number of years. A long history of this kind does not exclude a neoplastic disease such as chronic lymphocytic leukaemia or nodular lymphoma.

If a lymphoma is suspected, particular attention should be paid to the assessment of weight loss, if any, and whether or not the patient has had any episodes of fever or sweating, since the presence of 'B symptoms' has a major effect on the prognosis in non-Hodgkin lymphomas and will determine the approach to therapy in all types of lymphoma including Hodgkin's disease.

The distribution of superficial lymph nodes should be examined systematically to ascertain whether the node noted by the patient is single or there are nodes in other areas. The size of enlarged nodes should be noted, as should their texture and whether or not they are discrete, mobile or fixed. The throat should be examined for tonsillar enlargement or evidence of infection, and if the upper cervical nodes are involved a careful examination of the nasopharynx is necessary. The presence or absence of spleen and liver enlargement should be noted.

If it is thought that the lymphadenopathy may be due to an infection, throat swabs, screening for glandular fever, CMV and toxoplasma should be put in train. A blood count should be done, together with an ESR and examination of the blood film. The blood film may be diagnostic, e.g. in acute leukaemia or CLL, or it may show reactive lymphocytes compatible with the diagnosis of viral infection. A neutrophilia may suggest a bacterial infection, but does not exclude the diagnosis of a lymphoma: in occasional cases of Hodgkin's disease there may be quite a pronounced leucocytosis. Eosinophilia is seen very occasionally in Hodgkin's disease.

A chest X-ray may reveal bilateral hilar lymphadenopathy compatible with sarcoidosis, or mediastinal enlargement due to lymphomatous infiltration of nodes, or a T-cell tumour of the thymus. If the nodes are suspected of being involved with secondary neoplasm, bronchial carcinoma should be excluded.

All the preliminary investigations may leave the diagnosis in doubt, however, and a biopsy of the lymph node is then required; it is wise to do this sooner rather than later. The biopsy usually gives a definitive diagnosis but if it shows reactive changes only, the patient should be watched carefully for any sign of further lymphadenopathy, and if there is any serious suspicion of lymphoma another biopsy may be necessary.

If the biopsy shows Hodgkin's disease, it is important to ascertain the extent of the disease since this will determine further treatment. A lymphangiogram and liver and spleen scan should be done. If facilities are available a whole body CAT scan may give additional information. The bone marrow should be examined both by puncture and trephine. If the clinical staging following these investigations is IIIB or IV there is no need to proceed further, since chemotherapy is the treatment of choice. In the absence of B symptoms and in clinical stages I, II and III a staging laparotomy is indicated. This should, however, be carried out in a centre where there is special experience with the operation, otherwise there may be unacceptable morbidity associated with the procedure.

In the non-Hodgkin lymphomas there is either local involvement of only one group of nodes or the condition is widespread. If the condition is clinically stage IA, lymphangiography and bone-marrow examination are indicated. The lymphangiogram is useful both for staging and for following the progress of the disease when there is widespread involvement. A staging laparotomy is not indicated in the non-Hodgkin lymphomas.

HAEMORRHAGIC DISORDERS

A general disorder of haemostasis is suggested by spontaneous bleeding, often from multiple sites, or excessive post-traumatic haemorrhage. In addition, haemostatic defects may be suspected in patients with a family history of excessive bleeding or who have diseases known to be associated with an increased liability to haemorrhage. The most appropriate investigations to establish the presence and nature of a haemostatic abnormality are often indicated by the clinical setting.

Clinical assessment
The history and examination may indicate whether the disorder is hereditary or acquired, and whether it is associated with underlying diseases. These factors, together with the pattern of bleeding, often suggest the likely deficit, whether of blood vessels, platelets, coagulation, or a combined disorder.

Inherited defects. These are most commonly of the plasma protein clotting factors, and are strongly suggested by a positive personal and family history of excessive bleeding. Such a disorder may have declared itself in childhood, or have been sufficiently mild to escape detection until adult life. In the latter case, previous excessive bleeding under the stress of minor surgery, particularly tonsillectomy or dental extractions, may also suggest a longstanding disorder. Conversely, a normal haemostatic response to such challenges makes such a disorder most unlikely. The pattern of inheritance, whether sex-linked (as in haemophilia A and B), autosomal dominant (as in most cases of von Willebrand's disease) or recessive (as in the rare inherited abnormalities of other clotting proteins) may be diagnostically helpful. Inherited disorders of platelet function are rare but can be autosomal recessive (e.g. Glanzmann's thrombasthenia) or dominant (e.g. storage-pool deficiency). Hereditary haemorrhagic telangiectasia (Osler–Rendu–Weber disease), an autosomal dominant disorder of blood vessels, may be suspected from cutaneous telangiectatic lesions, particularly on the face.

Acquired defects. These are more likely with sudden unexpected bleeding, particularly if previous surgery has been well tolerated. They are also suggested by a history of recent drug exposure, including known anti-coagulants (e.g. heparin or coumarin derivatives), those with antiplatelet effect (e.g. aspirin), and the wide variety of agents that have been linked with marrow depression or selective thrombocytopenia. The presence of a disease known to be associated with haemostatic defects also suggests an acquired disorder and may be of help in deciding the most likely pathophysiology. Impaired synthesis of clotting factors is likely with underlying liver disease, and increased consumption of clotting factors may be suspected in situations known to be associated with disseminated intravascular coagulation (e.g. infections, malignancy or obstetric complications). A platelet deficit may be suspected with haematological malignancies, or a vascular purpura with a collagen-vascular disease. Combined defects of platelets and blood vessels may be expected in uraemia and with abnormal serum proteins (e.g. macroglobulinaemia and cryoglobulinaemia), where microvascular damage from hyperviscosity can add to interference with platelet function.

The pattern of bleeding. This provides additional information as to which part of the haemostatic mechanism is likely to be at fault. Platelet or blood-vessel disturbances are suggested by cutaneous petechial haemorrhages, though ecchymoses may also be present. Mucosal bleeding is characteristic of thrombocytopenia or platelet dysfunction, though it also occurs with vascular disorders. Retinal haemorrhages are common with thrombocytopenia, particularly when accompanied by severe anaemia [67]. The purpura associated with thrombocytopenia is usually flat and commonly most marked in dependent areas such as the lower legs where capillary hydrostatic pressure is high. In contrast, vasculitic petechiae are frequently raised.

Coagulation disorders are not associated with purpura, but may be suspected from spontaneous bruising, or muscle and joint haemorrhages. Acquired clotting defects are characterized by widespread ecchymoses and gastro-intestinal and urinary-tract bleeding, whereas single, large, recurrent haemorrhages are a more usual feature of the inherited disorders such as haemophilia. Prolonged, but delayed, bleeding after trauma in coagulation disorders contrasts with the immediate bleeding seen with platelet deficits, in which there is failure to form the primary haemostatic plug.

Initial laboratory investigation
In all patients, examination of the blood film, together with a blood count, forms an essential part of the initial investigations. Other tests may concentrate on screening for defects in primary haemostasis and/or coagulation as clinically appropriate (Table 36.11).

Blood examination
Changes in the number and morphology of platelets may be evident from the blood film. A rough estimate of platelet numbers may be made but must be confirmed by direct count (whether visual or automated). Decreased platelet numbers may be due to decreased production or increased destruction [68]. An increase in megathrombocytes (greater than 2·5 μm in diameter) is associated with compensatory increase in platelet production [59, 70] and may be helpful as an indication of increased platelet destruction.

A reactive thrombocytosis is part of the physiological response to infection, malignancies, iron deficiency and bleeding. A raised platelet count is also seen in myeloproliferative disorders, particularly essential thrombocythaemia and polycythaemia rubra vera, and more rarely myelofibrosis or CGL. A functional abnormality in platelets in these conditions can give rise to haemorrhage [71, 72].

Thrombocytopenia associated with anaemia and leucopenia suggests a generalized failure of haemopoiesis, as for example in aplastic anaemia, marrow infiltration or SLE. The presence of immature white cells may indicate a leukaemic marrow infiltrate, whereas an increase in lymphocytes may reflect a lymphoproliferative disorder producing a thrombocytopenia either by marrow replacement, an immune mechanism or, if there is splenomegaly, by splenic pooling of platelets. Megaloblastic haemopoiesis, which is associated with mild to moderate thrombocytopenia due to ineffective platelet production, may be suspected from the associated blood findings. Red-cell rouleaux formation may raise the question of a paraproteinaemia producing defective platelet function or, in the case of multiple myeloma, direct marrow infiltration.

No characteristic changes in the blood film are associated with the inherited coagulation disorders. However, the acquired defects may show evidence of accompanying disease, as in the macrocytosis and target-cell formation of liver disease, which may also be accompanied by thrombocytopenia if there is congestive splenomegaly. Fragmented red cells together with thrombocytopenia suggest a microangiopathic haemolytic anaemia and consumptive coagulopathy.

Defects of primary haemostasis

THROMBOCYTOPENIA
There is no detectable haemostatic defect when normal platelets are present in excess of 100×10^9/l [73], and spontaneous bleeding is unusual unless the platelet count falls below about $20–30 \times 10^9$/l. However, accompanying defects in platelet function (e.g. in uraemia), or local trauma or vascular lesions, may lead

Table 36.11. Investigation of haemorrhagic disorders

Screening tests
  Platelet count
  Blood count and film
  Prothrombin time (PT)
  Partial thromboplastin time (PTT)
  Thrombin clotting time (TCT)
  Bleeding time (in absence of thrombocytopenia)

Platelet disorders
  (1) Thrombocytopenia: Bone marrow
                         Platelet antibodies
  (2) Normal platelet count: Bleeding time
                              Aggregation studies
                              Clot retraction
                              Platelet-factor-3 availability

Coagulation disorders
  (1) Correction tests with normal plasma (? circulating anticoagulant)
  (2) If isolated PT prolongation, perform PT with Russell viper venom (? factor-VII deficiency)
  (3) Factor assays as indicated:
      Isolated prolongation of PTT—Factors VIII, IX, XI, XII
      Isolated prolongation of PT—Factor VII
      PTT and PT prolonged with normal TCT—Factors II, V, X
      Prolonged TCT—Reptilase time (? inhibitor such as heparin or FDP)
                  —Fibrinogen assay
  (4) Factor-XIII deficiency—Urea clot stability

Defibrination
  Fibrinogen assay
  Fibrin-degradation products
  Euglobulin clot lysis time
  Factor-V and -VIII assay

to bleeding at intermediate levels. When thrombocytopenia is present, a bone-marrow aspirate may be helpful in separating the basic mechanisms of increased loss or decreased production of platelets.

Impaired platelet production
A decrease in the number of megakaryocytes is indicative of impaired platelet production. This finding may need to be confirmed by examining histological sections from a marrow biopsy. Rarely there may be an isolated defect in platelet production as a result of drugs such as alcohol [74], gold, phenylbutazone or tolbutamide [75], in SLE [76], or as a congenital abnormality [77]. Much more frequently there are additional findings related to marrow damage (by drugs or irradiation), intrinsic marrow failure (e.g. in aplastic anaemia), or marrow infiltration by haematological or other malignancies.

The marrow may also show evidence of ineffective thrombopoiesis, as in most of the rare inherited thrombocytopenias and with megaloblastic haemopoiesis, whether due to vitamin-B_{12} or folate deficiency [78], or associated with erythroleukaemia. The megakaryocyte maturation defect typically results in increased numbers of micromegakaryocytes. This contrasts with the increase in size that often accompanies a reduced number of megakaryocytes in marrow failure [68].

Increased platelet loss
Increased peripheral loss of platelets, due either to immune destruction or consumption, is the commonest cause of an isolated thrombocytopenia. The resulting increased stimulus to thrombopoiesis results in the characteristic bone-marrow findings of normal or increased numbers of large megakaryocytes, as well as megathrombocytes in the blood.

Antibody-induced destruction of platelets is most commonly due to autoimmune antibodies as in idiopathic thrombocytopenic purpura (ITP) or SLE. In children especially, a recent history of viral infection may be obtained. Less commonly the antibodies may be drug-related, particular agents being quinine, quinidine and sulphonamide derivatives, though any drug ingestion must be suspect. Drug-related antibodies may be detected in *in-vitro* tests with the drug by their production of agglutination of normal platelets, complement fixation, antiglobulin consumption, ^{51}Cr release or inhibition of clot retraction [79–81]. The detection of autoantibodies is difficult and not routinely performed: many techniques have been used (see Chapter 25), but the most reliable method consists of the direct measurement of platelet-bound immunoglobulin and/or complement [81a–c]. In most cases, however, the diagnosis of ITP is based solely on the presence of thrombocytopenia with increased numbers and size of marrow megakaryocytes, in the absence of any other obvious cause of platelet destruction (particularly drugs) or consumption. Since ITP may be the harbinger of SLE and may also be associated with an immune haemolytic anaemia (Evan's syndrome), tests for LE cells and antinuclear factor should be performed, together with a direct antiglobulin test of the red cells in all patients with ITP. Splenomegaly is not a feature of ITP and if present may also suggest SLE.

Both autoantibodies and alloantibodies, that occasionally develop after multiple blood transfusions or pregnancies, may cross the placenta to produce neonatal thrombocytopenia. Alloantibodies may be detected by complement fixation or platelet agglutination tests.

Increased consumption of platelets is often suggested by the clinical context or blood changes associated with the thrombocytopenia. Thrombocytopenia in a febrile patient should raise the question of possible septicaemia and the need for blood cultures. Increased platelet destruction possibly accompanied by impaired platelet production occurs in a variety of bacterial, viral (e.g. varicella, mumps, adult cytomegalovirus and infectious mononucleosis) and rickettsial (e.g. typhus) infections, and may or may not be associated with evidence of disseminated intravascular coagulation (DIC); DIC may also be suspected from the association of haemorrhage and thrombocytopenia with obstetrical complications (amniotic fluid embolism, dead fetus syndrome and abruptio placentae), malignancies (particularly carcinoma of the prostate, lung and ovary, and acute myeloid leukaemia) and intravascular haemolysis. It may be confirmed by screening tests of coagulation and fibrinolysis (see below). Trauma or surgery produces local consumption of both platelets and fibrinogen related to the extent of the tissue injury. In addition, massive blood loss replaced by stored blood may produce a 'dilutional' thrombocytopenia.

Abnormal vascular surfaces may produce a more selective consumption of platelets [82]. This is a feature of the vasculitic diseases, of the haemolytic-uraemic syndrome and of thrombotic thrombocytopenic purpura, in which characteristic clinical features of the underlying disease, including renal dysfunction, may be combined with the blood findings of a microangiopathic haemolytic anaemia. The artificial vascular sufaces used in cardiac and arterial surgery, or in an extracorporeal bypass circulation, may also provoke a consumptive thrombocytopenia.

Congenital thrombocytopenias. These, associated with normal or increased numbers of megakaryocytes, are rare diseases that by virtue of the bone-marrow findings may occasionally be confused with the much more common acquired disorders of increased platelet destruction [83]. Most can be distinguished by a family and personal history combined with typical changes on the blood film, though platelet survival and function studies may sometimes be helpful (see below). In the May–Hegglin anomaly [84], large platelets are associated with a mild, absent, or intermittent thrombocytopenia. This autosomal dominant disorder is characterized by basophilic inclusions (Döhle bodies) in granulocytes, and is not usually associated with haemorrhage. In contrast, the giant platelets (greater than 4 μm in diameter compared with a normal of less than 3 μm) of the autosomal recessive Bernard–Soulier syndrome are associated with a severe bleeding tendency even though the platelet count is normal or only slightly reduced. Platelet survival is reduced in this disorder. The Wiskott–Aldrich syndrome is a sex-linked, recessive disorder characterized by thrombocytopenia, an immune deficit, multiple pyogenic infections and eczema. In this syndrome small platelets with a reduced lifespan are a diagnostic combination. Finally there is a group of autosomal dominant disorders in which the thrombocytopenia closely resembles ITP [83]; they are suggested, however, by the positive family history, an absence of demonstrable platelet antibodies, and in most cases a normal rather than a shortened platelet lifespan. In these circumstances the increase in megakaryocytes in the marrow suggests markedly ineffective thrombopoiesis.

Pooling of platelets in the spleen may also result in a mild thrombocytopenia accompanied by evidence of marrow compensation and increased megakaryocyte activity. This may be suspected whenever the spleen is moderately enlarged. Thrombocytopenia from this cause is rarely severe enough to cause bleeding on its own, but the underlying disease may itself be associated with impaired platelet production.

Platelet survival studies using ^{51}Cr-labelled platelets [85] have been useful in studies of the kinetics of thrombopoiesis and, as already discussed, in the characterization of the inherited thrombocytopenias. Their clinical application is limited, however. Most patients in whom such studies might be indicated have too low a platelet count to allow labelling of their own platelets, and ABO- and Rh-matched donor platelets must be used. Since nearly all disorders involving platelet destruction result from abnormalities extrinsic to the platelets, this is not usually an insuperable obstacle, and indeed decreased platelet survival is demonstrable in ITP. Surface counting over spleen and liver, however, has not proved helpful in predicting the response to splenectomy. Moreover, the presence of impaired platelet production (usually associated with a normal survival) is frequently clear from the examination of blood and bone marrow.

PLATELET DYSFUNCTION

When the platelet count is normal or only moderately reduced but the clinical picture is one of failure of primary haemostasis, further tests to screen platelet function may be indicated. These should not be performed within seven days of taking aspirin, or other drugs known to affect platelet function. An Ivy bleeding time [86], standardized by using a template method [87], is dependent on platelet numbers and function, as well as capillary function [73]. It is unnecessary if thrombocytopenia has already been demonstrated. When normal, the bleeding time can usually be taken as adequate evidence of normal platelet and capillary function. When it is prolonged, and there is no obvious reason for acquired platelet dysfunction (e.g. uraemia, dysproteinaemia, drug therapy, or myeloproliferative disease), or vascular abnormality (e.g. scurvy and inherited disorders of connective tissue), a genetic platelet defect is suggested. This will require more extensive tests of platelet function—particularly of aggregation—to establish a precise diagnosis. Tests of aggregation [88] and clot retraction [89] are extremely sensitive to minor variations of technique, and therefore of limited clinical value. Quantitative changes may be difficult to interpret, but qualitative changes are diagnostically helpful (see Chapter 26). Tests of platelet-factor-3 availability [90] are more easily standardized, but have little diagnostic precision.

Platelet function tests

Platelet aggregation in platelet-rich plasma can be measured in an optical aggregometer as an increase in light transmission on the addition of aggregating agents [88]. The most informative battery of aggregating agents for use in a clinical context consists of ADP, adrenaline, collagen, arachidonic acid and ristocetin. In thrombasthenia, no aggregation occurs in response to any of these but the latter, while in the Bernard–Soulier syndrome only the response to ristocetin is defective. In defects of the platelet-release reaction,

collagen-induced aggregation is defective and no second wave occurs in response to ADP or adrenaline. Defects of endoperoxide synthesis (e.g. due to aspirin) can be distinguished from storage-pool deficiency by the response to arachidonic acid, which is defective in the former but normal in the latter group. In thrombocythaemia and other myeloproliferative disorders, there may be a specific defect of adrenaline-induced aggregation; this is one of the features distinguishing this group of disorders from reactive thrombocytosis. In most patients with von Willebrand's disease, ristocetin fails to agglutinate the platelets in their own plasma [92]; when the patient's platelets are resuspended in normal plasma, a normal response to ristocetin is seen. Such a defect suggests the need for factor-VIII assays, including quantitative determination of the ristocetin cofactor (see below).

Clot retraction is measured as the volume of serum expressed after one hour by blood that has been allowed to clot at 37°C [89]. It is impaired in the inherited disorder of platelet function, Glanzmann's thrombasthenia, but also in any thrombocytopenia, in severe fibrinogen deficiency and when the PCV is raised.

Platelet-factor-3 availability may be indirectly reflected by the prothrombin consumption test (see below), and is determined by measuring the recalcification time [90] or Stypven time [91] after citrated platelet-rich plasma is incubated with aggregating agents or kaolin. It is severely impaired in thrombasthenia, and often moderately reduced in defects of the platelet-release reaction.

VASCULAR PURPURAS

The vascular purpuras are characterized by purpura or mucosal bleeding in the absence of platelet or coagulation disorders. The clinical context usually makes the diagnosis clear. Immunological vascular injury is the most important cause of vascular purpura and may be due to drugs, infections, insect bites or a collagen-vascular disease. The association of widespread vasculitis with platelet consumption has already been discussed. The disorders of vascular-supporting connective tissue (e.g. scurvy), mechanical vascular damage (e.g. by traumatic fat embolism or as a result of hyperviscosity with paraproteinaemias), and vascular damage resulting directly from infection (e.g. meningococcal), are reviewed in Chapter 26 and discussed there and in other chapters; they will not be considered further here.

Coagulation defects

In patients with chronic bleeding disorders or where

such a disorder is under suspicion, coagulation defects may be suggested by the clinical picture presented or by the exclusion of defects in platelet number and function.

However, combined platelet and coagulation deficiencies are common with sudden and unexpected bleeding and may demand an urgent screen of both aspects of haemostasis. Examples of combined defects may be found in acute myeloid leukaemias, where thrombocytopenia due to marrow infiltration may co-exist with DIC due to the disease or to accompanying infection; in the many other situations where a consumptive coagulopathy is likely; and in liver disease where complex pathophysiology is the rule.

COAGULATION SCREENING TESTS

The Lee–White whole-blood coagulation time [1] is dependent on technique, and is very insensitive. Even in moderately severe haemophilia or Christmas disease the coagulation time may be normal (4–9 minutes at 37°C). However, the type of clot formed may be helpful, being very poor or absent in defibrination syndromes. The sensitivity of this non-specific test of clotting efficiency can be somewhat improved by measuring the pro-thrombin consumption index at one hour. This compares the speed at which additional fibrinogen is clotted by the one-hour serum and by the patient's plasma. As much of the prothrombin is normally consumed by one hour, the serum time is normally much greater than that of the plasma.

Because of the insensitivity of these overall tests of coagulation, three overlapping screening tests are commonly used to assess different parts of the coagulation system (Fig. 36.4, Table 36.11). The one-stage prothrombin time (PT)—the time required for recalcified plasma to clot in the presence of brain thromboplastin—is a measure of the extrinsic coagulation pathway; the activated partial thromboplastin time (PTT)—the time required for platelet-poor citrated plasma to clot after incubation with cephalin and kaolin and subsequent recalcification—is a measure of the intrinsic coagulation pathway; and the thrombin clotting time (TCT)—the time required for conversion of fibrinogen to fibrin after addition of thrombin to plasma—is a measure of the final common pathway in the coagulation sequence. The thromboplastin-generation screening test is still occasionally used as an alternative measure of the intrinsic system. A prolonged TCT suggests severe depletion of fibrinogen (to a level below 1 g/l) or the presence of inhibitors of clot formation such as heparin or fibrin-degradation products. Hyperbilirubinaemia [93], dysproteinaemias (including multiple myeloma) [94], and impaired fibrinogen function (congenital dysfibrinogenaemia) are less common causes of an abnormally long TCT. When the TCT is long the PT and PTT will also be prolonged. Factors II, V and X are common to both intrinsic and extrinsic pathways and deficiencies or inhibitors of one or more of these factors will therefore prolong both PT and PTT (but not the TCT). Pro-

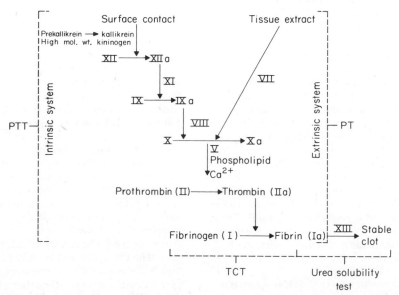

Fig. 36.4. Screening tests for coagulation defects. PTT: partial thromboplastin time; PT: prothrombin time; TCT: thrombin-clotting time.

longation of the PTT with normal TCT and PT suggests deficiency or inhibition of one or more of factors VIII, IX, XI and XII. An isolated prolongation of the PT indicates a factor-VII abnormality. Nearly all patients with coagulation disorders giving rise to clinical haemostatic deficiencies will be detected by one or more of these three screening tests. However, reduction of a single factor to below 30% of normal is required to prolong the appropriate clotting times, and in some patients where the history strongly suggests a coagulation disorder further investigation may be necessary despite normal screening tests. In von Willebrand's disease and mild haemophilia A, for example, with factor-VIII levels greater than 20% of normal, there may occasionally be a normal PTT. In addition, a deficiency of factor XIII (fibrin-stabilizing factor) is not detected by the three basic screening tests. This may be revealed by testing clot solubility in 5 M urea or 1% monochloracetic acid [95]. While mild defects are not detected by this test and can be shown only by specific assays, these mild abnormalities are not usually associated with bleeding.

DETECTION OF CIRCULATING ANTI-COAGULANTS

In all patients, whether with acute haemorrhage or chronic bleeding problems, the possibility of a circulating anti-coagulant should be considered. This may be exogenous heparin given as therapy, fibrin-degradation products resulting from consumption coagulopathy and fibrinolysis or, more rarely, spontaneously occurring inhibitors of specific coagulation factors. Detection of circulating anticoagulants is possible by repeating the screening tests (PT, PTT and TCT) with mixtures of normal and test plasma and comparing the clotting time with control mixtures of normal plasma and saline. Prolonged clotting times due to anticoagulants show little or no correction with equal volumes of normal plasma, whereas those due to factor deficiency are returned to normal. Most spontaneous inhibitors are antibodies directed against factor VIII and result in a prolonged PTT. They may be associated with multiple transfusions of factor-VIII preparations in haemophiliacs, with normal pregnancy, or with SLE, or they may occur spontaneously [96]. These inhibitors may require incubation with normal plasma prior to assay in the mixing tests [96, 97]. Another inhibitor resulting in a prolonged PT and PTT is found in 10% of patients with SLE and is probably responsible for an inhibition of prothrombin conversion to thrombin. However, it is not usually associated with clinically significant haemorrhage [98].

CHRONIC DISORDERS OF COAGULATION—FACTOR ASSAYS

In patients with chronic bleeding disorders with abnormal screening tests for coagulation and no evidence of inhibitors, the next step is the identification of the specific clotting-factor defect. The pattern of abnormalities in the screening tests, together with the clinical features, will identify the factor or group of factors in which a deficiency is likely (Table 36.11). Further discrimination is best obtained by measuring the ability of the patient's plasma to correct the prolonged clotting time of a known deficient plasma in either a qualitative test or an assay based on the PT, PTT or thromboplastin generation test. The reference plasma may be obtained from congenitally deficient patients. Where this is unavailable, reagents may be artificially prepared from normal plasma [99]. A comparison of the ability of the patient's test plasma and normal plasma to correct the clotting time of the known deficient plasma allows the factor activity of the test plasma to be expressed as a percentage of normal activity [1]. Immunoassay for the defective factor may also be possible, allowing the separation of functional from quantitative deficiencies.

As well as their diagnostic value, the quantitative factor assays are useful in prognosis and management of patients. For example, haemarthrosis is unlikely in haemophilia with factor-VIII concentrations of more than about 3–4 u/dl. In addition, the assays can be used to monitor the effectiveness of replacement therapy. However the intrinsic problems of most of the assays include labile reagents and the difficulty of establishing normal reference plasmas and standards [1]. These may lead to poor reproducibility and suggest that greater reliability may be obtained in laboratories undertaking the tests frequently.

Prolongation of the PTT

As factor-VIII deficiency associated with haemophilia A or von Willebrand's disease is the commonest cause of an isolated prolongation of the PTT, assay for this factor should be performed first, followed by factor IX (deficient in haemophilia B or Christmas disease). Factor-XI deficiency is rare and though absence of factor XII produces a prolongation of the PTT it does not result in clinical bleeding.

In mild cases of haemophilia A or B the PTT may be normal and as these patients are at risk of bleeding after trauma, clinical suspicion may necessitate factor assay. Factor-IX levels are low in the first weeks of life and the difficulties in obtaining adequate blood samples from infants mean that in any event the diagnosis should be confirmed later on during the first year. The differentiation of mild haemophilia A from von Willebrand's disease requires bleeding-time and platelet function studies, together with further analysis of the different properties of factor VIII which can be assayed. These properties can be identified as factor-

VIII procoagulant activity (VIIIC, measured in the standard clotting assay), factor-VIII-related antigen (VIIIR:Ag, the protein measured by reaction with xenogeneic antibodies raised against human factor VIII [100]), and von Willebrand factor activity (VIIIR:WF, or ristocetin cofactor activity, from its part in platelet agglutination). In von Willebrand's disease, all three properties may be reduced, in contrast to the functional deficit of VIIIC alone in haemophilia A. This combined deficit is typically manifest in a prolongation of the PTT with factor-VIIIC levels of five to 50% of normal, and defective platelet function as judged by a prolonged bleeding time, impaired ristocetin agglutination and defective platelet retention in glass-bead columns. However, there are several variants of the disease, with various patterns of deficiency of the factor-VIII complex [101, 102]. Impaired ristocetin cofactor activity appears to be the most consistent finding, though the platelet-rich plasma of some patients shows normal agglutination with ristocetin; a quantitative assay, using normal washed or formalin-fixed platelets, should be performed on the patient's platelet-poor plasma. It should be noted that VIIIC and VIIIR:Ag increase during pregnancy, with the use of oral contraceptives and sometimes after transfusion, and these should be excluded before performing tests for von Willebrand's disease. In general, the factor-VIII disorders can be separated on the basis of the family history, determination of VIIIC and VIIIR:Ag and, where indicated, ristocetin cofactor activity. A reduced VIIIC/VIIIR:Ag ratio is found in the majority of female carriers of haemophilia A, and provides the best available method for the identification of heterozygotes.

An isolated prolongation of the PTT may very rarely result from inherited deficiency of one of the contact activation factors, XII, XI, Fletcher factor (pre-kallikrein) and Fitzgerald factor (high-molecular-weight kininogen). These autosomal recessive disorders lead to extremely mild bleeding tendencies, or none at all. The assay of these factors is dependent on the use of known deficient substrate plasma in a modified PTT.

Deficiencies of factors II, V, VII and X

Isolated deficiencies of these factors are all rare autosomal disorders in which the bleeding tendency is usually mild. However, recurrent joint bleeding has been recorded with congenital prothrombin deficiency [103].

An abnormal PT with normal PTT suggests a factor-VII deficiency. As Russell's viper venom [104] directly activates factor X, bypassing factor VII, it may be used as an indirect screening test for factor-VII deficiency: a deficiency is suggested by a prolonged one-stage PT but a normal Russell's viper venom (Stypven) time. Specific assay may be impossible in the absence of factor-VII-deficient plasma for the substrate.

An abnormal PT and PTT combined with a normal TCT suggests isolated deficiency of factor II, V or X, or, more commonly, a combined deficiency of the vitamin-K-dependent factors, II, VII, IX and X. A two-stage prothrombin assay [105] may be used to assay prothrombin, but Taipan snake venom, which converts prothrombin directly to thrombin without the need for other clotting factors, is the basis of a simpler one-stage assay [106]. Factors V and X may be assayed in modified PT tests using factor-deficient plasmas as substrates. The scarcity of deficient human plasmas means these may have to be artificially prepared (e.g. oxalated plasma may be depleted of factor V by incubation at 37°C for 24 hours, and charcoal-filtered ox plasma is deficient in factor X).

Fibrinogen defects

A prolonged TCT (and thus also a long PT and PTT) may be due to congenital hypofibrinogenaemia (< 1 g/l), afibrinogenaemia or dysfibrinogenaemia. The latter two categories are associated with a lifelong bleeding tendency of variable severity, whereas there is often no clinical bleeding with hypofibrinogenaemias. The dysfibrinogenaemias are autosomal traits, with variable expression in heterozygotes, whereas afibrinogenaemia appears to be an autosomal recessive condition. The congenital disorders of fibrinogen need to be distinguished from acquired abnormalities (e.g. defibrination, or impaired fibrinogen synthesis in liver disease). Such distinctions are usually clear on clinical grounds. A prolonged TCT that is due to inhibitors—heparin or fibrin-degradation products—may be identified by the history and the normal clotting times when snake venoms, Reptilase or Arvin, are used in the place of thrombin. (The Reptilase and Arvin clotting times are prolonged together with the TCT where the defect is primarily of the fibrinogen.)

Fibrinogen can be assayed as thrombin-clottable protein measured quantitatively in a chemical assay [107], the normal range being 1·5–4·0 g/l. Simpler and more rapid semi-quantitative estimates are obtained by timing or turbidimetric measurement of the clot produced by thrombin [107a], or by using serial dilutions of normal and test plasmas and noting the highest dilution in which thrombin gives fibrin clots (normally up to 1/128) [108]. These rapid methods are useful in the emergency screening for defibrination syndrome. Further test dilutions in epsilon amino-caproic acid and protamine sulphate may be made to overcome the effects of excessive fibrinolysis and of fibrin-degradation products, respectively. These 'functional' assays give spuriously low results in congenital dysfibrinogenaemia, whereas physical precipitation methods [109], or immunoreactive assays [110] for fibrinogen usually give normal or even raised levels. This discrepancy is typical of the dysfibrinogenaemias which may be further characterized by immunoelectrophoresis of the plasma and other special tests (see Chapter 28).

INVESTIGATION OF ACUTE HAEMOSTATIC FAILURE
Further investigation of acute unexpected haemorrhage accompanied by abnormal coagulation screening tests frequently involves a search for evidence of consumptive coagulopathy, though impaired factor synthesis (e.g. in liver disease or neonates) and circulating anticoagulants must also be considered.

In acute DIC there may be prolongation of all three screening tests, due to consumption of factors and/or thrombin inhibition by fibrin-degradation products (FDP). Thrombocytopenia is also present and there may be evidence of red-cell destruction on the blood film. Confirmation involves detection of FDP and low levels of the group of clotting factors that are normally consumed in the process of clot formation—fibrinogen, and factors V and VIII. The FDP may be suspected if plasma gels on the addition of protamine sulphate [111], but are more sensitively detected by immunological methods. A simple slide agglutination test [112] uses latex particles coated with antibody to fibrinogen and test samples of serum in different dilutions to obtain a semi-quantitative assay of FDP (normal < 10 μg/ml). A more elaborate and quantitative haemagglutination-inhibition test uses fibrinogen-coated human red cells to probe the activity remaining in antifibrinogen serum after exposure to test serum [113]. Fibrinogen assay and assays for factor-V and -VIII activity have been described in previous sections.

Post-surgical coagulation abnormalities are often related to consumption of clotting factors. A situation in which this is especially likely to occur is open-heart surgery. Here the consumption may occur in the extracorporeal circulation. However, the defect is rarely severe, with a mild prolongation of the PT and thrombocytopenia [114]: a rebound in heparin activity due to the short half-life of the protamine used to neutralize the anticoagulant at the end of the operation may sometimes be responsible for a prolongation of the PT and PTT.

Excessive fibrinolysis is rarely if ever the cause of a haemostatic defect, though it occurs in patients receiving plasminogen activators (urokinase or streptokinase) for the treatment of thrombosis. Like DIC it produces high levels of FDP, prolonged TCT and low fibrinogen levels. The euglobulin clot lysis time and test of lysis of fibrin plates [1], though predominantly indicators of plasminogen-activator activity, may give paradoxical results if plasminogen itself is substantially depleted. It should also be recognized that patients with DIC may sometimes show increased plasminogen activity as the pathological process evolves, making it difficult to distinguish consumption of clotting factors from fibrinolysis as the primary cause. This emphasizes the difficulties that may be experienced in interpreting isolated test values in what are frequently transient and rapidly changing disturbances of coagulation.

Impaired synthesis of clotting factors may be suspected in acute or chronic liver disease where deficiencies of the vitamin-K-dependent factors II, VII, IX and and X may result in prolongation of the PT and PTT. Fibrinogen levels may be reduced due to impaired synthesis, but there may also be an element of increased consumption. As in DIC, thrombocytopenia is common in severe liver disease, though usually only when there is associated splenomegaly or folate deficiency. Impaired synthesis due to vitamin-K deficiency occurs in obstructive jaundice and other malabsorption states. Haemorrhagic disease of the newborn due to deficiency of vitamin-K-dependent clotting factors characteristically results in further prolongation of the PT and PTT beyond the normal neonatal values, which are longer than in adults because of the low levels of these factors at birth (see Chapter 3). Such bleeding may need to be distinguished from DIC in severely ill neonates and from the neonatal thrombocytopenias [115].

REFERENCES

1 DACIE J.V. & LEWIS S.M. (1975) *Practical Haematology*, 5th edn. Churchill, London.

2 GARBY L. (1970) The normal haemoglobin level. *British Journal of Haematology*, **19**, 429.

3 COOK J.D., ALVARADO A., GUTNISKY M., JAMRA J., LABARDINI J., LAYRISSE M., LINARES J., LORIA A., MASPES V., RESTREPO A., REYNAFARJE C., SANCHEZ-MEDAL L., VÉLEZ H. & VITERI F. (1971) Nutritional deficiency and anemia in Latin America: a collaborative study. *Blood*, **38**, 591.

4 HURTADO A., MERINO C. & DELGADO E. (1945) Influence of anoxemia on the hemopoietic activity. *Archives of Internal Medicine*, **75**, 284.

5 PRITCHARD J.A. (1960) Hematological aspects of pregnancy. *Clinical Obstetrics and Gynecology*, **3**, 378.

6 ADAMSON J. & HILLMAN R.S. (1968) Blood volume and plasma protein replacement following acute blood loss in normal man. *Journal of the American Medical Association*, **205**, 609.

7 WINTROBE M.M. (1934) Anemia—classification and treatment on the basis of differences in the average

volume and hemoglobin content of the red corpuscles. *Archives of Internal Medicine*, **54**, 256.

8 SHARP A.A. & BALLARD B.C.D. (1970) An evaluation of the Coulter S counter. *Journal of Clinical Pathology*, **23**, 327.

9 ZARKOWSKY H.S., OSKI F.A., SHA'AFI R., SHOHET S.B. & NATHAN D.G. (1968) Congenital hemolytic anemia with high sodium, low potassium red cells. I. Studies of membrane permeability. *New England Journal of Medicine*, **278**, 573.

10 PERROTTA A.L. & FINCH C.A. (1972) The polychromatic erythrocyte. *American Journal of Clinical Pathology*, **57**, 471.

11 HILLMAN R.S. & FINCH C.A. (1969) The misused reticulocyte. *British Journal of Haematology*, **17**, 313.

12 HILLMAN R.S. (1969) Characteristics of marrow production and reticulocyte maturation in normal man in response to anemia. *Journal of Clinical Investigation*, **48**, 443.

13 HILLMAN R.S. & FINCH C.A. (1974) *Red Cell Manual*, 4th edn, p. 60. Davis, Philadelphia.

14 HILLMAN R.S. & HENDERSON P.A. (1969) Control of marrow production by the level of iron supply. *Journal of Clinical Investigation*, **48**, 454.

15 BOTHWELL T.H., CHARLTON R.W., COOK J.D. & FINCH C.A. (1979) Clinical aspects of ferrokinetic measurements. In: *Iron Metabolism in Man*, p. 190. Blackwell Scientific Publications, Oxford.

16 CAVILL I., RICKETTS C. & JACOBS A. (1977) Radioiron and erythropoiesis: methods interpretation and application. *Clinics in Haematology*, **6**, 583.

17 RHYNER K. & GANZONI A. (1972) Erythrokinetics: evaluation of red cell production by ferrokinetics and reticulocyte counts. *European Journal of Clinical Investigation*, **2**, 96.

18 FREIREICH E.J., MILLER A., EMERSON C.P. & ROSS J.F. (1957) The effect of inflammation on the utilisation of erythrocyte and transferrin bound radioiron for red cell production. *Blood*, **12**, 972.

19 BAINTON D.F. & FINCH C.A. (1964) The diagnosis of iron deficiency anemia. *American Journal of Medicine*, **37**, 62.

20 LANGER E.E., HAINING R.G., LABBE R.F., JACOBS P., CROSBY E.F. & FINCH C.A. (1972) Erythrocyte protoporphyrin. *Blood*, **40**, 112.

21 RATH C.E. & FINCH C.A. (1948) Sternal marrow hemosiderin. A method for the determination of available iron stores in man. *Journal of Laboratory and Clinical Medicine*, **33**, 81.

22 JACOBS A., MILLER F., WORWOOD M., BEAMISH M.R. & WARDROP C.A. (1972) Ferritin in the serum of normal subjects and patients with iron deficiency and iron overload. *British Medical Journal*, **iv**, 206.

23 LIPSCHITZ D.A., COOK J.D. & FINCH C.A. (1974) A clinical evaluation of serum ferritin as an index of iron stores. *New England Journal of Medicine*, **290**, 1213.

24 BEUTLER E. (1959) The red cell indices in the diagnosis of iron deficiency anemia. *Annals of Internal Medicine*, **50**, 313.

25 ROWLEY P.T. (1976) The diagnosis of beta-thalassemia trait: a review. *American Journal of Hematology*, **1**, 129.

26 KATTAMIS C., LAGOS P., METAXOTOU-MAVROMATI A. &

MATSANIOTIS N. (1972) Serum iron and unsaturated iron-binding capacity in the β-thalassemia trait: their relation to the levels of hemoglobins A, A$_2$ and F. *Journal of Medical Genetics*, **9**, 154.

27 KUSHNER J.P., LEE G.R., WINTROBE M.M. & CARTWRIGHT G.E. (1971) Idiopathic refractory sideroblastic anemia. Clinical and laboratory investigation of 17 patients and review of the literature. *Medicine*, **50**, 139.

28 EICHNER E.R. & HILLMAN R.S. (1971) The evaluation of anemia in alcoholic patients. *American Journal of Medicine*, **50**, 218.

29 GRIGGS R.C. (1964) Lead poisoning: hematologic aspects. *Progress in Hematology*, **4**, 117.

30 MCPHEDRAN P., BARNES M.G., WEINSTEIN J.S. & ROBERTSON J.S. (1973) Interpretation of electronically determined macrocytosis. *Annals of Internal Medicine*, **78**, 677.

31 CHANARIN I., ENGLAND J.M. & HOFFBRAND A.V. (1973) Significance of large red blood cells. *British Journal of Haematology*, **25**, 351.

32 CHALMERS D.M., LEVI A.J., CHANARIN I., NORTH W.R.S. & MEADE T.W. (1979) Mean cell volume in a working population: the effects of age, smoking, alcohol and oral contraception. *British Journal of Haematology*, **43**, 631.

33 REYNOLDS E.H. (1976) Neurological aspects of folate and B$_{12}$ metabolism. *Clinics in Haematology*, **5**, 661.

34 COOPER B.A. & WHITEHEAD V.M. (1978) Evidence that some patients with pernicious anemia are not recognised by radiodilution assay for cobalamin in serum. *New England Journal of Medicine*, **299**, 816.

35 CORCINO J., ZALUSKY R. & GREENBERG M. (1971) Coexistence of pernicious anaemia and chronic myeloid leukaemia: an experiment of nature involving vitamin B$_{12}$ metabolism. *British Journal of Haematology*, **20**, 511.

36 HOFFBRAND A.V., NEWCOMBE B.F.A. & MILLIN D.L. (1966) Method of assay of red cell folate and the value of the assay as a test for folate deficiency. *Journal of Clinical Pathology*, **19**, 17.

37 COOPER B.A. & LOWENSTEIN L. (1964) Relative folate deficiency of erythrocytes in pernicious anemia and its correction with cyanocobalamin. *Blood*, **24**, 502.

38 TISMAN G. & HERBERT V. (1973) B$_{12}$ dependence of cell uptake of serum folate: an explanation for high serum folate and cell folate depletion in B$_{12}$ deficiency. *Blood*, **41**, 465.

39 SCHILLING R.F. (1953) Intrinsic factor studies. II. The effect of gastric juice on the urinary excretion of radioactivity after the oral administration of radioactive vitamin B$_{12}$. *Journal of Laboratory and Clinical Medicine*, **42**, 860.

40 MCINTYRE P.A. & WAGNER H.N. (1966) Comparison of the urinary excretion and 8 hour plasma tests for vitamin B$_{12}$ absorption. *Journal of Laboratory and Clinical Medicine*, **68**, 966.

41 CALLENDER S.T., WITTS L.J., WARNER G.T. & OLIVER R. (1966) The use of a simple whole-body counter for haematological investigations. *British Journal of Haematology*, **12**, 276.

42 ADAMS E.B. (1970) Anemia associated with protein deficiency. *Seminars in Hematology*, **7**, 55.

43 KINGSLEY PILLERS E.M., MARKS J. & MITCHELL J.S. (1956) The bone marrow in malignant disease. *British Journal of Cancer*, **10**, 458.

44 SCHMID J.R., KIELY J.M., HARRISON E.G. JR, BAYRD E.D. & PEASE G.L. (1965) Thymoma associated with pure red cell agenesis. *Cancer*, **18**, 216.

45 ESCHBACH J.W. JR, FUNK D., ADAMSON J., KUHN I., SCRIBNER B.H. & FINCH C.A. (1967) Erythropoiesis in patients with renal failure undergoing chronic dialysis. *New England Journal of Medicine*, **276**, 653.

46 CARTER M.E., HAWKINS J.B. & ROBINSON B.H.B. (1969) Iron metabolism in the anaemia of renal failure: effects of dialysis and of parenteral iron. *British Medical Journal*, iii, 206.

47 ESCHBACH J.W., COOK J.D., SCRIBNER B.H. & FINCH C.A. (1977) Iron balance in hemodialysis patients. *Annals of Internal Medicine*, **87**, 710.

48 HORTON L., COBURN R.J., ENGLAND J.M. & HIMS-WORTH R.L. (1976) The haematology of hypothyroidism. *Quarterly Journal of Medicine (New Series)*, **45**, 101.

49 TODD D. (1975) Diagnosis of hemolytic states. *Clinics in Hematology*, **4**, 63.

50 WHITE J.M. & DACIE J.V. (1971) The unstable hemoglobins—molecular and clinical features. *Progress in Hematology*, **7**, 69.

51 MILLER E.B., SINGER K. & DAMASHEK W. (1942) Use of the daily fecal output of urobilinogen and the hemolytic index in the measurement of hemolysis. *Archives of Internal Medicine*, **70**, 722.

52 OSTROW J.D., JANDL J.H. & SCHMID R. (1962) The formation of bilirubin from hemoglobin *in vivo*. *Journal of Clinical Investigation*, **41**, 1628.

53 BRUS I. & LEWIS S.M. (1959) The haptoglobin content of serum in hemolytic anaemia. *British Journal of Haematology*, **5**, 348.

54 OWEN J.A., SMITH R., PADANYI R. & MARTIN J. (1964) Serum haptoglobin in disease. *Clinical Science*, **26**, 1.

55 INTERNATIONAL COMMITTEE FOR STANDARDIZATION IN HAEMATOLOGY (1980) Recommended method for radio-isotope red-cell survival studies. *British Journal of Haematology*, **45**, 659.

56 GILLILAND B.C., BAXTER E. & EVANS R.S. (1971) Red cell antibodies in acquired hemolytic anaemia with negative antiglobulin serum tests. *New England Journal of Medicine*, **285**, 252.

57 DACIE J.V. (1975) Autoimmune hemolytic anemia. *Archives of Internal Medicine*, **135**, 1293.

58 EVANS R.S., TURNER E. & BINGHAM M. (1965) Studies with radio-iodinated cold agglutinins of ten patients. *American Journal of Medicine*, **38**, 378.

59 WORLLEDGE S.M. & ROUSSO C. (1965) Studies of the serology of paroxysmal cold haemoglobinuria (PCH) with special reference to its relationship with P blood group system. *Vox Sanguinis*, **10**, 293.

60 SELWYN J.G. & DACIE J.V. (1954) Autohemolysis and other changes resulting from the incubation *in vitro* of red cells from patients with congenital hemolytic anemia. *Blood*, **9**, 414.

61 BERLIN N.I. (1975) Diagnosis and classification of polycythemia. *Seminars in Hematology*, **12**, 339.

62 WEINREB N.J. & SHIH C.F. (1975) Spurious polycythemia. *Seminars in Hematology*, **12**, 397.

63 BALCERZAK S.P. & BROMBERG P.A. (1975) Secondary polycythemia. *Seminars in Hematology*, **12**, 353.

64 LICHTMAN M.A., MURPHY M.S. & ADAMSON J.W. (1976) Detection of mutant hemoglobins with altered affinity for oxygen. *Annals of Internal Medicine*, **84**, 517.

65 ADAMSON J.W., STAMATOYANNOPOULOS G., KONTRAS S., LASCARI A. & DETTER J. (1973) Recessive familial erythrocytosis: aspects of marrow regulation in two families. *Blood*, **41**, 641.

66 THORLING E.B. (1972) Paraneoplastic erythrocytosis and inappropriate erythropoietin production. *Scandinavian Journal of Haematology*, **17** (Suppl. 17), 1.

67 HOLT J.M. & GORDON-SMITH E.C. (1969) Retinal abnormalities in diseases of the blood. *British Journal of Ophthalmology*, **53**, 145.

68 HARKER L.A. & FINCH C.A. (1969) Thrombokinetics in man. *Journal of Clinical Investigation*, **48**, 963.

69 GARG S.K., AMOROSI E.L. & KARPATKIN S. (1971) Use of the megathrombocyte as an index of megakaryocyte number. *New England Journal of Medicine*, **284**, 11.

70 KARPATKIN S., GARG S.K. & SISKIND G.W. (1971) Autoimmune thrombocytopenic purpura and the compensated thrombocytolytic state. *American Journal of Medicine*, **51**, 1.

71 ZUCKER S. & MIELKE C.H. (1972) Classification of thrombocytosis based on platelet function tests: correlation with hemorrhagic and thrombotic complications. *Journal of Laboratory and Clinical Medicine*, **80**, 385.

72 SPAET T.H., LEJNIEKS I. GAYNOR E. & GOLDSTEIN M.L. (1969) Defective platelets in essential thrombocythemia. *Archives of Internal Medicine*, **124**, 135.

73 HARKER L.A. & SLICHTER S.J. (1972) The bleeding time as a screening test for evaluation of platelet function. *New England Journal of Medicine*, **287**, 155.

74 COWAN D.H. & HINES J.D. (1971) Thrombocytopenia of severe alcoholism. *Annals of Internal Medicine*, **74**, 37.

75 BOTTIGER L.E. & WESTERHOLM B. (1972) Thrombocytopenia. II. Drug induced thrombocytopenia. *Acta Medica Scandinavia*, **191**, 541.

76 GRINER P.F. & HOYER L.W. (1970) Amegakaryocytic thrombocytopenia in systemic lupus erythematosus. *Archives of Internal Medicine*, **125**, 328.

77 HALL J.G., LEVIN J., KUHN J.P., OTTENHEIMER E.J., VAN BERKUM K.A.P. & McKUSICK V.A. (1969) Thrombocytopenia with absent radius (TAR). *Medicine*, **48**, 411.

78 SMITH M.D., SMITH D.A. & FLETCHER M. (1962) Haemorrhage associated with thrombocytopenia in megaloblastic anaemia. *British Medical Journal*, i, 982.

79 ACKROYD J.F. (1962) The immunological basis of purpura due to drug hypersensitivity. *Proceedings of the Royal Society of Medicine*, **55**, 30.

80 WEINTRAUB R.M., PECHET L. & ALEXANDER B. (1962) Rapid diagnosis of drug-induced thrombocytopenic purpura. Report of three cases due to quinine, quinidine and dilantin. *Journal of the American Medical Association*, **180**, 528.

81 CIMO P.L., PISCIOTTA A.V., DESAI R.G., PINO J.L. & ASTER R.H. (1977) Detection of drug-dependent anti-

bodies by the Cr^{51} platelet lysis test: documentation of immune thrombocytopenia induced by diphenylhydantoin, diazepam and sulfisoxazole. *American Journal of Hematology*, **2**, 65.

81a DIXON R., ROSSE W. & EBBERT L. (1975) Quantitative determination of antibody in idiopathic thrombocytopenic purpura. *New England Journal of Medicine*, **292**, 230.

81b HAUCH T.W. & ROSSE W.F. (1977) Platelet-bound complement (C3) in immune thrombocytopenia. *Blood*, **50**, 1129.

81c CINES D.B. & SCHREIBER A.D. (1979) Immune thrombocytopenia. Use of a Coombs antiglobulin test to detect IgG and C3 on platelets. *New England Journal of Medicine*, **300**, 106.

82 HARKER L.A. & SLICHTER S.J. (1972) Platelet and fibrinogen consumption in man. *New England Journal of Medicine*, **287**, 999.

83 MURPHY S. (1972) Hereditary thrombocytopenia. *Clinics in Hematology*, **1**, 359.

84 OSKI F.A., NAIMAN J.L., ALLEN D.M. & DIAMOND L.K. (1962) Leucocytic inclusions—Döhle bodies—associated with platelet abnormality (the May–Hegglin anomaly). Report of a family and review of the literature. *Blood*, **20**, 657.

85 ASTER R.H. & JANDL J.H. (1964) Platelet sequestration in man. I. Methods. *Journal of Clinical Investigation*, **43**, 843.

86 IVY A.C., NELSON D. & BUCHER G. (1961) The standardisation of certain factors in cutaneous venostasis bleeding time technique. *Journal of Laboratory and Clinical Medicine*, **26**, 1812.

87 MIELKE C.H. JR, KANESHIRO M.M., MAHER I.A., WEINER J.M. & RAPAPORT S.I. (1969) The standardised normal Ivy bleeding time and its prolongation by aspirin. *Blood*, **34**, 204.

88 O'BRIEN J.R. (1962) Platelet aggregation. II. Some results from a new method of study. *Journal of Clinical Pathology*, **15**, 452.

89 MACFARLANE R.G. (1939) A simple method for measuring clot retraction. *Lancet*, **i**, 1199.

90 HARDISTY R.M. & HUTTON R.A. (1965) The kaolin clotting time of platelet-rich plasma: a test of platelet factor-3 availability. *British Journal of Haematology*, **11**, 258.

91 SPAET T.H. & CINTRON J. (1965) Studies on platelet factor-3 availability. *British Journal of Haematology*, **11**, 269.

92 HOWARD M.A., SAWERS R.J. & FIRKIN B.G. (1973) Ristocetin: a means of differentiating von Willebrand's disease into two groups. *Blood*, **41**, 687.

93 KOPÉC M., DAROCHA T., NIEWIAROWSKI J. & STACHURSKA J. (1961) The antithrombin activity of glucuronic esters of bilirubin. *Journal of Clinical Pathology*, **14**, 478.

94 LACKNER H. (1973) Hemostatic abnormalities associated with dysproteinemias. *Seminars in Hematology*, **10**, 125.

95 BRITTEN A.F.H. (1967) Congenital deficiency of factor XIII (fibrin stabilizing factor). Report of a case and review of the literature. *American Journal of Medicine*, **43**, 751.

96 SHAPIRO S.S. & HULTIN M. (1975) Acquired inhibitors to the blood coagulation factors. *Seminars in Thrombosis and Hemostasis*, **1**, 336.

97 ROBERTS H.R., SCALES M.B., MADISON J.T., WEBSTER W.P. & PENICK G.D. (1965) A clinical and experimental study of acquired inhibitors to factor VIII. *Blood*, **26**, 805.

98 RICK M.E. & HOYER L.W. (1975) Haemostatic disorders in systemic lupus erythematosus. *Clinics in Rheumatic Diseases*, **1**, 583.

99 INGRAM G.I.C., KNIGHTS S.F., AROCHA-PINANGO C.L., SHEPPARD J.P., PEREZ-REQUEJO J.L. & MILLS D.K. (1975) Simple screening tests for the diagnosis of isolated clotting factor defects. *Journal of Clinical Pathology*, **28**, 524.

100 ZIMMERMAN T.S., RATNOFF O.D. & POWELL A.E. (1971) Immunologic differentiation of classic hemophilia (factor VIII deficiency) and von Willebrand's disease. *Journal of Clinical Investigation*, **50**, 244.

101 WEISS H.J. (1975) Abnormalities of factor VIII and platelet aggregation—use of ristocetin in diagnosing von Willebrand's syndrome. *Blood*, **45**, 403.

102 NILSSON I.M. & HOLMBERG L. (1979) Von Willebrand's disease today. *Clinics in Haematology*, **8**, 167.

103 GIROLAMI A., STICCHI A., LAZZARIN M. & SCARPA R. (1970) Congenital hypoprothrombinaemia. Case report. *Acta Haematologica* (Basel), **44**, 164.

104 RAPAPORT S., AAS K. & OWREN P.A. (1956) The clotting action of Russell viper venom. *Blood*, **9**, 1185.

105 BIGGS R. & DOUGLAS A.S. (1953) The measurement of prothrombin in plasma. A case of prothrombin deficiency, *Journal of Clinical Pathology*, **6**, 15.

106 DENSON K.W.E., BORRETT R. & BIGGS R. (1971) The specific assay of prothrombin using the Taipan snake venom. *British Journal of Haematology*, **21**, 219.

107 RATNOFF O.D. & MENZIE C. (1951) A new method for the determination of fibrinogen in small samples of plasma. *Journal of Laboratory and Clinical Medicine*, **37**, 316.

107a CLAUSS A. (1957) Gerinnungsphysiologische schnellmethode zur bestimmung des fibrinogens. *Acta Haematologica*, **17**, 237.

107b ELLIS B.C. & STRANSKY A. (1961) A quick and accurate method for the determination of fibrinogen in plasma. *Journal of Laboratory and Clinical Medicine*, **58**, 477.

108 SHARP A.A., HOWIE B., BIGGS R. & METHUEN D.J. (1958) Defibrination syndrome in pregnancy: value of various diagnostic tests. *Lancet*, **ii**, 1309.

109 MILLAR H.R., SIMPSON J.G. & STALKER A.L. (1971) An evaluation of the heat precipitation method for plasma fibrinogen estimation. *Journal of Clinical Pathology*, **24**, 827.

110 WOLF P. & WALTON K.W. (1965) Investigation of a quantitative anomaly encountered in the assay of fibrinogen by immunodiffusion. *Immunology*, **8**, 6.

111 NIEWIAROWSKI S. & GUREWICH V. (1971) Laboratory identification of intravascular coagulation. The serial dilution protamine sulfate test for the detection of fibrin monomer and fibrin degradation products. *Journal of Laboratory and Clinical Medicine*, **77**, 665.

112 GARVEY M.B. & BLACK J.M. (1972) The detection of fibrinogen/fibrin degradation products by means of a

new antibody-coated latex particle. *Journal of Clinical Pathology*, **25,** 680.

113 MERSKEY C., LALEZARI P. & JOHNSON A.F. (1969) A rapid, simple, sensitive method for measuring fibrinolytic split products in human serum. *Proceedings of the Society for Experimental Biology and Medicine*, **131,** 871.

114 BACHMAN F., McKENNA R., COLE E.R. & NAJAFI H. (1975) The hemostatic mechanism after open heart surgery. *Journal of Thoracic Cardiovascular Surgery*, **70,** 76.

115 HATHAWAY W.E. (1975) The bleeding newborn. *Seminars in Hematology*, **12,** 175.

Index